Surgical Research

Edited by

Wiley W. Souba

Department of Surgery
Penn State College of Medicine
Hershey Medical Center
Hershey, Pennsylvania

Douglas W. Wilmore

Department of Surgery
Harvard Medical School
Brigham and Women's Hospital
Boston, Massachusetts

ACADEMIC PRESS

A Harcourt Science and Technology Company

San Diego • San Francisco • New York • Boston • London • Sydney • Tokyo

This book is printed on acid-free paper. ♾

Academic Press
A Harcourt Science and Technology Company
525 B Street, Suite 1900, San Diego, California 92101-4495, USA
http://www.academicpress.com

Academic Press
Harcourt Place, 32 Jamestown Road, London NW1 7BY, UK
http://www.academicpress.com

Library of Congress Catalog Card Number: 00-105499

International Standard Book Number: 0-12-655330-0

PRINTED IN THE UNITED STATES OF AMERICA
00 01 02 03 04 05 MM 9 8 7 6 5 4 3 2 1

Contents

55 Animal Models in Transplantation

I. L. Laskowski, J. B. Ames, M. Gasser, D. Whitley, and N. L. Tilney

56 Models to Study Surgical Nutrition and Metabolism

Wiley W. Souba and Douglas W. Wilmore

57 Stable Isotopes

Robert R. Wolfe

58 Body Composition

Lindsay D. Plank and Graham L. Hill

59 Energetics

Danny O. Jacobs and Takeaki Matsuda

60 Models of Protein Metabolism

Per-Olof Hasselgren, David R. Fischer, and Timothy A. Pritts

61 Membrane Transport of Nutrients

Bruce R. Stevens

62 Models of Wound Healing in Growth Factor Studies

Alexandrina Saulis and Thomas A. Mustoe

63 Animal Models of Sepsis and the Multiple Organ Dysfunction Syndrome

Mitchell P. Fink

Contributors

Numbers in parentheses indicate the pages on which the authors' contributions begin.

William M. Abbott (1011)
Division of Vascular Surgery, Massachusetts General Hospital, Boston, Massachusetts 02114

Steve F. Abcouwer (217)
Department of Biochemistry and Molecular Biology, University of New Mexico, School of Medicine, Albuquerque, New Mexico 87131

N. Scott Adzick (1065)
Division of Pediatric General, Thoracic and Fetal Surgery, The Children's Hospital of Philadelphia, Philadelphia, Pennsylvania 19104

Samuel S. Ahn (1001)
Division of Vascular Surgery, UCLA School of Medicine, Los Angeles, California 90095

David C. Allison (193)
Departments of Surgery, Medicine, and Physiology and Molecular Medicine, Medical College of Ohio, Toledo, Ohio 43614

J. B. Ames (757)
Surgical Research Laboratory, Harvard Medical School and Department of Surgery, Brigham and Women's Hospital, Boston, Massachusetts 02115

Keith D. Amos (497)
Department of Surgery, Washington University School of Medicine, St. Louis, Missouri 63110

Robert W. Anderson (1279)
Department of Surgery, Duke University Medical Center, Durham, North Carolina 27710

Jeffrey M. Arbeit (175)
Department of Surgery, UCSF/MT Zion Cancer Center, University of California, San Francisco, California 94115

Sonia Y. Archer (557)
Department of Surgery, Beth Israel Deaconess Medical Center, Boston, Massachusetts 02215

Arlene S. Ash (81)
Boston University School of Medicine and School of Public Health, Boston, Massachusetts 02218

Stanley W. Ashley (3)
Department of Surgery, Brigham and Women's Hospital, Boston, Massachusetts 02115

Anthony Atala (1107)
Laboratory for Tissue Engineering and Cellular Therapeutics, Department of Urology, Children's Hospital and Harvard Medical School, Boston, Massachusetts 02115

Alfred Ayala (317)
Center for Surgical Research and Department of Surgery, Brown University School of Medicine and Rhode Island Hospital, Providence, Rhode Island 02903

Matthew D. Bacchetta (137)
Department of Surgery, Anne and Max A. Cohen Surgical Intensive Care Unit, New York-Presbyterian Hospital–New York Weill Cornell Center, Weill Medical College of Cornell University, New York, New York 10021

Charles M. Balch (1237)
Departments of Surgery and Oncology, Johns Hopkins Medical Center, Baltimore, Maryland 21231

Anirban Banerjee (285)
Department of Surgery, University of Colorado Health Sciences Center, Denver, Colorado 80262

Adrian Barbul (1249)
Departments of Surgery, Sinai Hospital of Baltimore, and the Johns Hopkins Medical Institutions, Baltimore, Maryland 21215

Philip S. Barie (137)
Department of Surgery, Anne and Max A. Cohen Surgical Intensive Care Unit, New York-Presbyterian Hospital–New York Weill Cornell Center, Weill Medical College of Cornell University, New York, New York 10021

Clyde F. Barker (1261)
Department of Surgery, University of Pennsylvania, Philadelphia, Pennsylvania 19104

Jeffrey S. Barkun (155)
McGill University Health Centre, Montreal, Quebec, Canada H3A 1A1

Robert E. Barrow (367)
The University of Texas Medical Branch and Shriners' Burns Hospital, Galveston, Texas 77555

Harry D. Bear (415)
Division of Surgical Oncology, Department of Surgery, Medical College of Virginia at Virginia Commonwealth University, Richmond, Virginia 23298

Russell S. Berman (435)
Departments of Surgical Oncology and Cancer Biology, The University of Texas M. D. Anderson Cancer Center, Houston, Texas 77030

Walter L. Biffl (331)
Department of Surgery, Denver Health Medical Center, University of Colorado Health Sciences Center, Denver, Colorado 80204

Timothy R. Billiar (949)
Department of Surgery, University of Pittsburgh, Pittsburgh, Pennsylvania 15261

John D. Birkmeyer (101, 127)
VA Outcomes Group, VA Medical Center, White River Junction, Vermont 05009

Timothy G. Buchman (307, 1309)
Department of Surgery, Washington University School of Medicine, St. Louis, Missouri 63110

Eileen M. Bulger (893)
Department of Surgery, Harborview Medical Center and the University of Washington, Seattle, Washington 98104

Charles B. Cairns (285)
Department of Surgery, University of Colorado Health Sciences Center, Denver, Colorado 80262

Casey Calkins (1343)
Department of Surgery, University of Colorado, Denver, Colorado 80262

William G. Cance (253)
Department of Surgery and UNC Lineberger Comprehensive Cancer Center, University of North Carolina at Chapel Hill, Chapel Hill, North Carolina 27599

Irshad H. Chaudry (317, 357)
Center for Surgical Research, Department of Surgery, Brown University School of Medicine and Rhode Island Hospital, Providence, Rhode Island 02903

Cynthia S. Chin (415)
Division of Surgical Oncology, Department of Surgery, Medical College of Virginia at Virginia Commonwealth University, Richmond, Virginia 23298

Gyu S. Chin (1081)
Department of Surgery, New York University Medical Center, New York, New York 10016

Alexander W. Clowes (971)
Department of Surgery, University of Washington, Seattle, Washington 98195

Lisa Colletti (1349)
Department of Surgery, University of Michigan Medical School, Ann Arbor, Michigan 48109

Joy L. Collins (949)
Department of Surgery, University of Pittsburgh, Pittsburgh, Pennsylvania 15261

Suzy Conway (1319)
Francis A. Countway Library of Medicine, Harvard Medical School, Boston, Massachusetts 02115

Clay Cothren (1343)
Department of Surgery, University of Colorado, Denver, Colorado 80262

Christopher A. Crisera (613)
Department of Surgery, Children's Mercy Hospital, Kansas City, Missouri 64108

Joseph J. Cullen (507)
University of Iowa Hospitals and Clinics, Iowa City, Iowa 52242

P. William Curreri (1241)
Stratagem, Inc., Daphne, Alabama 36526

James C. Cusack, Jr. (457)
Division of Surgical Oncology, Massachusetts General Hospital, Boston, Massachusetts 02114

Roger E. De Filippo (1107)
Laboratory for Tissue Engineering and Cellular Therapeutics, Department of Urology, Children's Hospital and Harvard Medical School, Boston, Massachusetts 02115

Edwin A. Deitch (599)
Department of Surgery, UMD–New Jersey Medical School, Newark, New Jersey 07003

E. Patchen Dellinger (909)
Department of Surgery, University of Washington Medical Center, University of Washington School of Medicine, Seattle, Washington 98195

Achilles A. Demetriou (623, 709)
Department of Surgery, Cedars-Sinai Medical Center, Los Angeles, California 90048

Jeffrey A. Drebin (445)
Department of Surgery, Washington University School of Medicine, St. Louis, Missouri 63110

Soumitra R. Eachempati (137)
Department of Surgery, Anne and Max A. Cohen Surgical Intensive Care Unit, New York-Presbyterian Hospital–New York Weill Cornell Center, Weill Medical College of Cornell University, New York, New York 10021

Timothy J. Eberlein (497)
Department of Surgery, Washington University School of Medicine, St. Louis, Missouri 63110

David T. Efron (1249)
Departments of Surgery, Sinai Hospital of Baltimore, and the Johns Hopkins Medical Institutions, Baltimore, Maryland 21215

Nancy R. Ehrlich (1217)
The Recanati/Miller Transplantation Institute, New York, New York 10029

Theresa L. Eisenbraun (271)
University of Wisconsin Comprehensive Cancer Center, Madison, Wisconsin 53792

Lee M. Ellis (401, 435)
Departments of Surgical Oncology and Cancer Biology, The University of Texas M. D. Anderson Cancer Center, Houston, Texas 77030

Darwin Eton (1001)
Division of Vascular Surgery, University of Miami School of Medicine, Miami, Florida 33136

B. Mark Evers (23)
Department of Surgery, The University of Texas Medical Branch, Galveston, Texas 77555

Liane Feldman (155)
McGill University Health Centre, Montreal, Quebec, Canada H3A 1A1

Mitchell P. Fink (875)
Departments of Anesthesiology, Critical Care Medicine, and Surgery, University of Pittsburgh Medical School, Pittsburgh, Pennsylvania 15261

Joseph J. Fins (137)
Department of Medicine, Anne and Max A. Cohen Surgical Intensive Care Unit, New York-Presbyterian Hospital–New York Weill Cornell Center, Weill Medical College of Cornell University, New York, New York 10021

David R. Fischer (825)
Department of Surgery, University of Cincinnati College of Medicine, Cincinnati, Ohio 45267

Josef E. Fischer (63)
Department of Surgery, University of Cincinnati, Cincinnati, Ohio 45267

Alan W. Flake (207)
Department of Surgery and the Center for Fetal Diagnosis and Therapy, Children's Hospital of Philadelphia, University of Pennsylvania, Philadelphia, Pennsylvania 19104

Raquel M. Forsythe (599)
Department of Surgery, UMD—New Jersey Medical School, Newark, New Jersey 07003

Bradley D. Freeman (307)
Department of Surgery, Washington University School of Medicine, St. Louis, Missouri 63110

Fabia Gamboni-Robertson (285)
Department of Surgery, University of Colorado Health Sciences Center, Denver, Colorado 80262

R. Neal Garrison (1027)
Department of Surgery, University of Louisville, and Veterans Affairs Medical Center, Louisville, Kentucky 40292

James Garvey (1405)
Schroder Ventures International Life Science Fund, Boston, Massachusetts 02114

M. Gasser (757)
Surgical Research Laboratory, Harvard Medical School and Department of Surgery, Brigham and Women's Hospital, Boston, Massachusetts 02115; and Department of Surgery, University of Wuerzburg, 97080 Wuerzburg, Germany

Jonathan Gertler (1405)
Division of Vascular Surgery, Massachusetts General Hospital; Harvard Medical School; and Schroder Ventures International Life Science Fund, Boston, Massachusetts 02114

Anna Getselman (1319)
Francis A. Countway Library of Medicine, Harvard Medical School, Boston, Massachusetts 02115

George K. Gittes (613)
Department of Surgery, Children's Mercy Hospital, Kansas City, Missouri 64108

Matthew I. Goldblatt (721)
Department of Surgery, Medical College of Wisconsin, Milwaukee, Wisconsin 53226

Paul J. Gorman (1299)
Department of Surgery, Stanford University, Stanford, California 94043

Douglas W. Green (445)
Department of Surgery, Washington University School of Medicine, St. Louis, Missouri 63110

David G. Greenhalgh (379)
Department of Surgery, Shriners Hospitals for Children, Northern California, and University of California, Davis, Sacramento, California 95817

Jurgen Hannig (297)
Pritzker School of Medicine, The University of Chicago, Chicago, Illinois 60637

Alden H. Harken (1343)
Department of Surgery, University of Colorado, Denver, Colorado 80262

Per-Olof Hasselgren (825)
Department of Surgery, University of Cincinnati College of Medicine, Cincinnati, Ohio 45267

Julie Heimbach (1343)
Department of Surgery, University of Colorado, Denver, Colorado 80262

Peter K. Henke (989)
Jobst Vascular Research Laboratory, Section of Vascular Surgery, Department of Surgery, University of Michigan Medical Center, Ann Arbor, Michigan 48109

David N. Herndon (367)
The University of Texas Medical Branch and Shriners' Burns Hospital, Galveston, Texas 77555

Graham L. Hill (797)
University Department of Surgery, Auckland Hospital, Auckland 1001, New Zealand

Richard A. Hodin (557)
Department of Surgery, Beth Israel Deaconess Medical Center, Boston, Massachusetts 02215

Susan D. Horn (1393)
Institute for Clinical Outcomes Research, Salt Lake City, Utah 84109

Lisa I. Iezzoni (81)
Harvard Medical School and Division of General Medicine and Primary Care, Department of Medicine, Beth Israel Deaconess Medical Center, Boston, Massachusetts 02215

Daniel Inderbitzen (709)
Department of Surgery, Cedars-Sinai Medical Center, Los Angeles, California 90048

Svetlana Ivanova (1095)
Laboratory of Biomedical Science, North Shore University Hospital, Manhasset, New York 11030

Danny O. Jacobs (813)
Laboratories of Surgical Metabolism, Department of Surgery and Nutrition, Brigham and Women's Hospital, Harvard Medical School, Boston, Massachusetts 02115; and Creighton University Surgical Laboratories for Biomedical Investigation, Omaha, Nebraska 68131

Daniel B. Jones (573)
Southwestern Center for Minimally Invasive Surgery and Department of Surgery, The University of Texas Southwestern Medical Center, Dallas, Texas 75235

Mary Jane Kagarise (29)
Department of Surgery, The University of North Carolina School of Medicine, The University of North Carolina at Chapel Hill, Chapel Hill, North Carolina 27599

Gordon L. Kauffman, Jr. (71, 1201)
Department of Surgery, The Milton S. Hershey Medical Center, Penn State College of Medicine, Hershey, Pennsylvania 17033

Richard D. Kenagy (971)
Department of Surgery, University of Washington, Seattle, Washington 98195

Gregory D. Kennedy (271)
University of Wisconsin Comprehensive Cancer Center, Madison, Wisconsin 53792

Jerald J. Killion (435)
Department of Cancer Biology, The University of Texas M. D. Anderson Cancer Center, Houston, Texas 77030

Denise E. Kirschner (1309)
Departments of Microbiology and Immunology, The University of Michigan, Ann Arbor, Michigan 48109

Thomas M. Krummel (1299)
Department of Surgery, Stanford University, Stanford, California 94043

Alexander Sasha Krupnick (1065)
Division of Pediatric General, Thoracic and Fetal Surgery, The Children's Hospital of Philadelphia, Philadelphia, Pennsylvania 19104

I. L. Laskowski (757)
Surgical Research Laboratory, Harvard Medical School and Department of Surgery, Brigham and Women's Hospital, Boston, Massachusetts 02115; and Department of General and Transplant Surgery, Warsaw Medical University, 02-006 Warsaw, Poland

Robert D. Lasley (1119)
Department of Surgery, University of Kentucky College of Medicine, Lexington, Kentucky 40536

Stephen R. Lauterbach (1011)
Division of Vascular Surgery, Massachusetts General Hospital, Boston, Massachusetts 02114

Jeffrey H. Lawson (1279)
Department of Surgery, Duke University Medical Center, Durham, North Carolina 27710

Raphael C. Lee (297)
Pritzker School of Medicine, The University of Chicago, Chicago, Illinois 60637; and Burn Center, St. Mary's Medical Center, Hobart, Indiana 46342

David Lee-Parritz (47)
Center for Animal Resources and Comparative Medicine, Harvard Medical School, Boston, Massachusetts 02115

David C. Linehan (497)
Department of Surgery, Washington University School of Medicine, St. Louis, Missouri 63110

Jean Y. Liu (101)
VA Outcomes Group, VA Medical Center, White River Junction, Vermont 05009

Michael T. Longaker (1081)
Department of Surgery, Stanford University School of Medicine, Stanford, California 94305

Charles Lucey (1383)
21st Century Health Concepts, Houston, Texas 77061; and Dartmouth College, Hanover, New Hampshire 03755

Nancy R. Macdonald (1011)
Division of Vascular Surgery, Massachusetts General Hospital, Boston, Massachusetts 02114

Ronald V. Maier (893)
Department of Surgery, Harborview Medical Center and the University of Washington, Seattle, Washington 98104

Thomas S. Maldonado (613)
Department of Surgery, Children's Mercy Hospital, Kansas City, Missouri 64108

John C. Marshall (921)
Department of Surgery, University of Toronto, and University Health Network, Toronto, Ontario, Canada M5G 2C4

Takeaki Matsuda (813)
Laboratories of Surgical Metabolism, Department of Surgery and Nutrition, Brigham and Women's Hospital, Harvard Medical School, Boston, Massachusetts 02115; and Creighton University Surgical Laboratories for Biomedical Investigation, Omaha, Nebraska 68131

Jeffrey B. Matthews (533)
Department of Surgery, Beth Israel Deaconess Medical Center, Harvard Medical School, Boston, Massachusetts 02215

David T. Mauger (71, 1201)
Department of Health Evaluation Sciences, The Milton S. Hershey Medical Center, Penn State College of Medicine, Hershey, Pennsylvania 17033

Lucretia W. McClure (1319)
Francis A. Countway Library of Medicine, Harvard Medical School, Boston, Massachusetts 02115

Jonathan L. Meakins (155)
McGill University Health Centre, Montreal, Quebec, Canada H3A 1A1

Andreas H. Meier (1299)
Department of Surgery, Stanford University, Stanford, California 94043

Robert M. Mentzer, Jr. (1119)
Department of Surgery, University of Kentucky College of Medicine, Lexington, Kentucky 40536

Tanya K. Meyer (253)
Department of Surgery and UNC Lineberger Comprehensive Cancer Center, University of North Carolina at Chapel Hill, Chapel Hill, North Carolina 27599

Rebecca M. Minter (933)
Department of Surgery, University of Florida College of Medicine, Gainesville, Florida 32610

Lyle L. Moldawer (933)
Department of Surgery, University of Florida College of Medicine, Gainesville, Florida 32610

Ernest E. Moore (331)
Department of Surgery, Denver Health Medical Center, University of Colorado Health Sciences Center, Denver, Colorado 80204

Daniel Most (1249)
Departments of Surgery, Sinai Hospital of Baltimore, and the Johns Hopkins Medical Institutions, Baltimore, Maryland 21215

Caren M. Mulford (1119)
Department of Surgery, University of Kentucky College of Medicine, Lexington, Kentucky 40536

Michael W. Mulholland (9)
University of Michigan Medical Center, Ann Arbor, Michigan 48109

Joseph Murphy (583)
Department of Surgery, University of Texas Southwestern Medical Center and the Veterans Affairs North Texas Health Care System, Dallas, Texas 75216

Rene J. P. Musters (285)
Department of Surgery, University of Colorado Health Sciences Center, Denver, Colorado 80262

Thomas A. Mustoe (857)
Division of Plastic and Reconstructive Surgery, Northwestern University Medical School, Chicago, Illinois 60611

Daniel D. Myers, Jr. (989)
Jobst Vascular Research Laboratory, Section of Vascular Surgery, Unit for Laboratory Animal Medicine, University of Michigan Medical Center, Ann Arbor, Michigan 48109

Attila Nakeeb (721)
Department of Surgery, Medical College of Wisconsin, Milwaukee, Wisconsin 53226

Avery B. Nathens (893)
Department of Surgery, Harborview Medical Center and the University of Washington, Seattle, Washington 98104

Andrea L. Nestor (193)
Departments of Surgery, Medicine, and Physiology and Molecular Medicine, Medical College of Ohio, Toledo, Ohio 43614

John E. Niederhuber (271)
University of Wisconsin Comprehensive Cancer Center, Madison, Wisconsin 53792

Keith O'Rourke (167)
Department of Surgery and Clinical Epidemiology Unit, University of Ottawa, Ottawa Hospital, Ottawa, Ontario, Canada K1Y OK6

Marshall J. Orloff (637)
Department of Surgery, School of Medicine, University of California, San Diego, La Jolla, California 92093

Mary F. Otterson (507)
Medical College of Wisconsin, Milwaukee, Wisconsin 53226

Wayne R. Patterson (13)
The University of Texas Medical Branch, Galveston, Texas 77555

Timothy M. Pawlik (1349)
Department of Surgery, University of Michigan Medical School, Ann Arbor, Michigan 48109

Henry A. Pitt (721)
Department of Surgery, Medical College of Wisconsin, Milwaukee, Wisconsin 53226

Lindsay D. Plank (797)
University Department of Surgery, Auckland Hospital, Auckland 1001, New Zealand

Timothy A. Pritts (825)
Department of Surgery, University of Cincinnati College of Medicine, Cincinnati, Ohio 45267

R. Lawrence Reed II (347)
Department of Surgery, Loyola University Medical Center, Maywood, Illinois 60153

Robert V. Rege (573)
Southwestern Center for Minimally Invasive Surgery and Department of Surgery, The University of Texas Southwestern Medical Center, Dallas, Texas 75235

Robert S. Rhodes (1393)
University of Pennsylvania School of Medicine, Philadelphia, Pennsylvania 19103

Henry E. Rice (207)
Division of Pediatric Surgery, Department of Surgery, Duke University Medical Center, Durham, North Carolina 27710

Martin Riegler (533)
University Clinic of Surgery, Vienna General Hospital, A-1090 Vienna, Austria

Kyung M. Ro (1001)
Division of Vascular Surgery, UCLA School of Medicine, Los Angeles, California 90095

Thomas N. Robinson (285, 1343)
Department of Surgery, University of Colorado Health Sciences Center, Denver, Colorado 80262

John L. Rombeau (547)
Harrison Department of Surgical Research, University of Pennsylvania, Philadelphia, Pennsylvania 19104

Joseph M. Rosen (1383)
Plastic and Reconstructive Surgery, Dartmouth-Hitchcock Medical Center, Lebanon, New Hampshire 03756; and Thayer School of Engineering, Dartmouth College, Hanover, New Hampshire 03755

Ori D. Rotstein (1337)
Departments of Surgery, University Health Network, and University of Toronto, Toronto, Ontario, Canada M56 24C

Jacek Rozga (623, 703, 709)
Department of Surgery, Cedars-Sinai Medical Center, Los Angeles, California 90048

Justin T. Sambol (599)
Department of Surgery, UMD–New Jersey Medical School, Newark, New Jersey 07003

Michael G. Sarr (507)
Division of Gastroenterologic and General Surgery, Mayo Clinic, Mayo Medical School, Rochester, Minnesota 55902

Alexandrina Saulis (857)
Division of Plastic and Reconstructive Surgery, Northwestern University Medical School, Chicago, Illinois 60611

Mary C. Schuerman (1241)
Stratagem, Inc., Daphne, Alabama 36526

Martin G. Schwacha (357)
Center for Surgical Research, Department of Surgery, Brown University School of Medicine and Rhode Island Hospital, Providence, Rhode Island 02903

Patrica M. Scott (271)
University of Wisconsin Comprehensive Cancer Center, Madison, Wisconsin 53792

Patricia A. Sheiner (1217)
The Recanati/Miller Transplantation Institute, and the Mount Sinai School of Medicine, New York, New York 10029

George F. Sheldon (29)
Department of Surgery, The University of North Carolina School of Medicine, The University of North Carolina at Chapel Hill, Chapel Hill, North Carolina 27599

Michael Shwartz (81)
School of Management, Boston University, Boston, Massachusetts 02215

H. Hank Simms (393)
Division of Surgical Critical Care, Rhode Island Hospital, Providence, Rhode Island 02903

Marcus K. Simpson (1383)
Dartmouth College, Hanover, New Hampshire 03755

Clay Smith (207)
Center for Genetic and Cellular Therapy, Duke University Medical Center, Durham, North Carolina 27710

Scott D. Somers (1361)
Division of Pharmacology, Physiology, and Biological Chemistry, The National Institute of General Medical Sciences, Bethesda, Maryland 20892

Wiley W. Souba (773, 1375)
Department of Surgery, The Milton S. Hershey Medical Center, Penn State College of Medicine, Hershey, Pennsylvania 17033

David A. Spain (1027)
Department of Surgery, University of Louisville, and Veterans Affairs Medical Center, Louisville, Kentucky 40292

Jason A. Spector (1081)
Department of Surgery, New York University Medical Center, New York, New York 10016

Michael L. Steer (733)
Department of Surgery, Beth Israel Deaconess Medical Center, Harvard Medical School, Boston, Massachusetts 02215

Bruce R. Stevens (845)
Department of Physiology, College of Medicine, University of Florida, Gainesville, Florida 32610

Robert W. Storms (207)
Center for Genetic and Cellular Therapy, Duke University Medical Center, Durham, North Carolina 27710

Kenneth K. Tanabe (115, 457)
Division of Surgical Oncology, Massachusetts General Hospital, Boston, Massachusetts 02114

James C. Thompson (1)
Department of Surgery, The University of Texas Medical Branch, Galveston, Texas 77555

N. L. Tilney (757)
Surgical Research Laboratory, Harvard Medical School and Department of Surgery, Brigham and Women's Hospital, Boston, Massachusetts 02115

Daniel L. Traber (367)
The University of Texas Medical Branch and Shriners' Burns Hospital, Galveston, Texas 77555

Kevin J. Tracey (1095)
Laboratory for Tissue Engineering and Cellular Therapeutics, Department of Urology, Children's Hospital and Harvard Medical School, Boston, Massachusetts 02115

Richard H. Turnage (583)
Department of Surgery, University of Texas Southwestern Medical Center and the Veterans Affairs North Texas Health Care System, Dallas, Texas 75216

A. Simon Turner (1137)
Department of Clinical Sciences, Colorado State University, Fort Collins, Colorado 80523

Thomas C. Vary (747)
Department of Cellular and Molecular Physiology, Penn State University College of Medicine, Hershey, Pennsylvania 17033

Gus J. Vlahakes (1037)
Massachusetts General Hospital and Harvard Medical School, Boston, Massachusetts 02114

Yoram Vodovotz (949)
Department of Surgery, University of Pittsburgh, Pittsburgh, Pennsylvania 15261

Thomas W. Wakefield (989)
Jobst Vascular Research Laboratory, Section of Vascular Surgery, Department of Surgery, University of Michigan Medical Center; and Ann Arbor Veterans Administration Medical Center, Ann Arbor, Michigan 48109

Ping Wang (317, 357)
Center for Surgical Research, Department of Surgery, Brown University School of Medicine and Rhode Island Hospital, Providence, Rhode Island 02903

Glenn D. Warden (379)
Shriners Hospitals for Children—Cincinnati Burns Hospital, and University of Cincinnati, Cincinnati, Ohio 45229

Brad W. Warner (1047)
Division of Pediatric Surgery, Children's Hospital Medical Center, Cincinnati, Ohio 45229

Stephen M. Warren (1081)
Department of Surgery, Oregon Health Science University, Portland, Oregon 97201

James M. Watters (167)
Department of Surgery, Loeb Health Research Institute, University of Ottawa, Ottawa Hospital, Ottawa, Ontario, Canada K1Y OK6

Ronald J. Weigel (233)
Stanford University, School of Medicine, Stanford, California 94305

Frank J. Wessels (933)
Department of Surgery, University of Florida College of Medicine, Gainesville, Florida 32610

Edward E. Whang (3)
Department of Surgery, Brigham and Women's Hospital, Boston, Massachusetts 02115

D. Whitley (757)
University of Alabama, Birmingham, Alabama 35294

James Willey (193)
Departments of Surgery, Medicine, and Physiology and Molecular Medicine, Medical College of Ohio, Toledo, Ohio 43614

Douglas W. Wilmore (773, 1375)
Department of Surgery, Brigham and Women's Hospital, Boston, Massachusetts 02115

Robert R. Wolfe (789)
The University of Texas Medical Branch, Galveston, and Shriners Burns Hospital, Metabolism Unit, Galveston, Texas 77550

Shirley K. Wrobleski (989)
Jobst Vascular Research Laboratory, Section of Vascular Surgery, Department of Surgery, University of Michigan Medical Center, Ann Arbor, Michigan 48109

George P. Yang (233)
Stanford University, School of Medicine, Stanford, California 94305

Heidi Yeh (547)
Harrison Department of Surgical Research, University of Pennsylvania, Philadelphia, Pennsylvania 19104

Barbara A. Zehnbauer (307)
Departments of Pediatrics and Pathology, Washington University School of Medicine and St. Louis Childrens' Hospital, St. Louis, Missouri 63110

Moritz M. Ziegler (1287)
Department of Surgery, Children's Hospital Medical Center, Boston, Massachusetts 02115

Foreword

Surgical research probably offers better opportunities for success than it ever has before because of the advances in other sciences and in technology. Unfortunately, there seem to be forces in American medicine that discourage active participation in surgical research. Foremost among these factors are economic disincentives. First, medical schools have raised their tuitions to levels that leave the new M.D. buried under a burden of debt. Second, when he or she finally gets into practice, managed care can be a driving force to see more and more patients at lower and lower rates of remuneration. Not only does this affect the practitioner, but it affects the hospital where more and more patients and procedures are required to balance its budget. Most medical schools and hospitals with research departments look to those who do research not only to give their time and effort but to raise money through grants that provide heavy overhead funds in order to have the space and facilities to pursue their work. These pressures, some of which will be commented on later in this foreword, make a volume such as this most timely and important in the new millennium.

Upon learning of the plan to create a single-volume book for surgical research and receiving an invitation to write a foreword, I will admit that I cringed a bit, as the subject is so vast and potentially draws on a large number of scientific disciplines, each of which has its own distinctive and extensive set of contributions relating to research in the field of surgery. On second thought, however, I realized that with the capacity of the electronic media to make a vast array of reference material available, such a book would be an enormous help in particular to younger students entering areas that are relatively new to them. Thus, this volume can serve as a screen to show people whether or not their fresh ideas have already been explored and to what extent, and it can point the way to much relevant material in disciplines far removed from surgery, ranging from electrical engineering to the identification and enumeration of cancer cells in bone marrow or blood during the development of a clinical cancer.

Clearly, the value of such a book must depend on the insight and experience of its editors, Dr. Wiley Souba and Dr. Douglas Wilmore. Dr. Douglas Wilmore has long been known to me, first as a medical student and later as a teacher who brought me new information from his research and collective experience. Dr. Wilmore took his surgical residency at the Hospital of the University of Pennsylvania during the years I was chairman of that department. As a surgical resident he was superb in his approach to patients, his knowledge of surgery, his research endeavors during his residency, and, most importantly, his ability to teach. Even in those days, his thoroughness in research was evident in a lengthy study of the adaptability of duodenal mucosa to the loss of much of the jejuno-ileum in dogs. His interest in the short bowel syndrome stemmed at least in part out of the brilliant case that he and Dr. Stanley Dudrick managed at the Children's Hospital of Philadelphia of a female infant born with atresia of most of the jejuno-ileum and also the sigmoid. This patient and the subsequent report in the *Journal of the American Medical Association* probably did more to bring the attention of surgeons to the possibility of total parenteral nutrition than any other single article. It demonstrated so clearly that not only could life be maintained, but if sufficient nutrients were given, normal growth would occur even in an individual who could take nothing by mouth but water. It was typical of Dr. Wilmore's subsequent career that he took this problem to the laboratory to see how much jejunum and ileum could be sacrificed if TPN were given long enough for the duodenum to compensate maximally. He measured the weight of the duodenum per linear centimeter and the thickness of the mucosa and observed the architecture of the mucosa at various stages of its compensatory transformation. Thus, in dogs he established most of the criteria we now use in deciding whether a patient with a limited length of jejuno-ileum can compensate for the loss of much of the intestine. He went on to spend many valuable years with Dr. Basil Pruitt at the Surgical Research Center at Brooke Army Hospital in San Antonio. From there he was appointed to the faculty at Harvard, where he was entrusted with the very productive laboratory previously headed by Dr. Francis Moore and devoted to the study of the metabolism of surgical patients. Here he has continued to make important contributions showing that at least one of the nonessential amino acids, arginine, is really essential in the nourishment of the surgically stressed patient.

Dr. Wiley Souba has worked in several venues, a portion of the time with Dr. Dudrick and a portion of the time with Dr. Wilmore, and currently has assumed the chairmanship of the Department of Surgery at Pennsylvania State University in Hershey, formerly headed by Dr. John Waldhausen. His contributions to surgical research also have been highly significant. Dr. Souba has devoted himself to the study of parenteral nutrition and particularly to the metabolism of glutamine and the effects of inflammation and tumors on glutamine metabolism. He has gone on to study the means by which amino acids gain entrance to cells and he has also studied independent amino acid transport in endotoxemic rats, gaining evidence of selective stimulation of arginine transport. His papers constitute many pages in the *Journal of Parenteral and Enteral Nutrition* and a good number of contributions to the *Annals of Surgery*, *The Surgical Forum*, and many other prestigious journals. His bibliography shows beyond a doubt that he is familiar with many laboratory techniques and the various aspects of clinical investigation. The senior editors of this volume speak from a background of personal success in surgical research and they have selected a remarkable group of section editors and authors. Nearly every field of surgical research is discussed in detail in this volume by individuals who have been and are successfully engaged in investigative work. The volume is valuable for its overview of the whole field and equally valuable to the individual who has selected his field and wants to be updated on recent progress and the directions in which it seems to be going.

Drs. Souba and Wilmore not only have a rich background in surgical research themselves, but also have a remarkably broad knowledge of the leaders in various aspects of surgical research. They have been very fortunate to recruit such a fine group of editors and authors.

We speak of surgical research instead of surgical search. The purpose is to learn new things that will help the surgical patient. The term *research* implies that the results of the search must be repeatable. As remarked by Judah Folkman, "After a paper is published that contains new methods it may take some time before other researchers can learn the methods and reproduce the work. If a basic scientist receives a call from a colleague, who says, 'I cannot reproduce your work' this can be a terrifying experience for the basic scientist. However, for a surgeon it may be a source of pride and is called the 'Stradivarius problem' "[1].

In writing the beginning chapter of a textbook published by the J. B. Lippincott Company in 1957, edited by J. Garrott Allen, Henry N. Harkins, Carl Moyer, and myself [2], we emphasized the responsibility of those going into surgery not only to learn the science and art of surgery and to practice it as perfectly as possible, but also to enhance knowledge in the field of surgery, thus making an addition to surgical science, whether this be clinical or laboratory based. It is therefore most appropriate that this volume on surgical research draws together a large body of experience to help new surgical students find available resources and avoid some of the pitfalls that beset those of us who attempt surgical research.

It was my privilege to meet on several occasions the chairman of the Department of Physiological Chemistry at Harvard Medical School, Otto Folin, whose daughter later became my wife. He said that he thought that half of one's success in medical research was in the selection of the problem. He had worked seven years at a mental institution in an effort to see whether new biochemical techniques might throw light on the cause of mental illness. He employed these years to develop improved methods of urinalysis, many of which were used widely by other biochemists and clinical pathologists. However, he became convinced that the biochemistry then available was not likely to solve the problems of mental illness. He had the opportunity of changing his work to the Department of Physiological Chemistry at Harvard, where he worked on methods for most of his career. In short, he felt that one should select a problem that was likely to have an attainable solution.

Somewhat in contrast to this, my surgical mentor, I. S. Ravdin, often remarked that he had a particular respect for the individual who had worked on a difficult problem long and hard and had finally solved the problem. It seems to be a matter of judgment as to what to choose and how long to pursue the search. Undoubtedly, there are many people who stick with one problem and never achieve a solution. I have the temerity to suggest that the younger surgical scientists probably do well to undertake more straightforward problems at the beginning of their careers, as suggested by Folin. After this experience, which usually brings some recognition, they are in a better position to venture into more difficult fields and may have better judgment on the basis of their early experience as to whether the methods are available to solve the more difficult problems.

Surgeons have an unusual opportunity to see parts of the body that are hidden from the view of most specialists, even with the aid of modern radiologic techniques. Thus, observations in the operating room may often be the starting point for studies involving several disciplines.

Surgical research is often considered applied research, meaning that the underlying principles have been discovered in other areas and are simply being applied to surgical problems. For me this does not detract from its importance, as the increase in basic science knowledge would not benefit the surgical patient unless the means of applying it for the benefit of the patient is found. Furthermore, surgical techniques have in their turn contributed to the work of the preclinical scientist. An obvious example is the heart–lung apparatus developed by the late John Gibbon, Jr., which has made possible many studies of the heart that could not have been successful without this methodology. Surgical research is an umbrella term covering a great many approaches to the problems of surgical patients and their many diseases. The major categories are studies on the chemical environment of cells and organs, the immune system, and genetics; pathophysiology and pharmacology of organs affected by surgical diseases and surgical procedures; animal experimentation; statistical applications in clinical trials; and reevaluation of psychosocial problems. Surgeons are often in a unique position to explore and understand some of the latter. In the following pages you will see this categorization broken down more explicitly and indexed in a way that will permit readers to focus on the special aspects of the things in which they are interested.

When such studies suggest, they may bring the results back to the bedside and the operating room for evaluation. Patients are safeguarded in the United States and in many other countries. Regulations are imposed by both hospitals and government. These prescribe a stepwise approach to the introduction of new drugs, new methods, and new equipment, when the latter is to be introduced into the human body.

What are some of the major pitfalls in surgical research? One has already been alluded to: the attack on problems that are not likely to be solved by available methods. Another, undoubtedly, is the temptation as surgeons become busier in practice to relegate their research to assistants, employees, and collaborators, so they are not personally in a position to recognize the significance of findings that may turn up unexpectedly and so miss an important observation that could lead them to find an unexpected truth. Another pitfall is to focus too much on priority. This tendency often leads investigators to jump from one problem to another in the hope of adding something obvious that they can claim as a first. The tendency to start a new problem before one has finished the last was identified in the field of electricity by Faraday, whose motto is said to have been "work, finish, publish." We have all known people who are perfectionists and keep putting off publication until the original important findings are stale. Possibly the biggest sin of all is to claim more in one's conclusions than is the logical result of one's findings. One can go back to Aristotle and his list of ways in which false conclusions may be drawn. The use of statistical methods is a necessary evil in many types of biological research. While it quantitates the chances of error, it may lead the unwary to conclude that because a difference is not statistically significant there is no difference. The accepted borderline between statistical significance and the lack thereof is 5%. Thus, if the chances due to random sampling between experimental and control results have a probability of occurring by chance differences of less than 5%, one considers it statistically significant, whereas if it is over 5%, it is statistically insignificant. The author was pleased to learn some years ago that this figure was selected as the borderline because the great statistician Dr. C. Fisher said so. Perhaps no better borderline could be agreed upon, but it follows that if you reach 20 conclusions each at the 5% confidence level, the odds are that one of your conclusions will be false.

In the area of clinical trials one is confronted with the following ethical problem. If therapy A is shown to be better for patients than therapy B to the 5% confidence level (or to the 1% confidence level), how long is one justified in withholding therapy A from the control group of patients not receiving the apparently better therapy? Also, if one shows that therapy A is better than therapy B with a 10% confidence limit, does one declare that there is no difference between the two because there is no statistically significant difference, or does one persist in adding cases to the series in the hope of reaching statistical significance?

One additional pitfall in surgical and indeed medical research is the measurement of the value of a project by peer review for a grant such as an RO1 grant from the National Institutes of Health. The fact that one has submitted a grant request and that it has received sufficiently high priority from a carefully chosen group of people in the same field usually means that it is not very original, because it is in keeping with the thinking of the members of the study section group. Tremendous emphasis is attached to receiving a peer-reviewed grant from the NIH and this review process surely eliminates many ill-considered projects. However, the true measurement of success in research is not the extent of funding that supports it, but the actual discoveries that are made or the truths substantiated. There are many problems that cannot be successfully attacked solo or even with a small group of investigators and require major funding. However, if one achieves such funding and employs numerous people to participate, what becomes of these people if the problem is solved or the results are clearly negative? Rightly or wrongly, the leader of such a project feels under strong pressures to extend the study and maintain the jobs of the people that he has recruited. Although this is certainly fair from the standpoint of the persons recruited, it may not be in the best interest of science. In this day and age, the National Institutes of Health and many other funding agencies provide for the overhead expense of the institution; thus, in the case of large grants, this overhead becomes a significant part of the income on which the institution's budget is based. This also leads to a pressure to maintain continuity in a field of research whether or not there is great promise of important increments of knowledge.

These considerations add up to the proposition that the best years investigators have are before they become established, before their energies are consumed in practice or in administration of a large grant. Sometimes it seems as though the constraints of a limited budget or even of no budget led to important insights that led to a whole field of scientific advance. Again, the Gibbon heart–lung apparatus may be cited as an example. The idea came to Dr. Gibbon and his future wife while they were attending a patient who had had a pulmonary embolism and was dying of it. As the great inventor Thomas Edison said, "Discovery is 1% inspiration and 99% perspiration." The Gibbons worked for about two decades before they were able to demonstrate the value of the machine in clinical surgery.

In concluding this foreword, I commend the editors, the associates, and the authors for a prodigious contribution to persons engaged or desiring to become engaged in surgical research. One needs to be something of a gambler to invest years of effort in surgical research. It may lead to a Nobel Prize or it may lead to nothing. It is obvious, however, that if one does not try, one is sure not to learn anything new. If you do engage in surgical research, you may find something new and your life will be enriched by contacts with others active in the field. Sometimes you may experience the thrill of seeing a solution to a problem that had eluded you for a long time. If your independent work is "scooped" by another investigator who was a little ahead of you, you will lose some of the public recognition, but you can have the inward satisfaction that your work assured a future patient of the discovery. Sometimes it is the second paper that is required to establish the credibility of the first report. In short, I hope that this splendid volume will encourage many more young surgeons to pursue new knowledge and thus contribute to the welfare of future patients.

References

1. Judah Folkman, personal communication, March 2000.
2. *Surgery, Principles and Practice*, Lippincott, 1st ed., 1957, Chapter 1.
3. Academic Pitfalls in America—1907–1982. *J. Surg. Oncol.* 21:74–80, 1982.

Jonathan Rhoads

Preface

The field of surgery is slowly undergoing a quiet revolution. Utilizing newer methods of pain control, understanding and reducing the perioperative stress response, and adapting minimally invasive operative techniques to many procedures have greatly improved patient outcomes with fewer complications, shorter hospital stays, and reduced convalescent recovery. Academic surgery is also undergoing profound changes, brought about by the financial shortfall constantly facing hospitals and the decreased reimbursement provided for professional services. Surgeons have responded to these pressures by increasing the number of operations they perform, thus devoting more time to service (e.g., patient care) and less time to the academic pursuit of research.

For many reasons, surgeons are decidedly qualified to carry out research. As a general rule, they have an extraordinary capacity for hard work and tend to be problem-focused and solution-oriented. Their technical skills provide them with the opportunity to access blood and tissues as well as to master complex bench techniques. Surgical patients are among the most challenging to care for, posing an almost endless number of hypotheses that can be tested through basic, clinical, and translational research. In spite of pressures to spend more time in the operating room, we believe that advances in the understanding of the pathophysiology and treatment of diseases will be improved if the surgical-scientist is a front line investigator.

Several years ago it became apparent that surgical science was being deemphasized, and several of us sought remedies to decelerate and reverse these changes. A committee of the American Surgical Association was formed to make recommendations, a biannual teaching conference (Young Surgical Investigators) and a Clinical Trials Methods Course were organized by the American College of Surgeons, and the annual program on Fundamentals of Surgical Research was initiated by the Association for Academic Surgery. In addition, the senior editors of this book reviewed the general field of surgical research and suggested approaches to evaluating output and to improving and quantitating productivity by applying research methodologies developed and utilized in industry.

Finally, we concluded that a reference source on surgical research would provide the foundation for this academic endeavor and would serve to prevent erosion of this important intellectual basis of our specialty. Not only would such a volume be a place for young investigators to start when initiating their research projects, but it would reflect the philosophy, history, evolution, and ethical basis of this broad field.

Initially, we were hesitant to propose such a project, but we were greatly encouraged by members of the editorial staff of Academic Press; our thanks go to Jasna Markovac and Graham Lees for their help in initiating and completing this project. We contacted five recognized research leaders who would subsequently serve as co-editors, and they enthusiastically supported the concept of codifying the basics of surgical research. We then wrote to over 100 surgical scientists, recognized experts in diverse fields, and asked them if they would be willing to contribute to this effort; the response was a unanimous yes!

This work is organized so that the material required for designing and starting a research project is found at the front of the book, the methods and techniques required to perform the investigation are found in the middle of the volume, and the skills needed for analyzing, writing, and presenting the material follow. Overviews of research efforts in surgical subspecialties are also included, followed by chapters on the history of surgical research, the integration of research into a clinical department, biographies of surgeons who have been awarded the Nobel Prize, and a précis on converting an idea to a product.

The scope of the text is quite broad, and we have made every effort for the reader to use this information as a springboard to find new ideas and information by way of the Internet and traditional medical libraries.

The text is also supported by a Web site (http:\\www.academicpress.com/surgery), which will continue to provide updated information on new methodology and techniques in a variety of fields. We hope that this method of communication will keep our readers updated and current and will enhance the exchange of information within the surgical community.

Surgeons are in the best position to improve surgical care. By evaluating our outcomes and addressing our clinical problems, surgeons can use scientific methodology to enhance recovery of the surgical patient. We hope that *Surgical Research* will serve in some small way to support this effort.

Wiley W. Souba

Douglas W. Wilmore

1

Getting Started

James C. Thompson

Department of Surgery, The University of Texas Medical Branch, Galveston, Texas 77555

Nothing is more idiosyncratic than the start of a research career. Every established investigator has a different story, and each experience varies depending on the environment (geographic, intellectual, historic, biopolitical, and economic) that the new investigator faces. Practical considerations dictate many choices: if the investigator's mentor is a whiz at signal transduction or at molecular modeling, or in the flummoxing of cytokines, that will likely influence the candidate's early exposure.

Let us say that the person getting started has spent some time with a productive mentor and is now casting about for ways profitably to leave the nest. The general goal of research, of course, is to improve scientific productivity, to enlighten the world, and to establish a personal tradition of excellence.

In beginning to look at specific goals, a primary consideration is providing answers for important individual problems. Consider an example on a true megascale: about 30 years ago, the Chinese Academy of Science in Beijing decided to answer the question of why there was an epidemic of esophageal cancer in Lin County in Hunan Province. As a first step, they had to develop simple, reliable, and reproducible methods for the early diagnosis of esophageal cancer that could be carried out by doctors with extremely limited resources and supplies. They evolved the technique of having patients swallow balloons that had sand glued to the outside. Once passed into the stomach, these balloons, actually condoms, were inflated and then drawn back through the esophagus; the cells adherent to the surface of the balloon were then washed off for cytologic examination. In this manner more than one-half million samples were obtained for cytology. The Academy staff worked on the program for 12 years with epidemiologists, cytologists, surgeons, and biochemists and decided that the agent responsible for the induction of cancer was a fungus from pickled cabbage. The new investigator, of course, will not tackle a monumental problem such as this, but the problem that he/she chooses should be relevant.

It is important to exploit local advantages. When Dr. John H. Gibbon, Jr., the Philadelphia heart surgeon, developed his heart–lung bypass machine in the late 1940s, he had no grant support and, working at Harvard, Penn, and Jefferson Medical College, he shuttled between Boston and Philadelphia, scrounging equipment, technical help, and dogs. His initial success, a primative early incarnation, was a cumbersome Rube Golberg apparatus that filled a room. He met Tom Watson, the young president of International Business Machines (IBM) Corporation, who became fascinated with the potential of the machine and assigned a group of IBM engineers to the project. A year later, they produced a compact machine the size of a filing cabinet, descendants of which we are familiar. Another example, again in China, is when the Academy of Science exploited the principle of critical mass by gathering peptide chemists from all of China, sequestering them in an institution in Shanghai with the goal of synthesizing insulin. After a year and a half of minor success and major failure, they achieved synthesis of the full insulin molecule, the first successful effort anywhere.

On a local scale, my own group, led by Phil Rayford, had early success in developing radioimmunoassay techniques for measuring regulatory peptides of the gut. We were able to exploit that advantage by studying the role of these peptides in the study of gut secretion, absorption, motility, and growth (normal and neoplastic).

When a candidate is casting about for a career plan, therefore, the choice of a direction should meet several criteria:

1. The area of research to be addressed should be one of true importance, not just a passing fad. The evolution and disappearance of fads make a fascinating study . . . at a meeting of the College of Surgeons several years ago, two entire sessions (12 papers each) of the Surgical Forum were devoted to papers on gastric freezing. Where did they come from? Where did they go? The problem selected should be one of such enduring import that it will stand the test of time and that writing the "Significance" section of the grant proposal will be duck soup.

2. The research problem should be potentially solvable by the techniques and assets available to the investigator. Narrow the field. Most new investigators bite off more than they can chew. Initially, at least, the problem should be discreet, important, and capable of solution.

3. The problem chosen should have linkage to future studies. One of the major mysteries of the past decade was solved by the ingenious efforts of Richard Feynman, the great polymath, who concluded that the space shuttle ***Columbia*** exploded as the result of frozen O rings. A great contribution was made, but there were no follow-ups. An experiment is best designed so as to lead into a whole new area of potential productivity.

4. The investigator should avoid, if possible, attacking old, jaded controversies. Avoid fields that are strewn with the wrecks of shattered hypotheses and peopled by angry, opinionated champions. I once sought to address the question of whether acidification of the gastric antrum inhibited gastric acid secretion simply by cutting off release of the hormone, gastrin, or whether, in addition, a separate antral inhibitory hormone was released. At the time I started, five previous studies had weighed-in in favor of a separate agent, with six against it. My efforts, which I considered to be fairly spiffy, were lost in the reactivation of storms of old controversies. Two decades were to pass before we realized that the separate agent released by antral acidification is somatostatin.

5. The problem should be one to which research can bring a new light, not just a ditto mark. Confirmatory research is likely to give positive results, but is like dancing with your sister—that is, safe but without any great prospect.

6. A vital consideration is whether it is possible to elicit sufficient support so as to provide preliminary results on the problem the research will address, because the *sine qua non* of establishing your own credentials is to prove that you know how to do a project. Frame a proper question, perform the critical methodology, and analyze early results.

7. In line with exploitation of local advantages, search out and identify strong potential collaborators (local or within easy range) who can bring expertise and enthusiasm to your project. Enthusiasm for true collaboration, in my experience, is rarely found in famous, well-funded mavins. Much better is a young, bright, avid peer. Enthusiasm may be the secret of success in life; it certainly is in research. We have always worked closely with basic scientists in our department, and when asked how we have managed to maintain a happy relationship, the answer is that we ask the scientists what they want and then, if at all possible, we give it to them.

8. The investigator must be familiar with and plan to use the best current methodology. Just after one of our grants was approved in the middle 1980s, it occurred to us that this was likely the last grant NOT utilizing principles of molecular biology to be funded by the National Institutes of Health. We set about training folks, and their application of the new blots and dots allowed them to remain on or near the touted cutting edge. Change is the *leitmotiv* of our era; the Greek letter Δ could be the emblem on our research flag. We must be abreast of changes.

Once the problem is selected, the investigator should do a formal review of the literature and, in consequence, should narrow and renarrow and renarrow the field of interest so as to end up at the edge of what is known, to stand at the edge of knowledge peering out into darkness, with a plan of sending a ray of light into that gloom in order to illuminate a specific new phenomenon or mechanism.

I would suggest that, once a formal review is initiated, the investigator plan on writing a review article. A review article is a pain in the neck, but has many direct rewards, and significant halo effects:

1. It helps further to narrow the field—the author should plan on a critical comprehensive review of pertinent world literature that can be encompassed with no more than about 300 key references. Any more, and the topic is probably too large.
2. It allows critical appraisal of past efforts. What were the major successes and failures and how do they relate to the current state of the problem?
3. It may lead to discovery of errors or omissions in previous studies.

At this point, critical assessment of reviewed knowledge will lead the investigator to new research ideas, to the actual planning of a project, and to the submission of a grant proposal to the NIH, the literature-review section of which, *voila!*, has already been accomplished. Furthermore, the publication of a review by a relative newcomer will raise high the expectations of others and especially of the author, just adding in a little hubris.

Good luck.

2

Assessing Available Information

Edward E. Whang and Stanley W. Ashley

Department of Surgery, Brigham and Women's Hospital, Boston, Massachusetts 02115

I. Introduction

Technological advances have led to unprecedented increases in both the quantity of and the access to biomedical information. However, corresponding improvements in the validation protocol for such information represent a far greater challenge to the scientific community. Several initiatives that seek to diminish the role of peer review in biomedical publishing, such as the proposed PubMed Central (1), BioMed Central (2), and the British Medical Journal (3) Internet sites for completed but unreviewed studies, have the potential to dismantle the prevailing quality-assurance mechanism (4, 5). Therefore, the ability to appraise critically the validity of information, as a core skill of individual investigators, is likely to assume greater, rather than lesser, importance.

The important uses of published information (Table I) would suggest that surgical scientists, as well as clinical surgeons, have an obligation to acquire and practice peer-review skills with high proficiency. This chapter addresses strategies for evaluating available biomedical information. Sources of information and their relative merits are described. The discussion then focuses on the published literature, particularly original research reports, because they are the most important vehicle for transmitting new information in a format that can be critically appraised. Finally, limitations of currently available information are described, and suggestions for the future are offered.

II. Sources of Information

The most important sources of biomedical information play complementary roles, because the content of each is associated with particular strengths and weaknesses along

Table I Examples of Uses for Published Biomedical Information

Acquire new knowledge
Plan research
Prepare grant proposals
Plan management of patients or populations
Guide policy
Assess accomplishments in recruiting, promoting, and funding decisions

three dimensions: (1) validity, (2) accessibility, and (3) timeliness. Strategies for finding information in specific databases (e.g., MEDLINE) are detailed in a separate chapter in this textbook.

A. Journals

Major journals are the most important vehicle for communicating scientific information in a form that allows for critical evaluation. The validity of a journal's content is directly dependent on the rigor of its peer-review system. This quality-assurance mechanism serves two important functions: (1) eliminating obviously flawed studies from publication and (2) improving the quality of reports subsequently published. However, the rigor of peer review is limited by the skills and biases of individual reviewers and does not guarantee freedom from errors or fraud.

Relative to other information sources, the primary strength of journal articles is not that they are more valid, but that their validity can be determined most readily by each individual reader, and thus by the entire scientific community. The primary criterion for determining a journal's commitment to content validity is the degree to which it ensures that all necessary information is reported accurately in its articles. What information should be reported and how study validity can be assessed are discussed in a subsequent section of this chapter.

Journal contents are highly accessible through subscriptions, libraries, and, increasingly, electronically via the Internet in their full-text form. Although journals are published at regular intervals, delays due to the peer-review and editorial processes can result in significant time lags between study completion and publication.

B. Conference Proceedings and Abstracts

Summaries of work presented at scientific meetings are often published in the form of conference proceedings (e.g., *Surgical Forum*), which contain abbreviated manuscripts or abstracts. These publications are timely: they are usually distributed during the corresponding meeting. However, their accessibility is limited. They usually are not to be found in libraries, and they are not indexed in electronic databases such as MEDLINE. Posting meeting abstracts on Internet web sites (e.g., Society of University Surgeons meeting abstracts at www.sus.org) and publishing them in affiliated journals (e.g., Association for Academic Surgery meeting abstracts in *Journal of Surgical Research*) will increase the accessibility of these sources.

The validity of material contained in such conference proceedings is more difficult to evaluate than that of journal articles. These "minimanuscripts" and abstracts contain insufficient information to allow for assessment of study validity. Errors are particularly prevalent in meeting abstracts, which often are written hastily immediately prior to submission deadlines. These submissions undergo only an abbreviated form of peer review that tends to favor originality and positive outcomes rather than methodological rigor (6). A substantial percentage of abstracts presented are never published in full manuscript form, up to 50% in some disciplines, suggesting that these studies are withdrawn by the authors or that they do not meet the standards of full peer review (7, 8). Therefore, although conference proceedings and abstracts provide up-to-date information, they should be viewed with a level of skepticism even greater than that for journal articles.

C. Books

Book formats include (1) major general textbooks that cover entire fields, (2) specialized textbooks, (3) monographs of specific topics, and (4) review series that are updated annually. Books are appropriate sources for providing an introduction to a topic; however, in their current form they are associated with several weaknesses. Their contents reflect the biases of their authors and editors, and the validity of their contents cannot be assessed without reviewing the original source material. Books are available for purchase and in libraries, but they are not generally available electronically. Their contents usually lag behind information found in journals by several years. Methods for systematically reviewing and summarizing previously reported information are discussed in Section IV,B; some of the concepts described therein might be applicable to improving the quality of future books.

D. Other Sources

1. Conferences and Courses

Conferences can foster an interactive and timely exchange of information. The validity of such information should be approached with skepticism, as discussed above. Courses also allow for dialogue, but the material taught reflects the biases of the instructors. Relative to other information sources, conferences and courses are associated with high cost and low accessibility.

2. Colleagues and Personal Communications

The accessibility and timeliness of information from colleagues (from anywhere in the world) have improved dramatically with the advent of e-mail. Limitations of personal communications include, of course, bias and inaccuracy.

3. Internet Web Sites

Sources of information on the Internet are discussed in a separate chapter in this volume. Electronic versions of peer-reviewed journals are likely to become the most important scientific information source, replacing their print counterparts. Other sources should be approached with a high degree of skepticism.

III. Assessing Published Studies: External Measures of Quality

Commonly used criteria for judging the quality of a journal article include the reputation of the authors, the prestige of the institution from which the study arose, and the impact factor of the article and the journal in which it was published. These criteria often play a prominent role in promotion, funding, and award decisions for individual investigators. They also play a role in determining the perceived importance of a study's findings. However, these criteria are no substitute for a rigorous analysis of a study's internal validity. Their limitations are discussed below.

A. Authors and Institutions

Established investigators have a track record of productivity with particular methodologies or models. Large research institutions are likely to harbor a critical mass of skilled investigators, leading to an environment that fosters scientific rigor. However, even the most highly regarded investigators and institutions are not immune to errors in study execution or interpretation. In reports from multiple authors and/or institutions, the respective roles of each of the authors, and which author bears ultimate responsibility, often are ambiguous. All authors may not have reviewed the manuscript, and all authors may not even understand the entire study.

B. Journal

Major peer-reviewed journals should be distinguished from those that do not subscribe to this quality-control mechanism. Typically, the latter journals are sponsored by parties with commercial interests, arrive unsolicited in the mail, and are known as "throwaway journals." The primary purpose of these journals is to generate revenue through advertising rather than to disseminate scientific findings (4). Even the most prestigious journals, however, are subject to economic realities and depend on revenues from subscriptions and advertising for survival. They are not immune from overt bias either. For example, campaigns against smoking and gun ownership have been waged by the *Journal of the American Medical Association* and the *New England Journal of Medicine*, respectively (4).

C. Impact Factor

In response to the limitations of subjective measures, such as the ones discussed above, there has been an attempt to develop quantitative indices of scientific quality. These efforts have led to the development of **impact factors** for both individual articles and journals.

The Institute for Scientific Information (ISI) (9) maintains a database of all references found in the reference lists of selected scientific journals. This database is used to generate the Science Citation Index (SCI), which lists how many times the various references have been cited during the last year and by whom. The **journal impact factor,** published annually in the SCI Journal Citation Reports (9), is calculated as the mean number of reference citations, in a given year, to journal items published during the preceding 2 years.

These impact factors have been used for research evaluation, on the assumption that citations indicate scientific quality. However, this assumption is invalid for the following reasons: (1) authors select references for their manuscripts based not on their quality, but other factors, such as utility in research, (2) authors may have a poor knowledge of the primary literature in their field and may fail to cite seminal source material, (3) certain citing conventions distort the validity of impact factors (e.g., the originator of an analytic method is usually cited, but the discoverer of a useful chemical is not; biochemistry articles contain many citations, but mathematics articles contain few citations), (4) distortions within a field can also occur (in rapidly expanding areas citation rates will be high because the number of cites is high relative to the amount of citable material), and (5) citation rates are subject to manipulation (e.g., authors can inappropriately cite their own work, and journal editorials can inappropriately cite the journal's own articles) (10, 11). At best, impact factors remain an imperfect surrogate for quality, of either journals or individual studies.

IV. How to Read and Evaluate Published Studies

This section offers strategies for the critical analysis of published research studies. Each study should be approached with skepticism and assumed to be flawed until determined to be valid. In particular, the presence of bias, or systematic distortions away from truth, should be sought. [See Sackett (12) for a description of the most prevalent biases that infiltrate studies.]

The discussion below focuses on journal articles reporting the results of primary studies. Specific issues to scrutinize for each section of such articles are given. Secondary, or integrative, studies are discussed in Section IV,B.

A. Primary Studies

1. Title

The title is often written to catch the readers' attention. Its content may even be misleading and should not be assumed to reflect the results of the study (13).

2. Abstract

The abstract provides only a superficial amount of information with which the reader can decide if the paper is worth reading in greater detail. Because it does not provide enough information to assess study validity, conclusions should not be based on reading of the abstract alone.

3. Introduction

This section should contain (1) why the study was needed and (2) a clear statement of the study aims and hypotheses. The hypotheses should be formulated prior to data collection (*a priori*) and not afterward (*posteriori*). Hypothesis-generating studies (known as "fishing expeditions") can provide useful insights (e.g., in genomic expression profiling studies), but their conclusions should be considered preliminary until tested in subsequent studies.

4. Methods

The results of the study are not worth considering if the methodology was severely flawed. Specific methodological issues are described below.

a. Subjects For clinical studies, the population from which patients were selected should be described, as should strict inclusion and exclusion criteria. The reader should be able to state unequivocally whether any hypothetical patient would be included or excluded. Did all those eligible to enter the study enter? If not, why? All subjects who entered the trial should be accounted for at the conclusion of the trial. Withdrawals from trial (whether initiated by investigators or subjects) should be described. Detailed information on procedures used to follow-up patients should be described.

Rates of attrition for subjects from clinical studies greater than 10–15% should arouse concern about study validity. A strategy for assessing the possible effects of loss-of-subject bias (subjects lost to follow-up might be different from those who remain, and the groups studied might have different drop-out rates) is as follows: in a trial showing a more favorable outcome with treatment A than with treatment B, if all the patients lost from group A are assumed to have had a poor outcome and all those lost from group B are assumed to have had a favorable outcome, if the conclusions of the trial do not change using these assumptions, loss to follow-up was not excessive (14).

b. Models For experimental studies, it is important to determine whether the appropriate species and/or model was used. Detailed discussions of specific issues related to standard models of physiology and pathophysiology follow in subsequent chapters. As discussed below, results should not be extrapolated to species and models not studied.

c. Data Collection and Measurements Outcome parameters appropriate to the study aims should be selected. These parameters should be defined precisely (e.g., "mortality" is clear but "disease-free survival" is ambiguous unless criteria for its determination are clearly stated). Outcome assessment should be performed equivalently for all groups. Whether the act of measurement might have affected outcome should be considered.

Analytical instruments and assays should be described in detail and appropriate references given (many of the standard assays used in biomedical research are described in subsequent chapters). The limitations of these assays should be considered. Assessment of reliability should be given for measurements (e.g., intra- and interrater reliability for subjective determinations such as histology scores and X-ray interpretations). Coefficients of variation should be given for novel or unusual assays.

For studies in which experimental groups receive different treatments, blinding increases study validity by reducing the effects of *a priori* biases on the part of both investigators and subjects. If only the subjects are unaware of which treatment they are receiving, the study is called **blind.** If both subjects and investigators are unaware, it is called **double blind.**

d. Study Design The study design should be explicitly stated. Specific study designs are associated with different degrees of vulnerability to bias, or interference that produces results that are systematically removed from the truth. Clinical trials or experiments in which subjects are allocated to treatment/intervention and control groups using randomization techniques and are then evaluated prospectively (prospective randomized trial) are the least susceptible to bias. Case series, case reports, and expert opinions are the most susceptible to bias. Cohort studies (observational studies that prospectively follow groups to determine the relationship between risk factors and outcomes) and case control studies (observation studies that retrospectively examine risk factors for groups with known outcomes) carry an intermediate susceptibility to bias (15).

Randomization diminishes the potential for investigators selecting subjects in a way that would unfairly bias one treatment group over another (selection bias). Although studies with randomization are most likely to yield valid information on relative treatment efficacy and cause–effect relationships, they are associated with specific pitfalls. How the investigators actually performed the randomization should be described. Acceptable methods include the use a table of random numbers or a computer program that produces a random sequence. The outcomes of all subjects should be analyzed according to the groups to which they were randomized, even if they were noncompliant or switched groups. Such "intention-to-treat analysis" is likely to preserve the value of randomization, that relevant factors (both known and unknown) should be the same in both groups.

e. Statistics Statistical methods are discussed in greater detail in a separate chapter in this book. Three of the most prevalent statistical errors about which to be vigilant are (1) statistical analysis methods and sample size determinations being made after data collection (*posteriori*) rather than *a priori*, (2) lack of significance being interpreted to imply lack of difference [studies with negative (not statistically different) results must include power calculations so that the probability of type II errors (differences not detected when there are differences) can be assessed], and (3) multiple outcome measurements, multiple comparisons, and subgroup comparisons [in the absence of appropriate multivariable procedures and clear *a priori* hypotheses, suspect the presence of type I errors (differences concluded when there are no differences)].

5. Results

If the study was conducted appropriately, then the results should be scrutinized. The data presentation should be complete enough to allow quantitative and qualitative assessment of results; mere allusions to the data are insufficient. The authors' calculations and statistical analyses should be reproducible based on the data presented. Important visual data, such as *in situ* hybridization images, should be included so that their quality and interpretation can be assessed.

Quantitative data should consist of descriptive statistics (e.g., mean and standard deviation) and the results of statistical tests (the statistical test used should be clear; a p value without a specifying test is known as an "orphan p"). Sample size should be clearly stated for each result. Data from baseline measurements should be given for each study group, even for randomized studies. If the randomization procedure resulted in groups varying with respect to relevant factors, covariate methods are necessary.

6. Discussion

The reader should derive his or her own conclusions based on the data presented rather than rely on the authors' interpretation and opinions. There are two prevalent errors in study interpretation about which to be wary: (1) The *a priori* hypothesis was not addressed. The conclusions should be directly based on the study hypotheses. Study findings unrelated to the hypotheses should be the basis for further study, not firm conclusions. (2) Extrapolation beyond data analyzed in the study. The results should not be generalized to other models, other species, other patient populations, other drug dosages, other follow-up periods, etc.

The Discussion section should contain a review of the relevant literature. Previously published findings both concordant and discordant with the study results should be described. However, the reader should be aware that there is no assurance that citations were selected in a nonbiased way. Standards for conducting and reporting systematic literature reviews are discussed below.

B. Reviews

In their traditional form, reviews consist of summaries of an arbitrarily selected body of literature interspersed with the author's opinions. Such authoritative reviews are highly susceptible to bias, and the validity of the conclusions they contain usually cannot be assessed objectively. However, they are useful for obtaining background information and serve as a launching point for more detailed explorations on a given topic.

In contrast to authoritative reviews, systematic reviews attempt to answer focused questions through impartial compilation and rigorous analysis of available evidence. Systematic reviews can provide either qualitative or quantitative syntheses of evidence. Qualitative reviews do not provide statistical summaries of available data and may be the only option when the heterogeneity of available evidence precludes data pooling. Quantitative reviews (meta-analyses) combine the results of multiple studies to maximize statistical power. They evaluate the quality of available evidence, determine the similarity of results from different studies, evaluate the robustness of the pooled results, and attempt to relate these summary findings to the many individual studies (16).

Systematic reviews should be scrutinized as rigorously as original reports. Criteria for their evaluation are as follows: (1) The review should address a well-articulated, focused question (similar to a hypothesis or study aim). Broad overviews are rarely systematic. (2) The authors should describe methods for identifying reports included in the review in sufficient detail for the reader to nearly replicate the search. The reader should assess whether the authors may have missed pertinent literature or included irrelevant material. (3) The authors should describe strict inclusion/exclusion criteria for studies identified. Methods for assessing quality of the individual studies and their homogeneity (in quantitative reviews) should be detailed. The reader should realize that validity of the review conclusions is dependent on the quality of the original studies (17).

Clinical guidelines, closely related to systematic reviews, are designed to provide explicit recommendations for clinical practice, based on the synthesis and evaluation of available evidence. These guidelines should be judged using criteria similar to those for other types of systematic reviews. Because these guidelines are often prepared by professional organizations, they have the potential to carry the biases of these organizations and their sponsors (18).

V. Suggestions for the Future

Access to information should no longer be a limiting factor in scientific progress. Two implications of this assertion are as follows:

1. All the data generated in a study should be made available for scrutiny. Internet technology has made space limitations imposed by print journals obsolete. For example, data sets that are prohibitively large to be included in print form, such as those arising from DNA microarray studies, are being made available via Internet web sites. Similarly, comprehensive data sets should be made available for all studies, including clinical trials. All raw data and calculations should be made available, including those for individual experiments that "failed to work" for whatever reason. The practice of reporting data only from the subset of experiments that yielded data consistent with the hypothesis should be abandoned.

2. The results of all studies, even ones in which the null hypothesis was supported (negative studies), should be reported. Such negative results, assuming the study was conducted and interpreted correctly, provide valid and potentially important information. This should be a **requirement** for all studies conducted with public funds, even incorrectly conducted studies. This information would be useful in making funding decisions.

Regardless of how scientific information is communicated, its critical evaluation always will remain central to the scientific enterprise. This skill must be learned and practiced by its participants. Two types of errors will escape detection during even the most rigorous evaluation, however: (1) honest mistakes in execution and reporting and (2) outright fraud. Therefore, investigators must constantly strive for accuracy in their work, and the entire scientific community must remain ever vigilant in its search for truth.

References

1. http://www.pubmedcentral.nih.gov
2. http://www.biomedcnetral.com
3. http://clinmed.netprints.org/
4. Vandenbroucke, J. P. (1998). Medical journals and the shaping of medical knowledge. *Lancet* **352,** 2001–2006.
5. Bloom, F. E. (2000). Lunch selections expanding. *Science* **287,** 801.
6. Callaham, M. L., Wears, R. L., Weber, E. J., Barton, C., and Young, G. (1998). Positive-outcome bias and other limitations in the outcome of research abstracts submitted to a scientific meeting. *JAMA* **280,** 254-247.
7. Scherer, R. W., Dickersin, K., and Langenberg, P. (1994). Full publication of results initially presented in abstracts: A meta-analysis. *JAMA* **272,** 158–162.
8. Kelly, J. A. (1998). Scientific meeting abstracts: significance, access, trends. *Bull. Med. Libr. Assoc.* **86,** 68–76.
9. Garfield, E. (1994). "SCI Journal Citation Reports: A Bibliometric Analysis of Science Journals in the ISI Database." Institute for Science Information Inc., Philadelphia, PA.
10. Seglen, P. O. (1997). Citations and journal impact factors: questionable indicators of research quality. *Allergy* **52,** 1050–1056.
11. Vinkler, P. (1996). Ralationships between the rate of scientific development and citations. The change for a citedness model. *Scientometrics* **35,** 375–386.
12. Sackett, D. L. (1979). Bias in analytic research. *J. Chronic Dis.* **32,** 51–63.
13. Evans, M., and Pollock, V. (1984). Trials on trial. *Arch. Surg.* **119,** 109–113.
14. Guyatt, G. H., Sacket, D. L., and Cook, D. J. (1993). Users' guide to the medical literature. II. How to use an article about therapy or prevention. A. Are the results of the study valid? *JAMA* **270,** 2598–2601.
15. U.S. Preventive Services Task Force. Guide to clinical preventive services. Baltimore MD: William & Wilkins, 1989.
16. Lau, J., Ioannidis, J. P., and Schmid, C. H. (1997). Quantitative synthesis in systematic reviews. *Ann. Intern. Med.* **127,** 820–826.
17. Hunt, D. L., and McKibbon, K. A. (1997). Locating and apprasing systematic reviews. *Ann. Intern. Med.* **126,** 532–538.
18. Hayward, R. S. A., Wilson, M. C., Tunis, S. R., *et al.* (1995). User's guides to the medical literature: VIII. How to use clinical practice guidelines: A. Are the recommendations valid? *JAMA* **274,** 570–574.

3

Organizing and Preliminary Planning for Surgical Research

Michael W. Mulholland

University of Michigan Medical Center, Ann Arbor, Michigan 48109

I. Research as the Foundation of an Academic Surgical Career

Research is one of the cornerstones of an academic surgical career. In addition to caring for patients, teaching of medical students and residents, and service to the medical community, surgical research provides the motivation, and many of the rewards, for a career in academic surgery. Investigative efforts can take many forms, including activities as diverse as molecular biology, cell biology, epidemiology, patient-based outcomes studies, and financial analysis. The research should be judged in terms of its quality, originality, and impact in shaping the care and lives of future surgical patients. Success in an academic career based on research requires careful, thoughtful planning. Remember the Boy Scout motto: "Be prepared."

The recruitment of surgeons to investigative careers is a national priority. Data from the National Institutes of Health (NIH) indicate that progressively fewer young physicians are preparing for careers as independent NIH-funded investigators. In the 7-year period from 1989 through 1996, the proportion of medical students with a strong interest in research fell progressively from 14 to 10% (1). This decline in interest in research has been reflected, in subsequent years, by a decrease in the number of M.D. postdoctoral research fellows supported by NIH fellowships and training grants. Since 1992, the number of M.D. fellowship awardees has decreased by 51%. The Howard Hughes Medical Institute has noted similar trends. The result of these declines in physicians preparing for investigative careers has been an undersupply of motivated, highly qualified physician-scientists for junior faculty positions in American medical schools. This problem is most acute for surgical disciplines and is exacerbated by the flat rates of surgical graduate medical education enrollment and training graduation (2). For qualified investigative surgeons, employment opportunities abound.

II. Research Training

Most successful investigative surgeons have participated in research at some point during their training. In terms of timing, two main models have been employed. In the first model, research training has been acquired in the midst of the undergraduate general surgical residency. In the second model, research training is a component of Fellowship training. Both models can be applied to the benefit of the trainee. They both require an institutional commitment, exemplified by flexibility in training schedules, financial, personnel, and physical resources dedicated to the development of young surgical investigators, and a cadre of capable mentors.

The major consideration in preparing for an investigative career is the length of time dedicated to research training. A number of programs exist that are structured for 1-year, 2-year, and greater than 2-year experiences. The choice of timing is dependent on the trainee's research agenda. A 1-year block of time devoted to research is adequate to answer the question "Do I like research?" This period of time permits the trainee to participate in the scientific method, to develop a research protocol, and to accrue a body of data. It also permits the trainee to experience the inevitable frustrations that attend investigative work, and to experience the intellectual stimulation when experiments produce novel findings. A 1-year period is not usually, however, a sufficient period of time to perform a series of experiments, or to develop a line of investigation. For most trainees, 1-year experience is not an adequate period of time to develop fully as a biomedical investigator.

In the proper environment, a 2-year period of time provides a much more adequate experience. A series of experiments can be performed. It is the common observation of surgical investigators that data acquisition the second year more than doubles the output during the first year. This is an inevitable consequence of maturation of experimental judgment, improved efficiency in experimental technique, and the need to correct problems in experimental design. A 2-year period of time is often sufficient to develop a semiautonomous investigator. Papers can be written. Public presentations can be polished. Future collaborations can be established. A full range of research activities, including application for extramural funding, may not be accomplished within 2 years, however.

Research training extending for 3 or more years produces a more refined investigator. For many surgical trainees, the decision to extend the research training beyond 2 years represents a compromise. Long training periods for clinical subspecialties of general surgery place practical constraints on the amount of time that can be solely devoted to investigative work. In addition, external pressures, including constraints of funding of graduate medical education, limit an institution's flexibility in making prolonged periods of research training available.

III. Choosing a Research Mentor

The choice of a research mentor is the most important single decision that a research trainee will make. In his presidential address to the American Surgical Association, Dr. Clyde Barker [3] outlined his rules for a successful career in academic surgery, with rule #1 being "pick a good mentor." The choice of mentor requires an appropriate fit of personal and professional characteristics. This choice should be made by the trainee, rather than by the trainee's supervisor or potential mentor. The trainee should seek a mentor with whom he/she feels intellectually comfortable. The mentor should be approachable, open to intellectual discussions, and dedicated to the development of the trainee. Mentorship should not be chosen unless the potential mentor has the time, mental energy, physical resources, and financial flexibility to support the full development of the trainee.

A mentor–trainee relationship is not static. For most, the relationship begins with the mentor being directive in the development of the trainee. Techniques must be learned, intellectual discipline instilled, and projects proposed and provided. As the trainee becomes more adept scientifically, the mentorship must change to allow a greater degree of experimental independence. The trainee must be allowed to propose new research ideas and to test new techniques. Successes should be celebrated. Failures must be tolerated with equanimity. Under the proper circumstances, the trainee should eventually evolve into an independent investigator. At this point, the mentor should become supportive and advisory and should permit, even encourage, the trainee to move into new experimental directions.

IV. Choosing a Research Topic

In an ideal world, a fledgling investigator would pick a currently unsolved clinical problem as a research topic, and hope that a research program, narrowly focused on this clinical problem, could be combined with the clinical care of patients. This is an appealing concept. It provides relevance to the surgical research and intellectual gratification, which is both more immediate and less abstract. Unfortunately, a research career that is too narrowly focused can be stifling and sometimes unproductive. Research interests change. Basic scientific advances provide new understanding of disease pathology.

A better approach is to combine a clinically relevant research topic with a widely applicable level of scientific investigation. For example, the techniques used to investigate the molecular biology of colon cancer could be easily applied to examine the control of gastric acid secretion, or the pathogenesis of atherosclerosis, or the biology of solid organ rejection. The skills developed for the epidemiology of heart disease could equally well be applied to population studies of vehicular trauma or interpersonal violence.

V. General Preparation

Time is the most important ingredient in properly preparing for research training. To select a mentor properly, to develop a research topic, and to perform background reading in the midst of the demands of clinical patient care require sufficient lead time. If possible, a lead time of $1–1\frac{1}{2}$ years is recommend. Prior to entering the laboratory, a program of scientific reading should be undertaken. The reading program should be an introduction to the general scientific topic to be investigated. With time, the reading should become increasingly specific, and increasingly experimental. Primary sources should be sought. A sense of the direction of the experimental field, and its momentum, should be obtained. The relevance of the proposed research project to clinical care should be evaluated.

VI. Experimental Preparation

Experimental preparation begins by expression of hypotheses. A hypothesis forms the conceptual framework for the scientific work. The hypothesis must be broad enough to be scientifically important. It must also be focused narrowly enough to be expressed experimentally. The hypothesis must be testable. The discipline required to express, in written form, the hypothesis is a crucial first step in performing the experiment.

Hypothesis generation is the most important initial step in the research process. The hypotheses must be fully developed, yet succinct. The NIH and other scientific agencies do not fund great ideas–the NIH does fund systemic thinking.

Each of the hypotheses must be translated into an experimental aim. The experimental aim is the action plan for evaluating the hypothesis. In preparing specific aims, begin with a short statement of the contribution of the specific aim to the overall proposed study. Concisely state the aim, while being sure that the relationship to the overall hypothesis is clear. It is axiomatic that the time to limit the variables and delineate the controls is before the experiment is performed.

A young investigator should ask himself/herself the following questions before embarking upon a series of experiments:

1. Is the general question interesting, important, and original? Do other surgical scientists feel that the work is worth doing?
2. Have clear hypotheses been developed? Do the specific aims provide a logical test of the hypotheses?
3. Are the proposed studies feasible? Do the experiments utilize the most direct methods and experimental approaches?
4. Is the proposed mentor qualified to guide the work, as judged by academic credentials, preparation, and record of productivity?
5. Are facilities, equipment, and personnel adequate for the proposed work? Is the intellectual environment conducive to research?

The answers to all five questions must, of course, be affirmative.

At the outset of research training, it is advisable to adapt existing techniques. The experience of other seasoned investigators can thus be used as a yardstick of experimental competence. The development of new techniques is essential to mature scientists but represents a calculated risk. With new techniques, things do not always work smoothly. For most young investigators, the time constraints of the training period argue against starting with unproved techniques.

Before the experiment is conducted, an excellent intellectual exercise is to predict the results. State in plain English the expected observations. A second important intellectual exercise is to predict experimental problems. Experimental difficulties are of three major forms—technical, biological, and interpretive. Taking the time to articulate potential problems also provides an opportunity to articulate alternative methods or limits of interpretation of the data. An anticipated problem is usually a problem avoided.

Finally, young investigators should seek external critiques. The choice of mentor, the research plan, and the experimental details should all be discussed with a friendly, open, and scientifically sophisticated advisor. The purpose of the critique is not to seek affirmation of the choices. Instead, the critique should center on problems not anticipated, difficulties overlooked, potential problems to be remedied before they become real difficulties.

VII. Grant Preparation

At first consideration, it might seem inappropriate to include grant preparation as a topic related to "Organizing and Preliminary Planning." Most beginning investigators do not possess the experience or scientific sophistication to compose an extramural funding application. However, participation with a research mentor in grant preparation can be an unsurpassed method to crystallize experimental plans and to obtain state-of-the-art information.

For young surgical investigators, the American College of Surgeons is an invaluable resource. Most College resources can be accessed online. An excellent template for proposal preparation can be found at http://www.facs.org. Sources of surgical research funding are published each February in the *Bulletin of the American College of Surgeons*. This surgical research clearinghouse can also be obtained via the web at the above address. Recommendations for first time surgical grant writers are also included at that web site.

References

1. Rosenberg, L. E. (1999). Physician-scientists, endangered and essential. *Science* **283,** 331–332.
2. Kwalkwa, F., and Jonasson, O. (1999). The longitudinal study of surgical residents, 1994 to 1996. *J. Am. Coll. Surg.* **188,** 575–585.
3. Barker, C. F. (1997). Science, specialization, and the American Surgical Association. *Ann. Surg.* **226,** 1–18.

4

Writing a Protocol: Animals, Humans, and Use of Biologic, Chemical, and Radiologic Agents

Wayne R. Patterson

The University of Texas Medical Branch, Galveston, Texas 77555

I. Introduction

When utilizing animal or human subjects in research activities, it is necessary to write a specific animal or human use research protocol and submit it for review and approval before beginning the research. In fact, granting agencies will not fund (and may not even review) a proposal until it has received appropriate institutional approval. In addition, prior to accepting a manuscript for publication, many professional journals now require certification that the research was reviewed and approved by the appropriate institutional ethics and safety committees. These committees are concerned with ensuring that animal and human subjects are protected from unnecessary experimentation, as well as ensuring institutional compliance with a multitude of regulations governing the care and use of laboratory animals; human subject protections; biologic (including recombinant DNA), chemical, and radiologic safety; and radioactive drug research. Many times, the research must be reviewed by several committees, and although some institutions organizationally and physically colocate the committees, it is possible that the committees may not be directly associated with one another and may be located in separate offices. Therefore, in order to ensure a more efficient protocol review process, researchers must be aware of the committee associations and requirements.

In the United States, there are no standardized forms for ethics and safety committee review and approval, and most institutions require completion of their own customized protocol request form(s). The information requested and the questions asked on the institutional forms are designed to ensure that the committee is able to satisfy both the letter and the spirit of the regulatory requirements, thereby protecting the subjects, the investigators, and the institution. The intent of this chapter is to assist researchers in meeting their regulatory requirements by discussing what information must be supplied and explaining briefly why this information is required for review and subsequent approval of the research. Knowing the intent of a regulatory requirement may help researchers answer questions addressing specific requirements.

Because animal-related studies are often the starting point for researchers pursuing a specific line of investigation, the first discussion is of the requirements for laboratory animal protocol review and approval. This is followed by a discussion of human subject research and the issues and procedures involved when performing studies involving biologic hazards (including recombinant DNA, genetic engineering and gene therapy), hazardous chemicals, radioactive substances, and ionizing radiation. All of this is then tied together so that what appears at first glance to be a morass of regulations and requirements actually makes some sense, allowing researchers to navigate efficiently and successfully the research review and approval process.

II. Research Utilizing Laboratory Animals

A. General

From a philosophical and historical perspective, the framework of proper and humane care and use of laboratory animals emerged from scientists and from various groups concerned with protecting pets and other animals from abuse. At the National Institutes of Health (NIH), for example, the proper care and use of animals was strongly encouraged, on a voluntary basis, for about the first 70 years of the NIH's existence (1). An early organization, now known as the American Association for Laboratory Animal Science, published the first edition of the "Guide for the Care and Use of Laboratory Animals" (Guide) in 1963. The Guide, now published by the Institute for Laboratory Animal Research of the National Academy of Sciences, has been updated several times, and is the primary reference relating to laboratory animal care and use for the NIH and several other organizations (2). Three years after publication of the Guide and in response to public concerns regarding allegations that pets were being stolen and used in research, the Pet Protection Act of 1966, now more commonly known as the Animal Welfare Act (AWA), was passed by Congress (3). The requirements of the AWA are found in the Code of Federal Regulations (9 CFR, Parts 1, 2, and 3) and are implemented and enforced by the United States Department of Agriculture (USDA) (4). In addition to the Guide and the Animal Welfare Act, another document, the "Public Health Service Policy on Humane Care and Use of Laboratory Animals" (PHS Policy), became effective in 1986, applies to all institutions receiving PHS funds, and covers all live, vertebrate species (5). All three documents address the same concerns, but depending on several factors, e.g., the species used or the source of funding, an institution may be governed either by the USDA regulations, PHS Policy, or both. Although this is more of an institutional concern and does not usually affect researchers directly, an awareness of the laws and organization may help explain some of the hurdles that will have to be negotiated in preparing a protocol and in performing ongoing research.

The regulations require that the Chief Executive Officer of an institution at which studies using laboratory animals are performed must appoint an Institutional Animal Care and Use Committee (IACUC), "qualified through the experience and expertise of its members to oversee the institution's animal program, facilities, and procedures" (4, 5). Also, PHS Policy requires that an IACUC be composed of at least five members (the USDA requires a minimum of three members), some of whom must meet specific background and training requirements—i.e., one Doctor of Veterinary Medicine with training or experience in laboratory animal medicine, one practicing scientist, one nonscientist, and one member who is not affiliated with the institution except through the IACUC (5). The IACUC has the ultimate authority and responsibility for oversight of the animal care and use program and facilities at the institution, including reviewing new and ongoing research proposals and requests for modifications to protocols. Included with its oversight responsibilities is the IACUC's authority to suspend any animal-related research activity that does not conform to the regulations. Suspensions are rare, but it is important to note that, unlike many other institutional committees, there is no provision for an appeals process to an institutional executive administration. In other words, if the IACUC suspends an activity, that decision cannot be overturned by anyone at the institution.

As mentioned above, the IACUC is responsible for reviewing research proposals requesting to use laboratory animals and must determine that the proposed research conforms to the regulations. In doing so, IACUCs will require that principal investigators provide specific information. The information, and the rationale for requiring it, are discussed in the following section (4, 5).

B. Protocol Requirements

The IACUC requires the following information to be submitted:

1. *The name, departmental affiliation, and contact information of the principal investigator, and the names of all personnel who will be working with animals.* Obviously, the principal investigator must be identified, because this is the person who is ultimately responsible for the conduct of the research and for the actions of all staff involved with the animals. This information may also be used by the IACUC to determine if the personnel involved have the necessary training to handle the species that will be used, what training may be required before handling the animals, and who will be providing the training. In addition, person-

nel handling or having contact with nonhuman primates, dogs, cats, and sheep may be required to enroll in an Occupational Health monitoring program. For example, personnel in contact with nonhuman primates must be tested semiannually for tuberculosis. It often comes as a surprise to researchers that this requirement is for protection of the animals, not the humans.

2. *A brief summary or abstract, in lay terminology, describing the research, species used, and why the research will be beneficial to society.* This may be one of the toughest requirements for an investigator to complete, because researchers usually write for a scientific audience. Therefore, most lay summaries are neither brief nor in lay terminology. Perhaps the best way to approach this requirement is to think in terms of how you might explain your research to your grandmother, who has no scientific or medical training. Then simply, in one short paragraph, say what you will be doing (not too graphic), with what species of animal, and why the research is important. Some institutions may want to use this summary in press releases and other public relations announcements, so it is best to be rather general in describing your methods.

3. *The species and projected number of animals to be used.* This information is used by the IACUC to determine adequacy of housing and to assess whether the number of animals requested is the minimum necessary to obtain a scientifically valid answer to the research question. A power analysis is generally accepted and recommended as an appropriate justification for the number of animals requested.

4. *The rationale for using animals and why the species chosen is the most appropriate for the proposed experiments.* The principal investigator must justify why animals must be used and why the species chosen is the most appropriate species. This could be as simple as stating that an intact immune system is required that cannot be achieved in a lower order animal or by computer simulation or that all previous work has been performed in the selected species and that the species is the accepted animal model for this type of research. Be prepared to back this up with appropriate references.

5. *A description of the proposed use of the animals.* The IACUC will need to evaluate the proposed research. It is not technically a scientific review, because IACUCs are not supposed to perform this type of review, but rather is an evaluation of whether the proposed research is a valid and justifiable use of animals. This requirement could be achieved by attaching the Methods and Materials section of your grant proposal. Also, it is helpful (and may be required) to attach a flow chart illustrating the experimental groups, what will be done to each group, and at what time experimental manipulations and euthanasia will occur. A picture (diagram) may be worth a thousand words in this area.

6. *A description of procedures designed to assure that discomfort, distress, or pain to animals will be limited to what is unavoidable in the conduct of scientifically valuable research. Also, that analgesic, anesthetic, and tranquilizing drugs will be used where indicated and appropriate to minimize discomfort and pain to animals.* What the IACUC is looking for here is a description of anesthesia that will be used during the surgical procedure, the specific analgesic that will be administered postsurgery, the dose at which it will be given, and the duration for which it will be given. If administration of analgesics would interfere with data collection, withholding them must be scientifically justified. Also, the use of paralytics without the use of anesthesia is forbidden under any circumstances.

7. *A description of the method of euthanasia, the expected experimental endpoint, and criteria for a humane endpoint to experiments.* The method of euthanasia must follow the report of the AVMA Panel on euthanasia (6). This report lists methods of euthanasia appropriate for each species by dose and route of administration. Also important to describe to the IACUC are the criteria for a humane endpoint for those animals that become moribund prior to the expected experimental endpoint. Many IACUCs have specific criteria for each species and may even have a checklist to follow to determine if an animal should be humanely euthanized prior to the end of the experimental procedures.

8. *A written narrative description of the methods and sources used to identify alternatives to procedures that cause more than momentary or slight pain or distress to the animal, justifying the choice of species and methodology to be used.* The purpose of this item is to assure the IACUC that the principal investigator has considered and searched for alternatives to painful of distressful procedures. This is often interpreted to mean alternatives to the use of animals. This could be the case, but it also refers to a search for alternative, perhaps lower order, animals (e.g., invertebrates), whose use could also answer the research question, or alternative methods that are less stressful or painful. This will likely require a carefully constructed literature search and, possibly, assistance from the Animal Welfare Information Center of the National Agricultural Library (7).

9. *A written assurance that the experiments are not unnecessarily duplicative.* The scientist members of the IACUC will recognize that reproducing experimental data is sometimes necessary. What they are looking for is assurance that the investigator is not unnecessarily collecting data that has already been reported elsewhere. Again, a careful literature review will likely be necessary.

10. *A description of the housing location and location of actual use.* Housing of animals must be in facilities that meet all regulatory standards. If an institution has a Laboratory Animal Resources Center, this is not usually a problem. However, activities that involve surgical procedures must provide appropriate pre- and postsurgical care. In addition, all survival surgery must be performed using aseptic procedures and techniques, and surgeries on nonrodent species must be performed in an area dedicated only

for that purpose. At this time, surgery on rodents does not require a dedicated facility but must be performed using aseptic technique.

11. *A description of the level of training of all personnel handling the animals and any additional training that will be given prior to beginning the research.* It is the responsibility of the IACUC to ensure that all personnel involved in animal care and use are qualified to perform their tasks. If personnel have not received IACUC-approved training, it must be provided prior to beginning the research. Many institutions require specific training for certain species prior to conducting the research. The training may be offered by the IACUC, the Laboratory Animal Resources staff, or by some other method. Check with the IACUC to determine what needs to be done in this area.

12. *The type of medical or postsurgical care that will be given and who will give it.* The IACUC must also assure that medical care given to laboratory animals is readily available and provided by a qualified veterinarian. This is not usually a problem at larger institutions, but it must be clear who will provide this care.

13. *Assurance that no animal will be used in more than one major operative procedure from which the animal is allowed to recover.* This requirement is present to ensure that investigators do not recycle animals through several procedures in order to reduce costs. Multiple-survival surgeries can be approved by the IACUC, but they must be scientifically justified in writing by the principal investigator.

C. Continuing Review

Review and approval of ongoing research is another regulatory requirement. According to the USDA, ongoing research must be reviewed "at appropriate intervals as determined by the IACUC, but not less than annually" (4). PHS Policy requires continuing review every 3 years (5). In order to simplify the process and prevent confusion, most IACUCs take the more stringent stance and review ongoing research annually. IACUCs should notify investigators when continuing review is required and may have specific forms to be completed by the investigator.

D. Amendments

Changes to ongoing research must be approved by the IACUC prior to implementation, and, if minor, generally can take the form of a memo or e-mail to the IACUC office. Minor changes would likely include those in which the investigator is requesting approval of additional animals or changes to methods and procedures that do not affect the pain or distress level experienced by the animal. However, if the requested changes are significant, a new proposal must be submitted. The definition of significant may vary by institution, but examples might include an addition of a new species or a change in experimental methods that affects the animal's level of discomfort, distress, or pain. It is best to check with the IACUC office to determine which approach is appropriate.

E. Organizational Certification and Accreditation

Institutions that conduct a significant amount of animal research may be certified or accredited by federal or other agencies. Certification usually comes in the form of a Multiple Project Assurance (MPA) that is submitted to and approved by the Animal Welfare Division of the Office for Protection from Research Risks (5). Essentially, an MPA is a statement of the procedures used by an institution in order to meet federal regulatory requirements for animal research. If approved, the MPA is in effect for a period of 5 years and must be updated whenever there are changes to the animal care and use program or facilities, such as a change in IACUC membership or addition or deletion of an animal housing facility. Accreditation of institutional animal care and use programs is voluntary and is accomplished by the Association for Assessment and Accreditation of Laboratory Animal Care—International (AAALAC). AAALAC accreditation is considered to be the "gold standard" for animal research programs, and being accredited significantly reduces the paperwork required to be submitted in support of an NIH grant request.

F. Animal Rights Issues

It is perhaps appropriate to end this section with a brief discussion of animal welfare/animal rights organizations. IACUCs and federal agencies concerned with animal research usually have no problem working with animal welfare groups. Assuring and improving the welfare of laboratory animals is an appropriate goal for all. However, dealing with animal rights organizations is difficult, and in many cases not possible. The stated goal of animal rights groups is to stop unconditionally the use of animals in medical research entirely. Although scientists and the majority of the public agree that this is currently not possible, the difference of opinion is a significant issue. Therefore, incidents of animal facility break-ins and vandalism, with destruction of valuable equipment and research data, are likely to continue. Additionally, some investigators have been targeted and confronted by protesters at home and work, and in some cases received threats to their and their family's safety. Dealing with these groups, in what is usually an adversarial public relations event, is difficult and sometimes dangerous and better left to the institutional public relations or security departments.

III. Human Subject Research

A. General

Probably the first written and generally accepted principles for ethical human subject research are those known as the Nuremberg Code, written as part of the military tribunal and used as a standard to judge experiments performed by the Nazis on prisoners during World War II (8). The first principle states that "the voluntary consent of the human subject is absolutely essential." The other principles state that consent must be obtained without coercion, and address risk/benefit assessment, general qualifications of those conducting research, the ability of subjects to refuse to participate or to withdraw from participation, and the responsibility to explain risks of participation to the subjects. The World Medical Association made similar recommendations in 1964 in the Declaration of Helsinki: Recommendations Guiding Medical Doctors in Biomedical Research Involving Human Subjects (9). These recommendations have been revised twice and are distinct from the Nuremberg Code in that they distinguish therapeutic from nontherapeutic research. In 1966, the NIH issued its Policies for the Protection of Human Subjects that were eventually promulgated as regulations in 1974 (10). As a part of the National Research Act, the National Commission for the Protection of Human Subjects of Biomedical and Behavioral Research was established. The Commission issued many reports and recommendations on human subject research and, in 1979, described the basic ethical principles that should underlie human subject research in the Belmont Report (11). In 1981, the Department of Health and Human Services regulations were codified at Title 45 of the Code of Federal Regulations (CFR), revised several times, and in 1991 were promulgated by other federal agencies involved in human subject research as the so-called Common Rule (12). The Common Rule, or 45 CFR, Part 46, now includes three additional subparts providing additional protections for vulnerable classes of subjects, e.g., pregnant women, fetuses, prisoners, and children. Similar, and in many cases identical, regulations were promulgated by the FDA at Title 21 (13).

To assure compliance with the regulations, institutions conducting human subject research must appoint one or more Institutional Review Boards (IRBs) (12, 13). The IRB is then responsible for oversight and regulatory compliance of research involving human subjects. As is the case with the IACUC, the IRB is the ultimate authority regarding human subject research at the institution and IRB disapproval of a research activity cannot be overruled by executive administration at the institution. The regulations are specific in this area so as to prevent application of administrative pressure on IRB members to approve a potentially unethical or otherwise questionable study for fiscal or other politically motivated reasons. The decisions of an IRB must be based on ethical principles and seek to protect subjects from research risks to the extent possible and cannot, under any circumstances, be influenced by the amount of potential funding at stake.

Many IRBs require submission of specific institutional form(s) containing questions that address the regulatory requirements for review. In its review of a human subject research proposal, the IRB must determine that the requirements discussed in the following section are satisfied (12, 13).

B. Protocol Requirements

The IRB requires the following information to be submitted:

1. *The risks that will be experienced by the subjects are minimized.* This is accomplished by reviewing the research procedures for sound research design and minimization of subject's exposure to unnecessary risks.

2. *The risks to subjects are reasonable in relation to anticipated benefits.* The IRB should make a clear distinction between the risks and benefits associated with the research and those that are related to clinical care that would occur even if the subject were not participating in the research. The benefits to be considered do not necessarily have to relate to the individual subject, but may be more broad and societal. In some cases, there is no benefit to the individual but the knowledge from the study will have potential benefit to future patients. Many times, this is acceptable, depending on the level of risk to the subjects.

3. *Selection of subjects is equitable.* The selection of subjects cannot be discriminatory or exclude certain populations nor is it acceptable to target certain populations for the sake of convenience. It is justifiable, however, to limit the study to a certain population if the disease predominantly affects that population.

4. *Informed consent will be appropriately sought, obtained, and documented.* Written, informed consent for research procedures is required to be obtained from either the subject or the subject's legally authorized representative. Waivers and alterations to the consent process may be granted in certain cases and will be discussed later in this section.

5. *Where appropriate, data will be monitored to ensure the safety of subjects.* For industry-sponsored clinical research (drug or device studies) there is generally a requirement that the sponsor establish a Data Safety and Monitoring Board (DSMB) to provide ongoing review of data as related to subject safety. This is also performed at the local IRB level by the use of Adverse Event Reports. Even if a DSMB does not choose to stop a study for safety reasons, a local IRB may choose to do so.

6. *The privacy and confidentiality of subjects will be adequately protected.* The possibility of loss of confidentiality is a risk that is often overlooked. Subject confidentiality must be protected to the utmost levels. The use of

code numbers, with the key to the code kept secured by the principal investigator (PI) is an accepted method. For externally sponsored drug studies, names and other identifiable information should not be sent to the sponsor. If, for safety or follow-up reasons, a subject needs to be contacted, the proper procedure is for the sponsor to notify the PI of the code number(s) needing follow-up, and the PI contacts the subject. Some sponsor representatives can be very demanding of subject's identification so PIs need to be very diligent in this area.

7. *Where appropriate, vulnerable populations are protected from coercion and their rights and welfare are protected.* If there is a possibility that some subjects are likely to be vulnerable to coercion, PIs must explain the safeguards that will be used to prevent coercion and protect the rights and welfare of the subjects.

C. Consent Form Requirements

Federal regulations state that "no investigator may involve a human being as a subject in research . . . unless the investigator has obtained the legally effective informed consent of the subject or the subject's legally authorized representative. An investigator shall seek such consent only under the circumstances that provide the prospective subject or the representative sufficient opportunity to consider whether or not to participate and that minimize the possibility of coercion or undue influence" (12, 13). To accomplish this requirement, the regulations list several basic required elements of informed consent. The following elements are paraphrased from the regulations (12, 13):

1. The consent form must state that the study involves research. In addition, it must explain the purpose of the research, a description of the procedures to be followed and which ones are experimental, and the duration of the subject's participation.
2. A description of any reasonably foreseeable risks or discomforts to the subject.
3. A description with respect to the subject or to others of any benefits that can reasonably be expected from the research.
4. A disclosure of appropriate alternative procedures or courses of treatment, if any, that might be advantageous to the subject. One alternative is to not participate in the research and this should be clearly stated.
5. A statement describing how confidentiality will be protected and records maintained.
6. For studies of more than minimal risk, an explanation as to whether any compensation or medical treatments are available if injury occurs and, if so, what they consist of or where further information may be obtained.
7. An explanation of whom to contact for answers pertinent to the research, including whom to contact if an adverse event occurs (usually the investigator), or concerning their rights as a research subject (this should probably be a person associated with the IRB or IRB office).
8. A statement that the research is voluntary, that refusal to participate will involve no penalty or loss of benefits to which the subject is otherwise entitled, and that the subject may discontinue participation at any time without penalty or loss of benefits to which the subject is otherwise entitled.

In addition, when appropriate, one or more of the following elements should also be included in the consent form:

1. A statement that the research procedure may involve risks that are currently unforeseeable.
2. Circumstances under which the subject's participation may be terminated by the investigator without regard to the subject's consent.
3. Any additional costs to the subject that may result from participation.
4. Potential consequences of a subject's decision to withdraw from the research.
5. A statement that significant, new information obtained during the course of the research that may relate to the subject's willingness to continue participation will be provided to the subject.
6. The approximate number of subjects involved in the study.

Some Special Notes

Institutional IRBs often have a template consent form that must be used in order to maintain consistency of format and the ability to ensure that all the required elements are present. In any event, the consent form, with all of the appropriate elements, must be presented to the subject, or their representative, in a language that is understandable to the subject. It is recommended, if enrolled subjects do not speak English as a primary language, that a consent form translated into the subjects' first language be used. Inclusion of exculpatory language is not allowed. Subjects cannot be forced to waive their legal rights. Also, the use of "telephone consent" is not appropriate to a research study. The regulations are clear that written documentation of informed consent is required (12). Last, it is possible for an IRB to approve a waiver or alteration of the consent process. There are regulatory requirements that must be met, but willingness to waive or alter the consent process will vary between IRBs. It is best to contact the IRB to determine their specific policy in this area.

D. Adverse Event Reports

When a subject who is participating in a research study experiences an adverse reaction, the PI may be required to report the event to the IRB, the Office for Protection from

Research Risks at NIH, an industry sponsor, or the FDA. Institutional IRBs usually have specific procedures, and perhaps even specialized forms for reporting adverse events, so PIs should check with their local IRB, but as a rule of thumb, the following procedures generally apply (14):

1. If the adverse event or reaction was anticipated in the protocol and the subject was informed about the possibility of the event in the consent form, there is usually no requirement to inform the IRB, unless the event was unusually severe, life threatening, or fatal.
2. If the adverse event or reaction was unanticipated, unexpectedly serious, life threatening, or fatal, the PI must report the event to the IRB, usually within 24 hr.
3. If the research study is being supported by an industry sponsor, the PI is also responsible for notifying the sponsor. The sponsor will then notify the FDA.
4. If the PI holds the Investigational New Drug (IND) or Investigational New Device Exemption (IDE) in his/her name, he/she is considered to be the sponsor for purposes of reporting and must notify the IRB and FDA of the event within 24 hr.
5. The IRB may also require that the PI notify the hospital or institutional Risk Management Office, if appropriate.
6. For industry-sponsored research studies of drugs or devices, sponsors are required to inform investigators of adverse events that occur at other sites. PIs should review these reports and send a copy of the report to the IRB as soon as possible after their receipt.

E. Amendment and Revision Requests

Amendments or revisions to an approved research protocol must be reviewed and approved by the IRB prior to implementing the change(s). Many times the changes require revision of the consent form, which also must be reviewed and approved. The local IRB may have a specific procedure for requesting an amendment, but generally this can be accomplished by simply requesting the change via a letter or memo (e-mail requests may also be acceptable to the local IRB). If the changes are minor, they may be approved administratively by the IRB chair or the chair's designee. However, if the requested changes are significant, Federal regulations require review and approval by the entire IRB at a convened meeting.

F. Continuing Review of Ongoing Research

The Federal regulations require that "an IRB shall conduct continuing review . . . at intervals appropriate to the degree of risk, but not less than once per year" (12, 13). Many IRBs have a specified procedure and format for supplying the required information, but at a minimum the IRB is required to review the following documentation:

1. A status report on the progress of the research that includes (a) the number of subjects accrued, (b) a description of any adverse events or problems involving risks to subjects (if any), withdrawal of subjects from the research, or complaints about the research, (c) a summary of any recent literature, findings, or other relevant information (if any), especially if they affect the risks to the subjects.
2. A copy of the current informed consent document.

It is the responsibility of the IRB to perform this review, but it is the responsibility of the PI to supply the requested information when asked. Failure to supply the information leaves the IRB no choice but to suspend or terminate the research, even if it was unintentional. Most IRBs are willing to assist PIs in this effort and the process is rarely problematic.

G. Special Protections for Vulnerable Populations

As mentioned previously, the NIH regulations make provisions, in specific subparts of the regulation (12), for protecting several populations considered as vulnerable to coercion and/or special risks. The vulnerable populations are pregnant women, fetuses, prisoners, and children. In the future, in response to recommendations from the National Bioethics Advisory Commission, there may another subpart added for the mentally disabled and subjects who lack decision-making capacity (15). PIs wishing to include any of these vulnerable populations may be required by their IRB to provide additional justification for their inclusion.

H. Certification and Accreditation

At the time of this writing, there is no accreditation process in place for IRBs. There is, however, a form of certification required for those institutions receiving PHS funding. Certification is in the form of a Multiple Project Assurance (MPA) that is submitted to and approved by the Human Subjects Protection Division of the Office for Protection from Research Risks within the NIH. Essentially, an MPA is a statement of the procedures used by an institution in order to meet federal regulatory requirements for human subject research. If approved, the MPA is in effect for a period of 5 years and must be updated whenever there are changes to the program, such as a change in IRB membership or institutional official.

IV. Institutional Safety Committees

A. General

There are times when a research study proposes to use a biological agent, a hazardous chemical, or a radioactive substance, and the research will also have to be further reviewed by the appropriate safety committee. Institutions at which these types of agents are frequently used in research will generally have standing committees and institutional policies requiring review of the proposals. In addition, the committees are likely to have standard formats or forms to be submitted for review that, ideally, can occur simultaneously with IACUC or IRB review.

B. Biological Safety

Institutions at which biological agents are used in research generally establish a standing committee for the purpose of formulating and recommending institutional policies and procedures for the safe use of the agents. The charge of the committee is to ensure the safety of students, staff, faculty, and members of the surrounding community who, in many cases, may not be aware that such agents are in use at the institution. The committee will usually refer to the publications "Biosafety in Microbiological and Biomedical Laboratories" (16) and "Guidelines for Research Involving Recombinant DNA Molecules" (17) under the following circumstances:

1. When it establishes policies and procedures for the safe use of biological agents.
2. When it defines biosafety levels for activities involving biological agents.
3. When it reviews, recommends changes to, and approves research proposals involving biological agents or recombinant DNA molecules.
4. When it ensures that there are no undue hazards to researchers, students, staff, or the public.
5. When it verifies the appropriateness and adequacy of laboratory procedures.
6. When it reviews the qualifications of investigators and research staff.

When working with infectious agents, the following criteria will apply to the specific biosafety level (BSL) (16):

BSL 1—Not known consistently to cause disease in healthy adult humans.

BSL 2—Present in the community and associated with human disease following exposure by percutaneous injury, ingestion, or mucous membrane exposure.

BSL 3—Indigenous or exotic agents with the potential for aerosol transmission and/or causing a disease that may have serious or lethal consequences.

BSL 4—Dangerous and/or exotic agents that pose a high risk of life-threatening disease that may be aerosol-transmitted and for which there is no available vaccine or therapy; agents with unknown risk of transmission.

The laboratory and animal handling safety requirements for infectious agents become more stringent as the BSL increases. Investigators should review the specific requirements and consult with their biosafety office to determine the specific application or notification procedures for their institution. In order to conserve time, there is no regulatory requirement preventing concurrent biosafety, IACUC, or IRB proposal review.

C. Recombinant DNA

Institutions involved in recombinant DNA research that is funded by the NIH must obtain Institutional Biosafety Committee, IACUC, or IRB approval, and must adhere to the NIH Guidelines [17], which describes five categories of experiments, with examples of each, as follows:

1. Experiments that require Institutional Biosafety Committee (IBC) approval, Recombinant DNA Advisory Committee (RAC) review, and NIH Director approval before initiation.
   a. The deliberate transfer of a drug resistance trait to microorganisms that are not known to naturally acquire the trait, if such a transfer could compromise the use of the drug to control disease agents in humans, veterinary medicine, or agriculture.
   b. Human gene transfer experiments.
2. Experiments that require NIH/Office of Recombinant DNA Activities (ORDA), and IBC approval before initiation.
   a. Experiments involving the cloning of toxin molecules with LD50 of less than 100 ng per kilogram body weight.
3. Experiments that require IBC approval before initiation.
   a. Experiments involving introduction of recombinant DNA in to BSL 2, 3, 4, or restricted agents.
   b. Experiments in which DNA from BSL 2, 3, 4, or restricted agents is cloned into nonpathogenic prokaryotic or lower eukaryotic host–vector systems.
   c. Experiments involving the use of infectious DNA or RNA viruses or defective DNA or RNA viruses in the presence of a helper virus in tissue culture systems.
   d. Experiments involving whole animals or whole plants or those that involve more than 10 liters of culture.
4. Experiments that require IBC notification simultaneous with initiation.
   a. Experiments in which all components are derived from nonpathogenic prokaryotes and nonpathogenic lower eukaryotes.
   b. Experiments involving the formation of recombinant DNA molecules containing no more than two-thirds of the genome of any eukaryotic virus.
5. Experiments that are exempt from the NIH Guidelines.
   a. Experiments with DNA consisting entirely of segments from a single nonchromosomal or viral DNA source.

b. Experiments in which the DNA is not used in organisms or viruses.

The IBC should be contacted early in the proposal process to ensure that the proper formats, forms, and procedures are used. This is potentially a somewhat frustrating and certainly lengthy process, so it is better to be well informed at the outset.

D. Chemical Safety

At many institutions, executive management appoints a Chemical Safety Committee (CSC) to formulate and recommend policy concerning hazardous chemicals requirements:

1. Mechanisms for identifying and maintaining an inventory of hazardous chemicals and guidelines for safe handling, storage, and disposal of these chemicals.
2. Education and training programs for personnel who might become exposed to hazardous chemicals.
3. Review of hazardous chemical safety plans that might be required to be completed by investigators.

The definition or classification of risk associated with hazardous chemicals is left to the CSC and will likely vary somewhat from site to site. It is best to contact the office responsible for occupational health and safety at your institution to determine the exact procedures for review of hazardous chemical use, storage, and disposal. Some institutions will require submission of a standardized form(s) in which the investigator must describe the storage, use, location of use, and disposal of the hazardous chemical. The CSC then determines if the proposed plan complies with state and federal requirements. There is no regulatory requirement preventing concurrent CSC, IACUC, or IRB proposal review.

E. Radioactive Agents

In addressing some research questions, it may be necessary to use radioactively tagged tracers, drugs, or other chemicals, and use of these agents will cause both the administrative and the procedural aspects of the study to become more complex. Institutions that store and use radioactively tagged substances must be licensed (either at the state or federal level), are likely to have their own Radiation Safety Committee (RSC), and will have specific procedures and requirements for facilities, personnel training and certification, monitoring, and disposal of the substances. However, at any institution, there will be general concerns that must be addressed. Some of the concerns for both animal and human subject research will be discussed in the following sections.

For use of radioactive substances in animals, the proposal may have to be approved by the IACUC before it can be approved by the RSC, but simultaneous review may be possible. In a format specified by the RSC, the investigator may have to describe and specify protocols and conditions:

1. The facilities where injections or administration of the radioactive material will occur, and a description of the radionuclide that will be used regarding its volatility and dosage.
2. The procedures for restraining animals during administration and the methods for containing any spills or loss of radioactive material during its administration.
3. The type of caging that will be used and how the cages will be labeled.
4. Who will be handling, monitoring, and providing husbandry for the animals and their level of training and experience with radioactive materials.
5. The procedures for containment of contaminated materials (urine, feces, bedding, etc.).
6. The procedures for disposal of animal excreta and the animal carcasses.

Although many investigators fail to do so, consultation with the institution's attending veterinarian and the RSC early in the proposal development process will ultimately save time and frustration.

When using radioactively labeled materials in humans, the RSC is likely to have specific forms, formats, and procedures, some of which may be dictated by state or federal regulatory agencies (18), and all proposals will have to be approved by the IRB prior to official review by the RSC. Radiolabeled substances having a New Drug Application (NDA) or Investigational New Drug Exemption (INDE) approval from the FDA will only need approval from the IRB and RSC. Radiolabeled substances for research use in human subjects, not having NDA or INDE approval from the FDA, fit into either of two possible categories:

1. Those administered to human subjects for the purpose of obtaining basic information regarding the metabolism of the radiolabeled substance or regarding human physiology, pathophysiology, or biochemistry.
2. Those intended for immediate therapeutic, diagnostic, or similar purposes or to determine the safety and effectiveness of the radiolabeled substance for such purposes.

Radiolabeled substances falling into category 2 will need FDA approval before submission to the IRB or RSC. Those falling into category 1 can be approved by a local FDA-approved Radioactive Drug Research Committee (RDRC), not requiring submission to the FDA itself.

FDA regulations specify the membership requirements for the RDRC, and its members may or may not be the same individuals who serve on the RSC (18). In effect, the RDRC is considered to be a surrogate of the FDA in reviewing the proposed research and is required to evaluate under the following circumstances:

1. The pharmaceutical dose is appropriate and not likely to cause clinically detectable adverse pharmacological effects in the subjects.
2. The radiation dosage is the smallest possible to achieve the effect or answer the research question and does not exceed specified radiation exposure limits.
3. The radiation exposure is justified relative to the potential benefits. This is also an IRB review requirement, but the IRB may not have sufficient expertise to evaluate radiation risks. In these cases, the IRB will likely defer to the RDRC for evaluation of potential risks.
4. The investigator is appropriately qualified, licensed, and certified to administer the radioactive substances.

In both of the above cases (RSC or RDRC review), in order to assess risks to the subjects, radiation dose (including any X-ray exposures, if part of the research) to the whole body, target organs, and other radiation-sensitive organs that could be affected must be submitted as part of the approval request. Exposure limits for subjects and healthcare workers have been established by regulatory agencies and are used to evaluate actual and potential risks to the research subjects. In addition, the risk statements in the subject consent form should include appropriate information regarding the risk associated with the radiation dose to the subject. Efficient and effective review of research proposing to use radioactive substances by the various committees is dependent on a high degree of collaboration and rapport between the committees, and a high degree of interaction between the PI and the committees.

V. Summary

In this brief chapter, information has been presented that may prove valuable in assisting investigators in preparation of successful research proposals. An integral step in this process is the investigator's ability to navigate efficiently the institutional committees. Well-established, research-oriented institutions are likely to have associated with the various committees knowledgeable and helpful people who can and will assist in proposal preparation, but it never hurts to know and understand why some committees are so insistent or even dogmatic on certain issues. Perhaps the best advice would be to be proactive and to contact all the committees very early in the process. Doing so will enhance the probability that the process will go quite smoothly.

References

1. U.S. Department of Health and Human Services, National Institutes of Health. "Institutional Animal Care and Use Committee Guidebook." NIH Publication No. 92-3415. GPO, Washington, D.C. http://grants.nih.gov/grants/oprr/iacuc_guidebook/acuc_guidebook.htm
2. Institute of Laboratory Animal Resources, National Research Council (1996). "Guide for the Care and Use of Laboratory Animals." National Academy Press, Washington D.C. http://nap.edu/readingroom/books/labrats/
3. *The Animal Welfare Act.* Public Law 89-544, 1966, as amended (P.L. 91-579, P.L. 94-279, P.L. 99-198) 7 U.S.C. 2131 *et seq.* http://grants.nih.gov/grants/oprr/hrea1985.htm
4. *Code of Federal Regulations.* Title 9, Chapter 1, Subchapter A, Parts 1, 2, and 3. http://www.access.gpo.gov/nara/cfr/index.htm
5. Office for Protection from Research Risks (1986). "Public Health Service Policy on Humane Care and Use of Laboratory Animals." National Institutes of Health, Rockville, MD. http://grants.nih.gov/grants/oprr/phspol.htm
6. American Veterinary Medical Association (1993). Report of the AVMA Panel on euthanasia. *J. Am. Vet. Med. Assoc.* **202:** 229–249.
7. United States Department of Agriculture, National Agricultural Library, Animal Welfare Information Center: http://www.nal.usda.gov/awic.
8. U.S. Government Printing Office (1949). Permissible medical experiments. In "Trials of War Criminals Before the Nuremberg Military Tribunals," Vol. 2. GPO, Washington, D.C.
9. World Medical Association (1997). Declaration of Helsinki: Recommendations guiding physicians in biomedical research involving human subjects. *JAMA* **277,** 925–926.
10. Department of Health, Education, and Welfare (1974). Policies for the protection of human subjects. GPO, Washington, D.C.
11. Department of Health, Education, and Welfare (1978). The Belmont report: Ethical principles and guidelines for the protection of human subjects of research. DHEW Publication Nos. (OS) 78-0013 and (OS) 78-0014. GPO, Washington, D.C. http://grants.nih.gov/grants/oprr/humansubjects/guidance/belmont.htm
12. *Code of Federal Regulations.* Protection of Human Subjects (1981, revised 1991). Title 45, Part 46. http://grants.nih.gov/grants/oprr/humansubjects/45cfr46.htm
13. *Code of Federal Regulations.* Title 21, Chapter I, Food and Drug Administration, Subchapter A—General, Parts 50 and 56. http://www.fda.gov/cder/regguide.htm
14. *Code of Federal Regulations.* Title 21, Chapter I, Food and Drug Administration, Subchapter A—General, Parts 312 and 812. http://www.fda.gov/cder/regguide.htm
15. National Bioethics Advisory Commission (1998). Research involving persons with mental disorders that may affect decisionmaking capacity, Vol. I. Report and Recommendations of the National Bioethics Advisory Commission. http://bioethics.gov/capacity/TOC.htm
16. Department of Health and Human Services, Public Health Service (1999). "Biosafety in Microbiological and Biomedical Laboratories," 4th ed. Stock No. 017-040-00547-4. GPO, Washington, D.C.
17. National Institutes of Health, Office of Recombinant DNA Activities (1997). "Guidelines for Research Involving Recombinant DNA Molecules (NIH Guidelines)." GPO, Washington, D.C. http://nih.gov/od/orda
18. *Code of Federal Regulations.* Title 21, Chapter I, Food Drug Administration, Subchapter A—General, Part 361 and I. http://www.fda.gov/cder/regguide.htm

5

Grantsmanship

B. Mark Evers

Department of Surgery, The University of Texas Medical Branch, Galveston, Texas 77555

I. Introduction

The preparation and writing of a successful scientific grant is a true art form that requires meticulous attention to detail at every step of the process. The successful application requires not only a sound hypothesis, preliminary data to support this hypothesis, and a logical plan, but also a considerable amount of planning and time spent in the actual presentation of the material. No matter how logical a plan is when spoken, if it is not presented in a logical, straightforward, and easy to understand fashion, then the grant proposal will not be funded. Also, because it is a rare occurrence to have a first-time submission funded in the initial go-around, successful grant preparation requires patience, a trait not commonly found in most surgeons. The usual scenario is that the grant is returned for revisions and then may be funded on the next or subsequent rounds. Sometimes this process can take years from submission of the first grant to actual funding of the project. It should be, however, the goal of every young academic surgeon to obtain research funding as quickly as possible early in his or her academic career. The benefits of funding include the fact that the investigator is now recognized as a more independent investigator, and along with that recognition comes a certain amount of academic respect and creditability. This chapter addresses common misconceptions regarding grant submissions and presents various points of successful grant preparation. Obvious points, as well as more subtleties, will be discussed in an effort to demystify many of the aspects of grant preparation. Although there are multiple avenues of extramural support, the discussion in this chapter is predominantly based on experience with grant preparation for the National Institutes of Health (NIH), because this is the "gold standard" of peer review and should represent the goal of all scientific investigators.

II. Common Myths, Misconceptions, and Mistruths

There are a number of misconceptions regarding obtaining grant support that have persisted despite ample evidence to the contrary. These misconceptions are often quoted by young investigators as reasons for not applying for grant support. One common misconception is the widely held belief that surgeons and other physicians are writing a lot of grants but they are just not getting funded. Although this

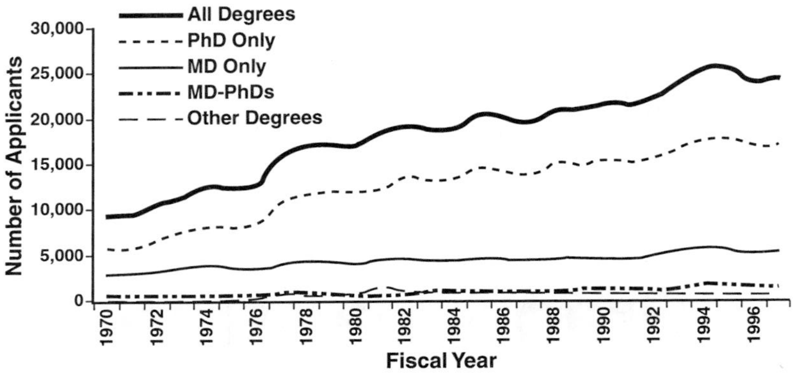

Figure 1 Numbers of National Institutes of Health research project applications by type of degree of principal investigator, 1970–1997. With permission, from Heinig *et al.* (1).

may be a commonly held belief, data obtained from the NIH demonstrates a decline over the past three decades in the percentage of grants submitted from physician-scientists (Fig. 1) (1–5). From 1970 to 1997 the number of NIH applications from Ph.D.s nearly tripled, but the number of applications from M.D.s only doubled. The number of applications from holders of dual M.D./Ph.D. degrees and other types of degrees increased only modestly during this interval. More worrisome are the indications that the number of first-time physician applicants has declined sharply during the past several years, as noted by a 31% drop from 1994 to 1997 (Fig. 2). As suggested by Rosenberg (5), if this trend persists, there would be no first-time M.D. applicants by 2003. Furthermore, if not funded on their first attempts, the M.D. applicants are far less likely than are Ph.D. applicants to resubmit their grant proposals (6).

A second misconception often expressed by physician-scientists is that individuals with M.D. degrees cannot compete effectively with Ph.D. scientists in successfully obtaining NIH support. Once again, as shown in Fig. 3, this statement is false. Since 1970, the success rates, or ratios, of awards to total applications have been approximately equivalent for physicians and Ph.D.s, thus indicating that research applications from these two groups have been of substantially similar quality and negating speculation of possible systematic bias against M.D. investigators in the peer review process (1, 5). In fact, in data obtained from fiscal year 1997, 30% of NIH grants submitted by Ph.D.s were successfully funded during this time period, whereas 35% of grants submitted by M.D.s were successfully funded. Those individuals with a combined M.D./Ph.D. degree faired somewhat worse, with only 23% of their grants funded.

A third misconception often expressed is that the NIH budget is so low that it is fruitless even to apply for grant support. Although this statement may have been more correct 10 years ago, the NIH budget has steadily grown over the past several years, thanks, in part, to several prominent Congressmen who have championed and supported the NIH mission. For fiscal year 1997, there was $12.8 billion in the budget for biomedical research; this increased 7% in 1998, for a total of $13.7 billion. In fiscal year 1999, the budget increased by 14.4% to $15.6 billion. Finally, there is discussion in Congress of further increasing the NIH budget within the next 5 years. Therefore, the next couple of years represent a golden opportunity for researchers who have sound ideas and good hypotheses to receive funding for their projects.

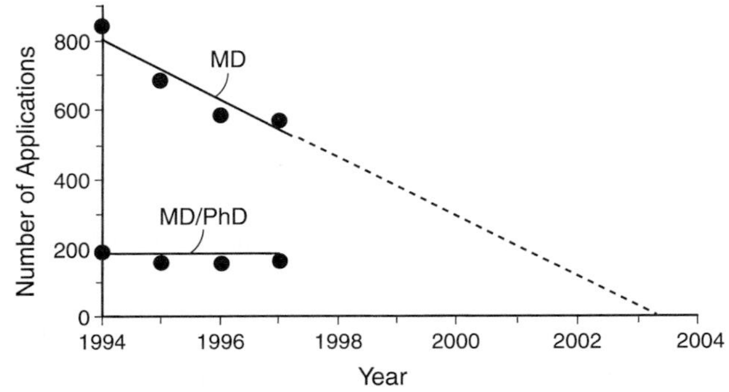

Figure 2 First-time applicants for NIH research project awards 1994–1997. From Rosenberg (5).

III. Grant Preparation—General Comments

The research proposal should follow a logical and specific hypothesis. If the hypothesis is not clearly elucidated as to the importance of the experiments and the logical endpoints that will be obtained, then reviewers will be less than enthusiastic about funding the proposal. In preparation for actually writing a grant proposal, it is important to read some successful and, probably more importantly, some unsuccessful grants in order to get some assessment as to how to construct the proposal and what constitutes a successful application.

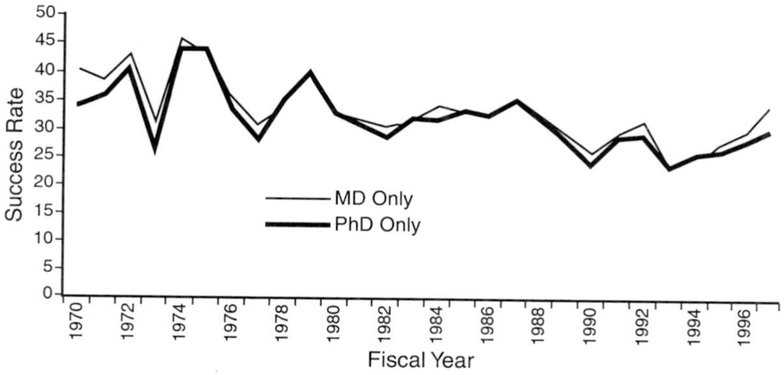

Figure 3 Success rates of National Institutes of Health research project applications by M.D.s only and by Ph.D.s only, 1970–1997. With permission, from Heinig *et al.* (1).

It is crucial that the applicant prepare well in advance of the actual deadline and that the proposal is written early enough so that it can be critically evaluated by scientifically knowledgeable colleagues. Care should be taken to identify experienced investigators who have been successful in obtaining grant support and ask that they provide you with a rigorous and critical review. It does the applicant no good to have his or her proposal evaluated by an individual who will simply give the grant a cursory review and write a few laudatory comments. It is critical to follow all of the rules as listed in the instructions. Strict adherence must be given to page limitations, font size, and margins. Finally, do not be sloppy. Attention to detail is as crucial to scientific investigation and grant preparation as it is to clinical practice. Poor typing, misspellings, faint copies, and disorganized layout all convey a negative impression and suggest a hasty, haphazard preparation. In the eyes of the reviewer, a sloppy and disorganized proposal equates to poor technique and careless thinking.

IV. Grant Preparation—Specific Comments

A. Title and Abstract

The title and abstract both require thought and represent important pieces of a grant proposal because this information will help decide which study section reviews the grant. The title should be broad enough so that the applicant is not locked into a very specific topic. This becomes most apparent when the time comes for the competitive renewal and it is obvious that the applicant has progressed from the original grant such that the current area of focus does not match the grant title. For example, a specific title such as "Analysis of Gastrin on Calcium Stimulation in Colonic Epithelial Cells," could be more appropriately and broadly titled, "Hormone-Mediated Signaling Pathways in Intestinal Cells." This then allows the applicant some flexibility when directions naturally change from the original submission.

The abstract also requires thoughtful preparation. The applicant should write the abstract last. In the abstract, the long-term objectives and specific aims should be clearly defined. There should be a concise description of the research design and it should make the reviewer excited about reading the remainder of the proposal.

B. Specific Aims

The first section of the actual body of the grant proposal is the section for specific aims. For this section the applicant should provide a brief but highly relevant background that describes the clear and testable hypothesis that will be studied throughout the proposal. A statement regarding long-term objectives and relevance to better patient care should also be given. Usually, no more than two or three specific aims should be listed, particularly for a first-time applicant. In fact, a common error for many first-time applicants is the inclusion of too many specific aims, which makes the proposal come across as either too global or too diffuse. An experienced investigator or mentor can help the applicant in defining the aims that could logically be tested during the grant period. This section, ideally, should be no more than one-half page long.

C. Background and Significance

The background and significance section is routinely three to four pages in length and should provide a concise and up-to-date review of the problem that is to be investigated. Not every reviewer will be an expert in this particular field, so it is important that the background is clearly delineated in terms of the importance of the problem and what gaps remain in our understanding of this problem. A careful, complete, and up-to-date literature search should be performed and the applicant needs to demonstrate clearly how the work of others supports his or her own proposal.

D. Preliminary Studies

Although the preliminary data section may not need to be as extensive for the first-time applicant as for the established investigator, this represents a very important section of the grant proposal. The applicant must convince the reviewers that he or she can, in fact, do the proposed work. The preliminary studies should flow and tell a clear story of how these experiments support and extend the overall hypothesis. Optimally, it would be advantageous to show preliminary results for all of the specific aims that are to be studied. The more the reviewers are convinced that this work is not only important, but that the applicant can clearly perform these studies, the more likely they are to recommend funding. Figures used in the preliminary data section should be clearly reproduced. If the blot or graph cannot be reproduced well, then consideration should be given to placing this particular piece of information in the appendix section so that it can be adequately evaluated.

E. Experimental Design and Methods

This section represents the real "meat" of the proposal. In this section the applicant will concisely describe the experiments to be performed in a logical and mature fashion. The purpose for each set of experiments should be clearly elucidated as to both design and importance. This section should be concise but yet yield sufficient details to ensure the reviewers that the applicant clearly understands the methodology. Most importantly, there needs to be a clear discussion of potential problems and alternative solutions in the event that the experiments do not turn out as expected. The applicant can rest assured that reviewers will be analyzing this section for potential problems; therefore, it is best to present these problems in a straightforward fashion, detailing the plan to address these problems should they occur. The mark of a truly mature application is the one in which the problems are anticipated and potential solutions offered.

F. Future Goals

After the experimental design and methods section, there should be a brief section on future goals. This section should briefly outline the goals for the next year or two after the period of funding. This allows for a refocusing on the long-range significance and directions of the work, thus bringing the reviewer to an intellectually satisfying breakpoint. Finally, this is the last opportunity to sell the reviewer on the project's significance.

G. Timetable

The instructions for many grants require inclusion of a timetable that demonstrates how and in what order the applicant plans on performing the studies. The timetable is another opportunity for the inexperienced investigator to expose their relative naivety. For example, the applicant should not underestimate the time required for experiments that are known to necessitate a considerable amount of time to set up and analyze the data.

H. Collaborators and Coinvestigators

It is important for both the first-time applicant and the seasoned investigator to identify collaborators or coinvestigators who can help in areas where the proposal may be weak or where the applicant lacks sufficient methodology to complete the aims. These collaborators should be recognized authorities, preferably with extramural funding, and the applicant should clearly state the roles of the collaborators or consultants on the particular project. With the sophistication of scientific technology, it is becoming almost impossible for any one investigator to perform all of the methodology required to address the questions and hypotheses posed by the proposal. Therefore, identifying good collaborators becomes a real must. In addition, collaboration makes the scientific investigation and discovery more fun and exciting.

I. Appendix Materials

Reprints from the investigator's laboratory that are pertinent to the proposal can be added as appendix materials. In addition, the applicant can put oversized figures in the appendix should more clarity be required to evaluate the material. However, the appendix should not be used as an extension of the proposal nor a place to put important material that could not fit into the page constraints of the actual proposal.

J. Biographical Sketches

Although the actual grant proposal is what the reviewers will be judging for scientific merit, the front pages, which include biographical sketches, budget, and other support, should not be put off, as they oftentimes are, to the very last minute. Considerable planning and preparation are required for these sections, particularly if the applicant has not previously submitted a grant proposal. The biographical sketch should be up to date for both the principal investigator as well as all collaborators. The biographical sketch should list everything that the applicant has published in the preceding 3 years and any publications that would be perceived as important in the overall evaluation of the proposal. Only publications that are published or in press should be included in the biographical sketch. This section should not be "padded" with publications that are submitted or in preparation.

K. Budget and Other Support

For applicants who have never filled out budget pages for grants, these can be quite tedious and time consuming and should be done well ahead of the submission date. The applicant should be accurate and act knowledgeable regarding the budget. The budget should not be inflated an inordinate amount. Conversely, the applicant should ask for what is needed to perform the experiments and not underestimate the costs. It is important that everything on the budget be justified, particularly with respect to personnel and large pieces of equipment, because both of these items tend to be the most costly portions of any proposal. All supplies, animals, and other items should likewise be justified and should conform to the experimental design. The role of each investigator should be clearly delineated with regard to their particular function and importance to the overall proposal.

The other support that an investigator may have should be listed in a straightforward fashion and any obvious areas of overlap (either with effort or experimental design) should be clearly addressed.

L. Research Involving Human Subjects and Vertebrate Animals

Any research performed on humans or vertebrate animals requires appropriate institutional review board (IRB) or institutional animal care and use committee (IACUC) approvals before this work can even be initiated. If human subjects are to be evaluated, then it must be clear that women and minorities are included.

V. Other Considerations

A. Directing the Proposal to the Appropriate Study Section

The applicant should be proactive and an active participant in deciding where the grant proposal is reviewed so that the group of study section members is composed of the appropriate and most knowledgeable individuals to review the particular proposal. This requires that the applicant be familiar with the various study sections and the members of these particular study sections. If the applicant is applying for an NIH grant, this information is readily available through the NIH website. There are three things that will help decide where the grant proposal is reviewed. The title and abstract of the proposal are key pieces of information that are used to help direct the proposal. In addition, the applicant is strongly encouraged to write a cover letter to accompany the grant proposal, stating the problem that is to be addressed and the appropriate study section that has the most expertise to evaluate the grant critically. To reiterate this point, all applicants should be active participants in this process and be proactive in directing the proposal to the most appropriate review section. If there are any questions regarding the appropriateness of a particular study section to review the proposal, the applicant should contact the scientific review administrator (SRA) of the particular study section so that these types of questions can be addressed.

B. Resubmission

Almost every investigator, at some point in his career, is faced with the unpleasant experience of finding that the grant proposal that he had spent the better part of 3 to 4 months of his life preparing did not achieve a score in the fundable range. This evokes natural and understandable reactions ranging from anger to self-pity. However, above all, the applicant should not simply throw up his or her hands and give up. The critique sheets should be critically evaluated and all criticisms addressed in a point-by-point fashion and the grant revised accordingly. The applicant should take the critique sheet as the "road map to success" and address every comment in a mature and nonconfrontational fashion. It is important that the grant be resubmitted with the next cycle so that momentum is not lost. The applicant should remember that persistence pays off in the long run and if all of the criticisms are adequately addressed, the likelihood of eventual funding is high.

VI. Conclusions

One of the most difficult things for an investigator to do is to prepare and submit a grant proposal. To write a competitive proposal requires much time, effort, and forethought. It is oftentimes tedious and not immediately gratifying in terms of seeing instant results. However, obtaining funding for projects is important to the applicant, the department, and the institution and is a clear affirmation of the importance and creditability of the work. Given the financial constraints of many clinical departments, it is no longer possible for an individual to perform "hobby research" with funding for projects derived from excess clinical funds, as was commonly done in the past.

To summarize some key points, it is important that the applicant has a testable, central hypothesis with well-defined goals and future directions. This hypothesis must clearly convey to the reviewers the specific problem, how the applicant plans on approaching the problem, and the long-term benefits that will be derived from studying this problem. Knowledgeable scientists and colleagues who have been successful in obtaining funding should be asked to provide a critical review of the proposal. This requires the applicant to actually have the proposal finished weeks ahead of time so that individuals will have enough time to critique the methods and design thoroughly. It is also crucial for the first-time applicant to identify collaborators and consultants who can provide additional expertise and fill in any potential holes in the experimental design. The applicant should take a proactive approach and specify which study section has the expertise to best review the proposal. Finally, if the grant is not funded the first time, the applicant should immediately revise and resubmit the proposal. The applicant may want to refer to additional literature regarding grant preparation (7–13) as well as the NIH web site (http://www.nih.gov/). In addition, the American College of Surgeons sponsors a Young Surgical Investigator's conference every 2 years to instruct junior surgical faculty in the preparation of grant proposals and provide an introduction to the various funding sources available, particularly the NIH. This has been a very successful program as demonstrated by the high percentage of funded grants obtained by previous attendees.

Surgeons are uniquely positioned as clinicians and scientists to raise important questions and bring basic research advances back to the bedside. Surgeons have a long and distinguished heritage of asking important questions and rigorously and critically performing the experiments that have resulted in a number of major breakthroughs in patient care. A few examples include transplantation, parenteral nutrition, and cardiovascular surgery (14). The value of the physician-scientist is becoming even more appreciated because it appears that physician-scientists are becoming fewer in number (1–5). Surgeons of the future must continue to ask the important and perceptive questions, because we provide a different perspective to the clinical problem compared with the nonphysician-scientist. To address these important clinical problems requires diligence, persistence, and hard work, not only to perform the experiments but also to secure the funding that is necessary to truly bridge the gap between the bench and bedside, as should be the goal and aspiration of all physician-scientists.

References

1. Heinig, S. J., Quon, A. S., Meyer, R. E., and Korn, D. (1999). The changing landscape for clinical research. *Acad. Med.* **74,** 726–745.
2. Wyngaarden, J. B. (1979). The clinical investigator as an endangered species. *N. Engl. J. Med.* **301,** 1254–1259.
3. Ahrens, E. H. (1992). "The Crisis in Clinical Research." Oxford Univ. Press, New York.
4. Goldstein, J. L., and Brown, M. S. (1997). The clinical investigator: Bewitched, bothered, and bewildered—but still beloved. *J. Clin. Invest.* **99,** 2803–2812.
5. Rosenberg, L. (1999). Physician-scientists—Endangered and essential. *Science* **283,** 331–332.
6. Nathan, D. G. (1997). The NIH Director's Panel on Clinical Research Report to the Advisory Committee of the Director: http://www.nih.gov/news/crp/97report/index.htm, accessed April 12, 1999. National Institutes of Health, Bethesda, MD.
7. National Institutes of Health (1995). Division of Research Grants. Helpful hints preparing an NIH research grant application. NIH, Bethesda, MD.
8. Eaves, G. N. (1984). Preparation of the research-grant application: Opportunities and pitfalls. *Grants Mag.* **7,** 151–157.
9. Eaves, G. N. (1982). Review of research grant applications at the National Institutes of Health. *In* "Proceedings from a Workshop on Thinking and Writing Clearly: Preparing an Application for Support." September 14, 1982.
10. Eaves, G. N., Pike, J. M., and Bernard, S. C. (1978). A successful grant application to the National Institutes of Health: Case history. *Grants Mag.* **1,** 263–286.
11. Gordon, S. L. (1989). Ingredients of a successful grant application to the National Institutes of Health. *J. Orthop. Res.* **7,** 138–141.
12. Novello, A. C. (1985). The peer review process: How to prepare research grant applications to the NIH. *Miner. Electrolyte Metab.* **11,** 282–286.
13. Rhein, R. (1996). Dollars & grants. Constructing a strong application. *J. NIH Res.* **8,** 29–30.
14. Thompson, J. C. (2000). Gifts from surgical research. Contributions to patients and to surgeons (Presidential address). *J. Am. Coll. Surg.* **190,** 509–521.

6

Informed Consent and the Protection of Human Research Subjects: Historical Perspectives and Guide to Current United States Regulations

Mary Jane Kagarise and George F. Sheldon

Department of Surgery, The University of North Carolina School of Medicine, The University of North Carolina at Chapel Hill, Chapel Hill, North Carolina 27599

I. History of Informed Consent

I will follow that system of regimes which according to my ability and judgment I consider for the benefit of my patients, and abstain from whatever is deleterious and mischievous.

THE HIPPOCRATIC OATH

A. Introduction

Experimentation involving human subjects, although complicated and sometimes controversial, is also very important. There are many examples of how experimentation involving human subjects has contributed to the understanding of diseases; without the involvement of these subjects, such advances would not have occurred. For example, understanding the mechanism of transmission of the yellow fever virus by a mosquito vector in the classic studies of William Gorgas, Walter Reed, and others made possible the control of the disease, in addition to advancing mosquito control and the building of the Panama Canal. It is likely that modern scourges, such as AIDS and cancer, will continue to require involvement of human subjects to achieve validation of therapy and breakthrough to cure.

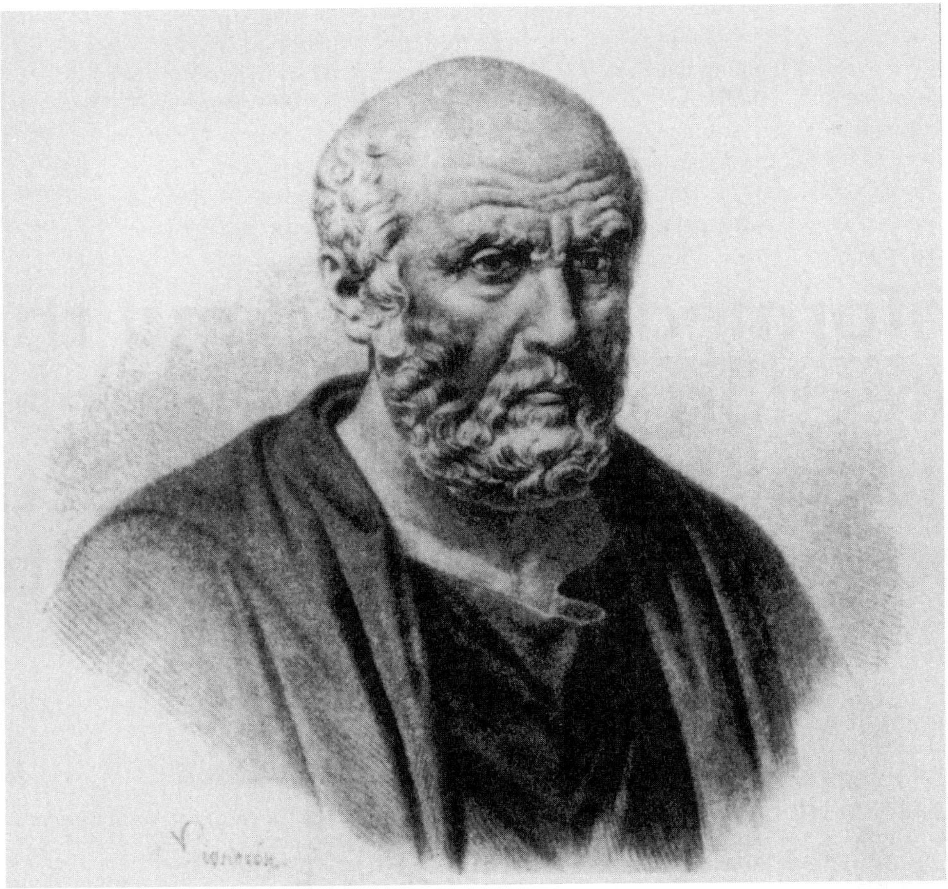

Figure 1 The Father of Medicine: Hippocrates. Hippocrates was born around 460 BC on the Isle of Cos in Asia Minor. The Hippocratic Oath is a code of professional behavior. Its elements are commitment to benefit patients, paternalism, and the admonition to "do no harm." It does not deal specifically with patients or humans as research subjects beyond the concept of the physician's first priority being to patients. Courtesy of Yale University, Harvey Cushing/John Hay Whitney Medical Library.

There have been occurrences of improper and unethical research involving human subjects. Examples are the Tuskegee (Alabama) syphilis experiments in which a number of black men were left untreated even after the advent of penicillin in order to observe the natural history of the disease. Other examples include the Willowbrook studies in which retarded children were administered hepatitis virus, and the New York Jewish Hospital study in which cancer cells were administered to patients.

Research involving human subjects is intimately linked to the ethics of medicine and the fiduciary responsibility of physicians to patients. The physician investigator assumes responsibility for furthering knowledge in order to serve the broader goal of improvement of health. The investigator involved in research using human subjects assumes responsibility for a minimization of risk to research subjects, as well as designing a competent experiment.

The ethical, legal, and regulatory dimensions of research involving human subjects have undergone change during the history of medical science. A number of landmarks have occurred that have resulted in specific requirements for the ethical conduct of research involving human subjects. The Nuremberg Doctors' Trial (1946–1947) and the subsequent Nuremberg Code, more than any other event, focused attention on the need for regulations and ethical standards.

B. Evolution of the Ethics of Research Involving Human Subjects

Celsus, in the First Century AD, discussed in "Medicine" the value of the common good being served by experimentation on cadavers. He expanded this rationale by citing and condemning practitioners who would further medical knowledge by opening the bodies of still living criminals (1).

Historically, most experiments involving humans were uncontrolled and unstandardized. The Hippocratic Oath has been viewed as tacitly giving advice on experimental diagnosis and therapy. By the year 1830, English law was interpreted as requiring the physician to obtain informed consent of the research subject when conducting therapeutic experiments, otherwise the physician might be expected to provide compensation (2). Over the centuries, human experimentation, including vivisection, had been performed on condemned prisoners. In England in 1721, condemned prisoners were offered a pardon if they participated in inoculation experiments for small pox.

An early ethical code was written by Thomas Percival (Fig. 2) in 1803 as a code of behavior for physicians, who had behaved poorly in an epidemic of typhus or typhoid. He labeled this code of behavior "medical ethics." It included specific directives to the physician planning to do research involving human subjects. Percival stressed the need to devise new therapies, but insisted that research be based on conscientious, scrupulous reasoning, careful investigation of fact, and consultation with fellow physicians. Percival's

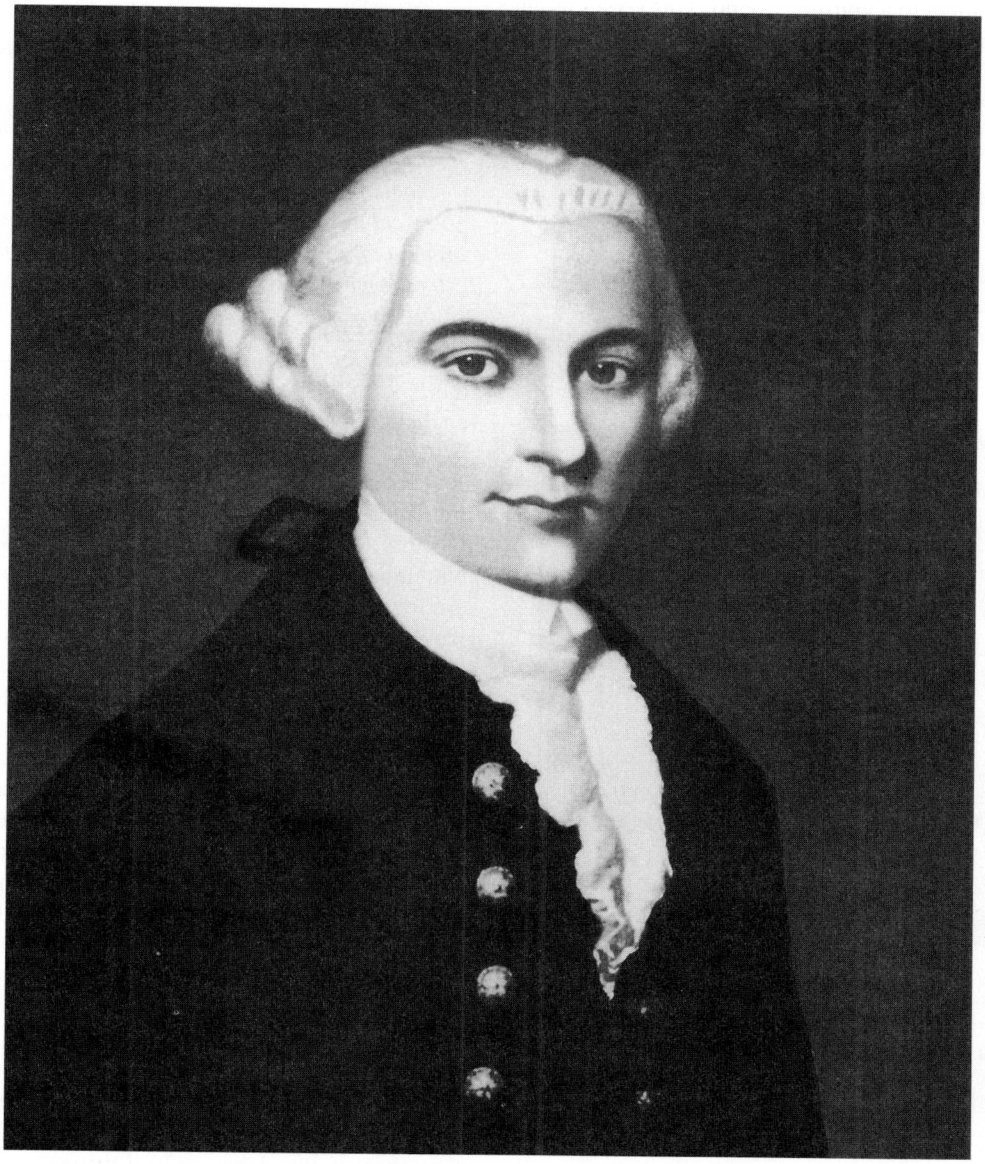

Figure 2 Thomas Percival (1740–1804). Thomas Percival was asked to write rules of behavior for physicians; he called these rules "medical ethics," which comprised some specific guidelines for physicians regarding human subjects in research, including the concept of consent. The guidelines were widely replicated in nascent American medical societies' codes of ethics, including that of the American Medical Association (1847), which adopted large portions of his guidelines, but did not officially mandate their implementation. Courtesy of The Manchester Literary and Philosophical Society.

code was highly influential to medical societies in the United States as they evolved in the nineteenth century. It provided the basis of the code of ethics of the American Medical Association (AMA) when it was founded in 1847. The initial AMA code did not include Percival's experimentation directives as an area of concern.

William Beaumont (Fig. 3) in 1833 wrote the oldest American document dealing with the ethics of human experimentation. Beaumont's research and classic experiment on the physiology of the stomach and digestion depended on experiments on his patient, Alexis St. Martin, who had a gastric fistula incident to a gunshot wound. This serves as an example of extensive nontherapeutic experimentation. Alexis St. Martin was in a dependent relationship with Beaumont and had difficulty escaping Beaumont when he wished to withdraw from the experiment. Beaumont actually had a contract with St. Martin to allow research. The Beaumont Principles (3) were as follows:

1. There must be recognition of an area where experimentation in man is needed.
2. Some experimental studies in man are justifiable when the information cannot otherwise be obtained.
3. The investigator must be conscientious and responsible . . . for a well-considered, methodological approach is required so that as much information as possible will be obtained whenever a human subject is used. No random studies are to be made.
4. The voluntary consent of the subject is necessary.
5. The experiment is to be discontinued when it causes distress to the subject.
6. The project must be abandoned when the subject becomes dissatisfied.

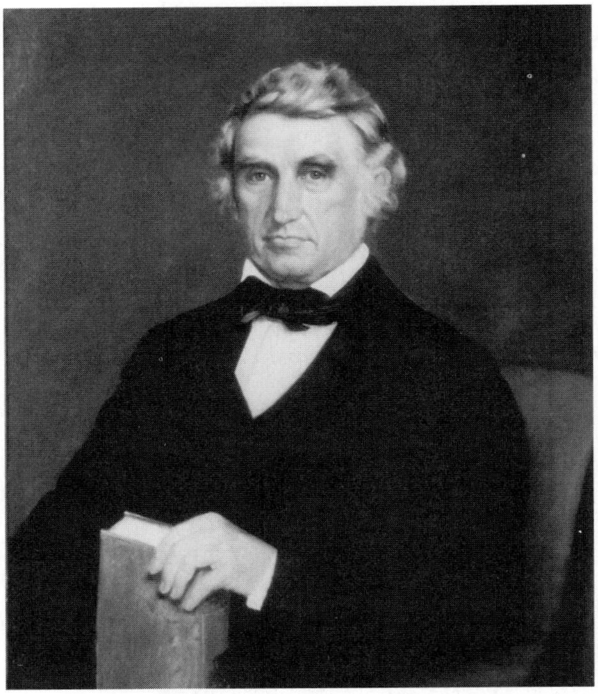

Figure 3 William Beaumont (1792–1866). The Beaumont Code, 1833, is sometimes cited as the oldest American document dealing with the ethics of human experimentation. The landmark experiments on gastric digestion and physiology were performed on Alexis St. Martin, who had a gastric fistula from a gunshot wound. Beaumont was an Army surgeon, and St. Martin was a soldier during the course of this experiment. Courtesy of the Bernard Becker Medical Library; Washington University School of Medicine, St. Louis.

Claude Bernard, the French physiologist, wrote of experimentation with human subjects (4). In his text, "An Introduction to the Study of Experimental Medicine," published in 1865, he wrote that

It is our duty and our right to perform an experiment on a man whenever it can save his life, cure him or gain him some personal benefit. The principle of medical and surgical mortality, therefore, consists in never performing on man an experiment which might be harmful to him to an extent, even though the result might be highly advantageous to the health of others.

Bernard's writing is a merger of patient care, innovative therapy, and therapeutic experimentation. He appears to exclude nontherapeutic research, by requiring the personal benefit of the patient.

The atrocities committed in Nazi Germany under the rubric of experimentation were the focus of the so-called Doctors' Trial, also called the Medical Case on the Second Nuremberg Trial. The Nuremberg Code ushered in the modern focus on research ethics involving human subjects. Ironically, Germany had been perhaps the most advanced country in the world regarding the regulation of research involving human subjects prior to the Nazi regime. The earliest legislation in Germany concerning ethics of human experimentation was a directive issued on December 29, 1900, by the Prussian Minister of Religious, Educational, and Medical Affairs. This three-part directive was to the directors of clinics, and mandated an absolute prohibition on medical interventions that were done for purposes other than diagnosis. Consent was a strong part of the directive that applied to diagnosis, therapy, or immunization. The Prussian directive, in contrast to the principles of Bernard, prohibited nontherapeutic research on minors or incompetents, i.e., those incapable of giving informed consent (5).

Medicine in prewar Germany was a respected academic and scholarly profession. Ethics and malpractice were handled through the German Medical Association, the Reich Chamber of Physicians. The German medical profession, however, was under criticism for alleged unethical conduct to a degree unparalleled in other countries. In the 1920s the criticism was in reaction to experiments on children. Moreover, hospitals were accused of working for the pharmaceutical industry.

On February 28, 1931, a Reich Circular issued guidelines entitled, "Regulations on New Therapy and Human Experimentation" (6). This document contained almost all of the points subsequently made in the Nuremberg Code. The document explicitly states that the individual physician and the chief physician are responsible for the well being of the patient or subject. The document had 14 points that included the obligation of a physician for the life and health of any persons on whom he undertakes innovative therapy or performs an experiment. The concept of unambiguous consent and prohibition of research on children or vulnerable populations was included. These guidelines were visionary and contained directives dealing with ethical standards of medicine, informed consent, documented justification of protocol deviation, risk–benefit analysis, etc.

Dr. Alexis Carrel, a French surgeon who won the Nobel Prize in 1912 for developing techniques to suture blood vessels and transplant organs, spent most of his career at the Rockefeller Institute. He collaborated with Charles Lindbergh and was influenced by Claude Bernard. Carrel respected science as a source of morality, and his work was cited by the lawyers defending Karl Brandt in the Nazi Doctors' Trial.

In 1907, Osler addressed the idea of experimentation in medicine and, as it related to human participation, superseded Bernard by anticipating the Nuremberg pronouncement advocating informed consent. Osler ruled out the concept of nontherapeutic research (7).

In 1886, a Boston physician, Charles Francis Whitington, published an "Essay on the Relation of Hospitals to Medical Education" and was awarded the prestigious Boylston Prize. He discussed the potential conflict between the rights of patients and the requirements of the investigation, and came down strongly on the side of a Patient's Bill of Rights. He stated that patients are "more than so much clinical material during their lives and so much more than pathological material after their death" (8). These writings draw a line between therapeutic and nontherapeutic research.

The implications today extend beyond these two distinctions—therapeutic and nontherapeutic research—first suggested by Claude Bernard. The line between therapeutic and nontherapeutic research is often unclear to the patient and to the physician. Today, patients with lethal diseases, such as AIDS and cancer, will clamor to be involved in clinical trials in the belief that they are being deprived of a potential cure if they are not allowed to participate.

C. The Nuremberg Code

In 1946 and 1947, the war crimes tribunals occurred in the Palace of Justice in Nuremberg, Germany. The second trial, the so-called Doctors Trial, indicted 23 physicians and health functionaries. Adolph Hitler's personal physician, Karl Brandt, was among the seven who were executed by hanging. The trial was unique in that the prosecutor, Brigadier General Telford Taylor (Fig. 4), in his opening statement noted that this was no mere murder trial, because the defendants were physicians sworn by the Hippocratic Oath to "do no harm" (9). Taylor held physicians to a higher standard than laymen due to the inviolable trust placed in physicians by patients, and he differentiated defensible medical research involving human subjects from criminal assault and battery. The chief United States witness, Dr. Andrew Ivy, vice president of the University of Illinois, was recommended to the tribunal by the American Medical Association. He referred to common practices of research that included Hippocratic ethical ideals, but also had specific recommendations for research codes formulated by the AMA, which were actually written after the trial began. Ivy's three principles (10) were that (1) the voluntary consent of the individual upon whom the experiment is to be performed must be obtained, (2) the danger of each experiment must be previously investigated by animal experiments, and (3) the experiment must be performed under proper medical protection and management.

From the trial, 10 principles for research involving human subjects were proposed as a "code" (Table I). The 10 Nuremberg principles evolving from the trial did not go unexamined. General Telford Taylor and Dr. Leo Alexander, the medical expert, hoped that the Nuremberg Code would become a useful educational guide for research involving human subjects.

Two Harvard professors critically examined different elements of the Code. The first was Professor of Anesthesia, Dr. Henry Beecher, who did not concede that the Code should be binding and eventually endorsed the Declaration of Helsinki. Dr. Francis Moore, Mosely Professor of Surgery at Harvard Medical School, entered the dialogue by criticizing Andrew Ivy in the context of Ivy's application of the research principles that he articulated at the Nuremberg Trials. The context was Ivy's involvement in the Krebiozen scandals. He had received an alleged wonder drug against cancer taken from the serum of hundreds of horses; Ivy had applied his principles of research involving human subjects in that he had tested it first in animal experiments, then on himself, and finally on patients (11).

In 1946, 32 national medical associations convened in London to create the World Medical Association (WMA). It was formed in response to the crimes committed by Nazi physicians, scientists, and other professionals in the name of the greater good of the state as opposed to the individual (12). They issued the Oath of Geneva, which was published in 1949 as the International Code of Medical Ethics. The declaration of Geneva was expressed in the Hippocratic tradition of the responsibility of the members of a profession and was felt to be an update of the Hippocratic Oath. The Hippocratic Oath is intended to be an oath of a code of honor of a profession, to be certain that it is ethically based. The

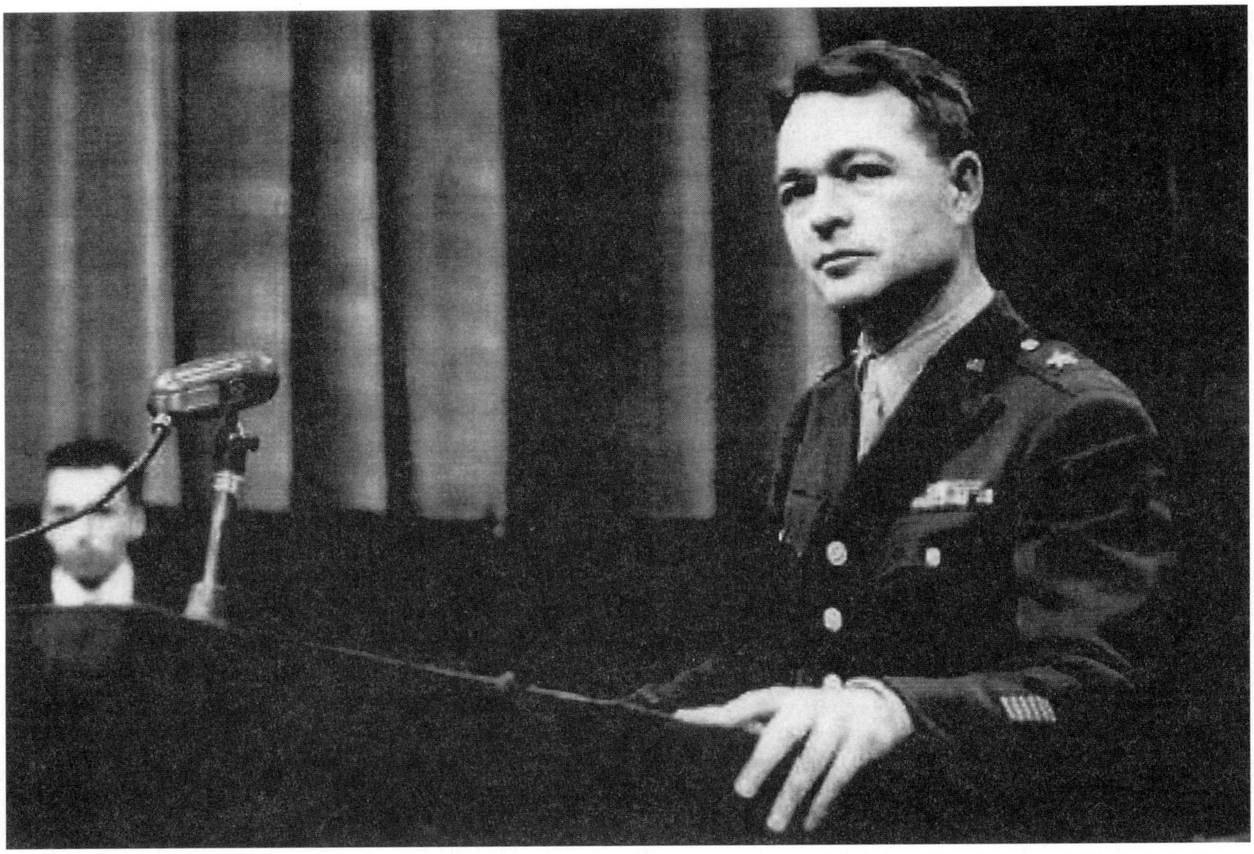

Figure 4 General Telford Taylor (1908–1998). A Harvard Law School graduate, Brigadier General Taylor delivered the opening statement at the Nuremberg Trials. The defendants (23 physicians and health personnel) were charged with murder, torture, and other atrocities in the name of medical science. Taylor considered these hearings to be much more than mere trials, because the defendants were physicians sworn by the Hippocratic Oath to "do no harm." Courtesy of United States Holocaust Memorial Museum.

World Medical Association declaration and pronouncements have been debated as to the degree that they were influenced by the Nuremberg Trial and the Nuremberg Code. It is clear that the Oath of Geneva was a reaction to the activities of the Nazi government. The Nuremberg Code is specific to the participation of human subjects in research. The World Medical Association's initial pronouncements are more specific to the behavior of the physicians as professionals.

During the first 10 years after its promulgation, the Nuremberg Code influenced the development of codes and guidelines, both in the general field of medicine and in human experimentation. In 1949, the WMA General Assembly adopted the International Code of Medical Ethics. It is noteworthy that there is again no mention of human experimentation.

There were four Geneva Conventions (13). The first, on April 12, 1949, showed the influence of the Nuremberg Code. Although a matter of some dispute, the Code is really a prescription to protect civilians from being subjected to biologic experiments. These conventions sequentially refined the ethic, as summarized in a commentary from the fourth convention: "The physician shall act only in the patient's interest while providing medical care that might have the effect of weakening the physical and mental condition of the patient" (14). In recent years, the Nuremberg Code has become recognized again as an important ethical standard of biomedical research. Seventy-four codes or regulations in 17 European and 15 Latin American countries have obvious language that reveals the influence of the Nuremberg Code (15).

In 1953, the National Institutes of Health (NIH) opened its clinical center and put in place regulations based on the Nuremberg Code. In that same year, the Secretary of Defense adopted the Nuremberg Code for all atomic, biologic, and chemical research done by the military; this is the earliest known adoption of the Nuremberg Code by a United States federal agency (16).

Senator Edward Kennedy's National Research Service Award Act endorsed new regulations that established the National Commission for the Protection of Human Subjects and of Biomedical and Behavior Research (National Commission). In the 1960s, there was an awakening of serious

Table I The Nuremberg Principles: The Nuremberg Code[a]

1. The voluntary consent of the human subject is absolutely essential. This means that the person involved should have legal capacity to give consent; should be so situated as to be able to exercise free power of choice, without the intervention of any element of force, fraud, deceit, duress, overreaching, or other ulterior form of constraint or coercion; and should have sufficient knowledge and comprehension of the elements of the subject matter involved as to enable him to make an understanding and enlightened decision. This latter element requires that before the acceptance of an affirmative decision by the experimental subject there should be made known to him the nature, duration, and purpose of the experiment; the method and means by which it is to be conducted; all inconveniences and hazards reasonably to be expected; and the effects upon his health or person which may possibly come from his participation in the experiment. The duty and responsibility for ascertaining the quality of the consent rest upon each individual who initiates, directs, or engages in the experiment. It is a personal duty and responsibility which may not be delegated to another with impunity.
2. The experiment should be such as to yield fruitful results for the good of society, unprocurable by other methods or means of study, and not random and unnecessary in nature.
3. The experiment should be so designed and based on the results of animal experimentation and a knowledge of the natural history of the disease or other problem under study that the anticipated results will justify the performance of the experiment.
4. The experiment should be so conducted as to avoid all unnecessary physical and mental suffering and injury.
5. No experiment should be conducted where there is an *a priori* reason to believe that death or disabling injury will occur, except, perhaps, in those experiments where the experimental physicians also serve as subjects.
6. The degree of risk to be taken should never exceed that determined by the humanitarian importance of the problem to be solved by the experiment.
7. Proper preparations should be made and adequate facilities provided to protect the experimental subject against even remote possibilities of injury, disability, or death.
8. The experiment should be conducted only by scientifically qualified persons. The highest degree of skill and care should be required through all stages of the experiment of those who conduct or engage in the experiment.
9. During the course of the experiment the human subject should be at liberty to bring the experiment to an end if he has reached the physical or mental state where continuation of the experiment seems to him to be impossible.
10. During the course of the experiment the scientist in charge must be prepared to terminate the experiment at any stage, if he has probable cause to believe, in the exercise of the good faith, superior skill, and careful judgment required of him, that a continuation of the experiment is likely to result in injury, disability, or death to the experimental subject.

[a]The major benchmark of human rights research involving human subjects was the Nuremberg Code. The Code was an outgrowth of the Nuremberg Trials, specifically from the so-called Doctors' Trial. It initiated the modern theme of patients' rights and the rights of human subjects in research. It was derived from writings of Thomas Percival, William Beaumont, Claude Bernard, and others. Its primary authors from the trial were Leo Alexander, Andrew Ivy, and Telford Taylor. From Shuster (10a).

thought about research practices and the concept of personal autonomy (17).

D. The United Nations

The founding of the United Nations included the establishment of a committee to write a Universal Declaration of Human Rights, which was chaired by Eleanor Roosevelt (Fig. 5). It incorporated four tenets: (1) human dignity rights, (2) civil and political rights, (3) economic, social, and cultural rights, and (4) solidarity rights. The first proposals regarding human experimentation are found in the proposition submitted by the United Kingdom representative on the drafting commission for the International Bill of Human Rights, submitted June 18, 1947, just 2 months after the judgment in the Nuremberg Medical Trial.

During the sixth session of the U.N. Commission on Human Rights, Eleanor Roosevelt, Chair, pointed out the draft International Covenant on Human Rights that had been introduced to the General Assembly. In 1952, the statement "against his will" was replaced by "without his free consent" (18).

Article 25 of the Universal Declaration mentions medical care as one of the means of assuring that a citizen has a standard of living adequate for his health and well being. The World Health Organization and Article 12 of the International Covenant on Civil and Political Rights of the United Nations speaks of the best state of health that one should be capable of attaining as a fundamental right. Article 13 of the European Social Charter states the right to achieve social and medical assistance. The parliamentary assembly of the Council of Europe adopted several recommendations related to healthcare rights. The first Declaration of Helsinski by the World Medical Association in 1962 set some new ethical rules of human experimentation, which somewhat superseded the Nuremberg Code. In 1975, the revised Declaration of Helsinski expanded the intent of the Nuremberg Code by recommending Institutional Review Boards. An important contribution was the shift in responsibility from the investigator to the institution in which the approval of the research protocol is entrusted. A subtle but important variation was the change from "voluntary consent" of the subject to "informed consent," later modernized to include the concept of "autonomy." In 1972, the American Hospital Association (AHA) published a Patient's Bill of Rights (19).

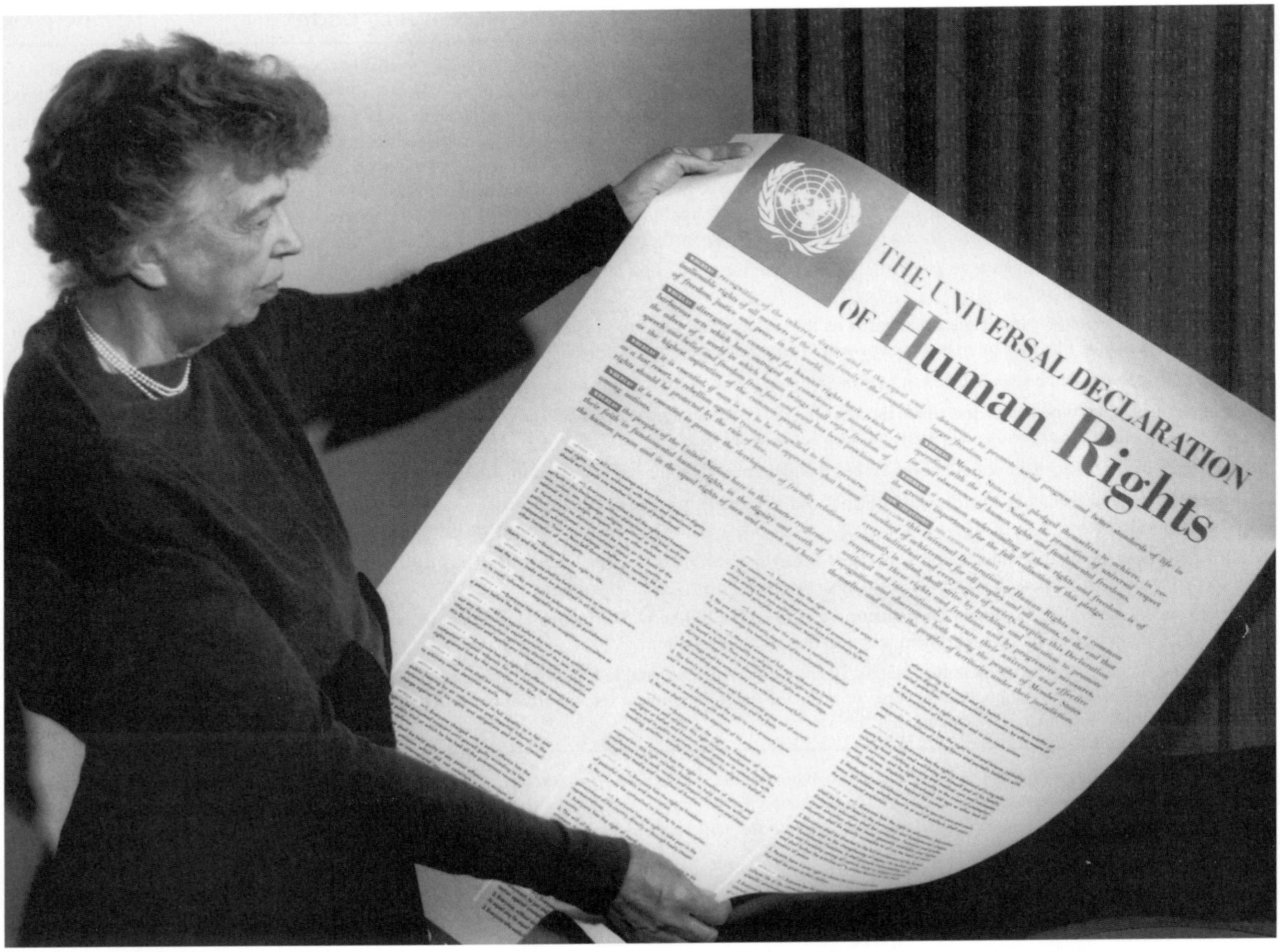

Figure 5 Eleanor Roosevelt (1884–1962). Eleanor Roosevelt was the Chair of the United Nations Commission on Human Rights. The document produced by the Commission, the Universal Declaration on Human Rights, was unanimously adopted. The document has sections that deal with healthcare and human rights. Courtesy of United Nations, Photo 23783, DOC WP/GAVAL2, New York, N.Y.

The research scandals in the United States in the 1970s resulted in the establishment of the National Commission for the Protection of Human Subjects of Biomedical and Behavioral Research. That commission produced *The Belmont Report* (1979), which in fact ultimately endorsed the universality of the Nuremberg Code (20). The Nuremberg principles of informed consent, responsibility of the research subject, and risk–benefit analysis were adopted and applied internationally. The word "informed" in the informed consent requirement has been criticized in that the researcher cannot possibly provide comprehensive information on every possible risk, and it is sometimes too technical for research subjects to understand the risk. Henry Beecher noted that the principle becomes the duty to disclose adequate information, not a duty to achieve full understanding in every subject.

II. United States Regulations Governing Informed Consent

Regulations in the United States (21) evolved from the first principle of "The Nuremberg Code on the Ethics of Human Research," developed by the International Military Tribunal, 1947:

The voluntary consent of the human subject is absolutely essential. This means that the person involved should have legal capacity to give consent; should be so situated as to be able to exercise free power of choice without the intervention of any element of force, fraud, deceit, duress, over-reaching, or other ulterior form of constraint or coercion; and should have sufficient knowledge and comprehension of the elements of the subject matter involved as to enable him to make an understanding and enlightened decision. This latter element requires that before the acceptance of an affirmative decision by the experimental subject there should be made known to him the nature, duration and purpose of the experiment; the method and means by which it is to be conducted; all inconveniences and hazards reasonably to be expected; and the effects upon his health or person which may possibly come from his participation in the experiment (22).

In 1966 the National Institutes of Health first issued Policies for the Protection of Human Subjects. The pursuant regulations issued by the Department of Health, Education, and Welfare (DHEW) became effective May 30, 1974, and first established the Institutional Review Board (IRB) as the primary mechanism to govern scientific investigation involving human subjects in the United States.

The National Commission for the Protection of Human Subjects of Biomedical and Behavioral Research (National Commission, 1974–1978) was established by the National Research Act, passed in July of 1974. The Commission's report, submitted on September 30, 1978, set forth the principles and guidelines that govern the protection of human subjects taking part in biomedical and behavioral research. It was named *The Belmont Report*, after the Belmont Conference Center at the Smithsonian Institution where the discussions were held.

Consistent with *The Belmont Report*, revised regulations for the protection of human subjects of research and for implementing a program of instruction and guidance in ethical issues associated with such research were issued in 1981 by the Department of Health and Human Services (DHHS, formerly DHEW). The DHHS regulations, later revised in 1983 and 1991, are codified at Title 45 Part 46 of the Code of Federal Regulations, Protection of Human Subjects (45 CFR 46, the Public Health Service Act).

After release of *The Belmont Report*, The President's Commission for the Study of Ethical Problems in Medicine and Biomedical and Behavioral Research (The President's Commission) was established by an Act of Congress on November 9, 1978. The President's Commission recommended that federal departments and agencies adopt a common set of regulations for the protection of human research subjects in order to promote uniformity and reduce confusion. In 1991, the standardized Federal Policy went into effect.

The Federal Policy of the United States regulates research involving living human subjects that is conducted, supported, or otherwise subject to regulation by the Department of Agriculture, Department of Energy, National Aeronautics and Space Administration, Department of Commerce, Consumer Product Safety Commission, International Development Cooperation Agency, Agency for International Development, Department of Housing and Urban Development, Department of Justice, Department of Defense, Department of Education, Department of Veterans Affairs, Environmental Protection Agency, Department of Health and Human Services, National Science Foundation, Department of Transportation, and Central Intelligence Agency. American investigators in foreign sites who are involved in DHHS-supported or DHHS-conducted research involving human subjects must abide by the federal regulations in all material respects. Any type of support provided by DHHS, even supplying a drug for research purposes, may trigger applicability of the regulations. The Office of Human Research Protection (OHRP), located within the DHHS, implements the regulations on behalf of the Secretary of DHHS. This unit, formerly known as the Office for Protection from Research Risks (OPRR), moved from NIH to DHHS in 2000.

Given that the regulatory mandate of the Food and Drug Administration (FDA) differs substantially from the research-supporting mandate of the other DHHS agencies, the FDA chose to make selected adjustments rather than adopting the Federal Policy in its entirety. Its IRB and informed consent regulations diverge from the Federal Policy. The FDA uses a system of inspections and audits, providing specific administrative action and sanctions for noncompliance, whereas DHHS relies on assurances of compliance that are negotiated prospectively by the OHRP. When a protocol is subject to review under both FDA and DHHS human subjects' regulations, both sets of regulations apply and must be met.

A. Conducting Ethical Research: Three Principles—Respect for Persons, Beneficence, and Justice

The Belmont Report declared three basic ethical principles that apply to the conduct of research involving human subjects (23, 24):

1. *Respect for persons*—a recognition of the personal dignity and autonomy of individuals, and special protection of those persons with diminished autonomy.
2. *Beneficence*—an obligation to protect persons from harm by maximizing anticipated benefits and minimizing possible risks of harm.
3. *Justice*—a requirement that the benefits and burdens of research be distributed fairly.

1. Ethical Principle One: Respect for Persons—Informed Consent

Informed consent has become the cornerstone for the ethical conduct of research involving human subjects. An ongoing educational process, "the requirement to obtain informed consent should be seen as not only a legal obligation, but also a moral one" (25). Informed consent, easier to describe than achieve, requires that (1) subjects be given sufficient information on which to decide whether to participate in the research protocol, (2) subjects be able to comprehend the information and understand it, and (3) consent be voluntarily given without coercion or undue influence. *The Belmont Report* suggests that a "reasonable volunteer" standard should be used in considering the extent and the nature of the information necessary.

a. Sufficient Information: First Requirement of Informed Consent Investigators are required by federal regulation to provide certain information to potential subjects [Federal Policy §__.116(a)] (26):

1. A statement that the study involves research, an explanation of the purposes of the research and the expected duration of the subject's participation, a description of the procedures to be followed, and identification of any procedures that are experimental.
2. A description of any reasonably foreseeable risks or discomforts to the subject.
3. A description of any benefits to the subject or to others that may reasonably be expected from the research.
4. A disclosure of appropriate alternative procedures or courses of treatment, if any, that might be advantageous to the subject.
5. A statement describing the extent, if any, to which confidentiality of records identifying the subject will be maintained.
6. If the research presents more than minimal risk, potential subjects must also be informed of the availability of medical treatment and compensation in the case of research-related injury, including who will pay for the treatment and the availability of other financial compensation [Federal Policy §__.116(a)(6); 21 CFR 50.25(a)(6)] (27).
7. An explanation of whom to contact for answers to pertinent questions about the research and the rights of the research subjects, and whom to contact in the event of a research-related injury to the subject.
8. Statements that participation is voluntary, refusal to participate will involve no penalty or loss of benefits to which the subject is otherwise entitled, and the subject may discontinue participation at any time without penalty or loss of benefits to which the subject is otherwise entitled.

The IRB judges the adequacy of the content of the information. Additional information may be required for certain protocols [Federal Policy §__.116(b)] (28):

1. A statement that the particular treatment or procedure may involve risks to the subject (or to the embryo or fetus, if the subject is or may become pregnant) that are currently unforeseeable.
2. Anticipated circumstances under which the subject's participation may be terminated by the investigator without regard to the subject's consent.
3. Any additional costs to the subject that may result from participation in the research.
4. The consequences of a subject's decision to withdraw from the research and the procedures for orderly termination of participation by the subject.
5. A statement that significant new findings developed during the course of the research that may relate to the subject's willingness to continue participation will be provided to the subject.
6. The approximate number of subjects involved in the study.

The consent document must be written in understandable language. It must describe the study design (including plans for randomization, use of placebos, and the probability that the subject will receive a given treatment) and the conditions for breaking the code, if the study is masked. The risks and benefits of each of the proposed interventions and of alternative courses available to the participants must be explained as well as the extent to which participation in the study precludes other therapeutic interventions (29).

The IRB may waive the regulatory requirement for written documentation of consent under the following circumstances (30):

1. The principal risks are those associated with a breach of confidentiality concerning the subject's participation in the research.
2. The consent document is the only record linking the subject with the research [Federal Policy §__.117(c)(1)].
3. The research presents no more than minimal risk and involves procedures that do not require written consent when they are performed outside of a research setting [Federal Policy §__.117(c)(2).
4. In selected record reviews (e.g., epidemiological studies) (a) the information is not particularly sensitive, (b) the investigator devised procedures to protect confidentiality of the information to be collected; or (c) the study could not practicably be carried out if consent were required.

Incomplete disclosure interferes with fully informed consent, though may be encountered in behavioral research. If an investigator plans to withhold any information about the real purpose of the research or give subjects false information about some aspect of the research, the information to be withheld from prospective subjects cannot be reasonably material to their decision whether to participate. It is justified only if it is clear that the goals of the research cannot be accomplished if full disclosure is made; the undisclosed risks are minimal; and, when appropriate, subjects will be debriefed and provided the research results (31). Debriefing is a mechanism that may be used to explain the deception involved and help subjects deal with any distress caused by the research. The decision whether to debrief becomes complicated if the debriefing could cause the subject pain, stress, or anxiety.

b. Comprehension: Second Requirement for Informed Consent The timing and setting for the explanation of the research must be conducive to good decision making, and the language and presentation need to be appropriate to the subject population. Potential subjects need to be informed as clearly as possible, in language they understand. Exculpatory language is not permitted; waivers or the appearance of waivers of any legal rights of the subject or any release of investigators, sponsors, or institutions from liability for negligence are prohibited. The potential subject must be afforded a sufficient opportunity to consider participation.

c. Voluntarism: Third Requirement for Informed Consent Informed consent must be given voluntarily by the potential subject, without coercion or undue influence. The IRB needs to know who the subjects will be, what incentives are being offered, and the conditions under which the offer will be made (32).

Recruitment procedures of potential subjects must be designed to assure that consent is freely given. Though federal regulations governing research with human subjects contain no specific guidance for IRB review of payment practices (33), it stands to reason that any incentives offered for participation should not be likely to unduly influence the potential subject's decision to participate. Otherwise, potential subjects could be tempted to conceal information that if known might disqualify their participation; or they could find their ability to evaluate risks impaired by especially attractive offers. Incentives need to be reasonable based on the complexities and inconveniences of the study and the particular subject population (34).

2. Ethical Principle Two: Beneficence

This principle requires that the risks and anticipated benefits of the research be accurately identified, evaluated, and described. Furthermore, in clinical research, the risks and benefits of the research interventions must be evaluated separately from those of the therapeutic interventions. Though the risks posed by the performance of investigational interventions and procedures may be more intuitively notable, many of the risks of research reside in the risks inherent in the methodologies of gathering and analyzing data (35).

Risk is "the probability of harm or injury (physical, psychological, social, or economic) occurring as a result of participation in a research study." Both the probability and magnitude of possible harm may vary from minimal to significant. Federal regulations define only minimal risk (36): "A risk is minimal where the probability and magnitude of harm or discomfort anticipated in the proposed research are not greater, in and of themselves, than those ordinarily encountered in daily life or during the performance of routine physical or psychological examinations or tests" [Federal Policy §__.102(1)] (37). There are strict limitations on research presenting more than minimal risk for research involving fetuses and pregnant women (45 CFR 46 Subpart B), research involving children (45 CFR 46 Subpart D), and research involving prisoners (45 CFR 46 Subpart C). The concepts of risk and benefit, then—having been classified as physical, psychological, social, and economic—incorporate all possible harms and advantages, not just the physical or psychological ones to an individual. For example, the societal benefits that might be gained from the research are to be considered.

The Belmont Report is concerned with the magnitudes and probabilities of possible risks and anticipated benefits in terms of defining their nature and scope, systematically assessing each one, assessing information on all aspects of the research, and systematically considering the alternatives. Five basic principles in making the risk–benefit analysis are cited (38):

1. Brutal or inhumane treatment of human subjects is never morally justified.
2. Risks should be minimized, including the avoidance of using human subjects if at all possible.
3. IRBs must be scrupulous in insisting upon sufficient justification for research involving "significant risk of serious impairment."
4. The appropriateness of involving vulnerable populations must be demonstrated.
5. The proposed informed consent process must thoroughly and completely disclose relevant risks and benefits.

The IRB performs six fundamental steps in risk-benefit analysis (39):

1. Identification of the risks associated with the research, as distinguished from the risks of therapies the subjects would receive even if not participating in research.
2. Determination that the risks will be minimized to the extent possible.
3. Identification of the probable benefits to be derived from the research, both to subjects and to society.
4. Determination that the risks are reasonable in relation to the anticipated benefits to subjects and the importance of the knowledge to be gained.
5. Assurance that potential subjects will be provided with an accurate and fair description of the risks or discomforts and the anticipated benefits.
6. Determination of the intervals of periodic review, and, where appropriate, determination that adequate provisions are in place for monitoring the data collected.

The process of distinguishing between the risks for potential human subjects associated with research and the risks associated with therapy requires that human subjects be defined and that research and practice be differentiated. The distinction between research and practice is often blurred in patient care situations as well as in some educational settings. Research and therapy may occur simultaneously, and experimental procedures do not necessarily constitute research (40).

Therapeutic practice consists of "interventions that are designed solely to enhance the well-being of an individual patient or client and that have a reasonable expectation of success. The purpose of medical or behavioral practice is to provide diagnosis, preventive treatment, or therapy to particular individuals" (41). Research is "an activity designed to test an hypothesis, permit conclusions to be drawn, and thereby to develop or contribute to generalizable knowledge (expressed, for example, in theories, principles, and statements of relationships). Research is usually described in a formal protocol that sets forth an objective and a set of procedures designed to reach that objective" (42). "Research itself is not therapeutic; for ill patients, research interventions may or may not be beneficial. Indeed, the purpose of evaluative research is to determine whether the test intervention is in fact therapeutic" (43). The federal regulations define research as "a systematic investigation, including research development, testing and evaluation, designed to develop or contribute to generalizable knowledge [Federal Policy §___.102(d)]" (44). Human subjects are "living individual(s) about whom an investigator (whether professional or student) conducting research obtains (1) data through intervention or interaction with the individual, or (2) identifiable private information [Federal Policy §___.102(f)]" (45).

Treatment of a single patient can constitute "research" if there is "a clear intent before treating the patient to use systematically collected data that would not ordinarily be collected in the course of clinical practice in reporting and publishing a case study. Treating with a research intent must be distinguished from the use of innovative treatment practices" (46).

Investigators are required to exercise due care to reduce and manage risks, including incorporating risk-reducing precautions, safeguards, and alternatives into the research protocol. The risk–benefit evaluation is the major ethical judgment required of the IRB (47). The IRB takes into consideration in its assessment the prevailing community standards, currently available information about the risks and benefits, the degree of confidence in this information, and whether the protocol involves the use of interventions that have the intent and reasonable probability of providing benefit for the individual patient or whether its procedures are performed only for research purposes (48).

Subjects always retain the right to withdraw from a research project, so continuing consent is important. Investigators must inform subjects of any important new information that might affect their willingness to continue participating (Federal Policy §___.116) (49). Thus it is necessary for the IRB to monitor whether the risk–benefit ratio has shifted, whether there are unanticipated findings involving risks to subjects, and whether any new information regarding the risks and benefits should be provided to subjects. IRBs are required [Federal Policy §___.108(e)] to reevaluate research projects on an annual basis plus at any additional intervals indicated by degree of risk (50).

3. Ethical Principle Three: Justice

The unjustified overutilization of certain segments of the population for research during the nineteenth and early twentieth centuries led to tragedies such as the Tuskegee syphilis study. Most clinical research involving human subjects during that era had been performed on indigent patients from "staff" hospital wards. This third principle prohibits vulnerable categories of the population from shouldering a disproportionate share of the burden of research. It relates to the potential subject as a member of social, racial, sexual, or ethnic groups and addresses issues of equity—"fairness in the distribution of the benefits and risks of research" (51).

The systematic selection of potential subjects who may be prone to undue influence because of their ready availability, compromised position, or susceptibility to manipulation (52) is prohibited. An order of preference for selecting subjects designates that adults rank before children, competent individuals before incompetent individuals, and noninstitutionalized before institutionalized persons.

Investigators must not overburden institutionalized and disabled persons by asking them to accept the additional burdens of research, unless the research concerns their particular disability or circumstance. In studies in which subjects are likely to be members of a vulnerable population, the IRB is charged with ensuring that appropriate additional safeguards are in place to protect their welfare. Many clinical studies, especially multicenter or double-masked trials, are assigned independent data and safety monitoring boards to fulfill this function.

Vulnerabilities may be subtle, but they can limit voluntarism. Vulnerable populations include children, prisoners, pregnant women, and persons who are economically or educationally disadvantaged or mentally or physically disabled. The latter, for example, may be overly compliant with requests to participate in research due to the effects of their illness or due to the prospect of relief from suffering (53). There are no specific regulations governing research with elderly subjects, because the elderly are recognized as a heterogeneous group not usually in need of special protections.

B. Responsibilities of the Institution Engaged in Research

Responsibilities that must be met prior to the conduct of research involving human subjects are specified by the DHHS. However (54),

> *DHHS regulations do not specify administrative actions for noncompliance with the human subject regulations, except to state that material failure to comply with the regulations can result in termination or suspension of support for department or agency projects, and that DHHS will take terminations or suspensions of funding due to noncompliance into consideration when making future funding decisions [45 CFR 46.123].*

The compliance oversight procedures of the OHRP, called compliance oversight evaluations, consist of site visits designed principally to instruct and educate, and of external investigations into credible reports of alleged noncompliance. "The need for site visits in connection with inquiries and investigations depends upon the seriousness and urgency of the circumstances, and whether on-site involvement is the most effective means of resolving the questions of noncompliance that have been raised" (55). Research sponsors may also regularly audit their research sites. Institutions are responsible for complying with all applicable regulations.

1. The Institutional Review Board

The OHRP describes the IRB as (56)

An administrative body established to protect the rights and welfare of human research subjects recruited to participate in research activities conducted under the auspices of the institution with which it is affiliated. The IRB has the authority to approve, require modifications in, or disapprove all research activities that fall within its jurisdiction as specified by both the federal regulations and local institutional policy.

The IRB ascertains the acceptability of proposed research in terms of institutional commitments and regulations, applicable law, and standards of professional conduct and practice (57). It determines the validity of the presuppositions of the research; distinguishes as clearly as possible the nature, probability and magnitude of risk; and determines whether the investigator's estimates of the probability of harm or benefits are reasonable, as judged by known facts or other available studies (58).

After reviewing the experiment's formal design, the IRB independently approves or disapproves the protocol, based on whether human subjects are adequately protected and all pertinent laws and regulations are observed. Institutional officials cannot approve research that has been disapproved by the IRB [Federal Policy §__.112] (59). Factors that must be evaluated by the IRB include the equitable selection of subjects, the qualifications and experience of the principal investigator; the collection, storage, and analysis of data to enable timely midcourse corrections and ensure validity; the quality assurance standards and mechanisms; scientific merit; and the timeliness and thoroughness by which the research will be monitored.

Clear criteria are not always available for every case, so the IRB may need to base some decisions on its members' sense of propriety and on the particular circumstances of the study (60). Some research protocols, such as in human genetics and transplantation, present complicated issues in that little may be known about the risks presented by the research or no consensus on the appropriate resolution of the problem may yet exist. The IRB also addresses nonvalidated procedures being used for therapeutic purposes within the institution. Through determining any indications requiring a formal research protocol for new procedures, the IRB works to avoid the dangers inherent in allowing untested procedures to come into widespread use without having been systematically validated in well-controlled trials.

Institutions must establish effective mechanisms for providing information to the IRB in the event that unexpected results are discovered that could raise the possibility of unanticipated risks to subjects, or agreed upon procedures are no longer in use: "It is only after research has begun that the real risks can be evaluated and the preliminary results used to compute the actual risk/benefit ratio; the IRB can then determine the correctness of the initial judgment" (61). Progress of the project together with the results of other new research may indicate that the IRB should relax special precautions or impose new ones. The leadership of the institution is responsible for maintaining open channels of communication at all levels. The staff, subjects, and other interested parties must have a means of communicating information to appropriate institutional officials, and IRB members, department heads, and others overseeing research must have "open and ready access to the highest levels of authority within the institution" (62).

The federal regulations do not clearly call for IRB review of the scientific validity of the research design (63). They do, however, require that IRBs make determinations comparing risks to the importance of the expected resulting knowledge. Flawed research methods cannot yield valid knowledge. As a general rule, other than looking for obvious flaws that place subjects at unnecessary risk, most IRBs leave rigorous evaluation of the science to the funding agency (64). In the absence of peer-reviewed scientific review, IRBs must review the research design more carefully. They may use consultants for this purpose to supply sufficient expertise.

The IRB must consist of at least five members from varying backgrounds who represent a diversity of heritage and sensitivities [Federal Policy §__.107]. It must include members with knowledge about institutional requirements, applicable law, and professional standards of conduct. If an IRB regularly reviews protocols involving a vulnerable category of subjects, at least one member should have expertise in working with those subjects. The IRB must include at least one member whose primary concerns are scientific and one whose primary concerns are in nonscientific areas. A member not affiliated with the institution should be drawn from the community at large. The IRB must not consist entirely of members of one profession nor of one gender.

The IRB must prepare and maintain adequate documentation of its activities [Federal Policy §__.115]. The records must be retained for at least 3 years (3 years after completion for conducted research), and "be accessible for inspection and copying by authorized representatives of the department or agency supporting or conducting the research at reasonable times and in a reasonable manner" [Federal Policy §___.115(b)] (65). The institution must provide the IRB "sufficient meeting space and staff to support the IRB's review and record keeping duties" [Federal Policy §___.103(b)(2)] (66).

The human subjects' policies of many institutions require that all research, even research that is exempt from review under the federal regulations, is to be reviewed by the IRB. In such cases, the IRB has jurisdiction over all research using human subjects, thereby providing broader protection for subjects than that required by the regulations. "It is crucial that IRBs keep in mind that their authority to approve, require modifications in, or disapprove research derives from both federal law and institutional policy" (67).

2. The Assurance

As stated in Federal Policy §___.103(b)(91) (68),

An institution involved in biomedical or behavioral research should have in place a set of principles and guidelines that govern the institution, its faculty, and staff, in the discharge of its responsibilities for protecting the rights and welfare of human subjects taking part in research conducted at, or sponsored by, the institution, regardless of the source of funding.

Federal Policy §46.103 (not adopted by the FDA) requires the leadership to provide an Assurance that the institution will comply with the requirements of 45 CFR 46. The Assurance is a written agreement negotiated with the OHRP, on behalf of the DHHS Secretary, that stipulates the method(s) by which the institution will protect the welfare of research subjects. It is a condition of receipt of DHHS support for research involving human subjects. Depending on the nature of the research and other considerations, Assurance documents may be one of three types: a Multiple Project Assurance (MPA), Single Project Assurance (SPA), or Cooperative Project Assurance (CPA). The Assurance must also be approved by the funding department or agency.

"As provided for in its Assurance, an institution must prepare written procedures and guidelines to be followed by the IRB when conducting its initial and continuing review of research, and for reporting its findings and actions to the investigator and the administration of the institution" (69). These procedures must include which projects will require review more often than annually and which projects require verification from sources other than the investigator that no material changes have occurred since the last IRB review. The procedures must ensure prompt reporting to the IRB by the investigator of proposed changes in a research activity, and that changes during the IRB existing approval may not be initiated without IRB approval, except when necessary to eliminate apparent immediate hazards to the subject [Federal Policy §___.103(b)(4)] (70).

The procedures must also ensure that the institution or the funding agency promptly report to the IRB any anticipated problems involving risks to subjects or others, any serious or continuing noncompliance with the Federal Policy or the requirements or determinations of the IRB, and any suspension or termination of IRB approval [Federal Policy §___.103(b)(5)] (71).

3. The Selection and Training of Personnel

The institutional leadership must select appropriate personnel not only to assure the protection of research subjects, but also to protect the institution. The institution's president serves as or appoints an "authorized institutional official" who has the legal authority to act and speak for the institution and who can ensure that the institution will effectively fulfill its research oversight function. Responsible officials must be designated.

The institution must adequately train its officials and personnel in the policies and procedures related to research with human subjects, and must support educational activities related to designing, conducting, and approving high-quality research. All personnel need to know the applicable institutional policies and mechanisms for approving research and reporting problems with research projects in progress. Personnel involved in the conduct of research and IRB members and others with responsibility for reviewing and approving research must receive additional training in the regulations, guidelines, and policies applicable externally and internally to human subjects research, and in good research practices and risk-minimizing methodologies (72).

4. The Audit System

An institution is responsible for maintaining an internal audit system "to assure the institution's administration that its policies and procedures are being adhered to and that they are proper in scope and content" (73). The institution must monitor its research and conduct audits of the research process to enable early identification and correction of problems. In order to ensure compliance, the leadership must adopt internal audit or self-assessment procedures and practices designed to assure proper protocol and consent preparation, proper protocol submission, proper review and approval by the IRB, and timely monitoring of protocol implementation.

5. Privacy and Confidentiality

The institution must ensure that information obtained by researchers about their subjects is not improperly divulged. Confidentiality of data concerns "safeguarding information that has been given voluntarily by one person to another" (74). It is usually a matter of taking standard precautions by following certain routine practices and procedures. However, more elaborate procedures may be needed in some sensitive studies that involve the following:

1. Information relating to sexual attitudes, preferences, or practices.

2. Information relating to the use of alcohol, drugs, or other addictive products.
3. Information pertaining to illegal conduct.
4. Information that, if released, could be damaging to an individual's financial standing, employability, or reputation within the community.
5. Information that would normally be recorded in a patient's medical record, and the disclosure of which could reasonably lead to social stigmatization or discrimination.
6. Information pertaining to an individual's psychological well being or mental health.
7. Information that divulges communicable disease.

Under state law, projects that intend routinely to determine whether its subjects have communicable diseases are required to report findings, with the following exceptions: the referring treating physician has already complied with the reporting requirements; the investigator has an agreement with the health department on procedures for cooperation; or disclosures of identifiable information comply with regulations on subject protection and are explained clearly to the subjects prior to their participation (75).

In 1977, the Privacy Protection Study Commission concluded and the National Commission endorsed that medical records can legitimately be used for biomedical and epidemiologic research without the explicit authorization of an individual as long as the treatment provider maintaining the record proceeds as follows (76):

1. Determines that such use or disclosure does not violate any limitations under which the record or information was collected.
2. Ascertains that use or disclosure in individually identifiable form is necessary to accomplish the research or statistical purpose.
3. Determines the importance of the purpose is such as to warrant the risk to the individual from additional exposure of the record/information.
4. Requires that adequate safeguards are established and maintained, including a program for removal or destruction of identifiers.
5. Obtains written consent before any further use or redisclosure in individually identifiable form is permitted.

The institution and IRB must also ensure the protection of the subject's privacy. "Invasion of privacy concerns access to a person's body or behavior without consent" (77):

Research involving survey or interview procedures with adult subjects is exempt from the federal regulations unless the information obtained is recorded in such a manner that the subjects can be identified, and the information obtained could reasonably place the subjects at risk of criminal or civil liability or be damaging to the subjects' financial standing, employability, or reputation [Federal Policy §___.101(b)(2)] (78).

Survey and interview research involving children is not exempt from IRB review (79).

Observational studies may involve covert observation and participant observation. Covert observation includes the use of concealed devices to record information for later analysis, and the concealment of the researcher while the behavior of subjects is being observed and recorded (80). Participant observation occurs when the researcher assumes a role in the setting or in the group being studied (81). Factors considered in IRB evaluation of privacy questions include the extent to which the behavior in question is public, and the reasonable expectation of privacy. Most observational research is exempt from the federal regulations, except when (1) the observations involve children and minors; (2) the observations are recorded in a manner that allows the subjects to be identified, directly or through identifiers linked to them; or (3) the observations recorded, if they became known outside the research, could reasonably place the subject either at risk of criminal or civil liability or cause damage to the subject's financial standing, employability, or reputation [Federal Policy §___.101(b)(2)] (82).

III. Conclusion

Arising from revulsion to the experiments conducted by Nazi doctors during World War II, the "Nuremberg Code on the Ethics of Human Research" in 1947 assimilated the legal and ethical conclusions of the deliberations of the Nuremberg Trials and established consent as the first of 10 principles of conduct expected of physicians in the performance of research involving human subjects. The long history of the ethics of research involving human subjects has evolved since then to resolutions in several areas. The concepts of different rules for therapeutic as opposed to nontherapeutic research, however, continue to blur and have now become nearly fused. Whereas in the past nontherapeutic research would presumably be less attractive than the implied potential benefit of therapeutic research, patients now view participation in research protocols as an opportunity—perhaps in desperation—to gain access to breakthrough medical science.

The concept of consent continues to evolve. Consent, initially thought to be a recommendation, is now an absolute requirement. In a sense, it is the lasting and most significant contribution of the Nuremberg Code. The terminology has also changed, from "voluntary" consent to "informed" consent. Informed consent now includes understanding as well as being informed. The concept continues to expand into the requirement of autonomy for the participating research subjects. The complexity of modern science mandates a responsible regulatory system. Even more, it requires that responsible investigators who experiment are competent.

References

1. Trohler, U., and Reiter-Theil, S. (1998). *In* "Ethics Codes in Medicine," p. 44. Ashgate Publishing Ltd., Aldershot.
2. Trohler, U., and Reiter-Theil, S. (1998). *In* "Ethics Codes in Medicine," p. 150. Ashgate Publishing Ltd., Aldershot.
3. Trohler, U., and Reiter-Theil, S. (1998). *In* "Ethics Codes in Medicine," p. 125. Ashgate Publishing Ltd., Aldershot.
4. Annas, G. J., and Grodin, M. A. (1992). *In* "The Nazi Doctors and the Nuremberg Code: Human Rights in Human Experimentation," pp. 125–126. Oxford University Press, New York.
5. Annas, G. J., and Grodin, M. A. (1992). *In* "The Nazi Doctors and the Nuremberg Code: Human Rights in Human Experimentation," p. 317. Oxford University Press, New York.
6. Trohler, U., and Reiter-Theil, S. (1998). *In* "Ethics Codes in Medicine," p. 318. Ashgate Publishing Ltd., Aldershot.
7. Trohler, U., and Reiter-Theil, S. (1998). *In* "Ethics Codes in Medicine," p. 65. Ashgate Publishing Ltd., Aldershot.
8. Trohler, U., and Reiter-Theil, S. (1998). *In* "Ethics Codes in Medicine," p. 53. Ashgate Publishing Ltd., Aldershot.
9. Annas, G. J., and Grodin, M. A. (1992). *In* "The Nazi Doctors and the Nuremberg Code: Human Rights in Human Experimentation," p. 68. Oxford University Press, New York.
10. Annas, G. J., and Grodin, M. A. (1992). *In* "The Nazi Doctors and the Nuremberg Code: Human Rights in Human Experimentation," p. 152. Oxford University Press, New York.

10a. Shuster, E. (1997). Fifty years later: The significance of the Nuremberg Code. *N. Engl. J. Med.* **337**(20), 1436.

11. Trohler, U., and Reiter-Theil, S. (1998). *In* "Ethics Codes in Medicine," p. 73. Ashgate Publishing Ltd., Aldershot.
12. World Medical Association web page (11 November, 1999): http://www.WMA.com.
13. Trohler, U., and Reiter-Theil, S. (1998). *In* "Ethics Codes in Medicine," p. 127. Ashgate Publishing Ltd., Aldershot.
14. Trohler, U., and Reiter-Theil, S. (1998). *In* "Ethics Codes in Medicine," p. 47. Ashgate Publishing Ltd., Aldershot.
15. Trohler, U., and Reiter-Theil, S. (1998). *In* "Ethics Codes in Medicine," p. 129. Ashgate Publishing Ltd., Aldershot.
16. Trohler, U., and Reiter-Theil, S. (1998). *In* "Ethics Codes in Medicine," p. 17. Ashgate Publishing Ltd., Aldershot.
17. Trohler, U., and Reiter-Theil, S. (1998). *In* "Ethics Codes in Medicine," p. 18. Ashgate Publishing Ltd., Aldershot.
18. Trohler, U., and Reiter-Theil, S. (1998). *In* "Ethics Codes in Medicine," p. 243. Ashgate Publishing Ltd., Aldershot.
19. Trohler, U., and Reiter-Theil, S. (1998). *In* "Ethics Codes in Medicine," p. 125. Ashgate Publishing Ltd., Aldershot.
20. Trohler, U., and Reiter-Theil, S. (1998). *In* "Ethics Codes in Medicine," p. 155. Ashgate Publishing Ltd., Aldershot.
21. Office for Protection from Research Risks (OPRR) (1993). "Protecting Human Research Subjects. Institutional Review Board Guidebook." GPO, Washington, D.C.
22. Office for Protection from Research Risks (OPRR) (1993). *In* "Protecting Human Research Subjects. Institutional Review Board Guidebook," 3–11. GPO, Washington, D.C.
23. Office for Protection from Research Risks (OPRR) (1993). *In* "Protecting Human Research Subjects. Institutional Review Board Guidebook," p. xxi. GPO, Washington, D.C.
24. Office for Protection from Research Risks (OPRR) (1993). *In* "Protecting Human Research Subjects. Institutional Review Board Guidebook," p. xxi. GPO, Washington, D.C.
25. Office for Protection from Research Risks (OPRR) (1993). *In* "Protecting Human Research Subjects. Institutional Review Board Guidebook," 3–11. GPO, Washington, D.C.
26. Office for Protection from Research Risks (OPRR) (1993). *In* "Protecting Human Research Subjects. Institutional Review Board Guidebook," 3–20. GPO, Washington, D.C.
27. Office for Protection from Research Risks (OPRR) (1993). *In* "Protecting Human Research Subjects. Institutional Review Board Guidebook," 3–5. GPO, Washington, D.C.
28. Office for Protection from Research Risks (OPRR) (1993). *In* "Protecting Human Research Subjects. Institutional Review Board Guidebook," 3–13. GPO, Washington, D.C.
29. Office for Protection from Research Risks (OPRR) (1993). *In* "Protecting Human Research Subjects. Institutional Review Board Guidebook," 4–25. GPO, Washington, D.C.
30. Office for Protection from Research Risks (OPRR) (1993). *In* "Protecting Human Research Subjects. Institutional Review Board Guidebook," 3–16. GPO, Washington, D.C.
31. Office for Protection from Research Risks (OPRR) (1993). *In* "Protecting Human Research Subjects. Institutional Review Board Guidebook," 3–19. GPO, Washington, D.C.
32. Office for Protection from Research Risks (OPRR) (1993). *In* "Protecting Human Research Subjects. Institutional Review Board Guidebook," 3–44. GPO, Washington, D.C.
33. Office for Protection from Research Risks (OPRR) (1993). *In* "Protecting Human Research Subjects. Institutional Review Board Guidebook," 3–44. GPO, Washington, D.C.
34. Office for Protection from Research Risks (OPRR) (1993). *In* "Protecting Human Research Subjects. Institutional Review Board Guidebook," 3–46. GPO, Washington, D.C.
35. Office for Protection from Research Risks (OPRR) (1993). *In* "Protecting Human Research Subjects. Institutional Review Board Guidebook," 3–3. GPO, Washington, D.C.
36. Office for Protection from Research Risks (OPRR) (1993). *In* "Protecting Human Research Subjects. Institutional Review Board Guidebook," 3–1. GPO, Washington, D.C.
37. Office for Protection from Research Risks (OPRR) (1993). *In* "Protecting Human Research Subjects. Institutional Review Board Guidebook," 3–1. GPO, Washington, D.C.
38. Office for Protection from Research Risks (OPRR) (1993). *In* "Protecting Human Research Subjects. Institutional Review Board Guidebook," p. xxiii. GPO, Washington, D.C.
39. Office for Protection from Research Risks (OPRR) (1993). *In* "Protecting Human Research Subjects. Institutional Review Board Guidebook," 3–2. GPO, Washington, D.C.
40. Office for Protection from Research Risks (OPRR) (1993). *In* "Protecting Human Research Subjects. Institutional Review Board Guidebook," p. xxi. GPO, Washington, D.C.
41. Office for Protection from Research Risks (OPRR) (1993). *In* "Protecting Human Research Subjects. Institutional Review Board Guidebook," p. xxi. GPO, Washington, D.C.
42. Office for Protection from Research Risks (OPRR) (1993). *In* "Protecting Human Research Subjects. Institutional Review Board Guidebook," p. xxi. GPO, Washington, D.C.
43. Office for Protection from Research Risks (OPRR) (1993). *In* "Protecting Human Research Subjects. Institutional Review Board Guidebook," 1–2. GPO, Washington, D.C.
44. Office for Protection from Research Risks (OPRR) (1993). *In* "Protecting Human Research Subjects. Institutional Review Board Guidebook," 1–1. GPO, Washington, D.C.
45. Office for Protection from Research Risks (OPRR) (1993). *In* "Protecting Human Research Subjects. Institutional Review Board Guidebook," 2–15. GPO, Washington, D.C.
46. Office for Protection from Research Risks (OPRR) (1993). *In* "Protecting Human Research Subjects. Institutional Review Board Guidebook," 2–15. GPO, Washington, D.C.
47. Office for Protection from Research Risks (OPRR) (1993). *In* "Protecting Human Research Subjects. Institutional Review Board Guidebook," 3–8. GPO, Washington, D.C.
48. Office for Protection from Research Risks (OPRR) (1993). *In* "Protecting Human Research Subjects. Institutional Review Board Guidebook," 3–9. GPO, Washington, D.C.

49. Office for Protection from Research Risks (OPRR) (1993). *In* "Protecting Human Research Subjects. Institutional Review Board Guidebook," 3–21. GPO, Washington, D.C.
50. Office for Protection from Research Risks (OPRR) (1993). *In* "Protecting Human Research Subjects. Institutional Review Board Guidebook," 3–9. GPO, Washington, D.C.
51. Office for Protection from Research Risks (OPRR) (1993). *In* "Protecting Human Research Subjects. Institutional Review Board Guidebook," 5–29. GPO, Washington, D.C.
52. Office for Protection from Research Risks (OPRR) (1993). *In* "Protecting Human Research Subjects. Institutional Review Board Guidebook," 3–23. GPO, Washington, D.C.
53. Office for Protection from Research Risks (OPRR) (1993). *In* "Protecting Human Research Subjects. Institutional Review Board Guidebook," 3–42. GPO, Washington, D.C.
54. Office for Protection from Research Risks (OPRR) (1993). *In* "Protecting Human Research Subjects. Institutional Review Board Guidebook," 1–13. GPO, Washington, D.C.
55. Office for Protection from Research Risks (OPRR) (1993). *In* "Protecting Human Research Subjects. Institutional Review Board Guidebook," 1–13. GPO, Washington, D.C.
56. Office for Protection from Research Risks (OPRR) (1993). *In* "Protecting Human Research Subjects. Institutional Review Board Guidebook," 1–1. GPO, Washington, D.C.
57. Office for Protection from Research Risks (OPRR) (1993). *In* "Protecting Human Research Subjects. Institutional Review Board Guidebook," 1–3. GPO, Washington, D.C.
58. Office for Protection from Research Risks (OPRR) (1993). *In* "Protecting Human Research Subjects. Institutional Review Board Guidebook," p. xxiii. GPO, Washington, D.C.
59. Office for Protection from Research Risks (OPRR) (1993). *In* "Protecting Human Research Subjects. Institutional Review Board Guidebook," 1–2. GPO, Washington, D.C.
60. Office for Protection from Research Risks (OPRR) (1993). *In* "Protecting Human Research Subjects. Institutional Review Board Guidebook," 3–35. GPO, Washington, D.C.
61. Office for Protection from Research Risks (OPRR) (1993). *In* "Protecting Human Research Subjects. Institutional Review Board Guidebook," 3–47. GPO, Washington, D.C.
62. Office for Protection from Research Risks (OPRR) (1993). *In* "Protecting Human Research Subjects. Institutional Review Board Guidebook," 1–6. GPO, Washington, D.C.
63. Office for Protection from Research Risks (OPRR) (1993). *In* "Protecting Human Research Subjects. Institutional Review Board Guidebook," 4–1. GPO, Washington, D.C.
64. Office for Protection from Research Risks (OPRR) (1993). *In* "Protecting Human Research Subjects. Institutional Review Board Guidebook," 4–1. GPO, Washington, D.C.
65. Office for Protection from Research Risks (OPRR) (1993). *In* "Protecting Human Research Subjects. Institutional Review Board Guidebook," 1–5. GPO, Washington, D.C.
66. Office for Protection from Research Risks (OPRR) (1993). *In* "Protecting Human Research Subjects. Institutional Review Board Guidebook," 1–6. GPO, Washington, D.C.
67. Office for Protection from Research Risks (OPRR) (1993). *In* "Protecting Human Research Subjects. Institutional Review Board Guidebook," 1–2. GPO, Washington, D.C.
68. Office for Protection from Research Risks (OPRR) (1993). *In* "Protecting Human Research Subjects. Institutional Review Board Guidebook," 1–6. GPO, Washington, D.C.
69. Office for Protection from Research Risks (OPRR) (1993). *In* "Protecting Human Research Subjects. Institutional Review Board Guidebook," 1–6. GPO, Washington, D.C.
70. Office for Protection from Research Risks (OPRR) (1993). *In* "Protecting Human Research Subjects. Institutional Review Board Guidebook," 1–7. GPO, Washington, D.C.
71. Office for Protection from Research Risks (OPRR) (1993). *In* "Protecting Human Research Subjects. Institutional Review Board Guidebook," 1–7. GPO, Washington, D.C.
72. Office for Protection from Research Risks (OPRR) (1993). *In* "Protecting Human Research Subjects. Institutional Review Board Guidebook," 1–7. GPO, Washington, D.C.
73. Office for Protection from Research Risks (OPRR) (1993). *In* "Protecting Human Research Subjects. Institutional Review Board Guidebook," 1–7. GPO, Washington, D.C.
74. Office for Protection from Research Risks (OPRR) (1993). *In* "Protecting Human Research Subjects. Institutional Review Board Guidebook," 3–4. GPO, Washington, D.C.
75. Office for Protection from Research Risks (OPRR) (1993). *In* "Protecting Human Research Subjects. Institutional Review Board Guidebook," 3–33. GPO, Washington, D.C.
76. Office for Protection from Research Risks (OPRR) (1993). *In* "Protecting Human Research Subjects. Institutional Review Board Guidebook," 3–29. GPO, Washington, D.C.
77. Office for Protection from Research Risks (OPRR) (1993). *In* "Protecting Human Research Subjects. Institutional Review Board Guidebook," 3–29. GPO, Washington, D.C.
78. Office for Protection from Research Risks (OPRR) (1993). *In* "Protecting Human Research Subjects. Institutional Review Board Guidebook," 4–9. GPO, Washington, D.C.
79. Office for Protection from Research Risks (OPRR) (1993). *In* "Protecting Human Research Subjects. Institutional Review Board Guidebook," 4–9. GPO, Washington, D.C.
80. Office for Protection from Research Risks (OPRR) (1993). *In* "Protecting Human Research Subjects. Institutional Review Board Guidebook," 3–30. GPO, Washington, D.C.
81. Office for Protection from Research Risks (OPRR) (1993). *In* "Protecting Human Research Subjects. Institutional Review Board Guidebook," 3–30. GPO, Washington, D.C.
82. Office for Protection from Research Risks (OPRR) (1993). *In* "Protecting Human Research Subjects. Institutional Review Board Guidebook," 3–30. GPO, Washington, D.C.

7

Animal Care and Maintenance

David Lee-Parritz

Center for Animal Resources and Comparative Medicine, Harvard Medical School, Boston, Massachusetts 02115

I. Introduction

Experimental use of animals is a vital part of biomedical research. Appropriate use of animal models allows prospective, controlled disease investigation that cannot be conducted in human patients or volunteers. Investigators must consider scientific, practical, and humane issues when developing studies that use animals. High-quality research requires close collaboration between veterinary and research professionals to provide humane care and use of laboratory animals, reducing animal pain and distress to the absolute minimum while maintaining the scientific goals of the project. This chapter briefly reviews ethical and regulatory issues and lists available information resources. Remaining sections address specific technical issues related to animal surgery, including design of surgical facilities, animal selection, anesthesia, and analgesia.

II. Ethical and Regulatory Overview

Investigators and research institutions have an ethical and legal responsibility to minimize pain and distress in research animals. Russell and Burch expressed the most widely understood ethical principles governing humane design of experiments using animals in 1959. Acknowledging that "we owe to animal experimentation many if not most of the benefits of modern medicine," these scientists reminded the research community that the most humane "possible treatment of experimental animals, far from being an obstacle, is actually a prerequisite" for high-quality research (1). Russell and Burch formulated the concept of the "three Rs" as a strategy to minimize experimental animal pain and distress. The first principle, *replacement*, states that nonanimal models should be used instead of animals to the maximum extent possible. Although inanimate models rarely allow examination of complex physiological processes often encountered in surgical research, suitable alternatives to the use of animals in surgical education may be appropriate. The principle of *reduction* states that investigators should use the minimum number of animals consistent with statistical power. The most important of the three Rs is the principle of *refinement*, which states that investigators should use the least invasive technique possible to minimize animal pain and distress (2). Continuous improvements in animal husbandry, diagnosis, and control of infectious disease have greatly reduced nonexperimental morbidity and mortality in modern research facilities. Advances in the development of animal anesthetics and analgesics have allowed further reduction and refinement of research animal use.

Widespread acceptance of the three Rs and continued public scrutiny of biomedical research now require investigators and institutions to comply with strict regulatory standards governing all aspects of research animal use. Several well-publicized incidents concerning mistreatment of research animals prompted Congress to enact the Animal Welfare Act (AWA) in 1966, requiring the federal government to develop a mechanism to assure humane treatment of animals. The Food and Drug Administration and the Good Laboratory Practices Act also regulate research conducted in direct support of new drugs or medical devices. In addition to compliance with governmental regulations, many research facilities in the United States and abroad seek voluntary accreditation by the Association for the Assessment and Accreditation of Laboratory Animal Care—International (AAALAC), an organization that promotes excellence in all phases of laboratory animal care.

The AWA regulates the treatment of animals used in research, for exhibition, and sold as pets in interstate commerce. The United States Department of Agriculture enforces the AWA through the Animal and Plant Health Inspection Service (APHIS). These regulations (Code of Federal Regulations, Title 9, Chapter 1, Parts 1–3) require research institutions to maintain an institutional animal care and use committee empowered to review and approve research protocols, oversee animal use, and investigate allegations of animal mistreatment. The regulations also describe standards for husbandry and veterinary care as well as acquisition, transportation, and disposal of animals. Additional regulations require facilities to provide for the psychological well-being of nonhuman primates and to assure that dogs have the opportunity for exercise and socialization. Although rare in biomedical research laboratories, the use of endangered species is further regulated by the Endangered Species Act. With few exceptions, research using endangered species must be done only for the direct benefit of animals with spontaneous disease (3).

The United States Public Health Service (PHS), through the National Institutes of Health, as the largest single sponsor of biomedical research using animals, has adopted regulations to assure humane and scientifically valid use of animals. The NIH Office for Laboratory Animal Welfare (OLAW), formerly known as the Office for Protection from Research Risks, develops and implements standards for animal care and use at recipient institutions, as formulated in Public Health Service Policy on Humane Care and Use of Laboratory Animals. Institutions receiving PHS support must file an "Animal Welfare Assurance" with OLAW indicating sufficient institutional resources to provide proper husbandry and veterinary care. Institutions must also indicate how they will approve and monitor research to assure scientific integrity and prevent inhumane treatment of animals. Assurances are approved for 5 years, after which a new application must be submitted (4).

The Association for the Assessment and Accreditation of Laboratory Animal Care—International is a nongovernmental organization that seeks to maintain the highest standards of laboratory animal care and use. Approximately 600 research facilities in the United States and in 10 other countries hold AAALAC accreditation. AAALAC policies are determined by the Board of Trustees, representing more than 50 scientific, educational, and professional organizations involved with biomedical research use of animals. The AAALAC Board appoints the Council on Accreditation, which reviews, grants, or suspends accreditation based on a triennial program review and site visit by at least one council member and ad hoc consultant. The OLAW accepts AAALAC accreditation as strong evidence that an institution's animal care and use program is in substantial compliance with the PHS Policy (3).

III. Available Resources

Although used to model human disease, research animals require specialized care that recognizes anatomic and physiologic differences between species. These differences determine routine husbandry and behavioral needs. Surgeons must also be aware of significant differences in gross and microscopic anatomy between the common laboratory species. Animals vary greatly in their response to anesthetics and other drugs, and anatomic differences often pose significant challenges to endotracheal intubation, surgical approach, and intravenous access.

Veterinarians offer important expertise to investigators using animals. Laboratory animal medicine is the specialty of veterinary medicine concerned with the care and use of animals in biomedical research. Laboratory animal medicine veterinarians specialize in the diagnosis and treatment of laboratory animal diseases and assist investigators in developing new experimental techniques and providing specialized preoperative, intraoperative, and postoperative care. Other veterinary specialties that surgical investigators may wish to utilize include surgery, anesthesia, pathology, and internal medicine (see Table I for contacts). Most large research institutions have at least one staff veterinarian trained and experienced in laboratory animal medicine. Smaller institutions may use the services of consultant veterinarians. Large research programs may include veterinarians as part of the research team.

Several information resources are valuable to surgical investigators. Print resources include textbooks and jour-

Table I Specialty Boards and Accrediting Agencies

Name	Address	Telephone number	Web site
American College of Laboratory Animal Medicine	Dr. Melvin W. Balk, Executive Director 96 Chester St., Chester, NH 03036	603 887-2467 (office) 603 887-0096 (fax)	www.aclam.org
American College of Veterinary Anesthesiologists	Dr. Richard Broadstone, Executive Secretary Virginia–Maryland Regional College of Veterinary Medicine, Duckpond Drive, Blacksburg, VA 24061-0442	540-231-9268 (office) 540-231-7367 (fax)	www.acva.org
American College of Veterinary Internal Medicine	Ms. June Pooley, Executive Director 1997 Wadsworth, Suite A, Lakewood, CO 80215-3327	800-245-9081 (office) 303-231-0880 (fax)	www.acvim.org
American College of Veterinary Pathologists	Susan Whitehouse, Executive Director 19 Manuta Rd., Mt. Royal, NJ 08061	856-423-0119 (office) 856-423-3240 (fax)	www.afip.org/acvp/index.html
American College of Veterinary Surgeons	Dr. Alan J. Lipowitz, Executive Secretary 4401 East West Hwy, Suite 205, Bethesda, MD 20814-4523	301-913-9550 (office) 301-913-2034 (fax)	www.acvs.org
Association for the Assessment and Accreditation of Laboratory Animal Care—International (AAALAC)	Dr. John Miller, Executive Director 11300 Rockville Pike, Suite 1211, Rockville, MD 20852-3035	301-231-5353 (office) 301-231-8282 (fax)	www.aaalac.org

nals. The "Guide for the Care and Use of Laboratory Animals" (3), commonly known as the "Guide," is the primary resource for standards and references concerning research administration and oversight, animal husbandry, veterinary care, and physical plant standards. Many groups, including AAALAC and OLAW, require institutional compliance with the Guide to maintain accreditation and eligibility for funding. Several excellent textbooks discuss general laboratory animal medicine (5, 6) and basic biology and methodology for rodents (7, 8, 9), rabbits (10, 11), cats (12), primates (13, 14), swine (15, 16), and other species (17, 18). Specialized texts provide detailed reviews of anesthetic techniques (19, 20), infectious disease (21, 22), and drug dosages (23) for experimental animals. Timely information on laboratory animal husbandry, diseases, and research techniques is available in several peer-reviewed journals (Table II). Finally, the World Wide Web has excellent resources for laboratory animal users, including reference material, bibliographical

Table II Laboratory Animal Medicine Journals

Name	Publisher	Telephone number	Web site
Contemporary Topics in Laboratory Animal Science	American Association for Laboratory Animal Science 9190 Crestwyn Hill Drive Memphis, TN 38125	901-754-8620 (office) 901-753-0046 (fax)	www.aalas.org
ILAR Journal	Institute for Laboratory Animal Research 2101 Constitution Avenue NW, Washington, D.C. 20418	202-334-2590 (office) 202-334-1687 (fax)	www4.nationalacademies.org/cls/ijhome.nsf
Lab Animal	Lab Animal P.O. Box 5054, Brentwood, TN 37024-5054	212-726-9200 (office)	www.labanimal.com
Laboratory Animals	The Royal Society of Medicine Press, Ltd. 1 Wimpole St., London W1M 8AE, UK	(+44) 171-290-2927 (office) (+44) 171-290-2929 (fax)	www.lal.org.uk
Laboratory Animal Science	American Association for Laboratory Animal Science 9190 Crestwyn Hill Drive, Memphis, TN 38125	901-754-8620 (office) 901-753-0046 (fax)	www.aalas.org

databases, and discussion groups on a variety of technical and regulatory topics (24). The NetVet portal is an excellent entry point to web-based laboratory animal resources (http://netvet.wustl.edu/vet.htm).

IV. Surgical Facility Design

High-quality surgical research requires the use of appropriately designed and equipped surgical facilities. The Guide requires the use of aseptic technique for all survival surgical procedures on laboratory animals. Components of aseptic technique include patient preparation (clipping and disinfection of the surgical site), surgeon preparation (surgical attire, surgical hand scrub, sterile gloves), and use of sterile instruments and techniques to reduce the chance of contamination (draping, traffic control) (3).

Design and configuration of operating room facilities require careful planning and cooperation on the part of research and veterinary staff. Nonrodent survival surgery may be performed only in dedicated facilities designed to minimize traffic and to provide for adequate patient and surgeon preparation. Rodent survival surgery does not require the use of a dedicated surgical suite as long as the conditions for asepsis are present.

Functional components of the survival surgery suite must include dedicated areas for surgery, animal preparation, surgeon's scrub, postoperative recovery, and surgical support. These areas should be in separate rooms, arranged to facilitate entry and exit of animals and staff while minimizing unnecessary traffic. In some cases, activities are consolidated as long as the ability to maintain aseptic conditions is intact. Clipping of animal hair in the operating room should never be allowed, because fur bears a high bacterial load and quickly contaminates every surface on which it settles. To maximize economy of scale and efficient use of skilled support staff, many research institutions maintain centralized experimental surgery suites. Smaller specialized facilities may be appropriate to accommodate unique experimental requirements. Principles of research animal operating room design have been described (3, 25).

V. Anesthesia

Anesthesia is the state of immobilization and elimination of pain, which is essential to all surgical procedures. The ideal anesthetic preserves cardiac output and other physiologic parameters, provides intraoperative analgesia that extends to the postoperative period, and is reversible and safe for the patient, operator, and environment. A variety of anesthetic agents are available for experimental surgery and may be administered parenterally or by inhalation. Several considerations should determine the selection of anesthetic agents for experimental surgery. The Guide requires an Institutional Animal Care and Use Committee (IACUC) to consider sedation, analgesia, and anesthesia when reviewing protocols. Consequently, most of these committees require advance approval of all anesthetic agents. Anesthesia for experimental surgery must be practical to implement by small research teams with minimal formal training in anesthesia.

Injectable anesthesia is popular in experimental surgery. The principal benefits of injectable anesthetic techniques are ease of administration and operator safety. Injectable techniques usually use a combination of agents given by the intramuscular or, for rodents, intraperitoneal routes. Intravenous anesthesia, by continuous or intermittent bolus infusion, may be appropriate in larger animals. Most injectable agents or combinations of agents provide 15 to 30 min of anesthesia. Injectable anesthetics are often used to allow endotracheal intubation for inhalation anesthesia. Muscle relaxation may be poor and excessive salivation may occur. Prolonged recovery and severe alteration of physiology result from repeated administration of injectable agents to maintain anesthesia during long procedures. Because reversal of injectable agents is often impossible, the operator must avoid administration of an accidental overdose. In addition, the operator must be careful not to breach aseptic technique when administering supplemental anesthetic. Many injectable anesthetic agents have a moderate to high abuse potential, therefore investigators who use these agents in research must register with the United States Drug Enforcement Administration and maintain proper records and storage facilities.

Inhalation anesthesia, usually with halothane or isoflurane, allows the operator a high degree of control over anesthetic depth and is the technique of choice for prolonged or invasive surgery. Inhalation anesthesia for major surgery requires a precision vaporizer and endotracheal intubation to allow proper control of anesthetic depth and the airway. Open-drop administration of highly volatile anesthetics for major procedures is not appropriate because rapid changes in anesthetic depth are likely and operator exposure to waste anesthetic gases is high. Anesthetic administration by facemask may be appropriate for brief or noninvasive procedures. Prolonged inhalation by mask is undesirable because it does not protect the airway from aspiration in the event of vomiting or allow positive pressure ventilation in an emergency. Ventilatory support is crucial for thoracotomy and to prevent hypoventilation during long procedures. Endotracheal intubation of some species requires special laryngoscopic equipment and knowledge of anatomic peculiarities that complicate accurate endotracheal tube placement.

A. Injectable Anesthetic Agents

1. Dissociative Anesthetics

Dissociative anesthetics are common in experimental surgery because they maintain cardiac output and provide good analgesia with a high margin of safety. Dissociative anesthetics produce unconsciousness and analgesia through selective disruption of ascending impulses to conscious brain centers rather than through generalized depression of the central nervous system. As sole agents, dissociative anesthetics usually produce unacceptable muscle rigidity and salivation and may cause seizures, especially in dogs (20, 26, 27).

Ketamine is the most commonly used dissociative agent. Ketamine is water soluble. Intramuscular (IM) or intraperitoneal (IP) administration is most common in small animals. Rapid anesthetic induction or supplementation occurs after intravenous administration. Because ketamine solutions are acidic, perivascular infiltration and large-volume intramuscular injection will produce pain and tissue irritation.

Xylazine is a common adjunct to ketamine anesthesia. Xylazine is an α-2 adrenergic agonist with potent sedative and analgesic activity, but is not acceptable as a sole agent for general anesthesia. Coadministration with ketamine provides up to 30 min of anesthesia with excellent muscle relaxation, smooth recovery, and a moderate degree of postoperative analgesia in many species. Ketamine/xylazine is also an excellent induction combination prior to endotracheal intubation and subsequent inhalation anesthesia. Intramuscular administration is preferable, because transient hypertension and cardiac arrythmia can occur after rapid intravenous boluses. Anticholinergic agents such as atropine or glycopyrrolate will control bradycardia in animals that receive xylazine (20).

There are a number of common side effects associated with xylazine. Xylazine commonly induces vomiting in many laboratory animal species. Xylazine also significantly depresses cardiac output at standard anesthetic doses. Cardiac depression is frequently subclinical in young healthy animals commonly used in experimental surgery. Decompensation may occur in aged animals or in those with clinical or experimentally induced illness.

Tranquilizers are common adjuncts in veterinary anesthesia to allay animal anxiety and to provide muscle relaxation. Acepromazine provides excellent sedation in many species, and protects the myocardium from catecholamine-induced arrythmias. Disadvantages of acepromazine include hypotension secondary to adrenergic blockade and prolonged recovery. Benzodiazepines such as diazepam, midazolam, and zolazepam provide excellent short-term sedation with little effect on blood pressure (20). Midazolam is relatively expensive and all benzodiazepines are controlled substances, which may limit their utility in some laboratories.

Telazol is a commercial mixture of the dissociative agent tiletamine and the benzodiazepine zolazepam. The product is supplied in a sterile vial, which is reconstituted with 5 ml of sterile water. Reconstituted vials contain 50 mg/ml of each agent and may be kept for 48 hr at room temperature or for 14 days in a refrigerator. Telazol has anesthetic efficacy similar to that of ketamine/xylazine or ketamine/diazepam. Telazol may also be combined with xylazine for greater anesthetic depth.

2. Barbiturates

The barbiturates are among the oldest anesthetic agents and remain useful for some experimental applications. Barbiturates act through general depression of the central nervous system. There is dose-dependent depression of respiration and cardiac output. Hepatic metabolism terminates the activity of long-acting oxybarbiturates such as sodium pentobarbital. Rapid redistribution to fat followed by hepatic detoxification characterizes the metabolism of the short-acting thiobarbiturates thiamylal and thiopental.

The principal advantage of sodium pentobarbital for general anesthesia is the ability to induce rapidly deep anesthesia with a single agent. Several disadvantages limit sodium pentobarbital's utility in prolonged or invasive procedures. Progressive cardiovascular depression occurs with prolonged anesthesia. Despite sleeping times of 5–15 hr, surgical anesthesia is often present only for 30–60 min in most species because this agent provides very little analgesia. Stormy recovery with vocalization and an unstable gait is common. Rapid-acting intravenous thiobarbiturates provide about 10 min of general anesthesia and are extremely useful for anesthetic induction. Barbiturate solutions are strongly alkaline and require intravenous or intraperitoneal administration to avoid pain and tissue necrosis (20).

3. Miscellaneous Injectable Anesthetics

Specific experimental situations may require the use of nonstandard anesthetics. These agents include chloral hydrate, α-chloralose, or urethane. Chloral hydrate and α-chloralose preserve motor and sensory nerve function but are poor anesthetics with minimal analgesic effect except at very high dosages. α-Chloralose and urethane result in stable cardiovascular performance during prolonged anesthesia. Urethane is mutagenic and carcinogenic in experimental animals and may be used only for nonsurvival procedures. Urethane may also be hazardous to research staff after prolonged contact. Because of these constraints, most IACUCs require investigators to justify the use of nonstandard agents on scientific grounds (26).

B. Inhalation Anesthetics

Inhalation anesthesia offers the experimental surgeon numerous advantages. The respiratory route of administration allows rapid and convenient adjustment of anesthetic depth. Delivery of the anesthetic in 100% oxygen assures excellent tissue oxygenation. Endotracheal intubation prior to anesthesia protects the airway and allows positive pressure ventilation when necessary.

The halogenated anesthetics are the agents of choice for clinical and experimental inhalation anesthesia. Although several halogenated anesthetics are available, isoflurane offers numerous advantages. Isoflurane is poorly soluble in blood and undergoes minimal metabolism. As a result, recovery after discontinuation of the anesthetic is rapid, even in animals with significant hepatic or renal impairment. Cardiac output remains normal even after prolonged procedures. Because dose-dependent cardiac depression occurs even with isoflurane anesthesia, a balanced anesthetic technique combining narcotic analgesics and muscle relaxants to reduce the required concentration of isoflurane is suggested for long procedures on animals with cardiac disease. Unlike halothane, isoflurane does not sensitize the myocardium to catecholamine-induced arrhythmias (29, 30).

Other halogenated anesthetics include halothane, methoxyflurane, desflurane, and sevoflurane. Halothane has a more pleasant odor and may engender less patient resistance than isoflurane when used for mask induction. Isoflurane and halothane are poor analgesics and require supplementary agents for intraoperative and postoperative pain control. Methoxyflurane has a much lower vapor pressure than isoflurane and halothane. When allowed to evaporate in a closed container, the steady-state concentration of methoxyflurane approximates the anesthetic dose. Methoxyflurane is the only halogenated agent suitable for the open-drop anesthetic technique. Although useful in many experimental settings, newer agents have supplanted methoxyflurane in clinical anesthesia. As a result, methoxyflurane is extremely expensive and difficult to obtain at present. The principal advantages of desflurane and sevoflurane are extremely rapid induction and recovery with essentially no patient metabolism. These agents are not in common usage because the agents and vaporizers remain very expensive. Halogenated anesthetics may be scavenged with activated charcoal canisters or by connection to an active exhaust circuit (29, 30).

Older inhalation anesthetics include diethyl ether and nitrous oxide. Like methoxyflurane, ether attains therapeutic anesthetic concentration in a closed container and has been used for bell jar and open-drop anesthesia of rodents. Ether is also inexpensive and readily available from chemical supply houses. Significant disadvantages to the use of ether include flammability and the risk of explosion if peroxides form when ether evaporates to dryness. Mask induction with ether is unpleasant for the patient. High lipid solubility prolongs recovery and analgesia is poor. Nitrous oxide provides slight analgesia when administered at high concentration but is not an effective anesthetic in animals. The maximum allowable concentration of nitrous oxide is 80% in oxygen, beyond which hypoxemia is likely. Activated charcoal does not absorb nitrous oxide, thus active exhaust scavengers are required when using nitrous oxide for anesthesia. Most institutions strongly discourage the use of these agents without specific scientific justification (30).

VI. Anesthetic Recommendations by Species

The following section will provide general recommendations for general anesthesia of the common laboratory animal species. Criteria for selection of healthy research subjects are also included. When appropriate, separate recommendations will be made for brief or noninvasive procedures. For detailed discussion of anesthesia for specific procedures or disease conditions, the reader is advised to consult the references or a veterinary specialist.

A. Rodent

1. Animal Selection and Preoperative Preparation

Specific-pathogen-free rodents should be used for all surgical procedures to reduce morbidity and mortality from chronic respiratory disease. Infectious agents commonly implicated in chronic respiratory disease of rodents include *Mycoplasma pulmonis*, Sendai virus, and cilia-associated-respiratory (CAR) bacillus (21). Other infectious agents may alter immune functions or impair detoxification of anesthetic or experimental drugs. Several commercial vendors supply common strains of laboratory rodents free from infection with these and other infectious agents. These animals are known as specific-pathogen-free (SPF) or virus-antibody-free (VAF) animals and should always be used for survival surgical procedures to minimize experimental variability and reduce surgical mortality. The specific panel of excluded agents may vary according to the vendor. The institution should adopt standard operating procedures to prevent introduction of rodent infectious agents and should regularly survey all holding areas for evidence of infection. Introduction of SPF animals to rooms with enzootic viral infection may result in rapid onset of severe clinical disease. Cedar or pine shavings commonly used for contact bedding contain aromatic compounds that induce hepatic microsomes and alter hepatic detoxification of anesthetics (31). To assure uniform response to anesthetics and experimental drugs, rodents should receive heat-treated wood chip, corncob, or cellulose bedding. A conditioning period of at least 3 days after purchase will minimize mortality associated with shipping stress and dehydration. Preoperative fasting in rodents should be kept to a minimum (2–3 hr) to avoid intraoperative hypoglycemia and shock (6).

2. General Anesthesia

Most surgical procedures in rodents are of short duration. Small body size and limited vascular access complicate anesthesia and intraoperative support of rodents. Nevertheless, skilled operators with appropriate instrumentation can accomplish delicate vascular surgery and other procedures in rats and mice with minimal postoperative mortality. Endotracheal intubation and positive pressure ventilation are also possible and require the use of customized equipment (31).

Several anesthetic combinations are appropriate for brief, noninvasive procedures in rodents. Tribromoethanol (Avertin) provides light anesthesia for 10–20 min in mice. Prepared solutions must be stored in the dark at 4°C to avoid production of gastric irritant decomposition compounds. The standard anesthetic dose is 0.2 ml/10 g of a 1.2% solution. This anesthetic is most appropriate for brief, nonpainful procedures in mice, such as retro-orbital blood sampling, embryo transfer, vasectomy, and tail biopsy (31). Tribromoethanol is contraindicated in rats because peritoneal fibrosis and peritonitis are common following intraperitoneal injection in this species (32). A recent report described the use of methohexitone (44 mg/kg of a 6.46 mg/ml solution IP) to achieve 2 min of chemical restraint for oral examination in C3H/Neu mice with recovery in 10–15 min. The major disadvantage of this technique was a very narrow therapeutic window: 40 mg/kg produced no immobility, whereas 50 mg/kg produced 40% mortality (33).

Intraperitoneal injection of ketamine (40–100 mg/kg) and xylazine (3–10 mg/kg) provides 20–60 min of surgical anesthesia in most rodent species. Muscle relaxation and analgesia are good. Duration of anesthesia varies in a dose-dependent manner. If necessary, supplemental administration of ketamine will provide additional anesthesia. Yohimbine (1–2 mg/kg IP) will reverse xylazine-associated sedation and speed recovery from anesthesia. Side effects of general anesthesia in rodents may include hypercarbia, hypoxemia, and hypotension, although these effects are less evident with ketamine and xylazine in comparison with sodium pentobarbital (31).

Many investigators use sodium pentobarbital (30–70 mg/kg IP) for general anesthesia of rodents. Disadvantages of this agent include brief periods of effective anesthesia (10–30 min), prolonged recovery, and poor analgesia. In addition to environmental factors discussed earlier, rodents also display marked individual and strain variability in the response to sodium pentobarbital. Pretreatment with buprenorphine prior to incision prolongs the period of effective anesthesia and lowers the effective dose of sodium pentobarbital required for anesthesia (34).

Isoflurane provides excellent anesthesia in rats and mice. This agent may be used for brief restraint and for procedures lasting several hours. Isoflurane requires the use of a precision vaporizer to provide the proper concentration of anesthetic. Rapid induction of anesthesia occurs following placement of animals into an induction chamber containing 3–4% isoflurane in oxygen. Most animals waken 1–2 min after removal from the chamber, which is sufficient time for retro-orbital blood sampling or tail biopsy. To maintain anesthesia for longer periods, the animal's head and nose may be placed into a customized nose cone connected to a nonrebreathing anesthetic circuit and scavenger. Concentrations of 2–3% isoflurane are commonly used for maintenance. The pedal withdrawal reflex is used to assess anesthetic depth. Rodent nose cones are easily fashioned from funnels or disposable syringe barrels. For procedures requiring positive pressure ventilation, endotracheal intubation is easily accomplished. Techniques for endotracheal intubation for rodents have been described (31).

B. Rabbit

1. Animal Selection and Preoperative Preparation

Infection with the respiratory pathogen *Pasteurella multocida* is extremely common in conventional rabbits. Colonization of the upper respiratory tract is often clinically silent, but spread to the lungs, middle ear, and brain occurs frequently and produces characteristic disease syndromes (6, 28). *Pasteurella*-negative rabbits flocks are available and should be used for all surgical protocols. Preoperative fasting should be limited to a maximum of 12 hr prior to anesthesia; longer periods of fasting may cause dehydration and subsequent intestinal motility disorders (28). Traumatic lower-back fracture is common when inexperienced staff handles rabbits. The best way to handle rabbits is to grasp the scruff of the neck with one hand while supporting the rump and hind legs with the other. Rabbits should never be lifted, moved, or restrained by the ears. Sudden onset of flaccid paraplegia in rabbits is almost always the result of lower-back fracture and warrants immediate euthanasia (6).

2. Brief Procedures

Combined administration of ketamine (35–50 mg/kg IM) and xylazine (5–10 mg/kg IM) provides excellent anesthesia for a variety of applications in the rabbit. General anesthesia lasts for 30 to 60 min and provides adequate analgesia and restraint for procedures of moderate intensity. Supplemental use of a narcotic analgesic such as buprenorphine (0.05 mg/kg IM) or butorphanol (0.1 mg/kg IM) prolongs anesthesia and improves analgesia. Telazol should not be used for survival procedures in rabbits because renal tubular damage is a common complication even at standard anesthetic dosages (27, 28).

3. Inhalation Anesthesia

The intramuscular ketamine/xylazine combination suggested for brief procedures is also an excellent induction agent prior to endotracheal intubation for inhalation anesthesia. Intravenous administration of ketamine and xylazine through the ear vein will achieve rapid induction but care is required to minimize skin irritation from perivascular infiltration. Mask induction is rarely indicated because apnea, breath holding, bradycardia, and struggling are common when unsedated rabbits are exposed to isoflurane and because operator exposure to waste anesthetic is difficult to avoid in this setting (35).

Endotracheal intubation of the rabbit may be difficult because of several distinctive anatomic features. The prominent incisor teeth, long oropharynx, and limited mobility of temporomandibular joint hinder direct visualization of the larynx from the front and require the use of a pediatric laryngoscope with a size 0–1 Wisconsin or size 1 Miller blade. Lidocaine spray on the vocal cords is necessary to prevent further narrowing of the larynx through laryngospasm. Benzocaine spray (Cetacaine) produces methemoglobinemia in rabbits and other species and should be avoided. The laryngeal opening is often smaller than the diameter of the trachea, requiring the use of a small endotracheal tube (2.5–4 mm). The tongue is short, friable, and difficult to grasp. Supine, prone, or lateral positions are all suitable for endotracheal intubation. Hyperextension of the neck will straighten the larynx and facilitate proper tube placement. Blind intubation of the trachea is easily accomplished with practice. The tube is placed in the supraglottic region and advanced toward the larynx in coordination with respiration. Identification of normal breath sounds, visualization of condensate on a dental mirror, or capnometry may be used to confirm proper tube placement (6, 28). Anesthetic maintenance with isoflurane usually requires a vaporizer setting of 1–4%. Ketamine and xylazine used for anesthetic induction will reduce the required amount of isoflurane during the initial period of anesthesia. Absence of the pinna and pedal withdrawal reflexes is the best indicator of a surgical anesthetic plane (28).

C. Dog and Cat

1. Animal Selection and Preoperative Preparation

Anesthesia of dogs and cats for experimental surgery is easily accomplished. Appropriate vendor selection and conditioning procedures are necessary to identify preexisting cardiovascular or renal diseases, malnutrition, or parasitism that can significantly complicate anesthesia and surgery. Heartworm disease, a result of *Dirofilaria immitis* infestation, causes eosinophilia and right heart failure. Intestinal parasites, including roundworms (*Toxocara canis*), hookworms (*Ancylostoma caninum*), and whipworms (*Trichuris vulpis*) cause eosinophilia, diarrhea, and general debilitation. All of these parasites are susceptible to common anthelmintics. A calm behavioral profile, reinforced by habituation to the research staff and regular training, is important for animals on long-term studies that call for frequent handling (blood sampling, drug administration, dressing changes). Purpose-bred dogs have a known pedigree and health history and often present a more consistent physiological profile compared to random-source dogs. Random-source dogs are significantly less expensive than purpose-bred dogs, but often have health and behavioral disorders that render them unsuitable for long-term studies (5).

2. Brief Procedures

Short-acting anesthetics may be required for brief procedures in dogs or cats. Calm dogs and cats may be trained to cooperate in noninvasive clinical procedures, thereby avoiding the need for sedatives or anesthetics. The best technique for short-term injectable anesthesia in dogs and cats is coadministration of a dissociative anesthetic with a sedative or tranquilizer and an anticholinergic drug. All of these drugs are suitable for intravenous administration to achieve rapid induction and recovery. Intravenous ketamine (10 mg/kg) and diazepam (0.5 mg/kg) or midazolam (0.5 mg/kg) provide 5–15 min of light anesthesia suitable for dressing changes, radiography, or other minor procedures. Intravenous Telazol (2.0–4.0 mg/kg IV) is an alternative drug for brief injectable anesthesia. Intramuscular administration of ketamine (10 mg/kg) and xylazine (0.7–1.0 mg/kg) produces 20–30 min of anesthesia. For longer procedures, Telazol (6–8 mg/kg), xylazine (0.7–1 mg/kg), and butorphanol (0.2 mg/kg) produce up to 1 hr of anesthesia. Anticholinergics (atropine 0.04 mg/kg) are often useful when using ketamine or xylazine to counteract excessive salivation or bradycardia. Supplemental administration of one-third to one-half of the original dose will usefully prolong the effective anesthetic period by 30–50%. Ketamine is not acceptable as a sole anesthetic in dogs because of excessive muscle tone, salivation, and the frequent occurrence of seizures. In cats, ketamine produces rigid catalepsy that allows minor clinical procedures, not endotracheal intubation or major surgery. The long-acting barbiturate sodium pentobarbital produces about 30 min of surgical anesthesia, but is not suitable for routine use because analgesia is poor and prolonged sleeping time and rough recovery are common. Short-acting barbiturates such as sodium thiopental (8–12 mg/kg IV) or methohexital (4–8 mg/kg IV) are inexpensive and provide about 15 min of light anesthesia, but have a lower margin of safety than dissociative anesthetics (36, 37).

3. Prolonged Procedures

Inhalant anesthetics such as isoflurane or halothane are most appropriate for prolonged or invasive procedures in the dog and cat. Because dogs and cats are prone to vomiting under anesthesia, proper preoperative fasting and endotracheal intubation are vital to prevent aspiration pneumonia. Premedication with sedative and analgesic drugs will allay anxiety, reduce postoperative pain, and reduce the required concentration of isoflurane or halothane for maintenance anesthesia. Rapid anesthetic induction may then be accomplished through intravenous administration of thiopental (8–12 mg/kg IV) or methohexital (4–8 mg/kg IV). Anesthetic induction by intramuscular administration of ketamine or Telazol plus xylazine, an anticholinergic, and an opioid is also appropriate. Mask induction is rarely indicated in dogs and cats, and should be used only in premedicated animals to reduce struggling.

Endotracheal intubation of dogs and cats is easily accomplished. A variety of endotracheal tube diameters should be available to accommodate individual and breed differences in tracheal diameter. Direct visualization and intubation of the larynx of most dogs and some cats is possible without a laryngoscope. A wire stylet and a laryngoscope with an appropriately sized Miller or Bizarri–Guiffrida blade should be available to accommodate unexpected difficulties. The animal is placed in sternal recumbency, and an assistant holds the mouth open and extends the tongue to expose the larynx. Judicious application of lidocaine spray to the vocal cords will prevent laryngospasm and facilitate intubation in cats and small dogs. Benzocaine (Cetacaine) spray will induce methemoglobinemia and should be avoided. After verifying accurate placement, the cuff is inflated and the tube is secured with gauze tied over the maxilla or behind the head (38).

Inhalant anesthesia with isoflurane or halothane may be maintained for several hours. The anesthetic concentration should be varied according to the animal's clinical status. In general, a vaporizer setting of 1–3% will produce adequate anesthesia in dogs and cats. There should be no flexor withdrawal or corneal blink reflexes in adequately anesthetized animals. Paralytic agents are rarely indicated for experimental surgery in dogs and cats. The heart rate and blood pressure should be monitored to assure adequate anesthesia of animals that receive paralytic agents. Ketamine and xylazine used for induction will wear off after 30 to 60 min and require an increase in isoflurane concentration to prevent sensation. Alternatively, small amounts of intravenous opioids such as fentanyl may be given to prevent isoflurane-induced myocardial depression. Isoflurane and halothane will accumulate in tissues during long procedures. The vaporizer setting may therefore be reduced toward the end of prolonged procedures, to avoid unnecessarily long recovery periods.

D. Pig

1. Animal Selection and Preoperative Preparation

Swine are commonly used in experimental surgery because of anatomic and physiologic similarity to humans in many models. Advantages of using pigs in the laboratory include low cost, ready availability, and ease of acclimation to the laboratory. Disadvantages include the uncooperative nature of pigs with respect to most clinical procedures, limited number of intravenous access sites, and relative difficulty of endotracheal intubation.

Because animals larger than 100 kg are difficult to handle in the laboratory, selective breeding has produced several types of miniature swine for research. The Gottingen minipig and the Yucatan micropig achieve a maximum bodyweight of 35–55 kg at 2 years of age. The Hanford and Yucatan minipigs are somewhat larger and weigh 70–90 kg at 2 years. By contrast, adult crossbred farm pigs weigh 90–110 kg at 6 months of age and weight 200–300 kg at 2 years of age (15, 16). Juvenile crossbred farm pigs are less expensive than minipigs or micropigs, and are often used for short-term surgical studies. Juvenile farm pigs gain 2–4 kg/week and require larger pens as they grow, to maintain facility compliance with the Guide (3). The choice of research subject should include practical considerations such as length of study and maximum allowable body size, as well as the physiological characteristics of the different breeds (15).

Careful evaluation of the vendor health program is required to reduce experimental morbidity from unrelated clinical conditions. Chronic respiratory disease is common in commercial swine operations. Although subclinical infections are common, transportation, anesthesia, and surgery may activate latent infections and result in excess morbidity and mortality. Causative agents in affected pigs include *Mycoplasma hyopneumoniae, Haeomophilus pleuropneumoniae, Bordetella bronchiseptica*, and *Actinobacillus pleuorpneumoniae* (22). Many commercial breeders of laboratory minipigs and micropigs maintain specific-pathogen-free herds that are free from infection with these agents. Rapid infection with respiratory pathogens occurs when SPF pigs are cohoused with conventional swine.

Malignant hyperthermia (MH) is an autosomal dominant trait that causes affected animals to develop hyperthermia and extensor muscle rigidity and necrosis after exposure to environmental extremes or halothane or isoflurane anesthesia. The disease has been described only in farm animals bred for rapid growth and is becoming increasingly rare as commercial breeders identify and cull carrier pigs. Affected pigs are still encountered sporadically in farm pigs used for experimental surgery. The condition has not been described in minipigs or micropigs. Known MH carriers should not be used for experimental surgery. Treatment of animals that develop MH during an experimental procedure requires immediate termination of anesthesia, whole-body cooling, and administration of corcticosteroids, sodium bicarbonate, and dantrolene sodium (3–5 mg/kg IV) (20, 39).

Food and contact bedding must be removed 6–8 hr prior to general anesthesia (16). Water may be offered until 2 hr before anesthesia. The presence of food in the stomach frequently results in gastric distension, hypoventilation, and tachycardia during prolonged general anesthesia, requiring prompt decompression through orogastric intubation (15).

2. Brief Restraint

The uncooperative nature of pigs in regard to handling frequently mandates the use of chemical restraint for minor clinical procedures. Slings and hammocks are available that will allow restraint of calm pigs up to 50 kg for up to several hours (16). Sedation may be necessary to facilitate initial placement of animals into the sling. Azaperone (4 mg/kg

IM) is a useful agent for this purpose. For more invasive procedures, a mixture of Telazol (4.4 mg/kg IM), xylazine (2.2 mg/kg IM), and atropine (0.05 mg/kg) provides approximately 30 min of anesthesia suitable for minor surgery, followed by smooth recovery. Endotracheal intubation for subsequent maintenance on isoflurane is also possible after Telazol and xylazine induction (15, 16). Alternative agents such as ketamine, ketamine/xylazine, or Telazol produce light anesthesia insufficient for surgery or intubation, characterized by rough recovery (40, 41).

3. Prolonged or Invasive Procedures

Prolonged or invasive procedures are best conducted under isoflurane anesthesia. Endotracheal intubation is warranted for general anesthesia in swine to protect the airway and allow for controlled ventilation when required. Required equipment for endotracheal intubation of swine includes a laryngoscope with a straight blade of 20–25 cm and a selection of cuffed tubes of appropriate size (4.5–8 mm). Endotracheal intubation is possible with the pig in dorsal, ventral, or lateral recumbency. There are two anatomic characteristics that can complicate the procedure. First, the soft plate is long and must be displaced dorsally for visualization of the larynx. Second, the laryngeal diverticulum distal to the larynx may "trap" the tip of the endotracheal tube unless the tube is gently twisted as it passes over the epiglottis. After intubation, maintenance anesthesia usually requires an isoflurane vaporizer setting of 1.5–2.5% in oxygen (15, 16, 39).

The actual concentration of isoflurane will vary according to the anesthetic induction regimen, type of procedure, and concurrent use of other narcotic and sedative agents. Administration of Telazol and xylazine for anesthetic induction has a substantial isoflurane sparing effect that may last for the first 30–60 min of anesthesia. Adequate surgical anesthesia is indicated by pedal withdrawal areflexia, absent jaw tone, and stable heart rate and blood pressure (15, 16, 39).

E. Small Ruminants

1. Animal Selection and Preoperative Preparation

Sheep and goats are desirable research animals because their adult body weight is comparable to that of humans and they are hardy, inexpensive, and have a calm disposition. Sheep are particularly useful for reproductive research because investigators may easily obtain cohorts of pregnant animals with known gestational age and hysterotomy, and fetal manipulation is possible with a low postoperative abortion rate. Cardiovascular research also uses sheep and goats because of similarities to humans in the ratio of the size and weight of the heart and other thoracic organs to body weight [42].

The quality of sheep and goats used in research often depends on the source. Vendors should avoid mixing multiple sources of animals in one flock. Surgical and transportation stress will reduce resistance to disease. Preventive health measures, including immunizations and anthelminthic treatments, should be provided at least 1 month before shipment. Recommended immunizations for sheep and goats include *Clostridia* spp, *Pasteurella multocida, Pasturella hemolytica*, contagious ecthyma, and parainfluenza III. A conditioning and quarantine period after arrival allows recovery from shipping stress, acclimation to the facility, and reduces transmission of infectious diseases to resident animals (42).

Facilities should adopt measures to prevent transmission of zoonoses from sheep and goats. Silent infection with *Coxiella burnetti*, the causative agent of human Q fever, is common in sheep. Fetal membranes and amniotic fluid from infected animals carry large numbers of hardy organisms. Human infection occurs from direct contact with infected materials or from fomites. Signs of Q fever infection in man range from subclinical disease to severe flulike symptoms, pneumonia, endocarditis, and death. Serologic evaluation of sheep is difficult because animals may shed large numbers of organisms in the absence of detectable antibody. Contagious ecthyma ("orf") is a poxvirus-induced papular disease of sheep and goats. Infected animals frequently have lesions on the mucocutaneous junctions of the head, which can spread to humans by direct contact. Affected animals and humans develop long-lasting immunity and usually recover in 10–14 days. Effective vaccines for sheep and goats are available (43).

Careful preoperative preparation of the rumen is required for safe anesthesia of sheep and goats. Adult animals require withdrawal of food and water for at least 24 hr to reduce rumen size and digestive activity. Rumen distension and hypoventilation are common when dorsal or lateral positioning of ruminants is required for anesthesia. Passage of a 1- to 2-cm-diameter thick-walled stomach tube into the rumen allows intraoperative aspiration of gas and fluid if required. Placement of a cuffed endotracheal tube should immediately follow anesthetic induction to prevent aspiration pneumonia. Aspiration pneumonia can be fatal after regurgitation because rumen fluid contains numerous anaerobic bacteria. Infant ruminants (<30 days of age) lack a functional rumen and do not require preoperative fasting (42).

2. Brief Procedures

Sheep and goats are docile and rarely require sedation for blood sampling, dressing changes, or other routine procedures. For more invasive procedures, animals may be sedated for 10–20 minutes with a low dose of xylazine (0.02–0.15 mg/kg IV or 0.05–0.3 mg/kg IM). Yohimbine (1 mg/kg IV) or atipamezole (0.02–0.06 mg/kg IV) (45) reverses xylazine-induced sedation when necessary. Animals in late pregnancy should not receive xylazine to avoid fetal hypo-oxygenation. The benzodiazepines diazepam (0.25 mg/kg

IV) and midazolam (1.3 mg/kg IV) produce muscle relaxation and sedation in sheep and goats with less depression of cardiac output than is seen with xylazine. Flumazenil (1 mg IV) reverses benzodiazepine-induced sedation. Ataxia and excitement are common following benzodiazepine administration (42).

3. General Anesthesia

Isoflurane is the anesthetic of choice for general anesthesia of sheep and goats. Intravenous administration of ketamine (2.75 mg/kg) and diazepam (0.2 mg/kg) or xylazine (0.1 mg/kg) rapidly induces light anesthesia lasting 10–20 min, suitable for endotracheal intubation. Thiopental (25 mg/kg IV) is an alternative induction agent; disadvantages include regurgitation, profuse salivation, and irritation from perivascular infiltration (42). Profuse salivation follows the administration of most anesthetic drugs in ruminants, hampering endotracheal intubation. Administration of atropine (0.04 mg/kg IV) or glycopyrrolate (0.022 mg/kg IV) is recommended to inhibit saliva production. In addition, anesthetized ruminants should be positioned with the head down to encourage drainage of saliva away from the airway (42).

Endotracheal intubation requires a laryngoscope with a 20- to 30-cm blade. Vinyl or silicone cuffed tubes 10–16 mm in diameter are suitable for most sheep and goats. An assistant positions the animal in sternal recumbency, extends the neck, and holds the mouth open. The anesthetist visualizes the epiglottis with the laryngoscope and intubates the trachea during inspiration. Prior application of 2% lidocaine spray to the vocal cords prevents laryngospasm. The use of a stylet may help deflect the tip of the tube into the larynx. A mouth gag is often necessary to prevent damage to the tube by sharp molar teeth. After inflation of the cuff, the tube is secured with gauze to the mandible. Isoflurane vaporizer settings of 0.75–1.0% are often sufficient to maintain general anesthesia in sheep and goats. Absence of chewing motions in response to stimulation indicates an adequate surgical plane. The presence of a centrally positioned eyeball with a dilated pupil and absent palpebral reflex indicates very deep anesthesia (42).

F. Nonhuman Primates

1. Animal Selection and Preoperative Preparation

Nonhuman primates have many anatomic, physiologic, and immunologic similarities to humans and are widely used in experimental surgery. Species commonly used in surgical research include the cynomolgus monkey (*Macaca fascicularis*), the rhesus monkey (*Macaca mulatta*), and the baboon (*Papio anubis*). Significant disadvantages to the use of primates include limited supply, high cost, and the possibility that primates may transmit zoonotic diseases to research staff. Bloodborne pathogens are especially important concerns in invasive procedures such as surgery.

All primates may be silent carriers of tuberculosis and enteric pathogens such as *Shigella* spp. and *Campylobacter* spp. Other zoonoses are limited to certain species. Macaques frequently harbor *Herpesvirus simiae* ("herpes B"), which may cause fatal encephalomyelitis in untreated humans. Transmission of herpes B may occur through bites, scratches, needle sticks, and splashes of body fluids to mucous membranes. Additional viral zoonoses of nonhuman primates include hepatitis B, simian immunodeficiency virus (a close relative of human immunodeficiency virus), and filoviruses such as Ebola virus or Marburg virus. Hemoparasites such as malaria and trypanosomiasis may also be present in laboratory primates. Although most primate plasmodia and trypanosomes cause mild disease and are species specific, zoonotic strains have been identified and cannot be distinguished for noninfectious strains morphologically (13, 14).

To assure the use of healthy animals and minimize the risk of zoonotic disease, research institutions must adopt a rigid quarantine program for all nonhuman primates. Minimum standards for nonhuman primate quarantine include testing for tuberculosis, enteric pathogens, and a species-specific panel of known viral zoonoses. The quarantine requires at least 6 weeks, to allow for all animals in the group to be tested for tuberculosis three times at 2-week intervals. All animals in the shipment must be negative on tuberculosis screening before any animal may be released from quarantine. Positive or equivocal skin tests require euthanasia of the suspect animal for definitive diagnosis. Confirmed diagnosis of tuberculosis in a quarantine shipment may require prolonged quarantine or euthanasia of the remaining animals. The quarantine period also allows for animals to overcome stress and physiologic disturbance related to capture and transportation and to become acclimated to the facility's husbandry program (5, 14).

Investigators should specify the use of animals that are free of known pathogens. Limited supply and high cost may complicate this goal. Particularly in the case of tuberculosis and herpes B virus, currently available tests have limited sensitivity and cannot absolutely exclude all infected animals. Therefore, universal precautions should be used with all nonhuman primates. All facilities using primates must have a written occupational health plan to cover primate-related injuries. The plan should be reviewed with research and animal care staff regularly. Prompt cleaning treatment of macaque bites and scratches effectively reduces the likelihood of infection. Bite kits should be available in all macaque rooms. Occupational health providers and veterinary staff should review and rehearse the emergency response plan regularly and provide for afterhours care (43).

Food and contact bedding must be removed at least 6 hr before anesthetic induction. Water must be withheld for at least 2 hr. Prolonged removal from water may predispose anesthetized primates to dehydration and hypovolemia.

Individually housed primates with free access to water often drink to excess and may be particularly sensitive to water deprivation because of renal medullary washout and impaired renal concentrating ability. Food stored in macaque cheek pouches should be removed after anesthetic induction to prevent possible aspiration during recovery.

2. Brief Procedures and Chemical Restraint

All nonhuman primates are wild animals and can inflict serious injuries to staff when resisting restraint. For this reason, most animals are chemically restrained for all clinical procedures. Intramuscular ketamine (10–20 mg/kg IM) provides 10–20 min of light anesthesia and allows physical examination, suturing of minor injuries, phlebotomy, intravenous infusion, or gavage. The use of Telazol (5–10 mg/kg IM) will provide longer duration anesthesia (20–40 min) with improved muscle relaxation and reduced salivation. Supplemental use of xylazine (1–2 mg/kg IM) induces a deeper state of anesthesia with improved analgesia to allow minor surgery (44).

When chemical restraint agents would interfere with research, many nonhuman primate species can be trained to allow conscious restraint, blood sampling, and drug administration. These procedures require the use of special equipment and carefully trained technicians and staff. Because of the increased likelihood of bites and scratches when working with conscious primates, the use of herpes B-negative macaques or a nonmacaque species is strongly advised.

3. General Anesthesia

Isoflurane is the inhalation agent of choice for prolonged general anesthesia of nonhuman primates. Anesthetic induction for endotracheal intubation of nonhuman primates requires a combination of a dissociative anesthetic and a sedative or tranquilizer. Appropriate combinations for this purpose include tiletamine/zolazepam (Telazol) (5–10 mg/kg IM) or ketamine (5–10 mg/kg IM) and xylazine (0.5–2 mg/kg) or medetomidine (0.1 mg/kg IM). An alternative approach for induction is to administer intravenous thiopental (3–5 mg/kg IV) or propofol (2–5 mg/kg) after light sedation with ketamine (5–10 mg/kg). Ketamine is not desirable as a sole agent for anesthetic induction because of excessive salivation and inadequate muscle relaxation (44).

Endotracheal intubation is readily accomplished with the animal in dorsal or lateral recumbency. A curved laryngoscope blade depresses the tongue and exposes the larynx. Gentle traction on the tongue will further expose the larynx if necessary. An assistant holds open the jaws using gauze loops behind the canine teeth. Topical lidocaine spray on the vocal cords prevents laryngospasm and laryngeal trauma. The anesthetist then introduces the tube into the trachea, verifies proper placement, inflates the cuff, and secures the tube. Maintenance anesthesia is with isoflurane between 1 and 3%. Palpebral and corneal areflexia, muscle relaxation, stable heart, and respiratory rate are indicators of a stable anesthetic plane (44).

VII. Analgesia

Prompt recognition and treatment of postoperative pain is a key responsibility of experimental surgeons. Experimental surgical procedures rarely, if ever, directly benefit the research subject and impose a substantial moral requirement on investigators to prevent or minimize any discomfort related to the experiment. Compliance with the AWA, PHS Policy, and the Guide (3, 4) requires investigators to relieve pain in experimental animals. Investigators must justify withholding of analgesics to the IACUC on scientific grounds.

Recognition of postoperative pain is difficult in most laboratory animal species. Anorexia, lethargy, piloerection, and wound hypersensitivity indicate the presence of moderate to severe pain. Behavioral and physiologic factors complicate the diagnosis of less severe pain, which may still require treatment to assure animal well-being. Rodents, for example, are nocturnal animals and are normally less active during the day than at night. Rodents typically receive a large amount of food each week, and nibble small amounts at frequent intervals. As a result, pain-induced inhibition of activity or feeding is difficult for research staff to recognize. In addition, rodents issue distress calls at ultrasonic frequencies that are inaudible to human beings (46). Most animals react to the presence of white-coated research staff with the "fight or flight" response, which effectively conceals subtle signs of pain and distress. For that reason, animal husbandry staff often notices subtle signs of pain or distress in research animals that are not apparent to investigators. Therefore investigators should consider that surgical procedures that would induce pain in a human would produce pain in an experimental animal, unless convincing evidence to the contrary exists (3).

Many effective analgesics for laboratory animals are available. Desirable qualities of the ideal analgesic for experimental surgery include effective pain relief; minimal adverse effect on respiration, appetite, or other physiologic parameters; ease of administration; and convenient dosing schedule. Broad categories of analgesic drugs include narcotics and nonsteroidal antiinflammatory drugs (NSAIDs) (47). Although investigators are often concerned that analgesic drugs may confound research data from experimental animals, these potential effects must be compared to the known adverse effect of unrelieved pain on physiology, mobility, and immune function in many species (48, 49).

Narcotics remain the analgesics of choice for severe pain in most species. Adverse effects of narcotics include dose-dependent sedation, hypoventilation, anorexia, and constipation. These effects are more pronounced with pure agonists such as morphine than with partial agonists such as butorphanol and buprenorphine. Buprenorphine is widely used in veterinary medicine because it provides excellent analgesia at a convenient dose interval (8–12 hr) and has minimal depressant effects on respiration and cardiac output (20, 51). Dosage and dose intervals of the narcotic analgesics vary widely between species because of the higher metabolic rate of the smaller species as well as species-specific responses to the agents. In comparison to larger animals, rodents require very high doses of most narcotics in proportion to their body weight for effective analgesia (31). Epidural administration of morphine or oxymorphone in dogs provides superior analgesia for up to 24 hr with excellent hemodynamic stability and slight respiratory depression (50). Limited experience indicates that epidural narcotic administration also provides effective analgesia in swine, sheep, and goats (20).

Nonsteroidal antiinflammatory drugs are most effective against moderate pain of musculoskeletal origin, including incisional pain from ventral abdominal incisions in swine and other large animals. The principal side effects of many NSAIDs include increased bleeding tendency from reduced platelet activity or gastric irritation because of prostaglandin inhibition. Although clinically significant, impairment of blood clotting ability is rare (52) and gastric toxicity remains a concern, particularly in dogs. Flunixin and ketoprofen are potent injectable NSAIDs with comparable clinical analgesic activity in many species (16, 53). Carprofen is a potent oral NSAID with minimal gastric toxicity that is very effective in dogs and other species (37, 52). Although analgesiometric testing indicates minimal analgesic effect from parenteral narcotics or flunixin in sheep (42), clinical experience shows substantial relief of postoperative pain following combination buprenorphine and flunixin therapy. Acetaminophen and aspirin have limited activity against surgical pain in animals and their use is not recommended.

Premedication with narcotic or nonsteroidal antiinflammatory agents reduces the impact of massive nociceptive impulse release during surgery, blunting the autonomic response to pain and minimizing intraoperative variations in blood pressure and heart rate. Ketamine, often used in anesthetic induction of laboratory animals, provides additional preemptive analgesic activity through blockade of *N*-methyl-D-aspartic acid receptors (52). Use of these agents often results in a significant reduction in the dose of general anesthetic required for surgery and a smoother recovery. This effect is especially pronounced with the use of newer inhalant agents such as isoflurane, which have relatively poor analgesic activity. Local, regional, and epidural anesthetic techniques also reduce intraoperative pain by blocking nociceptive afferents from the surgical site. In addition to reducing general anesthetic requirements, increasing evidence suggests that preemptive analgesic therapy limits postoperative pain and reduces analgesic requirements (54).

Table III contains the author's analgesic recommendations for the common laboratory animal species. For information on other agents, or for detailed discussion regarding mechanism or possible adverse effects, the reader should consult the references or a veterinary anesthesiologist. Combination therapy effectively relieves postoperative pain in

Table III Analgesics for Laboratory Animals

Species	Drug name	Type	Dose (mg/kg)	Route[a]	Interval (hours)
Rodent	Buprenorphine	Partial narcotic agonist	0.1	SQ	6–12
Rabbit	Buprenorphine	Partial narcotic agonist	0.01–0.05	SQ	6–12
Rabbit	Flunixin	NSAID	1	IM	12
Dog	Buprenorphine	Partial narcotic agonist	0.01–0.03	IM or SQ	12
Dog	Carprofen	NSAID	2–4	PO	12
Cat	Buprenorphine	Partial narcotic agonist	0.005–0.01	IM	12
Cat	Ketoprofen	NSAID	2	IM	12–24
Pig	Buprenorphine	Partial narcotic agonist	0.05–0.1	IM	12
Pig	Ketoprofen	NSAID	1–3	PO	8–12
Sheep	Buprenorphine	Partial narcotic agonist	0.003–0.005	IM	8–12
Sheep	Flunixin	NSAID	1–2	IM	12
Primate	Buprenorphine	Partial narcotic agonist	0.003–0.005	IM	12
Primate	Flunixin	NSAID	1	IM	12–24

[a]SQ, Subcutaneous; IM, intramuscular; PO, periorbital.

experimental animals with fewer side effects than with either class of drug as the sole agent. Narcotics are administered prior to and immediately after surgery, followed by NSAIDs for the next 2 or 3 days as necessary

VIII. Resources

Helpful information is available at the following Internet web sites:

1. American Association for Laboratory Science (*http://www.aalas.org*).
2. Lab Animal Homepage (*http://www.labanimal.com/*). Click on related links for information on vendors, species, regulatory guidelines, etc.
3. The American College of Laboratory Animal Medicine (*http://www.aclam.org/*).
4. Links in laboratory animal science (*http://www.ihh.kvl.dk/*).
5. World Wide Web Virtual Library: Veterinary medicine at Washington University, St. Louis, Missouri (*http://netvet.wustl.edu/vetmed/*).

References

1. Russell, W. M. S., and Burch, R. L. (1959). "The Principles of Humane Experimental Technique." Charles C. Thomas, Springfield.
2. Orlans, F. B., Beauchamp, T. L., Dresser, R., Morton, D. B., and Gluck, J. P (1998). "The Human Use of Animals: Case Studies in Ethical Choice." Oxford Univ. Press, New York.
3. National Research Council (1996). "Guide for the Care and Use of Laboratory Animals." National Academy Press, Washington, D.C.
4. Office for the Protection from Research Risks (1996). "Public Health Service Policy on Human Care and Use of Laboratory Animals." National Institutes of Health, Washington, D.C.
5. Fox, J. G., Cohen, B. J., and Loew, F. M., eds. (1984). "Laboratory Animal Medicine." Academic Press, San Diego.
6. Harkness, J. E., and Wagner, J. E., eds. (1995). "The Biology and Medicine of Rabbits and Rodents." Williams & Wilkins, Baltimore, MD.
7. Field, K., and Sibold, A. (1998). "The Laboratory Hamster and Gerbil." CRC Press, Boca Raton, FL.
8. Sharp, P., and LaRegina, M. (1998). "The Laboratory Rat." CRC Press, Boca Raton, FL.
9. Van Hoosier, G. L., and McPherson, C. W., eds. (1987). "Laboratory Hamsters." Academic Press, San Diego.
10. Manning, P. J., Ringler, D. H., and Newcomer, C. E., eds. (1994). "The Biology of the Laboratory Rabbit," 2nd Ed. Academic Press, San Diego.
11. Suckow, M. A., and Douglas, F. (1997). "The Laboratory Rabbit." CRC Press, Boca Raton, FL.
12. Martin, B. J. (1997). "The Laboratory Cat." CRC Press, Boca Raton, FL.
13. Bennett, B. T., Abee, C. R., and Henrickson, R., eds. (1998). "Nonhuman Primates in Biomedical Research: Diseases." Academic Press, San Diego.
14. Bennett, B. T., Abee, C. R., and Henrickson, R., eds. (1995). "Nonhuman Primates in Biomedical Research: Biology and Management." Academic Press, San Diego.
15. Bollen, J. A., Hansen, A. K., and Rasmussen, H. J. (2000). "The Laboratory Swine." CRC Press, Boca Raton, FL.
16. Swindle, M. (1998). "Anesthesia and Experimental Techniques in Swine." Iowa State University Press, Ames, IA.
17. Borkowski, G. L., and Allen, M. (1999). "The Laboratory Small Ruminant." CRC Press, Boca Raton, FL.
18. Terril-Robb, L., and Clemons, D. (1997). "The Laboratory Guinea Pig." CRC Press, Boca Raton, FL.
19. Kohn, D. F., Wixson, S. K., White, W. J., and Benson, G. J. (1997). "Anesthesia and Analgesia in Laboratory Animals." Academic Press, San Diego.
20. Thurmon, J. C., Tranquill, W. J., and Benson, G. J., eds. (1996). "Lumb and Jones' Veterinary Anesthesia," 3rd Ed. Williams & Wilkins, Baltimore, MD.
21. National Research Council (1991). "Infectious Diseases of Mice and Rats." National Academy Press, Washington, D.C.
22. Leman, A. D., Straw, B. E., Mengeling, W. L., D'Allaire, S., and Taylor, D. J., eds. (1992). "Diseases of Swine," 7th Ed. Iowa State University Press, Ames, IA.
23. Hawk, C. T., and Leary, S. L. (1995). "Formulary for Laboratory Animals." Iowa State University Press, Ames, IA.
24. Boschert, K. (1997). "Net Vet Mosby's Veterinary Guide to the Internet." Mosby, Philadelphia.
25. White, W. J., and Blum, J. R. (1997). Design of surgical suites and postsurgical care units. *In* "Anesthesia and Analgesia in Laboratory Animals," (D. F. Kohn, S. K. Wixson, W. J. White, and G. J. Benson, eds.), pp. 149–164. Academic Press, San Diego.
26. Fish, R. E. (1997). Pharmacology of injectable anesthetics. *In* "Anesthesia and Analgesia in Laboratory Animals" (D.F. Kohn, S. K. Wixson, W. J. White, and G. J. Benson, eds.), pp. 1–28. Academic Press, San Diego.
27. Lin, H. C. (1996). Dissociative anesthetics. *In* "Lumb and Jones' Veterinary Anesthesia," 3rd Ed. (J. C. Thurmon, W. J. Tranquill, and G. J. Benson, eds.), pp. 241–296. Williams & Wilkins, Baltimore, MD.
28. Lipman, N. S., Marini, R. P., and Flecknell, P. A. (1997). Anesthesia and analgesia of rabbits. *In* "Anesthesia and Analgesia in Laboratory Animals" (D. F. Kohn, S. K. Wixson, W. J. White, and G. J. Benson, eds.), pp. 205–232. Academic Press, San Diego.
29. Steffey, E. P. (1996). Inhalation anesthetics. *In* "Lumb and Jones' Veterinary Anesthesia," 3rd Ed. (J. C. Thurmon, W. J. Tranquill, and G. J. Benson, eds.), pp. 297–329. Williams & Wilkins, Baltimore, MD.
30. Brunson, D. (1997). Pharmacology of inhalation anesthetics. *In* "Anesthesia and Analgesia in Laboratory Animals" (D. F. Kohn, S. K. Wixson, W. J. White, and G. J. Benson, eds.), pp. 29–42. Academic Press, San Diego.
31. Wixson, S. K. and Smiler, K. L. (1997). Anesthesia and analgesia in rodents. *In* "Anesthesia and Analgesia in Laboratory Animals" (D. F. Kohn, S. K. Wixson, W. J. White, and G. J. Benson, eds.), pp. 165–204. Academic Press, San Diego.
32. Reid, W. C., Carmichael, K. P., Srinivas, S., and Bryant, J. L. (1999). Pathologic changes associated with use of tribromoethanol (Avertin) in the Sprague–Dawley rat. *Lab. Anim. Sci.* **49**, 665–667.
33. Dorr, W., and Weber-Frisch, M. (1999). Short-term immobilization of mice by methohexitone. *Lab. Anim.* **33**, 35–40.
34. Roughan, J. V., Ojeda, O. B., and Flecknell, P. A. (1999). The influence of pre-anesthetic administration of buprenorphine on the anaesthetic effects of ketamine/medetomidine and pentobarbitone in rats and the consequences of repeated anaesthesia. *Lab. Anim.* **33**, 234–242.
35. Flecknell, P. A., Roughan, J. V., and Hedenqvist, P. (1999). Induction of anaesthesia with sevoflurane and isoflurane in the rabbit. *Lab. Anim.* **33**, 41–46.
36. Bednarski, R. M. (1996). Anesthesia and immobilization of specific species: Dogs and cats. *In* "Lumb and Jones' Veterinary Anesthesia,"

3rd Ed. (J. C. Thurmon, W. J. Tranquill, and G. J. Benson, eds.), pp. 591–599. Williams & Wilkins, Baltimore, MD.

37. Harvey, R. C., Paddleford, R. R., Popilskis, S. J., and Wixson, S. K. (1997). Anesthesia and analgesia in dogs, cats and ferrets. *In* "Anesthesia and Analgesia in Laboratory Animals" (D. F. Kohn, S. K. Wixson, W. J. White, and G. J. Benson, eds.), pp. 257–280. Academic Press, San Diego.
38. Hartsfield, S. M. (1996). Airway management and ventilation. *In* "Lumb and Jones' Veterinary Anesthesia," 3rd Ed. (J. C. Thurmon, W. J. Tranquill, and G. J. Benson, eds.), pp. 515–556. Williams & Wilkins, Baltimore, MD.
39. Smith, A. C., Ehler, W. J., and Swindle, M. M. (1997). Anesthesia and analgesia in swine. *In* "Anesthesia and Analgesia in Laboratory Animals" (D. F. Kohn, S. K. Wixson, W. J. White, and G. J. Benson, eds.), pp. 313–336. Academic Press, San Diego.
40. Ko, J. C. H, Williams, B. L., Smith, V. L., McGrath, C. J., and Jacobson, J. D. (1993). Comparison of telazol, telazol-ketamine, telazol-xylazine, and telazol-ketamine-xylazine as chemical restraint and anesthetic induction combination in swine. *Lab. Anim. Sci.* **43**, 476–480.
41. Ko, J. C. H., Williams, B. L., Rogers, E. R., Pablo, L. S., McCaine, W. C., and McGrath, C. J. (1995). Increasing xylazine dose-enhanced anesthetic properties of telazol-xylazine combination in swine. *Lab Anim. Sci.* **45**, 290–294.
42. Riebold, T. W. (1996). Ruminants. *In* "Lumb and Jones' Veterinary Anesthesia," 3rd Ed. (J. C. Thurmon, W. J. Tranquill, and G. J. Benson, eds.), pp. 610–626. Williams & Wilkins, Baltimore, MD.
43. National Research Council (1997). "Occupational Health and Safety in the Care and Use of Research Animals." National Academy Press, Washington, D.C.
44. Popilskis, S. J., and Kohn, D. F. (1997). Anesthesia and analgesia in nonhuman primates. *In* "Anesthesia and Analgesia in Laboratory Animals" (D. F. Kohn, S. K. Wixson, W. J. White, and G. J. Benson, eds.), pp. 233–256. Academic Press, San Diego.
45. Dunlop, C. I., and Hoyt, R. F. (1997). Anesthesia and analgesia in ruminants. *In* "Anesthesia and Analgesia in Laboratory Animals" (D. F. Kohn, S. K. Wixson, W. J. White, and G. J. Benson, eds.), pp. 281–311. Academic Press, San Diego.
46. National Research Council (1992). "Recognition and Alleviation of Pain and Distress in Laboratory Animals." National Academy Press, Washington, D.C.
47. Carroll, G. L. (1999). Analgesics and pain. *Vet. Clin. North Am. Small Anim. Pract.* **29**, 701–718.
48. Liebeskind, J. C. (1991). Pain can kill [editorial]. *Pain* **44**, 3–4.
49. Page, G. G., Ben-Eliyahu, S., Yirmiya, R., and Liebeskind, J. C. (1993). Morphine attenuates surgery-induced enhancement of metastatic colonization in rats. *Pain* **54**, 21–28.
50. Skarda, R. T. (1996). Local and regional anesthetic and analgesic techniques. *In* "Lumb and Jones' Veterinary Anesthesia," 3rd Ed. (J. C. Thurmon, W. J. Tranquill, and G. J. Benson, eds.), pp. 426–514. Williams & Wilkins, Baltimore, MD.
51. Hermansen, K., Pedersen, L. E., and Olesen, H. O. (1986). The analgesic effect of buprenorphine, etorphine and pethidine in the pig: A randomized double blind cross-over study. *Acta Pharmacol. Toxicol.* **59**, 27–35.
52. Taylor, P. M. (1999). Newer analgesics: Nonsteroid anti-inflammatory drugs, opioids, and combinations. *Vet. Clin. North. Am. Small Anim. Pract.* **29**, 719–736.
53. Kopcha, M., and Ahl, A. S. (1989). Experimental uses of flunixin meglumine and phenylbutazone in food-producing animals. *J. Am. Vet. Med Assoc.* **194**, 45–49.
54. Hayes, J. H., and Flecknell, P. A. (1999). A comparison of pre- and post-surgical administration of bupivicaine or buprenorphine following laparotomy in the rat. *Lab. Anim.* **33**, 16–23.

8

Funding Strategies and Agencies: Academic–Industrial Relationships; Intellectual Property

Josef E. Fischer

Department of Surgery, University of Cincinnati, Cincinnati, Ohio 45267

I. Introduction

The extraordinary growth of research funding over the past four decades has been a marvel to behold. When I finished my residency in 1969, the halcyon days of the National Institutes of Health (NIH) were over. Prior to that, when one applied for a grant, usually the program director at the NIH would call up and say, "You asked for 3 years and $40,000. Would you like 5 years and $60,000?" It was just my luck, I thought, that as I finished, getting money from the NIH became very much more difficult. However, 30 years later, my laboratory still being funded by the NIH and other sources, the facts remain the same—the NIH is still a potent source of funds, as are other agencies. Funding from the NIH will increase to approximately $15 billion this year. The pay-line will remain between 20 and 30%, depending on the institute, and may be more stringent because of the large number of grants.

The following comments are some random thoughts concerning funding. There are a myriad of funding sources available. Actually, at present, industrial contributions to academic research now exceed contributions from the NIH. Consequently, one should take advantage of all of the opportunities for funding. A good balance is important, and when funding is lost from one grant, the presence of a wider net, as it were, will undoubtedly make life easier and mitigate against depression. Thus, a balance is very important.

II. Academic Agencies

A. The National Institutes of Health

A few suggestions concerning the NIH and suggestions concerning funding are appropriate.

1. Knowing the NIH

The NIH has a myriad of institutes, agencies, and programs. While it is true that the standard grant program R01 is still the coin of the NIH realm, there are many different programs. Indeed, to those who know the structure and function of the NIH, it is remarkable how many different types of approaches may be useful. Taking the time to sit down with the book concerning the NIH (or, more recently, carefully inspecting the web site) will reveal that, in addition to the traditional R01 programs, a number of programs may be available to the investigator. These include the following programs:

1. R03: A small planning grant with relatively small amounts of money, but rather easier to obtain and subject to a different review process. These are intended as planning grants.
2. The K series: By and large, these are intended as mentoring or transitional awards. In the K08 award, it is presumed that the individual cannot function as an independent investigator, but must seek a mentor, generally a basic scientist. Funding is reasonable but limited, yet provides for a committed period of time with the mentor preparing the individual for their own independent laboratory investigation and, presumably, funding.
3. Other K awards: A variety of K awards now exist and are intended to transition individuals to clinical research, allowing midcareer changes for individuals interested in clinical trials. In some cases, as in the K12 awards for obstetricians and gynecologists, awards are made to departments to develop academically inclined individuals within the departments to pursue academic careers. No such awards exist in surgery as yet.
4. A variety of technology-transfer and other approaches: A variety of these programs within the NIH deal with newer technologies, technology transfers, and certain activities that are not normally intended for the basic R01 mechanism.

2. The R01 Mechanism

With the disappearance of the first grant, or the R29, the R01 is the traditional grant for the new and established investigator. Presumably, the R01 for a first-time investigator is evaluated on a less rigorous basis than for the established investigator. Having said that, I have not observed such generosity or mercy for beginners in my attendance on study sections. A few words regarding the R01 are appropriate.

First, R01s are investigator-hypothesis driven—that is, there is a specific hypothesis that the investigator puts forth. The body of the grant should attempt to prove or disprove the proposed hypothesis. Thus, the first rule for R01 funding is that the grant must be hypothesis driven, not a "fishing expedition."

Second, most grant writers concentrate their efforts on the review of the literature and the section in which the experiments are described. Although these need attention, by far the most important page is the "specific aims" section. Second to this is the abstract. If these are weak, it is unlikely that the grant will be funded. Remember that those individuals who are reviewing the grants may have 10 or 15 grants to review for the study section. They do not have the time to do justice to each of the grants. Thus, they tend to look at the highlights, which are the specific aims and the abstract. A few suggestions:

1. Be certain that the hypothesis is clearly stated and in a way in which it can be specifically proven or disproved. If the hypothesis is interpreted as a fishing expedition, the grant is not likely to be funded.
2. Concentrate on two or three specific aims. Four, five, or more specific aims are not helpful to a grant, particularly to an early investigator, but rather are harmful. The two or three specific aims must refer back to the initial hypothesis in a way that either proves or disproves the hypothesis.
3. A common weakness of the relatively new investigator is a lack of enough preliminary data. A quandary about preliminary data is to put enough preliminary data so that the reviewers know that you can do the experiments, yet not giving too much data so that the reviewer can say that the grant has already been performed and there is no need for funding. Most experienced investigators have already done many of the experiments that they propose to do in the body of the next grant. They only reveal sufficient numbers of experiments within the preliminary data so that there is enough evidence for funding.
4. As one describes specific experiments, make certain that there is an interpretation section to each experiment. In other words, when experiments are designed, they must be able to be interpreted one way or another, and they must lead to something else, even if the results are not as expected. A common mistake is to put forth a grant in which there is a critical experiment that must come out a certain way. If that experiment turns out a different way, there is nothing further to do and the grant is over. This type of grant is usually not funded.
5. Make certain to put a sufficient amount of money for your own salary in the budget. A study section that sees that the budget is complete except for salary for the investigator is unlikely to be impressed that the investigator has sufficient money to provide enough time for performing the grant.
6. If the grant is not funded the first time, which is likely, pay attention to the critique and turn it in yet again, quickly, when the same individuals on the study section are likely to review it. If one waits a cycle or two, it is likely that there

will be mostly new reviewers, in which case the initial critique may not be paid attention to and you will get a whole series of other critiques.

3. Training Grants

Once a program is established and the nucleus of NIH-funded investigators is formed, a training grant should be submitted. The training grant, which may be in a variety of areas, i.e., cardiovascular, surgical oncology, trauma, and infection, to name but a few, is an essential part of a contemporary research-oriented department of surgery. Training grants provide support for residents going into the laboratory. The support is not total; that is, at least in our situation, the $35,000 salary from the NIH must be supplemented by approximately $11,000 or $12,000 for each resident so that the salary within the laboratory years is equivalent to the salary these residents would get if they remained within the training program. Nonetheless, one should not underestimate the amount of the benefit to a department from such a training grant. It provides an avenue for some of its residents as well as residents from other programs to go into well-established laboratories. Surgical residents are an excellent, hard-working, and an intellectually superior workforce, and training grants provide avenues for residents who want to take fellowships to publish a sufficient number of papers in order to be competitive for those fellowships.

4. Center Grants and Program Project Training Grants

Some surgical departments have a theme, such as transplantation or nitric oxide, with the prior being the regime of the Department of Surgery at the University of Minnesota, and the latter the regime of the Department of Surgery at the University of Pittsburgh, as examples. Under these circumstances, a large number of laboratories have been collected to participate in one intellectual area. Although this is the exception rather than the rule, it can be an extremely successful way of putting together a department of surgery. When one is successful in collecting such a group of individuals with external funding, then it is appropriate to put together either a program project grant or a center grant. The two are different, the rules for application are different, and the circumstances are different. The details may be obtained from the NIH web site. The purpose of these grants is to get a critical mass of seasoned investigators together and to have work that is related funded by the same mechanism. Although this is a tremendous amount of work, it has one benefit to a department, and that is that one can take a series of older, more established investigators and integrate younger investigators with their own laboratories in such a center. This may be accomplished by having such individuals within senior-investigator laboratories or, on occasion, with a mature investigator having the young investigator with his/her own laboratory.

In order to put together such a program project grant or a center grant, when and if the institutes that might be interested are still issuing these grants (some institutes prefer to concentrate on R01s or other types of funding mechanisms), a site visit will undoubtedly be necessary. One must prepare for such a site visit; that is, there must be a tremendous amount of attention devoted to the site visit, including rehearsal, careful planning, making certain that there is no overlap, and guiding younger investigators who have never experienced a site visit. In short, it is a tremendous effort, but it is well worthwhile if the grant is obtained.

5. Requests for Proposals

Periodically, the NIH will put forth Requests for Proposals (RFPs). These are prepared by a group of experts designated by the NIH for research in certain areas. Remember that the experts who have been so designated are part of a club that has been in existence for a long time. They have in general certain views about how the field should develop, and have probably prepared their RFP well in advance of its publication. Thus, the short time line: the investigator who is not part of the "club" is at a severe disadvantage, because the time line is short and the RFP vague enough so that if one does not know exactly what is required, one is at a disadvantage for funding. Second, the group that will review the responses to the RFP will likely consist of a major part of the original group that put together the RFP.

The only thing the investigator who is not part of the club can do, when there is rumor of such an RFP, is to prepare the grant well in advance. Thus, when the RFP is published, it is possible to meet the short time line. Because most RFPs have a limited number of awards, and because it is unlikely that the investigator who is not part of the club will get one of these awards, one must weigh the amount of effort put into the RFP by the nonmember as opposed to efforts that may be expended in other mechanisms in which funding is more likely to result.

B. The National Science Foundation

The National Science Foundation usually funds only basic science departments. However, they may occasionally fund construction costs when well justified, as well as pure bench research in clinical departments when these are deemed at a sufficiently molecular level to warrant their attention.

C. Other Agencies

There are numerous other agencies available for funding. Get to know these agencies and foundations and their application protocols. Examples include the Scottish Rite, the Whitaker Foundation, the Bristol Myers Foundation, and the Burroughs-Wellcome Foundation. All of these are available on web sites, and if there is an Associate Dean for Research within your institution, all of this information should be available within that office.

An unfortunate aspect of many of these awards, particularly for young investigators, is that surgeons, by dint of long training, may be excluded. Examples of such exclusions include year of graduation from medical school, which is often so recent that surgeons are excluded.

D. Nontraditional Foundations

An increasing number of foundations are interested in the delivery of healthcare. Although delivery of healthcare and outcome have not been a traditional activity in which surgeon-scientists have participated, an increased amount of such activity now borders on what is now commonly called "outcomes research." This is an area that can be funded through certain foundations. The Robert Wood Johnson Institute for Health Policy Research may in fact fund surgical studies in which some health policy is involved. A few charitable trusts have shown an interest in these areas as well. A number of fellowships for surgical residents in the area of outcomes research are now available.

E. Local and National Foundations

The number of foundations that may fund biomedical research is remarkable. There are usually books containing information about all the foundations within individual states. Become familiar with them. Both local and state foundations may exist for specific niche areas that may be of interest to either you or another member of your department.

III. Industry

A. Introduction

The turnaround with respect to the academic–industry relationship over the past three decades is remarkable. My own association with industry goes back to 1969. At that time, funds from industry never appeared on a curriculum vitae. Indeed, there was a general unwritten rule that if one had research funds from industry, one did not mention it, almost as if there were some associated shame. As the quality of science in industrial corporations has improved and evolved, and a number of first-rate scientists have begun to work for industry, the relationship between the academic community and industry has improved. Indeed, the collaboration has evolved to such an extent that in 1999 (prior to the $2 billion increase in NIH funding), industry supported biomedical research to a greater extent than the NIH and other government agencies combined.

Simultaneously there has evolved a change in the attitude of collaboration with industry in the academic community. Such funds are listed on one's curriculum vitae. Industry is openly courted by most universities, and relationships are openly promoted. Conversely, intellectual property has become an area into which universities have put increased resources. Scientists are now relatively free, with or without NIH support, to put together various companies and still maintain full-time faculty appointments.

B. Reasons for Improved Collaboration with Industry

The growth of biotechnology in the United States has been explosive. Industry has imported a great deal of academic talent, and indeed some universities may have difficulty in holding on to their own talent, owing to better facilities and much higher salaries in industry as compared to both basic and clinical science departments. Many industries spend between $1 and $2 billion annually on in-house research, much of which is carried out by teams of talented scientists within that company. For those projects that cannot be performed in-house, the research is contracted out, mostly to universities, in specific niche areas.

The explosion in genetic technology has resulted in a wholesale transfer of academics to industry. The lure of instant riches for academics with genetic technology expertise has certainly grown from a trickle to a flood. Many enlightened universities have attempted to keep their own talent by providing ever more generous arrangements as far as intellectual property, as will be discussed subsequently.

Other activities that generate an academic–industry connection include technical devices, clinical trials, and venture capital. These will be discussed in turn subsequently.

C. The Nature of Collaboration between the Academic Community and Industry

1. Outright Grants

As biotechnology has become one of the major growth areas in the United States, industry has attempted to take advantage (in the good sense) of the intellectual capital of various universities. In those situations in which bench research is required, and industry is increasingly cognizant of outstanding university bench research, industry gives outright grants to promising investigators within universities in exchange for the right of first refusal of product licensing. Thus, prominent investigators in genetic areas and common diseases, whose research may result in the genetic manipulation of certain disease states, are receiving outright large grants in exchange for the right to license.

2. Large-Scale Grants to Universities

Over the past 15 years, grants from certain industries to universities in exchange for the right to license have gone from being considered as ethically challenged to something that institutions pursue. Thus, company X may fund university Y with, for example, a $15–50 million outright grant. In exchange for this, certain aspects of work at the university, particularly in high-technology genetic manipulation, may be promised as collateral (as it were) to an industry for the right of first refusal in exchange for the grant. The grant might be used to support that laboratory, which is most common, or it might be used to support that laboratory and a number of other incipient laboratories that the university wishes to establish.

3. Venture Capital

Promising activities in a variety of laboratories may be the subject of investment by venture capital firms. These firms support the research in exchange for licensing and production of a given product that may result from such research.

4. Collaboration

A less common mechanism of industry–university association is collaboration. This is more likely in the area of devices, in which various companies have devices that they wish to test, and thus there is outright collaboration between industry and university researchers. In the traditional bench research area, such collaboration may take place between several laboratories, or several laboratories within the company may farm out certain aspects of their research to certain laboratories with whom they collaborate.

5. Clinical Trials

An increasing activity for various universities concerns clinical trials. Under such circumstances, these trials, which are generally directed at obtaining a Food and Drug Association (FDA)-approved product, become increasingly complex as individuals attempt to satisfy the needs of the FDA. Some universities have organized their own clinical trial groups, but industry has generally responded by farming out the requirement for clinical trials to third parties, which may then engage universities and university hospitals in specific arenas for the performance of clinical trials. These in general are less lucrative for universities than the traditional direct relationship with companies, because the intermediary generally takes a significant percentage of the amount of money that the company has set aside for such clinical trials.

IV. State Incubators and Local University Incubators

A. Introduction

With the growth of biotechnology as one of the hottest areas in the red-hot American economy, states have begun to take advantage of one of their principal assets, to which they have heretofore not paid a great deal of attention: the intellectual capital of their universities. Thus, states have funded incubators that are quasi-public foundations, in which collaborations with universities and state agencies take place.

B. State Incubators

A variety of states have been more or less aggressive in carrying out policies of intellectual development or capitalization on intellectual capital of universities. Thus, investigators with promising ideas that have commercial applicability may go to a state incubator and obtain funds to set up such companies in collaboration with the state. The royalty terms are generally fairly generous to both the individual investigator and the university. States with visionary arrangements have capitalized on such collaborations by encouraging development in their states of areas in which large numbers of companies coexist in the vicinity of a major research university (e.g., research parks or triangles), thus stimulating the state economy.

C. Local University Incubators

A number of universities have set aside funds from a variety of sources to create local incubators. In these arrangements, funding is obtained either from within the university, from state incubators, from venture capital, or through the use of National Institutes of Health Small Business Innovation Research or Small Business Technology Transfer awards. Universities that have incubators may provide offices, management expertise, secretarial support on a shared basis, and hard-to-obtain technical facilities such as "clean rooms" for certain types of biological research. The results of such successful collaborations will reward the universities, the individual collaborator, and the department in which the research originally takes place. Many of these ventures are NIH funded.

D. The Small Business Innovation Research and Small Business Technology Transfer

Two NIH-sponsored awards, Small Business Innovation Research (SBIR) and Small Business Technology Transfer (STTR), are usually set-asides in which (for example) 2.5% of the money available for a certain area must be given for such ventures. The purpose of these awards is to encourage innovation and to make certain that such products of bench research are available for the treatment of patients.

V. Intellectual Property

A. Introduction

Intellectual property has become a main focus of most, if not all, research universities. One of the by-products of the new biomedical technology and the spinoffs of various companies, both purely technical and biomedical, has been the realization that intellectual capital on the part of faculty is one of the most precious possessions of any university, and particularly a research university. Consequently, almost all universities have invested in intellectual property offices. As one might imagine in such a system, the quality of what transpires in those offices varies enormously. In addition, the contacts that such offices may have with patent attorneys, the familiarity of the intellectual property officer with patent law, and the energy level may spell the difference between a lucrative contract for investigator and university and the loss of such a patent for both the investigator and the university.

Another by-product of the current technological developments and biomedical technology explosion emanating from research universities is that the royalty agreements have become much more generous to the investigator. This is the direct result of some of the leading lights of major research universities leaving the university for private industry because of the perceived or real difficulties that the inventor has had in securing monetary rewards for his or her research. Consequently, most research universities now offer terms to the inventor (for example, 60% of the royalties up to a given figure) that would have horrified the university administration a decade ago. Furthermore, most intellectual property offices now are more aggressive, rather than less so, in attempting to establish novelty and in the ability to patent evolving technology and/or discoveries that they may have thought were very borderline a decade ago.

B. Investigator Responsibilities

For the investigator, who is usually not accustomed to thinking along these lines, the resultant largesse of research universities brings with it the following obligations on the part of the investigator:

1. Treat every potential discovery as something that is conceivably intellectual property, that is, intellectual property that can be treated as a novel discovery, as a mode of treatment, or as a patentable process that may have usefulness in industry.
2. The downside of this is that most investigators are accustomed to free exchange of information with their colleagues. This cannot be done as readily when there is a process that is patentable. Thus, in unaccustomed fashion, the investigator may have to withhold information from colleagues until the process is patented, at which point the information can be freely exchanged.
3. Remember the rules concerning patenting. In general, the investigator has 1 year from the time the material is published to establish priority with respect to a patent. This means that for that 1 year, there may have to be restraint of information exchange with respect to the remainder of the scientific world prior to publication and presentation. This may seem strange to some; however, remember your experience in submitting a paper to a quality journal and having the review delayed for 4 months, possibly because of the fact that one of the reviewers may be trying to repeat your experiment and publish it first as a rapid publication. Unfortunately, the scientific community does not appear bound, at least in some cases, by the ethics of priority.

C. Royalties

The take-home message is that a patented process/treatment/drug may not only result in personal wealth, but also, under most terms of intellectual property offices in research universities, may result in ongoing research support for the originating laboratory within the life of a patent.

For the investigator, the following advice applies:

1. Obtain your own legal advice. The better the quality of the attorney representing you, the more money you and your laboratory will get.
2. Make certain that if this is something with enormous potential, you are treated as such. In other words, the amount of money that goes to you personally should be increased over and above what the university ordinarily offers. Do not negotiate this yourself, but have your attorney negotiate this for you.
3. Make certain that this applies whether you leave the university or not. In other words, there should be no vesting policy concerning the amount of time you must remain within the university before the terms of the royalty agreement kick in. Remember, this is your property, not the university's. The support for this likely came from an external organization for which you applied. Nobody from the research office of the university helped you; indeed, they may have hindered you to a considerable extent.

4. Make certain that the provisions for support of your research laboratory include the possibility that you may shift the sites of your research. That means that at least part of the support for your laboratory must go with you to a new position. This may be most difficult to arrange, but a good attorney can negotiate this for you.

The bottom line for all of these stipulations is that support from inventions and patents of faculty is rapidly growing as a major source of support for most research universities. The operating hypothesis is that this intellectual property is the property of the inventor, not the university. If one thinks about it, the university has often had a minor role other than establishing a milieu and enabling the investigator to work within their property, something that the indirect costs of most grants cover amply and then perhaps more (yachts, large parties, President's home, etc.). There is no need to be bashful about this. The investigator is best protected by having an attorney negotiating with the university so that there is no personal rancor in any of these negotiations.

The potential income from a patent may permanently change the inventor's life for the better. Such opportunities are rare. Young investigators may not be prepared for the thinking that accompanies such negotiations. Thus, it is best that negotiations be carried out by a third party on the investigator's behalf.

9

Statistical Considerations

David T. Mauger* **and Gordon L. Kauffman, Jr.†**

**Department of Health Evaluation Sciences and*
†Department of Surgery, The Milton S. Hershey Medical Center, Penn State College of Medicine, Hershey, Pennsylvania 17033

I. Introduction

Inference is the means by which conclusions can be drawn either from logic or deduction. Statistical inference is the means by which conclusions about an underlying process can be drawn from observed data. Statistics may be viewed as a set of tools for making decisions in the face of uncertainty. Even though the data have been observed without doubt in a given experiment, uncertainty exists because of the stochastic (random) nature of the underlying process giving rise to the data. If the same experiment were repeated under exactly the same conditions, no one would be surprised if the observed data were not exactly the same. The amount of unexplainable variation that can be expected in any given experiment depends largely on the nature of the process being studied. In a physics lab, for example, one would expect to find very little variation in measurements of force or gravity. Similar repeatability might also be expected in a well-run chemistry lab. Biomedical research (particularly in humans), on the other hand, is highly susceptible to significant unexplainable or naturally occurring variation. For example, the concentration of glucose in human blood is conceptually quantifiable, but in practice, measurements of blood glucose are subject to substantial variability. Major components of this variability are variation between people, variation within a person over time, and variation induced by measurement error because glucose levels cannot be measured directly and must be estimated by assay.

In order to make statistical inference that can be meaningfully quantified, one must develop a framework for modeling natural variation. It is assumed that the randomness underlying the process being observed can be described mathematically. These mathematical models form the basis on which statistical theory is built. This chapter provides some insight into the statistical theory underlying quantitative issues in experimental design without going into mathematical detail or deriving results. From a practical point of view, the most important quantitative issues in experimental design are cost and benefit. The cost of a proposed study, in time and resources, is weighed against the expected gain in scientific knowledge. For example, suppose one is interested in studying the amount of time it takes to complete a cardiac bypass procedure. Not all cardiac bypass procedures take the same amount of time and no one, certainly no surgeon, would accept the time taken to complete the next procedure (or any one particular procedure) as a definitive answer. One might conceivably undertake to determine the lengths of all cardiac bypass procedures done in the United States last year, and assuming that surgical practices have not changed very much during that time, these data would provide much scientific knowledge about the duration of such procedures. Such an undertaking would be very costly, and one might reasonably ask whether (nearly) equivalent scientific knowledge could have been obtained based on only a sample of cardiac bypass procedures done in the United States last year. In particular, how many observations are required to arrive at a definitive answer, or at least an answer with some high degree of quantifiable confidence? Methods for answering questions like this are the subject of this chapter. For both practical and ethical reasons it is important to be able to answer such questions precisely. In this age of high competition for limited biomedical research funding it is critical that an investigator be able to convincingly justify their research plans.

There is another very important question to address: what method should be used to collect information on the proposed sample? Or in other words, what experimental design should be used? This question is at least partly qualitative in nature and in general cannot be answered based solely on a quantitative cost–benefit analysis. However, this question must be answered before one can proceed to address the issue of sample size. This is because all sample size questions are design dependent. Even though the general principle that larger sample size always results in greater scientific knowledge is true, the exact mathematical form of this relationship depends on the manner in which the sample will be obtained. This chapter does not provide a pathway for choosing an experimental design, but focuses rather on the rationale for determining an appropriate sample size for a chosen experimental design.

The primary reason to consider statistical issues during study design is to ensure judicious use of limited resources, and the importance of careful consideration cannot be overstated. In all cases, the cost of a research study (in both time and money) is directly related to the sample size. A study that is underpowered because the sample size is too small has little chance to provide useful results and is a waste of valuable resources. At the other extreme, an overpowered study is also a waste of resources because the same information could have been obtained with fewer observations. This chapter develops the rationale behind sample size calculations, presents some approximate formulas that can be used to get ballpark sample size estimates, and provides guidance for using these formulas appropriately.

II. Hypothesis Testing

In many research settings the question of interest is the acceptance or rejection of a posited hypothesis. Statistical inference of this sort is termed "hypothesis testing." In this setting, the statistical analysis done at the end of the study will lead to a decision to either accept or reject the null hypothesis. This approach is predicated on the use of a model that can be framed in terms of a pair of alternative hypotheses. For example, one may wish to determine which of two drugs should be used to minimize blood loss during surgery. A complete but rather lengthy description of one such model is as follows: If all patients undergoing surgery were given drug A, the distribution of blood loss in the population would be similar to the normal distribution, the mean of the distribution would be μ_A, and the standard deviation would be σ. Similarly, if all patients undergoing surgery were given drug B, the distribution of blood loss in the population would be similar to the normal distribution, the mean of the distribution would be μ_B, and the standard deviation would be σ. This model is displayed visually in Fig. 1. Statistical texts use shorthand notation to express models of this sort.

$$X_A \sim N(\mu_A, \sigma) \qquad \text{and} \qquad X_B \sim N(\mu_B, \sigma).$$

Here X stands for the outcome of interest (amount of blood lost during surgery), the symbol "$\sim$" means "is distributed as," and $N(\mu, \sigma)$ denotes the normal distribution with mean μ and standard deviation σ. In statistical terms, this model is fully characterized by the three parameters, μ_A, μ_B, and σ. That is, if one knows the numeric values for μ_A, μ_B, and σ, one knows everything possible about the model. This does not mean that the exact amount of blood loss for any particular patient is known because that is subject to unexplainable, natural variability. However, one could determine the probability that a particular patient's blood loss would be above a certain value.

If one accepts that this model is reasonable, then the research question at hand (is there any difference between the drugs with respect to blood loss?) can be addressed by considering two special cases of the model.

$$\text{(Case 1)} \quad X_A \sim N(\mu_A, \sigma) \quad \text{and} \quad X_B \sim N(\mu_B, \sigma) \quad \text{and} \quad \mu_A \neq \mu_B.$$

$$\text{(Case 2)} \quad X_A \sim N(\mu_A, \sigma) \quad \text{and} \quad X_B \sim N(\mu_B, \sigma) \quad \text{and} \quad \mu_A = \mu_B.$$

The second case can be written more simply as X_A and $X_B \sim N(\mu, \sigma)$; there is no need to distinguish between μ_A and μ_B because they are equal. In terms of the research question, μ_A and μ_B are the parameters of interest and σ is a nuisance parameter. By "nuisance parameter" it is meant that σ is not directly relevant to the research question. That is, the only thing that distinguishes between case 1 and case 2 is whether μ_A and μ_B are equal. It is important to note that case 1 and case 2 are competing models. If one accepts the general model, then either case 1 is true or case 2 is true, but they cannot both be true or both be false.

The question of whether μ_A and μ_B are equal can be phrased in terms of the following pair of competing hypotheses:

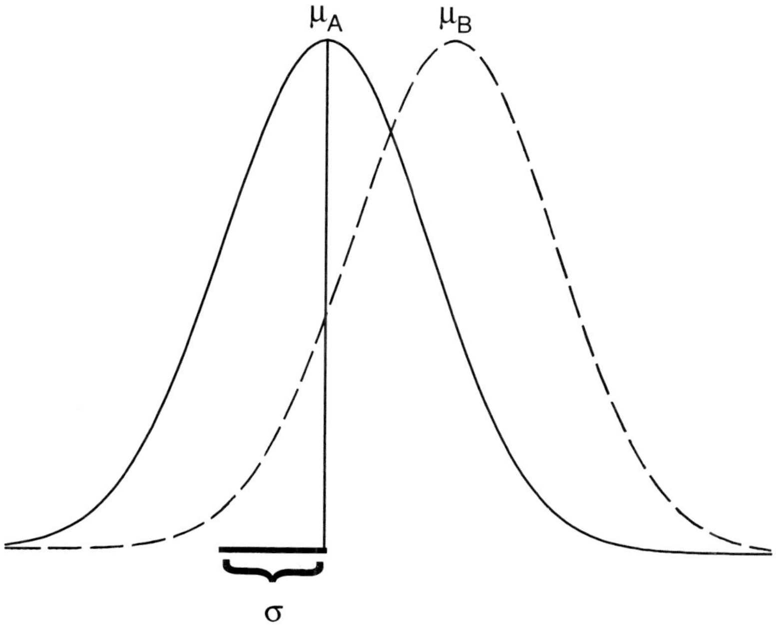

Figure 1 Illustration of the normal distribution model in the two-group setting. The standard deviation of the distribution is denoted by σ; μ_A and μ_B denote distribution means.

$$H_0: \mu_A = \mu_B \quad \text{versus} \quad H_a: \mu_A \neq \mu_B.$$

Once the data have been collected, a statistical analysis that directs a choice between these two hypotheses will be performed. In general terms, a statistical decision rule is stated as follows: reject the null hypothesis if the observed data are sufficiently inconsistent with it, otherwise do not reject the null hypothesis. This kind of decision rule is intuitively sensible, but there are many ways one could measure the inconsistency of the observed data with the null hypothesis leading to many different potential decision rules. It is necessary to have some quantifiable way of comparing potential decision rules so that the optimal can be identified. The situation is summarized in the following table.

	Reject H_0	*Do not reject H_0*
H_0 is true	*Type I error*	*Correct*
H_a is true	*Correct*	*Type II error*

Either H_0 or H_a is true and the decision will be to either reject or not reject H_0. The decision to reject H_0 when it is true is called a type I error and the decision not to reject H_0 when it is false is called a type II error. The behavior of a decision rule is quantified in terms of its type I and type II error rates. The type I error rate (denoted α) of a decision rule is the probability that using it will result in a type I error and likewise the type II error rate (denoted β) of a decision rule is the probability that using it will result in a type II error. The complement of the type II error rate $(1 - \beta)$ is called the power of the decision rule. Power is the probability of correctly rejecting the null hypothesis. It is conventional to quantify the behavior of decision rule in terms of its type I error rate (α) and its power $(1 - \beta)$. The hypothetical model presented here, that blood loss follows the normal distribution, is only one example of the kinds of models that can be used. All hypothesis tests are framed in terms of competing model-based hypotheses, but not all hypothesis tests are based on parameters, nor on the normal distribution.

One statistic that measures how consistent the observed data are with the null hypothesis is called the p value. So it is reasonable that the p value could form the basis for a decision rule to reject or not reject the null hypothesis. Methods for calculating p values will be taken up in a later chapter. It is often the case that there is more than one reasonable way to calculate p values for a given set of data (e.g., two-sample t test or Mann–Whitney test). For now it suffices to know that if the null hypothesis is true, the p value will follow the standard uniform distribution. That is, the p value is equally likely to take any value between zero and one. The left-hand panel in Fig. 2 shows the distribution of p-values that would be observed if the null hypothesis were true and the experiment were repeated many times. If the null hypothesis is not true, the p value will tend to be closer to zero than to one. For this reason, decision rules based on p values are constructed so that the null hypothesis is rejected if the observed p value is sufficiently small: reject the null hypothesis if the observed p value is less than some predetermined criteria, otherwise do not reject the null hypothesis. The type I error

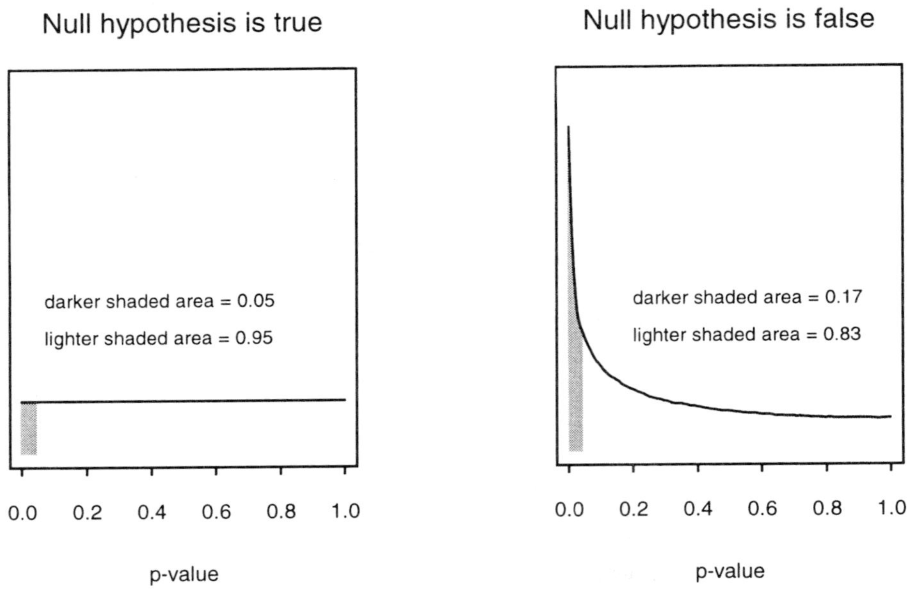

Figure 2 Illustration of the *p* value distribution under the null hypothesis (left panel) and under a particular instance of the alternative hypothesis (right panel).

rate for this decision rule can be determined from the left-hand panel in Fig. 2. The darker shaded area corresponds to the probability that the *p* value will be less than 0.05 if the null hypothesis is true; the darker shaded area is 0.05. It is an interesting property of *p* values that if the null hypothesis is true, the probability that the *p* value will be less than some number *X* is *X*. So the type I error rate of this decision rule is the value of the predetermined criteria. It has become standard to set this criteria equal to 0.05, i.e., $\alpha = 0.05$. This α is also sometimes called the significance level because *p* values less than α are termed "statistically significant" because they justify rejecting the null hypothesis. This decision rule is stated explicitly as follows: reject the null hypothesis if the *p* value for the observed data is less than 0.05, otherwise do not reject the null hypothesis.

It is important to understand that for decision rules based on *p* values the type I error rate is determined solely by the significance level of the decision rule; it is independent of study design, the method used to calculate it, sample size, and the amount of underlying variability. Power, on the other hand, depends on the distribution of the *p* value when the null hypothesis is false, which is directly influenced by study design, the method used to calculate it, sample size, and underlying variability. Determining the magnitude of power for this decision rule is quite complex. Part of the problem is that saying that the null hypothesis is false is not completely informative. The alternative hypothesis in this example is ambiguous in that it says only that the two means are not equal, but does not say anything about the magnitude of the difference. The degree to which the null hypothesis is not true is called the effect size. The alternative hypotheses (H_a: $\mu_A \neq \mu_B$) can be equivalently stated as H_a: $\mu_A - \mu_B \neq 0$. The difference, $\mu_A - \mu_B$, is the effect size.

A basic principle is that power is directly related to effect size. It is intuitively sensible that power, the probability of correctly rejecting the null hypothesis, should get larger as the degree to which the null hypothesis is false gets larger. In addition to effect size, power also depends on sample size (the amount of information collected), unexplained variability (the degree to which randomness dilutes the information collected), study design (how the information will be collected), planned statistical analysis (the method that will be used to calculate the *p* value), and type I error rate (the criteria for rejecting the null hypothesis). The relationship between power and type I error is illustrated in the right-hand panel of Fig. 2. The distribution curve shown is hypothetical, but is characteristic of the distribution of *p* values under the alternative hypothesis in that *p* values are likely to be closer to zero than to one. In this example, the darker shaded area corresponds to power, the probability that a *p* value will be less than 0.05. If the type I error rate were decreased, the power (area to the left of α) would also decrease.

Of all the quantities related to hypothesis testing, power and sample size are the two components that are under the unrestricted control of the investigator. Typically there are only a few study designs that can be used in any given setting, the appropriate analysis is generally determined by the study design, and α is usually set at 0.05 by convention. The other two pieces, effect size and unexplained variability, are determined by the nature of the process being studied. For example, one measuring device may be more precise than another, but no device can remove the natural variability between subjects in human research. Because of this, it is useful to pose the following question. "For a given study design, analysis, α level, effect size, and amount of variability, what is the relationship between power and sample size?" The exact mathematical form of the relationship between power and sample size is not always tractable. Relatively simple formulas are available in some cases (e.g., two-group mean comparison setting), but the use of computer software programs is unavoidable in many situations.

Inherent in the hypothesis testing approach is the assumption that the only possible explanation for inconsistency between the observed data and the null hypothesis is the alternative hypothesis. Another perfectly valid explanation is that the assumed model is incorrect, e.g., the outcome does not follow the normal distribution, the observed samples are not representative of the underlying population, there are differences between the groups other than simply which treatment they received. If the assumed model is incorrect, a small p value may be reflective of just that. The question of whether the null hypothesis is true cannot be reasonably addressed because the hypotheses themselves were predicated on the underlying model. Problems with the underlying model can sometimes be addressed by the statistical analysis so that the desired interpretation of the p value is preserved. However, some problems cannot be addressed by statistical analysis and therefore render the data incapable of yielding a conclusion. Most common among these problems are biases due to nonrepresentative sampling and lack of blinding. The validity of the assumption that the observed data are representative of the underlying population is absolutely critical to hypothesis testing. The best way of ensuring that the sample is representative is by taking a random sample. The use of selection criteria in determining the sample is separate from the issue of randomness. Selection criteria are used to define the population of interest; the relevant assumption is that the study participants represent a random sample of all persons who would fit the selection criteria. A related issue is that of randomization in a two-treatment design. A common design for a study comparing two treatments is to give one treatment to one-half of the subjects and the other treatment to the other half. A randomized study is one in which treatment assignment for each subject is random, i.e., does not depend on any characteristics of the individual. If treatment assignment is done in a nonrandom fashion (e.g., by gender), this produces a situation in which the two groups differ on some other factor in addition to treatment. In this case, the treatment effect is said to be confounded because it is impossible to determine the extent to which observed differences can be attributed to the treatment as opposed to the confounding factor. The purpose of randomization is to eliminate confounding factors. Another way in which a study can be confounded is lack of blinding. A fully blinded study is one in which neither the subject nor the investigator knows which treatment the subject is receiving. If there is lack of blinding, there is a possibility of intentionally biasing the results, particularly if the outcome is subjective in nature. Even if the outcome is completely objective, lack of blinding allows the possibility of bias in the way a subject is treated during the study. Surgical research is one area where blinding can be very difficult for both ethical and practical reasons and the issue of blinding must be carefully considered.

III. Sample Size Calculations

The usual way of expressing the relationship between power and sample size is to fix power at the desired level and then calculate the necessary sample size. The alternative approach is to fix the sample size and determine the resulting power. These two approaches are illustrated in Fig. 3. The two graphs shown in this figure are equivalent (i.e., the right-hand panel is the same as the left-hand panel rotated 90°), but it is instructional to consider the relationship both ways. Heuristically, the first approach is accomplished in the left-hand panel by choosing a point on the x axis (power) and then finding the associated sample size. In this hypothetical example, 90% power requires a sample size of approximately 21. Conversely, the right-hand panel illustrates the approach of first choosing the sample size (x axis) and then determining the resulting power. In this example, a sample size of 25 yields approximately 95% power. In biomedical research, adequate power is usually defined as anything greater than 80%. However, because power is the complement of the type II error rate, it might seem that 95% power would be more consistent with the standard 5% type I error rate.

Sample size calculations are very often done without direct consideration of the shape of the curve relating power and sample size. The investigator simply supplies the desired power and other parameters (α, effect size, variability, etc), and the computer software calculates the necessary sample size. However, Fig. 3 also illustrates another important feature of the relationship between power and sample size. The curve relating power and sample size has a hyperbolic shape. This is generally true, although the curve shown in Fig. 3 corresponds to a particular hypothetical example. The consequence of this fact is that it is critical for the investigator to consider the entire curve rather than just identifying the sample size required for the specified power. Considering the entire curve is analogous to a cost–benefit analysis. The cost of a study (in dollars and time) is directly related to the sample size, and power is an intuitive measure of the value of a study. Looking at the right-hand panel in Fig. 3, in this example power increases linearly with sample size up to about 15. Above 15 there is a diminishing return in power for equivalent increases in sample size. From the sample size calculation point of view, the left-hand panel indicates that for this particular example it is certainly reasonable to

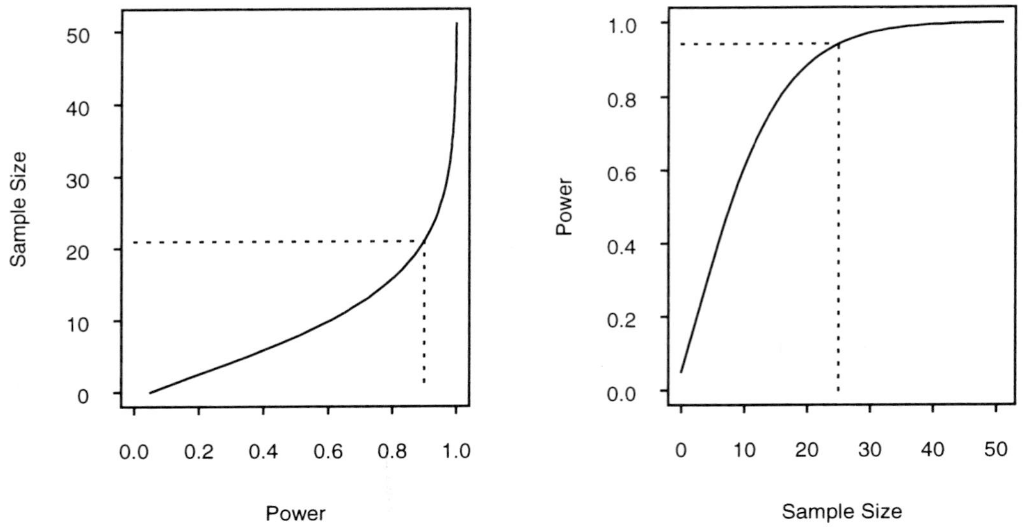

Figure 3 Hypothetical illustration of the relationship between sample size and power. Note the hyperbolic shape of the curve, indicating a nonlinear trade-off between sample size and power.

choose a sample size corresponding to 80–90% power. Whether it would be sensible to design the study with 95% power depends on other considerations. If sample size is not a budgetary constraint or if it is critical to have a very low type II error rate, then it may be sensible to consider 95% power or higher. A general rule of thumb is to choose a sample size that ensures 80–90% power unless this is beyond the point on the curve where sample size increases rapidly. If so, it may still be reasonable to consider 80% power or higher, but this should be done in light of all aspects of the study. Alternatively, one could consider using a different study design. Not all computer programs for calculating sample size are capable of producing graphs like those in Fig. 3. If one does not have access to such software, a rough outline of the sample size–power curve can be generated by calculating sample size for several different levels of power (e.g., 70, 75, 80, 85, 90, and 95%).

A. Two-Group Mean Comparison

The two-group design for which the planned analysis is to compare group means using the two-sample t test (see Chapter, this volume) is one setting for which the sample size formula is relatively simple and can be approximated well enough so that one can do reasonable "back of the envelope" calculations. The approximate sample size required for each group is

$$\frac{(\sigma_A^2 + \sigma_B^2)(z_{1-\alpha/2} + z_{1-\beta})^2}{(\mu_A - \mu_B)^2},$$

where (μ_A, σ_A) and (μ_B, σ_B) are the means and standard deviations of the two groups, and α and β are the type I and type II error rates. The value of z corresponding to the specified α and β can be obtained from a table of the cumulative normal distribution, available in most statistics texts and many scientific calculators. Several of the more commonly used values are provided as follows:

α	$z_{1-\alpha/2}$	Power	$z_{1-\beta}$
0.10	1.64	0.80	0.84
0.05	1.96	0.85	1.04
0.01	2.58	0.90	1.28

When it can be reasonably assumed that the standard deviation is same in each group ($\sigma_A = \sigma_B$) and for the standard $\alpha = 0.05$ and power $= 0.8$ ($\beta = 0.2$), this formula simplifies to

$$\frac{2\sigma^2(1.96 + 0.84)^2}{(\mu_A - \mu_B)^2} \approx 16 \times \left(\frac{\sigma}{\mu_A - \mu_B}\right)^2$$

or

$$\frac{2\sigma^2(1.96 + 1.28)^2}{(\mu_A - \mu_B)^2} \approx 21 \times \left(\frac{\sigma}{\mu_A - \mu_B}\right)^2,$$

for $\alpha = 0.05$ and power $= 0.9$ ($\beta = 0.1$). In these formulas, power is fixed and sample size is expressed as a function of unexplained variability (σ) and effect size under the alternative hypothesis ($\mu_A - \mu_B$). The ratio $(\mu_A - \mu_B)/\sigma$ is also called the relative effect size because it represents the magnitude of the effect size relative to the unexplained variability. Sample size is inversely proportional to the square of the relative effect size in the two-group setting. The relationship between sample size and power for several different relative effect sizes is shown in Fig. 4. This figure also demonstrates the potential for difference in shape of the sample size curve.

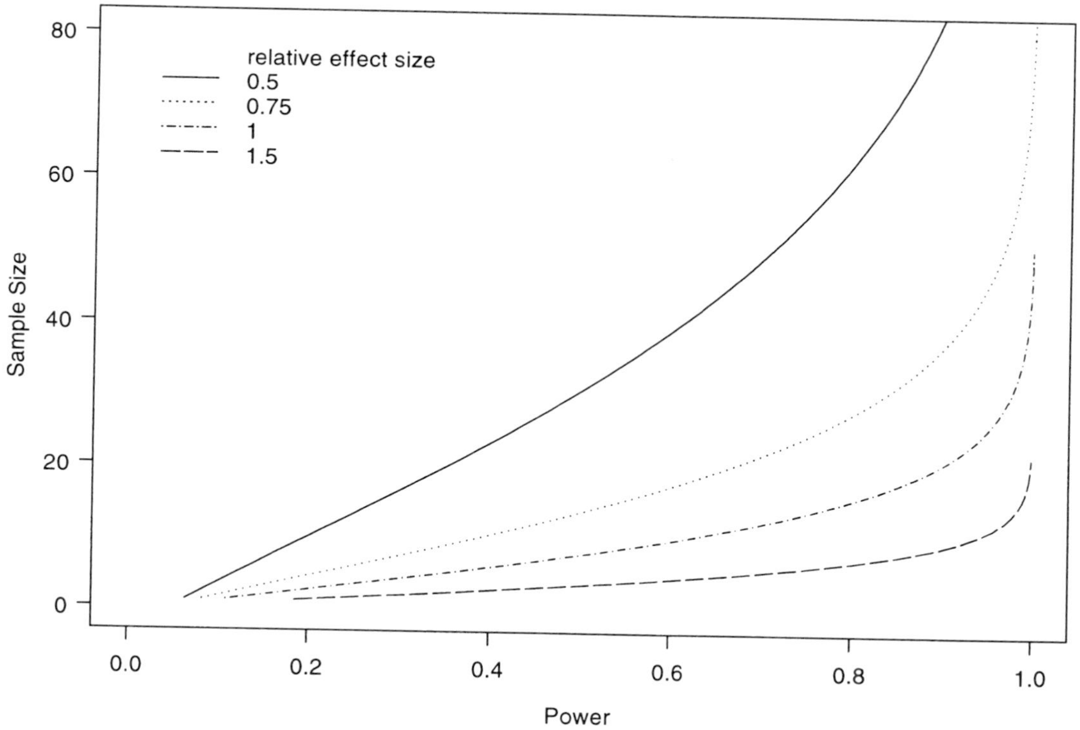

Figure 4 Hypothetical illustration of the difference between sample size/power curves for various relative effect sizes in the two-group setting.

When the relative effect size is 1.5, only a few more subjects are required to achieve 95% power instead of 80% power. On the other hand, when the relative effect size is 0.75, more than twice as many subjects are required to achieve 95% power instead of 80% power.

Two pieces of information must still be specified in order to use the formulas given above: unexplained variability (σ) and effect size under the alternative hypothesis ($\mu_A - \mu_B$). Generally speaking, only limited information about variability and effect size is available at the time of study design. The choice of values to use for the purpose of sample size calculation is more often based on an educated guess than on hard facts. After all, if the research area were so well understood that these quantities were already known, there would be little point in conducting the study. Selecting values for σ that are too small or values for $\mu_A - \mu_B$ that are too big are two of the more common pitfalls in sample size calculations. Sample size calculations are not analogous to income tax returns: the goal is not to minimize the required sample size. Figure 5 clearly demonstrates that either lowering σ or raising $\mu_A - \mu_B$ (i.e., raising the relative effect size) leads to a smaller sample size at the same level of power. The temptation to (intentionally) overestimate the relative effect size can be great, particularly for the investigator faced with insufficient resources. However, this strategy is doomed to failure because it artificially inflates the expected power of the planned study.

Selecting reasonable values for σ and $\mu_A - \mu_B$ is not always easy. Ideally, estimates should be based on previously published results or data from a pilot study. Even estimates based on published results typically require some extrapolation to the research question at hand, e.g., a slightly different dosing scheme or different eligibility criteria. In the absence of any relevant external data, values for $\mu_A - \mu_B$ can be determined based on minimal clinical relevance. For example if the primary outcome measure is amount of blood lost during surgery, the smallest difference in mean blood loss (between drug groups) that would be clinically relevant might by 0.5 units. By "clinically relevant" it is meant whether it is likely to impact clinical practice. One could certainly design a study to find a mean blood loss difference of 0.01 units, but even if such a difference were shown to be statistically significant, it is not likely that the result would influence clinical practice. It is important to use the minimal clinically relevant value. A study designed to have 80% power to find a mean blood loss difference of 2.0 units would have less than 80% power to find a difference of 0.5 units. If the true difference is 0.5, and that is clinically relevant, then the study should be designed for that difference. Determination of clinical significance is clearly not a

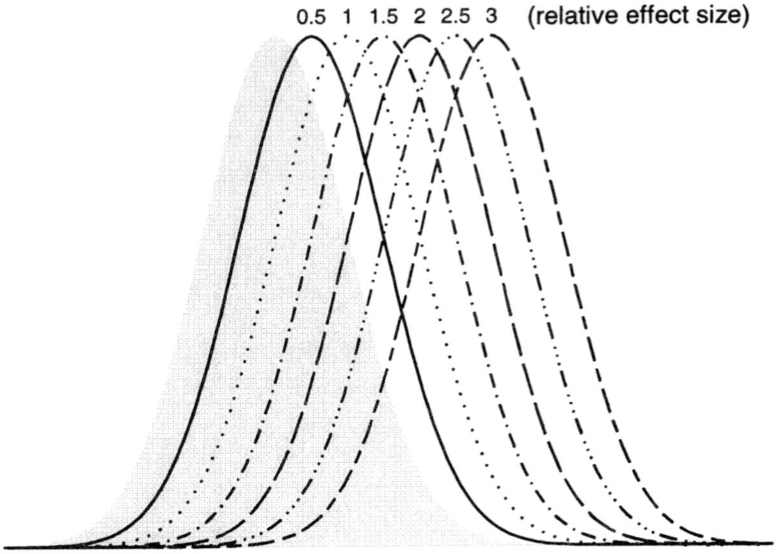

Figure 5 Illustration of the magnitude of the difference between underlying normal distributions associated with various relative effect sizes. Shaded curve is the reference group and dashed lines represent groups differing from the reference by the indicated amount.

statistical issue and must be based on expertise in the clinical setting under study.

Choosing values for σ in the absence of any relevant data is somewhat more difficult, and ideally a pilot study would be done at this point. If it is necessary to proceed without pilot data, the relative effect size $(\mu_A - \mu_B)/\sigma$ can be estimated directly instead of estimating both $\mu_A - \mu_B$ and σ separately. Relative effect size is unitless and does not have a direct clinical interpretation, but it may be possible to determine a reasonable value. Figure 5 illustrates one way of interpreting relative effect size. The shaded curve represents one of the treatment groups and the six curve outlines represent the amount of discrimination between the groups associated with various relative effect sizes. The tabulation below gives the amount of overlap between each outlined curve and the shaded curve.

Relative effect size	Percent overlap
0.5	80
1.0	62
1.5	45
2.0	32
2.5	21
3.0	13

As with minimal clinical relevance, choosing the relative effect size that is minimally relevant should be done by someone with expertise in the field. When sample size calculations are done without the benefit of external data, it is a good idea to do the calculations over a range of potential input values in order to determine how sensitive the results are to the assumed values. To quote John Tukey, "An approximate answer to the right question is worth a good deal more than an exact answer to the wrong question."

B. Multigroup Mean Comparison

When the goal of the study is to compare the mean outcome across more than two groups and the planned statistical analysis is analysis of variance (ANOVA; see Chapter 82, this volume), exact sample size calculations should be done using computer software. However, a reasonable approximation is to use the two-group formulas above to calculate the required sample size for each group based on the smallest effect size and then multiply by the number of groups. If the analysis will also include post hoc comparisons of individual groups, it is standard to adjust the significance level to account for the multiple testing (see Chapter 82, this volume). In this case, the adjustment must be taken into consideration at the design phase. For example, if post hoc analyses will be done at the 0.01 significance level instead of 0.05, sample size calculations must also be done using $\alpha = 0.01$.

C. Two-Group Mean Comparison—Paired Design

In some settings, a paired design can be used to compare two treatments. Here, each subject receives both treatments and the planned analysis is a paired *t* test (see Chapter 82, this volume). In terms of sample size, the paired design has two advantages over the unpaired design. The first is that fewer total subjects are needed because each subject will be measured twice, i.e., there will be twice as many outcomes as subjects. If the primary cost of the study is in obtaining the measurements (e.g., a very expensive assay must be done), then this benefit is of minor consequence to the overall cost of the study. If the primary cost is the recruitment of subjects or if eligible subjects are scarce, this benefit of the paired design can be substantial. The second benefit is due to the fact that observations on the same subject are often positively correlated with each other. The effect of this can be seen explicitly in the sample size formula for the paired design. The approximate total sample size required is

$$\frac{2(1-\rho)\sigma^2(z_{1-\alpha/2}+z_{1-\beta})^2}{(\mu_A-\mu_B)^2},$$

where $\mu_A - \mu_B$ is the effect size, σ is the standard deviation, and ρ is the correlation between the two measurements. For the standard $\alpha = 0.05$ and power $= 0.8$ ($\beta = 0.2$), this formula simplifies to

$$\frac{2(1-\rho)\sigma^2(1.96+0.84)^2}{(\mu_A-\mu_B)^2} \approx 16(1-\rho)\times\left(\frac{\sigma}{\mu_A-\mu_B}\right)^2$$

or

$$\frac{2(1-\rho)\sigma^2(1.96+1.28)^2}{(\mu_A-\mu_B)^2} \approx 21(1-\rho)\times\left(\frac{\sigma}{\mu_A-\mu_B}\right)^2,$$

for $\alpha = 0.05$ and power $= 0.9$ ($\beta = 0.1$). The larger the correlation, the smaller the sample size. In the absence of pilot data or previously published results on which to base estimates of ρ, it may be difficult to justify selecting values of ρ larger than zero. However, it is quite often the case that biomedical outcomes are positively correlated and using values for ρ in the neighborhood of 0.25 is not unreasonable. Note that if $\rho = 0$, the total sample size is exactly the same as that required for each group in the unpaired design. If $\rho = 0$ and the cost of the study is dependent only on the number of measurements taken (not the number of subjects), then the paired and unpaired design are equivalent in terms of cost.

D. Two-Group Comparison of Proportions

If the primary outcome is binary (e.g., yes/no), the population proportions will typically be compared using the χ^2 or Fisher's exact test (see Chapter 82, this volume). This is another setting for which the approximate sample size formula is relatively simple and close enough that one can do reasonable "back of the envelope" calculations. The approximate sample size required for each group is

$$\frac{[z_{1-\alpha/2}\sqrt{2\bar{\pi}(1-\bar{\pi})} - z_{1-\beta}\sqrt{\pi_1(1-\pi_1)+\pi_2(1-\pi_2)}]^2}{(\pi_1-\pi_2)^2},$$

where π_1 and π_2 are the are the expected proportions in each of the two groups and $\bar{\pi} = (\pi_1 + \pi_2)/2$. The quantity $(\pi_1 - \pi_2)$ corresponds to the expected effect size and the null hypothesis being tested in this case is H_0: $\pi_1 - \pi_2 = 0$. For example, a study into the effectiveness of a new prophylactic drug for preventing postoperative infection might utilize a two-group design. One group would receive the new drug and the other would receive a placebo. The estimated value for π in the placebo group could be reasonably based on the incidence of postoperative infection under the current standard of care, say 10%. If the minimal clinically relevant effect of the new drug were 5%, then $\pi_1 = 0.10$, $\pi_2 = 0.05$ (it does not matter which is which), and $\bar{\pi} = 0.075$. In order to ensure 80% power to detect this difference at the $\alpha = 0.05$ significance level, it would be necessary to enroll

$$\frac{[1.96\sqrt{2\times0.075(1-0.075)} - 0.84\sqrt{0.1(1-0.1)+0.05(1-0.05)}\,]^2}{(0.1-0.05)^2} \approx 71$$

subjects in each group. It is generally the case that larger sample sizes are required for binary outcomes than for continuous outcomes. This is because there is less information available (from a quantitative point of view) in a binary outcome than in a continuous outcome. It is advantageous, therefore, to utilize continuous outcomes whenever possible. This is not always possible, however, particularly when the primary outcome is presence or absence of some disease or symptom.

E. Confidence Intervals

Not all research questions can be phrased in terms of hypothesis testing. In some cases the goal of the study is to describe the population of interest with respect to some parameter. For example, one might wish to assess the sensitivity of a new diagnostic test in a population of patients known to have the disease of interest. The sensitivity of a diagnostic test is the proportion of diseased patients who have a positive test result. A rough approximation to the exact formula for calculating confidence intervals for proportions, suitable for "back of the envelope" calculations, is

$$p \pm z_{1-\alpha/2}\sqrt{p(1-p)/n},$$

where p is observed proportion and $100(1 - \alpha)$ is the desired confidence level, so that $\alpha = 0.05$ corresponds to a 95% confidence interval. The sample size of a proposed study can be chosen to yield a confidence interval with specified precision, e.g., $p \pm 0.05$. The necessary sample size can be obtained by setting the right side of the above equation equal to the desired precision and solving for n:

$$n = p(1-p)(z_{1-\alpha/2}/w)^2,$$

where w is desired precision of the interval. For example, the sample size required to yield a 95% confidence interval with precision $w = 0.05$ is

$$n = p(1 - p)(1.96/0.05)^2 = p(1 - p) \times 1537.$$

Note that the sample size depends on the observed proportion. Obviously, the observed proportion is unknown before the study is completed. It turns out that the most conservative (leading to the largest sample size) answer is obtained by using $p = 0.5$. In this case, that approach would give a sample size of 385 ($0.5 \times 0.5 \times 1537$). If it is safe to assume that the true proportion is different from 0.5, one might reasonably guess that the observed proportion will also be different from 0.5. For example, one might expect the diagnostic test to have sensitivity close to 0.9 because of its similarity to another well-established test with that sensitivity. Using $p = 0.9$ would give a sample size of 139 ($0.9 \times 0.1 \times 1537$), less than half the sample size required when using $p = 0.5$. Clearly, using $p = 0.5$ can be extremely conservative and should not be done if other reasonable estimates of p are available. On the other hand, using values for p that are either too close to one or too close to zero would lead to a study design with inadequate sample size. This example serves to underscore the fact that sample size calculations must be carefully and thoughtfully done if they are to be useful.

Another setting in which the confidence interval approach is useful is when the goal of the study is to measure the correlation between two outcomes. A rough approximation to the exact formula for calculating confidence intervals the correlation is

$$r \pm z_{1-\alpha/2}\sqrt{(1 - r^2)/n},$$

so that the sample size necessary to yield a confidence interval with precision w can be approximated by

$$n = (1 - r^2)(z_{1-\alpha/2}/w)^2.$$

The sample size is largest when $r = 0$ and decreases as r increases. As with proportions, sample sizes based on the confidence interval approach for correlations must be done carefully and with thoughtful consideration.

IV. Summary

This chapter was written for a wide readership of surgical investigators. The essential considerations required for the appropriate design of the proposed studies are available in many biostatistical texts. There is a list of references 1–9 at the end of this chapter. It is recommended that the serious investigator spend time reading the cited narratives, because the format is designed to lead the reader through the assumptions and logic underlying the application of sample size calculations. Crucial to the proposal is the clear statement of a testable hypothesis or desired confidence interval. The design of the study must reflect the investigator's attention to the trade-off between study cost (sample size) and benefit (power or precision). The formulas presented here are good approximations that can be used in relatively simple design settings. The reader is encouraged to seek consultation with an experienced applied biostatistician for help with more complex designs. There are many pitfalls in the use of sample size calculations for the inexperienced or unaware user.

References

1. Bland, M. (1995). "An Introduction To Medical Statistics," 2nd Ed. Oxford Univ. Press, London.
2. Wassertheil-Smoller, S. (1995). "Biostatistics and Epidemiology: A Primer For Health Professionals," 2nd Ed. Springer-Verlag, New York.
3. Campbell, M. J., and Machin, D. (1993). "Medical Statistics: A Commonsense Approach," 2nd Ed. John Wiley & Sons, New York.
4. Altman, D. G. (1991). "Practical Statistics For Medical Research." Chapman & Hall, London.
5. Fisher, L. D., and Van Belle, G. (1993). "Biostatistics: A Methodology For The Health Sciences." John Wiley & Sons, New York.
6. Clarke, G. M. (1994). "Statistics and Experimental Design." Edward Arnold, London.
7. Pocock, S. J. (1983). "Clinical Trials: A Practical Approach." John Wiley & Sons, New York.
8. Woolson, R. F. (1987). "Statistical Methods for the Analysis of Biomedical Data." John Wiley & Sons, New York.
9. Freidman, L. M., Furberg, C. D., and DeMets, D. L. (1998). "Fundamentals of Clinical Trials," 3rd Ed. Springer-Verlag, New York.

10

Use of Nonexperimental Studies to Evaluate Surgical Procedures and Other Interventions: The Challenge of Risk Adjustment

Michael Shwartz,* Arlene S. Ash,† and Lisa I. Iezzoni‡

* *School of Management, Boston University, Boston, Massachusetts 02215*
† *Boston University School of Medicine and School of Public Health, Boston, Massachusetts 02218*
‡ *Harvard Medical School and Division of General Medicine and Primary Care, Department of Medicine, Beth Israel Deaconess Medical Center, Boston, Massachusetts 02215*

I. Introduction

Randomized controlled trials (RCTs) are the "gold standard" for judging the efficacy of clinical interventions, i.e., the impact of an intervention in the controlled environment of a trial. If a large enough number of patients is randomly assigned to a study group that receives an intervention and a control group that does not, patients in each of the groups will be similar in terms of both measured and unmeasured baseline characteristics. Similarity of the two groups at baseline does not guarantee that differences in outcomes can be attributed to the intervention (1). For example, differences in how outcomes in the two groups are measured (something that "blinding" attempts to minimize) may introduce bias. Nevertheless, the balance on both known and unknown baseline characteristics that, on average, results from randomization significantly strengthens our confidence that differences in outcomes between the two groups are caused by the intervention.

Despite the value of RCTs, for a variety of reasons they have not been, and will not be, conducted for many interventions. First, because the investigator actively assigns patients to the study or control arm of the trial, there must be sufficient uncertainty about the benefit of the intervention to withhold it from some patients, but sufficient confidence in its potential to give it to others. Many interventions become widely adopted before RCTs are performed, creating a situation in which it may be difficult to recruit subjects because of preconceived ideas about effectiveness. This was the case when a randomized controlled trial to evaluate right heart catheterization was cancelled because most physicians refused to allow their patients to be randomized (2).

In order to increase the validity of findings from RCTs, patients who are acceptable candidates for randomization are often a narrow subset of those for whom the treatment will later be used, e.g., patients with substantial comorbidities may be excluded. Also, even among acceptable candidates, those that agree to participate may differ in important ways that are related to outcomes under consideration. For example, participants are likely to be a more healthy subset of the eligible cases, a bias referred to as the "healthy volunteer" effect. As a result, the generalizability of findings from RCTs to the types of patients seen in clinical practice is often of concern. There is some support for this concern, illustrated by the fact that perioperative mortality following carotid endarterectomy is substantially higher in actual practice than reported in randomized controlled trials, even in institutions that participated in the trials (3). RCTs are expensive, and often it takes many years before results are known. In the absence of RCT-based evidence to guide decisions, clinical practice must proceed, based on judgment drawn from case studies reported in the literature, observational evidence, and clinical logic.

In fact, most of what is "known" about the value of surgical interventions comes from nonexperimental observational studies in which there has been no randomization. For a variety of often poorly understood reasons, some patients receive a particular intervention and others do not. By examining the differences in baseline characteristics and outcomes between the two groups, nonexperimental studies seek insights into the effectiveness of interventions, i.e., the impact of interventions in actual clinical settings, as opposed to impact in the special circumstances of a trial.

The core problem in nonexperimental studies is that baseline risk factors differ in the two groups. Typically, the intervention is differentially given to those who have a much better (or worse) prognosis than average. This makes it difficult to determine the extent to which differences in outcomes are due to the intervention as opposed to differences in baseline risk. In analyzing data from observational studies, multivariate models are usually used to assess treatment effectiveness after "adjusting for" differences in baseline risk factors. If all important risk factors are measured and the relationship between the risk factors and outcome is correctly specified, such models provide an unbiased estimate of treatment effectiveness. In practice, however, we cannot measure all risk factors, nor can we be certain that the effect of risk factors on outcomes is correctly specified in the model.

In what follows, we (1) discuss major dimensions of risk in order to provide a framework for considering variables that should be included in models used to adjust for risk; (2) briefly discuss sources of data for risk factors; (3) present, for three different types of outcomes, the multivariate models most often used for risk adjustment and assessment of treatment effectiveness; (4) discuss issues in multivariate modeling of particular relevance to risk adjustment; and (5) illustrate with simple examples two approaches used to improve estimates of treatment effectiveness in nonexperimental studies when the relationship between risk and outcomes may not be correctly specified (matching or stratification on propensity score) or when there may be important unmeasured risk factors (instrumental variables).

II. Dimensions of Risk

Though the importance of risk adjustment in nonexperimental studies is unquestionable, the adequacy of risk adjustment in any particular study is often of concern. For example, despite the widespread use of transurethral resection of the prostate (TURP) to treat benign prostatic hyperplasia, several studies in the late 1980s using administrative data showed higher mortality rates from this procedure compared to open prostatectomy, even after adjusting for age and comorbidities. Concato *et al.* (4) demonstrated that when risk adjustment was based on more complete measures of comorbidity, mortality following TURP and open prostatectomy no longer differed.

To provide a basis for assessing the adequacy of adjustment for differences in risk, in what follows we briefly discuss the major dimensions of risk [see Iezzoni (5) for a more in-depth discussion]. In considering these dimensions, it is important to emphasize that which ones are of primary importance will depend on the outcomes of interest (see Chapter 11).

A. Age

After accounting for other patient attributes, age usually has an independent effect on outcomes. For example, even for seriously ill patients treated in intensive care units (ICUs), age is an important independent predictor of imminent death among those who are similar in terms of extent of organ system failure (6). This is particularly true for the oldest of the old (those above 80 or 85), who have lower physiologic reserves and usually have poorer outcomes than younger patients even if other characteristics are comparable.

As is true for many of the dimensions discussed below, it is rarely the case that age is related in a linear way to outcomes. Hence, the usual approach is to divide age into categories (60–64, 65–70, etc.) and use dummy variables (sometimes called indicator variables or 0/1 variables; see below) to model the relationship between age and outcomes as a step function (reflecting, for example, one mortality rate for those 60–64 years old, another for those 65–69, etc.). More sophisticated computer-based "smoothing techniques" are sometimes used to represent nonlinear relationships [e.g., see Le Gall *et al.* (7), who used the LOWESS (locally weighted least squares) smoothing function (8) or Knaus *et al.* (6), who considered the use of cubic splines when developing APACHE III (the Acute Physiology and Chronic Health Evaluation index, an index used to measure the severity of patients in the ICU). This approach assigns a continuously varying weight to a variable, though in Knaus' analysis, cubic splines did not increase explanatory power.] Sometimes the effect of age changes the effect of other risk factors. For example, in the Medicare Mortality Predictor System (MMPS), the APACHE II score is modified to take account of the increased likelihood of death among the elderly presenting with very low body temperatures (9). Though age by itself usually does not explain much of the variation in outcomes, it is usually included as a risk factor because of its availability and high level of face validity.

B. Gender

Anatomic, physiologic, and hormonal differences between men and women can result in different risks for certain outcomes. Unfortunately, efficacy trials of new treatments have often either excluded women or included too few women to perform separate analyses by gender. Hence, there are many unanswered questions about the effect of gender on outcomes and about the relative effectiveness of interventions in men versus women, questions that are often examined in observational studies. For example, several studies in the early 1990s reported lower use of and poorer results from invasive technologies for diagnosing and treating coronary artery disease in women (10–12). A more recent study that reflects advances in technology and improvements in techniques suggests that, after adjusting for the increased risk of women undergoing revascularization, women in fact have better outcomes than men (13).

Because of uncertainty about the relationship between gender and outcome, a dummy variable for gender is often included to take account of the possibility that outcomes are different in men and women.

C. Race and Ethnicity

Race and ethnicity are difficult to measure in a clear, consistent, and meaningful fashion. As LaVeist has noted (14),

> *Race is a social category, not a biological concept. It is a concept that has changed over time and is variable across societies. . . . Race is a concept that is determined fundamentally by political and social forces without regard to biogenetics or scientific rigor. . . . [In research], we must acknowledge that what is measured by the race dummy variable is not culture, biology, values or behavior. What is actually measured by the race variable is skin color.*

It is sometimes thought that race is primarily a proxy for differences in socioeconomic status. However, Williams (15) states that

> *Adjusting racial (black–white) disparities in health for socioeconomic status (SES) sometimes eliminates, but always substantially reduces, these differences. However, a frequent finding is that within each level of SES blacks still have worse health than whites. . . . This pattern clearly indicates that, while there is considerable overlap between race and SES, race reflects more than SES.*

Discrepancies in use of services and outcomes by race have been demonstrated. Wenneker and Epstein (16) reported that African-American patients were less likely than others to receive coronary angiography and coronary artery bypass graft (CABG) surgery; Ayanian *et al.* (17), in a study of over 27,000 Medicare beneficiaries, found an adjusted odds ratio of 1.78 for whites compared to blacks for obtaining revascularization procedures within 90 days after coronary angiography; a study involving hundreds of thousands of Medicare beneficiaries found that blacks were much less likely than whites to receive "referral-sensitive" surgeries (18). These differences could reflect differences in severity of presenting illness and appropriateness of the procedures, unmeasured differences in socioeconomic status, differences in patient attitudes, or, most troubling, racial discrimination. Their implications for adjusting for race as a risk factor is controversial, particularly when the purpose of the analysis is to compare provider performance. If risk is included, it holds providers "harmless" for differences in outcomes. To the extent that differences in outcomes reflect poorer quality of care provided to certain racial/ethnic groups, no incentives are created to reduce quality differentials. However, to the extent race/ethnicity is a proxy for unmeasured variables that are not related to quality of care but are related to outcomes, excluding race penalizes those providers with higher numbers of minorities. One way around the dilemma is to examine outcomes separately by race/ethnicity category, an approach referred to as stratification (in this case on race/ethnicity). In multivariate models to assess the effect of interventions, race is often included as a risk factor (often only making a distinction between white and black), though usually with little justification.

D. Acute Clinical Stability

The immediate physiologic functioning of the patient, measured by things such as vital signs, serum electrolytes, hematology findings (e.g., hematocrit, white blood cell count, clotting indices), arterial oxygenation, and levels of consciousness or neurologic functioning, is particularly crucial when examining outcomes of acutely ill patients in short time frames (e.g., during a hospitalization or within 30 days of admission). Because of their importance in the clinical management of acutely ill patients, most of these variables are routinely measured with minimal technologic intervention. However, it is often the case that a relatively small set of variables encompasses the most important predictors of risk of short-term mortality across both children and adults. For example, in the first revisions of APACHE, the initial set of 34 physiologic variables was reduced to a core group of 12 (which has since been expanded slightly) (16, 19, 20). A competing ICU severity measure (the Simplified Acute Physiology Score) uses even fewer variables (7).

Almost all studies that focus on procedure use in critically ill patients adjust for physiologic status. As in the case of age, nonlinear relationships between certain physiologic variables and outcomes can be captured by creating categories for the variable and entering dummy variables in the model for each category. For example, in the National Veterans' Administration (VA) Surgical Risk Study (discussed more fully below), serum sodium was divided into 3 categories (less than 136 mEq/ml, between 136 and 148 mEq/ml, and greater than 148 mEq/ml) to reflect the U-shaped relationship of this variable to outcomes.

E. Severity of Principal Diagnosis

"'Severity' is what sociologists term a 'folk wisdom' word like 'satisfaction' or 'happiness,' operationally indefinable in a way perfectly acceptable to all parties" (21). Nevertheless, at the core of severity is the notion of prognosis—expectations about clinical outcomes based on extent and nature of the disease. The types of outcomes that most often underlie notions of severity are in-hospital mortality, post-discharge mortality, cost, length of stay, and complications. Data are usually available from routine sources for these outcomes and provide the basis for our understanding of the relationship between patient characteristics and outcomes. When there is an interest in outcomes such as functional status and quality of life, defining severity is more problematic.

For some conditions, disease-specific clinical parameters related to severity have been more fully developed. For example, cancer staging methods are based on local tumor manifestations and the extent of lymphatic spread and distant metastases. The New York Heart Association developed a classification scheme based on the etiology, anatomy, physiologic function, and clinical manifestations of heart disease. But, for diseases with diverse presentations, defining severity can be more difficult. A variety of systems, many proprietary, have been developed to measure severity, some of which are described by Iezzoni (5, 22).

F. Extent and Severity of Comorbidities

Comorbidities are diseases unrelated in etiology or causality to the principal diagnosis (as distinguished from complications, which are sequelae of the principal diagnosis). The prototypical comorbidities are chronic conditions such as diabetes mellitus, chronic obstructive pulmonary disease, or chronic ischemic heart disease, though comorbid illnesses could also be acute (e.g., an acute myocardial infarction following admission to treat prostate disease). A large literature has shown that patients with significant comorbidities are at higher risk for poor outcomes. The extent of increased risk depends on the severity of the comorbid conditions.

Because of their higher risk, patients with significant comorbidities are often excluded from randomized controlled trials. However, such patients present frequently in the real world, particularly among the aged. Understanding the impact of comorbidities on outcomes, which is important for clinical management, is likely to come mainly from observational studies.

Several investigators have developed indices to measure the impact of comorbidities on outcomes, the most widely used being that developed by Charlson and co-workers (23). From the coefficients of a Cox proportional hazards model (discussed below) fit to 1-year survival data of 559 patients from New York Hospital, each comorbidity was assigned an integer weight ranging from 1 to 6. The resulting index, as well as an index constructed by simply counting the number of comorbidities, predicts 1-year mortality and has been shown to predict 5-year mortality (24). The Charlson index has been adapted for use with administrative data (25). Other studies have also found comorbidities to be important in predicting outcomes (4, 6, 26–28).

Often severity of principal diagnosis and of comorbidities are combined in one index. Most illustrative of this is the Physical Status Classification of the American Society of Anesthesiologists (ASA) that has been used for decades in the preoperative evaluation of surgical patients. ASA scores rate the risk of perioperative death on a global, subjective 5-point scale that attempts to capture all aspects of the patient's presentation. A study of patients undergoing cholecystectomy, total hip replacement, or transurethral prostatectomy found that increasing ASA scores were generally associated with longer hospital stays, higher complication rates, and more postoperative physician visits (29).

G. Physical Functional Status

Measures of functional status include assessment of basic activities of daily living (ADLs) (e.g., feeding, bathing, dressing, toileting, walking) and what are called instrumental ADLs (e.g., shopping, cooking, using transportation). More comprehensive measures encompass cognitive abilities (e.g., level of alertness, orientation, long- and short-term memory), affective health (e.g., happiness, anxiety), and social activities (e.g., visiting friends). Numerous functional status measures are available, and an extensive literature is available to help select relevant instruments (30–33).

Functional status can be an outcome as well as a risk factor. As a risk factor, it is closely linked to outcomes such as imminent death, postoperative complications, and future health service use. For example, in a study of 366 lung cancer patients, functional status in the month prior to admission was more predictive of in-hospital death (among the 24% dying) than were APACHE score, stage of cancer, and extent of comorbid disease (34). Davis, *et al.* (35) found that nursing assessments of patients' function were more predictive of in-hospital mortality than were most laboratory tests values and comorbid disease.

In regard to functional status, the following points are worth nothing, points that are also relevant to other quality-of-life-related dimensions discussed below. First, functional status is often largely independent of patient demographic characteristics and diagnoses. Second, specific functional status measures may not perform equally well across all types of conditions or types of patients (e.g., the elderly, the poorly educated, the impoverished, and patients with both medical and psychiatric comorbidities) (36). Third, the way in which data are collected (face-to-face interviews, mail with self-administration, telephone interviews) may influence the validity of the data (37). Fourth, though many measures are independent of disease, disease-specific measures are available for certain conditions. Condition-specific scales may be more sensitive to changes in specific functions than are generic measures. Finally, perceptions about functioning may depend on whom is asked—the physician or the patient.

H. Psychological, Cognitive, and Psychosocial Functioning

These characteristics, which include the capacity to understand information about one's healthcare needs and willingness to adhere to recommended treatment plans, can have a major impact on outcomes. Attempts to measure these aspects of functioning are often combined within scales of overall functioning. Even without sophisticated measurement, however, basic facts about how patients live can be related to outcomes in important ways. For example, after adjusting for variables such as New York Heart Association class, prior infarction, use of beta blockers, and education, patients living alone had a higher relative risk of poor outcomes than did those living with others—a relative risk of 1.54 for recurrent cardiac events and 1.58 for cardiac death (38). Another study that tracked over 1300 patients treated medically for coronary artery disease found that after controlling for "all known medical prognostic factors," social variables remained important predictors of risk of death (e.g., unmarried persons without confidants had a relative risk of 3.34 for cardiac death within 5 years) (39). As in the case of functional status, these variables become more important as the time frame for measuring outcomes becomes longer.

I. Socioeconomic Status

Many studies have found lower socioeconomic status is associated with higher mortality, due to a combination of delayed access to medical care, differences in attitudes toward the healthcare system, and chronic fundamental deprivations that subtly impair health. As Starfield (40) has noted in discussing the link between poverty and poor health, "The chain of events is complex. Predisposing factors involve environmental conditions, social conditions, and genetic risk factors. Some of these operate directly (such as housing with lead-based paint), and some operate indirectly through mediating factors involving induced behaviors, stress, social isolation, and decreased access to medical care. All risks interact in unknown ways in their effect on health." When available, measures of socioeconomic status are often included as risk factors. Sometimes the measures are not based on the socioeconomic status of the individual patient, but, because of the availability of census data, on the socioeconomic characteristics of the zip code where the patient lives. These types of ecological measures are most appropriate when one's interest is in the impact of immediate environment on things such as accessibility to individual physicians. As a proxy for individual socioeconomic characteristics, they obviously may be misleading.

J. Overall Assessment of Health Status and Health-Related Quality of Life

A large and growing literature describes numerous measures for a variety of populations and purposes (41–46). These measures, based on data collected directly from patients, assess attributes such as severity of illness, physical capabilities, psychosocial and emotional functioning, sense of well-being, and health-related quality of life. What really distinguishes these types of measures from other measures of health is that they incorporate patients' values and preferences (47). Like functional status, overall measures of health status and quality of life can be risk factors related to specific outcomes, or they can be outcomes.

K. Conclusions

In general, acute clinical stability and acute attributes of the principal diagnosis and comorbid conditions are the most important components of risk for studies involving short time frames. Chronic disability, physical functioning, and various types of nonclinical factors increase in importance as the time window within which outcomes are considered expands.

To move from dimensions of risk to operational measures of risk one proceeds roughly as follows: (1) Based on those dimensions judged important, define patient-specific risk factors that will be included in the analysis (e.g., cardiogenic shock, sepsis, liver failure, socioeconomic status, altered mental state, race); (2) for each factor, identify measures of their presence (e.g., low blood pressure, low cardiac output, positive blood cultures, prolonged prothrombin time, elevated bilirubin, decreased serum albumin, hepatic coma, median income of zip code of residence, abnormal mental status exam, white/black/other); (3) evaluate whether these measures can be reliably determined from available information or will require additional data collection. To answer this latter question takes us into the realm of the type of data available for risk adjustment. We briefly review this in the next section.

III. Data Sources

A. Administrative Databases

Administrative databases—large, computerized files generally compiled in billing for health services—are an important source of data for observational studies. Though not originally intended for this purpose, such databases have become the mainstay of an entire body of health services studies (48–51) and studies of outcomes (52–54).

Legislation establishing the federal Agency for Health Care Policy and Research (AHCPR) specified use of administrative files: "For facilitating research, the Secretary shall . . . (5) conduct and support research and demonstrations on the use of claims data . . . in determining outcome, effectiveness, and appropriateness of such treatment" (Omnibus Budget Reconciliation Act of 1989, P.L. 101–239, December, 19, 1989, Sec. 1142c).

The value of such studies has been mixed (55), in large part due to the limited clinical information available to control for differences in patient risk. In claims databases, clinical information is restricted to the World Health Organization's International Classification of Diseases, 9th Revision, Clinical Modification (ICD-9-CM) codes submitted as part of the billing process. Thus, to a large extent, the validity of studies of effectiveness using such databases depends on the credibility of ICD-9-CM codes as a source for risk adjustment (see Chapter 13).

B. The Medical Record

Although medical records contain a great deal of clinical information, even "objective" findings noted in medical records, such as diagnostic test results and physical examination findings, are often subject to wide variations among observers (56). Inter- and even intraobserver variability is common even for tests that are machine driven. Findings that reflect physician interpretation of patient experiences, e.g., patient functioning, are even less reliable (57). As Eddy (58) wrote, "Uncertainty creeps into medical practice through every pore . . . And the ambiguities grow worse as medical technology expands." The limited literature on the reliability of the medical record suggests that it is sufficient for certain purposes, but that it does not completely or accurately represent the care delivered to patients or certain aspects of their disease that could significantly affect risk (59–62).

If the purpose of an analysis is comparative (what institutions or providers more successfully perform certain procedures), difference in practice patterns may well result in biased assessments of risk. At the most basic level, if a physiologic value is not measured, it cannot be used to establish patient risk. This becomes particularly problematic when comparing results across institutions that differ in technological capabilities (e.g., academic medical centers vs. small community hospitals). Difficulties in comparisons are compounded by differences in medical record documentation.

Despite these problems, information from medical records is the best record of information used by providers to make diagnostic, therapeutic, and prognostic judgments, making data from records conceptually appealing as indicators of risk. In considering specific variables, the following questions are relevant:

1. Are most charts likely to contain the variable of interest? If data are missing, is there a basis for imputing a value (such as assuming that a missing temperature is normal)?
2. How reliably can the variable be abstracted from the records (i.e., how likely is it that different reviewers, or the same reviewer at different times, would obtain the same value)?
3. Related to the question of reliability, if the variable is recorded in several different places in the chart, which one should be used? How clearly can instructions be developed for locating the variable?

4. How sensitive is the particular variable to the characteristics of the person collecting it (e.g., physician vs. nurse) or the type of hospital at which records are being reviewed (teaching hospital vs. community hospital)?

C. Prospective Data Collection

In specially designed studies, data can be prospectively collected prior to treatment and then patients are followed for some time after treatment in order to monitor adverse outcomes and to assess changes in physical functioning and quality of life. To illustrate, the National VA Surgical Risk Study was initiated in 1991 with the goal of providing comparative risk-adjusted postoperative mortality rates for surgical services in the Veterans Health Administration (63). Inconsistent coding patterns across facilities and the inability to distinguish from discharge abstract data whether risk factors were present prior to surgery or occurred postoperatively limited use of the VA discharge abstract data. Abstracting data from medical charts suffered from poor reliability among the abstractors and the fact that important risk factors were not recorded in the charts. The result was a decision to collect data prospectively using consistent risk factor and outcome definitions. In the VA study, patients undergoing major surgery are identified preoperatively and selected risk factors assessed. Patients are then followed for 30 days postoperatively to determine mortality and the incidence of 21 predefined postoperative adverse events. As another example, in New York State, a patient-specific cardiac surgical report form is completed at discharge for all patients undergoing CABG, including data on variables such as ventricular ejection fraction, >90% narrowing of the left main coronary artery, diabetes mellitus requiring medication, and whether the CABG was a reoperation. These variables are then used for risk adjustment for the purpose of comparing the experiences of institutions and providers (64, 65).

Even when data are prospectively collected, certain variables may be unreliable. For example, across VA hospitals there was wide variability in the reporting of culture results, making collection of wound, blood, sputum, and urine culture bacteriology results unsuitable for risk adjustment. Results of cardiac, pulmonary, or vascular testing were not used to develop risk factors because only a small proportion of patients undergoing major surgery had these tests performed, interpretations across multiple facilities were judged to be inconsistent, and because obtaining results of such tests would have been time consuming.

Prospective collection of risk and outcome information overcomes many of the limitations of administrative data or retrospective medical chart review. However, special data are usually collected only on those undergoing a procedure, and not on those potentially eligible to receive the procedure who do not. Hence, such routinely collected prospective data are usually not available for studies to assess the effectiveness of a surgical intervention compared to no surgery, although they can be used in a comparison of two surgical procedures.

IV. Multivariate Modeling Framework

The goal of nonexperimental studies is to assess the effectiveness of an intervention after "controlling for" differences in baseline risk between those who receive the intervention and those who do not. Multivariate models are generally used to do this. We first illustrate the standard multivariate linear regression model for the situation in which the outcome is continuous. We then consider modifications when the outcome is dichotomous (such as whether a patient was alive 30 days posthospital admission) and, finally, when the outcome is duration of survival.

A. Modeling Continuous Outcomes

Let Y_i be the actual value of the outcome variable for the ith patient, and X_{ij} be the value of the jth independent variable for the ith person, $j = 1, \ldots, J$. These J independent variables are the risk factors for which adjustment is desired. Let I be a variable that is coded "1" if the patient receives the intervention and "0" if the patient does not. Such 0/1 variables are called "dummy" or "indicator" variables.

The standard multivariate linear regression model used to assess treatment effectiveness is

$$E(Y_i) = a + \sum_j b_j X_{ij} + c \cdot I,$$

where $E(Y_i)$ is the expected value of the outcome variable for the ith patient, a is a constant, the b_j values are coefficients that measure the effect of the risk factors (i.e., the X_{ij} values, on the outcome Y_i), and c is the coefficient that measures treatment effectiveness. Imagine two patients who have the same values for all risk factors, one of whom receives treatment ($I = 1$) while the other does not ($I = 0$). The expected outcome for the treated patient is c higher (or c lower, if c is negative) than for an untreated patient with the same risk factors. The coefficient b_j indicates how much the expected outcome changes for a one-unit increase in risk factor j. In many cases, the risk factors are also coded as dummy variables to capture nonlinear relationships between risk and outcomes. For example, age is often categorized and dummy variables are entered into the model for each age category except some reference category. The coefficient associated with a particular dummy variable indicates the expected effect on the outcome of being in that particular age range as opposed to the reference age category.

Models can be enriched by including "interaction" terms, which allow some variables to have a different effect on outcome depending on the value of another variable. Interactions of risk factors with the intervention variable are often of particular interest. Imagine a model that has a dummy variable for female, F, coded as 0 for men and 1 for women (with coefficient b_1), a dummy variable representing whether the patient receives the intervention (labeled I, with coefficient c) and an interaction between gender and receipt of the treatment, calculated as I times F (i.e., $I \cdot F$), with coefficient d. The interaction variable $I \cdot F$ is 1 for women who receive the intervention and 0 otherwise. The model then is

$$E(Y_i) = a + \text{other risk factors} + b_1 \cdot F + c \cdot I + \mathrm{d} \cdot (I \cdot F).$$

Among those who do not receive the intervention (i.e., $I = 0$ and $I \cdot F = 0$), the difference in expected outcome between men and women with otherwise similar risk factors is b_1. Among men (for whom $F = 0$ and $I \cdot F = 0$) the intervention adds c to the expected outcome; among women the intervention increases the expected outcome by $c + d$. The model is thus able to capture the possibility that the intervention may affect women and men by different amounts.

The model parameters—a, the b_j values, and c—are estimated from the data to make the predicted values, denoted by Y_i [which estimates $E(Y_i)$], as "close" as possible to the actual values, the Y_i values. Specifically, in ordinary least squares (OLS) regression, the "closest fit" is the one that minimizes the sum of the squared deviations (errors) between observed outcomes and predicted. That is, the OLS estimates are those that produce a set of Y_i values that minimize $\Sigma_i[Y_i - Y_i]^2$.

Associated with each parameter estimate is a 95% confidence interval (an interval that includes the "true" but unknown value of the parameter with probability 0.95) and a p value. A p value of, for example, 0.01 can be interpreted as follows: if the intervention really had zero effect on the outcome, then observed effects at least as large as the one we did observe would occur in under 1% of studies similar to this one. A common convention is to say that a p value less than 0.05 indicates a "statistically significant" effect. However, it is better to state p values explicitly, as in "this effect is statistically significant at the $p = 0.01$ level." In very small studies, even large observed effects may have nonstatistically significant p values (e.g., >0.05). On the other hand, if the sample size is very large, even very small effects can be highly statistically significant. Hence, it is also of value to consider whether the size of an effect is "clinically significant" (66).

Having estimated parameters to find the best fitting model, it is natural to ask how predictions compare to actual values. The most common summary measure of "goodness-of-fit" when predicting a continuous outcome is R^2, defined as

$$R^2 = 1 - \left\{\sum_i [Y_i - Y_i]^2 / \sum_i (Y_i - \overline{Y})^2\right\},$$

where $\overline{Y}$ is the average of all the Y_i values. $R^2 \cdot 100$ is often described as the percentage of the total variability in the outcome variable that is explained by differences in risk among cases used to build the model. Shwartz and Ash (67) discuss many issues to be considered when interpreting R^2 values.

B. Modeling Dichotomous Outcomes

Logistic regression is standard for modeling a dichotomous outcome. Here, the dependent variable is the "log of the odds" of an event of interest (e.g., being alive 30 days after hospital admission). If p_i is the probability of the event for the ith person, then the odds of the event for that person, O_i, is $p_i/(1 - p_i)$. A logistic regression model for assessing treatment effectiveness is

$$\ln O_i = \ln[p_i/(1 - p_i] = a + \sum_j b_j X_{ij} + c \cdot I,$$

where "ln" represents the natural (base "e") logarithm. Thus, the log odds of a person being alive increases by c when the intervention is present. The model can be rewritten as

$$O_i = e^{a + \Sigma_j b_j X_{ij} + c \cdot I} = e^{a + \Sigma_j b_j X_{ij}} \cdot e^{c \cdot I},$$

illustrating that the effect of the intervention is to multiply the odds of the event by e^c (a quantity that equals 1 when $c = 0$). An alternative interpretation is that e^c equals the odds of the event for a person with the intervention divided by the odds of the event for a person with similar risk factors who does not receive the intervention, a quantity referred to as the odds ratio (OR) for the event, given the treatment. Notice that the functional form of the model assumes that the effect is the same for all people, regardless of their characteristics. It is straightforward to compute the probability of the event from the odds:

$$p_i = O_i/(1 + O_i).$$

Model parameters are estimated using a maximum likelihood procedure—that is, coefficients are selected that maximize the likelihood of observing the data that actually were observed (technically, that maximize the likelihood function). Issues in specifying the relationships of independent variables to the log odds of the outcome are very similar to those in specifying the relationship of independent variables to a continuous outcome. As in the case of OLS multiple regression, 95% confidence intervals and p values are routinely computed for each parameter estimate.

The c statistic (68) is the most commonly reported summary measure of model performance when predicting a dichotomous outcome. One of several equivalent definitions of the c statistic is the following. Consider all pairs of cases such that one experiences the event and one does not. The c statistic is the proportion of all such pairs in which the predicted probability of the event based on the model is higher for the patient who experiences the event. Ash and Shwartz (69) discuss a range of issues related to evaluating the performance of models to predict a dichotomous outcome. Ash and Shwartz (70) also discuss the value of using R^2 as a measure of model performance with a dichotomous outcome.

C. Modeling Survival Time

When duration of survival is the outcome, we must consider the common situation in which not all cases are followed until death. Some are lost to follow-up and others are still alive when the study ends. Thus, for some patients, the time of death is known; for others, we only know that they were still alive at a particular time, but their actual time of death is unknown or "censored." The Cox proportional hazards model is standard for modeling survival data with censoring (71).

Survival time modeling relies on the fact that the probability that an event (e.g., death) occurs in a small interval of time (t to $t + \Delta t$) is the product of two probabilities: one, the probability that death does not occur prior to time t, and two, the conditional probability that a person who has survived until time t then dies prior to $t + \Delta t$. This latter probability is called a hazard rate. For example, consider 100 patients alive at time 0. In the first 6 months, 40 patients die. In the next week after the 6 months, 6 more patients die. The probability of surviving 6 months is 0.6 and the hazard rate at 6 months (for $\Delta = 1$ week) is 0.10 (6/60) per week, the probability of death during the next week among those 60 patients who make it to the start of the week. The product of the two probabilities ($0.6 \cdot 0.10 = 0.06$) is the observed probability of death in the interval 6 months to 6 months and 1 week.

The dependent variable in the Cox proportional hazard model is the "instantaneous" hazard rate at time t (i.e., the limit of the hazard rate in the interval t to $t + \Delta t$ as Δ shrinks to zero), denoted by $h(t)$. This is expressed as a function of some baseline hazard [$h_0(t)$, treated as a nuisance parameter] and other independent variables of interest. The model is as follows:

$$h(t) = h_0(t) \cdot e^{a + \Sigma_j b_j X_{ij} + c \cdot I} = h_0(t) \cdot e^{a + \Sigma_j b_j X_{ij}} \cdot e^{c \cdot I} = h_0(t) e^a e^{b_1 X_{i1}} e^{b_2 X_{i2}} \ldots e^{c \cdot I}.$$

The main assumption in this simple version of the model is that each independent variable affects the baseline hazard by a multiple that is the same for all patients regardless of their other characteristics and at all times t. In particular, the effect of the intervention on the hazard rate is multiplication by e^c. However, with many surgical interventions, patients experience a higher hazard perioperatively, but a lower hazard later. More complex time-dependent models are needed in this situation.

In proportional hazard models, as in logistic regression models, maximum likelihood procedures are used to produce model parameter estimates, 95% confidence intervals, and p values. From the hazard rates, survival functions (which plot the predicted probability of surviving different amounts of time) can be calculated and shown for patients with specific characteristics. There is no standard measure of model performance for the Cox proportional hazard model (72).

V. Incorporating Risk in Multivariate Models

Many books describe techniques for building and validating multivariate models [e.g., for multiple regression, (73–75), for logistic regression (76), and for survival time data (77, 78)]. In what follows, we briefly discuss a few issues particularly relevant to building models for risk adjustment.

First, a combination of clinical judgment and empiric modeling building is likely to result in models that make sense to clinicians (have face validity) and predict well in new data sets (are generalizable). Clinicians are best able to identify variables likely to be important, to suggest tentative hypothesis about the nature of relationships, and to suggest interactions that might be important. Further, they can identify relationships from empiric modeling that are not credible.

In developing the Medicare Mortality Prediction System (MMPS), a few of the clinical variables included in the models added little to predictive ability but were judged clinically important by the expert clinical panels (e.g., presence of positive blood cultures in pneumonia). Likewise, some variables that were removed from the model had predictive value, but the relationship contradicted clinical logic [e.g., in AMI, an elevated aspartate aminotransferase (formerly named serum glutamic oxalacetic transaminase) level was associated with a decreased likelihood of death] (9). In developing the RAND "sickness at admission" model, variables were rated 1, 2, 3, and 4 by clinicians (prior to looking at the data) based on the expected strength of their association with poor outcomes. Variables in the final model were strong predictors of outcomes (t statistic > 2.5, implying a p value of about 0.01) regardless of *a priori* judgments, medium predictors (t statistic > 2, implying a p value of about 0.05) with a clinical score of 1 or 2, or weak predictors ($t > 1.5$, implying a p value of about 0.13) if there was high face validity for clinicians (a clinical score of 3 or 4) (28).

Before analysis, data cleaning is important. This involves identifying values that are not plausible (such as a temperature of 102°C), identifying impossible occurrences (female patients admitted for prostate surgery), finding invalid data elements (e.g., illegal ICD-9-CM codes), and assessing frequencies of missing or poorly specified variables. Checking relationships between variables can also be important. Is systolic blood pressure always higher than diastolic pressure? Is the most extreme value during the first 24 hr of admission always higher (or lower) than the first recorded value?

Missing values require thought. In general, values that are missing for many patients are not good candidates for use in risk adjustment. But even variables that are routinely monitored, e.g., acute physiologic parameters, are sometimes missing. How best to handle such values depends on clinical context. Often, it is reasonable to substitute normal values for ones that are missing (9).

Sometimes missing values may be related to practice patterns. For example, among cerebrovascular disease cases at least one serum chemistry test used in the APACHE II severity system was missing in 2% of major teaching hospital cases, 10% of other teaching hospital cases, and 28% of nonteaching hospital cases (34), despite the comparability of cases across hospital types. Likewise, the availability of preoperative electrocardiograms (ECGs) depends on patient age and risk and hospital policies concerning the use of routine preoperative ECGs. Also, although functional status may be very predictive of outcomes, up to a third of patients may not have even a simple measure of functional status, such as ability to ambulate independently, recorded in their chart, even in the nursing notes (9).

Most statistical packages routinely drop cases with any missing values. Thus, if many predictors are used and the problem of missing values has not been addressed, a substantial fraction of cases likely will be eliminated from the analysis. This is undesirable because then models are fit to an unrepresentative subset of patients—those with no missing values.

Sophisticated statistical approaches for dealing with missing data elements exist. Though none of these are yet in common use in health services research, "multiple imputation" is beginning to be used to account properly for the greater variance associated with replacing missing values with imputed values (79, 80). The idea behind this approach is that rather than simply analyzing a single data set in which missing values have been replaced with imputed values and treated no differently than if they were real values, a small number of data sets (typically 3 to 5) are generated, each of which has different imputed values for the missing data elements. Imputed values are determined by random selection from estimated probability distributions for the missing variables, distributions that may depend on the values of the nonmissing variables. Multiple imputation analyzes the multiple data sets to obtain a single set of parameter estimates and standard errors that are appropriately inflated to reflect the contribution of having substituted for missing values. Much more common than any of the more sophisticated approaches, however, is to simply impute a single normal value for each missing data element, an approach used in both the APACHE III system (6) and the MMPS (9).

When there are many potential explanatory variables, model simplification is likely to be beneficial. Models that rely on too many variables typically "fit" the data set used for model development well, but predict less well when applied to new data (81).

In building a multivariate model, one first assembles a list of potential explanatory variables and then retains a subset of these variables that captures most of the stable explanatory power present in the larger set. The larger the sample size n, the larger the number of explanatory variables that can be considered. There is no exact relationship between n and k, the maximum number of potential explanatory variables whose relationship to the outcome can be explored reliably. However, modeling with fewer than $n = 10k$ observations is practically guaranteed to be unstable; n should probably be more like $20k$. With a dichotomous outcome, empirical modeling requires even larger samples. We recommend about 20 occurrences of the outcome for each potential predictor. For example, with $n = 10{,}000$ patients and a 2% problem rate (i.e., 200 occurrences of the outcome), it is reasonable to consider models with about 10 explanatory variables.

If an explanatory variable is "not very variable," it may not be a good predictor. For example, an indicator or dummy variable for a disease that is present for only 10 people is unlikely to be useful, no matter how large n is. If several variables each relate to "the same concept," such as compromised nutritional health, it is probably better to retain a single variable (such as a nutritional scale) that summarizes that concept than to retain each of the variables individually. Principal components or factor analysis, which create groups of highly correlated variables, might be of value in developing a composite of individual variables (68).

In seeking to pare down a long list of potential predictors, it is wisest to start with a list generated by "clinical wisdom," including variables identified by searching the literature. Variables that are statistically significantly related to the outcome (in bivariate analyses) are usually added to this list before empirical modeling is used to identify a final subset of important predictors. Empirical, clinical, and policy knowledge can all contribute when finalizing the multivariate model. Each retained variable should have independent explanatory power, its contribution to the model should make sense to clinicians, and the information needed to calculate it should be reliably available across the range of settings for which the model will be used. Many of the issues in building and validating multivariate models for risk adjustment to assess interventions are similar to those in other subject area domains. The references cited herein are to books that can provide guidance.

VI. Approaches for Improved Estimates of Treatment Effectiveness in Nonexperimental Studies: The Propensity Score and Instrumental Variables

Multivariate models will correctly adjust for differences in baseline risk between a study and a control group if (1) the important risk factors are measured and (2) the relationships between risk factors and the outcome of interest are correctly specified in the model. However, it is difficult to measure all important risk factors and to be sure that relationships are correctly specified (e.g., that there really is a linear relationship between a particular risk factor and the outcome). One should be particularly cautious about the validity of results from multivariate models when measured characteristics differ substantially between those who do and do not receive an intervention.

The first situation we consider assumes that all risk factors have been measured. The concern in this case in whether we have correctly specified the relationships between risk factors and the outcome. If risk factors have a strong relationship to the outcome and if risk factors are distributed very differently in the study and the control groups, model misspecification can lead to errors in estimating the effect of treatment.

If there are only a few important risk factors, one approach is to examine separately the effect of the intervention in each risk stratum. This eliminates the need to model the relationship between risk and the outcome. For example, if age and gender are the only two risk factors considered important, one might compare the outcome of those with and without the intervention separately by gender for each 10-year age category. However, with several risk factors, many of the strata may have too few cases for meaningful analysis. In what follows, we illustrate an approach—the propensity score—that reduces the need for a correctly specified model (82–85).

The second situation arises when important *unmeasured* risk factors are distributed differently for patients with and without the intervention. We illustrate the use of an instrumental variable to assess treatment effectiveness in the presence of such factors. Winship and Morgan (86) place both of these approaches in the more general framework of estimating causal effects from observational data.

A. The Propensity Score

We hypothesize a simple scenario to illustrate both the problem that can result from model misspecification and a "fix" for the problem. Assume that in a population of patients, there is a risk score (which may be derived from many individual risk factors) that varies uniformly between 0 and 2, i.e., a randomly selected person is equally likely to have any value between 0 and 2. Without treatment, we assume that the outcome is a number between 0 (worst outcome) and 10 (best) and is a decreasing function of risk. Specifically, we hypothesize the following relationship, where R denotes risk:

$$\text{outcome} = 1 - [e^{5\cdot(R-1)}/(1 + e^{5\cdot(R-1)})]\cdot 10. \quad (1)$$

Figure 1 is a plot of the relationship between outcome and risk.

We also assume that higher risk patients are more likely to be selected for treatment, leading to an imbalance in risk between the treated and control groups. In particular, we specify that the probability of being selected for treatment is

$$\text{probability of treatment} = e^{3\cdot(R-1)}/(1 + e^{3\cdot(R-1)}). \quad (2)$$

Figure 2 is a plot of the relationship between the probability of being selected for treatment and risk.

Finally, we assume that treatment increases each patient's outcome by 2. Our interest is in how well we are able to estimate this effect using standard analytic techniques.

We simulate a sample of 100 patients as follows:

1. For each patient, we select a random number between 0 and 2 from a uniform probability distribution (i.e., each number has an equally likely chance of selection) to be the patient's risk score, R.
2. Given R, we calculate the outcome from Eq. (1) and p = probability of treatment from Eq. (2).
3. We then use a random number generator to assign the patient to the treatment (with probability p) or the control group. If the patient is treated, 2 is added to outcome as computed in Eq. (1).

In the simulated sample, 49 patients receive the treatment. The average risk of the cases (those receiving treatment) is 1.36, over twice as high as the average risk of the controls, 0.64. As a result of the much higher risk of the cases, their average outcome (even though it is 2 higher than if they were not treated) is only 4.4, compared to 7.6 for the controls. Thus, a naive comparison that does not adjust for risk differences incorrectly suggests that treatment is harmful.

If the relationship between the risk score and the expected value of an outcome is correctly specified [e.g., as in Eq. (1)], then standard regression modeling techniques will estimate the treatment effect without bias. However, in most practical situations, particularly with many risk factors, we do not know the true relationship between the risk factors and the outcome. If the relationship is misspecified, then the standard analysis can lead to incorrect estimates of treatment effectiveness. To illustrate, assume that in our example the following model is fit to the data:

$$\text{expected (outcome)} = a + b \cdot R + \mathrm{c} \cdot \mathrm{I},$$

where R indicates the risk score and I is an indicator variable, which is 1 if the patient receives treatment and 0 otherwise. In the simulated sample, the coefficient c is calculated as 1.3, indicating that treatment increases the outcome by 1.3 units. As we know, the true impact of treatment is to increase the outcome 2.0 units. As a result of model misspecification (assuming a linear relationship between risk and the outcome when the relationship is nonlinear), we underestimate the effect of treatment. In 46 out of 50 simulated samples, the coefficient associated with treatment was below 2.0 (the mean coefficient was 1.7), illustrating the bias in this example toward underestimating treatment effectiveness.

Propensity score methods can be used to address concerns about model misspecification in the presence of risk factor imbalance by creating groups of treated and untreated

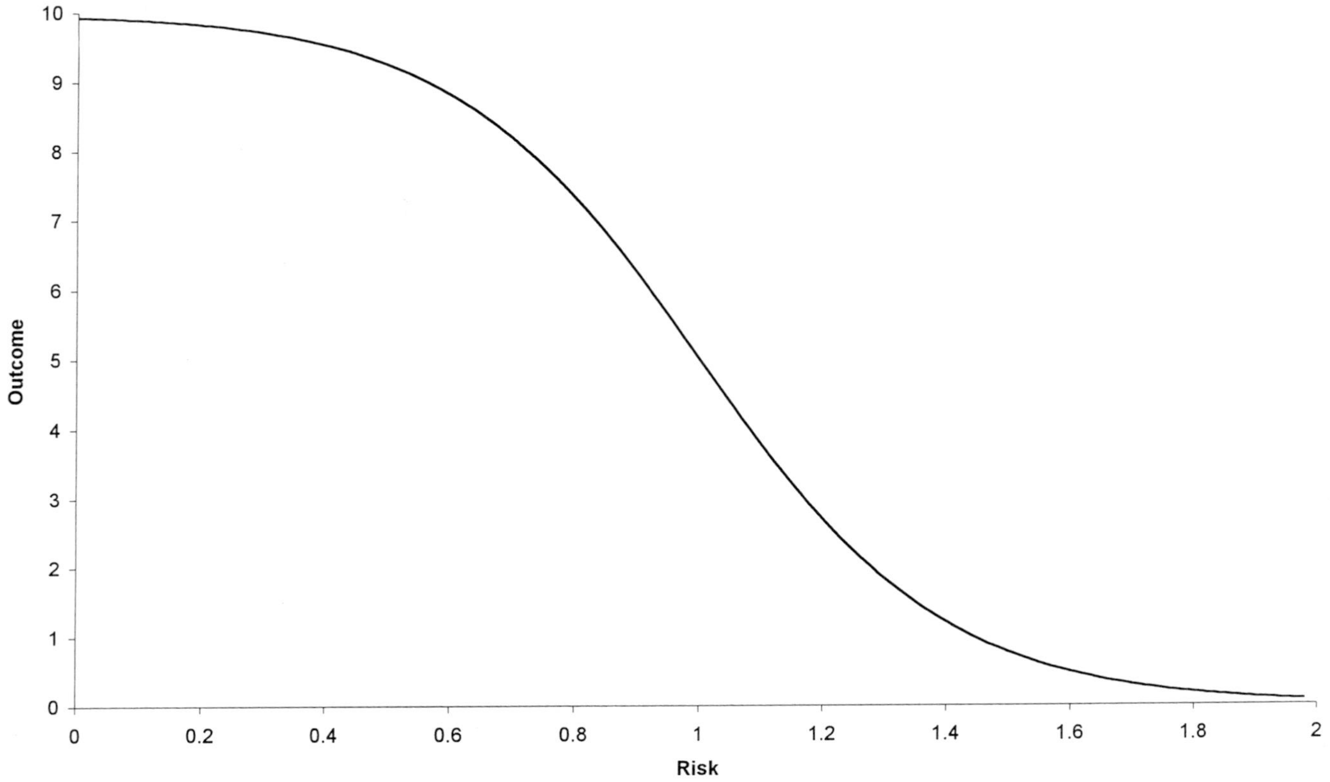

Figure 1 Relationship between risk and outcome.

patients that are more balanced in terms of measured risk factors (82–85). We illustrate one way of doing this, subsampling within propensity score category.

First, we fit a model to predict the probability of receiving treatment. The independent variables in this model could be any factors related to the likelihood of receiving treatment, although typically the same variables used for risk adjustment are used in this model. The model-predicted probability of receiving treatment is called the "propensity score." Groups of cases with similar propensity scores tend to have similar distributions across a range of the risk factors. In our example, suppose we (incorrectly) model the propensity score, PS (i.e., the probability of receiving treatment) as

$$\mathrm{PS} = a + b \cdot \mathrm{R}.$$

Figure 3 shows the propensity scores for cases (top line) and controls (bottom line). Notice that there are just a few treated cases with low propensity scores and a few untreated cases with high propensity scores. However, some cases do "look like" controls and some controls are like cases. There are 12 cases with propensity scores less than about 0.7, each of which can be matched to a control with a nearly similar propensity score, and there are 3 controls with a propensity score greater than 0.7 that can be matched with cases with a nearly similar propensity score. The result is a subset of 15 cases and 15 controls with closely matched propensity scores. In this subsample, the average risk score for the cases is 0.80 and for the controls, 0.81. When the (incorrectly specified) multiple regression model is fit to the subsample of 30 cases, c is correctly estimated as 0.20.

The propensity score approach reduces the need to "correctly" model the relationship between risk and outcome because the cases and controls that are used in the analysis are relatively similar in terms of the risk factors by which cases typically differ from controls. In our simple example, we could have subsampled cases based on risk score rather than propensity score. However, when there are several risk factors, the propensity score allows for matching along a single dimension in order to achieve approximate balance on each of the risk factors.

We used propensity score matching to compare outcomes for two modalities available to people seeking substance abuse detoxification through the publicly funded treatment system in Boston, Massachusetts: (1) acupuncture, which consists of daily acupuncture sessions during the acute

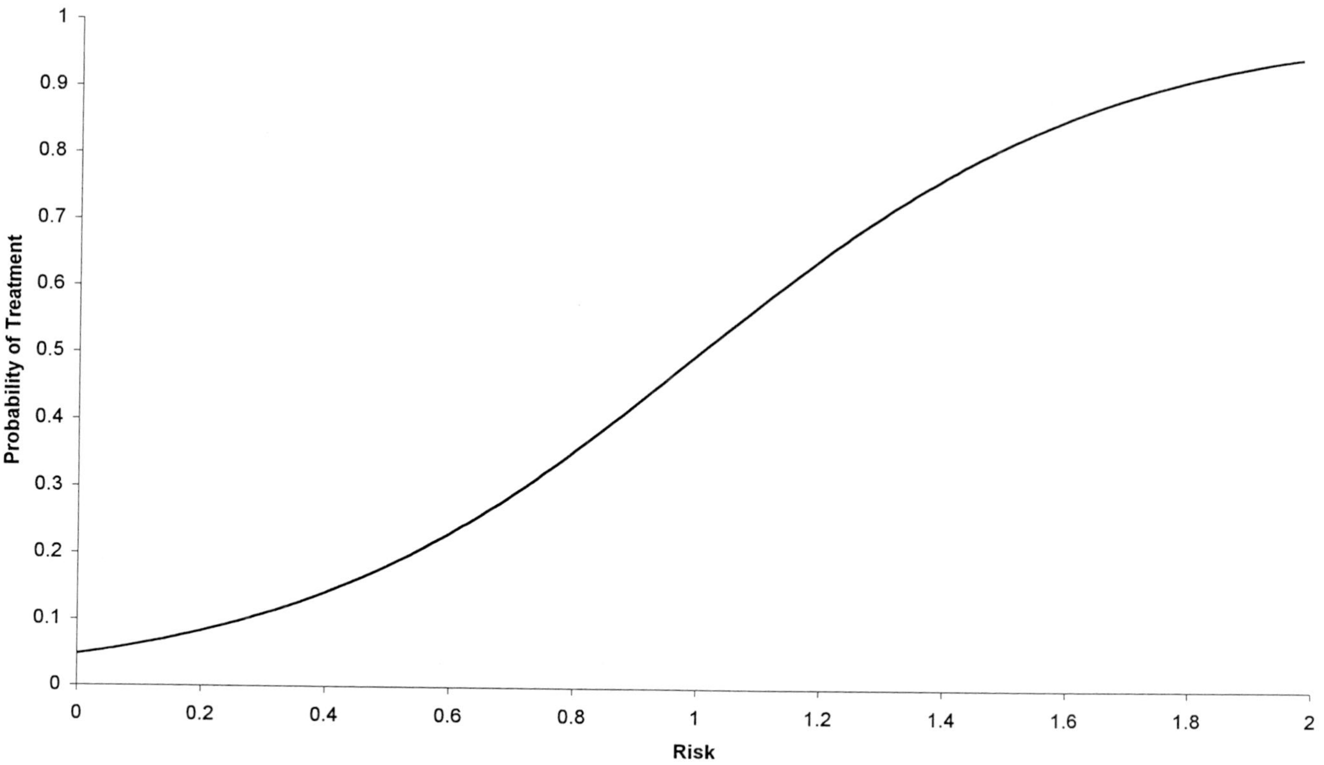

Figure 2 Relationship between risk and probability of treatment.

detoxification phase and then sessions 2 to 3 times per week (sessions include, in addition to acupuncture, maintenance and motivational counseling, usually in a group setting) for 3 to 6 months; and (2) residential detoxification, which lasts approximately 1 week, with encouragement on discharge to seek postdetox treatment (87).

Acupuncture clients were very different, and typically "better off" at baseline than those who received residential detox. For example, 13% of acupuncture patients, but only 4% of residential detox patients, were college graduates; 57% vs. 13% were employed; 15% vs. 3% had private insurance; 76% vs. 55% lived with others; 3% vs. 30% lived in a shelter; and 19% vs. 43% had previous detox admissions in the year prior to the index admission. Out of 1104 acupuncture cases and 6907 residential detox controls, we found 740 cases and 740 controls that could be matched on propensity score. These groups were largely balanced in terms of risk factors. For example, 7% of both types of patients were college graduates; 42% of acupuncture patients vs. 41% of residential detox patients were employed; 6% vs. 9% had private insurance; 77% vs. 72% lived with others; 4% vs. 5% lived in a shelter; 26% vs. 27% had previous detox admissions in the past year. In this particular example, the effectiveness of acupuncture as measured by 6-month readmissions for detox was relatively similar when the analysis was performed on the full sample (OR 0.71; 95% confidence interval 0.53–0.95) and the subsample matched on propensity score (OR 0.61; 95% confidence interval 0.39–0.94). This is because the original model fit to the full sample of cases had extremely good predictive power (*c* statistic 0.96), leaving little room for model misspecification.

Propensity score matching was used in a study of right heart catheterization [RHC, also called pulmonary artery (PA) catheterization], believed by many physicians to be necessary to guide therapy for certain critically ill patients. The widespread feeling that use of RHC is beneficial made it impossible to complete a randomized controlled trial of this procedure. Connors *et al.* (2) used the propensity score approach to examine the benefit of RHC during the first 24 hr of care in the ICU. The 38% of patients who received RHC within 24 hr in the ICU differed substantially from those not receiving RHC: they were more likely to be male; to have private insurance; to enter the study with acute respiratory failure, multiple organ system failure, congestive heart failure, or cancer; to have do-not-resuscitate orders within the first 24 hr of hospitalization; to have more abnor-

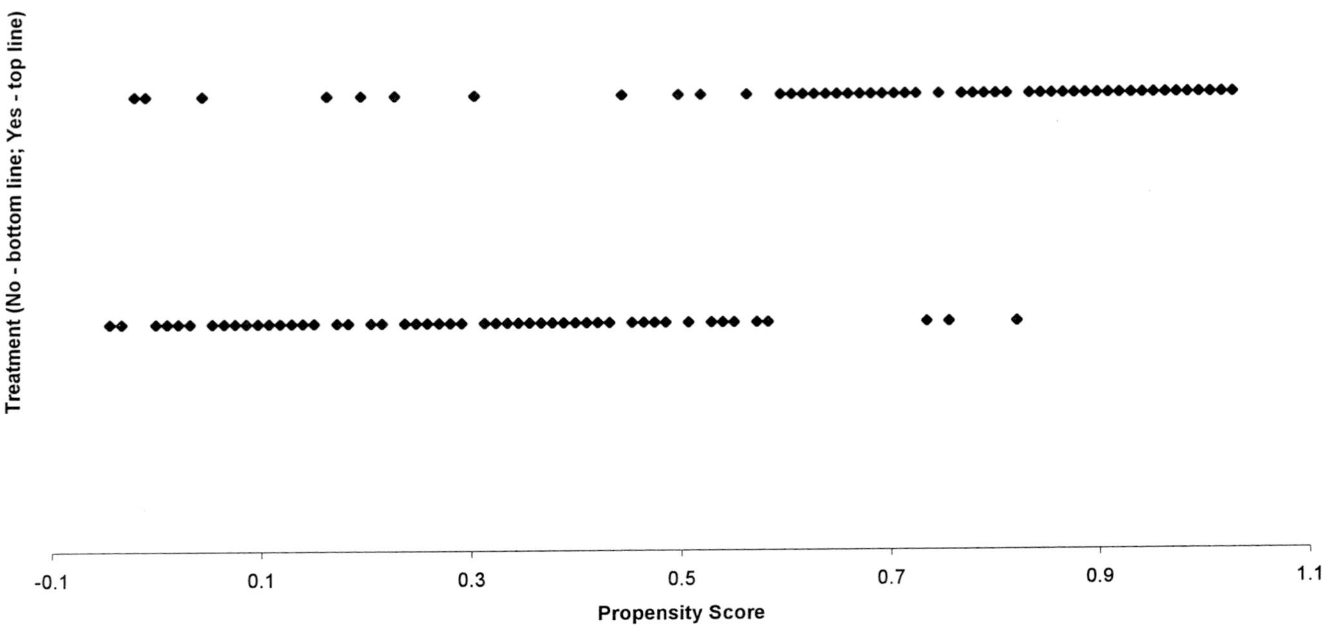

Figure 3 Relationship between propensity score and treatment status.

mal vital signs; and to have higher APACHE III scores and lower predicted probability of 2-month survival. They were also less likely to be over age 80 and had fewer comorbid conditions. Among 2184 patients receiving RHC and 3551 not receiving RHC, 1008 RHC patients were matched on propensity score with 1008 non-RHC patients. Risk factors were similar in the two subsampled groups. For the matched subsample, 30-, 60-, and 180-day survival was consistently worse for those receiving RHC. Dalen and Bone (88), in reviewing this study, felt "that these data clearly indicate that the higher mortality rate of patients receiving PA catheters cannot be explained by the fact that they were sicker."

An alternative to selecting matched samples based on the propensity score is to compare outcomes separately for those with and without the intervention within propensity score categories. Commonly, the propensity score is divided into quintiles (81), and the outcomes are compared for patients in the same propensity score quintile. This approach, to the extent that there are adequate numbers of both cases and controls within each quintile, allows for study of the possibility that the intervention's impact differs for people with different risk factors. Cooper *et al.* (89) used this approach to examine the value of upper endoscopy in an observational study of patients with upper gastrointestinal hemorrhage.

B. Instrumental Variables

Standard multivariate modeling and the propensity score are powerful tools for distinguishing the effect of an intervention from the effects of differential risk. However, they can still yield misleading results if some risk factors that strongly affect outcomes are unevenly distributed between cases and controls and are not available as predictors. Instrumental variables, a technique with some history in econometrics (90) but fairly new in health services research, is an approach for assessing effectiveness in the presence of unmeasured risk factors. We illustrate the method with a simple example.

Assume that a person with a particular medical condition can either have a "good" outcome or not, and that "I" is an intervention for treatment of the condition, which some people receive and some do not. Let $P(G)$ equal the probability of a good outcome and $P(I)$ equal the probability that a person receives the intervention. Assume a risk factor R that is not observed, but affects both $P(G)$ and $P(I)$. Further, assume a variable V that is associated with $P(I)$ but not with $P(G)$. Then V is called an "instrument" for studying the effect of the intervention on the probability of a good outcome. An example of an instrumental variable is the distance a patient lives from a hospital offering a particular type of treatment. Patients who live close to hospitals offering the treatment are more likely to receive it than are patients who live far from such hospitals. However, if unmeasured risk factors are distributed similarly for those who live close and those who live far from such hospitals, then the difference in patient outcomes is due only to the difference in the likelihood of receiving the treatment, not to differences in baseline risk.

Assume the following:

1. Half the patients are high risk (denoted by R) and half are not (denoted by $\sim R$).

2. Higher risk patients are more likely to receive the intervention. Specifically, for high-risk patients,

$$P(\mathrm{I}) = 0.8 \qquad (\text{i.e.,} \quad P(\mathrm{I} \mid R) = 0.8);$$

for others,

$$P(\mathrm{I}) = 0.2 \qquad (\text{i.e.,} \quad P(\mathrm{I} \mid \sim R) = 0.2);$$

Note: $P(\mathrm{I} \mid R)$ is read as "the probability of the intervention for a high-risk person."

3. Higher risk patients have worse outcomes. Specifically, for patients not receiving the intervention (i.e., ~I), if they are high risk,

$$P(\mathrm{G}) = 0.3 \qquad (\text{i.e.,} \quad P(\mathrm{G} \mid R, \sim\mathrm{I}) = 0.3);$$

for others,

$$P(\mathrm{G}) = 0.7 \qquad (\text{i.e.,} \quad P(\mathrm{G})\mid \sim R, \sim\mathrm{I}) = 0.7).$$

4. The intervention is somewhat helpful for low-risk patients, but more helpful for those at high risk. Specifically, for high-risk patients, the intervention increases the probability of a good outcome by 0.2, i.e., $P(\mathrm{G} \mid R, \mathrm{I}) = 0.5$; for others, the intervention increases the probability of a good outcome by 0.1, i.e., $P(\mathrm{G} \mid \sim R, \mathrm{I}) = 0.8$.

Assume 1000 patients are distributed by risk status and by whether they receive the intervention as follows:

	~*R*	*R*	Total
I	200	800	1000
~I	800	200	1000
Total	1000	1000	2000

By applying the probability of a good outcome to each risk/intervention category, we can calculate the number of patients expected to have a good outcome. Thus, among the 200 patients in category (~*R*, I), 160 (or 80%) will have a good outcome; among the 800 in category (*R*, I), 400 (50%) will have a good outcome. In total, 560 of 1000 patients who receive the intervention will have a good outcome, compared to 620 of 1000 patients who do not receive the intervention ($620 = 800 \cdot 0.7 + 200 \cdot 0.3$). Although the intervention improves outcomes, a simple comparison suggests that the intervention reduces the chances of a good outcome by 0.06 (from 0.62 to 0.56). As in our earlier example, the reason is "selection bias." Those at higher risk are both more likely to receive the intervention, and more likely to have a poor outcome. However, in the current example, we have assumed that the risk factor is not observed, and thus we cannot directly adjust for risk factor differences in our analysis.

Consider as our instrument information about the distance a patient lives from a hospital that offers the intervention. Assume that one-half of the patients live close and one-half live far, and that the distribution of risk factors does not depend on place of residence. Specifically, we assume the following distribution of the 2000 patients by risk and place of residence:

	Close	Far
R	500	500
~*R*	500	500

We will also assume that the effect of distance on the likelihood of receiving the intervention is larger for lower risk patients, as follows: Among high-risk patients, 70% of those who live far will receive the intervention [i.e., $P(\mathrm{I} \mid R, \text{far}) = 0.7$], rising to 90% for those who live close [i.e., $P(\mathrm{I} \mid R, \text{close}) = 0.9$]. Among low-risk patients, none of those who live far will receive the intervention [i.e., $P(\mathrm{I} \mid \sim R, \text{far}) = 0.0$], although 40% of those who live close do [i.e., $P(\mathrm{I} \mid \sim R, \text{close}) = 0.4$]

To further develop the example, we apply the probabilities of receiving the intervention to the distance/risk categories above to calculate the distribution of patients who receive the intervention. For example, of the 500 patients in the (close, *R*) category, 450 will receive the intervention and 50 will not. Continuing in this manner, we get the following numbers of patients by intervention status, place of residence, and risk:

	Close			Far		
	I	~I	Total	I	~I	Total
R	450	50	500	350	150	500
~*R*	200	300	500	0	500	500
Total	650	350	1000	350	650	1000

Remember, only the "Total" row in the above table is observed. Note that 65% of those who live close will receive the intervention versus only 35% of those who live far. Because unmeasured risk factors are assumed to be the same in each location group, differences in outcomes between those who live close and those who live far are due to the higher proportion of those receiving treatment in the close group.

Within each location category, we use our hypothesized probability of a good outcome in each risk/intervention category to determine the expected number of cases with a good outcome. For example, 50% of the 450 cases who live close and are in the (R, I) category and 50% of the 350 cases who live far and are in (R, I) will have a good outcome. This leads to the numbers 225 and 175 in the following table, which shows the number of patients with good outcomes by risk category and distance.

	Close			Far		
	I	~I	Total	I	~I	Total
R	225	15	240	175	45	220
~*R*	160	210	370	0	350	350
Total	385	225	610	175	395	570

Again, only the bottom row of this table is observed. From the bottom row of the previous table, we know that patients who live close more frequently get the intervention (650/1000 vs. 350/1000). From the bottom row of this table, we know that patients who live close more frequently have good outcomes (610/1000 vs. 570/1000). Because we assumed that underlying risk is the same for patients who live close and far, the better outcomes for nearby patients must be due to their higher rate of getting the intervention.

Effectiveness of the intervention is estimated as the ratio of the difference in the likelihood of a good outcome by location to the difference in the likelihood of receiving the intervention by location, or

$$\begin{aligned}\text{Effectiveness} &= [P(\text{G} \mid \text{close}) - P(\text{G} \mid \text{far})]/\\ &\quad [P(\text{I} \mid \text{close}) - P(\text{I} \mid \text{far})]\\ &= (0.610 - 0.570) / (0.650 - 0.350)\\ &= 40/300\\ &= 0.133.\end{aligned}$$

Associated with a change in the percentage of patients receiving the intervention from 35 to 65%, the chance of a good outcome increased by 0.04, which is an increase of 0.133 for each additional patient receiving the intervention. Note that we cannot conclude that the effect of the intervention is an increase in the probability of a good outcome of 0.133 for each additional patient, but rather that 0.133 is the average effect among patients whose treatment decision is affected by location.

Recall that among those at high risk, the intervention increased the likelihood of a good outcome by 0.2; among others, the intervention increased the likelihood of a good outcome by 0.1. Because half the cases were in each risk category, the true average effect of the intervention in the entire group of patients was 0.15, whereas our estimate of effectiveness from the instrumental variable analysis was 0.133. This lower estimate of effect reflects the particular mix of high- and low-risk patients in the group whose treatment decision is affected by location. In particular, because we constructed the example so that location has less impact on the decision to treat for high-risk patients, the estimated effect from the instrumental variable analysis is weighted toward the lower risk patients, for whom we postulated that the intervention is less effective.

A key assumption in our analysis was that the distribution of risk factors was similar across different values of the instrumental variable. For example, we assumed that 50% of the cases were high risk among both those who lived close to and those who lived far from hospitals offering the intervention. Results of an instrumental variable analysis can be very sensitive to this assumption. Suppose that (unknown to us) patients who live closer to the intervention hospitals really are sicker than those who live far away. For example, suppose 70% of the patients who live close are high risk versus only 30% of the patients who live far, but that all other assumptions remain the same. The instrumental variable analysis then yields an estimate of treatment effectiveness of −0.12, a seriously misleading finding.

Not only is the assumption of similarity in risk factors for different values of the instrument at the core of the validity of the analysis, it is an assumption that is not directly testable. That is because instrumental variables are used precisely when risk factors are not measured. In most practical situations, there are some measured risk factors and some unmeasured risk factors. To the extent that observable risk factors are distributed similarly across values of the instrument, it provides some confidence that unmeasured risk factors might be similarly distributed.

In more complex situations, a two-stage estimation procedure is used to estimate an intervention's effect. To illustrate, let RO be an observed risk factor, RU be an unobserved risk factor, and V be the instrument. In stage one, we predict the probability of the intervention, pred(I), as

$$\text{pred(I)} = a + b \cdot \text{RO} + c \cdot \text{V}.$$

In the second stage, we predict the probability of a good outcome as

$$\text{pred(G)} = d + e \cdot \text{RO} + f \cdot \text{pred (I)}.$$

The coefficient f is a measure of treatment effectiveness (comparable to the 0.133 we calculated above). Most statistical packages include two-stage model fitting for the situation in which the outcome is a continuous variable (as opposed to our example in which the outcome is dichotomous). When this is not the case, specialized techniques are needed (e.g., maximum-likelihood algorithms might be used to obtain unbiased estimates of parameters and correct standard errors).

A key report by McClellan *et al.* (91), stimulating interest in the use of instrumental variables to assess a healthcare intervention, motivated our example here. They wrote (p.859) that differential distances to hospitals that offer more intensive treatments for patients with AMI

> ... *approximately randomize patients to different likelihoods of receiving intensive treatments. Comparisons of patient groups that differ only in distances to source of intensive treatment suggest that the impact on mortality at 1 to 4 years after AMI of the incremental use of invasive procedures in Medicare patients was at most 5 percentage points; this gain was achieved during the first day of hospitalization and therefore appears attributable to treatments other than the procedures.*

Though instrumental variables offer the potential to assess interventions in the presence of unmeasured risk factors, the inability to test empirically the main assumption on which the validity of the approach rests, and the sensitivity of conclusions to violations of the assumption, suggest caution in its application.

VII. Conclusions

Despite the acknowledged value of randomized controlled trials, much of what we can infer about the clinical effectiveness of surgical interventions and procedures will come from nonexperimental studies. A major problem in such studies is that patient characteristics that are strongly related to treatment outcomes are often different for those receiving the intervention versus those not. It is important to both measure and adjust for these differences in risk factors when assessing effectiveness.

In the first part of this chapter, we described dimensions of risk that are related to a variety of outcomes—age; gender; race and ethnicity; acute clinical stability; severity of principal diagnosis; extent and severity of comorbidities; physical functional status; psychological, cognitive, and psychosocial functioning; socioeconomic status; and health status and quality of life. In any practical situation, it is unlikely that adequate measures for all dimensions of risk will be available. However, the list provides a guidepost for assessing the adequacy of the risk adjustment performed and the extent to which unmeasured risk factors may be contributing to potentially misleading findings.

Multivariate models are used to adjust for risk differences when assessing treatment effectiveness. We have illustrated the standard models for three widely used types of outcomes. In each case, some function of the outcome is modeled as a linear function of risk factors plus the intervention, thus allowing the effect of the intervention to be quantified after controlling for risk. In the case of a continuous outcome (e.g., length of hospital stay, cost), we predict the expected value of the outcome itself; in the case of a dichotomous outcome (e.g., death within 30 days), we predict the log of the odds of the outcome; in the case of survival time (for which time of death of those still alive at the end of the study is censored), we estimate the hazard rate.

Risk adjustment through multivariate models yields an unbiased estimate of treatment effect when all important risk factors have been measured and the relationship between risk and outcome is correctly specified. However, we rarely feel confident that these conditions are satisfied. If they are not, imbalances in risk between intervention and nonintervention groups can distort our perception of treatment effect. The propensity score is useful for dealing with imbalances when important measured risk factors differ between the treatment and control group. Because the analysis is conducted on subgroups with relatively similar risk factors, concerns about inadequate adjustment for differences in risk are much reduced. Instrumental variables have potential in situations in which important risk factors have not been measured. However, the sensitivity of conclusions to assumptions that are not empirically testable may limit the applicability of this approach.

References

1. Abel, U., and Koch, A. (1999). The role of randomization in clinical studies: Myths and beliefs. *J. Clin. Epidemiol.* **52**, 487–497.
2. Connors, A. F., Speroff, T., Dawson, N. V., *et al.* (1996). The effectiveness of right heart catheterization in the initial care of critically ill patients. *JAMA* **276**, 889–897.
3. Wennberg, D. E., Lucas, F. L., Birkmeyer, J. D., *et al.* (1998). Variation in carotid endarterectomy mortality in the Medicare population: Trial hospitals, volume and patient characteristics. *JAMA* **279**, 1278–1281.
4. Concato, J., Horwitz, R. I., Feinstein, A. R., *et al.* (1992) Problems of comorbidity in mortality after prostatectomy. *JAMA* **267**, 1077–1082.
5. Iezzoni, L. I. (1997). Dimensions of risk. *In* "Risk Adjustment for Measuring Healthcare Outcomes," 2nd Ed. Health Administration Press, Chicago.
6. Knaus, W. A., Wagner, D. P., Draper, E. A., *et al.* (1991). The APACHE III prognostic system: Risk prediction of hospital mortality for critically ill hospitalized adults. *Chest* **100**, 1619–1636.
7. Le Gall, J. R., Lemeshow S., and Saulnier, F. (1993). A new simplified acute physiology score (SAPS II) based on a European/North American multicenter study. *JAMA* **270**, 2957–2963.
8. Cleveland, W. S. (1979). Robust locally weighted regression and smoothing scatterplots. *J. Am. Stat. Assoc.* **74**, 829–836.
9. Daley, J., Jencks, S., Draper, D., *et al.* (1988). Predicting hospital-associated mortality for Medicare patients. A method for patients with stroke, pneumonia, acute myocardial infarction, and congestive heart failure. *JAMA* **260**, 3617–3624.
10. Weintraub, W. S., Craver J. M., Cohen C. L., *et al.* (1991). Influence of age on results of coronary artery surgery. *Circulation* **84** (Suppl. III), III-226–III-235.
11. Ayanian J. Z., and Epstein, A. M. (1991). Differences in the use of procedures between women and men hospitalized for coronary heart disease. *N. Engl. J. Med.* **325**, 221–225.
12. Udvarhelyi, I. S., Gatsonis, C., Epstein, A. M., *et al.* (1992). Acute myocardial infarction in the Medicare population: Process of care and clinical outcomes. *JAMA* **268**, 2530–2536.
13. Jacobs, A. K., Kelsey S. F., Brooks, M. M., *et al.* (1998). Better outcomes for women compared with men undergoing coronary revascu-

larization: A report from the bypass angioplasty revascularization investigation (BARI). *Circulation* **98**, 1279–1285.

14. LaVeist, T. A. (1994). Beyond dummy variables and sample selection: What health services researchers ought to know about race as a variable. *Health Serv. Res.* **29**, 1–16.
15. Williams, D. R. (1996). Race/ethnicity and socioeconomic status: Measurements and methodological issues. *Int. J. Health Serv.* **26**, 483–505.
16. Wenneker, M. B., and Epstein, A. M. (1989). Racial inequalities in the use of procedures for patients with ischemic heart disease in Massachusetts. *JAMA* **261**, 253–257.
17. Ayanian, J. Z., Udvarhelyi, I. S., Gatsonis, C. A., *et al.* (1993). Racial differences in the use of revascularization procedures after coronary angiography. *JAMA* **269**, 2642–2646.
18. McBean, A. M., and Gornick, M. (1994). Differences by race in the rates of procedures performed in hospitals for Medicare beneficiaries. *Health Care Financ. Rev.* **15**, 77–90.
19. Knaus, W. A., Zimmerman, J. E., Wagner, D. P. *et al.* (1981). APACHE—Acute physiology and chronic health evaluation: A physiologically based classification system. *Crit. Care Med.* **9**, 591–597.
20. Knaus, W. A., Draper, E. A., Wagner, D. P., and Zimmerman, J. E. (1985). APACHE II: A severity of disease classification system. *Crit. Care Med.* **13**, 818–829.
21. German, P. M., and Lowenstein, S. (1984). A research paradigm for severity of illness: Issues for the Diagnosis-Related Group system. *Health Care Financ. Rev.* (Annual Suppl.), 79–90.
22. Iezzoni, L. I. (1997). Risk and outcomes. *In* "Risk Adjustment for Measuring Healthcare Outcomes," 2nd Ed. Health Administration Press, Chicago.
23. Charlson, M. E., Pompei, P., Ales, K. L., and MacKenzie, C. R. (1987). A new method of classifying prognostic comorbidity in longitudinal studies: Development and validation. *J. Chronic Dis.* **40**, 373–383.
24. Krousel-Wood, M. A., Abdoh, A., and Re, R. (1996). Comparing comorbid-illness indices assessing outcome variation: The case of prostatectomy. *J. Gen. Intern. Med.* **11**, 32–38.
25. Deyo, R. A., Cherkin, D. C., and Ciol, M. A. (1992). Adapting a clinical comorbidity index for use with ICD-9-CM administrative databases. *J. Clin. Epidemiol.* **45**, 613–619.
26. Greenfield, S. G., Aronow, H. U., Elashoff, R. M., and Watanabe, D. (1988). Flaws in mortality data: The hazards of ignoring comorbid disease. *JAMA* **260**, 2253–2255.
27. Greenfield, S. G., Apolone, G., McNeil, B. J., and Cleary, P. D. (1993). The importance of co-existent disease in the occurrence of postoperative complications and one-year recovery in patients undergoing total hip replacement. Comorbidity and outcomes after hip replacement. *Med. Care* **31**, 141–154.
28. Keeler, E. B., Kahn, K. L., Draper, D., *et al.* (1990). Changes in sickness at admission following the introduction of the prospective payment system. *JAMA* **264**, 1962–1968.
29. Cullen, D. J., Apolone, G., Greenfield, S., *et al.* (1994). ASA physical status and age predict morbidity after three surgical procedures. *Ann. Surg.* **220**, 3–9.
30. McDowell, I., and Newell, C. (1987). "Measuring Health: A Guide to Rating Scales and Questionnaires." Oxford Univ. Press, New York.
31. Rubenstein, L. V., Calkins, D. R., Greenfield, S., *et al.* (1989). Health status assessment for elderly patients. Report of the society of general internal medicine task force on health assessment. *J. Am. Geriatr. Soc.* **37**, 562–569.
32. Spector, W. D. (1990). Functional disability scales. *In* "Quality of Life Assessments in Clinical Trials" (B. Spilker, ed.), Raven Press, New York.
33. Applegate, W. B., Blass, J. P., and Williams, T. F. (1990). Instruments for the functional assessments of older patients. *N. Engl. J. Med.* **322**, 1207–1214.
34. Iezzoni, L. I., Shwartz, M., Burnside, S., *et al.* (1989). "Diagnostic Mix, Illness Severity, and Costs at Teaching and Nonteaching Hospitals," National Technical Information Service (PB 89 184675/AS). U.S. Department of Commerce, Springfield, VA.
35. Davis, R. B., Iezzoni, L. I., Phillips, R. S., *et al.* (1995). Predicting in-hospital mortality. The importance of functional status information. *Med. Care* **33**, 906–920.
36. McHorney, C. A., Ware, J. E., Lu, J. F., and Sherbourne, C. D. (1994). The MOS 36-item short-form health survey (SF-36): III. Test of data quality, scaling assumptions, and reliability across diverse patient groups. *Med. Care* **32**, 40–66.
37. Weinberger, M., Oddone, E. Z., Samsa, G. P., and Landsman, P. B. (1996). Are health-related quality-of-life measures affected by the mode of administration? *J. Clin. Epidemiol.* **49**, 135–140.
38. Case, R. B., Moss, A. J., Case, N., *et al.* (1992). Living alone after myocardial infarction: Impact on prognosis. *JAMA* **267**, 515–519.
39. Williams, R. B., Barefoot, J. C., Califf, R. M., *et al.* (1992). Prognostic importance of social and economic resources among medically treated patients with angiographically documented coronary artery disease. *JAMA* **267**, 520–524.
40. Starfield, B. (1992). Effects of poverty on health status. *Bull. N.Y. Acad. Med.* **68**, 17–24.
41. Lohr, K., ed. (1989). Advances in health status assessment, conference proceedings. *Med. Care* **27** (Suppl.), S1–S294.
42. Lohr, K., (ed.) (1992). Advances in health status assessment: Fostering the application of health status measures in clinical settings: Proceedings of a conference. *Med. Care* **30** (Suppl.) MS1–MS293.
43. Stewart, A. L., and Ware, J. E., eds. (1992). "Measuring Functioning and Well-Being: The Medical Outcomes Study Approach." Duke Univ. Press, Durham.
44. Guyatt, G. H., Feeney, D. H., and Patrick, D. L. (1993). Measuring health-related quality of life. *Ann. Intern. Med.* **118**, 622–629.
45. Ware, J. E., Jr. (1995). The status of health assessment 1994. *Annu. Rev. Public Health* **16**, 327–354.
46. Streiner, D. L., and Norman, G. R. (1995). "Health Status Measurement Scales. A Practical Guide to Their Development and Use," 2nd Ed. Oxford Univ. Press, Oxford.
47. Gill, T. M., and Feinstein, A. R. (1994). A critical appraisal of the quality of quality-of-life measurements. *JAMA* **272**, 619–626.
48. Connell, F. A., Diehr, P., and Hart, L. G. (1987). The use of large data bases in health care studies. *Annu. Rev. Public Health* **8**, 51–74.
49. Wennberg, J. E., Roos, N., Sola, L., *et al.* (1987). Use of claims data systems to evaluate health care outcomes: Mortality and reoperation following prostatectomy. *JAMA* **257**, 933–936.
50. Anderson, G. E., Steinberg, E. P., Whittle, J., *et al.* (1990). Development of clinical and economic prognoses from Medicare claims data. *JAMA* **263**, 967–972.
51. Center for Evaluative Studies, Dartmouth Medical School. (1996). "The Dartmouth Atlas of Health Care." American Hospital Association, Chicago.
52. Sullivan, L. W., and Wilensky, G. R. (1991). "Medicare Hospital Mortality Information. 1987, 1988, 1989." U.S. Department of Health and Human Services, Health Care Financing Administration, Washington, D.C.
53. Lave, J. R., Pashos, C. L., Anderson, G. F., *et al.* (1994). Costing medical care: Using administrative data. *Med. Care* **32**, JS77–JS89.
54. Mitchell, J. B., Bubolz, T., Paul, J. E., *et al.* (1994). Using Medicare claims for outcomes research. *Med. Care* **32**, JS38–JS51.
55. Office of Technology Assessment, U.S. Congress (OTA). (1994). "Identifying Health Technologies That Work: Searching for Evidence." OTA-H-608. U.S. Government Printing Office, Washington, D.C.
56. Anderson, R. E., Hill, R. B., and Key, C. R. (1989). The sensitivity and specificity of clinical diagnostics during five decades: Toward an understanding of necessary fallibility. *JAMA* **261**, 1610–1617.
57. Calkins, D. R., Rubenstein, L. V., Cleary, P. D., *et al.* (1991). Failure of physicians to recognize functional disability in ambulatory patients. *Ann. Intern. Med.* **114**, 451–454.

58. Eddy, D. M. (1984). Variations in physician practice: The role of uncertainty. *Health Aff.* **3**, 74–89.
59. Starfield, B. D., Steinwachs, D., Morris, I., *et al.* (1979). Concordance between medical records and observations regarding information on coordination of care. *Med. Care* **17**, 758–766.
60. Romm, F. J., and Putnam, M. (1981). The validity of the medical record. *Med. Care* **19**, 310–315.
61. Kosecoff, J., Fink, A., Brook, R. H., and Chassin, M. R. (1987). The appropriateness of using a medical procedure: Is information in the medical record valid? *Med. Care* **25**, 196–201.
62. Feigl, P., Glaefke, G., Ford, L., *et al.* (1988). Studying patterns of cancer care: How useful is the medical record? *Am. J. Public Health* **78**, 526–533.
63. Khuri, S. F., Daley, J., Henderson, W., *et al.* (1997). Risk adjustment of the postoperative mortality rate for the comparative assessment of the quality of surgical care: Results of the national veterans affairs surgical risk study. *J. Am. Coll. Surg.* **185**, 315–327.
64. Hannan, E. L., Kilburn, H., Jr., O'Donnell, J. F., *et al.* (1990). Adult open heart surgery in New York State: An analysis of risk factors and hospital mortality rates. *JAMA* **264**, 2768–2774.
65. Hannan, E. L., Siu, A. L., Kumar, D., *et al.* (1995). The decline in coronary artery bypass graft surgery mortality in New York State. The role of surgical volume. *JAMA* **273**, 209–213.
66. Deyo, R. A., and Patrick, D. L. (1995). The significance of treatment effects: The clinical perspective. *Med. Care* **33**, AS286–AS291.
67. Shwartz, M., and Ash, A. S. (1997). Evaluating the performance of risk-adjustment methods: Continuous outcomes. *In* "Risk Adjustment for Measuring Healthcare Outcomes," 2nd Ed. Health Administration Press, Chicago.
68. Harrell, F. E., Jr., Lee, K. L., Califf, R. M., *et al.* (1984). Regression modeling strategies for improved prognostic prediction. *Stat. Med.* **3**, 143–152.
69. Ash, A. S. and Shwartz, M. (1997). Evaluating the performance of risk-adjustment methods: Dichotomous outcomes. *In* "Risk Adjustment for Measuring Healthcare Outcomes," 2nd Ed. Health Administration Press, Chicago.
70. Ash, A. S., and Shwartz, M. (1999). R^2: A useful measure of model performance for predicting a dichotomous outcome. *Stat. Med.* **18**, 375–384.
71. Cox, D. R. (1972). Regression models and life-tables. *J. R. Stat. Soc. B* **34**, 187–220.
72. Henderson, R. (1995). Problems and prediction in survival-data analysis. *Stat. Med.* **14**, 161–184.
73. Kleinbaum, D. G., Kupper, L. L., and Muller, K. E. (1988). "Applied Regression Analysis and Other Multivariate Methods," 2nd Ed. Duxbury Press, Pacific Grove, CA.
74. Neter, J., Wasserman, W., and Kutner, M. H. (1990). "Applied Linear Statistical Models: Regression, Analysis of Variance, and Experimental Design," 3rd Ed. Irwin, Chicago.
75. Draper, N. R., and Smith, H. (1998). "Applied Regression Analysis," 3rd Ed. John Wiley & Sons, New York.
76. Hosmer, D. W., and Lemeshow, S. (1989). "Applied Logistic Regression." John Wiley & Sons, New York.
77. Lee, E. T. (1992). "Statistical Methods for Survival Data Analysis," 2nd Ed. John Wiley & Sons, New York.
78. Collett, D. (1994). "Modelling Survival Data in Medical Research." Chapman & Hall, London.
79. Rubin, D. B. (1987). "Multiple Imputation for Nonresponse in Surveys." John Wiley & Sons, New York.
80. Rubin, D. B. (1993). Tasks in statistical inference for studying variation in medicine. *Med. Care* **31** (Suppl.), YS103–YS110.
81. Iezzoni, L. I., Ash, A. S., Coffman, G. A., and Moskowitz, M. A. (1992). Predicting in-hospital mortality. A comparison of severity measurement approaches. *Med. Care* **30,** 347–359.
82. Rosenbaum, P. R., and Rubin, D. B. (1983). The central role of the propensity score in observational studies of causal effect. *Biometrika* **76,** 41–55.
83. Rosenbaum, P. R., and Rubin, D. B. (1984). Reducing bias in observational studies using subclassification on the propensity score. *J. Am. Stat. Assoc.* **79,** 516–524.
84. Rosenbaum, P. R., and Rubin, D. B. (1985). Constructing a control group using multivariate matched sampling methods that incorporate the propensity score. *Am. Stat.* **39,** 33–38.
85. Rubin, D. B., and Thomas, N. (1996). Matching using estimated propensity scores: Relating theory to practice. *Biometrics* **52,** 249–264.
86. Winship, C., and Morgan, S. L. (1999). The estimation of causal effects from observational data. *Annu. Rev. Sociol.* **25,** 659–707.
87. Shwartz, M., Saitz, R., Mulvey, K., and Brannigan P. (1999). The value of acupuncture detoxification programs in a substance abuse treatment system. *J. Subst. Abuse Treat.* **17,** 305–312
88. Dalen, J. E., and Bone, R. C. (1996). Is it time to pull the pulmonary artery catheter? *JAMA* **276,** 916–918.
89. Cooper, G. S., Chak, A., Connors, A. F., *et al.* (1998). The effectiveness of early endoscopy for upper gastrointestinal hemorrhage: A community-based analysis. *Med. Care* **36,** 462–474.
90. Bowden, R. J., and Turkington, D. A. (1984). "Instrumental Variables." Cambridge Univ. Press, Cambridge.
91. McClellan, M., McNeil, B. J., and Newhouse, J. P. (1994). Does more intensive treatment of acute myocardial infarction in the elderly reduce mortality? Analysis using instrumental variables. *JAMA* **272,** 859–866.

11

Measuring Surgical Outcomes

Jean Y. Liu and John D. Birkmeyer

VA Outcomes Group, VA Medical Center, White River Junction, Vermont 05009

I. Introduction

There is increasing recognition that clinical research aimed at assessing the effectiveness of surgical interventions must consider their effects on patient quality of life. Intermediate outcomes (biologic or physiologic measures) and traditional clinical endpoints (morbidity and mortality) are clearly not sufficient for evaluating the increasing array of procedures whose primary purpose is to improve patient well-being. Although biologic or physiologic measures provide information to clinicians, they are of limited use to patients and often correlate poorly with functional ability and well-being. Researchers assessing the effectiveness of these procedures must therefore consider more "patient-centered" outcome measures. How are patients affected physically, mentally, or emotionally by surgery (or their disease)? How do patients value different health outcomes? How satisfied are they with their treatment decisions?

In this chapter, we review different tools and methodologic approaches to evaluating aspects of quality of life. We first review survey instruments available for assessing general health status, with specific emphasis on the Medical Outcomes Study short forms (SF-36 and modifications) (1, 2). We then discuss approaches to assess the effects of disabilities (e.g., activities of daily living) (3) and then address other instruments available for specific research needs, including tools for measuring pain and symptom scores for specific disease processes. Third, we review approaches to quantifying patient preferences (utility assessment), which, among other purposes, is necessary for calculating quality-adjusted life years (QALYs) for economic evaluation of surgical procedures. Finally, we review current approaches to assessing patient satisfaction with treatment.

II. Generic Measures of Health Status

A. General Considerations

Life has two dimensions: quantity and quality (4, 5). Measures of quantity of life (operative mortality, overall or disease-specific mortality, life expectancy, etc.) are standard features of most clinical research protocols assessing surgical interventions. Quality of life refers to how well people live. In the broadest sense, quality of life encompasses not only health, but standard of living, quality of housing, job satisfaction, and numerous other factors (6). However, medical researchers generally limit assessments to health-related quality of life (HRQOL) (7). According to the World Health Organization, health is defined as a "state of complete physical, mental, and social well-being and not merely the absence of disease or infirmity" (8). This definition implies the "dimensionality" of HRQOL and, in particular, the distinction between physical and mental components.

General health status surveys provide the broadest and most generalizable measures of HRQOL. They may be used for a variety of purposes. At the patient level, general health surveys are being used increasingly to detect problems with patient functioning or well-being usually missed during standard clinical encounters. In this context, the surveys have been described as the "new laboratory tests of medical practice" (7). General health surveys are also being used to assess and monitor the health status of populations. For example, the National Health Interview Surveys track aspects of HRQOL in the United States as U.S. Vital Statistics tracks mortality and life expectancy (9). At the population level, surveys are useful for evaluating the effects of specific changes in healthcare policy or reimbursement. For example, the Health Insurance Experiment used SF-36 surveys to assess the health and quality of life implications of two cost-containment strategies—cost sharing in a fee-for-service system and a prepaid health maintenance organization (HMO)-type group practice (10). With both strategies, health status declined in poorer and sicker study participants. Such harmful effects would not have been detected by mortality or other less precise measures.

In this section, we focus on the use of general health status surveys for clinical research and trials—a use midway between individual patients and populations. In this context, results of general health surveys may be used as (1) independent variables (i.e., to establish the "baseline" health of control and intervention groups) or (2) outcome measures. We next describe the wide range of survey instruments currently available and their basic attributes.

B. Overview of General Health Status Surveys

General health status is most commonly assessed using survey instruments. Several well-tested and well-known health status surveys are currently available for use in clinical research (Table I). Details, summaries, and critiques of the different survey instruments are available elsewhere (4, 11–13).

Although their content varies widely, health surveys measure health in three broad dimensions: physical health, mental health, and personal evaluations of health in general. Measures of physical and mental health account for a large proportion (80–85%) of the variance observed in overall assessments of general health (14–16). Surveys contain questions exploring specific domains of physical and mental health. For example, questions pertaining to patient mobility and self-care would be included in the physical functioning domain; questions about depression, anxiety, and sense of well-being would be included in the psychological well-being domain.

Questions exploring the different domains of physical and mental health take several forms. Most surveys rely on questions with the Likert method of summated ratings of responses (17). For example, when testing patient difficulties in bathing, the question can have five different responses: no difficulty, slight difficulty, moderate difficulty, severe difficulty, or cannot do this at all. Others [e.g., Sickness Impact Profile (SIP) (18); sections of the McMaster's Health Index Questionnaire (19)] use primarily questions with dichotomous or "yes/no" questions. Finally, several surveys [e.g., Uniscale (20); sections of the EuroQOL (21)] test a continuum by incorporating questions based on visual analog scales, whereby patients are asked to grade their responses on a 10-cm linear scale. These scales are generally bounded by two health extremes: worst health/death and perfect health/not bothered at all.

In addition to their basic content, researchers should consider details related to survey administration. For example, some surveys can be completed independently by patients, whereas others require a trained interviewer (Table I). Another important consideration is the complexity and time required to complete the different surveys, which vary considerably. For example, the Quality of Life Uniscale consists of a single question about global health, assessed using a visual analog scale, and takes less than a minute to complete (20). Conversely, the SIP is a very comprehensive survey and is considered the "gold standard" by many (11, 22). Although the SIP provides very precise estimates of quality of life in a number of domains, it contains 136 questions and requires at least 20–30 min to complete and takes 10 min to score. In selecting a general health status survey, researchers must consider these trade-offs between ease of administration and data precision. The right "balance" will usually depend on the specific research context.

C. Scoring Survey Responses

Scoring survey responses can be complex and will vary widely by survey. In general, data from specific questions are aggregated by domains. One score is calculated for each domain (e.g., a bodily pain score). A series of domain scores for an individual patient comprises a health profile. In many surveys [e.g, SF-36 (1)], information from questions in multiple, related domains can be collapsed into a broader summary score (e.g., a physical health summary score). Finally, some surveys [e.g., Quality of Life index (20); Quality of Well-Being Scale (23)] provide a single, overall score (a health index score) reflecting responses to all questions in

Table I Content and Other Characteristics of Different Health Status Surveys[a]

Content	Quality of well-being scale (short) (23)	Sickness impact profile (18)	McMaster's health index questionnaire (19)	Quality of life index (20)	Quality of life uniscale (20)	Nottingham health profile (41)	EuroQOL (21)	Medical outcomes study short form-36 (1)
Domains assessed								
Physical functioning	+	+	+	+		+	+	+
Social functioning	+	+	+	+		+	+	+
Role functioning	+	+	+	+		+	+	+
Psychological distress		+				+	+	+
General health perceptions			+	+	+	+	+	+
Bodily pain		+		+		+	+	+
Energy/ fatigue	+					+		+
Psychological well-being				+				+
Sleep		+				+		
Congnitive functioning		+						+
Reported health transition			+					+
Survey characteristics								
Number of items	18	136	59	6	1	45	5	36
Administration: (I, interviewer; S, self)	I	S, I	S, I	S, I	S	S, I	S	S, I
Time to complete (min)	7	20–30	20	2	1	10–15		5–10
Score calculation (R, raw; W, weighted)	W	W	R	R	R	Mixed	W	W

[a]See reference literature (number in parentheses given with each type of survey) for full discussion of each survey.

the survey. The use of health index scores for economic evaluations is reviewed later in the chapter.

Regardless of the level at which they are aggregated, survey scores are either "raw" or "weighted." Raw scores are derived solely from the subject's responses to the survey questions. For example, the McMaster's Health Index Questionnaire uses raw scores to give a profile on physical, social, and emotional function (19). The first section contains yes/no questions, where a "yes" or "no difficulty" is given one point. The second and third sections are categorical questions that are similarly scored, with the higher score given for a higher level of function. For example, for patients who do not wear a hearing aid, the question reads: "Do you have trouble hearing in a normal conversation with several other persons?" (1 = never, 2 = sometimes, and 3 = always). If the answer is "never," one point will be scored for the physical dimension. A score is obtained simply by summing the points accumulated for questions in the given domain.

Most surveys, however, rely on more complex, weighted scoring. Here, responses to each survey question are weighted according to their relative importance in determining overall health. Survey weights are empirically derived from previous applications of the given instrument to different populations and must be obtained from the survey developers before scores may be calculated. With some surveys, investigators may select weights from a variety of populations, e.g., patients with the disease of interest or a broader, nonselected population. Among the best known of the weighted surveys of general health status is the SF-36, which we discuss next.

D. The Medical Outcomes Study Short-Form Survey (SF-36)

Among the best known general health surveys is the Medical Outcomes Study Short Form. We describe it here in more detail because it has become a standard tool for assessing baseline health status and/or outcomes in clinical trials involving surgical interventions. Describing the SF-36 is also useful for illustrating the basic content and approaches to scoring health status surveys in general.

The SF-36 originated from research by the Rand Corporation; it was intended for use in the Health Insurance Experiment/Medical Outcomes Study. The 36-item question survey, currently the most widely used, was derived from results of a larger 245-item questionnaire administered to 22,000 patients aged 14–61 years in the Medical Outcomes Study (see the reprint of SF-36 at the end of this chapter, following the reference list). Two versions of the SF-36 are currently available: the standard version assessing health status within the past 4 weeks and an acute version that refers to problems within the past week. The SF-12 is a shorter version that may also be used. Although less comprehensive, the shorter version retains reasonable psychometric properties. Questions selected for the SF-12 account for approximately 90% of the variability in overall health status scores (2, 24), although the SF-12 may be less precise than the 36-item version. Licensing, scoring software, and forms are solely distributed by QualityMetric, Inc. (http://qmetric.com) in Lincoln, RI.

The SF-36, which takes 5–10 min to complete, may be self-administered or used in a personal or telephone interview (25). Administration may be via a mailed survey whereby answers are circled and then entered into a computer for analysis or answers are recorded on a machine-readable scan sheet. For surveys administered on site, a computerized touch screen by which responses are recorded directly can also be used. The 36 questions are distributed across eight health domains: physical functioning (10 questions), role limitations (4), bodily pain (2), general health (5), emotional functioning (4), social functioning (2), role limitations due to emotional problems (3), mental health (5), and a single item on perceptions of health changes over the past 12 months. Typical questions take the form: "In general, would you say your health is: excellent, very good, good, fair, or poor?"

In scoring the SF-36, "subscale" scores are calculated for each of the eight domains, creating a health profile. Summary scores for physical and mental function, based on broader aggregations of survey questions, are also computed. Table II describes subscale and summary scores for patients with four common medical conditions. Unlike some other health status surveys, however, the SF-36 does not provide a single, "global" health index score.

Scores are usually obtained using software from QualityMetric, Inc. Among several alternative (but analogous) approaches to computing scores, responses to individual questions are scaled on an ordinal 0 (worst response) to 100 (best) scale. For example, with the questions pertaining to lifting or carrying groceries, "yes, limited a lot" would score a 0, "yes, limited a little" would score a 50, and "no, not limited at all" would score a 100. Similarly, five category response scales are weighted in steps of 25: 0, 25, 50, 75, 100. Subscale scores are calculated by averaging scores for each question in that domain (missing responses are most often ignored).

Weighted scores are computed using weights specific for age, sex, and (where applicable) 13 specific medical conditions (1). In the context of clinical research or trials, weighted SF-36 scores are useful for accounting for the specific characteristics of the study population(s). When enough patients are enrolled, weighted scores for a study population can be compared to national norms.

III. Specific Measures of Health Status

A. Assessing Disability

Because they were developed to be applied to broad groups of patients, general health status surveys, including the SF-36, are not optimal for measuring severe disability.

Table II Examples of Comparison Scores as Adjusted Mean Scores for SF-36, PCS, and MCS[a]

Scale	Hypertension	Congestive heart failure	Recent myocardial infarction	Diabetes, type II
SF-36 domains				
Physical function	78.3	59.5	72.4	74.4
Physical role limitation	65.9	46.3	50.6	63.3
Bodily pain	75.1	69.6	76.2	73.6
General health	66.8	50.2	61.6	59.2
Vitality/ emotional function	61.6	47.2	56.1	59.1
Social function	90.1	78.6	87.7	86.5
Emotional role limitation	79.9	69.0	73.0	80.6
Mental health	80.4	78.5	76.3	78.8
PCS	45.9	38.3	43.5	43.9
MCS	53.4	51.4	51.7	53.0

[a]PCS, Physical Composite Score; MCS, Mental Composite Score; see Ware *et al.* (42).

Tools for this purpose would be needed in research protocols involving the very elderly, patients with major functional or mental limitations (e.g., after major limb amputations or stroke), and institutionalized patients.

Measure of disability can be divided into two general categories: activities of daily living and instrumental activities of daily living. The most widely used scale to measure activities of daily living is the Activities of Daily Living (ADL) scale developed by Katz (3). Designed primarily for elderly or institutionalized patients, this scale can be self-administered or assessed by a healthcare worker. It summarizes the degree of independence in bathing, dressing, using the toilet, moving around the house, continence, and eating, which are considered primary biologic functions. Each function is scaled on a three-point scale ranging from complete dependence to independence. The survey is scored according to the number of functions associated with dependence.

The instrumental activities of daily living scales are generally analagous, but intended for patients living in a community setting (26). Among surveys of this general type, the Health Assessment Questionnaire considers the effect of disease in terms of death, disability, discomfort, side effects of treatment, and cost (27). The Functional Status Index focuses on measures of dependence, pain, and difficulty experienced in daily activities (28).

B. Disease-Specific Symptom Scores

Clinical trials involving surgical interventions usually require instruments that measure symptoms and quality of life specific to the clinical condition under study. General health status surveys have the advantage of generalizability and capture broadly the implications of a given disease on overall health. However, they often lack the sensitivity and precision necessary to assess clinically meaningful changes in how patients experience a single clinical condition. For example, in a trial of therapy for gastroesophageal reflux disease, responses to physical and mental components of the SF-36 survey would reflect all health-related symptoms of patients in the study, not just those attributable to reflux disease. Also, heartburn symptoms that are bothersome to patients may not be sufficient to produce large effects on overall health-related quality of life.

For these reasons, clinical trials examining therapy for specific conditions should measure outcomes using both a general health status instrument and a disease-specific symptom score (29–31). A large number of symptom classification scores have been developed and widely tested for various clinical conditions. We provide a few examples of commonly used surveys in Table III. Most can be easily adapted for use in clinical research protocols. For conditions for which such instruments are not available "off the shelf," investigators may need to develop their own survey tools. Guidelines for developing survey instruments are beyond the scope of this chapter, but can be found elsewhere (4, 11–13).

C. Measuring Pain

Measuring pain is an essential component of many clinical trials assessing surgical interventions. For some clinical conditions, pain may be the primary outcome measure (e.g., surgery for sciatica, thoracic outlet syndrome, or carpal tunnel compression). Measuring pain, particularly procedure-related pain, is obviously essential for evaluating new minimally invasive technologies intended to replace existing surgical procedures (e.g., laparoscopic herniorraphy).

The most commonly used instruments assess pain in a unidimensional (or global) sense. These tools are very simple and short. Although they generally consist of a single question, responses are captured in several different but related ways. With the Verbal Rating Scales, patients are asked to grade their current pain on an ordinal scale, e.g., 0 = no pain, 1 = some pain, 2 = considerable pain, and 3 = pain that could not be more severe (32). With the Numerical Rating Scale and Box Scale (33), patients are asked to indicate a number between 0 and 10 (sometimes 100) that best represents their pain, where 0 represents no pain and 10 represents the worst pain ever experienced. The Visual Analogue Scale [VAS (34)] is a modification of this general approach: patients make a mark on a continuous 10-cm line with "no pain" on one end and "worst pain" on the other. Among these global pain assessment instruments, the VAS is the most widely used. An example of written approaches is presented in Fig. 1.

Other available instruments measure pain in different dimensions. For example, the McGill Pain Questionnaire (MPQ) assesses pain in three dimensions: sensory, affective, and evaluative (35). In this written evaluation, patients are presented 20 sets of word descriptors, each containing up to six words per set. One word is chosen from sets pertaining to sensory (e.g., sharp, cutting, lacerating), affective (e.g., fearful, frightful, terrifying), and evaluative (e.g., annoying, troublesome, miserable, intense, unbearable) dimensions. Scoring is based on the specific words chosen. The Present Pain Intensity scale is included as a part of the MPQ and is a global assessment of pain. Similar survey instruments include the Brief Pain Inventory scales (36). Although these instruments provide more comprehensive information than do global pain assessments, they take longer to complete (approximately 10–15 min). Thus, these instruments are probably best reserved for research protocols in which pain is a primary outcome measure.

IV. Utilities

Utilities are quantitative expressions of patient preferences for a particular state of health. Although both reflect

Table III Examples of Commonly Used Specific Surveys by System

System	Scale	Ref.
Eye	Activities of Daily Vision Scale	43
	VF-14	44
	National Eye Institute Visual Function Questionnaire	45
Cancer	Karnofsky Performance Index	46
	Functional Living Index—Cancer	47
Neurologic status	Glasgow Coma Score	48
	Mini Mental Status Examination	49
	Stroke Unit Mental Status Examination	50
Heart	New York Heart Association Functional Classification Scale	51
	Canadian Cardiovascular Society Functional Classification for Angina Pectoris	52
Gastrointestinal	Gastroesophageal Reflux Disease Health-Related Quality of Life Scale	53
	Rand Surgical Conditions Battery—Hemorrhoids	54
	Inflammatory Bowel Disease Questionnaire	31
	Colorectal Cancer Quality of Life Interview	55
Genital–urinary	International Prostate Symptom Score	56
	International Index of Erectile Function	57
Musculoskeleton	Arthritis Impact Measurement Scales	58
	Clinical Back Pain Questionnaire	59
	Oswestry Disability Index	60
Pulmonary	Rose Dyspnea Questionnaire	61
	Asthma Quality of Life Questionnaire	62
	6- and 12-minute walking tests	63
	Stair climbing	64
Vascular	Varicose Veins Questionnaire	65
	Walking Impairment Questionnaire	66

"quality of life," utilities should be distinguished from measures of health status described earlier in this chapter, which generally describe how patients are affected by a given clinical condition, what they can and cannot do, etc. Instead, utilities reflect how patients feel about or how they value living in a specific state of health. Utilities are typically assessed on a scale from 0 (death or worst health imaginable) to 1 (best health).

Utilities are perhaps most important for trials that include economic evaluations, particularly cost-effectiveness analyses. Results of cost-effectiveness analyses are expressed in terms of cost per unit benefit. Benefits are most often measured in quality-adjusted life-years (QALYs), a single measure that reflects both quality and quantity of life implications of a given intervention (37). QALYs are calculated by multiplying length of time spent in a given health state by the utility associated with state. For example, 10 years of life with a stroke (utility 0.5, hypothetically) would be credited as 5.0 QALYs in the cost-effectiveness model.

Patient utilities may be measured using a variety of techniques (Fig. 2). With the simplest approach, the visual analog scale, patients simply mark an "X" on a continuous scale between 0 and 1. Many investigators instead use survey-based methods for obtaining utilities. For example, the EuroQOL (21) and Quality of Well-Being Scale (23) are designed to provide a health index score—a single, summary score scaled from 0 to 1.

The most accepted approaches to utility assessment involve "iterative" techniques. These methods generally involve asking patients to make a series of choices to identify at what point they are indifferent between two options. There are two commonly used iterative approaches. With the time trade-off method, for example, a patient might be asked whether he would prefer (a) 10 years in good health or (b) 20 years living with a disabling stroke. If he choose (a), the choice might be modified to (a) 15 years in good health or (b) 20 years living with a disabling stroke. This iterative process would continue until the patient was "indifferent" between the

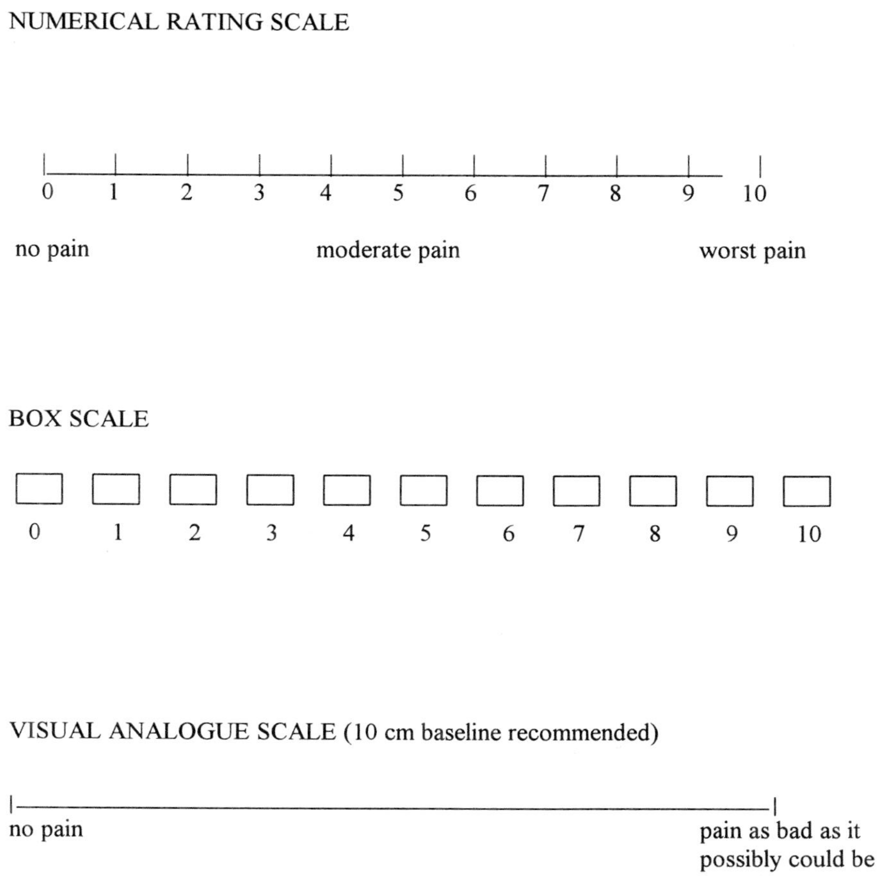

Figure 1 Methods of global assessment of pain.

two options, e.g., 12 years in good health was equivalent to 20 years living with a disabling stroke. In this case, his utility for stroke is the ratio of the two values: 12 / 20 = 0.6 (Fig. 2). With the standard gamble method, a patient is instead asked to choose between life with a specific condition and a gamble with variable probabilities of life without the condition and death. Several software packages are available for customized utility assessments using these iterative techniques.

Average utilities for a wide variety of clinical conditions or symptoms may also be obtained from the literature. One often-used "catalog" is the Beaver Dam study (38), a population-based study that describes utilities (by the Time Trade-Off method and Quality of Well-Being survey) for patients with a variety of common clinical conditions.

V. Patient Satisfaction

Patient satisfaction surveys assess what patients think about the actual healthcare or intervention, not the effects on an underlying disease process. Such assessments are most useful for trials comparing interventions believed to be associated with similar clinical outcomes, e.g., open versus laparoscopic appendectomy. In general terms, patient satisfaction surveys ask patients to judge their actual care against their underlying expectations. Each patient has an expectation of care from which actual care is judged: an ideal, a minimum expectation, an average of past experiences, or a sense of what one deserves (39). Relatively complex surveys assessing patient satisfaction in multiple dimensions have been developed for both office-based [e.g., Patient Satisfaction Questionnaire (40)] and inpatient care [e.g., Patient Judgements of Hospital Quality Questionnaire (40)]. However, for most surgical research protocols for which information about patient satisfaction is desired, a limited number of Likert-style questions will suffice—e.g., "How satisfied were you with your surgical procedure?" (not at all, somewhat satisfied, satisfied, or very satisfied). Alternatively, a visual analog scale specific to the intervention under study can be used.

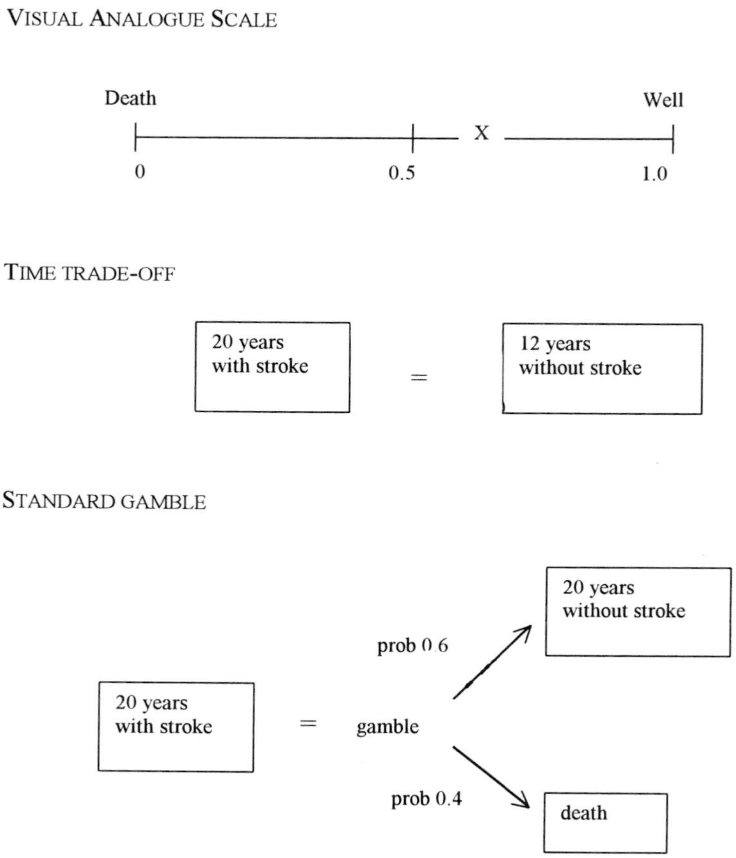

Figure 2 Three ways to measure or express a utility of 0.6 for a disabling stroke.

References

1. Ware, Jr., J. E., Snow, K. K., Kosinski, M., *et al.* (1993). "SF-36 Health Survey: Manual and Interpretation Guide." The Health Institute, New England Medical Center Hospitals, Boston.
2. Ware, Jr., J. E., Kosinski, M., and Keller, S. D. (1996). "SF-12: An even shorter health survey. *Med. Outcomes Trust Bull.* **2.**
3. Katz, S., Ford, A. B., Moskowitz, R. W., *et al.* (1963). Studies of illness in the aged: The index of ADL—A standardized measure of biological and psychosocial function. *JAMA* **185,** 914–919.
4. Patrick, D. L., and Rickson, P. (1993). "Health Status and Health Policy: Allocating Resources to Health Care." Oxford Univ. Press, New York.
5. Ware, Jr., J. E. (1992). "Measures for a New Era of Health Assessment." Duke Univ. Press, Durham, NC.
6. Campbell, A., Converse, P. E., and Rodgers, W. L. (1976). "The Quality of American Life: Perceptions, Evaluations, and Satisfaction." Russell Sage Foundation, New York.
7. Ware, Jr., J. E. (1995). "The Status of Health Assessment 1994." The Health Institute, New England Medical Center Hospitals, Boston.
8. World Health Organization (1948). World Health Organization constitution. *In* "World Health Organization, Basic Documents." WHO, Geneva.
9. National Center for Health Statistics (1996). Data file documentation, national health interview survey of topics related to the year 2000. Health objectives, 1992 [machine readable data file and documentation]. National Center for Health Statistics, Hyattsville, MD.
10. Patrick, D. L., Bush, J. W., and Chen, M. M. (1973). Methods for measuring levels of well-being for a health status index. *Health Serv. Res.* **8,** 229–234.
11. McDowell, I., and Newell, C. (1996). "Measuring Health: A Guide to Rating Scales and Questionnaires," 2nd Ed. Oxford Univ. Press, New York.
12. Bowling, A. (1995). "Measuring Disease." Open Univ. Press, Philadelphia.
13. Bowling A. (1997). "Measuring Health: A Review of Quality of Life Measurement Scales," 2nd Ed. Open Univ. Press, Philadelphia.
14. Hays, R. D., and Stewart, A. L. (1990). The structure of self-reported health in chronic disease patients. *Psychol. Assess. J. Consult. Clin. Psychol.* **2,** 22–30.
15. McHorney, C. A., Ware, J. E., and Raczek, A. E. (1993). The MOS 36-Item Short-Form Health Status Survey (SF-36): II. Psychometric and clinical tests of validity in measuring physical and mental health constructs. *Med. Care* **31,** 247–263.
16. Ware, Jr., J. E., Koniski, K., Bayliss, M. S., McHorney, C. A., Rogers, W. H., *et al.* (1995). Comparison of methods for the scoring and statistical analysis of SF-36 health profiles and summary measures: Results from the Medical Outcomes Study. *Med. Care* **33**(4), 264–279.

17. Likert, R. (1952). A technique for the development of attitude scales. *Educ. psychol. meas.* **12,** 313–315.
18. Bergner, M., Bobbitt, R. A., Kressel, S., Pollard, W. E., Gilson, B. S., *et al.* (1981). The Sickness Impact Profile: Development and final revision of a health status measure. *Med. Care* **19,** 787–805.
19. Chamber, L. W. (1984). The McMaster Health Index Questionnaire. *In* "Assessment of Quality of Life in Clinical Trials of Cardiovascular Therapies (N.K. Wenger, M.E. Mattson, C.D. Furberg, and J. Elinson, eds.). Le Jacq, New York.
20. Spitzer, W. O., Dobson, A. J., Hall, J., Chesterman, E., Levi, J., *et al.* (1981). Measuring the quality of life of cancer patients: A concise QL-index for use by physicians. *J. Chronic Dis.* **34,** 585–597.
21. EuroQOL group (1990). EuroQOL—A new facility for the measurement of health-related quality of life. *Health Policy* **16,** 199–208.
22. DeBruin, A. F., DeWitte, L. P., Stevens, F., *et al.* (1992). Sickness Impact Profile: The state of the art of a generic functional status measure. *Soc. Sci. Med.* **35,** 1003–1014.
23. Kaplan, R. M., and Anderson, J. P. (1988). "The Quality of Well-Being Scale: Rational for a Single Quality of Life Index." MTP Press, Lancaster.
24. Ware, Jr., J. E., Kosinski, M., and Keller, S. D. (1996). A 12-item short-form health survey construction of scales and preliminary tests of reliability and validity. *Med. Care* **34,** 220–233.
25. McHorney, C. A., Kosinski, M., and Ware, Jr., J. E. (1994). Comparison of the costs and quality of norms for the SF-36 health survey collected by mail versus telephone interview: Results from a national survey. *Med. Care* **32,** 551–567.
26. Fillenbaum, G. G. (1985). Screening the elderly: A brief instrumental activities of daily living measure. *J. Am. Geriatr. Soc.* **33,** 698–706.
27. Fries, J. F., Spitz, P. W., and Young, D. Y. (1982). The dimensions of health outcomes: The Health Assessment Questionnaire, disability and pain scales. *J. Rheumatol.* **9,** 789–793.
28. Jette, A. M. (1980). Functional capacity evaluation: An empirical approach. *Arch. Phys. Med. Rehabil.* **61,** 85–89.
29. Juniper, E. F., Guyatt, G. H., Epstein, R. S., Ferrie, P., Jaeschke, R., and Hiller, T. (1992). Evaluation of impairment of health related quality of life in asthma: Development of a questionnaire for use in clinical trials. *Thorax* **47,** 76–83.
30. Guyatt, G. H., Berman, L. B., Townsend, M., Pugsley, S. O., and Chambers, L. W. (1987). A measure of quality of life for clinical trials in chronic lung disease. *Thorax* **42,** 773–778.
31. Guyatt, G. H., Mitchell, A., Irvine, E. J., *et al.* (1989). A new measure of health status for clinical trials in inflammatory bowel disease. *Gastroenterology* **96,** 804–810.
32. Chapman, C. R., Casey, K. L., Dubner, R., Foley, K. M., Gracely, R. H., and Reading, A. E. (1985). Pain measurement: An overview. *Pain* **22,** 1–31.
33. Downie, W. W., Leatham, P. A., Rhind, V. M., Wright, V., Branco, J. A., and Anderson, J. A. (1978). Studies with pain rating scales. *Ann. Rheum. Dis.* **37,** 378–381.
34. Huskisson, E. C. (1974). Measurement of pain. *Lancet* **2,** 1127–1131.
35. Melzack, R., and Casey, K. (1968). Sensory, motivational, and central control determinants of pain: A new conceptual model. *In* "The Skin Senses" (D. Kenshalo, ed.). Charles C. Thomas, Springfield, IL.
36. Cleeland, C. S. (1991). Pain assessment in cancer. *In* "Effect of Cancer on Quality of Life (D. Osaba, ed.). CRC Press, Boca Raton, FL.
37. Torrance, G. (1987). Utility approach to measure health-related quality of life. *J. Chron. Dis.* **40,** 593–600.
38. Fryback, D. G., Dasbach, E. J., Klein, R., Klein, B. E., Dorn, N., Peterson, K., *et al.* (1993). The Beaver Dam Health Outcomes Study: Initial catalog of health-state quality factors. *Med. Decis. Making* **13,** 89–102.
39. Pascoe, G. (1983). Patient satisfaction in primary health care: A literature review and analysis. *Eval. Program Plann.* **6,** 185–210.
40. Ware, Jr., J. E., Snyder, M. K., Wright, W. R., *et al.* (1983). Defining and measuring patient satisfaction with medial care. *Eval. Program Plann.* **6,** 247–263.
41. Hunt, S. M., McKenna, S. P., McEwen, J., Williams, J., and Papp, E. (1981). The Nottingham Health Profile: Subjective health status and medical consultations. *Soc. Sci. Med.* **15a,** 221–229.
42. Ware, Jr., J. E., Kosinski, M., and Keller, S. D. (1994). "SF-36 Physical and Mental Health Summary Scales: A User's Manual," 2nd Ed. The Health Institute, New England Medical Center, Boston, MA.
43. Mangione, C. M., Phillips, R. S., and Seddon, J. M. (1992). Development of the Activities of Daily Vision Scale: A measure of visual functional status. *Med. Care* **30,** 1111–1126.
44. Steinberg, E. P., Tielsch, J. M., Schein, O. D., *et al.* (1994). The VF-14: An index of functional impairment in patients with cataract. *Arch. Ophthalmol.* **112,** 630–638.
45. Mangione, C. M., Berry, S., and Lee, P. P. (1998) Identifying the content area for the National Eye Institute Vision Function Questionnaire (NEI-VFQ): Results from focus groups with visually impaired persons. *Arch. Ophthalmol.* **116,** 227–238.
46. Karnofsky, D. A., Abelmann, W. H., Craver, L. F., *et al.* (1948). The use of nitrogen mustards in the palliative treatment of carcinoma. *Cancer* **1,** 634–656.
47. Schipper, H., Clinch, J., McMurray, A., *et al.* (1984). Measuring the quality of life of cancer patients: The Functional Living Index—Cancer: Development and validation. *J. Clin. Oncol.* **2,** 472–483.
48. Jennett, B., and Bond, M. (1975). Assessment of outcome after severe brain damage: A practical scale. *Lancet* **1,** 480–484.
49. Folstein, M. F., Folstein, S. E., and McHugh, P. R. (1975). Mini-mental state: A practical method for grading the cognitive state of patients for the clinician. *J. Psychiatr. Res.* **12,** 189–198.
50. Hajek, V. E., Rutman, D. L., and Scher, H. (1989). Brief assessment of cognitive impairment in patients with stroke. *Arch. Phys. Med. Rehabil.* **70,** 114–117.
51. Harvey, R. M., Doyle, E. F., and Ellis, K. (1974). Major changes made by the Criteria Committee of the New York Heart Association. *Circulation* **49,** 390.
52. Campeau, L. (1976). Grading of angina pectoris. *Circulation* **54,** 522–523.
53. Velanovich, V., Vallance, S. R., Gusz, J. R., Tapia, F. V., and Harkabus, M. A. (1996). Quality of life scale for gastroesophageal reflux disease. *J. Am. Coll. Surg.* **183,** 217–224.
54. Rubenstein, R. S., Beck, S., Lohr, K. N., *et al.* (1983). "Conceptualization and Measurement of Health for Adults." Rand Corporation, Santa Monica, CA.
55. Sprangers, M. A., te Velde, A., and Aaronson, N. K. (1999). The construction and testing of the EORTC colorectal cancer-specific quality of life questionnaire module (QLQ-CR38). European Organization for Research and Treatment of Cancer Study Group on Quality of Life. *Eur. J. Cancer* **35,** 238–247.
56. Cockett, A. T., Aso, Y., Denis, L., and Khoury, S. (1991). The international prostate symptom score (I-PSS) and quality of life assessment. *In* "Proceedings of the International Consultation of Benign Prostatic Hyperplasia; 1991," pp. 280–281. Paris.
57. Rosen, R. C., Riley, A., Wagner, G., Osterloh, I. H., Kirkpatrick, J., and Mishra, A. (1997). The international index of erectile function (IIEF): A multidimensional scale for assessment of erectile dysfunction. *Urology* **49,** 822–830.
58. Meenan, R. F. (1985). The AIMS approach to health status measurement: Conceptual background and measurement properties. *J. Rheum.* **9,** 785–788.
59. Ruta, D. A., Garratt, A. M., Wardlaw, D., and Russell, I. T. (1994). Developing a valid and reliable measure of health outcome for patients with low back pain. *Spine* **19,** 1887–1896.
60. Fairbank, J. C. T., Cooper, J., Davies, J. B., and O'Brien, J. P. (1980).

The Oswestry low back pain disability questionnaire. *Physiotherapy* **66,** 271–273.
61. Rose, G. A., Blackburn, H., Gillum, R. F., *et al.* (1982). "Cardiovascular Survey Methods." WHO Monograph No. 56, 2nd Ed. WHO, Geneva.
62. Juniper, E. F., Guyatt, G. H., Epstein, R. S., *et al.* (1992). Evaluation of impairment of quality of life in asthma: Development of a questionnaire for use in clinical trials. *Thorax* **47,** 76–83.
63. McGavin, C. R., Gupta, G. P., and McHardy, G. J. R. (1976). Twelve minute walking test for assessing disability in chronic bronchitis. *Brit. Med. J.* **i,** 822–823.
64. Johnson, A. N., Cooper, D. F., and Edwards, R. H. T. (1977). Exertion of stair climbing in normal subjects and in patients with chronic obstructive bronchitis. *Thorax* **32,** 711–716.
65. Garratt, A. M., Macdonald, L. M., Ruta, D. A., *et al.* (1993). Towards measurement of outcome for patients with varicose veins. *Qual. Health Care* **2,** 5–10.
66. Regensteiner, J. G., Steiner, J. F., Panzer, R. J., and Hiatt, W. R. (1990). Evaluation of walking impairment by questionnaire in patients with peripheral arterial disease. *J. Vasc. Med. Biol.* **2,** 142–150.

Appendix: The SF-36V$_2$ Health Survey Questionnaire

The SF-36V$_2$™ Health Survey

Instructions for Completing the Questionnaire

Please answer every question. Some questions may look like others, but each one is different. Please take the time to read and answer each question carefully by filling in the bubble that best represents your response.

EXAMPLE

This is for your review. Do not answer this question. The questionnaire begins with the section ***Your Health in General*** below.

For each question you will be asked to fill in a bubble in each line:

1. How strongly do you agree or disagree with each of the following statements?

	Strongly agree	Agree	Uncertain	Disagree	Strongly disagree
a) I enjoy listening to music.	○	●	○	○	○
b) I enjoy reading magazines.	●	○	○	○	○

Please begin answering the questions now.

Your Health in General

1. In general, would you say your health is:

Excellent	Very good	Good	Fair	Poor
○	○	○	○	○

2. **Compared to one year ago**, how would you rate your health in general now?

Much better now than one year ago	Somewhat better now than one year ago	About the same as one year ago	Somewhat worse now than one year ago	Much worse now than one year ago
○	○	○	○	○

Please turn the page and continue.

3. The following items are about activities you might do during a typical day. Does **your health now limit you** in these activities? If so, how much?

	Yes, Limited a lot	Yes, limited a little	No, not limited at all
a) **Vigorous activities**, such as running, lifting heavy objects, participating in strenuous sports	○	○	○
b) **Moderate activities**, such as moving a table, pushing a vacuum cleaner, bowling, or playing golf	○	○	○
c) Lifting or carrying groceries	○	○	○
d) Climbing **several** flights of stairs	○	○	○
e) Climbing **one** flight of stairs	○	○	○
f) Bending, kneeling, or stooping	○	○	○
g) Walking **more than a mile**	○	○	○
h) Walking **several hundred yards**	○	○	○
i) Walking **one hundred yards**	○	○	○
j) Bathing or dressing yourself	○	○	○

4. During the **past 4 weeks**, have you had any of the following problems with your work or other regular daily activities as a result of your physical health?

	All of the time	Most of the time	Some of the time	A little of the time	None of the time
a) Cut down on the **amount of time** you spent on work or other activities	○	○	○	○	○
b) **Accomplished less** than you would like	○	○	○	○	○
c) Were limited in the **kind** of work or other activities	○	○	○	○	○
d) Had **difficulty** performing the work or other activities (for example, it took extra effort)	○	○	○	○	○

5. During the **past 4 weeks**, have you had any of the following problems with your work or other regular daily activities as a result of any emotional problems (such as feeling depressed or anxious)?

	All of the time	Most of the time	Some of the time	A little of the time	None of the time
a) Cut down on the **amount of time** you spent on work or other activities	○	○	○	○	○
b) **Accomplished less** than you would like	○	○	○	○	○
c) Did work or other activities **less carefully than usual**	○	○	○	○	○

6. During the **past 4 weeks**, to what extent has your physical health or emotional problems interfered with your normal social activities with family, friends, neighbors, or groups?

Not at all	Slightly	Moderately	Quite a bit	Extremely
○	○	○	○	○

7. How much bodily pain have you had during the **past 4 weeks**?

None	Very mild	Mild	Moderate	Severe	Very severe
○	○	○	○	○	○

8. During the **past 4 weeks**, how much did pain interfere with your normal work (including both work outside the home and housework)?

Not at all	A little bit	Moderately	Quite a bit	Extremely
○	○	○	○	○

9. These questions are about how you feel and how things have been with you during the **past 4 weeks**. For each question, please give the one answer that comes closest to the way you have been feeling. How much of the time during the **past 4 weeks**...

	All of the time	Most of the time	Some of the time	A little of the time	None of the time
a) did you feel full of life?	○	○	○	○	○
b) have you been a very nervous person?	○	○	○	○	○
c) have you felt so down in the dumps nothing could cheer you up?	○	○	○	○	○
d) have you felt calm and peaceful?	○	○	○	○	○
e) did you have a lot of energy?	○	○	○	○	○
f) have you felt downhearted and depressed?	○	○	○	○	○
g) did you feel worn out?	○	○	○	○	○
h) have you been a happy person?	○	○	○	○	○
i) did you feel tired?	○	○	○	○	○

10. During the **past 4 weeks**, how much of the time has your physical health or emotional problems interfered with your social activities (like visiting friends, relatives, etc.)?

All of the time	Most of the time	Some of the time	A little of the time	None of the time
○	○	○	○	○

11. How TRUE or FALSE is each of the following statements for you?

	Definitely true	Mostly true	Don't know	Mostly false	Definitely false
a) I seem to get sick a little easier than other people	○	○	○	○	○
b) I am as healthy as anybody I know	○	○	○	○	○
c) I expect my health to get worse	○	○	○	○	○
d) My health is excellent	○	○	○	○	○

***THANK YOU* FOR COMPLETING THIS QUESTIONNAIRE!**

12

Design of Clinical Trials

Kenneth K. Tanabe

Division of Surgical Oncology, Massachusetts General Hospital, Boston, Massachusetts 02114

I. Introduction

Therapies are commonly accepted into clinical practice on the basis of well-designed and well-conducted clinical trials. For example, the acceptance of lumpectomy and radiation therapy as an alternative treatment to mastectomy was based on results of prospective randomized trials (1–3). Although results of clinical trials often provide the underpinnings to general acceptance of specific treatments, the conclusions that can be drawn from trial results are often limited because of poor trial design. This chapter highlights basic principles surrounding the development and design of clinical trials.

Statistical associations can be made during retrospective analyses of data sets. In contrast, a clinical trial is usually required to determine whether these statistical associations are causal. Strictly speaking, retrospective analysis of data sets (such as chart review studies) can at best help develop hypotheses, which should then be tested by an experimental trial. Similarly, the design of clinical trials should be based on information available in retrospective analyses.

One of the most important elements of a clinical trial is the written protocol. The elements of a written protocol are described in Table I. All aspects of a clinical trial flow from this document, including the length of time required to complete the trial, the manpower required to collect necessary data during conduct of the trial, and the power of the statistical observations. Accordingly, as the protocol is developed, this critical document should be carefully written, revised, and edited with the same care and attention to detail as a National Institutes of Health grant application. The style and form of a written protocol should satisfy many of the same requirements as in a grant application. All who read the protocol will not be experts in the specific area of study. The protocol should therefore be written clearly and concisely. The study endpoints must allow one to address the specific aims directly. Patient eligibility must be broad enough to allow extrapolation of the trial results to the intended patient population, but must be narrow enough to permit meaningful analysis of the data. The clinical and laboratory data recorded during the conduct of the study must be sufficient to measure the stated endpoints. Collection of unnecessary

Table I Elements of a Clinical Protocol

1. Brief summary
2. Introduction and scientific background
3. Hypotheses
4. Specific aims and endpoints
5. Patient eligibility
6. Design of study (including flow diagram and method of allocation to treatment group)
7. Treatment plan (including necessary dose modifications)
8. Drug formulations
9. Anticipated toxicities
10. Clinical and laboratory data required at specific time points
11. Criteria used to measure specific endpoints
12. Statistical considerations (including study size, duration, and methods of data analyses)
13. Informed consent form
14. Regulatory considerations (including record-keeping requirements, reports for adverse events, responsibilities of sponsor, accountability for investigational drugs or devices)
15. Data forms
16. References
17. Appendices (such as toxicity grading criteria)
18. Name, title, and address of study chairperson and all collaborating investigators

data raises the cost of a trial and increases the likelihood that important information will not be captured and recorded.

II. Hypotheses, Specific Aims, and Endpoints

Most hypotheses that are addressed in clinical trials are either based on observations made in the course of patient care or as a result of a retrospective chart review. For example, the observation that higher anastomotic leak rates occur in patients who have drains placed following low anterior resection compared to patients who do not have drains placed generates a hypothesis that can be examined experimentally (4, 5). The mere presence of a statistical association between drain usage and anastomotic leak rate observed in the course of a retrospective chart review does not imply a causal association. The absence of a causal association despite the presence of a statistical association in this example may be explained by the notion that surgeons more commonly place drains when they are concerned about the integrity of the anastomoses (for example, because of tissue tension or poor blood supply). Therefore, it would not be surprising that patients with drains are more likely to experience an anastomotic leak. Even when all known variables are taken into account for the analysis, the weakness of a retrospective study is its inability to address directly causal relationships that are implied by statistical associations.

Clinical trials may also arise from observations made in basic science laboratories. For example, the finding (6) that cells with absent or mutant p53 are more resistant to chemotherapy compared to cells with wild-type p53 has led to the development of gene therapy vectors to transduce tumor cells with the p53 gene (7). The safety and efficacy of these vectors can only be addressed in the context of a clinical trial.

Relevant published literature and the investigator's own unpublished data should be included in the written protocol to establish the basis for the hypotheses and to provide the rationale for the study. The specific aims should be precise and reflect the hypotheses. Specific aims should not be a fishing expedition, with the breadth and depth of data capture reflective of the broad, unstructured scope of the study. In the p53 example cited above, a poorly conceived specific aim may indicate the goal of "improving treatment of colon cancer." More precise specific aims may indicate goals of determining the toxicity of p53 gene administration and measurement of the objective response rate to a specific chemotherapy regimen following administration of the p53 gene.

The specific aims of a clinical trial should also reflect an understanding of the next clinical trial that will be conducted based on the results of the trial. It is most desirable to design a trial in such a way that whether the results demonstrate that the hypothesis is true or false, sufficient information will be obtained to design the next clinical trial in a logical manner.

"Endpoint" refers to a criterion by which the hypothesis of a trial will be examined. Careful selection of endpoints is necessary to ensure that they will permit the hypothesis to be examined. In addition, endpoints should be selected so that they represent a meaningful patient benefit. For example, design of a clinical trial endpoint consisting of detection of a 3% increase in the 5-year survival of patients with Dukes C rectal carcinoma may not be accepted by physicians as an endpoint that represents a meaningful benefit to the patient population at large. Response rates, duration of response, and disease-free survival are common endpoints in oncology trials, but it must be remembered that these endpoints allow only limited conclusions concerning therapeutic efficacy. Although the overall activity of a chemotherapy regimen can frequently be deduced from these endpoints, none of these endpoints reflects improvements to patient welfare. Overall survival and quality of life are endpoints that directly reflect improvements in patient welfare. Costs of therapy are also endpoints that are gaining popularity in clinical trials. Endpoints also determine the duration of a clinical trial. Data collection is longer for trials that measure survival as an endpoint compared to trials that are limited to measurement of perioperative complications, toxicity, or length of hospital stay as endpoints. The breadth of data collection required for measuring endpoints should be carefully considered in clinical trial design. The best guideline is summarized by Abramson's (8) advice to "choose as many as necessary and as few as possible."

III. Patient Eligibility

The definition of patient eligibility must take into consideration several competing goals. The inclusion criteria should be broad enough to permit sufficient patient enrollment to allow completion of the trial in a timely fashion. The inclusion criteria should also permit extrapolation of the results to the specific patient population in mind. If one is examining a particular therapy for Dukes C rectal carcinoma that has implications for all physicians treating patients with Dukes C rectal carcinoma, the eligibility criteria should not exclude the majority of patients. It is important to ensure that the results of the trial are meaningful for the general population of patients encountered. The eligibility criteria should also take into account the anticipated morbidity associated with the treatment program. If a particular antibiotic under study in a clinical trial may cause renal failure, eligibility should be limited to patients with adequate renal function, so that the incidence of this side effect can be determined. If one treatment arm of a prospective randomized trial requires intensive therapy, then all patients who are unable to tolerate this arm of the treatment should be excluded.

IV. Structure of Clinical Trials

Clinical trials in oncology and in other disciplines commonly fall into one of three categories. Phase I trials determine the relationship between toxicity and dose schedule. Phase II trials determine the types of diseases for which the treatment appears promising. Phase III trials determine whether the therapy is superior or equivalent to a standard reference therapy. The standard reference therapy may represent historical controls or another specific therapy. A slight variation on a phase III trial is determination whether the therapy is equivalent to a standard reference therapy but is associated with less morbidity.

A. Phase I Studies

These studies are designed to determine how the dose, route, or schedule of drug administration influences toxicity. Frequently used endpoints for these studies are determination of the maximum tolerated dose and determination of the dose-limiting toxicity. Most commonly for chemotherapy trials, the drug is initially administered at a dose representing a fraction of the lethal dose (LD_{10}) observed in animal studies. After sufficient time has passed to observe acute toxic side effects, the dose is escalated in subsequent cohorts of patients. A commonly used algorithm involves treatment of three patients in the initial cohort. If dose-limiting toxicity is not observed in any of the three patients, then the next three patients receive a higher dose level. In contrast, if one of three patients experiences dose-limiting toxicity, then up to three more patients are treated with the same dose level. If one or more of the three additional patients experiences dose-limiting toxicity, then the previous dose level is usually designated as the maximum tolerated dose (i.e., the dose level at which fewer than 33% of patients experience dose-limiting toxicity.) If none of the three additional patients experience dose-limiting toxicity, then the next three patients receive a higher dose level. Escalation of doses for subsequent courses in the same patient is generally not performed. Once the maximum tolerated dose is determined, it is common to treat an additional seven to ten patients at this dose level to confirm with a greater degree of statistical probability that the incidence of dose-limiting toxicity is less than 33% at this dose level. It is important to determine accurately the true maximum tolerated dose because this dose of medication will be administered to a larger cohort of patients in a phase II trial.

In cancer therapy trials, determination of dose-limiting toxicity and the maximum tolerated dose represent the principal endpoints of a phase I trial. Response rates, survival, and quality of life are not endpoints in most phase I trials. It is common for patients with various types of cancer to be enrolled into a phase I trial. In addition, by nature of the trial design, patients receive different dose schedules of the agent. These factors preclude meaningful analysis of survival or quality of life as endpoints. Because toxicity as a function of dose schedule serves as the primary endpoint for most phase I trials, it is important for eligibility to be limited to patients who are healthy enough to withstand toxicity and to allow measurement of toxicity. Patients for whom no effective therapies are known to exist are the ones most commonly enrolled in phase I cancer therapy trials. It is exceedingly important that phase I trial design place patient safety as the highest priority during conduct of the experimental therapy.

B. Phase II Studies

These trials are designed to determine the types of diseases for which the treatment appears promising, or alternatively, to determine the approximate efficacy of a treatment for a specific disease. Some hint of the types of cancers that may be responsive to an experimental chemotherapeutic regimen may be identified in the results of the preceding phase I trial. Alternatively, the experimental therapy may be naturally suited for a specific patient population. For example, experimental agents that are farnesyl transferase inhibitors and active against *ras*-activated cancers would logically be examined in patients with pancreatic carcinoma, a disease in which 85% of patients harbor activating mutations in the *ras* gene of their tumors. Phase II studies in oncology commonly treat a group of patients with one type of cancer with the maximum tolerated dose as defined in a phase I trial. Careful design of phase II trials is required to obtain meaningful results. It is important to avoid inadvertently declaring a therapy ineffective or inactive when it truly has therapeutic benefit. For example, a farnesyl transferase inhibitor may be effective against pancreatic carcinomas as first-line therapy, but will appear ineffective in a phase II clinical trial in which all patients enrolled had already been treated with numerous chemotherapy regimens. Similarly, it is important to avoid artificially favorable results, which lead to unnecessary costs in a phase III trial to compare the therapy against standard therapy. Investigators may knowingly or unknowingly significantly improve results of a phase II trial of an experimental therapy by selecting patients with a prognosis that is better than average for enrollment in trials. This leads to an all too common situation in which a phase II trial with favorable results is reported, but is then followed by similar trials performed at other institutions in which the results are far less promising (9, 10).

Phase II trials are frequently designed as two-stage studies. In the first stage, a specific number of patients are enrolled and the therapeutic value (based on defined endpoints) is measured. If fewer than a predetermined number of patients demonstrate benefit from the treatment, then the trial is terminated, realizing that the likelihood of discarding a therapy that is actually valuable is quite low. Alternatively, if the number of responders in this first cohort of patients is greater than this predetermined level, then the trial is continued and the remaining patients are enrolled. This two-stage design reduces the likelihood of enrolling a large number of patients in a phase II trial to receive a therapy that has no clinical value. The bar that must be cleared to continue to the second phase of the study can be set at any level, and depends on the minimum therapeutic response below which the therapy will be considered unhelpful. The higher the bar is set, the lower the likelihood that a large number of patients will receive a therapy that is of little or no benefit. However, the higher the bar is set, the higher the probability that a beneficial therapy will be discarded prematurely.

C. Phase III Studies

These trials are designed to determine whether an experimental therapy is more effective or associated with less morbidity, compared to a standard reference therapy. Phase III trials involve direct comparison of results observed in patients treated with the experimental therapy to those observed in patients treated with the standard therapy. In rare situations, the control group that serves as the basis for comparison will consist of case-matched controls or other historical controls. Use of matched historical controls has limitations because control patients can be matched only for known prognostic factors. Several additional prognostic factors presumably exist that are not yet understood, and will not be accounted for in case-matched controls. Because several undesirable biases are introduced when using historical controls, most phase III trials are conducted as randomized trials in which patients are allocated to either the experimental therapy or the standard reference therapy. Because patients are allocated randomly to one treatment arm or another, it is a statistical likelihood that the groups of patients will be similar in all aspects. This improves the probability that the observations are not influenced by patient selection biases. Even when unknown prognostic factors exist, it is likely that these factors will be distributed evenly throughout each of the treatment arms. Nonetheless, in some small, randomized trials, a process of stratified randomization is used to ensure that important prognostic factors are equally represented in the treatment groups (11, 12). A separate randomization list (or set of envelopes) is used for each subset. For example, if the value of lymph node dissection for treatment of patients with melanoma is to be evaluated, it may be helpful to stratify patients into subsets based on tumor thickness (13). This will ensure that the distribution of tumor thicknesses will be closely matched in the groups randomized to either lymph node dissection or control.

The process of randomization requires a mechanism that does not allow investigators to predict which treatment arm a particular patient will receive. For example, utilizing alternate days of the week or "even versus odd" patient medical record number is not adequate, because these mechanisms allow investigator bias in decisions on whether to enroll patients into the trial with foreknowledge of which treatment they will receive (14). The randomization process should occur as late as possible prior to the actual treatment. For example, when evaluating the potential value of a chemotherapy regimen that is administered following surgery, the randomization should be performed following recovery from surgery in an attempt to minimize biases that may be entered during the operation. This approach also reduces the number of patients that are disqualified because of postoperative morbidity that precludes them from receiving the chemotherapy regimen (15).

Some physicians believe that patient randomization is unethical because it is their obligation to provide patients with a choice of therapies based on an analysis of the risks and benefits of each treatment option. These physicians argue that an understanding of a patient's medical condition and personal preferences will always allow selection of the most suitable therapy. However, it is important to point out that experimental therapies are commonly only marginally better or worse than control therapies, yet it is common for competent physicians to hold widely divergent opinions concerning the relative value of each of the therapies. Insufficient data exist to support such opinions or hunches. Accordingly, an approach in which physicians counsel patients about the risks and benefits of each of the treatment arms, as well as the risks and benefits of a randomized trial that compares the two, is consistent with the highest standard of ethical study conduct.

Another device, employed to reduce the impact of physician bias on the results of a clinical trial, involves blinding physicians to the treatment allocation. A clinical trial designed to examine the efficacy of an antibiotic administered perioperatively to reduce wound infections may benefit from blinding of the investigators. The antibiotic solution can be made in the pharmacy and placed in a bag that does not reveal whether it is the study antibiotic or control antibiotic (or placebo). Physicians and research staff that evaluate the patients postoperatively for the presence or absence of wound infections will not know whether the patient received the study antibiotic. This type of trial is referred to as a double-blinded study, in which both the patients and the physicians are blinded to the treatment allocation. Some degrees of blindness are not feasible. For example, in a surgical trial that compares amputation to limb-sparing surgery, it is not possible to blind the participants (16). Blindness can also be employed in select portions of a clinical trial. For example, pathology slides, radiographs, or EKGs can be read and interpreted by physicians in a blind-coded fashion.

Factorial designs may be used to evaluate more than one treatment under study. For example, this approach was used to evaluate the efficacy of a 2-cm surgical margin versus a 4-cm surgical margin in patients with intermediate-thickness melanoma of the extremities. This same clinical trial evaluated the value of an elective lymph node dissection. Eligible patients who enrolled in this clinical trial were first randomized to undergo excision with either a 2-cm or a 4-cm surgical margin (17). All of the patients were then randomized to undergo elective lymph node dissection or observation of the regional lymph nodes. This factorial design allowed the clinical trial to address two hypotheses with the same number of patients required to address just one of the hypotheses. An important assumption that is made in this type of trial design is that the two sets of therapies administered to address each of the two hypotheses are completely independent of each other. In other words, the value of an elective lymph node dissection does not depend on whether the patient underwent a 2- or a 4-cm surgical margin excision. And it is also required to assume that the value of the width of surgical margin used to excise the melanoma does not depend on whether the patient undergoes an elective lymph node dissection.

V. Treatment Plan

The exact method of treatment should be clearly described within the body of the clinical protocol. In clinical trials that involve evaluation of an operation, it is important to ensure uniformity of the operation among participating surgeons and institutions. Every detail that may impact a measured endpoint, such as patient outcome, should be carefully described. For example, in a surgical trial designed to evaluate the effect of radical lymph node dissection on survival in patients with gastric cancer, it should be stipulated which lymph nodes should be resected (18). In a surgical trial designed to evaluate the accuracy of sentinel lymph node mapping for breast cancer, it is important to stipulate the volume and dose of injected isotope and the timing of isotope injection relative to the axillary incision (19). Mechanisms to monitor quality control are also frequently included in clinical trials involving surgery. The number of lymph nodes resected in a trial designed to evaluate the value of radical lymphadenectomy for gastric cancer may be monitored to ensure quality control (20). Alternatively, it may be necessary to design a run-in period in which the techniques of surgery are monitored for a specified number of patients prior to allowing surgeons to enroll patients.

For clinical trials designed to evaluate antibiotics or other medications (such as cancer chemotherapeutic agents), it is imperative that the exact formulation, dose, route, and schedule of administration be stipulated. It is equally important to use a mechanism to monitor adherence to the treatment plan. Chemotherapy trials often require dose reductions based on the observed toxicity. The dose reductions should be described in detail for each possible scenario. The types of toxicities that patients experience should also be clearly stated. Although these are included in the informed consent form, their inclusion in the written protocol is of great value because of their influence on trial design with respect to patient eligibility, treatment plan, anticipated dropout rate, and statistical analyses. As many elements of the treatment as possible should be included in the treatment plan to minimize variability that will impact on measured endpoints.

VI. Data Collection and Quality Assurance

The specific endpoints of a clinical trial will determine the scope of data collection required. It is important to remember that many endpoints require a baseline for comparison, and it is therefore necessary to obtain specific data prior to instituting a therapeutic intervention. These data also allow analysis on completion of the trial to ensure that groups of patients allocated to different treatment arms were equivalent at baseline. In addition, data to ensure eligibility and suitability for the treatment regimen must be collected and recorded. For example, if only patients with a forced expiratory volume (FEV_1) greater than 75% of predicted are eligible for a clinical trial of thoracoscopic surgery, it is important to collect and record the FEV_1 for all patients. Measurement of some parameters such as operative time, blood loss, or perioperative complications may seem obvious at first glance; however, the definition of each of these may differ between observers. Therefore, clear definitions should be used to describe variables.

The written protocol should include a table that specifies all of the required data and the time points at which these data are required (Table II). For example, a complete blood count (CBC) and urinalysis may be required on postoperative days 1, 7, 14, and 28 for purposes of the clinical trial. The inclusion of these items in a table allows treating physicians to quickly determine when to order specific tests and reduces the chances that important data points will be missing on completion of the trial.

To maximize accuracy of collected data, forms should be developed for each patient. These data forms should be simple and unambiguous. Data should be limited to those absolutely required to achieve the stated endpoints. Whenever possible, the forms should be designed such that data are easily entered in numerical format to facilitate subse-

Table II Example of a Table Summarizing Required Data

Data and observation	Prior to study	Days 8, 15, 22, and 29	Prior to each chemotherapy cycle	1 month after discontinuation of therapy
Signed informed consent	X			
History	X			
Physical examination	X	X	X	
Vital signs	X	X	X	
Height/weight/surface area	X		X	
Drug toxicity		X	X	X[a]
Performance status	X	X	X	
Laboratory tests				
CBC/platelets/differential	X[c]	X	X	
Creatinine	X[c]	X	X	
Alkaline phosphatase	X[c]	X	X	
Total bilirubin, aspartate aminotransferase	X[c]	X	X	
Carcinoembryonic antigen	X[c]		X	
Pregnancy test[b]	X[c]			
EKG[c]	X[c]			
Tumor measurements	X[d]		X[d]	

[a]Follow-up toxicity data will be obtained for patients experiencing dose-limiting toxicity until toxicity resolves.
[b]Only for female patients of childbearing potential within 72 hr of starting therapy.
[c]Labs within 14 days of therapy; EKG within 28 days of starting therapy.
[d]After every 2 cycles.

quent entry into a computerized database. For example, in a field used to capture data about a tumor, "0" could be entered for a well-differentiated tumor, "1" for a moderately differentiated tumor, and "2" for a poorly differentiated tumor. To reduce observer variation, training sessions for standardization of assessment of variables may be required. A group of qualified data collectors should be assembled. The time and date of data entry should be recorded and forms should be kept in a secure location. Security and confidentiality arrangements for data collection and storage should be addressed in the protocol and consent forms.

VII. Statistical Considerations in the Design of Clinical Trials

Investigators must address several questions concerning statistics during design and analysis of a clinical trial. How many patients are required? Is the trial designed to demonstrate equivalence in efficacy between two treatments, or designed to detect a difference between different treatments? How small of a difference between treatment groups is detectable? How many prognostic factors can be included in the analysis? How should patients who drop out from the trial be included in the statistical analysis? How often should the data be analyzed? A comprehensive primer in biostatistics is beyond the scope of this chapter—instead, some general guidelines and principles are presented.

Statistical significance is the degree of certainty with which an inference can be drawn. It is not a threshold level beyond which the inference clearly represents truth. For example, the statistical significance for comparing outcomes between two groups subjected to different treatments represents the statistical likelihood that differences as large as those observed could occur if the two treatments were actually equivalent, but differences in outcome occurred merely as a result of chance. Take, for instance, a study of patients with colon carcinoma in which administration of adjuvant therapy is associated with a reduction in mortality risk with a one-sided level of statistical significance of $p = 0.05$. This set of conditions implies that even if adjuvant therapy does not provide a reduction in mortality risk, these results would be observed by chance 5 times if the trial were conducted 100 times. If the desire is to analyze two groups for differences that may be either positive or negative in direction, the statistical equations used are two-sided, whereas, if probabilities are calculated only for differences in the same direction as that actually obtained, the statistical equations used are one-sided.

Several issues must be addressed when deciding how many patients to enroll in a clinical trial. The frequency of the endpoint in the control group and the magnitude of the difference in frequency that one is attempting to detect will influence sample size (Table III). The desired statistical confidence level with which inferences are made will also influence sample size. In addition, the equations used for dichotomous endpoints (e.g., success or failure) differ from those used for continuous endpoints.

The desired power of a study will also influence sample size. Power reflects the probability with which the absence of a measured treatment effect represents true equivalence of the treatments. The power of a study increases with larger sample size and greater treatment effect. For example, assume that a study is being designed with a sample size sufficient to detect a 20% improvement in 5-year survival in the treatment group. If survival of the treatment group does not demonstrate a 20% enhancement in survival with the desired level of statistical significance, then the null hypothesis is accepted as true (i.e., the treatment group and the control group are equivalent). If the sample size in this study is small, the ability to detect the 20% difference is decreased. In other words, with a small sample size, it is possible that a 20% improvement in survival will not be observed despite the presence of a true treatment effect. The power of the study reflects the statistical significance with which the absence of the minimum measured difference between the treatment groups represents the true absence of a treatment effect. It is all too common for clinical studies to be underpowered in design. In this situation authors report the absence of a treatment effect, but in reality the likelihood of the underpowered study to have identified the treatment effect with statistical significance was poor from the outset (low power). The greater the anticipated difference between the treatment and control groups, the higher the power of the study. The greater the sample size, the higher the power of the study. Using standard tables (Table III), one can determine that the number of patients required in a two-arm trial designed to detect the difference between a 15% success rate and 10% success rate with a significance level of 0.05 and power of 0.9 is 786 patients per arm! Take, for example, a prospective randomized trial designed to detect a reduction in wound infection rates following groin dissection from 15% to 10% with use of perioperative antibiotics. Such a trial would require 786 patients per arm in order to declare an absence of an effect by the antibiotic with a power of 0.9 if this difference in outcome is not observed. The number of patients required is even larger for a two-sided test (Table IV). The number of patients required for comparison between an experimental group and a historical control group is calculated from a different formula (Table V).

During the design of a clinical trial, it is important to account for anticipated loss of patients available for analysis following completion of therapy. Some patients may not tolerate the treatment regimen and will prematurely exit the trial. Some patients may drop out of the trial before its completion for other reasons, including a change of residence to

Table III Number of Patients Required in Each of Two Treatment Groups for Comparison Using a One-Sided Test[a]

Smaller success rate	Larger minus smaller success rate[b]									
	0.05	0.10	0.15	0.20	0.25	0.30	0.35	0.40	0.45	0.50
0.05	512	172	94	62	45	35	28	23	19	16
	381	129	72	48	35	27	22	18	15	13
0.10	786	236	121	76	54	40	31	25	21	17
	579	176	91	58	41	31	24	20	16	14
0.15	1026	292	144	88	60	44	34	27	22	18
	752	216	108	66	46	34	26	21	17	14
0.20	1231	339	163	98	66	48	36	29	23	19
	900	250	121	73	50	37	28	22	18	15
0.25	1402	377	178	105	70	50	38	29	23	19
	1024	278	132	79	53	38	29	23	18	15
0.30	1539	407	189	111	73	52	38	30	23	19
	1122	300	141	83	55	39	30	23	18	15
0.35	1642	429	197	114	74	52	38	29	23	18
	1196	315	146	85	56	40	30	23	18	14
0.40	1711	441	201	115	74	52	38	29	22	17
	1246	324	149	86	56	39	29	22	17	14
0.45	1745	446	201	114	73	50	36	27	21	16
	1271	327	149	85	55	38	28	21	16	13
0.50	1745	441	197	111	70	48	34	25	19	15
	1271	324	146	83	53	37	26	20	15	12

[a] Adapted from Simon (23). *In* "Cancer: Principles and Practice of Oncology" (V. T. DeVita, Jr., S. Hellman, and S. A. Rosenberg, eds.), pp. 418–440. J. B. Lippincott Company, Philadelphia, 1993.
[b] Upper figure: significance level 0.05, power 0.90; lower figure: significance level 0.05, power 0.80.

another geographic area, dissatisfaction with the treatment allocation, or death from causes unrelated to the disease or treatment under study. To reduce the chances of ending up with a data set that is inadequate to answer the proposed hypothesis, the number of patients that may be excluded from analysis during the conduct of the trial should be anticipated and factored into the design. The manner with which patients are excluded from analysis of a trial can also greatly alter the results. Patients who do not complete a therapy often have more substantial disease and a poorer prognosis compared to those who complete therapy. Exclusion of patients who do not complete therapy may distort results by falsely improving the results of the treatment group. Researchers may attempt to justify such an exclusion by claiming that their outcome was poor because they did not complete the specified therapy; however, this argument is not valid. Patients should be analyzed according to their treatment allocation ("intention-to-treat") regardless of the actual treatment administered. Results from trials analyzed in this rigorous fashion are most likely to be broadly applicable to the population at large. It is for this reason that clinical trials should be carefully designed to minimize protocol deviations.

Whenever possible, the distribution of important prognostic factors for the disease under study should be evenly distributed among treatment groups. This will improve the precision of the estimates of treatment differences. Even nonstatistically significant imbalances in important prognostic factors can dramatically alter the outcome of a clinical trial. Allocation to treatment groups by randomization usually will ensure that such important factors are evenly distributed; however, this strategy does not guarantee even distribution. It is safer to incorporate major prognostic factors as stratification variables in the randomization process to guarantee their even distribution.

The endpoints of a clinical trial establish the necessary comparisons and statistical analyses that are performed on completion of the trial. The analytic methods and comparison groups should be established before the trial commences. Analyses performed on subsets that are defined *post*

Table IV Number of Patients Required in Each of Two Treatment Groups for Comparison Using a Two-Sided Test[a]

Smaller success rate	Larger minus smaller success rate[b]									
	0.05	0.10	0.15	0.20	0.25	0.30	0.35	0.40	0.45	0.50
0.05	620	206	113	74	54	42	33	27	23	19
	473	159	88	58	43	33	27	22	18	16
0.10	956	285	146	92	64	48	38	30	25	21
	724	218	112	71	50	38	30	24	20	17
0.15	1250	354	174	106	73	53	41	33	26	22
	944	269	133	82	57	42	32	26	21	18
0.20	1502	411	197	118	79	57	44	34	27	22
	1132	313	151	91	62	45	34	27	22	18
0.25	1712	459	216	127	84	60	45	35	28	23
	1289	348	165	98	65	47	36	28	22	18
0.30	1880	495	230	134	88	62	46	36	28	22
	1414	375	175	103	68	48	36	28	22	18
0.35	2006	522	239	138	89	63	46	35	27	22
	1509	395	182	106	69	49	36	28	22	18
0.40	2090	537	244	139	89	62	45	34	26	21
	1571	407	186	107	69	48	36	27	21	17
0.45	2132	543	244	138	88	60	44	33	25	19
	1603	411	186	106	68	47	34	26	20	16
0.50	2132	537	239	134	84	57	41	30	23	17
	1603	407	182	103	65	45	32	24	18	14

[a]Adapted from Simon (23). *In* "Cancer: Principles and Practice of Oncology" (V. T. DeVita, Jr., S. Hellman, and S. A. Rosenberg, eds.), pp. 418–440. J. B. Lippincott Company, Philadelphia, 1993.
[b]Upper figure: significance level 0.05, power 0.90; lower figure: significance level 0.05, power 0.80.

hoc should be viewed with appropriate caution. The more subsets that are analyzed, the more it is likely that an observed difference will be observed solely on the basis of chance. It should be remembered that observation of a statistically significant difference ($p = 0.05$) implies that the outcome would be observed solely on the basis of chance (and not as a result of treatment) 1 in 20 times (5%). If one performs a second analysis on another subset, the same 5% chance of obtaining a false positive finding applies; but in combination, the probability of at least one of the two analyses representing a false positive is 9.7%. Similarly, if three analyses are performed on separate subsets, the probability that at least one of the analyses will represent a false positive is 14.3%. When 10 such comparisons are performed, the probability of at least one false positive is 40%! In order to minimize the need for subset analyses to account for prognostic factors, important prognostic variables should be incorporated into the randomization process to ensure even distribution. Subset analyses should be declared in advance, and statistical significance for these comparisons should reach a more stringent threshold (usually $p < 0.05/n$, where n = number of comparisons analyzed). Statistically significant associations observed in subset analyses are best used to formulate hypotheses that may be tested in a subsequent trial designed specifically for that subset (21, 22).

VIII. Informed Consent

Prospective clinical trials involve provision of the best known medical care to patients in a preplanned manner that allows reliable conclusions to be drawn from the observed outcomes. It is necessary for patients to be informed of the risks and benefits of participation in a clinical trial and for them (or their legal guardian) to sign a document indicating that they have been informed and they consent to participate in the trial. Standard elements included in an informed consent form are as follows:

1. A description of the purpose of the trial and a statement that the proposed treatment is experimental.

Table V Number of Patients Needed in an Experimental Group for 80% Power to Detect a Specified Difference in Success Rates[a]

Proportion of success for historical controls	Number of historical controls[b]						
	20	30	40	50	75	100	200
0.10	*	223†	108	80	58	50	42
	116	53±	40	35	29	27	24
	39	27‡	23	21	18	18	16
	22	17=	15	14	13	13	12
0.20	*	*	285	167	101	83	65
	385	98	67	55	44	40	35
	67	40	33	30	26	24	22
	31	23	21	19	18	17	16
0.30	*	*	554	259	137	108	80
	882	137	87	69	54	48	42
	86	49	39	35	30	29	26
	31	27	24	22	20	19	18
0.40	*	*	699	303	153	120	88
	913	147	92	74	58	52	44
	85	50	41	36	32	30	27
	36	27	24	22	21	20	19
0.50	*	*	538	267	145	115	86
	455	122	83	68	55	50	43
	67	44	37	34	30	28	26
	30	24	22	20	18	18	17
0.60	*	*	295	185	117	97	76
	179	83	63	55	46	42	38
	45	33	29	27	25	24	22
	22	19	17	17	15	15	15

[a]One-sided $\alpha = 0.05$. Adapted from Simon (23). *In* "Cancer: Principles and Practice of Oncology" (V. T. DeVita, Jr., S. Hellman, and S. A. Rosenberg, eds.), pp. 418–440. J. B. Lippincott Company, Philadelphia, 1993.

[b]Symbols: *, required sample size >1000; †, number of patients needed for the new treatment to detect a difference in success rate of 15 percentage points; ±, number of patients needed to detect a difference in success rate of 20 percentage points; ‡, number of patients needed to detect a difference in success rate of 25 percentage points; =, number of patients needed to detect a difference in success rate of 30 percentage points.

2. A description of the procedures and treatments involved in the experimental therapy, with clear identification of the components that are experimental.

3. A description of the risks and discomforts associated with the treatment, with clear identification of the components that are experimental.

4. A description of the anticipated costs associated with participation in the clinical trial. The costs for which the patient may be held responsible should be clearly outlined. Responsibility for costs that result from complications of the experimental therapy should also be described.

5. A description of benefits that are anticipated as a result of participation in the clinical trial. If no direct benefit to the patient is anticipated, this should be clearly stated.

6. A description of alternative procedures or treatments that are available.

7. A statement describing the confidentiality of the medical records, and a statement indicating that the study sponsor and Food and Drug Administration may inspect and copy the medical records in the course of carrying out their duties.

8. A description of individuals to contact to obtain further information about the study, patient's rights, or in case of an adverse event resulting from participation in the study.

9. A statement indicating that participation is voluntary, and that a decision to decline participation or subsequently drop out of the study will not affect present or future care by the treating physicians.

10. A statement describing whether compensation or treatment is available in the event of an injury resulting from participation in the clinical trial. The availability of treatment for injuries arising from participation in the clinical trial should also be described.

IX. Summary

Clinical trials represent an important research instrument, and patient participation in clinical trials is required to achieve progress in medicine. Poorly conducted clinical trials slow medical progress, waste the invaluable good will of participants, and erode public confidence. Poorly conducted clinical trials waste both time devoted to the conduct of the trial and time spent by subsequent investigators. It is important for physicians to study the fundamental principles of clinical trial design. A significant breakthrough has been made in public awareness and acceptance of clinical trials as a result of publicity surrounding trials demonstrating the safety and efficacy of breast conservation surgery compared to mastectomy. Physicians should make use of this opportunity and actively participate in and encourage patients to enroll in clinical trials. Moreover, these trials must be designed and conducted with proper attention to detail to produce meaningful and useful results.

References

1. Fisher, E. R., Anderson, S., Redmond, C., and Fisher, B. (1993). Pathologic findings from the National Surgical Adjuvant Breast Project protocol B-06. 10-year pathologic and clinical prognostic discriminants. *Cancer* **71**(8), 2507–2514.
2. Fisher, B., Wickerham, D. L., Deutsch, M., Anderson, S., Redmond, C., and Fisher, E. R. (1992). Breast tumor recurrence following lumpectomy with and without breast irradiation: An overview of recent NSABP findings. *Semin. Surg. Oncol.* **8**(3), 153–160.
3. Fisher, E. R., Redmond, C., Fisher, B., and Bass, G. (1990). Pathologic findings from the National Surgical Adjuvant Breast and Bowel Projects (NSABP). Prognostic discriminants for 8-year survival for node-negative invasive breast cancer patients. *Cancer* **65**(9), 2121–2128.
4. Scott, H., and Brown, A. C. (1996). Is routine drainage of pelvic anastomosis necessary? *Am. Surg.* **62**(6), 452–457.
5. Sagar, P. M., Hartley, M. N., Macfie, J., Mancey-Jones, B., Sedman, P., and May, J. (1995). Randomized trial of pelvic drainage after rectal resection. *Dis. Colon Rectum* **38**(3), 254–258.
6. Lowe, S. W., Bodis, S., McClatchey, A., *et al.* (1994). p53 status and the efficacy of cancer therapy *in vivo. Science* **266**(5186), 807–810.
7. Nielsen, L. L., Dell, J., Maxwell, E., Armstrong, L., Maneval, D., and Catino, J. J. (1997). Efficacy of p53 adenovirus-mediated gene therapy against human breast cancer xenografts. *Cancer Gene Ther.* **4**(2), 129–138.
8. Abramson, J. H. (1979). "Survey Methods in Community Medicine." Churchill-Livingstone, New York.
9. Wadler, S., Schwartz, E. L., Goldman, M., *et al.* (1989). Fluorouracil and recombinant α2a-interferon: An active regimen against advanced colorectal carcinoma [see comments]. *J. Clin. Oncol.* **7**(12), 1769–1775.
10. Kjaer, M. (1996). Combining 5-fluorouracil with interferon-α in the treatment of advanced colorectal cancer: Optimism followed by disappointment. *Anticancer Drugs* **7**(1), 35–42.
11. Ginsberg, R. J., and Rubinstein, L. V. (1995). Randomized trial of lobectomy versus limited resection for T1 N0 non-small cell lung cancer. Lung Cancer Study Group [see comments]. *Ann. Thorac. Surg.* **60**(3), 615–622.
12. Wolff, B. G., Pembeton, J. H., van Heerden, J. A., *et al.* (1989). Elective colon and rectal surgery without nasogastric decompression. A prospective, randomized trial. *Ann. Surg.* **209**(6), 670–673.
13. Balch, C. M., Soong, S. J., Bartolucci, A. A., *et al.* (1996). Efficacy of an elective regional lymph node dissection of 1 to 4 mm thick melanomas for patients 60 years of age and younger. *Ann. Surg.* **224**(3), 255–263.
14. Miller, E., Paull, D. E., Morrissey, K., Cortese, A., and Nowak, E. Scalpel versus electrocautery in modified radical mastectomy. *Am. Surg.* **54**(5), 284–286.
15. Gastrointestinal Tumor Study Group (1987). Further evidence of effective adjuvant combined radiation and chemotherapy following curative resection of pancreatic cancer. *Cancer* **59**(12), 2006–2010.
16. Rosenberg, S. A., Tepper, J., Glatstein, E., *et al.* (1982). The treatment of soft-tissue sarcomas of the extremities: Prospective randomized evaluations of (1) limb-sparing surgery plus radiation therapy compared with amputation and (2) the role of adjuvant chemotherapy. *Ann. Surg.* **196**(3), 305–315.
17. Balch, C. M., Urist, M. M., Karakousis, C. P., *et al.* (1993). Efficacy of 2-cm surgical margins for intermediate-thickness melanomas (1 to 4 mm). Results of a multi-institutional randomized surgical trial [see comments]. *Ann. Surg.* **218**(3), 262–267 [discussion 267–269].
18. Bonenkamp, J. J., Hermans, J., Sasako, M., and van de Velde, C. J. (1999). Extended lymph-node dissection for gastric cancer. Dutch Gastric Cancer Group [see comments]. *N. Engl. J. Med.* **340**(12), 908–914.
19. Krag, D., Weaver, D., Ashikaga, T., *et al.* (1998). The sentinel node in breast cancer—A multicenter validation study [see comments]. *N. Engl. J. Med.* **339**(14), 941–946.
20. Bunt, A. M., Hermans, J., Boon, M. C., *et al.* (1994). Evaluation of the extent of lymphadenectomy in a randomized trial of Western versus Japanese-type surgery in gastric cancer. *J. Clin. Oncol.* **12**(2), 417–422.
21. Laurie, J. A., Moertel, C. G., Fleming, T. R., *et al.* (1989). Surgical adjuvant therapy of large-bowel carcinoma: An evaluation of levamisole and the combination of levamisole and fluorouracil. The North Central Cancer Treatment Group and the Mayo Clinic [see comments]. *J. Clin. Oncol.* **7**(10), 1447–1456.
22. Moertel, C. G., Fleming, T. R., Macdonald, J. S., *et al.* (1995). Fluorouracil plus levamisole as effective adjuvant therapy after resection of stage III colon carcinoma: A final report. *Ann. Intern. Med.* **122**(5), 321–326.
23. Simon, R. (1993). Design and conduct of clinical trials. *In:* "Cancer: Principles and Practice of Oncology" (V. T. DeVita, Jr., S. Hellman, and S. A. Rosenberg, eds.), pp. 418–440. J. B. Lippincott Company, Philadelphia.

13

Using Administrative Data for Clinical Research

John D. Birkmeyer

VA Outcomes Group, VA Medical Center, White River Junction, Vermont 05009

I. Introduction

Administrative databases are being used increasingly in surgical research. Among many advantages for clinical and outcomes researchers, administrative databases usually contain information on large numbers of patients, which minimizes limitations associated with small sample size. They also tend to be population based, which avoids selection bias problems inherent in case series from large academic centers and allows assessment of outcomes in the "real world." For these reasons, administrative data are being used increasingly to study both utilization and patient outcomes after different surgical procedures.

Unfortunately, administrative (or "claims") databases were originally intended for administering health services and reimbursement, not performing clinical research. Thus, researchers must be aware of many methodologic challenges and limitations associated with this type of analysis. In particular, they must be aware of the accuracy of claims data in different contexts. Careful consideration of the limitations of administrative data for case-mix adjustment is particularly important for studies comparing outcome rates across providers (1, 2). In this chapter, administrative databases commonly used for clinical research, their basic content, and examples of research applications are reviewed and some of the pitfalls of administrative data analysis are considered.

II. Overview of Administrative Databases Used for Clinical Research

Large, administrative databases are produced and maintained by the federal government, state governments, and private health payers and providers. Table I summarizes several databases commonly used for clinical research; additional listings are available elsewhere (3). Research files pertaining to the Medicare program, maintained by the Health Care Financing Administration (HCFA), are among the most widely used data for clinical and outcomes research (4). These files contain information on acute care hospitalizations for Medicare enrollees (currently excluding the relatively small percentage enrolled in capitated managed care plans) and claims submitted by physicians or hospitals for outpatient care. HCFA's enrollment file contains demographic information on all patients eligible for Medicare benefits, including where they live. Thus, this file provides the "denominator" for studies exploring population-based utilization rates of surgical procedures.

In addition to its Medicare databases, the federal government is also responsible for data pertaining to patients receiving care by the Department of Veterans Affairs and Department of Defense healthcare systems. Finally, U.S. Health and Vital Statistics collects a broad range of clinically relevant information. One file—the National Death Index—collates death certificate information collected by states and is frequently used to determine long-term vital status for patients in clinical trials who are lost to follow-up.

State-level data often used for research include death certificate databases and utilization files for state Medicaid programs. Most frequently used is the Uniform Hospital Discharge Data Set (UHDDS), state-level databases of all acute care hospitalizations, regardless of payor (5). Among other research uses, UHDDS files frequently form the basis of state-wide trauma registries (6, 7). Though similar in nature to Medicare inpatient files, it contains information on all patient age groups. Unfortunately, UHDDS databases usually do not contain patient identifiers for "linking" with other data files or following patients over time. In addition, UHDDS files are not available in all states.

Large payors and insurers (e.g., Blue Cross/Blue Shield) and managed care networks (e.g., Kaiser-Permanente) maintain large administrative databases containing utilization and, to a lesser degree, patient outcome information (8). The content of these databases varies widely and, unlike state and federal data, they are proprietary.

A. Information Contained in Hospital Discharge Abstracts

Despite the large number and heterogeneity of administrative databases available for clinical research, most analyses focusing on surgery rely on hospital discharge abstract files (i.e., MEDPAR/Part A files for Medicare; UHDDS for individual states). Within each of these databases, a uniform set of information is collected for every patient experiencing acute care hospitalization. Of course, because hospitaliza-

Table I Overview of Administrative Databases Commonly Used for Clinical Research[a]

Federal level
Health Care Financing Administration (HCFA)/Medicare Research files
MEDPAR file (includes discharge abstracts for acute care hospitalizations)*
Part B file (contains claims for all physicians' services)
Provider files [information about all physicians with Uniform Physician Identification Numbers (UPINs)]
Enrollment file (demographic information on all Medicare enrollees, including vital status)*
Other files related to outpatient, home health, and skilled nursing facility care
Department of Veterans Affairs (VA)
Patient Treatment File (PTF)*
Outpatient File
Department of Defense
AQCESS in-patient data military
CHAMPUS healthcare data for dependents
Vital and Health Statistics Databases
National Death Index (collates death certificate information from states)*
State level
Medicaid management system
Uniform Hospital Discharge Data Set (UHDDS) (all-payor database of all hospitalizations, maintained by most but not all states)*
Birth and Death Certificate data
Private/proprietary databases
Large insurer databases, e.g., Blue Cross/Blue Shield
Provider network, managed care organization databases (content and availability vary widely)

[a]Note: This table lists examples only and does not represent all databases that could be used for research. Files most commonly used in studies of surgery utilization and outcomes are indicated by an asterisk*.

tion is required for inclusion, these files are generally useful only for studying surgical procedures with (at least) overnight hospital stays.

Data collected for each hospital discharge abstract includes demographic information—name and unique identifiers (Medicare only), age, sex, race/ethnicity, and patient residence. Administrative data include admission and discharge dates, total charges (and, for Medicare, amount reimbursed), expected payment source, admission type (elective, urgent, emergent), and discharge disposition (including vital status). Based on their Unique Physician Identification Numbers (UPINs), attending physicians and operating physicians are also identified. Finally, hospital discharge abstracts contain codes and dates for principal and other diagnoses and principal and other procedures. Table II displays a sample discharge abstract for an individual patient.

Clinical information from hospital discharge abstracts is represented by diagnosis codes from the "International Classification of Diseases, 9th Revision, Clinical Modification" (ICD-9-CM). Most discharge abstract formats now allow at least nine diagnosis codes. Coders in hospital medical records departments select ICD-9-CM codes to match primary (usually the admitting) clinical diagnoses indicated in the chart (e.g., 157.0, malignant neoplasm of head of pancreas; 410.0, acute myocardial infarction, anterolateral wall). Secondary diagnoses are also listed. These may reflect preexisting conditions (e.g., 401.9, essential hypertension, unspecified) or those arising during the index hospitalization (e.g., 482.0, pneumonia due to *Klebsiella pneumoniae*). Code modifiers (usually the last digit of the ICD-9-CM code) are often available for indicating illness severity or specific consequences of the underlying condition (e.g., 250.4, diabetes with renal manifestations).

ICD-9-CM codes are not restricted to clinical diagnoses, however. They may reflect instead patient symptoms (e.g., 789.0, abdominal pain), physical findings (e.g., 611.72, breast lump), or findings from laboratory tests (e.g., 276.2, acidosis). Personal and family history and miscellaneous socioeconomic variables are also reflected in ICD-9-CM codes (e.g., V16.0, family history of gastrointestinal tract cancer; V60.0, homelessness). Finally, an entire section of ICD-9-CM codes is devoted to complications of medical and surgical care (e.g., 998.1, hemorrhage or hematoma complicating a procedure). These latter codes are sometimes used as quality-of-care indicators.

Operations and other interventions occurring during the hospitalization, along with their dates of occurrence, are also identified in the hospital discharge abstract with ICD-9-CM codes. ICD-9-CM procedure codes do not precisely map to codes used by the American Medical Association's "Current Procedural Terminology" (CPT codes). CPT codes are used in claims (bills) for physician services and do not appear in hospital discharge abstract files.

B. Advantages of Administrative Databases

Typically based on observational (nonexperimental) study designs, clinical research based on administrative data has numerous advantages compared to research based on clinical data (Table III). Among the obvious practical reasons, administrative data have already been collected and, compared to clinical data, are very inexpensive to obtain. They also have numerous specific advantages for researchers interested in studying either surgical utilization or patient outcomes after procedures. These strengths are best illustrated with examples of how administrative data have been used in the past for research purposes. Reviewing common research applications also provides a useful context for later discussion of the major weaknesses of using administrative data for surgical research.

1. Studies of Surgery Utilization

Population-based administrative data are the only way to study utilization rates of surgical procedures. Calculating rates of a surgical procedure requires both a numerator (number of procedures performed) and a denominator (the number of persons "at risk" for surgery). For example, the rate of back surgery in the Wilmington, Delaware hospital referral region in 1994–1995 was 2.7 per 1000 Medicare enrollees (9). Surgery rates can only be calculated using population-based administrative databases that collect health-related information on all persons in a defined geographic area or population. Such databases allow measurement of the numerator because they include procedures performed at all hospitals in a defined region. Equally important, they provide the denominator of all members of the populations at risk for surgical intervention.

Population-based studies of surgery utilization can identify problems with surgical decision-making not apparent from patient-level or single hospital-level studies. Using administrative data, Wennberg has documented wide variation in rates of surgical procedures across geographic areas (small area analysis) (10, 11). For example, in 1994–1995, use of carotid endarterectomy in the Medicare population varied more than sevenfold across the 306 hospital referral regions from 1.0 per 1000 Medicare enrollees in Honolulu to 7.1 per 1000 in Houma, Louisiana (Fig. 1) (9). Variation of this magnitude could not be explained by regional variation in patient characteristics or illness rates or by variation in patient access to health services (all patients covered by Medicare). Instead, regional variation in use of carotid endarterectomy implied fundamental differences in physician practice style in the management of carotid artery disease.

With studies of regional variation in surgery rates, administrative data can be used to do more than just identify problems: they can help identify reasons for practice variation. With carotid artery disease, surgery rates were

Table II Information Contained in the Hospital Discharge Abstract[a]

Type of data	Information
Demographic	
Age	76 years
Sex	Female
Race	White
Zip code, state of residence	xxxxx, xx
Administrative	
Admission and discharge dates	dd-mm-yy, dd-mm-yy
Admission source	Hospital transfer
Admission type	Emergency
HMO enrollment	No
Provider	UPIN xxx
Total/reimbursed charges	$31,767/$33,788
ICU days/charges	2/$4,330
Discharge status	Alive
ICD-9-CM diagnosis codes	
414.01	Coronary atherosclerosis (native vessels)
428.0	Congestive heart failure
413.9	Other and unspecified angina pectoris
410.71	Subendocardial infarction (initial)
401.9	Essential hypertension (unspecified)
250.00	Adult-onset diabetes mellitus, without mention of complications
440.21	Atherosclerosis of extremities with claudication
244.9	Unspecified hypothyroidism
305.1	Tobacco use disorder
ICD-9-CM procedure codes	
36.12	Aortocoronary bypass of two coronary arteries (date)
36.15	Single internal mammary–coronary artery bypass (date)
37.61	Implantation of pulsation balloon (date)
39.61	Extracorporeal circulation auxiliary to open heart surgery
37.22	Left heart cardiac catheterization
88.56	Coronary arteriography using two catheters

[a]The example is an actual Medicare patient undergoing coronary artery bypass graft (CABG) surgery in 1996. Potentially identifying information has been omitted.

tightly correlated with regional rates of carotid duplex testing (Fig. 2) (12). Thus, rates of carotid endarterectomy varied not simply because surgical specialists disagreed about indications for surgery in patients with carotid stenosis. They varied because physicians disagreed about the use of carotid duplex testing and thus how hard to look for surgically treatable disease.

Finally, studies of surgery utilization can be used to make general inferences about efficacy of procedures. For example, Tunis *et al.* (13) studied the effectiveness of revascularization procedures for preventing lower extremity amputation in patients with peripheral vascular disease using Maryland (UHDDS) hospital discharge data. Between 1979 and 1989, annual rates of percutaneous transluminal angio-

Table III General Advantages of Using Administrative Data for Clinical Research and Specific Advantages for Studying Surgical Utilization or Patient Outcomes after Procedures

General advantages of administrative data
Inexpensive compared to clinical data
Data already collected; short time interval between study conception (or funding) and analysis
Advantages for studying surgical utilization
Only administrative data allow assessment of procedure utilization rates: contain information about both numerator (number of procedures performed) and denominator (population "at risk" for procedure) for surgery rates
Can assess regional use of surgical procedures (small area analysis) and explore reasons for variation in surgical practice style or intensity
Advantages for studying patient outcomes
Large sample size, critical for studying relatively infrequent outcome measures (e.g., postoperative mortality)
Outcomes of surgical procedures in the "real world"—provides data about effectiveness at all hospitals, not just large academic centers
Complete follow-up in cohort studies; by linking databases, can follow patients even if they transfer medical care to another facility or relocate

plasty increased from 1 to 24 per 100,000 residents. There was no evidence that angioplasty was reducing the need for lower extremity bypass surgery—bypass rates doubled from 32 to 65 per 100,000. During the same 10-year time period, however, annual rates of lower extremity amputation remained essentially unchanged. Thus, although revascularization procedures may have value for other purposes (e.g., improving claudication symptoms), this study found no evidence that increasing use of these procedures was preventing lower extremity amputations.

2. Patient Outcome Studies

Administrative databases have several advantages for researchers interested in studying patient outcomes after surgical procedures. First, because they are generally very large, studies have sufficient sample size and statistical power for almost any purpose. In studies of surgical outcomes, statistical power is often constrained by the relatively low frequency of the primary outcome measure, e.g., postoperative mortality. For example, to study surgeon-specific mortality rates with coronary bypass surgery (mean 3–5%), at least 500 patients per surgeon are needed for reasonable statistical precision. Administrative data may also be useful as a screening tool for identifying large numbers of patients with very infrequent surgical complications, e.g., major bile duct injury after laparoscopic cholecystectomy.

As a second major advantage, administrative databases provide the best insights into the risks and effectiveness of surgical procedures in the "real world." Traditionally, most surgical research based on clinical data relies on information from large academic centers—from case series from single institutions to large, multicenter trials. There is now broad agreement that data from these settings cannot be used to make inferences about the effectiveness of surgical therapy in the general community.

For example, Wennberg *et al.* (14) used the national Medicare database to study perioperative mortality with carotid endarterectomy, in 1992–1993. Mortality rates were substantially lower at high-volume centers (1.7%) than at low-volume hospitals (2.5%), confirming the well-known "volume-outcome" effect with this procedure (Fig. 3). Second, among high-volume hospitals, mortality rates were lower in those centers participating in the major clinical trials for this procedure (North American Symptomatic Carotid Surgery Trial and the Asymptomatic Carotid Artery Study) than in other high-volume centers (1.4 vs. 1.8%). Finally, at these trial hospitals, mortality rates were lower in patients enrolled in the trials (<0.5%) than in remaining patients not enrolled (1.5%). This study perhaps best illustrates the multiple levels at which selection bias (both patient and provider) can threaten the validity of non-population-based studies of surgical outcomes.

As a third major advantage, administrative databases can be used to ensure complete follow-up in studies of long-term outcomes after surgical procedures. Cohort studies based on clinical data are not only very expensive, but patients often become "lost" to follow-up when they move or even transfer their care to another local provider. Incomplete patient follow-up creates the potential for selection bias ("lost" patients may differ from other patients in important ways) and threaten the validity of the study's conclusions. Because many administrative databases contain information on patients regardless of where they move (or can be linked to databases that do), they can often ensure 100% follow-up rates rarely achievable in studies based on clinical data.

For example, using national Medicare data, Birkmeyer *et al.* (15, 16) studied the relationship between hospital procedural volume and patient outcomes after pancreaticoduodenectomy. Like many previous studies, they demonstrated much lower in-hospital mortality rates at high-volume hospitals (4%) than at low- and very low-volume hospitals (12

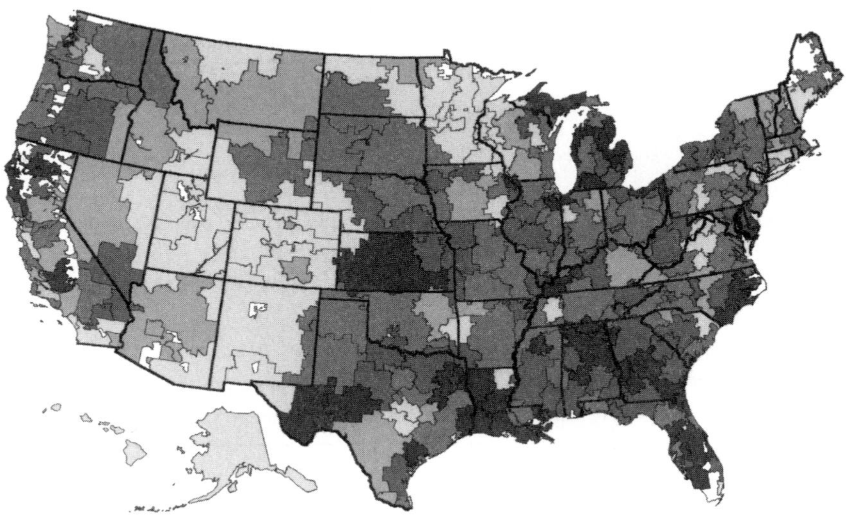

Figure 1 Map showing variation in rates of carotid endarterectomy in Medicare enrollees (1995–1996) across the 306 hospital referral regions of the United States. From Birkmeyer (12).

and 16%, respectively). However, their study was the first to demonstrate the relationship between increased hospital volume and lower mortality rates after hospital discharge—an analysis possible by linking Medicare's hospital discharge abstract file to patient vital status information contained in its enrollment (denominator) file.

III. Cautions about Using Administrative Databases for Research

Despite the many strengths of administrative databases, researchers must be aware of many serious limitations associated with these data sources (Table IV). Although the pitfalls of administrative data are manifest in different ways for different research applications, most are ultimately related to the precision and accuracy of ICD-9-CM codes for identifying surgical procedures and clinical diagnoses.

A. Accuracy for Classifying Surgical Procedures

The reliability of administrative data for classifying surgical procedures is essential for studies of procedure utilization. It is also important when procedure codes are used as the primary criteria for selecting subjects for study inclusion, e.g., all patients undergoing pancreaticoduodenectomy in the state of New York (17).

How well do administrative databases identify patients undergoing surgical procedures? As described earlier, hospital discharge abstract files do not include patients undergoing same-day/outpatient surgery. In some states, these files may also exclude patients admitted overnight on "observation" status. To correct these problems, many states are currently creating separate, outpatient files.

Administrative data are generally accurate, however, for classifying surgical procedures performed on an inpatient basis. In a 1985 coding validation study, Fisher *et al.* (18)

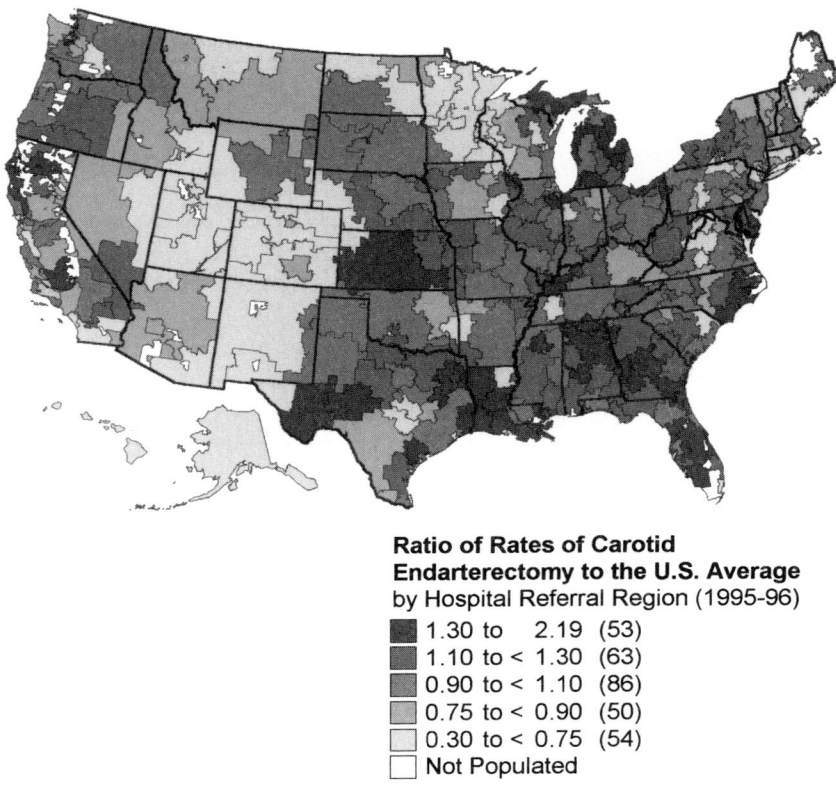

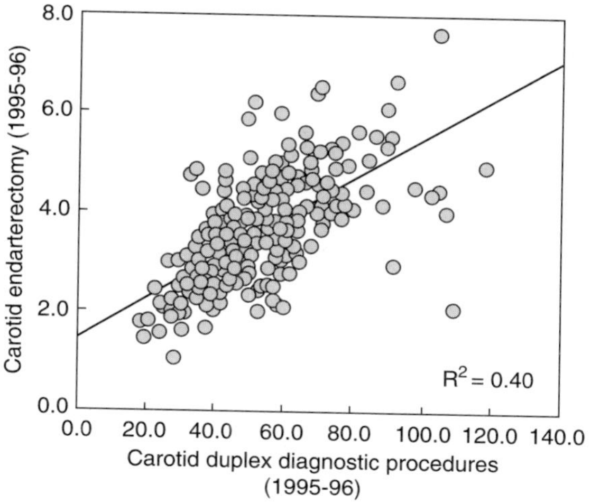

Figure 2 Relationship between regional rates of carotid duplex testing and carotid endarterectomy in Medicare patients. Each point reflects one of the 306 hospital referral regions of the United States. The strong correlation is reflected in the high R^2 (0.40). From Birkmeyer (12).

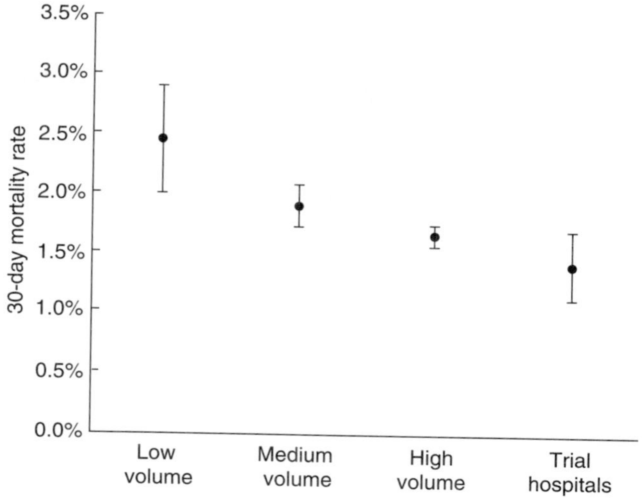

Figure 3 Relationship between hospital procedural volume and 30-day mortality with carotid endarterectomy. Mortality was lowest at centers participating in the major clinical trials of this procedure. From Ref. (14), Wennberg *et al.* (1998). *JAMA* **279**, 1278–1281. Copyrighted 1998 American Medical Association.

reviewed the accuracy of claims data for identifying 15 common procedures (all mainly performed as inpatient procedures at the time). Hospital charts for over 7000 randomly selected Medicare inpatients were reabstracted and compared to codes contained in the originally submitted discharge abstracts. Sensitivity rates (proportion of patients with the procedure who had the appropriate code) exceeded 0.95 for 10 of the 15 procedures. Positive predictive values (proportion of patients with the code who had the corresponding procedure) were similarly high, exceeding 0.99 for 7 of the 10 procedures.

Although ICD-9-CM coding of surgical procedures is generally reliable, the codes often lack specificity. For example, primary procedure codes do not distinguish between right vs. left or upper vs. lower extremity. (Modifier codes available for these distinctions are not used consistently.) Although admission acuity (elective vs. urgent/emergent) is captured in discharge abstracts, acuity for procedure(s) occurring after that admission is not.

B. Accuracy of Clinical Diagnoses

1. General Considerations

For surgery researchers, the reliability of administrative data for capturing clinical diagnoses is important for at least three reasons. First, clinical conditions are often part of the selection criteria for the study population. For example, researcher interested in long-term mortality rates after abdomino-perineal resection may wish to restrict the analysis to patients with rectal cancer. Second, the accuracy of diagnosis coding is important for researchers interested in describing rates of nonfatal endpoints after a given surgical procedure, e.g., incidence of stroke after carotid endarterectomy. Finally, primary admission diagnoses and secondary diagnoses (patient comorbidities) are necessary for case-mix adjustment. Ability to adjust for population characteristics is particularly crucial for studies comparing performance across providers (19).

The accuracy of ICD-9-CM coding for clinical conditions can first be considered in terms of its specificity, which determines the likelihood that patients get coded incorrectly for a condition they did not experience. (Specificity is 1 minus the false positive rate.) In general, the specificity of claims data for identifying clinical diagnoses is relatively good. In one validation study, specificity rates between 0.90 and 0.99 were documented for 12 acute and chronic conditions related to cardiovascular disease (20). Although relatively infrequent, false positives occur for numerous reasons (21, 22). With acute myocardial infarction, for example, false positive codes resulted when physicians (rather than coders) listed the acute myocardial infarction incorrectly, when the myocardial infarction occurred in previous admissions, or when myocardial infarctions were "ruled out."

Compared to specificity, the sensitivity of administrative data for clinical conditions—the rate at which patients with a given condition get coded for it—is somewhat lower. For primary (admitting) diagnoses, sensitivity rates range between 0.75 and 0.96 (18). Codes for relatively discrete,

Table IV Limitations of Using Administrative Data for Clinical and Outcomes Research

Identification of surgical procedures	
	Hospital discharge abstract databases miss procedures performed on outpatients
	Although sensitive for inpatient procedures, often lack specificity (e.g., right vs. left, upper vs. lower extremity)
Measuring nonfatal surgical outcomes	
	Difficult to determine and categorize reoperations
	Diagnostic codes lack information about timing of events, so difficult to differentiate between complications and preexisting conditions.
Risk adjustment	
	Inaccuracies and incompleteness of coding for comorbidities and preexisting conditions, particularly in most severely ill patients
	Difficult to grade illness severity
	May inadvertently adjust for surgical complications
	Variation in coding accuracy and completeness across providers

unambiguous conditions (hip fracture, colon cancer, and breast cancer) tend to be more reliable than codes for more "discretionary" diagnoses (congestive heart failure, chronic obstructive lung disease).

The sensitivity of administrative data for secondary diagnoses (including chronic, preexisting conditions) is much poorer, however. For example, among a cohort of patients with primary diagnosis of acute myocardial infarction, patient comorbidities listed less than half the time included cerebrovascular disease (sensitivity 0.14), peripheral vascular disease (0.29), and tobacco use (0.24) (20). Preexisting conditions are listed even less frequently for the most severely ill patients (e.g., patients with multiple postoperative complications). For these patients, chronic conditions are "crowded off" the hospital discharge abstract by acute events occurring during the hospitalization. The implications of this phenomenon for risk adjustment are discussed later.

Finally, even when diagnostic ICD-9-CM codes are used correctly, they often lack "clinical" specificity and fail to reflect the heterogeneity of patients with a given diagnosis. For example, the code for dissecting aortic aneurysm (ICD-9-CM 441.0) will not differentiate between an unstable patient with visceral ischemia and an asymptomatic patient noted to have dissection on a computerized tomography (CT) scan performed for other reasons.

2. Measuring Nonfatal Surgical Outcomes

Although most often used for studies assessing mortality (for which it is very accurate), administrative data are sometimes used to examine rates of nonfatal adverse events after surgical procedures (23, 24). Some of these events can be identified using procedure codes indicating reoperation (e.g., ICD-9-CM 54.12, reopening of recent laparotomy site). Although the reliability of reoperation codes has not been studied systematically, many reoperations are likely coded according the specific intervention (e.g., lysis of adhesions). Confirming that such events occurred at a second operation (instead of the first) is not always possible.

Using diagnosis codes to classify nonfatal postoperative events is also problematic. The coding of many complications after surgical procedures is no doubt prone to the same limitations described above for medical diagnoses. For example, very "discretionary" conditions such as pneumonia are unlikely to be coded reliably; pulmonary embolus codes may often be listed for "rule outs." Because diagnosis codes in the hospital discharge abstract lack information about the timing of events, it is frequently impossible to differentiate between preexisting conditions and new complications (25). As described earlier, there is a section of codes specific for complications of medical and surgical therapy (e.g., ICD-9-CM 998.3, disruption of operation wound). Unfortunately, the sensitivity of these codes for postoperative complications is suspect.

Given these concerns about coding, researchers interested in studying nonfatal outcomes often rely on more complex algorithms. For example, to study complications of carotid endarterectomy, Mitchell *et al.* (26) used an algorithm based on the use of head CT, head magnetic resonance imaging (MRI), or surgical exploration codes with 30 days of the index procedure. Alternatively, many researchers rely on simpler proxies for complications, such as length of stay (overall and intensive care unit) and 30-day readmission rates.

3. Case-Mix Adjustment with Administrative Data

As described previously (Chapter 10, this volume), studies comparing outcome rates among groups must account for any differences in patient case-mix between them. For example, hospital-specific mortality rates with coronary bypass surgery should be adjusted for the "risk profile" of patients at each hospital. The risk adjustment (most often multivariable logistic regression) model should include patient-level covariates known to affect surgical risks: (1) demographic information (e.g., age, sex, race), (2) preexisting patient comorbidities (e.g., diabetes, peripheral vascular disease), and (3) disease severity (e.g., acuity, ejection fraction, use of preoperative intraaortic balloon pump).

Individual comorbidities (e.g., diabetes) or illness severity measures, identified by their corresponding ICD-9-CM codes, may be used alone as independent variables in risk adjustment models. Alternatively, they may be compiled into a single comorbidity score, generally analogous to the Charlson comorbidity score, using a number of available claims-based classification schemes (27, 28). Among several advantages, comorbidity scores make use of highly predictive comorbidities (e.g., cirrhosis) that are too infrequent to be robust as independent variables in the risk adjustment model.

Unfortunately, risk adjustment with administrative data is no better than the information on which it is based. Although demographic information is very accurate in administrative databases, comorbidity data suffer from the sensitivity and (to a lesser extent) specificity problems of diagnostic coding described above (29). To better identify patient comorbidities, some have suggested using information from previous admissions and databases not requiring hospitalization (30). Although admission acuity is available, the same problems with diagnostic coding apply to assessing illness severity.

The limitations of use of administrative data for risk adjustment can lead to incorrect inferences. For example, one study based on Medicare claims data suggested that transurethral retrograde prostatectomy (TURP) was associated with higher perioperative mortality than open resection for benign prostatic hyperplasia (31). This observation was subsequently refuted by a study of these two procedures. Using clinical data, Concato *et al.* (32) noted that men undergoing TURP had a substantially greater number of comorbidities and were more likely to undergo urgent procedures—differences not apparent in the claims data. After accounting for these differences in patient case-mix, the TURP procedure was in fact associated with lower surgical risks.

Several studies have assessed the relative performance of clinical data and administrative data for case-mix adjustment. The two approaches often produce different results. For example, clinical and code-based adjustment methods often predicted very different odds of surgical mortality for patients undergoing coronary artery bypass surgery (33). However, empirical evidence that risk adjustment with clinical data has superior predictive or discriminative performance is lacking. One study compared the performance of several available severity measures for predicting in-hospital mortality with coronary bypass surgery and several acute medical conditions (34). The *C* statistics (which measure how well a severity measure discriminates between patients who lived and those who died) were very similar for adjustment methods based on clinical data and those using administrative data. One potential explanation for this finding may be that risk adjustment models using hospital discharge abstract codes often include complications occurring late in the hospitalization, as well as measures of illness severity at the time of admission. "Adjusting" for complications strongly related to mortality (e.g., cardiac arrest, renal failure) would lead to overestimation of the performance of risk adjustment models based on administrative data (25).

Researchers using administrative data for risk adjustment should be aware of other potential problems. As described above, the hospital discharge abstract has limited diagnosis fields. Patients who die during hospitalization often have "saturated" diagnosis fields. For example, in one analysis of mortality after Whipple procedures, 52% of in-hospital deaths had "saturated" diagnosis fields, compared to only 28% of survivors (15). For these patients, preexisting comorbidities may be "crowded off" the discharge abstract by acute events. Undercoding of comorbidities in patients experiencing in-hospital mortality (vs. survivors) is likely responsible for the paradox that comorbidities occasionally seem to reduce the risk of mortality (35). With Whipple procedures, for example, patients with diabetes, preexisting heart disease, and higher Charlson scores were less likely to die perioperatively.

Researchers using administrative data to compare outcomes across individual providers need to be particularly sensitive to case-mix adjustment issues. There is substantial variability in accuracy and thoroughness in coding practices between individual hospitals. One study examined the importance of coding accuracy in variation among California hospitals in risk-adjusted mortality rates with acute myocardial infarction (36). After reabstracting medical records, the study noted that at least one clinical risk factor was missing for 65% of patients (range 45 to 87% across hospitals). Conversely, overcoding, which occurred in 31.5% of records overall, varying from 10% in one "high"-mortality hospital to 74% at a "low"-mortality hospital. Variation in coding accuracy explained part of the variation in adjusted mortality rates between hospitals (36).

IV. Conclusions

Administrative data are being used increasingly to address important research questions in surgery. This interest can be explained in part by the obvious practical advantages of administrative databases—large amounts of longitudinal data that have already been obtained. From a scientific perspective, population-based administrative data permit investigations that would not be possible with clinical data alone. Studies of regional variation in the use of surgical procedures are just one example.

Although administrative databases are also valuable for studying patient outcomes after surgery, researchers must be aware of many methodologic challenges in this area, particularly those related to the accuracy of diagnostic coding and risk adjustment. Many of the most careful evaluations of administrative databases (reviewed in this chapter) were performed in the 1980s; there is evidence that coding practices have improved since then (18, 20). However, it is unlikely that information contained in administrative databases will ever replicate the clinical detail and specificity contained in medical charts. For these reasons, researchers using administrative data must be careful in how they select research questions. Studies most likely to suffer the pitfalls of administrative data will be those focusing on "ambiguous" clinical conditions and nonfatal clinical outcome measures. Researchers should also steer clear of comparisons between individual providers, particularly when there is a strong likelihood of confounding by patient case-mix.

References

1. Iezzoni, L. I. (1997). Assessing quality using administrative. *Ann. Intern. Med.* **127,** 666–674.
2. Williams, S. V., Nash, D. B., and Goldfarb, N. (1991). Differences in mortality from coronary artery bypass graft surgery at five teaching hospitals. *JAMA* **266,** 810–815.
3. Paul, J. E., Weis, K., and Epstein, R. A. (1993). Data bases for variations research. *Med. Care* **31,** S96–S102.
4. Mitchell, J. B., Bubolz, T., Paul, J. E., Pashos, C. L., Escarce, J. J., Mulbaier, L. H., *et al.* (1994). Using Medicare claims for outcomes research. *Med. Care* **32,** S38–S51.
5. Epstein, M. H. (1992). Guest alliance: Uses of state-level hospital discharge databases. *J. Am. Health Inf. Manage. Assoc.* **63,** 32–39.
6. Rutledge, (1995). The goals, development, and use of trauma registries and trauma data sources in decision making in injury. *Surg. Clin. North Am.* **75,** 305–326.
7. Mullins, R. J., and Mann, N. C. (1999). Population-based research assessing the effectiveness of trauma systems. *J. Trauma Inj. Infect. Crit. Care* **47,** S56–S66.
8. Selby, J. V. (1997). Linking automated databases for research in managed care settngs. *Ann. Intern. Med.* **127,** 719-24.
9. Wennberg, J. E., and Cooper, M. M. (1998). "Dartmouth Atlas of Health Care 1998." American Hospital Publishing, Chicago.
10. Wennberg, J. E., and Gittelsohn, A. (1973). Small area variations in health care delivery. *Science* **182,** 1102–1108.
11. Wennberg, J. E., Barnes, B. A., and Zubkoff, M. (1982). Professional uncertainty and the problem of supplier-induced demand. *Soc. Sci. Med.* **16,** 811–824.
12. Birkmeyer, J. D. (1999). Practice variations and the quality of surgical care for common conditions. *In* "The Darthmouth Atlas of Health Care 1999" (J.E. Wennberg and M.M. Cooper, eds.), pp. 139–174. American Hospital Publishing, Chicago.
13. Tunis, S. R., Bass, E. B., and Steinberg, E. P. (1991). The use of angioplasty, bypass surgery, and amputation in the management of peripheral vascular disease. *N. Engl. J. Med.* **325,** 556–562.
14. Wennberg, D. E., Lucas, F. L., Birkmeyer, J. D., Bredenberg, C. E., and Fisher, E. S. (1998). Variation in carotid endartectomy mortality in the Medicare population: Trial hospitals, volume, and patient characteristics. *JAMA* **279,** 1278–1281.
15. Birkmeyer, J. D., Finlayson, S. R. G., Tosteson, A. N. A., Sharp, S. M., Warshaw, A. L., and Fisher, E. S. (1999). Effect of hospital volume on in-hospital mortality with Whipple procedures. *Surgery* **125,** 250–256.
16. Birkmeyer, J. D., Warshaw, A. L., Finlayson, S. R. G., Grove, M. R., and Tosteson, A. N. A. (1999). Relationship between hospital volume and late survival after pancreaticoduodenectomy. *Surgery* (in press).
17. Lieberman, M. D., Kilburn, H., Lindsey, M., and Brennan, M. F. (1995). Relation of perioperative deaths to hospital volume among patients undergoing pancreatic resection for malignancy. *Ann. Surg.* **222,** 638–645.
18. Fisher, E. S., Whaley, F. S., Krushat, W. M., Malenka, D. J., Fleming, C., Baron, J. A., *et al.* (1992). The accuracy of Medicare's hospital claims data: Progress has been made, but problems remain. *Am. J. Public Health* **82,** 243–248.
19. Iezzoni, L. I. (1990). Using administrative diagnostic data to assess the quality of hospital care. *Int. J. Tech. Assess. Health Care* **6,** 272–281.
20. Jollis, J. G., Ancukiewicz, M., DeLong, E. R., Pryor, D. B., Muhlbaier, L. H., and Mark, D. B. (1993). Discordance of databases designed for claims payment versus clinical information services. Implications for outcomes research. *Ann. Intern. Med.* **119,** 844–850.
21. Iezzoni, L. I., Burnside, S., Sickles, L., Moskowitz, M. A., Sawitz, E., and Levine, P. A. (1988). Coding of acute myocardial infarction. Clinical policy implications. *Ann. Intern. Med.* **109,** 745–751.
22. van Walraven, C., Wang, B., Ugnat, A. M., and Naylor, C. D. (1990). False-positive coding for acute myocardial infarction on hospital discharge records: Chart audit results from a tertiary centre. *Can. J. Cardiol.* **6,** 383–386.
23. Iezzoni, L. I., Daley, J., Heeren, T., Foley, S. M., Fisher, E. S., Duncan, C., *et al.* (1994). Identifying complications of care using administrative data. *Med. Care* **32,** 700–715.
24. Norton, E. D., Garfinkel, S. A., McQuay, L. J., Heck, D. J., Wright, J. G., Dittus, R., *et al.* (1998). The effect of hospital volume on the in-hospital complication rate in knee replacement patients. *Health Serv. Res.* **33,** 1191–1210.
25. Roos, L. L., Stranc, L., James, R. C., and Li, J. (1997). Complications, comorbidities, and mortality: Improving classification and prediction. *Health Serv. Res.* **32,** 229–242.
26. Mitchell, J. B., Ballard, D. J., Whisnant, J. P., Ammering, C. J., Matchar, D. B., and Samsa, G. P. (1996). Using physician claims to identify postoperative complications of carotid endarterectomy. *Health Serv. Res.* **31,** 141–152.
27. Deyo, R. A., Cherkin, D. C., and Ciol, M. A. (1992). Adapting a clinical comorbidity index for use with ICD-9 administrative databases. *J. Clin. Epidemiol.* **45,** 613–619.
28. Romano, P. S., Roos, L. L., and Jollis, J. G. (1993). Adapting a clinical comorbidity index for use with ICD-9-CM administrative data: Differing perspectives. *J. Clin. Epidemiol.* **46,** 1075–1079.
29. Malenka, D. J., McLerran, D., Roos, N., Fisher, E. S., and Wennberg, J. E. (1994). Using administrative data to describe casemix: a comparison with the medical record. *J. Clin. Epidemiol.* **47,** 1027–1032.
30. Zhang, J. X., Iwashyna, T. J., and Christakis, N. A. (1999). The performance of different lookback periods and sources of information for Charlson comorbidity adjustment in Medicare claims data. *Med. Care* **37,** 1128–1139.
31. Roos, N. P., Wennberg, J. E., Malenka, D. J., Fisher, E. S., McPherson, K., Andersen, T. F., *et al.* (1989). Mortality and reoperation after open and transurethral resection of the prostate for benign prostatic hyperplasia. *N. Engl. J. Med.* **320,** 1120–1124.
32. Concato, J., Horwitz, R. I., Feinstein, A. R., Elmore, J. G., Schiff, S. F. (1992). Problems of comorbidity in mortality after prostatectomy. *JAMA* **267,** 1077–1082.
33. Iezzoni, L. I., Ash, A. S., Schwartz, M., Landon, B. E., and Mackiernan, Y. D. (1998). Predicting in-hospital deaths from coronary artery bypass graft surgery. *Med. Care* **36,** 28–39.
34. Iezzoni, L. I. (1997). The risks of risk adjustment. *JAMA* **278,** 1600–1607.
35. Iezzoni, L. I., Foley, S. M., Daley, J., Hughes, J., Fisher, E. S., and Heeren, T. (1992). Comorbidities, complications, and coding bias. Does the number of diagnosis codes matter in predicting in-hospital mortality? *JAMA* **267,** 2238–2239.
36. Wilson, P., Smoley, S. R., Werdegar, D. (1996). Office of Statewide Health Planning and Development. Second report of the California Hospital Outcome Project, 1996.

14

Research in the Intensive Care Unit: Ethical and Methodological Issues

Philip S. Barie, Matthew D. Bacchetta, Joseph J. Fins*, and Soumitra R. Eachempati

*Departments of Surgery and *Medicine, Anne and Max A. Cohen Surgical Intensive Care Unit, New York-Presbyterian Hospital—New York Weill Cornell Center, Weill Medical College of Cornell University, New York, New York 10021*

I. Introduction

The intensive care unit (ICU) is a fertile place for the conduct of clinical and translational research. Important questions abound, large numbers of potential study candidates are present in a defined space, clinical monitoring systems can be relied on to maximize patient safety during studies, and critical care practitioners are supportive and interested in advancing the science of critical care. That is not to say that research in the ICU is easy to perform, or even that it should be. The heterogeneity of disease processes inherent in a busy ICU can complicate the process of study design and confound the identification of patients for study. Instability of gas exchange or hemodynamics may characterize the target population for interventional studies, but may make observational studies or those involving multiple sequential measurements over time difficult to carry out and interpret. The ethical issues are complex when studying a vulnerable patient population such as critically ill patients; the ethical conduct of research must be respected to the utmost degree. This chapter discusses many ethical and methodologic issues that relate to the conduct of clinical research involving critically ill patients.

It is essential to recognize that several aspects affecting quality of care in an ICU can affect outcome (1). High-quality research in the ICU must be predicated on consistency of clinical management so as to minimize avoidable fluctuations of the stability of the patient/research subject. Several organizational characteristics of ICUs can affect the outcomes of critically ill patients, and it is recognized that there is variability in outcomes among ICUs (2). Characteristics of high-performance ICUs include the availability of new technologies, a culture of communication and cooperation, and participation of the ICU in hospital-wide quality management programs (3). Variability of outcomes (i.e., mortality) can complicate the design and interpretation of research studies, whether single center or multicenter. If mortality is low, then larger sample sizes must be planned. Studies may be difficult to fund if large numbers of patients must be enrolled: If mortality is unexpectedly low in the control group, then the study may be underpowered (i.e., too few patients are enrolled) and a Type-II or β-error may incorrectly identify no difference among groups. Conversely, control group mortality that appears to be too high (typically, compared with expectations generated by an assessment of severity of illness) may exaggerate the apparent effect of a treatment (1). Single-center studies are most susceptible to these types of errors, but multicenter trials are not immune.

Central to the conduct of research in the ICU is the protection of research subjects. Critically ill patients are a vulnerable population. Such patients are often unable to make their own decisions regarding participation and must have surrogates to act on their behalf. The surrogate often has not been designated in advance by the patient, and may be insecure in his or her knowledge of the patient's wishes. On the other hand, some studies are designed to test potentially lifesaving treatments in unstable patients, placing a premium on rapid decision making and rapid enrollment. Indeed, some studies incorporate time-sensitive enrollment criteria, raising the possibility of conflict or coercion between the patient (or surrogate), who may want to do "what is best" or "everything," or who may be hesitant to act out of insecurity, and the investigator, who has professional and financial interests at stake. Professional success is often predicated on success as a researcher, and increasingly, revenue from industry-sponsored studies are used to maintain the clinical research enterprise.

II. Spectrum of Research in the Intensive Care Unit

The ICU is a paradoxical environment that combines high technology with labor-intensive care. Research may be conducted to evaluate new technology, the patient–technology interface, therapies of many types, nontherapeutic drug interventions (e.g., pharmacokinetic studies), and the physiological responses to intervention. The psychological consequences of critical illness for patients, families, and staff, short- and long-term mortality, surrogate outcomes (e.g., length of stay in the ICU, the cost of care), and organizational issues in the unit may also be evaluated. Given these diverse possibilities, it can be challenging to develop and maintain a focused research program. It can also be challenging to parse a popular but finite patient population into various studies while maintaining a balance between investigator access and patient protection, especially for smaller units with ambitious research goals.

The type of research being performed will dictate many of the issues relating to the design of a study. The expertise of the study group and the nature of the patient population must be taken into account. The research question must be asked with precision and the study design and analysis plan must be defined in prospect. Although the "gold standard" for new biomedical research is the double-blind, randomized, controlled trial (RCT), such studies are expensive, cumbersome, and unsuited to several types of study. Whereas the RCT is indispensable to trials of new drug therapies or other treatment-related interventions, the RCT design is generally unsuited to epidemiologic or other outcomes research.

A. Defining the Research Question

Any research performed in the ICU setting should be hypothesis driven. A question cannot be answered unless it is asked correctly. A valid hypothesis can be generated by careful observation, systemic review of previously published trials, retrospective review of an existing database, or pilot prospective studies. Each source of background data has its own advantages and drawbacks. There are several essential prerequisites for the design of a clinical trial to maximize the likelihood of success. First is the clear enunciation of the hypothesis to be tested. Second, the patient population to be tested must be identified precisely, along with specific criteria for inclusion and exclusion and definition of the comparison group to be studied. The duration of the study must be defined. The duration is often defined as a result of several related factors, including whether the study will be conducted at one or several centers (thereby defining the rate of accrual), the endpoint chosen (mortality vs. a surrogate endpoint), the estimated prevalence of the endpoint in the study population (e.g., 40% mortality from standard care), and the estimated effect on the endpoint that the new treatment will have.

A good research question can arise from almost any source, including the investigator's imagination. However, to justify the risks involved in testing human subjects, especially a vulnerable population such as critically ill patients, there must usually be either some preliminary evidence that the intervention will have its intended effect, or the clinical condition must be so terrible and untreatable that even the glimmer of hope is adequate justification. The latter circumstances are increasingly few and far between as medicine advances progressively and protection of human research subjects is strengthened appropriately.

The hypothesis for a study can come from a review of the clinical literature, observations made in the basic or applied physiology laboratory (bench-to-bedside, or translational, research), preliminary clinical studies, or even the investigator's clinical experience. Systematic reviews include a thorough search for all existing data, an assessment of the quality of the primary source data, and a synthesis of available evidence regarding a focused query.

Retrospective database reviews have a high potential for the introduction of bias, but there can be value if carefully designed to reduce the chance of bias. Several techniques are available to minimize introduction of bias. The review of consecutive patient series without the opportunity to exclude selected patients, the evaluation of clinical databases rather than administrative data, and the use of case-matching methodology to maximize equivalence of comparison groups constructed post hoc may be employed. Prospective data collection and the examination of narrowly defined questions to avoid the chance identification of statistical significance by repetitive analyses *(data mining)* are well recognized. Administrative databases require a high degree of circumspection regarding the quality of the included data. Administrative databases are inherently limited because post hoc collection of data abstracted from charts (which may suffer from poor documentation), by observers (with variable training and credentials) who were not involved in the care of the patient at the time, introduces a substantial possibility of error.

Pilot prospective studies are commonly performed to establish safety as well as preliminary evidence of efficacy, especially for the evaluation of new pharmaceuticals. Safety studies (phase I) are usually performed in healthy volunteers outside of the critical care milieu. Phase II studies sometimes overlap the evaluation of safety along with an initial evaluation of efficacy, and may sometimes involve ICU patients. Establishment of a safety profile is paramount in such early-phase studies, but there also needs to be some rationale (evidence of benefit) beyond theoretical constructs or laboratory animal studies to justify the risk to the patient and the expense to the sponsoring organization. Pilot studies, by their very nature, do not always require the rigorous design (i.e., open-label as opposed to blinded studies) typical of prospective studies that are designed to produce unequivocal evidence of benefit (pivotal phase III studies).

There are times when the hypothesis needs only to be a prediction of equivalence, and other times when the superiority of a new intervention must be proved. Proof of equality is the usual standard when a new antibiotic is compared with an existing antibiotic, because it is assumed that both study arms will receive an effective drug. Adequate power to demonstrate the possibility of superiority must be ensured, lest a Type-II error be mistaken for true equivalence (see below). Comparison of monitoring devices (e.g., a new pulse oximeter) is also predicated on the substantial equivalence presumption for the introduction of similar technology under the Investigational Device Exception (IDE) regulations of the U.S. Food and Drug Administration (FDA). On the other hand, regulatory requirements for the introduction of novel therapies (e.g., immunomodulator therapy for sepsis) require that a treatment effect must be demonstrated beyond that of standard care provided to the control group. Traditionally, the applicable standard has been a reduction in mortality (usually 28-day, all-cause mortality), but increasingly it is argued that surrogate endpoints (e.g., reduced length of stay, reduced need for other therapies) are acceptable. This is an area of active debate.

In some cases, the research question may be addressed by an intervention that involves subtle or short-lived physiologic changes that are not expected to benefit patients directly. The risk to research subjects is inherently increased when there is no expectation of direct benefit, but the research may be able to go forward if there is an indirect benefit to be gained from the new knowledge and the risk is not to life or limb. Risks must be disclosed candidly so that potential subjects can provide informed consent, and there must be no improper inducements (e.g., a large cash payment) that could be considered coercive (see below). In other cases, human subject interaction may be minor and considered to be a minimal risk intervention (e.g., measurement of vital signs, data collection by cutaneous electrode, or the collection of small amounts of blood via venipuncture or a catheter placed for clinical indications). Because some researchers may inappropriately view patients in the ICU as a limitless source for blood samples, it is important that safeguards for the protection of research subjects are maintained. This is an area with strong federal regulatory oversight.

Outcomes research is a burgeoning area of research in the ICU, as the need increases to justify expensive and invasive interventions that have become the hallmark of modern surgical critical care. Observational studies that are often construed as outcomes research (true outcomes research analyzes the impact of a health intervention on a defined endpoint) are sometimes designed with a different standard for the hypothesis (e.g., "let's see what happens") and less quantifiable outcomes (e.g., a reduced incidence of "pneumonia"), especially in retrospective studies. This is regrettable, because rigorous prospective outcomes research can be performed. The reader is invited to look elsewhere in this volume for a detailed discussion of rigorous outcomes research methodology.

1. Patient Selection

The patient population to be selected for study is crucial; many studies have failed because inclusion criteria were nonspecific and patients without the disease in question were studied (5). The specificity of inclusion and exclusion criteria, stratification schemes, and methods to ensure equivalence among groups all play an important role in study design and will impact the power calculation. The correct identification of patients for inclusion can be challenging if either the at-risk population or the presenting symptoms of disease are heterogeneous. For example, if a study planned for acute respiratory distress syndrome (ARDS) captures as many patients as possible from all possible etiologies, the incidence of ARDS in the population at risk would be under

2%. However, if it was planned to study ARDS due to the most common causes, the incidence of ARDS would be closer to 30% but as many as one-third of total cases would be excluded (6). Thus, the study population must be understood as well as possible to minimize the chance of a fatal design flaw.

The issue of how to ensure that a patient does have the disease under study remains a conundrum because so many studies are now designed for early intervention. When a definitive diagnosis can be made based on physical findings alone or with a corroborating radiographic study, the issue is usually moot—there is no doubt when a patient develops cardiac arrest, as the most striking example. However, diagnostic insecurity inevitably leads to erroneous diagnosis in some cases, which must be addressed from a trial design standpoint. Patients with systemic inflammatory responsive syndrome (SIRS) (fever, leukocytosis, tachycardia, and tachypnea) may or may not have an infection (7). Even if purulent material is readily available for culture and gram stain, definitive characterization of the type of infection may take several days. In one example, a multicenter trial of an antiendotoxin monoclonal antibody failed in part because more than one-third of enrolled patients did not have gram-negative infection (5).

Studies of sepsis and septic shock exemplify the difficulty of patient selection for several reasons. Experiments to identify pharmacotherapy effective against sepsis and septic shock have been uniformly unsuccessful to date. Difficulty in patient selection has played a role in this. These patients are critically ill and unstable, therefore time to intervene is of essence. No specific bedside diagnostic test yet exists to make a definitive diagnosis. The biologic response to the insult is variable and unpredictable and is thus difficult to characterize and define rapidly and accurately. Given that mortality has proved difficult to reduce, there have been attempts to validate use of surrogate endpoints (see below).

Assuming that a study population is easy to identify, standard inclusion criteria are often defined by age, sufficient "proof" of diagnosis (e.g., microbiologic cultures), and good health prior to affliction. Defining inclusion based on gender should be avoided; evidence exists that discriminatory exclusion of females from clinical trials is common (8). Exclusion criteria are more variable, but standard to a degree. Standard exclusions may be based on age (pediatric or elderly patients), evidence that the disease under study is not present, pregnancy or unwillingness to practice effective birth control, receipt of (another) experimental drug within the previous 30 days, or a life expectancy less than 30–60 days due to the nature of the underlying disease or severity of illness. Exclusion criteria may also be study specific. For example, evidence of specific organ toxicity from preclinical or phase I–II trials often precludes enrollment of patients with even mild dysfunction of that organ.

2. Severity of Illness

The principles of study design require not only that appropriate patients be enrolled in adequate number, but that the groups being studied are comparable. Illness severity as an exclusion criterion cuts both ways. Set too low, the patient population may obscure a treatment effect because patients do not really need treatment, or small effects may be obscured by an underpowered study. Set too high, the illness severity may be so great as to nullify the effect of an intervention that might be effective if given sooner, before the disease has run its course and the patient has no chance of survival. The problem of high illness severity as an exclusion criterion for studies of new pharmaceuticals, where not only efficacy but safety must be demonstrated, is exemplified by studies of intraabdominal infection (9). The mortality rate of serious intraabdominal infections (about 15% of all such infections) exceeds 20%, yet such studies usually exclude severely ill patients in shock, yielding a study mortality rate of about 3%. Safety is proved, but effectiveness is not, unless demonstrated by a secondary outcome analysis (see below).

a. Illness Severity Scoring Of paramount importance in clinical trial design is ensuring that the groups being compared are equivalent in predefined ways (10). The equivalence criteria are often chosen to reflect patient characteristics that are likely to influence studies directly if equivalence is not achieved by the randomization process. The more equivalence criteria that must be met, the greater the statistical likelihood that groups will differ in a single criterion by chance alone. Randomization may be stratified by one or two key criteria to increase the likelihood of equivalence before the intervention. Illness severity scoring provides a quantifiable, reproducible means to assure comparability. Several schemes are available for use, and as acceptance has increased, some severity scores such as organ dysfunction scoring are garnering interest to quantify surrogate endpoints.

Among the many illness severity scores that have been described, by far the most popular is the second iteration of the Acute Physiology and Chronic Health Evaluation, or APACHE II (2). Described in 1985 for prediction of mortality in groups of patients as a 71-point scale, points are awarded based on age, defined severe chronic medical illness (e.g., New York Heart Association class IV heart disease), bidirectional acute physiologic derangements, and the Glasgow Coma Scale score. The APACHE II score as described is awarded at 24 hr after ICU admission based on the worst derangements observed during the preceding period. However, APACHE II has been adopted as an entry criterion for many studies, captured at a discrete point in time regardless of the antecedent duration of hospitalization or whether the patient requires ICU care. Such modified use, although not validated in a strict sense, appears to work and is certainly better than nothing. Another common tactic is to use only the acute physiologic derangement component of APACHE II, known as the Acute Physiology Score.

It is clear that APACHE II is an excellent predictor of mortality in groups of patients with systemic illness, such as systemic infections (11, 12) or pancreatitis. It is equally true that APACHE II substantially underestimates mortality and is therefore of limited use when applied to multiple trauma patients (13). Unfortunately, the poor reputation among surgeons that APACHE II garnered has tarnished unfairly its successor, APACHE III. In addition to "guilt by association," the developers of APACHE III have been criticized widely for keeping proprietary the disease-specific correction factors that are in the public domain for APACHE II. Regardless, the information necessary to calculate the APACHE III score is published (14), and correction factors are not needed to ensure equivalence in study groups, which are homogeneous compared with the general ICU population. Reported in 1991, and ironically developed in part as a result of the poor performance of APACHE II in trauma patients (particularly those with head injuries), APACHE III uses a 299-point scale. Among the notable differences incorporated in APACHE III, the neurologic assessment was revamped, renal and hepatic dysfunction are characterized with more precision, and chronic health points are not awarded after an elective admission to the ICU (e.g., for postoperative monitoring). Stated simply, APACHE III produces higher estimates of mortality compared to APACHE II in surgical patients (15), and therefore corrects some of the problems inherent in APACHE II. Moreover, APACHE III is superior to both APACHE II and specific injury severity scoring for mortality prediction in trauma patients (16). For most research-related purposes, APACHE II will suffice but APACHE III is worthy of use and deserves consideration.

Another alternative is the Therapeutic Intervention Scoring System (TISS), which quantifies various treatment interventions (e.g., transfusions, mechanical ventilation) (17). Designed originally as a tool to assess nurse staffing levels in the ICU, TISS has become a marker of intensity of therapy rather than severity of illness. Despite inherent problems, TISS is still used occasionally to describe patient groups (18). Among the difficulties in using TISS are that it has not been updated recently, so that many modern therapies are not accounted for. Moreover, it is unclear how severe illness and intensive care actually correlate. Therapeutic nihilism may lead to "undertreatment," whereas there is likely a certain severity of illness beyond which "more therapy" cannot be provided.

b. Illness-Specific Scores Many specific scoring systems are available, and may perform as well or better than even APACHE III in discrete patient populations. Investigators may sometimes choose to use one as an alternate to an APACHE score, or more likely will choose to use a second score to provide an extra degree of assurance. Examples of specific scores include the Injury Severity Score (19), the Penetrating Abdominal Trauma Index (20), and the Mangled Extremity Severity Score (21) for injured patients, and the Ranson score (22) among several used to quantify the severity of pancreatitis. The ARDS Score (23) and the Lung Injury Score (24) may be used to quantify acute lung injury. Scores are even available to describe specific morbidities such as decubitus ulcers. Not all of these scores are well validated. Therefore it would be preferable to make use of an existing scoring system whenever possible, assuming that it can be validated for use in the patient population being studied.

3. Organ Dysfunction—Entry Criterion, or Outcome?

Multiple organ dysfunction syndrome (MODS) is the leading cause of death in critically ill surgical patients. First described as multiple organ failure a quarter-century ago, understanding of MODS continues to evolve. It is now recognized that MODS develops much earlier than originally appreciated from early observations, and that substantial organ dysfunction may be present on admission. Therefore, the "window of opportunity" to intervene (e.g., with aggressive resuscitation) to ameliorate organ dysfunction may be narrow and may exist very early in the ICU course. Organ dysfunction may be either an entry criterion or an endpoint for evaluation.

Numerous schemes to quantify MODS have been published and validated. They differ in the organ derangements that are included, and how they are defined. Some describe organ dysfunction as "an all-or-nothing" phenomenon (25), whereas others describe gradations of organ dysfunction. Validated descriptions have been published by Marshall *et al.* (26), LeGall *et al.* (27), and Vincent *et al.* (28), although substantive head-to-head comparisons have not been published. Investigators should choose an established score when designing new studies.

Perhaps best characterized is the *MOD Score* of Marshall *et al.* (26). Six "organ" systems—cardiovascular, central nervous system (CNS), coagulation, hepatic, pulmonary, and renal—are awarded 0–4 points based on quantitative criteria (the exception is the CNS score, which is based on the subjective assessment of the Glasgow Coma Scale score, and itself subject to the vagaries of recovery from general anesthesia, sedative medication, and the inability to verbalize secondary to endotracheal intubation). The MOD score can be determined daily, on a cumulative basis (i.e., a patient who recovered from severe ARDS would have a pulmonary score of 4 points even after recovery), or as a change from baseline (ΔMODS). On a cumulative basis, a 30% mortality rate is associated with 9–12 points, 70% with 13–16 points, and >90% mortality occurs in patients who score ⩾17 points (26, 29). The cumulative MOD score is a better predictor of mortality than is APACHE III, and correlations also exist between the magnitude of organ dysfunction and surrogate outcomes such as prolonged length of stay (30).

4. Patient Selection in the Future

Rapid, accurate diagnosis and severity of illness assessment are needed at the bedside. Recent advances in molecular biology methods may be useful. It is known that individuals have differential tumor necrosis factor (TNF) responses to a standardized endotoxin challenge (4). This phenomenon may be explained by polymorphisms in the TNF gene (31); certain genotypes are associated with an adverse outcome from sepsis. These observations may be linked and could be useful, if determined as enrollment criteria in studies of sepsis. The emerging science of pharmacogenomics (32) is also providing a scientific explanation for differences in drug metabolism, the knowledge of which could be of great value in the design and conduct of future studies. Microarray technology or "gene chips" may allow rapid genotyping at the bedside in the future (33).

5. Outcomes and Endpoints

The *sine qua non* of ICU clinical research outcomes has been mortality. Although illness security scores were designed to be predictive of mortality for the hospitalization, most studies use 28-day mortality as an endpoint. However, it is recognized increasingly that mortality may not be a reasonable endpoint for many studies, especially when mortality is a rare event, such as in studies of intraabdominal infection.

Outcomes other than mortality are commonly referred to as surrogate outcomes. Other terminology refers to primary versus secondary endpoints. The primary endpoint refers to the main objective of the study—the question raised by the main hypothesis. Secondary endpoints are those of interest aside from the main hypothesis test. The primary endpoint may or may not be a surrogate, but a secondary endpoint invariably is represented by a surrogate. There is nothing inherently wrong with a secondary endpoint, as long as it is defined prospectively and accounted for in the analysis plan. A plan is essential, because as the number of secondary endpoints increases, the power of the study decreases.

Secondary endpoints give investigators, regulators, and journal editors pause, not only because of the potential for bias with post hoc testing, but also because they may be difficult to define or easy to manipulate. Mortality is a clear-cut dichotomous variable, but it can be difficult to make a confirmed diagnosis of pneumonia. Length of stay can be manipulated easily by practitioners—just "one more day" of therapy is often provided for "peace of mind" or medico-legal indemnification. In a variation of the length-of-stay theme, duration of mechanical ventilation has been used as a secondary endpoint (34), with the stipulation that there must be a strict adherence to a detailed, inflexible ventilator management and weaning protocol.

In studies of intraabdominal infection, the primary endpoint is clinical "cure," which is the eradication of all symptoms and signs of infection. The secondary endpoint is usually the eradication of microorganisms, which is often presumptive, given that there will be no follow-up material for culture from cases treated successfully. With such "soft" endpoints (35), there is the possibility for bias unless attention to detail is meticulous.

Investigators in general should identify surrogate endpoints that are defined rigorously, thereby minimizing the possibility of criticism over flawed design. Tactics to preserve the integrity of a study include blinding the study and maintaining the blind, controlling as many clinical care-related variables as possible (e.g., specified ventilator management protocols in studies of acute lung injury), and requiring the collection of the best available evidence (e.g., quantitative sputum microbiology in studies of pneumonia).

B. Analytical Considerations

The likelihood that a study will detect anticipated differences, in addition to the level of statistical significance with which the study will report its results, must be considered with care. These factors are incorporated into the power analysis, which is an essential exercise before embarking on any RCT. Power analysis defines the number of patients necessary to achieve the desired endpoint of the study with adequate statistical power. Typically, the power analysis is reported in a manner analogous to the study—for example, having an 80% chance to detect a 30% reduction in mortality at a p value <0.05. Higher power requires more patients to be accrued, as does a high anticipated dropout rate. A proper power analysis is essential for budgeting and to ensure that the time and expense of a complex study will not go for naught in a study that is too small (underpowered) to prove a point (Type II error) (36). Software is available to perform these calculations (37); for the active researcher involved in investigator-initiated studies, this represents an important tool.

It is also essential, and requisite to the power analysis, to have a predefined statistical analysis plan. This plan can be simple or complex, but it must be inclusive to eliminate bias, particularly with secondary endpoints. Powerful computers and software that are now available allow sophisticated analyses to be performed rapidly. If defined *a priori* in the plan of analysis, additional power can be designed into the study to counteract degradation inherent in post hoc analyses. However, unplanned post hoc testing has derisively been called "data dredging" or "data mining," and its results are inherently suspect. There are published examples in which the investigators were criticized for such post hoc testing (5). If the level of statistical significance has been set at $p < 0.05$ for a study, it connotes that a chance of a random event being misinterpreted as one of significance is less than 5%. It follows that the performance of 20 univariate statistical tests on a data set is highly likely to identify one "significant" difference at random. That is not to say that post hoc statistical testing is not valuable. It could be used to refine hypotheses or to generate new questions for further prospective testing. Another source of preliminary data for further trials can be the achievement of valid secondary endpoints (e.g., reduced mortality in extremely ill patients or those in whom a physiologic characteristic exists, such as renal failure) when the primary endpoint (e.g., reduced overall mortality) has not been achieved. However, preliminary evidence of efficacy by no means guarantees the results of confirmatory or redesigned trials (38).

Several statistical issues can impact the conduct of a blinded RCT. The methodology of randomization and allocation must be considered, including who will control the randomization documents and the circumstances under which the blinding may be broken. It is not mandatory for studies to be designed for equal allocation to groups, particularly when the characteristics of the comparison group are extremely well defined and its behavior can be predicted accurately. For example, a study comparing piperacillin/tazobactam with gentamicin and clindamycin for treatment of intraabdominal infection randomized patients to receive piperacillin/tazobactam on a 2:1 basis (39); this was valid in part because the response to gentamicin and clindamycin is well characterized and predictable in peritonitis and could be accounted for in the power analysis.

Randomization schemes may be simple or complex, but investigators must ensure that a randomization scheme is truly random and that it remains blinded before treatment group allocation occurs. One ersatz "randomization" scheme is to assign patients based on the last digit of their medical record number. Although at first glance such a method could achieve balanced allocation, it is actually rife with potential for bias. When the allocation is known before enrollment, as it would be from the record number, there is the potential that the patient would not be referred to the study if the referring physician believes that assignment of his or her patient to one particular treatment group is not what is desired.

Randomization can be accomplished simply by placing labeled cards in sealed opaque envelopes, mixing them thoroughly, and numbering the envelopes consecutively for accounting purposes. Alternatively, a randomization schedule may be derived from a computer program that generates random numbers. Complex randomization schemes may be designed to ensure that treatment groups are equivalent or that results from a single center in a multicenter trial are not biased. Potential bias in multicenter trials may arise when accrual occurs rapidly at one center, there is disproportionate enrollment for one type of patient where the population should be heterogeneous (i.e. "too many" appendicitis cases in an abdominal infection study) (39), or when a crucial treatment factor is not controlled for and inconsistent care occurs at one center (9) (Table I).

Allocation strategies include having the randomization schedule held at a central location by a disinterested person. Not only can the allocation for an individual enroller be provided by telephone while the blinding is kept secure, but eligibility screening may be confirmed prior to announcement of the allocation. Within a randomization scheme, allocation may be balanced by groups of patients (a block allocation scheme), allocations for individual centers, or stratification based on some critical patient characteristic, such as severity of illness. In a block allocation scheme, useful when a study is small or will be ended at a predetermined date rather

Table I Examples of Published Studies with Flawed Design

Protocol	Flaw	Ref.
Monoclonal antibody therapy of human endotoxemia	Poorly defined inclusion criteria—too many ineligible patients enrolled; post hoc testing not defined prospectively	5
Antibiotic treatment of intraabdominal infection	No control of wound management—large numbers of postoperative fasciitis cases at one center after primary closure of contaminated wounds	9
Antibiotic treatment of intraabdominal infection	No stratification for severity of illness	10
Surgical antibiotic prophylaxis	Type II error, followed by invalid post hoc testing	36
Antibiotic prophylaxis of severe pancreatitis	Rampant protocol violations	40
Effect of stress ulcer prophylaxis on the incidence of pneumonia	Rampant protocol violations	41
Use of discharge database to predict outcomes prospectively	Flawed hypothesis, flawed administrative data set	44
Retrospective estimation of the mortality risk of pulmonary artery catheterization	Statistical method to create equal comparison groups created unequal groups	47

than with a predetermined number of patients, an equal allocation is guaranteed within each group of four to six patients. Providing each center its own randomization schedule is less expensive than maintaining a central office or officer on call, but leaves open the possibility for the list to be compromised, for ineligible patients to be enrolled, or for some center-specific treatment bias uncontrolled for the overall design to call aberrant results from that center into question (9). Capping the enrollment from any given center after a predefined number of patients is enrolled is a valid design strategy (10).

Also valid are various stratification strategies to ensure that treatment groups are equivalent, especially when heterogeneous patient populations are studied. Stratification is often necessary to ensure that patient groups are equivalent and that the results will be interpretable (10) (Table I). It is most common to stratify for severity of illness, but in heterogeneous populations it may also be desirable to stratify for given diagnoses (e.g., perforated appendicitis in an intraabdominal infection study). In that example, the diagnosis and severity of illness issues are related, in that perforated appendicitis typically is less morbid and carries a lower risk of mortality compared to a colon perforation.

Evaluability

Invariably, some study subjects will fail to complete the protocol as specified. The potential reasons are numerous and not always under the control of the investigator. Patients may prove not to have the disease under study or to be ineligible for another reason. They may choose to withdraw, or may be withdrawn by the investigator because of a serious adverse event. An intervention may be omitted, the wrong intervention may be given (i.e., randomization occurs into one group, but the treatment for the other group is administered), or a crucial monitoring event may not occur at the proper time. The study subject may not comply with requirements for follow-up at specified points as an outpatient after the intervention ends, or other problems may develop. According to some protocols, this may make the patient unevaluable (10) and therefore excludable from the final analysis of the data. In studies with multiple endpoints, the analysis plan may render a subject evaluable for some endpoints, but not for others. For example, in a drug study with both safety and efficacy endpoints, administration of a single dose would qualify the subject for the safety analysis but not the efficacy analysis.

When evaluability criteria are stated prospectively this strategy may be used. However, there is potential for bias to enter the study when evaluability becomes subject to interpretation. For example, a research result might be excluded if a datum is determined to be a statistical "outlier," or if a failure of antibiotic therapy for peritonitis is believed to be due to an untimely or poorly performed operation. Leaving these decisions to a blinded *data monitoring and safety board* (DMSB) (see below) can minimize the potential for bias, but not eliminate it entirely.

Many investigators are designing "intention-to-treat" analyses into their protocols to minimize the problem of evaluation bias (10). This analysis eliminates almost all causes of nonevaluability as an issue, because any subject who receives the intervention, no matter how briefly, is retained in the analysis. Usually, the only cases excluded from an intention-to-treat analysis are those in which randomization occurs but the intervention does not (e.g., erroneous diagnosis, withdrawal of the subject). Analysis by intention-to-treat will not salvage a study replete with protocol violations, nor does it address specifically how to analyze an individual subject who has received the wrong intervention. In such a case, the decision to analyze the data according to the randomization or the actual treatment received, or to withdraw the patient, may best be made with professional statistical advice. Examples of studies published despite widespread, serious protocol violations are easy to find (40, 41).

C. Alternative Study Designs

Most of the present discussion has focused on the design and execution of a definitive clinical trial, the double-blind RCT. However, many questions can be answered in another valid manner. Most alternative designs retain the advantage of prospective conduct, although in some cases observations made in retrospect can serve as the basis for a confirmatory prospective trial of some sort. This discussion is largely limited to study designs where there is a comparison group; the design of purely retrospective studies is not considered beyond a brief discussion of their pitfalls.

1. Randomized Open-Label Studies

There are times when maintaining a blinded study is unnecessary or impossible. Blinding may be unnecessary for phase IV studies, for example, when an approved drug in a new dosage or administration schedule is being compared with itself given in standard fashion. A comparison with standard therapy may be valid for other studies as well. Blinding may be unnecessary on rare occasions for new a potential life-saving therapy of a disease without any known effective therapy; a valid comparison may be made with conventional treatment (that is, no treatment). Blinding may be impossible if no placebo drug or delivery mechanism or other comparable intervention can be identified. Blinding may be unethical in some circumstances also. For example, it would be unethical to administer a large volume of placebo liquid into the airway of a patient with acute lung injury who was receiving an experimental surfactant, because of potentially dangerous hypoxemia. A sham operation could not be performed ethically on a human subject under most circumstances.

Single-blind studies may also be appropriate for some designs. More an amalgam than a compromise, analgesic evaluations represent an area in which single-blind studies are performed. In most such cases, it is the patient who is blind to the study, but not invariably so. For example, a blinded comparison of analgesic requirements of inpatients after major laparoscopic abdominal operations would require identical bandages, pulmonary toilet regimens, and dietary management to maintain blinding of the caregivers administering the medication. Moreover, auscultation of the abdomen would not be permitted for study personnel, and even then the patient would know with certainty whether his or her pain derived from one large incision or several small ones. Conversely, for a comparison of analgesics after a standard operation, patient blinding is essential to obviate the known placebo effect (substantive analgesia after placebo administration). Parenthetically, placebo-controlled analgesic studies can be designed ethically. In one recent FDA-approved study, an effective dose of an analgesic was given initially, followed by the test analgesic versus placebo. The time interval until the patient self-administered a rescue dose of morphine from a patient-controlled analgesia machine was the primary endpoint.

2. Crossover Studies

Crossover studies are those in which an individual study subject will receive both interventions, and will serve as his or her own control. These studies are amenable to randomization and blinding; the random event is the order in which the interventions will occur. Crossover studies are usually used to evaluate the effect of an intervention at some physiologic endpoint (e.g., "is nitroprusside or nitroglycerin a more effective pulmonary vasodilator?") (42), rather than some outcome endpoint (Table II). Safety is a primary consideration in such studies if there is no potential benefit to a research subject. It is also essential for a research subject to be clinically stable during the study, lest the study conditions be different during the later phase. To the extent that the first intervention causes physiologic perturbation, a "washout" period should be included so that baseline conditions can be restored prior to the second intervention (42).

A crossover design may also be used for substantive therapeutic studies, provided both drugs are "effective" and the question is "Which one is better?" In one example, norepinephrine was compared to dopamine for vasopressor therapy of septic shock (43). After randomization, patients were crossed over to the alternate treatment only if the initial treatment was ineffective. The primary endpoint was the mortality rate from primary therapy, and the secondary endpoint was the salvage rate after crossover to the second intervention.

A variation in the crossover theme is a dose-ranging study, in which the minimum effective dose of a drug is determined in order to establish the dose to be tested in a large-scale phase III RCT. These are open-label, nonrandomized studies in which the drug dosage is increased according to protocol until the particular effect is observed. A study subject serves as his or her own control, but no washout period is employed. Such studies are seldom undertaken in the ICU.

3. Choice of Comparator in Nonrandomized Studies

Nonrandomized studies suffer by comparison to randomized ones, because of the perception that their design is less rigorous and that results are not as reliable. These "criticisms" are true to some extent, but nonrandomized prospective studies can provide important information. One key to their validity, and ultimately their acceptance, is the construction of the comparison group.

Least desirable are prospective cohort (consecutive patient enrollment) studies in which comparison is made to historical controls. The selection of a comparison population retrospectively from previously treated patients is fraught with bias, even when strict selection criteria are followed. Sometimes, new treatments over time may have improved outcomes to such a degree that historical outcomes become irrelevant, as is the case for mortality from ARDS. Flaws may exist in the database from which comparisons are made. Databases may be classified as clinical or administrative; the latter are problematic. Clinical databases are those maintained routinely by most clinicians; some quality control is maintained for the data. Administrative databases are

Table II Examples of High-Quality Study Design and Conduct

Protocol	Merit	Ref.
Low tidal volume ventilation of acute lung injury	Study stopped after interim analysis showed lower mortality in the treatment group	34
Dopamine vs. norepinephrine for therapy of septic shock	Excellent use of crossover design in a trial of therapy	43
Before/after antibiotic intervention to reduce antibiotic-resistant gram-negative pneumonia	Good example of an inherently limited study design	45
Case control study of the cost of nosocomial bloodstream infection	Superb example of careful case-matching methodology	46
Point-prevalence study of nosocomial infections in the ICU	A model of organization and conduct	47

those maintained by governmental or regulatory authorities (e.g., state trauma registries), whereby data are derived from hospital discharge data. Those data are captured by clerical personnel from patient medical records without knowledge of the context in which chart entries were made. Considering how difficult so many diagnoses are to make, there can be little confidence in any observations based on administrative data collection other than crude mortality or procedure rates (44).

Intermediate in value are "before and after" studies. A population is observed beginning at a point in time. After adequate characterization, an intervention is made and the effect of the intervention is observed in a population of presumably known behavior. The hypothesis is that the intervention, as an isolated change, will influence the population henceforth. The target characteristic must be stable throughout the "before" period, a challenge to achieve considering that the mere fact of observation is demonstrated to change behavior. Moreover, the intervention must be of limited complexity, to avoid the problem of determining which facet of a complex intervention actually caused the change in outcome. For example, it was hypothesized that a change of antibiotic prescribed empirically for gram-negative infection in cardiothoracic surgery patients would result in fewer antibiotic-resistant infections (45) (Table II). After a 6-month observation, ciprofloxacin was substituted for ceftazidime for an additional 6 months. The hypothesis was proved, but whether the improvement was due to the use of ciprofloxacin specifically, to the fact that a change was made, or to the avoidance of ceftazidime remains an important unanswered question.

Well executed case control studies can be quite powerful. Although not randomized, methods are employed to ensure, insofar as possible, that the comparison group resembles the study group. Such designs are particularly valuable for epidemiologic outcome studies. Ideally, the comparison cohort is constructed from concurrent patients who did not have the event in question. For low-prevalence events (e.g., afflicting 2% of patients), using the remaining 98% of patients as the comparison group would be uninformative, because it is likely that the smaller group will not resemble the larger group in one or more important characteristics. Simple comparisons can be based on a handful of characteristics, such as age, gender, and severity of illness. However, sophisticated comparisons are based on multiple relevant factors and also include an analysis of how effective the matching strategy was. As an example of case-matching methodology, the attributable mortality and excess cost associated with catheter-related blood stream infection were determined (46). The quantitative methodology used to assess the success of the case-matching algorithm added greatly to the acceptability of the study. In contrast, a less convincing example of case-matching methodology involved a retrospective assessment of pulmonary artery catheterization (47). Statistical methods were used to determine the likelihood that a catheter would be inserted, rather than a direct comparison of patient-derived data. The conclusion that pulmonary artery catheterization led to excess mortality is difficult to accept, considering that the catheterized group was more seriously ill, compared to the noncatheterized patients, in several important respects.

4. Observational Epidemiologic Studies

Prospective observation of groups can be very informative with respect to outcomes in several circumstances, even though there is neither an intervention being tested nor a comparison group. Revised descriptions of clinical syndromes may result, and entirely new hypotheses may be generated (48). The prevalence of disease within a population may be determined (49). Outcomes can be observed beyond the confines of the ICU or inpatient care (50).

Two types of these studies are commonly performed in the ICU setting. The first, the inception-cohort study, follows a defined population longitudinally to answer questions about an outcome or an intervention. Inception-cohort studies examine consecutive samples from time zero (the inception point) and can answer questions such as "how often will severe MODS develop in patients with a perforated viscus?" (12), or "are routine portable chest radiographs useful in the management of critically ill patients?" (51). The second type of study, the point-prevalence study, examines questions such as "what is the prevalence of nosocomial pneumonia in an ICU at any given time?" In one remarkable example of a point-prevalence study, the European Prevalence of Infection in Intensive Care (EPIC) study (49), the prevalence of nosocomial infection was determined on a single day for more than 10,000 patients in ICUs throughout Europe.

III. Site Selection and Investigator Responsibilities

All parties to a clinical investigation are responsible to ensure that a study is conducted accurately, honestly, and safely, with the rights of the research subject safeguarded. Many checks and balances exist to ensure that these goals are reached. Most clinical research in the ICU is sponsored, rather than investigator initiated, meaning that a corporation (usually, a pharmaceutical company) is testing an investigational drug or device in the hope that it will be approved for clinical use. The sponsor will seek assurances that a study site and its lead investigator have the facilities, personnel, expertise, and interest to conduct the study.

Increasingly, site selection and data collection functions are performed by a contract research organization (CRO) hired to act as the sponsor's agent. Once the sponsor has received the new drug application (NDA) or IDE number from the FDA, permitting research to proceed, the sponsor will begin finalizing the protocol and soliciting research sites. From the investigator's perspective, the process usually starts with the execution of a confidentiality agreement between investigator and sponsor so that information may be disclosed to ascertain the investigator's interest. Thereafter, a prequalification visit will be made to the investigator's site to assess the adequacy of laboratory and pharmacy resources, the security of record storage, the number of potential enrollees, and the qualifications of the investigator and the study coordinator (usually a registered nurse). Once selected, an "investigator's meeting" is held by the sponsor to renew the protocol, policies, and procedures. Enlightened sponsors encourage a critique of the protocol at this time, to strengthen it for finalization. Once a protocol is finalized, it is submitted to the institutional review board (IRB), which must approve it before enrollment can occur (see below). Concurrently, a budget and a contract (industrial agreement) are negotiated.

Use of CROs has allowed many more centers to be recruited. The expectation is that larger numbers of centers will allow more rapid completion of a study. However, hasty enrollment runs the risk that marginal candidates will be enrolled. The use of many centers invariably means that inexperienced centers and investigators will participate; each of these factors may degrade the quality of the study. With the realization that his or her own center may enjoy only modest enrollment for a particular study, an investigator may seek to run several studies concurrently to meet the fixed costs of the research program of a particular facility.

Once a protocol is active, the site will be monitored and data collected as accrued. Although online data submission is increasing, data are still usually entered manually into the case report form (CRF). The CRO representative will confirm the veracity of the data before transmitting the CRF to the sponsor, usually after each case has been closed. Queries from the sponsor to the investigator to resolve questions regarding the data may occur for a period thereafter.

When enrollment has ceased, the CRO conducts a "close-out" visit, during which the remaining data are collected, all drug supplies are accounted for and return shipment arranged, and study finances are reconciled. Throughout this entire series of events, the lead investigator assumes ultimate responsibility for all study-related activities at the site, except for the deliberations of the IRB and the legal aspects of budgeting and contracting. Obtaining IRB approval, the professional conduct of coinvestigators and support personnel, the conduct of the study, collection and transmission of accurate data, and secure, confidential storage of all records for production during rare but possible audits by the FDA are all the responsibility of the lead investigator at each site. Paramount among the investigators responsibilities is ensuring the integrity of the informed consent process (Table III) and subjugating all activities at all times to the welfare of the study subject.

IV. Ethical Issues

Although many of the ethical issues investigators are faced with in ICUs are common to the general practice of medicine, there are features of critical care and critical illness that are of heightened concern. Critical illness and the nature of intensive care complicate issues of clinical investigation, experimentation, resource allocation, end-of-life care, surrogate decision-making, and informed consent. The application of state-of-the-art medical technology in the insular environment of the ICU is both disconcerting and disorienting for patients and their families. It alters the dynamics of the patient–physician relationship in favor of the physician because of the increased dependence on expert opinion and invasive equipment, which can literally deprive a patient of his or her voice.

Of the many ethical issues in critical care, research that enlists ICU patients is fraught with more challenges than most. Foremost among these is meeting standards of ethically acceptable informed consent. There are a myriad of reasons why informed consent for research becomes more difficult in the ICU. Often, ICU patients lack the requisite decision-making capacity to understand the extent of their illness and current treatment, let alone a research proposal for which their enrollment is being sought. Furthermore, the dual roles of the physician/researcher and the potential for conflict of interest make consent difficult to be viewed as free of coercion, however unintended it may be on the part of the physician-investigator. Despite these quandaries, it is possible to comply with the requirements of informed consent for research involving ICU patients.

A. Background on Informed Consent

To understand current ethical challenges in the ICU, it is necessary to appreciate the historic development of informed consent in the law and medical ethics. The modern concept of informed consent was developed through several important cases over the past 100 years (52). The legal basis of informed consent in the United States finds its origin in a 1914 decision, *Schloendorff v. Society of New York Hospital* (53). In this case, a surgeon removed a uterine leiomyoma from a patient who had only agreed to an examination under anesthesia. Following complications from surgery, the

Table III Elements of Informed Consent

Consideration	Element
Process	
	Complete disclosure
	Purpose
	Risks/benefits (if any)/alternatives
	Recourse (questions, adverse events)
	Conflicts of interest on the part of the investigator
	Randomization and blinding (as appropriate)
	Consent is voluntary
	The subject has capacity to understand and decide
	Free of coercion
	Consent may be withdrawn at any time, for any reason
	Consent obtained by investigator/coinvestigator
	Not by subordinates
	Inducements
	Not inherently impermissible
	Commensurate with risk/inconvenience to subject
	Surrogate consent
	Avoid whenever possible (most circumstances)
	Permissible in life-threatening emergencies if approved in advance by IRB
Document	
	Oral consent permissible only for minimal-risk inventions (for example, electrocardiography and venipuncture)
	Approval and authentication by IRB prior to presentation
	Understandable at the sixth-grade reading level
	Simple declarative sentences
	Avoid medical/technical jargon, and define it simply when necessary
	Consider separate multilingual documents (depending on subject population)
	Explicit disclosure that the drug/device being tested is investigational (experimental)
	Explicit disclosure that the study is randomized or blinded, as appropriate
	Description of benefits
	Overstatement is a form of coercion
	There may be none for the subject, in some studies
	Description of risks
	"Prudent lay person" standard—what would a person usually want to know
	Rare events must be disclosed if they have serious consequences
	"Boilerplate"
	Disclosure of costs borne by subject, if any
	Disclosure of commercial sponsor, if any
	Liability clause
	Addresses and phone numbers for which investigator/IRB
	Permission to disclose data in patient nonidentifiable form to sponsor/FDA/journal, as appropriate
	Provision of a copy to the subject

patient initiated a lawsuit. Benjamin Cardozo, as Chief Judge of the New York State Court of Appeals, opined as follows:

> *Every human being of adult years and sound mind has a right to determine what shall be done with his own body; and a surgeon who performs an operation without the patient's consent commits an assault for which he is liable for damages. . . . This is true except in cases of emergency when the patient is unconscious and when it is necessary to operate before consent can be obtained.*

From this decision onward, the legal basis and definition were refined but the essential elements of informed consent were voiced in the Cardozo opinion. The decision recognized the universal right of informed consent and self-determination when patients were of sound mind (had *capacity*), and it stated clearly that a violation of these standards constituted an assault for which clinicians were liable. Furthermore, Cardozo anticipated the notion of the *emergency presumption* that allows treatment without consent when urgent medical intervention is needed and a patient is unable to provide informed consent. Subsequent legal opinions in the 1960s further codified the doctrine of informed consent, establishing reasonable person standards of disclosure and treatment options (54).

Without going into great detail, several important concepts in research ethics arose concurrently with the development of these clinical standards. Major influences on this consensus followed from the egregious disregard for the health of human research subjects, in studies ranging from the well intended to outright atrocities. Among those studies that had a major impact on the conceptualization of informed consent were the Nazi experiments on Holocaust victims, culminating in the Nuremberg Code (55), which stressed the centrality of informed and voluntary consent, and "The Tuskegee Study of Untreated Syphilis in the Negro Male" (56). Other landmark studies included the Willowbrook State School hepatitis studies on institutionalized, mentally retarded children, which greatly influenced the way in which children are protected in research studies, and Milgram's experiments on obedience (57–59). Henry Beecher, in his oft-cited essay published in 1966, criticized many experiments being conducted at that time for their disregard of obtaining informed consent of the research subjects (61). Beecher reported on 22 different experiments that had been conducted at distinguished universities and published in respected medical journals whereby informed consent had not been obtained. Beecher concluded further that this was the norm and not the exception of the state of affairs of clinical research. More recently, the U.S. government's sponsorship of radiation experiments on unknowing U.S. citizens came to light during the cold war (61).

In the Tuskegee study, subjects were recruited without knowledge of the aims of the study or their role in it. They were subjected to nontherapeutic procedures and were denied the standard of care for syphilis. The manner in which this study was conducted delayed treatment for patients and had adverse ramifications for both subjects and their families. The fact that this study continued for as many years as it did, even through the period of the Nuremberg trials and promulgation of the Nuremberg Code, is shocking. Although there are unique features to each of these cases, two common variables among them are the absence of informed consent and voluntary participation by the people who were subjected to these experiments, which is the *sine qua non* of conducting ethically acceptable research on humans.

Governmental actions, such as the National Research Act of 1974, which resulted in the Belmont Report, served to establish the current regulations regarding research on human subjects and further institutionalized the notion of informed consent (62–63). The principles established in the Belmont Report encompass respect for persons, beneficence, and justice. The principle of respect for persons rests on the idea that individuals ought to be treated as autonomous individuals. The principles of beneficence and its complement, nonmaleficence, express the idea that patients and research subjects ought to be protected against undue risks and harm as well as benefit whenever possible from the studies in which they participate. The principle of justice obligates researchers to distribute resources in a fair and nondiscriminatory manner so as not to overburden one segment of a population or to exclude another. In the case of research ethics, the Belmont Report asserted the importance of not using human subjects for research when they derive from a captive or available population, without clear justification for the use of vulnerable subjects.

From these principles, government agencies [the Office for Protection from Research Risk (OPRR), which is a unit of the Department of Health and Human Services (DHHS)] promulgated guidelines to protect research subjects through IRBs and a formalized informed consent process. Essential elements of informed consent as set forth in the Belmont Report and more recent statements include the provision of accurate information, language that is understandable, and a voluntary decision by the research subject (Table III). Although these conditions are simple conceptually, they present challenges to researchers who need to transform arcane technical language into lay terms free of sanguine or overly optimistic language. For example, it is important to avoid what is often described as the *therapeutic misconception,* in which an unproved clinical intervention is invested with presumed therapeutic efficacy. This can lead subjects to consent to investigational protocols under the mistaken belief that they are therapeutic (64). Patients who consider participating in research studies must understand the fundamental aspects of the study and the risks and benefits of their participation. Having attained this understanding, research subjects or their surrogates must consent voluntarily to partake in the study, an essential concept promulgated in the Nuremberg Code. It should be noted that this consent is not fixed and the patient retains the right to withdraw from a study at any point.

B. The Institutional Review Board

The IRB is responsible, under federal statute (52), to safeguard the welfare of research subjects. Every academic healthcare institution has one, and free-standing IRBs may review protocols for smaller facilities. At most institutions, the IRB is a diverse group of 20 or more people. Some diversity is mandated (lay people with no connection to the institution must participate), but many are constituted further to provide expertise in the areas of law, ethics, social sciences, humanities, and other disciplines in addition to the broad scientific expertise necessary for fair, in-depth review.

Each IRB requires a synopsis of the research protocol to be provided according to its own format, in addition to providing a copy of an unabridged protocol and the investigator's brochure (a detailed document that, in the case of an investigational drug study, contains background information on chemistry, pharmacology, toxicity, and preliminary data collected in humans). Time will not be saved by making the IRB submission prior to the availability of the final protocol, because the IRB will be unwilling to pass judgement on a preliminary document. The synopsis must be written in plain language, because the lay people on the IRB must be able to understand the proposed research as would a potential subject or his/her surrogate. The research plan, eligibility criteria, risks, benefits (including financial inducements), alternatives, and patient and data safeguards must be described. Even minor discrepancies between the unabridged document and the synopsis will require resolution, so it behooves the investigator to make the synopsis accurate from the onset. Any proposed advertising for recruitment must be reviewed and approved, even flyers intended for internal posting only.

The major focus of the IRB will be on the content and formatting of the consent form (Table III). Requirements for disclosure are explicit, although the language may vary from center to center. Approval of the document, which must occur prior to enrollment of anyone, often hinges on the understandability of the consent. This can be contentious, because the sponsor will provide a template consent form that contains language to its liking that the IRB may not accept.

Although the primary purview of the IRB involves a risk—benefit analysis on behalf of the research subject, the scientific merit of the study may also be scrutinized. If the study is devoid of merit, then any degree of risk, no matter if minimal, may become unacceptable if the benefit is zero. The risk–benefit ratio, in essence, becomes infinite and the study will not proceed.

Once a clinical protocol is approved, the investigator must submit to the IRB all reports of adverse events received from the sponsor. In some circumstances, there may also be an investigator obligation to report adverse events directly to the FDA. These will be reviewed, and if a pattern is discerned or a serious event attributable to the drug has occurred, the IRB may choose to amend the consent form or even to suspend accrual. Some studies generate numerous adverse event reports, but if the consent form has been crafted candidly, amendment is seldom necessary. The initial approval is valid for a period of 1 year from the initial IRB submission, so a protracted initial approval process may be followed by renewal shortly thereafter. The renewal process is a formal, thorough review. The investigator will be asked for the number of enrollees to date, and how many declined participation or withdrew their consent. Adverse events are reviewed again. Substantive changes in study design since the original approval must be described in detail. Preliminary results may be requested if the study is unblinded, and any resulting publications should be submitted. The finite life of an IRB protocol is usually 3 years, therefore a maximum of two annual renewals will be possible. Beyond 3 years an entirely new submission is required, if indeed such a long-term study is worthy of pursuit.

This background provides a framework from which to establish and analyze the informed consent process. Yet, this conceptualization often fails to capture the complexity of the clinical situation of patients and the competing demands of research in the critical care setting. The expectation that neatly packaged principles translate easily into workable guidelines for clinical research would be naive. The process of protecting research subjects relies on an informed pragmatic approach (65) to resolve specific ethical issues and conflicts.

C. Ethical Issues in Context

The ethics of informed consent rest on foundational notions of the right to self-determination and respect for autonomy. In their seminal text on biomedical ethics, Beauchamp and Childress suggest several elements that are required to meet ethically acceptable standards of informed consent (66). These include threshold elements or preconditions (such as competence to understand and decide and voluntariness to decide without coercive influences), information elements (which include accurate disclosure), a therapeutic recommendation, and understanding of the information disclosed and recommended course of action. On meeting these conditions, the patient must decide and authorize the recommended plan before a clinician can begin an intervention.

1. Equipoise

Clinical equipoise is an important concept concerning the state of knowledge about a particular research topic (67). In essence, it demands that true ambivalence toward the efficacy of a novel therapy exists among researchers. It serves as a minimum requirement to justify the investigation of a hypothesis, because any therapy believed by consensus to be efficacious should not be denied research subjects based on the principle of *beneficence,* whereas a therapeutic investigation considered harmful to subjects would violate the principle of *nonmaleficence*. Thus, any clinical investigation involving ICU patients must meet a standard of clinical equipoise.

2. Maintaining the Blinding

Principal investigators and the sponsors of blinded RCTs go to great lengths and expense to maintain the blinding of their study. The integrity of the study is preserved, making it more likely that external agencies will regard the result as convincing proof of efficacy. In the study of investigational pharmaceuticals, many millions of dollars are at stake. Maintaining the randomization schedule where the investigators do not have access, and the use of DMSBs for data resolution, are two standard maneuvers to maintain blinding.

Ethical investigators will not try to undermine the integrity of the blinding process. However, a lack of attention to ostensibly minor design details may make it possible to discern the study subject allocation as a result of casual observation. Particular attention must be paid to the placebo, if one is used. Differences in the color of parenteral solutions must be masked by an opaque covering. Differences in physical characteristics may result in foaming when a protein-containing solution is shaken, as opposed to no effect on a shaken saline solution. Other subtle differences, such as admixture incompatibilities and precipitation during infusion, must be anticipated.

Patient safety is paramount during a clinical trial, therefore it is always possible to break the blind and learn the allocation for an individual patient if it becomes necessary for the patient's welfare. To do so is not a trivial matter in terms of the interpretability of the study for the reasons discussed, and it is seldom indicated for reasons of patient safety. Virtually all commercially sponsored studies maintain constant access to a physician who serves as the medical monitor for the study. It is always stipulated in the study protocols that serious adverse events of any kind (those that jeopardize the patient's life or health, regardless of any association to study intervention) must be reported within 24 hr. Investigator-initiated requests for unblinding usually occur in that context, and are reviewed by the monitor before permission is granted.

3. Data Monitoring and Safety Boards

An interim analysis may be designed into a prospective trial at a predetermined point for many reasons. There may be a substantial question of whether the tested treatment may work, or whether it is safe. A decision to continue the study or to terminate it prematurely may result. Prospective planning is necessary because an interim analysis does affect power calculations, and the sample size may need to be increased if an interim analysis is planned. A decision to terminate a study may result when the interim analysis shows no treatment effect and it is unlikely that additional accrual will change the result. Such business decisions are unfortunate from a scientific perspective. Much more common is a decision to terminate a study because the interim analysis shows a statistically significant treatment result sooner than anticipated (34) (Table II). There may be excess mortality in one group, or it may be lower than expected. Ethical considerations should dictate the suspension of accrual while the interim analysis is performed if harm is suspected.

Alternatively, the DMSB may be asked to evaluate individual cases for adherence to the protocol, or to determine the response to therapy in equivocal cases where the assignation of an outcome requires the judgement of the investigator (i.e., "was the patient's infection cured?"). Protocol violations may render a case invalid, and cause it to be excluded from the final statistical analysis. Protocol violations may take many forms, including enrollment of an ineligible patient, randomization without the initiation of treatment (e.g., a patient reconsiders and rescinds his or her consent), administration of the wrong medication (pharmacy error), or failure to complete the required follow-up at the specified time point. In abdominal infection studies, it may be necessary to make a determination regarding the adequacy of the surgical procedure, because no antibiotic, however effective, can be expected to cure an intraabdominal infection if an undrained abscess or residual necrotic tissue remains after surgery.

Considering the high stakes, it is crucial for the DMSB to remain blinded during its deliberations, and equally important for the DMSB to be completely independent from the study. The composition of the DMSB may include experts in clinical trial design, statisticians, bioethicists, and experienced clinical investigators, but none should have a corporate or financial relationship to an industry sponsor or be an active investigator for the study in question.

4. Informed Consent in Context

Some of the most difficult aspects of achieving informed consent in the ICU are inherent to the nature of the critical care setting. Patients are isolated and highly dependent on intensive monitoring, mechanical and pharmacological means of life support, and the care of specially trained nurses and physicians. In essence, ICU patients represent a captive population. They remain tethered not only to medical devices but also to their clinicians, on whom they depend for life-sustaining interventions. This context creates the potential for an unintended coercive environment, which can threaten voluntary participation as a central element of informed consent. This is further complicated by uncertainty about a patient's prognosis, which can impede discussions about the relative risks and benefits of participation in clinical trials. This uncertainty makes complete disclosure difficult at best.

5. Surrogate Decision Making in the ICU

Surrogate decision making is a major issue in clinical research in the ICU setting and emergency situations (68). Patients with the capacity to make decisions relieve the informed consent process of the additional burden of surrogate decision making in which others—usually family members—make decisions on their behalf. Although some critically ill patients have the capacity to make decisions regarding invasive or intensive interventions, many being considered for experimental therapy and research in this setting rely on advance directives and surrogate decision-makers.

Surrogate decision making, as is the case with the informed consent process, has evolved over time and has its standards. These include, but are not limited to, *substituted judgment,* pure *autonomy,* the patient's best interest, and *minimal risk* or *appropriate incremental risk* (66, 69, 70). The standards of surrogate decision making have been tested in several court opinions; a complete analysis is beyond the scope of this chapter. However, the essential elements of surrogate decision making as they exist currently involve an appropriately designated surrogate who makes decisions for a patient/research subject without capacity in a manner consistent with the patient's expressed wishes. When the patient's expressed wishes are not known and cannot be ascertained, the surrogate must act in a manner consistent with the patients mores and values. In some cases, patients could facilitate this process with an advance directive for research that allows for prospective authorization of participation in a clinical trial (71). In the strict sense, an advance directive for research is separate and apart from the advance directives that inform clinical care (e.g., healthcare proxies, living wills). In fact, most investigators do not make this distinction (and need not, if surrogate consent has been approved by the IRB), provided that the person making the medical decisions for the potential research subject is in agreement with participation in the proposed research. However, IRBs in general have become increasingly skeptical of surrogate consent as protections for vulnerable subjects have strengthened. Many investigators are finding it increasingly difficult, if not impossible, to obtain IRB approval to seek the consent of a surrogate decision-maker to enroll subjects in research protocols.

In emergency situations, wherein the exigencies of the situation preclude time for a full discussion of treatment and its risks and benefits, the standards generally favor "a standard of care that would be rendered by a similar prudent practitioner offering a service under similar emergency circumstances" (68). This standard does not apply when considering research interventions in patients, not because the urgency is less, but because ICU research protocols by nature deviate from standards of care. Thus, the presumption to treat, which exists in emergency situations, does not apply to research, and informed consent is required to enlist patients into study protocols. The single exception to this rule involves enrollment in emergency research protocols, which may offer beneficial treatment for life-threatening conditions, and which have been IRB approved (72).

D. Physician–Investigator Role Conflict

Additional concerns that arise in research include potential conflicts of interest for the clinician-researcher who must balance the dual objectives of caring for a critically ill patient and conducting research designed to contribute to the advancement of medical science and clinical practice. Research activities focus on collecting data to test a hypothesis and draw conclusions about that hypothesis, which may or may not be therapeutic in nature. A conflict over what is in the patient's best medical interest and the researcher's best interest may arise, especially because of the facility with which "*clinical research becomes . . . conflated with treatment*" (73). Financial interests of researchers also represent challenges to ethically sound research generally and informed consent specifically.

Establishing the necessary checks and balances to protect research subjects and to promote and conduct good, ethical research is of paramount importance. Central to this idea is adequate disclosure to patients about the dual role of the clinician-researcher and risk of potentially nontherapeutic interventions. Some bioethicists have suggested that physician-investigators segregate these roles when conflicts between research and therapy become pronounced. This includes the use of independent consent monitors to ensure patients have the ability to provide consent, and the use of clinicians not affiliated with the research enterprise. Furthermore, when researchers have a financial stake in the outcome of their research, it exacerbates the potential for a conflict of interest on the part of the researcher. Most, if not all, of these concerns are best handled through complete and accurate disclosure to patients or their surrogates.

These important issues concerning the ethical conduct of research in ICUs are inherently complicated and challenging at all levels. The more relevant ethical issues relate primarily to the process of informed consent, most notably the appropriate disclosure of information, ensuring adequate understanding on the part of the patient or surrogate and voluntary agreement for participation. Meeting these standards requires awareness of the physician's potential conflict of interest and the vulnerability of critically ill patients and their families. An appreciation of these issues combined with a thorough and active review by the IRB can ensure that human subjects will be protected and medically useful research can be conducted in the surgical ICU.

References

1. Shortell, S. M., Zimmerman, J.E., Rousseau, D. M., *et al.* (1994). The performance of intensive care units: Does good management make a difference? *Med. Care* **32**;508–525.
2. Knaus, W. A., Draper, E. A., Wagner, D. P., and Zimmerman, J. E. (1985). APACHE II: A severity of disease classification system. *Crit. Care Med.* **13**;818–829.
3. Barie, P. S., Bacchetta, M. D., and Eachempati, S. R. (2000). The contemporary surgical intensive care unit: Structure, staffing, and issues. *Surg. Clin. North Am.* **80**;791–804.
4. Van Zee, K. J., Kohno, T. Fischer, E., *et al.* (1992). Tumor necrosis factor soluble receptors circulate during experimental and clinical inflammation and can protect against excessive tumor necrosis factor alpha *in vitro* and *in vivo*. *Proc. Natl. Acad. Sci. U.S.A.* **89**;4845–4849.
5. Ziegler, E. J., Fisher, C. J., Jr., Sprung, C. L., *et al.* (1991). Treatment of gram-negative bacteremia and septic shock with HA-1A human monoclonal antibody against endotoxin. A randomized, double-blind, placebo-controlled trial. The HA-1A Sepsis Study Group. *N. Engl. J. Med.* **324**; 429–436.
6. Barie, P. S. (1991). Respiratory distress syndrome in abdominal sepsis. *In* "Principles and Management of Surgical Infections" (J.M. Davis and G.T. Shires, eds.), 545–568. J.B. Lippincott, Philadelphia.
7. Meduri, G. U. (1993). Diagnosis of ventilator-associated pneumonia. *Infect. Dis. Clin. North Am.* **7**;295–329
8. Research neglects women, studies find. *The New York Times,* April 30, 2000; A18.
9. Solomkin, J. S., Dellinger, E. P., Christou, N. V., *et al.* (1990). Results of a multicenter trial comparing imipenem/cilastatin to tobramycin/clindamycin for intra-abdominal infections. *Ann. Surg.* **212**; 581–591.
10. Barie, P. S., Vogel, S. B., Dellinger, E. P., *et al.* (1997). A randomized, double-blind clinical trial comparing cefepime plus metronidazole with imipenem-cilastatin in the treatment of complicated intra-abdominal infections. Cefepime Intra-abdominal Infection Study Group. *Arch. Surg.* **132**; 1294–1302.
11. Christou, N. V., Barie, P. S., Dellinger, E. P., *et al.* (1993). Surgical Infection Society intra-abdominal infection study. Prospective evaluation of management techniques and outcome. *Arch. Surg.***128**; 193–198.
12. Barie, P. S., Hydo, L. J., and Fischer, E. (1996). Development of multiple organ dysfunction syndrome in critically ill patients with perforated viscus. Predictive value of APACHE severity scoring. *Arch. Surg.* **131**; 37–43.
13. Vassar, M. J., Wilkerson, C. L., Duran, P. J., *et al.* (1992). Comparison of APACHE II, TRISS, and a proposed 24-hour ICU point system for prediction of outcome in ICU trauma patients. *J. Trauma* **32**; 490–499.
14. Knaus, W. A., Wagner, D. P., Draper, E. A., *et al.* (1991). The APACHE III prognostic system. Risk prediction of hospital mortality for critically ill hospitalized adults. *Chest* **100**;1619–1636.
15. Barie, P. S., Hydo, L J., and Fischer, E. (1995). Comparison of APACHE II and III scoring systems for mortality prediction in critical surgical illness. *Arch. Surg.***130**; 77–82.
16. Vassar, M. J., Lewis, F. R., Jr., Chambers, J.A., *et al.* (1999). Prediction of outcome in intensive care unit trauma patients: A multicenter study of Acute Physiology and Chronic Health Evaluation (APACHE), Trauma and Injury Severity Score (TRISS), and a 24-hour intensive care unit (ICU) point system. *J. Trauma* **47**; 324–329.
17. Cullen, D. J., Civetta, J. M., Briggs, B. A., Ferrara, L. C. (1974). Therapeutic intervention scoring system: A method for quantitative comparison of patient care. *Crit. Care Med.* **2**; 57–60.
18. Bower, R. H., Cerra, F. B., Bershadsky, B., *et al.* (1995). Early enteral administration of a formula (Impact) supplemented with arginine, nucleotides, and fish oil in intensive care unit patients: Results of a multicenter, prospective, randomized, clinical trial. *Crit. Care Med.***23**; 436–449.
19. Osler, T. (1993). Injury severity scoring: perspectives in development and future directions. *Am. J. Surg.***165**; 43S–51S.
20. Moore, E. E., Dunn, E. L., Moore, J. B. and Thompson, J. S. (1981). Penetrating abdominal trauma index. *J. Trauma* **21**; 439–445.
21. Slauterbeck, J. R., Britton, C., Moneim, M. S., and Clevenger, F. W. (1994). Mangled extremity severity score: An accurate guide to treatment of the severely injured upper extremity. *J. Orthop. Trauma* **8**; 282–285.
22. Ranson, J. H., Rifkind, K. M., and Turner, J. W. (1976). Prognostic signs and nonoperative peritoneal lavage in acute pancreatitis. *Surg. Gynecol. Obstet.* **143**; 209–219.
23. Heffner, J. E., Brown, L., Barbieri, C. A., *et al.* (1995). Prospective validation of an acute respiratory distress syndrome predictive score. *Am. J. Respir. Crit. Care Med.***152**; 1518–1526.
24. Owens, C. M., Evans, T. W., Keogh, B. F., and Hansell, D. M. (1994). Computed tomography in established adult respiratory distress syndrome. Correlation with lung injury score. *Chest* **106**; 1815–1821.
25. Goris, R. J., Nuytinck, H. K., and Redl, H. (1987). Scoring systems and predictors of ARDS and MOF. *Prog. Clin. Biol. Res.* **236B**; 3–15.
26. Marshall, J. C., Cook, D. J., Christou, N. V. *et al.* (1995). Multiple organ dysfunction score: A reliable descriptor of a complex clinical outcome. *Crit. Care Med.* **23**; 1638–1652.
27. Le Gall, J. R., Klar, J., Lemeshow, S. *et al.* (1996). The Logistic Organ Dysfunction system. A new way to assess organ dysfunction in the intensive care unit. ICU Scoring Group. *JAMA* **276**; 802–810.
28. Vincent, J. L., Moreno, R., Takala, J., *et al.* (1996). The SOFA (Sepsis-related Organ Failure Assessment) score to describe organ dysfunction/failure. On behalf of the Working Group on Sepsis-Related Problems of the European Society of Intensive Care Medicine. *Intens. Care Med.* **22**; 707–710.
29. Barie, P. S., and Hydo, L. J. (2000). Epidemiology, risk factors, and outcome of multiple organ dysfunction syndrome in surgical patients. *In* "Multiple Organ Failure. Pathophysiology, Prevention, and Therapy" (A. E. Baue, E. Faist, and D. E. Fry, eds.), 52–67. Springer, New York.
30. Barie, P. S., and Hydo, L. J. (1996). Influence of multiple organ dysfunction syndrome on duration of critical illness and hospitalization. *Arch. Surg.* **131**; 1318–1323.
31. Mira, J. P., Cariou, A., Grall, F., *et al.* (1999). Association of TNF_2, a TNF-alpha promoter polymorphism, with septic shock susceptibility and mortality: A multicenter study. *JAMA* **282**; 561–568.
32. Evans, W. E., and Relling, M. V. (1999). Pharmacogenomics: translating functional genomics into rational therapeutics. *Science* **286**; 487–491.
33. Walker, J. and Rigley, K. (2000). Gene expression profiling in human peripheral blood mononuclear cells using high-density filter-based cDNA microarrays. *J. Immunol. Methods* **239**; 167–179.
34. The Acute Respiratory Distress Syndrome Network (2000). Ventilation with lower tidal volumes as compared with traditional tidal volumes for acute lung injury and the acute respiratory distress syndrome. *N. Engl. J. Med.* **342**; 1301–1308.
35. Solomkin, J. S., Hemsell, D. L., Sweet, R., *et al.* (1992). Evaluation of new anti-infective drugs for the treatment of intraabdominal infections. Infectious Diseases Society of America and the Food and Drug Administration. *Clin. Infect. Dis.* **15** (Suppl. 1); S33–S42.
36. Anderson, G., Boldiston, C., Woods, S., and O'Brien, P. (1996). A cost-effectiveness evaluation of 3 antimicrobial regimens for the prevention of infective complications after abdominal surgery. *Arch. Surg.* **131**; 744–748.
37. Shuster, J. J. (1993). Practical Handbook of Sample Size Guidelines for Clinical Trials. CRC Press, Boca Raton, Florida.

38. Opal, S. M., Fisher, C. J., Jr., Dhainaut, J. F., *et al.* (1997). Confirmatory interleukin-1 receptor antagonist trial in severe sepsis: A phase III, randomized, double-blind, placebo-controlled, multicenter trial. The Interleukin-1 Receptor Antagonist Sepsis Investigator Group. *Crit. Care Med.* **25;** 1115–1124.
39. Polk, H. C., Jr., Fink, M. P., Laverdiere, M., *et al.* (1993). Prospective randomized study of piperacillin/tazobactam therapy of surgically treated intra-abdominal infection. The Piperacillin/Tazobactam Intra-Abdominal Infection Study Group. *Am. Surg.* **59;** 598–605.
40. Sainio, V., Kemppainen, E., Puolakkainen, P., *et al.* (1995). Early antibiotic treatment in acute necrotising pancreatitis. *Lancet* **346;** 663–667.
41. Driks, M. R., Craven, D. E., Celli, B. R., *et al.* (1987). Nosocomial pneumonia in intubated patients given sucralfate as compared with antacids or histamine type 2 blockers. The role of gastric colonization. *N. Engl. J. Med.* **317;** 1376–1382.
42. Annest, S. J., Gottlieb, M. E., Rhodes, G. R., *et al.* (1981). Nitroprusside and nitroglycerine in patients with posttraumatic pulmonary failure. *J. Trauma* **21;** 1029–1031.
43. Martin, C., Papazian, L., Perrin, G., *et al.* (1993). Norepinephrine or dopamine for the treatment of hyperdynamic septic shock? *Chest* **103;** 1826–1831.
44. Osler, T., Rutledge, R., Deis, J. and Bedrick, E. (1996). ICISS: An international classification of disease-9 based injury severity score. *J. Trauma* **41;** 380–386.
45. Kollef, M. H., Vlasnik, J., Sharpless, L., *et al.* (1997). Scheduled change of antibiotic classes: A strategy to decrease the incidence of ventilator-associated pneumonia. *Am. J. Respir. Crit. Care Med.* **156;** 1040–1048.
46. Pittet, D., Tarara, D., and Wenzel, R. P. (1994). Nosocomial bloodstream infection in critically ill patients. Excess length of stay, extra costs, and attributable mortality. *JAMA* **271;** 1598–1601.
47. Connors, A. F., Jr., Speroff, T., Dawson, N. V., *et al.* (1996). The effectiveness of right heart catheterization in the initial care of critically ill patients. SUPPORT Investigators. *JAMA* **276;** 889–897.
48. Talmor, M., Hydo, L., and Barie, P.S. (1999). Relationship of systemic inflammatory response syndrome to organ dysfunction, length of stay, and mortality in critical surgical illness: Effect of intensive care unit resuscitation. *Arch. Surg.* **134;** 81–87.
49. Vincent, J. L., Bihari, D. J., Suter, P. M., *et al.* (1995). The prevalence of nosocomial infection in intensive care units in Europe. Results of the European Prevalence of Infection in Intensive Care (EPIC) Study. EPIC International Advisory Committee. *JAMA* **274;** 639–644.
50. Zenilman, M. E. (1998). Surgery in the elderly. *Curr. Prob. Surg.* **35;** 99–179.
51. Fong, Y., Whalen, G. F., Hariri, R. J., and Barie, P. S. (1995). Utility of routine chest radiographs in the surgical intensive care unit. A prospective study. *Arch. Surg.* **130;** 764–768.
52. Edgar, H., and Rothman, D. J. (1995). The institutional review board and beyond: Future challenges to the ethics of human experimentation. *Milbank Q.* **73;** 489–506.
53. Taubler, T. S., Viederman, M., and Fins, J. J. (1996). Ethical, legal and psychiatric issues in capacity, competency, and informed consent: An annotated bibliography. *Gen. Hosp. Psychiatr.* **18;** 155–172.
54. *Schloendorff v. Society of New York Hospital,* 105 N.E. 92 (N.Y. 1914).
55. Trials of war criminals before the Nuremberg military tribunals under control council law (1949). No. 10, Vol. 2. U.S. Government Printing Office, Washington, D.C.
56. Jones, J. (1993). Bad blood: The Tuskegee syphilis experiment. Free Press, New York.
57. Ingelfinger, F. J. (1973). Ethics of experiments on children. *N. Engl. J. Med.* **288;** 791–792.
58. Krugman, S. (1986). The Willowbrook hepatitis studies revisited: Ethical aspects. Rev. Infect. Dis. **8;** 157–162.
59. Milgram, S. (1974). Obedience to authority: An experimental view. Harper & Row, New York.
60. Beecher, H. (1966). Ethics and clinical research. N. Engl. J. Med. **274;** 1354–1360.
61. Faden, R. R., ed. (1996). United States Advisory Committee on Human Radiation Experiments. The human radiation experiments: The final report of the President's advisory committee. New Oxford University Press, New York.
62. Belmont Report: Ethical principles and guidelines for the protection of human subjects of research. (1979). Federal Register Document 79-12065.
63. OPRR IRB guidebook (1993). Protecting human research subjects. U.S. Government Printing Office, Washington, D.C.
64. Appelbaum, P. S., Roth, L. H., Lidz, C. W., *et al.* (1987). False hopes and best data: Consent to research and the therapeutic misconception. Hastings Center Rep. **17;** 20–24.
65. Fins, J. J. (2000). A proposed ethical framework for interventional cognitive neuroscience: A consideration of deep brain stimulation in impaired consciousness. *Neurol. Res.* **22;** 273–278.
66. Beauchamp, T. L., and Childress, J. F. (1994). "Principles of Biomedical Ethics," Fourth Ed., pp. 144–170. New Oxford University Press, New York.
67. Freedman, B. (1987). Equipoise and the ethics of clinical research. *N. Engl. J. Med.***317;** 141–145.
68. Mattox, K. L. and Engelhardt, H. T., Jr. (1998). Emergency patients: Serious moral choices with limited time, information, and patient participation. In "Surgical Ethics" (L. B. McCullough, J. W., Jones, and B. A. Brody, eds.). Oxford University Press, New York.
69. Karlawish, J. H. T., and Sachs, G. A. (1997). Research on the cognitively impaired: Lessons and warnings for the emergency research debate. *J. Am. Geriatr.* Soc. **45;** 474–481.
70. Sachs, G. A., and Siegler, M. (1991). Guidelines for decision making when the patient is incompetent. *J. Crit. Illness* **6;** 348–359.
71. National Bioethics Advisory Commission (1998). Research involving persons with mental disorders that may affect decision making capacity. Rockville, MD.
72. Biros, M. H., Lewis, R. J., Olsen, C. M., *et al.* (1995). Informed consent in emergency research: Consensus statement from the coalition conference of acute resuscitation and critical care researchers. *JAMA* **273;** 1283–1287.
73. Frader, J. E., and Caniano, D. A. (1998). Research and innovation in surgery. *In* "Surgical Ethics" (L. B. McCullough, J. W. Jones, and B. A. Brody, eds.). Oxford University Press, New York.

15

Research in the Operating Room

Liane Feldman, Jeffrey S. Barkun, and Jonathan L. Meakins

McGill University Health Centre, Montreal, Quebec, Canada H3A 1A1

I. Introduction and Overview

Surgical research is, in part, driven by the desire to find better ways of meeting the challenges encountered in the operating room (OR). For surgeons, every operation is a search for a better way, advancing individual knowledge and refining technique, and in that sense the OR is a research arena. Every teacher of surgical technique knows that a procedure taught to a student (staff or resident) evolves in its details. Surgeons put their own stamp on each operation. This individualism is characteristic of the "type" of person who becomes a surgeon. Most of these personal, unique technical approaches are never disseminated and represent unpublished or unpublishable new knowledge. In a sense, every surgeon is continually doing research, gaining new knowledge and developing new techniques.

Surgical research in this sense is in part hypothesis driven. However, the personalization of technique by surgeons often leads to new solutions to old problems, the development of surgical procedures for diseases previously treated in other ways, the invention of new procedures, and the utilization of new technology. All of these examples of progress and development require research in the operating room, not necessarily making the OR a laboratory but implicitly demanding some rules. Unquestioned enthusiasm for an improvement can lead to questionable practices. Examples include the multitude of inguinal hernia repairs, single surgeon's series of their operation, and many of the new laparoscopic procedures. The certainty with which some techniques are published approaches marketing. Key questions in this setting are how to evaluate new procedures and what are the appropriate outcome measures to incorporate into assessment. Do the principles of randomized controlled trials (RCTs) apply to testing surgical procedures? Is the RCT the correct approach to test new procedures or techniques?

Quite a different set of studies incorporate surgery either as a variable in a multiarmed trial, as a standard procedure with or without added forms of therapy, or as an operation versus a drug or other medical therapy. As will be seen, these types of studies (at least those that have been published) have achieved a high degree of quality, incorporating principles of study design and evaluation that improve their validity. These studies, in which surgery and the operating room are but a part, are almost always multisited and often multidisciplinary, often demanding by dint of size and complexity expensive external funding. Funding agencies, through peer review, have been useful drivers for quality of design, outcome variables, structure, and organization, much to the benefit of investigator and patient.

The third general means by which research is done in the OR involves utilizing the OR as a laboratory to study something around the operation. There are basically three concepts. First, the operation is standardized and some variable of technique (drains, cholangiography) is being examined. Second, the operation may be the basis by which either a therapeutic concept or an approach (prophylactic antibiotics, subcutaneous heparin, epidural anesthesia) is evaluated. Third, the operation is standardized and aspects of the conduct of the procedure are assessed. It is in this setting that the OR becomes the laboratory. Anesthesiologists have been aware of this for years as new techniques and variations of older approaches have been tested and evaluated. Surgeons too, often in collaboration with anesthesiologists and other OR personnel, have used the OR as a laboratory. Cardiac surgeons, addressing the many technical variables of open-heart surgery, have repeatedly tested and improved oxygenation, types of cardioplegia, and methods to control blood utilization.

Is research in the operating room fundamentally different from any other clinical investigation, or indeed research in general? Does this research demand a hypothesis, a clearly defined protocol, primary and secondary outcome measures, sample size calculation, informed consent, and an administrative structure? Indeed, does it require all of the organization and infrastructure of any good scientific study, independent of whether the operating room is an essential component? The answer to the first question is "no": OR research is not different. Furthermore, all of the criteria applied to research in general, and more, must be integrated into OR research. The principles applied to formulating and answering a research question, whether structured around a surgical technique or a basic molecular biology question, have to be delineated. The critical and complex issues around designing a clinical trial, including primary and secondary outcome measures, sample size, randomization, and consent, have been well described elsewhere in this text and will not be reiterated. Here we review the problems of randomized controlled trials and surgery, as well as approaches to the introduction of new techniques or new technology.

II. Randomized Controlled Trials in Surgery: Problems and Solutions

The randomized controlled trial is an invention of the twentieth century. At this point, a new drug will never be introduced into clinical practice without first being evaluated by an RCT. Conversely, new surgical procedures seem to emerge with little constraint. Although there is no question that a properly executed RCT is the best way to compare the efficacy of two medical therapies, the concept of the RCT as the "gold standard" has led to the general impression that new procedures should be similarly validated (1). Many have lamented, however, that surgeons do not seem to adhere to these rigorous standards when accepting new technologies into clinical practice. In an editorial in the *Lancet*, Horton (2) quoted the medical statistician Greenwood, who wrote in 1923 that "I should like to shame [surgeons] out of the comic opera performances which they suppose are statistics of operations." Horton argued that little has improved since then.

Surgeons have been implicitly and explicitly blamed for not doing more RCTs. However, imploring surgeons to squeeze the evaluation of all new technology into the "one-size-fits-all" randomized trial format, so well suited to the evaluation of new drugs, has not substantially moved the quality of surgical research forward. On the other hand, little has been written about observational study designs in surgical research. Nonexperimental designs are not meant to replace randomized trials, but to complement them (3). With the application of basic epidemiologic principles in design and analysis, observational studies have the ability to address many of the unanswered questions in surgery.

Why is clinical research in surgery held in such low esteem, and how can this be improved? In this chapter, the literature looking at the current state of clinical trials in surgery will first be reviewed. Some of the particular problems inherent in the performance of randomized surgical trials will then be discussed. Finally, a framework for the design of sound nonexperimental studies of new procedures will be suggested, paying particular attention to the estimation of risk and prognosis. Examples of studies we have done at McGill University to evaluate new procedures will be used.

A. Quantity and Quality of RCTs in Surgery

Only about 7% of original surgical research consists of RCTs (2, 4). It has been estimated that up to 40% of treatment questions in surgery could be answered by an RCT (5). However, only one-quarter of 202 RCTs in general surgery published in 1990 contained a surgical arm. Only one-third had a surgeon as principal author. In addition, the quality of these RCTs was found to be low (0.4 on a 0 to 1.0 scale) (6, 7).

Whether the quality of surgical trials has improved over time has been debated. McLeod's group (4) found no improvement in quality between 1980 and 1990. On the other hand, Schumm and co-workers (8) found that the frequency of reporting 11 basic elements of design and analysis in clinical trials improved from 59% in 1984 to 74% in 1996.

The explosion of minimally invasive surgery in the past decade provides a unique opportunity to assess a novel technology from its inception. The first laparoscopic cholecystectomy (LC) was performed in 1987; by 1992, 90% of cholecystectomies in the United States were performed laparoscopically (9). The fact that large RCTs were not done prior to the widespread acceptance of laparoscopic techniques has been widely decried. Examination of the RCTs that have been done since suggests that there has been little improvement in performance of RCTs when introducing new procedures. Slim and co-workers (10) retrieved forty RCTs involving at least one laparoscopic procedure. Only half the trials gave an adequate description of the randomization technique and demonstrated baseline equivalence of the treatment groups. Only 25% provided information about prospective evaluation of the sample size, whereas 15% described an unbiased assessment of the study endpoints. Although a major benefit of the laparoscopic approach is diminished pain and more rapid convalescence, only five trials assessed quality of life with established tools, and only eight examined cost-effectiveness of the procedures (10).

B. Problems of Randomized Controlled Trials in Surgery

Both the number and quality of surgical RCTs remain a significant concern. It has been surmised that this situation may be because "the personal attributes that go to make a successful surgeon differ from those needed for collaborative multicentre research" (2). Nonetheless, the unique pitfalls in the performance of RCTs in surgery may help explain their relative paucity, as well as underline the need for sound, nonexperimental studies. These problems have been discussed in detail by Bonchek (1) and McLeod (11), and what follows summarizes their work.

1. Drugs versus procedures: Several obvious differences between new drugs and new procedures affect how each is evaluated. Drugs do not change in composition after their introduction to the marketplace, and information about their side-effects increases with time. The effectiveness of a drug does not depend on the skill of the physician administering it. Placebos can be used for blinding in drug trials. Conversely, new surgical procedures evolve continuously and are not introduced in their final form. Complications and risks are greatest early on and decline with experience. Results can vary dramatically among different surgeons. Placebos ("sham operations") are not ethical and blinding is often impossible.

2. Standardization of the procedure: Unlike in medical trials employing standard drug preparations, surgical techniques can vary greatly from surgeon to surgeon. Surgeons involved in a trial may differ in their experience with a technique, even when required to demonstrate some minimal level of proficiency in order to participate. Surgeons develop technical tricks as a procedure evolves and often personalize aspects of the procedure. These variations are difficult to quantify. As well, the perioperative care, including anesthesia, nursing, etc, will vary from center to center.

3. Timing of a randomized trial: Chalmers argued that the first patient should be randomized. However, unlike with a new drug, there is a learning curve for every new technique, especially if the new operation requires considerable training (as did LC). Including the first patient in whom the technique is attempted would surely bias the trial against the new operation (12). On the other hand, if the trial is postponed, it may be impossible to begin an RCT for a procedure that has been accepted by patients and surgeons alike.

4. Bias in randomized trials: Although randomization minimizes both known and unknown sources of bias, it cannot account for patients who are never referred to the study in the first place. Although the validity of the trial may not be at issue, the ability to apply the trial to other patients will be affected. When a new procedure is being compared to an established technique, high-risk patients may be diverted away from the study. For example, Troidl's group (12) noted that of the first 100 patients referred to them for LC, 77 were classified as having mild disease, compared to only 10% of patients previously treated with open cholecystectomy. The validity of a surgical study is at risk from the difficulties in blinding patients and investigators, especially when medical and surgical treatments are being compared. When "hard" outcomes are of interest, such as well-defined complications or mortality, the lack of blinding may not be worrisome. However, more commonly, modern surgical trials seek differences in outcomes, such as length of hospitalization, time to oral intake, time to full recovery, pain, and quality-of-life. These outcomes are easily influenced by the patients' and investigators' prejudices. The importance of this was emphasized in the McGill RCT of LC versus minicholecystectomy. When the "duration of convalescence" of the LC patients as measured by the study nurses and treating surgeons was compared, the surgeon estimates were 4 days (15%) shorter than those of the nurses (14). Patient expectations are also influenced significantly by the lack of blinding. In a McGill trial comparing laparoscopic versus open inguinal hernia repair, patients randomized to the laparoscopic group were of the opinion that they would return to full activity on average 5.5 days sooner than their open surgery counterparts (13.7 versus 19.2 days) (15).

5. Feasibility issues: A randomized trial may not be feasible for a variety of reasons. First, the disease of interest may be very rare. Second, the outcome of interest may be unusual or take a long time to occur. It may take many years to obtain answers to questions facing us now. Third, RCTs are expensive, time consuming, and logistically complex. Finally, patients and their surgeons may decline randomization. Unlike in a trial of two medications whereby patients may be offered the other arm at the conclusion of the trial, surgical interventions are usually irreversible.

Patients may not like the idea of the decision being made by chance. Patient preferences play an increasingly large role in determining treatment strategy, and randomization by design eliminates these factors, which may not always be appropriate (3).

In addition to reluctance of patients to be randomized, surgeons contribute to difficulties in performing RCTs. Academic advancement in surgery has traditionally favored laboratory research over clinical research. Clinical surgical research has not been well funded. Surgeons may be reluctant to randomize patients referred for the "new operation" out of fear of alienating the referring doctors. There are also economic disincentives for performing new procedures, because they may take longer to perform.

C. Designing Sound Observational Studies in Surgery

There is no doubt that surgeons lag behind other physicians in the performance of RCTs. This is due in part to the fact that surgical trials may be more difficult to design and implement compared to drug trials, as discussed above. However, it is also true that surgeons seem to place more faith in the results of case series compared to other physicians. Unfortunately, due to biases in selection and follow-up of patients, these studies cannot be relied on to provide valid conclusions. When an RCT is not appropriate or feasible, it is the surgeon's responsibility to ensure that nonexperimental clinical studies are carried out in accordance with established epidemiologic principles. A quick browse through even the most prestigious surgical journals provides convincing evidence that we are currently falling short of that mark.

Although surgical questions may not lend themselves readily to the classic cohort or case-control designs, a great deal can be learned from a properly implemented consecutive series of patients. Analogous to a "prognostic" study in epidemiology (C. H. Infante-Rivard, personal communication), this provides an estimation of the probability of specified outcomes given a similar patient circumstance (age, sex, etc.) and a particular disease state or therapeutic intervention (16). "Rational clinical decision making requires sound estimates of the probabilities of various possible events occurring along each available therapeutic path" (16). Given an 80-year-old male patient with acute cholecystitis, what is the likelihood that an LC will be converted to a laparotomy? What is the likelihood that his course will be complicated by a bile duct injury? The early RCTs of LC excluded patients with acute cholecystitis, and were not designed to quantify rare outcomes such as bile duct injury. Although RCTs address the question of efficacy ("can it work under ideal circumstances?"), prognostic studies address effectiveness ("does it work in the real world?").

The RCT and prognostic study are complementary. The evaluation of the LC at McGill in the early 1990s provides an example. The first LC was performed on May 5, 1990. This patient and the next 1675 patients were entered into a database. The principal goal was to elucidate the basic outcomes of a new procedure: the complications, conversion rates, operating time, etc. Information from that database was used to answer several basic questions: What are the factors determining conversion to laparotomy (17)? Can LC be safely performed without routine cholangiography (18)? Can common bile duct stones be reliably predicted preoperatively (19)? What are the risks of blind insertion of the first trocar (20)? How are bile leaks managed (21)? Can LC be safely performed for acute cholecystitis (22)? Concurrently, an RCT was begun to compare LC and open minicholecystectomy. The principal outcome measures of this study were hospital stay and convalescence. This study of 70 patients remains one of the few studies comparing laparoscopic and open cholecystectomy. Although the trial stopped early because patient recruitment had become difficult, the superiority of the laparoscopic approach was established (14).

Thus, the RCT and prognostic studies can provide complementary information. However, we should be as rigorous in their design and implementation as we are with RCTs. The following basic principles of estimating risk and prognosis, summarized from Marion and Schecter (16), should be taken into account when such a study is considered:

1. Address an important therapeutic issue: Trials comparing different antibiotic combinations fill the literature. Yet we still do not know the most cost-effective way to treat common bile duct stones. We do not know how to reliably predict response to splenectomy in immune thrombocytopenia purpura. These questions will not be answered in an RCT.

2. Clarify the purpose of the study: Have a detailed protocol. Write down the main hypothesis early on and specify and endpoint. This will help in deciding which covariates will need to be collected. As well, it will make the study more credible than one in which data dictate which outcome will be emphasized ("fishing expedition") (16).

3. Think carefully about who to study and when to study them: Assembling a cohort of individuals who share a common "exposure" (a disease or intervention) and who will be followed over time is critical. Both who is studied and when they are studied are important considerations. Who is studied will determine the generalizability of the study. Is the cohort assembled from a referral center? If so, patients in the study may differ systematically from patients who did not require referral. Because a goal of the McGill LC database was to assess the safety of the procedure during its early stages, it included the very first patient. To maximize generalizability, an attempt was made to include every patient in whom a laparoscopic approach was undertaken.

Thus four different hospitals and over 20 surgeons were involved. If not all patients are to be studied, precise inclusion and exclusion criteria should be spelled out from the beginning. Choosing a time to begin collecting data on the members of the cohort ("time zero") is also important. The operation is a common inception point for the cohort. One does not want to risk missing patients undergoing the procedure. In the McGill study, surgeons were told to complete the data sheet at the completion of any attempted LC. One can verify that all patients have been included by cross-referencing the patients in the cohort with the operating room database. However, time zero is not necessarily the time of operation. In the LC database, enrolling patients at the time of operation, although very convenient, precluded collection of data on patients undergoing open cholecystectomy during the same time period, which would have provided an interesting comparison group.

4. Define what the endpoints will be: Decide early in the design of the study on the principal outcome of interest. All outcomes need to be rigorously defined. "Hard" outcomes, such as conversion to laparotomy, are not likely to be misclassified. Other outcomes require careful consideration. Does the diagnosis of a wound infection require a positive culture or simply the institution of treatment? Does the diagnosis of pneumonia require a positive sputum culture or simply a consistent chest X-ray? Quality of life and other such outcomes are even more complex and require the administration of previously validated questionnaires, which must be carefully chosen to be relevant for the disease or intervention of interest.

5. Determine how and when endpoints will be monitored: Endpoints need to be measured in the same way for all members of the cohort to reduce the possibility of bias. For example, a surgeon may decide to see a patient converted to laparotomy more often in the perioperative period because of a concern about the development of a wound complication. This differential follow-up may result in the performance of more diagnostic tests in the converted group and the discovery of outcomes that would not otherwise have been found. If patients who have undergone an operation for gastroesophageal reflux disease are seen in clinic more often than patients who remained on medical therapy, comparing quality of life in the two groups may be biased. The timing of the determination of the endpoint is also important. In the LC database, for example, a patient who presented with a retained stone 6 months postoperatively would have been less likely to be included as a complication than one who presented at 1 week postoperatively, because the surgeons would have already handed in their study sheets. Surveillance bias can be further minimized by having an individual who is unaware of the patient's risk factors determine the outcome. For example, in a study about recurrence rates after different types of inguinal hernia repair, evaluation of the patient is best done by an individual who is unaware of the treatment status.

6. Do everything possible to minimize losses to follow-up: Losses to follow-up are the "Achilles heel" of cohort studies. How many of the original cohorts were lost to follow-up and at what point are critical pieces of information not reported. In a mobile society, particularly when studying a disease or procedure that is not life threatening (e.g., hernia, gallbladder disease, gastroesophageal reflux disease) patients may move away from the hospital region or be unwilling to participate in further evaluation once they have recovered from their operation. A protocol for contacting patients regularly may help in tracking them. If patients who are lost to follow-up differ systematically from those who are followed completely, the study may be biased. For example, in studying the platelet response to splenectomy, patients who have had a good response may be more readily lost to follow-up compared to those whose platelets are low, requiring frequent blood tests and medication adjustments.

7. Understand the measures of risk that will be generated by the study: We are interested in determining the probability of an outcome of interest in our cohort over time. For example, we may be interested in studying recurrence rates of thrombocytopenia after splenectomy. The time aspect is critical here. The probability of recurrent thrombocytopenia faced at the outset by all patients at month 12 is not quite the same as that faced at month 12 by patients who began month 11 without a recurrence. In calculating the latter probability, individuals who have developed a recurrence or are lost to follow-up between months 1 and 11 are removed from the denominator. This "hazard" rate, calculated by including only persons at risk at the start of the time interval, is a more accurate measure of risk than a regular proportion (16). In other cases, the time interval is not crucial. For example, in the LC database, one important outcome was conversion to laparotomy. Conversion obviously occurs at the same time for all patients and there are no censored patients.

8. Have a strategy to deal with incomplete follow-up: Recruitment into the study may be staggered, with patients at various stages of follow-up at the termination date of the study. For example, in studying quality of life at 1 year in a consecutive group of patients undergoing laparoscopic Nissen fundoplication, patients who were operated on earlier in the study were followed longer (23). Excluding patients who did not complete the follow-up would waste a lot of useful data. Techniques of survival analysis (e.g., Kaplan and Meier) can be used to estimate risk from incomplete data. In survival analysis, patients who are lost to follow-up are assumed to be similar to patients followed completely. That assumption can be tested using best- and worst-case scenarios (i.e., all losses are assumed to have optimal outcomes on one hand or the worst outcomes on the other) (16).

9. Consider the role of covariates: Determinants of the outcome in the cohort will depend both on the intervention or disease of interest and the individual profiles of the patients (e.g., age, sex, comorbidities). Think about the outcome of interest and what is known through previous studies and expert opinion to be important predictors. Make sure information about these factors is reliably collected in the study. Regression models can then be used to account for important prognostic covariables and can enable clinicians to assess risk for individuals with particular sets of predictor variables. Logistic regression is used when the focus is on cumulative risk, whereas Cox regression is used to compare rates (16). Collaboration with an epidemiologist is best done in the design phase of the study.

As surgeons, we have been accused of sloppy research. We seem to be more complacent in accepting the results of poorly designed case series compared to our nonsurgical peers. We have been implored to perform more RCTs to study the efficacy of our procedures. Although there are many methodologic and feasibility issues unique to RCTs in surgery, many of these hurdles could undoubtedly be overcome. Why, then, is the number of well-performed RCTs not rapidly increasing? Surgeons may be aware of the need for trials in the evaluation of new technologies, but still seem to put their faith in case series, particularly from reputable individuals or institutions. Surgeons value individual contributions highly, and the "how I do it" paper remains an important source of information that should not be discarded. Nonetheless, there is an important role for more rigorous observational studies in surgery. In this review, only one kind of cohort study, the prognostic study, has been discussed in detail, because it is related to the well-loved case series but provides much more valid information on which to base clinical decisions. As Pollock (24) concludes in a discussion of "surgical evaluation at the crossroads," "important advances will increasingly depend on compete, accurate and objective reporting of the outcome of consecutive series based on apparently logical scientific foundations."

III. Randomized Controlled Trials in Surgery: What Works and Why

Although there are substantial difficulties with RCTs and surgical procedures, there have been some notable successes that have dramatically changed clinical practice. It is worth looking at some of these trials to see what components have contributed to their success. Single-center studies are most suitable to a small trial of a very clear question regarding a clinical problem for which there will be a big difference in the outcome and for which the single outcome (endpoint) is easy to define and clinically relevant. The recent study of use of neostigmine compared to colonoscopy and standard care in the management of Ogilvie's syndrome demonstrated the clear superiority of drug therapy. The differences were so great that early termination of the study was an easy decision (26). Our own experience with RCTs in surgical questions has been somewhat different. The comparison of laparoscopic compared to open cholecystectomy had to be terminated because of difficulty in recruiting patients, even though we were using the hospitals in our network and the surgeons were all a part of the same academic operation. Patients did not like being randomized, the surgeons wanted to do the laparoscopic operation, and the patients wanted the new procedure. We discovered as we analyzed the data that the operators could not be the evaluators. In addition, the difficulty in blinding the patient to the procedure might have biased the results. (14) In another study of hernias, the endpoints we selected were all patient-centered and the sample size was adequate (15). However, the surgical community was as interested in long-term results as we were in the short-term results, and for recurrence and pain data at a year the sample was too small. In an ongoing study of laparoscopic compared to open tension-free inguinal hernia repairs in the Veterans Administration system, the sample size for a primary endpoint of specific patient-centered outcomes and secondary outcome of recurrence was over 2000 enrollees. Clearly this is a study that has to be done as a multicentered program with a coordinating center, monitoring committees, safety monitoring committee, and site directors and patient coordinators. All of this requires elaborate organization and adequate funding. Although the proliferation of types of hernia repairs points out that the surgical community has not solved this problem and also the weakness of a series of repairs from a single surgeon or institution, the methodology and funding mechanisms, it turns out, have only recently been delineated.

If, to properly evaluate an operation or a new technique, a large-scale program, well funded and focused, is required, the National Adjuvant Surgical Breast and Bowel Project (NSABP) is an excellent example. Their studies have not only changed surgical clinical practice in a major way but also have led the way in how to think about and how to do trials involving a surgical procedure. The initial study (protocol B04) of the operative management of breast cancer compared radical mastectomy to total mastectomy with and without radiation (27). Operations were reasonably well described but were pretty standard and were monitored by review of the operative reports. Slight variations in technique were considered balanced by the large sample size and were not seen to be crucial to the overall outcome. When protocol B06 was developed, the approach to the surgical procedure was very carefully monitored (28). The protocol was to compare segmental mastectomy and axillary dissection with and without radiation of the breast and total mastectomy and axillary dissection. Technique was now a critical part of the protocol. The segmental mastectomy had to be done in a very standard manner and had to meet clearly defined pathologic criteria. Only in this manner could the question be answered in a way that would satisfy everyone, because there were strong opinions expressed about the reduction in surgical approach supported by protocol B04, and this study was even less radical surgically and flew in the face of classic Halstedian oncologic surgical principles. The result has, of course, changed our thinking about breast cancer, not only from a surgical point of view but also in terms of our understanding of its biology.

Today, the ongoing NSABP surgical trial is comparing sentinel node resection to conventional axillary dissection in clinically node-negative breast cancer patients. The criteria for surgeons to be able to participate in this study are strict, requiring an ability to do the procedure repeatedly with confirmation by pathology of the ability to identify and remove the sentinel node consistently. Specific goals must be achieved before a surgeon can become a participant. The same will be true for the protocol defined by the American College of Surgeons Clinical Oncology Group (ACSCOG). A surgeon's performance will be strictly monitored to ensure that the procedure is being done correctly. This approach of a standardized surgical technique is offensive to some surgeons, because they are sure they know how to do the operation. However, it is obvious that if the procedure is not done the same way by everyone, the question will not be answered nor will, in the best circumstances, the operation be shown efficacious, a concept to be discussed subsequently. Because the reconstruction of the breast has not been properly evaluated, despite many claims, in our patient-centered view this will be one of the next surgical questions to be addressed.

The NSABP has applied the same concepts to surgical studies in colon and rectal cancer. In C-02, the evaluation of portal vein infusion in the prevention of liver metastases, the technique was monitored very closely, ensuring equivalence of patients managed in different centers in both arms of the trial (29). In the ongoing surgical trial CI-64 (laparoscopic-assisted colectomy versus open colectomy), definitions of the procedure, training of the surgeons, and monitoring the of technique will be adhered to very closely. The laparoscopic operations can be monitored by videotape, clearly a very effective way to guarantee compliance with the protocol. In the Veterans Administration study of tension-free hernia repair, there was a meeting of all involved surgeons and the exact procedure was defined. There will be monitoring and the use of videotapes to ensure adherence to the surgical protocol.

A number of other surgical studies have had significant impact, either because the operation did what it was supposed to do or it was shown that the operation did not succeed and should be abandoned. It is not important to enumerate all of the areas in which RCTs have been of value, although a few examples will emphasize the power of these studies and the impact that they have on clinical behavior. Carotid endarterectomy (CEA) has been available since the 1960s yet it was not until 1991 that its value was clearly defined. Publication of the NASCET trial (30) comparing optimal medical therapy to CEA in symptomatic patients supported CEA. These results have been confirmed by two other large RCTs (31, 32). By 1995, the value of CEA was clarified in asymptomatic patients who had a stenosis of 70% (33). It is now clear that moderate stenosis (58–69%) in the presence of symptoms is also an indication for CEA (34). These well-done studies have established the criteria for CEA and in addition have defined the acceptable complication rates for surgery. If the level of adverse outcomes exceeds those described for optimal medical therapy, also published as part of the trials, that center or surgeon should not be doing the operation. Similarly well-designed studies have defined the indications and value of coronary artery bypass and the criteria for the surgery of small aortic aneurysms.

The extracranial to intracranial bypass for the management or prevention of stroke is an example of a procedure that was eliminated following RCT analysis. This was an operation with powerful adherents and a very fashionable status in the surgical community, but when tested in an RCT was found to provide no benefit to those who underwent the procedure (35). The importance of these trials in defining surgical therapy and standards cannot be overemphasized. For instance, in the case of peptic ulcer disease surgery, gastrojejunostomy was very popular in the 1920s and early 1930s until the recurrence rates were actually determined to be in the range of 30%. The subsequent controversy, with competing schools advocating either subtotal gastrectomy or subsequently antrectomy with a truncal vagotomy, compared to the advocates of some form of vagotomy with a drainage procedure or the highly selective vagotomies, seemed important at the time. The arrival of pharmacologic acid suppression almost eliminated the surgical option, which disappeared following discovery that peptic ulcers in many instances were an infectious disease cured with antibiotics.

IV. The Operating Room as Laboratory

The operating room can be a laboratory. Data can be collected on how different types of surgeries are performed and details of the procedures (variations regarding drugs, drains, or process, pre- or postoperative). Weisel and colleagues (36) very nicely outline issues around studying the details of developing and evolving the techniques of open heart surgery, focusing primarily on methods of myocardial protection using metabolic, functional, and clinical endpoints. Of particular importance, they outline the principle that this research is not different from any other research of quality involving patients. In particular, a study must be hypothesis driven and protocol based, using established methodology, evaluation techniques, sample size calculation, etc. There are, in addition, all of the ethical considerations associated with clinical research, and risk versus benefit must be evaluated and appropriate informed consent must be obtained.

An additional consideration for this type of OR research is the organization of the studies. The hospital must recognize that the increased time these operations will take and the loss of productivity that will result will increase cost. Specific physical requirements or equipment requirements may result in increased space requirement and additional costs. The long view is that this research will lead to improvements in care and therefore cost savings that are realized in better patient outcomes, as Weisel has noted, and/or savings in the actual surgical procedure, as studies of laparoscopic cholecystectomy and hernia repair have shown. It becomes very important to assess costs in a global way, looking at all of the areas that are affected by major changes in the way clinical care is delivered. Hospital and procedure costs must, therefore, be integrated with broader employment costs (days a patient misses work, employer costs, workman's compensation issues, etc.) as well health insurance-related expenses and other costs not normally considered in the evaluation of a surgical procedure or how it is performed. In the long run, the ability of a hospital to perform procedures in a way that will reduce overall societal costs will have a powerful marketing advantage.

Although not strictly OR research, during some surgical procedures the study variable is a drug or other approach to a clinical problem and the outcome of the operation or some component of the operation is the primary outcome variable. Examples include studies of prophylactic antibiotics to prevent wound infection or subcutaneous heparin for reduction of deep vein thrombophlebitis and pulmonary embolism, both of which have dramatically changed clinical practice. There have also been important trials that have provided evidence of perioperative care that was fashionable but that did not help. Our own study on the effect of protein-sparing therapy and major surgery showed that the nutritional support had no beneficial effect on any outcome variable (36). The Veterans Administration trial on perioperative total parenteral nutrition, in a similar way, subsequently defined which patients would benefit from this form of therapy, those who did not meet the criteria had an adverse outcome. The striking common denominator in these trials is that they meet the basic criteria of trial design.

V. Technology Assessment

Research in the operating room can be interpreted in the broader context of technology assessment, for which the ultimate goal is to assess any existing or emerging healthcare technology that will be administered by a surgeon. This typically targets the use of innovative surgical equipment, but also can characterize the development of new indications for previously developed technology. For example, although diagnostic laparoscopy has been part of the realm of the surgeon for many years, its use and test performance (sensitivity, specificity) in the staging of pancreatico-biliary tumors have only recently been more formally evaluated (37).

A. Definition of Technology Assessment in the OR

Technology assessment can be defined as a paradigm whereby new technology is thoroughly assessed from the time of its first development (*in vitro* or in animal models) until the time of its widespread acceptance in the routine medical care of patients. Most clinicians are familiar with this process in the context of the introduction of a new drug and the phases I to IV of drug trial development (38). The introduction of a new technology in surgery, however, also involves unique aspects related to issues of operator dependency, the existence of a "learning curve" phenomenon, the amortised cost of equipment and its maintenance, and the need for operator accreditation, to name but a few.

B. Clinicians' Perception of Technology Assessment

The first misconception by clinicians is the perception that the whole process of technology assessment represents but an exercise in "cost effectiveness." In addition cost-effectiveness studies are usually perceived by clinicians as a bureaucratic *deus ex machina* with a strict view to saving healthcare payer money. Certainly, if technology was free, there would not be a need for technology assessment, but another fundamental premise of technology assessment is that the quality of healthcare delivery is not a simple function of the level of technological sophistication applied. Therefore, both the cost and the effectiveness of new technology represent a quagmire of riddles that technology assessment attempts to resolve simultaneously. This is in fact the main balancing act of technology assessment.

The second misconception is that the process of technology assessment has a start and an end. In fact, it can be more appropriately described as a never-ending loop whereby feedback from an applied technology leads to a refinement in the instrumentation or its application, which in turn leads to new evaluation of that modified technology.

C. Cost-Effectiveness in Healthcare

Administrative exercises in costing outside of healthcare have often led to the concept of "budget neutrality," whereby a new policy is instituted only if it is, at most, no more expensive than a previous one. Such a situation is, however, almost never the case following the introduction of a new technology, because there is almost always an incremental cost for improvements in the delivery of care. With this in mind, the more appropriate question to ask is usually whether a new technology represents "acceptable value for money" (39). This will often be expressed as "years of life saved per thousand dollars," or "quality of life years gained per thousand dollars." The onus is therefore to demonstrate the added value for clinical practice provided by the adoption of a new technology. Accordingly, technology assessment is preoccupied with the generation of both effectiveness and costing data. In order to gain information on both, techniques in study design are borrowed from the realms of epidemiology, experimental surgery, and economics. Ultimately, both health technology assessment as a whole and healthcare economics in particular attempt to provide information so that three key factors can be balanced: access to healthcare (equity), quality of healthcare (effectiveness), and cost or cost-efficiency of healthcare provision (40). In this exercise, the priority of clinician scientists should remain that of demonstrating effectiveness, i.e., quality of care over cost (41).

D. Dimensions of Technology Assessment

Technology assessment was initially viewed according to a simplified paradigm as driven by scientific progress ("science push"), or induced by market demand ("demand pull") (42). Yet it is now recognized that the process of technology assessment has become infinitely more sophisticated and includes a multitude of political and social influences that may explain some of its inherent shortcomings (42). This exercise eventually leads to the concept of performing technological trade-offs, which can be addressed from numerous viewpoints: political, administrative, and ethical (43). These trade-offs are often socially and politically sensitive, and include equity among age groups, social classes, concept of need, and legitimacy of therapeutic goal. Regardless of the conceptual model adopted, the ultimate success of a technology assessment exercise will lie in the successful popularization, or "diffusion," of worthwhile technology. The process of diffusion of a technology will thus ultimately determine whether it gets accepted as a standard of care or gets condemned as just another gimmick (44). This is discussed in more detail below.

E. Generating Information for Technology Assessment

As a rule, the assessment of new devices—for example, those used in novel laparoendoscopic techniques—has lagged behind the performance of pharmacologic trials. One reason for this discrepancy relates to differing regulatory requirements (45, 46). Additional factors may include institutional structure variations within which development decision-making takes place. Indeed, in the case of surgical procedures, such as in the initial development and popularization of laparoscopy, the process is often carried out by physicians in clinical practice as opposed to corporate, academic, and government clinical research settings, which is usually the case for the development of new drugs. Whatever the reason, comparative evaluations in the surgical literature have been, in general, less frequent than in the medical literature (47, 48), and their number did not increase significantly from 1980 to 1990 (49). Although this trend is now clearly reversing, the quality of reported comparative trials has recently been questioned (50) (see Section II). In particular, the quality of economic evaluations has not always been constant. For example, in a review of economic evaluations on knee arthroplasty available from 1966 to 1996, none of 40 studies met established criteria to form a comprehensive economic evaluation (51).

F. Stages in Technology Assessment

As described above, technology assessment is the necessary link between health science and health policy (52). In general terms, there are primary technology assessments through which new data are generated, including feasibility studies, epidemiologic observational studies, and trials yielding data on efficacy and effectiveness (randomized controlled trials and medical effectiveness studies) (53). Secondary health technology assessments make use of existing data and include such methods as cost-effectiveness and cost–benefit analyses, computer modeling, systematic literature synthesis, and meta-analysis, as well as ethical, legal, and social assessments (53).

1. Feasibility

Early on, laboratory and, usually, animal studies will establish technical feasibility and preliminary data on the safety of a technique. The technique is then applied to a small or medium-sized series of selected patients, thus yielding preliminary results based on observational studies. Unfortunately, new techniques are often unjustifiably adopted at this stage without further evaluation, even though efficacy and effectiveness have yet to be assessed. Additionally, premature adoption of the technology at this point often represents a missed opportunity for truly objective evaluation.

2. Efficacy and Effectiveness

Efficacy refers to the performance of a technology when measured under ideal circumstances: ideal patients, expert technicians, perfectly clear and appropriate indications, etc., thus limiting the external validity or generalizability of the trial. Effectiveness relates to the application of the novel technology when the assessment is performed under real-life conditions that would usually include a more heterogeneous group of patients and varied operator expertise (54).

3. Cost-Effectiveness Analyses

Most often, these studies are carried out as a form of secondary technology assessment, whereby the effectiveness component is derived from existing data in the literature (such as in decision modeling). It is often at this stage of the evaluative process that the assessment moves from an individual to a societal perspective (cost-effectiveness or cost–benefit analyses can also view aggregate costs from other perspectives, including the provider's or the insurer's). The unit of interest is at this stage no longer an individual patient, but rather a group of patients undergoing the technology, which intuitively is counter to a clinician's perspective. Perhaps for this reason, as well as the previously stated inherent mistrust by physicians, most cost-effectiveness reports have not been associated with changes in surgeon behavior. Other factors have also played a role: many healthcare providers display a short-term parochial financial perspective whereas cost-effectiveness analyses often require a long-term view to capture all costs, benefits, and hazards (55). There also has been poor standardization of methodology, and unrealistic expectations that fundamental ethical and political questions could be answered. Mostly though, there has been a failure of society to accept the need for allocating scarce resources more judiciously (55).

4. Outcomes Research

At the later stages of technological development, methods of assessment usually employ large databases (56), practice variation data, and decision-modeling techniques—all with the not always implicit goal of developing practice guidelines or clinical management tools. Monitoring systems such as quality assurance and maintenance programs (57) provide clinicians with feedback and education and aim to modify behavior and improve guidelines. A typical example is the assessment of regional practice variations with respect to cholecystectomy. Outcomes research can therefore be seen to complete the initial cycle of technology assessment (58) by providing feedback once it has been widely accepted and used.

5. Nonclinical Assessments

The need for additional assessments is increasingly recognized and includes ethical, legal, and social evaluations (59). This poses significant methodological problems, and requires a range of methods, both quantitative and qualitative, as well as a different set of skills from those required for clinical evaluation. It has been suggested that much can be learned from interviewing relevant people, including those receiving treatment, their relatives, friends, and those providing care (53). As an example of this type of analysis, there has been a suggestion to carry out more structured "error analyses" as are used in airplane accidents. This recommendation is, however, a trade-off between possible legal consequences and the hope of further improving surgical care provided with new technologies (60).

G. Diffusion of the Results of Technology Assessment

Experience has shown that there is not a direct relationship between the quality of a given technology evaluation and the subsequent popularity of its results in healthcare delivery. This is not surprising when one considers that there is often no formal way in which technology evaluation results are reported, applied, or taught. In fact, many factors other than the conclusions of a technology evaluation will primarily influence the impact of study conclusions on clinical practice. These include societal pressures, remuneration considerations, actual comprehension of study conclusions, and parochialism. Even more, different factors may be more important in different geographical areas or physician groups. Occasionally, the poor diffusion of a novel technology may be traced back to an assessment for which the "significant" conclusions were based primarily on statistical considerations rather than on clinical relevance. Such seems to have been the case for laparoscopic appendectomy, for which postoperative wound infection, according to a recent meta-analysis, seems to have been the only meaningful clinical benefit over open appendectomy (61). It is increasingly clear that physician education alone is probably not sufficient to bring about changes in clinical practice, be it from a costing or quality-of-care point of view (62, 63). In fact, probably as important as the quality of the trials generated in the phases of technology assessment are the ability to change clinical practice and the ability to establish a lasting change in clinical practice. In effect, there is a significant difference between providing information and imparting knowledge (64). One little-studied yet crucial factor may be what the new technology brings as benefits (ease of use, operating room time) to the surgeons who will be applying it. For example, a tedious operative technique, which is associated with marginal yet statistically significant benefits, may not be expected to gain widespread approval among clinicians. This may well be the case for laparoscopic inguinal hernia repair, which contrasts starkly with the technological ease of an open tension-free herniorrhaphy (65,66).

VI. Summary and Conclusions

Research in the operating room is not fundamentally different from hypothesis-driven research done in any other setting. The particularities of validating new procedures, introducing new techniques, and evaluating new technology bring very specific problems to the investigator. The difficulties of the randomized controlled trial in surgical settings have been outlined, but also clearly have a role but usually require large numbers and multiple centers. Cohort studies and registries have an important role in the introduction and evaluation of new approaches to surgical care. A new field in which surgeons must become involved is technology evaluation. If we do not, the risk is that government or its agencies will be doing the assessments for us and our input will be lost. Although this area of investigation is not yet fashionable for surgeons, it is ideally suited to our work patterns. The data are collected and organized by coordinators, but are studied and conclusions are drawn by surgeons outside of the usual working hours.

References

1. Bonchek, L. I. (1997). Randomized trials of new procedures: Problems and pitfalls. *Heart* **78,** 535–536.
2. Horton, R. (1996). Surgical research or comic opera: Questions, but few answers. *Lancet* **347,** 984–985.
3. Black, N. (1996). Why we need observational studies to evaluate the effectiveness of health care. *BMJ* **312,** 1215–1219.
4. Solomon, M. J., and McLeod, R. S. (1993). Clinical studies in surgical journals—Have we improved? *Dis. Colon Rectum* **36,** 43–48.
5. Solomon, M. J., and McLeod, R. S. (1995). Should we be performing more randomized controlled trials evaluating surgical operations? *Surgery* **11,** 459–467.
6. Solomon, M. J., Laxamana, A., Devore, L., and McLeod, R. S. (1994). Randomized controlled trials in surgery. *Surgery* **115,** 707–712.
7. Hall, J. C., Platell, C., and Hall, J. L. (1998). Surgery on trial: An account of clinical trials evaluating operations. *Surgery* **124,** 22–27.
8. Schumm, L. P., Fisher, J. S., Thisted, R., and Olak, J. (1999). Clinical trials in general surgical journals: Are methods better reported? *Surgery* **125,** 41–45.
9. Hunter, J. G., and Trus, T. (1997). "Laparoscopic Cholecystectomy, Intraoperative Cholangiography, and Common Bile Duct Exploration. Mastery of Surgery," 3rd Ed. (L. M. Nyhus, R. J. Baker, and J. E. Fischer, eds.). Little, Brown & Co, New York.
10. Slim, K., Bousquet, J., Kwiatkowski, F., Pezet, D., and Chipponi, J. (1997). Analysis of randomized controlled trials in laparoscopic surgery. *Br. J. Surg.* **84,** 610–614.
11. McLeod, R. S., Wright, J. G., Solomon, M. J., Hu, X., Walters, B. C., and Lossing, A. (1996). Randomized controlled trials in surgery: Issues and problems. *Surgery* **119,** 483–486.
12. Neugebauer, E., Troidl, H., Spangenberger, W., Dietrich, A., Lefering, R., and The Cholecystectomy Study Group (1991). Conventional versus laparoscopic cholecystectomy and the randomized controlled trial. *Br. J. Surg.* **78,** 150–154.
13. The Department of Veterans Affairs Gastroesophageal Reflux Disease Study Group (1992). Comparison of medical and surgical therapy for complicated gastroesophageal reflux disease in veterans. *N. Engl. J. Med.* **326,** 786–792.
14. Barkun, J. S., Barkun, A. N., Sampalis, J. S., Fried, G., Taylor, B., Wexler, M. J., Goresky, C. A., and Meakins, J. L. (1992). Randomized controlled trial of laparoscopic versus mini cholecystectomy. *Lancet* **340,** 1116–1119.
15. Barkun, J. S., Wexler, M. J., Hinchey, E. J., Thibeault, D., and Meakins, J. L. (1995). Laparoscopic versus open inguinal herniorrhaphy: Preliminary results of a randomized controlled trial. *Surgery* **118,** 703–710.
16. Marion, S. A., and Schechter, M. T. (1998). Estimating risk and prognosis. *In* "Surgical Research: Basic Principles and Practice" (H. Troidl, M. F., McKneally, D. S., Mulder, *et al.*, eds.), 3rd Ed., pp. 243–256. Springer-Verlag, New York.
17. Fried, G. M., Barkun, J. S., Sigman, H. H., Joseph, L., Clas, D., Garzon, J., Hinchey, E. J., and Meakins, J. L. (1994). Factors determining conversion to laparotomy in patients undergoing laparoscopic cholecystectomy. *Am. J. Surg.* **167,** 35–41.
18. Barkun, J. S., Fried, G. M., Barkun, A. N., Sigman, H. H., Hinchey, E. J., Garzon, J., Wexler, M. J., and Meakins, J. L. (1993). Cholecystectomy without operative cholangiography. Implications for common bile duct injury and retained common bile duct stones. *Ann. Surg.* **218,** 371–379.
19. Barkun, A. N., Barkun, J. S., Fried, G. M., Ghitulescu, G., Steinmetz, O., Pham, C., Meakins, J. L., and Goretsky, C. A. (1994). Useful predictors of bile duct stones in patients undergoing laparoscopic cholecystectomy. *Ann. Surg.* **220,** 32–39.
20. Sigman, H. H., Fried, G. M., Garzon, J., Hinchey, E. J., Wexler, M. J., Meakins, J. L., and Barkun, J. S. (1993). Risks of blind versus open approach to celiotomy for laparoscopic surgery. *Surg. Lap. Endosc.* **3,** 296–299.
21. Barkun, A. N., Rezieg, M., Mehta, S. N., Pavone, E., Landry, S., Barkun, J. S., Fried, G. M., Bret, A., and Cohen, A. (1997). Post cholecystectomy bile leaks in the laparoscopic era: Risk factors, presentation and management. *Gastrointest. Endosc.* **45,** 277–282.
22. Feldman, L. S., Sigman, H. H., Barkun, J. S., Garzon, J., Antoniuk, M., and Fried, G. M. (1999). Complications of laparoscopic cholecystectomy for acute cholecystitis: A prospective study. *Can. J. Surg.* **42,** A140.
23. Feldman, L. S., Mayrand, S., Antoniuk, M., and Fried, G. M. (1999). Patient-centered outcomes of laparoscopic Nissen fundoplication for gastroesophageal reflux disease. *Can. J. Surg.* **42,** A133.
24. Pollock, A. V. (1993). Surgical evaluation at the crossroads. *Br. J. Surg.* **80,** 964–966.
25. Ponec, R. J., Saunders, M. D., and Kimmey, M. B. (1999). Neostigmine for the treatment of acute colonic pseudo-obstruction. *N. Engl. J. Med.* **341,** 137–141.
26. Fisher, B., Redmond, C., Fisher, E. R., *et al.* (1985). Ten-year results of a randomized clinical trial comparing radical mastectomy and total mastectomy with or without radiation. *N. Engl. J. Med.* **312,** 674–681.
27. Fisher, B., Bauer, M., Margoliese, R., *et al.* (1985). Five-year results of a randomized clinical trial comparing total mastectomy and segmental mastectomy with or without radiation in the treatment of breast cancer. *N. Engl. J. Med.* **312,** 665–673.
28. Wolmark, N., Rockette, H., Wickerham, D. L., *et al.* (1990). Adjuvant therapy of Duke's A, B, and C adenocarcinoma of the colon with portal-vein fluorouracil hepatic infusion: Preliminary result of national surgical adjuvant breast and bowel project protocol C-02. *J. Clin. Oncol.* **8,** 1466–1475.
29. North American Symptomatic Carotid Endarterectomy Trial Collaborators (1991). The beneficial effects of carotid endarterectomy in symptomatic patients with high-grade carotid stenosis. *N. Engl. J. Med.* **325,** 445–453.
30. European Carotid Surgery Trialists Collaborative Group (1998). Randomised trial of endarterectomy for recently symptomatic carotid stenosis: Final results of the MRC European Carotid Surgery Trial (ECST) *Lancet* **351,** 1379–1387.
31. Mayberg, M. R., Wilson, S. E., Yatsu, F., *et al.* (1991). Carotid endarterectomy and prevention of cerebral ischemia in symptomatic carotid stenosis: Veterans Affairs Cooperative Studies Program 309 Trialists Group. *JAMA* **266,** 3289–3294.
32. Executive Committee for the Asymptomatic Carotid Atherosclerosis Study (1995). Endarterectomy for symptomatic carotid artery stenosis. *JAMA* **273,** 1421-8.
33. Barnett, H. J. M., Taylor, D. W., Eliasziw, M., *et al.* (1998). Benefit of carotid endarterectomy in patients with symptomatic moderate or severe stenosis. North American Symptomatic Carotid Endarterectomy Trial Collaborators. *N. Engl. J. Med.* **339,** 1415–1425.

34. Rao, V., Christakis, G. T., and Weisel, R. D. (1998). The operating room as a laboratory. *In* "Principles and Practice of Research: Strategies for Surgical Investigators," 3rd Ed. (H. Troidl, *et al.*, eds.), pp. 471–480. Springer-Verlag, New York.
35. The EC/IC Bypass Study Group (1985). Failure of extracranial-intracranial arterial bypass to reduce the risk of ischemic stroke. *N. Engl. J. Med.* **313,** 1191–1200.
36. Christou, N. V., Superina, R., Brodhead, M., and Meakins, J. L. (1982). Postoperative depression of host resistance: Determinants and effect of peripheral protein-sparing therapy. *Surgery* **92,** 786–792.
37. Beger, H. G., and Schoenberg, M. H. (1997). The Role of laparoscopy and ultrasonography in pancreatic head carcinoma. *HPB Surg.* **10,** 186–188.
38. Jadad, A. R. (1998). Types of randomized controlled trials, pages 14–16. *In* "Randomized Controlled Trials—A User's Guide," pp. 14–16. BMJ Publishing Group, London.
39. Weinstein, M. (1999). Editorial. *Ann. Intern. Med.* **130,** 857.
40. Horl, W. H., de Alvaro, F., and Williams, P. F. (1999). Healthcare systems and end-stage renal disease (ESRD) therapies—An international review: Access to ESRD treatments. *Nephrol. Dial. Transplant.* **14**(Suppl. 6), 10–15.
41. Barkun, J. S. (2000). Editorial. *J. Am. Coll. Surg.* **191,** 192.
42. Blume, S. (1998). Early warning in the light of theories of technological change. *Int. J. Technol. Assess. Healthcare* **14,** 613–623.
43. Giacomini, M. K. (1999). The which-hunt: Assembling health technologies for assessment and rationing [see comments]. *J. Health Polit. Policy Law* **24,** 715–758.
44. Traverso, L. (1996). Technology and surgery: Dilemma of the gimmick, true advances, and cost effectiveness. *Surg. Clin. N. Am.* **76,** 129–138.
45. American College of Physicians. (1990). Access to health care. *Ann. Intern. Med.* **112,** 641–661.
46. United States General Accounting Office—Report to Congressional committees. Medical device reporting. (Jan 1997.) GAO/HEHS-97-21, http://www.fda.gov/cdrh/hes9721.pdf.
47. Colditz, G. A., Miller, N. J., and Mosteller, F. (1989). How study design affects outcomes in comparisons of therapy. I and II: Medical. *Stat. Med.* **8,** 441–454, 455–466.
48. Gray, D. T., Hewitt, P., and Chalmers, T. C. (1989). The evaluation of surgical therapy. *In*: Rutkow I.M., Ed., "The Socioeconomics of Surgical Health Care Delivery" (I. M. Rutkow, ed.), pp. 228–256. CV Mosby Co, St. Louis, MO.
49. Solomon, M. J., and McLeod, R. S. (1993). Clinical studies in surgical journals—Have we improved? *Dis. Colon Rectum* **36,** 43–48.
50. Bell, P. R. (1997). Surgical research and randomized trials. *Br. J. Surg.* **84,** 737–738.
51. Saleh, K. J., Fagni, A., Macaulay, W. B., Miric, A., Saleh, L., and Schatzker, J. (1999). Understanding economic evaluations: A review of the knee arthroplasty literature. *Am. J. Knee Surg.* **12,** 55–60.
52. Barkun, J. S., Barkun, A. N., Mulder, D. S., and Battista, R. N. (1991). Technology assessment. *In* "Principles and Practice of Research: Strategies for Surgical Investigators," 2nd Ed., pp. 313–321. Springer-Verlag, New York.
53. Mowatt, G., Bower, D. J., Brebner, J. A., Cairns, J. A., Grant, A. M., and McKee, L. (1998). When is the 'right' time to initiate an assessment of a health technology? *Int. J. Technol. Assess. Health Care* **14,** 372–386.
54. Bond, J. H. (1992). Outcomes and effectiveness of endoscopic procedures. *Gastrointest. Endosc.* **38,** 725–727.
55. Berger, M. L. (1999). The once and future application of cost-effectiveness analysis. *Jt. Comm. J. Qual. Improv.* **25,** 455–461.
56. Steiner, C. A., Bass, E. B., Talamini, M. A., Pitt, H. A., and Steinberg, E. P. (1994). Surgical rates and operative mortality for open and laparoscopic cholecystectomy in Maryland. *N. Engl. J. Med.* **330,** 403–408.
57. Sapienza, P. E., Levine, G. M., Pomerantz, S., Davidson, J. H., Weinryb, J., and Glassman, J. (1992). Impact of a quality assurance program on gastrointestinal endoscopy. *Gastroenterology* **102,** 387–393.
58. Bouchard, S., Barkun, A. N., Barkun, J. S., and Joseph, L. (1996). Technology assessment in laparoscopic general surgery and gastrointestinal endoscopy—Science or convenience? *Gastroenterology* **110,** 915–925.
59. Dolan, A., and Zingg, W. (1993). Health care technology: How can we tell if we can afford it? A Canadian viewpoint. *J. Long Term Eff. Med Implants* **3,** 277–282.
60. Troidl, H. (1999). Disasters of endoscopic surgery and how to avoid them: Error analysis. *World J. Surg.* **23,** 846–855.
61. Fingerhut, A., Millat, B., and Borrie, F. (1999). Laparoscopic versus open appendectomy: Time to decide. *World J. Surg.* **23,** 835–845.
62. Eisenberg, J. M. (1986). "Doctors' Decisions and the Cost of Medical Care: The reasons for Doctors' Practice Patterns and Ways to Change Them." Health Administration Press, Ann Arbor, MI.
63. Greco, P. J., and Eisenberg, J. M. (1993). Changing physicians' practices. *N. Engl. J. Med.* **329,** 1271–1274.
64. Lowe, P. F., and Eisenberg, J. M. (1997). Can information on cost improve clinicians' behavior? *Int. J. Technol. Assess. Health Care* **13,** 553–561.
65. Liem, M. S., van der Graaf, Y., van Steensel, C. J., *et al.* (1997). Comparison of conventional anterior surgery and laparoscopic surgery for inguinal-hernia repair. *N. Engl. J. Med.* **336,** 1541–1547.
66. Meakins, J. L., and Barkun, J. S. (1997). Old and new ways to repair inguinal hernias. *N. Engl. J. Med.* **336,** 1596–1597.

16

Effects of Age and Gender

James M. Watters* and Keith O'Rourke†

**,†Department of Surgery, *Loeb Health Research Institute, and †Clinical Epidemiology Unit, University of Ottawa, Ottawa Hospital, Ottawa, Ontario, Canada K1Y OK6*

I. Importance of Age and Gender

It is essential from several perspectives that the potential effects of age and gender be considered in the design, analysis, and/or appraisal of clinical studies. Either variable or both may be an important predictor or determinant of the outcomes of interest. Aging is accompanied by (1) physiologic changes that alter host responses to surgical illness, (2) changing patterns of disease (e.g., a preponderance of perforated vs. nonperforated appendicitis), (3) changing disease frequency (e.g., increased incidence of many types of cancer), and (4) greater morbidity and mortality following surgery, trauma, and critical illness (1, 2). Gender-dependent differences in clinical outcomes from trauma, sepsis, and other conditions have been identified in a number of studies, although such findings are not universal or fully consistent (3–10). Additionally, menstrual phase may influence outcomes: survival rates in premenopausal women with breast cancer have been reported to be significantly influenced by the timing of surgery within their menstrual cycle (11).

Age and gender, on reflection, are somewhat vague and ill-defined descriptors that need to be made as precise as possible in research, and especially so in comparative research (12). Age and gender effects may be due to cultural, training, and/or biologic factors. Both age and gender are surrogates for other variables. Age is correlated with the prevalence of comorbidity, muscle mass, and functional status, whereas gender predicts differences in body composition, hormonal environment, etc. Whether age or gender is of primary interest in a study, recognizing the effects and associations of each factor may allow the investigator to account statistically for some or much of the variability in clinical data sets and to focus better on the primary outcomes.

The concept of justice is central among the ethical principles that guide the conduct of research in human subjects. It concerns, in part, the distribution of the benefits and the burdens of research. Distributive justice requires that those who may benefit from the advances of research are not neglected or denied such benefits, and that no individuals or groups should bear an unfair burden or risk related to the conduct of research (13). Women of childbearing age have been excluded from participation in some research because of concern about possible harm to the fetus or the newborn or to reproductive capacity, or questions about the effects of hormonal cycles. However, such exclusion fails to address potential differences in diseases and responses to treatment between men and women, raises questions about generalizability, and leaves data for women to be inferred. Women may thereby be denied the potential benefits of research or may be exposed to increased risk from inaccurate inferences. Advanced age has also been an exclusion criterion for some research and, despite widely recognized demographic changes in North America, there is a relative paucity of research information pertaining to the elderly in important clinical areas (14). Questions of competence and consent may be challenging in individuals with cognitive impairments. However, concerns about possible vulnerability and exploitation as research subjects do not negate the obligation to conduct research in such individuals because their automatic exclusion would be unjust in denying the potential benefits of research to populations who may be most in need.

II. Age and Gender as Surrogates

The concept that age and gender are subject to a variety of definitions and are surrogates for other variables is essential to focusing the research question. The investigator's interest needs to be thought out carefully: for example, does it lie in elucidating fundamental aspects of biology or disease, or more simply in studying the problems of patients typical of those who present for surgical care? If the former, then the effects of age- and gender-associated variables must be excluded to the fullest extent possible in order that basic mechanisms or causality can be examined. In the latter, a knowledge of age- and gender-related variables is valuable to allow judgments about generalizability, but is less critical when prediction or prognostication is the goal of the research.

Age and gender are surrogates for biologic, clinical, social, and other variables. Age and gender effects on comorbidity, functional status, and educational exposure may be very relevant to the research problem. Some diagnoses are more common in older patients whereas others are influenced by gender, and the likelihood of requiring an urgent rather than elective surgical procedure is greater in older patients for a number of surgical conditions. The potential relevance of these variables needs to be considered when designing a study, and their measurement then incorporated in the methods as appropriate. Numerous instruments have been used in clinical studies of age and aging to evaluate comorbidity, physical function, cognitive function, physical and instrumental activities of daily living, and health-related quality of life (15–25). These may take the form of direct testing of subjects, questionnaires, data abstraction, etc. The details of their development, validation, scope, and usefulness for a specific study are highly variable. Of particular note for clinical studies is the Charlson comorbidity index (26, 27). This classification of comorbidity developed for use in longitudinal studies has been employed to adjust for the confounding effect of comorbid conditions on overall survival. It has also been adapted for use with "International Classification of Diseases, 9th Revision, Clinical Modification" (ICD-9-CM) administrative data sets (28). The effects of age and gender are heterogeneous, and the method by which research subjects are selected will have a major impact on the observations of clinical studies (29). For example, studies involving institutionalized elderly patients with multiple comorbidities and impaired physical and cognitive function are likely to yield very different findings compared to studies of active, community-dwelling elderly free of coexisting disease. Depending on the specific research question, screening may be appropriate to minimize, or avoid, effects of comorbidity on the outcomes of interest. For example, conclusions about age-associated changes in resting cardiac index vary considerably with the subjects studied: there is relatively little change with age when subjects free of cardiac disease are studied, but a significant decline when the study population has not been screened (30). Undue stringency in screening, or restriction, can result in the selection of individuals who are not representative of the population of interest. Sources of bias in the selection of subjects and the concept of restriction (choosing subjects with specific attributes in order to minimize imbalances in covariates between groups) are discussed below.

III. Design Issues for Randomized Controlled Trials

Randomized trials offer the strongest evidence about causation, in that they attempt to assemble groups that are similar in every respect except for the intervention under study. Ideally, variables other than the intervention are allocated independently of the intervention and similarly in the groups. Simple comparison between groups is then sufficient to evaluate causation. Because it is impractical to randomize individuals to being young or old or male or female, we must employ nonrandomized (observational) designs in clinical studies in which age or gender is the principal concern. These designs are discussed below. However, age and gender are often important covariates and thus very relevant to randomized trials. In order to avoid imbalances in age and gender between groups, consideration should be given to stratifying randomization on these variables when they may have a significant influence on the outcomes of interest. Kernan *et al.* suggest that stratification is "a simple method . . . that is harmless always, useful frequently, and important rarely" (31).

IV. Design Issues for Observational Studies

Prospective cohort or observational studies represent a practical alternative when randomized clinical studies are not feasible, i.e., when age and/or gender are the primary "interventions" or variables of interest. Observational studies are especially useful for description and prognostication and are more challenging and ultimately less satisfactory in defining causal relationships.

A. Description and Prognostication

Descriptive and prognostic analyses of observational (nonrandomized) data are fairly uncontroversial and straightforward, using regression analysis techniques (e.g., 32). When the research objective is to determine whether age and/or gender are useful predictors of an outcome, a prediction rule is developed in one setting or group of subjects. Its performance is then evaluated in another setting or group of subjects (validation or test set), as a measure of the generalizability of the rule (33). There is no direct concern about a possible causal relationship, the principal concerns being how well the outcome can be predicted and how generalizable is the performance of the prediction rule. Of course, knowledge of causal relationships will assist in making better predictions and in assessing generalizability. There are numerous methods of developing prediction rules, both statistical (often termed "data mining" in recent literature) and nonstatistical ("judgmental") (34). Determining the best approach is often empiric.

When only one data set is available, validation data sets can be simulated using cross-validation and bootstrap methods. In cross-validation, a part of the data is set aside to be treated as the validation set, often selected at random. The prediction rule is developed on the remaining data, and the rule is then tested on the data set aside. When a specific variable (such as age or gender) is expected to have significant potential influence, then the generalizability of the rule with respect to the variable can be investigated by developing it in one group (e.g., females or older subjects), and then examining its predictive performance in the other group (e.g., males or young subjects). If the rule does not perform well, then its generalizability to other populations with different age and gender distributions may be questioned. This issue may also be investigated by adding interaction terms between the variable of interest (e.g., age or gender) and all other variables for which data have been collected to a multivariate model, but cross-validation is likely to be less ambiguous, especially if there is a small number of subjects within one value of the variable (e.g., few males). More usually, cross-validation generates a number (n) of estimates of how well the prediction rule performs. In n-fold cross-validation, the data set is divided randomly into n subsets. Each subset is omitted and used in turn as a validation set for the prediction rule developed from the remaining data. These methods are helpful in suggesting how generally applicable a prediction rule will be, but the ideal remains testing the rule on a new (and thereby slightly different) data set.

B. Causation

To evaluate age or gender as a causative factor, we must assemble subjects of differing ages or genders and compare them. Unfortunately, as a result of our inability to assign subjects randomly to being young or old or male or female, study groups that differ in age or gender by design will also unavoidably differ in terms of other variables (covariates). The covariates may be recognized (and amenable to evaluation) or not. They are critical in the evaluation of causation because of their potential effect on the outcomes of interest in the study. Confounding occurs when an outcome seems to be associated with a variable (e.g., age) but the relationship exists only because the variable is associated with other variables (e.g., muscle mass) and not because the relationship is a causal one (35). Confounding issues arise whenever a causal relationship is postulated on the basis of a comparison of groups that were not formed by random assignment (36). For most aspects of age and gender that we wish to study clinically, randomization is simply not possible. As a result, the guarantee that random assignment gives—of groups that are comparable except with respect to the intervention or condition under study—will always be missing, and the resulting imbalance in covariates between groups must be addressed. There is no fully adequate way to accomplish this, not least because we will never have complete information about all of the variables on which the groups may differ.

Nonetheless, there are several strategies relevant to study design and analysis that attempt to minimize or to adjust for imbalances among groups. In terms of design, the choice of research setting and subjects ("restriction") can minimize the imbalances among groups. At the stage of analysis, matching/stratification, multivariate modeling, and propensity score techniques can adjust for them. Specific expertise in nonrandomized comparison studies is necessary to avoid designs that give rise to large uncertainties (i.e., do not hold up under sensitivity analysis), statistical adjustments that are not well thought out, and causal inferences which are not well founded (35, 37, 38, 43). Consultation with an individual with such expertise, at the stage of study design, is strongly recommended.

1. Restriction

Restriction selects for study subjects whose inclusion is expected to result in groups that are not unduly different. For instance, if one was studying age or gender effects on the risk of motor vehicle crash, one might choose to restrict the analysis to patients not taking benzodiazepines (39). Restriction may avoid extreme inequalities between groups or inequalities in covariates that are difficult to measure, but seldom, if ever, does it fully address the problem of imbalance. Selection of subjects can also have the unintended consequence of introducing bias to the study, as is discussed in Section V,C.

2. Matching/Stratification

Matching/stratification ensures that comparisons are made among like subjects (matching) or subgroups (stratification), these comparisons then being pooled. For example, a gender effect on some outcome following surgery might be evaluated by comparison of the outcome between males and females stratified as those who underwent the procedure electively and those who had emergency surgery. Matching/stratification works well if the subgrouping is truly uniform and discrete (i.e., without gradation within strata), and if there are few subgroups. The presence or absence of cancer is an example of a discrete variable. Grip strength is not discrete or uniform when stratified, for example, because there will be gradations within any stratum. Stratification on more than a few confounders rapidly becomes impractical: two variables each having two strata result in four subgroups whereas five variables each with three strata yield 243 subgroups. With a large number of strata, most strata will have observations from only one group, and no comparison can be made from strata that do not have observations from all groups.

3. Multivariate Modeling

Multivariate modeling mathematically models the outcome of interest using a subset of the variables available and mathematical functions thereof (i.e., interaction terms, power or log functions, etc.), yielding an equation describing the model. This allows interpolation and extrapolation of what the outcome would have been in hypothetical cases over a range of variable values. A variety of mathematical models is available. These include linear regression, logistic regression, nonlinear regression, continuous adaptive regression trees (CART), multivariate adaptive regression splines (MARS), additive models, neural nets, and others. The selection of variables incorporated in the model is important: unfortunately no methods are generally accepted as definitive, and judgment is required. Evaluating the effect of a covariate essentially involves a comparison between the outcomes as interpolated and extrapolated by the mathematical model with the values of all other variables held equal among groups or set to some common values. The techniques of multivariate modeling are often highly automated in statistical software packages, but the method of variable selection and how best to guard against a model that fits the data poorly or extrapolates inappropriately (and hence results in poor comparisons) are far from straightforward (37, 40, 41, 43).

4. Propensity Score Techniques

Multivariate modeling methods are not ideal and propensity score techniques are arguably the best currently available techniques to address confounding and support causal inferences in observational studies, e.g., when attributing differences in outcomes to differences in age or gender (42–44). Propensity score techniques are an extension of discriminant matching. They are less sensitive to modeling variations (e.g., variable selection and transformations) than regression techniques and they provide an assessment of whether the groups overlap sufficiently in terms of covariates to allow comparisons among groups. Propensity scores represent a single, composite stratifying variable that simultaneously controls for bias due to the measured covariates (44). Stratification on propensity scores thus balances covariates so that, within each stratum, direct comparison of treated and control (or young and old or male and female) subjects allows causal inferences to be drawn. The techniques of propensity score analysis are straightforward to implement. Propensity score techniques address the effects of differing prediction models on within-stratum covariate balance, multivariate comparability of comparison groups, and constancy of comparisons across strata. Similar issues can be addressed in the multivariate modeling approach, at least in theory, but often are not. Both stratification and matching variants of propensity score analysis have been described (45).

Regardless of the statistical approach, there remains the issue of age and gender as surrogates or intermediate variables. For example, if by aging one means to include gradual but predictable decreases in glucose tolerance, then restricting, matching, multivariate adjustment and propensity score adjustment on the basis of glucose tolerance will inappropriately remove that part of the age effect. If, on the other hand, the definition of aging does not encompass decreasing glucose tolerance, the age effect that is determined will be biased unless glucose tolerance is separately addressed.

C. Standardization of Rates

When binary outcomes such as mortality are compared between groups or populations, standardization of rates in terms of age and/or gender is common. Standardization on these variables (or others) is undertaken because of their influence on mortality (or other outcomes), and its techniques are therefore somewhat related to those described above for addressing imbalances in covariates between groups (46). In direct standardization, the observed rates (e.g., of mortality) for subjects in specific age/gender categories of the study population are applied to the numbers of subjects in the same categories of a standard population that has been identified, yielding a summary (or "standardized") rate that would be observed in the standard population. In indirect standardization, the rates for specific age/gender categories of a standard population are extrapolated to the observed age/gender distribution of the study population. In small samples the observed rates and observed age/gender distribution can be highly variable, with the result that the standardized rates are highly unstable (i.e., change considerably for modest changes in rates or distribution). Some investigators have argued for the use of multivariate modeling of the observed rates to obtain fitted rates that are less unstable (47). These more stable fitted rates could be used in place of the observed rates in the direct standardization approach. The overall standardized rate can be seen as a particular multivariate modeling summary for the chosen standard population and would also be more stable. The distinctions from the multivariate modeling discussed above are the extrapolation of the fitted rates to a chosen standard population, and the calculation of an overall summary rate.

D. Sample Size Estimation

The conventional strategy for estimating sample size requirements considers the magnitude of the postulated difference between groups in the outcome of interest, variability in that outcome, and acceptable levels of type 1 and type 2 errors. However, such an approach presumes that the groups are comparable (i.e., randomized), fails to account for imbalances between them in covariates, and is inappropriate for observational studies (35). The most satisfactory approach to sample size estimation in observational studies is mathematical simulation of potential imbalances, which yields information about how reliably bias is removed and real effects detected. Such simulations can be carried out in many modern standard statistical software packages. If one is planning on using propensity score techniques, a useful starting point is to estimate sample size on the basis of the number of degrees of freedom in the covariates (48). For example, an observational study comparing physical function in young and older patients following elective resection for colorectal cancer might include covariates such as gender, preoperative physical function, Charlson comorbidity index, and tumor location and stage. A conservative assumption is that from 10 to 15 observations are required per group to address adequately each degree of freedom in the covariates (48). We have developed a simulation study of this particular example (see our web site, http://www.lri.ca/programs/ceu/orourke/default.htm), which, because it also entails doing the propensity score analysis repeatedly, may provide useful detail for carrying out such analyses.

V. Other Issues in Study Design

A. Choice of Outcomes

Whereas mortality is generally unambiguous, other outcomes may not be, and the importance that individuals give to various outcomes may be, in part, a function of their age and gender. For example, older patients with serious surgical illness may be less concerned about prolonging their survival than with maintenance of function and relief of symptoms. Similarly, expectations about and self-rating of health-related quality of life may vary with age (49). Thus care must be given to selecting outcomes that are important in relation to the age and gender of the subjects, and attention paid to the effects of variation in age and gender on their measurement. Care must also be taken in choosing the most appropriate denominator when expressing physiologic or metabolic values that vary with age and/or gender, e.g., body weight (which changes little with age) versus lean body mass (which is typically lower in women and which declines with age) (50).

B. Age as a Continuous or Categorical Variable

Most age-related changes in biologic and clinical variables occur progressively and it is usually reasonable to assume linearity (1, 51). Two reasonably defined groups will identify linear effects whereas nonlinear relationships (especially nonmonotonic) will require more. Cutoff values among groups may be arbitrary but should be established *a priori*, ideally on the basis of existing knowledge of the relationship being examined, or as the midpoint of the age range, etc. It may be appropriate to adopt a different cutoff value after acquiring and examining the data, but experimental conclusions will be less strong. Some statisticians would argue for always treating age as a continuous variable, respecting the "scale" of the analysis (i.e., nominal, ordinal, ratio, or absolute), whereas others are more open to treating it pragmatically (52, 53).

C. Bias in Subject Selection

Bias occurs when flaws in study design lead to a misrepresentation of the relationship between a variable and an outcome (35, 54). The selection of subjects is a common source of bias and several considerations are especially relevant to age. Older subjects are survivors from an original young cohort, some of whom have died. They may therefore not be fully representative of all members of the original cohort, and are likely to be those who are especially fit. A related problem is that of selective mortality: if one is studying a variable that is a risk factor (or has a protective effect), then a cross-sectional study (see below) will tend to demonstrate age differences in the factor when none exists, because prior mortality in an older group will have been increased (or decreased) by the risk (or protective) factor (29). Additionally, given the passage of years, a contemporary young cohort may not be comparable to the original, larger young cohort from which current older subjects have been drawn. Referral bias may also occur and take several forms (54). For example, elderly patients may be perceived as unsuitable in some way for surgical therapy and not referred unless they are particularly fit representatives of the larger population with the same condition. For this reason and others, reports of outcomes of elderly patients cared for in tertiary centers or single institutions may not accurately reflect the outcomes that would be defined in population-based data. The risks identified in a tertiary institutional experience would be underestimated if patients referred from some distance were relatively fit (55). By contrast, risks might be overestimated if unfit patients were preferentially directed to a referral center while more fit patients with the same surgical problem were managed in a secondary setting. Referral bias occurs also in relation to gender: for example, less frequent referral for invasive procedures has been described in women with coronary artery disease (56).

The likelihood of bias from these sources and others will vary considerably from one study to another. Those that represent specific, credible threats to the validity of a study's conclusions should be acknowledged and assumed to be present. Their presence should be investigated by whatever means are available or can be devised. A clear description of the source of subjects and the basis on which they came to be studied will allow others to make judgments about bias and generalizability. Many forms of bias may be minimized by careful and imaginative study designs. As in all empirical research, more than one study will usually be required to arrive at firm conclusions. Considering multiple studies in a meta-analysis may also allow many forms of bias to be ruled out. Unlike the meta-analysis of randomized studies, the observations of nonrandomized studies are not combined per se, but are compared and contrasted to appraise the likely effects of various biases (38, 57, 58).

D. Longitudinal, Cross-Sectional, and Retrospective Designs

In general, studies of human aging can be cross-sectional or longitudinal in design. In cross-sectional studies, subjects of various ages are assembled and observations made at one point in time. Such studies must be designed and interpreted with care because of the possibilities of confounding and bias, as described above and elsewhere (29). In longitudinal studies, a cohort is assembled and followed prospectively, with observations being made at planned times. Changes in the outcomes of interest as a function of changes in age are determined for each individual. For practical reasons, cohorts of subjects of varying ages are often studied concurrently over periods of time much shorter than the usual complete or adult life-span. Although not without drawbacks, longitudinal studies are uniquely valuable and have yielded fundamental information about human aging (29, 51). However, studies of the healthcare of older persons (geriatrics) and especially of the problems of surgical illness are most often, of necessity, cross-sectional in design.

Retrospective studies are often attractive in terms of time, effort, and cost, but data collected retrospectively from charts or other sources are typically less complete and accurate compared to prospective collection. Data collected prospectively in a study designed for another purpose are generally superior to retrospective data, but are less satisfactory than if collected prospectively for a specific purpose (59).

VI. Animal Models

Animal models are used extensively to study both the biologic processes of aging and the illnesses that are common in old age (e.g., atherosclerosis). Experimental research into the biology of aging requires the use of animal models, which are usually chosen as mimics of some aspects of human physiology, function, or behavior (60). In general, the considerations in selecting an appropriate animal model include specificity (the trait of interest, i.e., aging, is exhibited in the model), generality (applicability of findings to other species or strains), and feasibility (e.g., availability, cost, well-characterized attributes) (60). It is likely that the processes of aging are similar in a given class of animals, e.g., mammals, but this assumption must be examined when a specific question is being addressed (61). The genetic structure of the population (inbred, F_1 hybrid, or outbred) is also relevant (60). Longevity is a heritable trait and the use of inbred strains allows experiments to be repeated without concern for genetic background. The use of outbred animals allows generalizability with respect to genetic background to be evaluated but may also have disadvantages. Desirable attributes of animal models of aging are that life-span is relatively short (to facilitate longitudinal studies) and well characterized, age-related disease characteristics are well defined, genetic characteristics are well defined, environmental factors influencing aging are well understood, and availability and cost are reasonable (61). Among its resources for investigators, the National Institute on Aging (NIA) of the U.S. National Institutes of Health (http://www.nih.gov/nia/) maintains colonies of animals, including genetically altered and calorie-restricted animals, utilized as models for research on aging processes and specific age-related diseases. These range from rodents, which are used most frequently, to nonhuman primates.

In the context of surgical illness, animal models have been employed more often to study gender effects. For example, interest in gender-related differences in outcome following trauma and sepsis is reflected in the publication of a number of animal and clinical studies (3, 6, 8, 9, 62–64). Gender-related hormonal effects can be manipulated in animal models by a variety of means, which include castration, administration of hormones (e.g., androgen administration to females) or inactive metabolites (dihydroepiandrostenedione), and receptor blockade (e.g., testosterone receptor blockade by flutamide). Interestingly, gender-related changes in the immune response of young mice in a trauma–hemorrhage model are reversed in aged mice, coincident with decreased sex hormone levels (63). The relationship of gender effects identified in animal models to the clinical setting is complex: for example, improved survival in female mice in a sepsis model is related to the state of estrus, whereas such information is often lacking in clinical studies, and cycles stop once the physiologic insult occurs (65).

VII. Summary

Age and gender are important variables relevant to the design and analysis of many clinical studies. However, they are nonspecific descriptors in that they convey a range of biologic, cultural and other influences, and are surrogates for other variables. The investigator must focus and formulate the research question carefully with this in mind. When age or gender is the primary variable, human studies are necessarily observational, because randomization on age and gender are not feasible. Descriptive and prognostic analyses of such studies are straightforward; establishing causal inferences requires careful study design and planning of the statistical analysis.

References

1. Kenney, R. A. (1989). "Physiology of aging: A synopsis," 2nd Ed. Chicago. Year Book,
2. Watters, J. M., and McClaran, J. C. (1996). The elderly surgical patient. *In* "Scientific American Surgery" (D. W. Wilmore, L. Y. Cheung, A. H. Harken, J. W. Holcroft, and J. L. Meakins, eds.). Scientific American, New York.
3. Crabtree, T. D., Pelletier, S. J., Gleason, T. G., Pruett, T. L., and Sawyer, R. G. (1999). Gender-dependent differences in outcome after the treatment of infection in hospitalized patients. *JAMA* **282,** 2143–2148.
4. Maynard, C., Litwin, P. E., Martin, J. S., and Weaver, W. D. (1992). Gender differences in the treatment and outcome of acute myocardial infarction. Results from the Myocardial Infarction Triage and Intervention Registry. *Arch. Intern. Med.* **152,** 972–976.
5. Stone, P. H., Thompson, B., Anderson, H. V., Kronenberg, M. W., Gibson, R. S., Rogers, W. J., *et al.* (1996). Influence of race, sex, and age on management of unstable angina and non-Q-wave myocardial infarction: The TIMI III registry. *JAMA* **275,** 1104–1112.
6. Eachempati, S. R., Hydo, L., and Barie, P. S. (1999). Gender-based differences in outcome in patients with sepsis. *Arch. Surg.* **134,** 1342–1347.
7. Stewart, R. D., Blair, J. L., Emond, C. E., Lahey, S. J., Levitsky, S., and Campos, C. T. (1999). Gender and functional outcome after coronary artery bypass. *Surgery* **126,** 184–190.
8. Offner, P. J., Moore, E. E., and Biffl, W. L. (1999). Male gender is a risk factor for major infections after surgery. *Arch. Surg.* **134,** 935–940.
9. Schroder, J., Kahlke, V., Staubach, K. H., Zabel, P., and Stuber, F. (1998). Gender differences in human sepsis. *Arch. Surg.* **133,** 1200–1205.
10. Ziser, A., Plevak, D. J., Wiesner, R. H., Rakela, J., Offord, K. P., and Brown, D. L. (1999). Morbidity and mortality in cirrhotic patients undergoing anesthesia and surgery. *Anesthesiology* **90,** 42–53.
11. Cooper, L. S., Gillett, C. E., Patel, N. K., Barnes, D. M., and Fentiman, I. S. (1999). Survival of premenopausal breast carcinoma patients in relation to menstrual cycle timing of surgery and estrogen receptor/progesterone receptor status of the primary tumor. *Cancer* **86,** 2053–2058.
12. Rubin, D. (1986). Which ifs have causal answers: Comment on statistics and causal inference. *J. Am. Stat. Assoc.* **81,** 961–962.
13. Medical Research Council of Canada, Natural Sciences and Engineering Research Council of Canada, Social Sciences and Humanities Research Council of Canada (1998). Tri-Council Policy Statement. Ethical Conduct for Research Involving Humans. Report No. MR21-18/1998E. Public Works and Government Services, Canada. http://www.mrc.gc.ca/publications/publications.html
14. Hutchins, L. F., Unger, J. M., Crowley, J. J., Coltman, C. A., Jr., and Albain, K. S. (1999). Underrepresentation of patients 65 years of age or older in cancer-treatment trials. *N. Engl. J. Med.* **341,** 2061–2067.
15. Mahoney, F., and Barthel D. (1965). Functional evaluation: The Barthel Index. *Md State Med. J.* **14,** 45–55.
16. Folstein, M. F., Folstein, S. E., and McHugh, P. R. (1975). Mini-mental state. A practical method for grading the cognitive state of patients for the clinician. *J. Psychiatr. Res.* **12,** 189–198.
17. Spector, W. D., Katz, S., Murphy, J. B., and Fulton, J. P. (1987). The hierarchical relationship between activities of daily living and instrumental activities of daily living *J. Chronic Dis.* **40,** 481–489.
18. Katz, S., Ford, A. B., Moskowitz, R. W., Jackson, B. A., and Jaffe, M. W. (1963). Studies of illness in the aged. The index of ADL: A standardized measure of biological and psychosocial function. *JAMA* **185,** 914–919.
19. Katz, S., and Akpom, C. A. (1976). A measure of primary sociobiological functions. *Int. J. Health Serv.* **6,** 493–507.
20. Osoba, D., Aaronson, N., Zee, B., Sprangers, M., te Velde, A., and the Symptom Control and Quality of Life Committees of the NCI of Canada Clinical Trials Group (1997). Modification of the EORTC QLQ-C30 (version 2.0) based on content validity and reliability testing in large samples of patients with cancer. *Qual. Life Res.* **6,** 103–108.
21. Ware, J. E., Jr., and Sherbourne, C. D. (1992). The MOS 36-Item Short-Form Health Survey (SF-36). I. Conceptual framework and item selection. *Med. Care* **30:** 473–483.
22. Moller, J. T., Cluitmans, P., Rasmussen, L. S., Houx, P., Rasmussen, H., and Canet, J., *et al.* (1998). Long-term postoperative cognitive dysfunction in the elderly: ISPOCD1 study. *Lancet* **351,** 857–861.
23. Guralnik, J. M., Ferrucci, L., Simonsick, E. M., Salive, M. E., and Wallace, R. B. (1995) Lower-extremity function in persons over the age of 70 years as a predictor of subsequent disability. *N. Engl. J. Med.* **332,** 556–561.
24. Podsiadlo, D., and Richardson, S. (1991). The timed "Up & Go": A test of basic functional mobility for frail elderly persons. *J. Am. Geriatr. Soc.* **39,** 142–148.
25. Rubenstein, L. V., Calkins, D. R., Young, R. T., Cleary, P. D., Fink, A., Kosecoff, J., *et al.* (1989). Improving patient function: a randomized

trial of functional disability screening. *Ann. Intern. Med.* **111,** 836–842.
26. Charlson, M. E., Ales, K. A., Pompei, P., and Mackenzie, C. R. (1987). A new method of classification of prognostic comorbidity for longitudinal studies: development and validation. *J. Chron. Dis.* **40,** 373–383.
27. Charlson, M. E., Szatrowski, T. P., Peterson, J., and Gold, J. (1994). Validation of a combined comorbidity index. *J. Clin. Epidemiol.* **47,** 1245–1251.
28. Romano, P. S., Roos, L. L., and Jollis, J. G. (1993). Adapting a clinical comorbidity index for use with ICD-9-CM administrative data: Differing perspectives. *J. Clin. Epidemiol.* **46,** 1075–1079.
29. Elahi, D., Muller, D. C., Rowe, J. W. (1996). Design, conduct, and analysis of human aging research. *In* "Handbook of the Biology of Aging," 4th Ed. (E. L. Schneider and J. W. Rowe, eds.), pp. 24–36. Academic Press, San Diego.
30. Lakatta, E. G. (1990). Changes in cardiovascular function with aging. *Eur. Heart J.* **11** (Suppl. C), 22–29.
31. Kernan, W. N., Viscoli, C. M., Makuch, R. W., Brass, L. M., Horwitz, R. I. (1999). Stratified randomization for clinical trials. *J. Clin. Epidemiol.* **52,** 19–26.
32. Harrell, F. E., Lee, K. L., and Mark, D. B. (1996). Tutorial in biostatistics multivariable prognostic models: issues in developing models, evaluating assumptions and adequacy, and measuring and reducing errors. *Stat. Med.* **15,** 361–387.
33. Christou N. V., Tellado-Rodriguez, J., Chartrand, L., Giannas, B., Kapadia, B., Meakins, J., *et al.* (1989). Estimating mortality risk in preoperative patients using immunologic, nutritional, and acute-phase response variables. *Ann. Surg.* **210,** 69–77.
34. Loeb, M., Walter, S. D., McGeer, A., Simor, A. E., McArthur, M. A., and Norman G. (1999). A comparison of model-building strategies for lower respiratory tract infection in long-term care. *J. Clin. Epidemiol.* **52,** 1239–1248.
35. Brennan, P., and Croft, P. (1994). Interpreting the results of observational research: Chance is not such a fine thing. *BMJ* **309,** 727–730.
36. Sacristan, J. A., Soto, J., Galende, I., and Hylan, T. R. (1998). Randomized database studies: A new method to assess drugs' effectiveness? *J. Clin. Epidemiol.* **51,** 713–715.
37. Freedman, D. (1999). From association to causation: Some remarks on the history of statistics. *Stat. Sci.* **14,** 243–258.
38. Rosenbaum, P. R. (1999). Choice as an alternative to control in observational studies. *Stat. Sci.* **14,** 259–304.
39. Hemmelgarn, B., Suissa, S., Huang, A., Boivin, J. F., and Pinard, G. (1997). Benzodiazepine use and the risk of motor vehicle crash in the elderly. *JAMA* **278,** 27–31.
40. Greenland, S., Robins, J. M., and Pearl, J. (1999). Confounding and callapsibility in causal inference. *Stat. Sci.* **14,** 29–46.
41. Maldonado, G., and Greenland, S. (1993). Simulation study of confounder-selection strategies. *Am. J. Epidemiol.* **138,** 923–936.
42. Rosenbaum, P., and Rubin, D. B. (1983). The central role of the propensity score in observational studies for causal effects. *Biometrika* **70,** 41–45.
43. Rubin, D. B. (1997). Estimating causal effects from large data sets using propensity scores. *Ann. Intern. Med.* **127,** 757–763.
44. McIntosh, M. W., and Rubin, D. B. (1999). On estimating the causal effects of DNR orders. *Med. Care* **37,** 722–726.
45. Rubin, D. B., and Thomas, N. (1996). Matching using estimated propensity scores: Relating theory to practice. *Biometrics* **52,** 249–264.
46. Mosteller, F., and Tukey, J. W. (1977). Data analysis and regression. Addison-Wesley, New York.
47. Joffe, M. M., and Greenland, S. (1995). Standardized estimates from categorical regression models. *Stat. Med.* **14,** 2131–2141.
48. Harrell, Jr., F. E., Lee, K. L., and Mark, D. B. (1996). Multivariable prognostic models: Issues in developing models, evaluating assumptions and adequacy, and measuring and reducing errors. *Stat. Med.* **15,** 361–387.
49. Mor, V., Malin, M., and Allen, S. (1994). Age differences in the psychosocial problems encountered by breast cancer patients. *J. Natl. Cancer Instit. Monogr.* **16,** 191–197.
50. Watters, J. M., Norris, S. B., and Kirkpatrick, S. M. (1997). Endogenous glucose production following injury increases with age. *J. Clin. Endocrinol. Metab.* **82,** 3005–3010.
51. Shock, N. W., Greulich, R. C., Andres, R., Arenberg, D., Costa, P. T., Jr., Lakatta, E. G., *et al.*, eds. (1984). "Normal Human Aging: The Baltimore Longitudinal Study of Aging." NIH Publication No. 84-2450. U.S. Government Printing Office, Washington, D.C.
52. Sarle, W. S. (1995). Measurement theory: Frequently asked questions. *In* "Disseminations of the International Statistical Applications Institute," 4th Ed.
53. Ripley, B. (1999). "Modern Data Analysis in S-PLUS. 1999 International User Conference Workshop." Mathsoft, New Orleans.
54. Sackett, D. L. (1979). Bias in analytic research. *J. Chronic Dis.* **32,** 51–63.
55. Warner, M. A., Hosking, M. P., Lobdell, C. M., and Melton III, L. J. (1990). Effects of referral bias on surgical outcomes: A population-based study of surgical patients 90 years of age or older. *Mayo Clin. Proc.* **65,** 1185–1191.
56. Travin, M. I., and Johnson, L. (1997). Assessment of coronary artery disease in women. *Curr. Opin. Cardiol.* **12,** 587–594.
57. Egger, M., Schneider, M., and Smith, G. D. (1998). Spurious precision? Meta-analysis of observational studies. *BMJ* **316,** 140–144.
58. O'Rourke, K., and Wells, G. (1999). "Meta-analysis of Clinical Trials: Likelihoods, GLMs, HGLMs & Bayes." ASA Joint Statistical Meetings, Baltimore, Maryland.
59. Laupacis, A., Sekar, N., and Stiell, I. G. (1997). Clinical prediction rules. A review and suggested modifications of methodological standards. *JAMA* **277,** 488–494.
60. Sprott, R. L., and Austad, S. N. (1996). Animal models for aging research. *In* "Handbook of the Biology of Aging," 4th Ed. (E. L. Schneider and J. W. Rowe, eds.), pp. 3–23. Academic Press, San Diego.
61. Masoro, E. J. (1990). Animal models in aging research. *In* "Handbook of the Biology of Aging," 3rd Ed. (E. L. Schneider and J. W. Rowe, eds.), pp. 72–94. Academic Press, San Diego.
62. Zellweger, R., Wichmann, M. W., Ayala, A., Stein, S., DeMaso, C. M., and Chaudry, I. H. (1997). Females in proestrus state maintain splenic immune functions and tolerate sepsis better than males *Crit. Care Med.* **25,** 106–110.
63. Kahlke, V., Angele, M. K., Ayala, A., Schwacha, M. G., Cioffi, W. G., Bland, K. I., *et al.* (2000). Immune dysfunction following trauma-haemorrhage: Influence of gender and age. *Cytokine* **12,** 69–77.
64. Angele, M. K., Xu, Y. X., Ayala, A., Schwacha, M. G., Catania, R. K., Cioffi, W. G., *et al.* (1999). Gender dimorphism in trauma-hemorrhage-induced thymocyte apoptosis. *Shock* **12,** 316–322.
65. Chaudry, I. H. (1999). Gender-based differences in outcome in patients with sepsis. *Arch. Surg.* **134,** 1342–1347.

17

Strategies, Principles, and Techniques Using Transgenic and Knockout Mouse Models

Jeffrey M. Arbeit

Department of Surgery, UCSF/MT Zion Cancer Center, University of California, San Francisco, California 94115

I. Introduction

Creation of transgenic and knockout mice by genetic manipulation of the mouse genome stands at the cross-roads of molecular biology and pathophysiology. Experiments using genetically manipulated mice range from determination of function for a particular molecule, to modeling human disease, to testing drugs in biologically relevant systems. Growing funding support for grant proposals using these genetically manipulated mice highlight their importance for surgical research. The use of transgenic and knockout models of surgical disease has been assessed recently (1). Here, the focus is on strategies underlying the use of transgenic and knockout mice in both individual experiments and in research programs. Overviews and rationales for both basic and more complex molecular genetic manipulations of the mouse genome are also explained, so the reader can understand the scope of both scientific resources and funding support necessary to accomplish experiments using these animals.

II. Design of Basic Experiments

In this section the basic principles of using transgenic and knockout mice are described. In the following section more complex genetic manipulations are presented. Moreover, because each experiment presents potential roadblocks along with opportunities for discovery, problems that arise preventing successful completion of transgenic and knockout mouse experiments are also enumerated. Fortunately, many of the roadblocks using basic strategies can be circumvented by using more complex manipulations of the mouse genome.

A. Strategies for Transgenic and Knockout Mouse Experiments

A paramount question is what type of research questions are appropriate for transgenic or knockout technology. In general, transgenic technology models gain of gene function, whereas knockout technology models loss of gene function, although there are special instances in which the reverse conditions may apply for both techniques. Application of either transgenic or knockout technology depends on the type and form of research question at hand, and many times both gain and loss of molecular function are pursued to obtain complementary views of the same gene. Two general principles guiding experimental strategy are (1) determination of biological function and molecular pathway analysis of a previously unknown gene, or (2) testing the contribution of a known or unknown gene to a normal or disease process. When an unknown gene is considered, there is a choice to either pursue transgenic or knockout technology. In general, the "purer" functional test is to knock out the gene, and then determine the resulting phenotype. The investigator must be aware that the gene in question may control a critical stage of development and that loss of its function may lead to embryonic lethality at any stage of gestation (see Section IV). To test the function of components of a molecular pathway, genetic manipulation creates a mouse in which the component is either overexpressed or deleted in the function. Next, another component immediately downstream of the first molecular function is either overexpressed or deleted in a second independent genetically manipulated mouse. Mice representing both components of this pathway are then bred to bring both alterations together in the cells of the offspring and the phenotype is analyzed by a variety of methods (see Section V). Importantly, in many instances the choice of cell types or tissues to target for manipulation in these experiments centers more on the type of information required to define functionality or tissue accessibility, and may not have any relevance to a specific disease.

The other general approach is centered on the role of a known gene in a particular disease or normal process. Here, research strategy is driven by whether the molecular function encoded by the gene is gained or lost, and the relevant cell type from which the normal or disease process originates and progresses. First, the biology of gain or loss of molecular function is determined using transgenic or knockout mice in isolation, in the absence of the myriad of potentially confounding additional genetic and epigenetic changes that also occur during the course of the normal biological process or in disease. Second, the role of the gene in the normal process or disease is specifically determined by initiating the process or the disease in genetically manipulated mice and testing whether either is altered by gain or loss of gene function.

A similar but distinct research goal is modeling a specific disease using transgenic or knockout mice. Initially, research options in this strategy are narrow and focus on manipulation of gene expression toward relevant cell types in specific tissues. If a reasonably close replica of the disease is created, secondary questions encompassing both previous strategies emerge: new genes of unknown function may be cloned or gain of function of known genes may be uncovered at specific stages of the disease model. At this point future work focuses both on delineating the function of the genes in question in isolation of, or in conjunction with, the original model. The latter strategy determines whether the gene regulates or contributes to disease progression or whether its alteration in function is merely associated and ancillary during the course of the disease.

An example of application of these strategies has occurred in our own work. First we created models of human papillomavirus (HPV) squamous carcinogenesis in skin and cervix using transgenic mice overexpressing the viral oncogenes in basal keratinocytes (2–4). Next, we identified gain of expression of a candidate gene with a previously described function, in both multistage skin and cervical carcinogenesis, and also in wound healing. We now have four distinct questions encompassing most of the strategies outlined in the previous paragraphs. First, what skin phenotype is mediated by gain of function of this molecule in isolation from the original multistage model? To answer this question, we have created transgenic mice using a targeted gene expression approach (see Section II,C). Second, is this molecule required for wound healing? Here, because the "standard" gene knockout is embryonic lethal, we have collected a series of mice with selected functions and engineered a "tissue-specific" knockout of the gene in specific keratinocyte cell populations of the epidermis (see Section III,D). We will wound these mice to determine whether there is a delay in wound healing. Third, we can ask how does gain of function of this gene contribute to the original disease or normal process? Here, we use the newly created transgenic mice expressing our gene in question to go back and ask if gain of function will accelerate multistage carcinogenesis in the original transgenic model or wound healing in nontransgenic mice. Finally, our newly created transgenic mice develop a secondary skin phenotype. This additional phenotype is known to be activated by a downstream target of the transgene. We now ask if this "secondary" phenotype is mediated by the downstream target. We will inhibit the function of this downstream target, and determine whether the phenotype in question remains or disappears.

This discussion illuminates an underlying principle in the biological study of genes: in many instances a comprehensive investigation involving multiple approaches may be required to determine gene function in the cells and tissues of living animals. To plan and organize this comprehensive approach involves knowledge of strategies, techniques, limitations, and pitfalls associated with each of these avenues of investigation.

B. Design and Technical Aspects of Experiments Using Transgenic Mice

Both transgenic and knockout technologies involve insertion of foreign DNA into the mouse germline (5, 6), and the DNA construct used in each technique has a particular form and principle of construction (Fig. 1). In transgenic technology, the transgene must contain all the DNA elements necessary for gene expression. These components are ordered along the DNA from beginning to end (from 5′ to 3′) and include a regulatory region, termed an enhancer/promoter (see below), the coding sequence of the expressed gene, and a DNA fragment encoding a polyadenylation signal for the encoded mRNA. Most often the gene coding sequence is provided by cDNA, but occasionally genomic DNA [containing exons (coding sequences) and introns (non coding intervening sequences), spliced out of the final mRNA] is used. Moreover, in special circumstances, larger genomic DNA fragments of 50–200 kilobases (kb) or 250 kb to 1.5 Mb are used to create transgenic mice (7). These large DNA fragments are carried on vectors such as P1s, bacteria artificial chromosomes (BACs) (8), or yeast artificial chromosomes (YACs), respectively. When cDNA is used as the coding sequence, short intron segments are almost always added either in front (5′) or behind (3′) the cDNA, because transgene expression appears to be enhanced by gene splicing (Fig. 1). The transgene is then rigorously purified and the concentration of the DNA solution is precisely adjusted and then injected into one cell, 12- to 16-hr-old mouse embryos in which the sperm and oocyte nuclei, termed pronuclei, are

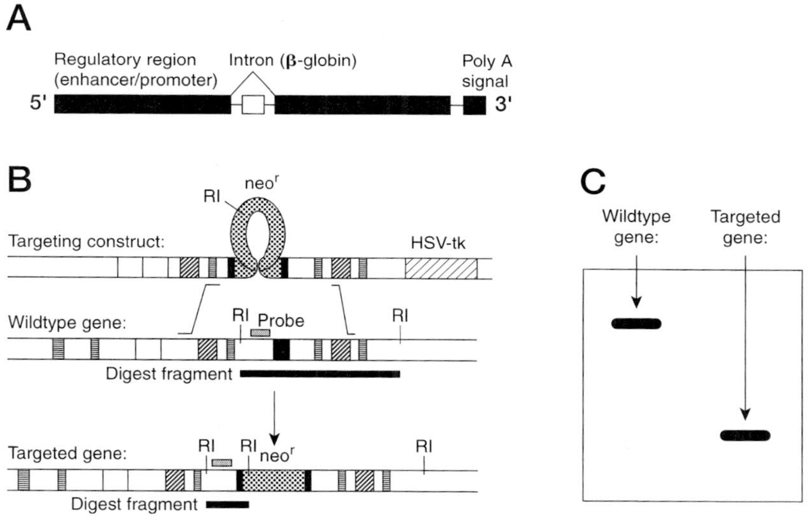

Figure 1 DNA constructs used for transgenic and knockout mice and Southern blotting. A transgenic construct (A) contains a 5′ region that activates gene expression, an enhancer/promoter or regulatory region, the gene-coding element, which is most commonly cDNA, and a 3′ signal for addition of a "tail" of adenine bases [poly(A) signal]. Splicing is important to achieve high-level expression from cDNA, therefore a "generic" intron, usually from rabbit β-globin, is used either 5′ or 3′ to the cDNA. A targeting construct is a replica of genomic DNA, containing coding (exons) and noncoding (introns) regions, and an antibiotic resistance gene that is used for gene function ablation by disrupting an exon and also for selection of clones containing the construct (B). The targeting construct contains a marker used for negative selection, usually the thymidine kinase gene from herpes simplex virus (HSV). This element is lost during homologous recombination, thus cells that randomly incorporate the targeting vector will be killed when exposed to gangcyclovir. Southern blotting is a hybridization procedure used to detect fragments of DNA that are of different length following restriction enzyme digest (C). Southern blotting is used to detect ES cells with targeted as opposed to random insertion of the vector, and also to confirm the presence and copy number of a transgene. Modified from Ref. (1), J. Arbeit and R. Hirose. Murine mentors: Transgenic and knockout models of surgical disease. *Annals of Surgery* **229**(1), 21–40.

visible under 40× power. The injection procedure requires an indirect microscope with attached micromanipulators that control holding and injection pipettes, and Nomarski optics (1). The volume of injected DNA solution is not controlled; injection is continued until visible swelling of the pronucleus occurs, rather than adjustment of the concentration. Most importantly the "cleanliness" of the DNA solution is absolutely critical for successful transgene incorporation. Insertion of the transgene occurs randomly, and most frequently at a single place in the genome, although multiple copies (1–>100) usually integrate as a head-to-tail array, concatenate, of the transgene. Following successful microinjection, the embryos are transferred into the oviducts of pseudopregnant females (Fig. 2). This procedure is done under 5× power using a dissecting microscope. Mice born 20 days later are screened for the presence of the transgene using the polymerase chain reaction (PCR).

C. Strategies of Gene Expression in Transgenic Mice

There are several strategies for manipulating gene expression in transgenic mice. Two basic strategies are presented here (see Section III for three others). Two alternative strategies in basic experiments are to express the transgene in all tissues of the mouse or to express the transgene in selected cell types within specific tissues. Ubiquitous transgene expression utilizes the enhancer/promoter of a gene expressed on every cell, such as β-actin, MHC class I, or RNA polymerase II (Table I). Targeted gene expression uses enhancers/promoters specific for a range of tissues and cell types (1); a representative collection of these cell type-specific promoters are listed in Table I. The rationale underlying the use of ubiquitous expression is that the sensitivity of a range of tissues and cell types to the gain of gene func-

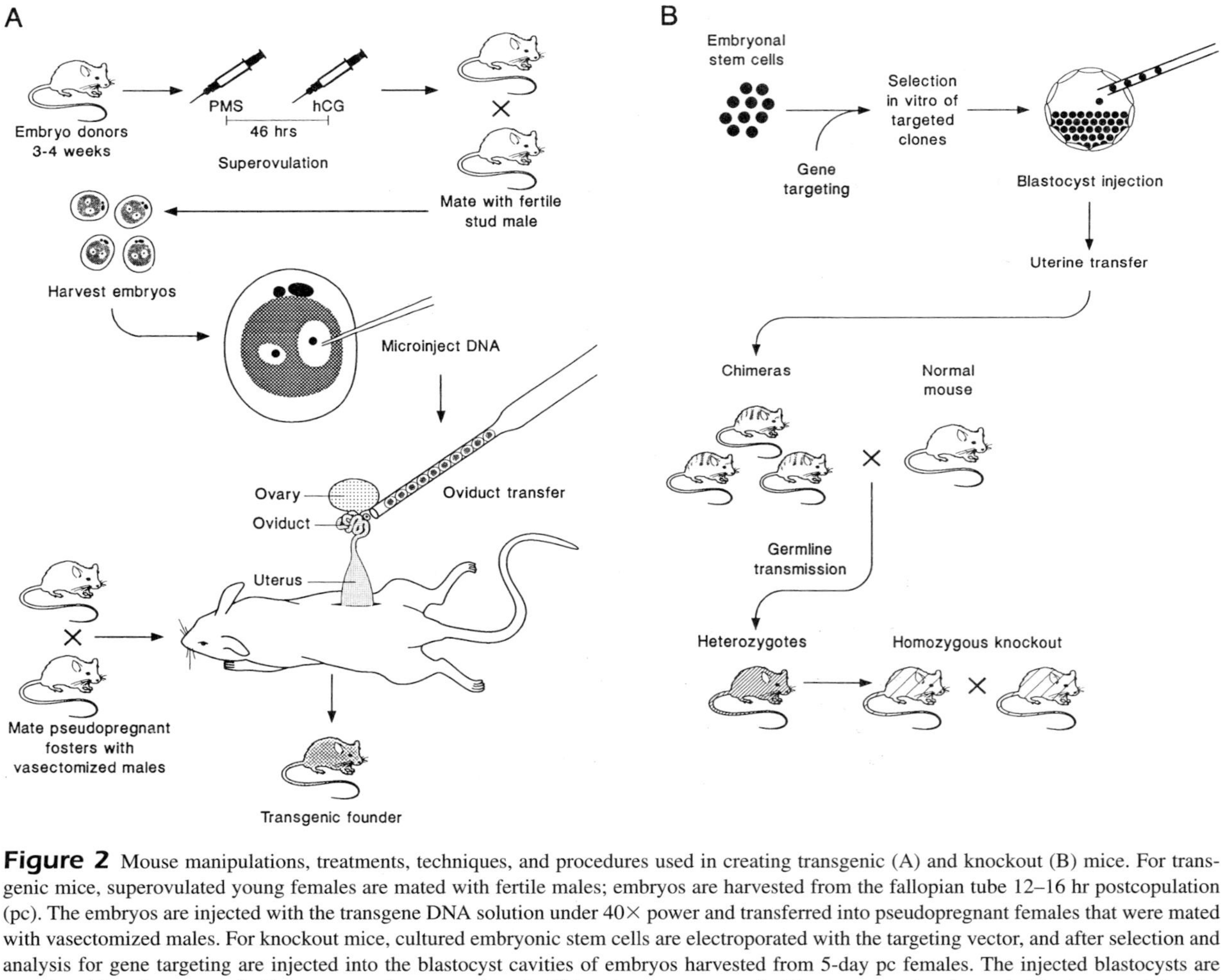

Figure 2 Mouse manipulations, treatments, techniques, and procedures used in creating transgenic (A) and knockout (B) mice. For transgenic mice, superovulated young females are mated with fertile males; embryos are harvested from the fallopian tube 12–16 hr postcopulation (pc). The embryos are injected with the transgene DNA solution under 40× power and transferred into pseudopregnant females that were mated with vasectomized males. For knockout mice, cultured embryonic stem cells are electroporated with the targeting vector, and after selection and analysis for gene targeting are injected into the blastocyst cavities of embryos harvested from 5-day pc females. The injected blastocysts are transferred into the uterus of a 5-day pc pseudopregnant female. Chimeric mice are mated with nontransgenic mice and offspring containing the targeted vector have "gone germline." Heterozygous targeted mice are mated together, producing the homozygous gene knockout. Reproduced from Ref. (1), J. Arbeit and R. Hirose. Murine mentors: Transgenic and knockout models of surgical disease. *Annals of Surgery* 229(1), 21–40.

Table I DNA Regulatory Elements Used for Ubiquitous or Targeted Gene Expression in Transgenic Mice

Ubiquitous	Cell type/tissue specific
β-Actin (human and chicken)	**Mammary gland**
MHC class I	Mouse mammary tumor virus (MMTV), whey acidic protein (WAP)
Metallothionein	**Epidermis**
RNA polymerase II	Keratins 14 and 6, HK-1, transglutaminase, loricrin
	Liver
	Albumin, antithrombin III
	Heart
	Myosin light chain (MLC), myosin heavy chain (MHC)
	Colon/small bowel
	Liver fatty acid binding protein (LFABP)
	Pancreas
	Rat insulin promoter (RIP)
	Brain
	Nestin, glial fibrillary acidic protein (GFAP)
	Neuroendocrine/melanocytes
	Catechol-*o*-methyltransferase (COMT), tyrosinase
	Lung
	Keratin-19
	Thyroid
	Rat thyroglobulin
	Hematopoietic/lymphatic/immunolog
	Eμ-immunoglobin heavy chain, T cell receptor (TCR)

tion can be compared and contrasted. In contrast, targeted gene expression determines the effect of gain of gene function on a specific type of cell. The particular cell type chosen for transgene expression will have a characteristic that the investigator wishes to probe via gain of gene function, or will be the site of gain of function of an endogenous gene during disease. Another motivation for targeted versus ubiquitous transgene expression is that transgene expression in all cells and tissues of the animal may be lethal either in embryonic or neonatal development. However, targeted gene expression can also produce early death and reproductive failure, secondary to systemic effects of transgene gain of function in certain cell types, particularly stem or transient amplifying cells whose population may expand, or can lead to developmental phenotypes in the targeted organs or tissues. Fortunately, most organ systems contain cell types at different stages of development, and if expression in a stemlike progenitor is lethal, more differentiation cells can be targeted for transgene expression and subsequent biological characterization of genetic function in the particular target tissue. For instance, in skin, basal keratinocytes are the proliferative, stemlike cells, whereas the suprabasal cells are at various stages of terminal differentiation (9). Occasionally targeted expression in basal keratinocytes will produce neonatal lethality, whereas expression in suprabasal cells may perturb differentiation, but will still yield a viable adolescent or adult mouse for additional experimentation.

D. Design and Technical Aspects of Experiments Using Knockout Mice

Two overarching requisite areas of expertise in order to perform gene knockout studies are (1) design, cloning, and construction of a "targeting vector" and (2) cell culture, gene transfection, selection, and identification of targeted genes using embryonic stem (ES) cells (see below) (10). Investigators must also become facile mouse embryologists because frequently gene knockouts produce developmental phenotypes and lethality.

Knockout technology relies on replacement of a segment of an endogenous gene with a construct that is almost an exact replica of its target, by the process of homologous recombination (5). However, this construct, the "targeting vector," has a mutation inserted into the DNA such that one or more DNA coding segments (exons) are deleted; the end result is ablation of gene function when the targeting vector replaces the endogenous gene. The "standard" targeting vector encodes for gene deletion by replacement of exons critical for gene function by an antibiotic resistance gene, usually encoding for neomycin (NEO) or hygromycin phosphotransferase (Fig. 1). Unmanipulated mammalian cells can be killed by the aminoglycoside G418, whereas the NEO gene renders cells resistant to the antibiotic. Thus cells containing insertions of the targeting vector can be "selected" for NEO resistance by growth in G418, and clones of these cells can be isolated and analyzed (see below). A variation of the standard gene deletion knockout is termed a gene "knockin." Here, instead of deletions, single base-pair mutations are introduced into the targeting vector, such that gene function is maintained, albeit in an abnormal way. In these cases the antibiotic resistance cassette is located in an intron, or is deleted in the cloning procedure. Targeting vectors are approximately 6–9 kilobase pairs (kbp) in size. For precise insertion into the host genome and replacement of endogenous genes, they must contain "regions of homology," that is, be exact copies of the endogenous genomic DNA. Thus targeting vectors, in contrast to transgenes, contain both exons (coding regions) and introns (intervening sequences "spliced out" of the final mRNA message). Regions of homology in the targeting vector are located on its flanks or arms. In order to manipulate the DNA to create the targeting vector, genomic DNA containing the gene of interest must be isolated from a mouse 129sv embryonic stem cell library (10). The strain of the library is important because introns are markedly different (highly polymorphic) in different mouse strains. The strain 129 mouse embryonic stem cells have the highest propensity to "go germline" (see below), hence they are used for the targeting vector isolation and creation. Genomic libraries are usually carried in bacteriophages, because these vectors can accommodate larger fragments of DNA (25- to 100-kb inserts) compared to bacterial cDNA libraries. The phages are spread onto a lawn of bacteria growing on a plate, and after incubation plaques or clear areas form where bacterial colonies containing phage have been lysed. Filters are placed on, and oriented exactly to, the position of the plaques on the plate, and part of the phage DNA is transferred to the filter. The filter is hybridized with a probe for the gene of interest and a positive colony is then located on the original plate. Phages from the positive plaque are scraped and used to infect other bacteria. After several rounds of selection the entire plaque plug is removed from the plate, and genomic DNA is purified from the phage DNA. A smaller restriction fragment, 6–9 kb, is isolated from the genomic DNA corresponding to the region most critical for function of the gene. A detailed restriction map is then constructed for this fragment of genomic DNA; exons and introns are identified from previous data regarding the gene (usually the cDNA has been cloned first). The exon(s) to be deleted are identified, and "in-frame" insertion of the NEO cassette is accomplished via use of previously identified restriction sites. The completed targeting vector is then sequenced to confirm that no rearrangements occurred during cloning.

The second cornerstone of gene knockouts are ES cells, which possess two properties critical for success of the technique (10). First, they possess a very high rate of homologous recombination, allowing replacement of endogenous genes with targeting vectors. Second, they are totipotent and have a marked propensity to contribute to each organ and tissue of the embryonic mouse. Hence, the degree of "chimerism" (see below) is high. Mouse embryonic stem cells are isolated from the inner cell mass of a blastocyst. They are cultured in special media to prevent differentiation and loss of totipotency, are expanded in cell number, and stocks are tested for germline transmission and then frozen for later use. The targeting vector is introduced (transfected) into the embryonic stem cells by electroporation, which is a short electric shock that opens pores in the membrane, allowing ingress of DNA. After recovery, the ES cells are grown in 96-well plates in the presence of G418. Surviving clones have integrated the vector, but not necessarily into the location of the endogenous gene. Therefore, Southern blotting of restriction-digested DNA isolated from embryonic stem cells must be performed to determine if there was "gene targeting," as opposed to random insertion of the vector (Fig. 1). Once ES cells with correct gene targeting are identified, they are expanded and microinjected into the coelom of blastocysts, which in mice are 5-day-old embryos (Fig. 2). The microinjection setup is similar to that used for transgenic mice except that the holding pipette is wider and is beveled in a specific manner (11). Injected blastocysts are transferred into pseudopregnant females 5 days postcoitus. The blastocysts are transferred into the uterus rather than the ostium of the fallopian tube. Subsequently (3 weeks later), chimeric mice are born. Because the ES cells have been incorporated into blastocysts they make a variable contribution to each tissue of the mouse. Thus the number of cells containing the targeted allele is different in cells within the same organ, and between different cell types and tissues. Because chimerism is also present in the germline, the next major hurdle is whether the targeted allele can be passed through the germline. Thus the chimeric mice are mated to wild-type nontransgenic mice. Once germline transmission occurs in the heterozygote, there is one copy of the targeted allele in each and every cell of the mouse. The goal is to assess complete loss of gene function, thus two heterozygotes are bred together and the progeny of this cross assessed (see below) for a homozygous gene knockout (Fig. 2). In many instances the litters of a heterozygous cross will not contain homozygotes. This indicates that complete loss of gene function is lethal *in utero*. Moreover, these data also indicate that the gene may control a critical stage of embryonic development, motivating timed matings, serial sacrifice, and embryo harvesting to determine the developmental phenotype resulting from loss of gene function.

III. Design of Advanced Experiments

There are several goals of more complex genetic manipulations in transgenic and knockout mouse technology. The most obvious rationale is that either gain or loss of gene function is lethal, or produces mortality in adolescent mice either prior to sexual maturity, to maintain a permanent line, or prior to development of disease in the original model. Alternatively, more control over gene expression may be the focus of experimentation. Examples include the ability to either turn genes on or off in adult mice, or to sequentially turn a gene on, then off, testing which component of an induced phenotype is independent of, or dependent on, continued transgene expression. The promise of temporal control of gene expression is particularly suited to multistage processes such as carcinogenesis or atherogenesis, wherein activation of a gene at a precise stage of progression can specifically determine its role in disease.

A. Inducible Transgene Expression

Two strategies are available to turn transgenes on or off at will. The first approach is the tetracycline repressor/operator system (tetR/op) (12, 13). The system can work in two ways, dependent on the type of repressor used. The wild-type tetR is, as the name implies, a repressor and inhibitor of gene function when bound to tetracycline. Using this approach, pregnant mice are placed on tetracycline to keep the gene off during gestation, neonatal, and early adult life, and then are withdrawn from the drug, activating the transgene function in mature animals. The alternative system uses a mutant form of the repressor that is an activator (rtTA), turning gene function on when bound to tetracycline (14). In this system, the transgene is off until tetracycline is administered, initiating transcription. The advantage of the wild-type tetR repressor system is tighter gene regulation and greater induction of expression compared to the mutant rtTA. The down side of the wild-type tetR repressor is the requirement for continuous tetracycline administration to keep the gene off until the time of activation.

The overall scheme for creation of the tetR-inducible system is outlined in Fig. 3A. This system is termed "bitransgenic." It involves creation of two transgenic mouse lines and their subsequent intercross to yield double or "bitransgenic mice." One mouse line contains the transgene whose expression is to be inducible. This transgene is composed of a cDNA linked to a minimal promoter whose expression is not turned on or off unless the attached enhancer element, a "tet operator," is engaged by either wild-type or mutant tetR, respectively. The second type of transgenic mouse contains the cDNA for the tetR, either wild-type or mutant rtTA, linked most frequently to a tissue-specific promoter for targeted gene expression, or less frequently to a ubiquitous promoter. The power of targeted expression of the tetR is that the investigator can control gene expression within a specific cell type or tissue (see above). Intercrossing both of these mice yields the completed system, which is screened by PCR for the presence of both transgenes. In actual experi-

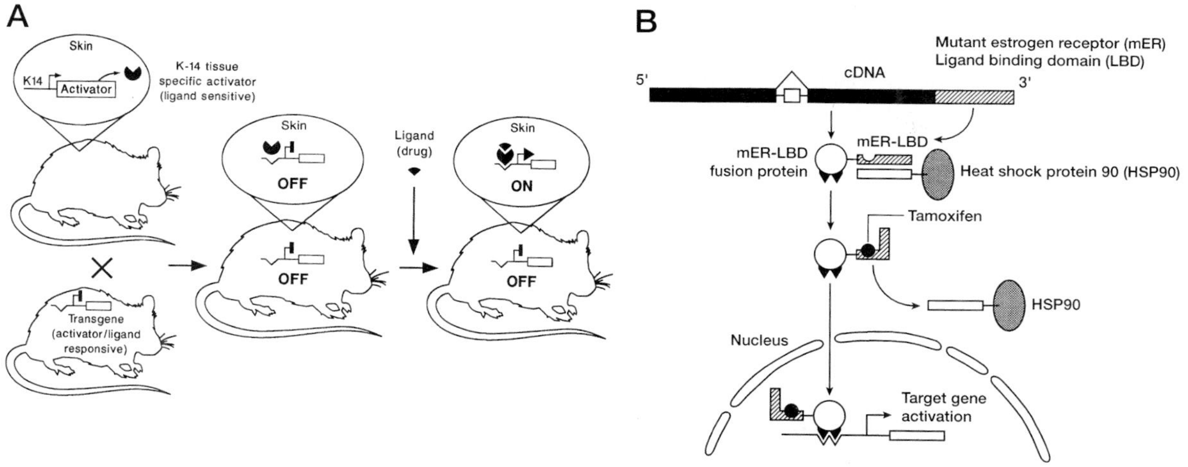

Figure 3 Strategies for inducible transgene expression. The drug-inducible system is based on creating double-transgenic mice by breeding (A). One transgenic mouse has the "responder" transgene containing a DNA element that requires or is inhibited by the ligand-responsive activator/repressor, and controls gene expression. The second transgenic mouse expresses the ligand-sensitive activator/repressor, usually in a tissue-specific and cell type-specific manner. The two types of transgenic mice are bred together, and the double-transgenic progeny will have transgene expression that is controlled by the ligand. Some systems are inhibited by the ligand and others are activated by it. An alternative strategy is expression of a transgene cDNA fused to a mutant estrogen receptor responsive to tamoxifen (B). In the absence of hormone the transgenic protein is sequestered in an inactive complex with HSP90, whereas following tamoxifen administration, the transgenic protein is activated, allowing or permitting nuclear translocation. Modified from Ref. (1), J. Arbeit and R. Hirose. Murine mentors: Transgenic and knockout models of surgical disease. *Annals of Surgery* **229**(1), 21–40.

ments several independent mouse lines of targeted tetR expression and inducible transgene must be created and screened. The former is screened for expression of wild-type or mutant rtTA in the cell type targeted for expression. These tetR mice can be then be used in all subsequent experiments of inducible gene expression in that cell type. For the wild-type tetR system, transgenic lines containing the inducible transgene are then tested for inhibition by tetracycline and induction by antibiotic withdrawal. For the mutant rtTA system the absence of expression without tetracycline, and moderate to high-level induction of expression in response to antibiotic, are tested. Obviously, these experiments are costly and labor intensive, but provide a unique opportunity to investigate temporal control of gene expression.

There are two other approaches to inducible transgene expression. The ecdysone activator system uses the insect molting hormone ecdysone, myristerone, or cheaper insecticides to activate a hormone binding transcription factor specific for a regulatory region in a target transgene (15). This concept is similar to the tetR/activator system. Another, simpler system can be used, but it is less versatile. Here, the transgene cDNA is fused in-frame to a mutant form of the estrogen receptor hormone-binding domain, specific for tamoxifen rather than estradiol. The transgene is expressed in either a tissue-specific or ubiquitous manner, although the most straightforward experiments with this system use targeted expression to the skin (16) (see below). In the absence of tamoxifen, the transgene is expressed but is bound to heat shock protein 90 (HSP90) (Fig. 3B). In the presence of tamoxifen, the transgene dissociates from HSP90 and is activated. The down side of this approach to inducible gene expression is that transgene expression requires the continuous administration of tamoxifen. Although the drug can be administered orally in the drinking water, the side effects of this partial estrogen agonist/antagonist complicate certain experiments. Alternatively, if transgene expression is targeted to the skin, tamoxifen can be topically applied in a dimethyl sulfoxide (DMSO) or ethanol solvent and local gene expression can be activated without the confounding variable of prolonged systemic hormone administration.

B. Inhibition of Gene Function Using Dominant-Negative Transgenic Mice

In general, transgenic technology is used to test the biology of gain of gene function, although transgenic expression of a "dominant-negative" form of a gene can be used to inhibit function of its endogenous counterpart (17). Dominant-negative gene function is dependent on two principles. One is dimerization or oligomerization of encoded molecules. The second is the partition of protein function into discrete domains or modules (Fig. 4) (18). Many cellular proteins, such as tyrosine kinase growth factor receptors or transcription factors, fall into this classification. These molecules either bind with their identical counterparts (homodimerization) or with related members of the same gene family (heterodimerization). They both contain distinct domains. Transcription factors are composed of a transactivation domain, a dimerization domain, and a DNA-binding region. Tyrosine kinase growth factor receptors contain an extracytoplasmic ligand-binding domain, which also is the main region of dimerization, an α-helical transmembrane region, and an intracytoplasmic domain containing ATPase and signal transduction protein binding sites. To create a dominant-negative form of each of these genes, the dimerization domains are left intact but either the transactivation (transcription factor) or the intracytoplasmic (growth factor receptor) regions are deleted (19). When these truncation mutants are expressed in cells they bind to their respective normal counterparts and produce an inactive complex,

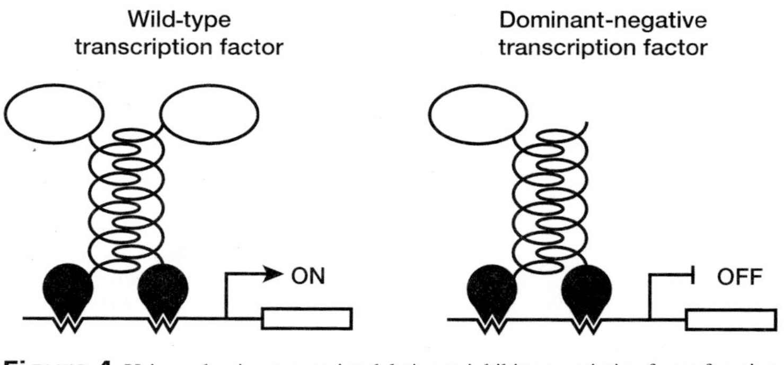

Figure 4 Using a dominant-negative deletion to inhibit transcription factor function. Dominant-negative mutants are based on proteins that contain modular elements mediating different functions and on their property to pair (dimer formation). A dominant-negative mutant protein must contain the dimerization domain (represented by a coil), and may also contain a domain such as the DNA binding element (circles with two protruding triangles) to ensure protein stability. The mutant lacks a critical function, here the transactivation domain of this transcription factor (oval at top of coil). Dimerization of the dominant-negative gene inhibits function of the endogenous transcription factor.

resulting in inhibition of target gene transcription, or signaling via the particular growth factor receptor pathway. Dominant-negative inhibition is usually used in combination with a tissue-specific promoter to achieve diminution or loss of target gene function in specific cell types (Fig. 4) (19). A major caveat of the dominant-negative approach is heterodimerization with multiple members of a gene family. In this case, function of the whole family can be inhibited, rather than one specific targeted molecule (20). Inhibition of an entire gene family prevents testing loss of one discrete molecular target, and the converse investigation of molecular redundancy.

C. BAC, P1, and YAC Transgenic Mice

Gene regulation is complex, and in most instances DNA elements modulating endogenous gene expression can be found long distances either upstream (5′) or downstream (3′) of their endogenous coding sequences. Moreover, some regulatory elements exist in the noncoding introns. Thus a more representative study of gain of function of an endogenous gene, concomitantly preserving regulation of expression similar to that of the endogenous counterpart, is to create transgenic mice with large pieces of genomic DNA encompassing long stretches of 5′, 3′ sequence, and the entire genomic DNA, encompassing all of the exons and introns. For this approach, which can involve DNA segments ranging from 100 kb to 1.5 Mb, plasmid or cosmid vectors (which can contain up to 50 kb) are insufficient. There are, however, "artificial" chromosome vectors, containing centromeres and telomeres, which can be normally segregated to bacterial or yeast progeny that can accommodate DNA segments of this size range. Bacterial artificial chromosomes or P1 phagemid bacterial chromosomes can hold up to 200 kb of insert DNA, whereas yeast artificial chromosomes can accommodate DNA segments up to 2 Mb. Transgenic mice have been created using all three types of vectors (7, 8); subsequent characterization demonstrates normal gene regulation of these large inserts in response to various physiologic perturbations. BACs or P1s are more preferable because their DNA inserts are more "stable" than those of YACs, which are prone to deletions or rearrangements (chimerism). Creation of BAC or YAC transgenic mice has also been used in positional cloning to narrow a candidate locus to a 100- to 500-kb interval (21), which using modern technology can be completely sequenced expeditiously.

D. Tissue-Specific Knockouts

Gene knockout studies are highly informative regarding gene function, but they may be unable to test gene function in a particular tissue or cell type, due to either embryonic lethality or an unexpected effect of deletion of the gene in every tissue of the mouse. The strategy of tissue-specific knockouts enables the investigator to test gene function in selected tissues or cell types. This approach also involves the use of bitransgenic mice to achieve the desired selective gene rearrangement (Fig. 5). One transgenic mouse line expresses a DNA recombinase targeted to the cell type of interest (see below) and the second transgenic mouse contains the target gene to be deleted (Fig. 5).

There are several time-consuming aspects to establishment of mouse systems for tissue-specific knockouts. The most complex is generation of mice carrying the targeted gene. The techniques are the same as for standard gene knockout procedures, except the goal is to "knock in" an altered but still functional allele, replacing the endogenous wild-type gene. The system is based on a DNA recombinase enzyme that activates an intramolecular recombination between two specific 34-bp recognition sequences, with the resulting deletion of the intervening DNA segment (Fig. 5A). There are two DNA recombinases, each with a specific recognition sequence, in current use in mouse genome manipulation—Cre recombinase derived from bacteriophage, or flp recombinase cloned from yeast. Cre recognizes *loxP* sites, whereas flp recombinase binds to *frt* sites. In the past, the Cre system appeared to be more efficient; however, recent manipulations of the flp enzyme (changing the sequence to mammalian nucleotide usage) have been optimized, potentially rendering it as potent as Cre.

Based on the dual requirements of functionality, yet responsiveness to a DNA recombinase, the design of the targeting vector for gene knockin has two outstanding features. First, the segment of gene to be deleted, one or more exons, is flanked by recombinase sites. This procedure has been assigned the name "floxed" (flanked by *loxP*, for targeted gene deletion using the Cre–*lox* system), or "flrted" (pronounced "flirted") when using the flp–*frt* system (22). Second, the NEO cassette for selection of targeted ES clones is inserted into an intron to maintain gene functionality in the absence of recombination. (Fig. 5). Most investigators also flank the NEO cassette either with *frt* sites or with additional *loxP* sites such that after the targeted ES clones are identified, flp or Cre can be transfected into these cells to excise NEO. Excision of NEO is desirable, because the resistance cassette contains "cryptic" splice sites that can produce truncations of the endogenous gene in the absence of tissue-specific recombination, generating a "hypomorphic" gene phenotype (22). In sum, there is considerably more technical maneuvers on the DNA to create a targeting vector for tissue-specific knockouts, along with additional ES cell manipulations to ensure normal gene function in the absence of the DNA recombinase. Thus production of knockin mice takes longer and is less efficient than standard knockout experiments.

The second component of tissue-specific knockouts is generation of transgenic mice with targeted expression of

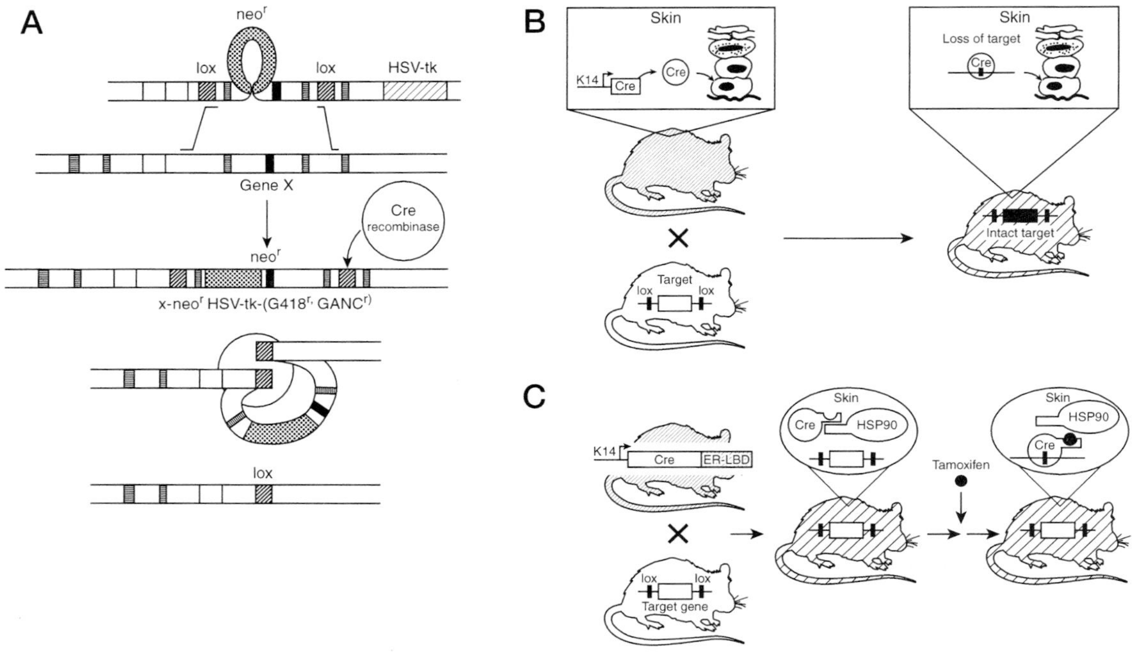

Figure 5 Concepts and strategies used to create tissue-specific knockout mice. In contrast to conventional knockouts, the tissue-specific knockout targeting vector locates the antibiotic resistance element in an intron as well as placing *loxP* DNA recombinase sites (here the Cre–*lox* system is depicted) in introns flanking the exon to be deleted (A). Cre protein catalyzes recombination across the *loxP* sites, leading to excision of the intervening sequence (A). Tissue-specific knockouts are created by breeding (see Fig. 6) the "knockin" mice containing the "floxed" targeted gene with transgenic mice expressing Cre in specific cell types (B). Activation of the Cre transgene at the appropriate time during development leads to cell type-specific gene exon excision. Using inducible transgene expression mediated by fusing Cre to the mutant estrogen receptor ligand binding domain, a tissue-specific gene knockout can be induced at any time in postnatal life by treatment of composite mice with tamoxifen (C). Modified from Ref. (1), J. Arbeit and R. Hirose. Murine mentors: Transgenic and knockout models of surgical disease. *Annals of Surgery* **229**(1), 21–40.

the DNA recombinase (Fig. 5B). Here, standard transgenic technology is used to microinject a transgene with the Cre or flp recombinase linked to a tissue-specific promoter (Table I). The most frequent difficulty in creating the appropriate transgenic line for tissue-specific knockouts is that in many instances the enhancer/promoter used, although tissue specific in adult mice, will "fire" at the one- or two-cell stage of embryonic development, obviating tissue specificity. Therefore, multiple DNA recombinase transgenic mouse lines must be screened to ascertain that (1) recombination takes place at the same time in embryonic development as does the promoter of the endogenous tissue-specific gene, (2) Cre is expressed in the appropriate cell type and tissue, and (3) the percentage recombination is adequate to produce ablation or marked reduction in gene function in the tissue of interest. To screen these recombinase transgenic lines, each is mated with a "reporter" transgenic mouse line containing a β-galactosidase transgene linked to an upstream intron flanked by recombinase sites and a ubiquitous promoter (23). The intron is deleted by the recombinase, juxtaposing the β-galactosidase gene to the promoter. β-Galactosidase encodes for a gene that turns cells deep blue on incubation with the appropriate substrate. The number of blue cells in a tissue compared to unstained cells is indicative of the efficiency of the DNA recombinase. Ultimately, careful screening of DNA recombinase transgenic lines yields one or two lines with a recombinase activity that is activated at the appropriate time in development. Once characterized, DNA recombinase transgenic lines can be maintained and used in all future experiments to knock out sequentially whole gene repertories in selected tissues. In most instances, the efficiency of Cre recombinase ranges from 80 to 100%, when recombination is activated during development (see Section III,E). This degree of loss of gene function is usually sufficient to elicit a phenotype, particularly in carcinogenesis experiments whereby cells with loss of function are further selected for expansion during neoplastic progression.

The final point regarding tissue-specific knockouts is that the breeding scheme to generate these mice is complex. Thus both the tissue-specific recombinase and the targeted allele must be brought together in the same cell by breeding (Fig. 6). Moreover, because the mammalian genome is diploid, both copies of the floxed or flrted alleles must be in the same cell as the DNA recombinase. Alternatively, a standard knockout is generated and, if homozygous lethal, is maintained as a heterozygote. Via three rounds of subse-

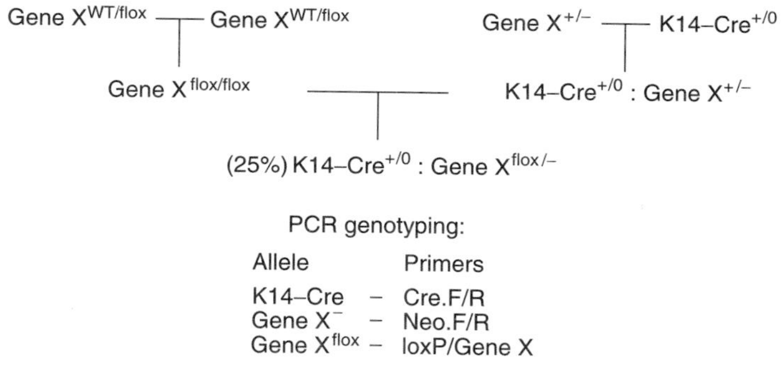

Figure 6 Breeding plan for generating tissue-specific knockout mice. To create tissue-specific knockouts, three genes must be brought together in the same mouse (see Fig. 5). First, heterozygous conventional knockouts are placed together with transgenic mice with targeted Cre expression (right top). These composite mice are bred with a "knockin" mouse homozygous for both "floxed" targeted genes. A quarter of the progeny can be expected to have tissue-specific gene deletion.

quent breeding the standard knockout, floxed allele, and the DNA recombinase, are brought together in the same cell type. This approach prevents potential intermolecular recombination across the paternal and maternal DNA strands containing the recombinase recognition sequences, generating a large DNA rearrangement rather than gene excision.

Ultimately, despite the time, expense, and technical hurdles, tissue-specific gene knockouts greatly increase the precision of genetic manipulations in the mouse, and in many instances are the only way to study loss of gene function in specific tissues in the face of early embryonic lethality.

E. Inducible Tissue-Specific Knockouts

In some instances deletion of gene function, even in a tissue-specific fashion, is either lethal or leads to a severe phenotype incompatible with reaching adulthood. In other instances, the investigator may specifically want to determine the effect of loss of gene function in adult tissues of the mouse, or at precise stages in a disease model. The technique of inducible tissue-specific knockouts fulfills this goal (Fig. 5C).

Inducible tissue-specific knockouts can be achieved by a combination of techniques for tissue-specific knockouts, and by inducible gene expression. Knockin techniques of the floxed or flrted targeting vector are the same as outlined in the previous section. The transgene used for tissue-specific DNA recombinase expression is different. Here, the recombinase cDNA is fused to a mutant estrogen receptor hormone-binding domain. Because the DNA recombinase is a nuclear enzyme, and in the presence of tamoxifen, it is released from cytoplasmic HSP90, translocating to the nucleus and producing DNA recombination across recombinase sites. Transgenic mouse lines containing the hormone-inducible tissue-specific recombinase are generated and screened for using β-galactosidase reporter mice. After determination of the transgenic line with the highest recombination frequency and tamoxifen induction, this transgenic line can also be used in all future experiments. The breeding schemes for these experiments are the same as for "standard" tissue-specific knockouts, and the targeted allele is placed over gene deficiency, as described in the previous section. The major difference in this type of experiment, compared to "standard" inducible transgene expression, is that induction of DNA recombinase need only be transitory to achieve permanent gene ablation in the targeted cell. In most instances bitransgenic mice containing the targeted allele and the inducible recombinase need only one systemic dose of tamoxifen in order to achieve DNA recombination and deletion of the targeted allele. More doses only enhance toxicity without achieving more efficient gene deletion. Topical tamoxifen application is also an option in studies of gene deletion in accessible epithelial tissues such as the skin, mouth, tongue, and anorectum. The overall efficiency of inducible gene knockouts in adult tissues appears to be less than that achieved during early development, and may range from 40 to 60%. However, this efficiency is more than adequate when there is selection for loss of gene function as in carcinogenesis.

IV. Pitfalls in Transgenic and Knockout Experiments

The problems and roadblocks encountered during transgenic and knockout experiments have been alluded to in the preceding discussions. A specific list is presented in Table II. Fortunately, due to the development of the advanced techniques of genome manipulation, also presented above, most of these roadblocks can be circumvented. Each of these problems and solutions is briefly discussed in the following sections.

Table II Problems and Pitfalls in Transgenic and Knockout Experiments

Transgenic and Knockouts	
	Embryonic lethality
	Death before reproduction
	Sterile transgenic founder or chimera
	No germline transmission, persistent mosaicism
	Death before phenotype
	No phenotype despite transgene expression or homozygous gene knockout
Transgenic	
	No transgene expression
Knockout	
	Aberrant splicing, creating truncated but functional partial knockout protein
	Unable to produce heterozygous mice due to haploinsufficiency (death with only one gene copy)
	Limited selection of genetic background for embryonic stem cells

A. Failure of Transmission of the Genetic Manipulation

Establishment of permanent lines of transgenic or knockout mice is a major achievement, because each member of the lineage will have the same phenotype for as long as the line is maintained. There are several roadblocks to attaining permanent lines of genetically manipulated mice. Embryonic lethality can occur following either transgenic or knockout technology. As discussed above, embryonic lethality may reveal a novel role for a gene in development. A particularly vexing problem occurs when gene deletion is embryonic lethal even when heterozygous; this is termed the "gene dosage" effect, or haploinsufficiency. Genetically manipulated mice may be born, but die either as neonates or prior to sexual maturation. In transgenic technology neonatal death occurs as a result of a phenotype produced by gain of function that is too severe to be compatible with survival. Frequently mothers will cannibalize pups they perceive as abnormal. Genetically manipulated mice may also be sterile, either as a result of random insertional mutagenesis caused by the transgene, or because of a specific gene knockout such as deletion of the estrogen receptor-α. Sterility induced by homozygous gene deletion can be obviated by carrying the knockout allele as a heterozygote and relying on continual breeding to generate homozygotes. Both founder transgenic and chimeric knockout mice may never pass the altered allele through the germline. In both instances the mice have a low level of chimerism in the germline, although both transgenic founder and chimeric mice should produce approximately 50–100 pups before accepting this diagnosis.

B. Transmission without a Phenotype

In transgenic technology, founder mice may pass the transgene to offspring, establishing a permanent line, yet the transgene is never expressed. One explanation for this result is transgene integration into heterochromatin, a silent region of the genome. Alternatively, the phenotype mediated by the transgene is so severe that negative *in utero* selection produces pups lacking transgene expression. Most frequently, lack of a knockout phenotype is due to genetic redundancy, with multiple members of a family of homologous but separate genes, each located on different chromosomes.

C. Problem Solving

Using combinations of experimental iteration, combinatorial genetic manipulations, advanced techniques, or biological provocation, most of these roadblocks can be bypassed. In transgenic mice, embryonic or neonatal lethality can be solved either by switching gene promoters to specifically target transgene expression or by changing the cell type wherein expression is activated, or by inducible systems that leave the transgene "off" during development and turn it "on" after sexual maturation. Similarly, embryonic lethality in knockout studies can be addressed by tissue-specific or inducible tissue-specific knockouts. This approach may also work for the rare cases of haploinsufficiency. If the transgene is not passed to subsequent generations, then one or two more rounds of embryo microinjection, with more stringent efforts at cleaning and purifying the transgene DNA, are warranted. The approach to lack of a phenotype in either transgenic or knockout mice can be tackled by several approaches. In some cases one can anticipate latency of the initial genetic modification, such that an informative phenotype is evident only when either a second genetic lesion is added or, a biological perturbation is applied, such as wounding, graft transplantation, infectious challenge, or exposure to carcinogens. Lack of a knockout phenotype due to genetic redundancy can be approached by knocking out another family member and crossing the two different knockout mice. Here the double-knockout mice may have a phenotype such that each single-knockout mouse appears normal.

V. Stepwise Analysis of Genotype, Gene Expression, and Phenotypes in Transgenic and Knockout Mice

Methods of analysis of transgenic and knockout mice share many similarities. The major difference is that knockout mice frequently display development phenotypes that also illuminate gene function, and must be carefully analyzed and characterized.

For transgenic mice the initial analysis starts with the birth of the first litter subsequent to oviduct transfer into pseudopregnant females. This litter will contain "founder" transgenic mice. Founder transgenic mice are special because each mouse represents a unique transgene insertion site. Transgene expression and hence phenotype elaboration can be strikingly influenced by insertion site. To be certain that a phenotype is due to transgene expression rather than to a cryptic effect of transgene insertion into a particular chromosomal locus, at least two transgenic lines must display the same phenotype in order to establish the validity of the findings. At best, 25–30% of an entire injection series of 150–250 embryos, implanted into 4–6 pseudopregnant females and yielding 30–100 pups, will contain founder transgenic mice. Usually the number is more in the range of 15–20%. Founder transgenic mice are identified by analysis for the presence of the transgene in genomic DNA isolated from clipping a 1-cm piece of tail at the time of weaning of the mice, at 3 weeks of age. At that time each mouse is assigned a number that is either clipped from the ear or tattooed on the proximal tail. The genomic DNA isolated from the tail clipping is first screened by the polymerase chain reaction using primers specific for the transgene and generating a fragment of specified length (usually 250–500 bp for best PCR efficiency) on ethidium-stained gels. A positive band indicates a transgenic founder. In many instances it is desirable to confirm the PCR results with a hybridization procedure, also specific for the transgene sequence. Either DNA dot–blot or Southern hybridization following restriction digestion of the DNA will provide PCR confirmation, and will also indicate the relative copy number of the transgene and document independent transgene insertion sites for each individual founder. For knockout mice, chimeras are easily identified without the need for PCR, based on coat color. The 129sv ES cells used in these experiments come from albino white mice; they are implanted into C57BL/6 blastocyst cavities, and mice of this strain have black coat colors. Thus the extent of chimerism may be estimated by the extent of white patches in the fur of mice born after uterine transfer. This estimate usually, but not always, reflects percentage of germline chimerism. Similar to transgenic experiments, knockout mice from two independent ES cell clones should be initially characterized to determine that the phenotype is independent of changes within a single ES cell clone.

After establishing the presence of founder transgenic mice and identification of chimeric knockout mice, the next goal of breeding founders is to establish permanent heterozygous transgenic and knockout mouse lines. Unlike founder mice, all of the subsequent transgenic mice derived from an individual founder have the same transgene insertion site and essentially the same phenotype. Approximately 5–10% of transgenic founders are either sterile or do not pass the transgene in the germline due to transgene integration after the first embryonic division, resulting in germline chimerism. A major goal in knockout technology is to determine if the knockout allele has "gone germline." Heterozygous knockout allele germline passage is a major event toward establishment of a complete gene knockout. Identification of heterozygous knockout mice is also determined by either PCR using primers specific for the NEO cassette used to disrupt the gene, or Southern blotting of restriction-digested DNA to detect a restriction fragment polymorphism between the targeted and genomic allele (Fig. 1). The next step is to cross the heterozygous knockout mice to attempt to generate homozygous knockout mice.

Following establishment of permanent transgenic lines and potentially homozygous knockout mice, the next step is determination of the extent and level of transgene expression and the degree of loss of gene function in the knockout mice. For transgenic mice, the form of this analysis depends on the strategy employed for transgene expression. Experiments using ubiquitous promoters are more challenging because the extent and level of transgene expression must be determined for a range of tissues and organs of the mouse. In contrast, for targeted transgene expression, the specific tissues in question and a limited number of control tissues wherein expression is not anticipated are sampled and analyzed. Acquisition and handling of the tissues are different, depending on the type of analysis and tissue location. For internal organs, the mouse must be sacrificed, but the form of sacrifice depends on the planned molecular analysis of the tissues. For histopathology, mRNA *in situ* hybridization, and immunohistochemistry, we prefer intracardiac perfusion with iced saline and 3.75% paraformaldehyde, which both flushes blood from the capillaries and provides near instant fixation, leading to optimal mRNA preservation. The tissues can then either be frozen in embedding matrix for frozen sectioning, or processed for paraffin embedding. The former is used for immunohistochemistry of protein epitopes destroyed by paraffin embedding, whereas paraffin provides optimal tissue architecture, can be used for most immunohistochemical assays, and is excellent for mRNA *in situ* hybridization. Transgene expression or lack of expression in knockout mice can be determined at the level of protein by either immunohistochemistry (see above) or Western blotting of tissue extracts. Western blotting demonstrates a discrete band on a gel running at a specific relative molecular weight and with immunoaffinity for the detecting antibody. It is also semiquantitative because the amount of total protein loaded in each lane is controlled. Moreover, relative levels of protein expression can be inferred by comparisons of tissue extracts with stable transfected cell lines expressing known quantities of the gene in question. Moreover, in some instances, available antibodies may recognize epitopes only in Western blots, but not in tissues, therefore protein extracts are the only way to document and estimate the level of transgene protein expression. In the absence of available antibodies, transgene mRNA can be determined in tissues. RNA can be analyzed using reverse transcription polymerase chain reaction (RT-PCR), RNase protection, or Northern blotting. Both RT-PCR and RNase protection have the advantage that they do not require full-length mRNA, but can detect expression in the face of partial degradation, which is important because mRNA is extremely labile due to endogenous tissue RNases, and some tissues, such as pancreas, are loaded with this enzyme. RNase protection is quantitative whereas RT-PCR is only semiquantitative. In contrast, RT-PCR is easy to perform and does not require radioactivity. Thus, RT-PCR is particularly useful for screening a panel of tissues for transgene expression. The information gleaned from Northern blotting is similar to that of the Western blot. It is quantitative and generates a band containing a specific number of base pairs, confirming the identity of the transgene mRNA. The power of both mRNA *in situ* hybridization and immunohistochemistry is that transgene expression, or lack of expression in knockout mice, can be localized to specific cell types in selected tissues. A rough estimate of changes in expression level can be gleaned from a visual grading of the silver grain density for *in situ* hybridization (we and others find the [^{35}S]UTP method most sensitive compared to nonradioactive detection methods) or the intensity of chromogen development in immunohistochemistry.

The same analytical techniques are also applicable to knockout mice. In general, the "standard" gene knockout studies, wherein the gene is deleted from every tissue in the body, present two challenges: the possibility of an embryonic lethal developmental abnormality must be anticipated, and each organ and tissue of adult homozygous knockout mice should be sampled for unanticipated phenotypes. An embryonic lethal phenotype is first suspected by analysis of the frequency of homozygous knockout mice generated from an intercross of heterozygous mice. Frequencies of knockout mice significantly lower than 25% indicate embryonic lethality. The precise characterization of the embryonic lethal phenotype can yield important insight into the function of the gene in development, and may provide hints at its role in the adult animal. To determine the developmental stage of the embryonic phenotype, timed matings between heterozygous knockout mice are set up. The morning after copulation there is a "plug" of coagulated ejaculate at the orifice or within the vagina. "Plugged" females are considered to be 0.5-day postcoitus (pc). "Plugged" females can then be serially sacrificed on each pc day to determine the embryonic phenotype. For pc days 1–8 the uterus is embedded and the embryos are visualized by serial section, whereas the embryos can be individually identified and removed from later stages and embedded separate from the uterus.

There are two additional concepts regarding elucidation and characterization of phenotypes in transgenic and knockout mice. First, there are additional analyses appropriate for some types of genetic manipulation compared to others. Examples include lymphocyte subpopulation analysis by fluoresence-activated cell sorting, transplantation of various types of grafts, or challenges with infectious agents in genetic manipulations involving the immune system, or cardiac function tests in mice in which gene expression has been manipulated in the heart (1). Second, some phenotypes may not be evident in unchallenged mice, but require some provocation to be apparent. Examples include uncovering latent atherogenesis by "Western" diets in mice in which genes affecting lipoprotein analysis have been perturbed, and wound-healing experiments in mice with altered clotting factors, adhesion or extracellular matrix molecules, or proteinases. Moreover, some mice with genetic alterations that modulate tumorigenesis must be investigated by additional perturbations, such as chemical or radiation carcinogenesis (24, 25). Finally, phenotypes may not emerge in young adult mice but may require prolonged periods of aging or even repetitive backcrossing (26) to become evident. Most investigators will age a small cohort of genetically manipulated mice for up to 1.5–2 years.

VI. Modification of Phenotype by Genetic Differences in Inbred Strains

An emerging principle in genetic manipulation of the mouse is modulation of phenotype by different inbred mouse strains. The degree of modulation can range from embryonic lethality in one strain to its absence in another. Slightly less subtle effects have been identified in tumorigenesis experiments in both transgenic and knockout mice wherein selected strains or even just one mouse strain will be permissive for carcinogenesis, but other strains are totally resistant or at best develop intermediate neoplastic lesions that fail to convert to malignancy. Changes in transgene or knockout gene phenotype induced by inbred strains are caused by one or usually several "modifier" genes. These genes can be of diverse function, ranging from members of the same molecular pathway as the transgene or knockout, to genes controlling metabolism or gene expression of ancillary genes that ultimately feedback to the original genetic lesion created by the investigator. In cancer research, these modifier genes are the subject of intense investigation because they may lead to identification of human homologs controlling resistance or susceptibility to malignancy. Excellent reviews and texts have described the generation and genetic marker analysis of interspecific backcross mice that are required to identify chromosomal loci potentially containing modifier genes (27, 28).

VII. Combinatorial Genetic Manipulations in Mice

There are several instances wherein creation of genetically manipulated mice with more than one genetic alteration is desirable. There are two contexts wherein this approach is particularly appropriate. In some biological systems there are either redundant genetic controls encompassing at least two regulatory genes or a family of related but distinct genes. This redundancy can lead to the absence of a phenotype when only a family member is knocked out due to compensatory un-regulation of other members. Straightforward examples are the *myc* family, composed of c-, L-, and N-*myc*, and the retinoic acid or retinoid receptors, which contain six family members each. An extreme example is the *Hox* gene clusters, for which there are 13 family members for each of four families! Second, one genetic network or signaling pathway may not mediate an entire phenotypic response, but instead may require the combinatorial contribution of a cascade of molecular networks. Here an example is transplant graft rejection, and this system has been approached by interbreeding mice lacking both MHC class I and MHC class II responses. Third, some biological processes are characterized by an accumulation of genetic lesions acquired by individual somatic stem or proliferative cells. The paramount example is multistage carcinogenesis. Here, multiple genetic lesions can be emulated by bringing at least two if not three distinct genetic changes together in the same cell by a combination of multiple transgenes coupled with standard or tissue-specific knockouts. Finally, some biological processes such as wound healing involve temporal and transitory changes in gene expression during distinct acute, intermediate, reepithelialization, and dermal remodeling stages. Here inducible gene expression systems, possibly involving two different pharmacologic inducers alone or in combination with tissue-specific knockouts, can be combined in intercross mice to investigate perturbation of sequential activation and inactivation of genetic networks.

A. Creation of Double Transgenic Mice by Mating

The simplest example is the generation of mice containing two different transgenes by interbreeding two independent transgenic lines. Approximately 25% of the offspring will contain both transgenes. One potential impediment to this approach is if each individual transgene elicits a moderate or severe phenotype in the tissue of interest. Neonatal double-transgenic mice may not be viable, or may not appear in litters at all due to embryonic lethality. A second disadvantage to this simplistic approach occurs if three genes, two transgenes, and a knockout gene are targeted for manipulation in the same cell type. Using this approach would require segregation of three different genes and a very low percentage of desired composite mice from a large number of repetitive breedings.

B. Creation of Double Transgenic Mice by Transgene Coinjection

One way to circumvent the problem of segregating three genes is to coinject two different transgenes as a 1:1 mixture directly into one-cell embryos. Most often both transgenes integrate as a multicopy head-to-tail linked array (concatenate). In subsequent breeding, the two cointegrated transgenes segregate together, as a single genetic trait.

C. Single Composite Transgenic/Knockout Mice

To place a transgene together with a knockout gene is straightforward, but somewhat time consuming, depending on whether the knockout is sterile or lethal as a homozygote. If the homozygous knockout is viable and fertile, it is more expeditious to first generate transgenic mice that are also homozygous for the knockout allele and repeatedly backcross the composite mice with homozygous knockout mice. In this case, once homozygosity for the knockout gene is established, only the transgene needs to be screened for. Cases in which homozygous knockout mice are sterile require that both the composite transgenic/knockout and the index knockout lines are heterozygous for the deleted gene. Here the desired transgene over homozygous knockout mice must be generated from each individual cross, and at best 12.5% of pups will possess the desired genotype.

D. Composite Double-Transgenic/Knockout Mice

The best approach to place two transgenes together with a gene knockout is to first generate double-transgenic mice by coinjection, and then segregate the "single" double-transgenic locus over the knockout gene by breeding. The yield in this cross can range from 25 to 50% if composite transgene/homozygous knockout mice can first be created and serially backcrossed to single homozygous knockout mice.

VIII. Conclusions

Transgenic and knockout mouse models are powerful experimental tools at several levels. They can decipher the biology of individual molecules or test upstream and downstream members of a pathway in the context of intact tissues and organs. Although there are potential roadblocks using genetically manipulated mice, these obstacles can usually be overcome with additional genetic manipulations to more precisely control location, timing, or level of gene function. They can also test the response of a biological perturbation, either a normal process or a disease, subsequent to gain or loss of a specific molecule or a molecular pathway. Transgenic or knockout mouse models of disease can also be created, and then used to first screen for differential expression of candidate genes at specific stages of pathological progression. Promising candidates can then be introduced by creating new genetically manipulated mice, wherein expression of the candidate is perturbed, breeding these new mice into the original disease model. Ultimately, increased understanding of the function of molecules within tissues will lead to identification and development of targeted drugs selective for a particular aspect of molecular function.

Acknowledgment

The author thanks Terry Schoop for rendering Figs. 1–6.

References

1. Arbeit, J., and Hirose, R. (1999). Murine mentors: Transgenic and knockout models of surgical disease. *Ann. Surg.* **229**(1), 21–40.
2. Arbeit, J., Münger, K., Howley, P., and Hanahan, D. (1994). Progressive squamous epithelial neoplasia in K14-human papillomavirus type 16 transgenic mice. *J. Virol.* **68,** 4358–4368.
3. Arbeit, J., Howley, P., and Hanahan, D. (1996). Chronic estrogen induced cervical and vaginal squamous carcinogenesis in HPV16 transgenic mice. *Proc. Natl. Acad. Sci. U.S.A.* **93,** 2930–2935.
4. Arbeit, J., Riley, R., Huey, B., Porter, B., Kelloff, G., Lubet, R., Ward, J., and Pinkel, D. (1999). DFMO chemoprevention of epidermal carcinogenesis in K14-HPV16 transgenic mice. *Cancer Res.* **59,** 3610–3620.
5. Hasty, P., and Bradley, A. (1993). Gene targeting vectors for mammalian cells. *In* "Gene Targeting: A Practical Approach" (A. Joyner, ed.), pp. 1–31. Oxford University Press, New York.
6. Hogan, B., Beddington, R., Costantini, F., and Lacy, E., eds. (1994). "Manipulating the Mouse Embryo," 2nd Ed. pp. 217–257. Cold Spring Harbor Press, Cold Spring Harbor, New York.
7. Lamb, B., and Gearhart, J. (1995). YAC transgenics and the study of genetics and human disease. *Curr. Biol.* **5,** 342–348.
8. Nielsen, L., McCormick, S., Pierotti, V., Tam, C., Gunn, M., Shizuya, H., and Young, S. (1997). Human apolipoprotein B transgenic mice generated with 207- and 145-kilobase pair bacterial artificial chromosomes. Evidence that a distant 5′-element confers appropriate transgene expression in the intestine. *J. Biol. Chem.* **272**(47), 29752–29758.
9. Arbeit, J. (1996). Transgenic models of epidermal neoplasia and multistage carcinogenesis. *Cancer Surv.* **26,** 7–34.
10. Wurst, W., and Joyner, A. (1993). Production of targeted embryonic stem cell clones. *In* "Gene Targeting: A Practical Approach" (A. Joyner, ed.), pp. 33–61. Oxford University Press, New York.
11. Papaioannou, V., and Johnson, R. (1993). Production of chimeras and genetically defined offspring from targeted ES cells. *In* "Gene Targeting: A Practical Approach" (A. Joyner, ed.), pp. 107–146. Oxford University Press, New York.
12. Baron, U., Gossen, M., and Bujard, H. (1997). Tetracycline-controlled transcription in eukaryotes: Novel transactivators with graded transactivation potential. *Nucleic Acids Res.* **25,** 2723–2729.
13. Furth, P. A., St. Onge, L., Boger, H., Gruss, P., Gossen, M., Kistner, A., Bujard, H., and Hennighausen, L. (1994). Temporal control of gene expression in transgenic mice by a tetracycline-responsive promoter. *Proc. Natl. Acad. Sci. U.S.A.* **92,** 9302–9306.
14. Gossen, M., Freundlieb, S., Bender, G., Muller, G., Hillen, W., and Bujard, H. (1995). Transcriptional activation by tetracyclines in mammalian cells. *Science* **268,** 1766–1768.
15. No, D., Yao, T., and Evans, R. (1996). Ecdysone-inducible gene expression in mammalian cells and transgenic mice. *Proc. Natl. Acad. Sci. U.S.A.* **93,** 3346–3351.
16. Pelengaris, S., Littlewood, T., Khan, M., Elia, G., and Evan, G. (1999). Reversible activation of c-Myc in skin: Induction of a complex neoplastic phenotype by a single oncogenic lesion. *Mol. Cell* **3**(5), 565–577.
17. Herskowitz, I. (1987). Functional inactivation of genes by dominant-negative mutations. *Nature (London)* **329**(6136), 219–222.
18. Arbeit, J. (1990). Molecules, cancer, and the surgeon. *Ann. Surg.* **212**(1), 3–13.
19. Werner, S., Weinberg, W., Liao, X., Peters, K. G., Bledding, M., Yuspa, S. H., Weiner, R. L., and Williams, L. T. (1993). Targeted expression of a dominant-negative FGF receptor mutant in the epidermis of transgenic mice reveals a role of FGF in keratinocyte organization and differentiation. *EMBO J.* **12,** 2635–2643.
20. Werner, S., Smola, H., Liao, X., Longaker, M., Krieg, T., Hofschneider, P., and Williams, L. (1994). The function of KGF in morphogenesis of epithelium and reepithelialization of wounds. *Science* **266**(5186), 819–822.
21. Antoch, M. P., Song, E. J., Vitaerna, M. H., Zhao, Y., Wilsbacher, L. D., Sangoram, A. M., King, D. P., Pinto, L. H., and Takahashi, J. S. (1997). Functional identification of the mouse circadian Clock gene by transgenic BAC rescue. *Cell* **89**(4), 655–667.
22. Meyers, E., Lewandoski, M., and Martin, G. (1998). An Fgf8 mutant allelic series generated by Cre- and Flp-mediated recombination. *Nature Genet.* **18**(2), 136–141.
23. Akagi, K., Sandig, V., Voorijs, M., Van der Valk, M., Giovanni, M., Strauss, M., and Berns, A. (1997). Cre-mediated somatic site-specific recombination in mice. *Nucleic Acids Res.* **25**(9), 1766–1773.
24. Kemp, C., Donehower, L., Bradley, A., and Balmain, A. (1993). Reduction of p53 gene dosage does not increase initiation or promotion but enhances malignant progression of chemically induced skin tumors. *Cell* **74,** 813–822.

25. Saez, E, Rutbert, S., Mueller, E., Oppenheim, H., Smoluk, J., Yuspa, S. H., and Spiegelman, B. M. (1995). c-fos is required for malignant progression of skin tumors. *Cell* **82,** 721–732.
26. Rudolph, K. L., Chang, S., Lee, H. W., Blasco, M., Gottlieb, G. J., Greider, C., and DePinho, R. A. (1999). Longevity, stress response, and cancer in aging telomerase-deficient mice. *Cell* **86**(5), 701–712.
27. Kemp, C., Fee, F., and Balmain, A. (1993). Allelotype analysis of mouse skin tumors using polymorphic microsatellites: Sequential genetic alterations on chromosomes 6, 7 and 11. *Cancer Res.* **53,** 6022–6027.
28. Silver, L. (1995). "Mouse Genetics: Concepts and Applications," pp. 44–52. Oxford University Press, New York.

18

Tissue Culture, Cell Growth, and Analysis

Andrea L. Nestor, James Willey, and David C. Allison

Departments of Surgery, Medicine, and Physiology and Molecular Medicine, Medical College of Ohio, Toledo, Ohio 43614

I. Introduction and Environment

Tissue culture is one of the most important research tools in cell biology. Nontransformed mammalian cells can be cultured for ~35 generations, or to the "Hayflick limit," before generalized senescence and cell death set in because of telomeric shortening. However, about 1 in 10^6 cells in such senescent cultures will spontaneously "transform" and become immortal. There seems to be no limit to the number of divisions possible for such spontaneously transformed lines, or for cell lines initially derived from malignant cells. Indeed, HeLa cells, derived from a human cervical cancer, have been in continuous passage for more than 50 years.

It is necessary to have the proper laboratory environment and equipment to perform tissue culture successfully. Ideally, the tissue culture area should be physically isolated from the general traffic flow of the laboratory. All precautions (see below) must be employed continuously to avoid contamination of the dedicated tissue culture work area, which should have at least three air changes per hour and contain the following equipment: a tissue culture incubator; laminar flow high-efficiency particulate air (HEPA)-filtered hood; centrifuge; inverted phase microscope; and a hemocytometer/light microscope and/or a Coulter counter for cell counting. Also, a refrigerator, autoclave, standard freezer (−4°C), ultralow freezer (−80°C), and a liquid nitrogen storage system (−130°C) for the long-term preservation of frozen cell lines should be available (1).

II. Sterilizing Techniques

Tissue culture supplies and work areas must be sterile. This is difficult when many people are working in the laboratory. Access to the area of the facility dedicated to tissue culture should be limited to those people who are actually culturing cells. Solutions or subcultures of cell lines should not be shared among different users. Sterile techniques necessary for cell culture include autoclaving and glassware cleaning, UV irradiation and HEPA filtration of gases, chemical disinfection of work surfaces, and the filtration of media.

Solutions that are not inactivated by heat, as well as most glassware, can be sterilized by autoclaving. Autoclaves remove the ambient atmosphere and replace it with superheated steam. They are equipped with preset cycles for air removal, sterilization, and drying (2). The particular cycle employed depends on whether the load to be sterilized is plastic, glass, liquid, or biologic waste. Autoclaving cannot be used for liquids requiring exact solute concentrations. Items placed in an autoclave are identified with indicator tape to ensure that sterilization has actually occurred. Pipettes, micropipette tips, and other small items are placed into glass containers and covered with aluminum foil for autoclaving. Single plastic items should be tested to see whether they can withstand autoclaving before batch processing is performed. Some bottle caps contain seals and plugs that melt, or are sucked into the bottle, during autoclaving. Thus, a test run with one type of each capped item should be made to determine whether the caps can simply be loosened, or whether cap removal and covering with aluminum foil are necessary for autoclaving. The autoclave should be checked periodically to ensure that it is generating the proper sterilization temperatures and pressures.

UV lights kill microbial organisms by causing DNA strand breaks and are often used in biologic safety cabinets (BSCs). UV light can also be used to sterilize surfaces that cannot withstand autoclaving. The sterilization power of a given UV bulb is dependent on its number of burn hours. UV bulbs should be changed routinely after the hours of use recommended in the manufacturer's specifications. Direct exposure to UV light is harmful to the eyes and skin, and the UV lights should turn off automatically when the BSC is in use or when people are in the tissue culture facility.

Solutions available for chemical disinfection include 70% ethanol, hypochlorite (bleach), and phenol. Ethanol is used most commonly because it is not toxic. Concentrations of ethanol higher than 80% are not as effective as 70% because of spore encapsulation. Ethanol can be used on the hands (directly or gloved), the insides of BSCs and incubators, and the outsides of containers and other objects used for cell culture. Ethanol is usually stored in a "gardening" bottle for spraying of surfaces, which are thoroughly saturated and then allowed to air dry. Ethanol vapors are very flammable and must be evaporated completely before a flame can be used. Hypochlorite (bleach) is normally used for wiping down of surfaces of laboratory bench tops and for cleaning of glassware, with exposures of at least 30 min to overnight needed to be effective. Most solutions of hypochlorite are ~2500 ppm and are stable for about 24 hr (13). Bleach is inexpensive and less toxic than phenol or formaldehyde, but does leave a residue that should be washed off after disinfection. Bleach is also corrosive and should not be used on metal surfaces. Phenol is occasionally used for disinfection of surfaces and incubators, but is corrosive and toxic and contains carcinogenic benzene rings. Also, phenol does not neutralize the endospores of many organisms.

Filters of cellulose nitrate, cellulose acetate, or nylon are used for sterilizing media. Single-use filters are available through a number of manufacturers (Millipore, Gelman, Schleicher & Schuell, etc.) and are ideal for use in small laboratories. Polyethersulfone or polyvinylidene fluoride filters have relatively low protein binding and fast filtration rates. A filter pore size of 0.2 μm is generally used for removing bacteria and fungi, although 0.1-μm filters remove these microorganisms as well as the smaller mycoplasma. One must make sure that the specific filter employed is capable of handling the amount of liquid to be filtered. Most manufacturers' catalogs (e.g., Fisher Scientific, Inc. catalog) will list the filtration capabilities for each unit. Filters are available as complete units containing both the filter and sterile bottle, or as single-use bottle-top filters. For smaller units, 50-ml filter tops for conical tubes and aerodiscs for syringes are available.

III. Handling of Media and Cells

Ideally, one should use 18 MΩ filtered "ultrapure" water to produce tissue culture media if one is going to make media from commercially obtained powder mixtures and other ingredients. The still employed, or another type of apparatus used to produce pure water, should be dedicated to the tissue culture laboratory and kept meticulously clean and free of residue. The distilled water and other media ingredients should be brought together under a sterile, laminar-flow, HEPA-filtered hood. Alternatively, one can directly buy sterile balanced salt solutions (BSSs) or other partially reconstituted liquid media from tissue culture supply companies (e.g., Gibco, Hyclone, Atlanta Biologicals, Mediatech). Regardless of the source of media ingredients, fastidious attention must be paid to the use of sterile technique to avoid contamination. Autoclaved glass pipettes with filter plugs, or disposable plastic pipettes, are used for transfer of liquids. It is advisable to "flame" all glassware appropriately, even under the hood. After the constituents of a medium are combined (usually in 1-liter volumes) the medium is filtered and aliquoted into 10 100-ml bottles, which are kept frozen until use. The medium in one of these 100-ml bottles should be thawed out and placed in a tissue culture flask in a 37°C, 5% CO_2 incubator for 1 week as a check for contamination. Bacteria and fungi can be seen with a ×32 phase lens, and contamination also leads to cloudiness and acidification of the test medium. If this test bottle is free of contaminates, the remaining bottles of medium can be used for culture experiments.

Cell lines from known repositories are often supplied with a list giving the optimal media constituents for their growth (see Section IX,A). However, for new cells or for incompletely described culture lines, it may be necessary experimentally to find the optimal nutrients required for successful growth. This is tedious work, but there are excellent literature sources giving specific methods (4). A "final medium" is a combination of amino acids, inorganic salts, serum, vitamins, growth factors, hormones, buffers, and a pH indicator that allows the growth of a particular cell type. Antibiotics may also be added to minimize contamination. Once a satisfactory medium is found for a given cell type, the cells are placed at a temperature with oxygen and carbon dioxide concentrations that support growth. Usually, 37°C with O_2 and CO_2 concentrations of 95 and 5%, respectively, are employed.

Media of a number of different compositions can be purchased in powder or liquid form; some of these include minimum essential medium (MEM), Dulbecco's minimum essential medium (DMEM), RPMI 1640, Media 199, and Ham's F-12 (5–9). A convenient resource for looking up the composition of formulated media is the "Gibco BRL Products & Reference Guide" (Life Technologies, Rockville, MD). All media contain BSS, buffers, a pH indicator, nutrients, and growth factors. BSS and buffers are needed to maintain the correct pH and osmolality and consist of varying mixtures of inorganic ions (Na^+, K^+, Mg^{2+}, Cl^-, SO_4^{2-}, Ca^{2+}, PO_4^{3-}, and HCO_3^-): Dulbecco's phosphate-buffered saline (PBS), Hanks' BSS, Eagle's spinner salt solution, and Earle's BSS are commonly used. BSSs lack serum supplements that provide essential growth factors and other hormonal ingredients needed for cell growth (4, 10).

Phosphate and hydroxyethyl piperazineethane sulfonic acid (HEPES) buffers are not sensitive to the CO_2 concentration of the ambient atmosphere. However, for media or BSS buffered with sodium bicarbonate, exposure to ambient atmospheres of <5% CO_2 will allow CO_2 to "blow off," leading to the rapid development of a "basic" medium or BSS, with a pH of 8 or higher. High pH is indicated by a purple color of the phenol indicator dye and is very detrimental to cell survival. Acidic pH changes of the media occur with cell culture growth because of the metabolism of glucose into lactic acid. Acidity causes the phenol red indicators to assume a yellowish color. However, within limits, cells seem to tolerate acidic media reasonably well. The optimal pH for cell growth (7.2–7.5) turns the phenol red indicator a pink/red color. The pH indicator system of a medium can be rigorously standardized by the method of Freshney (2).

Nutrients must be added to the BSS to allow cell growth. These include the essential (cysteine and tyrosine) and nonessential amino acids. Sugars, usually glucose, are also added to the nutrient mixture as an energy source, as is the amino acid L-glutamine. L-Glutamine must be used immediately after thawing because it deteriorates rapidly. Fresh serum is usually added to the culture medium and contains adhesion factors, insulin, hydrocortisone, and triiodothyronine; it also may contain epidermal, fibroblast, and platelet-derived growth factors (EGF, FGF, and PDGF), as well as other factors needed for cell growth. Aliquots of calf, fetal bovine, or horse serum are stored at −20°C, thawed in a 37°C water bath with gentle agitation for use in culture, and placed into the medium generally at concentrations between 10 and 20%. The frozen serum should be thawed only once and not refrozen, so that denaturation is avoided. Unused, thawed serum should be stored in a refrigerator; it retains activity for approximately 2 weeks. Most commercially obtained serums are filtered and can be used directly for tissue culture. However, if there is any question of possible contamination, the serum can be added to the final medium and refiltered, taking care to minimize "bubbling," which causes protein denaturation. This is followed by aliquoting and freezing. Serum-containing medium filtered in this manner should be tested to ensure that it can support cell growth before it is used in experiments.

Cells can also be grown in serum-free media containing growth factors, vitamins, trace elements, attachment factors, and protease inhibitors. Some of the commonly used additives are insulin, hydrocortisone, epidermal growth factor, fibroblast growth factor, and nerve growth factor. A good introduction to this technique can be found in the cell culture methods series by Sato *et al.* and Barnes *et al.* (11, 12). In general, a specific formulation for serum-free growth is good for only one cell type or culture line. Thus, this approach often initially proves to be time consuming while the right combinations and concentrations of nutrients for growing a new cell type are developed. Cells grown in serum-free media are very sensitive to pH, osmolality, and trypsinization.

Antibiotics are often used for cell culture, but should not be used on a continuous basis so that the development of antibiotic-resistant microorganisms is prevented. High doses and prolonged antibiotic levels in tissue culture may also change cell growth and function and may delay the detection of contamination until complete antibiotic resistance has developed. This delay in the detection of contamination from continuous antibiotics may create serious problems, especially if low-level contaminated cells from such cultures are unknowingly used as "frozen stocks." Thus, if careful procedures for developing a proper "pyramid" of frozen stocks from clean cultures have not previously been employed (see Section IV), the whole cell line may be lost.

IV. Maintaining Frozen Stocks and Record Keeping

It is necessary to perform a "primary" and "secondary" freeze of a new cell line when it arrives. The line is then expanded from the tertiary passage for experimental use (Fig. 1). This strategy protects the original stock if a contamination problem should arise in later passages. Meticulous records should be kept of the passage number of each culture employed experimentally. Also, the karyotype, DNA fingerprint, and/or the PSO enzyme electrophoretic analysis of the "working stock" should be reconfirmed at least yearly to make certain that chromosomal or other genetic changes have not occurred in the line (13–15).

Freezing medium contains the basic growth media normally used for a given cell line with the addition of 20% serum and 10% dimethyl sulfoxide (DMSO) or glycerol (16). The DMSO and glycerol are used to inhibit the formation of ice crystals by permeabilization of the plasma membrane so that water can flow out during the freezing process (1). Once cells are resuspended in freezing medium, they are aliquoted into cryovials for storage in liquid nitrogen, or in a −80°C ultralow freezer. The cryovials are slowly cooled at a rate of 1°C/min in freezing canisters, which are available from most cell tissue culture supply companies (e.g., Fisher). Short-term storage of frozen cells in a −80°C ultralow freezer can be used for up to 2 weeks; for long-term storage, however, cells should be kept below −130°C in a liquid nitrogen system.

For reculture, the frozen cells in the cryovials are quickly thawed by gentle shaking in a 37°C water bath (1, 16). The outsides of the cryovials are then dried and sprayed with 70% ethanol to minimize contamination risk after thawing. The thawed cells are then transferred into a T25 culture flask (Corning, Falcon, etc.) with complete growth medium under the tissue culture hood and allowed to grow for 24 hr. The medium is then changed to remove the remaining cryopreservatives. However, some cell lines do better if the cryopreservatives are removed immediately after thawing. This is done by adding complete medium and cells to a 15-ml tube, followed by centrifugation for 10 min at 1500 rpm (~400 *g*). The cells are then resuspended in complete growth medium, plated in a T25 flask, and placed in the incubator at 37°C and 5% CO_2. Records of freeze dates, as well as the medium used, passage number, and location in the freezer, should be kept in a separate laboratory notebook for frozen stocks.

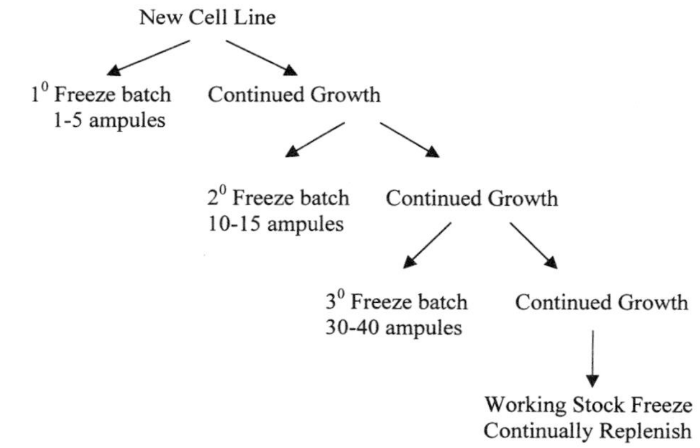

Figure 1 "Freezing pyramid" to protect a new cell line from contamination.

V. Basic Cell Culture

Monolayer cultures, which are possible with mesenchymal or epithelial cells, attach to the tissue culture flasks or to slide surfaces in some culture systems. The cells are usually plated at a density of (1.3–5) × 10^6 cells/5 ml of medium in a T25 flask, giving an average of 5.2 × 10^4 to 2.0 × 10^5 cells/cm^2 of flask surface area. The average volume of medium is 0.2 ml/cm^2. Monolayer cultures can also be grown directly on microscope slides by use of single or multichamber removable plastic wells bonded to the slides (Nalge Nunc, Int., 75 Panorama Creek Drive, Rochester, NY). Alternatively, cells can be grown on coverslips placed in petri dishes, which are subsequently placed on microscope slides (1, 16). Both of these system allow the cultured cells to be fixed *in situ* for subsequent microscopic examination.

After the cell suspensions are placed into culture, the cells attach to the bottom of the flask or slide surface within 12 hr (lag period; Fig. 2A). Failure to attach within the first 24 hr may mean that the culture is contaminated. The monolayer cultures then enter the exponential growth phase, during which rapid doubling of the cell numbers occurs (Figs. 2B and 3A). After exponential growth, the cells become confluent and enter the plateau phase of growth (Figs. 2C and 3B), with no further increase in cell number observed despite the availability of fresh medium. If the cells are left in depleted medium, actual loss of cell numbers occurs and the cultures are said to be in the "starved phase" (Fig. 3C). It is best to passage monolayer cells grown for continued growth just before they reach confluence or the plateau phase (Fig. 3A/B).

Harvesting cells to seed new cultures is called a "passage" or "subculture." It is necessary to detach the monolayer cells from the bottom of the tissue culture flask for harvest. Monolayer cells attach by producing an extracellular matrix (ECM) consisting of laminin, fibronectin, and attachment proteins. The attached monolayer cells must be released from the ECM proteins by treatment with trypsin in order to create suspensions of living cells for subsequent subcultures, freezing, or experimental use. For trypsinization, the monolayer cultures are first washed with protein and Ca^{2+}-free BSS for removal of any protease inhibitors or

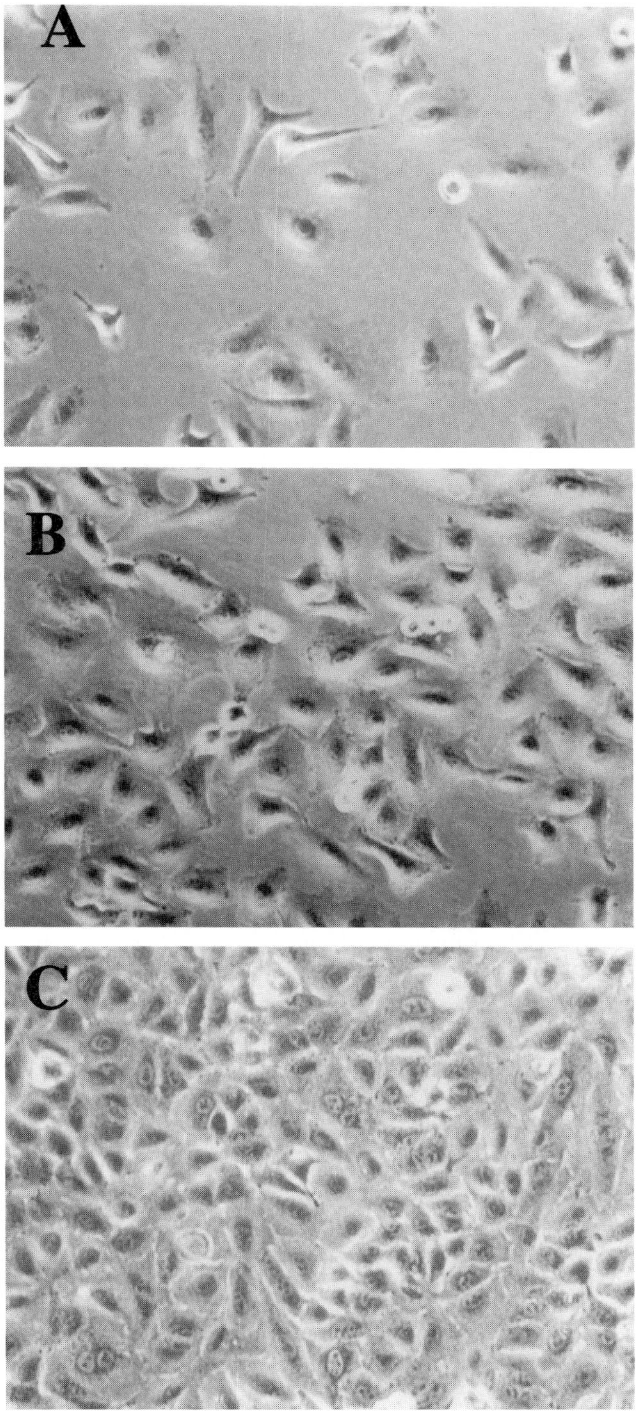

Figure 2 Photomicrograph of an A549 lung carcinoma monolayer culture that has just attached to the culture plate and is in the lag period (A); an A549 culture in exponential growth (B) and confluent or plateau growth (C).

Ca^{2+} that might inhibit the trypsin activity. This is done by carefully drawing off the supernatant media of the culture with a sterile pipette under the tissue culture hood and replacing it with an identical volume of serum and Ca^{2+}-free BSS. This BSS solution is, in turn, removed, and the monolayer cultures are then treated with BSS containing trypsin under experimental conditions worked out for each cell line. Specifically, too little trypsinization will not detach the cells, and too much trypsinization can lead to cell lysis and death. Generally, treatment with 0.25% of trypsin-EDTA in phosphate-buffered saline at 37°C for 20 min with gentle tapping of the flask can be used safely for most cell types.

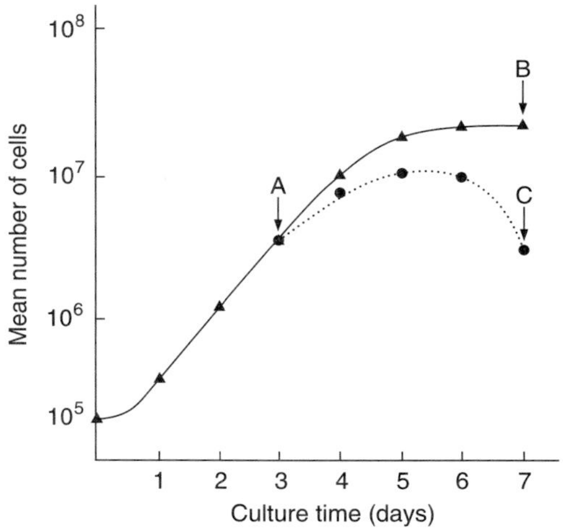

Figure 3 Growth curves for exponential (A), plateau (B), and starved (C) MCa-11 monolayer cultures. With permission, from Allison *et al.* (35).

After trypsinization, the bottom of the flask can also be gently wiped with a sterile rubber "policeman," which further detaches the cells. For subculturing, the now-suspended monolayer cells are drawn from the flask with a sterile pipette and centrifuged down (1500 rpm or ~400 $g \times 10$ min) and resuspended ino complete, fresh medium. The cells are counted and plated at an appropriate density into new culture flasks. Care must be taken to record the culture passage number in the experimental notebook. Finally, if one wants to prepare an enriched population of mitotic cells from exponential monolayer cultures, the "mitotic shake" technique can be employed. This involves sharply tapping the tissue culture flask three or four times to detach the mitotic cells selectively (17).

One specialized tissue culture model of malignant growth is worthy of note. Coating the bottoms of plastic tissue culture flasks with agar prevents cell attachment (18). Under these conditions, certain malignant cell lines, primarily derived from epithelial cancers, have the capacity to grow in suspension above the agar as freely floating "tissue culture spheroids." Spheroids start as microscopic aggregates of a few cells and grow from the center outward up to a diameter of 1000 μm or more. Tissue culture spheroids are important because they mimic all of the stages of solid tumor growth *in vivo*. For example, Fig. 4 shows an autoradiograph of a section of a 500-μm MCa-11 spheroid, which had been incubated in [^{3}H] thymidine for 24 hr prior to fixation (19).

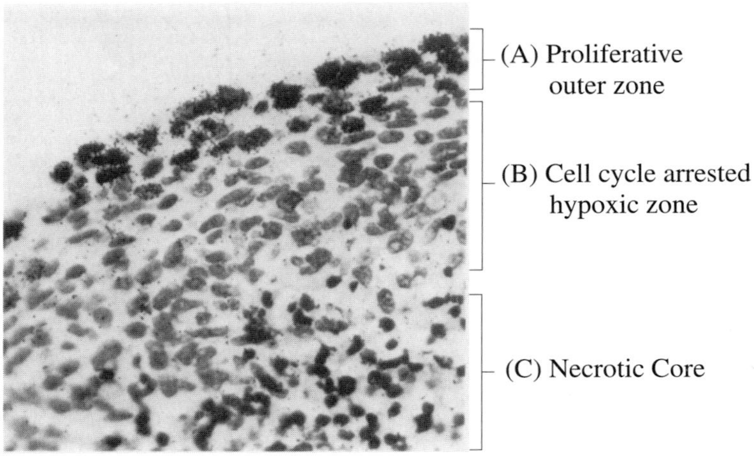

Figure 4 Autoradiograph of an MCa-11 spheroid labeled continuously for 24 hr with 2 μCi/ml of [^{3}H]thymidine. The preferential labeling of the periphery of the viable rim is apparent (A). Beneath the proliferating cells on the outside of the spheroid (A) is a viable layer of cell cycle-arrested, hypoxic cells (B) and a centrally located necrotic core (C). With permission, from Allison *et al.* (19).

It can be seen that the spheroid has a viable rim of proliferating cells covered by autoradiographic grains (Fig. 4A). Beneath this proliferating zone is an area of viable, hypoxic-arrested cells that are not labeled (Fig. 4B), and the center of the spheroid consists of pynotic and necrotic cells (Fig. 4C).

VI. Primary Cultures

A. Peripheral Blood Culture

Human lymphocytes are a readily available source of nontransformed cells for short-term culture experiments (14). Human blood (5–10 ml) drawn into a 3% heparinized syringe is diluted 1:1 with 0.9% sterile saline. Of this solution, 10 ml is placed on top of 8 ml of a Ficoll/sucrose gradient solution in a 50-ml conical centrifuge tube. The tube is centrifuged at 1500 rpm (~400 *g*) for 20 min to separate the white blood cells (WBCs) from the red blood cells (RBCs). The gradient band containing the WBCs is taken off with a pipette, placed into a clean 15-ml centrifuge tube, diluted with 8 ml of washing medium, pelleted, and resuspended in 3–5 ml of complete bicarbonate-buffered RPMI-1640 with 10% fetal calf serum containing 1% phytohemagglutinin (PHA, Amersham Pharmacia Biotech, Inc., 800 Centennial Avenue, Piscataway, NJ), a T cell mitogen. Exponential growth continues for 72 hr, at which time the cells are at a sufficient number for experimental study.

B. Culture of Nontransformed Solid Tissues

Different types of solid tissues are made of varying proportions of epithelial, mesenchymal, and hematogenous cells. Specialized techniques are needed to culture purified cell populations of these different cell types. For example, placing disaggregated normal tissues into complete media with serum favors the growth of the fibroblasts present in the tissue fragments. Epithelial cells are preferentially grown in a media with relatively low calcium (150 μ*M*) and no serum. The following protocol is an example of the culture technique employed to grow normal human bronchial epithelial cells (20, 21).

Normal bronchial epithelium is a single-layer, pseudostratified tissue that lines the airways. Typically, the epithelial cells are isolated from normal airway tissues that were unavoidably removed during surgical resection of diseased (cancerous or infected) lung, or airway tissues obtained at immediate autopsy. As with culture of any normal cell type, it is first necessary to isolate the cells of interest from the other cells they are combined with to form a complex tissue. The two primary approaches for selective isolation of normal human bronchial epithelial cells include scraping or digesting the epithelial cells off the airway, or placing pieces of airway tissue into explant culture and allowing the epithelial cells to grow as an outgrowth off the explant and onto the culture substrate. In the latter approach, the explant outgrowth is a pure culture of epithelial cells that can be subsequently transplanted to another culture vessel.

The optimal media for selective culture of epithelial cells from airway tissues contains a relatively low concentration of calcium (150 μ*M*) and no serum. This is because bronchial epithelial cells tolerate low levels of calcium but fibroblasts and endothelial cells do not. Media and attachment factors that are optimized for the culture of human bronchial epithelial cells are commercially available: bronchial epithelial basal medium (BEBM) from Clonetics

(9245 Brown Deer Rd., San Diego, CA), or LHC-9 from Biofluids (1146 Taft St., Rockville, MD). Terminal squamous differentiation is accelerated in human bronchial epithelial cells when high levels (1 m*M*) of calcium are present in the medium (21). When bronchial epithelial cells are allowed to grow to confluence, they also rapidly undergo terminal squamous differentiation and a marked decrease in the population doubling potential (22). The population doubling potential of normal human bronchial epithelial cells varies from one sample to another. Under ideal conditions, a culture of these cells may undergo as many as 15 population doublings. Although the limit to continuous proliferation of normal human bronchial epithelial cells is invariably stopped by terminal metaplastic squamous differentiation, in rodent models it is possible to define media that maintain these cells in their normal ciliated, mucus-secreting phenotype (23). Efforts to define such media for human bronchial epithelial cells have not been successful.

1. Explant Culture of Normal Human Bronchial Epithelial Cells

Explant outgrowth culture is most commonly used for culture of normal human bronchial epithelial cells when it is necessary to produce as many cells as possible. In explant cultures, the epithelial cells undergo more population doublings than they do when the cells are simply scraped or digested away from the airway and placed directly in culture. It is hypothesized that growth or nutrition factors contained within the explant tissues contribute to maintenance of epithelial cells in culture, but such tissue factors have not yet been identified.

For explant culture, bronchial tissues obtained at immediate autopsy or surgery are placed in ice-cold L15 medium for transport to the laboratory. The airways are then carefully dissected from the pulmonary vessels and lung parenchyma. Scissors and scalpel are used to dissect the airway into approximately 0.5×0.5 cm^2 explants. Tissue culture dishes (100 mm in diameter) are prepared by using a needle to scratch seven areas (six areas arranged in a hexagon around the dish and a seventh in the middle) onto the tissue culture surface. Each scratched area is slightly less than the size of the explant. If the scratched area is bigger than the explant, it will prevent the outgrowth of the epithelial cells from the surface of the explant onto the dish. The culture surfaces are then coated with a solution containing fibronectin (Collaborative Biomedical Products, a division of Becton Dickinson, Franklin Lakes, NJ), human type I collagen (Vitrogen 100, Cohesion Technologies, Palo Alto, CA), and bovine serum albumin (BSA) (Miles Laboratories, Kankakee, IL). The coated dishes should be incubated at 33°C for 2–3 hr prior to use. These attachment factors are critical for optimal culture of the bronchial epithelial cells. Attachment factors other than those described here (e.g., laminin) either add nothing to, or actually inhibit, growth of the bronchial epithelial cells.

The explants are placed onto the dish with the epithelial side up and incubated at room temperature for 3–5 min without tissue culture media. This allows the explants to attach firmly to the scratched area. Then 7 ml of LHC-9 (21) or BEBM medium is added to the dishes and the explants are incubated at 36.5°C in a humidified CO_2 (4.5%) incubator. The medium is replaced with fresh medium every 3–4 days. After 8–11 days of incubation the epithelial cell outgrowths radiate from the tissue fragments more than 0.5 cm. Fibroblastic or endothelial contamination is rare due to the selective nature of the culture medium. The tissue explants are transferred to a new dish prepared as above. The postexplant outgrowth cultures may be incubated for a further 2–4 days, followed by dissociation with trypsin. The dissociated cells may be placed back in culture, cryopreserved, or used in experiments. High-density outgrowth cultures should be subcultured before they become confluent, because confluent cultures rapidly undergo terminal squamous differentiation.

2. Culture of Bronchial Epithelial Cells by Cell Dissociation and Subculturing

The details of this procedure are described in Lechner and LaVeck (21). Isolation of epithelial cells from airway tissue prior to culture is preferable to explant culture in certain situations, such as for epithelial cell samples obtained through bronchoscopic biopsy (brush or forceps) from normal volunteers or patients. Although the numbers obtained through this approach are far smaller than those obtained through explant culture, they are sufficient for many molecular and cytogenetic studies.

The tissue samples containing the bronchial epithelial cells are first rinsed twice with calcium-free HEPES-buffered saline, as even low levels of calcium inhibit trypsin. The cultures are then placed in polyvinylpyroolidine (PVP)/EDTA/trypsin (PET) solution. The EDTA in the PET solution chelates any remaining calcium. The cultures then are incubated with PET at room temperature until cells begin to detach from the surface of the culture dish, as monitored by phase microscopy. This usually takes ~5–10 min. The dissociated single cells are suspended by adding 1 volume of LHC-9 basal medium containing 10% FBS and gently triturating with a pipette. The suspended cells are counted (using a hemacytometer), pelleted (125 *g* at 4°C for 5 min), and resuspended in fresh LHC-9 medium.

C. Immortalization of Normal Human Bronchial Epithelial Cells

As described above, normal bronchial epithelial cells grow in culture for only 15–20 population doublings before they undergo terminal squamous differentiation. This severely restricts studies attempting to produce malignant transformation of normal cells, because repeated exposures to a carcinogen over many passages may be required to damage the DNA. The population doubling potential may be indefinitely extended in a process called "immortalization." Normal human bronchial epithelial cells have been immortalized by stable introduction of either SV40 adenovirus transfection, giving rise to the BEAS2B line (24), or human papillomavirus 16 or 18 transfection giving rise to the BEP2D and BEP3D cell lines (25). In general, the media requirements of these immortalized cells are considerably less stringent than those of nontransformed human bronchial epithelial cells. For example, immortalized cells will grow in moderate concentrations of serum with less growth factors and do not require attachment factors.

Although immortal, these lines are not tumorigenic when injected into immunosuppressed mice, making them useful in carcinogenesis experiments. BEAS2B has given rise to malignant transformants following treatment with cigarette smoke condensate, 4-methylnitrosamino-1-(3-pyridyl)-1-butanone (NNK), and benzo[*a*]pyrene (26). BEP2D has given rise to tumorigenic lines following treatment with radon and asbestos (27, 28).

D. Culture of Malignant Bronchial Epithelial Cells

There are many uses for well-characterized cultures of malignant human bronchial epithelial (also termed bronchogenic carcinoma) cells. Conditions for culturing the two major histologic categories of bronchogenic carcinoma cells, small cell and nonsmall cell, have been described (29, 30). More than 200 human small or nonsmall cell lung cancer cell lines were established using the serum-free, hormone and growth factor-supplemented, defined media HITES and ACL4 (31). Characterization of these lines has extended our knowledge of lung cell biology and allowed direct comparisons of genetic markers that differentiate normal from malignant human bronchial epithelial cells (32).

VII. Contamination and Decontamination

In almost every tissue culture laboratory, there are occasional episodes of mass contamination. This is usually due to poor technique, but contamination can also be secondary to the unsuspected introduction of infected new lines into the laboratory or to the breakdown of sterilization procedures or products. For example, a nonworking autoclave, the acquisition of a batch of contaminated fetal calf serum, or even an institutional problem with the sterile air supply can all lead to contamination. Although the isolated contamination of an occasional culture is not a great loss, failure of early recognition of low-level contamination in one line can lead to the contamination of the tissue culture hoods and incubators, and thereby to the subsequent infection of the subcultures of other, previously sterile lines.

Two methods are used for detecting contamination early and preventing its spread throughout the facility. The importance of "growing out" reagents and cell lines in test cultures without antibiotics has already been mentioned. Also, frequent microscopic screening of the cultures with a 32× phase-contrast objective allows early detection of bacteria and fungi in the cultures, which can be differentiated from inanimate particles by their non-Brownian movements and their division. If contamination is found in a subculture of a cell line, that culture is discarded, and the suspect line is regrown from a sterile stock without antibiotics. If this and other sterile test cultures subsequently become contaminated, then a generalized laboratory contamination is probable (see below). The most important means of minimizing the effects of such a contamination episode after it is contained is to have well-documented, noncontaminated frozen stocks of all cell lines available (Fig. 1) to rebuild the experimental cell lines for the laboratory.

Decontaminating a tissue culture laboratory is an arduous and time-consuming project. First, it is necessary to check all individual components of the media and cell lines to make certain that there is not a simple solution to the problem, which might involve a defective batch of Millipore filters, a nonfunctioning autoclave, contaminated fetal calf serum, etc. If, as is sometimes the case, one cause cannot be clearly identified to provide a simple solution to the problem, then a general decontamination of the facility will be necessary. This includes checking and possibly reworking the airflow into the laboratory, and checking and/or professionally replacing all of the HEPA filters and the UV sterilization systems of the laboratory. The insides of the hoods and incubators must also be professionally fumigated, usually by burning of formaldehyde (3). All walls and surfaces of the laboratory must be chemically decontaminated, and new stocks of media, fetal calf serum, and filters must be obtained.

The newly cleaned laboratory should be restarted with clean cultures, either from a frozen stock or from primary lymphocyte cultures. If successful, cultures from the primary freeze (Fig. 1) of initially clean stocks can be carefully reintroduced one at a time for experimental use. Also, if one suspects a possible low level of contamination in a given culture, it is sometimes possible to "clean" the culture by treatment with three or four passages of antibiotics, followed by further passages in antibiotic-free medium to ensure that the contamination has been eliminated. However, there is no guarantee of success for such attempts to "clean" contaminated cultures.

VIII. Cell Growth Analysis

Direct cell counts are the most easily interpreted method for measuring the growth of cultured cells. The cell counts, preferably in triplicate, must be measured by a standardized method, the simplest being the use of a hemacytometer and a light microscope. The hemacytometer contains two chambers, each chamber having nine ruled squares. One square can be viewed completely with a 10 × objective for 100 × total magnification and contains 1.0×10^{-4} ml of fluid when coverslipped (Fig. 5). For counting the number of cells in a square, any cells touching the boundary lines of the left and top are counted, but cells touching the right and bottom boundaries are excluded. By counting the number of cells in 10 squares (the 4 corner squares and the center square of both chambers of the hemacytometer) (Fig. 5), one measures the total number of cells in 1×10^{-3} ml. This value is used to calculate the final cell concentration by the following formula:

$$\text{Total number of cells/ml} = \text{\# measured in 10 squares} \times 1000 \times \text{dilution factor.}$$

After use, the hemacytometer is rinsed with distilled water followed by 70% ethanol, dried with lens paper, and stored. Electronic cell-counting instruments, such as Coulter counters, must be calibrated frequently against known standards to ensure the comparability of counts performed at different times.

Epithelial and mesenchymal cells grown as monolayers typically show a triphasic growth curve after the lag period: (1) exponential growth, when the cells are plated at a low density in fresh medium and are proliferating at the maximum possible rate (Fig. 3A), (2) plateau growth, after the cells have become confluent with no net increase in cell number despite the availability of fresh medium (Fig. 3B), and (3) starved growth, in which an actual decrease in cell number occurs when the cells are left in nutritionally depleted medium (Fig. 3C). Studies of cultured cells in these growth phases help in the interpretation of measurements of the DNA distributions of cultured cells and radionucleotide incorporation, two commonly employed methods for quantifying cellular proliferation.

Flow cytometry (FCM), or image analysis, allows measurement of the cellular DNA content of a large number of individual cells or nuclei. For FCM, cells taken from monolayer or spheroid cultures must be carefully disaggregated to ensure that clumped nuclei and debris do not lead to measurement artifacts, although this is a greater problem when one works with nuclei disaggregated from solid tissues (33). Individual cellular DNA measurements are plotted on an *XY* graph (*X* axis, DNA content; *Y* axis, cell number), the so-called DNA distribution (Fig. 6). The DNA distributions of single cell populations generally have G_0/G_1 and G_2/M peaks, and the cells between the G_0/G_1 and G_2/M peaks are in S phase (Fig. 6, solid black areas). It had previously been assumed that all "noncycling" cells in monolayer cultures in exponential, plateau, or starved-growth phases arrest in the G_0/G_1 peak, and that the cells in all three types of cultures committed to replication go through S and G_2/M phases at relatively rapid and uniform rates. If this were correct, then

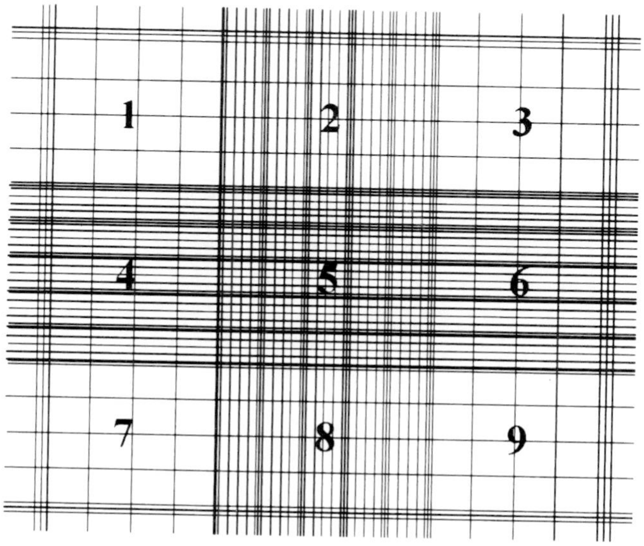

Figure 5 Diagram of one chamber of a hemacytometer. The volume of fluid in one of the numbered squares is 1×10^4 ml.

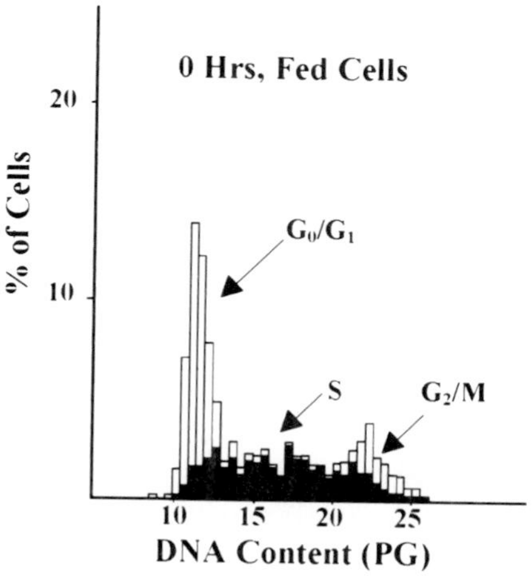

Figure 6 DNA distribution and [^{3}H]thymidine labeling at time 0 of exponential MCa-11 monolayer cultures. Black areas show the percentage of labeled cells in each 0.5-pg interval of cellular DNA content. It can be seen that all of the S phase cells, between the G_0/G_1 and G_2/M peaks, are labeled. With permission, from Allison *et al.* (36).

the proliferative rate of a cell population would be directly proportional to its percentage of S and G_2/M phase cells in the DNA distribution.

The assumption that replicating cells go through S and G_2/M phases at rapid and uniform rates may be true only for cultured cells in exponential growth (Fig. 3A) (34–36). This is shown in Fig. 7, which depicts a series of bivariate DNA distributions of MCa-11 tumor cells grown in exponential monolayer cultures. The DNA of the S phase cells in these cultures was pulse labeled for 5 min with [^{3}H]thymidine at time 0 (Fig. 7A) (37). The isotope was then removed and the cells were grown in fresh medium without isotope. The DNA content and isotopic labeling (determined by autoradiography; see below) of the same cells were then measured at 2, 4, 6, 8, and 10 hr after the initial labeling pulse (B–F, Fig. 7). The labeled cells flow smoothly through S phase into G_2/M phase at 2–4 hr (B and C). At 6 hr, the labeled cells are all in G_2/M, or have divided and returned to G_0/G_1 (Fig. 7D). At 8–10 hr (E and F), many of the labeled cells have reentered early S phase from G_0/G_1 to begin another round of DNA replication.

However, the perturbations of the growth rates of cultured cells by crowding, nutrient deprivation, chemical imbalances, pH changes, or physical change such as temperature variations or radiation are much more complex than the simple model of G_0/G_1 arrest. Quite simply, the transit rates of cells through all phases of the cell cycle can be lengthened by these environmental factors. It is probable that cell arrest or death can also occur in any phase of the cell cycle (34–36). Figure 8 (A–C) shows the flow cytometric DNA distributions of the exponential (A), plateau (B), and starved (C) MCa-11 tumor cells whose growth curves are shown in Fig. 3. The flow cytometric DNA distributions of the experimental, plateau, and starved cultures are all relatively similar (Fig. 8, A–C), although the growth rates of these cultures vary greatly (Fig. 3, A–C). It can also be seen that the proportion of S phase cells labeled with [^{3}H]thymidine varies directly with the growth rate of the culture (Fig. 8, A–C).

In summary, a cultured cell population whose FCM or image analysis DNA distribution shows all cells to be in G_0/G_1 is obviously not proliferating, although this is rarely observed unless an artifactual G_0/G_1 block has been induced. However, the corollary that a cultured cell population with a high fraction of S and G_2/M phase cells must be rapidly replicating is not true. Thus, each individual culture system must have its DNA distributions calibrated against changes in the actual cell numbers (Fig. 3) or the results of other kinetic assays to be discussed below.

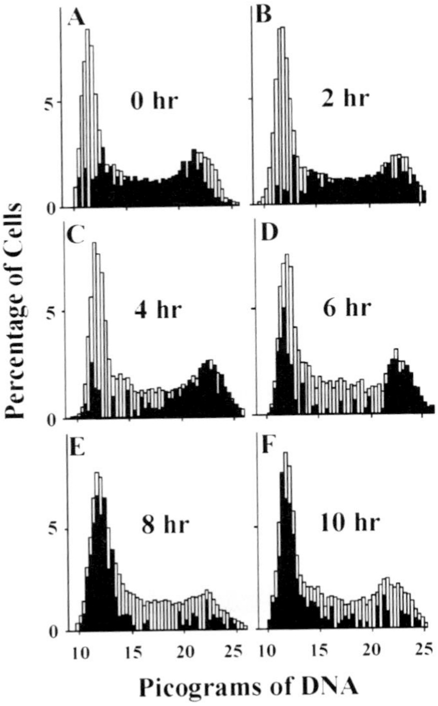

Figure 7 Exponential monolayer cultures of MCa-11 cells were pulse-chase labeled with [^{3}H]thymidine at time 0 (A) and then placed into fresh medium without isotope. There is a clear progression of almost all of the labeled cells through the cell cycle over the next 10 hr (B–F). With permission, from Allison *et al.* (37).

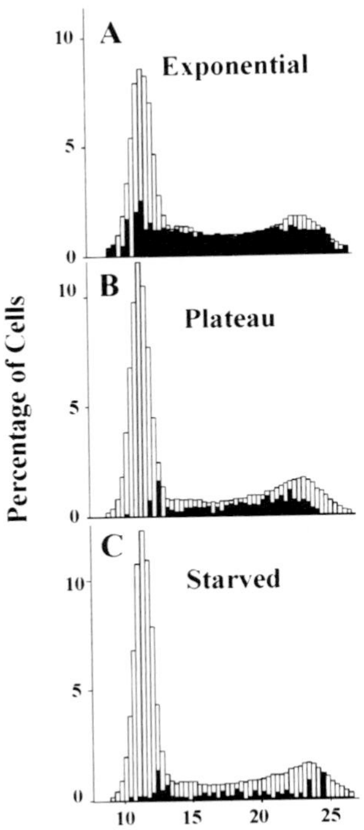

Figure 8 Flow-cytometric DNA distributions and [^{3}H]thymidine labeling of MCa-11 tumor cells in exponential (A), plateau (B), and starved (C) monolayer cultures. Although the FCM distributions are similar for all three types of cultures, there are significant decreases in the proportions of labeled S phase cells in the plateau and starved cultures. With permission, from Allison *et al.* (35).

The amount of radiolabeled nucleotides, usually [^{3}H]thymidine, incorporated into DNA can be measured directly by scintigraphy of DNA extracted from cultured cells. Although this assay is commonly used as an index for cellular proliferation, several variables make its interpretation quite complex. Exogenous [^{3}H]thymidine is incorporated into DNA through the thymidine salvage pathway. However, most cells produce thymidine for DNA replication from deoxyuridine through the thymidylate synthetase pathway. Thus, the relative activities of the thymidine salvage and the thymidylate synthetase enzymatic pathways in a given cell type can influence the amount of exogenous [^{3}H]thymidine incorporation. Variations in the size of the different intracellular nucleotide pools can also influence the amount of exogenous [^{3}H]thymidine incorporated. Finally, the amount of radioactivity incorporated per cell is, in itself, a meaningless number, which gives no information on what proportion of cells in the culture are actually replicating, or how fast they are going through the cell cycle. Thus, [^{3}H]thymidine incorporation measurements must be carefully calibrated by growth curves (Fig. 3), DNA distributions (Figs. 6–8), and/or the autoradiographic assays described below to provide meaningful estimates of cell proliferation.

One can prepare autoradiographs by covering microscopic slides of [^{3}H]thymidine-labeled cells with photographic emulsion (38). The emulsion-covered slides are exposed in the dark for variable time periods, followed by photographic development of the emulsion. The cells covered with silver grains are assumed to have incorporated the isotope into their newly replicated DNA (Fig. 9). A similar technique uses monoclonal antibodies (mAbs) to detect incorporation of bromodeoxyuridine (BrdU), a compound that is stable when incorporated into DNA through the thymidine salvage pathway (39). The BrdU technique has the advantages of rapidity and of being applicable to bivariate flow cytometry, in which the DNA content and labeling are measured for the same cells. Similar bivariate techniques can be applied to cells fixed on slides by the use of image analysis measurements of both cellular DNA content and [^{3}H]thymidine or BrdU grains (40), as shown in Fig. 7. Autoradiographs or BrdU-labeling techniques can also be used with simple light microscopy to determine the labeling index (LI), or the percentage of [^{3}H]thymidine or BrdU-labeled cells. The LI is proportional to the size of the S phase compartment and the proliferative rate of many culture systems. If these assays are used, it may be necessary to use "plateau labeling times" to obtain accurate LIs for [^{3}H]thymidine autoradiographs (41). One must also carefully calibrate the BrdU–mAb labeling to eliminate nonspecific staining. Both of these methods can be used for timing the appearance of labeled mitotic figures in the "percentage labeled mitosis method" (PLM) to obtain rough estimates of the rates of transit through all phases of the cell cycle for cultured cell populations. The classic PLM method can be performed without the use of complex imaging equipment (42, 43) and is still valid for many experimental systems (44).

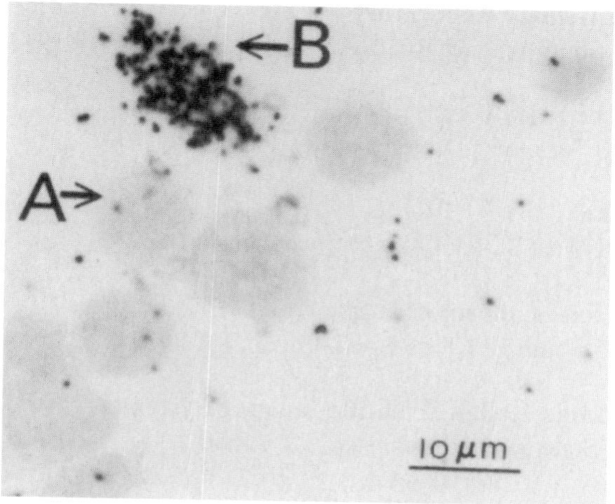

Figure 9 Autoradiograph of an unlabeled Ca-26 cell (A) with S phase DNA content adjacent to a labeled S phase cell (B). With permission, from Allison *et al.* (34).

IX. Resources

A. Cell Repositories

American Type Culture Collection (ATCC)
10801 University Boulevard
Manassas, VA 20110-2209
Telephone (703) 365-2700
http://www.atcc.org/

Coriell Cell Repositories (CCR)
(NIA) Aging Cell Culture Repository
(NIGMS) Human Genetic Cell Repository
(ADA) American Diabetes Association
(HBDI) Human Biological Data Interchange
Coriell Institute for Medical Research
401 Haddon Ave.
Camden, NJ 08103
Telephone (800) 752-3805
Fax (856) 757-9737
http://locus.umdnj.edu

Department of Human and Animal Cell Cultures (DSMZ)
DSMZ-German Collection of Microorganisms and Cell Cultures
Department of Human and Animal Cell Cultures
Mascheroder Weg 1b

D-38124 Braunschweig, Germany
Phone: +49-531-2616.161
Fax: +49-531-2616.150
http://www.dsmz.de/index.html

European Collection of Animal Cell Cultures (ECACC)
European Collection of Cell Cultures Centre for Applied Microbiology and Research
Salisbury, Wiltshire SP4 0JG, England
Tel: +44 (0) 1980 612512
Fax: +44 (0) 1980 611315
http://fuseii.star.co.uk/camr/

Japanese Collection of Research Bioresources (JCRB)
Health Science Research Resources Bank (HSRRB)
Hoenzaka 1-1-43, Chuo-ku,
Osaka 540, Japan
Fax: +81-6-6945-2872
http://www.jhsf.or.jp/English/index_gc.html

National Laboratory for the Genetics of Israeli Populations (NLGIP)
Sackler Faculty of Medicine
Tel-Aviv University
Tel-Aviv 69978, Israel
Telephone: ++972-3-640-7611
Fax: ++972-3-640-7611
http://www.tau.ac.il/medicine/NLGIP/nlgip.htm

Riken Gene Bank
The Institute of Physical and Chemical Research (RIKEN)
3-1-1 Koyadai
Tsukuba Science City, 305, Japan
Telephone +81-298-36-9124
Fax +81-298-36-9130

The University of Michigan Human Breast Cell/Tissue Bank and Data Base
Stephen P. Ethier, Ph.D., Sofia Merajver, M.D., Ph.D., and Tom Giordano, M.D., Ph.D.
Departments of Radiation Oncology, Internal Medicine and Pathology
The University of Michigan Medical School
1331 E. Ann Street
Rm # 3034
Ann Arbor, MI 48109
http://www.cancer.med.umich.edu/umbnkdb.html

B. Manufacturers

Amersham Pharmacia Biotech, Inc.
800 Centennial Avenue, P.O. Box 1327, Piscataway, NJ 08855-1327

Atlanta Biologicals
1425 Oakbrook Drive, Suite 400, Norcross, GA 30093

Becton Dickinson
1 Becton Drive, Franklin Lakes, NJ 07417-1883

Bio-Whittaker
8830 Biggs Ford Rd., Walkersville, MD 21793-0127

Biofluids
1146 Taft St., Rockville, MD 20850

Calbiochem-Novabiochem Corporation
P.O. Box 12087, La Jolla, CA 92039-2087

Chemicon International, Ltd.
28835 Single Oak Drive, Temecula, CA 92590

Clonetics
9245 Brown Deer Rd, San Diego, CA 92121

Cohesion Technologies
2500 Faber Place, Palo Alto, CA 94303

Collaborative Biomedical Products
A division of Becton Dickinson

Corning Scietific Products
P.O. Box 5000, Corning, NY 14830

Difco Laboratories
P.O. Box 14B, Central Avenue, West Molesey, Surrey, KT8 2SE UK

Falcon
A division of Becton Dickinson

Pall Gelman Laboratory
600 South Wagner Road, Ann Arbor, MI 48103-9019

Fisher Scientific
4500 Turnberry Drive, Hanover Park, IL 60103

Fluka
1001 West St. Paul Ave., Milwaukee, WI 53233

Hyclone Laboratories Inc.
1725 South HyClone Road, Logan, UT 84321

Eastman Kodak Scientific Imaging Systems
343 State Street, Rochester, NY 14650

Life Technologies/Gibco-BRL
9800 Medical Center Drive, P.O. Box 6482, Rockville, MD 20849-6482

Mediatech
13884 Park Center Road, Herndon, VA 20171

Miles Laboratories
195 West Birch Street, Kankakee, IL 60901

Millipore Corporation
80 Ashby Road, Bedford, MA 01730-2271

Nalge Nunc International
75 Panorama Creek Drive, P.O. Box 20365, Rochester, NY 14602-0365

Pharmacia
See Amersham Pharmacia Biotech, Inc.

Roche Bioscience
3401 Hillview Avenue, P.O. Box 10850, Palo Alto, CA 94304-1397

Schleicher & Schuell Inc
10 Optical Avenue, P.O. Box 2012, Keene, NH 03431

Sigma
P.O. Box 14508, St. Louis, MO 63178

Stratagene
11011 North Torrey Pines Road, La Jolla, CA 92037 USA

Whatman International Ltd.
St. Leonard's Road, 20/20 Maidstone, Kent, ME 16 OLS UK

Wheaton Science Products
1501 N. 10th Street, Millville, NJ 08332-2093

Zeiss
One Zeiss Drive, Thornwood, NY 10594

Acknowledgments

This work was supported by the Cancer Biology Fund of the Medical College of Ohio Foundation. We thank Kay Langenderfer for her help in preparing this manuscript.

References

1. McAteer, J. A., and Davis, J. (1994). Basic cell culture technique and the maintenance of cell lines. *In* "Basic Cell Culture: A Practical Approach" (J. M. Davis, ed.), pp. 109–143. Oxford Univ. Press, New York.
2. Freshney, R. I. (1987). "Culture of Animal Cells: A Manual of Basic Technique". 2nd Ed. Alan R. Liss, New York.
3. Roberts, P. L. (1994). Sterilization. *In* "Basic Cell Culture: A Practical Approach" (J.M. Davis, ed.), p. 46. Oxford Univ. Press, New York.
4. Cartwright, T., and Shah, G. P. (1994). Culture media. *In* "Basic Cell Culture: A Practical Approach" (J.M. Davis, ed.), pp. 57–89. Oxford Univ. Press, New York.
5. Morgan, J. G., Morton, H. J., and Parker, R. C. (1950). Nutritional Studies of Animal Cells in Culture. I. Initial Studies on a Synthetic Medium. *Proc. Soc. Exp. Biol. Med.* **73,** 1.
6. Dulbecco, R., and Freeman, G. (1959). Plaque formation by the polyoma virus. *Virology* **8,** 396–397.
7. Eagle, H. (1959). Amino acid metabolism in mammalian cell cultures. *Science* **130,** 432.
8. Ham, R. G. (1965). Clonal growth of mammalian cells in a chemically defined synthetic medium. *Proc. Natl. Acad. Sci. U.S.A.* **53,** 288.
9. Moore, G. E., Gerner, R. E., and Franklin, H. A. (1967). Culture of normal human leukocytes. *J. Am. Med. Assoc.* **199,** 519–524.
10. Grady, K. (1999). How basal media provide the optimal environment for cell culture. *Focus* **21,** (3), 76.
11. Barnes, W. D., Sirbasku, D. A., and Sato, G. H., eds. (1984). Methods for preparation of media, supplements, and substrata for serum-free animal cell culture. "Cell Culture Methods for Molecular and Cell Biology," Vol. 1. Alan R. Liss, New York.
12. Sato, J. D., Hayashi, I., Hayaski, J., Hoshi, H., Kawamoto, T., McKeehan, W. L., Matsuda, R., Matsuzaki, K., Mills, K. H. G., Okamoto, T., Serrero, G., Sussman, D. J., and Kan, M. (1994). Specific cell types and their requirements. *In* "Basic Cell Culture: A Practical Approach" (J. M. Davis, ed.), pp. 181–217. Oxford Univ. Press, New York.
13. Hsu, T. C. (1979). "Human and Mammalian Cytogenetics An Historical Perspective." Springer-Verlag, New York.
14. Barch, M. J., Lawce, H. J., and Arshma, M. S. (1991). Peripheral blood culture. *In* "The ACT Cytogenetics Laboratory Manual," 2nd Ed. (M.J. Barch., ed.), pp. 17–66. Raven Press, New York.
15. Doyle, A., and Bolton, B. J. (1994). The quality control of cell lines and the prevention, detection, and cure of contamination. *In* "Basic Cell Culture: A Practical Approach" (J.M. Davis, ed.), pp. 243–248. Oxford Univ. Press, New York.
16. Spector, D. L., Goldman, R. D., and Leinwald, L. A. (1998). Culture and biochemical analysis of cells. "Cells: A Laboratory Manual," Vol. 1, pp. 2.11–2.13. Cold Spring Harbor Laboratory, Cold Spring Harbor, New York.
17. Lawce, H. J., and Brown, G. (1991). Harvesting, slide-making, and chromosome elongation techniques. *In* "The ACT Cytogenetics Laboratory Manual," 2nd Ed. (M. J. Barch, ed.), pp. 31–66. Raven Press, New York.
18. Yuhas, J. M., Li, A. P., Martinex, A. G., and Landman, A. J. (1977). A simplified method for production and growth of multicellular tumor spheroids. *Cancer Res.* **37,** 3639–3647.
19. Allison, D. C., Yuhas, J. M., Ridolpho, P. F., Anderson, and S. L., Johnson, T. S. (1983). Cytophotometric measurement of the cellular DNA content of (^{3}H)thymidine-labeled spheroids: Direct demonstration of non-labeled cells with S and G_2 DNA content. *Cell Tissue Kinet.* **16,** 237–246.
20. Lechner, J. F., Haugen, A., McClendon, I. A., and Pettis, E. W. (1982). Clonal growth of normal adult human bronchial epithelial cells in a serum-free medium. *In Vitro* **18,** 633–642.
21. Lechner, J. F., and LaVeck, M. A. (1985). A serum-free method for culturing normal human bronchial epithelial cells at clonal density. *J. Tissue Culture Methods* **9,** 43–48.
22. Lechner, J. F., Haugen, A., and McClendon, I. A. (1984). Induction of differentiation of normal bronchial epithelial cells by small amounts of serum. *Differentiation* **25,** 229–237.
23. Wu, R., Groelke, J. W., Chang, L. Y., Porter, M. E., Smith, D., and Nettesheim, P. (1982). Effects of hormones on the multiplication and differentiation of tracheal epithelial cells in culture. *In* "Growth of Cells in Hormonally Defined Media" (D. Sirbasku, G. H. Sato, and A. Pardee, eds.), p. 641. Cold Spring Harbor Laboratory, Cold Spring Harbor, New York.

24. Reddel, R. R., Ke, Y., Gerwin, B. I., McMenamin, M. G., Lechner, J. F., Su, R. T., Brash, D. E., Park, J. B., Rhim, J. S., and Harris, C. C. (1988). Transformation of human bronchial epithelial cells by infection with SV40 or adenovirus-12SV40 hybrid virus, or transfection via strontium phosphate coprecipitation with a plasmid containing SV40 early region genes. *Cancer Res.* **48,** 1904–1909.
25. Willey, J. C., Broussoud, A., Sleemi, A., Bennett, W. P., Cerutti, P., and Harris, C. C. (1991). Immortalization of normal human bronchial epithelial cells by human papillomaviruses 16 or 18. *Cancer Res.* **51,** 5370–5377.
26. Klein-Szanto, A. J, Iizasa, T., Momiki, S., Garcia-Palazzo, I., Caamano, J., Metcalf, R., Welsh, J., and Harris, C. C. (1992). A tobacco-specific *N*-nitrosamine or cigarette smoke condensate causes neoplastic transformation of xenotransplanted human bronchial epithelial cells. *Proc. Natl. Acad. Sci. U.S.A.* **89,** 6693–6697.
27. Hei, T. K., Piao, C. Q., Willey, J. C., and Hall, E. J. (1994). Malignant transformation of human bronchial epithelial cells by radon-simulated alpha particles. *Carcinogenesis* **15,** 431–437.
28. Hei, T. K., Wu, L. J., and Piao, C. Q. (1997). Malignant transformation of immortalized human bronchial epithelial cells by asbestos fibers. *Environ. Health Perspect.* **105,** (5),.
29. Simms, E., Gazdar, A. F., Abrams, P. G., and Minna, J. D. (1980). Growth of human small cell (oat cell) carcinoma of the lung in serum-free growth factor supplemented medium. *Cancer Res.* **40,** 4356–4363.
30. Oie, H. K., Russell, E. K., Carney, D. N., and Gazdar, A. F. (1996). Cell culture methods for the establishment of the NCI series of lung cancer cell lines. *J. Cell. Biochem. Suppl.* **24,** 24–31.
31. Phelps, R. M., Johnson, B. E., Ihde, D. C., Gazdar, A. F., Carbone, D. P., McClintock, P. R., Linnoila, R. I., Matthews, M. J., Bunn, P. A., Jr., Carney, D., Minna, J. D., and Mulshine, J. L. (1996). NCI-Navy Medical Oncology Branch cell line data base. *J. Cell. Biochem. Suppl.* **24,** 32–91.
32. DeMuth, J. P., Jackson, C. M., Weaver, D. A., Crawford, E. L., Durzinsky, D. S., Durham, S. J., Zaher, A., Phillips, E. R., Khuder, S. A., and Willey, J. C. (1998). The gene expression index c-*myc* x E2F-1/p21 is highly predictive of malignant phenotype in human bronchial epithelial cells. *Am. J. Respir. Cell Mol. Biol.* **19,** 25–31.
33. Bose, K., Curley, S., Smith, W., and Allison, D. C. (1989). Differences in the flow and absorption cytometric DNA distributions of mouse hepatocytes and tumor cells. *Cytometry* **10,** 388–393.
34. Allison, D. C., Ridolpho, P. F., Anderson, S., and Bose, K. (1985). Variations in the (^{3}H)thymidine-labeling of S-phase cells in solid mouse tumors. *Cancer Res.* **45,** 6010–6016.
35. Allison, D. C., Anderson, S., Meyne, J., Ridolpho, P. F., and Robertson, J. (1988). Alterations in the DNA metabolism of MCa-11 mouse mammary tumor cells grown *in vivo* and *in vitro*. *Cancer Res.* **46,** 3951–3957.
36. Allison, D. C., Bose, K. B., Anderson, S., Curley, S., and Robertson, J. (1989). Slowing of cell cycle traverse for cells in exponential monolayer cultures placed into plateau-fed and starved medium. *Cancer Res.* **49,** 1456–1464.
37. Allison, D. C., Chakerian, M., Ridolpho, P., Curley, S., Wilder, M., Anderson, S., and Robertson, J. (1987). Combined flow and absorption DNA measurements of (^{3}H)thymidine labeled tumor cells. *Cell Tissue Kinet.* **20,** 273–290.
38. Allison, D. C., Meyne, J., Ridolpho, P. F., Bose, K., Chakerian, M., and Robertson, J. (1984). Computerized measurement of the DNA content areas and autoradiographic grains of the same nuclei. *J. Histochem. Cytochem.* **32,** 1197–1203.
39. Gratzner, H. G. (1982). Monoclonal antibiody to 5-bromo- and 5-iodo-deoxyuridine: A new reagent for detection of DNA replication. *Science* **218,** 474.
40. Lin, P., and Allison, D. C. (1993). Measurement of DNA content and of tritiated thymidine and bromodeoxyurdine incorporation by the same cells. *J. Histochem. Cytochem.* **41,** 1435–1439.
41. Simpson-Herren, L., Sanford, A. H., Holinquist, J. P., Springer, T. A., and Lloyd, H. A. (1976). Ambiguity of the thymidine index. *Cancer Res.* **36,** 4705–4709.
42. Allison, D. C., Lawrence, G. N., O'Grady, B. J., Rasch, R. W., and Rasch, E. M. (1984). Increased accuracy and speed of absorption cytometric DNA measurements by automatic correction for nuclear darkness. *Cytometry* **5,** 217–227.
43. Allison, D. C., Mayall, B. H., Levin, F., and Levin, J. (1988). Comparison of absorption measurements of DNA stain content by utilizing video and scanning image cytometers. *Cytometry* **9,** 573–578.
44. Dooley, W. C., Allison, D. C., Lin, P., and Paul, M. (1993) Evidence for altered cell-cycle traverse of the non-model cells of the heteroploid MCa-11 line. *Cell Prolif.* **26,** 349–360.

19

Hematopoietic Stem Cells: Basic Concepts and Applications to Surgical Research

Henry E. Rice,* Robert W. Storms,† Clay Smith,† and Alan W. Flake‡

** Division of Pediatric Surgery, Department of Surgery, and †Center for Genetic and Cellular Therapy, Duke University Medical Center, Durham, North Carolina 27710*

‡ Department of Surgery and the Center for Fetal Diagnosis and Therapy, Children's Hospital of Philadelphia, University of Pennsylvania, Philadelphia, Pennsylvania 19104

I. Introduction

Although over 40 years have passed since the first transplants of hematopoietic stem cells (HSCs), applications of stem cell transplantation continue to expand. In many areas of medical and scientific research, the use of hematopoietic and other stem cell-based strategies has revolutionized clinical treatment and opened new areas of basic research investigation. For the surgical investigator, the use of stem cell-based applications has supported many exciting and novel approaches to surgical disease.

At present in the United States, over 20,000 hematopoietic stem cell transplants are performed annually, usually for the treatment of hematologic and solid organ malignancies. New areas of investigation include the use of HSCs to induce tolerance for solid organ transplantation, to serve as a vehicle for gene therapy, and to treat a fetus *in utero* for a variety of inherited conditions. Given the wide range of applications for stem cell transplantation, it is no surprise that these areas are receiving a great deal of interest by the National Institutes of Health. An understanding of the biology of stem cells and their potential application to surgical research is of increasing importance to the surgical investigator.

II. Historical Review

In the early twentieth century, through the work of Alex Carrel and others, it was clear that a transplanted solid organ or skin allograft would function for a short period of time before the graft would be lost. Owen first observed that freemartin bovine dizygotic cattle twins, who shared placental circulation of blood, were chimeric for their siblings blood type (1). This observation of nature paved the way for subsequent studies by Billingham, Brent, and Medawar, who demonstrated that donor-specific tolerance could be induced by injection of donor hematopoietic stem cells into newborn mice tolerant for solid organ or skin grafts from their twins (2).

Recognition of the biologic basis for hematopoietic cell transplantation began with the studies of Jacobson, who demonstrated that transplantation of spleen or marrow cells would protect a mouse from lethal irradiation (3). The finding that cellular reconstitution was responsible for irradiation protection following marrow transfusion was shown by Main and Prehn (4). Early murine studies defined many of the factors responsible for a successful marrow graft, and demonstrated that allogeneic donor marrow cells could mount an immune attack against the host, resulting in a wasting disease, now recognized as graft-versus-host disease (GVHD). It was soon established that the severity of GVHD was controlled by genetic factors, later defined as histocompatability (human leukocyte) antigens (5).

The first clinical attempts at bone marrow transplantation were characterized by a series of successive treatment failures. In 1959, Thomas reported the first successful bone marrow transplant using an identical twin donor (6). However, early allogeneic transplants were unsuccessful prior to the full understanding of human leukocyte antigen (HLA) typing. The modern era of marrow transplantation began in the late 1960s, when a number of investigators began using marrow from HLA-matched siblings for treating leukemia or aplastic anemia. Eight of the first 100 transplant recipients were alive more than 20 years later, demonstrating that at least some patients with leukemia could be cured of their disease using bone marrow transplantation.

After the initial success with bone marrow transplantation for advanced leukemia, marrow transplantation became accepted for earlier stage leukemia. In the 1980s, hematopoietic stem cell transplantation became one of the standard treatment options for a range of malignant diseases that all had in common a high mortality with conventional therapy. Furthermore, hematopoietic stem cell transplantation began to be advocated for nonmalignant conditions such as immunodeficiencies, aplastic anemia, and hemoglobinopathies.

III. Hematopoiesis

Hematopoiesis is a dynamic process in which various blood elements are developed in bone marrow and other hematopoietic sites, and are maintained at physiologic levels. This process is carefully regulated by multiple control mechanisms, and results in a balance between cell proliferation and cell death. Hematopoiesis is maintained by pluripotent hematopoietic stem cells, with each HSC capable of either self-renewal or differentiation into any hematopoietic cell lineage (Fig. 1).

Although true human HSCs have never been definitively identified, current data suggest that the number of HSCs in a human is relatively small compared to the number of other hematopoietic progenitor cells. Studies by Abkowitz *et al.* (7) in cats suggest that the majority of HSCs are quiescent, and at any one time only a small number of HSCs are contributing to hematopoiesis. Animal models of hematopoiesis in immunodeficient mice suggest that the frequency of HSCs capable of contributing to all hematopoietic cell lineages is present at approximately 1–5 cells per million cells of bone marrow.

After transplantation, HSCs home to the recipient hematopoietic stromal environment. If conditions are favorable, hematopoietic stem cells engraft in these spaces and then are able under strict physiologic control to differentiate and proliferate into all hematopoietic lineages. An understanding of this complex process of HSC engraftment and control is important for the investigation of HSC transplantation for clinical purposes.

IV. Embryonic Stem Cells

Embryonic stem (ES) cells are self-renewing pluripotent stem cells of embryonic origin, first isolated from the inner cell mass of developing mouse blastocysts. These cells are characterized both by their capacity to be maintained in an undifferentiated state indefinitely *in vitro* and by their potential to differentiate into all cell lineages when implanted back into a blastocyst. In the presence of a differentiation inhibitory factor known as leukemia inhibitory factor (LIF), ES cells can be maintained indefinitely in an undifferentiated state in culture. When LIF is withdrawn, ES cells differentiate to form embryoid bodies (EBs) that contain elements of all three embryonic germ layers: ectoderm, mesoderm, and endoderm. As differentiation continues, a wide range of cell types, including hematopoietic, endothelial, muscle, and neuronal cells, develop within the EBs (8).

Potential applications of ES cell-based research include both basic research and clinically directed therapies. ES cells provide an opportunity to study the genetic events regulating lineage commitment and tissue development. The

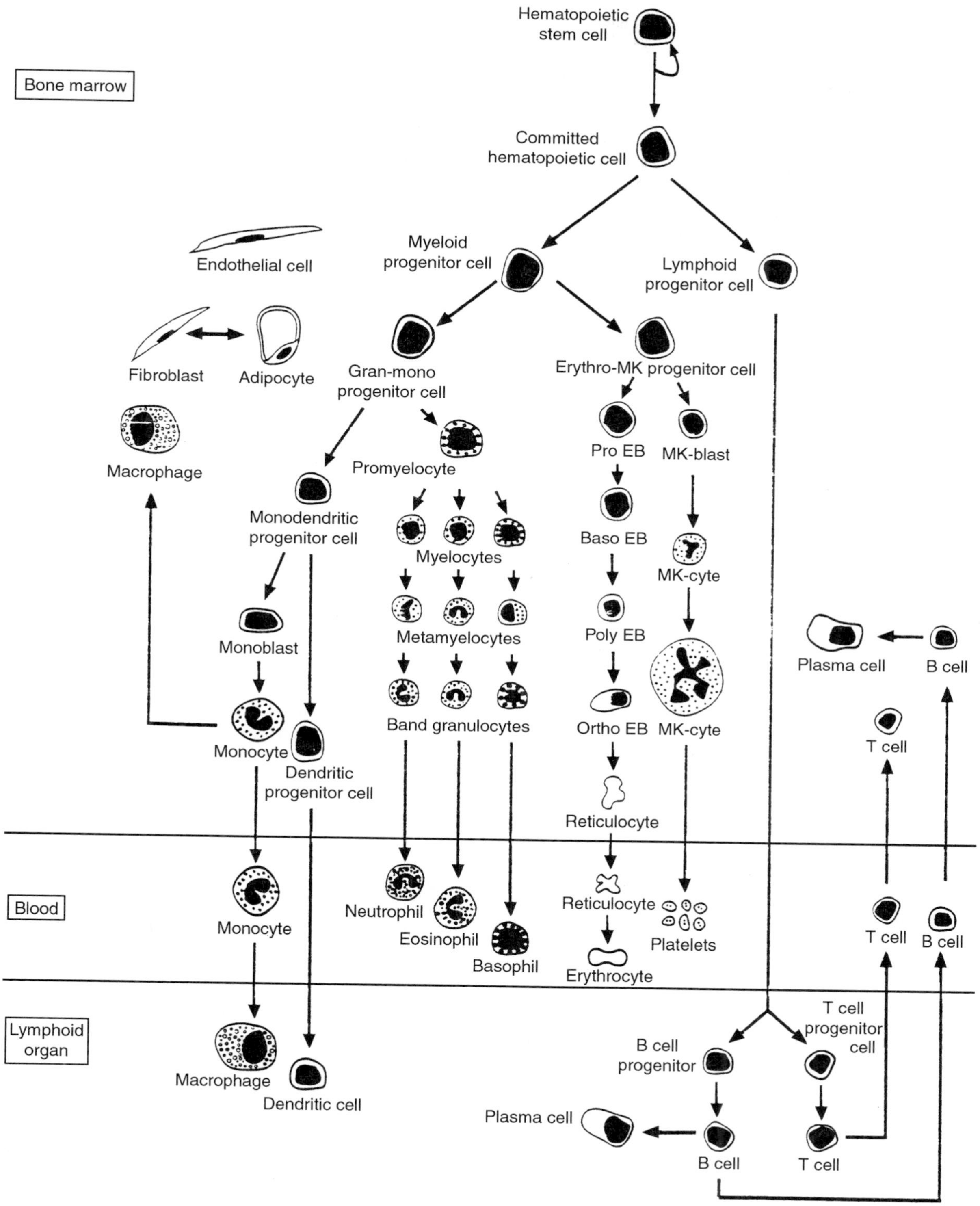

Figure 1 Onotogeny of hematopoietic stem cells. Cells originate from putative primitive, totipotent stem cells and differentiate into various hematopoietic cell lineages. With permission, from "Wintrobe's Clinical Hematology," 10th Ed., Williams & Wilkins, Baltimore, 1998.

control of ES cell differentiation can be used to develop a rapid assay for the study of most genes, offering an *in vitro* assay to complement the long-term *in vivo* mouse transgenic systems currently used to examine many genes. In theory, EBs could provide an unlimited supply of specific cell types for transplantation. To date, ES cell-derived cardiomyocytes, neural precursors, and hematopoietic precursors have been transplanted into recipient animals. (9–11). Finally, human ES cells can be used to evaluate the toxicity of new drugs, because many of the cell types and mutations in cell development will mimic the effect of these drugs on human or animal growth.

Current limitations to the application of ES cell-based therapies include donor/recipient incompatibility and graft rejection. Several novel lines of investigation are addressing these limitations, including cloning studies in which nuclear transfer could be used to produce starting material that would allow the isolation of individualized ES cell lines (12). These cell lines would be genetically identical to those of the patient, thereby limiting the immunologic rejection of the graft. Two major developments in ES biology have greatly enhanced the use of these cells for research purposes. Gearhart and colleagues have developed a human embryonic germ cell line that functions as totipotent ES cells (13). As well, Thomson and others have described the isolation of human cells with the properties of ES cells (14).

V. Mesenchymal Stem Cells

Adult bone marrow contains a number of cellular elements, including the major source of hematopoietic stem cells. However, bone marrow stroma also contains mesenchymal stem cells (MSCs), which contribute to the regeneration of bone, cartilage, muscle, tendon, adipose tissue, and stroma (15). This multipotentiality, in combination with their ease of expansion and the relative efficiency of genetic manipulation of MSCs, suggests clinical applications in tissue engineering, cellular transplantation, and gene therapy. In addition, the complex interaction between recipient bone marrow stroma and donor hematopoietic cells is fundamental for hematopoietic stem cell engraftment following transplantation. Therefore, MSC transplantation may be effective as a method to augment the engraftment of donor hematopoietic cells or hasten hematopoietic reconstitution after bone marrow transplantation.

Putative MSCs have been isolated from human bone marrow by density centrifugation and selective cell culture in a medium that supports mesenchymal cells (16). The colony-forming unit-fibroblast (CFU-F) assay has been used to confirm the role of MSCs in stromal cell formation *in vitro* and has been used to evaluate stromal progenitors for clinical and research applications. These cells are characterized by their ability to proliferate in culture with an attached, well-spread morphology, by the presence of a consistent set of marker proteins on their surface, and by their differentiation to multiple mesenchymal lineages under controlled *in vitro* conditions. The successful isolation and characterization of human MSCs may allow the potential use of these cells for the restoration of damaged or diseased mesenchymal tissue.

VI. In Utero HSC Transplantation

The *in utero* transplantation of HSCs is developing as an alternative to postnatal transplantation of HSCs for the treatment of various congenital disorders that can be diagnosed during fetal development. Advances in prenatal diagnosis now allow the diagnosis of many hematologic, immunologic, and metabolic disorders by analysis of trophoblastic tissue obtained by amniocentesis or chorionic villus sampling. The evolution of high-resolution ultrasound and other fetal imaging and surgical techniques has overcome many of the obstacles to performing early-gestation cellular therapy.

The biologic rationale for *in utero* HSC transplantation is compelling. As originally observed by Owen (1), the early-gestation fetus is relatively immunologically immature and uniquely tolerant to foreign antigens. Under specific conditions, the fetal environment may be permissive for the engraftment of foreign HSCs without the need for extensive myeloablation. The successful *in utero* engraftment of HSCs could prevent the development of severe clinical manifestations of several diseases that occur during gestation, thus limiting morbidity due to the underlying disease.

Although *in utero* HSC transplantation may offer theoretical advantages over postnatal transplantation for various inherited diseases, the clinical experience to date has suggested that an *in utero* HSC transplantation is quite difficult to accomplish. In over 25 attempts to transplant human fetuses with HSCs for a number of conditions, the only clear successful and long-lasting transplants are in the few fetuses with inherited immunodeficiencies (17). Thus the concept that an *in utero* HSC transplant might be the ideal cure for all inherited hematologic or metabolic diseases has been transformed into the recognition that in most diseases, there is no selective advantage for the engraftment of allogeneic donor cells in the fetal environment. Further clinical attempts with *in utero* HSC transplantation are being approached cautiously, as questions are being addressed to define the barriers to *in utero* HSC engraftment.

Surgical models to examine the engraftment of HSCs after *in utero* transplantation have had a variable degree of success. Normal immunocompetent animals have been used to accept the transplant of either allogeneic or xenogeneic hematopoietic stem cells, the most successful of which is the fetal lamb model. In contrast to the fetal lamb, the level of engraftment of HSCs in other animals is relatively low, and below what might be expected to be therapeutic for most diseases.

In contrast to normal animals, it is clear that animal models in which there is a selective advantage for the engraftment of donor cells demonstrate a high level of donor engraftment. This phenomenon was first demonstrated by Fleishman and Mintz (18), who demonstrated that *in utero* transplantation of HSCs in w/w mutant anemic mice can result in complete hematopoietic reconstitution. The degree of erythroid replacement is dependent on the severity of the anemia, and donor myeloid engraftment is less than that of red cells. This phenomenon has been demonstrated in several other models of murine immunodeficiencies or anemias, including those involving severe combined immune-deficient and nonobese diabetic (SCID, NOD/SCID) mice and β-thalassemia.

To overcome the barriers for donor HSC engraftment *in utero*, a number of strategies are currently being studied. One common approach may be to increase the donor cell number by increasing the dose of HSCs in a single transplant or by performing repeated donor cell transplants. Other approaches may be to use specific subpopulations of donor cells or to "condition" the recipient by performing MSC or stromal cotransplants. Finally, methods to achieve minimal nontoxic myeloablation or to actively suppress the immunologic response are possible and may allow increased application of *in utero* HSC transplantation in the future.

VII. Stem Cell Transplantation to Induce Tolerance

One of the most potentially exciting applications of stem cell transplantation is for the facilitation of immunologic tolerance to solid organ grafts. The basis for this work dates to the original observation that freemartin cattle twins who shared placental circulation of blood were tolerant of the siblings' skin grafts after birth (1). Tolerance induction for solid organ grafts has been the "holy grail" of transplantation research for many years, and data now suggest that the induction of tolerance may be facilitated by the creation of hematopoietic chimerism between the donor and host.

Immunologic tolerance for grafts following stem cell transplantation is based on a complex series of thymic central and peripheral processes resulting in both clonal deletion and clonal reactivity of host cells to donor tissue. Sykes and others have shown in B6 mice that received a nonlethal transplant regimen of both depleting anti-CD4 and anti-CD8 monoclonal antibodies as well as local thymic irradiation that the transplantation of MHC-mismatched B10 bone marrow results in permanent, multilineage mixed chimerism, donor-specific skin graft tolerance, and *in vitro* tolerance (19). Flake and others have shown that after *in utero* HSC transplantation in mice, the tolerant state is characterized by partial clonal deletion of donor-reactive T cells combined with clonal anergy of nondeleted donor-reactive T cells (20).

In clinical practice, the induction of tolerance after hematopoietic stem cell transplantation has been difficult to achieve. In some human cases, immunologic tolerance has been reported in patients after withdrawal of immunosuppression, by the persistent function of a solid allograft. This tolerance may be due to the presence of donor hematopoietic micro chimerism related to "passenger" hematopoietic elements in the graft, although the relationship of chimerism to tolerance has not been conclusively demonstrated. To enhance the acceptance of organs, perioperative infusion of donor bone marrow has been attempted with variable success. It has been suggested that established microchimerism is not only associated with long-term acceptance of the graft, but it also plays an active role in induction and maintenance of donor-specific unresponsiveness (21). However, the mechanisms responsible for prolonged graft survival in this setting remain speculative. In the future, optimization of this strategy to achieve higher levels of mixed chimerism may overcome the immunologic barriers to allogeneic organ and cellular transplantation.

VIII. In Vitro Techniques

A variety of laboratory techniques are critical to understanding stem cell biology. A few of the essential techniques are summarized below.

A. Cluster Designation and Stem Cell Nomenclature

Beginning in the 1980s, lineage-specific monoclonal antibodies began to be used to characterize antigens present on hematopoietic cells at various stages of differentiation. In 1982, the first International Workshop on Human Leukocyte Differentiation Antigens led to the basis for the identification of cluster designation (CD) to group antibodies, which will recognize the same protein or carbohydate antigen on a cell surface. Now over 100 CD designations are applied commonly to hematopoietic cells and form the basis of flow cytometry analysis and sorting of hematopoietic cells. Current studies are focused on the function of antigens defined by a given CD marker. CD markers useful for studying human hematopoietic stem cells include CD34, CD38, and CD33.

B. Flow Cytometry

Flow cytometry is an indispensable tool for identifying and isolating hematopoietic and other stem cells. This technique is based on the measurement of various cellular properties as cells move in a fluid stream, and is capable of rapid, quantitative, multiparameter analysis of heterogeneous cell populations on a cell-by-cell basis. Although any more than a cursory introduction to flow cytometry is beyond this text, several principles of flow cytometry are basic to the understanding of this technology.

Cytometers use a laser light source, usually an argon beam, for two purposes. First, the laser can be used to quantify various intrinsic cellular parameters. Once a cell is injected into a fluid stream, light from the beam at the incident wavelength will be scattered by the cell, and the dynamics of this light scatter can be detected. Two parameters, termed forward and side scatter, reflect the cell size and granularity, respectively. Thus a given cell suspension will result in a typical light-scatter profile that will reflect these intrinsic cellular characteristics.

A second process, which occurs after a laser beam has intersected with a cell, is based on the ability of fluorochromes present in or bound to the cell to absorb the laser light and re-emit the light at a different wavelength, a property known as fluorescence (Table I). The amount of emitted light is proportional to the amount and strength of the fluorochrome. This emitted light is separated into its constituent wavelengths, and each is directed to a different photodetector. Light from several different fluorochromes can be physically separated and individually quantitated by cytometry analysis computer systems. Computer software can then process each individual signal and develop patterns that reflect the cellular constituents.

Table I Hematopoietic Stem Cell Processing from Human Umbilical Cord Blood or Bone Marrow for Research Purposes

1. Collect human umbilical cord blood with sterile technique from umbilical vein after passage of human placenta. Collect blood or bone marrow (30–75 ml) in sterile container with 25 ml of ACD as anticoagulant. Transfer to sterile tissue culture hood for processing. Use universal precautions for all tissue handling.
2. Dilute blood 1:1 with phosphate-buffered saline (PBS) and place 40 ml in a 50-ml conical tube.
3. Add 8 ml of 6% hetastarch and gently invert to mix (final concentration, 1% hetastarch). Incubate at room temperature for 60 min to agglutinate red blood cells. Transfer top 25–30 ml of supernatent to new conical tube. Wash twice with 25–30 ml of PBS. Spin at 1200 *g* for 5–6 min at room temperature.
4. Wash pellet with 10 ml of lysis buffer (0.17 *N* ammonium chloride, 20 m*M* TRIS, 0.2 m*M* EDTA, pH 7.2). Spin at 1200 *g* for 5–6 min.
5. Resuspend pellet in 30 ml of lysis buffer. Incubate at 37°C for 30–60 min to allow lysis of red blood cells.
6. Spin at 1200 *g* for 5–6 min. Wash pellet twice with PBS and enumerate.
7. Pellet at this stage will include all primitive and mature hematopoietic progenitors. Usual yield is (2–3) × 10^8 cells/umbilical cord. Usual fraction of cells expressing CD34 is 1–2%.

Table II Fluorochromes Commonly Used in Flow Cytometry

	Wavelength (nm)	
Fluorochrome	Excitation	Emission
Fluorescein isothiocyanate	488	530
Phycoerythrin	488	580
Peridinin chlorophyll	488	670
Allophycocyanin	633	670

C. Purification of Human HSC Cells

Human hematopoietic stem cells can be harvested from a number of sources, including bone marrow, peripheral blood, and umbilical cord blood. Each cell source has its particular merits for clinical and research purposes. To isolate stem cells from each of these tissues, a variety of strategies have been developed. For example, our protocol for the isolation of human HSCs is based on a series of steps to enrich the tissue for hematopoietic progenitors (Table II). First, red blood cells are removed using agglutination and lysis. The resultant mononuclear cells are then treated to remove lineage-committed cells via a variety of techniques, such as a negative-selection cell separation column (StemSep; StemCell Technologies, Vancouver, Canada) (Fig. 2). This technique is based on the staining of the mononuclear cells with a mixture of lineage-specific antibodies (CD2, CD3, CD14, CD16, CD19, CD24, CD56, CD66b, glycophorin A), followed by the addition of secondary antibody conjugated to metal colloid. Unwanted cells are immunomagnetically labeled, and then eluted through a magnetized column in order to enrich for cells not expressing the lineage markers (Lin^-). Advantages of a negative-selection separation column include the rapidity of the technique, allowing the recovery of cells that have not been previously labeled.

If a very purified cell population is required, further depletion of committed progenitors can be performed using fluorescence-activated cell sorting (FACS). After the depletion of Lin^+ cells using a StemSep column, the resultant Lin^- cells can be stained with a variety of antibodies, such as CD34 and CD38, to separate cells expressing these surface antigens. The stained cells can then be sorted by using a high-flow automated cell sorter, equipped with 5-W and 30-mW helium neon lasers (Fig. 3). The use of cell sorters typically results in sorted cell fractions with high levels of purity (98–99%).

D. Colony-Forming Assays

Insights into hematopoietic stem cell precursors have been provided in large part by *in vitro* colony techniques. Hematopoietic cells can be plated in semisolid media, usual-

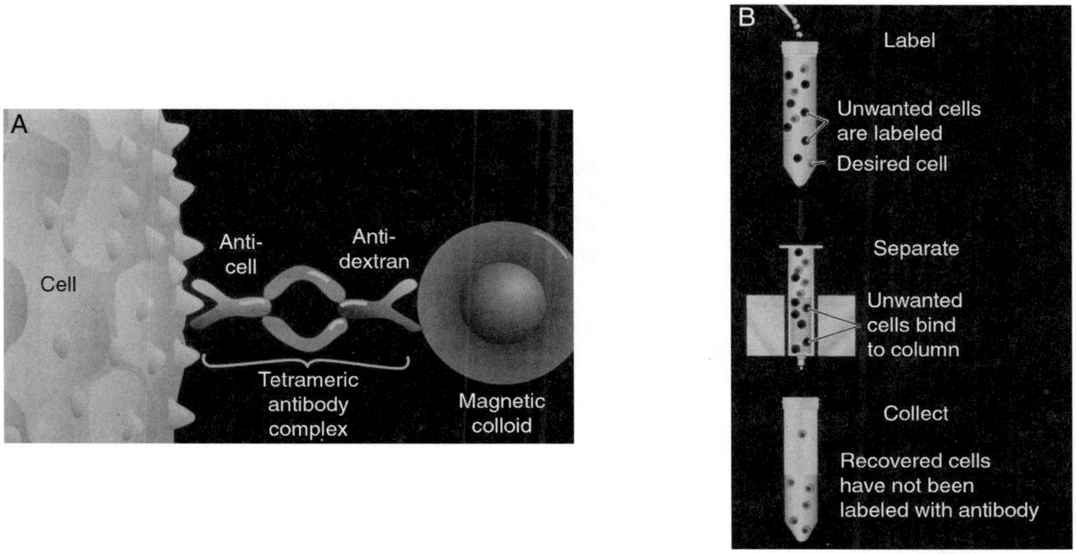

Figure 2 (A) StemSep method for negative selection of human hematopoietic stem cells. Human cells are directly labeled with magnetic particles using a cocktail of tetrameric antibody complexes representing various lineage-committed cell markers. Human cells are cross-linked to dextran iron particles using tetrameric antibody complexes composed of two murine IgG monoclonal antibodies. (B) The cell separation is then passed through a high-gradient magnetic column of stainless-steel mesh. The magnetically labeled cells (Lin^+) bind to the column while the unlabeled cells (Lin^-) pass through. With permission, from StemCell Technologies, Vancouver, Canada.

ly methlycellulose, which has been supplemented with species-specific growth factors. After 14–16 days, the cells proliferate and differentiate into isolated colonies that can be distinguished as granulocyte/macrophage or erythroid lineages. The colony progenitors are hierarchically organized; undifferentiated blast colonies can terminally differentiate into all types of myeloid and erythroid colonies, including those of early multilineage colony-forming units (CFU-GEMM). Applications for methlycellulose progenitor assays include the characterization of hematopoietic progenitors from cord blood or other source of interest, quality control for stem cell processing, the confirmation of cell viability following cryopreservation, and the quantitation of progenitors following *ex vivo* expansion.

The earliest hematopoietic progenitor cells can be assayed *in vitro* in a variety of culture systems, including long-term culture initiating cell (LTC-IC) culture systems, originally described in the 1970s (22). These long-term cultures require an adherent stromal layer of either primary or cell line-derived mesenchymal cells to be used with the hematopoietic cell population. This stroma supports the growth and differentiation of myeloid colonogenic progenitors for many weeks, provided that an appropriate medium is available. Common approaches to LTC-IC include the use of limiting dilution analysis to determine the frequency of LTC-ICs as well as the number of colony-forming cells (CFCs) in a cell population. Human LTC-ICs appear to originate from $CD34^+$ cells, and are a heterogeneous cell population.

IX. In Vivo Techniques

In addition to *in vitro* techniques for studying human hematopoietic stem cells, a variety of *in vivo* transplant models exist as well.

A. Xenogeneic Models of Human Hematopoiesis

The most conclusive way to identify stem cells is to document the repopulation of the cells in an animal model after transplantation. Animal models of human hematopoiesis, which are limited by xenogeneic rejection of foreign cells, have been relatively difficult to establish. The first murine models of human hematopoiesis used irradiated, athymic nude (nu/nu) mice, which resulted in relatively poor engraftment due to the retention of functional B cells, complement, and natural killer (NK) cells. The development of bg/nu/xid (BNX) mice and severe combined immune-deficient mice improved the engraftment of human HSCs (23). SCID mice are homozygous for a mutation in the *scid* gene, which results in unsuccessful DNA rearrangements and prevents the productive rearrangement of immunoglobulin and T cell receptor genes. These SCID mice are deficient in both T cell and B cell function. However, the residual NK cells and complement function limits the degree of engraftment of human cells.

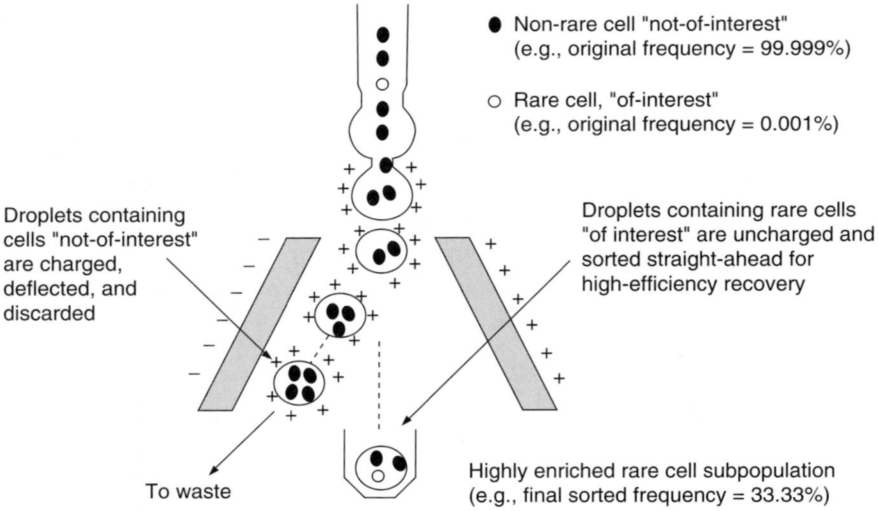

Figure 3 Fluorescence-activated cell sorting using flow cytometry for enrichment of rare cell populations. All cells are stained with fluorochrome-labeled monoclonal antibodies and then passed through a flow cytometer. This example shows "straight ahead" sorting, by which droplets containing rare cells of interest are uncharged and pass through for high-efficiency recovery. This sorting may be based on multiple parameters through the cytometer. From "Current Protocols in Cytometry," John Wiley & Sons, Inc., New York, 1997. Copyright © 1997 John Wiley & Sons, Inc. Reprinted by permission of Wiley-Liss, Inc., a subsidiary of John Wiley & Sons, Inc.

B. NOD/SCID Mice

Murine models of human HSC engraftment have been greatly improved by the development of the nonobese diabetic (NOD/SCID) mouse. These mice have less residual immunity than do SCID mice, because NOD mice have defects in the complement pathway and macrophage function (24). Transplantation of human bone marrow or umbilical cord blood into sublethally irradiated NOD/SCID mice results in low levels of long-term multilineage engraftment. This engraftment occurs 4–8 weeks after the intravenous injection of human cells, suggesting that primitive cells had engrafted. These cells have been termed SCID-repopulating cells (SRCs). Currently the NOD/SCID mouse is the most frequently used animal model to document the presence of human hematopoietic stem cells, and offers a relatively inexpensive and reproducible method to support many areas of research in human hematopoiesis.

C. Fetal Sheep Model

Efforts to reproduce "natural" chimerism in the laboratory by the *in utero* transplantation of allogeneic or xenogeneic HSCs have had variable degrees of success. The most successful animal model is the fetal lamb as described by Flake, Zanjani, and co-workers (25). In this model, the transplantation of allogeneic fetal liver-derived HSCs into early-gestation fetal lambs results in a high rate of sustained multilineage hematopoietic chimerism that is typically in the range of 10–15% of bone marrow cells and peripheral blood (26).

The fetal lamb model is also permissive for widely disparate xenogeneic engraftment, and is the best immunocompetent animal model to document the presence of human HSCs. Multilineage hematopoietic chimerism has been documented after transplantation of human fetal liver-derived HSCs, umbilical cord blood-derived HSCs, and adult bone marrow cells (25, 27). In this model, engraftment of true human HSCs is confirmed by repopulation following transplantation of recipient marrow into second-generation fetal lamb recipients. The major limitation to the use of this model to study human hematopoietic stem cells is primarily the cost. Other normal immunocompetent animals have been shown to accept the engraftment of human xenogeneic HSCs after *in utero* transplantation, although the engraftment rates and the reliability of these models are greatly inferior compared to the fetal lamb.

Acknowledgments

Supported in part by the Wagensteen Fund for Surgical Research of the American College of Surgeons, and by the Children's Miracle Network Foundation.

References

1. Owen, R. D. (1945). Immunologic consequences of vascular anastomoses between bovine twins. *Science* **102**, 400.
2. Billingham, R. E., Lampkin, G. H., Medawar, P. B., *et al.* (1952). Tolerance to homografts, twin diagnosis, and the freemarting condition in cattle. *Heredity* **6**, 201.

3. Jacobson, L. O., Marks, E. K., Robson, M. J., *et al.* (1949). Effect of spleen protection on mortality following x-irradiation. *J. Lab. Clin. Med.* **34**, 1538–1543.
4. Main, J. M., and Prehn, R. T. (1955). Successful skin homografts after the administration of high dosage X radiation and homologous bone marrow. *J. Natl. Cancer Inst.* **15**, 1023–1029.
5. Uphoff, D. E. (1957). Genetic factors influencing irradiation protection by bone marrow. *Proc. Soc. Exp. Biol. Med.* **92**, 123–125.
6. Thomas, E. D., Lochte, H. L., Jr., Cannon, J. H., *et al.* (1959). Supralethal whole body irradiation and isologous marrow transplantation in man. *J. Clin. Invest.* **38**, 1709–1716.
7. Abkowitz, J. L., Catlin, S. N., and Guttorp P. (1996). Evidence that hematopoiesis may be a stochastic process *in vivo. Nat. Med.* **2**, 190–197.
8. Keller, G. (1995). *In vitro* differentiation of embryonic stem cells. *Curr. Opin. Cell Biol.* **7**, 862–869.
9. Klug, M. G., Soonpaa, M. H., Koh, G. Y., *et al.* (1996). Genetically selected cardiomyocytes from differentiating embryonic stem cells from stable intracardiac grafts. *J. Clin. Invest.* **98**, 216–224.
10. Brustle, O., Spiro, A. C., Karram, K., *et al.* (1997). *In vitro*-generated neural precursors participate in mammalian brain development. *Proc. Natl. Acad. Sci. U.S.A.* **94,** 14809–14814.
11. Potocnik, A. J., Kohler, H., and Eichmann, K. (1997). Hematolymphoid *in vivo* reconstitution potential of subpopulations derived from *in vitro* differentiated embryonic stem cells. *Proc. Natl. Acad. Sci. U.S.A.* **94,** 10295–13000.
12. Kato, Y., Tani, T., Sotomaru, Y., *et al.* (1998). Eight calves cloned from somatic cells of a single adult. *Science* **282,** 2095–2098.
13. Shamblott, M. J., Axelman, J., Wang, S., *et al.* (1998). Derivation of pluripotent stem cells from cultured human primordial germ cells. *Proc. Natl. Acad. Sci. U.S.A.* **95,** 13726–13731.
14. Thomson, J. A., Itskovitz-Eldor, J., Shapiro, S. S., *et al.* (1998). Embryonic stem cell lines derived from human blastocysts. *Science* **282,** 1145–1147.
15. Haynesworth, S. E., Goshima, J., Goldberg, V. M., *et al.* (1992). Characterization of cells with osteogenic potential from human marrow. *Bone* **13,** 81–88.
16. Pittenger, M. F., Mackay, A. M., Beck, S. C., *et al.* (1999). Multilineage potential of adult human mesenchymal stem cells. *Science* **284,** 143–147.
17. Flake, A. W., and Zanajani, E. D. (1997). *In utero* hematopoietic stem cell transplantation. A status report. *JAMA* **278,** 932–937.
18. Fleischman, R. A., and Mintz, B. (1979). Prevention of genetic anemias in mice by microinjection of normal hematopoietic stem cells into the fetal placenta. *Proc. Natl. Acad. Sci. U.S.A.* **76,** 5736–5740.
19. Nikolic, B., and Sykes, M. (1997). Bone marrow chimerism and transplantation tolerance. *Curr. Opin. Immunol.* **9,** 634–640.
20. Kim, H. B., Shaaban, A. F., Milner, R., *et al.* (1999). *In utero* bone marrow transplantation induces donor-specific tolerance by a combination of clonal deletion and clonal anergy. *J. Pediatr. Surg.* **34,** 726–730.
21. Rao, A. S., Thomson, A. W., Shapiro, R., *et al.* (1994). Chimerism after whole organ transplantation: Its relationship to graft rejection and tolerance induction. *Curr. Opin. Nephrol. Hypertens.* **33:6,** 589–595.
22. Dexter, T. M., Allen, T. D., and Lajtha, L. G. (1977). Conditions controlling the proliferation of haemopoietic stem cells *in vitro. J. Cell Physiol.* **91,** 335–344.
23. Greiner, D. L., Hesselton, R. A., and Shultz, L. D. (1998). SCID mouse models of human stem cell engraftment. *Stem Cells* **16,** 166–177.
24. Kataoka, S., Satoh, J., Fujiya, H., *et al.* (1983). Immunologic aspects of the nonobese diabetic (NOD) mouse. *Diabetes* **32,** 247–253.
25. Zanjani, E. D., Flake, A. W., Rice, H., *et al.* (1994). Long-term repopulating ability of xenogeneic transplanted human fetal liver hematopoietic stem cells in sheep. *J. Clin. Invest.* **93,** 1051–1055.
26. Flake, A. W., Harrison, M. R., Adzick, N. S., *et al.* (1986). Transplantation of fetal hematopoietic stem cells *in utero:* The creation of hematopoietic chimeras. *Science* **233,** 776–778.
27. Srour, E. F., Zanjani, E. D., and Brandt, J. E., *et al.* (1992). Sustained human hematopoiesis in sheep transplanted in utero during early gestation with fractionated adult human bone marrow cells. *Blood* **79,** 1404–1412.

20

Basic Molecular Biological Methods in Surgical Research: Genetic Library Construction, Screening, and DNA Sequencing

Steve F. Abcouwer

Department of Biochemistry and Molecular Biology, University of New Mexico, School of Medicine, Albuquerque, New Mexico 87131

I. Introduction

What constitutes surgical research? Sometimes surgical research is inspired by a problem or phenomenon associated with a surgical procedure, but this is not the norm. Rather, surgical research encompasses any research performed in a surgical department, conducted by surgeons, conceived by surgeons, or financed by surgeons. Thus, surgical research is simply medical research that benefits from the views and experience of surgeons as well as from the financial resources of surgical departments. Consequently, surgical research is now in direct competition with all facets of medical research conducted by medical and basic science departments. Thus, when seeking to publish results, the surgical researcher may find that reviewers hold their work to a higher standard, set outside the realms of surgical departments. Such reviewers may suggest that work is "phenomenological" and not "mechanistic." This can lead to manuscript rejection because many scientific and medical journals are eagerly seeking to focus more on molecular bases. Often such rejection stems from the fact that the reviewers come from a molecular background and have grown accustomed to research that answers molecular rather the medical questions. However, it can also stem from the fact that reviewers often realize that additional experiments of a molecular nature can provide much-needed insights into biological phenomena. What is more, reviewers may view experiments that utilize molecular techniques as commonplace, and therefore think nothing of suggesting that they be completed before deeming the manuscript worthy of publication.

Given that medical research is increasingly focusing on molecular analysis, the surgical researcher must contend with the rapidly developing field of molecular biology. This may seem a daunting task for the clinically busy surgeon, especially now that molecular biology is undergoing a technological revolution with the advent of genomics, functional genomics, expression profiling, and proteomics. These disciplines represent technology-driven science, rather than hypothesis-driven science, with the goal of gathering huge amounts of information on the sequence, expression, and function of genes. The information gleaned from this research will soon render it possible to perform many biological experiments on the Internet rather than in the laboratory. Some have predicted that such a capability will render more traditional molecular biological methods obsolete. However, there will always be a need for hypothesis-driven biological research aimed at solving medical problems, and basic molecular biological methods will still be needed for these studies. The information obtained from genomics, functional genomics, expression profiling, and proteomics will only help us to conceive more appropriate hypotheses and to more easily test these hypotheses. Surgeons possess unique medical knowledge that allows them to propose highly relevant hypotheses. However, without knowledge of molecular processes, a surgical researcher cannot even envision what mechanistic questions are feasible to answer. Reading this chapter cannot substitute for gaining experience and knowledge of molecular biological processes and the methods to monitor them. The information here, however, provides a framework for further study and perhaps for communication with those who can help facilitate the adoption of molecular methods into the surgical research laboratory.

Consider that such a framework as can be provided by this chapter is not sufficient to enable the utilization of the potential of molecular biology. Then consider that the use of molecular biological methods is commonly viewed to be as easy as opening the right catalog. Today, it might even be said that it is as easy as contracting the right molecular biology service company. This is increasingly true for a subset of molecular techniques such as library screening, sequencing, and antibody production. However, molecular biology is both a set of methods and a discipline. The effective use of molecular methods to answer medical hypotheses requires a good deal of knowledge. The knowledge base consists of what methods are available, what methods are appropriate, how easy or difficult each method is to master, how quantitative and reliable a given method is, the sources of error associated with a method, the costs, and the equipment that is needed. Obtaining a kit from a catalog will often greatly facilitate the utilization of a molecular method. However, no kit is truly complete and instruction manuals are notoriously wanting. Often very subtle but crucial bits of information can only be obtained from experience. There is no substitute for understanding the content of each reagent and the purpose and operation of each step in a procedure. Such knowledge enables troubleshooting when the results are not as advertised. More importantly, knowledge of a procedure is often crucial for correctly evaluating the results obtained. A principal investigator should not rely on the data interpretations presented by an associate or even a colleague. Rather, a principal investigator must have sufficient knowledge of the methods used in the conduction of his or her research project to provide an interpretation of data.

II. Genetic Library Construction, Screening, and DNA Sequencing

As the name implies, molecular biology involves the study of biological processes on the molecular level. This includes genes, ribonucleic acids (RNAs), proteins, peptides, carbohydrates, lipids, and ions. Most often, and in this discussion, molecular biology refers to the study of genes, messenger RNAs (mRNAs), and proteins, as well as the production, function, and interactions of these molecules. In this context, molecular biology includes the study of three main areas: molecular genetics, gene expression, and molecular interactions. A technological revolution has given birth to the fields of genomics, functional genomics, expression profiling, and proteomics. These fields are rapidly changing the way that molecular genetics, gene expression, and molecular interactions are studied. This is not to say that basic molecular biological techniques are no longer useful. Rather, these methods remain indispensable and knowledge of the basic principles on which they are based is crucial to understanding the emerging technologies. This chapter represents an introduction to three methods that have made this revolution possible—genetic library construction, library screening, and DNA sequencing.

Often when one thinks of molecular biology, one thinks of gene discovery. In reality, gene hunting is a relatively small part of molecular biology. Furthermore, with progression of genomic technology, including sequencing of the entire human genome, mouse genome, and soon the rat genome, gene discovery as we now know it will become less and less necessary. All genes will have been sequenced and catalogued (although perhaps not discovered). What will become increasingly important is the study of gene expression and function made possible by this revolution in genomics. Surgical research will benefit from the ability to identify and obtain genetic clones in ways much more expedient than traditional library construction and screening followed by clone isolation and sequencing. However, these methods will still be useful, and a knowledge of these techniques indispensable. Furthermore, it is important to be aware of the utility of genetic informatics as a cloning tool.

A. Genetic Libraries

Genetic libraries are the keys to the genomic revolution taking place today. Simply stated, a library is a population of DNA molecules containing all the necessary sequence information to allow DNA propagation in a cellular host. Also in the library are molecules that carry inserts representing a complex genome or a complex mRNA population from a cell or tissue. Libraries are of two main types, genomic and cDNA. Genomic libraries are created by isolating genomic DNA from a cell or tissue, cleaving it into relatively small pieces (usually by the use of restriction enzymes), and inserting these pieces into the carrier DNA molecule, called a vector, by a process called ligation. These libraries are then introduced into hosts, which supply the machinery needed to duplicate these DNA molecules and pass them along to their progeny. Hosts include bacteria, viruses, and yeast. Initially, circular plasmid vectors propagated in bacteria were used (1–4). Bacteriophage vectors that took advantage of a lytic viral life cycle in bacteria soon displaced these (5–7). The most common bacteriophage vector is a family of filamentous phage vectors called lamda (λ). Today, most genomic libraries are constructed using bacterial artificial chromosome (BAC) and yeast artificial chromosome (YAC) vectors (8). As the names imply, these vectors masquerade as chromosomes in these cells, being duplicated and distributed equally between daughter cells during synthesis, cytokinesis, and mitosis. These vectors are preferred because they have the ability to carry DNA inserts many times longer than the largest inserts carried by plasmid and bacteriophage vectors.

B. cDNA Library Construction

Well-constructed cDNA libraries carry inserts that represent the population of mRNA molecules within the cells or tissue of interest. For several reasons. cDNA libraries are much more difficult to construct than genomic libraries. Several detailed protocols have been published (9–11). All these procedures have common basic steps (Fig. 1) (12). First, intact mRNA must be isolated and purified. There are many RNA and mRNA purification protocols suitable for various types of cells and tissues (9, 11, 13, 14). It is essential that the mRNA used as starting material to produce a cDNA library is both pure and undegraded. The mRNA must be free of chemical contaminants that may inhibit subsequent reactions during the library construction process. The mRNA must be free of contaminating DNA, which would be incorporated into the library more efficiently than the mRNA sequences. Any mRNA degradation will result in a library that is not representative of the mRNA population present in the original sample, and may cause the complete loss of rare mRNA species.

Once isolated and purified the mRNA is reverse transcribed, producing single-stranded DNA complementary to the mRNA molecules in a process deemed "first-strand synthesis." This is done using an RNase H-deficient reverse transcriptase enzyme in the presence of an oligonucleotide primer, buffer, salts, and deoxynucleotide triphosphates (dNTPs) (15). Various primers are used, depending on the library construction scheme. Usually, the primer sequence includes a "linker" and a stretch of thymine DNA bases (oligo-dT) (16). The linker contains a restriction site that will be utilized when inserting the cDNA into a library vector. The oligo-dT stretch of the primers is intended to anneal to the 3′-poly(A) tails of the mRNA molecules. The annealed DNA primes the reverse transcriptase polymerization reaction, which adds complementary dNTPs to the 3′ end of the primer in accordance with the sequence of the mRNA. The primer is extended until the enzyme reaches the 5′ cap of the mRNA, or until the enzyme is halted or inhibited in some fashion. Partial cDNAs that are less than full-length will result if a primer anneals to an internal poly(A) group or if the reverse transcriptase enzyme is blocked by secondary structure in the mRNA. Proper annealing temperatures and denaturants that inhibit RNA secondary structure are used to reduce the incidence of truncated cDNAs. Often, 5-methyl-dCTP is used in place of unmodified dCTP during reverse transcription to produce hemimethylated first strands, which are resistant to restriction enzymes used in subsequent construction steps.

Before insertion into a vector, the RNA–DNA hybrid created by first-strand synthesis must be converted to double-stranded DNA in a process termed "second-strand synthesis." To do this, the mRNA template must be removed and the second strand must be primed and synthesized. One method of accomplishing this is initiated by treating the hybrid with RNase H, followed by DNA polymerase I. RNase H nicks the mRNA strand and DNA polymerase I synthesizes the second DNA strand using the nicked RNA as multiple primers. The DNA polymerase replaces the ribonucleotides of the mRNA strands with deoxyribonucleotides and then repairs the nicks between strands, resulting in an intact secondary strand. This double-strand complementary DNA (ds-cDNA) is then tipped with adapter sequences that allow digestion with specific restriction enzymes and insertion into a cloning vector. After restriction digestion of the cDNA ends, excess adapters, cleaved adapter pieces, and deoxyribonucleotides must be completely removed from the cDNA molecules. This is usually accomplished by size-exclusion chromatography, using a flow, push, or spin column filled with a porous gel matrix. Once prepared and purified, the cDNAs are ligated into cloning vector molecules. When using λ phage, each cDNA end is attached to a different phage DNA "arm," resulting in a library of recombinant phage DNA molecules. Before this library can be replicated, however, the DNA must be "packaged" into phage particles.

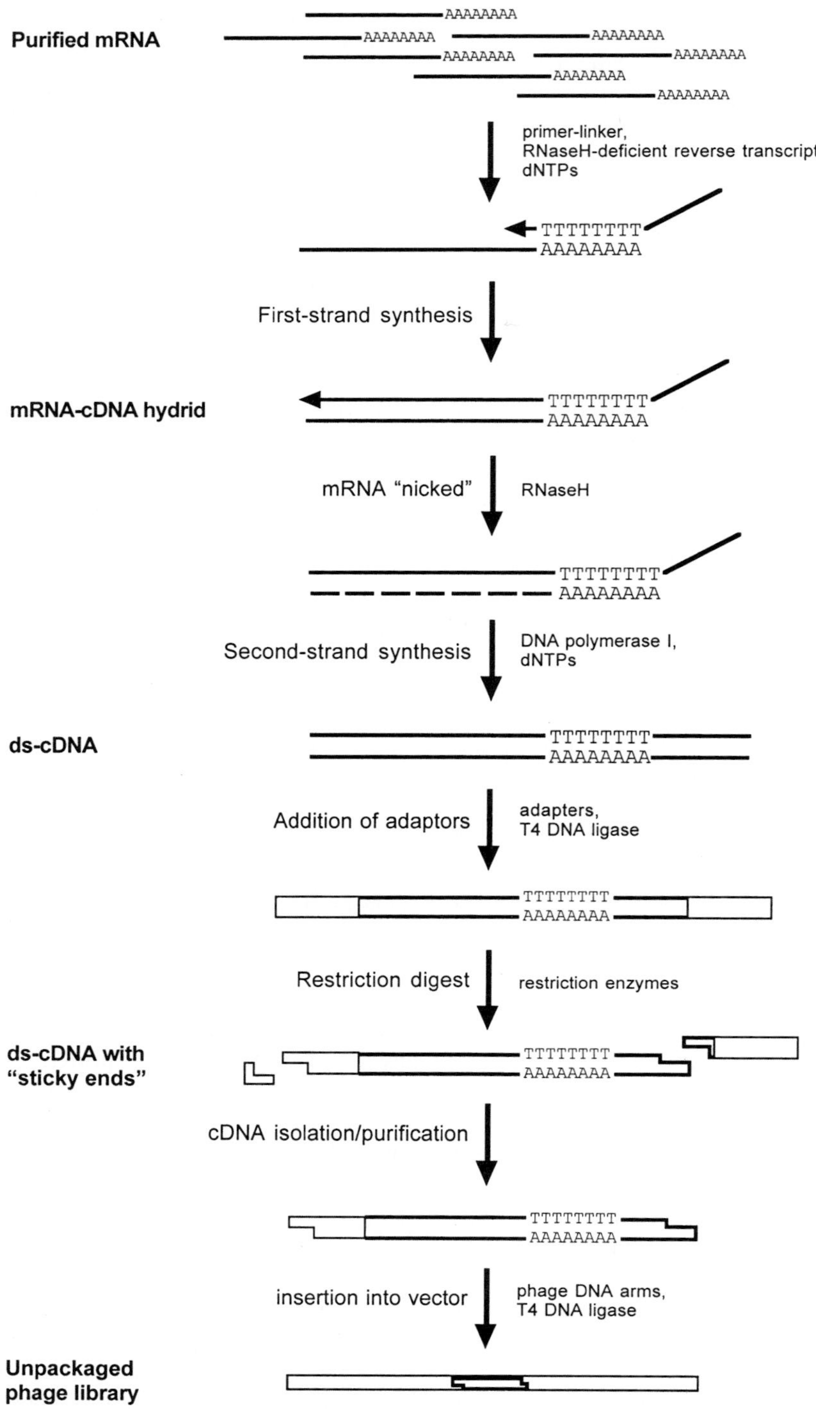

Figure 1 Construction of a cDNA library. Schematic representation of the construction of an unpackaged phage cDNA library from isolated mRNA. The linear phage DNA with cDNA inserts is next packaged into viral particles and then used to infect a bacterial culture, resulting in an expanded phage cDNA library.

This is done *in vitro* by combining the DNA with a "packaging extract." Packaging extracts are commercially produced lysates of phage-infected *Escherichia coli.* These extracts contain ATP, empty phage heads, unattached phage tails, and all the phage-encoded proteins required to insert DNA molecules into the heads and attach the tails. Once packaged, infecting a culture of *E. coli* hosts expands the library. The resulting lysate is cleared by centrifugation and stored refrigerated in the presence of chloroform.

C. Commercial versus Custom Libraries

As the preceding discussions illustrate, library construction is a complex procedure. Furthermore, each step must be performed with a high efficiency in order to obtain a cDNA library that is truly representative of the mRNA population originally present in the cellular sample. This is especially important if the library is to be used to isolate a cDNA that corresponds to a relatively scarce mRNA, or if a cDNA that represents a full-length copy of a mRNA is desired. Fortunately, library construction kits that greatly facilitate this process are commercially available. Even so, researchers now seldom construct their own genetic libraries. This is because library construction is very demanding and because numerous libraries are available both noncommercially and commercially at prices that are comparable to the cost of creating a library in the research lab. However, often a custom cDNA library is needed that is not available commercially. For example, to clone a relatively rare mRNA it may be best to construct a library from a sample that contains a relative abundance of that mRNA. The source may be an unusual cell line, a cell line subjected to a particular treatment, a particular tissue, or a tissue subjected to disease or treatment. A library constructed from such starting material will increase the chances of isolating the rare mRNA of interest. In this case, the researcher can construct a library, using one of several commercially available library construction kits, or the researcher can hire out the library construction. This is typically done by sending a total RNA or mRNA sample to one of several molecular biology service companies. Unfortunately, custom cDNA construction services are relatively expensive. On the other hand, the quality of a commercially obtained library is often superior to that obtained in research laboratories. Either way, it should be noted that the mRNA isolation procedure is crucial because a good cDNA library cannot be made from a degraded mRNA sample.

Subtractive hybridization is another cloning strategy that requires custom library construction. This procedure is used to isolate differentially expressed mRNAs. It requires mRNA from a source that contains a relative large amount of the species to be cloned and a cDNA population derived from an mRNA source that is similar, but relatively lacking in the mRNA to be cloned. Such populations may be derived from diseased and healthy tissue, from cells treated with a drug and their untreated counterparts, or any pair of experimental and control mRNA sources that one believes will contain significantly different amounts of a limited number of mRNA species. Numerous subtractive hybridization procedures have been published (17, 18). In most of these schemes, the target mRNA is enriched by combining and annealing the experimental mRNA and control cDNA populations and removing mRNA–cDNA hybrids, thus leaving an mRNA population enriched in species specific to or in greater abundance in the experimental population. This subtracted mRNA population is then used to produce an enriched cDNA library, or is used to generate probe to screen a library derived from the unsubtracted experimental mRNA. The latter is often done because the subtraction procedure may result in mRNA that is slightly degraded, and therefore incapable of producing a high-quality library.

D. Electronic Cloning

More and more, researchers are able to identify desired cDNA and genomic clones using the Internet. This is due to recent mass sequencing efforts to compile the entire sequence of several genomes and to identify and catalogue huge numbers of expressed sequence tags (ESTs). (ESTs are short sequences derived from cDNA clones picked at random from cDNA libraries.) The availability of huge amounts of sequence information in searchable formats, and the computing power to quickly search these sequences, allow the identification of genes and cDNAs of interest without ever screening a library. A comprehensive list of sequence databases has been published (19) and is available on the Internet (http://www.oup.co.uk/nar/Volume_27/Issue_01/summary/gkc105_gml.html). For example, perhaps the most comprehensive and useful source of sequence information is GenBank (http://www.ncbi.nim.nih.gov/Web/Genbank/index.html). Genbank contains sequence information from numerous international sources as well as sequence similarity searching capabilities using BLAST database search programs (20).

The power of electronic cloning can be illustrated by comparing traditional cDNA cloning with the identification of an EST clone from the dbEST database (21). ESTs represent short portions of cDNA clones picked at random from cDNA libraries and subjected to automated sequencing. The information in each EST represents a single sequencing run from a primer site within the library construction vector into the unknown cDNA insert. Therefore, ESTs seldom contain more than 200 or 300 bases of reliable sequence information. ESTs were originally intended to provide tags to be used to identify expressed regions within the genomic sequence (22). Given that the majority of eukaryotic DNA is not transcribed into RNA, such tags enable the identification of active genes within a sea of seemingly inactive genome. ESTs also enable the identification of active portions of the genome—that is, regions that contain a relatively high density of transcribed gene sequences. Now, ESTs are beginning to fulfill another role in molecular biology, that of a substitute for screening cDNA libraries. This is because there is now a sufficient number of ESTs within public databases to enable the identification of many cDNA clones by computer (23). For example, to clone the human homolog of a cDNA previously identified only in yeast, traditionally the yeast cDNA would be obtained from a colleague and then used to perform a low-stringency screen of a human cDNA library, hoping to isolate homologous human cDNAs. Now, the prudent researcher will first use a computer and the Internet to obtain the published yeast cDNA sequence and then perform a BLAST search comparing the yeast cDNA to the human dbEST database. Very often, the ESTs identified will exhibit significant sequence homology to the yeast cDNA. Most cDNA clones from which ESTs were derived are available to researchers at a minimal cost through such companies as Genome Systems (http://www.genomesystems.com) and Research Genetics (http://www.resgen.com) or directly from the Integrated Molecular Analysis of Genomes and Their Expression (IMAGE) Consortium (24). Of course, it is up to the researcher to confirm the identity of the human cDNAs containing the homologous ESTs and to prove that they truly represent functional human homologs of the yeast cDNA. Another consideration is the fact that cDNA clones obtained from EST libraries seldom contain inserts that represent full-length mRNA species. Several EST cDNA clones may be needed to piece together a full-length cDNA. But this is also often the case when screening a conventional library. Partial length is of little consequence if a cDNA is needed only to serve as a probe for hybridization in techniques such as Northern blotting and *in situ* hybridization. For these purposes, a partial cDNA clone is sufficient. In fact, perhaps the greatest utility of the dbEST database and associated cDNA libraries to a surgical researcher is as a readily available source of cDNA clones to use as probes in hybridization experiments.

E. RT-PCR Cloning

There is another simple method of obtaining a partial cDNA for use as probe for hybridization experiments without library screening. Reverse transcription followed by polymerase chain reaction (RT-PCR) can easily be used to generate portions of cDNAs, provided sufficient sequence data to design flanking PCR oligonucleotide primers. Oligonucleotide primers are short strands of single-stranded DNA (15 to 30 base pairs) that are complementary to the mRNA or to the corresponding cDNA at either end of the portion to be amplified. Usually these "oligos" are ordered from a service company or a core facility by stipulating the sequence of bases needed. Thus, once a gene is cloned and its sequence is published, this information can be used to design primers and to generate, amplify, and clone a portion of this cDNA from any RNA sample that contains the corresponding mRNA. This RT-PCR product can then be used directly to generate probe for hybridization experiments, or can be inserted into a plasmid vector to create an RT-PCR clone for further use. Several alternative methods of amplification and cloning of RT-PCR products have been devised (11). Regardless of the methods used, the identity of an RT-PCR product should be carefully verified before it is utilized in an experiment, because even the most well-designed PCR primers can lead to inadvertent RT-PCR products. Amplification of the desired RT-PCR product can be better assured by performing repeated PCR with nested oligonucleotide primers (primers that anneal to flanking sequences found within the original PCR product). This procedure will ensure that the RT-PCR product obtained came from an mRNA species containing sequences complementary to both these primers pairs. Once obtained, the identity of an RT-PCR product can be verified by restriction mapping, Southern hybridization with an oligomer probe complementary to an internal sequence of the desired product, and, ultimately, sequencing a portion of the product. The entire sequence of an RT-PCR clone should be confirmed if the clone is to be used to express the corresponding protein, because mutations can be introduced during each round of PCR amplification. PCR mutations can be all but avoided by using thermostable polymerase enzymes with greater fidelity than Taq polymerase (a number of these are now commercially available). However, because these enzymes often owe their fidelity to proofreading 3′–5′ exonuclease activity, it is often more difficult to obtain a product with small amounts of template. Furthermore, due to the complex nature of cellular RNA samples, the specific target template in RT-PCR reactions represents a very small fraction of all reverse-transcribed molecules. However, new generations of genetically engineered thermostable polymerase enzymes promise high fidelity and efficiency, as well as increased processivity, allowing for the efficient and accurate amplification of large templates.

F. RACE Techniques

Often, it is difficult to obtain a cDNA representing the entire full length of an mRNA molecule. In particular, the nature of cDNA library construction often disallows finding cDNA clones with intact 5′ and 3′ ends. However, a PCR technique termed rapid amplification of cDNA ends (RACE) enables the 5′ and 3′ ends of full-length cDNAs to be identified and cloned (25). These methods are based on the construction of cDNA molecules with PCR primer sites attached to either the 5′ or 3′ ends (26). For 5′-RACE, first-strand cDNA synthesis is primed with random hexamers, in order to obtain internally primed cDNAs with a good chance of containing intact 5′ ends. Then linker molecules are ligated to the 5′ ends of these cDNAs. For 3′-RACE, first-strand synthesis is primed with poly(dT) and linker sequence-containing primers. The linkers contain a sequence designed to provide optimal primer annealing sites for subsequent PCR. Desired cDNA ends are then amplified by PCR using primers that anneal to the linker and to a sequence unique to the cDNA being sought. Usually, two rounds of PCR are performed, the second with nested primers that anneal to an internal linker site and an internal cDNA-specific site. The PCR products obtained are then cloned into a plasmid vector for further analysis and sequencing. If both 5′-RACE and 3′-RACE are successfully performed, resulting in both ends of a cDNA, RT-PCR can be used to amplify the internal cDNA region from an mRNA source. Thus, an entire cDNA clone can be obtained quickly, without screening a library. However, because PCR amplification can lead to the introduction of point mutations, the sequence of cDNAs derived as RT-PCR clones should be confirmed or viewed with suspicion. Often the RACE technique is used to complete a partial cDNA obtained by screening a library. 5′ -RACE is often used for this purpose because clones derived from poly(dT)-primed cDNA libraries seldom contain complete 5′ ends.

G. Library Screening

There are still uses for traditional library screening—for example, when homology searches of dbEST databases do not identify clones with significant homology or when screening is to be performed using protein interaction rather than nucleotide sequence homology. The goal of any screening process is the identification and isolation of clones that possess a selectable property from a mixture of millions of clones that compose a library. Selectable properties include homology with a known DNA sequence, or expression of a protein or peptide with a given property. Homology screens usually exploit the ability of a DNA probe molecule to anneal to sequences within a library by complementary base pairing. Examples of screening for homology include using a cDNA from one species to screen for the corresponding cDNA from another species, using a cDNA to screen for cDNAs that represent additional members of a gene family, using degenerate oligomers to screen for a cDNA that encodes a peptide sequence, and using a cDNA to probe a genomic library to obtain the corresponding gene. Expression library screens are usually based on the ability of a cDNA-encoded amino acid sequence to bind to a protein or a double-stranded DNA probe. Examples of expression screens include using an antibody raised against a novel protein to screen for a cDNA that encodes that protein and using a DNA probe corresponding to a gene promoter region to screen for a cDNA that encodes a transcription factor.

1. Using a Phage Library

The principles and major steps of screening a phage library are relatively simple in theory, but somewhat demanding in practice. Detailed protocols are available from several sources (9, 11, 27). Screening of phage libraries takes advantage of the lytic infection cycle of the phage, which culminates in the bursting of infected bacteria and release of multiple viral particles as well as naked phage DNA and phage-encoded proteins (28). A phage library exists in the form of a suspension containing millions of viral particles per milliliter. Each phage contains inserted genomic DNA or cDNA derived from a cellular source. In order to screen the library, each phage must be separated from the population and made to present the DNA insert or the peptide encoded by the DNA insert in a fashion allowing it to be probed, identified, and isolated.

Once a phage library is obtained or constructed, the viral titer, or the concentration of viable phage particles, must be determined prior to library screening (Fig. 2). This is done by infecting a number of identical bacterial cultures with serial dilutions of a known volume of the viral stock. These cultures are then diluted in top-agar and spread on media-agar plates and incubated. If the ratio of bacteria to virus is within a certain range, a plate will become covered with a continuous opaque lawn of growing bacteria that eventually develops tiny translucent circles, or plaques. These plaques represent spreading regions of viral infection that each originated from a single infected bacterium at the center. As the virus completes its life cycle, the infection spreads outward and results in a "cleared" region of bacterial lysis. If the ratio of viral particles to bacteria is too high, the entire plate will clear. If the ratio is appropriate, the plate will contain a countable number of separate, clear plaques. By counting these and referring to the dilution of viral stock used to produce that plate, the concentration of viral particles in the original suspension can be calculated. To facilitate screening the library, this viral titer is used to calculate the amount of viral stock needed to create plates with a desired density of plaques. The more plaques per plate, the harder to identify and isolate positive clones. The fewer plaques per plate, the more plates needed to screen an appreciable number of clones. The number of clones to be screened is usually determined by the abundance of the corresponding mRNA species and the number of clones desired. For example, to obtain at least 10 cDNAs corresponding to a relatively scarce mRNA, it may be wise to screen 10^6 clones. This may be accomplished by screening 20 plates, each containing 50,000 plaques per plate.

Once a desired number of plates containing an appropriate density of viral plaques are created, the process of

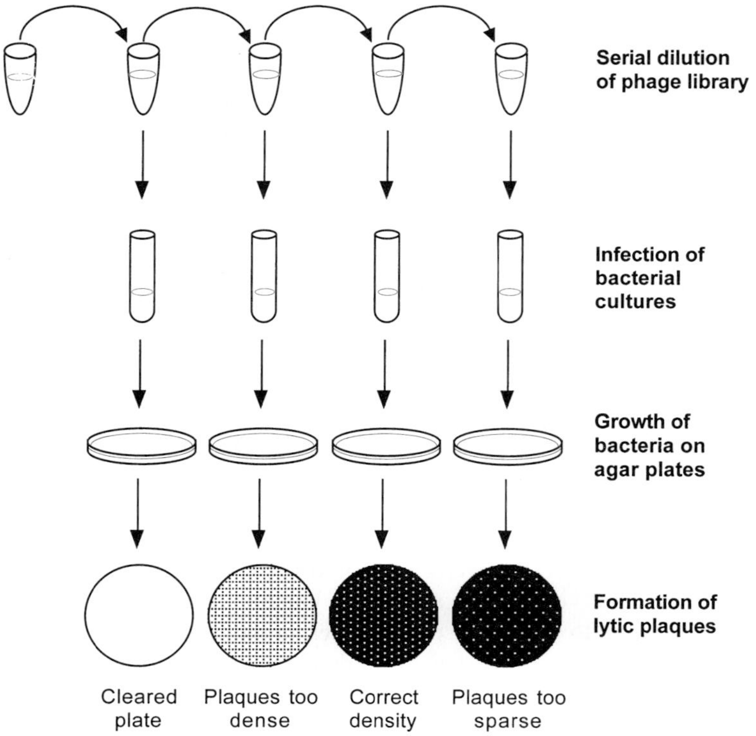

Figure 2 Titering of a phage library. Schematic representation of the process used to estimate the concentration of plaque-forming units (PFU) in an expanded phage library. This information is then used to determine the amount of phage suspension to use to produce bacterial plates with a suitable density of plaques for screening.

screening these plates can begin (Fig. 3). Bringing a separate charged nitrocellulose or nylon membrane filter into contact with the surface of each plate starts this process. A dry circular filter is gently placed on the bacterial lawn and allowed to set until it becomes fully wetted. Before separating, filter and plate are marked to record the relative orientation for future reference. The filters are then gently lifted from the plate. They now contain adhered phage particles, phage DNA, phage-encoded proteins, as well as bacterial debris and proteins, creating a mirror image of the viral plaques. This lifting process is usually repeated to obtain a confirmatory set of duplicate filters. The filters are then used to screen the library, and the associated bacterial lysis plates are safely stowed in the refrigerator. For example, if a homology screen is to be performed, then a process that is directly analogous to the probing portion of Southern blotting (29) is used to screen the filter lifts for homologous cDNAs. All the filters are placed on filter paper containing sodium hydroxide to destruct the phage particles, spill the viral DNA on the membrane, and to denature the dsDNA. Because the membranes are charged, the single-stranded DNA molecules and proteins adhere via electrostatic forces. The membranes are removed from the alkali, neutralized in a strong buffer, and then heated or exposed to ultraviolet light to fix the viral DNA onto the filters. The membranes are then washed to remove bacteria and debris and are "prehybridized" by incubating them in a complex mixture of buffer, salts, detergent, polymers, and nucleic acids. This is done to block unoccupied charged sites on the membrane. The filters are then hybridized with a radioactive probe, usually in the same complex mixture used during prehybridization. Hybridization is done at an elevated temperature (45–70°C) and for an extended time (4 to 24 hr), thus enabling the probe to anneal the membrane-attached viral DNAs that possess appreciable homology. (Because the filters are blocked, the probe will not bind to the membrane, but only to homologous DNA that is fixed to the membrane.) The membranes are then repeatedly washed in warm solutions containing buffer, salt, and detergent to remove unhybridized and weakly hybridized probe. Finally, the filters are exposed to X-ray films in a known orientation. If all went well, on developing, dark circular spots that correspond to a subset of plaques on the plates will be apparent on the resulting autoradiographs. These spots may represent positive plaques that contain phage with cDNA inserts that have significant homology to the probe sequence. The autoradiographs of the like-treated duplicate set of filter lifts are used to confirm that each spot is a true positive. By comparing the

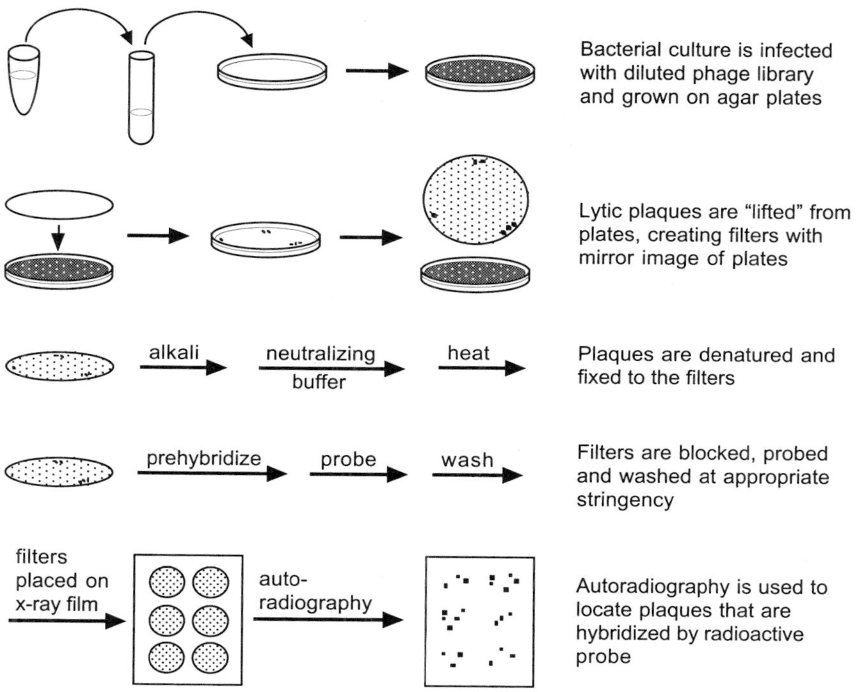
Bacterial culture is infected with diluted phage library and grown on agar plates
Lytic plaques are "lifted" from plates, creating filters with mirror image of plates
alkali
neutralizing buffer
heat
Plaques are denatured and fixed to the filters
prehybridize
probe
wash
Filters are blocked, probed and washed at appropriate stringency
filters placed on x-ray film
auto-radiography
Autoradiography is used to locate plaques that are hybridized by radioactive probe

Figure 3 Screening a phage library. Schematic representation of the steps involved in plating and screening a phage library with a radioactive probe (such as a ^{32}P-labeled complimentary cDNA probe). Proper dilution of the phage library is calculated from the PFU concentration obtained from titering the library. A bacterial culture is infected and then plated on several agarmedia plates. After incubation and appearance of separated lytic plaques, replicates of the plates are produced by contacting a filter membrane to each plate (usually performed in duplicate). These filter lifts are processed and probed to identify phage that contain molecules with affinity to the probe (inserted cDNA or cDNA-encoded peptide). The positive plaques are identified as spots on film after autoradiography, and this information is used to locate these plaques on the original bacterial plates.

films to the original plates, positive plaques are located. (At this point, the importance of marking and retaining the orientations of plates, membranes, and film becomes apparent.)

After identification, positive plaques are "picked" by removing agar plugs that contain the corresponding regions on the plate. Plugs are cut and removed in one step, using the broad end of a sterile Pasteur pipette or a sterile wide-barreled plastic pipetter tip in a cookie-cutter fashion. These plugs are placed in solution to release the phage particles by diffusion. The resulting phage suspensions contain not only positive clones, but also unwanted phage that resided in plaques neighboring the positive clones. (The number of neighbors depends on the density of the plate and the size of the plug.) For this reason, these phage suspensions must be subjected to a process termed "plaque purification" (30). The phage suspensions are each used to reinfect a culture of host bacteria that is then replated and rescreened with probe. A tertiary screen will follow this secondary screen, and so on, until plugs containing only single positive plaques are picked. The pure phage populations are then amplified and stored for safekeeping. The cDNA inserts contained in these phage are usually "subcloned" into a phagmid or an M13 plasmid vector for analysis (see Section II, H). To do this, viral DNA is purified; cDNA inserts are excised by restriction digest, separated from viral DNA, and ligated into the desired vector (9, 11, 27).

2. Screening for Homology

When screening for homology, the most important factor is stringency, or the extent to which only perfect annealing partners will be tolerated and retained. Stringency is determined by temperature, by salt content, and by the presence of chaotropic agents (such as detergents and formamide). High stringency is obtained at relatively high temperatures, low salt content, and with the use of chaotropic agents during annealing and/or during subsequent washing steps. A high-stringency screen will detect only clones that have a high degree of homology with the probe sequence. This includes clones with perfect homology and clones with long, uninterrupted stretches of homology. The use of high stringency is appropriate when using a cDNA to screen for the corresponding cDNA of a closely related species and when using a cDNA to screen a genomic library for the corresponding gene. As stringency is lowered, clones with increasingly imperfect homology and clones with shorter stretches of uninterrupted homology will be detected. The use of lesser stringency is appropriate when using a cDNA to screen for the corresponding cDNA of an unrelated species, when screening for members of gene families, and when using an oligonucleotide as probe. Because of their small size, oligomer probes will succeed only when medium or low stringencies are used. Both because of small size and base mismatches, degenerate oligomer probes require low stringencies.

Often, the appropriate stringency cannot be accurately predicted. The use of too high a stringency will lead to no clones being detected. The use of too low a stringency will detect numerous clones, including clones with insignificant relationships to the probe. Such a screen would necessitate the isolation and analysis of many useless clones. Fortunately, the washing steps can dictate the stringency of a screen and these steps can be performed in a progressively stringent manner. The hybridization step can be performed at a relatively low stringency, leading to annealing of probe to both related and unrelated clones. The membranes can then be washed at low stringency, and the clones that are annealed to probe under those conditions identified. The membranes can then be rewashed at higher stringency, and those clones that retain annealed probe are identified. This can be repeated at increasing stringencies until no positive clones remain. One can then begin to isolate and analyze clones that retained hybridized probe at a relatively high stringency. If desired, additional clones more distantly related to the probe sequence can then be identified from a lower stringency wash and detection step. However, in practice one may observe the number of clones detected by the probe rapidly transition from profuse, to scarce, to none as the appropriate stringency is bracketed.

3. Screening for Protein Interactions

Certain types of genetic libraries can also be screened on the basis of protein–protein or protein–DNA interactions. For example, a bacteriophage λgt-11 enables the expression of cDNA fused to the coding sequence of the enzyme β-galactosidase (27). If the cDNA contains an open reading frame inserted in the correct orientation and a codon reading frame, a fusion protein is expressed and released during lytic infection. A λgt-11 expression library can be screened with any probe that may attach to the cDNA-encoded peptide. Expression libraries can be used to identify and clone protein—protein binding partners by using a radioactively labeled, enzymatically labeled, or bacterial-produced fusion protein as probe. For example, such a technique is now used to rapidly identify antigen-binding Fab fragments of antibodies expressed by B cells, by constructing a cDNA expression library using RNA from B cells of an immunigenized animal and screening the library with antigen as probe (31). The Fab-encoding cDNAs thus isolated are used to produce the Fab fragments or to produce a humanized antibody. Expression libraries have often been used to clone the cDNAs encoding newly isolated proteins. To do this, the protein is first used as an antigen to produce antibodies or antisera. These antibodies are then used to probe filters from an expression library, in a manner directly analogous to the antibody-probing portion of Western blotting (32, 33). Expression libraries can also be used to identify transcription factors by screening with end-labeled dsDNA probes that correspond to a promoter element (34).

Expression libraries must be constructed in such a way as to present cDNA sequences translated in all three codon reading frames. This is accomplished by placing cDNAs into three separate vectors that contain insertion sites offset by zero, one, and two nucleotide bases. The three possible reading frames and two possible orientations of the cDNA necessitate that six times as many library clones must be screened with probe to obtain the same number of positive clones as would be obtained by a homology screen. Because presented peptides most often will not contain the entire amino acid sequence of the native protein, and because they are presented as fusion proteins, there is a significant chance that a clone will not retain the binding ability of the native protein. If this is so, an expression screen is doomed to failure.

4. Screening with the Yeast *n*-Hybrid Systems

Additional methods used to screen for protein interactions include the interaction trap, or yeast two-hybrid system (35), and its many novel interactions (36, 37). Together, the two-hybrid method and its variations are often referred to as yeast *n*-hybrid systems. These methods are all based on functional genetic complementation in yeast cells, leading to transcriptional activation or deactivation of reporter gene expression. In this method, an expression library and a reporter gene are both inserted into yeast cells. In the simplest version of this method, all the yeast cells are made to express a "bait" protein as a fusion with a DNA-binding protein called LexA. The yeast cells also contain a reporter gene fused to a gene promoter that is responsive to the LexA protein. The promoter contains a LexA operator, which turns on transcription if LexA is brought into close proximity. The expression library used in this system is designed to express the peptides encoded by genomic DNA fragments or cDNAs as fusion proteins attached to a stretch of acidic amino acids (often called and "acid blob"). This acid blob has the ability to bind the reporter gene's promoter region tightly, at a spot just upstream of the LexA operator. Thus, if a library-expressed fusion protein forms a hybrid with the LexA-fused bait protein, LexA will be trapped adjacent to the LexA operon and the reporter gene will be turned on.

Expression of the reporter gene may cause the yeast colony to turn a color or allow it to grow in a nutrient-deficient media, so that positive clones can be identified and isolated.

Although somewhat complex, yeast *n*-hybrid systems have many advantages over conventional expression libraries. These methods accomplish expression of both the probe protein (as bait) and the library insert-encoded peptides. There is no need to produce, purify, and label a protein probe. In the *n*-hybrid system, the protein–protein interactions are formed *in vivo* rather than *in vitro,* which is advantageous if the intracellular environment is essential to facilitate the protein–protein interaction of interest. Variations of the two-hybrid system can be used to screen library-encoded proteins involved in complex interactions that could never be screened for using conventional expression libraries. These variations include a scheme to screen for encoded proteins involved in tripartite protein–protein–protein interactions (36, 37). Other variations, known as reverse-*n*-hybrid systems, can be used to clone genes or cDNAs encoding proteins that disrupt protein–protein complexes (36, 37). On the other hand, these methods suffer from a high frequency of false positives. Thus, once positive clones are identified they must be carefully analyzed to identify true positives. Often, this cannot be accomplished without production and purification of the fusion protein and testing of the putative interaction by *in vitro* methods.

5. Library Screening Services

It should be noted that screening a library is only the first and perhaps the least labor-intensive step in the process of isolating and analyzing a cDNA or genomic clone. As mentioned above, once positive clones have been identified by a primary screen they must be isolated from all other clones in the library in a process called clone purification. During the initial screen, clones will be located in close proximity to one another. Therefore, when first picked, clones will still be among tens or hundreds of other clones. The clones are isolated by repeatedly picking, replating, and rescreening the clone until a pure population is obtained. Each round in this process takes several days to complete. The number of iterations required depends on the density at which the library was initially plated and the efficiency at which clones are picked. Once purified, each clone must be subcloned, analyzed, and compared.

Because this process of screening and isolating clones is time and resource intensive, library-screening services are now popular. These services can very efficiently identify and provide purified clones from select genetic libraries using patron-provided probe or PCR primers. These services can screen libraries very efficiently using robotics and a process of clone pooling. In this process, all the clones that comprise a library are initially separated and catalogued. Thus, clone isolation is already complete. In order to identify which clone is related to a probe, clones are pooled into subgroups and groups. For homology screens, reusable membranes are prepared and screened. Membranes dotted with DNA from groups of clones are screened by hybridization to determine which group contains one or more positive clones. Membranes containing dotted subgroups of positive groups are subsequently screened. Smaller and smaller positive subgroups are identified until membranes containing dots of DNA from individual members of the final subgroup are screened to identify positive clones. Pools can also be screened using PCR. In this case, DNA from groups, subgroups, and ultimately clones are not screened as dots on membranes, but rather are subjected to PCR reactions with primers that amplify a portion of the desired cDNA or genomic DNA insert. Positive pools and clones are identified by successful amplification of the expected PCR product. After completing the screening process, all that remains to be done is to send a culture of the positive clones to the customer. Most companies will contract to send a certain number of positive clones and will refund all or a portion of their fee if the screening process is unsuccessful. Because the library and its groups, subgroups, and isolated clones preexist, and because this process is highly automated, this service can be provided at a price comparable to or even less than the cost of isolating clones in a research laboratory. Of course, even if the library screening and clone isolation are contracted, the researcher must analyze the resulting clones.

H. DNA Sequencing

Molecular biology would not be possible if not for DNA sequencing. In recent years, colossal effort has been expended to improve and automate the process of DNA sequencing. The resulting technological advances have made possible revolutions in genomics, such as the Human Genome Project. Whether automated or manual, all sequencing procedures are based on two fundamental methods, the chemical degradation method and the chain termination method. These methods were invented more or less simultaneously at Harvard and Cambridge and both were published in 1977 (38, 39). Because of recent advances in the chain termination method that allow sequencing of longer strands in a single reaction, this method is now more common and only this method is described here.

The fundamental steps in the chain termination method include template-directed DNA polymerase extension of an oligonucleotide primer, random termination of extension, and detection of the terminated molecules (Fig. 4). Chain termination DNA sequencing reactions require a single-stranded DNA template to be sequenced, an oligonucleotide primer, DNA polymerase, standard deoxynucleotide triphophates, and termination nucleotides. Single-stranded

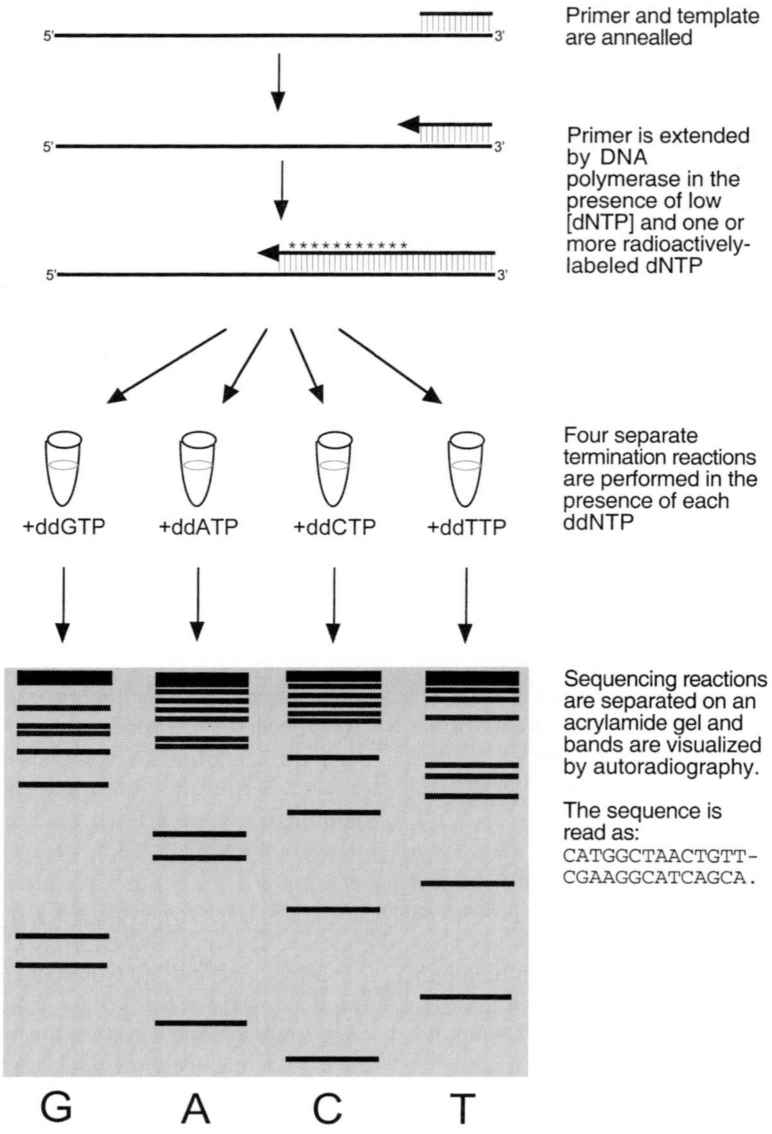

Figure 4 DNA sequencing. The fundamental steps of sequencing with separate strand labeling and termination reactions. The resulting autoradiograph is read from bottom to top to obtain the sequence, which reads CATGGCTAACTGTTCGAAGGCATCAGCA. Note that the autoradiographic bands become closer together at the top of the gel, until the sequence can no longer be discerned.

templates are obtained either by denaturization of dsDNA, by production of single-stranded bacteriophage DNA using M13mp cloning vectors, by production of single-stranded bacteriophage DNA with phagemid cloning vectors and superinfection by helper phage, or by asymmetric PCR (11). The oligonucleotide primers used for sequencing are short strands of single-stranded DNA (usually 15 to 20 base pairs) designed to be complementary to a single sequence on the template that is positioned 40 or 50 bases 3′ (downstream) of the portion to be sequenced. Termination nucleotides are modified nucleotides that, once incorporated into a DNA polymer, do not allow the attachment of additional nucleotides to the chain. For example, 2′, 3′-dideoxyribonucleotides (ddNTPs) function as terminators because they lack the 3′ hydroxyl group on the ribose backbone, to which subsequent ribonucleic acid molecules would be attached.

Combining the template and sequencing primer and allowing them to anneal initiates the sequencing process. Once the primer has annealed, DNA polymerase begins to extend the 5′ end of the primer by adding nucleotides that are complementary to the template. Because a sequencing reaction contains millions of DNA templates and primers, multiple DNA strands complementary to the template are simultaneously being extended. In manual sequencing, four sequencing reactions are prepared for each template and primer pair. To each of the four reactions all four standard nucleotides are added (dATP, dCTP, dGTP, and dTTP) but only one dideoxyribonucleotide is added (ddATP, ddCTP, ddGTP, or ddTTP). DNA polymerase shows no preference for dNTPs over ddNTPs. Therefore, the ddNTP is incorporated into growing DNA strands at random and in accordance with the template sequence and the relative abundance of the ddNTP and its corresponding dNTP. Thus in a reaction containing ddATP, a number of strands are terminated at each point where the template sequence contained a thymine base and the DNA polymerase incorporated an adenosine base that just happened to be a ddATP. Each reaction will proceed until all initiated DNA extensions are terminated. What results are populations of complementary DNA chains of varying lengths, but all corresponding to lengths that have the same base (either A, C, G, or T) at their termini. The ratio of ddNTP to dNTP can be increased or decreased to obtain shorter or longer mean chain lengths, respectively.

1. Obtaining the Sequence

The next step in sequencing is the separation and detection of the synthesized DNA strands of different lengths, and reading of the sequence. In manual sequencing, separation is accomplished by polyacrylamide gel electrophoresis in a large and thin format gel. The synthesized strands of DNA are separated from template DNA by heating in the presence of a denaturant, and then each reaction is loaded in adjacent wells at the top of the gel. DNA strands of increasing lengths exhibit decreasing electrophoretic mobilities and therefore migrate shorter distances down the gel as the voltage is applied from top to bottom. Molecules corresponding to each termination site lead to separate bands in the gel. Autoradiography is the most common method of visualizing the bands. This is done by including radioactive nucleotides in the sequencing reaction and detecting the radioactive DNA strands by exposure of the gel to X-ray film. Usually ^{32}P or ^{35}S isotopes are used. With its greater energy particle emission, ^{32}P has the advantage of requiring shorter film exposure times. With its lower energy particle emission, ^{35}S gives greater band resolution because radioactive particles traveling at an angle from the bands have less chance to convert silver particles in the film. Although relatively expensive, ^{33}P, with its intermediate energy particle emission, can produce both desirable exposure times and band resolution (40).

The incorporation of a radiolabeled dNTP during the sequencing reaction has a disadvantage. Short DNA strands contain little radioactivity and are therefore less easily detected by autoradiography. This problem can be avoided by 5′-end labeling the oligonucleotide primer before using it in the sequencing reactions (41). The primer is labeled using [λ-^{32}P]ATP or [λ-^{35}S]ATP and the enzyme T4 polynucleotide kinase, which transfers the radioactive λ-phosphate or λ-sulfur to the 5′ end of the primer's deoxyribose backbone (42). Because each DNA strand produced by the sequencing reaction contains only one primer, incorporation of radioactive primers produces DNA chains that are equally radioactive regardless of length. Therefore, after separation and autoradiography, these reactions produce bands with intensities proportional only to the number of chains of a given length. A similar result can be obtained by performing separate labeling and sequencing reactions (43). In this method, an initial prelabeling reaction is performed that includes polymerase, template, primer, and small amounts of dNTPs, including one or more radioactive dNTP. This reaction extends the primer for only a short distance, but incorporates a good deal of radioactivity into each strand. This initial reaction is then divided into four sequencing reactions containing ample dNTPs and one ddNTP each. The resulting DNA strands contain similar amounts of radioactivity, regardless of the point at which they are terminated, and therefore are equally detectable by autoradiography. There are also alternative methods of detecting sequencing bands that avoid the use of radioisotopes. These include silver staining (44) and chemiluminescence (45).

Manual sequencing requires manual reading of sequence from the gel or autoradiographic image of the gel. This is made possible by the fact that the four termination reactions (A, T, G, and C) are loaded in adjacent wells of the sequencing gel and electrophoresed simultaneously. Thus, each reaction runs in adjacent lanes within the gel at the same overall speed, and the distance that each individual band has run can be compared to others in all four lanes. The sequence can be read by starting at the bottom of the gel and identifying the lowest visible band. This is the shortest terminated DNA strand. If this band is in the A lane, the sequence begins with A. Moving up the gel, toward the wells, the next band and its lane is identified. If this band is in the T lane, then the sequence is AT. This process is continued up the sequencing ladder until the bands become indiscernible. At the bottom of a sequencing gel, where the strands are short, bands are well spread and easy to read. Toward the top of a sequencing gel, where the strands are long, bands become very close together and hard to differentiate. This is because the absolute size difference between bands is always one nucleotide base. Thus, the relative difference in sizes becomes less as the total length increases. Eventually, bands become so close to one another that it is impossible to determine with certainty which comes next.

In order to increase the length of sequence obtained from each set of four reactions, reactions are reloaded on a gel at time intervals, so that the DNA strands are electrophoresed for different periods. The progression of electrophoresis is continuously visualized by the addition of two marker dyes, bromophenol blue and xylene cyanol, to each reaction mixture prior to loading on the gel. (Depending upon the acrylamide content and cross-linking, these dyes migrate down the gel along with DNA strands approximately 25 and 100 nucleotides in length, respectively.) Voltage is applied until many of the shortest DNA strands in the first-loaded reactions have electrophoresed right out of the bottom of the gel. By electrophoresing these reactions for an extended time, bands corresponding to very long DNA strands are better separated, and thus become readable. The sequence information corresponding to short strands, which ran off the bottom of the gel in the first-loaded lanes, can be obtained by reading lanes loaded at a later time. In this way, a much greater length of sequence can be obtained from a single set of reactions. Optimally, a set of sequence reactions from a single primer should provide 300 to 400 bases of sequence information. Once read, it is important to remember that the sequence obtained is that of the DNA strand complementary to the template. The template sequence is the reverse complement of the sequence obtained.

2. Automated Sequencing

Although the principles and process of sequencing are relatively simple, in practice, manual sequencing can be quite difficult to do well. Although it is advisable that every molecular biology laboratory possesses the capability to perform manual sequencing, automated sequencing is now much faster and more efficient than manual sequencing. One reason for this speed and efficiency is the use of dye-termination reactions. In these reactions, the termination nucleotides are modified further to incorporate a fluorescent dye (46). Terminated DNA strands can then be detected by the excitation and emission of these dyes. By including four termination nucleotides each with different dyes attached, a single sequencing reaction can take the place of four reactions in manual sequencing. An automated detector can then establish the identity of each band as it progresses down an electrophoretic gel or as it proceeds along an electrophoretic capillary (47). The sequence is "read" as each dye marker passes the fluorescence detector. The sequence data are then recorded in real time by a computer. Much of the process of reaction, loading, separating, reading, and data entry can be fully automated. Most institutions now have sequencing core facilities that offer sequencing service at a price far less than the material and labor costs of manual sequencing. The researcher must provide the template and sequencing primers. Each facility will have its own preference for template and primer form and purity. It is best to contact the facility in advance and obtain guidelines for production, purification, and dilution of each. A good facility will provide accurate sequence in a timely manner if provided starting materials of sufficient quality. In-laboratory sequencing is necessary only when the local core facility does not provide sufficient accuracy or acceptable turnover times.

3. Sequence Walking

Whether done in the research laboratory or by a core facility, the applications of sequencing reactions to obtain the sequence of a genomic or cDNA clone are the same. A common method of obtaining the sequence of an entire genomic or cDNA clone is termed "walking." For example, when sequencing a cDNA obtained by screening a phage library, the insert is removed from the phage and cloned in forward and reverse orientations in a phagmid or M13 vector pairs. Having the insert in both orientations allows production of single-stranded DNA templates corresponding to both complementary strands. These two strands can then be used to obtain sequence simultaneously from each end of the cDNA insert. To initiate sequencing of the unknown cDNA, primers complementary to the known sequence of the vectors and 40 to 50 bases 3′ of the cDNA insert are used in the first round of sequence reactions. Information obtained from each of these initial reactions will start with sequence within the vectors, proceed through the restriction site used for subcloning the insert, and end with a portion of the cDNA. The cDNA sequence obtained is then used to design a new pair of oligos to prime the next round of sequence reactions. Sequencing rounds are continued in this way until they have "walked" through the entire insert from either direction. The two reverse-complementary sequences are then compared. Often, bases that are difficult to read in one direction can be read from the reverse way. If the sequences from each direction have common trouble spots, an additional pair of primers should be designed and complementary reactions run and read. In this way, sequence ambiguities can be worked out, resulting in a fully accurate cDNA sequence.

III. Conclusion

Embracing molecular biological techniques and embarking on a research plan that involves cloning of a novel gene or cDNA are ambitious steps for any investigator who is not a trained molecular biologist. On the other hand, when successful, the rewards of such a plan are great. Cloning and studying a novel gene, mRNA, and protein will be viewed as novel and unique research, two key ingredients for obtaining research funding. Fortunately, the advent of molecular biology kits and service companies has made this process easier and more expedient. However, it is crucial to understand the principles and methods used to complete the many tasks that must be accomplished before bringing such a research plan to fruition. In other words "If you do not know how you got there, then you cannot truly know where you are."

References

1. Ish-Horowitz, D., and Burke, J. F. (1981). Rapid and efficient cosmid vector cloning. *Nucleic Acids Res.* **9,** 2989–2999.
2. Clark, L., and Carbon, J. (1976). A colony bank containing synthetic *Col/El* hybrids representative of the entire *E. coli* genome. *Cell* **9,** 91–99.
3. Okayama, H., and Berg, P. (1982). High-efficiency cloning of full-length cDNA. *Mol. Cell. Biol.* **2,** 161–170.
4. Seed, B., Parker, R. C., and Davidson, N. (1982). Representation of DNA sequences in recombinant DNA libraries prepared by restriction enzyme partial digestion. *Gene* **19,** 201–209.
5. Williams, B. G., and Blattner, F. R. (1980). Bacteriophage lambda vectors for DNA cloning. *In* "Genetic Engineering" (J. K. Setlow and A. Mullander, eds,), Vol. 2, p. 201. Plenum, New York.
6. Frischauf, A.-M., Lehrach, H., Poustka, A., and Murray, N. (1983). Lambda replacement vectors carrying polylinker sequences. *J. Mol. Biol.* **170,** 827–842.
7. Huynh, T., Young, R., and Davis, R. (1984). Construction and screening cDNA libraries in λgt10 and λgt11. *In* "DNA Cloning, Vol. 1: A Practical Approach" (D. Glover, ed.), pp. 49–78. IRL Press, Oxford, UK.
8. Monaco, A. P., and Larin, Z. (1994). YACs, BACs, PACs and MACs: Artificial chromosomes as research tools. *Trends Biotechnol.* **12,** 280–286.
9. Sambrook, J., Fritsch, E. F., and Maniatis, T., ed. (1989). "Molecular Cloning: A Laboratory Manual." Cold Spring Laboratory Press, Cold Spring Harbor, NY.
10. Sneed, M. A., Alting-Mees, M. A., and Short, J. M. (1997). cDNA library construction for the lambda ZAP®-based vectors. *In* "cDNA Library Protocols" (I. G. Cowell and C. A. Austin, eds.), pp. 39–51. Humana Press. Totowa, NJ.
11. Ausubel, F. M., Brent, R., Kingston, R. E., Moore, D. D., Seidman, J. G., Smith, J. A., and Struhl, K., eds. (2000). "Current Protocols in Molecular Biology." John Wiley & Sons, Inc., New York.
12. Kimmel, A. R., and Berger, S. L., (1989). Preparation of cDNA and the generation of cDNA libraries: Overview. *Methods Enzymol.* **152,** 307–316.
13. Chirgwin, J. M., Przbyla, A. E., MacDonald, R. J., and Rutter, W. J. (1979). Isolation of biologically active ribonucleic acid from sources enriched in ribonuclease. *Biochemistry* **18,** 5294–5299.
14. Chomczynski, P., and Sacchi, N. (1987). Single-step method of RNA isolation by acid quanidinium thiocyanate-phenol-chloroform extraction. *Anal. Biochem.* **162,** 156–159.
15. Gerard, G. (1989). cDNA synthesis by cloned Moloney murine leukemia Virus reverse transcriptase lacking RNase activity. *Focus* **11,** 66.
16. Krug, M. S., and Berger, S. L. (1989). First strand cDNA synthesis primed with oligo (dT). *Methods Enzymol.* **152,** 316–325.
17. Aasheim, H.-C., Logtenberg, T., and Larsen, F. (1997). Subtractive hybridization for the isolation of differentially expressed gene using magnetic beads. *In* "cDNA Library Protocols" (I. G. Cowell and C. A. Austin, eds.), pp. 115–128. Humana Press, Totowa, NJ.
18. Scheinfest, C. W., Nelson, P. S., Graber, M. W., Demopoulos, R. I., and Papas, T. S. (2000). Subtraction hybridization cDNA libraries. *In* "The Nucleic Acid Protocol Handbook" (R. Rapley, ed.), pp. 305–318. Humana Press, Totwa, NJ.
19. Burks, C. (1999). Molecular biology database list. *Nucleic Acids Res.* **27,** 1–9.
20. Benson, D. A., Boguski, M. S., Lipman, D. J., Ostell, J., Ouellette, B. F. F., Rapp, B. A., and Wheeler, D. L. (1999). GenBank. *Nucleic Acids Res.* **27,** 12–17.
21. Boguski, M. S. (1993). dbEST—Database for "expressed sequence tags." *Nature Genet.* **4,** 332–333.
22. Adams, M. D., Kelly, J. M., Gocayne, J. D., Dubnick, M., Polymeropoulos, M. H., Xia, H., Merril, C. R., Wu, A., Olde, B., Moreno, R. F., Kervelage, A. R., McCombie, W. R., and Venter, J. C. (1991). Complementary DNA sequencing: Expressed sequence tags and the human genome project. *Science* **252,** 1651–1656.
23. Rodriguez-Tome, P. (1997). Searching the dbEST database. *In* "cDNA Library Protocols" (I. G. Cowell and C. A. Austin, eds.), pp. 269–283. Humana Press, Totowa, NJ.
24. Lennon, G., Auffray, C., Polymeropoulos, M., and Soarse, M. B. (1996). The I.M.A.G.E. Consortium: An integrated molecular analysis of genomes and their expression. *Genomics* **33,** 151–152.
25. Frohman, M. A., Dush, M. K., and Martin, G. R. (1988). Rapid production of full length cDNAs from rare transcripts: Amplification using a single gene-specific oligonucleotide primer. *Proc. Natl. Acad. Sci. U.S.A.* **85,** 8998–9002.
26. Zhang, Y., and Frohman, M. A. (1997). Using rapid amplification of cDNA ends (RACE) to obtain full-length cDNAs. *In* "cDNA Library Protocols" (I. G. Cowell and C. A. Austin, eds.), pp. 61–87. Humana Press, Totowa, NJ.
27. Arber, W., Enquist, L., Hohn, B., Murray, N., and Murray, K. (1983). Experimental methods for use with lambda. *In* "Lambda II" (R. W. Hendrix, J. W. Roberts, F. W. Stahl, and R. A. Weisberg, eds.), pp. 433–466. Cold Spring Harbor Laboratory, Cold Spring Harbor, NY.
28. Benton, W. D., and Davis, R. W. (1977). Screening λgt recombinant clones by hybridization to single plaques *in situ.* *Science* **196,** 180–182.
29. Southern, E. M. (1975). Detection of specific sequences among DNA fragments separated by gel electrophoresis. *J. Mol. Biol.* **98,** 503–517.
30. Kaiser, K., and Murray, N. E. (1984). The use of phage lambda replacement vectors in the construction of representative genomic DNA libraries. *In* "DNA Cloning: A Practical Approach, Vol. 1" (D. M. Glover, ed.), pp. 1–47, IRL Press, Oxford, UK.
31. Engberg, J., Andersen, P. S., Nielsen, L. K., Dziegiel, M., Johansen, L. K., and Albrechtsen, B. (1996). Phage-display libraries of murine and human antibody Fab fragments. *Mol. Biotechnol.* **6,** 287–310.
32. Burnette, W. N. (1981). Western blotting: Electrophoretic transfer of proteins from sodium dodecyl sulfate–polyacrylamide gels to unmodified nitrocellulose and radiographic detection with antibody and radioiodinated protein A. *Anal. Biochem.* **112,** 195–203.
33. Peluso, R. W., and Rosenberg, G. H. (1987). Quantitative electrotransfer of proteins from sodium dodecyl sulfate polyacrylamide gels onto positively charged nylon membranes. *Anal. Biochem.* **162,** 389–398.
34. Cowell, I. G. (1997). Cloning sequence-specific DNA-binding factors from cDNA expression libraries using oligonucleotide binding site probes. *In* "cDNA Library Protocols" (I. G. Cowell and C. A. Austin, eds.), pp. 161–170. Humana Press, Totowa, NJ.
35. Cowell, I. G. (1997). Yeast two-hybrid library screening. *In* "cDNA Library Protocols" (I. G. Cowell and C. A. Austin, eds.), pp. 185–202. Humana Press, Totowa, NJ.
36. Drees, B. L. (1999). Progress and variations in two-hybrid and three-hybrid technologies. *Curr. Opin. Chem. Biol.* **3,** 64–70.
37. Videl, M., and Legrain, P. (1999). Yeast forward and reverse *'n'*-hybrid systems. *Nucleic Acids Res.* **27,** 919–929.
38. Maxam, A. M., and Gilbert, W. (1977). A new method for sequencing DNA. *Proc. Natl. Acad. Sci. U.S.A.* **74,** 560–564.
39. Sanger, F., Nicklen, S., and Coulson, A. R. (1977). DNA sequencing with chain-terminating inhibitors. *Proc. Natl. Acad. Sci. U.S.A.* **74,** 5463–5467.
40. Zagursky, R. J., Conway, P. S., and Kashdan, M. A. (1991). Use of ^{33}P for Sanger DNA sequencing. *BioTechniques* **11,** 36–38.

41. Slatko, B. E. (1991). Protocols for manual dideoxy DNA sequencing. *In* "Methods in Nucleic Acids Research" (J. L. Karam, L. Chao, and G. Warr, eds.), pp. 83–129. CRC Press, Boca Raton, FL.
42. Chaconas, G., and van de Sande, J. H. (1980). 5′-^{32}P labeling of RNA and DNA restriction fragments. *Methods Enzymol.* **65,** 75–88.
43. Tabor, S., and Richardson, C. C. (1987). DNA sequence analysis with a modified bacteriophage T7 DNA polymerase. *Proc. Natl. Acad. Sci. U.S.A.* **84,** 4767–4771.
44. Kruchinina, N. G., and Gresshoff, P. M. (1994). Detergent affects silver sequencing. *BioTechniques* **17,** 280–282.
45. Beck, S., O'Keefe, T. O., Coull, J. M., and Koster, H. (1989). Chemiluminescent detection of DNA: Application for DNA sequencing and hybridization. *Nucleic Acids Res.* **17,** 5115–5123.
46. Prober, J., Trainor, G., Dam, R., Hobbs, F., Robertson, C., Zagursky, R., Cocuzza, R., Jensen, M., and Baumeister, K. (1987). A system for rapid DNA sequencing with fluorescent chain-terminating dideoxynucleotides. *Science* **238,** 336–341.
47. Zagursky, R., and McCormick, R. (1990). DNA sequencing separations in capillary gels on a modified commercial DNA sequencing instrument. *BioTechniques* **9,** 74–79.

21

Transcription

George P. Yang and Ronald J. Weigel

Stanford University, School of Medicine, Stanford, California 94305

I. Introduction

Transcriptional regulation plays a critical role in orchestrating many aspects of physiology. As research questions in surgical disciplines have progressed to a molecular level, the study of gene regulation has come to center stage. Cell processes as diverse as tumor growth, atherosclerosis, cellular rejection, and shock involve alterations in gene regulation and, in most cases, alterations of gene transcription. This chapter is aimed at providing an understanding of basic aspects of transcriptional regulation germane to the surgical investigator. The sections will address general features of the control of gene transcription, methods to examine gene expression in cells and tissues, methods to identify differentially expressed genes, approaches to study eukaryotic promoters, and methods to identify cellular factors involved in transcriptional regulation. Throughout the text we have drawn on examples from our own work in estrogen receptor (ER) control of gene expression to illustrate particular points.

II. General Aspects of Eukaryotic Transcription

Much of our understanding of the details of eukaryotic gene regulation has been derived from studies in yeast. Yeast have been helpful in this regard because the genome has been fully sequenced and genetic manipulation and selection using yeast cells can be performed easily in comparison to animal cells. Where experiments in yeast can be compared to higher organisms, there has been good evidence that transcriptional mechanisms have been highly conserved in evolution. Therefore, results in yeast genetics have facilitated advances in human systems.

Gene expression requires a number of complex cellular processes that convert genetic information in the chromosomes to proteins that have the physiologic effect. The genes are embedded in the structure of the chromosomes, which in humans encode approximately 50,000–100,000 genes. Transcription is a process that converts the DNA chromosome sequence into a complimentary RNA molecule known as heteronuclear RNA (hnRNA). The location where the RNA molecule begins is called the cap site. The transcription process is controlled by the promoter of the gene. Eukaryotic promoters are DNA sequences that are normally found upstream of the cap site and are high-affinity binding sites for nuclear factors called transcription factors. Important promoter elements can also be found downstream of cap sites, often within the gene introns. Binding of transcription factors to the DNA promoter elements initiates the process of transcription, which results in the synthesis of a molecule of hnRNA. In eukaryotic cells, the hnRNA molecule is processed prior to export to the cytoplasm. RNA processing includes the addition of a methylated guanine residue to the 5′ end (called the cap), removing segments (introns) of the RNA internally by a process called RNA splicing, and adding 100–200 adenine nucleotides to the 3′ end (a process called polyadenylation). The processed RNA is called messenger RNA (mRNA), which is transported to the cytoplasm where it is translated into a protein.

A. Core Promoter Elements

Transcription of genes encoding proteins utilizes RNA polymerase II (RNA pol II), which is an enzyme that builds the hnRNA transcript. A eukaryotic promoter can be functionally divided into core elements and regulatory elements. The core promoter elements encompass the site of the promoter where the general transcription factors (GTFs) form a preinitiation complex (PIC) responsible for accurate basal-level transcription initiation (1). The promoter regulatory elements are regions of the promoter that direct proper temporal and tissue-specific gene transcription. Regulatory elements can be activating or repressing and may also involve a complex interplay of several factors. Regulatory factors are linked to the GTFs at the core promoter element through TATA binding protein-associated factors (TAFs) (see Fig. 1 for schematic). Mechanisms linking regulatory elements to the general transcriptional machinery are currently some of the most intriguing aspects of gene regulation. Besides protein–protein interactions, this process is also likely to involve alterations of chromatin structure.

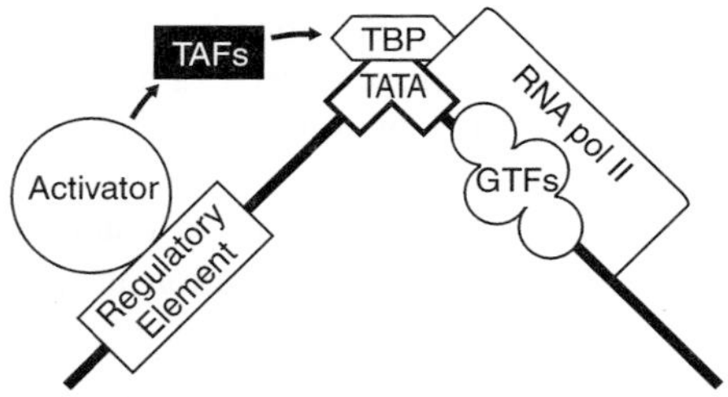

Figure 1 Schematic of transcriptional machinery. The general transcriptional machinery binds at the TATA element of the DNA. The general transcriptional machinery includes TATA binding protein (TBP) and a number of general transcription factors (GTFs) involved in bringing RNA polymerase II (RNA pol II) to the promoter. Interaction of GFTs with the TATA element induces a sharp bend in the DNA template. Activator proteins bind to regulatory elements and are linked to the general transcription machinery through TATA binding protein-associated factors (TAFs).

The core promoter elements include the TATA sequence located 20–30 bp upstream of the initiator (Inr) sequence, which is located at the cap site (start site) of transcription. TATA binding protein (TBP) recognizes the TATA sequence and this DNA–factor association forms the core of the PIC (1, 2). TBP is critical for assembly of the PIC even in so-called TATA-less promoters. A set of TBP-associated factors is recruited to the promoter through interactions with TBP or the Inr sequence forming the TFIID multisubunit complex (2, 3). Additional GTFs are recruited in a defined order to generate the PIC and include TFIIB, TFIIF, TFIIE, TFIIH, and RNA pol II. The formation of this multiprotein complex initiates gene transcription. The activity of a promoter is regulated by the rate of PIC formation, which is controlled largely through factors interacting with regulatory elements.

B. Regulatory Promoter Elements

There is a diverse set of transcriptional regulatory factors responsible for coordinating the promoter activity of genes. These transcription factors are composed of multiple domains, each performing one of the functions that is required of the whole protein. For example, the estrogen receptor (ER) is a member of the family of nuclear hormone receptors that includes the thyroid hormone receptor, retinoic acid receptor, and the steroid hormone receptors (4) (see Fig. 2). Each member displays a characteristic arrangement of three separate domains. From amino to carboxy terminus, the domains are an A/B region that is cell and promoter specific, containing a transcriptional activation region, a DNA-binding domain (C), and a hormone-binding and dimerization domain (E).

Every transcription factor works by recognizing a specific DNA sequence, the enhancer element, which it binds with high affinity. After binding that site, the transcription factor is then capable of initiating transcription from associated promoters. Enhancer elements have fairly specific DNA sequences, but some variation is allowed. For example, the transcription factor may accept either purine nucleotide at one position, while at other positions any mutation will prevent binding. Each enhancer has a consensus sequence that represents the sequence the transcription factor binds to with the greatest affinity. Certain protein sequences, or motifs, have been identified in transcription factors that form structures involved in DNA binding. These motifs are useful in analyzing the protein sequence of a transcription factor to identify what part of the protein may be involved in that function. In the case of the ER, the protein contains what is known as a zinc finger. In this particular protein motif, the protein folds around a central molecule of zinc through ionic bonds and forms a tertiary structure capable of binding to the palindromic estrogen response element (ERE) DNA sequence (5).

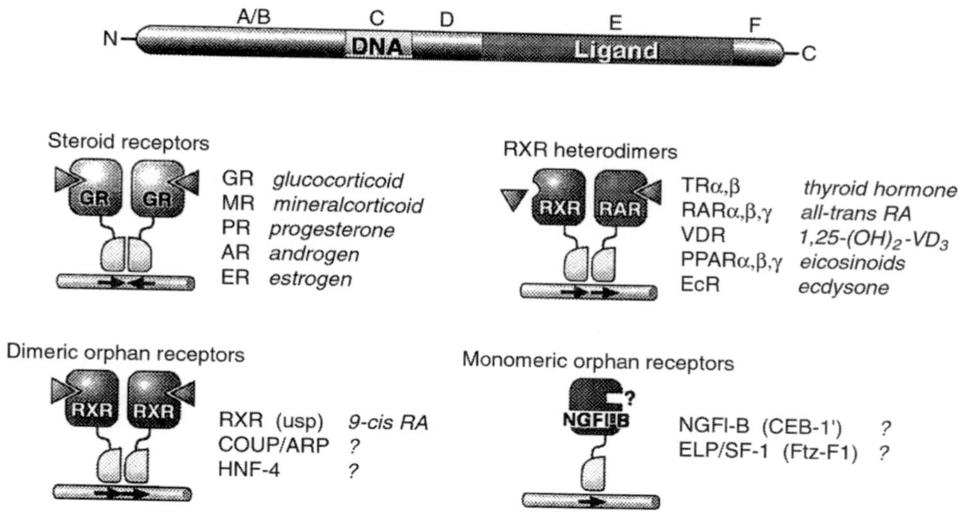

Figure 2 Schematic of nuclear hormone receptors. Schematic representation demonstrates conserved regions of nuclear receptors: a variable N-terminal region (A/B), a conserved DNA binding domain (C), a variable hinge region (D), a ligand-binding domain (E), and a variable C-terminal region (F). The nuclear hormone receptors can be grouped into four categories: steroid receptors, RXR heterodimers, dimeric orphan receptors, and monomeric orphan receptors. From Ref. (4), with permission from Cell Press.

The dimerization domain is what allows the ER to bind other proteins. It is now known that the ER binds to its enhancer site as a homodimer. In other circumstances, it is believed that the ER binds as a heterodimer with other nuclear hormone receptors. The interaction between the ER and other transcription factors allows for an additional mechanism of regulation that does not require the ER to bind to DNA. A recurring theme in molecular biology is that transcription factors can form complexes with other transcription factors to create a transcriptional complex with unique properties. This added level of regulation helps the cell to tailor transcriptional responses using the same transcription factor. Certain protein motifs have been identified, such as the so-called leucine zipper, that can help identify a dimerization domain.

The transcriptional activation domain is the portion of the ER that interacts with other components of the basal transcriptional complex that permits RNA polymerase to begin transcription of the mRNA. Multiple protein motifs have been identified that can identify a transcriptional activation domain and include regions of strong negative charge (acid blobs or acidic tails). These regions interact with the basic transcriptional machinery in ways that are yet to be fully defined to activate transcription, but are likely to be mediated through TAFs (3).

Transcription is a highly regulated event within the cell and multiple mechanisms exist to control the activity of factors. Some transcription factors may require a ligand, estradiol in the case of the ER, in order to bind the enhancer site. Another method of control is through phosphorylation. Within the cell there are multiple kinases and phosphatases that are capable of modifying other proteins (these are discussed in greater detail in other chapters). The act of phosphorylation or dephosphorylation can change the ionic charge status and affect protein function (6). Finally, there are known intracellular inhibitors of transcription factors. These are proteins that are capable of binding the transcription factor and rendering it incapable of transactivating. NFκB is a transcription factor that is normally bound by an inhibitor, IκB. These mechanisms often work in conjunction; it is phosphorylation of IκB that causes it to dissociate from NFκB, which is then capable of transactivation (7).

III. Methods to Identify Gene Expression

The first step to understanding the regulation of a gene is to determine the conditions under which the gene is expressed. The complexity of genetic regulation is what allows tissue-specific gene expression. Transcription may also be controlled in a time-dependent manner, as is seen in tissue development, differentiation, or during changes of the cell cycle.

A. Northern Blot

One of the first steps is to define the steady-state level of the expression of a gene. Northern blot can be used to examine the abundance of a mRNA derived from cell lines or tissues (8). A number of cell lines that have been established from different tissue types have been studied for years and have well-known characteristics. It is equally important to recognize that cell culture can be a very artificial system. Typically, results found from one model system should be confirmed in another cell line derived from the same lineage or in another similar model system. Finding the same results in multiple cell lines enhances the likelihood that the results are relevant to the tissue.

The first step of Northern blot analysis is isolation of RNA from the cell line or tissue. RNA is highly susceptible to RNases that exist practically everywhere, including in human skin, and great care is needed in preparation to ensure that the RNA is not degraded. Several kits are commercially available to facilitate RNA extraction. Trizol (Gibco BRL) is based on cell lysis in the presence of chemicals that denature proteins. This technique is rapid and provides total cell RNA, which is mostly composed of ribosomal RNA. Other kits such as Fast Track Kit 2.0 (Invitrogen Corp., Carlsbad, CA) provide an easy method to extract RNA enriched for poly(A)$^+$ mRNA utilizing oligodeoxythymidine (dT) cellulose.

The next step of a Northern blot is separation of hundreds of thousands of RNA species within any sample based on size using gel electrophoresis. The RNA must be denatured to eliminate secondary structure that will result in anomalous migration. Formamide is commonly used for this purpose. If total RNA is used, the 18S and 28S ribosomal RNAs can be visualized in an ethidium bromide-stained gel on an ultraviolet light box. This helps to confirm proper migration; it also suggests that adequate RNA was loaded in the well and that the RNA has not been degraded, but it is not conclusive. The agarose gel is then placed in contact with the membrane support, and the RNA is transferred by capillary action. Traditionally, the supports have been sheets of nitrocellulose. These functioned well, but are brittle when dried and are not durable for multiple hybridizations. Newer supports using nylon or other similar synthetics are available and do not have those failings. The RNA is then bound to the support either by baking in an oven or by cross-linking with UV radiation.

The blot is hybridized with a DNA probe that is complementary to the RNA of interest. DNA probes are commonly labeled with ^{32}P, but nonradioactive methods for detection are also available. After washing, the membrane is exposed to radiographic film. Highly expressed mRNAs such as actin can be detected after only an hour of exposure. Commonly, it requires 1 to 3 days of exposure for low-abundance mRNAs. Message abundance and amount of RNA loaded affect signal intensity. To control for the amount of RNA loaded, the blot is hybridized with a housekeeping gene such as β-actin. The intensity of the housekeeping gene can be used to correct for amount of RNA and allow a relative quantitation of mRNA abundance. Normally a fivefold or more difference of RNA levels as measured by this method will be reliable. Methods to quantify the signal intensity include densitometer reading of the autoradiograph and phosphor imaging of the radioactive blot. Of these two methods, phosphor imaging is more accurate, especially when dealing with values that range over several orders of magnitude.

B. RNase Protection

Northern blot has great utility, but it is often not sensitive enough for many RNA species that may be expressed at only approximately one copy per cell. Other assays exist that provide more sensitive measures of RNA levels. One such assay is the RNase protection assay (9). This utilizes RNases with the known property of digesting single-stranded RNAs while leaving double-stranded RNAs intact. A radiolabeled RNA probe is generated by *in vitro* synthesis from a cDNA template using RNA polymerase and [α-^{32}P]UTP. The probe is then added to a pool of RNA and will hybridize only with its complementary strand. This mixture is then treated with single-strand-specific RNases that will degrade any single-stranded RNA, including unhybridized probe. Multiple RNases are available and each different probe must be tested to determine which RNase works best with it in an empiric manner. The result of that reaction is electrophoresed on a polyacrylamide gel that will separate out fragments based on size. The gel is dried and exposed to film. The protected fragment of the expected size can be measured and is an accurate assessment of mRNA abundance. However, this assay is more difficult to perform and each different RNA probe requires optimized assay conditions. Even probes that recognize different portions of the same mRNA may not function with the same RNase.

C. Reverse Transcriptase–Polymerase Chain Reaction

A technique that has become increasingly popular to identify rare mRNAs is reverse transcription and polymerase chain reaction (RT–PCR) (10, 11). This procedure utilizes a two-step reaction to amplify a fragment of the gene of interest. In the first step of the procedure, cDNA is generated from the RNA using reverse transcriptase and oligo-dT or random oligonucleotides as primer. In the second step, the cDNA of the gene of interest is amplified with gene-specific primers by PCR. In addition to providing an answer about whether the mRNA is present, it can also be used in a quantitative manner. Quantitative PCR can be done only if proper controls are used. Known amounts of a control DNA are added to the reaction along with a set of primers that will amplify that sequence. This is added to each PCR reaction and serves as an internal control for the amount of amplification that is taking place. If the same amount of the control is in each reaction, then the detectable product of that PCR reaction will be ascribed a value of 1, to which the intensity of other PCR products can be compared. Even under the most careful controls, quantitative PCR is fraught with potential errors and artifacts and the results are to be interpreted with caution.

D. Nuclear Run-on

All of the above techniques examine steady-state levels of a particular mRNA species, but do not determine whether any changes in these levels are the result of altered transcription or altered stability or processing. Nuclear run-on is a method to examine rates of gene transcription directly (12). Cells are harvested under the conditions of interest and are gently lysed while preserving the nuclei. The nuclei are then collected by centrifugation and incubated in the presence of [α-^{32}P]UTP, which will be incorporated into newly synthesized mRNAs. The labeled mRNA is isolated and hybridized to immobilized DNA from the genes of interest. Signal intensity is an indication of the relative rate of transcription from that gene under those conditions. This is a difficult assay to perform, but it remains the most sensitive method of determining the rate of gene transcription.

The half-life of an mRNA species can be determined with the use of actinomycin D. The addition of actinomycin D will inhibit new RNA synthesis. RNA is isolated from cells at various time points after they have been treated. The levels of the mRNA of interest are examined by any of the above methods. The comparison of mRNA levels at various times following treatment will provide a sense of the speed at which mRNA is being degraded.

E. In Situ Hybridization

The above methods can be used for cells in culture or for tissue. However, when working with tissue, it is not possible to have a pure cell population as it is in cell culture. A question may arise about whether the mRNA being detected is being synthesized by breast ductal epithelium, for example, or by the stromal cells or vascular endothelial cells present in the same specimen. *In situ* hybridization is a technique capable of defining which cell types are expressing the gene (13). The technique can be performed in either frozen or permanent sections. It is possible that for some genes one technique will work better than another. The process of tissue fixation and slide preparation must be individualized empirically for each tissue and gene being studied (the further discussion of these subtle differences is beyond the scope of this chapter). A DNA or RNA probe that hybridizes to the sequence of interest is used to detect expression. Traditionally, hybridization was detected by placing specialized film or emulsion radiography to detect a radiolabeled probe. These detection methods often took long exposure times to see a result. Newer detection methods using immunohistochemical and immunofluorescent techniques promise faster results and greater sensitivity. *In situ* hybridization is a powerful technique that allows analysis of gene expression in complex tissues and can also follow temporal and spatial expression of a gene during development. Determination of the reaction conditions required for each gene must be done empirically and can be time consuming.

IV. Methods of Identifying Differentially Expressed Genes

There are a number of situations in which it may be useful to compare patterns of gene expression with the intent of identifying differentially expressed genes. This approach is based on the hypothesis that physiologic differences between two cell types or between cells under different conditions are determined by differences in the pattern of gene expression. Often differences in the pattern of gene expression are explained by differences of gene transcription. Examples where one may want to examine differential gene expression are cancer cells versus normal cells, quiescent cells versus growth-stimulated cells, and primary tumor cells versus metastatic cells. The value of the approach is not limited to cancer but is germane to many physiologic processes, including angiogenesis, atherosclerosis, gastrointestinal physiology, and shock. A number of techniques can be used to compare patterns of gene expression with the intent of identifying a gene or genes that are differentially expressed. Early techniques relied on the construction of subtracted cDNA libraries, which are difficult to construct and time consuming to make. Recent developments in molecular biology have offered new approaches to the isolation of differentially expressed genes. These techniques include differential screening, differential display, serial analysis of gene expression, representational difference analysis, suppression subtractive hybridization, and cDNA arrays.

A. Differential Screening

The technique of differential screening is outlined in Fig. 3. In this example, the pattern of gene expression in differentiated F9 teratocarcinoma cells was compared to undifferentiated F9 cells (14). Poly(A)$^+$ mRNA was isolated from undifferentiated and differentiated F9 cells and cDNA was synthesized from the mRNA. A cDNA library was constructed from the differentiated F9 cDNA and duplicate plaque lifts were prepared from the plated library. The duplicate plaque lifts were hybridized with total cDNA prepared from the undifferentiated and differentiated F9 cDNA. The pattern of hybridization is compared and plaques are identified that hybridize to the differentiated F9 cDNA probe but not the undifferentiated cDNA probe. The plaques are purified and the inserts are recovered and can be used as probes for Northern blots. In the example shown in Fig. 3, genes

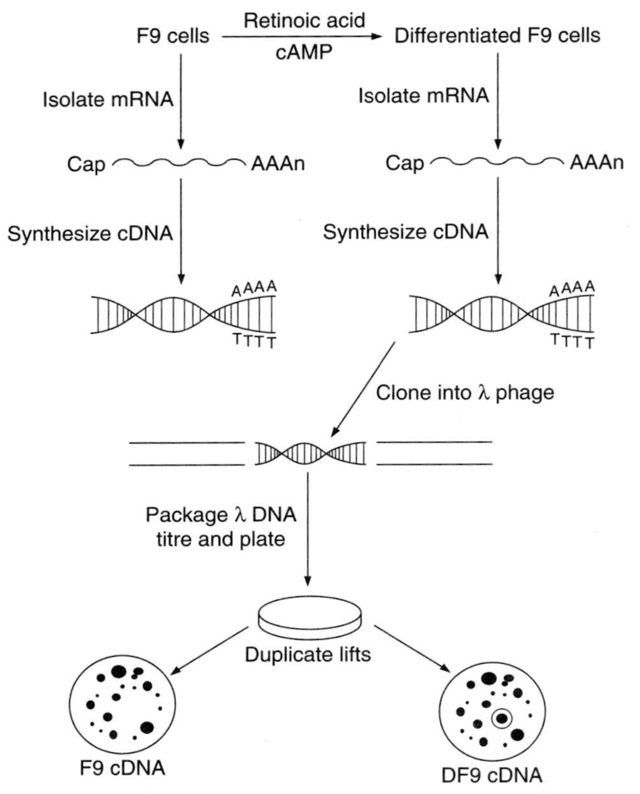

Figure 3 Differential screening. Schematic representation for differential cloning strategy. RNA is isolated from two cell types (F9 cells and differentiated F9 cells). cDNA is synthesized and cloned into a lambda phage vector. Duplicate lifts are performed and probed with either the F9 or differentiated F9 cDNA. Differentially expressed genes are identified by comparing patterns of hybridization (14).

induced during differentiation by retinoic acid in F9 cells were successfully cloned.

Genes of relatively high abundance will be isolated by this method. It is theoretically possible to perform three-way (or more) comparison by performing triplicate (or more) plaque lifts. However, comparison of more than two cell types on primary plaque lifts is tedious and this comparison is better done after phage isolation either by hybridizing purified phage or by Northern blot. In general, genes with differential expression of greater than 5–10 can be isolated. One additional advantage of this technique is that if the library is correctly constructed, full-length cDNA clones are obtained in the course of the screening procedure. The disadvantage of this technique is that abundantly expressed genes tend to be reisolated multiple times. Less abundantly expressed genes are also missed by this technique.

B. Differential Display

Differential display utilizes reverse transcriptase–polymerase chain reaction to randomly amplify a subset of mRNAs in a cell (15, 16). The amplification is performed in the presence of radioactive nucleotides so that the amplified products can be resolved on sequencing gels and visualized by autoradiography. The pattern of amplified products is compared using templates from various cell sources. Differences in the pattern of gene expression are represented by differences in the amplified products. Discordant bands are excised from the sequencing gel and recovered by reamplification. The recovered PCR products are commonly used as probes on Northern blots to confirm the differential pattern of gene expression.

There have been a number of technical refinements in differential display over the past few years. Originally, amplification was performed with "anchored" primers in which oligo-dT primers with one or two base substitutions at the 3′ end were used to amplify subsets of mRNAs. The 5′ oligonucleotide was a random primer of 10–20 bp. Purified cDNA has been used with random oligonucleotides with good success. Testing various PCR conditions to optimize reaction times, temperatures, and number of cycles is necessary to determine conditions that yield an appropriate number of bands. After reamplification of an interesting band from the differential display gels, multiple independent clones are often examined because a single band can give rise to multiple different clones (17). The amplification process allows isolation of low-abundance mRNAs. In addition, because each lane on the differential display gel is from a reaction with a different template, this technique readily lends itself to a multicell line comparison. The main disadvantage found by most investigators is the discouraging number of false positive clones.

C. Serial Analysis of Gene Expression

Serial analysis of gene expression (SAGE) is based on the principle that an oligonucleotide sequence of 9–10 bp can uniquely identify a gene (18). In this technique, 9-bp oligonucleotides of cDNAs are cloned in a long, concatenated string with "punctuations" between the cDNA oligonucleotides. Figure 4 outlines this procedure. The long string is sequenced and the sequence of each oligonucleotide is compared to the GenBank or other sequence database. Abundantly expressed cDNAs turn up more frequently in the string whereas less abundant transcripts are less frequent. SAGE provides a statistical analysis of the frequency of expressed genes. A comparison by performing SAGE on a normal and a cancer cell can provide information on the differences in the pattern of gene expression. SAGE requires extensive sequencing and sequence analysis capability. Automated sequencing is mandatory. In addition, novel genes will not match known sequences and obtaining a full-length cDNA with a 10-bp oligonucleotide probe can be difficult.

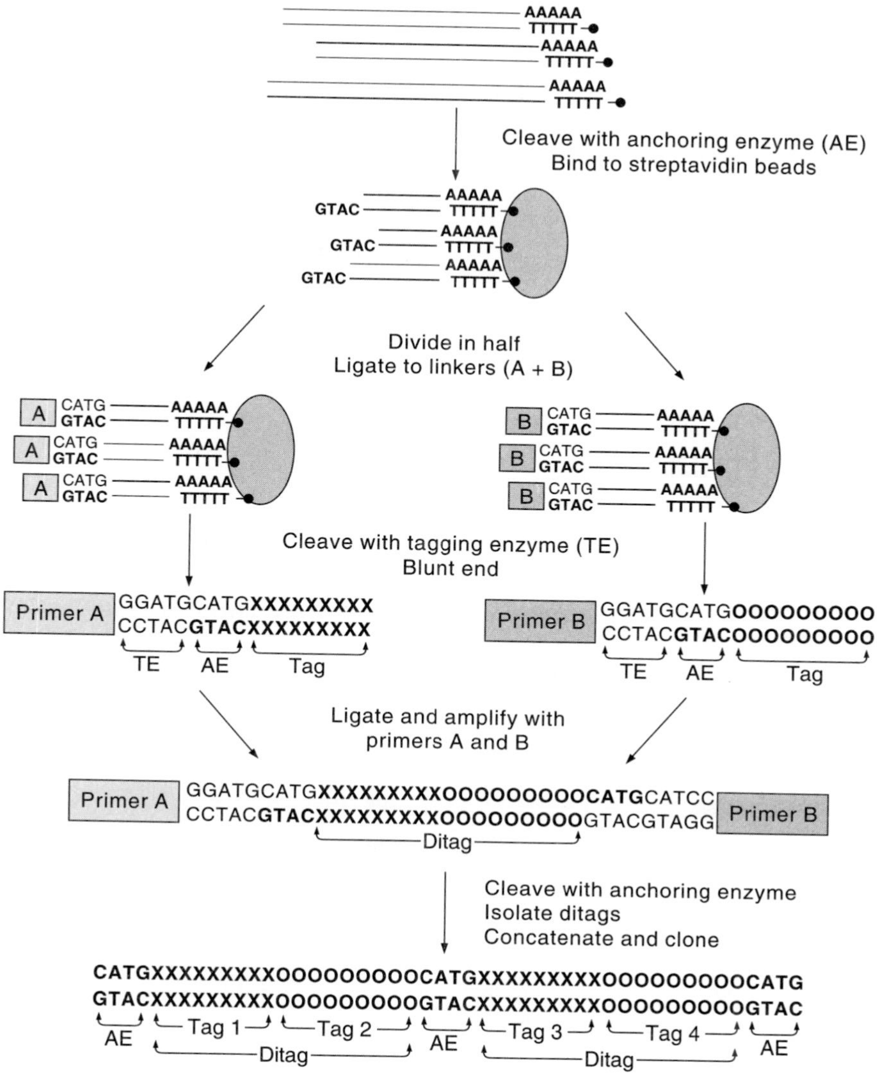

Figure 4 Serial analysis of gene expression. Diagram of SAGE technique resulting in a concatenated string of sequence tags. Reprinted with permission from Ref. (18), Velculescu, V. E., *et al.* (1995). Serial analysis of gene expression. *Science* **270**(5235), 484–487. Copyright 1995 American Association for the Advancement of Science.

D. Representational Difference Analysis and Suppression Subtractive Hybridization

Representational difference analysis (RDA) is a PCR-based technology in which sequences that differ between two sources are selectively amplified (19). Suppression subtractive hybridization (SSH) is a similar technique that uses multiple primers to increase the yield of differentially expressed sequences (20). The SSH procedure is shown schematically in Fig. 5. The cDNA that contains the differentially expressed gene is referred to as the "tester" and the reference cDNA is the "driver." The tester cDNA is ligated separately to two different primers. Two hybridizations are performed with excess driver cDNA. These two hybridizations are mixed under hybridization conditions and the ends extended with polymerase. In the second hybridization, cDNAs of differentially expressed genes are able to form and have a different primer at each end. PCR is used to amplify the hybridization products. Sequences present in the tester that are absent or minimally expressed in the driver are selectively amplified.

This technique has several advantages. Compared to differential screening, SSH is able to identify transcripts of much lower abundance and the rate of false positive clones is less than with differential display (21). Novel and known

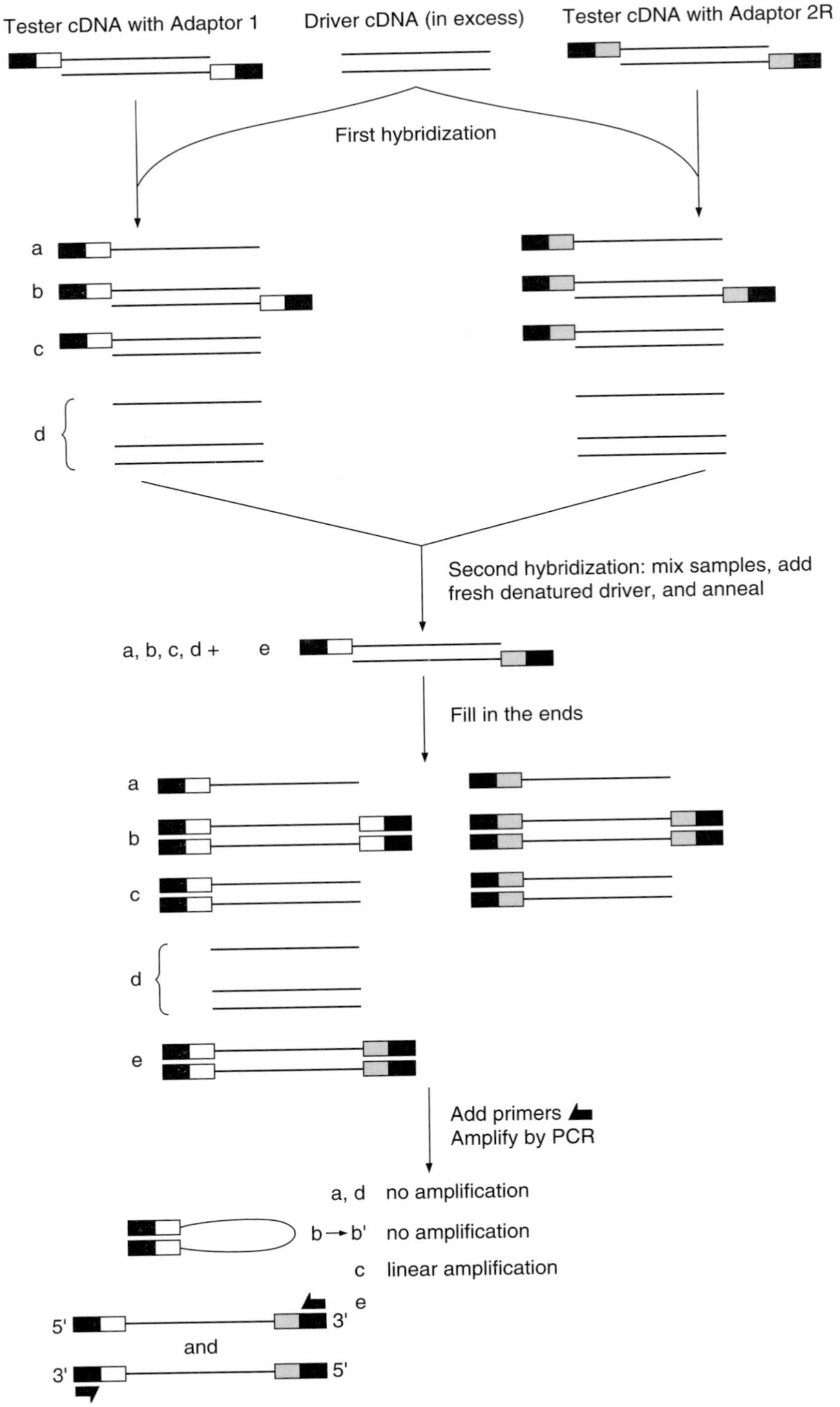

Figure 5 Suppression subtractive hybridization. Diagram of SSH technique, which allows identification of differentially expressed genes. Two sequential hybridizations with amplification of specified primers result in identification of differentially expressed genes (from the Clontech manual). Reprinted from Ref. (20), Diatchenko, L., *et al.* (1996). Suppression subtractive hybridization: A method for generating differentially regulated or tissue-specific cDNA probes and libraries. *Proc. Nat. Acad. Sci. U.S.A.* **93**(12), 6025–6030. Copyright 1996 National Academy of Sciences, U.S.A.

genes are both identified and in the case of novel clones a cDNA fragment sufficient for library screening is obtained. In addition, multiple cell lines can be compared by pooling cDNAs to form the driver.

E. cDNA Arrays

In this technology, cDNA clones are placed on a solid substrate in a defined order. The "array" is hybridized with cDNA from a number of sources and the pattern of hybridization is compared. The comparison is used to identify differentially expressed genes. These data are usually confirmed by Northern blot or RT–PCR. Two broad categories of cDNA arrays are available. Conventional arrays can be commercially obtained (22). These arrays have known cDNAs spotted on nitrocellulose and are ready for hybridization. Newer methods using microarray technology have been developed (23, 24). Two-color hybridizations are used to determine the relative degree of expression, and the intensity of fluorescence indicates the abundance. The advantage of this technology is that thousands of cDNAs can be screened for expression on a single glass slide. Examples of conventional arrays and microarrays are shown in Fig. 6.

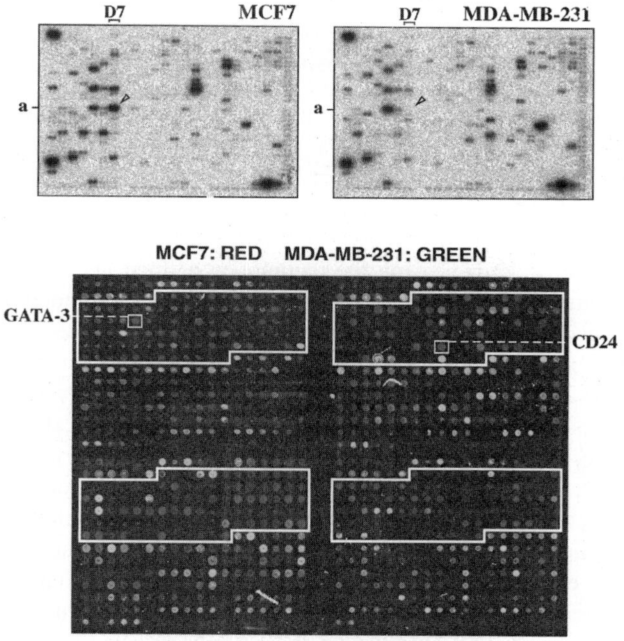

Figure 6 cDNA arrays. Shown are two examples of conventional arrays (top) and microarrays (bottom) identifying differentially expressed genes comparing MCF7 and MDA-MB-231. In the top panel, the arrow indicates the clone GATA-3 at position D7a. In the bottom panel, GATA-3 is identified on microarrays. (Top) Reprinted from Ref. (22), Hoch, R. V., *et al.* (1999). GATA-3 is expressed in association with estrogen receptor in breast cancer. *Int. J. Cancer* **84**(2), 122–128, copyright © 1999 John Wiley & Sons. Reprinted by permission of Wiley-Liss, Inc., a subsidiary of John Wiley & Sons, Inc. (Bottom) Reprinted from Ref. (24), Yang, G. P., *et al.* (1999). Combining SSH and cDNA microarrays for rapid identification of differentially expressed genes. *Nucleic Acids Research* **27**(6), 1517–1523, by permission of Oxford University Press. (See color plates.)

V. Mapping a Eukaryotic Promoter

This section addresses the issue of how to identify the promoter region of a gene and the regulatory factors controlling transcription. Promoter analysis is a routine part of many expression studies but unfortunately the regulation of most promoters remains a mystery. Regions controlling expression can be far removed from the transcriptional start or cap site. Multiple cap sites are also often found and these can be separated by thousands or in some cases hundreds of thousands of base pairs. The factors involved in regulation interact with the DNA and each other adding additional complexity. In some cases these factors can alter chromosomal structure, thereby altering accessibility of the promoter. Having said this, there are some general guidelines in approaching promoter analysis. First, it is important to determine if transcription is a mechanism likely to be controlling the gene under study. Approaches discussed in the preceding sections will help to determine if transcriptional regulation seems likely.

A. Genomic Clones and Genomic Structure

It is important to have a reasonable area of the genomic area under study (called the contig). A sufficient region of genomic DNA can be obtained by screening genomic libraries. Human genomic libraries are commercially available. A lambda phage library will yield 15–25 kbp of sequence. Bacterial artificial chromosomes (BACs) will provide 100–200 kbp inserts. Promoter elements can exist several kilobases from the actual transcriptional start site as well as in introns of the gene. Multiple overlapping clones are often needed to obtain a sufficient contig of the region of interest. It is anticipated that in a few years the human genome will be sequenced and will facilitate this line of investigation. Prior to having this information, a restriction map is generated using standard restriction enzymes. It allows for rapid identification of potential introns by comparison to the restriction map of the cDNA clone and it provides a guide to further genetic manipulations that will be necessary. These techniques are well described elsewhere. Sequencing of the gene is done with the standard Sanger protocol. Once the sequence is known, a wealth of information can be gained. Much is known about specific sequences that are involved in transcription. There are consensus sites known for the initiation of transcription and for the addition of a polyadenosine tail. Comparison of the genomic and cDNA sequences will reveal the presence of introns. Many enhancer sites are already known and characterized and these can be detected using sequence analysis software that search for the consensus sequences. Doing this provides a great deal of information about potential transcription factors that may be acting to control transcription and may help to focus future directions for experimentation.

B. Identification of a Gene Cap Site

In most cases promoter analysis should begin with identification of the mRNA cap site(s), intron/exon boundaries, and polyadenylation sites. The intron/exon locations and polyadenylation sites are easily determined by cloning the cDNA and comparing the sequence to genomic sequence. However, it is difficult to know if the 5′ end of the cDNA clone represents the cap site of the mRNA or premature termination by reverse transcriptase. S1 nuclease, primer extension, and 5′ rapid amplification of cDNA ends (RACE) can be used to map the cap sites of mRNAs. The S1 nuclease is an enzyme capable of digesting single-stranded DNA (25). A DNA probe with a sequence based on the genomic DNA sequence that has been end labeled is hybridized to mRNA. The mRNA will hybridize to those parts of the probe that are complementary but will leave single-stranded DNA overhangs. Treatment with S1 nuclease will create a uniquely sized digestion product that can be visualized on an acrylamide gel. This protocol provides information about the location of 5′ and 3′ ends, and can be used to map introns depending on the design of the probe and the end that is labeled. The products of S1 digestion are electrophoresed with a sizing ladder that will allow specific determination of the size of the resulting fragment. The size of the fragment maps the distance of the end of the RNA relative to the end of the DNA probe. S1 nuclease determines the end of complementary sequence between mRNA and genomic DNA. Therefore, the results do not discriminate between a 5′ splice site and a cap site of the message. Cap site locations determined by S1 mapping should be confirmed by primer extension or 5′ RACE.

For primer extension, a DNA primer of 30–50 bp is chosen that will hybridize 100–300 bp downstream from the predicted 5′ end of the RNA (26). The primer is labeled, hybridized to the mRNA, and reverse transcriptase (RT) is used to extend the primer. The enzyme will extend the primer to the end of the mRNA. Resolving the product on a polyacrylamide gel allows quantitation of the size of the product and a determination of the location of the 5′ end of the mRNA. Artifacts resulting from premature termination (strong RT stops) can occur. However, mRNA ends mapped by S1 and primer extension are likely to be correct. Primer extension is difficult when used to map scarce mRNAs. The related technique known as 5′ RACE is an alternative that works well for most genes (27). A primer of 20 bp is annealed to the mRNA and extended with RT. The cDNA product is tailed using terminal deoxynucleotidyl transferase. The cDNA is amplified once or twice with a set of nested primers and cloned. The 5′ RACE products are sequenced and the sequences compared to genomic sequences to determine the structure of the 5′ end of the mRNA.

C. DNase I Hypersensitive Sites

Identifying regions of the gene that are hypersensitive to DNase digestion can help to locate important regulatory elements (28). This is based on the theory that regulatory regions of genes actively transcribed have more accessible chromosomal structure. In this technique, nuclei are prepared from cells that are discordant for expression of the gene under study. The intact nuclei are treated with various concentrations of DNase I and subsequently harvested and the DNA purified. The DNA is digested with restriction enzymes and analyzed by Southern blot. The location of the DNase I sites is determined relative to the restriction site. These regions should be included in a promoter analysis.

D. Using Promoter Constructs in a Transient Assay

Once a fragment of genomic DNA has been identified and is believed to include the promoter region, it is necessary to prove that that piece of DNA is able to direct synthesis of RNA under the conditions expected. By this time, an accurate picture of the transcriptional response of the gene should be known using the techniques defined above. The fragment of the gene believed to contain the promoter is placed 5′ to a reporter gene. The reporter gene encodes for a protein that can be readily assayed and serves as a surrogate marker for transcriptional activity. Three common reporter genes are the chloramphenicol acetyltransferase (CAT) gene, the β-galactosidase gene, and the firefly luciferase gene. These genes have enzymatic activity that can be detected by a simple assay. In the case of CAT, chloramphenicol is placed in the presence of ^{14}C-labeled acetate. The enzyme will catalyze transfer of the radioactivity to chloramphenicol, and this is easily detected using thin-layer chromatography. The β-gal gene is easily detected in a colorimetric assay. Luciferase will generate a chemiluminescent product in the presence of substrate that can be detected with a specialized spectrophotometer.

To perform the assays, the promoter being tested is cloned 5′ to the reporter gene. This construct is transfected into a cell line that is known to express the gene in an appropriate fashion. Comparing expression in a cell that does not express the gene or under conditions that are known to alter expression is helpful to determine that the reporter assay expression is recapitulating the native pattern of gene expression. Cotransfection of an alternate basal promoter construct [e.g., cytomegalovirus (CMV)-β-gal] can be used to control for transfection efficiency. Although these techniques are highly sensitive, differences of less than fivefold are difficult to interpret. Finally, it is important to remember that it is the enzymatic activity of a protein that is being measured. This activity is several steps removed from the actual process of transcription; these assays do not measure transcription directly.

The previously described techniques of Northern blot, RNase protection, and S1 nuclease mapping can also be used to detect the mRNA transcribed from the reporter constructs. These assays are significantly more difficult to perform compared to the enzymatic assays. It is common to use the enzymatic assays to gain broad information about transcriptional activation whereas the more direct measures are used to do more detailed promoter analysis and confirm accurate transcriptional initiation.

E. Identifying Regulatory Elements

Once a promoter has been defined, the next step is to identify the portions of the promoter that are necessary and sufficient for the transcriptional responses being studied. Although sequence analysis can often give a great deal of information, it is still necessary to test fragments of the promoter for their ability to stimulate transcription. In our laboratory, we were interested in the transcriptional regulation of the estrogen receptor (ER) gene. We had used the ER-positive MCF-7 and T47-D breast cancer cell lines for our promoter analysis (29). Figure 7 shows results for an analysis of the human ER promoter. We were interested in finding a transcription factor that stimulated ER transcription in ER-positive breast tumors. The first step is to create deletion mutants of the promoter to study how much of the promoter is necessary for the transcriptional response being studied. Deletion mutants were made from both the 5′ and the 3′ ends of the promoter to define the 5′ and 3′ limits of the necessary promoter regions.

One of the early techniques for generating deletion mutants was the use of Bal31, an enzyme that will digest DNA from any free end (30). By stopping the reaction at selected time points, it is possible to get a variety of deletion mutants. The difficulty is in controlling the reaction. It is not possible to precisely gauge how far the enzyme will digest, and it is by sheer luck and brute force that a researcher would finally be able to accumulate an adequate series of deletion mutants that spanned the entire promoter sequence.

The development of PCR has now made the process of generating a series of deletion mutants a trivial task. Once the sequence of the promoter is known, oligonucleotides can be synthesized that allow the exact fragment desired to be generated for promoter analysis. One caveat is that all of these fragments must be completely sequenced to ensure that the process of PCR did not place any point mutations within the sequence, because these may be critical in a promoter analysis.

The use of deletion mutants allowed us to narrow down from over 3 kb to a roughly 75-bp segment of the promoter that appeared to be necessary for ER expression (29) (see Fig. 7). To identify the specific site, a technique called linker scanning can be used to further narrow down the site of interest. This uses PCR to generate known mutations. By incorporating known areas of mutation into oligonucleotides used to PCR amplify a fragment, you can incorporate specific mutations into a sequence. By spacing the areas of mutation, the enhancer element needed for transcription can be defined to the precise base pair.

VI. Identifying and Cloning Transcription Factors

Once a regulatory element has been identified, the next important step is to understand how that promoter element regulates gene expression. In most cases, this DNA element interacts in a sequence-specific fashion with nuclear proteins called transcription factors. The following section addresses methods to identify and study factors controlling gene transcription.

A. Identifying Factors Binding Regulatory Elements

The above studies are needed to demonstrate that a small sequence of DNA is necessary for gene transcription. The next step is to identify the protein responsible for the transcriptional activity. The gel mobility-shift assay is used to demonstrate that a protein binds to the area of DNA that has been identified (31). Although it may be that this gel shift activity is found in the cell line in which transcription is present and not in the other one, it is also possible that the gel shift activity is present in both cell lines, but is simply not functionally active in one. This technique relies on the theory that the binding of protein to DNA will create a complex that will migrate through a polyacrylamide gel at a different rate than the DNA alone. To perform the assay, a fragment of DNA containing the suspected binding site is labeled by the addition of ^{32}P using T7 DNA kinase. The radiolabeled probe is incubated with a cellular extract containing transcription factors. If the transcription factor that will bind to that site is present, a new band will be visualized by autoradiography that will correspond to the protein–DNA complex. In our studies, the ERF-1/AP2γ factor was first identified by gel shift analysis using the ER promoter regulatory element as a probe (29), as shown in Fig. 8.

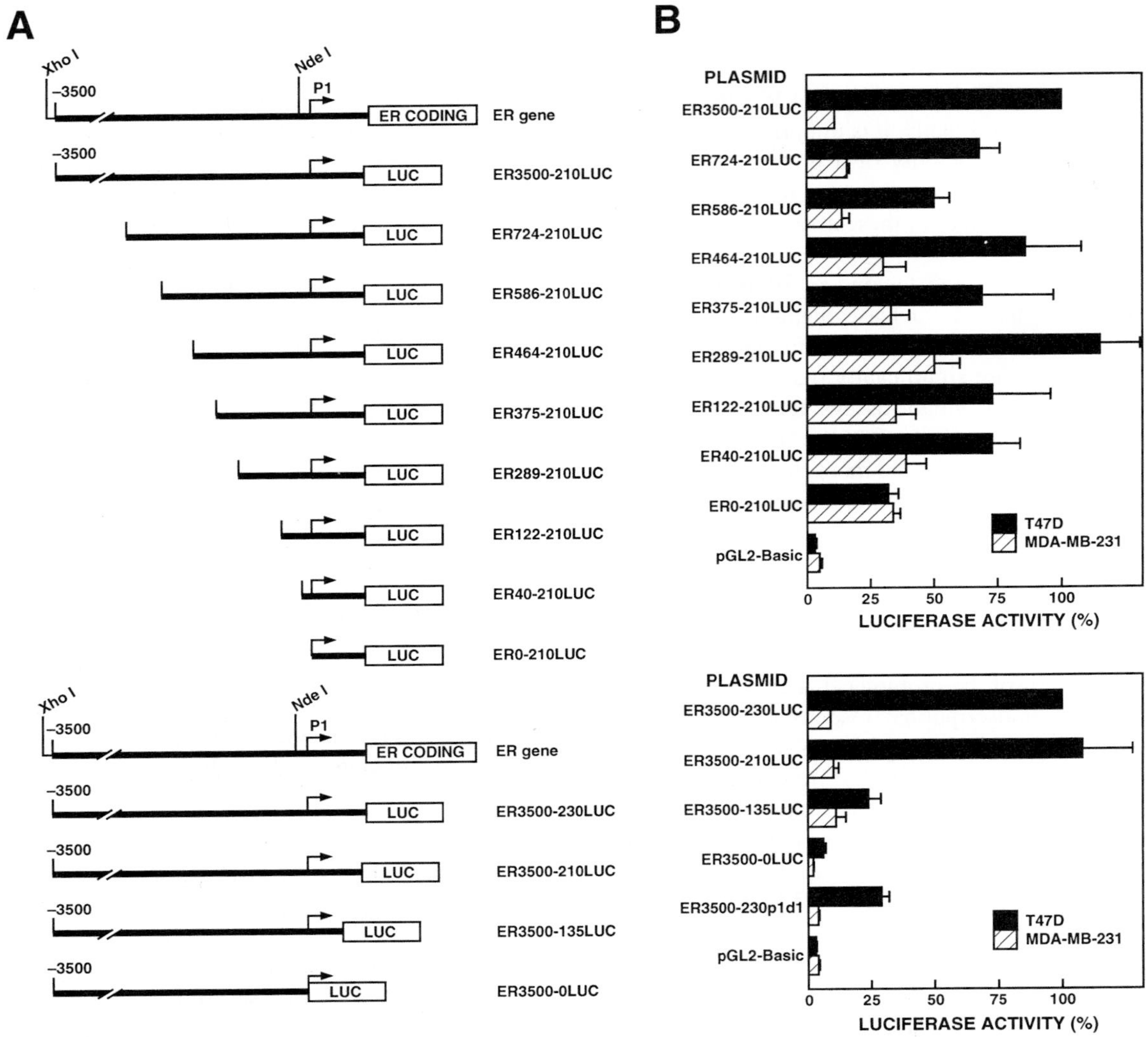

Figure 7 ER promoter analysis. Promoter analysis of the human ER gene is shown with 5′ and 3′ deletion constructs. (A) Schematic representation showing each construct cloned upstream of the luciferase reporter. (B) Corrected luciferase activity for each construct in T47D and MDA-MB-231 cells. These studies identified the ER-specific regulatory element in the 3′ region from +135 to +210 (29).

To confirm that this is a sequence-specific interaction, competition with excess unlabeled probe should eliminate the complex band whereas the use of a mutated or random fragment of DNA will not. Additionally, the protein binding to the DNA can be specifically identified if there is an antibody available to the transcription factor that is believed to bind to the site. The addition of antibody to the reaction will result in what is termed a supershift of the specific protein–DNA complex. The combined antibody–protein–DNA interaction forms an even larger complex that will migrate at a higher point in the gel.

The gel mobility-shift assay can also be used to identify optimal sequences for binding. Every transcription factor has a consensus sequence to which the factor will bind with the greatest avidity. Once the enhancer site has been identified, oligonucleotides can be constructed with single mutations in known sites. The ability of the transcription factor to bind with these sequences on gel mobility-shift assays is one measure of the strength of binding. In addition, the different oligonucleotides can be used as cold competitors to binding with other sequences (see Fig. 8). The ability of one sequence to compete for binding with another indicates that the transcription factor has a preference for one sequence over the other. Defining a consensus binding site can be helpful to identify a transcription factor.

Although the gel mobility-shift assay can show that a transcription factor will bind to a sequence, the DNase footprinting is needed to identify the specific nucleotides that are important for the binding interaction. This technique takes advantage of the fact that binding of DNA by protein

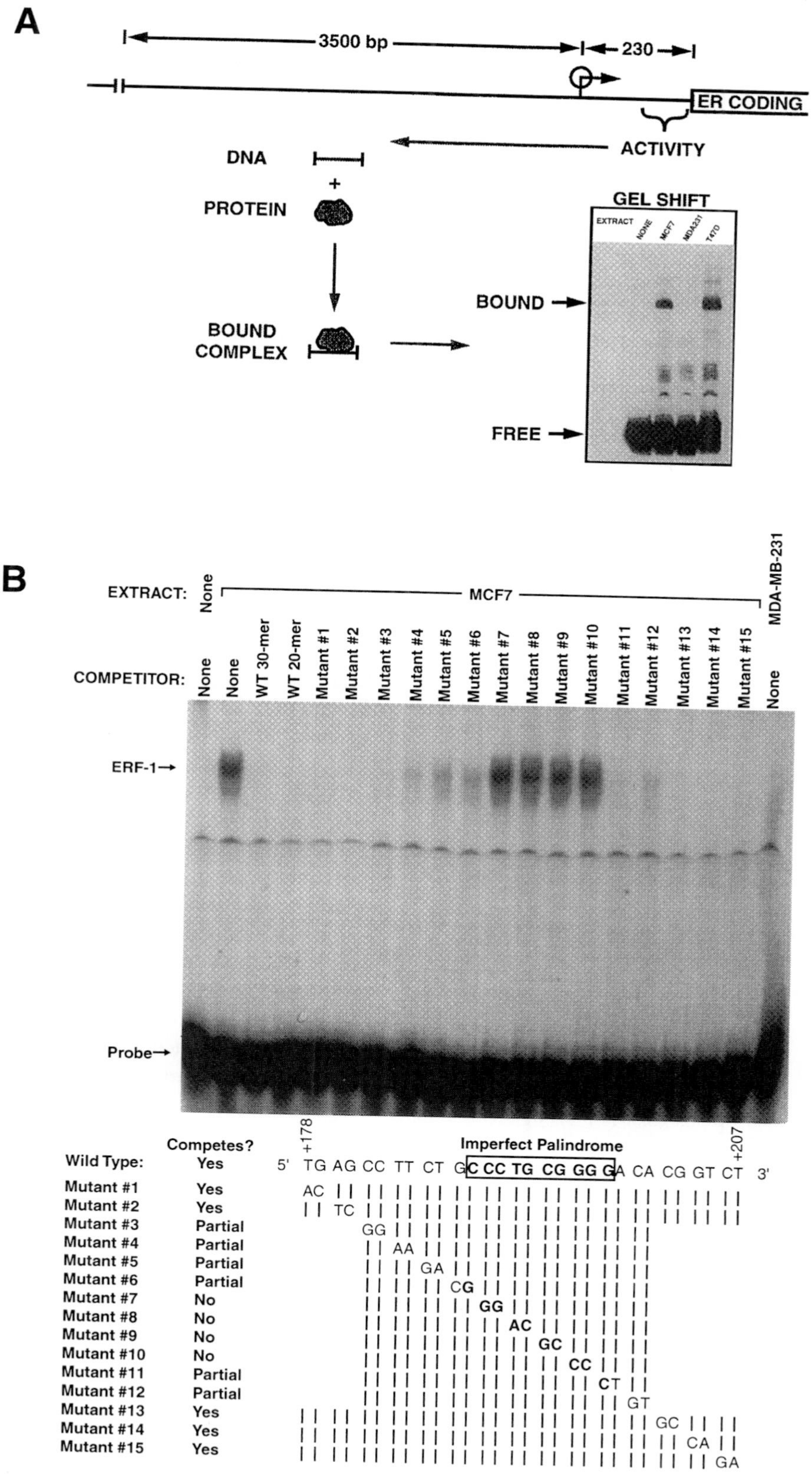

Figure 8 Gel shift analysis. Demonstration of gel shift activity of ERF-1/AP2γ binding to a region of the ER promoter. (A) Schematic of gel shift in which protein binding to the DNA probe generates a complex identified as a band with slower mobility than the free probe. Gel insert demonstrates ERF-1/AP2γ activity in MCF7 and T47D. (B) Gel shift competition identifying a binding site as an imperfect palindrome in the region of the probe. From Ref. (29) and from Ref. (37), McPherson, L. A., *et al.* (1997). Identification of ERF-1 as a member of the AP2 transcription factor family. *Proc. Nat. Acad. Sci. U.S.A.* **94**(9), 4342–4347. Copyright 1997 National Academy of Sciences, U.S.A.

will protect it from digestion by DNase (32). A DNA fragment is labeled at one end with [γ-^{32}P]ATP. The fragment is bound by the transcription factor prior to the addition of DNase. Digestion conditions are selected so that each piece of DNA is randomly cleaved at one point. In a large population of DNAs, this generates a ladder of DNA fragments of various sizes except for those sizes that correspond to the points where the DNA is bound by the transcription factor. Identification of the binding site of the transcription factor can be known to the specific base pair with this method, as shown in Fig. 9.

Methylation interference is a very similar method (33). This takes advantage of the ability of dimethyl sulfate (DMS) to methylate guanine (G) residues on DNA. These methylated guanine residues can then be cleaved with piperidine. The G residues that are methylated are not bound by protein. The methylation reaction is done under conditions such that on average only one G per DNA molecule is methylated. After performing gel shift with the methylated probe, the bound and free probe are recovered and cleaved with piperidine. The products are analyzed on sequencing gels. The free probe should have all G residues equally represented. Because methylated G residues will not bind protein, G residues involved in binding the protein will not be present in the lane derived from the bound probe. This will be evident by gaps in the ladder and will correspond to G residues involved in protein contact. Obviously this method will not be useful in AT-rich DNA binding sites.

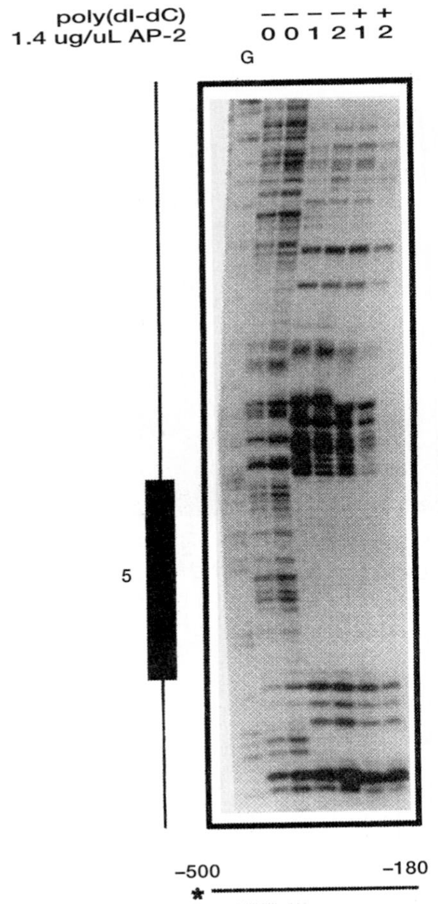

Figure 9 Footprint analysis. Example of a footprint analysis of AP2 binding to the region of DNA with the binding site. AP2 binding to DNA protects the region of binding from digestion with DNase I. The binding region is identified by a space in the ladder on the gel. Figure provided by Dr. Devon Thompson, Stanford University.

Methylation interference has also been modified to generate *in vivo* information. The previous methods are done *in vitro*, which can leave questions about which sites are actually important in living cells. Cells are fully permeable to DMS, and the identical methylation interference reaction can be performed in intact cells. Instead of having labeled fragments, PCR is then used to amplify the fragments after cleavage. A missing PCR product will indicate a protected G residue.

After the identification of an enhancer site, it is useful to determine a consensus sequence for that site. As described above, the consensus sequence represents the DNA sequence that binds the transcription factor with the greatest avidity. There are a number of methods to do so. If the particular enhancer site has been described in multiple genes, a simple sequence analysis can determine which nucleotide residues are most highly conserved. For example, it may be found that in one position, only an A will allow binding, whereas at other residues, a purine will suffice. Some residues within the enhancer may tolerate any nucleotide, which would suggest that this is not a specific point of contact of the transcription factor, even though it may be only two nucleotides from a highly conserved residue.

However, sequence analysis will not define a strict consensus based on hard data. A number of techniques exist to define a consensus. One technique mentioned above is the use of different oligonucleotides in gel mobility-shift assays. With the current ease of oligonucleotide synthesis, it is possible to synthesize every given permutation of a site for analysis by gel mobility shift. However, this can be tedious and there can be considerable expense in synthesizing so many oligonucleotides.

There are multiple ways of generating mutants to test for their ability to bind the transcription factor. However, a short 10-bp sequence has a potential of 4^{10} different permutations and it becomes impractical to simply make mutants without a guide. With the use of DNase footprinting as described above, it is possible to identify critical nucleotide residues and then to focus mutants at those sites.

One elegant method to test all possible sites in a rapid manner is termed PCR-assisted binding-site selection (34). An oligonucleotide is synthesized that has a random sequence inserted between restriction enzyme cloning sites.

The length of the random sequence corresponds to the length of the enhancer. Statistically, every possible sequence permutation is represented in that population. This pool of oligonucleotides is incubated with the transcription factor and electrophoresed on an acrylamide gel as if a gel mobility-shift assay is being performed. The band on the gel corresponding to the DNA–transcription factor complex is then excised out of the gel, purified, and cloned into a sequencing vector. Multiple fragments are sequenced and the resulting sequences are analyzed. The frequency with which each nucleotide is represented at each site is calculated and the result represents the consensus binding site. This technique was recently used to demonstrate that AP2α and AP2γ have the same DNA consensus site (35).

B. Identification of a Known Transcription Factor

Once a DNA binding site has been identified, the next step is to identify the transcription factor that binds to it. If the consensus site matches a previously identified factor, this protein becomes a candidate for the regulatory element under study (36). However, multiple transcription factors can act on the same sequence. This reflects the potential for tissue-specific gene expression and the multiple layers of transcriptional regulation that exist in complex organisms. Although it may be known that one particular transcription factor binds at a given site, the researcher who finds that same site in another model system cannot assume the same transcription factor is involved.

The first step in confirming that a known transcription factor is regulating transcription from a newly defined promoter is to identify the presence of the transcription factor in that cell line. Published transcription factors will have a cDNA sequence known and specific antibodies may also be available. Northern blot analysis will confirm that mRNA for this transcription factor is present and a Western blot will identify the protein. Furthermore, it is necessary to show that the protein is functional by doing a gel mobility supershift as described above.

C. Identification of a Novel Transcription Factor

If the enhancer site has not been previously identified, or the transcription factor believed to bind to that site is novel, then it is necessary to identify the protein that binds to the site. One of the first techniques described to purify a transcription factor involves the use of a DNA affinity column. The ability of a transcription factor to bind its cognate DNA binding site is no different from any other chemical affinity reaction. Multiple copies of the binding site are covalently linked to a support, typically agarose beads. Cellular lysates are made under nondenaturing conditions from the appropriate cell lines or tissue. The source chosen should have what is believed to be a relatively high level of the transcription factor. It is important in using whole tissue to know whether another transcription factor is present in an unrelated cell type within the specimen that also binds to the same site. This approach was successfully used to clone the ERF-1/AP2γ transcription factor (37), as outlined in Fig. 10.

The lysate is first tested on a gel mobility-shift assay to ensure that the binding activity is present within the sample. It is often helpful to obtain an estimate of the factor size using UV cross-linking. In this technique, the factor is covalently linked to the radiolabeled probe and the complex recovered by gel shift. The protein–DNA complex is analyzed by SDS–PAGE and the protein molecular weight is estimated by subtracting the weight of the probe DNA. The factor is purified from the nuclear extract using ion affinity and DNA affinity chromatography. The gel mobility shift

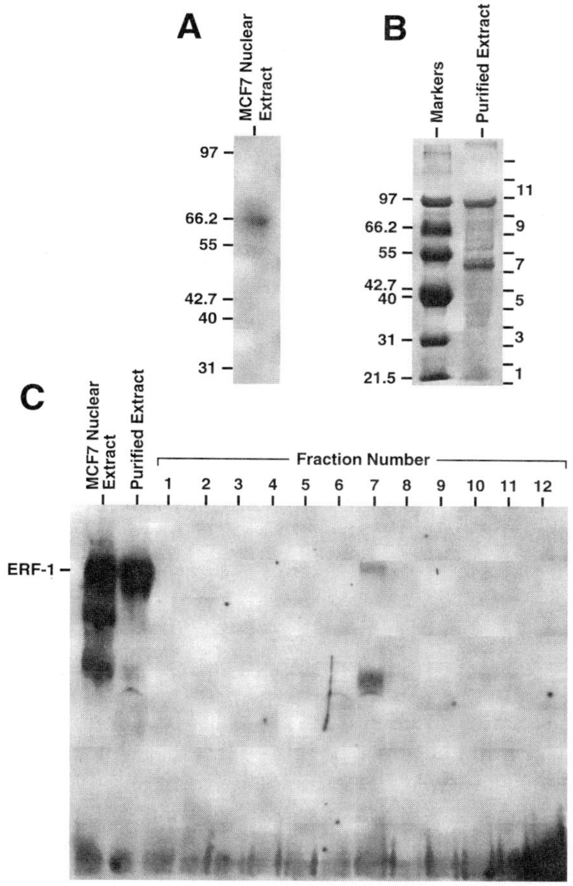

Figure 10 UV cross-link and protein purification. (A) UV cross-link experiment identifying ERF-1/AP2γ as a 50-kDa protein. The complex with DNA migrates at approximately 66 kDa. (B) Silver stain of purified extract. (C) Renatured ERF-1 activity is identified in fraction 7. From Ref. (37), McPherson, L. A., *et al.* (1997). Identification of ERF-1 as a member of the AP2 transcription factor family. *Proc. Nat. Acad. Sci. U.S.A.* **94**(9), 4342–4347. Copyright 1997 National Academy of Sciences, U.S.A.

becomes the functional assay used in following purification. It is usually useful to first partially purify the sample using some nonspecific separation columns such as Sepharose, heparin agarose, and/or DNA–cellulose. The partially purified lysate is then passed over a DNA affinity column with subsequent elution of the binding proteins. The eluted proteins are separated by SDS–PAGE and visualized. Multiple bands may be present, and the various proteins can be eluted, renatured, and tested for DNA binding. All bands, no matter how minor, must be examined. Each band is excised from the gel followed by elution of the protein. The protein is partially sequenced by conventional technology to obtain peptide sequences. The peptides are compared to known sequences to determine if there is correspondance to a known protein. If the sequences are unique, then degenerate oligonucleotides are synthesized corresponding to the peptide sequence and RT–PCR are used to generate a fragment of the gene. This fragment can be used to screen a cDNA library to obtain the gene for the factor. The importance of examining every band is highlighted by our experience with ERF-1/AP2γ. During the purification process, a single major band was eluted that corresponded to a protein with no known transcriptional function. Further examination identified a minor band of almost the same molecular weight that was found by direct protein sequencing to be the ERF-1/AP2γ transcription factor.

This method remains one of the best for purifying a transcription factor. However, it is a technically demanding and time-consuming process that can often be marked by multiple missteps and false leads. Another approach to identifying the transcription factor is to use a labeled oligonucleotide containing the binding site to probe a lambda phage expression library. This approach requires that the protein be made by the bacteria in sufficient quantity and in a conformation capable of binding DNA. There are no tests that can show this other than to attempt to identify the clone in this manner. At least 1–3 million recombinant phages need to be screened in this process.

D. Confirming the Function of a Transcription Factor

Once the transcription factor has been purified and cloned, it still remains to be proved that this is the transcription factor involved in the biologic process that was being studied in the first place. It is not uncommon to go through an elaborate identification and purification process as described above only to find that there is no apparent transactivation of the promoter being studied by the transcription factor that has been found.

The simplest method for initially establishing that a transcription factor is capable of activating a particular promoter is to perform cotransfection assays. The promoter is cloned behind a reporter gene such as luciferase or CAT. On a separate plasmid, the cDNA for the transcription factor is cloned downstream from a constitutively active promoter. When these two plasmids are cotransfected into a reporter cell line, one should be able to detect significant transcriptional activity using the reporter assay. It is necessary to demonstrate that the reporter cell line does not contain any activity that can transactivate from the enhancer. As controls, the promoter–reporter plasmid can be cotransfected with a second plasmid that does not contain the cDNA for the transcription factor. A more elegant control is to introduce an early translational stop codon that results in a severely truncated protein. This allows the control plasmid to be nearly identical to the experimental plasmid with the exception of a single base pair. The reverse can also be done, with the plasmid containing the transcription factor unaltered, but the enhancer in the promoter is mutated to a site that is known not to bind the transcription factor based on earlier experimentation. This approach was used to provide additional evidence that the AP2 proteins transactivate the human ER promoter (35) (see Fig. 11).

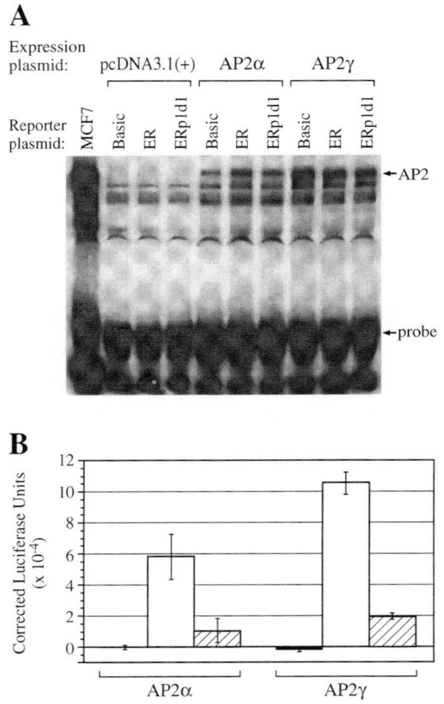

Figure 11 Activation of the ER promoter by AP2α and ERF-1/AP2γ. (A) AP2 activity is demonstrated by gel shift following transfection of AP2α or AP2γ into MDA-MB-231 cells. (B) Transactivation of the cloned ER promoter by AP2α and AP2γ. The black bar with basal activity is vector with no promoter; the clear bar is the cloned ER promoter construct and the striped bar is the ER promoter construct with mutated AP2 sites. From Ref. (35), McPherson, L. A., and Weigel, R. J. (1999). AP2alpha and AP2gamma: A comparison of binding site specificity and transactivation of the estrogen receptor promoter and single site promoter constructs. *Nucl. Acids Res.* **27**(20), 4040–4049, by permssion of Oxford University Press.

By necessity this work is done in a cell line that is usually unrelated to the original physiologic process being studied. In addition, cloned promoters can respond quite differently than endogenous chromosomal genes. It remains to be demonstrated that the transcription factor that has been purified has a significant role in the original disease process. Most of the approaches involve disrupting the function of the transcription factor to demonstrate loss of transcriptional activity. This serves to prove that this transcription factor is necessary for expression of the gene of interest. One way to eliminate expression of the factor is with the use of antisense oligonucleotides. Down-regulation of the protein should decrease expression of the target gene.

A more efficient way to eliminate the activity of a transcription factor is with the use of a dominant negative mutant (38). A dominant negative mutant is one that will suppress the function of wild-type protein that may be present. Many of these act as dominant negatives because they have a high affinity for the enhancer site but do not stimulate transactivation. By binding to the enhancer site, they prevent the wild-type protein from binding and functioning. These mutants can be powerful tools in dissecting the function of a transcription factor and the role of this factor in gene regulation.

E. Identifying Transcriptional Cofactors

One feature of transcription factors that must be remembered is that they often function as complexes. There is a reasonable likelihood that the transcription factor that binds an enhancer site is actually a complex of multiple proteins. One of the prototypes is the AP-1 transcription factor that is composed of the fos and jun proteins. There are two methods commonly employed to identify transcriptional coactivators—coimmunoprecipitation and the yeast two-hybrid system.

In coimmunoprecipitation experiments, an antibody to the factor is used to precipitate complexes from cell extracts. The proteins precipitated are recovered and identified. If a reasonable guess can be made as to the protein identity, a Western blot or coimmunoprecipitation with antibody to the other protein will confirm the hypothesis. Alternatively the other protein will need to be purified and sequenced.

The yeast two-hybrid system takes advantage of the fact that yeasts (*Saccharomyces cerevisiae*) are eukaryotic, unicellular organisms that share the same basic transcriptional machinery as mammals (39–41). We have successfully used this technique to identify proteins that interact with ER in a ligand-dependent fashion, as shown in Fig. 12. The GAL4 transcription factor has two domains—a DNA binding and an activation domain. These domains can be separated and produced as chimeric proteins. If two regions of the chimeric proteins interact, then the activation and DNA binding domains will be brought into close enough proximity to generate an active GAL4 complex. There are many strains of yeasts that will not grow in the absence of specific nutrients.

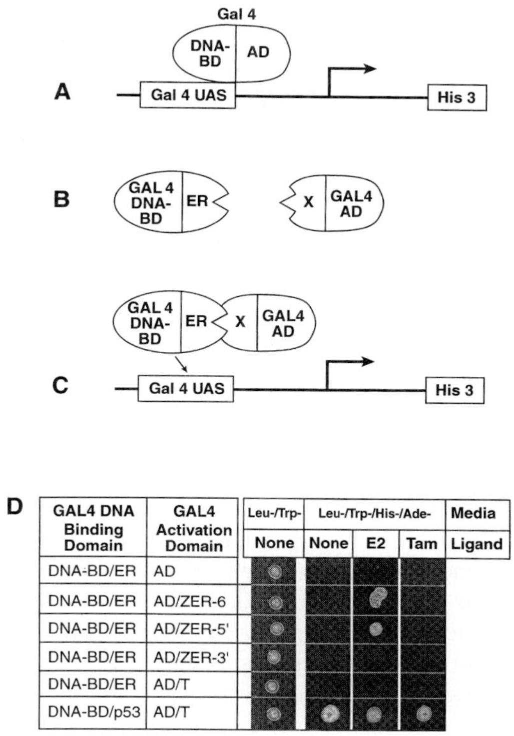

Figure 12 Yeast two-hybrid system for identification of coactivators. (A) The GAL4 transcription factor activates transcription of a HIS reporter. (B) The GAL4 DNA binding region cloned as a chimera with human estrogen receptor. The human cDNA library of multiple genes (X) cloned as a chimera with GAL4 activation domain. (C) Interaction of ER with X brings the GAL4 activation domain to the promoter, activating HIS expression. (D) Demonstration of ligand-dependent interactions of the estrogen receptor with ZER6 protein. The 5′ end of ZER6 that contains a zinc finger domain is the region of activation; p53 and T antigen interaction is demonstrated to be ligand independent (unpublished results).

These strains can grow under those restrictive conditions if they produce an enzyme capable of generating that nutrient (for example, histidine). The enzyme is cloned downstream from a GAL4-dependent promoter. The transcription factor under study is engineered as a chimeric protein with the GAL4 DNA binding domain. A cDNA library is engineered as a chimeric protein with the GAL4 activation domain. The two sets of constructs are transfected into yeast under selective growth conditions. Only those yeasts that have a protein able to bind to the factor are able to grow. The plasmids are recovered from the yeasts and sequenced. This technique is widely used as a method to identify coactivating proteins.

F. Examining Transcriptional Regulation in Tissues

The series of experiments outlined above are directed at identifying and characterizing regulatory elements and transcription factors that may control the expression of a gene.

However, the processes identified in the cell culture model may not hold true at the organ or organism level. Tissues are composed of a complex variety of different cell types that can often have significant interactions with each other. We will briefly discuss some methods that allow for the study of transcriptional control in complex tissues.

In situ hybridization has already been discussed as a method for identifying mRNAs in whole tissue. Once a cDNA for a transcription factor has been cloned, it is possible to engineer bacteria genetically to make large amounts of protein that can be used to generate antibody. Using either monoclonal antibodies or affinity-purified polyclonal antibodies it is possible to perform immunohistochemistry to look at protein expression in tissue. This is important when dealing with proteins that have long half-lives. *In situ* hybridization may not demonstrate the presence of a scarce mRNA, but the protein may be identified with this technique.

Transgenic mice have provided a valuable and powerful tool for genetic analysis. As we noted earlier, promoters can respond to different stimuli in mature tissues or during embryogenesis. The temporal and spatial regulation of a promoter in development provides significant clues as to the role of the gene in morphogenesis. A great deal of information can be gained by the use of the promoter deletion mutants that were generated for basic promoter analysis. These fragments are cloned proximal to a reporter gene such as *lacZ*, a bacterial gene that encodes β-galactosidase. When given the proper substrate, the resulting enzymatic reaction produces a blue compound that is visible. This bacterial protein will be produced wherever the promoter is active. With this technique it is possible to identify the tissues in which the promoter is active. By making different transgenic mouse lines with different fragments of the promoter, it is possible to see which portions are responsible for expression at particular points in development.

Transgenic animals can be helpful in determining the physiologic function of gene expression. Transgenic mice can be generated in which the gene under study is overexpressed in a given tissue. The gene is cloned downstream of a tissue-specific promoter and introduced into the mouse oocytes. Animals expressing the gene can be examined for alterations in phenotype.

Knockout mice are another important tool to study the function of a transcription factor in the whole animal. Knockout mice are animals in which the gene of interest has been ablated on both chromosomes and the animal is therefore homozygous null/null. Once a transcription factor is identified, a great deal about its importance can be discovered by creating a genetic knockout. A number of known mutations are kept in a few laboratories around the world that specialize in cataloging mouse strains; one of the most accessible is the Jackson Laboratories in Bar Harbor, Maine. A catalog of mouse strains is kept with as much genetic information as is known about each animal. One of the first steps to save the time and expense of generating a knockout mouse is to check existing lines to see if by chance a null mutant already exists. In most instances, one does not and generating a knockout is the simplest method to gain this information. Knockouts are capable of telling you what physiologic processes are dependent on the gene of interest. Additionally, knockouts may be prone to developing particular malignancies, suggesting that the gene may perform a tumor suppressor role.

We have outlined a series of experiments that are meant to act as a guide to studying a promoter. The techniques mentioned above are by no means exhaustive, and serve only to frame a path of experimentation for the researcher. Furthermore, many of the same experiments can be performed concurrently. As many of us are all too aware, experiments seem to fail more often than they succeed, and the more ways a problem is approached, the greater the chance of success. If more than one approach is successful, then it is simply more support for a hypothesis.

References

1. Hampsey, M. (1998). Molecular genetics of the RNA polymerase II general transcriptional machinery. *Microbiol. Mol. Biol. Rev.* **62**(2), 465–503.
2. Lee, T. I., and Young, R. A. (1998). Regulation of gene expression by TBP-associated proteins. *Genes Dev.* **12**(10), 1398–1408.
3. Barberis, A., and Gaudreau, L. (1998). Recruitment of the RNA polymerase II holoenzyme and its implications in gene regulation. *Biol. Chem.* **379**(12), 1397–1405.
4. Mangelsdorf, D. J., *et al.* (1995). The nuclear receptor superfamily: The second decade. *Cell* **83**(6), 835–839.
5. Gronemeyer, H. (1991). Transcription activation by estrogen and progesterone receptors. *Annu. Rev. Gene.* **25**(5), 89–123.
6. Hunter, T. and Karin, M. (1992). The regulation of transcription by phosphorylation. *Cell* **70**(3), 375–387.
7. Simeonidis, S., *et al.* (1999). Mechanisms by which IκB proteins control NF-κB activity. *Proc. Nat. Acad. Sci. U.S.A.* **96**(1), 49–54.
8. Irwin, N. (1987). Electrophoresis of RNA through gels containing formaldehyde. *In* "Molecular Cloning, A Laboratory Manual" (E. F. Fritsch and T. Maniatis, eds.), pp. 7.43–7.57. Cold Spring Harbor Laboratory Press, Cold Spring Harbor, New York.
9. Irwin, N. (1987). Mapping of RNA with ribonuclease and radiolabeled RNA probes. *In* "Molecular Cloning, A Laboratory Manual" (E. F. Fritsch and T. Maniatis, eds.), pp. 7.71–7.78 Cold Spring Harbor Laboratory Press, Cold Spring Harbor, New York.
10. Greenberg, M. E., and Bender, T. P. (1987). Enzymatic amplification of RNA by PCR. *In* "Current Protocols in Molecular Biology" (I. Ausubel and M. Frederick, eds.) pp. 15.4.1–15.4.5. John Wiley & Sons, New York.
11. Thompson, D. A., Carmeci, C., and Weigel, R. J. (1998). RT-PCR using formalin-fixed, paraffin-embedded (FFPE) archival tumor specimens. *In* Gene Cloning and Analysis by RT-PCR" (P. Siebert and J. Larrick, Eds.), pp. 3–17. Bio Techniques Books, Natick, MA.
12. Greenberg, M. E., and Bender, T. P. (1987). Identification of newly transcribed RNA. *In* "Current Protocols in Molecular Biology" (I. Ausubel and M. Frederick, Eds.), pp. 4.10.1–4.10.10. John Wiley & Sons, New York.
13. Greenberg, M. E., and Bender, T. P. (1987). Whole-mount *in situ* hybridization and detection of RNAs in vertebrate embryos and isolated organs. *In* "Current Protocols in Molecular Biology" (I. Ausubel

and M. Frederick, Eds.), pp. 14.9.1–14.9.14. John Wiley & Sons, New York.
14. Weigel, R. J., and Nevins, J. R. (1990). Adenovirus infection of differentiated F9 cells results in a global shut-off of differentiation-induced gene expression. *Nucleic Acids Res.* **18**(20), 6107–6112.
15. Liang, P., *et al.* (1994). Differential display using one-base anchored oligo-dT primers. *Nucleic Acids Res.* **22**(25), 5763–5764.
16. Liang, P., *et al.* (1992). Differential display and cloning of messenger RNAs from human breast cancer versus mammary epithelial cells. *Cancer Res.* **52**(24), 6966–6968.
17. Callard, D., Lescure, B., and Mazzolini, L. (1994). A method for the elimination of false positives generated by the mRNA differential display technique. *Biotechniques* **16**(6), 1096–1097, 1100–1103.
18. Velculescu, V. E., *et al.* (1995). Serial analysis of gene expression [see comments]. *Science* **270**(5235), 484–487.
19. Hubank, M., and Schatz, D. G. (1994). Identifying differences in mRNA expression by representational difference analysis of cDNA. *Nucleic Acids Res.* **22**(25), 5640–5648.
20. Diatchenko, L., *et al.* (1996). Suppression subtractive hybridization: A method for generating differentially regulated or tissue-specific cDNA probes and libraries. *Proc. Nat. Acad. Sci. U.S.A.* **93**(12), 6025–6030.
21. Kuang, W. W., *et al.* (1998). Differential screening and suppression subtractive hybridization identified genes differentially expressed in an estrogen receptor-positive breast carcinoma cell line. *Nucleic Acids Res.* **26**(4), 1116–1123.
22. Hoch, R. V., *et al.* (1999). GATA-3 is expressed in association with estrogen receptor in breast cancer. *Int. J. Cancer* **84**(2), 122–128.
23. Schena, M., *et al.* (1996). Parallel human genome analysis: Microarray-based expression monitoring of 1000 genes. *Proc. Nat. Acad. Sci. U.S.A.* **93**(20), 10614–10619.
24. Yang, G. P., *et al.* (1999). Combining SSH and cDNA microarrays for rapid identification of differentially expressed genes. *Nucleic Acids Res.* **27**(6), 1517–1523.
25. Greenberg, M. E., and Bender, T. P. (1987). Analysis of RNA structure and synthesis. *In* "Current Protocols in Molecular Biology" (I. Ausubel and M. Frederick, Eds.) pp. 4.6.1–4.6.11. John Wiley & Sons, New York.
26. Greenberg, M. E., and Bender, T. P. (1987). Primer extension. *In* "Current Protocols in Molecular Biology" (I. Ausubel and M. Frederick, Eds.), pp. 4.8.1–4.8.4. John Wiley & Sons, New York.
27. Greenberg, M. E., and Bender, T. P. (1987). Amplification of regions upstream (5′) of known sequence. *In* "Current Protocols in Molecular Biology," (I. Ausubel and M. Frederick, eds.), pp. 15.64–15.66. John Wiley & Sons, New York.
28. Wu, C., (1980). The 5′ ends of *Drosophila* heat shock genes in chromatin are hypersensitive to DNase I. *Nature* **286** (5776), 854–860.
29. deConinck, E. C., McPherson, L. A., and Weigel, R. J. (1995). Transcriptional regulation of estrogen receptor in breast carcinomas. *Mol. Cell. Biol.* **15**(4), 2191–2196.
30. Greenberg, M. E., and Bender, T. P. (1987). Endonucleases. *In* "Current Protocols in Molecular Biology" (I. Ausubel and M. Frederick, eds.), pp. 3.12.1–3.12.2. John Wiley & Sons, New York.
31. Greenberg, M. E., and Bender, T. P. (1987). Mobility shift DNA-binding assay using gel electrophoresis. *In* "Current Protocols in Molecular Biology" (I. Ausubel and M. Frederick, eds.), pp. 12.2.1–12.2.7. John Wiley & Sons, New York.
32. Greenberg, M. E., and Bender, T. P. (1987). DNase I footprint analysis of protein–DNA binding. *In* "Current Protocols in Molecular Biology" (I. Ausubel and M. Frederick, eds.), pp. 12.4.1–12.4.11. John Wiley & Sons, New York.
33. Greenberg, M. E., and Bender, T. P. (1987). Methylation and uracil interference assays for analysis of protein–DNA interactions. *In* "Current Protocols in Molecular Biology" (I. Ausubel and M. Frederick, eds.), pp. 12.3.1–12.3.5. John Wiley & Sons, New York.
34. Greenberg, M. E., and Bender, T. P. (1987). Determination of protein–DNA sequence specificity by PCR-assisted binding-site selection. *In* "Current Protocols in Molecular Biology" (I. Ausubel and M. Frederick, eds.), pp. 12.11.1–12.11.8. John Wiley & Sons, New York.
35. McPherson, L. A., and Weigel, R. J. (1999). AP2α and AP2γ: A comparison of binding site specificity and trans-activation of the estrogen receptor promoter and single site promoter constructs. *Nucleic Acids* Res. **27**(20), 4040–4049.
36. Faisst, S., and Meyer, S. (1992). Compilation of vertebrate-encoded transcription factors. *Nucleic Acids Res.* **20**(1), 3–26.
37. McPherson, L. A., Baichwal, V. R., and Weigel, R. J. (1997). Identification of ERF-1 as a member of the AP2 transcription factor family. *Proc. Natl. Acad. Sci. U.S.A.* **94**(9), 4342–4347.
38. Pestov, D. G., and Lau, L. F. (1994). Genetic selection of growth-inhibitory sequences in mammalian cells. *Proc. Natl. Acad. Sci. U.S.A.* **91**(26), 12549–12553.
39. Fields, S., and Song, O. (1989). A novel genetic system to detect protein-protein interactions. *Nature* **340**(6230), 245–246.
40. Chien, C. T., *et al.* (1991). The two-hybrid system: A method to identify and clone genes for proteins that interact with a protein of interest. *Proc. Natl. Acad. Sci. U.S.A.* **88**(21), 9578–9582.
41. Chevray, P. M., and Nathans, D. (1992). Protein interaction cloning in yeast: Identification of mammalian proteins that react with the leucine zipper of Jun. *Proc. Natl. Acad. Sci. U.S.A.* **89**(13), 5789–5793.

22

Signal Transduction and Apoptosis

Tanya K. Meyer and William G. Cance

Department of Surgery and UNC Lineberger Comprehensive Cancer Center, University of North Carolina at Chapel Hill, Chapel Hill, North Carolina 27599

The artist knows that the stroke of ink or color left by a brush takes on meaning only when viewed in relationship to the stroke that went before and after. And to the musician, a note, no matter how beautiful, is not music except in the context of other notes.

KYUDO MASTER

The signal transduction literature is overwhelming with respect to the sheer number of proteins implicated, the complexity of cascades, and the amount of redundancy and cross-talk between cascades. This point is exemplified in Fig. 1, which is a simplified schematic of selected members in the c-erbB–2/Her-2/*neu* pathway (1). This pathway has been shown to have significance in human tumor systems. Although such cascades include many different proteins, it is important to realize that selective techniques are used to isolate one particular arm of the pathway for study at any time. Thus the importance of one pathway in the context of the whole signaling response can be emphasized. The purpose of this chapter is to describe some common techniques in the signaling field and to identify the importance and limitation of each technique. Once a technique has been described it is followed with a specific experimental example.

I. Expression of Signal Transduction Proteins

Western Blots Quantitatively Detect Protein Expression

Crucial to the study of signal transduction is the ability to quantitatively assay the presence of any given signaling

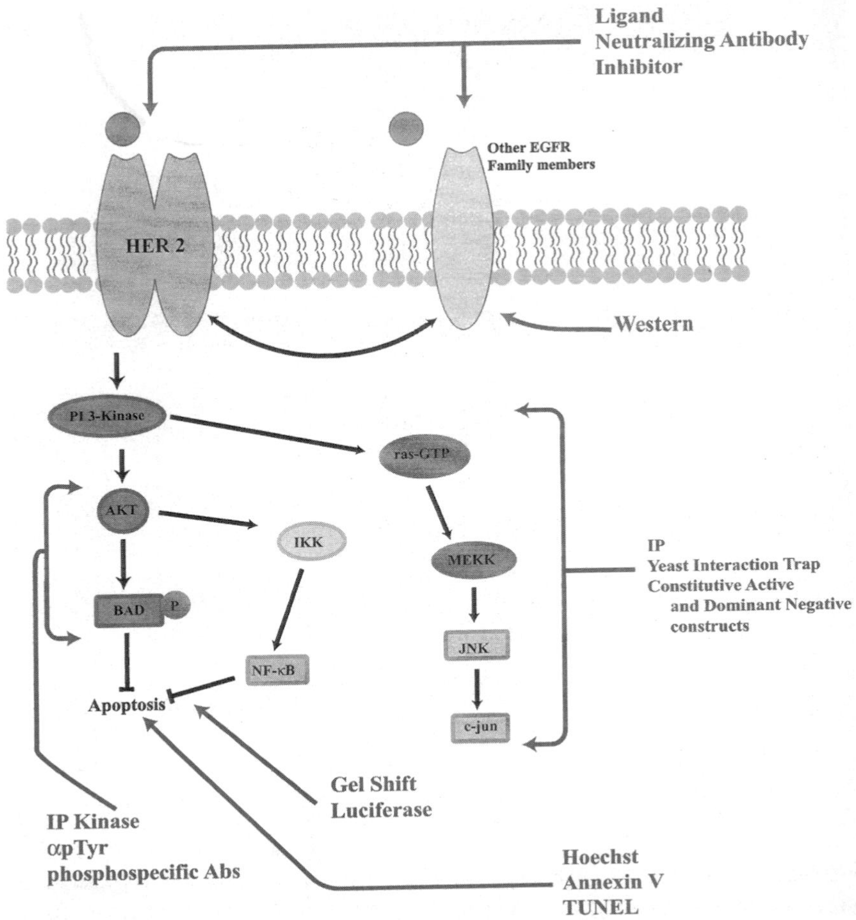

Figure 1 The Her-2/*neu* signaling cascade. Various signal transduction methodologies can be used to dissect this complex cascade (1). (See color plates.)

molecule. When a specific antibody to the molecule of interest is available, this question can be easily answered using a Western blot (Fig. 2). Western blotting detects protein expression levels in lysates of clinical specimens, cell cultures, or cellular fractions using sodium dodecyl sulfate–polyacrylamide gel electrophoresis (SDS–PAGE) to resolve the proteins by size and immunoblotting with an antibody to detect the protein of interest. Briefly, aliquots of the samples to be analyzed are mixed with a buffer solution containing β-mercaptoethanol (to reduce disulfide bonds) and the detergent sodium dodecyl sulfate (to apply a uniform negative charge to the surface of the protein). The proteins are then denatured by boiling. In this manner the proteins are unfolded into linear extended polypeptide chains coated with the negatively charged SDS. The detergent not only releases the proteins from association with other cellular components, but its negative charge masks the intrinsic charge of the polypeptide. When the solution is loaded onto an SDS–PAGE gel and exposed to current, proteins will migrate toward the anode at rates relative to their size.

The proteins are transferred from the gel to a nitrocellulose or polyvinylidene fluoride (PVDF) membrane, again using current. After transfer, any membrane binding sites not occupied by protein are "blocked" with nonspecific protein. This is typically a solution of low-fat milk or bovine serum albumin (BSA). Blocking inhibits nonspecific binding of antibodies to the membrane. Finally, the membrane is probed for the presence of a particular protein by incubating with a specific primary antibody. The primary will typically be either mouse monoclonal or rabbit polyclonal. A secondary antibody (based on the species of the primary), which recognizes the constant region of the primary antibody and is conjugated to a detection agent, is then used to identify the primary antibody. The detection agent on the secondary antibody (such as horseradish peroxidase) is chemically activated to produce light, which is visualized by exposure to film (enhanced chemiluminescence, ECL). Alternatively, the secondary may be conjugated to a radioactive marker. Western blots are quantitative in that the intensity of the

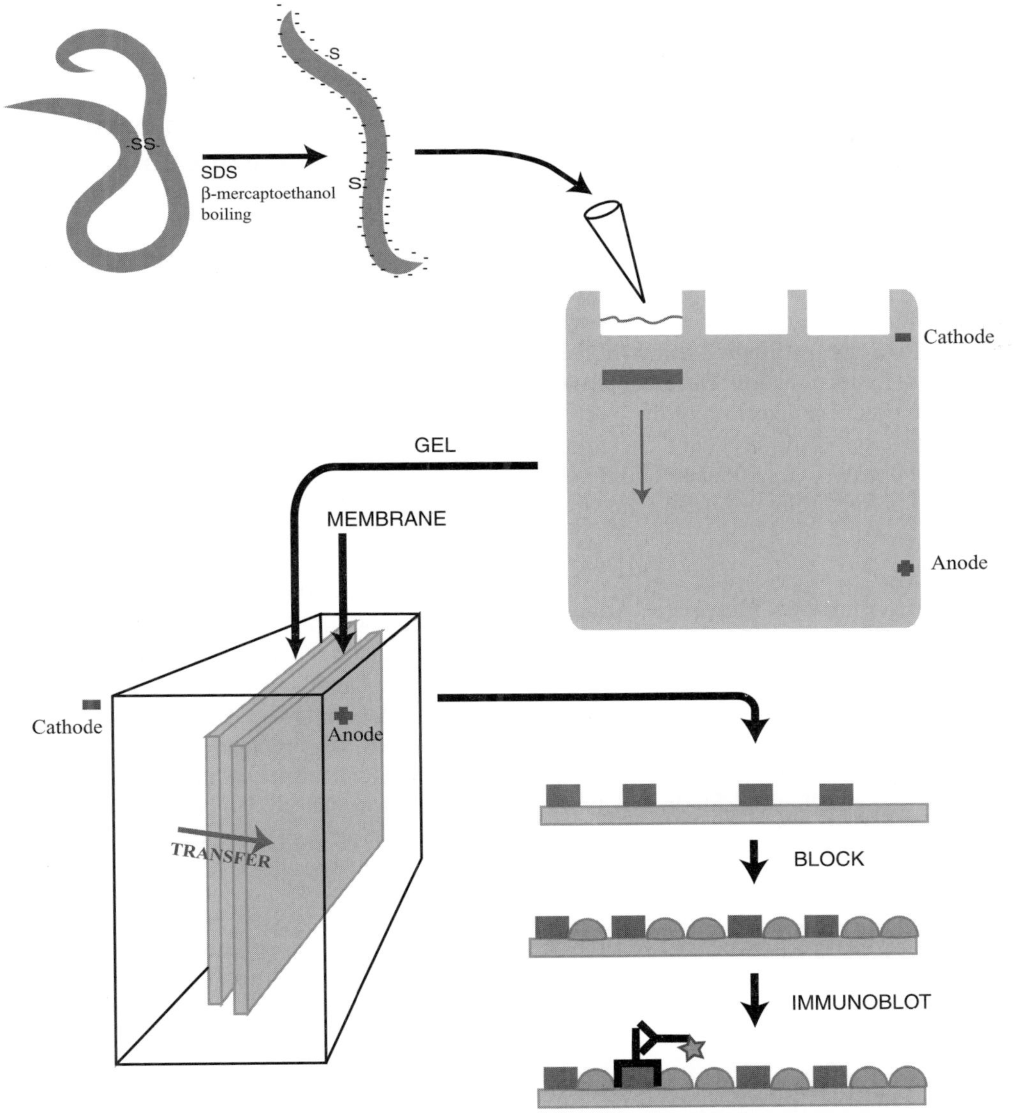

Figure 2 General methodology of Western blotting. Denatured proteins are loaded onto a polyacrylamide gel and resolved with current. The proteins in the gel are transferred to a membrane. Available protein-binding sites on the membrane are blocked and the membrane is immunoblotted with a primary, then secondary, antibody. In this schematic, bands are detected using enhanced chemiluminescence.

band on the film correlates with the amount of bound antibody, which correlates with the amount of protein. The intensity of the band can be measured densitometrically.

Care should be taken during the preparation of lysates to prevent protein degradation. All steps should be done expediently on ice and protease inhibitors such as phenylmethylsulfonyl fluoride (PMSF), aprotinin, leupeptin, and pepstatin must be added. In addition, phosphatase inhibitors such as sodium vanadate, sodium fluoride, or β-glycerolphosphate may be considered if preservation of protein phosphorylation is important. Cells can be fractionated and either the nuclear or cytoplasmic fraction assayed if the subcellular localization of the protein is known.

If protein expression between lysates is to be compared, one must ensure that the quantity of total protein loaded into each well is similar by not only loading equal amounts of protein onto the gel, but also with the use of internal controls. The protein concentration of lysates can be determined using standard methods such as the Bradford assay. To confirm equal loading using internal controls, a blot can be stripped of antibody (a β-mercaptoethanol buffer will "strip" the blotting antibodies from the membrane while leaving, for the most part, the denatured proteins in the membrane intact) and reprobed with an antibody to a ubiquitously expressed protein such as actin or tubulin. Lanes with discrepant concentrations of actin (bands of different intensity) suggest differential loading and would not permit quantitative comparison.

No matter how carefully the lysate is prepared or the gel run, the resultant blot can only be as sensitive/specific as the primary antibody. Western blots are limited by the quality of the antibodies used. Because a Western blot is performed under denaturing conditions, the antibody must recognize denatured protein motifs. Some antibodies will only recognize proteins in their native conformation. Different blocking solutions can be tried to optimize detection of the particular protein/antibody combination while reducing background. Finally, the Western blot is only a tool of quantitation; it does not give direct information regarding enzymatic function or interaction partners.

Example of Western Blotting: The Focal Adhesion Kinase Is Overexpressed in Invasive Human Tumors

Western blots have been used extensively to search for proteins that become differentially expressed during the process of oncogenesis. The focal adhesion kinase (FAK) is a 125-kDa protein tyrosine kinase that resides in focal adhesions and plays a role in cell adhesion. Studies of protein expression in human tumors have shown that FAK expression is elevated in the majority of invasive colon tumors and breast tumors (2) (Fig. 3).

II. Interactions between Signal Transduction Proteins

A. Immunoprecipitation Can Detect Interactions between Two Known Partners

Signal transduction involves protein–protein interactions. When an interesting protein has been identified, the next logical step is to identify putative interacting molecules. Immunoprecipitation (IP) is a powerful method to detect protein–protein interactions *in vitro*. This method uses an antibody to recognize and isolate a known partner and relies on protein–protein interactions to precipitate, or "bring down," associated interacting partners (Fig. 4). Cellular lysates are prepared that contain the protein of interest along with its binding partners. An antibody that binds to the protein in its native conformation (the precipitating antibody) is added to the lysate under nondenaturing conditions. Included in the incubation are *Staphylococcus* protein A/G-coated agarose beads. Protein A/G binds the Fc portions of the precipitating antibody. Thus, the immune complexes formed consist of bead, antibody, and protein with attached binding partners. The beads are collected by centrifugation and washed several times in an appropriate buffer to remove proteins not specific

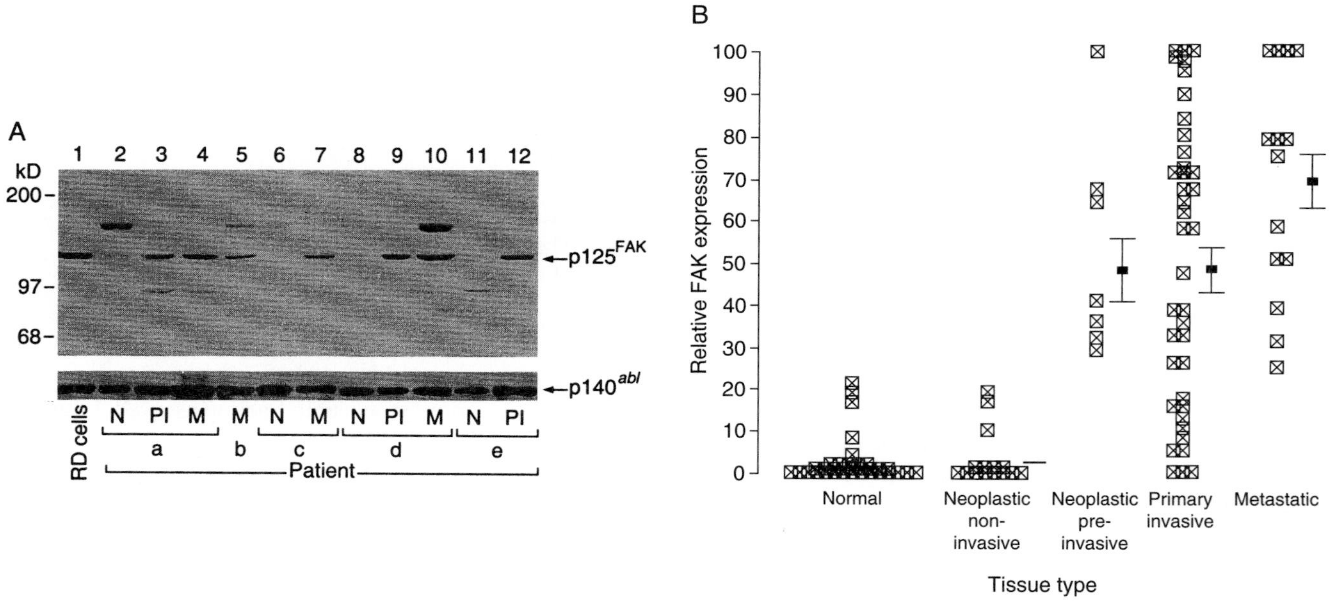

Figure 3 (A) Western blot of p125^{FAK} expression in human tissue preparations demonstrates up-regulation of FAK expression in primary and metastatic tumors in comparison to normal tissue. p140^{abl} is an alternate tyrosine kinase and is used as a loading control. The positions of p125^{FAK} and p140^{abl} are indicated. Other bands reflect nonspecific cross-reactivity of the antibody. N, Normal tissue; PI, primary invasive tumor; M, metastasis; RD, rhabdomyosarcoma cell lysate as a positive control of FAK expression. Rhabdomyosarcoma cells overexpress FAK constitutively. (B) Densitometry of the relative p125^{FAK} expression by Western blot of 119 human tissue samples. From Owens *et al.* (2), with permission.

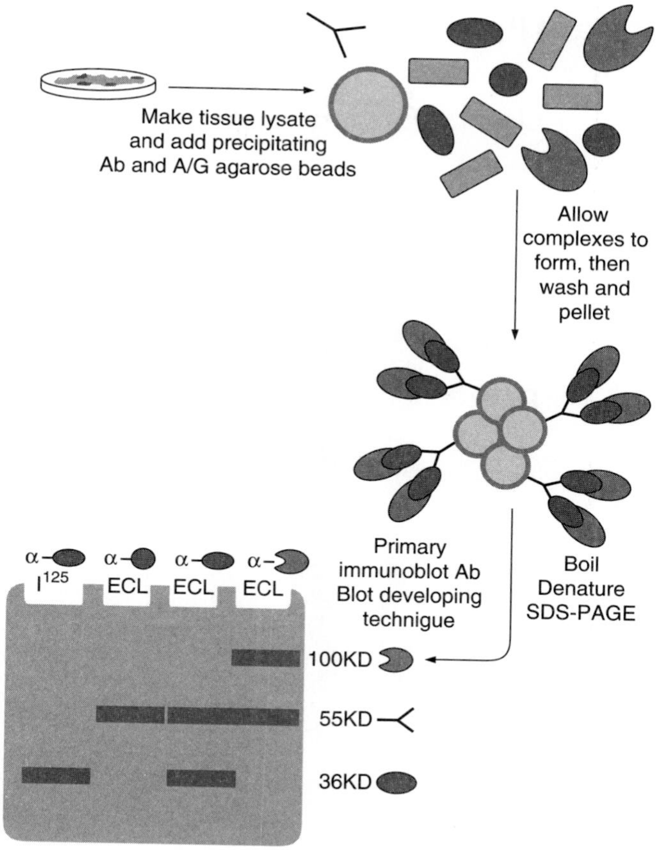

Figure 4 Immunoprecipitation. The precipitating antibody (IP-Ab) and protein A/G agarose beads are added to a cell or tissue lysate. Complexes consisting of *bead/IP-Ab/protein/binding partners* then form. These complexes are pelleted, washed, and the individual species are resolved by SDS–PAGE. The schematic Western blot in this figure demonstrates the difference between using a ^{125}I-labeled primary immunoblotting antibody versus ECL with a horseradish peroxidase-labeled secondary immunoblotting antibody detecting the primary Ab. ECL develops faster (several minutes as compared to 18–24 hrs for ^{125}I) and avoids radioactivity, but the secondary Ab will recognize the IP-Ab and give a heavy band around 55 kDa. In lane 1 the primary Ab is conjugated to ^{125}I and there is no cross-reactivity with the IP-Ab. In lane 2 a primary Ab is used that is not specific for any protein found in the IP complexes. No bands are detected by the primary Ab, but the secondary Ab has recognized the precipitating antibody at 55 kDa. Lanes 3 and 4 are blotted with primary Ab to proteins in the IP complexes—bands are evident representing the proteins and immunoglobulin.

to the IP complex. The samples are boiled in a denaturing buffer, which separates the bead–antibody–protein complex into individual species, and the samples are resolved by SDS–PAGE. The subsequent blot can be probed by a variety of antibodies with the implication that detected proteins are binding partners of the immunoprecipitated protein.

The most important component in the success of an IP is the choice of the precipitating antibody. As noted previously, the precipitating antibody in the IP is recognizing proteins in their native conformation—as opposed to Western blots, in which the antibodies recognize denatured peptide motifs. Some antibodies can be used for both IP and Western blots, but this is not always the rule. Care must also be taken in the proper preparation of lysates, as described above for Western blots. All steps must be done expediently on ice to minimize degrading reactions. Nonionic detergents are added to the buffers to establish stringency, and protease and phosphatase inhibitors are added to preserve proteins and their phosphorylation status. To reduce nonspecific binding of proteins to the beads, the lysates should be precleared: the lysates are incubated for 45 min with just the beads and the resultant supernatant (after the beads have been pelleted and removed) is then used for the immunoprecipitation proper. To control for nonspecific binding of proteins to the precipitating antibody, an unrelated isotype-matched control antibody (e.g., MOPC-21, an IgG_1 myeloma protein to control for IgG_1 monoclonal antibodies) is used in place of the precipitating antibody. Any proteins precipitated by both the precipitating antibody and MOPC-21 likely represent nonspecific binding.

It is important to have some hypothesis of which proteins may be interaction partners in order to choose the correct blot developing technique. If using ECL, it will be difficult if not impossible to detect proteins around the 50-kDa range, because this is the size of the precipitating antibody IgG heavy chain, which will be present on all blots because it is a member of the immune complex (Fig. 5). Thus, if there may be proteins in this region of interest it will be necessary to use ^{125}I-labeled immunoblotting antibodies to avoid use of a secondary antibody preparation.

Alternatively, all proteins in a cell culture can be labeled with ^{35}S by directly placing the isotope in the culture medium. After IP and separation by electrophoresis, these proteins can be detected by radiography without the need for immunoblotting.

Example of Immunoprecipitation: FAK Binds to the SH2 Domains of the Oncoprotein Src

Proteins in the Src family were the first transforming proteins of the kinase type to be isolated, and the first examples of tyrosine kinases to be studied. FAK and Src are both present in cellular focal adhesions and have been shown to be binding partners using the technique of immunoprecipitation (3) (Figs. 6 and 7).

B. The Yeast Two-Hybrid System: A Method to Identify Protein–Protein Interactions

Although immunoprecipitation is a reliable method to identify protein–protein interactions, it has several limitations. It is an assay done entirely *in vitro* and depends on the quality of a reagent—the precipitating antibody. Another useful method to detect specific protein–protein interactions is the yeast two-hybrid analysis, or interaction trap. Using

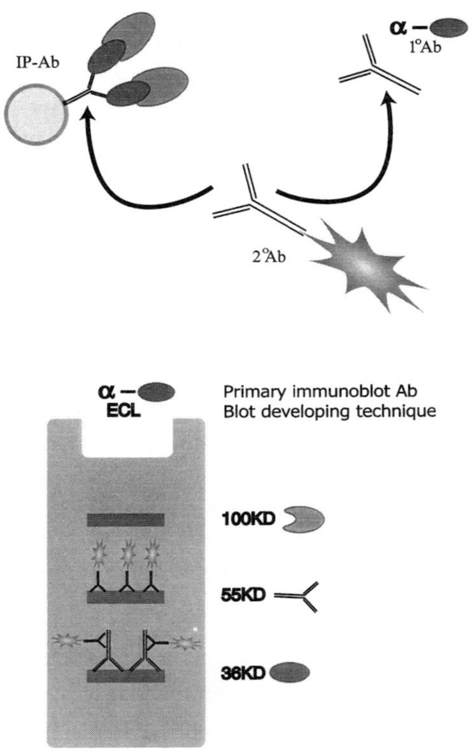

Figure 5 ECL detects the Ig heavy chain and is not optimal for development of Western blots of immunoprecipitated proteins in the 55-kDa range. IP with resolution of the complexes by SDS–PAGE, detection by immunoblotting, and development by ECL require the use of up to three separate antibodies: the precipitation antibody (IP-Ab), the primary immunoblotting antibody (1° Ab), and the secondary immunoblotting or developing antibody (2°Ab). The 2° Ab recognizes not only the 1° Ab but also the IP-Ab that is sedimented with the agarose bead.

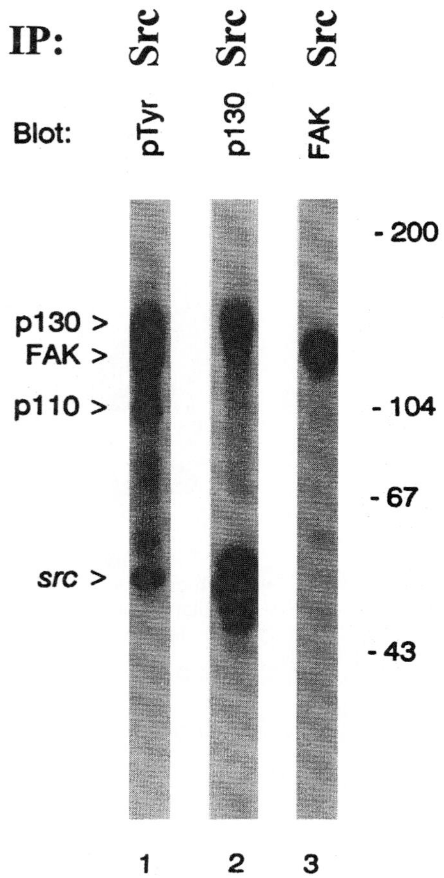

Figure 6 Immunoprecipitation (IP) of activated Src reveals association with p130, FAK, and p110. Chicken embryo cells were stably transformed with a constitutively active mutant of Src [pp60^{527F}; tyrosine 527 mutated to phenylalanine (F)] and lysed in RIPA buffer. Src immune complexes were isolated with an Src-specific monoclonal antibody (mAb). The immune complexes were resolved by SDS–PAGE and Western blotted with antibody to phosphotyrosine (lane 1), pp130-specific mAb (lane 2), and p125^{FAK}-specific rabbit antibody (polyclonal). In lanes 1 and 3 ^{125}I-labeled protein A was used as the detection reagent. In lane 2 an ^{125}I-labeled goat antimouse secondary antibody was used; it yielded a labeled band with an apparent molecular mass of 60 Da as the heavy chain of the primary antibody. This experiment demonstrates the association of activated Src with p130 and with FAK. It also shows that p130, FAK, and activated Src are all phosphorylated. From Cobb *et al.* (3), with permission.

the yeast organism as a test system, putative binding partners are heterologously expressed and the interaction is detected using a reporter gene readout such as *lacZ* (Fig. 8).

Many eukaryotic transcription factors consist of two modular domains. The DNA binding domain (BD) localizes the transcription factor to the promoter region of the gene, and the acidic transcriptional activation domain (AD) directs the RNA polymerase II complex to transcribe the downstream gene. Both domains can act independently of each other when separated into individual proteins, but both domain activities are also required to effect gene transcription. The two domains must be brought into physical association for proper function. So if each domain is fused to two individual proteins (e.g., protein X and Y) that bind to each other, the BD and the AD will be brought into physical proximity by the interaction of X and Y and thus will be able to localize to the promoter and direct gene transcription. In the case of the interaction trap, a reporter gene such as *lacZ* is used to screen for gene transcription.

The protein under study is termed the bait protein and is fused to the DNA binding domain. Other chosen proteins or an array of proteins from a cDNA library, collectively termed prey, are fused to the acidic domain. An interactor hunt involves expression of these constructs in yeast. If the prey takes the bait (binding of prey–AD to bait–BD), the complex will localize to the promoter region and direct transcription of *lacZ* with subsequent growth of blue yeast colonies.

The interaction trap is an elegant tool to detect *in vivo* protein interactions. In the ideal setting, the identification of binding proteins can take as little as 4 weeks, and depending on the bait protein anywhere from zero to hundreds of specific interactors may be obtained. Whereas other methods to identify protein interactions require stable associations, the

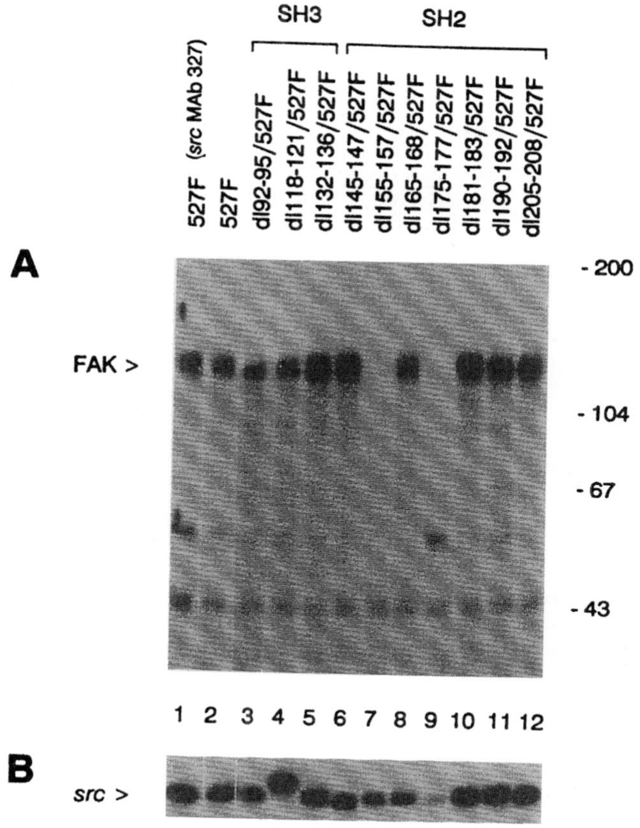

Figure 7 The association between FAK and Src requires an intact SH2 domain in Src. Src was immunoprecipitated from chicken embryo cells expressing deletion constructs of activated Src in the SH2 and SH3 domains. The immune complexes were divided and Western blotted for either FAK (top) or Src (bottom). Activated Src only (lanes 1 and 2) and all the SH3 domain deletion constructs of Src (lanes 3–5) successfully coimmunoprecipitated pp125^{FAK}. Two of the SH2 domain deletion constructs (lanes 6–12) were unable to coimmunoprecipitate FAK. These results imply that FAK binds to Src through the SH2 domain (when the SH2 domain is mutated, FAK can no longer bind to Src and will not come down with the immunoprecipitation of Src). Note that Src was Western blotted from the IP, thus confirming that the precipitating antibody still recognized the deletion mutants. 527F refers to Src with tyrosine 527 mutated to phenylalanine (F). dl92-95/527F refers to Src with the 527 phenylalanine substitution and amino acids 92–95 deleted. From Cobb *et al.* (3), with permission.

yeast two-hybrid can be used to detect transient interactions that may not survive a coprecipitation.

III. Protein Phosphorylation Plays a Key Role in Enzyme Activity Regulation

Most proteins undergo some type of posttranslational modification to influence trafficking, target for secretion, or regulate catalytic activity. Protein phosphorylation, one of the more important forms of modification, provides a sensitive and quick method of influencing enzymatic activity. Protein phosphorylation (by kinases) and dephosphorylation (by phosphatases) function together in signal transduction to modify the activity of a pathway (4). Signals can be received, amplified, and implemented very quickly. The cascades are like an enzymatic relay race: all the runners are on standby for their respective kinase, to phosphorylate and activate them. Most peptide growth factors and cytokines induce phosphorylation on binding to their receptors (5), and mitosis is regulated in all nucleated organisms by cyclin-dependent protein kinases (6).

A. Phosphotyrosine and Phosphopeptide Antibodies Can Detect Levels of Protein Phosphorylation

The most straightforward method to detect protein phosphorylation is via an antiphosphotyrosine antibody (α-pTyr) (7, 8). Phosphotyrosine in proteins is a reversibly modified amino acid that fortuitously acts as a strong hapten. However, multiple proteins in any given lysate will contain phosphotyrosines, and one protein may contain multiple phosphotyrosine residues. Although the α-pTyr antibody is a good tool, the identity of the detected proteins must be inferred from their size in relation to the marker (see Fig. 6). For more exact verification, the α-pTyr blot can be stripped (as described above) and reprobed with antibodies specific to proteins of potential interest. If the Western blot from an immunoprecipitation is developed using ECL, bands representing the heavy and light chains of the antibody used in the immunoprecipitation will be present—and this will not represent phosphorylation.

Serine and threonine phosphorylation is a different matter and there has not been good success at generating antibodies to these phosphoamino acids. However, if the sequence flanking these residues is known, phospho-specific antibodies can be produced (9, 10). This allows monitoring of phosphorylation at a specific residue (α-pTyr monitors phosphorylation at any tyrosine) of a specific protein. There are many phospho-specific antibodies commercially available that recognize known serine and threonine residues in a variety of specific protein contexts.

B. Kinase Assays Can Detect Phosphorylation Activity in Vivo or in Vitro

To detect kinase activity as opposed to its endpoint—phosphorylation—there are multiple kinase assays that can be employed (Fig. 9). *In vivo* kinase activity can be detected with the addition of [^{32}P]orthophosphate ($^{32}P_i$) to the media of the cell culture. The stimulus of interest (e.g., adding growth factors) is applied to the cell culture in the presence of $^{32}P_i$, lysate is prepared, and the protein of interest is immunoprecipitated. If the protein has been phosphorylated, it will be detected by autoradiography. This assay will measure kinase activity exerted on a protein in response to a given stimulus, but gives

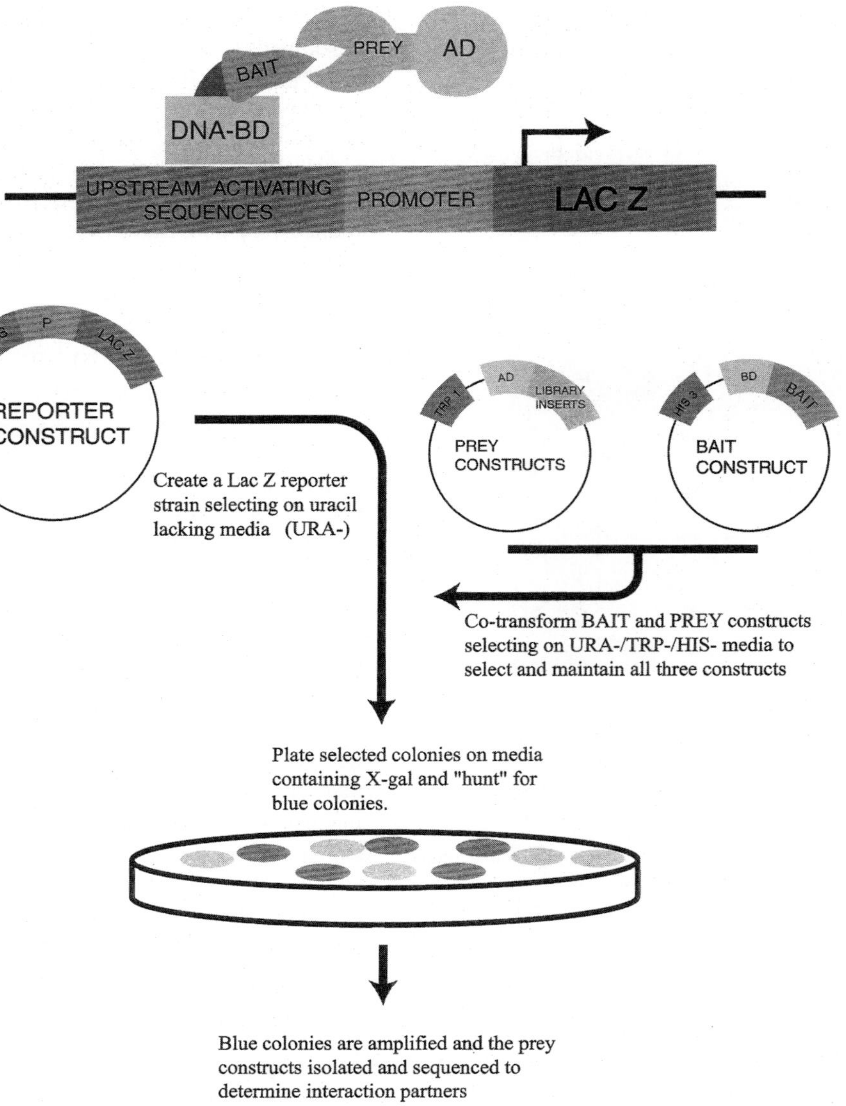
PREY
AD
BAIT
DNA-BD
UPSTREAM ACTIVATING SEQUENCES
PROMOTER
LAC Z
UAS
P
LAC Z
URA 3
REPORTER CONSTRUCT
Create a Lac Z reporter strain selecting on uracil lacking media (URA-)
TRP 1
AD
LIBRARY INSERTS
PREY CONSTRUCTS
HIS 3
BD
BAIT
BAIT CONSTRUCT
Co-transform BAIT and PREY constructs selecting on URA-/TRP-/HIS- media to select and maintain all three constructs
Plate selected colonies on media containing X-gal and "hunt" for blue colonies.
Blue colonies are amplified and the prey constructs isolated and sequenced to determine interaction partners

Figure 8 Yeast two-hybrid system. The prey–AD fusion protein interacts with the bait–DNA BD protein, allowing transcription of *lacZ*. AD, Activation domain; DNA BD, DNA binding domain; UAS, upstream activating sequences; P, promoter. (See color plates.)

no insight as to the responsible kinase. The strength of the assay is that it is performed *in vivo*, and not in a test tube.

The immune complex kinase assay is a different procedure designed to detect autophosphorylation of the immunoprecipitated protein or phosphorylation between members of the immune complex. A protein is immunoprecipitated and the resultant complexes are resuspended in a kinase buffer containing [γ-^{32}P]ATP. Any kinase activity in the immune complex will allow incorporation of ^{32}P. After a set reaction time, the samples are denatured, separated by SDS-PAGE, and detected by autoradiography. In this assay, phosphorylation could reflect either autophosphorylation (a protein exerts kinase activity on itself) or the kinase activity of a binding partner.

Finally, a substrate kinase assay can be used to determine specific phosphorylation of a known kinase substrate. Here the same general principle is employed, but with the addition of a substrate. The immunoprecipitation is performed and the complexes resuspended in kinase buffer with both [γ-^{32}P]ATP and substrate (such as histone 2B). The sample is resolved by SDS-PAGE. The incorporation of [γ-^{32}P]ATP into the substrate can be detected by autoradiography as a measure of the kinase activity of the immunoprecipitated enzyme. Densitometry can be used to quantitate the kinase activity.

These assays can reveal kinase activity in response to a physiologic stimulus *in vivo*, autophosphorylation *in vitro*, or substrate phosphorylation *in vitro*.

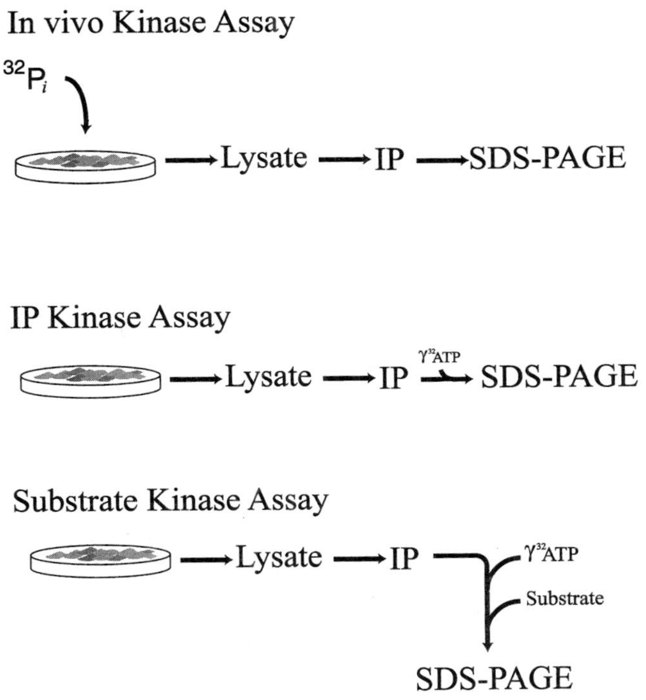

Figure 9 Three types of kinase assays.

An Example of Kinase Assays: The Insulin Receptor and Jun N-Terminal Kinase

Insulin is one of the most extensively studied hormones and is involved in numerous biological processes, including glycemic control, growth, and the stress response. The insulin receptor, on binding insulin, is known to first autophosphorylate both of its β subunits and then to phosphorylate substrate. Figure 10 shows an *in vivo* kinase assay using orthophosphate and an IP kinase assay using [γ-^{32}P]ATP.

Other proteins implicated in the stress response are Jun N-terminal kinase (JNK), a member of the JNK/Jun cascade, and angiotensin II, a peptide hormone. Using a Jun kinase assay, as diagrammed in Figs. 11 and 12, the activation of JNK can be measured in response to angiotensin II treatment (11).

IV. Receptor Agonist and Antagonist with Blockade

The simplest method of studying receptors involved in signaling mechanisms is assaying for downstream effects after manipulation with ligand. For instance, if insulin is

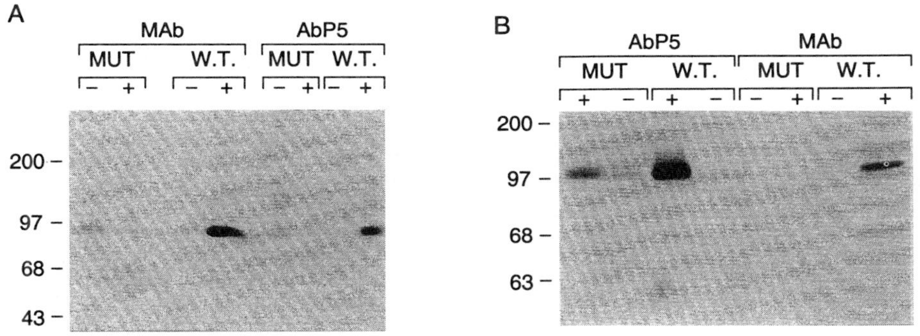

Figure 10 (A) Mutant insulin receptors lacking tyrosine kinase activity show no insulin-stimulated receptor phosphorylation *in vivo*. Expression of human wild-type insulin receptors (W.T.) and mutant receptors lacking kinase activity (MUT) were established in Chinese hamster ovary cell lines. Where indicated (−, +), the cells were exposed to 0.1 μ*M* insulin for 10 min in the presence of [^{32}P]orthophosphate ($^{32}P_i$). The insulin receptors were then immunoprecipitated with two different monoclonal antibodies specific for insulin receptors (MAb and AbP5), separated by SDS–PAGE, and autoradiographed. Only wild-type receptors evidenced phosphorylation when stimulated with insulin only. Mutant receptors showed no phosphorylation in response to insulin stimulation. This experiment demonstrates *in vivo* the phosphorylation status of a protein in response to ligand stimulation, but gives no information regarding the responsible kinase. (B) Insulin receptors lacking tyrosine kinase activity are unable to autophosphorylate with ligand stimulation. Wild-type and mutant human insulin receptors were immunoprecipitated from Chinese hamster ovary cell lines by either MAb or AbP5. IP complexes were resuspended in kinase buffer containing [γ-^{32}P]ATP in the presence or absence of (+, −) of 0.1 μ*M* insulin. Samples were resolved by SDS–PAGE and autoradiographed. In the MAb immunoprecipitation, only wild-type receptors evidenced insulin-dependent autophosphorylation. The immune complex kinase assay allows speculation as to the responsible kinase. In the AbP5 immunoprecipitation the mutant receptors also showed a low level of autophosphorylation—this was felt to actually represent wild-type receptors that were endogenous to the Chinese hamster ovary cells. MAb is human species specific; AbP5 has cross-reactivity between human and hamster. This demonstrates the importance of proper antibody selection. From Chou *et al.* (23), with permission.

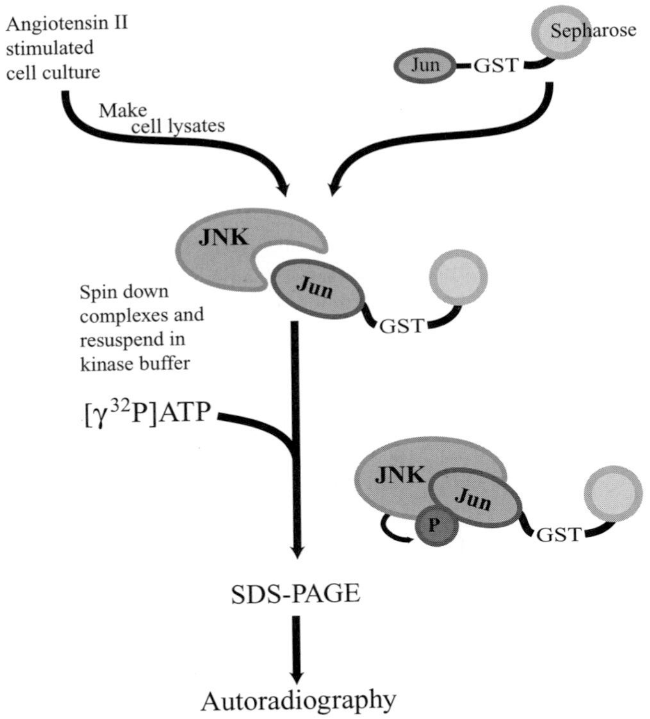

Figure 11 GST–Jun kinase assay. JNK and Jun are unique in that there is a strong enough interaction between substrate and kinase that they will coprecipitate. When Jun is made into a glutathione-*S*-transferase (GST) fusion protein, it will bind to a Sepharose bead. When incubated with a cell lysate, GST–Jun will "bring down" JNK. If the JNK has been activated by a prior stimulus (such as angiotensin II), then the JNK will phosphorylate Jun. Thus the incorporation of radioactive phosphate into Jun is a measure of the activation of JNK.

added to cells, an increase in insulin receptor autophosphorylation and kinase activity can be measured. Antibodies to receptors can also be used to block or enhance function. Antibodies to the epidermal growth factor receptor (EGFR) bring receptor monomers into proximity, simulating ligand-induced receptor dimerization, which leads to an increase in EGFR activity (12).

An interesting example with direct clinical relevance involves the oncogene c-erbB-2/Her2/*neu*, a member of the EGFR family. The Her-2/*neu* receptor is overexpressed in many human cancers, including breast, ovarian, lung, gastric, and oral cancers (13, 14), and serves as a tumor marker for poor prognosis (15). Heregulin is one of the ligands for the c-erbB-3 and c-erbB-4 receptors, and through unspecified mechanisms results in an increased kinase activity of c-erbB-2/Her2/*neu* (16). Antibodies to the Her-2/*neu* receptor may be inhibitory or stimulating for the signaling cascade. One particular antibody to Her-2/*neu*, herceptin, exerts inhibitory activity and decreases receptor phosphorylation (17, 18). Herceptin is currently undergoing clinical trials as an anticancer therapeutic.

V. Constitutively Active and Dominant Negative Proteins Elucidate the Importance of Signal Transduction Cascades

Of all of the techniques described thus far, the use of biological constructs encoding dominant negative or constitutively active proteins has contributed the most useful information toward identifying the importance of signaling cascades. Signaling can be thought of as a process in which one molecule becomes activated and subsequently is responsible for stimulating multiple additional effector molecules. Signal amplification occurs when these effector molecules activate additional pathways. The importance of a particular protein in the signaling cascade can be determined through the use of dominant negative and constitutively active proteins. Constitutively active proteins contain a gain-of-function mutation that allows the encoded protein to stimulate effector pathways independent of upstream signals normally required to activate the wild-type protein. Conversely, dominant negative proteins contain a loss-of-function mutation that interferes or prevents further downstream signaling,

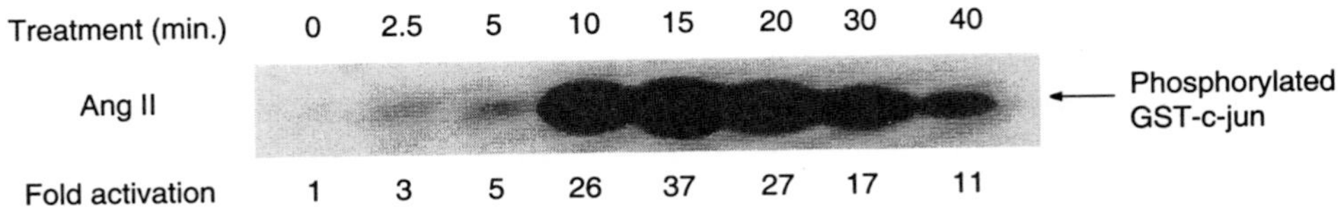

Figure 12 Angiotensin II stimulates Jun N-terminal kinase (JNK). Rat liver epithelial cells were treated with 1 μM angiotensin II for the indicated time points. Cell lysates were incubated with GST–c-Jun linked to Sepharose beads. Jun is both the substrate for JNK and also binds tightly to JNK. The beads are pelleted and washed and the resultant JNK–Jun–GST–Sepharose complex is resuspended in a kinase buffer containing [γ-^{32}P]ATP for 10 min at 30°C, then chilled to stop the kinase reaction. The complexes are separated by SDS–PAGE and analyzed by autoradiography. The fold activation of JNK as measured by Jun–GST phosphorylation was determined by PhosphorImager analysis. From Li *et al.* (11), with permission.

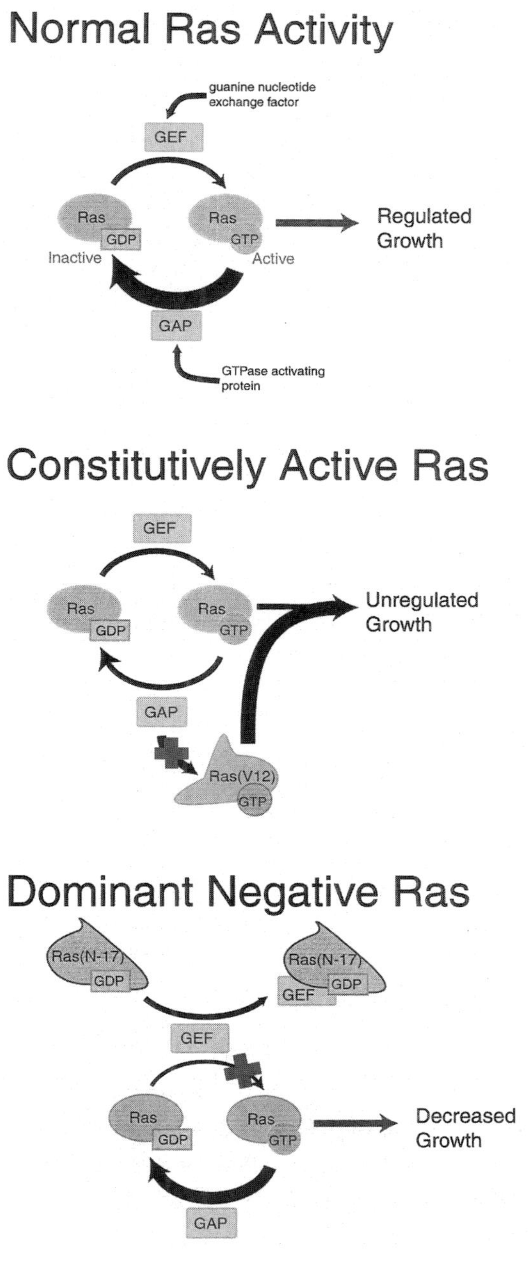

Figure 13 H-Ras(V12) and H-Ras(N17) are examples of constitutively active and dominant negative proteins. The top panel illustrates wild-type Ras and regulated growth. Ras–GDP is inactive and through the activity of guanidine nucleotide exchange factors (GEFs) the GDP is exchanged for GTP, leading to activation of Ras. GTPase-activating proteins (GAPs) stimulate the intrinsic GTPase activity of Ras, thereby leading to the hydrolysis of GTP to GDP and the deactivation of Ras. H-Ras(V12) contains a single amino acid mutation (Gly to Val at position 12) that renders Ras insensitive to GAPs. So the protein always remains activated because the bound GTP is never hydrolyzed to GDP. H-Ras(N17) contains a different mutation (Ser to Asn at position17) that gives Ras a preferential affinity for GDP. In this case, Ras(N17)-GDP binds all available GEFs, sequestering them from wild-type Ras. Both mutant Ras (N17) and wild-type Ras remain in the GDP-bound state in this situation, leading to down-regulation of the Ras pathway. (See color plates.)

usually by sequestering other effector molecules required by the wild-type protein for activation (Fig. 13).

Thus, the delivery of plasmids encoding a constitutively active construct into cells will establish whether this signaling molecule can elicit the same biological response as observed when the endogenous proteins become activated through a physiologic response. Although constitutively active constructs are commonly used to study signaling cascades, the biologic consequences of the expression of such mutant proteins in cells must be interpreted with care. These mutant proteins may stimulate other pathways not involved in the wild-type response. This is most likely due to the fact that constitutively active mutants are always stimulating their effector molecules. Moreover, gain-of-function mutations in some signaling proteins can cause loss of specificity for effector targets. For these reasons, dominant negative constructs have proved to be very useful at elucidating the importance of signaling molecules in the cascade. This stems from the observation that loss-of-function mutations usually display specificity to the signaling pathway in question.

Examples of Constitutively Active and Dominant Negative Proteins: H-Ras(V12) and H-Ras(N17)

The Ras family of GTP-binding proteins is responsible for mediating cellular proliferation, differentiation, and apoptosis (Fig. 13). The *ras* proto-oncogene is frequently mutated in human tumors. Mutations at amino acid position 12 that convert leucine to valine result in a loss of Ras-mediated GTPase activity (19). Thus, the H-Ras(V12) chronically binds GTP, resulting in the constitutive activation of downstream MAPK, MAPK-like, and MAPK-independent signaling cascades. Expression of H-Ras(V12) has been shown to rescue PDGF-responsive cells from growth factor-induced cell death and to stimulate proliferation. However, to establish whether PDGF requires Ras signaling to mediate cell proliferation and survival, a dominant negative H-Ras(N17) mutant was employed. A mutation in H-Ras that replaces an asparagine for serine residue at position 17 creates a mutant protein that functions to block the guanine nucleotide exchange factor required for wild-type Ras signaling (20). In other words, the dominant negative construct interrupts the signaling cascade by competing with the wild-type protein for required effector molecules. Thus, PDGF-induced cell survival and proliferation was shown to require Ras-mediated signaling, because the expression of the dominant negative H-Ras(N17) blocked wild-type Ras and caused cell death even in the presence of PDGF.

VI. Regulation of Signal Transduction Gene Expression

A. The Transient Expression Reporter Assay Allows Identification of Upstream Regulators of Gene Transcription

If the promoter sequence of a gene has been identified and isolated, a transient expression reporter assay can be employed to identify upstream regulators of the pathway (Fig. 14). In this assay, the promoter of the gene under study is fused to the luciferase gene (other reporters can also be used). Luciferase, an enzyme originally isolated from the North American firefly (*Photinus pyralis*), when mixed with its substrates luciferin, ATP, and Mg^{2+}, creates a temporal burst of light that can be quantified by a luminometer. Hence any events that activate the promoter and cause gene transcription can be artificially measured by quantifying luciferase activity. Typically, a plasmid encoding the promoter–luciferase fusion gene and a plasmid encoding other proteins that might directly or indirectly interact with the promoter are cotransfected. After a specified time period (24–48 hr, for example) the cells are harvested and lysates prepared. Aliquots of each sample normalized for protein concentration are mixed with the luciferin reagent and the generated light is measured.

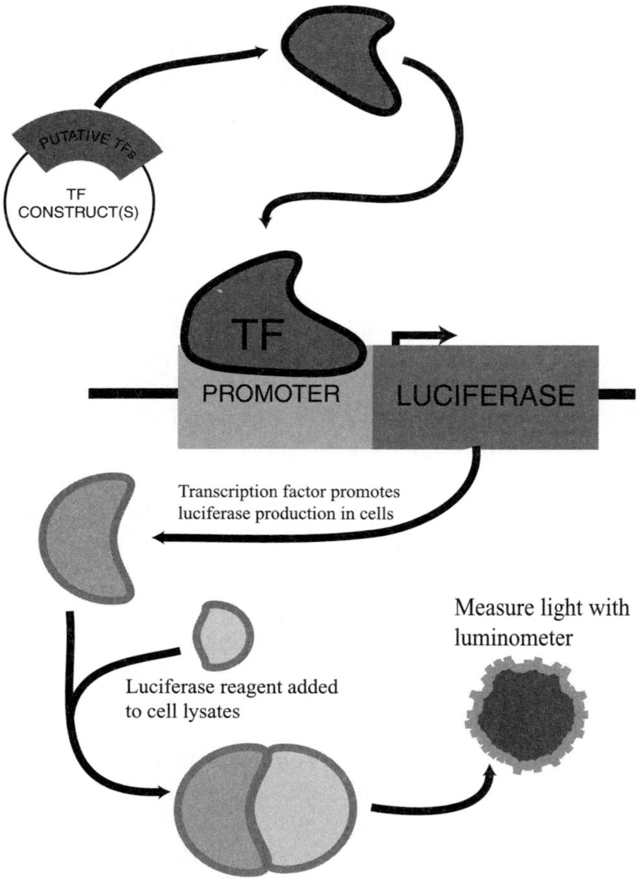

Figure 14 Luciferase assay.

Reporter readout (i.e., luciferase-generated light) requires several sequential processes: the production of the cotransfected proteins/transcription factors (10 min–4 hr) to activate transcription of the promoter–luciferase fusion gene (1–12 hr), with subsequent production of luciferase (1 hr). The luciferase protein has a half-life of 4–6 hr, so a time course is needed to allow measurement of light at the time of maximal activation.

An Example of the Transient Expression Reporter Assay: The Wilms' Tumor Supressor Gene Product, WT1

The Wilms' tumor suppressor gene product WT1 is a transcription factor that transcriptionally up-regulates the bcl-2 promoter and negatively regulates several growth factor promoters. In Denys–Drash syndrome (in which there is a marked predisposition to develop Wilms' tumor), nearly all patients exhibit either a deletion or mutation of WT1. However, WT1 is also required to inhibit apoptosis *in vivo* and *in vitro*, and consistent with this observation, 90% of all sporadic Wilms' tumors continue to express this protein. Thus, in different contexts, WT1 can act as a tumor supressor, or provide survival advantage through antiapoptotic effects.

Figure 15 shows how the luciferase assay has been employed to detect WT1 up-regulation of the bcl-2 promoter (21).

B. The Gel Shift Assay Will Detect Protein Binding to Specific DNA Sequences

The gel shift analysis [also called electrophoretic mobility-shift assay (EMSA)] is used to demonstrate specific binding of putative transcription factors (TFs) to DNA consensus sequences—sites in a promoter known to be specific for transcription factor binding (Fig. 16). A radiolabeled double-stranded oligonucleotide probe is created that mimics the DNA consensus sequence. This probe is then incubated with nuclear extracts from stimulated and unstimulated cells. If the TF that binds to the probe is present in the extract, a TF–DNA duplex will form. The extracts are then resolved by nondenaturing PAGE (the TF–DNA complexes must remain bound to each other) and assessed for radioactivity. Unbound oligonucleotides are quite small and will run as a free probe front to the bottom of the gel. TFs that do not bind the sequence will not be radioactive and thus will be present in the gel, but undetected. Transcription factors that recognize the DNA will form TF–DNA complexes that will run much slower than free probe and be observed as a shift in the mobility of the radiolabeled DNA.

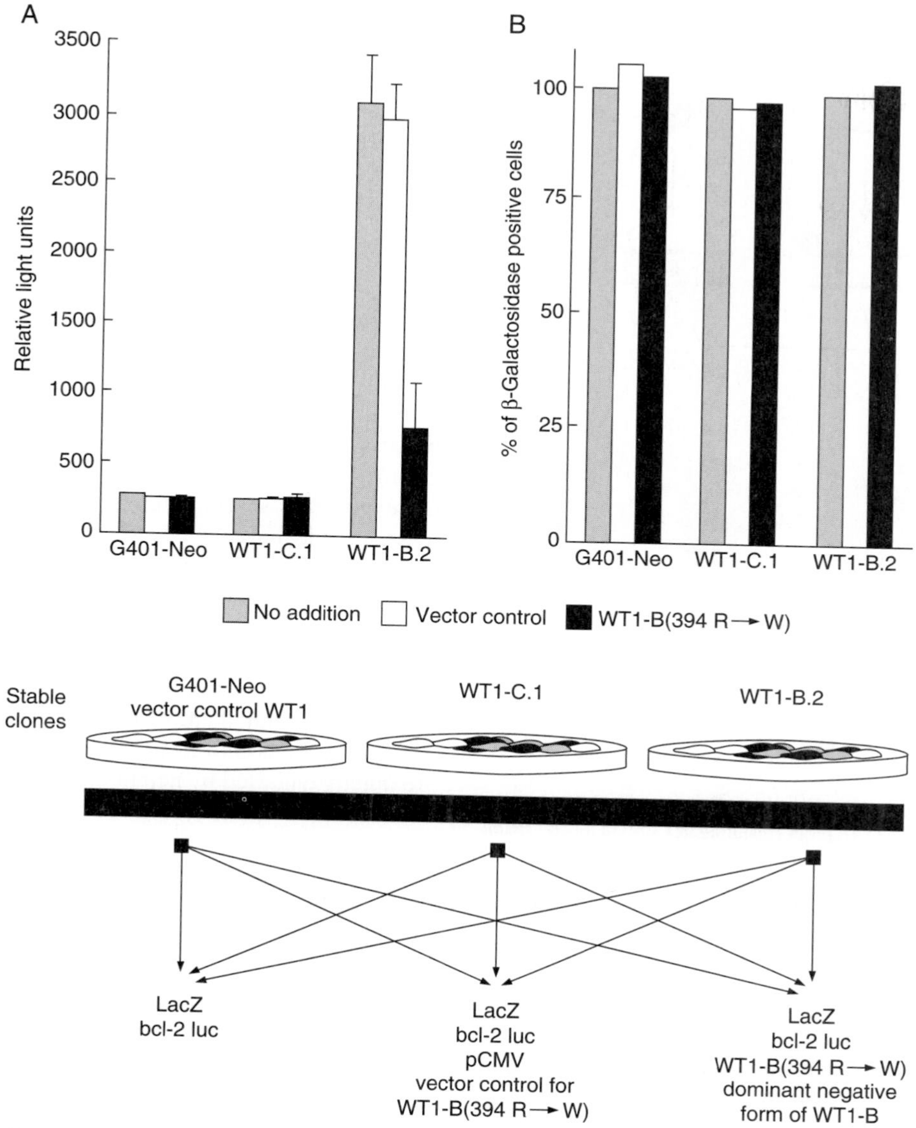

Figure 15 WT1-B.2 form of the WT1 protein up-regulates the bcl-2 promoter through a transcriptional mechanism. Stably transfected clones containing vector control (G401-Neo) and two forms of WT1 (WT1-C.1 and WT1-B.2) were transfected with both the bcl-2-luc and LacZ reporter plasmids. Some groups were additionally transfected with a dominant negative form of WT1 (WT1-B 394R-W) and its vector control (pCMV). Cell lysates were harvested 40 hr after transfection and assayed for luciferase activity as a measurement of WT activation of transcription via the bcl-2 promoter. LacZ was used as a control of both the transfection efficiency and toxicity of the assay. (A) Only WT1-B activates transcription of luciferase via bcl-2; this activity is abrogated with the presence of the dominant negative WT1-B (394R-W). The vector control (G401-Neo) and WT1-C show no transcription of luciferase. (B) In all groups there is equal LacZ activity, implying that the differential transcription of luciferase was not due to toxicity of WT1-C or to better transfection of WTl-B, but rather to the ability of the dominant negative form to repress the DNA-binding ability of wild-type WT1-B.2. From (21), Mayo *et al.* (1999), *Embo J.* **18** (14), 3990–4003; reproduced by permission of Oxford University Press.

Supershift Analysis and Competition Controls Help Confirm the Specificity of the Gel Shift

How do we know that the TF–DNA complex causing the gel shift is representing interactions between the probe and the specific transcription factor we are investigating? In other words, how do we know that it is not a different protein that just happens to bind to the DNA? If there is an antibody available that recognizes the transcription factor, then

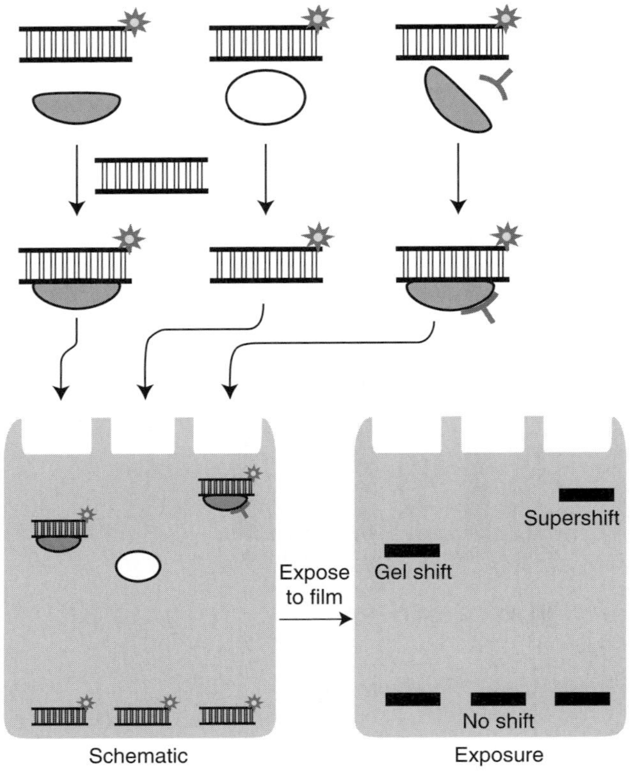

Figure 16 Gel shift. The first lane shows a DNA-binding protein interacting with the radiolabeled DNA probe, resulting in a shift in the migration of the radiolabeled probe. In the second lane the protein does not bind and there is no shift. In the third lane, an antibody recognizing the DNA-binding protein is added, resulting in a larger complex. This is a supershift.

a supershift analysis can be performed to confirm the specificity of the TF–DNA interaction. A gel shift assay is performed as above with the addition of antibody to a separate aliquot of cellular extract/probe mix, allowing complexes of TF–DNA–Ab to form. These complexes will run still slower than just TF–DNA complexes due to the bound antibody. These TF–DNA–Ab complexes are said to be supershifted. Nonspecific protein binding to oligonucleotides are not recognized by the antibody and subsequently are not supershifted. Not all antibodies are able to supershift TF–DNA complexes, so the absence of supershift does not necessarily preclude a specific interaction.

To further confirm specificity, competition controls can be employed that involve incubation with a cold probe (no radiolabel) or a mutant probe (site-specific mutation within the oligo that precludes TF binding). If an excess of cold probe is preincubated with the transcription factor, all DNA binding sites will be saturated and subsequently added hot probe will be unable to bind. This implies specific binding between DNA and transcription factor. If a mutant probe is preincubated with the transcription factor, the DNA binding sites will remain available and subsequently added hot probe will be able to bind. This implies the absence of nonspecific binding.

Figure 17 (21) shows an elegant example of how a gel shift assay can demonstrate transcription factor binding to a DNA consensus sequence within a promoter. Note the copious use of controls to ensure the specificity of the finding.

VII. Signal Transduction and Apoptosis

Although many of the signal transduction pathways illustrated in this chapter thus far have been involved in response of cells to their extracellular environment and regulation of cellular growth, signaling cascades are also prominent in the process of cellular death. Cell death can occur by two mechanisms—necrosis or apoptosis. Necrosis occurs after cells are exposed to severe external trauma, noxious stimuli, or lethal chemical events. Necrosis is characterized by cellular swelling, mitochondrial dysfunction, uncontrolled lysis of the cell membrane, and release of cellular contents into the surrounding tissues, thereby inciting a marked inflammatory response. In contrast, apoptosis is a regulated sequence of energy-requiring events throughout which membrane integrity is maintained, resulting in the dissolution of the cell and nucleus into neat membrane-bound packages that are quietly engulfed by neighboring phagocytes.

The term apoptosis (pronounced with the second p silent) has Greek origins and describes the process of leaves falling from trees or petals from flowers. As autumn occurs during the natural progression of the seasons, apoptosis occurs during the many developmental and housekeeping cellular processes. Programmed cell death is used by an organism during development in the sculpting of limbs (deletion of interdigital cells during development of hands and feet) and in the elimination of dangerous or unwanted cells (creation of tolerance in thymocytes). Anoikis (Greek meaning "homeless") describes the process of cells undergoing forced apoptosis due to loss of cell anchorage or adhesion. This phenomenon is seen in enterocytes that are sloughed into the lumen of the gut. If these cells remained viable despite detachment, an organism would eventually suffer dire consequences from cells randomly reattaching and growing. In the mature organism, apoptosis is the predominant mechanism allowing organs to maintain cell mass while simultaneously deleting cells that have become aged or damaged. It is also the mechanism by which cytotoxic T cells kill tumor target cells.

Apoptosis is an energy-demanding process; therefore, the mitochondrial machinery of the cell must remain intact and functional. During apoptosis, cells undergo organized cytoplasmic and nuclear condensation with DNA cleavage between nucleosomes. The plasma membrane blebs and finally the entire cell degenerates into apoptotic bodies.

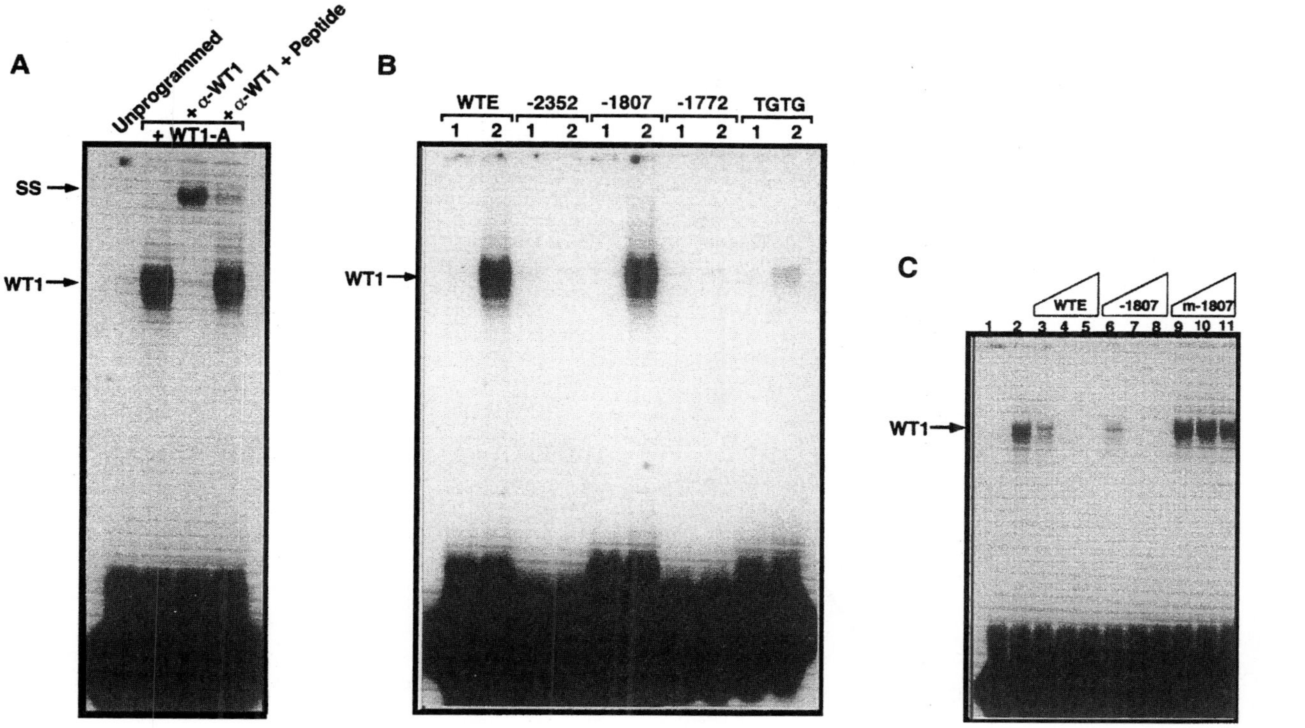

Figure 17 (A) EMSA shows that WT1-A interacts with the WT1 element (WTE) DNA consensus sequence. Unprogrammed reticulocyte lysate (lane one) or WT1-A protein preparations (lanes 2–4) were incubated with the ^{32}P-labeled double-stranded DNA probe WTE. The unprogrammed lysate has negligible WT1 and thus there is no gel shift. The WT1-A protein preparations bind to WTE and shifts. To demonstrate specificity of the gel shift, the DNA–protein complexes were incubated with anti-WT1-specific antibody either alone (lane 3) or in combination with a WT1-specific immune peptide inhibitor (lane 4). α-WT1 is able to supershift (SS) the DNA–protein complex, and the supershift is blocked by the immune peptide inhibitor as expected. (B) EMSA demonstrates that WT1 directly binds to DNA elements located in the bcl-2 promoter region. Unprogrammed lysate (lane 1) or WT1-A protein preparations (lane 2) were incubated with ^{32}P-labeled double-stranded DNA oligonucleotides corresponding to the positive control WTE or to four potential DNA-binding sites located within the bcl-2 promoter (−2352, −1807, −1772, TGTG) and EMSA was performed. Only WTE and oligo −1807 allow TF binding and shifts. (C) Competition assays using cold and mutant −1807 oligo prove specificity of the WT1-A TF binding. Lanes 1 and 2 show EMSA with unprogrammed or with WT1-A protein preparations and the labeled −1807 oligo. Lanes 3–11 demonstrate competition assays performed by preincubating WT1-A protein preparations with increasing concentrations (50-, 100-, and 200-fold excess) of unlabeled, double-stranded DNA probes corresponding to WTE (lanes 3–5), −1807 (lanes 6–8), and mutated −1807 unable to bind TF (lanes 9–11) before the addition of 40,000 c.p.m. of ^{32}P-labeled −1807 DNA probe. Cold WTE and −1807 successfully compete with labeled −1807. Mutant −1807 is unable to bind to WT1-A and thus gel shift is seen at all concentrations. From (21), Mayo *et al.* (1999), *Embo J.* **18**(14); 3990–4003; reproduced by permission of Oxford University Press.

Apoptosis requires the activity of specific groups of proteins (Fig. 18). The cascade can be initiated by a receptor–ligand event such as the binding of TNF or the Fas ligand. The receptors for TNF and the Fas ligand share common domains (death domains) that, when activated, trigger the apoptosis cascade. Aggregation of death domains and recruitment of other proteins result in death-inducing signaling complex (DISC) formation, which activates members of the caspase family. This family of intracellular proteases cleaves targets following aspartic acid residues (*cysteine aspartases*). Fourteen members of the family have been reported, and the number is still growing. The caspases catalyze a series of events peculiar to apoptosis, including the rearrangement of the phospholipid bilayer, which forms the basis for a common assay to detect cellular suicide.

The following discussions describe three different methods to detect apoptosis in cells (see Table I).

A. An Early Event in Apoptosis: Migration of Phosphatidylserine from the Inner to the Outer Leaflet of the Plasma Membrane

In normal, healthy cells, the phospholipid phosphatidylserine (PS) is maintained on the inner surface of the cell membrane. Two enzymes are involved in the movement of PS in membranes: scramblases, which move PS from the inner to the outer leaflet, and translocases, which return the PS from the outer leaflet back to the inner leaflet (Fig. 19). In the normal cell, scramblases are inhibited and translocases are active, thus maintaining all PSs on the inner leaflet. During the early

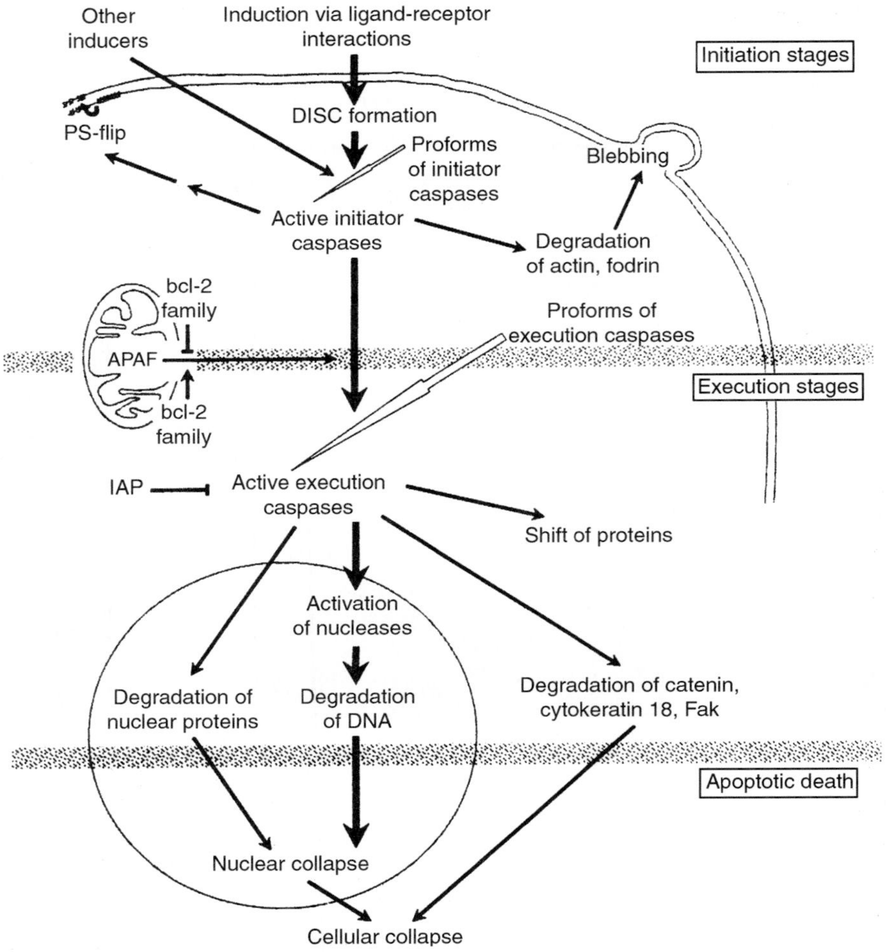

Figure 18 Apoptosis cascade. Apoptotic death is the result of a complex cascade of events that finally leads to the collapse of the cell and nucleus. Even in this final stage the cell does not release intracellular components, thus avoiding inflammatory reactions. From (24); B. Huppertz, H. G. Frank, and P. Kaufmann (1999). The apoptosis cascade—Morphological and immunohistochemical methods for its visualization. *Anat. Embryol.* (Berl.) **200**(1), 1–18, Fig. 1, © Springer-Verlag.

stages of apoptosis, caspases inactivate translocases and/or activate scramblases, allowing PS to accumulate on the outer surface of the cell membrane. Thus PS can be used as a marker for apoptotic cells and can be detected by phospholipid-binding proteins such as annexin V (AV). Annexin V has an avid and specific affinity for PS. It is found on macrophages *in vivo* and allows phagocytes to identify apoptotic cells. When conjugated to a chromophore, AV can be detected by fluorescence (using microscopy or flow cytometry) or when conjugated to streptavidin it can be detected colorimetrically.

Care must be taken when using AV to detect apoptosis. The specificity of the assay relies on the fact that apoptotic cells maintain the integrity of their cellular membrane. A membrane-impermeable dye, propidium iodide (PI) or 7-aminoactinomycin D (7AAD), is used as a counterstain to distinguish apoptotic from necrotic cells. Therefore, apoptotic cells are AV positive and PI negative. In contrast, necrotic cells are AV positive and PI positive, because loss of membrane integrity allows entrance of PI into the nucleus and access of AV to the inner leaflet. Unfortunately, in cell culture, where there are no phagocytes, apoptotic cells also eventually undergo necrosis—termed secondary necrosis—and become AV positive and PI positive. As a result it becomes impossible to differentiate necrosis from late apoptosis with this technique.

B. Late Events of Apoptosis Include DNA Fragmentation Detectable by the TUNEL Assay

Caspases also activate endonucleases, which clip chromosomes into nucleosome-sized DNA fragments, leading to the characteristic ladder of DNA fragmentation seen on

Table I Markers of Apoptosis and Tools for Their Identification[a]

Protein/event	Tools	Putative source
Fas/FasL	Various antibodies	Upstate Biotechnology, R&D Systems
TNF-R1/TNFα	Various antibodies	R&D Systems
Caspases	Antibodies against pro- and active forms	Santa Cruz, Clontech
Cytoskeletal proteins	Various antibodies	ICN
Membrane blebbing	Light and electron microscopy	
Phosphatidyl serine flip	Annexin V	Clontech
Bcl-2 proteins	Various antibodies	Sigma, Upstate Biotechnology
PARP	Various antibodies	Upstate Biotechnology
Lamin B	Various antibodies	Oncogene/Calbiochem
DNA single-strand breaks	TUNEL	Calbiochem, Enzo Diagnostics
Annular chromatin condensation—nuclear morphology	Light and electron microscopy with the aid of nuclear dyes	

[a]From (24). B. Huppertz, H. G. Frank, and P. Kaufmann (1999). The apoptosis cascade—Morphological and immunohistochemical methods for its visualization. *Anat. Embryol. (Berl.)* **200**(1), 1–18, Table 1, © Springer-Verlag.

agarose gel. Terminal deoxynucleotidyl transferase (TdT) can be used *in vitro* to covalently label the exposed 3′OH termini strand breaks with modified nucleotides—typically digoxinin-conjugated nucleotides (22). The digoxinin can then be detected with a specific antibody. Although a baseline level of DNA strand breaks exists in all cells, this proportion is usually miniscule in comparison to breaks generated by apoptosis. Nevertheless, a careful inspection of samples and controls should ensue to correlate TdT-mediated & UTP nick end labeling (TUNEL) positivity with apoptotic nuclear morphology.

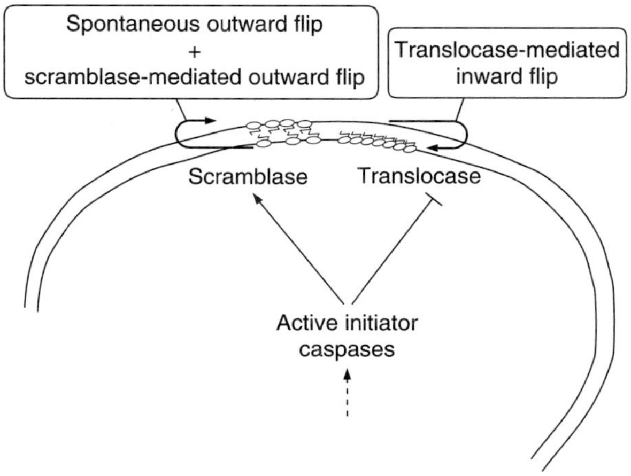

Figure 19 Mechanisms regulating the distribution of phosphatidylserine in the inner and outer leaflet of the plasma membrane. In healthy cells, PS is maintained on the inner leaflet by ATP-dependent translocases. During the early stages of apoptosis, caspases inactivate translocases and activate scramblases resulting in a flip of PS from the inner to the outer leaflet. From (24); B. Huppertz, H. G. Frank, and P. Kaufmann (1999). The apoptosis cascade—Morphological and immunohistochemical methods for its visualization. *Anat. Embryol. (Berl.)* **200**(1), 1–18, Fig. 5, © Springer-Verlag.

C. Hoechst 33342 Dye Allows Visualization of Nuclear Morphology

Hoechst dye is membrane permeable and binds avidly to DNA. It is visible with UV light. Apoptotic nuclear morphology is characteristic and proceeds from annular chromatin condensation to fragmentation of DNA with dispersion into discrete droplets distributed throughout the cytoplasm, and finally cellular dissolution into small membrane-bound apoptotic bodies consisting of cytoplasmic and nuclear elements. Although Hoechst staining can quickly and accurately determine apoptotic morphology, cells must be examined individually for the progression of apoptotic nuclear anatomy.

VIII. Key Resources

The following resources are invaluable in the field of signal transduction.

1. "Current Protocols in Molecular Biology" (1997, John Wiley & Sons, Inc.). Most of the methods described in this text are examined thoroughly, with detailed protocols. This is certainly one of the best references for specific methods.
2. "Cell Biology: A Laboratory Handbook" (edited by Julio E. Celis, 1998, Academic Press).
3. "Molecular Cloning: A Laboratory Manual" (edited by J. Sambrook, E.F. Fritsch, and T. Maniatis, 1989, Cold Spring Harbor Laboratory Press).
4. An extensive body of information is available from the Internet in manufacturers' sites. Technical help can easily be obtained via e-mail (or with a phone call).
5. The Signal Transduction Society homepage: http://www.sigtrans.de/start.shtml.

Acknowledgments

We thank Dr. Marty Mayo for invaluable assistance in the preparation of this manuscript, Drs. Keith Burridge, Albert Baldwin, Channing Der, Shelton Earp, Kevin Pruitt, Michael Schaller, and Wendell Yarbrough for helpful discussions, and Drs. Steven Gross and Charles Smith for critical evaluation of the manuscript.

References

1. Hung, M. C., and Lau, Y. K. (1999). Basic science of HER-2/neu: A review. *Semin. Oncol.* **26**(4, Suppl. 12), 51–59.
2. Owens, L. V., Xu, L., Craven, R. J., *et al.* (1995). Overexpression of the focal adhesion kinase (p125FAK) in invasive human tumors. *Cancer Res.* **55**(13), 2752–2755.
3. Cobb, B. S., Schaller, M. D., Leu, T. H., and Parsons, J. T. (1994). Stable association of pp60src and pp59fyn with the focal adhesion-associated protein tyrosine kinase, pp125FAK. *Mol. Cell. Biol.* **14**(1), 147–155.
4. Hunter, T. (1995). Protein kinases and phosphatases: The yin and yang of protein phosphorylation and signaling. *Cell* **80**(2), 225–236.
5. Tan, Y. H. (1993). Yin and yang of phosphorylation in cytokine signaling. *Science* **262**(5132), 376–377.
6. Doree, M., and Galas, S. (1994). The cyclin-dependent protein kinases and the control of cell division. *FASEB J.* **8**(14), 1114–1121.
7. Kamps, M. P., and Sefton, B. M. (1988). Identification of multiple novel polypeptide substrates of the v-src, v-yes, v-fps, v-ros, and v-erb-B oncogenic tyrosine protein kinases utilizing antisera against phosphotyrosine. *Oncogene* **2**(4), 305–315.
8. Morla, A. O., and Wang, J. Y. (1986). Protein tyrosine phosphorylation in the cell cycle of BALB/c 3T3 fibroblasts. *Proc. Natl. Acad. Sci. U.S.A.* **83**(21), 8191–8195.
9. Nairn, A. C., Detre, J. A., Casnellie, J. E., and Greengard, P. (1982). Serum antibodies that distinguish between the phospho- and dephospho- forms of a phosphoprotein. *Nature* (*London*) **299**(5885), 734–736.
10. Doolittle, R. F. (1986). "Of Urfs and Orfs: A Primer on How to Analyze Derived Amino Acid Sequences." University Science Books, Mill Valley, California.
11. Li, X., Yu, H., Graves, L. M., and Earp, H. S. (1997). Protein kinase C and protein kinase A inhibit calcium-dependent but not stress-dependent c-Jun N-terminal kinase activation in rat liver epithelial cells. *J. Biol. Chem.* **272**(23), 14996–5002.
12. Spaargaren, M., Boonstra, J., de Laat, S. W. (1991). Biological signal transduction. *In* "Biological Signal Transduction," Vol. 52 (E. Wirtz, ed.), pp. 45–58. Springer-Verlag, New York.
13. Schneider, P. M., Hung, M. C., Chiocca, S. M., *et al.* (1989). Differential expression of the c-erbB-2 gene in human small cell and non-small cell lung cancer. *Cancer Res.* **49**(18), 4968–4971.
14. Yokota, J., Yamamoto, T., Miyajima, N., *et al.* (1988). Genetic alterations of the c-erbB-2 oncogene occur frequently in tubular adenocarcinoma of the stomach and are often accompanied by amplification of the v-erb A homologue. *Oncogene* **2**(3), 283–287.
15. Slamon, D. J., Clark, G. M., Wong, S. G., *et al.* (1987). Human breast cancer: Correlation of relapse and survival with amplification of the HER-2/neu oncogene. *Science* **235**(4785), 177–182.
16. Peles, E., Bacus, S. S., Koski, R. A., *et al.* (1992). Isolation of the neu/HER-2 stimulatory ligand: A 44 kd glycoprotein that induces differentiation of mammary tumor cells. *Cell* **69**(1), 205–216.
17. Shak, S. (1999). Overview of the trastuzumab (Herceptin) anti-HER2 monoclonal antibody clinical program in HER2-overexpressing metastatic breast cancer. Herceptin Multinational Investigator Study Group. *Semin. Oncol.* **26**(4, Suppl. 12), 71–77.
18. Sliwkowski, M. X., Lofgren, J. A., Lewis, G. D., *et al.* (1999). Nonclinical studies addressing the mechanism of action of trastuzumab (Herceptin). *Semin. Oncol.* **26**(4, Suppl. 12), 60–70.
19. Feig, L. A., and Cooper, G. M. (1988). Inhibition of NIH 3T3 cell proliferation by a mutant ras protein with preferential affinity for GDP. *Mol. Cell. Biol.* **8**(8), 3235–3243.
20. Stacey, D. W., Roudebush, M., Day, R., *et al.* (1991). Dominant inhibitory Ras mutants demonstrate the requirement for Ras activity in the action of tyrosine kinase oncogenes. *Oncogene* **6**(12), 2297–2304.
21. Mayo, M. W., Wang, C. Y., Drouin, S. S., *et al.* (1994). WT1 modulates apoptosis by transcriptionally upregulating the bcl-2 proto-oncogene. *Embo J.* **18**(14), 3990–4003.
22. Sgonc, R., and Wick, G. (1994). Methods for the detection of apoptosis. *Int. Arch. Allergy Immunol.* **105**(4), 327–332.
23. Chou, C. K., Dull, T. J., Russell, D. S., *et al.* (1987). Human insulin receptors mutated at the ATP-binding site lack protein tyrosine kinase activity and fail to mediate postreceptor effects of insulin. *J. Biol. Chem.* **262**(4), 1842–1847.
24. Huppertz, B., Frank, H. G., and Kaufmann, P. (1999). The apoptosis cascade—Morphological and immunohistochemical methods for its visualization. *Anat. Embryol. (Berl.)* **200**(1), 1–18.

23

Mechanisms and Regulation of Eukaryotic Protein Synthesis

Theresa L. Eisenbraun, Patricia M. Scott, Gregory D. Kennedy, and John E. Niederhuber

University of Wisconsin Comprehensive Cancer Center, Madison, Wisconsin 53792

I. Introduction

The central dogma of molecular biology is the inheritance of genetic information encoded in specific sequences of nucleic acid known as genes, and the conversion of this encoded information into specific proteins—a concept often referred to as "one gene/one protein." Inheritance of the information encoded in the nucleic acid sequence occurs by exact replication of the double-stranded DNA. Expression of the information encoded in the nucleic acid sequence involves two sequential processes—transcription and translation. Transcription is the mechanism by which the cell generates a single strand of RNA identical in sequence to one strand of the double-stranded DNA. Translation is the process by which one form of RNA, messenger (mRNA), is used as the template for the synthesis of specific proteins. This chapter focuses on the mechanisms controlling protein synthesis and the relevance of the regulation of protein synthesis to biomedical research and disease. The chapter also reviews the techniques used to study protein synthesis.

II. Overview of Protein Synthesis

Until recently, study of the mechanisms controlling gene expression was focused mainly on transcription. Because the majority of eukaryotic mRNAs are monocistronic, i.e., contain only one coding region, regulation of gene expression at the level of translation was not seriously considered. The discovery of mRNAs with 5′ ends that contain more than one possible reading frame, as well as viruses that usurp the host cell translation machinery to preferentially translate their own proteins, provided the first clues that regulation of gene expression could also occur during translation.

Translation can be divided into three sequential components: initiation, elongation, and termination. Although each of these steps in the process of translation is addressed in this chapter, the majority of translation research in eukaryotes has focused on initiation, the rate-limiting step of protein synthesis.

A. Initiation

Initiation is the process during which a 40S ribosomal subunit, in conjunction with various initiation factors, binds to an mRNA and, after recognition of an appropriate initiator codon, is joined by a 60S ribosomal subunit to form an elongation-competent 80S ribosome (1).

1. Components of the Translation Machinery

a. The Ribosome The ribosome is a ribonucleoprotein complex consisting of two subunits, designated 40S and 60S, based on their approximate rates of sedimentation. These two subunits join together to form a complex with a sedimentation coefficient of 80S. [The unit of sedimentation, S, stands for Svedberg. One Svedberg (1S) is equivalent to 10^{-13} sec.] Each of the ribosomal subunits is composed of protein and RNA. The 40S subunit contains approximately 33 proteins and the 18S ribosomal RNA (rRNA); the 60S subunit contains approximately 49 proteins and three species of rRNA, 5S, 5.8S, and 28S. [For a more thorough description of the ribosome, the reader is referred to "The Ribosome: Structure, Function, Antibiotics, and Cellular Interactions" (2).]

b. Initiation Factors Associated with the 40S ribosomal subunit are proteins called initiation factors. A brief description of the role each of these factors plays in initiation is included in Table I. [For a more thorough description of the roles and regulation of each of the initiation factors, readers are referred to reviews by Pestova and Hellen (3), McKendrick *et al.* (4), Raught and Gingras (5), Keiper *et al.* (6), Lawrence and Abraham (7), and Kimble (8).]

c. Met-tRNA$_i$ Transfer RNA (tRNA) molecules serve as adapters that translate a three-nucleotide code (codon) in the messenger RNA into an amino acid. The codons and the amino acids they code for are outlined in Table II. The tRNA that specifically serves as the initiator is aminoacylated with methionine to form Met-tRNA$_i$. What distinguishes the Met-tRNA$_i$ complex from the Met tRNA complexes that are incorporated during elongation is its ability to associate with the eukaryotic initiation factor-2 (eIF2). Met-tRNA$_i$ associates with mRNA through interaction of its anticodon (5′-CAU-3′) with the codon for methionine (5′-AUG-3′).

Table I The Eukaryotic Translation Initiation Factors

Initiation factor (eIF)	Role in initiation
1	With eIF1A, helps 43S initiation complex reach the initiation codon
1A	Stabilizes binding of mRNA to the 40S ribosomal subunit; helps 43S initiation complex reach the initiation codon
2	Forms ternary complex with GTP and Met-tRNA$_i$; positions Met-tRNA$_i$ on the 40S ribosomal subunit
2B	Guanine nucleotide exchange factor that catalyzes the exchange of GDP associated with eIF2 for GTP
3	Interacts with both mRNA and eIF4G to promote association of the 43S initiation complex with the mRNA cap structure
4A	The helicase component of eIF4F; binds eIF4G
4B	Aids in helicase activity of eIF4F
4E	Cap-binding component of eIF4F
4G	Recruitment of mRNA to the 43S initiation complex; binds eIF4E and PABP [poly(A) binding protein]
4F	Cap-binding complex composed of eIF4A, eIF4E, and eIF4G
5	Catalyzes hydrolysis of GTP in the eIF2–GTP–Met-tRNA$_i$ complex

2. Mechanisms of Translation Initiation

a. The Scanning Model of Translation Initiation For the majority of eukaryotic mRNAs, initiation occurs by the process described in Fig. 1. Briefly, a ternary complex of eIF2, GTP, and Met-tRNA$_i$ is recruited to a 40S ribosomal subunit that is already associated with eIF3, eIF1A, and possibly, eIF1 (1, 9). Collectively, this is called the 43S preinitiation complex. An mRNA molecule is then bound at its 5′ terminus through interaction of its $7^{m}G$ cap structure with the eIF4E component of the cap-binding complex, eIF4F (1, 4). The eIF4F also contains the initiation factors eIF4A and eIF4G. Attachment of the cap-binding complex to the mRNA cap structure requires hydrolysis of ATP and is augmented by another initiation factor, eIF4B (9). Formation of the 48S preinitiation complex occurs when the mRNA is then recruited to the 43S complex through the interaction of eIF4G and eIF3 (6). An additional level of complexity is added with the interaction of eIF4G and poly(A) binding protein (PABP), a protein that binds to the 3′ poly(A) tail of the mRNA (10, 11). The 40S ribosomal subunit then scans in a 5′ to 3′ direction on the mRNA until an appropriate initiator codon is reached. Generally, the initiator codon is the nucleotide sequence AUG, but there are instances in which alternative codons such as CUG have been utilized as translation start sites (12). ATP is hydrolyzed during scanning by eIF4A in its role as an RNA helicase (3). However, it is not known if ATP hydrolysis is also necessary for the actual movement of the 40S ribosome. After recognition of an appropriate initiator codon, the GTP that is associated with eIF2 is hydrolyzed to GDP in a reaction that is catalyzed by yet another initiation factor, eIF5 (8). The resulting eIF2–GDP complex and eIF3 are released and the 40S ribosomal subunit is joined by the 60S ribosomal subunit to form the elongation-competent 80S ribosome. The fate of the other initiation factors after joining of the 40S and 60S ribosomal subunits is still under investigation.

The basic scanning mechanism calls for translation to initiate at the first AUG codon that the 40S ribosomal subunit reaches (3, 13). However, experimental evidence indicates that this is not always the case. Many mRNAs contain AUG codons upstream of known translation start sites. One reason these codons may not be recognized, or are recog-

Table II Codons and Their Amino Acids

Amino acid	One-letter symbol	Three-letter symbol	Codons
Alanine	A	Ala	GCA GCC GCG GCU
Cysteine	C	Cys	UGC UGU
Aspartic acid	D	Asp	GAC GAU
Glutamic acid	E	Glu	GAA GAG
Phenylalanine	F	Phe	UUC UUU
Glycine	G	Gly	GGA GGC GGG GGU
Histidine	H	His	CAC CAU
Isoleucine	I	Ile	AUA AUC AUU
Lysine	K	Lys	AAA AAG
Leucine	L	Leu	UUA UUG CUA CUC CUG CUU
Methionine	M	Met	AUG
Asparagine	N	Asn	AAC AAU
Proline	P	Pro	CCA CCC CCG CCU
Glutamine	Q	Gln	CAA CAG
Arginine	R	Arg	AGA AGG CGA CGC CGG CGU
Serine	S	Ser	AGC AGU UCA UCC UCG UCU
Threonine	T	Thr	ACA ACC ACG ACU
Valine	V	Val	GUA GUC GUG GUU
Tryptophan	T	Trp	UGG
Tyrosine	Y	Tyr	UAC UAU

nized inefficiently as initiation codons, is that they appear to reside within sequence contexts that are suboptimal for initiation. Kozak (14) has determined experimentally that the consensus sequence for initiation is A/GNNAUGG, where the A of AUG is numbered as +1. The sequence of the nucleotides in the −3 and +4 positions is most important, with optimal initiation occurring when a purine (preferably an A) is present in the −3 position and G is present in the +4 position. When an AUG codon is found in a suboptimal context, 40S ribosomal subunits may bypass this AUG codon and continue scanning until an AUG codon in a sequence context more appropriate for initiation is reached. This variation of the scanning mechanism is called "leaky scanning" [(14), and references therein].

Many viral and some cellular mRNAs are known to have more than one coding region translated from the same mRNA. There are at least two mechanisms by which this occurs. The first mechanism is leaky scanning, as mentioned above. Initiation occurs at a downstream AUG codon because an upstream AUG codon is inefficiently used as a translation start site. The second mechanism involves ribosomes that have translated the upstream reading frame but are then able to continue scanning and reinitiate translation at the downstream AUG codon. The ability of ribosomes to reinitiate translation at downstream AUG codons appears to be influenced by the distance between initiator codons as well as the efficiency with which translation of the upstream reading frame was terminated (15, 16).

In addition to mRNAs that contain upstream AUG codons and/or reading frames, many mRNAs have 5′ ends that are unusually long, i.e., contain greater than 200 nucleotides. These 5′ ends have the potential to form complex secondary structures that are predicted to inhibit translation initiation by scanning 40S ribosomes. Accordingly, in a subset of these mRNAs, translation initiation by scanning 40S ribosomes does not occur efficiently under normal cellular conditions. However, under conditions in which the limiting component of the cap-binding complex, eIF4E, is synthesized at higher levels and/or phosphorylation is enhanced, translation of some members of this subset of mRNAs increases (5, 17, 18). Interestingly, many of the mRNAs that have unusually long and potentially structured 5′ ends and appear to be regulated at translation initiation are cellular growth control factors, including fibroblast growth factor-2 (FGF-2) (19, 20), transforming growth factor-β (TGF-β) (19, 21), and ornithine decarboxylase (ODC) (22, 23). Therefore, translation of these mRNAs may have evolved to be less efficient during normal cellular conditions to avoid deleterious effects on the cell.

b. Initiation via Internal Ribosomal Entry Sites An alternative mechanism whereby translation is initiated on

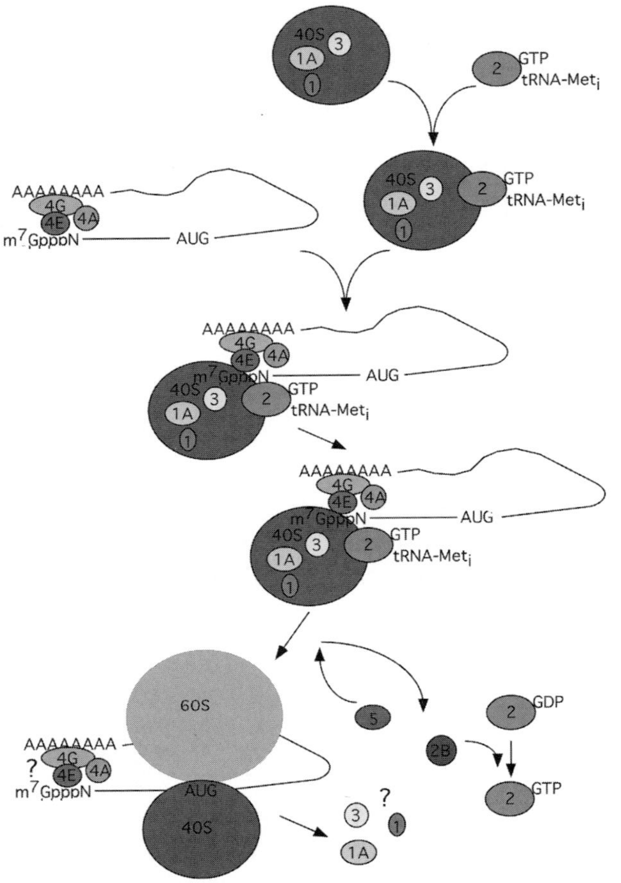

Figure 1 Translation initiation. (See color plates.)

eukaryotic mRNAs was first demonstrated in picornavirus-infected cells (24), but has been found subsequently to occur on a subset of cellular mRNAs for factors that are involved in cellular growth control and oncogenesis, including platelet-derived growth factor (PDGF) (19, 25), vascular endothelial growth factor VEGF (26, 27), and c-myc (28, 29). These viral and cellular mRNAs are similar in that they both have unusually long and highly structured 5′ ends. The basic mechanism by which initiation occurs in this subset of mRNAs is through the binding of ribosomes to internal ribosomal entry sites (IRES), independent of the 5′ 7^m G cap structure. Although the details of this mechanism are still being worked out, in the picornavirus family, ribosomes appear to bind specific structures within the 5′ end (30). Ribosomes likely bind to specific structures in the 5′ ends of cellular mRNAs, but whether these structures have any obvious homology with the structures predicted to form in the picornaviral mRNA 5′ ends is not clear (31).

3. Links between Initiation and Other Cellular Processes

a. The Cell Cycle Regulation of the level and activity of eIF4E is correlated with effects on cell cycle progression. During mitosis, translation rates are low and eIF4E is underphosphorylated. Alternatively, an increase in eIF4E phosphorylation, which apparently results in an increase in affinity of eIF4E for the mRNA cap structure, is observed after treatment of cells with growth factors or cytokines (5, 32). One enzyme implicated in eIF4E phosphorylation is MNK1 kinase, a substrate of the ERK and p38 MAPKs (33, 34). eIF4E activity is also regulated by its association with a family of repressor proteins called the eIF4BPs. Binding of eIF4E by members of the eIF4BP family prevents the association of eIF4E with eIF4F and subsequently results in the inhibition of cap-dependent translation (4, 7, 35). Phosphorylation of the eIF4BPs by an antiapoptotic kinase, Akt/PKB, which is involved in a PI3 kinase-dependent signaling pathway, disrupts the eIF4E/eIF4BP complex to allow eIF4E to associate with the cap-binding complex (36). Other kinases may also be involved in the phosphorylation of the eIF4BPs.

b. Cellular Proliferation and Apoptosis Regulation of protein synthesis at initiation is observed in many mRNAs that are involved in cell proliferation. For example, synthesis of the two rate-limiting enzymes of the polyamine biosynthetic pathway, ornithine decarboxylase (ODC) and *S*-adenosylmethionine decarboxylase (AdoMetDC), is regulated at initiation, but the mechanisms by which this occurs are different. Regulation of AdoMetDC synthesis is controlled by a mechanism involving translation of an upstream reading frame. What is unusual about the regulation of AdoMetDC synthesis is that the sequence of the upstream reading frame is important. It appears that there is a sequence-dependent stalling of ribosomes during translation of the upstream reading frame resulting in a decrease in efficiency of AdoMETDC translation (23). On the other hand, the ODC mRNA contains a fairly structured 5′ end but is still translated via scanning of ribosomes. However, efficient translation of ODC appears to depend on the availability of active eIF4E (22, 23).

A more global control of protein synthesis involves the initiation factor eIF2. After Met-tRNA$_i$ has been transferred to the ribosome, the GTP bound to eIF2 is hydrolyzed to GDP and the eIF2–GDP complex is released from the ribosome. In order for eIF2 to become competent again for initiation, GDP has to be exchanged for GTP, a reaction that is mediated by the initiation factor eIF2B (see Fig. 1). The exchange of GDP for GTP can be prevented by phosphorylation of the α subunit of eIF2, a process that converts eIF2 from a substrate into a competitive inhibitor of eIF2B (37). Phosphorylation of eIF2α can be mediated by several different kinases, including the double-stranded, RNA-activated, serine/threonine protein kinase, PKR (38). There is some evidence in mouse cell lines that correlates activation of PKR and phosphorylation of eIF2α with an increase in protein levels of the proapoptotic protein, Bax (38). A more thorough discussion involving PKR and eIF2α phosphorylation will be undertaken in the section that describes the links between intiation and tumorigenesis.

c. Cell Growth and Differentiation Translation initiation of many growth factor mRNAs is regulated specifically during differentiation and growth including VEGF (26), PDGF2 (39, 40), FGF-2 (41), and TGF-β (42). In addition, changes in efficiency of translation initiation of many of these mRNAs have been implicated in the progression of various forms of cancer (17, 43).

d. DNA Repair A recent study by Ting *et al.* (44) showed that the α, β, and γ subunits of eIF2 interacted with DNA-dependent protein kinase (DNA-PK) in a complex also consisting of the DNA-binding protein, Ku. This study also showed that the eIF2β subunit was phosphorylated by DNA-PK and that a portion of eIF2 localizes to the nucleus. These results suggest that eIF2, in addition to its role in translation, may play a role in DNA repair.

4. Initiation and Disease

a. Initiation and Viral Infection Infection by certain viruses, including the picornavirus and orthomyxovirus families, results in the preferential translation of viral mRNAs, although the mechanisms by which this occurs are quite different. On infection by picornaviruses, a protease is activated that specifically cleaves eIF4G near its amino terminus. Because the amino terminus of eIF4G contains the eIF4E binding site, this results in the loss of cap binding activity for eIF4F and, subsequently, the inhibition of cellular protein synthesis (6). Picornaviral mRNAs are then preferentially translated because they do not contain cap structures (45). Alternatively, orthomyxovirus mRNAs are preferentially translated by a cap-dependent mechanism that is mediated by the 5′ end of the orthomyxovirus mRNAs. There is some evidence now for a specific enhancement of translation by the binding of cellular factors to the viral 5′ ends (46). In addition, these viruses utilize a unique mechanism for capping their mRNAs, i.e., "cap-stealing." The mRNA synthesis in orthomyxovirus-infected cells is initiated with 10–15 nucleotide capped primers that have been cleaved from a subset of cellular mRNAs by a virally encoded nuclease, PB2 (47).

b. Initiation and Tumorigenesis There are now several links between the regulation of translation initiation and the progression of certain forms of cancer. Because many tumors demonstrate higher rates of protein synthesis than the corresponding normal tissue, metabolic screening methods using positron emission tomography have been developed for several solid tumors (48).

In carcinomas of the breast (49) and head and neck (50) and in various tumor cell lines (51) elevated levels of the initiation factor eIF4E have been found. In addition, overexpression of this factor in mammalian cells lines leads to rapid proliferation and malignant transformation (52). In cell lines in which eIF4E is overexpressed, translation of many mRNAs involved in cellular growth control, including c-myc, cyclin D1, ODC, and VEGF, is up-regulated (18).

As mentioned previously, there is also a connection between induction of the double-stranded RNA-activated serine/threonine protein kinase, PKR, and phosphorylation of the initiation factor, eIF2α, with breast cancer (53). Normally, high levels of PKR expression correlate with a decrease in protein synthesis. However, PKR levels in several breast cancer cell lines are abnormally high compared to the levels seen in normal breast cells. The solution to this paradox is that the PKR from the breast cancer cell lines has minimal activity as judged by its ability to phosphorylate eIF2α or respond to dsRNA (53). This may be the first evidence that implicates PKR in the pathogenesis of human cancer.

B. Elongation

Elongation is the process by which amino acids are added to a peptide chain as the protein is assembled (1) (see Fig. 2). The amino acids are added by the formation of peptide bonds in an order dictated by the mRNA sequence. The information in the mRNA sequence is contained in three base units arranged sequentially. The key requirements for translating this information to a peptide molecule are that each codon be matched to a specific amino acid and that each codon be read sequentially, without overlap. The amino acids and their corresponding codons are shown in Table II. The process of elongation contains several regulatory mechanisms to ensure accuracy.

1. Elements Involved in Elongation

The three base codons of the mRNA sequence are matched to a specific amino acid by adapter molecules known as transfer RNAs (tRNAs) (see Table II). In the simplest case, a given species of tRNA binds one specific amino acid and one specific mRNA codon. An amino acid is covalently attached to its cognate tRNA in an acylation reaction that creates an aminoacyl-tRNA. This reaction is catalyzed by a specific aminoacyl-synthetase. The basis of amino acid–tRNA recognition is not completely understood, but is known to depend on the three-dimensional tRNA structure. Additional specificity is provided by the proofreading capability of the synthetases. Each tRNA binds mRNA noncovalently through complementary base pairing between the mRNA codon and a three-base anticodon sequence in the tRNA (1).

Elongation takes place on the ribosome assembled around the mRNA. The ribosome contains two sites for tRNA binding: the P site, which holds the peptidyl-tRNA whose amino acid has already formed a bond with the growing

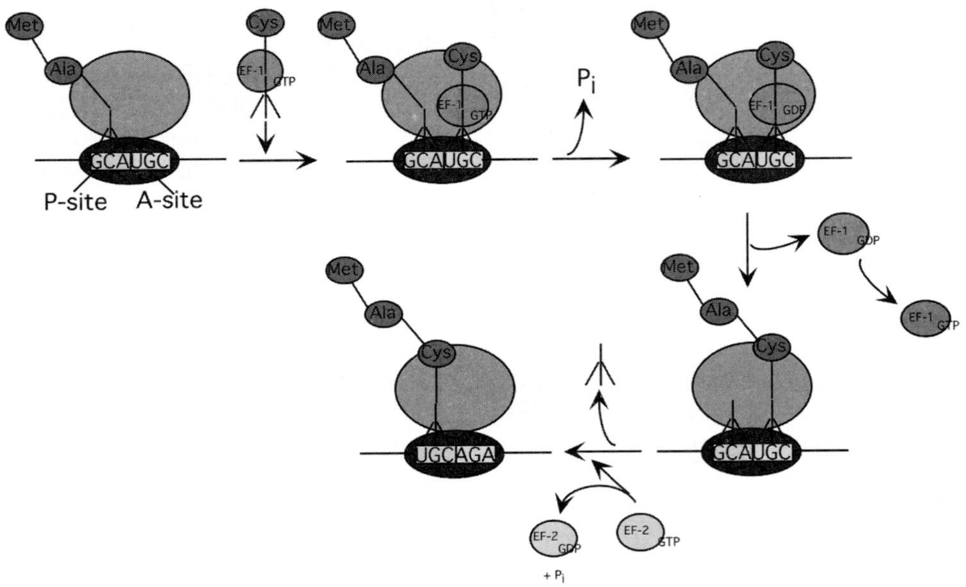

Figure 2 Translation elongation. (See color plates.)

peptide chain, and the A site, which holds the incoming aminoacyl-tRNA. The P and A sites are positioned so that the tRNAs occupying them are bound to adjacent codons.

Two GTP-binding factors participate in elongation: eEF-1 and eEF-2 (54). eEF-1 is a complex required for binding of the aminoacyl-tRNA to the ribosome. eEF-1 is a multisubunit complex consisting of the GTPase subunit eEF-1α, and the eEF-1 β, γ, and δ subunits whose guanine nucleotide exchange activity regulates the regeneration of eEF-1α by promoting the exchange of GDP for GTP. eEF-2 is a monomeric GTPase that is required for translocation of the ribosome along the mRNA.

2. Elongation Cycle

At the start of the elongation cycle, a peptidyl-tRNA covalently linked to a peptide chain (or initiating methionine) occupies the P site (55). An incoming aminoacyl-tRNA moves into the A site. A regulatory mechanism involving eEF-1 ensures that only the cognate tRNA binds to the mRNA (54).

With the two tRNAs aligned on adjacent mRNA codons, the amino group of the incoming amino acid attacks the acyl bond holding the peptide chain to the tRNA in the P site, leading to formation of a new peptide bond. As a consequence the peptide chain is transferred to the incoming tRNA.

Finally, the new peptidyl-tRNA complex is translocated to the P site, in a process that moves the ribosome exactly three bases down the mRNA, freeing the A site for a new aminoacyl-tRNA. The energy for the elongation step ultimately comes from GTP hydrolysis catalyzed by eEF-2 (55).

3. Fidelity of Codon Recognition

Accuracy of elongation depends on the interaction between the tRNA anticodon and the mRNA codon. However, the differences in binding energy of cognate versus noncognate anticodons are not sufficient in and of themselves to guarantee accuracy, so an additional mechanism known as kinetic proofreading is used to amplify the effect of correct initial recognition (56). After the initial recognition step, stable association of the aminoacyl tRNA in the A site with the mRNA requires GTP hydrolysis catalyzed by the eEF-1α subunit of eEF-1. Following hydrolysis, eEF-1α is released and peptide bond formation can proceed. Only the interaction between codon and cognate anticodon is sufficiently strong to ensure that the aminoacyl tRNA remains in the A site long enough for GTP hydrolysis to take place. Thus, only cognate aminoacyl-tRNAs associate stably with the mRNA in a fashion that allows the formation of a peptide bond. In *Escherichia coli* and in yeast, mutations or increases in the level of eEF-1α (or the prokaryotic equivalent, EF-Tu) increase the frequency of mutation.

4. Links between Elongation and Other Cellular Processes

The ribosomal elongation cycle is considered to be constitutive, requiring input of energy but not a specific signal for induction. However, this cycle is linked to other processes in the cell through eEF-1 and eEF-2.

a. The Cytoskeleton Studies have shown that many elements of the translational machinery associate with the cytoskeleton, including eEF-1α, tRNA synthetases, mRNA, and polyribosomes (57, 58). In addition, eEF-1α has been demonstrated to have F-actin binding and bundling characteristics and a microtubule-severing activity (59, 60). One model that links eEF-1α's cytoskeletal association with its translational role is that eEF-1α is sequestered by its association with the cytoskeleton, thus providing a means to regulate its availability for elongation.

Another model in which cytoskeletal association plays a role is the channeling model, in which ribosomal elongation is directly linked to the aminoacylation of tRNAs through the eEF-1 complex. Classically, the role of eEF-1 is to promote aminoacyl-tRNA association with the correct mRNA codon. However, eEF-1βγδ has been found to be physically associated with the val-tRNA synthetase. eEF-1a has been shown to stimulate activity of valyl, phenylalanyl, and aspartyl synthetases and to associate physically with val-tRNA-synthetase (58). In permeabilized CHO cells it has been shown that exogenously added amino acids are not incorporated into newly synthesized proteins and that repeated cycles of protein synthesis can occur without exogenously added tRNAs (61, 62). These results have led to the proposal that tRNA may be physically transferred from synthetase to ribosome and back to synthetase, in a macromolecular complex associated with eEF-1 and the cytoskeleton (58). Because cytoskeletal organization is altered by many cellular processes and extracellular signals, links between the elongation apparatus and the cytoskeleton may link elongation to these processes as well.

b. Growth Factor Signaling and the Cell Cycle Experimental manipulation of eEF-1α levels in murine fibroblast cell lines has been reported to alter cellular sensitivity to apoptosis. An increase in eEF-1α levels through overexpression leads to increased sensitivity to apoptosis, whereas a decrease in eEF-1α levels through antisense expression leads to decreased sensitivity (63). Further, it has been reported that eEF-1α associates with a zinc finger protein, ZPR-1, and is translocated to the nucleus in response to epidermal growth factor stimulation in A431 cells and in response to starvation in yeast. Mutation of the ZPR-1/eEF-1α interaction region leads to G_2/M arrest in yeast (64). Other elongation factors have also been linked to the cell cycle. eEF-1γ is a substrate for maturation-promoting factor, which regulates entry into the M phase of the cell cycle (65). eEF-1δ has been reported to be phosphorylated by casein kinase I, cdc2 kinase, and PKC (65–67). It is thought that phosphorylation increases eEF-1δ activity. In support of this model, phosphorylation by cdc2 kinase correlates with an increase in translation (65, 68–70). eEF-2 activity is increased in response to insulin stimulation in CHO cells. eEF-2 activity is down-regulated by phosphorylation on threonine by calcium–calmodulin kinaseIII/EF2 kinase. eEF-2 activity can be up-regulated directly by the phosphatase PP-2A or indirectly by insulin, which decreases the activity of EF-2 kinase. Insulin treatment has been shown to lead to an increase in rate of elongation, but the relationship of the rate of elongation to overall rate of protein synthesis is unclear (71, 72).

5. Links between Elongation and Disease

Malfunction of the elongation machinery can play a role in disease either by blocking elongation and thus protein synthesis, or by affecting fidelity. In addition, many viruses appropriate elongation factors at some point in their life cycles. Mutations that abrogate the activity of elongation factors might be expected to be lethal. In fact, the perinatal-lethal murine mutation, *wasted*, has been characterized as a defect in a tissue-specific isoform of eEF-1α (73). Similarly, bacterial toxins, such as diptheria toxin and *Pseudomonas* exotoxin A, which inactivate eEF-2 by ADP-ribosylation, block translation with potentially lethal results (74).

a. Elongation and Viral Infection Factors involved in elongation may play a role in disease in more subtle ways as well. Interaction of viral proteins with elongation factors plays a role in several viral life cycles. The GAG-derived MA protein of HIV-1 binds eEF-1α. It has been proposed that accumulation of GAG leads to inhibition of translation and thus release of viral RNA from polysomes, freeing these RNAs for packaging (75). The vesicular stomatitis virus (VSV) RNA polymerase requires association with eEF-1α for its activity (76). In the case of HSV-1, the viral protein ICP0 interacts with eEF-1δ, altering its activity (77). Further, the viral kinase U_L13 phosphorylates eEF-1δ, with increased phosphorylation of this factor correlating with increased protein synthesis (78).

b. Elongation and Tumorigenesis Elongation factors have also been linked to transformation and tumorigenesis. eEF-1α has been linked to carcinogenesis in several ways. eEF-1α was identified as a transformation-promoting factor in a screen for factors that increased susceptibility of murine fibroblasts to transformation (79). It has been proposed that eEF-1α plays a role in metastasis based on a study showing that this factor binds actin less closely in a metastatic breast carcinoma line than in a nonmetastatic line. It is proposed that decreased eEF-1α binding could affect metastasis either by altering cytoskeletal organization, and thus cell mobility; or by releasing cytoskeletal sequestration of eEF-1α, and thus promoting increased translation (80). The evidence for EF-1α involvement is strongest for the gene *PTI-1*. *PTI-1* was cloned based on its differential expression in a human prostate cancer cell line, LNCaP. The *PTI-1* cDNA consists of a 5′ untranslated region fused to a truncated, mutated human EF-1α coding sequence. Transfection with this cDNA leads to transformation *in vitro* and tumor formation in nude mice. Further, expression of an antisense construct blocks transformation and tumor formation. The mechanism by which *PTI-1* induces transformation is not known. It has been proposed that it may act as a defective version of EF-1α to interfere with translation efficiency or accuracy, or to disrupt cytoskeletal organization. Further support for a role for *PTI-1* in human cancer comes from studies in which *PTI-1* transcripts have been detected in human prostate, breast, colon, and lung cancer cell lines, as well as in patient-derived prostate cancer tissue, but not in normal or benign prostate hyperplastic tissue (81–84). Overexpression of other EF-1 subunits in malignancies has also been reported, but no causal connections have been demonstrated. EF-1γ transcript is reported to be overexpressed in colorectal adenoma carcinomas and in pancreatic cancers. EF-1γ protein has been detected in higher levels in colorectal adenomas than in surrounding normal tissue (85–88). In addition, human EF-1δ transcripts were detected by subtractive hybridization in a breast cancer cell line (89).

C. Termination

Termination is the least understood step in translation. Although the existence of eukaryotic activities involved in termination was demonstrated in 1977 (90), these factors have only recently been cloned and characterized. Their mechanism of action is still not completely understood.

1. Elements Involved in Termination

The information signaling the end of translation is contained in each mRNA sequence in the form of one of three specific stop codons, UAA, UAG, or UGA (1) (see Fig. 3). These codons have no cognate tRNAs or amino acids. Instead they are recognized by the factors involved in termination, which promote the release of the peptide chain from the ribosome.

The factors essential for eukaryotic termination are eRF-1 and eRF-3. eRF-1 specifically recognizes the stop codon and alters the activity of the ribosomal peptidyl transferase. eRF-3 is a GTP-binding protein required for activity of eRF-1 (91–94).

When a stop codon appears in the A site of the ribosome, eRF-1 occupies this site. In this position, eRF-1 interacts with the peptidyl transferase activity of the ribosome such that the transferase catalyzes addition of a molecule of water instead of an amino acid to the peptide chain (1). As a result, the bond between the peptide chain and the tRNA is broken and the polypeptide is released from the ribosome. eRF-3 in its GTP-bound state is thought to promote association of eRF-1 with the A site and the peptidyl transferase (90). eRF-3 GTP to GDP hydrolysis is required for the release of eRF-1 and eRF-3 from the ribosome to allow another round of activity. The activities of eRF-1 and eRF-3 are interdependent. eRF-1 activity requires eRF-3. In turn, the GTPase activity of isolated eRF-3 is minimal. This GTPase activity requires the presence of both eRF-1 and the ribosome.

Specificity of the termination step is provided by eRF-1 recognition of stop codons (90). It is thought that eRF-1 specifically recognizes these codons through a small segment of the protein that mimics the structure of the anticodon of the tRNA.

2. Links between Termination and Other Cellular Processes

a. Termination and the Cell Cycle eRF-3 has been linked to the cell cycle in yeast. *Sup35*, the yeast gene coding for eRF-3, was independently isolated as GST1, a factor required for cell cycle progression from G_1 to S (95). In the mouse as well, there may be a link between eEF-3 and the cell cycle. Two forms of murine eRF-3 have been cloned: GSPT1 and GSPT2. Both forms associate with eRF-1. They differ in that GSPT1 is up-regulated during the G_1 to S transition, whereas the levels of GSPT2 are constant throughout the cycle. However, the relationship between the role of eRF-3 in cell cycle and its role in translation in either yeast or mammals is unknown (96).

b. Termination and RNA Surveillance Point mutations or frameshift mutations can introduce premature stop codons in an mRNA sequence, creating a nonsense mRNA. Nonsense mRNAs would be expected to produce truncated proteins, but, in fact, such truncated proteins are seldom detected in the cell. It is thought that the cell is protected by an mRNA surveillance mechanism known as nonsense-mRNA mediated decay (NMD), which mediates the rapid degradation of nonsense mRNAs.

The mechanism of this process is still being worked out. However, it is thought to involve the linkage of translational termination to mRNA degradation. Most mRNA coding regions contain multiple versions of a short, degenerate sequence known as the downstream sequence element (DSE) (97). Thus, a nonsense stop codon, but not a legitimate stop codon, would be expected to occur in conjunction with a DSE. When a stop codon occurs in the context of a DSE, additional factors assemble with the termination complex. In yeast, three genes associated with NMD have been identified, *Upf1*, *Upf2*, and *Upf3*, and in humans, one gene, *RENT1/HUPF1* (98). It is proposed that these factors recognize that a stop codon is inappropriate through its position upstream of a DSE. Further, once translation has been terminated by the releasing factors, the NMD factors disrupt RNA structure through their helicase activity. This disruption exposes the 5' cap, leading to rapid degradation.

RNA surveillance through NMD has at least two implications for disease. First, many human genetic diseases and

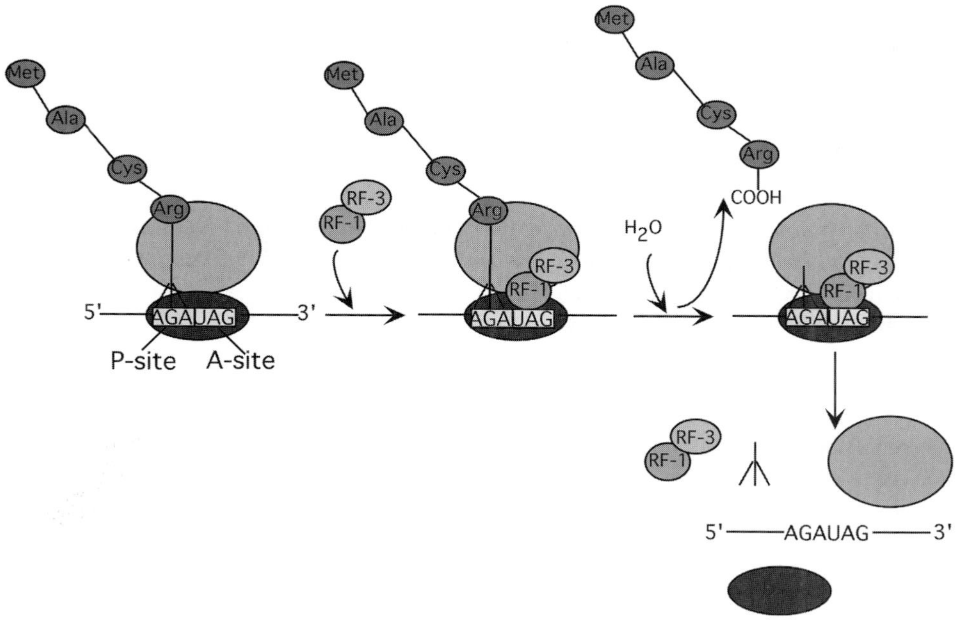

Figure 3 Translation termination. (See color plates.)

inherited cancers involve mutations that lead to premature chain termination, including 89% of mutations in *ATM*, leading to ataxia telangiectasia, and 77% of mutations in *BRCA1*, leading to breast cancer (99). Although in some cases mRNA degradation may protect from synthesis of a deletrious mutant protein, in others overriding the nonsense mutation might allow a functional protein to be made. Second, NMD, by preventing the expression of mutant genes, would be expected to have a tumor suppressor function. Thus defects in this pathway might contribute to tumorigenesis. In addition, specific activation of this pathway could conceivably be tailored to prevent expression of specific mutant proteins.

III. Methods for Studying Protein Synthesis

Generally, many of the molecular and biochemical methods that are used to study other cellular processes are also used to study the mechanisms and regulation of translation. The following section of this chapter will briefly describe some of the methods that are used in translation research. A more detailed description of the majority of methods and techniques used in the study of protein synthesis can be found in "Current Protocols in Molecular Biology" (100). There are also useful sites on the Internet for translation research and brief descriptions of these sites and addresses have been included.

A. In Vitro

1. Initiation

Eukaryotic translation initiation can be studied *in vitro* in extracts of wheat germ or in reticulocyte lysates. Both are available commercially from Promega (Madison, WI) and Ambion (Austin, TX) in the form of translation-only or coupled transcription/translation systems. These systems are useful (1) for determining the order in which factors interact, providing that the system can be depleted of the factors in question and that the factors can be added back successfully to the systems; (2) for characterizing gene products; and (3) for characterizing proteins that have been mutated by either site-specific or random mutagenesis. In addition, the *in vitro* systems can be used to test whether a specific mRNA relies on a $7^{m}G$ cap structure for translation initiation. However, one needs to be aware that mechanisms of protein synthesis may not be accurately represented in either *in vitro* system.

The source of mRNA for the translation-only systems is mRNA that is transcribed *in vitro* using SP6, T7, or T3 RNA polymerases. Kits specifically designed for *in vitro* transcription of mRNA are available from Promega, Invitrogen (Carlsbad, CA), and Ambion. Depending on the kit selected, the templates for mRNA synthesis in the coupled transcription/translation systems can be either supercoiled or linear plasmid DNA, or PCR fragments that contain the promoters for either the SP6, T7, or T3 RNA polymerases. Protocols for *in vitro* transcription and translation are available with all of these kits and alternative protocols for these processes can be found (100).

2. Elongation

The efficiency of translation elongation has been estimated using an assay in which poly(U)-directed incorporation of [^{3}H]polyphenylalanine into a polypeptide is measured (101, 102). The elements required for elongation are purified from rabbit reticulocyte lysate and supplied at saturating concentrations. The factors being investigated, i.e., eEF-1 and/or eEF-2, are isolated from the cells of interest as the postribosomal fraction and supplied at suboptimal concentrations. Thus, cellular conditions that alter the activity of eEF-1 and/or eEF-2 will alter the efficiency of elongation in this system. This assay has been used to study the effect of insulin on elongation and the effect of phorbol myristic acid (PMA) on eEF-1 activity, and is described in detail by Venema *et al.* (101).

3. Termination

An *in vitro* assay has been utilized to identify and characterize release factors and to determine the cellular conditions that alter the activity of the release factors. To accomplish this goal, an artificial mRNA containing an internal in-frame stop codon was used as the template for *in vitro* translation. In the presence of efficient release factors, the short form of the protein was synthesized. This method was used to characterize human eRF-1A, and a detailed description of this assay can be found in Drugeon *et al.* (91).

B. In Vivo

1. Mammalian Reporter Plasmids and Cell Lines

In order to study the regulation of translation initiation in mammalian cell lines it is often wise to substitute the coding region of the gene of interest with a reporter gene. This not only alleviates problems associated with endogenous protein, but makes it easy to assay the effects of mutations on gene expression. There are many reporter genes available commercially from several different sources, including three different species of luciferase, chloramphenicol acetyltransferase, the multicolored (green, red, yellow, blue) fluorescent protein family (GFP, RFP, YFP, and BFP), and secreted alkaline phosphatase (SEAP). Which reporter gene is chosen depends on individual preference and whether more than one reporter is being assayed at the same time. For example, if the goal of the experiment is to determine if the 5′ untranslated region of a particular gene contains an IRES, a bicistronic reporter plasmid with two forms of luciferase is a good choice because the same cell lysate can be tested for both luciferase activities. As an alternative, we constructed a bicistronic reporter plasmid using SEAP as the upstream reporter gene but found that the background level of SEAP activity was extremely high, at least in the B cell lines that we employ.

Assaying expression of the reporter genes described in the previous paragraph is generally straightforward. The companies that sell the reporter plasmids sell kits that can be used to assay appropriate gene expression. In addition, additional protocols for assaying expression of the majority of reporter genes can be found (100).

As far as the actual cell lines used in translation research, generally, if a mRNA is expressed in specific cell types, then translation should be studied in lines derived from those cells. However, it may be necessary to carry out some experiments in cell lines in which the mRNA may not be expressed. For example, if the goal is to determine if a mRNA can be translated in a cap-independent fashion, then a picornaviral-infected cell line may be the line of choice to use. Alternatively, a cell line that expresses an excess of eIF4E would be the cell line of choice if the goal is to determine if an mRNA with a highly structured 5′ end is translated more efficiently.

2. Transfection of Mammalian Cell Lines

Mammalian cells can be transfected either transiently or stably. In a transient transfection, cells are harvested within days after introduction of DNA or RNA and assayed for gene expression. In a stable transfection, DNA is introduced along with a selectable marker into the cell line of choice. Depending on the plasmid vector, the DNA either integrates into the chromosomal DNA or is stably propagated as episomal DNA. The choice of either transient or stable transfection and the method by which the DNA is introduced into the cells depends on the cell line in which the translation studies are being done and the goal of the transfection. For example, we transfect mammalian B cell lines both transiently and stably by the method of electroporation. Cell lines such as CV1 or COS cells (monkey kidney cell lines) are more amenable to transfection with either calcium phosphate or DEAE-dextran. A detailed description of these and other methods used in the transfection of mammalian cells can be found (100).

3. Polysome Profiles

This methodology is useful for assessing not only the efficiency with which an mRNA is translated *in vivo*, but also for assessing the interaction of factors associated with the translation machinery at all stages of protein synthesis. The main problem associated with this protocol is that it is tedious and time consuming. However, this is a small price to pay for the amount of information that can be gleaned.

Briefly, extracts must first be prepared from the cells being used. How the extracts are prepared depends on the type of cell, but generally, procedures for making extracts are available (100). The extracts are then centrifuged at high speeds through sucrose gradients and fractions are collected. A very thorough description of this process can be found in a paper by Mangus and Jacobson (103). The mRNA present

Table III Internet Sites for Translation Research

Application	URL	Comments
Structure	http://rnadraw.base8.se/#wwwRnadrawIndex	"Free-ware" that requires the Windows OS (104)
	http://mfold2.wustl.edu/~mfold/rna/form1.cgi	Well-maintained, useful background information (105, 106)
	http://www.ibc.wustl.edu/~zuker/rna/energy/	Links from Dr. Zuker's homepage (107)
	http://ndbserver.rutgers.edu:80/	Biological structure database focusing on nucleic acids; well-maintained with useful background information
	http://www.tbi.univie.ac.at/cgi-bin/RNAfold.cgi	New folding server; not as much background information as others, but easy to navigate
RNA modification	http://medlib.med.utah.edu/RNAmods/rnaopen.htm	Copious background information; easy to navigate
Sequences	http://www.uni-bayreuth.de/departments/biochemie/trna/	All tRNAs known are located in this database; free downloads
	http://ncbi.nlm.nih.gov/Genbank/GenbankOverview.html	GenBank; searchable database for proteins, DNA, or cDNA; cornerstone of the sequence databases
Miscellaneous sites	http://paris.chem.yale.edu/extinct.html	Calculate melting temperature and extinction coefficients of single-stranded nucleotides
	http://www.rcsb.org/pdb/	Protein database may be helpful in identification of RNA binding proteins
	http://www.imb-jena.de/RNA.html	"RNA World"—list of web sites with potential application for the study of RNA
	http://www.dartmouth.edu/artsci/bio/ambros/protocols/molbio.html	Collection of molecular biology protocols
	http://www.cup.org/Default.htm	Publishers of the *RNA Journal*
	http://www.pitt.edu/~rnal/	Homepage of the RNA Society

in each of the fractions can then be assayed by a method such as primer extension, S1 mapping, or RNase protection after removal of sucrose and proteins. Alternatively, Western blotting can be performed on the fractions to determine if a specific protein is associated with polyribosomes.

C. Translation on the Internet

There are literally hundreds and maybe thousands of Internet-based databases that can now be browsed by the scientist looking for molecular biology data. The ease of accessing these databases over locally installed web browsers has made data retrieval a relatively trivial process. However, the reliability of these databases can at times be problematic. The goal here is to provide the clinician scientist with a relatively short but reliable list of databases that will perform tasks and retrieve data relevant to the study of translation (see Table III). In addition, the Internet addresses of companies that sell products related to translation research (see Table IV) have been included.

Table IV Biotech Companies with Products Applicable to Translation Research

Name	URL	Utility
Qiagen	http://www.qiagen.com	RNA/DNA isolation kits
Promega	http://www.promega.com	RNA isolation, RT–PCR, enzymes
Ambion	http://www.ambion.com	"The RNA company," many utilities on this site
Santa Cruz Biotech	http://www.scbt.com	Antibodies
Transduction Laboratories	http://www.translab.com	Antibodies
Life Technologies	http://www.lifetech.com	Basic supplies, transfection systems, much more
American Type Culture Collection	http://www.atcc.org	Cell lines, hybridomas, other resources
Integrated DNA Technologies	http://www.idtdna.com	Oligonucleotides, primer labeling systems, more
Fisher Scientific	http://www1.fishersci.com	Basic lab supplies and reagents
Perkin-Elmer	http://www.pebio.com	RT–PCR, DNA/RNA synthesis

1. RNA Folding

Prediction of RNA secondary structure is based on identification of regions of potential complementary base pairing within the RNA sequence. Needless to say, the prediction of RNA secondary structure can be quite complex, yet is very important to the actual translation into protein product. Dr. Michael Zuker of Washington University maintains a very well-designed Internet site (http://www.ibc.wustl.edu/~zuker/). This site contains a lot of background information as well as rules for RNA folding and a link to the RNA folding *mfold* server. This site is a very user friendly, well-maintained interface that is not cluttered with irrelevant information.

2. RNA Sequences

Databases of known RNA sequences are quite easy to find and include tRNA, 5S rRNA, small RNA, and mRNA sequences. The GenBank web site (http://www.ncbi.nlm.nih.gov/Genbank/GenbankSearch.html) includes links to the BLAST sequence similarity search database, as well as to the "Entrez" browser. The Entrez browser database allows the scientist to search for cDNAs by name whereas the BLAST database allows one to search for matches according to partial sequences.

References

1. Alberts, B., Bray, Lewis, J., Raff, M., Roberts, K., and Watson, J. D. (1994). "Molecular Biology of the Cell." Garland Publishing, Inc., New York & London.
2. Garrett, R. A., Douthwaite, S. R., Lilgas, A., Matheson, A. T., Moore, P. B., and Noller, H. (2000). "The Ribosome: Structure, Function, Antibiotics, and Cellular Interactions," 1st Ed. American Society for Microbiology Press, Washington, D.C.
3. Pestova, T. V., and Hellen, C. U. T. (1999). Ribosome recruitment and scanning: what's new? *Trends Biochem. Sci.* **24,** 85–87.
4. McKendrick, L., Pain, V. M., and Morley, S. J. (1999). Translation initiation factor 4E. *Int. J. Biochem. Cell Biol.* **31,** 31–35.
5. Raught, B., and Gingras, A.-E. (1999). eIF4E activity is regulated at multiple levels. *Int. J. Biochem. Cell. Biol.* **31,** 43–57.
6. Keiper, B. D., Gan, W., and Rhoads, R. E. (1999). Protein synthesis initiation factor 4G. *Int. J. Biochem. Cell Biol.* **31,** 37–41.
7. Lawrence, J. C., Jr., and Abraham, R. T. (1997). PHAS/4E-BPs as regulators of mRNA translation and cell proliferation. *Trends Biochem. Sci.* **22,** 345–349.
8. Kimble, S. R. (1999). Eukaryotic initiation factor eIF2. *Int. J. Biochem. Cell Biol.* **31,** 25–29.
9. Pestova, T. V., Borukhov, S. I., and Hellen, C. U. T. (1998). Eukaryotic ribosomes require initiation factors 1 and 1A to locate initiation codons. *Nature (London)* **394,** 854–859.
10. Wells, S. E., Hillner, P. E., Vale, R. D., and Sachs, A. B. (1998). Circularization of mRNA by eukaryotic translation initiation factors. *Mol. Cell* **2,** 135–140.
11. Imataka, H., Gradi, A., and Sonenberg, N. (1998). A newly-identifed N-terminal amino acid sequence of human eIF4G binds poly(A)-binding protein and functions in poly(A)-dependent translation. *EMBO J.* **17,** 7480–7489.
12. Kozak, M. (1989). Context effects and (inefficient) initiation at non-AUG codons in eucaryotic cell-free translation systems. *Mol. Cell Biol.* **9,** 5073–5080.
13. Kozak, M. (1989). The scanning model for translation: an update. *J. Cell Biol.* **108,** 229–241.
14. Kozak, M. (1997). Recognition of AUG and alternative initiator codons is augmented by G in position +4 but is not generally affected by the nucleotides in positions +5 and +6. *EMBO J.* **16,** 2482–2492.
15. Peabody, D. S., and Berg, P. (1986). Termination-reinitiation occurs in the translation of mammalian cell RNAs. *Mol. Cell. Biol.* **6,** 2695–2703.
16. Miller, P. F., and Hinnebusch A. G. (1989). Sequences that surround the stop codons of upstream open reading frames in GCN4 mRNA determine their distinct functions in translational control. *Genes Dev.* **3,** 1217–1225.
17. Clemens, M. J., and Bommer, U.-A. (1999). Translational control: the cancer connection. *Int. J. Biochem. Cell Biol.* **31,** 1–23.
18. De Benedetti, A., and Harris, A. L. (1999). eIF4E expression in tumors: its possible role in progression of malignancies. *Int. J. Biochem. Cell Biol.* **31,** 59–72.
19. Willis, A. E. (1999). Translational control of growth factor and proto-oncogene expression. *Int. J. Biochem. Cell Biol.* **31,** 73–86
20. Kevil, C., Carter, P., Hu, B., and DeBenedetti, A. (1995). Translational enhancement of of FGF-2 by eIF-4 factors, and alternate utilization of CUG and AUG codons for translation initiation. *Oncogene* **11,** 2339–2348.
21. Arrick, B. A., Lee A. L., Grendell, R. L., and Derynck, R. (1991). Inhibition of translation of transforming growth factor-β3 m RNA by its 5′ untranslated region. *Mol. Cell. Biol.* **11,** 4306–4313.
22. Grens, A., and Scheffler, I. E. (1990). The 5′- and 3′-untranslated regions of ornithine decarboxylase mRNA affect the translational efficiency. *J. Biol. Chem.* **265,** 11810–11816.
23. Shantz, L. M., and Pegg, A. E. (1999) Translational regulation of ornithine decarboxylase and other enzymes of the polyamine pathway. *Int. J. Biochem. Cell Biol.* **31,** 107–122.
24. Pelletier, J., and Sonenberg, N. (1988). Internal initiation of translation of eukaryotic mRNA directed by a sequence derived from poliovirus RNA. *Nature (London)* **334,** 320–325.
25. Sella, O., Gerlitz, G., Le, S. -Y., and Elroy-Stein, O. (1999). Differentiation-induced internal translation of c-*sis* mRNA: Analysis of the *cis* elements and their differentiation-linked binding to the hnRNP C protein. *Mol. Cell. Biol.* **19,** 5429–5440.
26. Stein, I., Itin, A., Einat, P., Skaliter, R., Grossman, Z., and Keshet, E. (1998). Translation of vascular endothelial growth factor mRNA by internal ribosome entry: implications for translation under hypoxia. *Mol. Cell. Biol.* **18,** 3112–3119.
27. Huez, I., Créancier, L., Audigier, S., Gensac, M.-C., Prats, A.-C., and Prats, H. (1998). Two independent internal ribosome entry sites are involved in translation initiation of vascular endothelial growth factor mRNA. *Mol. Cell. Biol.* **18,** 6178–6190.
28. Nanbru, C., Lafon, I., Audigier, S., Gensac, M.-C., Vagner, S., Huez, G., and Prats, A.-C. (1997). Alternative translation of the proto-oncogene c-*myc* by an internal ribosome entry site. *J. Biol. Chem.* **272,** 32061–32066.
29. Carter, P. S., Jarquin-Pardo, M., and DeBenedetti, A. (1999). Differential expression of Myc1 and Myc-2 isoforms in cells transformed by eIF4E: Evidence for internal ribosome repositioning in the human c-*myc* 5′ UTR. *Oncogene* **18,** 4326–4335.
30. Le, S.-Y., Siddiqui, A., and Maizel Jr., J. V. (1996). A common structural core in the internal ribosome entry sites of picornavirus, hepatitus C virus, and pestivurus. *Virus Genes* **12,** 135–147.
31. Le, S.-Y., and Maizel, Jr., J. V. (1997). A common RNA structural motif involved in the internal initiation of translation of cellular mRNAs. *Nucleic Acids Res.* **25,** 362–369.
32. Minich, W. B., Balasta, M. L., Goss, D. J., and Rhoads, R. E. (1994). Chromatographic resolution of in vivo phosphorylated and nonphos-

phorylated eukaryotic translation initiation factor eIF4E: Increased cap affinity of the phosphorylated form. *Proc. Natl. Acad. Sci. U.S.A.* **91,** 7668–7672.

33. Wang, X., Flynn, A., Waskiewicz, A. J., Webb, B. L. J., Vries, R. G., Baines, I. A., Cooper, J. A., and Proud, C. G. (1998). The phosphorylation of eukaryotic initiation factor eIF4E in response to phorbol esters, cell stresses, and cytokines is mediated by distinct MAP kinase pathways. *J. Biol. Chem.* **273,** 9373–9377.
34. Pyronnet, S., Imataka, H., Gingras, A. C., Fukunaga, R., Hunter, T., and Sonenberg, N. (1999). Human eukaryotic translation initiation factor 4G (eIF4G) recruits mnk1 to phosphorylate eIF4E. *EMBO J.* **18,** 270–279.
35. Pause, A., Belsham, G. J., Gingras, A.-C., Donzé, O., Lin, T.-A., Lawrence, Jr., J. C., and Sonenberg, N. (1994). Insulin-dependent stimulation of protein synthesis by phosphorylation of a regulator of 5′ cap function. *Nature (London)* **371,** 762–767.
36. Gingras, A.-C., Kennedy, S. G., O'Leary, M A., Sonenberg, N., and Hay, N. (1998). 4E-BP1, a repressor of mRNA translation, is phosphorylated and inactivated by the Akt(PKB) signaling pathway. *Genes Dev.* **12,** 502–513.
37. Kimball, S. R., Fabian, J. R., Pavitt, G. D., Hinnebusch, A. G., and Jefferson, L. S. (1998). Regulation of guanine nucleotide exchange through phosphorylation of eukaryotic initiation factor eIF2α. *J. Biol. Chem.* **273,** 12841–12845.
38. Jagus, R., Joshi, B., and Barber, G. N. (1999). PKR, apoptosis, and cancer. *Int. J. Biochem. Cell Biol.* **31,** 123–138.
39. Bernstein, J., Shefler, I., and Elroy-Stein, O., (1995). The translational repression mediated by the platelet-derived growth factor 2/*c-sis* mRNA leader is relieved during megakaryocyte differentiation. *J. Biol. Chem.* **270,** 10559–10565.
40. Wang, C., and Stiles, C. D. (1993). Regulation of platelet-derived growth factor A messenger RNA translation in differentiating F9 teratocarcinoma cells. *Cell Growth Diff.* **4,** 871–877.
41. Bugler, B., Amalric, F., and Prats, H. (1991). Alternative initiation of translation determines cytoplasmicor nuclear localization of basic fibroblast growth factor. *Mol. Cell. Biol.* **11,** 573–577.
42. Kim, S.-J., Park, K., Koeller, D., Kim, K. Y., Wakefield, L. M., Sporn, M. B., and Roberts, A. B. (1992). Post-transcriptional regulation of the human transforming growth factor-β1 gene. *J. Biol. Chem.* **267,** 13702–13707.
43. Van der Velden, A. W., and Thomas, A. A. M. (1999). The role of the 5′ untranslated region of an mRNA in translation regulation during development. *Int. J. Biochem. Cell Biol.* **31,** 87–1061.
44. Ting, N. S. Y., Kao, P. N., Chan, D. W., Lintott, L. G., and Lees-Miller, S. P. (1998). DNA-dependent protein kinase interacts with antigen receptor response element binding proteins, NF90 and NF45. *J. Biol. Chem.* **273,** 2136–2145.
45. Sonenberg, N. (1991). Picornavirus RNA translation continues to surprise. *Trends Genet.* **7,** 105–106.
46. Park, Y. W., Wilusz, J., and Katze, M. G. (1999). Regulation of eukaryotic protein synthesis: Selective influenza viral mRNA translation is mediated by the cellular RNA-binding protein GRSF-1. *Proc. Natl. Acad. Sci. U.S.A.* **96,** 6694–6699.
47. Lamb, R. A., and Horvath, C. M. (1991). Diversity of coding strategies in influenza viruses. *Trends Genet.* **7,** 261–266.
48. Koh, W. J., Griffin, T. W., Rasey, J. S., and Laramore, G. E. (1994). Positron emission tomography: A new tool for characterization of malignant disease. *Acta Oncol.* **33,** 323–3271.
49. Kerekatte, V., Smiley, K., Hu, B., Smith, A., Gelder, F., and De Benedetti, A. (1995). The proto-oncogene/translation initiation factor eIF4E: A survey of its expression in breast carcinomas. *Int. J. Cancer* **64,** 27–31.
50. Nathan, C. A. O., Liu, L., Li, B. D., Abreo, F. W., Nandy, I., and De Benedetti, A. (1997). Detection of the proto-oncogene eIF4E in surgical margins may predict recurrence in head and neck cancer. *Oncogene* **15,** 579–584.
51. Miyagi, Y., Sugiyama, A., Asai, A., Okazaki, T., Kuchino, Y., and Kerr, S. J. (1995). Elevated levels of eukaryotic translation initiation factor eIF-4E mRNA in a broad spectrum of transformed cell lines. *Cancer Lett.* **91,** 247–252.
52. Lazaris-Karatzas, A., Montine, K. S., and Sonenberg, N. (1990). Malignant transformation by a eukaryotic initiation factor subunit that binds to mRNA 5′ cap. *Nature (London)* **345,** 544–547.
53. Savinova, O., Joshi, B., and Jagus, R. (1999). Abnormal levels and minimal activity of the dsRNA-activated protein kinase, PKR, in breast carcinoma cells. *Int. J. Biochem. Cell Biol.* **31,** 175–189.
54. Riis, B., Rattan, S. I. S., Clark, B. F. C., and Merrick, W. C. (1990). Eukaryotic protein elongation factors. *Trends Biochem. Sci.* **15,** 420–424.
55. Merrick, W. C. (1992). Mechanism and regulation of eukaryotic protein synthesis. *Microbiol. Rev.* **56,** 291–315.
56. Green, R., and Noller, H. (1997). Ribosomes and translation. *Annu. Rev. Biochem.* **66,** 679–716.
57. Gray, N., and Wickens, M. (1998). Control of translation initiation in animals. *Annu. Rev. Cell Dev. Biol.* **14,** 399–458.
58. Negrutskii, B. S., Shalak, V. F., Kerjan, P., El'skaya, A. V., and Mirande, M. (1999). Functional interaction of mammalian valyl-tRNA synthetase with elongation factor EF-1α in the complex with EF-1H. *J. Biol. Chem.* **274,** 4545–4550.
59. Umikawa, M., Tanaka, K., Kamei, T., Shimizu, K., Imamura, H., and Sasaki, Y. (1998). Interaction of Rho1p target Bni1p with F-actin-binding elongation factor 1alpha: Implication in Rho1p-regulated reorganization of the actin cytoskeleton in *Saccharomyces cerevisiae. Oncogene* **16,** 2011–2016.
60. Moore, R. C., Durso, N. A., and Cyr, R. J. (1998). Elongation factor-1 alpha stabilizes microtubules in a calcium/calmodulin-dependent manner. *Cell Motil. Cytoskel.* **41,** 168–180.
61. Stapulionis, R., and Deutscher, M. P. (1995). A channeled tRNA cycle during mammalian protein synthesis. *Proc. Natl. Acad. Sci. U.S.A.* **92,** 7158–7161.
62. Negrutskii, B. S., Stapulionis, R., and Deutscher, M. P. (1994). Supramolecular organization of the mammalian translation system. *Proc. Natl. Acad. Sci. U.S.A.* **91,** 964–968.
63. Duttaroy, A., Bourbeau, D., Wang, X. L., and Wang, E. (1998). Apoptosis rate can be accelerated or decelerated by overexpression or reduction of the level of elongation factor-1 alpha. *Exp. Cell Res.* **238,** 168–76.
64. Gangwani, L., Mikrut, M., Galcheva-Gargova, Z., and Davis R. J. (1998). Interaction of ZPR1 with translation elongation factor-1α in proliferating cells. *J. Cell. Biol.* **143,** 1471–1484.
65. Mulner-Lorillon, O., Minella, O., Cormier, P., Capony, J.-P., Cavadore, J.-C., Morales, J., Pouhle, R., and Belle, R. (1994). Elongation factor EF-1δ, a new target for maturation-promoting factor in *Xenopus* oocytes. *J. Biol. Chem.* **269,** 20201–20207.
66. Palen, E., Venema, R. C., Chang, Y.-W. E., and Traugh, J. A. (1994). GDP as a regulator of phosphorylation of elongation factor 1 by casein kinase II. *Biochemistry* **33,** 8515–8520.
67. Venema, R. C., Peters, H. I., and Traugh, J. A. (1991). Phosphorylation of elongation factor 1 (EF-1) and valyl-tRNA synthetase by protein kinase C and stimulation of EF-1 activity. *J. Biol. Chem.* **266,** 12574–12580.
68. Minella, O., Cormier, P., Morales, J., Poulhe, R., Belle, R., and Mulner-Lorillon, O. (1994). cdc2 kinase sets a memory phosphorylation signal on elongation factor EF-1δ during meiotic cell division, which perdures in early development. *Cell Mol. Biol.* **40,** 521–525.
69. Richter, J. D., Wasserman, W. J., and Smith, L. D. (1982). The mechanism for increased protein synthesis during *Xenopus* oocyte maturation. *Dev. Biol.* **89,** 159–167.

70. Wasserman, R. C., Richter, J. D., and Smith, L. D. (1982). Protein synthesis during maturation promoting factor- and progesterone-induced maturation in *Xenopus* oocytes. *Dev. Biol.* **89,** 152–158.
71. Chang, Y.-W., and Traugh, J. A. (1998). Insulin stimulation of phosphorylation of elongation factor 1 (eEF-1) enhances elongation activity. *Eur. J. Biochem.* **251,** 201–207.
72. Proud, C. G., and Denton, R. M. (1997). Molecular mechanisms for the control of translation by insulin. *Biochem. J.* **328,** 328–341.
73. Chambers, D. M., Peters, J., and Abbott, C. M. (1998). The lethal mutation of the mouse wasted (*wst*) is a deletion that abolishes expression of a tissue-specific isoform of translation elongation factor 1α, encoded by the *Eefla2* gene. *Proc. Natl. Acad. Sci. U.S.A.* **95,** 4463–4468.
74. Iglewski, W. J. (1994). Cellular ADP-ribosylation of elongation factor 2. *Mol. Cell. Biochem.* **138,** 131–133.
75. Cimarelli, A. and Luban, J. (1999). Translation elongation factor 1-alpha interacts specifically with the human immunodeficiency virus type 1 Gag polyprotein. *J. Virol.* **73,** 5388–5401.
76. Das, T., Mathur, M., Gupta, A. K., Janssen, G. M. C., and Banerjee, A. K. (1998). RNA polymerase of vesicular stomatitis virus specifically associates with translation elongation factor-1 αβγ for its activity. *Proc. Natl. Acad. Sci. U.S.A.* **95,** 1449–1454.
77. Kawaguchi, Y., Matsumura, T., Roizman, B., and Hirai, K. (1999). Cellular elongation factor 1 delta is modified in cells infected with representative alpha-, beta-, or gammaherpesviruses. *J. Virol.* **73,** 4456–4460.
78. Kawaguchi, Y., Van Sant, C., and Roizman, B. (1998). Eukaryotic elongation factor 1δ is hyperphosphorylated by the protein kinase encoded by the U_L13 gene of Herpes Simplex Virus 1. *J. Virol.* **72,** 1731–1736.
79. Tatsuka, M., Mitsui, H., Wada, M., Nagata, A., Nojima, H., and Okayama, H. (1992). Elongation factor-1 alpha gene determines susceptibility to transformation. *Nature (London)* **359,** 333–336.
80. Edmonds, B. T., Wyckoff, J., Yeung, Y-G., Wang, Y., Stanley, E. R., Jones, J., Segall, J., and Condeelis, J. (1996). Elongation factor-1α is an overexpressed actin binding protein in metastatic rat mammary adenocarcinoma. *J. Cell Sci.* **109,** 2705–2714.
81. Su, Z. -Z., Goldstein, N. I., and Fisher, P. B. (1998). Antisense inhibition of the PTI-1 oncogene reverses cancer phenotypes. *Proc. Natl. Acad. Sci. U.S.A.* **95,** 1764–1769.
82. Gopalakrishnan, R. V., Su, Z.-Z., Goldstein, N. I., and Fisher, P. B. (1999). Translational infidelity and human cancer: Role of the PTI-1 oncogene. *Int. J. Biochem. Cell Biol.* **31,** 151–62.
83. Sun, Y., Katz, A. E., and Fisher, P. B. (1997). Human prostatic carcinoma oncogene PTI-1 is expressed in human tumor cell lines and prostate carcinoma patient blood samples. *Cancer Res.* **57,** 18–23.
84. Shen, R., Su, Z -Z., Olsson, C. A., and Fisher, P. B. (1995). Identification of the human prostatic carcinoma oncogene PTI-1 by rapid expression of cloning and differential display. *Proc. Natl. Acad. Sci. U.S.A.* **92,** 6778–6782.
85. Lew, Y., Jones, D. V., Mars, W. M., Evans, D., Byrd, D., and Frazier, M. L. (1992). Expression of elongation factor-1 gamma-related sequence in human pancreatic cancer. *Pancreas* **7,** 144–152.
86. Chi, K., Jones, D. V., and Frazier, M. L. (1992). Expression of an elongation factor 1 gamma-related sequence in adenocarcinoma of the colon. *Gastroenterology* **103,** 98–102.
87. Ender, B., Lynch, P., Kim, Y. H., Inamdar, N. V., Cleary, K. R., and Frazier, M. L. (1993). Overexpression of an elongation factor-1 gamma-hybridizing RNA in colorectal adenomas. *Mol. Carcinog.* **7,** 18–20.
88. Mathur, S., Cleary, K. R., Inamdar, N., Kim, Y. H., Steck, P., and Frazier, M. L. (1998). Overexpression of elongation factor-1 gamma protein in colorectal carcinoma. *Cancer* **82,** 816–821.
89. Kolettas, E., Lymboura, M., Khazaie, K., and Lugmani, Y. (1998). Modulation of elongation factor-1 delta (EF-1 delta) expression in human epithelial cells. *Anticancer Res.* **18,** 385–392.
90. Nakamura, Y., Ito, K., and Isaksson, L. A. (1996). Emerging understanding of translation termination. *Cell* **87,** 147–150.
91. Drugeon, G., Jean-Jean, O., Frolova, L., Le Goff, X., Philippe, M., Kisselev, L., and Haenni, A. -L. (1997). Eukaryotic release factor 1 (eRF1) abolishes readthrough and competes with suppressor tRNAs at all three termination codons in messenger RNA. *Nucleic Acids Res.* **25,** 2254–2258.
92. Stansfield, I., Eurwilaichitr, L., Akhmaloka, and Tuite, M. F. (1996). Depletion in the levels of the release factor eERF1 causes a reduction in the eficiency of translation termination in yeast. *Mol. Microbiol.* **20,** 1135–1143.
93. Frovola, L., Le Goff, X., Zhouravleva, G., Davydova, E., Philippe, M., and Kisselev, L. (1996). Eukaryotic polypeptide chain release factor eRF3 is an eRF1-and ribosome-dependent guanosine triphosphatase. *RNA* **2,** 334–341.
94. Stansfield, I., Kushnirov, W., Jones, K. M., and Tuite, M. F. (1997). A conditional-lethal translation termination defect in a sup45 mutant of the yease *Saccharomyces cerevisiae. Eur. J. Biochem.* **245,** 557–563.
95. Kikuchi, Y., Shimatake, H., and Kikuchi, A. (1988). A yeast gene required for the G1-to-S transition encodes a protein containing an A-kinase target site and GTPase domain. *EMBO J.* **7,** 1175–1182.
96. Hoshino, S., Imai, M., Kikuchi, Y., Hanaoka, F., Ui, M., and Katada, T. (1998). Molecular cloning of a novel member of the eukaryotic polypeptide chain-releasing factors (eRF). *J. Biol. Chem.* **273,** 22254–22259.
97. Zhang, S., Ruiz-Echevarria, M., Quan, Y., and Peltz, S. W. (1995). Identification and characterization of a sequence motif involved in nonsense-mediated mRNA decay. *Mol. Cell. Biol.* **15,** 2231–2244.
98. Czaplinski, K., Ruiz-Echevarria, M., Paushkin, S. V., Han, I., Weng, Y., Perlick, H. A., Dietz, H. C., Ter-Avanesyan, M. D., and Peltz, S. W. (1998). The surveillance complex interacts with the translation release factors to enhance termination and degrade aberrant mRNAs. *Genes Dev.* **12,** 1665–1677.
99. Culbertson, M. R. (1999). RNA surveillance: unforseen consequences for gene expression, inherited genetic disorders and cancer. *Trends Genet.* **15,** 74–80.
100. Brent, R., Moore, D., and Kingston, R. E. (1993). "Current Protocols in Molecular Biology" (F. M. Ausubel, ed.). John Wiley and Sons, Inc., New York.
101. Venema, R. C., Peters, H. I., and Traugh, J. A. (1991). Phosphorylation of valyl-tRNA synthetase and elongation factor 1 in response to phorbol esters is associated with stimulation of both activities. *J. Biol. Chem.* **266,** 11993–11998.
102. Merrick, W. C. (1979). Assays for eukaryotic protein synthesis. *In* "Methods in Enzymology" (S. P. Colowick, and N. O. Kaplan, eds.), Vol. LX, pp. 108–123. Academic Press, New York.
103. Mangus, D. A., and Jacobson, A. (1999). Linking mRNA turnover and translation: Assessing the polyribosomal association of mRNA decay factors and degradative intermediates. *Methods* **17,** 28–37.
104. Matzura, O., and Wennborg, A. (1996). RNAdraw: An integrated program for RNA secondary structure calculation and analysis under 32-bit Microsoft Windows. *Comput. Appl. Biosci. (CABIOS)* **12,** 247–249.
105. Zuker, M., Mathews, D. H., and Turner, D. H. (1999). Algorithms and thermodynamics for RNA secondary structure prediction: A practical guide. *In* "RNA Biochemistry and Biotechnology" (J. Barciszewski and B. F. C. Clark, eds.), pp 11–43. Kluwer.
106. Mathews, D. H., Sabina, J., Zuker, M., and Turner, D. H. (1999). Expanded sequence dependence of thermodynamic parameters provides robust prediction of RNA secondary structure. *J. Mol. Biol.* **288,** 911–9401.
107. Frier, S. M., Kierzak, R., Jaeger, J. A., Sugimoto, N., Caruthers, M. H., Nielson, T., and Turner, D. H. (1986). Improved free-energy parameters for predictions of RNA duplex stability. *Proc. Natl. Acad. Sci. U.S.A.* **83,** 9373–9377.

24

Organelle Studies: Mitochondria, Golgi, and Endoplasmic Reticulum

Anirban Banerjee, Thomas N. Robinson, Fabia Gamboni-Robertson, Charles B. Cairns, and Rene J. P. Musters

Department of Surgery, University of Colorado Health Sciences Center, Denver, Colorado 80262

I. The Mitochondria

The mitochondria of human cells are descendants of ancient protobacteria that were engulfed by and drawn into a symbiotic relationship with eukaryotic cells some 3 billion years ago (1, 2). By reversing the flow of the photosynthetic cycle that combined solar energy, CO_2, and water to make organic compounds and oxygen, mitochondria evolved the citric acid cycle, which "burns" small organic compounds to make CO_2, water, and chemical energy (Fig. 1) (3). In humans, mitochondria are the major oxygen consumers and the predominant organelles of aerobic organs such as brain, heart, and red skeletal muscle (colored by the high concentration of mitochondrial cytochrome contents). In contrast, liver mitochondria may be mostly committed to biosynthesis, and neutrophils usually do not contain any (4, 5). Mitochondria still retain a small fraction of their original genome and unique double-walled structure, testimony to the engulfment of the ancient protobacteria (the present-day inner membrane and matrix) and their entrapment within intracellular vacuoles (the outer mitochondrial membrane) (1). The impermeable inner membrane contains special iron–sulfur and ancient heme-containing proteins that extrude H^+ ions, creating a "charged halo" that distinguishes the symbionts biophysically (3, 6, 7). The energy of the proton gradient, up to 2 pH units higher than cytosol (or -200 mV, matrix negative), is used to make ATP and to transport ions and substrates. Of the few ancient genes remaining in human mitochondria ($\sim$17), several encode components of the electron transport chain (ETC) and unique (bacteria-like) tRNAs (1, 2). Thus, import of proteins from the cytosol and placement into membranes or matrix are challenging but hot topics of research (8). The reader should note that the outer mitochondrial wall (relatively permeable) is fused to the inner membrane (very impermeable, even to small ions) at select spots. Here, protein insertion into either membrane or matrix is allowed. The process involves leader sequences, transporter proteins (of the inner and outer membranes, called TIMS and TOMS), protease cleavage, and refolding by specialized chaperones (e.g., mtHsp70) (8).

Glucose, pyruvate, lactate, ketones, fats, amino acids

$$4\text{Acetyl-CoA} + 11O_2 + 48\text{ADP} + 48\text{Pi} \longrightarrow 8CO_2 + 6H_2O + 4\text{CoA} + 48\text{ATP}$$

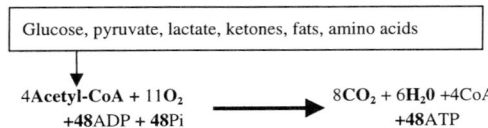

Figure 1 Ingested foods are converted by separate metabolic pathways to acetyl-CoA (and also NADH and FADH). The two-carbon acetyl-CoA is decarboxylated by the Kreb's cycle reactions, producing three NADH and one FADH (and one GTP) per cycle. These are ultimately used to reduce oxygen to water. The equation sums the span of dozens of reactions to highlight the concept of fuel burning.

II. Surgically Relevant Questions

The major surgical questions concern how mitochondria in different tissues are linked to the needs of specific cells and organs. Given the importance of mitochondria in oxidizing various fuels by consuming oxygen, how are these activities chosen to fulfill the energy demands of the cell (Fig. 2)? Simultaneously, mitochondria produce many of the raw materials that cells need to survive. How is this biosynthesis mission balanced against energy production? Last, what happens to mitochondria during apoptosis?

The long evolution of the symbiosis between mitochondria and cells has led to an extremely complex relationship. Basic science efforts have characterized the protein machinery that guides flow of energy and substrates into the mitochondrion while high-energy phosphates, essential building blocks (encompassing gluconeogenesis, fatty acids, porphyrins, nucleic bases, and amino acids) are transported out (4, 5, 9–11). The mitochondria also secrete reactive oxygen species (12, 13) and buffer cations (mostly Ca^{2+}) (14). This contributes to cell signaling and to apoptotis (programmed cell death) (13, 15). Indeed, the importance of intramitochondrial proteins such as cytochrome *c* and apoptosis inducing factor (AIF) in activating caspases and degrading nuclear DNA, respectively, has proved to be a surprising revelation (15). Certain inflammatory ligands such as TNFα absolutely require mitochondrial participation to induce apoptosis (13).

The essential mitochondrial role in extracting ATP by oxidizing sugars with high efficiency (compared to glycolysis) needs no recounting (5, 6). It enables the existence of excitable tissues and accounts for the exquisite sensitivity of heart and brain to ischemia. Occasionally the ETC will spit out partially (one-, two-, or three-electron) reduced oxygen species (ROS) as oxygen is continually reduced to water (Fig. 3) (6, 16). This has led cells to elaborate antioxidant defenses, including a dedicated manganese–superoxide dismutase (Mn–SOD) found only on mitochondria (16). The ROS may also promote cell signaling by kinases and nuclear transcription factors (3, 14). TNFα and other stimuli promote ROS production, both for signaling and apoptosis (13), but excess ROS released by the ETC can precipitate cell death (secondary necrosis) (15).

Although it is extremely well characterized biochemically, the role of mitochondria in supporting biosynthesis has been overlooked (Fig. 4). The fact that acetyl-CoA produced by mitochondrial pyruvate dehydrogenase complex is the starting point of several amino acids, nucleic acids, sterols, and fatty acids has serious implications for wound repair, posttraumatic catabolism, and surgical nutrition (4, 6, 10, 17, 18) (see also Chapter 56).

A. In Vivo Studies

Although the mitochondria consume the bulk of oxygen delivered to tissue, and are crucial to biosynthesis and maintenance of every cell, indicators of oxygen consumption *in vivo* are hard to interpret (5) (see also Chapter 56). This is because mitochondria in different tissues of the body (e.g., liver vs. heart) can be engaged in utterly different missions (4, 10) (see Chapters 60 and 61). Biosynthesis might require minimal oxygenation, whereas uncoupled mitochondria can consume vast amounts of oxygen without making ATP (5, 19). Oxygen delivery issues caused by shunting or poor perfusion add another layer of uncertainty in gauging whether persistent lactic acidosis indicates mitochondrial dysfunction in a patient. Increasing demand with exercise or catecholamines can be useful for evaluating chronic changes

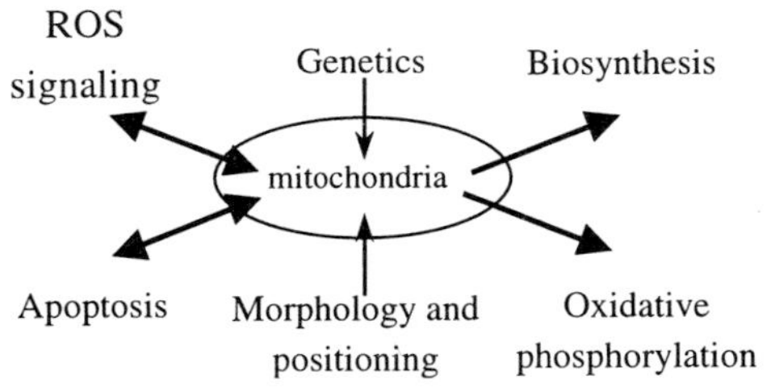

Figure 2 The mitochondria integrate a large number of cellular cues and also direct the cell fate over short-term and longer term scales. (See also Chapters 18, 46, 49, 58, 59, 62, and 63.)

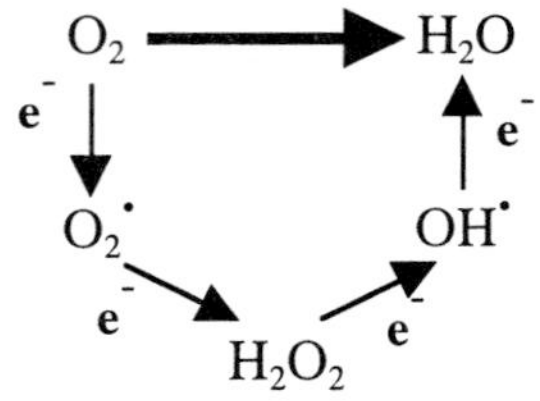

Figure 3 Normally the four-electron reduction of oxygen to water occurs in one concerted step at cytochrome *aa3*. However, if other electron-rich centers cause reduction, then a variety of toxic, partially reduced species can be formed.

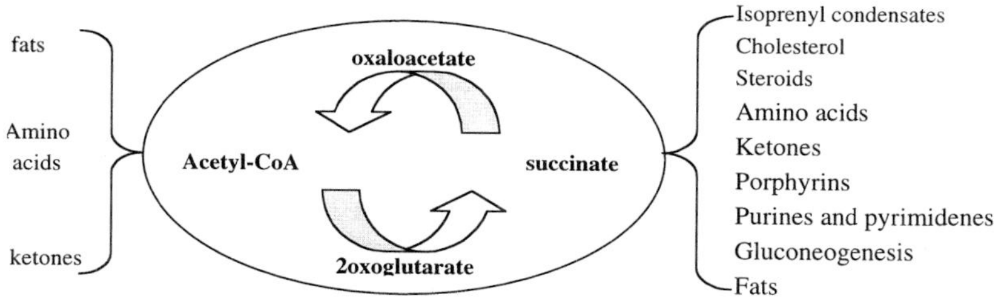

Figure 4 Circulating fuels are transformed by the mitochondria to enter the Kreb's cycle as small two to six-membered carbon chains. These same molecules are used as the feedstock for a variety of building blocks the cell needs to survive.

(e.g., diabetics), but this is not applicable to an intensive care unit (ICU) patient.

The arterial ketone body ratio (KBR) is one technique that can be exploited to discern the state of hepatic mitochondria (20, 21) in animal models and patients. Ketone body production and their systemic ratio directly reflect the redox state of hepatic mitochondria. Enhanced ketone production after trauma can reflect diversion of the Kreb's cycle toward gluconeogenesis, under control of insulin catecholamines and glucagon (22). KBRs might detect hepatic rejection and oxidative injury before other tests (20–22), indicating early mitochondrial damage.

The status of the highly colored heme-containing proteins of the ETC (6) can be directly studied by their absorption in the deep red wavelengths. This technology is called near infrared reflectance spectroscopy (NIRS) (23) and exploits the ability of near infrared wavelengths to penetrate 10–50 mm into tissue without harm. These devices are small, portable, and similar to pulse oximeters. By monitoring several wavelengths (using various pattern extraction algorithms) these can specifically detect the state of the heme ring in hemoglobin (oxidized/reduced, or complexed to CO or cyanide) and the oxidation state of other hemes in the ETC. Cytochrome *aa3*, the last complex of the ETC (which actually transfers 4 electrons to oxygen), is particularly well studied. This methodology not only reveals tissue oxygenation but also how well the mitochondria in the light path are actually consuming oxygen.

In patients dying of multiple organ failure, oxygen consumption can become independent of perfusion (oxygenation), despite persisting acidosis. Here, discrepancies between hemoglobin saturation and cytochrome reduction can be clearly seen (23) in topical recordings made from the shoulder (skeletal muscle) or brain. The use of NIRS to assess therapy quickly and noninvasively is likely to become extensive, and detection of other colored compounds within cells is imminent.

B. Isolated Mitochondria from Tissues and Cells

Study of isolated cellular and tissue mitochondria is the oldest and most popular approach for research (24). Isolation is important, because this eliminates interference from other cellular organelles, and removal of the impermeable cell plasma membrane gives the investigator access. The major disadvantage is that regulation by cytoplasmic signaling pathways and cytoskeleton is lost.

The general details of isolation procedures have been given in excellent specialized monographs (24), but these are starting points that need to be optimized in each laboratory. It is crucial to break cells without severely damaging the mitochondria. Mechanical breakage and cautious enzymatic digestion are favored because hypotonic lysis disrupts mitochondrial membranes. In tough tissues such as myocardium, there is a trade-off between retaining yield and mitochondrial integrity. Centrifugal separation from lighter organelles is usually followed by further purification by fractionation in a density gradient (Percoll) when very pure preparations are desired (24). Because yields are low, it is not clear what kinds of mitochondria are enriched or lost. Organelle-associated protein or lipid complexes may also be stripped.

Isolated mitochondria are commonly used to study the functionality of the ETC system (9, 24). Oxygen consumption before and after ADP indicates the P:O ratio (ATP produced per oxygen atom consumed, normally about 3). Substrates (glutamate, malate, succinate) and drugs (rotenone) can be combined to assess the electron flow through portions of the ETC (6,9,19). Other drugs that decouple the transmembrane potential, or block ADP to ATP conversion, can measure the maximum flux of electrons to oxygen through the ETC, or membrane leakiness, respectively (6, 9, 19). Curiously many drugs (bongkrekic acid, atractyloside) and endotoxin (25) inhibit the all-important exchange of ATP from mitochondrial matrix and cytosol (9). Such mitochondria are unresponsive to the energy needs of the cell. This exchanger is being recognized for its importance during apoptosis (15). The rates of oxygen consumption in the presence of different substrates and drugs can be analyzed to obtain a model of the thermodynamic efficiency (19). Thus the different roles of mitochondria in heart, brain, or liver (producing large amounts of ATP, maintaining high levels of ATP/ADP potential, or performing oxidative phosphorylation with the highest efficiency) can now be distinguished (19).

Isolated mitochondria form the starting point for further subfractionation to determine their characteristic proteins and nucleic acids and abundance. Progressive detergent lysis of outer and inner membranes has revealed the protein composition of these subcompartments. Antibody tags and protease digestion are used to determine the orientation of protein epitopes at the inner and outer faces of each membrane.

The study of mitochondrial DNA constitutes a discipline on its own (1, 2). mtDNA is entirely derived from the maternal egg cell and is subject to faster mutation compared to nuclear DNA. Pathologic mutations give rise to inherited diseases that can manifest in childhood and that can get worse if the mutant DNA accumulates (26). Peripheral vascular disease and diabetes both show changes in mtDNA. Interestingly, the same mutation can give rise to different symptoms within the same family, depending on the fluctuating percentages of mutant mtDNA the individual inherits (26).

Subfractionation of isolated mitochondria and biochemical characterization permitted earlier workers to decipher the complex metabolic transformations of the Kreb's cycle, fatty acid oxidation, and the ETC (9, 27). The individual enzymes have been mostly characterized, including their allosteric regulation. These regulatory factors (including hormones, Kreb' cycle substrates, and ions) help the mitochondria choose between fuels used for either ATP production or biosynthesis (gluconeogenesis, fatty acid, amino acids, etc.) (9, 22, 24). Biosynthesis shunts carbon substrates from the Kreb's cycle to the cytosol. Biosynthesis also requires reducing reactions (always by NADPH, because NADH carries the electrons of catabolism into the ETC) and high-energy ATP and GTP. Tropic hormones (luteinizing hormone and adrenocorticotropic hormone) produce a marked increase in steroid hormone synthesis within minutes (18). The rate-limiting step in this acute steroidogenic response is the transport of cholesterol from the outer to the inner mitochondrial membrane, where the first committed step in steroid synthesis is performed by the side-chain cleavage enzyme system (P450scc), resulting in the production of pregnenolone (18).

Fractionation of matrix constituents, including biologic cations (Na^+, K^+, Ca^{2+}), allowed the first measurements of the transmembrane potential (ΔV or $\Delta\Psi$, about -200 mV at maximum) (9, 24). Subfractionation of membrane into matrix and intermembrane constituents showed that the outer membrane (topologically the remnant of the engulfing plasma membrane vacuole) is fairly porous (<1000 Da), but the inner membrane is impervious to ions as small as H^+ (9, 24). Indeed, the extrusion of protons is the fundamental power source of mitochondria. Controlled entry of charge down the pH gradient allows ATP synthesis and also entry of cations (K^+, Ca^{2+}) through specialized channels and subsequent export by H^+ linked antiporters (9, 24). Both K^+ and Ca^{2+} exert powerful regulatory effects on the flow of mitochondrial metabolism. A mitochondrial sulfonylurea-regulated K_{ATP} channel has drawn interest because it appears to be a final effector of cardiac preconditioning signaling (28–30). The transmembrane gradient is also used to transport substrate anions (phosphate citrate, glutamate, malate) against their chemical concentration gradients by specialized exchanger proteins (9).

C. Mitochondria in Intact Cells

Most of our concepts of mitochondria derive from electron microscopic (EM) images (9). Many textbooks show the classic elliptic slipper shapes (from liver, about 0.5×1.4 μm). EM images also reveal the double-membraned structure and the cristae formed by deep invaginations of the inner membrane. Antibodies carrying gold particles have been used to localize proteins to each subcompartment. However, EM has several shortcomings: the harshness of preparation, the sampling of more than a few mitochondria per cell, and the repertoire of cell types that have been studied. Using fixed cells with optical microscopes eliminates some of these drawbacks but sacrifices resolution (100–200 nm at best with confocal methods) (31–35). However, many antibodies (which would not survive the EM sample preparation process) can be imaged quantitatively with fluorescence staining techniques. Cells 10–20 μm thick can be easily visualized. Both EM and light microscopy can use appropriately labeled antibodies to visualize the marvelous arrangements of the mitochondrion and its proteins in thin frozen or fixed tissue sections. Recently it has become possible to study live mitochondria in intact cells (31–35). However, at present it is not easy to study mitochondria in tissues without fixing (34).

In the past decade fluorescent dyes that select for mitochondrial membranes have become available (see the Internet sites at www.probes.com/ and www. piercenet.com/ for extensive information). Continuing improvements have produced cationic fluorophores such as JC-1 (Molecular Probes), which distribute about the charged inner membrane according to the Nernst equation (7, 36). Unlike previously used dyes (e.g., rhodamine or rosamine), JC-1 aggregates above 160 n*M*, or when the local transmembrane potential (ΔV) exceeds 20 mV. The aggregates emit an increasingly brighter fluorescence in the red wavelengths (540 nm) and the monomer emission stays constant after loading (about 1 hr)

These dyes can be used for isolated mitochondria, but are most powerful (and easy) when applied to live cells and studied with a digital epifluorescence microscope (7, 32, 36). This differs from a true confocal microscope in that it does not use lasers to excite fluorescence within a small voxel. Rather, small steps off the stage move the plane of focus (optical sectioning). The stacks of images so obtained are deconvolved by computer to remove out-of-focus light. Photoexcitation can lead to extensive dye bleaching and can be cytotoxic by photosensitizing oxygen in live cells. In addition, lasers are expensive and wavelengths cannot be changed easily.

These studies show that in a number of cultured cells (mostly transformed cells to date), mitochondria are not distributed evenly around the cell (7, 36–38). Nor are they all of the commonly imagined elliptical shapes. Many mitochondria appear as elongated (about 0.5 × >3–20 μm), snaky cylinders that can be pinched off to form the smaller, familiar elliptical shapes. These reticulated mitochondria are most common around the nucleus (and have also been seen in EM images) (Fig. 5) (37). JC-1 staining shows that the smaller mitochondria tend to have the highest charge (red fluorescence), and the longer reticulated mitochondria have lower

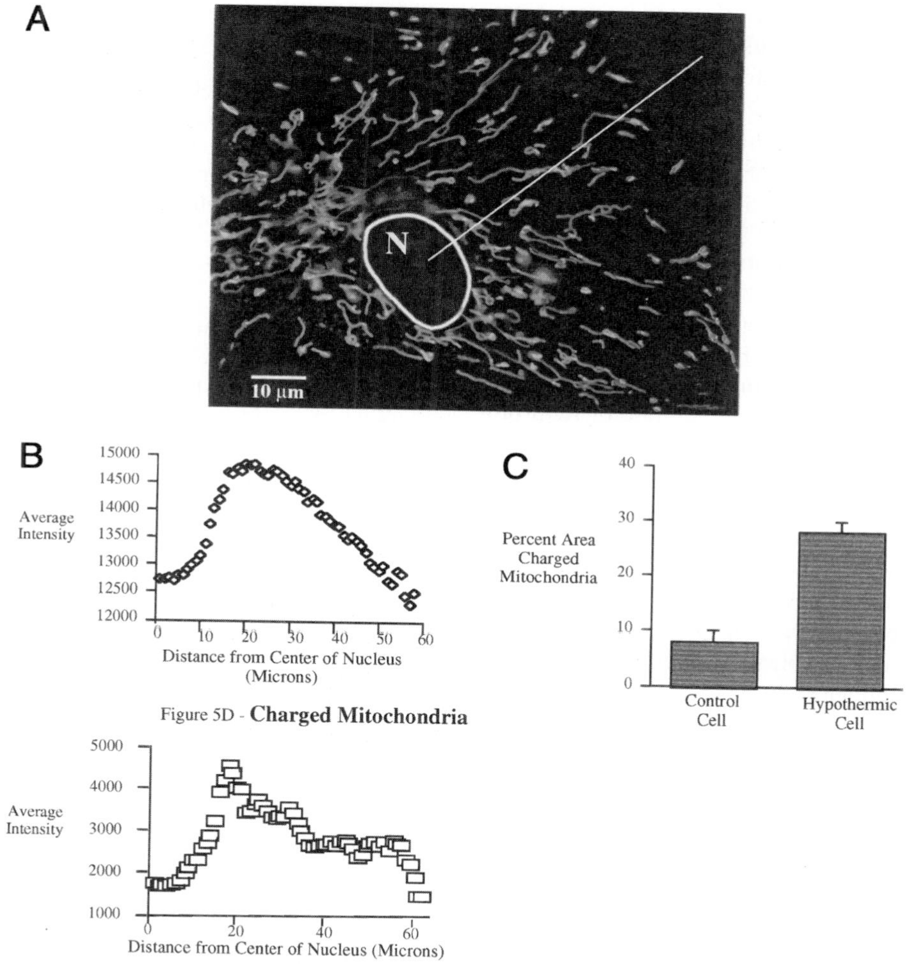

Figure 5 JC-1-loaded mitochondria show areas of low transmembrane voltage (20 mv, JC-1 monomers only, green) and areas at a high potential (JC-1 aggregates, red). Areas at intermediate potential appear yellow to orange. The nucleus (N) and the cell edge were first found by enhancing the low-intensity autofluorescence. Then the cell body was spanned by a line extending from the nuclear center to 5 μm outside the cell (shown in white). The intensity values for each pixel along the line samples were averaged over 16 lines, each from a different cell, and are presented in panels B and C for the green and red channels, respectively. Generally, all mitochondrial membranes (B) are abundant in the nuclear periphery, and rarer at the cell edge. In contrast, the charged mitochondria plateau (D, note greater density) just near the cell edge. The total number of red pixels (charged mitochondria) can also be expressed as percentage of the total number of green pixels (all mitochondria). (C) Reducing cellular energy demand by cooling to 23°C increases the charged area ($p < 0.01$). (See color plates.)

charge (staining green with the selective JC-1 monomer, but unable to cause aggregate formation and thus not emitting red fluorescence). However, within a long snaking strand there can be patches of membrane that are highly polarized. In some cell types all mitochondria are small and highly charged (cardiac myocytes, breast cancer) (7, 36, 38); in others both populations are present in different proportions, and in yet others there are no areas of high charge at all. The reasons for this heterogeneity in a cell and even within a strand are unclear. Mitochondrial dyes also reveal that the different structures are interconverted on a time scale of minutes, consistent with the evidence that cytoskeletal elements are involved in positioning mitochondria within the cell (39, 40). A number of kinesin isoforms (ATP-dependent motor proteins that travel along microtubules in either outward or inward directions) (40) have been found. Certain myosin isoforms may also be involved in positioning (39).

Other vital stains that are useful to study live mitochondria include dyes that detect ROS (see www.probes.com/, for extensive information). These permeable dyes enter the cell in dihydro form, and on oxygenation change fluorescence emission color. Newer variants leak out slowly and so permit longer observations. Mitochondria typically produce a small amount of ROS during normal respiration. Drugs that interfere with the ETC, signaling lipids such as ceramide, fatty acids, and sudden metabolic jumps, e.g., during ischemia reperfusion (12) elevate the rate of ROS production (15). Some receptor signals such as TNFα may directly affect portions of the ETC and create leakage of electrons prior to transfer to oxygen at cytochrome *aa3* (13). These effects may synergize with changes in cytoskeletally guided transport because TNFα causes clusters of mitochondria on one side of the nucleus (41). For TNFα, these mitochondrial changes appear to precede caspase activation and cell death. Microtubule-destabilizing drugs such as vinblastine and colchicine can augment the cytotoxicity of TNFα, whereas other apoptotic stimuli (e.g., Fas) are unaffected.

Live microscopy of mitochondria is most useful for surgical research. Many of the other approaches were developed to characterize specific aspects of oxidative respiration, transport, carbon metabolism, or genetics. Newer insights into aspects of mitochondrial symbiosis include the positioning of mitochondria to suit the need of polarized cells in tissues and the novel integrative functions leading to apoptosis (15, 37, 41). The core issues of surgical research—inflammation, cell death, oxygen consumption, nutrition, ischemia reperfusion, or diabetic degeneration—impact all aspects of mitochondrial function simultaneously. Live mitochondria in intact cells may be essential to study problems that involve the integration of mitochondria with cell metabolism, or those that evaluate cytokine signals or test therapeutic maneuvers. Newer dyes and probes will enhance our ability to study these various aspects readily. Most surgical issues require primary cells, preferably human, to provide clinically relevant answers. Live microscopy can be conducted on just a few thousand cells from a biopsy, no matter how short lived the cell.

The requirements for live microscopy of mitochondria are similar those for the endoplasmic reticulum and golgi (ER–golgi) (see below). A good camera and friendly image-processing software are critical. Dye bleaching in live cells (presence of oxygen and water) is a severe problem with many dyes, including JC-1. Therefore it is hard to image the same cell over time (repeated measures). With heterogeneous mitochondria within a cell, different cells in a dish, and variance between runs and cell passage, the experimenter should be well versed in nested analysis of variance to make statistical statements about treatments.

D. The Endoplasmic Reticulum—Golgi–Endosome Circuit

Animal tissues consist of cells that must replenish themselves constantly, while ensuring that newly synthesized proteins are placed correctly. In a range of animal cells, the rates of protein turnover (days to hours) and membrane turnover (hours) are phenomenally fast, placing great burdens on energy systems and resynthesis mechanisms. Moreover the newly synthesized proteins must be positioned correctly at apical or basolateral cell faces, because most animal cells within tissues are polarized. Cell polarization is maintained by using the cytoskeleton to guide correct positioning of mature proteins. Polarized cells within organs perform numerous secretory and uptake or clearance functions. Although these functions performed by macrophages, hepatocytes, gut, pancreas, thyroid, and neurons are clearly recognized, other specialized cells and tissues, as diverse as myocytes, endothelium, and connective tissues, also secrete powerful signaling peptides. With a few exceptions these are translated into the ER, modified within the golgi, and released from vesicles that fuse to the plasma membrane.

III. Areas of Surgical Interest: How to Study

The major surgical questions concern how well patients are able to maintain the normal turnover in healthy tissues, especially while repairing injury. The entire equilibrium between cellular breakdown and resynthesis is changed after surgical stress/trauma (44), but it remains unclear as to how counterregulatory hormones and inducible cytokines accomplish this specific regulation in different tissues. Moreover, how do growth factors, cytokines, and other circulating stress proteins enter into the circulation? Last, what is the impact of accelerated membrane/protein turnover on signal transduction and infection?

The fundamental processes underlying these questions involve the molecular mechanisms of vesicle formation and its progressive modification (including cargo sorting), followed by fusion with a target compartment. These intracellular processes transport material from the ER to the golgi, from the golgi to the plasma membrane, and back from the plasma membrane to the lysozomes or the golgi. This field of study is in its infancy but several textbooks and monographs have outlined and integrated newly acquired knowledge of these processes (42, 43). Often the studies are accomplished with transformed cells or lower life forms. However, there is every reason to suspect that these multiple steps are highly regulated by intra- and extra cellular determinants.

The balance between protein anabolism (i.e., translation, maturation, and externalization) and catabolism (internalization and processing of ingested matter) is a very basic aspect of all surgical care (44). The stress of anesthesia and surgery alters the normal balance of protein turnover. Although the mechanisms remain complex, nutritional support is valuable for aiding patient recovery. For both shock and sepsis the receptor- and cell-signaling pathways that alter protein expression and turnover are being worked out. Ischemia, too, appears to involve TNFα and other cytokines that alter gene expression and metabolism (45). The hormones and peptides that are responsible for causing postsurgical changes are either stored within secretory vesicles or manufactured *de novo*.

Elevated levels of catecholamines, neuropeptides, cytokines, and bactericidal enzymes all attest to stimulated exocytotic secretion (44). Secreted proteins or receptors whose cell surface presentation can be quickly up-regulated are often stored in storage vesicles and are released at either constitutive rates or at accelerated rates. Normal secretion must occur at the correct cell face (apical or toward a lumen; basolateral; etc.) (43). The molecular biology of transcriptional control has revealed a powerful machinery that can enhance peptide synthesis (e.g., acute phase proteins, TNFα) very rapidly (43, 44). The ER–golgi system then conducts the appropriate postranslational modifications, followed by vesicular storage/secretion.

In addition to the forward traffic of material, in all cells there is a retrograde half of cellular transport involving endocytosis, inward trafficking, and cargo sorting toward either recycling or incorporation into lysozomes for degradation. This circuit is revealed by the disappearance of liganded receptors from the cell surface, or by the clearance of drugs and substrates from the circulation. Receptor internalization affects surface availability and can produce tachyphylaxis (desensitization). More importantly, most ligand-bound receptors appear to continue signaling after they have been internalized. For example, the activation of MAPK pathways by β-adrenergic receptors, and activation of apoptotic pathways by TNFα, occur after internalization (46, 47). Therapeutically, interrupting endosome maturation could abrogate certain downstream sequlae of receptor signaling. Moreover, many viruses and bacteria utilize the endocytotic processes to gain entry into cells (48, 49).

A. Isolated Studies in Cultured Cells

The ER–golgi system is much too dynamic to be studied by centrifugal isolation techniques alone. Although such approaches have been valuable for defining the basic machinery, it is the dynamic regulation of this system during acute injury and healing that is of primary interest to surgical researchers. Established techniques involving crushing and grinding of cells still provide useful adjunct data.

Any cell system that can be placed in a dish for the duration of an experiment is open to study. The problem of studying dynamic organelles that constantly bud and fuse with new compartments has driven most basic investigators into eschewing studies on tissues. Further, because most cell biologists have used genetic and molecular biology approaches to characterize the protein machinery surrounding ER–golgi and endosomal transport, they have selected stably transformed mammalian cell lines or lower animals such as yeast or insects (42).

The individual proteins and the associated regulatory mechanisms deciphered from these simpler models offer the opportunity for surgical researchers to ask important questions:

1. How the circuit works in a cell line of clinical interest.
2. How postsurgical trauma alters the flow and sorting of material in and out of the cell.
3. How signaling via hormones, substrates, and drugs can elicit desirable outcomes.

B. Synthesis and Posttranslational Modifications in the ER and Golgi

The cell makes several proteins for secretory export, whereas others are localized to the cell surface. Such proteins are first imported into the ER from the cytosol. In the ER lumen the peptides fold and oligomerize; disulfide bonds are added and a special N-linked oligosaccharide is added. In all eukaryotes selected asparagine residues gain a tag consisting of two *N*-acetylglucosamines followed by nine mannoses. COP II coated vesicles bud from specialized areas of the ER, where they are modified to into larger tubules, the ER–golgi intermediate (ERGIC), and then into the cisternae of the cis-golgi stack. The COP II coatomer coat is removed and recycled with other ER resident proteins, and new enzymes are added. These enzymes modify the original glycosylated protein by adding phosphates or trimming terminal mannose sugars (mannosidase I is a marker for cis-golgi). At this point the *N*-acetylglucosamine residues become resistant to the specific endoglycosidase, Endo H.

Perhaps due to their structure and folding, some proteins are not modified at all, retaining their original high mannose content; others are now ready for further glycosylation. After mannose cleavage, sugars are added one at a time, including variable amounts of *N*-acetylglucosamine, sialic acid, and fucose. These proteins are called complex oligosaccharides and include the familiar receptors, integrins, and iontransporters. Resistance to Endo H also forms the basis of an enzymatic digestion protocol to distinguish high-mannose oligosaccharides from the extensively modified complex oligosaccharides. Secreted proteoglycans that form the extracellular matrix, including basement membranes, are the most heavily glycolsylated of all. These processes, as revealed by a variety of drugs, are becoming available to block the individual enzymes that modify glycosylation. Similarly, there is an ever-increasing range of commercial products that determine the glycosylation and phosphorylation status of numerous proteins. These are being developed at so rapid a rate that the annual number of catalogs and flyers from specialty companies outstrips the information contained in the latest reviews (see Table I). Searching databases for products can be incomplete if a researcher is unaware of the mechanistic relevance of a product. Indeed, many critical developments come from research areas (yeast, *Drosophila*, plants) that surgical researchers are likely to overlook. This simply attests to the fact that much of the machinery of the ER–golgi–endosomal circuit arose with the first multicellular organisms and is still basically retained in humans, with extensive regulatory modifications.

New enzymes and sugar nucleotide transporters are added to the maturing golgi stack, giving it new biochemical identities (medial-golgi, trans-golgi). The original idea that cisternae mature with the addition of new cargo-modifying enzymes while other enzymes are recycled back to the start of the cis-golgi has been recently substantiated (42). Theories based largely on electron microscopic images showing vesicles budding between golgi stacks postulated that cargoes progressed by a series of vesicle budding and fusing steps, leading from cis- to medial- to trans-golgi cisternae (Fig. 6). Evidence that procollagen fibrils (>300 nm) that are too large to fit inside any vesicle (50) are correctly folded after proline hydoxylation steps as they transit the golgi stacks in fibroblasts refurbishes this controversy.

C. Secretion

Some of the earliest advances in the study of the ER–golgi and endosomal circuit documented the fact that the trans-golgi network (TGN) produces at least two populations of vesicles. One carries constitutively produced proteins. Another distinct pathway under signaling control leads to a variety of storage granules that can be released on stimulation. As outlined above these cargoes probably differ in some detail of their molecular structure (localization tags or domains).

In culture the secretion of inducible proteins (such as cytokines, interferons, and peptide hormones) in response to a pathological or receptor-mediated stimulus can be easily

Table I Sources of Commercial Products

Vendor	Phone	Internet source
EY Labs	800-821-0044	www.eylabs.com
Vector Labs	800-227-6666	www.vectorlabs.com
Amersham	800-526-3593	www.apbiotech.com
Biorad	800-4BIORAD	www.bio-rad.com
Calbiochem	800-854-3417	www.calbiochem.com
Chemicon	800-437-7500	www.chemicon.com
Toronto	800-727-9240	www.trc-canada.com
Alexis	800-900-0065	alexis-usa@alexis-corp.com
Glyko	800-334-5956	www.glyco.com
Upstate	800-520-3011	www.upstatebiotech.co
Sigma	800-325-3010	www.sigma-aldrich.com
ICN Biomedicals	800-854-0530	www.icnbiomed.com
New England Biolabs	800-632-5227	www.neb.com
Pierce	800-874-3723	www.piercenet.com
ProZyme	800-457-9444	www.prozyme.com
Seikagaku America	800-237-4512	www.seikagaku.com
Vector Laboratories	800-227-6666	www.vectorlabs.com

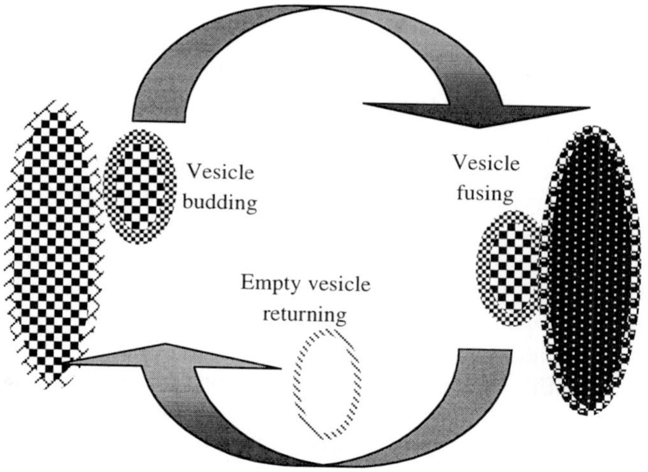

Figure 6 Cargoes are recognized by special coat protein complexes; a chain of events leads to formation of vesicles and separation from the parent compartment. The membrane lipids undergo complex changes and driving energy is obtained from the hydrolysis of ATP and GTP. The process of fusion is still unclear. Empty vesicles with a characteristic coat return and replenish the parent compartment.

followed. The molecules can be detected in the cell supernatants by one of the new commercial ELISA kits. Production of the molecules can be documented within the cell by using specific antibodies on fixed cells. Flow cytometric analysis offers superb statistical quantitation on thousands of cells and digital light microscopy can provide spatial intracellular location. In both immunofluorescent techniques, the use of several antibodies (or lectins), each labeled with different dyes, can provide ratiometric data. This can be useful for identifying a particular phenotype or, in the case of digitized images, for quantitating subcompartmentation, by virtue of signal colocalization.

A range of inhibitors provide useful tools for documenting the life cycle of proteins as they are synthesized, matured, and released from the cell. At the earliest stage, the N-glycosylated (high-mannose) proteins in the ER can be quantitated and blocked by the nojirimycin series (51) and related drugs. The tools of glycobiology rely chiefly on specialized sugar-binding proteins called lectins, which are often derived from plants (wheat germ agglutinin, peas, potatoes, etc.). The drugs that block specific glycosylation steps are also derived from plants or fungi, but more quirky antibodies are becoming available. Both labeled lectins and antibodies can be used to visualize glycosylated proteins in cells or on gels. In many cases the activity of the glycosylase or glycosyl transferase can be measured with good sensitivity (often using fluorescence methodology).

Further demannosylation followed by extensive N- or O-linked glycosidic modification occurs in the golgi stacks. Again a variety of products for detecting and perturbing the transformations are becoming available. Many established and specialty companies are staking a future in glycobiology.

Dynamic studies of ER–golgi transport took a leap in the mid-1980s when it was realized that at 15°C, vesicular transport into the golgi is blocked and cargoes accumulate in the pregolgi intermediate compartment (42). At 20°C traffic from the trans-golgi is still inhibited and cargoes accumulate in the trans-golgi network. These reversible temperature barriers are commonly used to synchronize traffic that occurs above the permissive temperature. Such temperatures are reached during organ preservation or cardiac bypass and could block cell traffic.

This review cannot cover the enormous progress that is being made in defining how the cell sorts protein cargoes to their right places, and how the vesicles carrying these cargoes are actually fused to the target compartment. Interested readers should be aware of the SNARE hypothesis of paired docking proteins that confer recognition and specificity between fusing vesicle and target membrane (52). Researchers should also be aware that developments in proteomics are constantly revealing new motifs and sequences that confer placement recognition and specificity (see Table II). Not all of the cellular proteins that bind to the targeting motif have yet been found. Several Web sites are dedicated to upgrading and updating this information (see www.expasy.ch/sprot/prosite.html and http://psort.nibb.ac.jp/). PROSITE and PSORT are two of many computer programs for the prediction of protein localization sites in cells. An input sequence is analyzed by applying the stored rules for various sequence features of known protein sorting signals. Finally, the important motifs and the possibility for the input protein to be localized at each candidate site are reported with additional information.

The most vexing problem in translating basic research on cell biology to surgical problems (i.e., the biology of stressed human cells) is the understanding of protein structure and function. Computerized proteomics indicate that the number of regulatory proteins, such as protein and phospholipid kinases or phosphatases, has multiplied severalfold since the evolutionary appearance of specialized tissues in early nematodes and insects. In many cases this reflects solutions to cargo sorting and direction-specific presentation

Table II Proteomics Research

Amino acid sequence	Cellular action
KFERQ	Degradation in lysozomes
KDEL	Retention in ER
YXXPhi(L)	Endocytosis; binds AP-2 μ2 subunit
LL-COOH	Endocytosis; binds clathrin?
NPxY	Endocytosis; binds clathrin?

of surface molecules and secreted products in these complex tissues (e.g., heart, liver, immune system, neurons). Surgical biology is rarely about discovering novel proteins and their functions in human disease, and more often about exploiting existing basic science developments to figure out how mechanisms described in transformed cell or lower eukaryotic models play out in humans cell phenotypes, especially during acute disease.

Efforts have focused on understanding the signaling proteins that regulate vesicle fission and fusion to a target membrane (53). Early observations indicated that Gα subunits of the heterotrimeric G-proteins were located on golgi membranes and regulated degranulation of mast cells, neutrophils, neurons, and many other cells. Other small GTPases have also been implicated. These include the Rab isoforms that are present in the different types of golgi and endosomal vesicles (54, 55).

Different areas of research are revealing how the ER–golgi systems are positioned within the cell, by the cytoskeleton. Specific motors (ATP-using protein complexes) bind appropriate membrane vesicles and by riding cytoskeletal filament "tracks" conduct either retrograde or anterograde transport of their bound cargo to proper locations within the cell. After fusing with the next compartment and emptying the cargo, the empty vesicles are transported back (Fig. 7). Surprisingly, the ER remains spread throughout the cell, especially the periphery, while the golgi system occupies a preferred area close to the nucleus. This is a remarkable circuit, where ER-derived vesicles travel inward, maturing along with their contained cargoes. These evolve into maturing golgi vesicles, which are transported outward for final placement. Simultaneously, at each step, empty vesicles cycle back to the immediate precursor compartment. The ER–golgi–endosome circuit shows intrinsic repair capability (56). There are conserved systems to reclaim coat proteins or constitutive vesicle proteins that have become displaced. Videos of golgi traffic in living cells are recommended viewing (see http://mecko.nichd.nih.gov/CBMB/pb1labob.html or http://www.molbiolcell.org/cgi/content/full/9/7/1617?view=full&pmid=9658158#FN182).

The ER uses a variety of motor protein mechanisms including myosins (riding the actin filaments) or kinesins (large complexes that travel toward the juxtanuclear (−) end of microtubules (anchored at the centromere) (57). The treadmilling activity of microtubule at the (+) end is also utilized to position organelles. Similarly, golgi vesicles containing cargoes and coated with COP proteins use microtubules for forward transport, while empty vesicles are recycled back to a more proximal compartment by oppositely directed motors (57). A range of drugs that either stabilize or depolymerize actin and tubulin are listed in annual specialty catalogs. Some of these, such as the *Vinca* alkaloids, are currently approved for therapeutic use.

Researchers should also be aware that vesicle maturation is associated with profound changes in lipid constituents (see also Chapter 25). Moreover, it is known that a number of proteins involved in lipid transformation (such as

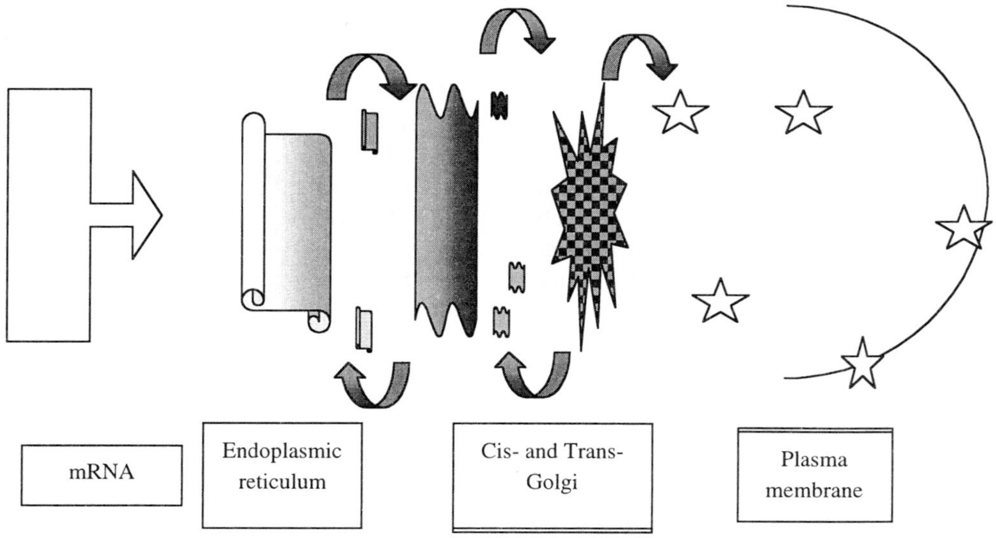

Figure 7 A schematic showing the flow of proteins destined either for insertion at the plasma membrane or for secretion. Newly synthesized mRNA bearing the appropriate tags enters a series of compartments leading from the ER to the golgi to secretory vesicles. Many intermediate compartments are not shown. Cargo-containing vesicles bud off and fuse with subsequent compartments. After dumping their contents, the empty vesicles return to the parent compartment.

phospholipases, phosphatidyl kinases, and phosphatases) are found on various intercellular vesicles (58).

D. In Vivo and Isolated Studies

Virtually all organs secrete characteristic proteins and peptides. Detecting secreted molecules in the plasma means that exocytosis is active. Failure to detect secreted products could indicate defects in exocytosis or defects in the sequence between synthesis, maturation in the golgi, and formation of storage vesicles. Northern blots or RT-PCR on biopsy samples could reveal whether mRNA transcription has occurred successfully. Tissue samples might also indicate whether the peptide was synthesized. However, depletion of circulating levels (e.g., of peptide hormones, coagulation factors, or albumin) could simply mean enhanced uptake and degradation in some tissue beds.

Pulse labeling an organ with radiolabeled essential amino acids followed by either Western blotting or microautoradiography can provide crude estimates of cellular uptake, retention, and incorporation into new proteins. The main problems besides perfusion variables (which can be controlled by using nonmetabolized markers or tracer dyes) are related to metabolic degradation (see also Chapters 57 and 60).

Its is useful to keep in mind that few products of the cell are secreted without the ER–golgi stacks. A notable example is IL-1 (α and β isoforms) (59). These can be useful controls, representing peptide synthesis. The biggest problem that has kept investigators from studying ER–golgi traffic in animals or organs is the multicellular nature of these tissues. If production or secretion of a protein exclusively by a single cell type can be identified, there is no reason why the techniques described for studying ER–golgi and endosomal transport in individual cells could not be applied to arteriovenous gradients in any animal.

References

1. Gray, M. W., Burger, G., and Lang, B. F. (1999). Mitochondrial evolution. *Science* **283,** 1476–1481.
2. Yaffe, M. P. (1999). The machinery of mitochondrial inheritance and behavior. *Science* **283,** 1493–1497.
3. Saraste, M. (1999). Oxidative phosphorylation at the fin de siecle. *Science* **283,** 1488–1493.
4. Jungas, R. L., Halperin, M. L., and Brosnan, J. T. (1992). Quantitative analysis of amino acid oxidation and related gluconeogenesis in humans. *Physiol. Rev.* **72,** 419–448.
5. Rolfe, D. F., and Brown, G. C. (1997). Cellular energy utilization and molecular origin of standard metabolic rate in mammals. *Physiol. Rev.* **77,** 731–758.
6. Hatefi, Y. (1985). The mitochondrial electron transport and oxidative phosphorylation system. *Annu. Rev. Biochem.* **54,** 1015–1069.
7. Reers, M., Smiley, S. T., Mottola-Hartshorn, C., Chen, A., Lin, M., and Chen, L. B. (1995). Mitochondrial membrane potential monitored by JC-1 dye. *Methods Enzymol.* **260,** 406–417.
8. Neupert, W. (1997). Protein import into mitochondria, *Annu. Rev. Biochem.* **66,** 863–917.
9. Lehninger, A. L., Nelson, D. L., and Cox, M. M. (1993). "Principles of Biochemistry," 2nd Ed. Worth Publishers, New York.
10. Hers, H. G., and Hue, L. (1983). Gluconeogenesis and related aspects of glycolysis. *Annu. Rev. Biochem.* **52,** 617–653.
11. Kovacevic, Z., and McGivan, J. D. (1983). Mitochondrial metabolism of glutamine and glutamate and its physiological significance. *Physiol. Rev.* **63,** 547–605.
12. Vanden Hoek, T. L., Becker, L. B., Shao, Z., Li, C., and Schumacker, P. T. (1998). Reactive oxygen species released from mitochondria during brief hypoxia induce preconditioning in cardiomyocytes. *J. Biol. Chem.* **273,** 18092–18098.
13. Wallach, D., Boldin, M., Varfolomeev, E., Beyaert, R., Vandenabeele, P., and Fiers, W. (1997). Cell death induction by receptors of the TNF family: Towards a molecular understanding. *FEBS Lett.* **410,** 96–106.
14. Chakraborti, T., Das, S., Mondal, M., Roychoudhury, S., and Chakraborti, S. (1999). Oxidant, mitochondria and calcium: An overview. *Cell Signal.* **11,** 77–85.
15. Kroemer, G., Dallaporta, B., and Resche-Rigon, M. (1998). The mitochondrial death/life regulator in apoptosis and necrosis. *Annu. Rev. Physiol.* **60,** 619–642.
16. Kiningham, K. K., Oberley, T. D., Lin, S., Mattingly, C. A., and St. Clair, D. K. (1999). Overexpression of manganese superoxide dismutase protects against mitochondrial-initiated poly(ADP-ribose) polymerase-mediated cell death. *FASEB J.* **13,** 1601–1610.
17. Hegardt, F. G. (1999). Mitochondrial 3-hydroxy-3-methylglutaryl-CoA synthase: A control enzyme in ketogenesis. *Biochem. J.* **338,** 569–582.
18. Kallen, C. B., Arakane, F., Christenson, L. K., Watari, H., Devoto, L., and Strauss, J. F., 3rd. (1998). Unveiling the mechanism of action and regulation of the steroidogenic acute regulatory protein. *Mol. Cell. Endocrinol.* **145,** 39–45.
19. Cairns, C. B., Walther, J., Harken, A. H., and Banerjee, A. (1988). Mitochondrial oxidative phosphorylation thermodynamic efficiencies reflect physiological organ roles. *Am. J. Physiol.* **274,** R1376–R1383.
20. Poggetti, R. S., Moore, E. E., Moore, F. A., Koike, K., Tuder, R., Anderson, B. O., and Banerjee, A. (1995). Quantifying oxidative injury in the liver. *Am. J. Physiol.* **268,** G471–G479.
21. Morimoto, T., Ukikusa, M., Taki, Y., Koizumi, K., Yokoo, N., Tanaka, A., Noguchi, M., Yamamoto, S., Nitta, N., Kamiyama, Y., *et al.* (1988). Changes in energy metabolism of allografts after liver transplantation. *Eur. Surg. Res.* **20,** 120–127.
22. Poggetti, R. S., Moore, E. E., Moore, F. A., Bensard, D. D., Parsons, P., Anderson, B. O., and Banerjee, A. (1992). Gut and liver coordinated metabolic response following major torso injury. *J. Surg. Res.* **52,** 27–33.
23. Cairns, C. B., Moore, F. A., Haenel, J. B., Gallea, B. L., Ortner, J. P., Rose, S. J., and Moore, E. E. (1997). Evidence for early supply independent mitochondrial dysfunction in patients developing multiple organ failure after trauma. *J. Trauma* **42,** 532–536.
24. Darley-Usmar, V. M., Rickwood, D., and Wilson, M. T. (1987). "Mitochondria, a Practical Approach." IRL Press, Oxford, Washington, D.C.
25. Takeda, H., and Liu, M. S. (1980). Effect of *Escherichia coli* endotoxin on adenine nucleotide translocation in canine heart mitochondria. *Arch. Biochem. Biophys.* **204,** 153–160.
26. Wallace, D. C. (1999). Mitochondrial diseases in man and mouse. *Science* **283,** 1482–1488.
27. Sies, H. (1982). "Metabolic compartmentation." Academic Press, London, New York.
28. Liu, Y., Sato, T., Seharaseyon, J., Szewczyk, A., O'Rourke, B., and Marban, E. (1999). Mitochondrial ATP-dependent potassium channels. Viable candidate effectors of ischemic preconditioning. *Ann. N.Y. Acad. Sci.* **874,** 27–37.

29. Garlid, K. D., Paucek, P., Yarov-Yarovoy, V., Murray, H. N., Darbenzio, R. B., D'Alonzo, A. J., Lodge, N. J., Smith, M. A., and Grover, G. J. (1997). Cardioprotective effect of diazoxide and its interaction with mitochondrial ATP-sensitive K^+ channels. Possible mechanism of cardioprotection. *Circ. Res.* **81,** 1072–1082.
30. Cleveland, J. C., Jr., Meldrum, D. R., Cain, B. S., Banerjee, A., and Harken, A. H. (1997). Oral sulfonylurea hypoglycemic agents prevent ischemic preconditioning in human myocardium. Two paradoxes revisited [see comments]. *Circulation* **96,** 29–32.
31. Bkaily, G., Jacques, D., and Pothier, P. (1999). Use of confocal microscopy to investigate cell structure and function. *Methods Enzymol.* **307,** 119–135.
32. Rizzuto, R., Carrington, W., and Tuft, R. A. (1998). Digital imaging microscopy of living cells. *Trends Cell Biol.* **8,** 288–292.
33. Bastiaens, P. I., and Squire, A. (1999). Fluorescence lifetime imaging microscopy: Spatial resolution of biochemical processes in the cell. *Trends Cell Biol.* **9,** 48–52.
34. Piston, D. W. (1999). Imaging living cells and tissues by two-photon excitation microscopy. *Trends Cell Biol.* **9,** 66–69.
35. Ellenberg, J., Lippincott-Schwartz, J., and Presley, J. F. (1999). Dual-colour imaging with GFP variants. *Trends Cell Biol.* **9,** 52–56.
36. Diaz, G., Setzu, M. D., Zucca, A., Isola, R., Diana, A., Murru, R., Sogos, V., and Gremo, F. (1999). Subcellular heterogeneity of mitochondrial membrane potential: Relationship with organelle distribution and intercellular contacts in normal, hypoxic and apoptotic cells. *J. Cell Sci.* **112,** 1077–1084.
37. Bereiter-Hahn, J. (1990). Behavior of mitochondria in the living cell. *Int. Rev. Cytol.* **122,** 1–63.
38. Salvioli, S., Ardizzoni, A., Franceschi, C., and Cossarizza, A. (1997). JC-1, but not DiOC6(3) or rhodamine 123, is a reliable fluorescent probe to assess delta psi changes in intact cells: Implications for studies on mitochondrial functionality during apoptosis. *FEBS Lett.* **411,** 77–82.
39. Mermall, V., Post, P. L., and Mooseker, M. S. (1998). Unconventional myosins in cell movement, membrane traffic, and signal transduction. *Science* **279,** 527–533.
40. Hirokawa, N. (1998). Kinesin and dynein superfamily proteins and the mechanism of organelle transport. *Science* **279,** 519–526.
41. De Vos, K., Goossens, V., Boone, E., Vercammen, D., Vancompernolle, K., Vandenabeele, P., Haegeman, G., Fiers, W., and Grooten, J. (1998). The 55-kDa tumor necrosis factor receptor induces clustering of mitochondria through its membrane-proximal region. *J. Biol. Chem.* **273,** 9673–9680.
42. Farquhar, M. G., and Palade, G. E. (1998). The Golgi apparatus: 100 years of progress and controversy. *Trends Cell Biol.* **8,** 2–10.
43. Alberts, B. (1994). "Molecular Biology of the Cell," 3rd Ed. Garland Publishing, New York.
44. Greenfield, L. J., and Mulholland, M. W. (1997). Surgery: Scientific Principles and Practice," 2nd Ed. Lippincott-Raven Publishers, Philadelphia.
45. Meldrum, D. R., and Donnahoo, K. K. (1999). Role of TNF in mediating renal insufficiency following cardiac surgery: Evidence of a post-bypass cardiorenal syndrome. *J. Surg. Res.* **85,** 185–199.
46. Lefkowitz, R. J. (1998). G protein-coupled receptors. III. New roles for receptor kinases and beta-arrestins in receptor signaling and desensitization. *J. Biol. Chem.* **273,** 18677–18680.
47. Lichtman, S. N., Wang, J., and Lemasters, J. J. (1998). Lipopolysaccharide-stimulated TNF-alpha release from cultured rat Kupffer cells: Sequence of intracellular signaling pathways. *J. Leukoc. Biol.* **64,** 368–372.
48. Haas, A. (1998). Reprogramming the phagocytic pathway—intracellular pathogens and their vacuoles (review). *Mol. Membr. Biol.* **15,** 103–121.
49. Carrasco, L. (1994). Entry of animal viruses and macromolecules into cells. *FEBS Lett.* **350,** 151–154.
50. Bonfanti, L., Mironov, A. A., Jr., Martinez-Menarguez, J. A., Martella, O., Fusella, A., Baldassarre, M., Buccione, R., Geuze, H. J., Mironov, A. A., and Luini, A. (1998). Procollagen traverses the Golgi stack without leaving the lumen of cisternae: Evidence for cisternal maturation [see comments]. *Cell* **95,** 993–1003.
51. Zeng, Y., Pan, Y. T., Asano, N., Nash, R. J., and Elbein, A. D. (1997). Homonojirimycin and *N*-methyl-homonojirimycin inhibit N-linked oligosaccharide processing. *Glycobiology* **7,** 297–304.
52. Pfeffer, S. R. (1999). Transport-vesicle targeting: Tethers before SNAREs. *Nature Cell Biol.* **1,** E17–E22.
53. Nuoffer, C., and Balch, W. E. (1994). GTPases: Multifunctional molecular switches regulating vesicular traffic. *Annu. Rev. Biochem.* **63,** 949–990.
54. Schimmoller, F., Simon, I., and Pfeffer, S. R. (1998). Rab GTPases, directors of vesicle docking. *J. Biol. Chem.* **273,** 22161–22164.
55. Martinez, O., and Goud, B. (1998). Rab proteins. *Biochim. Biophys. Acta* **1404,** 101–112.
56. Bannykh, S. I., Nishimura, N., and Balch, W. E. (1998). Getting into the Golgi. *Trends Cell Biol.* **8,** 21–25.
57. Lippincott-Schwartz, J. (1998). Cytoskeletal proteins and Golgi dynamics. *Curr Opin. Cell Biol.* **10,** 52–59.
58. Corvera, S., D'Arrigo, A., and Stenmark, H. (1999). Phosphoinositides in membrane traffic, *Curr. Opin. Cell Biol.* **11,** 460–45.
59. Dinarello, C. A. (1996). Biologic basis for interleukin-1 in disease. *Blood* **87,** 2095–2147.

25

Membrane Biology and Biophysics

Raphael C. Lee*,† and Jurgen Hannig*

**Pritzker School of Medicine, The University of Chicago, Chicago, Illinois 60637*
†Burn Center, St. Mary's Medical Center, Hobart, Indiana 46342

I. Medical Relevance

A significant part of the energy required to sustain cellular function is expended in maintaining the large differences in electrolyte ion concentrations across the cell membrane. The lipid bilayer, formed through the spontaneous self-assembly of amphiphilic phospholipids, provides the necessary ionic diffusion barrier that makes it energetically possible to maintain large transmembrane ion concentration gradients. The lipid bilayer serves this role remarkably well by establishing a nonpolar region through which an ion must pass to cross the membrane. Because water is one of the most polar substances on Earth, the energy, referred to as the Born energy, required to move a hydrated ion from the aqueous phase into the nonpolar lipid phase is extremely high, ranging between 68 and 100 k_BT. Here k_B is the Boltzman constant and T is the absolute temperature in Kelvin. This is reflective of the strong impediment to passive ion diffusion across the lipid bilayer (1). However, cell membranes typically include 30% protein. Many membrane proteins facilitate and regulate membrane ion transport, including the gated ion-selective channels, ionic pumps, or other hydrophilic transport pathways. These protein effects combine to make the mammalian cell membrane approximately 10^6 times more conductive to ions compared to the pure lipid bilayer (2).

The mammalian cell membrane lipid bilayer is a two-dimensional structured fluid. It is held intact only by differential hydration forces. There are no chemical bonds. Phospholipids exhibit rotational and lateral diffusion within the plane of the membrane. Occasionally, small separations in the lipid packing order occur, producing transient structural defects that have lifetimes on the order of nanoseconds. This is sufficient to permit passage of small solutes, including water. The lifetime and size of these transient pores are influenced by temperature, the electric field strength in the membrane, and polymers that adsorb onto the membrane interface.

The structural integrity of the lipid bilayer component of the cell membrane is essential for facilitating the maintenance of physiological transmembrane ionic concentration gradients at a metabolic energy cost that is affordable. Despite the effectiveness of the lipid bilayer in restricting diffusive ionic transport, approximately 85–95% of cellular metabolic energy is used to maintain the gradients by specialized ion pumps. The sodium–potassium pump may serve as an example. It simultaneously transports potassium into and sodium out of the cell, against the transmembrane ionic concentration gradients, with ATP as the energy source.

It is ironic that despite its critical role in supporting life, the lipid bilayer is quite fragile in comparison to other biologic macromolecular structures. Permeabilization and disruption of the membrane lipid bilayer is a major component of massive radiation injury, reperfusion injury, thermal burns, frostbite, electrical shock, and many other forms of trauma-mediated tissue injury. Thus, the biology and biophysics of cell membrane damage and subsequent sealing are central to the science of surgery.

II. Methodology—General Considerations

One of the basic biologic design considerations, which is reflected in successful adaptation of biologic systems, is "operating temperature." Across the animal kingdom, cell membrane composition is found to be dependent on the temperature range in the species' habitat. Thus, proper choice of an *in vitro* cell model to match the system of interest is an important consideration in surgical research. Furthermore, experimental conditions must be tightly temperature controlled. For example, thresholds for transmembrane ionic diffusion are very temperature dependent. The same is true for other biophysical phenomena, such as membrane receptor binding and cross-link kinetics. Finally, binding of membranes to surfaces or to solutes in the bathing media can have a major impact on physical state of the lipid bilayer and thus influence measurements. It is reasonable to expect that the kinetics of all processes that depend on membrane protein and lipid movement will change when the cell environment temperature changes.

III. Methodology—Assessing Membrane Integrity

Structural integrity of the cell membrane governs its transport properties. The extent of structural alteration of the membrane is reflected in the kinetics and molecular size of the solutes that permeate it. Assessment of the transport properties of the cell membrane is commonly made by measurement of the kinetics of transmembrane transport of various tracers. Tracers in this case means substances that can be located inside or outside the cell and can be quantified or have their transmembrane movement monitored, either qualitatively or quantitatively. Radioisotope-labeled molecules, absorbent or fluorescent molecules, and charge-carrying atoms (ions) fall into this category.

Transmembrane transport studies can be performed either on artificial membrane systems (pure lipid bilayers) or cellular membranes that typically contain 30–40% protein by weight. There are advantages and limitations to either method.

A. Membrane Systems

1. Lipid Bilayer Models

Large varieties of pure lipids [e.g., dipalmitoylphosphatidylethanolamine (DPPE)] and of lipid mixtures [e.g., egg phosphatidylcholine (egg-PC)] are readily obtained from specialized vendors. Obviously, lipid bilayers provide a simplified model of a cellular membrane because any "impurities" in the form of proteins are missing. Nevertheless, if for a particular cell type the lipid composition of its membrane is known, mixed lipid bilayers can be produced that mimic quite closely the lipid bilayer sections of the cell membrane. If desired, even the cholesterol content (by weight percent) can be adjusted. Artificial lipid bilayers can be produced either planar (lamellar bilayers) or spherical (lipid vesicles or liposomes).

a. Planar Lipid Bilayers Typically, a planar bilayer is formed across an aperture in a hydrophobic partition separating two aqueous compartments. There are two simple ways to get the lipids to form the bilayer across the hole:

1. Dissolve the amphiphilic lipids in an appropriate organic solvent and "paint" this over the aperture; the resulting planar film forms a bilayer with the hydrophilic head groups pointing toward both aqueous compartments (3).
2. The two aqueous compartments are filled just below the hole; lipids are added to both compartments, forming a monolayer on the air–water interface, and then the water level is raised above the hole, causing each monolayer to cover its side of the hydrophobic hole in the partition, leaving a planar bilayer (folding method, Fig. 1) (4).

Using the second method a destroyed bilayer can easily be reformed by lowering and again raising the water level in the two compartments, allowing repetitive measurements under similar conditions. Because in both cases the planar lipid bilayer separates two hydrophilic compartments, transport measurements across the bilayer can easily be performed by adding the desired tracer into one side and observing its appearance on the other under the conditions to be tested.

b. Vesicles or Liposomes Multiple methods have been described to produce lipid vesicles in aqueous environments. For a systematic review, see the work of Szoka and Papahadjopoulos (5). In general, the idea is to create a large interface between the lipid and the aqueous phase. An example is the "peeling" method. Lipids (pure or mixed) dried onto the inner surface of a glass flask by organic solvent evaporation are dissolved by repeatedly rinsing the surface with a small amount of water. The result is multi-

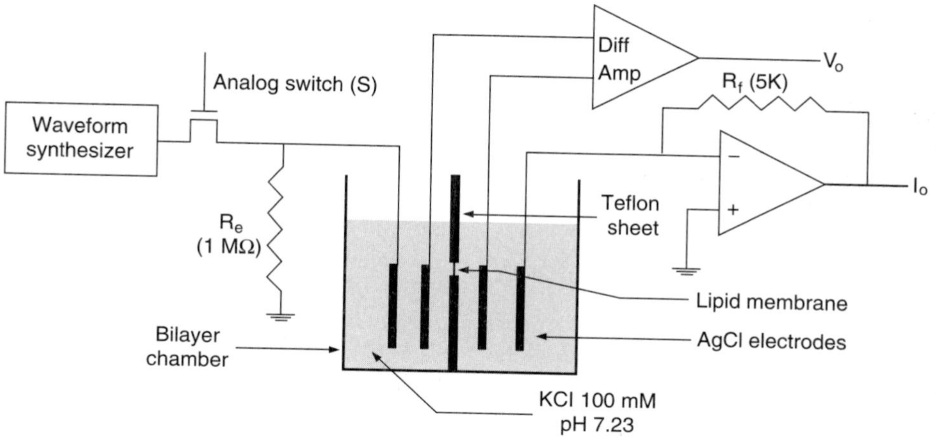

Figure 1 Schematic illustration of voltage clamp setup of a lipid bilayer formed across a hole in the Teflon sheet using the folding method (see text). Two of the four Ag–AgCl electrodes were used to measure the transmembrane voltage V_0 and the other two were used to apply voltage pulses for electroporation experiments and successive transmembrane current I_0 measurements. From Sharma *et al.* (14), with permission.

lamellar liposomes consisting of many concentric water compartments separated from each other by lipid bilayers. For many physical studies, including transmembrane transport, it is more appropriate and useful to employ unilamellar vesicles (UVs) having only a single continuous lipid bilayer enclosing an aqueous volume. There are again a number of methods available for the preparation of UVs from multilamellar vesicles. Prolonged ultrasonic irradiation is the most commonly used technique to produce a dispersion of small UVs (SUVs) with radii of 10–50 nm. Repeated freezing and thawing of SUVs in solution is widely used to create large UVs (LUVs), up to 1 mm, as desired.

Tracers can be introduced into the vesicles by adding them to the aqueous phase, so that they are entrapped during the vesicle formation. If the "natural" transbilayer transport kinetics of the tracer is slow enough, the composition of the aqueous phase outside the vesicles can be changed by dialysis. Sufficient removal e.g., of all ions from the solution for conductance measurements requires at least 24 hr using a tightly timed dialysis buffer exchange schedule (at least three times). Centrifugation of the vesicles and supernatant exchange can be applied when the transmembrane transport is in the range of minutes. Typically, monosaccharides are used as a substitute for ionic solutes to maintain isoosmolality.

A disadvantage of vesicles can be, depending on the experiments to be performed, their size dispersion and, depending on the lipid(s) used, their mechanical instability. Centrifugation, for example, is known to sometimes reproduce multilamellar vesicles and change size dispersion. The mechanical instability can cause the tracer to leak in (or out) during vesicle fusion and separation.

2. Cellular Membranes

Although artificial bilayers serve as a well-defined model for the lipid bilayer properties of a cell membrane, only investigations on natural cellular membranes include the complexity of mixed protein–lipid bilayer interactions. Most transport studies are performed in isolated cells *in vitro*, but a few methods are feasible for *in vivo* studies as well.

a. In Vitro Models Generally, *in vitro* transport studies can be separated into two major categories: (1) cells studied as a large population, expressing results by means of percentage of cells; and (2) studies on single cells, providing access to kinetic and quantitative data that are then averaged over several cells. Whichever system is chosen depends on the particular experimental method. Large population studies are preferably performed on proliferating cell lines cultivated in one's own laboratory to fulfill the demand of, e.g., dye-exclusion-based live/dead assays or flow cytometric studies (see Section III, B, 2). Although all sorts of very fine instrumentation for microscopic use is available, for single-cell studies the cell object is preferably large in size, e.g., quantitative fluorescence dye loss of myocytes (6).

b. In Vivo Models Many of the methods available to study membrane transport *in vitro* are not suitable for *in vivo* studies because of physical constraints. Light-based measurements, for instance, have only a very limited depth (think of a laser doppler flow meter). Again, *in vivo* studies can generally be separated into two groups: (1) noninvasive methods such as clinical diagnostic spectroscopy and (2) nonsurvival studies whereby a particular tracer is detected histopathologically. The first methods allow time-resolved survival studies to monitor damage progression and healing. Histopathologic tissue analysis postmortem often provides only "yes/no" answers to a problem and quantitative analysis is rarely possible (slide ranking by blinded pathologist). We therefore prefer noninvasive diagnostic spectroscopy, including quantitative image analysis, and use histology for qualitative damage conformation purposes.

B. Techniques to Assess Membrane Integrity

The basic strategy to assess membrane transport properties is to measure the transport of tracer molecules across the membrane. The tracers are typically charged. Because of the Born energy barrier, charged probes do not readily permeate an intact membrane. In addition, they are too large to permeate gated ion channels. Rather, they traverse the cell membrane through transient aqueous pores in the membrane. Deficiencies in the structural integrity of a membrane lead to either increase in number or enlargement of these transient pores, observed by an enhanced intracellular accumulation or increased uptake kinetics of these molecules.

1. Tracers

a. In Vitro Models The general strategy for studying transmembrane transport with tracers *in vitro* consists of adding a quantitatively known amount of the ionic, membrane-impermeable, labeled substance into the suspension medium (before or shortly after the physicochemical membrane insult), separation of the vesicles or cells from the medium after a certain amount of time by centrifugation, and quantitative analysis of the activity remaining in the removed supernatant and in the resuspended vesicles or cells. The tracer can be a spin-labeled or radioactive substance. The activity can be determined quantitatively by either electron spin resonance (ESR) or scintigraphy, where by the radioactivity in a fluid is converted into a proportional fluorescence signal (scintillation counter). If cells have been grown attached to a culture plate, their radioactive uptake can be determined by exposing a film with the plate, with successive gray-scale image analysis, providing quantitative data. An example of a radioactive test substance is ^{45}Ca for indication of ion homeostasis loss due to membrane permeabilization.

If the incubation time of the vesicles or cells with the radioactive substance is kept constant, the amount of radioactivity found in the vesicles or cells is proportional to the membrane diffusivity of the compound, which in turn depends on the structural integrity of the membrane. Varying the incubation time under otherwise constant conditions allows determination of the transmembrane diffusion kinetic.

b. In Vivo Models For *in vivo* measurements ionic tracers are injected into the subject after the physicochemical insult and the region of interest is imaged after a few hours, using the appropriate instrument: gamma camera for gamma-emitting, typically short-lived, radiotracers such as ^{99m}Tc; magnetic resonance imaging for image contrast enhancers such as gadolinium-labeled agents; and ESR for spin-labeled compounds. The activities remaining in the tissue (proportional to the amounts of tracer captured within the cell) are indications for the amount of cell membrane damage (7, 8). Uptake kinetics can be monitored by taking serial images over several hours after the injection. The serial images are converted into time–activity curves (TACs) using commercial or purpose-written image analysis programs. Typically, such TACs show an exponential decline of the activity in the tissue due to kidney clearance. The kinetics of the decline and the activity remaining in the tissue are again indications of the degree of cell membrane damage (7, 9).

In the case of radiolabeled tracers, another option is to track their accumulation in the tissue postmortem by dissecting and fixing the appropriate tissue through immediate deep freezing. Thin thaw-mounted histologic slices can be "imaged" with photographic emulsion-coated slides (10) and analyzed as described in detail by Stumpf and Solomon (11). As stated above, quantitative histopathologic tissue analysis is not easy and here the precision of the tracer localization on the cellular level is, in addition, dependent on the granularity of the emulsion.

A more indirect variation of tracer detection is the use of reporter genes. Once the gene is able to permeate the membrane due to structural deficiencies it is expressed in the cell. Depending on the gene, uptake can be monitored as resistivity to antibiotics, antibody binding after membrane protein expression, or certain enzymatic activities (e.g., luciferase).

2. Fluorescence

a. In Vitro Models Two basic approaches are used: measuring dye transport into the cells and dye transport out of the cells. When measuring dye transport into the cells, the methods used are similar to the tracer methods described above. Fluorescent cells can be either counted using a microscope on the basis of percentage fluorescent/nonfluorescent or, more quantitatively, by flow cytometry. A classical example is the dye-exclusion-based assay that uses membrane permeabilization as the ultimate result of cell death to distinguish between live/dead status. Dyes used in this category include trypan blue (blue indicates cell death) and ethidium bromide (red fluorescence, death). In some cases, the sensitivity of the assay is enhanced due to the binding of the fluorescent molecules to intracellular molecules such as DNA, which is associated with a drastic increase of fluorescence intensity and is very distinguishable from the faint fluorescent background. More accurate live/dead assays use double-fluorescence staining, as shown in Fig. 2. Here, a mem-

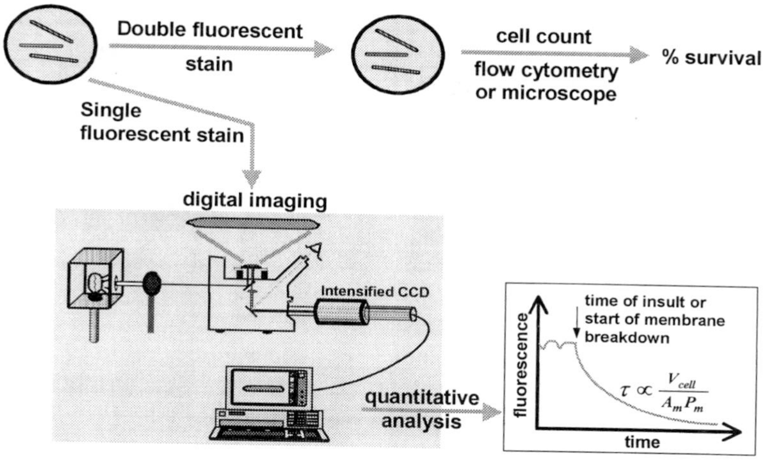

Figure 2 Schematic illustration of membrane permeability studies based on either double-fluorescence live/dead assays or quantitative fluorescence dye leakage measurements using digital microscopic image analysis (gray inset). Generally, the fluorescence intensity integrated over the entire cell decreases exponentially with time. Curve fitting provides a value for the time-constant τ for the dye leakage. For a given cell with the volume V_{cell} and the membrane area A_{m}, τ is a measure of the cell membrane's permeability P_{m} to the dye.

brane-permeant dye precursor (calcein-AM) is converted inside living cells to the green fluorescent dye calcein by ATP-requiring nonspecific esterases (green indicates living cells); dead cells take up the normally nonpermeant fluorescence dye (red, cell death). A large variety of these dyes are commercially available, and very detailed descriptions on their use can be found in the catalogs.

To measure fluorescent dye efflux from cells, normally membrane-impermeant dyes can be loaded into intact cells in three ways: (1) transient permeabilization of the membrane (e.g., scrape loading of cells in monolayer culture or by electroporation), (2) esterification of the charged side groups with a nonpolar moiety that will be cleaved by many different ATP-requiring esterases in the cytoplasm, and (3) transfection of the cell with genes for fluorescent proteins. All three methods are commonly employed. Once the fluorescent probe is loaded into the cytoplasm, dye leakage can be measured by flow cytometry at certain time intervals or by integrating the point (i.e., pixel) intensities within a single cell boundary using quantitative two-dimensional light microscopy (Fig. 2, gray inset). Techniques of quantitative fluorescence microscopy are well developed and are reviewed in depth in microscopy literature (12). Confocal methods can be used to separate out image information from a specific object plane perpendicular to the central optical path (13).

A break in membrane structural integrity is followed by diffusion of the fluorescent molecules out of the cell. This is manifested by a decrease in the intracellular fluorescence intensity. If the concentration of the fluorophore is high enough such that all protein binding is saturated, meaning there is an excess of fluorophore available for diffusion, then the transport kinetics reflects the membrane permeability to the fluorophore. One type of such experiment is further described in Section IV,A.

3. Electrical Measurements

a. In Vitro Models Electrical measurements across a planar lipid bilayer can easily be performed by placing two electrodes into the aqueous compartments on each side of the hydrophobic partition containing the bilayer (see Section III,A,1). Two circuitry methods are commonly used. In the charge-pulse method the membrane is very quickly charged through ion accumulation on its surface by applying a short direct current pulse, and the decay of the induced transmembrane voltage is monitored. Increased bilayer permeability to ions is indicated by shorter decay times. The second method requires a more complex circuitry and is called a voltage clamp. Here, a constant voltage is applied across the bilayer and the current measured is dependent on the permeability of the bilayer to ions (14). Using specific, commercially available, ion-sensitive electrodes, the permeability to a particular ion can be determined. This setup is suitable for electric field-mediated membrane permeabilization as shown in Fig. 1, less suitable for irradiation-induced permeabilization, and even less suitable for heat-damage investigations, because the two compartments do not easily allow for controlled, rapid temperature rise. Salt-filled vesicles have been used to study ion efflux from vesicle suspensions after electroporation (15). Measurements require a low-conductive suspension medium to increase the sensitivity to changes in the conductance across the suspension (see Section III,A,1).

Time-resolved measurements of the conductance allow determination of the degree of permeabilization and, if the ion concentration in the medium never reaches an equilibrium with the concentration inside the cell, the resealing kinetics of the pores after the membrane damage. As for electrical measurements on planar bilayers, this method is best suited to assess electric field-mediated membrane damage.

The first challenge in measuring ion transport properties of natural cellular membranes *in vitro* is to decide which solutes are of interest to the research question. If the substance is an ion that can pass through membrane ion channels, then it is critical to distinguish which transmembrane pathways are to be investigated. Voltage-gated and ligand-gated channels typically have high specificity for a specific ion species. To eliminate their effect on transmembrane transport, they can often be blocked with toxins that bind strongly to these channels and block passage of the specific ion species. For example, voltage-gated K^+ channels can be blocked with tetraethylammonium (TEA), voltage-gated Na^+ channels can be blocked using tetrodotoxin (TTX), and calcium channels can be blocked with cobalt. There are other specific ion channel blockers as well. With the gated channels blocked it is possible to measure transport of ions through the remainder of the membrane.

The electrode placement, particularly inside a small cell, is challenging as well. Typically, a microelectrode, insulated by a very fine glass capillary, is inserted into the cell under the microscope and the counter electrode is placed into the suspension medium. A slightly different approach uses a glass capillary, which is softly placed against the cell membrane, and by applying a very brief vacuum burst the membrane area covering the capillary end is ripped out of the membrane. By filling the capillary beforehand with a desired solution and an electrode wire, this capillary can be dipped carefully into any solution containing the counter electrode, creating a setup similar to that for the planar bilayer method described above.

A much more elegant setup, the double petroleum jelly gap chamber shown in Fig. 3, has been described by Chen and Lee (16). Elongated cells, here isolated myocytes, are placed across two petroleum jelly bridges that divide the cell bath. By adding a mild surfactant to the solution in the connected outer compartments, the cell membranes at both ends are dissolved. This results in a setup wherein the outer compartment fluid is connected to the cytoplasm and the solution in the center compartment is separated from it only by the cell membrane (= interstitial fluid), allowing quite easy electrode placement for ion transport measurements. Although so far used only for the investigation of electroporation, this method could be adapted to test other membrane damage mechanisms.

b. In Vivo Models In tissue, resistivity measurements can be, in principle, used to follow cell membrane permeabilization as the resistivity decreases when the intracellular fluid contributes to current flow. But the electrode placement is invasive and causes side effects that are difficult to control. Bhatt *et al.* (17) employed impedance measurements to isolated muscle flaps in electrical injury experiments.

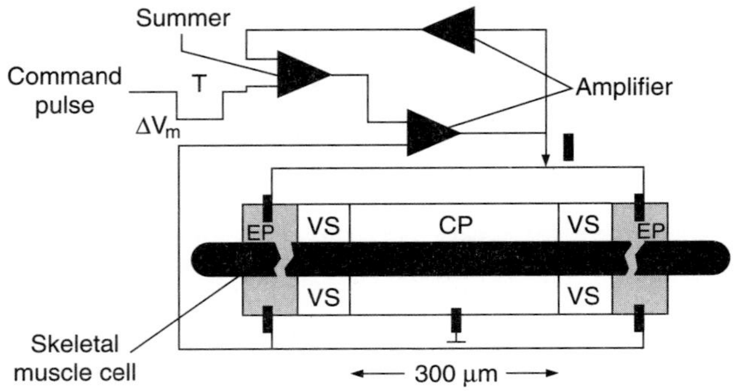

Figure 3 Schematic illustration of a skeletal muscle cell in the double petroleum jelly gap voltage clamp arrangement. The central pool (CP) and end pools (EP) are separated by the petroleum jelly seal (VS). Voltage monitoring and current injection for electroporation experiments occur at both ends.

A more elegant method uses neurophysiologic measurements. Because nerve signal transport and muscle stimulus are dependent on induced transmembrane potentials, an ion-permeable membrane does not conduct the signal. Thus motor nerve and sensory nerve functions are decreased after cell membrane damage. Stimulating surface electrodes based on magnetic field pulses and surface recording electrodes provide a noninvasive methodology for these tests and have high sensitivity to membrane barrier function damage.

IV. Cell Membrane Injury

A. Heat-Mediated Membrane Permeabilization

Cell membrane disruption can be caused by exposure to supraphysiologic temperatures (18–21). It has been well demonstrated that at temperatures in excess of 42.5°C, structural alteration of mammalian membranes develops. Employing membrane transport experiments based on the dye leakage technique, Cravalho *et al.* (22) subjected cells loaded with the cell membrane-impermeant fluorescent dye carboxyfluorescein to a series of temperature-clamp experiments. These fluorescence-labeled cells were brought to room temperature equilibrium, then the temperature was suddenly elevated from room temperature to 45°, 50°, 55°, and 60°C using a custom temperature-clamp epifluorescent microscopy stage. The fluorescence intensity of a cell was monitored during the exposure protocol and changes in the cell membrane permeability were quantified by digital video image analysis as illustrated in Fig. 2. The investigators found that the higher the temperature, the more rapidly the dye left the cytoplasm, suggesting that the extent of membrane damage was temperature dependent. These results were later corroborated by Bischof *et al.* (23) using the same technique.

B. Electroporation

Electric field-mediated membrane permeabilization, a result of field-induced supranatural transmembrane potential, is now widely used as an application to introduce foreign molecules, such as DNA, cytostatica, and antibodies, into cells by overcoming the natural diffusion barrier. Although electroporation is widely used, the precise mechanism is still under intense investigation using almost all of the above-described techniques. Sharma *et al.* measured electrically induced planar bilayer breakdown using both charge-pulse and voltage-clamp techniques (14). Gift and Weaver's flow cytometric quantifications of calcein uptake by yeast cells after electroporation exemplify fluorescent dye uptake (24). Kakorin and Neumann used salt-filled vesicle and cell electroporation in a low-conductive medium to measure the kinetics of pore formation and resealing as well as bilayer deformations (25). Gowrishankar *et al.* used the double petroleum jelly gap chamber and the voltage-clamp technique to investigate membrane permeabilization of isolated skeletal muscle cells and their pore sealing kinetics (26).

Besides these fundamental mechanistic investigations, *in vivo* electroporation has attracted major interest for two reasons: (1) electric field-induced membrane permeabilization has been identified as a major cause of tissue damage in electrical shock victims, in addition to heat damage (Joule heating), and (2) the electric field-enhanced delivery of cytostatica into tumors, and genes into skeletal muscle tissue, show promising therapeutic results.

Block *et al.* (9) and Matthew *et al.* (7) measured electric field-induced membrane damage in hind limb muscle tissue using an *in vivo* rat model in which nonthermal direct current electrical pulses (4 msec duration, 2 A, 150 V/cm) were applied through cuff-type electrodes placed on the ankle and the tail. They used the radiotracer ^{99m}Tc pyrophosphate (and others), which is known to follow calcium, and monitored tissue uptake and retention using a small custom-made gamma camera (7, 9, 27). Their results indicate that the tissue damage, as seen by increased tracer uptake in the shocked hind limb, is electric field dose dependent. The increase in tracer uptake is a consequence of cell membrane permeabilization, leading to calcium and tracer flux into the damaged cells. The tissue damage in this *in vivo* electrical injury model has been confirmed qualitatively by hypercontraction band formation apparent in histologic sections. Using the same *in vivo* model, it was also shown that contrast-enhanced magnetic resonance imaging (MRI) can be used to diagnose the extent of tissue damage, based on the increase in contrast agent distribution volume when the cells become electroporated (8).

In electrochemotherapy the membrane structural damage caused by the applied electric field is actually desired to achieve enhanced drug delivery into tumor cells. Invasive needle arrays for deep or flat electrode pairs for subcutaneous tumors have been used *in vivo* and the extent of membrane damage is assessed by either tumor cell survival or reporter gene expression (28, 29). Gene delivery methods to treat muscle disorders and for the systemic secretion of therapeutic proteins have also used the reporter gene and radiotracer techniques (30, 31).

C. ROS-Mediated Membrane Lysis

Another important factor in the structural integrity of the cell membrane is the three-dimensional structure of the lipid molecule that allows the condensed self-assembly necessary to achieve restricted diffusive ionic transport. Mammalian membrane phospholipids usually contain unsaturated fatty acid residues, which can be subject to peroxidation. Membrane lipid peroxidation by reactive oxygen species (ROS) is presumed to be the basic mechanism of radiation and ischemia reperfusion-induced membrane permeability.

Numerous studies have produced results indicating that cell membrane peroxidation is an important mechanism of cell damage from ionizing irradiation (32). Both major constituents of cell membranes, phospholipids and proteins, are affected by exposure to ionizing irradiation. The relative contribution of damage to each component to cell membrane radiopermeabilization remains to be defined and is perhaps cell type specific. Both effects are mediated by superoxide free-radical interactions, leading to structural changes of the membrane constituents. Subsequent permeabilization of the plasma membrane has been well documented using a large variety of the transport methodologies, as described above. A few examples are given below.

Konings (33) irradiated bovine erythrocytes and measured efflux amounts of cytoplasmic K^+ (up to 50%) by flame photometry, and hemoglobin spectrophotometrically, in the supernatant. Gwozdzinski *et al.* (34) and Jozwiak (35) measured the irradiation-induced permeability of erythrocyte membranes by following the transport of spin-labeled anionic, cationic, and nonelectrolyte compounds into the cells. In another study Konings (36) employed trypan blue influx measurements to characterize the irradiation dose-membrane permeabilization relationship in lymphocytes. Canaday *et al.* performed kinetic fluorescent dye efflux studies on irradiated isolated skeletal muscle cells after loading them with the neutral membrane-permeable precursor calcein-AM (6).

Ischemia reperfusion injuries such as myocardial infarction, cerebrovascular stroke, cerebral palsy from difficult childbirth, and testicular torsion represent another large group of injuries in which cell membrane permeability increases are based on reactive oxygen species production.

V. Sealing of Permeabilized Membranes

At present, the most promising compounds for therapeutic use in resealing membrane "pores" caused by any of the above-described physicochemical insults are in a class of triblock copolymers of propylene oxide and ethylene oxide. Propylene oxide, having a tertiary methyl group, is relatively hydrophobic, whereas the ethylene oxide is more hydrophilic. By manipulation of the relative proportions of the ethylene/propylene oxide content as well as their location and arrangement in a compound, it is possible to control the physical properties of the molecule (37).

As an initial attempt to understand the physical properties important in allowing these molecules to act as membrane sealants, our research has focused on the hydrophile/hydrophobe ratio. To date only one poloxamer has been tested extensively in terms of its efficacy in sealing "electropores," poloxamer 188. We base our discussion on this molecule. Poloxamer 188 has 75 ethylene oxide (EO) units on either side (MW, 3317) of 30 propylene oxide (PO) units (MW, 1710), for a total molecular weight of approximately 8400. Poloxamer 188 is a solid at room temperature and dissolves in buffer to form a stock solution of 100 mg/ml. It is suggested that the therapeutically relevant concentration is around 1 mg/ml, which is its critical micelle concentration—the concentration at which micelles spontaneously form. By taking the C–C bond to be 1.75 Å, and the C–O bond length to be 1.35 Å, we see that each poly ethylene oxide and each poly propylene oxide subunit is about 3 Å. Thus, each molecule has a 210 Å hydrophilic chain on either side of a 90 Å (but bulky) hydrophobic chain. Like other nonionic surfactants, it seems that the poloxamers do not interact with normal, undamaged cell membranes. Instead, they form small micelles in solution or, alternatively, single molecule structures in which the hydrophilic part wraps around the hydrophobic part. A proposed mechanism of action is that the poloxamer interacts with the cell when membrane exposes hydrophobic domains.

In order to determine the mechanism of poloxamer 188 action and whether utilizing solely the hydrophobic or hydrophilic portions of poloxamer 188 was sufficient to arrest calcein leakage, *in vitro* heat injury experiments were conducted with polyethylene glycol (PEG) at 20 mg/ml and polypropylene glycol (PPG) at 10 mg/ml. PEG was used at a concentration of 20 mg/ml in order to appropriately represent each poloxamer 188 molecule containing two hydrophilic ethylene oxide tails at a concentration of 10 mg/ml. Neither PEG nor PPG alone was able to arrest or even retard calcein leakage as effectively as poloxamer 188 at 42° and 50°C. This suggests that both the hydrophilic and hydrophobic portions of poloxamer 188 must function together to arrest calcein leakage (22).

This study has demonstrated the effectiveness of poloxamer 188 in arresting and retarding transmembrane calcein leakage from skeletal muscle cells exposed to 40°–60°C. The specificity of poloxamer 188 was demonstrated by the ineffectiveness of neutral dextran in arresting calcein leakage as compared to poloxamer 188. Other studies, which showed the ineffectiveness of PPG and PEG as compared to poloxamer 188, suggested that both the hydrophilic and hydrophobic components of poloxamer 188 were needed to arrest calcein leakage. It is noteworthy to mention that, in this study, cells were exposed to poloxamer 188 just prior to the thermal insult. Obviously, this is not the case for the clinical application, and further studies should investigate the efficacy of poloxamer 188 infused following a thermal insult. Nevertheless, the success of poloxamer 188 in sealing thermally damaged cell membranes is very encouraging and certainly merits additional investigation to determine the precise nature of the thermal damage process and the mechanism of poloxamer 188 action. This information should aid in the development of better therapeutic treatment schemes for electrical trauma and burn victims and in the design of more effective copolymer surfactants.

References

1. Parsegian, A. (1969). Energy of an ion crossing a low dielectric membrane: Solutions to four relevant problems. *Nature (London)* **221,** 844–846.
2. Schanne, P. F., and Ceretti, E. R. P. (1978). "Impedance Measurements in Biological Cells." Wiley, New York.
3. Mueller, P., and Rudin, D. O. (1968). Action potentials induced in bimolecular lipid membranes. *Nature (London)* **217,** 713–719.
4. White, S. H. (1986). The physical nature of planar bilayer membranes. *In* "Ion Channels Reconstitution" (C. Miller, ed.), pp. 3–32. Plenum Press, New York.
5. Szoka, F., and Papahadjopoulos, D. (1980). Comparative properties and methods of preparation of lipid vesicles (liposomes). *Annu. Rev. Biophys. Bioeng.* **9,** 467–508.
6. Canaday, D. J., Li, P., Weichselbaum, R., Astumian, R. D., and Lee, R. C. (1994). Membrane permeability changes in gamma-irradiated muscle cells. *Ann. N.Y. Acad. Sci.* **720,** 153–159.
7. Matthews II, K. L., Aarsvold, J. N., Mintzer R. A., Chen, C.-T., Capelli-Schellpfeffer, M., Cooper, M., and Lee, R. C. (1999). Radiotracers for imaging electroporation. *Ann. N.Y. Acad. Sci.* **888,** 285–299.
8. Hannig, J., Kovar, D. A., Abramov, G. S., Zhang, D., Zamora, M., Karczmar, G. S., and Lee, R. C. (1999). Contrast enhanced MRI of electroporation injury. *Proc. First Joint BMES/EMBS Conference, Atlanta, GA, Oct. 13–16* [on CD #1078].
9. Block, T. A., Aarsvold, J. N., Matthews II, K. L., Mintzer, R. A., River, L. P., Capelli-Schellpfeffer, M., Wollmann, R. L., Tripathi, S., Chen, C.-T., and Lee, R. C. (1995). Nonthermally mediated muscle injury and necrosis in electrical trauma. *J. Burn Care Rehabil.* **16**(6), 581–588.

10. Stumpf, W. E. (1976). Techniques for the autoradiography of diffusible compounds. *In* "Methods in Cell Biology" (D. M. Prescott, ed.), pp. 171–193. Academic Press, New York.
11. Stumpf, W. E., and Solomon, H. E., eds. (1994). "Autoradiography and Correlative Imaging." Academic Press, New York.
12. Kohen, E., and Hirschberg, J. G. (1990). "Cell Structure and Function by Microspectrofluorometry." Academic Press, New York.
13. Matsumoto, B., ed. (1993). "Cell Biological Applications of Confocal Microscopy." Academic Press, New York.
14. Sharma, V., Stebe, K., Murphy, J. C., and Tung, L. (1996). Poloxamer 188 decreases susceptibility of artificial lipid membranes to electroporation. *Biophys. J.* **71,** 3229–3241.
15. Kakorin, S., Redeker, E., and Neumann, E. (1996). Electroporative deformation of salt filled vesicles. *Eur. Biophys. J.* **27,** 43–53.
16. Chen, W., and Lee, R. C. (1994). An improved double vaseline gap voltage clamp to study electroporated skeletal muscle fibers. *Biophys. J.* **66,** 700–709.
17. Bhatt, D. L., Gaylor, D. C., and Lee, R. C. (1990). Rhabdomyolysis due to pulsed electric fields. *Plast. Reconstr. Surg.* **86,** 24–34.
18. Moussa, N. A., Tell, E. N., and Cravalho, E. G. (1979). Time progression of hemolysis of erythrocyte populations exposed to supraphysiologic temperatures. *J. Biomech. Eng.* **101,** 213–217.
19. Gershfeld, N. L., and Murayama, M. (1968). Thermal instability of red blood cell membrane bilayers: Temperature dependence of hemolysis. *J. Membr. Biol.* **101,** 62–72.
20. Moussa, N. A., McGrath, J. J., Cravalho, E. G., and Asimacopoulos, P. J. (1977). Kinetics of thermal injury in cells. *J. Biomed. Eng.* **99,** 155–159.
21. Mixter, G., Delhery, Jr., G. P., Derksen, W. L., and Monahan, T. I. (1963). The influence of time on the death of HeLa cells at elevated temperatures. *In* "Temperature: Its Measurement and Control in Science and Industry" (J. D. Hardy, ed.), Vol. 3, pp. 177–182. Reinhold, New York.
22. Cravalho, E. G., Toner, M., Gaylor, D., and Lee, R. C. (1992). Response of cells to supraphysiologic temperatures: Experimental measurements and kinetic models. *In* "Electrical Trauma: The Pathophysiology, Manifestations, and Clinical Management" (R. C. Lee, E. G. Cravalho, and J. F. Burke, eds.), pp. 281–300. Cambridge Univ. Press, Cambridge.
23. Bischof, J. C., Padanilam, J., Holmes, W. H., Ezzell, R. M., Lee, R. C., Tompkins, R. G., Yarmush, M. L., and Toner, M. (1995). Dynamics of cell membrane permeability changes at supraphysiological temperatures. *Biophys. J.* **68**(8), 2608–14.
24. Gift, E. A., and Weaver, J. C. (1995). Observation of extremely heterogeneous electroporative molecular uptake by *Saccharomyces cerevisiae* which changes with electric-field pulse amplitude. *Biochim. Biophys. Acta* **1234**(1), 52–62.
25. Kakorin, S., and Neumann, E. (1998). Kinetics of electroporative deformation of lipid vesicles and biological cells in an electric field. *Ber. Bunsenges. Phys. Chem.* **102,** 670–674.
26. Gowrishankar, T. R., Chen, W., and Lee, R. C. (1998). Non-linear microscale alterations in membrane transport by electropermeabilization. *Ann. N.Y. Acad. Sci.* **858,** 205–16.
27. Aarsvold, J. N., Mintzer, R. A., Yasillo, Y. N., Heimsath, S. J., Block, T. A., Matthews, K. L., Pan, X., Wu, C., Beck, R. N., Chen, C.-T., and Cooper, M. (1994). A miniature gamma camera. *Ann. N.Y. Acad. Sci.* **720,** 192–205.
28. Jaroszeski, M. J., Gilbert, R. A., and Heller, R. (1997). *In vivo* antitumor effects of electrochemotherapy in a hepatoma model. *Biochim. Biophys. Acta* **1334,** 15–18.
29. Mir, L. M., and Orlowski, S. (1999). Mechanisms of electrochemotherapy. *Adv. Drug Deliv. Rev.* **35**(1), 107–118.
30. Mir, L. M., Bureau, M. F., Gehl, J., Rangara, R., Rouy, D., Caillaud, J. M., Delaere, P., Branellec, D., Schwartz, B., and Scherman, D. (1999). High-efficiency gene transfer into skeletal muscle mediated by electric pulses. *Proc. Natl. Acad. Sci. U.S.A.* **96**(8), 4262–4267.
31. Gehl, J., and Mir, M. L. (1999). Determination of optimal parameters for *in vivo* gene transfer by electroporation, using a rapid *in vivo* test for cell permeabilization. *Biochem. Biophys. Res. Commun.* **261,** 377–380.
32. Leyko, W., and Bartosz, G. (1986). Membrane effects of ionizing radiation and hyperthermia. *Int. J. Radiat. Biol.* **49,** 743–770.
33. Konings, A. W. T. (1981). Radiation-induced efflux of potassium ions and haemoglobin in bovine erythrocytes at low doses and low doserates. *Int. J. Radiat. Biol.* **40,** 441–444.
34. Gwozdzinski, K., Bartosz, B., and Leyko, W. (1981). Effect of gamma irradiation on the transport of spin-labeled compounds across the erythrocyte membrane. *Radiat. Environ. Biophys.* **19,** 275–285.
35. Jozwiak, Z. (1983). Effect of ionizing radiation on the transport of spin-labeled compounds across the porcine erythrocyte membrane, II. *Int. J. Radiat. Biol.* **43,** 201–205.
36. Konings, A. W. T. (1984). The involvement of polyunsaturated fatty acid chains of membrane phospholipids to radiation induced cell death of mammalian cells. *In* "Oxygen Radicals in Chemistry and Biology (W. Bors, M. Saran, and D. Tait, eds.), pp. 593–602, Walter de Gruyter, Berlin.
37. Schmolka, I. R. (1994). Physical basis for poloxamer interactions. *Ann. N.Y. Acad. Sci.* **720,** 92–97.

26

Molecular Epidemiology: Beyond Gene Discovery to Clinical Diagnostic Tools

Barbara A. Zehnbauer,* Bradley D. Freeman,† and Timothy G. Buchman†

**Departments of Pediatrics and Pathology and †Department of Surgery, Washington University School of Medicine and *St. Louis Childrens' Hospital, St. Louis, Missouri 63110*

I. Introduction

Molecular variants in genetic markers (alleles) contribute to expression of disease conditions (phenotype). The interplay of environmental factors with this genetic potential (genotype) to determine the range and frequency of expression of clinical disease is the study of genetic epidemiology. Characterization of genotype by molecular methods further defines molecular genetic epidemiology. Included in this discipline (1) are elements of molecular biology diagnostic techniques, epidemiological study design and population characteristics, population genetics to assess allele frequency and association with disease incidence, and biostatistics to determine validity and significance of the correlations among events and genetic traits.

The integrated use of these practices is essential to translating the enormous potential of the gene discoveries of the Human Genome Project into more effective clinical tools for diagnosis, prognosis, treatment, and prevention strategies. These perspectives are required for understanding the complex interactions of the multiple gene products that contribute to the manifestation of common, multigenic human diseases. Although the research field of genetic epidemiology is oriented to gene identification and characterization, it is essential to the characterization of the effects of genes in populations. Incorporating this population perspective is necessary to translate research molecular genetic findings to significant tools in clinical care practice. This chapter outlines the central tenets of implementing molecular genetic testing in medical/surgical care delivery. Another goal of this chapter is to elucidate the current and future importance of molecular genetics to the clinical practice and/or research of surgery and to indicate strengths and weaknesses of current tools.

A. Importance of Molecular Genetics in the Practice/Research of Surgery

The explosion of genetic information from the Human Genome Project investigations easily demonstrates the impact of gene discovery on the practice of medical genetics. Beyond this discipline, identification of multiple genetic factors that contribute to common diseases, presymptomatic diagnosis of inherited and sporadic tumors, and the genetic susceptibility to disease or drug reactions will lend significant genetic tools to the practice of many medical disciplines. How will these genetic discoveries impact the care of the surgical patient? What tools applied in the laboratory can be translated to the bedside? In this chapter we discuss ways in which the genetic diagnosis, prognosis, and predisposition to disease can direct the course of patient care. Definition of genetic terms that will increasingly find their way into other medical disciplines are explained. We emphasize the current and future methodologies of molecular genetics that will facilitate the timely application of genetic analysis in the clinical setting.

B. Background

In order to understand the current and potential impact of clinical molecular genetics on surgical care, it is valuable to distinguish inherited characteristics from acquired characteristics, and gene structure from gene expression. Surgeons deal with a relatively few but important inherited genes linked directly to disease. Examples include breast cancer, Marfan syndrome, lymphoma, medullary thyroid carcinoma (multiple endocrine neoplasia type 2), Von Hippel–Lindau disease, and polycystic kidney disease, among others. The mechanism by which the abnormal allele produces a disease phenotype has been established in many cases. Some alleles cause an abnormal protein to be expressed in normal quantity (multiple endocrine neoplasia type 2). Others cause an abnormal expression level of an otherwise normal protein (β-thalassemia). Deletion of part of a protein, compared to a single amino acid substitution, may create a more severe clinical expression. However a single amino acid substitution at a residue that interacts with a ligand or substrate molecule or a crucial cofactor may also inactivate or reduce the function of the target protein molecule. Although diseases caused by inherited characteristics will continue to be important to surgeons, it now appears that two evolving applications of clinical molecular genetics will be integrated into general surgical care.

The first evolving application relates to oncologic care. It now appears that many if not most solid tumors referred to surgeons for care result from the acquisition of one or more genetic abnormalities. The best-studied example of this process is colorectal cancer, in which acquisition of genetic abnormalities in phenotypically normal tissues appears to predict predisposition to the malignant phenotype (2). Increasingly, surgeons will face the challenge of discerning meaningful from meaningless changes in gene expression. The rapid infiltration of "chip" technology into research laboratories merely presages its extension to clinical use. In this chapter we discuss the strengths and limitations of such analyses.

The second evolving application relates to critical care (3). The complex regimens of drugs administered to critically ill patients predispose to unexpected effects and interactions. Studies begun in the discipline of oncology point to gene-dependent variation in drug metabolism. Such analysis [often termed pharmacogenomics (4)] is presently being tested for extension into the critical care environment. It appears that as few as a dozen genes may determine the metabolic fate of nearly all commonly administered medications in the intensive care unit (ICU).

The surgical investigator (and the surgical clinician) must assimilate genetic information at a high rate. The applicability of a specific technique and the relevance of a particular report are not always clear on initial inspection. Our purpose in this chapter is to provide direction, illuminating common pitfalls and establishing a basis for determining how molecular genetics may integrate into a comprehensive research program.

II. Utility of Molecular Genetic Testing

Molecular genetic testing has applications in diagnosis, in monitoring treatment efficacy to detect minimal residual disease, in stratifying treatment to optimize clinical outcome, in assessing prognostic indicators, and in screening at-risk relatives.

A. Sporadic Tumors

Perhaps the most well-documented utility of genetic testing is reflected in the significant role that clinical molecular pathology of tumors has provided for improvements in diagnosis, prognosis, and monitoring of cancer treatment efficacy. Leukemia and lymphoma are hematologic malignancies frequently classified by the acquired development of specific, clonal gene rearrangements (5) that define diagnostic subgroups. These molecular signatures can be used as markers of minimal residual disease in monitoring treatment efficacy because the genetic variants are characteristic only of tumor cells and do not identify normal cells of the same lineage. Frequently the biologic consequences of the abnormal gene configuration may correlate with prognosis or predict response to treatment. The category of genetic alteration(s) may then be used to stratify patients to different treatment regimens. Tumor cells of follicular lymphoma have reciprocal rearrangements of chromosomes 14 and 18 involving the

BCL2 gene, with a role in apoptosis control. Polymerase chain reaction (PCR) assays provide both identification of the altered DNA in this region and sensitive detection of the molecular signature as evidence of minimal residual disease. This allows specific and sensitive monitoring of treatment efficacy in lymph node, bone marrow, or peripheral blood.

Another example, a form of acute leukemia, acute promyelocytic leukemia (APL), is also diagnosed by a tumor-specific chromosomal and molecular rearrangement, this time involving chromosomes 15 and 17. PCR detection of this aberrant rearrangement identifies patients with leukemia cells that specifically respond to a treatment regimen of all-*trans*-retinoic acid. These patients are stratified to this treatment rather than to routine AML chemotherapy regiments based on the molecular diagnostic detection of the 15 and 17 translocations. One of the genes interrupted by this rearrangement is a receptor for retinoic acid. The biological reasoning is that the retinoic acid treatment stimulates the tumor cells to differentiate to a mature and terminal cell type. Patients with AML without this chromosomal change do not respond to this retinoic acid treatment. Other genetic changes in this same disease, such as loss of specific genetic material, indicate progression to aggressive leukemia subtypes that are less responsive to traditional therapies. Minimal residual APL cells can also be monitored with this PCR methodology.

Genetic characterization of solid tumors is progressing along the lines of the hematologic malignancies. In some gliomas loss of chromosome 1p sequences may be detected by chromosomal loss (fluorescent *in situ* hybridization, FISH) or loss of DNA sequences in tumor cells (PCR loss of heterozygosity, LOH). This loss has been correlated with a better response to therapy and this diagnostic assay serves as a prognostic marker for favorable treatment response. Specific treatment strategies directed toward unusual, tumor-specific patterns of gene expression will be developed.

B. Familial Cancer Syndromes

Inherited predisposition or increased risk for tumor development is a feature of tumors that are specifically observed with higher frequency in particular families—both in multiple individuals and multiple generations. Usually the tumor types observed in affected kindreds exhibit an earlier age of onset compared to sporadic incidences of the same tumor type in the general population. The tumors may also be bilateral or multifocal, depending on the affected organ. These familial cancer syndromes have characteristic genetic mutations in a single gene in all cells of the body, inherited as an autosomal dominant trait. Cancers are observed in target organs when gene function in cells that require the specific gene expression is lost from the first and second alleles of the same gene. This loss of gene function in the tumor tissue defines tumor suppressor gene functions of the altered gene. Loss of both functional copies (alleles) results in a loss of normal growth regulation. The carrier tumor cells develop a proliferative growth advantage over neighboring normal cells, which maintain regulated growth control. For some familial cancer syndromes the types of tumors expressed or the severity of the clinical symptoms can be correlated with particular regions of the gene that contain the mutation or particular types of gene mutations.

An example of an autosomal dominant familial cancer syndrome is multiple endocrine neoplasia type 2 (MEN2). Patients with MEN2A usually develop medullary thyroid carcinoma (MTC; 90%), pheochromocytoma (PHEO; 50%), and/or parathyroid hyperplasia (10–15%). Nearly all (>98%) of families with MEN2 carry a mutation in a single gene, the *RET* protooncogene, usually at one of a number of well-conserved amino acid residues and always as a missense mutation (single-base change) with the result of an amino acid substitution. Diagnosis of the specific missense mutation in the *RET* gene of these patients is more specific and sensitive than the biochemical screening for MTC (pentagastrin stimulation of calcitonin release from hyperplastic C cells of the MTC), particularly in asymptomatic relatives at risk for inheriting MEN2 (6). The genetic assay is not affected by physiologic changes that may raise calcitonin levels in the absence of MTC.

Genotype may also contribute to the definition of the phenotypic expression of the disease (genotype–phenotype correlations). In Von Hippel–Lindau (VHL) disease, which is a syndrome of hypervascularized tumors (including renal cell carcinoma, retinal hemangioma, and/or pheochromocytoma), the type and location of mutations in the VHL gene correlate with the observation of PHEO (7). Most of the mutations in the VHL gene that are associated with PHEO are missense mutations in surface amino acid residues. Other mutations, such as deletions or insertions, which affect the structural integrity of the VHL protein, are rarely observed when PHEOs are part of the diagnosis (8, 8a).

C. Genetic Predisposition Polymorphisms

Future public health roles for molecular genetics will include assessing genetic markers that do not confer constitutional expression of clinical symptoms. Rather these variations demonstrate gene and environment interactions and will be observed only when a carrier individual is challenged with particular environmental agents, drugs, or physiologic stimuli (9).

1. Pharmacogenetics

Probably one of the more exciting future roles of molecular genetics is the identification of genetic markers that predispose carriers to adverse drug reactions or treatment outcomes (4). Adverse drug reactions with genetic basis have been recognized for many years, but only with the more comprehensive definition of gene sequences through the advances of the Human Genome Project has it now become feasible to test for functional genetic polymorphisms affecting the activity of drug-metabolizing enzymes. Cytochrome P450 enzymes metabolize a majority of drugs (10). Polymorphic genetic variations in the genes for these enzymes may abolish, alter quantitatively or qualitatively, or enhance metabolism of drug substrates. As a result, patients may demonstrate lack of drug response attributable to ultrarapid metabolism or failure to convert to the active metabolite. Also observed is extreme drug sensitivity due to reduction in the rate of drug clearance and prolonged, high levels of drug. Knowledge of the functional polymorphism status at the genes for drug-metabolizing enzymes (DMEs) can be utilized in clinical practice (choice of drug, dosing algorithms) and drug development. Examples are (1) *CYP2C9* missense polymorphisms that produce reduced metabolism of *S*-warfarin, phenytoin, tolbutamide, and nonsteroidal antiinflammatory drugs (NSAIDS); (2) *CYP2D6*, which catalyzes the oxidation of many drug categories—debrisoquine, beta blockers, antidepressants, and codeine—and has more than 17 allelic variants ranging from poor metabolizers to ultrarapid metabolizers; and (3) *CYP2A6* variants, which are complete gene deletions or a single-base change, both resulting in the absence of functional enzyme activity and failure to metabolize coumarin compounds (4, 10).

Thus treatment efficacy may be drastically influenced by a patient's genetic potential for metabolism, increased or decreased, of pharmacologic agents. Hyperthermia reactions to anesthesia, polymorphisms in clotting factors that predispose to increased risk of thromboembolism, cytochrome P450 drug-metabolizing enzymes, and many other pharmacogenetic associations will bring more specific treatment options to each patient. Many pharmaceutical companies are using these genetic data to develop treatment alternatives tailored to prevalent genotypes, in hopes of shortening the time line for effective drug development/approval and minimizing the number of individuals who do not benefit from a particular agent.

2. Sepsis

Increasing evidence from animal and human studies demonstrates that susceptibility to severe sepsis or outcome from sepsis is partly determined by genetic variants in cytokine and inflammatory response genes (11). Genetic polymorphisms have been identified in many genes coding for the molecules that effect immunologic response to infection, including IL-1α, IL-1β, IL-1 receptor antagonist, IL-6, IL-10, TNFα, and TNFβ (11, 12). Many of the polymorphisms are located in the promoter or regulatory regions of these genes and probably produce higher levels of synthesis of cytokines. These have been implicated in the increased susceptibility to sepsis or increased mortality from sepsis. Conflicting data have been published regarding the role of these polymorphisms in regulating incidence of immunologic disease.

III. State of the Science

In the following sections we present examples of how each category of clinical molecular genetic testing has and will continue to influence surgical practice. Details of current and future methodologies are also presented, with particular attention to clinical diagnostic implementation.

Illustrating the association of genetic markers with clinical conditions in research studies usually focuses on case control or population association methods. Translating these findings to clinically relevant and feasible genetic assays necessitates much further consideration of many facets of genetic epidemiology and clinical laboratory practice.

Genetic research studies typically center on families or populations with high incidence of disease in order to maximize the likelihood of identification of causative genes. These "idealized" kindreds may not be representative of the same genetic background or disease mechanisms that predominate in the general clinical patient population. Apart from a "yes–no" or "mutation–no mutation" assessment, one must consider the context of the findings and, when possible, reconsider the relative risk for any carrier (penetrance), the range of different mutations (allelic heterogeneity), and the ability of the molecular method to detect the range of mutations (sensitivity), plus the spectrum of symptoms that an aberrant gene product may induce (expressivity) (see Table I). Some mutations are predictive of severity of phenotype or response to treatment. Other mutations are acted on by separate gene functions to elaborate different phenotypes in carriers of the same marker gene alteration, requiring a cohort of interacting genotypes to be considered for accurate prognosis.

For example, identification of a mutation in the *BRCA1* gene in a woman with a strong family history of breast cancer in several first-degree relatives presents a compelling scenario for a very high lifetime risk for development of breast cancer. Similar screening and *BRCA1* mutation detection, in the absence of a marked family incidence of breast cancer, may confer a somewhat higher risk for breast cancer in comparison to women in the general population (sporadic incidence), but not as high a risk as the same mutation in a high-risk kindred with multiple, affected close relatives (13). We may not always be able to extrapolate directly from research risk assessments to clinical practice.

Genetic screening techniques (Table II) are used for broad-based population screening for genetic alterations associated with a particular disorder regardless of family or medical history of the disorder. Mutation screening specifically refers to the total survey of the gene(s) for any

Table I Glossary of Genetic Terms

Term	Definition
Chromosome	Structure in cell on which genes are located, consisting of densely organized DNA and protein
Gene	Region of DNA that specifies a functional polypeptide
Mutation	A heritable change in DNA sequence
Allele	One of many forms of DNA sequence of a gene
Polymorphism	Two or more alleles for a gene that occur frequently (>1%) in the population
Genetic marker	DNA polymorphism with a specific location, inherited in stable fashion, and used in genetic mapping
Linkage	Joint inheritance of gene and marker due to their physical proximity on the chromosome
Association	Nonrandom occurrence of disorder and genetic marker
Genotype	Constitution of specific genetic alleles
Phenotype	Physical characteristics determined by specific genetic alleles
Penetrance	Frequency of altered phenotype in presence of mutant genotype
Expressivity	Range of phenotypic variability of a genetic trait
Genetic predisposition	Inherited increased risk for altered phenotype

Table II Mutation Screening

Method	Description	Advantages	Disadvantages
Genomic Southern hybridization (GSH)	DNA rearrangements detected by size changes as hybrid molecules form by complementary pairing between one filter-bound DNA strand and one radiolabeled DNA strand in solution; detected by autoradiography	Long-range/large size alterations detectable; gene sequence not required	Laborious; specimen requirements = 10^6 cells; large molecular weight DNA (>30 kb)
Gene sequencing	DNA nucleotide sequence determined by *in vitro* resynthesis using fluorescent dideoxynucleotides	Detects all base changes; automated	Laborious; limited to DNA segments 100–1000 bp long; excessive information; only some sequence changes produce altered function; error prone
Heteroduplex analysis	Detects mismatch between normal and mutant allele(s) in double-stranded hybrid DNA	Simple and rapid gel shift assay	Short DNA regions (<200 bp); limited sensitivity; does not identify position or base change of mutation
Single-strand conformation polymorphism or variance (SSCP or V)	Detects sequence-dependent structural differences between normal and mutant allele(s)	Simple and rapid gel shift assay	Limited to DNA regions <400 bp; does not identify position or base change of mutation
Denaturing gradient gel electrophoresis (DGGE)	Detects sequence differences as changes in partial melting behavior of double-stranded DNA	Very specific melting profiles on denaturing gels; high sensitivity for detection of base changes	Choice of primers sequence is critical; GC clamp design expensive and difficult to optimize; does not identify position or base change of mutation
Protein truncation test (PrTT)	*In vitro* synthesis of radiolabeled polypeptides by coupled transcription and translation [TnT] from PCR fragment	Very specific for stop mutations that produce shortened polypeptide; position of termination is determined	Laborious and expensive; does not detect missense or regulatory mutations; technically challenging; *in vitro* TnT lysate is not well-defined
Mismatch cleavage, chemical or enzymatic	Recognition and cleavage of normal-mutant hybrid DNA at nonmatching base pair(s)	Very sensitive; cleavage position localizes mismatch	Toxic chemicals used; technically challenging

alteration that may be associated with or predictive of an abnormal phenotype. This is to be compared with mutation testing, which is the specific search for known, pathogenic alteration(s) in an individual with symptoms or strong family history of the genetic disorder.

A. Analytic Approaches

The application of molecular genetics requires careful selection to match a tool to a specific clinical problem. For example, genotyping or even RT-PCR experiments to quantitate messenger RNA content will be unhelpful if the underlying genetic defect results in truncation during transcription. A key step in the application of molecular genetic tools to a research study is to understand not only the location of a particular mutation but also its specific effect on cell function. Table III relates mutations, their effects, analytic approaches, and strengths and limitations. Each technique is discussed with respect to the general ease of getting the method "up and running" in a research lab, as well as the typical human and dollar resources consumed. Most of these methods have been utilized extensively in molecular research labs but are not as suitable for clinical lab use because they are quite laborious and expensive and they do not distinguish between base changes that are pathogenic and those that are functionally silent.

Table III Direct Mutation Testing

Method	Description	Advantages	Disadvantages
Allele-specific oligonucleotide hybridization (ASO)	Separate oligonucleotide probes hybridize specifically to detect normal and mutant DNA sequences	Very specific; may be multiplexed; reverse dot-blot format may be used	Difficult to optimize oligonucleotide hybridization conditions to distinguish both normal and mutant sequences
Polymerase chain reaction *plus* restriction fragment length polymorphism (PCR-RFLP)	Site of base change creates specific alteration in enzyme digestion profile of PCR products in normal and mutant alleles	Simple; specific sequence change associated with the mutation alters enzyme recognition	Requires knowledge of sequence at/around variable site; mutations may not create change in enzyme recognition site; gel electrophoresis required
Amplification refractive mutation systems (ARMS)	PCR amplification primers specific for normal or mutant allele	High specificity; may be multiplexed	Stringent amplification conditions required for optimal discrimination
Oligonucleotide ligation assay	Enzymatic linkage of two annealed oligonucleotides flanking position of sequence variation between normal and mutation	Specific mismatch detection; high throughput; rapid	Requires hybridization conditions optimal for both sequences; limited to single base changes
Cleavase and Invader (Third Wave Technologies)	Endonuclease cleavage of triple-strand DNA structure; released oligonucleotide detected by fluorescence signal change	Sequence specific; rapid; high throughput; amplifies signal not target; does not require PCR	Requires knowledge of sequence at/around variable site; proprietary design of oligonucleotides around site; expensive fluorescent primers
Template-directed extension (TDI) with fluorescence resonance energy transfer (FRET)	Minisequencing single-nucleotide extension detected by change in fluorescence signal	Very sequence specific; single tube, homogeneous reaction; rapid, high throughput	Requires knowledge of sequence at/around variable site
TaqMan (Perkin Elmer Corp.)	ASO + enzymatic mismatch cleavage	Rapid; specific; sensitive, real-time fluorescent detection	Difficult to optimize oligonucleotide hybridization conditions; expensive, proprietary reagents
Mass spectrometry	Detection of physical mass of strands of DNA	Detects small insertions, deletions, and missense base changes	Limited to DNA fragments <100 bp; requires extensive comparative database to deduce fragment composition; novel fragments may not be defined
DNA chips/microarrays (Affymetrix)	Sequence-specific oligonucleotides arrayed by computer on a silicon chip base at very high-density; complementary sequence hybridization detected by fluorescent signals	High-density, simultaneous assay of many sequence changes ($>10^5$)	Excessive information; inflexible to addition of new alleles; expensive, single-use chips; confocal fluorescent microscopy for interpretation; extensive informatics programs required for scoring and sorting signals

Nearly all methods have been adapted to PCR approaches, at least when adequate gene sequence information is available to specify primer sequences. This is rarely possible when large (>10 kb) or long-range DNA rearrangements (chromosome inversions, DNA duplications or deletions) produce mutant alleles. Many of these methods lend themselves to a variety of physical detection formats. Changes in size or mobility of DNA fragments as identified by gel electrophoresis are used in many different assay types. The current trend is for detection of specific genetic variations to be identified as a change in the intensity or spectrum of fluorescent emissions. The fluorescent resonance energy transfer (FRET) detection method uses two fluorescent dyes in close proximity (usually at the ends of a relatively short, ~20-bp, oligonucleotide); the transfer of energy from the donor dye to the acceptor fluorophore decreases or quenches the emission from the donor but increases the specific emission intensity of the acceptor dye. When the donor dye is separated from the acceptor dye, the donor emission is detected. Some methods identify the release and accumulation of the donor fluorescence (Taqman) (14) and others rely on the specific detection of the increase in acceptor signal (template-directed extension FRET) (15). Reactions can be monitored in real time, providing quantitative assessment of the number of cells carrying the mutation or numerical aberrations, such as deletions, duplications, unbalanced translocations, or loss of heterozygosity. The reactions may be performed in a liquid state or have solid-phase components fixed in reaction tubes. Eliminating post-PCR handling prevents product contamination concerns. Fluorescence detection can be very sensitive, especially for small amounts of nucleic acid or PCR product. Detection may also be very rapid, such as with capillary electrophoresis, and high throughput (adapted to a 96-well plate format). With appropriate equipment it is possible to detect the real-time accumulation of specific fluorescent products or emission signals to produce a rapid, clinically relevant, "point-of-care" testing alternative.

B. Practical Concerns for Organization

Clinical laboratories, including those that perform molecular genetic testing, are distinctly different from research laboratory investigations in operation, structure, quality control, quality assurance, financing, and regulatory oversight. Many molecular biology methods that are preferred in research labs must be significantly revised and standardized for routine clinical lab use. The cost, reproducibility, accuracy, and oversight of the activities of clinical genetics lab are comparable to clinical service entities. Standards of training and qualifications are being certified and applied by professional societies. The American Board of Medical Genetics is the accreditation body for training programs and the certifying body for medical geneticists. The American College of Medical Genetics is the standards and practice arm of the medical genetics community, whereas the parent organization, the American Society of Human Genetics, is the scientific research arm of the field (17). The College of American Pathologists (CAP) and the United States Health Care Financing Administration (HCFA) provide the Laboratory Accreditation Program (LAP) through on-site lab inspections and proficiency testing. This is done under the Clinical Laboratory Improvement Amendments (CLIA) of 1988 and is recognized by the Joint Commission on Accreditation of Healthcare Organizations (JCAHO). More than 3500 checklist questions are used for field evaluation.

The following criteria are considered in most clinical lab applications but have been restated specifically with the challenges of molecular diagnostics in mind.

C. "Seven Deadly Sins" of Molecular Genetic Testing

1. Genotype Does Not Affect Clinical Course

Variable penetrance of the genetic variant describes the pattern of heritable gene expression when more individuals carry the variant than actually exhibit clinical symptoms of the disease phenotype. Variable phenotypic expression of the variant genotype does not predict a certainty of clinical features. Other gene functions are likely involved that influence the range of abnormal expression of the marker being studied.

2. No Predictable Intervention to Alter Clinical Course

No treatment is available to alter the clinical course of the condition diagnosed by molecular genetics. Treatments available have unknown efficacy with regard to different genotype classifications. Genetic predisposition conditions may not respond in the same manner as treatment for sporadic disease. Alternatively, the presence of a marker that indicates genetic predisposition implies only an increased risk of phenotype, not a certainty of disease development or the current presence of abnormal gene function.

3. A Specific Screening Test Is Not Available

Most diseases are associated with many different abnormal alleles with different mutation mechanisms, either in the same gene (allelic heterogeneity) or in different genes (genetic heterogeneity). These alleles frequently have very different effects on the protein function and therefore a range of phenotypes may result. The challenge to molecular diagnostics is to design testing formats that can, at least, detect the most common alleles associated with disease expression. In many instances a combination of the assay formats described in Tables II and III is required to detect with sensitivity the majority of disease-producing alleles for a single disorder. Negative test results must always be interpreted within the limits of sensitivity and specificity of the validated assay. Thus negative test results may not be equivalent to normal phenotype or to zero risk of disease phenotype.

The frequency of different mutant alleles usually varies in different ethnic populations, with the extreme being represented by founder effects in which some genetic disorders are rarely observed outside a distinct ethnic subgroup. Also, the rate at which new mutations arise in the population in the marker studied must be considered, because this significantly alters the assessment of family history, recurrence risk, and feasibility of carrier testing. Functional genetic polymorphisms may have not been identified in any family members because they have not experienced the eliciting stimulus, such as a inflammatory reaction, sepsis, or drug reaction.

4. No Clinical Service Resources Available for Genetic Counseling

Informed consent may not be possible, e.g., in surgical ICU or trauma patients. The inheritance pattern may be unknown or not discerned from a single index case in the ICU. Meaningful risk assessment for other relatives or for recurrence to the patient may not be attainable in these circumstances. Genetic counseling is usually provided prior to testing to explain both the risks of the test and the possible findings, both positive and negative, as well as the limitations of the test methodology. This is presented in a nondirective style in order that the patient or family may make an informed decision about whether to participate in the genetic testing procedure. After consent, specimen collection, and testing, the genetic counselor also conveys the findings to the patient or family in a confidential, supportive setting with considerable explanation of options and implications of the findings. These sessions help put the results in context and include recognition of personal, cultural, ethnic, family, and cognitive elements of each patient's circumstances to help the patient make the choice that is most suitable for him or her.

5. Test Is neither Cost-Effective nor Cost-Beneficial

Current molecular genetic testing methods are usually more laborious and expensive compared to traditional clinical lab testing. "STAT" may mean several days for turnaround. Therefore one should be certain that the genetic test findings will significantly add to the assessment or care of a critically ill patient. This may include the avoidance of less specific or more costly or invasive or risky surveillance procedures. Molecular findings may be instrumental in stratifying a patient to an optimal course of treatment.

6. Clinicians Fail to Accept Test as Worthwhile

Existing test methodology is sufficient and concordant with molecular genetic techniques. Presymptomatic or prenatal screening may not be appropriate, practical, or necessary. Diagnosis and/or treatment are unaltered by molecular genetic findings. Again genetic predisposition implies increased risk but does not equate to certainty of disease development. Prevention strategies, environmental risk factors, and increased surveillance for early signs of disease may play an increased role in maintaining a healthy condition.

7. Risk of Social Implications of Genetic Profiling

Potential for discrimination in employment opportunities or health insurance restrictions may result from genetic testing and associated or implied risk of disease or sensitivity. This may extend to the offspring of the tested individual. Ethnic stigma may be exhibited particularly when founder-effect gene-disease correlations are manifested. An individual's self-image or relationship with family members may be adversely impacted due to increased risk for chronic or debilitating disease. Survivor guilt may even result when negative test findings indicate that the tested individual has a reduced risk but other relatives are/will be affected. Dynamics within a family are significantly influenced when any single individual participates in genetic testing.

IV. Recommendations to Surgical Investigators

A. Quality Control

Researchers embarking on molecular genetics voyages soon find themselves awash in a sea of data. Unless rigorous quality controls are established at the outset, the validity of data will sooner or later become suspect. The reason is that many of the analytic techniques depend on PCR amplification, which is very sensitive to trace contamination. Specimen quality and contamination become suspect as soon as an unexpected result appears. Quality control programs have been developed (16–19). The novice is advised to seek out the local clinical molecular genetics laboratory because such laboratories must conform to the highest standards of quality control. Although the research laboratory often does not meet these high standards, simply knowing the difference between best practice and actual practice can often help troubleshoot problems as they crop up during the study.

B. Research

Research what is already known about the genetics of the disease in question. In addition to literature databases such as MEDLINE, genetic databases contain helpful syntheses of genetic information and reference sources. One compendium is the Online Mendelian Inheritance in Man OMIM (20), an Internet version of the series originally developed by Victor McKusick of Johns Hopkins, whom many consider the father of medical genetics. Many databases also exist for particularly well-studied genes and the mutations that have been reported as associated with disease incidence. Internet links for many of these (21–23) are provided by OMIM.

Gene Tests, an on-line resource (24) for many medical genetics professionals, is operated from the University of Washington and lists labs that perform genetic testing for many disorders, either for research or clinical purposes. They also have a Genetics Clinics feature, which reviews and summarizes many clinical features of genetic disease diagnosis, treatment, molecular testing, and prognosis produced by leading geneticists specializing in each disorder. Nicholas *et al.* have a web site for animal model studies (22), as does Jackson Labs (25). Mouse–human homologies are imperfect and mouse knockout or overexpressor strains frequently do not mimic or provide a mechanism for the human disease.

C. Value Assessment

The human genetics component should add significantly to the value of your study. Gratuitous genetics ("because we can") in this decade is not better than the gratuitous molecular biology or cell biology of past decades. Remember the "Seven Deadly Sins" (Section III, C) in assessing the added value that genetics analyses will bring to your investigations. Once a particular mutant or polymorphic allele with functional consequences and disease phenotype has been identified, it is usually important to stratify patients to risk groups. Defects in a number of other alleles or separate genes may independently confer disease susceptibility beyond the alterations being screened (9). If a study does not require stratification of patient populations, there may not be a significant influence from genetic factors.

D. Statistics

Consider the statistical components and power calculations to provide meaningful data now and consult a biostatistician or epidemiologist with experience in genetic study design (1, 26, 27). Information about allele frequency, penetrance, or expression of phenotype and the range of symptoms in the study population are crucial to calculate the size of study population required to provide statistically significant correlations and meaningful import on clinical care.

E. Regulatory and Practical Considerations

Become familiar with the rules, regulations, and requirements of genetics testing specified by the local IRB and federal laboratory accreditation bodies (28–29). The documentation and quality measures far exceed those commonly in use in most research labs. Consider allying with a clinical lab that already has this certification if it is desired to use test results to make decisions about patient care or to give written reports in consultation with patient or families. Outsourcing to an active clinical or research genetics lab or shared resource component frequently saves time and money in the long run. The expertise can alleviate many mistakes and expedite a study. Development, validation, and implementation of a new genetic test (including labor) may cost $5000–20,000 depending on the methodology, the anticipated sample volume, existing facilities, and availability of standards. This means it will cost this amount to analyze the first specimen and a few dollars afterward to process and analyze each succeeding specimen. Researchers need to incorporate these funds into grant or clinic budgets up front rather than assume that the collaborating facility will begin testing in the hope of finding a payment source later.

Spend the money to consult with an experienced medical geneticist to determine the best molecular method to achieve the genetic information required. DNA sequencing of the entire gene may be the gold standard but is not feasible for a large population study. Focus on a few more common mutations or those with a particularly severe phenotype. If the number of different alleles is large and the types of mutations observed are diverse, sequencing may be required but in a more limited population. It also helps to discuss the possible impact or changes in clinical care or lifestyle patterns the patient participating in the testing should consider as a result of a positive or negative genetic test finding. Consider whether effective therapy is available to change the disease course or whether the family could lose medical coverage when these findings are interpreted to indicate a preexisting condition.

F. Data Management

Data management is complex. Investigators who are used to recording studies and their outcomes in traditional laboratory notebooks quickly discover that molecular genetics requires decidedly different documentation tools. The importance of a searchable specimen log (typically a relational database) cannot be overemphasized. Selection of data recording formats today may have ramifications 5 years later because specific data must be recovered from an archive. The "original data" are often no longer actual autoradiographic images but rather density files from phosphorimaging plates, fluorescent readers, and so on. The need to establish a nonviolable system of recording and archiving data should be obvious. The need to establish a system of backup data files and archives in a distant location is clear but often unheeded until disaster strikes. "Caveat investigator."

Acknowledgment

This work was supported in part by a grant from the National Institutes of Health to B.D.F. (K08-GM00691-01).

References

1. Schork, N. J., Cardon, L. R., and Xu, X. (1998). The future of genetic epidemiology. *Trends Genet.* **14,** 266–272.
2. Kinzler, K. W., and Vogelstein, B. (1998). Colorectal tumors. *In* "The Genetic Basis of Human Cancer" (B. Vogelstein and K.W. Kinzler, eds.), p. 565. McGraw-Hill, New York.
3. Zehnbauer, B. A., Romkes, M., and Carcillo, J. A. (1999). Genetic influences on critical illness. *In* "Textbook of Critical Care," 4th Ed. (W. C. Shoemaker, S. M. Ayres, A. Grenvik, and P. R. Holbrook, eds.), pp. 613–620. W.B. Saunders Co., Philadelphia.
4. Evans, W. E., and Relling, M. V. Pharmacogenomics: Translating functional genomics into rational therapeutics. *Science* **286,** 487–491.
5. Look, A. T. (1998). Genes altered by chromosomal translocations in leukemias and lymphomas. *In* "The Genetic Basis of Human Cancer" (B. Vogelstein and K. W. Kinzler, eds.) p. 109. McGraw-Hill, New York.
6. Lips, C. J. M., Landsvater, R. M., Hoppener, J. W. M., *et al.* (1994). Clinical screening as compared with DNA analysis in families with multiple endocrine neoplasia type 2A. *N. Engl. J. Med.* **331,** 828–835.
7. Kaelin, W. G., and Maher, E. R. (1998). The VHL tumor-suppressor gene paradigm. *Trends Genet.* **14,** 423–426.
8. Stebbins, C. E., Kaelin, W. G., and Pavletich, N. P. (1999). Structure of the VHL-ElonginC–ElonginB complex: Implications for VHL tumor suppressor function. *Science* **284,** 455–461.

8a. Pavletich, N. P. (2000). 21st Rhoads Lecture, 91st Annual AACR Meeting, April 2000. AACR, San Francisco, CA.

9. Schork, N. J. (1997). Genetics of complex disease: Approaches, problems, and solutions. *Am. J. Resp. Crit. Care Med.* **156,** S103–S109.
10. Ingelman-Sundberg, M., Oscarson, M., and McLellan, R. A. (1999). Polymorphic human cytochrome P450 enzymes: An opportunity for individualized drug treatment. *Trends Pharmacol. Sci.* **20,** 342–349.
11. Zehnbauer, B. A., Romkes, M., and Carcillo, J. A. (1999). Genetic influences on critical illness. *In* "Textbook of Critical Care," 4th Ed. (W. C. Shoemaker, S. M. Ayres, A. Grenvik, and P. R. Holbrook, eds.), pp. 613–620. W.B. Saunders Co., Philadelphia.
12. Freeman, B. D., and Zehnbauer, B. A. (2000). "Genetic Susceptibility to Infection and Sepsis, in Evolving Concepts in Sepsis and Septic Shock" (P.Q. Eichacker and J. Pugin, eds.). In press.
13. Fitzgerald, M. G., *et al.* (1996). Germ-line BRCA1 mutations in Jewish and non-Jewish women with early-onset breast cancer. *N. Engl. J. Med.* **334,** 143–149.
14. Livak, K. J., Flood, S. J., Marmaro, J., *et al.* (1995). Oligonucleotides with fluorescent dyes at opposite ends provide a quenched probe system useful for detecting PCR product and nucleic acid hybridization. *PCR Methods Appl.* **4,** 357–362.
15. Chen, X., Zehnbauer, B. A., Gnirke, A., and Kwok, P.-Y. (1997). Fluorescence energy transfer detection as a homogeneous DNA diagnostic method. *Proc. Natl. Acad. Sci. U.S.A* **94,** 10756–10761.
16. Mark, H. F. L., Kelly, T., Watson, M. S., *et al.* (1995). Current issues of personnel and laboratory practices in genetic testing. *J. Med. Genet.* **32,** 780–786.
17. Laboratory Improvement and Laboratory Accreditation Program, College of American Pathologists (2000). World Wide Web URL: http://www.cap.org.
18. Pence, E. M. (1999). A practical guide for the validation of genetic tests. *Gene. Testing* **3,** 201–205.
19. Standards and Guidelines for Clinical Genetics Laboratories. American College of Medical Genetics (2000). World Wide Web URL: http://www.faseb.org/genetics/acmg/stds/stdsmenu.htm.
20. Online Mendelian Inheritance in Man (OMIM) (2000). McKusick–Nathans Institute for Genetic Medicine, Johns Hopkins University (Baltimore, MD) and National Center for Biotechnology Information, National Library of Medicine (Bethesda, MD). World Wide Web URL: http://www.ncbi.nlm.nih.gov/omim/.
21. Krawczak, M., and Cooper, D. N. (1997). The Human Gene Mutation Database. *Trends Genet.* **13,** 121–122. World Wide Web URL: http://www.uwcm.ac.uk/uwcm/mg/hgmd0.html.
22. Nicholas, F. W., Brown, S. C., and Le Tissier, P. R. (2000). Online Mendelian Inheritance in Animals. World Wide Web URL: http://www.angis.su.oz.au/Databases/BIRX/omia/.
23. Entrez (2000). Search and Retrieval System, National Center for Biotechnology Information, National Library of Medicine and National Institutes of Health. World Wide Web URL: http://www3.ncbi.nlm.nih.gov/Entrez/.
24. GeneTests (2000). Genetic Testing Resource [database online]. Copyright, Children's Health Care System, Seattle, WA, 1999–2000. Updated continually. World Wide Web URL: http://www.genetests.org. Accessed May, 2000.
25. Mouse Genome Informatics at The Jackson Laboratories (2000). World Wide Web URL: http://www.informatics.jax.org/.
26. Khoury, M. J., Beaty, T. H., and Cohen, B. H. (1993). "Fundamentals of Genetic Epidemiology." Oxford University Press, Cambridge.
27. Weiss, K. M. (1994). "Genetic Variation and Human Disease: Principles and Evolutionary Approaches." Cambridge University Press, Cambridge.
28. CLIA Final Rules (2000). Amendments to and Clarifications of Regulations and Clinical Laboratory Improvement Advisory Committee (CLIAC) Recommendations, College of American Pathologists Advocacy Network. World Wide Web URL: http://www.cap.org/HTML/ADVOCACY/capdocs/cliachrt.html.
29. Office for Protection from Research Risks (2000). NIH Office of Extramural Research. World Wide Web URL: http://grants.nih.gov/grants/oprr/.

27

Shock Models: Hemorrhage

Alfred Ayala, Ping Wang, and Irshad H. Chaudry

Center for Surgical Research and Department of Surgery, Brown University School of Medicine and Rhode Island Hospital, Providence, Rhode Island 02903

I. Introduction

Hemorrhagic shock, defined as life-threatening blood loss, remains a common complication of traumatic injury arising from soft-tissue or bony injuries. With respect to traumatic shock, it has been reported that up to 50% of the deaths occur from exsanguination or central nervous system complications within the first hour, and another 30% are lost to major internal organ injury during the next 1–2 hr (1). Of those who survive the initial insult, approximately 50% succumb to infections and multiple organ failure. Although trauma ranks fifth on the list of causes of death in the United States (behind heart disease and cancer), the cost in patient care dollars is ~\$335,000/individual. This cost is about 2.4 times more per trauma-related death than the cost associated with treatment of a cancer or cardiovascular patient (per the 1996 Centers for Disease Control National Center for Health Statistics). Intensive experimental efforts will continue to be needed if we are to understand the effect(s) of hemorrhagic and/or hypovolemic shock alone or in the presence of various forms of traumatic tissue injury and if we are to understand the pathophysiologic changes manifested in these patients. For this review we have selected studies that are representatives of the different hemorrhagic shock models. Although experimental hypovolemic shock can and has been produced in a wide array of different animal species (which have specific advantages and disadvantages) (2–5), we have chosen to confine the discussion here to models of hemorrhagic shock utilized in rodents.

Advantages to using rats and mice over other animal species include rapid reproduction, the low cost of surgical instrumentation/monitoring, low acquisition and per diem animal costs, and the ability to manipulate/regulate inheritable genetic backgrounds (primarily with respect to mice). Compared to traumatically injured or shocked patients, animals offer direct access to a wide array of tissues and organs that cannot be readily studied in humans. Comparative costs of assessment and/or isolation of organs and/or tissues from rodents are substantially lower than they are for larger animals. With respect to mice, the most significant advantages are the availability of a wide number of inbred strains (many of which exhibit various defined genetic alterations that have arisen spontaneously) and the burgeoning number of mice that carry various induced mutations/deficiencies (knockouts) or express various transgenes (transgenic mice). This ability to manipulate the genetic background of these animals has fostered the development of an extensive array of biologic and immunologic tools (bioassays, cytokines, antibodies, molecular probes, etc.) that can be applied in this species.

The biggest disadvantage beyond species dissimilarities between humans and rodents is the small size of rats and mice. The best example of this disadvantage relates to peripheral blood: the primary sample taken at one time from most human volunteers or patients is commonly 50–100 ml, but in a mouse only 20–30 μl can be taken at a single tail bleed or from the orbital fissure. However, even with the arterial access, repeated bleeding of volumes much greater than 100 μl in a mouse can produce deleterious events such as hypovolemic shock. Although this is somewhat less of a problem in rats, repeated bleeding volumes beyond 1 ml are unusual even in this animal model. Thus, a direct response of observed cells or mediators present in peripheral (systemic) blood samples of humans is difficult to compare in mice and rats.

II. Models of Hemorrhagic Shock

Shock is defined as a state resulting from dyshomeostasis in tissue perfusion, which leads to an inability to maintain normal organ functions (5, 6). The shock state, with respect to hemorrhage, is due to an inadequacy of circulating blood volume (2, 5). Hemorrhagic shock, unlike other forms of shock, i.e., toxic/toxin shock, septic shock, traumatic shock (related to tissue injury), and cardiogenic shock, appears to be the result of an organized programmed series of responses, which distinguishes it from other forms of shock (2, 5). However, the nature of the pathophysiologic mechanism and its nidus in the shock state still remain to be determined.

What then are the criteria for an ideal model of hemorrhagic–hypovolemic shock? The most significant aspect of model choice relates to how well the chosen model produces the sequellae commonly encountered in trauma victims who have developed hypovolemic shock (2, 7). For example, does the model of hemorrhagic shock produce dyshomeostasis in tissue perfusion and does this result in the development of organ system dysfunction (i.e., altered gut, liver, kidney, and immune system)? If the model does so, from a scientific viewpoint one would also want to know if these events occur in a consistent (predictable) and readily reproducible fashion. From a clinical perspective, one might ask to what extent this model of shock compares to events that typically occur in the surgical and/or traumatized patient. It is this latter aspect of modeling that brings up a common problem with all models. Do we choose our model based solely on outcome, or is our choice to be driven by emulating the injury?

It is important to utilize a model that is clinically relevant/comparable, but this can also confound the interpretation of the endpoints to be assessed if the variables that are included are not properly controlled. For example, if one is looking for immune system alterations similar to those seen in the critically ill trauma patient, such as depressed major histocompatibility complex (MHC) class II expression (8, 9) or suppression of lymphoid/macrophage responsiveness (10–12), does the model of hemorrhage chosen produce these in a consistent and comparable fashion? How do variables such as the administration of anesthesia, heparinization, resuscitation (with blood, colloids, crystalloids, or combinations, as well as aspects of rate and volume of resuscitant), and tissue (surgical) trauma affect the model? Each variable must be considered not only when choosing a given shock model but also in the interpretation of data generated (see model discussions below). Therefore, it is important to address the contributions these variables may make to the model outcomes by running appropriate controls (e.g., inclusion of untreated/unmanipulated animals, animals subjected to heparin or anesthesia) and/or, where possible, by eliminating confounding variables.

The species of animal chosen, as well as its age, gender, and endocrine and nutritional status, must be considered relative to the hypothesis one wishes to test. For example, if the question concerns the contribution of inducible nitric oxide production to the macrophage cytokine production following shock, it is important to realize that macrophages from rats produce significantly more nitric oxide and inducible nitric oxide synthase compared to humans. This divergence in NO production is due in part to differences in species-specific regulation of the related gene (13, 14). Such factors must be considered in drawing conclusions relative to the human condition. Even basic differences, such as the knowledge that mice are nocturnally active and feed during that period (15), in contrast to humans, should be considered when choosing/designing a shock model, because this carries significant implications with regard to nutritional condition (16) as well as endocrine status in these animals (17). Although there are advantages to using mice and rats, validation of the mechanisms relative to the pathophysiology of clinical hemorrhagic shock need to be examined in other mammalian species, as well as in humans, before these findings are applied to the shock and trauma patient.

From a practical standpoint, the expense of the animals and their housing and care is lower for small animals, but the cost of the materials and equipment required to conduct the experiments still needs to be considered. Similarly, the experiment/model that one intends to use needs to stay within the standards of humane animal care set by the National

Institutes of Health Guidelines for Animal Care (18) and by local animal care facilities and use committees. It is also critical that the laboratory make the appropriate occupational health and safety considerations with respect to the precautions that must also be taken when handling animals (18). For a more thorough discussion of these topics the reader is directed to earlier chapters on animal care.

In this chapter we describe three basic models that have been used in the study of hemorrhagic shock, i.e., fixed-volume bleed, fixed-pressure hemorrhage, and uncontrolled bleeding, and discuss some of the advantages/disadvantages of these models. Modifications (inclusion of tissue injury, fracture, alcohol exposure, etc.) have been and continue to be applied to these models in an attempt to make them more clinically comparable to the status of the shock seen in the traumatized patient (2). However, in an effort to not overcomplicate the initial discussion of the various advantages and disadvantages of given models, we have chosen to focus here on these basic hemorrhagic shock models. We also provide detailed methodological descriptions of a few models of simple hemorrhage (Section VIII).

III. Anesthetized and Unanesthetized Fixed-Volume Bleed-Out Models of Hemorrhage

Anesthetized fixed-volume bleed-out models have been utilized by a number of investigators with varying results (19–24). In these models the animal, typically a rat, is bled between 2 and 50% of its total calculated blood volume over a set period of time under pentobarbital anesthesia. The animal is then allowed to compensate for a set period of time, at the end of which the animal is either returned to its housing or is resuscitated. If the animal is resuscitated it usually receives shed blood with or without an accompanying volume of a resuscitation fluid [lactated Ringer's solution (LRS) or normal saline]. The primary advantage of this model is that the potential contribution of the animal's homeostatic (compensatory) mechanisms can be addressed following acute blood volume loss. In this respect, this model has been utilized to study a variety of processes in the shocked host, such as carbohydrate and protein metabolism (25, 26), changes in blood glucose as well as liver glycogen levels (27), general histopathology (28), survival (29), and various therapeutic interventions (30, 31). The primary drawback to such an approach is that the extent of hypotension induced is typically unknown, so its impact cannot be assessed. The use of anesthesia has significant cardiovascular (suppressive) effects that need to be considered (32–34). If the animals' shed blood is to be returned, usually an anticoagulant, such as heparin sulfate, is provided (see detailed discussion of heparinization later in this chapter).

Lapage (35) was one of the first to study hypovolemic shock in the absence of the complicating side effects of anesthesia. In his model, the animal was transiently anesthetized with ether and restrained in a sling; on awakening, the tail of the rat was cut at the end and allowed to bleed until a predetermined volume was reached. However, this model lacked control over the depth of the hypotensive insult and the rate at which the bleeding took place. As an alternative to this, Collins and Stechenberg (36) initially inserted femoral arterial catheters under volatile anesthesia and heparinized the animals, on full awakening, a fixed volume of blood was removed to induce shock. The investigators then resuscitated these animals with their own shed blood. Using this model they assessed both the role of changing hemoglobin levels and the effect of hypovolemia on survival. Later, others (37–39) applied a comparable model of fixed 30% calculated blood volume bleed (see Section VIII,A for a detailed description of this model in mice), initially in a catheterized rat but later using a cardiac stick under light, volatile anesthesia, to assess the impact of hypovolemic shock on immune response. This latter model has the advantage of inducing minimal surgical injury, hypothetically, although some degree of cardiac contusion may be present in these animals. As with the other models of fixed-volume bleeding, the contribution of hypotension to the process is not known.

IV. Anesthetized and Unanesthetized Fixed-Pressure Models of Hemorrhage

Although many of the models of fixed-volume hemorrhage described above were designed to address the contribution of hypovolemia, dependent on the degree of blood loss, it was not always clear to what degree these models produce marked hypotension. Typically the duration of the hypotensive state produced is variable, thus further complicating the investigator's capacity to determine the contribution of pressure to the development of shock and its associated organ dysfunction. With respect to this, as early as 1919, Penfield (40) initially described a model in which maintenance of a set pressure was the objective. His goal was "to bleed the animals until the arterial pressure reached 40 mmHg and to maintain this pressure as nearly as possible by repeated hemorrhage or if necessary, small saline infusions." Based on this, Wiggers (41) put forward the fixed-pressure model of hemorrhagic shock in which animals were catheterized under anesthesia, then heparinized and bled to a predetermined pressure and maintained at that pressure for a given period of time. Following these early classic studies, a number of investigators have used modifications of the classic anesthetized fixed-pressure Wiggers model (41). Typically, in this model the animal is catheterized under anesthesia, such as pentobarbital, then heparinized so as to maintain catheter patency. Arterial access allows the investigator the ability to draw blood and infuse agents and to monitor the extent of hypotension. While still under general anesthesia the animal is bled to the desired mean blood pressure, which has been varied by investigators from 70 to 35 mmHg) (42–59). This hypotensive shock state has been maintained for as little as 30 min or in some studies as long 5 hr (42–59). Most of these investigations also provide some index of the degree of blood volume (hypovolemia) that must be withdrawn to initially induce this state of hypotension and to maintain it. Investigators using this model have examined a number of questions concerning hypotensive shock induced in the anesthetized animal; these are summarized in Table I. However, as mentioned earlier, the contribution of anesthesia is a potential concern, because it is documented to lower metabolic demand (17, 60–63), depress cardiovascular response (32–34), and in some cases alter microbial translocation (64).

Sayeed and Baue in 1971 (65) developed a modification of the above model of hypotensive shock in conscious animals. In this model, the rat was initially fasted overnight, then lightly anesthetized with ether, and restrained in the supine position; both femoral arteries were cannulated and the animal was then heparinized. While still restrained, the animal was allowed to awaken, at which point the rat was bled spontaneously into a reservoir until the pressure reached 40 mmHg. This pressure was maintained by the withdrawal/infusion of small amounts of blood until 25% of the maximum shed blood volume had been returned. Typically the hypotensive period was maintained for 1–2 hr. The

Table I General Summary of Studies Utilizing Fixed-Pressure Anesthetized Hemorrhage Models

Topic	Ref.
Assessment of glucose uptake in the diaphragm as well as changes in various metabolic pathways	42, 43
Examination of the changes of the adenine nucleotide pool in the liver	42
Assessment of lactate and pyruvate levels as indexes of the severity of acute circulatory failure produced by shock	44
Assessment of the effect of shock on mitochondrial metabolism	45
Ultrastructural assessment of mitochondrial changes following shock	114
Determination of the extent of mitochondrial dysfunction and hypoglycemia	46
Examination of the impact of shock on hepatic energy charge and changes in membrane potential	47, 48
Examination of the effects of shock on glucagon metabolism	49, 115
Determination of the impact of hypotension on nuclear DNA	49
Assessment of shock's capacity to predispose the host to subsequent infection	50
Investigation of shock's capacity to predispose the host to subsequent bacterial translocation	52
Shock-induced change in adrenegric vascular compensatory mechanisms	51
Contribution of various vasoactive molecules as therapy in shock	53
Examination of the capacity of shock to alter bone marrow function	54
Examination of changes in intestinal microvascular blood flow	56
Addressed the role of nitric oxide in liver injury following hemorrhage	58, 116
Assessed the contributions of peroxynitrite to shock-induced mortality	59, 117, 118
Examination of the role of calcium in shock	55
Assessed the contributions of prostacylins in hemorrhage	119
Addressed the contribution of platelet-activating factor in hypotension	56
Investigated the role of tumor necrosis factor in shock	120
Determination of the role of IL-6 and granulocyte colony-stimulating factor in hemorrhage	57, 121, 122
The role of different mediators in the model of fixed-pressure anethetized hemorrhage	
Calcium	55
Prostacyclin	119
Platelet-activating factor	56
Tumor necrosis factor	120
Granulocyte colony-stimulating factor and IL-6	57, 121, 122

animal's resuscitation was then begun by returning the shed blood followed by a volume of LRS sufficient to equal twice the maximum bleed-out volume. This model has been utilized to assess organelle and cellular functions, which are briefly outlined in Table II. However, although the animal is not subjected to the effects of anesthesia during shock, this model still involves preheparinization and restraint stress.

In our own laboratory, we have used a modification of the conscious fixed-pressure hemorrhage model in mice. This model in mice was initially described by Stephan *et al.* (66). Details of the actual experimental protocol are provided in Section VIII,B. In brief, this model also requires the application of light anesthesia in the form or Metofane or ether, followed by restraint in the supine position, catheterization of the femoral arteries, and then administration a of low dose of heparin (1–2 units/mouse). Once the animal is fully awake it is bled to a mean pressure of ~35 mmHg, which is maintained typically for 1 hr, although varying time periods (15–90 min) have been used (67). At the end of the hypotensive episode the mouse is resuscitated, first with its own shed blood then typically with LRS (volume based on twice the shed blood volume). This model is typically nonlethal in nature; however, in our laboratory (68, 69) as well as in others (70, 71) it produces a wide array of derangements in both immune and certain organ functions, which culminate in the animal exhibiting a markedly reduced capacity to ward off subsequent lethal septic challenge (also see Table II). To the extent that many of the changes that have been reported in these models are a response to resuscitation (a reperfusion event), we (72, 73) and others (70) have shown that many of these pathologic process are initiated during the hypotensive episode prior to the provision of fluids. Nonetheless, fluid resuscitation (74–76) as well as the type of resuscitant (71, 77–80) also have modulating effects on the pathophysiologic changes induced by hemorrhage. However, although this model is reproducible and predictable, it remains one of restraint (because the size of the experimental subject at present prohibits easy maintenance of long-term tunneled arterial catheter access) and the animals are still heparinized, although the dosage is low.

Machiedo and colleagues (81) modified the fixed-pressure hemorrhage model in the rat by tunneling the catheters back out through the skin behind the neck through a tether, which allowed hemorrhage (40 mmHg for 180 min) to be reproduced in a unrestrained model. Utilizing this approach they where able to examine the effect of ATP-$MgCl_2$ as a adjuvant in resuscitation fluids on hepatic cell membrane permeability and metabolism. However, the contributions of heparinization and shorter periods of hypotension are not known.

A more extensively catheterized version of this unrestrained model has been used by Koziol *et al.* (82), in which they documented that rats subjected to hypotensive (40 mmHg) periods showed evidence of bacteremia but typically only have 2–3 hr of sustained shock. Using the same model Rush *et al.* (83) subsequently showed in germ-free animals that mortality was reduced but not absent when compared to shocked animals containing normal gut flora. Here again these animals, although conscious, were still heparinized (~500 units of heparin/kg body weight).

V. Heparin as a Possible Confounding Variable

As is evident from the discussion above, in essentially all of these models, especially the fixed-pressure models (where catheterization is a component of the protocol), heparinization was utilized in the experimental animal. In this respect, heparin has been shown, at high dosage

Table II General Summary of Studies Utilizing Fixed-Pressure Unanesthetized Hemorrhage Models

Topic	Ref.
Rats	
Assessment of mitochondrial dysfunction following shock	123
Demonstration of changes in membrane transport	124
Determination of alteration in adenine nucleotide cellular pool	125
Examination of the changes in *in vivo* of hepatocyte transmembrane potential following shock	126
Impact of ATP-$MgCl_2$ administration on survival	127
Mice	
Assessment of immune responsiveness following hemorrhage	66, 67, 69, 70–73, 128–131
Examination of the effects of various resuscitation protocols and/or resuscitants on immune cell function following shock	71, 74–80
Determination of effect of gender on immune function following simple hemorrhage	105, 132–13
Established the presence of apoptosis in the thymus and gut following shock	135, 136

(1000–500 units/kg body weight), to have a wide array of effects (84–92). However, work by Rana *et al.* (93) has illustrated that preheparinization markedly improves microvascular patency during shock. This is in keeping with the findings of a number of other laboratories, which observed that heparin administration in itself had salutary effects on mortality encountered with severe hemorrhagic shock (84–87). The mechanisms for this are still debated, but heparin has been shown to alter the release of vasoactive agents such as catecholamines (88), to alter cytokine levels (89, 90), to affect blood viscosity (91), to alter endothelial cell interaction (91, 92), and to directly and indirectly affect the coagulation cascade and the release of various of its bioactive components (91).

This raises concerns about heparin's role as a potentially confounding variable in a number of the models that have been described (2, 94), because the pharmacokenetics of the delivery of investigational agents can be markedly altered by this agent as well as the general pathophysiologic response of the animal to the hypotensive/hypovolemic insult.

In light of these issues, we have (95) established a model of fixed-pressure hemorrhage in the rat that does not utilize heparin; instead, the animal, once catheters are placed (under Metofane or isoflurane anesthesia) and tunneled, is conscious and unrestrained (see Section VIII,C). Combined with simple trauma in the form of a midline laparotomy prior to hemorrhage, we have carried out a wide array of studies addressing mortality, liver function, renal function, gut absorptive capacity, adrenal/endocrine function, cardiovascular function, and inflammatory mediator changes seen following hemorrhagic shock (95–104). A modification of this model has been applied in the mouse to address a number of questions concerning gender and immune response (68, 69, 105), as well as some aspects of organ function (106); however, these subjects remain restrained due the limitations of catheter flexibility and relative size, as mentioned earlier (74).

VI. Uncontrolled Hemorrhage Models

Although much can be learned from volume- or pressure-controlled models of hemorrhage, because of their well-defined nature, the trauma victim experiencing hemorrhagic shock represents a situation of initially uncontrolled hemorrhage. Thus, when resuscitation is typically initiated the process of blood loss may still be ongoing and the pathophysiologic response may differ from that seen in the aforementioned models. Some investigators have attempted to address the effects of ongoing shock by applying various versions of arterial or venous models of uncontrolled hemorrhage. Using a canine model of uncontrolled hemorrhage, Canon *et al.* reported in 1918 (107) that simply raising blood pressure by provision of fluids, without stopping the ongoing hemorrhage, increased mortality. In subsequent studies examining the physiologic effects of uncontrolled hemorrhage, investigators directed efforts at maintaining a near normal blood pressure (80 mmHg or greater) in a swine model of uncontrolled hemorrhage and found this also worsened acidosis in the animals while decreasing survival (108, 109). Capone *et al.* (110, 111), using an alternative rat model, in which 75% of the tail is amputated to induce uncontrolled hemorrhage, observed animals that were resuscitated back to a mean arterial pressure of only 40 mmHg as opposed to near normal mean blood pressure approaching 80 mmHg, prior to controlling the bleeding; survival over 3 days following shock was nearly 60% as opposed 0%, respectively. In keeping with these findings, Smail *et al.* (112) found that moderate to low volume as opposed to higher volume resuscitation in a rat model of uncontrolled venous hemorrhage also provided a greater benefit in the maintenance of organ blood flow and varying aspects of cardiac function. These findings, taken together, have contributed to active debate concerning the approach to resuscitating trauma victims, with respect to volume, rate, indices used to define adequacy, and timing, when the site of bleeding remains uncontrolled (1, 113). However, because these models have remained significantly less predictable, their application in the laboratory, with respect to understanding how hypovolemia and/or hyptension produce the pathophysiology seen in patients or animal models, remains limited (5).

VII. Summary

It is our hope that discussion of models of the pathophysiology of hemorrhagic shock has provided some insight into both the nature and variety of shock models and their respective advantages and disadvantages. Furthermore, it is our hope that this discussion and the examples given will serve as a basis for choosing a useful model and the technical foundations for their use. In the following section, three animal model protocols are presented in detail.

VIII. Animal Models

A. Fixed-Volume Hemorrhage (Shock) Model in Mice via Cardiac Puncture

See Abraham and Freitas (39) and Shenkar *et al.* (137) for details.

Animals

Virtually any inbred mouse strain: present source Jackson Laboratories, Bar Harbor, ME, or Charles River Laboratories, Wilmington, MA. Male and/or females, typically at least 6 to 8 weeks old, weighing 20–25 g. Note: Prior to hemorrhage procedure, animals are fasted overnight but are allowed water *ad libitum*.

Materials

1. Metofane [methoxyflurane; 2,2-dichloro-1,1-difluoroethyl methyl ether BHT (butylated hydroxytoluene, 0.01%, w/w), Schering-Plough Animal Health Corp., Union, NJ]. Used in jar with wire mesh over gauze at bottom and in plastic cone with gauze at the end. Note: Isoflurane can be used as a replacement anesthetic if methoxyflurane unavailable. However, an appropriate vaporizor/scavenger system is required (Viking Medical Products, Inc., Medford, NJ).
2. Lactated Ringer's solution (LRS), for resuscitation.
3. Plexiglass board (4″ × 6″), to secure/restrain mouse.
4. Syringe, 1 ml, containing 0.1 ml of heparin (50 units/ml stock) with an attached 30-gauge needle.

Hemorrhage Procedures

1. *Operative preparation:* Lightly anesthetize the mouse with Metofane (use a jar with gauze at the bottom) and place animal onto a plexiglass board in supine position. The mouse can be kept anesthetized by placing a "Metofane cone" above its nose. Note: Care should be taken not to soak the mouse with Metofane or the animal will stick to the board.
2. *Hypovolemic shock*
   a. Holding the syringe in the palm of your hand with your thumb on the plunger (so it can be withdrawn), insert the needle (bevel side facing down) into the mouse chest just below and slightly to the left of the xiphoid cartilage at the base of the sternum. The needle should enter at about a 15–20° angle.
   b. Slowly advance the needle while simultaneously applying a slight negative pressure to the syringe via withdrawal of the the plunger. Blood will flow into the tip of the syringe when the right atrium is properly encountered. Continue to aspirate blood for about 60 sec until the predetermined blood volume has been removed, e.g., ~30%, or ~0.5 ml (39, 138). Typically the blood volume to be removed can be calculated based on the total body weight. For a mouse this is reportedly ~75 ml/kg body weight or 1.5–1.9 ml for a mouse weighing 20–25 g. For a rat the estimated total blood volume is closer to ~61 ml/kg body weight (139–141).
   c. The animal is then returned to its cage and allowed to awaken; it should be kept there until it recovers and then is returned to the animal care facility.
3. *Resuscitation*
   a. If the animal is to be subsequently resuscitated with its shed blood [which is retained in a sterile syringe with heparin sulfate (5 units/mouse) at 37°C], the blood is typically returned through the orbital plexus (137). This requires a second exposure to Metofane to produce light general anesthesia, typically about 1 hr after initial blood withdrawal.
   b. Place the anesthetized animal on its side. Grasp the mouse by the neck and head with the index finger and thumb of one hand. Using the index finger to apply pressure to the jugular vein, use the thumb to push the superior eyelid dorsally, exposing the base of the eye.
   c. Insert the syringe into the lateral canthus of the eye, moving it in a medial direction (not anteriorly, because the orbital sinus is located posteriorly in the orbit of the eye). The blood can then be reinfused with gentle pressure on the syringe plunger.
   d. Following reinfusion remove the syringe needle and apply pressure over the eye to prevent the development of a hematoma.
   e. So as not to permanently damage the eye it is suggested that resuscitants such as lactated Ringer's solution and/or experimental drugs be provided separately by a subcutaneous route.
   f. Monitor recovery for 20–30 min to assure that animals return to a near normal state of locomotion/arousal. Animals are then returned to the animal facility. Note: If the animals are resuscitated with blood and/or fluids, the total anesthesia period is ~10–15 min (two periods of 5–8 min each).

B. Fixed-Pressure Hemorrhage (Shock) Model in Mice

See Ayala *et al.* (67) and Stephan *et al.* (142) for details.

Animals

See Section VIII,A for sources and fasting information for inbred mouse strains.

Materials

1. Dissecting microscope and stand; optical capacity must be between 60 and 250× magnification, with an appropriate fiber-optic light source.
2. MicroMed or Grass physiograph with pressure manometer for calibration.
3. Metofane or isoflurane for general anethesia (see Section VIII,A).

4. Betadine solution (topical antiseptic bactericide/ virucide)

5. Hypotears ointment (eye lubricant).

6. Lidocaine, 1% (10 mg/ml).

7. Heparin sodium injection, dilute to 20 U/ml in 0.9% NaCl injection.

8. Lactated Ringer's solution, for resuscitation.

9. Electrical cordless pet trimmer (Wahl model #8980).

10. Plexiglass board (4″ × 6″), to secure/restrain mouse.

11. ~0.3″ × 2″–3″ pieces of adhesive tape (four pieces/ animal) for securing mouse to board.

12. Silk pieces (5-0), 3″–4″, six/animal.

13. 30G $\frac{1}{2}$″ needle.

14. Suture (6.0), black monofilament nylon, with cutting P-1.

15. Cotton-tipped applicators (6″).

16. Two catheters/animal [polyethylene tubing (PE-10)] attached to a 27G $\frac{1}{2}$″ needle (tip ground) and in turn attached to a 1-ml syringe filled with heparin NaCl (20 U/ml).

17. Sterilized surgical pack containing 4″ microdissecting scissors, 4″ serrated straight forceps, 4″ serrated curved forceps, 4″ mosquito forceps, Hayman microspatula (6$\frac{1}{2}$″), microdissecting hook finger (6″), silk pieces (5-0), needle holder, gauze sponges (2 × 2 8ply), and cotton swabs.

Hemorrhage Procedures

1. *Operative preparation:* Lightly anesthetize the mouse with Metofane (use a jar with gauze at the bottom) and restrain with thin tape tethers in supine position on a plexiglass board. The mouse can be kept anesthetized by placing a "Metofane cone" above its nose. Shave off fur in the inguinal area (both sides) and apply Betadine solution with a cotton-tipped applicator. Apply eye ointment (Hypotears).

2. *Catheterization*

a. Elevate the inguinal fold and make an incision with microscissors, cutting only the skin layer. With the aid of the dissecting microscope, use the microforceps to dissect the areolar tissue down to the femoral vessel bundle. Note: Lidocaine (xylocaine; local analgesic) should be applied periodically to the incision area alternately with saline to keep the vessels and tissue moist and to maintain localized anesthesia.

b. Using the hook-finger or smoothed curved forceps, carefully separate the femoral nerve from the venous tissue and lift aside. At this point the artery may be either separated from the vein or retained intact for stability purposes.

c. The three (5-0) silk ties can be passed under the vessels by gently lifting the vessels from underneath using bent forceps. The three silk ties are placed as follows: *Distal* (for decanulation): place most distally in relation to the spatula and have "tie-ready" but not tied at this time. *Medial* (catheter security): place just caudal to the distal tie and have "tie-ready" but not tied at this time. *Caudal* (venous cannulation and tension control): place most caudal (relative to the spatula) and securely tie. Note: When securing a suture tie on any mouse vessel it is important to apply force laterally and downward toward the vessel. Never pull upward or vessel may rupture.

d. Once all ties are in place, slide the Hayman microspatula underneath the vessels (for support) by gently lifting the blood vessels with the medial tie.

e. Gently stretch the vessel by placing moderated tension on the distal tie by taping tie ends to the board. Be sure that medial and caudal ties are slipped back off the caudal edge of spatula surface. Note: No ties should remain on the spatula surface because this impedes catheter movement.

f. Using a 30G needle (bent at a ~45° angle) make a small puncture incision in the femoral artery just above the distal tie knot (to avoid puncturing through both sides of the vessel, advance the needle at a slight angle, nearly parallel). If tension is adequate on the vessel from the distal tie, little or no blood should seep from the vessel.

g. Using serrated straight or curved forceps advance the catheter into the vessel with its bevel facing down (this allows the catheter to catch the hole/incision) at about a 45° angle. Note: It is important to stretch and recut the catheter before inserting it into the artery. This will allow the catheter to slide in easier [to stretch PE-10 tubing, hold between hand (wearing latex gloves) and pull with moderate strength until the catheter is about two-thirds to one-half its original diameter].

h. When the catheter is inside the artery, blood should back up into the catheter. At this point the catheter can be gently advanced with one hand while keeping the spatula flattened with the other hand (the advancement is approximately 1–2 cm without force).

i. Once the catheter is in place, carefully slide the medial tie distally just above the catheter insertion point and tie a secure knot. For extra security, it is sometimes useful to criss-cross the ends of the distal tie with the medial tie. The caudal tie, however, should still be "tie-ready" (but not tied tight) and pushed caudally (close to the peritoneal wall) away from the arterial incision.

j. The spatula now can be backed out from underneath the vessels. Note: Again, it is important to keep the vessels moist.
k. This same procedure is repeated on the opposite side of the mouse. Note: One side will be used for monitoring the blood pressure via a polygraph and the other side will be for blood withdrawal.
l. Before connecting the mouse to the physiograph give 0.5 ml heparin (20 U/ml NaCl) in each femoral artery via catheter injection (total volume of ~0.1 ml).
m. Once the catheters are connected to the polygraph allow the mouse to stabilize (awaken fully) for about 5–10 min (stabilizing pressure should be in the range of 90–98 mmHg) before beginning the hemorrhage procedure.

3. *Hemorrhage and Resuscitation*
a. Blood should be withdrawn at a steady but slow rate (~30–45 sec/0.1 ml) until a mean arterial pressure between 40–30 mmHg is achieved. Note: Sham's undergo the same surgical protocol and period of board stress as hemorrhaged mice; however, they are not bled or resuscitated (they have no significant fluid loss).
b. The mouse is left to stabilize at this point for a predetermined period of time without anesthesia (the time and amount of shed blood are recorded). Note: The rapid bleeding of the animals to induce hemorrhage (~5 min) produces a state of depressed sensibility in the absence of anesthetic, thus minimizing stress and discomfort during the hypotensive state.
c. At the end of the selected period of hemorrhage (typically 1 hr, but shorter/longer periods of 15–30 or 90 min have also been used) the final shed blood volume is recorded, then given back (via catheter injection) at a slow but steady rate (15–30 sec/0.1 ml). The mouse is then resuscitated with LRS (equivalent to twice the volume of shed blood) and disconnected from the polygraph; the mouse is now ready for decannulation.

4. *Catheter removal*
a. Before decannulation, check the position of the caudal tie (the piece should be tie-ready and placed above the arterial catheter entrance, clear of any tissues). With the aid of the scope, gently and slowly pull the catheter back while holding the artery in place by grasping the medial tie with the forceps (less tension is applied to the artery by holding the medial tie). When the tip of the catheter can be seen just above the opening in the artery (and is clear of the caudal tie), the caudal tie can quickly be secured.
b. After both decannulations have been achieved the incisions are sutured in a single layer with (6-0) black monofilament nylon (cutting P-1 needle) (this should be done after lightly anesthetizing animal).
c. Animal is then untethered (unrestrained) and returned to its cage. The cage should be lined with a paper towel so as to avoid laying animals directly into bedding material while in recovery.
d. Recovery is then monitored for 20–30 min to assure that animals return to a near normal state of locomotion/arousal. Animals are then returned to the animal facility following recovery. Note: Total restraint time is ~30 min anesthetized and 1.25 hr unanesthetized.

C. Unrestrained, Unheparinized, Conscious, Fixed-Pressure Model of Trauma Hemorrhage (Shock) in Rats

See Wang *et al.* (95) for details.

Animals

Typically any strain of rat: present source, Charles River Laboratories, Wilmington, MA. Male and/or females, typically at least 6 to 8 weeks old, weighing 250–300 g. Note: Prior to hemorrhage procedure, animals are typically fasted overnight (14–16 hr) but are allowed water *ad libitum.*

Materials

1. MicroMed or Grass physiograph with pressure manometer for calibration.
2. Metofane or isoflurane for general anesthesia (see Section VIII, A).
3. Betadine solution (topical antiseptic bactericide/virucide)
4. Lidocaine, 1% (10 mg/ml).
5. Lactated Ringer's solution, for resuscitation.
6. Electrical small animal trimmer (Oster, model A-1).
7. Wood board (4″ × 6″), to secure/restrain.
8. ~1″ × 2″–3″ pieces of adhesive tape (four pieces/animal) for securing mouse to board.
9. Silk pieces (5-0), 3″–4″, six/animal.
10. Suture (6.0), black monofilament nylon, with cutting P-1.
11. Cotton-tipped applicators (6″).
12. Three catheters/animal [polyethylene tubing (PE-50)] attached to a 23G $\frac{1}{2}$″ stub adapter and in turn attached to a syringe filled with LRS.
13. Sterilized surgical pack containing 4″ microdissecting scissors, 4″ serrated straight forceps, 4″ serrated curved

forceps, 4″ mosquito forceps, microspatula (8″), microdissecting hook finger (6″), silk pieces, (5-0), needle holder, gauze sponges (2 × 2 8ply), and cotton swabs.

Hemorrhage Procedures

1. *Operative preparation:* Lightly anesthetize the rat with Metofane (use a jar with gauze at the bottom) and shave off fur from the base of the head (the neck); shave the abdomen and clip the hair of the inguinal area (both sides) and apply Betadine solution with a cotton-tipped applicator. The rat is then restrained with tape tethers in supine position onto a wood board for surgery. The rat can be kept anesthetized by placing a "Metofane cone" above its nose.

2. *Soft tissue trauma*
   a. Make a snip incision (cutting only the skin layer) on midline just below the diaphragm. With forceps lift skin and advance scissors under the skin and separate the two layers by spreading scissors. After separating the layers, make a cut along the midline distal to the incision. The cut should be about 4–5 cm long.
   b. Make another snip incision into the muscle layer, also just below the diaphragm. Be careful not to cut into any organs underneath. Locate the linea-alba and cut along this distally. This cut should be a little smaller than the previous one.
   c. Suture both the muscle layer and the epidermal layer separately with (6-0) monofilament nylon. The wound is bathed in lidocaine.

3. *Catheterization*
   a. Elevate the inguinal fold and make an incision with microscissors, cutting only the skin layer. Use the forceps to dissect the areolar tissue down to the femoral vessel bundle. Note: Lidocaine (xylocaine; local analgesic) should be applied periodically to the incision area.
   b. Using the smoothed curved forceps, carefully separate the femoral nerve from the venous tissue and lift aside. At this point the artery is also separated from the vein.
   c. The two (5-0) silk ties can be passed under the vessels by gently lifting the vessels from underneath using bent forceps. The two silk ties are placed as follows: *Distal* (for decanulation): place most distally in relation to the spatula and have "tie-ready" but not tied at this time. *Caudal* (venous cannulation and tension control): place most caudal and securely tie.
   d. Once all ties are in place, slide the microspatula underneath the vessels for support by gently lifting the blood vessels with the medial tie.
   e. Gently stretch the vessel by placing moderated tension on the distal tie by taping tie ends to the board. Be sure that medial and caudal ties are slipped back off the caudal edge of the extended forceps.
   f. Using a microscissor, make a small incision in the respective artery or vein just above the distal tie knot. If tension is adequate on vessel from the distal tie, little or no blood should seep from the vessel.
   g. Using serrated straight or curved forceps the catheter can then be advance into the vessel with its bevel facing down (this allows the catheter to catch the hole/incision) at about a 45° angle.
   h. When the catheter is inside the artery, blood should back up into the catheter (Note: this will not occur with the vein). At this point the catheter can be gently advanced with one hand while keeping the spatula flattened with the other hand (the advancement is approximately 1–2 cm, without force).
   i. Once the catheter is in place secure the caudal tie with a knot. For extra security, it is sometimes useful to criss-cross the ends of the distal tie with the caudal tie.
   j. The spatula now can be backed out from underneath the vessels. Note: Again it is important to keep the vessels moist.
   k. This same procedure is repeated on the opposite side of the rat and one vein is also catheterized. One artery will be used for monitoring the blood pressure via polygraph, the other artery will be for blood withdrawal and the vein will be for resuscitation.
   l. The catheters are then tunneled underneath the skin and brought out through a small incision made in the back of the nape of the neck (dorsal side).
   m. The catheters are connected to the polygraph and the rat is allowed to stabilize (awaken fully) for about 5–10 min (stabilizing pressure should be in the range of 105–110 mmHg) before beginning the hemorrhage procedure.

4. *Hemorrhage and resuscitation*
   a. The animal is then allowed to bleed from the remaining arterial catheter into a reservoir over a 10-min period until the mean arterial pressure, ~40 mmHg, is achieved.
   b. The rat is maintained at this mean arterial pressure of 40 mmHg by the further withdrawal of small volumes of blood until the animal can no longer maintain this blood pressure (decompensates) without the provision of fluids. This point is considered as the maximum bleed-out. The time required to reach this point is typically about 50 min, at which point the shed blood volume is recorded. Note: The rapid bleeding of the animals to induce hemorrhage (~10 min) produces a state of depressed sensibility in the absence of anesthet-

ic, thus minimizing stress and discomfort during the hypotensive state.

c. The mean arterial pressure is maintained at 40 mmHg until 40% of the maximum bleed-out volume has been returned to the animal in the form of lactated Ringer's solution (this typically takes another ~45 min).

d. At the end of this hypotensive period the rat is then resuscitated with LRS (equivalent four times the maximum bleed-out volume) over a 60-min period and disconnected from the polygraph; the catheters are sealed and the excess trimmed away.

e. Recovery is then monitored for 20–30 min. to assure that the animals return to a near normal state of locomotion/arousal. Animals are then returned to the animal facility following recovery. Note: Total restraint time is ~30 min anesthetized and 2.5 hr unanesthetized.

Acknowledgments

We would like to express our sincerest thanks to Ms. Joanne Lomas for editorial assistance with the development of this manuscript. This work was supported by the National Institutes of Health Grant R01-GM37127 and Grant R01-GM39519.

References

1. Pope, A., French, G., and Longnecker, D. E. (1999). Fluid resuscitation. State of the science for treating combat casualties and civilian injuries.
2. Chaudry, I. H., Wang, P., Singh, G., Hauptman, J. G., *et al.* (1993). Rat and mouse models of hypovolemic-traumatic shock. *In* Pathophysiology of Shock, Sepsis, and Organ Failure" (G. Schlag and H. Redl, eds.), pp. 371–383. Springer-Verlag, Berlin.
3. Chaudry, I. H., and Ayala, A. (1992). "Immunological Aspects of Hemorrhage." R. G. Landes Company, Austin, Texas.
4. Schlag, G., and Redl, H. (1993). "Pathophysiology of Shock, Sepsis, and Organ Failure." Springer-Verlag, Berlin.
5. Peitzman, A. B., Billiar, T. R., Harbrecht, B. G., Kelly, E., Udekwu, A. O., and Simmons, R. L. (1995). Hemorrhagic shock. *Curr. Prob. Surg.* **32,** 927–1002.
6. MacLean, L. D. (1977). Causes and management of circulatory collapse. *In* "Davis–Christopher Textbook of Surgery" (D. C. Sebastian, ed.) pp. 65–94. Saunders, Philadelphia.
7. Deitch, E. A. (1998). Animal models of sepsis and shock: A review and lessons learned. *Shock* **9,** 1–11.
8. Livingston, D. H., Apel, S. H., Wellhausen, S. R., Sonnenfeld, G., and Polk, H. C. (1988). Depressed interferon-gamma production and monocyte HLA-DR expression after severe injury. *Arch. Surg.* **123,** 1309–1312.
9. Miller-Graziano, C. L., Szabo, G., Takayama, T., and Wu, J. Y. (1989). Alterations of monocyte function following major injury. *In* "Immune Consequences of Trauma, Shock, and Sepsis: Mechanisms and Therapeutic Approaches" (E. Faist, J. Ninnemann, and D. Green, eds.), pp. 95–108. Springer-Verlag, Berlin.
10. Livingston, D. H., and Malangoni, M. A. (1989). An experimental study of susceptibility to infection after hemorrhagic shock. *Surg. Gynecol. Obstet.* **168,** 138–142.
11. Livingston, D. H., and Malangoni, M. A. (1987). Prolonged susceptibility to infection exists after hemorrhagic shock despite resuscitation and antibiotics. *Surg. Forum* **38,** 64–67.
12. Miller-Graziano, C. L., Szabo, G., Kodys, K., and Mehta, B. (1993). Interactions of immunopathological mediators (tumor necrosis factor-α, TGF-β, prostaglandin E_2) in traumatized individuals. *In* "Host Defense Dysfunction in Trauma, Shock and Sepsis: Mechanisms and Therapeutic Approaches" (E. Faist, J. L. Meakins, and F. W. Schildberg, eds.), pp. 637–650. Springer-Verlag, Berlin.
13. Denis, M. (1994). Human monocytes/macrophages: NO or NO? *J. Leukoc. Biol.* **55,** 682–684.
14. Zhang, X., Laubach, V. E., Alley, E. W., Edwards, K. A., Sherman, P. A., Russell, S. W., and Murphy, W. J. (1996). Transcriptional basis for hyporesponsiveness of the human inducible nitric oxide synthase gene to lipopolysaccharide/interferon-gamma. *J. Leukoc. Biol.* **59,** 575–585.
15. Ebong, S. J., Call, D. R., Bolgos, G., Newcomb, D. E., Granger, J. I., O'Reilly, M., and Remick, D. G. (1999). Immunopathologic responses to non-lethal sepsis. *Shock* **12,** 118–126.
16. McCarter, R. J., and McGee, J. R. (1989). Transient reduction of metabolic rate by food restriction. *Am. J. Physiol.* **257,** E175–E179.
17. Meijerink, W. J. H. J., Molina, P. E., and Abumrad, N. N. (1999). Mammalian opiate alkaloid synthesis: Lessons derived from plant biochemistry. *Shock* **12,** 165–173.
18. Anonymous (1996). "Guide for the Care and Use of Laboratory Animals." Institute of Laboratory Animal Resources, Commission on Life Sciences, National Research Council.
19. Baker, C. H., Wilmoth, F. R., Sutton, E. T., and Price, J. M. (1988). Microvascular responses of intact and adrenal medullectomized rats to hemorrhagic shock. *Circ. Shock* **26,** 203–218.
20. Bitterman, H., Smith, B. A., and Lefer, A. M. (1988). Beneficial actions of antagonism of peptide leukotrienes in hemorrhagic shock. *Circ. Shock* **24,** 159–168.
21. Blum, H., Schnall, M. D., Renshaw, P. F., and Buzby, G. P. (1988). Metabolic and ionic changes in muscle during hemorrhagic shock. *Circ. Shock* **26,** 341–351.
22. Ikai, I., Ozaki, N., Shimahara, Y., Wakashiro, S., Tokunaga, Y., Tanaka, A., and Ozawa, K. (1989). Significance of hepatic mitochondrial redox potential on the concentrations of plasma amino acids following hemorrhagic shock in rats. *Circ. Shock* **27,** 63–72.
23. Sato, T., Kamiyama, Y., Kamano, T., Rutkowski, J., Cowley, R. A., Trump, B. F., and Jones, R. T. (1985). Pathophysiology of hemorrhagic shock. A model for studying the effects of acute blood loss in the rat. *Virchow's Arch. B Cell Pathol.* **48,** 361–375.
24. van der Meer, C., Valkenburg, P. W., Snijders, P. M., Wignans, M., and van Eck, P. (1987). A method for hemorrhagic shock in the rat. *J. Pharm. Methods* **17,** 75–82.
25. Russell, J. A., Long, C. N. H., and Engel, F. L. (1944). Biochemical studies on shock. II. The role of the peripheral tissues in the metabolism of protein and carbohydrate during hemorrhagic shock in the rat. *J. Exp. Med.* **79,** 1–7.
26. Schumer, W. (1968). Localization of the energy pathway block in shock. *Surgery* **64,** 55–59.
27. Strawitz, J. G., Hift, H., Ehrhardt, A., and Cline, D. W. (1961). Irreversible hemorrhagic shock in rats: Changes in blood glucose and liver glycogen. *Am. J. Physiol.* **200,** 261–263.
28. Ukikusa, M., Kamiyama, Y., Sato, T., Tanaka, J., Jones, R. T., Cowley, R. A., and Trump, B. F. (1981). Pathophysiology of hemorrhagic shock. II. Anoxic metabolism of the rat liver following acute blood loss in the rat. *Circ. Shock* **8,** 483–490.
29. Cunningham, J. N., Shires, G. T., and Wagner, Y. (1971). Cellular transport defects in hemorrhagic shock. *Surgery* **70,** 215–222.
30. Altura, B. M. (1976). Microcirculatory approach to the treatment of circulatory shock with a new analog of vasopressin, [2-phenylalanine, 8-ornithine]vasopressin. *J. Pharmacol. Exp. Ther.* **198,** 187–196.

31. Hershey, S. G., Guccrone, I., and Zweifach, B. (1953). Beneficial action of pretreatment with chlorpromazine on survival following graded hemorrhage in the rat. *Surg. Gynecol. Obstet.* **101,** 431–436.
32. Hauser, G. J., Dayao, E. K., and Zukowska-Grojec, Z. (1995). Effect of pentobarbital anesthesia on the pressor response to agonists *in vivo* in normal and endotoxemic rats. *Res. Commun. Chem. Pathol. Pharmacol.* **90,** 289–300.
33. Hassen, A. H., Feruerstein, G., and Faden, A. I. (1984). Selective cardiorespiratory effects mediated by mu opiod receptors in the nucleus ambiguus. *Neuropharmacology* **23,** 407–415.
34. Sawyer, D. C., Lumb, W. W., and Stone, H. L. (1971). Cardiovascular effects of halothane, methoxyflurane, pentobarbital, and thiamylal. *J. Appl. Physiol.* **30,** 36–43.
35. LePage, G. A. (1946). The effects of hemorrhage on tissue metabolites. *Am. J. Physiol.* **147,** 446–453.
36. Collins, J. A., and Stechenberg, L. (1979). The effects of the concentration and function of hemoglobin on the survival of rats after hemorrhage. *Surgery* **85,** 412–418.
37. Abraham, E., Richmond, J. N., and Chang, Y. H. (1988). Effects of hemorrhage on interleukin-1 production. *Circ. Shock* **25,** 33–40.
38. Giovine, F. S., and Duff, G. W. (1990). IL-1: The first interleukin. *Immunol. Today* **11,** 13–20.
39. Abraham, E., and Freitas, A. A. (1989). Hemorrhage produces abnormalities in lymphocyte function and lymphokine generation. *J. Immunol.* **142,** 899–906.
40. Penfield, W. G. (1919). The treatment of severe and progressive hemorrhage by intravenous injections. *Am. J. Physiol.* **48,** 121–132.
41. Wiggers, C. J. (1942). The present status of the shock problem. *Physiol. Rev.* **22,** 74–123.
42. Drucker, W. R., and DeKiewiet, J. C. (1964) Glucose uptake by diaphragms from rats subjected to hemorrhagic shock. *Am. J. Physiol.* **206,** 317–320.
43. Drucker, W. R., Schlatter, J., and Drucker, R. P. (1968). Metabolic factors associated with endotoxin-induced tolerance for hemorrhagic shock. *Surgery* **64,** 75–84.
44. Weil, M. H., and Afifi, A. A. (1970). Experimental and clinical studies on lactate and pyruvate as indicators of the severity of acute circulatory failure. *Circulation* **XLI,** 989–1001.
45. Mela, L., Bacalzo, L. V., Jr., and Miller, L. D. (1971). Defective oxidative metabolism of rat liver mitochondria in hemorrhagic and endotoxin shock. *Am. J. Physiol.* **220,** 571–577.
46. Rhodes, R. S., and Depalma R. G. (1980). Mitochondrial dysfunction of the liver and hypoglycemia in hemorrhagic shock. *Surg. Gynecol. Obstet.* **150,** 347–352.
47. Ozawa, K., Ida, T., Kamano, T., Garbus, J., and Cowley, R. A. (1976). Different response of hepatic energy change and adenine nucleotide concentrations to hemorrhagic shock. *Res. Exp. Med.* **169,** 145–153.
48. Holliday, R. L., Illner, H. P., and Shires, G. T. (1981). Liver cell membrane alterations during hemorrhagic shock in the rat. *J. Surg. Res.* **31,** 506–515.
49. Lazarus, H. M., and Hopfenbeck, A. (1979). Effects of hemorrhagic shock on nuclear DNA. *Surgery* **85,** 297–302.
50. Esrig, B. C., Frazee, L., Stephenson, S. F., Polk, H. C., Jr., Fulton, R. L., and Jones, C. E. (1977). The predisposition to infection following hemorrhagic shock. *Surg. Gynecol. Obstet.* **144,** 915–917.
51. Schaumloffel, V., Pugh, V., and Bealer, S. L. (1990). Preoptic hypothalamic lesions reduce adrenergic vascular compensation during hemorrhagic shock. *Circ. Shock* **31,** 193–202.
52. Deitch, E. A., Bridges, W., Baker, J., Ma, J., Ma, L., Grisham, M. B., Granger, N., Specian, R. D., and Berg, R. (1988). Hemorrhagic shock-induced bacterial translocation is reduced by xanthine oxidase inhibition or inactivation. *Surgery* **104,** 191–198.
53. Altura, B. M. (1976). DPAVP: A vasopressin analog with selective microvascular and RES actions for the treatment of circulatory shock in rats. *Eur. J. Pharmacol.* **37,** 155–167.
54. Livingston, D. H., Gentile, P. S., and Malangoni, M. A. (1990). Bone marrow failure after hemorrhagic shock. *Circ. Shock* **30,** 255–263.
55. Maitra, S. R., Krikhely, M., Dulchavsky, S. A., Geller, E. R., and Kreis, D. J. J. (1991). Beneficial effects of diltiazem in hemorrhagic shock. *Circ. Shock* **33,** 121–125.
56. Stahl, G. L., Bitterman, H., Terashita, Z., and Lefer, A. M. (1988). Salutary consequences of blockade of platelet activating factor in hemorrhagic shock. *Eur. J. Pharmacol.* **149,** 233–240.
57. Hierholzer, C., Kalff, J. C., Billiar, T. R., and Tweardy, D. J. (1998). Activation of STAT proteins in the lung of rats following resuscitation from hemorrhagic shock. *Arch. Orthop. Trauma Surg.* **117,** 372–375.
58. Tsukada, K., Omert, L. A., Menezes, J., Harbrecht, B. G., Miyagishima, M., and Billiar, T. R. (1999). Neutrophil accumulation and damage to the gastric mucosa in resuscitated hemorrhagic shock is dependent on inducible nitric oxide synthase. *Shock* **11,** 319–324.
59. Zingarelli, B., Ischiropoulos, H., Salzman, A. L., and Szabo, C. (1997). Amelioration by mercaptoethylguanidine of vascular and energetic failure in haemorrhagic shock in the anesthetised rat. *Eur. J. Pharmacol.* **338,** 55–65.
60. Stenseth, R., Berg, E. M., Bjella, L., Christensen, O., Levang, O. W., and Gisvold, S. E. (1993). The influence of thoracic epidural analgesia alone and in combination with general anesthesia on cardiovascular function and myocardial metabolism in patients recieving beta-adrenergic blockers. *Anesth. Analg.* **77,** 463–468.
61. Todd, M. M., and Drummond, J. C. (1984). A comparison of cerebrovascular and metabolic effects of halothane and isoflurane in the cat. *Anesthesiology* **60,** 276–282.
62. Crosby, G., Crane, A. M., and Sokoloff, L. (1982). Local changes in cerebral glucose utilization during ketamine anesthesia. *Anesthesiology* **56,** 437–443.
63. Brunner, E. A., Cheng, S. C., and Berman, M. L. (1975). Effects of anesthesia on intermediary metabolism. *Annu. Rev. Med.* **26,** 391–401.
64. Hillburger, M. E., Adler, M. W., Taunt, A. L., Meissler, J. J., Satishchandran, V., Rogers, T. J., and Eisenstein, T. K. (1997) Morphine induces sepsis in mice. *J. Infect. Dis.* **176,** 183–188.
65. Sayeed, M. M., and Baue, A. E. (1971). Mitochondrial metabolism of succinate, β-hydroxybutyrate, and α-ketoglutarate in hemorrhagic shock. *Am. J. Physiol.* **220,** 1275–1281.
66. Stephan, R. N., Ayala, A., Harkema, J. M., Dean, R. E., Border, J. R., and Chaudry, I. H. (1989). Mechanism of immunosuppression following hemorrhage: Defective antigen presentation by macrophages. *J. Surg. Res.* **46:** 553–556.
67. Ayala, A., Perrin, M. M., and Chaudry, I. H. (1990). Defective macrophage antigen presentation following haemorrhage is associated with the loss of MHC class II (Ia) antigens. *Immunology* **70,** 33–39.
68. Chaudry, I. H., Wichmann, M. W., and Ayala, A. (1997). Immunological alterations following hemorrhagic shock: Considerations for resuscitation with blood substitutes. *In* "Fundamental Principles and Clinical Applications of Red Blood Cell Substitutes" (R. Rabinovici, G. Feuerstein, and A. S. Rudolph, eds.), pp. 165–188.
69. Ayala, A., Ertel, W., and Chaudry, I. H. (1996). Trauma-induced suppression of antigen presentation and expression of major histocompatibility class II antigen complex. *Shock* **5**(2), 79–90.
70. Hierholzer, C., Harbrecht, B., Menezes, J. M., Kane, J., MacMicking, J., Nathan, C. F., Peitzman, A. B., Billiar, T. R., and Tweardy, D. J. (1998). Essential role of induced nitric oxide in the initiation of the inflammatory response after hemorrhagic shock. *J. Exp. Med.* **187,** 917–928.
71. Coimbra, R., Hoyt, D. B., Junger, W. G., Angle, N., Wolf, P., Loomis, W., and Evers, M. F. (1997). Hypertonic saline resuscitation decreases susceptibility to sepsis after hemorrhagic shock. *J. Trauma* **42,** 602–607.
72. Ayala, A., Perrin, M. M., Meldrum, D. R., Ertel, W., and Chaudry, I. H. (1990). Hemorrhage induces an increase in serum TNF which is not associated with elevated levels of endotoxin. *Cytokine* **2,** 170–174.

73. Ayala, A., Wang, P., Ba, Z. F., Perrin, M. M., Ertel, W., and Chaudry, I. H. (1991). Differential alterations in plasma IL-6 and TNF levels following trauma and hemorrhage. *Am. J. Physiol.* **260,** R167–R171.
74. Schmand, J. F., Ayala, A., and Chaudry, I. H. (1994). Effects of trauma, duration of hypotension, and resuscitation regimen on cellular immunity following hemorrhagic shock. *Crit. Care Med.* **22,** 1076–1083.
75. Knoferl, M. W., Angele, M. K., Ayala, A., Cioffi, W. G., Bland, K. I., and Chaudry, I. H. (1999). Do different rates of fluid resuscitation adversely or beneficially influence immune responses after trauma-hemorrhage? *J. Trauma* **46,** 23–33.
76. Angle, N., Hoyt, D. B., Cabello-Passini, R., Herdon-Remelius, C., Loomis, W., and Junger, W. G. (1998). Hypertonic saline resuscitation reduces neutrophil margination by suppressing neutrophil L selectin expression. *J. Trauma* **45,** 7–13.
77. Schmand, J. F., Ayala, A., Morrison, M. H., and Chaudry, I. H. (1994). Dextran 70 administration after trauma-hemorrhagic shock does not impair cellular immune functions. *J. Crit. Care* **9,** 244–254.
78. Schmand, J. F., Ayala A., Morrison, M. H., and Chaudry, I. H. (1995). Restoration of macrophage integrity and prevention of increased circulating interleukin-6 levels. *Crit. Care Med.* **23,** 806–814.
79. Fan, J., Marshall, J. C., Jimenez, M., Shek, P. N., Zagorski, J., and Rotstein, O. D. (1998). Hemorrhagic shock primes for increased expression of cytokine-induced neutrophil chemoattractant in the lung: Role in pulmonary inflammation following lipopolysaccaride. *J. Immunol.* **161,** 440–447.
80. Rizoli, S. B., Kapus, A., Fan, J., Li, Y. H., Marshall, J. C., and Rotstein, O. D. (1998). Immunomodulatory effects of hypertonic resuscitation on the development of lung inflammation following hemorrhagic shock. *J. Immunol.* **161,** 6288–6296.
81. Machiedo, G. W., Ghuman, S., Rush, B. F., Kraven, T., and Dikdan, G. (1981). The effect of ATP-$MgCl_2$ infusion on hepatic cell permeability and metabolism after hemorrhagic shock. *Surgery* **90,** 328–335.
82. Koziol, J. M., Rush, B. F., Smith, S. M., and Machiedo, G. W. (1988). Occurrence of bacteremia during hemorrhagic shock. *J. Trauma* **28,** 10–16.
83. Rush, B. F., Redan, J. A., Flanagan, J. J., Heneghan, J. B., Hsieh, J., Murphy, T. F., Smith, S., and Machiedo, G. W. (1989). Does the bacteremia observed in hemorrhagic shock have clinical significance? A study in germ-free animals. *Ann. Surg.* **210,** 342–347.
84. Crowell, J. W., and Read, W. I. (1955). *In vivo* coagulation—A probable cause of irreversible shock. *Am. J. Physiol.* **183,** 565–569.
85. Coalson, J. J., Benjamin, B., Archer, L. T., Beller, B., Gilliam, C. L., Taylor, F. B., and Hinshaw, L. B. (1978). Prolonged shock in the baboon subjected to infusion of *E. coli* endotoxin. *Circ. Shock* **5,** 423–437.
86. Rush, B. F., Sori, A. J., Murphy, T. F., Smith, S., Flanagan, J. J., and Machiedo, G. W. (1988). Endotoxemia and bacteremia during hemorrhagic shock. The link between trauma and sepsis? *Ann. Surg.* **207,** 549–554.
87. Fry, D. E., Hanschen, S. R., Ratcliff, D. J., and Garrison, R. N. (1984). The effects of heparin on hemorrhagic shock. *Circ. Shock* **13,** 60–61.
88. Devereux, D. F., Michas, C. A., and Rice S. (1977). Heparin pretreatment suppresses norepinephrine concentrations in dogs in endotoxic shock. *Clin. Chem.* **23,** 1346–1347.
89. McBride, W. T., Armstrong, M. A., and McMurray, T. J. (1996). An investigation of the effects of heparin, low molecular weight heparin, protamine and fentanyl on balance of pro- and anti-inflammatory cytokines in *in-vitro* monocyte cultures. *Anaesthesia* **51,** 634–640.
90. Call, D. R., and Remick, D. G. (1998). Low molecular weight heparin is associated with greater cytokine production in a stimulated whole blood model. *Shock* **10,** 192–197.
91. Coon, W. W., and Willis P. W. (1966). Some side effects of heparin, heparinoids, and their antagonists. *Clin. Pharmacol. Therap.* **7,** 379–398.
92. Chopra, P. S., Srinivasan, S., and Lucas, T. (1967). Effect of low molecular weight dextran, heparin and protamine on the surface charge of blood vessels. *Surg. Forum* **18,** 195–197.
93. Rana, M. W., Singh, G., Wang, P., Ayala, A., Zhou, M., and Chaudry, I. H. (1992). Protective effects of preheparinization on the microvasculature during and after hemorrhagic shock. *J. Trauma* **32,** 420–426.
94. Rocko, J. M., Tikellis, J., Barillo, D., Barbalinardo, R., and Rush, B. F. (1986). A non-heparinized muscle model for studies of ischemia-reperfusion. *J. Surg. Res.* **41,** 574–579.
95. Wang, P., Singh, G., Rana, M. W., Ba, Z. F., and Chaudry, I. H. (1990). Preheparinization improves organ function after hemorrhage and resuscitation. *Am. J. Physiol.* **259,** R645–R650.
96. Wang, P., Ba, Z. F., and Chaudry, I. H. (1992). ATP-$MgCl_2$ restores the depressed cardiac output following trauma and severe hemorrhage even in the absence of blood resuscitation. *Circ. Shock* **36,** 277–283.
97. Wang, P., Ba, Z. F., Ayala, A., and Chaudry, I. H. (1992). Hepatocellular dysfunction persists during early sepsis despite increased volume of crystalloid resuscitation. *J. Trauma* **32,** 389–397.
98. Wang, P., Ayala, A., Dean, R. E., Hauptman, J. G., Ba, Z. F., DeJong, G. K., and Chaudry, I. H. (1991). Adequate crystalloid resuscitation restores but fails to maintain the active hepatocellular function following hemorrhagic shock. *J. Trauma* **31,** 601–608.
99. Hauptman, J. G., Wang, P., DeJong, G. K., and Chaudry, I. H. (1991). Improved methodology for the evaluation of the velocity of clearance of indocyanine green in the rat. *Circ. Shock* **32,** 26–32.
100. Wang, P., Tait, S. M., Ba, Z. F., and Chaudry, I. H. (1994). ATP-$MgCl_2$ administration normalizes macrophage cyclic AMP and β-adrenergic receptors after hemorrhage and resuscitation. *Am. J. Physiol.* **267,** G52–G58.
101. Wang, W. Y., Smail, N., Wang, P., and Chaudry, I. H. (1998). Increased gut permeability after hemorrhage is associated with upregulation of local and systemic IL-6. *J. Surg. Res.* **79,** 39–46.
102. Wang, P., Ba, Z. F., and Chaudry, I. H. (1994). Chemically modified heparin improves hepatocellular function, cardiac output, and microcirculation after trauma-hemorrhage and resuscitation. *Surgery* **116,** 169–176.
103. Wang, P., Ba, Z. F., Lu, M. -C., Ayala, A., Harkema, J. M., and Chaudry, I. H. (1994). Measurement of circulating blood volume *in vivo* after trauma-hemorrhage and hemodilution. *Am. J. Physiol.* **266,** R368–R374.
104. Dorraid, J., Chaudry, I. H., and Wang, P. (1999). Organ dysfunction following hemorrhage and sepsis: Mechanisms and therapeutic approaches (review). *Int. J. Mol. Med.* **4,** 575–583.
105. Zellweger, R., Ayala, A., and Chaudry, I. H. (1998). Predisposing factors: Effects of sex, nutrional factors and age on immunity following shock and sepsis. *In* "Cytokines in Severe Sepsis and Septic Shock" (H. Redl and G. Schlag, eds.), pp. 57–77.
106. Wang, P., Ba, Z. F., Burkhardt, J., and Chaudry, I. H. (1993). Trauma-hemorrhage and resuscitation in the mouse: Effects on cardiac output and organ blood flow. *Am. J. Physiol.* **264,** H1166–H1173.
107. Cannon, W. B., Fraser, J., and Cowell, E. M. (1918). The preventive treatment of wound shock. *JAMA* **70,** 618–621.
108. Bickell, W. H., Bruttig, S. P., Millnamow, G. A., O'Benar, J., and Wade, C. E. (1991). The deterimental effects of crystalloid after aortotomy in swine. *Surgery* **110,** 529–536.
109. Stern, S. A., Dronen, S. C., and Wang, X. (1995). Multiple resuscitation regimens in a near-fatal porcine aortic injury hemorrhage model. *Acad. Emerg. Med.* **2,** 89–97.
110. Capone, A. C., Safar, P., Stezoski, W., Tisherman, S., and Peitzman, A. B. (1995). Improved outcome with fluid resuscitation in treatment of uncontrolled hemorrhagic shock. *J. Am. Coll. Surg.* **180,** 49–56.
111. Marchall, H. P. J., Capone, A., Courcoulas, A. P., Harbrecht, B. G., Billiar, T. R., Udekwu, A. O., and Peitzman, A. B. (1997). Effects of hemodilution on long-term survival in an uncontrolled hemorrhagic shock model in rats. *J. Trauma* **43,** 673–679.

112. Smail, N., Wang, P., Cioffi, W. G., Bland, K. I., and Chaudry, I. H. (1998). Resuscitation after uncontrolled venous hemorrhage: Does increased resuscitation volume improve regional perfusion? *J. Trauma* **44,** 701–708.
113. Bickell, W. H., Wall, M. J. J., Pepe, P. E., Martin, R. R., Ginger, V. F., Allen, M. K., and Mattox, K. L. (1994). Immediated versus delayed fluid resuscitation for hypotensive patients with penetrating torso injuries. *N. Engl. J. Med.* **331,** 1105–1109.
114. White, R. R., Mela, L., Bacalzo, L. V., Jr., Olofsson, K., and Miller, L. D. (1973). Hepatic ultrastructure in endotoxemia, hemorrhage, and hypoxia: Emphasis on mitochondrial changes. *Surgery* **73,** 525–534.
115. Nagler, A. L., and McConn, R. (1976). The role of humoral factors in shock. *In* "Shock" (L. A. Ledingham, ed.), pp. 79–109. Excerpta Medica, Amsterdam.
116. Szabo, C., and Billiar, T. R. (1999). Novel roles of nitric oxide in hemorrhagic shock. *Shock* **12,** 1–9.
117. Szabo, C. (1998). Potential role of peroxynitrate-poly (ADP-ribose) synthetase pathway in a rat model of severe hemorrhagic shock. *Shock* **9,** 341–344.
118. Szabo, A., Hake, P., Salzman, A. L., and Szabo, C. (1998). 3-Aminobenzamide, an inhibitor of poly (ADP-ribose) synthetase, improves hemodynamics and prolongs survival in a porcine model of hemorrhagic shock. *Shock* **10,** 347–353.
119. Myers, S. I., and Small, J. (1991). Prolonged hemorrhagic shock decreases splanchnic prostacyclin synthesis. *J. Surg. Res.* **50,** 417–420.
120. Pellicane, J. V., DeMaria, E. J., Leeper-Woodford, S., Lee, R. B., *et al.* (1992). Tumor necrosis factor antibody improves survival following hemorrhagic shock in awake rats. *Circ. Shock* **37,** 54 (abstract).
121. Hierholzer, C., Kalff, J. C., Bednarski, B., Memarzadeh, F., Kim, Y. M., Billiar, T. R., and Tweardy, D. J. (1999). Rapid and simultaneous activation of STAT3 and the production of interleukin 6 in resuscitated hemorrhagic shock. *Arch. Orthop. Trauma Surg.* **119,** 332–336.
122. Hierholzer, C., Kelly, E., Tsukada, K., Loeffert, E., Watkins, S., Billiar, T. R., and Tweardy, D. J. (1997). Hemorrhagic shock induces G-CSF expression in bronchial epithelium. *Am. J. Physiol.* **273,** L1058–L1064.
123. Baue, A. E., Chaudry, I. H., Wurth, M. A., and Sayeed, M. M. (1974). Cellular alterations with shock and ischemia. *Angiology* **25,** 31–41.
124. Baue, A. E., Wurth, M. A., Chaudry, I. H., and Sayeed, M. M. (1973). Impairment of cell membrane transport during shock and after treatment. *Ann. Surg.* **178,** 412–422.
125. Chaudry, I. H., Sayeed, M. M., and Baue, A. E. (1974). Effect of hemorrhagic shock on tissue adenine nucleotides in conscious rats. *Can. J. Physiol. Pharmacol.* **52,** 131–137.
126. Sayeed, M. M., Adler, R. J., Chaudry, I. H., and Baue, A. E. (1981). Effect of hemorrhagic shock on hepatic transmembrane potentials and intracellular electrolytes, *in vivo. Am. J. Physiol.* **240,** R211–R219.
127. Chaudry, I. H., Sayeed, M. M., and Baue, A. E. (1974). Effect of adenosine triphosphate-magnesium chloride administration in shock. *Surgery* **75,** 220–227.
128. Zellweger, R., Ayala, A., Schmand, J. F., Morrison, M. H., and Chaudry, I. H. (1995). PAF-antagonist administration after hemorrhage-resuscitation prevents splenocyte immunodepression. *J. Surg. Res.* **59,** 366–370.
129. Zellweger, R., Ayala, A., Zhu, X., Holme, K. R., DeMaso, C. M., and Chaudry, I. H. (1995). A novel nonanticoagulant heparin improves splenocyte and peritoneal macrophage immune function after trauma-hemorrhage and resuscitation. *J. Surg. Res.* **59,** 211–218.
130. Zhu, X., Zellweger, R., Zhu, X., Ayala, A., and Chaudry, I. H. (1995). Cytokine gene expression in splenic macrophages and Kupffer cells following haemorrhage. *Cytokine* **7,** 8–14.
131. Zhu, X., Ayala, A., Zellweger, R., Morrison, M. H., and Chaudry, I. H. (1994). Peritoneal macrophages show increased cytokine gene expression following hemorrhagic shock. *Immunology* **83,** 378–383.
132. Zellweger, R., Ayala, A., Zhu, X. H., DeMaso, C. M., and Chaudry, I. H. (1996). Prolactin improves cell-mediated immune function, normalizes plasma corticosteroid levels and decreases susceptibiltiy to sepsi after hemorrhagic shock in mice. *J. Immunol.* **157,** 5748–5754.
133. Wichmann, M. W., Zellweger, R., DeMaso, C. M., Ayala, A., and Chaudry, I. H. (1996). Mechanism if immunosuppression in males following trauma-hemorrhage: Critical role of testosterone. *Arch. Surg.* **131,** 1186–1192.
134. Angele, M. K., Schwacha, M. G., Ayala, A., and Chaudry, I. H. (2000). Effect of gender and sex hormones on immune responses following shock. *Shock* **14,** 81–90.
135. Ayala, A., Xu, Y. X., Ayala, C. A., Sonefeld, D. E., Karr, S. M., Evans, T. A., and Chaudry I. H. (1998). Increased mucosal B-lymphocyte apoptosis during polymicrobial sepsis is a Fas ligand but not an endotoxin mediated process. *Blood* **91,** 1362–1372.
136. Xu, Y. X., Ayala, A., Monfils, B., Cioffi, W. G., and Chaudry, I. H. (1997). Mechanism of intestinal mucosal immune dysfunction following trauma-hemorrhage: Increased apoptosis associated with elevated Fas expression in Peyer's patches. *J. Surg. Res.* **70,** 55–60.
137. Shenkar, R., Chang, Y., and Abraham, E. (1994). Cytokine expression in Peyer's patches following hemorrhage and resuscitation. *Shock* **1,** 25–30.
138. Abraham, E., and Freitas, A. A. (1989). Hemorrhage in mice induces alterations in immunoglobulin-secreting B-cells. *Crit. Care Med.* **17,** 1015–1019.
139. Hauptman, J. G., DeJong, G. K., Blasko, K. A., and Chaudry, I. H. (1989). Measurement of hepatocellular function, cardiac output, effective blood volume and oxygen saturation in the rat. *Am. J. Physiol.* **257,** R439–R444.
140. Harkness, J. E., and Wagner, J. E. (1989). Biology and husbandry. *In* "The Biology and Medicine of Rabbits and Rodents," 3rd Ed., pp. 9–54. Lea & Febiger, Philadelphia.
141. Flecknell, P. A. (1993). Anaesthesia of animals for biomedical research. *Brit. J. Anesth.* **71,** 885–894.
142. Stephan, R. N., Kupper, T. S., Geha, A. S., Baue, A. S., and Chaudry, I. H. (1987). Hemorrhage without tissue trauma produces immunosuppression and enhances susceptibility to sepsis. *Arch. Surg.* **122,** 62–68.

28

Scoring Systems for Trauma Research

Walter L. Biffl and Ernest E. Moore

Department of Surgery, Denver Health Medical Center, University of Colorado Health Sciences Center, Denver, Colorado 80204

I. Introduction

Scoring systems in clinical research provide a language to facilitate decisions and offer an investigative basis for this decision-making. For example the tumor, node, metastasis (TNM) classification for malignancies standardizes the reporting of clinical data for cancer. Many trauma scoring systems have been developed over several decades with the goal of quantitatively describing injuries, ascribing to them relative severities, and facilitating prognosis. Scoring systems are meant to promote the evaluation of trauma care quality and efficiency and validate predictors of outcome. In this chapter we provide an overview of the Injury Severity Score (ISS), an Organ Injury Scaling (OIS) system, and a Multiple Organ Failure (MOF) score.

II. The Abbreviated Injury Scale and Injury Severity Score

The first organized effort to develop a taxonomy for injuries was cosponsored by the Association for the Advancement of Automotive Medicine (AAAM), the American Medical Association, and the Society of Automotive Engineers (1–3). The project goal was to define the impact of changes in automobile structure on the injuries sustained by its occupants. This charge was delegated to the Committee on Medical Aspects of Automotive Safety, a group composed predominantly of epidemiologists, biomechanical engineers, and orthopedic surgeons. Their product, the Abbreviated Injury Scale (AIS), was introduced in 1971 (2). The original AIS was a progressive grading scale of injury severity—ranging from 1 (minor) to 6 (maximum)—for each body region but, with the expertise of the subcommittee, focused more on the degree of disability associated with fractures and soft tissue injury than on the degree of injury. The AIS has undergone several revisions, with the most recent being updated in 1998 (1). Although AIS assigns a (relative severity to each injury, it does not allow characterization of the overall status of a multiply injured patient.

Baker and colleagues (4) subsequently employed AIS as the foundation for the ISS in an attempt to predict survival.

The ISS is an anatomic system, based on six body regions—head and neck, face, thorax, abdomen and visceral pelvis, bony pelvis and extremities, and external structures. The highest AIS score in each body region is squared, and the ISS is equal to the sum of the three highest values:

$$\text{ISS} = \text{AIS}^2_{\text{Region 1}} + \text{AIS}^2_{\text{Region 2}} + \text{AIS}^2_{\text{Region 3}}.$$

The ISS may range from 0 to 75. An AIS value of 6 in any body region—considered a lethal injury—is automatically assigned an ISS of 75. Although the ISS represented an improved model for survival probability, the limited perspective of the original ISS (i.e., only one injury per region is considered) became evident when applied to complex multisystem trauma as well as penetrating wounds.

III. The New Injury Severity Score

In an attempt to improve the prognostic ability of injury severity scoring, Osler and colleagues (5) proposed a simple modification called the New Injury Severity Score (NISS). The NISS considers the three most severe injuries, irrespective of body region, and is calculated by adding the squared AIS scores of these injuries:

$$\text{NISS} = \text{AIS}_1^2 + \text{AIS}_2^2 + \text{AIS}_3^2.$$

Osler and colleagues (5) found that NISS is not only easier to calculate than ISS, but was more predictive of survival in two large independent data sets.

IV. The Abdominal Trauma Index

The Penetrating Abdominal Trauma Index (PATI) was developed in 1979 (6) as a result of the inadequacies of ISS to assist in clinical investigation of penetrating wounds, and was subsequently modified to the Abdominal Trauma Index (ATI) (7). The ATI was based on (1) the individual organ severity and (2) the relative risk of early morbidity and mortality estimated for each organ. Specific injuries were graded from 1 to 5, and a complication risk factor x was assigned to each organ, ranging from 1 (lowest risk) to 5 (highest risk) (Table I). The ATI is calculated by multiplying each organ injury grade by that organ's complication risk factor, and summing the scores for all of the individual injuries:

$$\begin{aligned}\text{ATI} = {} & (\text{Injury Grade}_1 \times \text{Complication Risk Factor}_1) + \\ & (\text{Injury Grade}_2 \times \text{Complication Risk Factor}_2) \\ & + \ldots + (\text{Injury Grade}_n \times \text{Complication Risk Factor}_n).\end{aligned}$$

Simplistic in design, the ATI has demonstrated prognostic value: patients with a PATI score >25 had a complication rate of 46%, compared with 7% for those with PATI ≤25 (6). The risk grading concept was validated in our institution (7) and others (8).

Table I Complication Risk Factors for Individual Organs Used in Calculating the Abdominal Trauma Index[a]

Injured organ	Complication risk factor
Colon, pancreas, major vascular	5
Duodenum, liver	4
Spleen, stomach	3
Kidney, ureter	2
Bladder, bone, diaphragm, extrahepatic biliary, small bowel, minor vascular	1

[a]Adapted from Ref. (7), B.C. Borlase, E. E. Moore, and F. A. Moore (1990). The abdominal trauma index: A critical reassessment and validation. *J. Trauma* **30,** 1340–1344.

V. Organ Injury Scaling

In 1987 the American Association for the Surgery of Trauma (AAST) appointed an OIS committee with the singular goal of developing a comprehensive scaling of specific organ injuries (9). The OIS committee members, surgeons representing trauma, neurosurgery, urology, and orthopedics, had published experience in injury scaling. The individual organ injuries were graded I (minimal), II (mild), III (moderate), IV (severe), V (massive), and VI (lethal), similar to the AIS. The scale, however, was based on the magnitude of anatomic disruption similar to the ATI. Specifically, the OIS did not consider estimated blood loss or therapeutic interventions in the scaling. The exclusion of procedures was believed to be important for the OIS to be used for management decisions. The process of generating a specific OIS involved a review of available injury scales, a stratification of injury severity ranked against morbidity and mortality, and discussion within the OIS committee (10). A consensus-derived OIS was drafted and matured with further consideration by the OIS committee members as well as consultants representing other disciplines, e.g., obstetrics and gynecology. The final draft was submitted to the AAST Board of Managers for review, comment, and approval prior to publication in *The Journal of Trauma* (10–16). A correlative listing of AIS-90 (1) grades as well as International Classification of Disease (ICD) 9-CM (17) codes was included for comparison in the OIS tables.

The AAST/OIS Committee has developed OISs for visceral, vascular, and soft tissue injuries of the neck, chest, abdomen and extremities. These were published in the sequence in which they were completed (10–16), and include the following anatomic groups: cervical vascular (Table II); chest wall (Table III); heart (Table IV); lung (Table V); thoracic vascular (Table VI); diaphragm (Table

Table II Cervical Vascular Organ Injury Scale[a]

Grade[b]	Description of injury	ICD-9	AIS-90
I	Thyroid veins	900.8	1–3
	Common facial vein	900.8	1–3
	External jugular vein	900.81	1–3
	Unnamed arterial/venous branches	900.9	1–3
II	External carotid arterial branches (ascending pharyngeal, superior thyroid, lingual, facial, maxillary, occipital, posterior auricular)	900.8	1–3
	Thyrocervical trunk or primary branches	900.8	1–3
	Internal jugular vein	900.1	1–3
III	External carotid artery	900.02	2–3
	Subclavian vein	901.3	3–4
	Vertebral artery	900.8	2–4
IV	Common carotid artery	900.01	3–5
	Subclavian artery	901.1	3–4
V	Internal carotid artery (extracranial)	900.03	3–5

[a]Adapted from Ref. (16), E. E. Moore, M.A. Malangoni, T. H. Cogbill, *et al.* (1996). Organ injury scaling VII: Cervical vascular, peripheral vascular, adrenal, penis, testis, and scrotum. *J. Trauma* **41,** 523–524.

[b]Increase one grade for multiple grade III or IV injuries involving >50% vessel circumference. Decrease one grade for <25% vessel circumference disruption for grade IV or V.

Table III Chest Wall Organ Injury Scale[a]

Grade[b]	Injury type	Description of injury	ICD-9	AIS-90
I	Contusion	Any size	911.0/922.1	1
	Laceration	Skin and subcutaneous	875.0	1
	Fracture	<3 ribs, closed	807.01/.02	1–2
		Nondisplaced clavicle, closed	810.00-.03	2
II	Laceration	Skin, subcutaneous, and muscle	875.1	1
	Fracture	≥3 adjacent ribs, closed	807.03–807.09	2–3
		Open or displaced clavicle	810.10–807.13	2
		Nondisplaced sternum, closed	807.2	2
		Scapular body, open or closed	811.00–807.19	2
III	Laceration	Full thickness, including pleural penetration	862.29	2
	Fracture	Open or displaced sternum; flail sternum	807.2/.3	2
		Unilateral flail segment (<3 ribs)	807.4	3–4
IV	Laceration	Avulsion of chest wall tissues with underlying rib fractures	807.10–807.19	4
	Fracture	Unilateral flail chest (≥3 ribs)	807.4	3–4
V	Fracture	Bilateral flail chest (≥3 ribs on both sides)	807.4	5

[a]This scale is confined to the chest wall alone and does not reflect associated internal thoracic or abdominal injuries. Therefore, further delineation of upper versus lower or anterior versus posterior chest wall was not considered, and a grade VI was not warranted. Specifically, thoracic crush was not used as a descriptive term; instead, the geography and extent of fractures and soft tissue injury were used to define the grade. Adapted from Ref. (12), E. E. Moore, T. H. Cogbill, G.J. Jurkovich, *et al.* (1992). Organ injury scaling III: Chest wall, abdominal vascular, ureter, bladder, and urethra. *J. Trauma* **33,** 337–339.

[b]Upgrade by one grade for bilateral injuries.

Table IV Cardiac Organ Injury Scale[a]

Grade[b]	Description of injury	ICD-9	AIS-90
I	Blunt cardiac injury with minor ECG abnormality (nonspecific ST or T wave changes, premature atrial/ventricular contraction, or persistent sinus tachycardia)	861.01	3
	Blunt or penetrating pericardial wound without cardiac injury, cardiac tamponade, or cardiac herniation	861.01	3
II	Blunt cardiac injury with heart block (right or left bundle branch, left anterior fascicular, or atrioventricular) or ischemic changes (ST depression or T wave inversion) without cardiac failure	861.01	3
	Penetrating tangential myocardial wound up to, but not extending through endocardium, without tamponade	861.12	3
III	Blunt cardiac injury with sustained (≥5 beats/min) or multifocal ventricular contractions	861.01	3–4
	Blunt or penetrating cardiac injury with septal rupture, pulmonary or tricuspid valvular incompetence, papillary muscle dysfunction, or distal coronary arterial occlusion without cardiac failure	861.01	3–4
	Blunt pericardial laceration with cardiac herniation	861.01	3–4
	Blunt cardiac injury with cardiac failure	861.01	3–4
	Penetrating tangential myocardial wound up to, but not extending through, endocardium, with tamponade	861.12	3
IV	Blunt or penetrating cardiac injury with septal rupture, pulmonary or tricuspid valvular incompetence, papillary muscle dysfunction, or distal coronary arterial occlusion producing cardiac failure	861.12	3
	Blunt or penetrating cardiac injury with aortic or mitral valve incompetence	861.12	3
	Blunt or penetrating right ventricular, right atrial, or left atrial perforation	861.03/.13	5
V	Blunt or penetrating cardiac injury with proximal coronary arterial occlusion	861.03/.13	5
	Blunt or penetrating left ventricular perforation	861.03/.13	5
	Stellate injuries with <50% tissue loss of the right ventricle, right atrium, or left atrium	861.03/.13	5
VI	Blunt avulsion of the heart; penetrating wound producing >50% tissue loss of a chamber	861.03/.13	6

[a]Adapted from Ref. (13), E. E. Moore, M. A. Malangoni, T. H. Cogbill, *et al.* (1994). Organ injury scaling IV: Thoracic vascular, lung, cardiac, and diaphragm. *J. Trauma* **36,** 299–300.
[b]Advance one grade for multiple penetrating wounds to a single chamber or multiple chamber involvement.

Table V Lung Organ Injury Scale[a]

Grade[b]	Injury type	Description of injury	ICD-9	AIS-90
I	Contusion	Unilateral, <1 lobe	861.12/.31	3
II	Contusion	Unilateral, single lobe	861.20/.30	3
	Laceration	Simple pneumothorax	860.0/1, 860.4/5	3
III	Contusion	Unilateral, >1 lobe	861.20/.30	3
	Laceration	Persistent (> 72 hr) air leak from distal airway	860.0/1, 860.4/5	3–4
	Hematoma	Nonexpanding intraparenchymal	861.30/862.0	3–4
IV	Laceration	Major (segmental or lobar) air leak	862.21/861.31	4–5
	Hematoma	Expanding intraparenchymal	862.21/861.31	4–5
	Vascular	Primary branch intrapulmonary vessel disruption	901.40	3–5
V	Vascular	Hilar vessel disruption	901.41/.42	4
VI	Vascular	Total, uncontained transection of pulmonary hilum	901.41/.42	4

[a]Adapted from Ref. (13), E. E. Moore, M. A. Malangoni, T. H. Cogbill, *et al.* (1994). Organ injury scaling IV: Thoracic vascular, lung, cardiac, and diaphragm. *J. Trauma* **36,** 299–300.
[b]Advance one grade for bilateral injuries up to grade III; hemothorax is graded according to thoracic vascular OIS.

Table VI Thoracic Vascular Organ Injury Scale[a]

Grade[b]	Description of injury	ICD-9	AIS-90
I	Intercostal artery/vein	901.81	2–3
	Internal mammary artery/vein	901.82	2–3
	Bronchial artery/vein	901.89	2–3
	Esophageal artery/vein	901.9	2–3
	Hemiazygos vein	901.89	2–3
	Unnamed artery/vein	901.9	2–3
II	Azygos vein	901.89	2–3
	Internal jugular vein	900.1	2–3
	Subclavian vein	901.3	3–4
	Innominate vein	901.3	3–4
III	Carotid artery	900.01	3–5
	Innominate artery	901.1	3–4
	Subclavian artery	901.1	3–4
IV	Thoracic aorta, descending	901.0	4–5
	Inferior vena cava (intrathoracic)	902.10	3–4
	Pulmonary artery, primary intraparenchymal branch	901.41	3
	Pulmonary vein, primary intraparenchymal branch	901.42	3
V	Thoracic aorta, ascending and arch	901.0	5
	Superior vena cava	901.2	3–4
	Pulmonary artery, main trunk	901.41	4
	Pulmonary vein, main trunk	901.42	4
VI	Uncontained total transection of thoracic aorta or pulmonary hilum	901.0 901.41/.42	5 4

[a]Adapted from Ref. (13), E. E. Moore, M. A. Malangoni, T. H. Cogbill, *et al.* (1994). Organ injury scaling IV: Thoracic vascular, lung, cardiac, and diaphragm. *J. Trauma* **36,** 299–300.

[b]Increase one grade for multiple grade III or IV injuries if >50% circumference; decrease one grade for grade IV and V injuries if <25% circumference.

VII); spleen (Table VIII); liver (Table IX); extrahepatic biliary (Table X); pancreas (Table XI); esophagus (Table XII); stomach (Table XIII); duodenum (Table XIV); small bowel (Table XV); colon (Table XVI); rectum (Table XVII); abdominal vascular (Table XVIII); adrenal (Table XIX); kidney (Table XX); ureter (Table XXI); bladder (Table XXII); urethra (Table XXIII); uterus nonpregnant (Table XXIV); uterus, pregnant (Table XXV); fallopian tube (Table XXVI); ovary (Table XXVII); vagina (Table XXVIII); vulva (Table XIX); testis (Table XXX); scrotum (Table XXXI); penis (Table XXXII); and peripheral vascular (Table XXXIII) (18). Because these OISs represent the first attempt at consolidating diverse views on scaling, revision is anticipated with clinical experience and testing for validity. The spleen and liver OISs are currently in their second generation (10, 14).

OIS has proved useful in clinical investigation. Perhaps the best examples are the evolution of nonoperative management for solid-organ injuries (19–22) and operative decision-making for hollow visceral wounds (23). The ability to characterize liver injuries has provided compelling support for nonoperative treatment of major lesions, whereas a description of splenic trauma has underscored the potential risks of bleeding from relatively minor splenic injuries. The indications for primary repair of colonic wounds expanded quickly with the availability of uniform descriptors (23). Organ injury scaling has also provided a template for

Table VII Diaphragm Organ Injury Scale[a]

Grade[b]	Description of injury	ICD-9	AIS-90
I	Contusion	862.0	2
II	Laceration ≤2 cm	862.1	3
III	Laceration 2–10 cm	862.1	3
IV	Laceration >10 cm with tissue loss ≤25 cm^2	862.1	3
V	Laceration with tissue loss >25 cm^2	862.1	3

[a]Adapted from Ref. (13), E. E. Moore, M. A. Malangoni, T. H. Cogbill, *et al.* (1994). Organ injury scaling IV: Thoracic vascular, lung, cardiac, and diaphragm. *J. Trauma* **36,** 299–300.

[b]Advance one grade for bilateral injuries.

Table VIII Spleen Organ Injury Scale (1994 Revision)[a]

Grade[b]	Injury type	Description of injury	ICD-9	AIS-90
I	Hematoma	Subcapsular, <10% surface area	865.01/.11	2
	Laceration	Capsular tear, <1 cm parenchymal depth	865.02/.12	2
II	Hematoma	Subcapsular, 10–50% surface area; intraparenchymal, <5 cm in diameter	865.01/.11	2
	Laceration	Capsular tear, 1–3 cm parenchymal depth that does not involve a trabecular vessel	865.02/.12	2
III	Hematoma	Subcapsular, >50% surface area or expanding; ruptured subcapsular or parenchymal hematoma; intraparenchymal hematoma >5 cm or expanding	865.01/.11	3
	Laceration	>3 cm parenchymal depth or involving trabecular vessels	865.03/.13	3
IV	Laceration	Laceration involving segmental or hilar vessels producing major devascularization (>25% of spleen)	865.04/.14	4
V	Laceration	Completely shattered spleen	865.04/.14	5
	Vascular	Hilar vascular injury which devascularizes spleen	865.04/.14	5

[a]Adapted from Ref. (14), E. E. Moore, T. H. Cogbill, G. J. Jukovich, *et al.* (1995). Organ injury scaling: Spleen and liver (1994 revision). *J. Trauma* **38,** 323–324.
[b]Advance one grade for multiple injuries, up to grade III.

improving the AIS, particularly in emphasizing the need for greater scoring detail in specific organs. Finally, OIS can be insinuated into outcome-based scoring systems (e.g., the ATI) (6, 7) for the purposes of identifying and stratifying injured patients for clinical trials.

A substantial challenge for the OIS system is to incorporate neurologic and orthopedic trauma into a comparable scaling format. Despite a number of ongoing multilateral efforts, there has been slow progress in reaching a working consensus. In part, this is due to the complexities of these injuries. Fractures are systematically characterized in the Arbeitsgemeinschaft für Osteosynthesfragen (AO) classification, but this scheme does not rank fractures according to magnitude of injury. Fracture injury scaling is complicated by the associated soft tissue disruption. There is no available scaling system for central nervous system injuries, largely because of the difficulty in deriving an anatomic classification with outcome specificity.

Another major goal for OIS is to achieve international consensus. For example, the Japanese Association for the Surgery of Trauma has developed a separate organ scaling system (24). Trauma is a worldwide epidemic and care of the injured can be improved from sharing information based on a common language. Meaningful trauma outcome assessment

Table IX Liver Organ Injury Scale (1994 Revision)[a]

Grade[b]	Type of injury	Description of injury	ICD-9	AIS-90
I	Hematoma	Subcapsular, <10% surface area	864.01/.11	2
	Laceration	Capsular tear, <1 cm parenchymal depth	864.02/.12	2
II	Hematoma	Subcapsular, 10–50% surface area; intraparenchymal, <10 cm in diameter	864.01/.11	2
	Laceration	1–3 cm parenchymal depth, <10 cm in length	864.03/.13	2
III	Hematoma	Subcapsular, >50% surface area or expanding; ruptured subcapsular or parenchymal hematoma; intraparenchymal hematoma >10 cm or expanding	864.01/.11	3
	Laceration	>3 cm parenchymal depth	864.04/.14	3
IV	Laceration	Parenchymal disruption involving 25–75% of hepatic lobe or 1–3 Couinaud's segments within a single lobe	864.04/.14	4
V	Laceration	Parenchymal disruption involving >75% of hepatic lobe or >3 Couinaud's segments within a single lobe	864.04/.14	5
	Vascular	Juxtahepatic venous injuries; i.e., retrohepatic vena cava/central major hepatic veins	864.04/.14	5
VI	Vascular	Hepatic avulsion	864.04/.14	6

[a]Adapted from Ref. (14), E. E. Moore, T. H. Cogbill, G. J. Jukovich, *et al.* (1995). Organ injury scaling: Spleen and liver (1994 revision). *J. Trauma* **38,** 323–324.
[b]Advance one grade for multiple injuries up to grade II.

Table X Extrahepatic Biliary Tree Organ Injury Scale[a]

Grade[b]	Description of injury	ICD-9	AIS-90
I	Gallbladder contusion	868.02	2
	Portal triad contusion	868.02	2
II	Partial gallbladder avulsion from liver bed; cystic duct intact	868.02	2
	Laceration or perforation of the gallbladder	868.12	2
III	Complete gallbladder avulsion from liver bed	868.02	3
	Cystic duct laceration/transection	868.12	3
IV	Partial or complete right hepatic duct laceration	868.12	3
	Partial or complete left hepatic duct laceration	868.12	3
	Partial common hepatic duct laceration (≤50%)	868.12	3
	Partial common bile duct laceration (≤50%)	868.12	3
V	>50% transection of common hepatic duct	868.12	3–4
	>50% transection of common bile duct	868.12	3–4
	Combined right and left hepatic duct injuries	868.12	3–4
	Intraduodenal or intrapancreatic bile duct injuries	868.12	3–4

[a]Adapted from Ref. (15), E. E. Moore, G. J. Jukovich, M. M. Knudson, *et al.* (1995). Organ injury scaling VI: Extrahepatic biliary, esophagus, stomach, vulva, vagina, uterus (non pregnant), uterus (pregnant), fallopian tube, and ovary. *J. Trauma* **39,** 1069–1070.

[b]Advance one grade for multiple injuries up to grade III.

Table XI Pancreatic Organ Injury Scale[a]

Grade[b]	Type of injury	Description of injury	ICD-9[c]	AIS-90
I	Hematoma	Minor contusion without duct injury	863.81–863.83	2
	Laceration	Superficial laceration without duct injury	863.91–863.93	2
II	Hematoma	Major contusion without duct injury or tissue loss	863.81–863.83	2
	Laceration	Major laceration without duct injury or tissue loss	863.91–863.93	3
III	Laceration	Distal transection or parenchymal injury with duct injury	863.92–863.93	3
IV	Laceration	Proximal[d] transection or parenchymal injury involving ampulla	863.91	4
V	Laceration	Massive disruption of pancreatic head	863.91	5

[a]Adapted from Ref. (11), E. E. Moore, T. H. Cogbill, M. A. Malangoni, *et al.* (1990). Organ injury scaling II: Pancreas, duodenum, small bowel, colon, and rectum. *J. Trauma* **30,** 1427–1429.

[b]Advance one grade for multiple injuries.

[c]Codes: .81 and .91, head; .82 and .92, body; .83 and .93, tail.

[d]Proximal pancreas is to the patients' right of the superior mesenteric vein.

Table XII Esophagus Organ Injury Scale[a]

Grade[b]	Description of injury	ICD-9	AIS-90
I	Contusion/hematoma	862.22/.32	2
	Partial thickness laceration	862.22/.32	3
II	Laceration ≤50% circumference	862.22/.32	4
III	Laceration >50% circumference	862.22/.32	4
IV	Segmental loss or devascularization ≤2 cm	862.22/.32	5
V	Segmental loss or devascularization >2 cm	862.22/.32	5

[a]Adapted from Ref. (15), E. E. Moore, G. J. Jukovich, M. M. Knudson, *et al.* (1995). Organ injury scaling VI: Extrahepatic biliary, esophagus, stomach, valva, vagina, uterus (not pregnant), uterus (pregnant), fallopian tube, and ovary. *J. Trauma* **39,** 1069–1070.

[b]Advance one grade for multiple injuries up to grade III.

Table XIII Stomach Organ Injury Scale[a]

Grade[b]	Description of injury[c]	ICD-9	AIS-90
I	Contusion/hematoma	863.0/.1	2
	Partial-thickness laceration	863.0/.1	2
II	Laceration ≤2 cm in GE junction or pylorus	863.0/.1	3
	≤5 cm in proximal one-third of stomach	863.0/.1	3
	≤10 cm in distal two-thirds of stomach	863.0/.1	3
III	Laceration >2 cm in GE junction or pylorus	863.0/.1	3
	>5 cm in proximal one-third of stomach	863.0/.1	3
	>10 cm in distal two-thirds of stomach	863.0/.1	3
IV	Tissue loss or devascularization ≤2/3 stomach	863.0/.1	4
V	Tissue loss or devascularization >2/3 stomach	863.0/.1	4

[a]Adapted from Ref. (15), E. E. Moore, G. J. Jukovich, M. M. Knudson, *et al.* (1995). Organ injury scaling VI: Extrahepatic biliary, esophagus, stomach, vulva, vagina, uterus (non pregnant), uterus (pregnant), fallopian tube, and ovary. *J. Trauma* **39,** 1069–1070.

[b]Advance one grade for multiple injuries up to grade III.

[c]GE, Gastro esophageal.

Table XIV Duodenum Organ Injury Scale[a]

Grade[b]	Type of injury	Description of injury[c]	ICD-9	AIS-90
I	Hematoma	Involving single portion of duodenum	863.21	2
	Laceration	Partial thickness, no perforation	863.21	3
II	Hematoma	Involving more than one portion	863.21	2
	Laceration	Disruption <50% of circumference	863.31	4
III	Laceration	Disruption 50–75% of circumference of D2	863.31	4
		Disruption 50–100% of circumference of D1, D3, D4	863.31	4
IV	Laceration	Disruption >75% circumference of D2	863.31	5
		Involving ampulla or distal common bile duct	863.31	5
V	Laceration	Massive disruption of duodenopancreatic complex	863.31	5
	Vascular	Devascularization of duodenum	863.31	5

[a]Adapted from Ref. (11), E. E. Moore, T. H. Cogbill, M. A. Malangoni, *et al.* (1990). Organ injury scaling II: Pancreas, duodenum, small bowel, colon, and rectum. *J. Trauma* **30,** 1427–1429.

[b]Advance one grade for multiple injuries up to grade III.

[c]D1, First portion of duodenum; D2, second portion of duodenum; D3, third portion of duodenum; D4, fourth portion of duodenum.

Table XV Small Bowel Organ Injury Scale[a]

Grade[b]	Type of injury	Description of injury	ICD-9	AIS-90
I	Hematoma	Contusion or hematoma without devascularization	863.20	2
	Laceration	Partial thickness, no perforation	863.20	2
II	Laceration	Laceration <50% of circumference	863.30	3
III	Laceration	Laceration ≥50% of circumference without transection	863.30	3
IV	Laceration	Transection	863.30	4
V	Laceration	Transection with segmental tissue loss	863.30	4
	Vascular	Devascularized segment	863.30	4

[a]Adapted from Ref. (11), E. E. Moore, T. H. Cogbill, M. A. Malangoni, *et al.* (1990). Organ injury scaling II: Pancreas, duodenum, small bowel, colon, and rectum. *J. Trauma* **30,** 1427–1429.

[b]Advance one grade for multiple injuries.

Table XVI Colon Organ Injury Scale[a]

Grade[b]	Type of injury	Description of injury	ICD-9[c]	AIS-90
I	Hematoma	Contusion or hematoma without devascularization	863.40–863.44	2
	Laceration	Partial thickness, no perforation	863.40–863.44	2
II	Laceration	Laceration <50% of circumference	863.50–863.54	3
III	Laceration	Laceration ≥50% of circumference without transection	863.50–863.54	3
IV	Laceration	Transection	863.50–863.54	4
V	Laceration	Transection with segmental tissue loss	863.50–863.54	4
	Vascular	Devascularized segment	863.50–863.54	4

[a]Adapted from Ref. (11), E. E. Moore, T. H. Cogbill, M. A. Malangoni, *et al.* (1990). Organ injury scaling II: Pancreas, duodenum, small bowel, colon, and rectum. *J. Trauma* **30,** 1427–1429.
[b]Advance one grade for multiple injuries.
[c]Code: .41 and .51, ascending; .42 and .52, transverse; .43 and .53, descending; .44 and .54, rectum.

demands a complete description of the injured patient that encompasses the essential components: (1) anatomic disruption, (2) physiologic status, and (3) preexisting host factors. The OIS represents a critical step in approaching this goal and, in the interim, serves as an important tool for improving care of the injured.

VI. Multiple Organ Failure Scoring

The dysfunction and failure of organs following trauma have been the focus of a great deal of surgical research over the past two decades. Recognizing the significance of MOF as a clinical endpoint, we developed an MOF score in order to characterize the syndrome quantitatively, and to identify victims for purposes of epidemiologic studies and enrollment in therapeutic clinical trials (25). Difficulty in the practical application of this MOF score in a multicenter trial resulted in its revision (26). Gastrointestinal, hematologic, neurologic, and metabolic failure were eliminated because their definitions were subjective and, more importantly, they did not substantially contribute to identifying MOF. Additionally, the definitions of pulmonary, renal, hepatic, and cardiac failure were revised to facilitate their consistent application at multiple centers (Table XXXIV). Organ failure is defined by a score of 2 or more for an individual organ; MOF is defined as a score of 4 or more, 48 hr after admission (to avoid overdiagnosing MOF in the presence of reversible derangements or incomplete resuscitation). Alternative MOF scores exist (27, 28) and a consensus conference would be helpful to standardize definitions and identify alternative variables to quantify organ failure. However, the scores are similar and, when compared, identify a similar group of patients.

VII. Conclusions

One of the objectives of injury severity scoring is the ability to stratify patients for clinical trials. The ATI and PATI have found their greatest utility in predicting infectious complications, and thus have been useful in selecting high-risk patients for studies of nutritional support (6, 7, 29). In epidemiologic studies we previously identified ISS to be a predictor of MOF, but more recently have found that NISS is a more accurate predictor of MOF (30). The NISS may supplant the ISS as a tool in studying patients with multisystem trauma.

Table XVII Rectal Organ Injury Scale[a]

Grade[b]	Type of injury	Description of injury	ICD-9	AIS-90
I	Hematoma	Contusion or hematoma without devascularization	863.45	2
	Laceration	Partial-thickness laceration	863.45	2
II	Laceration	Laceration <50% of circumference	863.55	3
III	Laceration	Laceration ≥50% of circumference	863.55	4
IV	Laceration	Full-thickness laceration with extension into the perineum	863.55	5
V	Vascular	Devascularized segment	863.55	5

[a]Adapted from Ref. (11), E. E. Moore, T. H. Cogbill, M. A. Malangoni, *et al.* (1990). Organ injury scaling II: Pancreas, duodenum, small bowel, colon, and rectum. *J. Trauma* **30,** 1427–1429.
[b]Advance one grade for multiple injuries.

Table XVIII Abdominal Vascular Injury Scale[a]

Grade[b]	Description of injury	ICD-9	AIS-90[c]
I	Unnamed superior mesenteric artery or superior mesenteric vein branches	902.20/.39	NS
	Unnamed inferior mesenteric artery or inferior mesenteric vein branches	902.27/.32	NS
	Phrenic artery/vein	902.89	NS
	Lumbar artery/vein	902.89	NS
	Gonadal artery/vein	902.89	NS
	Ovarian artery/vein	902.81/.82	NS
	Other unnamed small arterial or venous structures requiring ligation	902.90	NS
II	Right, left, or common hepatic artery	902.22	3
	Splenic artery/vein	902.23/.34	3
	Right or left gastric artery	902.21	3
	Gastroduodenal artery	902.24	3
	Inferior mesenteric artery, trunk or inferior mesenteric vein, trunk	902.27/.32	3
	Primary named branches of mesenteric artery (e.g., ileocolic artery) or mesenteric vein	902.26/.31	3
	Other named abdominal vessels requiring ligation/repair	902.89	3
III	Superior mesenteric vein, trunk	902.31	3
	Renal artery/vein	902.41/.42	3
	Iliac artery/vein	902.53/.54	3
	Hypogastric artery/vein	902.51/.52	3
	Vena cava, infrarenal	902.10	3
IV	Superior mesenteric artery, trunk	902.25	3
	Celiac axis proper	902.24	3
	Vena cava, suprarenal and infrahepatic	902.10	3
	Aorta, infrarenal	902.00	4
V	Portal vein	902.33	3
	Extraparenchymal hepatic vein	902.11	3/5
	Vena cava, retrohepatic or suprahepatic	902.19	5
	Aorta, suprarenal, subdiaphragmatic	902.00	4

[a]Adapted from Ref. (12), E. E. Moore, T. H. Cogbill, G.J. Jurkovich, *et al.* (1992), Organ injury scaling III: Chest wall, abdominal vascular, ureter, bladder, and urethra. *J. Trauma* **33,** 337–339.

[b]This classification system is applicable to extraparenchymal vascular injuries. If the vessel injury is within 2 cm of the organ parenchyma, refer to specific organ injury scale. Increase one grade for multiple grade III or IV injuries involving >50% vessel circumference. Downgrade one grade if <25% vessel circumference laceration for grades IV or V.

[c]NS, Not scored.

Table XIX Adrenal Organ Injury Scale[a]

Grade[b]	Description of injury	ICD-9	AIS-90
I	Contusion	868.01/.11	1
II	Laceration involving only cortex (<2 cm)	868.01/.11	1
III	Laceration extending into medulla (≥2 cm)	868.01/.11	2
IV	>50% parenchymal destruction	868.01/.11	2
V	Total parenchymal destruction (including massive intraparenchymal hemorrhage)	868.01/.11	3
	Avulsion from blood supply	868.01/.11	3

[a]Adapted from Ref. (16), E. E. Moore, M.A. Malangoni, T. H. Cogbill, *et al.* (1996). Organ injury scaling VII: Cervical vascular, peripheral vascular, adrenal, penis, testis, and scrotum. *J. Trauma* **41,** 523–524.

[b]Advance one grade for multiple injuries up to grade V.

Table XX Renal Injury Scale[a]

Grade[b]	Type of injury	Description of injury	ICD-9	AIS-90
I	Contusion	Microscopic or gross hematuria; urologic studies normal		2
	Hematoma	Subcapsular, nonexpanding without parenchymal laceration	866.01/.11	2
II	Hematoma	Nonexpanding perirenal hematoma confined to renal retroperitoneum	866.01/.11	2
	Laceration	<1.0 cm parenchymal depth of renal cortex without urinary extravasation	866.02/.12	2
III	Laceration	>1.0 cm parenchymal depth of renal cortex without collecting system rupture or urinary extravasation	866.02/.12	3
IV	Laceration	Parenchymal laceration extending through renal cortex, medulla, and collecting system		4
	Vascular	Main renal artery or vein injury with contained hemorrhage		4
V	Laceration	Completely shattered kidney	866.03	5
	Vascular	Avulsion of renal hilum, which devascularizes kidney	866.13	5

[a]Adapted from Ref. (10), E. E. Moore, S. R. Shackford, H. L. Pachter *et al.* (1989). Organ injury scaling: Spleen, liver, and kidney. *J. Trauma* **29,** 1664–1666.
[b]Advance one grade for multiple injuries.

Table XXI Ureter Organ Injury Scale[a]

Grade[b]	Type of injury	Description of injury	ICD-9	AIS-90
I	Hematoma	Contusion or hematoma without devascularization	867.2/.3	2
II	Laceration	<50% transection	867.2/.3	2
III	Laceration	≥50% transection	867.2/.3	3
IV	Laceration	Complete transection with <2 cm devascularization	867.2/.3	3
V	Laceration	Avulsion with ≥2 cm of devascularization	867.2/.3	3

[a]Adapted from Ref. (12), E. E. Moore, T. H. Cogbill, G.J. Jurkovich, *et al.* (1992). Organ injury scaling III: Chest wall, abdominal vascular, ureter, bladder, and urethra. *J. Trauma* **33,** 337–339.
[b]Advance one grade for multiple injuries.

Table XXII Bladder Organ Injury Scale[a]

Grade[b]	Type of injury	Description of injury	ICD-9	AIS-90
I	Hematoma	Contusion, intramural hematoma	867.0/.1	2
	Laceration	Partial thickness	867.0/.1	3
II	Laceration	Extraperitoneal bladder wall laceration <2 cm	867.0/.1	4
III	Laceration	Extraperitoneal (≥2 cm) or intraperitoneal (<2 cm) bladder wall laceration	867.0/.1	4
IV	Laceration	Intraperitoneal bladder wall laceration ≥2 cm	867.0/.1	4
V	Laceration	Intra- or extraperitoneal bladder wall laceration extending into the bladder neck or ureteral orifice (trigone)	867.0/.1	4

[a]Adapted from Ref. (12), E. E. Moore, T. H. Cogbill, G.J. Jurkovich, *et al.* (1992). Organ injury scaling III: Chest wall, abdominal vascular, ureter, bladder, and urethra. *J. Trauma* **33,** 337–339.
[b]Advance one grade for multiple injuries.

Table XXIII Urethra Organ Injury Scale[a]

Grade[b]	Type of injury	Description of injury	ICD-9	AIS-90
I	Contusion	Blood at urethral meatus; urethrography normal	867.0/.1	2
II	Stretch injury	Elongation of urethra without extravasation on urethrography	867.0/.1	2
III	Partial disruption	Extravasation of urethrography contrast at injury site with contrast visualization in the bladder	867.0/.1	2
IV	Complete disruption	Extravasation of urethrography contrast at injury site without visualization in the bladder; <2 cm of urethral separation	867.0/.1	3
V	Complete disruption	Complete transection with ≥2 cm urethral separation, or extension into the prostate or vagina	867.0/.1	4

[a]Adapted from Ref. (12), E. E. Moore, T. H. Cogbill, G.J. Jurkovich, *et al.* (1992). Organ injury scaling III: Chest wall, abdominal vascular, ureter, bladder, and urethra. *J. Trauma* **33,** 337–339.
[b]Advance one grade for multiple injuries.

Table XXIV Uterus (Nonpregnant) Organ Injury Scale[a]

Grade[b]	Description of injury	ICD-9	AIS-90
I	Contusion/hematoma	867.4/.5	2
II	Superficial laceration (≤1 cm)	867.4/.5	2
III	Deep laceration (>1 cm)	867.4/.5	3
IV	Laceration involving uterine artery	902.55	3
V	Avulsion/devascularization	867.4/.5	3

[a]Adapted from Ref. (15), E. E. Moore, G. J. Jukovich, M. M. Knudson, *et al.* (1995). Organ injury scaling VI: Extrahepatic biliary, esophagus, stomach, vulva, vagina, uterus (non pregnant), uterus (pregnant), fallopian tube, and ovary. *J. Trauma* **39,** 1069–1070.

[b]Advance one grade for multiple injuries up to grade III.

Table XXV Uterus (Pregnant) Organ Injury Scale[a]

Grade[b]	Description of injury	ICD-9	AIS-90
I	Contusion/hematoma (without placental abruption)	867.4/.5	2
II	Superficial laceration (≤1 cm) or partial placental abruption <25%	867.4/.5	3
III	Deep laceration (>1 cm) occurring in second trimester or placental abruption >25% but <50%	867.4/.5	3
	Deep laceration (>1 cm) in third trimester	867.4/.5	4
IV	Laceration involving uterine artery	902.55	4
	Deep laceration (>1 cm) with >50% placental abruption	867.4/.5	4
V	Uterine rupture—second trimester	867.4/.5	4
	Uterine rupture—third trimester	867.4/.5	5
	Complete placental abruption	867.4/.5	4–5

[a]Adapted from Ref. (15), E. E. Moore, G. J. Jukovich, M. M. Knudson, *et al.* (1995). Organ injury scaling VI: Extrahepatic biliary, esophagus, stomach, vulva, vagina, uterus (non pregnant), uterus (pregnant), fallopian tube, and ovary. *J. Trauma* **39,** 1069–1070.

[b]Advance one grade for multiple injuries up to grade III.

Table XXVI Fallopian Tube Organ Injury Scale[a]

Grade[b]	Description of injury	ICD-9	AIS-90
I	Hematoma/contusion	867.6/.7	2
II	Laceration ≤50% circumference	867.6/.7	2
III	Laceration >50% circumference	867.6/.7	2
IV	Transection	867.6/.7	2
V	Vascular injury; devascularized segment	902.89	2

[a]Adapted from Ref. (15), E. E. Moore, G. J. Jukovich, M. M. Knudson, *et al.* (1995). Organ injury scaling VI: Extrahepatic biliary, esophagus, stomach, vulva, vagina, uterus (non pregnant), uterus (pregnant), fallopian tube, and ovary. *J. Trauma* **39,** 1069–1070.

[b]Advance one grade for bilateral injuries up to grade III.

Table XXVII Ovary Organ Injury Scale[a]

Grade[b]	Description of injury	ICD-9	AIS-90
I	Contusion/hematoma	867.6/.7	1
II	Superficial laceration (depth ≤0.5 cm)	867.6/.7	2
III	Deep laceration (depth >0.5 cm)	867.6/.7	3
IV	Partial disruption of blood supply	902.81	3
V	Avulsion or complete parenchymal destruction	902.81	3

[a]Adapted from Ref. (15), E. E. Moore, G. J. Jukovich, M. M. Knudson, *et al.* (1995). Organ injury scaling VI: Extrahepatic biliary, esophagus, stomach, vulva, vagina, uterus (non pregnant), uterus (pregnant), fallopian tube, and ovary. *J. Trauma* **39,** 1069–1070.

[b]Advance one grade for bilateral injuries up to grade III.

Table XXVIII Vagina Organ Injury Scale[a]

Grade[b]	Description of injury	ICD-9	AIS-90
I	Contusion/hematoma	922.4	1
II	Laceration, superficial (mucosa only)	878.6	1
III	Laceration, deep into fat/muscle	878.6	2
IV	Laceration, complex, into cervix or peritoneum	878.7	3
V	Injury into adjacent organs (anus/rectum/urethra/bladder)	878.7	3

[a]Adapted from Ref. (15), E. E. Moore, G. J. Jukovich, M. M. Knudson, *et al.* (1995). Organ injury scaling VI: Extrahepatic biliary, esophagus, stomach, vulva, vagina, uterus (non pregnant), uterus (pregnant), fallopian tube, and ovary. *J. Trauma* **39,** 1069–1070.
[b]Advance one grade for multiple injuries up to grade III.

Table XXIX Vulva Organ Injury Scale[a]

Grade[b]	Description of injury	ICD-9	AIS-90
I	Contusion/hematoma	922.4	1
II	Laceration, superficial (skin only)	878.4	1
III	Laceration, deep (into fat/muscle)	878.4	2
IV	Avulsion; skin/fat/muscle	878.5	3
V	Injury into adjacent organs (anus/rectum/urethra/bladder)	878.5	3

[a]Adapted from Ref. (15), E. E. Moore, G. J. Jukovich, M. M. Knudson, *et al.* (1995). Organ injury scaling VI: Extrahepatic biliary, esophagus, stomach, vulva, vagina, uterus (non pregnant), uterus (pregnant), fallopian tube, and ovary. *J. Trauma* **39,** 1069–1070.
[b]Advance one grade for multiple injuries up to grade III.

Table XXX Testis Organ Injury Scale[a]

Grade[b]	Description of injury	ICD-9	AIS-90
I	Contusion/hematoma	911.0/922.4	1
II	Subclinical laceration of tunica albuginea	922.4	1
III	Laceration of tunica albuginea with <50% parenchymal loss	878.2	2
IV	Major laceration of tunica albuginea with ≥50% parenchymal loss	878.3	2
V	Total testicular destruction or avulsion	878.3	2

[a]Adapted from Ref. (16), E. E. Moore, M.A. Malangoni, T. H. Cogbill, *et al.* (1996). Organ injury scaling VII: Cervical vascular, peripheral vascular, adrenal, penis, testis, and scrotum. *J. Trauma* **41,** 523–524.
[b]Advance one grade for bilateral injuries up to grade V.

Table XXXI Scrotum Organ Injury Scale[a]

Grade	Description of injury	ICD-9	AIS-90
I	Contusion	922.4	1
II	Laceration <25% of scrotal diameter	878.2	1
III	Laceration ≥25% of scrotal diameter or stellate	878.3	2
IV	Avulsion <50%	878.3	2
V	Avulsion ≥50%	878.3	2

[a]Adapted from Ref. (16), E. E. Moore, M.A. Malangoni, T. H. Cogbill, *et al.* (1996). Organ injury scaling VII: Cervical vascular, peripheral vascular, adrenal, penis, testis, and scrotum. *J. Trauma* **41,** 523–524.

Table XXXII Penis Organ Injury Scale[a]

Grade[b]	Description of injury	ICD-9	AIS-90
I	Cutaneous laceration/contusion	911.0/922.4	1
II	Buck's fascia (cavernosum) laceration without tissue loss	878.0	1
III	Cutaneous avulsion	878.1	3
	Laceration through glans/meatus		
	Cavernosal or urethral defect <2 cm		
IV	Partial penectomy	878.1	3
	Cavernosal or urethral defect ≥2 cm		
V	Total penectomy	878.1	3

[a]Adapted from Ref. (16), E. E. Moore, M.A. Malangoni, T. H. Cogbill, *et al.* (1996). Organ injury scaling VII: Cervical vascular, peripheral vascular, adrenal, penis, testis, and scrotum. *J. Trauma* **41,** 523–524.
[b]Advance one grade for multiple injuries up to grade III.

Table XXXIII Peripheral Vascular Organ Injury Scale[a]

Grade[b]	Description of injury	ICD-9	AIS-90
I	Digital artery/vein	903.5	1–3
	Palmar artery/vein	903.4	1–3
	Deep palmar artery/vein	904.6	1–3
	Dorsalis pedis artery	904.7	1–3
	Plantar artery/vein	904.6	1–3
	Unnamed arterial/venous branches	903.8/904.7	1–3
II	Basilic/cephalic vein	903.8	1–3
	Saphenous vein	904.3	1–3
	Radial artery	903.2	1–3
	Ulnar artery	903.3	1–3
III	Axillary vein	903.02	2–3
	Superficial/deep femoral vein	903.02	2–3
	Popliteal vein	904.42	2–3
	Brachial artery	903.1	2–3
	Anterior tibial artery	904.51/.52	1–3
	Posterior tibial artery	904.53/.54	1–3
	Peroneal artery	904.7	1–3
	Tibioperoneal trunk	904.7	2–3
IV	Superficial/deep femoral artery	904.1/904.7	3–4
	Popliteal artery	904.41	2–3
V	Axillary artery	903.01	2–3
	Common femoral artery	904.0	3–4

[a]Adapted from Ref. (16), E. E. Moore, M.A. Malangoni, T. H. Cogbill, *et al.* (1996). Organ injury scaling VII: Cervical vascular, peripheral vascular, adrenal, penis, testis, and scrotum. *J. Trauma* **41,** 523–524.
[b]Increase one grade for multiple grade III or IV injuries involving >50% vessel circumference. Decrease one grade for <25% vessel circumference disruption for grades IV or V.

Table XXXIV Denver Multiple Organ Failure Score[a]

Organ	Grade 0	Grade 1 dysfunction	Grade 2 dysfunction	Grade 3 dysfunction
Pulmonary	Normal	ARDS score >5	ARDS score >9	ARDS score >13
Renal	Normal	Creatinine >1.8 mg/dl	Creatinine >2.5 mg/dl	Creatinine >5 mg/dl
Hepatic[b]	Normal	Bilirubin >2 mg/dl	Bilirubin >4 mg/dl	Bilirubin >8 mg/dl
Cardiac[c]	Normal	Minimal inotropes	Moderate inotropes	High inotropes

ARDS score = A + B + C + D + E

A. Pulmonary findings by plain chest radiography
- 0 = Normal
- 1 = Diffuse, mild interstitial marking/opacities
- 2 = Diffuse, marked interstitial/mild airspace opacities
- 3 = Diffuse, moderate airspace opacities
- 4 = Diffuse, severe airspace consolidation

B. Hypoxemia (P_{ao_2}/F_{io_2})
- 0 = Normal
- 1 = 175–250
- 2 = 125–174
- 3 = 80–124
- 4 = <80

C. Minute ventilation (liters/min)
- 0 = <11
- 1 = 11–13
- 2 = 14–16
- 3 = 17–20
- 4 = >20

D. Positive end expiratory pressure (cm H_2O)
- 0 = <6
- 1 = 6–9
- 2 = 10–13
- 3 = 14–17
- 4 = >17

E. Static compliance (ml/cm H_2O)
- 0 = >50
- 1 = 40–50
- 2 = 30–39
- 3 = 20–29
- 4 = <20

[a] Adapted from Sauaia *et al.* (26).

[b] Biliary obstruction and resolving hematoma excluded.

[c] Cardiac index <3.0 liters/min/m^2 requiring inotropic support. Minimal dose, dopamine or dobutamine <5 μg/kg/min; moderate dose, dopamine or dobutamine 5–15 μg/kg/min; high dose, greater than moderate doses of above agents.

References

1. Committee on Injury Scaling (1998). The Abbreviated Injury Scale, 1990 Revision, Update 98. Association for the Advancement of Automotive Medicine, Des Plaines, IL.
2. Committee on Medical Aspects of Automotive Safety (1971). Rating the severity of tissue damage: I. The abbreviated scale. *JAMA* **215,** 277–280.
3. Committee on Medical Aspects of Automotive Safety (1972). Rating the severity of tissue damage: II. The comprehensive scale. *JAMA* **220,** 717–720.
4. Baker, S. P., O'Neill, B., Haddon, W., Jr., *et al.* (1974). The injury severity score: A method for describing patients with multiple injuries and evaluating emergency care. *J. Trauma* **14,** 187–196.
5. Osler, T., Baker, S. P., and Long, W. (1997). A modification of the injury severity score that both improves accuracy and simplifies scoring. *J. Trauma* **43,** 922–926.
6. Moore, E. E., Dunn, E. L., Moore, J. B., *et al.* (1981). Penetrating abdominal trauma index. *J. Trauma* **21,** 439–445.
7. Borlase, B. C., Moore, E. E., and Moore, F. A. (1990). The abdominal trauma index: A critical reassessment and validation. *J. Trauma* **30,** 1340–1344.
8. Croce, M. A., Fabian, T. C., Stewart, R. M., *et al.* (1992). Correlation of abdominal trauma index and injury severity score with abdominal septic complications in penetrating and blunt trauma. *J. Trauma* **32,** 380–388.
9. Trunkey, D. D. (1988). Trauma care at mid-passage: A personal viewpoint. *J. Trauma* **28,** 889–895.
10. Moore, E. E., Shackford, S. R., Pachter, H. L., *et al.* (1989). Organ injury scaling: Spleen, liver, and kidney. *J. Trauma* **29,** 1664–1666.
11. Moore, E. E., Cogbill, T. H., Malangoni, M. A., *et al.* (1990). Organ injury scaling II: Pancreas, duodenum, small bowel, colon, and rectum. *J. Trauma* **30,** 1427–1429.
12. Moore, E. E., Cogbill, T. H., Jurkovich, G. J., *et al.* (1992). Organ injury scaling III: Chest wall, abdominal vascular, ureter, bladder, and urethra. *J. Trauma* **33,** 337–339.
13. Moore, E. E., Malangoni, M. A., Cogbill, T. H., *et al.* (1994). Organ injury scaling IV: Thoracic vascular, lung, cardiac, and diaphragm. *J. Trauma* **36,** 299–300.
14. Moore, E. E., Cogbill, T. H., Jurkovich, G. J., *et al.* (1995). Organ injury scaling: Spleen and liver (1994 revision). *J. Trauma* **38,** 323–324.
15. Moore, E. E., Jurkovich, G. J., Knudson, M. M., *et al.* (1995). Organ injury scaling VI: Extrahepatic biliary, esophagus, stomach, vulva,

vagina, uterus (nonpregnant), uterus (pregnant), fallopian tube, and ovary. *J. Trauma* **39,** 1069–1070.

16. Moore, E. E., Malangoni, M. A., Cogbill, T. H., *et al.* (1996). Organ injury scaling VII: Cervical vascular, peripheral vascular, adrenal, penis, testis, and scrotum. *J. Trauma* **41,** 523–524.
17. U.S. Department of Health and Human Services (1994). "International Classification of diseases, 9th revision, Clinical Modification." St. Anthony Publishing, Reston, VA.
18. Moore, E. E., Cogbill, T. H., Malangoni, M. A., *et al.* (1996). Scaling system for organ specific injuries. *Curr. Opin. Crit. Care* **2,** 450–462.
19. Cogbill, T. H., Moore, E. E., Jurkovich, G. J., *et al.* (1989). Nonoperative management of blunt splenic trauma: A multicenter experience. *J. Trauma* **29,** 1312–1317.
20. Croce, M. A., Fabian, T. C., Menke, P. G., *et al.* (1995). Nonoperative management of blunt hepatic trauma is the treatment of choice for hemodynamically stable patients: Results of a prospective trial. *Ann. Surg.* **221,** 744–755.
21. Mucha, P., Daly, R. C., and Farnell, M. B. (1986). Selective management of blunt splenic trauma. *J. Trauma* **26,** 970–979.
22. Pachter, H. L., Knudson, M. M., Esrig, B., *et al.* (1996). Status of nonoperative management of blunt hepatic injuries in 1995: A multicenter experience with 404 patients. *J. Trauma* **40,** 31–38.
23. Burch, J. M., Martin, R. R., Richardson, R. J., *et al.* (1991). Evolution of the treatment of the injured colon in the 1980s. *Arch. Surg.* **126,** 979–984.
24. Yamamoto, S., Yoshii, H., Maekawa, K., *et al.* (1991). New concept for classification of hepatic injury [Japanese]. *Surg. Therap. (Geka Chiryo)* **65,** 507–511.
25. Moore, F. A., Moore, E. E., Poggetti, R., *et al.* (1991). Gut bacterial translocation via the portal vein: A clinical perspective with major torso trauma. *J. Trauma* **31,** 629–638.
26. Sauaia, A., Moore, F. A., Moore, E. E., *et al.* (1994). Early predictors of postinjury multiple organ failure. *Arch. Surg.* **129,** 39–45.
27. Goris, R. J., te Boekhorst, T. P., Nuytinck, J. K., *et al.* (1985). Multiple-organ failure: Generalized autodestructive inflammation? *Arch. Surg.* **120,** 1109–1115.
28. Marshall, J. C., Christou, N. V., Horn, R., *et al.* (1988). The microbiology of multiple organ failure: The proximal gastrointestinal tract as an occult reservoir of pathogens. *Arch. Surg.* **123,** 309–315.
29. Moore, F. A., and Moore, E. E. (1996). The benefits of enteric feeding. *Adv. Surg.* **30,** 141–154.
30. Balogh, Z., Offner, P. J., Moore, E. E., *et al.* (2000). The NISS predicts postinjury multiple organ failure better than the ISS. *J. Trauma* **48,** 624–628.

29

Blunt Trauma Models

Fractures, Chest Trauma, Head Injury, Soft-Tissue Trauma, and Abdominal Trauma

R. Lawrence Reed II

Department of Surgery, Loyola University Medical Center, Maywood, Illinois 60153

I. Introduction

Injury is a major problem in modern health care. Trauma continues to be the leading cause of death for individuals who are between 1 and 44 years of age. Thus, for two-thirds of the normal life span, the most likely cause of death is from injury. The annual costs of trauma care are estimated to exceed $250 billion annually in the United States alone.

Trauma is far from a single mechanism of disease, but constitutes a very heterogeneous group of etiologies and disease processes. Trauma classification schemes are based upon intentionality (intentional vs unintentional), primary injuring mechanism (blunt, penetrating, thermal), type of injury produced (contusion, laceration, burn, etc.), and others.

Trauma models seek to mimic the nature of human injuries to elucidate the pathophysiologic mechanisms of dysfunction involved and/or to determine the effectiveness of various types of therapy. Acceptable models must fulfill specific goals to be useful in this regard. First, the model must accurately represent the injury as seen in humans. Second, the degree of injury must be measurable. Finally, the model must be reproducible.

The accuracy of the representation of the human injury by the model is first developed through accurate recording of the characteristics seen in injured humans. Extensive reporting of injury types has filled the trauma literature for the past several decades. Additionally, objective scoring systems of various anatomic injuries have been developed, such as the injury severity score (ISS), that help to stratify the degree of injuries among various individuals and injury mechanisms. Injuries in various body areas can be categorized by type as abrasions, contusions, lacerations, dislocations, fractures, and hematomas. The degree within each of these categories, in turn, can be objectively determined through these scoring systems. Application of such clinically developed descriptions to injury models should allow for better extrapolation of findings produced by the models to those expected to occur in the injured human.

Similarly, measurement of the degree of injury can occur in an anatomic manner, similar to those that have been developed for clinical scoring systems (length or depth of lacerations, percentage of an organ replaced by hematoma, etc.). In addition to anatomic alterations, however, the direct impact of the injury on physiology should also be measurable. For example, a pulmonary contusion model can be assessed by the degree of change in intrapulmonary shunt. A soft-tissue trauma model could be assessed by the quantity of circulating volume lost into the parenchyma. More indirectly, various indirect physiologic responses to injury can be assessed, such as the quantity of specific cytokines or other acute-phase reactants released. However, such responses are frequently the focus of the investigation itself; correlation to a specific degree of injury is usually necessary to determine the character of the physiologic response.

Reproducibility is frequently the Achilles' heel of blunt trauma models. Despite careful attention to ensuring that exactly the same energy, trajectory, and other conditions occur each and every time, variability in the subject's body habitus, relative fat and muscle content, tissue integrity, and other factors can profoundly influence the degree of the resulting injury. Thus, variable results can frequently occur despite great attention to consistency.

To help overcome this weakness in blunt trauma models, accurate measurement of the nature or degree of the injury produced is extremely helpful. By stratifying the experimental results according to the severity or nature of the actual injury produced, more reliable conclusions can often be drawn than when such controls are not applied. For example, a blunt impact to the abdomen may or may not produce uncontrolled intra-abdominal hemorrhage, depending on whether certain organs such as the spleen or liver were ruptured and how severely they were injured. Using such a model by itself to determine the effectiveness of a variety of resuscitation techniques could produce variable and nearly uninterpretable results. However, quantitation of the amount of blood lost into the abdomen at the conclusion of the experiment would provide an additional useful control on the experimental design. By stratifying the results according to the volume of blood lost, the relationship between the resuscitation regimen and outcome would likely be more clearly elucidated.

II. Blunt Head Injury Models

Traumatic brain injury (TBI) and spinal cord injury (SCI) together are responsible for serious mortality and morbidity, producing approximately 90,000 disabled individuals annually. TBI alone is responsible for an estimated 500,000 hospitalizations annually in the United States (1). Several *in vivo* models of central nervous system (CNS) injury have been developed and characterized over the past several decades to improve patient care and reduce costs. The primary types of injuries managed clinically include cerebral contusions and lacerations.

In vitro models of neuronal injury have also been developed to complement the ability of *in vivo* models to reproduce the sequella of human CNS injury. For example, a large proportion of cells in a contusion die immediately following traumatic brain injury, but a still higher number of cells will often die over the next several hours. This second wave of neuronal death is induced by phenomena such as secondary axotomy and brain edema. Many aspects of posttraumatic sequella are faithfully reproduced in cultured cells, including ultrastructural changes, ionic derangements, electrophysiological alterations, and free radical generation (2). The data generated with *in vitro* systems can be then compared and contrasted with data from *in vivo* models of CNS injury (3).

Modern brain injury models started with the work of Denny-Brown and Russell in 1941 (4). They categorized head injury types as either "acceleration concussion" or "percussion concussion." These are roughly consistent with more modern models currently described, although there are more varieties within these categories. An extensive review of animate models of head injury was published by Gennarelli in 1994 (5) and more recently by Laurer and McIntosh in 1999 (1).

Fluid percussion involves injecting a small fluid volume into the subdural space, usually using an impacted fluid column or via rapid pump infusion (6). The injury is produced by the brief fluid pressure pulsed to the intact dural surface. This force then moves in the epidural space concentrically, leading to a more diffuse loading injury to the brain. A variety of animal species have been subjected to the model, including dogs, sheep, swine, rabbits, cats, rats, and mice (1). The percussion can be applied either centrally or laterally. Central percussion tends to produce a smaller and more variable contusion than does lateral percussion. Lateral percussion tends to produce a unilateral injury, although occasionally the contralateral side can sustain some injury (5). Both are characterized by brief unconsciousness, metabolic alterations, and disturbances in cerebral blood flow and blood-brain barrier permeability. Long-lasting impairments in motor function, cognitive deficits, and necrosis have been observed, as well as traumatic axonal injury (TAI) in the subcortical white matter that is actually somewhat remote from the actual area of injury.

Rigid indentation models are performed with a solid indenter rapidly impacting the dura at controllable speeds and depths of tissue indentation (7). It produces injury to the intact dura and underlying gray and white matter with the head of the animal restrained. These models can also be delivered both centrally and laterally. Central rigid indentation can produce coma of variable duration in the ferret (8) and the rat (11). On the other hand, lateral rigid indentation produces a relatively brief coma. Because rigid indentation can be closely controlled for deformation parameters, such as duration, velocity, and depth of impact, it offers the potential for greater reproducibility. A pneumatically driven impact device is often recommended over methods where the impactor is driven by a free-falling weight because the risk of rebound is eliminated (9,10). Rigid indentation typically produces edema, cerebral blood flow changes, cortical damage, gray matter ablation, occasional white matter ablation, cell death, TAI, and deficits in cognitive and motor function.

Both lateral fluid percussion and lateral rigid indentation models (11) have been employed by Gennarelli in combination with a contralateral dural opening (5). This enables isolation of the damage produced from the ipsilateral, or "coup," injury from any pathophysiology resulting from injury to the contralateral, or "contracoup," side.

Weight drop models of brain injury employ the use of a free-falling weight onto the exposed skull of a restrained or unrestrained animal. The models are characterized by derangement of the blood-brain barrier, edema, intracranial pressure increases, contusion, and frequent skull fractures. Impairments in motor and cognitive function have been described (1). Reproducibility is not likely to be high with these types of models, however, especially in unrestrained animals.

Inertial acceleration models produce rotational movement of the head. If the loading conditions exceed a particular threshold, rotation and deformation of the brain result, leading to injuries mostly involving the axons deep in the white matter (12,13). The models can also produce relatively pure acute subdural hematomas, coma, and diffuse axonal injury (14,15).

Impact acceleration models were developed to help avoid skull fractures in rodents subjected to traumatic brain injury. A stainless steel protection helmet is provided over the skull to help protect it from fracturing while the head is impacted. The unrestrained head is placed on a foam bed with a known spring constant to allow movement after the impact (i.e., the acceleration). The model produces traumatic axonal injury, edema, cortical neuronal shrinkage, subarachnoid hemorrhages, and intraventricular hemorrhages. Motor and cognitive impairments are noted. Unfortunately, variable skull fracturing does occur, compromising the model's specificity and reproducibility (5).

III. Blunt Chest Trauma Models

Firearms of various types have been used for creation of blunt trauma models, especially of the chest. The protective rib cage helps to diffuse injuries to the intrathoracic organs that can develop from the concussive force provided by a firearm. Two major firearm types exist. One employs a handgun loaded with blank cartridges. This was the model initially reported in a series of landmark experimental studies of pulmonary contusion conducted by Trinkle *et al.* (16,17). After the establishment of general anesthesia, endotracheal intubation, and controlled mechanical ventilation, a quarter is taped to the lower thorax. A .38 special revolver with a blank cartridge is then held firmly against the quarter and fired. This model produces a nonpenetrating, localized, and reproducible contusion of the lung. The major weakness of this model is the potential for the quarter to become dislodged upon firing, making it a projectile and carrying the risk of injury to the investigative team.

The other version of the model employs a captive-bolt pistol (Koch Supplies, Kansas City, MO) (18). Captive-bolt weapons are usually employed in slaughterhouses for the humane processing of large animals. A charge much like a blank is fired in the chamber of the pistol-like device. However, no projectile is released from the muzzle. Instead, the blast propels a metal rod (the "bolt") which is held captive within the chamber by a recoil rim, preventing it from going any more forward than 7.5 cm. Thus, the captive bolt never leaves the pistol, but its surface advances and recoils rapidly, moving forward at a speed of 51.8 m/s.

Moseley and colleagues described the use of a captive-bolt pistol in the production of pulmonary contusion in a canine model (19). The projectile's blast was diffused over the chest wall by placing a 2-in.-thick foam rubber pad over the chest and covering the pad with a 3-in.-diameter steel plate. The captive-bolt pistol was then fired against the steel plate, producing a pulmonary contusion with a characteristic radiologic appearance and a reproducible alteration in pulmonary and cardiac function.

Myocardial contusion can be studied while using the Langendorff-perfused rabbit heart model (20). This enables accurate assessment of the physiologic impact of the contusion on the working myocardium. It also employs smaller and less expensive animals than larger contusion models using firearms. In this model, the contusion can be reproducibly and simply applied by a single blow from a ball dropped from a predefined height directly onto the surface of the heart (21).

A potentially useful technique for studying pulmonary contusion is the use of the lithotripsy device. Chapman *et al.* described the impact of extracorporeal shockwave lithotripsy in a canine model (22). They carried out a series of acute and chronic studies in dogs exposed to varying numbers of shockwaves directed at the gallbladder wall via a transthoracic or transabdominal targeting approach. When shockwaves were directed transthoracically, pulmonary hemorrhagic contusions resulted, some relatively large. In contrast, when a transabdominal approach was used, only focal areas of hemorrhage were found in the gallbladder wall and adjacent liver, with no alterations in postlithotripsy pancreatic or liver enzymes, and normal cholecystokinin octapeptide stimulated oral cholecystograms were obtained 6 days after treatment. Although this model is intriguing, few have used it for the study of pulmonary contusion.

IV. Blunt Abdominal Trauma Models

Blunt abdominal trauma can produce a variety of injuries in an infinite number of combinations of nature and severity. Models that produce generalized blunt abdominal trauma are relatively unpredictable in terms of the specific organs that are injured. Consistent patterns of injury can be observed, however, with enough control and focus on the process of blunt energy transmission.

Very generalized traumatic models may or may not produce abdominal injury. For example, the rotating drum model applied to rodents can be used to evaluate the results of a generalized injury on the circulation's effectiveness (23). However, in this model, there is a significant lack of control over the nature and degree of injuries sustained. Therefore, reproducibility from the standpoint of blunt abdominal trauma is a problem with such a technique.

A more focused blast can be generated against the abdominal wall. Jaffin *et al.* describe a model for studying blunt truncal energy employing a blast generator on rodents (24). Lesions were produced by pressure waves of short duration (0.5–1.0 ms) within a range of high intensity (60–375 psi). The animals were divided into three groups: the first group was exposed to midthoracic blasts, the second group was exposed to abdominal blasts, and the third group was the control group, exposed only to a gentle stream of gas. Group I showed gross and microscopic evidence of lung blast injury of "rib imprint" hemorrhages, intra-alveolar hemorrhage, marked increase in lung weight, prolonged apnea, and bradycardia. Group II showed typical blunt abdominal trauma at the closest ranges but characteristic submucosal hemorrhages up to 4.0 cm from the blast nozzle. In both groups, a protective effect was seen in heavier animals. The lung and bowel lesions induced were grossly and microscopically similar to injuries of blast exposure seen in injured patients. Thus, it appears that a device such as a blast wave generator can reproducibly create blast injury in the laboratory that is safe and clinically relevant.

Because one of the most serious consequences of blunt abdominal trauma is uncontrolled intra-abdominal hemorrhage, models have been created to mimic this situation. For example, Silbergleit *et al.* used a porcine model in which the animals were bled through a flow-monitored shunt placed between the femoral artery and the peritoneal cavity (25,26). The shunt could be connected to catheters of varying diameters placed in the femoral artery to create three rates of hemorrhage. Blood flow through the shunt was measured with an in-line Doppler probe. This system offers the advantage of modeling a contained hemorrhage, different from that of any model of hemorrhage resulting in external blood loss. Moreover, it enables quantification of the rate of hemorrhage so that its impact on outcome and response to therapy can be determined.

In order to study the specific effects of blunt abdominal trauma on individual organs, injury models for each organ have been used. Such models include those of isolated splenic injuries, isolated hepatic injuries, isolated hollow viscus injuries, renal injuries, and so forth. In the models that have been described, the individual study interests are widely divergent. Thus, there are no models that are used widely enough to be considered standards. Instead, necessity, feasibility, and innovation have influenced the models that have been employed.

Because of the significant clinical challenge presented by severe liver injuries, models of blunt hepatic trauma are among the most commonly studied. A model for complex hepatic injury using an external blast was successfully used by Cohn *et al.* to study the ability of fibrin glue to arrest hemorrhage (27). A standardized liver injury in rats can be produced through a midline celiotomy incision. The rat liver has four lobes. Approximately 65% of the median and left lateral lobes are removed by sharp dissection. The cut edge of the liver is allowed to bleed freely into the peritoneal cavity, and the celiotomy incision is closed with running suture. For standardization control of the model, the resected portions of liver are weighed (28). A similar model has been described in dogs by Fleisher *et al* (29). In that model, a resection of 45–55% of the right median hepatic lobe was performed followed by immediate closure of the laparotomy incision.

Splenic trauma has been specifically studied in a variety of models. Ali and colleagues used a model of crushed splenic injury in dogs that initially seems to be a very appropriate model for studying splenic trauma. (30) However, standardization of the injury and response to injury is likely problematic with this particular model. Controlling for the degree of injury with a crush is significantly more difficult than if the injury is produced by a laceration. A crush can produce parenchymal injuries with or without major vascular injuries, thereby leading to widely divergent blood losses and stress responses. Also, the applicability of the model to the human situation is a particular problem in the case of canine models because of the significantly more contractile nature of the spleen in that species (31).

Solomonov *et al.* produced uncontrolled hemorrhagic shock from a standardized model of massive splenic injuries by creating two transverse incisions in rat spleens (32). The same group recently described a modification of the technique for producing a moderate splenic injury by creating a single transverse splenic incision. After anesthesia and cannulation, a midline laparotomy is performed (33). The splenic parenchyma is sharply transected transversely in the middle of the spleen between the entrance of the major branches of the splenic artery into the spleen. Care is taken to avoid injury to the branches of the splenic artery, thereby producing a purely parenchymal injury. The cut edges of the spleen are allowed to bleed freely into the peritoneal cavity while the laparotomy incision is closed with a continuous suture. This model enables the study of various resuscitative regimens for the treatment of uncontrolled hemorrhagic shock. Upon completion of the experimental protocol, the abdomen can be reopened, and free intraperitoneal blood can be collected onto preweighed pieces of cotton. The amount of blood loss can then be determined by the difference in wet and dry weights. The blood loss can be proportioned to the rat's total blood volume, typically considered to be 6.0 mL/g of body weight.

Intestinal injuries can be simulated by re-creating them in a controlled surgical manner in the case of serosal tears or free perforations (34). Contusions and hematomas can also be created from indirect external injuries, which are more difficult to control, or by direct internal injury.

Mesenteric injuries have been studied as a means of evaluating the process of tissue repair. A commonly used model entails the creation of standardized mesenteric perforations in the abdomens of rats (35). The perforations are made to a consistent size and number, improving the reproducibility of the experimental results.

Both blunt and penetrating injury to the peritoneal cavity typically results in a repair process that can lead to the development of intra-abdominal adhesions. Because of the serious postoperative morbidity that such adhesions can produce over an individual's lifetime, the mechanisms for their production and potential preventative strategies have been the subject of a number of investigations. Two rat models have commonly been employed in the study of intra-abdominal adhesions. One involved the production of a controlled cecal abrasion (36,37). Another is a side wall-uterine horn abrasion model (38,39). The uterine horn abrasion model has also been used in ewes (40,41).

Diaphragmatic injuries can be produced by creating a controlled laceration in the diaphragms of anesthetized laparotomized animals, such as swine (42), and can consistently produce the injury desired. However, depending on the focus of a set of experimental studies, the diaphragm could be approached for such a laceration from either the thoracic or the abdominal aspect, thereby helping to avoid potentially confounding findings resulting from the surgical procedure itself.

V. Fracture Models

A. General and Extremity

Several animal species have been used as models to study fracture production and healing. Fractures are produced through either closed or open means or by way of isolated or segmental osteotomies. Fracture healing is usually evaluated through histologic, mechanical, chemical, or biological studies. Experimental models can involve a variety of therapeutic interventions, primarily various types of internal fixation, external fixation, or even no fixation. As with most blunt trauma models, standardization of the injury is often difficult, leading often to variable results.

The majority of fracture models have been applied through relatively simple techniques. In the most controlled circumstances, an osteotomy or a bone gap is surgically created at a specific point in a specific bone in an experimental animal, such as in the rabbit humerus (43). The size of the defect is variable, depending primarily on the size of the species studied. For example, 2-mm-long fibular defects have been described in rats (44), 13-mm femoral diaphyseal gaps have been produced in rabbits (45), and 21- to 25-mm femoral diaphyseal gaps have been created in dogs (46,47). Such models have been found useful for studying the nature and rate of fracture healing, with or without various efforts at repair or fixation.

The advantage of such surgical bone gaps is that they can be highly controlled, thus helping to lead to reproducible results. However, a major disadvantage is that only the bone injury itself can be evaluated with such a model. The influences of injuries to associated ligaments, tendons, and other soft tissues on loss of function and responses to therapy are less reliably assessed with such models, or are not addressed at all. Also, a bone defect is also a relatively artificial model for trauma. Pathologic fractures resulting from neoplastic demineralization could potentially be modeled by such a technique; however, such fractures are also profoundly influenced by the seriously abnormal physiology at the site resulting from the neoplastic process.

A more relevant clinical model for blunt trauma, therefore, is that of the three-point bending technique (48–50). This type of model applies a controllable amount of force to three points perpendicular to the long axis of a bone until the bone is bent beyond its compliance limit, resulting in a fracture. In some descriptions, a small (e.g., 1.5-mm diameter) hole is drilled through the lateral cortex of the bone to be fractured to act as a stress riser and fracture initiation site. This also minimizes the influence of the loading rate on the fracture characteristics. Transverse fractures or oblique fractures at any desired angle can be produced by variations of the position of the cortical drill hole relative to the central loading point. The three-point bending model has the advantages of potentially incorporating associated soft-tissue injuries into the analytical process. Thus, local cytokines and other inflammatory mediators that initiate the response to injury and set the stage for repair could potentially reflect those changes that occur in the clinical setting. An arguable disadvantage is that variable amounts of force must be applied to fracture bones from different animals, although the cortical hole can help to reduce such variability.

Arguably, the variability in force necessary to produce the fracture may be seen as an advantage in the model, in that only the amount of force necessary to produce a fracture can be imparted. This actually mimics the clinical scenario fairly accurately: injured patients can be inflicted with variable amounts of force. Some forces can produce fractures in some frail patients, but may not result in fractures in others with stronger and/or thicker bones.

Another technology that has been applied to produce fractures actually seeks to assess the structural integrity of various bones. For example, Sugawara and colleagues performed a number of experiments on a variety of bones in rats to assess bone strength following spinal cord injury (51). This was performed by determining the torque and compressive load necessary to produce structural failure in the bone. While this model certainly relates to a clinically relevant issue, it is most appropriate in the study of osteoporosis and not specifically blunt trauma. When compressive loads are encountered in the modern trauma setting, they typically occur as a result of jumps or falls. The impact is absorbed by more than the bone alone, as joints, tendons, muscles, and ligaments are all strained to variable degrees, depending on the load and the direction of impact. For example, a compressive force may actually produce a joint dislocation instead of a fracture. Thus, modeling a compressive load is much more complicated than the simple assessment of bone strength. Again, stratification of the experimental results according to the nature and degree of injury actually sustained can go a long way to improving the interpretability of the findings.

Impact loading is an important parameter in the understanding of skeletal injuries. Borrelli and colleagues conducted an *in vitro* investigation using mature bovine cartilage and bone, as well as isolated cartilage explants, to study the biological and mechanical effects of a single-impact load on articular cartilage (52). Each specimen was impacted with a single load applied with a specially designed impactor. This allowed for analysis of force–displacement curves and determination of failure–stress points.

Axial loading of the spine is an important mechanism that warrants extensive study, given its clinical importance due to falls. In animal models, however, this often requires an *ex vivo* analysis of the physical forces, as most animals do not use their spine for bearing weight axially. Rather, the spine in four-legged creatures is typically employed as a suspensory structure. Despite such obvious drawbacks, axial loading of excised spines has been used as a biologic model. Lim and colleagues excised 15 fresh calf spines (L2-L5) and loaded them with pure unconstrained moments in flexion, extension, axial rotation, and lateral bending directions (53). Evaluation of the biomechanical flexibility before and after creation of an anterior and middle column defect and fixation by anterior and posterior instrumentation was then undertaken.

An important aspect of fractures in the multiply injured or critically injured patient is the potential for pulmonary insufficiency, typically thought to be associated with fat embolism following long-bone fractures. Models re-creating this entity involve reaming long bones, such as the tibia or the femur, to release bone marrow products into the circulation. The resulting effects on pulmonary function can then be studied (54,60).

B. Spinal Injury

Spinal instability can also be modeled by surgical transection of the longitudinal ligaments and/or partial resection of the intervertebral discs. This can be performed in fresh cadavers, in animal models, or in biomechanical models (55). Aprahamian *et al.* created a model of cervical spine injury in a human cadaver by transecting the anterior and posterior longitudinal, intertransverse, and articular capsular ligaments, as well as the ligamentum flavum at the level of C_5–C_6 (56). With this severely unstable model, they found that all maneuvers to establish an airway produced some positional changes in the vertebral elements, especially with no cervical collar in place. The presence of a normal-sized soft cervical collar or a rigid Philadelphia collar offered no protection, but the placement of a larger-than-normal soft collar appeared to minimize the displacement that occurred. Nasopharyngeal tube and a "blind" nasotracheal tube insertion appeared to be the safest maneuvers. Similarly, Bivins *et al.* documented significant osseous distraction in recently deceased trauma patients with known cervical injuries when traction (6.8 kg by head halter) was employed during intubation attempts (57). The similarity of these models to the clinical scenario is speculative, given the severity of the neck instabilities studied and the absence of muscle spasm in the fresh cadaver. Although intriguing, these studies probably represent the extremes that can be encountered with intubation attempts.

Many experimental preparations that study musculoskeletal trauma may not even employ a fracture, or for that matter, an instability. For example, studies of spinal fusion have been performed where the bones are fused with bone graft or with a control media, but no fracture has actually been performed (58,59). Alternatively, various screws, plates, pins, or other fixation devices can be placed in intact spinal columns or other bones to assess the degree of immobilization applied or the strength provided. Although, strictly speaking, these are not fracture models, they can certainly be an effective means of studying various aspects of treating fractures.

C. Pelvic Fractures

Because of the unique shape and function of the human pelvis in comparison with other animals, it has often been necessary to employ cadaver models for the evaluation of pelvic fractures, instabilities, and fixation techniques

(61,62). Loading of a one-leg-stance model is typically employed to produce a relatively consistent injury. The pelvises are loaded in the upright position with weights calibrated to some percentage of body weight; in one study, Pohlemann used weights ranging from 50 to 130% of body weight (63). Ghanayem and colleagues used a cadaveric model to compare the efficacy of pelvic fracture reduction and stabilization using an external fixator with that of two experimental devices, the pelvic stabilizer and the pelvic c-clamp (64). A similar process was used to evaluate the effect of laparotomy and external fixator stabilization on pelvic volume in an unstable pelvic injury (65).

VI. Soft-Tissue Trauma Modeling (5)

Few reports or reviews specific for modeling soft-tissue injury exist. However, soft-tissues models are employed in a variety of global and focal models of injury. In fact, one of the earliest studies of soft-tissue injury was conducted by Dr. Alfred Blalock in the late 1920s. At that time, the cause of hypotension and shock following blunt traumatic injury was mysterious. Blalock reproducibly produced blunt muscle injury to the canine hindlimb using blows from a padded mallet. He then performed bilateral hindquarter excisions and compared the weights of the injured and uninjured extremities. The sequestration of blood and fluid into the injured tissue constituted a circulating volume loss in excess of 50%, easily accounting for the observed hypotension (66).

Specific injuries that can develop from either blunt or penetrating trauma are modeled using soft tissues. In most models of blunt soft-tissue trauma, a surgical dissection is involved to create the specific injury sought. This is especially important for soft-tissue elements that have structural roles, such as muscles, tendons, and ligaments. For example, studies of ligamentous instability and fixation frequently employ cutting the ligaments directly to produce the desired instability, as was conducted in cadaveric studies of cervical spine stability (56,57).

Other soft-tissue injuries, such as contusions and hematomas, can be produced by a variety of devices. Dropped weights, captive-bolt pistols, and other impactors can all produce variable types and degrees of soft-tissue injury. Depending upon the measurable endpoint of study sought, the degree of control and reproducibility required should be assessed before a method of soft-tissue injury production is chosen.

For example, Cardany and colleagues studied the cellular and inflammatory response to crush injury (67). They used a standardized experimental impact injury model to produce soft-tissue trauma that simulated impact injuries to soft tissue overlying the cranium. An aluminum impact instrument was constructed that delivered a measurable amount of energy to a finite area of soft tissue over a specific area. Impact injury resulted in readily demonstrable changes in the morphology of the tissue and its blood flow as measured by the distribution of fluorescein dye (57).

VII. Mathematical and Inanimate Modeling of Blunt Trauma

Because of the fundamental influence of physical forces in generating traumatic conditions, it is natural that a great deal of research in blunt trauma has been conducted with the aid of mathematical models. For example, Lau and colleagues constructed mathematical models relating the height of falls to the injuries sustained for a sample of 416 individuals who had fallen from known heights ranging from 3.0 to 69.6 m. Bivariate analysis of this group was able to correlate the injury severity score (ISS) with both the height of fall and age. A model was constructed that related the height of fall with age, ISS, and the extent of injury (mostly AIS ≥ 3). Conceptually, such statistical models could be designed and used to assess any apparent discrepancy between injury severity as determined at autopsy and the suspected or alleged height of fall (68).

Similarly, several mathematical models have been developed to describe the impact of blast injuries to various parts of the body, such as to the chest and lungs (69,70), to determine the potential for blast injury to an anatomic structure from measured or computed pressure traces of a blast without additional animal testing. Thus, improved occupational exposure criteria could follow from such methodology (71).

Computerized models have also been used in a variety of applications evaluating blunt trauma. This is most useful in evaluation of skeletal trauma, where evaluation of the interaction between structural and mechanical forces can be accurately represented. These types of studies have been remarkably aided in recent years through the use of computerized tomography and magnetic resonance image data. For example, Dawson and colleagues evaluated the structural behavior of the pelvis during lateral impact using data created from computerized tomography (72). Importantly, as is necessary with this type of approach, the authors compared their findings to published experimental results for validation.

Because motor vehicle collisions are responsible for a large proportion of the blunt trauma experienced in our society, crash dummies provide a mechanism for studying the potential forces impacting the body. Pearlman and colleagues studied crash dummies fitted with a pregnancy insert to study the effects of various restraint conditions on energy transmission to both the mother and fetus (73). The model consisted of an elasticized vinyl uterine shell, simulated silicone amniotic fluid, and a 28-week simulated fetus attached to a female crash dummy. The fetus was instrumented with accelerometers in the head and thorax and a transducer to measure force transmission through the uterus.

Computerized, mathematical, and other inanimate types of models can therefore improve the quantity and quality of information related to injury. A specific area where such types of models can prove superior to animate models includes structural design and planning to reduce the potential incidence of injury. However, while such models allow for excellent evaluation of the forces that can be applied during a collision or other traumatic event, the actual impact on living human tissues cannot yet be determined from inanimate modeling; the molecular, cellular, hormonal, and physiologic response is thus far too complex and incompletely understood to model with absolute assurance of accuracy. To understand the physiologic effects and responses produced from blunt trauma, animate models are still essential components of the research effort.

VIII. Conclusion

Blunt trauma can produce a variety of injuries to any number and combination of human organs and tissues. The severity and consequences of such injuries can vary from innocuous to debilitating to fatal. A variety of animate and inanimate models have been developed and employed to improve our understanding of the mechanisms, consequences, and potential therapeutics involved in the life of the injured patient. Because of the variety of potential injuries and the various issues under consideration, few standard models of injury exist. The surgical researcher studying blunt trauma should have a keen sense of the nature of his or her question. The model or models chosen (or developed) should provide the required reproducibility, objectivity, and quantifiability to provide measurable endpoints sufficient to provide meaningful answers.

References

1. Laurer, H. L., and McIntosh, T. K. Experimental models of brain trauma. *Curr Opin Neurol* **12**(6), 715–721 (1999).
2. Morrison, B., 3rd, Saatman, K. E., Meaney, D. F., and McIntosh, T. K. *In vitro* central nervous system models of mechanically induced trauma: A review. *J Neurotrauma* **15**(11), 911–928 (1998).
3. McIntosh, T. K., Juhler, M., and Wieloch, T. Novel pharmacologic strategies in the treatment of experimental traumatic brain injury. *J. Neurotrauma* **15**(10), 731–769 (1998).
4. Denny-Brown, D., and Russell, W. R. Experimental cerebral concussion. *Brain* **64,** 93–164 (1941). [Abstract]
5. Gennarelli, T. A. Animate models of human head injury. *J Neurotrauma* **11**(4), 357–368 (1994).
6. Toulmond, S., Duval, D., Serrano, A., Scatton, B., and Benavides, J. Biochemical and histological alterations induced by fluid percussion brain injury in the rat. *Brain Res.* **620,** 24–31 (1993). [Abstract]
7. Sutton, R. L., Lescaudron, L., and Stein, D. G. Unilateral cortical contusion injury in the rat. Vascular disruption and temporal development of cortical necrosis. *J. Neurotrauma* **10,** 135–149 (1993). [Abstract]
8. Lighthall, J. W. Controlled cortical impact: A new experimental brain injury model. *J Neurotrauma* **5**(1), 1–15 (1988).
9. Dail, W. G., Feeney, D. M., Murray, H. M., Linn, R. T., and Boyeson, M. G. Responses to cortical injury: II. Widespread depression of the activity of an enzyme in cortex remote from a focal injury. *Brain Res* **211**(1), 79–89 (1981).
10. Feeney, D. M., Boyeson, M. G., Linn, R. T., Murray, H. M., and Dail, W. G. Responses to cortical injury: I. Methodology and local effects of contusions in the rat. *Brain Res* **211**(1), 67–77 (1981).
11. Dixon, C. E., Clifton, G. L., Lighthall, J. W., Yaghmai, A. A., and Hayes, R. L. A controlled cortical impact model of traumatic brain injury in the rat. *J Neurosci Methods* **39**(3), 253–262 (1991).
12. Smith, D. H., Chen, X. H., Xu, B. N., McIntosh, T. K., Gennarelli, T. A., and Meaney, D. F. Characterization of diffuse axonal pathology and selective hippocampal damage following inertial brain trauma in the pig. *J Neuropathol Exp Neurol* **56**(7), 822–834 (1997).
13. McGowan, J. C., McCormack, T. M., Grossman, R. I., Mendonca, R., Chen, X. H., Berlin, J. A., Meaney, D. F., Xu, B. N., Cecil, K. M., McIntosh, T. K., and Smith, D. H. Diffuse axonal pathology detected with magnetization transfer imaging following brain injury in the pig. *Magn Reson Med* **41**(4), 727–733 (1999).
14. Gennarelli, T. A., and Thibault, L. E. Biomechanics of acute subdural hematoma. *J Trauma* **22**(8), 680–686 (1982).
15. Gennarelli, T. A., Thibault, L. E., Adams, J. H., Graham, D. I., Thompson, C. J., and Marcincin, R. P. Diffuse axonal injury and traumatic coma in the primate. *Ann Neurol* **12**(6), 564–574 (1982).
16. Trinkle, J. K., Furman, R. W., Hinshaw, M. A., Bryant, L. R., and Griffen, W. O. Pulmonary contusion: Pathogenesis and effect of various resuscitative measures. *Ann Thor Surg* **16**(6), 568–573 (1973).
17. Richardson, J. D., Franz, J. L., Grover, F. L., and Trinkle, J. K. Pulmonary contusion and hemorrhage—Crystalloid versus colloid replacement. *J Surg Res* **16,** 330–336 (1974).
18. Graeber, G. M., Belville, W. D., and Sepulveda, R. A. A safe model for creating blunt and penetrating ballistic injury. *J Trauma* **21**(6), 473–476 (1981).
19. Moseley, R. V., Vernick, J. J., and Doty, D. B. Response to blunt chest injury: A new experimental model. *J Trauma* **10**(8), 673–683 (1970).
20. Robert, E., de la Coussaye, J. E., Aya, A. G., Bertinchant, J. P., Polge, A., Fabbro-Peray, P., Pignodel, C., and Eledjam, J. J. Mechanisms of ventricular arrhythmias induced by myocardial contusion: A high-resolution mapping study in left ventricular rabbit heart. *Anesthesiology* **92**(4), 1132–1143 (2000).
21. Bertinchant, J. P., Robert, E., Polge, A., de la Coussaye, J. E., Pignodel, C., Aya, G., Fabbro-Peray, P., Poirey, S., Ledermann, B., Eledjam, J. J., and Dauzat, M. Release kinetics of cardiac troponin I and cardiac troponin T in effluents from isolated perfused rabbit hearts after graded experimental myocardial contusion. *J Trauma* **47**(3), 474–480 (1999).
22. Chapman, W. C., Parish, K. L., Kaufman, A. J., Stephens, W. H., Anderson, S., Woodward, S., and Williams, L. F., Jr. Pathophysiologic effects of biliary shockwave lithotripsy in a canine model. *Am Surg* **57**(1), 34–38 (1991).
23. Purro, A., Appendini, L., De Gaetano, A., Gudjonsdottir, M., Donner, C. F., and Rossi, A. Physiologic determinants of ventilator dependence in long-term mechanically ventilated patients. *Am J Respir Crit Care Med* **161**(4 Pt 1), 1115–1123 (2000).
24. Jaffin, J. H., McKinney, L., Kinney, R. C., Cunningham, J. A., Moritz, D. M., Kraimer, J. M., Graeber, G. M., Moe, J. B., Salander, J. M., and Harmon, J. W. A laboratory model for studying blast overpressure injury. *J Trauma* **27**(4), 349–356 (1987).
25. Silbergleit, R., Satz, W., McNamara, R. M., Lee, D. C., and Schoffstall, J. M. A new model of uncontrolled hemorrhage that allows correlation of blood pressure and hemorrhage. *Acad Emerg Med* **3**(10), 917–921 (1996).

26. Silbergleit, R., Satz, W., McNamara, R. M., Lee, D. C., and Schoffstall, J. M. Effect of permissive hypotension in continuous uncontrolled intra-abdominal hemorrhage. *Acad Emerg Med* **3**(10), 922–926 (1996).
27. Cohn, S. M., Cross, J. H., Ivy, M. E., Feinstein, A. J., and Samotowka, M. A. Fibrin glue terminates massive bleeding after complex hepatic injury. *J Trauma* **45**(4), 666–672 (1998).
28. Matsuoka, T., Hildreth, J., and Wisner, D. H. Liver injury as a model of uncontrolled hemorrhagic shock: Resuscitation with different hypertonic regimens. *J Trauma* **39**(4), 674–680 (1995).
29. Fleisher, G., Templeton, J., and Delgado-Paredes, C. Fluid resuscitation following liver laceration: A comparison of fluid delivery above and below the diaphragm in a pediatric animal model. *Ann Emerg Med* **16**(2), 147–152 (1987).
30. Ali, J., and Duke, K. Pneumatic antishock garment decreases hemorrhage and mortality from splenic injury. *Can J Surg* **34**(5), 496–501 (1991).
31. Risoe, C., Hall, C., and Smiseth, O. A. Blood volume changes in liver and spleen during cardiogenic shock in dogs. *Am J Physiol* **261**(6 Pt 2), H1763-H1768 (1991).
32. Solomonov, E., Hirsh, M., Yahiya, A., and Krausf, M. M. The effect of vigorous fluid resuscitation in uncontrolled hemorrhagic shock after massive splenic injury. *Crit Care Med* **28**(3), 749–754 (2000).
33. Krausz, M. M., Bashenko, Y., and Hirsh, M. Crystalloid or colloid resuscitation of uncontrolled hemorrhagic shock after moderate splenic injury. *Shock* **13**(3), 230–235 (2000).
34. Parker, M. M. Predicting success of extubation in children. *Crit Care Med* **24**(9), 1429–1430 (1996).
35. Franzen, L. E. The perforated mesentery of the rat: A novel model for the study of genuine connective tissue contraction. *J Surg Res* **60**(1), 91–100 (1996).
36. Burns, J. W., Skinner, K., Colt, J., Sheidlin, A., Bronson, R., Yaacobi, Y., and Goldberg, E. P. Prevention of tissue injury and postsurgical adhesions by precoating tissues with hyaluronic acid solutions. *J Surg Res* **59**(6), 644–652 (1995).
37. Burns, J. W., Colt, M. J., Burgees, L. S., and Skinner, K. C. Preclinical evaluation of Seprafilm bioresorbable membrane. *Eur J Surg* (Suppl 577), 40–48 (1997).
38. Bakkum, E. A., Dalmeijer, R. A., Verdel, M. J., Hermans, J., van Blitterswijk, C. A., and Trimbos, J. B. Quantitative analysis of the inflammatory reaction surrounding sutures commonly used in operative procedures and the relation to postsurgical adhesion formation. *Biomaterials* **16**(17), 1283–1289 (1995).
39. Korell, M., Scheidel, P., and Hepp, H. Experimental animal model for readhesion formation study. *J Invest Surg* **7**(5), 409–415 (1994).
40. Moll, H. D., Wolfe, D. F., Schumacher, J., and Wright, J. C. Evaluation of sodium carboxymethylcellulose for prevention of adhesions after uterine trauma in ewes. *Am J Vet Res* **53**(8), 1454–1456 (1992).
41. Fukasawa, M., Abe, H., Masaoka, T., Orita, H., Horikawa, H., Campeau, J. D., and Washio, M. The hemostatic effect of deacetylated chitin membrane on peritoneal injury in rabbit model. *Surg Today* **22**(4), 333–338 (1992).
42. Israel, R. S., McDaniel, P. A., Primack, S. L., Salmon, C. J., Fountain, R. L., and Koslin, D. B. Diagnosis of diaphragmatic trauma with helical CT in a swine model. *AJR Am J Roentgenol* **167**(3), 637–641 (1996).
43. Lowry, K. J., Hamson, K. R., Bear, L., Peng, Y. B., Calaluce, R., Evans, M. L., Anglen, J. O., and Allen, W. C. Polycaprolactone/glass bioabsorbable implant in a rabbit humerus fracture model. *J Biomed Mater Res* **36**(4), 536–541 (1997).
44. Chakkalakal, D. A., Strates, B. S., Mashoof, A. A., Garvin, K. L., Novak, J. R., Fritz, E. D., Mollner, T. J., and McGuire, M. H. Repair of segmental bone defects in the rat: An experimental model of human fracture healing. *Bone* **25**(3), 321–332 (1999).
45. Baltzer, A. W., Lattermann, C., Whalen, J. D., Braunstein, S., Robbins, P. D., and Evans, C. H. A gene therapy approach to accelerating bone healing. Evaluation of gene expression in a New Zealand white rabbit model. *Knee Surg Sports Traumatol Arthrosc* **7**(3), 197–202 (1999).
46. Kraus, K. H., Kadiyala, S., Wotton, H., Kurth, A., Shea, M., Hannan, M., Hayes, W. C., Kirker-Head, C. A., and Bruder, S. Critically sized osteo-periosteal femoral defects: A dog model. *J Invest Surg* **12**(2), 115–124 (1999).
47. Hupel, T. M., Aksenov, S. A., and Schemitsch, E. H. Cortical bone blood flow in loose and tight fitting locked unreamed intramedullary nailing: A canine segmental tibia fracture model. *J Orthop Trauma* **12**(2), 127–135 (1998).
48. Macdonald, W., Skirving, A. P., and Scull, E. R. A device for producing experimental fractures. *Acta Orthop Scand* **59**(5), 542–544 (1988).
49. Probst, A., Jansen, H., Ladas, A., and Spiegel, H. U. Callus formation and fixation rigidity: A fracture model in rats. *J Orthop Res* **17**(2), 256–260 (1999).
50. Fujita, M., Matsui, N., Tsunoda, M., and Saura, R. Establishment of a non-union model using muscle interposition without osteotomy in rats. *Kobe J Med Sci* **44**(5–6), 217–233 (1998).
51. Sugawara, H., Linsenmeyer, T. A., Beam, H., and Parsons, J. R. Mechanical properties of bone in a paraplegic rat model. *J Spinal Cord Med* **21**(4), 302–308 (1998).
52. Borrelli, J., Jr., Torzilli, P. A., Grigiene, R., and Helfet, D. L. Effect of impact load on articular cartilage: Development of an intra-articular fracture model. *J Orthop Trauma* **11**(5), 319–326 (1997).
53. Lim, T. H., An, H. S., Hong, J. H., Ahn, J. Y., You, J. W., Eck, J., and McGrady, L. M. Biomechanical evaluation of anterior and posterior fixations in an unstable calf spine model. *Spine* **22**(3), 261–266 (1997).
54. Schemitsch, E. H., Jain, R., Turchin, D. C., Mullen, J. B., Byrick, R. J., Anderson, G. I., and Richards, R. R. Pulmonary effects of fixation of a fracture with a plate compared with intramedullary nailing. A canine model of fat embolism and fracture fixation. *J Bone Joint Surg Am* **79**(7), 984–996 (1997).
55. Abumi, K., Panjabi, M. M., and Duranceau, J. Biomechanical evaluation of spinal fixation devices. Part III. Stability provided by six spinal fixation devices and interbody bone graft. *Spine* **14**(11), 1249–1255 (1989).
56. Aprahamian, C., Thompson, B. M., Finger, W. A., and Darin, J. C. Experimental cervical spine injury model: Evaluation of airway management and splinting techniques. *Ann Emerg Med* **13**(8), 584–587 (1984).
57. Bivins, H. G., Ford, S., Bezmalinovic, Z., Price, H. M., and Williams, J. L. The effect of axial traction during orotracheal intubation of the trauma victim with an unstable cervical spine [see comments]. *Ann Emerg Med* **17**(1), 25–29 (1988).
58. Kanayama, M., Cunningham, B. W., Sefter, J. C., Goldstein, J. A., Stewart, G., Kaneda, K., and McAfee, P. C. Does spinal instrumentation influence the healing process of posterolateral spinal fusion? An *in vivo* animal model. *Spine* **24**(11), 1058–1065 (1999).
59. Curylo, L. J., Johnstone, B., Petersilge, C. A., Janicki, J. A., and Yoo, J. U. Augmentation of spinal arthrodesis with autologous bone marrow in a rabbit posterolateral spine fusion model. *Spine* **24**(5), 434–438; discussion 438–439 (1999).
60. Duwelius, P. J., Huckfeldt, R., Mullins, R. J., Shiota, T., Woll, T. S., Lindsey, K. H., and Wheeler, D. The effects of femoral intramedullary reaming on pulmonary function in a sheep lung model. *J Bone Joint Surg Am* **79**(2), 194–202 (1997).
61. Hak, D. J., Hamel, A. J., Bay, B. K., Sharkey, N. A., and Olson, S. A. Consequences of transverse acetabular fracture malreduction on load transmission across the hip joint. *J Orthop Trauma* **12**(2), 90–100 (1998).
62. Pohlemann, T., Angst, M., Schneider, E., Ganz, R., and Tscherne, H. Fixation of transforaminal sacrum fractures: A biomechanical study. *J Orthop Trauma* **7**(2), 107–117 (1993).
63. Pohlemann, T., Culemann, U., and Tscherne, H. [Comparative biomechanical studies of internal stabilization of trans-foraminal sacrum fractures]. *Orthopade* **21**(6), 413–421 (1992).

64. Ghanayem, A. J., Stover, M. D., Goldstein, J. A., Bellon, E., and Wilber, J. H. Emergent treatment of pelvic fractures. Comparison of methods for stabilization. *Clin Orthop* **318,** 75–80 (1995).
65. Ghanayem, A. J., Wilber, J. H., Lieberman, J. M., and Motta, A. O. The effect of laparotomy and external fixator stabilization on pelvic volume in an unstable pelvic injury. *J Trauma* **38**(3), 396–400; discussion 400–401 (1995).
66. Blalock, A. Experimental shock: The cause of low blood pressure caused by muscle injury. *Arch Surg* **20,** 959 (1930).
67. Cardany, C. R., Rodeheaver, G., Thacker, J., Edgerton, M. T., and Edlich, R. F. The crush injury: A high risk wound. *JACEP* **5**(12), 965–970 (1976).
68. Lau, G., Ooi, P. L., and Phoon, B. Fatal falls from a height: The use of mathematical models to estimate the height of fall from the injuries sustained. *Forensic Sci Int* **93**(1), 33–44 (1998).
69. Axelsson, H., and Yelverton, J. T. Chest wall velocity as a predictor of nonauditory blast injury in a complex wave environment. *J Trauma* **40** (Suppl 3), S31-S37 (1996).
70. Cooper, G. J., Pearce, B. P., Sedman, A. J., Bush, I. S., and Oakley, C. W. Experimental evaluation of a rig to simulate the response of the thorax to blast loading. *J Trauma* **40** (Suppl 3), S38-S41 (1996).
71. Stuhmiller, J. H., Ho, K. H., Vander Vorst, M. J., Dodd, K. T., Fitzpatrick, T., and Mayorga, M. A model of blast overpressure injury to the lung. *J Biomech* **29**(2), 227–234 (1996).
72. Dawson, J. M., Khmelniker, B. V., and McAndrew, M. P. Analysis of the structural behavior of the pelvis during lateral impact using the finite element method. *Accid Anal Prev* **31**(1–2), 109–119 (1999).
73. Pearlman, M. D., and Viano, D. Automobile crash simulation with the first pregnant crash test dummy. *Am J Obstet Gynecol* **175**(4 Pt 1), 977–981 (1996).

30

Trauma Models for Studying the Influence of Gender and Aging

Martin G. Schwacha, Ping Wang, and Irshad H. Chaudry

Center for Surgical Research, Department of Surgery, Brown University School of Medicine and Rhode Island Hospital, Providence, Rhode Island 02903

I. Introduction

Trauma is the leading cause of death in the United States for those between the ages of 1 and 38 years (1). Despite advances in patient care that have resulted in increased short-term survival, sepsis and multiple organ failure account for upward of 60% of the deaths in the intensive care unit (2–4). Traumatic injury leading to these complications usually produces alterations in various systems in an integrated manner and as such is considered a multisystem disease.

A number of risk factors for traumatic injury have been identified (lifestyle, alcoholism/drug abuse, economic background, employment, etc.). Several epidemiologic studies also suggest the importance of age and gender as additional risk factors in traumatic injury (5). The majority of trauma victims are young males (6). These young males have higher mortality following trauma, compared to females, and are also more susceptible to septic complications (6–8). Therefore, gender differences exist in both the prevalence of traumatic injury and the susceptibility to subsequent complications, such as sepsis. The reasons for these gender differences are unclear, although several studies have implicated the effects of sex steroids in the immune dysfunction associated with trauma, shock, and sepsis (9–13). Because aging is associated with a decrease in circulating sex steroids in both males and females, this hormonal change may influence the response to traumatic injury. The sexually dimorphic immune response following trauma and hemorrhage appears to reverse with aging (10, 11). Nonetheless, the majority of experimental trauma models have used young male animals and only limited studies have focused on the role of gender or age. This is a potentially fruitful area for experimental study that may have important clinical implications. For example, advances in this area of trauma research may contribute to the development of gender-specific therapeutic regimes for trauma victims, leading to decreased morbidity and mortality. The focus of this chapter is on experimental techniques that take into consideration the impact of gender and aging on traumatic injury.

II. Experimental Trauma Models

Trauma occurs in many forms. Various experimental trauma models, including blunt trauma, bone fracture, soft-tissue trauma (i.e., laparatomy), hemorrhagic shock, septic shock, and thermal injury, are described in other chapters of this volume and hence will not be covered here. An additional consideration with trauma models is the use of "single-hit" or "double-hit" models. A single-hit model simply investigates the impact of simple trauma (bone fracture only, burn only, etc.). In contrast, a double-hit model is used to study the impact of successive insults. Examples include soft-tissue trauma with hemorrhage (14, 15), bone fracture with hemorrhage (16, 17), hemorrhage followed by subsequent sepsis (18, 19), and thermal injury followed by subsequent sepsis (20, 21). In general, the initial insult "primes" the experimental animal for an abnormal or enhanced response to the second insult (22). Combination of simple trauma models with more complex double-hit models should take into consideration the insults that are being combined. For example, the combination of hemorrhage with burn injury is impractical, because it would be highly uncommon. In contrast, the combination of penetrating blunt trauma, bone fracture, or soft-tissue trauma with hemorrhage more accurately reflects the clinical situation.

The impact of gender and aging can be easily assessed in these models by using appropriate gender- and age-matched animals. With regard to gender, sex steroids have been shown to influence both immunologic and physiologic responses following traumatic injury (12, 13, 23, 24). With aging, sex steroid levels decline and thus aging impacts the response to trauma due to this hormonal change (10, 11). In males sex steroid levels remain relatively constant, with a slow decline in testosterone levels with advanced age; however, female laboratory animals have an estrus cycle in which estrogen and progesterone (the primary female sex steroids) markedly fluctuate over a short period of time. Therefore, an important consideration with regard to studying gender differences following trauma is the stage of the estrus cycle in females. Table I shows basic information on the estrus cycle of animals commonly used in experimental studies.

Androgens and estrogens are potent modulators of the immune response (25). With aging, the sex steroid's profile changes and cellular immunity is concurrently altered (26–28). Thus, the influence of aging can be applied to trauma models by comparing animals of different ages and levels of sexual maturity. Table II shows the average life expectancy of various laboratory animals and humans. The ratio of life expectancy between laboratory animals and humans allows the scientist to calculate the "relative age" of the laboratory animal in "human years." With regard to sex steroid levels, application of this relative age principle gives reasonable results when comparing animals to humans. However, other factors such as metabolic rate are not similar between relative aged animals and humans. Thus, aged laboratory animals have some limitations in modeling the human condition and caution in interpretation of experimental results should be exercised.

An important consideration in developing a trauma model to study the effect of gender and/or aging is species selection. With regard to aging, many of the larger species, such as primates, sheep, and pigs, are not practical due to their expense of purchase, high per diem costs, and longer life-span. In contrast, the smaller species, specifically rodents, are well suited to study gender and aging. Their short life-span allows them to reach a geriatric age within a short period of time (18–24 months). Laboratory animals of intermediate size and life-spans (4–6 years), such as rabbits and guinea pigs, have applicability in trauma models requiring complicated and/or involved measurements that cannot be routinely performed on small rodents. Their life-span is still relatively short, allowing them to reach geriatric age within 3–5 years. Larger animals, such as cats and dogs, require up to 13 years to reach the same relative age. Based on cost alone these species are of limited applicability in the study of aging.

III. Methodology

The methodology detailed below will focus on rodents (rats and mice), because these are the species most commonly used to study immune function (mice), cardiovascular

Table I Estrus Cycle Features for Various Laboratory Animals

Species	Age of puberty	Cycle type	Cycle length
Mice	28–49 days	Polyestrus; all year	4–5 days
Rats	37–67 days	Polyestrus; all year	4–5 days
Rabbits	5–9 months	Induced ovulation; nonseasonal	No regular cycles
Guinea pigs	55–70 days	Polyestrus; all year	16.5 days
Cats	4–12 months	Induced ovulation; seasonally polyestrus	14–21 days
Dogs	5–24 month	Monoestrus; nonseasonal	3.5–13 months

Table II Average Life Expectancy of Various Laboratory Animals

Species	Average life expectancy (years)	Ratio to human life expectancy
Mice	1.5–3	26
Rats	2.5–3.5	23
Rabbits	5–6	13
Guinea Pigs	4–5	16
Cats	16	5
Dogs	12	7
Humans	~80	—

responses (rats), and organ function (rats). Detailed descriptions of procedures for larger animals (i.e., rabbits, cats, and dogs) can be found in veterinarian surgical textbooks. Surgical procedures such as castration and ovariectomy effectively deplete the animal of testosterone and estrogen, respectively, thereby allowing for the mechanistic analysis of the effects of sex steroids. The effect of female sex steroids can be further determined by using females in different stages of the estrus cycle.

In addition to surgical manipulation of sex steroid levels, a number of pharmaceutical agents have been developed that act as androgen and estrogen receptor antagonists, and these effectively castrate or ovarectomize the animal. The understanding of the mechanism of sex steroid action in normal and pathologic states has expanded greatly, due to the identification of specific receptors in cells for these hormones and elucidation of the cascade of events leading to sex steroid effects on cell differentiation and proliferation (29, 30). In general, the cascade begins by binding of the sex steroid to its specific intracellular receptor and proceeds through signal transduction events that produce the final hormone action, which is genomic. The activated sex steroid receptor acts as a nuclear transcription factor, which regulates gene expression. Interestingly, some studies have suggested the existence of a plasma membrane form of the estrogen receptor, the actions of which are nongenomic (31, 32). Unlike surgical manipulation of sex steroid levels, pharmaceutical agents can be administered in a posttrauma regimen.

A. Male Animal Models

1. Surgical Orchidectomy (Castration)

The testes are oval-shaped organs enclosed in the scrotum and are the primary site of testosterone synthesis. Orchidectomy, or castration, involves the removal of the two testes from the animal using a simple surgical procedure (33). Surgical castration prior to experimental trauma can be used to deplete circulating androgen levels, allowing study of the effect of androgens on the immunologic and physiologic responses under such conditions. Castration should be carried out at least 2 weeks prior to the trauma procedure to allow for reduction of body testosterone levels. The procedure begins by placing the animal under anesthesia, positioned on its back with the its tail facing the surgeon. As shown in Fig. 1, the scrotum is cleaned of all fecal matter and an incision (5–10 mm) is made at the tip of the scrotum (A). Subcutaneous tissue is cleared away, exposing the muscular sacs that contain the testes. Application of pressure to the lower abdomen of the animal will push the testes down, allowing for clearer viewing (B). A small incision (2–5 mm) is made in each scrotal sac at the tip. The cauda epididymis is pulled out along with the testes. This is followed by the capud epididymis, the vas deferens, and the spermatic blood vessels (C and D). A single ligature is placed around the vas deferens and spermatic blood vessels (E and F). The vas deferens and blood vessels are cut distal to the ligature and removed from the animal. The remaining vas deferens and fat are pushed back into the scrotal sac, which is closed with a single suture. The scrotum is then closed with sutures or wound clips.

2. Pharmacological Castration with Antiandrogenic Agents

Obviously, surgical castration is not a viable option in the treatment of the deleterious effects of trauma; however, nonsteroidal pharmacologic agents that block the action of androgens at the receptor level have been developed (Table III).

Flutamide (Schering) is a nonsteroidal agent that has potent antiandrogenic activity by inhibiting androgen uptake or nuclear binding of the activated androgen receptor to nuclear response elements in the nucleus. It is used clinically for the treatment of androgen-sensitive prostatic carcinoma. Animal studies have shown that flutamide is effective, in a posttreatment regime, in preventing the deleterious effects of hemorrhagic shock on cell-mediated immunity (34, 35) and cardiovascular and hepatocellular depression (36). Administration of flutamide (25 mg/kg) subcutaneously in 1,2-propanediol has been shown to have optimal antiandrogenic effects in animal trauma models (34, 35).

Another common antiandrogenic compound is bucalutamide (Zeneca) (37, 38). It is nonsteroidal and related to flutamide in its mechanism of action. It competitively inhibits the binding of androgen to its cytosolic receptor in target tissues and is used clinically in the treatment of prostate cancer. Interestingly, in dogs it is approximately 50 times more potent than flutamide in causing atrophy of the prostate and has a fourfold higher affinity for the androgen receptor (38). Unlike flutamide, which can elevate circulating testosterone levels, it has little effect on serum testosterone levels. Optimal dosage is 25 mg/kg daily, orally. However, oral administration of pharmacologic agents is not desirable because gut absorptive capacity is impaired

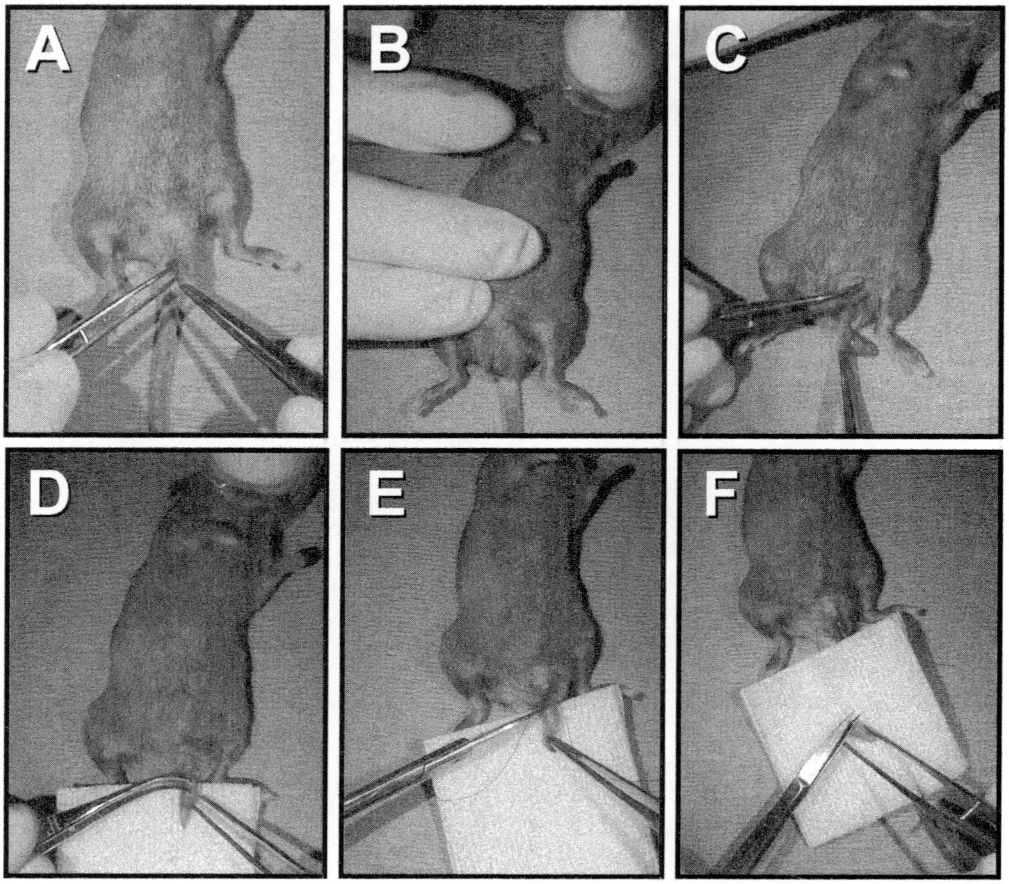

Figure 1 Surgical castration of the mouse. (A) Scrotal incision. (B) Exposure of the muscular sacs containing the testes. (C) Removal of the testes, epididymis, and vas deferens. (D) Isolation of the testes. (E) Placement of ligature around the blood vessels and vas deferens. (F) Removed testes. (See color plates.)

following trauma (39). Nonetheless, although this agent has promise in the application in male trauma models, studies have yet to be conducted to determine its efficacy under such conditions, by nonoral administrative routes.

If different doses of flutamide or bucalutamide are employed it is important to determine the degree of antiandrogenic activity. A simple method by which antagonism of the androgen receptor can be determined is to measure the wet weight of androgen-sensitive tissues, such as the seminal vesicles and prostate. Antagonism of androgen activity will dose dependently decrease the wet weight of these tissues, which can be assessed quantitatively (37, 40).

B. Female Animal Models

1. Estrus Cycle Stage Determination

The cellular contents of the vagina undergo cyclic changes during the estrus cycle. Observation of these changes in vaginal smears allows for determination of the successive stages of the estrus cycle (41).

The estrus cycle of the mouse or rat can be divided into four stages; diestrus, proestrus, estrus, and postestrus (Table IV). Proestrus and estrus are anabolic stages with active growth, postestrus is a catabolic stage characterized by degenerative changes in the genital tract, and diestrus is

Table III Nonsteroidal Antiandrogenic Compounds

Name (source)	Mechanism of action	Dose	Route of administration
Flutamide (Schering)	Inhibition of androgen uptake and/or nuclear binding of androgen in target tissues	25 mg/kg	Subcutaneous
Bicalutamide (Zenaca)	Inhibition of androgen binding to receptor in target tissues	25 mg/kg	Oral

a quiescent stage with slow growth. The different stages of the cycle are also paralleled by marked changes in the sex steroid environment (Table IV). In general, estrogen is high during proestrus and declines during estrus to low levels at post- and diestrus. Progesterone levels are low at the beginning of proestrus, but peak during estrus following ovulation. Progesterone remains elevated during postestrus and declines to low levels at diestrus.

The method to determine the stage of the estrus cycle is visual inspection of vaginal smears for changes in cellular composition. The lavage method is most common and least stressful to the animal. A small pipette, the tip of which has been flamed to a smooth aperture, or an eye-dropper containing a few drops of isotonic saline, is inserted into the vagina; the fluid is ejected and immediately withdrawn. The saline, with its cellular content, is transferred to a microscope slide. A drop of methylene blue is added for contrast and to bring out the nuclei. Examination is carried out under low-power, then high-power magnification, with reduced lighting.

Three types of cells are found in vaginal smears: polymorphonuclear cells, nucleated epithelial cells, and cornified epithelial cells. Polymorphonuclear cells are small, round, highly refractive cells with an irregularly shaped nucleus. Nucleated epithelial cells are round or oval-shaped cells, larger than polymorphonuclear cells, that have a clear cytoplasm and a centrally located nucleus that stains strongly with methylene blue. Cornified epithelial cells are the largest cells in the smear. They are flattened and angular in outline. Unlike nucleated epithelial cells and polymorphonuclear cells, cornified epithelial cells lack a nucleus. Typical vaginal smears from female mice at the various stages of the estrus cycle are shown in Fig. 2. Table IV contains information on the vaginal smear characteristics.

2. Surgical Ovariectomy (Spaying)

The ovaries are small, irregularly shaped organs found on each side of the abdomen. The are attached to the uterine horn via the oviduct or fallopian tubes. They are the primary site of estrogen and progesterone synthesis in the female. Ovariectomy, or spaying, involves the removal of both ovaries from the animal by a basic surgical procedure that is only slightly more involved than castration (33). Surgical ovariectomy prior to experimental trauma can be used to deplete circulating estrogen levels, and thereby to study the effect of estrogens on the immunologic and physiologic responses under such conditions. Ovariectomy should be carried out at least 2 weeks prior to the trauma procedure to allow body estrogen levels to decline. The procedure begins by placing the animal under anesthesia, positioned on its ventral surface with its tail facing the surgeon. As shown in Fig. 3, the dorsal surface is shaved and prepared with alcohol or similar antiseptic (i.e., betadine). A dorsal midline incision (1–2 cm) is made approximately half-way between the back hump and the base of the tail (A). The skin incision is retracted to one side to remove one ovary and then to the other side to remove the second ovary. The peritoneal cavity is entered via a small incision in the muscle just posterior to the last rib, about two-thirds the way down the side of the animal and only a few millimeters off the spinal muscles (B). The ovary is surrounded by a fat pad and is located approximately two-thirds of the way into the peritoneal cavity. The ovary should be pulled out through the muscle incision, by the surrounding fat pad (C and D). It should not be touched, because small pieces may become detached and reimplanted in the animal. A single ligature is placed around the oviduct, blood vessels, and fat (E). The junction between the oviduct and the uterine horn, along with blood vessels and fat, is severed with a single cut (F). The uterine horn is returned to the peritoneal cavity. The procedure is repeated on the opposite side and the muscle and skin layers are closed with sutures.

3. Pharmacologic Ovariectomy with Antiestrogenic Agents

Similar to androgens, agents have been developed that block the action of estrogens at the receptor level. Antiestrogenic agents were initially developed for the treatment of estrogen-sensitive breast cancer. However, tamoxifen, the only widely used antiestrogen, has a mixed agonist/antagonist estrogen action (42), thus limiting its effectiveness in the treatment of breast cancer and its experimental application as

Table IV The Estrus Cycle in the Mouse[a]

Cycle stage	Stage length	Vaginal smear characteristics[b]	Hormonal profile
Diestrus	2–4 days	Very few cells, all types	Low estrogen, low progesterone
Proestrus	1–1.5 days	Primarily nucleated ECs with a few cornified ECs	High estrogen, low progesterone
Estrus	1–3 days	Primarily cornified ECs with few nucleated ECs	Decreasing estrogen, high progesterone
Post (met)estrus	1–5 days	Primarily PMNs with a few nucleated and cornified EC	Low estrogen, high progesterone

[a]Total estrus cycle length is 4.5 to 5 days.
[b]ECs, Epithelial cells; PMNs, polymorphonuclear leukocytes.

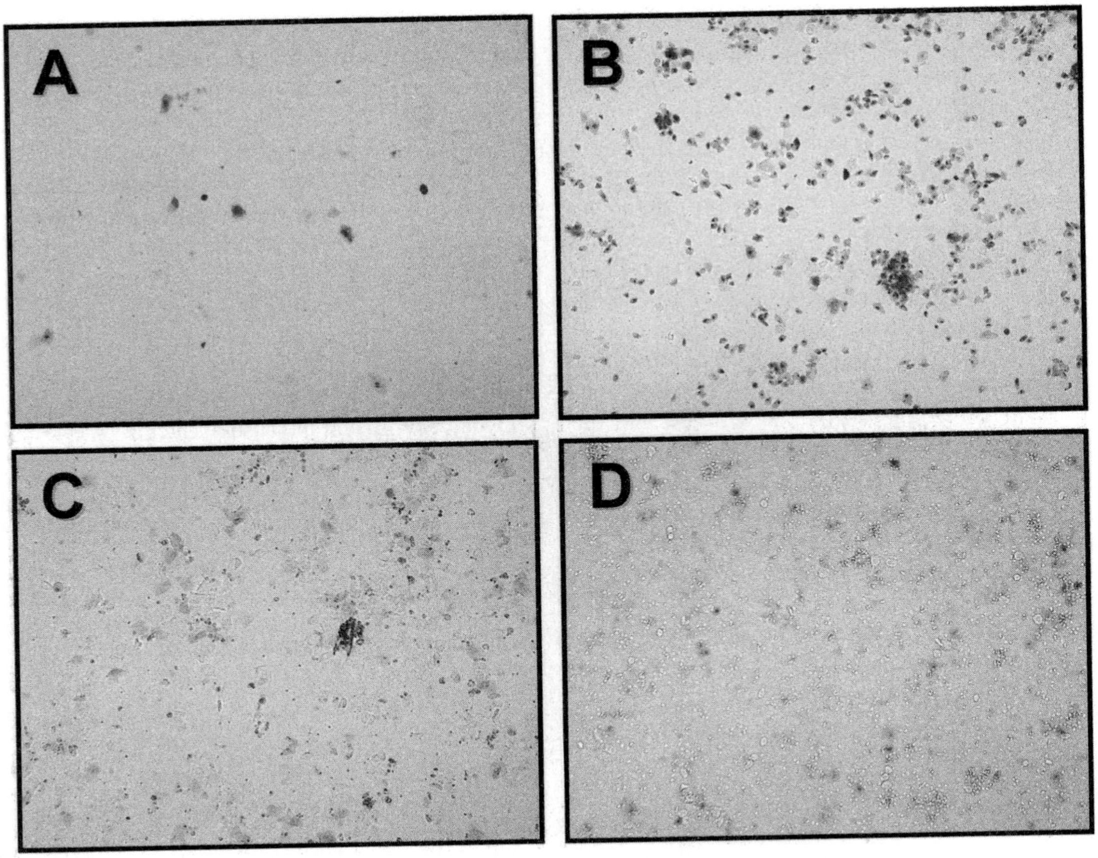

Figure 2 Vaginal smears from mice at different stages of the estrus cycle. (A) Diestrus, few cells of all types. (B) Proestrus, large numbers of nucleated epithelial cells. (C) Estrus, large numbers of cornified epithelial cells with some nucleated epithelial cells. (D) Postestrus, large numbers of highly refractive polymorphonuclear cells. (See color plates.)

an antiestrogenic agent. Other agents have been developed that have "pure" and potent antiestrogenic activity in both *in vivo* and *in vitro* systems (43, 44). Two of these agents, which are nonsteroidal in nature, are listed in Table V.

EM-800 (Schering) is an estrogen receptor antagonist that blocks the transcriptional functions of estrogen receptors α and β (45). Daily oral doses of 50 to 400 μg completely prevented estrogen-sensitive tumor growth in mice (46). Furthermore, long-term treatment of mice (24 weeks) with EM-800 decreased uterine and vaginal wet weight by approximately 75% (47). Interestingly, this treatment regime (3–100 μg/day, given orally) was more effective than ovariectomy in inducing uterine atrophy, thus indicating that EM-800 has pure antiestrogenic activity. EM-800 also did not affect circulating estrogen levels; however, estrogen receptor expression was reduced (47).

Daily subcutaneous administration of EM-800 (0.3–10 μg/mouse) can also significantly decrease uterine and vaginal wet weight (48). Treatment of animals by this method may be more convenient and accurate than oral gavage. Preparation of EM-800 for subcutaneous treatment requires that the drug be dissolved in a 50:50 (vol:vol) mixture of polyethylene glycol 600 and ethanol and administered in a 1% (wt/vol) gelatin–0.9% saline solution. The final concentration of polyethylene glycol 600/ethanol should be 8% (48).

Another pure antiestrogen that can be obtained commercially is ICI 182,780 (Tocris). ICI 182,780 inhibits estrogen binding to the estrogen receptor complex. However, ICI 182,780 is approximately 10 times less potent than EM-800 as determined by inhibition of estrone-stimulated uterine weight in ovariectomized mice (48). ICI 182,780 can be administered orally or subcutaneously. Preparation of ICI 182,780 for subcutaneous administration is the same as that described by EM-800.

If different doses of these agents are employed, the degree of antiestrogenic activity can be determined by measuring the wet weight of estrogen-sensitive tissues, such as the uterus and vagina. Antagonism of estrogen activity will dose-dependently decrease the wet weight of these tissues, which can be assessed quantitatively (48).

To date, published studies have not examined the effects of EM-800 and ICI 182,780 on either immunologic or phys-

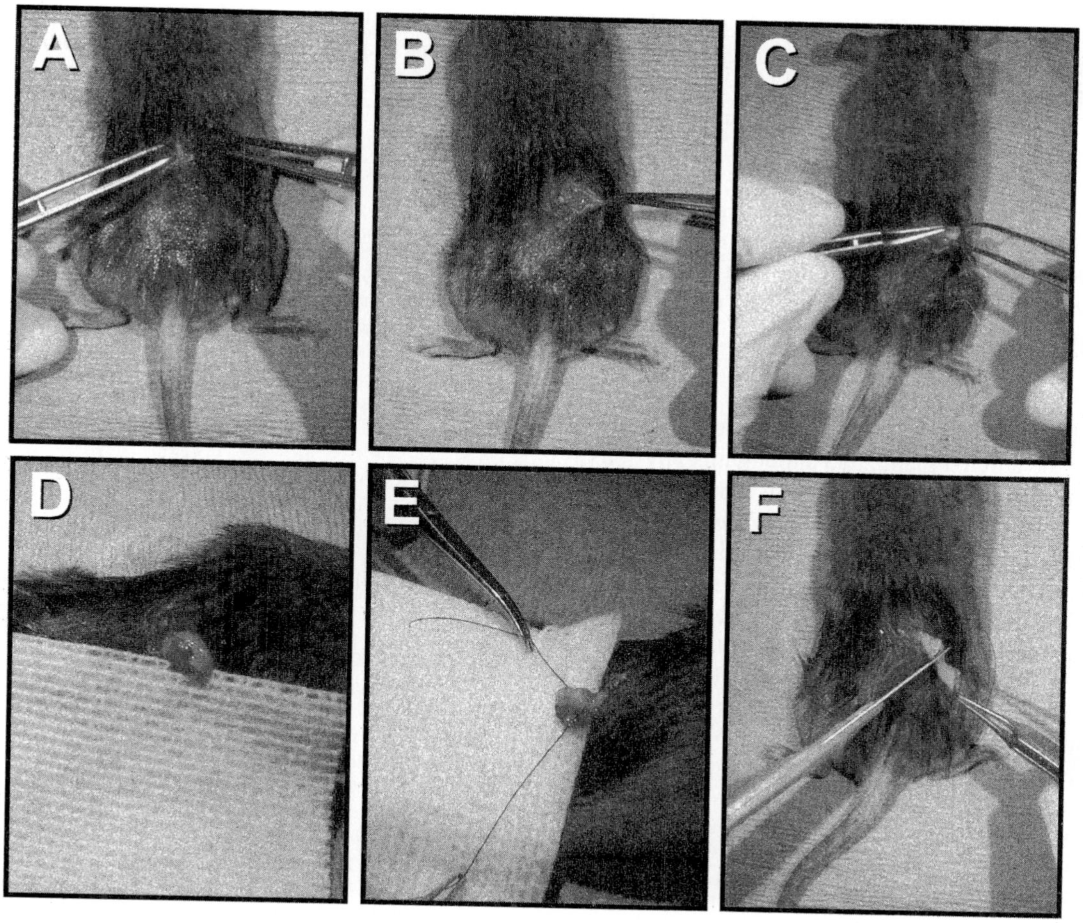

Figure 3 Surgical ovariectomy of the mouse. (A) Proper placement of midline incision. (B) Retraction of skin incision to one side. (C) Removal of ovary and surrounding fat pad. (D) Isolation of the ovary and fat pad. (E) Placement of ligature around the oviduct and blood vessels. (F) Removal of ovary. (See color plates.)

iologic parameters in animal trauma models. Nonetheless, these agents, due to their "pure" antiestrogenic activity, hold promise in determining the role of estrogens in the gender dimorphic response to trauma that has been previously observed (10–13, 49, 50).

C. Nongonadal Sex Hormones

1. Prolactin

Although prolactin is a pituitary hormone, the heterogeneous nature of prolactin-producing cells, and the expression of prolactin receptors in almost all tissues and the existence of a signal transduction pathway common with cytokines, support the role of prolactin as a cytokine in pleiotrophic functions. The involvement of prolactin in the regulation of the immune system is evident (51, 52). Furthermore, prolactin release from the pituitary is stimulated by estrogen, linking this hormone to gender differences. With regard to trauma, studies have shown that administration of prolactin following hemorrhagic shock in males improves many aspects of cell-mediated immunity and decreases susceptibility to sepsis (53–56). In those studies, prolactin was administered subcutaneously at a dose of

Table V Nonsteroidal Antiestrogenic Compounds

Name (source)	Mechanism of action	Dose	Route of administration
ICI 182,780 (Tocris)	Inhibition of estrogen binding to the receptor complex	3 mg/kg	Subcutaneous
EM-800 (Schering)	Inhibition of estrogen receptor complex activities	3 mg/kg	Subcutaneous

4 mg/kg body weight daily. These studies suggest that prolactin may play an important role in the regulation of the immune response to traumatic injury.

Prolactin secretion is suppressed by dopamine and studies have shown that dopamine antagonists will increase prolactin production (57, 58). In this regard, the dopamine antagonist metoclopramide, when administered subcutaneously (4 mg/kg body weight) following trauma-hemorrhage, has been reported to restore immune function (59). Thus, agents that modulate dopamine can be used indirectly to regulate prolactin levels.

2. Dehydroepiandrosterone

Dehydroepiandrosterone (DHEA) is a steroid hormone produced by the adrenal gland, and although its physiological role in humans remains controversial, it has been shown to possess potent immunomodulatory properties (60). Administration of DHEA in experimental trauma models has been shown to improve a number of aspects of immune function (61, 62) and to decrease susceptibility to subsequent sepsis (63). Furthermore, DHEA administration following trauma-hemorrhage normalized circulating corticosterone levels and the effect on T lymphocytes was direct and independent of androgen receptor activity (61). DHEA can be administered subcutaneously in propylene glycol. A daily dosage of 4 mg/kg in mice has been shown to be optimal for modulation of immune parameters (63).

D. Measurement of Sex Hormone Levels

A number of techniques can be employed to measure circulating levels of sex hormones. These include enzyme-linked immunoabsorbent assay (ELISA), radioimmunoassay (RIA), and high-performance liquid chromatography (HPLC). Kits, both ELISA and RIA, are commercially available for many of the sex hormones (testosterone, estrogen, prolactin, DHEA, etc.) and are relatively easy to perform. In contrast, HPLC methodology is more complicated, but provides wider flexibility. The drawback to HPLC is the initial cost of the equipment and level of technical expertise required to operate it properly.

IV. Conclusions

The techniques discussed in this chapter can provide the basis for the development of experimental systems to study the effect of gender and aging in trauma models. As new agents become available and as new insights into the role of these factors are elucidated, trauma models will need to be modified accordingly. This area of experimental study is in its infancy. Application of these methods is far ranging and includes subsequent study of immunologic, physiologic, biochemical, and metabolic parameters. Limitations are only in the ability of the investigator to design experimental models/systems that are relevant and that accurately mimic the clinical setting. It is hoped that information gained from experimental study in this area will lead to the development of safe and useful therapeutic approaches for the treatment of trauma victims, leading to decreased morbidity and mortality.

Acknowledgments

This work was support by Grant R01 GM 37127 from the National Institutes of Health. The authors wish to thank Drs. Christian Schneider and Eike Nickel for their technical assistance in the preparation of the figures.

References

1. Barton, R. G. and Cerra, F. B. (1990). Initial management of trauma. The first 5 minutes. *Postgrad. Med.* **88,** 83–90.
2. Baue, A. E. (1990). "Multiple Organ Failure. Patient Care and Prevention." Mosby, St. Louis.
3. DeCamp, M. M., and Demling, R. H. (1988). Post-traumatic multisystem organ failure. *JAMA* **260,** 530–534.
4. Deitch, E. A. (1990). Multiple organ failure: Summary and overview. *In* "Multiple Organ Failure" (E. A. Deitch, ed.), pp. 285–299. Thieme Medical Publishers, New York.
5. Meyers, B. R., Sherman, E., Mendelson, M. H., Valsquez, G., Srulevitch-Chin, E., Hubbard, M., and Hirschman, S. Z. (1989). Bloodstream infections in the elderly. *Am. J. Med.* **86,** 379–384.
6. Schroder, J., Kahlke, V., Staubach, K. H., Zabel, P., and Stuber, F. (1998). Gender differences in human sepsis. *Arch. Surg.* **133,** 1200–1205.
7. McGowan, J. E., Barnes, M. W., and Finland, N. (1975). Bacteremia at Boston City Hospital: Occurrence and mortality during 12 selected years (1935–1972) with special reference to hospital-acquired cases. *J. Infect. Dis.* **132,** 316–335.
8. Bone, R. C. (1992). Toward an epidemiology and natural history of SIRS (systemic inflammatory response syndrome). *JAMA* **268,** 3452–3455.
9. Altura, B. M. (1976). Sex and estrogens in protection against circulatory stress reactions. *Am. J. Physiol.* **231,** 842–847.
10. Kahlke, V., Angele, M. K., Ayala, A., Schwacha, M. G., Cioffi, W. G., Bland, K. I., and Chaudry, I. H. (2000). Immune dysfunction following trauma-hemorrhage: Influence of gender and age. *Cytokine* **12,** 69–77.
11. Kahlke, V., Angele, M. K., Schwacha, M. G., Ayala, A., Cioffi, W. G., Bland, K. I., and Chaudry, I. H. (2000). Reversal of sexual dimorphism in splenic T-lymphocyte responses following trauma-hemorrhage with aging. *Am. J. Physiol.* **278,** C509–C516.
12. Wichmann, M. W., Zellweger, R., DeMaso, C. M., Ayala, A., and Chaudry, I. H. (1996). Enhanced immune responses in females as opposed to decreased responses in males following hemorrhagic shock. *Cytokine* **8,** 853–863.
13. Zellweger, R., Ayala, A., Stein, S., DeMaso, C. M., and Chaudry, I. H. (1997). Females in proestrus state tolerate sepsis better than males. *Crit. Care Med.* **25,** 106–110.
14. Chaudry, I. H., Wang, P., Ba, Z. F., and Burkhardt, J. (1992). Trauma-hemorrhage and resuscitation in mice: Effects on cardiac output and organ blood flow. *FASEB J.* **6,** A2040.
15. Chaudry, I. H., Wang, P., Singh, G., Hauptman, J. G., and Ayala, A. (1993). Rat and mouse models of hypovolemic-traumatic shock. *In* "Pathophysiology of Shock, Sepsis, and Organ Failure" (G. Schlag and H. Redl, eds.), pp. 371–383. Springer-Verlag, Berlin.
16. Wichmann, M. W., Arnoczky, S. P., DeMaso, C. M., Ayala, A., and Chaudry, I. H. (1996). Depressed osteoblast activity and increased

osteocyte necrosis following closed bone fracture and hemorrhagic shock. *J. Trauma* **41,** 628–633.
17. Wichmann, M. W., Zellweger, R., Williams, C., Ayala, A., DeMaso, C. M., and Chaudry, I. H. (1996). Immune function is more compromised following closed bone fracture and hemorrhagic shock than hemorrhage alone. *Arch. Surg.* **131,** 995–1000.
18. Ertel, W., Morrison, M. H., Meldrum, D. R., Ayala, A., and Chaudry, I. H. (1992). Ibuprofen restores cellular immunity and decreases susceptibility to sepsis following hemorrhage. *J. Surg. Res.* **53,** 55–61.
19. Ayala, A., Lehman, D. L., Herdon, C. D., and Chaudry, I. H. (1994). Mechanism of enhanced susceptibility to sepsis following hemorrhage: Interleukin (IL)-10 suppression of T-cell response is mediated by eicosanoid induced IL-4 release. *Arch. Surg.* **129,** 1172–1178.
20. Moss, N. M., Gough, D. B., Jordan, A. L., Grbic, J. T., Wood, J. J., Rodrick, M. L., and Mannick, J. A. (1988). Temporal correlation of impaired immune response after thermal injury with susceptibility to infection in a murine model. *Surgery* **104,** 882–887.
21. O'Riordain, M. G., Collins, K. H., Pilz, M., Saporoschetz, I. B., Mannick, J. A., and Rodrick, M. L. (1992). Modulation of macrophage hyperactivity improves survival in a burn-sepsis model. *Arch. Surg.* **127,** 152–158.
22. Deitch, E. A. (1992). Multiple organ failure: Pathophysiology and potential future therapy. *Ann. Surg.* **216,** 117–134.
23. Jarrar, D., Wang, P., Cioffi, W. G., Bland, K. I., and Chaudry, I. H. (1999). The female reproductive cycle is an important variable in the response to trauma-hemorrhage. *Shock* **11** (Suppl. 1), 70.
24. Slimmer, L. M. and Blair, M. L. (1996). Female reproductive cycle influences plasma volume and protein restitution after hemorrhage in the conscious rat. *Am. J. Physiol.* **271,** R626–R633
25. Olsen, N. J., and Kovacs, W. J. (1996). Gonadal steroids and immunity. *Endocr. Rev.* **17,** 369–384.
26. Caruso, C., Candore, C., Cigna, D., DiLorenzo, G., Sireci, G., Dieli, F., and Salerno, A. (1996). Cytokine production pathway in the elderly. *Immunol. Res.* **15,** 84–90.
27. Bonello, R. S., Marcus, R., Bloch, D., and Stroder, S. (1996). Effects of growth hormone and estrogen on T lymphocytes in older women. *J. Am. Geriatr. Soc.* **44,** 1038–1042.
28. Proust, J. J., Quadri, R. A., Arbogast, A., and Phelouzat, M. A. (1996). Molecular mechanism of age-related lymphocyte dysfunction. *Pathol. Biol.* **44,** 729–736.
29. Beato, M. (1989). Gene regulation by steroid hormones. *Cell* **56,** 335–344.
30. Beato, M., Chavez, S., and Truss, M. (1996). Transcriptional regulation by steroid hormones. *Steroids* **61,** 240–251.
31. Norfleet, A. M., Thomas, M. L., and Watson, C. S. (1999). Estrogen receptor-alpha detected on the plasma membrane of aldehyde-fixed GH3/B6/F10 rat pituitary tumor cells by enzyme-linked immunocytochemistry. *Endocrinology* **140,** 3805–3514.
32. Stevis, P. E., Deecher, D. C., Suhandolnik, L., Mallis, L. M., and Frail, D. E. (1999). Differential effects of estradiol and estradiol-BSA conjugates. *Endocrinology* **140,** 5455–5458.
33. Waynforth, H. B. (1980). "Experimental and Surgical Technique in the Rat." Academic Press, London.
34. Wichmann, M. W., Angele, M. K., Ayala, A., Cioffi, W. G., and Chaudry, I. (1997). Flutamide: A novel agent for restoring the depressed cell-mediated immunity following soft-tissue trauma and hemorrhagic shock. *Shock* **8,** 1–7.
35. Angele, M. K., Ayala, A., Cioffi, W. G., Bland, K. I., and Chaudry, I. H. (1998). Testosterone: The culprit for producing splenocyte immune depression after trauma hemorrhage. *Am. J. Physiol.* **274,** C1530–C1536
36. Remmers, D. E., Wang, P., Cioffi, W. G., Bland, K. I., and Chaudry, I. H. (1997). Testosterone receptor blockade after trauma-hemorrhage improves cardiac and hepatic functions in males. *Am. J. Physiol.* **273,** H2919–H2925
37. Luo, S., Martel, C., Chen, C., Labrie, C., Candas, B., Singh, S. M., and Labrie, F. (1997). Daily dosing of flutamide or casodex exerts maximal antiandrogenic activity. *Urology* **50,** 913–919.
38. Furr, B. J. (1996). The development of Casodex (bicalutamide): Preclinical studies. *Eur. Urol.* **29,** 83–95.
39. Kerner, J., Wang, P., and Chaudry, I. H. (1995). Impaired gut lipid absorptive capacity after trauma-hemorrhage and resuscitation. *Am. J. Physiol.* **269,** R869–R873
40. Marchetti, B., and Labrie, F. (1998). Characteristics of flutamide action on prostatic and testicular functions in the rat. *J. Steroid Biochem.* **29,** 691–698.
41. Snell, G. D. (1956). Reproduction. *In* "Biology of the Laboratory Mouse" (G. D. Snell, ed.), pp. 55–88. Dover Publications, Inc., New York.
42. Furr, B. J., and Jordan, V. C. (1984). The pharmacology and clinical uses of tamoxifen. *Pharmacol. Ther.* **25,** 127–205.
43. Wakeling, A. E., and Bowler, J. (1988). Biology and mode of action of pure antiestrogens. *J. Steroid Biochem.* **30,** 141–147.
44. Labrie, C., Martel, C., Dufour, J. M., Levesque, C., Merand, Y., and Labrie, F. (1992). Novel compounds inhibit estrogen formation and action. *Cancer Res.* **52,** 610–615.
45. Tremblay, A., Tremblay, G. B., Labrie, F., and Giguere, V. (1998). EM-800, a novel antiestrogen, acts as a pure antagonist of the transcriptional functions of estrogen receptors alpha and beta. *Endocrinology* **139,** 111–118.
46. Couillard, S., Gutman, M., Labrie, C., Belanger, A., Candas, B., and Labrie, F. (1998). Comparison of the effects of the antiestrogens EM-800 and tamoxifen on the growth of human breast ZR-75-1 cancer xenografts in nude mice. *Cancer Res.* **58,** 60–64.
47. Luo, S., Souria, A., Labrie, C., Gauthier, S., Merand, Y., Belanger, A., and Labrie, F. (1998). Effect of twenty-four-week treatment with the antiestrogen EM-800 on estrogen-sensitive parameters in intact and ovariectomized mice. *Endocrinology* **139,** 2645–2656.
48. Martel, C., Labrie, C., Belanger, A., Gauthier, S., Merand, Y., Li, X., Provencher, L., Candas, B., and Labrie, F. (1998). Comparison of the effects of the new orally active antiestrogen EM-800 with ICI 182 780 and toremifene on estrogen-sensitive parameters in the ovariectomized mouse. *Endocrinology* **139,** 2486–2492.
49. Angele, M. K., Xu, Y.-X., Ayala, A., Schwacha, M. G., Catania, R. A., Cioffi, W. G., Bland, K. I., and Chaudry, I. H. (1999). Gender dimorphism in trauma-hemorrhage induced thymocyte apoptosis. *Shock* **12,** 316–322.
50. Zellweger, R., Wichmann, M. W., Ayala, A., Stein, S., DeMaso, C. M., and Chaudry, I. H. (1997). Females in proestrus state maintain splenic immune functions and tolerate sepsis better than males. *Crit. Care Med.* **25,** 106–110.
51. Walker, S. E. (1993). Prolactin: An immune-stimulating peptide that regulates other immune-modulating hormones. *Lupus* **2,** 67–69.
52. Viselli, S. M., Stanek, E. M., Mukherjee, P., and Hymer, W. C. (1991). Prolactin-induced mitogenesis of lymphocytes from ovariectomized rats. *Endocrinology* **129,** 983–990.
53. Zellweger, R., Zhu, X.-H., Wichmann, M. W., Ayala, A., DeMaso, C. M., and Chaudry, I. H. (1996). Prolactin administration following hemorrhagic shock improves macrophage cytokine release capacity and decreases mortality from subsequent sepsis. *J. Immunol.* **157,** 5748–5754.
54. Zellweger, R., Wichmann, M. W., Ayala, A., DeMaso, C. M., and Chaudry, I. H. (1996). Prolactin: A novel and safe immunomodulating hormone for the treatment of immunodepression following severe hemorrhage. *J. Surg. Res.* **63,** 53–58.
55. Zhu, X.-H., Zellweger, R., Wichmann, M. W., Ayala, A., and Chaudry, I. H. (1997). Effects of prolactin and metoclopramide on macrophage cytokine gene expression in late sepsis. *Cytokine* **9,** 437–446.
56. Zellweger, R., Zhu, X.-H., Wichmann, M. W., Ayala, A., DeMaso, C. M., and Chaudry, I. H. (1996). Prolactin administration following

hemorrhagic shock improves macrophage cytokine release capacity and decreases mortality from subsequent sepsis. *J. Immunol.* **157,** 5748–5754.

57. Brouwers, J. R. B. J., Assies, J., Wiersinga, W. M., Huizing, G., and Tytgat, G. N. (1980). Plasma prolactin levels after acute and subchronic oral administration of domperidone and of metoclopramide: A crossover study in healthy volunteers. *Clin. Endocrinol.* **12,** 435–440.
58. Harrington, R. A., Hamilton, C. W., Brogden, R. N., Linkewich, J. A., Romankiewicz, J. A., and Heel, R. C. (1983). Metoclopramide. An updated review of its pharmacological properties and clinical use. *Drugs* **25,** 451–494.
59. Zellweger, R., Wichmann, M. W., Ayala, A., and Chaudry, I. H. (1998). Metoclopramide: A novel and safe immunomodulating agent for restoring the depressed macrophage function following trauma-hemorrhage. *J. Trauma* **44,** 70–77.
60. Daynes, R. A., Dudley, D. J., and Araneo, B. A. (1990). Regulation of murine lymphokine production *in vivo*. II. Dehydroepiandrosterone is a natural enhancer of interleukin 2 synthesis by helper T cells. *Eur. J. Immunol.* **20,** 793–802.
61. Catania, R. A., Angele, M. K., Ayala, A., Cioffi, W. G., Bland, K. I., and Chaudry, I. H. (1999). Dehydroepiandrosterone restores immune function following trauma-haemorrhage by a direct effect on T lymphocytes. *Cytokine* **11,** 443–450.
62. Araneo, B. A., Shelby, J., Li, G. Z., Ku, W., and Daynes, R. A. (1993). Administration of dehydroepiandrosterone to burned mice preserves normal immunologic competence. *Arch. Surg.* **128,** 318–325.
63. Angele, M. K., Catania, R. A., Ayala, A., Cioffi, W. G., Bland, K. I., and Chaudry, I. H. (1998). Dehydroepiandrosterone: An inexpensive steroid hormone that decreases the mortality due to sepsis following trauma-induced hemorrhage. *Arch. Surg.* **133,** 1281–1288.

31

Animal Models of Burn Injury

Daniel L. Traber, Robert E. Barrow, and David N. Herndon

The University of Texas Medical Branch and Shriners' Burns Hospital, Galveston, Texas 77555

I. Introduction

Nearly 3.5 million people receive a thermal injury in the United States annually, with over 80,000 requiring hospitalization and care by specialized burn services. Both adults and children suffer the dire consequences associated with the application of thermal energy to the skin, most commonly from an open flame or direct contact with hot liquids or objects. Injury from toxic chemicals or high-voltage electrical current is less common.

The depth of a thermal injury is dependent on the temperature of heat applied, the rate of thermal energy released, the duration of application, and the thermal conductivity of the tissues involved. Thermal injuries result in marked derangement in homeostasis and metabolic function. As the basis of body regulation of homeostasis is better understood, this knowledge is being applied to understanding the pathophysiology that underlies thermal injury.

Animal models are used to study burn injury to assess whether experimental interventions will compromise or improve the status of a burn patient. As the pathophysiology of burn injuries is better understood, more therapeutic interventions can be tested in animal models. If the proper model has been established, the efficacy as well as serious side effects of the treatment can be identified, and thus the safest and most effective therapeutic intervention can be identified for testing in the thermally injured patient.

Burns are easy to model and the degree of injury can be controlled without difficulty. Consequently, the burn model is also frequently used to investigate multiple traumas, which have similar pathophysiology but are difficult to model. Multiple traumas present major surgical problems, and despite surgical skill, a surgeon treating a multiple trauma victim may induce iatrogenic trauma. Thus the burn model makes an important contribution toward improving treatment for trauma patients.

Burn patients frequently have other associated injuries, such as smoke inhalation pneumonia or sepsis, and these can also be modeled in animals. These models are important because they allow study of situations that are associated with great clinical morbidity and mortality.

Whatever model is used, it is important that the clinical situation be duplicated. Many of the clinical trial failures in the area of trauma and sepsis have been the result of the use of inappropriate modeling. Such failures have wasted resources available for investigation, contributed to increase in patient mortality, and reduced the support available for research.

II. Animal Rights Considerations

Investigators who work in the area of thermal injury must be especially cautious to ensure that the animals that they are studying are not in pain. Investigators in burn research are easy targets of animal rights groups. It is very important that every effort be made to ensure absolute adherence to the spirit and letter of the principles for care and use of animals in research as expressed by the American Physiological Society and the National Institutes of Health (NIH). These can be found online (http://faseb.org/aps/animal.html#policy and http://www.nap.edu/readingroom/books/labrats/). Experiments involving burns should never be attempted in the absence of an experienced investigator. The investigational staff should be trained in the proper induction of an injury and, if the animal is to be awakened, the staff should also be trained and experienced in recognizing pain in the animal species that they are studying.

In preparation for the burn injury model protocol, a thorough search of the literature should be performed. We accomplish this using the NIH search engine, PubMed (http://www.ncbi.nlm.nih.gov/PubMed/). This is a very important step in the mind of most Institutional Committee Members and shows that you are a seasoned investigator who knows the ropes. Proposals for funding should begin and end with emphasis on the clinical importance of burn research.

As you continue your protocol, be very careful to include all the steps to ensure that every measure has been taken to see that the animal is comfortable and free from pain, that you are collecting data in a professional manner, and that the study will result in information that is scientifically important and of clinical relevance. As part of your proposal invite the committee or one of the representatives to visit your lab and observe you doing the study. Ensure them that you are prepared to terminate the experiment at any time that a member observes that the animals suffer.

III. Methodology

The experimental methodology for producing burn injuries varies. (In all cases, the animals are protected from undue suffering, as discussed in the following sections.) Many investigators induce burn injury with a flame, because the most severe burns seen clinically are the result of flame injury (1–5). The body surface area of an animal can be determined from its size and weight (Table I) (6). Based on body weight, the area to be experimentally burned is measured and marked. The injury is usually performed with a Bunsen burner. As the flame is applied to the skin it contracts; at this point a third-degree (full-thickness) burn is obtained. The flame is then moved to a new area of skin. After completion of the burning procedure the skin is observed and those areas that are pink in color are considered to be second degree. These are given additional injury. In this way a standardized injury can be induced (7). The wounds are induced in mice with a cutout through a flame-retardant material (Fig. 1) (8).

Table I Mammalian Body Surface Area[a]

Animal	*K*-Value constant
Mouse	0.090
Rat	0.091
Cat	0.100
Guinea pig	0.090
Rabbit	0.0975
Dog	
Over 4 kg	0.112
Under 4 kg	0.101
Sheep (sheared wt.)	0.084
Swine	0.090
Cow and steer	0.090
Horse	0.100
Monkey	0.118
Human	0.11
Bird	0.10

[a]Surface area (m^2) = K[(body weight)$^{2/3}$] (kg). Data from Dubois (6).

The scald burn is easier to standardize. The animals are placed into specially constructed templates based on the size of burn that is to be produced (Fig. 2). They are then placed in water at different temperatures and for various time periods, depending on the depth of burn that is desired (9, 10). For a third-degree burn the animals are placed in water at 99°C for 10 sec (10).

Standardized burn injury can also be created with heated brass or aluminum templates (11, 12). The metal templates are heated to varying temperatures in order to produce partial or full-thickness burns. Because the templates allow burns over a given surface area, a very consistent injury can be made in a very rapid order. This is especially useful when the research plan calls for a large number of burned animals.

IV. Large Animals

The great advantage of using large animals is that the clinical situation is easy to duplicate, and the same sort of measurements made in humans can be correlated with more invasive techniques. For example, the animals' cardiopulmonary function can be monitored, and flow probes may be placed on the vessels of the major organs, such as kidney (13), gastrointestinal tract (14, 15), or brain (16, 17) and lung (18, 19). Blood flow to the various organs can be validated

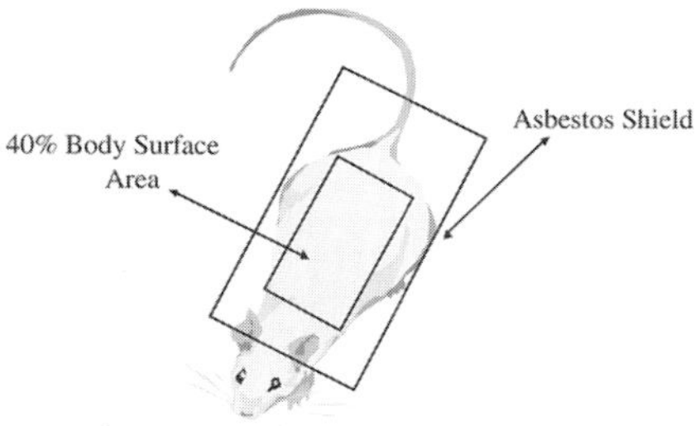

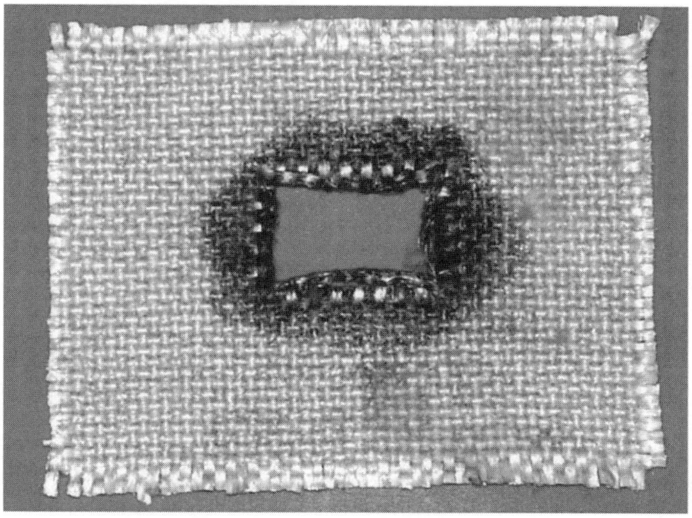

Figure 1 Asbestos template used for inducing flame injury in small animals. Animals of similar body weights are obtained. Their body surface area is calculated using the equation for body weight/body surface area constant given in Table I. Depending on the size of the burn the investigator wants to induce, an appropriate opening is cut in the asbestos material. This technique is most frequently used in mice and rats.

using radioactive (16, 20) or colored microspheres (21), urinary output and renal function can be gauged (22), and the animals can be resuscitated to specific endpoints. Efficacy of treatment can be evaluated in terms of improvement of measured respiratory, vascular, or renal function. Samples of exhaled gas, urine, blood, or other body fluids can be obtained for study without compromising homeostasis. Because of the accuracy and lack of variability of the data obtained, fewer animals are needed to accomplish a study.

There are problems with the use of large animals in burn research. These animals are expensive. A sheep in the Galveston–Houston (Texas) area costs $200, and swine cost $175. In addition, the animals require additional care and a relatively large space for housing. Size is also an important factor in studying drugs. Experimental compounds are expensive, and the larger the animal, the more compound is required, and thus, the more expensive the experiment. Many of the antibodies that are available for analytical procedures do not cross-react with materials from large animals. Another great disadvantage of large animals is their long gestational period, which makes it difficult to develop transgenic animals. However, rapid advances are being made in cell biology and genetics in sheep and swine (23–26). Most notably, in recent times cloned sheep have been developed (27). In the future, more and more cell biological reagents for swine and sheep will become available.

A. Dog

The dog has been used as a model for burn injury. Healthy dogs, however, have become difficult to obtain in most areas and, where available, they are usually quite expensive. Of all the animal kingdom, the general public is least likely to accept the use of the dog in research settings that involve trauma. In addition, barking dogs have a disruptive effect on vivariums. Thus it is becoming increasingly difficult to find

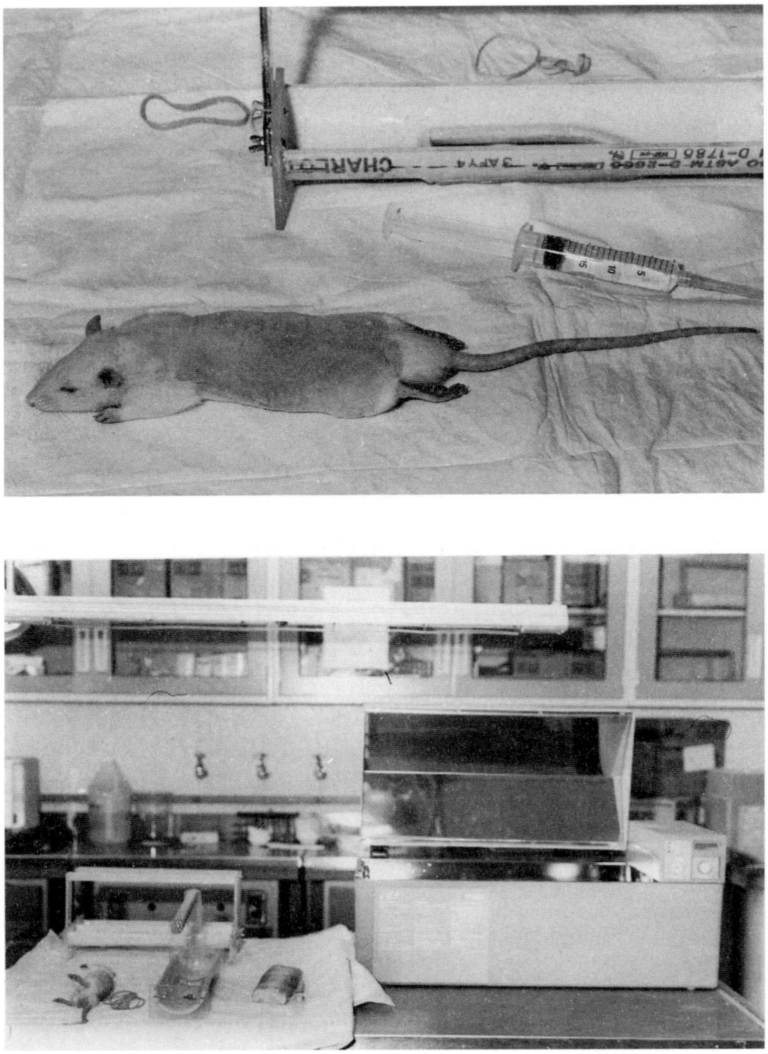

Figure 2 Plastic template used for inducing a scald burn (9). As in Fig. 1, animals of similar weights are used for the study. (Top) The anesthetized animal is placed into the device. (Bottom) The animal is then placed into heated water at a set temperature to produce the desired depth of burn.

animal care facilities in academic settings that house dogs. During the past year there has only been one publication from western Europe and the United States that reported the use of dogs in burn research (28). There were four such reports 10 years ago and 12 reports 20 years ago.

B. Sheep

Sheep have become one of the most widely used of the large animals in trauma and burn research. Most of the animals used in research are either yearling males that have been castrated or older females that have been culled from the flock. Reproducing ewes are the main variety used in animal husbandry; the placenta may carry Q fever, a highly contagious microbiologic vector. The advantage of using young males is that they are somewhat smaller (~20 kg). The disadvantage is that they are rambunctious and noisy. The older females are larger (~40 kg), docile, and quiet. Ewes live in flocks and are very uncomfortable when not in the presence of another sheep. For study, the sheep are placed into metabolic cages (Fig. 3). The animals, especially the older ewes, appear content in these cages as long as they are with another sheep and have food and water. The animals are easily fed with pellets and hay. Hay is important because it stimulates gastrointestinal motility. If sheep do not eat they lose gastrointestinal tone; gas will form in their rumen. This can occur rapidly and is referred to as bloat; if it occurs the animal's rumen has to be decompressed.

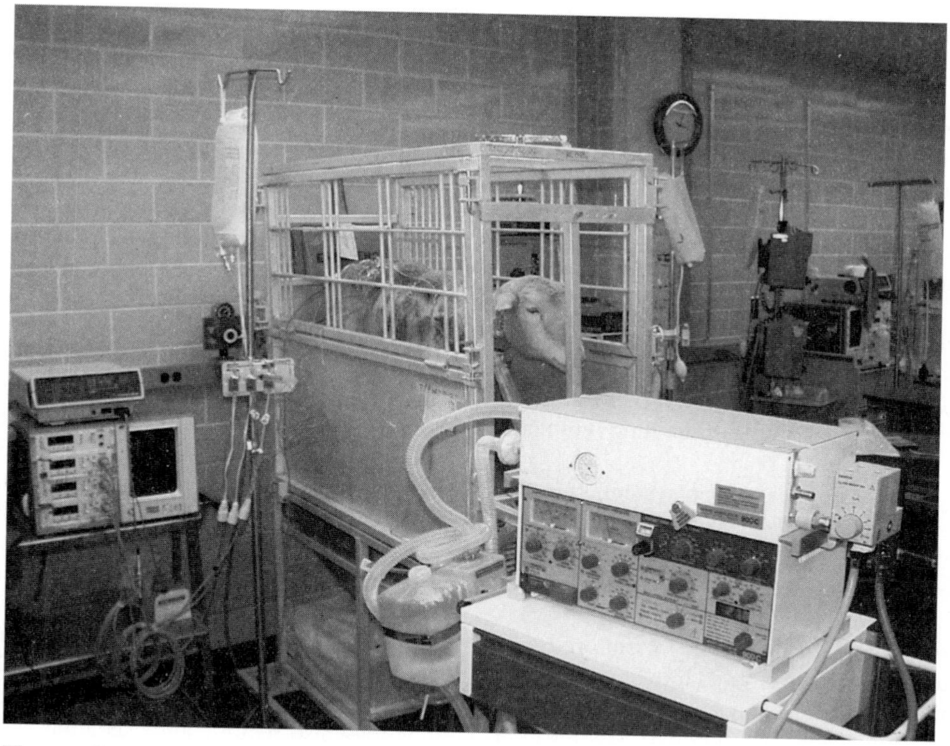

Figure 3 A sheep in a metabolic cage. Sheep placed in metabolic cages are easily accessible for study, and the monitoring devices are less likely to be disrupted. Occasionally, the sheep will try to chew the catheters, and for this reason a collar can be placed around their neck, preventing them from turning around to bite their catheters. In the cage the feces and urine are easily collected; for more precise urinary values a Foley urinary retention catheter can be used. Food and oral water intake can be controlled and monitored. The sheep tolerate assisted ventilation without sedation.

Sheep are easy to anesthetize. They have a sensitivity to anesthetics similar to that of humans. Ketamine in these animals is a good, short-acting anesthetic for induction and for short procedures. Sheep do not appear to have hallucinations with this agent, as do humans. Some agents used in anesthesia are to be avoided. Nitrous oxide diffuses into the rumen and can cause bloat. All depolarizing muscle relaxants are long acting in the sheep and should be avoided. Long-acting agents such as dexamethonium may paralyze the animals for days. Before anesthesia, food (but not water) should be withdrawn. Some may feel uncomfortable about not withdrawing water, but the gastrointestinal tract of the sheep is such that if the animals do not drink, water will still flow into the lumen. Lack of drinking water can lead to a reduction in motility and to distension.

If the sheep are to be studied postprocedure in the unanesthetized state, induction with ketamine and anesthesia with an agent such as halothane or isoflurane should be used. This anesthetic technique will result in an awake, alert animal within an hour or two of the operative procedure, depending on the duration of the anesthesia and the skill of the surgeon. When large operative procedures are performed, it is advisable to infiltrate the wound with a local anesthetic. Postoperatively, pain is detectable if the animals grit their teeth and appear to be uncomfortable (getting up and sitting down repeatedly, refusing to stand), and if their pupils are narrowed. Buprenorphine (0.3mg/kg/12 hr, intravenous) is a very effective analgesic. Ibuprofen (800 mg, periorbital) may also be effective.

If the studies are to be performed in the anesthetized state, the animals must be placed on a ventilator. Their central control of ventilation is very sensitive to anesthetics, similar to human sensitivity. The animals should be placed in a prone position to remove the weight of the abdominal viscera from the inferior vena cava and the diaphragm. As is the case with most animals, the body temperature must be supported. It should be noted that the body temperature of most animals is between 38° and 39°C (29). As is the case in all animals, it is important to be generous in fluid administration. This is especially true during the time periods when the body cavities are opened. Sheep, like humans, are very sensitive to endotoxin. Even when the experiments are performed on an acute basis, sterile pyrogen-free fluids should be used. Clean, aseptic conditions should be utilized.

Perhaps the reason why the ovine species was selected for study initially was that these animals have a lung that is most similar to the human lung (30). The sheep has a single efferent that drains its lungs and can be cannulated (31). The flow in this lymphatic is equal to the transvascular fluid flux from the pulmonary circuit. The factors that are responsible for fluid movement across the microvasculature are represented in the Starling equation: lung lymph flow $= K_f[(P_c - P_i) - \sigma(\pi_p - \pi_i)]$. Here K_f is the filtration coefficient, an index of permeability to small molecular weight; P_c and P_i are the hydrostatic pressures in the microvasculature and interstitial spaces respectively; σ is the reflection coefficient, an index of permeability to large molecular weight materials such as protein; π_p and π_i are the oncotic and protein osmotic pressures. These parameters can be determined in the ovine chronic lung lymphatic preparation (32).

The ovine lung also has rather unique systemic circulation because sheep have a single bronchial artery for the lung systemic blood supply (33, 34). Flow probes can be placed on this vessel (19). The animals can be placed on ventilators and studied for prolonged time periods (7, 35), and the ventilation settings can be easily monitored with blood gases because the animals have a large blood volume. Pulmonary compliance and resistance can be determined (36). The animal is thus ideal for pulmonary studies (37). The veins of the bronchial circulation drain into the pulmonary microvasculature (34). Mediators released from an injured airway would enter into the pulmonary areas. This bronchial venous blood flow can be measured and the mediators determined (38). Occluders can be placed on the left pulmonary artery and veins, and a catheter can be placed in the left pulmonary artery distal to the pulmonary arterial occluder. When the occluder is activated, the pulmonary arterial inflow and venous outflow are sealed and the inflow into the pulmonary vasculature is thus isolated from the bronchial vasculature, and blood flow can be determined in the pouch (38).

In addition to the lung lymphatic, sheep have in the flank a lymphatic that drains the dermal surface of the animal, the prefemoral lymphatic (39). This preparation has been used to study the cutaneous microvascular permeability of both burned and unburned skin (7, 40, 41). Systemic fluid balance can also be evaluated in sheep and other large animals by intake and output studies. The urethra of the sheep is easily cannulated (7). Most sheep tolerate Foley retention catheters with few problems.

The size of sheep, dogs, and swine allows the placement of Swan–Ganz catheters that are of the same gauge as those used in humans. Thus, it is relatively easy to determine cardiac output, heart rate, and pulmonary, right atrial, and systemic arterial pressures in these animals (1, 42, 43). In addition, manometers can be placed into the heart for the determination of the left ventricular pressure (44, 45). The volume of the heart can be determined by ultrasound or thermal dilution (46, 47). Using these variables one can assess myocardial contractility in these animals (48, 49). The sheep has also been used to evaluate extracorporeal support devices (50–53).

C. Swine

As was noted above, swine can also be used in a number of cardiopulmonary studies. Although there was a trend to use miniature swine in the past (54), no burn studies have utilized these animals in the past year; investigators are now using immature swine in their studies (55) because they are more accessible and much cheaper. Studies with swine have included both anesthetized and unanesthetized models. Unlike sheep, swine that are studied in the unanesthetized state usually need to be moderately restrained (Fig. 4). Restraint is usually accomplished by placing the animals into slings (56). In studies of wound healing (57) or studies of skin flaps (58), this may be necessary only until the animals have reacted to the anesthetic. After the animals have recovered from the anesthetic they can be placed in pens that will allow them to walk. Mobility is preferable in these cases because it helps to reduce pain. Pain medication for swine is similar to that used in sheep. When the animals are in slings they may also require some sedation, and will also need to be fed by jejunostomy (59).

Virtually all that was said in regard to sheep cardiopulmonary and renal function is also true for swine. Because the gastrointestinal tract of the swine is more similar to that of humans, they are used for evaluating gut functions (20). Also, the skin of swine is similar to human skin, thus swine are frequently used in wound healing studies (57, 60). Swine have a fat metabolism similar to that seen in humans and are therefore suitable for metabolic studies of lipid metabolism. The formation of surfactant has been studied in swine with a 40% burn injury (61).

In one model of burn injury in swine, hepatic blood flow was determined by placing ultrasonic flow probes on the superior mesenteric and hepatic arteries. Catheters are placed into the portal and hepatic veins (59). Thus in this model the uptake and production of materials by the liver, as well as hepatic oxygen consumption, can be determined. Given the similarity in metabolism between the swine and humans, this model should be very important for future metabolic studies.

D. Rabbit

Although the rabbit is a relatively small animal (2–5 kg), it is large enough for instrumentation in order to determine cardiac outputs and vascular filling pressure (62). The lung of the rabbit is small and can be used in isolated perfusion experiments (63). Rabbit experiments have been performed for the study of burn injury (5) and smoke inhalation (62). As was the case with sheep and swine, cell biological mate-

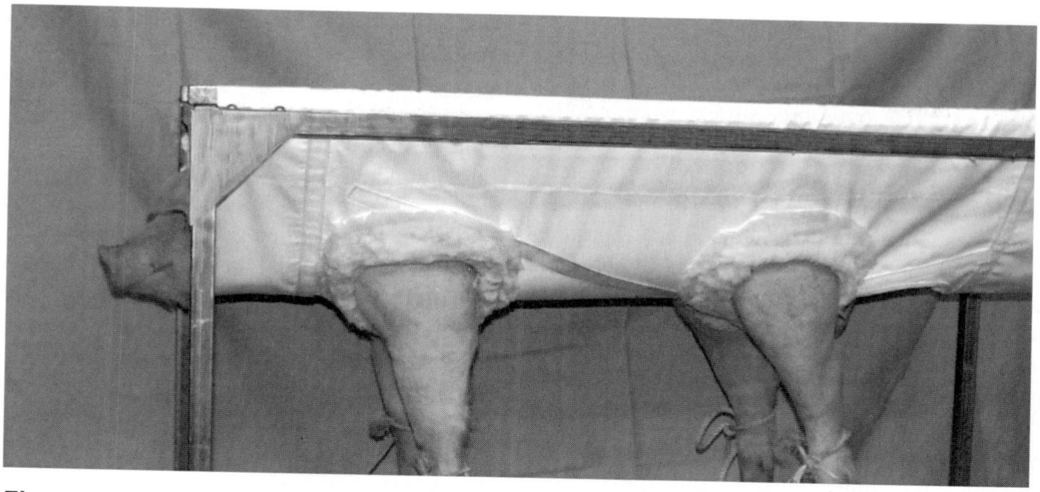

Figure 4 A pig in a sling. Unlike sheep, swine require additional restraint when studied. This is accomplished by placing them in slings. The animals may be maintained and studied in this manner for several days. If they are to be studied for prolonged time periods, a feeding tube must be inserted. In many instances the swine may require sedation. We have found that diazepam is appropriate for this purpose.

rials are also available in lagomorphs (64–66). In addition to the lung, the rabbit is also studied because of its ears. The ear has an artery and a vein and the structure is almost pure skin, consequently the rabbit ear is used to evaluate metabolic changes in burned skin (67). Similarly, rabbit ears are used to evaluate the effects of various materials on metabolism (68, 69).

The great advantage of the rabbit is the fact that it is smaller than many of the other animals, thus housing is cheaper. In addition, rabbits cost much less. The disadvantage of using rabbits is that their size limits the amount of blood that can be drawn for samples. Much of the instrumentation that is used in the rabbit has to be specially designed, so equipment costs are greater. However, smaller size means lower housing and drug costs.

V. Small Animals

A. Mouse

The mouse is by far the most popular animal for study because of the ready availability of transgenic and knockout animals. There were some 42 publications related to mice and thermal injury during the past 12 months. The mouse burn model has been used in a host of studies, including gut barrier function (70, 71), bacterial killing (72), angiotensin converting enzyme inhibition (73), T cell function and immune suppression (74), virus infection (75), and many others.

In the mouse, a thermal injury produces a severe hypermetabolic response that is characterized by catabolism, protein wasting, and increased oxygen consumption. This hyperdynamic state causes loss of body weight and lean body mass and impaired wound healing, which cause prolonged recovery times and increases in morbidity and mortality. Major trauma has been shown in clinical and laboratory studies to have profound effects on immune function and has enhanced the severity of viral and bacterial infections, the clinical effect of which would increase mortality in patients suffering severe trauma.

A thermal injury is experimentally produced in mice using a gas flame. Before being subjected to the burn injury, the mice are anesthetized with pentobarbital (40 mg/kg) administered intraperitoneally (IP). The hair is removed from the back with an electric clipper. An asbestos cloth with a 3-cm × 4-cm window is pressed firmly against the shaved back, and for 10 sec the area is exposed to the flame of a Fisher burner. This procedure results in the production of a third-degree (30% of the total body surface area) burn in a 26-g mouse. Just after the burn injury, 4 ml of physiological saline is administered IP to each mouse for fluid resuscitation

Although the problem with mice is that their size limits the ability to monitor them, many techniques are being developed to determine various aspects of murine function. Techniques have been developed to determine the degree of hypoxic pulmonary vasoconstriction (76), ventricular volume and cardiac output (77), blood gases and arterial pressure (78), and myocardial contractility (79). Intravital microscopy can be performed (80). Pulmonary arterial pressure and pulmonary wedge pressure can be determined and pulmonary vascular resistance can be calculated (81). More and more techniques are being developed that will enable the investigator to perform burn experiments in animals that are resuscitated to endpoints.

B. Guinea Pig

Many burn studies have been performed on guinea pigs (10, 82), but in the past year only three studies were reported by MEDLINE. These are studies related to wound healing, nutrition, and myocardial contractility in the isolated perfused guinea pig heart after thermal injury (83, 84). Studies of experimental chemical burns have also been reported (85, 86). Guinea pigs, as is the case for humans, cannot produce ascorbic acid (87). For this reason the guinea pig will probably remain an important model when it comes to studies involving this vitamin. The guinea pig is used in nutrition studies because enteral and parenteral feeding can easily be administered to the animals (87).

Guinea pigs used in burn studies are treated similar to rats. The advantages of the guinea pig as a small animal burn model are that they are more docile and tolerate in-dwelling catheters and enteral feeding. The guinea pig burn model also simulates the human response to thermal injury and thus may be utilized as a suitable model for investigating a variety of responses to severe burns.

C. Rat

The burned rat model was originally used to investigate burn management with different air temperatures and relative humidities, and to follow the metabolic response of a thermal injury under these conditions. This model has expanded in its use to study the mechanisms of wound healing, kidney and liver changes, inhalation injury concomitant with a thermal injury, cardiovascular responses, and neurological changes associated with a severe thermal injury.

Rats are anesthetized with either ketamine (40–90 mg/kg IP) plus xylazine (8 mg/kg IP) or ketamine (60 mg/kg IP) plus pentobarbital (20 mg/kg IP) and buprenorphine or butorphanol (0.1 mg/kg SC). Analgesia is used when pain becomes evident: buprenorphine (0.05–0.1 mg/kg SC tid to bid) for 5 days or butorphanol (5–10 mg/kg SC). The hair on the back and abdomen is clipped and 1 ml/% burn/kg body weight of Ringer's lactate solution is given by IP injection.

Placing the animals in molds (Fig. 2b) that expose an area on the dorsum equal to 25% of the total body surface produces scald burns. The area is then immersed in 99°C water for 10 sec; 50% total body surface area (TBSA) burns are produced by placing the animals with back burns in the molds with their abdomens exposed and subjecting this area to water at 99°C. A 10-sec eßxposure to the dorsum produces a full-thickness burn; 3 sec produces a partial-thickness burn. Histologic examinations have demonstrated that uniform full-thickness injuries are obtained without damage to the visceral organs. At 8 hr following injury, all animals receive a second intraperitoneal injection of 1 ml/% Ringer's lactate solution burn/kg body weight. On removal from the water, the dorsum is quickly dried to prevent additional burning. This procedure produces a uniform burn with sharp margins. Animals can survive a 20% burn without resuscitation; however, animals with larger burns need to be resuscitated. The scald burns do not interfere too greatly with mobility or the animal's ability to easily eat and drink. A large number of burned animals can be prepared by this technique within a reasonable time, using only simple equipment. The technique has been particularly useful for studies of burn infection and treatment and for metabolism studies (9, 10).

The burned rat shows a dose response relationship between burn size and oxygen consumption similar to that observed in humans and thus this model may be suitable in studying thermal injuries. It is suggested that the mature rat be used when weight stability during the study period is important, because in older rats most correction for body weight is unnecessary.

Despite the great advantages of working with mice, rats continue to be the most popular animal for burn research. Rats are relatively inexpensive ($12–15) and many of their antibodies will cross-react with murine antigens. The size of the rat makes housing easy and inexpensive and the animals are large enough to attach to instrumentation. Techniques are available for determining cardiac output by thermal dilution (88). Arterial pressures can be measured accurately and on a chronic basis (89). The rat has been used in experiments involving would healing and gene transfer of growth factors (90). The thoracic duct of the rat can be cannulated and its flow measured, and mediators may be measured in the lymph (91,92). Myocardial contractility can be determined in the intact rat (93) and the isolated perfused rat lung can be evaluated (94).

VI. Conclusion

Many techniques and preparations are available to study burn models in several animal species. The protocols used depend on the expertise and experience of the investigator and the information that is to be obtained.

References

1. Turner, R., Carvajal, H. F., and Traber, D. L. (1977). Effects of ganglionic blockade upon the renal and cardiovascular dysfunction induced by thermal injury. *Circ. Shock* **4,** 103.
2. Arturson, G. (1969). The plasma kinins in thermal injury. *Scand. J. Clin. Lab. Invest.* **24** (Suppl. 107), 1.
3. Baxter, C. R., Marvin, J. A., and Curreri, P. W. (1974). Early management of thermal burns. *Postgrad. Med.* **55,** 131.
4. Asch, M. J., Feldman, R. J., Walker, H. L., Foley, F. D., Popp, R. L., Mason, A. D., Jr., and Pruitt, B. A., Jr. (1982). Systemic and pulmonary hemodynamic changes accompanying thermal injury. *Ann. Surg.* **178,** 218.
5. Hartl, W. H., Herndon, D. N., and Wolfe, R. R. (1990). Kinin/prostaglandin system: Its therapeutic value in surgical stress. *Crit. Care Med.* **18,** 1167.

6. Dubois, E. F. (1936). The estimation of the surface area of the body. *In* "Basal Metabolism in Health and Disease" (E.F. DuBois, ed.), pp. 125–144. Lea & Febiger, Philadelphia.
7. Sakurai, H., Schmalstieg, F. C., Traber, L. D., Hawkins, H. K., and Traber, D. L. (1999). Role of L-selectin in physiological manifestations after burn and smoke inhalation injury in sheep. *J. Appl. Physiol.* **86,** 1151.
8. Takagi, K., Suzuki, F., Barrow, R. E., Wolf, S. E., and Herndon, D. N. (1998). Recombinant human growth hormone modulates Th1 and Th2 cytokine response in burned mice. *Ann. Surg.* **228,** 106.
9. Walker, H. L., and Mason, A. D., Jr. (1968). A standard animal burn. *J. Trauma* **8,** 1049.
10. Herndon, D. N., Wilmore, D. W., and Mason, A. D., Jr. (1978). Development and analysis of a small animal model simulating the human postburn hypermetabolic response. *J. Surg. Res.* **25,** 394.
11. Noormohamed, S. E., Kumar, V., and Min, D. I. (1994). Evaluation of traditional African medicine "Compound R" for the treatment of thermal burn wounds in fuzzy rats. *J. Burn Care Rehabil.* **15,** 519.
12. Bucky, L. P., Vedder, N. B., Hong, H. Z., Ehrlich, H. P., Winn, R. K., Harlan, J. M., and May, J. W., Jr. (1994). Reduction of burn injury by inhibiting CD18-mediated leukocyte adherence in rabbits. *Plast. Reconstr. Surg.* **93,** 1473, 1994.
13. Herndon, D. N., Morris, S. E., Coffey, J. A., Milhoan, R. A., Barrow, R. E., Traber, D. L., and Townsend, C. M. (1989). The effect of mucosal integrity and mesenteric blood flow on enteric translocation of microorganisms in cutaneous thermal injury. *Prog. Clin. Biol. Res.* **308,** 377.
14. Morris, S. E., Navaratnam, N., and Herndon, D. N. (1990). A comparison of effects of thermal injury and smoke inhalation on bacterial translocation. *J. Trauma* **30,** 639.
15. Tokyay, R., Loick, H. M., Traber, D. L., Heggers, J. P., and Herndon, D. N. (1992). Effects of thromboxane synthetase inhibition on postburn mesenteric vascular resistance and the rate of bacterial translocation in a chronic porcine model. *Surg. Gynecol. Obstet.* **174,** 125.
16. Meyer, J., Stothert, J., Pollard, V., Hinder, F., Herndon, D., and Traber, D. L. (1993). Increased organ blood flow in sepsis and its reversal with the nitric oxide synthase inhibitor L-NAME. *Crit. Care Med.* **21,** S280 (abstract).
17. Garzon, A. A., Seltzer, B., Song, I. C., Bromberg, B. E., and Karlson, K. E. (1970). Respiratory mechanics in patients with inhalation burns. *J. Trauma* **10,** 57.
18. Fischer, S. R., Deyo, D. J., Bone, H. G., McGuire, R., and Traber, L. D. (1997). Nitric oxide synthase inhibition restores hypoxic pulmonary vasoconstriction in sepsis. *Am. J. Respir. Crit. Care Med.* **156,** 833.
19. Abdi, S., Herndon, D., Mcguire, J., Traber, L., and Traber, D. L. (1990). Time course of alterations in lung lymph and bronchial blood flows after inhalation injury. *J. Burn Care Rehabil.* **11,** 510.
20. Tokyay, R., Zeigler, S. T., Traber, D. L., Stothert, J. C., Loick, H. M., Heggers, J. P., and Herndon, D. N. (1993). Postburn gastrointestinal vasoconstriction increases bacterial and endotoxin translocation. *J. Appl. Physiol.* **74,** 1521.
21. Schenarts, P. J., Bone, H. G., Traber, L. D., and Traber, D. L. (1996). Effect of severe smoke inhalation injury on systemic microvascular blood flow in sheep. *Shock* **3,** 201.
22. Hinder, F., Matsumoto, N., Traber, L. D., and Traber, D. L. (1994). Nitric oxide synthase inhibition during experimental sepsis increases urine output in the presence of chronically elevated atrial natriuretic peptide. *Crit. Care Med.* **22,** A123 (abstract).
23. Cahill, C. M., Holder, A. T., Lawton, T. L., Butcher, G. W., and Taussig, M. J. (1997). Recognition of porcine growth hormone by a panel of monoclonal antibodies. *Hybridoma* **16,** 371.
24. Vernersson, M., Pejler, G., Kristersson, T., Alving, K., and Hellman, L. (1997). Cloning, structural analysis, and expression of the pig IgE epsilon chain. *Immunogenetics* **46,** 461.
25. Moore, C., Jie, R., Shulkes, A., and Baldwin, G. S. (1997). Molecular cloning and sequence of the ovine gastrin gene. *DNA Seq.* **8,** 39.
26. Chooback, L., Price, N. E., Karsten, W. E., Nelson, J., Sundstrom, P., and Cook, P. F. (1998). Cloning, expression, purification, and characterization of the 6-phosphogluconate dehydrogenase from sheep liver. *Protein Expr. Purif.* **13,** 251.
27. Wells, D. N., Misica, P. M., Day, T. A., and Tervit, H. R. (1997). Production of cloned lambs from an established embryonic cell line: a comparison between *in vivo-* and *in vitro*-matured cytoplasts. *Biol. Reprod.* **57,** 385.
28. Gabazza, E. C., Taguchi, O., Tamaki, S., Murashima, S., Kobayashi, H., Yasui, H., Kobayashi, T., Hataji, O., and Adachi, Y. (1999). Role of nitric oxide in airway remodeling. *Clin. Sci.* (in press).
29. Traber, D. L., and Traber, L. D. (1989). Sheep as a cardiopulmonary model. *Prog. Clin. Biol. Res* **299,** 253.
30. Halmagyi, D. F. J., Starzeki, B., and Horner, G. J. (1963). Mechanism and pharmacology of endotoxin shock in sheep. *J. Appl. Physiol.* **(18)3,** 544.
31. Staub, N. C., Bland, R. D., Brigham, K. L., Demling, R., Erdmann, A. J., and Woolverton, W. C. (1975). Preparation of chronic lung lymph fistulas in sheep. *J. Surg. Res.* **19,** 315.
32. Isago, T., Noshima, S., Traber, L. D., Herndon, D. N., and Traber, D. L. (1991). Analysis of pulmonary microvascular permeability after smoke inhalation. *J. Appl. Physiol.* **71,** 1403.
33. Magno, M. G., and Fishman, A. P. (1982). Origin, distribution, and blood flow of bronchial circulation in anesthetized sheep. *J. Appl. Physiol.* **53,** 272.
34. Charan, N. B., Turk, G. M., and Dhand, R. (1984). Gross and subgross anatomy of bronchial circulation in sheep. *J. Appl. Physiol.* **57,** 658.
35. Kimura, R., Traber, L. D., Herndon, D. N., Linares, H. A., Lübbesmeyer, H. J., and Traber, D. L. (1988). Increasing duration of smoke exposure induces more severe lung injury in sheep. *J. Appl. Physiol.* **64,** 1107.
36. Goldfarb, R. D., Nightingale, L. M., Kish, P., Weber, P. B., and Loegering, D. J. (1986). Left ventricular function during lethal and sublethal endotoxemia in swine. *Am. J. Physiol.* **251,** H364.
37. King, M. (1998). Experimental models for studying mucociliary clearance. *Eur. Respir. J.* **11,** 222.
38. Hinder, F., Matsumoto, N., Booke, M., Bradford, D. W., Traber, L. D., and Traber, D. L. (1997). Inhalation injury increases the anasstomotic bronchial blood flow in the pouch model of the left ovine lung. *Shock* **8,** 131.
39. Demling, R. H., Smith, M., Gunther, R., Wandzilak, T., and Pederson, N. C. (1981). Use of a chronic prefemoral lymphatic fistula for monitoring systemic capillary integrity in unanesthetized sheep. *J. Surg. Res.* **31,** 136.
40. Kramer, G. C., Gunther, R. A., Nerlich, M. L., Zweifach, S. S., and Demling, R. H. (1982). Effect of dextran-70 on increased microvascular fluid and protein flux after thermal injury. *Circ. Shock* **9,** 529.
41. Montero, K., Lübbesmeyer, H. J., Traber, D. L., Kimura, R., Traber, L. D., and Herndon, D. N. (1989). Inhalation injury increases systemic microvascular permeability. *Surg. Forum* **38,** 303.
42. Battigelli, M. C., Halbritter, K. A., and Parker, J. E. (1989). Smoke inhalation. *W. V. Med. J.* **85,** 427.
43. Tokyay, R., Zeigler, S. T., Kramer, G. C., Rogers, C. S., Heggers, J. P., Traber, D. L., and Herndon, D. N. (1992). Effects of hypertonic saline dextran resuscitation on oxygen delivery, oxygen consumption, and lipid peroxidation after burn injury. *J. Trauma* **32,** 704.
44. Sugi, K., Newald, J., Traber, L. D., Maguire, J. P., Herndon, D. N., Schlag, G., and Traber, D. L. (1991), Cardiac dysfunction after acute endotoxin administration in conscious sheep. *Am. J. Physiol.* **260,** H1474.
45. Goldfarb, R. D., Lee, K. J., Andrejuk, T., and Dziuban, S. W. (1990). End-systolic elastance as an evaluation of myocardial function in shock. *Circ. Shock* **30,** 15.
46. Nishida, K., Matsumoto, N., Kikuchi, Y., Herndon, D. N., Traber, L. D., and Traber, D. L. (1995). Effect of phenytoin on smoke inhalation injury in sheep. *Shock* **4,** 211.

47. Redl, G., Abdi, S., Traber, L. D., Nichols, R. J., Flynn, J. T., Herndon, D. N., and Traber, D. L. (1991). Inhibition of thromboxane synthesis reduces endotoxin-induced right ventricular failure in sheep. *Crit. Care Med.* **19,** 1294.
48. Sugi, K., Theissen, J. L., Traber, L. D., Herndon, D. N., and Traber, D. L. (1990). Impact of carbon monoxide on cardiopulmonary dysfunction after smoke inhalation injury. *Circ. Res.* **66,** 69.
49. Goldfarb, R. D., Glock, D., Kumar, A., McCarthy, R. J., Mei, J., Guynn, T., Matushek, M., Trenholme, G., and Parrillo, J. E. (1996). A porcine model of peritonitis and bacteremia simulates human septic shock. *Shock* **6,** 442.
50. Zapol, W. M., Jones, R., Brown, M., Traber, D. L., Herndon, D. N., Oldham, K. T., and Traber, L. D. (1987). Vascular components of ARDS. Clinical pulmonary hemodynamics and morphology. The use of venovenous extracorporeal membrane oxygenation in sheep receiving severe smoke inhalation injury. *Am. Rev. Respir. Dis.* **13,** 34.
51. Zwischenberger, J. B., Nguyen, T. T., Tao, W., Bush, P. E., Cox, C. S., Traber, D. L., Herndon, D. N., and Bidani, A. (1994). IVOX with gradual permissive hypercapnia: A new management technique for respiratory failure. *J. Surg. Res.* **57,** 99.
52. Zwischenberger, J. B., Cox, C. S., Minifee, P. K., Traber, D. L., Traber, L. D., Flynn, J. T., Linares, H. A., and Herndon, D. N. (1993). Pathophysiology of ovine smoke inhalation injury treated with extracorporeal membrane oxygenation. *Chest* **103,** 1582.
53. Brunston, R. L., Jr., Zwischenberger, J. B., Tao, W., Cardenas, V. J.,Jr., Traber, D. L., and Bidani, A. (1997). Total arteriovenous CO_2 removal: Simplifying extracorporeal support for respiratory failure [see comments]. *Ann. Thorac. Surg.* **64,** 1599.
54. Iglesias, G., Zeigler, S. T., Lentz, C. W., Traber, D. L., and Herndon, D. N. (1994). Thromboxane synthetase inhibition and thromboxane receptor blockade preserve pulmonary and circulatory function in a porcine burn sepsis model. *Surg. Gynecol. Obstet.* **179,** 187.
55. Tao, W., Zwischenberger, J. B., Nguyen, T. T., Vertrees, R. A., McDaniel, L. B., Nutt, L. K., and Kramer, G. C. (1995). Gut mucosal ischemia during normothermic cardiopulmonary bypass results from blood flow redistribution and increased oxygen demand. *J. Thorac. Cardiovasc. Surg.* **110,** 819.
56. Tokyay, R., Ziegler, S. T., Traber, D. L., Stothert, J. C., Jr., Loick, H. M., Heggers, J. P., and Herndon, D. N. (1992). Postburn selective splanchnic vasoconstriction is associated with increased bacterial translocation and endotoxin absorption from the gut. *J. Appl. Physiol.* **74,** 1521.
57. Livesey, S. A., Herndon, D. N., Hollyoak, M. A., Atkinson, Y. H., and Nag, A. (1995). Transplanted acellular allograft dermal matrix. Potential as a template for the reconstruction of viable dermis. *Transplantation* **60,** 1.
58. Mann, R., Phillips, L. G., Heggers, J. P., Linares, H. A., Traber, L. D., and Robson, M. C. (1990). The effect of venous obstruction in infected pedicle flap. *Arch. Surg.* **125,** 1177.
59. Baron, P., Traber, L. D., Traber, D. L., Nguyen, T., Hollyoak, M., Heggers, J. P., and Herndon, D. N. (1994). Gut failure and translocation following burn and sepsis. *J. Surg. Res.* **57,** 197.
60. Bowes, L. E., Jimenez, M. C., Hiester, E. D., Sacks, M. S., Brahmatewari, J., Mertz, P., and Eaglstein, W. H. (1999). Collagen fiber orientation as quantified by small angle light scattering in wounds treated with transforming growth factor-beta2 and its neutalizing antibody. *Wound Repair Regen.* **7,** 179.
61. Martini, W. Z., Chinkes, D. L., Barrow, R. E., Murphey, E. D., and Wolfe, R. R. (1999). Lung surfactant kinetics in conscious pigs. *Am. J. Physiol.* **277,** E187.
62. Laffon, M., Pittet, J. F., Modelska, K., Matthay, M. A., and Young, D. M. Interleukin-8 mediates injury from smoke inhalation to both the lung endothelial and the alveolar epithelial barriers in rabbits. *Am. J. Respir. Crit. Care Med.* **160,** 1443.
63. Carter, E. P., Umenishi, F., Matthay, M. A., and Verkman, A. S. Developmental changes in water permeability across the alveolar barrier in perinatal rabbit lung. *J. Clin. Invest.* **100,** 1071.
64. Nwariaku, F., Sikes, P., Lightfoot, E., McIntyre, K., and Mileski, W. J. (1996). Role of CD14 in hemorrhagic shock-induced alterations of the monocyte tumor necrosis factor response to endotoxin. *J. Trauma* **40,** 564.
65. Kubo, H., Doyle, N. A., Graham, L., Bhagwan, S. D., Quinlan, W. M., and Doerschuk, C. M. (1999), L- and P-selectin and CD11/CD18 in intracapillary neutrophil sequestration in rabbit lungs. *Am. J. Respir, Crit. Care Med.* **159,** 267.
66. Folkesson, H. G., Matthay, M. A., Hebert, C. A., and Broaddus, V. C. (1995). Acid aspiration-induced lung injury in rabbits is mediated by interleukin-8-dependent mechanisms. *J. Clin. Invest.* **96,** 107.
67. Zhang, X. J., Sakurai, Y., and Wolfe, R. R. (1996). An animal model for measurement of protein metabolism in the skin. *Surgery* **119,** 326.
68. Zhang, X. J., Chinkes, D. L., Wolf, S. E., and Wolfe, R. R. (1999). Insulin but not growth hormone stimulates protein anabolism in skin wound and muscle. *Am. J. Physiol.* **276,** E712.
69. Zhang, X. J., Chinkes, D. L., Doyle, D., Jr., and Wolfe, R. R. (1998). Metabolism of skin and muscle protein is regulated differently in response to nutrition. *Am. J. Physiol.* **274,** E484.
70. Eaves-Pyles, T., and Alexander, J. W. (1998). Rapid and prolonged impairment of gut barrier function after thermal injury in mice. *Shock* **9,** 95.
71. Wolf, S. E., Ikeda, H., Matin, S., Debroy, M. A., Rajaraman, S., Herndon, D. N., and Thompson, J. C. (1999). Cutaneous burn increases apoptosis in the gut epithelium of mice. *J. Am. Coll. Surg.* **188,** 10.
72. Eaves-Pyles, T., and Alexander, J. W. (1996). Granulocyte colony-stimulating factor enhances killing of translocated bacteria but does not affect barrier function in a burn mouse model. *J. Trauma* **41,** 1013.
73. Gennari, R., Alexander, J. W., Boyce, S. T., Lilly, N., Babcock, G. F., and Cornaggia, M. (1996). Effects of the angiotensin converting enzyme inhibitor enalapril on bacterial translocation after thermal injury and bacterial challenge. *Shock* **6,** 95.
74. Utsunomiya, T., Kobayashi, M., Herndon, D. N., and Pollard, R. B. (1997). A relationship between the generation of burn-associated type 2 T cells and their antagonistic ceells in thermally injuryed mice. *Burns* **23,** 281.
75. Kobayashi, H., Kobayashi, M., McCauley, R. L., Herndon, D. N., Pollard, R. B., and Suzuki, F. (1999). Cadaveric skin allograft-associated cytomegalovirus transmission in a mouse model of thermal injury. *Clin. Immunol.* **92,** 181.
76. Ullrich, R., Bloch, K. D., Ichinose, F., Steudel, W., and Zapol, W. M. (1999). Hypoxic pulmonary blood flow redistribution and arterial oxygenation in endotoxin-challenged NOS2-deficient mice. *J. Clin. Invest.* **104,** 1421.
77. Scherrer-Crosbie, M., Steudel, W., Ullrich, R., Hunziker, P. R., Liel-Cohen, N., Newell, J., Zaroff, J., Zapol, W. M., and Picard, M. H. (1999). Echocardiographic determination of risk area size in a murine model of myocardial ischemia. *Am. J. Physiol.* **277,** H986.
78. Kline, D. D., Yang, T., Huang, P. L., and Prabhakar, N. R. (1998). Altered respiratory responses to hypoxia in mutant mice deficient in neuronal nitric oxide synthase. *J. Physiol. (Lond).* **511,** 273.
79. Cross, H. R., Steenbergen, C., Lefkowitz, R. J., Koch, W. J., and Murphy, E. (1999). Overexpression of the cardiac beta(2)-adrenergic receptor and expression of a beta-adrenergic receptor kinase-1 (betaARK1) inhibitor both increase myocardial contractility but have differential effects on susceptibility to ischemic injury. *Circ. Res.* **85,** 1077.
80. Hickey, M. J., Sharkey, K. A., Sihota, E. G., Reinhardt, P. H., MacMicking, J. D., Nathan, C., and Kubes, P. (1997). Inducible nitric oxide synthase-deficient mice have enhanced leukocyte-endothelium interactions in endotoxemia. *FASEB J.* **11,** 955.

81. Champion, H. C., Bivalacqua, T. J., D'Souza, F. M., Ortiz, L. A., Jeter, J. R., Toyoda, K., Heistad, D. D., Hyman, A. L., and Kadowitz, P. J. (1999). Gene transfer of endothelial nitric oxide synthase to the lung of the mouse *in vivo*. Effect on agonist-induced and flow-mediated vascular responses. *Circ. Res.* **84,** 1422.
82. Herndon, D. N., Wilmore, D. W., Mason, A. D., Jr., and Curreri, P. W. (1979). Increased rates of wound healing in burned guinea pigs treated with L-thyroxine. *Surg. Forum* **30,** 95.
83. Horton, J. W., White, D. J., Maass, D., Sanders, B., Thompson, M., and Giroir, B. (1999). Calcium antagonists improve cardiac mechanical performance after thermal trauma. *J. Surg. Res.* **87,** 39.
84. Murphy, J. T., Giroir, B., and Horton, J. W. (1999). Thermal injury alters myocardial sarcoplasmic reticulum calcium channel function. *J. Surg. Res.* **82,** 244.
85. Jobin, J., Heng, M. K., Martin, J., Wyatt, H. L., and Lee, P. L. (1985). Clinical evaluation of left ventricular function using the cardiac helical fiber model: An echocardiographic study. *Am. Heart J.* **110,** 1226.
86. Raichlen, J. S., Trivedi, S. S., Herman, G. T., St John, S. M. G., and Reichek, N. (1986). Dynamic three-dimensional reconstruction of the left ventricle from two-dimensional echocardiograms. *J. Am. Coll. Cardiol.* **8,** 364.
87. Sakurai, M., Tanaka, H., Matsuda, T., Goya, T., Shimazaki, S., and Matsuda, H. (1997). Reduced resuscitation fluid volume for second-degree experimental burns with delayed initiation of vitamin C therapy (beginning 6 h after injury). *J. Surg. Res.* **73,** 24.
88. Gulati, A., Sharma, A. C., and Singh, G. (1996). Role of endothelin in the cardiovascular effects of diaspirin crosslinked and stroma reduced hemoglobin. *Crit. Care Med.* **24,** 137.
89. Nelson, C. L. (1987). Prevention of sepsis. *Clin. Orthop.* **66.**
90. Jeschke, M. G., Barrow, R. E., Hawkins, H. K., Chrysopoulo, M. T., Perez-Polo, J. R., and Herndon, D. N. (1999). Effect of multiple gene transfers of insulinlike growth factor I complementary DNA gene constructs in rats after thermal injury. *Arch. Surg.* **134,** 1137.
91. Upperman, J. S., Deitch, E. A., Guo, W., Lu, Q., and Xu, D. (1998). Post-hemorrhagic shock mesenteric lymph is cytotoxic to endothelial cells and activates neutrophils [see comments]. *Shock* **10,** 407.
92. Magnotti, L. J., Upperman, J. S., Xu, D. Z., Lu, Q., and Deitch, E. A. (1998). Gut-derived mesenteric lymph but not portal blood increases endothelial cell permeability and promotes lung injury after hemorrhagic shock. *Ann. Surg.* **228,** 518.
93. Schertel, E. R., Pratt, J. W., Schaefer, S. L., Valentine, A. K., and McCreary, M. R. (1996). Effects of acid aspiration-induced lung injury on left ventricular function. *Surgery* **119,** 81.
94. Heller, A., Fiedler, F., Schmeck, J., Luck, V., Iovanna, J. L., and Koch, T. (1999). Pancreatitis-associated protein protects the lung from leukocyte-induced injury. *Anesthesiology* **91,** 1408.

32

Wound Care Models

David G. Greenhalgh* and Glenn D. Warden†

**Department of Surgery, Shriners Hospitals for Children, Northern California, and University of California, Davis, Sacramento, California 95817*

†Shriners Hospitals for Children—Cincinnati Burns Hospital, and University of Cincinnati, Cincinnati, Ohio 45229

I. Introduction

Tissue repair is essential for any type of surgery. Failure to heal is one of the initial steps that leads to many surgical complications. If an incision breaks down, such as after fascial dehiscence, then the patient is at risk for evisceration. If a bowel anastomosis breaks down, then the resulting leakage leads to an abscess and potentially the systemic inflammatory response syndrome. In essence, the ultimate result of impaired tissue repair is multiple organ failure and death. If healing occurrs promptly and completely, then sepsis and multiple organ failure may not occur. Investigators have been studying tissue repair in order to understand the processes that control normal healing. Clinically, however, most healthy patients have no abnormalities in healing; patients with some form of impairment (malnutrition, infection, diabetes, steroid use) tend to be at high risk for altered tissue repair. Many models of tissue repair attempt to reproduce these forms of impairment. In addition, a great deal of knowledge has been gained regarding the factors that accelerate healing. In reality, however, compared to impaired wound repair, more pathology results from excessive healing or scarring. Clearly, scarring is a major problem for burn patients, but scarring affects other tissues besides skin. For example, peritoneal adhesions lead to obstruction, liver damage leads to cirrhosis, and lung injury leads to pulmonary fibrosis. Models are also needed to understand the mechanisms of scar formation. This review examines current models of normal and impaired tissue repair, and assesses methods to study scar formation.

It is important to remember that all models have limitations. One should not automatically assume that a model correlates with a human clinical condition. For instance, there are many models of altered tissue repair in diabetic animals. Many of the problems of these diabetic animals resemble the human situation but there are also many differences. Healing in a diabetic rodent model is impaired but contraction is the major form of healing. In a nonhealing diabetic foot ulcer, hyperglycemia plays a role, but, in addition, impaired blood supply, neuropathy, and infection also are key factors. One should choose a model that can best answer a hypothesis-driven question. Weaknesses exist in all models. These weaknesses should be remembered when trying to correlate the clinical situation to the results of healing in a model.

II. In Vitro Models of Tissue Repair

In vitro models have the advantage of being able to isolate one cell type and determine whether isolated factors affect those cells. For instance, one can isolate fibroblasts and determine whether the addition of a growth factor will increase their proliferation. In other words, the *in vitro* models break down the healing process into multiple individual questions. These studies are important for answering specific mechanistic questions, but tissue repair is a multiple cell process that is profoundly influenced by the milieu of the extracellular matrix (ECM). For instance, after exposure to epidermal growth factor, keratinocytes will migrate freely on type I collagen but will not move extensively on laminin (1). The *in vitro* models usually examine the role of external factors on specific cell types.

When utilizing these models, one must keep in mind that there are types and phases of healing that are dominated by specific cell types. In recreation of a scar, there is an inflammatory phase that involves leukocytes and normal inflammation. That phase will not be covered here. The second phase is the proliferative phase, when fibroblasts deposit the ECM and endothelial cells recreate the blood supply (angiogenesis and vasculogenesis). Fibroblasts are also the key cell in the final maturation phase, and are also involved in the second type of healing, contraction. They appear to develop characteristics of muscle cells and are often called "myofibroblasts." *In vitro* models that examine contraction are used quite frequently. The final type of healing is reepithelialization. The control of reepithelialization is a major focus of many laboratories. The techniques developed by these *in vitro* models have led the way to the methodologies used to develop skin substitutes, whereby many of the key cells of skin are grown in culture and transferred to a patient.

Most *in vitro* models isolate a specific cell and determine whether an external factor (such as a growth factor) increases that cell's proliferation, stimulates migration (chemotaxis), or induces production of a specific protein that is related to healing (such as collagen). Fibroblasts are easy to grow from explants of skin and wounds. Dozens of investigators have used this strategy to isolate fibroblasts from wounds that have impaired healing (2–5), or from hypertrophic scars and keloids (6–8). The growth characteristics and responses to external stimuli of cells from keloids are compared with fibroblasts isolated from normal skin. Many differences have been observed by comparing fibroblasts from these different tissues. In other words, phenotypic differences exist for fibroblasts isolated from wounds that heal abnormally when compared to one that healed normally. One must be careful to review these results critically. Differences may exist for cells isolated from different tissues, but there are many other factors that influence healing. For instance, if a cell is taken from the wound of a diabetic patient, the hyperglycemia that previously existed is lost. Are we to assume that there are genetic differences between these different cells isolated from the different tissues? If differences do exist, then how long will they exist if the cell is removed from the abnormal wound environment? How many passages in culture will be needed before the phenotypic differences are lost? Clearly, once the cell is removed from the milieu of the wound, then many factors change that are difficult to relate to the clinical situation.

A popular model of wound contraction is the fibroblast-populated collagen lattice (FPCL). Fibroblasts are cultured in a collagen gel and then the extent of lattice contracture is easy to measure (9). The model can be used to measure the effects of mediators on the extent of contraction *in vitro* (10, 11). It is also of value in studies examining factors that influence the development of the myofibroblast phenotype (12–14). As for any study, one must not extend the interpretation of any results beyond the limitations of the model. Contraction in the FPCL occurs within a matter of hours, not days as occurs for contraction of a wound. It is also important to remember that the model has very little resemblance to the formation of scar contractures. Contractures develop over a matter of months and involve collagen remodeling in addition to cell contraction. The FPCL model is very useful for determining which factors influence myofibroblast migration and contraction.

Angiogenesis is another important factor for normal healing. In addition, angiogenesis is involved in carcinogenesis and other disease processes. In tissue repair, vasculogenesis (the development of new vessels from stem cells) is also important (15). Several *in vitro* models of angiogenesis can be performed (16–21). Endothelial cells can be isolated and cultured; there may be cell differences, dependent on where the cells are isolated. Many studies utilize human umbilical vein endothelial cells (HUVECs) because they are easy to obtain (16). One must ask if these cells are the same as those isolated from a diseased aorta or from capillaries. Proliferation and chemotaxis studies can be performed on these cells as for any other cell. Endothelial cells will form a tubelike structure in the proper environment (17). Endothelial cells may also be cultured onto vascular conduits in order to decrease thrombotic tendencies in grafts (18).

To determine whether a protein is "angiogenic," a few well-established models exist. A factor may be injected into the chorioallantoic membrane (CAM) of a chicken egg (19). Blood vessels can be easily observed migrating toward the injection site for angiogenic factors. Another method is not really an *in vitro* model but will be described in this section. The rabbit cornea model has also been extensively used for determining angiogenesis (20). The angiogenic factor is injected into the cornea of the rabbit eye. Any factor that induces angiogenesis leads to the ingrowth of new vessels. Both models have been used extensively for years and are reliable. One must make certain when determining whether a factor is angiogenic that there is a difference between a factor that attracts endothelial cells and one that stimulates inflammatory cells that, in turn, increase angiogenesis (indirect angiogenesis) (21).

The final type of healing is recreation of the epithelial barrier that covers the external surface of many organs. Most studies examine keratinocytes as the key cell of the epidermis. Reepithelialization involves the migration of a sheet of keratinocytes across a flat, viable surface. Therefore, most studies examine keratinocyte migration. One method is to "scrape" away a linear path of keratinocytes from a culture plate. The rate of keratinocyte migration across the gap can be determined. It is important to remember that the surface the keratinocyte contacts influences the ability for that cell to migrate. Keratinocytes tend to stay put when in contact with proteins of the basement membrane (collagen type IV, laminin) and migrate when in contact with proteins commonly seen in the wound (collagen type I, fibronectin). Woodley examined keratinocyte migration by coating plates with gold particles (1, 22). As the keratinocyte migrated, the gold particles were consumed and left a "record" of the migratory pathways. Another technique is to examine keratinocyte migration using a time-lapse video to record keratinocyte migration (23, 24).

A technique for investigating healing is through the use of organ culture. An "explant" model has been developed for examining fetal healing (25). Forelimbs from animals can be grown in organ culture. Wounds can be created in the forelimbs and tissue repair can be studied as though being performed in adult animals. In a similar technique, composite skins, consisting of a bilayer of keratinocytes and fibroblast-populated neodermis, can be used for these kinds of "explant" studies (26–28). In some studies, the composite skin received a thermal burn (29–30). The healing and cellular response of the composite tissue were then examined.

III. Animal Models

In vitro models are designed to answer specific questions that involve one or two cell types in response to one or a few stimuli. Normal healing is far more complex. There are multiple cell types, with each playing a different role at different times during the healing process. In addition, there are multiple physical factors, such as the ECM, the multiple serum hormones and proteins, pH, oxygenation, temperature, nutritional status, overall health, plus many other factors, that influence tissue repair. Animal models are essential to examine factors that influence healing in this complex environment. The following discussion is divided into two sections. The first discusses wound types that are often examined in the line of wound healing research. The second presents models of impaired tissue repair. The focus of the review is on healing in skin. There are many models of healing in other tissues that will not be discussed here.

A. Granuloma Models

Granuloma models were developed to test whether a "factor" could increase either inflammation or collagen deposition in a material placed in the subcutaneous tissue of animals. An early technique was to simply inject the substance under the skin. Transforming growth factor-β (TGF-β) was found to increase collagen deposition in this manner (31). Eventually, inert materials that could act as carriers of potential healing stimulators were placed in subcutaneous pockets. Polyvinyl alcohol (PVA) sponges have been utilized most frequently (32–33). Cellulose sponges have also been utilized (34, 35). These sponges can be soaked with known concentrations of materials to test whether they stimulate inflammation, collagen formation, or angiogenesis. These sponges are valuable to determine whether a factor can attract specific cell types and induce collagen production. Usually, hydroxyproline is measured as a rough estimate of collagen deposition.

Another model has involved placing a porous (usually wire mesh) cylinder in the subcutaneous tissue. The most well-known example is the "Hunt–Schilling" chamber (36, 37). The chamber has rubber stoppers at each end, allowing for the injection of the test "factor." An advantage to the model is that the chamber can be aspirated at different time points *in situ* so that cells and proteins can be detected at various time points. It is important to remember that each time a needle is introduced, a minor local injury may also be introduced. Another variation on the subcutaneous model is the use of polytetrafluoroethylene (PTFE) tubes (38, 39). The PTFE is porous and thus allows for the ingrowth of the wound-healing cells. The major drawback with these models is that they involve a foreign body that will elicit some form of chronic inflammation, thus the name "granuloma" model. These models simulate an artificial wound that usually does not exist clinically.

B. Incision Models

Another often utilized model is the incision model (40–43). An incision is made through the skin and is usually closed with sutures or staples. Alternatively, the incision may be left open and allowed to close spontaneously. The main question that is answered with the incision model is the strength of the incision. At different time points, the animals are sacrificed and a template of skin is cut out of the pelt. There has been a significant amount written as to the physics of disrupting an incision (44). "Tensile strength" is the breaking strength per cross-sectional area. The skin is stretched at a constant rate and a strain gauge measures the force created until the incision breaks. In addition, the degree of extensibility is also plotted as the skin is stretched. To control for the length of the incision that is tested, the template is used to cut a uniform piece of skin. The difficult part is to determine the thickness of the skin. Special calipers have been used, but they often compress the incision and thus are not accurate. They also may disturb a fresh incision. Photographic techniques are also used, but again are not very accurate. An alternative is to assume that there is little variation of incision thickness and simply measure the "breaking strength." Most studies just measure this parameter because it is easy to determine and has clinical value. A surgeon wants to know whether an incision will disrupt irrespective of the thickness of the wound. For the best accuracy, the breaking strength should be measured when the tissue is fresh. In addition, the wound may be placed in formalin before determining the breaking strength. Formalin creates cross-links between the collagen molecules and thus can be a rough measure of intercollagenous bonds (45, 46).

Another variation of this technique is to determine the "bursting strength" of the incision (47, 48). A balloon is placed inside the peritoneal cavity and is filled with gas. The pressure that it takes to burst the incision is then determined. This model has obvious clinical significance and this technique is also used for other types of tissues—for example, muscle, tendon, and ligaments (49, 50). Any organ with a lumen can be "burst open" with a balloon. Many studies on the various portions of the gut utilize this technique (51).

The incision models are good for testing whether a systemic factor can either strengthen or weaken healing. Many of the factors that impair tissue repair were initially tested with this model. The breaking strength can be obtained in many animals at any time point. The absolute value allows for easy statistical analysis. Histology is also easy to perform on these incisions and affords insight into mechanisms of healing impairment. Unfortunately, this model has its limits. Many investigators have attempted to dissect out the incision and perform biochemical analyses. It is difficult to know whether such assays detect what is going on in the incision or in the nearby skin. To avoid this pitfall, many investigators will place a PVA sponge or Hunt–Schilling chamber in, but away from, the incision. Another problem with the model was appreciated after the isolation of growth factors. Most growth factors are designed to be given locally. Delivering a growth factor over a prolonged period to an incision is difficult.

C. Open Wound Models

The use of an open wound for measuring wound healing has been used for decades (23). Very simply, a wound is created in the skin and is either left open or covered with a dressing. All aspects of healing, reepithelialization, granulation tissue formation, scar formation, contraction, and angiogenesis can be investigated. These wounds also allow for the study of topical applications of wound-healing agents. It is important to distinguish partial-thickness from full-thickness wounds. A partial-thickness wound leaves part of the dermis and thus the skin adnexa (52). This type of wound is used to measure the rate of reepithelialization of a wound. Because rodent skin is so thin, it is less difficult to create these wounds in larger animals, which are often used. The porcine model is most often utilized because pig skin very closely resembles to human skin, more so any other animal skin (53–55). Multiple wounds are created on the backs of pigs by using a dermatome. The rate of reepithelialization is then determined by examination of the wound. Techniques that allow for clinically accurate assessment of reepithelialization are somewhat subjective. One technique is to measure the surface electrical capacitance as a determinant of recreation of the epithelial barrier (56). The use of devices that determine evaporative water loss are also utilized (57). Finally, some investigators use a dermatome set at a thick setting to harvest the entire wound (54). The degree of reepithelialization can then be determined by separating the epithelium from the dermis.

Most nonimpaired full-thickness wound models measure contraction as the main type of healing. From 80 to 90% of healing in any large, open wound in a rodent is by contraction (41, 58, 59). This fact is important to remember when trying to relate any findings with healing in patients. Clinically, contraction is important for areas of the body with loose skin, such as the buttocks. In wounds with little room for movement (such as the medial malleolus) contraction plays a much smaller role. The same principle may apply when designing models of closure in rodents. Mustoe's group has reported creating a mouse wound model that might have delayed healing as a result of "splinting" of the wound. He created an open wound on the top of the head, where contraction was limited by the tightness of the skin in that region (T.A. Mustoe, personal communication). The extent of contraction appeared to be inhibited. This model was developed to take advantage of the many transgenic mice that are available.

These open wounds are amenable to treatment with topical agents by placing the agent under a dressing (60, 61). Another strategy is to cover the wound with a transparent polyurethane dressing that allows visualization of the healing wound (62). The agent can be injected through the dressing and onto the wound. The wound size can be measured by tracing the wound edge onto clear plastic or a glass microscope slide. Alternatively, the wound can be photographed over time. The wound size is then determined by planimetry by using an image analysis system. The wound is also easy to harvest for histology and molecular biologic assays. Investigators have been able to measure mRNA, proteins, and cell signaling cascades in these wounds (63–65).

Full-thickness wounds are also amenable to skin grafting techniques (66). Split-thickness or full-thickness grafts can be placed without difficulty. A rough estimate of graft "take" can be made subjectively or the size of the wound edge can be followed over time. A graft that "takes" tends not to contract and thus wounds with less contraction have better "take." Meshed skin grafts are also used as an animal model of reepithelialization (67, 68). The rate of epithelial filling of the interstices is used as a measure of reepithelialization.

The full-thickness wound is also used for the preclinical evaluation of composite skins (69, 70). Usually, athymic (nude) mice are utilized because they accept tissues from foreign species. A block of skin is excised down to the panniculus carnosus and the graft is sutured in place. The extent of take is measured as for any other type of graft. This technique has been utilized for the development of better topical nutrients and antibiotics for these composite skins (71).

The same principle has been used for the transfer of scars to athymic animals (72–74). There are no good models for chronic scarring in animals (with the possible exception of a chronic rabbit model, see below). In order to determine factors that might reduce scar formation, investigators have transferred human hypertrophic scars and keloids to these animals. Unfortunately, the scars tend to regress over time. There has been the development of a modification of the rabbit ear model that appears to result in a hypertrophic scar. When a large wound is created in the ear and allowed to remain open for a prolonged period, then some fibrous and epithelial hypertrophy does result. The extent and duration of this hypertrophy still needs to be elucidated. Finally, the ultimate test of this model will be to determine whether antiscarring therapies have any effect in the model (75).

D. Burn Models

Burn models of various types have been documented for many years (23, 76–86). Both partial-thickness (second-degree) and full-thickness (third-degree) burn models have been described. The depth of the burn is dependent on the temperature of the contacting agent, the duration of contact, the thickness of the skin, and the blood supply to that skin. Heated metal bars that are held in contact with the skin of an anesthetized animal for a set time will produce a reproducible burn (80). The contact model has been modified to create three parallel burns that leave a small space of unburned skin (84, 85). The purpose of this burn model is to examine factors that prevent the usual progression of a burn injury. Without any treatment, the spared areas eventually undergo necrosis. In one study, treatment with antibodies against adhesion molecules spared these areas (84).

Contact burn models produce relatively small burns. To create larger burns, scald (76, 77) or flame (79, 86) injuries are used. Usually, a template is created to isolate a section of skin and the animal is placed in scalding water, or a flammable liquid is placed on the area and ignited. These models result in reproducible burns. It is important to remember two facts about these burn models. First, the estimate of the total body surface area (TBSA) tends to be exaggerated in small animals. With rodents, for example, a large proportion of the body is covered with ears, tails and toes, so that trunk burns are on relatively small areas. There are formulas that estimate the TBSA of most species. Second, be careful to examine appropriate forms of healing with the model. Clinically, burn doctors do not wait for burn eschars to separate, granulation to form, and then contraction to occur. In contrast, the opposite is desired. Prolonged exposure of granulation tissue tends to lead to increased scarring. Instead, most burn surgeons believe in early excision and grafting to treat a burn wound. The larger models are useful, however, for examining the systemic responses of a major wound (86).

IV. Impaired Healing Models

Healing in the healthy population is rarely a clinical problem, but patients with some form of impairment have a tendency to develop complications. The factors that impair healing have been well described. Altered tissue repair results from malnutrition, diabetes, infection, hypoxia, venous stasis, or after treatment with steroids, chemotherapy agents, or radiation (87). In order to develop strategies to deal with these clinical problems, models that mimic these problems have been developed. As mentioned earlier, it is important to remember that all models have limitations and they do not totally represent the clinical situation.

A. Malnutrition

One of the earliest factors that was found to influence tissue repair was malnutrition (46, 88–93). Probably all types of healing are impaired by limiting nutritional input. Models can mimic total protein/calorie (88) or only protein (89–90) malnutrition (marasmus or kwashiorkor). Total protein/calorie malnutrition can be induced by limiting the food that is available for the animal model. Wound breaking strength is reduced in proportion to the extent of nutritional restriction and weight loss (92). For protein malnutrition, diets are available that give adequate calories but have minimal protein content. Wound healing is, again, markedly impaired in these animals. The role of nutritional intake is important when using other models of impaired tissue repair, because if the animal becomes sick, as with an infection, the resulting anorexia may contribute as much to the altered healing as does the other cause (46). It is always important to weigh the animals during any wound healing study to ensure that there is no nutritional impairment that contributes to the healing deficiency. To some extent, growth factors have been able to reverse the healing abnormality (93).

In addition to general malnutrition, many studies have been performed to test whether a specific nutrient alters tissue repair. One of the earliest agents to be tested was vitamin C (94). Other vitamins have also been found to be essential to normal tissue repair, including vitamin A (95, 96) and thiamine (97). Trace minerals such as zinc (98) and copper (99) are also essential for healing. Several investigators have examined the question whether specific amino acids are essential. Periodically there is the "favorite" amino acid to examine. In the past, methionine and cysteine were found to be essential (100, 101). More recent work has demonstrated that arginine is essential (102). Glutamine is important for many stress-related processes but has not been found to accelerate healing to an excessive degree (103). Many other nutrients have an influence on healing (including essential fatty acids) (104, 105), but the clinical significance of giving extra amounts of these nutrients is less clear.

B. Infection

Although it seems that infection would be an obvious model of altered healing, the experimental evidence has been surprising. Studies of bacteria or bacterial products would often lead to accelerated tissue repair (106–108). At other times, tissue repair would be markedly impaired (108–111). One current theory is that if a relatively small number of bacteria are introduced into a wound, then an accelerated inflammatory response results in an increase in the number of macrophages and other cells that release growth factors and will augment wound healing. In support of this concept, several studies have demonstrated that many mild inflammatory stimuli will accelerate tissue repair (112). If, on the other hand, there are a large number of especially virulent organisms introduced into a wound, then the destructive enzymes of the bacteria lead to impaired tissue repair. Infection models have also been studied in open wounds (113–115) and burns (79), with reproducible results.

Infections at sites distant from the wound will also lead to altered healing (46, 113). For instance, creation of an abscess with cecal ligation and puncture in a mouse will lead to decreased incisional strength (46). Caution must be taken because these animals also developed anorexia and lost a significant amount of weight. When control animals were pair-fed the same amounts as the infected animals, then wound healing was not that different from the control healing. As mentioned above, nutritional intake needs to be followed closely.

C. Ischemia

It is well documented that healing is altered when there is inadequate delivery of oxygen to the wound (116, 117). Clinically relevant models have been developed to mimic ischemia. One method is to develop flaps of skin on the backs of rodents (118). Longer flaps tend to have less perfusion in the distal segment. The healing in these flaps can be tested for incisional strength. These models have been well described but are not always reproducible. Many variations of the flap technique are possible. Vessels can be clipped to reduce the blood supply. Bipedical or musculocutaneous flaps can be performed. Make certain that these models answer the specific question that is being asked.

One of the best models of reproducible delayed and ischemic healing was created by Mustoe's group. They create an open wound in the skin of a rabbit ear (119). The wound is created to the level of the cartilage. Because cartilage is relatively avascular, it has significant delays in wound closure. The amount of granulation tissue formation and reepithelialization that occurs is relatively easy to determine. The model can be modified to increase the extent of ischemia by ligating two of the three arteries supplying the rabbit ear. The model has been used extensively to test the activities of topical growth factors and effects of hyperbaric oxygen (75, 120–122). The model is relatively easy to use and quite reproducible. In addition, a modification on the model will lead to a temporary hypertrophic scar (see above).

D. Diabetes

Diabetes mellitus is commonly associated with altered healing. Three factors contribute to the altered healing in human diabetes (123–124). First, there is often some degree of alteration in the blood supply to the limb. Atherosclerosis is accelerated, affecting larger vessels, and microvascular supply is also altered. Second, peripheral neuropathy leads to the inability to feel minor wounds and pressure, which will lead to the progression of minor wounds. In addition, neuropathy of the feet leads to altered muscular feedback that maintains the normal arch of the foot. These patients often develop a foot deformity that places increased weight over the metatarsal heads, and the resulting pressure leads to ischemia and breakdown. Finally, once a wound develops, the resistance to infection is altered. Diabetic patients have a much higher amputation rate because of this problem.

Because of the magnitude of the problem related to diabetes, several models have been developed. It is important to remember that no model can totally reproduce all of the vascular, neuropathologic, and infection problems that people suffer. When choosing a model, one should always try to choose a model that has the best chance for answering the hypothesis-driven question. In addition, the type of diabetes (insulin dependent or insulin resistant) that one wishes to investigate should also be kept in mind. In animals, diabetes mellitus is produced either chemically or exists genetically. Chemical diabetes is produced by medicines that destroy the beta cells within the pancreas (125). Alloxan and streptozotocin both selectively eliminate nearly all of the beta cells to produce an insulin-dependent diabetes (125). There are numerous studies that demonstrate impaired breaking strength and collagen deposition in wounds (126, 127). Growth factors (128) and glucose control with insulin (126) reverse at least some of the deficits in repair. A problem with the chemical agents is that they produce inconsistent degrees of hyperglycemia (125). Some animals become profoundly diabetic while others appear almost normal. Most studies will describe screening the animals for hyperglycemia before including them in studies. In addition, the drugs do induce other changes in the animals including altered T cell function and decreased macrophage phagocytosis (125). The diabetic animals also lose weight, and one may ask whether nutritional alterations play a role in the altered healing.

Several strains of genetically diabetic rodents have been used for tissue repair investigations. The most commonly used animal has been the genetically diabetic "db/db" mouse (C57BL/KsJ-db/db) (62, 129–132). The homozygous mutants (db/db) become massively obese and develop marked hyperglycemia (average, 900 g/dl) and insulin resistance (62). In other words, the animals develop diabetes that resembles type 2 (insulin-resistant diabetes). The underlying defect in these animals is that they lack the receptor for leptin and thus are never satiated. The heterozygous litter mates (db/+) have no observable defect and thus can serve as a control. The most common model has been an open wound that is followed for the degree of closure (62, 129–132). The author created a 1.5 × 1.5-cm full-thickness wound on the back of the animals and covered it with a transparent polyurethane dressing (62). Topical agents are easily injected through the dressing and spread over the wound. At the same time, the rate of wound closure can be followed. Nondiabetic litter mates rapidly close their wound, within 10–14 days, with 80–90% of the closure resulting from contraction. In diabetic animals, wound closure was delayed for 4–6 weeks. The delay in healing was related to an impairment in the migration of inflammatory cells and fibroblasts into the wound. In other words, the inflammatory phase of tissue repair was prolonged. Once these cells arrived, tissue repair appeared to proceed relatively normally. In addition, contraction contributed to only 40–50% of the closure. The rest of the healing involved granulation tissue formation and reepithelialization. It has been found that these wounds have a significant delay in growth factor expression of at least IGF-I, IGF-II, KGF, and TGF-β (133, 134). Although this model may not have all of the characteristics of human diabetes, it has been very useful for testing whether topical agents can stimulate tissue repair by attracting the early cells of wound healing (inflammatory cells, fibroblasts, and endothelial cells).

Other genetically diabetic models have been described and used for healing studies. The ob/ob mouse lacks the gene to produce leptin, leading to obesity but with less severe diabetes than in the db/db mouse (135, 136). Healing is impaired in these animals. Several other models produce insulin-resistant diabetes [Agouti mice, New Zealand Obese mice, Spiny mice, Djungarian hamsters, and Zucker obese ("fatty") rats] (137). These animals have not been studied to the same extent as the db/db animals. Finally, there are animal strains that develop diabetes without the obesity. These strains include the Nonobese diabetic (NOD) mice, BB Wister rats, Chinese hamsters, Yucatan miniature swine, several dog species, and primates (138–142). There have been some wound healing studies in these animals but they are less well characterized.

E. Steroid Treatment

It has been known for decades that steroids impair tissue repair (143–145). Almost any wound model can be used after treatment of steroids. Steroids may be given as a single dose or over a prolonged period. The degree of impairment is also dependent on the type of steroid that is given to the animal. The steroid models do have some similarities to changes that occur in humans. The major mechanism of action is through the impairment of cellular proliferation. The effects of steroids have been at least partially reversed with vitamin A (95) and some growth factors (145, 146).

F. Chemotherapy Agents

Chemotherapy agents kill rapidly proliferating cells. Unfortunately, rapid proliferation is required for all forms of tissue repair. As would be expected, most of these agents lead to some degree of altered wound healing (148–151). The agents can be given systemically to mimic the clinical situation (42). Several agents have been found to reproducibly alter healing. The degree of impairment may be affected by the malnutrition that is induced by the typical postchemotherapy anorexia (92). Chemotherapy agents may be injected into tissue to create a chronic, nonhealing wound that resembles an extravasation from an intravenous infusion (151). Several agents can produce these wounds and the animal model can assist with developing strategies for local treatment of the wound.

G. Radiation

Radiation is used for the treatment of cancer because it kills cells that are undergoing rapid growth. As for chemotherapy agents, radiation inhibits tissue repair by inhibiting the activities of inflammatory cells, endothelial cells, and fibroblasts in the wound (152, 153). Radiation can be given locally or as a total body treatment (154, 155). There have been some successes with treating radiated wounds with vitamin A (96) and growth factors (155).

H. Pressure-Related Wounds

Several investigators have tried to develop models that more closely resemble the problem wounds in patients. Pressure sores are probably the most common chronic wound that clinicians deal with. An animal model that could be used for analyzing the pathophysiology and potential treatments would be of value. Several models of pressure sores have been designed in rats, rabbits, dogs, guinea pigs, and pigs (156–159). Although the pressure induces a wound in these models, the degree of chronicity is not of the degree that we see in patients.

I. Venous Stasis Ulcers

Studies of venous stasis ulcer models have elucidated some of the characteristics of human venous stasis ulcers (160). One of the best models reproduced the pericapillary deposits, pigment deposition, and venous hypertension after creating arteriovenous fistulas in greyhounds (160). The problem with animal models is that venous hypertension is difficult to produce over a long time. Venous stasis is a problem of larger animals that stand for prolonged periods after damage to valves. It is likely that a large animal would be required to create a really clinically relevant model.

V. Transgenic Models

In order to determine whether a specific protein plays a role in tissue repair, it makes sense to either increase or eliminate that one protein. In the past, investigators have added factors to the wound or animal model to increase the protein's effect. Eliminating the effects of a protein was much more difficult. Antibodies can be given in the hope of blocking the action of a factor, but the effects may not truly represent the elimination of that factor. Investigators are now able to either eliminate or overexpress a specific gene (161–164). Transgenic changes are usually introduced into mice. The genes are either eliminated or introduced into embryonic cells, which are then introduced into "pseudo" pregnant females. The gene can also be attached to a specific promoter in order to target a specific cell type. The classic example is the use of specific keratin promoters to target keratinocytes. The transgenic changes are then tested to determine whether the elimination or up-regulation of that protein affects tissue repair.

The surprising thing about transgenic models is the often unexpected results. Some mutations are lethal whereas others tend to show very little changes from the normals. The results of one transgenic model can demonstrate these findings. TGF-β1 knockouts were found to be born relatively normal but would die of an overwhelming and invasive inflammatory response at 2–3 weeks of age (164). Tissue repair in the pups seemed to be normal until the animals became moribund (165). It appeared that the other TGF-β isoforms "covered" for TGF-β1. It turned out that this supposition was wrong. TGF-β1 was found to be transferred in the milk and the animals died when they were weaned (166). To confuse matters more, TGF-β1 was eliminated from severe-combined immunodeficiency (SCID) mice (167). These animals lack lymphocytes and thus were not capable of initiating an invasive inflammatory response. The knockout animals could now grow to adulthood. Tissue repair in the SCID animals lacking TGF-β1 was significantly impaired when compared to "normal" SCID animals. There was a decrease in the cellularity of the wounds and marked delay in closure. Apparently, the tie between lymphocytes, inflammation, tissue repair, and TGF-β1 is quite complex. This example demonstrates that transgenic studies must be carefully scrutinized prior to making any global conclusions.

VI. Tissue Repair Models in Patients

To evaluate the effects of various potential agents in patients, several models of healing have been introduced. All potential agents must undergo preclinical testing, followed by clinical testing. Most studies are performed in patients with problem wounds. Essentially, two types of wounds have been used for clinical trials: chronic nonhealing ulcers and split-thickness donor sites (168). The trials with chronic nonhealing ulcers are important because such wounds are a major clinical problem and are the major targets for treatments using growth factors. Growth factors have been tested in pressure sores (169–171), diabetic ulcers (172), and in venous stasis ulcers (173–174). The problem with these wounds is that they have a huge degree of variation among different patients. For instance, it is difficult to compare a pressure sore in a malnourished, incontinent 85-year-old patient with one in a healthy 17-year-old paraplegic. The other problem is that the treatment does not eliminate the source of the problem. Growth factors, for instance, will not eliminate venous stasis and there will be a high tendency to recur.

Donor sites have been used for many other studies. Donor site studies have the greatest ability to control the study (175–177). Two donor sites can be harvested from similar areas (i.e., two thighs) and at the same depth. Treatment can be randomized and blinded to test the agent properly. The problem with the donor site studies is that the wounds tend to heal rapidly irrespective of treatment. There have been many studies that show a "statistically significant" difference in closure by 1–2 days. Unfortunately, the clinical relevance of 1–2 days in a small donor site is negligible when they can be allowed to heal at home. A growth factor would be cost effective if it shortened hospital stay. Herndon *et al.* (177) did demonstrate that he could shorten hospital stay by systemic treatment with growth hormone in children with large burns. The major lesson is that donor site healing is most likely slowed when the patient has a massive burn. These factors allow for rapid reepithelialization over multiple reharvests and thus shorten hospital stays.

There have also been other models of tissue repair evaluation in patients. Most of these models mimic animal models. There have been several investigators who have placed reservoirs into the subcutaneous tissue of patients (178–181). PTFE tubes (178, 179) and silicone reservoirs (180, 181) have been used to test the ability of an agent to increase cellularity and hydroxyproline deposition. Tissue has also been taken from biopsies to test for the same factors. There are some problems with performing biopsies on wounds that patients are trying to heal. Each biopsy creates a new wound and may potentially lead to further delays and an increased tendency to scar. Finally, some investigators have reported the testing of breaking strengths in small incisions (182). There may be difficulty in finding patients to participate in this type of study.

VII. Conclusion

Tissue repair is essential for all surgical procedures that we perform. Inadequate healing is one of the first components of complications such as sepsis, systemic inflammatory response syndrome, and multiple organ dysfunction syndrome. Models have been designed to examine all forms of healing. The greatest weakness in the models is in the evaluation of scar formation. With the development of modern molecular biologic techniques, we now have the capability of influencing the genes that control tissue repair. These techniques will eventually help us to have a better control of healing failures and excessive scar formation.

References

1. Woodley, D. T., O'Keefe, E. J., and Prunieras, M. (1985). Cutaneous wound healing: A model for cell-matrix interactions. *J. Am. Acad. Dermatol.* **12,** 420–433.
2. al-Khateeb, T., Stephens, P., Shepherd, J. P., and Thomas, D. W. (1997). An investigation of preferential fibroblast wound repopulation using a novel *in vitro* wound model. *J. Periodontol.* **68,** 1063–1069.
3. Garner, W. L. (1998). Epidermal regulation of dermal fibroblast activity. *Plast. Reconstr. Surg.* **102,** 135–139.
4. Fray, T. R., and Wood, E. J. (1996). Effect of growth factors on fibroblast migration in a simplified wound healing model. *Biochem. Soc. Trans.* **24,** 258S.
5. Carrel, A., and Eberling, A. H. (1921). Age and multiplication of fibroblasts. *J. Exp. Med.* **34,** 599–623.
6. Harrop, A. R., Ghahary, A., Scott, P. G., *et al.* (1995). Regulation of collagen synthesis and mRNA expression in normal and hypertrophic scar fibroblasts *in vitro* by interferon-γ. *J. Surg. Res.* **58,** 471–477.
7. Ghahary, A., Shen, Y. J., Nedelec, B., *et al.* (1995). Interferons gamma and alpha-2b differentially regulate the expression of collagenase and tissue inhibitor of metalloproteinase-1 messenger RNA in human hypertrophic and normal dermal fibroblasts. *Wound Rep. Regen.* **3,** 176–184.
8. Bettinger, D. A., Yager D. R., Diegelmann, R. F., and Cohen, I. K. (1995). The effect of TGF-β on keloid fibroblast proliferation and collagen synthesis. *Plast. Reconstr. Surg.* **98,** 827–833.
9. Bell, E., Ivanson, B., and Merrill, C. (1979). Production of a tissue-like structure by contraction of collagen lattice by human fibroblasts of different proliferative potential *in vitro. Proc. Natl. Acad. Sci. U.S.A.* **76,** 1274–1278.
10. Guidry, C., and Grinnell, F. (1985). Studies on the mechanism of hydrated collagen gel reorganization by human skin fibroblasts. *J. Cell Sci.* **79,** 67–81.
11. Grinnell, F. (1994). Fibroblasts, myofibroblasts, and wound contraction. *J. Cell. Biol.* **124,** 401–404.
12. Grinnell, F., Zhu, M., Carlson, M. A., and Abrams, J. M. (1999). Release of mechanical tension triggers apoptosis of human fibroblasts in a model of regressing granulation tissue. *Exp. Med. Res.* **248,** 608–619.
13. Fluck, J., Querfeld, C., Cremer, A., *et al.* (1998). Normal human primary fibroblasts undergo apoptosis in three-dimensional contractile gels. *J. Invest. Dermatol.* **110,** 153–157.
14. Garner, W. L., Rittenberg, T., Ehrlich, H. P., *et al.* (1995). Hypertrophic scar fibroblasts accelerate collagen gel contraction. *Wound Rep. Regen.* **3,** 185–189.
15. Carmeliet, P. (2000). Mechanisms of angiogenesis and arteriogenesis. *Nature Med.* **6,** 389–395.
16. Folkman, J. (1985). Towards an understanding of angiogeneis: Search and discovery. *Perspect. Biol. Med.* **29,** 10–36.
17. Fajardo, L. F., Kowalsi, J., Kwan, H. H., *et al.* (1988). Methods in laboratory investigation. The disc angiogenesis system. *Lab. Invest.* **58,** 718–724.
18. Culliton, B. J. (1989). Gore Tex organoids and genetic drugs. *Science* **246,** 747–749.
19. Auerback, R., Kubai, L., Knighton, D., and Folkman, J. (1974). A simple procedure for the long term cultivation of chicken embryos. *Dev. Biol.* **41,** 391–394.
20. Friedlander, M., Brooks, P. C., Shaffer, R. W., *et al.* (1995). Definition of two angiogenic pathways by distinct α_v intregrins. *Science* **270,** 1500–1502.
21. Roesel, J. F., and Nanney, L. B. (1995). Assessment of differential cytokine effects on angiogenesis using an *in vivo* model of cutaneous wound repair. *J. Surg. Res.* **58,** 449–459.
22. Woodley, D. T., Wynn, K. C., and O'Keefe, E. J. (1990). Type IV collagen and fibronectin enhance human keratinocyte thymidine incorporation and spreading in the absence of soluble growth factors. *J. Invest. Dermatol.* **94,** 139–143.
23. Svedman, C., Hammarlund, C., Kutlu, N., and Svedman, P. (1991). Skin suction blister wound exposed to u.v. irradiation: A burn wound model for use in humans. *Burns* **17,** 41–46.
24. Walmod, P. S., Foley, A., Berezin, A., *et al.* (1998). Cell motility is inhibited by the antiepileptic compound, valproic acid and its teratogenic analogues. *Cell Motil. Cytoskeleton* **40,** 220–237.

25. Adzick, N. S., and Longaker, M. T. (1991). Animal models for the study of fetal tissue repair. *J. Surg. Res.* **51,** 216–221.
26. Strande, L. F., Foley, S. T., Doolin, E. J., and Hewitt, C. W. (1997). *In vitro* bioartificial skin culture model of tissue rejection and inflammatory/immune mechanisms. *Transplant. Proc.* **29,** 2118–2119.
27. O'Leary, R., Arrowsmith, M., and Wood, E. J. (1997). The use of an *in vitro* wound healing model, the tri-layered skin equivalent, to study the effects of cytokines on the repopulation of the wound defect by fibroblasts and keratinocytes. *Biochem. Soc. Trans.* **25,** 369S.
28. Kratz, G. (1998). Modeling of wound healing processes in human skin using tissue culture. *Microsc. Res. Tech.* **1,** 345–350.
29. Gallin, W. J., and Hepperle, B. (1998). Burn healing in organ cultures of embryonic chicken skin: A model system. *Burns* **24,** 613–620.
30. Emanualsson, P., and Kratz, G. (1997). Characterization of a new *in vitro* burn wound model. *Burns* **23,** 32–36.
31. Roberts, A. B., Sporn, M. B., Assoian, R. K., *et al.* (1986). Transforming growth factor type beta: Rapid induction of fibrosis and angiogenesis *in vivo* and stimulation of collagen formation *in vitro. Proc. Natl. Acad. Sci. U.S.A.* **83,** 4167–4171.
32. Paulini, K., Korner, B., Beneke, G., and Endres, R. (1974). A quantitative study on the growth of connective tissue: Investigations on implanted polyester-polyurethane sponges. *Connect. Tissue Res.* **2,** 257–265.
33. Diegelmann, R. F., Lindblad, W. J., and Cohen, I. K. (1986). A subcutaneous implant for wound healing studies in humans. *J. Surg. Res.* **40,** 229–237.
34. Holm-Pedersen, P., and Zederfeldt, B. (1971). Granulation tissue formation in subcutaneous implanted cellulose sponges in young and old rats. *Plast. Reconstr. Surg.* **5,** 13–16.
35. Kurkinen, M., Vaheri, A., Roberts, P. J., and Stenman, S. Sequential appearance of fibronectin and collagen in experimental granulation tissue. *Lab. Med.* **43,** 47–51.
36. Schilling, J. A., Joel, W., and Shurby, H. M. (1959). Wound healing: A comparative study of the histochemical changes in granulation tissue contained in stainless steel wire mesh cylinders and polyvinyl sponges. *Surgery* **46,** 702–710.
37. Hunt, T. K., Twomey, P., Zedrefeldt, B., and Dunphy, J. E. (1967). Respiratory gas tensions and pH in healing wounds. *Am. J. Surg.* **114,** 302–307.
38. Goodson, W. H., and Hunt, T. K. (1982). Development of a new miniature method for the study of wound healing in human subjects. *J. Surg. Res.* **33**, 394–401.
39. Sprugel, K. H., Mcpherson, J. M., Clowes, A. W., *et al.* (1987). Effects of growth factors *in vivo*: I. Cell ingrowth into porous subcutaneous chambers. *Am. J. Pathol.* **129,** 601–613.
40. Viljanto, J. (1964). Biochemical basis of tensile strength in wound healing. *Acta. Chir. Scand.* (Suppl.) **333,** 6–101.
41. Levenson, S. M., Geever, E. F., Crowley, L. V., *et al.* (1965). The healing of rat skin wounds. *Ann. Surg.* **161,** 293–308.
42. Van Winkle, W., Jr. (1969). The tensile strength of wounds and factors that influence it. *Surg. Gynecol. Obstet.* **127,** 819–842.
43. Charles, D., Williams, K., Perry, L. C., *et al.* (1992). An improved method of *in vivo* wound disruption and measurement. *J. Surg. Res.* **52,** 214–218.
44. Paul, R. G., Tarlton, J. F., Purslow, P. P., *et al.* (1997). Biomechanical and biochemical study of a standardized wound healing model. *Int. J. Biochem. Cell. Biol.* **29,** 211–220.
45. Greenhalgh, D. G., Gamelli, R. L., Foster, R. S., Jr., and Chester, A. (1986). Inhibition of wound healing by *Corynebacterium parvum. J. Surg. Res.* **41,** 209–214.
46. Greenhalgh, D. G., and Gamelli, R. L. (1987). Is impaired wound healing caused by infection or nutritional depletion? *Surgery* **102,** 306–312.
47. Kobak, M. W., Benditt, E. P., Wissler, R. W., and Steffee, C. H. (1947). The relation of protein deficiency to experimental wound healing. *Surg. Gynecol. Obstet.* **85,** 751–777.
48. Haxton, H. (1965). The influence of suture materials and methods on the healing of abdominal wounds. *Br. J. Surg.* **52,** 372–383.
49. Steiner, M. (1982). Biomechanics of tendon healing. *J. Biomech.* **15,** 951–958.
50. Woo, S. L.-Y. (1982). Mechanical properties of tendons and ligaments. *Biorheology* **19,** 385–396.
51. Cronin, K., Jackson, D. S., and Dunphy, J. E. (1968). Changing bursting strength and collagen content of the healing colon. *Surg. Gynecol. Obstet.* **126,** 747–753.
52. Greenhalgh, D. G. (1996). The healing of burn wounds. *Dermatol. Nursing* **8,** 13–25.
53. Montagna, W., and Yun, J. S. (1964). The skin of the domestic pig. *J. Invest. Dermatol.* **43,** 11–21.
54. Eaglstein, W. H., and Mertz, P. M. (1978). New method for assessing epidermal wound healing: The effects of triamcinolone and polyethylene film occlusion. *J. Invest. Dermatol.* **71,** 382–384.
55. Roesel, J. F., and Nanney, L. B. (1995). Assessment of differential cytokine effects on angiogenesis using an *in vivo* model of cutaneous wound repair. *J. Surg. Res.* **58,** 449–459.
56. Goretsky, M. J., Supp, A. P., Greenhalgh, D. G., Warden, G. D., and Boyce, S. T. (1995). Surface electrical capacitance (SEC) as an index of epidermal barrier properties of composite skin substitutes and skin autografts. *Wound Rep. Reg.* **3,** 419–425.
57. Surinchak, J. S., Malinowski, J. A., Wilson, D. R., and Maibach, H. I. (1985). Skin wound healing determined by water loss. *J. Surg. Res.* **38,** 258–262.
58. Montandon, D., D'Andiran, G., and Gabbiani, G. (1977). The mechanism of wound contraction and epithelialization. *Clinics Plast. Surg.* **4,** 325–346.
59. Tranquillo, R. T., and Murray, J. D. (1993). Mechanistic model of wound contraction. *J. Surg. Res.* **55,** 233–247.
60. Ksander, G. A., Ogawa, Y. A. M., Chu, G. H., *et al.* (1990). Exogenous transforming growth factor-beta 2 enhances connective tissue formation and wound strength in guinea pig dermal wounds by secondary intent. *Ann. Surg.* **211,** 288–294.
61. Wu, L., Siddiqui, A., Morris, D. E., *et al.* (1997) Transforming growth factor β3 (TGF-β) accelerates wound healing without alteration of scar prominence. *Arch. Surg.* **132,** 753–760.
62. Greenhalgh, D. G., Sprugel, K. H., Murray, M. J., and Ross, R. (1990). PDGF and FGF stimulate wound healing in the genetically diabetic mouse. *Am. J. Pathol.* **136,** 1235–1246.
63. Werner, S., Breeden, M., Greenhalgh, D. G., Hofschneider, P. H., and Longaker, M. T. (1994). Induction of keratinocyte growth factor is reduced and delayed during wound healing in the genetically diabetic mouse. *J. Invest. Dermatol.* **103,** 469–472.
64. Frank, S., Hubner, G., Breier, G., Longaker, M. T., Greenhalgh, D. G., and Werner, S. (1995). Regulation of vascular endothelial growth factor expression in cultured keratinocytes. *J. Biol. Chem.* **270,** 12607–12613.
65. Brown, D. L., Kane, C. D., Chernausek, S. D., and Greenhalgh, D. G. (1997). Differential expression and localization of IGF-I and IGF-II in cutaneous wounds of diabetic versus nondiabetic mice. *Am. J. Pathol.* **151,** 715–724.
66. Boyce, S. T., Greenhalgh, D. G., Kagan, R. J., *et al.* (1993). Skin anatomy and antigen expression after burn wound closure with composite grafts of cultured skin cells and biopolymers. *Plast. Reconstr. Surg.* **91,** 632–641.
67. Cooper, M. L., Hansbrough, J. F., Foreman, T. J., *et al.* (1991). The effects of epidermal growth factor and basic fibroblast growth factor on epithelialization of meshed skin graft interstices. *Prog. Clin. Biol. Res.* **365,** 429–442.
68. Harries, R. H., Rogers, B. G., Leitch, I. O., and Robson, M. C. (1995). An *in vivo* model for epithelialization kinetics in human skin. *Aust. N.Z. J. Surg.* **65,** 600–603.

69. Hansbrough, J. F., Dore, C., and Hansbrough, W. B. (1992). Clinical trials of a living dermal tissue replacement placed beneath meshed, split-thickness skin grafts on excised burn wounds. *J. Burn Care Rehabil.* **13,** 519–529.
70. Hansbrough, J. F., Morgan, J. L., Greenleaf, G. E., and Bartel, R. (1993). Composite grafts of human keratinocytes grown on a polyglactin mesh-cultured fibroblast dermal substitute function as a bilayer skin replacement in full-thickness wounds on athymic mice. *J. Burn Care Rehabil.* **14,** 485–94.
71. Boyce, S. T., Supp, A. P., Harriger, M. D., Greenhalgh, D. G., and Warden, G. D. (1995). Topical nutrients promote engraftment and inhibit wound contraction of cultured skin substitutes in athymic mice. *J. Invest. Dermatol.* **104,** 345–349.
72. Robb, E. C., Waymack, J. P., Warden, G. D., *et al.* (1987). A new model for studying the development of human hypertrophic burn scar formation. *J. Burn Care Rehabil.* **8,** 371–375.
73. Kischer, C. W., Pindur, J., Shetlar, M. R., and Shetlar, C. L. (1989). Implants of hypertrophic scars and keloids into the nude (athymic) mouse: Viability and morphology. *J. Trauma* **29,** 672–677.
74. Polo, M., Kim, Y.-J., Kucukcelebi, A., *et al.* (1998). An *in vivo* model of human proliferative scar. *J. Surg. Res.* **74,** 187–195.
75. Marcus, J. R., Tyrone, J. W., Bonomo, S., *et al.* (2000). Cellular mechanisms for diminished scarring with aging. *Plast. Reconstr. Surg.* **105,** 1591–1599.
76. Arturson, G. (1964). The infliction and healing of a large standard burn in rats. *Acta Pathol. Microbiol. Scand.* **61,** 353–370.
77. Walker, H. L., and Mason, A. D., Jr. (1968). A standard animal burn. *J. Trauma* **8,** 1049–1060.
78. Schildt, B., and Nilsson, A. (1970). Standardized burns in mice. *Eur. Surg. Res.* **2,** 23–37.
79. Stieritz, D. D., and Holder, I. A. (1975). Experimental studies of the pathogenesis of infections due to *Pseudomonas aeruginosa*: Descriptions of a burned mouse model. *J. Inf. Dis.* **131,** 688–698.
80. Greenhalgh, D. G., and Gamelli, R. L. (1987). Immunomodulators and wound healing. *J. Trauma* **27,** 510–514.
81. Breuing, K., Eriksson, E., Liu, P., and Miller, D. R. (1992). Healing of partial thickness porcine skin wounds in a liquid environment. *J. Surg. Res.* **52,** 50–58.
82. Cribbs, R. K., Luquette, M. H., and Bessner, G. E. (1998). A standardized model of partial thickness scald burns in mice. (1998). *J. Surg. Res.* **80,** 69–74.
83. Knabl, J. S., Bayer, G. S., Bauer, W. A., *et al.* (1999). Controlled partial thickness burns: An animal model for studies of burn wound progression. *Burns* **25,** 229–235.
84. Mileski, W., Borgstrom, D., Lightfoot, E., *et al.* (1992). Inhibition of leukocyte-endothelial adherence following thermal injury. *J. Surg. Res.* **52,** 334–339.
85. Bucky, L. P., Vedder, J. B., Hong, H. Z., *et al.* Reduction of burn injury by inhibiting CD18-mediated leukocyte adherence in rabbits. *Plast. Reconstr. Surg.* **93,** 1473–1478.
86. Cho, K., Zipkin, R. I., Adamson, L. K., *et al.* (2000). Differential regulation of c-Jun expression in liver and lung of mice after thermal injury. *Shock* **14**(2), 182–186.
87. Greenhalgh, D. G. (1996). The role of growth factors in wound healing. *J. Trauma* **41,** 159–167.
88. Howes, E. L., Briggs, H., Shea, R., *et al.* (1933). Effect of complete and partial starvation on the rate of fibroplasia in the healing wound. *Arch. Surg.* **26,** 846–858.
89. Rhoads, J. E., Fliegelman, M. T., and Panzer, L. M. (1942). The mechanism of delayed wound healing in the presence of hypoproteinemia. *J. Am. Med. Assoc.* **118,** 21–25.
90. Daly, J. M., Vars, H. M., and Dudvich, S. J. (1972). Effects of protein depletion on strength of colonic anastomoses. *Surg. Gynecol. Obstet.* **134,** 15–21.
91. Irvin, T. T. (1978). Effects of malnutrition and hyperalimentation on wound healing. *Surg. Gynecol. Obstet.* **146,** 33–37.
92. Greenhalgh, D. G., and Gamelli, R. L. (1988). Do nutritional alterations contribute to adriamycin-induced impaired wound healing? *J. Surg. Res.* **45,** 261–265.
93. Albertson, S., Hummel, R. P., III, Breeden, M., and Greenhalgh, D. G. (1993). PDGF and FGF reverse the healing impairment in protein malnourished diabetic mice. *Surgery* **114,** 368–373.
94. Bartlett, M. K., Jones, C. M., and Ryan, A. E. (1942). Vitamin C and wound healing. I. Experimental wounds in guinea pigs. *N. Engl. J. Med.* **226,** 469–473.
95. Ehrlich, H. P., and Hunt, T. K. (1968). Effects of cortisone and vitamin A on wound healing. *Ann. Surg.* **167,** 324–328.
96. Levenson, S. M., Gruber, C. A., Rettura, G., *et al.* (1984). Supplemental vitamin A prevents the acute radiation-induced defect in wound healing. *Ann. Surg.* **200,** 494–512.
97. Alvarez, O. M., and Gilbreath, R. L. (1982). Thiamine influence on collagen during the granulation of skin wounds. *J. Surg. Res.* **32,** 24–31.
98. Pories, W. J., *et al.* (1967). Acceleration of healing with zinc oxide. *Ann. Surg.* **165,** 432–436.
99. Pinnell, S. R., and Martin, G. R. (1968). The cross linking of collagen and elastin. *Proc. Natl. Acad. Sci. U.S.A.* **61,** 708–714.
100. Localio, S. A., Morgan, M. E., and Hinton, J. W. (1948). The biological chemistry of wound healing. The effect of methionine on the healing of wounds in protein-depleted animals. *Surg. Gynecol. Obstet.* **86,** 582–589.
101. Williamson, M. B., and Fromm, H. J. (1955). The incorporation of sulphur amino aids into proteins of regenerating wound tissue. *J. Biol. Chem.* **212,** 705–712.
102. Seifter, E., Rettura, G., Barbul, A., *et al.* (1978). Arginine: An essential amino acid for injured rats. *Surgery* **84,** 224–230.
103. McCauley, R., Platell, M. B., Hall, J., and McCulloch, R. (1991). Effects of glutamine on colonic anastomotic strength in the rat. *JPEN J. Parenter. Enteral Nutr.* **15,** 437–439.
104. Hulsey, T. K., O'Neill, J. A., Neblett, W. R., *et al.* (1980). Experimental wound healing in essential fatty acid deficiency. *J. Pediatr. Surg.* **15,** 505–508.
105. Albina, J. E., Gladden, P., and Walsh, W. R. (1993). Detrimental effects of an ω-3 fatty acid-enriched diet on wound healing. *JPEN J. Parenter. Enteral Nutr.* **17,** 519–521.
106. Tenorio, A., *et al.* (1976). Accelerated healing in infected wounds. *Surg. Gynecol. Obstet.* **142,** 537–543.
107. Raju, D. R., *et al.* (1977). A study of the critical inoculum to cause a stimulus to wound healing. *Surg. Gynecol. Obstet.* **144,** 347–350.
108. Levenson, S. M., *et al.* (1983). Wound healing accelerated by *Staphylococcus aureus*. *Arch. Surg.* **118,** 310–320.
109. Smith, M., and Enquist, I. F. (1967). A quantitative study of impaired healing resulting from infection. *Surg. Gynecol. Obstet.* **125,** 965–973.
110. Irvin, T. T. (1976). Collagen metabolism in infected colonic anastomoses. *Surg. Gynecol. Obstet.* **143,** 220–224.
111. Bucknall, T. E. (1980). The effect of local infection upon wound healing. *Br. J. Surg.* **67,** 851–855.
112. Hayward, P., Hokanson, J., Heggars, J., *et al.* (1992). Fibroblast growth factor reverses the bacterial retardation of wound contraction. *Am. J. Surg.* **163,** 288–293.
113. DeHaan, B. B., Ellis, H., and Wilks, M. (1974). The role of infection on wound healing. *Surg. Gynecol. Obstet.* **138,** 693–700.
114. Houck, J. C., and Jacob, R. (1961). Connective tissue. II. Distant dermal response to local inflammation. *Proc. Soc. Exp. Biol. Med.* **106,** 145–147.
115. Freihoffer, U., *et al.* (1969). The effect of bacterial endotoxin on connective tissue growth and wound tensile strength. *Surg. Forum* **11,** 293–295.

116. Hunt, T. K., and Pai, M. P. (1972). The effect of varying ambient oxygen tensions on wound metabolism and collagen synthesis. *Surg. Gynecol. Obstet.* **135,** 561–567.
117. LaVan, F. B., and Hunt, T. K. (1990). Oxygen and wound healing. *Clin. Plast. Surg.* **17,** 463–472.
118. Chen, C., Schultz, G. S., Bloch, M., *et al.* (1999). Molecular and mechanistic validation of delayed healing rat wounds as a model for human chronic wounds. *Wound Rep. Regen.* **7,** 486–494.
119. Mustoe, T. A., Pierce, G. F., Morishima, C., and Deuel, T. F. (1991). Growth factor-induced acceleration of tissue repair through direct and inductive activities in a rabbit dermal ulcer model. *J. Clin. Invest.* **87,** 694–703.
120. Wu, L., and Mustoe, T. A. (1995). Effect of ischemia on growth factor enhancement of incisional wound healing. *Surgery* **117,** 570–576.
121. Corral, C. J., Siddiqui, A., Wu, L., *et al.* (1999). Vascular endothelial growth factor is more important than basic fibroblastic growth factor during ischemic wound healing. *Arch. Surg.* **134,** 200–205.
122. Zhao, L. L., Davidson, J. D., Wee, S. C., *et al.* (1994). Effect of hyperbaric oxygen and growth factors on rabbit ear ischemic ulcers. *Arch. Surg.* **129,** 1043–1049.
123. McMurry, J. F., Jr. (1984). Wound healing with diabetes mellitus. *Surg. Clin. N. Am.* **64,** 769–778.
124. Goodson, W. H., III, and Hunt, T. K. (1979). Wound healing and the diabetic patient. *Surg. Gynecol. Obstet.* **149,** 600–608.
125. Rerup, C. C. (1970). Drugs producing diabetes through damage of insulin secreting cells. *Pharmacol. Rev.* **22,** 485–518.
126. Goodson, W. H., III, and Hunt, T. K. (1977). Studies of wound healing experimental diabetes mellitus. *J. Surg. Res.* **22,** 221–227.
127. Seifter, E., Rettura, G., Padawer, J., *et al.* (1981). Impaired wound healing in streptozotocin diabetes. Prevention by supplemental vitamin A. *Ann. Surg.* **194,** 42–50.
128. Grotendorst, G. R., Martin, G. R., Pencev, D., *et al.* (1985). Stimulation of granulation tissue formation by platelet-derived growth factor in normal and diabetic rats. *J. Clin. Invest.* **76,** 2323–2329.
129. Greenhalgh, D. G., Hummel III, R. P., Albertson, A., and Breeden, M. P. (1993). Synergistic actions of platelet-derived growth factor and the insulin-like growth factors *in vivo*. *Wound Rep. Regen.* **1,** 69–81.
130. Brown, R. L., Breeden, M. P., and Greenhalgh, D. G. (1994). PDGF and TGF-α act synergistically to improve healing in the genetically diabetic mouse. *J. Surg. Res.* **56,** 562–570.
131. Tsuboi, R., and Rifkin, D. B. (1990). Recombinant basic fibroblast growth factor stimulates wound healing in healing-impaired db/db mice. *J. Exp. Med.* **172,** 245–251.
132. Klingbeil, C. K., Cesar, L. B., and Fiddes, J. C. (1991). Basic fibroblast growth factor accelerates tissue repair in models of impaired wound healing. *Prog. Clin. Biol. Res.* **365,** 443–458.
133. Brown, D. L., Kane, C. D., Chernausek, S. D., and Greenhalgh, D. G. (1997). Differential expression and localization of IGF-I and IGF-II in cutaneous wounds of diabetic versus nondiabetic mice. *Am. J. Pathol.* **151,** 715–724.
134. Werner, S., Breeden, M., Greenhalgh, D. G., *et al.* (1994). Induction of keratinocyte growth factor is reduced and delayed during wound healing in the genetically diabetic mouse. *J. Invest. Dermatol.* **103,** 469–472.
135. Goodson III, W. H., and Hunt, T. K. (1979). Deficient collagen formation by obese mice in a standard wound model. *Am. J. Surg.* **138,** 692–694.
136. Goodson III, W. H., and Hunt, T. K. (1986). Wound collagen accumulation in obese hyperglycemic mice. *Diabetes* **35,** 491–495.
137. Coleman, D. M. (1982). Other potentially useful rodents as models for the study of human diabetes mellitus. *Diabetes* **31** (Suppl. 1), 24–25.
138. Like, A. A., Butler, L., Williams, R. M., *et al.* (1982). Spontaneous autoimmune diabetes mellitus in the BB rat. *Diabetes* **31** (Suppl. 1), 7–13.
139. Gerritsen, G. C. (1982). The chinese hamster as a model for the study of diabetes mellitus. *Diabetes* **31** (Suppl. 1), 14–23.
140. Phillips, R. W., Panepinto, L. M., Spangler, R., and Westmoreland, N. (1982). Yucatan swine as a model of human diabetes mellitus. *Diabetes* **31** (Suppl. 1), 30–36.
141. Engerman, R. L., and Kramer, J. W. (1982). Dogs with induced or spontaneous diabetes as models for the study of human diabetes mellitus. *Diabetes* **31** (Suppl. 1), 26–29.
142. Howard, C. F., Jr. (1982). Nonhuman primates as models for the study of human diabetes mellitus. *Diabetes* **31** (Suppl. 1), 37–42.
143. Howes, E. L., *et al.* (1950). Retardation of wound healing by cortisone. *Surgery* **28,** 177–181.
144. Sandberg, N. (1964). Time relationship between administration of cortisone and wound healing in rats. *Acta Chir. Scand.* **127,** 446–455.
145. Laato, M., Heino, J., Kahari, V. M., *et al.* (1989). Epidermal growth factor (EGF) prevents methylprednisolone-induced inhibition of wound healing. *J. Surg. Res.* **47,** 354–359.
146. Pierce, G. F., Mustoe, T. A., Lingelbach, J., *et al.* (1989). Transforming growth factor β reverses the glucocorticoid-induced wound healing deficit in rats: Possible regulation in macrophages by platelet-derived growth factor. *Proc. Natl. Acad. Sci. U.S.A.* **86,** 2229–2233.
147. Beck, L. S., DeGuzman, L. Lee, W. P., *et al.* (1991). TGF-β1 accelerates wound healing: Reversal of steroid-impaired healing in rats and rabbits. *Growth Factors* **5,** 295–300.
148. Ferguson, M. K.. (1982). The effects of antineoplastic agents on wound healing. *Surg. Gynecol. Obstet.* **154,** 421–429.
149. Falcone, R. E., and Napp, J. F. (1984). Chemotherapy and wound healing. *Surg. Clin. N. Am.* **64,** 779–795.
150. Lawrence, W. T., Sporn, M. B., Gorschboth, C., *et al.* (1986). The reversal of an Adriamycin induced healing impairment with chemoattractants and growth factors. *Ann. Surg.* **203,** 142–147.
151. Bland, K. I., Palin, W. E., vonFraunhofer, J. A., *et al.* (1984). Experimental and clinical observations of the effects of cytotoxic chemotherapy drugs on wound healing. *Ann. Surg.* **199,** 782–790.
152. Reinisch, J. F., and Puckett, C. L. (1984). Management of radiation wounds. *Surg. Clin. N. Am.* **64,** 795–802.
153. Luce, E. A. (1984). The irradiated wound. *Surg. Clin. N. Am.* **64,** 821–829.
154. Schwentker, A., Evans, S. M., Partington, M., *et al.* (1988). A model of wound healing in chronically radiation-damaged rat skin. *Cancer Lett.* **128,** 71–78.
155. Mustoe, T. A., Purdy, J., Gramates, P., *et al.* (1989). Reversal of impaired wound healing in irradiated rats by platelet-derived growth factor-BB. *Am. J. Surg.* **158,** 345–350.
156. Daniel, R. K., Wheatley, D. C., and Priest, D. L. (1985). Pressure sores and paraplegia: An experimental model. *Ann. Plast. Surg.* **15,** 41–49.
157. Constantine, B. E., and Bolton, L. L. (1986). A wound model for ischemic ulcers in the guinea pig. *Arch. Dermatol. Res.* **278,** 429–431.
158. Hyodo, A., Reger, S. I., Negami, S., *et al.* (1995). Evaluation of a pressure sore model using monoplegic pigs. *Plast. Reconstr. Surg.* **96,** 421–428.
159. Peirce, S. M., Skalak, T. C., and Rodeheaver, G. T. (2000). Ischemia-reperfusion injury in chronic pressure ulcer formation: A skin model in the rat. *Wound Rep. Regen.* **8,** 68–76.
160. Burnand, K. G., Clemenson, G., Whimster, I., *et al.* (1982). The effect of sustained venous hypertension on the skin capillaries of the canine limb. *Br. J. Surg.* **69,** 41–44.
161. Arbeit, J. M., and Hirose, R. (1999). Murine mentors: Transgenic and knockout models of surgical disease. *Ann. Surg.* **229,** 21–40.
162. Abbott, R. E., Corral, C. J., MacIvor, D. M., *et al.* (1998). Augmented inflammatory responses and altered wound healing in cathepsin G-deficient mice. *Arch. Surg.* **133,** 1002–1006.
163. Bullard, K. M., Lund, L., Midgett, J. S., *et al.* (1999). Impaired wound contraction in stromelysin-1-deficient mice. *Ann. Surg.* **230,** 260–265.

164. Shull, M. M., Ormsby, I., Kier, A. B., *et al.* (1992). Targeted disruption of the mouse transforming growth factor-β1 gene results in multi focal inflammatory disease. *Nature (London)* **35,** 693–699.
165. Brown, R. L., Ormsby, I., Doetschman, T. C., and Greenhalgh, D. G. (1995). Wound healing in the transforming growth factor-β1-deficient mouse. *Wound Rep. Regen.* **3** 25–36.
166. Letterio, J. J., Geiser, A. G., Kulkarni, A. B., *et al.* (1994). Maternal rescue of transforming growth factor-β1 null mice. *Science* **264,** 1936–1938.
167. Crowe, M. J., Doetschman, T., and Greenhalgh, D. G. (2000). Delayed wound healing in immunodeficient TGF-beta 1 knockout mice. *J. Invest. Dermatol.* **115**, 3–11.
168. Greenhalgh, D. G. (1996). The role of growth factors in wound healing. *J. Trauma* **41,** 159–167.
169. Robson, M. C., Phillips, L. G., Thomason, A., *et al.* (1992). Platelet-derived growth factor BB for the treatment of chronic pressure ulcers. *Lancet* **339,** 23–25.
170. Robson, M. C., Phillips, L. G., Lawrence, W. T., *et al.* (1992). The safety and effect of topically applied recombinant basic fibroblast growth factor on the healing of chronic pressure sores. *Ann. Surg.* **216,** 401–410.
171. Mustoe, T. A., Cutler, N. R., Allman, R. M., *et al.* (1994). A phase II study to evaluate recombinant platelet-derived growth factor-BB in the treatment of stage 3 and 4 pressure ulcers. *Arch. Surg.* **129,** 213–218.
172. Steed, D. L., and The Diabetic Study Group. (1995). Clinical evaluation of recombinant human platelet-derived growth factor for the treatment of lower extremity diabetic ulcers. *J. Vasc. Surg.* **21,** 71–77.
173. Robson, M. C., Phillips, L. G., Cooper, D. M., *et al.* (1995). Safety and effect of transforming growth factor-beta2 for the treatment of venous stasis ulcers. *Wound Rep. Regen.* **3,** 157–163.
174. Falanga, V., Eaglstein, W. H., Bucalo, B., *et al.* (1992). Topical use of human recombinant epidermal growth factor (h-EGF) in venous ulcers. *J. Dermatol. Surg. Oncol.* **18,** 604–610.
175. Brown, G. L., Nanney, L. B., Griffin, J., *et al.* (1989). Enhancement of wound healing by topical treatment with epidermal growth factor. *N. Engl. J. Med.* **321,** 76–83.
176. Greenhalgh, D. G., and Rieman, M. (1994). Effects of basic fibroblast growth factor on the healing of partial-thickness donor sites: A prospective, randomized, double-blinded trial. *Wound Rep. Regen.* **2,** 113–121.
177. Herndon, D. N., Barrow, R. E., Kunkel, K. R., *et al.* (1990). Effects of human growth hormone on donor-site healing in severely burned children. *Ann. Surg.* **212,** 424–432.
178. Jorgensen, L. N., Kallehave, F., Karlsmark, T., *et al.* (1994). Evaluation of the wound healing potential in human beings from the subcutaneous insertion of expanded polytetrafluoroethylenen tubes. A methodologic study. *Wound Rep. Regen.* **4,** 20–30.
179. Wicke, C., Halliday, B. J., Scheuenstuhl, H., *et al.* (1995). Examination of expanded polytetrafluoroethylene wound healing models. *Wound Rep. Regen.* **3,** 284–291.
180. Viljanto, J. (1976). Cellstick: A device for wound healing studies in man. Description of the method. *J. Surg. Res.* **20,** 115–119.
181. Diegelmann, R. F., Kim, J. C., Lindblad, W. J., *et al.* (1987). Collection of leukocytes, fibroblasts, and collagen within an implantable reservoir tube during tissue repair. *J. Leukoc. Biol.* **42,** 667–672.
182. Lindstedt, E., and Sandblom, P. (1975). Wound healing in man: Tensile strength of healing wounds in some patient groups. *Ann. Surg.* **181,** 842–846.

33

Models of Adult Respiratory Distress Syndrome—Aspiration

H. Hank Simms

Division of Surgical Critical Care, Rhode Island Hospital, Providence, Rhode Island 02903

I. Introduction

The purpose of this chapter is to define various models of acute lung injury that result in adult respiratory distress syndrome (ARDS). The advantage and disadvantages of each model will be documented along with salient findings that a multiplicity of authors have documented. Where possible the clinical relevance of each model will also be discussed. In general, models of acute lung injury can be divided into two broad categories: models that utilize direct pulmonary insults to produce lung injury and models that rely on distant noxious stimuli to produce lung injury. The models employing distant noxious stimuli are generally intraabdominal vs. extremity ischemia-reperfusion models. These models will be discussed first.

II. Intraabdominal Models

Intraabdominal models that induce lung injury generally fall into two categories: sterile inflammation and endotoxin/sepsis. Representative examples of each group are discussed here, and the advantages/disadvantages are compared in Table I.

One of the most common models of sterile inflammation producing acute lung injury (ALI) is cerulein-induced pancreatitis (1, 2). This model is generally employed in rats and utilizes cerulein, a cholecystokinin analog infused intravenously in supramaximal doses (5 μg/kg/hr) to induce acute pancreatitis. Although this model produces reversible edematous pancreatitis as opposed to rapidly progressive lethal pancreatitis, histologic and physiologic changes in the lung are very similar in patients with ARDS. In this model, significant lung injury is produced anywhere from 3 to 6 hr after cerulein infusion is started. Classically, cerulein infusion produces increased pulmonary microvascular permeability and wet lung weights, intraalveolar hemorrhage, endothelial cell disruption, and neutrophil sequestration. Further, cerulein-induced acute lung injury can also be seen using *ex vivo* heart–lung perfusion models (3).

Table I Advantages/Disadvantages of Intraabdominal Models[a]

Pros	Cons
Cerulein infusion consistently produces ALI	Intrapancreatic infusion is not seen clinically
Zymosan IP injection is easy technically	Lethal models; delayed onset of ALI
LPS IP injection is easy technically; consistently produces ALI	Cecal ligation and puncture induce lethality, require laparotomy
Cecal ligation and puncture consistently produce ALI	Technically more difficult, mortality rate 18–25%, increased expense
Mesenteric ischemia–reperfusion consistently produce ALI; in sheep, an added benefit is hemodynamic and pulmonary function	

[a]Abbreviations: ALI, acute lung injury; IP, intraperitoneal; LPS, lipopolysaccharide.

Another model of sterile peritonitis that induces acute lung injury is the intraperitoneal injection of zymosan (4). Zymosan administration produces a prolonged activation of the alternative complement pathway. In this model, 0.6 mg/kg of zymosan is injected under direct vision using a 14-gauge needle; rabbits are the most frequently utilized animals in this model. As opposed to the model discussed above, intraperitoneal (IP) injection of zymosan produces a 24-hr mortality rate of 35–45%. Further, although acute lung injury is seen, the sequelae are usually seen within days, rather than hours, after zymosan administration. Intraperitoneal injection of zymosan results in marked hypoxemia, pulmonary neutrophil sequestration, and interstitial edema (5).

Although cecal ligation and puncture protocols have been the most commonly used model of intraperitoneal sepsis used to induce acute lung injury, intraperitoneal administration of endotoxin/lipopolysaccharide will also produce acute lung injury. Intraperitoneal lipopolysaccharide (LPS) administration has been performed in both murine and rat models. In murine models, animals are typically 12–15 weeks old and receive 200–300 μg of LPS intraperitoneally. This results in a model of peripheral leukopenia with neutrophils sequestrated in the lung and liver. In this particular model, neutrophil sequestration within the lung is dependent on CD11b/CD18 (6), and physiologic changes (i.e., hypoxemia, hypercarbia) occur within 24 hr (7). Rat models of intraperitoneal LPS generally involve larger amounts of endotoxin. Typically, 500 μg/kg of LPS is administered intraperitoneally in rats, with the majority of the acute lung injury changes seen in 6–12 hr. These changes include transient neutrophil sequestration within the lung, increased lung microvascular permeability as measured using ^{125}I-labeled albumin and elastase release from pulmonary neutrophils (8).

The commonly used means of inducing intraabdominal sepsis via cecal ligation and puncture also leads to acute lung injury. This technique has been described by Chaudry *et al.* (9) and Bohnen *et al.* (10) in detail. In this model, a midline laparotomy is performed and the cecum is ligated. Various puncture wound sizes have been used, but most frequently two separate puncture wounds on the antimesenteric border using 18-gauge needles are utilized. Cecal ligation and puncture (CLP) procedures produce mortality rates of 20–25% at 24 hr and 65–75% at 7 days after CLP. Cecal ligation and puncture will reproducibly lead to increases in lung wet/dry weight ratios, atelectasis, hyaline membrane formation, and neutrophil sequestration. Hypoxemia is seen within 2–3 days in those animals that survive (11–13).

III. Ischemia–Reperfusion Models

Two models of ischemia–reperfusion injury that lead to acute lung injury are mesenteric and hind limb ischemia–reperfusion injury. Mesenteric ischemia–reperfusion models frequently employ a murine model; in general, Sprague–Dawley rats (~500 g) are utilized. Collateral vessels from the caudal mesenteric and celiac axis are ligated and the superior mesenteric artery is occluded. Occlusion times vary from 30 to 90 min but mesenteric ischemia of 90 min followed by reperfusion results in an 18–25% mortality rate (14). Following reperfusion (1–3 hr), pulmonary insults are seen. These include neutrophil sequestration within the lung and increased lung microvascular permeability, which is prevented when monoclonal antibodies to CD11b/CD18 are used (15). Extremity ischemia–reperfusion models have been widely described but will be reviewed here in both rat and sheep models.

In rat models of extremity ischemia–reperfusion, animals weighing 300–350 g are used and tourniquets, causing pressure to block arterial blood flow, are placed on both hind limbs proximal to the trochanter major. Frequently, 4 hr of ischemia followed by 1–4 hr of reperfusion will be used in this model. Laser doppler velocimeters should be used to confirm the absence of blood flow during the period of ischemia. In this model, significant lung injury is reproducibly seen and includes increased vascular permeability using ^{125}I-labeled albumin and intrapulmonary hemorrhage using ^{51}Cr-labeled erythrocytes (16–17). As opposed to integrin-dependent lung injury in other models, here lung injury is primarily L- and E-selectin dependent.

Sheep models of extremity reperfusion injury are similar to that described above, except that, because of their increased size, Swan–Ganz catheter, left atrial pressure, and lung lymph data can be measured. In sheep, tourniquets are applied to both hind limbs and inflated to 300 mmHg for 0–2 hr (18). In this model, acute lung injury is seen with ischemia alone: these changes include increases in mean pulmonary arterial pressure, thromboxane B_2, and lung lymph flow. Lung histology consistently demonstrates leukosequestration and endothelial cell barrier disruption (19).

IV. Models of Hemorrhage That Induce Acute Lung Injury

Models of hemorrhage that induce acute lung injury have been described in mice, rats, and pigs. Variations in these animal models and the changes seen in lung physiology are described here, and advantages/disadvantages are compared in Table II.

Murine models of hemorrhage generally involve animals that are 8–12 weeks old. Cardiac puncture is used to remove approximately 35% of the calculated blood volume (0.55 ml for a 20-g mouse). This procedure has a mortality rate of 10–15% (21). Femoral artery catheters are used to monitor blood pressure and the removal of 30% blood volume decreases mean arterial blood pressure to approximately 40 mmHg, with restoration to normal levels over the 60 min following hemorrhage (21). In this model, neutrophil sequestration, endothelial cell disruption, and interleukin (IL-1β) production from sequestrated pulmonary neutrophils are seen. In those models involving reinfusion of red blood cells, a retroorbital plexus injection is used.

Following hemorrhage and resuscitation in mice, histopathologic changes are seen in the lung maximally at day 3. These changes include intraalveolar hemorrhage, vascular congestion, interstitial edema, and neutrophil infiltrates (22). Further, therapy with monoclonal antitumor necrosis factor (anti-TNFα) antibodies significantly attenuates vascular sequestration and cytokine gene expression for IL-1β, IL-6, and IL-10. Hemorrhage can also be induced in a controlled fashion by withdrawing blood from preplaced catheters.

In mice, following the induction of general anesthesia, femoral artery catheters are placed and the animals are heparinized (40 U/kg body weight) until they awaken. Blood is withdrawn until the desired blood pressure (often mean arterial pressure) of 40 mmHg is reached. Ischemic periods of 1–3 hr have been utilized and animals are resuscitated with isotonic or hypertonic crystalloid solution. Isotonic crystalloid resuscitation requires 2–3 times the volume of shed blood to restore mean arterial pressure. After resuscitation, catheters are removed and femoral arteries are ligated. Mortality rates in the model are low and acute lung injury is reliably produced (23–24). Following hemorrhage and resuscitation in this model, intraalveolar hemorrhage, interstitial edema, and cellular infiltrates are seen. Lung myeloperoxidase levels increase and bronchoalveolar lavage fluid demonstrates significant increases in neutrophils.

The use of hemorrhage to induce acute lung injury has also been performed in rats. Classically, Sprague–Dawley rats (300–500 g) are anesthetized and again systemic hypotension [mean arterial pressure (MAP), 40 mmHg] is induced by blood withdrawal via carotid artery catheterization for 1 hr (25–26). A multiplicity of changes in the lung are seen following these procedures, including enhanced neutrophil sequestration and transpulmonary albumin flux. In porcine models of hemorrhage, pigs of both sexes (approximately 20 kg weight) are bled to a MAP of 40–45 mmHg for 1 hr. Resuscitation can be accomplished with crystalloid or blood. Potential advantages of the larger animal model include the ability to measure arterial and venous blood gases, to place Swan–Ganz catheters, and to assess cardiac dP/dT readings (27).

In addition to hemorrhage alone, hemorrhagic shock plus the administration of LPS have been used to induce acute lung injury (28). In rat models (300–350 g) mean arterial pressure is brought to 40 mmHg for 1 hr; following resuscitation, LPS is administered intratracheally at multiple times. Generally LPS is given from 1 to 18 hr after resuscitation. In these "two-hit" models, early (4 hr) neutrophil sequestration within the lung is seen along with intraalveolar hemorrhage and interstitial edema. Importantly, this is a nonlethal model, with animal survival exceeding 90% with this protocol.

A variant to the hemorrhage model is that of mesenteric ischemia–reperfusion to induce acute lung injury. Although

Table II Advantages/Disadvantages of Hemorrhage Models

Pros	Cons
Cardiac puncture produces consistent changes in blood pressure	Elevated mortality rate; limited blood volume to be withdrawn and assayed
Femoral artery is accessible for blood withdrawal and stable blood pressure	Controlled hemorrhage with defined resuscitation is not identical to clinical situations
Lung injury is consistently produced	

the mesenteric ischemia–reperfusion models do not involve hemorrhage, these models clearly rely on intestinal ischemia–reperfusion to provide noxious stimuli to the lung.

In those models involving rats, ~300-g animals are used. Following general anesthesia with intraperitoneal ketamine (50 mg/kg), collateral vessels from the inferior mesenteric artery and celiac axis are ligated and the superior mesenteric artery is occluded with a microvascular clip. Following 1 hr of ischemia, the clip is removed and reperfusion is confirmed by the return of pulsations in the mesenteric arcade. Following closure of the incision, animals are sacrificed from 30 to 240 min following reperfusion (29). This model reproducibly leads to acute lung injury as evident by neutrophil sequestration, pulmonary microvascular leak, and intrapulmonary hemorrhage. Further, this model leads to early pulmonary physiologic changes, including increased intrapulmonary shunt and dead space (30).

V. Models Using Intravenous Injections

Multiple substances have been injected intravenously to induce acute lung injury. Four commonly employed agents are endotoxin (LPS), live bacteria, cobra venom factor (immune complexes), and cytokines, particularly IL-2. The physiologic effects and experimental paradigms of each agent are discussed below, and advantages/disadvantages are compared in Table III.

In murine models of intravenous (IV) endotoxin, BALB/c mice(18–20 g) generally receive a single IV injection of LPS from *Escherichia coli* 0111:B4 at 3 mg/kg. Saline injections are used as a control: in general this is a nonlethal model and IV LPS induces the extravascular accumulation of albumin, neutrophil sequestration, and endothelial cell barrier dissruption. Interestingly, many of these changes are ablated when neutrophil adherence is limited using monoclonal antibodies to CD11b/CD18 (31).

In contrast to murine models, rat models of endotoxemia-induced acute lung injury require larger amounts of endotoxin. Rats (185–250 g) are used for study and a 4-hr continuous intravenous infusion of *E. coli* LPS (0127:B8) in a total dose of 100 mg/kg is used. Although this is also a nonlethal model, more immediate and pronounced changes in lung function are seen. Animals become tachypneic and develop a respiratory alkalosis and lung microvascular permeability, and lung wet/dry weight ratios are increased. These changes are seen immediately following the cessation of endotoxin infusion until at least 4 hr postinfusion (32). In rats, *Salmonella typhosa* LPS (20 mg/kg) may also be used to induce acute lung injury (33). Rabbit models of intravenous endotoxin-induced acute lung injury have also been described.

In this model, animals generally undergo tracheostomy and receive 0.9 mg/kg of *E. coli* LPS intravenously over 30 min. Four hours later, animals are sacrificed and subsequent pathologic changes within the lung are seen. These changes include neutrophil sequestration, alveolar proteinaceous fluid, pulmonary vascular congestion, edema, and necrotic cell debris (34). During the intravenous infusion of *E. coli* endotoxin, pressor support or hetastarch is often needed to maintain blood pressure. Further, the use of rabbits allows for the placement of arterial lines in the central ear artery. Larger animals models of acute lung injury following administration of endotoxin levels have also been described.

In sheep, animals receive 2 mg/kg of *E. coli* endotoxin (often serotype 055:B5) and changes in lung pathology can be measured as early as 15 min out to 24 hr after endotoxin administration. Changes consistently seen include increases in pulmonary artery pressure and lung lymph flow mediated primarily by thromboxane B_2 (35). In porcine models of endotoxemia, animals receive *E. coli* LPS over 20 min at dosages up to 250 μg/kg. Larger animal models allow for Swan–Ganz catheter, flow probe, and tonometer placement. Intravenous LPS in pigs induces hypotension, with decreases in SVR and cardiac output. Hypoxemia is secondary to increased intrapulmonary shunting, with the above changes occurring within 3 hr of endotoxin administration (36).

The intravenous infusion of cobra venom factor (CVF) activates complement and produces a lung injury model that is neutrophil dependent and oxygen-radical mediated (37). Usually pathogen-free, adult rats are used; animals receive 2 U cobra venom factor intravenously, and 30 min after infusion, consistent lung injury is found. Using ^{125}I-labeled bovine serum albumin (BSA) and ^{51}Cr-labeled rat red cells, increased lung microvascular permeability, intrapulmonary hemorrhage, and neutrophil sequestration are seen. In the

Table III Advantages/Disadvantages of Intravenous Models

Pros	Cons
Multiplicity of agents will induce acute lung injury	Tracheostomy is required in multiple models
Generally, models are nonlethal	Variable degrees of hypotension are produced, requiring pressor support
Consistently produce acute lung injury	Marked variability in time frame for acute lung injury
Applicable in small to larger animal models	

CVF model of acute lung injury, L- and P-selectin expression are required (38).

The most commonly used bacterial species infused intravenously to produce acute lung injury is *Pseudomonas aeruginosa*. This model has been utilized almost exclusively in porcine models with the infusion of 5×10^8 colony-forming units intravenously over 1 hr (39). Changes consistent with acute lung injury are reproducibly seen within 60 min. These changes include increases in peak inspiratory pressures, pulmonary artery pressure, and hypoxemia. Bronchoalveolar lavage protein levels, neutrophils, and lung myeloperoxidase levels increase significantly. Further, these changes continue through at least a 5-hr experimental protocol; in general, this is a nonlethal model of acute lung injury (40).

Last, acute lung injury has been produced with cytokine infusion, most commonly IL-2. In rats, animals receive 10^6 U IL-2 and are sacrificed from 0 to 6 hr after the infusion, which takes place over 1 hr. IL-2 infusion induces an increase in lung wet/dry weight ratios, lung permeability, and neutrophil sequestration (41). A similar procedure may used in sheep; animals are infused with 10^5 U/kg of IL-2 and acute lung injury is seen over the next 5 hr. Peak airway pressure and lung lymph flow increase along with peripheral neutropenia and thrombocytopenia (42).

VI. Aspiration-Induced Models

There are several models based on aspiration-induced acute lung injury. Advantages/disadvantages are given in Table IV. Aerosolized LPS has been used to induce acute lung injury. In this model, adult rats weighing between 250 and 350 g are used. Following general anesthesia and in the upright position, aerosolized LPS (7 mg/kg) dissolved in 0.5 ml of phosphate-buffered saline (PBS) is administered intratracheally. The rats usually regain consciousness within 1 hr, although lethality in this model is 30–40% (43). Lung injury is seen within 24 hr and includes increases in wet/dry lung weight ratios, intrapulmonary hemorrhage, and neutrophil sequestration. Alternatively, rats may be injected intratracheally with an aqueous preparation of endotoxin. Typically, 5.0 μg of *S. typhosa* is administered, with acute lung injury being seen from 1 to 24 hr after the intratracheal injection of LPS (44). This model leads to a marked increase in neutrophil recovery in bronchoalveolar lavage (BAL) fluid. IL-1β expression increases, and histology consistent with an organizing pneumonia is seen.

Acute lung injury may also be induced by repeat lung lavages with normal saline. In tracheostomized rabbits, 25 ml/kg of warmed 0.9% normal saline is instilled followed by the injection of 1–3 cm^3 of air. Typically the procedure is repeated four to six times and will produce $P_{aO}2$ less than 60 torr (45). Lung injury is consistently seen almost immediately, with most protocols ending from 4 to 6 hr after completion of lung lavage. Lung lavage with normal saline produces hypoxemia, decreased dynamic lung compliance, hyaline membrane formation, and leukocyte infiltration.

Cytokine instillation into the lung also produces acute lung injury, with IL-1β being the most commonly utilized agent. In adult rats, intratracheal IL-1β (50 μg) is administered followed by two puffs of air with a 3-ml syringe. Total injection volume equals 0.5 ml. In general, this is a nonlethal model of acute lung injury at least out to 4 hr postprocedure. Changes in pulmonary physiology include elevated lavage cytokine-induced neutrophil chemoattractant (CINC) levels, lavage neutrophil counts, and lung myeloperoxidase (46).

Last, the intrapulmonary instillation of IgG immune complexes produces an aspiration-induced acute lung injury. In this model, pathogen-free rats have immune complex-induced lung injury by using the intratracheal instillation of 2.5 mg anti-BSA in 300 μl saline followed by IV injection of 10 mg BSA (47). Rats are sacrificed 4 hr later and acute lung injury is seen. Changes include increased pulmonary permeability, hemorrhage, and neutrophil sequestration.

A prospective, randomized controlled animal study has provided details of the physiologic effects of four different animal models. In this study, four separate porcine models of acute lung injury were studied (48). These included (1) intrapulmonary arterial infusion of *E. coli* endotoxin, (2) bronchoalveolar instillation of 0.05 *N* hydrochloric acid, (3) repeated bronchoalveolar lavage with warmed saline, and (4) intrapulmonary arterial intravenous infusion of oleic acid. Changes consistent with acute lung injury were seen as early as 60 min after injury and continued for at least

Table IV Advantages/Disadvantages of Aspiration Models

Pros	Cons
Technically easy, relatively inexpensive	Significant mortality rates in a variety of aspiration models
Multiplicity of agents can be used to induce acute lung injury	Variable production of pathophysiologic changes (i.e., hypoxemia)
Prospective randomized study completed to allow for comparison of models	

165 min. Salient findings were lack of tachycardia or changes in SVR in any model. Second, hydrochloric acid instillation and saline lavage produce hypoxemia. Third, endotoxin infusion increases mean pulmonary artery pressure (PAP) and pulmonary vascular resistance (PVR), contributing to decreases in cardiac output and MAP. Hypoxemia was not produced in this model. Last, oleic acid infusion produces marked hypoxemia and increases mean PAP and PVR. Interestingly, none of the models led to the production of TNFα within the lung.

VII. Summary

In summary, acute lung injury may be produced in a variety of ways and in multiple experimental models. The ultimate model to be used by an investigator will likely depend on technical expertise, reagent availability, quantity of blood and tissue needed for analysis, and expense. In general, larger animal models allow for the acquisition of greater amounts of data, which needs to be balanced against the cost of the model.

References

1. Guice, K. S., Oldham, K. T., Johnson, K. J., Kunkel, R. G., Morganroth, M. L., and Ward, P. A. (1988). Pancreatitis induced acute lung injury. An ARDS model. *Ann. Surg.* **208**(1), 71–77.
2. Steer, M. L. (1985). Workshop on experimental pancreatitis in the rat induced by excessive doses of a pancreatic secretagogue. *Dig. Dis. Sci.* **30,** 575–581.
3. Guice, K. S., Oldham, K. T., Wolfe, R. R., and Simmons, R. H. (1987). Lung injury in acute pancreatitis: Primary inhibition of pulmonary phospholipid synthesis. *Am. J. Surg.* **153,** 54–61.
4. Chiara, O., Giomarelli, P. P., Borrelli, E., Alseeandro, C., Segala, M., and Grossi, A. (1991). Inhibition by methylprednisolone of leukocyte-induced pulmonary damage. *Crit. Care Med.* **19**(2) 260–265.
5. Goris, R. J. A., Boekholtz, W. K. F., VanBebber, I. P. T., *et al.* (1986). Multiple organ failure and sepsis without bacteria. An experimental model. *Arch. Surg.* **121,** 896.
6. Morisaki, T., Goya, T., Toh, H., Nishihara, K., and Torisu, M. (1991). The anti mac-1 monoclonal antibody inhibits neutrophil sequestration in lung and liver in a septic murine model. *Clin. Immunol. Immunopathol.* **61,** 365–376.
7. Vedder, N. B., Fouty, B. W., Winn, R. K., Harlan, J. M., and Rice, C. L. (1989). Role of neutrophils in generalized reperfusion injury associated with resuscitation from shock. *Surgery* **106,** 509–516.
8. Anderson, B. S., Brown, J. M., Bensard, D. D., Grosso, M. A., Banerjee, A., Patt, A., Whitman, G. J., and Harken, A. H. (1990). Reversible lung neutrophil accumulation can cause lung injury by elastase-mediated mechanisms. *Surgery* **108**(2), 262–268.
9. Chaudry, I. H., Wichterman, K. A., and Baue, A. E. (1979). Effect of sepsis on tissue adenine nucleotide levels. *Surgery* **85,** 205–211.
10. Bohnen, J. M., Matlow, A. G., Mustard, R. A., *et al.* (1988). Antibiotic efficacy in intraabdominal sepsis: A clinically relevant model. *Can. J. Microbiol.* **34,** 323–326.
11. Villar, J., Ribeiro, S. P., Mullen, B. M., Kuliszewski, M., Post, M., and Slutsky, A. S. (1994). Induction of the heat shock responses reduces mortality rate and organ damage in a sepsis-induced acute lung injury model. *Crit. Care Med.* **22**(6), 914–921.
12. Katzenstein, A. A., and Askin, F. B. (1982). Diffuse alveolar damage. *In* "Surgical Pathology of Nonneoplastic Lung Disease," Vol. 13. (J. L. Bennington, ed), pp. 9–42. W.B. Saunders, Philadelphia.
13. Ribeiro, S. P., Villar, J., Downey, G. P., Edelson, J. D., and Slutsky, A. S. (1994). Sodium arsenite induces heat shock protein-72 kilodalton expression in the lungs and protects rats against sepsis. *Crit. Care Med.* **22**(6), 922–929.
14. Hill, J., Lindsay, T., Rusche, J., Valeri, R., Shepro, D., and Hechtman, H. B., (1992). A Mac-1 Antibody reduces liver and lung injury but not neutrophil sequestration after intestinal ischemia-reperfusion. *Surgery* **112**(2), 166–172.
15. Kishimoto, T. K., Jutila, M. A., Berg, E. L., and Buthcer, E. C. (1989). Neutrophil Mac-1 and MEL-14 adhesion proteins inversely regulated chemotatic factors. *Science* **245,** 1238–1241.
16. Seekamp, A., Till, G. O., Mullilgan, M. S., Paulson, J. C., Anderson, D. C., Miyasaka, M., and Ward, P. A. (1994). Role of selectins in local and remote tissue injury following ischemia and reperfusion. *Am. J. Pathol.* **144**(3), 592–598.
17. Mulligan, M. S., Lowe, J. B., Larsen, R. D., Paulson, J., Zheng, Z., DeFrees, S., Maemura, K., Fukuda, M., and Ward, P. A. (1993). Projective effects of sialylated oligosaccharides in immune complex-induced acute lung injury. *J. Exp. Med.* **178,** 623–631.
18. Kluasner, J. M., Anner, H., Paterson, I. S., Kobzik, L., Valeri, C. R., Shepro, D., and Hechtman, H. B. (1988). Lower torso ischemia-induced lung injury is leukocyte dependent. *Ann. Surg.* **208**(6), 761–767.
19. Anner, H., Kaufman, R. P., Kobzik, L., *et al.* (1987). Pulmonary leukoseuqestration induced by hind limb ischemia. *Ann. Surg.* **206,** 162–167.
20. Parsey, M. V., Tuder, R. M., and Abraham, E. (1998). Neutrophils are major contributors to intraparenchymal lung IL-1β expression after hemorrhage and endotoxemia. *J. Immunol.* **160**(2), 1007–1013.
21. Shenkar, R., Coulson, W. F., and Abraham, E. (1994). Hemorrhage and resuscitation induce alterations in cytokine expression and the development of acute lung injury. *Am. J. Respir. Cell Mol. Biol.* **10,** 290.
22. Abraham, E., Jesmok, G., Tuder, R., Allbee, J., and Chang, Y. (1995). Contribution of tumor necrosis factor-α to pulmonary cytokine expression and lung injury after hemorrhage and resuscitation. *Crit. Care Med.* **23**(8), 1319–1326.
23. Angle, N., Hoyt, D. B., Coimbra, R., Liu, F., Herdon-Remelius, C., Loomis, W., and Junger, W. G. (1998). Hypertonic saline resusciation diminishes lung injury by suppressing neutrophil activation after hemorrhagic shock. *Shock* **9**(3), 164–170.
24. Hampton, M., Chambers, S., Vissers, M., and Winterbourn, C. C. (1994). Bacterial killing by neutrophils in hypertonic environments. *J. Infect. Dis.* **169,** 839–846.
25. Fan, J., Marshall, J. C., Jimenez, M., Shek, P. N., Zagorski, J., and Rotstein, O. D. (1998). Hemorrhagic shock primes for increased expression of cytokine-induced neutrophil chemoattractant in the lung: Role in pulmonary inflammation following lipopolysaccharide. *J. Immunol.* **161**(1), 440–447.
26. Rizoli, S. B., Kapus, A., Fan, J., Li, Y. H., Marshall, J. C., Rotstein, O. D. (1998). Immunomodulatory effects of hypertonic resuscitation on the development of lung inflammation following hemorrhagic shock. *J. Immunol.* **161**(11), 6288–6296.
27. Hardaway, R. M., Williams, C. H., Marvasti, M., Farias, M., Tseng, A., Pinon, I., Yanez, D., Martinez, M., and Navar, J. (1990). Prevention of adult respiratory distress syndrome with plasminogen activator in pigs. *Crit. Care Med.* **18**(12), 1413–1418.
28. Rizoli, S. B., Kapus, A., Parodo, J., Fan, J., Rotstein, O. D., Hypertonic immunomodulation is reversible and accompanied by changes in CD11b expression. *J. Surg. Res.* **83,** 130–135.

29. Sorkine, P., Setton, A., Halpern, P., Miller, A., Rudick, V., Marmor, S., Klausner, J. M., and Goldman, G. (1995). Soluble tumor necrosis factor receptors reduce bowel ischemia-induced lung permeability and neutrophil sequestration. *Crit. Care Med.* **23**(8), 1377–1381.
30. Koike, K., Moore, E. E., Moore, F. A., Carl, V. S., Pitman, J. M., and Banerjee, A. (1992). Phospholipase A_2 inhibition decouples lung injury from gut ischemia-reperfusion. *Surgery* **112**(2), 173–180.
31. Miotla, J. M., Williams, T. J., Hellewell, P. G., and Jeffery, P. K. (1996). A role for the β_2 integren CD11b in mediating experimental lung injury in mice. *Am. J. Respir. Cell Mol. Biol.* **14,** 363–373.
32. Schneider, J., Friderichs, E., Heintze, K., and Flohe, L. (1990). Effects of recombinant human superoxide dismutase on increased lung vascular permeability and respiratory disorder in endotoxemic rats. *Circ. Shock* **30,** 97–106.
33. Aaron, S. D., Valenza, F., Volgyesi, G., Mullen, J. B. M., Slutsky, A. S., and Steward, T. E. (1998). Inhibition of exhaled nitric oxide production during sepsis does not prevent lung inflammation. *Crit. Care Med.* **26**(2), 309–314.
34. Rotta, A. T., and Steinhorn, D. M. (1998). Partial liquid ventilation reduces pulmonary neutrophil accumulation in an experimental model of systemic endotoxemia and acute lung injury. *Crit. Care Med.* **26**(10), 1707–1715.
35. Wisner, D., Sturm, J., Sutter, G., Ellendorf, B., and Nerlich, M. (1988). Thromboxane receptor blockade in an animal model of ARDS. *Surgery* **104**(1), 91–97.
36. Cohn, S. M., Kruithoff, K. L., Rothschild, H. R., Wang, H., Antonsson, J. B., and Fink, M. P. (1991). Beneficial effects of LY203647, a novel leukotriene C_4/D_4 antagonist, on pulmonary function and mesenteric perfusion in a porcine model of endotoxic shock and ARDS. *Cir. Shock* **33,** 7–16.
37. Mulligan, M. S., Polley, M. J., Bayer, R. J., Nunn, M. F., Paulson, J. C., and Ward, P. A. (1992). Neutrophil-dependent acute lung injury. *J. Clin. Invest.* **90,** 1600–1607.
38. Mulligan, M. S., Watson, S. R., Fennie, C., and Ward, P. A. (1993). Protective effects of selectin chimeras in neutrophil-mediated lung injury. *J. Immunol.* **151**(11), 6410–6417.
39. Bloomfield, G. L., Holloway, S., Ridings, P. C., Fisher, B. J., Blocher, C. R., Sholley, M., Bunch, T., Sugerman, H. J., and Fowler, A. A. (1997). Pretreatment with inhaled nitric oxide inhibits neutrophil migration and oxidative activity resulting in attenuated sepsis-induced acute lung injury. *Crit. Care Med.* **25**(4), 584–593.
40. Ridings, P. C., Bloomfield, G. L., Holloway, S., Windsor, A. C. J., Jutila, M. A., Fowler, A. A. and Sugerman, H. J. (1995). Sepsis-induced acute lung injury is attenuated by selectin blockade following the onset of sepsis. *Arch. Surg.* **130,** 1199–1208.
41. Welbourn, R., Goldman, G., Kobzik, L., Paterson, I., Shepro, D., Hechtman, H. B. (1991). Interleukin-2 induces early multisystem organ edema mediated by neutrophils. *Ann. Surg.* **214**(2), 181–186.
42. Klausner, J. M., Paterson, I. S., Goldman, G., Kobzik, L., Lelcuk, S., Skornick, Y., Eberlein, T., Valeri, R., Shepro, D., and Hechtman, H. B. (1991). Interleukin-2-induced lung injury is mediated by oxygen free radicals. *Surgery* **109**(2), 169–175.
43. Turner, C. R., Lackey, M. N., Quinlan, M. F., Griswold, D. E., Schwartz, L. W., and Wheeldon, E. B. (1991). Therapeutic intervention in a rat model of adult respiratory distress syndrome: II. Lipoxygenase pathway inhibition. *Circ. Shock* **34,**263–269.
44. Tang, W. W., Yi, E. S., Remick, D. G., Wittwer, A., Yin, S., Qi, M., and Ulich, T. R. (1995). Intratracheal injection of endotoxin and cytokines. IX. Contribution of CD11a/ICAM-1to neutrophil emigration. *Am. Physiol. Soc.* **269**(5, Pt. 1), L653–L659.
45. Rimensberger, P. C., Fedorko, L., Cutz, E., and Bohn, D. J. (1998). Attenuation of ventilator-induced acute lung injury in an animal model by inhibition of neutrophil adhesion by leumedins (NPC 15669). *Crit. Care Med.* **26**(3), 548–555.
46. Koh, Y., Hybertson, B. M., Jepson, E. K., Cho, O. J., and Repine, J. E. (1995). Cytokine-induced neutrophil chemoattractant is necessary for interleukin-1-induced lung leak in rats. *Am. Physiol. Soc.* **79**(2), 472–478.
47. Mulligan, M. S., Vaporciyan, A. A., Warner, R. L., Jones, M. L., Foreman, K. E., Miyasaka, M., Todd, R. F., and Ward, P. A. (1995). Compartmentalized roles for leukocytic adhesion molecules in lung inflammatory injury. *J. Immunol.* **154**(3), 1350–1363.
48. Rosenthal, C., Caronia, C., Quinn, C., Lugo, N., and Sagy, M. (1998). A comparison among animal models of acute lung injury. *Crit. Care Med.* **26**(5), 912–916.

34

Tumor Angiogenesis

Lee M. Ellis

Departments of Surgical Oncology and Cancer Biology, The University of Texas M. D. Anderson Cancer Center, Houston, Texas 77030

I. Biology of Angiogenesis

A. Introduction

Currently, no other field in cancer research is undergoing such explosive growth as that of tumor angiogenesis. More than 600 papers were published on aspects of angiogenesis in 1998, and this field of research is closely scrutinized by scientists, clinicians, and patients. Patients are highly attuned to information as regards the initiation of antiangiogenic trials. Unfortunately, little information other than toxicity data is available regarding the efficacy of antiangiogenic therapy. However, the basic biology of the process of angiogenesis must be understood before effective antiangiogenic therapy can be developed.

By definition, "angiogenesis" is the establishment of a neovascular blood supply derived from preexisting blood vessels—specifically, from postcapillary venules. In contrast, "vasculogenesis" is the embryonic establishment of a blood supply from mesodermal precursors such as angioblasts or hemangioblasts. The processes of angiogenesis and vasculogenesis are very similar; it is now apparent that the process of tumor angiogenesis is, in reality, a combination of the above, in which the main blood supply to a tumor is derived from preexisting blood vessels, but circulating endothelial cell precursors may contribute to the growing endothelial cell mass.

Pioneering work from the laboratory of Folkman and colleagues over the past 30 years has established that tumor growth depends on angiogenesis (1–3). Direct observation of tumor growth demonstrates that the rapid exponential growth of a tumor does not occur until neovascularization occurs. Furthermore, tumor growth in organs in which blood vessels do not proliferate is limited to the distance that oxygen can diffuse (1–2 mm). Further evidence to support the dependence of tumor growth on angiogenesis is the fact that the proliferative index of tumor cells decreases with increasing distance from the nearest capillary blood vessel. The proliferation of tumor cells is directly proportional to the labeling index of vascular endothelial cells in the tumor. Last, some angiogenic inhibitors can inhibit tumor growth *in vivo* yet have no effect on tumor cells *in vitro*. These principles, established by Folkman and colleagues, have provided the foundation for our understanding of the biology of tumor angiogenesis as well as the development of potential antineoplastic therapies (3).

Angiogenesis is an essential step both in the growth of primary tumors and in metastasis (see Chapter 36, Fig. 1) (4). For a tumor to become clinically relevant, angiogenesis must occur to provide nutrients to the growing tumor mass.

This neovascular blood supply is also essential for increasing the chance that tumor cells will gain access to the circulation and thus embolize to form a metastasis at a different site. Once a tumor establishes an invasive phenotype in the organ of metastasis, it must establish its own neovascular blood supply to grow there. Numerous investigators have established the association of tumor angiogenesis with metastasis. A landmark publication from Weidner *et al.* (5) in 1991 brought to the forefront the principle that tumor vascularity could be used to predict the biologic aggressiveness of individual tumor types. In that study, breast cancer specimens were stained for factor VIII-related antigen (FVIII-RA), which highlights endothelial cells; these investigators were able to demonstrate that the vascularity of breast cancers directly correlated with metastatic formation. This landmark study led the way to several other studies in which tumor vascularity and aggressiveness were examined in numerous tumor systems (6). The vast majority (~90%) of investigations have demonstrated a direct correlation between tumor vascularity and tumor aggressiveness; however, given that some have not demonstrated such an association, individual studies must be carefully evaluated to determine how patient selection and other study methods affect the conclusions drawn.

B. Historical Evolution of Angiogenic Concepts

Until Folkman's studies provided evidence that tumors depend on angiogenesis, tumors were thought to derive their blood supply from preexisting blood vessels. However, histologic analysis of tumors revealed that the morphology of the tumor vasculature was quite different than that of normal blood vessels. Furthermore, *in vivo* microscopy studies revealed that the blood supply of tumors was disorganized, with blood flow highly variable and even bidirectional (7). Thus, it became clear that the characteristics and phenotype of the tumor vasculature were quite different than those of the normal preexisting blood vessels.

Subsequent studies established that specific factors released from tumor cells could induce blood vessel formation. A simple model was developed in which a tumor cell would release a soluble factor that would then bind to an endothelial cell and induce endothelial cell proliferation, leading to a neovascular blood supply. A refinement of this model was proposed by Bouck (8), who hypothesized that the process of angiogenesis was actually the outcome of the balance between the effects of stimulatory and inhibitory molecules on this process, and that that balance may be regulated by oncogenes and tumor suppressor genes. According to this model, pathologic angiogenesis occurs when the effect of stimulatory molecules outweighs the effect of inhibitory molecules. A better understanding of the process of angiogenesis led to the realization that this process involves more than endothelial cells simply proliferating, but rather involves those cells dividing, invading the basement membrane, migrating, and eventually undergoing differentiation and capillary tube formation. This process is driven not only by angiogenic molecules, but also by other factors such as degradative enzymes that enhance the abovementioned processes. Interestingly, the processes of tumor angiogenesis and tumor cell invasion are very similar; in fact, these two processes are mediated by many of the same factors (Table I).

A hypothesis on the regulation of tumor angiogenesis suggests that tumor angiogenesis involves the use of preexisting blood vessels (cooption) as well as vascular regression and neovascularization (9). Initially, tumors coopt or use existing blood vessels within an organ for their nutrient blood supply. However, shortly thereafter, the existing vasculature becomes destabilized, most likely through the release of angiopoietin-2 (Ang-2) by endothelial cells. This loss of vascular integrity leads to relative hypoxia within the tumor. This hypoxia leads to up-regulation of vascular endothelial growth factor (VEGF) in the remaining tumor cells, which then leads to a robust angiogenic response. At that stage, the newly developed endothelial cells require stabilization, which is achieved through diffuse expression of angiopoietin-1 (Ang-1) by tumor cells and possibly through continued response to VEGF. Thus, the process of angiogenesis depends on the temporal coordination of factors that regulate pathways necessary for the establishment of stable conduits to provide a nutrient blood supply to the tumor (Fig. 1).

C. Angiogenic Effector Molecules

As alluded to previously, the process of angiogenesis is driven by the production of positive angiogenic factors that override the effect of inhibitory angiogenic factors

Table I Similarities between Angiogenesis and Tumor Cell Invasion

Process	Angiogenesis	Tumor invasion
Proliferation	X	X
Degradation of basement membrane	X	X
Invasion	X	X
Survival	X	X
Differentiation/tube formation	X	
Recruitment of supportive cells	X	
Genetic instability/defects		X

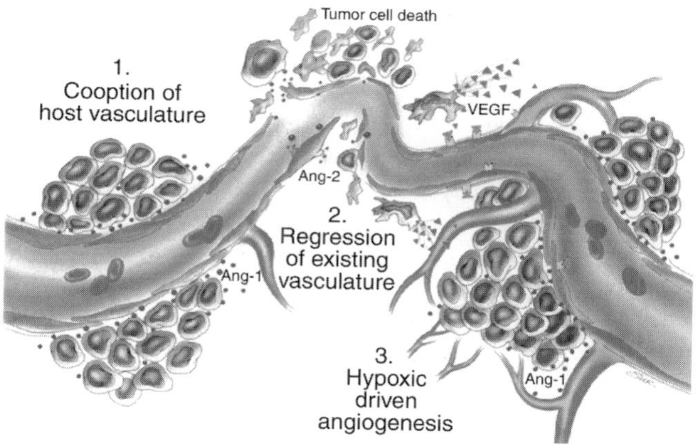

Figure 1 Host vessel cooption and induction of angiogenesis by tumors. A current hypothesis on tumor angiogenesis suggests that tumors initially use the existing vasculature for a nutrient blood supply. Endothelial cells then release Ang-2, which leads to vessel destabilization and relative hypoxia, which in turn lead to the release of VEGF and robust angiogenesis. (See color plates.)

(Table II). There are two basic classes of angiogenic factors, one being the specific factors released by numerous cell types that bind specifically to receptors on endothelial cells and the other being proangiogenic factors that not only bind to endothelial cells but also can affect the function of other cell types.

There are two important subclasses of specific angiogenic effector molecules. The most well characterized is the vascular endothelial growth factor family, which consists of the five VEGF molecules, designated A, B, C, D, and E, and the placenta growth factor (PlGF). The best characterized of these factors is VEGF-A, which will be referred to as VEGF in the remainder of this review. VEGF is known to be angiogenic in numerous *in vivo* and *in vitro* angiogenic models. In addition, VEGF has been associated with the aggressive phenotype in numerous solid malignancies (10–15). The importance of VEGF in tumor progression and angiogenesis is supported by the fact that numerous antiangiogenic strategies target VEGF activity.

Table II Endogenous Pro- and Antiangiogenic Factors

Proangiogenic	Antiangiogenic
Acidic and basic FGF	Angiostatin
Angiogenin	Antithrombin fragment
Hepatocyte growth factor	Endostatin
IL-8	Vasculostatin
Placenta growth factor	Interferon-α, -β, -γ
Platelet-derived endothelial cell growth factor	Platelet factor-4
Transforming growth factor-α, -β	Prolactin fragment
Tumor necrosis factor-α	Thrombospondins-1/2
Vascular endothelial growth factor/vascular permeability factor	TIMPs-1/2/3
Others	Others

VEGF is a 32- to 44-kDa protein secreted by nearly all cells. VEGF is expressed as four isoforms derived from alternate splicing of the mRNA (16). The smaller isoforms, VEGF-121 and VEGF-165 (the numbers denote the number of amino acids), are secreted from cells. The larger isoforms, VEGF-189 and VEGF-205, are cell-associated, and their functions are not well known at this time. Preliminary evidence suggests that overexpression of various isoforms of VEGF may have differential effects on tumor angiogenesis.

One distinguishing factor of VEGF is its ability to induce vascular permeability. In fact, this factor was originally named vascular permeability factor (VPF) and was subsequently found to be homologous to VEGF (17–19). The extent of vascular permeability induced by VEGF is 50,000 times that of histamine, the gold standard for induction of permeability. This action by VEGF allows proteins to diffuse into the interstitium and to form the lattice network onto which endothelial cells migrate.

VEGF-C is most commonly associated with lymphangiogenesis, but its expression has been associated recently with tumor angiogenesis in several systems (20–25). VEGF-C binds preferentially to the VEGF receptor 3 (as described further below). VEGF-B most likely plays an important role in vasculogenesis, but may also have other functions such as activating invasive enzymes on endothelial cells (26, 27). The role of VEGF-D is less well defined, but it may bind to the VEGF receptors 2 and 3 and may induce *in vivo* angiogenesis (28, 29). Little is known about VEGF-E except that it binds to the VEGF receptor 2 and can induce endothelial cell mitosis and angiogenesis (30, 31).

Receptors for VEGF are expressed almost exclusively on endothelial cells. Expression of the various VEGF receptors has been demonstrated on cells of neural origin, Kaposi's sarcoma cells, hematopoietic precursor cells, and other rare tumor cell types (32, 33). The current nomenclature for the VEGF receptors lists three receptors: VEGFR-1 (Flt-1), VEGFR-2 (Kdr/Flk-1), and VEGFR-3 (Flt-4). These tyrosine kinase receptors require dimerization to induce intracellular signaling; they bind to specific ligands as shown in Fig. 2. The receptors for VEGF may mediate distinct functions within the endothelial cell; e.g., VEGFR-1 may be important in migration whereas VEGF-R2 may be important in the induction of permeability and cell proliferation. The recent discovery of VEGF receptors on angiogenic precursors such as angioblasts and hemangioblasts as well as on other progenitor cells (32) may suggest that these precursor

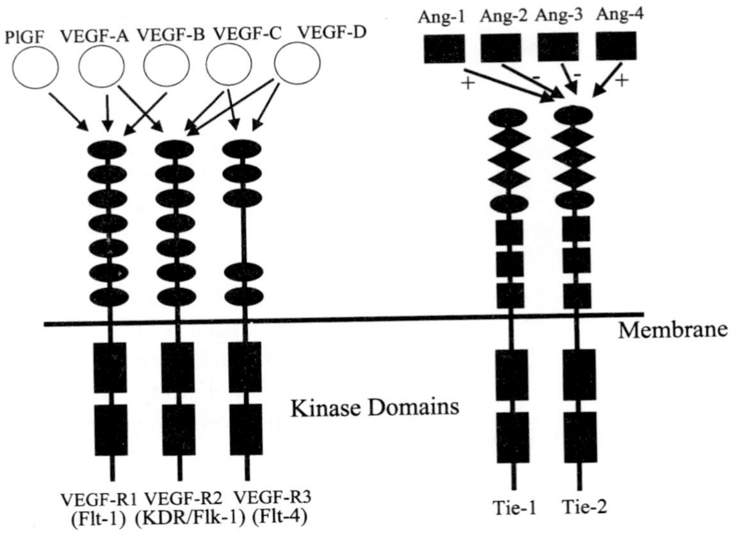

Figure 2 VEGF and angiopoietin family members and their receptors. At least five members of the VEGF family bind with different affinities to specific tyrosine kinase receptors, as discussed in the text. The angiopoietins bind to the Tie-2 tyrosine kinase receptor but have different downstream effects. Ang-1 activates the receptor and leads to vessel stability, whereas Ang-2 binds to the receptor, competitively inhibits Ang-1, and leads to vessel instability. Modified from Gale and Yancopoulos (38), *Genes & Development.*

cells may have a role in therapeutic angiogenesis for patients with vascular insufficiency. Another recently recognized receptor for VEGF, neuropilin, is typically expressed on neural cells but has also been identified on endothelial cells. Neuropilin binds only to VEGF-165 as a coreceptor to VEGF-R2 (34).

Another family of endothelial cell-specific molecules is the angiopoietin family. At present, the members of this family are designated angiopoietins 1 through 4, and the best characterized are Ang-1 and Ang-2. Ang-1 and -2 bind to the specific tyrosine kinase receptor Tie-2 on endothelial cells. Ang-1 acts as an agonist and is involved in endothelial cell differentiation and stabilization (35). In contrast, Ang-2 binds to Tie-2 and blocks the binding of Ang-1 to this receptor (36, 37). This blockade leads to endothelial cell destabilization and vascular regression (9). Although Tie-1 has been identified on endothelial cells, its ligand remains to be identified.

An insightful way to study the function of various molecules is to develop mice in which the gene in question has been "knocked out." Mice with homozygous knockout of the VEGF gene or any of the VEGF receptor genes die in the embryonic stage (38) from lethal defects in vascular development. Similarly, knockouts for Ang-1, Ang-2, Tie-1, or Tie-2 also lead to embryonic lethality from defective vascular development (39, 40). Thus, these factors are critical for vasculogenesis and are likely to play an essential role in tumor angiogenesis as well.

In addition to the specific angiogenic effector molecules described above are numerous nonspecific angiogenic molecules that affect the growth of other cell types in addition to that of endothelial cells. These factors include the fibroblast growth factors (acidic and basic), transforming growth factor-α and EGF (both of which bind to the EGF receptor), platelet-derived growth factor, platelet-derived endothelial cell growth factor (PD-ECGF), angiogenin, and the CXC chemokines IL-8, MIP, PF-4, and GRO (41). These factors are known to be angiogenic in *in vivo* models but are not specific for endothelial cells. However, the process of angiogenesis is probably not driven by a single molecule or family of molecules but rather depends on the cooperation and integration of various factors that lead to endothelial cell proliferation, migration, invasion, differentiation, and capillary tube formation. It is yet to be determined whether inhibiting the activity of a single angiogenic factor would lead to vascular compromise of significant duration. More likely, the redundancy in the angiogenic process would allow up-regulation of other angiogenic factors when a specific angiogenic factor is targeted with antiangiogenic therapy.

In addition to angiogenic factors that may induce the formation of new blood vessels, the newly developed blood vessels also must be able to survive under adverse conditions. Because the tumor microenvironment is low in oxygen tension and is acidic, angiogenic survival factors are necessary for endothelial cells to maintain their integrity under these conditions. VEGF has been shown to act as a survival factor for endothelial cells under various stress conditions, including serum starvation and hypoxia (42, 43). In addition, the integrins αvβ3 and αvβ5 have been shown to act as survival factors for endothelial cells, and disruption of the binding between integrins and the extracellular matrix may lead to endothelial cell death (44–46). Down-regulation of the function of these endothelial cell survival factors is currently being investigated as a therapeutic strategy (47). Furthermore, in the absence of other endothelial cell survival factors, pericytes may enhance survival of newly formed endothelial cells (48).

The development of a neovascular blood supply is a series of interlinked processes that is undoubtedly regulated by various angiogenic factors (49). For example, basic fibroblast growth factor (bFGF) is the most potent mitogen for endothelial cells, followed in potency by VEGF and PD-ECGF. VEGF and bFGF are also the most potent survival factors for endothelial cells, although bFGF also enhances the activity of degradative enzymes. Hepatocyte growth factor enhances motility to a greater extent than do other angiogenic factors. The roles of Ang-1 and Ang-2 in endothelial cell stabilization suggest that these molecules are most important in endothelial cell survival.

D. Upstream Regulation of Angiogenesis

Because the process of angiogenesis is driven by the production of angiogenic molecules, it is essential to understand the cascade of events leading to up-regulation of angiogenic factor expression and secretion. Signals that up-regulate angiogenic factors include extracellular signals, intrinsic up-regulation of signal transduction activity, and loss of tumor suppressor genes. Examples of these signals are discussed further below.

External signals that lead to induction of angiogenic factor expression include environmental stimuli such as hypoxia or a decrease in pH (50–52). In fact, hypoxia is the most potent stimulus for inducing angiogenic factors, especially VEGF. Hypoxic induction of VEGF is probably mediated through Src kinase activity, which then leads to downstream induction of signaling cascades and eventually an increase in the activity of hypoxia-inducible factor-1α (HIF-1α) (53, 54). This factor then increases the transcription of the VEGF gene, which in turn leads to the induction of angiogenesis. Other external factors that increase the angiogenic response include various cytokines and growth factors. Insulin growth factors 1 and 2, epidermal growth factor, hepatocyte growth factor, interleukin-1, and the platelet-derived growth factors have all been shown to up-regulate VEGF (55–57). Thus, antiangiogenic therapy could involve down-regulation of upstream targets of the angiogenic factors rather than targeting the angiogenic factors (54, 58).

Once a growth factor or a cytokine binds to its receptor, a cascade of intracellular signaling events is initiated. Two specific signal transduction pathways are well known to mediate the up-regulation of angiogenic factors—the PI3 kinase/Akt signal transduction pathway, which eventually leads to stabilization of HIF-1α (59, 60), and the MAP kinase pathway, in which activation of Erk-1/2 activated factors that increase transcription of the VEGF gene (61). Activated Ras and Src also have been shown in *in vivo* models to be associated with increased VEGF production and angiogenesis (62). Again, therapeutic strategies that target the upstream effector molecules in angiogenesis may be a rational means for inducing antiangiogenesis. Inhibitors to signal transduction molecules have been shown to inhibit angiogenesis in *in vivo* tumor models (54).

Protein products of tumor suppressor genes such as the Von-Hippel–Lindau (VHL) or p53 genes also regulate angiogenesis. The wild-type VHL protein represses transcriptional regulation of the VEGF gene (63–65). A loss of heterozygosity with a mutation in the remaining VHL allele leads to loss of transcriptional control of the VEGF gene and overexpression of VEGF. Mutant p53 has also been associated with an increase in angiogenesis (66). Reinsertion of the wild-type p53 gene into cells with mutant p53 can down-regulate VEGF expression and angiogenesis (58). Thus, the process of angiogenesis is driven by external forces (including environmental stimuli), aberrations in internal signaling, and alterations in tumor suppressor gene function.

II. Models of Angiogenesis

A. Techniques for Examining Angiogenic Activity in Tumor Specimens

Studying the process of angiogenesis requires that angiogenic activity be analyzed in tumors or tissues. Historically, angiogenesis in tumor specimens has been examined by using standard radiographic techniques such as angiography, computed tomography scanning, or magnetic resonance imaging. However, these techniques provide only general estimates of the degree of angiogenesis from tumor type to tumor type; they cannot be used to assess variations in angiogenesis among patients with similar tumors. Studying angiogenesis in tumor specimens requires that tissue be obtained for histologic evaluation. For the evaluation of human tumor specimens, the gold standard technique is to highlight the tumor endothelium with antibodies that differentiate endothelial cells from other cells within the tumor (67). The first such antibody to be used for this purpose, FVIII-RA, is still in use; other endothelial cell-specific antibodies include CD31/PECAM, CD34, CD36, TEC-11, and

UEA, with the most common at present being FVIII-RA, CD31, and CD34.

Once a slide is prepared, then the level of angiogenesis must be quantified within the tumor. Such quantifications require systematic analysis by one of several possible means. For example, the five most vascularized areas in a tumor can be scanned at low power and the number of vessels in these areas counted under higher magnification. In certain tumors, such as colon or gastric cancers, the location at which the vessels were counted must be defined, because vessel counts can differ depending on their distance from the invading edge of the tumor (11, 12). The number of blood vessels can be quantified either in a single high-power field or in several high-power fields and the number averaged for the individual tumor specimen (Fig. 3).

In addition to counting blood vessels in a high-power field, the degree of vasculature can also be graded on a scale of 0 to 3+, where 3+ indicates the most vascularity. This subjective approach is prone to problems with reproducibility. Another method for analyzing tumor angiogenesis involves highlighting the vessels with an endothelial cell-specific antibody as described above and using computer-aided image analysis to determine the proportion of the area occupied by positively stained cells. Computer software and access to imaging systems are necessary for this technique. Another method for quantifying the degree of angiogenesis is to count the number of branch points in vessels within a tumor. Last, the Chalkley grid method (68), common in Europe, involves the use of an eyepiece with imprinted crossbars that overlap the examining field of a tumor that has been stained with an endothelial-specific antibody. The areas in which an endothelial cell intersects a crossbar in the eyepiece are counted, and the total sum in a high-power field of these counts equals the "Chalkley score."

Why is angiogenesis associated with metastasis? The study of angiogenic activity within a tumor has demonstrated that increased angiogenic activity is associated with increased aggressiveness of a particular tumor type. This association holds true in numerous tumor types, including melanoma; breast, colon, and rectal cancers; central nervous system malignancies; ovarian, cervical, and uterine malignancies; lung cancer; thyroid cancer; testicular, prostate, and bladder cancers; head and neck cancers; squamous cell carcinomas; sarcomas; gastric cancers; and other malignancies (6). In more than 90% of reported studies, an association has been found between high angiogenic activity and poor survival in patients with the above-mentioned tumors. However, exceptions have been reported as well. These exceptions beg the question of why angiogenesis would be associated with metastasis. The answer to this question has three components. First, the number of tumor cells released into the circulation correlates with the chance that a clinically relevant metastasis will develop; the greater the number of blood vessels in a primary tumor, the greater the tumor mass and the greater the number of cells that can be shed into the circulation. Second, for tumor cells to embolize within the circulation, a large surface area must be available where tumor cells and endothelial cells can interact. The greater the number of blood vessels in a primary tumor, the greater the surface area by which tumor cells may be able to invade into endothelial cell channels and thus embolize to a distant site. Third, evidence exists to suggest that endothelial cells secrete factors that serve as growth factors for tumor cells. Thus, the greater the number of endothelial cells, the greater the stimulus for tumor cell proliferation.

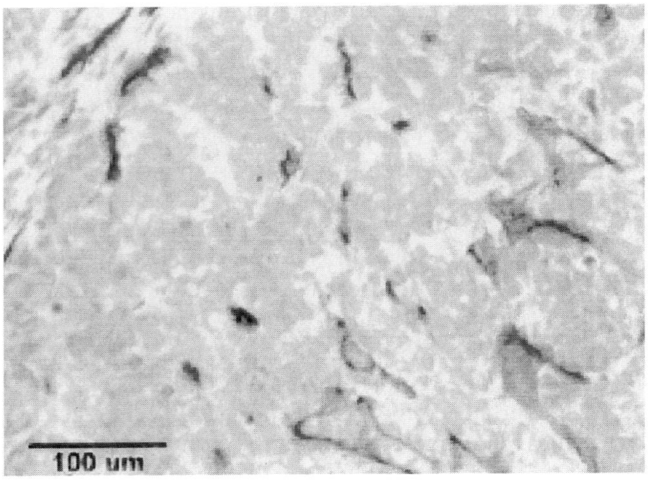

Figure 3 Examination of tumors for vessel counts. Tumors are harvested and frozen or paraffin embedded. Sections are then stained with an endothelial cell-specific marker and quantified as described in the text. From Shaheen *et al.* (84), with permission. (See color plates.)

B. Experimental Models of Angiogenesis

For the study of angiogenesis in experimental systems, numerous *in vivo* and *in vitro* models have been established. Among the *in vivo* models is the corneal micropocket assay (69). In this system, a polymer pellet is implanted in a micropocket made within the cornea of the experimental animal several millimeters from the limbus region. The polymer is usually impregnated with an angiogenic factor such as bFGF or VEGF. After several days, an influx of blood vessels becomes apparent from the limbus region toward the pellet. Using this assay in combination with systemic administration of an antiangiogenic agent provides a means of detecting antiangiogenic activity. This assay was conducted with rabbits, but rat and mouse models have been developed as well (Fig. 4).

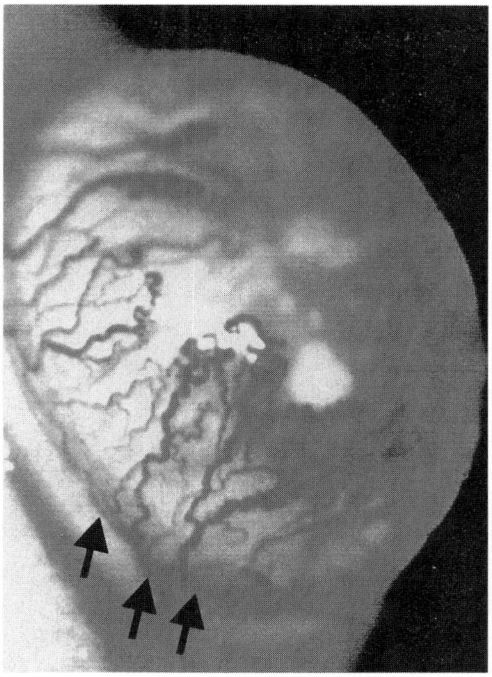

Figure 4 Mouse corneal assay for angiogenesis. A micropocket is created in the mouse cornea and a pellet impregnated with an angiogenic factor is implanted therein. Angiogenesis will commence from the corneal margin (arrows). This assay can be used to test systemic inhibitors of angiogenesis by examining the ability of agents to block this neovascularization. From (69), Kenyon *et al.* (1996). A model of angiogenesis in the mouse cornea. *Invest. Ophthalmol. Vis. Sci.* **37,** 1625–1632, with permission from the Association for Research in Vision and Ophthalmology. (See color plates.)

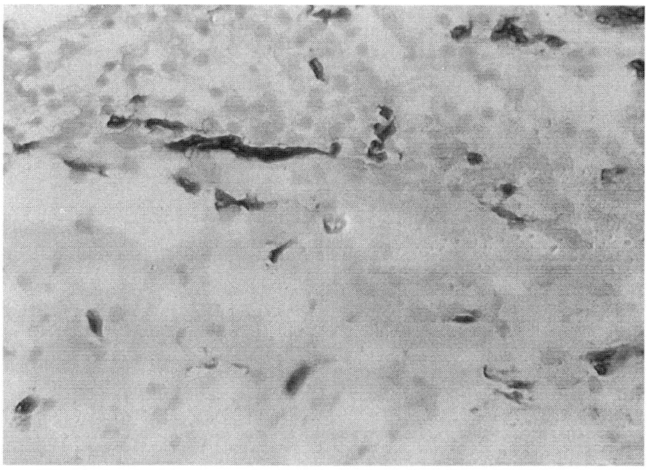

Figure 5 Matrigel plug assay for angiogenesis. A Matrigel plug (usually mixed with an angiogenic agent) is implanted subcutaneously, harvested (typically 7–10 days later), and processed for immunohistochemistry for the study of newly formed blood vessels. In this specimen, the sample was stained for CD31 (brown) to denote the ingrowth of endothelial cells from the host. Courtesy of Marya McCarty, The University of Texas M. D. Anderson Cancer Center, Houston, Texas. (See color plates.)

Another method for evaluating the activity of angiogenic factors or antiangiogenic agents is to inject a Matrigel plug beneath the skin of mice (70, 71). Matrigel is a liquid at 4°C, but at body temperature it forms a gelatin plug into which vessels grow within 8–10 days after injection. The Matrigel plug can be harvested and processed for immunohistochemical staining for endothelial cell markers; alternatively, hemoglobin, which provides an indirect measure of angiogenic activity, can be extracted from the plug and quantified (Fig. 5).

In the dorsal air sac chamber assay, air is injected subcutaneously on the backs of mice for several days in order to create a pocket. After this air injection, tumor cells grown on semipermeable Millipore filters are implanted within this dorsal air sac chamber and the skin is closed (58). Several days later, the superior skin flap is raised, and angiogenic activity can be observed directly through this transparent chamber (Fig. 6).

Another more complex method for examining angiogenesis is *in vivo* microscopy. Jain has established numerous models of glass chamber assays in which a window is created in the dorsum or cranium of a mouse (72, 73). A tumor can be implanted in this window, and the angiogenic activity as it grows can be visualized directly with *in vivo* microscopy. This technique can also be used to measure blood flow dynamics, permeability, and adherence of cells to the tumor microvasculature.

Numerous *in vitro* models of angiogenesis have various merits as well. The simplest angiogenesis model is that of endothelial cell proliferation (74). Among the endothelial cell lines commonly used are human umbilical vein endothelial cells, human dermal microvascular endothelial cells, and cells from other sources such as the aorta or pulmonary artery. Several other cell lines, such as bovine aortic endothelial cells, have been established from other species. These cells can be used in standard proliferation assays. Similarly, these endothelial cells, which are not immortalized, can be used to assay cell invasion or migration through collagen gels or in Boyden chambers (75).

Another *in vitro* assay involving endothelial cells is the tube formation assay. Endothelial cells will grow on an underlying matrix such as Matrigel or collagen gels, but will form tubes only in the presence of appropriate angiogenic factors (Fig. 7). This process is thought to represent differentiation like that which occurs in tumor angiogenesis. However, numerous cell types have been shown to form tubes under appropriate growth conditions, and thus this system may not be specific for endothelial cell differentiation (76).

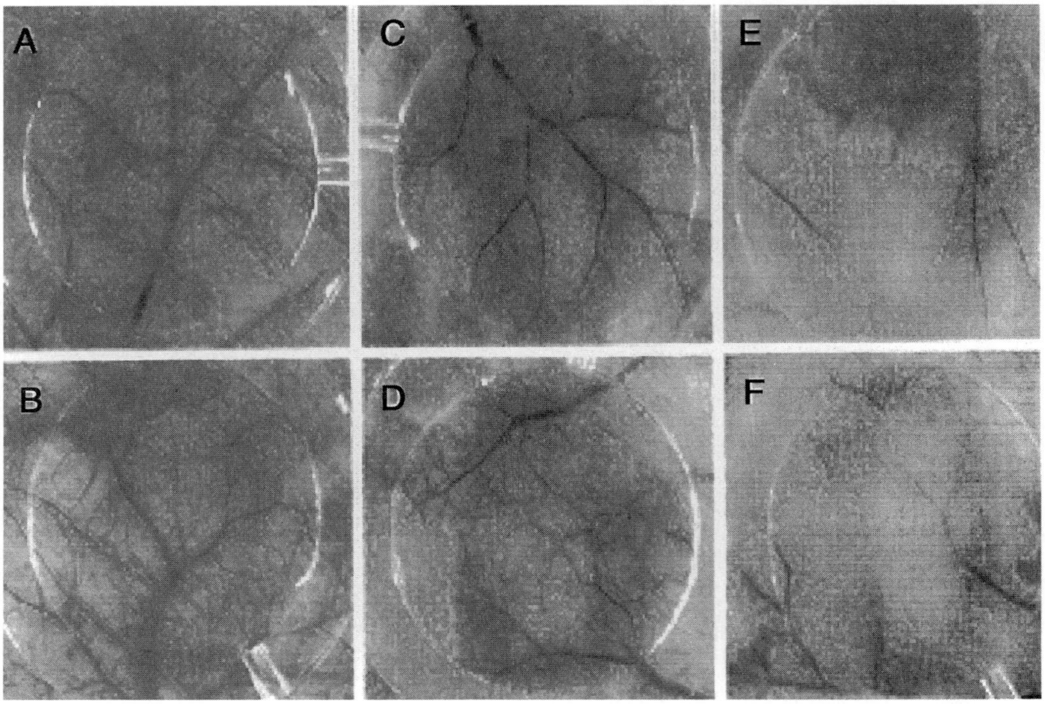

Figure 6 Dorsal air sac chamber assay for angiogenesis. A subcutaneous pocket is created on the back or flank of mice by repeated injections of air. Cells are then grown on a semipermeable membrane, the membrane is implanted in this pocket, and 7–10 days later the skin flap is retracted and the density of blood vessels observed. In this experiment, the cells on the right (panels E and F) were infected with the wild-type p53 gene, which down-regulated VEGF expression. The cells in panels A–D were controls. From Bouvet *et al.* (58), with permission. (See color plates.)

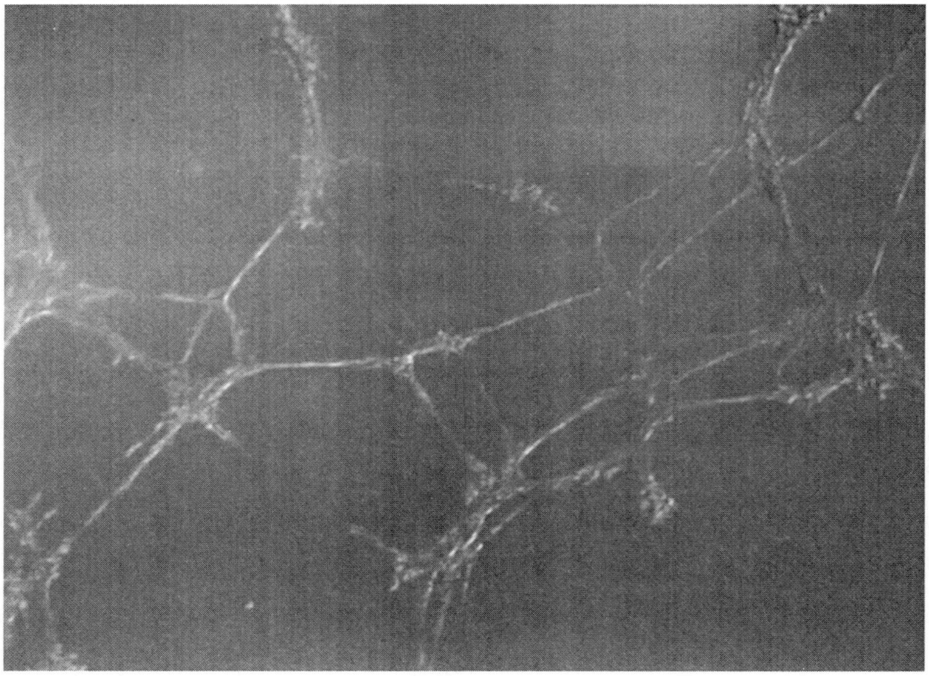

Figure 7 Capillary tube formation. In this assay, endothelial cells are plated on a collagen matrix or Matrigel with or without additional angiogenic or antiangiogenic factors. The ability to form tubelike structures as shown here suggests differentiation and tube formation. Courtesy of Marya McCarty, The University of Texas M. D. Anderson Cancer Center, Houston, Texas.

A standard angiogenesis assay that has been used over many years has been the chorioallantoic membrane (CAM) assay (77, 78), which involves the use of fertilized chicken eggs. This assay can be done in several ways. In one, a square window of a fertilized egg is carefully excised, and a sterile polymer disk containing angiogenic or antiangiogenic agents is placed within the membrane; angiogenesis is then observed over the ensuing 2–3 days. Another way of using the CAM assay is to extract the CAM and the chick embryo, place them in a dish, apply a polymer disk onto the CAM, and observe the angiogenic activity over the next several days.

A final example of an *in vitro* angiogenesis assay is the rat aortic ring assay. In this technique, a ring of a rat aorta is flushed and any surrounding tissue removed. The aortic ring is then placed in a collagen/thrombin gel that maintains its integrity and orientation and provides a latticework for the migration of endothelial cells. Conditioned media or media containing various angiogenic or antiangiogenic factors can then be added to the superficial portion of the gel and allowed to migrate through the gel. The outgrowth of capillary sprouts can then be examined, either subjectively or objectively, with the aid of computer analysis (79, 80) (Fig. 8).

III. Antiangiogenic Therapy: Issues and Expectations

The knowledge that angiogenesis is essential for tumor growth and the formation of metastases has led to one of the largest research efforts ever undertaken in an attempt to discover effective antiangiogenesis compounds. Angiogenesis is not only a pathologic process, but also is essential for homeostasis. Physiologic angiogenesis is important in reproduction, wound healing, menses, and vascular diseases such as coronary artery and peripheral vascular diseases. Thus, as always, a balance must be obtained in which angiogenesis in tumors is limited while the host is protected from toxic effects.

In addition to potential toxicity, the duration of therapy is another issue to be considered in antiangiogenic therapy. Because most antiangiogenic therapy is intended to decrease the development of new blood vessels, the endpoints for treatment success or failure must be redefined. For example, a desirable response for standard chemotherapy is to decrease the cross-sectional area of a tumor by 50%; however, the desired endpoint after antiangiogenic therapy might be no further tumor growth. Thus, criteria for the

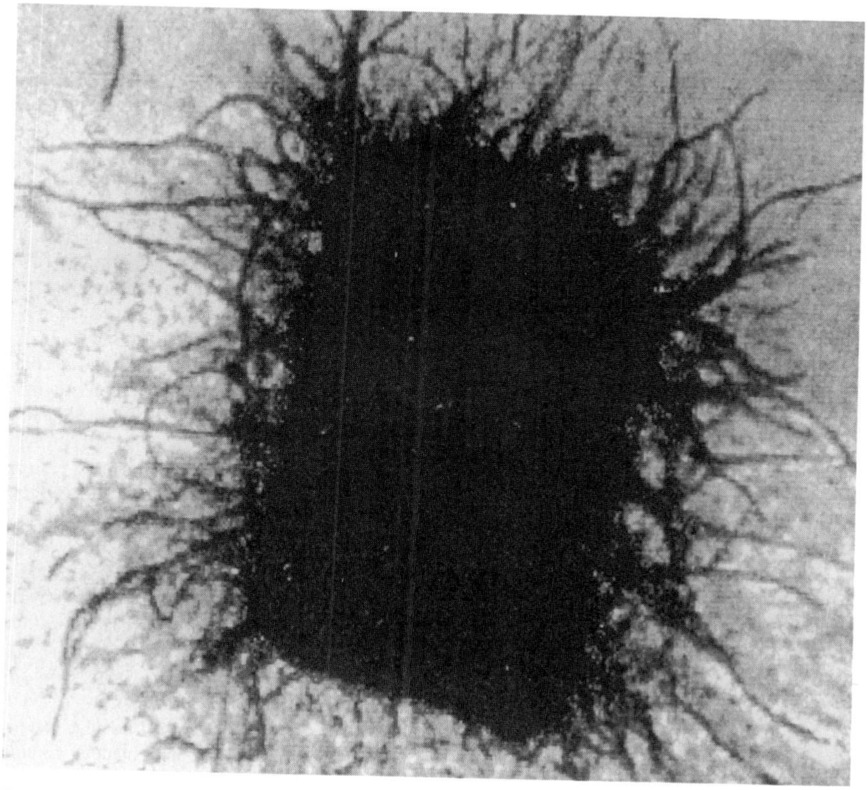

Figure 8 Rat aortic ring assay for angiogenesis. Rat aorta (either a ring or a fragment) is embedded in a plasmin gel. The addition of angiogenic or antiangiogenic factors will affect outgrowth of endothelial cells from the edge of the embedded tissue. To confirm that these cells are of endothelial origin (and not fibroblasts), these outgrowths can be stained for endothelial cell markers.

effectiveness of antiangiogenic therapy, whether in the clinic or in the laboratory, must be considered from a new perspective relative to those for conventional therapies.

Because one-time doses of antiangiogenic agents may not decrease tumor growth, antiangiogenic therapy will probably need to be delivered on a chronic basis. Chronic administration will require that the agent be easily delivered (i.e., by the oral route) and have few long-term effects. Moreover, the effect of antiangiogenic therapy may require longer evaluation intervals, because stability of disease may be difficult to determine at short intervals.

Although some reports exist of tumor regression in experimental models of angiogenesis (81, 82), such findings are rare; the vast majority of studies in this field demonstrate that antiangiogenic therapy leads to an inhibition of tumor growth rather than to a regression of established tumors (83, 84). The ability to interpret experimental studies appropriately is critical to ensure that extrapolations to the clinical setting are not fraught with unrealistic expectations. In designing experiments or in reading the literature, it is important to determine whether antiangiogenic therapy is being used as a chemopreventive agent (i.e., delivered before or at the time of tumor inoculation), as adjuvant therapy (i.e., delivered when the tumor is at a relatively small volume, such as shortly after tumor injection), or as a therapeutic modality (i.e., delivered to animals with established tumors).

If the response to antiangiogenic therapy is to be evaluated appropriately, the endpoints must be defined before the study is begun. Typically, tumor size or mass is determined at initiation of therapy and at termination of the study. Tumors can be harvested for immunohistochemical staining to determine vessel counts, rates of tumor cell proliferation and apoptosis, and even rates of endothelial cell proliferation and apoptosis. Survival studies will give important clues as to the long-term effectiveness of antiangiogenic therapy. The toxicity of the intended therapy to the host always must be assessed.

The site of tumor injection is critical in experimental antiangiogenesis studies. Endothelium from different organs clearly is phenotypically distinct (85), and therefore therapy that is effective at one site may be ineffective at another. The growth and patterns of metastases also depend on the site of injection (86). Hence, the most relevant model for evaluating antiangiogenic therapy will be an orthotopic one in which the tumor is growing in the appropriate host environment.

The constant evolution of new agents being introduced into clinical trials makes written reviews of clinical trials of antiangiogenic agents impractical. However, up-to-date information on clinical trials can be accessed from the National Cancer Institute's web site at http://cancertrials.nci.nih.gov/NCI_CANCER_TRIALS/zones/PressInfo/Angio/table.html. In addition, an overview of anti-angiogenesis can be viewed at http://cancertrials.nci.nih.gov/NCI_CANCER_TRIALS/zones/PressInfo/Angio/.

Acknowledgments

Supported by The Gillson-Longenbaugh Foundation and the Jon and Suzie Hall Fund for Colon Cancer Research. The author thanks Joan Small and Christine Wogan for editorial assistance.

References

1. Folkman, J., and Tyler, K. (1977). Tumor angiogenesis: Its possible role in metastasis and invasion. *In* "Cancer Invasion and Metastasis: Biologic Mechanisms and Therapy" (S. B. Day, W. P. L. Myers, P. Stansly, S. Gerattini, and M. G. Lewis, eds.), pp. 95–103. Raven Press, New York.
2. Folkman, J. (1986). How is blood vessel growth regulated in normal and neoplastic tissue?—G.H.A. Clowes Memorial Award Lecture. *Cancer Res.* **46,** 467–473.
3. Folkman, J. (1989). What is the evidence that tumors are angiogenesis dependent? *J. Natl. Cancer Inst.* **82,** 4–6.
4. Fidler, I. J., and Ellis, L. M. (1994). The implications of angiogenesis to the biology and therapy of cancer metastasis. *Cell* **79,** 185–188.

4a. Fidler, I. J. (1997). Molecular biology of cancer: Invasion and metastasis. *In* "Cancer Principles and Practice of Oncology," 5th Ed. (J. R. De Vita, S. Hellman, and S. A. Rosenberg, eds.), pp. 135–152. Lippincott-Raven, Philadelphia.

5. Weidner, N., Semple, J. P., Welch, W. R., and Folkman, J. (1991). Tumor angiogenesis and metastasis-correlation in invasive breast cancer. *N. Engl. J. Med.* **324,** 1–8.
6. Weidner, N. (1995). Tumor angiogenesis: Review of current applications in tumor prognostication. *In* "New Cancer Strategies: Angiogenesis Antagonists," Washington, D.C.
7. Jain, R. K. (1994). Barriers to drug deliver in solid tumors. *Sci. Am.* **271,** 58–65.
8. Bouck, N. (1990). Tumor angiogenesis: The role of oncogenes and tumor suppressor genes. *Cancer Cells* **2,** 179–185.
9. Holash, J., Maisonpierre, P. C., Compton, D., Boland, P., Alexander, C. R., Zagzag, D., Yancopoulos, G. D., and Wiegand, S. J. (1999). Vessel cooption, regression, and growth in tumors mediated by angiopoietins and VEGF. *Science* **284,** 1994–1998.
10. Takahashi, A., Sasaki, H., Kim, S. J., Tobisu, K., Kakizoe, T., Tsukomoto, T., Kumamoto, Y., Sugimura, T., and Terada, M. (1994). Markedly increased amounts of messenger RNA's for vascular endothelial growth factor and placenta growth factor in renal cell carcinoma associated with angiogenesis. *Cancer Res.* **54,** 4233–4237.
11. Takahashi, Y., Kitadai, Y., Bucana, C. D., Cleary, K. R., and Ellis, L. M. (1995). Expression of vascular endothelial growth factor and its receptor, KDR, correlates with vascularity, metastasis, and proliferation of human colon cancer. *Cancer Res.* **55,** 3964–3968.
12. Takahashi, Y., Cleary, K. R., Mai, M., Kitadai, Y., Bucana, C. D., and Ellis, L. M. (1996). Significance of vessel count and vascular endothelial growth factor and its receptor (KDR) in intestinal-type gastric cancer. *Clin. Cancer Res.* **2,** 1679–1684.
13. Brown, L. F., Berse, B., Jackman, R. W., Tognazzi, K., Manseau, E. J., Senger, D. R., and Dvorak, H. F. (1993). Expression of vascular permeability factor (vascular endothelial growth factor) and its receptors in adenocarcinomas of the gastrointestinal tract. *Cancer Res.* **53,** 4727–4735.
14. Brown, L. F., Berse, B., Jackman, R. W., Tognazzi, K., Manseau, E. J., Dvorak, H. F., and Senger, D. R. (1993). Increased expression of vascular permeability factor (vascular endothelial growth factor) and its receptors in kidney and bladder carcinomas. *Am. J. Pathol.* **143,** 1255–1262.
15. Toi, M., Kondo, S., Suzuki, H., Yamamoto, Y., Inada, K., Imazawa, T., Taniguchi, T., and Tominaga, T. (1996). Quantitative analysis of vascular endothelial growth factor in primary breast cancer. *Cancer* **77,** 1101–1106.

16. Tischer, E., Mitchell, R., Hartman, T., Silva, S., Gospodarowicz, D., Fiddes, J. C., and Abraham, J. A. (1991). The human gene for vascular endothelial growth factor. Multiple protein forms are encoded through alternate exon splicing. *J. Biol. Chem.* **266,** 11947–11954.
17. Dvorak, H. F., Dvorak, A. M., Manseau, E. J., Wiberg, L., and Churchill, W. H. (1979). Fibrin-gel investment associated with line 1 and line 10 solid tumor growth, angiogenesis, and fibroplasia in guinea pigs. Role of cellular immunity, myofibroblasts, microvascular damage, and infarction in line 1 tumor regression. *J. Natl. Cancer Inst.* **62,** 1459–1472.
18. Senger, D. R., Galli, S. J., Dvorak, A. M., Perruzzi, C. A., Harvey, V. S., and Dvorak, H. F. (1983). Tumor cells secrete a vascular permeability factor that promotes accumulation of ascites fluid. *Science* **219,** 983–985.
19. Dvorak, H. F., Nagy, J. A., Berse, B., Brown, L. F., Yeo, K. T., Yeo, T. K., Dvorak, A. M., Van De Water, L., Sioussat, T. M., and Senger, D. R. (1992). Vascular permeability factor, fibrin, and the pathogenesis of tumor stroma formation. *Ann. N.Y. Acad. Sci.* **667,** 101–111.
20. Tsurusaki, T., Kanda, S., Sakai, H., Kanetake, H., Saito, Y., Alitalo, K., and Koji, T. (1999). Vascular endothelial growth factor-C expression in human prostatic carcinoma and its relationship to lymph node metastasis. *Br. J. Cancer* **80,** 309–313.
21. Veikkola, T., and Alitalo, K. (1999). VEGFs, receptors and angiogenesis. *Semin. Cancer Biol.* **9,** 211–220.
22. Valtola, R., Salven, P., Heikkila, P., Taipale, J., Joensuu, H., Rehn, M., Pihlajaniemi, T., Weich, H., deWaal, R., and Alitalo, K. (1999). VEGFR-3 and its ligand VEGF-C are associated with angiogenesis in breast cancer. *Am. J. Pathol.* **154,** 1381–1390.
23. Salven, P., Lymboussaki, A., Heikkila, P., Jaaskela-Saari, H., Enholm, B., Aase, K., von Euler, G., Eriksson, U., Alitalo, K., and Joensuu, H. (1998). Vascular endothelial growth factors VEGF-B and VEGF-C are expressed in human tumors. *Am. J. Pathol.* **153,** 103–108.
24. Cao, Y., Linden, P., Farnebo, J., Cao, R., Eriksson, A., Kumar, V., Qi, J. H., Claesson-Welsh, L., and Alitalo, K. (1998). Vascular endothelial growth factor C induces angiogenesis in vivo. *Proc. Natl. Acad. Sci. U.S.A.* **95,** 14389–14394.
25. Lymboussaki, A., Partanen, T. A., Olofsson, B., Thomas-Crusells, J., Fletcher, C. D., deWaal, R. M., Kaipainen, A., and Alitalo, K. (1998). Expression of the vascular endothelial growth factor C receptor VEGFR-3 in lymphatic endothelium of the skin and in vascular tumors. *Am. J. Pathol.* **153,** 395–403.
26. Aase, K., Lymboussaki, A., Kaipainen, A., Olofsson, B., Alitalo, K., and Eriksson, U. (1999). Localization of VEGF-B in the mouse embryo suggests a paracrine role of the growth factor in the developing vasculature. *Dev. Dyn.* **215,** 12–25.
27. Olofsson, B., Korpelainen, E., Pepper, M. S., Mandriota, S. J., Aase, K., Kumar, V., Gunji, Y., Jeltsch, M. M., Shibuya, M., Alitalo, K., and Eriksson, U. (1998). Vascular endothelial growth factor B (VEGF-B) binds to VEGF receptor-1 and regulates plasminogen activator activity in endothelial cells. *Proc. Natl. Acad. Sci. U.S.A.* **95,** 11709–11714.
28. Marconcini, L., Marchio, S., Morbidelli, L., Cartocci, E., Albini, A., Ziche, M., Bussolino, F., and Olivero, S. (1999). c-fos-induced growth factor/vascular endothelial growth factor D induces angiogenesis *in vivo* and *in vitro*. *Proc. Natl. Acad. Sci. U.S.A.* **96,** 9671–9676.
29. Achen, M. G., Jeltsch, M., Kukk, E., Makinen, T., Vitali, A., Wilks, A. F., Alitalo, K., and Stacker, S. A. (1998). Vascular endothelial growth factor D (VEGF-D) is a ligand for the tyrosine kinases VEGF receptor 2 (Flk1) and VEGF receptor 3 (Flt4). *Proc. Natl. Acad. Sci. U.S.A.* **95,** 548–553.
30. Meyer, M., Clauss, M., Lepple-Wienhues, A., Waltenberger, J., Augustin, H. G., Ziche, M., Lanz, C., Buttner, M., Rziha, H. J., and Dehio, C. (1999). A novel vascular endothelial growth factor encoded by Orf virus, VEGF-E, mediates angiogenesis via signalling through VEGFR-2 (KDR) but not VEGFR-1 (Flt-1) receptor tyrosine kinases. *EMBO J.* **18,** 363–374.
31. Ogawa, S., Oku, A., Sawano, A., Yamaguchi, S., Yazaki, Y., and Shibuya, M. (1998). A novel type of vascular endothelial growth factor, VEGF-E (NZ-7 VEGF), preferentially utilizes KDR/Flk-1 receptor and carries a potent mitotic activity without heparin-binding domain. *J. Biol. Chem.* **273,** 31273–31282.
32. Ziegler, B. L., Valtieri, M., Porada, G. A., De Maria, R., Muller, R., Masella, B., Gabbianelli, M., Casella, I., Pelosi, E., Bock, T., Zanjani, E. D., and Peschle, C. (1999). KDR receptor: A key marker defining hematopoietic stem cells. *Science* **285,** 1553–1558.
33. Ferrer, F. A., Miller, L. J., Lindquist, R., Kowalczyk, P., Laudone, V. P., Albertsen, P. C., and Kreutzer, D. L. (1999). Expression of vascular endothelial growth factor receptors in human prostate cancer. *Urology* **53,** 567–572, 1999.
34. Soker, S., Takashima, S., Miao, H. Q., Neufeld, G., and Klagsbrun, M. (1998). Neuropilin-1 is expressed by endothelial and tumor cells as an isoform-specific receptor for vascular endothelial growth factor. *Cell* **92,** 735–745.
35. Papapetropoulos, A., Garcia-Cardena, G., Dengler, T. J., Maisonpierre, P. C., Yancopoulos, G. D., and Sessa, W. C. (1999). Direct actions of angiopoietin-1 on human endothelium: Evidence for network stabilization, cell survival, and interaction with other angiogenic growth factors. *Lab Invest.* **79,** 213–223.
36. Lauren, J., Gunji, Y., and Alitalo, K. (1998). Is angiopoietin-2 necessary for the initiation of tumor angiogenesis? *Am. J. Pathol.* **153,** 1333–1339.
37. Davis, S., and Yancopoulos, G. D. (1999). The angiopoietins: Yin and Yang in angiogenesis. *Curr. Top. Microbiol. Immunol.* **237,** 173–185.
38. Gale, N. W., and Yancopoulos, G. D. (1999). Growth factors acting via endothelial cell-specific receptor tyrosine kinases: VEGFs, angiopoietins, and ephrins in vascular development. *Genes Dev.* **13,** 1055–1066.
39. Patan, S. (1998). TIE1 and TIE2 receptor tyrosine kinases inversely regulate embryonic angiogenesis by the mechanism of intussusceptive microvascular growth. *Microvasc. Res.* **56,** 1–21.
40. Suri, C., Jones, P. F., Patan, S., Bartunkova, S., Maisonpierre, P. C., Davis, S., Sato, T. N., and Yancopoulos, G. D. (1996). Requisite role of angiopoietin-1, a ligand for the TIE2 receptor, during embryonic angiogenesis. *Cell* **87,** 1171–1180.
41. Moore, B. B., Arenberg, D. A., Addison, C. L., Keane, M. P., and Strieter, R. M. (1998). Tumor angiogenesis is regulated by CXC chemokines. *J. Lab. Clin. Med.* **132,** 97–103.
42. Gerber, H. P., McMurtrey, A., Kowalski, J., Yan, M., Keyt, B. A., Dixit, V., and Ferrara, N. (1998). Vascular endothelial growth factor regulates endothelial cell survival through the phosphatidylinositol 3'-kinase/Akt signal transduction pathway. Requirement for Flk-1/KDR activation. *J. Biol. Chem.* **273,** 30336–30343.
43. Gerber, H. P., Dixit, V., and Ferrara, N. (1998). Vascular endothelial growth factor induces expression of the antiapoptotic proteins Bcl-2 and A1 in vascular endothelial cells. *J. Biol. Chem.* **273,** 13313–13316.
44. Eliceiri, B. P., and Cheresh, D. A. (1999). The role of alphav integrins during angiogenesis: Insights into potential mechanisms of action and clinical development. *J. Clin. Invest.* **103,** 1227–1230.
45. Eliceiri, B. P., Klemke, R., Stromblad, S., and Cheresh, D. A. (1998). Integrin alphavbeta3 requirement for sustained mitogen-activated protein kinase activity during angiogenesis. *J. Cell Biol.* **140,** 1255–1263.
46. Scatena, M., Almeida, M., Chaisson, M. L., Fausto, N., Nicosia, R. F., and Giachelli, C. M. (1998). NF-kappaB mediates alphavbeta3 integrin-induced endothelial cell survival. *J. Cell Biol.* **141,** 1083–1093.
47. Wu, H., Beuerlein, G., Nie, Y., Smith, H., Lee, B. A., Hensler, M., Huse, W. D., and Watkins, J. D. (1998). Stepwise *in vitro* affinity maturation of Vitaxin, an alphav beta3-specific humanized mAb. *Proc. Natl. Acad. Sci. U.S.A.* **95,** 6037–6042.
48. Hirschi, K. K., and D'Amore, P. A. (1997). Control of angiogenesis by the pericyte: Molecular mechanisms and significance. *EXS* **79,** 419–428.
49. Kumar, R., Yoneda, J., Bucana, C. D., and Fidler, I. J. (1998). Regulation of distinct steps of angiogenesis by different angiogenic molecules. *Int. J. Oncol.* **12,** 749–757.

50. Levy, A. P., Levy, N. S., Wegner, S., and Goldberg, M. A. (1995). Transcriptional regulation of the rat vascular endothelial growth factor gene by hypoxia. *J. Biol. Chem.* **270,** 13333–13340.
51. Shweiki, D., Neeman, M., Itin, A., and Keshet, E. (1995). Induction of vascular endothelial growth factor expression by hypoxia and by glucose deficiency in multicell spheroids: implications for tumor angiogenesis. *Proc. Natl. Acad. Sci. U.S.A.* **92,** 768–772.
52. Shweiki, D., Itin, A., Stoffer, D., and Keshet, E. (1992). Vascular endothelial growth factor induced by hypoxia may mediate hypoxia-initiated angiogenesis. *Nature (London)* **359,** 843–845.
53. Mukhopadhyay, D., Tsiokas, L., Zhou, X. M., Foster, D., Brugge, J. S., and Sukhatme, V. P. (1995). Hypoxic induction of human vascular endothelial growth factor expression through c-*src* activation. *Nature (London)* **375,** 577–581.
54. Ellis, L. M., Staley, C. A., Liu, W., Fleming, R. Y. D., Parikh, N., Bucana, C. D., and Gallick, G. E. (1998). Down-regulation of vascular endothelial growth factor in a human colon carcinoma cell line transfected with an antisense expression vector specific for c-src. *J. Biol. Chem.* **273,** 1052–1057.
55. Akagi, Y., Liu, W., Xie, K., Zebrowski, B., and Ellis, L. M. (1998). Regulation of vascular endothelial growth factor expression in human colon cancer by insulin-like growth factor-I. *Cancer Res.* **58,** 4008–4014.
56. Akagi, Y., Liu, W., Xie, K., Zebrowski, B., Shaheen, R. M., and Ellis, L. M. (1999). Regulation of vascular endothelial growth factor expression in human colon cancer by interleukin-1. *Br. J. Cancer* **80,** 506–1511.
57. Tsai, J. C., Goldman, C. K., and Gillespie, G. Y. (1995). Vascular endothelial growth factor in human glioma cell lines: induced secretion by EGF, PDGF-BB, and bFGF. *J. Neurosurg.* **82,** 864–873.
58. Bouvet, M., Ellis, L. M., Nishizaki, M., Fujiwara, T., Liu, W., Bucana, C. D., Fang, B., Lee, J. J., and Roth, J. A. (1998). Adenovirally-mediated wild-type p53 gene transfer down-regulates vascular endothelial growth factor expression and inhibits angiogenesis in human colon cancer. *Cancer Res.* **58,** 2288–2292.
59. Mazure, N. M., Chen, E. Y., Laderoute, K. R., and Giaccia, A. J. (1997). Induction of vascular endothelial growth factor by hypoxia is modulated by a phosphatidylinositol 3-kinase/Akt signaling pathway in Ha-ras-transformed cells through a hypoxia inducible factor-1 transcriptional element. *Blood* **90,** 3322–3331.
60. Maxwell, P. H., Dachs, G. U., Gleadle, J. M., Nicholls, L. G., Harris, A. L., Stratford, I. J., Hankinson, O., Pugh, C. W., and Ratcliffe, P. J. (1997). Hypoxia-inducible factor-1 modulates gene expression in solid tumors and influences both angiogenesis and tumor growth. *Proc. Natl. Acad. Sci. U.S.A.* **94,** 8104–8109.
61. Jung, Y. D., Nakano, K., Liu, W., Gallick, G. E., and Ellis, L. M (1999). Extracellular signal-regulated kinase activation is required for upregulation of vascular endothelial growth factor by serum starvation in human colon carcinoma cells. *Cancer Res.* **59,** 4804–4807.
62. Rak, J., Mitsuhashi, Y., Bayko, L., Filmus, J., Shirasawa, S., Sasazuki, T., and Kerbel, R. S. (1995). Mutant ras oncogenes upregulate VEGF/VPF expression: Implications for induction and inhibition of tumor angiogenesis. *Cancer Res.* **55,** 4575–4580.
63. Pal, S., Claffey, K. P., Dvorak, H. F., and Mukhopadhyay, D. (1997). The von Hippel–Lindau gene product inhibits vascular permeability factor/vascular endothelial growth factor expression in renal cell carcinoma by blocking protein kinase C pathways. *J. Biol. Chem.* **272,** 27509–27512.
64. Mukhopadhyay, D., Knebelmann, B., Cohen, H. T., Ananth, S., and Sukhatme, V. P. (1997). The von Hippel–Lindau tumor suppressor gene product interacts with Sp1 to repress vascular endothelial growth factor promoter activity. *Mol. Cell. Biol.* **17,** 5629–5639.
65. Levy, A. P., Levy, N. S., and Goldberg, M. A. (1996). Hypoxia-inducible protein binding to vascular endothelial growth factor mRNA and its modulation by the von Hippel–Lindau protein. *J. Biol. Chem.* **271,** 25492–25497.
66. Takahashi, Y., Bucana, C. D., Cleary, K. R., and Ellis, L. M. (1998). p53, vessel count, and vascular endothelial growth factor expression in human colon cancer. *Int. J. Cancer* **79,** 34–38.
67. Vermeulen, P. B., Gasparini, G., Fox, S. B., Toi, M., Martin, L., McCulloch, P., Pezzella, F., Viale, G., Weidner, N., Harris, A. L., and Dirix, L. Y. (1996). Quantification of angiogenesis in solid human tumours: an international consensus on the methodology and criteria of evaluation. *Eur. J. Cancer* **32A,** 2474–2484.
68. Makris, A., Powles, T. J., Kakolyris, S., Dowsett, M., Ashley, S. E., and Harris, A. L. (1999). Reduction in angiogenesis after neoadjuvant chemoendocrine therapy in patients with operable breast carcinoma. *Cancer* **85,** 1996–2000.
69. Kenyon, B. M., Voest, E. E., Chen, C. C., Flynn, E., Folkman, J., and D'Amato, R. J. (1996). A model of angiogenesis in the mouse cornea. *Invest. Ophthalmol. Vis. Sci.* **37,** 1625–1632.
70. Ito, Y., Iwamoto, Y., Tanaka, K., Okuyama, K., and Sugioka, Y. (1996). A quantitative assay using basement membrane extracts to study tumor angiogenesis in vivo. *Int. J. Cancer* **67,** 148–152.
71. Passaniti, A., Taylor, R. M., Pili, R., Guo, Y., Long, P. V., Haney, J. A., Pauly, R. R., Grant, D. S., and Martin, G. R. (1992). A simple, quantitative method for assessing angiogenesis and antiangiogenic agents using reconstituted basement membrane, heparin, and fibroblast growth factor. *Lab. Invest.* **67,** 519–528.
72. Sckell, A., Safabakhsh, N., Dellian, M., and Jain, R. K. (1998). Primary tumor size-dependent inhibition of angiogenesis at a secondary site: An intravital microscopic study in mice. *Cancer Res.* **58,** 5866–5869.
73. Gohongi, T., Fukumura, D., Boucher, Y., Yun, C. O., Soff, G. A., Compton, C., Todoroki, T., and Jain, R. K. (1999). Tumor-host interactions in the gallbladder suppress distal angiogenesis and tumor growth: involvement of transforming growth factor beta1. *Nature Med.* **5,** 1203–1208.
74. Ellis, L. M., Liu, W., and Wilson, M. (1996). Downregulation of vascular endothelial growth factor in human colon carcinoma cell lines by antisense transfection decreases endothelial cell proliferation. *Surgery* **120,** 871–878.
75. Fernandez, H. A., Kallenbach, K., Seghezzi, G., Grossi, E., Colvin, S., Schneider, R., Mignatti, P., and Galloway, A. (1999). Inhibition of endothelial cell migration by gene transfer of tissue inhibitor of metalloproteinases-1. *J. Surg. Res.* **82,** 156–162.
76. Maniotis, A. J., Folberg, R., Hess, A., Seftor, E. A., Gardner, L. M., Pe'er, J., Trent, J. M., Meltzer, P. S., and Hendrix, M. J. (1999). Vascular channel formation by human melanoma cells *in vivo* and *in vitro*: Vasculogenic mimicry. *Am. J. Pathol.* **155,** 739–752.
77. Jakob, W., Jentzsch, K. D., Mauersberger, B., and Heder, G. (1978). The chick embryo choriallantoic membrane as a bioassay for angiogenesis factors: Reactions induced by carrier materials. *Exp. Pathol. (Jena)* **15,** 241–249.
78. Knighton, D., Ausprunk, D., Tapper, D., and Folkman, J. (1977). Avascular and vascular phases of tumour growth in the chick embryo. *Br. J. Cancer* **35,** 347–356.
79. Nicosia, R. F., and Ottinetti, A. (1990). Growth of microvessels in serum-free matrix culture of rat aorta. A quantitative assay of angiogenesis in vitro. *Lab. Invest.* **63,** 115–122.
80. Nicosia, R. F., Nicosia, S. V., and Smith, M. (1994). Vascular endothelial growth factor, platelet-derived growth factor, and insulin-like growth factor-1 promote rate aortic angiogenesis *in vitro*. *Am. J. Pathol.* **145,** 1023–1029.
81. O'Reilly, M. S., Boehm, T., Shing, Y., Fukai, N., Vasios, G., Lane, W. S., Flynn, E., Birkhead, J. R., Olsen, B. R., and Folkman, J. (1997). Endostatin: An endogenous inhibitor of angiogenesis and tumor growth. *Cell* **88,** 277–285.

82. Lode, H. N., Moehler, T., Xiang, R., Jonczyk, A., Gillies, S. D., Cheresh, D. A., and Reisfeld, R. A. (1999). Synergy between an antiangiogenic integrin alphav antagonist and an antibody-cytokine fusion protein eradicates spontaneous tumor metastases. *Proc. Natl. Acad. Sci. U.S.A.* **96,** 1591–1596.
83. Warren, R. S., Yuan, H., Matli, M. R., Gillett, N. A., and Ferrara, N. (1995). Regulation by vascular endothelial growth factor of human colon cancer tumorigenesis in a mouse model of experimental liver metastasis. *J. Clin. Invest.* **95,** 1789–1797.
84. Shaheen, R. M., Davis, D. W., Liu, W., Zebrowski, B. K., Wilson, M. R., Bucana, C. D., McConkey, D. J., McMahon, G., and Ellis, L. M. (1999). Antiangiogenic therapy targeting the tyrosine kinase receptor for vascular endothelial growth factor receptor inhibits the growth of colon cancer liver metastasis and induces tumor and endothelial cell apoptosis. *Cancer Res.* **59,** 5412–5416.
85. Pasqualini, R., and Ruoslahti, E. (1996). Organ targeting *in vivo* using phage display peptide libraries. *Nature (London)* **380,** 364–366.
86. Takahashi, Y., Mai, M., Wilson, M. R., Kitadai, Y., Bucana, C. D., and Ellis, L. M. (1996). Site-dependent expression of vascular endothelial growth factor, angiogenesis and proliferation in human gastric carcinoma. *Int. J. Oncol.* **8,** 701–705.

35

Approaches to Adoptive Immunotherapy

Harry D. Bear and Cynthia S. Chin

Division of Surgical Oncology, Department of Surgery, Medical College of Virginia at Virginia Commonwealth University, Richmond, Virginia 23298

I. Introduction

Surgery, chemotherapy, and radiation therapy are the conventional modalities used for the treatment of cancer. Despite the use of one, two, or even all three options, some cancers persist uncontrolled and cause devastating morbidity and mortality. The manipulation of the immune system has emerged as a promising fourth modality for cancer treatment. Modes of immunomodulation can be divided into two broad categories, passive and active. Passive immunotherapy involves the transfer of antibodies or cells with antitumor capabilities to a tumor-bearing host; active vaccination requires immunization of a tumor-bearing host with forms of antigen that elicit an immune reaction capable of eliminating the tumor. Such active therapies, involving peptides, bacterial adjuvants, gene manipulation, cytokines, and tumor cell vaccines, are discussed elsewhere in this volume. This chapter focuses on attempts to augment the immune system using the passive approach.

It was originally believed that the humoral component of the immune response (i.e., antibodies) was the most important for antitumor defense. Unfortunately, cancer patients have a high frequency of tumor-specific antibodies that do not correlate well with the disease state (1). Interestingly, a study by Syrengelas and Levy (2) suggests that the effects of DNA vaccination against an idiotype expressed on a murine B cell lymphoma could be due to a humoral rather than a cellular response. Monoclonal antitumor antibodies, produced *ex vivo* and infused into patients with cancer, may require the assistance of other components of the immune system to produce significant tumor damage. Various materials have been conjugated to monoclonal antibodies, including radionuclides and toxins, to increase their antitumor effectiveness. However, cellular immunity has a more consistent antitumor activity, and we focus here on the use of cellular adoptive immunotherapy (AIT).

Adoptive immunotherapy involves the transfer of cells with antitumor activity to a tumor-bearing host. The term "adoptive immunotherapy" was coined when lymph node cells from mice with skin allografts were used to transfer allograft immunity to normal mice (3). In 1976 Hewitt *et al.* (4), after reviewing data showing 27 murine tumors were apparently nonimmunogenic, deduced that tumor cells could not be distinguished by the immune system and, therefore, that the use of immunotherapy in the treatment of cancer was futile. This was clearly discouraging to those working in this field. However, in 1982, Boon *et al.* (5) showed that an apparently nonimmunogenic murine tumor could elicit a protective immune response, and concluded that the lack of an immune response might not be due to a lack of a tumor antigen but rather to an insufficient stimulation of the immune system by tumor cells. After many promising results in animals, Rosenberg *et al.* (6) reported the first successful clinical study of cellular therapy in humans.

The first half of this chapter is structured to help the reader develop useful adoptive immunotherapy models, which can fulfill two main purposes. First, the development of methods for inducing tumor regression in animals with adoptive transfer of cells helps with the rational design of clinical AIT protocols. Second, investigating the immunologic mechanisms that mediate tumor regression in animal models provides important clues as to what immunologic endpoints are likely to predict the effectiveness of immunologic manipulations in humans, including vaccines (7). The second half of this chapter is devoted to discussions on the *in vitro* and *in vivo* techniques used to evaluate these models.

II. Immunology Background

This section is designed to give a brief background on the immune system, necessary to understand the subsequent discussion of tumor immunotherapy models, although detailed explanations of the mechanisms of the immune system are beyond the scope of this chapter. Janeway's "Immunobiology" text (8) is an excellent reference for a more in-depth discussion of basic immunology. The goal of the immune system is to be able to distinguish nonself from self-molecules and cells and then to destroy these intruders, employing effector cells that have specific responsibilities for maintaining host defenses (see Fig. 1).

A. Adaptive vs. Innate Immunity

1. Innate Immunity

The immune system can be broadly divided into innate and adaptive immunity. The innate immune system involves physical and chemical barriers as well as cells such as granulocytes and natural killer cells. These are important in the early phases of a host response to a pathogen. However, they cannot discriminate between different pathogens, and the response does not change with repeated exposure to the same pathogen. The effectors of innate immunity can, however, be stimulated by cytokines released from T lymphocytes (see below).

2. Adaptive Immunity

Adaptive immune responses are mediated by B and T lymphocytes that are able to produce an antigen-specific reaction to a pathogen, leading to the development of memory cells that mediate a swifter and stronger response to repeated exposure to the same pathogen. The difference in the mechanism of action of these two cell types leads to a differentiation between humoral and cell-mediated immune responses.

a. Humoral Immunity The B cell is stimulated when it encounters an antigen that binds to its membrane-bound immunoglubulin receptor. B cell activation, augmented by T helper cells, leads to differentiation of B cells into plasma cells (antibody producers) and memory B cells. As stated earlier, antibodies require activation of complement and/or other cells in order to produce tissue damage. Macrophages, for example, can destroy antibody-coated pathogens or tumor cells.

b. Cellular Immunity T cells are derived from bone marrow stem cells, but mature in the thymus and can be divided into two main subsets based on surface markers, CD8 and CD4. $CD8^+$ cells, also known as cytotoxic T lymphocytes (CTLs), are able to interact with target cells and initiate their demise. Conversely, most $CD4^+$ lymphocytes are unable to kill target cells directly. They direct other cells to react and thus have been referred to as T helper (TH) cells. In 1986, two subsets of $CD4^+$ cells, TH1 and TH2, were identified, each with a distinct pattern of cytokine production (9). TH1 cells secrete cytokines such as interleukin-2 (IL-2), tumor necrosis factor-β (TNFβ), and interferon-γ (IFN-γ), which regulate cell-mediated immunity against intracellular pathogens as well as delayed hypersensitivity reactions. The TH1 cells, via cytokine production, amplify macrophage and $CD8^+$ CTL responses against foreign cells or infected self-cells. The TH2 subset, on the other hand, stimulates B cell growth and differentiation by release of IL-4. TH2 cells also produce additional cytokines, IL-5, IL-10, and IL-13, which in conjunction with IL-4 inhibit macrophage functions. The stimulation of TH1 and down-regulation of TH2 response are believed to be beneficial for tumor rejection; therefore

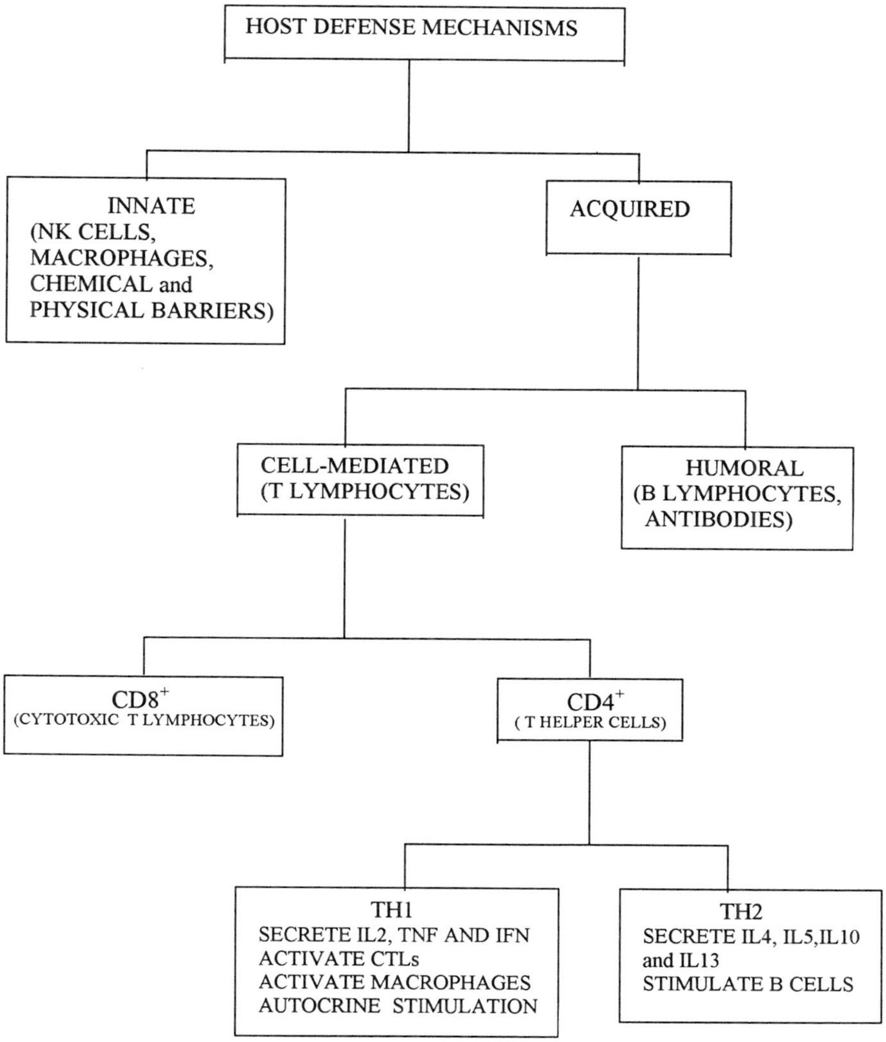

Figure 1 The immune system.

attempts have been made to manipulate these subsets in tumor-bearing hosts by administering either cytokines, such as interleukin-12 (IL-12) (10), or pharmacologic agents (11).

T cells have a membrane-bound antigen-specific receptor, which recognizes a complex of antigenic peptides bound to major histocompatibility complex molecules (MHCs) on antigen-presenting cells. There are two types of MHC molecules, MHC class I and class II. MHC I complexes, found on all nucleated cells except sperm, generally bind endogenous peptides derived from intracellular proteins, and are able to stimulate $CD8^+$ T cells. The MHC II complex is located on professional antigen-presenting cells (APCs), which include B cells, macrophages, and dendritic cells. $CD4^+$ T cells recognize MHC class II-associated epitopes, usually derived from extracellular proteins.

A signal derived from antigen-dependent binding to the T cell receptor (TCR) is necessary, but not sufficient, to activate a T cell. Additional antigen-independent, costimulatory signals are required for optimal T cell activation. This costimulation can be provided by the binding of ligands present on APCs to CD28 and other molecules on the T cell. Tumor cells often do not have the appropriate ligands and therefore may not be capable of producing a costimulatory signal to activate T cells directly.

As with B cells, T lymphocytes can also develop into memory cells. Ideally, adoptive immunotherapy to a tumor-bearing host would generate a rejection of the tumor as well as long-lasting immunity against future tumor challenges. Therefore, there is much interest in the identification and separation of memory $CD4^+$ and $CD8^+$ cells from other lymphocytes (12–14).

III. Tumor Evasion of the Immune System

It was once believed that tumor cells did not differ enough from normal cells to be recognized as foreign structures by mediators of the immune system. As previously stated, Boon *et al.* (5) in 1982 observed that tumors could be antigenic but not necessarily immunogenic. Patients with solid tumors or lymphomas are known to have impaired immune systems (15). T cells from cancer patients are less responsive than T cells in healthy controls to *in vitro* stimulation (16). Observance of the ability of tumor cells to evade the body's sophisticated immune system has resulted in an abundance of research in this area. Possible reasons for the lack of immunogenicity include a lack of effective costimulation of CTLs (17, 18), secretion of inhibitory factors (e.g., TGF-β or IL-10) (19–21), down-regulation of MHC expression (22–24), physiological barriers secondary to tumor location (25, 26), defects in T cell signal transduction (27, 28), and the development of peripheral tolerance to tumor antigen (29). CTLs depend on the presence of MHC class I expression on the target cell in order to initiate cytotoxic killing, and therefore tumor cells lacking MHC class I expression could escape a cytotoxic death. Costimulation of T cells activated by antigens requires additional stimulation, which is available from a variety of cells; the lack of costimulatory signals on tumor cells may lead to anergy or tolerance. As we further uncover the revelant events behind tumor-associated immunosuppression, pharmacologic and biologic approaches can be developed to increase tumor immunogenicity.

IV. Developing Models for AIT

A number of points must be considered when planning a model for AIT, including (1) tumor type, (2) route of AIT, (3) stage or size of tumor to be treated, (4) tumor site, (5) immune effector cells to be transferred, (6) source of effector cells, (7) mechanism for *ex vivo* stimulation of effector cells, and (8) which, if any, additional drugs or cytokines will be used.

A. Tumor and Species

A number of tumor models are available in different species. Syngeneic rodent strains (highly inbred strains with all of the individuals genetically identical) make it possible to transplant tumors and infuse immunologically active cells to individuals without inciting responses to foreign MHC antigens. Because the murine immune system has been well characterized and is very similar to that in humans, AIT experiments are most commonly carried out in mice, although rat models are also used by some investigators. The murine immune system has been widely studied and thus many murine tumor lines and reagents, including monoclonal antibodies and cytokines, are available for delineation and manipulation of immune response components.

Although it is impossible to design a murine model that can translate directly to human pathology, intuitively it is best to study a model that simulates the human disease as much as possible. Human tumors are believed to be very weakly, if at all, immunogenic, and thus a relevant model should use a poorly immunogenic tumor. A tumor strain that is too immunogeneic will be rejected by the animal without any intervention. Clearly this model is not representative of human cancer progression. Immunogenic models, however, can be used to develop methods that can then be applied to weakly immunogenic or nonimmunogenic models. In general, murine tumors can be induced by one of four methods: (1) UV light, (2) chemical carcinogens, (3) oncogenic viruses, or (4) spontaneously. UV light and virally induced tumors are the most immunogenic, with chemically induced tumors having moderate immunogenicity. Spontaneous tumors are considered the least immunogenic and probably are most ideal to study. If the immunogenicity of a tumor strain is unknown, it can be elucidated by several traditional experiments in which an immunized host is rechallenged with the tumor. Methods of immunization include (1) inoculation of tumor cells followed by excision of the resulting tumor, (2) inoculation with irradiated tumor cells, or (3) inoculation with tumor cells and a bacterial adjuvant (e.g., *Corynebacterium parvum*). Immunity to tumor rechallenge indicates a moderately to strongly immunogenic tumor, whereas tumor growth with the rechallenge suggests weaker immunogenicicity (30).

It is also important to remember that tumor cells in long-term culture may mutate and develop another clonal population of tumor cells. To avoid spontaneous mutations *in vitro*, cells should not be kept in culture for long periods of time. Similarly, repeated passage in mice can lead to alterations in the tumor, and should be limited as much as possible. The experimenter should freeze tumor cells in liquid nitrogen for future use rather than keep the same cell line growing in culture or passage *in vivo* for long periods of time.

B. Route of AIT

Theoretically, AIT of immune effector cells can be given by intravenous (IV), intraperitoneal (IP), or intradermal (ID) routes. We believe IV administration gives the greatest assurance that the cells will be incorporated into the systemic immune system. Conversely, subcutaneous injections may not encounter tumor cells at a different site. Intraperitoneal AIT has been used in some models. However, we strongly advise against administering IP AIT in models in which the tumor is given IP as well. The immune cells and the tumor cells may only interact because they were both injected into the peritoneal cavity. This is really not very different from mixing cells in a culture flask, and even though the effector cells may eliminate the tumor, the results may not accurately reflect a systemic response. The mouse ends up being a glorified and expensive petri dish.

C. Tumor for Rejection: Sites and Stages

Successful immunization of mice against a subsequent tumor challenge is not a likely scenario in humans. This model does not translate well to effects of immunotherapy on tumor growth, because the strength of an immunization to prevent initial tumor establishment is probably less than that required to inhibit growth or cause regression of an established tumor. However, it may be useful first to establish that an AIT protocol can lead to protection against tumor challenge in a naive host. If AIT does not protect against a tumor in this setting, it is unlikely to be effective against an established tumor.

If a naive mouse receiving AIT can reject a tumor challenge, the next step would be to determine the effects of AIT on established tumors. In some models, tumor cells are infused IV, which allows the tumor cells to circulate through the bloodstream and deposit in the lungs, creating pulmonary nodules. AIT-induced regression of these nodules can be evaluated after mice are euthanized by quantitating the tumors in the lungs. In at least one tumor model (P815 mastocytoma in DBA/2 mice), IV inoculation resulted in liver metastases, which could be treated with AIT (31). Liver metastases can also be "seeded" by splenic injection of tumor cells and splenectomy. The use of ID tumor inoculations into the flank is advantageous in that it allows the experimenter to observe tumor regression (or progression) throughout the experiment. A final possibility is the use of a metastasizing tumor line for establishment of spontaneous pulmonary metastases.

The stage or size of the established tumor to be treated depends on the growth characteristics of the tumor. When using fast-growing, aggressive tumors, the use of more advanced tumors may not be appropriate because the mice may need to be euthanized secondary to large tumor mass before any clinical benefit can be observed. It must be emphasized that the appropriate stage of the tumor for AIT experiments may vary from one tumor to another. Although very early tumors may be more readily treated by AIT, they may not be as relevant to clinical AIT. However, very advanced tumors may profoundly depress host immune effector mechanisms that may be critical for the success of AIT. Furthermore, large tumors may be poorly vascularized, so that immune effector cells do not have access to the whole tumor.

D. Choosing an Immune Effector for AIT

The bulk of the discussion in this chapter is on T lymphocytes, because these cells have the most potent and specific antitumor activity. Other cells will be briefly mentioned in this section (see Table I).

1. Lymphokine-Activated Killer Cells

In an effort to stimulate T cell growth with high doses of IL-2, lymphokine-activated killer (LAK) cells were inadvertently discovered (32). LAK cells are predominantly of natural killer cell origin and induce a nonspecific, non-MHC-restricted cytotoxic death of tumor cells. After observing promising results, in murine AIT models, clinical trials of LAK with IL-2 were started. Unfortunately, clinical trials for the treatment of melanoma and renal cell carcino-

Table I Cells for Cellular AIT

Method	Advantages	Disadvantages	Ref.
Lymphocyte-activated killer cells	High cytotoxic activity after culture with IL-2	Non-MHC-restricted lysis of tumor cells; no significant difference seen between LAK/IL-2 therapy vs. IL-2 alone	32–34
Tumor-infiltrating lymphocytes	Lymphocytes with tumor-specific activity; 50–100 times more potent than LAK; usually antigen-specific T cell lines	Long periods for *ex vivo* culture; not all tumor types will have sufficient TILs; may require high-dose IL-2 at time of AIT	39–45
Draining lymph nodes	High percentage of tumor-specific lymphocytes; expand *ex vivo* with low-dose IL-2 after appropriate stimulation; can confer immunologic memory in the host	Poorly immunogenic tumor lines will not adequately sensitize T cells; aggressive tumors may grow too fast in relation to time needed for sufficient DLN sensitization	40, 46–49
Spleen	Large number of lymphocytes	Low proportion of tumor-specific T cells; sensitization of the spleen requires strong systemic reaction to the tumor	51, 52
Monocytes/macrophages	Variety of antitumor activities, including contact cell death and release of TNF	Non-MHC-restricted tumor destruction; difficult to obtain in large numbers	37–38

ma (RCC), comparing IL-2 and LAK cells to IL-2 alone, did not appear to show any advantage for the use of LAK cells (33, 34). Attention has since refocused on using tumor-specific T cells for AIT after the clinical disappointment with LAK cells.

2. T Lymphocytes

T cells have a broad range of functions, including the lysis of tumor cells, production of tumoricidal cytokines (IFN-γ and TNFα), and stimulation of macrophage-mediated tumor cell death, which make them highly effective for AIT. With regard to AIT, T lymphocytes have a number of advantages over LAK cells, including antigen specificity, smaller IL-2 requirement, lower amount of cells needed for transfer, and potential for production of memory cells for long-term protection (35). Murine tumor models have shown regression with T lymphocyte-based AIT. In fact, these therapeutic effects remain long after the treatment has concluded (36). The sources and methods for expansion of T cells for AIT will be discussed later in this chapter.

3. Monocytes and Macrophages

Monocyte/macrophage tumoricidal activities, which are not MHC antigen restricted, are a result of direct cell contact and the release of the tumor necrosis factor and other mediators such as nitric oxide (37). After observing regression in tumor-bearing animals using activated macrophages in AIT, clinical trials were undertaken. A phase I clinical trial showed that AIT using activated macrophages was tolerated by nine cancer patients, with one case having a minor tumor response and the other eight having progression of their disease (38). Only a few publications focus on macrophages as primary cells for AIT, although many nonspecific immunologic stimulants "target" macrophages. Activated macrophages may be better used as *ex vivo* APCs to stimulate T cell cultures (see below).

E. Sources of T Lymphocytes for AIT

T cells circulate in the bloodstream, taking up residence in the spleen, lymph nodes, and other lymphoid tissues that may be useful sources of cells for AIT. These organs, as well as the tumors, may be sources for tumor-reactive T cells (see Table I).

1. Tumor-Infiltrating Lymphocytes

Shortly after clinical trials with LAK cells, attention was refocused on T cells. Tumor-infiltrating lymphocytes (TILs), as the name indicates, are T cells found in tumors. It was assumed that TIL cells may have an advantage over peripheral circulating lymphocytes because they have migrated to and/or proliferated within the tumor. Thus, it was also felt to be likely that the T cells present in TILs contained a high proportion of tumor antigen-specific clones.

TIL cells, isolated from solid tumors and grown in single-cell suspensions with interleukin-2 (39), were found to be 50–100 times more potent than LAK cells in the regression of pulmonary sarcoma micrometastases in experimental animals (40). Clinical response rates in patients with metastatic melanoma or renal cell carcinoma treated with TILs and IL-2 have been in the range of 15–20% (41–43).

Unfortunately, the use of TILs in AIT has drawbacks. TIL antitumor activities may require *in vivo* coadministration of high-dose IL-2. Toxicities associated with this level of IL-2 administration (see Section IV,F) severely limit the therapeutic use of TILs for AIT. Another disadvantage is related to the time required for *ex vivo* expansion of TILs. The optimal therapeutic dose of TILs was determined to be $>10^{11}$ cells. Expansion to the appropriate level requires at least 30–45 days. Furthermore, cultured cells between days 15 and 25 often exhibit non-MHC-restricted lysis of tumor cells. It is postulated that immune specificity is acquired by TILs as the culture time passes (44). Unfortunately, some patients' disease progressed during the required culture period and they became too ill to receive the therapy.

TIL cells have been used as a key "reagent" in the identification of some tumor-associated antigens (TAAs). Genomic DNA or cDNA of tumor cells has been transfected into cells expressing the appropriate MHC molecules. These cells with MHC–tumor antigen complexes are mixed with TIL cells. TILs will lyse the target cells or release cytokines when presented the appropriate tumor antigen by the transfected cells. This "scanning" of genetic libraries with tumor-specific TIL cells has led to identification of the majority of known human tumor antigens (45).

2. Draining Lymph Nodes

Preeffector T cells that are not functionally capable of tumor rejection at the time of harvest have been shown to be present in regional lymph nodes draining the primary tumor site. After stimulation *in vitro* with tumor cells and low-dose IL-2, T cells, derived from draining lymph nodes (DLNs), develop antitumor activity (46, 47). DLNs can be primed *in vivo* by tumor or a vaccine of irradiated tumor cells. It has been our experience that the most reliable method of priming well-defined DLNs in mice is to inject the tumor cells into a footpad for priming of popliteal lymph nodes. However, others have used ipsilateral inguinal or axillary nodes after ID inoculation of tumor or vaccine into the flank. With poorly immunogeneic tumors, the development of antigen-specific T cells in the DLN may not occur without the aid of an adjuvant. In some cases, tumor lines have been transfected with genes for immune-enhancing cytokines, such as IL-1, IL-2, IL-4, IL-6, TNF-α, IFN-γ, or granulocyte–macrophage colony-stimulating factor (GM-CSF) to facilitate the generation of tumor-specific T cells for AIT. The cytokines (e.g., IL-1, IL-2, or GM-CSF) can also be injected directly into the footpad with the tumor or tumor vaccine with similar results (48–50). Bacterial adjuvants such as the bacillus of Calmette–Guérin (BCG), a vaccine used for immunity against tuberculosis, and *Corynebacterium parvum* can also help stimulate an immune response.

The time period for DLN harvest will depend on the tumor type and its rate of growth and/or spread. DLNs harvested early (3–8 days) may not have had enough time to develop significant preeffector T cells. Conversely, DLNs that are harvested late (>12 days) may have been affected by tumor-induced immunosuppression. Additionally, DLNs need to be harvested before the footpad tumor becomes too large and the animal must be euthanized for humane reasons. The growth of the tumor, in relation to the development of sufficient DLN T cell sensitization, is related to the inoculation size as well as tumor characteristics such as aggressiveness and immunogenicity. When working with a new tumor line, the appropriate dose can be determined by injecting the footpads of several groups of mice with various concentrations of tumor cells and harvesting DLNs at different intervals (usually 8–12 days after tumor inoculation). If a nonviable tumor vaccine is used or the tumor has been genetically modified such that spontaneous regression occurs, DLN T cells will remain active for AIT at longer intervals, sometimes up to 1 month after inoculation.

3. Spleen

The spleen is a lymphoid organ that can also be a source of T lymphocytes. The inoculation of the vaccine can be at any site, but IP or ID inoculation into the flank is usually used. However, for spleen cells to be active, the immunizing tumor cells or vaccine must generally be capable of inducing strong systemic immunity, not just regional sensitization. The percentages of $CD4^+$ and $CD8^+$ T cells in the spleen are approximately 24 and 11%, respectively, compared to 55 and 25% of the cells in lymph nodes (51). Nylon wool adherence can enrich a lymphoid tissue suspension for T cells [outlined steps for this procedure have been given by Hathcock (52)].

F. Options for Ex Vivo Activation and Expansion

Effective AIT also requires practical methods for *ex vivo* activation and expansion of T cells. T cells require antigen stimulation in order to proliferate in physiologic concentrations of IL-2. Historically, stimulation and expansion were done with tumor cells. However, unlike murine models, there is only a finite number of human cancer cells, from a given patient, available for *in vitro* stimulation; therefore, it is a priority to develop alternative methods for T cell stimulation. Stimulators that can be used for expansion, in addition to tumor cells, include synthetic peptides (plus APCs), monoclonal antibodies specific for a variety of T cell ligands, and pharmocologic agents (see Table II).

1. Tumor Cells or Tumor Antigens

Stephenson *et al.* (47) cultured DLNs, primed with MCA 105, with irradiated (2000 rads) tumor cells in 24-well tissue culture plates at a ratio of 1:1 in media containing IL-2 at a concentration of 1000 IU/ml. After 12 days in culture, these stimulated and expanded tumor-specific T cells could induce tumor regression *in vivo*. This model has limited use in human clinical trials, because tumor cells are not often available in quantities sufficient for *ex vivo* expansion. The identification of tumor-specific antigens has been a major development for tumor immunology. The discussion of methods for detection of tumor antigens is beyond the scope of this chapter, and the reader is directed to an excellent review article by Rosenberg (53). Defined tumor antigens have the potential to increase tumor immunity in several ways. Tumor peptide epitopes can be used as vaccine *in vivo* to sensitize T cells or *in vitro* to activate T cells for AIT (54). Synthetic peptides, modeled after tumor antigens, have been used successfully to expand *in vitro* tumor-reactive CTLs for AIT. TAAs used to expand antigen-specific lymphocytes *in vitro* can give rise to T lymphocytes 50–100 times more potent than TILs (55).

The discovery of dendritic cells and their spectrum of functions with regard to the immune system has been an important advancement. Dendritic cells reside in the periphery (e.g., skin), where they interact with, take up, and process antigens. They carry these foreign particles to the regional lymph nodes, where B or T lymphocytes with the appropriate specificity for the antigen are stimulated to proliferate and differentiate. Dendritic cells are "professional" APCs, which gives them advantages over tumor cells with regard to T cell stimulation. First of all, dendritic cells display a much greater number of the MHC class I–antigen complexes compared to tumor cells, as well as MHC class II molecules, which are usually absent on tumor cells. Second, dendritic cells have important costimulatory molecules that tumor cells usually lack.

Several methods of *ex vivo* incorporation of a tumor antigen onto a dendritic cell are being considered (56). These include "feeding" defined peptides or tumor cell lysates to dendritic cells in culture or transducing dendritic cells with genes encoding tumor-specific proteins

2. T Cell Stimulation with Monoclonal Antibodies

As mentioned, the TCR/CD3 complex initiates intracellular signal transduction after the binding of an antigen (peptide–MHC complex). Stimulation of primed DLNs *ex vivo* by anti-CD3 monoclonal antibodies (mAbs), followed by culture with IL-2 in the absence of tumor antigens, can produce tumor-reactive T cells that are capable of inducing regression of established tumors. Without *in vitro* activation, these "preeffector" cells were inactive for AIT. Despite polyclonal activation, tumor regression was tumor specific (57). Other mAbs, such as CD28 and anti-CD3 mAbs, have

Table II ***In Vitro*** **Stimulation of T Lymphocytes for AIT**

Stimulant	Advantages	Disadvantages	Ref.
Tumor cells	Not necessary to know exact antigen epitope; widely available for murine tumors	Limited availability of human tumor cells	48
Tumor antigens (natural or synthetic)	Can be pulsed onto dendritic cells for more potent antigen presentation; synthetic peptides may be important in human clinical trials	Tumor epitope must be known	53–56
Monoclonal antibodies against TCR/CD3 and/or costimulatory receptors	Knowledge of tumor epitope is not necessary; can provide important costimulatory signals for T cells; can cross-link T cell receptors; tumor cells not necessary for efficient stimulation and expansion; can amplify sensitized T cell population into a tumor-specific population	Stimulation of naive lymphocytes or "nonsensitized" T cells leads to non-MHC-restricted activation; expensive	57–58
Pharmacologic agents	Can amplify T cell receptor signaling cascade; tumor cells not necessary for efficient stimulation and expansion; can amplify sensitized T cell population into a tumor-specific population	Agents with potential side effects, including some with tumor-promoting activity; may also activate nonspecific T cells	59–64

been found to be useful in similar expansion of peripheral blood mononuclear cells. Garlie *et al.* (58) showed that this population of T lymphocytes, coined COACTS, can exhibit cytotoxic killing of several tumor lines. However, this was non-MHC-restricted cytotoxicity. This combination of mAbs may also be useful to expand a population of tumor-specific T lymphocytes.

3. Pharmacologic Activation

The intracellular cascade leading to T cell activation involves an intracellular enzyme, phospholipase C. Phospholipase C is activated by the binding of an antigen to the T cell receptor/CD3 complex (see Fig. 2). Phospholipase C (PLC) then catalyzes the cleavage of phosphotidylinositol biphosphate into inositol triphosphate (IP_3) and diacylglycerol (DG). IP_3 stimulates an increase in intracellular calcium, whereas DG activates protein kinase C (PKC). PKC activity in conjunction with calcium increases transcription of certain genes, which ultimately leads to increased expression of high-affinity IL-2 receptors and increased T cell proliferation, especially if exogenous IL-2 is provided. Calcium ionophores, such as ionomycin (Io), have been shown to mimic the effects of IP_3 (59). Phorbol dibutyrate (PDBu), as well as other phorbol esters, can activate PKC. The combination of Io and PDBu with IL-2 can activate T-cells for *in vitro* growth, even in the absence of accessory cells (60). DLNs primed with MCA 105 sarcoma cells, pulsed with PDBu/Io for 18 hr and cultured with IL-2, expanded 500-fold over 21 days. Despite nonspecific stimulation, the resulting lymphocytes could induce tumor-specific regression of established sarcoma lung metastases (61).

Unfortunately, PBDu may have potentially adverse effects in humans. Although care is taken with removing these substances from the media before performing AIT, the theoretical dangers are still worrisome. PBDu is known to be a tumor-promoting agent, leading us to experimental protocols involving bryostatin. Bryostatin 1, a macrocyclic lactone derived from a marine invertebrate, *Bugula neritina*, has not been observed to have tumor-promoting qualities (62). In combination with a calcium ionophore and IL-2, bryostatin (Bryo) can also stimulate proliferation of primed lymphocytes that can mediate the regression of pulmonary metastases (63). AIT with these Bryo/Io-stimulated cells also confers immunologic memory on the host such that the

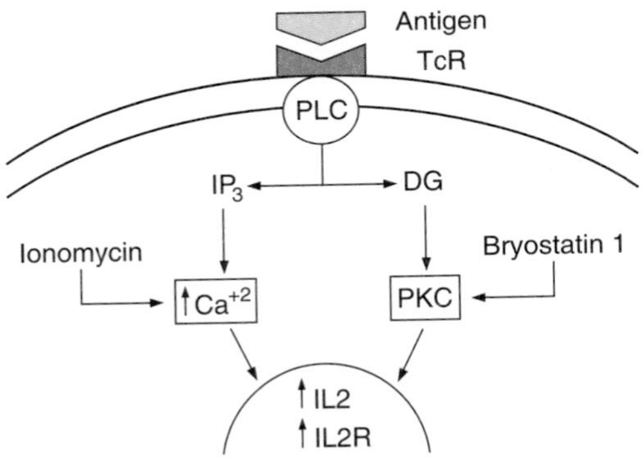

Figure 2 Depiction of the intracellular cascade that is initiated by binding of antigen to T cell receptor (TCR). Binding of antigen to TCR initiates a cascade involving phospholipase C (PLC) that leads to production of ionositol triphosphate (IP_3) and diacylglycerol (DG). Bryostatin 1 can substitute for DG by activating protein kinase C (PKC), and ionomycin mimics IP_3 effects on intracellular calcium. The use of these agents together leads to increased IL-2 production as well as up-regulation of the IL-2 receptor on the T cell.

recipient animals had tumor-specific resistance to rechallenge for up to 23 weeks, even without any prior exposure of the host to the tumor antigens (64).

G. Roles of Cytokines and Chemotherapy

The effect AIT has on a tumor-bearing host may be amplified or augmented by administration of cytokines. Unfortunately, a thorough discussion of cytokines is beyond the scope of this chapter. IL-2 and IFN-α are briefly mentioned here, and a more in-depth discussion of the functions of the known cytokines can be found in the referenced immunobiology text.

IL-2, produced by activated T cells, does not have any direct antitumor effects. Rather, it serves as an activation and proliferative factor for T cells and, to a lesser degree, for macrophages, natural killer (NK) cells, and B cells. Recombinant technology in the 1980s made available mass quantities of IL-2 for experimental and clinical protocols. IL-2 therapy in tumor-bearing animals induced the regression of established metastases (65), which led to great enthusiasm for the use of IL-2 in human clinical trials. IL-2 therapy was shown to have significant positive effects in patients with metastatic melanoma or renal cell carcinoma (42, 43). IL-2 administration has also been shown to increase the survival and proliferation of adoptively transferred T cells (66, 67).

Unfortunately, the high doses IL-2 that were often used had significant side effects, with the most dangerous including fluid gain and capillary leak syndrome, leading to hypotension, respiratory distress, and rarely death in humans (65, 67–70). Fortunately, nonfatal toxic effects of IL-2 reversed with cessation of treatment. In 1992, after experimental dosage adjustments, IL-2 was approved by the FDA for treatment of renal cell carcinoma.

IFN-α is another cytokine that can significantly enhance the effects of AIT. This family of cytokines, discovered in the 1950s, was the first to be used for therapeutic purposes (71). IFN-α may render a tumor more immunogenic by up-regulating the expression of the MHC–antigen complexes on tumor cells (72). Exogenously administered IFN-α appears to have synergistic effects with TILs and IL-2 (73). Van der Woude *et al.* (74) showed similar enhanced effects of AIT when IFN-α was given in conjunction with tumor-activated DLNs.

In addition to cytokines, cytotoxic chemotherapy drugs, such as cyclophosphamide (CYP), have been used successfully in conjunction with AIT to augment tumor regression (75). Several mechanisms account for the efficacy of CYP as an "adjuvant" to AIT. First, CYP in a tumor-bearing host may have a direct effect of tumor "debulking." This may be particularly important for rapidly growing tumors that may progress too quickly relative to the time required for the adoptively transferred cells to proliferate and "traffic" to tumor sites. Second, CYP has been shown to eliminate tumor-induced suppressor cells (76,77). Third, administration of CYP has been shown to induce secretion of cytokines that stimulate T cell growth *in vivo* (75). This effect, along with the elimination of many existing host lymphocytes, provides an "environment" that is very favorable for the growth and differentiation of the adoptively transferred cells. Finally, it has been postulated that the antitumor effects of CYP are related to its ability to shift the host immune system in a direction favoring TH1 (78)

The development of a working AIT model requires several successful steps (see Table III). The failure of any one of the listed steps can lead to failure of tumor regression in an AIT model. Some of these obstacles can be overcome using the experimental protocols described above. For instance, a weakly immunogenic tumor line may be able to stimulate adequate T cells in the DLN when used in conjunction with cytokines or when transduced with a cytokine gene. Because many of the obstacles listed in Table IV are common in human clinical trials, development of methods to overcome these impediments can be valuable in clinical trials.

V. Methods for Evaluation of Lymphocytes for Adoptive Immunotherapy

Lymphocytes for AIT can be evaluated either *in vivo* or *in vitro*. Each can provide information on the effectiveness of the model and possibly identify the effectors of the immune system involved in tumor regression. One can also perform *in vivo* and *in vitro* cell depletion experiments that can be used to determine which subsets of the adoptively transferred and/or host cells are critical for tumor regression.

A. In Vivo Monitoring of AIT

After developing a mechanism for sensitizing, obtaining, restimulating, and expanding cells for AIT, the experimenter must next determine which method will be used for deter-

Table III Requirements for Successful Immunotherapy of Cancer with T Lymphocytes

1. Tumor antigens recognized by T cells
2. Successful *in vivo* sensitization of T cells
3. Stimulation and activation of T cells *in vitro*
4. Sufficient expansion of tumor-specific T cells in culture
5. Adequate trafficking of T cells to tumor site
6. Potent antitumor effect at tumor site

Table IV Obstacles to T Cell AIT for Cancer Therapy

1.	Weakly immunogenic antigens
2.	Inadequate T cell sensitization before harvest
3.	Insufficient T cell expansion
4.	Inability of T cells to traffic to tumor site.
5.	Inability of adoptively transferred cells to survive and proliferate *in vivo*

mining the effectiveness of the cellular AIT. The four possible choices for evaluating AIT *in vivo* are depicted in Fig. 3 and discussed in detail below.

1. AIT to a Naive Host

A naive mouse (one that has never been exposed to tumor) can be given AIT and then challenged with tumor cells at a later date. This experiment may be a good first step in evaluating the efficacy of an AIT regimen, because the strength of immunity required to protect against tumor establishment is generally less than that required to cause regression in an established tumor. Failure of an AIT protocol to prevent tumor growth in this setting may be an indication that the sensitization method does not stimulate a significant immune response to the tumor cells. This model can also be used to evaluate immunologic memory. Immunity to a tumor challenge 1 month or more after the adoptive transfer of effector cells into naive mice indicates the development of memory cells from the adoptively transferred cell population.

2. Primary Tumor Regression

Serial measurements of ID flank tumors (using calipers to measure the two perpendicular diameters) can be used to evaluate the effectiveness of an AIT regimen. This can be done biweekly until tumors have regressed and are no longer palpable or the animals have to be euthanized for humane reasons. The animals with complete tumor regression can be kept and rechallenged at a later date. The results could be subject to the experimenter's bias, but this can be overcome by devising double-blind experiments with the same person, who is unaware of the treatments, measuring tumor size throughout. Data can be expressed as tumor size (usually expressed as the product of the two diameters) or as a percentage of mice with or without tumors vs. time (see Fig. 4). Complete tumor regression and resistance to rechallenge are fairly strong evidence that the immune system, the adoptively transferred cells, and/or the host cells are contributing to antitumor host defenses. Remember, though, that cure of an established tumor by any means (e.g., surgery or chemotherapy) can result in immunization of the host. Thus, one must establish that the transferred cells are responsible for subsequent immunity. This can be accomplished either by selective depletion of transferred or host cells prior to challenge (see below), or by AIT to naive mice followed by challenge with viable tumor cells.

3. Experimental Metastases

Pulmonary nodules, as discussed earlier, were originally induced with IV injections of tumor cells. After the development of microscopic pulmonary nodules (~3 days), AIT is given to these mice. Based on "pilot" experiments, all of the mice in the experiment are euthanized at the same time (usually about 10–14 days after tumor inoculation) and lung nodules are enumerated. To assess metastases, the thoracic cavity of a euthanized mouse is opened and the trachea is injected with a biologic stain (such as Nigrosian stain or 15% India ink), the lungs are removed *en bloc*, and the specimen is fixed in Fekete's solution (79). The injected ink travels down the trachea into the lungs, following the path of the bronchi and bronchioles. It will be unable to reach diseased areas and therefore these areas will appear white after counterstaining with Fekete's (see Fig. 5). An alternative method for quantitating lung metastases is based on weight, which is proportional to tumor load (80).

4. Spontaneous Metastatic Disease

Some tumor strains, such as 4T1, metastasize spontaneously from a primary site. Flank tumors can be induced and excised and then the animals can be treated with AIT. The appropriate timing of the excision depends on the aggressiveness of the tumor. Tumors will vary as to when metastatic seeding occurs. Removing a tumor too early will result in a lack of metastatic seeding and therefore no therapeutic effect of AIT can be determined. The best time for excision (usually 10–14 days) can be easily determined by inoculating mice ID and then euthanizing and counting metastases (using the previously described procedure) at different time points. AIT can be administered after excision of the tumor. Mice are observed for signs of disease progression such as dehydration (the coat will lose its shiny, healthy look), edema, weight loss, and/or tachypnea. For humane reasons, it is important to recognize these signs so the mouse can be euthanized. When sick, the mice are euthanized and the pulmonary metastases are enumerated. All mice should be sacrificed and evaluated for pulmonary metastases at the conclusion of the experiment. Also, gross examination of the abdominal cavity as well as the incision site should be done to ensure that the local tumor has not recurred. It should be noted that pulmonary metastases of some tumors, such as melanoma, can be seen without the biologic stain. The nodules should be enumerated by a colleague blinded to the treatment groups. The results of such an experiment can be

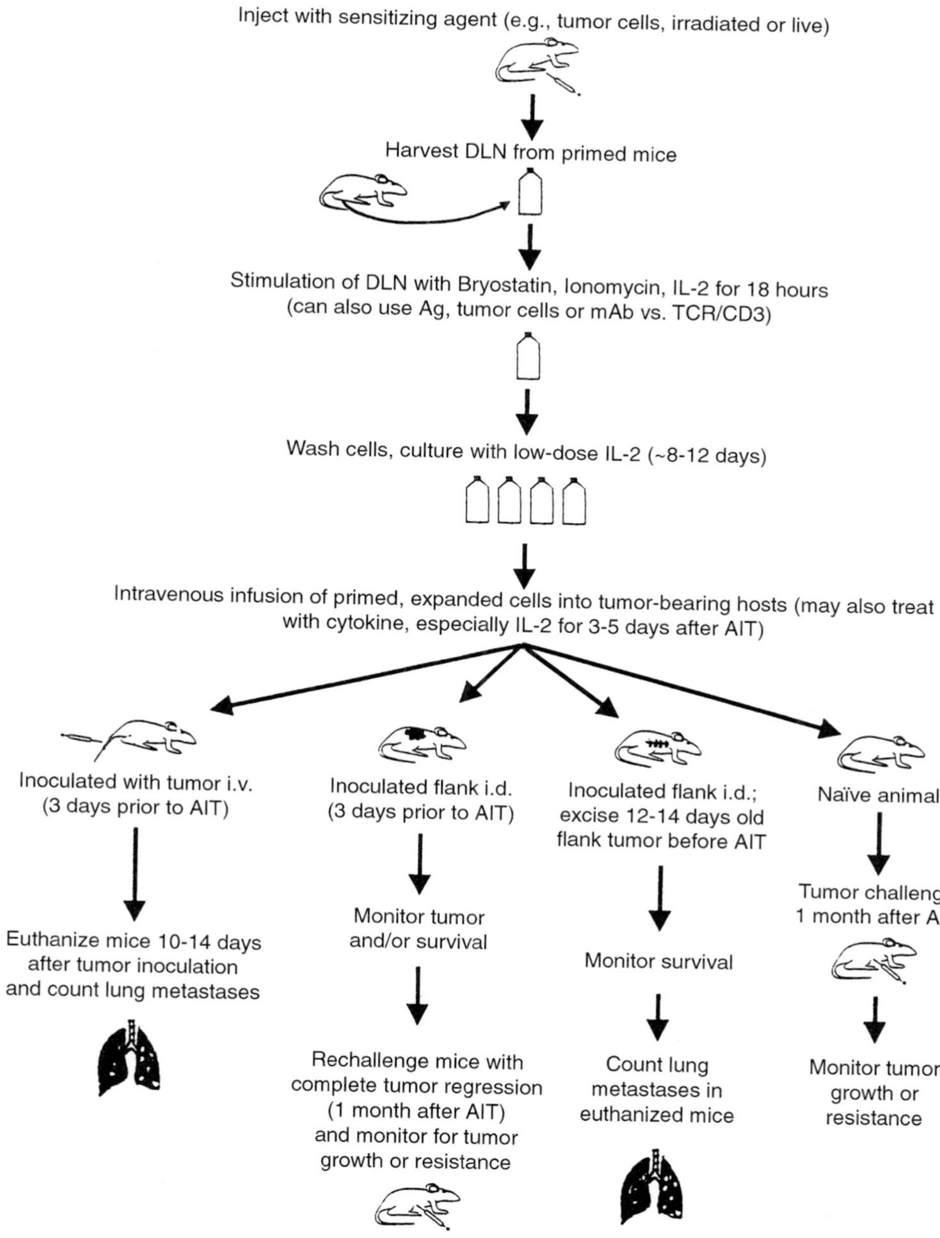
Inject with sensitizing agent (e.g., tumor cells, irradiated or live)
Harvest DLN from primed mice
Stimulation of DLN with Bryostatin, Ionomycin, IL-2 for 18 hours
(can also use Ag, tumor cells or mAb vs. TCR/CD3)
Wash cells, culture with low-dose IL-2 (~8-12 days)
Intravenous infusion of primed, expanded cells into tumor-bearing hosts (may also treat with cytokine, especially IL-2 for 3-5 days after AIT)
Inoculated with tumor i.v. (3 days prior to AIT)
Euthanize mice 10-14 days after tumor inoculation and count lung metastases
Inoculated flank i.d. (3 days prior to AIT)
Monitor tumor and/or survival
Rechallenge mice with complete tumor regression (1 month after AIT) and monitor for tumor growth or resistance
Inoculated flank i.d.; excise 12-14 days old flank tumor before AIT
Monitor survival
Count lung metastases in euthanized mice
Naïve animal
Tumor challenge 1 month after AIT
Monitor tumor growth or resistance

Figure 3 Adoptive immunotherapy in murine models.

presented as number of metastatic nodules at a fixed time, or survival curves can be made, as long as mice are euthanized when they become ill.

B. Protocols for Depletion of T Cell Subtypes

Once an AIT model has been established, different immune cells can be manipulated to see the effects on tumor regression. By depleting subsets of cells, it can be determined whether they are required for the observed antitumor effect. Using *in vivo* and *in vitro* depletion methods, for example, we have shown that depletion of $CD8^+$ T cells, in the MCA105 murine sarcoma model, results in a markedly reduced antitumor effect of AIT (63). Conversely, depletion of $CD4^+$ cells did not alter the immunotherapeutic effect. Other experimenters, using T cell subset depletion methods, have shown that $CD8^+$ cells are vital in the AIT-mediated regression of experimental murine colon cancer (81). In this

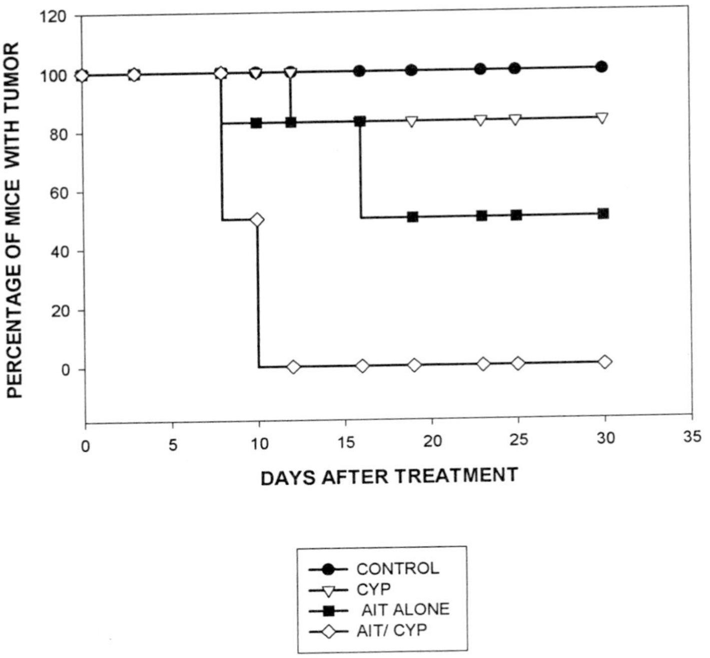

Figure 4 Theoretical example of a disease-free survival curve used to present data obtained from an experiment using mice with 3-day old 4TO7 flank tumors treated with 1 of four regimens: (1) control, no treatment; (2) CYP, given 100 mg/kg cyclophosphamide on day 3; (3) AIT, on day 4 given 1 × 10^6 expanded lymphocytes (DLNs obtained from 4TO7–IL-2-primed mice, stimulated with bryostatin and ionomycin overnight, and expanded for 10 days in media containing low-dose IL-2); and (4) AIT and CYP, given the CYP on day 3 and AIT on day 4. It appears that the group receiving AIT and CYP had an increased tumor-free survival compared to controls or CYP alone.

model, $CD4^+$ depletion lessened, but did not extinguish, tumor regression by AIT. Various techniques are available that allow for *in vivo* and *in vitro* depletions for specific populations of cells. This section provides a short discussion on some of these protocols.

1. *In Vitro* Depletion

In vitro depletions that are pertinent to this chapter involve antibodies against cell surface markers. The first step is to obtain either monoclonal antibodies or antisera that will target the desired population. Cells tagged with monoclonal antibodies can be sorted or depleted by various techniques involving panning, fluorescence-activated cell sorting (FACS), complement-mediated lysis, or immunomagnetic sorting (see Table V).

The panning technique was first described by Mage *et al.* in 1977 (82). When panning for a T cell subset, granulocytes, adherent cells (monocytes and macrophages), and B cells must first be removed from the suspension, often by a physical method such as adherence to nylon wool columns. Alternatively, the mouse cell suspension may be added to a polystyrene tissue culture plate coated with antimouse Ig antibodies. After incubation, the supernatant will contain only nonplastic adherent and Ig^- cells, which are then mixed with monoclonal antibody against Thy-1, CD4, or CD8. The suspension is then added to a new antimouse (or antirat, depending on the origin of the primary antibody), Ig antibody-coated polystyrene tissue culture plate. The marker-positive cells will be adherent to the plate and the marker-negative cells will be in the fluid suspension. After washing the plates, the positive cells can then be recovered by forcefully pipetting them off the plate (83). The negative and positive subsets can then be tested for antitumor activity in the AIT model being studied. Done properly, "panning" provides a very enriched population of marker-positive cells in the adherent population, but is not a very effective method for depleting cells in a given subset.

The fluorescence-activated cell sorter is a flow cytometer that detects and sorts subsets of fluorescently labeled T cells into various groups, depending on the number of markers used. This procedure is very accurate and reliable and sever-

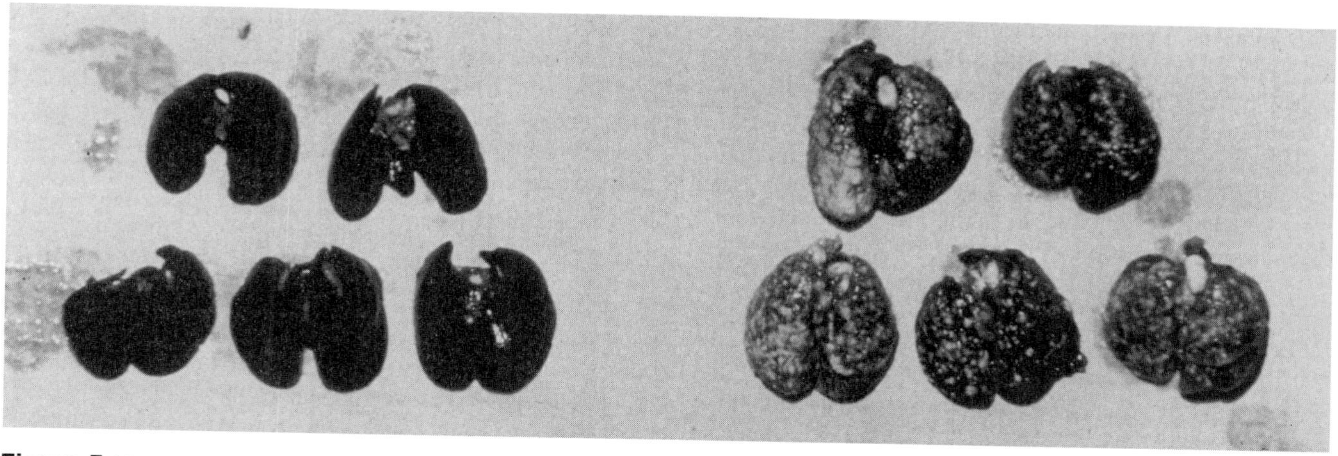

Figure 5 Metastatic pulmonary nodules. This is a photograph of murine lungs stained with 15% India Ink and counterstained with Fekete's solution. However, on the right the lungs have nodular white areas that represent pulmonary metastases induced by IV inoculation of sarcoma cells. The ink is not able to reach the areas with tumor due to bronchi or bronchiole blockage by tumor. Lungs on the left, with no tumor nodules, are from mice treated with AIT, using bryostatin/ionomycin–activated DLN cells from donor mice inoculated in the footpad with the same sarcoma 10 days prior to harvest of popliteal nodes.

al subsets can be separated at one time. However, FACS is not ideal for sorting large quantities of cells, because it is a very slow process.

In complement-mediated lysis, subsets are negatively selected or depleted *in vitro* by antibody-dependent, complement-mediated lysis. That is, antibodies are added that target the cell type to be removed. To deplete $CD8^+$ cells, anti-CD8 monoclonal antibodies (51) or hybridoma ascites (84) are added to the suspension. Cell suspensions with mAbs should be kept on ice because lower temperatures decrease CD4 and CD8 mobility and maximize antibody binding. After incubation, complement (in the form of rabbit or guinea pig serum specifically for this purpose, available from Cedarlane Laboratories) is added to the suspension and incubated at 37°C for 30–60 min. Antibody-coated cells will be lysed by complement and the remaining cells can then be used for AIT. For some primary antibodies that do not fix complement efficiently, a secondary anti-Ig antibody may be needed.

This protocol is simple, rapid, and accurate if care is taken in selecting appropriate antibodies and complement. One must be careful about conclusions made from such experiments. If depletion of one subset abrogates antitumor activity, one should not conclude that this subset alone is responsible for tumor regression, unless depletion of other subsets has no effect. In some models, for example, both $CD4^+$ and $CD8^+$ T cells may be required for optimal antitumor effects.

2. *In Vivo* Depletion with Monoclonal Antibodies

Similar to *in vitro* depletions, *in vivo* depletions with monoclonal antibodies will follow the same principles. However, with *in vivo* depletions, the subsets may only be negatively selected. That is, the antibody that is added will bind to the particular cell type and cause destruction of these cells in the adoptive host, via complement-dependent lysis and/or opsonization of the target cells. Purified monoclonal antibodies will have the greatest specificity, but the greatest cost. Specificity and reactivity of the chosen mAb should be tested *in vitro* prior to *in vivo* use. One should also carry out FACS analysis of the spleens and/or peripheral blood lymphocytes of treated mice 7–10 days after antibody injection to validate the depletion technique.

Table V Methods for in Vitro Depletion of T Cell Subsets

Method	Advantages	Disadvantages	Ref.
Panning	Can enrich marker-positive cells	Not very efficient for direct subset depletion; labor intensive, time consuming	82–83
Fluorescence-activated cell sorter	Accurate and reliable; ability to separate more than one subset at a time	Not efficient for sorting large quantities of cells; requires access to and knowledge of expensive equipment	93–94
Monoclonal antibodies	Accurate and reliable; widely available mAb for murine T cell surface antigens	Expensive; may need to add a secondary antibody if primary unable to bind and activate complement efficiently	51, 84

Similar in concept to *in vivo* depletion of T cell subsets, depletion of cytokines can be carried out *in vivo* to determine their role in AIT-induced tumor regression. For example, using mAbs against IFN-γ was critical for AIT of a metastatic sarcoma (85). Cytokine gene knockout mice, which can be either AIT cell donors or the tumor-bearing recipient, have been used to clarify the role of specific cytokines in AIT models (86).

3. Thy-1 Congenic Strains

Thy-1 is a T cell-specific surface marker that can be altered in congenic strains such that there exist Thy1.1$^+$ and Thy1.2$^+$ murine strains. These mice, which are identical at all gene loci other than the Thy-1 gene, are an important tool for discrimination between effects mediated by AIT-transferred cells vs. host cells. We have used Thy-1 congenics to show that tumor immunity was dependent on transferred T cells, but not on host T cells (85, 87). Briefly, Thy1.1$^+$ mice were sensitized with MCA105 sarcoma cells and the DLNs were harvested, stimulated with bryostatin and ionomycin, and cultured for 10 days with low-dose IL-2 before being adoptively transferred to a naive Thy1.2$^+$ host. These mice had a protective immunity when challenged with MCA105 1 or 5 weeks later. If an anti-Thy1.1 mAb was administered to the Thy1.2$^+$ host before tumor challenge, immunologic protection was abolished. Anti-Thy1.2 Ab had no effect and long-term memory appeared to be mediated by the adoptively transferred cells (Thy-1$^+$) and independent of the host cells (Thy-2$^+$). Similar results were observed when these cells were used to treat established lung metastases (85). Congenic strains, when available, can be an extremely useful tool for evaluating effects of transferred cells on the host.

C. In Vitro Experimental Procedures

In vitro assessment of cell functions that can induce tumor regression *in vivo* provides important information about the possible mechanisms involved (see Table VI). Moreover, the results of such studies can guide future clinical immunotherapy trials (passive or active) by suggesting the appropriate intermediate immunologic endpoints that should be monitored.

1. Chromium (^{51}Cr)-Release Cytotoxicity Assay

The simplest and most direct antitumor effector mechanism is cell contact-mediated killing. In 1968, Brunner *et al.* (88) described this simple assay, which gives a qualitative and quantitative indication of cytotoxic activity. Briefly, the cytotoxicity of an effector is measured by its ability to lyse target cells, which have been prelabeled with radioactive chromium (^{51}Cr). Effectors are cultured with target cells at different ratios (usually 5:1 to 100:1). In order to avoid a high degree of nonspecific lysis, the effector:target ratio should not exceed 100:1. Cell lysis results in the release of ^{51}Cr into the supernatant, which can be measured with a gamma-counter. The corrected percentage of lysis is determined by the equation below, which corrects for any spontaneous release of ^{51}Cr (89). Maximum release is determined by lysis of labeled target cells in distilled water and a detergent.

$$\frac{(\text{test } ^{51}\text{Cr release}) - (\text{spontaneous } ^{51}\text{Cr release})}{(\text{maximum } ^{51}\text{Cr release}) - (\text{spontaneous } ^{51}\text{Cr release})}.$$

As an example, one can test whether 4T07 (a BALB/c murine mammary tumor line)-primed DLNs contain CTLs that can lyse 4T07 targets. Furthermore, antigen specificity should be determined by using another syngeneic target cell. CTLs that have antigen-specific cytotoxic activity will lyse only 4T07 cells. The cytotoxicity of the cultured DLN cells could be a result of non-MHC-restricted killer cells. This can be detected by assaying lysis of YAC-1 target cells, which are sensitive to NK cell lysis.

This is a very easy and reproducible experiment that can be carried out over the course of a day. The effectors and the targets should not be incubated together longer than 4–6 hr. Longer incubation times increase the likelihood of detecting other types of activity, such as macrophage-mediated killing. In general, the problems that arise from the assay are easily overcome by familiarity with the protocol. A limitation of this assay is that cytotoxicity at the single-cell level is not evaluated. And, even though a single CTL effector can recycle after each "hit" and kill multiple target cells during incubation, the assay is relatively insensitive for detection of small numbers of effector cells.

Romero *et al.* (90) have optimized this technique to provide semiquantitative assessment of CTL activity in cancer patients. Essentially, they devised a multiple microculture procedure, which involves magnetic cell sorting of peripheral blood mononuclear cells (PBMCs). The highly enriched CD8$^+$ cells obtained after sorting are plated out at 10^4 cells per microtiter well (0.25-ml wells in 96-well plates). The CD8$^+$-depleted suspension is pulsed with antigenic peptide, then added to the wells as the APC stimulators. The microcultures are restimulated twice and then tested twice for specific CTL activity. The designers claim a 1 in 2×10^6 PMBC sensitivity when a total of 2×10^5 CD8$^+$ cells are studied. Unfortunately, this assay is both labor intensive and time consuming.

2. Limiting Dilution Analysis

The limiting dilution analysis (LDA) technique allows quantification of antigen-specific "preeffector" lymphocytes. LDA can be used to estimate precursor frequency for cytotoxic T cells, for T cells that proliferate in response to antigen, or for T cells producing cytokines in response to antigen. The assay differentiates between positive and negative responses in the individual wells of the experiment. An arbitrary level is set to distinguish between the two

Table VI In Vitro Methods for Detecting Lymphocyte Antitumor Activity

Method	Function	Advantages	Disadvantages	Ref.
Chromium-release cytotoxicity assay	Detection of T cell cytotoxicity	Reliable and reproducible; simple and quick assay	Measures activity of a population, not the single cell level; insensitive for detection of small number of effectors; involves radioisotype handling	88–90
Limiting dilution analysis	Detection of T cell cytotoxicity or cytokine release	Used to statistically estimate CTL precursor frequency	Evaluation of a population of cells, not single-cell activity; labor and time intensive; requires *ex vivo* T cell proliferation	91–92
Tetrameric MHC–peptide complex	Identification of antigen-specific T cells	Increased avidity of label antigen to TCR, allowing for flow cytometry analysis	Not yet available commercially	96
ELISA	Detection of cytokine release	Inexpensive, simple, sensitive, and reproducible	Detects activity of a population, not single cells	97–99
ELISPOT	Detection of cytokine release	Detects cytokines at the single-cell level; 20–200× more sensitive than ELISA	Potential ambiguity of spots decreases reliability; detects presence of only one cytokine at a time	89, 97–99
In situ hybridization	Detection of cytokine production	Detects cytokine mRNA production in cells	Expensive, labor intensive	101
Intracellular cytokine assay	Detection of cytokine presence within a cell	Detects accumulation of multiple cytokines; allows simultaneous detection of cytokines and cell surface markers	Requires sophisticated flow cytometer; difficult to distinguish cytokines produced by a cell from cytokines that are taken up	102–103
Immunohistochemistry	Visualization of immune effector cells	Enables observation of tumor infiltration patterns and cytokine production by those cells	Technically difficult; detects presence of cells, not activity	78, 104, 105

responses. Serial dilution of cells down to a theoretical level of one antigen-specific precursor cell per well is performed, and cells are cultured for several days before assaying effector function. Poisson statistics are employed to estimate the proportion of lymphocytes with a certain functional response (91, 92). A drawback is that the analysis of cells plated with this method and grown up into a clone may not reflect the killing activity of a single cell and depends on the avidity, potency, and clonal "burst" size of proliferation.

3. Tetrameric MHC–Peptide Complex

Unlike B cells, which have high-affinity antigen receptors that bind free antigen, T cell receptors do not bind to free peptide epitopes and dissociate rapidly from soluble peptide–MHC complexes. The identification, enumeration, and separation of T cells based on their antigen specificity would be difficult to achieve with soluble antigens. A more suitable method involving use of fluorochrome-labeled tetrameric peptide–MHC complexes has been described.

Altman *et al.* (93) have developed a method to determine antigen-specific T cell frequency in a population of cells using binding of a synthetic tetrameric MHC–peptide complex. This tetramer may be able to bind to more than one TCR on a T cell. Intuitively, the greater the number of TCRs bound, the higher the avidity of the receptor–ligand interaction. With a slower dissociation rate, the complex is more stable for analysis with FACS. Unlike LDA, this method does not require the *in vitro* stimulation and proliferation of a population of T cells to obtain results. This allows a more rapid and direct method for phenotypic analysis of T cells. However, the use of this tetrameric MHC–peptide complex requires knowledge of the specific tumor peptide epitope. These tetramers will also be MHC restricted, which will limit their use in humans. The major drawback to the application of this technique is that tetramers are not readily available commercially at this time.

4. Techniques for Cytokine Detection

The observation that T cells of different subsets produce distinct groups of cytokines, which relate to their antitumor activity, has led to the need for experimental protocols that study cytokine production by a cell. The development of such methods is particularly important for the analysis of $CD4^+$ T cell activity. Unlike CTLs, the activity of $CD4^+$ cells cannot usually be quantitated by observing target cell lysis, although MHC class II-restricted cytotoxic $CD4^+$ cells have been described. In order to detect the activity of effector $CD4^+$ T cells, cytokine production needs to be measured. These methods may also be a very sensitive technique for assessment of $CD8^+$ T cell responses. The use of two enzyme-linked assays, *in situ* hybridization, and intracellular cytokine staining for evaluation of T cell functions will be briefly discussed here.

a. Enzyme-Linked Immunosorbent Assay The sandwich enzyme-linked immunosorbent assay (ELISA) is most commonly used to detect cytokines. In this method, an unlabeled antibody to the cytokine is bound to a plastic well and the culture medium or animal serum to be tested is added and incubated for 4 hr. For example, after incubating antitumor effector cells with tumor cells or tumor antigen for 24–48 hr, the supernatant would be harvested and tested for specific cytokine release in an ELISA. The excess medium is then rinsed away and a second anticytokine antibody, which is chemically coupled to an enzyme that catalyzes a reaction with later reagents to form a colored compound, is added. Again, the well is rinsed to remove any unbound secondary antibodies and the plate is incubated with a colorless substrate that will become a colored reaction product in the presence of labeled antibody. A microplate reader, which can analyze light absorption in each well at a specific wavelength, is used to quantitate the color of the wells (94).

This method is simple, sensitive, easily reproducible, and relatively inexpensive. However, it cannot distinguish within the population the frequency of cells that are producing the cytokine. ELISA assays are only able to quantitate the composite amount of cytokines made by a population of cells in response to an antigen (e.g., tumor cells). Several other methods, including ELISPOT, enable the detection of cytokine production at the single-cell level.

b. ELISPOT This method is similar in principle to the ELISA, but begins with the plating of lymphoid cells on nitrocellulose-lined microtiter plates that have been precoated with a cytokine-specific monoclonal antibody. The cells are then stimulated with antigen (e.g., tumor cells or peptide and APC complexes). After an appropriate incubation period (~48 hr), the cells are washed away with phosphate-buffered saline and biotinylated rat antimouse antibody against the desired cytokine is added, followed by alkaline phospatase-conjugated streptavidin. After adding substrates that are converted to a colored compound by the enzyme's activity, the released cytokine is detected as discrete spots, which can be viewed with a stereomicroscope. Each spot, theoretically, represents activity of a single cell. ELISPOT does not rely on growth of a cell clone and therefore is a more reliable indicator of individual cell activity. However, when T cells of the relevant specificity are very infrequent, repeated cycles of antigen and growth factor stimulation may be required to expand these clones to sufficient numbers to be detected even in an ELISPOT assay. ELISPOT is very fast and efficient. ELISPOT is 20–200 times more sensitive than ELISA, on culture supernatants, in detecting cytokine production (95, 96). It can also measure the activity of $CD8^+$ T cells with a 30–100 times greater sensitivity compared to the chromium-release assay (90).

Unfortunately, the quantification of a large number of spots, or ambiguity in shape, shade, and size of spots, can make this process tedious and less reliable. Small, dark spots, which do not reflect the presence of cytokine, usually appear when there is inadequate removal of cells. Another problem is diffuse darkening of the nitrocellulose paper caused by too much cytokine being released. If there are too many cytokine-secreting cells, the cytokines accumulate in the media rather than adhering to a spot on the paper. This problem can be avoided by decreasing the number of cells or the duration of incubation. Occasionally, few or no spots are seen after the cells are properly stimulated. This is related to a loss of activity of the labeled antibody or substrate solution. To recognize this problem, positive controls, such as cells that produce cytokines regardless of the presence of stimuli, should be used (97). Another disadvantage is that ELISPOT can measure only one cytokine at a time. *In situ* hybridization and intracellular staining are methods that enable detection of more than one cytokine.

c. In Situ Hybridization This technique is designed to detect the presence of cytokine mRNA in cultured cells or excised tissue. This can be used to assess the activity of effector cells infiltrating a tumor after immunotherapy. First, the organ or cells need to be flash frozen, then cryostat sectioned, followed by fixation with paraformaldehyde. The sections are then probed with labeled cDNA. Different probes can be used to detect different cytokine mRNA species (98). This method is labor intensive as well as expensive. The cDNA probe can be costly.

d. Intracellular Cytokine Staining Another method, intracellular staining, can detect the presence of more than one cytokine at the cellular level with considerably less time and fewer financial demands. This method involves the stimulation of cells in the presence of brefeldin A (BFA) or monensin. These agents disable the golgi complex, thus preventing secretion of cytokines, which will accumulate in the cytoplasm. Next, the cells need to be permeabilized with a detergent so that anticytokine antibodies may enter. The cells can also be labeled for surface markers, allowing analysis by FACS (99, 100).

Once familiarized with the protocol, this technique can be simple, reliable, and reproducible. This is an excellent method for observing cytokine activity in a large population at the cellular level. As with ELISA and ELISPOT, intracellular cytokine staining usually does not require *in vitro* clonal expansion. This technique, like ELISPOT, also gathers data on individual cells. However, this method produces more objective results compared to ELISPOT. An added advantage in this protocol is that flow cytometry can simultaneously analyze the intracellular cytokine production as well as determine the cell phenotype based on cell surface markers.

As with all methods, this has its drawbacks as well. The number of cytokines and cell subsets that can be distinguished with this protocol relies on the sophistication of the flow cytometer. Another disadvantage is the fact that the fixation and permeabilizaton of the cell membrane preclude the further use of these cells in culture or for AIT *in vivo*. Finally, it is not possible to distinguish cytokines produced in a cell from cytokines taken up from the surrounding environment by that cell.

5. Immunohistochemistry

This technique allows for the visualization of immune cells present in a tumor. Tumors at different time periods in the course of an AIT experiment can be excised and analyzed in hope of observing an infiltration pattern associated with tumor regression. Simply, a tumor is excised, flash frozen in liquid nitrogen, and then subjected to cryostat sectioning. The sections are placed on slides, stored in a cardboard box, and air-dried in a −4°C freezer overnight. These slides can be kept for up to 7 days in the −4°C freezer without loss of antigenicity. The staining protocol, involving commercially produced monoclonal antibodies to a variety of immune cells, takes about 6 hr (101). The availability of antibodies for a particular effector cell is animal dependent. For example, there is an absence of a highly specific antibody for NK cell staining in BALB/c mice. In general, however, finding the right antibodies is not very difficult.

Properly freezing the tissue is vital to the quality of the staining. If tissues are not properly frozen or allowed to thaw, significant tissue damage can occur. Ice crystals may develop and cause fracture lines, which tend to be a source of artifactual staining. As with any other protocol involving antibodies, care must be taken to ensure that the reagents have not lost specificity or reactivity. Normal tissue can be used as a positive control.

The results will be qualitative rather than quantitative. Another theoretical concern is that the staining will delineate which cells are present, but this does not necessarily translate to cell activity nor does it prove that any particular subset of cells found in the tumor is actually playing a key role in tumor regression. Despite its limitations, this technique is valuable in observing cellular patterns at the tumor site and providing clues for more definitive studies (e.g., *in vitro* depletion) (78, 102).

VI. Conclusion

The reader is reminded that the goals of using animal AIT models are twofold. Ideally, the model can be translated into human clinical therapy. However, these models can serve another equally important function. AIT models can be manipulated in a variety of ways to help define the importance of different parts of the immune system in tumor regression. For example, work pertaining to the importance of $CD4^+$ and $CD8^+$ cells in antitumor defense have used AIT models (81). The importance of many cytokines, such as IFN-γ, has also been recognized through the use of AIT models (86). A well-thought out model can be very useful in teasing out various components of the immune system, the results of which may have a significant impact on tumor immunotherapy in humans.

There are many new avenues to be investigated using adoptive immunotherapy, including (1) ways to up-regulate tumor immunogenicity with genetic manipulations to increase T cell stimulation, such as expression of cytokines or costimulatory molecules on tumor cells; (2) methods to select tumor-reactive T cell subsets, especially those with memory potential; (3) techniques to develop more effective and/or rapid *ex vivo* expansion of T cells; (4) investigation into genetic alteration of T cells into more effective mediators of tumor destruction; and (5) development of protocols involving tumor vaccines for the sensitization of effector T cells. Each new development with adoptive immunotherapy gives rise to a new "family" of protocols that will hopefully lead to results that may impact clinical cancer treatment.

References

1. Disis, M. L., and Cheever, M. A. (1996). Oncogenic proteins as tumor antigens. *Curr. Opin. Immunol.* **8,** 637–642.
2. Syrengelas, A. D., and Levy, R. (1999). DNA vaccination against the idiotype of a murine B cell lymphoma: Mechanism of tumor protection. *J. Immunol.* **162,** 4790–4795.
3. Billingham, R. E., Brent, L., and Medowar P. B. (1954). Quantitative studies on tissue transplantation. *Proc. R. Soc. Biol.* **143,** 58.
4. Hewitt, H., Blake, E., and Walder, A. (1976). A critique of the evidence for active host defense against cancer, based on personal studies of 27 murine tumors of spontaneous origin. *Br. J. Cancer* **33,** 241–259.
5. Van pel, A., and Boon, T. (1982). Protection against a nonimmunogenic mouse leukemia by an immunogenic variant obtained by mutagenesis. *Proc. Natl. Acad. Sci. U.S.A.* **79,** 4718–4722.
6. Rosenberg, S. A., Lotze, M. T., Muul, L. M., Leitman, S., Chang, A. E., Ettinghausen, S. E., Matory, Y. L., Skibber, J. M., and Vetto, J. T. (1985). Observations on the systemic administration of autologous lymphokine-activated killer cells and recombinant interleukin-2 to patients with metastatic cancer. *N. Engl. J. Med.* **313,** 1485–1492.

7. Slingluff, C. L. (1996). Tumor antigens and tumor vaccines: Peptides as immunogens. *Semin. Surg. Oncol.* **12,** 446–453.
8. Janeway, C. A., Travers, P., Walport, M., and Capra, D. J. (1999). "Immunobiology: The Immune System in Health and Disease," 4th Ed. Elsevier Science Ltd. Garland Publishing, New York.
9. Mosmann, T. R., Chervinshi, H., Bond, M. W., Giedlin, M. A., and Coffman, R. L. (1986). Two types of murine helper T-cell clone. I. Definition according to profiles of lymphokine activities and secreted proteins. *J. Immunol.* **136,** 2348–2357.
10. Tsung, K., Meko, J. B., Peplinski, G. R., Tsung, Y. L., and Norton, J. A. (1997). IL-12 induces T helper 1-directed antitumor response. *J. Immunol.* **158,** 3359–3365.
11. Sredni, B, Tichler, T, Shani, A, Catane, R., Kaufman, B., Strassmann, G., Albeck, M., and Kalechman, Y. (1996). Predominance of THI response in tumor-bearing mice and cancer patients treated with AS101. *J. Natl. Cancer Inst.* **18,** 1276–84.
12. Bell, E. B., Sparshott, S. M., and Bunce, C. (1998). $CD4^+$ T-cell memory, CD45R subsets and the persistence of antigen- a unifying concept. *Immunol. Today* **19,** 60–64.
13. Hamann, D., Baars, P. A., Rep, M., Hooibrink, B., Kerkhof-Garde, S., Klein, M. R., and van Lier, R. A. (1997). Phenotypic and functional separation of memory and effector human $CD8^+$ T cells. *J. Exp. Med.* **186,** 1407–1418.
14. Mackay, C. R. (1999). Dual personality of memory T cells. *Nature* (London). **401,** 659–660.
15. Broder, S., and Waldmann, T. A. (1978). The suppressor-cell network in cancer. *N. Engl. J. Med.* **299,** 1281–1284.
16. Miescher, S., Whiteside, TL., Carrel, C. V., and Fledner, V. (1986). Functional properties of tumor-infiltrating and blood lymphocytes in patients with solid tumors: Effects of tumor cells and their supernatants on proliferative responses of lymphocytes. *J. Immunol.* **136,** 1899–1907.
17. Chen, L., Ashe, S., Brady, W. A., Hellstrom, I., Hellstrom, K. E., Ledbetter, J. A., McGowan, P., and Linsley, P. S. (1992) Co-stimulation of antitumor immunity by the B7 counterreceptor for the T lymphocyte molecules CD28 and CTLA-4. *Cell* **71,** 1093–1102.
18. Townsend, S. E., and Allison, J. P. (1993). Tumor rejection after direct costimulation of $CD8^+$ T cells by B7-transfected melanoma cells. *Science* **259,** 368–370.
19. Inge, T. H., Hoover, S. K., Susskind, B. M., Barrett, and Bear, H. D. (1992). Inhibition of tumor-specific cytotoxic T-lymphocyte responses by transforming growth factor β_1. *Cancer Res.* **52,** 1386–1392.
20. Wang, Q., Redovan, C., Tubbs, R., Olencki, T., Klein, E., Kudoh, S., Finke, J., and Bukowski, R. M. (1995). Selective cytokine gene expression in renal cell carcinoma tumor cells and tumor infiltrating lymphocytes. *Int. J. Cancer* **61,** 780–785.
21. Sulitzeanu, D. (1993). Immunosuppressive factors in human cancer. *Adv. Cancer Res.* **60,** 247–267.
22. Cromme, F. V., Airey, J., Heemels, M. Y., Ploegh, H. L., Keating, P. J., Stern, P. L., Meijer, C. J. L. M., and Walboomers, J. M. M. (1994). Loss of transporter protein, encoded by the TAP-1 gene, is highly correlated with loss of HLA expression in cervical carcinomas. *J. Exp. Med.* **179,** 335–340.
23. Garrido, F., Ruiz-Cabello, F., Cabera, T., Perez-Villar, J. J., Lopez-Botet, M., Duggan-Keen, M., and Stern, P. L. (1997). Implications for immunosurveillance of altered HLA class I phenotypes in human tumors. *Immunol. Today* **18,** 89–95.
24. Weber, J. S., and Rosenberg, S. A. (1983). Modulation of murine tumor major histocompatability antigens by cytokines *in vivo* and *in vitro.* *Cancer Res.* **48,** 5818–5824.
25. Speiser, D. E., Miranda, R., Zakarian, A., Bachmann, M. F., McKall-Faienza, K., and Odermatt, B. (1997). Self antigens expressed by solid tumors do not efficiently stimulate naïve or activated T cells: implications for immunotherapy. *J. Exp. Med.* **186,** 645–653.
26. Ando, K., Guidotti, L. G., Cerny, A., Ishikawa, T., and Chisari, F. V. (1994). CTL access to tissue antigen is restricted *in vivo. J. Immunol.* **153,** 482–488.
27. Alexander, J. P., Kudph, S., Melsop, K. A., Hamilton, T. A., Edinger, M. G., Tubbs, R. R., Sica, D., Tuason, L., Klein, E., Bukowski, R. M., and Finke, J. H. (1993). T-cells infiltrating renal cell carcinoma display a poor proliferative response even though they can produce interleukin-2 and they express interleukin-2 receptors. *Cancer Res.* **53,** 1380–1387.
28. Mizoguchi, H., O'Shea, J. J., Longo, D. L., Loeffler, C. M., Mc Vicar, D. W., and Ochoa, A. C. (1992). Alteration in signal transduction molecules in T-lymphocytes from tumor-bearing mice. *Science* **258,** 1795–1798.
29. Ye, X., McCarrick, J., Jewett, L., and Knowles, B. B. (1994). Timely immunization subverts the development of peripheral nonresponsiveness and suppressor tumor development in simian virus 40 tumor antigen-transgenic mice. *Proc. Natl. Acad. Sci. U.S.A.* **91,** 3916–3920.
30. Chang, A. E., and Shu, S. (1996). Current status of adoptive immunotherapy of cancer. *Crit. Rev. Oncol. Hematol.* **22,** 213–228.
31. Tuttle, T. M., Inge, T. H., Wirt, C. P., Frank, J. L., McCrady, C. M., and Bear, H. D. (1992). Bryostatin 1 activates T cells that have antitumor activity. *J. Immunotherap.* **12,** 75–81.
32. Grimm, E. A., Robb, R. J., Roth, J. A., Neckers, L. M., Lachman L. B., Wilson D. J., and Rosenberg S. A. (1983). Lymphokine-activated killer cell phenomenon III. Evidence that IL-2 is sufficient for direct activation of peripheral blood lymphocytes into lymphokine-activated killer cells. *J. Exp. Med.* **158,** 1356–1361.
33. Rosenberg, S. A., Lotze, M. T., Yang, J. C., Topalian, S. L., Chang, A. E., Schwartzenruber, D. J., Aebersold, P., Leitman, S., Linehan, W. M., and Seipp, C. A. (1993). Prospective randomized trial of high-dose interleukin-2 alone or in conjunction with lymphokine-activated killer cells for the treatment of patients with advanced cancer. *J. Natl. Cancer Inst.* **85,** 622–632.
34. Koretz, M. J., Lawson, D. H., York, R. M., Graham, S. D., Murray, D. R., Gillespie, T. M., Levitt, D., and Sell, K. M. (1991). Randomized study of interleukin-2 (IL-2) alone vs. IL-2 plus lymphokine-activated killer cells for the treatment of melanoma and renal cell cancer. *Arch. Surg.* **126,** 898–903.
35. Rosenberg, S. A., Yang, J. C., Topalian, S. L., Schwartenruber, D. J., Weber, J. S., Parkinson, D. R., Seipp, C. A., Einhorn, J. H., and White, D. E. (1994). Treatment of 283 consecutive patients with metastatic melanomas or renal cell cancer using high-dose bolused interleukin-2. *JAMA* **271,** 907–913.
36. Tuttle, T. M., Inge, T. H., Lind, D. S., and Bear, H. D. (1992). Adoptive transfer of bryostatin 1-activated T cells provides long-term protection from tumor metastases. *Surg. Oncol.* **1,** 299–307.
37. Hasday, J. D., Shah, E. A., and Lieberman, A. P. (1990). Macrophage tumor necrosis factor-alpha release is induced by contact with some tumors. *J. Immunol.* **145,** 371–379.
38. Hennemann, B., Beckmann, G., Eichelmann, A., Rehm, A., and Andreesen, R. (1998). Phase I clinical trial of adoptive immunotherapy of cancer patients using monocyte-derived macrophages activated with interferon gamma and lipopolysaccharide. *Cancer Immunol. Immunother.* **45,** 250–256.
39. Rosenberg, S. A., Spiess, P., and Lafeniere, R. (1986). A new approach to the adoptive immunotherapy of cancer with tumor-infiltrating lymphocytes. *Science* **233,** 1318–1321.
40. Spiess, P. J., Yang, J. C., and Rosenberg, S. A. (1987). *In vivo* antitumor activity of tumor-infiltrating lymphocytes expanded in recombinant interleukin-2. *J. Natl. Cancer Inst.* **79,** 1067–1075.
41. Taneja, S. S., Pierce, W., Figlin, R., and Belldegrun, A. (1995). Immunotherapy for renal cell carcinoma: The era of interleukin-2 based treatment. *Urology* **45,** 911–924.
42. Rosenberg, S. A., Packard, B. S., Aebersold, P. M., Solomon, D., Topalian, S. L., Toy, S. T., Simon, P., Lotze, M. T., Yang, J. C., Seipp, C. A., *et al.* (1988). Use of tumor-infiltrating lymphocytes and inter-

leukin-2 in the immunotherapy of patients with metastatic melanoma: A preliminary report. *N. Engl. J. Med.* **319,** 1676–1680.

43. Goedegebuure, P. S., Douville, L. M., Li, H., Richmond, G. C., Schoof, D. D., Scavone, M., and Eberlein, T. J. (1995). Adoptive immunotherapy with tumor-infiltrating lymphocytes and interleukin-2 in patients with metastatic malignant melanoma and renal cell carcinoma: A pilot study. *J. Clin. Oncol.* **13,** 1939–1949.
44. Yannelli, J. R., Hyatt, C., McConnell, S., Hines, K., Jacknin, L., Parker, L., Sanders, M., and Rosenberg, S. A. (1996). Growth of tumor-infiltrating lymphocytes from human solid cancers: Summary of a 5-year experience. *Int. J. Cancer* **65,** 413–421.
45. Boon, T. (1993). Tumor antigens recognized by cytolytic T lymphocytes: Present perspectives for specific immunotherapy. *Int. J. Cancer* **54,** 177–180.
46. Lynch, D. H., and Miller, R. E. (1991). Immunotherapeutic elimination of syngeneic tumors *in vivo* by cytotoxic T lymphocytes generated *in vitro* from lymphocytes from the draining lymph nodes of tumor-bearing mice. *Eur. J. Immunol.* **21,** 1403–1410.
47. Stephenson, K. R., Perry-Lalley, D., Griffith, K. D., Shu, S., and Chang, A. E. (1989). Development of antitumor reactivity in regional lymph nodes from tumor-immunized and tumor bearing murine hosts. *Surgery* **105,** 523–528.
48. Shu, S., Chou, T., and Rosenberg, S. A. (1987). Generation from tumor-bearing mice of lymphocytes with *in vivo* therapeutic efficacy. *J. Immunol.* **139,** 295–304.
49. Chou, T., Chang, A. E., and Shu, S. (1988). Generation of therapeutic T lymphocytes from tumor-bearing mice by *in vitro* sensitization: Culture requirements and characterization of immunologic specificity. *J. Immunol.* **140,** 2453–2461.
50. Shondak, V. K., Tuck, M. K., Shu, S., Yoshizawa, H., and Chang, A. E. (1991). Enhancing effects of interleukin-1α administration on antitumor effector T cell development. *Arch. Surg.* **126,** 1503–1509.
51. Hathcock, K. S. (1996). T cell depletion by cytotoxic elimination. *In* "Current Protocols in Immunology" (J. E. Coligan, A. M. Kruisbeek, D. H. Margulies, E. M. Shevach, and W. Strober, eds.), pp. 3.4.1–3.4.3. John Wiley & Sons, Inc., New York.
52. Hathcock, K. S. (1996). T cell enrichment by nonadherence to nylon. *In* "Current Protocols in Immunology" (J. E. Coligan, A. M. Kruisbeek, D. H. Margulies, E. M. Shevach, and W. Strober, eds.), pp. 3.2.1–3.2.4. John Wiley & Sons, Inc., New York.
53. Rosenberg, S. A. (1999). A new era for cancer immunotherapy based on the genes that encode cancer antigens. *Immunity* **10,** 281–287.
54. Jaeger, E., Bernhard, H., Romero, P., Ringhoffer, M., Arand, M., Karbach, J., Ilsemann, C., Hagedorn, M., and Knuth, A. (1996). Generation of cytotoxic T-cell responses with synthetic melanoma-associated peptides *in vivo*: Implications for tumor vaccines with melanoma-associated antigens. *Int. J. Cancer* **66,** 162–169.
55. Rivoltini, L., Kawakami, Y., Sakaguchi, K., Sountwood, S., Sette, A., Robbins, P. F., Marincola, F. M., Salgaller, M. L., Yannelli, J. R., Appella, E., *et al.* (1995). Induction of tumor-reactive CTL from peripheral blood and tumor-infiltrating lymphocytes of melanoma patients by *in vitro* stimulation with an immunodominant peptide of the human melanoma antigen MART-1. *J. Immunol.* **154,** 2257–2265.
56. Banchereau, J., and Steinman, R. M. (1998). Dendritic cells and the control of immunity. *Nature* (London) **392,** 245–252.
57. Yoshizawa, H., Chang, A. E., and Shu, S. (1991). Specific adoptive immunotherapy mediated by tumor-draining lymph node cells sequentially activated with anti-CD3 and IL-2. *J. Immunol.* **147,** 729–737.
58. Garlie, N. K., LeFever, A. V., Sienbenlist, R. E., Levine, B. L., June, C. H., and Lum, L. G. (1999). T cell coactivated with immobilized anti-CD3 and anti-CD28 as potential immunotherapy for cancer. *J. Immunother.* **22,** 336–345.
59. Chatila, T., Silverman, L., Miller, R., and Geha, R. (1989). Mechanisms of T cell activation of by calcium inonophore, ionomycin. *J. Immunol.* **143,** 1283–1289.
60. Kumagai, N., Benedict, S. H., Mills, G. B., and Gelfand, E. W. (1988). Induction of competence and progression signals in human T lymphocytes by phorbol esters and calcium ionophores. *J. Cell Physiol.* **137,** 329–336.
61. Tuttle, T. M., Inge, T. H., McCrady, C. M., Bethke, K. P., and Bear, H. D. (1992). Activation of $CD8^+$ murine T cells from tumor-draining lymph nodes by phorbol dibutyrate plus calcium ionophore. *J. Immunother.* **12,** 32–40.
62. Blumberg, P. M., Pettit, G. R., Takayama, H., Hu-Li, J., and Sitkovsky, M. V. (1989). "Skin Carcinogenesis: Mechanisms and Human Relevance," pp. 201–212. Alan R Liss, New York.
63. Tuttle, T. M., Inge, T. H., Bethke, K. P., McCrady, C. W., Pettit, G. R., and Bear, H. D. (1992). Activation and growth of murine tumor-specific T-cells which have *in vivo* activity with bryostatin 1. *Cancer Res.* **52,** 548–553.
64. Tuttle, T. M., Inge, T. H., Lind, D. S., and Bear, H. D. (1992). Adoptive transfer of bryostatin 1-activated T cells provides long-term protection from metastases. *Surg. Oncol.* **1,** 299–307.
65. Rosenberg, S. A. (1997). Principles of cancer management. *In* "Cancer Principles and Practice of Oncology," pp. 349–372. Lippincott, Philadelphia.
66. Cheever, M. A., Greenberg, P. D., Fefer, A., and Gillis, S. (1982). Augmentation of the anti-tumor therapeutic efficacy of long-term cultured T lymphocytes by *in vivo* administration of purified interleukin-2. *J. Exp. Med.* **155,** 968–980.
67. Cheever, M. A., Greenberg, P. D., Irle, C., Thompson, J. A., Urdal, D. L., Mochizuki, D. Y., Henney, C. S., and Gillis, S. (1984). Interleukin-2 administration *in vivo* induces the growth of cultured T cells *in vivo. J. Immunol.* **132,** 2259–2265.
68. Atkins, M. B. (1998). Immunotherapy and experimental approaches for metastatic melanoma. *Hematol. Oncol. Clin. N. Am.* **12,** 877–903.
69. Bukowski, R. M. (1997). Natural history and therapy of metastatic renal cell carcinoma: The role of IL-2. *Cancer* **80,** 1198–1220.
70. Bear, H. D., Hamad, G. G., and Kostuchenko, P. J. (1996). Biologic therapy of melanoma with cytokines and lymphocytes. *Semin. Surg. Oncol.* **12,** 436–445.
71. Sella, A., Swanson, D. A., Ro, J. Y., Putnam, J. B., Amato, R. J., Markowitz, A. B., and Logothetis, C. J. (1993). Surgery following response to interferon-alpha-based therapy for residual renal cell carcinoma. *J. Urol.* **149,** 19–21.
72. Wallach, D., Fellous, M., and Revel, M. (1982). Preferential effect of gamma interferon on the synthesis of HLA antigens and their mRNAs in human cells. *Nature (London)* **299,** 833–836.
73. Rosenberg, S. A., Schwartz, S. L., and Spiess, P. J. (1988). Combination immunotherapy for cancer: Synergistic antitumor interactions of interleukin-2, interferon alpha, and tumor-infiltrating lymphocytes. *J. Natl. Cancer Inst.* **80,** 1393–1397.
74. Vander Woude, D. L., Wagner, P. D., Shu, S., and Chang, A. E. (1991). Enhanced antitumor reactivity of tumor-sensitized T-cells by interferon alpha. *Arch. Surg.* **126,** 307–313.
75. Proietti, E., Greco, G., Garrone, B., Baccarini, S., Mauri, C., Venditti, M., Carlei, D., and Belardelli, F. (1998). Importance of cyclophosphamide-induced bystander effect on T cells for successful tumor eradication in response to adoptive immunotherapy in mice. *J. Clin. Invest.* **2,** 429–441.
76. Awwad, M., and North, R. J. (1988). Cyclophosphamide (Cy)-facilitated adoptive immunotherapy of a Cy-resistant tumour. Evidence that Cy permits the expression of adoptive T-cell mediated immunity by removing suppressor T cells rather than by reducing tumour burden. *Immunology* **65,** 87–92.

77. Tuttle, T. M., Fleming, M. D., Hogg, P. S., Inge, T. H., and Bear, H. D. (1994). Ability of low-dose cyclophosphamide to overcome metastasis-induced immunosuppression. *Ann. Surg. Oncol.* **1,** 53–58.
78. Tsung, K., Meko, J. B., Tsung, Y. L., Peplinski, G. R., and Norton, J. A. (1998). Immune response against large tumors eradicated by treatment with cyclophoshamide and IL-12. *J. Immunol.* **160,** 1369–1377.
79. Wexler, H. (1966). Accurate identification of experimental pulmonary metastases. *J. Natl. Cancer Inst.* **36,** 641–645.
80. Coveney, E., Clary, B., Iacobucci, M., Philip, R., and Lyerly, K. (1996). Active immunotherapy with transiently infected cytokine-secreting tumor cells inhibits breast cancer metastases in tumor-bearing animals. *Surgery* **120,** 265–272.
81. Abrams, S. I., Hodge, H. W., McLaughlin, J. P., Steinberg, S. M., Kantor, J. A., and Schlom, J., (1997). Adoptive immunotherapy as an in vivo model to explore antitumor mechanisms induced by a recombinant anticancer vaccine. *J. Immunother.* **20,** 48–59.
82. Mage, M. G., McHugh, L. L., and Rothstein, T. L. (1977). Mouse lymphocytes with and without surface immunoglobulin: preparative scale separation in polystrene tissue culture plates coated with specifically purified anti-immunoglobulin. *J. Immunol. Methods* **15,** 47–56.
83. Mage, M. G. (1996). Fractionation of T cells and B cells. *In* "Current Protocols in Immunology" (J. E. Coligan, A. M. Kruisbeek, D. H. Margulies, E. M. Shevach, and W. Strober, eds.), pp. 3.5.1–3.5.6. John Wiley & Sons, Inc., New York.
84. Yokoyama, W. M. (1996). Monoclonal antibody supernatant and ascites fluid production. *In* "Current Protocols in Immunology" (J. E. Coligan, A. M. Kruisbeek, D. H. Margulies, E. M. Shevach, and W. Strober, eds.), pp. 2.6.1–2.6.7. John Wiley & Sons, Inc., New York.
85. Tuttle, T. M., McCrady, C. W., Inge, T. H., Salour, M., and Bear H. D. (1993) γ-Interferon plays a key role in T-cell-induced tumor regression. *Cancer Res.* **53,** 833–839.
86. Nagoshi, M., Goedegebuure, P. S., Burger, U. L., Sadanaga, N., Chang, M. P., and Eberlein, T. J. (1998). Successful adoptive cellular immunotherapy is dependent on induction of a host immune response triggered by cytokine (IFN-γ and granulocyte/macrophage colony-stimulating factor) producing donor tumor-infiltrating lymphocytes. *J. Immunol.* **160,** 334–344.
87. Tuttle, T. M., Inge, T. H., Lind, D. S., and Bear, H. D. (1992). Adoptive transfer of bryostatin 1-activated T cells provides long-term protection from tumour metastases. *Surg. Oncol.* **1,** 299–307.
88. Brunner, K. T., Mauel, J., Cerottini, J. C., and Chapuis, B. (1968). Quantitative assay of lytic action of immune lymphoid cells on ^{51}Cr-labelled allogeneic target cells *in vitro*: Inhibition by isoantibody and by drugs. *Immunology* **14,** 181–196.
89. Wunderlich, J., and Shearer, G. (1996). Induction and measurement of cytotoxic T lymphocyte activity *In* "Current Protocols in Immunology" (J. E. Coligan, A. M. Kruisbeek, D. H. Margulies, E. M. Shevach, and W. Strober, eds.), pp. 3.11.1–3.11.15. John Wiley & Sons, Inc., New York.
90. Romero, P., Cerottini, J. C., and Waanders, G. A. (1998). Novel methods to monitor antigen-specific cytotoxic T-cell responses in cancer immunotherapy. *Mol. Med. Today* **4,** 305–312.
91. Sharrock, C. E. M., Kaminski, E., and Man, S. (1990). Limiting dilution analysis of human T cells: A useful clinical tool. *Immunol. Today* **11,** 281–286.
92. Miller, R. A. (1996). Quantitation of functional T cells by limiting dilution. *In* "Current Protocols in Immunology" (J. E. Coligan, A. M. Kruisbeek, D. H. Margulies, E. M. Shevach, and W. Strober, eds.), pp. 3.15.1–3.15.12. John Wiley & Sons, Inc., New York.
93. Sharrow, S. O. (1996). Overview of flow cytometry. *In* "Current Protocols in Immunology" (J. E. Coligan, A. M. Kruisbeek, D. H. Margulies, E. M. Shevach, and W. Strober, eds.), pp. 5.1.1–5.1.8. John Wiley & Sons Inc., New York.
94. Sharrow, S. O. (1996). Analysis of flow cytometry data. *In* "Current Protocols in Immunology" (J. E. Coligan, A. M. Kruisbeek, D. H. Margulies, E. M. Shevach, and W. Strober, eds.), pp. 5.2.1–5.2.10. John Wiley & Sons Inc., New York.
95. Schmid, I., and Giorgi, J. V. (1996). Preparation of cells and reagents for flow cytometry. *In* "Current Protocols in Immunology" (J. E. Coligan, A. M. Kruisbeek, D. H. Margulies, E. M. Shevach, and W. Strober, eds.), pp. 5.3.1–5.3.22. John Wiley & Sons Inc., New York.
96. Altman, J. D., Moss, P. A. H., Goulder, P. J. R., Barouch, D. H., McHeyzer-Williams, M. G., Bell, J. I., McMichael, A. J., and Davis, M. M. (1996) Phenotypic analysis of antigen-specific T lymphocytes. *Science* **274,** 94–96.
97. Hornbeck, P. (1996). Enzyme-linked immunosorbent assay. *In* "Current Protocols in Immunology" (J. E. Coligan, A. M. Kruisbeek, D. H. Margulies, E. M. Shevach, and W. Strober, eds.), pp. 2.1.1–2.1.22. John Wiley & Sons, Inc., New York.
98. Tanguay, S., and Killion, J. (1994). Direct comparison of ELISPOT and ELISA-based assays for detection of individual cytokine-secreting cells. *Lymphokine Cytokine Res.* **13,** 259–263.
99. Shirai, A., Holmes, K., and Klinman, D. M. (1993). Detection and quantitation of cells secreting IL-6 under physiologic conditions in BALB/c mice. *J. Immunol.* **150,** 793–799.
100. Klinman, D. M., and Nutman, T. B. (1996). ELISPOT assay to detect cytokine-secreting murine and human cells. *In* "Current Protocols in Immunology" (J. E. Coligan, A. M. Kruisbeek, D. H. Margulies, E. M. Shevach, and W. Strober, eds.), pp. 6.19.1–6.19.8. John Wiley & Sons, Inc., New York.
101. Carter, L. L., and Swain, S. L. (1997). Single cell analyses of cytokine production. *Curr. Opin. Immunol.* **9,** 177–182.
102. Jung, T., Schauer, U., Heusser, C., Neumann, C., and Rieger, C. (1993). Detection of intracellular cytokines by flow cytometry. *J. Immunol. Methods* **159,** 197–207.
103. Prussin, C., and Metcalfe, D. D. (1995). Detection of intracytoplasmic cytokine using flow cytometry and directly conjugated anti-cytokine antibodies. *J. Immunol. Methods* **188,** 117–128.
104. Jaffe, E. S., and Raffeld, M. (1996). Identification of cells in tissue sections. *In* "Current Protocols in Immunology" (J. E. Coligan, A. M. Kruisbeek, D. H. Margulies, E. M, Shevach, and W. Strober, eds.), pp. 5.8.1–5.8.8. John Wiley & Sons, Inc., New York.
105. Cavallo, F., Di Carlo, E., Butera, M., Verrua, R., Colombo, M. P., Musiani, P., and Forni, G. (1999). Immune events associated with the cure of established tumors and spontaneous metastases by local and systemic interleukin 12. *Cancer Res.* **59,** 414–421.

36

Metastasis: Biology and Experimental Models

Russell S. Berman,[*,†] Jerald J. Killion,[†] and Lee M. Ellis[*,†]

[*]Departments of Surgical Oncology and [†]Cancer Biology,
The University of Texas M. D. Anderson Cancer Center, Houston, Texas 77030

I. Introduction

Metastasis is the major cause of death from cancer. Many cancers have already metastasized from the primary tumor site by the time they are diagnosed, and multiple metastases are nearly impossible to eradicate by surgery, radiation, chemotherapy, or biotherapy. Current therapies for distant metastases have had minimal effects on outcome. Therefore, a better understanding of the biology of metastasis and of the molecular events leading to the metastatic phenotype is essential if new and innovative antineoplastic therapeutic approaches are to be developed. This chapter highlights the molecular and biologic alterations that lead to the development of metastasis and will describe some of the model systems used to study this process.

II. Biology of Metastasis

A. The Metastatic Cascade

Metastasis is a highly selective, nonrandom process consisting of a series of linked, sequential steps that favor the survival of a subpopulation of metastatic cells that exist within the primary tumor mass (1) (Fig. 1). For a tumor cell to be able to form a metastasis, it must express a complex phenotype that begins with the invasion of the surrounding normal stroma, either by a single tumor cell with increased motility or by groups of cells from the primary tumor. Once the invading cells penetrate the vascular or lymphatic channels, the cells can detach from the walls of those channels and be transported within the circulatory system. Such tumor "emboli" must be able to survive the host's immune defenses and the turbulence of the circulation, stop in the capillary bed of compatible organs, extravasate into the organ parenchyma, proliferate, and establish a micrometastasis. Continued growth of these small lesions requires the development of a vascular supply (angiogenesis) and continuous evasion of host defense cells. Failure to complete one or more steps of this process (e.g., inability to grow in a distant organ's parenchyma) will eliminate the cells. Thus, to produce clinically relevant metastases, the successful metastatic cell must exhibit a complex phenotype that is regulated by transient or permanent changes in different genes at the level of the DNA, the mRNA, or both (1, 2).

It is now widely accepted that many malignant tumors contain heterogeneous subpopulations of cells. This heterogeneity is exhibited in a wide range of genetic, biochemical, immunologic, and biologic characteristics such as growth rate, antigenic and immunogenic status, cell surface receptors and products, enzymes, karyotypes, cell morphology, invasiveness, drug resistance, and metastatic potential. Specific tumor cells or colonies within the larger heterogeneous tumor specimen probably are the forerunners of distant metastases (3).

Successful metastasis depends in part on the interaction of favored tumor cells with a compatible milieu provided by a particular organ environment (4). In humans and in experimental rodent systems, numerous examples exist in which malignant tumors metastasize to specific organs (1). Two arguments were advanced long ago to explain organ-specific metastasis. In 1889, Paget proposed that the growth of metastases is influenced by the interaction of particular tumor cells (the "seed") with unique organ environments (the "soil") and thus that metastases result only when the seed and soil are compatible (5). Forty years later, Ewing challenged Paget's "seed and soil" theory and hypothesized that metastatic dissemination occurs by purely mechanical factors reflecting the anatomic structure of the vascular system (6). These explanations have been evoked, separately or together, to explain the secondary site preference of certain types of neoplasms. In a 1981 review of clinical studies on this topic, Sugarbaker concluded that common regional metastasis could be attributed to anatomic or mechanical considerations, such as efferent venous circulation or lymphatic drainage to regional lymph nodes, but that distant

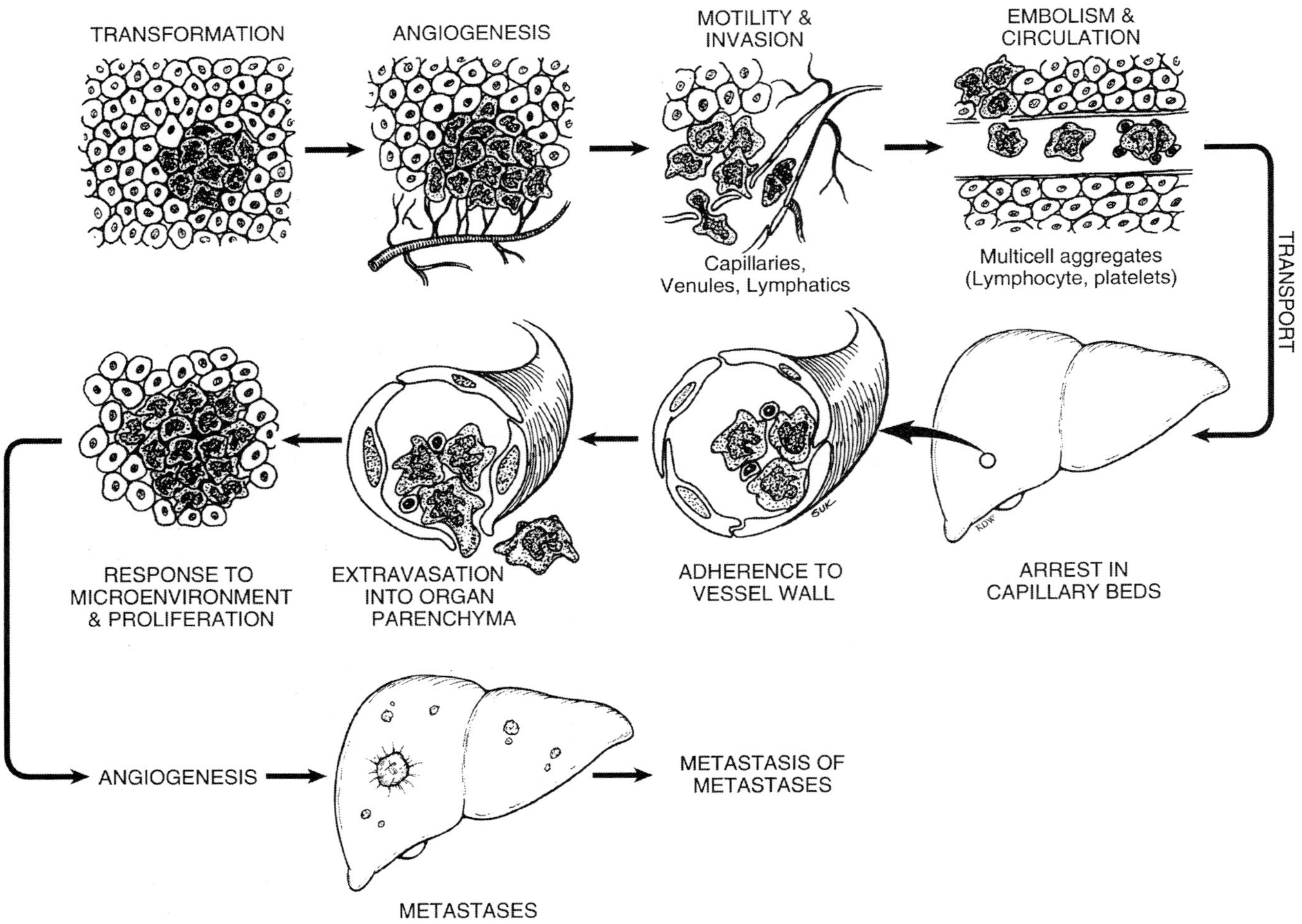

Figure 1 The pathogenesis of cancer metastasis. To produce metastases, tumor cells must detach from the primary tumor, invade the extracellular matrix and enter the circulation, survive in the circulation to arrest in the capillary bed, adhere to subendothelial basement membrane, gain entry into the organ parenchyma, respond to paracrine growth factors, proliferate and induce angiogenesis, and evade host defenses. The pathogenesis of metastasis is therefore complex and consists of multiple sequential, selective, and interdependent steps, the outcome of which depends on the interaction of tumor cells with homeostatic factors. Modified from Ref. (1a), I.J. Fidler (1997). Molecular biology of cancer: Invasion and metastasis. In "Cancer Principles and Practice of Oncology" (J.R. De Vita, S. Hellman, and S.A. Rosenberg, Eds.), pp. 135–152. Lippincott, Williams & Wilkins, Philadelphia, PA.

organ colonization by metastatic cells from various cancers was attributable to the cells' own patterns of site specificity (7). These observations have been confirmed, both experimentally (8) and clinically (9), by other investigators. Thus, the microenvironment of each organ can influence the implantation, invasion, survival, and growth of particular tumor cells; the importance of each individual interaction varies among different tumor systems.

B. Steps in the Metastatic Process

1. Angiogenesis

The realization that both the growth and the spread of tumors depend on angiogenesis has created new avenues of research designed to help improve the understanding of cancer biology and to facilitate the development of new therapeutic strategies. Since Folkman's initial discovery of the dependence of tumors on angiogenesis (10), myriad positive and negative regulators of angiogenesis have been discovered. Tumor survival and metastasis depend on a shift in the balance of endogenous angiogenic and antiangiogenic factors (Table I) such that the outcome favors increased angiogenesis (11). Of the angiogenic factors identified to date, vascular endothelial growth factor (VEGF) has been the most frequently associated with tumor progression and metastasis (12, 13).

Angiogenesis consists of sequential processes emanating from microvascular endothelial cells (10). To generate capillary sprouts, endothelial cells must proliferate, migrate toward the source of angiogenic molecules, and eventually penetrate host stroma. The capillary sprout subsequently expands and undergoes morphogenesis to yield a capillary. Although most solid tumors are highly vascular, their vessels differ from those in normal tissue in cellular composition, permeability, stability, and regulation of growth (10).

Numerous antiangiogenic agents are currently under clinical investigation, including those that inhibit matrix breakdown, block activators of angiogenesis, inhibit endothelial cell survival signals or growth, or inhibit angiogenesis through unknown mechanisms. More detailed descriptions of angiogenesis are provided in Chapter 34 (this volume).

2. Growth Factors and Growth Factor Receptors

The presence of a tumor cell in a distant organ does not automatically lead to the development of a clinically relevant metastasis. Less than 1% of all circulating cancer cells are capable of forming a metastatic focus. For a tumor cell that has implanted at a distant site to form a viable metastatic lesion, it must be able to respond appropriately to environmental stimuli. Proliferation, a necessary step in the development of clinically relevant metastases, may occur in response to constitutively activated oncogenes such as k-*ras* or *src* or microenvironmental stimuli such as growth factors. Growth factors act by binding to specific tyrosine kinase receptors. Activation of these receptors produces intracellular signals that ultimately lead to the transcription of genes that regulate cellular proliferation and metastatic tumor growth.

Tyrosine kinase receptors are cell membrane proteins composed of three domains: an extracellular domain responsible for binding the receptor's ligand, a transmembrane domain that anchors the protein to the membrane, and a cytosolic domain with catalytic activity that leads to tyrosine phosphorylation and activation. Binding between a receptor and its ligand at the extracellular domain causes the tyrosine kinase receptor to dimerize. This dimerization stimulates the protein kinases located on each receptor monomer to phosphorylate a distinct set of tyrosine residues in the cytoplasmic portion of its dimerized partner. The phosphorylation of

Table I Endogenous Angiogenic and Antiangiogenic Factors

Stimulatory	Inhibitory
Acidic and basic fibroblast growth factor	Angiostatin
Angiogenin	Antithrombin III fragment
Hepatocyte growth factor	Endostatin
Interleukin-8	Interferon-α, -β
Placenta growth factor	Interferon-inducible protein-10
Platelet-derived endothelial cell growth factor	Platelet factor 4
Pleiotrophin	Prolactin fragment
Transforming growth factor-α, -β	Thrombospondin
Tumor necrosis factor-α	Tissue inhibitor of metalloproteinase
Vascular endothelial growth factor/vascular permeability factor	Vasculostatin
Others	Others

tyrosine residues of the activated receptor leads to downstream effects that can alter cell function (14). Several families of tyrosine kinase receptors involved in metastasis have been identified, including those for epidermal growth factor (including Her2/neu), fibroblast growth factor, hepatocyte growth factor (HGF), insulin-like growth factor-I (IGF-I), and platelet-derived growth factor families.

3. Invasion and Migration

The ability of tumor cells to invade tissues is a prerequisite for successful metastasis. Invasion requires that the tumor cell be able to traverse the basement membrane (BM) and extracellular matrix (ECM). The process of invasion is so critical to tumor progression that the histologic depth of tumor penetration is a major determinant in tumor staging and treatment algorithms.

The complex interaction between tumor cells and the host microenvironment can significantly influence tumor progression and metastatic potential (15). Numerous mechanisms by which tumor cells invade host tissue have been described (16). The mechanical pressure induced by a rapidly growing neoplasm may force tumor cells along tissue planes that offer minimal resistance (17). Increased cell motility may also increase tumor cell invasiveness (16). A third mechanism for invasion involves degradation of the BM and ECM, which function as barriers between epithelial cells and the stroma. This degradation of the ECM and BM is the focus of intense research on the invasive mechanisms involved in tumor progression and metastasis. The ECM and BM are a mixture of connective tissue components including collagen, laminin, proteoglycans, and other molecules (18) and are produced not only by host epithelial and stromal cells but also by tumor cells. Collagen acts as the structural support for the BM, whereas laminin plays a role in cellular adhesion (18). The BM and ECM are generally believed to act as a barrier between tumor cells and normal host cells; tumor cells must be able to invade these structures to spread locally (i.e., through the bowel wall to contiguous structures) or to metastasize (by gaining access to blood or lymphatic vessels).

Among the most extensively studied of the degradative enzymes are the matrix-degrading metalloproteinases (MMPs) (Table II). The MMPs constitute a family of enzymes that degrade the ECM and BM at physiologic pH and are produced both by host connective tissue and by tumor cells (19). The MMPs play a role in normal tissue turnover as well as in pathologic conditions such as arthritis and malignancy. To date, at least 17 MMPs have been identified in four subfamilies: the collagenases, the gelatinases, the stromelysins, and the metalloelastases (20). Three MMP-specific inhibitors, tissue inhibitors of metalloproteinases (TIMPs), have also been identified. The balance of activity of MMPs and TIMPs is likely to influence the invasive phenotypes of both normal cells and tumor cells.

Table II Major Matrix-Degrading Metalloproteinases

Collagenases	Gelatinases	Stromelysins	Metalloelastase
MMP-1	MMP-2	MMP-3	MMP-12
MMP-5	MMP-9	MMP-10	
		MMP-11	
		MMP-7	

Migration is critical for allowing cells to gain access to the circulation and is regulated by factors that affect cell motility. The migration and motility of cells are stimulated by cytokines known as scatter factors. The prototype protein of this group of factors is hepatocyte growth factor (HGF) (21), a naturally occurring peptide produced in large quantities by the liver, mainly by cells of mesodermal origin. The receptor for HGF (c-met) is located in the cellular membrane and has intrinsic tyrosine kinase activity. Studies suggest that overexpression of the c-*met* gene is important in the selection of cells that can migrate and form distant metastases.

4. Adhesion

Adhesion molecules play vital roles at several stages of tumor progression and metastasis formation. On the basis of their biochemical structure, adhesion molecules can be classified into four groups: integrins, cadherins, selectins, and immunoglobulin-like proteins. Invasion of the BM and ECM cannot take place without adhesion. Although invasion is considered one step of the metastatic cascade, it can be divided into numerous substeps in which adhesion molecules play distinct and differing roles. First, tumor cells must attach to the BM and ECM to initiate degradation through mechanisms discussed elsewhere (22). The integrin family of adhesion molecules can act as cell surface receptors that bind to the laminin, fibronectin, and collagen component of the ECM, and many integrins are expressed on the surface of human cancer cells (23–25). Tumor cell adhesion to BM laminins has been recognized as a critical step in the invasion process; recent studies show that in many carcinomas, the invading front is rich in the expression of certain laminins (26). Laminin-5 has also been shown to increase cell migration (27).

Adhesion is also critical for tumor cells to arrest in the microvasculature of the distant metastatic site. Embolized tumor cells often circulate as clumps of cells that adhere to other tumor cells or to platelets. This ability to clump during tumor cell embolization may increase trapping of tumor cells in the microcirculation of distant organs such as the liver, thereby increasing metastatic potential. However, arrest of tumor cells alone does not guarantee survival and formation of metastasis (28); cell surface adhesion molecules must also attach the arrested tumor cells to the endothelial cells or the ECM of the distant organ. Tumor cells in which specific adhesion molecules are up-regulated may have an advantage in the metastatic process. Members of the integrin family have also been shown to facilitate dynamic attachment and detachment of tumor cells to endothelial cells under the laminar flow conditions present in the microcirculation, a process known as "rolling" (29).

5. Survival (Evasion of Apoptosis)

On a simple level, cancer can be viewed as the result of an inappropriate net gain of transformed cells. Recognition of the role of apoptosis in both normal and abnormal physiology has resulted in the revision of the traditional cancer model that centered exclusively on cellular proliferation. Uncontrolled cell proliferation, decreased cell death, or both are responsible for the net gain of abnormal cells known as cancer. The term "apoptosis" was first used to introduce a distinct physiologic process of cellular suicide or "programmed cell death." Apoptosis is critical for normal homeostasis, and the apoptotic machinery is present in almost all eukaryotic cells. Either the activation of death-inducing factors or the withdrawal of survival factors can trigger the apoptotic process (Fig. 2).

Although different triggers of apoptosis may result in activation of distinct intracellular apoptotic signaling pathways, the cysteine aspartate proteases, known as caspases, are responsible for both the initiation and the execution of apoptosis. To do so, both initiator and effector caspases cleave substrates at aspartate residues and are themselves activated by cleavage on aspartate residues, resulting in a proteolytic cascade. This caspase cascade leads to cellular disassembly (30). Finally, apoptotic bodies form and are eliminated through phagocytosis by neighboring cells and macrophages; the presence of intact plasma membranes allows this removal of apoptotic bodies to take place without inflammatory reactions (31).

A complex set of pro- and antiapoptotic factors tightly controls the process of apoptosis (Table III). Cancer cells can exploit these factors to bypass the normal physiologic checkpoints that would trigger defective cells to undergo apoptosis. The elaborate array of mechanisms used by tumors to evade apoptosis was summarized by Reed (30). As described briefly below, the up-regulation of antiapoptotic genes and the down-regulation of proapoptotic genes are mechanisms by which cells avoid apoptosis. Alterations in Bcl-2 proteins, which play a major role in apoptosis regulation, are often present in cancers. Currently, approximately 16 members of the Bcl-2 family, both pro- and antiapoptotic, have been identified in humans. Some factors may mediate both pro- and antiapoptotic pathways, depending on their activation by phosphorylation. An additional mechanism by which proapoptotic genes are down-regulated is the phosphorylation of the proapoptotic protein BAD by Akt, thereby preventing BAD from dimerizing with Bcl-2/Bcl-X_L (30). Other ways that tumors suppress apoptosis include expression of proteins that inhibit apoptosis. One such protein, survivan, is overexpressed in human cancers (32). Tumor cells can also avoid apoptosis by overexpressing antiapoptotic death effector domains (33), by down-regulating Fas receptors, by mutating Fas, or by increasing the expression of decoy receptors (30).

Tumor progression to the metastatic phenotype has been associated with alterations in apoptosis. Highly metastatic breast (human) and melanoma (human and mouse) cell lines are more resistant to apoptosis than are their poorly metastatic counterparts (34). Also, murine melanoma cells that overexpress the antiapoptotic protein Bcl-2 form more pulmonary metastases than do parental cells, which have low Bcl-2 expression and low metastatic potential (35). Changes in apoptotic pathways in metastatic colon cancer have not been as clear-cut; in fact, rates of apoptosis in lymph node and liver metastases from colon cancer have actually been higher than those in primary lesions (36).

Current data on apoptosis in metastatic cancer are inconclusive and occasionally contradictory. Studying the matrix-independent survival of metastatic cells may help to clarify the role of apoptosis in the metastatic process. As alluded to earlier in this chapter, cancer cells must establish ECM-independent survival during their passage through the circulation in order to form a metastatic focus at a distant site. Therefore, studying cancer cells in suspension may be more informative than studying already established metastatic foci *in vivo* or adherent metastatic cells *in vitro*. Anoikis, or detachment-induced apoptosis, is a normal physiologic mechanism first discovered in epithelial cells that were experimentally dissociated from their ECM (37). Anoikis

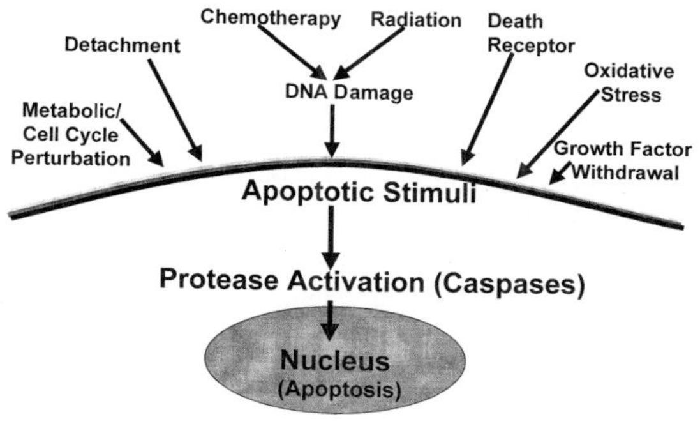

Figure 2 Common triggers of apoptosis. Apoptosis is essential in both physiologic and pathologic processes, including cancer. Numerous extrinsic and intrinsic triggers of apoptosis result in activation of common intracellular pathways that lead to a caspase cascade, which ultimately leads to DNA fragmentation and cellular disassembly. Reprinted from (29a), *Surg. Onc.*, Vol. **7**; C.A. Portera, R.S. Berman, and L.M. Ellis; Molecular determinants of metastasis, pp. 183–195. Copyright 1999, with permission from Elsevier Science.

Table III Apoptotic Factors

Apoptosis suppressors	Apoptosis promoters
Bcl-2	Bax
Bcl-X_L	Bak
Bcl-ω	BAD
Mcl-1	Bik
Bfl-1	Bid
Brag-1	Bcl-X_S
A-1	Hrk

normally prevents cells from colonizing elsewhere after they have been detached (37). Hence, resistance to anoikis may enhance the ability to survive independent of attachment to the ECM.

III. Experimental Models for Studying the Biology of Metastasis

The first requirement for studying tumor metastasis *in vivo*, such as in rodent models of malignancy, is that the host system allow tumor cells or fragments to grow. Primary tumors can develop spontaneously or in response to genetic manipulations (e.g., transgenic or knockout mice) or carcinogens. Tumor cells derived from a particular strain of host animal will not be rejected by syngeneic (genetically identical) animal strains. However, the study of human tumors in animal models requires that the animal's immune system does not reject the human tumor xenografts. Many animal models for this purpose are available and representative models are presented in Table IV. Two of the most commonly used mouse strains are nude mice, which are deficient in T cells, or severe combined immunodeficiency (SCID) mice, which are deficient in both B and T cells.

Traditional models for the study of metastasis involve injecting tumor cells into tail veins or implanting them under the skin or into organs of interest. More recent models have taken advantage of advances in molecular biology to manipulate the function or expression of specific genes in intact organisms. Aspects of these models are reviewed briefly below.

A. Tumor Cell Injection Models

The study of metastasis in murine and other animal systems depends on both the intrinsic characteristics of the cells and the route by which the tumor cells are introduced into the host. Assuming that the cell type possesses the molecular machinery necessary to induce metastasis (as described earlier in this chapter), tumor cells injected via the tail vein will lead to lung metastases, and tumor cells injected into the portal vein will produce liver metastases. Injection of tumor cells is an imperfect model of metastasis, because the first several steps of the metastatic cascade are bypassed. However, the first few steps of that cascade are similar to those that allow growth in the organ of metastasis, and these models are adequate for studying tumors that are known to metastasize to the lung or liver. An alternative to portal vein injection for producing liver metastasis is to inject tumor cells beneath the splenic capsule. This technique is both easier technically and carries less risk of blood loss than injection into a portal vein.

B. Orthotopic and Ectopic Implantation Models

Orthotopic implantation refers to the technique of implanting tumor cells into the organ from which those cells were derived. For example, colon cancer cells may be implanted in the wall of the colon, and breast cancer cells may be injected into the mammary fat pad. Most published studies have involved the use of ectopic models such as injection of tumor cells into subcutaneous tissues. This injection site is orthotopic only for melanoma or soft tissue tumors; it is not relevant for studying primary tumor growth or metastasis. However, subcutaneous implantation may be a reasonable starting point for studying tumor progression, because growth of tumors implanted there can be measured easily over time. Nevertheless, for the reasons discussed below, orthotopic implantation is greatly preferable over ectopic implantation for studying tumor systems.

Several lines of evidence have shown that interactions between the tumor cells and the host microenvironment are critical for tumor development and metastasis. Early clinical observations that specific tumors metastasize to specific sites (5) led to subsequent investigations of the effect of implantation site on tumor growth and the formation of metastases. Implantation of human tumor cells into orthotopic sites in nude mice was found to provide an environment more conducive to growth and metastasis formation than was implantation at ectopic sites. For example, SN12C human renal cell carcinoma cells implanted in the kidneys of nude mice grew and metastasized faster than did cells injected intravenously, intraperitoneally, subcutaneously, or intrasplenically (38, 39). Similarly, implantation of human colon carcinoma cells into the cecal wall produced both regional and liver metastases, but subcutaneous implantation of these cells produced no metastases (40).

Other experiments have shown that the site at which tumor cells are implanted also affects their resistance to chemotherapeutic agents. For example, implants of the UV-2237 murine fibrosarcoma cell line in the subcutis and

Table IV Commonly Used Models of Tumor Growth and Metastasis[a]

Tumor type	Organ of metastasis	Cell lines frequently used	Description of method	Ref.
Colon	Liver, lymph nodes	KM12L4, KM12SM, HT29, CT-26	Injection into the cecum, splenic injection (produces liver metastases)	58–61
Breast	Lymph nodes, lungs	MDA-MB-435, MDA-MB-231	Injection into the mammary fat pad, IV	Reviewed in 62
Endometrial	Liver, lymph nodes, lungs	SPEC-2, SPEC-2, LIV1, SPEC-2, LU1	Injection into the uterus	63
Ovarian	Peritoneal cavity	SKOV 3ip1, HEY-A8, 2274-C10, OCCI	Injection into the ovary, IP injection	64
Renal cell	Lymph nodes, lungs	SNI2pm6, RENCA, SNI2C, KG-2	Injection beneath the renal capsule, IV surgical attachment	56, 65
Pancreas	Liver, lymph nodes	COLO-357, L3.6sl, L3.7pl	Injection into the tail of the pancreas	66
Prostate	Lymph nodes, lung, lymph node	LNCaP, PC-3MMZ, LNCaP-LN3	Injection into the ventral lobe of the prostate	56, 67–69
Bladder	Lymph nodes	ZS3JBV, MBT-2	Injection into the wall of the dome of the bladder	70, 71
Melanoma	Brain, lungs??	B16, K1735, LIV2237, A375, DM-4, SK-MELZ	Intracarotid artery, SQ or IV	72–74; reviewed in 75
Sarcoma	Lungs	L-1, Bp8, COS31	Soft tissues, IV, intraperitoneal	76–78
Lung	Lung, brain	PC-14, PC-14 PM4, 3LL	Intrabronchial injection, IV	79, 80
Gastric	Lymph nodes, liver	KKLS	Injection into the gastric wall	81

[a]Sites of metastasis are dependent on site of injection and cells used; please see individual references for details.

spleen of mice was sensitive to systemic doxorubicin (Adriamycin), but lung metastases were not (41). A follow-up study assessed the sensitivity of CT-26 (a syngeneic murine colon carcinoma cell line) injected intravenously (to produce lung lesions), subcutaneously, into the cecal wall, and into the spleen (to produce liver lesions) to systemic administration of 5-fluorouracil (5-FU) and doxorubicin (42). The tumors in the cecum and spleen were the most sensitive to 5-FU; the subcutaneous tumors were the most sensitive to doxorubicin; and the tumors in the liver were highly resistant to both drugs. Later studies demonstrated that the site of tumor-cell implantation greatly influences expression of the *MDR-1* gene, which encodes for p-glycoprotein (43). These studies demonstrate the importance of the interaction between tumor cells and the host microenvironment in the regulation of specific genes and hence the phenotype of tumor cells.

Further justification for the use of orthotopic models in the study of metastasis comes from observations that the site of injection alters gene expression by the tumor cells. As alluded to earlier in this chapter, the expression of many of the genes involved in metastasis is affected by cytokines and growth factors. Each organ expresses distinct cytokines and growth factors that mediate homeostasis for that organ. The liver, for example, expresses high levels of HGF and IGF-I, two factors that are implicated in hepatic regeneration. Therefore, the study of colon cancer metastases, which appear most often in the liver, should involve a model that produces metastases in the liver rather than in other sites, because the expression of cytokines and growth factors would be different at those other sites.

Organ-derived cytokines and growth factors can affect tumor growth directly by inducing cell proliferation, or they can affect the regulation of gene expression, which mediates other processes such as angiogenesis or survival. For example, expression of basic fibroblast growth factor, a potent angiogenic factor, was 10 to 20 times higher in human renal cell tumors implanted in the kidneys of nude mice than in tumors implanted in the subcutaneous tissues (44). In another study of the organ-specific expression of IL-8, an angiogenic growth factor associated with metastatic potential of melanoma cells, both parental A375P and metastatic A375SM human melanoma cells produced the greatest amounts of IL-8 when implanted subcutaneously, followed by lung lesions (induced by tail vein injection) and finally by liver metastases (induced by intrasplenic injection) (45). These and other results underscore the importance of host microenvironment on the expression of tumor cell genes.

C. Transgenic Models

The standard models for the study of metastasis described above have involved either implanting tumor cells or injecting them via tail vein or portal vein. More recent models have incorporated molecular biology techniques to allow investigations to be targeted more specifically to the biologic function of specific genes. One such model, the transgenic model, involves the insertion of new or modified genes into the host genome through the microinjection of germ-line cells. Experiments with transgenic mice have shown that overexpression of activated oncogenes may be associated with both primary tumor growth and metastasis formation (46–48). In early transgenic mouse models, the inserted gene eventually becomes incorporated in somatic and germ-line cells throughout the entire organism; thus, the gene of interest could be expressed at sites not desired by the investigator. More recent transgenic mouse models have incorporated tissue-specific promoters that limit overexpression of a specific oncogene to a specific organ (49–52). For example, placement of the *neu* protooncogene downstream of the mouse mammary tumor virus promoter/enhancer region in transgenic mice has led to a model in which overexpression of the *neu* gene is limited to cells derived from the mammary gland (53).

D. Tracking Metastatic Tumor Cells

Another aspect of studying metastasis involves following the formation and progression of metastatic lesions after the tumor cells are established in the host. In some models, metastases are visible on the surface of the liver or lung; these lesions can be counted with the aid of a dissecting microscope. However, the presence of micrometastatic disease, whether in animal models or in patients, significantly influences survival. Thus, evaluations of therapeutic protocols require a means of detecting micrometastatic tumor cells within the host organism.

In animal models, one relatively straightforward way of determining whether micrometastatic tumor cells exist in a particular organ is to radiolabel the tumor cells before injecting them. After the experiment is completed, organs can be harvested, homogenized, and the tissues analyzed for relative radioactivity (40). One drawback of this method is that it cannot distinguish live tumor cells from dead ones that still maintain some radioactivity. An alternative technique that can detect the presence of living cells is to use reverse transcriptase–polymerase chain reaction (RT–PCR) for the presence of a tumor-specific gene in an organ or in blood samples.

In the 1980s, investigators began transfecting tumor cells with plasmids that express genes such as *lac z* (54, 55) that can be identified by colorimetric analysis. Stably transfected clones of these cells are injected into mice; after the experimental period is complete, the tissues are harvested and stained with a colorimetric substrate to visualize tumor cells. Green fluorescent protein (GFP) has also been used as a marker of micrometastatic disease. In this technique, tumor cells are transfected with a plasmid encoding GFP (56), and the stable transfectants are injected into the animals. Transfected cells within tumors can be visualized with fluorescent light; large tumor deposits can even be visualized *in vivo* (38, 39). Finally, videomicroscopy can be used to track the dynamics of metastatic cells in organs such as the lung or liver in living animals, thus providing a means of examining tumor–host interactions in detail, in "real time" (57).

Acknowledgments

Supported by The Gillson–Longenbaugh Foundation, the Jon and Suzie Hall Fund for Colon Cancer Research, NIH Grant CA74821 (LME), and NIH Grant CA09599-11 (RSB). The authors thank Christine Wogan and Joan Small for editorial assistance.

References

1. Fidler, I. J. (1990). Critical factors in the biology of human cancer metastasis: Twenty-eighth G.H.A. Clowes Memorial Award Lecture. *Cancer Res.* **50,** 6130–6138.

1a. Fidler, I. J. (1997). Molecular biology of cancer: Invasion and metastasis. *In* "Cancer Principles and Practice of Oncology," 5th Ed. (J. R. De Vita, S. Hellman, and S. A. Rosenberg, eds.), pp. 135–152.

2. Fidler, I., and Radinsky, R. (1990). Genetic control of cancer metastasis (editorial). *J. Natl. Cancer. Inst.* **82,** 166–168.

3. Kerbel, R. (1990). Growth dominance of the metastatic cancer cell: Cellular and molecular aspects. *Adv. Cancer Res.* **55,** 87–132.

4. Fidler, I. J. (1995). Modulation of the organ microenvironment for treatment of cancer metastasis. *J. Natl. Cancer Inst.* **87,** 1588–1592.

5. Paget, S. (1889). The distribution of secondary growths in cancer of the breast. *Lancet* **1,** 571–573.

6. Ewing, J. (1928). "Neoplastic Diseases." W.B. Saunders, Philadelphia.

7. Sugarbaker, E. (1981). Patterns of metastasis in human malignancies. *Cancer Biol. Rev.* **2,** 235–278.

8. Hart, I. (1982). "Seed and soil" revisited: Mechanisms of site specific metastasis to specific secondary sites. *Cancer Metastasis Rev.* **1,** 5–17.

9. Tarin, D., Price, J., *et al.* (1984). Mechanisms of human tumor metastasis studied in patients with peritoneovenous shunts. *Cancer Res.* **44,** 3584–3592.

10. Folkman, J. (1986). How is blood vessel growth regulated in normal and neoplastic tissue?—G.H.A. Clowes Memorial Award Lecture. *Cancer Res.* **46,** 467–473.

11. Fidler, I. J., and Ellis, L. M. (1994). The implications of angiogenesis to the biology and therapy of cancer metastasis. *Cell* **79,** 185–188.

12. Takahashi, Y., Kitadai, Y., Bucana, C. D., Cleary, K. R., and Ellis, L. M. (1995). Expression of vascular endothelial growth factor and its receptor, KDR, correlates with vascularity, metastasis, and proliferation of human colon cancer. *Cancer Res.* **55,** 3964–3968.

13. Warren, R. S., Yuan, H., Matli, M. R., Gillett, N. A., and Ferrara, N. (1995). Regulation by vascular endothelial growth factor of human colon cancer tumorigenesis in a mouse model of experimental liver metastasis. *J. Clin. Invest.* **95,** 1789–1797.

14. Yarden, Y., and Ullrich, A. (1988). Growth factor receptor tyrosine kinases. *Annu. Rev. Biochem.* **57,** 443.

15. Radinsky, R. (1993). Paracrine growth regulation of human colon carcinoma organ-specific metastasis. *Cancer Metastasis Rev.* **12,** 345–361.

16. Gutman, M., and Fidler, I. J. (1995). Biology of human colon cancer metastasis. *World J. Surg.* **19,** 226–234.

17. Gabbert, H. (1985). Mechanisms of tumor invasion: Evidence from *in vivo* observations. *Cancer Metastasis Rev.* **4,** 293–309.

18. Liotta, L. A. (1986). Tumor invasion and metastases—Role of the extracellular matrix: Rhoads Memorial Award lecture. *Cancer Res.* **46,** 1–7.

19. Matrisian, L. M. (1992). The matrix-degrading metalloproteinases. *BioEssays.* **14,** 455–463.
20. Matrisian, L. M., Wright, J., Newell, K., and Witty, J. P. (1994). Matrix-degrading metalloproteinases in tumor progression. *Princess Takamatsu Symp.* **24,** 152–161.
21. To, C. T. T., and Tsao, M. S. (1998). The roles of hepatocyte growth factor/scatter factor and Met receptor in human cancers (review). *Oncol. Rep.* **5,** 1013–1024.
22. Stetler-Stevenson, W. G., Aznavoorian, S., and Liotta, L. A. (1993). Tumor cell interactions with the extracellular matrix during invasion and metastasis. *Annu. Rev. Cell Biol.* **9,** 541–573.
23. Koretz, K., Schlag, P., Boumsell, L., and Moller, P. (1991). Expression of VLA-alpha 2, VLA-alpha 6, and VLA-beta 1 chains in normal mucosa and adenomas of the colon, and in colon carcinomas and their liver metastases. *Am. J. Pathol.* **138,** 741–750.
24. Hemler, M. E., Crouse, C., and Sonnenberg, A. (1989). Association of the VLA alpha 6 subunit with a novel protein. A possible alternative to the common VLA beta 1 subunit on certain cell lines. *J. Biol. Chem.* **264,** 6529–6535.
25. Pignatelli, M., Smith, M. E., and Bodmer, W. F. (1990). Low expression of collagen receptors in moderate and poorly differentiated colorectal adenocarcinomas. *Br. J. Cancer* **61,** 636–638.
26. Pyke, C., Salo, S., Ralfkiaer, E., Romer, J., Dano, K., and Tryggvason, K. (1995). Laminin-5 is a marker of invading cancer cells in some human carcinomas and is coexpressed with the receptor for urokinase plasminogen activator in budding cancer cells in colon adenocarcinomas. *Cancer Res.* **55,** 4132–4139.
27. Kikkawa, Y., Umeda, M., and Miyazaki, K. (1994). Marked stimulation of cell adhesion and motility by ladsin, a laminin-like scatter factor. *J. Biochem. (Tokyo)* **116,** 862–869.
28. Barbera-Guillem, E., Smith, I., and Weiss, L. (1992). Cancer-cell traffic in the liver. I. Growth kinetics of cancer cells after portal-vein delivery. *Int. J. Cancer* **52,** 974–977.
29. Morris, V. L., Schmidt, E. E., MacDonald, I. C., Groom, A. C., and Chambers, A. F. (1997). Sequential steps in hematogenous metastasis of cancer cells studied by *in vivo* videomicroscopy. *Invasion Metastasis* **17,** 281–96.
29a. Portera, C. A., Berman, R. S., and Ellis, L. M. (1999). molecular determinants of metastasis. *Surg. Oncol.* **7,** 183–195.
30. Reed, J. C. (1999). Mechanisms of apoptosis avoidance in cancer. *Curr. Opin. Oncol.* **11,** 68–75.
31. Hetts, W. H. (1998). Apoptosis and its role in disease. *JAMA* **279,** 300–307.
32. Ambrosini, G., Adida, C., and Altieri, D. C. (1997). A novel anti-apoptosis gene, survivin, expressed in cancer and lymphoma. *Nature Med.* **3,** 917–21.
33. Irmler, M., Thome, M., Hahne, M., Schneider, P., Hofmann, K., Steiner, V., Bodmer, J. L., *et al.* (1997). Inhibition of death receptor signals by cellular FLIP. *Nature (London)* **388,** 190–195.
34. Glinsky, G. V., Glinsky, V. V., Ivanova, A. B., and Hueser, C. J. (1997). Apoptosis and metastasis: Increased apoptosis resistance of metastatic cancer cells is associated with the profound deficiency of apoptosis execution mechanisms. *Cancer Lett.* **115,** 185–193.
35. Takaoka, A., Adachi, M., Okuda, H., Sato, S., Yawata, A., Hinoda, Y., Takayama, S., *et al.* (1997). Anti-cell death activity promotes pulmonary metastatis of melanoma cells. *Oncogene* **14,** 2971–2977.
36. Tatebe, S., Ishida, M., Kasagi, N., Tsujitani, S., Kaibara, N., and Ito, H. (1996). Apoptosis occurs more frequently in metastatic foci than in primary lesions of human colorectal carcinomas: Analysis by terminal-deoxynucleotidyl-transferase-mediated dUTP-biotin nick end labeling. *Int. J. Cancer* **65,** 173–177.
37. Frisch, S. M., and Francis, H. (1994). Disruption of epithelial cell-matrix interactions induces apoptosis. *J. Cell Biol.* **124,** 619–26.
38. Naito, S., von Eschenbach, A. C., Giavazzi, R., and Fidler, I. J. (1986). Growth and metastasis of tumor cells isolated from a human renal cell carcinoma implanted into different organs of nude mice. *Cancer Res.* **46,** 4109–4115.
39. Naito, S., von Eschenbach, A. C., and Fidler, I. J. (1987). Different growth pattern and biologic behavior of human renal cell carcinoma implanted into different organs of nude mice. *J. Natl. Cancer Inst.* **78,** 377–385.
40. Morikawa, K., Walker, S. M., Jessup, J. M., and Fidler, I. J. (1988). *In vivo* selection of highly metastatic cells from surgical specimens of different primary human colon carcinomas implanted into nude mice. *Cancer Res.* **48,** 1943–1948.
41. Staroselsky, A. N., Fan, D., O'Brian, C. A., Bucana, C. D., Gupta, K. P., and Fidler, I. J. (1990). Site-dependent differences in response of the UV-2237 murine fibrosarcoma to systemic therapy with adriamycin. *Cancer Res.* **50,** 7775–7780.
42. Wilmanns, C., Fan, D., O'Brian, C. A., Bucana, C. D., and Fidler, I. J. (1992). Orthotopic and ectopic organ environments differentially influence the sensitivity of murine colon carcinoma cells to doxorubicin and 5-fluorouracil. *Int. J. Cancer* **52,** 98–104.
43. Dong, Z., Radinsky, R., Fan, D., Tsan, R., Bucana, C. D., Wilmanns, C., and Fidler, I. J. (1994). Organ-specific modulation of steady-state *mdr* gene expression and drug resistance in murine colon cancer cells. *J. Natl. Cancer Inst.* **86,** 913–920.
44. Singh, R. K., Bucana, C. D., Gutman, M., Fan, D., Wilson, M. R., and Fidler, I. J. (1994). Organ site-dependent expression of basic fibroblast growth factor in human renal cell carcinoma cells. *Am. J. Pathol.* **145,** 365–374.
45. Gutman, M., Singh, R. K., Xie, K., Bucana, C. D., and Fidler, I. J. (1995). Regulation of interleukin-8 expression in human melanoma cells by the organ environment. *Cancer Res.* **55,** 2470–2475.
46. Broome Powell, M., Gause, P. R., Hyman, P., Gregus, J., Lluria-Prevatt, M., Nagle, R., and Bowden, G. T. (1999). Induction of melanoma in TPras transgenic mice. *Carcinogenesis* **20,** 1747–1753.
47. Garabedian, E. M., Humphrey, P. A., and Gordon, J. I. (1998). A transgenic mouse model of metastatic prostate cancer originating from neuroendocrine cells. *Proc. Natl. Acad. Sci. U.S.A.* **95,** 15382–15387.
48. Lifsted, T., Le Voyer, T., Williams, M., Muller, W., Klein-Szanto, A., Buetow, K. H., and Hunter, K. W. (1998). Identification of inbred mouse strains harboring genetic modifers of mammary tumor age of onset and metastatic progression. *Int. J. Cancer* **77,** 640–644.
49. Ambartsumian, N. S., Grigorian, M. S., Larsen, I. F., Karlstrom, O., Sidenius, N., Rygaard, J., Georgiev, G., *et al.* (1996). Metastasis of mammary carcinomas in GRS/A hybrid mice transgenic for the *mts1* gene. *Oncogene* **13,** 1621–1630.
50. Perez-Stable, C., Altman, N. H., Mehta, P. P., Deftos, L. J., and Roos, B. A. (1997). Prostate cancer progression, metastasis, and gene expression in transgenic mice. *Cancer Res.* **57,** 900–906.
51. Webster, M. A., and Muller, W. J. (1994). Mammary tumorigenesis and metastasis in transgenic mice. *Semin. Cancer Biol.* **5,** 69–76.
52. Searle, P. F., Thomas, D. P., Faulkner, K. B., and Tinsley, J. M. (1994). Stomach cancer in transgenic mice expressing human papillomavirus type 16 early region genes from a keratin promoter. *J. Gen. Virol.* **75,** 1125–37.
53. Guy, C. T., Webster, M. A., Schaller, M., Parsons, T. J., Cardiff, R. D., and Muller, W. J. (1992). Expression of the neu protooncogene in the mammary epthelium of transgenic mice induces metastatic disease. *Proc. Natl. Acad. Sci. U.S.A.* **89,** 10578–10582.
54. Culp, L. A., Lin, W., Kleinman, N. R., O'Connor, K. L. and Lechner, R. (1998). Earliest steps in primary tumor formation and micrometastasis resolved with histochemical markers of gene-tagged tumor cells. *J. Histochem. Cytochem.* **46,** 557–568.
55. Dooley, T. P., Stamp-Cole, M., and Ouding, R. J. (1993). Evaluation of a nude mouse tumor model using beta-galactosidase-expressing melanoma cells. *Lab. Anim. Sci.* **43,** 48–57.
56. Hoffman, R. M. (1998-99). Orthotopic transplant mouse models with

green fluorescent protein-expressing cancer cells to visualize metastasis and angiogenesis. *Cancer Metastasis Rev.* **17,** 271–277.
57. Naumov, G. N., Wilson, S. M., MacDonald, I. C., Schmidt, E. E., Morris, V. L., Groom, A. C., Hoffman, R. M., *et al.* (1999). Cellular expression of green fluorscent protein, coupled with high-resolution *in vivo* videomicroscopy, to monitor steps in tumor metastasis. *J. Cell Sci.* **112,** 1835–1842.
58. Morikawa, K., Walkeer, S. M., Jessup, J. M., and Fidler, I. J. (1988). *In vivo* selection of highly metastatic cells from surgical specimens of different primary human colon carcinoma implanted into nude mice. *Cancer Res.* **48,** 1943–1948.
59. Schackert, G., and Fidler, I. J. (1988). Development of *in vivo* models for studies of brain metastasis. *Int. J. Cancer* **41.**
60. Schackert, H. K., and Fidler, I. J. (1989). Development of an animal model to study the biology of recurrent colorectal cancer originating from mesenteric lymph system metastases. *Int. J. Cancer* **44,** 177–181.
61. Yoon, S. S., Carroll, N. M., Chiocca, E. A., and Tanabe, K. K. (1998). Cancer gene therapy using a replication-competent herpes simplex virus type 1 vector. *Ann. Surg.* **228,** 366–374.
62. Price, J. E. (1996). Metatasis from human breast cancer cell lines. *Breast Cancer Res. Treat.* **39,** 93–102.
63. Berry, K., Siegal, G. P., Boyd, J. A., Singh, R. K., and Fidler, I. J. (1994). Development of a metastatic model for human endometrial carcinoma using orthotopic implantation in nude mice. *Int. J. Oncol.* **4.**
64. Yoneda, J., Kuniyasu, H., Crispens, M. A., Price, J. E., Bucana, C. D., and Fidler, I. J. (1998). Expression of angiogenesis-related genes and progression of human ovarian carcinomas in nude mice. *J. Natl. Cancer Inst.* **90,** 447–454.
65. Killion, J. J., and Fidler, I. J. (1998). Treatment of metastasis by tumoricidal activation of tissue macrophages using liposome-encapsulated immunomodulators. *Pharmacol. Ther.* **78.**
66. Bruns, C. J., Harbison, M. T., Kuniyasu, H., Eue, I., and Fidler, I. J. (1999). *In vivo* selection and characterization of metastatic variants from human pancreatic adenocarcinoma by using orthotopic implantation in nude mice. *Neoplasia* **1.**
67. Stephenson, R. A., Dinney, C. P. N., Gohji, K., Ordonez, N. G., Killion, J. J., and Fidler, I. J. (1992). Metastatic model for human prostate cancer using orthotopic implantation in nude mice. *J. Natl. Cancer Inst.* **84,** 951–957.
68. Pettaway, C. A., Pathak, S., Greene, G., Ramirez, E., Wilson, M. R., Killion, J. J., and Fidler, I. J. (1996). Selection of highly metastatic variants of different human prostatic carcinomas using orthotopic implantation in nude mice. *Clin. Cancer Res.* **2.**
69. Balbay, M. D., Pettaway, C. A., Kuniyasu, H., Inoue, K., Ramirez, E., Li, E., Fidler, I. J., *et al.* (1999). Highly metastatic human prostate cancer growing within the prostate of athymic mice overexpresses vascular endothelial growth factor. *Clin. Cancer Res.* **4,** 783–789.
70. Dinney, C. P., Tanguay, S., Bucana, C. D., Eve, B. Y., and Fidler, I. J. (1995). Intravesical liposomal muramyl tripeptide phosphatidylethanoloamine treatment of human bladder carcinoma growing in nude mice. *J. Interferon Cytokine Res.* **15,** 585–592.
71. Dinney, C. P., Bielenberg, D. R., Perrotte, P., Reich, R., Eve, B. Y., Bucana, C. D., and Fidler, I. J. (1998). Inhibition of basic fibroblast growth factor expression, angiogenesis, and growth of human bladder carcinoma in mice by systemic interferon-alpha administration. *Cancer Res.* **58,** 808–814.
72. Schackert, G., and Fidler, I. J. (1988). Site-specific metastasis of mouse melanomas and a fibrosarcoma in the brain or meninges of syngeneic animals. *Cancer Res.* **48,** 3478–3484.
73. Zhang, R. D., Price, J. E., Schackert, G., Itoh, K., and Fidler, I. J. (1991). Malignant potential of cells isolated from lymph node or brain metastases of melanoma patients and implications for prognosis. *Cancer Res.* **51,** 2029–2035.
74. Jean, D., Gershenwald, J. E., Huang, S., Luca, M., Hudson, M. J., Tainsky, M. A., and Bar-Eli, M. (1998). Loss of AP-2 results in up-regulation of MCAM/MUC18 and an increase in tumor growth and metastasis of human melanoma cells. *J. Biol. Chem.* **273,** 16501–16508.
75. Luca, M. R., and Bar-Eli, M. (1998). Molecular changes in human melanoma metastasis. *Histol. Histopathol.* **13,** 1225–1231.
76. Beuth, J., Ko, H. L., Gabius, H. J., and Pulverer, G. (1991). Influence of treatment with the immunomodulatory effective dose of the beta-galactoside-specific lectin from mistletoe on tumor colonization in BALB/c-mice for two experimental model systems. *In Vivo* **5,** 29–32.
77. Lewin, F., Skog, S., Tribukait, B., and Ringborg, U. (1990). Effect of combined treatment with cisplatin and 5-fluorouracil on cell growth and cell cycle kinetics of a mouse ascites tumor growing *in vivo. In Vivo* **4,** 277–282.
78. Shoieb, A. M., Hahn, K. A., and Barnhill, M. A. (1998). An *in vivo/in vitro* experimental model system for the study of human osteosarcoma: Canine osteosarcoma cells (COS31) which retain osteblastic and metastatic properties in nude mice. *In Vivo* **12,** 463–472.
79. Li, L. M., Shin, D. M., and Fidler, I. J. (1990). Intrabronchial implantation of the Lewis lung tumor does not favor tumorigenicity and metastasis. *Invasion Metastasis* **10,** 129–141.
80. Yano, S., Nokihara, H., Hanibuchi, M., Parajuli, P., Shinohara, T., Kawano, T., and Soue, S. (1997). Model of malignant pleural effusion of human lung adenocarcinoma in SCID mice. *Oncol. Res.* **9.**
81. Takahashi, Y., Mai, M., Wilson, M. R., Kitadai, Y., Bucana, C. D., and Ellis, L. M. (1996). Site-dependent expression of vascular endothelial growth factor, angiogenesis and proliferation in human gastric carcinoma. *Int. J. Oncol.* **8,** 701–705.

37

Cancer Genetics

Douglas W. Green and Jeffrey A. Drebin

Department of Surgery, Washington University School of Medicine, St. Louis, Missouri 63110

I. Introduction

Cancer is a disorder of cellular growth resulting from the sequential accumulation of genetic alterations in a clonal population of cells. The scientific study of cancer genetics involves the identification and characterization of the specific genetic alterations that lead to the development of particular types of cancer. The field of cancer genetics is broad and has benefited from an explosion of scientific information over the past two decades. Cancer genetics can be conveniently broken down into three distinct, complementary areas of study: population genetics, cytogenetics, and molecular genetics. This chapter briefly reviews each of these separate areas of study, discusses research methodology of particular use in studying cancer genetics, and provides specific examples in which human malignancies have been characterized at the population, cytogenetic, and molecular genetic levels.

A. Population Genetics

The observation that members of some families seem to be unusually prone to the development of particular forms of cancer has led to the description of a number of familial cancer syndromes. Population genetics, as applied to cancer research, refers to the identification and characterization of inherited cancer syndromes in particular families or other genetically restricted populations. The goals of studying cancer genetics at the population level are to define cancer syndromes in which transmission of a genetic trait from parent to child leads to an increased risk of the child developing specific tumor types and to define the mechanism of inheritance of the genetic trait (i.e., dominant or recessive).

B. Cytogenetics

Chromosomal abnormalities have been associated with the development of cancer for over 100 years (Table I). Cancer cytogenetics refers to the identification of specific chromosomal abnormalities in cancer cells. These may be relatively simple abnormalities, such as chromosomal breakage, duplication, or loss, or may be complex reciprocal translocations between chromosomes. The goals of studying cancer cytogenetics are to identify specific regions of specific chromosomes that are reproducibly altered in the development of particular tumor types.

Table I Cancer and Chromosomal Abnormalities[a]

Researcher	Year	Observation
Von Hausemann	1894	Tumor cells noted to have abnormal nuclei
Boveri	1914	Postulated that cancer resulted from genetic aberrations
Levan and Tijo	1954	Established human chromosome number at 46
Levan	1956	Demonstrated chromosomal anomalies in human tumor cells
Nowel and Hungerford	1960	Described first specific chromosomal abnormality in chronic myeloid leukemia (the Philadelphia chromosome)

[a]Adapted from Glassman (62).

C. Molecular Genetics

The tremendous advances in molecular biology that have occurred over the past 50 years have led to the ability to clone, sequence, and study the function of specific genes. Cancer molecular genetics refers to the characterization at the DNA level of specific genes that play a role in the etiology of cancer. Advances in studying the molecular genetics of cancer have also led to advances in population and cytogenetic studies, in some cases by defining the specific gene that is responsible for an inherited cancer family syndrome or that resides at the site of a particular chromosomal abnormality (Table II).

Although the protein products of most genes are thought to play defined roles in normal cellular growth and development, mutations or other alterations in certain genes have been specifically linked to carcinogenesis. Three distinct classes of genes have been identified as playing a role in the development of cancer: oncogenes, tumor suppressor genes, and genes that function to preserve genomic fidelity. A large number of different cancer genes have been sufficiently well characterized to be identified as members of each of these three classes; some genes may be appropriately linked to more than one class.

Oncogenes are genes that contribute to neoplastic transformation by excessive activity of their encoded protein products. This may result from expressing abnormally large amounts of a normal protein product, or from expressing normal levels of a structurally altered protein product with enhanced biological activity. Many oncogenes encode proteins that are elements in mitogenic signal transduction cascades and serve to stimulate cell cycle progression. Enhanced expression or activity of the particular oncogene-encoded protein then results in increased mitogenic signaling, leading to increased cellular proliferation. Other oncogenes encode proteins that are elements of antiapoptotic cell survival pathways. Elevated activity of such proteins results in cellular resistance to apoptotic signaling that normally functions to prevent the survival of neoplastically transformed cells. Regardless of their specific mechanism of action, oncogenes are characterized by excessive activity in cancer cells.

In contrast to the activity of oncogenes, tumor suppressor genes encode proteins that normally serve as regulators of cell cycle progression or that normally induce apoptotic cell death in cells displaying DNA damage or disordered growth. As a result of mutation or chromosomal deletion, both copies of a particular tumor suppressor gene are lost in the

Table II Inherited Cancer Family Syndromes[a]

Cancer syndrome	Chromosome region	Gene
Li–Fraumeni syndrome	17p	p53
Breast	17p	BRCA1
Hereditary nonpolyposis colorectal cancer		
Lynch I	18q	MSH2
Lynch II	2p	LCF2
MEN 2a	10q	MEN2a
Familial adenomatous polyposis	5q	APC
Retinoblastoma	13q	RB1
Wilm's tumor	11p	WT1
Dysplastic nevus syndrome	1p	CMM1

[a]Adapted from *Eur. J. Cancer* **33**, G.H. Lyman and N.M. Kuderer, Basic population and cancer genetics and their use in the assessment of cancer risk, pp. 2160–2167. Copyright 1997, with permission from Elsevier Science.

process of oncogenesis, resulting in a cell that has lost one of the critical mechanisms that normally serve to regulate cell growth. Thus the activity of tumor suppressor gene product is absent in cancer cells. It is apparent that alterations in oncogenes and tumor suppressor genes can be complementary—one increases the cancer cells' stimulus to proliferate while the other results in loss of the ability to inhibit aberrant cell proliferation.

The final class of cancer genes includes those that function to preserve genomic fidelity. Proteins encoded by a complex network of genes are involved in arresting cell growth and identifying and repairing mutations involving specific nucleotide bases in cellular DNA. It is now clear that in some cases an initial alteration in a particular DNA repair pathway can lead, in turn, to the successive accumulation of mutations in other genes, resulting in the eventual activation of oncogenes and loss of tumor suppressor genes.

It is apparent that the study of cancer genetics is scientifically broad, potentially involving research at the population, chromosomal, and molecular levels. Furthermore, there may be multiple genetic abnormalities involved in the etiology of specific types of cancer, rendering the study of such malignancies even more complicated. In the remainder of this chapter, experimental methods and approaches relevant to the study of cancer genetics are reviewed, and illustrative examples in which particular malignancies have been linked to familial syndromes, chromosomal abnormalities, and/or specific DNA mutations are presented. Finally, some speculations on the impact of the complete sequencing of the human genome on the study of cancer genetics will be presented.

II. Experimental Methods

A. Population Genetics

A number of genes important in the etiology of cancer have been initially characterized by identifying familial cancer syndromes. Identification of a potential familial cancer syndrome first and foremost requires an accurate family history involving multiple generations. It is important to distinguish a higher than expected incidence of a particular type of cancer resulting at random, or due to a shared environmental risk factor, from a true inherited trait. The occurrence of the particular tumor across multiple generations, following a Mendelian inheritance pattern, is strongly suggestive of an inherited genetic trait. Malignancies resulting from inherited cancer syndromes frequently occur several decades earlier in affected family members than is typical for sporadic tumors of the same type, and are more likely to be multifocal. Complex statistical analysis, beyond the scope of this chapter, may be required to definitively link an inherited genetic trait to a particular cancer phenotype (1).

The chromosomal position of genes relevant to familial cancer syndromes can be further mapped through the use of restriction fragment length polymorphism (RFLP) analysis of linked chromosomal markers. In this manner, the mutated gene can be traced through affected family members. For example, if a DNA marker and the gene in question lie on different chromosomes, the probe and the gene will segregate in a random fashion among different family members. However, if they lie on the same chromosome they will segregate together unless a recombination occurs between the marker and the gene. The closer the marker and gene lie together, the less likely it becomes that a recombination event will occur. Identifying these events and mapping sites lying close to either side of the gene is the goal. Following the characterization of such closely linked markers, the gene of interest can be cloned and sequenced, a relatively straightforward but often labor-intensive task (2).

B. Cytogenetics

Cytogenetic analysis of tumor cells has been a frequent starting point leading to the identification of genes involved in tumorigenesis. Initial cytogenetic analysis begins with karyotyping, a procedure wherein the overall number and structure of individual chromosomes within a cell are analyzed (Fig. 1). Tumor cells frequently have multiple abnormal chromosomes. In order to be of real interest a particular chromosomal abnormality must occur in a significant fraction of tumors of a particular type, and must not be present in nonmalignant cells from affected individuals. Nowell and Hungerford used karyotype analysis to successfully describe the first specific chromosomal abnormality associated with cancer—the Philadelphia chromosome (3).

Karyotype analysis is performed on cultured cells by blocking cells in mitosis and staining their condensed chromosomes with Giemsa dye. This dye stains regions of DNA that are rich in the base pairs adenine and thymine, producing a reproducible series of dark bands along the length of the chromosome. Each band contains over a million base pairs and potentially hundreds of genes. Karyotype analysis involves comparing chromosomes for length, position of centromeres, and the location and size of bands. Karyotype analysis requires fairly extensive training and experience. Such expertise in most cases is best obtained by arranging a collaboration with an experienced cytogeneticist, rather than by the investigator attempting to develop this expertise within their own laboratory. Traditional karyotyping methodology is also limited by the need to work with cells growing in tissue culture.

New techniques have allowed cytogenetic analysis of tumors to advance beyond simple karyotyping, by combining molecular biologic techniques with chromosomal imaging. Methods such as fluorescence *in situ* hybridization

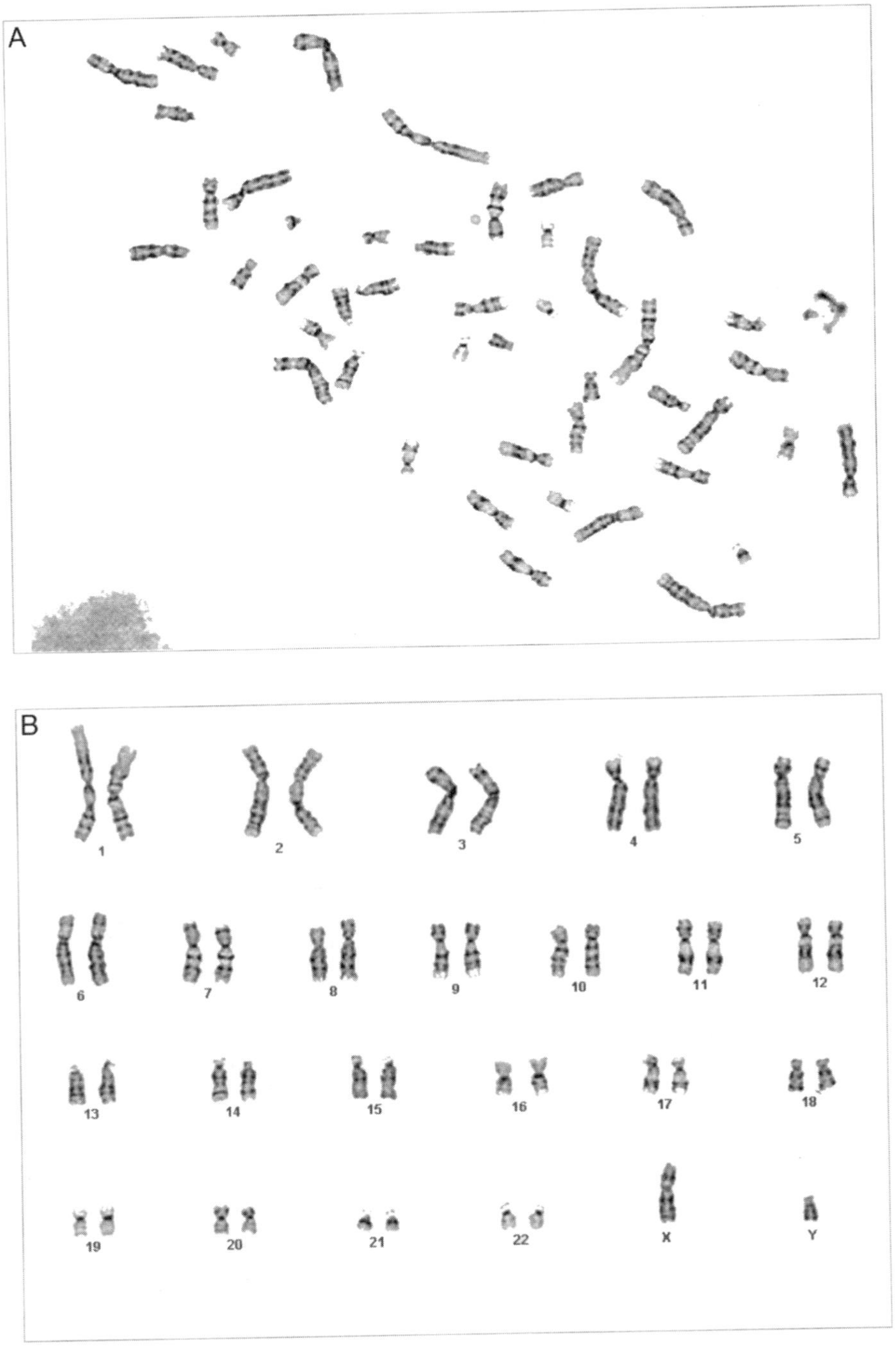

Figure 1 Karyotype analysis of human chromosomes. (A) Photomicrograph shows a Giemsa-stained metaphase chromosome spread as initially obtained following cell lysis. (B) Formal karyotype profile demonstrating each of the 23 pairs of human chromosomes.

(FISH) allow an investigator to identify the presence and location of a region of cellular DNA within morphologically preserved chromosome preparations, fixed cells, or tissue sections (4). This technology is based on the hybridization between target sequences of chromosomal DNA with complementary DNA probes labeled with fluorochrome compounds or antibodies. The DNA probes will bind uniquely to the specific site on the chromosome at which the complementary DNA is located, and can be visualized using fluorescence microscopy. FISH can be used for many purposes, including the chromosomal localization of specific genes, morphologic detection of genetic defects, and chromosomal rearrangements. Even newer techniques, such as M-FISH, comparative genomic hybridization, and spectral karyotyping have been developed, which further extend the investigator's ability to obtain cytogenetic information from tumor specimens. A detailed discussion of such methodology is beyond the scope of this chapter, but has been reviewed (5).

C. Molecular Genetics

Cloning and sequencing of genes implicated in cancer allow the precise characterization of such genes. These genes may be initially identified by linkage analysis in familial cancer syndromes or at sites of karyotypic abnormalities, as described above. More commonly genes implicated in tumorigenesis have been isolated based on their expression or biologic activity in tumor specimens or cultured cells. The number of oncogenes, tumor suppressor genes, and genes responsible for genomic fidelity that have been implicated in cancer is already sizable. Advances in the molecular analysis of gene expression, using methods such as microarray hybridization, will undoubtedly reveal even larger numbers of genes that are differentially expressed in cancer cells.

However, the cloning and sequencing of a potential cancer gene represents only the first step in its experimental characterization. The ultimate goal of molecular genetics, as applied to cancer, is to define the mechanism (or mechanisms) by which a particular gene contributes to the neoplastic behavior of the cancer cell. To perform these experiments it is necessary to express the gene of interest in an appropriate cellular milieu, permitting the identification of biologic changes resulting from the action of the expressed gene. Such experiments may require a number of experimental techniques, including analysis of the neoplastic phenotype, cell cycle studies, characterization of effects on apoptotic cell death, and transgenic mouse methodologies. Alternatively, the activity of the gene may be inhibited and the resulting biologic changes used to infer the gene's underlying function. For these studies the use of antisense oligonucleotides or gene "knockout" mice may be critical. An overview of these approaches is presented below and summarized in Table III.

1. Transformed Phenotype

Cancer cells display a variety of biologic properties distinct from nonmalignant cells, collectively referred to as the transformed phenotype (6). These properties include the ability to grow to high density, reflecting the loss of normal mechanisms of contact inhibition; the ability to grow in low concentrations of serum, reflecting autocrine synthesis of growth factors and/or intrinsic activation of mitogenic signaling cascades; the ability to grow when suspended in a semisolid medium (anchorage-independent growth), reflecting loss of the normal requirements for cell attachments to the extracellular matrix; secretion of proteases, which mediate cellular invasiveness and migration; and secretion of growth factors that promote the development of blood vessels, facilitating tumor angiogenesis. Studies suggest that the ability of cells to grow in the absence of anchorage is the aspect of the transformed phenotype that correlates most closely with the ability to form a tumor on implantation into immunodeficient mice (6). However, the ability of a particular gene to mediate any aspect of the transformed phenotype may suggest a mechanistic link to the etiology of cancer.

Analysis of the contribution of a particular gene to the transformed phenotype requires stable expression of that gene in a cell line not already neoplastically transformed. Rodent fibroblasts, such as murine NIH 3T3 cells or the rat fibroblast line Rat-1, have been commonly used in such experiments. However, it is worth noting that the ability of some genes to mediate aspects of the transformed phenotype is critically dependent on the cellular background in which the gene is expressed. Thus a gene implicated in cancer may not alter the biologic behavior of fibroblasts, but may be able to induce anchorage-independent growth *in vitro* and tumorigenic growth *in vivo* when expressed in a nontransformed epithelial cell line (7).

2. Cell Cycle Analysis

Aberrant cellular proliferation is one of the hallmarks of cancer. Many cancer genes interact with, or are part of, regulatory pathways that normally serve to control cell cycle progression. The analysis of the effects of a particular gene on cell proliferation can be relatively simple, such as the measurement of the incorporation of labeled thymidine into DNA. A more sophisticated analysis can be performed using flow cytometry (8). Cells permeabilized and stained with a compound such as propidium iodide (PI), which binds to DNA, will fluoresce in proportion to the amount of DNA in the cell. Using the flow cytometer it is possible to quantitate the DNA content of individual cells. If a population of cells is analyzed, there will be two peaks of cellular DNA, corresponding to the G_0/G_1 (normal diploid genome content) and G_2/M (quadruploid precell division genome content) fraction of cells. There will also be a percentage of cells showing an intermediate DNA content; these correspond to cells in the process of replicating their DNA (S phase). Computer software packages are available to measure the area under the curves of the G_0/G_1–S–G_2/M peaks allowing an accurate determination of the proportion of cells in each phase of the cell cycle.

Table III Comparison of Molecular Genetic Techniques

Technique	Advantage	Disadvantage
Cloning and sequencing	A necessity in analyzing gene expression and function; sequencing inexpensive using automated sequencers	May be time consuming and technically difficult; cloning ranges from inexpensive to expensive
Transformed phenotype	Identifies genetically controlled traits critical to neoplastic cell growth; inexpensive	Critically dependent on cellular background; not all cancer genes alter the transformed phenotype
Cell cycle analysis	Simple, rapid. Many cancer genes alter cell cycle control; experiments are inexpensive	Limited by aneuploidy; not all cancer genes alter cell cycle control; start-up costs for flow cytometry apparatus, software are high
Apoptosis	Many cancer genes alter apoptotic cell death	Not all cancer genes alter apoptotic cell death
Tunel	Can be performed on fixed specimens; inexpensive	Requires subjective evaluation of immunohistochemical staining
DNA laddering	Rapid, specific; inexpensive	Relatively insensitive, not evident in all systems
Flow cytometry	Rapid, sensitive, specific; inexpensive	Requires flow cytometric equipment
Annexin V staining	Sensitive, rapid	Requires flow cytometric equipment
Caspase activity analysis	Sensitive, rapid	Must be performed on cultured cells; kits are moderately expensive
Evaluation of tumor suppressor genes	Straightforward cell culture methods; inexpensive to moderately expensive	Must be expressed in appropriate cell lines; difficult to evaluate lethal or cytostatic genes
Transgenic mice	Allows *in vivo* evaluation of gene function	Mouse systems are expensive and have long time courses relative to *in vitro* systems; transgenes may have lethal effects
Antisense ODNs	Highly specific and selective; useful both *in vitro* and *in vivo; in vitro* experiments inexpensive	Experiments must be carefully designed; nonspecific effects can be difficult to exclude; *in vivo* experiments expensive
Knockout mice	Particularly useful for tumor suppressor gene evaluation and evaluating gene function in normal development	Oncogene analysis may not reveal the gene's function in cancer; mouse systems are expensive and have long time courses relative to *in vitro* systems

One limitation of using such approaches on cancer cells is the fact that many such cells are aneuploid. However, even for aneuploid cell populations, PI staining and cytometric analysis will demonstrate a peak (modal) DNA content, corresponding to the G_0/G_1 population, and a second peak corresponding to twice the G_0/G_1 content, which reflects the G_2/M population. The use of computer algorithms to determine the fraction of S phase cells in such aneuploid populations may be less accurate due to irregularities in the shoulders of the G_0/G_1 and G_2/M curves resulting from variable DNA content. A higher degree of accuracy can be obtained by briefly pulsing the cells with bromodeoxyuridine (BrdU) prior to processing, and performing simultaneous analysis of DNA content using PI, and of DNA synthesis by BrdU staining using a fluorochrome-coupled anti-BrdU antibody (9).

3. Apoptosis

Many genes implicated in cancer play a role in antiapoptotic cell survival mechanisms. Apoptosis is a complex, energy-dependent cell process in which a variety of stimuli trigger signaling cascades that activate endogenous proteases (caspases), resulting in cellular death. The first such cancer gene to be shown definitively to inhibit apoptotic tumor cell death was the Bcl-2 gene, identified at the site of chromosomal rearrangements in some B cell lymphomas (10). Subsequent studies have demonstrated that many oncogenes interfere with apoptotic mechanisms and contribute to tumor cell survival. A number of distinct assays are useful in detecting apoptosis in cell populations (11). These include evaluating intranucleasomal DNA cleavage, using techniques such as the Tunel assay, measurement of DNA laddering on ethidium-stained agarose gels, and measurement of subdiploid DNA content using flow cytometry; evaluating membrane alterations in phosphotidylserine expression, as determined by Annexin V staining; and direct measurement of caspase activity, which has been greatly facilitated by the commercial availability of assay kits. Because caspase-3 activation represents the final common pathway by which virtually all apoptotic mechanisms appear to activate cell death (12), caspase-3 activation assays are particularly useful.

4. Evaluation of Tumor Suppressor Gene Function

Although the strategies outlined above, using nontransformed cell lines, are useful in analyzing the mechanisms by which excessive gene function may contribute to the etiology of cancer, they may be less useful in evaluating suppressor gene function. In order to evaluate the function of a putative tumor suppressor gene, it must be introduced and expressed in a tumor cell line in which the gene is inactivated. Furthermore, because many tumor suppressor genes trigger cell cycle arrest and/or apoptosis, the establishment of growing lines expressing such potentially lethal or cytostatic genes can be problematic. A successful strategy for the evaluation of such genes is to use tightly regulated inducible promoter systems to control the expression of the target gene. In this way, the gene can be introduced into the appropriate cell line without deleterious effects. Its expression can then be triggered and effects on tumor cell biology evaluated. This approach has been useful in evaluating the mechanisms of action of a number of tumor suppressor genes (13).

5. Transgenic Mice

The introduction of specific genes into cultured cells is an extremely useful strategy to determine the mechanisms by which a gene contributes to the etiology of cancer, but this approach is somewhat artificial and may not be sensitive to all of the potential oncogenic activities of a specific gene in a variety of cellular backgrounds. A distinct approach is to target the gene for expression in the tissues of transgenic mice (14). In this way, the role of a specific gene in the etiology of cancer can be evaluated *in vivo*, and the full range of interactions of the gene with distinct cell types and stages of differentiation can be obtained. If a relatively ubiquitously expressed promoter is used in the construction of the transgene, the gene of interest will be widely expressed. Although this may be advantageous in yielding the widest array of potential phenotypes, it may be problematic, in that aberrant expression of a gene may result in lethal developmental abnormalities.

One approach to studying the function of a specific gene in a particular tissue is the use of tissue-specific promoters in transgene construction. The use of promoter or enhancer elements that will selectively direct expression of the target gene to a particular tissue may eliminate problems with developmental lethality, and still permit transgenic study of gene function in the tissue of greatest interest. Numerous studies have been performed using such approaches, and tissue-specific promoters selective for the breast (15), pancreas (16), bowel (17), and other organs (18, 19) have been successfully utilized to study the function of cancer-related genes in transgenic animals.

6. Suppression of Gene Expression Using Antisense Oligonucleotides

Short (10–30 bases) DNA oligonucleotides (ODNs) complementary to sequences in a particular target mRNA can catalyze the degradation of the mRNA molecule by the endogenous nuclease RNase H (20). Such small DNA fragments are referred to as "antisense" because they are complementary to the "sense" sequences that encode a specific protein in the mRNA target. By selectively down-regulating the mRNA expression of a particular target gene, antisense treatment may alter cellular growth, differentiation, or the activity of apoptotic cell death programs. A role for the target gene in these processes may then be inferred. Antisense oligonucleotides represent a potent method of selectively inhibiting gene expression *in vitro* and *in vivo*. However, antisense studies are fraught with a variety of problems relating to experimental design and interpretation, which must be overcome if this technology is to be accurately utilized to characterize the function of a particular target gene.

The need to achieve adequate levels of ODNs despite the potential degradation of DNA oligonucleotides by endogenous and serum-derived nucleases has led some investigators to use extremely high concentrations of ODNs in an attempt to achieve antisense effects. Concentrations of up to 100 μM have been used in some studies, with resulting nonantisense-related toxic effects. Even at more physiologic or pharmacologic dose levels, antisense molecules may exert nonspecific or sequence-specific effects related to protein binding rather than this being due to effects on the intended mRNA target. For example, some ODNs have been shown to bind growth factors or their receptors (20). Alterations in biologic systems resulting from such ODN–protein interactions have been erroneously attributed to specific antisense effects on gene expression in several cases. Furthermore, certain ODN sequences may trigger nonspecific immunologic activation and cytokine release if administered *in vivo* (20). Again, effects resulting from the administration of such ODNs to tumor-bearing mice may be mistakenly assumed to be the result of specific inhibition of the mRNA target.

Many of the limitations to antisense experiments, described above, have been relatively easily overcome. The substitution of phosphorothioate linkages for the normal phosphodiester linkages between nucleotide bases dramatically enhances ODN resistance to nuclease-mediated degradation (20). The use of cationic lipids, such as Lipofectin (Life Technologies), to facilitate delivery of ODNs in tissue culture allows experiments to be performed at concentrations of 1 μM and below (20). Interestingly, the *in vivo* delivery of ODNs appears to be more efficient than that occurring *in vitro* (20). Target mRNA sequences that would require a complementary antisense ODN containing sequences associated with nonspecific effects on cell growth, or that have been associated with nonspecific immunologic activation, can be avoided in selecting mRNA target sequences. Although still controversial (21), available data suggest that carefully designed antisense experiments can be useful in defining the mechanisms by which a particular cancer gene alters cancer cell biology.

7. Knockout Mice

The ability to delete both copies of a particular gene in a target cell by the process of homologous recombination, in concert with advances in stem cell biology and transgenic technology, has led to the widespread adoption of "gene knockout" experiments as an approach to analyzing gene function (22). Knockout mice are animals in which both copies of a particular gene have been inactivated; the gene is thus not expressed in the organism. This type of analysis is of the greatest use in assessing the function of tumor suppressor genes, because the knockout phenotype exactly mimics the inactivation of both gene copies seen in tumors. Knockout analysis of oncogene function will generally not define the mechanism by which excessive activity of a particular gene leads to neoplastic transformation, but may shed light on the normal role the putative oncogene plays in embryonic development or tissue homeostasis.

In many cases organisms homozygous for a genetic deletion of interest are nonviable, generally as a result of developmental anomalies. In such cases analysis of heterozygous animals containing a single normal gene allele and a single knockout allele may be useful. If such animals display an increased incidence of a particular tumor type, and if those tumors have undergone an additional genetic alteration inactivating the normal allele, a tumor suppressor role for the gene of interest is strongly supported. It is worth noting, however, that in many cases the specific neoplastic histology associated with a particular tumor suppressor gene may be different in humans than in knockout mice.

III. Genetic Abnormalities in Human Cancer

The clinical syndromes described below represent malignancies with well-characterized genetic etiologies. These disorders may have been initially identified based on familial syndromes, chromosomal abnormalities, or the identification of genes capable of inducing the transformed phenotype following transfer into appropriate cells. These examples have been chosen for the breadth of experimental analysis required for the identification of the responsible cancer genes, and for the diverse methods utilized to characterize their biological functions. This list is by no means comprehensive, and the reader is referred to several excellent texts (23, 24) for additional information.

A. Retinoblastoma—The Rb Gene

Retinoblastoma is the most common eye tumor in the pediatric population, affecting approximately 1 live birth in 20,000 (25). Retinoblastoma has been the prototypic example of the genetic predisposition to cancer and the model for a tumor suppressor gene. The majority of retinoblastoma tumors occur with no preceding family history, but this malignancy may also occur as part of a familial cancer syndrome. Mutations involving Rb, the gene responsible for retinoblastoma, occur in both familial and sporadic forms. With few exceptions, the familial form of the disease is transmitted in a typical mendelian autosomal dominant pattern. Therefore, offspring of gene carriers stand a 50% chance of inheriting the mutant allele. However, pedigree analysis has demonstrated a penetrance (development of retinoblastoma) of less than 100% in individuals who inherit the mutant allele. Thus, only the predisposition to cancer formation is inherited and a second event is required to develop a retinoblastoma. Subsequent work has shown that in most cases this second event is loss of function of the remaining wild-type Rb allele, resulting from a somatic mutation.

This observation led to the realization that, although retinoblastoma is inherited like an autosomal dominant genetic disorder, genes like Rb are actually recessive at the cellular level—tumor development does not occur if one normal copy of the gene is present. For this reason, such genes have been labeled "tumor suppressor genes"—the normal copy suppresses tumor formation. In 1971, Knudsen proposed his now famous theory that retinoblastoma is the result of mutational events in both alleles of a single gene (26, 27). In sporadic cases, both of these "hits," or mutational events, occur as random events in the same retinal cell, a statistically very rare event. In familial cases all somatic cells already contain a single mutated retinoblastoma allele, and retinoblastoma development is much more likely (and occurs earlier in development) because only a single additional genetic mutational event is required to render a cell malignant.

The majority of mutations described to date have occurred around a common region, band 14 of 13q, near the marker gene esterase D. The analysis of restriction length polymorphisms (RFLPs) demonstrated loss of heterozygosity in tumors and eventually resulted in localization and cloning of the gene (28). The increasing resolution of cytogenetic technology and use of DNA probes to detect loci immediately surrounding the retinoblastoma gene have demonstrated previously undetected genomic rearrangements, perhaps explaining nonpenetrance in individuals carrying mutations in the retinoblastoma susceptibility locus.

B. Familial Adenomatous Polyposis—The APC Gene

Familial adenomatous polyposis (FAP) is a dominantly inherited cancer predisposition with an incidence of approximately 1:10,000. Patients affected with FAP develop multiple benign colorectal adenomas. The likelihood that one or more of these lesions will progress to malignancy is high. FAP families have been extensively studied with the aim of identifying the causative gene. Initial clues to the location of the gene followed chromosomal analysis of a patient with FAP (29). This analysis demonstrated a large deletion in the region of 5q21–22. This location was later confirmed as the site of the gene through the use of RFLP analysis (30, 31). To do this, the investigators researched large numbers of FAP-affected families by probing DNA with a series of polymorphic DNA probes mapping to regions of chromosome 5. A close linkage was noted with one probe to region 5q21. The adenomatous polyposis coli (APC) gene has since been cloned and sequenced, and maps to the 5q21 locus. Interestingly, adenomas in patients with FAP show evidence of having a second inactivating event involving the noninherited allele of the APC gene, suggesting that the gene plays a tumor suppressor role analogous to that of the Rb gene.

Loss of APC gene function appears to be common in sporadic (noninherited) colon adenomas and carcinomas as well. Studies of such sporadic colorectal neoplasms were initially performed by RFLP analysis with polymorphic DNA probes mapping to chromosome 5. In one series 29% of sporadic adenomas and 36% of sporadic carcinomas were found to have deletions in the region of the APC gene (32). Subsequent analysis using genetic sequencing suggests that up to 80% of colon adenomas and carcinomas have undergone inactivating events involving both alleles of the APC gene (33); more than 300 different mutations of the APC gene have been described (34). Interestingly, several strains of mice have been identified that are heterozygous for an inactivating mutation of the APC gene (35); such mice have a high incidence of spontaneous intestinal adenomas, and thus appear to mimic accurately the FAP phenotype.

C. Li–Fraumeni Syndrome—The p53 Tumor Suppressor Gene

In 1969, Li and Fraumeni reported four families with an autosomal dominant predisposition to soft tissue sarcoma, breast cancer, and other tumors (36). Many reports have since followed. Although the syndrome, now known as the Li–Fraumeni syndrome, is rare, its importance lies in the unusual range of cancer predisposition and the fact that it is caused by a cancer gene implicated in the majority of noninherited sporadic carcinomas—the p53 gene.

The p53 gene and its encoded protein were originally identified in 1979 by virtue of their expression in cells infected with tumor viruses (37). During initial studies, the cellular p53 gene was thought to be an oncogene, in part because of its ability to transform rat embryo fibroblasts (38). However, molecular evidence for a role of the p53 gene in human tumors initially came from the study of allelic loss, and suggested that the gene was more likely to function as a tumor suppressor (34). Comparison of heterozygous alleles present in tumor tissue with those in normal tissue allows the identification of deletions as loss of heterozygosity (LOH) (39). The frequent identification of loss of a specific chromosomal marker in tumor tissue has been taken to represent one step in the inactivation of a tumor suppressor gene residing on the lost chromosome. Studies of multiple human tumors suggested that a tumor suppressor gene located on chromosome 17p was commonly inactivated—subsequent studies demonstrated that this gene was in fact the p53 gene. Sequencing of p53 alleles from multiple tumors has confirmed that inactivating mutations involving this gene, as well as loss of entire alleles, are common in tumors, confirming a tumor suppressor-type rather than an oncogene-type function.

The p53 gene has been implicated in over half the cancers occurring in the Li–Fraumeni syndrome by previous mutation and deletion studies. Examination of normal somatic cells of affected and unaffected members of five families was undertaken through amplification of the genomic region encompassing the majority of mutations found in p53. The region was then sequenced using multiple primers. Affected members from all five families were found to have mutations lying within this region (40).

The p53 gene plays an important role in regulating genomic fidelity, by inhibiting cell replication in cells that have received DNA damage until such damage can be repaired (41). In some cases, if irreparable DNA damage or other cellular stresses have occurred, p53 directs cellular apoptosis. It is apparent why the loss of this important mechanism of preserving genomic fidelity should be so common in human tumors, because the loss of p53 results in cells unable to repair genetic damage and resistant to apoptotic cell death. Interestingly, p53 knockout mice are viable and have a marked propensity to develop a variety of malignancies (42), similar to the analogous human syndrome.

D. Chronic Myelogenous Leukemia—The Philadelphia Chromosome

The discovery of the Philadelphia chromosome and its consistent involvement in chronic myeloid leukemia (CML) was the first demonstration of a relationship between a cytogenetic abnormality and a particular malignancy. CML is a myeloproliferative disease that originates in a hematopoietic stem cell. No strong familial links to the development of CML have been established, but an increased incidence has been observed among survivors of atomic bomb blasts.

Nowell and Hungerford described a specific chromosomal abnormality in CML cells in 1960 (3). They noted a shortened chromosome 22, which came to be known as the Philadelphia chromosome, and a lengthened chromosome 9. Later, banding techniques would demonstrate that the Philadelphia chromosome was the result of a reciprocal recombination event between chromosomes 9 and 22. The Philadelphia chromosome has been detected in more than 90% of patients afflicted with CML (43). The Philadelphia chromosome rearrangement creates a novel gene containing elements from two distinct genes, known as *bcr* and *abl* (44). Interestingly, the *abl* gene encodes an oncogene that has been previously linked to the etiology of certain murine leukemias. The *bcr–abl* fusion gene leads to expression of a novel *bcr–abl*-encoded hybrid protein product. It appears that the protein encoded by *bcr-abl* provides a growth advantage to CML cells by virtue of increased protein kinase activity that may amplify normal proliferative signals (44).

E. Breast Cancer—The HER2/neu Oncogene

The HER2/*neu* gene was originally identified as an oncogene in rat neuroblastoma cells capable of inducing neoplastic transformation of NIH 3T3 cells in DNA transfection assays (45). A substantial body of evidence supports a role for HER2/*neu* in human cancer as well. HER2/*neu* is overexpressed in approximately 30% of patients with breast cancer (46, 47), and this overexpression has been shown to correlate with a worse prognosis (47). Additionally, HER2/*neu* is overexpressed in ovarian carcinoma (48), pancreatic carcinoma (49), gastric carcinoma (50), endometrial carcinoma (51), and non-small-cell lung carcinoma (52), and generally predicts a poor prognosis.

HER2/*neu* overexpression often results from gene amplification; such chromosomal gene amplification can be readily detected in tumor specimens using FISH analysis, as previously described (53). The HER2/*neu* gene encodes a cell surface protein product that can serve as a target for monoclonal antibody-mediated therapeutics (54, 55); the success of such monoclonal antibody-based treatments represents the prototype for the targeted therapy of cancer. Tissue-specific expression of HER2/*neu* in the mammary glands of transgenic mice results in mammary carcinogenesis, which can be treated with anti-HER2/*neu* monoclonal antibodies (56), closely mimicking human disease. HER2/*neu* knockout animals are nonviable due to cardiac and neuromuscular abnormalities in embryogenesis (57), suggesting that normally HER2/*neu* plays a critical role in the development of these organs.

F. Multiple Endocrine Neoplasia Type 2—The RET Oncogene

The multiple endocrine neoplasia (MEN) syndromes consist of two distinct clinical entities: MEN type 1 and MEN type 2. These syndromes encompass a wide range of endocrine problems but are the result of just two heritable genetic defects. MEN 1, characterized by parathyroid hyperplasia, pancreaticoduodenal neuroendocrine tumors, and pituitary adenomas, is due to a defect in the MEN 1 tumor suppressor gene (2, 58). MEN 2 syndromes are characterized by medullary thyroid cancer (MTC). The various subtypes of the syndrome differ in their variable expression of pheochromocytomas, hyperparathyroidism, and other clinical features. These syndromes are the result of mutations in the RET oncogene.

MEN 2 syndromes consist of MEN IIa, MEN IIb, and familial non-MEN medullary thyroid carcinoma (FMTC). MEN 2a patients variably develop parathyroid hyperplasia and pheochromocytomas in addition to MTC. MEN 2b patients are also prone to pheochromocytomas and invariably suffer from MTC, although these tumors occur at a younger age and grow more aggressively than in MEN 2a patients. MEN 2b patients also develop neural gangliomas, particularly of the digestive tract. They do not develop hyperparathyroidism. FMTC patients demonstrate only MTC with no other associated endocrine anomalies.

Initial pedigree analysis of affected kindreds revealed an autosomal dominant inheritance pattern. Cytogenetic studies utilizing linkage analysis identified the susceptibility gene for MEN 2 and localized it to chromosome 10q 11.2 (59). Further analysis of this region revealed a gene encoding a transmembrane tyrosine kinase, later named the RET gene. Several mutations have been described within the RET gene (60). The final result of these various mutations is a gain of function for the RET protein product, defining RET as an oncogene. The importance of identification of the several mutations in RET is that a direct DNA test can be performed to test possible affected kindred members, permitting early detection and in some cases prophylactic thyroidectomy (61). Such treatment represents a life-saving advance in the management of patients with MEN-2 syndromes.

IV. The Future

Cancer genetics has been a broad and fertile area of research. Over the past several decades a large number of cancer genes have been identified and characterized. This has led to improvements in genetic testing and diagnostics, as well as more accurate prognostic information; advances in cancer genetics are just beginning to impact cancer therapeutics. The impending complete sequencing of the human genome by the Human Genome Project, in combination with further advances in techniques such as microarray expression analysis, will dramatically enhance progress in the study of cancer genetics. Sites of chromosome breakage, once identified, will be readily cloned based on the known genes residing at the specific chromosomal position. Similarly, an enlarging pool of RFLP markers will greatly facilitate the localization of genes linked to familial cancer syndromes. Again, consultation of chromosomal maps to delineate genes closely linked to a particular site may substitute for laborious positional cloning methodology.

However, the completion of the Genome Project will largely facilitate descriptive studies—identifying and cloning specific cancer-related genes. Mechanistic experiments to determine the molecular basis by which particular genes facilitate the process of tumorigenesis will still need to be performed, and may be rendered more complex by the increasing volume of background genetic information obtainable. Furthermore, the ability to study patterns of gene expression in which tens of thousands of distinct genes are analyzed simultaneously will require new approaches to experimental design. Collectively these advances should make the study of cancer genetics even more intellectually appealing, because researchers will be able to spend less time identifying the pieces and more time trying to put the puzzle together.

References

1. Lyman, G. H., and Kuderer, N. M. (1997). Basic population and cancer genetics and their use in the assessment of cancer risk. *Eur. J. Cancer* **33,** 2160–2167.
2. Chandrasekharappa, S. C., Guru, S. C., Manicham, P., Olufemi, S.-E., Collins, F. S., *et al.* (1997). Positional cloning of the gene for multiple endocrine neoplasia type I. *Science* **276,** 404–407.
3. Nowell, S., and Hungerford, D. A. (1960). A minute chromosome in human chronic granulocytic leukemia. *Science* **132,** 1497.
4. Pinkel, D., Straume, T., and Gray, J. W. (1986). Cytogenetic analysis using quantitative, high-sensitivity, fluorescence hybridization. *Proc. Natl. Acad. Sci. U.S.A.* **83,** 2934–2938.
5. Patel, A. S., Hawkins, A. L., and Griffin, C. A. (2000). Cytogenetics and cancer. *Curr. Opin. Oncol.* **12,** 62–67.
6. Pollack, R., Chen, S., Powers, S., and Verderame, M. (1984). Transformation mechanisms at the cellular level. *In* "Advances in Viral Oncology," Vol. 4 (G. Kleine, ed.), pp. 3–28. Raven Press, New York.
7. Kolligs, F. T., Hu, G., Dang, C. V., and Fearon, E. R. (1999). Neoplastic transformation of RK3E by mutant β-catenin requires deregulation of Tcf/Lef transcription but not activation of c-myc expression. *Mol. Cell. Biol.* **19,** 5696–5706.
8. Gille, H., and Downward, J. (1999). Multiple ras effector pathways contribute to G1 cell cycle progression. *J. Biol. Chem.* **274,** 22033–22040.
9. Dolbeare, F., Gratzner, H., Pallavicini, M., and Gray, J. W. (1983). Flow cytometric measurements of total cellular DNA content and incorporated bromodeoxyuridine. *Proc. Natl. Acad. Sci. U.S.A.* **80,** 5573–5577.
10. Korsmeyer, S. J. (1992). Bcl-2 initiates a new category of oncogenes: Regulators of cell death. *Blood* **80,** 879–881.
11. Reed, J. C. (2000). Dysregulation of apoptosis in cancer. *J. Clin. Oncol.* **17,** 2941–2953.
12. Roh, H., Pippin, J., and Drebin, J. A. (2000). Down-regulation of HER2/neu expression induces apoptosis in human cancer cells that overexpress HER2/neu. *Cancer Res.* **60,** 560–565.
13. Morin, P. J., Vogelstein, B., and Kinzler, K. W. (1996). Apoptosis and APC in colorectal tumorigenesis. *Proc. Natl. Acad. Sci. U.S.A.* **93,** 7950–7954.
14. Gordon, J. W., Harold, G., and Leila, Y. (1993). Transgenic animal methodologies and their applications. *Hum. Cell* **6,** 161–169.
15. Dankort, D. L., and Muller, W. J. (2000). Signal transduction in mammary tumorigenesis: A transgenic perspective. *Oncogene* **19,** 1038–1044.
16. MacDonald, R. J., Hammer, R. E., Swift, G. H., Ornitz, D. M., Davis, B. P., Palmiter, R. D., and Brinster, R. L. (1986). Tissue-specific expression of pancreatic genes in transgenic mice. *Ann. N.Y. Acad. Sci.* **478,** 131–146.
17. Kim, S. H., Roth, K. A., Moser, A. R., and Gordon, J. I. (1993). Transgenic mouse models that explore the multistep hypothesis of intestinal neoplasia. *J. Cell Biol.* **123,** 877–893.
18. DelaCoste, A., Romagnolo, B., Billuart, P., Renard, C. -A., Buendia, M.-A., *et al.* (1998). Somatic mutations of the β-catenin gene are frequent in mouse and human hepatocellular carcinomas. *Proc. Natl. Acad. Sci. U.S.A.* **95,** 8847–8851.
19. Strasser, A., O'Connor, L., Huang, D. C., O'Reilly, L. A., Stanley, M. L., *et al.* (1996). Lessons from bcl-2 transgenic mice for immunology, cancer biology and cell death research. *Behring Inst. Mitt.* **97,** 101–117.
20. Green, D. W., Roh, H., Pippin, J., and Drebin, J. A. (2000). Antisense oligonucleotides: An evolving technology for the modulation of gene expression in human disease. *J. Am. Coll. Surg.* **191,** 93–105.
21. Stein, C. A. (1995). Does antisense exist? *Nature Med.* **1,** 1119–1121.
22. Majzoub, J. A., and Muglia, L. J. (1996). Knockout mice. *N. Engl. J. Med.* **334,** 904–907.
23. Vogelstein, B., and Kinzler, K. W., eds. (1998). "The Genetic Basis of Human Cancer." Mcgraw-Hill, New York.
24. Bishop, J. M., and Weinberg, R. A., eds. (1996). "Molecular Oncology." Scientific American, New York.
25. Pendergrass, T. W. (1980). Incidence of retinoblastoma in the United States. *Arch. Ophthalmol.* **98,** 1204–1210.
26. Knudson, A. G. (1971). Mutation and cancer: Statistical study of retinoblastoma. *Proc. Natl. Acad. Sci. U.S.A.* **68,** 820.
27. Hetcote, H. W., and Knudson, A. G. (1978). Model for the incidence of embryonal cancers: Application to retinoblastoma. *Proc. Natl. Acad. Sci. U.S.A.* **75,** 2453.
28. Friend, S. H., Bernards, R., and Rogers, S. (1986). A human DNA segment with properties of the gene that predisposes to retinoblastoma and osteosarcoma. *Nature (London)* **323,** 643–646.
29. Herrera, L., Kakati, S., Gibas, L., Pietrzak, E., and Sandberg, A. A. (1986). Gardner's syndrome in a man with an intestinal deletion in 5q. *Am. J. Med. Genet.* **25,** 473–476.
30. Bodmer, W. F., Bailey, C. J., and Bodmer, J. (1987). Localization of the gene for familial adenomatous polyposis within a small region of chromosome 5. *Nature (London)* **328,** 614–616.
31. Leppert, M., Dobbs, M., and Scrambler, P. (1987). The gene for familial polyposis coli maps to the long arm of chromosome 5. *Science* **238,** 1411–1413.
32. Vogelstein, B., Fearon, E. R., and Hamilton, S. R. (1988). Genetic alterations during colorectal tumor development. *N. Engl. J. Med.* **319,** 525–531.
33. Miki, Y., Nishisho, I., and Myoshi, Y. (1991). Frequent loss of heterozygosity at the MCC locus on chromosome 5q21-22 in sporadic colorectal cancer. *Jpn. J. Cancer Res.* **82,** 1003–1007.
34. Beroud, C., and Soussi, T. (1996). APC gene: Database of germline and somatic mutations in human tumors and cell lines. *Nucleic Acid Res.* **24,** 121–124.
35. Halberg, R. B., Katzung, D. S., Hoff, P. D., Moser, A. R., Cole, C. E., *et al.* (2000). Tumorigenesis in the multiple intestinal neoplasia mouse: redundancy of negative regulators and specificity of modifiers. *Proc. Natl. Acad. Sci. U.S.A.* **97,** 3461–3466.
36. Li, F. P., and Fraumeni, J. E. (1969). Soft tissue sarcomas, breast cancer and other neoplasms: A familial syndrome? *Ann. Intern. Med.* **71,** 747–752.
37. Lane, D. P., and Crawford, L. V. (1979). T antigen is bound to a host protein in SV40-transformed cells. *Nature (London)* **278,** 261.
38. Eliyahu, D., Raz, A., Gruss, P., Givol, D., and Oren, M. (1984). Participation of p53 cellular tumor antigen in transformation of normal embryonal cells. *Nature (London)* **312,** 646.
39. Baker, S. J., Preisinger, A. C., Jessup, J. M., Parasheva, C., Markowitz, S., *et al.* (1990). p53 gene mutations occur in combination with 17p allelic deletions as late events in colorectal tumorigenesis. *Cancer Res.* **50,** 7717–7722.

40. Malkin, D., Li, F. P., and Strong, L. C. (1990). Germ line p53 mutations in a familial syndrome of breast cancer, sarcomas and other neoplasms. *Science* **250,** 1233–1238.
41. May, P., and May, E. (1999). Twenty years of p53 research: structural and functional aspects of the p53 protein. *Oncogene* **18,** 7621–7636.
42. Finlay, C. A. (1992). p53 loss of function: Implications for the process of immortalization and tumorigenesis. *BioEssays* **14,** 557–560.
43. Rowley, J. D. (1973). A new consistent chromosomal abnormality in chronic myelogenous leukemia identified by quinacrine and giemsa staining. *Nature (London)* **243,** 290–293.
44. Chissoe, S. L., Bodenteich, A., Wang, Y. F., Burian, D., *et al.* (1995). Sequence and analysis of the human abl gene, the bcr gene, and the regions involved in the Philadelphia chromosomal translocation. *Genomics* **27,** 67–82.
45. Schecter, A. L., Stern, D. F., and Vaidyanathan, L. (1984). The neu oncogene: An erb-B-related gene encoding a 185,000-Mr tumor antigen. *Nature (London)* **312,** 513–516.
46. Coussens, L., Yang-Feng, T. L., Liao, Y.-C., Chen, E., Gray, A., McGrath, J., Seeburg, P. H., Liebermann, T. A., Schlessinger, J., Francke, U., Levinson, A., and Ullrich, A. (1985). Tyrosine kinase receptor with extensive homology to EGF receptor shares chromosomal location with neu oncogene. *Science* **230,** 1132–1139.
47. Slamon, D. J., Clark, G. M., Wong, S. G., Levin, W. J., Ullrich, A., and Mcguire, W. L. (1987). Human breast cancer: Correlation of relapse and survival with amplification of the HER-2/neu oncogene. *Science* **235,** 177–182.
48. Berchuck, A., Kamel, A., Whitaker, R., Kerns, B., Olt, G., Kinney, R., Soper, J. T., Dodge, R., Clarke-Pearson, D. L., and Marks, P. (1990). Overexpression of HER-2*neu* is associated with a poor survival in advanced epithelial ovarian cancer. *Cancer Res.* **50,** 4087–4091.
49. Williams, T. M., Weiner, D. B., Greene, M. I., and Maguire, H. C. (1991). Expression of c-erbB-2 in human pancreatic adenocarcinomas. *Pathobiology* **59,** 46–52.
50. Yonemura, Y., Ninomiya, I., Ohoyama, S., Kimura, H. M., Yamaguchi, A., Fushida, S., Kosaka, T., Miwa, K., Miyazaki, I., and Endou, Y. (1991). Expression of c-erbB-2 oncoprotein in gastric carcinoma. Immunoreactivity for c-erbB-2 protein is an independent indicator of poor short-term prognosis in patients with gastric carcinoma. *Cancer* **67,** 2914–2918.
51. Berchuck, A., Rodriguez, G., Kinney, R. B., Soper, J. T., Dodge, R. K., Clarke-Pearson, D. L., and Bast, R. C. (1991). Overexpression of HER-2*neu* in endometrial cancer is associated with advanced stage disease. *Am. J. Obstet. Gynecol.* **164,** 15–21.
52. Kern, J. A., Schwartz, D. A., Nordberg, J. E., Weiner, D. B., Greene, M. I., Tourney, L., and Robinson, R. A. (1990). P185neu expression of human lung adenocarcinomas predicts shortened survival. *Cancer Res.* **50,** 5184–5187.
53. Jimenez, R. E., Wallis, T., Tabsczka, P., and Visscher, D. W. (2000). Determination of HER2/neu status in breast carcinoma: Comparative analysis of immunohistochemistry and fluorescent *in situ* hybridization. *Mod. Pathol.* **13,** 37–45.
54. Drebin, J. A., Link, V. C., Weinberg, R. A., and Greene, M. I. (1986). Inhibition of tumor growth by a monoclonal antibody reactive with an oncogene-encoded tumor antigen. *Proc. Natl. Acad. Sci. U.S.A.* **83,** 9129–9133.
55. Baselga, J., Tripathy, D., Mendelsohn, J., Baughman, S., Benz, C. C., *et al.* (1996). Phase II study of weekly intravenous recombinant humanized anti-p185HER2 monoclonal antibody in patients with HER2/neu-overexpressing metastatic breast cancer. *J. Clin. Oncol.* **14,** 737–744.
56. Katsumata, M., Okudaira, T., Samanta, A., Clark, D. P., Drebin, J. A., *et al.* (1995). Prevention of breast tumor development *in vivo* by downregulation of the p185neu receptor. *Nature Med.* **1,** 644–648.
57. Lin, W., Sanchez, H. B., Deerinck, T., Morris, J. K., Ellisman, M., *et al.* (2000). Aberrant development of motor axons and neuromuscular synapses in erbB2-deficient mice. *Proc. Natl. Acad. Sci. U.S.A.* **97,** 1299–1304.
58. Marx, S. J. (1998). Multiple endocrine neoplasia type 1. *In* "The Genetic Basis of Human Cancer" (B. Vogelstein and K.W. Kinzler, eds.), pp. 489–506. McGraw-Hill, New York.
59. Gardner, E., Papi, L., Easton, D. F., *et al.* (1993). Genetic linkage studies map the multiple endocrine neoplasia type 2 loci to a small interval on chromosome 10q11.2. *Hum. Mol. Genet.* **2,** 241–246.
60. Phay, J. E., Moley, J. F., and Lairmore, T. C. (2000). Multiple endocrine neoplasias. *Semin. Surg. Oncol.* **18,** 324–332.
61. Wells, S. A., and Skinner, M. A. (1998). Prophylactic thyroidectomy, based on direct genetic testing, in patients at risk for the multiple endocrine neoplasia type-2 syndromes. *Exp. Clin. Endocrin. Diabetes* **106,** 29–34.
62. Glassman, A. B. (1998). Cytogenetics, *in situ* hybridization and molecular approaches in the diagnosis of cancer. *Ann. Clin. Lab. Sci.* **28,** 324–330.

38

Cancer Gene Therapy

Kenneth K. Tanabe and James C. Cusack, Jr.

Division of Surgical Oncology, Massachusetts General Hospital, Boston, Massachusetts 02114

I. Introduction

The past decade has been witness to numerous advances in molecular biology, genetics, immunology, virology, and tumor biology that have contributed to the rapid growth of human gene therapy. Gene therapy involves the introduction of genetic material into a cell to achieve a desired therapeutic effect. Historically, diseases that result from inheritance of a single gene presented the first targets for human gene therapy. Severe combined immune deficiency, which arises from a genetic defect in the adenosine deaminase gene, was the first human disease treated by introduction of a gene (1). Treatment of this type of inherited disease necessitates long-term expression of a normal copy of the defective gene. Unfortunately, currently existing gene delivery and expression systems are relatively inefficient and do not produce long-term gene expression. Nonetheless, current gene transfer technology is suitable for cancer gene therapy.

In 1990, Fearon and Vogelstein proposed a model that linked malignant transformation to a combination of specific genetic errors (2). This contributed to the development of cancer gene therapy strategies based on replacement of defective tumor suppressor genes and inactivation of oncogenes. Several other cancer gene therapy strategies have been explored, including transfer of specific genes that, although not necessarily involved in tumorigenesis, may (1) enhance response to conventional therapies, (2) augment host immune responses, (3) express proteins that are cytotoxic, or (4) express genes that protect stem cells from cytotoxic chemotherapy. Because transient transgene expression lends itself well to the treatment of cancer (3), a disproportionate percentage of human gene therapy trials that have been approved are for cancer patients. As of January, 2000, 218 of 340 (64%) human therapeutic gene transfer protocols approved by the Office of Recombinant DNA Activities of the National Institutes of Health (NIH) are for the treatment of cancer (4).

II. Gene Transfer

Gene delivery vehicles differ in their gene transfer efficiency, target specificity, longevity of transgene expression, integration into host cell chromosomes, ease of vector production, immunogenicity, and transgene capacity. Several different biologic vectors and non biologic delivery systems have been developed, and properties of the most commonly used gene therapy vehicles are listed in Table I. Biologic vectors are used in approximately 80% of clinical trials approved by the Recombinant DNA Advisory Committee because of their ability to transfer nucleic acids efficiently to

Table I Gene Delivery Systems for Cancer Gene Therapy

Vector (size)	Advantages	Disadvantages	Insert size
Retrovirus (10 kb)	Small genome Stable colinear integration Efficient gene transfer Nontoxic to host cells Infects dividing cells	Requires actively dividing cells Small insert capacity Low titer Transient expression Insertional mutagenesis Random integration Labile *in vivo*	9–12 kb
Adenovirus (36 kb)	High viral titers can be produced Highly efficient gene transfer Nontoxic to host cells Infects dividing and nondividing cells Replication-competent mutants useful for oncolysis	Transient expression Small insert capacity Viral antigenicity produces immune response	7.5 kb
Adeno-associated virus (5 kb)	Small genome Specific integration site in chromosome 19 Efficient gene transfer Nonpathogenic to humans Infects dividing and nondividing cells Weakly immunogenic	Small insert capacity Safety not yet demonstrated in clinical trials Loss of nonrandom integration over time Low viral titers	5 kb
Vaccinia virus (187 kb)	Transient gene expression Highly efficient gene transfer and expression Replication-competent mutants useful for oncolysis Large transgene capacity	Strongly immunogenic Safety concerns in immunosuppressed patients Viral antigenicity produces immune response	25 kb
Herpes simplex virus type 1 (152 kb)	Infects dividing and nondividing cells Neurotropic Replication-competent mutants useful for oncolysis High viral titers can be produced Very large transgene capacity Potential for prolonged gene expression	Possibility of herpes encephalitis Viral antigenicity produces immune response	40–50 kb
Protein/DNA complexes	Cell-specific targeting Very large transgene capacity	Inefficient gene transfer	No limit
Liposomes	Synthetic Very large transgene capacity	Inefficient gene transfer No specific targeting mechanism	No limit
Nonviral plasmid	Transient gene expression Few safety concerns Very large transgene capacity	Inefficient gene transfer	No limit

host cells (Table II). As a result of evolutionary forces, viruses have necessarily evolved efficient mechanisms to deliver their genetic material into cells, avoid cellular defenses, and induce host cells to transcribe and translate viral genes. Viruses therefore serve as ideal vehicles for delivery of foreign genes. Recombinant viral vectors generally have been rendered incapable of replication outside of specific packaging cells by genetic engineering. This strategy maintains the gene transfer capabilities of the native virus while attempting to minimize virus-induced pathogenicity. Several nonviral vectors have also been developed. These vehicles lack many of the mechanisms that have evolved in viruses to protect the transferred DNA or RNA from degradation by the host cell. However, this disadvantage is offset by the absence of a host immune response to these types of vectors and the relatively low cost of vector production. The ideal gene delivery system has not yet been constructed, and development of safer and more efficient gene delivery systems is necessary for gene therapy to benefit patients. Emerging technologies such as manipulation of the surface charge of liposomes (5, 6) and restriction of gene expression by incorporation of transcriptional response elements (7) should yield more effective gene transfer vectors in the future.

A. Retrovirus

Retroviruses are diploid positive-strand RNA viruses that may infect cells that express surface receptors specific for retroviral envelope glycoproteins (8). The genome contains approximately 10,000 base pairs (10 kb) of DNA and can carry approximately 9–12 kb of transgene sequence. Infection with these viruses have been associated with a variety of diseases, including lymphoma, leukemia, murine

Table II Approved Cancer Gene Therapy Clinical Trials

Cancer	RAC protocol approval number[a]	Principal investigator, institution, contact numbers	Protocol title	Gene transduction	Target cell	Therapeutic gene	Delivery vehicle
Melanoma							
Melanoma	9007-003, open	Rosenberg, S.A. NIH Tel.301-496-4164 FAX 301-402-1738	Gene therapy of patients with advanced cancer using tumor infiltrating lymphcytes transduced with gene coding for tumor necrosis factor	*In vitro*	TILs	TNF	Retrovirus
Melanoma: renal, colon, breast	9110-010, open	Rosenberg, S.A. NIH Tel. 301-496-4164 FAX 301-402-1738	Immunization of cancer patients using autologous cancer cells modified by insertion of the gene for tumor necrosis factor	*In vitro*	Autologous tumor cells	TNF	Retrovirus
Melanoma	9110-011, open	Rosenberg, S.A. NIH Tel. 301-496-4164 FAX 301-402-1738	Immunization of cancer patients using autologous cancer cells modified by insertion of the gene for interleukin-2	*In vitro*	Autologous tumor cells	IL-2	Retrovirus
Melanoma	9206-021, closed	Gansbacher, B. Memorial Sloan Kettering Cancer Center Tel. 212-639-6667 FAX 212-794-5813	Immunization with HLA-A2-matched allogeneic melanoma cells that secrete interleukin-2 in patients with metastatic melanoma	*In vitro*	Irradiated allogenic HLA-A2-matched tumor cells	IL-2	Retrovirus
Melanoma	9202-013, closed	Nabel, G.I. Univ. of Michigan Tel. 313-647-4798 FAX 313-647-4730	Immunotherapy of malignancy by *in vivo* gene transfer into tumors	*In vivo*	Autologous tumor cells	HLA-B7/β_2-microglobulin	Liposome
Melanoma	9306-043, open	Seigler, H.F. Duke University Medical Center Tel. 919-684-3942 FAX 919-684-6070	A phase I trial of human γ-interferon-transduced autologous tumor cells in patients with disseminated malignant melanoma	*In vitro*	Autologous tumor cells	δ-IFN	Retrovirus
Melanoma	9309-058, open	Economou, J.S. Univ. of CA Medical Center Tel. 310-825-2644 FAX 310-825-7575	Genetically engineered autologous tumor vaccines producing interleukin-2 for the treatment of metastatic melanoma	*In vitro*	Autologous tumor cells	IL-2	Retrovirus
Melanoma	9312-065, open	Chang, A.E. Univ. of Michigan Tel. 313-936-4392 FAX 313-936-9647	Adoptive immunotherapy of cancer in vivo with activated lymph node cells primed with autologous tumor cells transduced with GM-CSF gene	*Ex vivo*	Autologous tumor cells	GM-CSF gene	Retrovirus

continues

Table II *continued*

Cancer	RAC protocol approval number[a]	Principal investigator, institution, contact numbers	Protocol title	Gene transduction	Target cell	Therapeutic gene	Delivery vehicle
Melanoma	9312-063, open	Sznol, M. NIH Tel. 301-496-8798 FAX 301-402-0428	A phase I trial of B7-transfected lethally irradiated allogeneic melanoma cell lines to induce cell-mediated immunity against tumor-associated antigens presented by HLA-A2 or HLA-A1 in patients with stage IV melanoma	*In vitro*	Allogeneic tumor cells	B7 (CD80), HLA-B7	Liposome
Melanoma	9309-058, open	Economou, J.S. UCLA Tel. 310-825-2644 FAX 310-825-7575	Genetically engineered autologous tumor vaccines producing interleukin-2 for the treatment of metastatic melanoma	*In vitro*	Allogeneic tumor cells	IL-2	Retrovirus
Melanoma	9309-056, open	Das Gupta, T.K. Univ. of Illinois at Chicago Tel. 312-996-6666 FAX 312-996-9365	Immunization of malignant melanoma patients with interleukin-2-secreting melanoma cells expressing defined allogeneic histocompatibility antigens	*In vitro*	Allogeneic tumor cells	IL-2	Retrovirus
Melanoma	9411-093, open	Dranoff, G. Dana Farber Cancer Institute, Boston Tel. 617-632-5051 FAX 617-632-5167	A phase I study of vaccination with autologous, irradiated melanoma cells engineered to secrete human granulocyte–macrophage colony-stimulating factor	*In vitro*	Autologous tumor cells	GM-CSF	Retrovirus
Melanoma: lymphoma, breast, head and neck	9406-081, open	Lotze, M.T. Univ. of Pittsburgh Tel. 412-692-2852 FAX 412-648-6761	IL-12 gene therapy using direct injection of tumor with genetically engineered autologous fibroblasts	*In vitro*	Autologous fibroblasts	IL-12	Retrovirus
Melanoma	9403-072, closed	Hersh, E. Arizona Cancer Center, Tucson Tel. 520-626-2250 FAX 520-626-2225	Phase I study of immunotherapy of malignant melanoma by direct gene transfer	*In vivo*	Autologous tumor cells	HLA-B7/β_2-microglobulin	Liposome
Melanoma	9512-140, open	Rosenberg, S.A. NIH Tel. 301-496-4164 FAX 301-402-1738	Phase I trial in patients with metastatic melanoma of immunization with a recombinant adenovirus encoding the MART-1 melanoma antigen	*In vivo*	Melanoma tumor cells	MART-1 melanoma antigen	Adenovirus
Melanoma	9511-136, open	Yee, C. Univ. of Washington, Seattle Tel. 206-285-1704 FAX 206-285-8883	Phase I study to evaluate the safety of cellular adoptive immunotherapy using autologous unmodified and genetically modified $CD8^+$ tyrosinase-specific T cells in patients with metastatic melanoma	*In vitro*	Autologous $CD8^+$ tyrosinase-specific T cells	HSV-TK	Retrovirus

Melanoma	9508-120, open	Chang, A.E. Univ. of Michigan Tel. 313-936-4392 FAX 313-936-9647	Phase I study of tumor-infiltrating lymphocytes derived from *in vivo* HLA-B7 gene modified tumors in the adoptive immunotherapy of melanoma	*In vivo*	Autologous tumor cells	TIL/HLA-B7	Liposome
Melanoma: breast, renal, colorectal, non-Hodgkins lymphoma	9508-115, open	Chang, A.E. Univ. of Michigan Tel. 313-936-4392 FAX 313-936-9647	Phase II study of immunotherapy of metastatic cancer by direct gene transfer	*In vivo*	Autologous tumor cells	HLA-B7/β_2-microglobulin	Retrovirus
Melanoma	9506-108, open	Fox, B.A. Chiles Research Institute, Providence Medical Center, Portland Tel. 503-215-6311 FAX 503-215-6841	Adoptive cellular therapy of cancer combining direct HLA-B7/β_2-microglobulin gene transfer with autologous tumor vaccination for the generation of vaccine-primed anti-CD3 activated lymphocytes	*In vitro*	Autologous tumor cells	HLA-B7/β_2-microglobulin	Liposome
Melanoma	9503-102, open	Gansbacher, B. Motzer, R. Memorial Sloan Kettering Cancer Center Tel. 212-639-6667 FAX 212-794-5813	Phase I/II study of immunization with MHC class I-matched allogeneic human prostatic carcinoma cells engineered to secrete interleukin-2 and interferon-γ	*In vitro*	HLA-matched allogeneic tumor cells	IL-2	Retrovirus
Melanoma	9503-101, closed	Economou, J.S. UCLA Tel. 310-825-2644 FAX 310-825-7575	A phase I testing of genetically engineered interleukin-7 melanoma vaccines	*In vitro*	Allogeneic tumor cells	IL-7/HSV-TK	Retrovirus
Melanoma	9611-168, open	Hersh, E. Arizona Cancer Center, Tucson Tel. 520-626-2250 FAX 520-626-2225	Phase II study of immunotherapy of metastatic melanoma by direct gene transfer	*In vivo*	Autologous tumor cells	HLA-B7/β_2-microglobulin	Liposome
Melanoma	9611-166, open	Rosenberg, S.A. NIH Tel. 301-496-4164 FAX 301-402-1738	Phase I trial in patients with metastatic melanoma of immunization with a recombinant vaccinia virus encoding the MART-1 melanoma antigen	*In vivo*	Melanoma cells	MART-1 melanoma antigen	Vaccinia virus
Melanoma	9611-165, open	Rosenberg, S.A. NIH Tel. 301-496-4164 FAX 301-402-1738	Phase I trial in patients with metastatic melanoma of immunization with a recombinant fowlpox virus encoding the GP100 melanoma antigen	*In vivo*	Melanoma cells	gp 100 melanoma antigen	Fowlpox virus
Melanoma	9610-163, open	Rosenberg, S.A. NIH Tel. 301-496-4164 FAX 301-402-1738	Phase I trial in patients with metastatic melanoma of immunization with a recombinant fowlpox virus encoding the MART-1 melanoma antigen	*In vivo*	Melanoma cells	MART-1 melanoma antigen	Fowlpox virus

continues

Table II *continued*

Cancer	RAC protocol approval number[a]	Principal investigator, institution, contact numbers	Protocol title	Gene transduction	Target cell	Therapeutic gene	Delivery vehicle
Melanoma, sarcoma	9608-158, open	Mahvi, D.M. Univ. of Wisconsin Tel. 608-263-1383 FAX 608-263-7652	Phase I/IB study of immunization with autologous tumor cells transfected with the GM-CSF gene by particle-mediated transfer in patients with melanoma or sarcoma	*In vitro*	Autologous tumor cells	GM-CSF	Plasmid
Melanoma	9604-151, open	Rosenberg, S.A. NIH Tel. 301-496-4164 FAX 301-402-1738	Phase I trial in patients with metastatic melanoma of immunization with a recombinant adenovirus encoding the GP100 melanoma antigen	*In vivo*	Autologous tumor cells	Serotype 2/GP100 melanoma antigen/concurrent IL-2	Adenovirus
Melanoma	9707-202, open	Dranoff, G. Dana-Farber Cancer Institute, Boston Tel. 617-632-5051 FAX 617-632-5167	A phase I study of vaccination with autologous lethally irradiated melanoma cells engineered by adenoviral mediated gene transfer to secrete human granulocyte-macrophage colony stimulating factor	*In vitro*	Autologous tumor cells	GM-CSF	Adenovirus
Melanoma	9709-210, open	Gonzalez, R. University of Colorado Cancer Center, Denver Tel. 303-372-6651 FAX 303-372-6554	Compassionate use protocol for retreatment with allovectin-7 immunotherapy for metastatic cancer by direct gene transfer	*In vivo*	Autologous tumor cells	HLA-B7/β_2-macroglobulin	Liposome
Melanoma	9709-212, open	Gonzalez, R. University of Colorado Cancer Center, Denver Tel. 303-372-6651 FAX 303-372-6554	Phase I study of direct gene transfer of HLA-B7 plasmid DNA/DMRIE/DOPE lipid complex (allovectin-7) with IL-2 plasmid DNA/DMRIE/DOPE lipid complex (leuvectin) as an immunotherapeutic regimen in patients with metastatic melanoma	*In vivo*	Autologous tumor cells	HLA-B7/β_2-microglobulin	Liposome
Melanoma	9706-197, open	Conry, R.M. Univ. of Alabama, Birmingham Tel. 205-934-7167 FAX 205-934-1608	Phase Ib trial of intratumoral injection of a recombinant canarypox virus encoding human B7.1 (ALVAC-hB7.1) or a combination of ALVAC-hB7.1 and a recombinant canarypox virus encoding human interleukin-12 (ALVAC-HIL-12) in patients with surgically incurable melanoma	*In vivo*	Autologous melanoma cell	B7(CD80), IL-12	Canarypox virus
Melanoma	9704-185, open	Conry, R.M. Univ. of Alabama, Birmingham Tel. 205-934-7167 FAX 205-934-1608	Phase Ib trial of intratumoral injection of a recombinant canarypox virus encoding the human interleukin-12 gene (ALVAC-hIL-12) in patients with surgically incurable melanoma	*In vivo*	Autologous melanoma cell	IL-12	Canarypox virus

Melanoma	9701-174, open	Das Gupta, T.K. Univ. of Illinois at Chicago Tel. 312-996-6666 FAX 312-996-9365	A pilot study using interleukin-2-transfected irradiated allogeneic melanoma cells encapsulated in an immunoisolation device in patients with metastatic malignant melanoma	*In vitro*	Allogeneic tumor cells	IL-2	Retrovirus
Melanoma	9802-233, open	Dreicer, R. University of Iowa Hospitals and Clinics Tel. 319-356-8722	Phase II study of direct gene transfer of HLA-B7 plasmid DNA/DMRIE/DOPE lipid complex (allovectin-7) as an immunotherapeutic agent in patients with stage III and IV melanoma with no treatment alternatives	*In vivo*	Autologous tumor cells	HLA-B7	Liposome
Melanoma	9802-234, open	Thompson, J.A. University of Washington Tel. 206-548-4251 FAX 206-548-4509	A controlled, randomized, phase III trial comparing the response to dacarbazine with and without allovectin-7 in patients with metastatic melanoma	*In vivo*	Autologous tumor cells	HLA-7/β_2-microglobulin	Liposome
Melanoma	9804-244, open	Walsh, P. University of Colorado Health Sciences Center, Denver Tel. 303-315-7738 FAX 303-315-8272	A phase I study using direct combination DNA injections for the immunotherapy of metastatic melanoma	*In vivo*	Autologous tumor cells	IL-2, *Staphylococcus enterotoxin B*	Plasmid, liposome
Melanoma, breast	9804-248, open	Schuchter, L. University of Pennsylvania School of Medicine Tel. 215-662-7907 FAX 215-349-5326	Phase I trial of therapeutic cancer vaccine using intratumoral injections of B7-1 (H5.030CMVhB7) in patients with metastatic melanoma or metastatic breast cancer	*In vivo*	Autologous tumor cells	B7.1(CD80)	Adenovirus
Melanoma	9805-254, open	Rosenberg, S.A. NIH Tel. 301-496-4164 FAX 301-402-1738	Immunization of patients with metastatic melanoma using DNA encoding the GP100 melanoma antigen	*In vivo*	Autologous fibroblasts	gp 100 melanoma antigen	Plasmid
Melanoma	9806-256, open	Suzuki, T. University of Kansas Medical Center Tel. 913-588-6724 FAX 913-588-7295	Autologous, irradiated, melanoma cells transduced *ex vivo* with an adenovirus vector (Adv/GM-CSF) expressing granulocyte–macrophage colony-stimulating factor gene	*In vitro*	Autologous tumor cells	GM-CSF	Adenovirus

continues

Table II *continued*

Cancer	RAC protocol approval number[a]	Principal investigator, institution, contact numbers	Protocol title	Gene transduction	Target cell	Therapeutic gene	Delivery vehicle
Melanoma	9806-260, open	Hersh, E. Arizona Cancer Center, Tucson Tel. 520-626-2250 FAX 520-626-2225	Phase I study of HLA-B7/β2M plasmid DNA/DMRIE/DOPE lipid complex (leuvectin) as an immunotherapeutic regimen in patients with metastatic renal cell carcinoma	*In vivo*	Autologous tumor cells	HLA-7/β^2-microglobulin	Liposome
Melanoma	9810-267, open	Morris, J.C. NIH Tel. 301-402-0161 FAX 301-402-2373	A phase I study of intralesional administration of an adenovirus vector expressing the HSV-1 thymidine kinase gene (AdV.RSV-TK) in combination with escalating doses of ganciclovir in patients with cutaneous metastatic malignant melanoma	*In vivo*	Autologous tumor cells	HSV-TK	Adenovirus
Melanoma	9811-269, open	Economou, J.A. UCLA Medical Center Tel. 310-825-2644 FAX 310-825-7575	A phase I trial testing MART-1 genetic immunization in malignant melanoma	*In vitro*	Autologous dendritic cells	MART-1 melanoma antigen	Adenovirus
Melanoma	9901-278, open	Conry, R.M. University of Alabama at Birmingham Tel. 205-934-7167 FAX 205-934-1608	Phase I dose escalation trial of polynucleotide immunization with plasmid DNA encoding MART-1 (melanoma antigen recognized by T cells-1) in patients with resected melanoma at significant risk for relapse	*In vivo*	Autologous fibroblasts	MART-1 melanoma antigen	Plasmid
Nervous system							
Astrocytoma	9306-050, open	Raffel, C. Mayo Clinic Tel. 507-284-8167 FAX 507-284-5206	Gene therapy for the treatment of recurrent pediatric malignant astrocytomas with *in vivo* tumor transduction with the herpes simplex thymidine kinase gene	*In vivo*	Tumor site in brain	HSV-TK	Retrovirus
Astrocytoma	9502-099, open	Fetell, M. Columbia Presbyterian Medical Center, NY, NY Tel. 212-305-5571 FAX 212-305-7365	Stereotaxic injection of herpes simplex thymidine kinase vector producer cells (PA-317/G1TkSvNa.7) and intravenous ganciclovir for the treatment of recurrent malignant glioma	*In vivo*	Autologous tumor cells	PA317/HSV-TK	Retrovirus
Brain	9206-019, closed	Oldfield, E. NIH Tel. 301-496-5728 FAX 301-402-0380	Gene therapy for the treatment of brain tumors using intratumoral transduction with the thymidine kinase gene and intravenous ganciclovir	*In vivo*	Autologous tumor cells	PA317/HSV-TK	Retrovirus

Brain	9309-055, open	Kun, L.E. St. Jude Children's Research Hospital, Memphis Tel. 901-495-3565 FAX 901-495-3113	Gene therapy for recurrent pediatric brain tumors	*In vivo*	Autologous tumor cells	HSV-TK	Retrovirus
Glioma	9512-138, open	Black, K.L. UCLA Tel. 310-206-5687 FAX 310-206-9486	A phase I study of the safety of injecting malignant glioma patients with irradiated TGF-β_2 antisense gene modified autologous tumor cells	*In vitro*	Autologous tumor cells	TGF-β_2 gene	Plasmid
Brain	9605-154, open	Harsh IV, G.R. Harvard Medical School Tel. 617-724-3804 FAX 617-724-8769	Phase I study of retroviral-mediated incorporation of the HSV-thymidine kinase gene and gancliclovir in malignant gliomas	*In vivo*	Autologous tumor cells	HSV-TK	Retrovirus
CNS	9409-089, open	Eck, S.M. Univ. of Pennsylvania Medical Center Tel. 215-898-4178 FAX 215-573-8606	Treatment of advanced CNS malignancy with the recombinant adenovirus H5.020RSVTK; a phase I trial	*In vivo*	Autologous tumor cells	HSV-TK	Adenovirus
CNS	9412-098, open	Grossman, R. Methodist Hospital, Houston, TX Tel. 713-790-3980 FAX 713-798-3739	Phase I study of adenoviral vector delivery of the HSV-TK gene and the intravenous administration of ganciclovir in adults with malignant tumors of the central nervous system	*In vivo*	Autologous tumor cells	HSV-TK	Adenovirus
Glioblastoma	9303-037, open	VanGilder, J.C. Univ. of Iowa Tel. 319-356-2772	Gene therapy for the treatment of recurrent glioblastoma multiforme with *in vivo* tumor transduction with the herpes simplex thymidine kinase gene/ganciclovir system	*In vivo*	Autologous tumor cells	HSV-TK	Retrovirus
Glioblastoma	9306-052, open	Ilan, J. Case Western Reserve Univ. Tel. 216-368-3590 FAX 216-368-1357	Gene therapy for human brain tumors using episome-based antisense cDNA transcription of insulin-like growth factor I	*In vitro*	Autologous tumor cells	Antisense insulin-like growth factor	Liposome
Glioblastoma	9406-080, open	Sobol, R. San Diego Regional Cancer Center Tel. 619-552-8585 FAX 619-450-3251	Injection of glioblastoma patients with tumor cells genetically modified to secrete interleukin-2; a phase I study	*In vitro*	Autologous fibroblasts/ in combination with untransduced autologous tumor cells	IL-2	Retrovirus

continues

Table II *continued*

Cancer	RAC protocol approval number[a]	Principal investigator, institution, contact numbers	Protocol title	Gene transduction	Target cell	Therapeutic gene	Delivery vehicle
Glioma	9502-099, open	Fetell, M. Columbia Presbyterian Medical Center, NY, NY Tel. 212-305-5571 FAX 212-305-7365	Stereotaxic injection of herpes simplex thymidine kinase vector producer cells (PA317/G1 TkSvNa.7) and intravenous ganciclovir for the treatment of recurrent malignant glioma	*In vivo*	Autologous tumor cells	HSV-TK	Retrovirus
Malignant glioma	9508-116, open	Bozik, M. Univ. of Pittsburgh Cancer Center Tel. 412-692-2600 FAX 412-692-2610	Gene therapy of malignant gliomas; a phase I study of IL-4 gene-modified autologous tumor to elicit an immune response	*In vitro*	Autologous tumor cells glioma)	IL-4	Retrovirus
Glioblastoma	9608-157, open	Maria, B. Univ. of Florida, Gainesville Tel. 352-392-6442 FAX 352-392-9802	Prospective, open-label, parallel-group, randomized multicenter trial comparing the efficacy of surgery, radiation, and injection of murine cells producing herpes simplex thymidine kinase vector followed by intravenous ganciclovir against the efficacy of surgery and radiation in the treatment of newly diagnosed, previously untreated glioblastoma	*In vivo*	Autologous tumor cells	HSV-TK	Retrovirus
Glioblastoma	9611-167, open	Maria, B. Univ. of Florida; Gainesville Tel. 352-392-6442 FAX 352-392-9802	Prospective, open-label, multicenter, extension trial for the treatment of recurrent glioblastoma multiforme with surgery and injection of murine cells producing herpes simplex thymidine kinase vector followed by intravenous ganciclovir for patients with disease progression following standard treatment on protocol GTI-0115	*In vivo*	Autologous tumor cells	HSV-TK	Retrovirus
Brain	9701-173, open	Croop, J. Indiana Univ. School of Medicine Tel. 317-274-8960 FAX 317-274-8679	A pilot study of dose intensified procarbazine, CCNU, vincristine (PCV) for poor prognosis pediatric and adult brain tumors utilizing fibronectin-assisted, retroviral-mediated modification of $CD34^+$ peripheral blood cells with O^6-methylguanine DNA methyltransferase	*In vitro*	$CD34^+$ peripheral blood cells	Peripheral blood $CD34^+$ cells	Retrovirus
Glioblastoma	9701-175, open	Lieberman, F. Mt. Sinai Medical Center, NY, NY Tel. 212-241-7581 FAX 212-987-3301	Gene therapy for recurrent glioblastoma multiforme; phase I trial of intraparenchymal adenoviral vector delivery of the HSV-TK gene and intravenous administration of ganciclovir	*In vivo*	Autologous tumor cells	HSV-TK	Adenovirus

Neuroblastoma	9712-223, open	Bowman, L. St. Jude Children's Research Hospital, Memphis Tel. 901-495-3410	Phase I study of chemokine and cytokine gene modified allogeneic neuroblastoma cells for treatment of relapsed/refractory neuroblastoma using a retroviral vector	*In vitro*	Allogeneic neuroblastoma cell lines	IL-2	Retrovirus
Neuroblastoma	9712-224, open	Bowman, L. St. Jude Children's Research Hospital, Memphis Tel. 901-495-3410	Phase I study of chemokine and cytokine gene modified autologous neuroblastoma cells for treatment of relapsed/refractory neuroblastoma using an adenoviral vector	*In vitro*	Autologous tumor cells	IL-2	Adenovirus
Leptomeningeal carcinomatosis	9312-059, closed	Oldfield, E.H. NIH Tel. 301-496-5728 FAX 301-402-0380	Intrathecal gene therapy for the treatment of leptomeningeal carcinomatosis	*In vivo*	Autologous tumor cells	HSV-TK	Retrovirus
Multiple myeloma	9506-107, open	Munshi, N.C. Univ. of Arkansas for Medical Sciences Tel. 501-686-5222 FAX 501-686-6442	Thymidine kinase (TK) transduced donor leukocyte infusions as a treatment for patients with relapsed or persistent multiple myeloma after T cell-depleted allogeneic bone marrow transplant	*In vitro*	Allogeneic T lymphocytes	HSV-TK	Retrovirus
Neuroblastoma	9206-018, open	Brenner, M.K. St. Jude Children's Research Hospital, Memphis Tel. 901-522-0410 FAX 901-521-9005	Phase I study of cytokine-gene modified autologous neuroblastoma cells for treatment of relapsed/refractory neuroblastoma	*In vitro*	Autogenous neuroblastoma cells	IL-2	Retrovirus
Neuroblastoma	9403-068, open	Rosenblatt, J. Univ. of Rochester, NY Tel. 716-275-0842 FAX 716-273-1051	A phase I study of immunization with g-interferon transduced neuroblastoma cells	*In vitro*	Autologous tumor cells/allogeneic tumor cells	IFN-γ	Retrovirus
Neuroblastoma	9511-133, open	Brenner, M.K. St. Jude Children's Research Hospital, Memphis Tel. 901-522-0410 FAX 901-521-9005	Phase I study of cytokine gene modified autologous neuroblastoma cells for treatment of relapsed/refractory neuroblastoma using an adenoviral vector	*In vitro*	Autologous tumor cells	IL-2 gene	Adenovirus
Glioblastoma	9802-235, open	Markert, J. University of Alabama Tel. 205-934-7170 FAX 205-975-3203	A dose escalating phase I study of the treatment of malignant glioma with G207, a genetically engineered HSV-1	*In vivo*	Autologous tumor cells	Tumor lysis	HSV-type 1

continues

Table II *continued*

Cancer	RAC protocol approval number[a]	Principal investigator, institution, contact numbers	Protocol title	Gene transduction	Target cell	Therapeutic gene	Delivery vehicle
Glioma	9808-263, open	Lang, Jr., F.F. University of Texas MD Anderson Cancer Center Tel. 713-792-2400 FAX 713-794-4950	Phase I trial of adenovirus-mediated wild-type p53 gene therapy for malignant gliomas	*In vivo*	Autologous tumor cells	p53	Adenovirus
Breast							
Breast	9409-086, open	Lyerly, H.K. Duke Univ. Tel. 919-681-8350 FAX 919-681-7970	A pilot study of autologous human interleukin-2 gene modified tumor cells in patients with refractory or recurrent metastatic breast cancer	*In vitro*	Autologous tumor cells	IL-2	Liposome
Breast	9309-054, open	O'Shaughnessy, J.A. Kentucky Medical Oncology Assoc. Tel. 502-582-3735 FAX 502-582-9968	Retroviral-mediated transfer of the human multidrug resistance gene (MDR-1) into hematopoietic stem cells during autologous transplantation after intensive chemotherapy for breast cancer	*In vitro*	$CD34^+$ autologous peripheral blood cells	MDR-1	Retrovirus
Breast, ovarian	9512-137, open	Hortobagyi, G. M.D. Anderson Cancer Center Tel. 713-792-2933 FAX 713-794-4535	Phase I study of E1A gene therapy for patients with metastatic breast or epithelial ovarian cancer that overexpresses HER-2/neu	*In vivo*	Autologous tumor cells	E1A gene	Liposome
Breast	9409-084, open	Holt, J.T. Vanderbilt Univ. Tel. 615-343-4730 FAX 615-343-4539	Gene therapy for the treatment of metastatic breast cancer by in vivo infection with breast-targeted retroviral vectors expressing antisense c-fos or antisense c-myc RNA.	*In vivo*	Autologous tumor cells	c-fos antisense, c-myc antisense	Retrovirus
Breast	9601-143, open	Cowen, K.H. NIH Tel. 301-496-4916 FAX 301-402-0172	Antimetabolite induction, high-dose alkylating agent consolidation, and retroviral transduction of the MDR1 gene into peripheral blood progenitor cells followed by intensification therapy with sequential paclitaxel and doxorubicin for stage 4 breast cancer	*In vitro*	Autologous CD341 peripheral blood lymphocytes	MDR-1	Retrovirus
Breast	9608-156, open	Urba, W.J. Providence Portland Medical Center Tel. 503-215-6014 FAX 503-215-6841	Phase I trial using a CD80-modified allogeneic breast cancer line to vaccinate HLA-A2-positive women with breast cancer	*In vitro*	Allogeneic tumor cells	B7 (CD80)	Liposome

Breast	9709-216, open	VonMehren, M. Fox Chase Cancer Center, Philadelphia Tel. 215-728-3545	Phase I/pilot study of p53 intralesional gene therapy with chemotherapy in breast cancer	*In vivo*	Autologous	p53	Adenovirus
Breast	9811-272, open	Kufe, D.W. Dana-Farber Cancer Institute, Boston Tel. 617-632-3141 FAX 617-632-2934	A phase I trial of recombinant vaccinia virus that expresses DF3/MUC1 in patients with metastatic adenocarcinoma of the breast	*In vivo*	Autologous fibroblasts	MUC-1	Vaccinia virus
CEA-positive malignancies							
CEA-expressing malignancies	9703-179, open	Lyerly, H.K. Duke Univ. Tel. 919-681-8350 FAX 919-681-7970	A phase I study of active immunotherapy with carcinoembryonic antigen RNA-pulsed autologous human cultured dendritic cells in patients with metastatic malignancies expressing carcinoembryonic antigen	*In vitro*	Autologous dendritic cells	mRNA for carcinoembryonic antigen	Uptake by dendritic micropinocytosis
CEA-expressing malignancies	9706-195, open	Conry, R.M. Univ. of Alabama, Birmingham Tel. 205-934-7167 FAX 205-934-1608	A phase I trial of a recombinant vaccinia-CEA (180 kDa) vaccine delivered by intradermal needle injection versus subcutaneous jet injection in patients with metastatic CEA-expressing adenocarcinoma	*In vivo*	Skin of upper arm	CEA	Vaccinia virus
CEA-expressing malignancies	9508-122, open	Hawkins, M.J. Georgetown Univ. Tel. 202-687-2198 FAX 202-687-2249	A study of recombinant ALVAC virus that expresses carcinoembryonic antigen in patients with advanced cancers	*In vivo*	Autologous muscle cells	CEA	Canarypox virus
CEA-expressing malignancies	9706-193, open	Marshall, J.L. Vincent T. Lombardi Cancer Research Center, Washington, D.C. Tel. 202-687-2198 FAX 202-687-4429	A pilot study of sequential vaccinations with ALVAC-CEA and vaccinia-CEA with the addition of IL-2 and GM-CSF in patients with CEA-expressing tumors	*In vivo*	Autologous muscle cells	IL-2, GM-CSF	Canarypox virus, vaccinia virus
CEA-expressing malignancies	9709-215, open	VonMehren, M. Fox Chase Cancer Center, Philadelphia Tel. 215-728-3545 FAX 215-728-3639	Phase I/pilot study of ALVAC-CEA-B7.1 immunization in patients with advanced adenocarcinoma expressing CEA	*In vivo*	Autologous cancer cells	B7.1(CD80)	Canarypox virus

continues

Table II *continued*

Cancer	RAC protocol approval number[a]	Principal investigator, institution, contact numbers	Protocol title	Gene transduction	Target cell	Therapeutic gene	Delivery vehicle
CEA-expressing malignancies	9804-249, open	Junghans, R.P. Beth Israel Deaconness Medical Center, Boston Tel. 617-632-0943 FAX 617-632-0998	Phase I study of T cells modified with chimeric anti-CEA immunoglobulin-T cell receptors (IgTCR) in adenocarcinoma	*In vitro*	Autologous T lymphcytes	Anti-CEA SFV-Zeta T cell receptor	Retrovirus
Hematologic							
CML	9705-188, open	Verfaillie, C. Univ. of Minnesota Tel. 612-624-3921 FAX 612-626-4074	Autologous transplantation for chronic myelogenous leukemia with stem cells transduced with a methotrexate-resistant DHFR and anti-BCR/ABL-containing vector and posttransplant methotrexate administration	*In vitro*	Autologous peripheral blood	Anti-b3a2BCR/ABL gene	Retrovirus
Hematologic malignancies	9602-146, open	Link, C.J. Human Gene Therapy Research Institute, Des Moines Tel. 515-241-8787 FAX 515-241-8788	Adoptive immunotherapy for leukemia: donor lymphocytes transduced with the herpes simplex thymidine kinase gene for remission induction	*In vitro*	Allogeneic peripheral blood lymphocytes	HSV-TK	Retrovirus
Gastrointestinal							
Colon	9312-060, open	Sobol, R.E. San Diego Regional Cancer Center Tel. 619-450-5990 FAX 619-450-3251	Injection of colon carcinoma patients with autologous irradiated tumor cells and fibroblasts genetically modified to secrete interleukin-2	*In vitro*	Autologous fibroblasts/ in combination with untransduced autologous tumor cells	IL-2	Retrovirus
Colon, hepatic metastasis	9312-064, closed	Rubin, J. Mayo Clinic Tel. 507-284-3902 FAX 507-284-1803	Phase I study of immunotherapy of advanced colorectal carcinoma by direct gene transfer into hepatic metastases	*In vivo*	Autologous tumor sites in liver	HLA-B7/β_2-microglobulin	Liposome
Colon	9406-073, open	Curiel, D. Univ. of Alabama Tel. 205-934-8627 FAX 205-975-7476	Phase I trial of a polynucleotide augmented anti-tumor immunization to human carcinoembryonic antigen in patients with metastatic colorectal cancer	*In vivo*	Autologous tumor cells	CEA plasmid expression vector	Plasmid
Colon	9509-125, open	Crystal, R.G. NY Hospital—Cornell, Medical Center Tel. 212-746-2258 FAX 212-746-8383	A phase I study of direct administration of replication-deficient adenovirus vector containing the *E. coli* cytosine deaminase gene to metastatic colon carcinoma of the liver in association with the oral administration of the pro-drug 5-fluorocytosine	*In vivo*	Autologous tumor cells	*Escherichia coli* cytosine deaminase	Adenovirus

Colorectal	9707-198, open	Venook, A.P. Univ. of California, San Francisco Tel. 415-476-3745 FAX 415-476-0467	A phase I/II study of autologous CC49-Zeta gene-modified T cells and a-interferon in patients with advanced colorectal carcinomas expressing the tumor-associated antigen, TAG-72	*In vitro*	Autologous $CD8^+$ and $CD4^+$ T lymphocytes	CC49-Zeta T cell receptor	Retrovirus
Colorectal	9708-207, open	Kaufman, H.L. Albert Einstein Cancer Center, Bronx, NY Tel. 718-430-3517 FAX 718-430-3099	Phase I clinical trial of a recombinant ALVAC-CEA-B7 vaccine in the treatment of advanced colorectal carcinoma	*In vivo*	Autologous tumor cells	B7.1(CD80)	Canarypox virus
GI breast, lung	9510-128, open	Cole, D.J. Medical Univ. of South Carolina Tel. 803-792-3276 FAX 803-792-2048	Phase I study of recombinant CEA vaccinia virus vaccine with postvaccination CEA peptide challenge	*In vivo*	Antigen presenting cells	CEA	Vaccinia virus
Liver metastases	9610-164, open	Sung, M.W. Mt. Sinai Medical Center, New York Tel. 212-241-6368 FAX 212-423-0522	Phase I trial of adenoviral vector delivery of the herpes simplex thymidine kinase gene by intratumoral injection followed by intravenous ganciclovir in patients with hepatic metastases	*In vivo*	Autologous tumor cells	HSV-TK	Adenovirus
Primary and metastatic liver tumors	9412-097, open	Venook, A.P. Univ. of California, San Francisco Tel. 415-476-3745 FAX 415-476-0467	Gene therapy of primary and metastatic malignant tumors of the liver using ACN53 via hepatic artery infusion; a phase I study	*In vivo*	Autologous tumor cells	p53	Adenovirus
Bladder	9710-219, open	Pagliaro, L.C. University of Texas MD Anderson Cancer Center Tel. 713-792-2830 FAX 713-745-1625	A phase I trial of intravesical Ad-p53 treatment in locally advanced and metastatic bladder cancer	*In vivo*	Autologous tumor cells	p53	Adenovirus
Hepatic metastasis/ colorectal	9802-239, open	Bergsland, E.K. Univ. of California, San Francisco Tel. 415-476-8277 FAX 415-731-3612	A phase I/II study of hepatic infusion of autologous CC49-Zeta-gene-modified T cells in patients with hepatic metastasis from colorectal cancer	*In vitro*	Autologous $CD4^+$ and $CD8^+$ lymphocytes	CC49-zeta T cell receptor	Retrovirus
Colorectal	9805-252, open	Sobol, R.E. San Diego Regional Cancer Center Tel. 619-450-5990 FAX 619-450-3251	A phase I study of allogeneic tumor cells genetically modified to express B7.1 (CD80) mixed with allogeneic fibroblasts genetically modified to secrete IL-2 in patents with colorectal carcinoma	*In vitro*	Allogeneic tumor cells and fibroblasts	IL-2, B7.1(CD80)	Plasmid

continues

Table II *continued*

Cancer	RAC protocol approval number[a]	Principal investigator, institution, contact numbers	Protocol title	Gene transduction	Target cell	Therapeutic gene	Delivery vehicle
Head and neck							
Head and neck SCC	9412-096, open	Clayman, G.J. M.D. Anderson Cancer Center Tel. 713-792-8837 FAX 713-794-4662	Clinical protocol for modification of tumor suppressor gene expression in head and neck squamous cell carcinoma with an adenovirus vector expressing wild-type p53	*In vivo*	Autologous tumor cells	p53	Adenovirus
Head and neck SCC	9512-142, open	Gluckman, J.L. Univ. of Cincinnati Medical Center Tel. 513-558-3272 FAX 513 558-5203	Allovectin-7 in the treatment of squamous cell carcinoma of the head and neck	*In vivo*	Autologous tumor cells	HLA-B7/β_2	Liposome
Head and neck SCC	9602-148, open	O'Malley, B.W. Johns Hopkins Tel. 410-955-8409 FAX 410-955-0035	Phase I study of adenoviral vector delivery of the HSV-TK gene and the intravenous administration of ganciclovir in adults with recurrent or persistent head and neck cancer	*In vivo*	Autologous tumor cells	HSV-TK	Adenovirus
Head and neck SCC	9705-190, open	O'Malley, B.W. Johns Hopkins Tel. 410-955-8409 FAX 410-955-0035	A double-blind, placebo-controlled, single rising dose study of the safety and tolerability of formulated hIL-2 plasmid in patients with squamous cell carcinoma of the head and neck (SCCHN)	*In vivo*	Autologous tumor cells	IL-2	Liposome
Head and neck SCC	9706-191, open	Gluckman, J.L. Univ. of Cincinnati Medical Center Tel. 513-558-3272 FAX 513 558-5203	Phase II study of immunotherapy by direct gene transfer of allovectin-7 for the treatment of recurrent or metastatic squamous cell carcinoma of the head and neck	*In vivo*	Autologous tumor cells	HLA-B7/β_2	Liposome
Head and neck SCC	9709-214, open	Breau, R.L. University of Arkansas for Medical Sciences, Little Rock Tel. 501-686-5017 FAX 501-686-8029	A phase II, multicenter, open-label, randomized study to evaluate effectiveness and safety of two treatment regimens of Ad5CVM-p53 administered by intratumoral injections in 78 patients with recurrent squamous cell carcinoma of the head and neck (SCCHN)	*In vivo*	Autologous tumor cells	p53	Adenovirus
Head and neck SCC	9712-226, open	Dreicer, R. University of Iowa College of Medicine, Iowa City Tel. 319-356-8722	A phase II, multicenter, open-label study to evaluate effectiveness and safety of Ad5CMV-p53 administered by intratumoral injections in 39 patients with recurrent squamous cell carcinoma of the head and neck	*In vivo*	Autologous tumor cells	p53	Adenovirus

Head and neck	9801-227, open	Lotze, M.T. University of Pittsburgh Cancer Institute Tel. 412-692-2852 FAX 412-648-6761	IL-12 gene therapy using direct injection of tumors with genetically engineered autologous fibroblasts (a phase II study)	*In vitro*	Autologous fibroblasts	IL-12	Retrovirus
Head and neck SCC	9804-246, open	Yoo, G.H. Wayne State University School of Medicine Tel. 313-577-0804 FAX 313-577-8555	A multicenter phase II study of E1A lipid complex for the intratumoral treatment of patients with recurrent head and neck squamous cell carcinoma	*In vivo*	Autologous tumor cells	DC-chol-DOPE E1A	Liposome
Head and neck SCC	9811-270, open	Hanna, E. University of Arkansas for Medical Sciences Tel. 501-686-514 FAX 501-686-8029	Phase II study of the safety, efficacy, and effect on quality of life of allovectin-7 immunotherapy for the treatment of recurrent or persistent squamous cell carcinoma of the head and neck	*In vivo*	Autologous tumor cells	HLA-B7/β_2-microglobulin	Liposome
Lung							
Lung NSCLC	9309-053, open	Cassileth, P. Univ. of Miami Tel. 305-243-4929 FAX: 305-243-9161	Phase I study of transfected cancer cells expressing the interleukin-2 gene product in limited stage small cell lung cancer	*In vitro*	Autologous tumor cells	IL-2	Liposome
Lung NSCLC	9403-031, open	Roth, J.A. M.D. Anderson Cancer Center Tel. 713-792-6932 FAX 713-794-4901	Clinical protocol for modification of oncogene and tumor suppressor gene expression in non-small-cell lung cancer	*In vivo*	Autologous tumor cells	p53/antisense K-ras	Retrovirus
Lung NSCLC	9406-079, closed	Roth, J.A. M.D. Anderson Cancer Center Tel. 713-792-6932 FAX 713-794-4901	Clinical protocol for modification of tumor suppressor gene expression and induction of apoptosis in non-small-cell lung cancer with an adenovirus vector expressing wild-type p53 and cisplatin	*In vivo*	Autologous tumor cells	p53	Adenovirus
Lung small cell	9609-161, closed	Antonia, S.J. H. Lee Moffitt Cancer Center, Tampa, FL Tel. 813-979-3883 FAX 813-979-3893	Treatment of small cell lung cancer patients in partial remission or at relapse with B7-1 gene-modified autologous tumor cells as a vaccine with systemic interferon-γ	*In vitro*	Autologous tumor cells	B7-1(CD80)	Liposome
Lung NSCLC	9707-203, open	Dranoff, G. Dana-Farber Cancer Institute, Boston Tel. 617-632-5051 FAX 617-632-5167	A phase I study of vaccination with autologous, lethally irradiated non-small-cell lung carcinoma cells engineered by adenoviral-mediated gene transfer to secrete human granulocyte–macrophage colony-stimulating factor	*In vitro*	Autologous tumor cells	GM-CSF	Adenovirus

continues

Table II *continued*

Cancer	RAC protocol approval number[a]	Principal investigator, institution, contact numbers	Protocol title	Gene transduction	Target cell	Therapeutic gene	Delivery vehicle
Lung NSCLC	9808-264, open	Gitlitz, B.I. University of California at Los Angeles Tel. 310-206-5713 FAX 310-267-1491	Phase I/II trial of antigen-specific immunotherapy in MUC-1 positive patients with advanced non-small-cell lung cancer using vaccinia virus-MUC1-IL2 (TG1031)	*In vivo*	Autologous fibroblasts	MUC-1 IL-2	Vaccinia virus
Lung	8708-209, open	Harvey, B.G. New York Hospital/Cornell Medical Center Tel. 212-746-5353 FAX 212-746-8824	Systemic and respiratory immune response to administration of an adenovirus type 5 gene transfer vector (AdGVCD10)	*In vivo*	Bronchial epithelial cells	*Escherichia coli* cytosine deaminase	Adenovirus
Mesothelioma	9409-090, open	Albelda, S.M. Univ. of Pennsylvania Tel. 215-662-3307 FAX 215-349-5172	Treatment of advanced mesothelioma with the recombinant adenovirus H5.010RSVTK; a phase I trial	*In vivo*	Autologous tumor cells	Serotype 5/HSV-TK	Adenovirus
Mesothelioma	9708-208, open	Schwarzenberger, P. Louisiana State Univ. Tel. 504-568-5843 FAX 504-568-3694	The treatment of malignant pleural mesothelioma with a gene-modified cancer vaccine; a phase I study	*In vivo*	Allogeneic tumor cells	HSV-TK	Retrovirus
Lung NSCLC	9710-220, open	Dobbs, T.W. Tennessee Oncology/ Hematology, P.C., Knoxville Tel. 423-632-5122 FAX 423-632-5116	A phase II gene therapy study in patients with non-small-cell lung cancer using SCH 58500 (rAd/p53) in combination with chemotherapy for multiple cycles	*In vivo*	Autologous tumor cells	p53	Adenovirus
Lung NSCLC	9803-240, open	Rom, W.N. New York University School of Medicine Tel. 212-263-6479 FAX 212-263-8442	Phase I trial of adenoviral vector delivery of the herpes simplex thymidine kinase gene by intratumoral injection followed by intravenous ganciclovir in patients with advanced non-small-cell lung cancer	*In vivo*	Autologous tumor cells	HSV-TK	Adenovirus
Lung NSCLC	9804-250, open	Swisher, S. University of Texas MD Anderson Cancer Center Tel. 713-792-6932 FAX 713-794-4901	An efficacy study of adenoviral vector expressing wild-type p53 (Ad5CVM-p53) administered intralesionally as an adjunct to radiation therapy in patients with non-small-cell lung cancer	*In vivo*	Autologous tumor cells	p53	Adenovirus

Ovarian							
Ovarian	9202-016, open	Freeman, S.M. Tulane Univ. Tel. 504-588-5224 FAX 504-587-7389	Gene transfer for the treatment of cancer	*In vitro*	Allogeneic tumor cells	HSV-TK	Retrovirus
Ovarian	9506-110, open	Berchuck, A. Duke Univ. Tel. 919-684-3618 FAX 919-684-8719	A phase I study of autologous human interleukin-2 gene modified tumor cells in patients with refractory metastatic ovarian cancer	*In vitro*	Autologous tumor cells	IL-2	Liposome
Ovarian	9306-044, open	Deisseroth, A.B. Yale Univ. Tel. 203-737-5608 FAX 203-737-5698	Use of safety-modified retroviruses to introduce chemotherapy-resistance sequences into normal hematopoietic cells for chemoprotection during the therapy of ovarian cancer; a pilot trial	*In vivo*	$CD34^+$ hematopoietic cells	MDR-1	Retrovirus
Ovarian, breast, brain	9306-051, open	Hesdorffer, C.S. Columbia Univ. Tel. 212-305-4907 FAX 212-305-6798	Human MDR gene transfer in patients with advanced cancer	*In vitro*	Autologous bone marrow cells	MDR-1	Retrovirus
Ovarian	9503-100, open	Link, C.J. Human Gene Therapy Research Institute, Des Moines, Iowa Tel. 515-241-8787 FAX 515-241-8788	A phase I trial of *in vivo* gene therapy with herpes simplex thymidine kinase/ganciclovir system for the treatment of refractory or recurrent ovarian cancer	*In vivo*	Autologous tumor cells	HSV-TK	Retrovirus
Ovarian	9506-109, open	Hwu, P. NIH Tel. 301-402-1156 FAX 301-435-5167	Treatment of patients with advanced epithelial ovarian cancer using anti-CD3 stimulated peripheral blood lymphocytes transduced with a gene encoding a chimeric T cell receptor reactive with folate-binding protein	*In vitro*	Autologous peripheral blood lymphocytes	Mov-γ T cell receptor	Retrovirus
Ovarian	9506-110, open	Berchuck, A. Duke Univ. Tel. 919-684-3618 FAX 919-684-8719	A phase I study of autologous human interleukin-2 gene modified tumor cells in patients with refractory metastatic ovarian cancer	*In vitro*	Autologous tumor cells	IL-2	Liposome
Ovarian	9509-124, open	Curiel, D.T. Univ. of Alabama Tel. 205-934-8627 FAX 205-975-7476	A phase I study of recombinant adenovirus vector-mediated delivery of an anti-erbB-2 single chain (sFv) antibody gene for previously treated ovarian and extraovarian cancer patients	*In vivo*	Autologous tumor cells	Anti-erbB-2 single-chain antibody	Adenovirus
Ovarian	9511-135, open	Alvarez, R.D. Univ. of Alabama Tel. 205-934-4986 FAX 205-934-4986	A phase I study of recombinant adenovirus vector-mediated intraperitoneal delivery of herpes simplex thymidine kinase-TK gene and intravenous ganciclovir for previously treated ovarian and extraovarian cancer patients	*In vivo*	Autologous tumor cells	HSV-TK gene	Adenovirus

continues

Table II *continued*

Cancer	RAC protocol approval number[a]	Principal investigator, institution, contact numbers	Protocol title	Gene transduction	Target cell	Therapeutic gene	Delivery vehicle
Ovarian	9603-149, open	Holt, J.T. Vanderbilt Univ. Tel. 615-343-4730 FAX 615-343-4539	Ovarian cancer gene therapy with BRCA-1	*In vivo*	Autologous tumor cells	BRCA-1 gene	Retrovirus
Ovarian	9605-155, open	Freeman, S.M. Tulane Univ. Tel. 504-588-5224 FAX 504-587-7389	Tumor vaccination with HER-2/Neu using a B7-expressing tumor cell line prior to treatment with HSV-TK gene-modified cells	*In vitro*	Allogeneic tumor cells	B7 (CD80), HSV-TK	Liposome/ retrovirus
Ovarian	9707-201, open	Freedman, R. M.D. Anderson Cancer Center Tel. 713-792-2764 FAX 713-792-7586	Intraperitoneal autologous therapeutic tumor vaccine (AUT-OV-ALVAC-hB7.1) plus IP r1FN-γ for patients with ovarian cancer; a pilot study	*In vitro*	Autologous tumor cells	B7.1	Canarypox virus
Ovarian	9801-228, open	Kieback, K.G. Baylor College of Medicine, Houston Tel. 713-798-7675 FAX 713-798-5333	Phase I study of concomitant adenovirus-mediated transduction of ovarian cancer with HSV-TK gene followed by intravenous administration of acyclovir and chemotherapy with topotecan in patients after optimal debulking surgery for recurrent ovarian cancer	*In vivo*	Autologous tumor cells	HSV-TK	Adenovirus
Ovarian	9806-255, open	Muller, C.Y. University of Texas Southwestern Medical School Tel. 214-648-3026 FAX 214-648-8404	Phase I trial of intraperitoneal adenoviral p53 gene therapy in patients with advanced recurrent or persistent ovarian cancer	*In vivo*	Autologous tumor cells	P53	Adenovirus
Ovarian	9807-262, open	Wolf, J.K. University of Texas MD Anderson Cancer Center Tel. 713-792-7310 FAX 713-792-7586	A phase I study of Ad-p53 (NCS#683550) for patients with platinum and paclitaxel-resistant epithelial ovarian cancer	*In vivo*	Autologous tumor cells	p53	Adenovirus
Prostate							
Prostate	9408-082, open	Simons, J. Johns Hopkins Tel. 410-614-1662 FAX 410-614-3695	Phase I/II study of autologous human GM-CSF gene-transduced prostate cancer vaccines in patients with metastatic prostate carcinoma	*In vitro*	Autologous tumor cells	GM-CSF	Retrovirus
Prostate	9509-123, open	Steiner, M.S. Vanderbilt Univ. Tel. 901-448-5868 FAX 901-448-8758	Gene therapy for the treatment of advanced prostate cancer by in vivo transduction with prostate-targeted retroviral vectors expressing antisense c-myc RNA	*In vivo*	Autologous tumor cells	Antisense c-myc	Retrovirus

Prostate	9509-126, open	Chen, A.P. National Naval Medical Center Tel. 301-496-0901 FAX 301-496-0047	A phase I study of recombinant vaccinia that expresses prostate-specific antigen in adult patients with adenocarcinoma of the prostate	*In vivo*	Antigen-presenting cells	PSA	Vaccinia virus
Prostate	9510-132, open	Paulson, D. Duke Univ. Tel. 919-684-5057 FAX 919-684-4611	A phase I study of autologous human interleukin-2 gene modified tumor cells in patients with locally advanced or metastatic prostate cancer	*In vitro*	Autologous tumor cells	IL-2	Liposome
Prostate	9601-144, open	Scardino, P.T. Baylor College of Medicine, Houston Tel. 713-798-4287 FAX 713-798-8185	Phase I study of adenoviral vector delivery of the HSV-TK gene and the intravenous administration of ganciclovir in men with local recurrence of prostate cancer after radiation therapy	*In vivo*	Autologous tumor cells	HSV-TK	Adenovirus
Prostate	9609-160, open	Kufe, D.W. Dana Farber Cancer Institute, Boston Tel. 617-632-3141 FAX 617-632-2934	A phase I trial of recombinant vaccine virus that expresses PSA in patients with adenocarcinoma of the prostate	*In vivo*	Antigen-presenting cells	PSA	Vaccinia virus
Prostate	9702-176, open	Sanda, M.G. Univ. of Michigan Tel. 313-647-5644 FAX 313-647-9271	A phase I/II clinical trial evaluating the safety and biologic activity of recombinant vaccinia-PSA vaccine in patients with serological recurrence of prostate cancer following radical prostatectomy	*In vivo*	Antigen-presenting cells	PSA	Vaccinia virus
Prostate	9703-184, open	Belldegrun, A. UCLA Tel. 310-206-1434 FAX 310-206-5343	A phase I study evaluating the safety and efficacy of interleukin-2 gene therapy delivered by lipid mediated gene transfer (leuvectin) in prostate cancer patients	*In vivo*	Autologous tumor cells	IL-2	Liposome
Prostate	9705-187, open	Hall, S.J. Mt. Sinai School of Medicine, New York Tel. 212-824-7751 FAX 212-803-6740	Phase I trial of adenoviral-mediated herpes simplex thymidine kinase gene transduction in conjunction with ganciclovir therapy as neoadjuvant treatment for patients with clinically localized (stage T1c and T2b and c) prostate cancer prior to radical prostatectomy	*In vivo*	Autologous tumor cells	HSV-TK	Adenovirus
Prostate	9706-192, open	Belldegrun, A. UCLA School of Medicine Tel. 310-206-1434 FAX 310-206-5343	A phase I study in patients with locally advanced or recurrent adenocarcinoma of the prostate using SCH58500 (rAd/p53) administered by intratumoral injection	*In vivo*	Autologous tumor cells	p53	Adenovirus
Prostate	9708-205, open	Simons, J.W. Johns Hopkins Tel. 410-614-1662 FAX 410-614-3695	Phase I/II study of allogeneic human GM-CSF gene-transduced irradiated prostate cancer cell vaccines in patients with prostate cancer	*In vitro*	Allogeneic tumor cells	GM-CSF	Retrovirus

continues

Table II *continued*

Cancer	RAC protocol approval number[a]	Principal investigator, institution, contact numbers	Protocol title	Gene transduction	Target cell	Therapeutic gene	Delivery vehicle
Prostate	9710-217, open	Logothetis, C.J. University of Texas MD Anderson Cancer Center Tel. 713-792-2830 FAX 713-745-1625	A tolerance and efficacy study of intraprostatic INGN 201 followed by pathologic staging and possible radical prostatectomy in patients with locally advanced prostate cancer	*In vivo*	Autologous cancer cells	p53	Adenovirus
Prostate	9801-229, open	Kadmon, D. Baylor College of Medicine, Houston Tel. 713-798-4842	Neoadjuvant preradical prostatectomy gene therapy (HSV-TK gene transduction followed by ganciclovir) in patients with poor prognostic indicators	*In vivo*	Autologous tumor cells	HSV-TK	Adenovirus
Prostate	9802-236, open	Simons, J.W. Johns Hopkins University School of Medicine, Baltimore Tel. 410-614-1662 FAX 410-614-3695	A phase I study of the introprostatic injections of CN706, a prostate-specific antigen gene-regulated cytologic adenovirus, in patients with locally recurrent cancer following definitive radiotherapy	*In vivo*	Autologous tumor cells	CN706	Adenovirus
Prostate	9805-251, open	Figlin, R. UCLA Tel. 310-825-5788 FAX 310-267-1491	Phase I/II trial of antigen-specific immunotherapy in MUC-1 positive patients with adenocarcinoma of the prostate using vaccinia virus-MUC1-IL-2 (TG 1031)	*In vitro*	Autologous fibroblasts	MUC-1, IL-2	Vaccinia virus
Prostate	9812-276, open	Gardner, T.A. University of Virginia Tel. 804-243-6787 FAX 804-243-6648	Phase I study of Ad-OC-TK plus valacyclovir for the treatment of metastatic or recurrent prostate cancer	*In vivo*	Autologous tumor cells	HSV-TK	Adenovirus
Renal							
Renal	9206-022, open	Gansbacher, B. Memorial Sloan Kettering Cancer Centre Tel. 212-639-6667 FAX 212-794-5813	Immunization with interleukin-2-secreting allogeneic HLA-A2-matched renal cell carcinoma cells in patients with advanced renal cell carcinoma	*In vitro*	Allogeneic tumor	IL-2	Retrovirus
Renal	9209-033, open	Lotze, M.T. Univ. of Pittsburgh Tel. 412-692-2852 FAX 412-648-6761	Gene therapy of cancer; a pilot study of IL-4 gene-modified antitumor vaccines	*In vitro*	Autologous fibroblasts in combination with untransduced autologous tumor cells	IL-4	Retrovirus

Renal	9303-040, open	Simons, J. Johns Hopkins Tel.410-614-1662 FAX 410-614-3695	Phase I study of nonreplicating autologous tumor cell injections using cells prepared with or without granulocyte–macrophage colony-stimulating factor gene transduction in patients with metastatic renal cell carcinoma	*In vitro*	Autologous tumor cells	GM-CSF	Retrovirus
Renal	9508-121, open	Figlin, R.A. UCLA Tel. 310-825-5788 FAX 310-267-1491	Phase I study of HLA-B7 plasmid DNA/DMRIE/DOPE lipid complex as an immunotherapeutic agent in renal cell carcinoma by direct gene transfer with concurrent low-dose bolus IL-2 protein therapy	*In vivo*	Autologous tumor cells	HLA-B7	Liposome
Renal	9705-189, open	Belani, C.H. University of Pittsburgh Medical Center Tel. 412-648-6619 FAX 412-648-6579	Phase I study of percutaneous injections of adenovirus p53 construct (adeno-p53) for hepatocellular carcinoma	*In vivo*	Autologous tumor cells	p53	Adenovirus
Renal cell	9806-259, open	Figlin, R. UCLA Tel. 310-825-5788 FAX 310-267-1491	Phase II study of direct gene transfer of IL-2 plasmid DNA/DMRIE/DOPE lipid complex (leuvectin) as an immunotherapeutic regimen in patients with metastatic renal cell carcinoma	*In vivo*	Autologous tumor cells	IL-2	Liposome
Renal cell	9810-268, open	Antonia, S.J. H. Lee Moffitt Cancer Center, Tampa, FL Tel. 813-979-3883 FAX 813-979-3893	Treatment of patients with stage IV renal cell carcinoma with B7-1 gene-modified autologous tumor cells and systemic IL-2	*In vitro*	Autologous tumor cells	B7.1(CD80)	Adenovirus
Solid tumors							
Solid tumors	9306-045, open	Nabel, G.J. Univ. of Michigan Tel. 313-647-4798 FAX 313-647-4730	Immunotherapy for cancer by direct gene transfer into tumors	*In vivo*	Autologous tumor cells	HLA-B7 and β_2-microglobulin	Liposome
Solid tumors	9412-095, open	Hersh, E. Arizona Cancer Center, Tucson Tel. 520-626-2250 FAX 520-626-2225	Phase I trial of interleukin-2 plasmid DNA/DMRIE/DOPE lipid complex as an immunotherapeutic agent in solid malignant tumors or lymphomas by direct gene transfer	*In vivo*	Autologous tumor cells	IL-2	Liposome
Solid tumors	9610-162, open	LaFollette, S. Presbyterian/ St.Luke's Medical Center, Chicago Tel. 312-942-5904 FAX 312-942-3192	A phase I multicenter study of intratumoral E1A gene therapy for patients with unresectable or metastatic solid tumors that overexpress HER-2/neu	*In vivo*	Autologous tumor cells	E1A	Liposome

continues

Table II *continued*

Cancer	RAC protocol approval number[a]	Principal investigator, institution, contact numbers	Protocol title	Gene transduction	Target cell	Therapeutic gene	Delivery vehicle
Solid tumors	9611-169, open	Hersh, E. Arizona Cancer Center, Tucson Tel. 520-626-2250 FAX 520-626-2225	Phase I/II trial of interleukin-2 DNA/DMRIE/DOPE lipid complex as an immunotherapeutic agent in cancer by direct gene transfer	*In vivo*	Autologous tumor cells	IL-2	Liposome
Solid tumors	9709-199, open	Park, C.H. Samsung Medical Center, Korea Tel. 2-3410-3450 FAX 2-3410-2860	IL-12 gene therapy using direct injection of tumors with genetically engineered autologous fibroblasts	*In vitro*	Autologous fibroblasts	IL-12	Retrovirus
Solid tumors	9806-257, open	Suzuki, T. University of Kansas Medical Center Tel. 913-588-6724 FAX 913-588-7295	Autologous, irradiated, cancer cells (breast cancer, colon cancer, head and neck cancer, and soft tissue sarcoma) transduced *ex vivo* with an adenovirus vector (Adv/GM-CSF) expressing granulocyte–macrophage colony-stimulating factor gene	*In vitro*	Autologous tumor cells	GM-CSF	Adenovirus
Solid tumors	9809-265, open	Gerson, S.L. Case Western Reserve University Tel. 216-368-1176 FAX 216-368-1166	Mutant MGMT gene transfer into human hematopoietic progenitors to protect hematopoiesis during O^6-benzylguanine (BG, NSC 637037) and BCNU therapy of advanced solid tumors	*In vitro*	Peripheral blood $CD34^+$ cells	O^6-Methylguanine DNA methlytransferase	Retrovirus
Testicular							
Testicular germ cell	9701-172, open	Cornetta, K. Indiana Univ. Tel. 317-274-0843 FAX 317-278-2262	High-dose carboplatin and etoposide followed by transplantation with peripheral blood stem cells transduced with the MDR gene in the treatment of germ cell tumors; a pilot study	*In vitro*	G-CSF-mobilized autologous $CD34^+$	MDR-1	Retrovirus
Lymphoma							
Lymphoma non-Hodgkin B cell/mantle cell lymphoma	9707-200, open	Levy, R. Stanford Univ. School of Medicine Tel. 650-725-6452 FAX 650-725-1420	Phase I/II study of vaccine therapy for B cell lymphoma utilizing plasmid DNA coding for tumor idiotype	*In vivo*	Muscle tissue	Tumor idiotype	Plasmid

[a]Recombinant DNA advisory committe (RAC) protocol approval numbers are the year and month approved (first 4 digits) followed by the number in consecutive order approved by the RAC.

mammary cancer, avian sarcoma, and AIDS (9). Recombinant retroviral vectors used in gene therapy applications are commonly engineered to remove viral structural genes (*gag, pol, env*) that are required for the production of replication-competent viruses. These genes are replaced with therapeutic genes (transgenes), which are transferred by the virus to the target cells (10). The genetically engineered virus can deliver transgenes to target cells but cannot produce progeny virions in these cells because they lack the genes that encode critical viral structural proteins. Retrovirus vectors are produced for experimental and human applications in a packaging cell line that has been engineered to produce the necessary viral structural proteins. The resulting packaging cell line produces replication-defective retroviral particles that can transfer therapeutic genes but cannot replicate in infected target cells (Fig. 1).

Since the report of the first retroviral vector in 1981 (11), this vector has become the most widely used gene delivery system in clinical gene transfer protocols. The popularity of this vector in early clinical trials was based primarily on the propensity of these viruses to infect dividing cells, stably integrate into a wide variety of host cell types, and produce moderate levels of transgene expression for sustained periods (12–14). The selectivity of retroviral vectors for target cells that are actively dividing suggests that these vectors are well suited to cancer gene therapy applications, because cancer cells are generally rapidly dividing cells. However, the development of improved vectors based on other viruses, the relatively low *in vivo* transduction efficiency of retroviral vectors, and safety concerns arising from their chromosomal integration have limited their use (15, 16). Gene therapy strategies that rely on *in vivo* retroviral gene transfer have been plagued by relatively low levels of gene transfer. Consequently, retroviruses are better suited to *ex vivo* gene transfer, in which transgenes are delivered to cells that have been harvested and maintained outside the body. Examples that use this approach include transfer of immunostimulatory genes into harvested tumor cells prior to administration to patients as gene-modified tumor cell vaccines (17), *ex vivo* modification of tumor-infiltrating lymphocytes (TILs) (18, 19), and transduction of bone marrow stem cells with marker genes or the multidrug resistance (MDR) gene (20).

With use of retroviral vectors, there is the possibility of unwanted insertional mutagenesis in the host cell or recombination between genetically engineered retrovirus and wild-type retrovirus to yield a replication-competent retro-

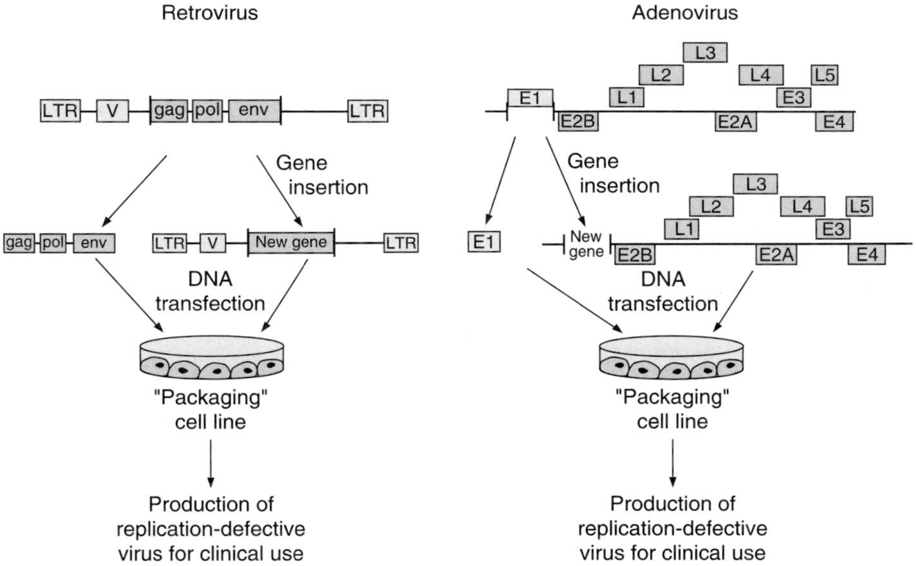

Figure 1 Replication-defective viral vector systems. (Left) Retroviral vectors are generated by replacing the essential viral genes (*gag, pol,* and *env*) with transgenes. Packaging cell lines have been engineered to express the deleted essential viral genes. Accordingly, introduction of the recombinant retrovirus vector into the packaging cell line results in production of viral particles that can deliver the transgene, but cannot replicate in target cells because they do not express the deleted essential viral genes. (Right) First-generation adenovirus vectors are constructed by replacing the essential *E1* early genes with transgenes. Packaging cell lines have been engineered to express the *E1* gene, and, accordingly, introduction of the recombinant adenovirus vector into the packaging cell line results in production of viral particles that are capable of transgene delivery but incapable of replication in infected target cells. LTR, Long terminal repeat of the retrovirus-encoding gene regulatory sequences; ψ, the packaging signal required to direct incorporation of viral RNA into the retroviral particles. From (197), G. Dranoff (1998). Cancer gene therapy: Connecting basic research with clinical inquiry. *J. Clin. Oncol.* **16**, 2548–2556. (See color plates.)

virus. Integration of the retroviral vector into the host cell genome is a random process, and could theoretically result in activation of oncogenes or inactivation of tumor suppressor genes. Despite these safety concerns, there have been no reports of malignant transformation resulting from the use of replication-incompetent retroviral vectors in humans to date, and the growing body of experience with recombinant retroviral vectors suggests that this is a highly unlikely event.

Future advances in recombinant retrovirus production technology will incorporate (1) engineering of the viral envelope to contain proteins to improve specificity of infection (21, 22), (2) incorporation of tissue-specific enhancers and promoters (23, 24), and (3) high-titer packaging cell lines. However, despite the progress in retroviral vector technology and their documented safety record, development of better gene transfer vehicles has significantly reduced the use of retroviruses in gene therapy applications.

B. Adenovirus

The adenovirus genome consists of approximately 36 kb of double-stranded DNA. Adenoviral tropism for specific epithelial tissues is based on binding of the adenovirus to specific cell surface receptors. Infection in humans is typically confined to the respiratory epithelium, cornea, and gastrointestinal tract, and typically manifests as an upper respiratory infection, hemorrhagic cystitis, or keratoconjunctivitis (8, 25). These infections are generally self-limited and have not been associated with the development of malignancy in humans (26).

Recombinant adenovirus vectors have been based most commonly on the serotype 5 (Ad-5) or serotype 2 (Ad-2) genome. In first-generation replication-defective vectors the *E1A* and *E1B* adenoviral early genes that encode essential regulatory proteins are replaced with transgene sequences (Fig. 1) (27–30). Lacking E1A and E1B proteins, these vectors are replication incompetent. Production of this type of recombinant adenovirus vector requires packaging cell lines that are transformed to express *E1* gene products (31). More extensive deletion of both the *E1* and *E3* adenoviral genes results in a recombinant vector that may accommodate up to 7.5 kb of transgene sequence.

Adenoviral vectors have rapidly become one of the most widely used gene transfer vehicles because they possess several favorable properties. These vectors possess a large transgene capacity and can achieve high levels of *in vivo* gene transfer in a variety of benign (28, 32–40) and malignant (41–51) cell types. Adenoviral vectors infect both dividing and nondividing cells (25) and can be produced in large volumes and high plague-forming unit (pfu) titers (10^{11}–10^{12} pfu/ml) with relative ease. Adenoviral genes do not integrate into the host cell genome, and, accordingly, adenoviral (and transgene) DNA is lost after a few cell divisions. Adenovirus-mediated gene transfer results in peak transgene expression within several days of infection, with a rapid decrease in expression occurring over 1–4 weeks.

Adenovirus infection elicits strong cellular and humoral immune responses that reduce the duration of transgene expression and render readministration of these vectors potentially less effective (8, 52–54). Viral gene expression following infection with recombinant adenovirus vectors leads to presentation of viral proteins by major histocompatibility (MHC) class I molecules to $CD8^+$ T cells with subsequent activation of cytotoxic T lymphocytes (CTLs) directed at the host cell (52–54). Presentation of adenoviral proteins by MHC class II molecules leads to activation of $CD4^+$ T helper cells and production of neutralizing antibodies (52–54). In an attempt to reduce these immune responses, several vector modifications have been incorporated in later generation adenoviral vectors. The *E2A* region has been deleted in second-generation vectors, which decreases antigenicity and results in longer transgene expression (55, 56). Third-generation vectors, deleted in *E1* and *E4*, express even lower levels of viral proteins and are currently under investigation in clinical trials (57). Alternative strategies such as sequential utilization of different adenovirus serotypes to circumvent sensitization-induced inflammatory toxicity and immunoreactivity have been proposed to achieve persistently high levels of transgene expression after repeat vector administration (58). In contrast to development of replication-incompetent adenoviral vectors, some researchers have examined use of replication-competent adenovirus mutants in a strategy in which cancer cell destruction is achieved specifically by adenoviral replication within the cancer cells (59). These vectors and this strategy are discussed in greater detail in Section III,D.

C. Herpes Simplex Virus Type 1

The herpes simplex virus type 1 (HSV1) genome consists of approximately 152 kb of double-stranded DNA, of which as much as 30 kb may be replaced by transgene sequences (60). Viral infection is initiated by attachment of the viral envelope to specific cell surface receptors that are present on a wide variety of cells. Clinical infection with HSV1 typically manifests as vesicular lesions of the mouth and lips, local ulcerations of the genitalia, or keratoconjunctivitis. HSV1 can remain latent in specific tissues and then resume replication after prolonged periods of latency (61). HSV1 is capable of replication in a variety of animal tumor cell lines *in vitro*; however, significantly higher multiplicities of infection (MOIs) are required to infect these cell lines compared to human tumor cell lines. Tropism for particular species and tissues has resulted in significant limitations in the ability to test HSV1 vectors in tumor-bearing rodents.

One of the most important and useful properties of HSV1 became evident in studies examining gene transfer into the CNS, in which significant cytotoxicity from cellular lysis was observed (62). These lytic properties of HSV1 vectors have been adapted for therapeutic purposes in the treatment of cancer. Entry of wild-type HSV1 into cells leads to a sequential cascade of viral gene expression that ultimately results in the production of multiple progeny virions together with cell lysis and death. Consequently, tumor cells infected with HSV1 are ultimately destroyed by HSV1 replication. Recombinant HSV1 vectors that are defective in ribonucleotide reductase expression selectively replicate in mitotically active tumor cells but not in nondividing cells such as neurons (47, 63, 64). Replication-competent, attenuated HSV1 mutants can replicate within and destroy human malignant meningioma xenografts without producing neurologic dysfunction or pathologic changes in the surrounding brain tissue (65).

Another property of HSV1 that makes it suitable for cancer gene therapy is its expression of viral thymidine kinase (HSV-TK), which initiates conversion of ganciclovir into a toxic metabolite that inhibits DNA synthesis (66, 67). Because ganciclovir is normally nontoxic to mammalian cells, only cells that have been transduced to express HSV-TK are susceptible to ganciclovir treatment. HSV-TK is normally expressed in the course of HSV1 infection, thereby rendering infected cells susceptible to ganciclovir. The HSV-TK gene has also been cloned into other vectors to render infected cells susceptible to ganciclovir. This gene therapy approach is discussed in Section III,E.

Another type of HSV1 vector, an amplicon vector, is derived from plasmids that bear an *Escherichia coli* origin of DNA replication, an antibiotic resistance gene for propagation in bacteria, an HSV1 origin of DNA replication and packaging signal, and additional desired transgenes (68). Recent advances have allowed production of HSV1 amplicons with lower levels of contamination by helper virus. HSV1 genes that are cytotoxic to normal cells have been deleted from HSV1 amplicons, thereby enhancing the safety of these vectors. Two principal advantages of amplicons are their ease of construction and the fact that promoter elements introduced into these amplicons to achieve tissue-specific gene expression retain more specificity than do similar promoters introduced into the herpes simplex virus genome (61).

In summary, several biologic properties support the use of HSV1 in cancer gene therapy. First, tumor cell destruction results from HSV1 replication and does not require transgene expression. Second, cancer cell death and tumoricidal response induced by HSV1 infection may be enhanced by the addition of the prodrug ganciclovir. Third, HSV1 vectors can carry up to 30 kb of transgene sequence. And fourth, HSV1 is a common pathogen in humans, yet very rarely causes serious medical illness. Further development of the recombinant HSV1 vectors will facilitate broader application of this gene delivery system for the purpose of transferring potentially larger genes to central nervous system malignancies as well as other malignancies.

D. Vaccinia Virus

The development of vaccinia viruses for human gene therapy applications has benefited from the vast experience with this virus for vaccination of humans against smallpox. These viruses have now been modified to function as expression vectors and vaccines against other infectious diseases and cancer (69). Similar to herpes simplex virus, vaccinia virus is a large double-strand DNA virus that contains 186 kb of DNA, and can accommodate up to 25 kb of DNA transgene sequence (70). Similar to adenovirus and herpes simplex virus, vaccinia virus is capable of infecting and replicating in both dividing and nondividing cells. Cellular infection with vaccinia virus results in virus replication within the cytoplasm until the infected cell is destroyed. Vaccinia viral infection elicits a strong cytotoxic T lymphocyte response, thereby making it an ideal vehicle for cancer vaccines (71). Other biologic properties of vaccinia virus that make it a good candidate for gene delivery in humans include (1) relative ease of vector construction (2) wide range of infectivity, (3) relatively high levels of transgene expression, and (4) ability to produce high titers of recombinant vaccinia virus. Several strains of vaccinia virus that are highly attenuated and replication deficient have been developed for clinical applications (71). Replication-competent vaccinia viral vectors have also been developed to destroy cancer cells in the course of viral replication.

Vaccinia virus has been used as an adjuvant for preparation of a melanoma oncolysate vaccine using human melanoma cell lines (72). In addition, several poxvirus-based vectors have been used to develop vaccines against tumor-associated antigens (73) and modify autologous tumor cells for subsequent vaccination (74–76). The enthusiasm for vaccinia virus for gene therapy is in large part a result of its versatility (77).

E. Adeno-Associated Virus

Adeno-associated viruses (AAVs) are small, linear, single-stranded DNA viruses that contain very few viral genes, and are therefore dependent on helper viruses (e.g., adenovirus, vaccinia, or herpes virus) to provide the proteins required for completion of its life cycle. Similar to adenovirus vectors, AAV vectors infect both dividing and nondividing cells with relatively high efficiency (78). These viruses integrate into the target cell genome in a predictable and site-specific manner and produce prolonged transgene expression without known human pathogenicity (79). Integration of AAV into the genome differs in two specific ways from that of retrovirus. First, AAV integrates in a nonrandom fashion into chromosome 19 (80), thereby reducing the risk of insertional mutagenesis compared to that associated with the random integration of the retrovirus genome. Second, recombinant AAV virus vectors lose their ability to integrate over time (81), but continue to express the transgene from a chromosomal and epichromosomal location for up to 10 months (82). In addition, the ability to engineer recombinant AAV vectors with much of the viral genome replaced by therapeutic genes has resulted in low immunogenicity and therefore decreased immunoreactivity associated with repeat vector administrations. Unfortunately, enthusiasm for this gene delivery system has been tempered by the inability to produce large volumes of high-titer vector that are needed for clinical applications. Development of packaging cell lines that can produce the high titers of virus that are required for clinical applications is a prerequisite to broader use of AAV vectors in cancer gene therapy.

F. Nonviral Gene Delivery Systems

Although viruses serve as excellent gene delivery vehicles, many methods have been developed to transfer DNA directly into host tissues without the aid of viruses. These methods include (1) gene gun injection, in which DNA is coated onto gold particles and is shot into cells (83), (2) direct injection of "naked DNA" into soft tissues, (3) injection of DNA that is contained within lipid vesicles (liposomes), and (4) injection of DNA that is conjugated to a molecule that facilitates targeted, receptor-mediated uptake of the DNA. Nonviral methods of gene transfer face several host defense mechanisms. These include a low-grade immune response, sequestration of liposomes by reticuloendothelial cells, and rapid degradation of lipid–DNA complexes by lysosomal nucleases. Because of these challenges, nonviral gene transfer techniques have been plagued by low-efficiency gene transfer and expression. Large quantities of vehicle can be used in an attempt to compensate for these limitations and can accomplish higher levels of gene expression.

Liposomes and DNA–protein conjugates represent two nonviral gene transfer vehicles that have been applied to the treatment of cancer. Plasmid DNA (pDNA) can be internalized within lipid bilayers known as liposomes, which are capable of delivering the pDNA to a variety of cell types (84). Fusion between liposomes and cytoplasmic membranes facilitates passage of the plasmid DNA into target cells. The DNA is then transported to the nucleus, where it is transiently expressed prior to degradation by host cell endonucleases. Liposomes consisting of the two most commonly used lipid molecules, *N*-[1-(2,3-dioleoyloxy)propyl]-*N,N,N*-trimethyl-ammonium methylsulfate (DOTAP) and *N*-[1-(2,3-dioleyloxy)propyl]-*N,N,N*-trimethylammonium-chloride (DOTMA), are readily generated and relatively simple to use (77). However, targeting by liposomal-mediated gene transfer is typically non-specific and relatively less efficient compared to virus-mediated gene transfer. Techniques to improve the target specificity of liposomes include development of "stealth" liposomes that utilize a coating of sialic acid residues on the liposomes to evade detection and uptake by reticuloendothelial cells (85). Other improvements include construction of the liposomal membrane with glycolipids that traffic selectively to the liver (86) and use of cationic liposomes that are complexed to site-specific monoclonal antibodies (87). One example of a clinical trial in which a liposomal vector is used involves *in vivo* gene transfer of foreign HLA antigens in an attempt to enhance systemic antitumor immune responses in the host (88).

DNA–protein conjugates represent another nonviral gene delivery vehicle that has been used to facilitate gene transfer to specific target cells. DNA–protein complexes display enhanced tissue specificity by virtue of a coupling between plasmid DNA and a tissue-specific ligand or antibody (89–91). Interaction between the complexes and a receptor on the cell membrane leads to internalization of the DNA by receptor-mediated endocytosis (90). Simultaneous administration of defective adenovirus particles stabilizes the DNA–protein complex against lysosomal degradation and improves transgene expression (92, 93). One application of this approach involves specific targeting of epidermal growth factor (EGF) receptors using EGF/DNA complexes (94).

The advantages of nonviral gene transfer are the ability to transduce quiescent cells, to deliver transgenes of unlimited size, and to readminister the complexes because of their relatively low immunogenicity. Further improvements in target specificity, gene transfer efficiency, and gene expression should result in broader inclusion of liposomal vectors in gene therapy applications.

III. Cancer Gene Therapy Techniques

Many cancer gene therapy strategies use gene transfer techniques to enhance previously existing therapies. For example, although adoptive immunotherapy strategies have been examined for decades, the more recent development of gene transfer vehicles has permitted investigators to genetically engineer the lymphocytes prior to their administration back into patients. Another strategy by which gene therapy may enhance immunotherapy involves *in vivo* transduction of tumor cells with genes to up-regulate expression of MHC molecules. Gene therapy has also been used to improve traditional chemotherapy and radiation therapy. The recent explosion of knowledge into the molecular events that lead to malignant transformation has provided investigators with a wealth of new targets for cancer therapy, many of which are prime targets for gene therapy. A better understanding of the molecular biology of cancer combined with recent developments in gene transfer technology have enabled investigators to manipulate abnormal growth regulatory mechanisms, susceptibility to chemotherapeutic agents, or host immune responses to cancer. The shear number of novel cancer gene therapy approaches described each year precludes an inclusive description of each approach. Instead, some of the most common approaches that are currently under examination in clinical trials are summarized.

A. Genetically Modified Tumor Vaccines

The ability to manipulate the host immune system to cause significant tumor regression represents a significant medical advance (95). Unfortunately, the antitumor host response fails to prevent tumor progression in most patients. Where tumor vaccines have failed, further improvements may come as a result of the ability to modulate cell function with gene transduction. Mechanisms behind the inadequate host immune response to vaccines have been studied and include improper antigen presentation, insufficient recruitment of $CD4^+$ cells, and inadequate immune costimulation. Gene therapy has been used to try to overcome each of these problems. Gene transfer to modulate cancer immunotherapy presently represents the most commonly used cancer gene therapy approach (Table III).

T cell receptor engagement of a tumor-associated peptide within an MHC complex is generally insufficient for efficient activation of T cells (Fig. 2). Costimulatory molecules such as those in the B7 family enhance this activation response by binding to CD28 and CTLA-4 and providing costimulation (96, 97). However, unlike professional antigen-presenting cells such as macrophages and dendritic cells, tumor cells generally do not express these costimulatory molecules. It has been demonstrated in animal models that gene transfer to induce tumor cell expression of costimulatory molecules such as B7 enhances the efficacy of tumor vaccines (74, 75, 98).

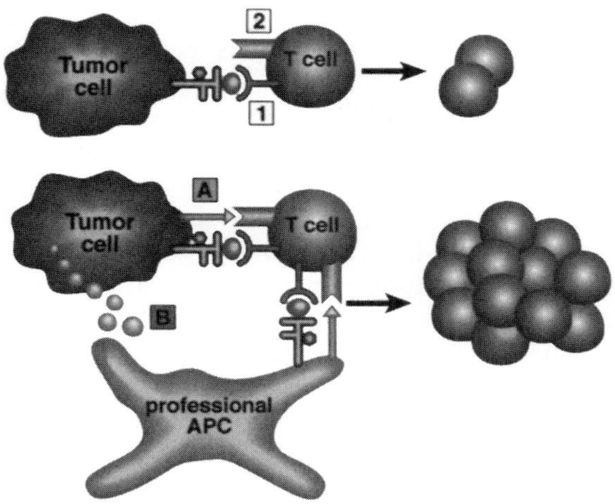

Figure 2 T cell tolerance occurs when tumor cells present tumor antigens on MHC molecules (1) to T cells without a second costimulatory signal (2). Genetically engineered tumor cells express either costimulatory molecules on their cell surface (A) to activate T cells directly or release cytokines (B) to attract professional APCs, which subsequently activate antigen-specific T cells. From (198), T. F. Greten and E.M. Jaffe (1999). Cancer vaccines. *J. Clin. Oncol.* **17**, 1047–1060. (See color plates.)

Table III Human Gene Transfer Protocols for Cancer[a]

Therapeutic approach	Number of approved protocols
Antisense	4
Chemoprotection	9
Immunotherapy/*in vitro* transduction	56
Immunotherapy/*in vivo* transduction	51
Prodrug/HSV-TK and ganciclovir	28
Tumor suppressor gene	18
Single-chain antibody	2
Oncogene down-regulation	3
Vector-directed cell lysis	2
Total	173

[a]Source: National Institutes of Health, Office of Recombinant DNA Activities, Bethesda, MD; updated 2/10/99.

Another possible mechanism of immune tolerance involves the environment in which the interaction occurs. The absence of appropriate cytokines in the tumor microenvironment may reduce the immune response to tumor antigens. Granulocyte–macrophage colony-stimulating factor (GM-CSF) is a potent cytokine that can enhance the host immune response to tumor antigens. In experiments in which mice were immunized with irradiated melanoma cells that express one of a number of cytokines as a result of retrovirus-mediated cytokine gene transfer, the efficacy of vaccination was most enhanced by melanoma cell expression of GM-CSF (17). These preclinical results were used to design a phase I clinical trial in which patients with melanoma were vaccinated with irradiated autologous tumor transduced with a retrovirus to express GM-CSF (99).

IL-2 and interferon are known to stimulate the immune system effectively and, accordingly, investigators have examined therapeutic strategies to transfer the genes for these cytokines into tumor cells (100–104). Animals that are vaccinated with irradiated tumor cells that have been transduced with the interferon-γ gene or interleukin-2 (IL-2) gene are protected against subsequent tumor challenge. Several clinical trials using this approach are being conducted for a variety of tumors, including breast cancer, melanoma, renal cell carcinoma, and malignant brain tumors (Table II). Among the many cytokines identified to date, IL-2, IL-12, and GM-CSF have demonstrated the most potential (100,

105). Other cytokines that have been transduced into tumor cells for vaccination in clinical trials include IL-7, TNFα, IL-4, and TGF-β2 (77, 106).

One of the most labor-intensive and expensive components required for this type of cancer gene therapy is surgical harvesting of autologous tumor cells combined with *in vitro* propagation and gene transfer. Vaccination would be a more practical and less costly strategy if allogeneic tumor cells could be used for the immunizations. The presence of tumor antigens that are shared between different patients' tumors supports the feasibility of this approach. This strategy has been examined using adenovirus or vaccinia viruses that have been genetically engineered to express tumor-associated antigens (e.g., CEA, MART-1, gp100) for vaccination (107–109), and these vectors are currently being tested in phase I trials (77, 106). Skin fibroblasts are an alternative source of inexpensive cells for vaccine development. These cells can be obtained from a skin biopsy, transduced to express a tumor-associated antigen such as CEA, and then readministered as a vaccine. This approach has the advantage of using target cells that are much simpler and less costly to obtain than are tumor cells (105).

B. Genetically Modified Immune Effector Cells

Adoptive immunotherapy involves administration of immune effector cells into a patient to produce antitumor effects. The first effector cells that gained notoriety in adoptive immunotherapy were autologous lymphocytes activated by IL-2, i.e., lymphokine-activated killer (LAK) cells. LAK cells were generated from peripheral blood lymphocytes and cultured in the presence of IL-2 (110). Lymphocytes harvested from tumor biopsies (tumor-infiltrating lymphocytes) were subsequently demonstrated to be more effective immune effector cells than were LAK cells (111, 112). Although LAK cells and TILs have been effective in the eradication of tumors in mice, clinical trials of adoptive cellular immunotherapy have not been as successful. Moreover, this approach has been of limited value in the treatment of tumors that are less immunogenic than melanoma and renal cell carcinoma (113). Several mechanisms that lead to inadequate tumor eradication with TILs have been identified, some of which may be addressed using gene transfer techniques. For example, the microenvironment in which the adoptively transferred TILs interact with tumor cells may not be optimal to achieve tumor destruction and may be enhanced by transduction of the TILs to express specific cytokines such as IL-2. Transduction of TILs with the IL-2 gene may enhance therapeutic efficacy by two mechanisms: increased TIL propagation *in vivo* and enhanced antitumor activity (114). Transduction of TILs with other genes may also enhance their antitumor activity. TILs transduced with the TNFα gene produce impressive antitumor responses in animal models (115). In an alternative approach, transduction of TILs with genes encoding receptors for activation factors such as IL-3 or GM-CSF enhances their propagation and activation *in vivo* (116).

Analogous to the inability of tumor cells serving as a vaccine to activate T cells, tumor cells may not possess the relevant antigens and costimulatory molecules required to generate TILs optimally. Investigators have used gene transfer techniques to study this problem. Some weakly immunogenic tumors may be converted into more immunoreactive ones by up-regulation of their MHC class I molecules. *In vivo* transduction of tumors with allogeneic MHC class I genes by liposomal delivery has been demonstrated to enhance tumor reactivity of TILs and tumor regression (117). These results have stimulated a clinical trial of *in vivo* transfer of the HLA-B7 MHC class I gene for patients with metastatic melanoma. In a model of poorly immunogenic murine fibrosarcoma, TIL cells that were generated from tumor cells were more effective when the tumor cells had first been transduced to secrete interferon-γ (IFN-γ) and up-regulate MHC class I molecules (118). In yet another approach involving genetic engineering of immune effector cells, the GM-CSF gene has been transfected into tumor cells followed by inoculation of mice with the genetically altered tumor cells to elicit T cells in draining lymph nodes (119). The expression of GM-CSF resulted in effective priming of T cells in draining lymph nodes such that they are capable of eradicating tumor in adoptive transfer experiments. These results have been used to develop a clinical trial for melanoma patients (120). As a final example, gene transfer approaches have been used to mark T cells prior to adoptive transfer into patients to enable investigators to perform lymphocyte trafficking studies.

C. Targeting Tumor Suppressor Genes and Oncogenes

Cellular transformation requires an accumulation of genetic defects (2, 121). Fearon and Vogelstein first proposed the multistep genetic model to describe the transformation of benign colonic mucosa into colon carcinoma (2). These investigators proposed that malignant transformation results from an accumulation of defects leading to inactivation of tumor suppressor genes and activation of oncogenes. Similar genetic models of tumor progression have been described for other malignancies (122). Mutations in a third type of gene, known as DNA damage recognition and repair genes, can also contribute to malignant transformation by creating genetic instability and an accumulation of mutations in both tumor suppressor genes and oncogenes (123, 124). Patients with hereditary nonpolyposis colorectal cancer (HNPCC) are known to harbor germ-line defects in this class of gene. Persistent expression of telomerase also contributes to malignant transformation by maintaining chomosomal ends (121).

The multistep genetic model for malignant transformation involves a combination of oncogene activation, tumor suppressor gene inactivation, and telomerase activation (121, 124). For example, activation of the K-*ras* oncogene and loss of function of the *DCC* (deleted in colorectal cancer), *APC* (adenomatous polyposis coli), and *p53* genes contribute to transformation of normal colonic mucosa to colon carcinoma (2). It is the accumulation of mutations rather than the order with respect to one another that determines the tumor's biologic properties. Because gene delivery vehicles will probably never achieve 100% efficiency of *in vivo* transduction, it is unlikely that it will be possible to correct every genetic defect in every cancer cell to restore normal growth control. Nonetheless, correction of only one of the multiple genetic defects in a cancer cell may inhibit its tumorigenicity (125). Indeed, clinical trials of cancer gene therapies in which only a single type of genetic defect has been corrected have produced promising results (126).

The p53 gene is one of the most commonly mutated genes identified in cancers, and this gene has served as a target for gene therapy strategies. Loss or functional inactivation of p53 is a critical component of tumorigenesis (2, 124), and replacement of deleted or mutant p53 restores normal growth control mechanisms and sensitivity to chemotherapy and radiotherapy (125, 127, 128). Adenovirus-mediated transfer of the wild-type p53 gene inhibits growth *in vivo* in a wide variety of tumor models, including rat glioma (129), head and neck cancer (126, 130), and colon cancer (49). Introduction of p53 into tumor cells restores cellular mechanisms of apoptosis in response to chemotherapy or ionizing radiation. One of the most important uses of p53 gene transduction may be to restore sensitivity of cancer cells to chemotherapeutic agents (131). The success of preclinical studies has led to the clinical application of this approach to treat patients with lung cancer, head and neck cancers, and primary and metastatic liver cancers (132). Tumor growth *in vivo* may also be inhibited by transfer of other tumor suppressor genes, including p16 and a truncated retinoblastoma (Rb) gene (133–135). Tumor suppressor gene replacement alone may induce apoptosis in some cancers (131), whereas concurrent administration of chemotherapeutic agents (48) or radiotherapy may be necessary to induce apoptosis in others (77).

Cancer gene therapy strategies designed to inactivate oncogenes necessarily rely on strategies other than those designed to replace defective tumor supressor genes. Some of the gene therapy strategies that have been investigated for inactivation of oncogenes involve use of antisense DNA, ribozymes, intracellular antibodies, or dominant-negative proteins. Binding of antisense sequences to sense sequences of target oncogenes by Watson–Crick base pairing inhibits messenger RNA (mRNA) splicing, transport, and translation, and thereby blocks synthesis of the targeted protein (77, 136). For example, growth of human lung cancers can be inhibited *in vitro* and *in vivo* by selective blockage of mutant K-*ras* mRNA with an antisense K-*ras* construct (137–139). A different approach to inactivate oncogenes involves use of ribozymes, which recognize and cleave specific oncogene mRNA sequences (140–144). Another clever gene therapy strategy to target protooncogene protein products involves vectors that encode intracellular antibodies that are targeted against cytoplasmic oncoproteins (intrabodies) (145,146). The rapid advances in our understanding of oncogenes and tumor suppressor genes will undoubtedly produce additional targets for cancer gene therapy.

D. Oncolysis by Replication-Competent Viruses

Viruses used for gene delivery generally have been genetically engineered such that they are incapable of replication. To accomplish this, packaging cell lines have been developed that can produce engineered viruses, which are incapable of viral replication outside of the special packaging cell lines (Fig. 1). These packaging cell lines are created by deleting from viruses critical genes that are essential for replication, and then integrating these genes into the genome of the packaging cell line. Development of packaging cell lines has enabled investigators to produce viruses that are incapable of replication outside of the packaging cell line.

Importantly, the replication cycle of several wild-type viruses, including adenovirus, reovirus, and HSV1, is toxic to cells and leads to cell death. Accordingly, investigators have developed mutant viruses that selectively replicate in tumor cells rather than normal cells (63). Tumor cells infected by virus are destroyed in the process of viral replication, which simultaneously produces progeny virions that can infect adjacent tumor cells. The major advantage of this approach is that it relies on an extremely effective method of tumor destruction, namely, viral oncolysis. Another advantage of this strategy is that it does not require prolonged transgene expression. This strategy thereby avoids an inherent problem with most viral gene delivery vectors, which is the ability to achieve transgene expression in target cells for only a limited period of time. Nonetheless, the strategy of viral oncolysis does require viral genetic engineering to ensure that viral replication proceeds selectively in tumor cells and not elsewhere in the host.

The strategy of oncolysis by viral replication was first examined in clinical trials using an adenovirus that is defective in viral E1B expression (59). Adenovirus E1B protein aids in viral replication putatively by binding to and inactivating wild-type p53. Wild-type p53 protein has at least two important functions in the maintenance of cellular integrity and growth control. It plays a role in preventing cells from passing normally through the cell cycle when damaged or foreign DNA is present; p53 also enables cells to undergo programmed cell death (apoptosis) under specific conditions of cellular stress. Therefore, adenoviral replication may theoretically proceed more robustly following inactivation of p53 by adenoviral E1B, and an adenovirus that is defective in E1B expression should replicate poorly in cells that have wild-type p53. However, if cells are deficient in p53 function, an E1B-defective adenovirus should replicate robustly. Accordingly, an E1B-defective adenovirus should replicate selectively in tumor cells with deficient p53 but not in normal cells (59). It is estimated that approximately 50% of tumors are deficient in p53 function. Replication of one specific E1B-deleted adenovirus, Onyx-015, has been examined in normal cells and in several tumors with mutant or deleted p53 (59). Wild-type adenovirus replicates in all cells robustly, whereas the absence of E1B in Onyx-015 prevents efficient replication in cells with wild-type p53. The notion that Onyx-015 replication proceeds selectively in p53-deficient cells has been challenged by some investigators (147–149). Chemotherapy agents such as cisplatin and 5-fluorouricil (5-FU) augment the antitumor effects of Onyx-015 (150). Early results from clinical trials also appear promising (151).

The importance of the interaction between adenovirus E1B and cellular p53 in the process of viral replication suggests that the intracellular environment is a critical factor that dictates the outcome of cellular infection by a virus. Another example of this relationship is provided by reovirus. Interestingly, reovirus can replicate efficiently in NIH 3T3 cells only after they have been transformed with *ras* (152). Because activating *ras* mutations occur in about 30% of human tumors, including pancreatic, colorectal, and lung carcinomas, reovirus has been examined as a potential oncolytic virus that can selectively replicate in cells with an activated *ras* pathway (153). Experiments in preclinical models have demonstrated significant regression of tumors with *ras*-activated pathways after direct intratumoral inoculation of reovirus (153).

Another virus that has been used to achieve oncolysis through viral replication is HSV1. HSV1 entry into a cell leads to a cascade of viral gene expression that ultimately results in production of progeny virion and cell death (60). HSV1 vectors have been engineered such that they replicate preferentially in tumor cells rather than in normal cells (63, 64, 154). One strategy has been to delete viral ribonucleotide reductase, which is an enzyme responsible for the synthesis of DNA precursors and is critical for viral replication. HSV1 mutants that are deficient in expression of this viral enzyme can replicate only in mitotically active cells that provide ribonucleotide reductase in complementation (155). One such HSV1 mutant, designated hrR3, replicates poorly in nondividing cells, such as cells of the central nervous system, but also dramatically inhibits the growth of experimental gliomas and carcinomas in animal models (47). The increased mitotic activity of these tumors compared to the relatively quiescent surrounding normal tissues serves as the basis for selective replication of hrR3 in the tumors. Similar to the brain, the normal liver has very little mitotic activity and consequently expresses very little ribonucelotide reductase, whereas liver metastases have significantly higher mitotic activity and express high levels of ribonucleotide reductase (156). Accordingly, when introduced into the portal vein, hrR3 replicates selectively in the metastases and produces significant antitumor effects (63, 157). HSV1 vectors have been developed in which genes encoding for neurovirulence factors have been deleted (65). Clinical trials using HSV1 vectors for brain tumors are presently examining the safety of this approach.

E. Gene Transfer and Chemotherapy

Although chemotherapy has served as the most common cancer therapy for decades, it has achieved only very limited success. Very few chemotherapeutic agents are specific for tumor cells and are usually toxic to some normal cells. The cytotoxicity against normal cells results in undesirable side effects and also limits the dose of chemotherapy that may be administered. Several gene therapy strategies have been developed to address these problems. One strategy involves introduction into cancer cells a gene that is required to convert an otherwise innocuous agent into an active chemotherapeutic agent. The objective of this approach is to modify the tumor cells such that they are sensitized to a systemically administered prodrug. Drug sensitization is typically accomplished by transfer of a gene that encodes an exogenous enzyme capable of converting a nontoxic prodrug into a toxic metabolite. Only cells that express the transferred gene are then susceptible to the cytotoxic effects of the prodrug, and, accordingly, these genes have been referred to as "suicide" genes. Another strategy used to enhance the efficacy of traditional chemotherapy involves gene therapy to modulate resistance to chemotherapy of either normal cells or tumor cells. Both types of cells rely on several mechanisms to avoid cell death induced by chemotherapeutic agents. Accordingly, gene transfer has been used to either enhance the resistance of normal cells to chemotherapy or conversely reduce the resistance of cancer cells to chemotherapy.

Suicide gene therapy involves transfer of a gene into tumor cells, after which administration of a prodrug results in the production of high concentrations of the cytotoxic metabolite specifically in the transduced tumor cells with relatively low systemic levels of the active metabolite (158–160). HSV-TK and ganciclovir served as the prototypical suicide gene and prodrug combination. This strategy relies on known differences between the substrate specificity of HSV-TK and mammalian cellular TK (161). Phosphorylation of thymidine by cellular TK represents a salvage pathway for DNA synthesis. Whereas cellular TK displays a highly restricted range of substrates, HSV-TK exhibits a much less restricted range. The prodrug ganciclovir is monophosphorylated by HSV-TK but not by cellular TK. Monophosphorylated ganciclovir is further phosphorylated by cellular enzymes to the di- and triphosphate forms. When incorporated into DNA, ganciclovir triphosphate inhibits chain elongation by DNA polymerase. In contrast to phosphorylated ganciclovir, unphosphorylated ganciclovir is nontoxic. Accordingly, when exposed to ganciclovir, only cells that express HSV-TK undergo apoptosis.

The HSV-TK gene has been cloned into various gene delivery vehicles to treat experimental animal tumors with HSV-TK and ganciclovir (42, 47, 162–167). Several cancer gene therapy clinical trials have been designed to examine the efficacy of this strategy in humans (Table II). Most of these clinical trials involve direct intratumoral inoculation of either an adenovirus or a retrovirus that expresses the HSV-TK gene.

The observed antitumor activity of suicide gene therapy in cultured cells and in rodent tumor model systems exceeds that which would be expected based on the fraction of tumor cells that are transduced with the suicide gene. For example, with some suicide gene–prodrug combinations, transduction of as few as 10% of tumor cells is sufficient to destroy 100% of the tumor on exposure to the prodrug (168). This enhanced cytotoxicity results from "bystander killing," a term that refers to the death of untransduced tumor cells located adjacent to transduced tumor cells (168–173). Several mechanisms have been reported that may contribute to bystander killing. These involve transfer of prodrug metabolites from untransduced to transduced cells, host immune responses, transfer of apoptotic vesicles from untransduced to transduced cells, and local cytokine release within the tumors (168, 174–176). It remains to be determined whether the magnitude of bystander killing observed in animal models will be observed in clinical trials. However, because it is unlikely that any gene delivery vehicle will be able to transduce 100% of tumor cells, the bystander effect observed in prodrug activation therapies may be extremely important. Gene therapy strategies that produce bystander killing have a significant advantage over gene therapy strategies that require transduction of all tumor cells.

Other suicide gene–prodrug combinations have been developed. The gene encoding cytosine deaminase (CD) is present in some bacteria and fungi but absent in mammalian cells. CD is responsible for conversion of cytosine to uracil in times of nutritional stress. This enzyme also catalyzes conversion of the prodrug 5-fluorocytosine (5-FC) into 5-fluorouracil, which is further metabolized within cells into metabolites that inhibit RNA and DNA synthesis (177, 178). The potential benefit of this prodrug–suicide gene combination is being examined in a clinical trial for patients with colon carcinoma liver metastases (Table II). Xanthine–guanine phosphoribosyltransferase (XGPRT) is encoded by the *gpt* gene and is normally found in *E. coli* but not in mammalian cells. XGPRT converts the prodrug 6-thioxanthine into 6-thioxanthine nucleoside monophosphate, which inhibits DNA synthesis (179). A unique feature of the *gpt* gene is its ability to confer resistance to specific agents, such as the combination of mycophenolic acid, xanthine, and hypoxanthine. This trait permits selection of cells that express XGPRT (180). Other prodrug–suicide gene combinations include *E. coli* purine nucleoside phosphorylase activation of the prodrugs 6-methylpurine-2′-deoxyriboside and arabinofuranosyl-2-fluoroadenine monophosphate (181), *E. coli* nitroreductase activation of the prodrug CB1954 (182), cytochrome P450 activation of the prodrug cyclophosphamide (183), and *E. coli* carboxypeptidase G2 activation of the prodrug 4-[(2-chloroethyl)(2-mesyloxyethyl)amino]benzoyl-L-glutamic acid (184).

Gene therapy has been used in other ways to enhance the efficacy of traditional chemotherapy. Several studies have demonstrated that the absence of p53 or the presence of mutant p53 renders cells resistant to chemotherapy by loss of p53-dependent apoptosis pathways (131). To overcome this mechanism of resistance, the wild-type p53 gene can be introduced into cancer cells to restore their susceptibility to chemotherapeutic agents. In a clinical trial in which p53 was introduced into non-small-cell lung carcinomas with a retrovirus, significant tumor regression was observed in some injected tumor nodules (185). (This cancer gene therapy strategy was discussed in Section III,C.)

Another gene therapy strategy designed to enhance chemotherapy involves enhancement of drug resistance of normal bone marrow precursor cells in patients receiving bone marrow transplants. These rapidly dividing cells are inherently sensitive to the cytotoxic effects of chemotherapeutic agents such as vinca alkaloids, anthracyclines, podophyllins, and paclitaxel. However, transduction of marrow cells with the multiple-drug-resistance (MDR) gene may reduce their sensitivity to these types of chemotherapeutic agents, thereby reducing the chances that bone marrow suppression will be a dose-limiting toxicity. The feasibility of this chemoprotective gene therapy approach has been examined in a clinical trial using a retrovirus to transduce marrow cells prior to reinfusion after high-dose chemotherapy (186). Although this approach proved to be safe, prolonged high-level MDR expression was not observed in most patients.

F. Targeting Gene Expression

The ability to destroy tumor cells effectively without destruction of normal cells lies at the heart of any cancer therapy, including approaches involving gene therapy. With some gene therapy strategies, indiscriminate transduction of both normal cells and tumors cells may produce unacceptable toxicity. For example, suicide gene transfer followed by systemic exposure to prodrugs may destroy any cells that have also been transduced with the suicide gene. Several techniques exist to target tumor cells specifically. The first involves introduction of the therapeutic gene only into specific cell populations (e.g., malignant cells). An example of this approach exploits the known tropism of certain viruses for specific types of cells. Herpes simplex viruses are neurotropic, retrovirus infection is limited to cells that are dividing, and adenoviruses are highly hepatotropic. Viruses can also be engineered to alter their natural tropism for specific cell types. For example, the cell recognition domain of adenovirus fibers can be modified to direct this virus to specific cell types (187). Another strategy used to direct gene transfer to specific populations of target cells involves confining vector exposure to specific tissues. The most obvious example of this approach involves inoculation of vectors directly into tumors to reduce transduction of normal tissues (51). Another approach involves harvesting tumor cells for *ex vivo* gene transfer to produce vaccines (75). Similarly, immune effector cells have been isolated and tranduced *ex vivo* (188).

An alternative approach to target specific cell populations does not require this type of selective transduction. Instead, nonspecific cell transduction is combined with strategies to restrict transgene expression to specific cell populations. The most commonly used strategy to accomplish this form of regulation relies on gene promoters that restrict gene expression to a specific cell type. Promoters are segments of DNA that regulate gene transcription by interaction with specific cellular proteins (transcriptional activators). A promoter linked to a gene will permit expression of the gene only in cells that express specific proteins required by that particular promoter. This strategy has been referred to as "transcriptional targeting." As an example, the promoter for carcinoembryonic antigen (CEA) has been incorporated into vectors to selectively limit expression of the *E. coli* cytosine deaminase gene to colon cancer cells that express CEA (7, 189). When the CEA promoter is linked to the cytosine deaminase gene, expression of cytosine deaminase will occur only in cells that possess the necessary proteins to activate CEA expression. In this scenario, cytosine deaminase conversion of 5-FC to 5-FU will occur to the greatest extent in cells that express CEA. The CEA promoter has also been used to restrict HSV-TK gene expression to CEA-positive lung cancer cells (162). Similarly, α-fetoprotein (AFP) is commonly overexpressed in hepatocellular cancers, which makes the AFP promoter ideal for gene therapy applications that target hepatocellular carcinoma (190). The AFP enhancer has been used together with the albumin promoter to restrict HSV-TK expression to hepatocellular cancer cells (191). The AFP promoter and enhancer have been used in a retrovirus vector to restrict expression of the wild-type p53 gene (192). As another example, the promoter for prostate-specific antigen (PSA) has also been used to target transgene expression to prostate cancer cells (193, 194).

Some promoters have been identified that activate gene transcription in response to specific inducing agents such as heat, high-frequency ultrasound, or ionizing radiation. Numerous genes are expressed in response to radiation, and the promoters for these genes can be used to direct gene expression. For example, the EGR1 gene is up-regulated in response to ionizing radiation (195). In a novel gene therapy strategy, human glioma xenografts were treated with an adenovirus vector containing the EGR1 promoter linked to the TNFα gene and then subjected to ionizing radiation (196). TNFα enhances the effect of ionizing radiation on tumors. The tumor regression observed in mice treated in this fashion was significantly greater than in mice that received the vector without radiation, radiation alone, or radiation combined with a control adenovirus vector. Further development of gene delivery systems that incorporate transcriptional regulatory sequences to selectively produce high levels of transgene expression may reduce the nonspecific toxicity of cancer gene therapy applications.

IV. Summary

Gene therapy has rapidly emerged as a new tool to treat human diseases. Cancer gene therapy represents a natural by-product of the numerous advances made in the fields of cancer biology, molecular biology, immunology, molecular genetics, and virology. In many instances, gene therapy approaches to cancer have been designed to augment currently existing therapies, such as chemotherapy and immunotherapy. In other instances, gene therapy has provided the tools necessary to exploit newly gained insight into the role of oncogenes and tumor suppressor genes. The past decade has produced many promising leads in the field of cancer gene therapy, many of which are being examined in clinical trials. Unfortunately, gene therapy has yet to produce its first cancer cure. Successful cancer gene therapy approaches will require development of vectors with (1) improved target-specificity, (2) higher *in vivo* transduction efficiency, (3) the ability to induce long-term transgene expression, and (4) decreased vector toxicity. The rapid discovery of novel targets for cancer therapy combined with improvements in gene transfer technology will undoubtedly lead to more effective cancer treatments in the near future.

References

1. Blaese, R. M., and Culver, K. W. (1992). Gene therapy for primary immunodeficiency disease. *Immunodefic. Rev.* **3,** 329–349.
2. Fearon, E. R., and Vogelstein, B. (1990). A genetic model for colorectal tumorigenesis. *Cell* **61,** 759–767.
3. Roth, J. A. (1998). Restoration of tumour suppressor gene expression for cancer. Forum. *Trends Exp. Clin. Med.* **8,** 368–376.

4. Jenks, S. (2000). Gene therapy death—Everyone has to share in the guilt. *J. Natl. Cancer Inst.* **2000,** 98–100.
5. Allen, T. M., and Hansen, C. (1991). Pharmacokinetics of stealth versus conventional liposomes: Effect of dose. *Biochim. Biophys. Acta* **1068,** 133–141.
6. Vaage, J., Donovan, D., Wipff, E., *et al.* (1999). Therapy of a xenografted human colonic carcinoma using cisplatin or doxorubicin encapsulated in long-circulating pegylated stealth liposomes. *Int. J. Cancer* **80,** 134–137.
7. Richards, C. A., Austin, E. A., and Huber, B. E. (1995). Transcriptional regulatory sequences of carcinoembryonic antigen: Identification and use with cytosine deaminase for tumor-specific gene therapy. *Human Gene Ther.* **6,** 881–893.
8. Wivel, N. A., and Wilson, J. M. (1998). Methods of gene delivery. *Hematol. Oncol. Clin. North Am.* **12,** 483–501.
9. Coffin, J. M. (1996). "Retroviridae," 3rd Ed. Raven Press, New York.
10. Miller, A. D., Miller, D. G., Garcia, J. V., and Lynch, C. M. Use of retroviral vectors for gene transfer and expression. *Methods Enzymol.* **217,** 581–599.
11. Wei, R. M., Gibson, M., Spear, P.G, and Scolnick, E. M. (1981). Construction and isolation of a transmissible retrovirus containing the src gene of Harvey murine sarcoma virus and the thymidine kinase gene of herpes simplex virus type 1. *J. Virol.* **39,** 935–944.
12. van Beusechem, V.W, Kukler, A., Heidt, P.J, and Valerio, D. (1992). Long-term expression of human adenosine deaminase in rhesus monkeys transplanted with retrovirus-infected bone marrow cells. *Proc. Natl. Acad. Sci. U.S.A.* **89,** 7640–7644.
13. Dai, Y., Roman, M., Naviaux, R., and Verma, I. M. (1992). Gene therapy via primary myoblasts: Long-term expression of factor IX protein following transplantation *in vivo. Proc. Natl. Acad. Sci. U.S.A.* **89,** 10392–10895.
14. Blaese, R. M. (1993). Development of gene therapy for immunodeficiency: Adenosine deaminase deficiency. *Pediatr. Res.* **33** (Suppl.), 549–555.
15. Hodgson, C. P. (1995). The vector void in gene therapy: Can viral vectors and transfection be combined to permit safe, efficacious, and targeted gene therapy? *Biotechnology* **13,** 222–225.
16. Hermann, F. (1995). Cancer gene therapy: Principles, problems, and perspectives. *J. Mol. Med.* **73,** 157–163.
17. Dranoff, G., Jaffee, E., Lazenby, A., *et al.* (1993). Vaccination with irradiated tumor cells engineered to secrete murine granulocyte-macrophage colon-stimulating factor stimulates potent, specific, and long-lasting anti-tumor immunity. *Proc. Natl. Acad. Sci. U.S.A.* **90,** 3539–3543.
18. Simons, J. W. (1994). Phase I/II study of autologous human GM-CSF gene transduced prostate cancer vaccines in patients with metastatic prostate carcinoma. RAC Report #9408-082.
19. Rosenberg, S. A., Aebersold, P., Cornetta K., *et al.* (1990). Gene transfer into humans—Immunotherapy of patients with advanced melanoma, using tumor-infiltrating lymphocytes modified by retroviral gene transduction [see comments]. *N. Engl. J. Med.* **323,** 570–578.
20. Deisseroth, A., Guo, D., Wang, T., *et al.* (1998). Molecular therapy for cancer. *Cancer J. Sci. Am.* **4** (Suppl 1), S5–7.
21. Huber, B. E., Richards, C. E., and Austin, E. A. (1994). Virus-directed enzyme/prodrug therapy (VDEPT) selectively engineering drug sensitivity into tumors. *N.Y. Acad. Sci.* **716,** 104–114.
22. Somia, N. V., Zoppé, M., and Verma, I. M. (1995). Generation of targeted retroviral vectors by using single-chain variable fragment: An approach to *in vivo* gene delivery. *Proc. Natl. Acad. Sci. U.S.A.* **92,** 7570–7574.
23. Episkopou, V., Murphy, A. J. M., and Efstratiadis, A. (1984). Cell-specified expression of a selectable hybrid gene. *Proc. Natl. Acad. Sci. U.S.A.* **81,** 4657–4661.
24. Dzierzak, E. A., Papayannopoulou, T., and Mulligan, R. C. (1988). Lineage-specific expression of a human β-globin gene in murine bone marrow transplant recipients reconstituted with retrovirus-transduced stem cells. *Nature (London)* **331,** 35–41.
25. Horwitz, M. (1990). Adenoviridae and their replication. *In* "Virology," 2nd ed. (B. Fields and D.M. Knipe, eds.), pp. 1679–1712. Raven Press, New York.
26. Green, M., Wold, W. S. M., Brackmann, K. H., *et al.* (1980). Human adenovirus transforming genes: Group relationships, integration, expression in transformed cells and analysis of human cancers and tonsils. *Cold Spring Harb. Symp. Quant. Biol.* **44** (Pt. 1), 457–469.
27. Stratford-Perricaudet, L. D., Levrero, M., Chasse, J. -F., Perricaudet, M., and Briand, P. (1990). Evaluation of the transfer and expression in mice of an enzyme-encoding gene using a human adenovirus vector. *Human Gene Ther.* **1,** 241–256.
28. Rosenfeld, M. A., Siegfried, W., Yoshimura, K., *et al.* (1991). Adenovirus-mediated transfer of a recombinant α1-antitrypsin gene to the lung epithelium *in vivo. Science* **252,** 431–434.
29. Mittal, S. K., McDermott, M. R., Johnson, D. C., Prevec, L., and Graham, F. L. (1993). Monitoring foreign gene expression by a human adenovirus-based vector using the firefly luciferase gene as a reporter. *Virus Res.* **28,** 67–90.
30. Ballay, A., Levrero, M., Buendia, M. -A., Tiollais, P., and Perricaudet, M. (1985). *In vitro* and *in vivo* synthesis of the hepatitis B virus surface antigen and of the receptor for polymerized human serum albumin from recombinant human adenoviruses. *EMBO J.* **4,** 3861–3865.
31. Ghosh-Choudhury, G., Haj-Ahmad, Y., Brinkley, P., Rudy, J., and Graham, F. L. (1986). Human adenovirus cloning vectors based on infectious bacterial plasmids. *Gene* **50,** 161–171.
32. Rosenfeld, M. A., Yoshimura, K., Trapnell, B. C., *et al.* (1992). *In vivo* transfer of the human cystic fibrosis transmembrane conductance regulator gene to the airway epithelium. *Cell* **68,** 143–155.
33. Stratford-Pericaudet, L. D., Makeh, I., Perricaudet, M., and Briand, P. (1992). Widespread long-term gene transfer to mouse skeletal muscles and heart. *J. Clin. Invest.* **90,** 626–630.
34. Setoguchi, Y., Jaffe, H. A., Chu, C. -S., and Crystal, R. G. (1994). Intraperitoneal *in vivo* gene therapy to deliver alphal-antitrypsin to the systemic circulation. *Am. J. Respir. Cell. Mol. Biol.* **10,** 369–377.
35. Quantin, B., Perricaudet, L. D., Tajbakhsh, S., and Mandel, J. -L. (1992). Adenovirus as an expression vector in muscle cells *in vivo. Proc. Natl. Acad. Sci. U.S.A.* **89,** 2581–2584.
36. Jaffe, H. A., Danel, C., Longenecker, G., *et al.* (1992). Adenovirus-mediated *in vivo* gene transfer and expression in normal rat liver. *Nature Genet.* **1,** 372–378.
37. Li, Q., Kay, M. A., Finegold, M., Stratford-Perricaudet, L. D., and Woo, S. L. (1993). Assessment of recombinant adenoviral vectors for hepatic gene therapy. *Human Gene Ther.* **4,** 403–409.
38. Davidson, B. L., Allen, E. D., Kozarsky, K. F., Wilson, J. M., and Roessler, B. J. (1993). A model system for *in vivo* gene transfer into the cnetral nervous system using an adenoviral vector. *Nature Genet.* **3,** 219–223.
39. Zabner, J., Peterson, D. M., Puga, A. P., Graham, S. M., and Welsh, M. J. (1994). Safety and efficacy of repetitive adenovirus-mediated transfer of CFTR cDNA to airway epithelia of primates and cotton rats. *Nature Genet.* **6,** 75–83.
40. Vincent, N., Ragot, T., Gilgenkrantz, H., *et al.* (1993). Long-term correction of mouse dystrophic degeneration by adenovirus-mediated transfer of a minidystrophin gene. *Nature Genet.* **5,** 130–134.
41. Chen, S. -H., Shine, H. D., Goodman, J. C., Grossman, R. G., and Woo, S. L. (1994). Gene therapy for brain tumors: Regression of experimental gliomas by adenovirus-mediated gene transfer *in vivo. Proc. Natl. Acad. Sci. U.S.A.* **91,** 3054–3057.
42. Smythe, W. R., Hwang, H. C., Elshami, A. A., *et al.* (1995). Treatment of experimental human mesothelioma using adenovirus transfer of the herpes simplex thymidine kinase gene. *Ann. Surg.* **222,** 78–86.
43. Hirschowitz, E. A., Ohwada, A., Pascal, W. R., Russi, T. J., and Crystal, R. G. (1995). *In vivo* adenovirus-mediated gene transfer of the

Escherichia coli cytosine deaminase gene to human colon carcinoma-derived tumors induces chemosensitivity to 5-fluorocytosine. *Human Gene Ther.* **6,** 1055–1063.
44. Brody, S. L., Jaffe, H. A., Han, S. K., Wersto, R. P., and Crystal, R. G. (1994). Direct *in vivo* gene transfer and expression in malignant cells using adenovirus vectors. *Human Gene Ther.* **5,** 437–447.
45. Boviatsis, E. J., Chase, M., Wei, M. X., *et al.* (1994). Gene transfer into experimental brain tumors mediated by adenovirus, herpes simplex virus, and retrovirus vectors. *Human Gene Ther.* **5,** 183–191.
46. Boviatsis, E. J., Scharf, J. M., Chase, M., *et al.* (1994). Antitumor activity and reporter gene transfer into rat brain neoplasms inoculated with herpes simplex virus vectors defective in thymidine kinase or ribonucleotide reductase. *Gene Ther.* **1,** 323–331.
47. Boviatsis, E. J., Park, J. S., Sena-Esteves, M., *et al.* (1994). Long-term survival of rats harboring brain neoplasms treated with ganciclovir and a herpes simplex virus that retains an intact thymidine kinase gene. *Cancer Res.* **54,** 5745–5751.
48. Fujiwara, T., Grimm, E. A., Mukhopadhyay, T., Zhang, W. -W., Owen-Schaub, L. B., and Roth, J. A. (1994). Induction of chemosensitivity in human lung cancer cells *in vivo* by an adenoviral-mediated transfer of the wild-type p53 gene. *Cancer Res.* **54,** 2287–2291.
49. Spitz, F. R., Nguyen, D., Skibber, J. M., Cusack, J. C., Roth, J. A., and Cristiano, R. J. (1996). *In vivo* adenovirus-mediated p53 tumor suppressor gene therapy for colorectal cancer. *Anticancer Res.* **16,** 3415–3422.
50. Tanaka, T., Fumihiko, K., Okabe, S., *et al.* (1996). Adenovirus-mediated prodrug gene therapy for carcinoembryonic antigen-producing human gastric carcinoma cells *in vitro. Cancer Res.* **56,** 1341–1345.
51. Cusack, J. C., Spitz, F. R., Nguyen, D., Zhang, W. -W., Cristiano, R. J., and Roth, J. A. (1996). High levels of gene transduction in human lung tumors following intralesional injection of recombinant adenovirus. *Cancer Gene Ther.* **3,** 245–249.
52. Yang, Y., Nunes, F., Berencsi, K., Furth, E. E., Gonczol, E., and Wilson, J. M. (1994). Cellular immunity to viral antigens limits E1-deleted adenoviruses for gene therapy. *Proc. Natl. Acad. Sci. U.S.A.* **91,** 4407–4441.
53. Yang, Y., Ertl, H. C., and Wilson, J. M. (1994). MHC class I-restricted cytotoxic T lymphocytes to viral antigens destroy hepatocytes in mice infected with E1-deleted recombinant adenoviruses. *Immunity* **1,** 433–442.
54. Yang, Y., Li, Q., Ertl, H. C., and Wilson, J. M. (1995). Cellular and humoral immune responses to viral antigens create barriers to lung-directed gene therapy with recombinant adenoviruses. *J. Virol.* **69,** 2004–2015.
55. Englehardt, J. F., Litzky, L., and Wilson, J. M. (1994). Prolonged transgene expression in cotton rat lung with recombinant adenoviruses defective in E2a. *Human Gene Ther.* **5,** 1217–1229.
56. Englehardt, J. F., Ye, X., Doranz, B., and Wilson, J. M. (1994). Ablation of E2A in recombinant adenoviruses improves transgene persistence and decreases inflammatory response in mouse liver. *Proc. Natl. Acad. Sci. U.S.A.* **91,** 6196–6200.
57. Gao, G. P., Yang, Y., and Wilson, J. M. (1996). Biology of adenovirus vectors with E1 and E4 deletions for liver-directed gene therapy. *J. Virol.* **70,** 8934–8943.
58. Crystal, R. G. (1995). Transfer of genes to humans: early lessons and obstacles to success. *Science* **270,** 404–410.
59. Bischoff, J. R., Kirn, D. H., Williams, A., *et al.* (1996). An adenovirus mutant that replicates selectively in p53-deficient human tumor cells. *Science* **274,** 373–376.
60. Roizman, B., and Sears, A. E. (1996). Herpes simplex viruses and their replication. *In* "Fields Virology," 3rd Ed. (B.N. Fields, D.M. Knipe, and P.M. Howley, eds.), pp. 2231–2295. Lippincott–Raven Publ., Philadelphia.
61. Breakefield, X. O., Kramm, C. M., Chiocca, E. A., and Pechan, P. A. (1995). Herpes simplex virus vectors for tumor therapy. *In* "The Internet Book of Gene Therapy" (R.E. Sobol and K.J. Scanlon, eds.), pp. 41–56. Appleton and Lange, Stamford.
62. Johnson, P. A., Miyanohara, A., Levine, F., Cahil, T., and Friedmann, T. (1992). Cytotoxicity of a replication-defective mutant of herpes simplex virus type 1. *J. Virol.* **66,** 2952–2965.
63. Yoon, S. S., Nakamura, H., Carroll, N. M., Bode, B. P., Chiocca, E. A., and Tanabe, K. K. (2000). An oncolytic herpes simplex virus type 1 vector selectively treats diffuse liver metastases from colon carcinoma. *FASEB J.* **14**(2), 301–311.
64. Mineta, T., Rabkin, S. D., and Martuza, R. L. (1994). Treatment of malignant gliomas using ganciclovir-hypersensitive, ribonucleotide reductase-deficient herpes simplex viral mutant. *Cancer Res.* **54,** 3963–3966.
65. Yazaki, T., Manz, H. J., Rabkin, S. D., and Martuza, R. L. (1995). Treatment of human malignant meningiomas by G207, a replication-competent multimutated herpes simplex virus 1. *Cancer Res.* **55,** 4752–4756.
66. McGeoch, D. J., Dalrymple, M. A., Davison, A. J., *et al.* (1988). The complete DNA sequence of the long unique region in the genome of herpes simplex virus type 1. *J. Gen. Virol.* **69,** 1531–1574.
67. Moolten, F. L., and Wells, J. M. (1990). Curability of tumors bearing herpes thymidine kinase genes transferred by retroviral vectors. *J. Natl. Cancer Inst.* **82,** 297–300.
68. Geller, A. I., and Breakefield, X. O. (1988). A defective HSV-1 vector expresses *E. coli* beta-galactosidase in cultured rat peripheral neurons. *Science* **241,** 1667–1669.
69. Moss, B. (1996). Genetically engineered poxviruses for recombinant gene expression, vaccination, and safety. *Proc. Natl. Acad. Sci. U.S.A.* **93,** 11341–11348.
70. Moss, B. (1990). Poxviridae and their replication. *In* "Virology," 2nd Ed. (B.N. Fields and D.M. Knipe, eds.), pp. 2644–2655. Raven Press, New York.
71. Paoletti, E. (1996). Applications of pox virus vectors to vaccination: An update. *Proc. Natl. Acad. Sci. U.S.A.* **93,** 11349–11353.
72. Wallack, M. K., Sivanandham, M., Ditaranto, K., *et al.* (1997). Increased survival of patients treated with a vaccinia melanoma oncolysate vaccine. *Ann. Surg.* **226,** 198–206.
73. Kantor, J., Irvine, K., Abrams, S., Kaufman, H., DiPietro, J., and Schlom, J. (1992). Antitumor activity and immune responses induced by a recombinant carcinoembryonic antigen-vaccinia virus vaccine. *J. Natl. Cancer Inst.* **84,** 1084–1091.
74. Peplinski, G. R., Tsung, K., Whitman, E. D., Meko, J. B., and Norton, J. A. (1995). Construction and expression in tumor cells of a recombinant vaccinia virus encoding human interleukin-1 beta. *Ann. Surg. Oncol.* **2,** 151–159.
75. Hodge, J. W., Abrams, S., Schlom, J., and Kantor, J. A. (1994). Induction of antitumor immunity by recombinant vaccinia viruses expressing B7-1 or B7-2 costimulatory molecules. *Cancer Res.* **54,** 5552–5555.
76. Qin, H., and Chatterjee, S. K. (1996). Recombinant vaccinia expressing interleukin-2 for cancer gene therapy. *Cancer Gene Ther.* **3,** 163–167.
77. Roth, J. A., and Cristiano, R. J. (1997). Gene therapy for cancer: what have we done and where are we going? *J. Natl. Cancer Inst.* **88,** 21–39.
78. Flotte, T. R., Afione, S. A., Conrad, C., *et al.* (1993). Stable *in vivo* expression of the cystic fibrosis transmembrane conductance regulator with an adeno-associated virus vector. *Proc. Natl. Acad. Sci. U.S.A.* **90,** 10613–10617.
79. Berns, K. I., Cheung, A., Ostrove, J., and Lewis, M. (1982). Adeno-associated virus latent infection. *In* "Virus Persistence," (B.W.J. Mahy, A.C. Minso, and G.K. Darby, eds.), p. 249. Cambridge University Press, Cambridge.
80. Samulski, R. J., Zhu, X., Xiao, X., *et al.* (1991). Targeted integration of adeno-associated virus (AAV) into human chromosome 19. *EMBO J.* **10,** 3941–3950 [published erratum appears in *EMBO J.* **11**(3), 1228].

81. Halbert, C. L., Alexander, I. E., Wolgamot, G. M., and Miller, A. D. (1995). Adeno-associated virus vectors transduce primary cells much less efficiently than immortalized cells. *J. Virol.* **69,** 1473–1479.
82. Kessler, P. D., Podsakoff, G. M., Chen, X., *et al.* (1996). Gene delivery to skeletal muscle results in sustained expression and systemic delivery of a therapeutic protein. *Proc. Natl. Acad. Sci. U.S.A.* **93,** 14082–14087.
83. Yang, N. S., Burkholder, J., Roberts, B., Martinell, B., and McCabe, D. (1990). *In vivo* and *in vitro* gene transfer to mammalian somatic cells by particle bombardment. *Proc. Natl. Acad. Sci. U.S.A.* **87,** 9568–9572.
84. Nabel, E. G., Gordon, D., Yang, Z. Y., *et al.* (1992). Gene transfer *in vivo* with DNA–liposome complexes: Lack of autoimmunity and gonadal localization. *Human Gene Ther.* **3,** 649–656.
85. Lasic, D. D., Martin, F. J., Gabizon, A., Huang, S. K., and Papahadjopoulos, D. (1991). Sterically stabilized liposomes: A hypothesis on the molecular origin of the extended circulation times. *Biochim. Biophys. Acta* **1070,** 187–192.
86. Wagner, E., Zenke, M., Cotten, M., Beug, H., and Birnstiel, M. L. (1990). Transferrin-polycation conjugates as carriers for DNA uptake into cells. *Proc. Natl. Acad. Sci. U.S.A.* **87,** 3410–3414.
87. Kao, G. Y., Change, L. J., and Allen, T. M. (1996). Use of cationic liposomes in enhanced DNA delivery to cancer cells. *Cancer Gene Ther.* **3,** 250–256.
88. Nabel, E. G., Tang, Z., Muller, D., *et al.* (1994). Safety and toxicity of catheter delivery to the pulmonary vasculature in a patient with metastatic melanoma. *Human Gene Ther.* **5,** 1089–1094.
89. Gao, L., Wagner, E., Cotten, M., *et al.* (1993). Direct *in vivo* gene transfer to airway epithelium employing adenovirus–polylysine-DNA complexes. *Human Gene Ther.* **4,** 17–24.
90. Cristiano, R. J., Smith, L. C., Kay, M. A., Brinkly, B. R., and Woo, S. L. Hepatic gene therapy: Efficient gene delivery and expression in primary hepatocytes utilizing a conjugated adenovirus–DNA complex. *Proc. Natl. Acad. Sci. U.S.A.* **90,** 11548–11552.
91. Bunnell, B. A., Askari, F. K., and Wilson, J. M. (1992). Targeted delivery of antisense oligonucleotides by molecular conjugates. *Somat. Cell Mol. Genet.* **18,** 559–569.
92. Cotten, M., Wagner, E., Zatloukal, K., Philips, S., Curiel, D. T., and Birnstiel, M. L. (1992). High-efficiency receptor mediated delivery of small and large (48 kilobase) gene constructs using the endosome-disruption activity of defective or chemically inactivated adenovirus particles. *Proc. Natl. Acad. Sci. U.S.A.* **89,** 6094–6098.
93. Curiel, D. T., Wagner, E., Cotten, M., *et al.* (1992). High-efficiency gene transfer mediated by adenovirus coupled to DNA-polylysine complexes. *Human Gene Ther.* **3,** 147–154.
94. Cristiano, R., and Roth, J. (1996). Epidermal growth factor mediated DNA delivery into lung cancer cells via the epidermal growth factor receptor. *Cancer Gene Ther.* **3,** 4–10.
95. Rosenberg, S. A., Yannelli, J. R., Yang, J. C., *et al.* (1994). Treatment of patients with metastatic melanoma with autologous tumor-infiltrating lymphocytes and interleukin 2. *J. Natl. Cancer Inst.* **86,** 1159–1166.
96. Sobol, R. E., Shawler, D., Dorigo, O., Gold, D., Royston, I., and Fakhrai, H. (1995). Immunogene therapy of cancer. *In* "The Internet Book of Gene Therapy" (R.E. Sobol and K.J. Scanlong, eds.), pp. 175–180. Appleton and Lange, Stanford.
97. Guinan, E. C., Gribben, J. G., Boussiotis, V. A., Freeman, G. J., and Nadler, L. M. (1994). Pivotal role of the B7:CD28 pathway in transplantation tolerance and tumor immunity. *Blood* **84,** 3261–3282.
98. Townsend, S. E., and Allison, J. P. (1993). Tumor rejection after direct costimulation of CD8+ T cells by B7-transfected melanoma cells. *Science* **259,** 368–370.
99. Soiffer, R., Lynch, T., Mihm, M., *et al.* (1997). A phase I study of vaccination with autologous, irradiated melanoma cells engineered to secrete human granulocyte-macrophage colony stimulating factor. *Human Gene Ther.* **8,** 111–123.
100. Fearon, E. R., Pardoll, D. M., Itaya, T., *et al.* (1990). Interleukin-2 production by tumor cells bypasses T helper function in the generation of an antitumor response. *Cell* **60,** 397–403.
101. Gansbacher, B., Zier, K., Daniels, B., Cronin, K., Bannerji, R., and Gilboa, E. (1990). Interleukin 2 gene transfer abrogates tumorigenicity and induces protective immunity. *J. Exp. Med.* **172,** 1217–1224.
102. Porgador, A., Gansbacher, B., Bannerji, R., *et al.* (1993). Anti-metastatic vaccination of tumor-bearing mice with IL-2-gene-inserted tumor cells. *Int. J. Cancer* **53,** 471–477.
103. Gansbacher, B., Bannerji, R., Daniels, B., Zier, K., Cronin, K., and Gilboa, E. (1990). Retroviral vector-mediated gamma-interferon gene transfer into tumor cells generates potent and long lasting antitumor immunity. *Cancer Res.* **50,** 7820–7825.
104. Watanabe, Y., Kuribayashi, K., Miyatake, S., *et al.* (1989). Exogenous expression of mouse interferon gamma cDNA in mouse neuroblastoma C1300 cells results in reduced tumorigenicity by augmented anti-tumor immunity. *Proc. Natl. Acad. Sci. U.S.A.* **86,** 9456–9460.
105. Tahara, H., Zeh, H., Jr., Storkus, W. J., *et al.* Fibroblasts genetically engineered to secrete interleukin 12 can suppress tumor growth and induce antitumor immunity to a murine melanoma *in vivo. Cancer Res.* **54,** 182–189.
106. Rosenberg, S. A., Blaese, R. M., Brenner, M. K., *et al.* (1999). Human gene marker/therapy clinical protocols. *Human Gene Ther.* **10,** 3067–3123.
107. Cole, D. J., Wilson, M. C., Baron, P. L., *et al.* (1996). Phase I study of recombinant CEA vaccinia virus vaccine with post vaccination CEA peptide challenge. *Human Gene Ther.* **7,** 1381–1394.
108. Kim, C. J., Prevette, T., Cormier, J., *et al.* (1997). Dendritic cells infected with poxviruses encoding MART-1/Melan A sensitize T lymphocytes *in vitro. J. Immunother.* **20,** 276–286.
109. Salgaller, M. L., Marincola, F. M., Cormier, J. N., and Rosenberg, S. A. (1996). Immunization against epitopes in the human melanoma antigen gp100 following patient immunization with synthetic peptides. *Cancer Res.* **56,** 4749–4757.
110. Rosenberg, S. A., Lotze, M. T., Muul, L. M., *et al.* (1985). Observations on the systemic administration of autologous lymphokine-activated killer cells and recombinant interleukin-2 to patients with metastatic cancer. *N. Engl. J. Med.* **313,** 1485–1492.
111. Rosenberg, S. A., Spiess, P., and Lafreniere, R. (1986). A new approach to the adoptive immunotherapy of cancer. *Science* **223,** 1318–1321.
112. Rosenberg, S. A., Packard, B. S., Aebersold, P. M., *et al.* (1988). Use of tumor-infiltrating lymphocytes and interleukin-2 in the immunotherapy of patients with metastatic melanoma. A preliminary report. *N. Engl. J. Med.* **319,** 1676–1680.
113. Spiess, P. J., Yang, J. C., and Rosenberg, S. A. (1987). *In vivo* antitumor activity of tumor-infiltrating lymphocytes expanded in recombinant interleukin-2. *J. Natl. Cancer Inst.* **79,** 1067–1075.
114. Karasuyama, H., Tohyama, N., and Tada, T. (1989). Autocrine growth and tumorigenicity of interleukin 2-dependent helper T cells transfected with IL-2 gene. *J. Exp. Med.* **169,** 13–25.
115. Rosenberg, S. A. (1993). Newer approaches to cancer treatment. In "Cancer: Principles and Practice of Oncology" (D.T.J. De Vita, S. Hellman, and S.A. Rosenberg, eds.), pp. 2598–2613. J.B. Lippincott Co., Philadelphia.
116. Kitamura, T., and Miyajima, A. (1992). Functional reconstitution of the human interleukin-3 receptor. *Blood* **80,** 84–90.
117. Plautz, G. E., Yang, Z. Y., Wu, B. Y., Gao, X., Huang, L., and Nabel, G. J. (1993). Immunotherapy of malignancy by *in vivo* gene transfer into tumors. *Proc. Natl. Acad. Sci. U.S.A.* **90,** 4645–4649.
118. Restifo, N. P., Spiess, P. J., Karp, S. E., Mule, J. J., and Rosenberg, S. A. (1992). A nonimmunogenic sarcoma transduced with the cDNA for interferon gamma elicits CD8+ T cells against the wild-type tumor: Correlation with antigen presentation capability. *J. Exp. Med.* **175,** 1423–1431.

119. Arca, M. J., Krauss, J. C., Aruga, A., Cameron, M. J., Shu, S., and Chang, A. E. (1996). Therapeutic efficacy of T cells derived from lymph nodes draining a poorly immunogenic tumor transduced to secrete granulocyte-macrophage colony-stimulating factor. *Cancer Gene Ther.* **3,** 39–47.
120. Chang, A. E., Sondak, V. K., Bishop, D. K., Nickoloff, B. J., Mulligan, R. C., Mule, J. J. Adoptive immunotherapy of cancer with activated lymph node cells primed *in vivo* with autologous tumor cells transduced with the GM-CSF gene. *Human Gene Ther.* **7,** 773–792.
121. Hahn, W. C., Counter, C. M., Lundberg, A. S., Beijersbergen, R. L., Brooks, M. W., and Weinberg, R. A. (1999). Creation of human tumour cells with defined genetic elements [see comments]. *Nature (London)* **400,** 464–468.
122. Sikora, K., and Pandha, H. (1993). Gene therapy for prostate cancer. *Br. J. Urol.* **79,** 64–68.
123. Aaltonen, L. A., Peltomaki, P., Leach, F. S., *et al.* (1993). Clues to the pathogenesis of familial colorectal cancer. *Science* **260,** 812–816.
124. Fearon, E. R., Molecular genetics of colorectal cancer. *Ann.* N.Y. *Acad. Sci.* **768,** 101–110.
125. Goyette, M. C., Cho, K., Fasching, C. L., *et al.* (1992). Progression of colorectal cancer is associated with multiple tumor suppressor gene defects but inhibition of tumorigenicity is accomplished by correction of any single defect via chromosome transfer. *Mol. Cell. Biol.* **12,** 1387–1395.
126. Clayman, G. L., El-Naggar, A. K., Lippman, S. M., *et al.* (1998). Adenovirus-mediated p53 gene transfer in patients with advanced recurrent head and neck squamous cell carcinoma. *J. Clin. Oncol.* **16,** 2221–2232.
127. Takahashi, T., Carbone, D., Nau, M. M., *et al.* (1992). Wild-type but not mutant p53 suppresses the growth of human lung cancer cells bearing multiple genetic lesions. *Cancer Res.* **52,** 2340–2343.
128. Wang, J., Bucana, C. D., Roth, J. A., Zhang, W. W. (1995). Apoptosis induced in human osteosarcoma cells is one of the mechanisms for the cytocidal effect of Ad5CMV-p53. *Cancer Gene Ther.* **2,** 9–17.
129. Badie, B., Drazan, K. E., Kramer, M. H., Shaked, A., and Black, K. L. (1995). Adenovirus-mediated p53 gene delivery inhibits 91 glioma growth in rats. *Neurol. Res.* **17,** 209–216.
130. Clayman, G. L., El-Naggar, A. K., Roth, J. A., *et al.* (1995). *In vivo* molecular therapy with p53 adenovirus for microscopic residual head and neck squamous carcinoma. *Cancer Res.* **55,** 1–6.
131. Lowe, S. W., Ruley, H. E., Jacks, T., and Housman, D. E. (1993). p53-dependent apoptosis modulates the cytotoxicity of anticancer agents. *Cell* **74,** 957–967.
132. Cusack, Jr., J. C., and Tanabe, K. K. (1998). Cancer gene therapy. *Surg. Oncol. Clin. North Am.* **7,** 421–469.
133. Xu, H. J., Zhou, Y., Seigne, J., *et al.* (1996). Enhanced tumor suppressor gene therapy via replication-deficient adenovirus vectors expressing an N-terminal truncated retinoblastoma protein. *Cancer Res.* **56,** 2245–2249.
134. Fueyo, J., Gomez-Manzano, C., Yung, W. K., *et al.* (1996). Adenovirus-mediated p16/CDKN2 gene transfer induces growth arrest and modifies the transformed phenotype of glioma cells. *Oncogene* **12,** 103–110.
135. Jin, X., Nguyen, D., Zhang, W. W., Kyritsis, A. P., and Roth, J. A. (1995). Cell cycle arrest and inhibition of tumor cell proliferation by the p16INK4 gene mediated by an adenovirus vector. *Cancer Res.* **55,** 3250–3253.
136. Calabretta, B. (1991). Inhibition of protooncogene expression by antisense oligodeoxynucleotides: Biological and therapeutic implications. *Cancer Res.* **51,** 4505–4510.
137. Zhang, Y., Mukhopadhyay, T., Donehower, L. A., Georges, R. N., and Roth, J. A. (1993). Retroviral vector-mediated transduction of K-ras antisense RNA into human lung cancer cells inhibits expression of the malignant phenotype. *Human Gene Ther.* **4,** 451–460.
138. Mukhopadhyay, T., Tainsky, M., Cavender, A. C., and Roth, J. A. (1991). Specific inhibition of K-ras expression and tumorigenicity of lung cancer cells by antisense RNA. *Cancer Res.* **51,** 1744–1748.
139. Georges, R. N., Mukhopadhyay, T., Zhang, Y., Yen, N., and Roth, J. A. (1993). Prevention of orthotopic human lung cancer growth by intratracheal instillation of a retroviral antisense K-ras construct. *Cancer Res.* **53,** 1743–1746.
140. Feng, M., Cabrera, G., Deshane, J., Scanlon, K. J., and Curiel, D. T. (1995). Neoplastic reversion accomplished by high efficiency adenoviral-mediated delivery of an anti-ras ribozyme. *Cancer Res.* **55,** 2024–2028.
141. Kashani-Sabet, M., Funato, T., Florenes, V. A., Fodstad, O., and Scanlon, K. J. (1994). Suppression of the neoplastic phenotype *in vivo* by an anti-ras ribozyme. *Cancer Res.* **54,** 900–902.
142. Scanlon, K., Jiao, L., Funato, T., Wang, W., and Tone, T. (1991). Ribozyme-mediated cleavages of c-fos mRNA reduce gene expression of DNA synthesis enzymes and metallothionein. *Proc. Natl. Acad. Sci. U.S.A.* **88,** 10591–10595.
143. Parthasarathy, R., Cote, G. J., and Gagel, R. F. (1999). Hammerhead ribozyme-mediated inactivation of mutant RET in medullary thyroid carcinoma. *Cancer Res.* **59,** 3911–3914.
144. Abounader, R., Ranganathan, S., Lal, B., *et al.* (1999). Reversion of human glioblastoma malignancy by U1 small nuclear RNA/ribozyme targeting of scatter factor/hepatocyte growth factor and c- met expression. *J. Natl. Cancer Inst.* **91,** 1548–1556.
145. Marasco, W. A. (1997). Intrabodies: Turning the humoral immune system outside in for intracellular immunization. *Gene Ther.* **4,** 11–15.
146. Chen, S. Y., and Marasco, W. A. (1996). Novel genetic immunotoxins and intracellular antibodies for cancer therapy. *Semin. Oncol.* **23,** 148–153.
147. Hall, A. R., Dix, B. R., O'Carroll, S. J., and Braithwaite, A. W. (1998). p53-dependent cell death/apoptosis is required for a productive adenovirus infection. *Nature Med.* **4,** 1068–1072.
148. Goodrum, F. D., and Ornelles, D. A. (1998). p53 status does not determine outcome of E1B 55-kilodalton mutant adenovirus lytic infection. *J. Virol.* **72,** 9479–9490.
149. Rothmann, T., Hengstermann, A., Whitaker, N. J., Scheffner, M., and zur Hausen, H. (1998). Replication of Onyx-015, a potential anticancer adenovirus, is independent of p53 status in tumor cells. *J. Virol.* **72,** 9470–9478.
150. Heise, C., Sampson-Johannes, A., Williams, A., McCormick, F., Von Hoff, D. D., and Kirn, D. H. (1997). ONYX-015, an E1B gene-attenuated adenovirus, causes tumor-specific cytolysis and antitumoral efficacy that can be augmented by standard chemotherapeutic agents. *Nature Med.* **3,** 639–645.
151. Kirn, D., Mermiston, T., and McCormick, F. (1998). Onyx-015: Clinical data are encouraging [letter to the editor]. *Nature Med.* **4,** 1341–1342.
152. Strong, J. E., Coffey, M. C., Tang, D., Sabinin, P., and Lee, P. W. K. (1998). The molecular basis of viral oncolysis: Usurpation of the ras signaling pathway by reovirus. *EMBO J.* **17,** 3351–3362.
153. Coffey, M. C., Strong, J. E., Forsyth, P. A., and Lee, P. W. K. (1998). Reovirus therapy of tumors with activated ras pathways. *Science* **282,** 1332–1334.
154. Martuza, R. L., Malick, A., Markert, J. M., Ruffner, K. L., and Coen, D. M. (1991). Experimental therapy of human glioma by means of a genetically engineered virus mutant. *Science* **252,** 854–856.
155. Goldstein, D. J., and Weller, S. K. (1988). Herpes simplex virus type 1-induced ribonucleotide reductase activity is dispensable for virus growth and DNA synthesis: Isolation and characterization of an ICP6 lacZ insertion mutant. *J. Virol.* **62,** 196–205.
156. Carroll, N. M., Chiocca, E. A., Takahashi, K., and Tanabe, K. K. (1996). Enhancement of gene therapy specificity for diffuse colon carcinoma liver metastases with recombinant herpes simplex virus. *Ann. Surg.* **224,** 323–330.

157. Yoon, S. S., Carroll, N. M., Chiocca, E. A., and Tanabe, K. K. (1998). Cancer gene therapy using replication-competent herpes simplex virus type 1. *Ann. Surg.* **228,** 366–374.
158. Harris, J. D., Gutierrez, A. A., Hurst, H. C., Sikora, K., and Lemoine, N. R. (1994). Gene therapy for cancer using tumor-specific prodrug activation. *Gene Ther.* **1,** 170–175.
159. Gutierrez, A. A., Lemoine, N. R., and Sikora, K. (1992). Gene therapy for cancer. *Lancet* **339,** 715–721.
160. Mullen, C. A. (1994). The use of suicide vectors for the gene therapy of cancer. *Pharmacol. Ther.* **63,** 199–207.
161. Ezzeddine, Z. D., Martuza, R. L., Platika, D., *et al.* (1991). Selective killing of glioma cells in culture and *in vivo* by retrovirus transfer of the herpes simplex virus thymidine kinase gene. *New Biol.* **3,** 608–614.
162. Osaki, T., Tanio, Y., Tachibana, I., *et al.* (1994). Gene therapy for carcinoembryonic antigen-producing human lung cancer cells by cell type specific expression of herpes simplex virus thymidine kinase gene. *Cancer Res.* **54,** 5258–5261.
163. Takamiya, Y., Short, M. P., Moolten, F. L., *et al.* (1993). An experimental model of retrovirus gene therapy for malignant brain tumors. *J. Neurosurg.* **79,** 104–110.
164. DiMaio, J. M., Clary, B. M., Via, D. F., Coveney, E., Pappas, T. N., and Lyerly, H. K. (1994). Directed enzyme pro-drug gene therapy for pancreatic cancer *in vivo*. *Surgery* **116,** 205–213.
165. Calvez, V., Rixe, O., Wang, P., *et al.* (1996). Virus-free transfer of the herpes simplex virus thymidine kinase gene followed by ganciclovir treatment induces tumor cell death. *Clin. Cancer Res.* **2,** 47–51.
166. Yoshida, K., Kawami, H., Yamaguchi, Y., *et al.* (1995). Retrovirally transmitted gene therapy for gastric carcinoma using herpes simplex virus thymidine kinase gene. *Cancer* **75,** 1467–1471.
167. Caruso, M., Panis, Y., and Gagandeep, S. (1993). Regression of established macroscopic liver metastases after *in situ* transduction of a suicide gene. *Proc. Natl. Acad. Sci. U.S.A.* **90,** 7024–7028.
168. Freeman, S. M., Abboud, C. N., Whartenby, K. A., *et al.* The "bystander effect": Tumor regression when a fraction of the tumor mass is genetically modified. *Cancer Res.* **53,** 5274–5283.
169. Freeman, S. M., Ramesh, R., Shastri, M., Munshi, A., Jensen, A. K., and Marrogi, A. J. (1995). The role of cytokines in mediating the bystander effect using HSV-TK xenogeneic cells. *Cancer Lett.* **92,** 167–174.
170. Chen, C. Y., Chang, Y. N., Ryan, P., Linscott, M., McGarrity, G. J., and Chiang, Y. L. (1995). Effect of herpes simplex virus thymidine kinase expression levels on ganciclovir-mediated cytotoxicity and the "bystander effect." *Human Gene Ther.* **6,** 1467–1476.
171. Bi, W. L., Parysek, L. M., Warnick, R., and Stambrook, P. J. (1993). *In vitro* evidence that metabolic cooperation is responsible for the bystander effect observed with HSV tk retroviral gene therapy. *Human Gene Ther.* **4,** 725–731.
172. Colombo, B. M., Benedetti, S., Ottolenghi, S., *et al.* (1995). The "bystander effect": Association of U87 cell death with ganciclovir-mediated apoptosis of nearby cells and the lack of effect in athymic mice. *Human Gene Ther.* **6,** 763–772.
173. Kuriyama, S., Nakatani, T., Masui, K., *et al.* (1995). Bystander effect caused by suicide gene expression indicates the feasibility of gene therapy for hepatocellar carcinoma. *Hepatology* **22,** 1838–1846.
174. Mesnil, M., Piccoli, C., Tiraby, G., Willecke, K., and Yamasaki, H. (1996). Bystander killing of cancer cells by herpes simplex virus thymidine kinase gene is mediated by connexins. *Proc. Natl. Acad. Sci. U.S.A.* **93,** 1831–1835.
175. Fick, J., Barker, F. G., Dazin, P., Westphale, E. M., Beyer, E. C., and Israel, M. A. (1995). The extent of heterocellular communication mediated by gap junctions is predictive of bystander tumor cytotoxicity *in vitro*. *Proc. Natl. Acad. Sci. U.S.A.* **92,** 11071–11075.
176. Elshami, A. A., Saavedra, A., Zhang, H., *et al.* (1996). Gap junctions play a role in the bystander effect of the herpes simplex virus thymidine kinase ganciclovir system *in vitro*. *Gene Ther.* **3,** 85–92.
177. Mullen, C. A., Kilstrup, M., and Blaese, R. M. (1992). Transfer of bacterial gene for cytosine deaminase to mammalian cells confers lethal sensitivity to 5-fluorocytosine: a negative selection system. *Proc. Natl. Acad. Sci. U.S.A.* **89,** 33–37.
178. Mullen, C. A., Coale, M. M., Lowe, R., and Blaese, R. M. (1994). Tumors expressing the cytosine deaminase suicide gene can be eliminated *in vivo* with 5-fluorocytosine and induce protective immunity to wild type tumor. *Cancer Res.* **54,** 1503–1506.
179. Mroz, P. J., and Moolten, F. L. (1993). Retrovirally transduced *Escherichia coli gpt* genes combine selectability with chemosensitivity capable of mediating tumor eradication. *Human Gene Ther.* **4,** 589–595.
180. Tamiya, T., Ono, Y., Wei, M. X., Mroz, P. J., Moolten, F. L., and Chiocca, E. A. (1996). *Escherichia coli gpt* gene sensitizes rat glioma cells to killing by 6-thioxanthine or 6-thioguanine. *Cancer Gene Ther.* **3,** 155–162.
181. Parker, W. B., King, S. A., Allan, P. W., *et al.* (1997). *In vivo* gene therapy of cancer with *E. coli* purine nucleoside phosphorylase. *Human Gene Ther.* **8,** 1637–1644.
182. Bridgewater, J. A., Springer, C. J., Knox, R. J., Minton, N. P., Michael, N. P., and Collins, M. K. (1995). Expression of the bacterial nitroreductase enzyme in mammalian cells renders them selectively sensitive to killing by the prodrug CB1954. *Eur. J. Cancer* **31a,** 2362–2370.
183. Wei, M. X., Tamiya, T., Chase, M., *et al.* (1994). Experimental tumor therapy in mice using the cyclophosphamide-activating cytochrome P450 2B1 gene. *Human Gene Ther.* **5,** 969–978.
184. Marais, R., Spooner, R. A., Light, Y., Martin, J., and Springer, C. J. (1996). Gene-directed enzyme prodrug therapy with a mustard prodrug/carboxypeptidase G2 combination. *Cancer Res.* **56,** 4735–4742.
185. Roth, J. A., Nguyen, D., Lawrence, D. D., *et al.* (1996). Retrovirus-mediated wild-type p53 gene transfer to tumors of patients with lung cancer [see comments]. *Nature Med.* **2,** 985–991.
186. Hesdorffer, C., Ayello, J., Ward, M., *et al.* (1998). Phase I trial of retroviral-mediated transfer of the human MDR1 gene as marrow chemoprotection in patients undergoing high-dose chemotherapy and autologous stem-cell transplantation. *J. Clin. Oncol.* **16,** 165–172.
187. Krasnykh, V. N., Mikheeva, G. V., Douglas, J. T., and Curiel, D. T. (1996). Generation of recombinant adenovirus vectors with modified fibers for altering viral tropism. *J. Virol.* **70,** 6839–6846.
188. Weijtens, M. E., Willemsen, R. A., Hart, E. H., and Bolhuis, R. L. (1998). A retroviral vector system 'STITCH' in combination with an optimized single chain antibody chimeric receptor gene structure allows efficient gene transduction and expression in human T lymphocytes. *Gene Ther.* **5,** 1195–1203.
189. Richards, C. A., Wolberg, A. S., and Huber, B. E. (1993). The transcriptional control region of the human carcinoembryonic antigen gene: DNA sequence and homology studies. *DNA Seq.* **4,** 185–196.
190. Sakai, M., Morinaga, T., Urano, Y., Watanabe, K., Wegmann, T. G., and Tamaoki, T. (1985). The human α-fetoprotein gene. *J. Biol. Chem.* **260,** 5055–5060.
191. Su, H., Chang, J. C., Xu, S. M., and Kan, Y. W. (1996). Selective killing of AFP-positive hepatocellular carcinoma cells by adeno-associated virus transfer of the herpes simplex virus thymidine kinase gene. *Human Gene Ther.* **7,** 463–470.
192. Xu, G. W., Sun, Z. T., Forrester, K., Wang, X. W., Coursen, J., and Harris, C. C. (1996). Tissue-specific growth suppression and chemosensitivity promotion in human hepatocellular carcinoma cells by retroviral-mediated transfer of the wild-type p53 gene. *Hepatology* **24,** 1264–1268.
193. Lee, C. -H., Liu, M., Sie, K. -L., and Lee, M. -S. (1996). Prostate-specific antigen promoter driven gene therapy targeting DNA polymerase-α and topoisomerase IIα in prostate cancer. *Anticancer Res.* **16,** 1805–1812.

194. Pang, S., Taneja, S., Kaboo, R., *et al.* (1994). Gene therapy: Prostate tissue specificity of the promoter for prostate specific antigen (PSA): Potential approach for the development of target specific gene therapy. Cold Spring Harbor Symposium on Quantitative Biology, Vol. 59; pp. 677–707. Cold Spring Harbor, Cold Spring Harbor Laboratory.
195. Datta, R., Rubin, E., Sukhatme, V., *et al.* (1992). Ionizing radiation activates transcription of the EGR1 gene via CArG elements. *Proc. Natl. Acad. Sci. U.S.A.* **89,** 10149–10153.
196. Staba, M. J., Mauceri, H. J., Kufe, D. W., Hallahan, D. E., and Weichselbaum, R. R. (1998). Adenoviral TNF-alpha gene therapy and radiation damage tumor vasculature in a human malignant glioma xenograft. *Gene Ther.* **5,** 293–300.
197. Dranoff, G. (1998). Cancer gene therapy: Connecting basic research with clinical inquiry. *J. Clin. Oncol.* **16,** 2548–2556.
198. Greten, T. F., and Jaffee, E. M. (1999). Cancer vaccines. *J. Clin. Oncol.* **17,** 1047–1060.

39

Active Immunotherapy for Cancer

Keith D. Amos, David C. Linehan, and Timothy J. Eberlein

Department of Surgery, Washington University School of Medicine, St. Louis, Missouri 63110

I. Introduction

The role of the immune system in the recognition and regression of cancers has recently been an area of intense study. Throughout the twentieth century, the interactions between the immune system and tumor cells have been investigated as a treatment for cancer. In 1890, Dr. William Coley, a surgeon at the New York Cancer Hospital, began to review the case histories of sarcoma patients. Dr. Coley found that, with few exceptions, sarcoma patients had a rapid recurrence of the disease after treatment. Among the few success stories described, he noticed that some infection was almost always present (1). This association had been previously documented by others. Samuel Gross noted this phenomenon in an analysis of long bone sarcoma written in 1879. In 1813, others believed that there was an antagonistic relationship between gangrene and cancer. Other associations were noted between cancer regression and malaria and tuberculosis.

The core of Dr. Coley's research was a review of the cases of sarcoma patients treated over a 15-year period at the New York Hospital and the New York Cancer Hospital. One particular case stood out from the 90 cases reviewed. A 29-year-old male patient had undergone surgery five times for a round-cell sarcoma of the neck. The tumor had recurred after each of the first four resections. On the fifth resection, the tumor was only partially resected. The patient developed a severe erysipelas infection in the wound postoperatively. Remarkably, he recovered from the infection, and the remnant of the unresected tumor spontaneously regressed. With 7 years of follow-up, there was no recurrence of tumor. Coley reasoned that if an accidental infection of erysipelas could trigger the body to eradicate a sarcoma, then a deliberate inoculation of erysipelas should accomplish similar results. Coley began his experimental treatments by "giving injections of bouillon cultures of erysipelas directly into the tumor of the neck" of another patient with a recurrent neck sarcoma. This study formed the beginning of Coley's toxins and the foundations for the study of immunotherapy for cancer.

Early immunotherapists followed Coley's lead and nonspecific immune stimulation strategies were supplanted by novel methods aimed at generating a tumor-specific immune response. Most initial attempts involved vaccines using autologous or allogeneic cancer cells or cancer cell lysates together with a variety of adjuvants (2). The field has since evolved dramatically as a result of the molecular identification of tumor antigens and an advanced understanding of the molecular biology of antigen presentation and recognition and the antitumor immune response.

Active cancer immunotherapies are divided into three broad categories: (1) nonspecific immune system stimulation, (2) adoptive transfer of *ex vivo* expanded immune effector cells, and (3) immunization with vaccine. This is in contrast to passive immunotherapy, whereby immunoglobulins (sometimes conjugated to chemotherapeutic agents) specific for tumor-associated antigens (TAAs) expressed on the cell surface are infused into patients. This strategy has shown some promise in hematologic malignancies (3). The distinction revolves around the role of the host in tumor rejection, although, in some cases, even with passive transfer of immunoglobulins, host effectors are necessary for the generation and sustenance of an antitumor response. In this chapter we focus on cell-mediated, tumor-specific approaches to immunotherapy with emphasis placed on developing vaccine strategies. Because this text is devoted to surgical research, we focus on the current state of cancer vaccine research examining the laboratory methods that are fundamental to TAA identification and assessment of immune effector recognition, activation, proliferation, and cytolytic activity.

Several examples of nonspecific immune stimulants used in cancer treatment can be cited. Nonspecific activation of the immune system with adjuvants, such as bacillus Calmette–Guérin (BCG) and lipopolysaccharide (LPS), has shown success in the treatment of certain tumors. BCG has been shown to be superior to chemotherapy in the treatment of superficial bladder cancer (4). The endotoxin LPS has been shown to have antitumor activity (5). Direct intratumoral injection of LPS causes tumor regression; however, the toxicity of this agent has limited its use. Other nonspecific immune stimulants have been used successfully in the treatment of cancer, most notably the use of adjuvant levamisole in combination with 5-fluorouracil in the adjuvant treatment of resected, node-positive colon cancer, although the mechanism of its action is poorly understood (6).

Most studies of adoptive immunotherapy have focused on the cell-mediated immune response and the transfer of *ex vivo* activated tumor-specific cytotoxic T lymphocytes or lymphokine-activated killer (LAK) cells (7–10). Early melanoma immunotherapies used expanded *ex vivo* populations of tumor-infiltrating lymphocytes (TILs) from melanoma lesions. With advances in T cell culture technique, T cells isolated from patients' tumors (which presumably have a high prevalence of tumor specific cytotoxic T lymphocytes) are isolated, expanded *ex vivo* to large numbers, and reinfused into patients with measurable metastasic disease. Initial results showed some dramatic regression of tumor in select patients, but the majority of patients showed little or no clinical response.

Vaccine therapy implies the immunization of a tumor-bearing host with an antigen to induce a host T cell or an antibody-mediated immune response to tumor cells. The goal of all vaccination therapy is to induce a sustained tumor-specific immunity that causes tumor regression and/or prevents recurrence. There are a variety of vaccination methods to initiate cell-mediated tumor recognition, as shown in Table I (11). Clinical trials have evolved considerably, from initial studies using irradiated whole tumor cell vaccines (12) or tumor cell lysates, to current protocols using vaccination with synthetic antigenic peptides, antigen-presenting cells, naked DNA, or genetically modified

Table I Categories of Cancer Vaccines[a]

Type	Description
Whole cancer cells	Inactivated cancer cells and their extracts can jump-start the immune system. Cancer cells engineered to secrete cytokines, such as IL-2 or GM-CSF, similarly heighten antitumor immunity. Cells designed to express costimulatory molecules, such as B-7, enhance the ability of T cells to recognize tumor cells
Peptides	Tumor peptides, fragments of tumor proteins recognized by T cells, are injected alone or with immune-boosting adjuvants
Proteins	Antigen-presenting cells take up injected tumor proteins and break them down into a range of peptide fragments recognized by T cells
Dendritic cells	These antigen-presenting cells are isolated from the blood, exposed to tumor peptides, or engineered to produce tumor proteins and then reinjected
Gangliosides	Humans can produce antibodies to these molecules, such as GM2, found on the surface of tumor cells. Clinical studies have shown that melanoma patients with GM2 antibodies have a better prognosis
Heat-shock proteins	These cellular constituents ordinarily bind peptides. Injecting heat-shock proteins isolated from tumors rouses antitumor immunity in mice
Viral and bacterial vectors	Genes coding for tumor antigens are incorporated into viral or bacterial genomes. When injected, these altered infectious agents draw immunity against themselves and the encoded antigens
Nucleic acids	DNA and RNA coding for tumor antigens prompt normal cells to begin producing these antigens

[a]Cancer vaccines are intended to induce T cells or other components of the immune system to recognize and vigorously attack malignant tissue. From (11), with permission.

(cytokine-secreting) tumor cells (13–). For example, T lymphocyte sensitization and clinical responses of tumor regression have been documented in melanoma patients treated with dendritic cells transfected with tumor-associated peptide antigens (15). However, the number of patients treated in these vaccination trials has been small and controlled trials are lacking.

Vaccines are being tested that elicit a humoral response against aberrantly expressed cell surface molecules such as the ganglioside GM2. Humans can produce antibodies to these cell surface molecules. It has been shown that naturally occuring or vaccine-induced antibodies to GM2 are associated with a better prognosis in melanoma patients (19, 20). From these preliminary clinical trials, more antigen-specific vaccines are being designed for future protocols.

Immunotherapy research over the past decade has focused on the activation of tumor-specific T cells. We know from early results of clinical trials and *in vivo* experimentation that this, by itself, is insufficient, although essential, for a clinically relevant antitumor immune response. It is clear that other factors such as the cytokine milieu, costimulatory molecules, and other immune effector cells are important to the complex interaction that culminates in the immune recognition and destruction of tumor cells. The challenge remains to take lessons learned at the research bench regarding the immunobiology of the antitumor immune response and design rational, sound, hypothesis-driven clinical trials for cancer patients.

Methods to identify molecules produced by cancer cells that can be recognized by antigen-specific T lymphocytes are fundamental to the development of new anticancer vaccines. The rapidity with which anticancer vaccine trials have been developed is due to the fact that powerful new methods of TAA identification have emerged over the past decade (21). In this chapter, we describe experimental methods of tumor antigen identification, methods for measuring tumor-specific cytotoxic T lymphocyte (CTL) activation and effector function, and research strategies for the development of anti-cancer vaccine trials.

II. Methods of Antigen Identification

Figure 1 shows a simplistic schematic of the complex interaction between immune effector cells and a tumor antigen presented on the cell surface by a major histocompatibility complex (MHC) molecule. These molecules bind 8–10 amino acid peptides that are fragments of the cellular protein repertoire produced by that particular cell. The MHC/peptide complex is presented to T cells for recognition by the T cell receptor (TCR). Key to this interaction between CD8$^+$ T cell and target cell is the 9- to 10-amino acid peptide antigen that differentiates tumor cells from normal cells. Though understanding of the complex interaction of costimulatory molecules, cytokines, and other immune effector cells (such as helper CD4$^+$ T cells and antigen-presenting cells) is important, the identification of relevant tumor antigens is the critical first step in manipulating the immune system to reject tumors. We therefore focus on the methodology and strategy of TAA identification. Table II depicts the currently defined cancer antigens and their allele-specific MHC restriction.

A. cDNA Expression Cloning

The earliest method used to identify tumor antigens was pioneered by Boon and colleagues at the Ludwig Institute for Cancer Research in Belgium (22, 23). Starting with tumor-specific CTLs generated from tumor-stimulated peripheral blood lymphocytes or TILs, a cDNA library of a tumor or tumor cell line is screened to identify and isolate genes that encode TAAs. This method involves the transfection of genomic DNA or a cDNA library from tumor cells recognized by cytotoxic T lymphocytes into other cell lines expressing a matching major histocompatibility complex. MHC molecules are extracellular proteins that are present on the surface of nucleated cells. Before transfection, the target cell line is not recognized by the tumor-specific cytotoxic T lymphocytes. Clones that expressed genes encoding

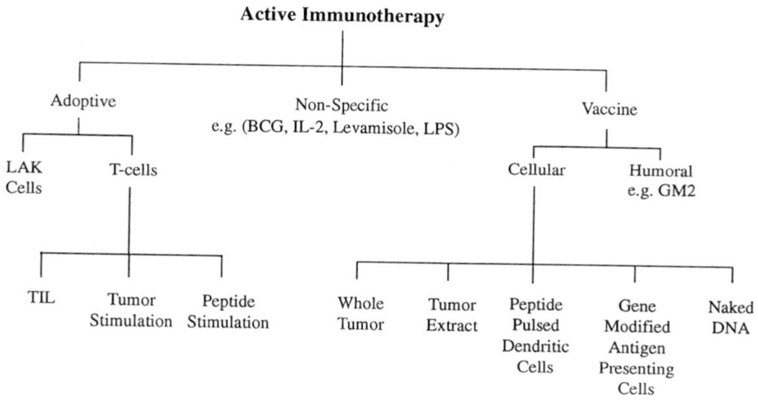

Figure 1 Classification of methods of active immunotherapy.

for tumor antigens are selected on the basis of their ability to stimulate cytokine release or cytolytic activity from TILs or CTLs. The approach was improved by transiently transfecting cDNA pools into COS-7 or 293 cells with a cDNA of an HLA-matched molecule to the CTL. These highly transfectable cell lines provided immediate testing of clones recognized by CTLs. The cDNA pools could be easily subcloned until a single gene (encoding the TAA) was identified and sequenced.

The majority of human tumor-associated antigens were identified using this approach and novel TAAs continue to be discovered with this method. This method was used by the Boon and Rosenberg groups to identify tumor-associated antigens in melanoma and other cancers. Antigens identified using this method include the MAGE family of proteins, MART-1, tyrosinase, gp75, CDK4, and p15(21). This group of antigens has expanded to include several other melanoma and nonmelanoma antigens and the list of novel TAAs continues to grow.

Although this is a powerful method for antigen identification, there are several drawbacks to cDNA expression cloning:

1. One must be able to isolate large numbers of tumor-specific lymphocytes for clone screening. Tumor-specific lymphocytes can be isolated from solid tumors, lymph nodes, metastatic effusions, and peripheral blood. Although there are several sources for tumor-specific lymphocytes, it is often difficult to isolate enough lymphocytes from certain solid tumor types. The majority of T cells are not tumor specific, even if screening is performed with TILs.

2. There is the likelihood that there will be identification of cDNA clones that encode cross-reactive peptides recognized by T lymphocytes due to the high expression level in the COS system.

3. Although the gene encoding the antigen is identified, one will need to perform further studies to obtain the amino acid sequence of the antigen epitope.

Table II Defined Cancer Antigens[a]

Tumor antigen category	Antigen	MHC restriction
Melanocyte differentiation	MART-1/MelanA	A2, B45
	gp100	A2, A3, A24
	Tyrosinase	A1, A2, A24, DR4
	TRP-1	A31
	TRP-2	A2, A31, A68
Cancer, testis	MAGE-1	A1, Cw16
	MAGE-3	A1, A2, B44
	GAGE-1/2	Cw16
	BAGE	Cw16
	RAGE	B7
	NY-ESO-1	A2, A31
Tumor specific	CDK-4	A2
	β-Catenin	A24
	MUM-1	B44
	Caspase-8	B35
	KIAA0205	B44
	HPVE7	A2
	HER2/neu	A2
	PSMA	A2
Widely expressed	SART-1	A26
	PRAME	A24
	p15	A24
	Mucin	Unrestricted

[a]From (21), copyright 1999 Cell Press.

B. In Vitro Sensitization against Candidate Tumor Antigens

When tumor antigens are known or suspected, *in vitro* sensitization of T cells can be employed to generate tumor-specific CTLs and thus prove antigenicity (24, 25). A candidate tumor antigen is selected or identified based on tumor-specific expression, tumor-specific overexpression, or the gene cloning method described previously. The amino acid sequence of the candidate protein is screened for known HLA binding epitopes (26, 27). These epitopes are selected based on anchor residues that promote noncovalent binding between peptides and MHC molecules. The anchor residue positions are at positions two, nine, or ten. Allele-specific peptide motifs are known and candidate antigen proteins can be screened for binding affinity, synthesized, and pulsed onto allele-specific APCs to test for their ability to generate peptide-specific, tumor-specific CTLs.

After synthesis, the crude peptide must be purified and analyzed for quality. Purification is performed by gel filtration (GF) chromatography or reversed-phased high-performance liquid chromatography (HPLC). HPLC more thoroughly purifies crude peptides. The purification process removes any cleavage reaction scavengers, truncated peptide sequences, and peptides with side-chain protecting groups. After purification is performed, peptide molecular weight can be verified with mass spectometry.

To screen for reactivity, the synthetic peptide is pulsed onto antigen-presenting cells expressing the appropriate HLA type. Ebstein–Barr virus (EBV)-transformed B lymphoblasts, T2 cells, and dendritic cells have been used as antigen-presenting cells. These APCs are favored due to high level of MHC and costimulatory molecules expressed on the cell surface. The expression of these molecules is required for proper T cell activation and the avoidance of anergy. The peptide-pulsed APCs are then irradiated and cocultured with lymphocytes. The lymphocytes are restimulated with peptide-pulsed APCs on a weekly basis. After the third or fourth stimulation, the lymphocytes are assessed for cytotoxic activity and/or cytokine release. Cytotoxic activity is measured through the ^{51}Cr release assay, and enzyme-linked immunosorbent assays (ELISAs) are used to measure cytokines such as interferon-γ and granulocyte–macrophage colony-stimulating factor (GM-CSF). Any lymphocyte activity should be observed by week three of stimulation. In our experience, optimal CTL activity is seen after the third stimulation.

There are several potential problems with this method.

1. Each peptide sequence selected is only a prediction. The actual peptide sequence may not be expressed by MHC on living cells.
2. Large proteins may contain hundreds of potential peptides. It may be necessary to screen a large number of candidate peptides to identify one immunogenic sequence. A large screening process can be time consuming and costly.
3. Synthesis and purification of peptides by biotechnology companies is expensive. For a nonameric peptide, costs can range up to $600.
4. Peptide binding affinity may not correlate with CTL activity or tumor antigenicity.

C. Peptide Elution

Peptides expressed on MHC molecules on tumor cells can be isolated by acid (28, 29). For this method, *in vitro* tumor lines are washed in an acidic citrate–phosphate buffer. The acid wash is removed and centrifuged to remove cell debris. The supernatant is passed through a C18 column. The peptides are eluted from the column and lyophilized. After reconstitution in the citrate–phosphate buffer, the peptides are filtered through an ultrafiltration device. The filtrate is injected onto a C18 analytical column. Reverse-phase liquid chromatography is used to separate the peptides, which are finally collected in 1-ml fractions. These peptide fractions are lyophilized and reconstituted in Hank's balanced salt solution (HBSS). The fractions are then used in peptide-pulsed cytotoxic assays. Fractions that are capable of generating tumor-specific CTLs undergo sequence identification by mass spectrometry. Problems with this method include (1) the need for highly specialized, expensive equipment; (2) requirement for specific peptides present in sufficient amounts on tumor cells to undergo the series of elution and identification steps; (3) need for massive numbers of tumor cells to elute an adequate amount of peptide for sequencing; and (4) need for large numbers of T cells to screen candidate peptides.

D. Heat-Shock Protein-Associated Peptides

Heat-shock proteins (HSPs) are a ubiquitously expressed superfamily of proteins. Certain HSPs are known to associate with a broad array of cellular peptides that are generated during protein degradation, such that the HSPs chaperone the antigenic repertoire of the cells from which they are purified. It has been shown by Srivastava and colleagues that purified HSP70 and HSP90 carry a range of noncovalently associated endogenous peptides and that HSP fractions of any given cell type contain the peptide repertoire of that particular cell type (30, 31). Studies from Srivastava *et al.* have shown that vaccination of mice and rats with HSP–peptide complexes leads to a strong antigen-specific cellular response against peptides (mediated by $CD4^+$ and $CD8^+$ CTLs), but not against HSP molecules.

The HSP–peptide complexes are stable and withstand conventional biochemical fractionation. There are several methods to isolate HSPs from cells, the most common of which is adenosine 5′-triphosphate affinity chromatography (32). The HSP preparations obtained from tumor cells can be used to generate antigen-specific, MHC class I-restricted, cytotoxic T lymphocytes. Mice are immunized twice weekly with subcutaneous injections of HSP preparations. Injections are performed without adjuvant. After final injection on day seven, spleens are harvested. Splenocytes are cocultured with the cognate stimulator cells for 5 to 7 days. T cells are then tested for cytotoxicity with a chromium release assay or cytokine release assay.

Similarly, vaccination with tumor-derived HSP70 in a murine metastatic tumor model has shown a reduction in progression of primary tumors, diminished metastases, and prolongation of survival when compared with HSP derived from nonautologous tumors. The advantage of such a vaccination method is that immunotherapy can be delivered without the need to identify specific antigenic epitopes and specific MHC alleles. There are, however, two major problems with this technique:

1. HSP isolation is difficult. There are several protocols for isolation that include several reagents and a multitude of steps. Fresh tumor specimen is required.
2. HSP–peptide immunization avoids identification of antigenic peptide sequences. Therefore, HSP–peptide complexes isolated from a patient's cancer can serve as only customized, patient-specific therapeutic vaccines. Generation of a unique vaccine for each patient would be labor intensive and costly and would depend on successful HSP isolation from each patient's tumor cells.

E. SEREX

In 1995, Sahin *et al.* (33) introduced a method for identification of human tumor antigens that elicit a humoral immune response. The method is called serological identification of antigens by recombinant expression cloning (SEREX). Novel and previously defined tumor antigens have been identified using this method. SEREX uses diluted serum from cancer patients to screen cDNA libraries prepared from autologous tumors for immune recognition. Although this method uses antibodies from the patient's humoral response for screening, it is assumed that helper T cell activity stimulates antibody production, and therefore a humoral response correlates with a cell-mediated response. SEREX is therefore able to identify antigens recognized by both B and T cells. SEREX analysis of several human tumor types has identified a number of novel tumor antigens, including the class of antigens described as "tumor–testis antigens," which are expressed in normal testis and tumor (e.g., SSX2/HOM-MEL-40 and NY-ESO-1) (34).

Briefly, the method involves the extraction of mRNA from autologous tumor samples. The mRNA is then used to generate a cDNA expression library in a bacteriophage. Serum is obtained from the tumor-bearing host. The bacteriophages are used to infect bacteria, resulting in expression of the recombinant proteins in the bacteria and capture on a nitrocellulose membrane. Membranes are incubated with autologous sera to permit antibodies to bind to unique, tumor-derived proteins or protein fragments. This is followed by a secondary enzyme-labeled antihuman antibody and the membranes are then developed. Serum-positive clones are subcloned and retested. The plasmid DNA is purified and restriction enzyme digested to cut out the candidate gene. The cDNA inserts are then sequenced for identification.

Of the methods described in this chapter for antigen identification, the SEREX method does not initially require T cells for antigen identification. There is no need to establish stable *in vitro* CTLs for TAA identification. In addition, there is also no need to establish autologous tumor lines. This is a particular advantage to the study of prostate, breast, and colon cancer lines, which are generally very difficult to maintain in culture.

A problem with the SEREX method includes the lack of identification of the specific class I peptide antigen sequence. This method assumes that there is a class II or helper (CD4) T cell response that promotes antibody formation. There is not always a strong correlation between cytotoxic (CD8) T cell response to tumor and antibody formation.

III. Assays of Cytotoxic T Lymphocyte Activation and Function

Activation of T cells requires a cell-to-cell interaction involving the T cell receptor and its putative antigen expressed by an antigen-presenting cell (APC). This interaction has been difficult to study for many reasons, not the least of which is the complex interaction between several accessory and costimulatory molecules that is required to cause activation and proliferation (see Fig. 2). Cloning tumor-specific T cells can be difficult because their prevalence is low for any given antigen, and, hence, the elucidation of this very specific and complex interaction is a daunting task. Furthermore, even if the TCR finds its antigen, if the appropriate accessory and costimulatory molecules are absent, anergy results (35, 36).

Assays that measure the tumor specificity and cytotoxicity of tumor-specific CTLs are the foundation of tumor immunology research. Here we review the standard assays used to assess *in vitro* T cell activation and function. CTLs are defined by their unique ability to destroy target cells by one of two mechanisms: (1) TCR-mediated granule exocytosis of perforins and other cellular toxins or (2) cross-linking of fas ligand (FasL) or similar molecules to specific receptors on the target cell, resulting in target cell apoptosis (37). Tumor specificity of CTLs has been assessed by examining various steps along this pathway that include initial T cell activation by TCR/antigen binding, proliferation of CTLs in response to binding, cytokine release as a result of this specific interaction, and, finally, through direct measures of target cell destruction in CTL/target cell coculture.

Lymphocyte effector function has been characterized and quantitated using these *in vitro* assays, but the *in vivo* relevance of such antigen recognition and target cell killing does not always correspond with *in vitro* findings. However, the design of many *in vivo* studies in both animal and human studies is based on tumor specificity and cytotoxicity observed in these *in vitro* assays. In addition, non-MHC-restricted cytotoxicity can be observed with other immune effectors such as natural killer (NK) cells and macrophages, but the majority of research in the area of active immunotherapy has focused on the very specific CTL/tumor cell interaction.

A. Activation

CTL activation is a complex, specific interaction whereby the TCR of a quiescent T cell encounters its putative antigen presented on the cell surface of a target cell (class I) or an APC (class I and II) in the context of a specific major histocompatability complex. This interaction results in T cell activation if the appropriate costimulatory and adhesion molecules (e.g., B-7, ICAM-1, LFA-3) are present to facilitate activation (38). In the absence of these molecules, anergy develops. Professional antigen-presenting cells such as dendritic cells (DCs) have the requisite cell surface costimulatory proteins to promote T cell activation and not anergy when the TCR/MHC/antigen interaction occurs. Both preclinical and clinical studies have focused on the use of DCs as APCs and multiple strategies are being tested, including gene-modified and or peptide-pulsed DCs as vaccines (18, 39). Molecular characterization of the complex ligand–receptor interactions that occur during antigen presentation and T cell activation continues to be elucidated, and, certain-

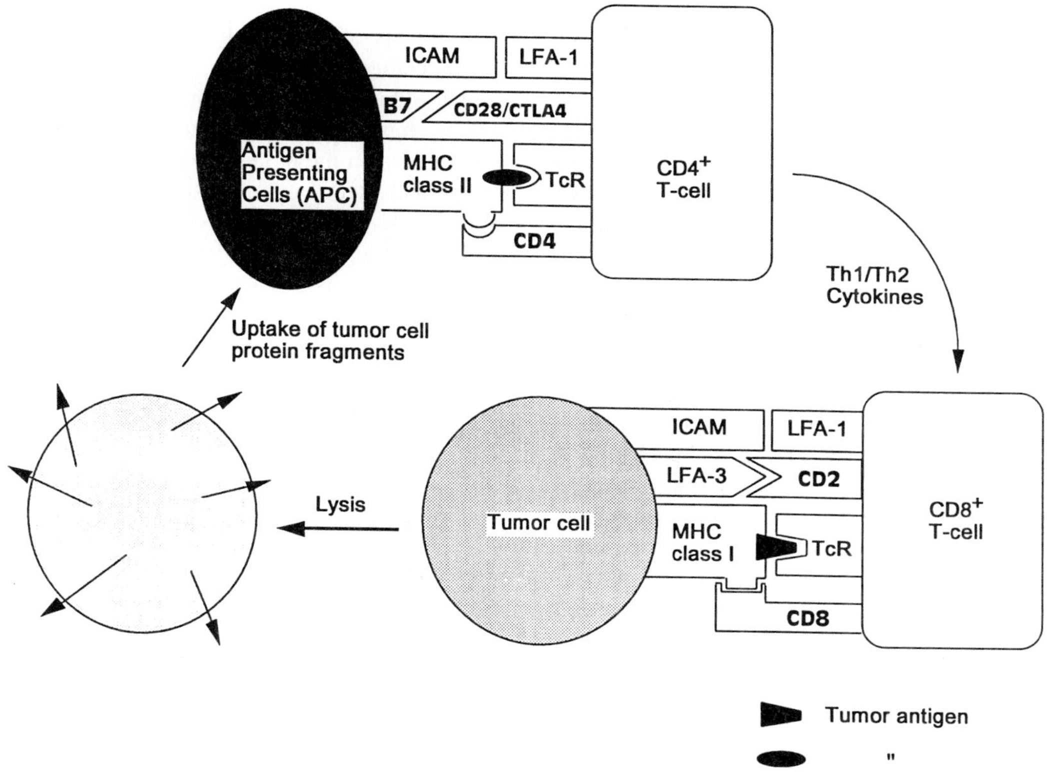

Figure 2 Schematic overview of the general activation pathways of tumor-specific $CD4^+$ and $CD8^+$ T cells. $CD4^+$ T cells recognize TAAs by HLA class II molecules on APCs. Costimulation is provided by the B7/CTLA4 interaction. Activated $CD4^+$ T cells produce cytokines that regulates cytotoxic T lymphocytes ($CD8^+$). The $CD8^+$ cells directly interact with the HLA class I molecules presenting TAAs on tumor cells. Lysed tumor cell fragments are taken up by APCs and are processed for recognition by $CD4^+$ T cells. From (34a), with permission.

ly, complex sets of triggers and counterregulatory controls govern this process, which protects the organism from autoimmunity.

Many studies have used techniques of nonspecific T cell activation prior to antigen-specific stimulation in order to generate a population of tumor-specific or antigen-specific CTLs. Early studies in adoptive immunotherapy (including our own) used large numbers of *ex vivo* expanded CTLs. Nonspecific activation followed by antigen-specific stimulation and culture in IL-2-enriched medium resulted in up to 10,000-fold expansion of T cells obtained from tumors (TILs). In our laboratory, we have accomplished nonspecific stimulation using solid-phase anti-CD3 activation by incubating T cells on antibody-coated flasks containing anti-CD3 mAb for 12 to 24 hr. This results in a nonspecific proliferative response of naive T cells, which are then stimulated with tumor-specific peptide antigen or intact irradiated tumor cells to elicit a tumor-specific response. Using this technique, we have been able to generate tumor-specific CTLs against tumor-specific peptides (derived from a tumor-associated, overexpressed protooncogene, HER2/neu) in breast, ovarian, lung, and pancreas cancer (24, 40–43).

Experimental models designed to study T cell activation have included (1) measurement of signal transduction events such as calcium flux or tyrosine phosphorylation or (2) increase in cell surface expression of markers of activation such as interleukin-2 receptor (IL-2R) or class II MHC molecules (37). These markers appear early and are nonspecific and their presence or absence does not always correlate with a cellular response. Most would agree that a downstream marker, such as cytokine production or cytotoxicity, is a better experimental measurement to test to assure that an antigen-specific activation of T cells has occurred. Calcium flux or tyrosine phosphorylation is a nonspecific marker because other interactions besides TCR/antigen binding can cause these events, and hence this is a rarely used measure of a tumor-specific CTL response.

B. Proliferation

Proliferation of T cells is easily measured after T cell activation. The simplest method is simple cell counting using trypan blue exclusion and a hemacytometer. Typically, a 10- to 100-fold increase in the number of viable T cells is seen after activation, in the first 3–7 days. A more precise and quantifiable measurement of T cell proliferation involves the uptake of [^{3}H]thymidine, because rapidly proliferating cells will incorporate the radiolabeled thymidine into their DNA, and the amount can be quantified using a beta counter. This is a widely used proliferation assay that can quantify increased cell division, but again is not specific for CTL induction and proliferation.

C. Cytokine Release

The most sensitive measure of CTL tumor specificity is the demonstration of tumor-specific cytokine release, which occurs when CTLs and target cells are coincubated. Tumor-specific cytokine release (e.g., interferon-γ, interleukin-2, tumor necrosis factor) by CTLs is easily measured and can be used to demonstrate a specific TCR/antigen interaction. Enzyme-linked immunosorbent assays are used to quantify cytokine release in the supernatant of mixed CTLs and target cell coculture (44). Using an antibody-coated microtiter well for the cytokine of interest, the cytokine is bound to the solid-phase antibody. Finally, a second antibody, linked to enzyme, is added and enzyme activity is quantitated by absorbance. This gives a precise measurement of the amount of a specific cytokine released by CTLs in response to a target cell.

A more sensitive variation of the measurement of cytokine production has been advocated as an assay to demonstrate tumor specificity of CTLs. This method, real-time polymerase chain reaction (PCR), measures mRNA production for a specific cytokine as the result of the interaction of CTLs and target cells (45). There are two major advantages of this method: (1) it measures an upstream step to cytokine production that can be used to identify TCR/ligand binding at a very early phase in the interaction and (2) it can be performed on biopsy material or small tumor fragments. Translation of cytokine mRNA, processing, and extracellular secretion are required to detect the tumor-specific interaction when ELISA is used, but with real-time PCR, the TCR binding ligand elicits an immediate up-regulation of cytokine mRNA that can be measured quickly and directly.

D. Cytotoxicity

In vitro cytotoxicity assays have played a major role in the development of clinical trials in active immunotherapy. The advantage of these assays over cytokine release assays is that they require measurable target cell destruction by CTLs and therefore may be more likely to mimic the *in vivo* biology of tumor-specific CTL function. Target cell death can be measured by two different methods related to two different cellular dysfunctions seen as the target cells die: (1) the loss of plasma membrane integrity and (2) DNA fragmentation.

The standard technique in the field for measuring target cell death is the chromium release assay, which relates to the loss of plasma membrane integrity of target cells mediated by the activated T cell in response to TCR/antigen binding (46). Target cells are loaded with ^{51}Cr, an isotope that is reduced intracellularly to $^{51}Cr^{3+}$ and complexes with intracellular anions. When plasma membrane integrity is disrupted, these complexes are released into the supernatant and cannot be taken up by other living cells in the reaction mixture. Gamma emission can then be quantitated as an indirect measure of cell death.

Another measure of cell death that has been advocated is an assay that measures DNA fragmentation as an early step in cell death in response to activated CTLs (47). The characteristic pattern of apoptotic target cell death associated with CTLs is characterized by early DNA fragmentation by endonucleases, and a commitment to cell death that can be measured prior to perforin-mediated cell membrane instability. Apoptosis can be measured using annexin V/propidium iodide staining (48). However, we do not commonly use this type of assay in our laboratory and we find the chromium release assay to be simple, inexpensive, and reproducible.

Although CTLs are defined by their *in vitro* characteristics, *in vivo* studies that have shown antitumor activity have been a major impetus to the development of active immunotherapy clinical trials. Many murine models have been used where adoptive transfer of tumor-stimulated or antigen-stimulated CTLs has resulted in measurable antitumor activity (most commonly in pulmonary metastasis models) (49). Similarly, such adoptive transfer has conveyed protective immunity against subsequent challenge with wild-type tumor, again suggesting *in vivo* efficacy. In addition, multiple murine studies have shown that vaccination with gene-modified tumor cells can result in protective immunity to subsequent challenge with tumor and to the eradication of established tumors (50, 51). The most commonly used experimental models include simple measurement of subcutaneously injected tumor implants and pulmonary metastasis counting models.

In the case of adoptive transfer of *ex vivo* generated CTLs, the mechanism of tumor cell death, however, is a complex process that involves other host factors. Using a congenic mouse model that allows us to differentiate between host and adoptively transferred immune effector cells, our group has been able to show that adoptively transferred cells are able to initiate an antitumor immune response, but host effectors are necessary to sustain the response. It is the host effectors, that are important for detectable target cell death (52, 53). Because CTLs are major sources of interferon-γ and other cytokines, the contribution of host effector cells stimulated by the cytokine milieu created by CTLs needs to be considered. Thus, although adoptively transferred cells may be required to initiate a series of events resulting in tumor cell destruction, the *in vivo* mechanism of cell death is not simplistic and likely does not correlate with the artificial environment created in *in vitro* assays.

E. Pitfalls of Assays Measuring CTL Function

There are several examples by which tumor-specific cytokine release or cytotoxicity can be demonstrated, but *in vitro* cytotoxicity assays show no lytic activity. This emphasizes the point that T cell antigen recognition, activation, proliferation, cytokine release, and ultimate target cell lysis are a complex series of reactions that are difficult to measure. *In vitro* measurements cannot mimic the *in vivo* situation wherein a specific microenvironment composed of many cell types and cytokines results in T cell activation, proliferation, and tumor destruction. Despite the popularity of these assays in demonstrating tumor specificity, the complexity of the interaction and the sensitivity of the test are such that the biological relevance of the model remains questionable.

IV. Summary

Powerful new methods to identify tumor-associated antigens have renewed enthusiasm for the testing of active immunotherapies for cancer. Similarly, our ever-improving knowledge of the biology of antigen presentation and T cell activation has stimulated interest in the development of cancer vaccines that can elicit a sustained antitumor response. Many different clinical trials employing diverse strategies of active immunotherapy have been recently commenced. The most promising vaccines include cell-based vaccinations using professional antigen-presenting cells, such as dendritic cells that have been gene modified or exogenously loaded with known tumor antigens. Cell culture techniques have been perfected and dendritic cells can be grown for *in vitro* or *in vivo* use. Such promising new techniques, which combine novel tumor antigens and lessons learned from studying the biology of antigen presentation, are currently being tested.

Active immunotherapy has evolved rapidly over the past decade and in a short time we have progressed from simple strategies using whole tumor cell vaccines (with no knowledge of the important tumor rejection antigens) to sophisticated gene-modified dendritic cell vaccines based on specific, known tumor antigens. This is a perfect example whereby lessons learned at the laboratory bench (many of which have been pioneered by surgeons) can be rapidly used in translational research in order to design sound, focused clinical trials.

References

1. Coley, W. B. (1891). Contribution to the knowledge of sarcoma. *Ann. Surg.* **14,** 199–220.
2. Slingluff, C. L., Jr., and Seigler, H. F. (1992). Immunotherapy for malignant melanoma with a tumor cell vaccine. *Ann. Plast. Surg.* **28,** 104–107.
3. Sievers, E. L., *et al.* (1999). Selective ablation of acute myeloid leukemia using antibody-targeted chemotherapy: A phase I study of an anti-CD33 calicheamicin immunoconjugate. *Blood* **93,** 3678–3684.
4. Lamm, D. L., *et al.* (1991). A randomized trial of intravesical doxorubicin and immunotherapy with bacille Calmette–Guerin for transitional-cell carcinoma of the bladder. *N. Engl. J. Med.* **325,** 1205–1209.
5. Nowotny, A, and Butler, R. C. (1979) Studies on the endotoxin induced tumor resistance. *Adv. Exp. Med. Biol.* **121B,** 455–469.
6. Moertel, C. G., *et al.* (1990). Levamisole and fluorouracil for adjuvant therapy of resected colon carcinoma [see comments]. *N. Engl. J. Med.* **322,** 352–358.
7. Oettgen, H., and Old, L. (1991). The history of cancer immunotherapy. *In* "Biologic Therapy of Cancer" (V. DeVita, S. Hellman, and S. A. Rosenberg, eds.), pp. 87–119. Lippicott, Philadelphia.
8. Topalian, S. L., and Rosenberg, S. A. (1987). Therapy of cancer using the adoptive transfer of activated killer cells and interleukin-2. *Acta Haematol.* **78** (Suppl. 1), 75–76.
9. Lotze, M. T., and Rosenberg, S. A. (1986). Results of clinical trials with the administration of interleukin 2 and adoptive immunotherapy with activated cells in patients with cancer. *Immunobiology* **172,** 420–437.
10. Goedegebuure, P. S., *et al.* (1995). Adoptive immunotherapy with tumor-infiltrating lymphocytes and interleukin-2 in patients with metastatic malignant melanoma and renal cell carcinoma: A pilot study. *J. Clin. Oncol.* **13,** 1939-1349.
11. Old, L. J. (1996). Immunotherapy for cancer. *Sci. Am.* **275,** 136–143.
12. Eton, O., *et al.* (1998). Active immunotherapy with ultraviolet B-irradiated autologous whole melanoma cells plus DETOX in patients with metastatic melanoma. *Clin. Cancer Res.* **4,** 619–627.
13. Salgaller, M. L., Marincola, F. M., Cormier, J. N., and Rosenberg, S. A. (1996). Immunization against epitopes in the human melanoma antigen gp 100 following patient immunization with synthetic peptides. *Cancer Res.* **56,** 4749–4757.
14. Overwijk, W. W., *et al.* (1999). Vaccination with a recombinant vaccinia virus encoding a "self" antigen induces autoimmune vitiligo and tumor cell destruction in mice: Requirement for CD4(+) T lymphocytes. *Proc. Natl. Acad. Sci. U.S.A.* **96,** 2982–2987.
15. Kim, C. J., *et al.* (1997). Dendritic cells infected with poxviruses encoding MART-1/Melan A sensitize T lymphocytes *in vitro. J. Immunother.* **20,** 276–286.
16. Restifo, N. P., and Rosenberg, S. A. Developing recombinant and synthetic vaccines for the treatment of melanoma. *Curr. Opin. Oncol.* **11,** 50–57.
17. Morse, M. A., *et al.* (1999). A phase I study of active immunotherapy with carcinoembryonic antigen peptide (CAP-1)-pulsed, autologous human cultured dendritic cells in patients with metastatic malignancies expressing carcinoembryonic antigen. *Clin. Cancer Res.* **5,** 1331–1338.

18. Gilboa, E., Nair, S. K., and Lyerly, H. K. (1998). Immunotherapy of cancer with dendritic-cell-based vaccines. *Cancer Immunol. Immunother.* **46,** 82–87.
19. Wolchok, J. D., Livingston, P. O., and Houghton, A. N. (1998). Vaccines and other adjuvant therapies for melanoma. *Hematol. Oncol. Clin. North Am.* **12,** 835–848, vii.
20. Livingston, P. O., *et al.* (1987). Vaccines containing purified GM2 ganglioside elicit GM2 antibodies in melanoma patients. *Proc. Natl. Acad. Sci. U.S.A.* **84,** 2911–2915.
21. Rosenberg, S. A. (1999). A new era for cancer immunotherapy based on the genes that encode cancer antigens. *Immunity* **10,** 281–287.
22. Van Den Eynde, B. J., and Boon, T. (1997). Tumor antigens recognized by T lymphocytes. *Int. J. Clin. Lab. Res.* **27,** 81–86.
23. Boon, T., van der Bruggen, P. (1996). Human tumor antigens recognized by T lymphocytes. *J. Exp. Med.* **183,** 725–729.
24. Peoples, G. E., *et al.* (1995). Breast and ovarian cancer-specific cytotoxic T lymphocytes recognize the same HER2/neu-derived peptide. *Proc. Natl. Acad. Sci. U.S.A.* **92,** 432–436.
25. Linehan, D. C., Goedegebuure, P. S., Peoples, G. E., Rogers, S. O., and Eberlein, T. J., (1995). Tumor-specific and HLA-A2-restricted cytolysis by tumor-associated lymphocytes in human metastatic breast cancer. *J. Immunol.* **155,** 4486–4491.
26. Falk, K., Rotzschke, O., Stevanovic, S., Jung, G., and Rammensee, H. G. (1991). Allele-specific motifs revealed by sequencing of self-peptides eluted from MHC molecules. *Nature (London)* **351,** 290–296.
27. Rotzschke, O., *et al.* (1990). Isolation and analysis of naturally processed viral peptides as recognized by cytotoxic T cells [see comments]. *Nature (London)* **348,** 252–254.
28. Cox, A. L., *et al.* (1994). Identification of a peptide recognized by five melanoma-specific human cytotoxic T cell lines. *Science* **264,** 716–719.
29. Engelhard, V. H., *et al.* (1993). Mass spectrometric analysis of peptides associated with the human class I MHC molecules HLA-A2.1 and HLA-B7 and identification of structural features that determine binding. *Chem. Immunol.* **57,** 39–62.
30. Tamura, Y., Peng, P., Liu, K., Daou, M., and Srivastava, P. K. (1997). Immunotherapy of tumors with autologous tumor-derived heat shock protein preparations *Science* **278,** 117–120 [erratum appears in *Science* **283**(5405), preceding 1119].
31. Suto, R., and Srivastava, P. K. (1995). A mechanism for the specific immunogenicity of heat shock protein-chaperoned peptides. *Science* **269,** 1585–1588.
32. Srivastava, P. K. (1997). Purification of heat shock protein–peptide complexes for use in vaccination against cancers and intracellular pathogens. *Methods* **12,** 165–171.
33. Sahin, U., Tureci, O., and Pfreundschuh, M. (1997). Serological identification of human tumor antigens. *Curr. Opin. Immunol.* **9,** 709–716.
34. Chen, Y., *et al.* (1998). Identification of multiple cancer/testis antigens by allogenic antibody screening of a melanoma cell line library. *Proc. Natl. Acad. Sci. U.S.A.* **95,** 6919–6923.
34a. Goedegebuure, P. S., Spanjaard, R. A., and Eberlein, T. J. (1997). T cells and tumor-infiltrating lymphocytes. *In* "Encyclopedia of Cancer," Vol. III, p. 1736. Academic Press, San Diego.
35. Old, L. J. (1996). Cancer immunology. *Sci. Am.* **236,** 62–63, 76, 79.
36. Linehan, D. C., Goedegebuure, P. S., and Eberlein, T. J. (1996). Vaccine therapy for cancer. *Ann. Surg. Oncol.* **3,** 219–28.
37. Henkart, P. A. (1999). Cytotoxic T lymphocytes. *In* "Fundamental Immunology" (W.E. Paul, ed.), pp. 1021–1049. Lippincott-Raven, Philadelphia.
38. Krummel, M. F., Heath, W. R., and Allison, J. (1999). Differential coupling of second signals for cytotoxicity and proliferation in CD8+ T cell effectors: Amplification of the lytic potential by B7. *J. Immunol.* **163,** 2999–3006.
39. Nair, S. K., *et al.* (1999). Induction of carcinoembryonic antigen (CEA)-specific cytotoxic T-lymphocyte responses *in vitro* using autologous dendritic cells loaded with CEA peptide or CEA RNA in patients with metastatic malignancies expressing CEA. *Int. J. Cancer* **82,** 121–124.
40. Peoples, G. E., *et al.* (1995). Shared T cell epitopes in epithelial tumors. *Cell Immunol.* **164,** 279–286.
41. Linehan, D. C., *et al.* (1995). *In vitro* stimulation of ovarian tumour-associated lymphocytes with a peptide derived from HER2/neu induces cytotoxicity against autologous tumour. *Surg. Oncol.* **4,** 41–49.
42. Yoshino, I., *et al.* (1994). HER2/neu-derived peptides are shared antigens among human non-small cell lung cancer and ovarian cancer. *Cancer Res.* **54,** 3387–3390.
43. Peiper, M., *et al.* (1997). The HER2/neu-derived peptide p654-662 is a tumor-associated antigen in human pancreatic cancer recognized by cytotoxic T lymphocytes. *Eur. J. Immunol.* **27,** 1115–1123.
44. Pass, H. A., Schwarz, S. L., Wunderlich, J. R., and Rosenberg, S. A. (1998). Immunization of patients with melanoma peptide vaccines: Immunologic assessment using the ELISPOT assay [see comments]. *Cancer J. Sci. Am.* **4,** 316–323.
45. Kammula, U., *et al.* (1999). Functional analysis of antigen-specific T lymphocytes by serial measurements of gene expression in peripheral blood mononuclear cells and tumor specimens. *J. Immunol.* **163,** 6867–6875.
46. Martz, E. (1993). The 51-chromium release assay for CTL-mediated target cell lysis. *In* "Cytotoxic Cells: Recognition, Effector Function, Generation and Methods" (M. Sitkovsky and P. Henkart, eds.), pp. 457–467. Birhauser, Boston.
47. Duke, R. C., and Cohen, J. J. (1988). The role of nuclear damage in lysis of target cells by cytotoxic T-lymphocytes. *In* "Cytolytic Lymphocytes and Complement: Effectors of the Immune System" (E. R. Podack, ed.), pp. 35–37. CRC Press, Boca Raton.
48. Matteucci, C., Grelli, S., De Smaele, E., Fontana, C., and Mastino, A. (1999). Identification of nuclei from apoptotic, necrotic, and viable lymphoid cells by using multiparameter flow cytometry. *Cytometry* **35,** 145–153.
49. North, R. J. (1982). Cyclophosphamide-facilitated adoptive immunotherapy of an established tumor depends on elimination of tumor-induced suppressor T cells. *J. Exp. Med.* **155,** 1063–1074.
50. Hodi, F. S., and Dranoff, G. (1998). Genetically modified tumor cell vaccines. *Surg. Oncol. Clin. North Am.* **7,** 471–485.
51. Matory, Y. L., Chen, M., Goedegebuure, P. S., and Eberlein, T. J. (1995). Anti-tumor effects and tumor immunogenicity following IL2 or IL4 cytokine gene transfection of three mouse mammary tumors. *Ann. Surg. Oncol.* **2,** 502–511.
52. Nagoshi, M., Sadanaga, N., Joo, H. G., Goedegebuure, P. S., and Eberlein, T. J. (1999). Tumor-specific cytokine release by donor T cells induces an effective host anti-tumor response through recruitment of host naive antigen presenting cells. *Int. J. Cancer* **80,** 308–314.
53. Nagoshi, M., *et al.* (1998). Successful adoptive cellular immunotherapy is dependent on induction of a host immune response triggered by cytokine (IFN-gamma and granulocyte/macrophage colony-stimulating factor) producing donor tumor-infiltrating lymphocytes. *J. Immunol.* **160,** 334–344.

40

Gastrointestinal Motility

Michael G. Sarr,* Joseph J. Cullen,† and Mary F. Otterson‡

*Division of Gastroenterologic and General Surgery, Mayo Clinic, Mayo Medical School, Rochester, Minnesota 55902
†University of Iowa Hospitals and Clinics, Iowa City, Iowa 52242
‡Medical College of Wisconsin, Milwaukee, Wisconsin 53226

I. Introduction

Investigation of gastrointestinal (GI) motility allows research primarily into the physiology and pathophysiology of one aspect of GI function—i.e., movement of intestinal content through the gut. Depending on the topic of interest when addressing techniques, methodology, and models to study GI motility, one needs to be cognizant of both *in vitro* and *in vivo* processes—both have their strengths and limitations.

Ultimately, GI motility depends on the presence of contractile activity within the gut to create the forces that move intestinal content distally (or proximally during vomiting). One might choose to measure contractile activity either directly or indirectly, or to measure the movement/transit of luminal content out of the stomach (gastric emptying), through the small and/or large intestine (intestinal transit), and/or finally its discharge from the gut (defecation). Each of these parameters may be studied in animals or in humans.

This chapter first discusses briefly the physiology of smooth muscle contraction of the gut, with special reference to aspects of the techniques to measure contractile activity. Last, models of *in vitro* and *in vivo* preparations to study GI motility are addressed. The focus of the discussion concentrates on techniques and methodologies and their individual advantages and limitations.

II. Physiology of Intestinal Contractions

GI motility ultimately depends on intestinal smooth muscle contractions that generate the force needed to move intraluminal content along the gut. The final common pathway of intestinal smooth muscle contractions depends on intracellular release of calcium. Once liberated, the intracellular calcium induces the intracellular mechanisms controlling interaction of contractile proteins leading to cell shortening; this biochemistry of contraction will not be the focus of this chapter.

However, the release of intracellular calcium is ultimately controlled by the intracellular electrical potential of the smooth muscle cell, which coordinates the timing and organization of contraction. The intracellular electrical potential of a smooth muscle cell of the gut undergoes a cyclic depolarization/repolarization referred to as the action potential or slow wave. This cyclic variation in cell potential is likely driven by the pacemaker cells of the gut—the interstitial cells of Cajal. The changes in cell potential are the result of selective opening and closing of specific ion channels in the membrane, which are gated by voltage (cell potential), intracellular calcium, and various extracellular chemical stimuli (neurotransmitters, hormones, etc.). For instance, opening of inward-directed sodium and calcium channels leads to depolarization (the normal resting cell potential of gut smooth muscle cells is -40 to -80 mV as controlled by active outward sodium pumps) or to repolarization/hyperpolarization by opening of outward potassium channels. Because contractions can occur only during depolarization and only when the depolarization reaches a threshold potential, the regular cyclic changes in cell potential "pace" the onset and ultimate timing of contractions. The aborad vector of contractions (i.e., distal spread of contractions down the gut) occurs because the layers of smooth muscle of the gut are functionally electrical syncytiums. The cyclic changes in cell potential are driven from separate pacemakers in the proximal stomach and the proximal duodenum and are propagated down the stomach and small bowel, respectively, from smooth muscle cell to adjacent smooth muscle cell. Thus, if one were able to measure cell potential in immediately adjacent regions along the stomach or small bowel, one would see a wave of depolarization and subsequent repolarization that begins proximally and propagates in an orderly sequential manner aborad down the bowel. All extrinsic forces that modulate contractile activity (neural, hormonal, humoral) act via local effects on this cyclic electrical activity of the smooth muscle. Although similar cyclic changes in cell potential occur in the large intestine, they are not as clearly organized in a global proximal-to-distal orientation and appear to arise from multiple, wandering "pacemakers." The organization of cyclic activity in the colon remains poorly understood.

Superimposed on these cycle-to-cycle changes in cell potential (and thus individual contractions) are more global mechanisms controlling patterns of contractions occurring over minutes to hours. For instance, during the interdigestive (fasting) period in most mammals, the stomach and small bowel undergo a cyclic pattern of global contractile activity consisting of four phases of different contractile activity (1, 2). These four phases, the most characteristic of which is phase III (often called the activity front), cycle monotonously. This cycle pattern, likely controlled by a complex interplay of regulatory peptide hormones with the enteric nervous system, begins in the lower esophageal sphincter and stomach, then appears in the proximal duodenum, after which this characteristic pattern of contractile activity migrates down the entire small bowel in a very orderly fashion. The cycle recurs about every 2 hr in humans and the larger mammals, but the pattern is more frequent in smaller animal models, i.e., in rats occurring about every 30 min. Because of its characteristic migrating pattern, this interdigestive pattern has been called the migrating motor complex.

With feeding and the establishment of the postprandial period, the cyclic interdigestive motor pattern is disrupted and is replaced by a postprandial pattern of intermittent, ostensibly irregular contractions that persist for a variable length of time, dependent on the number of calories and form of nutrients ingested. The interdigestive pattern of contractions involves intensive peristaltic contractions that spread over short segments of the small intestine (10–30 cm only) that strip the lumen of nondigestive debris, bacteria, and desquamated cells, thereby "preparing" the gut for the anticipated ingested food. In contrast, the postprandial contractions are believed to mix intestinal content to maximize absorption while still moving intraluminal content distally. These global patterns of contractions are present only *in vivo* because they require the integration of numerous neural and hormonal systems of the entire organism, and thus the study of these global patterns requires *in vivo* preparations. In contrast, individual control of contractions can be studied either *in vivo* or *in vitro*.

Global patterns of colonic motility are less well understood. Contractile activity within the colon is organized (1) to optimize appropriate absorption of water and electrolytes, (2) to store fecal material, and (3) to expel fecal material at socially acceptable times. The colonic contractile activity of different species is organized differently. Nonhuman primates and rats have individual phasic contractile activity that is rarely organized into groups of contractions. Canine contractile activity is organized as groups of contractions with interspersed periods of quiescence. Human colonic contractile activity resembles both, with random contractions interspersed between groups of contractions.

In humans, there are two types of colonic contractions—individual phasic contractions and giant migrating contractions. As in the rest of the digestive tract, individual phasic contractions are the primary unit of contractile activity. They may be organized into clusters of contractions or contractile states. By definition, a colonic migrating motor complex is said to occur when colonic contractile states propagate over greater than half the length of the colon. Colonic migrating motor complexes may propagate in an orad or caudad direction but the vast majority are caudally migrating. Giant migrating contractions occur infrequently and result in the mass movement of feces. When giant migrating contractions occur in the distal colon, they are associated with defecation. The control of individual phasic contractions is maintained via three distinct mechanisms: myogenic, neural, and chemical. Control mechanisms for the giant migrating contractions of the colon are less well defined.

It is with this brief background that the following section addresses basic techniques of studying contractile activity and/or movement of intestinal content.

III. Techniques of Measuring Contractile Activity

A. In Vitro Methodology

Basically, one can measure changes in (1) length or tension of segments of smooth muscle suspended in a tissue bath, (2) intracellular electrical potential of smooth muscle cells within a segment of smooth muscle, (3) changes in transmembrane current, or (4) changes in length of individual dispersed smooth muscle cells.

1. Isolated Segments of Gut

Several attempts have been designed to study motility in isolated organs such as the stomach, small bowel, and colon (3). These types of experiments have used the same methodology and techniques utilized when studying contractile activity *in vivo*—intraluminal manometry, changes in pressure within an intraluminal balloon, and serosal strain gauges. These techniques will be discussed in depth below (Section III,B)

2. Smooth Muscle Strips

Most experimental setups designed to study contractile activity of various strips of gut muscle do so in tissue baths designed to maintain the muscle strip within a physiologic, temperature-controlled, buffer solution bubbled with an oxygen/carbon dioxide gas mixture. This technique involves harvesting smooth muscle directly into a controlled environment designed to maintain viability of the muscle strip such that contractility can be measured, while individual parameters (temperature, oxygen content, changes in electrolyte composition, concentration of putative regulatory substances, etc.) are changed in a controlled fashion independent of all the other neural, hormonal, and humoral stimuli unable to be fully controlled in an *in vivo* preparation.

a. Contractile Force (Isometric, Isotonic) The muscle strip is fixed at one end and connected either to a force transducer at the other end, if measuring isometric force, or to a fixed weight (tone), if measuring isotonic contractions (4). When measuring isometric force by a force transducer, one measures the force of contraction at a fixed length. In contrast, isotonic conditions measure contractile force indirectly by measuring changes in length of the muscle strip against a constant force. The exact muscle group studied (i.e., the circular muscle layer or the longitudinal muscle layer) depends on either the orientation of the strip with the axis of the strain gauge or via specific dissections with isolation of longitudinal or circular smooth muscle strips from one another. By adding various chemical or biologically active substances to the bath solution, the investigator can determine effects of various chemical parameters on contractile activity in a controlled fashion. Similarly, by subjecting the muscle strip to electrical field stimulation at differing voltages, stimulus durations, and/or frequencies delivered by electrodes within the chamber, one can evaluate the effects of neurally mediated phenomena.

Advantages/limitations. Because the bath solution is isolated and not subject to all the variations of an organ *in situ* (e.g., changes in blood flow, hormones, extrinsic neural innervation, humoral substances, external mechanical forces), the investigator can vary the conditions in a controlled fashion, determining the effect(s) of changing one variable (ion concentration, regulatory substances, temperature, oxygen content, etc.) on contractile response. Similarly, one can study separately each muscular layer as a whole by selectively excising other anatomic layers of the gut wall. In contrast, the study of muscle strips has limitations. Just the fact that the muscle strip has to be excised and isolated in a tissue bath means that it is acutely denervated extrinsically and lacks intrinsic neural continuity with the remainder of the adjacent gut from where it was harvested. By isolating the muscle strip in the tissue chamber without nutrients, the viability of the muscle strip is necessarily limited to hours. Use of electrical field stimulation allows the investigator to study neurally mediated events acting via neurotransmitters or neurokine agents. However, electrical field stimulation excites nondiscriminately all nerves within the muscle strip, and thus the effect measured may represent a "net" effect of the release of both excitatory and inhibitory agents. The study of specific neurotransmitters requires both specific agonists and antagonists. Overall, muscle strips can be used to address specific questions concerning variables of local contractility, but the experimental conditions are far from "physiologic," and effects of humoral, neural, or hormonal agents on "global" motor patterns are not possible *in vitro*.

b. Intracellular Electrical Potential Study of smooth muscle cell transmembrane potential is attractive because ultimately it is the changes in cell potential which induce contractions. Technically, a smooth muscle cell is impaled intracellularly with a "microelectrode" filled with various ion-containing conductive solutions to allow measurement of electrical forces (5). The recordings of electrical potential are amplified and measured in relation to a grounded source and displayed on an oscilloscope; these changes in cell potential take place over milliseconds. This technique of intracellular recording is both sophisticated and very delicate and requires immobilization of the region of study, usually by pinning the muscle strip to an immobile background on which the muscle strip lies. Although ideally one would want to monitor simultaneously contraction and changes in cell potential in the same region, contractile activity will displace the microelectrode from the cell. One experimental preparation involves pinning and immobilizing one end of the strip to record intracellular activity while leaving the other end free to record simultaneous changes in isometric force or isotonic length. With this technology, again the environment is well controlled. The investigator can alter the bath solution or inject current into the cell via the microelectrode, thereby externally altering the cell potential to determine the response in membrane potential.

Advantages/disadvantages. As with muscle strip techniques, this methodology allows control of the environment to which the cell being studied is exposed, allowing one parameter at a time to be varied. In contrast, the disadvantages include the "nonphysiologic" and artificial environment of the tissue bath, the isolation of the cell being studied from the whole organism, the delicacy of the intracellular electrode and the ease with which the microelectrode is displaced, and, finally, the observation that only one individual cell within the strip is studied with observations generalized to all the remaining cells within that layer. We know, for instance, that the latter generalization is not accurate for the various depths of smooth muscle cells within the circular muscle of the stomach and small bowel.

c. Patch Clamp Techniques The concept with this approach is to measure directly current exiting or entering the cell across a limited segment (or patch) of membrane. This technique requires use of very sophisticated software to measure rapid and very small changes in current (picoamps), as well as highly insulated, electrically shielded recording systems. Depending on experimental conditions, one can study changes in whole cell current or opening/closing of individual ion channels.

The concept with patch clamping is that a micropipette is slowly advanced until it contacts the cell membrane. A slight negative pressure is applied to the microelectrode such that the cell membrane spans the tip of the electrode and forms a mechanically stable electrical "seal" as determined by the presence of a measurable capacitance, usually in the range of gigaohms. The high resistance of this electrical seal ensures that the small currents originating within the membrane "patch" will flow into the micropipette and from there into the circuitry that measures current flow.

Several basic techniques are used (6,7). **Cell-attached recordings** allow measurement of current across the membrane patch subject to opening and closing of channels as mediated either by changes in the external environment (e.g., ion concentrations, neuroregulatory substances), effects on the cell at a distant site not within the patch, or events mediated by the intracellular environment. The **perforated patch technique** involves subjecting the cell to a substance such as amphotericin, which permeabilizes the membrane. With this approach, the ionic composition of the bath solution can be modified and thereby will directly affect the intracellular ionic composition because the membrane has been permeabilized, e.g., intracellular calcium or second-messenger systems. The patch micropipette will then be able to measure changes in current related to these controllable changes in the intracellular compartment while maintaining the intracellular milieu in contact with the membrane patched. **Whole cell recordings** can be obtained by first attaining a cell-attached configuration, and then applying either a pulse of suction or voltage to disrupt the membrane patch but keeping the micropipette sealed to the cell. This configuration provides a direct, low-resistance access to the cell interior that allows recording of cell potential and voltage clamping of the cell, similar in principle to intracellular recordings of cell potential. The **excised patch technique** involves patching a segment of the membrane, but then "ripping" this patch of membrane off the cell yet maintaining the electrical seal. There are two variations. The first involves the **inside-out patch.** With this technique, the membrane's inner surface is exposed directly to the bath solution, allowing one to measure opening and closing of individual ion channels within that segment of the cell membrane independent of the intracellular microenvironment. With this excised inside-out patch technique, one can determine the effects of "intracellular" substances on the "inside" of the membrane by varying the composition of the bath. Similarly, by adding a substance to the solution within the micropipette, the investigator can evaluate the response to the substance on the "outside" of the membrane independent of the intracellular microenvironment. The second variation, the **outside-out patch**, is created by conditions that first lead to a whole cell configuration, but pulling the micropipette "off" the cell in such a way that a membrane patch forms to seal the micropipette tip, but now with the outside aspect of the membrane exposed to the bath. In contrast to the inside-out patch, with the outside-out patch the membrane can be exposed to changes in the bath that will affect the outside aspect of the membrane patch.

Because channels are either "open" or "closed," current conducted across an open channel is of a unit value; when two identical channels are open, the current is double what it would be with one open channel. Thus, changes in current occur as quantum increases. By "clamping" the electrical potential across the patch at different holding potentials, the investigator can determine the voltage dependence of the channel (probability of the channel being "open" at a given potential). This technique is especially useful for channels that open or close at various cell voltages (e.g., voltage-gated channels). By varying the ionic concentration of the bath, one can determine the effect of varying concentrations of specific ions on open-channel probability independent of membrane voltage, i.e., calcium-dependent channels that open when intracellular concentration reaches a threshold value.

Advantages/limitations. By studying one small patch of membrane, the effects of varying the concentration of ions or chemical substances in the bath solution, changing the cell voltage, or altering the intracellular environment can be determined on individual types of ion channels. Of most interest for the GI physiologist, these channels ultimately regulate cell potential and thereby contractile activity. Because most of the channels are proteins, they are subject to mutations that alter expression or activity, which can lead to hereditary disorders. The limitations of patch clamping, however, are that this is a very difficult and delicate technology and a theoretical concept requiring many months to learn and understand, the equipment is expensive, and the experimental conditions are artificial and far from the physiologic world. This is not a technique that can be rapidly developed by otherwise naive investigators to study one aspect of motility.

3. Isolated Smooth Muscle Cells

This methodology first requires the ability to dissociate and disperse mechanically and/or chemically individual smooth muscle cells from a specific region of the gut wall within a buffer solution (8). Once individual muscle cells are successfully isolated and appear viable and able to contract, the investigator can then directly measure cell shortening under phase-contrast microscopy by altering the bath solution (9). Similarly, as described above, the cells can be impaled with microelectrodes to measure changes in cell potential or can be patched to measure channel currents.

Advantages/limitations. The primary advantage of this technique is that cell contraction is visualized and measured directly in response to various experimental conditions. The effect of drugs directly on the muscle cell, devoid of other confounding influences (nerves, tissue enzymes, passive forces of interstitial connective tissue, etc.), is an attractive concept. In contrast, there are many limitations. First, the isolation/dispersion technique may injure the cell or disrupt poorly understood critical intercellular mechanisms of cell-to-cell control, both electrical and physical. Also, it is difficult (or impossible) to determine the true viability of the cells and whether important mechanisms regulating contractility are maintained. In addition, to examine relaxation, the muscle cells may first require application of a procontractile agonist to "precontract" them in order to measure relaxation; similarly, to measure contraction, the muscle cells may need to be "prerelaxed."

B. In Vivo Methodology

In vivo measurements of motility have their advantages and disadvantages. Although the experimental conditions cannot be as well regulated as with many *in vitro* conditions, motor activity in the living organism does involve a complex interplay of many variables not able to be reproduced *in vitro*. Knowledge of many of these forces is limited, and thus study of the whole organism involves a more "integrative" physiology. *In vivo* techniques are, of course, limited in several respects in order to maintain the viability of the organism. Contractile activity is measured either by changes in extracellular intraluminal pressure, changes in length or wall tension within a segment, changes in myoelectric potential, or changes in either distance between fixed points (longitudinal muscle contractions) or in circumferential diameter reflecting changes in luminal diameter (circular muscle contractions).

1. Intraluminal Pressure

By measuring changes in intraluminal pressure, implications about muscular contractions can be inferred. However, for intraluminal pressure to increase within a hollow viscus secondary to contraction of its surrounding musculature, the lumen containing the recording device must be a closed system. For instance, if the gallbladder contracts and the diameter of the organ decreases, intraluminal pressure will increase, provided that the cystic duct and the sphincter of Oddi are closed; the intraluminal pressure will then be a function of the strength of the contraction. In contrast, if the cystic duct and the sphincter of Oddi are wide open (and offer no significant resistance to flow of bile out of the gallbladder), intraluminal pressure within the gallbladder may not change appreciably despite contraction of the wall musculature, because it is not a "closed" system. Fortunately, most parts of the GI tract, except possibly the proximal stomach, act as closed systems due to occlusive, segmenting contractions, and thus changes in intraluminal pressure reflect contractile activity.

Intraluminal pressure can be recorded by open-tipped manometry catheters or by solid-state manometry catheters (10). Open-tipped catheters are filled with a noncompressible fluid (usually water) that is in continuity with an external strain gauge transducer, which can be calibrated to known pressures. The best methodology for open-tipped manometry incorporates a closed, noncompliant system that perfuses the catheter at a very slow rate to avoid adherence of the wall of the organ to the tip of the catheter; response rates to changes in pressure should be very rapid (<100 msec). Solid-state "manometry" catheters are really miniature force transducers (strain gauges) imbedded within the catheter system. These catheter systems can be either surgically implanted for chronic usage or introduced into the lumen of the gut segment when needed, the experiment conducted, and the manometric assembly then removed when the experiment is over. A now outdated methodology of placing a fluid-filled balloon or bladder into the lumen and monitoring pressure within this balloon or bladder is much less reliable.

Advantages/limitations. The primary advantages of manometric measurements are that they reflect the effect of muscular contraction of the entire organ on the intraluminal pressure at that level, and they are cheap to make and use. The former concept is important because movement of intraluminal content ultimately depends on changes in intraluminal pressure between adjacent segments (and is usually a function of contractile activity). Other methodologies involving fixed measurements at a specific point on the gut wall (e.g., strain gauges, electrodes; see below) reflect contraction at that specific site but may not be indicative of contractions in the remainder of the adjacent musculature in the bowel circumference and do not measure any direct effects of these contractions on intraluminal pressure. The advantages of open-tipped manometry catheters are that they can be maintained *in vivo* in an active state for months at a time, and measurements of pressure are absolute and not relative. Solid-state transducers are better utilized as single experiment intubations. Another advantage of manometry catheters are that they can measure intraluminal effects of both tonic and phasic activity.

Limitations of manometric technology are primarily related to the indirect nature of their measurements. Manometry measures intraluminal pressure and is not a direct measurement of muscular contraction (i.e., muscular shortening). For instance, in the proximal stomach, contractions that occur in one region may be associated with relaxation elsewhere in the proximal stomach, with the end result measured by manometric techniques as little or no change in intraluminal pressure (e.g., during gastric emptying). Also, changes in intraluminal pressure at the tip of the manometer do not necessarily reflect contractile activity at that site, but only an increase in pressure at that site; the contraction leading to an increase in pressure within the segment acting as a closed system could be proximal or distal to the recording site.

2. Serosal Strain Gauges

These recording devices measure changes in length between the ends of the strain gauge by measuring changes in capacitance across the strain gauge during the deformation caused by the contraction. As the underlying muscle contracts, the distance between the ends of the strain gauge shortens, and the capacitance changes. These devices are basically a form of Wheatstone bridge, one resistance of which varies with deformation of the strain gauge (11, 12). This change in capacitance is converted to an electrical signal that can be measured and quantitated. Strain gauge measurements can be calibrated to known forces, but the measurements are relative measures as opposed to absolute measurements. The direction of orientation of the strain gauge (i.e., the direction of the force vector measured) determines the layer of muscular contraction measured. For instance, longitudinal orientation measures longitudinal muscle contraction (longitudinal shortening), whereas a circular orientation measures circular contraction (decreased luminal diameter).

Advantages/limitations. Serosal strain gauges represent a direct measure of muscular shortening independent of any changes in intraluminal events. Also, they will reflect relaxation (lengthening) as well as contraction (shortening). Strain gauges are especially suited for parts of the GI tract where contractions might not be well estimated by changes in intraluminal pressure because the system (viscus cavity) may not be a closed system—e.g., the proximal stomach during gastric emptying, the gallbladder during gallbladder emptying, and the distal colon/rectum during defecation.

The limitations are in some respects a reflection of the advantages of the serosal strain gauges and depend on what aspect of smooth muscle contraction the investigator wishes to monitor. These strain gauge measurements do not measure changes in the intraluminal environment; if the investigator were most interested in movement of intraluminal content secondary to intraluminal forces, serosal strain gauges would not be the best methodology. In addition, because the measurements are relative, it is difficult to compare different regions on an absolute basis. Moreover, strain gauges are quite difficult to make or are expensive when purchased. Their functional half-life *in vivo* is only 2–6 months, primarily related to the need to keep the strain gauge elements electrically isolated from body fluids. Changes in the passive resistance needed to deform the strain gauge secondary to the fibrosis generated by the body's reaction to this foreign device may alter the absolute measurements over time and thus the ability to correlate the strength of contractions at that site over time. One additional limitation is that a strain gauge measures only what happens specifically over the span of the strain gauge and is not a function of the entire gut wall or even the immediately adjacent muscle.

3. Barostats

The barostat was designed to measure, indirectly, changes in tone or wall tension of a hollow viscus. In brief, a barostat consists of a thin-walled bag that (in theory) has infinite compliance, completely fills the viscus cavity, and conforms to whatever shape the cavity assumes. Using an external servomechanism connected to the lumen of the bag, the pressure within the bag is kept constant and just above (usually 1–2 mmHg) resting pressure to ensure that the bag remains inflated and fills the cavity. Through inflation or deflation of the bag, the volume of the bag is thus a measure, indirectly, of contractile activity, and because the pressure is kept constant at a baseline pressure, a function of wall tension or tone. For instance, as the proximal stomach increases its tone during the emptying phase of the postprandial period (when the stomach empties), a barostat system would measure a decrease in bag volume as the tone in the proximal stomach increases. Intraluminal pressure in the proximal stomach physiologically would vary very little compared to the magnitude of change in dimension of the proximal stomach secondary to contraction of the proximal gastric musculature, because the proximal stomach during gastric emptying is not a closed system.

Advantages/limitations. The barostat concept is the only methodology available to measure, albeit indirectly, wall tension or tone. Functionally, it reflects changes in the entire organ and not just at one point as measured by a strain gauge. However, there are multiple limitations to use of a barostat. First, it is a very artificial system because the intraluminal pressure environment is fixed and maintained at a constant level. The intraluminal bag must also have an "infinite" compliance and will need to conform fully to the shape of the viscus cavity if it is to reflect accurately changes in tone. Luminal contents outside the bag will alter the volume measurements and especially so if chyme enters or leave the viscus. Finally, because the bag is so delicate, for each experiment it usually needs to be introduced into the viscus and then removed at the end. Thus, the organ needs to be readily accessible to intubation.

4. Serosal Electrodes/Mucosal Suction Electrodes

As explained in Section II, each smooth muscle cell of the gut undergoes a cyclic change in cell potential called the action potential or intracellular slow wave. This cyclic change is driven by pacemaker regions, for the stomach in the midbody region, for the small bowel in the proximal duodenum, and for the colon in many differing regions that appear to vary over time. The pacemaker rates are greater than the "inherent" rate of depolarization/repolarization of the individual smooth muscle cells at sites distant to the pacemaker. Because the gut smooth muscle functions as an electrical spectrum, this cyclic change in cell potential generated by the pacemaker region is "myoelectrically" conducted from cell to cell in a proximal-to-distal orientation. By fixing an electrode to the serosal surface (or a suction electrode onto the mucosal surface—the suction holds it in place), the electrical potential at the electrode site will be a measure of the summation of all the smooth muscle cells underlying the electrode. If the individual smooth muscle cell does not reach threshold during its cyclic depolarization, no contraction occurs, yet the subthreshold cyclic depolarization/repolarization still occurs and will be measurable by an extracellular electrode. Serosal or mucosal electrodes measure the summation of cyclic changes in electrical potential of the underlying smooth muscle cells. These cyclic changes have been called the slow wave (14–16), the pacesetter potential, the basic electrical rhythm, or the electrical control activity; all are synonyms for this cyclic extracellular change in potential. In contrast, when some population of underlying smooth muscle cells reach their threshold potential, a more marked increase in potential occurs; this, when summated by the overlying serosal electrode, appears as a series of "spike potentials" (also called action potentials or electrical response activity). These spike potentials are the (indirect) myoelectric correlates of smooth muscle contractions.

These serosal or mucosal extracellular electrodes, which may be unipolar or bipolar, measure changes in the surrounding (myoelectric) potential relative to another point. Unipolar electrodes record their electrical potential measured in relation to an indifferent, grounded electrode, such as a subcutaneous electrode (whose electrical potential does not change over time). Bipolar electrodes measure the change in potential between the two electrodes; because the slow wave (depolarization/repolarization) propagates from proximal to distal along the bowel, bipolar electrodes also record the cyclic change in potential as well as spike activity indicative of contractions.

Serosal electrodes can be constructed from stainless steel, Ag^{+}/AgCl, platinum, or any metal that can measure a change in electrical potential. The electrode tip is exposed to the point on the tissue where the activity is to be measured, but the wire connecting the electrode to the recording device requires electrically secure insulation from surrounding tissues.

Advantages/limitations. Serosal electrodes are quite easy to construct or obtain commercially (e.g., cardiac pacing wires). They can be reliably sewn onto a fixed point on the stomach, small bowel, or colon, connected to an electrical socket, and their output easily recorded by a chart recorder able to measure millivolt dimensions; most chart recorders require, however, a preamplifier to further amplify the signal. One major advantage of serosal electrodes is that they measure the slow wave independent of contractile activity and thereby can measure the maximum frequency of contraction. Any changes in frequency of the slow wave reflect maximal contraction frequency. Such changes may occur related to proximal intestinal transection (which separates the bowel distally from the proximal pacemaker), changes in temperature, or overall disorganization of the aborad vector of propagation that ultimately controls direction of contractions and thus direction of transit. Serosal electrodes are easy to implant, can be inserted in such a fashion as to be easily removed postoperatively, especially in humans, and are easy to access and use repetitively. Mucosal suction electrodes are more troublesome, because they are designed to be inserted and removed on a daily basis. Their fixation within the lumen of the gut is less secure because their use requires maintenance of a suction seal; gut motility attempts to displace the electrode, and it may be difficult to reposition the electrode in the exact site repetitively.

Electrodes have many limitations that must be acknowledged. First, they do not measure contractile activity directly but only indirectly via recording of spike activity. Second, the strength of the myoelectric signal is not absolutely proportional to the strength of the underlying myoelectric signal, and thus anatomically separate electrodes cannot be compared on an absolute basis. Similarly, the amplitude of contractile activity that leads to spike activity is not directly absolutely proportional to the amount of spike activity measured at different electrodes, but is only a "relative" indication of the strength of the associated contraction. Third, electrodes measure the changes in potential at that one site; these changes may not necessarily be indicative of the remainder of the bowel wall. Fourth, serosal electrodes have a relatively short functional lifetime *in vivo* (2–4 months). In the esophagus, proximal stomach, gallbladder, and large intestine, the pattern of serosal electrodes is less regular, less well organized, and currently less well understood.

5. Cutaneous Electrodes—Electrogastrogram

Just as serosal electrodes can measure the underlying changes in electrical potential of the intestine, and cutaneous electrodes can record the electrocardiogram, cutaneous electrodes over the anterior epigastric area can record the underlying changes in potential from the stomach, i.e., the electrogastrogram (EGG) (17). This technique is possible because (1) all the gastric smooth muscle cells that generate a slow wave have the same frequency of change and (2) no other cyclically active tissues in this region (small bowel, heart) harbor a frequency near that of the stomach (4–5 cycles/min). The signals recorded from the cutaneous electrodes, however, must be subjected to a type of Fourier transformation to recognize the dominant frequencies of the underlying stomach and their individual amplitudes. With this type of analysis, one can look for more than one dominant frequency (suggestive of gastric dysrhythmia) and monitor the relative amplitude of the dominant frequency (18), although the latter parameter is less well characterized.

Advantages/limitations. Universal acceptance of the importance of the EEG remains controversial and is not fully endorsed as a useful or significantly meaningful technique. Its advantage lies in its noninvasive nature and may be best considered more as a diagnostic test looking for disorders of electrical organization of the distal, electrically active stomach. Limitations are that this technique requires sophisticated software and considerable experience in its interpretation, and important established or universally accepted uses for determining therapy or investigating physiology are notably lacking. Moreover, the EGG provides no information about the proximal stomach. Because the proximal stomach does not generate a cyclic electrical activity, the EGG cannot measure any parameter of proximal stomach function.

6. Ultrasonic Microtransducer Crystals

Using modern ultrasound technology and knowing the speed of sound within tissue, distances between emitting and recording microtransducer crystals can be determined accurately. This technology has been used extensively in the heart for many years to monitor changes in geometry of the heart wall, but it is quite new in the GI tract. Previous preliminary work has centered on making measurements across the pylorus as a measure of the pylorus being either open or closed (19).

Advantages/limitations. Although this technology measures contractile activity only indirectly, in theory, one could follow changes in bowel diameter and bowel circumference (using an array of crystals) as an indicator of circular muscle contraction and relaxation; similarly, longitudinal length would be a measure of longitudinal muscle contraction/relaxation (20). However, these measurements are subject to active as well as passive changes. The ultrasound signal passes through the tissue by the shortest tissue route. In theory, the signal should be transmitted preferentially through the wall of the bowel and not across the lumen; thus, if two microcrystals are positioned at 180° apart on opposite sides of the intestinal wall, the distance between crystals (as a measure of the bowel circumference) should vary indirectly with circular contractions. However, if the lumen is empty and the mucosa of each side of the bowel wall are touching one another, the signal preferentially goes through the shortest possible tissue distance—i.e., mucosa to mucosa and not around the circumference of the bowel wall. Also, differing lumen contents appear to conduct the ultrasonic signal across the lumen to a variable extent as well, thereby making certain measurements less reliable. Similarly, for longitudinal distances, if the loop of bowel is bent back on itself and the serosal surfaces touch one another, the distance measured will be falsely shortened because the ultrasound signal takes the shortest tissue pathway. Although this technique may work well in a fixed motile organ such as the heart, which is always filled with blood, the reliability of this technology in the gut in which the luminal content may contain liquid, solid, or gas remains questionable. Thus, use of these miniature ultrasonic crystals as a measure of GI motility remains of questionable benefit.

IV. Techniques of Measuring Gastric Emptying

A. Physiology

The primary motor functions of the stomach are to act as a receptive reservoir for ingested foods and as a grinder and mechanical digester (triturater) of ingested solids. The former function is largely governed by the proximal stomach and the latter by the antropyloric region.

1. Proximal Stomach

The ingestion of food into the normal stomach leads to receptive relaxation of the proximal stomach (fundus and corpus), which accommodates to the incoming volume such that intraluminal pressure remains low. This receptive relaxation/

accommodation, mediated by vagal innervation, allows the proximal stomach to store the ingested meal early postprandially. Thereafter, the tone in the proximal stomach gradually increases over the first several postprandial hours, leading to slight increases in intraluminal pressure causing gastric emptying of liquids. The rate of increase in proximal gastric tone varies with the type and caloric content of the meal and is also influenced by feedback mechanisms from the small intestine. The proximal stomach does not exhibit phasic contractile activity but rather more chronic slow changes in tone. By these mechanisms, the proximal stomach in large part regulates the rate of gastric emptying of liquids through its changes in tone and thus volume. Vagotomy denervates the proximal stomach, inhibits receptive relaxation and accommodation, leads to an increase in baseline and postprandial tone, and serves to speed the gastric emptying of liquids.

2. Distal Stomach

In contrast with the proximal stomach, there is no reservoir function offered by the antropyloric region, but rather this region largely regulates the rate of emptying of solids. With a normally innervated, intact stomach, solid particles leaving the stomach are $\leq$1 mm in diameter. The "antropyloric pump" serves to triturate the intraluminal solid matter in the postprandial period through the regular peristaltic contractile waves that spread down the antrum to the pylorus. As the contractile wave, again mediated in part by vagal innervation, sweeps solid content distally toward the pylorus, particles $>$1 mm in diameter meet a relatively closed pylorus and are retropelled back into the proximal stomach. This pumplike action in conjunction with the limited enzymatic actions of gastric secretions leads to a mechanical breakdown of larger, solid "digestible" particles into smaller solids that then can leave the stomach when they reach a diameter of $\leq$1 mm (21). This trituration assures maximal ability of the small intestine to be able to digest the solid matter enzymatically. Vagotomy tends to decrease the amplitude and regularity of these antral waves, thereby slowing the gastric emptying of solids. Nondigestible solid matter of $>$1 mm diameter remains in the stomach during the postprandial period but is emptied during the high-amplitude peristaltic contractions of phase III of the migrating motor complex during the "interdigestive" period.

B. Luminal Sampling

One can monitor gastric emptying by ingesting or instilling a marker into the stomach and then at a designated time afterward aspirating all the gastric content, analyzing for marker recovery, and calculating amount of instilled marker emptied. This technique is the easiest, least expensive technique of assessing gastric emptying but yields the least information about the dynamics of gastric emptying.

Advantages/limitations. This technique is quick, easy, and inexpensive and in certain conditions is a perfectly acceptable gross estimate of efficiency and speed of gastric emptying of liquids. There are many limitations, however. This technique is not appropriate for most solids because of the inability of an orgogastic tube to evacuate accurately all solid material remaining in the stomach. For liquid recovery, one needs to assume that the orogastric tube allows complete aspiration of *all* gastric content. Most importantly, however, is that luminal sampling is a one-time, static measurement of the percentage of gastric emptying at the time of luminal aspiration; one cannot determine real-time or dynamic changes in emptying with this technique. In theory, one can reinstill the aspirate and resample later; however, this repeated aspiration/reinstillation may alter the intragastric milieu and thus the mechanics of gastric emptying.

C. Radiographic and Dynamic Fluoroscopy

As with luminal sampling, radiographic markers (to estimate solid emptying) or liquid contrast agents (to estimate liquid emptying) can be ingested or instilled into the stomach and emptying monitored either by repeated abdominal radiographs or by real-time fluoroscopy (22). The latter technique allows a more subjective evaluation of movement of content within the stomach as well as an indirect assessment of gastric contractions and gastric peristalsis. This technique also allows assessment of gastric trituration.

Advantages/limitations. Both radiographic and fluoroscopic methodologies are readily available, the technique is easy, and sophisticated hardware and software are not needed. However, both techniques require radiation exposure, both to the subject and, when using fluoroscopy, to the investigator. Although radiographic emptying of solid markers can be "quantitated," these markers are, however, not similar to normal, mechanically digestible solid food. Similarly, emptying of oral contrast agents from the stomach can be monitored (subjectively) by fluoroscopy, but quantification over time is very difficult and crude at best. Moreover, the specific gravities of the iodine-containing contrast agents are much greater than that of water (which has a value of one, similar to most meals), and gastric emptying is altered significantly by the specific gravity of the intraluminal content.

D. Scintigraphy

Use of an external gamma camera revolutionized the accurate measurement of gastric emptying of solid and/or liquid meals and currently represents the "gold standard" (23, 24). By ingesting a nutrient meal labeled with a gamma-emitting radionuclide (e.g., ^{99m}Tc, ^{111}In, ^{131}I, or ^{57}Co) incorporated into the solid or liquid phase of the meal, the investigator can "scan" the abdomen at multiple time points postprandially and thereby quantitate dynamically the rate of emptying of the meal. Gamma-emitting radionuclides are necessary, in contrast to beta-emitting labels, because the latter do not have high enough energy to penetrate the abdominal wall to be measured externally.

Advantages/limitations. The major advantage of the scintigraphic technique is the ability to measure gastric emptying at multiple time points postprandially to generate a dynamic emptying curve; moreover, one can also measure $t_{1/2}$—the time needed to empty half the maker. Probably the best characterization of gastric emptying (especially for solids) involves calculation of the lag time (time for emptying to begin) as well as the slope of the emptying curve. Liquids empty exponentially, whereas solids empty linearly. Thus, this technique allows estimates of early, mid, and late trends in gastric emptying, each of which may be altered by disease states. A major advantage of scintigraphy is that gastric emptying of both solids and liquids can be measured simultaneously. By selecting radionuclide markers that give off different energies of gamma radiation (e.g., ^{99m}Tc and ^{111}In) to label the solid and liquid phases, the gamma camera can be collimated to quantitate each marker individually, thereby determining the selective emptying of each marker simultaneously.

The limitations of scintigraphic emptying involve primarily the technology (hardware/software) needed to carry out the test. Although this technique requires gamma-labeled radionuclides, the amount of radiation exposure is virtually negligible. The investigator must be careful in choosing the solid marker to be certain that the radiolabel stays in the solid phase during mechanical trituration and does not leach out of the solid phase to empty with the liquid phase. A notable limitation of scintigraphy is that contraction-to-contraction correlation of scintigraphy with another direct measure of contractile activity is impossible due to the time needed to image the stomach by the gamma counter.

E. Magnetic Resonance Imaging and Computed Tomography

Using a multiple array of two-dimensional images and complex software to transform the data into three-dimensional reconstructions, an accurate assessment of gastric emptying of the intraluminal content of the stomach can be calculated from magnetic resonance imaging (MRI) and radiographic imaging (25, 26). Complex but available software can reconstruct gastric volume measurements both over the stomach as a whole as well as in individual definable regions (e.g., antrum, proximal stomach).

Advantages/limitations. Both MRI and computed tomography (CT) techniques allow a reliable quantification of gastric volumes dynamically in the postprandial period. However, the limitations must be acknowledged. First, unlike scintigraphic measurements, this approach does not allow the investigator to measure emptying of a meal but rather the changes in gastric volume postprandially. Gastric volume is a function of both ingested meal and gastric secretion; the latter may be significant if the meal contains protein or is hyperosmolar. Second, repeated CT measurements involve considerable radiation exposure, and, although repeated MR imaging is radiation free, availability of CT and MRI technology for these types of research utilizations is scarce. Finally, the expense of these techniques would make CT and MRI unrealistic in most research arenas.

F. Ultrasonography

Ultrasonography represents a relatively new, noninvasive, radiation-free technique for following gastric emptying indirectly by monitoring changes in the luminal diameter of the stomach (27). Real-time monitoring is possible continuously during the postprandial period.

Advantages/limitations. The major advantage lies in its radiation-free ability to monitor changes in gastric shape dynamically and continuously. However, quantification of gastric emptying requires numerous assumptions of the relationship between diameter and gastric shape (conversion from one measurement to three-dimensional shape as a cylinder, sphere, ellipsoid, etc.) that are far from accurate. Unlike computed tomography, which utilizes multiple arrays of radiographic imaging allowing three-dimensional reconstruction, as of yet ultrasonographic analyses remain as a single source with a one-dimensional measurement. As with fluoroscopic observations, ultrasonography is more of a subjective monitor of changes in diameter after various stimuli or perturbations. Directional flow can be evaluated as well using real-time duplex ultrasonography.

G. Flowmetry

Use of low probes placed across the pylorus have been used to monitor transpyloric flow (28). As with many of the above techniques, quantification of gastric emptying is quite limited. However, this approach allows real-time monitoring of volume of the bolus emptied and bidirectional flow, i.e., gastric emptying and duodenal reflux, especially after certain surgical maneuvers or other chemical or physical manipulations; this concept represents its major advantage. Because flow probes require surgical implantation and are thus invasive, their use is limited to select indications.

H. Duodenal Absorption

Certain chemical substances, once emptied from the stomach into the duodenum, are rapidly absorbed into the bloodstream, such as acetaminophen (29), or into the breath, such as [^{13}C]octacnoic acid (30). Monitoring their dynamic appearance can reflect the rate of gastric emptying.

Advantages/limitations. This approach is quite attractive because it involves little sophisticated hardware or software, necessitates no significant radiation exposure, and only requires collection of blood samples. There are several limitations. First the volume of distribution of the chemical after absorption (circulating plasma volume, extracellular fluid, total body water, etc.) must be known, and second, the rate of plasma disappearance/metabolism may vary between individuals. Although this technique is useful on a relative basis within individuals before and after certain experimental conditions, it is a bit too crude for most studies of gastric emptying.

I. Marker Dilution Technique

This approach to the measurement of gastric emptying is invasive and requires insertion of catheters or cannulas, and thus obviously is of primary utilization in animal studies. The basic concept is quite simple: quantitative recovery of an orally ingested or intragastrically instilled, nonabsorbable marker from the duodenum will reflect gastric emptying (31, 32). One approach is to place in the proximal duodenum a cannula that can be reversibly converted to a functional end "stoma," collect all gastric efflux, and measure dynamic marker recovery. The problem with this approach is that duodenal and small bowel content stimulates multiple neural and hormonal mechanisms that feed back on gastric motility to modulate regulation of gastric emptying. Another more common technique is to establish a constant duodenal perfusion with a second nonabsorbable marker. Quantitative recovery of this second marker allows calculation of duodenal flow; by knowing duodenal flow (ml/min) and the concentration of the orally ingested marker (marker/ml) in the duodenal content, one can quantitate marker recovery and thereby calculate gastric emptying.

Advantages/limitations. This perfusion technique using dual markers and the concept of marker dilution can be used repeatedly in the same animal on many occasions. Quantitative analyses of nonabsorbable markers are relatively standard (e.g., polyethylene glycol, phenol red, Evans blue, ^{3}H- or ^{14}C-labeled compounds such as polyethylene glycol) and the perfusion apparatus is readily available. The limitations are primarily the invasive nature of implanting and maintaining patency of the catheters and/or cannulas and the need for a duodenal infusion.

J. Impedance

This methodology has been evaluated as a noninvasive and accurate technique for monitoring the volume of various organs and in the gut as a function of contractile activity and gastric emptying (33). Impedance measures changes in conductance of low current densities between electrodes placed externally "across" the organ of interest. As the stomach fills, the impedance increases, and as the stomach empties, the impedance decreases.

Advantages/limitations. The primary advantage of this technology is that the technique is noninvasive and requires no specific marker or radionuclide, and thus involves no radiation exposure. However, this methodology has never become popular or universally accepted. Limitations include the need for a certain upright position (45° angle) to maximize measurements and the notable variation across individuals in the position of the stomach (33). Probably its best use is in monitoring relative differences between experimental conditions within each individual subject.

V. Techniques of Measuring Intestinal Transit

A. Physiology

Ultimately intestinal content moves through the gut secondary to external and internal forces that normally propel content distally (or proximally during vomiting). Implications about transit through a segment of gut can be obtained by measuring contractile activity (directly or indirectly). However, direct measurements of the movement of intestinal content from one region to another may provide the investigator with the information desired without need to monitor or measure the actual active and/or passive forces (contractions, gravity, diaphragmatic or pelvic floor excursions) that lead to transit.

Why does intestinal content preferentially move distally (aborad)? As discussed above, there is an aborad vector to the direction of spread of contractions. This vector is largely controlled by the pacemaking region of the proximal duodenum, which drives the spread of the depolarizing slow wave distally. Because the smooth muscle cell can contract only during depolarization, the slow wave not only controls when the muscle contracts, but also the directional spread of the slow wave determines the direction of spread of contractions. Movement of intestinal content along the gut depends on the vectors of force and pressure differential created by active forces (e.g., intestinal contractions) or passive forces (e.g., inflow of content from proximally) or potentially external forces on certain regions that are relatively fixed and thus subject to compression from external forces (and thus leading to increases in intraluminal pressure). Ultimately, intestinal content moves from higher to lower pressures. Although content within a segment of gut may "slosh" back and forth during nonperistaltic, segmenting contractions, the greater frequency of contractions in the proximal small intestine and the aborad direction of the spread of peristaltic contractions eventuate in aborad transit.

The large intestine appears to act differently from the small intestine. In general, most colonic contractile activity is not coordinated between adjacent segments; groups of propagating contractions that move aborally occur only occasionally. This lack of a true aborad vector of spread leads to individual segmenting contractions, which tend to allow for maximal mixing and exposure of luminal content to the mucosa.

However, overall aborad transit through the large intestine does occur; several forces account for this movement. The inflow of content from the ileum into the cecum may serve as an intraluminal force that tends to move content distally in the large intestine. Another active propulsive force is related to the colonic migrating motor complexes (MMCs). These groups of organized contractions may spread in an orad or aborad direction, but the vast majority are oriented aborad. By definition, a colonic migrating motor complex occurs when a group of related contractions spread in an organized fashion over at least one-half of the large intestine. The third active force in the large intestine is the giant migrating contraction, also known as a mass movement. These high-amplitude "peristaltic" contractions spread rapidly aborad along the large intestine and propel intraluminal content distally. When they involve the distal large intestine, they are usually associated with defecation. Colonic giant migrating contractions are quite unusual and occur only a few times a day.

In vivo methodology. Because transit involves a truly integrated set of forces, most all uses of measuring transit are appropriate only for the *in vivo* state. There are two major problems involved in determining intestinal transit. First, the marker needed to study transit has to be placed or delivered at the starting point of the segment to be studied. Unless gastric emptying is being studied as well (see above), intubation or chronic cannulation of the small intestine or colon must be accomplished. The second major problem involves collecting or quantitatively monitoring the marker either within or at the end of the segment through which transit is being evaluated. Most of the quantitative techniques, except for scintigraphy, involve intestinal intubation/cannulation or sacrifice of the animal to retrieve the marker, unless one adopts a more subjective technique such as radiopaque markers or fluoroscopic techniques of imaging.

B. Radiographic Markers

Ingestion of radiopaque markers allows one to monitor the distal passage of these markers by repeatedly taking abdominal radiographs to determine their position in the small (34) and large (35) intestine. The "holdup" of these markers in certain regions of the gut implies problems with transit at that site or distally. This static technique represents one of the simplest yet still useful techniques for measuring segmental colonic transit in humans.

Advantages/limitations. The primary advantage of this technique is its simplicity and almost universal availability—all that is required is the ability to obtain an abdominal radiograph. But its simplicity also defines its many limitations. Although quite good for defining abnormalities in colonic transit because of the relatively fixed sites in the colon defining anatomic segments (cecum, hepatic flexure, splenic flexure, sigmoid colon, and rectum), this technique is of no use for small bowel transit. Also, it may take several days for the markers to reach and travel through the large intestine. Similarly, each radiograph represents a static time point in a dynamic process. Although a good test for gross global abnormalities in colonic transit, the radiograph marker technique is generally too crude for research interests.

C. Dynamic Fluoroscopy

Real-time imaging of movement of intestinal content is probably best done with direct fluoroscopic monitoring. Injection of a nonabsorbable radiographic contrast agent into the gut will allow the investigator to watch the movements of the contrast agent in real time as it is subjected to different forces. Cannon (22), early in the twentieth century, was one of the first investigators to use this technique to look at intestinal contractions and transit. Because the contrast outlines the bowel lumen, contractions can be visualized by changes in diameter of the bowel. Peristaltic contractions, leading to distal propulsion of the contrast, are readily recognized, as are segmenting contractions, which lead to a more "sloshing about," back-and-forth movement of luminal content.

Advantages/limitations. This technique is currently the only one that allows real-time "imaging" of transit; although good for looking at the actual subjective movement of chyme, quantitative measurements are limited. Quantitating speed of transit from point A to point B is fraught with error because the anatomic position of the segment of gut will change on the screen. Imaging requires repeated instillation of contrast agents, and as the bowel fills with contrast, segments of gut overlap one another, making recognition of the segment of interest difficult or impossible. Also, most contrast agents, contain iodine and their specific gravities far exceed those of water and most natural chyme, which have specific gravities of near one. For these reasons, most investigators relegate this technique for subjective impressions of luminal movement of chyme but not for quantitative measurements of transit. Moreover, the amount of radiation exposure both to subject and to investigator limits the duration of study and the number of studies possible within each individual subject/patient.

D. Breath Tests

In humans, the small intestine is relatively inaccessible, often requiring use of indirect methods to assess transit. Bond and Levitt (36) first introduced the measurement of orocecal transit by utilizing the hydrogen breath test. Selected disaccharides (e.g., lactulose) and complex carbohydrates pass through the small intestine undigested and are broken down into hydrogen by colonic bacteria only when they enter the cecum. The hydrogen produced in the colon rapidly diffuses into the blood and then is exhaled from the lungs. Thus, the time for orocecal transit can be determined by ingestion of these carbohydrates and measuring and quantitating (on a relative basis) the excretion of hydrogen in the breath. Simplified methods to sample hydrogen and to determine hydrogen concentrations have led to widespread use of hydrogen breath tests not only in motility studies primarily aimed to calculate orocecal transit time, but also in studies of carbohydrate malabsorption and in the diagnosis of bacterial overgrowth, which may also reflect a motility disorder.

Advantages/limitations. The hydrogen breath test remains a useful physiologic and clinical test to determine intestinal transit when more expensive and laborious methods such as scintigraphy are unavailable. Advantages of this technique are that it is noninvasive and there is no radiation exposure. The primary use is to recognize gross abnormalities in orocecal transit. The limitations, however, are many. First, the method does not distinguish between gastric emptying and intestinal transit unless the marker is placed directly into the intestine. The hydrogen breath test cannot be used for measurement of orocecal transit time in individuals with an altered intestinal bacterial flora, either in individuals with abnormal flora proximal to the colon, e.g. patients with bacterial overgrowth secondary to achlorhydria of the stomach and/or the small intestine, or in patients with an abnormal colonic flora that fails to ferment the carbohydrate rapidly, e.g., those patients recently treated with antibiotics. Similarly, this test cannot differentiate segmental abnormalities in specific regions of the small bowel and is difficult to quantitate across individuals. Most investigators use breath tests as a function of the initial appearance of the leading edge of the marker into the cecum. Breath tests remain useful as clinical tests to determine intestinal transit when more detailed and/or expensive methods such as scintigraphy are unavailable or unnecessary.

E. Scintigraphy

Just as radiographic markers can be visualized by static radiography or fluoroscopy, an ingested meal containing radionuclide-labeled compounds can be followed using an external gamma camera as the meal travels out of the stomach, into the small bowel, and eventually into the large intestine (37). Although the individual images are "static," multiple repeated images can be taken over several hours without the radiation exposure required by repeated radiographs or prolonged fluoroscopy. Scintigraphy has been shown to correlate well with simultaneous hydrogen breath tests (38). A novel technique has been designed specifically to measure colonic transit. By developing a capsule whose external wall is dissolved only when it reaches the distal ileum, this approach will allow release of radionuclide directly into the cecum, which then allows transit through the colon to be imaged and quantitated directly.

Advantages/limitations. The primary strengths of this radionuclide technique are that the radiotracers are more physiologic than are radiographic contrast agents, multiple static images can be obtained without added risk to the subject, and the computer-assisted software allows an easy and accurate quantification of movement of the radionuclide marker. Limitations are that unless the marker is placed into the duodenum by a transpyloric tube, gastric emptying represents another variable; although gastric emptying can be accounted for, the resolution is decreased. Similar to other techniques of total small bowel transit, scintigraphy is limited by the relative inability to recognize accurately separate regions of the small bowel (e.g., proximal/distal jejunum and ileum) and the need to monitor radioactivity in an anatomically fixed region (e.g., cecum). In addition, the scintigraphic equipment is expensive, and although the amount of radiation exposure is relatively low, multiple studies in humans may not be feasible.

F. Multilumen Catheter Assemblies Using Marker Dilution Techniques

Many of the original studies on absorption and secretion involved intestinal perfusion/recovery studies using either surgically implanted catheters or intestinal intubation catheter assemblies (39, 40). After beginning a constant infusion of a test solution and achieving a steady state (amount of a nonabsorbable marker infused per unit of time into the segment equals the mean amount of marker recovered per unit of time from the end of the segment), transit through the perfused segment could easily be measured by injecting a bolus of a second marker and quantitating its recovery from the end of the segment by simple marker dilution techniques. The perfusion was established in an attempt to mimic the postprandial state with intraluminal flow of intestinal content.

Advantages/limitations. Marker dilution techniques can be used to monitor changes in transit through defined segments of the small or large intestine and not necessarily the entire small or large intestine. Moreover, quantitation is more accurate than most of the other more global techniques discussed above, and more subtle differences can be studied.

However, the numerous limitations require acknowledgment. First, this is an invasive technique because the catheter system needs to be either implanted surgically or repeatedly inserted into the segment to be studied. Second, the infusion of the perfusate is given as a constant infusion, which differs from the bolus-type propulsion of luminal content that occurs physiologically—this constant infusion may alter normal mechanisms of transit. Third, a steady state must be established before transit experiments can be performed; any acute change in motor pattern that alters the characteristics of the steady state cannot be accurately studied until a new steady state has been established.

G. Acute Marker Transit Using Geometric Center

This technique, described by Summers *et al.* (41, 42), involves injecting a nonabsorbable marker (dye, chemical substance such as polyethylene glycol, fluorescent tag, or a radionuclide) either into the stomach, duodenum, or colon, waiting an appropriate duration of time, and then rapidly killing the animal (usually a rodent), dividing and ligating the intestinal segment to be studied into multiple defined segments, and quantitating the amount (usually percentage) of marker in each segment. Transit can then be expressed as the geometric center of the distribution of the marker, calculated as the sum of the percentage of marker per segment multiplied by the segment number. The segment representing the geometric center represents the mean transit.

Advantages/limitations. This technique almost always uses rodents because of cost considerations. The results are reproducible across animals and are known to reflect changes in transit accurately, as measured by other techniques that are less quantifiable. However, the limitations are that this technique requires killing of the test animal and thus is not appropriate in large animal models. Additionally, each animal (or time point) is a static measure of transit at one time point and the technique requires a means of injecting the marker at the proximal end of the segment of interest; should the investigator wish to determine small bowel or colonic activity specifically, an infusion catheter will need to be surgically implanted in the test animal several days before the day of the experiment.

VI. Techniques of Measuring Defecation

A. Physiology

The physiology of defecation is a complex, multifactorial process (43) involving both autonomic and skeletal muscles and nerves, as well as modulation by the central nervous system (CNS). This interplay of autonomic (involuntary) and voluntary (skeletal) muscles and nerves differs from gastrointestinal contractions, which are all autonomic. Timing of defecation in humans and many animals is heavily modulated by the CNS to occur at a time when it is "socially acceptable." At this point, the abdominal wall musculature contracts, the pelvic floor (levator ani) and perineum descend, the rectoanal angle straightens, the distal colonic wall musculature contracts, and the puborectalis and anal sphincters relax. Defecation involves CNS input from afferent signals from the mid to distal rectum, which "sample" the characteristics of luminal content, and reflex arcs through the pelvic nerves, which allow activation of the pelvic floor, contraction of the distal colon, and relaxation of the puborectalis muscle and anal sphincters. Distal to the oropharynx, this physiologic GI process is the only motor event that reliably requires the integration of voluntary and involuntary muscles. Although (possibly) not as subjectively appealing to the naive investigator as other functions of GI motility, defecation represents one of the more interesting, complex, but poorly understood areas of GI physiology.

B. Anorectal Manometry

Anorectal manometry represents the most frequently utilized test of anorectal motor function (44). Utilizing measurement of intraluminal pressure, the investigator can quantitate anal resting pressure (internal anal sphincter tone), squeeze pressure (maximum external anal sphincter tone), and the anorectal reflex. The latter reflex involves relaxation of the internal anal sphincter during distention of a balloon in the rectum. This reflex suggests the presence of enteric ganglion cells in the rectum (which are absent in Hirschsprung's disease) and a functional interaction of the intrinsic nerves of the distal rectum and anal canal, which are anatomically distinct from one another.

Advantages/limitations. Although this technique represents one of the diagnostic tests of choice for Hirschsprung's disease, its use in patients with other abnormalities of defecation (constipation, incontinence) has been disappointing. The 24-hr or nighttime monitoring of anal canal tone and intrarectal pressure has led to some interesting observations of nocturnal motor activity, but most of the uses of anorectal manometry from a research standpoint involve study of measurable parameters before and after operative procedures in the pelvis and perineum.

C. Anorectal Angle

The anorectal angle is defined as the angle between the anal canal and the rectum (45). Normally, the puborectalis muscle sling surrounds the junction of the rectum and the anal canal. As one defecates, this angle widens (becoming more obtuse) because the puborectalis relaxes, the perineum descends, and the junction of the rectum and anal canal straightens. This angle can be measured during a Valsalva maneuver or during a defecating proctogram (see below). As with anorectal manometry, this measurement, indicative of one aspect of anorectal motility, has been a poor discriminator of specific defects in defecation and represents just one of the multiple measurements necessary to characterize motor function during defecation.

D. Defecating Proctography

This technique involves videofluoroscopy of changes in rectal and anal canal anatomy during defecation (46). The rectum is filled with radiopaque contrast and the patient is asked to defecate. Fluoroscopically, one can monitor subjectively and indirectly rectal contraction, relaxation of the puborectalis and anal sphincters, and the efficiency of stool evacuation. Objective measurement of the anorectal angle can be made as well as the extent of perineal descent. Other disorders such as intrarectal intussusception and rectal prolapse can be noted as well. This test may be the best overall functional test of defecation and can be evaluated repeatedly after surgical, mechanical, or psychological (biofeedback) interventions.

E. Efficiency of Defecation

Several techniques to measure efficiency of evacuation of the rectum have been evaluated, including quantification of evacuation of artificial stool (47) and the amount of external weight needed to expel an intrarectal balloon (48). The former technique has involved intrarectal instillation of artificial stool labeled with a radiolabeled marker. The patient is asked to defecate under scintigraphy; efficiency of evacuation is measured as well as the anorectal angle. The latter technique involves inserting a balloon into the rectum and determining how much weight attached to the balloon is needed by the patient to allow transanal expulsion. As with many of the other techniques, these tests are primarily used before and after various interventions.

F. Rectal Compliance

Evaluation of rectal compliance is a measure of the distensibility and indirectly the tone of the rectum (49). A balloon of potentially "infinite" volume is inserted in the rectum and slowly inflated with air. The investigator can quantitatively measure either the volume needed to induce the sensations of rectal "fullness," urgency to defecate, or "pain," or the intraluminal pressure induced by a certain volume. Volume/pressure curves can be constructed. Again, this technique is most useful when an individual subject is used as his/her own control before and after various interventions.

G. Electromyography of Puborectalis

As with peripheral neuromuscular studies, the puborectalis muscle and external anal sphincter can be evaluated by inserting a needle "electrode" into the muscle and recording the electromyogram (EMG) (50). Experience with accurate interpretation is limited. One should be able to evaluate the muscle recordings for changes indicative of denervation, abnormal response to stimuli that normally lead to muscle relaxation or contraction, etc. The primary limitation of this technique is that a thorough understanding of normal and abnormal EMG recordings from puborectalis and external anal sphincter is largely lacking; moreover, the test is quite uncomfortable for the patient.

VII. Models for Studying Gastrointestinal Motility

This section addresses the most commonly used models for studying various aspects of GI motility. No attempt will be made to discuss all the models because the basic models are often modified in various ways to address selected aspects of physiology, pathophysiology, etc.

A. In Vitro Models

1. Contractile Force

Most models measuring contractile force involve isolating a segment or strip of muscle in a temperature-controlled bath within which the muscle is exposed to a buffered bath solution. The strip can be suspended vertically or horizontally (Fig. 1). The bath solution is either perfused continuously through the study chamber or the chamber can be filled statically with the bath solution, which is changed at various intervals (51, 52). The perfusion system prevents the buildup in the bath of metabolites or other noxious substances from the muscle strip, but also requires more buffer solution. Similarly, when a test substance is administered as a bolus into the perfusate, the effective concentration to which the muscle strip is exposed changes as the substance enters the chamber, reaches its maximum concentration, and is then washed out by further inflow of perfusate. An option to avoid this crescendo/decrescendo concentration phenomenon is to make up a new perfusate containing the substance of interest and perfusing the chamber with the new perfusate; this approach, however, requires a larger amount of test substance and may be impractical with various hormones/neurotransmitters, etc. In contrast, with the static chamber model, the test substances can be administered directly into the chamber, reach their final concentration very rapidly (depending on the chamber volume), and can be washed out almost immediately by emptying the chamber completely and refilling with new bath buffer.

This setup can measure either isometric or isotonic force. When measuring isometric force, the muscle strip does not actually contract in length, but exerts a contractile "force" on the strain gauge during contraction. To measure isotonic force, other systems will "hang" a fixed force (or weight, usually ~1 g) on the muscle strip and, in an isotonic manner, measure change in length of the muscle strip as a function of contractile force.

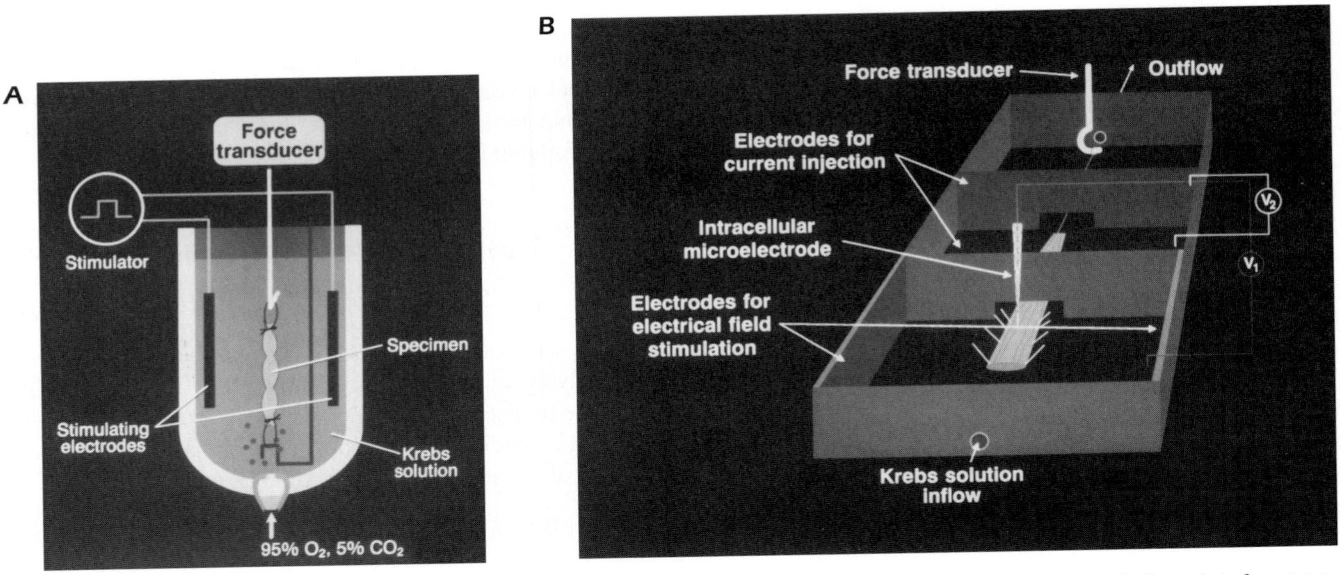

Figure 1 *In vitro* tissue chambers to record contractile activity. (A) Vertically "hung" muscle strip; note connection of upper end of muscle to force transducer and electrodes for electrical field stimulation. (B) Horizontally supported muscle strip; this modification involves pinning out half of the strip to prevent contraction, to allow intracellular puncture of smooth muscle cells by a microelectrode and simple fixation of the other half to permit measurement of contractile force.

2. Patch Clamp Models

The experimental setup for patch clamping is complex and involves special micropipettes (a type of microelectrode) that are advanced to abut the cell membrane (Fig. 2). By maintaining a slight negative pressure on the lumen of the micropipette, the membrane becomes electrically sealed (10 to 15 GΩ) to the tip of the micropipette. When in this configuration, the technique provides the cell-attached recordings. When the membrane within the tip of the micopipette is disrupted, it allows whole-cell recordings. The patch of membrane can also be "excised" and in practice "ripped" off the cell, but maintaining its electrical seal on the micropipette. With this configuration, it represents a so-called inside-out patch or and outside-out patch, depending on the experimental conditions, or excised patch, whereby the inside or outside aspect, respectively, of this membrane patch is now exposed to the bath solution rather than to the intracellular environment.

Electrical current is then measured across the membrane patch as channels "open," allowing the flow of ions (current) across the membrane. Recording systems must have a very high fidelity and use complex software that allows quantum measurements of individual channel openings and closings. The types of ion channels measured (K^+, Ca^+, Na^+, Cl^-, etc) depend on experimental conditions, the ions present in the micropipette and buffer, the presence of specific inhibitor or agonists/antagonists of various channels, and the membrane studied. Complex electrical theory is necessary to derive measurements of cell membrane potential and channel conductance (53). [For further theory, the reader should refer to Hamill *et al.* (6) or DeFelice (7).]

3. Intracellular Potential

This model can be used for many areas of the GI tract. The smooth muscle (or neural plexus) of interest is immobilized in a tissue bath. Specially made microelectrodes are advanced into the muscle or nerve layer of interest until the potential measured becomes a negative value, implying an intracellular location (Fig. 1B). Changes in cell potential (i.e., the electrical potential across the membrane) are then recorded dynamically during various experimental conditions, such as electrical field stimulation to release neuroactive substances from nerves, administration of various substances either into the bath solution or "spritzed" into the tissue in close approximation to the tip of the microelectrode, or in response to "injecting" current into the cell via the microelectrode.

B. In Vivo Models—Animals

1. Contractile Activity

a. Direct Recording Devices Whether the investigator is using intraluminal manometric catheters, serosal strain gauges, serosal electrodes, or serosal ultrasonic microtransducers, the wires attached to the device must somehow exit

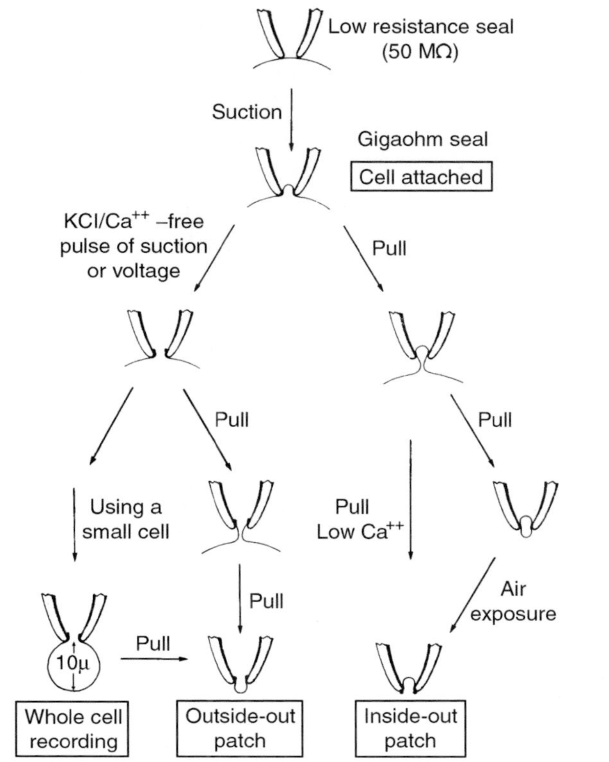

Figure 2 Patch clamp models of cell-attached, whole-cell, excised outside-in, and excised inside-out patches. From Ref. (6), O. P. Hamill, A. Marty, E. Neber, S. Sakmann, and F. G. Sigworth (1981). Improved patch clamp techniques for high resolution current recordings from cells and cell-free membrane patches. *Pflugers Arch. Eur. J. Physiol.* **391,** 85–100, Fig. 9. Copyright © 1981 Springer-Verlag.

the body to allow the recordings to be obtained. The recording devices can be sewn to stomach, small intestine, large intestine, or even the gallbladder. In large animals, many investigators (54, 55) have cemented the wires within a metal cannula, which is imbedded within the abdominal wall, thereby exteriorizing the cannula for electrical connection to the recorder (Fig. 3). Exteriorization in the abdominal wall prevents the animal from being able to cause physical disruption of the cannula with its mouth/teeth or extremities. In small animals (e.g., rodents, etc), many researchers exteriorize the wires between the scapula; the wires are often put in a bag and the animal is kept (if possible) in a type of external jacket that prevents physical trauma to the wires. Other systems utilize a swivel connection that allows the animal free movement within the cage. Typical recordings from manometric catheters of intraluminal pressure, strain gauges of change in force, and serosal electrodes measuring electrical potential are shown in Fig. 4.

b. Barostat Models Use of the barostat (Fig. 5) was initially in the stomach (13), but any hollow organ with contractile properties can be studied, such as the small bowel (56), colon (57), rectum (49), and gallbladder (58). Each model requires an access to the organ of study for introduction of the barostat bag. For instance, the stomach and proximal small bowel can be intubated either per os or via a cannula in the stomach; similarly, the colon and rectum can be intubated transanally. In contrast, the gallbladder requires an intraluminal cannula for barostat bag insertion. Initially the barostat recorders were made individually by the research unit using this technology, but currently there are commercial units available through several biotechnology companies.

c. Electrogastrogram The electrogastrogram is similar in principle to the electrocardiogram. Cutaneous electrodes are placed across the epigastrium, and the underlying signals are recorded (59). The recordings of these changes in electrical potential, however, are much more complex than for the heart and require a computer-assisted analysis to isolate out the multiple concurrent frequency oscillations that occur simultaneously but out of phase (multiple points along the stomach).

2. Gastric Emptying

Intubation Models Most animal models of gastric emptying utilize either a bolus gavage of nonabsorbable marker, a radionuclide, or a perfusion system. The bolus gavage of a nonabsorbable marker can be used in small or large animal models. In rodents, gastric emptying is most often monitored by gavage of the marker, with sacrifice of multiple animals at various time points and quantification of amount of marker remaining in the stomach (60–63). This technique is feasible for inexpensive animal models (rats, mice, etc.) in which numerous pharmacologic agents are to be tried; the models are quite reproducible for both solid and liquid markers. In large animal models, however, this approach is not practical. A more appropriate static technique is to instill the marker by tube gavage and then to later aspirate the stomach at a specific time and to quantitate recovery of the marker as a function of the amount emptied. Because complete aspiration of gastric content by a tube is not always reliable, especially for solid markers, a second, different marker can be instilled immediately before aspirating gastric content. The efficiency of gastric aspiration can be measured by immediate quantification of recovery of this second marker; recovery of the original marker can then be "corrected" appropriately.

Radionuclides to be measured scintigraphically (Fig. 6A) are administered in a meal eaten by the animal or as a solution administered intragastrically via a tube/catheter system inserted into the stomach either by mouth or via a gastric cannula or tube gastrostomy. The animal is immobilized in a type of Pavlov-like sling or is trained to be quiet while the

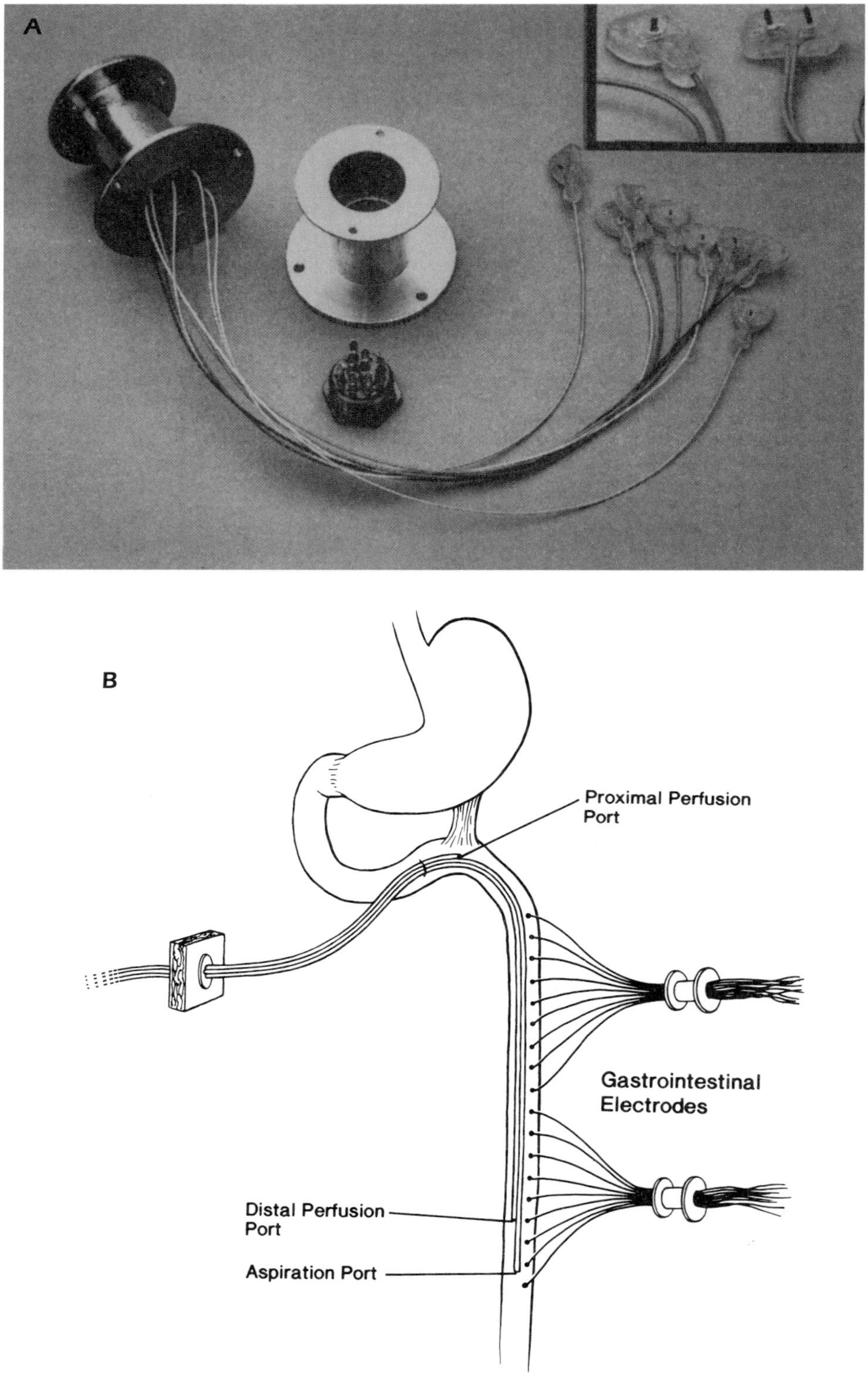

Figure 3 *In vivo* model for recording of basic motor activity. The wires from the recording devices (in this case gastrointestinal electrodes) are cemented within a metal cannula (A) imbedded within the abdominal wall (B). Also shown is an intraluminal catheter assembly with three ports, to be used for measurement of transit by a bolus, marker dilution technique. (A) From Soper and Sarr (55a), in "An Illustrated Guide to Gastrointestinal Mobility" (D. Kumar and S. Gustavson, eds.), 1988. Reproduced by permission of John Wiley & Sons Limited. (B) From Cullen *et al.* (40), with permission.

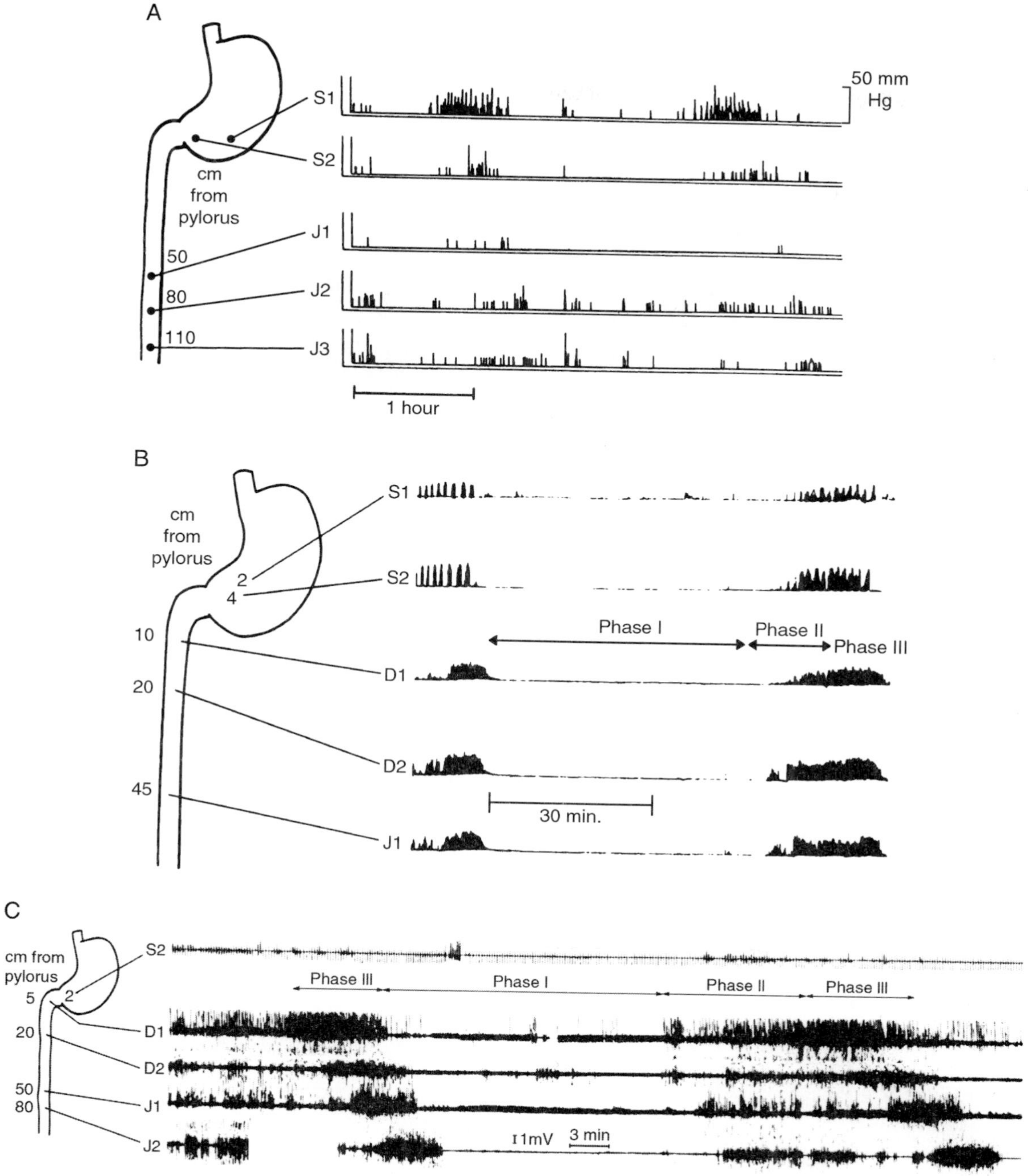

Figure 4 Typical recordings using a model as in Fig. 3. (A) Manometric intraluminal pressure. (B) Strain gauge changes in force. (C) Serosal electrodes measuring change in serosal electrical potential.

gamma camera records images of the stomach. This technique is most appropriate for large animals, not only in terms of resolution and accuracy, but also because it is difficult to immobilize a small animal without the added confounding factor of stress and its potential effects on gastric emptying; also, the resolution of imaging is much less with small animals. Scintigraphic studies allow multiple measurements of gastric emptying of solids, liquids, or both on the same animal and allow a real-time dynamic depiction of gastric emptying rather than a static measurement; this technique currently is the gold standard.

Gastric emptying measured by a constant perfusion system has been utilized in large animal models for many years. It has the main advantage of not requiring an external

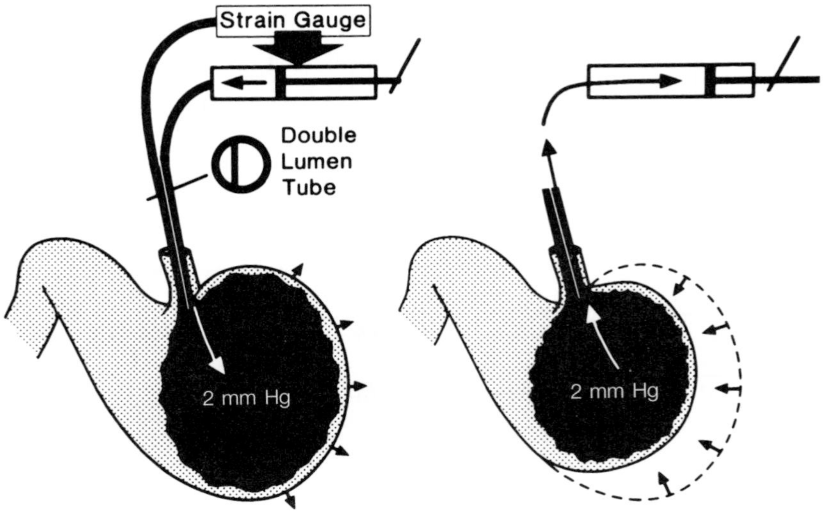

Figure 5 Barostat as used in the stomach. The barostat "bag" is introduced into the stomach either by mouth or via a gastric cannula and is connected to the servomechanism of the barostat machine. From Apiroz and Malagelada (13), with permission.

gamma camera. Numerous types of models can be used, but the basic concept involves intragastric instillation of a nonabsorbable marker and recovery of this marker (emptied from the stomach) by aspiration of duodenal content (64) (Fig. 6B). Because complete recovery of duodenal content is not reliable, a second nonabsorbable marker is perfused proximally into the duodenum. By the dilution of this duodenal marker secondary to gastric emptying and pancreatobiliary secretions, one can calculate duodenal flow rate. Knowing duodenal flow rate (ml/min) and measuring the concentration of the gastric marker in the duodenal aspirate (mg/ml) allows the investigator to calculate gastric emptying of the gastric marker (32). This need for a duodenal marker can be obviated by the use of a functional end duodenostomy cannula that diverts all duodenal content externally. Using this model, gastric emptying of the marker can be measured directly. However, complete duodenal diversion by this technique is far from physiologic, because it dissociates control of gastric emptying from duodenal receptors and short and long neural reflexes that modulate gastric emptying from the duodenal and small bowel mucosa; this method is rarely used currently.

3. Intestinal Transit

a. Small Animal Models Most animal models of transit using rodents (usually rats) involve operative placement of an intraluminal catheter 2 to 5 days prior to the experiment (42). Intraduodenal cannulas are used for measuring small bowel transit, and intracecal catheters are used for colonic transit. After recovery from this minioperative procedure, a

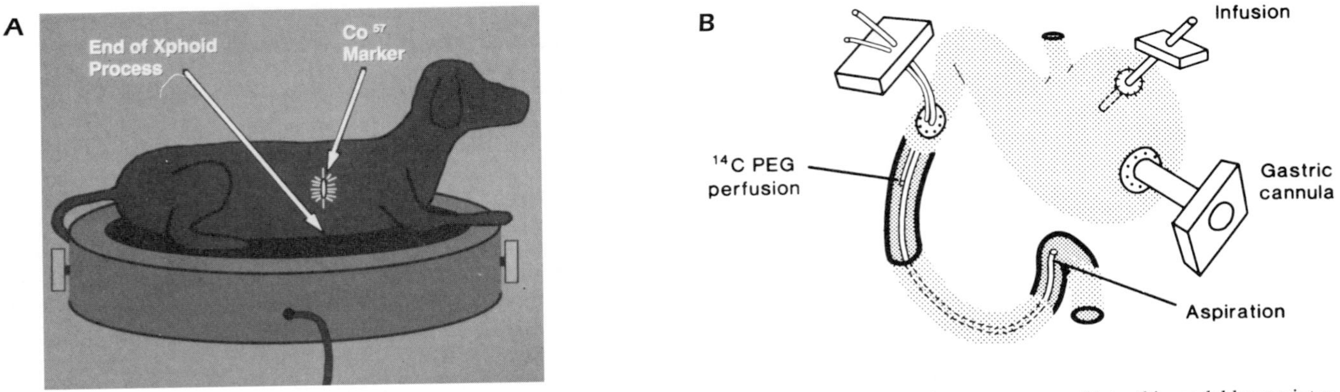

Figure 6 Models of gastric emptying. (A) Scintigraphic recording of gastric emptying using an external gamma camera. Note: this model has an internal marker (^{57}Co) to help localize area of interest. (B) Example of an intragastric/duodenal perfusion model; note separate gastric and duodenal catheters for marker dilution calculations. (B) From Kholeif *et al.* (64), with permission.

nonabsorbable marker (radionuclide, dye, chemical reactant, fluorescent agent) is instilled intraluminally as a bolus, and the animal is killed at various times after marker instillation. The region of gut to be studied is divided into segments of interest, and the amount of marker in each segment is quantitated. This model is relatively inexpensive but requires multiple rodents to evaluate transit. The major limitation is that each animal can be studied only once, and thus it is not appropriate for large animals. Although small bowel transit can be evaluated after intragastric administration (see Section VII,B,2), other assumptions and corrections for gastric emptying are necessary.

b. Large Animal Models Similar in principle to the model for small animals, catheters can be placed operatively within the duodenum and colon to measure transit of the small and large bowel, respectively (65); however, instead of killing the animal and excising the gut, a radionuclide can be given and transit quantitated using an external gamma camera. Small bowel transit is usually expressed as the time necessary for a certain percentage of the marker to reach the right colon (which has a relatively fixed anatomic location). For colonic transit, the various anatomic segments that are relatively fixed can be analyzed separately and a geometric center of the mean determined.

Other models used to measure transit *in situ* involve creation of an enterically isolated segment, such as a Thiry–Vella loop (or similar modification) (66,67), or a catheter-based, marker dilution technique (40,68) (Fig. 7). With the enterically isolated loop, all the liquid infused into the loop will exit distally, giving a reliable, 100% recovery of marker. With the perfusion-based marker dilution techniques in which flow (and thereby transit) is measured by "sampling" intestinal content downstream from the site of marker instillation, a second marker may be needed to calculate efficiency of recovery, etc. The benefits of these techniques are that multiple evaluations of transit can be performed within the same animals. Moreover, this technique is relatively inexpensive.

4. Defecation

There are very few reliable animal models of defecation. Because the control of active defecation is governed by social customs, subjective cerebral initiation and inhibition, and other factors, animal models are poor models of defecation. Although rectal compliance, rectal manometry, and some reflexes via puborectalis electromyography can be monitored in selected animal models, these techniques address specific questions but cannot adequately measure or quantitate defecation (see the following discussion of human models).

C. In Vivo Models—Humans

1. Contractile Activity

As with animal models, direct recording of contractile activity can be accomplished using intraluminal manometric

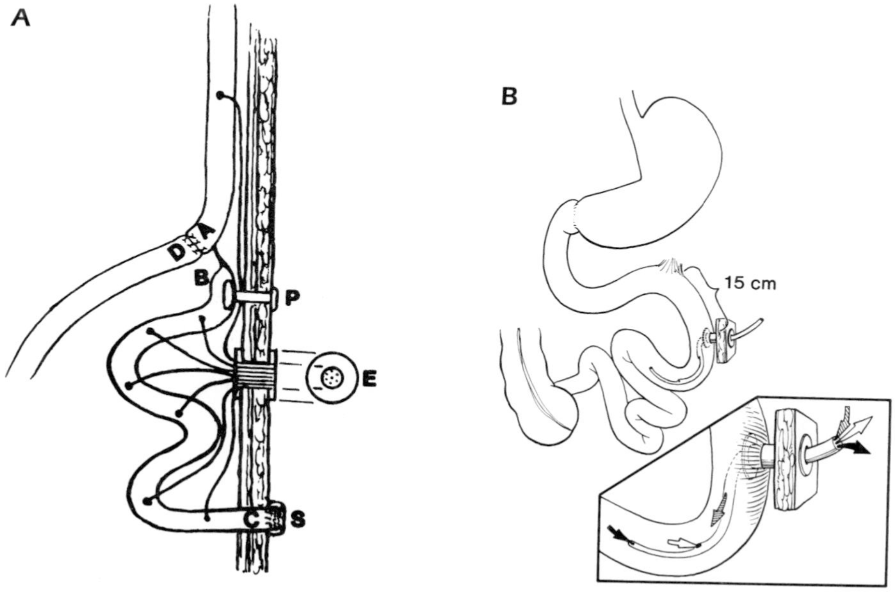

Figure 7 Large animal models of *in situ* intestinal transit. (A) Thiry–Vella type, enterically isolated loop. Note infusion cannula (P) and stoma (S) for collection of perfusate, and the metal cannula (E) for wires from serosal electrodes. (B) Marker dilution technique with intestinal perfusion—triple lumen model. Nonabsorbable marker given at second port of catheter system. (B) From Herkes *et al.* (68a), with permission.

catheter systems (Fig. 8A) (68b) introduced either transorally for measurement of gastric or intestinal manometry (69–71) or transanally under colonoscopic guidance for colonic manometry (72). Either solid-state transducers or luminally perfused, open-tip manometric systems can be used. For chronic prolonged recordings (73), radiotelemetry capsules have been developed to measure contractile activity and to transmit the electrical signals to an external, wireless recording device (74).

For myoelectric recordings of changes in electrical potential, "serosal" electrodes can be placed at the time of intraabdominal surgery, to be removed postoperatively (75–78). Usually these electrodes are "wire" electrodes implanted intramurally in the region of interest (Fig. 8B)

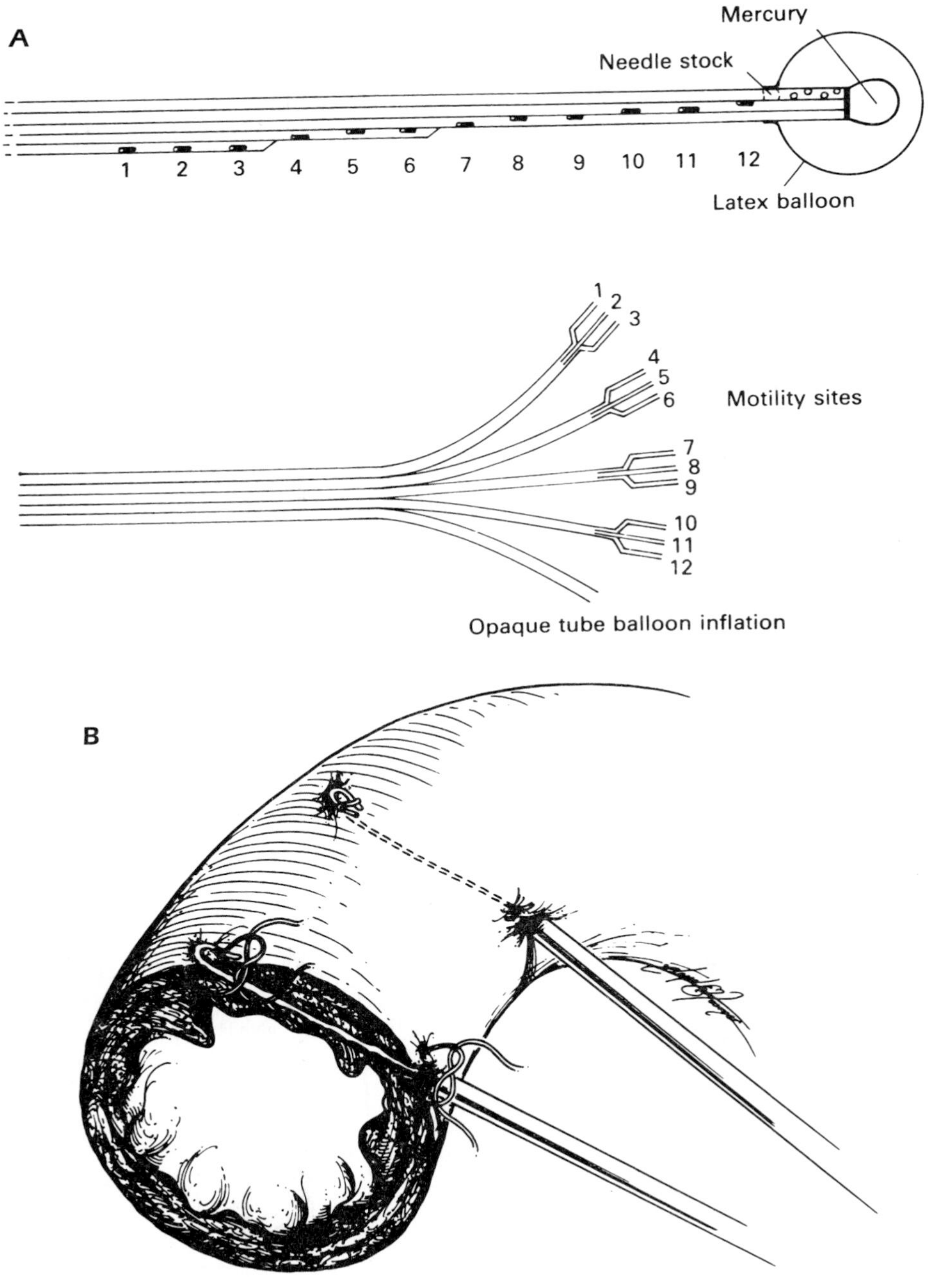

Figure 8 Direct recording devices for measuring contractile activity in man. (A) Manometric catheter assembly—13-lumen tube. Latex balloon filled with mercury aids distal propulsion of tube. (B) Temporary intestinal electrodes—note the exposed wire placed intramurally, allowing electrodes to be pulled out transabdominally several days postoperatively. (A) From Gustavsson and Tucker (68b), in "An Illustrated Guide to Gastrointestinal Mobility" (D. Kumar and S. Gustavson, eds.), 1988. Reproduced by permission of John Wiley & Sons Limited. (B) From Soper *et al.* (68c), with permission.

and are brought out through a stab wound or drain site in the anterior abdominal wall. Because these wires need to be covered with plastic or silastic insulation in the areas not within the muscle of interest, the electrodes can be easily removed postoperatively with gentle traction. Typical electrodes utilized include the commercially available cardiac surgery epicardial pacing wires (75). Other electrode techniques include suction electrodes (79, 80) and ring electrodes (81). Electrodes have also been placed directly on bowel exposed to a stoma.

Barostat recordings offer another model for measuring GI contractility in humans. The barostat balloons are placed either in the proximal stomach (82) or upper small bowel by a transoral route or in the colon or rectum by a transanal approach (99). This model measures more closely the tone of the bowel wall rather than actual contractile activity.

2. Gastric Emptying

Currently, most models of gastric emptying in humans are based on scintigraphic techniques. Intubation techniques are too cumbersome, involve too many assumptions, are uncomfortable to the patient or subject, and are not as accurate as scintigraphy. Liquid markers used include ^{99m}Tc or ^{111}In labels in the liquid phase, often using DTPA diethylene triaminepentaacetic acid (DTPA) or ^{99m}Tc-labeled sulfur colloid as the liquid vehicle (83). Solid markers used include labeling chicken liver with either ^{99m}Tc or ^{113m}In colloidal particles or with [^{57}Co]cyanocobalamin and then using the labeled liver as the solid marker (84). Eggs can now be labeled with ^{99m}Tc without much loss of label into the aqueous phase (85); ^{131}I-labeled fiber is another solid marker used (86). ^{111}In-Labeled Amberlite resin beads of 0.5 to 1.8 mm diameter are now also used as a marker of solid emptying (87).

3. Intestinal Transit

A rather crude model of intestinal transit in humans involves ingestion of lactulose with measurement of breath hydrogen (88). This technique suffers from dependence on gastric emptying, which cannot be measured simultaneously with this technique alone. Intubation techniques using dye or radionuclide dilution can be utilized in the proximalmost gut, but this model is cumbersome and uncomfortable for the patient.

Scintigraphy has all but replaced other models of measuring intestinal transit in humans (90–93). Most markers of small bowel transit are administered as an oral meal; by separately quantitating gastric emptying, small bowel transit can be determined and expressed as the amount of time for a given percentage of marker emptied to reach the cecum. Direct intraluminal instillation of the radionuclide marker by a transoral duodenal tube is possible and is ultimately more accurate, but adds an additional level of complexity and patient discomfort.

Colonic transit is a bit more difficult to measure accurately. The typical orally administered markers may take a long time (several days) to reach the colon, small bowel radioactivity overlaps the colonic region of interest, and the marker is not delivered as a bolus, making the calculations of delivery of marker into the colon and its subsequent transit difficult; accuracy is markedly affected. Transorally or transanally positioned tubes into the cecum for bolus instillation of radionuclide marker are also not practical.

For these reasons, Proano *et al.* (94) developed a gelatin capsule filled with radionuclide but coated with a pH-sensitive polymer (methacrylate) that dissolves in the distal ileum. This model allows a relative bolus-type delivery of marker into the ascending colon without significant overlap of gastric or small bowel radioactivity. Currently, this technique represents the gold standard for measuring colonic transit dynamically. By using two different radionuclides with different energy disintegrations and appropriately collimating the gamma camera, the investigator can simultaneously measure gastric emptying, small bowel transit, and colonic transit (i.e., whole gut transit) (95).

References

1. Sarna, S. K. (1985). Cyclic motor activity: Migrating motor complex. *Gastroenterology* **89,** 894–913.
2. Clench, M. H., Pineiro-Carrero, V. M., and Mathias, J. R. (1989). Migrating myoelectric complex demonstrated in four avian species. *Am. J. Physiol.* **256,** G598–G603.
3. Weems, W. A., and Weisbrodt, N. S. (1984). Comparison of colonic and ileal propulsive capabilities under conditions requiring hydrostatic work. *Am. J. Physiol.* **246,** G587–G593.
4. Murr, M. M., Miller, V. M., and Sarr. M. G. (1996). Contractile properties of enteric smooth muscle after small bowel transplantation in rats. *Am. J. Surg.* **171,** 212–218.
5. Lu, G., Sarr, M. G., and Szurszewski, J. H. (1997). Effect of extrinsic denervation in a canine model of jejunoileal autotransplantation on mechanical and electrical activity of jejunal circular smooth muscle. *Dig. Dis. Sci.* **42,** 40–46.
6. Hamill, O. P., Marty, A., Neher, E., Sakmann, S., and Sigworth, F. J. (1981). Improved patch clamp techniques for high resolution current recordings from cells and cell-free membrane patches. *Pflugers Arch.* **391,** 85–100.
7. DeFelice, L. J. (1997). "Electrical Properties of Cells: Patch Clamp For Biologists." Plenum Press, New York.
8. Lu, G., Sarr, M. G., and Szurszewski, J. H. (1998). Effect of motilin and erythromycin on calcium-activated potassium channels in rabbit colonic myocytes. *Gastroenterology* **114,** 748–754.
9. McHenry, L., Murthy, K. S., Grider, J. R., and Makhlouf, G. M. (1991). Inhibition of muscle cell relaxation by somatostatin: Tissue-specific, cAMP-dependent, pertussis toxin sensitive. *Am. J. Physiol.* **261,** G45–G49.
10. Malagelada, J.-R., Camilleri, M., and Stanghellini, V. (1986). "Manometric Diagnosis of Gastrointestinal Motility Disorders." Thieme Medical Publishers, Inc., New York.
11. Bass, P., and Wiley, J. N. (1972). Contractile force transducer for recording muscle activity in unanesthetized animals. *J. Appl. Physiol.* **32,** 567–572.
12. Cowles, V. G., Condon, R. E., Schulte, W. J., Woods, J. H., and Sillin, L. F. (1978). A quarter Wheatstne bridge strain gauge force transducer for recording gut motility. *Am. J. Dig. Dis.* **23,** 936–939.

13. Azpiroz, F., and Malagelada, J.-R. (1985). Physiological variations in canine gastric tone measured by an electronic barostat. *Am. J. Physiol.* **248,** G229–G237.
14. Alvarez, W. C., and Mahoney, L. J. (1922). Action currents in stomach and duodenum. *Am. J. Physiol.* **58,** 476.
15. Bass, P., and Wiley, J. N. (1965). Effects of ligation and morphine on electric and motor activity of the dog duodenum. *Am. J. Physiol.* **208,** 908–916.
16. Dusdieker, N., aand Summers, R. W. (1979). Patterns of smooth muscle contractions in the jejunum. *Gastroenterology* **76,** 1126 (abstract).
17. Hamilton, J. W., Bellahsene, B. G., Reichelderfer, M., Webster, J. G., and Bass, P. (1986). Human elecrogastrogams: Comparison of surface and mucosal recordins. *Dig. Dis. Sci.* **31,** 33–39.
18. Abell, T. L., and Malagelada, J.-R. (1985). Glucagon-evoked gastric dysrhythmias in humans shown by an improved electrogastrographic technique. *Gastroenterology* **88,** 1932–1940.
19. Mondrek, K. (1991). Diameter and wall thickness recording of canine pylorus with implantable miniature ultrasonic transducers. *Dig. Dis.* **9,** 325–331.
20. Chiba, T., Sarr, M. G., Bharucha, A. E., Kendrick, M. L., Tanaka, T., Zyromski, N. J., and Phillips, S. F. (2000). Implantable ultrasonic transducers measure canine jejunal wall motion *in vivo. Gastroenterology* (abstract) **118,** A152.
21. Meyer, J. H., Ohashi, H. Jehn, D., and Thomson, J. B. (1981). Size of liver particles emptied from the human stomach. *Gastroenterology* **80,** 1489–1496.
22. Cannon, W. B. (1905). The passage of different food-stuffs from the stomach and through the small intestine. *Am. J. Physiol.* **12,** 387–418.
23. Camilleri, M., Malagelada, J.-R., Brown, M. L., Becker, G., and Zinsmeister, A. R. (1985). Relation between antral motility and gastric emptying of solids and liquids in humans. *Am. J. Physiol.* **249,** G580–G585.
24. Elashoff, J. D., Reedy, T. J., and Meyer, J. H. (1982). Analysis of gastric emptying data. *Gastroenterology* **83,** 1306–1312.
25. Feinle, C., Kunz, P., Boesige, P., Fried, M., and Schwizer W. (1999). Scintigraphic validation of magnetic resonance imaging method to study gastric emptying of a solid meal in humans. *Gut* **44,** 106–111.
26. Seide, K., and Ritman, E. L. (1984). Three dimensional dynamic x-ray-computed tomography imaging of stomach motility. *Am. J. Physiol.* **247,** G574–G581.
27. King, P. M., Heading, R. C., and Pryde, A. (1985). Coordinated motor activity of the human gastroduodenal region. *Dig. Dis. Sci.* **30,** 219–224.
28. Malbert, C. H., and Ruckebush, Y. (1989). Duodenal bulb control of the flow rate of digesta in the fasted and fed dog. *J. Physiol.* **409,** 371–384.
29. Sanaka, M., Koike, Y., Yamamoto, T., Mineshita, S., Yamaoka S., Hirama, S., Tanaka, H., Kuyama, Y., and Yamanaka, M. (1997). A reliable and convenient parameter of the rate of paracetamol absorption to measure gastric emptying of liquids. *Int. J. Clin. Pharmacol. Ther.* **35,** 509–513.
30. Choi, M.-G., Camilleri, M., Burton, D. D., Zinsmeister, A. R., Forstrom, L. A., Nair, K. S. (1997). ^{13}C-Octanoic acid breath test for gastric emptying of solids: Accuracy, reproducibility and comparison with scintigraphy. *Gastroenterology* **112,** 1155–1162.
31. Miller-Lissner, S. A., Fimmel, C. J., Will, N., Muller-Puysin, W., Heinzel, F., and Blum, A. L. (1982). Effect of gastic and transpyloric tubes on gastric emptying and duodenogastric reflux. *Gastroenterology* **83,** 1276–1279.
32. Tohno, H., Sarr, M. G., and DiMagno, E. P. (1995). Intraileal carbohydrate regulates canine postprandial pancreaticobiliary secretion and upper gut motility. *Gastroenterology* **109,** 1977–1985.
33. Sutton, J. A., Thompson, S., and Sobnack, R. (1985). Measurement of gastric emptying rates by radioactive isotope scanning and epigastric impedance. *Lancet* **1,** 898–900.
34. Cullen, J. J., Eagon, J. C., Dozois, E. J., and Kelly, K. A. (1993). Treatment of acute postoperative ileus with octreotide. *Am. J. Surg.* **165,** 113–120.
35. O'Brien, M. D., and Phillips, S. F. (1996). Colonic motility in health and disease. *Gastroenterol. Clin. North Am.* **25,** 113–145.
36. Bond, J. H., and Levitt, M. D. (1975). Investigation of small bowel transit time in man utilizing pulmonary hydrogen (H_2) measurements. *J. Lab. Clin. Med.* **85,** 546–555.
37. Read, N. W., Miles, C. A., Fisher, D., Holgate, A. M., Kim, N. D., Mitchell, M. A., Reeve, A. M., Roche, T. B., and Walter, M. (1980). Transit of a meal through the stomach, small intestine and colon in normal subjects and its role in the pathogenesis of diarrhoea. *Gastroenterology* **79,** 1276–1282.
38. Caride, V. G., Prokop, E. K., Trncale, F. J., Buddoura, W., Winchenbach, K., and McCallum, R. W. (1984). Scintigraphic determination of small intestinal transit time: Comparison with the hydrogen breath technique. *Gastroenterology* **86,** 714–720.
39. Dillard, R. L., Eastman, H., and Fordtran, J. S. (1965). Volume–flow relationship during the transport of fluid through the human small intestine. *Gastroenterology* **49,** 58.
40. Cullen, J. J., Eagon, J. C., Hould, F.-S., Hanson, R. B., and Kelly, K. A. (1995). Ectopic jejunal pacemakes after jejunal transection and their relationship to transit. *Am. J. Physiol.* **268,** G959–G967.
41. Summers, R. W., Kent, T. H., and Osborn, J. W. (1976). Effects of drugs, ileal obstruction, and irradiation on rat gastrointestinal propulsion. *Gastroenterology* **70,** 731–739.
42. Kelley, M. C., Hocking, M. P., Marchand, S. D., and Sninsky, C. A. (1993). Ketorolac prevents postoperative small intestinal ileus in rats. *Am. J. Surg.* **165,** 107–111.
43. Kalff, J. C., Buchholz, B. M., Eskandari, M. K., Hierholzer, C., Schraut, W. H., Simmons, R. L., and Bauer, A. J. (1999). Biphasic response to gut manipulation and temporal correlation of cellular infiltrates and muscle dysfunction in rat. *Surgery* **126,** 498–509.
43. Rasmussen, O. O. (1994). Anorectal function. *Dis. Colon Rectum* **37,** 386–403.
44. Hancock, B. D. (1975). Measurement of anal pressure and motility. *Gut* **17,** 645–651.
45. Barkel, D. C., Pemberton, J. H., Phillips, S. F., Kelly, K. A., and Brown, M. L. (1986) Scintigraphic assessment of the anorectal angle in health and after operation. *Surg. Forum* **37,** 183–186.
46. Mahieu, P., Pringot, J., and Bodart, P. (1984). Defecography. I: Description of a new procedure and results in normal patients. *Gastrointest. Radiol.* **9,** 247–252.
47. Ambroze, W. L., Pemberton, J. H., Bell, A. M., Brown, M. L., and Zinsmeister, A. R. (1991). The effect of stool consistency on rectal and neorectal emptying. *Dis. Colon Rectum* **34,** 1–7.
48. Henry, M. M., Snooks, S. J., Barnes, P. R. U., and Swash, M. (1985). Investigation of disorders of the anorectum and colon. *Ann. R. Coll. Surg.* **67,** 355–360.
49. Hammer, H. F., Phillips, S. F., Camilleri, M., and Hanson, R. B. (1998). Rectal tone, distensibility, and perception: Reproducibility and response to different distensions. *Am. J. Physiol.* **274,** G584–G590.
50. Bartolo, D. C. C., Jarratt, J. A., and Read, N. W. (1983). The use of conventional EMG to assess external anal sphincter neuropathy in man. *J. Neurol. Neurosurg. Psychiatry* **46,** 1115–1118.
51. Shibata, C., Murr, M. M., Balsiger, B., Anding, W. J., and Sarr, M. G. (1998). Contractile activity of circular smooth muscle in rats 1 year after small bowel transplantation: Differing adaptive response of the jejunum and ileum to denervation. *J. Gastrointest. Surg.* **2,** 463–472.
52. Shibata, C., Balsiger, B. M., Anding, W. J., Duenes, J. A., Miller, V. M., and Sarr, M. G. (1998). Functional changes in non-adrenergic noncholinergic inhibitory neurons in ileal circular smooth muscle after small bowel transplantation in rats. *Dig. Dis. Sci.* **43,** 2446–2454.

53. Lu, G., Mazet, B., Sarr, M. G., and Szurszewski, J. H. (1998). Effect of nitric oxide on calcium-activated potassium channels in colonic smooth muscle of rabbits. *Am. J. Physiol.* **274,** G848–G856.
54. Sarr, M. G., and Kelly, K. A. (1981). Myoelectric activity of the autotransplanted canine jejunoileum. *Gastroenterology* **81,** 303–310.
55. Akwari, O. E., Kelly, K. A., Steinbach, J. H., and Code, C. F. (1975). Electrical pacing of intact and transected canine small intestine and its computer model. *Am. J. Physiol.* **229,** 1188–1197.
55a. Soper, N. J., and Sarr, M. G. (1988). Electromyography. *In* "An Illustrated Guide to Gastrointestinal Mobility" (D. Kumar and S. Gustavsson, eds.), p. 105. John Wiley & Sons, Chichester.
56. Rouillon, J. M., Azpiroz, F., Malagelada, J.-R. (1991). Reflex changes in intestinal tone: Relationship to perception. *Am. J. Physiol.* **261,** G280–G286.
57. O'Brien, M. D., Camilleri, M., von der Ohe, M. R., Phillips, S. F., Pemberton, J. H., Prather, C. M., Wiste, J. A., and Hanson, R. B. (1996). Motility and tone of the left colon in constipation: a role in clinical practice? *Am. J. Gastroenterol.* **91,** 2523–2538.
58. Tanaka, M., Sarr, M. G., Miller, L. J., and Malagelada, J.-R. (1990). Change in tone of canine gallbladder measured by an electronic pneumatic barostat. *Am. J. Physiol.* **259,** G314–G320.
59. van der Schee, E. J., and Grashins, J. L. (1983). Contraction-related, low-frequency components in canine electrogastrographic signals. *Am. J. Physiol.* **245,** G470–G475.
60. Derblom, H., Johansson, H., and Nylander, G. (1966). A simple method of recording quantitatively certain gastrointestinal motility functions in the rat. *Acta Chir. Scand.* **132,** 154.
61. Purdon, R. A., and Bass, P. (1973). Gastric and intestinal transit in rats measured by a radioactive test meal. *Gastroenterology* **64,** 968–976.
62. Summers, R. W., Kent, T. H., and Osborne, J. W. (1970). Effects of drugs, ileal obstruction, and irradiation on rat gastrointestinal propulsion. *Gastroenterology* **59,** 731–739.
63. Nilssen, F., Jung, B., and Lundqvist, H. (1973). Gastric evacuation and small bowel propulsion measured with a double isotope technique. *Acta Chir. Scand.* **139,** 71–723.
64. Kholeif, H., Larach, J., Thomforde, G. M., Dozois, R. R., and Malagelada, J.-R. (1983). A canine model for the study of gastric secretion and emptying after a meal. *Dig. Dis. Sci.* **28,** 633–640.
65. Davies, W., Kollmorgen, C. F., Tu, Q. M., Thompson, G. B., Nelson, H., and Sarr, M. G. (1997). Laparoscopic colectomy shortens postoperative ileus in a canine model. *Surgery* **121,** 550–555.
66. Sarr, M. G., Kelly, K. A., and Phillips, S. F. (1980). Canine jejunal absorption and transit during interdigestive and digestive motor states. *Am. J. Physiol.* **239,** G167–G172.
67. Sarr, M. G., Kelly, K. A., and Gladen, H. E. (1981). Electrical control of canine jejunal propulsion. *Am. J. Physiol.* **240,** G355–G360.
68. Johnson, C. P., Sarna, S. K., Baytiyeh, R., Zhu, Y. R., Cowles, V. E., Telford, G. L., Roza, A. M., and Adams, M. B. (1997). Postprandial motor activity and its relationship to transit in the canine ileum. *Surgery* **121,** 182–189.
68a. Herkes, S. M., Smith, C. D., Prabhakar, L. P., Phillips, S. F., and Sarr, M. G. (1993). Effect of α-methylnorepinephune, an α_2-adrenergic agonist, on jejunal absorption in the neurally intact concious dog. *Dig. Dis. Sci.* **38,** 1645–1650.
68b. Gustavsson, S., and Tucker, R. (1988). Manometry. *In* "An Illustrated Guide to Intestinal Motility" (D. Kumar and S. Gustavsson, eds.), p. 68. John Wiley & Sons, Chichester.
68c. Soper, N. J., Sarr, M. G., and Kelly, K. A. (1990). Human duodenal myoelectric activity after operation and with pacing. *Surgery* **107,** 63–68.
69. Ahluwalia, N. K., Thompson, D. G., Barlow, J., and Heggie, L. (1994). Human small intestinal contractions and aboral traction forces during fasting and after feeding. *Gut* **35,** 625–630.
70. Frank, J. W., Sarr, M. G., and Camilleri, M. (1994). Use of gastroduodenal manometry to differentiate mechanical and functional intestinal obstruction: An analysis of clinical outcome. *Am. J. Gastroenterol.* **89,** 339–344.
71. Camilleri, M. (1993). Study of human gastroduodenojejunal motility: Applied physiology in clinical practice. *Dig. Dis. Sci.* **38,** 785–794.
72. von der Ohe, M., Hanson, R. B., and Camilleri, M. (1994). Comparison of simultaneous recordings of human colonic contractions by manometry and a barostat. *Neurogastroenterol. Motil.* **6,** 213–222.
73. Husebye, E., Skar, V., Aalen, O. O., and Osnes, M. (1990). Digital ambulatory manometry of the small intestine in healthy adults: Estimates of variation within and between individuals an statistical management of incomplete MMC periods. *Dig. Dis. Sci.* **35,** 1057–1065.
74. Thompson, D. G., Wingate, D. L., Archer, L., Benson, M. J., Green, W. J., and Hardy, R. J. (1980). Normal patterns of human upper small bowel motor activity recorded by prolonged radiotelemetry. *Gut* **21,** 500–506.
76. Duthe, H. L., Kwong, N. K., Brown, B. H., and Whittaker, G. E. (1971). Pacesetter potential of the human gastroduodenal junction. *Gut* **12,** 250–256.
77. Pezzolla, F., Riezzo, G., Maselli, M. A., and Giorgio, I. (1991). Gastric electrical dysrhythmia following cholecystectomy in humans. *Digestion* **49,** 134–139.
78. Sarna, S. K., Bardakjian, B. L., Waterfall, W. E., and Lind, J. F. (1980). Human colonic electrical control activity (ECA). *Gastroenterology* **78,** 1526–1536.
79. Schang, J.-C., and Devroede, G. (1983). Fasting and postprandial myoelectric spiking activity in the human sigmoid colon. *Gastroenterology* **85,** 1048–1053.
80. Latimer, P., Sarna, S., Campbell, D., Latimer, M., Waterfall, W., and Daniel, E. E. (1981). Colonic motor and myoelectrical activity: A comparative study of normal subjects, psychoneurotic patients, and patients with irritable bowel syndrome. *Gastroenterology* **80,** 893–901.
81. Fleckenstein, P. (1978). A probe for intraluminal recording of myoelectric activity from multiple sites in the human small intestine. *Scand. J. Gasroenterol.* **13,** 767–774.
82. Azpiroz, F., and Malagelada, J.-R. (1987). Gastric tone measured by an electronic barostat in health and postsurgical gastroparesis. *Gastroentrology* **92,** 934–943.
83. Thomforde, G. M., Brown, M. L., and Malagelada, J.-R. (1985). Practical solid and liquid phase markers for studying gastric emptying in man. *J. Nucl. Med. Tech.* **13,** 11–14.
84. Meyer, J. H., MacGregor, I. L., Guellar, R., Martin, P., and Cavalieri, R. (1976). ^{99m}Tc-tagged chicken liver as a marker of solid food in the human stomach. *Am. J. Dig. Dis.* **21,** 296–304.
86. Malagelada, J.-R., Carter, S. E., Brown, M. L., and Carlson, G. L. (1980). Radiolabelled fiber: A physiologic marker for gastric emptying and intestinal transit of solids. *Dig. Dis. Sci.* **25,** 81–87.
87. Camilleri, M., Colemont, L. J., Phillips, S. F., Brown, M. L., Thomforde, G. M., Chapman, N. J., and Zinsmeister, A. R. (1989). Human gastric emptying and colonic filling of solids characterized by a new method. *Am. J. Physiol.* **257,** G284–G290.
88. LaBrooy, S. J., Male, P.-J., Beavis, A. K., and Misiewicz, J. J. (1983). Assessment of the reproducibility of the lactulose H_2 breath test as a measure of mouth to caecum transit time. *Gut* **24,** 893–896.
89. Barreiro, M. A., McKenna, R. D., and Beck, I. T. (1968). Determination of transit time in the human jejunum by the single injection indicator-dilution technique. *Am. J. Dig. Dis.* **13,** 222–233.
90. Caride, V. J., Prokop, E. K., Troncale, F. J., Buddoura, W., Winchenbach, K., and McCallum, R. W. (1984). Scintigraphic determination of small intestinal transit time: Comparison with the hydrogen breath technique. *Gastroenterology* **86,** 714–720.
91. Malagelada, J.-R., Robertson, J. S., Brown, M. L., Remington, M., Duenes, J. A., Thomforde, G. M., and Carryer, P. W. (1984). Intestinal

transit of solid and liquid components of a meal in health. *Gastroenterology* **87,** 1255–1263.

92. von der Ohe, M. R., and Camilleri, M. (1992). Measurement of small bowel and colonic transit: Indications and methods. *Mayo Clin. Proc.* **67,** 1169–1179.
93. Camilleri, M., Zinsmeister, A. R., Greydanus, M. P., Brown, M. L., Proano, M. (1991). Towards a less costly but accurate test of gastric emptying and small bowel transit. *Dig. Dis. Sci.* **36,** 609–615.
94. Proano, M., Camilleri, M., Phillips, S. F., Brown, M. L., and Thomforde, G. M. (1990). Transit of solids through the human colon: Regional quantification in the unprepared bowel. *Am. J. Physiol.* **258,** G856–862.
95. Charles, F., Camilleri, M., Phillips, S. F., Thomforde, G. M., and Forstrom, L. A. (1995). Scintigraphy of the whole gut: clinical evaluation of transit disorders. *Mayo Clin. Proc.* **70,** 113–118.
96. Sagar, P. M., and Pemberton, J. H. (1996). The assessment and treatment of anorectal incontinence. *In* "Advances in Surgery" (J. L. Cameron, ed.), pp. 1–20. Mosby-Year Book, Inc., St. Louis.
97. Nyam, D. C. N. K., Frizelle, F., and Pemberton, J. H. (1998). Physiologic derangements of the rectum and anus. *In* "Modern Surgical Care: Physiologic Foundations" (T. A. Miller, ed.), pp. 702–727. Quality Medical Publishers, St. Louis.
98. Sagar, P. M., and Pemberton, J. H. (1996). Anorectal and pelvic floor function: Relevance to continence, incontinence, and constipation. *In* "Gastroenterology Clinics of North America" (M. Camilleri, ed.), pp. 163–182. W.B. Saunders Co., Philadelphia.

41

Models of Intestinal Secretion and Absorption

Martin Riegler* and Jeffrey B. Matthews†

*University Clinic of Surgery, Vienna General Hospital, A-1090 Vienna, Austria

†Department of Surgery, Beth Israel Deaconess Medical Center, Harvard Medical School, Boston, Massachusetts 02215

I. Introduction

The intestinal epithelium represents the site of fluid and nutrient exchange between the gut lumen and the bloodstream. Many gastrointestinal diseases are associated with disorders of gut secretory or absorptive function. A variety of experimental models and techniques are available to investigate the mechanisms underlying such disorders. Epithelial absorptive and secretory function are under continuous neurohumoral regulation. Under physiologic conditions the amount of fluid absorption and secretion is balanced. In contrast, disease-induced imbalances between absorption and secretion may lead to conditions characterized by increased fluid secretion into the gut lumen (e.g., diarrhea associated with inflammation, benign and malignant epithelial tumors, endocrine tumors, hypoxia, toxins, drugs) or impaired intestinal secretion (constipation as seen in cystic fibrosis and hypothyroidism). Nutrient absorption is impaired under a variety of clinical disorders, and identifying means to enhance gut absorptive capacity may lead to new approaches in the treatment of short bowel syndrome.

In this chapter we provide an overview of experimental techniques designed to study absorptive and secretory function of intestinal epithelia and to model disorders associated with imbalance of absorptive/secretory function. Models presented range from the molecular to the intact tissue level and from *in vitro* to *in vivo* models. Experimental techniques for investigation of epithelial absorptive/secretory function include electrophysiologic and ion flux studies, which can be performed either *in vitro* (Ussing chamber studies, patch clamp studies) or *in vivo* (animal loop models). Cultured epithelial cell lines or native human or animal tissue can be used to model epithelial physiology/pathophysiology. Although molecular mechanisms are often best investigated in cell culture studies, studies using native tissue *in vitro* or animals *in vivo* are necessary in order to understand the integrated complexity of the *in vivo* situation. Each technique has limitations, advantages, and disadvantages; therefore, a combination of *in vitro* and *in vivo* approaches often provides the most comprehensive picture of the transport process being studied.

II. In Vitro Studies

Prerequisites for an *in vitro* model for investigation of mechanisms of secretion and absorption by intestinal epithelia are design of a model epithelium and availability of physiologic parameters for measuring transepithelial electrolyte and fluid transport. Both demands are met by a two-half-chamber system (Ussing chamber system) (1) into which either monolayers of cultured epithelial cell lines (2) or sheets of native intestinal mucosa (3–5) can be mounted for electrophysiologic and ion flux studies. Application of similar principles at the level of the plasma membrane underlies the patch clamp technique, whereby ionic movement over a specific area of cell membrane is measured as flux of electrical current (6). *In vitro* methods for investigation of intestinal secretion/absorption are based on the physiology (structure and function) of an intestinal epithelium (7). Individual epithelial cells form a single layer (sheet), which is attached to the mucosa (subepithelial compartment) via the basal lamina. Apical and basolateral epithelial cell membranes and the apical intercellular junction belt (TJ) represent the rate-limiting structures for transepithelial fluid movement (Fig. 1). Net vectorial transport (absorption or secretion) results from active and passive transepithelial fluid movement.

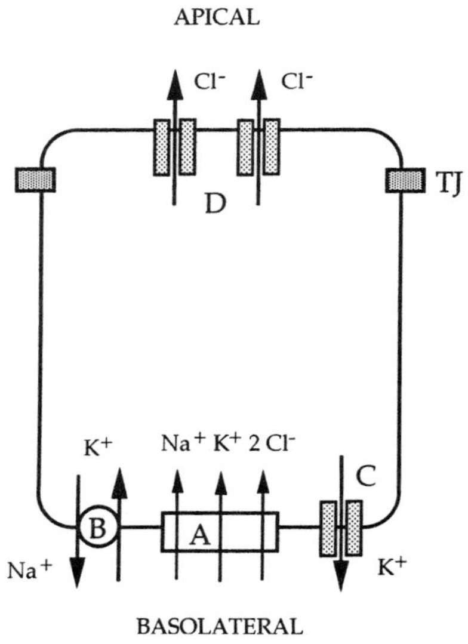

Figure 1 Model of active chloride secretion based on studies in T_{84} cells. Chloride entry across the basolateral membrane occurs via $Na^+/K^+/2Cl^-$ cotransport (A) and is driven by the Na^+ gradient that is maintained by Na^+/K^+ ATPase (B). Potassium is recycled via the basolateral membrane via Ba^{2+}-sensitive cAMP/GMP-dependent or Ba^{2+}-insensitive calcium-dependent K^+ channels (C). Apical chloride conductances are activated by cAMP or cGMP (D). TJ, Tight junction.

A. Ussing Chamber Technique

The Ussing chamber, originally designed by Ussing and Zerhan (1) for studies of frog skin, represents an important tool to study intestinal epithelial barrier function, permeability, and transepithelial fluid movement. Monolayers of cultured intestinal epithelial cells (2) and mucosal sheets of native intestine (animal or human) (3–5) are mounted into Ussing chambers for electrophysiologic and ion flux studies.

B. Ussing Chamber Design

An Ussing chamber is made up of two half-chambers with openings between, in which a sheet of tissue is mounted in vertical orientation. Half-chambers are filled with buffer, which is heated and gassed. Depending on size, volume, and orientation of the half-chamber, two types of plexiglas chambers are commercially available: a cylindrical or tubelike half-chamber, distributed by World Precision Instruments (WPI) (8) (Fig. 2A), or a cuboidal-shaped half-chamber (Costar; Precision Instruments) (9) (Fig. 2B). The half-chamber volume ranges from 1 to 10 ml for cuboidal-shaped chambers, and up to 40 ml for the cylindrical half-chambers, which are connected to a buffer reservoir that is thermoregulated by a waterjacket. Temperature of the cuboidal-type chamber is regulated via a heating block into which the chamber is mounted. The half-chamber opening, i.e., area of tissue, ranges from 0.2 to 2 cm^2 for both systems. Tissues are mounted between the half-chambers, which are held together either by metal rings (cuboidal chamber; Fig. 2B) or by lateral holding screws (cylindrical chamber; Fig. 2A). Gentle contact will avoid edge damage. Half-chambers can be filled with buffer and gassed independently.

C. Model Epithelia

Monolayers of cultured intestinal epithelial cells are used to model epithelial physiology. A number of intestinal epithelial cell lines are commercially available and are suitable for studies in Ussing chambers. In addition to cell lines of malignant origin (T_{84}, HT29, $Caco_2$ cells) (2, 10–12), "normal" (nontransformed) human colonic epithelial cells derived from transverse colon have been successfully passaged in culture (13). In order for a cell line to be suitable for the Ussing chamber technique, the cells must grow to confluence, form intercellular junctional complexes, and display apical–basolateral membrane polarity.

1. Cultured Cell Lines

Major progress in understanding the cellular basis and molecular regulation of intestinal epithelial secretion was made possible with the introduction of cultured epithelial cell lines such as human colonic T_{84} cells, which were initially derived from a lung metastasis of colonic cancer

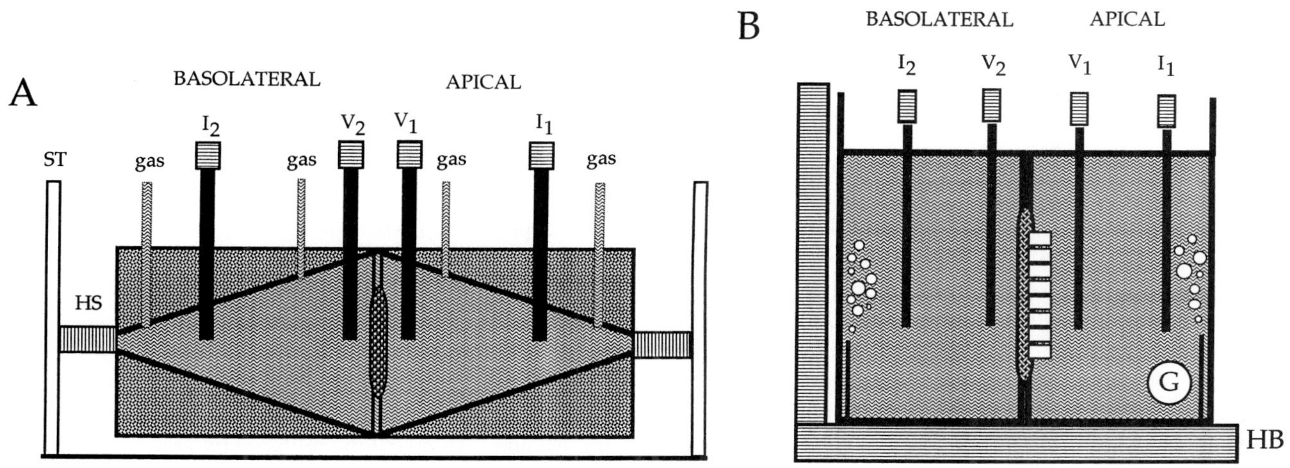

Figure 2 Schematic drawing of Ussing chamber made up of (A) cylindrical/tubelike half-chambers (World Precision Instruments), or (B) cuboidal-shaped half-chambers (Costar, Precision Instruments). Model epithelium grown on plastic insert or intestinal mucosa is mounted between half-chambers. Half-chambers are filled with buffer and gassed. V_1 and V_2 indicate apical (luminal) and basolateral (serosal) voltage-sensing electrodes, respectively. I_1 and I_2 indicate apical and basolateral current-passing electrodes, respectively. Gas, tubes connecting half-chamber to gas-lift apparatus/reservoir containing buffer heated by waterjacket; HS, holding screws for fixation and approximation of half chambers; ST, stand; G, gassing by built-in gas-lift oxygenation system; HB, heating block.

injected subcutaneously into nude mice (14, 15). The major advantage of T_{84} cells is due to the fact that the short-circuit current (I_{sc}) generated by these cells when mounted in a Ussing chamber is equivalent to net chloride secretion (Fig. 1) (10, 14, 15). Because T_{84} cells perhaps represent the most widely used model of epithelial secretion and barrier function, methodological aspects of these cells are described below in detail. In general, the techniques of cell culture and electrophysiologic assays as described for T_{84} cells can be adapted to other cultured intestinal cell lines. T_{84} cells, originally characterized by Dharmsathaporn (14, 15) are available from the American Type Culture Collection (ATCC), Rockville, MD (cat. no. CCL 248). For electrophysiologic studies, there is occasionally some variability of cells between passages. In our experience, up to 20 passages of T_{84} cell will show consistent electrophysiologic profiles.

2. Preparation of T_{84} Cell Monolayers

T_{84} cells are grown as monolayers in a 1:1 mixture of Dulbecco–Vogt modified Eagle's (DME) medium and Ham's F12 medium supplemented with 15 m*M* Na^+ HEPES buffer, pH 7.5, 1.2 g $NaHCO_3$, 40 mg/liter penicillin, 8 mg/liter ampicillin, 90 mg/liter streptomycin, and 5% newborn bovine serum (14, 15, 16). Care must be taken when growth factors are added to the buffer because growth factors may affect the polarized phenotype and secretory apparatus of T_{84} cells (17). Thus some experimental conditions may require the use of serum-free media (17). Confluency of T_{84} cells is monitored under the light microscope. Cells are split near confluency by incubation in 0.1% trypsin and 0.9 m*M* EDTA in Ca^{2+}- and Mg^{2+}-free phosphate-buffered saline for about 30 min. T_{84} cells grow best when split 1:2. Lower cell densities may retard growth. After splitting, confluency is achieved within 5 to 8 days, after which T_{84} cells should be used for experiments.

For experiments, monolayers of T_{84} cells can be grown on commercially available insert systems, which are polycarbonate filters with varying thickness and pore size, that can be mounted into Ussing chambers (Costar). Pore size can be varied dependening on the experimental set up. Larger pore sizes are recommended for inflammatory cell transmigration assays (18), and smaller pore sizes, for secretion studies (19). The larger pore size has the disadvantage of multilayer formation because cells may protrude through large filter pores (5 μm). Permeable supports are coated with collagen I, which enhances attachment of T_{84} cells. Thus collagen I and the cells are added to the filter and allowed to attach for 5 hr before mounting the monolayers into 24-well plates. Monolayers of different cell types grown on permeable supports are now commercially available (Costar).

For electrophysiologic assays T_{84} cell-coated monolayers are lifted from the 24-well holding plate, drained of media, gently rinsed by dipping in a 200-ml container of Hank's balanced salt solution (HBSS), and mounted into Ussing chambers (see below) and buffered with HBSS, without bicarbonate or phenol red, to which 10 m*M* HEPES is added, pH 7.4.

Interaction of epithelial cells with cells of the subepithelial layer (fibroblasts, immune cells) can be modeled using coculture systems. Monolayers of T_{84} cells are mounted into 24-well plates as described above in the presence of other cell types, which are placed either into the luminal or serosal side of the monolayer (18, 20).

Because T_{84} cells are transformed cells, data obtained with T_{84} cells should be compared with native intestinal mucosa of either animal or human origin, where practical.

3. Transport Studies in Other Epithelial Cell Lines

A number of other cultured intestinal cell lines are commercially available for studies of epithelial physiology (HT29 cells, Caco2 cells). The parent HT29 cell line is unpolarized, but several polarized subclones have been derived that are useful for studies of epithelial secretion. In addition, because HT29 cells can be induced to differentiate in culture, this cell line is occasionally useful to examine molecular regulation of specific transport proteins in response to growth factors or other manipulations. Caco2 cells spontaneously differentiate in culture into an absorptive phenotype and have been used to study elements of active Na^+, nutrient, and drug absorption.

Because of possible differences in regulation of fluid secretion in normal human colonocytes vs. cultured (human and animal) colonic cell lines, and the short-term availability of primary cultured human colonocytes (>72 hr), great emphasis has focused on the development of a passageable "normal" human intestinal cell line. A new model to study ion transport using an immortalized, nontransformed, human colonic cell line (NCM460), derived from normal human transverse colon, has been introduced (13). When compared to normal colonocytes, NCM460 cells exhibit similar mechanisms of chloride secretion and fluid absorption (Na^+/H^+ exchanger expression). Thus, NCM460 cells are a new, suitable *in vitro* model for fluid absorption and chloride secretion in human colon (13). NCM460 cells are commercially available from In Cell (San Antonio, TX) and cultured in M3:10 culture medium (In Cell) containing 10% fetal bovine serum and antibiotics. NCM460 colonocytes are counted and plated at a density of $\sim 2 \times 100{,}000$ cells/ml in Costar flasks (75 ml) at 37°C with 6% CO_2. The cells are passaged by using a cell scraper and splitting them 1:2. The epithelial origin of the cells is confirmed by immunofluorescent detection of cytokeratin, villin, the colon specific glycoprotein 5E113, and intermediate filament as described by Yang *et al.* (21).

4. Preparation of Native Intestinal Mucosa

Native animal or human small and large intestinal mucosa may be used in the Ussing chamber apparatus (3–5). The intestinal segment is opened longitudinally at the antimesenteric border, placed on a wax plate, mucosal side facing downward, and rinsed with gassed ice-cold nutrient buffer. Tissue viability is acceptable if the interval until tissue mounting does not exceed 10 min. Tissue preparation can be performed either by blunt dissection using forceps or sharp dissection using a razor blade or a pair of scissors. Preparation of native intestinal mucosa is recommended to be performed under the dissecting microscope to avoid mucosal damage and to ascertain the right plane of dissection between the mucosal and the submucosal layer, resulting in a sheet of intestinal mucosa, which is then mounted between two half-chambers (3–5).

D. Buffers

Composition of buffer and gassing depends on the experimental setup. Typical buffer and gassing for incubation of T_{84} cell monolayers (14–19) and native tissues (3–5, 22–24) are shown in Table I. Ion substitution may be a useful manipulation to determine the contribution or ion dependency of a given transport process. For example, chloride may be replaced by isethionate (4, 17, 25) or other monovalent anions, and sodium can be replaced by *N*-methyl glucamine or choline (4). Temperature and pH of buffer are kept at 37°C and 7.4, respectively.

E. Heating and Gassing

Chamber fluids can be either heated and gassed separately or collectively. We prefer the use of a heating block with gassing devices for six Ussing chambers. Heating and gassing are achieved by connecting the heating block to a waterbath (37°C) and a gas cylinder, respectively.

F. Electrophysiologic Measurements

Transepithelial movement of ions and/or nutrients can be either electrogenic or electroneutral. Electrophysiologically, an intestinal epithelium can be simply modeled as a sheet of epithelial cells (resistors) in parallel, which separate charge between the luminal and serosal side (2). The Na^+/K^+ ATPase pump generates the driving force for active transepithelial movement of ions (i.e., current), which is normally neutralized by passive movement of ions and solutes via the transcellular or paracellular pathway. Transcellular routes are ion conductances (channels, cotransports, ion exchangers) that are inserted into the epithelial cell membrane (see above). The tight junctions represent the rate-limiting step for paracellular movement of ions and solutes (7). Electrophysiologically an epithelium mounted in a Ussing chamber is characterized by potential difference (PD), short-circuit current (I_{sc}), and resistance (R). The capability of an epithelium to separate charges (PD) and net active electrogenic transepithelial movement of ions (I_{sc}) are measured using the four-electrode technique. Using Ohm's law, resistance to passive ion flux is calculated. Because tight junctions represent the major route for passive ion flux, R represents a good measure for tight junction function and directly correlates with tight junction structure (2, 7).

A PD-sensing and a current-passing electrode are introduced into each buffered and gassed half-chamber; the PD-sensing electrode is placed next to the tissue plane while the

Table I Ionic Composition of Buffers Used for Ussing Chamber Experiments for T84 Cells and Native Intestinal Mucosa[a]

T84 cell monolayer buffers					Native intestinal mucosa buffers						
Component	HEPES buffer (14)	Component	Ringer's (15)	Cl free (17)	Component	A (3)	B (5)	C (22)	D (8, 23)	E (24)
NaCl	135	Na	140	145	NaCl	114	122	113	113, 6	125
KCl	5	K	5, 2	5, 2	KCl	5	5	4, 5	5, 4	5
NaH_2PO_4	3, 33	Ca	1, 2	1, 2	$CaCl_2$	1, 25	2	1, 25	1, 2	1, 2
$CaCl_2$	1	Mg	1, 2	1, 2	$MgCl_2$	1, 1	—	1	1, 2	—
$MgCl_2$	1	Cl	119, 8	—	Na_2HPO_4	1, 65	—	0, 2	—	—
L-Glucose	10	HCO_3	25	25	NaH_2PO_4	0, 3	—	—	—	2
HEPES	5	H_2PO_4	2, 4	2, 4	$NaHCO_3$	25	25	25	21	22
		HPO_4	0, 4	0, 4	Glucose	10	20	—	10	10, 2
		Glucose	10	10	$MgSO_4$	—	1, 3	—	—	1, 2
		SO_4	—	2, 4	Mannitol	—	—	10	—	—
		Isethionate	—	120, 1	β-OH-butyrate	—	—	—	0, 5	—
					L-Glutamine	—	—	—	2, 5	—
					D(+)-Mannose	—	—	—	10	—
					O_2	95%	95%	95%	95%	—
					CO_2	5%	5%	5%	5%	—

[a]Note: Concentrations of electrolytes and substrates are given in millimoles/liter; reference numbers are given in parentheses.

current passing electrode is placed at the largest vertical distance from the horizontal plane of the tissue to maximally compensate for fluid resistance (see below) (Fig. 2) (1, 3–5, 16). In high-resistance tissues (>1000 $\Omega\cdot cm^2$), such as human colonic T_{84} cell monolayers, positional effects are minimal (14–19), but become significant in low-resistance tissues, such as native intestine (<100 $\Omega\cdot cm^2$) (3–5). Electrodes are connected to a voltage/current clamp.

Under open-circuit conditions potential difference (PD) is measured and given in millivolts. In order to measure net active transepithelial current PD has to be nullified by activating the clamp mode of the voltage/current clamp, i.e., the tissue is short-circuited to zero. During clamping the amount of current required to abolish open-circuit PD is passed over the tissue via the current-passing electrodes. The current required to clamp the tissue PD to zero equals the net active current generated by the epithelium (i.e., in the absence of potential difference passive ion movement equals zero) and is termed short-circuit current (I_{sc}, $\mu A/cm^2$). Using Ohm's law (resistance $R = PD/I_{sc}$), tissue resistance is calculated and given in $\Omega\cdot cm^2$. Ion substitution experiments and inhibitor sensitivity may be used to further define the ionic basis of the short-circuit current.

PD-sensing and current-passing electrodes are Ag/AgCl electrodes. Bathing solution is connected to the silver wire either via agar bridges or glass tubes (with ceramic tip) filled with KCl solution. Because agar bridges have the disadvantage of air bubble formation, we recommend the use of glass tubes. However, agar bridges are advantageous for serial resistance records from 24-well plates of cultured cell monolayers.

A voltage/current clamp allows clamping of transepithelial PD (sensed by PD electrodes) to estimated values by passage of respective currents: The current required to nullify a given PD is termed short-circuit current (see above). Voltage/current clamps are commercially available either as individual clamp units or as two-, four-, or six-clamp units from several companies (WPI; Iowa Dual Voltage clamps, University of Iowa; Precision Instruments, San Diego, CA).

Before mounting the monolayer or tissue, the system should be calibrated for PD and the resistance of the bulk gassed fluid (fluid resistance). Electrodes are introduced into buffered chambers without tissue or monolayer. If PD deflects more than 5 mV by 10 min after equilibration, PD electrodes should be checked for technical problems or exchanged. Major causes for PD deflections during equilibration are air bubbles or lack of fluid or agar from glass electrodes or agar bridges, respectively, damage of silver wire, and oxidation of silver wire (best detected and removed under the light microscope by use of a small forceps). Fluid resistance should not exceed 2–4 $\Omega\cdot cm^2$. When monolayers of cultured cell lines are used the system should be corrected for the resistance of fluids and permeable supports, i.e., equilibration has to be performed in the presence of gassed buffer and permeable support. When a voltage current clamp is used for the first time, equilibration is performed as suggested by the manufacturer. Quality of current-passing electrodes is tested as recommended by the producer of the voltage/current clamp. The principle of electrode testing represents passage of a defined current via the electrodes. If this current decreases by 10% over subsequent 60 sec, current-passing electrodes should be changed or checked for technical problems as suggested for PD electrodes (see above). PD-sensing electrodes should not be used for passing current and vice versa (George Grass, personal communication). Positioning of the electrodes should not be restricted to one side of the monolayer/tissue, preventing early damage of electrodes. If used on a daily basis electrodes are recommended to be exchanged every 1 to 1.5 years.

G. Epithelial Permeability Studies

The intestinal epithelium represents the barrier between the gut lumen and the bloodstream. Impairment of epithelial barrier function is characterized by an increase in epithelial permeability. Transepithelial flux of various permeability markers of different radius (e.g., horseradish peroxidase, mannitol, inulin, polyethylene glycol) serves to assess epithelial permeability (2, 5, 26–28).

Following mounting of the model epithelium in the Ussing chamber and equilibration, 10 μM of horseradish peroxidase or 5–10 μCi of tritiated permeability marker ([^{3}H]mannitol, [^{3}H]inulin, or [^{3}H]PEG 4000) is administered to one side of the monolayer/tissue (final concentration, approximately 10 μM). Thereafter samples are taken every 10 to 15 min from the opposite compartment. Amount of marker is determined by fluid scintillation counting or high-performance liquid chromatography. Experiments are performed under short-circuited conditions to exclude PD-induced passive transepithelial movement of the permeability marker.

H. Transepithelial Ion Flux Studies

Transepithelial movement of ions such as Na^+ and Cl^- can be determined by flux of their respective radioisotopes ^{22}Na and ^{36}Cl. In such experiments, ^{22}Na and ^{36}Cl are added to known specific activity either to the mucosal or serosal half-chamber and the tissues (monolayers or mucosal sheets) are short-circuited by voltage clamping (see above) and bathed by symmetric solutions to exclude PD-driven, passive transepithelial ion movement. Tissues are paired by matching resistances. If resistances of paired tissues differ by >30%, the experiments should be discarded. A sample-and-replace technique is used to obtain aliquots from the trans-compartment. Following an initial flux period of approximately 15 to 30 min, additional flux periods should last at least 15 to 20 min, to allow sufficient accumulation of the isotope in the respective half-chamber. Unidirectional fluxes (mucosa to serosa, or serosa to mucosa) and the net fluxes of Cl^- and Na^+ are calculated from aliquots taken at the beginning and end of each flux period. To calculate the unidirectional ion fluxes, steady-state rates of isotope transfer are divided by the specific activity of the initially labeled side and by the surface area of exposed tissue. The net flux is calculated as the difference between oppositely directed unidirectional fluxes of tissue pairs ($J_{net} = J_{m\text{-}s} - J_{s\text{-}m}$).

III. In Vitro Models of Intestinal Transport

A. Transepithelial Transport in T_{84} Epithelial Cell Monolayers

Electrophysiologically T_{84} cell monolayers are characterized by PD, I_{sc}, and R values of approximately 5–20 mV (lumen negative), 0.1–2 μA/cm^2, and 600–2000 $\Omega\cdot$cm^2, respectively, when incubated in Ussing chambers under baseline conditions. The basal and agonist-stimulated I_{sc} produced by T_{84} cells has been shown to approximate net electrogenic Cl^- secretion under a wide variety of experimental conditions. Thus, the T_{84} model represents a widely used approach for studying mechanisms of Cl^- secretion (14–20). Cl^- secretion can be induced by secretagogues that increase of intracellular cAMP (i.e., forskolin or cholera toxin) or calcium (i.e., the acetylcholine analogue carbachol) (10). Typical time course experiments show that forskolin (cAMP)-mediated chloride secretion is characterized by a sustained dose-dependent I_{sc} increase, which peaks by 20 to 30 min and is subsequently maintained over at least the next 60 min (10, 13–20, 29). In contrast, intracellular Ca^{2+}-mediated chloride secretion by carbachol is characterized by a rapid I_{sc} rise, which peaks within about 1–5 min and returns to baseline approximately 10–20 min following agonist administration (10, 14, 29).

1. Isolation of Individual Transport Pathways

Transepithelial transport (secretion or absorption) requires the coordinated activities of multiple specific transport pathways at both the apical and the basolateral membranes. A variety of techniques may be used to isolate the activity of an individual transport pathway to more closely study its regulation. For example, the activity of the basolateral $Na^+/K^+/2Cl^-$ cotransporter can be studied by isotopic flux analysis, using ^{86}Rb as a tracer for K^+ and bumetanide (50 μM) as an inhibitor of cotransport. Thus, for example, the activity of the cotransporter can be studied by adding 1–2 μCi/ml ^{86}Rb to the basolateral buffer, and, after a specified time has elapsed (typically 3 min, during which uptake is linear), monolayers are rapidly removed and uptake is stopped in ice-cold buffer. Radioactivity is extracted and counted by standard scintillation techniques. The difference between uptake of ^{86}Rb measured in the absence and presence of bumetanide in paired monolayers reflects the activity of the cotransporter (12). In analogous fashion, the activity of the Na^+/K^+ ATPase can be estimated as ouabain-inhibitable, bumetanide-insensitive ^{86}Rb uptake. This principle can be adapted to study the activity of a wide variety of salt and nutrient transporters involved in active secretion and absorption. For example, influx of radiolabeled glucose or amino acids in the presence and absence of specific inhibitors of Na^+-coupled nutrient transporters may be studied.

Flux studies can be used in certain instances to examine the activity of ion channels. These are usually in the form of radioisotopic efflux experiments. For example, using ^{125}I as a tracer for Cl^-, efflux from cells preloaded with ^{125}I can be used to assess the relative Cl^- conductance of the plasma membrane. Precise quantification of ion conductances by this method is difficult, due to inability to control ion gradients and membrane potential, but can be used to screen for the presence of regulated ion channel function (12).

2. Ion Transport Studies in Asymmetrically Permeabilized Cells

Apical and basolateral membrane transport processes can be studied in isolation by the technique of selective membrane permeabilization (29). This technique functionally eliminates the contralateral membrane from the electrical circuit by permeabilization with monovalent ionophores such as nystatin or amphotericin B. Application of a transepithelial (apical to basolateral or vice versa) chemical gradient under zero voltage clamp conditions will yield a current that reflects the conductance of the nonpermeabilized membrane to that ionic species. Thus agonist-stimulated conductance changes for monovalent ions at either the apical or basolateral cell membrane can be modeled. This technique has been used to measure basolateral membrane K^+ conductance (29).

Both apical and basolateral chambers are initially filled with low K^+ solution containing 10 m*M* sodium gluconate, 135 m*M* *N*-methylglucamine gluconate, 5 m*M* potassium gluconate, 1 m*M* $MgSO_4$, 1.0 m*M* calcium gluconate, 10 m*M* glucose, and 10 m*M* HEPES, at pH 7.4 until electrical parameters stabilize. The K^+ gradient is then applied by replacing the original apical low-K^+ solution with a high-K^+ solution that substitutes 5 m*M* potassium gluconate and 135 m*M* *N*-methylglucamine gluconate with 140 m*M* potassium gluconate. Nystatin (500 U/ml) is administered to the apical solution to permeabilize the apical cell membrane. To inhibit electrogenic movement of K^+ via the basolateral cell membrane, Na^+/K^+ ATPase is inhibited by basolateral administration of 100 μM of ouabain. Under these conditions I_{sc} equals the K^+ conductance via the basolateral cell membrane and the paracellular pathway. Because of the stable nature of paracellular conductance during experimental conditions, the agonist-induced change in K^+ conductance is mainly due to changes in K^+ permeability of the basolateral membrane.

Apical Cl^- conductance is measured using a similar approach involving a high basolateral to low apical gradient of Cl^- followed by basolateral membrane permeabilization with nystatin. Both apical and basolateral chambers are initially filled with a Cl^--free/high-K^+ solution containing 10 m*M* sodium gluconate 140 m*M* potassium gluconate, 1 m*M* calcium gluconate, 10 m*M* L-glucose, and 10 m*M* HEPES, at pH 7.4. After equilibration, the basolateral solution is replaced with a high-Cl^-/high-K^+ solution containing 10 m*M* NaCl, 140 m*M* KCl, 1 m*M* $MgSO_4$, 1 m*M* $CaCl_2$, 10 m*M* L-glucose, and 10 m*M* HEPES, at pH 7.4. Nystatin (500 U/ml) is then added to the basolateral solution to permeabilize the basolateral membrane. The resultant current (I_{Cl}) thus reflects the isolated apical membrane Cl^- conductance.

B. Ussing Chamber Studies in Native Intestinal Mucosa

In vivo, chloride secretion from epithelial cells is mediated by numerous secretagogues released from lamina propria cells (nerve cells, mast cells, immune cells, fibroblasts) and epithelial cells (enterocytes, M cells) (30). Agonist-dependent activation of enterocyte receptor(s) induces a signal transduction cascade resulting in elevation of second messengers (cAMP, Ca^{2+}) and opening of ion channels required for transepithelial movement of chloride (10, 17). Exposure of animal or human intestinal mucosa to agonists of chloride secretion enables modeling of interactions between lamina propria and epithelial cells. A wide range of pharmacologic tools are commercially available to study the role of nerve cells, mast cells, and various secretagogues in the modulation of intestinal transepithelial fluid movement and to establish models of transmucosal signal transduction (22, 31).

Human colonic mucosa mounted in Ussing chambers exhibits PD, I_{sc}, and *R* of approximately -20 to 30 mV (lumen negative), 150 to 200 $\mu A/cm^2$, and 80 to 120 $\Omega \cdot cm^2$, respectively. When compared to distal colon, proximal colonic mucosa exhibits higher resistances, indicating that the proximal colonic epithelium is a "tighter" barrier to transepithelial passive ion movement (3, 22, 32). In addition to electrophysiologic studies, transepithelial movement of ions can be established by measurement of isotopic fluxes (3, 4). Because availability of human intestinal mucosa is limited, animal tissue is used more widely. Rabbit (33) and porcine colon (8) exhibit similar electrophysiologic values when compared to human colon (3). Although electrophysiologic values of guinea pig (34), mouse (35), and rat colon (4) are significantly lower when compared to human (3, 5, 22), rabbit (33), or porcine colon (8), agonist-induced electrophysiologic responses are similar.

Further insights into transepithelial electrolyte transport are achieved by the use of isotopic flux studies, as described above (3). Following equilibration of animal/human colonic mucosa, ^{22}Na and ^{36}Cl are administered either to the mucosal or serosal half-chamber and the tissues are short-circuited by voltage clamping (see above).

C. Pharmacologic and Neural Stimulation of Intestinal Transport

In vivo intestinal secretion is under neurohumoral control (30). Using the T_{84} cell monolayer model the effect of various secretagogues on epithelial cell has been established (see above). Mounting animal/human colonic mucosa in Ussing chamber enables the investigator to model the complexity of interactions between epithelial and lamina propria cells. In agreement with the observations made in T_{84} cell monolayers, luminal and/or serosal administration of secretagogues to Ussing chambered native tissue induces changes of I_{sc} . The ionic basis of agonist-induced I_{sc} changes is established using ion substitution experiments (chloride-, sodium-free solution) or by administration of pharmacologic inhibitors of ion transport pathways such as amiloride (blocker of Na^+ channels and Na^+–H^+ exchange), ouabain (inhibitor of Na^+/K^+ ATPase), and bumetanide (inhibitor of $Na^+/K^+/2Cl^-$ cotransport), or chloride channel blockers (i.e., *N*-phenylanthranilic acid) (10–20). In animal/human colonic mucosa carbachol- and forskolin-stimulated I_{sc} increase is inhibited by the presence of the above-described inhibitors of chloride secretion and Cl^--free buffer, indicating that the electrical response reflects stimulation of chloride secretion (4, 31).

Involvement of lamina propria cells in the mediation of secretagogue-induced I_{sc} changes can be deduced by sensitivity to 10^{-5} to 10^{-9} *M* of the neuronal blocker tetrodotoxin, the mast cell inhibitor lodoxamide, and/or the prostaglandin synthesis inhibitor indomethacin (31). Involvement of receptors in the mediation of a secretagogue-induced response can be tested by administration of specific receptor antagonists. Morphologic confirmation of receptor location can be obtained using immunofluorescence microscopy (31). Taken together, inhibitor sensitivity and morphologic evidence may yield critical information regarding the mechanism of action of a given secretory stimulus.

In addition to the pharmacologic techniques described above, electrical field stimulation (36, 37) and mechanical stroking (38) of the mucosal surface of Ussing-chambered intestinal mucosa may be used to investigate the involvement of neural reflex pathways in the mediation of secretory responses. Animal or human intestinal mucosa is mounted into the Ussing chamber and buffered, and electrophysiologic parameters (PD, I_{sc}) are measured as described above. For electrical field stimulation two aluminum foil ribbon electrodes juxtaposed between the flux chamber halves and the submucosal surface of the colon are attached to the output of a electronic stimulator (Grass SD9 or S88; Grass Instruments, Quincy, MA). Repetitive bipolar rectangular stimulus pulses are passed parallel to the plane of the submucosa. The stimulus parameters have a pulse duration of 0.5 msec, an amplitude range of 2–35 V (0.5–11 mA), and a frequency range of 1–15 Hz. Electrical field stimulation is applied for 2–10 min, and the maximum change in short-circuit current is recorded on a polygraph.

Mucosal stroking can also induce transport responses. Intestinal mucosa is mounted horizontally into a modified Ussing chamber, with the mucosal side oriented upward. Tissue is buffered and electrophysiologic parameters are measured. A 2-mm-wide brush attached to a micromanipulator is lowered onto the mucosal surface. Repetitive stroking of the mucosa is carried out at 1 stroke/5 min for up to 1 hr. After three strokes during the first 15 min, drugs or vehicle are added to the serosal or mucosal side to assess their effects on the mucosal stroking response. Using this technique, Cooke and co-workers demonstrated that electrical field stimulation and mucosal stroking activate specific neuronal reflexes, involving the release of mediators from nerve cells and lamina propria cells (substance P, serotonin, acethylcholine, calcitonin gene-related peptide, vasoactive intestial peptide, adenosine), which induce chloride secretion by acting on epithelial cells (36–38).

D. Colonic Crypt Perfusion Model

The use of native tissue *in vitro* or *in vivo* does not allow discrimination between transepithelial fluid movement or ion transport from either crypt or surface epithelial cells. This issue has been elegantly addressed by an isolated colonic crypt perfusion model, introduced by Singh and co-workers (24) by adaptation of a model originally designed to study fluid transport in renal tubules. Following hand dissection, rat colonic crypts are placed in a temperature-controlled superfusable 0.25-ml chamber on the stage of an inverted microscope. The blind end of the crypt is held by an assembly of concentric glass micropipettes and is punctured by a perfusion pipette to introduce the perfusate containing 10 μCi/ml of methoxy[^{3}H]inulin (New England Nuclear, Boston, MA) into the crypt lumen. A second set of micropipettes is used to cannulate the open end of the crypt for collection of the effluent. Thus the crypt lumen is continuously rinsed with a collection rate of 4 nl/min. Simultaneously the serosal/blood side bath of the crypt is superfused at a rate of 3 ml/min. Aliquots of effluent are sampled with a volume-calibrated pipette, net fluid movement (J_v) is calculated from the rate at which the effluent accumulates in the collection pipette and the concentration of methoxy[^{3}H]inulin in the perfusate and effluent. Methoxy[^{3}H]inulin concentration is determined with a liquid scintilation spectrometer (Model 6892; Tracor Analytic, Elk Grove Village, IL). The bathing solution contains 125 m*M* NaCl, 5 m*M* KCl, 1.2 m*M* CaCl2, 1.2 m*M* $MgSO_4$, 2 m*M* NaH2PO_4, 10.2 m*M* glucose, and 22 m*M* $NaHCO_3$. The solution is equlibrated with 5% CO_2, and adjusted to an osmolality of 300–310 mOsm/kg. The pH of all solutions is 7.4; temperature is 37°C. In Na^+-free buffer, NaCl and $NaHCO_3$ are replaced with equivalent amounts of choline-C and choline-HCO_3.

The absence of nonepithelial cells in rat crypt preparation is revealed by immunohistochemistry for localization of myofibroblasts using a monoclonal antibody that reacts with myofibroblasts in the pericryptal sheath. Using this model it was demonstrated that rat colonic crypts absorb fluid in the basal, unstimulated state, and that secretagogues [dibutyryl cAMP, vasoactive intestinal peptide (VIP), and acethylcholine (ACh)] induce net fluid secretion from colonic crypts. Furthermore, experiments performed in the presence of Na^+-free buffer indicated that fluid absorption in the crypt is Na^+ dependent.

E. Isolated Membrane Transport Studies

Ion absorption processes can be studied using isolated membrane vesicles. Nutrient absorption and other Na^+-coupled absorptive processes are suitable for this model. For example, in intestinal epithelial cells sodium is absorbed through solute-coupled electrogenic transporters (i.e., Na^+/K^+ ATPase; see Section III,A) and an electrically neutral Cl^--dependent process. The Cl^--dependent process is mediated via two coupled neutral exchangers, the Na^+/H^+ and Cl^-/HCO_3 antiporter. Na^+/H^+ antiport activity has been studied by Donowitz and co-workers, using intestinal brush border vesicle membranes (39, 40).

A variety of techniques have been used to prepare membrane vesicles. For example, to prepare small intestinal epithelial brush border membranes, New Zealand white male rabbits are sacrificed by IV injection of sodium pentobarbital; an ileal segment is resected, opened longitudinally at the antimesenteric border, and rinsed with iced 154 m*M* NaCl containing 0.5 m*M* phenylmethylsulfonylfluoride (PMSF) and 0.003 TIU/ml aprotinin, and then gently scraped to provide mostly villus cells (39, 40). The collected cells are then homogenized at high speed in a blender for 3 min in a solution containing 60 m*M* mannitol, 2.4 m*M* Tris (hydroxymethyl)-aminomethane HCl, pH 7.1, and 1 m*M* EGTA, along with the protease inhibitors 0.32 m*M* PMSF, 0.09 *N*-(αrhamnopyranosyloxyhydroxyphosphinyl)-L-leucine-tryptophan (phosphorhamidone) and 0.003 TIU/ml aprotinin. The homogenization and subsequent procedures of membrane preparation are performed at 4°C. The homogenate is then treated with 10 m*M* $MgCl_2$ for 15 min and centrifuged at 12,000 *g* for 15 min. Following pellet discharge, the supernatant is centrifuged at 27,000 *g* for 30 min. The pellet is then resuspended in 60 m*M* mannitol, 5 m*M* EGTA, and 10 m*M* Tris, at pH 7.1. The 10 m*M* $MgCl_2$ precipitation steps are repeated and the membranes are resuspended in 300 m*M* mannitol, 5 m*M* Mg(gluconate)$_2$, and 20 m*M* HEPES/Tris, at pH 7.4, and centrifuged at 30,000 *g* for 40 min. The final pellet is resuspended in the same buffer using a 25-gauge needle. The membrane is stored in liquid nitrogen and is generally used less than 1 week after preparation.

A freeze–thaw procedure may be used to incorporate compounds into brush border vesicles (39). Using this technique enables the investigator to incorporate compounds required for transvesicular absorption/secretion into brush border vesicle preparations prior to transport studies (see below). Frozen aliquots of brush border vesicles are thawed and homogenized in a glass–Teflon homogenizer at high speed in a membrane buffer consisting of 200 m*M* mannitol, 5 m*M* Mg (gluconate)$_2$, 2 m*M* EGTA, and 40 m*M* Mopso/Tris, at pH 6.5, 4°C. The vesicles are then resuspended in the membrane buffer to a concentration of 10 mg/ml. Then 350-μl aliquots of the membranes along with 36 μl of additives are rapidly frozen in liquid nitrogen for 5 min, and thawed slowly in an ice-water slurry at 4°C for 1 hr. Usually all additions are made immediately prior to freezing, except creatine phosphate, which is added immediately after the aliquot is removed from the ice-water slurry. After thawing, the vesicles are kept at 30°C for 2 min and then at 4°C for an additional 15 min.

As typical examples of studies using membrane vesicles, ^{22}Na and [^3H]glucose initial rate uptake studies can be measured in the following manner. Mix 15 μl of membrane suspension with 30 μl of transport buffer at 25°C. At 3, 5, or 8 sec after mixing the membrane and transport buffers, the uptake is stopped by electronically timed injection of 1 ml of ice-cold stop solution. Equilibrium uptake values are determined after 90 min at 25°C. The reaction mixture is then rapidly vacuum filtered through nitrocellulose filters, 0.45-μm pore size (Millipore Corp., Bedford, MA), and rinsed with 6 ml of ice-cold stop solution. The filters are then dissolved in 3 ml of scintillation fluid and radioactivity measured in a liquid scintillation spectrometer. Initial uptake rates are expressed in Picomoles/milligram protein per second computed by linear regression analyses of data obtained in individual experiments.

Na^+/H^+ antiport activity is stimulated by alterations of intracellular pH (pH_i). Thus the Na^+ transport buffer used in the acid inside pH gradient-stimulated Na^+ uptake studies contains (in final concentration): 180 m*M* mannitol, 1.8 m*M* EGTA, 4.5 m*M* Mg(gluconate)$_2$, 1.0 m*M* NaCl (0.02 μCi/μl ^{22}NaCl), and 36 m*M* Tris/Mes such that the final combined pH of the transport and membrane buffers is 8.0. The stop solution contains 40 m*M* mannitol, 90 m*M* K gluconate, and 20 m*M* Tris/Mes at pH 8.0. The sodium transport buffer used in experiments not involving a pH gradient contains 180 m*M* mannitol, 1.8 m*M* EGTA, 4.5 m*M* Mg(gluconate)$_2$, 1.0 m*M* NaCl (0.04 μCi/μl ^{22}NaCl), and 36 m*M* Mopso/Tris such that combined pH is 6.5. The stop solution contains 40 m*M* mannitol, 90 mM K gluconate, and 20 mM Mopso/Tris, pH 6.5. Sodium-concentration dependence of Na^+ uptake is determined in the presence and absence of an acid inside pH gradient (pH 6.5 in/pH 8.0 out). Initial rates of Na^+ uptake are determined at concentrations of Na gluconate between 2 and 24 mM. For analysis, precise Na^+ concentrations in the combinations of transport and membrane buffers are determined by atomic absorption spectrometry.

The glucose uptake buffer contains 20 mM mannitol, 2 mM EGTA, 5 mM $Mg(gluconate)_2$, and 40 mM Mopso/Tris, pH 6.5, 90 mM NaCl, and 0.15 mM D-[^{3}H]glucose (0.03 μCi/μl). The stop solution is the same as that used in the Na^+ transport experiments without pH gradient (see above). Using this technique, the effect of Ca^{2+}/calmodulin/ATP on ileal brush border Na^+/H^+ exchange and on Na^+-dependent glucose uptake has been investigated (39, 40). Intestinal brush border vesicle membranes have also been used to identify and kinetically characterize various isoforms of Na^+/H^+ exchangers (41). In addition, brush border vesicle membranes represent a good model to study distribution, mechanism, and regulation of other transmembrane transport systems in native tissue or cultured intestinal epithelial cells.

F. Patch Clamp Studies

The patch clamp technique is designed to investigate ionic movement/current(s) over an individual cell membrane (a whole-cell recording) or an excised patch of cell membrane of single cultured epithelial cells (42). This approach requires extensive training and expertise and cannot be fully discussed here. As described for Ussing chamber studies (see above), the ionic basis of currents can be assessed by ion substitution experiments or pharmacologic inhibition of ion conductances (see above). In addition, characteristics such as voltage dependence and time dependence as well as individual channel conductance can be determined. For whole-cell recordings, a patch glass pipette produced by a patch pipette puller (Axon Instruments, Burlingame, CA; Dow Corming, Midland, MI) is manipulated against the plasma membrane of an individual cultured epithelial cell under light microscopic guidance and a gigaohm seal is made (42). Applying moderate suction to the pipette lumen will rupture the seal and allow current measurement between the inside of the patch pipette (reflecting the cytosol) and the outside bath (reflecting the extracellular space), a configuration known as "whole cell." Alternatively, after formation of the gigaohm seal, a patch of cell membrane can be excised; in this configuration, the pipette solution is "extracellular" and the bath is "intracellular," the so-called inside-out configuration, which allows electrophysiologic characterization of the properties of single-ion channels. Depending on the technique used to obtain the patch of membrane, these studies can also be performed in the outside-in configuration (42).

IV. In Vivo Models

A. Intestinal Loop Model

The isolated intestinal loop model is used to examine transport in a neurovascularly intact segment of intestine *in vivo* and to determine the effects of drug, toxin, or other experimental manipulations on intestinal permeability, secretion, and morphology (43). An abdominal incision is performed in animals (mice, rats, rabbits, hamsters, and guinea pigs are suitable for this technique) after an intraperitoneal injection of pentobarbital (40 mg/kg), and two 5-cm loops are isolated in the investigated intestinal segment (distal ileum or colon). Both renal pedicles are ligated to prevent renal excretion of injected tracers. For permeability studies, 10 μCi of [^{3}H]mannitol are injected into the inferior vena cava. In a typical experiment the lumen of each loop would be perfused with 0.4 ml of 50 mM tris(hydroxymethyl)aminomethane (Tris) buffer (pH 7.4) containing the compound to be tested: e.g., a bile salt or bacterial toxin or buffer alone control loop). The abdomen is then sutured (single or double layer), and animals are maintained under light anesthesia. After a suitable interval, animals are sacrificed by bolus injection of intraperitoneal pentobarbital sodium (120 μg/kg). The loops are removed, weighed, and measured, and their content is aspirated and assayed for volume and radioactivity. Mucosal permeability to mannitol [given in disintegrations per minute (dpm/cm loop)] is assessed by fluid scintillation counting and fluid secretion [loop weight (mg)/length (cm)] is measured. Following the end of *in vivo* experiments tissues can be processed for light or electron microscopy for morphologic studies (5, 43).

Using the intestinal loop model it has been demonstrated that low concentrations of bile salts do not have an effect on rat colonic water absorption (44). However, higher concentrations inhibit water absorption. Similar results were obtained in rabbit colon *in vivo* (45). *Clostridium difficile* toxin action has been investigated in the intestinal loop model (43, 46, 47). Luminal administration of toxin A induces increase of fluid secretion and intestinal permeability for mannitol in rat distal ileum *in vivo* (46). Castagliuolo *et al.* (48) used this model to demonstrate that *Saccharomyces boulardii* attenuates fluid secretion and permeability changes induced by *C. difficile* toxin A in rat ileum *in vivo*.

B. Transgenic Animal Models

The use of transgenic mice represents a novel approach to examine the involvement of specific proteins in biologic pathways (43, 49). Genetically manipulated mice lacking genes encoding specific proteins (i.e., CFTR, substance P NK-1 receptor, VIP) or cell types (mast cells, dendritic cells) have been developed. Cystic fibrosis research represents an important example in which "knockout" mice are suitable to model and investigate the pathophysiology of disease. Cystic fibrosis is a genetic exocrine disease affecting a variety of epithelial tissues (lungs, pancrease, intestine). The product of the gene causing the disorder, the cystic fibrosis transmembrane conductance regulator (CFTR), is a cAMP-regulated chloride channel. Various "cystic fibrosis" transgenic mice expressing either no (null) or mutant CFTR have been developed, as reviewed by Grubb *et al.* (49).

Substance P (SP) NK-1 receptor knockout mice are used to study the involvement of SP in the mediation of intestinal inflammation (43). Thus it has been demonstrated that toxin A of *C. difficile* does not induce inflammation and secretion in mice lacking the SP NK-1 receptor. Mast cell-deficient mice are used in different *in vivo* and *in vitro* models of intestinal secretion (25). Intestinal mucosa from mice lacking mast cells do not respond to administration of substance P. However, the secretory response to substance P is restored after mast cell administration (25). Using mucosal preparations from mast cell-deficient mice it has been demonstrated that mast cells and histamine contribute to bile acid-stimulated colonic secretion (35).

C. In Vivo Studies of Intestinal Fluid Absorption

1. Transport Studies in Humans

This technique is suitable for measurement of human jejunal (50), colonic (51, 52), and rectal (53, 54) electrolyte (sodium, potassium, chloride, bicarbonate) and water absorption *in vivo*, and to study the effect of compounds (i.e., amiloride, glucocorticoids) in those processes.

a. In Vivo Transport Studies in Human Colon Subjects are incubated with a double-lumen mercury-weighted polyvinyl tube under fluoroscopic guidance. This tube has an infusion site and one collection site located 30 cm beyond the infusion site. The collection site is allowed to pass to the cecum, placing the infusion site in the distal ileum. An additional tube is placed in the rectum as a second collecting site. With this arrangement there is a 30-cm mixing segment in the distal ileum and the test segment includes the entire colon.

In other studies (modification) an additional collection port is placed at the descending colon–sigmoid colon junction by means of a flexible endoscope. An endoscope (Olympus) is introduced through the anus without sedation and advanced an average of 55 ± 3 cm into the colon. A wash catheter is then placed through the biopsy channel of the endoscope so that fluid can be aspirated from this point. When this arrangement is used there is a 30-cm mixing segment in the distal ileum and two colonic test segments, the first including the cecum, ascending, transverse, and descending colon and the second including the sigmoid colon and rectum. An electrolyte solution containing polyethylene glycol (PEG), as a nonabsorbable marker, is infused into the ileum at a rate of 20 ml/min. Once watery diarrhea develops, the rectal tube and endoscope (if used) are positioned and the infusion restarted. Following a 60-min equilibration period (approximately five times the mean transit time through the colon at this rate of infusion), a 2-hr test period is started. During this time fluid is aspirated from the collection site in the cecum (and from the descending colon–sigmoid junction when this is intubated; see above). Rectal effluent is collected by gravity drainage.

Samples of fluid are then analyzed for electrolyte concentrations and PEG, and net water and electrolyte absorption rates are calculated by means of correlation between PEG and electrolyte concentration in the collected samples. If the colon is divided into two segments by use of the colonoscope (see above), absorption rates are calculated for each segment separately and added to give the result for the entire colon.

In four segmental colon perfusion studies, tritiated water (^3H_2O), 5 μCi/liter, is administered to the perfusate to estimate the relative surface area of the two segments. Radioactivity in samples of perfusate and luminal fluid from the sampling site is measured with a liquid scintillation counter and expressed as specific activity (dpm/ml). Absorption is calculated by standard nonabsorbable marker equations and expressed as a percentage of the radioactivity entering the test segment.

b. In Vivo Transport Studies in Human Rectum Rates of net electrolyte and water transport are measured using a dialysis technique (53, 54). Dialysis bags are constructed from 6- to 8-cm lengths of Visking tubing (1.43 cm diameter; Medicell International, London). One end is sealed using silk thread and epoxy resin, and after turning the bag inside out, two polyethylene tubes are introduced into the bag before sealing the other end around the tubes in a similar manner. One tube (Portex; internal diameter 3 mm) acts as an electrical bridge and contains 4% agar in Ringer's solution. The other tube (internal diameter 1 mm) allows Ringer's solution to be introduced into the bag *in situ*. With the subject in the left lateral position, the bag is paced in the rectum via a sigmoidoscope after ensuring the mucosa is free of fecal material, such that the lower end is 8 cm from the anus. Studies are performed using Ringer solution containing PEG as a nonabsorbable marker.

For ion transport studies the dialysis bag remains in the rectum for 60 min; rectal potential difference is measured every 5 to 10 min. At the end of the dialysis period, the solution is removed from the bag for subsequent analysis. Sodium, chloride, and bicarbonate are measured by autoanalyzer and PEG is assayed turbidimetrically.

The volume of solution in the dialysis bag at time zero (V_0, in milliliters, assuming a specific gravity of 1) is calculated as

$$V_0 = [(A_1 - A_2)(5/\mathrm{PEG}_0)] - (B_1 - B_2),$$

and the volume after a 60-min dialysis period (V_{60}) is

$$V_{60} = V_0 \,(\text{PEG}_0/\text{PEG}_{60}),$$

where A_1 is the weight (in grams) of syringe A filled with Ringer solution, A_2 is the weight of syringe A empty, B_1 is the weight of syringe B containing Ringer solution at time zero, B_2 is the weight of syringe B empty, PEG_0 is the PEG concentration (grams/liter) at time zero, and PEG_{60} is the PEG concentration after a 60-min dialysis. The volume change in the bag is calculated as ($V_0 - V_{60}$). Changes in content of individual electrolytes are calculated from V_0, V_{60}, and electrolyte concentrations at the end of dialysis. The area of the bag (calculated from its length and radius) is assumed to equal the area of mucosa in contact with the solution, and the net fluxes of water and electrolytes are therefore expressed as μl/cm²/hr and μmol/cm²/hr, respectively. Positive values indicate loss from the bag—that is, net absorption; negative values indicate addition to the bag—that is, net secretion.

Using this method it has been demonstrated that single pharmacologic doses of glucocorticoids stimulate rectal sodium and water absorption in control subjects and in patients with ulcerative colitis (53, 54).

2. *In Vivo* Measurement of Colonic Electrophysiology

PD is measured between a subcutaneous reference electrode placed either in the forearm or on the lateral aspect of the thigh, and an electrode placed into the lumen of the colon or rectum (via colonoscope or sigmoidoscope) by means of agar bridges, matched calomel half-cells (Radiometer Copenhagen, Model K 401), and a voltmeter (Avometer, Model DA 211), and KCI (4 *M*). Normal colonic and rectal PD is lumen negative (approximately −20 to −40 mV) (51–54).

3. *In Vivo* Studies of Water Absorption/Secretion in Animal Intestinal Loops

This method is suitable for *in vivo* studies of intestinal water absorption and secretion in animals (e.g., pigs, dogs, rabbits, rats, mice) (55). Under general anesthesia, a midline abdominal incision is performed and an intestinal segment is ligated proximally and distally, resulting in the formation of an intestinal loop (small or large intestine). The length of the intestinal loop ranges from 1 cm (mouse) to 10 cm (dog, pig). After introduction of plastic tubes (diameter, 0.2–2 cm) the intestinal loop is perfused with Ringer's buffer solution containing (in mmol/liter) Na, 142.6; K, 5.0; Cl, 123.8; Mg, 1.2; Ca, 1.3; HCO_3, 25; HPO_4, 17; H_2PO_4, 0.3; and glucose, 5.0. The solution also contains 1 μCi/liter of [^{14}C]polyethylene glycol (mol wt. 4000) as a nonabsorbed dilution marker of water flux and 5 g/liter of unlabeled polyethylene glycol 4000 as a carrier.

The intestinal segment is perfused at a constant rate (6 ml/hr), and the effluent is collected during consecutive 15-min periods over a total period of 240 min, with the first 2 hr corresponding to the equilibration period. The ^{14}C activity in collected samples is determined by liquid scintillation. Water flux for each 15-min interval is calculated by the following formula: $1 - \text{cpmS}/\text{cpmX} \times P/L$ = net water flux, where cpmS and cpmX are the ^{14}C activity in buffer solution and effluent, respectively, expressed as counts per minute (cpm); P is the rate (μl/hr) of perfusion, L is the length (cm) of the intestinal segment, and net water flux is expressed in μl/cm/hr.

Water fluxes occuring over two consecutive 15-min intervals are averaged to obtain a mean net flux of water over a 30-min period. Positive values represent net absorption; negative values indicate net secretion of water. This technique has been used to study the effect of drugs and toxins on intestinal secretion/absorption *in vivo* (55).

V. Conclusion

To date numerous experimental techniques are available to study the mechanisms involved in the regulation of fluid/nutrient absorption and secretion in the intestine. Experimental systems ranging from molecular and cell levels (*in vitro*) to studies in whole organisms (*in vivo*) were designed to study intestinal physiology and to model conditions of intestinal disease. Being aware of the advantages and disadvantages of each model aids in finding the appropriate experimental system for investigation of specific issues of intestinal physiology.

References

1. Ussing, H. H., and Zerahn, K. (1951). Active transport of sodium as the source of electric current in the short-circuited isolated frog skin. *Acta Physiol. Scand.* **23,** 110.
2. Madara, J. L., Dharmsathaporn, K. (1985). Occluding junction structure-function relationships in a cultured epithelial monolayer. *J. Cell Biol.* **101,** 2124–2133.
3. Sellin, H. J., De Soignie, R. (1987). Ion transport in human colon *in vitro*. *Gastroenterology* **93,** 441–448.
4. Binder, H. J., Foster, E. S., Budinger, M. E., and Hayslett, J. P. Mechanism of electroneutral sodium chloride absorption in distal colon of the rat. *Gastroenterology* **93,** 449–455.
5. Riegler, M., Sedivy, R., Pothoulakis, C., Hamilton, G., Zacherl, J., Bischof, G., Cosentini, E., Feil, W., Schiessel, R., LaMont, J. T., and Wenzl, E. (1995). *Clostridium difficile* toxin B is more potent than toxin A in damaging human colonic epithelium *in vitro*. *J. Clin. Invest.* **95,** 2004–2011.
6. Devor, D. C., and Frizzell, R. A. (1993). Calcium-mediated agonists activate an inwardly rectified K channel in colonic secretory cells. *Am. J. Physiol.* **265,** C1271–C1280.
7. Madara, J. L. (1990). Warner-Lambert/Parke-Davis award lecture: Pathobiology of the intestinal epithelial barrier. *Am. J. Pathol.* **137** (6), 1273–1281.
8. Hegel, U., Fromm, M., Kreusel, K. M., and Widerholt, M. (1993). Bovine and porcine large intestine as model epithelia in a student lab course. *Am. J. Physiol.* **265** (10), S10–S19.

9. Grass, G. M., and Sweetana, S. A. (1988). *In vitro* measurements of gastrointestinal tissue permeability using a new diffusion cell. *Pharm. Res.* **5,** 372–376.
10. Vajanaphanich, M., Schultz, C., Tsien, R. Y., Traynor, Kaplan, A. E., Pandol, S. J., and Barrett, K. E. (1995). Cross-talk between calcium and cAMP-dependent intracellular signaling pathways. Implications for synergistic secretion in T84 colonic epithelial cells and rat pancreatic acinar cells. *J. Clin. Invest.* **96,** 386–393.
11. Vaandrager, A. B., Berghe, N. V., Bot, A. G. M., and de Jonge, H. R. (1992). Phorbol esters stimulate and inhibit Cl-secretion by different mechanisms in a colonic cell line. *Am. J. Physiol.* **262,** G249–G256.
12. Matthews, J. B., Smith, J. A., Tally, K. J., Awtrey, S., Nguyen, H., Rich, J., and Madara, J. L. (1994). Na-K-2Cl cotransport in intestinal epithelial cells Influence of chloride efflux and F-actin on regulation of cotransporter activity and bumetanide binding. *J. Biol. Chem.* **269**(22), 15703–15709.
13. Sahi, J., Nataraja, S. G., Layden, T. J., Goldstein, J. L., Moyer, M. P., and Rao, M. C. (1998). CI transport in an immortalized human epithelial cell line (NCM460) derived from the normal transverse colon. *Am. J. Physiol.* **275,** C1048–C1057.
14. Dharmsathaporn, K., McRoberts, J. A., Mandel, K. G., Tisdale, L. D., and Masui, H. M. (1984). A human colonic tumor cell line that maintains vectorial electrolyte transport. *Am. J. Physiol.* **246,** G204–G208.
15. Dharmsathaporn, K., and Pandol, S. J. (1986). Mechanism of chloride secretion induced by charbachol in a colonic epithelial cell line. *J. Clin. Invest.* **77,** 348–354.
16. Madara, J. L., Colgan, S., Nusrat, A., Delp, C., and Parkos, C. (1992). A simple approach to measurement of electrical parameters of cultured epithelial monolayers: Use in assessing neutrophil–epithelial interactions. *J. Tissue Culture Methods* **14,** 209–216.
17. Uribe, J. M., Gelbmann, C. M., Traynor-Kaplan, A. E., and Barett, K. E. (1996). Epidermal growth factor inhibits Ca-dependent Cl transport in T84 human colonic epithelial cells. *Am. J. Physiol.* **271,** C914–C922.
18. Nash, S., Parkos, C., Nusrat, A., Delp, C., and Madara, J. L. (1991). *In vitro* model of intestinal crypt abscess. A novel neutrophil-derived secretagogue activity. *J. Clin. Invest.* **87,** 1474–1477.
19. Prasad, M., Smith, J. A., Resnick, A., Awtrey, C. S., Hrnjez, B. J., and Matthews, J. B. (1995). Ammonia inhibits cAMP-regulated intestinal Cl transport. *J. Clin. Invest.* **96,** 2142–2151.
20. Berschneider, H. M., and Powell, D. W. (1992). Fibroblasts modulate intestinal secretory responses to inflammatory mediators. *J. Clin. Invest.* **89,** 484–489.
21. Yang, H. Y., Lieska, N., Goldman, A. E., and Goldman, R. D. (1985). A 300,000 mol. wt. intermediate filament associated protein in baby hamster kidney (BHK-21) cells. *J. Cell Biol.* **100,** 620–631.
22. Hubel, K. A., Renquist, K., and Shirazi, S. (1987). Ion transport in human cecum, transverse colon, and sigmoid colon *in vitro*. Baseline and response to electrical stimulation of intrinsic nerves. *Gastroenterology* **92,** 501–507.
23. Schmitz, H., Fromm, M., Bode, H., Scholz, P., Riecken, E. O., and Schulzke, J. D. Tumor necrosis factor alpha induced Cl and K secretion in human distal colon driven by prostaglandin E2. *Am. J. Physiol.* **271,** G669–G674.
24. Singh, S. K., Binder, H. J., Boron, W. F., and Geibel, J. P. (1995). Fluid absorption in isolated perfused colonic crypts. *J. Clin. Invest.* **96,** 2373–2379.
25. Wang, L., Stanisz, A. M., Wershil, B. K., Galli, S. J., and Perdue, M. H. (1995). Substance P induces ion secretion in mouse small intestine through effects on enteric nerves and mast cells. *Am. J. Physiol.* **269,** G85–G92.
26. Bulsma P. B., Peeters, R. A., Groot, J. A., Dekker, P. R., Taminiau, J. A. J. M., and van der Meer, R. (1995). Differential *in vivo* and *in vitro* intestinal permeability to lactulose and mannitol in animals and humans: A hypothesis. *Gastroenterology* **108,** 687–696.
27. Prasad, M., Ito, S., and Silen, W. (1997). Functional studies of *in vitro* rat distal colon before and after restitution. *Surgery* **121,** 430–439.
28. Stein, J., Ries, J., and Barrett, K. (1998). Disruption of intestinal barrier function associated with experimental colitis: possible role of mast cells. *Am. J. Physiol.* **274,** G203–G209.
29. Mun, E., Mayol, J. M., Riegler, M., O'Brien T. C., Farokhazad, O. C., Song, J. C., Pothoulakis, C., Hrnjez, B. J., and Matthews, J. B. (1998). Levamisole inhibits intestinal Cl secretion via basolateral K channel blockade. *Gastroenterology* **114,** 1257–1267.
30. Cooke, H. J. (1994). Neuroimmune signaling in regulation of intestinal ion transport. *Am. J. Physiol.* **266,** G167–G178.
31. Riegler, M., Castagliuolo, I., So, P. T., Lotz, M., Wang, C., Wlk, M., Sogukoglu, T., Cosentini, E., Bischof, G., Hamilton, G., Teleky, B., Wenzl, E., Matthews, J. B., and Pothoulakis, C. (1999). Effects of substance P on human colonic mucosa *in vitro*. *Am. J. Physiol.* **276,** G1473–G1483.
32. Sandle, G. I., Wills, N. K., Alles, W., and Binder, H. J. (1986). Electrophysiology of the human colon: Evidence of segmental heterogeneity. *Gut* **27,** 999–1005.
33. Clauss, W., Schäfer, H., Horch, I., and Hörnicke, H. (1985). Segmental differences in electrical properties and Na transport of rabbit caecum, proximal and distal colon. *Pflügers Arch.* **403,** 278–282.
34. Yajima, T., Suzuki, T., and Suzuki, Y. (1988). Synergism between calcium-mediated and ccyclic AMP-mediated activation of chloride secretion in isolated guinea pig distal colon. *Jpn. J. Physiol.* **38,** 427–443.
35. Gelbmann, C. M., Schteingart, C. D., Thompson, S. M., Hofmann, A. F., and Barrett, K. E. (1995). Mast cells and histamine contribute to bile acid-stimulated secretion in the mouse colon. *J. Clin. Invest.* **95,** 2831–2839.
36. Kuwahara, A., Bowen, S., Wang, J., Condon, C., and Cooke, H. J. (1987). Epithelal responses evoked by stimulation of submucosal neurons in guinea pig distal colon. *Am. J. Physiol.* **252,** G667–G674.
37. Kuwahara, A., Cooke, H. J., Carey, H. V., Mekhjian, H., Ellison, E. C., and McGregor, B. (1989). Effects of enteric neural stimulation on chloride transport in human left colon *in vitro*. *Dig. Dis. Sci.* **34,** 206–213.
38. Sidhu, M., and Cooke, H. J. (1995). Role for 5-HT and ACh in submucosal reflexes mediating colonic secretion. *Am. J. Physiol.* **269,** G346–G351.
39. Emmer, E., Rood, R. P., Wesolek, J. H., Cohen, M. E., Braithwaite, R. S., Sharp, G. W. G., Murer, H., and Donowitz, M. (1989). Role of calcium and calmodulin in the regulation of the rabbit ileal brush border membrane Na/H antiporter. *J. Membr. Biol.* **108,** 207–215.
40. Cohen, M. E., Reinlib, L., Watson, A. J. M., Gorelick, F., Rys-Sikora, K., Tse, M., Rood, R. P., Czernik, A. J., Sharp, G. W. G., and Donowitz, M. (1990). Rabbit ileal villus cell brush border Na/H exchange is regulated by Ca++/calmodulin-dependent protein kinase II, a brush border membrane protein. *Proc. Natl. Acad. Sci. U.S.A.* **87,** 8990–8994.
41. Cavet, M. E., Akhter, S., Sanchez de Medina, F., Donowitz, M., and Tse, C. M. (1999). Na/H exchangers (NHE1-3) have similar turn over numbers but different percentages on the cell surface. *Am. J. Physiol.* **277,** C1111–C1121.
42. Cliff, W. H., and Frizell, R. A. (1990). Separate Cl conductances activated by cAMP and Ca++ in Cl secreting epithelial cells. *Proc. Natl. Acad. Sci. U.S.A.* **87,** 4956–4960.
43. Castagliuolo, I., Riegler, M., Pasha, A., Nikulasson, S., Lu, B., Gerard, G., Gerard, N. P., and Pothoulakis, C. (1998). Neurokinin-1 (NK-1) receptor is required in *Clostridium difficile*-induced enteritis. *J. Clin. Invest.* **101,** 1547–1550.
44. Saunders, D. R., Hedges, J. R., Sillery, J., Esther, L., Matsumura, K., and Rubin, C. E. (1975). Morphological and functional effects of bile salts on rat colon. *Gastroenterology* **68,** 1236–1245.
45. Gaginella, T. S., Chadwick, V. S., Debongnie, J. C., Lewis, J. C., and Phillps, S. F. (1977). Perfusion of rabbit colon with ricinoleic acid:

dose-related mucosal injury, fluid secretion, and increased permeability. *Gastroenterology* **73,** 95–101.

46. Triadafilopoulos, G., Pothoulakis, C., O'Brien, M. J., and LaMont, J. T. (1987). Differential effects of *Clostridium difficile* toxins A and B on rabbit ileum. *Gastroenterology* **93,** 273–279.
47. Castagliuolo, I., Kelly, C. P., Qiu, B. S., Nikulasson, S. T., LaMont, J. T., and Pothoulakis, C. (1997). IL-11 inhibits *Clostridium difficile* toxin A enterotoxicity in rat ileum. *Am. J. Physiol.* **273,** G333–G341.
48. Pothoulakis, C., Kelly, C. P., Joshi, M. A., Gao, N., O'Keane, C. J., Castagliuolo, I., and LaMont, J. T. (1993). *Saccharomyces boulardii* inhibits *Clostridium difficile* toxin A binding and enterotoxicity in rat ileum. *Gastroenterology* **104,** 1108–1115.
49. Grubb, B. R., and Gabriel, S. E. (1997). Intestinal physiology and pathology in gene-targeted mouse models of cystic fibrosis. *Am. J. Physiol.* **273,** G258–G266.
50. Davis, R. G., Santa Ana, C. A., Morawski, S. G., and Fordtran, J. S. (1980). Active chloride secretion in normal human jejunum. *J. Clin. Invest.* **66,** 1326–1333.
51. Davis, G. R., Morawski, S. G., Santa Ana, C. A., and Fordtran, J. S. (1983). Evaluation of chloride/bicarbonate exchange in the human colon in vivo. *J. Clin. Invest.* **71,** 201–207.
52. Schiller, L. R., Santa Ana, C. A., Morawski, S. G., and Fordtran, J. S. (1988). Effect of amiloride on sodium transport in the proximal, distal, and entire human colon *in vivo*. *Dig. Dis. Sci.* **33,** 969–976.
53. Sandle, G. I., Hayslett, J. P., Binder, H. J. (1986). Effect of glucocorticoids on rectal transport in normal subjects and patients with ulcerative colitis. *Gut* **27,** 309–316.
54. Rampton, D. S., Sladen, G. E., and Youlten, L. F. J. (1980). Rectal mucosal prostaglandin E2 release and its relation to disease activity, electrical potential difference, and treatment in ulcerative colitis. *Gut* **21,** 591–596.
55. Theodorou, V., Eutamene, H., Fioramonti, J., Junien, J. L., and Bueno, L. (1994). Interleukin 1 induces a neurally mediated colonic secretion in rats: involvement of mast cells and prostaglandins. *Gastroenterology* **106,** 1493–1500.
56. Mintenig, G. M., Monaghan, A. S., and Sepulveda, F. V. (1992). A large conductance K-selective channel of guinea pig villus enterocytes is Ca++ independent. *Am. J. Physiol.* **262,** G369–G374.

42

Surgical Models of Inflammatory Bowel Disease

Heidi Yeh and John L. Rombeau

Harrison Department of Surgical Research, University of Pennsylvania, Philadelphia, Pennsylvania 19104

I. Introduction

Inflammatory bowel disease (IBD) is categorized into two distinct entities by clinical and pathologic findings: Crohn's disease and ulcerative colitis. The causes of IBD remain unknown. Although the management of Crohn's disease and ulcerative colitis is largely medical, surgeons are also closely involved with the care of many IBD patients. Approximately 70% of Crohn's patients require surgery for complications such as obstruction, perforation, fistula formation, intractable disease, weight loss (or significant growth retardation in children), and, less commonly, bleeding, toxic megacolon, and cancer. Of note, extraintestinal manifestations often subside with resection of grossly involved intestine. Disease recurs most commonly at, or proximal to, the anastomosis or stomal site (1). On the other hand, surgery is the definitive cure for ulcerative colitis. Surgical indications more frequently include hemorrhage, toxic megacolon, acute episodes that do not respond to intravenous steroids, obstruction, cancer, weight loss (growth retardation), and failure to respond to medical therapy (2).

There is significant morbidity and impact on quality of life associated with both of these disorders and with the drugs and surgical techniques used for their treatment. It is important to gain a better understanding of the pathogenesis of IBD in order to design more specific therapies and better regimens for prevention, and to decrease both the complications of and the need for surgery.

It is necessary to understand the histology and clinical findings in Crohn's disease and ulcerative colitis in order to compare the available animal models. Crohn's disease presents most often with chronic, relapsing pain, diarrhea, and weight loss. Extraintestinal manifestations include polyarthritis, ankylosing spondylitis, erythema nodosum, clubbing of fingertips, uveitis, hepatic pericholangitis, and systemic amyloidosis. Any part of the gastrointestinal (GI) tract can be affected by aphthous ulcers, fissures, cobblestoning, and creeping fat. It is characteristic of Crohn's to have intervening segments of normal bowel. Microscopically, there are transmural neutrophilic infiltrates, distortion of crypt architecture, ulcerations, atrophy, and the distinguishing sarcoidlike granulomas. Crohn's patients may have increased intestinal permeability to polyethylene glycol. The disease is linked to the HLA-B27 haplotype when associated with ankylosing spondylitis (3).

Ulcerative colitis patients also present with cramping pain, bloody diarrhea, and weight loss. Extraintestinal manifestations again include polyarthritis, ankylosing spondylitis, uveitis, pericholangitis and primary sclerosing cholangitis, and a variety of skin lesions. However, only the colon is affected in continuous fashion from distal, progressing proximal, with friable mucosa, broad-based ulcerations, and pseudopolyps. The inflammatory infiltrate is usually limited to the lamina propria and there are no granulomas. Ulcerative colitis patients have been found to have circulating antibodies (to normal colonic epithelium) that cross-react with enterobacterial lipopolysaccharide antigens, and IgG levels five times those of normal patients. There are alterations in mucin glycoprotein levels in mucosal colonocytes and a protein-loss enteropathy along with other malabsorption syndromes. The HLA AW24 and BW35 haplotypes are found in Israeli Jews of European origin who have ulcerative colitis (3).

This chapter reviews the animal models of IBD with an emphasis on their relevancy to surgical research (Table I).

II. Spontaneous Models

A. Cotton-Top Tamarin Colitis

Spontaneous colitis in cotton-top tamarins is one of the most widely accepted models of ulcerative colitis (UC). Sometimes referred to (incorrectly) as marmosets, the tamarin species *Saguinas oedipus* has been best characterized. Up to 80% of tamarins in captivity will develop colitis

Table I Models of Inflammatory Bowel Disease

Model	Advantages	Disadvantages	Potential surgical utilities
Cotton-top tamarin	Large animals; similarity to human UC; spontaneous	Difficult access; expensive care	Pouchitis; wound healing
C3H/HEJBir mice	Easy access and care; spontaneous	Small; short life span	Use necropsy rather than biopsy for data points
SAMP1/Yit mice	Easy access and care; spontaneous; extraintestinal manifestations	Small; very short life span; unclear if CD or UC model	Immunologic studies; immediate postoperative complications; relation of intestinal disease to extraintestinal manifestations
Equine granulomatous enteritis	Similarity to human Crohn's disease; large animals; spontaneous	No access	—
HLA-B27 rats	Extraintestinal manifestations; cancer incidence	Questionable applicability to IBD not associated with spondyloarthropathy	Relation of intestinal and systemic disease; cancer risk stratification
IL-2 knockout mice	Extraintestinal manifestations; attenuated course in germ-free environments	Small animals; very short life-span	Use of antibiotics and postoperative complications; relation of intestinal and systemic disease
IL-10 knockout mice	Involvement of entire GI tract; attenuated course in germ-free environments	Small animals	Techniques for bowel conservation; avoidance of recurrence; use of antibiotics and postoperative complications
TCR/MHCII knockout mice	Extraintestinal manifestations	Small animals	Immunologic studies; relation of intestinal and systemic disease
N-Cadherin chimeric mice	Very specific abnormality	Small animals; technically difficult to produce	Role of epithelium; mucosal protection and IBD
TNBS (mice, rats, guinea pigs, cats)	Well-characterized; large animals available; easy administration	Short time course	Postoperative complications; short-term pharmacologic screening
PG–PS (rats)	Similarity to CD; extraintestinal manifestations	Tedious preparation	Techniques for bowel conservation; avoidance of recurrence; relation of intestinal and systemic disease
Indomethacin (rats/dogs)	Easy administration	Poor resemblance to human IBD	—
DSS (mice)	Easy administration; chronic course	—	Pouchitis
Immune complex (rabbits)	—	Poor resemblance to human IBD; multiple-step administration	—
Oxazolone (mice)	Easy administration	Short-time course	Short-term pharmacologic screening

(4). From 25 to 40% of animals develop colonic adenocarcinoma, predominantly right-sided (5, 6).

Clinically, cotton-tops develop weight loss, diarrhea, and anorexia in a pattern of relapse and remission, starting as early as 18 days of age (7). Grossly, the colonic mucosa appears congested and thickened, with areas of hemorrhage, ulceration, and pseudopolyps. Histologically, there is inflammatory cell infiltration in the lamina propria, mucosal atrophy, crypt distortion, goblet cell depletion, and crypt abscesses (5, 6, 8). Unlike human colitis, cotton-top colitis affects primarily the ascending colon, and lesions are occasionally seen in the jejunum and ileum, rather than progressing from the rectum to the cecum (7). There is a change in the sulfation of mucins in the colon and their binding to lectins and eicosanoid levels is increased (5, 8). Systemically, CD4/CD8 ratios are altered and antibodies to components of colonic epithelial cells are increased (8).

As mentioned, cotton-tops develop adenocarcinoma, most frequently mucinous or signet-ring types, which are unusual in human UC patients (9). Cancer in cotton-tops is less often preceded by dysplasia compared to humans, and metastasis to the liver has not been shown to occur (5, 10). A small number of animals have been noted at necropsy to have periportal chronic inflammation resembling human sclerosing cholangitis (5).

Chronic cotton-top colitis responds to both 5-aminosalicylate (5-ASA) and steroids, relapsing when treatment stops (9). Systemic administration of antibodies to integrin $\alpha 4\beta 7$, crucial in recruiting lymphocytes to the intestines, also results in resolution of clinical symptoms and histologic inflammation within 72 hr (11). Although cotton-tops seem to have a decreased incidence of colitis when reared in isolation, an extensive search for a transmissible agent was negative (9) and the response to immunosuppression makes infection an unlikely cause. It should be noted that only 15% of animals in the wild develop colitis of a much milder variety (no carcinoma has been found in wild animals), and the previous observation may simply be the result of housing conditions (10).

One of the difficulties with the cotton-top tamarin is difficult access, because it is an endangered species, further complicating the usual limitations of using primates for large-scale studies (the expense and space required for their maintenance). In addition, the cotton-top appears to develop four other types of colitis, including infective colitides associated with *Campylobacter jejuni* and *Klebsiella pneumoniae*, pseudomembranous colitis, and rare cases that histologically resemble Crohn's more than UC, in that they have skip lesions and microgranulomas (5, 6). Due to the previously described concerns, the utility of this model for surgical research is limited. However, the large size of cotton-tops does make them better candidates for surgical interventions and endoscopic surveillance. This makes them ideal for investigating postoperative complications such as pouchitis and healing impairment secondary to the use of immune suppressants such as cyclosporine and steroids.

B. C3H/HeJBir Mice

C3H/HeJ mice at Jackson Laboratory (Bar Harbor, Maine) have a higher incidence of colitis than do other strains, despite negative routine testing for pathogens at necropsy. A severely affected female was bred with a normal male and the substrain is maintained by brother–sister mating, with at least one parent positive for the disease. C3H/HeJ are known to differ from other strains in having mother's milk containing mouse mammary tumor virus, which encodes a superantigen that causes the initial stimulation of and then deletion of certain T cell receptor subsets. The strain also carries a mutation that reduces the response to bacterial lipopolysaccharide (LPS). The new substrain has a higher frequency of antibodies to proteins present in normal enteric bacterial flora when compared to the founding C3H/HeJ colony.

Approximately 80% of animals are positive for occult blood, 25% for diarrhea, and 8% of females and 27% of males are positive for perianal ulcerations. Histologically, lesions in the cecum and proximal colon show large numbers of inflammatory cells in the lamina propria, crypt abscesses, ulcerations, regenerative hyperplasia, and submucosal scarring. Lesions first appear at 14 days, and progress to a peak at 3–6 weeks, slowly healing to regenerative crypts and chronic inflammatory infiltrates at 10 weeks. Of note, mice wean at 2 weeks and this is the point of initial colonization of the gut with intestinal flora, being most concentrated in the cecum and right colon (12). Extraintestinal manifestations, progression to cancer, and response to drugs are not well defined in C3H/HeJBir mice.

Although mice are more distantly related to humans than are primates or horses, and this colitis is not as well characterized, the easy availability and maintenance of mice makes them a far more attractive model to use for surgical experimentation. Another problem is the difficulty of endoscopy in small animals and their short life-span. However, they are remarkably resilient to open surgical manipulation, and deserve further characterization. Because it is possible to use large numbers of animals, one solution to the technical difficulties is to use necropsy to take data points rather than biopsy, and follow a group of animals at one time point each rather than the same animal at several time points. It is unclear what to make of the unusual distribution of inflammation as compared to human ulcerative colitis in C3H/HeJBir mice, but this may be related to differences in distribution of colonic flora in humans and mice.

C. SAMP1/Yit Mice

SAMP1 mice, derived from the AKR/J colony at Jackson Laboratory, have a short life-span (9 months), spontaneous amyloidosis, alopecia, and osteoporosis. In addition, they have defects in their T-dependent antibody response due to decreased T helper cell activity. Matsumoto *et al.* (13) bred a new subline of SAMP1 mice by selecting for mating mice with a spontaneous skin ulceration. The new substrain has a normal life-span and no amyloidosis, but does have inflammation of the gut in association with the skin lesions. Several serologic tests, cultures, and smears were negative for a large variety of pathogens. None of the standard genetic markers showed any difference from the original strain. Animals kept in a germ-free environment do not develop inflammation until 10 weeks after being moved back to conventional housing conditions.

At about 10 weeks of age, discontinuous thickening of the intestinal wall occurs, maximal in the terminal ileum, but restricted to the distal jejunum, ileum, and ileocecal valve. Histologically, there is inflammatory infiltration into the lamina propria and submucosa, with epithelial cell hyperplasia, villous atrophy, and crypt abscesses. There are abnormalities in myeloperoxidase and nitric oxide synthase levels in the mice, but current research is insufficient to determine whether this is a cause or a result of the chronic inflammation.

Skin lesions occur on the back and eyelids, with loss of epidermis and infiltration of inflammatory cells into the dermis. In addition, focal clusters of lymphocytes were scattered throughout the hepatic acini. The other body tissues are otherwise histologically normal (13).

This model suggests again that inflammatory bowel disease is secondary to an aberrant immune response to endemic antigens. It is difficult to categorize as a Crohn's disease or an ulcerative colitis model because it lacks the granulomas and fissures of Crohn's, but does have the distribution, skin lesions, and intestinal wall thickening. The surgical utility of this model appears to be best suited for short-term studies addressing immunologic hypotheses and postoperative complications. Because of the presence of skin and liver lesions, this model may also be useful for investigating the effects of surgery on extraintestinal manifestations.

D. Equine Granulomatous Enteritis

Although the lack of horse colonies to provide experimental material makes them a difficult study subject, the wealth of information collected from sporadic cases makes equine granulomatous enteritis worth a brief discussion. Like human Crohn's, equine granulomatous enteritis is idiopathic, occurring in multiple breeds, with age of diagnosis anywhere from 1 to 13 years. Horses have chronic weight loss for several months despite normal appetite and intermittent diarrhea characterized by decreased xylose absorption and intestinal protein loss. Grossly, the bowel wall is thickened, with linear ulcerations and serosal adhesions. Disease extends from the stomach to the colon with transmural inflammatory cell infiltrate, squamous cell metaplasia, linear ulcerations, thickened mucosa, villous atrophy, and well-defined granulomas. Extraintestinal manifestations include dermatitis, arthritis, spondylitis, linear erosions of the vulva, and portal fibrosis in the liver without distortion of the remaining parenchyma (14).

The search for an infectious etiology unearthed only *Mycobacterium avium* in some affected horses (15) and cyasthostomes in others (16), with unclear causal relationships. Later reports of disease remission with dexamethasone (17) makes an infectious cause even more unlikely and attempts to transfer colitis by injecting diseased tissue homogenates into unaffected animals have been unsuccessful (14). Two attempts at surgical cure have been reported; one horse remained disease-free up to 13 months after resection of the affected segment while the other died of volvulus secondary to adhesions (18). There has been no further follow-up on the surviving horse as to whether it developed disease in a different segment.

Equine granulomatous enteritis bears remarkable similarities to human Crohn's. Unfortunately, there is as yet no good source of experimental subjects. Otherwise, horses would be ideal for following short- and long-term studies of pharmacologic and surgical therapies and their effects on intestinal and extraintestinal disease.

III. Transgenic Rodent Models

A. HLA-B27 Rats

The HLA-B27 haplotype is known to be associated with the human spondyloarthropathies, which sometimes include IBD. HLA-B27 transgenic rats on the Fischer 344 (F344) background have a 95% incidence of chronic colitis. They also develop proliferative lesions ranging from inflammatory hyperplasia to invasive carcinoma. HLA-B27 transgenics on the Lewis background also develop IBD, but no cancer (19). All stool cultures are negative and nontransgenics or nonaffected littermates do not contract the disease despite living in close proximity.

Clinically, rats develop diarrhea at about 10 weeks of age (21). Histologically, there is diffuse mucosal inflammation throughout the colon and rectum, primarily restricted to the lamina propria. Crypts contain regenerative atypia and abscesses. Lesions occur occasionally in the stomach and small bowel. Inflammation also affects the peripheral and vertebral joints, male genital tract, skin, nails, and heart. Over 5 months of age, F344 rats develop a progression of hyperplasia, adenoma, then carcinoma through polyp formation, unlike in human ulcerative colitis, where it occurs via flat dysplastic mucosa (19, 20).

Being of larger size than mice, rats are a more attractive surgical model. Although neoplastic indications for surgery in human ulcerative colitis are fairly well accepted, the two different rat strains and their propensity to develop cancer may offer some insight into both risk stratification and the molecular basis for progression from hyperplasia to dysplasia to carcinoma in ulcerative colitis. The presence of extraintestinal manifestations allows the surgical researcher to study any relationship between intestinal disease and systemic disease.

B. IL-2, IL-10, T Cell Receptor, and MHC Class II Knockouts

Several transgenic mice models were originally used to investigate the molecular regulation of T cell development and function; these models serendipitously resulted in gut inflammation models.

1. IL-2 Knockout

Mice homozygous for an IL-2 mutation (21) completely abrogating function have normal thymic structure and normal thymocyte and peripheral T cell subset compositions. *In vitro* responses to T cell mitogens are reduced but not eliminated. Serum measurements show a skewing of T helper cells toward TH2 isotypes, IL-$2^{-/-}$ mice having higher levels of IgG_1 and IgE.

Mice appear normal until about 3–4 weeks of age. About 50% then die in the next 5–6 weeks of a disease characterized by splenomegaly, lymphadenopathy, and severe anemia. The remaining 50% develop chronic diarrhea, intermittent intestinal bleeding, and rectal prolapse. These animals die within 10–25 weeks. Multiple serologic and culture tests were negative for an infectious cause and there was no evidence of horizontal disease transmission to normal littermates. However, in germ-free environments, there is no clinical evidence of IBD and microscopic and immunologic signs of inflammation are delayed until 17–20 weeks.

Histologically, there is infiltration of the mucosa with inflammatory cells, thickening of the mucosa and submucosa with mucosal ulcerations, crypt abscesses, loss of goblet cells, and destruction of crypt architecture with epithelial dysplasia. Disease increases in intensity from the rectum to the cecum and there is no involvement of the small bowel. Systemically, there is amyloidosis of the liver, spleen, and kidneys.

In addition to the advantages of any other mouse model, IL-2 knockout mice can be used to study the effect of normal bacterial exposure and antibiotics on postoperative complications, because a germ-free environment has already been noted to slow disease progression. This model also offers the opportunity to elucidate the relationship between extraintestinal inflammation and GI involvement at the site of antigen exposure.

2. IL-10 Knockout

IL-10, on the other hand, is associated (22) with the TH2 helper subset (stimulating B cells to mature into plasma cells and produce antibody) and suppresses macrophage activation. In mice with the IL-10 gene inactivated by targeted mutation, the T cell compartments in the thymus and spleen are normal. The B cell distribution and antibody response seem normal, too. However, IL-10-deficient mice produce a TH1 response to nematodes, which is normally suppressed in wild-type mice. The mice therefore appear to have normal TH2 response, but have inappropriate TH1 responses, which it appears IL-10 is necessary to suppress.

About 90% of mice are affected by intestinal inflammation characterized by anemia and weight loss, with growth retardation evident at 3–4 weeks, the time of weaning and colonization of the gut with normal flora. The enterocolitis affects the entire gastrointestinal tract, with the duodenum, proximal jejunum, and proximal colon most severely affected. Histologically, inflammatory cells infiltrate the lamina propria and submucosa resulting in hyperplasia of mucosa, abnormal crypt structures, superficial erosions, and thickening of subepithelial basement membranes. There is also MHC class II expression in epithelial cells that normally do not express MHC class II in wild-type mice, spurring speculation that aberrant expression of class II in colonic epithelium could be the cause of IBD in humans. Under specific pathogen-free conditions, disease is limited to the colon and does not affect the small intestine.

Because of the involvement of the entire GI tract, this model may be similar enough to Crohn's disease (although there are no granulomas) to be used for studies of recurrence and attempts at bowel conservation by strictureplasty or proximal diversion rather than resection.

3. TCR and Class II Knockouts

Two T cell receptor mutants (TCR-α and TCR-β) (23) appear normal for 3–4 months. Subsequently, about 30% will develop chronic diarrhea, wasting, and anorectal prolapse. Few mice survive beyond 1 year. This does appear to be related to an absolute T cell deficiency, because RAG1 mice, which have neither B cells nor T cells, have no disease (although they do die of pneumonia and abscesses). Disease occurred even under specific pathogen-free conditions. One mouse developed rectal adenocarcinoma.

Grossly, there is thickening and dilation of the rectum extending continuously up to the cecum, but the boundary between macroscopically normal and diseased bowel is sharp. The small intestine is normal. Histologically, there is infiltration of inflammatory cells into the lamina propria and submucosa, but there is no muscle involvement. Crypt distortion, depletion of goblet cells, and crypt abscesses are found, but no granulomas or transmural fissures. No analysis of the joints has been performed, but there are focal mixed inflammatory cell infiltrates in the livers.

Several other similar knockouts exist: TCR-β × TCR-σ double mutants, class II MHC mutants, TCR-α × class II double mutants, and TCR-β × class II MHC double mutants. Colitis is most severe in the class II mutants and TCR-α mutants. This is the opposite of what one would expect based on the findings of the IL-10 knockout, and implies multiple causes of inflammatory bowel disease in humans as well as mice. This group of models would be especially useful in comparing immunologic abnormalities in IBD.

IV. Other Models

A. N-Cadherin Mutants

Cadherins are essential for the regulation of cell adhesion. Alterations in cell adhesion are associated with the ability of tumor cells to invade and metastasize, and culture studies suggest that complexes with catenins regulate cell polarity, junctional complexes, migration, and proliferation. Chimeric mice were engineered by transfecting 129/Sv embryonic stem cells with a dominant negative N-cadherin mutant whose expression is driven by a promoter active in the duodenum to ileum, maximal activity being in the proximal jejunum. Production of this mutant results in disruption of cell–cell and cell–matrix contacts, increased rates of cell migration, and precocious entry of enteroctyes into apoptosis. Transfected embryonic stem cells were then introduced into a normal B6 blastocyst, from which they could be distinguished by differential lectin *Ulex europeaus* agglutinin type 1 binding. Because of the organization of small intestinal epithelium, all stem cells in each crypt of an adult chimeric mouse share an identical genotype.

All chimeric mice generated develop inflammatory bowel disease. By 6 weeks of age, lymphoid aggregates are increased in the 129/Sv, but not in normal B6 epithelium. MHC class II concentrations are also markedly increased in 129/Sv crypt–villus units. By 3 months of age, inflammatory foci within 129/Sv patches become transmural, including crypt abscesses, neutrophilic infiltrates, goblet cell depletion, Paneth cell hyperplasia, and aphthoid and linear mucosal ulcers. These changes continue to progress and worsen through the 18 months of life. However, changes remain confined to 129/Sv-derived epithelium, ruling out the presence of autoimmune disease. Nontransgenic chimeras raised in the same isolator do not acquire inflammatory bowel disease, confirming the absence of an infectious particle. Expression of the dominant negative is required along the entire crypt–villus axis; restriction to the epithelium results in a minimal increase of lymphocytes in the lamina propria without progression to features of inflammatory bowel disease. Bacterial passage through poorly adherent cells is similar in both instances. This suggests that it is not only the abnormal stimulus of the disrupted epithelium that is responsible for inflammatory bowel disease, but also an abnormal immune response that is involved, mediated either by the lack of N-cadherin or the resultant abnormal crypt–villus architecture. Adenomas are common, beginning as early as 3 months of life, but no progression to adenocarcinoma has been observed during the first 19 months of life (24).

This model would be particularly interesting in studying problems of infection and healing after surgery for IBD. In addition, the association of immunologic abnormalities with deficiencies in adhesion molecules is important. The major drawback of this model is the technical expertise required in producing chimeras.

B. Chemical Induction

There are several models involving either the topical application of or injection of various chemicals into the colons of animals, resulting in chronic inflammation. Only a few of them seem to be worthwhile models, but a brief mention is made of several others that have been in use for many years.

C. Trinitrobenzene Sulfonic Acid

Rectal administration (25) of 10–30 mg of trinitrobenzene sulfonic acid (TNBS) in 0.25 ml of 50% ethanol results in colonic injury in mice, rats, rabbit, cats, and guinea pigs. Injury peaks at 1 week but persists for at least 8 weeks. Inflammatory cells infiltrate in the external muscle and serosa with granulomas in the mucosa. About 3% of animals will die. Interestingly enough, only certain strains of mice (C3H/HeN and BALB/c) are susceptible to chronic colitis and DBA/2 mice are resistant, suggesting that it is not a purely caustic phenomenon. In addition, EtOH or TNBS alone results in only transient, nongranulomatous colitis. However, TNBS can reactivate inflammation if given alone after the initial combination enema. A direct subserosal injection of TNBS alone also produces chronic granulomatous disease, giving rise to theories that ethanol disrupts the mucosal barrier, allowing the TNBS to be absorbed.

Prostaglandins, prednisone, and 5-ASA are all effective in ameliorating colitis if given within 24 hr of the enema. Soluble mediator and cytokine profiles are similar to those seen in Crohn's disease. Anti-IL-12 antibodies abolish colitis (26), possibly via apoptosis of $CD4^+$ TH1 cells (27), linking this chemical induction model with the previously discussed transgenic models. Other evidence of the involvement of the immune system includes increase or decrease in inflammation with prior sensitization or tolerization and the ability to reactivate inflammation with systemic rather than direct colonic exposure (8, 28).

This is a widely used, well-characterized model that is convenient to use for several species, including larger ones on which surgery is easier. However, the short span of inflammation makes it useful only for short-term studies on immediate postoperative complications rather than for questions of how to prevent recurrence or issues of bowel conservation for small bowel strictures. Again, the different susceptibilities of different strains present an opportunity to examine genetic factors involved in the development of IBD.

D. Peptidoglycan–Polysaccharide Polymers

Injection of sonicated peptidoglycan–polysaccharide (PG–PS) polymers (29) derived from group A or D streptococci in the distal ileum and cecum of Sprague–Dawley rats results in acute and chronic granulomatous inflammation at the site of the injection and draining lymph nodes. Acute inflammation resolves in 2 weeks, but the reinjection of enterococcal PG–PS results in chronic inflammation for at least 6 months. There is, again, a difference in the susceptibility among strains. Lewis rats develop granulomas in the liver and biliary tract, anemia, and arthritis, with serosal nodules and dense adhesions at sites distant from the injection. Approximately 70–80% of Lewis rats will develop chronic colitis, whereas only 10–20% of buffalo rats will. Fischer 344 rats, which are MHC identical to Lewis rats, are nevertheless low responders. Histologically, rats develop transmural inflammation with granulomas, crypt abscesses, linear fissures, fibrosis, and hyperplasia of smooth muscle cells.

The main disadvantage of this model is the difficulty in purifying PG–PS and the requirement for laparotomy to inject the material. It is otherwise very similar to Crohn's disease in humans, especially with the constellation of extraintestinal manifestations. The longer disease course also makes it more attractive in studying long-term effects of diversion for distal disease and recurrence following surgical resection.

E. Indomethacin and Acetic Acid

An oral indomethacin dose of 3–4 mg/kg/day for 4–14 days and a subcutaneous dose of 7.5 mg/kg/day for 2 days results in chronic inflammation in rats and dogs, resolving over 6 weeks (30). Clinically, rats have anemia and weight loss, but little diarrhea. Grossly, the disease begins with multiple round punctate ulcers throughout the small intestine, especially in the midjejunum along the mesenteric border (or the ileum in dogs), in the cecum, and in the stomach. There is thickening of the jejunum with adhesion formation and frequent obstruction. Microscopically, inflammatory cells infiltrate transmurally and diseased areas are interspersed with normal areas. Germ-free rats develop minimal small intestinal ulcers and no colonic ulcers, but continue to have gastric ulcers at the same rate. Cincophen has been used in dogs with definite granuloma formation.

This model responds to broad-spectrum antibiotics, prostaglandin agonists, sucralfate, and naloxone, but not to steroids. Nonsteroidal antiinflammatory drugs (NSAIDs) are found to cause an increase in epithelial permeability and higher concentrations of small intestinal concentrations of bacteria, especially *Bacteroides* species. Both could lead to higher exposure of the mucosa to antigenic stimuli.

This model does not offer the chronicity that other chemical induction models do; is complicated by gastric ulcers, which seem to have a different mechanism of formation than do the enterocolitic ulcers; and its pharmacologic profile does not closely match human inflammatory bowel disease. For the ease of oral administration, the dextran sulfate sodium model may be preferable. The acetic acid model more closely resembles ischemic colitis than inflammatory bowel disease.

F. Carageenan

Carageenan, an extract of red seaweed (*Eucheuma spinosum*), is composed of sulfated polysaccharides. It is known to injure colonic epithelial cells and destroy intraepithelial tight junctions, leading to increased mucosal permeability. The partially degraded form (30 kDa) has been added to the drinking water of guinea pigs, rabbits, rats, mice, and monkeys to form a 5% solution that produces colitis after 3–4 weeks of administration, continuing up to 1–2 weeks after cessation (31). Native polymers (100–800 kDa) take up to 6 months to induce colitis. Germ-free animals do not develop colitis.

There are superficial ulcers grossly, and inflammatory infiltrate in the lamina propria, epithelial atrophy, and crypt abscesses microscopically. Immunization with *Bacteroides* outer membrane proteins enhances colitis and Flagyl attenuates inflammation if given before the carageenan (28). It may be that increased uptake of normally present *Bacteroides* antigens is the irritating factor in this model. This model lacks the self-perpetuating features, which are the hallmark of human IBD, although it may be useful in studying the role of altered membrane permeability in chronic colitis.

G. Dextran Sulfate Sodium

Dextran sulfate sodium (3–10%) in the drinking water of rodents results in weight loss and diarrhea after about 10 days (32). Three to five cycles of treatments suffices to start a chronic colitis that does not require further administration. The colitis is characterized acutely by mucosal inflammation and ulcers, worse in the left colon than in the right. Chronic colitis is distinguished by leukocyte infiltration in the mucosa, high-grade epithelial cell dysplasia, and colonic shortening. As in carageenan administration, colonic counts of *Bacteroides* are noted to be elevated. This model requires further characterization, but the long time course makes it useful for issues such as pouchitis in UC patients following colectomy.

H. Immune Complex Colitis

A 1% formalin enema in rabbits increases the vascular permeability of the rectum, allowing localization of immune complexes injected intravenously (33). The enema is followed 2 hr later by IV injection of preformed human serum albumin immune complexes, with the antigen in excess. Inflammatory cell infiltration begins as soon as 3 hr after immune complex injection and continues out to 3 months. This is followed by crypt distortion and rectal mucosal ulceration. Sulfasalazine can improve the colitis, but, unfortunately, steroids do not. Sensitization to ubiquitous bacterial antigens prolongs the length of inflammation. This model, too, has not been widely used, perhaps because of the multiple steps involved.

I. Oxazolone

The administration of 6 mg of oxazolone (OXZ) in 50% ethanol intrarectally into normal SLJ/J mice leads to weight loss and superficial colitis involving only the distal 50% of the colon (34). IL-4 and TGF-β levels are high in lymphocytes purified from the lamina propria, but histologic changes of inflammatory infiltration, goblet cell depletion, and epithelial cell loss last for only 10 days. Extent, duration, and severity of disease can be modified with anti-IL-4 and anti-TGF-β antibodies, but in the absence of additional immunologic manipulation, SLJ/J mice seem to have the intrinsic capability of down-regulating inflammation, which patients with IBD lack. It may be that a different strain of mice would have chronic colitis following the same treatment and exploring the genetic differences between the two would provide valuable clues to the etiology of inflammatory bowel disease. This is indeed true of all the chemical induction models that have varying susceptibilities from one strain to the next.

This model might be useful for pharmocologic screening and short-term immunologic studies, but the short time course makes it inappropriate for investigating outcomes for surgical treatment except for questions of the immediate effects on the stress and immune response. In addition, this model is relatively new and, to date, poorly characterized.

V. Conclusions

It is most appealing to use spontaneous models of colitis, because they seem to have the same idiopathic etiology as seen in human disease. However, as we move toward thinking of inflammatory bowel disease as an uncontrolled immune response to ubiquitous antigens, it becomes more appropriate to make use of transgenics with altered immune systems. The broad spectrum of genetic disruptions that result in a similar phenotype suggests that a similar range of genes may be responsible for inflammatory bowel disease in humans. The models that do not develop colitis in sterile conditions point to the interaction of heredity and the environment. Chemically induced models are useful if we think of inflammatory bowel disease as being initiated by an unusual exposure to antigens inducing a physiologic immune response, rather than the immune system being abnormal. Such models may also pertain more to abnormalities in permeability and mucosal proteins found in human inflammatory bowel disease, although there has not been much in the way of characterization of colonocytes in the transgenic mice.

As our understanding of inflammatory bowel disease progresses, the use of infectious agents, obstruction of lymphatic drainage or arterial supply, and mechanical trauma as models becomes irrelevant. There nevertheless remains a plethora of models available, many of which await comparison to human inflammatory bowel disease in terms of reaction to pharmacologic agents, systemic and local biochemical and immunologic markers, and colonocyte characteristics before further experimental studies can be considered valid.

References

1. Kelly, K. A., and Wolff, B. G. (1997). Crohn's disease (regional enteritis). *In* "Textbook of Surgery" (D. J. Sabiston and H. K. Lyerly, eds.), pp. 923–932. W.B. Saunders, Philadelphia.
2. Becker, J. M., and Moody, F. G. (1997). Ulcerative colitis. *In* "Textbook of Surgery" (D. I. Sabiston and H. K. Lyerly, eds.), pp. 1001–1014. W.B. Saunders, Philadelphia.
3. Crawford, J. M. (1994). The gastrointestinal tract. *In* "Pathologic Basis of Disease" (R. S. Cotran, V. Kumar, and S. L. Robbins, eds.), pp. 755–830. W.B. Saunders, Philadelphia.
4. Wood, J. D., Peck, O. C., Tefend, K. S., Rodriguez-M., M. A., Rodriguez-M., J. V., Hernandez-C., J. I., Stonerook, M. J., and Sharma, H. M. (1998). Colitis and colon cancer in cotton-top tamarins (*Saguinus oedipus oedipus*) living wild in their natural habitat. *Dig. Dis. Sci.* **43,** 1443–1453.
5. Warren, B. F., and Watkins, P. (1997) Animal models—naturally occurring. *In* "Inflammatory Bowel Disease" (R. N. Allan, J. M. Rhodes,

S. B. Hanauer, M. R. B. Kingsley, J. Alexander-Williams, and Fazio, V .F., eds.), pp. 157–165. Churchill Livingstone, New York.
6. Chalifoux, L. V., Hunt, R. D., and King, N. W. (1985). Adenocarcinoma of the colon and chronic colitis in *Saguinas oedipus*: A possible model for analagous human disease. *In* "Animal Models for Intestinal Disease" (C. J. Pfeiffer, ed.), pp. 69–78. CRC Press, Boca Raton.
7. Beeken, W. L. (1992). Experimental inflammatory bowel disease. *In* "Inflammatory Bowel Disease" (J. B. Kirsner and R. G. Shorter, eds.), pp. 37–49. Lea and Febiger, Philadelphia.
8. Sartor, R. B. (1992). Animal models of intestinal inflammation. *In* "Inflammatory Bowel Disease" (R. P. MacDermott and W. F. Stenson, eds.), pp. 237–353. Elsevier, New York.
9. Johnson, L. D., Ausman, L. M., Prabhat, K. S., and King, N. W. (1996). A prospective study of the epidemiology of colitis and colon cancer in cotton-top tamarins. *Gastroenterology* **110,** 102–115.
10. Clapp, N. K., Henke, M. L., Lushbaugh, C., Humason, G. L., and Gangaware, B. L. (1988). Effect of various biological factors on spontaneous marmoset and tamarin colitis. A retrospective histopathologic study. *Dig. Dis. Sci.* **33,** 1013–1019.
11. Hesterberg, P. E., Winsor-Hines, D., Briskin, M. J., Soler-Ferran, D., Merrill, C., Mackay, C. R., Newman, W., and Ringler, D. J. (1996). Rapid resolution of chronic colitis in the cotton-top tamarin with an antibody to a gut-homing integrin alpha 4 beta 7. *Gastroenterology* **111,** 1373–1380.
12. Sundberg, J. P., Elson, C. O., Bedigian, H., and Birkenmeier, E. H. (1994). Spontaneous, heritable colitis in a new substrain of C3H/HeJ mice. *Gastroenterology* **107,** 1726–1735.
13. Matsumoto, S., Okabe, Y., Setoyama, H., Takayama, K., Ohtsuka, J., Funahashi, H., Imaoka, A., Okada, Y., and Umesaki, Y. (1998). Inflammatory bowel disease-like enteritis and caecitis in a senescence accelerated mouse P1/Yit strain. *Gut* **43,** 71–78.
14. Cimprich, R. E. (1985). Equine granulomatous enteritis. *In* "Animal Models for Intestinal Disease" (C. J. Pfeiffer, ed.), pp. 134–145. CRC Press, Boca Raton.
15. Buergelt, C. D., Green, S. L., Mayhew, I. G., Wilson, J. H., and Merritt, A. M. (1998). Avian mycobacteriosis in three horses. *Cornell Vet.* **78,** 365–380.
16. Jasko, D. J., and Roth, L. (1984). Granulomatous colitis associated with small strongyle larvae in a horse. *J. Am. Vet. Med. Assoc.* **185,** 553–554.
17. Duryea, J. H., Ainsworth, D. M., Mauldin, E. A., Cooper, B. J., and Edwards, 3rd R. B. (1997). Clinical remission of granulomatous enteritis in a standardbred gelding following long-term dexamethasone administration. *Equine Vet. J.* **29,** 164–167.
18. Schumacher, J., Moll, H. D., Spano, J. S., Barone, L. M., Powers, R. D. (1990). Effect of intestinal resection on two juvenile horses with granulomatous enteritis. *J. Vet. Intern. Med.* **4,** 153–156.
19. Hammer, R. E., Richardson, J. A., Simmons, W. A., White, A. L., Breban, M., and Taurog, J. D. (1995). High prevalence of colorectal cancer in HLA-B27 transgenic F344 rats with chronic inflammatory bowel disease. *J. Invest Med.* **43,** 262–268.
20. Hammer, R. E., Maika, S. D., Richardson, J. A., Tang, J. P., and Taurog, J. D. (1990). Spontaneous inflammatory disease in transgenic rats expressing HLA-B27 and human beta 2m: An animal model of HLA-B27-associated human disorders. *Cell* **63,** 1099–1112.
21. Sadlack, B., Merz, H., Schorle, H., Schimpl, A., Feller, A. C., and Horak, I. (1993). Ulcerative colitis-like disease in mice with a disrupted interleukin-2 gene. *Cell* **75,** 253–61.
22. Kuhn, R., Lohler, J., Rennick, D., Rajewsky, K., and Muller, W. (1993). Interleukin-10-deficient mice develop chronic enterocolitis. *Cell* **75,** 263–274.
23. Mombaerts, P., Mizoguchi, E., Grusby, M. J., Glimcher, L. H., Bhan, A. K., and Tonegawa, S. (1993). Spontaneous development of inflammatory bowel disease in T cell receptor mutant mice. *Cell* **75,** 274–282.
24. Hermiston, M. L., and Gordon, J. I. (1995). Inflammatory bowel disease and adenomas in mice expressing a dominant negative N-cadherin. *Science* **270,** 1203–1207.
25. Morris, G. P., Beck, P. L., Herridge, M. S., Depew, W. T., Szewczuk, M. R., and Wallace, J. L. (1989). Hapten-induced model of chronic inflammation and ulceration in the rat colon. *Gastroenterology* **96,** 795–803.
26. Neurath, M. F., Fuss, I., Kelsall, B. L., Stuber, E., and Strober, W. (1995). Antibodies to interleukin 12 abrogate established experimental colitis in mice. *J. Exp. Med.* **182,** 1281–1290.
27. Strober, W., Fuss, I. J., Ehrhardt, R. O., Neurath, M., Boirivant, M., and Ludviksson, B. R. (1998). Mucosal immunoregulation and inflammatory bowel disease: new insights from murine models of inflammation. *Scand. J. Immunol.* **48,** 453–458.
28. Wallace, J. L., and Hogaboam, C. M. (1997). Animal models of inflammatory bowel disease—Experimental. *In* "Inflammatory Bowel Diseases" (R. N. Allan, J. M. Rhodes, S. B. Hanauer, M. R. B. Keighley, J. Alexander-Williams, and V. F. Fazio, eds.), pp. 167–171. Churchill Livingstone, New York.
29. Sartor, R. B., Cromartie, W. J., Powell, D. W., and Schwab, J. H. (1985). Granulomatous enterocolitis induced in rats by purified bacterial cell wall fragments. *Gastroenterology* **89,** 587–595.
30. Kent, T. H., Cardelli, R. M., and Stamler, F. W. (1969). Small intestinal ulcers and intestinal flora in rats given indomethacin. *Am. J. Pathol.* **54,** 237–249.
31. Marcus, A. J., Marcus, S. N., Marcus, R., and Watt, J. (1989). Rapid production of ulcerative disease of the colon in newly-weaned guinea-pigs by degraded carrageenan. *J. Pharm. Pharmacol.* **41,** 423–426.
32. Okayasu, I., Hatakeyama, S., Yamada, M., Ohkusa, T., Inagaki, Y., and Nakaya, R. (1990). A novel method in the induction of reliable experimental acute and chronic ulcerative colitis in mice. *Gastroenterology* **98,** 694–702.
33. Hodgson, H. J., Potter, B. J., Skinner, J., and Jewell, D. P. (1978). Immune-complex mediated colitis in rabbits. An experimental model.' *Gut* **19,** 225–232.
34. Boirivant, M., Fuss, I. J., Chu, A., and Strober, W. (1998). Oxazolone colitis: A murine model of T helper cell type 2 colitis treatable with antibodies to interleukin 4. *J. Exp. Med.* **16,** 1929–1939.

43

Intestinal Regeneration and Adaptation Models

Sonia Y. Archer and Richard A. Hodin

Department of Surgery, Beth Israel Deaconess Medical Center, Boston, Massachusetts 02215

I. Introduction

In mammals, the gut undergoes constant growth and regeneration throughout the lifetime of the organism, and has the capacity to adapt to a variety of stresses. In fact, the small intestinal epithelium is the most rapidly proliferating tissue in the body, with a turnover time of 2 to 3 days in mice and rats, and 3 to 6 days in humans (1, 2). This turnover rate is so rapid that cells do not normally enter the prolonged G_0 phase seen in other, more slowly dividing tissues. This renewal is critical for maintenance of the functional integrity of the gut and is very tightly regulated along the crypt–villus axis through the migration of pluripotent stem cells located within the crypts of Lieberkuhn. Crypt and villus architecture is controlled, in part, by stromal and epithelial elements. The cells acquire a differentiated phenotype as they migrate toward the villus tip (absorptive enterocyte, goblet, and enteroendocrine cells), and are eventually extruded into the lumen (1, 3). Paneth cells do not migrate, however, but differentiate within the base of the crypts, eventually degenerate, and are lost through phagocytosis (3). Thus, a steady-state equilibrium is maintained between cell production and cell loss (see Fig. 1). Villus height follows a gradient from duodenum, where it is greatest, to the ileum, where the shortest villi are encountered. Accordingly, there is a proximal-to-distal gradient in villus height, cell number, and absorptive surface area in the small intestine. These anatomic differences depend not only on the larger amount of ingested nutrients encountered by the proximal gut, but also on an intrinsic genetic program (4). Thus, the processes of replication, migration, and differentiation are innate characteristics of the intestinal epithelium, and these processes can be modified by a variety of external stimuli.

The sheath of fibroblasts surrounding crypts of the intestine within the lamina propria of the bowel has also been shown to undergo rapid turnover, similar to that of the epithelial cells (5). Zajicek proposed the term "intestinal proliferon," referring to the structural and functional coordination that exists among epithelial, connective tissue, neural, and vascular elements within the gut (6).

Mechanisms controlling the gut renewal process are complex, involving both endogenous and exogenous factors, most notably luminal nutrients. Additionally, maturation of specific epithelial cell functions may be regulated by unique control mechanisms, distinct in the proximal versus distal

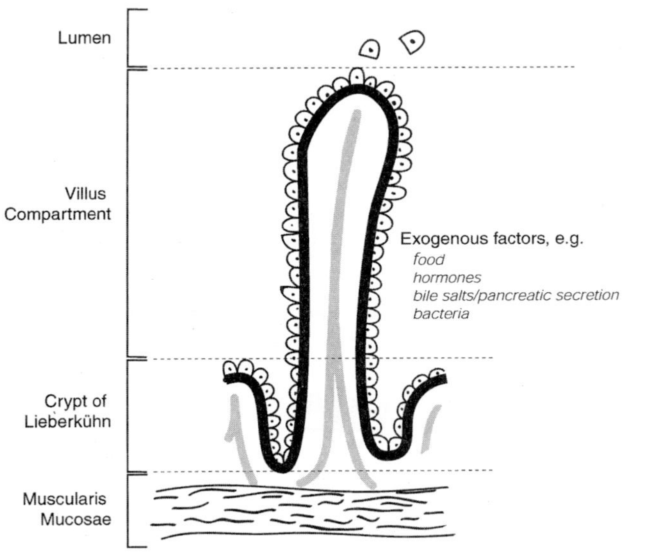

Figure 1 Villus architecture. Depiction of normal small intestinal villus architecture.

small intestine. The adult colon lacks true villi but does have crypt cells that give rise to the surface epithelium, similar to that seen in the small intestine. So too, the stomach is lined by a glandular epithelium containing many differentiated cells of specified function. However, again, there are no villi and the glands penetrate deeply into the mucosal lining.

Disruptions in the normal process of cellular growth are commonly observed in the clinical setting. For example, decreased crypt cell proliferation occurs with prolonged fasting, Crohn's disease, radiation enteritis, defunctioned bypassed segments of small intestine, small bowel lymphoma, burns, and sepsis. These conditions are characterizd by villus atrophy and are often associated with diarrhea, malabsorption, and impairment in gut barrier function, leading to significant morbidity and mortality in affected patients (7, 8). The diarrhea and malabsorption may be related in part to decreased absorptive area, but the etiology of the barrier dysfunction is not known, because anatomic defects in the cellular architecture have not been detected.

Conversely, increased cell proliferation is commonly seen after massive enterectomy (short bowel syndrome) or colectomy, in functional segments after intestinal bypass procedures, postfasting refeeding, lactation, celiac sprue disease, and administraton of various trophic hormones (thyroxine, testosterone, growth hormone, glucagon-like polypeptide-2, epidermal growth factor, etc.). In order to understand and better treat these conditions, the processes of intestinal adaptation/regeneration have been extensively studied, utilizing experimental model systems that address distinct aspects of gut physiology. Most of these models have focused on the small intestine, given its great capacity to regenerate and adapt and its critical role in maintaining adequate nutrient absorption, which is vital to overall health.

It is important to have a clear understanding of the terms "regeneration," "adaptation," and "restitution." Regeneration refers to a process whereby damaged components of the intestine are replaced by cells from the surviving components, resulting in a return to normal structure and function. Intestinal adaptation refers to a more generalized response that occurs when there is a substantial loss in gut absorptive surface area, e.g., following massive resection or bypass. Adaptation may involve changes in cell production, migration, and/or function. Clearly, the processes of intestinal adaptation and regeneration can occur simultaneously. In contrast to regeneration and adaptation, restitution refers to a process by which a locally damaged area of the epithelium is replaced from the adjacent epithelium, with the more remote regions of the gut remaining unaltered.

II. In Vivo Models

A. Models of Intestinal Restitution

Superficial epithelial damage is a frequent occurrence along the alimentary tract (9). Under normal conditions, epithelial integrity is rapidly reestablished by restitution, a process first described by Hollander in 1954 (10). Restitution has been studied in a variety of species, including rodents, frogs, rabbits, and humans. Additionally, this process has been examined in all regions of the alimentary tract: stomach, duodenum, small intestine, and colon. From these studies, it appears that rapid epithelial restitution is a fundamental process in the repair of the gastrointestinal mucosa.

The molecular mechanisms that govern the process of epithelial restitution are not well understood. Calcium and collagen are known to be required for restitution (11). An acidic environment has been shown to inhibit the restitution process, but this can be overcome by basic fibroblast growth factor (12). As expected, given the rapidity of the process, manipulation of protein synthesis and cell division do not appear to inhibit restitution (11). Several models have been used to study restitution in different areas of the G.I. tract. We will describe only one per section.

1. Stomach

a. Ethanol-Induced Injury Rats are fasted overnight with water *ad libitum*. General anesthesia is administered and the stomach is exposed through a small incision in the left upper quadrant. The esophagus and duodenum are ligated to obstruct their lumina, with care to avoid ligating adjacent arteries and nerves. Fluids are injected by hypodermic syringe through the nonglandular (squamous-lined forestomach) stomach wall. Approximately 4 ml of 70–100% ethanol is injected into the gastric lumen, distending the stomach so that the entire mucosal surface is exposed to the alcohol. After 30 to 45 sec, the ethanol is quickly removed with the syringe and the stomach is fixed with 2.5% formaldehyde, 5% glutaraldehyde, and 0.06% picric acid in 0.1 *M* cacodylate buffer, pH 7.4, or rinsed with 4 ml of warmed (37°C) physiologic saline (0.85% NaCl). Fresh warmed saline (4 ml) is again injected, and the stomach is returned to the abdominal cavity. At various time intervals, e.g., 3, 7, 15, 30, or 60 min, the stomach is exteriorized following anesthesia and the saline is removed and replaced with fixative. The abdomen is closed and the rats are sacrificed 5–10 min after placing the fixative within the stomach (13).

b. Hypertonic Saline Injury to the Stomach After making the left upper quadrant incision, 1 ml of 4.5 *M* NaCl is instilled into the stomach with a gastric tube. Control animals receive 1 ml of 0.9% saline. The animals are then sacrificed, the mucosa immediately fixed by instillation of 10 ml of Bouin's solution for 10 min, and the stomach is then excised (14).

2. Duodenum

The duodenal response to injury has been studied in rabbits using luminal acid to induce mucosal damage. Nonfasted animals are anesthesized and a 5-cm segment of proximal (distal to the entry of the common bile duct) and/or distal duodenum (approximately 10–15 cm from the pylorus) is isolated, with care taken to avoid impairing the blood supply. Each duodenal segment is intubated on both ends with a polyvinyl cannula and perfused *in situ* with isotonic saline solution via a pump, which is used to recirculate solutions. The perfusate is maintained at 37°C and gassed with 100% O_2 in the reservoir. After 20 min to ensure equilibrium, the duodenal segment is perfused with 200 m*M* HCl for 30 min. The remaining acid is washed out with saline for 10 min, and the perfusion is continued for additional time periods, as necessary. This model produces uniform mucosal damage within the duodenal segment (15).

3. Colon

a. Bile Salt Injury Rats are fasted overnight with free access to water. After induction of anesthetic, the abdomen is opened and a cannula is secured within the lumen of the large intestine, approximately 6 cm from the anus. The segment of bowel is flushed clean with Krebs buffer (pH 7.1) and the anus is clipped. A 1-ml solution of 25 m*M* sodium deoxycholate in Krebs buffer is introduced into the *in situ* loop via the indwelling catheter. During a 20-min period, the loop is emptied and filled on three occasions with fresh bile salt solution. The segment is then emptied and flushed once with fresh buffer. The animals are then sacrificed at 30 min, 1 hr, and 2 hr after treatment, and the affected tissue is excised for study (16).

4. Rectum

Injury within the rectum has been accomplished using a physical method involving scraping the mucosa onto a gelatin-coated glass slide. The coating on the slides can be made from the gelatin of drug capsules dissolved in boiling water at a concentration of 10%. This gelatin is used because it is not easily dissolved by the warm rectal mucosa, thus allowing the cells to adhere. In anesthesized mice, the anterior wall of the lower rectum is exposed by manipulation of the perianal skin, and the slide is pressed on the mucosa and then pulled away, selectively removing superficial epithelial cells from the mucosa near the anal junction. Using a fresh part of the slide, the process is repeated several times. Animals are then sacrificed at varying time intervals after the stripping procedure (17).

5. Morphologic Changes Involved in Restitution

In the stomach, the process of restitution depends on the severity of damage to the mucosa (18). Although a variety of agents have been used to induce injury (9), the type of agent does not appear to be as important as its strength and the length of time that it is in contact with the mucosa. In rat models using 70–100% ethanol as the injurious agent, various histologic changes have been described (13). Immediately after brief ethanol exposure (30–45 sec), nearly all of the epithelial cells lining the interfoveolar and upper gastric pit regions (exclusively mucous cells) are extensively and irreversibly damaged. The necrotic epithelium lifts off the basal lamina, but remains contiguous with viable deeper cells along the sides of the gastric glands. Very little damage occurs to the lamina propria. As the necrotic epithelium detaches from the mucosa, a protective mucoid layer is formed with adjacent mucus and cellular debris. By 7 min, restitution begins, with viable epithelial cells lining the lower gastric pits assuming a flattened shape and extending lamellipodia over the bare, denuded basal lamina. Lamellipodia from cells in adjacent gastric pits make contact at the interfoveolar region and form tight junctions. The flattened mucous cells then return to cuboidal shape and again become polarized. The restitution is completed by reformation of the gastric epithelial barrier. This entire process occurs over a period of approximately 1 hr.

Similar studies have examined the mucosal repair mechanisms in duodenum using injurious agents such as 200 m*M* HCl (15). Similar to that seen in the stomach, there is a cycle of villus damage and repair. However, some differences exist between stomach and duodenum. For example, in the damaged duodenal mucosa, the first sign of repair is seen at approximately 3 hr, when damaged epithelial cells became detached from the underlying basal lamina, whereas in the stomach, this process begins much earlier. Also, epithelial coverage in the duodenum involves enterocytes, whereas mucous cells participate in restitution of the stomach. Another difference is that in the stomach, migrating cells follow the contour of denuded basal lamina until they make contact with other migrating cells, then forming tight junctions, whereas in the duodenum, the necrotic debris is pinched off and extruded into the lumen. Detachment of these portions of parenchyma results in significantly reduced villus height 9 hr after injury. Migration of the epithelial cells, however, proceeds in a fashion similar to that in the stomach (9).

Rapid restitution occurs in the rectum, similar to that observed in the stomach, although the process is somewhat slower, beginning at 20 min after damage with near completion by 4 hr (17). In the rabbit colon exposed to 100 m*M* HCl for 5 min, onset of repair begins by 15 min and is 90% completed by 2 hr. After exfoliation of superficial epithelial cells, colonocyte lamellipodia form, and the cells migrate over the denuded basal lamina, forming tight junctions on contact and restablishing the surface epithelium, similar to that seen in the stomach (19). Again, a similar process was noted in rat colon following superficial injury with bile salts (16). In this model, cell migration began at 30 min and reestablishment of the surface epithelium was seen at 2 hr. After bile salt injury, neither a continuous contact between migrating cells and basal lamina, nor a complete covering of secreted mucus, appeared necessary for restitution to occur.

B. Models of Intestinal Regeneration/Adaptation

1. Intestinal Resection, Bypass, Transposition, and Patching

Massive resection of the small intestine is among the strongest of all stimuli for intestinal regeneration and adaptation, and such models have provided much insight into gut physiology. These studies generally examine morphologic, physiologic, and/or biochemical changes in the residual tissue following resections of varying lengths of intestine.

a. Intestinal Resection Rodents, rabbits, and dogs have been used in these experiments. Mice can also be used, but the mouse intestine is quite small, making resection and anastomosis technically more challenging. Adult animals are fasted overnight and the procedures are performed in rooms with laminar air flow and under sterile conditions. Anesthesia is usually achieved with either intramuscular ketamine (25–35 mg/kg) and xylazine (7 mg/kg), or pentobarbital (50–60 mg/kg). The animals are placed supine on the operating table, the abdomen is shaved and cleansed with antiseptic solution, and a midline incision is made, first through the skin and then through the abdominal wall. The ligament of Treitz is identified and the precise region (proximal or distal) and length of intestine (generally between 30 and 80% of small intestine) to be resected are chosen (Fig. 2). Following resection, an anastomosis is created, generally using interrupted fine silk stitches, and the abdominal wall and skin are closed. Animals are initially given liquids and returned to normal chow diet by postoperative day 2 (20).

As a control for the resected group, a simple transection followed by reanastomosis is generally used. Transection is an excellent control for the resection group because obstruction proximal to the anastomosis can cause hyperplasia, and this should be the same for the resection and transected groups.

b. Intestinal Bypass Jejunoileal and biliopancreatic bypass procedures were originally used clinically as treatments for morbid obesity, and have been used experimentally to study the effects of exposure of areas of small intestine to different environments within the gastrointestinal tract.

For the jejunoileal bypass, anesthetized animals undergo a midline laparotomy and the small intestine is transected just beyond the ligament of Treitz; the proximal jejunum is then anastomosed to the ileum. Alternatively, duodenoileal bypasses can be performed via a side-to-side anastomosis (21).

For the biliopancreatic bypass, after making a midline laparotomy, a gastrectomy, including slightly less than the distal half of the stomach, is performed. The duodenal stump is occluded and the intestinal tract from the ligament of Treitz to the ileocecal valve is exteriorized. The small intestine is transected at its midpoint and a gastroenterostomy is per-

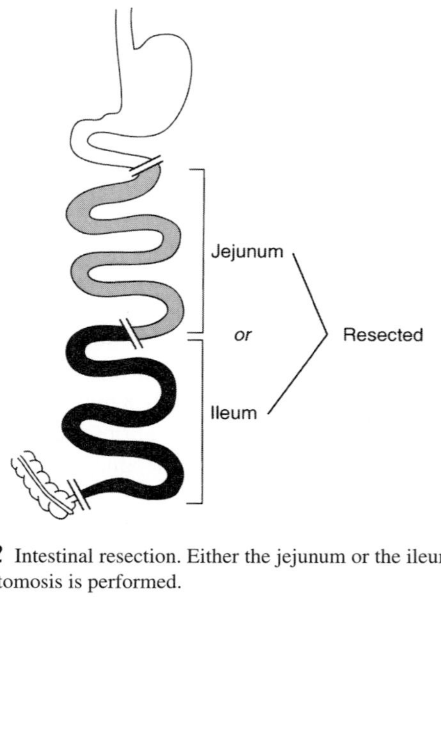

Figure 2 Intestinal resection. Either the jejunum or the ileum is resected and anastomosis is performed.

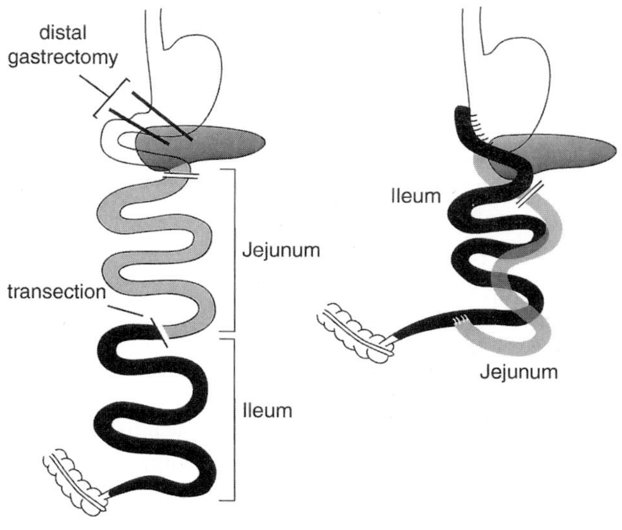

Figure 3 Biliopancreatic bypass.

formed with the distal segment. The excluded loop (duodenum and jejunum) is anastomosed in an end-to-side fashion to the terminal ileum, 5 cm from the ileocecal valve (Fig. 3). In this way, the distal ileum receives higher concentrations of nutrients and biliopancreatic secretions. A sham (control) operation is performed in which transections and reanastomoses are made in the gastric antrum, first part of duodenum, midsmall intestine, and terminal ileum (22).

The Thiry–Vella loop/fistula model was originally described by Vella and consists of a loop of bowel removed from continuity with the remainder of the intestine, but with intact nerves, blood supply, and lymphatic drainage. The ends of the loop are generally brought to the skin surface of the abdomen by creation of two stomas. As such, this model has been commonly used for studying the effects of complete deprivation of luminal nutrition and digestive juices and specific gut hormones on intestinal regeneration and adaptation. Alternatively, Thiry–Vella loops have been used to examine the physiology of epithelial transport, digestion, and absorption.

For creation of a jejunal fistula in the rat, the small bowel is divided at 10 and 30 cm distal to the ligament of Treitz, leaving the mesentery intact. The two ends of this 20-cm segment are brought out through the left side of the abdominal wall and sutured to the abdominal skin with silk sutures. Intestinal continuity is restored by performing an end-to-end anastomosis (Fig. 4). The midline abdominal wound is then closed. An ileal Thiry–Vella fistula is created using a similar procedure, but a segment of distal ileum 10–30 cm proximal to the cecum is used (23).

c. Intestinal Transposition These procedures are also used to study the effects of exposure of areas of small intestine to different luminal environments. Here, segments of intestine are excised and transposed with intact mesentery to different sites, e.g., ileum to jejunum and vice versa (24) (Fig. 5).

d. Intestinal Patching This technique involves the creation of a full-thickness small intestinal defect, e.g., in the ileum, which is then patched, using the serosal side of adjacent colon, e.g., cecum. Healing of this defect occurs by contraction of the wound as well as the development of a neomucosa by proliferation and migration of adjacent cells

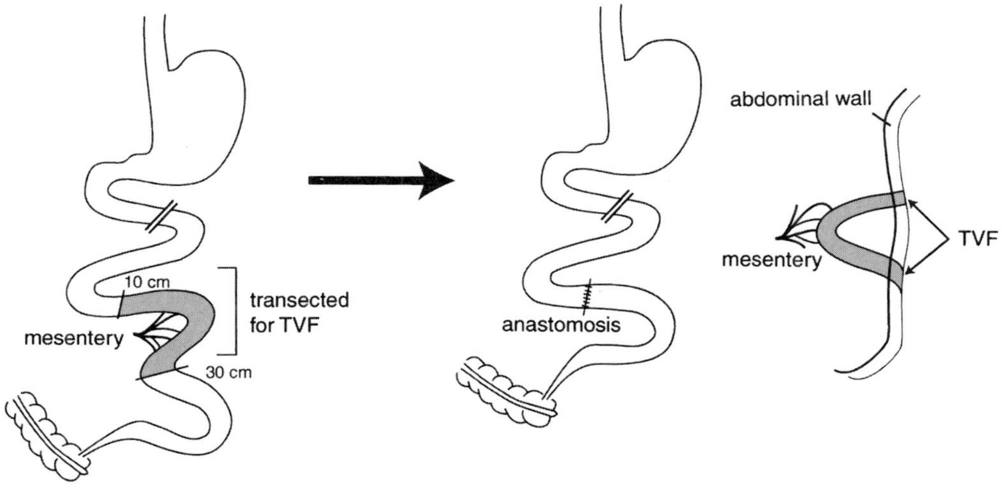

Figure 4 Jejunal Thiry–Vella fistula (TVF). A segment of jejunum between 10 and 30 cm from the ligament of Treitz is transected and the ends are brought out to the abdominal wall as stomas. A similar procedure is performed for ileal Thiry–Vella fistulas.

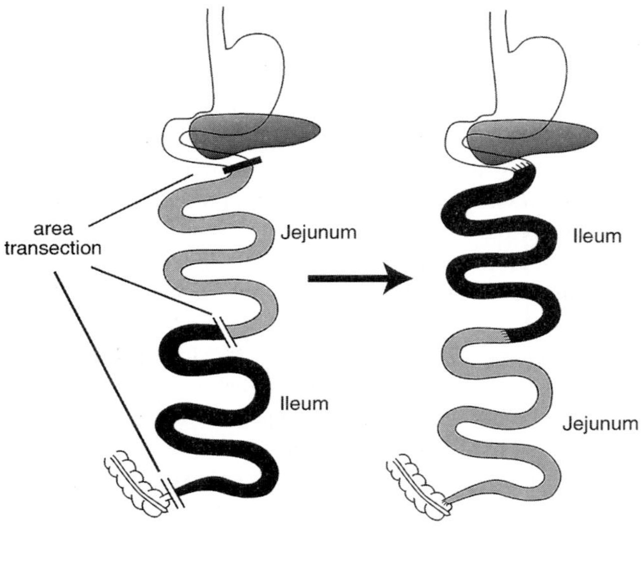

Figure 5 Intestinal transposition. Segments of jejunum and ileum are transected and transposed.

over the cecal serosa. The model allows the study of mechanisms involved in regeneration of the small intestine and is also being evaluated as a potential treatment for the short bowel syndrome, because a new mucosal segment can be created.

After an overnight fast, the animals (rabbits or rats) are anesthesized and the abdomen is opened by a midline incision and the terminal ileum 10 cm proximal to the ileocecal valve (rabbits) is opened along the antimesenteric border. The margins of incised ileum are then sutured onto the serosal surface of the cecum, generally using a continuous nonabsorbable (silk) inverted suture (Fig. 6). This technique results in an elliptical patch of 2 × 5 cm in rabbits and 1 × 4 cm in rats. The nonabsorbable sutures provide the advantage of clearly demarcating the patch outline, and therefore its size at autopsy. Care should be taken to avoid approximating Peyer's patches to the ileocecal patch. Approximately 28 days in the rabbit and 12 days in the rat are needed for complete reepitheliazation to occur (25).

e. Morphologic Changes Following partial small bowel resection, the residual intestine undergoes structural and functional changes. These changes are more marked in the ileum than in the jejunum, i.e., greater after proximal than after distal small bowel resections. In addition, the adaptation response is directly related to the amount of tissue removed; the more tissue removed, the stronger the response in the remaining intestine. Interestingly, the response is maximal near the anastomosis, and tapers off distally (26, 27). It appears that there is an initial period of hypoproliferation after operation, but within 1–3 weeks there is compensatory growth involving all layers of the bowel wall. The increase in mucosal thickness is primarily due to crypt cell hyperplasia, resulting in increased villus height and crypt depth (27, 28). These changes are followed by dilatation and lengthening of the intestinal remnant. Increases in intestinal dry weight as well as in amounts of DNA, RNA, and protein confirm the increased number of cells. The number of crypts per unit length of intestine does not change, but the size of each crypt increases, i.e., there is an increase in the number of cells per crypt (27, 29). Additionally, no gross changes in villus shape have been reported after bowel resection by ultrastructural evaluation.

There is an increase in cell proliferation in the ileal mucosa within 48 hr after jejunectomy. A shortening of the cell cycle time results primarily from a shortening of the S phase, and the height of the crypt proliferative compartment increases (28). This increase in the size of the proliferative compartment appears to be due to an increase in output from the stem cell zone, not from an increase in the number of transit cell divisions within the proliferative zone (20). The growth of the proliferative compartment is proportional to the growth of the entire crypt, so that when expressed as a fraction of the total crypt population, the relative size of the proliferative compartment does not change (27, 28). Simi-

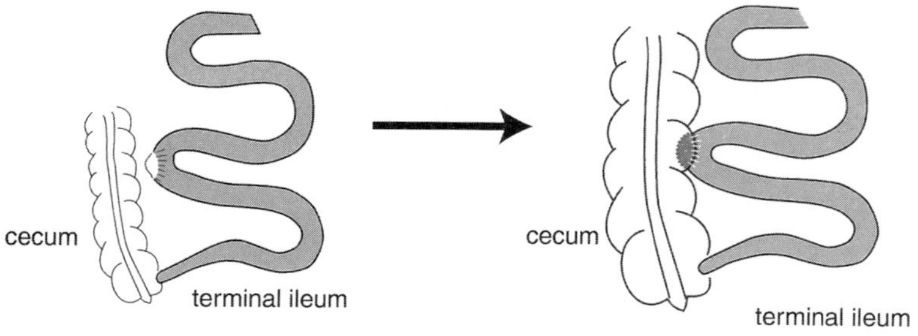

Figure 6 Intestinal patching. The terminal ileum is opened and patched to the serosa of the adjacent cecum.

larly, the labeling index remains constant. Additionally, the height of the stem cell zone remains the same and the transit time of a cell through the stem cell compartment is decreased, indicating an increase in cell migration and through-put (20). Although the cells migrate faster after resection, they have a greater distance to travel along the elongated villi. As such, a new steady state is reached whereby augmented villus height is maintained by accelerated cell migration. This mucosal hyperplasia persists for several months and results in an overall improvement in bowel function.

Intestinal bypasses with self-emptying blind loops, jejunoileal transposition, pancreaticobiliary diversion, and intestinal isolation with Thiry–Vella fistulas all share common morphologic and physiologic changes in the remaining bowel, similar to that seen after partial intestinal resection. In these nonresection models, however, the functional adaptation in the remaining bowel is often negated by bacterial colonization of the excluded loop, resulting in diarrhea and steatorrhea. In general, within the defunctionalized segment of bowel there is hypoplasia and villus atrophy along with eventual luminal narrowing and thinning of the bowel wall (30). There may be regional differences in the hypoplastic response in that jejunal villi have been shown to be particularly apt to undergo atrophy. This discrepancy may be related to bacterial colonization of the ileal sac. Within a period of 1–2 weeks, Thiry–Vella loops exhibit a decrease in the number of crypt cells, leading to a proportionate decrease in the size of the villus compartment. Additionally, there is a decrease in the rate of cell migration and cell turnover. This hypoplasia is associated with a progressive reduction in the absorption of glucose and amino acids (31). Interestingly, the atrophy and its functional effects are fully reversible if normal intestinal continuity is restored.

f. Functional Adaptation After small bowel resection, there appears to be an increase in uptake of normally absorbed substances such as mono- and disaccharides, calcium, amino acids, water, and electrolytes. Additionally, within the ileum there is an increase in transepithelial transport of bile acids and vitamin B_{12} (26, 32, 33). The increase in glucose and water absorption correlates with the increased cell number, the rates being unchanged when considered in relation to mucosal weight or protein. In other words, it appears that functional adaptation after small bowel resection occurs via an increase in the number of epithelial cells in which individual absorptive capacity is not increased. Interestingly, some specific disaccharidase and dipeptidase activities are normal or decreased after resection, e.g., lactase (34), suggesting that the differentiated cells of the hyperplastic epithelium may be "immature." Similar to the small intestine, the absorptive function of colonic epithelium is also enhanced. As such, overall gut mucosal absorption returns to normal if enough bowel remains and the adaptive process is not impaired by the presence of other diseases or inadequate nutrition.

g. Mechanisms Involved in Intestinal Adaptation The mechanisms responsible for intestinal adaptation after bowel resection or bypass are felt to be multifactorial and include luminal nutrients, pancreatic and biliary secretions, endocrine and paracrine factors, neural factors, and increased blood flow. Of these mechanisms, the most important appears to be the effect of luminal nutrition, with the most potent stimulus being long-chain triglycerides. The remnant small intestine is bathed in chyme containing high levels of carbohydrates, fat, and protein. This theory may explain the greater intestinal adaptation after proximal, compared to distal, resections, because the ileum is not normally exposed to these rich nutrients. Additionally, the normal crypt–villus thickness is greatest in the proximal intestine, raising the possibility that the ileum may have more growth "potential." The nutrient theory would also explain why maximal changes in adaptation occur in the bowel closest to the anastomosis (35, 36). Additional support for this theory comes from the finding that the atrophy seen with models in which the intestine is isolated, e.g., Thiry–Vella fistulas, is fully reversible by restoration of intestinal continuity, and can be prevented by perfusion of the excluded segment with glucose and amino acids. In addition to the nutritional component, mechanical stimulation may also play a role, because even nonnutritive substances induce cell proliferation in the isolated segment.

Bile and pancreatic secretions also influence small intestinal adaptation after resection and bypass. For example, the ileum is brought closer to the stomach and duodenum after jejunal resection, and it appears that although gastric and duodenal juices cause villus hyperplasia, the pancreatic and biliary secretions have an even more potent trophic effect (37).

In addition to these local influences, it appears that humoral or systemic factors are important in the adaptation response. Parabiotic experiments have confirmed this phenomenon because villus hyperplasia is seen in the unoperated partners of animals undergoing intestinal resection (38). Additionally, humoral factors are likely responsible for the hyperplasia of ileal mucosal fragments transplanted beneath the renal capsule in rats who have undergone intestinal resection (39). Investigators have yet to identify the key endogenous circulating humoral factor(s) that may underlie the adaptation response. A variety of trophic substances have been used exogenously in order to enhance the adaptive response. For example, epidermal growth factor (EGF), fibroblast growth factor (FGF), transforming growth factor (TGF), thyroxine, glucagon-like polypeptide-2 (GLP-2), and short-chain fatty acids (acetate, proprionate, and butyrate), among others, have all been shown to augment the adaptive hyperplasia.

GLP-2, one of the proglucagon-derived peptides, may be a particularly important growth factor. This recently characterized 33-amino acid peptide is produced throughout the intestine by enteroendocrine cells located mostly in the ileum. Its trophic effect appears to be highly specific for the intestine. GLP-2 has been shown to enhance dramatically normal rat small intestine mucosal mass (small bowel weight and crypt–villus height) as well as absorption (40). Epidermal growth factor is another extremely potent gut trophic factor. EGF is found in saliva and mother's milk, suggesting physiologically important roles in the processes of gastrointestinal growth and development. Because adult jejunal crypt cells are able to bind, internalize, and degrade EGF, it has been proposed that EGF may play a role in the maintenance and proliferative response of the adult intestinal epithelium. This growth factor has been shown to have effects on both the stimulation of crypt cell proliferation (41) and the migration of epithelial cells. Both intraluminal and intravenous routes of administration are effective (42).

The importance of EGF in intestinal adaptation is suggested by experiments performed in *waved-2* mice. These mice possess a defective EGF receptor as a result of a spontaneous point mutation (T $\rightarrow$ G), causing a substitution of glycine for the highly conserved valine at position 743 in the tyrosine kinase domain. After a 50% proximal small bowel resection, these mutant mice do not gain weight to the same extent as their wild-type controls, and also exhibit less pronounced increases in villus height and crypt cell proliferation. In addition, apoptosis has been shown to be much increased in the *waved-2* mice following 50% small bowel resection (43, 44). These studies suggest that endogenous EGF likely plays an important role in the gut adaptation following massive resection.

In contrast to the growth-promoting effect of these various peptides and hormones, somatostatin is a regulatory peptide that has a number of inhibitory roles in the gastrointestinal tract, and has been shown to block the adaptive hyperplasia that normally occurs following massive intestinal resection. In addition, somatostatin is able to block induction of protooncogene expression by EGF in intestinal IEC-6 cells (45). In a rabbit model of full-thickness patched intestinal defects, the somatostatin analog, octreotide, has been shown to inhibit EGF-stimulated proliferative activity, but not EGF-stimulated migration (46). Thus, prolonged administration of octreotide may adversely affect normal and adaptive intestinal regeneration.

Finally, changes in intestinal blood flow and peripheral nerve activity likely play a role in intestinal adaptation. For example, sympathectomy has been shown to inhibit crypt cell proliferation, whereas cholinergic drug stimulation of mesenteric nerves increases intestinal cell proliferation.

h. Clinical Applications The adaptational changes after resection have been documented in patients, including small bowel dilatation and hypertrophy. Epithelial cell hyperplasia and increased absorption of water, electrolytes, and glucose have also been seen. As might be predicted from experiments in animals, distal resections are not tolerated as well as proximal resections, due to poorer adaptation of the jejunum. In addition, ileal resections lead to a loss of the enterohepatic circulation of bile salts. Additionally, absence of the ileocecal valve allows bacterial overgrowth in the remaining small bowel segment, leading to diarrhea and steatorrhea due to deconjugation of bile salts. Patients who have undergone massive distal resection may benefit from intravenous hyperalimentation and elemental diets to allow adequate time for intestinal adaptation to occur. A gradual return to oral feeding can often be accomplished in such patients, depending on the extent of resection. Wilmore *et al.* (47) have shown that by administering a combination of the trophic agents growth hormone and glutamine, along with a modified diet high in complex carbohydrates and low in fat, 58% of patients with jejunal–ileal remnants less than or equal to 50 cm were able to be free of total parenteral nutrition (TPN) after a 4-week period. However, given the limitations of the adaptive response in many cases, effective methods for intestinal transplantation are currently being developed.

Serosal patching of the small intestine has been examined as a possible treatment of short bowel syndrome, as well as a means of understanding the processes of cellular proliferation and migration during regeneration. In this model, intestinal regeneration begins with migration of epithelial cells from the edge of the defect onto the serosa of the cecum. An increase in proliferation in the mucosa adjacent to, or even distant from, the defect then follows. These processes are regulated at least in part by EGF. Crypts develop later as invaginations of the epithelium into the underlying connective tissue, and eventually villi are formed with connective tissue covered by epithelium. Additionally, the muscularis mucosa regenerates deep into the epithelium. However, there is eventual contraction of the defect such that the defect is 40% of the original size by 8 weeks (25, 46, 48, 49).

2. Atrophy/Growth Factors

a. Fasting/Refeeding Model The fasting/refeeding model is quite commonly used for inducing gut atrophy and studying the regeneration process that occurs with refeeding. Rodents are commonly used for these experiments and are housed in cages with wire mesh floors to prevent coprophagia. Food is generally withdrawn for a period of 2–4 days, but the animals are allowed to drink water. Refeeding is accomplished by providing free access to standard chow (50).

I. Effects on Intestinal Morphology and Function Prolonged fasting leads to decreases in the weight of the whole animal, as well as each individual organ, but there is a preferential effect of fasting on the small intestine. Short-term starvation (1–2 days) leads to similar changes, though less profound. Atrophy of the small intestine and a proportional decrease in villus height and crypt depth occur due to a decrease in the rate of crypt cell growth, and the result is a decrease in total mucosal thickness (51). These changes are considerably more pronounced in the jejunum than in the ileum. In fact, ileal mucosa may exhibit some degree of hyperplasia during starvation. Changes in function accompany the mucosal atrophy induced by starvation. There is an increase in mucosal permeability as well as changes in brush border enzyme expression that to some extent mimic the suckling, preweaned phenotype. For example, with atrophy, intestinal alkaline phosphatase (IAP) is decreased but lactase is increased. In other words, in intestinal atrophy, there is a decrease in the number of cells and an overall decrease in absorptive capacity and function, but within individual cells, enzyme expression is differentially regulated (50).

Refeeding reverses the histologic changes caused by fasting by inducing crypt cell proliferation within a period of 9–12 hr, in conjunction with significant increases in the expression of the growth-associated protooncogenes c-*fos* and c-*jun*. Brush border gene expression also returns to normal (50). Similar proliferative changes are seen in colonic crypts 12 hr or more after refeeding.

II. MECHANISMS INVOLVED IN MUCOSAL CHANGES ASSOCIATED WITH FASTING/REFEEDING Both luminal and systemic factors may underlie the intestinal response to starvation. In addition to the luminal factors, the hormone gastrin may play a role in the trophic response to refeeding, because its levels are increased as food intake is reestablished. Furthermore, gastrin is known to block partially the mucosal atrophy associated with starvation. Other gut hormones, such as bombesin, EGF, thyroid hormone, and neurotensin, have also been shown to inhibit partially the mucosal atrophy induced by fasting. Bombesin may be of particular interest, because it was shown to prevent the alterations in gut permeability that normally occur in starved (TPN-fed) animals.

b. Hypo/Hyperthyroidism Model Thyroid hormone (triiodothyronine, T3) is a gut trophic factor that has been studied in both developing and adult animals. The thyroid hormone model offers a unique advantage over other gut trophic factors, because hypothyroidism can be induced via administration of a drug, propylthiouracil. As such, the effects of both the presence and absence of T3 can be examined. Such studies cannot be accomplished with other gut growth factors because there are no means of decreasing their levels. Exceptions to this rule include the *waved* mice (defective EGF receptor).

I. METHOD Adult male Sprague–Dawley rats (250–300 g) are maintained on standard chow and are water supplemented with 0.05% (wt/vol) propylthiouracil for a 7-week period to induce hypothyroidism. Daily intraperitoneal injections of either saline (hypothyroid group) or 30 μg/100 g body weight T3 (hyperthyroid group) are begun at the end of 6 weeks, and the animals are sacrificed on day 7. Untreated rats are used for control purposes (52) (Fig. 7).

II. EFFECTS ON SMALL INTESTINAL MUCOSAL MORPHOLOGY AND FUNCTION Hypothyroidism causes atrophy whereas thyroid hormone administration leads to mucosal hyperplasia throughout the small intestine. Thyroid hormone induces crypt mitoses, resulting in significant increases in total mucosal thickness. In addition to these histologic changes, T3 also causes a decrease in lactase and an increase in intestinal alkaline phosphatase (IAP) levels in adult rats, similar to what has been shown with the fasting/refeeding model (52).

3. Ischemia

Intestinal ischemia followed by reperfusion is a relatively frequent clinical event with important local and systemic consequences. Examples include occlusive and nonocclusive mesenteric ischemia, midgut volvulus, and necrotizing enterocolitis.

a. Method Adult animals are fasted overnight. The animals are anesthesized and a midline laparotomy is performed. The superior mesenteric artery is isolated, and total (central occlusive) or partial (segmental occlusive) mesenteric occlusion is achieved by placement of a microvascular clip (see Fig. 8). Groups of animals can be separated according to length of mesenteric occlusion time (30 min to 2 hr). Reperfusion of the ischemic intestine is achieved by removal

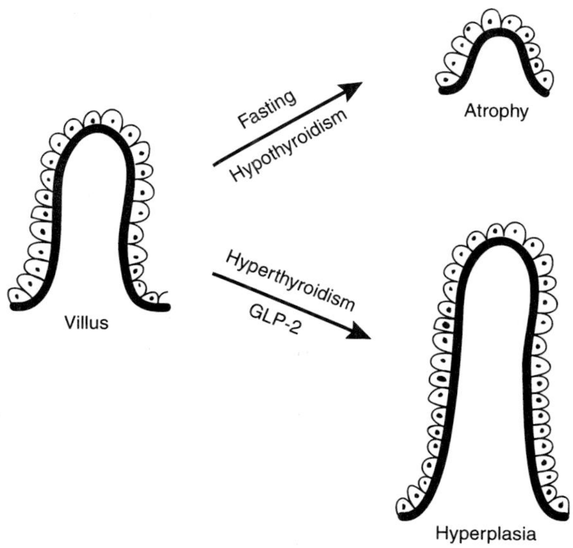

Figure 7 Summary of atrophy/growth factor models. GLP-2, Glucagon-like polypeptide-2.

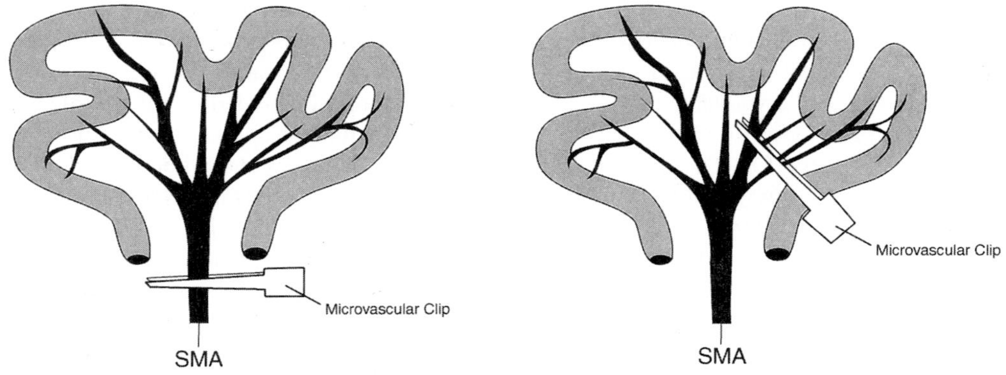

Figure 8 Ischemia models. Central occlusive (left) or segmental occlusive (right) intestinal ischemia may be obtained by appropriate placement of a microvascular clamp. SMA, Superior mesenteric artery.

of the microvascular clip. The animals are given fluids on the first postoperative day and a standard chow diet by the second postoperative day, being sacrificed at varying intervals after surgery (53).

b. Effects of Ischemia on Intestinal Morphology and Function The intestinal villus microcirculation is supplied by a central arteriole. Branching of this vessel near the tip of the villus forms a subepithelial network of capillaries and venules. Flows in these capillaries and venules are closely approximated and opposite to the direction of the central arteriole. Thus, a countercurrent arrangement is achieved such that arterial–venous diffusional shunting of oxygen occurs, resulting in a lower oxygen tension at the villus tip compared to the base, and making this compartment more sensitive than the crypts to warm ischemia. In cases of systemic hypotension or vasospasm, this countercurrent shunting of oxygen is more pronounced (54–56). Intestinal mucosal damage due to ischemia thus begins at the tips of the villi, progressing to the crypts as ischemia time is prolonged. Mucosal damage can also occur as a result of reperfusion injury, perhaps due to the presence of reactive oxygen metabolites (57).

Structural damage to the small intestine occurs remarkably soon after the onset of ischemia. Ultrastructural studies have shown alterations in the villus tips 3–5 min after total circulatory arrest. First, epithelial cells detach from the basement membrane in the apical regions of the villi with the formation of subepithelial blebs. After 30 min of ischemia in the rat and 60 min in the dog, the upper two-thirds of the villi are completely denuded of epithelial cells, but the lower villi and crypts remain intact. The subepithelial blebs are thought to result from seepage of cytoplasmic fluid from cells deprived of energy, causing detachment of enterocytes from the basement membrane. The intact cells are then lost into the gut lumen, where they are destroyed by hydrolases (58). In the rat, by 2 hrs of ischemia, the villi are completely stripped of epithelial cells, the villus stroma becomes necrotic, and the basement membrane ruptures and is shed along with the stroma into the intestinal lumen (59). During the ischemic insult, a reduced rate of cell proliferation is seen. After ischemia lasting for 5 hr, almost the entire intestinal wall is necrotic and survival rates of the animals markedly decrease (60).

There is good correlation between the structural abnormalities and the functional derangements associated with intestinal ischemia, although an impairment in barrier function actually occurs prior to the morphologic changes. In guinea pigs, it has been shown that the movement of glucose across the ischemic small intestine is greatly reduced at 1 hr. In rats, 30 min of ischemia results in a complete loss of the capacity to accumulate sugars and amino acids against a concentration gradient *in vitro*. In the dog, similar changes are noted after 1 hr of ischemia, and there is a net secretion of water and electrolytes across the damaged mucosa, possibly resulting from the lack of absorptive epithelial cells in the villus compartment (58).

c. Regeneration of the Intestine after Ischemia Following an ischemic insult, the intestinal mucosa recovers in a rapid fashion. In the dog, 24 hr after a period of ischemia for 1 hr, the villi are covered with an almost normal epithelium, with only rare defects at the villus tips. In the rat, recovery of normal epithelium occurs after 48–72 hr. If the ischemia is prolonged to 2 hr, it may take up to 1 week for normalization of the epithelium to occur, in both rat and dog (58). Assuming the animal has survived, the gut mucosa is capable of recovery from up to 7 hr of ischemia.

Following ischemic damage, reepithelialization of the villi initially occurs through an increase in cell division and output of cells from the residual crypts. However, increased proliferation does not fully account for the rapid reepithelialization of the villi; migration of crypt cells is also of importance. After an ischemic episode lasting 2 hr in the rat, few crypts are noted by 12 hr of regeneration. At this time, there is a flat epithelium without a brush border and the basement membrane is absent. After 24 hr, the crypt zone is wider than normal, but again with narrow lumina. On the mucosal surface, flat protuberances of lamina propria are seen, and nascent villi are covered with cuboid and columnar epithelium. The basement membrane begins to form at this time, and in some areas a well-developed brush border is again seen. By 3 days, the mucosa has a dense population of villi with enlarged villus tips and a well-formed brush-border that is fully covered by a surface coat. By 8 days of repair, the mucosa has fully returned to its normal appearance (59).

There is a close correlation between restoration of function and morphologic appearance of the tissue. After 12 hr of regeneration, alkaline phosphatase activity cannot be demonstrated in the reepithelialized mucosa, but activity is noted in the brush border after 24 hr, mostly in epithelial cells at the base of the villi. After 3 days of regeneration, alkaline phosphatase is demonstrated in the brush border of all villus epithelia, but with weaker activity as compared to normal values. By 8 days, the intracellular localization of this enzyme returns to normal. Similar changes are seen in regard to other enzymes, such as α-glucosidase and nonspecific esterase. These findings suggest that a correct qualitative differentiation of individual enterocytic enzymes depends not only on mature villus structures, but also the correct development of the differentiation compartment. Interestingly, the levels of the oxidoreductases succinate and malate dehydrogenase return to normal much earlier (24 hr) compared to the brush border enzymes. Because these oxidoreductases are part of the citric acid cycle and are linked to energy metabolism, early normalization of their levels would be necessary for the maintenance of cells as well as the increased proliferation in the crypts (59).

It is of interest that regeneration of the mucosa following ischemia does not appear to be greatly influenced by luminal factors. For example, in dogs, intestine that had been obstructed was able to regenerate with the same rapidity as nonobstructed intestine (58).

The colonic mucosa is much less sensitive to ischemia than is the small intestine, and, once damaged, the colonic mucosa appears to regenerate more slowly. As in the small intestine, there is a close correlation between functional events and histological appearance. Two hours of ischemia in the dog required 7 days for complete functional recovery in the colon (transmural sodium transport), but is inadequate for morphologic recovery, e.g., discrete mucosal ulcers were still visible at 1 week (58).

4. Irradiation

With increasing use of radiation therapy for treatment of abdominopelvic and retroperitoneal tumors, and because the tolerance level of much of the alimentary tract is close to the dose necessary to control many tumors, complications of radiation are increasingly encountered by the clinician. It is estimated that 5–25% of all patients undergoing abdominopelvic radiotherapy will develop radiation-induced intestinal injury (61). Moreover, many of these patients will require surgical intervention and long-term total parental nutrition for complications such as perforation, fistula, malabsorption, and stricture.

a. Method Rodents are commonly used in these studies. Adult animals are anesthesized and then subjected to whole body or focal abdominal irradiation using a conventional X-radiation source, e.g., Varian 4/100 (Milpitas, CA) or a 137Cs γ-irradiator. The radiation dose is delivered at a rate of approximately 137.5 cGy/min at the center of the radiation field. A dose of 1100 rads has been shown to produce radiation enteritis in rats, although dose–response curves may be performed, depending on the goal of the studies. Antibiotic coverage is important to prevent early sepsis associated with the intestinal injury. After recovery from anesthesia, the animals are allowed free access to food and drinking water (61).

b. Effects of Radiation on Intestinal Morphology and Function An important determinant of the effect of abdominal radiation on the intestine is intestinal mobility or fixation. Mobile regions are relatively protected whereas fixed areas are more prone to injury, because these segments will tend to receive the entire dose. The duodenum, upper jejunum at the ligament of Treitz, and terminal ileum (because of its attachment to the cecum) are immobile areas of the small intestine. For this reason, and because radiation is most often applied to the lower abdomen to treat pelvic malignancies, the terminal ileum is the portion of the small intestine most often involved in radiation injury. Also, adhesions from prior operations or inflammatory conditions increase the risk of radiation injury (62).

Ionizing radiation preferentially affects cells during the G_2 and M phases of the cell cycle. Most of the acute and some delayed changes of radiation injury depend on turnover rates of the target cells. As such, the enteric mucosa is among the most radiosensitive tissues in the body. However, the rapid turnover also increases the capacity of the gut to recover completely from the acute radiation injury. In contrast, cells in the underlying submucosa, e.g., blood vessels, are less resilient and tend to develop fibrosing lesions, resulting in narrowing and chronic ischemic damage (63).

The phases of radiation injury can be divided into acute (early) and chronic (delayed). Acute radiation lesions are rarely biopsied in humans and therefore much of our knowledge of the histopathologic changes comes from experimental animals. Within 2–3 hr of a significant whole body dose of radiation, pyknosis and karyorrhexis are seen in the replicating stem cells of the intestinal crypts, progressing to rapid cell death. These cells appear morphologically identical to apoptotic cells. Maximal, acute cell death and sloughing of dead cells into crypt lumina occur by about 8 hr. Further mitosis is inhibited, or mitosis may lead to cell death, therefore replacement of the cells in the upper crypt and villus does not take place, leading to loss of the mucosa by denudation within a few days. Paneth cells persist in the crypt base, however. Death of the victim appears to be related to the fluid–electrolyte derangements resulting from the denuded or damaged surface epithelium, as well as the sepsis that results from coincident leukopenia (62).

Following therapeutic doses of radiation (150–300 rads), acute cell changes with some necrosis in the crypt cells are also seen by about 12–24 hr, suggesting that these rapidly dividing cells are the most radiosensitive. The mitotic rate of crypt epithelial cells decreases with an apparent mitotic block and accumulation of cells in the G_2 phase. In fact, by day 2 after irradiation, cell numbers in the crypts are reduced by more than 50%. In addition, though cell migration continues in the first 24 hr, velocity is markedly reduced, leading to a progressive loss of villus-associated cells, villus atrophy (proportional decrease in crypt and villus size), and cystic crypt dilatation within the following days to weeks. Atypical cells and mitoses within the crypts are also seen. The remaining cells flatten and spread over the surfaces in an attempt to maintain a continuous epithelial cover. Frank ulceration may be absent, but focal erosions can be seen. After completion of the radiation treatment, cells within the proliferative zone of the crypts begin to regenerate. By 22 hr after radiation, expansion of clonogenic cells within the crypts begins, followed by a shortening of the cell cycle time, and by 2 days, cell migration has returned to normal. Given that these early changes in crypt cells are seen even before changes in villus cellularity, Paulus *et al.* (64) suggested that control of cellular regeneration within intestinal crypts is based solely on local stem cells rather than on feedback signals from the villus. Within 2–3 weeks, the entire mucosa may appear normal. With higher doses of radiation or in immobile segments of intestine, recovery may be incomplete, resulting in persistent villus atrophy and stunted or cystic crypts (64).

In the delayed phase of radiation injury, the mucosal folds may be nearly normal, but are often irregular, cobblestone-like, and may contain focal ulcerations. These ulcers are most often at the point of the most severe stricture. At the microscopic level, the mucosa is often atrophic with absent or blunt villi thickened by edema or fibrosis of the lamina propria. Mucosal cells are flattened and goblet cells are sparse.

The colon may exhibit responses to irradiation similar to that of the small intestine. Because of architectural, anatomic, and cellular differences compared to the small intestine, the frequency and severity of colonic lesions are distinct. In the colon, crypt cell proliferation is slower, many cells remain in prolonged interphase, and true villi are lacking, such that there are less epithelial cells at risk to radiation injury. On the other hand, the colon, especially the rectum, is more fixed, making it more susceptible to injury (62). Acute changes include atypical cells in the crypts, decreased mitoses, and mild atrophy. Healing of injuries after therapeutic doses of radiation occurs within 1 month.

Several agents have been studied in the hopes of accelerating intestinal healing after radiation-induced intestinal injury. For example, Klimberg *et al.* (65) found that oral glutamine, the principal fuel used by the intestinal tract, resulted in improved intestinal mucosal morphometrics and overall morbidity and mortality in rats exposed to 10 Gy whole abdominal radiation. Specifically, there was improved survival, diminished diarrhea, and a decrease in the incidence of bowel perforation in treated animals. In addition, there was a marked increase in villus height and number, as well as in the number of mitoses per crypt (65). Another study by Gurbuz *et al.* revealed that supplemental dietary arginine accelerates intestinal mucosal regeneration and enhances bacterial clearance following radiation enteritis in rats. They found that when the diets were supplemented with 4% arginine, there was enhancement of bacterial clearance from mesenteric lymph nodes, as well as significant increases in mucosal and villus heights 7 days after 1100 rads of whole body X-radiation. Because intestinal mucosal damage due to radiation may be due to toxic free radicals, and nitric oxide, which is synthesized from arginine, has been shown to inactivate superoxide ion, the authors conclude that increased arginine may better protect the mucosal lining from reactive oxygen metabolites. Also, because arginine is a precursor of the polyamines, which are required for optimum growth of the intestinal mucosa, this may be a mechanism for its protective effects.

III. In Vitro Models

Several *in vitro* model systems are used to study intestinal restitution and regeneration. These *in vitro* models offer the advantage of being able to test specific factors in a controlled, isolated environment.

A. Models of Intestinal Restitution

1. Ussing Chamber Intestinal Mucosal Preparations

This model is commonly used for electrophysiologic and solute flux studies of epithelia, but has also been used to assess the process of intestinal epithelial restitution following direct injury. In these studies, mucosa is examined in an *in vitro* chamber, where specific components of its environment can be controlled. The chamber is constructed with luminal and serosal reservoirs, and contains current-passing and voltage-sensitive electrodes such that transmucosal potential electrical differences can be measured (67).

Mucosa of any type can be used, e.g., stomach, small intestine, or colon. The peritoneal cavity is opened in nonfasted animals, and an approximate 2–5 cm of the segment of bowel for study is removed. The tissue is immediately placed in ice-cold buffer solution (Ringer's), then gassed with 95% O_2/5% CO_2. The tissues are rapidly stripped of serosa and muscularis externa under a dissecting microscope, leaving the mucosa behind. Adjacent segments are mounted between Lucite half-chambers with an exposed mucosal surface area of 0.64 cm^2. Tissues are mounted in pairs, one for control and the other for experimental studies, with luminal surface up. Luminal and nutrient sides of the tissue are each incubated with solution in water-jacketed reservoirs maintained at 37°C. Bathing solutions consist of a buffer aerated with 95% O_2/5% CO_2 at pH 7.4.

Once mounted, the mucosa can be exposed to various treatment regimens on the luminal side, then transmucosal electrical differences are measured. For studies on small intestinal restitution, a model using guinea pig ileal mucosa has been described by Moore *et al.* (67). In this model, injury and denudation of the villus tip epithelium is induced by a 5-min exposure to Triton X-100 solution (0.06%), after which the detergent is removed from the chamber. Electrophysiologic and solute flux studies are then performed during the time of epithelial repair. Results from these studies showed that denudation of the epithelium occurred at the tips of 86% of villi, and this was associated with increased permeability and decreased transepithelial potential difference. Electron microscopic studies showed that during recovery, the absorptive cells shouldering the foci of denudation rapidly changed shape after injury, becoming flattened and sending projections over the denuded basement membrane. By 60 min after injury, cells from opposite shoulders of the denudation abutted, resealing the defect. These structural changes were associated with return of transepithelial resistance, potential difference, and permeability to control values. These studies confirm that a rapid restitution, similar to that seen in the duodenum *in vivo*, occurs in the small intestine *in vitro*.

Models for evaluation of colonic restitution have employed hypertonic saline (1.5 mol/liter) for 10 min (68) or the bile salt sodium deoxycholate (0.5 m*M* for 10 mins).

2. Human Intestinal Cell Lines

Nusrat *et al.* (69) described an *in vitro* model of restitution using the T84 human colon carcinoma cell line; these cells closely resemble small intestinal crypt cells, e.g., they are polarized and exhibit electrogenic chloride secretion. In this model, T84 cells are grown as monolayers on translucent permeable supports of rat tail type 1 collagen in a culture dish, in the absence of any filter support. These disks of collagen are attached via a collagen gluing method to holes made in the roughened base of a ring of polycarbonated tube. The bottom of this chamber is therefore formed by the collagen membrane supporting the T84 monolayer. The polycarbonate rings are suspended to allow basolateral access to media. Wounds are made in the monolayers by micropipettes (beveled tip diameter of 0.5–0.6 mm) controlled by a micromanipulator. The pipette is brought to the epithelial surface and a disk of epithelium is removed by suction without disturbing the underlying matrix. For imaging, the ring is placed in a glass-bottom petri dish and examined by microscopy. Alternatively, monolayers can be transferred to a Ussing chamber for functional studies. Using this model, it has been shown that wounding is accompanied by a decrease in resistance and an increase in monolayer permeability. Mimicking the *in vivo* changes, cells shouldering the wounds migrate by extension of lamellipodia-like processes to reseal wounds, as defined by structural and functional criteria. This model provides an easy and reproducible way to examine the structural and functional processes occurring with restitution.

Another restitution model using T84 cells has been described by Lotz *et al.* (70). The cells are grown on type 1 collagen-coated 12-mm × 12-mm glass coverslips for 10–14 days. Circular wounds are made in the monolayers by suction, using 0.5-mm beveled micropipette tips, which are controlled by a micromanipulator. Restitution of the monolayer can then be examined over time.

Rat IEC-6 cells have also been used to examine restitution (71). IEC-6 cells were originally established from small intestinal crypt cells. In the restitution model, confluent monolayers of IEC-6 cells are grown in 60-mm plastic dishes. Generally, two or more 10- to 25-mm wounds are made and separated by about 1.5 cm. Cells are then washed with fresh media to remove any residual cell debris. The cells may then be treated with various agents, including growth factors, and assessed for processes such as proliferation and migration. Migration of the IEC-6 cells is determined by counting the number of cells across the wound border in a standardized wound area. Wound areas are standardized by taking photomicrographs at 100-fold magnification using an inverted microscope and camera.

This IEC-6 model has been particularly useful in dissecting out the events of restitution *in vitro*. For example, it has been shown that various cytokines promote epithelial restitution through increased production of TGF-β (72). In addition, the importance of trefoil peptides and extracellular matrix in promoting restitution has been demonstrated (73).

B. Models of Intestinal Regeneration

In Vitro Models of Atrophy/ Hyperplasia

Certain aspects of the molecular mechanisms that govern cellular recovery from starvation can be studied using intestinal epithelial cell lines. A useful cell line is the human carcinoma cell line, HT-29, which closely resembles small intestinal crypt cells. These cells undergo into enterocyte-like differentiation, with development of apical microvilli and expression of brush border-associated enzymes, in response to treatment with the short-chain fatty acid sodium butyrate, or glucose deprivation. Serum starvation can be used to mimic the effects of fasting *in vivo*, because in both cases the crypt cells undergo cell cycle arrest. One can then induce differentiation of these cells by treatment with sodium butyrate. Under such conditions, the phenotype is similar to that seen *in vivo* with fasting, i.e., there is a specific defect in intestinal alkaline phosphatase expression. Replacement of serum, like refeeding of the animals, results in reversal of these changes (74).

The intestinal cell lines have also been used to study proliferative processes. For example, IEC-6, HT-29, and Caco-2 cells have been used to study effects of various gut trophic factors, such as gastrin, EGF, FGF, TGF-α and -β, and keratinocyte growth factors. These studies have been instrumental in advancing our understanding of the molecular mechanisms by which extracellular signals alter intestinal epithelial proliferation (75).

IV. Summary

A variety of excellent *in vivo* and *in vitro* model systems have been used to address distinct aspects of gut physiology related to regeneration and adaptation. These models have been instrumental in advancing our understanding of the events that occur under these conditions. For a given research project, the specific model(s) should be chosen only after careful consideration is given to all of its advantages and drawbacks, as well as the precise question that one is trying to answer.

References

1. Leblond, C. P. (1948). The constant renewal of the intestinal epithelium in the albino rat. *Anat. Rec.* **100,** 357–377.
2. Lipkin, M., Sherlock, P., and Bell, B. (1963). Cell proliferation kinetics in the gastrointestinal tract of man. II. Cell renewal in stomach, ileum, colon, and rectum. *Gastroenterology* **45,** 721–729.
3. Gordon, J. I. (1989). Intestinal epithelial differentiation: New insights from chimeric and transgenic mice. *J. Cell Biol.* **108**(4), 1187–1194.
4. Sprinz, H. (1971). Factors influencing intestinal cell renewal: A statement of principles. *Cancer* **28,** 71–74.
5. Parker, F. G., Barnes, E. N., and Kaye, G. I. (1974). The pericryptal fibroblast sheath. IV. Replication, migration, and differentiation of the subepithelial fibroblasts of the crypts and villus of the rabbit jejunum. *Gastroenterology* **67,** 607–621.
6. Zajicek, G. (1977). The intestinal proliferon. *J. Theor. Biol.* **67,** 515–521.
7. Earnest, D. (1988). Gastrointestinal changes from starvation and stress. "The Report of The Eighth Ross Conference On Medical Research," pp. 11–16. Ross Laboratories, Ohio.
8. Alverdy, J. C., Aoys, E., and Moss, G. S. (1988). Total parenteral nutrition promotes bacterial translocation from the gut. *Surgery* **104**(2), 185-90.
9. Lacy, E. R. (1988). Epithelial restitution in the gastrointestinal tract. *J. Clin. Gastroenterol.* **10**(Suppl. 1), S72–S77.
10. Hollander, F. (1954). The two-component mucous barrier. *Arch. Intern. Med.* **93,** 107–120.
11. Critchlow, J., Magee, D., Ito, S., Takeuchi, and K., Silen, W. (1985). Requirements for restitution of the surface epithelium of frog stomach after mucosal injury. *Gastroenterology* **88,** 237–249.
12. Paimela, H., Goddard, P. J., Carter, K., *et al.* (1993). Restitution of frog gastric mucosa *in vitro*: Effect of basic fibroblast growth factor. *Gastroenterology* **104**(5), 1337–1345.
13. Lacy, E. R., and Ito, S. (1984). Rapid epithelial restitution of the rat gastric mucosa after ethanol injury. *Lab. Invest.* **51**(5), 573–583.
14. Sorbye, H., Svanes, C., Stangeland, L., Kvinnsland, S., Svanes, K., and Srbye, H. (1988). Epithelial restitution and cellular proliferation after gastric mucosal damage caused by hypertonic NaCl in rats. *Virchows Arch. A Pathol. Anat.* **413,** 445–455.
15. Feil, W., Wenzl, E., Vattay, P., *et al.* (1987). Repair of rabbit duodenal mucosa after acid injury *in vivo* and *in vitro. Gastroenterology* **92**(6), 1973–1986.
16. Waller, D. A., Thomas, N. W., and Self, T. J. (1988). Epithelial restitution in the large intestine of the rat following insult with bile salts. *Virchows Arch. A Pathol. Anat.* **414,** 77–81.
17. Buck, R. (1986). Ultrastructural features of rectal epithelium of the mouse during the early phases of migration to repair a defect. *Virchows Arch. [B]* **51,** 331–340.
18. Lacy, E. R. (1987). Gastric mucosal defense after superficial injury. *Clin. Invest. Med.* **10**(3), 189–200.
19. Feil, W., Lacy, E. R., Wong, Y. M., *et al.* (1989). Rapid epithelial restitution of human and rabbit colonic mucosa. *Gastroenterology* **97**(3), 685–701.
20. Bjerknes, M., and Cheng, H. (1981). The stem cell zone of the small intestinal epithelium. IV. Effects of resecting 30% of the small intestine. *Am. J. Anat.* **160,** 93–103.
21. Tilson, M. D., and Wright, H. K. (1970). Adaptation of functioning and bypassed segments of ileum during compensatory hypertrophy of the gut. *Surgery* **67**(4), 687–693.
22. Evrard, S., Aprahamian, M., Hoeltzel, A., *et al.* (1993). Trophic and enzymatic adaptation of the intestine to biliopancreatic bypass in the rat. *Int. J. Obes. Relat. Metab. Disord.* **17**(9), 541–547.
23. Chung, D. H., Evers, B. M., Shimoda, I., *et al.* (1992). Effect of neurotensin on gut mucosal growth in rats with jejunal and ileal Thiry–Vella fistulas. *Gastroenterology* **103**(4), 1254–1259.
24. Altmann, G. G., and Leblond, C. P. (1970). Factors influencing villus size in the small intestine of adult rats as revealed by transposition of intestinal segments. *Am. J. Anat.* **127,** 15–36.
25. Thompson, J. S., Saxena, S. K., and Sharp, J. G. (1988). Effect of urogastrone on intestinal regeneration is dose-dependent. *Cell Tissue Kinet.* **21**(3), 183–191.
26. Dowling, R. H., and Booth, C. C. (1967). Structural and functional changes following small intestinal resection in the rat. *Clin. Sci.* **32,** 139–149.
27. Hanson, W. R., Osborne, J. W., and Sharp, J. G. (1977). Compensation by the residual intestine after intestinal resection in the rat. I. Influence of amount of tissue removed. *Gastroenterology* **73,** 692–700.
28. Hanson, W. R., and Osborne, J. W. (1971). Epithelial cell kinetics in the small intestine of the rat 60 days after resection of 70 percent of the ileum and jejunum. *Gastroenterology* **60,** 1087–1097.
29. Nygaard, K. (1967). Resection of the small intestine in rats. III. Morphological cahnges in the intestinal tract. *Acta Chir. Scand.* **133,** 233–248.
30. Fenyo, G., Backman, L., and Hallberg, D. (1976). Morphological changes of the small intestine following jejuno-ileal shunt in obese subjects. *Acta Chir. Scand.* **142,** 154–159.
31. Gleeson, M. H., Cullen, J., and Dowling, R. H. (1972). Intestinal structure and function after small bowel bypass in the rat. *Clin. Sci.* **43,** 731–742.

32. Urban, E., and Pena, M. *In vivo* calcium transport by rat small intestine after massive small bowel resection. *Am. J. Physiol.* **226**(6), 1304–1308.
33. Bury, K. D. (1972). Carbohydrate digestion and absorption after massive resection of the small intestine. *Surg. Gynecol. Obstet.* **135**(2), 177–187.
34. Bochenek, W. J., Narczewska, B., and Grzebieluch, M. (1973). Effect of massive proximal small bowel resection on intestinal sucrase and lactase activity in the rat. *Digestion* **9**(3), 224–230.
35. Altmann, G. G., and Enesco, M. (1967). Cell number as a measure of distribution and renewal of epithelial cells in the small intestine of growing and adult rats. *Am. J. Anat.* **121**(2), 319–336.
36. Levine, G. M., Deren, J. J., Steiger, E., and Zinno, R. (1974). Role of oral intake in maintenance of gut mass and disaccharide activity. *Gastroenterology* **67**(5), 975–982.
37. Williamson, R. C., Bauer, F. L., Ross, J. S., and Malt, R. A. (1978). Contributions of bile and pancreatic juice to cell proliferation in ileal mucosa. *Surgery* **83**(5), 570–576.
38. Williamson, R. C., Buchholtz, T. W., and Malt, R. A. (1978). Humoral stimulation of cell proliferation in small bowel after transection and resection in rats. *Gastroenterology* **75**(2), 249–254.
39. Tilson, M. D., and Livstone, E. M. (1975). Radioautography of heterotopic autografts of ileal mucosa in rats after partial enterectomy. *Surg. Forum* **26,** 393–394.
40. Kato, Y., Yu, D., and Schwartz, M. Z. (1999). Glucagonlike peptide-2 enhances small intestinal absorptive function and mucosal mass *in vivo. J. Pediatr. Surg.* **34**(1), 18–20; discussion, 20–21.
41. Duncan, M. D., Korman, L. Y., and Bass, B. L. Epidermal growth factor primes intestinal epithelial cells for proliferative effect of insulin-like growth factor I. *Dig. Dis. Sci.* **39**(10), 2197–2201.
42. Thompson, J. S., Saxena, S. K., Greaton, C., *et al.* (1989). The effect of the route of delivery of urogastrone on intestinal regeneration. *Surgery* **106**(1), 45–51.
43. Helmrath, M. A., Erwin, C. R., and Warner, B. W. (1997). A defective EGF-receptor in waved-2 mice attenuates intestinal adaptation. *J. Surg. Res.* **69**(1), 76–80.
44. Helmrath, M. A., Shin, C. E., Erwin, C. R., and Warner, B. W. (1998). The EGFEGF-receptor axis modulates enterocyte apoptosis during intestinal adaptation. *J. Surg. Res.* **77**(1), 17–22.
45. Hodin, R. A., Saldinger, P., and Meng, S. (1995). Small bowel adaptation: Counterregulatory effects of epidermal growth factor and somatostatin on the program of early gene expression. *Surgery* **118**(2), 206–210; discussion, 210–211.
46. Thompson, J. S., Nguyen, B. L., and Harty, R. F. (1993). Somatostatin analogue inhibits intestinal regeneration. *Arch. Surg.* **128**(4), 385–389.
47. Wilmore, D. W., Lacey, J. M., Soultanakis, R. P., *et al.* (1997). Factors predicting a successful outcome after pharmacologic bowel compensation. *Ann. Surg.* **226**(3), 288–292; discussion, 292–293.
48. Thompson, J. S., Bragg, L. E., and Saxena, S. K. (1990). The effect of intestinal resection and urogastrone on intestinal regeneration. *Arch. Surg.* **125**(12), 1617–1621.
49. Thompson, J. S. (1992). Effect of a smooth muscle antagonist on contraction of patched intestinal defects. *J. Surg. Res.* **53**(3), 257–262.
50. Hodin, R. A., Graham, J. R., Meng, S., and Upton, M. P. (1994). Temporal pattern of rat small intestinal gene expression with refeeding. *Am. J. Physiol.* **266**(1 Pt. 1), G83–G89.
51. Clarke, R. M. (1975). The time-course of changes in mucosal architecture and epithelial cell production and cell shedding in the small intestine of the rat fed after fasting. *J. Anat.* **120**(2), 321–327.
52. Hodin, R. A., Chamberlain, S. M., and Upton, M. P. (1992). Thyroid hormone differentially regulates rat intestinal brush border enzyme gene expression. *Gastroenterology* **103**(5), 1529–1536.
53. Zheng, S., Jin, B., Caty, M. G., and Tjota, A. (1997). Mucosa cell regeneration following intestinal ischemia/reperfusion injury in rats. *Chin. Med. J. (Engl.)* **110**(5), 338–340.
54. Kampp, M., Lundgren, O., and Nilsson, N. J. (1968). Extravascular shunting of oxygen in the small intestine of the cat. *Acta Physiol. Scand.* **72**(4), 396–403.
55. Bohlen, H. G. (1980). Intestinal tissue PO_2 and microvascular responses during glucose exposure. *Am. J. Physiol.* **238**(2), H164–H171.
56. Lundgren, O., and Svanvik, J. (1973). Mucosal hemodynamics in the small intestine of the cat during reduced perfusion pressure. *Acta Physiol. Scand.* **88**(4), 551–563.
57. Granger, D. N., Hollwarth, M. E., and Parks, D. A. (1986). Ischemia-reprfusion injury: Role of oxygen-derived free radicals. *Acta Physiol. Scand.* (Suppl.), S48–S63.
58. Robinson, J. W., Mirkovitch, V., Winistorfer, B., and Saegesser, F. (1981). Response of the intestinal mucosa to ischaemia. *Gut* **22**(6), 512–527.
59. Gabbert, H., Wagner, R., Aust, P., and Hohn, P. (1978). Ischemia and post-ischemia regeneration of the small intestinal mucosa. An enzyme-histochemical investigation. *Acta Histochem.* **63**, 197–213.
60. Wagner, R., Gabbert, H., and Hohn, P. (1979). The mechanism of epithelial shedding after ischemic damage to the small intestinal mucosa. A light and electron microscopic investigation. *Virchows Arch. B Cell. Pathol.* **30**, 25–31.
61. Earnest, D. L., and Trier, J. S. (1989). Radiation enteritis and colitis. In "Gastrointestinal Disease" (M. H. Sleisinger and J. S. Ford, Eds.), pp. 1360–1382. W. B. Saunders, Philadelphia.
62. Berthrong, M., and Fajardo, L. F. (1981). Radiation injury in surgical pathology. Part II. Alimentary tract. *Am. J. Surg. Pathol.* **5**(2), 153–178.
63. Berthrong, M. (1986). Pathologic changes secondary to radiation. *World J. Surg.* **10**(2), 155– 170.
64. Paulus, U., Potten, C. S., and Loeffler, M. (1992). A model of the control of cellular regeneration in the intestinal crypt after perturbation based solely on local stem cell regulation. *Cell Prolif.* **25**(6), 559–578.
65. Klimberg, V. S., Salloum, R. M., Kasper, M., *et al.* (1990). Oral glutamine accelerates healing of the small intestine and improves outcome after whole abdominal radiation. *Arch. Surg.* **125**(8), 1040–1045.
66. Gurbuz, A. T., Kunzelman, J., and Ratzer, E. E. (1998). Supplemental dietary arginine accelerates intestinal mucosal regeneration and enhances bacterial clearance following radiation enteritis in rats. *J. Surg. Res.* **74**(2), 149–154.
67. Moore, R., Carlson, S., and Madara, J. L. (1989). Rapid barrier restitution in an *in vitro* model of intestinal epithelial injury. *Lab. Invest.* **60**(2), 237–244.
68. Prasad, M., Ito, S., and Silen, W. (1997). Functional studies of *in vitro* rat distal colon before and after restitution. *Surgery* **121**(4), 430–439.
69. Nusrat, A., Delp, C., and Madara, J. L. (1992). Intestinal epithelial restitution. Characterization of a cell culture model and mapping of cytoskeletal elements in migrating cells. *J. Clin. Invest.* **89**(5), 1501–1511.
70. Lotz, M. M., Nusrat, A., Madara, J. L., *et al.* (1997). Intestinal epithelial restitution. Involvement of specific laminin isoforms and integrin laminin receptors in wound closure of a transformed model epithelium. *Am. J. Pathol.* **150**(2), 747–760.
71. Ciacci, C., Lind, S. E., and Podolsky, D. K. (1993). Transforming growth factor beta regulation of migration in wounded rat intestinal epithelial monolayers. *Gastroenterology* **105**(1), 93–101.
72. Dignass, A. U., and Podolsky, D. K. (1993). Cytokine modulation of intestinal epithelial cell restitution: Central role of transforming growth factor beta. *Gastroenterology* **105**(5), 1323–1332.
73. Dignass, A., Lynch-Devaney, K., Kindon, H., *et al.* (1994). Trefoil peptides promote epithelial migration through a transforming growth factor beta-independent pathway. *J. Clin. Invest.* **94**(1), 376–383.
74. Hodin, R. A., Meng, S., Archer, and S., Tang, R. (1996). Cellular growth state differentially regulates enterocyte gene expression in butyrate-treated HT-29 cells. *Cell Growth Differ.* **7**(5), 647–653.
75. Dignass, A. U., Tsunekawa, S., and Podolsky, D. K. (1994). Fibroblast growth factors modulate intestinal epithelial cell growth and migration. *Gastroenterology* **106**(5), 1254–1262.

44

Minimally Invasive Surgery

Daniel B. Jones and Robert V. Rege

Southwestern Center for Minimally Invasive Surgery and Department of Surgery, The University of Texas Southwestern Medical Center, Dallas, Texas 75235

I. Introduction

Technology has propelled surgery into an age of minimally invasive (or "minimal access") operations. Surgeons in different specialties use this approach to operate on the abdominal cavity, chest, pelvis, and extremities by means of access ports placed through small incisions. For access to the abdomen, laparoscopy, a method of viewing the peritoneal cavity by means of an endoscope introduced through a small incision in the abdominal wall, has revolutionized the field of general surgery. Similarly, an operation guided by a 15-fold magnification telescope that is placed through a small incision in the chest is called thoracoscopy. Procedures performed using thoroscopes are termed video-assisted thoracic surgery. Procedures using scopes in the pelvis or in joints are termed pelvicoscopy and arthroscopy, respectively. The first laparoscopic cholecystectomy was performed in France in 1987, and the first in the United States in 1988 (1). Since then, there has been an upsurge in the popularity of laparoscopic surgery, and many other operations have been reported.

The rapid evolution in surgery toward minimal invasion has been driven by the demand for more cosmetic and less painful incisions. Many procedures decrease length of hospital stay and time to full recovery. However, questions concerning which approach is medically the best, ultimate outcomes, and relative costs of each method remain unanswered. Industry has responded to powerful market forces with new equipment and a substantial investment for research and development. Consequently, scientific and technological advances in minimally invasive surgery have been exponential. Surgeons have had to learn new surgical techniques, and hospitals have been forced to redesign operating suites and retrain nurses to keep pace with technological changes. Still, long-term follow-up and randomized outcome studies are needed to prove which minimally invasive operations are truly safer and more cost effective.

Although many of the advances in minimally invasive surgery have come from the private sector, the responsibility is now for the academic centers to evaluate the proposed advantages and disadvantages of these new techniques. Surgeons are asked to be cost effective as technology advances. It is no longer adequate to say simply that new procedures are feasible; surgeons must demonstrate that new techniques and procedures are beneficial to patients and offer cost savings to the hospital and to society. This chapter examines methodology for addressing these questions.

II. Models and Methodology

Basic science, clinical outcomes, product/procedure development, and education research have been carried out for minimally invasive surgery. The type of model used depends on the studies performed and includes inanimate models, small animals, large animals, and humans.

In this chapter, we exemplify models of active investigation in minimally invasive surgery by investigators throughout the world, describing the authors' experience with basic science and clinical research conducted at the Southwestern Center for Minimally Invasive Surgery (SCMIS) at The University of Texas Southwestern Medical Center at Dallas, Texas, and the Washington University Institute for Minimally Invasive Surgery (WUIMIS) at St. Louis, Missouri. Contributions from other institutions are also included.

A. Small Animals

Small animals such as mice and hamsters are particularly useful in studies of minimally invasive surgery when basic questions are addressed and large numbers of data points are required to prove small but important differences. For example, the hamster model has been used to study the effects of pneumoperitoneum on tumor implantation at trocar sites (2). Using inhalational anesthesia, four trocars are inserted through the abdominal wall and the abdominal cavity is insufflated with carbon dioxide to a pressure of 10 mmHg (Fig. 1). With this model, investigators have been able to vary pneumoperitoneum pressure and inoculum of tumor cells, and apply topical chemotherapy and tumoricidal agents to better understand how to prevent tumor implantation during laparoscopy for cancer (3, 4, 5). The disadvantage of small animal models relates to the usual question about whether one can reliably extrapolate data on rodents to humans. In addition, actual performance of laparoscopic procedures can be technically difficult and are not necessarily analogous to those performed in humans.

Other investigators have also used small animals to further understand the physiologic effects of pneumoperitoneum, immunology, and tumor implantation. At Duke University, in Raleigh, North Carolina, researchers have used a well-established *Listeria monocytogenes in vivo* model to study cell-mediated immune responses (6). Mice received carbon dioxide or helium insufflation prior to sublethal inoculation of the intracellular pathogen, *Listeria*. Liver and spleen were harvested at 3 and 5 days. Tissue was homogenized and plated on agar. Investigators found that carbon dioxide pneumoperitoneum impaired cell-mediated intraperitoneal immunity more than helium pneumoperitoneum after 3 days, but by 5 days intraperitoneal immuno-

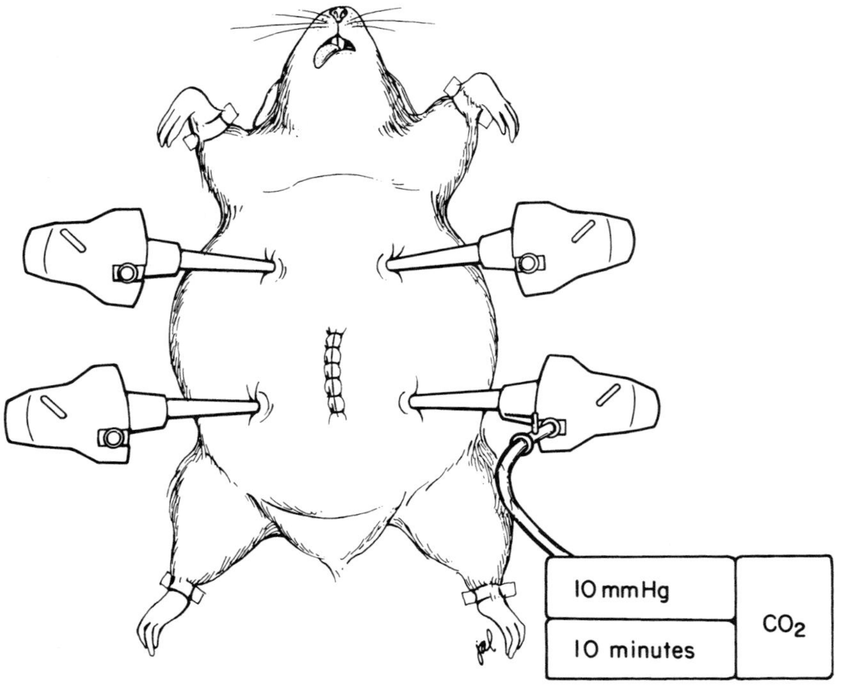

Figure 1 Hamster model using pneumoperitoneum to assess impact of tumor implantation at port sites. Pneumoperitoneum is established at an insufflation pressure of 10 mmHg for a 10-min duration. From Ref. (38), S. B. Jones and D. B. Jones (1998). Extending the limits: Minimally invasive surgery. *Curr. Opin. Anesthesiol.* **11**, 629–636.

suppression resolved. The investigators, however, were not able to control the systemic effects of pneumoperitoneum (i.e., blood pH measurement) due to the animals small size. The investigators acknowledge that delayed bacterial clearance may be due to systemic acidosis in the carbon dioxide group. Further study is needed to elucidate the specific immune mechanism and its correlation to clinical science.

Gleason *et al.* (7) established a practical and reliable mouse model to test immunomodulating drugs and therapies. C3H/HeN mice were given three serial delayed-type hypersensitivity challenges of phytohemagglutinin before and after the test procedure. All challenges were administered via subcutaneous injection. Skin thickness immediately before and 24 hr after injection represented response, and could be used for open and minimal access procedures in a simple and cost-effective manner.

This group then demonstrated that more cell-mediated immunosuppression occurs after full laparotomy compared to either pneumoperitoneum or anesthesia alone (8). Furthermore, postoperative immunosuppression was associated with the length of the incision. Other investigators questioned whether immunosuppression was really secondary to exposure of the peritoneal cavity to air contamination (small amounts of lipopolysaccharides found in circulating air).

Other investigators have chosen to work with midsize animal models. The rabbit model has been used to investigate the effect of CO_2 pneumoperitoneum on cancer cells implanted in the portal vein (9). Compared with laparotomy, CO_2 pneumoperitoneum enhanced the development of liver metastases. Further studies are needed to elucidate the pathomechanisms involved in the enhancement of liver metastasis caused by CO_2 pneumoperitoneum.

Less commonly used models have included the opossum and prairie dog. The opossum model has been used to study esophageal motility following laparoscopic fundoplication (10). Investigators have developed topographic esophageal manometric methods for studying the effects of laparoscopic fundoplication in the opossum model. The prairie dog model has been used to evaluate the effects of retained gallstones following laparoscopic cholecystectomy (11).

B. Large Animals

Large animals may also be used to answer basic questions, but are more expensive. They are most useful for physiological studies, for product/procedure development studies, and for training of surgeons, because procedures are quite similar to those in humans. In many respects, responses by large animals to minimally invasive techniques are more similar to the human response. Use of large animals requires animal operating rooms and equipment similar to that used in the hospital.

Palombo *et al.* (12) established a sepsis model in pathogen-free Hanford pigs by injecting *Escherichia coli* intraperitoneally. These investigators sought to determine if laparoscopic irrigation of the abdominal cavity was as effective as that achieved during laparotomy. Furthermore, their model allowed characterization of the effect of pneumoperitoneum in patients with cardiopulmonary insufficiency and endotoxemic shock. The gram-negative bacterial peritonitis model described in this study simulates generalized peritonitis without evidence of shock, as might be observed clinically in patients with appendicitis or pelvic inflammatory disease. Results of their study found that laparoscopic treatment of *E. coli* peritonitis is as effective as that achieved by laparotomy. Investigators subsequently assessed specific interventions to improve cardiopulmonary hemodynamics during laparoscopy in their sepsis model (13).

Animal models have also been used to establish the effectiveness of novel concepts such as use of a micropump that aerosolizes therapeutic substances to be distributed into the pneumoperitoneum (14). In a porcine model, precise determination of total quantity of drug administered was possible. Investigators used cytostatic and bacteriostatic drugs and adhesion-modulating agents. The microvaporisator may have applications for locoregional cancer therapy, prevention of port site recurrences, immunomodulation, analgesia, peritonitis, and prevention of postoperative adhesions.

Large animals are ideal for assessing the feasibility of a new operation in living tissues. Larger animals can simulate laparoscopic trocar placement, retraction, and positioning in humans. After the first laparoscopic Whipple procedure was reported clinically (15), investigators turned to the animal laboratory prior to advocating this technique. In the dog model, laparoscopic pancreaticoduodenectomy could be performed; however, investigators identified several reasons why this application of laparoscopic surgery exceeded reason (16).

Swine serve as good models for many laparoscopic procedures because porcine anatomy is generally similar to human anatomy (17). Practice on porcine models may refine operative technique and most continuing medical education (CME) courses at UT Southwestern and nationally use this model. At SCMIS, investigators compared laparoscopic and hand-assisted techniques advocated by others in the porcine model prior to embarking on the laparoscopic roux-en-Y gastric bypass for morbid obesity (18). Several subtle modifications to the technique simplified the operation and facilitated surgeons being able to offer this investigational procedure to patients (19). In other procedures, the dog model has suggested that new procedures are feasible and safe in acute and chronic survival studies, such as endoscopic neck exploration and parathyroidectomy (20); nonetheless, convincing clinical data to support the procedure are lacking.

Large animals are often preferred to assess the changes in operative exposure that occur with pneumoperitoneum and extremes of positioning required of laparoscopy. The pig has been used to compare transperitoneal and retroperitoneal approaches to laparoscopic-assisted aortic bypass surgery (21). With the transperitoneal technique, very steep Trendelenberg positioning is required for adequate gravity-aided retraction of small bowel (Fig. 2). Meanwhile, other technologies have advanced endovascular surgery to overcome many of these limitations of laparoscopy.

Minimally invasive surgery has spread beyond the conventional body cavities to new applications and disease processes. In general, human cadaver studies, in addition to animal studies, are important before animal data can be extrapolated to patients clinically. In the dog, for example, hernia balloon inflation of the axilla can create a working space for endoscopic axillary dissection. However, because the dog has few axillary nodes, a cadaver endoscopic dissection was necessary to assess port placement (Fig. 3) and the completeness of endoscopic axillary dissection (22).

With the rapid introduction of new technology, investigators are evaluating advances in biologic glues (23), radiofrequency ablation of liver (24), and performance of a three-dimensional camera system in the animal laboratory (25). At WUIMIS technology used for teleconferencing has been evaluated for teleproctoring during continuing medical education courses (26). At SCMIS, robots are being compared to surgeons in the animal operating room using human performance measures. At the Imperial College School of Medicine in London investigators are studying the feasibility of performing laparoscopic surgery with intraoperative imaging within an interventional magnetic resonance (MR) unit (27). The exact indications for the application of this new technology await development, but the investigators predict that MR combined with laparoscopy may be used for the staging of intraabdominal malignancy, laparoscopically assisted MR-guided interstitial thermotherapy techniques, and MR-guided laparoscopic hepatic/retroperitoneal tumor resection.

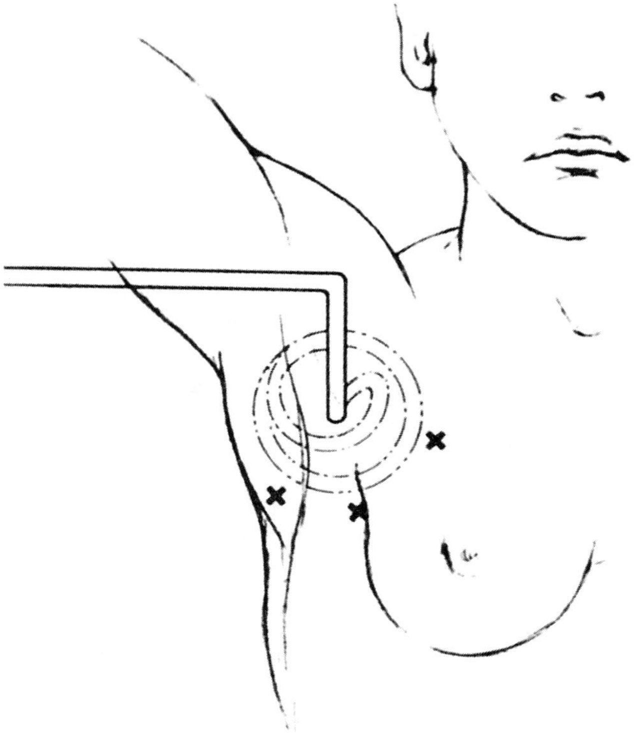

Figure 3 Cadaver model of endoscopic axillary lymph node excision using balloon dissection to create a working space, showing port sites (X). From Ref. (21).

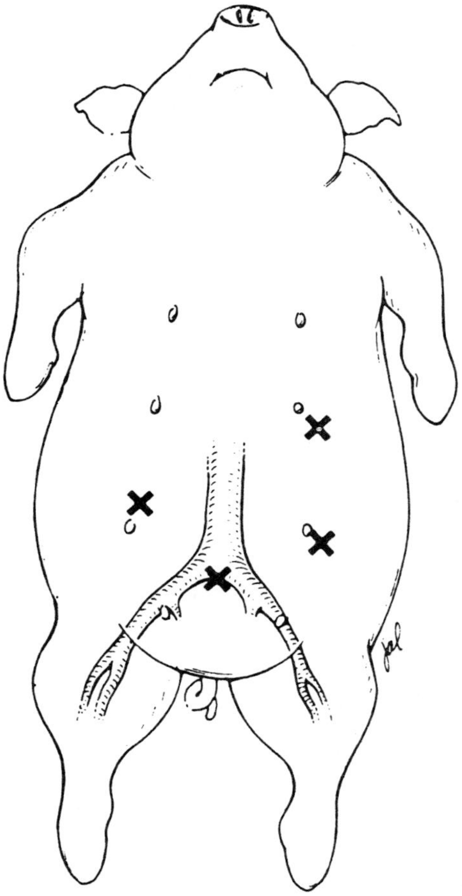

Figure 2 Pig model comparing effects of gravity displacement of intraabdominal organs with extremes of animal position during laparoscopic-assisted aortic bypass. From Ref. (2), D. B. Jones, L. W. Guo, M. K. Reinhard, N. J. Soper, G. W. Philpott, J. Connett, and J. W. Fleshman (1995). Impact of pneumoperitoneum on trocar site implantation of colon cancer in hamster model. *Dis. Colon. Rectum* **38** (11), 1182–1188.

C. Human Cadavers

Patients and families who donate their bodies make a valuable contribution to science and surgical education. The human cadaver models are ideal for learning complex anatomy. At SCMIS, we have preferentially used cadaver models to teach practicing surgeons (who are often unfamiliar with pelvic anatomy) the totally extraperitoneal (TEP) hernia repair. Anatomical relationships are crucial to the successful

TEP repairs and cannot be extrapolated from animal models. Similarly, orthopedic surgeons have used cadaver models to teach laparoscopic spine surgery, and colorectal surgeons have used cadaver models to teach advanced colorectal operations.

The major disadvantage of cadavers is the lack of normal vascular response and rigid tissue. Moreover, cadaver models have limited availability and exorbitant costs (greater than $1000 each) associated with body preparation and appropriate disposal of remains. Working with cadavers may also be emotionally stressful for investigators.

At SCMIS, surgeons, teamed with modeling artists, have built a silicone/rubber pelvis to teach laparoscopic TEP hernia procedures (28). After casting a cadaver's pelvis, a crude model was produced. The model was then brought to the operating room during actual hernia operations to better refine key anatomical relations. A single, reusable, realistic, working model was not only expensive to design, but took over 12 months to develop.

D. Inanimate Models

Animal studies have been important to developing applications of laparoscopy and to better understanding the physiology of pneumoperitoneum. It is hoped that inanimate models will be proved reliable for research and training and will render animal models obsolete. This is especially true for resident education. Developing technical skills is essential to surgical resident training. Historically this has been done in the operating room. The substantial costs associated with prolonged operative time make this system expensive and inefficient. Laparoscopy poses a new obstacle to skill acquisition because significant experience is required before competency is achieved.

Laparoscopic skills may be effectively taught outside the operating room. Inanimate models on a videotrainer (Fig. 4) may provide a safe, reproducible, effective, efficient and controlled environment for the acquisition and refinement of laparoscopic skills. At WUIMIS, skill performance

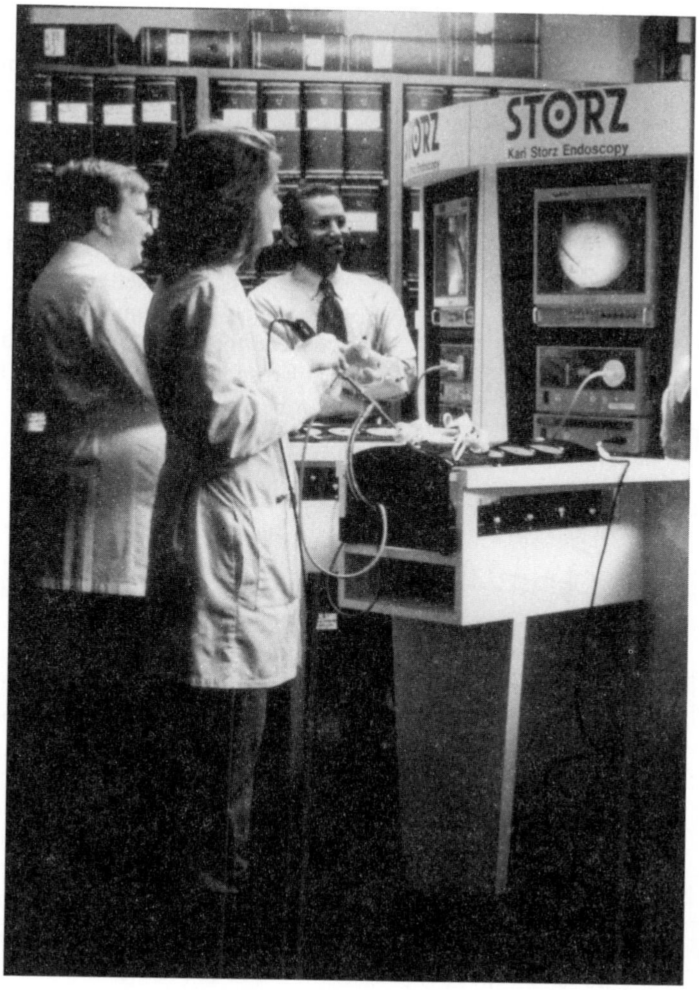

Figure 4 Videotrainer developed for group learning of laparoscopic skills. From Ref. (22). Reprinted with permission from the American College of Surgeons (Journal of the American College of Surgeons, 1998, Vol. 187, pp. 158–163).

improved with repetition of five tasks (Fig. 5) using two-dimensional and three dimensional camera systems (25). At SCMIS, investigators have found that as little as 30 min of training daily for 10 days on a videotrainer can demonstrate improved performance in the operating room using previously validated global assessments (29,30). Based on these dramatic findings, UT Southwestern established a Technical Skills Laboratory to investigate alternative teaching modalities such as virtual reality simulators, silicon models to practice laparoscopic hernia repair, interactive CD ROMS for laparoscopic ultrasound, and haptic feedback for computer simulation. Washington University, on the other hand, encourages surgery residents to practice on a videotrainer but does not have a technical skill curriculum. Several other universities are currently developing a technical skills training program (see Chapter 90, Research on Surgical Education).

Although simplistic, computer-based virtual reality models are improving; combinations of haptic (force-feedback) input, improved computer graphics, and rapidly increasing computer speeds and memory (and thus improved response times when instruments are used) portend well for realistic virtual reality-based models in the future. Currently, the use of realistic inanimate models and multimodality teaching techniques (video, interactive CD-ROM, computer-based learning programs) is increasing and their effectiveness is being tested. Skill training is enhanced by observation of an instructive video and an interactive CD ROM program. Efficacy of this curriculum is currently underway by comparing performance of residents in the human operating room with respect to residents who have and have not been trained.

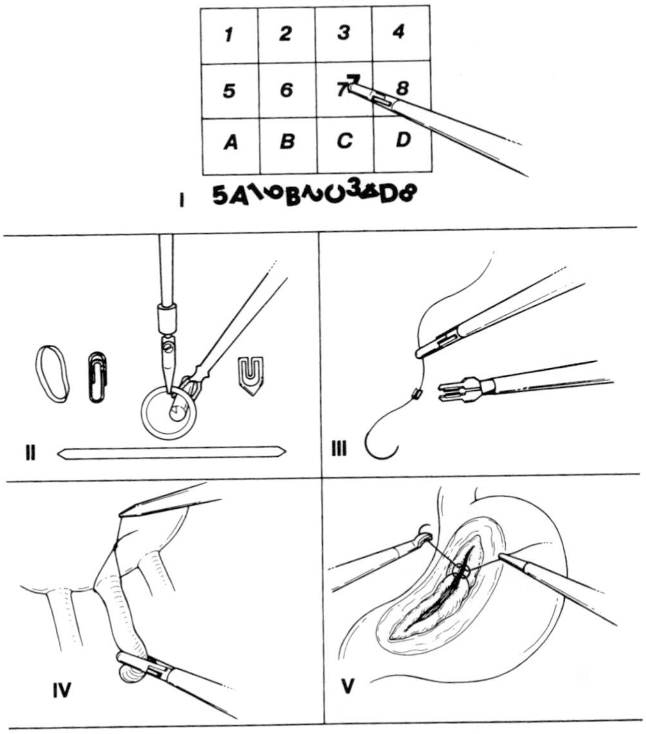

Figure 5 Five tasks performed in a videotrainer. (I) Checkerboard. Lead numbers and letters are arranged on a flat surface. (II) Loop pass. Objects are passed through a suspended ring. (III) Lapra-Ty. Suture is clipped. (IV) Loop ligature. Foam pedicle is loop ligated. (V) Simple suture.

Inanimate trainers clearly improve skills measured on the device. Thus, students improve (decreased time to complete tasks and improved accuracy). However, it should be understood that ultimately the utility of these devices must be measured by demonstrating improved performance in the operating room and improvement in patient outcomes.

E. Clinical Studies

The feasibility of an operation is not an indication for its performance; consequently, clinical studies are needed prior to recommending a procedure to patients. Case reports of technological successes and complications have been important. For example, reports of strangulated bowel encourage surgeons routinely to close port sites greater than 5 mm (31). Reports of tumor implantation at port sites sparked investigators to study this question in the laboratory and in practice because of its implications to cancer patients (32).

Retrospective studies may also give us insight into the effectiveness of new laparoscopic procedures. For example, with laparoscopic colorectal surgery for malignancy, the Clinical Outcomes of Surgical Therapy (COST) group retrospectively assessed patient benefit after a laparoscopic approach (33). Importantly, in 372 patients with colorectal cancer, the COST group found that port-site recurrence after laparoscopic colectomy was not as dire a consequence as formerly considered, thereby opening the door to prospective studies.

Similarly, anecdotal cases of abscesses after spillage of bile during laparoscopic cholecystectomy were reported in the literature. It used to be thought that spillage of bile and stones would place patients at high risk for infection. However, a review of several hundred laparoscopic cholecystectomy patients challenged this concern and suggested that the risk was overstated (34). Intraoperative gallbladder perforation occurred in one-third of patients, and contrary to traditional dogma, a drain was not necessary after laparoscopic cholecystectomy.

Most importantly, randomized prospective multiinistutional studies are needed to determine whether new laparoscopic procedures are beneficial and cost effective. Comparisons between laparoscopic and open procedures, as well as between laparoscopic procedures and medical treatment, are both important. For example, initial studies have shown that the laparoscopic colectomy achieves adequate margin of resection, nodal dissection, and anastomotic creation (35). Definitive questions regarding laparoscopic surgery will be answered by a prospective randomization of 1200 patients in an ongoing National Cancer Institute-sponsored trial (36). Clinical trials are ongoing and designed to answer whether cancer-free survival following laparoscopic colectomy is different than after open colectomy.

Multiinstitutional studies have also suggested a benefit of laparoscopic herniorrhaphy (37), and the Veterans Affairs is currently funding a randomized prospective multiinstitutional outcome study to compare the Lichtenstein "tension-free" repair to the laparoscopic herniorrhaphy (see Chapter 11, Measuring Surgical Outcomes).

III. Setup and Equipment

At the University of Texas Southwestern Medical Center, for example, the medical school has dedicated one animal operating room for ongoing research in minimally invasive surgery. Unrestricted educational grants from industry have allowed the space to be converted into a state-of-the-art endosuite (Fig. 6) (38). Color monitor, carbon dioxide insufflator, laparoscopic ultrasound, and videocassette recorder are kept on adjustable booms that spider from the ceiling. Motorized operating room tables allow the extremes of position required of advanced laparoscopic operations. Cameras and recorders are digitally enhanced for the best visualization and capturing of results. Lighting is critical for video imaging and for autopsy assessments. Technologies such as ultrasonic coagulation, radiofrequency ablation, and biologic glues supplement the investigator's armamentarium in the operating room facility. Standard human anesthesia machines and monitors are used routinely. The animal operating room is essentially the same as endosuites used in human operating rooms.

Personnel are crucial to success. Ideally, the goal is to simulate the level of support in an actual operating room. For most large animal investigation this requires a dedicated person for anesthesia to assure depth of anesthesia and adequate ventilation. Most operations are best performed by two investigators—a surgeon and an assistant surgeon—with the aid of a scrub nurse to pass instruments. A circulating technician is helpful to retrieve equipment and record results. For new procedures that will ultimately be performed on patients, it's best to have several surgeons involved in animal research who can then transition as a team to the clinical practice. In our facility, we have a full-time technician for anesthesia and animal preparation, a nurse, laparoscopy fellow, medical student, and at least one attending surgeon whenever possible for large animal laparoscopic research.

Acquiring space and resources is a formidable obstacle for a young investigator beginning any research program. It is even more difficult to establish a program in minimally invasive surgery. The department of surgery and medical center will need to allocate space to conduct research. Although renting space may be adequate, ideally the institution will need to dedicate space. Animal endosuites maintain

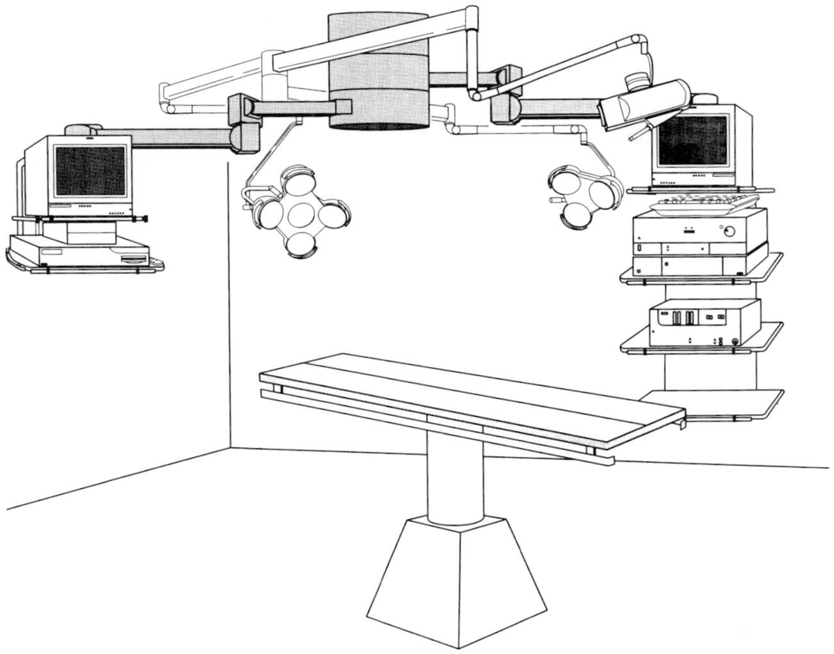

Figure 6 Animal endosuite. Monitors, carbon dioxide insufflator, laparoscopic ultrasound, and electrocautery are stored on booms hanging from the ceiling. From Ref. (25), D. B. Jones, J. D. Brewer, and N. J. Soper (1996). The influence of three-dimensional video systems on laparoscopic task performance. *Surg. Laparosc. Endosc.* **6** (3), 191–197.

expensive high-tech equipment that requires installation and maintenance, and the equipment is not easily transportable.

IV. Funding

Corporate sponsors, such as United States Surgical and Ethicon Endosurgery, have established unrestricted educational grants to create "Centers of Excellence" throughout the United States. The grants differ by institution, but in general there is funding to support education, research, and resident training. Other companies are also receptive to supporting minimally invasive surgery research. At the Southwestern Center for Minimally Invasive Surgery, for example, Storz supplies cameras, insufflators, and monitors. Heraeus installed booms to hold equipment, Steris motorized tables are used, Marquet monitors enable sophisticated anesthesia, laparoscopic ultrasound by B&K Medical provides "hands-on" technological advances to the animal laboratory, and smaller companies such as Mediflex donate mechanical retractors for improved operative exposure. Specific research projects may in some cases use loaned equipment, such as the AESOP robot by Computer Motion (see Chapter 8, Funding Strategies and Agencies).

Several surgical societies have awarded grants for investigation in minimally invasive surgery. The Society of American Gastrointestinal Surgeons (SAGES) has several awards each year. In 1999 SAGES funded the following investigations:

1. Assessment of esophageal autonomic functioning GERD and influence of laparoscopic antireflux surgery.
2. Randomized prospective trial of laparoscopic Nissen fundoplication versus laparoscopic modified Toupet fundoplication in patients with failed esophageal body peristalsis.
3. Esophageal clearance and gastroesophageal reflux following laparoscopic Heller myotomy.
4. Standardized evaluation of improved instrumentation for laparoscopic surgery using a combined task performance and ergonomic measure.
5. Role of endothelin in the oliguria induced by prolonged CO_2 pneumoperitoneum.
6. Intraperitoneal immune response to laparotomy and laparoscopy.
7. A phase I/II trial of submucosal colonic injection with onyx-015 to treat metastatic lymph nodes in patients with colorectal cancer.

In 2000, SAGES has funded the following surgical studies:

1. Using multichannel intraluminal impedance to predict postoperative outcomes in patients with symptomatic foregut disease.
2. The effect of fundoplication on sleep architecture and nocturnal gastroesophageal reflux.
3. Hypoxic pneumoperitoneum enhancing tumor metastatic potential.
4. Short- and long-term impact of pneumoperitoneum on renal function and histomorphology in donors and recipients.
5. Development of a web-based system for evaluating laparoscopic skills of surgical residents.
6. Comparison of robotic versus human laparoscopic camera control: impact on surgeon efficiency.
7. The effect of antireflux surgery on gene expression in Barrett's esophagus.

Other organizations, such as The American Society of Colon and Rectal Surgeons (ASCRS), have funded animal studies addressing the concern of tumor implantation at trocar sites during laparoscopic colectomy. The Association of Surgical Education (ASE) has awarded funding for laparoscopic technical skills training. The Veteran Affairs Hospitals has funded a clinical multiinstitutional study to evaluate laparoscopic hernia repair.

V. Conclusion

Advances in minimally invasive surgery came forth from the private sector. Academic surgery was at first slow to embrace laparoscopy, even though it seemed intuitive that a small incision was preferable to a large incision. Today, academic surgeons are asked to prove the benefits of laparoscopy using bench-top and clinical outcome measures. What are the physiologic changes that occur with pneumoperitoneum compared with a laparotomy? Is it cost-effective to use a robotic arm? And how will we teach advanced laparoscopy to the next generation of surgeons? Minimally invasive surgery research is an exciting area of investigation that applies surgical research to today's clinical practice.

VI. Resources

A. General References

Eubanks, W. S., Swanstrom, L. L., and Soper, N. J. (2000). "Mastery of Endoscopic and Laparoscopic Surgery." Lippincott Williams & Wilkins, Philadelphia.

Jones, D. B., Wu, J., and Soper, N.J. (1997). "Laparoscopic Surgery: Principles and Procedures." Quality Medical Publishing, St. Louis.

MacFadyen, B. V., and Ponsky, J. L. (1996). "Operative Laparoscopy and Thoracoscopy." Lippincott-Raven, Philadelphia.

Wexner, S. D. (1999). "Protocols in General Surgery: Laparoscopic Colorectal Surgery." John Wiley & Sons, New York.

B. Grants

Society of American Gastrointestinal Endoscopic Surgeons
Kelly Wettengel
2716 Ocean Park Blvd., Suite 3000
Santa Monica, CA 90405
(310) 314-2404; fax (310) 314-2585

The American Society of Colon and Rectal Surgeons
Herand Abcarian, M.D.
85 West Algonquin Rd., Suite 550
Arlington Heights, IL 60005
(847) 290-9184; fax (847) 290-9203

Association of Surgical Education
University of Cincinnati Medical Center
Fred A. Luchette, M.D., F.A.C.S.
P.O. Box 670558
Cincinnati, OH 45267-0558
(513) 558-5661; fax (513) 558-3136

C. Corporate Contacts

United States Surgical Corporation
Tyco Healthcare Group LP
150 Glover Avenue
Norwalk, CT 06856
(800) 722-8772

Karl Storz Endoscopy
600 Corporate Pointe
Culver City, CA 90230-7600
(800) 421-0837; fax (800) 321-1304

Ethicon Endo-Surgery
4545 Creek Road
Cincinnati, OH 45242-2839
(513) 483-8223; fax (513) 483-8310

STERIS Corporation
North America Healthcare Division
5960 Heisley Road
Mentor, OH 44060-1834
(440) 354-2600; fax (440) 639-4450

GE Marquette Medical Systems
P. O. Box 414
Milwaukee, WI 53201

Heraeus Medical Inc.
6764-A Preston Avenue
Livermore, CA 94550
(800) 227-8372

B-K Medical Systems, Inc.
267 Boston Road, Bldg. A
North Billerica, MA 01862
(800) 876-7226 fax (978) 262-0596

Mediflex
250 Gibbs Road
Islandia, NY 11722-2697
(800) 879-7575; fax (516) 582-8487

Computer Motion
130-B Cremona Drive
Goleta, CA 93117
(805) 968-9600; fax (805) 685-5170

D. Other

Human Performance Institute-UTA
George V. Kondraske, Ph.D.
P. O. Box 19180
Arlington, TX 76019-0180
(817) 272-2335; fax (817) 272-2548

References

1. Soper, N. J., Brunt, L. M., and Kerb, K. (1994). Laparoscopic general surgery. *N. Engl. J. Med.* **330,** 409–419.
2. Jones, D. B., Guo, L. W., Reinhard, M. K., Soper, N. J., Philpott, G. W., Connett, J., and Fleshman, J. W. (1995). Impact of pneumoperitoneum on trocar site implantation of colon cancer in hamster model. *Dis. Colon. Rectum* **38**(11), 1182–1188.
3. Wu, J. S., Brasfield, B. S., Guo, Li-Wu, Ruiz, M., Connett, J. M., Philpott, G. W., Jones, D. B., and Fleshman, J. W. (1997). Implantation of colon cancer at trocar sites is increased by low-pressure pneumoperitoneum. *Surgery* **122,** 1–7.
4. Wu, J. S., Jones, D. B., Guo, L. W., Brasfield, E. B., Ruiz, M. B., Connett, J. M., and Fleshman, J. W. (1998). Effects of pneumoperitoneum on tumor implantation with decreasing tumor inoculum. *Dis. Colon Rectum* **41,** 141–146.
5. Simmang, C., and Jones, D. B. (1999). Wound implantation of cancer after laparoscopic colectomy: Clinical and basic research. *In*: "Seminars in Colon and Rectal Surgery," Vol. 10. (D. J. Schoetz, ed.), pp. 1–9. W. B. Saunders, Philadelphia.
6. Chekan, E. G., Nataraj, C., Clary, E. M., Hayward, T. Z., Brody, F. J., *et al.* (1999). Intraperitoneal immunity and pneumoperitoneum. *Surg. Endosc.* **13,** 1135–1138.
7. Gleason, N. R., Blanco, I., Allendorf, J. D., Lee, S. W., Bessler, M., and Whelan, R. L. (1999). Delayed-type hypersensitivity response is better preserved in mice following insufflation than after laparotomy. *Surg. Endosc.* **13,** 1032–1034.
8. Lee, S. W., Southall, J. C., Gleason, N. R., Huang, E. H., Bessler, M., and Whelan, R. L. (2000). Lymphocyte proliferation in mice after a full laparotomy is the same whether performed in a sealed carbon dioxide chamber or in room air. *Surg. Endosc.* **14,** 235–238.
9. Ishida, H., Murata, N., Yamada, H., Nakada, H., Takeuchi, I., Shimomura, K., Fujioka, M., and Ideezuki, Y. (2000). Pneumoperitoneum with carbon dioxide enhances liver metastases of cancer cells implanted into the portal vein in rabbits. *Surg. Endosc.* **14,** 239–242.

10. Underwood, R. A., Prakash, C., Horoian, L., *et al.* (1999). *Didelphis virginiana:* A useful model for the study of upper gut motility. *Surg. Endosc.* **13,** S83.
11. Bonar, J. P., Bowyer, M. W., Welling, D. R., and Hirsch, K. (1998). The fate of retained gallstones following laparoscopic cholecystectomy in a prairie dog model. *JSLS* **2**(3), 263–268.
12. Palombo, J. D., Liu, K., Greif, W. M., Rawn, J. D., Boyce, P. J., and Forse, R. A. (1999). Effects of laparoscopic vs laparotomy treatment of *E. coli* peritonitis on hemodynamic responses in a porcine model. *Surg. Endosc.* **13,** 1001–1006.
13. Grief, W. M., and Forse, R. A. (1999). Interventions to improve cardiopulmonary hemodynamics during laparoscopy in a porcine sepsis model. *J. Am. Coll. Surg.* **189**(5), 450–458.
14. Reymond, M. A., Hu, B., Garcia, A., Reck, T., Kockerling, F., Hess, J., and Morel, P. (2000). Feasibility of therapeutic pneumoperitoneum in a large animal model using microvaporisator. *Surg. Endosc.* **14,** 51–55.
15. Gagner, M. (1994). Laparoscopic duodenopancreatectomy. *In* "Minimally Invasive Surgery and New Technology" (F. M. Steichen and R. Welter, eds.), pp. 192–199. Quality Medical Publishing, St. Louis.
16. Jones, D. B., Wu, J. S., and Soper, N. J. (1997). Laparoscopic pancreaticoduodenectomy in the porcine model. *Surg. Endosc.* **11,** 326–330.
17. Srinivasan, A., Trus, T. L., Conrad, A. J., and Scarbrough, T. J. (1999). Common laparoscopic procedures in swine: A review. *J. Invest. Surg.* **12**(1), 5–14.
18. Scott, D. J., Provost, D. A., Huber, P. J., Guo, W. A., Tesfay, S. T., and Jones, D. B. (1999). Comparison of laparoscopic versus hand-assisted Roux-Y gastric bypass. *8th Int. Mtg. Laparoendoscopic Surgeons, SLS Ann. Mtg. Endo Expo 4 December, 1999*, New York, New York.
19. Scott, D. J., Provost, D. A., and Jones, D. B. (2000). Laparoscopic Roux-en-Y bypass for morbid obesity. *Surg. Rounds* **23**(4), 177–189.
20. Brunt, L. M., Jones, D. B., Wu, J. S., Quasebarth, M. A., Meininger, T., and Soper, N. J. (1997). Experimental development of an endoscopic approach to neck exploration and parathyroidectomy. *Surgery* **122**(5), 893–901.
21. Jones, D. B., Thompson, R. W., Olin, J. M., Meininger, T. A., Soper, N. J., and Rubin, B. G. (1996). Comparison of transperitoneal and retroperitoneal approaches of laparoscopic-assisted aorta-femoral bypass in a porcine model. *J. Vasc. Surg.* **23**(3), 466–471.
22. Brunt, L. M., Jones, D. B., Wu, J. S., Brunt, E. M., and Radford, D. M. (1998). Endoscopic axillary lymph node dissection: An experimental study in human cadavers. *J. Am. Coll. Surg.* **187,** 158–163.
23. Jones, D. B., Brewer, J. D., Meininger, T. A., and Soper, N. J. (1995). Sutured or fibrin-glued laparoscopic choledochojejunostomy. *Surg. Endosc.* **9,** 1020–1027.
24. Scott, D. J., Young, W. N., Watumull, L. M., *et al.* (2000). Development of an *in vivo* tumor mimic model for learning radiofrequency ablation. *Surg. Endosc.* **14,** 217.
25. Jones, D. B., Brewer, J. D., and Soper, N. J. (1996). The influence of three-dimensional video systems on laparoscopic task performance. *Surg. Laparosc. Endosc.* **6**(3), 191–197.
26. Luttmann, D. R., Jones, D. B., and Soper, N. J. (1996). Teleproctoring laparoscopic operations, off-the-shelf technology. *In* "Transforming Medicine" (S. J. Weghorst, H. B. Sieburg, and K. S. Morgan, eds.), pp. 313–318. IOS Press and Ohmsha, Amsterdam.
27. Gould, S. W. T., Gedroyce, W., and Darzi, A. (1999). Laparoscopic surgery in a 0.5-t interventional magnetic resonance unit. *Surg. Endosc.* **13,** 604–610.
28. Scott, D. J., Rege, R. V., Tesfay, S. T., and Jones, D. B. (2000). Development of a laparoscopic TEP hernia repair simulator for training surgery residents. *Surg. Endosc.* **14,** 217.
29. Scott, D. J., Bergen, P. C., Euhus, D. M., Guo, W. A., Jeyarajah, R., Laycock, R., Rege, R. V., Tesfay, S. T., Thompson, W. M., Valentine, R. J., and Jones, D. B. (1999). Intense laparoscopic skills training improves operative performance of surgery residents. *Surg. Forum* **L,** 670–671.
30. Reznik, R., Regehr, G., MacRae, H., *et al.* (1997). Testing technical skill via an innovative "bench station" examination. *Am. J. Surg.* **173,** 226-30.
31. Jones, D. B., Callery, M. P., and Soper, N. J. (1996). Strangulated incisional hernia at trocar site. *Surg. Laparosc. Endosc.* **6**(2), 152–154.
32. Alexanader, R. J. T., Jaques, B. C., and Mitchell, K. G. (1993). Laparoscopically assisted colectomy and wound recurrence. *Lancet* **341,** 249–250.
33. Fleshman, J. W., Nelson, H., Peters, W. R., *et al.* (1996). Early results of laparoscopic surgery for colorectal cancer: retrospective analysis of 372 patients treated by clinical outcomes of surgical therapy (COST) study group. *Dis. Colon Rectum* **39,** 53–58.
34. Jones, D. B., Dunnegan, D. L., Brewer, J. D., and Soper, N. J. (1995). The influence of intraoperative gallbladder perforation on long-term outcome after laparoscopic cholecystectomy. *Surg. Endosc.* **9,** 977–980.
35. Milsom, J. W., Bohm, B., Hammerhofer, K. A., Fazio, V., Steiger, E., and Elson, P. (1998). A prospective randomized trial comparing laparoscopic versus conventional techniques in colorectal cancer surgery: A preliminary report. *J. Am. Coll. Surg.* **187,** 46–54.
36. Stocchi, L., and Nelson, H. (1998). Laparoscopic colectomy for colon cancer: Trial update. *Surg. Oncol.* **68,** 255–267.
37. Fitzgibbons, R. J., Camps, J., Cornet, D., Nguyen, N. X., *et al.* (1998). Laparoscopic inguinal herniorrhaphy: Results of a multicenter trial. *Ann. Surg.* **221,** 3–13.
38. Jones, S. B., and Jones, D. B. (1998). Extending the limits: Minimally invasive surgery. *Curr. Opin. Anesthesiol.* **11,** 629–636.

45

Experimental Models and Endpoints for Studies of Intestinal Ischemia–Reperfusion Injury

Joseph Murphy and Richard H. Turnage

Department of Surgery, University of Texas Southwestern Medical Center and the Veterans Affairs North Texas Health Care System, Dallas, Texas 75216

I. Overview

Ischemia–reperfusion injury is an important cause of morbidity and mortality for surgical patients and thus it is a particularly relevant topic for research by surgical investigators. In its simplest terms, ischemia is defined as a reduction in blood flow to a given tissue or organ that results in an imbalance between oxygen and nutrient consumption and delivery. Restoration of perfusion, termed reperfusion, restores the flow of oxygen and nutrients to the ischemic tissue and facilitates the clearance of metabolic waste. Depending principally on the duration of ischemia (and the metabolic requirements of the tissue), the restoration of blood flow either may abrogate the ischemic injury or, in the case of longer periods of ischemia, may enhance the local inflammatory response and exacerbate tissue loss.

At rest, the gastrointestinal tract receives 10–15% of the total cardiac output, 70–90% of which supplies the mucosa and submucosa. Under normal conditions, splanchnic perfusion is regulated by local mediators such as the vasodilators adenosine, nitric oxide, prostaglandins E_2 and I_2, and histamine. Stimulation of the sympathetic nervous system activates adrenergic receptors within the splanchnic circulation, resulting in vasoconstriction. Circulating mediators such as the gastrointestinal hormones gastrin, cholecystokinin, and glucagon increase splanchnic blood flow whereas angiotensin II is a potent vasoconstrictor. During reperfusion inflammatory mediators may directly impair splanchnic microvascular perfusion by mechanically occluding the microvasculature (e.g., neutrophils or platelets) or they may alter the release of paracrine vasoconstrictive and vasodilatory mediators to favor local vasoconstriction.

II. Clinical Relevance

The reactivity of the splanchnic vascular bed to circulating and local paracrine vasoconstrictors and the sensitivity of the intestinal mucosa to reduced oxygen and nutrient delivery makes it particularly susceptible to hypoperfusion and subsequent reperfusion injury. Classically reperfusion injury follows the restoration of blood flow to the intestine on removal of a vascular clamp from the aorta or the superior mesenteric artery (SMA) during vascular reconstructive operations. Perhaps a more important cause of reperfusion injury is the restoration of systemic perfusion in patients suffering hypovolemic or cardiogenic shock.

The clinical manifestations of intestinal ischemia–reperfusion injury are primarily dependent on the duration and severity of the underlying ischemia. The classic clinical presentation of midabdominal pain out of proportion to the physical findings has been well described for patients with acute intestinal ischemia (e.g., following embolic occlusion of the SMA). Prolonged ischemia (with or without reperfusion) may be associated with transmural necrosis of the intestinal wall with perforation, peritonitis, and death.

Even relatively modest periods of ischemia (e.g., 1 hr) may be associated with altered intestinal epithelial integrity (1). This finding has lead to a hypothesis relating splanchnic ischemia–reperfusion injury to the pathogenesis of the systemic sepsis syndrome and multiple organ failure in critically ill patients (2–4). This hypothesis has been supported by several clinical studies demonstrating enhanced intestinal permeability following injury (5, 6) and numerous laboratory studies (7, 8) demonstrating the translocation of enteric flora into the mesenteric lymphatics sand systemic circulation following injury.

III. Characteristics of Intestinal Ischemia–Reperfusion Injury

A. Intestinal Injury

1. Functional Characteristics

The principal physiologic characteristics of intestinal ischemia–reperfusion injury are impaired microvascular and epithelial barrier function. As such, investigators have targeted these parameters as endpoints in studies examining the pathophysiology of intestinal reperfusion injury and the effectiveness of therapeutic interventions. Commonly employed parameters (and corresponding assays) of intestinal reperfusion injury are described in subsequent sections of this chapter and are shown in Table I.

2. Morphologic Characteristics

The histologic features of intestinal ischemia–reperfusion injury have been well described (9) and are shown in Fig. 1. As is apparent from these photomicrographs, the principal morphologic site of intestinal ischemia–reperfusion injury is the mucosa, with epithelial sloughing from the villi, mucosal edema, neutrophil infiltration, and hemorrhage into the lumen (10, 11). Although various grading scales have been utilized to describe, compare, and quantitate the degree of mucosal injury associated with ischemia–reperfusion injury, most are based on the original observations of Chiu *et al.* (9) (Table II).

B. Systemic Inflammatory Response and Remote Organ Injury

Intestinal ischemia–reperfusion incites a generalized inflammatory response characterized by the appearance of activated complement fragments, neutrophils, eicosanoids, endotoxin, and cytokines within the circulation (12–15). In addition to exacerbating the local intestinal injury, these mediators lead to the generation of paracrine proinflammatory and vasoactive substances in remote organs. As such, animal models of intestinal ischemia–reperfusion injury have been used to study the pathophysiology of systemic sepsis syndrome and multiple organ failure syndrome. Some of the mediators that have been most commonly incriminated in the pathophysiology of intestinal ischemia–reperfusion injury are enumerated in Table III. Many of these substances direct, amplify, and disseminate the local and systemic inflammatory response. For example, in addition to directly injuring tissue through the peroxidation of plasma membranes, oxygen-derived free radicals (ODFRs) have been shown to be important chemotactic substances for neutrophils, contribute to the activation of complement, and are at least in part responsible for the impairment of the compensatory release of the potent vasodilator prostacyclin (PGI_2). These relationships highlight the redundancy in these proinflammatory systems and serve to reiterate the difficulties in devising therapeutic strategies to abrogate the systemic consequences of this and other "local" inflammatory states.

This generalized inflammatory state culminates in injury to the lungs, liver, heart, and kidneys (12). The pathophysiologic effects of intestinal ischemia–reperfusion injury on the function of these organs are summarized in Fig. 2a–c. Of these remote organ injuries, the pulmonary injury is best

Table I Functional Parameters of Intestinal Ischemia–Reperfusion Injury and Commonly Used Techniques for Their Measurement

Dysfunction	Measurement technique
Microvascular	
Enhanced permeability	
	Quantitation of fluid and protein extravasation
	Edema indices
	Evans Blue dye
	^{125}I-labeled albumin
	Permeability coefficients
	Osmotic reflection coefficient
	Capillary filtration coefficient
	Wet to dry weight ratio
Altered microvascular integrity	
	Quantitation of red blood cell extravasation
	Extravasation of radiolabeled red blood cells
Impaired perfusion	
	Quantitation of superior mesenteric artery blood flow
	Doppler flow probes
	Quantitation of tissue perfusion
	Radiolabeled or colorimetric microspheres
Epithelial barrier	
Altered epithelial permeability	
	Quantitation of intravascular or interstitial markers in the intestinal lumen
	Flux of ^{51}Cr-labeled EDTA into the intestinal lumen
	Flux of radiolabeled albumin into the intestinal lumen
Translocation of enteric bacteria	
	Culture of enteric organisms from the systemic circulation or mesenteric lymph nodes
	Presence of radiolabeled enteric organisms in the systemic circulation or mesenteric lymph nodes

characterized with pathophysiologic and ultrastructural features of the acute lung injury and acute respiratory distress syndrome seen in critically ill patients (13,16).

IV. In Vivo Models of Intestinal Ischemia–Reperfusion Injury

Animal studies of the pathophysiology of intestinal ischemia–reperfusion injury have included models of global ischemia–reperfusion (e.g., hemorrhagic shock and resuscitation), visceral and skeletal muscle ischemia–reperfusion (e.g., occlusion of the suprarenal aorta with a microvascular clip), and isolated intestinal ischemia–reperfusion (e.g., occlusion of the superior mesenteric artery with a microvascular clip). These experimental models are summarized in Table IV; endpoints utilized in these studies include measures of intestinal epithelial barrier integrity, microvascular permeability, and blood flow. Commonly used assays for each of these endpoints are shown in Tables I and V.

A. Feline in Vivo Perfused Intestine Model

This commonly used experimental preparation allows for the relatively precise quantitation of splanchnic microvascular permeability and splanchnic arterial blood flow. Furthermore, it is a commonly used preparation for intravital microscopy. In this model, adult cats (2 to 3 kg) are fasted for 24 hr and then anesthetized initially with ketamine hydrochloride. Central venous access is obtained by placing a cannula in either the femoral vein or the jugular vein, after which anesthesia is maintained by the intravenous administration of pentobarbital sodium. A tracheostomy is performed to facilitate breathing and mechanical ventilation should the animal become apneic. Systemic arterial pressure is monia b c

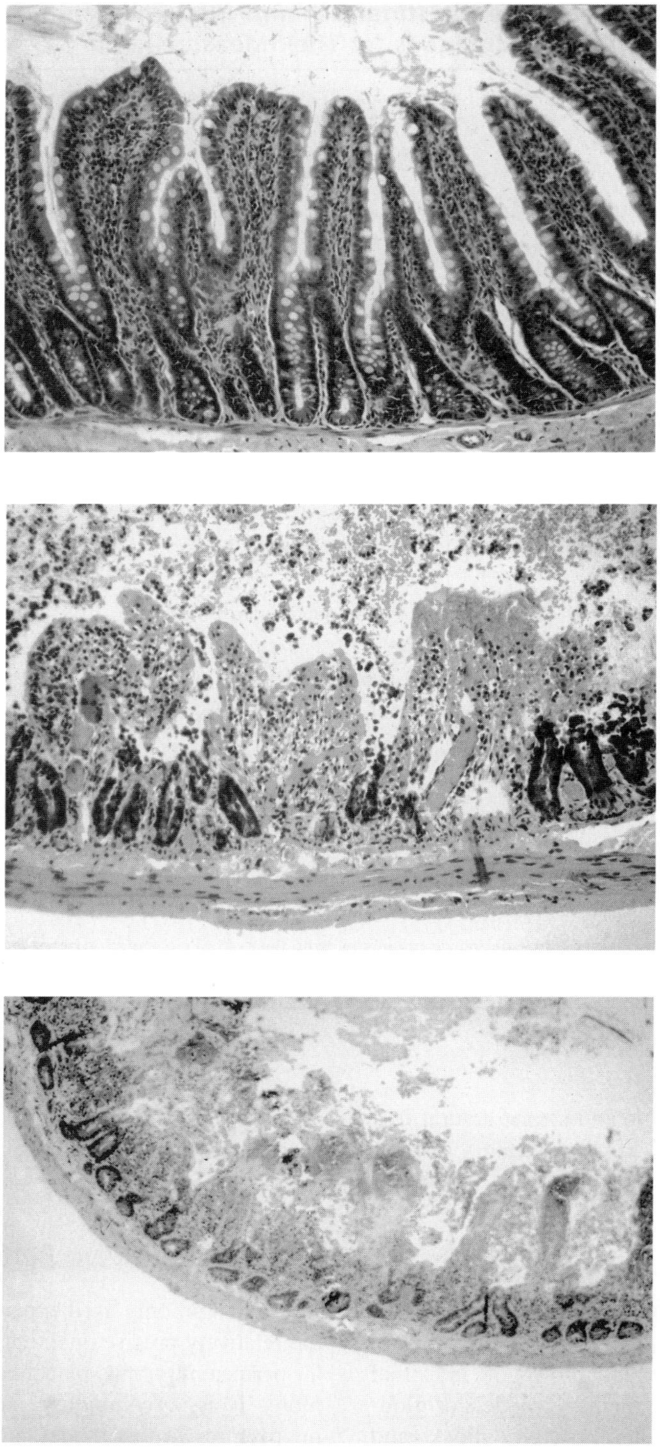

Figure 1 Histologic features of intestinal ischemia–reperfusion injury. (a) Photomicrograph of normal rat ileum. (b) Photomicrograph of rat ileum following 120 min of intestinal ischemia induced by occluding the superior mesenteric artery with a microvascular clip; release of the clip allowed reperfusion for 60 min. (c) Photomicrograph of rat ileum following hemorrhage and resuscitation in which a rat was bled to an arterial blood pressure of 30 mmHg. This was maintained for 30 min, after which the shed blood was reinfused; 60 min later the intestine was sampled. Hematoxylin–eosin staining.

Table II Morphologic Grading Scale for Intestinal Ischemia–Reperfusion Injury[a]

Scale	Characteristic
Grade 0	Normal mucosal villi
Grade 1	Development of subepithelial space usually at the apex of the villus, with capillary congestion
Grade 2	Extension of the subepithelial space with moderate lifting of the epithelial layer from the lamina propria
Grade 3	Massive epithelial lifting down the sides of villi; a few tips may be denuded
Grade 4	Denuded villi with lamina propria and dilated capillaries exposed; increased cellularity of lamina propria may be noted
Grade 5	Digestion and disintegration of lamina propria; hemorrhage and ulceration

[a]From Chiu *et al.* (9).

tored via a catheter in the right femoral artery. The animal's body temperature is maintained at 37°C with a thermistor-controlled infrared lamp. The animal is heparinized by the intravenous administration of 1000 units/kg of heparin.

A midline laparotomy is performed and a segment of ileum is delivered through the incision. An arterial circuit is established between the SMA and the femoral artery. Superior mesenteric artery blood flow is continuously monitored by an electromagnetic flowmeter connected to a probe positioned within the arterial circuit; SMA pressure is measured via a transducer attached to a side port in the flow probe or via a T-tube interposed within the arterial circuit. Partial occlusion of the arterial circuit with a C-clamp results in ischemia; release of the clamp allows reperfusion. Commonly utilized durations of ischemia and reperfusion range from 60 to 240 min of ischemia and 60 to 240 min of reperfusion. Commonly utilized ischemic perfusion pressures range from 0 to 30 mmHg.

B. Feline Model of Splanchnic Artery Occlusion

Aoki *et al.* (25) utilized a feline model of visceral ischemia–reperfusion injury in which the celiac, SMA, and inferior mesenteric arteries of adult cats were occluded by atraumatic vascular clamps. This preparation has the benefits of a large animal model but avoids the technical manipulations required to establish an arterial circuit as described above. In this model, adult male cats (2.5–3.5 kg) are anesthetized with pentobarbital sodium (30 mg/kg IV) and a tracheostomy is performed to facilitate mechanical ventilation. Polyethylene catheters (PE-90) are placed into the right femoral vein and artery. A midline laparotomy is performed and the celiac, SMA, and inferior mesenteric arteries are isolated near their aortic origins. The animals are then heparinized and each of these arteries are occluded with atraumatic vascular clamps for 120 min; removal of the

Table III Proinflammatory and Vasoactive Mediators Postulated to Be Involved in the Pathophysiology of Local and Remote Organ Injury during Intestinal Ischemia–Reperfusion Injury

Factor	Description
Paracrine	
	Oxygen-derived free radicals (superoxide anion, hydrogen peroxide, hydroxyl radical, nitric oxide)
	Arachidonic acid derivatives (prostacyclin, thromboxane, leukotrienes C4 and B4)
	Platelet-activating factor
	Cytokines (tumor necrosis factor-α, interleukin-1, -6, and -8)
Circulating	
	Neutrophils
	Complement
	Lipopolysaccharide
	Platelets

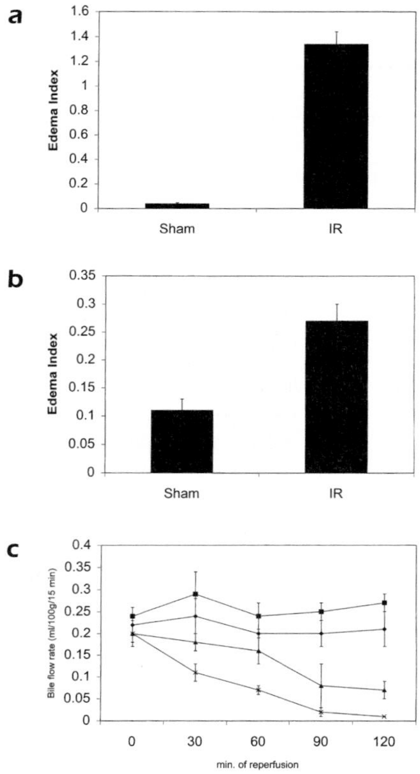

Figure 2 Local and remote organ injury associated with intestinal ischemia–reperfusion injury. In each of these studies a Sprague–Dawley rat underwent 120 min of intestinal ischemia by placing a microvascular clip across the origin of the superior mesenteric artery. At 60 min after release of the clip, injury was assessed in the intestine, lung, and liver. The intestinal injury (a) and pulmonary injury (b) were assessed by measuring the extravasation of radiolabeled albumin into the interstitium of these organs. An edema index was derived by determining the ratio of radioactivity within the intestine or lung to that of 1 ml of blood. Hepatic injury (c) was determined by quantitating bile flow rates for animals undergoing 120 (x), 90 (△), 60 (◇), or 0 (□) min of intestinal ischemia.

occlusive clamps allows reperfusion for 120 min prior to sampling of blood and tissue.

C. Rat Model of SMA Occlusion

This is the most commonly employed model of intestinal ischemia–reperfusion injury and involves occlusion of the SMA of a rat with a microvascular clip. There have been numerous permutations of this protocol and those most commonly employed are outlined below. In general these protocols vary according to the duration of ischemia and reperfusion, the anesthetic chosen, the use of heparin, and ligation of collateral vascular arcades. The most appropriate model for a given experiment depends on the pathophysiologic process of most interest to the investigator. For example, shorter periods of ischemia are most appropriate to study the local intestinal injury whereas longer periods of ischemia–reperfusion injury allow examination of the resultant systemic inflammatory response and remote organ injury.

1. Guice–Oldham–Turnage Group

In this protocol (12,13,15,16,26–29) pathogen-free male Sprague–Dawley rats (100–150 g) undergo 120 min of intestinal ischemia and 60 min of reperfusion. In early experiments the animals were anesthetized with ketamine hydrochloride; subsequent studies employed pentobarbital and most recently we have utilized methoxyflurane. In this protocol a midline laparotomy is performed and the proximal SMA is occluded with a microvascular clip. The intestine is rendered ischemic for 120 min, after which the clip is released, allowing reperfusion for 60 min. Reperfusion is confirmed by observing the return of pulsations within the vasa recta. This degree of intestinal reperfusion injury has been consistently associated with activation of the systemic inflammatory response and intestinal, hepatic, renal, and pulmonary injury (Fig. 2a–c). The 12-hr mortality rate for this model of severe intestinal reperfusion injury is 100%. Time-matched, sham-operated animals serve as controls; these animals undergo laparotomy and dissection of the proximal SMA without occlusion.

2. Hechtman Group

These investigators (30) have employed a model of 1 hr of intestinal ischemia and 3 hr of reperfusion. In their studies, 500-g male Sprague–Dawley rats are anesthetized with pentobarbital sodium, after which the tail vein and right carotid artery are cannulated. A midline laparotomy is performed and collateral vessels from the caudal mesenteric and celiac axis are ligated. The proximal SMA is occluded with a microvascular clip and the incision is closed. After 1 hr the abdomen is opened and the microvascular clip is removed. The incision is again closed and the animals are kept supine for the duration of the experiment. Body temperature is maintained with warming pads and blood sampling losses are replaced volume for volume with 0.9% saline. These investigators indicated that a 60-min period of ischemia was chosen because there was no mortality during the 3-hr period of reperfusion, whereas a 90-min period of ischemia resulted in a 20% mortality. Sham-operated animals were treated in an identical fashion with the omission of vascular occlusion.

3. Horton Group

This group (32–35) utilizes a very brief period of ischemia (20 min) followed by 30–120 min of reperfusion. In this experimental model, adult Sprague–Dawley rats are anesthetized with methoxyflurane anesthesia and polyethylene cannulas are inserted into the left carotid artery (to measure arterial pressure) and the external jugular vein (for

Table IV Summary of Advantages and Disadvantages of Commonly Employed Models of Intestinal Ischemia–Reperfusion Injury

Model	Common uses	Advantage	Disadvantage	Expense
Feline *in vivo* perfused intestine	Studies of the physiologic effects of reperfusion on the bowel	Allows quantitation of the permeability characteristics of the intestinal microvasculature	Increased expense; technically demanding and labor-intensive preparation	$$$$
Rat model of superior mesenteric artery occlusion	Studies of the systemic inflammation and local intestinal and remote organ injury	Technically easy to perform; local and remote organ effects and systemic inflammatory response well characterized	Difficult to precisely quantitate the permeability characteristics of the microvasculature; unable to serially sample blood	$$
Mouse model of supraceliac aortic occlusion	Remote organ injury model	Allows use of genetically manipulated populations, e.g., gene knockouts	Technically difficult to perform due to small animal size; relatively little published description of systemic inflammatory response and local and remote organ injury	$$
Rat model of hemorrhage and resuscitation	Global ischemia–reperfusion injury; studies of intestinal contribution to systemic inflammation associated with hemorrhagic shock	Technically easy to perform; systemic inflammatory response and remote organ effects well characterized; models a common clinical phenomenon	Global injury, not localized to the intestine; difficult to serially sample blood	$$

Table V Summary of Advantages and Disadvantages of Commonly Employed Endpoints for Studying Intestinal Ischemia–Reperfusion Injury

Endpoint	Common uses	Advantage	Disadvantage	Expense
Microvascular injury				
Edema index ^{125}I-labeled albumin Evans Blue dye	Simultaneous assessment of local and remote organ microvascular protein leak	Ease of performance, reproducibility, long published record of its use	Does not separate microvascular permeability effects from other causes of edema formation—hydrostatic and oncotic effects; radiation exposure	$–$$
Edema index Intravital microscopy	Simultaneous assessment of neutrophil–endothelial cell interaction and microvascular protein leak	Allows simultaneous assessment of leukocyte–endothelial interaction and protein leak	Technically demanding; large startup costs for intravital microscopy; relatively few laboratories have requisite equipment	$$$$
Permeability coefficients Osmotic reflection coefficient Capillary filtration coefficient	Quantitation of the effect of ischemia–reperfusion on microvascular protein permeability	"Precise" estimate of microvascular permeability	Technically demanding experimental preparation; requires large animal model; relatively few laboratories have requisite equipment and expertise	$$$$
Epithelial injury				
Light microscopy and morphometrics	Quantitation of light microscopic findings associated with ischemia–reperfusion injury	Ease of performance	Subjective unless carefully performed; descriptive, not functional	$$$
Blood to lumen clearance of 51Cr-labeled EDTA	Quantitation of the functional effect of ischemia–reperfusion injury on epithelial barrier function	Ease of performance; describes functional integrity of mucosal barrier	Radiation exposure; unclear how this relates to the translocation of endotoxin, bacteria	$$

acquisition of blood samples and the administration of drugs and fluid). Heparin (5000 units/kg) is then injected intravenously and the animals undergo a midline laparotomy. A loop of intestine is exposed and the collateral vascular arcades to this segment of bowel are ligated. The SMA is occluded with an atraumatic microvascular clip; 20 min later the clip is released and perfusion is reestablished.

D. Mouse Model of Supraceliac Aortic Occlusion

This experimental model (36) seeks to reproduce the profound visceral and skeletal muscle reperfusion injury (and hence systemic inflammatory response) associated with cross-clamping of the supraceliac aorta. The use of a murine experimental model allows one to take advantage of the availability of genetically manipulated animals. Unfortunately the small size of these animals presents significant technical limitations not associated with larger animals, including the rat.

In the studies described by Welborn *et al.* (36), male and female C57BL/6 mice (20–25 g) are anesthetized with sodium pentobarbital (35 mg/kg intraperitoneally) and undergo a midline laparotomy. The intestine is exteriorized and the supraceliac aorta, the celiac axis, and the SMA are identified. The supraceliac aorta is dissected just as it emerges from below the diaphragm and is occluded by a microvascular clip. Visceral ischemia is confirmed by noting a cessation of pulsations in the mesenteric arcades as well as the loss of liver volume, blanching of the liver, and darkening of the spleen. The abdominal wall is then closed to minimize evaporative fluid loss and the animals receive 50 ml/kg of an isotonic salt solution subcutaneously. After 30 min of visceral ischemia, the abdomen is reopened and the supraceliac aortic clip is removed. Reperfusion is confirmed by noting a return of pulsatile blood flow to the abdominal viscera. The abdominal incisions are again closed and the animals are given an additional 50 ml/kg of isotonic salt solution. After 2–4 hr the animals are sacrificed and blood and tissue are sampled. Controls for these experiments include animals undergoing laparotomy and aortic dissection without supraceliac aortic occlusion and those undergoing laparotomy with occlusion of the infrarenal aorta. In all cases, the animals receive the same volume of normal saline and are treated in a manner identical to the animals undergoing supraceliac ischemia–reperfusion.

E. Rat Model of Hemorrhage and Resuscitation

The contribution of intestinal reperfusion injury to the systemic inflammatory state associated with global ischemia–reperfusion injury (such as that accompanying resuscitation from hemorrhage) has received considerable interest (37–42). In these studies investigators have rendered animals hypotensive for varying periods of time and then evaluated the contribution of the intestinal injury to the systemic inflammatory response.

In this model, Sprague–Dawley rats are anesthetized with methoxyfluorane inhalation and the femoral artery is cannulated with a polyethylene catheter (PE-20) for constant monitoring of arterial pressure. The animals are heparinized and randomized to either a hemorrhage and resuscitation group or a control group. The experimental group consists of animals that are bled via the femoral arterial cannula to a mean arterial pressure of 30 mmHg. The animal is maintained hypotensive for 30 to 45 min, after which the shed heparinized blood is reinfused to restore systemic blood pressure to normal levels. The animals are then observed for up to 120 min, after which measurements are taken. The control group consists of animals that are instrumented but not bled. These animals receive identical amounts of anesthetic and are time-matched compared with the experimental group.

V. Considerations for Experimental Models of Intestinal Ischemia–Reperfusion Injury

A. Anesthetics

It is well recognized from clinical practice that anesthetic agents influence cardiac function and splanchnic blood flow. A variety of investigators have demonstrated that pentobarbital, isoflurane, and halothane decrease cardiac output whereas the reported effects on splanchnic perfusion have been variable (43–46). Myers *et al.* (46) compared methoxyflurane inhalation and the intraperitoneal administration of pentobarbital in the rat model of hemorrhage and resuscitation described earlier. They found that both methoxyflurane and pentobarbital decreased systemic arterial blood pressure and SMA and aortic blood flow by 50% in control animals, whereas arterial pressure and SMA blood flow were significantly less in those animals receiving pentobarbital when compared to those receiving methoxyflurane. This finding was consistent with an earlier report from their laboratory in which they found that bacterial translocation was more likely to occur following hemorrhagic shock if the experimental animal had been anesthetized with pentobarbital in comparison to methoxyflurane (47).

B. Collaterals

Collateral arterial pathways may maintain, at least in part, perfusion to segments of the small intestine despite occlusion of the SMA (48). This becomes important as one attempts fine control of the amount of perfusion to a specific segment of the intestine, particularly at the extremities of the ischemic injury. Horton *et al.* (32–35) and Hechtman *et al.* (30) have considered this in their experimental models by ligating potential sites of collateral arterial flow. As alluded to by Horton *et al.* (32–35) this has allowed a much more severe degree of intestinal ischemia despite a significantly shortened period of arterial occlusion. Regardless of the approach one takes, it is important to standardize the segment of bowel studied. In our laboratory this is performed by routinely taking tissue samples from a segment of intestine a fixed distance from the ileocecal valve (generally 2 cm).

C. Hypovolemia

Intestinal ischemia–reperfusion injury is characterized by activation of a systemic inflammatory response and a diffuse microvascular "leak." The extravasation of fluid and protein from the vascular space results in intravascular volume depletion—a condition that has been previously shown to exacerbate the local and remote organ effects of intestinal ischemia–reperfusion injury (49). In our studies involving the rat model of SMA occlusion we found that the provision of 40 ml/kg/hr (about 6 ml/hr) was required to restore intravascular volume to preinjury levels. This volume of lactated Ringer's solution reduced the intestinal injury by 50% and restored bile flow rates to preinjury levels (49).

VI. Endpoints for in Vivo Studies of Intestinal Ischemia–Reperfusion Injury

A. Measurement of Microvascular Injury

1. Edema Index

Reperfusion-induced intestinal (and pulmonary) microvascular dysfunction has been quantitated by measuring the movement of labeled proteins from the intravascular to the interstitial compartments. The two most commonly employed markers are radiolabeled albumin (^{125}I-labeled albumin) and Evans Blue dye. In either case, an edema index is derived by relating the concentration of labeled protein in the interstitial space of an injured tissue to that within the blood. The principal advantage of this methodology is the ease of performance with standard laboratory equipment and the ability to assess the protein "leak" in several tissues simultaneously. The principal disadvantage is that this methodology describes only the movement of protein across the microvascular barrier and does not define the permeability characteristics of the microvasculature. It should be recalled that the movement of fluid and protein into the interstitium compartment is determined by both the permeability characteristics of the microvascular membrane as well as the overall balance of Starlings forces (hydrostatic and oncotic pressures) between the interstitial and vascular compartments. Edema indices describe the overall flux of protein without determining the factor responsible for this movement.

2. Radiolabeled Albumin

This assay has been used most commonly with small animal models such as the rat model of tissue ischemia–reperfusion injury (13, 14, 30, 50–54). At 30 to 60 min prior to the time in which the injury is to be assessed, the animal receives 800,000 to 1,000,000 counts per minute ^{125}I-labeled bovine serum albumin intravenously in 1 ml of sterile saline. At the conclusion of the experiment, 1 ml of blood is drawn from the aorta or vena cava, and the small intestine and its supporting mesentery are excised *en bloc*. The SMA is cannulated and the blood retained within the splanchnic microvasculature is removed by gently infusing 10 ml of 0.9% saline solution. The radioactivity in a uniform segment of intestine (1–2 cm) and 1 ml of blood is then determined in a gamma scintillation counter and the ratio of intestine to blood counts per minute is determined. The advantages of this technique include the ease of performance and reproducibility, although the use of radioactivity detracts somewhat from the appeal of this methodology.

3. Evans Blue Dye

The use of Evans Blue dye as a marker of plasma protein flux has been shown to compare favorably both *in vivo* and *in vitro* with techniques utilizing ^{125}I-labeled albumin (55–57). Evans Blue dye is a vital dye that, when injected intravenously, binds avidly to plasma proteins. As such, it has been used as a marker for protein extravasation in models of altered microvascular permeability.

The assay is performed by infusing 30 mg/kg of Evans Blue dye intravenously about 30 min prior to the time at which microvascular permeability is to be measured. At the completion of the experiment, 1 ml of blood is withdrawn from the abdominal aorta and the intestine is excised *en bloc* as described above. The SMA is then cannulated and the blood remaining within the vasculature is removed by gently infusing 10 ml of saline. A uniform segment of intestine (2 cm) is excised and then weighed. The tissue is then placed in 5 ml of formamide and homogenized for 2 min. The tissue suspension is then incubated at 37°C for 16 hr and centrifuged at 5000 *g* for 30 min. The dye concentration of the eluate is measured spectrophotometrically at 620 nm and expressed as milligrams of dye per gram of wet (or dry) tissue weight. A permeability index can also be calculated as described above in which the concentration of dye within the intestine is standardized to the serum concentration.

B. Estimation of Microvascular Permeability Coefficients

Larger animal models (particularly the feline model) have been employed to describe the effect of inflammation or injury on the permeability characteristics of a particular microvascular bed. In general these models have been utilized to determine the osmotic reflection coefficient and the capillary filtration coefficient of isolated, perfused organ preparations.

1. Osmotic Reflection Coefficient

The osmotic reflection coefficient (σ_d) (58–61) estimates the selectivity of the microvascular barrier to solutes (generally proteins) and is one of the best indicators of microvascular permeability (61). It is estimated using the steady-state relationship between lymph to plasma protein concentration ratio (C_L/C_P) and lymph flow. As lymph flow increases, C_L/C_P decreases rapidly (filtration dependent) and becomes relatively constant as C_L/C_P approaches a minimal value (filtration independent), during which time lymph flow is high. Theoretical and experimental evidence suggests that $\sigma_d = 1 - C_L/C_P$ when C_L/C_P is filtration rate independent (59, 60).

The experimental preparation was described earlier (feline *in vivo* perfused intestine model). Briefly, mesenteric lymph is collected for measurement of lymph volume and protein concentration by cannulating the large lymphatic vessel draining the mesentery of the isolated intestinal segment. The remaining portions of the mesenteric pedicle are ligated to ensure that venous and lymphatic outflow represents total organ values. The superior mesenteric vein is cannulated with a large polyethylene catheter and the venous outflow is passed into a reservoir before being returned to the animal. The end of the venous outflow cannula is attached to a vertically positioned pulley system that allows venous outflow pressure to be set by adjusting the height of the reservoir. This pressure is monitored from a T connector located in the venous circuit. Heparinized blood from a freshly killed donor cat is used to prime the extracorporeal venous and arterial circuits.

In the studies described by Granger *et al.* (19), pressure within the SMA arterial circuit was reduced to 30–40 mmHg using an adjustable C clamp interposed within the arterial circuit. Arterial pressure was maintained at this level for 60 min, during which time lymph flow and C_L and C_P were determined at 15-min intervals. After 60 minutes of local arterial hypotension, the arterial clamp was released and the mesenteric lymph flow rate was increased by elevating the mesenteric venous pressure in 10-mmHg increments up to 40 mmHg. At each pressure level, intestinal venous pressure was maintained constant until all parameters were in a steady state, at which time lymph and plasma samples were acquired for protein concentration determination and lymph flow rates were measured to calculate $1 - \sigma$.

2. Intravital Microscopy

Neutrophils are an important pathogenic mediator of intestinal reperfusion injury and intravital microscopy has proved to be an invaluable tool in understanding the interaction between activated neutrophils and the microvascular endothelium (62–64). In these studies, the movement of fluorescently labeled albumin across the microvasculature into the interstitium is used to calculate an edema index relating the amount of extravasated protein to that remaining within the microvasculature (62).

The basic experimental preparation of large animals such as cats has been described by House and Lipowsky (63), whereas Gaboury *et al.* (64) modified the technique for rats. Regardless of the animal utilized the fundamentals of the procedure are similar. Briefly, the mesentery is draped over an optically clear viewing pedestal that allows for the transillumination of a 2- to 3-cm segment of tissue. The exposed bowel is draped with saline-soaked gauze while the remainder of the mesentery is covered with a plastic sheet. The exposed mesentery is suffused with warmed bicarbonate-buffered saline (pH 7.4) that is bubbled with a mixture of 5% O_2, 5% CO_2, and 90% N_2. The mesentery is transilluminated and viewed with an intravital microscope (×40 objective lens and ×10 eyepiece). Single unbranched venules (diameter 25–35 μm, length 250 μm) are observed through the microscope and the images are projected onto a color video monitor via a video camera mounted on the microscope.

To quantify albumin leakage across the mesenteric venule, 50 mg/kg fluorescein isothiocyanate (FITC)-labeled rat albumin is administered to the animals 10 min before each experiment. Fluorescence intensity (excitation wavelength, 420–490 nm; emission wavelength, 520 nm) is detected with a silicone-intensified target camera. The fluorescence intensities of FITC–albumin within three segments of the venule and three contiguous areas of perivenular interstitium are measured at various times after administration of FITC–albumin using a computer-assisted digital imaging processor. An index of vascular albumin leakage (edema index) is determined from the ratio of fluorescent intensity within the interstitium to that within the venule.

3. Measurement of Splanchnic Blood Flow

The reperfusion of ischemic intestine has important effects on microvascular blood flow, such that within minutes of reperfusion there is a profound reduction in splanchnic blood flow. Intestinal perfusion has been quantitated utilizing a variety of techniques, most commonly radiolabeled microspheres, intravital microscopy, and laser doppler velocimetry (techniques are discussed in detail in Chapter 73.

C. Measurement of Epithelial Injury

1. Morphometrics

The most commonly utilized method of characterizing the mucosal injury associated with intestinal ischemia–reperfusion injury is to describe the histopathologic findings seen with light microscopy. As indicated earlier, most injury grading scales are based on the original work of Chiu *et al.* (9) (Table II).

Careful and objective performance of tissue morphometry allows the investigator to discern relatively subtle differences in the epithelial injury that may result from a specific therapy or intervention. This is performed by prospectively identifying a uniform segment of intestine that is to be assessed (generally this is related to a specific distance from the ileocecal valve or the ligament of Treitz). The segment is excised and placed in 10% buffered formalin. It is embedded in paraffin, sectioned, and stained with hematoxylin and eosin. The tissues are then examined by a pathologist with experience in gastrointestinal pathology, and the injury is graded according to the scale established by Chiu *et al.* (9). The tissues are delivered to the pathologist such that there is no awareness of from which experimental group the sample is derived. In general, the pathologist will utilize a grid pattern to choose which fields to score. Five to 10 sections are examined per experimental animal and there are three to five animals in each experimental group. In addition to the morphometric description of the epithelial injury, representative photomicrographs are obtained and used to illustrate the relevant histopathologic findings to the reviewer.

2. Blood to Lumen Clearance of 51Cr-Labeled EDTA

Kubes *et al.* (65) have physiologically quantitated the integrity of the epithelial barrier by measuring the movement of ^{51}Cr-labeled EDTA from the intravascular space into the lumen of the injured bowel. The intravenous administration of ^{51}Cr-labeled EDTA results in almost instantaneous equilibration between the vascular and the interstitial spaces; disruption of the mucosal barrier results in the movement of ^{51}Cr-labeled EDTA into the intestinal lumen. This methodology has been employed in both large (21, 65) and small animal (35, 66) models. The animal preparation is as described above except that a segment of small intestine (10 to 15 cm for both the rat and the feline models) is isolated along with its vascular and lymphatic pedicle. The remainder of the small and large intestine is excised and both renal pedicles are ligated to prevent the excretion of ^{51}Cr-labeled EDTA into the urine. The isolated intestine and its mesenteric pedicle are kept moist with saline-soaked gauze and covered with a clear plastic sheet to minimize evaporation and tissue desiccation. The intestinal loop is cannulated and perfused with warmed Tyrode solution at a rate of 1 ml/min. ^{51}Cr-Labeled EDTA (100–150 μCi/kg) is injected intravenously 1 hr prior to the onset of ischemia to allow tissue equilibration of the ^{51}Cr-labeled EDTA. Immediately prior to the onset of ischemia the luminal perfusate is collected over three 10-min control periods, after which blood flow to the isolated segment of intestine is reduced. Following reperfusion, plasma and 2-ml aliquots of perfusate are collected and assayed for ^{51}Cr-labeled EDTA activity. The intestinal loop is then removed, rinsed, and weighed. The plasma to lumen clearance of ^{51}Cr-labeled EDTA is calculated as

$$\text{Clearance} = \frac{\text{cpm}_\text{p} \times \text{PR} \times 100}{\text{cpm}_\text{pl} \times \text{WT}},$$

where the clearance of ^{51}Cr-labeled EDTA is given in milliliters per minute per unit of tissue weight, cpm_p is the counts per minute per milliliter of perfusate, PR is perfusion rate, and WT is the weight of the intestinal segment in grams or milligrams, depending on the animal used.

VII. In Vitro Models of Intestinal Ischemia–Reperfusion Injury

Investigators have utilized cell culture systems to overcome the complexity of whole organ or *in vivo* models of tissue ischemia–reperfusion injury. There are advantages and uses of these experimental models:

1. Allow determination of the effects of ischemia–reperfusion injury on a specific cell type (e.g., epithelial versus endothelial).
2. Allow determination of the effect of ischemia–reperfusion injury on a particular cellular function (e.g., signal transduction, cellular metabolism, the synthesis of a particular protein).
3. Allow isolation of the specific effects of hypoxia–reoxygenation, distinct from effects of secondary pro- and antiinflammatory mediators.
4. Provide a uniform injury by precisely controlling oxygen and nutrient delivery to a specific population of cells.
5. Provide a mechanism to study the interaction between two specific cell types (e.g., neutrophils and endothelial cells).

Most of the studies to date have involved the use of either intestinally derived cells [e.g., Caco-2 (67), HT29 (68), or IEC-6 (69) cells] or vascular endothelial cells (e.g, human umbilical vein endothelial cells) that have been studied in either monolayer cultures and cell suspensions. The cells are rendered hypoxic by incubating them in an anaerobic incubator in which an oxygen tension near 0% can be maintained. Cell culture medium and buffers can be made hypoxic by bubbling 85% N_2, 10%H_2, and 5% CO_2 through the solution for 20–30 min. It generally takes about 20 min for oxygen levels in 100 ml of buffer to reach 0.1%. A pipette port/glove box and an airlock permit the maintenance of hypoxia during manipulation and sampling of the cells and their media. The media is maintained under hypoxic conditions by blowing O_2-free gas over its surface. It should be noted that this experimental preparation is more accurately defined as hypoxic (rather than anoxic) because of the difficulty in achieving and maintaining a truly anoxic environment. This necessitates the use of an oximeter to measure the amount of oxygen within the media during the experiments. Other biochemical characteristics of ischemia (e.g., acidosis, hypoglycemia, and the accumulation of metabolic wastes) can be mimicked *in vitro* by manipulation of the culture media. Reoxygenation is achieved by replacing the hypoxic media with one containing oxygen. Furthermore, exchange of the culture media allows the reintroduction of glucose, restoration of a normal pH, and the removal of metabolic wastes.

VIII. Endpoints for in Vitro Studies of Intestinal Ischemia–Reperfusion Injury

A. Cellular Injury

A variety of commonly used assays for quantitating cell injury and viability are applicable to models of *in vitro* ischemia–reperfusion injury. The most commonly employed assays are based on the uptake of vital dyes and the release of cytosolic enzymes by injured or dead cells.

B. Vital Dyes

The uptake of vital dyes, such as Trypan blue and Erythrosine B, is a commonly used assay to assess the integrity of the cell membrane (70). It is based on the ability of intact membranes to exclude these dyes. The principal limitations of these techniques include nonspecific staining of nuclear proteins and the binding of the stains to cell surfaces or culture media proteins.

C. Fluorescent Dyes

A variety of fluorescent compounds allow the discrimination of viable and nonviable cells (70, 71). In general, they are more reliable than vital dyes because of their simplicity of use, insensitivity to protein in the culture medium, and ultimately less interobserver variability. Fluorescein diacetate is a commonly used fluorescent dye that is cleaved by esterases within viable cells to liberate the fluorescent compound fluorescein. Thus viable cells retain the dye and fluoresce whereas nonviable cells do not. Fluorescein diacetate is not cytotoxic.

Another technique involving the use of two fluorescent dyes has been described: Hoechst 33258 (0.25 to 2 μg/ml) causes dead cells to fluoresce a brilliant blue and acridine orange (1.0 to 5.0 μg/ml) causes living cells to fluoresce green. These dyes permit the simultaneous observation of viable and nonviable cells. They are not cytotoxic and are unaffected by the presence of protein in the culture media.

D. Release of Lactate Dehydrogenase

Lactate dehydrogenase (LDH) is a ubiquitous intracellular cytoplasmic enzyme of high molecular weight. This property inhibits movement across the cell membrane unless the integrity of the cell is compromised. Thus an increase in extracellular LDH suggests cell membrane disruption and cell death. In that LDH is very easily measured, it is a very commonly used index of cell viability *in vitro*.

E. Mitochondrial Reduction of Tetrazolium Salt MTT

Cell viability can also be measured based on the reduction of the tetrazolium salt MTT [3-(4,5-dimethylthiazol-2-yl)-2,5 diphenyl tetrazolium bromide] to a formazan by the mitochondrium (72); formazan can then be measured spectrophotometrically. This assay is useful for the rapid determination of either intact cell viability or isolated mitochondrial function because tetrazolium salt reduction depends on a mitochondrial succinate tetrazolium reductase system.

F. Monolayer "Permeability"

The movement of labeled solutes across an intact cell monolayer has been used to model *in vitro* the effect of various proinflammatory substances on epithelial (69) and endothelial (73) barrier permeability. It should be noted, however, that *in vivo* the integrity of the endothelial and epithelial barriers is determined by many factors in addition to the continuity of the cell monolayer (e.g., basement membrane, composition of the interstitial compartment). Thus these models tend to overestimate the permeability of the microvascular membrane when compared with *in vivo* physiologic assessments (74). Nevertheless, the simplicity of these models and the ability to relate changes in cell shape, cytoskeleton, and function to monolayer integrity, and hence "permeability", have led to their frequent use.

To assess monolayer integrity *in vitro*, cells are typically grown to confluence on semiporous polycarbonate or polyester membranes of known pore size (0.3–0.45 μm) within the upper chamber of a "well within a well" or bicameral culture plate (67,69,75,76). The membranes are often coated with type 1 collagen, transferrin, albumin, or fibronectin to facilitate adhesion and confluent growth. "Permeability" of the monolayer may be quantitated by measuring the transepithelial or transendothelial electrical resistance across the cells or by measuring the movement of labeled proteins across the monolayer.

Transepithelial or transendothelial electrical resistance is measured in $\Omega \cdot cm^2$ as an alternating current is applied (160 μA) across the cells. Resistance across cell monolayers is calculated by subtracting the resistance for the membranes alone from the resistance from the membrane/monolayer and multiplying by the area of the membrane. Confluent monolayers of Caco-2 cells typically have resistance values of greater than 130 $\Omega \cdot cm^2$.

Monolayer integrity may be assessed by measuring the flux of labeled reagents across the confluent monolayers on the membrane. Typically transmonolayer migration of radiolabeled or fluorescently labeled proteins (albumin, inulin), complex carbohydrates (dextran), bacterial colony-forming foci, or dyes (phenol red) are assessed by sampling of the lower culture chamber media. Results of *in vitro* permeability investigations are reported in a multitude of forms: a percentage of the total label initially placed in the upper cell culture chamber; the absolute optical density of the lower chamber media sample; the milligrams/milliliter of accumulated labeled protein in the lower chamber; or by formula [permeability index (%) = experimental clearance − spontaneous clearance/clearance of membrane alone − spontaneous clearance] × 100.

IX. Summary

Intestinal ischemia–reperfusion injury induces both a local and systemic inflammatory response resulting in intestinal and remote organ injury. Reperfusion injury is a component of the pathophysiology of a variety of diseases commonly treated by surgeons and hence it is a very relevant topic for surgical investigators to study. Locally the intestinal injury is characterized by microvascular dysfunction (impaired perfusion, enhanced permeability, altered vascular integrity) and epithelial injury (enhanced permeability and morphologic change). A variety of large and small animal models have been developed to investigate the pathophysiology of intestinal ischemia–reperfusion. In general the larger animal models allow for the precise physiologic quantitation of microvascular barrier function; however, their expense and the technically demanding nature of these preparations have limited their widespread usage. In contrast, small animal models (most notably, rat models) are technically easy to perform; however, it is difficult to quantitate the physiologic forces responsible for edema formation. *In vitro* systems are available to assess the effect of various proinflammatory mediators on the integrity of a cell monolayer, but how this relates to *in vivo* conditions is speculative. The availability of these experimental models allows surgical investigators the capability to examine tissue reperfusion injury utilizing a variety of experimental systems with complementary degrees of control and clinical relevance.

References

1. Payne, D., and Kubes, P. (1993). Nitric oxide donors reduce the rise in reperfusion-induced intestinal mucosal permeability. *Am. J. Physiol.* **265,** G189–G195.
2. Deitch, E. A. (1992). Multiple organ failure: Pathophysiology and potential future therapy. *Ann. Surg.* **216,** 117–134.
3. Paterson, I. S., Klausner, J. M., Pugatch, R., Allen, P., Mannick, J. A., Shepro, D., and Hechtman, H. B. (1989). Non-cardiogenic pulmonary edema after abdominal aortic aneurysm surgery. *Ann. Surg.* **209,** 231–236.
4. Huber, T. S., Harward, T. R., Flynn, T. C., Albright, J. L., and Seeger, J. M. (1995). Operative mortality rates after elective infrarenal aortic reconstructions. *J. Vasc. Surg.* **22,** 287–293.
5. Ziegler, T. R., Smith, R. J., O'Dwyer, S. T., Demling, R. H., and Wilmore, D. W. (1988). Increased intestinal permeability associated with infection in burn patients. *Arch. Surg.* **123,** 1313–1319.
6. Deitch, E. A. (1990). Intestinal permeability is increased in burn patients shortly after injury. *Surgery* **107,** 411–416.
7. Deitch, E. A., Berg, R. D., and Specian R. D. (1988). Endotoxin promotes the translocation of bacteria from the gut. *Arch. Surg.* **122,** 185–190.
8. Baker, J. W., Deitch, E. A., Li, M., Berg, R. D., and Specian, R. D. (1988). Hemorrhagic shock induces bacterial translocation from the gut. *J. Trauma* **28,** 896–906.
9. Chiu, C. J., McArdle, A. H., Brown, R., Scott, H. J., and Gurd, F. N. (1970). Intestinal mucosal lesion in low-flow states. I. A morphologic, hemodynamic, and metabolic reappraisal. *Arch. Surg.* **101,** 478–483.
10. Parks, D. A., and Granger, D. N. (1982). Contributions of ischemia and reperfusion to mucosal lesion formation. *Am. J. Physiol.* **250,** G749–G753.
11. Mangino, M. J., Andeson, C. B., Murphy, M. K., Brunt, E., and Turk, J. (1989). Mucosal arachidonate metabolism and intestinal ischemia-reperfusion. *Am. J. Physiol.* **257,** G299–G307.
12. Oldham, K. T., Guice, K. S., Turnage, R. H., *et al.* (1993). The systemic consequences of intestinal ischemia/reperfusion injury. *J. Vasc. Surg.* **93,** 136–137.
13. Schmeling, D. J., Caty, M. G., Oldham, K. T., *et al.* (1989). Evidence for neutrophil-related acute lung injury after intestinal ischemia-reperfusion. *Surgery* **106,** 195–202.
14. Poggetti, R. S., Moore, F. A., Moore, E. E., *et al.* (1992). Liver injury is reversible neutrophil-mediated event following ischemia. *Arch. Surg.* **127,** 175–179.
15. Kadesky, K. M., Turnage, R. H., Rogers, T. E., Inman, L., and Myers, S. I. (1995). *In vitro* evidence of neutrophil mediated lung injury after intestinal reperfusion. *Shock* **4,** 102–106.
16. Turnage, R. H., LaNoue, J. L., Kadesky, K. M., Meng, Y., and Myers, S. I. (1997). Thromboxane A_2 mediates increased pulmonary microvascular permeability after intestinal reperfusion. *J. Appl. Physiol.* **82,** 592–598.
17. Oliver, M. G., Specian, R. D., Perry, M. A., and Granger, D. N. (1991). Morphologic assessment of leukocyte-endothelial cell interactions in mesenteric venules subjected to ischemia and reperfusion. *Inflammation* **15,** 331–346.
18. Grisham, M. B., Hernandez, L. A., and Granger, D. N. (1986). Xanthine oxidase and neutrophil infiltration in intestinal ischemia. *Am. J. Physiol.* **251,** G567–G574.
19. Granger, D. N., Rutili, G., and McCord, J. M. (1981). Superoxide radicals in feline intestinal ischemia. *Gastroenterology* **81,** 22–29.

20. Suzuki, M., Inauen, W., Kvietys, P. R., Grisham, M. B., Meininger, C., Schelling, M. E., Granger, H. J., and Granger, D. N. (1989). Superoxide mediates reperfusion-induced leukocyte-endothelial cell interactions. *Am. J. Physiol.* **257,** H1740–H1745.
21. Kanwar, S., Tepperman, B. L., Payne, D., Sutherland, L. R., and Kubes, P. (1994). Time course of nitric oxide production and epithelial dysfunction during ischemia/reperfusion of the feline small intestine. *Circ. Shock* **42,** 135–140.
22. Zimmerman, B. J., Grisham, M. B., and Granger, D. N. (1990). Role of oxidants in ischemia/reperfusion-induced granulocyte infiltration. *Am. J. Physiol.* **258,** G185–G190.
23. Schoenberg, M. H., Fredholm, B. B., Haglund, U., Jung, H., Sellin, D., Younes, M., and Schildberg, F. W. (1985). Studies on the oxygen radical mechanism involved in the small intestinal reperfusion damage. *Acta Physiol. Scand.* **124,** 581–589.
24. Schoenberg, M. H., Poch, B., Younes, M., Schwarz, A., Baczako, K., Lundberg, C., Haglund, U., and Beger, H. G. (1991). Involvement of neutrophils in postischaemic damage to the small intestine. *Gut* **32,** 905–912.
25. Aoki, N., Johnson, G., and Lefer, A. M. (1990). Beneficial effects of two forms of NO administration in feline splanchnic artery occlusion shock. *Am. J. Physiol.* **258,** G275–G281.
26. Rothenbach, P., Turnage, R. H., Iglesias, J., Riva, A., Bartula, L., and Myers, S. I. (1997). Downstream effects of splanchnic ischemia-reperfusion injury on renal function and eicosanoid release. *J. Appl. Physiol.* **82,** 530–536.
27. Turnage, R. H., Kadesky, K. M., Myers, S. I., Guice, K. S., and Oldham, K. T. (1996). Hepatic hypoperfusion following intestinal reperfusion injury. *Surgery* **119,** 151–160.
28. Turnage, R. H., Bagnasco, J., Berger, J., *et al.* (1991). Hepatocellular oxidant stress following intestinal ischemia-reperfusion injury. *J. Surg. Res.* **51,** 467–471.
29. LaNoue, J. L., Turnage, R. H., Kadesky, K. M., Guice, K. S., Oldham, K. T., and Myers, S. I. (1996). The effect of intestinal reperfusion on renal function and perfusion. *J. Surg. Res.* **64,** 19–25.
30. Hill, J., Lindsay, T. F., Ortiz, F., Yeh, C. G., Hechtman, H. B., and Moore, F. D., Jr. (1992). Soluble complement receptor type 1 ameliorates the local and remote organ injury after intestinal ischemia-reperfusion in the rat. *J. Immun.* **149,** 1723–1728.
31. Hill, J., Lindsay, T., Valeri, C. R., *et al.* (1993). A CD18 antibody prevents lung injury but not hypotension following intestinal ischemia-reperfusion. *J. Appl. Physiol.* **74,** 659–664.
32. Horton, J. W., and White, D. J. (1993). Lipid peroxidation contributes to cardiac deficits after ischemia and reperfusion of the small bowel. *Am. J. Physiol.* **264,** H1686–H1692, 1993.
33. Horton, J. W., and Walker, P. B. (1993). Oxygen radicals, lipid peroxidation, and permeability changes after intestinal ischemia and reperfusion. *J. Appl. Physiol.* **74,** 1515–1520.
34. Megison, S. M., Horton, J. W., Chao, H., and Walker, P. B. (1990). Prolonged survival and decreased mucosal injury after low-dose enteral allopurinol prophylaxis in mesenteric ischemia. *J. Pediatr. Surg.* **25,** 917–921.
35. Vaughan, W. G., Horton, J. W., and Walker, P. B. (1992). Allopurinol prevents intestinal permeability changes after ischemia-reperfusion injury. *J. Pediatr. Surg.* **27,** 968–973.
36. Welborn III, M. B., Douglas, W. G., Abouhamze, Z., *et al.* (1996). Visceral ischemia-reperfusion injury promotes tumor necrosis factor (TNF) and interleukin-1 (IL-1) dependent organ injury in the mouse. *Shock* **6,** 171–176.
37. Turnage, R. H., Kadesky, K. M., Rogers, T., Hernandez, R., Bartula, L., and Myers, S. I. (1995). Neutrophil regulation of splanchnic blood flow after hemorrhagic shock. *Ann. Surg.* **222,** 66–72.
38. Myers, S. I., Reed, M. K., Taylor, B., *et al.* (1990). Splanchnic prostanoid production: Effect of hemorrhagic shock. *J. Surg. Res.* **48,** 579–583.
39. Myers, S. I., and Small, J. (1991). Prolonged hemorrhagic shock decreased splanchnic prostacyclin synthesis. *J. Surg. Res.* **50,** 417–420.
40. Myers, S. I., and Hernandez, R. (1993). Exaggerated splanchnic PGI_2 release following acute hemorrhage is due to new protein synthesis. *Prostaglandins Leukot. Essent. Fatty Acids* **48,** 207–210.
41. Myers, S. I., and Hernandez, R. (1992). Oxygen free radical regulation of rat splanchnic blood flow. *Surgery* **112,** 347–354.
42. Myer, S. I., Hernandez, R., and Miller, T. A. (1994). Differing effects of anesthetics on splanchnic arterial blood flow during hemorrhagic shock. *J. Appl. Physiol.* **76,** 2304–2309.
43. Gelman, S., Fowler, K. C., and Smith, L. R. (1984). Regional blood flow during isoflurane and halothane anesthesia. *Anesth. Analg.* **63,** 557–565.
44. Lee, S. S., Girod, C., Valla, D., Geoffroy, P., and Lebrec, D. (1985). Effects of pentobarbital sodium anesthesia on splanchnic hemodynamics of normal and portal-hypertensive rats. *Am. J. Physiol.* **249,** G528–G532.
45. Miller, E. D., Kistner, J. R., and Epstein, R. M. (1980). Whole-body distribution of radioactively labelled microspheres in the rat during anesthesia with halothane, enflurane, or ketamine. *Anesthesiology* **52,** 296–302.
46. Myers, S. I., Hernandez, R., and Miller, T. A. (1994). Differing effects of anesthetics on splanchnic arterial blood flow during hemorrhagic shock. *J. Appl. Physiol.* **76,** 2304–2309.
47. LaRocco, M. R., Rodriguez, L. F., Chen, C. Y., Smith, G. S., Russell, D. H., Cocanour, C. S., Reed, R. L., Myers, S. I., and Miller, T. A. (1993). Reevaluation of the linkage between acute hemorrhagic shock and bacterial translocation in the rat. *Circ. Shock* **40,** 212–220.
48. Bulkley, G. B., Womack, W. A., Downey, J. M., Kvietys, P. R., and Granger, D. N. (1986). Collateral blood flow in segmental intestinal ischemia: Effects of vasoactive agents. *Surgery* **100,** 157–166.
49. Turnage, R. H., Guice, K. S., and Oldham, K. T. (1994). The effects of hypovolemia on multiple organ injury following intestinal reperfusion. *Shock* **1,** 408–413.
50. Guice, K. S., Oldham, K. T., Caty, M. G., *et al.* (1989). Neutrophil-dependent, oxygen-radical mediated lung injury associated with acute pancreatitis. *Ann. Surg.* **210,** 740–747.
51. Till, G. O., Beauchamp, C., Menapace, D., *et al.* (1984). Oxygen radical dependent lung damage following thermal injury of rat skin. *J. Trauma* **23,** 269–277.
52. Turnage, R. H., Guice, K. S., and Oldham, K. T. (1994). Endotoxemia and remote organ injury following intestinal reperfusion. *J. Surg. Res.* **56,** 571–578.
53. Guice, K. S., Oldham, K. T., Johnson, K. J., Kunkel, R. G., Morgenroth, M. L., and Ward, P. A. (1988) Pancreatitis-induced lung injury: An ARDS model. *Ann. Surg.* **208,** 71–77.
54. Till, G. O., Johnson, K. J., and Kunkel, R. G. (1982). Intravascular activation of complement and acute lung injury: Dependency on neutrophils and toxic oxygen metabolites. *J. Clin. Invest.* **69,** 1126–1135.
55. Iglesias, J. L., LaNoue, J. L., Rogers, T. E., Inman, L., and Turnage, R. H. (1998). Physiologic basis of pulmonary edema during intestinal reperfusion. *J. Surg. Res.* **80,** 156–163.
56. Green, T. P., Johnson, D. E., Marchssault, R. P., and Gatto, C. W. (1988). Transvascular flux and tissue accrual of Evans blue: Effects of endotoxin and histamine. *J. Lab. Clin. Med.* **111,** 173–183.
57. Patterson, C. E., Rhoades, R. A., and Garcia, J. G. N. (1992). Evans blue dye as a marker of albumin clearance in cultured endothelial monolayer and isolated lung. *J. Appl. Physiol.* **72,** 865–873.
58. Kubes, P., Granger, D. N. (1992). Nitric oxide modulates microvascular permeability. *Am. J. Physiol.* **262,** H611–H615.
59. Granger, D. N., and Taylor, A. E. (1980). Permeability of intestinal capillaries to endogenous macromolecules. *Am. J. Physiol.* **238,** H457–H464.
60. Granger, D. N., Taylor, A. E. (1980). Permselectivity of intestinal capillaries. *Physiologist* **23,** 47–52.

61. Drake, R. E., and Laine, G. A. (1988). Pulmonary microvascular permeability to fluid and macromolecules. *J. Appl. Physiol.* **64,** 487–501.
62. Kurose, I., Kubes, P., Wolf, R., *et al.* (1993). Inhibition of nitric oxide production: Mechanisms of vascular albumin leakage. *Circ. Res.* **73,** 164–171.
63. House, S. D., and Lipowsky, H. H. (1987). Leukocyte-endothelium adhesion: Microhemodynamics in mesentery of the cat. *Microvasc. Res.* **34,** 363–379.
64. Gaboury, J., Woodman, R. C., Granger, D. N., Reinhardt, P., and Kubes, P. (1993). Nitric oxide prevents leukocyte adherence: role of superoxide. *Am. J. Physiol.* **265,** H862–H867.
65. Kubes, P. (1993). Ischemia-reperfusion in feline small intestine: A role for nitric oxide. *Am. J. Physiol.* **264,** G143–G149.
66. Nylander, O., Kvietys, P., and Granger, D. N. (1989). Effects of hydrochloric acid on duodenal and jejunal mucosal permeability in the rat. *Am. J. Physiol.* **257,** G653–G660.
67. Baker, R., Baker, S., and LaRosa, K. (1995). Polarized Caco-2 cells. Effect of reactive oxygen metabolites on enterocyte barrier function. *Dig. Dis. Sci.* **40,** 510–518.
68. Huet, C., Sauquillo-Merino, C., Coudrier, E., and Louvard, D. (1987). Absorptive and mucus-secreting subclones isolated from a multipotent intestinal cell line (HT-29) provide new models for cell polarity and terminal differentiation. *J. Cell. Biol.* **105,** 345–357.
69. Xu, D-Z, Lu, Q., Kubicka, R., and Deitch, E. (1999). The effect of hypoxia/reoxygenation on the cellular function of intestinal epithelial cells. *J. Trauma* **46,** 280–285.
70. Singh, N. P., and Stevens, R. E. (1986). A novel technique for viable cell determinations. *Stain Tech.* **61,** 315–318.
71. Rotman, B., and Papermast, B. W. (1966). Membrane properties of living mammalian cells as studied by enzymatic hydrolysis of fluorogenic esters. *Proc. Natl Acad. Sci. U. S.A* **55,** 134–141.
72. Muniswamy, M., Bhaskar, L., and Balasubramanian, K. A. (1997). Enterocyte viability and mitochondrial function after graded intestinal ischemia and reperfusion in rats. *Mol. Cell Biochem.* **167,** 81–87.
73. Vouret-Craviari, V., Boquet, P., Pouyssegur, J., and Obberghen-Schilling E. (1998). Regulation of the actin cytoskeleton by thrombin in human endothelial cells: Role of rho proteins in endothelial barrier function. *Mol. Biol. Cell* **9,** 2639–2653.
74. Michel, C. C., and Curry, F. E. (1999). Microvascular permeability. *Physiol. Rev.* **79,** 703–761.
75. Murphy, E., and Horrocks, L. (1993). Mechanism of hypoxic and ischemic injury. Use of cell culture models. *Mol. Chem. Neuropathol.* **19,** 95–106.
76. Wells, C. L., Jechorek, R. P., and Olmsted, S. B. (1993). Effect of LPS on epithelial integrity and bacterial uptake in the polarized human enterocyte-like cell line Caco-2. *Circ. Shock* **40,** 276–288.

46

Gut Barrier Failure

Justin T. Sambol, Raquel M. Forsythe, and Edwin A. Deitch

Department of Surgery, UMD—New Jersey Medical School, Newark, New Jersey 07003

I. Introduction

The gastrointestinal tract is a complex organ that performs important metabolic, immunologic, and barrier functions in addition to its role in the digestion and absorption of nutrients. Failure of intestinal barrier function leading to the escape of bacteria or endotoxin from the gut—bacterial translocation—has been implicated in the pathogenesis of systemic infection and the multiple organ failure syndrome in high-risk surgical patients (1). These patient populations include burn and trauma victims, immunocompromised patients, and those who have prolonged intensive care unit stays. Although the exact clinical implications of gut barrier failure remain to be fully determined, this area has been a focus of intense research for many years. Because of the complexities of studying gut barrier function, numerous approaches utilizing different models and methods have been developed and employed over the past 15 years. In this chapter, we review the biology of gut barrier defenses as well as discuss the principles of the major techniques that we and others have used to investigate gut barrier function.

In our own work, we have chosen to study the process of gut barrier failure and bacterial translocation directly utilizing three different experimental systems. This is because in no one system is it possible to characterize or elucidate adequately the various potential mechanisms involved in normal intestinal barrier function or how these defenses are altered under conditions of gut barrier failure. The three experimental systems are (1) *in vivo* animal models, (2) *in vitro* cultured intestinal epithelial cells models, and (3) the *ex vivo* Ussing chamber system. In the Ussing chamber system, the barrier function of intestinal mucosa harvested from normal animals or animals subjected to various *in vivo* insults can be tested *in vitro*. Each of these systems has advantages and disadvantages and the data obtained from each can be combined to help better understand the complexities of the gut barrier.

Because direct studies in humans are difficult or impossible to perform, *in vivo* animal models are the most biologically relevant models. However, due to technical limitations and the complexity of the *in vivo* system, it is not always possible to carry out the definitive mechanistic studies required to clarify the biology of the translocation process or the mechanisms underlying gut barrier dysfunction. Thus, *in vitro* and *ex vivo* model systems are necessary. Regardless of the model systems used, knowledge of the biology of gut barrier defenses is a critical starting point.

II. The Gut Barrier

It is important to understand the normal mechanisms utilized by the gut to maintain barrier function in order to understand better how these protective mechanisms may fail during periods of stress or illness. Because the gut contains high concentrations of bacteria and endotoxin that must be excluded, in addition to nutrients that must be absorbed, the host has developed multiple defense mechanisms that function together to prevent intestinal bacteria and endotoxin from crossing the mucosal barrier and/or reaching systemic organs and tissues. These defenses include the stabilizing influences of a normal intestinal microflora, plus mechanical and immunologic defenses as well as bile acids and gastric acidity (Table I). However, under certain experimental and clinical circumstances, this intestinal barrier function becomes overwhelmed or impaired, resulting in the translocation of bacteria to the mesenteric lymph nodes (MLNs) and other tissues. We have previously shown that the three major mechanisms promoting bacterial translocation are (1) intestinal bacterial overgrowth, (2) deficiencies in host immune defenses, and (3) increased permeability or damage to the intestinal mucosal barrier (2). Many, if not all, of the defenses that prevent bacterial translocation are impaired in critically ill or injured patients. These patients are frequently immunosuppressed and the antibiotic regimens they receive may disrupt the normal ecology of the gut flora, resulting in bacterial overgrowth with potential pathogens. For example, H-2 blockers by alkalinizing the stomach may result in gastric and distal intestinal colonization of orally ingested bacteria. Parenteral feedings may disrupt not only the normal bacterial ecology of the gut, but may also result in mucosal atrophy and altered intestinal mechanical defenses, and the hypoalbuminemia and capillary leak syndrome that commonly occur in these patients can result in intestinal edema, impaired jejunoileal peristalsis, intestinal stasis, bacterial overgrowth, and altered intestinal permeability. Last, decreased gut perfusion during shock states or in response to systemic insults can lead to an ischemia/reperfusion-mediated gut mucosal injury.

Table I Components of the Gut Barrier

Microbial	
	Microflora
	Colonization resistance
Mechanical	
	Mucus layer
	Gastric acidity
	Epithelial barrier
	Peristalsis
	Junctional complexes
Intestinal immune system	
	Gut-associated lymph tissue
	Secretory immunoglobulins
Gut–liver axis	
	Bile salts
	Reticuloendothelial function

The role of gut barrier defenses in preventing the escape of bacteria from the intestine is best illustrated by breaking down the process of bacterial translocation into several steps. The first step in bacterial translocation begins with the association and then adherence of the translocating bacteria to the epithelial cell surface or to ulcerated areas of the intestinal mucosal surface. One of the most important defense mechanisms preventing potential pathogens colonizing the gut from adhering directly to the intestinal mucosa is the presence of a normal gut microflora. Van Der Waaij first recognized the importance of the normal gut microflora, especially the strict anaerobic bacteria, in the gut's resistance to infection by potential bacterial pathogens. He coined the term "colonization resistance" to describe this protective role of the normal intestinal microflora, notably the obligate anaerobes, and showed that this resistance is altered by the administration of antibiotics (3). It is now clear that the obligate anaerobic bacteria are responsible for colonization resistance, because they form a barrier that limits the direct attachment or intimate association of potential translocating bacteria, such as *Escherichia coli*, to the mucosa.

Mechanical defenses are the second constituent of the gut barrier and include the mucosal surfaces, the mucus layer, and peristalsis. The mucosal layer is composed of many cell types including columnar epithelium, goblet cells, Paneth cells, and intraepithelial lymphocytes. These epithelial cells are joined together by junctional complexes and desmosomes, which under normal conditions prevent the passage of intraluminal bacteria into the systemic circulation. The intestinal mucosa is covered by a 30- to 50-μm-thick mucus layer. This mucus layer is secreted by the goblet cells and assists in nutrient absorption and, at the same time, impedes the adherence of bacteria to the mucosal layer and thereby blocks bacterial translocation (4,5). Additionally, in the small intestine, normal peristalsis prevents prolonged stasis of bacteria in close proximity to the intestinal mucosa and thereby reduces the chance that bacteria will have adequate time to penetrate the mucus layer and attach to the epithelium. Together, these mechanical defenses limit the ability of bacteria to reach and then cross the epithelial mucosal barrier.

The intestinal immune system, termed the gut-associated lymphoid tissue (GALT), consists of Peyer's patches, lymphoid follicles, lamina propria lymphocytes, intraepithelial lymphocytes, and cells of the MLN. The immune cells of the GALT, as well as secretory immunoglobulins, act to limit the passage of bacteria and toxic antigens into the systemic circulation. For example, on exposure to bacteria, the B cells located within the Peyer's patches differentiate into IgA-producing plasma cells, and the secretory IgA (sIgA) produced by these B cells binds bacteria, preventing their adherence to the mucosa. Studies by Diebel (6) documenting that secretory IgA significantly reduces bacterial translocation *in vitro* when enterocyte monolayers were exposed to bacteria support a protective role for sIgA.

The final components of the gut barrier are bile salts and the hepatic reticuloendothelial system. The bile salts are thought to be important in preventing portal and systemic endotoxemia, but have also been shown to be important in limiting bacterial translocation (7). They act by binding endotoxin and preventing its absorption from the intestinal lumen through the formation of insoluble complexes (8). Despite the ability of bile salt to clear intraluminal endotoxin, a small amount may be absorbed systemically. Once in the portal circulation, the hepatic reticuloendothelial cells clear these gut-derived bacterial products, preventing the development of systemic endotoxemia.

III. Models for Studying Barrier Function

A. Animal Models of Bacterial Translocation

Multiple models have been used to study the phenomenon of bacterial translocation, including animals subjected to hemorrhagic shock, burn injury, trauma, nutritional perturbations, and inflammatory insults (2). In the best of these studies, the animals are subjected to actual or sham injury (insult) and then are sacrificed at various times after the insult. At sacrifice, the degree of bacterial translocation is determined by culturing the MLN (primary site of bacterial translocation) and other organs, such as the spleen, liver, lung, and kidney as well as the portal and systemic blood. The exact organs and tissues to culture will vary based on the experimental design or model used. However, the MLN is always cultured, because it is the initial tissue involved in the process of bacterial translocation. Furthermore, because the MLNs are normally sterile, the presence of bacteria in these nodes is a sensitive marker of bacterial translocation. Intestinal bacterial overgrowth can promote bacterial translocation, thus the effect of the experimental manipulation on the ecology of the indigenous gastrointestinal (GI) microflora is determined by quantitating the population levels of resident bacteria within the cecum. Similarly, sections of the ileum and/or cecum are examined histologically to determine whether the gut mucosa has been physically damaged.

Remember, when studying the phenomenon of bacterial translocation in animal models, it is important to measure not just bacteria in the animal's tissues, but also to quantitate intestinal bacterial population levels and determine whether there is evidence of mucosal damage. These additional measurements are necessary, because intestinal bacterial overgrowth and mucosal injury both promote bacterial translocation. Most of the experimental work has been done in rodent (mice and rat) models, thus we will illustrate the details of measuring bacterial translocation in rodents.

1. Animal Husbandry

Changes in the gut flora can influence the results of experiments, therefore it is important to use only specific pathogen-free (SPF) animals. SPF means that the company selling the animals has tested them to be sure that they do not contain enteric pathogens.

The animals are housed under barrier-sustained conditions to prevent bacterial contamination and are housed in a room with controlled temperature (22°C), humidity, and 12-hr light–dark cycles. For the majority of experiments, the animals are fed standard laboratory chow *ad libitum*. Specific experiments involving diet-induced bacterial translocation with oral or intravenous total parenteral nutrition (TPN) require specific dietary formulas and will not be addressed here. Parenteral diet protocols for rats can be found in Deitch *et al.* (9).

The availability of different genetic strains of mice has greatly improved our ability to perform mechanistic studies. However, caution must be exercised when inbred strains of mice or rats are used, because the sensitivity of these strains to specific insults may vary. This concept is illustrated by studies documenting that certain inbred strains of mice are more susceptible to burn-induced bacterial translocation and gut-origin sepsis than are other strains (BALBc more sensitive than C57 black mice) and that both inbred strains are more sensitive than outbred mice (10, 11). Because transgenic and knockout mice are derived from inbred strains, it is critical that the investigator consider the possibility that some of the changes observed may relate to the strain of the animal used as well as to the gene being studied. Additionally, in performing animal studies, it is important to note the increasing body of information indicating that males and females may respond differently to a similar insult (12). Last, studies investigating the gut flora can be carried out in germ-free animals (13). However, because germ-free animals must be kept in a germ-free (sterile) environment, studies using germ-free animals are technically difficult and complex.

2. Method of Measuring Bacterial Translocation

Depending on the experiment, the animals are either sacrificed or anesthetized. If the rats are to be anesthetized, we use either an intraperitoneal (IP) injection of pentobarbital (50 mg/kg) or ketamine (80 mg/kg) plus xylazine (8 mg/kg). Complete anesthesia occurs in approximately 5 min and lasts between 30 min and 1 hr.

Following anesthesia, the skin is cleaned with 70% ethanol. Using sterile instruments, an abdominal incision is made and flaps are retracted laterally. The abdominal muscles are treated with ethanol and the peritoneum is opened.

First, the peritoneal cavity is swabbed with sterile cotton-tipped applicators and cultured in brain–heart infusion medium (BHI) or tryptic soy broth to determine accidental bacterial contamination. Samples of portal venous and systemic blood (1 ml) are then obtained and incubated with 5 ml of BHI at 37°C for 48 hr. Bacterial growth is assessed at both 24 and 48 hr. The mesenteric lymph node complex is identified in the base of the mesentery of the ascending colon by reflecting the bowel to the left with a moist sterile gauze (Fig. 1). The MLN is sharply excised, weighed, and homogenized in sterile grinding tubes containing 0.5 ml of tryptic soy broth with 0.05% dithiothreitol to reduce oxygen contamination. Next, the spleen and liver are removed, weighed, placed in sterile grinding tubes containing 1.0 ml of tryptic soy broth, and homogenized as above. Once the MLN is removed, the peritoneum is again swabbed with sterile applicators for accidental contamination. Last, the cecum is removed, weighed, and placed in grinding tubes containing either sterile PBS or BHI. Then 0.1 ml of the MLN or 0.2 ml of the organ homogenates is cultured in duplicate on blood agar plates to quantitate both gram-positive and gram-negative enteric bacteria, as well as on MacConkey's agar, which is specific for gram-negative enteric bacilli. Due to the large number of bacteria in the cecum, the cecal homogenate is serially diluted (1:100 and 1:1000 or more) and 0.1 ml is plated. The plates are examined at 24 and 48 hr for bacterial growth, at which time the number of colony-forming units (CFU) present is counted. The numbers of viable bacteria are determined per gram of organ or per whole organ using the following formula:

$$\text{CFU/gram} = (\text{CFU} \times \text{dilution})/\text{sample weight}.$$

After the specimens are harvested for bacterial translocation, sections of ileum are prepared for histologic examination. Specimens are fixed by luminal perfusion and immersion in 2% paraformaldehyde and 4% glutaraldehyde in 0.1 mol/liter phosphate buffer at pH 7.4 overnight at 4°C. The tissue is dehydrated in 95% ethanol and embedded in methyl methacrylate. Sections are cut on glass knives at a thickness of 2–3 μm and stained with toluidine blue. Sections are then examined by a blinded examiner and scored for villus damage using the scale developed by Chiu (14). The system is a five-step grading scale to measure intestinal mucosal damage and is highly reproducible. Table II describes the grading scale.

3. Pitfalls

There are several important points to remember when performing this procedure. First, the last piece of tissue harvested is the intestine, because removing the intestine will lead to peritoneal contamination. Second, it is important to culture essentially all of the MLN and organ homogenates to ensure that bacterial translocation is not missed. To count accurately the number of bacteria on a plate, the number of bacterial colonies should be less than 250. Because the cecum can contain up to 10^8 CFU/g of tissue, it is important to ensure that adequate dilutions are made. Last, it is important to culture the entire MLN complex, especially the small segment next to the bowel (usually separate from the main body of the complex), because the greatest number of translocating bacteria are present in this small segment of the MLN complex (15) (Fig. 2).

4. Advantages and Disadvantages

The major advantage of any model of bacterial translocation is that infection occurs via a natural route that requires the translocating bacteria to invade the host and survive in

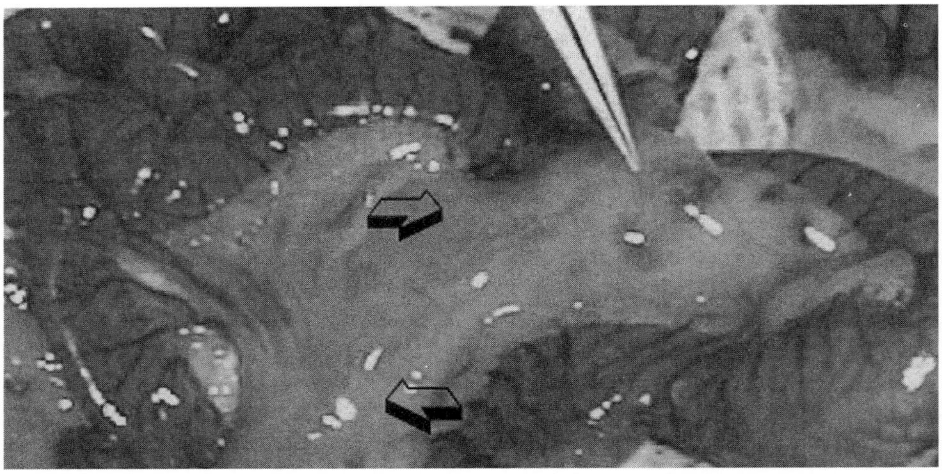

Figure 1 The mesenteric lymph node complex. The forceps are pointing to segment one of the MLN. The arrows demonstrate the remainder of the MLN chain. (See color plates.)

Table II

Grade	Histologic appearance[a]
0	Normal mucosal villi
1	Development of subepithelial space (Greunhagen's space) at villus tips; capillary congestion may be seen
2	Extension of subepithelial space with separation of epithelial layer from the lamina propria
3	Massive extension of subepithelial space, extending down the sides of the villi; may begin to see denuded tips of villi
4	Denuded villi with exposed lamina propria and dilated capillaries
5	Destruction of lamina propria with frank hemorrhage and ulceration

[a]From Chiu *et al.* (14).

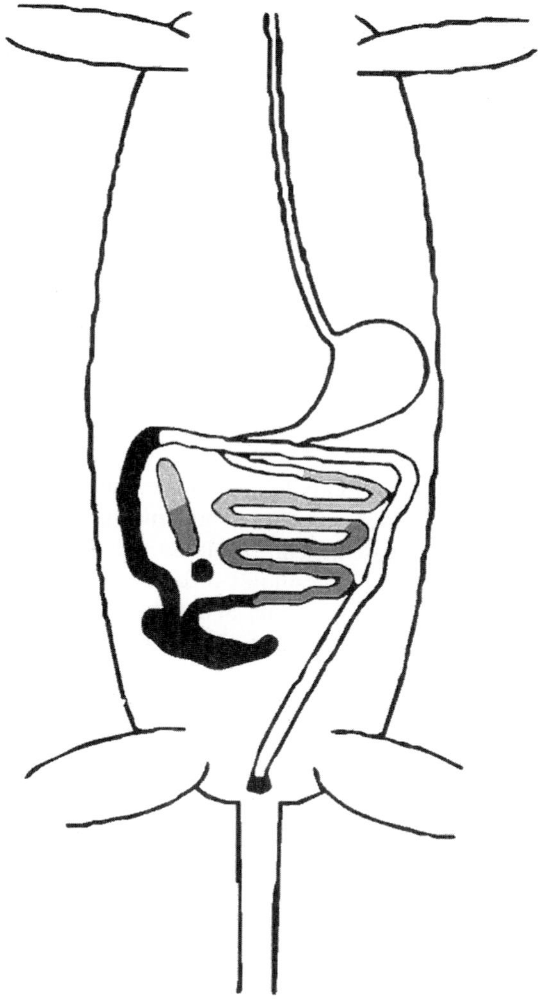

Figure 2 The MLN consists of three distinct segments of the MLN complex, each of which drains a region of the gut. The distal ileum, cecum and ascending colon drain into segment 1 (black). The proximal ileum drains into segment 2 (dark gray), and the jejunum drains into MLN segment 3 (light gray).

systemic organs and tissues. Consequently, it represents a natural route of infection and is less artificial than infection models in which the bacteria are injected intravenously. A second advantage is the ability to model clinically common events (burn injury, shock, endotoxemia, etc.) as well as the ability to mimic the clinical situation by using combinations of insults. Thus, models of bacterial translocation allow investigation of two-hit phenomena.

The major disadvantage of any model of bacterial translocation is the limited sensitivity of the culture techniques used in identifying translocating bacteria. Alexander *et al.* (16) documented that bacteriologic techniques, which only quantitate viable bacteria, grossly underestimate the magnitude of bacterial translocation by over a thousandfold as compared to radiolabeling techniques that quantitate both viable and nonviable translocated bacteria. Culture techniques therefore may fail to detect or may underestimate the degree of bacterial translocation secondary to the fact that the translocating bacteria may have been killed by macrophages, or, in the case of clinical studies, by the administration of preoperative antibiotics. Thus, in certain circumstances the use of radiolabeled bacteria as described by Alexander *et al* (16) may be necessary.

5. Modulation of the Gut Flora

Intestinal bacterial overgrowth is associated with commonly used clinical therapies (TPN, broad spectrum antibiotics, H-2 blockers) as well as the development of ileus, and bacterial overgrowth potentiates bacterial translocation, thus it is necessary to be able to test the effects of various insults in animals with bacterial overgrowth. Likewise, in order to test the influence of alterations in the gut flora on certain parameters, it may be necessary to study animals with reduced as well as increased bacterial population levels. Therefore, we have developed a strategy to decrease or increase the gut flora (Fig. 3).

The technique of antibiotic decontamination is used to decrease the indigenous gut microflora. We have had success using each of the following antibiotic regimens to

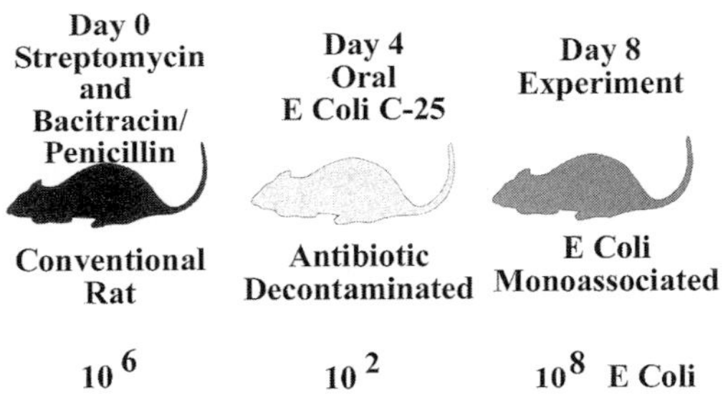

Figure 3 Illustration of the technique of antibiotic decontamination as well as *E. coli* monoassociation in the rat model. The numbers at the bottom represent the cecal population level of gram-negative enteric bacteria.

antibiotically decontaminate mice and rats. In regimen 1, SPF animals are given drinking water containing 4 mg/ml of streptomycin and 4 mg/ml of bacitracin for 4 days (17). In regimen 2, SPF animals are given drinking water containing 4 mg/ml of streptomycin and 2 mg/ml of penicillin for 4 days (18). Some animals may not drink the water because of the taste of the antibiotics. This problem can be overcome by adding a small amount of saccharine to the water. After 4 days of antibiotics, feces are gram-stained and examined to verify that the indigenous flora have been eliminated or at least greatly reduced. These antibiotic regimens typically reduce the total aerobic cecal bacterial population levels from $>10^6$ to $<10^2$ CFUs per gram of cecum. At this point, the antibiotically decontaminated animals can be employed in any experiments desired or colonized with a particular strain of bacteria.

If we desire to examine the effect of bacterial overgrowth in the proposed experiments, we colonize the antibiotically decontaminated animals with an antibiotic-resistant bacteria. We have used *E. coli* C25 as our test bacteria, because it is not enteropathogenic, it is streptomycin resistant, and it has been shown to translocate *in vivo* without causing overt disease. The fact that it is resistant to streptomycin allows for increased technical flexibility. Once colonized with *E. coli* C25, the animals are termed monoassociated. To monoassociate the animals, first *E. coli* C25 cultures are grown overnight in brain–heart infusion medium, washed, and resuspended in sterile Dulbecco's modified Eagle's medium (DMEM), at a concentration of 4.2×10^{10} CFU/ml. The antibiotically decontaminated animals are then monoassociated by oral intragastric inoculation of 3×10^8 *E. coli* C25 using a 6.35-cm 22-gauge feeding needle with a 2-mm stainless-steel bulb on the tip. The *E. coli* C25 can also be added to the drinking water as well. After inoculation, the animals continue to receive streptomycin in their drinking water for a total of 4 days to prevent the regrowth of their indigenous flora.

To measure bacterial translocation (BT) in these monoassociated animals, samples are collected as described in Section III, A,2. Once collected, samples are homogenized in grinding tubes containing either tryptic soy broth or BHI. Aliquots are cultured on MacConkey's agar plates containing streptomycin at 37°C (streptomycin inhibits the growth of the normal gut flora) and are examined at 24 and 48 hr for bacterial growth.

Monoassociated animals are useful for studying the effects of intestinal bacterial overgrowth by itself or in conjunction with other models. Because bacterial overgrowth-induced bacterial translocation does not rely on gut injury, but rather exclusively on the degree of intestinal bacterial overgrowth, the variables of susceptibility of the animal to injury as well as the degree of injury are avoided. The disadvantages are similar to those of the bacterial translocation methods described previously. That is, the assessment of the magnitude of bacterial translocation is limited by culture techniques and may underestimate the extent of translocation as compared with immunofluorescence or radiolabeling techniques.

B. In Vitro and ex Vivo Systems

It is not always possible to carry out specific mechanistic studies using *in vivo* models, thus *in vitro* and *ex vivo* models have been developed or adapted to the study of gut barrier function. The two major systems used are cell culture models and studies using harvested intestines from normal or manipulated animals. The advantages of using a cultured epithelial monolayer is that the system is physiologically simple, it is relatively easy to manipulate, and is optimal for morphologic and basic cellular and mechanistic studies. Furthermore, because the cultured intestinal monolayer does not contain goblet cells, studies of epithelial cell function and physiology are not confounded by the presence of mucus. The main disadvantage of this system is that it lacks the complexity of the *in vivo* state. The *ex vivo* intestinal membrane Ussing chamber model, although more complex and time consuming than the tissue culture model, has the advantage that mucosal specimens harvested from animals subjected to various insults can be tested directly. Additionally, because the intestinal mucosa contains the entire repertoire of intestinal cells, responses are more likely to reflect *in vivo* intestinal responses. However, because the goblet cells present in the tissue samples secrete mucus during the investigative period, it is not possible to study isolated epithelial cell function in the absence of mucus. In addition, tissue samples placed in the Ussing chambers begin to deteriorate after 4–6 hr. Thus, each of these systems has their own advantages and disadvantages and the results obtained in these systems should be interpreted in light of whole animal studies.

1. Cell Culture Models

The concept that gut permeability increases and bacterial translocation occurs in stress states has been documented in both human and animal studies. However, due to limitations of human and whole animal studies, it has been difficult to examine adequately the mechanisms by which these phenomena occur. It is for this reason that in addition to animal models, our laboratory has worked to develop cell culture *in vitro* systems to better assess the physiology of intestinal barrier function and the pathophysiology of bacterial translocation. Although there are numerous cell lines available for the study of intestinal epithelium, primarily four cell lines are used for studies of the gut barrier. These are the Caco-2, HT29, T84, and the IEC-6 cell lines, all of which are available from the American Type Culture Collection (Manassas, VA; Internet web site: www.atcc.org). Each of these cell lines has different characteristics that are useful for different studies. The characteristics as well as the pros and cons of each cell line are summarized in Table III.

It is because the Caco-2 cells most closely mimic normal intestinal epithelium when grown in standard conditions (19) that we initially chose to use them for studying gut dysfunction under variable conditions (20). In addition to Caco-2 cells, we often use the rat intestinal epithelial IEC-6 cell line to control for species differences when studying rodent factors (21). In addition, the IEC-6 cell line has the added advantages that it is not a transformed cell line and that the majority of the animal work in this field has been done in rodents.

To investigate bacterial–enterocyte interactions and the effects of various insults on intestinal permeability, we have employed a two-compartment system where Caco-2 or IEC-6 cells are grown as polarized monolayers on collagen-coated membranes in bicameral chambers (Transwell, 3-μm pore membranes, Costar Corp., Cambridge, MA.) (Figs. 4 and 5). Prior to seeding the Transwell filters, the Caco-2 cells are maintained in Dulbecco's modified Eagle's medium supplemented with 10% fetal bovine serum, nonessential amino acids, 0.5 mg/ml L-glutamine, and antibiotics (100 U/ml penicillin-G, 100 U/ml streptomycin, 250 ng/ml amphotericin), whereas the IEC-6 cells are maintained in DMEM with 5% fetal bovine serum, 0.1 U/ml insulin, and a similar antibiotic regimen. The cells are then cultured in 75 cm^2 tissue culture flasks at 37°C in a humidified 5% carbon dioxide atmosphere. Once a sufficient number of cells have been grown in these culture flasks to seed the Transwell filters, they are detached from the flasks by trypsinization and washed and resuspended in DMEM.

The Caco-2 or IEC-6 cells are then seeded at 10,000 cells per insert onto type 1 collagen-coated membranes (3.0-μm pore size) contained in the apical chamber of the bicameral system (Fig. 5). The cells are grown on the apical chamber until a sealed monolayer is formed. Based on studies correlating permeability of the monolayer to differ-

Table III Cell Lines

Cell lines	Characteristics	Pros	Cons
Caco-2[a]	Grows confluent monolayer when grown on collagen matrix; forms microvilli; appearance of desmosomes; expresses brush border enzymes; forms domes, which suggests polarity	Spontaneously expresses enterocyte differentiation when grown in standard conditions; human cell line	Must be grown on coated matrix to form monolayer; derived from transformed colon adenocarcinoma
HT29[b, c]	When grown in glucose, undifferentiated; no glucose, differentiates into polarized absorptive enterocytes and mucus-secreting goblet cells	Human cell line; expresses features of enterocytes when grown in glucose-free medium	Differentiation modulated by culture conditions; goblet cells may confound results; derived from transformed adenocarcinoma
T84[d]	Grows to confluent monolayers; tight junctions and desmosomes present; retained structural polarity	Human cell line; expresses some features of enterocytes when grown in serum	Must be grown in serum to develop these properties; grows three times faster in serum-free medium but does not form confluent monolayers; derived from transformed adenocarcinoma
IEC-6[e]	Epithelial cells with larger nuclei; grows as tight colonies of polygonal, closely opposed cells; numerous microvilli; cytologic features typical of crypt cells; tight junctions link adjacent cells	Easily stored in liquid nitrogen; derived from small intestinal crypt cell	Rat cell line

[a]From Pinto *et al.* (18a).
[b]From Wells *et al.* (18b).
[c]From Pinto *et al.* (18c).
[d]From Dharmsathaphorn *et al.* (32).
[e]From Quaroni *et al.* (18d).

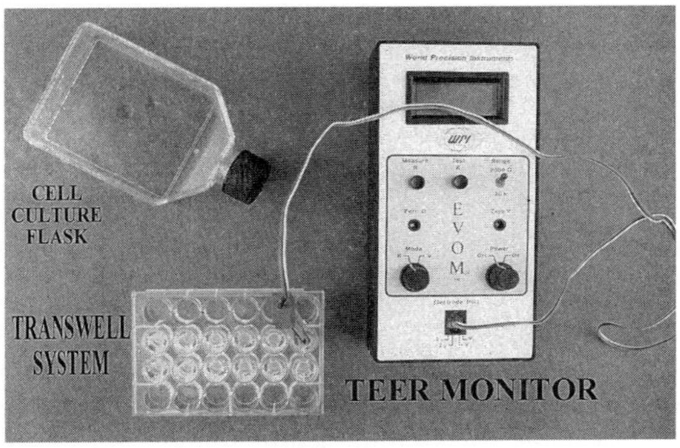

Figure 4 The components used in the cell culture model: a typical cell culture flask, in which primary enterocytes are grown, the Transwell System plate, in which the cells are seeded and the TEER voltmeter used to measure monolayer resistance.

ent size permeability probes with electrical measurements of membrane resistance, we established that monolayer tight junction integrity was established when the transepithelial electrical resistance (TEER) of the IEC-6 cell monolayer was above 42 $\Omega \cdot cm^2$ and the Caco2 monolayer TEER values were above 136 $\Omega \cdot cm^2$ (21, 22). Typically 14–18 days are needed to reach these TEER levels, during which time the cells differentiate, form microvilli, and become polarized (22).

Once the monolayer is sealed, studies can be performed investigating the phenomenon of bacterial translocation as well as the effects of various insults, agents, or conditions on monolayer permeability. Whether one is measuring bacterial translocation or permeability, the approach is similar. Bacteria, a permeability probe of the desired size (such as flourescent dextran), or both are placed in the apical chamber. At the desired times, samples from the basal chamber are collected. Bacterial translocation is quantitated by plating an aliquot of fluid from the basal chamber on blood agar plates and counting the number of bacterial colonies present after a 24- and 48-hr incubation period. Permeability is quantitated by measuring the amount of the permeability probe that has crossed the enterocyte monolayer from the apical to the basal chamber. Measurements can be made serially (i.e., each hour) or at specifically defined time periods. We generally measure bacterial translocation 3 hr after inoculating the apical chamber with bacteria.

We have used this cell culture monolayer model to quantitate the threshold of the bacterial inoculum required to observe bacterial translocation, to determine the ability of various bacterial species to translocate (23), and to determine the ability of various interventions to limit bacterial translocation (24), as well as to study the biology of bacterial–enterocyte interactions (25). Because of our interests in endotoxin-induced gut permeability and ischemiareperfusion-mediated gut injury, we have modeled these conditions in this cell culture system (21, 26).

This cell culture system is also excellent for investigating the effects of specific proinflammatory factors or bacteria on enterocyte metabolism, viability, and factor production (e.g., cytokines, complement) (27). By having a pure enterocyte cell culture without other contaminating cells present, it is possible to better define the response of enterocyte populations to various stimuli. Thus, this *in vitro* cell culture model has been quite useful in the study of epithelial cell function

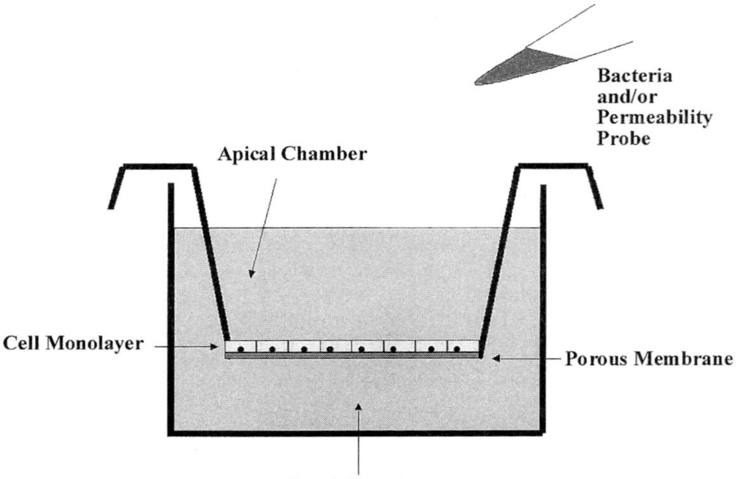

Figure 5 Schematic diagram of the Transwell System demonstrating inoculation of the apical chamber with bacteria or a permeability probe. The cell monolayer is grown on a porous membrane as shown; the samples are then withdrawn from the basal chamber and measured using techniques described in the text.

and dysfunction. It offers many advantages, including its ease of use, lack of other cell types, and the model's ability to be subjected to variable conditions. One disadvantage is the time required to grow the cells to confluence (6–20 days, depending on cell type). In addition, although enterocytes are the primary cell type in the gut, the lack of other cell types and the nature of the *in vitro* environmental conditions make it hazardous to extrapolate cell culture results directly to animal models or human disease. Nonetheless, basic mechanistic questions can be addressed in this system that cannot be studied in any other way.

2. *Ex Vivo* System: The Ussing Chamber

The Ussing system was developed by Hans Ussing in 1949 (28) to study electrolyte fluxes in frog skin. It has been described as an *ex vivo* system, bridging the gap between the simpler *in vitro* cell culture models and more complex *in vivo* animal models. It allows for precise control of the experimental conditions in studies of the gut barrier, while maintaining the normal intestinal mucosal architecture. The Ussing chamber (Figs. 6 and 7) allows for constant conditions of intestinal perfusion and oxygenation. The system allows addition of mediators to either the mucosal or serosal side of the system or sampling of medium from either side (Fig. 7). We have used the system to study mucosal permeability induced by diet (29), endotoxin (30), and ischemia/reperfusion (31). A variety of gut barrier function parameters can be examined, such as bacterial translocation, permeability to various probes, and the production of nitric oxide or cytokines.

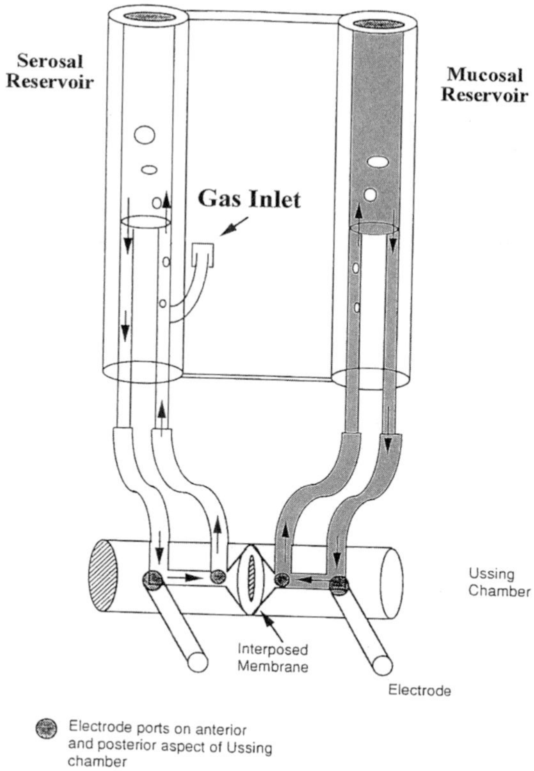

Figure 6 Schematic diagram of the Ussing chamber system. The intestinal sample is placed with the mucosal side of the intestine facing the mucosal reservoir and the serosal side facing the serosal reservoir. The mucosal reservoir on the left contains DMEM alone; the mucosal reservoir on the right contains DMEM with phenol red (shaded area). The electrodes monitor the transepithelial electrical potential difference.

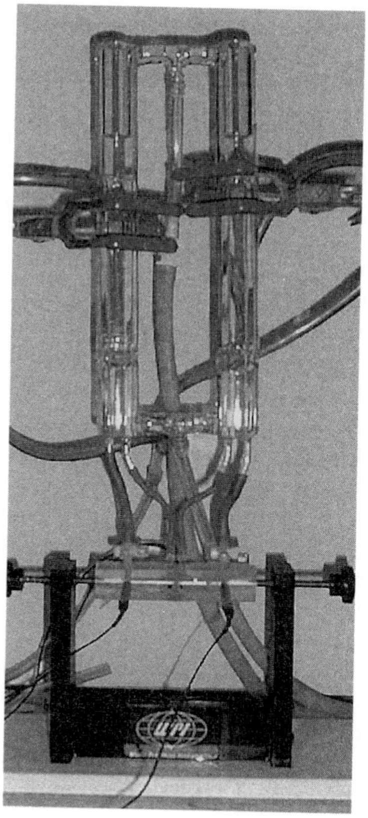

Figure 7 The Ussing chamber system.

The system is prepared as follows. A 2-cm segment of Peyer's patch-free ileal (or other intestinal segment) mucosa is harvested, opened along the mesenteric border, and washed in medium to remove luminal contents. The serosa and external longitudinal muscle layers are removed by blunt dissection. The mucosa is mounted between the two chambers of a sterilized Ussing system with a 1.12-cm^2 opening. Two calomel voltage-sensitive electrodes and two Ag–AgCl current-passing electrodes are connected to the Ussing chamber via agar bridges. Both the mucosal and serosal chambers are connected to sterilized circulating reservoirs containing sterile Dulbecco's modified Eagle's medium supplemented with 20 m*M* glutamine. The mucosal reservoir is filled with DMEM containing phenol red (or other permeability probe), whereas the serosal reservoir contains phenol red-free DMEM alone. Each reservoir has ports for sample collection and various test substances can be added to either side. The reservoir fluid is oxygenated and driven by a gas lift column of 95% O_2/5% CO_2 to ensure adequate oxygenation of the tissue. Temperature is maintained at a constant 37°C by a jacketed circulating water bath. This system also allows electrical parameters of the intestinal segment to be monitored, such as the potential difference and the resistance of the intestinal mucosal segment. The transepithelial electrical potential difference (millivolts) is measured directly across the ileal mucosal membrane and is an indicator of tissue viability. The transmembrane resistance ($\Omega \cdot cm^2$) is determined using Ohm's law by passing a 50-μA current through the membrane. The resistance of the tissue sample reflects membrane integrity.

Once mounted, the mucosal membranes are allowed to stabilize for 15 min prior to any experimental manipulation. This stabilization period verifies proper functioning of the system and ensures that the membranes are not damaged. At the end of the 15-min period, a sample is taken from each reservoir for culture to verify sterility of the system. In our studies, mucosal membranes are excluded from further study if any of four conditions occur: (1) If the length of time between ileal harvest and mounting in the Ussing chamber is more than 10 min, (2) if the initial potential difference value of the mounted membrane is less than 3.0 mV, (3) if the potential difference values decrease during the initial 15-min stabilization period, and (4) if visible clouding of the serosal perfusate occurs during the experimental period, in which case the membranes are not used, because this indicates injury of the ileal mucosal membrane.

Advantages of the Ussing system include the ability to have rigorous control over experimental conditions. This eliminates the confounding variables of gut perfusion and oxygenation. The system also offers considerable technical flexibility, because it can be adapted to a variety of experimental conditions. For example, the system can be modified to test cell monolayers (32).

The major drawback to the Ussing system is that despite an intact mucosal architecture, the system may not behave in experimental conditions as would intact gut. Additionally, the system is complex and can be difficult to set up properly and the mucosal membranes are very fragile and to prepare them without damage requires skill. Despite the technical difficulties in the use of the Ussing system, we have found that the advantage of using a controlled *ex vivo* system outweighs these drawbacks.

C. Human Studies

Although the majority of this work has been performed in animal models, there is evidence that this phenomenon can be directly studied and does occur in humans. For example, lymph nodes harvested at surgery can be cultured for translocating bacteria using the methods described earlier. Results from a study by Deitch *et al.* (33), which looked at bacterial translocation in patients with small bowel obstruction by culturing MLNs harvested at the time of surgery, showed that 59% of patients with intestinal obstruction had viable bacteria culture from their mesenteric lymph nodes vs. 4% of operated patients without bowel obstruction. It is likely that small bowel obstruction induced bacterial translocation in these patients by promoting bacterial overgrowth, inhibiting peristalsis, increasing intestinal permeability, and disrupting the mucosal layer. Similarly, a study by O'Boyle showed that translocation occurred in MLNs sampled from 15.4% of surgical patients, and 41% of the patients with evidence of bacterial translocation were found to have septic complications compared with just 14% of those with culture-negative nodes (34). Thus, studies have demonstrated bacterial translocation in the MLNs of humans with bowel obstruction (33), Crohn's disease (35), and other conditions (34). In humans, just as in the animal studies, there is evidence that simple culturing techniques grossly underestimate the magnitude of bacterial translocation, because they only measure viable bacteria. Using immunofluorescence to the bacterial enzyme β-galactosidase, Brathwaite (36) found evidence of bacterial translocation in all of 20 trauma patients studied, although only one patient had culturable bacteria recovered from the MLNs or portal blood.

Indirect studies of gut barrier function, using permeability probes, performed in several high-risk surgical patient populations indicate that gut permeability is increased (37, 38). Most of these studies have used the nonmetabolizable sugars lactulose and mannitol, because after oral ingestion they are excreted unchanged in the urine and they have previously been documented to be effective markers of increased intestinal permeability in patients with inflammatory bowel disease. Additionally, in patients with increased intestinal permeability, the absorption of disaccharides, such as lactulose, is significantly increased, whereas absorption of monosaccharides, such as mannitol, is either unchanged or impaired. In fact, because many variables may influence the results of tests in which a single permeability probe is used, differential permeability techniques that involve the simultaneous use of two markers is optimal. That is, a major advantage of the dual-marker technique is that the confounding effects of variables that may influence results based on a single marker can be overcome by expressing absorption as a ratio of the two markers. For example, factors, such as intestinal motility, surface area of absorption, renal clearance and the accuracy of urine collection, that may alter the results obtained with a single marker of permeability will not alter the absorption ratio of two markers because both markers will be equally affected. In summary, because the amount of lactulose and mannitol excreted in the urine directly reflects the amount absorbed, and lactulose, in contrast to mannitol, is not normally absorbed, an increase in the urinary lactulose:mannitol ratio indicates increased intestinal permeability, even in patients with an ileus.

D. Gut Permeability Techniques

Other permeability markers can be used, some of which in human and all of which in animal studies include ^{51}Cr-labeled EDTA, polyethylene glycols (PEGs) of various sizes, horseradish peroxidase (HRP), and fluorecent-labeled dextran. These markers have the advantage that they are not degraded by intestinal bacteria and therefore can be used to evaluate colonic permeability. ^{51}Cr-labeled EDTA can be used in combination with lactulose, which is absorbed in the small bowel, to provide a correction for the permeability contribution of the small bowel (39). PEG 400 is the most commonly used polyethylene glycol. It contains at least nine distinct polymeric units with molecular masses between 242 and 594 Da (average, 400 Da) (40). Urinary analysis is done by high-pressure liquid chromatography (HPLC), which determines the fraction of each sized PEG separately. HRP is a 40,000-Da probe that crosses the intestinal barrier transcellularly. It has the advantage of detection either cytochemically or quantitatively with a sensitive enzymatic assay (41), but has the disadvantage of requiring tissue samples. Fluorescent-labeled dextran is transported via a paracellular pathway. It can be measured either spectrophotometrically or by fluorescence microscopy. Table IV summarizes the permeability probes discussed above.

Permeability techniques specific to animal studies include everted gut sacs and intestinal isolation. To prepare everted gut sacs (42), sections of the desired intestinal segment are resected and irrigated with cold saline to clear luminal contents. The gut is everted and the ends are tied to form closed sacs. The sacs, filled with buffer, are placed in a solution of the same buffer with a permeability marker. The sacs are then incubated at 37°C on a shaker, with a continuous infusion of O_2 for the desired length of time. When the sac is removed from the buffer, the contents can then be aspirated and analyzed for the permeability probe.

An *in vivo* technique for measuring intestinal permeability is the study of isolated intestinal loops. In this technique, isolated intestinal loops are prepared by incising both ends of a desired segment of bowel (generally 10–15 cm in length) and anastamosing the ends to restore bowel continuity (43). The isolated loop is then cannulated at either end with silastic tubing. The loop is then flushed gently with warm (37°C) saline to remove intestinal contents and is returned to the peritoneal cavity with the ends of the catheter outside the body. Using this method, bidirectional permeability can be assessed by injecting different radiolabeled markers. For example, ^{125}I-labeled albumin can be injected intravenously while ^{131}I-labeled albumin is flushed through the isolated loop. Blood samples and intestinal effluent are sampled simultaneously and permeability is measured using the following formulas (43):

$$\text{Clearance}_{(\text{blood to lumen})} = \frac{\text{perfusate (cpm/ml)} \times \text{perfusion rate (ml/min)} \times 100}{\text{plasma (cpm/ml)} \times \text{sample weight (g)}}$$

$$\text{Clearance}_{(\text{lumen to blood})} = \frac{\text{plasma (cpm/ml)} \times \text{perfusion rate (ml/min)} \times 100}{\text{perfusate (cpm/ml)} \times \text{sample weight (g)}}$$

IV. Conclusion

Gut barrier failure cannot be adequately studied by using a single method or model. Rather, gut barrier defenses are best studied by using a combination of model systems and experimental designs that, when taken together, help to give a picture of the role of the intestinal defenses in preventing systemic illness after injury. In this chapter we have provided some insight into several types of experimental systems

Table IV Permeability Probes

Probe	Advantages	Disadvantages
Lactulose/manntitol[a]	Utilizes ratio of absorption of each molecule to minimize error (dual marker); nontoxic	Sugars can be degraded by intestinal bacteria (especially in stasis); cannot assess colonic permeability
^{51}Cr-Labeled EDTA[b]	Resistant to bacterial degradation; easily measured	Use of radioactivity; single marker test; ^{51}Cr short half-life (27 days) limits uses
Polyethylene glycol[c]	Resistant to bacterial degradation; multiple-sized polymers available; nontoxic	Question of lipid solubility (diffusion through membrane) creating variable results; single marker

[a]From Deitch (37).
[b]From Maxton *et al.* (41a).
[c]From Chadwick *et al.* (40).

that can help to better understand the complex function of the gut barrier.

References

1. Deitch, E. A. (1992). Multiple organ failure. Pathophysiology and potential future therapy. *Ann. Surg.* **216,** 117–134.
2. Deitch, E. A. (1990). Bacterial translocation of the gut flora. *J. Trauma* **30,** S184–S189.
3. Van Der Waaij, D., Berghuis-De Vries, J. M., and Lekkerkerk-Van Der Wees, J. E. C. (1971). Colonization resistance of the digestive tract in conventional and antibiotic-treated mice. *J. Hyg.* **69,** 405–411.
4. Katayama, M., Xu, D., Specian, R., and Deitch, E. (1997). Role of bacterial adherence and the mucus barrier on bacterial translocation: Effects of protein malnutrition and endotoxin in rats. *Ann. Surg.* **225,** 317–326.
5. Rozee, K. R., Cooper, D. Lam, K., and Costerton, J. W. (1982). Microbial flora of the mouse ileum mucus layer and epithelial surface. *Appl. Environ. Microbiol.* **43,** 1451–1463.
6. Diebel L., Liberat, D., Dulchavsky, S., Diglio, C., and Brown, W. (1999). Synergistic effect of hyperoxia and immunoglobulin A on mucosal barrier defense. *J. Trauma* **46,** 374–379.
7. Slocum, M., Sittig, K., Specian, R., and Deitch, E. (1992). Absence of intestinal bile promotes bacterial translocation. *Am. Surg.* **58,** 305–310.
8. Bertok, L. (1977). Physico-chemical defense of vertebrate organisms: The role of bile aids in defense against bacterial endotoxins. *Perspect. Biol. Med.* **21,** 70–76.
9. Deitch, E. A., Xu, D., Naruhn, M., Deitch, D., Lu, Q., and Marino, A. (1995). Elemental diet and IV-TPN-induced bacterial translocation is associated with loss of intestinal mucosal barrier function against bacteria. *Ann. Surg.* **221,** 299–307.
10. Deitch, E. A., Ma, L., Ma, J., and Berg, R. D. (1989). Lethal burn-induced bacterial translocation: Role of genetic resistance. *J. Trauma* **25,** 385–391.
11. Ma, L., Ma, J., Deitch, E. A., Specian, R. D., and Berg, R. D., (1989). Genetic susceptibility to mucosal damage leads to bacterial translocation in a murine burn model. *J. Trauma* **29,** 1245–1251.
12. Wichmann, M. W., Zellweger, R., DeMaso, C., Ayala, A., and Chaudry, I. (1996). Enhanced immune responses in females as opposed to decreased responses in males after hemorrhagic shock. *Cytokine* **8,** 853–863.
13. Berg, R. D., and Garlington, A. W. (1979). Translocation of certain indigenous bacteria from the mouse gastrointestinal tract to the mesenteric lymph nodes and other organs in a gnotobiotic mouse model. *Infect. Immun.* **23,** 403–411.
14. Chiu, C., McArdle, A., Brown, R., Scott, H., and Gurd, F. (1970). Intestinal mucosal lesion in low flow states. I. A morphological hemodynamic, and metabolic reappraisal. *Arch. Surg.* **101,** 478–483.
15. Gautreaux, M., Deitch, E., and Berg, R. (1994). Bacterial Translocation from the gastrointestinal tract to various segments of the mesenteric lymph node complex. *Infect. Immun.* **62,** 2132–2134.
16. Alexnder, J. W., Gianotti, L., Pyles, T., Carey, M. A., and Babcock, G. F. (1991). Distribution and survival of *Escherichia coli* translocating from the intestine after thermal injury. *Ann. Surg.* **213,** 558–567.
17. Berg, R. D. (1980). Inhibition of *Escherichia coli* translocation from the gastrointestinal tract by normal cecal flora in gnotobiotic or antibiotic decontaminated mice. *Infect. Immun.* **29,** 1073–1081.
18. Gu, W., Ding, J., Huang, Q., Jerrells, T., and Deitch E. A. (1995). Alterations in intestinal bacterial flora modulate the systemic cytokine response to hemorrhagic shock. *Am. J. Physiol.* **269,** G827–G832.

18a. Pinto, M., Robine-Leon, S., Appay, M. D., Kedinger, M., Triadou, N., Dusaulx, E., Lacroix, B., Simon-Assmann, P., Haffen, K., Fogh, J., and Zweibaum, A. (1983). Enterocyte-like differentiation and polarization of the human colon carcinoma cell line Caco-2 in culture. *Biol. Cell.* **47,** 323–330.

18b. Wells, C., Van de Westerlo, E., Jechorek, R., and Erlandsen, S. (1996). Intracellular survival of enteric bacteria in cultured human enterocytes. *Shock* **6,** 27–34.

18c. Pinto, M., Appay, M., Simon-Assmann, P., Chevalier, G., Dracopoli, N., Fogh, J., and Zweibaum, A. (1982). Enterocytic differentiation of cultured human colon cancer cells by replacement of glucose by galactose in the medium. *Biol. Cell.* **44,** 193–196.

18d. Quaroni, A., Wands, J., Trelstad, R., and Isselbacher, K. (1979). Epithelioid cell cultures from rat small intestine: Characterization by morphologic and immunologic criteria. *J. Cell Biol.* **80,** 248–265.

19. Rousset, M. (1986). The human colon carcinoma cell line HT-29 and Caco-2: Two *in vitro* models for the study of intestinal differentiation. *Biochimie* **68,** 1035–1040.
20. Cruz, N., Lu, Q., Alvarez, X., Berg, R., and Deich, E. (1994). The Caco-2 cell monolayer system as an *in vitro* model for studying bacterial-enterocyte interactions and bacterial translocation. *J. Burn Care Rehabil.* **15,** 207–212.
21. Xu, D., Lu, Q., Swank, G., and Deitch, E. (1996). Effect of heat shock and endotoxin stress on enterocyte viability apoptosis and function varies based on whether the cells are exposed to heat shock or endotoxin first, *Arch. Surg.* **131,** 1222–1228.
22. Hidalgo, I., Raub, T., and Borchardt, R. (1989). Characterization of the human colon carcinoma cell line (Caco-2) as a model system for intestinal epithelial permeability. *Gastroenterology* **96,** 736–49.
23. Cruz, N., Lu, Q., Alvarez, X., and Deitch, E. (1994). Bacterial translocation is bacterial species dependent: Results using the human Caco-2 intestinal cell line. *J. Trauma* **36,** 612–616.
24. Katayama, M., Xu D., Specian, R., and Deitch E. (1997). Role of bacterial adherence and the mucus barrier on bacterial translocation: Effects of protein malnutrition and endotoxin in rats. *Ann. Surg.* **225,** 317–326.
25. Cruz, N., Alvarez, X., Berg, R., and Deitch, E. (1994). Bacterial translocation across enterocytes: Results of a study of bacterial-enterocyte interactions utilizing Caco-2 cells. *Shock* **1,** 67–72.
26. Xu, D., Lu, Q., Kubicka, R., and Deitch, E. (1999). The effect of hypoxia/reoxygenation on the cellular function of intestinal epithelial cells. *J. Trauma,* **46,** 280–285.
27. Michalsky, M. P., Deitch, E. A., Ding, J., Lu, Q., and Huang, Q. (1997). Interleukin-6 and tumor necrosis factor production in an enterocyte cell model (Caco-2) during exposure to *Eschericia coli. Shock* **7,** 139–146.
28. Ussing, H. H. (1949). The active ion transport through the isolated frog skin in the light of tracer studies. *Acta Physiol. Scand.* **17,** 1–37.
29. Deitch, E. A., Xu, D., Naruhn, M. B., Deitch, D. C., Lu, Q., and Marino, A. A. (1995). Elemental diet and IV-TPN-induced bacterial translocation is associated with loss of intestinal mucosal barrier function against bacteria. *Ann. Surg.* **221,** 299–307.
30. Mishima, S., Xu, D., and Deitch, E. A. (1999). Increase in endotoxin-induced mucosal permeability is related to increased nitric oxide synthase activity using the Ussing chamber. *Crit. Care Med.* **27,** 880–886.
31. Grotz, M. R. W., Deitch, E. A., Ding J., Xu, D., Huang, Q., and Regel, G. (1999). The intestinal cytokine response after gut ischemia—Role of gut barrier failure. *Ann. Surg.* **229,** 478–486.
32. Dharmsathaphorn, K., McRoberts, J., Mandel, K., *et al.* (1984) A human colonic tumor cell line that maintains vectorial electrolyte transport. *Am. J. Physiol.* **246,** G204–208.
33. Deitch, E. A. (1989). Simple intestinal obstruction causes bacterial translocation in man. *Arch. Surg.* **124,** 699–701.
34. O'Boyle, C. J., MacFie, J., Mitchell, C. J., Johnstone, D., Sagar, P., and Sedman, P. (1998). Microbiology of bacterial translocation in humans. *Gut* **42,** 29–35.
35. Ambrose, N. S., Johnson, M., Burdon, D. W., and Keighley, M. R. B.

(1984). Incidence of pathogenic bacteria from mesenteric lymph nodes and ileal serosa during Crohn's disease surgery. *Brit. J. Surg.* **71,** 623–625.

36. Brathwaite, C. E., Ross, S. E., Nagele, R., Mure, A. J., O'Malley, K. F., and Garcia-Perez, F. A. (1993). Bacterial translocation occurs in humans after traumatic injury: Evidence using immunofluorescence. *J. Trauma* **34,** 586–589.
37. Deitch, E. (1990). Intestinal permeability is increased in burn patients shortly after injury. *Surgery* **107,** 411–416.
38. Brooks, A. D., Hochwald, S. N., Heslin, M. J., Harrison, L. E., Burt, M., and Brennan, M. (1999). Intestinal permeability after early post-operative enteral nutrition in patients with upper gastrointestinal malignancy. *JPEN* **23,** 75–79.
39. Jenkins, R. T., Trew, D. R., Crump, B. J., Nukajam, W. S., Foley, J. A., Menzies, I. S., and Creamer, B. (1991). Do non-steroidal anti-inflammatory drugs increase colonic permeability? *Gut* **32,** 66–69.
40. Chadwick, V. S., Phillips, S. F., and Hoffman, A. F. (1977). Measurements of intestinal permeability using low molecular weight polyethylene glycols. *Gastroenterology* **73,** 241–246.
41. Warshaw, A. L., Walker, W. A., Cornell, R., and Isselbacher, K. (1971). Small intestinal permeability to macromolecules: Transmission of horseradish peroxidase into mesenteric lymph and portal blood. *Lab. Invest.* **25,** 675–684.

41a. Maxton, D., Bjarnason, I., Reynolds, A., Catt, S., Peters, T., and Menzies, I. (1986). Lactulose, ^{51}Cr-labelled ethylenediaminetetia-acetate, L-rhamnose, and polyethylene glycol 500 as probe markers for assessment *in vivo* of human intestinal permeability. *Clin. Sci.* **71,** 71–80.

42. Carter, E. A., Bloch, K. J., Cohen, S., Isselbacher, K. J., and Walker, W. (1981). Use of hydrogen gas (H_2) analysis to assess intestinal absorption. *Gastroenterology* **81,** 1091–1097.

42. Sun, Z. W., Wang, X. D., Deng, X. M., Wallen, R., Gefors, L., Hallberg, E., and Andersson, R. (1997). The influence of circulatory and gut luminal changes on bidirectional intestinal barrier permeability in rats. *Scand. J. Gastroenterol.* **32,** 995–1004.

47

Developmental Studies in the Gastrointestinal Tract

George K. Gittes, Thomas S. Maldonado, and Christopher A. Crisera

Department of Surgery, Children's Mercy Hospital, Kansas City, Missouri 64108

I. Introduction

Developmental biology is rapidly evolving as a field, due to progress in molecular biology, as well as in tissue culture and cell biology. The field is becoming more interesting to surgeons as we begin to understand how the processes of morphogenesis and differentiation that occur in the embryo may mirror processes seen in tissues both abnormally, as in cancer, or else normally in a venue of tissue engineering. This chapter focuses on concepts and techniques pertinent to gastrointestinal development, as well as development of the pancreas.

In general, developmental studies can be focused on different levels involved in organogenesis. In the gastrointestinal tract, we can specifically look at morphogenesis of tissues, such as the formation of the crypts and villi of the intestine, as well as the morphogenesis of the pancreatic ducts, acini, and endocrine islets. These morphogenetic processes can be studied both by simple histology, as well as by studying the controlling patterning genes that influence this morphogenesis. Along a different line, a process of cell-specific differentiation can be studied by simply looking at the ontogeny of these expressions, or else by manipulating the process of differentiation using transgenic animals or by manipulating gene expression *in vitro* in a tissue culture system. Alternatively, we can look at the nature in which cell differentiation is guided between different cell lineages within the developing organ. Lineage selection is of particular importance for tissue engineering because lineage selection pathways are responsible for guiding stem cells into fully differentiated cells (1–6). Tissue engineers wish to use these forces to guide *in vitro* stem cells to recreate organs for clinical use.

Last, diseased or abnormal tissue, modified by transgenic technology or by toxins, can be studied developmentally in tissue culture or through simple histology. These diseased or abnormal tissues can give us insight into disease processes that we see clinically.

II. Working with Embryonic Tissues

In order to perform studies in developmental biology, it is necessary to gain access to embryonic tissues. Many laboratories have focused predominantly on mice, given the availability of transgenic animals to study the role of different genes and gene products in embryonic development. Alternatively, chick embryos have been used historically by embryologists because these embryos can be cultured whole in a dish, allowing for direct surgical manipulation of these developing embryos with tissue transfers, introduction of foreign objects/tissues, or addition of exogenous molecules without difficulty. Obviously, the choice of the type of embryo in particular must strike a balance between closeness to humans and technical facilitation. For this chapter, we focus on mouse and rat embryos because of their frequent use in the biomedical literature.

In general, the age of the embryo is a very important aspect of using these embryos. Precise time-dated mating of mice or rats can be performed by obtaining females that are over 4–5 weeks of age and examining them for the presence of estrous. Estrous corresponds to the time of ovulation and is specifically defined by a pink and somewhat edematous vaginal mucosa, which occurs periodically. Females housed together in a cage frequently become uniform in their cycling to estrous and this greatly facilitates determining which mice are in estrous for timed mating. These females should be placed in the cage (in groups of 1–3) with one male mouse that is at least 5 weeks old and has been singly housed for at least 1 week prior to mating. In addition, newly arrived males frequently will yield a false-positive plug in the female. Thus, avoiding younger males that have not been singly housed and have not arrived from the vendor within the past 7 days will give a higher yield of pregnancy. Generally, the mice will mate within the first hour or two after the lights are turned off in the animal facility, but there is added variability in the age of the embryos given the exact time of fertilization, as well as the rate of growth of different strains of mice. Typically, inspection of the females the next morning will show a mucous plug present in the vagina. This usually (approximately 80–90%) indicates pregnancy. For the purpose of uniformity, noon of the day of discovering a vaginal plug is used as time 0.5 days of gestation, which assumes that fertilization of the egg occurred at approximately midnight. Due to the aforementioned variability within this time-dated mating system, an internal aging of the embryos is also very important. Between days 8 and 12 in mice, and approximately days 9 and 13 in rats, the age of the embryo can be precisely determined by counting somites. Typically, each additional somite adds 2 hr to the age of the embryo during this time. Outside of these time windows, however, specific markers of the exact age of the embryo have been outlined by various scaling systems. These systems employ markers such as the eyes turning black, the paddles of the limbs becoming subdivided, return of the intestines into the abdomen, etc.

In general, embryos are harvested by performing a cervical dislocation on the pregnant mother and then removing the hair and skin from the abdomen to avoid any contamination of the embryos with hair. This is most rapidly done by a pinch-and-pull technique after washing the abdomen with 95% ethanol. Once the skin and hair have been pulled out of the way, the gloves are then changed and the abdominal muscles are opened with sterile scissors, taking care to avoid nicking the intestine, which obviously would lead to contamination. The uterine horns are then harvested and placed into cold tissue culture medium. The embryos are then removed from the uterine segments individually as quickly as possible to cool off the embryo and therefore slow metabolism. The removal of the embryo from the uterine segments is nontrivial and requires carefully opening up the uterine sac and then extruding the embryo slowly to avoid tearing or rupture of the embryo, particularly at younger ages (days 9–11). At very young ages (less than day 9) the embryo and amniotic fluid sack are not directly visible through the uterine wall, and it is best to dissect slowly through the uterine wall with microdissection under direct visualization with a dissecting microscope. Once the embryo is removed, the head should be amputated to avoid any pain sensation by the embryo or fetus. In general, the tissue dissection should then be performed rapidly, with a focus on reducing the amount of time that the whole embryo is in the tissue culture medium, because diffusion of nutrients into the whole embryo is minimal. Preparation for experiments through extensive practice of dissection should be performed before conducting actual experiments, to facilitate the speed with which these dissections are performed. Speed is of particular importance when considering harvesting tissue for RNA isolation, because of the relative instability of mRNA. The tissue dissections should be done in medium that contains serum and glucose to avoid any unnecessary metabolic stress for the embryonic tissues. Embryonic tissue dissections are highly variable depending on the organ that is being dissected and the age of the embryo. Of note, older embryos tend to have thicker tissues and in general the dissections may not lend themselves to transmitted light. Specifically, the whole mouse embryo after day 12 does not transilluminate and the initial part of the dissection must be done with light from above. As the individual organ or blocks of tissue of interest are removed from the embryo, even at day 12 or later, the light should then be switched to posterior lighting to allow transillumination of the tissues. Transillumination can be done throughout the dissection for younger embryos. Transillumination is of particular advantage because it allows the dissector to visualize subtle tissue planes in three-dimensional structures much more easily.

In addition to the lighting techniques, dissection instruments are also very important. Typically, a larger pair of tissue scissors is used for removing the embryo from the uterine sac. However, a smaller, preferably iridectomy, scissors is also needed, as well as very fine-tipped (#4 or #5) jeweler's forceps. In addition, a spear or sharp-pointed tip (small-gauge needles can be used here) is also very helpful. In general, the approach in embryo dissection is to safely remove tissue that you are sure is not the tissue of interest. This approach can be used to slowly whittle down the embryonic tissue. Once the tissue of interest is isolated, a hand-held pipette-man is best for transferring the tissue. Embryonic tissues are extremely sticky and the commercially available "slick" pipette tips for the hand-held pipettes are best. All handling of embryonic tissue at the organ level should be done under direct visualization with a dissecting microscope. Once the tissue of interest is placed into the pipette it should then be placed into a second petri dish with the media, again under direct visualization, by removing the dish that contains the excess embryonic tissue and putting the new petri dish under the dissecting microscope view. Then the organ in the pipette can be directly placed into the new petri dish. This use of direct visualization is extremely important to avoid the common problem of the tissue mysteriously disappearing during transfers. As will be outlined below, occasionally it is necessary for experimental purposes to separate the epithelium and the mesenchyme in the embryonic tissues (see Fig. 1). In general, the earlier the gestational time point at which tissues are being worked with, the easier it is to separate the mesenchyme. Epithelium and mesenchyme are usually separated by a basement membranelike layer, which is sensitive to trypsin. Other enzymes such as collagenase type IV can be used, but traditionally trypsin has had the best results. In general, however, trypsinization is best performed by exposing the tissue to a 1% trypsin solution at 4°C instead of either at room temperature or in an incubator. The reason is that at colder temperatures the enzyme is much less active and can penetrate into the tissue to act specifically on what appears to be the preferred substrate, the basement membrane. In this way, a more precise cleavage plane appears to develop between the epithelium and the mesenchyme in most organs. If the trypsin is exposed to the tissue at warmer temperatures, the enzyme tends to digest all of the connections between tissues and cells as it diffuses through the tissue, and therefore by the time the basement membrane is lysed by the trypsin, other potentially important aspects of the embryonic tissue are also digested. The amount of time for exposure to the 1% trypsin solution is highly variable, and dependent on both the age of the tissue and the type of tissue being dissected. For example, for an 11- or 12-day mouse intestine, roughly 15–20 min of 1% trypsin at 4°C is necessary to develop a cleavage plane. Intestine mesenchyme tends to be easy to remove, compared with pancreas.

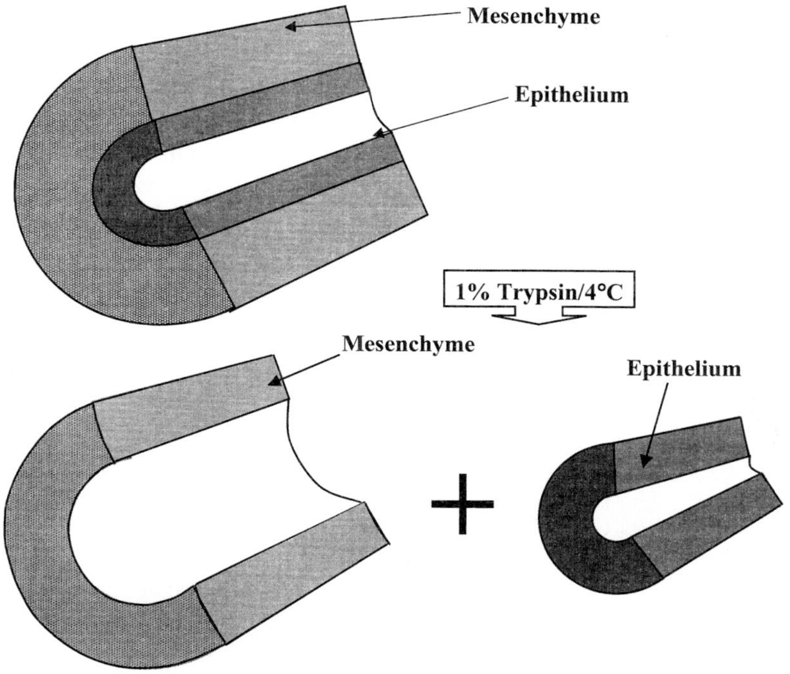

Figure 1 Frequently it is necessary to separate epithelium from its surrounding mesenchyme in developing gastrointestinal tissues, including the intestine and pancreas. Here it is shown that using 1% trypsin at 4°C, the epithelium and mesenchyme can usually be separated along a clean plane. This trypsinization requires careful attention to the amount of time the tissues are exposed to trypsin and also reversal of the trypsinization using serum at the end of the dissection.

III. Tissue and Organ Culture

Broadly speaking, we can study morphogenesis and cell-specific differentiation in two ways, using *in vitro* culture systems and using *in vivo* ontogeny studies. Each provides us with unique insight into developmental processes.

Various approaches exist for embryonic tissue culture. These approaches include intestinal cultures, either whole intestine for different regions of the gut, or else a disbursed cell culture with monolayer, or even cells grown in apposition to mesenchyme to test epithelial–mesenchymal interactions. These cultures can be done either in gel matrices or on various substrata, such as submucosa devoid of cells (7, 8) (see Fig. 2). For pancreas, options again include monolayer culture or three-dimensional culture with epithelium alone or with mesenchyme (9–12).

The three-dimensional culture system consists of embedding the organ of interest in a gel matrix on a 12-mm diameter 4-μm pore size filter-well insert. The organ is then grown in culture media, typically composed of Dulbecco's modified Eagle's medium (DMEM) with 10% fetal calf serum (FCS) and antimycotic/antibiotic, for up to 7 days. This system can be further varied by using collagen or basement membrane gels. Alternatively, organs can also be grown at the air–fluid interface in two dimensions on a filter as an organ culture system. The intestine or pancreas can also be grown under the renal capsule of a syngenic or athymic adult mouse to give an *in vivo* environment for development (12).

Epithelial mix-and-match studies can be done in a gel culture or in a feeder layer system (7, 13–16). Special care must be taken to approximate epithelium and mesenchyme when performing mix-and-match experiments in a gel culture system. Fortuitously, tissues placed in gel matrices tend to gravitate toward each other over time, probably due to specific cell adhesion molecules (17–20). Nevertheless, collagen gels usually solidify within 1 hr at 37°C, thus epithelium and mesenchyme should be checked for juxtaposition after 1 hr, immediately prior to placing them in the incubator. Similarly, cell lines such as intestinal epithelial crypt (IEC) cells can be used for intestinal differentiation studies, with exposure to different components or even mesenchyme, to test differentiation pathways (21, 22).

One goal for working with mouse and rat embryonic tissues *in vitro* is to establish a culture model that parallels the normal *in vivo* growth and development of the particular organ of interest. To ascertain the *in vitro* validation of *in vivo* developmental patterning, one should start with an appropriately early gestational age, which contains undifferentiated cells. For example, in our pancreas culture system, E11.5 represents a gestational age that is relatively undifferentiated and has not undergone appreciable morphogenesis. Typically E11.5 embryonic organs are grown for 7 days *in vitro* because this represents full-term *in vivo* growth. Moreover, exocrine organs, such as the pancreas, tend to lyse due to autodigestion if grown for more than 7 days (10–12). A three-dimensional gel culture system is preferred when establishing *in vitro* models of development for embryonic organs, because the matrix provides a framework for growth and differentiation in all directions (as *in vivo*), without allowing for flattening of the pancreas or intestine on the filter.

Once an *in vitro* model is established one can validate the system by determining if the system parallels that which is known to occur *in vivo* during development. In particular,

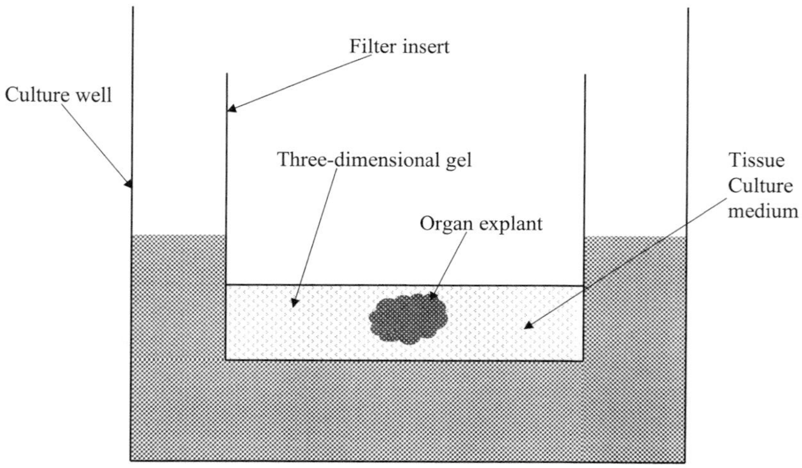

Figure 2 A schematic representation of the embryonic organ culture system. A filter insert that contains a layer of gel within the insert that contains the organ explant is placed into a well that contains normal tissue culture medium, typically in a 6-well or 24-well plate. Alternatively, no gel can be used and the tissue can be grown in a flat, two-dimensional plane on the filter at the air–media interface.

morphogenesis, as determined by histology and cell differentiation, as described through cell markers at the genetic and protein level, serve to validate the *in vitro* model.

A. Methods of Analysis

Analysis of embryonic organs grown *in vitro*, as well as *in vivo*, can be performed using a variety of standard techniques, including histology, immunohistochemistry, *in situ* hybridization, as well as RNA and protein analysis of tissue grind-ups with Northern hybridization techniques, reverse transcriptase–polymerase chain reaction (RT-PCR), Western blotting, or enzyme-linked immunosorbent assay (ELISA). Typical histology of embryonic tissues using hematoxylin and eosin staining provides for fundamental analyses of morphogenesis. These histologic studies are particularly important when studying complex organs such as pancreas and liver whose architecture often dictates function. Immunohistochemistry (IHC) can be of further use in examining morphogenesis. For instance, IHC can be employed to examine pancreatic islet architecture, normally consisting of central insulin and peripheral glucagon and somatostatin cells. The use of monoclonal primary antibodies has traditionally been problematic when studying mouse or rat adult tissues because of significant background staining. Although various monoclonal antibody IHC kits are commercially available to circumvent this, in our experience embryonic tissues tend to be less immunogenic and often do not necessitate such measures.

In addition to studying morphogenesis, immunohistochemistry is perhaps most often used for studying cell differentiation. This study of differentiation becomes especially important when studying embryonic tissues containing purported pluripotential cells or stem cells, because these cells are generally not well characterized for gut, liver, and pancreas (2, 5, 23, 24). In our laboratory we have used double or triple immunofluorescent techniques to identify such pluripotential cells in the embryonic pancreas, which express markers of both exocrine and endocrine pancreatic markers. Moreover, these cells have been manipulated *in vitro*, as discussed below, to undergo selective differentiation, thus confirming their pluripotentiality.

In situ hybridization provides yet another important tool for studying embryonic tissues both *in vivo* and *in vitro*. This technique can be difficult to perform in exocrine digestive organs, such as pancreas, because of autolysis. However, early embryonic ages (prior to E16.5) are less difficult to work with using *in situ* hybridization, because these tissues have not yet developed zymogen granules with RNases (25). Nonetheless, all tissues subject to *in situ* hybridization should be handled using strict RNase precautions.

Preparing specimens for immunohistochemistry can be challenging given the small size (as low as 100 μm in some cases) of early gestational-aged embryonic organs. Specimens should be fixed in 2% paraformaldehyde for 2 hr followed by 2 hr in 30% sucrose, embedded in OCT media, and flash frozen in liquid nitrogen. Care must be taken to place the specimens in the center of embedding molds and swirled to ensure that the OCT media percolates into the specimen, thus preventing fracturing of the specimen when cutting frozen sections. Furthermore, specimens may be briefly dipped in eosin prior to embedding in order to facilitate finding them when cutting. However, eosin dipping must be avoided if immunofluorescent IHC is planned due to the autofluorescence of eosin.

In addition to histology and other staining techniques, such as immunohistochemistry and *in situ* hybridization, one can use tissue homogenates to study RNA and protein expression of both *in vivo* specimens (for the purposes of describing ontogeny) and *in vitro* specimens grown in culture. Northern and Western analyses are best performed by pooling embryonic specimens because each requires a minimum of 15–30 μg of RNA and 100 μg of protein, respectively. In particular, pancreas can be difficult to analyze using Northern or Western analyses because the yield from each pancreas for RNA and protein is in the range of nanograms. Instead, RT-PCR can be employed when analyzing RNA from such low-yield organs as pancreas. Basic RT-PCR can offer information about the presence or absence of a given mRNA, but it cannot be used for quantitative analysis (26–28). New modified PCR techniques in which the amplification of a gene product can be monitored in "real-time," with respect to a control gene product via a luminometric assay, can be used for quantitative data analysis (29). These modified systems may offer a significant breakthrough in studies involving microscopic embryonic structures in which Northern analysis is impossible.

ELISA systems do have some utility in the study of embryonic structures, because they are exquisitely sensitive. Mid to late gestational gastrointestinal structures can be used to effectively condition media for ELISA quantification of protein expression. ELISA kits are commercially available for a variety of growth factors and cytokines, which are known to be biologically active in gastrointestinal organogenesis.

B. Simple Ontogeny Studies

Simple ontogeny studies are often the foundation of developmental research. Ontogeny studies are commonly designed with specific target factors in mind. These target factors may represent genes or proteins specific to the organ of interest. They may be transcription factors implicated in the patterning of that organ. They may be transcription factors or cytokines that regulate gene expression and function in the organ as it develops. The distribution of the target factor in the organ of interest at various gestational time points often provides the investigator with clues to its specific role(s) in that organ. For example, the localization of a given protein to the developing endocrine cells of the mid to late gestation embryonic pancreas might suggest that this factor plays some role in endocrine lineage selection. These observations frequently translate into secondary studies entailing perturbation of the factors in culture systems or in transgenic animals.

To begin studying the ontogeny of a given factor it is, of course, necessary to create a bank of tissue specimens from various time points of embryonic development. The level of investigation of the gene of interest (i.e., mRNA vs. protein/gene product) will dictate the manner in which the bank of gestational specimens is gathered (RNA isolation, histologic specimens, protein isolation, etc). Regardless, it is vital that the investigator is able to recognize developmental landmarks to age-date embryos and that he is facile with embryonic dissections (as discussed in Section II) to isolate the developing organs of interest.

The methods of analysis in ontogeny studies are identical to those mentioned in Section III,A. This similarity is fortunate because it provides an opportunity to validate the *in vitro* culture system as a truly appropriate model of *in vivo* organogenesis. Being able to correlate the identical steps of differentiation and morphogenesis histologically, or on the mRNA level via RT-PCR, Northern blots, and *in situ* hybridization, or on the protein level via immunohistochemistry, Western blot analysis, and ELISA, sets the stage for further studies in which the *in vitro* model is manipulated to derive insights into the specific roles of the critical target factors in organogenesis.

C. Manipulation of Cultures

The establishment of a reliable culture system for studying embryonic organ development *in vitro*, or the growth characteristics of a gastrointestinal-derived cell line, affords the investigator great power and flexibility to begin elucidating specific molecular mechanisms in organogenesis. For example, recognizing the association of the expression of a candidate factor with the timing of a specific developmental step (morphogenesis or cytodifferentiation) in the embryo might lead the investigator to question what effect the misexpression (inhibition or overexpression) of that factor would have on the normal developmental process. Subsequent analysis of the organ or cells grown in the manipulated culture system should yield insights into the specific function of the perturbed factor in the growing tissue, and possibly its relationship to other critical regulatory or patterning factors.

With an appropriately valid and reliable *in vitro* model, this type of educated "candidate factor" approach, in which the expression of specific genes or proteins is perturbed in a developing culture system, is easier, cheaper, and arguably cleaner, with respect to the quality of the data it generates, than other molecular means of deriving similar information, such as the creation of transgenic or knockout mice. Altering the expression of a factor globally in a developing embryo, via transgenic methods, may allow for confounding epiphenomena or nonspecific signaling compensations throughout the embryo, making the interpretation of the effects of the manipulation on a specific organ difficult. Thus, manipulation of the factor in an isolated organ or cell culture model may provide a truer understanding of the biological role of this factor in the developing system.

In general, manipulation of a culture system involves either augmenting or blocking the endogenous expression of a target factor in a growing system. There are numerous research strategies to accomplish these ends *in vitro* (see Table I).

1. Blocking Studies

One major benefit of recent advances in biotechnology has been the proliferation of commercial sources that manufacture antibodies against most target factors of interest. These antibodies are commonly designed for immunohistochemical staining and Western analyses, but often they can function to bind to and functionally block the activity of a factor in a growing culture system. The effectiveness of this method of inhibiting endogenous activity of a target factor is obviously dependent on the specificity and affinity of the antibody for the target protein. Nonetheless, blocking activity at the functional level is an efficient way to study the role of a target protein in a developing system. Frequently, preliminary experiments must be conducted to establish the optimal dosage of the antibody in the culture system. A major potential pitfall of performing blocking manipulations with antibodies in embryonic gastrointestinal organ culture models (particularly the pancreas) is the ability of the antibody to penetrate throughout the growing three-dimensional organ. The embryonic mesenchyme, which enshrouds these growing organs, can act as a barrier to the penetration of the antibodies into the epithelium of the structures. Thus, the

Table I Culture Manipulation Strategies[a]

Blocking	Activation
Antisense oligonucleotides	Exogenous proteins
Neutralizing antibody	Transgenic mice with high expression
Null mutant mice	Blocking inhibitors
Dominant negative transgenic System	

[a]Many techniques are available for manipulating embryonic tissues in culture, or *in vivo*. The various strategies for either blocking or activating/enhancing signaling or expression are shown in the table.

risk of partial blockade must be recognized as one attempts to interpret data from antibody-blocking studies. One final caution about using antibodies to perform blocking manipulations is their expense. The concentrations required to perform adequate blockage frequently are quite high. Although the antibodies are readily available commercially, this convenience has a price. In general, for these antibody blocking experiments, proper controls should include preincubation of the antibody with free protein, if available, to rule out nonspecific binding of the antibody.

Another effective means of blocking expression of a target factor *in vitro* is the utilization of antisense strategies. Antisense involves inhibition of expression at the mRNA level. The means through which this is accomplished is via the addition of single-stranded fragments of oligodeoxynucleotides, about 20 base pairs in length, which are manufactured to be complementary (hence "antisense") to the start region of the target factor's mRNA sequence (30). Inhibition seems to be accomplished in two ways. The binding of the antisense fragment to the mRNA blocks translation of the target factor. It also appears to activate ribonucleases (specifically RNase H) that degrade the mRNA–antisense complex. To assure that the effect of the antisense manipulation is specifically attributable to the antisense fragment, a critical control for such studies is the parallel addition of a "missense" oligodeoxynucleotide fragment to the growing culture system. The missense fragment is the same length as the antisense fragment, but rather than having a specific base pair sequence, it is just a random sequence. Thus, it should not bind to the target, or any other mRNA sequence, and it will not activate ribonucleases. Antisense manipulations can be very effective at blocking expression of a target gene. Antisense seems to work better against targets that are not abundantly expressed in a normal developing tissue. Advances in antisense technology have helped to overcome some of the inherent flaws in such strategies. Most significant have been the modifications to the oligodeoxynucleotide fragments to minimize their susceptibility to intracellular degradation, such as substituting sulfur moieties for oxygen on the oligo backbone (31, 32). Because of the potential for interaction (binding) with elements of serum in culture media, antisense manipulations are best performed in serum-free culture systems. The optimal concentration of antisense must be determined for each system in titration experiments. Regardless, the antisense solute must be replenished in the media every 2 to 3 days for ongoing blockage. In addition to analyzing the global effects of the antisense manipulation on the growing organ or cells (see Section III,A), efforts should also be made to assay the target-specific effectiveness of blocking of the manipulation, if possible. Finally, when using a culture system in which the organ or cells are growing within a well-filter insert (see Section III), care must be taken to use an insert with a filter pore size large enough (usually 1.0 μm or greater) to allow for easy passage of the antisense or missense fragments across the filter to the growing tissue(s).

2. Augmentation Studies

The easiest means of analyzing the effect of overexpression of a target factor in a developing system is to add increasing concentrations of the protein exogenously to the growth medium. The availability of exogenous factors is the primary limitation to this strategy. Many common growth factors are available commercially, but this technique is certainly not applicable to the study of transcription factors. When purified factors can be obtained, examining the effect of exposing the growing organ or cells to a spectrum of concentrations of the factor will often yield a dose–response phenomenon in the growing structure. In this way, insights into the normal role of the factor can become apparent.

Another popular technique for augmenting the endogenous level of expression of a target factor is through viral delivery of DNA encoding the factor. Replication-deficient adenoviruses and retroviruses have been used extensively for this type of gene therapy *in vivo* and *in vitro* (33–37). Viral delivery to cells in culture is relatively straightforward and is discussed in greater detail elsewhere in this text. The level of expression of the target gene in the virus is dependent on factors such as the strength of the promoter of the gene construct. This is particularly true when dealing with embryonic tissues, because the activity of specific promoters has been noted to be affected by the unique embryonic environment. Viral delivery to growing embryonic gastrointestinal organ culture systems has been quite problematic. This difficulty is primarily due to the inability of the virus to penetrate the peripheral mesenchyme of these structures and infect the entire organ. Work with nonviral mechanisms of delivery, such as cationic liposomes, has shown some promise, but is often complicated by the same problems of penetrance (38–41).

Clearly, experiments in which a developmental system is manipulated are very valuable for illuminating the role(s) of specific regulatory factors in organogenesis. The potential for an even greater value to these types of experiments cannot be understated. The ability to isolate early embryonic structures and then orchestrate their subsequent development to desired ends has huge implications for the growing field of tissue engineering. It is not unreasonable to believe that soon relatively simple *in vitro* manipulations will allow us to amplify pools of cells from the early embryonic foregut and steer them toward a β-cell phenotype or toward hepatocyte maturation. The essential data foundation for such cellular engineering will undoubtedly arise from basic ontogeny studies, blocking and augmentation culture studies, and transgenic mouse studies.

IV. Transgenic Animals in Studies of Developmental Biology

In the past 20 years, the technology of creating transgenic and knockout mice has greatly changed the ways in which we can study developmental processes in mammals. As discussed elsewhere in this book, transgenic technology allows the tissue specific or else global expression of transgenes introduced into the fertilized egg, so that the embryo or mouse that develops has had a specific manipulation of gene expression. Using this promoter-driven concept, we can then test the effect of genetic manipulations on the development of specific tissue. In general, these techniques can be applied to developmental studies as discussed above, either by examining tissue culture specimens, or else by studying simple ontogeny of these transgenic tissues. There are two provisos with working with transgenic animals for the developmental studies outlined above. First is that the speed of development of embryos varies greatly for different transgenically altered animals. In particular, certain strains of mice will develop more slowly. In addition, there is also the potential for embryonic lethal phenotypes. Embryonic developmental studies offer a particular advantage in these embryonic lethal phenotypes in that postnatal studies are obviously not possible. If the embryonic lethality is relatively late in gestation (commonly occurring in the 9- to 12-day range), then the specific culture of earlier prelethal tissues can be performed for specific manipulations and studies as outlined above. An intrinsic problem with transgenic systems is that they are perturbed systems, and usually do not reliably indicate the true developmental biology that occurs normally. In addition, transgenic systems typically require overexpression analysis. Overexpression is more easily induced by using highly expressed promoters. Alternatively, to use the transgenic system to allow blockage of signaling, dominant-negative receptors can be induced to be expressed at high levels either in a tissue-specific way, or globally, to test the effect of blocking the signaling of a specific pathway (42). Dominant-negative receptors typically work through a normal extracellular domain of the receptor that lacks the normal intracellular signaling component, and therefore no intracellular signaling is conducted. If these receptors are expressed at a high level, they functionally block the normal signaling by serving as a competitive antagonist of normal signaling.

Specific phenotypes in transgenic animals can be secondarily examined by mix-and-match strategies, for example, if we wish to look at epithelial–mesenchymal interactions, the epithelium of a wild-type organ can be recombined with the mesenchyme of a transgenic animal or vice versa. This recombination approach allows the direction of specific signaling (epithelium-to-mesenchyme, or vice-versa) and the source of signaling in a genetically altered system to be carefully analyzed. A last way of using transgenic systems is either heterotopic expression of genes (rather than overexpression or dominant-negative expression) or heterochronic expression of transgenes. This use of altered expression can facilitate studies in development wherein one wishes to sort out lineage selection or else to isolate the role of a specific transgene in various tissues by using tissue-specific promoters. Heterochronic expression is performed by using a promoter that is expressed earlier or later than the normal expression period of a gene in question, though in the proper organ or location. Heterotopic expression is easily performed by using a tissue-specific promoter different than the tissue that normally expresses the transgene. Collectively, these transgenic systems obviously allow for a great deal of flexibility in different approaches to studying these systems. As outlined elsewhere in this book, the transgenic technology, though very sophisticated, has become streamlined now to allow the procedures to be commonplace in medical research.

The technique of gene knockout in studying mouse development is predicated on initial observations of mutations or deletions in lower animals such as *Drosophila*, in which interesting mutations could then be ascribed to a specific genetic defect. In mice the gene knockout technology allows us to ablate the gene of interest in all of the cells of the embryo, or else in specific cells beginning at a specific time in gestation using a special splicing cre–lox system. Obviously, the effects of these knockouts are frequently manifested during development and make for very interesting developmental studies. As outlined elsewhere in this text book, the basic technique is to generate embryonic stem cells with a homozygous deletion of the gene in question by using homologous recombination. These embryonic stem cells are then injected into a blastocyst and founders are established in which the injected embryonic stem cells are incorporated into the germ line and the progeny therefore have the same deletion.

The power of these knockouts over the past few years has been quite dramatic, however there are several problems with this system. The greatest problem is the time and cost necessary for generating a knockout mouse. In general it takes 2–3 years and typically \$20,000–\$30,000 to generate a knockout with a verified phenotype. Another problem is the questionable nature of the phenotype. In general, after this extensive investment of time and money, there is a high risk of creating a knockout mouse that has an absolutely normal phenotype. Alternatively, there may be phenotypes that are unique and interesting, but may not truly reflect the most important functions of the gene in question. In general, this unpredictable nature of the phenotype from these knockout mice is due to the extensive redundancy and overlap of gene function that normally occurs, especially in mammalian systems. The mammalian genome is replete with multiple isoforms or family members of certain families that may all signal through one or a related receptor. It is quite clear that the absence of a gene from the genome from the initial point of fertilization allows for multiple potential pathways of redundancy to easily accommodate this gene defect. The most dramatic effect of this redundancy and compensation effect was shown recently wherein a knockout mouse for the myoglobin gene was found to have near normal muscle function, with no defect in any measurable aspect of the muscle (43). Also, in our laboratory, we have shown an interesting example of how the mix-and-match or recombination strategy can uncover this overlap. In pancreatic development, the epithelium and mesenchyme have an important function together. We showed that a mouse with blocked TGF-β signaling, using a dominant-negative transgenic system, had a relatively normal phenotype if the embryonic pancreas is cultured. However, when epithelium of a wild-type mouse was recombined with the mesenchyme of this transgenic TGF-β dominant-negative, or vice-versa, the entire pancreas underwent complete apoptosis (unpublished data). Thus, the wild-type tissues, which have developed in an environment with normal TGF-β signaling, were not able to adapt to a potential lack of TGF-β, and therefore, when suddenly exposed to an epithelial–mesenchymal interaction in which there was unidirectional absence of TGF-β signaling, the tissues responded by total apoptosis.

These systems all represent a complex interplay of genomics with phenotype. There is an important power to these tools, but they must be taken with a critical view if proper interpretation is to be performed.

References

1. Brook, F. A., and Gardner, R. L. (1997). The origin and efficient derivation of embryonic stem cells in the mouse. *Proc. Natl. Acad. Sci. U.S.A.* **94**(11), 5709–5712.
2. Hermiston, M. L., and Gordon, J. I. (1995). Organization of the crypt-villus axis and evolution of its stem cell hierarchy during intestinal development. Am J Physiol, **268**(5 Pt 1), G813–G822.
3. Mason, R. J., *et al.* (1997). Stem cells in lung development, disease, and therapy. *Am. J. Respir. Cell. Mol. Biol.* **16**(4), 355–363.
4. Matapurkar, B. G., *et al.* (1998). Organogenesis by desired metaplasia of autogenous stem cells. *Ann. N.Y. Acad. Sci.* **857,** 263–267.
5. Sigal, S. H., *et al.* (1992). The liver as a stem cell and lineage system. *Am. J. Physiol.* **263**(2 Pt 1), G139–G148.
6. Solter, D., and Gearhart, J. (1999). Putting stem cells to work [see comments]. *Science* **283**(5407), 1468–1470.
7. Simon-Assmann, P., *et al.* (1988). Epithelial-mesenchymal interactions in the production of basement membrane components in the gut. *Development* **102,** 339–347.
8. Kedinger, M., *et al.* (1998). Intestinal epithelial-mesenchymal cell interactions. *Ann. N.Y. Acad. Sci.* **859,** 1–17.
9. Spooner, B. S., Cohen, H. I., and Faubion, J. (1977). Development of the embryonic mammalian pancreas: The relationship between morphogenesis and cytodifferentiation. *Dev. Biol.* **61**(2), 119–130.
10. Gittes, G., and Galante, P. (1993). A culture system for the study of pancreatic organogenesis. *J. Tiss. Cult. Meth.* **15,** 23–28.
11. Gittes, G. K. (1994). Studies of early events in pancreatic organogenesis. *Ann. N.Y. Acad. Sci.* **733,** 68–74.
12. Gittes, G. K., *et al.* (1996). Lineage-specific morphogenesis in the developing pancreas: Role of mesenchymal factors. *Development* **122**(2), 439–447.
13. Rose, M. I., *et al.* (1999). Epithelio-mesenchymal interactions in the developing mouse pancreas: Morphogenesis of the adult architecture. *J. Pediatr. Surg.* **34**(5), 774–779; discussion, 780.
14. Haffen, K., Kedinger, M., and Simon-Assmann, P. (1987). Mesenchyme-dependent differentiation of epithelial progenitor cells in the gut. *J. Pediatr. Gastroenterol. Nutr.* **6**(1), 14–23.
15. Stein, B., and Andrew, A. (1989). Differentiation of endocrine cells in chick allantoic epithelium combined with pancreatic mesenchyme. *Cell Differ. Dev.* **26**(3), 173–180.
16. Kedinger, M., *et al.* (1988). Epithelial-mesenchymal interactions in intestinal epithelial differentiation. Scand. J. Gastroenterol. **151,** 62–69.
17. Cirulli, V., *et al.* (1998). KSA antigen Ep-CAM mediates cell-cell adhesion of pancreatic epithelial cells: Morphoregulatory roles in pancreatic islet development. *J. Cell Biol.* **140**(6), 1519–1534.
18. Dahl, U., Sjodin, A., and Semb, H. (1996). Cadherins regulate aggregation of pancreatic beta-cells *in vivo. Development* **122**(9), 2895–2902.
19. Sastry, S. K., and Horwitz, A. F. (1996). Adhesion-growth factor interactions during differentiation: An integrated biological response. *Dev. Biol.* **180**(2), 455–467.
20. Zisch, A. H., and Pasquale, E. B. (1997). The Eph family: A multitude of receptors that mediate cell recognition signals. *Cell Tissue Res.* **290**(2), 217–226.
21. Ferretti, E., *et al.* (1996). Mesenchymal regulation of differentiation of intestinal epithelial cells. *J. Pediatr. Gastroenterol. Nutr.* **23**(1), 65–73.
22. Kedinger, M., *et al.* (1986). Fetal gut mesenchyme induces differentiation of cultured intestinal endodermal and crypt cells. *Dev. Biol.* **113**(2), 474–483.
23. Nagy, P., Bisgaard, H. C., and Thorgeirsson, S. S. (1994). Expression of hepatic transcription factors during liver development and oval cell differentiation. *J. Cell Biol.* **126**(1), 223–233.
24. Rao, M. S., Yeldandi, A. V., and Reddy, J. K. (1990). Stem cell potential of ductular and periductular cells in the adult rat pancreas. *Cell Differ. Dev.* **29**(3), 155–163.
25. Han, J. H., Rall, L., and Rutter, W. J. (1986). Selective expression of rat pancreatic genes during embryonic development. *Proc. Natl. Acad. Sci. U.S.A.* **83**(1), 110–114.
26. Gittes, G. K., and Rutter, W. J. (1992). Onset of cell-specific gene expression in the developing mouse pancreas. *Proc. Natl. Acad. Sci. U.S.A.* **89**(3), 1128–1132.
27. Gittes, G. K., Rutter, W. J., and Debas, H. T. (1993). Initiation of gastrin expression during the development of the mouse pancreas. *Am. J. Surg.* **165**(1), 23–25; discussion, 25–26.
28. Wang, X. M. and Evers, B. M. (1999). Characterization of early development pattern of expression of neurotensin/neuromedin N gene in foregut and midgut. *Dig. Dis. Sci.* **44**(1), 33–40.
29. Uehara, H., *et al.* (1999). Detection of telomerase activity utilizing energy transfer primers: Comparison with gel- and ELISA-based detection. *Biotechniques* **26**(3), 552–558.
30. Wagner, R. W., *et al.* (1993). Antisense gene inhibition by oligonucleotides containing C-5 propyne pyrimidines. *Science* **260**(5113), 1510–1513.
31. Marcusson, E. G., *et al.* (1999). Preclinical and clinical pharmacology of antisense oligonucleotides. *Mol. Biotechnol.* **12**(1), p. 1–11.
32. Leaman, D. W., and Cramer, H. (1999). Controlling gene expression with 2-5A antisense. *Methods* **18**(3), 252–265.
33. Csete, M. E., *et al.* (1995). Efficient gene transfer to pancreatic islets mediated by adenoviral vectors. *Transplantation* **59**(2), 263–268.
34. Blau, H. M., and Hughes, S. M. (1990). Retroviral lineage markers for assessing myoblast fate *in vivo. Adv. Exp. Med. Biol.* **280,** 201–203.
35. Duprez, D. M., *et al.* (1996). Activation of Fgf-4 and HoxD gene expression by BMP-2 expressing cells in the developing chick limb. *Development* **122**(6), 1821–1828.

36. Raper, S. E., and DeMatteo, R. P. (1996). Adenovirus-mediated in vivo gene transfer and expression in normal rat pancreas. *Pancreas* **12**(4), 401–410.
37. Kasahara, N., Dozy, A. M., and Kan, Y. W. (1994). Tissue-specific targeting of retroviral vectors through ligand-receptor interactions [see comments]. *Science* **266**(5189), 1373–1376.
38. Denham, W., *et al.* (1998). Cationic liposome-mediated gene transfer during acute pancreatitis: Tissue specificity, duration, and effects of acute inflammation. *J. Gastrointest. Surg.* **2**(1), 95–101.
39. Miller, N., and Vile, R. (1995). Targeted vectors for gene therapy. *FASEB J.* **9**(2), 190–199.
40. Wheeler, C. J., *et al.* (1996). A novel cationic lipid greatly enhances plasmid DNA delivery and expression in mouse lung. *Proc. Natl. Acad. Sci. U.S.A.* **93**(21), 11454–11459.
41. Schmid, R. M., *et al.* (1998). Direct gene transfer into the rat pancreas using DNA-liposomes. *Eur. J. Clin. Invest.* **28**(3), 220–226.
42. Bottinger, E. P., *et al.* (1997). Expression of a dominant-negative mutant TGF-Beta type II receptor in transgenic mice reveals essential roles for TGF-Beta in regulation of growth and differentiation in the exocrine pancreas. *EMBO J.* **16**(10), 2621–2633.
43. Garry, D. J., *et al.* (1998). Mice without myoglobin. *Nature* (*London*) **395**(6705), 905–908.

48

Animal Models of Liver Failure

Jacek Rozga and Achilles A. Demetriou

Department of Surgery, Cedars-Sinai Medical Center, Los Angeles, California 90048

I. Introduction

The availability of suitable animal models reproducing at least some of the typical clinical features of acute and chronic liver disease in humans would facilitate studies of liver pathophysiology and the design and evaluation of new treatments. Unfortunately, with the exception of hereditary enzyme deficiencies and acetaminophen poisoning, only a few animal models of liver failure appear to meet this requirement. Additionally, in fulminant hepatic failure (FHF) models, the hepatic injury should be potentially reversible and death should occur within a well-defined interval as the direct consequence of FHF and its complications, including coma and brain swelling (1). For practical reasons, the animal should have a blood volume large enough to permit serial sampling and use of therapeutic interventions such as hemoperfusion (2).

None of the currently available toxic-induced [e.g., carbon tetrachloride (CCl_4), thioacetamide, D-galactosamine], virus-induced, or surgically induced (hepatic devasularization, total hepatectomy) models meet these criteria. In addition, hypothermia, acidosis, uremia, weight loss, dehydration, and starvation due to anorexia are all factors that need to be considered as potential contributors to any behavioral (hepatic encephalopathy) or laboratory changes observed in these models. As noted by Mullen *et al.* (3), these types of problems are rarely published and may account for some controversy in the literature.

Despite these limitations, the majority of acute liver failure animal models are useful in either testing a specific hypothesis or evaluating safety and efficacy of a particular therapeutic modality. This chapter examines many of the models described in the literature, including those developed and used by the authors.

II. Models of Hereditary Liver Defects

Animal models of hereditary defects of liver metabolism have provided a wealth of information on physiologic, biochemical, and molecular mechanisms of several enzymatic defects. Experiments in defective animals have also contributed to the development of specific therapies (dietary, pharmacologic, gene therapy, replacement by organ and hepatocyte transplantation).

A. The Gunn Rat—Crigler–Najjar Syndrome

In 1938, C. H. Gunn described a colony of mutant Wistar rats with recessively inherited hyperbilirubinemia (4). At that time, the existence of uridine diphosphoglucuronate glucuronosyltransferase (UGT) and the significance of bilirubin glucuronidation were unknown. Twenty years passed before the lack of bilirubin glucuronidation was reported in the Gunn rat (5) and another 15 years passed before it was recognized as a phynotypic model of human Crigler–Najjar syndrome, Type I (6). Much of our current knowledge of bilirubin toxicity clinically and its treatment has come from studies performed in these rats.

In normal rats, only small amounts of unconjugated bilirubin are present in bile and there is a great reserve capacity for biliary excretion in response to intravenous infusion of bilirubin. In contrast, bilirubin excreted in Gunn rat bile and plasma is unconjugated and biliary excretion does not increase significantly after administration of bilirubin. Depending on the background strain, serum bilirubin varies from 5 mg/dl to over 20 mg/dl (7). A detailed description of this model has been published by Roy-Chowdhury *et al.* (8).

B. Hyperbilirubinemia—Dubin–Johnson Syndrome

In 1983, a Wistar strain of rats with autosomal recessively inherited conjugated hyperbilirubinemia was described (9). These rats were named TR^- rats (transport-negative rats) because of impaired hepatobiliary secretion of bilirubin glucuronides, various glutathione conjugates, and many other organic ions (9, 10). Rats with a similar defect were found in Groningen [GY, or Groningen yellow; also a Wistar strain (11)] and in Japan [Eisai rats; a Sprague–Dawley strain (12)]. The mechanism of the canalicular excretion defect in these rats remains unclear. When TR^- rats are maintained on normal laboratory chow, their livers look normal. However, when TR^- rats are fed a diet enriched with tryptophan, tyrosine, and phenylalanine, impaired secretion of anionic metabolites of these amino acids results in their retention, oxidation, polymerization, and lysosomal accumulation (13). A similar black pigment is seen in livers of mutant Corriedale sheep (14) and, more importantly, in patients with the Dubin–Johnson syndrome (15). A detailed description of these models is given by Jansen and Oude Elferink in their excellent review (16).

C. The Nagase Analbuminemic Rat

In the late 1970s, a strain of mutant albumin-deficient rats was found among Sprague–Dawley rats from Clea Japan (Kanagawa, Japan) (17). The strain was named after Sumi Nagase and has since been widely used in studies of hepatocellular transplantation. The genetic abnormality of the Nagase analbuminemic rat (NAR) is the deletion of the 7 bp downstream from the exon H, G + H, or H + I during pre-mRNA processing (18, 19). Baseline plasma albumin levels in these animals are negligible (0.001–0.003 g/dl) and on liver sections less than 1% of parenchymal cells can be identified as albumin positive (20, 21). After transplantation of normal albumin-producing hepatocytes, it is possible to follow the functional effect of cell therapy by measuring plasma albumin levels and to identify transplanted cells using immunostaining for albumin in liver sections (20–22). It is worth noting, however, that in NAR rat livers, occasional albumin-positive cells may appear through aging or after carcinogen treatment (23).

D. A Model of Infantile Scurvy

The $ODS^{od/od}$ rat is a mutant rat unable to synthesize ascorbic acid in the liver because of lack of L-gulonolactone oxidase in the liver microsomes. Unless fed with ascorbic acid, the rat dies from rapid weight loss, resulting in inability to stand up or move due to deformity of the extremities (24). Attempts were made to treat $ODS^{od/od}$ rats with hepatocellular transplantation (25).

E. The Heritable Hyperlipidemic Rabbit

The genetic defect in the Watanabe heritable hyperlipidemic (WHHL) rabbit is the counterpart of familial hypercholesterolemia in humans (26, 27). Homozygous animals have a mutation in the low-density lipoprotein (LDL) receptor gene and express almost no functional LDL receptors. As a result, intermediate-density lipoproteins (IDLs) and LDLs accumulate in the plasma, leading to accelerated development of atherosclerosis and premature death. Attempts have been made to treat familial hypercholesterolemia using gene therapy. One strategy involved harvesting of "defective" hepatocytes, transduction of hepatocytes *in vitro* using a retroviral vector carrying the normal LDL receptor gene, and transplantation of "repaired" hepatocytes back into the patient (28). This experiment has been carried out in WHHL rabbits and has also been attempted clinically (29). More recently, direct intraportal injection of a recombinant adenoviral vector containing rabbit LDL receptor cDNA has been introduced (30). Both strategies resulted in modest and transient reductions in serum cholesterol and LDL levels. In our laboratory, selective transplantation of a small number of normal allogeneic hepatocytes into the right lateral liver lobe of WHHL rabbits and subsequent induction of regeneration of the transplanted lobes resulted in dramatic and sustained decreases in serum cholesterol and LDL levels. Of great importance was the finding of near total lack of atherosclerotic changes in the aortas of hepatocyte WHHL recipients (31).

F. Dalmatian Dogs with Hyperuricemia

There exists a strain of Dalmatian dogs that lacks a normal transport system for uric acid into the hepatocyte. As a result, conversion of uric acid to allantoin is impaired, leading to high blood uric acid levels and lower blood levels of allantoin. In this model, heterotopic auxiliary liver transplantation resulted in successful prolonged correction of metabolic defect (32).

III. Toxic Liver Injury

Intravenous administration of the selective hepatotoxin remains the simplest technique of inducing fulminant hepatic failure in small (mouse, rat) and large (rabbit, dog, pig) laboratory animals. Unfortunately, the simplicity of hepatotoxic models is not paralleled by reliability and reproducibility. For example, hepatotoxic effects of agents such as acetaminophen, CCl_4, and D-galactosamine depend on the type of toxin used, animal species, strain and age, dose, route of administration, nutritional status of the animal, toxic effects on other organs, and other factors (33, 34). As a result, the extent of liver necrosis and/or functional impairment is difficult to predict and there is significant variability from experiment to experiment. In general, when using such animal models, investigators rely on the serum activity of liver enzymes and/or degree of neurologic dysfunction (35).

A. D-Galactosamine

Hepatic metabolism of this substance through the galactose pathway results in intracellular deficiencies of uridine moieties (36). Whether this mechanism alone can cause hepatic necrosis or cooperation with other factors such as endotoxemia is needed is not certain (37).

1. In Rats

Lo *et al.* (38) administered galactosamine hydrochloride intraperitoneally to rats (250–350 g; 3 g/kg of body weight) as a 0.28 *M* solution in bacteriostatic water and adjusted to pH 7.4 with 1 *M* NaOH (37). Animals were fed standard laboratory chow and a 10% dextrose solution was added to the drinking water to prevent development of hypoglycemia. The clinical and laboratory signs of hepatic failure developed within 24 hrs posttreatment and at 36 and 42 hrs animals were stuporous, but not comatose. No data on animal mortality were reported. In the studies by Baumgartner *et al.* (39) intraperitoneal injection of a much smaller dose of 0.5 g/kg of D-galactosamine in male Fisher 344 rats (170–300 g) resulted in 95% lethal acute hepatic necrosis. All deaths occurred 30–65 hrs after injection. All rats alive at 65 hrs postinjection survived indefinitely.

2. In Rabbits

Blitzer *et al.* (2) used intravenous injection of galactosamine hydrochloride to 1- to 2-kg rabbits in a dose of 4.25 m*M*/kg of body weight. The toxin was dissolved in 9 ml of 5% dextrose in water and the pH of the solution was made acidic (pH 6.8) in view of the known instability of amino sugars in alkaline media. The solution was administered slowly over 2 min via an ear vein. The authors also advocate the use of genetically uniform animals to improve reproducibility of the proposed model.

3. In Dogs

Diaz-Buxo *et al.* (40) used dogs (~30 kg; $n = 10$) and infused D-galactosamine intravenously in a dose of 1.0–1.5 g/kg of body weight. The agent was dissolved in 5% dextrose in water to a concentration of 0.05 g/liter and the pH adjusted to 6.8 with 1 *M*/liter NaOH. The solution was filter sterilized and injected via a jugular vein catheter. After D-galactosamine infusion, lactated Ringer's with KCl (35 mEq/liter) was administered at 100 ml/hr as the maintenance fluid. Blood lactate levels were determined at 3-hr intervals and when they were higher than 1.5 m*M*/liter, the maintenance fluid was replaced by 5% dextrose in normal saline with KCl. If the blood glucose concentration exceeded 175 mg/dl, the fluid was switched to normal saline with KCl. In this model, 8/10 animals died between 40 and 72 hr. No correlation was observed between the D-galactosamine dose and duration of animal survival. In 5/7 animals, grand mal seizures started 24 hr after infusion of the hepatotoxin. Coagulation parameters (prothrombin and partial thromboplastin times, fibrinogen) became abnormal 12–24 hr postinfusion, whereas transaminases, ammonia, and bilirubin began to rise at 24 hr and remained elevated until the end of the study. All dogs remained normoglycemic throughout. At necropsy, hepatic edema, congestion, and hemorrhage were common findings. Although destruction of the hepatic parenchyma was common, the degree of necrosis was not homogeneous. Results of these studies illustrate well the difficulty in developing a highly standardized and reproducible large animal model of acute hepatic failure.

B. Thioacetamide

This hepatotoxin has been used to induce liver cirrhosis or acute hepatic encephalopathy rather than fulminant hepatic failure. In treated rats, behavioral, biochemical, and histologic abnormalities (including increase in brain ammonia and octopamine concentrations and spongy degeneration of cerebral cortex white matter) as well as electroencephalographic abnormalities are similar to those found in other models of hepatogenic encephalopathy (41, 42). In rats (150–300 g), intraperitoneal injection of thioacetamide at a dose of 250 mg/kg of body weight (2.5% solution in 0.15 *M* NaCl) is given every 24 hr for 2–3 days (42, 43).

C. Carbon Tetrachloride

Carbon tetrachloride, a classic hepatotoxin, is thought to induce cellular injury through metabolites that are generated by a cytochrome P450-dependent step. Briefly, injury results initially from activity of highly reactive trichloromethyl radicals, which trigger lipid peroxidation, resulting in damage to hepatocellular membranes. Secondary liver damage occurs from exposure to the products of activated Kupffer cells, which release chemoattractants and activators of neutrophils. The resulting inflammatory response promotes extensive tissue damage through the release of reactive oxygen radicals (44).

1. Acute Liver Injury

Oral, intraperitoneal, or subcutaneous administration of CCl_4 results in acute, reversible liver injury. It is characterized by centrilobular (zone 3) necrosis, followed by its resolution and tissue repair (regeneration). In mice (22–28 g), this type of acute liver injury may be induced with a single intraperitoneal dose of CCl_4 (0.1 ml/kg of body weight) following dilution in corn oil (44). The same dose of CCl_4 diluted with olive oil ($\times 10$) is recommended for rats (45). A more severe injury of the rat liver was induced after administration of 4 ml/kg of CCl_4 (1:1 vol/vol mixture with olive oil) by way of a nasogastric tube (46).

2. Induction of Liver Cirrhosis

Several decades ago, Cameron and Karunaratne (47) described liver cirrhosis in rats treated with CCl_4 subcutaneously twice weekly over a period of 6 months. However, due to a large variation in the response to CCl_4 in the rat, it was not possible to obtain a consistent and satisfactory degree of cirrhosis (47). Of equal importance was frequent regression of the cirrhotic changes after cessation of CCl_4 administration (48). The efficiency of the model was significantly improved with the use of phenobarbital (PhB) during the induction period (49). This was based on the observation that PhB-dependent stimulation of microsomal hydroxylating enzyme systems in the liver enhanced CCl_4 hepatotoxicity (50). Ultimately, Proctor and Chatamra (51) introduced a body weight/CCl_4 dose calibration, which resulted in the induction of irreversible ascitic form of micronodular cirrhosis in more than two-thirds of PhB/CCl_4-treated rats. We have further improved this model by a more precise adjustment of each subsequent weekly dose of CCl_4 (52). For intragastric administration, a fine intravenous cannula (Blue Luer 3FG, Portex Ltd., Hythe, Kent, England) was inserted into the lumen of the feeding tube (CH5 Argyle). Rats were not starved before treatment and the first dose of CCl_4 was 0.08 ml. In 30 male Wistar rats, there was a need of treatment with CCl_4 for 10 to 18 weeks (mean 15 $\pm$ 3) until ascites developed.

3. Induction of Fulminant Hepatic Failure

In 1987, Alp and Hickman (53) described a model of fulminant hepatic failure in pigs, which consistently produced irreversible hepatic coma and death within a narrowly defined time period. Pigs (15–20 kg) were given phenobarbital, 8 mg/kg orally for 3 days. Thereafter, a laparotomy was performed and all ligamentous attachments of the liver were transected except the portal triad. The hepatic artery was then occluded for 2 hr and after revascularization CCl_4 (0.5 ml/kg) was injected into the stomach. Sixteen untreated pigs survived from 16 to 52 hr (mean 32 hr). Death was preceded by 6–18 hr of deepening coma and occasional convulsions. Levels of plasma bilirubin, serum transaminases, ammonia, and prothrombin index were all abnormal.

D. Acetaminophen

Animal models for acetaminophen-induced FHF are useful in the development and evaluation of potential medical therapies for patients who attempt to commit suicide by ingesting excessive amounts of this widely available analgesic agent. The liver injury is thought to involve a chemically reactive metabolite, which resembles *N*-acetyl-*p*-benzoquinoneimine (54) and, perhaps, contributions from thiol oxidation and lipid peroxidation (55, 56).

Zieve *et al.* (57) and Leonard *et al.* (58) induced FHF in rats using acetaminophen. In the former studies (57), acetaminophen (1400 mg/kg) was given to fasted (20–22 hr) Sprague–Dawley rats (200 $\pm$ 25 g) by gastric instillation. The mortality was 4.3% and at autopsy the livers showed extensive necrosis spreading outward from the central veins. In the latter series of experiments (58) male Fischer 344 rats (170–250 g) were given a lower dose of acetaminophen (750 mg/kg, PO) but also displayed massive hepatic necrosis 24 hr after treatment, as assessed by transaminase activity and histopathologic changes.

In theory, a large animal model for acetaminophen poisoning would allow for serial observations to be made in animals that may be recovering. In 1989, Francavilla *et al.* (59) reported that multiple subcutaneous injections of acetaminophen dissolved in dimethyl sulfoxide consistently produced FHF in dogs, some of which (10%) fully recovered. The first injection of acetaminophen (750 mg/kg of body weight) was given at noon, the second injection (200 mg/kg) was given 9 hr later, and the third dose (200 mg/kg) was administered 24 hr after the initial dose. This dosing schedule maintained a concentration of acetaminophen in serum of $>$140 μg/ml for a period of at least 20 hr. Previous clinical studies showed that the maintenance of such high blood levels of the drug for a period of 24 hr is necessary to produce consistent panlobular necrosis (60). No animals died within the first 36 hr. By 72 hr after initial drug administration, mortality was 90%. All of the animals demonstrated a histopathologic, biochemical, and clinical picture consistent with FHF.

IV. Immune Liver Injury

Concanavalin A

It is generally believed that activated T lymphocytes are involved in the pathogenesis of some forms of acute and chronic hepatitis (61). A murine hepatitis model has been developed in which T cell-mediated liver-specific inflammatory lesions were induced by the injection of concanavalin A (62). Several endogenous mediators such as tumor necrosis factor-α, interferon-γ, interleukin-12, perforin, intercellular adhesion molecule-1, and lymphocyte function-associated antigen-1, were activated (63–65). Mice (8–12 weeks old) should be injected intravenously with concanavalin A (10–20 mg/kg; Sigma Chemical Co., St. Louis, MO) dissolved in either 300 μl phosphate-buffered saline or RPMI 640 medium without serum.

V. Spontaneous Hepatitis

Hepatitis in Long–Evans Cinnamon Rats

This unique animal model is characterized by spontaneous onset of acute hepatitis followed by chronic hepatitis, hepatic fibrosis, and, in rats surviving for more than 1 year, development of a hepatoma (66–68). Because of abnormal accumulation of copper in the liver, marked reduction in serum ceruloplasmin levels, and homologous genetic abnormality (69), the Long–Evans cinnamon rat represents an animal model of Wilson's disease.

VI. Lethal Hepatocyte Apoptosis in Mice

Apoptosis is a form of cell death that plays an important role in deleting damaged, senescent, or unwanted cells from tissues. Perturbations of this process have been implicated in a wide range of diseases, including viral and toxic liver injury, where both necrosis and apoptosis may contribute to liver cell death. Fas antigen (CD95/APO-1) (70), a member of the tumor necrosis factor (TNF) receptor family, has been shown to trigger cell death on specific ligand or antibody binding. Treatment of mice with an anti-Fas monoclonal antibody causes early and massive apoptosis of hepatocytes, leading to the death of animals within a few hours (71). The sequence of pathologic changes is similar to those found in fulminant toxic or viral hepatitis in humans. This model appears to offer unique insights into cellular and molecular mechanisms of liver cell death in acute and chronic hepatobiliary diseases. It may also help design new therapeutic strategies. In the studies by Lacronique *et al.* (72), a purified hamster monoclonal anti-Fas antibody (10 μg of Jo2; Pharmigen) was administered intravenously in mice. Fulminant hepatic failure occurred in all animals within 40 hr, with a 90% mortality rate at 6 hr.

VII. Surgical Models of Hepatic Failure

Most of the surgical animal models of hepatic failure do not reproduce the full gamut of metabolic and physiologic derangements seen clinically in severe acute liver failure. In addition, there is significant variation in the physiologic, biochemical, and survival effects. This baseline variation in outcome makes evaluation of the effects of the various forms of therapeutic intervention difficult.

The major surgical models studied include acute transient or permanent liver ischemia, sometimes in combination with Eck's fistula (portacaval shunt; PCS) or partial liver resection. In these preparations, however, it is difficult to standardize the degree of liver injury. Complete liver devascularization, an experimental approach used by most investigators, although it appears to be more consistently reproducible, it is followed by a degree of rapid and severe deterioration of all vital functions and sepsis, which is rarely seen clinically. Thus what could be achieved with artificial liver support using the devascularized liver animal model is at best a decrease in the rate of deterioration of various metabolic and physiologic parameters, i.e., acidosis, hypoglycemia, hyperammonemia, and coagulopathy.

Theoretically, the "cleanest" *in vivo* model that could be used to test artifical liver support function would be an anhepatic animal, because in these animals there is a rapid accumulation in the blood of substances normally metabolized by the liver, including ammonia, bilirubin, bile acids, lactate, and aromatic amino acids, to name but a few. Additionally, any liver-specific function detected during the study would be attributed to the support system. The anhepatic animal, however, does not reproduce the clinical setting of severe acute liver failure, i.e., massive liver necrosis and cerebral edema, and it cannot be used to predict how a specific liver support system will function in the liver failure environment.

A. Anhepatic Rat

Various techniques for creating an anhepatic rat have been described, but in general, their complexity resulted in high mortality and inability to obtain consistently reproducible data (73–75). In the rat, adherence of the posterior liver lobes to the inferior vena cava (IVC) mandates replacement of a segment of the IVC with a prosthesis whenever complete liver removal is attempted. To avoid grafting, multistage procedures have been devised, where initially either partial constriction of both the portal vein and vena cava or ligation of the IVC alone were carried out to establish adequate collateral circulation. At a second stage, about 2 months later, a portacaval shunt (PCS) was constructed; liver resection was usually carried out at a third stage (74, 76, 77). We have previously described a two-stage technique of total hepatectomy (78) whereby initially acute and progressive atrophy of the posterior liver lobes was induced by selective portal venous branch ligations, as described elsewhere (79). Two weeks later, when these lobes comprised approximately 3% of the total liver mass, the hepatic artery was ligated and the enlarged anterior liver lobes were resected. An end-to-side PCS was then carried out to ensure vascular integrity of the splanchnic area (Fig. 1). This procedure in skilled hands can be carried out without operative mortality and glucose-supplemented rats have a mean survival time of 20 ± 5 hr. However, technical problems have been frequently encountered during dissection for portasystemic shunting due to the presence of peritoneal adhesions caused by earlier surgical manipulations.

Single-stage techniques for total hepatectomy in the rat were described by Yamaguchi *et al.* (80), Lorenzo *et al.* (80), and Azoulay *et al.* (75). All variants utilized either a custom-made vascular prosthesis or homologous vein graft (80) and therefore were time consuming and required use of advanced microsurgical techniques (75, 80).

We have described a simple, rapid, and safe (no blood loss) single-stage technique of total hepatectomy in the rat (82). It requires only basic microsurgical skills and produces an anhepatic rat that rapidly recovers from anesthesia and shows remarkable hemodynamic stability. Briefly, the operation is performed with the aid of an operating microscope (OPMI MD, Carl Zeiss Inc., Germany). The rat abdomen is entered through a midline incision, the portal vein is dissected, and an end-to-side PCS is created with 8/0 Ethilon (Ethicon Inc., Somerville, NJ) suture, as described previously (78). Next, the hepatic artery and bile duct are ligated and divided and a 4- to 5-cm-long piece of a 14-gauge Angiocath (Becton Dickinson, Sandy, UT) is inserted into the lumen of the inferior vena cava (IVC) *via* direct puncture at the level between the left renal and the right iliolumbar vein. Once in the IVC lumen, the stent is secured using 4-0 silk ligatures at two points: just above the PCS and between the diaphragm and liver dome (Fig. 2). After stenting, the whole liver, including the tissue surrounding the intrahepatic IVC portion, is resected and the abdomen is closed. The entire procedure is completed within 30–35 min. Following recovery from anesthesia, rats were kept at 21°C and received intravenous glucose infusion (20 mg/100 g/hr) via a jugular vein cannula (Silastic Medical Grade Tubing, Dow Corning Co., Midland, MI) using an infusion pump (Harvard Apparatus, South Natick, MA). Survival time in untreated anhepatic rats ($n = 16$) was 22.4 ± 5.2 hr. Animals reached stages 3–4 encephalopathy after 16.6 ± 5.7 hr.

B. Anhepatic Rabbit

A seemingly simple technique of total hepatectomy in rabbits was described by Takahashi *et al.* (83). After cutting the portal vein and IVC above and below the liver, the remaining ends of the vessels were connected with a three-way silicone tube. During the procedure, portal blood was

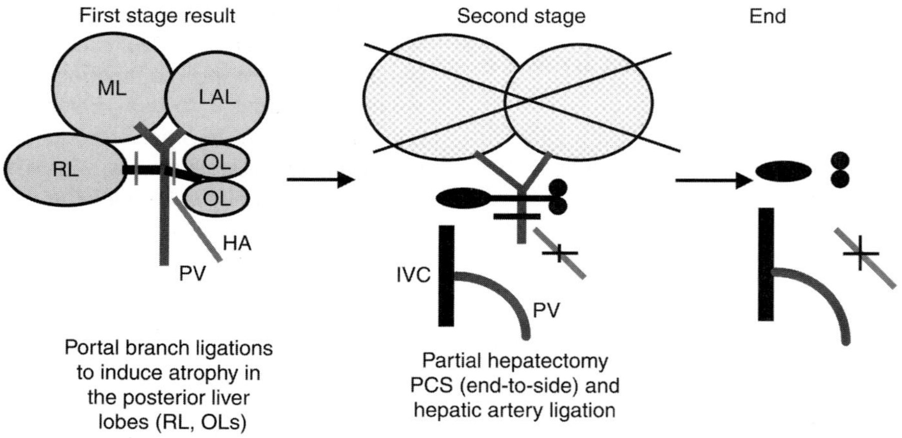

Figure 1 Schematic illustration of the first and the second stages of the total hepatectomy (ML, median liver lobe; LAL, left anterior lobe; RL, right lobes; OL, omental lobes; PV, portal vein; IVC, inferior vena cava; HA, hepatic artery; PCS, portacaval shunt).

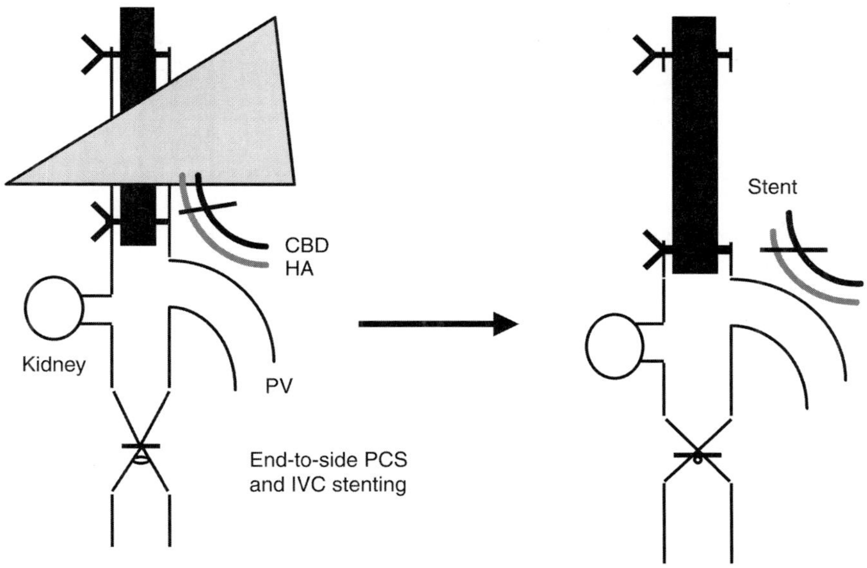

Figure 2 Schematic representation of the surgical technique used to induce the anhepatic state in rats. A piece of 14-gauge Angiocath (stent) has replaced part of the inferior vena cava that was resected during hepatectomy (CBD, common bile duct; HA, hepatic artery; PV, portal vein; PCS, portacaval shunt; IVC, inferior vena cava).

returned through an external jugular vein. Survival time in untreated rabbits was determined in only two animals and it was 13 and 18 hr, respectively.

C. Anhepatic Pig

It is difficult to extrapolate small animal data to the clinical setting. In large animal studies, dogs were first studied because their livers could be removed after ligation of the individual hepatic veins (84). In the pig, the liver envelopes the IVC, thus after hepatectomy caval continuity must be restored (85). The elegant technique described by Hickman *et al.* (86, 87) involves performance of a side-to-side PCS for portal decompression during caval reconstruction with a straight synthetic graft. Subsequently, the side-to-side PCS is converted to end-to-side by ligation of the distal portal vein and removal of the liver with anastomosis of the upper end of the synthetic graft to the transected suprahepatic caval vein.

We have developed a simple technique to induce the anhepatic state in the pig, which has resulted in significant prolongation of postoperative survival (88). Briefly, after creating an end-to-side PCS at the level of the left renal vein, the hepatoduodenal ligament was transected and the liver removed between two clamps. Inferior vena cava continuity was reconstituted with an 18-mm polytetrafluoroethylene graft (Gore-Tex Stretch, W.L. Gore & Associates Inc., Flagstaff, AZ) (Fig. 3). Heparin administration and veno-venous bypass were not utilized. Using this technique, the two episodes of splanchnic venous stasis (portacaval shunt and vena cava grafting) lasted only 10–15 min each and were separated by a 10-min interval during transection of hepatoduodenal ligament. After surgery, pigs were maintained on continuous intravenous infusion of 5% dextrose in lactated Ringer's solution (Abott Laboratories, Chicago, IL; 0.07 ml/kg/min). No other supportive measures were used and no attempts were made to correct respiratory, hemodynamic, or metabolic abnormalities. In normothermic animals, body core temperature was maintained at 37°C through external heating (heating pad, blanket, and lamp) and through warming of intravenously administered fluids (Spectratherm, Cobe BCT, Inc., Lakewood, CO). Hypothermic animals were kept in a temperature-controlled environment at 21°C so that their body temperature was allowed to decrease to 25.4 ± 0.5°C. In hypothermic animals ($n = 20$) survival time was 44 ± 4 hrs; this compares favorably with 19 ± 8 hr reported in pigs by Hickman *et al.* (87) and 22 ± 5 hr reported in dogs by Drapanas *et al.* (89). Onset of hepatic coma was late (22–28 hr) and all hypothermic animals showed remarkable hemodynamic stability until 30–36 hr posthepatectomy. The intracranial pressure (ICP) remained within the normal range throughout the study period, including the prolonged period of low (<40 mmHg) cerebral perfusion pressure seen during the preterminal hemodynamic collapse. Considering that our normothermic anhepatic pigs ($n = 27$) had a shorter survival time (33 ± 11 hr; $P < 0.01$), it is possible that hypothermia contributes to the prolonged

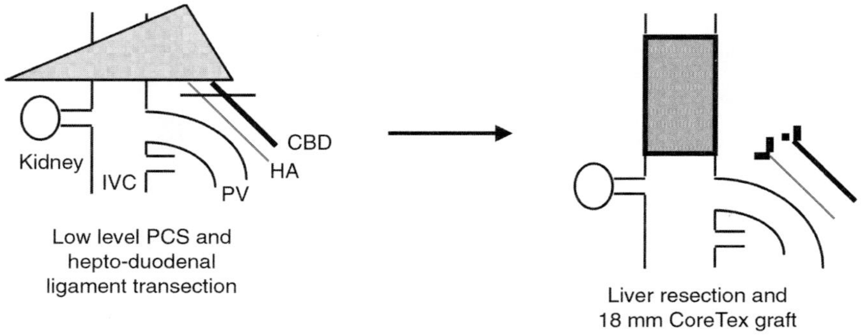

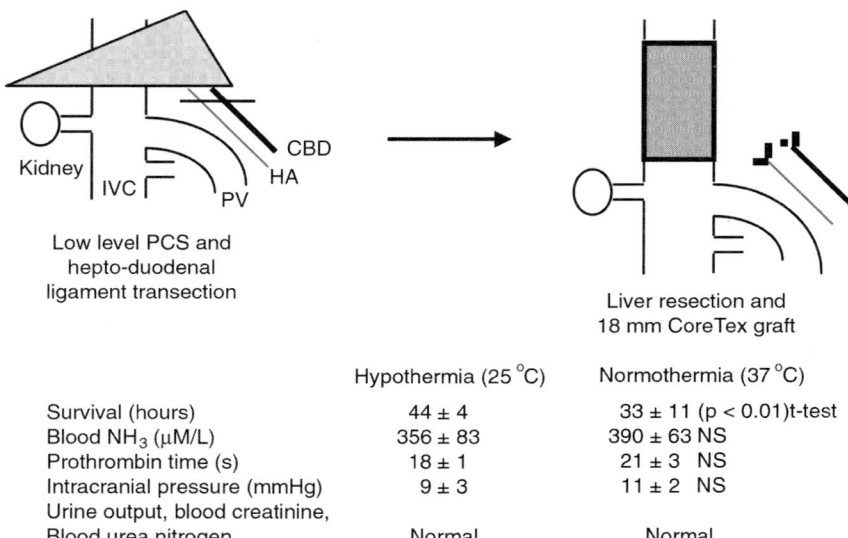

	Hypothermia (25 °C)	Normothermia (37 °C)
Survival (hours)	44 ± 4	33 ± 11 (p < 0.01)t-test
Blood NH_3 (μM/L)	356 ± 83	390 ± 63 NS
Prothrombin time (s)	18 ± 1	21 ± 3 NS
Intracranial pressure (mmHg)	9 ± 3	11 ± 2 NS
Urine output, blood creatinine, Blood urea nitrogen	Normal	Normal

Figure 3 Diagram depicting the technique used to produce an anhepatic pig. A low-level portacaval shunt (PCS) was created, the liver was rapidly removed, and inferior vena cava continuity was restored using a straight graft (IVC, inferior vena cava; PV, portal vein; HA, hepatic artery; CBD, common bile duct). In normothermic pigs, body core temperature was maintained at 37°C through external heating and warming of intravenously administered fluids. Hypothermic animals were kept in a temperature-controlled environment at 21°C so that their body temperature was allowed to decrease.

survival time in the anhepatic animals (Fig 3). Significantly, normothermic anhepatic pigs did not develop intracranial hypertension, either. The latter finding is of particular interest, because the anhepatic state was found to be associated with a rapid and progressive hyperammonemia, hyperbilirubinemia, metabolic acidosis with hyperlactic acidemia, and elevated levels of aromatic amino acids. Other findings included decreasing albumin and fibrinogen levels and a steady increase in the activity of LDH and transaminases, presumably from extrahepatic sites. Renal function was well preserved throughout the experimental period and, surprisingly, there was only slight prolongation of prothrombin time (PT) without development of overt bleeding, even as late as 61 hr posthepatectomy (PTs in the two longest survivors were 17 and 18 sec, respectively) (Fig. 3).

A new technique of total hepatectomy in pigs was described by Filipponi *et al.* (90). It involves *en bloc* caval resection and vascular reconstruction with use of bifurcated prosthesis and pump-assisted caval–portal–jugular bypass (CPJB). Mean survival time was 16.9 hr (range 10–26 hr; $n = 7$) and the time needed to complete the operation ranged from 2 to 3 hr .

D. Subtotal (90%) Hepatectomy

In theory, a near total liver removal may be an ideal model when liver insufficiency without ongoing hepatocyte necrosis is desired (91). In practice, other complications, including portal venous stasis, cerebral edema, hypothermia, hypoglycemia, endotoxemia, sepsis, proteinuria, and apoptosis (92) may all interfere with metabolic measurements under investigation.

1. Subtotal Hepatectomy in Rats

In rats, the mass of each liver lobe remains in direct proportion to the total body and liver weight (79, 93). Thus, removal of the two anterior liver lobes, which is achieved after placement of only single ligature, results in highly standardized (~68%) partial hepatectomy. After resecting the right liver lobes, an additional 22–24% of the liver is eliminated. What are left "intact" are the two omental liver lobes representing approximately 10% of the total liver mass. This technique has been used by many investigators, including ourselves (94–97). We have observed that some variability seen with this model was due to individual variations in the amount of liver tissue surrounding the intrahepatic portion of the caval vein and "bridging" the right and omental liver lobes; thus the extent of hepatectomy can vary anywhere from 83 to 87%. The common right lobes' pedicle is so wide that complete removal of these lobes without damaging the IVC is not feasible. Therefore, we now perform subtotal hepatectomy in rats by first placing a ligature around the portal triad supplying the right lobes and only then removing the anterior lobes and the devascularized right lobes. After this procedure, a clear demarcation line separates the ischemic liver tissue from viable parenchyma and the extent of hepatectomy is 90 ± 1% ($n = 20$).

Whatever technique of subtotal hepatectomy is used, animals should be maintained on postoperative glucose supplementation to prevent hypoglycemia and, therefore, to prolong survival time. In rats, 20% glucose solution can be given in tap drinking water. In comatose animals, glucose may be given subcutaneously or intravenously (20 mg/hr/100 g of body weight). Rats should be kept in individual cages and maintained at 35–37°C during and after the operation using a heating pad and a heating lamp.

2. Subtotal Hepatoctomy in Rabbits

Rabbits are difficult laboratory animals to handle and it is not surprising that very few investigators choose to use this species to study the effects of 90% hepatectomy (91, 98).

E. Transient Liver Ischemia

In an attempt to develop a model of temporary acute hepatic failure, several groups of investigators induced ischemia of the liver for periods ranging from 1 to 6 hr (99–103). The choice of species seemed important because, in dogs, 60 min of hepatic ischemia was always fatal (99). For pigs, the tolerable period was longer and animals subjected to a 4-hr or even 6-hr ischemia had a potential for full recovery (103).

F. Permanent Liver Ischemia

Portacaval shunt with permanent disruption of arterial blood supply to the liver in one or two stages (104, 105) is often criticized for lack of potential reversibility and too rapid development of laboratory and clinical signs of FHF. Other factors, such as endotoxemia, sepsis, and early hemodynamic instability, may also influence outcome. Despite these reservations, permanent liver devascularization has been the most frequently used animal model in studies of new therapies for human FHF, perhaps because of its relative simplicity and high reproducibility.

1. Ischemic Liver Failure in Rats

In rats, the construction of an end-to-side PCS requires microsurgical skills. In addition, delayed dearterialization may necessitate relaparotomy and may be difficult to perform due to local inflammation (adhesion formation). For these and other reasons (e.g., small blood volume), PCS is frequently combined with other procedures such as common bile duct ligation (106) and partial hepatectomy (3, 107). These and other manipulations (e.g., blood gavage, feeding with ammonium acetate) (108) have been introduced primarily to produce a more severe form of hepatic encephalopathy. In 1987, Chamuleau *et al.* (109) induced complete liver ischemia in PCS rats by tightening up a wire around the coeliac trunk. This wire was left *in situ* during the portacaval shunt procedure on the previous day. Combination of PCS and 75% hepatectomy (removal of the two anterior and both omental lobes) is another interesting and overlooked procedure. In the experience of Demma *et al.* (107) hepatic failure had >80% mortality rate within 24–48 hr, but was potentially reversible. Intrasplenic or intraperitoneal injection of 20 million isolated fresh hepatocytes was shown to reduce the mortality rate significantly in this model (110).

2. A Rat Model of FHF

We have developed a model of acute liver failure, which reproduces in rats a number of clinical, biochemical, histologic, and molecular biological features of the clinical FHF syndrome, including severely impaired ability of the residual liver tissue to regenerate. In this simple and highly reproducible preparation, resection of the two anterior liver lobes (68% liver mass) is combined with ligation of the common right liver lobes pedicle (22–24% liver mass) (Fig. 4). As a result, the functional liver mass is greatly reduced, there is a significant amount of liver tissue undergoing necrosis, and animal survival is dependent on the ability of the residual omental liver lobes (~10% liver mass) to

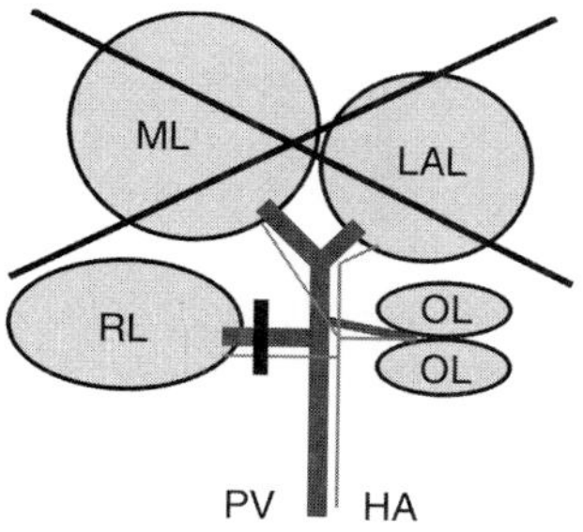

Figure 4 Diagram depicting the technique used to induce fulminant hepatic failure in rats. Two anterior lobes [~68%; median lobe (ML) and left anterior lobe (LAL)] were resected and the right lobes (RL; 22–24%) were rendered necrotic. Only the omental lobes (OL; 8%) and part of the liver tissue surrounding the intrahepatic portion of the inferior vena cava (~2%) remained intact and received the entire portal venous flow.

mass) to regenerate. More than 90% of untreated FHF rats died between 24 and 48 hr postoperatively (mean: 39 ± 11 hr), all with biochemical signs of progressive liver failure, coma, and brain swelling. Interestingly, even though they had less than 10% of functional liver mass in place, none developed profound hypoglycemia and survival was not affected by postoperative supplementation with 5% dextrose (single vs. repeated subcutaneous injections). All FHF rats died with no signs of liver regeneration. A slight increase in liver weight was caused by edema and no parenchymal cells stained positive for bromodeoxyuridine or showed mitotic figures (111). To better understand the cause of impaired regeneration response in FHF rats, we studied the plasma profile of two important growth modulators, hepatocyte growth factor (HGF) and transforming growth factor-β1 (TGF-β1), along with mRNA expression of HGF and c-met (HGF receptor) in residual omental liver lobes. In FHF rats, plasma HGF and TGF-β1 levels were greatly elevated throughout the postinduction period, a finding that is in agreement with the clinical data on FHF (112). Additionally, FHF rat livers showed delayed HGF and c-met expression.

3. Ischemic Liver Failure in Dogs and Pigs

Over the years, we have developed a hybrid hepatocyte-based artificial liver and evaluated it in several large animal (dog, pig) models of permanent liver ischemia (113–115) (Fig. 5).

Adult mongrel dogs underwent end-to-side PCS and placement of exteriorized ligatures around the common hepatic and gastroduodenal arteries. The crucial difference of this technique from others previously described is the ligation of the gastroduodenal artery. We found that retrograde flow through this vessel following ligation of the hepatic artery proper in these animals was associated with recovery of liver function. This could account for inconsistent results obtained with that model in the past. Animals were allowed to recover for 72 hr, at which time, they were reanesthetized and supported by mechanical ventilation. Jugular venous and femoral arterial cannulas were placed for fluid administration and pressure monitoring, respectively. The exteriorized arterial ligatures were applied after collection of baseline blood sample for serum glucose, ammonia, lactate, transaminases, and pH determinations. Each animal included in the study was administered 0.5 mg/kg indocyanine green (ICG) and its clearance was determined before shunting and at 2 hrs following arterial ligation. Prior to the PCS, there was rapid clearance of ICG at 20 min (absorbency at 280 nm: 1.90 ± 0.08 to 0.52 ± 0.08); following arterial ligation, clearance was significantly decreased (2.0 ± 0.10 to 1.80 ± 0.09). At 5 hrs following hepatic devascularization, significant metabolic derangement was noted. Serum glucose decreased (94.7 ± 12.7 to 22.5 ± 4.31 mg/dl; $P < 0.02$), ammonia increased (6.43 ± 0.6 to 16.3 ± 0.8 μg/liter; $P < 0.05$), lactate increased (1.91 ± 0.3 to 11.3 ± 1.4 μg/liter; $P < 0.05$), and pH decreased (7.34 ± 0.07 to 7.02 ± 0.05; $P < 0.05$). In addition, there was a significant increase in the activity of serum transaminases following hepatic devascularization. Random liver biopsies at the end of the experiments (6–7 hr) revealed massive necrosis.

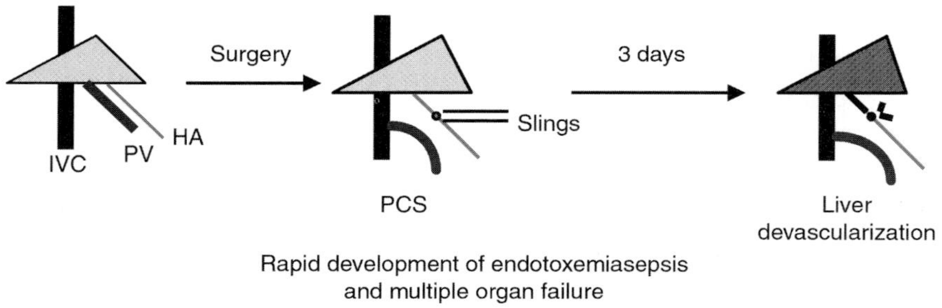

	Hypothermia (25 °C)	Normothermia (37 °C)
Survival (hours)	29 ± 1	22 ± 2
Intracranial pressure (mmHg)	10 ± 4	29 ± 4
Blood NH_3 (μM/L)	364 ± 113	490 ± 163

Figure 5 Diagram depicting the technique used to induce liver ischemia. An end-to-side portacaval shunt (PCS) was created and two slings were placed around the hepatic artery and the common bile duct, as described in the text. After 3–4 days, the slings were removed. In normothermic pigs, body core temperature was maintained at 37°C through external heating and warming of intravenously administered fluids. Hypothermic animals were kept in a temperature-controlled environment at 21°C so that their body temperature was allowed to decrease. Differences in survival time, intracranial pressure, and blood ammonia level between the two groups were statistically significant ($P <$ 0.01–0.001; paired *t*-test).

In pigs, ischemic liver failure is also achieved after PCS (to ensure decompression of the splanchnic vascular bed) and interruption of arterial blood supply to the liver. Dearterialization can either be performed at the time of shunting, or later (hours, days) by tying off tourniquets that have been placed around the common hepatic and gastroduodenal arteries and the common bile duct at the time of shunting and brought out into a subcutaneous pocket. We have evaluated these two techniques while searching for an optimal large animal model of brain edema as a cause of death in FHF.

In the first series of experiments, the liver was devasacularized at the time of PCS. Unfortunately, only 6 out of 10 liver failure pigs developed intracranial hypertension (unpublished data). In the second study, 20 adult pigs (40–55 kg) underwent a two-stage procedure (dearterialization after 3 days). During the second stage, a subdural bolt was inserted for ICP monitoring. After recovery from anesthesia, eight pigs were kept at ambient (21°C) room temperature and became hypothermic (25.0 ± 0.1°C at 20 hr). In the remaining 12 pigs, body temperature was maintained >36°C using a warming pad and a heating lamp. All pigs were maintained on intravenous glucose (5 g/hr) supplementation. We found that hypothermic pigs lived longer than normothermic ones (29 ± 1.6 hr versus 22 ± 2 hr; $P < 0.05$). Significant and persistent intracranial hypertension developed only in normothermic pigs with liver necrosis (29 ± 4 mmHg). Characteristically, ICP showed fluctuations exceeding 30 mmHg on stimulation, which is widely seen clinically, and all pigs died from brain stem herniation. Only half of the hypothermic pigs had a transient rise in ICP at 18–22 hours postinduction (33 ± 9 mmHg); in the remaining ones the ICP remained normal (10 ± 4 mmHg). These results show that pigs with liver ischemia develop brain edema early (6–12 hr) and consistently provided that they are maintained normothermic throughout the postoperative period. Furthermore, this study suggests that in FHF pigs with liver necrosis, hypothermia prolongs survival time and exerts a protective effect against intracranial hypertension. Review of the literature reveals that hypothermia lowers metabolic demands, slows accumulation of compounds normally metabolized by the liver, and reduces neurotoxicity of ammonia (116). It also prevented increase in brain water content in rats with complete liver ischemia (117).

References

1. Terblanche, J., Hickman, R., Miller, D., *et al.* (1975). Animal experience with support systems: Are there appropriate animal models of fulminant hepatic necrosis? *In* "Artificial Liver Support" (R. Williams and I. Murray-Lyon, eds.), pp. 163–172. Pittman, London.
2. Blitzer, B. L., Waggoner, J. G., Jones, E. A., Gralnick, H. R., Towne, D., Butler, J., Weise, V., Kopin, I. J., Walters, I., Teychenne, P. F., Goodman, D. G., and Berk, P. D. (1978). A model of fulminant hepatic failure in the rabbit. *Gastroenterology* **74,** 664–671.
3. Mullen, K. D., Birgisson, S., Gacad, R. C., Conjeevaram, H. (1994). Animal models of hepatic encephalopathy and hyperammonemia. *In* "Hepatic Encephalopathy, Hyperammonemia, and Ammonia Toxicity" V. Felipo and S. Grisolia, eds.), pp. 1–21. Plenum Press, New York.
4. Gunn, C. H. (1938). Hereditary acholuric jaundice in a new mutant strain of rats. *J. Hered.* **29,** 137–139.
5. Carbone, J. V., and Grodsky, G. M. Constitutional non-hemolytic hyperbilirubinemia in the rat: Defect of bilirubin conjugation. *Proc. Soc. Exp. Biol. Med.* **94,** 461–463.
6. Cornelius, C. E., and Arias, I. M. (1972). Animal model of human disease. Crigler–Najjar syndrome animal model: Hereditary nonhemolytic unconjugated hyperbilirubinemia in Gunn rats. *Am. J. Pathol.* **69,** 369–372.
7. Johnson, L., Sarmiento, F., Blanc, W. A., and Day, R. Kernicterus in rats with an inherited deficiency in glucuronyl transferase. *AMAJ Dis. Child* **99,** 591–608.
8. Roy-Chowdhury, J., Kondapalli, R., and Roy Chowdhury, N. (1993). Gunn rat: A model for inherited deficiency of bilirubin conjugation. *In* "Animal Models in Liver Research. Advances in Veterinary Science and Comparative Medicine" (C. E. Cornelius, ed.), pp. 149–164. Academic Press, San Diego
9. Jansen, P. L. M., Peters, W. H. M., and Lamers, W. H. (1985) Hereditary chronic conjugated hyperbilirubinemia in mutant rats caused by defective hepatic anion transport. *Hepatology* **5,** 573–579.
10. Jansen, P. L. M., Groothuhis, G. M. M., Peters, W. H. M., and Meijer, D. K. F. (1987). Selective hepatobiliary transport defectfor organic anions and neutral steroids in mutant rats with hereditary conjugated hyperbilirubinemia. *Hepatology* **7,** 71–76.
11. Kuipers, F., Enserink, M., Havinga, R., van der Steen, A. B. M., Hardonk, M. J., Fevery, J., and Vonk, R. J. (1988). Separate transport systems for biliary secretion of sulfated and unsulfated bile acids in the rat. *J. Clin. Invest.* **81,** 1593–1599.
12. Takikawa, H., Sano, N., Narita, T., Uchida, Y., Yamanaka, M., Horie, T., Mikami, T., and Tagaya, O. (1991). Biliary excretion of bile acid conjugates in a hyperbilirubinemic mutant Sprague–Dawley rat. *Hepatology* **14,** 352-60.
13. Kitamura, T., Alroy, J., Gatmaitan, Z., Inoue, M., Mikami, T., Jansen, and P., Arias, I. M. (1992). Defective biliary excretion of epinephrine metabolites in mutant (TR-) rats: Relation to the pathogenesis of black liver in the Dubin-Johnson syndrome and Correidale sheep with an analogous excretory defect. *Hepatology* **15,** 1154–1159.
14. Cornelius, C. E., Arias, I. M., and Osburn, B. I. (1965). Hepatic pigmentation with photosensitivity: A syndrome in Corriedale sheep resembling Dubin-Johnson syndrome in man. *J. Am. Vet. Med. Assoc.* **146,** 709–713.
15. Dubin, I. N., and Johnson, F. B. (1954). Chronic idiopathic jaundice with unidentified pigment in liver cells. *Medicine* **33,** 155–197.
16. Jansen, P. L. M., and Oude Elferink, R. P. J. (1993). Hereditary conjugated hyperbilirubinemia in Wistar rats: A model for the study of ATP-dependent hepatocanalicular organic anion transport. *In* "Animal Models in Liver Research. Advances in Veterinary Science and Comparative Medicine" (C. E. Cornelius, ed.), pp. 175–195. Academic Press, San Diego.
17. Nagase, S., Shimamune, K., and Shumiya, S. (1979). Albumin-deficient rat mutant. *Science* **205,** 590–591.
18. Esumi, H., Takahashi, Y., Sato, S., Nagase, S., and Sugimura, T. (1983). A seven-base-pair deletion in an intron of the albumin gene of analbuminemic rats. *Proc. Natl. Acad. Sci. U.S.A.* **80,** 95.
19. Shalaby, F., and Schafritz, D. A. (1990). Exon skipping during splicing of albumin mRNA precursors in Nagase analbuminemic rats. *Proc. Natl. Acad. Sci. U.S.A.* **87,** 2652–2656.
20. Holzman, M., Rozga, J., Moscioni, A. D., and Demetriou, A. A. (1993). Selective intraportal hepatocyte transplantation in analbuminemic and Gunn rats. *Transplantation* **55,** 1213–1219.

21. Rozga, J., Holzman, M., Moscioni, A. D., Fujioka, H., Morsiani, E., and Demetriou, A. A. (1995). Repeated intraportal hepatocyte transplantation in analbuminemic rats. *Cell Transplant.* **4,** 237–243.
22. Moscioni, A. D., Rozga, J., Chen, S., Naim, A., Scott, H. S., and Demetriou, A. A. (1996). Long-term correction of albumin levels in the Nagase analbuminemic rat: Repopulation of the liver by transplanted normal hepatocytes under a regeneration response. *Cell Transplant.* **5,** 499–503.
23. Ogawa, K., Ohta, T., Inagaki, M., and Nagase, S. (1993). Identification of F344 rat hepatocytes transplanted within the liver of congenic analbuminemic rats by the polymerase chain reaction. *Transplantation* **56,** 9–15.
24. Makino, S., and Katagiri, K. (1980). Osteogenic disorder rat. *Exp. Anim.* **29,** 374–385.
25. Onodera, K., Kasai, S., Kato, K., Sawa, M., Mito, M., and Nozawa, M. (1994). Effects of intrfasplenic hepatocyte transplantation in rats congenitally deficient in ascorbic acid biosynthetic enzyme. *Cell Transplant.* **3**(Suppl. 1), 31–34.
26. Watanabe, Y. (1980). Serial inbreeding of rabbits with hereditary hyperlipidemia (WHHL-rabbit). *Arteriosclerosis* **36,** 261–270.
27. Kita, T., Brown, M. S., Watanabe, Y., Goldstein, J. L. (1981). Deficiency of low density lipoprotein receptors in liver and adrenal gland of the WHHL rabbit, an animal model of familial hypercholesterolemia. *Proc. Natl. Acad. Sci. U.S.A.* **78,** 2268.
28. Wilson, J. M., Johnston, D. E., Jefferson, D. M., and Mulligan, R. C. (1988). Correction of the genetic defect in hepatocytes from the Watanabe heritable hyperlipidemic rabbit. *Proc. Natl. Acad. Sci. U.S.A.* **85,** 4421–4425.
29. Grossman, M., Raper, S. E., Kozarsky, K., *et al.* (1994). Successful *ex vivo* gene therapy directed to liver in a patient with familial hypercholesterolemia. *Nature Genet.* **6,** 335–341.
30. Li, J., Fang, B., Eisensmith, R. C., Li, X. H. C., *et al.* (1995). *In vivo* gene therapy for hyperlipidemis: Phenotypic correction in Watanabe rabbits by hepatic delivery of the rabbit LDL receptor gene. *J. Clin. Invest.* **95,** 768.
31. Eguchi, S., Rozga, J., Chen, S., Wang, C.-C., Rosenthal, R., Hewitt, W. R., Middleton, Y., Lebow, L. T., and Demetriou, A. A. (1996). Treatment of Hypercholesterolemia in the Watanabe Rabbit using allogeneic hepatocellular transplantation under a regeneration stimulus. *Transplantation* **62,** 1–6.
32. Provoost, A. P., Madern, G. C., Sinaasappel, M., Terpstra, O., and Molenaar, J. C. (1993). Successful prolonged correction of an inborn metabolic defect by heterotopic auxiliary liver transplantation in a dog model. *Transplant. Proc.* **215,** 1950–1951.
33. Terblanche, J., and Hickman, R. (1991). Animal model of fulminant hepatic failure. *Dig. Dis. Sci.* **6,** 15–22.
34. Mullen, K. D., Schafer, D. F., Maynard, T. F., DeKnegt, R., Jones, D. B., Roessle, M., and Jones, E. A. (1986). Galactosamine induced fulminant hepatic failure in the rat may be an unsuitable model for acute hepatic encephalopathy; a comparison with the rabbit model. *Gastroenterology* **90,** 1750–1758.
35. Tabata, Y., and Chang, T. M. S. (1980). Comparisons of six artificial liver support regimens in fulminant hepatic failure rats. *Trans. Am. Soc. Artif. Intern. Organs* **26,** 394–399.
36. Decker, K., and Keppler, D. (1972). Galactosamine induced liver injury. *In* "Progress in Liver Diseases" (H. Popper and F. Schaffner, eds.), Vol. 4, pp. 183–196. Grune & Stratton, New York.
37. Grun, M., Liehr, H., and Rasenack, U. (1976). Significance of endotoxemia in experimental "galactosamine hepatitis" in the rat. *Acta Hepatogastroenterol. (Stuttg.)* **23,** 64–81.
38. Lo, W. D., Ennis, S. R., Goldstein, G. W., McNeely, D. L., and Betz, A. L. (1987). The effects of galactosamine-induced hepatic failure upon blood-brain barrier. *Hepatology* **7,** 452–456.
39. Baumgartner, D., LaPlante-O'Neill, P. M., Sutherland, D. E. R., and Najarian, J. S. (1983). Effects of intrasplenic injection of hepatocytes, hepatocyte fragments and hepatocyte culture supernatants on D-galactosamine-induced liver failure in rats. *Eur. Surg. Res.* **15,** 129–135.
40. Diaz-Buxo, J. A., Blumenthal, S., Hayes, D., Gores, P., and Gordon, B. (1997). Galactosamine-induced fulminant hepatic necrosis in unanesthetized canines. *Hepatology* **25,** 950–957.
41. Hilgier, W., Albrecht, J., and Krasnicka, Z. (1983). Thioacetamide-induced hepatogenic encephalopathy in the rat. *Neuropathol. Pol.* **45,** 7–10.
42. Albrecht, J., and Hilgier, W. (1986). Arginine in thioacetamide-induced hepatogenic encephalopathy in rats: Activation of enzymes of arginine metabolism to glutamate. *Acta Neurol. Scand.* **73,** 498–501.
43. Maddison, J. E., Dodd, P. R., Johnston, G. A. R., and Farrell, G. C. (1987). Brain γ-aminobutyric acid receptor binding is normal in rats with thioacetamide-induced hepatic encaphalopthy despite elevated plasma γ-aminobutyric acid-like activity. *Gastroenetrology* **93,** 1062–1068.
44. Bruccoleri, A., Gallucci, R., Germolec, D. R., Blackshear, P., Simeonova, P., Thurman, R. G., and Luster, M. I. (1997). Induction of early-immediate genes by tumor necrosis factor a contribute to liver repair following chemical-induced hepatotoxicity. *Hepatology* **25,** 133–141.
45. Liu, K.-X., Kato, Y., Yamazaki, M., Higuchi, O., Nakamura, T., and Sugiyama, Y. (1993). Decrease in the hepatic clearance of hepatocyte growth factor in carbon tetrachloride-intoxicated rats. *Hepatology* **17,** 651–660.
46. Lindroos, P. M., Zarnegar, R., and Michalopoulos, G. K. (1991). Hepatocyte growth factor (hepatopoietin A) rapidly increases in plasma before DNA synthesis and liver regeneration stimulated by partial hepatectomy and carbon tetrachloride administration. *Hepatology* **13,** 743–749.
47. Cameron, G. R., and Karunaratne, W. A. E. (1936). Carbon tetrachloride cirrhosis in relation to liver regeneration. *J. Pathol. Bact.* **42,** 1–10.
48. Quinn, P. S., and Higginson, J. (1965). Reversible and irreversible changes in experimental cirrhosis. *Am. J. Pathol.* **47,** 353–361.
49. McLean, A. E. M., McLean, E. K., and Sutton, P. M. (1969). Instant cirrhosis. *Br. J. Exp. Pathol.* **50,** 502–509.
50. McLean, A. E. M., and McLean, E. K. (1966). The effect of diet and 1,1,1-trichloro-2,2-bis(p-chlorophenyl) ethane (DDT) on microsomal hydroxylating enzymes and on sensitivity of rats to carbon tetrachloride poisoning. *Biochem. J.* **100,** 564–569.
51. Proctor, E., and Chatamra, K. (1982). High yield micronodular cirrhosis in the rat. *Gastroenterology* **83,** 1183–1191.
52. Rozga, J., Foss, A., Alumets, J., Ahren, B., Jeppsson, B., and Bengmark, S. Liver cirrhosis in rats: Regeneration and assessment of the role of phenobarbital. *J. Surg. Res.* **51,** 329–335.
53. Alp, M. H., and Hickman, R. (1987). The effect of prostaglandins, branched-chain amino acids and other drugs on the outcome of experimental acute porcine hepatic failure. *J. Hepatol.* **4,** 99–107.
54. Miner, D. J., and Kissinger, P. T. (1979). Evidence for the involvement of *N*-acetyl-*p*-quinoneimine in acetaminophen metabolism. *Biochem. Pharmacol.* **28,** 3285–3290.
55. Tirmenstein, M., and Nelson, S. D. (1990). Acetaminophen-induced oxidation of protein thiols. *J. Biol. Chem.* **265,** 3059–3065.
56. Jaeschke, H. R. (1990). Glutathione disulfide formation and oxidant stress during acetaminophen-induced hepatotoxicity in mice *in vivo*: The protective effect of allopurinol. *J. Pharmacol. Exp. Ther.* **255,** 935–941.
57. Zieve, L., Dozeman, R., LaFontaine, D., and Draves, K. (1985). Kinase activity and ornithine decarboxylase activity after massive necrosis with acetaminophen in the rat. *J. Lab. Clin. Med.* **106,** 583–588.
58. Leonard, T. B., Morgan, D. G., and Dent, J. G. (1985). Ranitidine-acetaminophen interaction: Effects on acetaminophen-induced hepatotoxicity in Fischer 344 rats. *Hepatology* **5,** 480–487.
59. Francavilla, A., Makowka, L., Polimeno, L., Barone, M., Demetris, J., Prelich, J., Van Thiel, D. H., and Starzl, T. E. (1989). A dog model for

acetaminophen-induced fulminant hepatic failure. *Gastroenterology* **96,** 470–478.

60. Prescott, L. F., Roscoe, P., and Wright, N., *et al.* (1971). Plasma-paracetamol half-life and hepatic necrosis in patients with paracetamol overdosage. *Lancet* **i,** 519–521.
61. Wermers, G. W., Band, H., and Yunis, E. J. (1988). "Role of the HLA System in Antigen Recognition and Disease," 2nd Ed. Raven, New York.
62. Tiegs, H., Hentschel, J., and Wendel, A. (1992). A T cell-dependent experimental liver injury in mice inducible by concanavalin A. *Am. J. Clin. Invest.* **90,** 196–203.
63. Louis, H., Le Moine, O., Peny, M.-D., Quertinmont, E., Fokan, D., Goldman, M., and Deviere, J. (1997). Production and role of interleukin-10 in concanavalin A-induced hepatitis in mice. *Hepatology* **25,** 1382–1389.
64. Mizuhara, H., O'Neill, E., Seki, N., Ogawa, T., Kusunoki, C., Otsuka, K., Satoh, S., *et al.* (1994). T cell activation-associated hepatic injury: mediation by tumor necrosis factors and protection by interleukin 6. *J. Exp. Med.* **179,** 1529–1537.
65. Watanabe, Y., Morita, M., and Akaike, T. (1996). Concanavalin A induces perforin-mediated but not Fas-mediated hepatic injury. *Hepatology* **24,** 702-10.
66. Yoshida, M. C., Masuda, R., Sasaki, M., Takeichi, N., Kobayashi, H., Dempo, K., and Mori, M. (1987). Ne mutation causing hereditary hepatitis in the laboratory rat. *J. Hered.* **78,** 361–365.
67. Takeichi, N., Kobayashi, H., Yoshida, M. C., Sasaki, M., Dempo, and K., Mori, M. (1988). Spontaneous hepatitis in Long-Evans rats: A potential animal model for fulminant hepatitis in man. *Acta. Pathol. Jpn.* **38,** 1369–1375.
68. Masuda, R., Yoshida, M. C., Sasaki, M., Dempo, K., and Mori, M. (1988). High susceptibility to hepatocellular carcinoma development in LEC rats with hereditary hepatitis. *Jpn. J. Cancer Res.* **79,** 828–835.
69. Wu, J., Forbes, J. R., Chen, H. S., and Cox, D. W. (1994). The LEC rat has a deletion in the copper transporting ATPase gene homologous to the Wilson disease gene. *Nature Genet.* **7,** 541–545.
70. Nagata, S., and Golstein, P. The Fas death factor. *Science* **267,** 1449–1456.
71. Ogasawara, J., *et al.* (1993). Lethal effect of the anti-Fas antibody in mice. *Nature (London)* **364,** 806–809.
72. Lacronique, V., Mignon, A., Fabre, M., *et al.* (1996). Bcl-2 protects from lethal hepatic apoptosis induced by an anti-Fas antibody in mice. *Nature Med.* **2,** 80–86.
73. Vogels, B. A. P. M., Mass, M. A. W., Bosma, A., and Chamuleau, A. F. M. (1996). Significant improvement of survival by intrasplenic hepatocyte transplantation in totally hepatectomized rats. *Cell Transplant.* **5,** 369–378.
74. Meehan, F. P. (1954). Total hepatectomy in the rat. *Am. J. Physiol.* **179,** 282–284.
75. Azoulay, D., Astarcioglu, I., Astarcioglu, H., Lemoine, A., Majno, P., and Bismuth, H. (1997). A new technique of one stage total hepatectomy in the rat. *Surgery* **121,** 219–222.
76. Bollman, J. L., and Van Hook, E. (1968). A simplified two-stage hepatectomy in the rat. *J. Appl. Physiol.* **24,** 722–723.
77. Holmin, T., Alinder, G., and Herlin, P. (1982). A microsurgical method for total hepatectomy in the rat. *Eur. Surg. Res.* **14,** 420–427.
78. Rozga, J., Jeppsson, B., Bengmark, S., and Demetriou, A. A. (1992). A simple two-stage technique of total hepatectomy in the rat. *J. Surg. Res.* **52,** 46–49.
79. Rozga, J., Jeppsson, B., and Bengmark, S. (1986). Portal branch ligation in the rat. Re-evaluation of a model. *Am. J. Pathol.* **125,** 300–308.
80. Yamaguchi, Y., Bollinger, R. R., DeFaria, E., Landis, B., and Quarfordt, S. (1989). A simplified single stage total hepatectomy in the rat with maintenance of gastrointestinal absorptive function. *Hepatology* **9,** 69–74.
81. Lorenzo, M., Ventriglia, R., Angrisani, L., Spagnuolo, S., and Di Salvo, E. (1994). Ratto anepatico, tecnica di ricostruzione della circolazione venosa. *Ann. Ital. Chir.* **60,** 365–368.
82. Arkadopoulos, N., Lilja, H., Suh, K. S., Demetriou, A. A., and Rozga, J. (1998). Intrasplenic transplantation of allogeneic hepatocytes prolongs survival in anhepatic rats. *Hepatology* **28,** 1365–1370.
83. Takahashi, M., Matsue, H., Matsushita, M., Sato, K., Nishikawa, M., Koike, M., Noto, H., Nakajima, Y., Uchino, J., Komai, T., and Hashimura, E. (1992). Does a porcine hepatocyte hybrid artificial liver prolong the survival time of anhepatic rabbits? *ASAIO J.* **38,** M468–M472.
84. Starzl, T. E., Bernhard, V. M., Benvenuto, R., and Cortes, N. (1959). A new method for one-stage hepatectomy for dogs. *Surgery* **46,** 880–886.
85. Lempinen, M., Soyer, T., and Eiseman, B. (1973). A new technique for preparing totally hepatectomized pigs. *Surgery* **73,** 463–467.
86. Hickman, R., Dent, D. M., and Terblanche, J. (1974). The anhepatic model in a pig. *S. Afr. Med. J.* **48,** 263–264.
87. Hickman, R., Bracher, M., Tyler, M., Lotz, Z., and Fourie, J. (1992). Effect of total hepatectomy on coagulation and glucose homeostasis in the pig. *Dig. Dis. Sci.* **37,** 328–334.
88. Arkadopoulos, N., Chen, S., Khalili, T. M., Detry, O., Hewitt, W. R., Lilja, H., Kamachi, H., Demetriou, A. A., and Rozga, J. (1998). Transplantation of hepatocytes for prevention of intracranial hypertension in pigs with ischemic liver failure. *Cell Transplant.* **7,** 357–363.
89. Drapanas, T., McMenamy, R. H., Adler, W. J., and Vang, J. O. (1965). Intermediary metabolism following hepatectomy in dogs. *Ann. Surg.* **162,** 621–633.
90. Filipponi, F., Boggi, U., Meacci, L., Burchielli, S., Vistoli, F., Bellini, R., Prota, C., Colizzi, L., Kusmic, C., Campani, D., Gneri, C., Trivella, M. G., and Mosca, F. (1999). A new technique for total hepatectomy in the pig for testing liver support devices. *Surgery* **125,** 448–455.
91. Berlinger, W. G., Stene, R. A., Spector, R., and Al-Jurf, A. S. (1987). Plasma and cerebrospinal fluid nucleosides and oxypurines in acute liver failure. *J. Lab. Clin. Med.* **110,** 137–144.
92. Eguchi, S., Matsuzaki, S., Fujioka, H., Koji, T., Higami, Y., and Kanematsu, T. (1998). The Fas/Fas-ligand system functions in hepatocytes in the early stage of fulminant hepatic failure in rats. *Hepatol. Res.* **11,** 103–114.
93. Higgins, G. M., and Anderson, R. M. (1931). Restoration of the liver of the white rat following partial surgical removal. *AMA Arch. Pathol.* **12,** 186–202.
94. Weinbren, K., and Tarsh, E. (1964). The mitotic response in the rat liver after different regenerative stimuli. *Br. J. Exp. Pathol.* **45,** 475–480.
95. Gaub, J., and Iverson, J. (1984). Rat liver regeneration after 90% partial hepatectomy. *Hepatology* **4,** 902–904.
96. Sarac, T. P., Sax, H. C., Doerr, R., Yuksel, U., Pulli, R., and Caruana, J. (1994). Preoperative fasting improves survival after 90% hepatectomy. *Arch. Surg.* **129,** 729–733.
97. Demetriou, A. A., Reisner, A., Sanchez, J., Levenson, S. M., Moscioni, A. D., and Roy Chowdhury, J. (1988). Transplantation of microcarrier-attached hepatocytes into 90% partially hepatectomized rats. *Hepatology* **8,** 1006–1009.
98. McMaster, P. D., and Drury, D. R. (1929). The production of partial liver insufficiency in rabbits. *J. Exp. Med.* **49,** 745–758.
99. Misra, M. K., P'eng, E. K., Sayhoun, A., *et al.* (1972). Acute hepatic coma: A canine model. *Surgery* 634–642.
100. Fischer, M., Stotter, L., Schmahl, W., *et al.* (1976). Acute liver failure due to temporary hepatic ischemia in the pig. *Acta Hepato-Gastroenterol.* **23,** 241–249.
101. Nordlinger, B., Douvin, D., Javaudin, L., *et al.* (1980). An experimental study of survival after two hours of normothermic hepatic ischemia. *Surg. Gynecol. Obstet.* **150,** 859-64.

102. Harris, K. A., Wallace, A. C., and Wall, W. J. (1982). Tolerance of the liver to ischemia in the pig. *J. Surg. Res.* **33,** 524–530.
103. DeGroot, G. H., Reuvers, C. B., Schalm, S. W., Boks, A. L., Terpstra, O. T., Jeekel, H., Ten Kate, F. W. J., and Bruinvels, J. (1987). A reproducible model of acute hepatic failure by transient ischemia in the pig. *J. Surg. Res.* **42,** 92–100.
104. Rappaport, A. M., Malcolm, H., MacDonald, H., *et al.* (1953). Hepatic coma following ischemia of the liver. *Surg. Gynecol. Obstet.* **97,** 748–762.
105. Tonnesen, K. (1976). Total devascularization of the liver: An experimental model of acute liver failure. *Scand. J. Gastroenterol.* **11** (Suppl. 37), 23–26.
106. Maddison, J. E., Dodd, P. R., Morrison, M., and Farrell, G. C. (1987). Plasma GABA, GABA like activity and the brain GABA-benzodiazepine receptor complex in rats with chronic hepatic encephalopathy. *Hepatology* **7,** 621–628.
107. Demma, I., Houssin, D., Capron, M., Minato, M., Morin, J., Gigou, M., Szekely, A. M., and Bismuth, H. (1986). Therapeutic efficacy of the transplantation of isolated hepatocytes in rats with surgically induced acute hepatic failure: A study of the mechanism. *Eur. Surg. Res.* **18,** 12–18.
108. Hindtfeldt, B., Plum, F., and Duggy, T. E. (1977). Effect of acute ammonia intoxication or cerebral metabolism in rats with portacaval shunts. *J. Clin. Invest.* **49,** 386–396.
109. Chamuleau, R. A. F. M., Deutz, N. E. P., de Haan, J. G., and van Gool, J. (1987). Correlation between electroencephalographic and biochemical indices in acute hepatic encephalopathy rats. *J. Hepatol.* **4,** 299–306.
110. Minato, M., Houssin, D., Demma, I., Morin, J., Gigou, M., Szekely, A. M., and Bismuth, H. (1984). *Eur. Surg. Res.* **16,** 162–169.
111. Eguchi, S., Kamlot, A., Ljubimova, J., Hewitt, W. R., Lebow, L. T., Demetriou, A. A., and Rozga, J. (1996). Fulminant hepatic failure in rats: Survival and effect on blood chemistry and liver regeneration. *Hepatology* **24,** 1452–1459.
112. Tsubouchi, H., Hirono, S., Gohda, E., Nakayama, H., Takahashi, K., Sakiyama, O., Miyazaki, H., *et al.* (1989). Clinical significance of human hepatocyte growth factor in blood from patients with fulminant hepatic failure. *Hepatology* **9,** 875–881.
113. Rozga, J., Holzman M. D., Ro, M. S., Griffin, D. W., Neuzil, D. F., Giorgio, T., Moscioni, A. D., and Demetriou, A. A. (1993). Hybrid bioartificial liver support treatment of animals with severe ischemic liver failure. *Ann. Surg.* **217,** 502–511.
114. Rozga, J., Williams, R. F., Moscioni, A. D., Giorgio, T., Ro, M. S., Daniel, N., Hakim, R., and Demetriou, A. A. (1993). Development of a bioartificial liver support system. *Hepatology* **17,** 258–264.
115. Khalili, T., Navarro, A., Ting, P., Arkadopoulos, N., Kamohara, Y., Mullon, C. J.-P., Demetriou, A. A., and Rozga, J. (1998). Bioartificial liver (BAL) treatment prevents development of intracranial hypertension in pigs with fulminant hepatic failure. *Hepatology* **28** (4, Pt.2), 171A.
116. Schenker, S., and Warren, K. S. (1960). Effect of temperature variation on toxicity and metabolism of ammonia in mice. *J. Lab. Clin. Med.* **60,** 291–296.
117. Traber, P., DalCanto, M., Ganger, D., and Blei, A. T. (1989). Effect of body temperature on brain edema and encephalopathy in the rat after hepatic devascularization. *Gastroenterology* **96,** 885–891.

49

Portal Hypertension and Portacaval Shunt*

Marshall J. Orloff

Department of Surgery, School of Medicine, University of California, San Diego, La Jolla, California 92093

I. Portal Hypertension

Portal hypertension (PH) is the complication of liver disease that most frequently involves the surgeon. In normal subjects at rest, portal pressures range from 4 to 10 mm Hg (60–140 mm saline) while inferior vena caval pressures range from 0.5 to 4 mm Hg (7–55 mm saline) (1,2). Clinically meaningful PH may be defined as a portal vein (PV)–inferior vena cava (IVC) gradient of 10 mm Hg (135 mm saline) or greater in the presence of a patent IVC. Several studies of the relationship of the PV–IVC pressure gradient to bleeding from esophagogastric varices have reported that bleeding did not occur below a level of 12 mm Hg (3–7). More important than the specific numbers, PH may be defined in terms of the pathologic disturbances it produces that compromise health and threaten life. Some of these disorders, such as bleeding esophagogastric varices and hypersplenism, are a direct reflection of the high pressure in the portal circulation and its collateral communications. Others such as ascites, hepatic encephalopathy, and hepatorenal syndrome are complicated manifestations of a number of factors, including the PH, the underlying liver disease, and the required treatment.

The splanchnic vascular bed includes all of the abdominal organs except the kidney. It receives 25% of the cardiac output. This flow, in turn, is conducted by the PV to the liver, 60% from the intestine, 20% from the stomach, 10% from the spleen, and 10% from the pancreas. The PV supplies about 75% of total hepatic blood flow and the hepatic artery supplies about 25%. Hepatic blood volume is very large, accounting for 12% of the total blood volume of the body and representing about 30% of liver volume. The other splanchnic organs contain about 21% of total blood volume so that altogether the splanchnic bed, the venous pressure of which is regulated by the liver, contains about one-third of total blood volume. Sinusoidal pressure in the liver and pressure in the PV are similar. Almost all of the pressure drop from the PV to the IVC occurs across sphincter-like areas in the hepatic veins that can be stimulated by sympathetic nerves and vasoconstrictors in the blood.

The hepatic circulation is altered in all forms of liver disease. Hepatic arterial flow is regulated by an adenosine washout mechanism in order to maintain total hepatic blood flow at relatively constant levels. This hepatic arterial buffer

*Supported by NIH Grants A3048, A5919, AM07315, AM07511, AM1228, AM19875, AM12280, AM17103, and DK41920.

response, which involves dilatation in response to reduced portal flow, also plays a role in regulation of intrahepatic and portal pressure and may be a major factor in determining the viability of diseased livers in which portal blood flow is diverted through portal-systemic collaterals or surgically created shunts. Total venous flow is not directly controlled by the liver, and changes in hepatic vascular resistance lead only to changes in portal pressure. In alcoholic cirrhosis most of the elevated vascular resistance appears to be localized to the hepatic veins, particularly to the hepatic vein sphincters.

A. Causes of Portal Hypertension

The causes of PH are shown in Table I. Except for the rare splanchnic arteriovenous fistulas, obstruction to portal blood flow is the main mechanism by which all of the conditions produce PH. The various diseases may be divided into two broad categories: those that originate in the blood vessels outside the liver and those that stem from within the liver.

Table I Causes of Portal Hypertension

Extrahepatic disease
Portal vein obstruction
Thrombosis due to infection, or trauma, or coagulopathy, or unknown
Cavernomatous transformation
Congenital atresia or stenosis
Extrinsic compression
Hepatic vein or IVC (outflow) obstruction
Budd–Chiari syndrome
Constrictive pericarditis
Excessive portal blood flow
Arteriovenous fistula between hepatic artery and portal vein
Arteriovenous fistula between splenic artery and vein
Intrahepatic obstructive disease
Alcoholic cirrhosis
Postnepatitic cirrhosis
Biliary cirrhosis (primary and secondary)
Toxic (chemical or drug) cirrhosis
Metabolic (genetic) cirrhosis (hemochromatosis)
Nutritional cirrhosis (after intestinal bypass)
Other forms of cirrhosis (cryptogenic, congestive, etc.)
Alcoholic hepatitis
Neoplasms and granulomas
Schistosomiasis (portal venules)
Veno-occlusive disease (hepatic venules)
Congenital hepatic fibrosis
Hepatoportal sclerosis

Extrahepatic obstruction of the PV (EHPH) is responsible for 8.4% of the cases of PH in our large series. It is most often caused by thrombosis. Often the event responsible for thrombosis cannot be determined. Cavernomatous transformation is the end result of thrombosis and recanalization of the PV. The clinical manifestations of EHPH usually develop in childhood or early adult life. Furthermore, the patients usually do not have liver damage, are otherwise in good health, and usually tolerate both the complications of their circulatory disorder and the required surgical therapy quite well.

Extrahepatic obstruction of the hepatic venous outflow system occurs in a group of conditions called the Budd-Chiari syndrome. The obstruction involves thrombosis of the hepatic veins and, sometimes, of the adjacent IVC. The etiology of the process is sometimes obscure, although many cases are associated with use of oral contraceptives, polycythemia rubra vera, or other thrombogenic hematologic disorders. Marked hepatomegaly and massive ascites are the most striking clinical findings. When the occlusion is confined to the hepatic veins, the condition has been relieved consistently by construction of a side-to-side portacaval shunt.

Intrahepatic obstructive diseases account for more than 90% of cases of PH. Of these, cirrhosis associated with chronic alcoholism is by far the most common cause in the United States. Cirrhosis due to viral hepatitis is an increasingly common cause of PH, whereas the incidence of biliary cirrhosis due to extrahepatic bile duct obstruction or primary intrahepatic disease is low. The other forms of intrahepatic obstruction are uncommon in the United States. Because cirrhosis is largely a disease of adulthood and, particularly with alcoholic cirrhosis, because it develops slowly over many years, patients with PH of the intrahepatic type are most often in the fifth or sixth decade of life. Moreover, they are usually in poor health because of the underlying liver disease, and the risk of operative treatment is significant.

A more detailed analysis of the causes of PH based on hemodynamic studies is shown in Table II, which identifies three categories, namely, prehepatic, intrahepatic, and posthepatic (12). The intrahepatic category is subdivided, whenever possible, according to the site of obstruction, i.e., presinusoidal, sinusoidal, and postsinusoidal. However, the largest subcategories bear the designation "mixed" because there is more than one site of obstruction.

B. Consequences of Portal Hypertension

The etiologic agents that cause cirrhosis of the liver produce widespread destruction of the hepatic parenchyma, which leads to an overgrowth of fibrous tissue and the formation of regenerative nodules in a pathologic rearrangement of liver architecture (8). As a result, the hepatic blood vessels are compressed and distorted. Because of their low

Table II Classification of Portal Hypertension Based on Hemodynamic Studies

Prehepatic	
Portal vein thrombosis	Idiopathic tropical splenomegaly
Splenic arteriovenous fistula	Splenic capillary hemangiomatosis

Intrahepatic					
Presinusoidal		Sinusoidal		Postsinusoidal	
Pure	Mixed	Pure	Mixed	Pure	Mixed
Schistosomiasis Sarcoidosis Myeloproliferative diseases? Metastatic malignancy Intrahepatic arteriovenous fistula Congenital hepatic fibrosis Idiopathic portal hypertension	Idiopathic portal hypertension Primary biliary cirrhosis (early) Congenital hepatic fibrosis Schistosomiasis (late) Chronic active hepatitis Vinyl chloride toxicity	Idiopathic portal hypertension?	Alcoholic cirrhosis Primary biliary cirrhosis (late) Cryptogenic cirrhosis (late) Peliosis hepatis? Fulminant viral hepatitis? Methotrexate Idiopathic portal hypertension?	Hepatic vein thrombosis (Budd–Chiari syndrome) Veno-occlusive disease Partial nodular transformation	Alcoholic hepatitis Hypervitaminosis A?

Posthepatic
Inferior vena cava thrombosis (Budd–Chiari syndrome)
Inferior vena cava web
Constrictive pericarditis
Tricuspid insufficiency
Severe heart failure

pressure and thin protective coat of connective tissue, the branches of the hepatic vein are often affected more than the other components of the vasculature, and hepatic venous outflow obstruction develops. Our studies suggest that this postsinusoidal obstruction is the fundamental hemodynamic lesion in alcoholic cirrhosis (9–11). Outflow obstruction leads to an increase in sinusoidal pressure, which, in turn, is reflected in an elevation of portal pressure and a decrease in portal blood flow to the liver. In extreme stages of postsinusoidal obstruction, the valveless PV may become an outflow tract and conduct blood in a retrograde manner away from the liver, leaving the hepatic artery alone to nourish the parenchyma. An additional consequence of the disruption of hepatic integrity is the development of communications between the intrahepatic branches of the hepatic artery and PV and between the tributaries of the PV and hepatic vein. The arteriovenous shunts contribute to the PH. Moreover, both types of shunts divert blood away from the hepatic parenchyma and compromise the nutrition of the liver cells. In an unsuccessful attempt to compensate for the reduction in portal flow to the liver, hepatic artery flow increases and the liver becomes dependent upon the hepatic artery for a major portion of its blood supply.

The elevated pressure in the PV leads to an enlargement of all the collateral venous connections between the portal and systemic circulations and to the development of varicosities (Fig. 1). In addition, splenomegaly develops. Blood flow through the collaterals is away from the liver, which further impairs hepatic nutrition. Despite their large size, the portal-systemic anastomoses are insufficient to accommodate the volume flow of portal blood and to overcome PH. Most prominent among the collaterals are those in the submucosa of the lower esophagus and upper stomach and those around the umbilicus and anterior abdominal wall. Rupture of the esophageal or gastric varices often causes massive hemorrhage and is associated with a high mortality rate.

Table III lists the main consequences of PH. In addition to those discussed above, ascites is a predictable consequence of PH because of the permeability of the sinusoids and the greatly increased formation of hepatic interstitial fluid that results from increases in intrasinusoidal pressure. Much of the excess interstitial fluid is returned to the bloodstream by the hepatic lymphatics but the remainder escapes into the peritoneal cavity to produce ascites.

Whether the cause of portal-systemic encephalopathy proves ultimately to be ammonia or some more complex

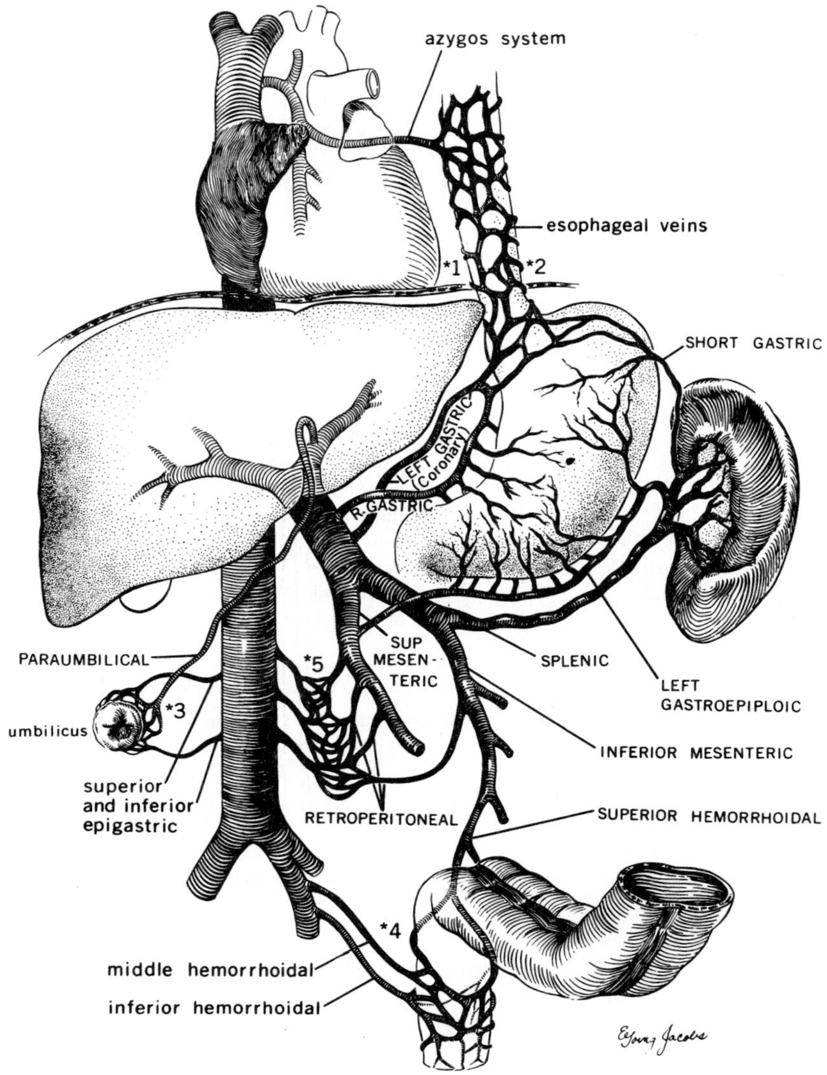

Figure 1 Sites of portal-systemic anastomoses, labeled *1 to *5. [From Orloff, M.J. (1981). The liver. *In* Davis–Christopher Textbook of Surgery (Sabiston, D.C., Jr., Ed), 12th ed., pp. 1131–1194. Saunders, Philadelphia.]

Table III Consequences of Portal Hypertension

Development of portal-systemic collaterals and bleeding from esophagogastric varices
Splenomegaly and hypersplenism
Reduced portal inflow to the liver
Increased hepatic artery flow
Ascites
Portal-systemic encephalopathy
Altered metabolism of splanchnic substances
Altered drug metabolism

nitrogenous substance, there is strong evidence that it is produced in the colon, normally extracted from the portal blood by the liver, and reaches the brain in unusual amounts by way of portal collateral veins. Therefore, the term "portal-systemic encephalopathy" is appropriate.

The pharmacokinetics of many drugs and the metabolism of endogenous substances produced in the splanchnic area are markedly affected by portal-systemic collateral circulation. Orally administered drugs like nitroglycerin and propranolol that are normally highly extracted by the liver on their first pass through the portal circulation will reach the systemic circulation in greatly increased concentrations. Gut hormones that enter the portal blood and are normally metabolized by the liver will likewise have the potential for systemic effects.

The scientific literature on PH is vast and the number of research studies is far too extensive to summarize here. Instead, some examples of research in this field will be presented to illustrate important research questions and approaches.

C. Animal Models of Portal Hypertension

1. Intrahepatic Portal Hypertension

Excellent animal models of prehepatic and posthepatic PH have existed for some years, but an ideal experimental model of intrahepatic PH has yet to be developed. The common forms of cirrhosis of the liver found in humans have not been reproduced in experimental animals by practical and consistent methods. The criteria for an ideal model should include the following (13). (1) duplication of morphologic features seen in human disease; (2) gradual and discrete progression of pathologic changes; (3) high reproducibility and low mortality; (4) reversibility and irreversibility of fibrotic changes; (5) development of pathophysiologic sequelae. Animal models of hepatic fibrosis can be categorized by etiologic agent, as shown in Table IV (13): (1) toxic; (2) nutritional; (3) immunologic; (4) biliary; (5) alcoholic; and (6) genetic.

Various toxic chemical agents have been used to produce necrosis of hepatocytes followed by fibrosis and what has been called cirrhosis in rats, hamsters, rabbits, mice, dogs, monkeys, and baboons. Included among these are carbon tetrachloride (CCl_4) (14–19), dimethylnitrosamine (20,21), thioacetamide (22–24), monocrotaline (25), alcohol (26–31), and an extract of the plant *Senecio discolor*, which contains hepatotoxic pyrrolizidine alkaloids and causes veno-occlusive disease in humans (32,33). In addition, experimental liver damage has been produced by common bile duct ligation, which results in biliary cirrhosis (34–39), and by feeding a choline-deficient or methionine-deficient diet (40). Some of the problems with the use of these agents have been inconsistency, a high mortality rate of the animals, difficulties in arriving at sublethal dosages that cause cirrhosis, and obtaining significant PH that is long lasting and does not disappear when administration of the toxic agent is discontinued.

The most widely used animal model of cirrhosis and PH has been the rat exposed to CCl_4. Extensive studies of the hemodynamics of PH, drug treatment of PH, ascites, renal function, hepatic encephalopathy, abnormal hepatic collagen synthesis, and treatment of esophageal varices have been performed in rats with CCl_4-induced cirrhosis. CCl_4 has been administered by gastric lavage, by injection, or by inhalation. Induction of liver damage is hastened by addition of phenobarbital to the drinking water, which has become standard practice in this model. In general, chronic administration of CCl_4 in the presence of phenobarbital in the drinking water has caused loss of body weight, extensive cirrhosis in 4–6 weeks, ascites, and finally death of the animal. One widely used method of CCl_4 administration is that described by McLean *et al.* (15) and modified by López-Novoa *et al.* (16–18) in which rats are placed in a chamber receiving air flow that previously has been bubbled through a bottle containing CCl_4. The rats are exposed to the air flow twice a week for periods of 1–5 min.

2. Prehepatic Portal Hypertension

Partial PV ligation (PVL) in various animals, but particularly in the rat, has been used widely for studies of PH. However, PVL does not produce liver damage, and there is some question about the relationship of prehepatic PH to the hemodynamic abnormalities associated with cirrhosis of the liver such as are found in over 90% of humans with PH. A common technique of partial PVL involves simply ligating the PV over a 20-gauge needle which is then removed, allowing the PV to reexpand to the predetermined size (40). Simplicity and reproducibility are the attractive features of partial PVL.

3. Posthepatic Portal Hypertension

Animal models of posthepatic PH have been used extensively for studies of ascites, Budd-Chiari syndrome, and congestive cirrhosis. In 1728, Lower first described the experimental production of ascites by occlusion of the thoracic IVC (41). In 1907, Bolton confirmed Lower's studies (42), and in 1948 McKee *et al.* clearly established this technique as a simple and reliable method of producing ascites (43). Results of a number of studies indicate that the ascites arising from partial occlusion of the thoracic IVC is derived largely from the surface of the liver and is a consequence of obstruction of hepatic venous outflow (44–46). Some evidence suggests that much of the ascitic fluid originates directly from the hepatic lymphatics (46–48). The technique of IVC occlusion was improved by our development of a method of gradually occluding the suprahepatic IVC below the diaphragm with an ameroid constrictor (49). The ameroid constrictor is a hygroscopic casein plastic disc encased in a steel rim. Both the disc and the rim contain an opening to allow placement around the IVC. After the ameroid is inserted around the IVC, it is locked in place by rotating the opening in the plastic disc away from the slit in the steel rim. At the time of insertion, the ameroid does not constrict the IVC. However, as the hygroscopic casein plastic takes up fluid and swells centrally, the lumen in the ameroid gradually narrows until, after 25–30 days, it completely occludes the IVC and produces severe hepatic outflow block, PH, and massive, intractable ascites typi-

Table IV Experimental Models of Hepatic Fibrosis/Cirrhosis[a]

	Species	Method	Lesion	Duration	
				Fibrosis	Cirrhosis
Toxic					
Carbon tetrachloride (CCl_4)	Rats 150–200 g	Subcutaneous injection, 0.1–0.2 mL/100 g of body weight twice weekly	Centrilobular, central–portal	>6 weeks	>12 weeks
	Rats 150–200 g	Inhalation twice weekly plus sodium phenobarbital in drinking water	Central–portal	>1–2 weeks	>4 weeks
Dimethylnitrosamine (DMNA)	Rats 150–200 g	Intraperitoneal injection 3 days weekly	Central–portal	>4 weeks	>13 weeks
	Dogs 10–30 kg	Oral adminstration 2 days weekly	Central–portal	>3–4 weeks	>13 weeks
Thioacetamide (TAA)	Rats 200 g	TAA in drinking water (300 mg/Liter)	Portal–portal, portal–central	>2–3 months	>3 months
Nutritional					
	Rats/mice 100–150 g	High-fat/low-choline, low-protein diet	Centrilobular, central–central, central–portal	>6 weeks	>12–24 weeks
Immunologic					
Heterologous serum	Rats 150–200 g	Low-protein/low-methionine diet plus ethionine (0.5%)	Diffuse	>4 weeks	>12 weeks
		Swine serum, intraperitoneal injection twice weekly	Periportal, portal–central	>5 weeks	>10 weeks
Bacterial cell wall	Rats 150–200 g	Streptococcal cell wall, single intraperitoneal injection (20 mg/g of body weight)	Periportal, granulomatous	>6 weeks	—
Murine schistosomiasis	Mice 20 g	Subcutaneous injection, 50 cercariae of *Schistosoma mansoni*	Periportal, granulomatous	>6 weeks	—
Endotoxin	Rabbits 2.5–3.0 kg	*Escherichia coli* endotoxin injection into the common bile duct (0.2/mg) followed 24 h later by 0.1/mg via the marginal ear vein	Periportal portal–portal, portal–central	—	>9 days
Biliary					
	Rats 150–300 g	Common bile duct ligation	Periportal	>4 weeks	—
	Dogs 10–25 kg	Common bile duct ligation	Periportal centrilobular	>4 weeks	—
	Monkeys 3–6 kg	Common bile duct ligation	Portal–portal, portal–central	>2 months	>6 months
Alcoholic					
	Baboons	Ethanol-containing liquid diet, *ad lib.*	Centrilobular, central–central	>6 months	>24 months
	Rats 350–400 g	Continuous intragastric infusion of ethanol and a high-fat diet	Centrilobular, central–central	>3 months	—
Genetic					
	Rhino mice	Mutant with the antosomal recessive gene	Periportal	>6 months	—

[a]From Ref. (13).

cal of the type of Budd-Chiari syndrome caused by IVC occlusion.

In 1961 we sought to develop a method of producing hepatic venous outflow obstruction that more closely mimicked the hemodynamic lesion of cirrhosis and did not obstruct the IVC. Initially, we developed a technique of gradually occluding the hepatic veins by inserting a polyvinyl cannula into the IVC opposite the orifices of the hepatic veins in dogs (50). Subsequently, we made a series of improvements in the creation of hepatic venous outflow obstruction by direct ligation of all of the hepatic veins except the large superior hepatic vein, which was gradually occluded, initially with a fiberglass ligature, then with a hepatic vein choker, and, in the final model, with an ameroid constrictor (51–55). The technique of hepatic vein ligation has been used in hundreds of dogs and rats and has proven to be a highly reliable method of producing hepatic venous outflow obstruction, congestive cirrhosis, and massive intractable ascites without alterations of pressure and blood flow in the IVC. Figure 2 is a drawing of the method of hepatic vein ligation using an ameroid constrictor around the superior hepatic vein (54). Figure 3 is a picture of an ameroid constrictor before and 35 days after insertion in a dog (54). Figure 4 is a picture of a typical dog with ascites 30 days after hepatic vein ligation (51).

D. Methods of Assessment of Portal Hypertension

1. Wedged Hepatic Vein Pressure

Catheterization of the hepatic veins was first reported in 1944 (56). Seven years later, Myers and Taylor described a technique for wedging a catheter in a hepatic vein and measuring the pressure (57). Subsequently, wedged hepatic vein pressure (WHVP) was shown to be approximately equal to PV pressure in the common forms of cirrhosis and normal in presinusoidal PH, such as occurs in schistosomiasis and PV thrombosis (58–60). More important than WHVP alone is the pressure gradient between WHVP and free hepatic vein pressure or IVC pressure, called the hepatic venous pressure gradient (HVPG). The development of a balloon catheter for measuring wedged and free hepatic vein pressures has facilitated the performance of serial measurements of HVPG and its response to therapy of PH, particularly treatment with pharmacological agents (61). Hepatic vein catheterization has been used widely in research on portal hemodynamics and as a predictor of survival in patients with cirrhosis (4,62–64).

2. Splenic Pulp Pressure

Because there are no valves in the portal venous system, portal pressure can be measured at any point in the system.

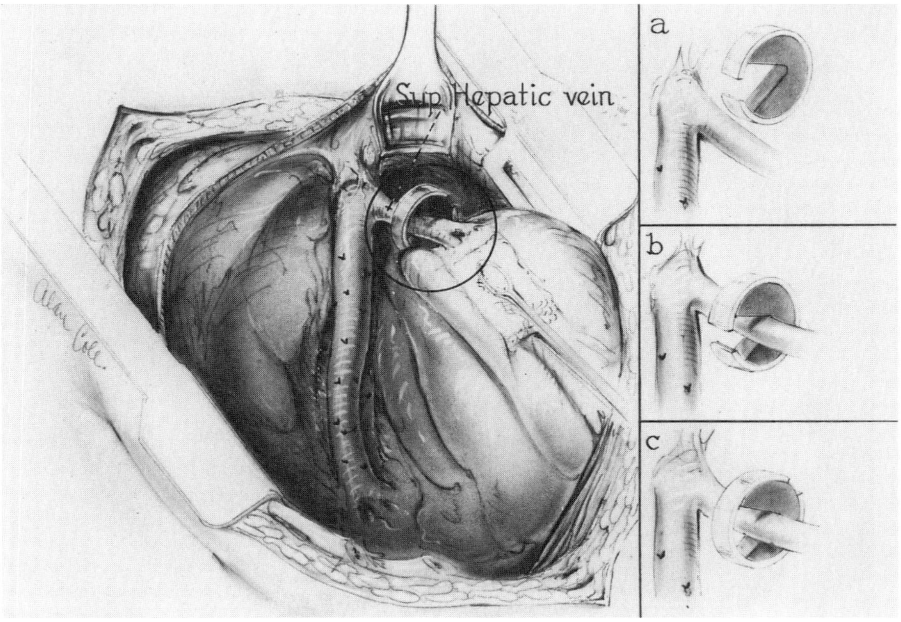

Figure 2 Technique of induction of Budd–Chiari syndrome in dogs by ligation and division of all hepatic veins except the large superior hepatic vein (left hepatic vein), which was surrounded by an ameroid constrictor.

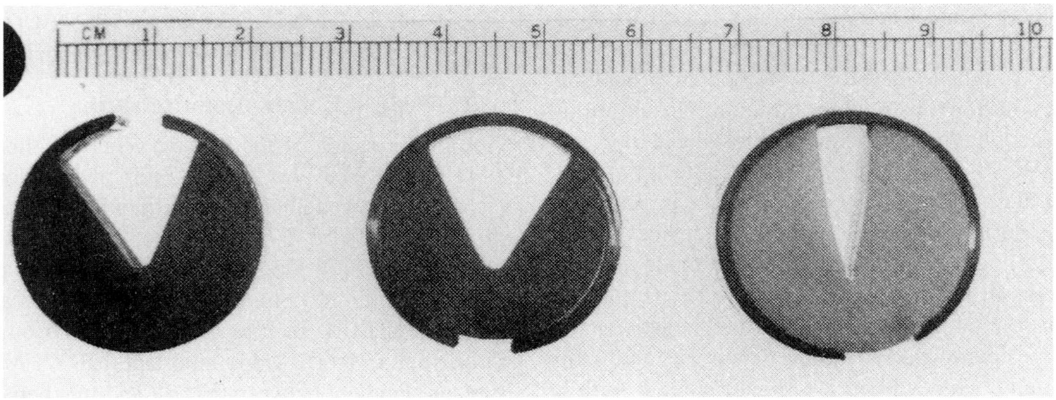

Figure 3 Ameroid constrictor made of a casein plastic disc surrounded by a stainless steel rim used for gradual occlusion of the left hepatic vein. On the left the ameroid is in position for insertion around the vein. In the middle the ameroid is in the locked position (after insertion around the vein), with the plastic disc rotated so that its slit is at a distance from the slit in the steel rim. On the right is an ameroid removed 35 days after insertion in a dog; the hygroscopic casein plastic has swelled, resulting in narrowing of the slit and occlusion of the vein.

Measurement of portal pressure by percutaneous puncture of the spleen with a needle is a highly accurate method of evaluating PH (65–67). Usually the technique is combined with venography of the portal system. Splenic pulp pressure is elevated in all forms of PH and does not define the site of origin of the underlying disease. Because of the small risk of bleeding from the splenic puncture and the development of other methods of visualizing the portal system, splenic pulp pressure measurements are used infrequently today.

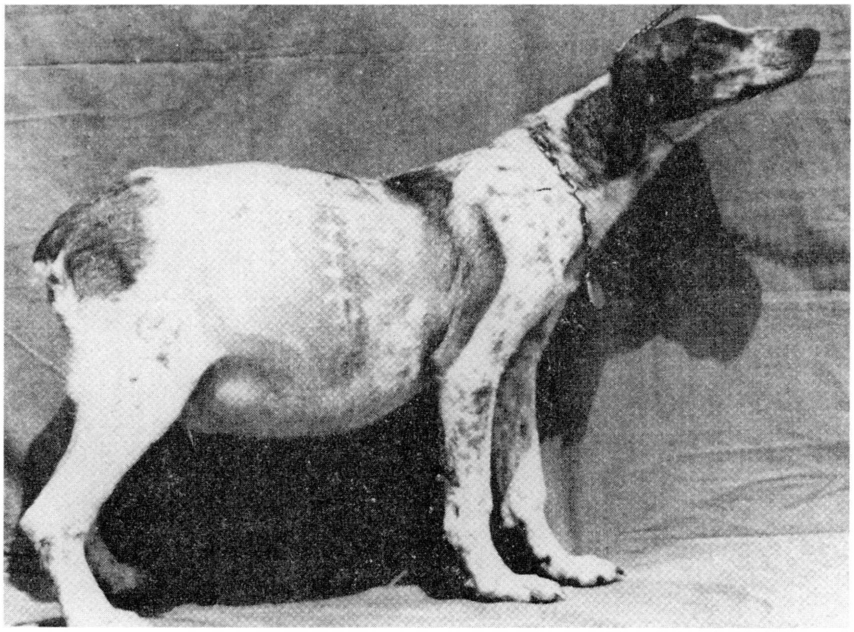

Figure 4 Photograph of Dog No. 62–223, taken 30 days after hepatic vein ligation and 21 days after a sham operation, shows massive reaccumulation of ascites. The portal pressure measured during the sham procedure was 226 mm saline. [From Ref. (51), Orloff, M.J., *et al.* (1963). *Surgery* **54,** 627–639.]

3. Transhepatic Portal Pressure

Transhepatic cannulation of an intrahepatic branch of the PV with a "skinny needle" makes it possible to measure portal pressure directly (68). Portal pressure is increased in all forms of intrahepatic and posthepatic PH, but is normal in prehepatic portal obstruction. The technique has the disadvantage of not having an internal zero reference point that permits determination of the gradient between the PV and IVC. This disadvantage can be overcome by inserting the needle into a hepatic vein or catheterizing the IVC.

4. Other Methods of Measuring Portal Pressure

Forcefully recanalizing the occluded umbilical vein for pressure measurements and portal venography has been used for research studies of PH, but is rarely used in clinical practice. Transjugular intrahepatic portal pressure measurements can be obtained by passing a catheter down the internal jugular vein into the liver. This method is used regularly as part of transjugular intrahepatic portosystemic shunt (TIPS) and can be combined with liver biopsy.

5. Radiographic Imaging of the Portal Venous System

Imaging of the portal venous system by various radiographic techniques provides information about portal venous anatomy, patency, direction of blood flow, and size and direction of collateral vessels.

Arterial portography currently is the most widely used method of visualizing the portal system. After contrast medium injection into the celiac axis and superior mesenteric artery, delayed films will usually show the splenic, superior mesenteric, and portal veins and their collaterals. With modern angiographic equipment and the use of subtraction techniques, if necessary, visualization of the portal venous system is satisfactory in over 90% of patients. This method is particularly useful in special situations such as the splenectomized patient or suspected splanchnic arteriovenous fistula.

Splenoportography was the first method used for opacification of the portal system and it has provided important information about portal hemodynamics, portal-systemic collateral formation, and hepatic encephalopathy (65–67,69,70). Splenic venography shows the splenic and portal veins well because it is easy to obtain a relatively high concentration of contrast medium in the splenic and, to a lesser extent, portal blood. It has some disadvantages; about 1–2% of patients have significant splenic bleeding, forceful injection of contrast medium can result in artificial flow patterns, and in patients with very large collaterals, the contrast may be entirely diverted prior to entry into the PV, causing the phenomenon known as "false thrombosis of the PV."

Ultrasonography using duplex Doppler ultrasound is a valuable technique for determining PV patency, direction of portal blood flow, presence of portal collateral vessels, flow in the splenic, superior mesenteric, and hepatic arteries, presence and amount of ascites, size of the liver and spleen, and presence of masses in the liver suggestive of hepatoma in patients with cirrhosis (71–78). Its great advantages are that it can be performed at the bedside, even in acutely bleeding patients, is noninvasive, and requires only a small amount of time.

Computerized tomography provides some of the same information as ultrasonography, but is superior in demonstrating liver masses.

Umbilical portography provides portal venograms of excellent quality if the umbilical vein can be forcefully recanalized and a catheter can be threaded through the umbilical vein into the main portal trunk. Prior upper abdominal surgery often destroys the umbilical vein remnant in the falciform ligament, which precludes the use of the umbilical vein route.

Percutaneous transhepatic portography was pioneered in 1975 by Lunderquist and Vang, who showed that it was possible to pass a catheter transhepatically into the intrahepatic PV over a guide wire inserted through a small needle (78). It is technically difficult and carries some risk of bleeding from the liver surface because of the frequent necessity of multiple punctures before successful PV entry. Remarkably good portograms are obtainable because of achievement of high density of contrast in the portal blood. Portography can be combined with portal pressure measurement and attempts to occlude portal collateral vessels with sclerosing solutions or coils. Smith-Laing *et al.* published one of the largest series of patients studied by this method, which includes data on portal pressure and collateral flow patterns and their correlations with variceal bleeding (79,80).

E. Hepatic Blood Flow

1. Total Hepatic Blood Flow

Quantitative hemodynamic data regarding hepatic perfusion under varying pathologic circumstances have potentially important diagnostic and therapeutic implications, particularly in PH, where the degree of hepatic perfusion before and after various forms of treatment could determine the response to therapy. In 1945, Bradley *et al.* described measurement of total hepatic blood flow (HBF) based on the indirect Fick principle involving selective removal of bromsulphthalein (BSP) dye by hepatocytes from blood perfusing the liver (81). BSP was injected into a peripheral vein and sampled via a catheter in a hepatic vein. Application of the Fick principle involves knowledge of the concentration of BSP in blood entering the liver, the concentration of BSP in blood leaving the liver, and the total amount of BSP removed per minute by the organ. With these values known, blood flow through the liver may be calculated by dividing the total amount of BSP removed per minute by the amount of BSP removed from each milliliter of blood passing through the liver. Since the concentration of BSP entering the liver was not directly measured, this value was indirectly approached by varying the infusion rate to maintain a constant peripheral blood concentration of BSP. The rationale was that BSP infusion rate was then equal to the hepatic extraction rate. The concentration of BSP entering the liver was then calculated as being equal to the peripheral concentration, and the concentration of BSP leaving the liver was determined by the hepatic venous catheter.

Clearance techniques such as that pioneered by Bradley *et al.* have become the most widely used methods of measuring total HBF in humans and experimental animals. Yet, to this day, it is uncertain whether any technique can produce reliable data on total HBF under all circumstances. Table V, taken from Bradley *et al.* (82), lists the methods used to measure total HBF, arranged in three broad categories: (1) techniques relying on hepatic clearance of a substance such as BSP from the circulation; (2) techniques depending upon indicator dilution methodology; and (3) a group of miscellaneous techniques applying a form of physical measurement.

Clearance techniques using agents that depend on hepatocyte extraction have replaced BSP, which is no longer available for use in humans. Caesar *et al.* used indocyanine green dye, which they believed was more reliable than BSP (83). Combes was an early advocate of ^{131}I-labeled rose bengal (84). Others have described clearance methods that depend on hepatocyte uptake and metabolism of agents such as ethanol, galactose, and propranolol (85,86). No doubt other materials specifically removed from the circulation by the hepatocyte can be used to determine total HBF.

The accuracy of all clearance techniques dependent upon hepatocyte extraction is based upon several assumptions: the material is removed from the blood *only* by the liver, single hepatic vein sampling is representative of the total venous efflux, extrahepatic shunting does not exist, and, most importantly, the efficiency of hepatocyte clearance is not spontaneously variable or affected by the presence of hepatic disease. While the validity of solitary hepatic vein sampling as representative of total hepatic venous concentration has been established (87,88), many of the other assumptions are not valid. Some materials supposedly extracted solely by the liver are subject to varying amounts of extrahepatic removal (83). The occurrence of spontaneous extrahepatic portosystemic shunts in cirrhosis is well known. Under these circumstances, marker concentration in the hepatic vein will be artificially low, resulting in an underestimation of hepatic flow if the marker is not lost in a concentration equal to that remaining in the PV. Finally, the major limitation to these techniques is that hepatocyte extraction diminishes markedly and becomes quite variable in the presence of hepatocellular disease (89,90).

Recognizing some of the problems inherent in clearance techniques that depend on extraction by hepatocytes, Dobson and Jones formulated a method of determining total HBF related to hepatic reticuloendothelial cell function (91). They observed that following intravenous injection of a particulate material, chromic ^{32}P, clearance of the circulating concentration of the substance at any given time could be described by an exponential function. Since the original description of this method, many other colloidal and particulate materials have been used to measure HBF in this fashion: ^{198}Au, ^{59}Fe-labeled saccharate, ^{99m}Tc-sulfur colloid, and ^{131}I-labeled heat denatured serum albumin (88,92–94). In addition to this method, others have related the hepatic accumulation rate of colloidal material as measured by external counting to total HBF (95,96).

Because approximately 90% of reticuloendothelial cells are found lining the liver sinusoids under normal conditions, particulate clearance methods would seem quite applicable to volumetric determination of HBF. However, the accuracy of this form of clearance methodology is dependent upon several assumptions: all of the marker is removed on the first pass through the liver or the extraction efficiency can be accurately measured by hepatic vein catheter; extrahepatic portosystemic shunting does not occur, particulate material is cleared from the blood only by the liver; the disappearance constant is independent of the initial colloid concentra-

Table V Methods for the Determination of Total Hepatic Blood Flow[a]

Clearance techniques
Hepatocyte excretory clearance
Bromsulphthacin
Indocyanine green
^{131}I-labeled rose bengal
Hepatocyte metabolic clearance
Ethanol
Galactose
Reticuloendothelial particle clearance
^{33}P-labeled chromic colloid
^{198}Au
^{99m}Tc-labeled sulfur colloid
^{131}I-labeled heat-denatured serum albumin
Miscellaneous
^{133}Xe
Indicator dilution techniques
^{131}I-labeled serum albumin
^{51}Cr-labeled red blood cells
Miscellaneous physical techniques
Electromagnetic flowmetry
Lipiodol velocity
Heat transfer

[a]From Ref. (82).

tion; and reticuloendothelial cell function is not affected by the presence of hepatic disease. However, these assumptions have not been validated, so clearance techniques that depend on reticuloendothelial cell function are not reliable.

Indicator dilution techniques of measuring total HBF were introduced by Reichman *et al.*, who applied the Stewart-Hamilton principle to the volumetric determination of HBF (97). The indicator, ^{131}I-labeled serum albumin, was injected into the spleen and monitored in a hepatic vein. Other studies based upon indicator dilution principles but using ^{51}Cr-labeled red blood cells were subsequently reported (87). This method is an extension of the Fick principle and requires knowing only the total amount of indicator injected and the ability to determine the concentrations of the indicator immediately after it has passed through the organ. Results are based upon integration of the concentrations of the specific indicator appearing at a hepatic vein catheter during the first circulation through the liver. Several assumptions underlie this method. Two of the most important are that the indicator remains in the vascular space and is neither metabolized nor excreted prior to reaching the sampling site and that the hepatic circulation is in a steady state. The existence of spontaneous or surgically induced extrahepatic portosystemic shunting permits indicator to bypass the hepatic vein sampling site. In order to permit meaningful calculations under these circumstances, the amount of indicator lost through shunts must be similar in concentration to that remaining in the PV and subsequently sampled at the hepatic vein. Data supporting this assumption are not available. Secondly, the accuracy of indicator dilution methodology in general has been questioned. Marked discrepancies between actual flow values and those determined by indicator dilution techniques have been noted in carefully controlled model systems (98). Visscher and Johnson showed that the Fick principle assumes that blood flow is constant, i.e., steady state, and not pulsatile (99). Under these circumstances, in order to apply Fick techniques to calculations, it is necessary to postulate that either the flow or the marker concentrations are equal on each side of the organ at each instant of time. Such a set of conditions is highly unlikely. Finally, this method permits only estimation of total volumetric HBF but the fraction of hepatic perfusion actually nourishing cells is of greater importance than total HBF rates. It is conceivable that organ dysfunction may exist as a result of inadequate cellular perfusion while maintaining "normal" total HBF rates. Since both venovenous and arteriovenous shunts are numerous in cirrhosis (100), total HBF values may not be meaningfully comparable among cirrhotic patients without the nutritive perfusion fraction being known.

Physical techniques for measuring total HBF are generally cumbersome and often impractical. Placement of electromagnetic flowmeters around the hepatic artery and PV provides reliable data on HBF, but the necessity for operative exposure restricts repeatability and clinical usefulness (101). Moreover, the need for anesthesia represents an uncontrolled variable. Reichle *et al.* suggested a method for quantitation of portal blood flow involving determination of the cross-sectional area of the PV by biplane fluoroscopy and multiplying this value by the velocity of portal venous flow obtained by cineradiographic mapping of Lipiodol droplets introduced into the portal system via umbilical vein catheterization (102). While theoretically acceptable, the complexity of this method and the need for umbilical vein catheterization have limited its widespread clinical use. Graf applied thermodynamic principles to the determination of total HBF (103). An almost linear relationship exists between thermal conductivity and vascular perfusion when thermocouples are placed in the liver. However, it was also shown that hepatic temperatures are not solely dependent upon blood flow. It is important to stress that none of these techniques is capable of measuring nutritive, or effective, hepatic perfusion.

2. Portal Vein and Hepatic Artery Flow

Much more difficult than measurement of total HBF has been the measurement of the volume of the separate portal venous and hepatic arterial components. A number of methods have been used, all with some theoretical and practical problems. PV flow has been of particular interest because its preservation might be of prognostic importance in chronic liver disease. One method of measurement employs the Stewart-Hamilton principle of recording an indicator dilution curve both from the hepatic vein and from the PV near its entrance into the liver after injection of a bolus of nonmetabolizable indicator (^{131}I-labeled albumin or ^{51}Cr-labeled red blood cells) downstream. The bolus must mix evenly in the entire portal blood before reaching the sampling site. Total HBF is calculated from the hepatic venous indicator dilution curve, and portal blood flow from the portal venous indicator dilution curve (104). The indicator can be injected into the spleen or distal splenic vein, or the superior mesenteric artery (87). In PH there may be loss of indicator via portal collaterals between the injection site and the PV sampling site, in which case only the portal fraction of total HBF, rather than the actual blood flow, can be calculated. Results from using this method in patients with cirrhosis and PH show a wide range of values for the portal fraction of total HBF, from 0 to 95%, averaging about 50%.

The most direct assessment of hepatic artery and PV flow comes from electromagnetic flowmeter measurements at surgery. Reported results in patients with chronic liver disease average about 425 mL/min for hepatic arterial flow and about 450 mL/min for PV flow, with a wide range. The most extensive series of measurements have come from Burchell *et al.* (105,106) Portal flow was stagnant or minimal in 8% of patients undergoing portacaval shunt. Disappointingly, no relationship was found between portal flow and prognosis after portacaval shunt, but the data did support the concept that a substantial rise in hepatic artery flow after PV clamping was a good prognostic sign.

External counting over the liver after intravenous injection of a radionuclide usually shows two different slopes of isotope arrival in the liver, corresponding to the hepatic arterial and portal venous circulations. Mena *et al.* (107) used this observation to measure the "cardioportal circulation time." Ueda *et al.*, (96) Biersack *et al.*, (108) and Rypins *et al.* (109) reported that computer analysis of the isotope accumulation slopes could be used to calculate the relative hepatic arterial and portal venous fractions of total HBF. This noninvasive method could be a useful tool in PH for assessing prognosis, suitability for surgical shunt, and course after shunt.

Recently, radiographic imaging techniques for measuring portal venous and hepatic arterial blood flow have been introduced. These include the use of duplex Doppler ultrasonography and position emission tomography (PET) (110,111).

3. Portal Collateral Flow

Portal collateral flow can be estimated from pharmacokinetic data utilizing drugs that have virtually no bioavailability when given orally in small doses. These drugs are almost completely extracted from portal blood on passing through the liver. If appreciable quantities of such a drug appear in the blood after a small oral dose, shunting of portal blood, either extrahepatically or intrahepatically, is implied. A tracer dose of radioactively labeled ursodeoxycholic acid given orally has been used to measure the shunt fraction of portal flow by this principle (112). After oral administration of nitroglycerin, its shunt fraction was estimated by digital plethysmography, providing a noninvasive assessment of portal shunting (113). Intrahepatic anatomical shunts between portal and hepatic veins can be measured by the method of Hoefs *et al.* (114). Labeled microspheres 25 microns in diameter are injected in an intrahepatic PV branch in a known ratio with a reference material, ^{131}I-labeled albumin. Recovery of microspheres in hepatic vein blood indicates the presence of anatomical shunts large enough to accommodate the microspheres. Quantitation is achieved by comparison with the concentration of the reference substance. The average intrahepatic portal shunt in 52 patients with chronic alcoholic liver disease calculated by this method was 12%. Bosch and Groszmann introduced a technique that measures only the portion of portal collateral flow that goes to the esophagus by quantitating blood flow in the azygous vein with a double-thermistor catheter (115). Azygous blood flow averaged 597 mL/min in patients with large esophageal varices, compared to 305 mL/min in patients with no varices and prior portacaval shunt.

F. Hemodynamic Studies of Portal Hypertension

PH is a hemodynamic disorder and, therefore, has been the subject of a vast number of hemodynamic studies. The pressure gradient between the PV and the hepatic veins or IVC represents the hepatic perfusion pressure and is the result of the interaction between portal blood flow and the vascular resistance that opposes that flow. This relationship is expressed by Ohm's law: $\Delta P = Q \times R$, where ΔP is the portal pressure gradient, Q is the blood flow within the portal venous system (including the portal-systemic collaterals), and R is the vascular resistance in the portal system. It follows that portal pressure may increase because of an increase in vascular resistance, an increase in portal blood flow, or a combination of both. For many years it was generally believed that obstruction to portal blood flow, with the consequent increase in resistance, was the sole cause of PH. Moreover, in cirrhosis the increased intrahepatic vascular resistance was thought to be due to a fixed, architectural distortion of the liver microcirculation caused by fibrosis, scarring, and nodule formation. Recent studies, however, suggest that there is a dynamic component to intrahepatic obstruction due to active contraction of the vascular smooth muscle cells, myofibroblasts, and other contractile elements within the hepatic microcirculation. Furthermore, recent evidence indicates that increased portal venous inflow plays a contributory role in aggravating PH. These observations have stimulated a new debate over the relative importance of resistance ("backward flow" theory) versus flow ("forward flow" theory) in the pathogenesis of PH.

1. Increased Resistance

An early view of vascular resistance in cirrhotic livers hypothesized that PH is the consequence of a vascular obliterative process, with scar tissue and regenerative nodules both occluding and compressing vascular structures (116,117). These morphological changes are undoubtedly the most important factor causing the increased intrahepatic resistance. However, recent data suggest a role of functional factors that lead to increased vascular tone, similar to that which is seen in arterial hypertension. In chronic liver disease and also during acute liver injury, hepatic stellate cells acquire contractile properties and may contribute to the dynamic modulation of intrahepatic resistance (118). These cells may act as pericytes, a type of cell that has been shown to regulate blood flow in other organs. The hepatic stellate cells, which also are the main source of collagen synthesis, may contribute to the regulation of hepatic blood flow at the microcirculatory level. Stellate cells are strategically located in the sinusoids, with perisinusoidal and interhepatocellular branching processes containing actin-like filaments. They also express the α smooth muscle actin gene, which is characteristic of vascular smooth muscle cells. The characteristics of these cells make them similar to myofibroblasts. Myofibroblasts are intermediate in structure between smooth muscle cells and fibroblasts. Myofibroblast-like cells have been shown to exist in fibrous septa around the sinusoids and terminal hepatic venules in cirrhotic livers (119). These cells are postulated to play a role in the regulation of vascular resistance in the cirrhotic rat liver (120).

The vascular endothelium synthesizes vasodilators such as nitric oxide, prostacyclins, hyperpolarizing factor, and vasoconstrictors such as endothelins and prostanoids (121,122). These vasoactive substances act in a paracrine fashion on the underlying vascular smooth muscle and modulate vascular tone. Normal vascular tone is maintained by a delicate balance between these vasodilatory and vasoconstrictive substances. Perturbation of this balance leads to abnormal vascular tone. Increased vascular tone, seen in cirrhotic livers, could be due to a deficit of endothelial vasodilators or an increase in vasoconstrictors, or a combination of both. Nitric oxide (NO) is a potent endothelial vasodilator shown to play an important role in the modulation of intrahepatic vascular tone in normal livers (123). The observation that the hepatic response to norepinephrine, a well-known vasoconstrictor, was markedly enhanced after NO inhibition further suggested a role for NO in modulating hepatic vascular tone (124). Similarly, NO has also been shown to attenuate the portohepatic response to endothelin (124). Therefore, NO may be important in counterbalancing vasoconstrictor influences on the intrahepatic resistance and, therefore, on portal perfusion pressure in normal livers. In the cirrhotic liver, it has been shown that synthesis of NO is decreased and unable to compensate for the abundance of vasoconstrictor stimuli found in cirrhosis (125). This deficit of NO release at the intrahepatic circulation occurs despite normal eNOS mRNA expression and normal eNOS protein levels (126,127). The reason for the decreased activity of hepatic eNOS in cirrhosis has been related to an increased caveolin content, which has been shown to result in decreased eNOS activity in other conditions (128). Such a decreased hepatic NO generation is suspected of being a major factor contributing to the increase in intrahepatic vascular resistance in experimental cirrhosis. It is possible that both a deficit of vasodilators and an increase in vasoconstrictors may be responsible for the increased vascular tone. In summary, there are multiple factors that may lead to increased resistance to portal blood flow. Some of these are irreversible, such as fibrosis, capillarization, and regenerating nodules, and some are quite dynamic, such as the imbalance between endothelial factors that leads to increased vascular tone.

2. Hyperdynamic Circulation in Portal Hypertension

Almost a half century ago, Kowalski and Abelman described a hyperdynamic circulatory syndrome in patients with advanced liver disease (129). This syndrome, characterized by vasodilatation with decreased arterial pressure, increased cardiac output, and regional organ blood flow, is also observed in animal models of PH. More recently, hemodynamic assessment of the severity of the hyperdynamic state has been used to predict survival in patients with cirrhosis and PH (130–132). In rats with PH, peripheral vasodilatation initiates the development of the classic profile of decreased systemic vascular resistance and mean arterial pressure, plasma volume expansion, elevated splanchnic blood flow, and elevated cardiac index that characterizes this state (133). At least three mechanisms are thought to contribute to the peripheral vasodilation: (1) increased concentrations of circulating vasodilators; (2) increased endothelial production of local vasodilators; and (3) decreased vascular responsiveness to endogenous vasoconstrictors. The relative importance of each of these potential causes of peripheral vasodilation is unknown.

a. Increased Circulating Vasodilators In PH, there is an increase in both endothelium-dependent and endothelium-independent vasodilators. Possible etiologies for increased circulatory concentrations of vasodilatory substances include increased production, decreased catabolism secondary to impaired hepatic function, and portosystemic shunting.

Circulating bile acids and glucagon increase splanchnic flow. Circulating bile acids, routinely cleared by the liver, are present in elevated concentrations when liver function is impaired. Bile acid depletion has been shown to be associated with a decrease in splanchnic hyperemia. However, experimental evidence suggests that an increase in circulating bile acids is not essential for maintaining the hyperdynamic state in PH. More specifically, cholestyramine-induced reduction of bile acids to concentrations seen in placebo-treated controls did not ameliorate the hemodynamic changes of the hyperdynamic circulatory state in animals with PH (134).

Glucagon is the humoral vasodilator for which there is the most evidence of a significant role in promoting splanchnic hyperemia in PH (135–138). Many studies have demonstrated that plasma glucagon levels are elevated in patients with cirrhosis as well as in experimental models of PH. Hyperglucagonism results, in part, from decreased hepatic clearance of glucagon, but more importantly from an increased secretion of glucagon by pancreatic α cells (139,140). Support for a role of glucagon in modulating splanchnic blood flow comes from physiological studies in rats with experimental PH, where normalization of circulating glucagon by means of glucagon antibodies or by somatostatin infusion partially reversed the increased splanchnic blood flow (137,138). This response could be specifically blocked by preventing the fall in circulating glucagon by a concomitant glucagon infusion (141). Conversely, other studies showed that increasing the circulating glucagon levels of normal rats to values similar to those observed in PH caused a significant increase in splanchnic blood flow (135). On the basis of these studies, it has been suggested that hyperglucagonism may account for as much as 30–40% of the splanchnic vasodilation of chronic PH (135). However, other studies have yielded divergent results, suggesting that in experimental PH, splanchnic vasodilation is not necessarily associated with hyperglucagonism (142). One such study failed to demonstrate increased levels of glucagon in cirrhotic patients or a correlation between changes in glucagon levels and changes in forearm hemodynamics (143).

b. Increased Production of Endothelial Vasodilators Recent evidence has pointed toward a major role for the endothelium in the maintenance of basal vascular tone and the development of local and generalized vasodilatation in PH. The endothelium produces at least two substances that are believed to contribute to the development of systemic and splanchnic vasodilatation in PH: nitric oxide (NO) and prostaglandins (144). Experimental studies using specific NO inhibitors have shown that NO is involved in the regulation of splanchnic and systemic hemodynamics in animals with PH (145–148). Administration of specific NO antagonists caused splanchnic and systemic vasoconstriction. This vasoconstrictive effect was significantly greater in portal hypertensive than in control animals, suggesting that an excessive production of NO may be responsible, at least in part, for the vasodilation observed in PH (145,146,148). In addition, NO inhibition has been shown to correct the characteristic vascular hyporesponsiveness to vasoconstrictors that is present in PH and which is thought to contribute to the systemic and splanchnic vasodilation (149–156). This has been further demonstrated in *in vitro* perfused mesenteric artery preparations from portal hypertensive rats (157). These studies have demonstrated an overproduction of NO in the mesenteric arterial bed from portal hypertensive animals. Interestingly, NO production correlated with the degree of shear stress and with the magnitude of the baseline vasodilation and impaired vasoconstrictor response (157). Since shear stress is the main factor activating endothelial NO synthase (or eNOS), these findings support the suggestion that such NO overproduction occurs in the vascular endothelium through the activation of eNOS.

The recent finding that patients with cirrhosis have increased serum and urinary concentrations of nitrite and nitrate, which are products indicative of NO oxidation, also supports a role for NO in the genesis of the circulatory disturbances of PH (158). However, it has been shown that NO inhibition attenuates, but does not entirely normalize, the hyperkinetic syndrome of PH. Moreover, although chronic NO inhibition by specific antagonists precludes the development of systemic vasodilation (159–161), it delays, but does not prevent, the development of splanchnic vasodilation, suggesting that other factors, different from NO, may also be involved in the pathogenesis of the hyperdynamic circulation (161).

Which NO synthase is responsible for the increased NO activity of PH has been a subject of controversy for several years (147,162). The original hypothesis proposed that overproduction of NO would be due to an increased expression of the inducible NO synthase (iNOS) due to endotoxemia. However, there is no evidence indicating that the increased NO activity observed in PH is due to a hyperstimulation of the constitutive NO synthase, which is normally present in the endothelium (eNOS or NOS-3) (153,154,162–168). Factors likely to activate eNOS include shear stress, circulating vasoactive factors such as endothelin, angiotensin II, vasopressin, norepinephrine, and cytokines, such as LPS and TNFα (169,170).

Several studies have also supported a role for prostaglandins in the hyperdynamic circulation of PH (171–173). Animal studies showed a partial reversion of the splanchnic vasodilation after prostacyclin blockade (174). This effect was independent of that of NO (174). It has been further shown that patients with cirrhosis may have increased systemic levels of prostacyclin (173). In addition, inhibition of prostaglandin biosynthesis by indomethacin reduced the hyperdynamic circulation and portal pressure in patients with cirrhosis and PH (175). Thus, available evidence supports the idea that prostaglandins may contribute to the vasodilation of PH.

Finally, recent studies have suggested that cyclooxygenase (CO) may also be involved in modulating splanchnic blood flow in PH (176). CO is a powerful vasodilator produced by the heme oxygenases (HOs). It promotes vasodilation by a mechanism similar to that of NO. It has been shown that splanchnic tissues from portal hypertensive animals have an increased expression of HO-2, which is not expressed in normal animals (176).

c. Decreased Response to Vasoconstrictors Basal vascular tone is regulated by the complex balance between endogenous vasodilators and vasoconstrictors. A blunted response to vasoconstrictors, therefore, could also contribute to vasodilation and, subsequently, hyperdynamic flow. In PH, *in vitro* hyporesponsiveness to the endogenous vasopressors norepinephrine, arginine vasopressin, and angiotensin II has been reported to contribute to the hyperdynamic circulation (177,178). This hyporeactivity to vasopressors appears to be mediated largely by NO. In rats with PH, inhibition of NO in isolated, perfused superior mesenteric artery beds has been shown to prevent the development of vascular hyporeactivity to the endogenous vasoconstrictors norepinephrine and vasopressin (177), the exogenous α agonist methoxamine, and the receptor-independent vasoconstrictor potassium chloride (178). These observations are consistent with the hypothesis

Table VI Results of Two Studies of the Survival Rates of Patients Admitted to General Hospitals Because of Cirrhosis

Authors	Sources of cases and years	Number of cases	Manifestations of cirrhosis	Survival (%) 1 year	Survival (%) 2 years	Survival (%) 5 years
Ratnoff and Patek (179)	Five New York hospitals (1916–1938)	296	Ascites	32	17	7
		245	Jaundice	26	23	5
		106	Hematemesis	28	25	20
Boston Inter-Hospital Liver Group (180)	Seven Boston hospitals (1959–1961)	467	Varices	34	21	5.5
		288	Varices without bleeding	43	25	8
		179	Varices with bleeding	21	14	1.5

that the decreased response to vasoconstrictors in PH is mediated by receptor-independent mechanisms.

In rats with PH, a role for prostaglandins in hyporesponsiveness to vasoconstrictors has not been substantiated. In fact, cyclooxygenase inhibition with indomethacin did not ameliorate vascular hyporeactivity in superior mesenteric artery preparations in partial PV ligated rats (177). Therefore, at least in the rat model of PH, NO appears to cause the vascular hyporeactivity to endogenous and exogenous vasoconstrictors that contributes to the generalized vasodilation seen in the hyperdynamic state.

G. Treatment of Portal Hypertension

The most frequent cause of death in patients with cirrhosis of the liver and PH is bleeding from esophagogastric varices. Table VI shows the results of two studies of the survival rates of patients admitted to general hospitals because of cirrhosis (179,180). The exact mortality rate from alcoholic cirrhosis in the United States today is difficult to determine because studies of this matter have involved different populations of patients, but there is no question that it is a highly lethal disease. The results of the two studies shown in Table VI indicate that once a patient entered the hospital for treatment of cirrhosis, the chances of living for 1 year were similar to those of a patient with acute lymphocytic leukemia, and the chances of surviving 5 years were about the same as those observed in most untreated cancers.

The most frequent cause of death from upper gastrointestinal bleeding is rupture of an esophageal varix with hemorrhage. Until recently, approximately three out of four cirrhotic patients who entered the hospital with their first episode of bleeding varices failed to leave the hospital alive. Table VII, which shows the results of a number of studies conducted during the past half century, indicates that as of 1962, the immediate mortality rate of the first variceal hemorrhage averaged 73% (179,181–187). From these statistics, it is apparent that the emergency treatment of bleeding esophageal varices is a very important aspect of the therapy of PH.

The precipitating cause of rupture of esophageal varices is increased hydrostatic pressure which causes a "blowout", (188,190). It is important to point out that only 35–50% of patients with proven varices ultimately bleed from the

Table VII Mortality Rate of First Episode of Bleeding from Esophageal Varices in Patients with Cirrhosis

Authors	Year reported	Type of hospital	Number of patients	Mortality rate (%)
Ratnoff and Patek (179)	1942	Five private teaching	106	40
Higgins (183)	1947	City indigent	45	76
Atik and Simeone (181)	1954	City indigent	59	83
Nachlas *et al.* (185)	1955	City indigent	102	59
Cohn and Blaisdell (182)	1958	City indigent	456	74
Taylor and Jontz (186)	1959	Veterans	102	45
Merigan *et al.* (184)	1960	City indigent	74	76
Orloff (187)	1966	City indigent	87	84
			Total 1031	Mean 73

varices (182). However, once bleeding has occurred, the patient is almost certain to bleed again, usually within a year of the first bleeding episode. The prognosis and therapeutic implications of esophageal varices depend on whether or not bleeding has occurred.

Treatment of esophagogastric varices due to intrahepatic PH has been applied as *prophylactic* therapy in patients with varices who have never bled, as *emergency* therapy in patients who are actively bleeding, and as *elective* treatment to prevent recurrent bleeding in patients who have recovered from a bout of hemorrhage. Treatment modalities can be considered in three categories: (1) direct attacks on the varices by endoscopic, radiographic, or surgical methods; (2) pharmacological agents that affect portal hemodynamics; and (3) portal decompression by portal-systemic shunts constructed surgically or by radiographic methods. Laboratory and clinical research in PH has resulted in major advances in all three of these categories. Much of the research that has been conducted in patients who have serious complications of PH has consisted of randomized clinical trials (RCTs), prospective unrandomized studies, reviews of accumulated clinical experience, and retrospective case reviews.

1. Direct Attacks on the Varices

a. Esophageal Balloon Tamponade The most widely used nonoperative measure of therapy during the past 50 years has been esophageal balloon tamponade, which stops variceal bleeding initially in a large percentage of the patients in whom it is used (190–199). However, the results have been discouraging because many of the patients resumed bleeding when the balloons were deflated. Moreover, we and others have observed frequent and sometimes lethal complications of balloon tamponade (191,193,200). Most important, data indicate that balloon tamponade has not measurably influenced the mortality rate of bleeding esophageal varices during a trial of 50 years. For these reasons, we use balloon tamponade only on infrequent occasions as a temporary measure to prepare patients for operation when massive bleeding cannot initially be controlled by other means.

b. Endoscopic Sclerotherapy and Variceal Band Ligation Endoscopic sclerotherapy (EST) was first reported in 1939, but it was not used widely until the 1970s, when technological advances in endoscopic instrumentation were responsible for revival of interest in this mode of therapy. Today EST is used throughout the world as a primary emergency and long-term treatment (201–220). Numerous studies have shown that emergency EST is associated with cessation of bleeding in 70–90% of patients. However, if used alone, the majority of patients have rebled and there has been no improvement in survival rate. Elective (chronic, repetitive, long-term) EST has been associated with rebleeding in 40–72% of patients. Most RCTs of long-term EST in selected patients have shown a reduction in the frequency of subsequent bleeding episodes compared to conventional therapy, but no improvement in survival (203,206,207,211,214,217). Prophylactic EST in patients who have never had variceal bleeding has failed to reduce the incidence of subsequent bleeding or to influence the survival rate in several RCTs (221–228). In the VA cooperative RCT, prophylactic EST actually *increased* the risk of both bleeding and dying (221). EST is not applicable to all types of PH-related bleeding. EST cannot be used for portal hypertensive gastropathy and is often not feasible or is of limited effectiveness in bleeding gastric varices (229–236).

EST has been associated with a number of complications, including necrosis and perforation of the esophagus and esophageal stricture. Complication rates have been higher in prospective studies (e.g., 30, 51, and 63%) than in retrospective reviews (10–46%). Approximately 10–15% of patients have had a serious complication of the procedure. Hemorrhage from esophageal erosions is one of the most frequent complications and may result in massive bleeding. The most common late sequela is esophageal stricture, which usually responds to dilation.

In the late 1980s, as an alternative to EST, endoscopic band ligation of esophageal varices was introduced, particularly in the elective treatment setting, and is now used widely (237–248). In actively bleeding patients, endoscopic variceal band ligation appears to be equal in effectiveness to EST (237,238,240,244). A meta-analysis of a number of RCTs was reported to show that band ligation is superior to EST when used in the elective setting to prevent recurrent bleeding (244). Band ligation reportedly required fewer sessions to achieve variceal ablation and had a lower incidence of esophageal stenosis and other complications. On the other hand, a higher incidence of recurrent varices has been reported in a recent randomized comparison of band ligation and EST (245).

c. Percutaneous Transhepatic Obliteration of Varices Radiologists have attempted to obliterate esophageal varices by percutaneous transhepatic catheterization of the PV and its branches and injection of blood clots, hemostatic polymers, or sclerosing solutions into the coronary vein and the varices (249–257). This method has been used in actively bleeding patients as emergency treatment and as elective therapy in patients who have recovered from a bleeding episode. Substantial experience with the percutaneous transhepatic technique has accumulated, although many of the results reported in the literature are anecdotal. The incidence of rebleeding has been high, and there has been a substantial number of complications directly related to the procedure. Moreover, the procedure has failed to improve the survival rate of patients with varix hemorrhage. There is little question that the varices, if obliterated, will invariably recur; hence, the potential of this approach lies in the temporary control of active hemorrhage in the expectation of preparing the patient for definitive treatment.

d. Transesophageal Varix Ligation (TVL) Transesophageal ligation of esophageal varices, shown in Fig. 5, was first described in 1949 (258). The mortality rate has ranged from 15 to 86% (258–261). The largest reported series involved 72 selected patients, with an operative mortality rate of 50%. Because the value of this procedure was not clearly established, some years ago we undertook a prospective comparison of emergency TVL and medical therapy (262). Every cirrhotic patient admitted to the hospital with varix bleeding was included in the study, with no attempt at selection. The diagnostic workup was completed within 6 h and, in the surgical group, the operation was performed within 8 h of admission to the hospital. When feasible, the patients who survived emergency surgical or medical therapy were prepared for and underwent an elective portacaval shunt at a later date.

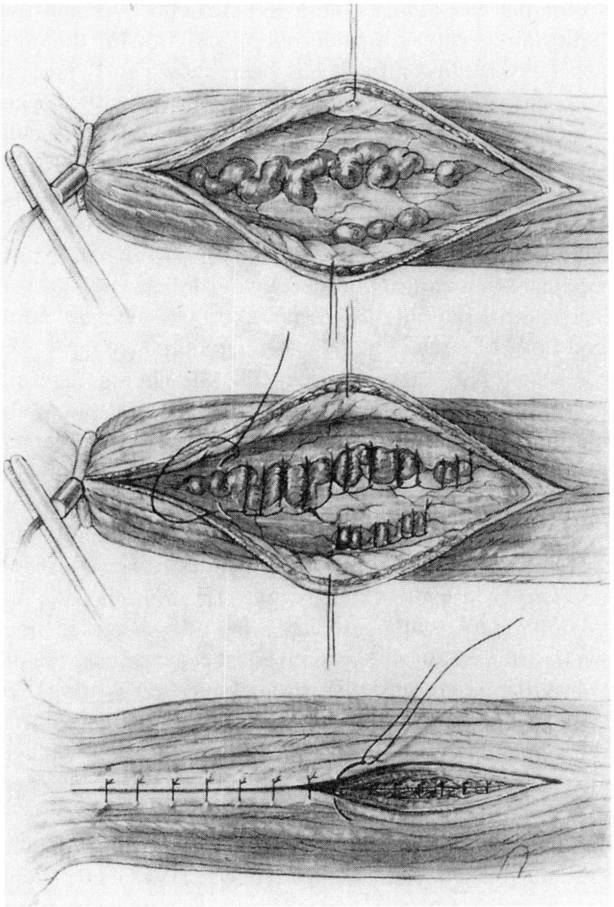

Figure 5 Technique of transesophageal varix ligation. [From Ref. (262), Orloff, M.J. (1962). *Surgery* **52,** 102–116.]

Emergency TVL consistently controlled bleeding. The early survival rate was 54% following operative ligation, compared with 14% in the medically treated patients. The 5-year survival rate was 21% in the surgical group and 3% in the medical group; the 10-year survival rates were 11% and 0, respectively. Our experience showed that TVL is not a definitive procedure but rather must be considered the first of two stages in treatment, the second stage of which is elective portal decompression. The refusal of some patients to undergo a subsequent elective shunt was invariably associated with rebleeding and played a major role in the declining survival rate.

e. Esophagogastric Devascularization Procedures Various esophagogastric devascularization procedures have been used as both emergency and elective treatment of bleeding esophageal varices (263–277). Included among these are (1) gastric or esophageal transection and reanastomosis, often done with the aid of a stapling gun, which is sometimes combined with splenectomy and extensive ligation of the veins around the distal esophagus and upper stomach; (2) esophagogastrectomy and pyloroplasty with or without interposition of a segment of colon or jejunum and with or without ligation of collateral veins and splenectomy; (3) splenectomy alone or with coronary vein ligation; and (4) ligation of the hepatic, left gastric, and splenic arteries. By and large, these operations involve transection of the esophagus and/or resection of parts of the lower esophagus and upper stomach and/or extensive ligation of collateral veins that connect with the esophageal varices. The results of these procedures are difficult to evaluate because most of the series are small, involve highly selected patients with many types of PH, and are retrospective in nature. By far the greatest experience with these operations has been in Japan, where surgeons have largely abandoned portal-systemic shunting in favor of esophagogastric devascularization, which they have performed prophylactically, electively, and emergently (263,266,267,275). The Japanese have reported favorable results, but their reports do not lend themselves readily to analysis, and the results have not been verified in other countries. Moreover, in several reports, the long-term survival rate of cirrhotic patients has been low. In the United States, esophagogastric devascularization procedures in cirrhotic patients have been associated with substantial mortality rates and a high incidence of recurrent varix bleeding.

2. Pharmacological Therapy

During the past decade, laboratory experiments and clinical research have produced marked progress in knowledge of the pathophysiology of PH which, in turn, has opened the door to expanding pharmacological therapy. Table VIII summarizes current and potential future pharmacological treatment of PH (278). Increased resistance to portal blood flow is the primary factor in the pathophysiology of PH and is mainly determined by the morphological changes occurring in chronic liver diseases. This is aggravated by a dynamic component in the form of active, potentially reversible contraction of different elements of the intrahepatic portal bed. Decreased synthesis of NO in the intrahepatic circulation appears to be the main determinant of this dynamic component. This provides a rationale for the use of vasodilators to reduce intrahepatic resistance and portal pressure. Another factor contributing to PH is a significant increase in portal blood flow caused by splanchnic arteriolar vasodilation and hyperkinetic circulation. Most pharmacological treatments have been aimed at correcting the increased portal blood inflow by the use of splanchnic vasoconstrictors, such as β blockers, vasopressin derivatives, and somatostatin. Several studies have demonstrated that changes in the hepatic venous pressure gradient (HVPG) during maintenance therapy are useful to identify those patients who are going to have variceal bleeding or rebleeding. A priority for research in the forthcoming years is to develop accurate noninvasive methods to assess prognosis, which can be used to substitute or as surrogate indicators of the HVPG response. In the clinical management of PH, β blockers are at present the only accepted treatment for the prevention of variceal bleeding.

Table VIII Pharmacological Treatment of Portal Hypertension[a]

Drugs that reduce intrahepatic resistance
Increasing intrahepatic NO production
Present possibilities
Nitrovasodilators: nitroglycerin, isosorbide 5-mononitrate and dinitrate
Future possibilities
Enhanced expression of NO synthase
Targeted delivery of NO
α-Adrenergic antagonists
Prazosin (α_1 antagonist)
Clonidine (central α_2 agonist)
Carvedilol (α_1 antagonist and nonselective β blocker)
Blockade of the renin–angiotensin system
Losartan (angiotensin II antagonist)
Spironolactone
Drugs that decrease splanchnic blood flow
Nonselective β blockers
Propranolol, nadolol, timolol, carvedilol
Vasopressin and its analoguest
Vasopressin, terlipressin, F-180
Somatostatin and its analogues
Somatostatin, octreotide, lantreotide
Agents that reduce splanchnic blood volume
Spironolactone
Drugs that increase lower esophageal sphincter pressure
Metoclopramide, domperidone
Drug combinations
β blockers + nitrates, β blockers + prazosin
β blockers + spironolactone

[a]From Ref. (278). © 2000 EASL, the European Association for the Study of the Liver.

a. Drugs That Reduce Intrahepatic Resistance

I. Increasing intrahepatic NO production Some alternative treatments of PH were tested even before it was known that they may act by correcting the increased intrahepatic vascular resistance. This is the case of nitrovasodilators, such as nitroglycerin, isosorbide dinitrate, or isosorbide 5-mononitrate (Is5Mn) (279). It is now known that these agents, through their capacity to release NO, may compensate for the NO deficit within the cirrhotic liver and thus reduce intrahepatic vascular resistance. Is5Mn, the most extensively studied nitrate, has been shown to reduce the HVPG in patients with cirrhosis without reducing hepatic blood flow, which suggested a reduction in hepatic vascular resistance (280). However, the vasodilatory action of these drugs extends to the systemic circulation, where it causes arterial hypotension and may elicit reflex splanchnic vasoconstriction with ensuing reduction in portal blood flow. Vasodilators also usually decrease cardiac preload and hence cardiac output, which may further decrease portal blood flow. Moreover, many vasodilators reduce the vascular resistance at the portocollateral circulation, diverting portal blood flow through the portal collaterals, a potentially undesirable effect. Finally, in some instances, the beneficial effects of decreasing intrahepatic resistance are offset by the splanchnic vasodilatory effect of the drug, which may result in increased portocollateral blood flow and hinder any decrease in portal pressure (281). Thus, in some cases a vasodilator will cause changes not only in the hepatic and portocollateral vascular resistance but also in portal blood flow. In addition, in patients with advanced cirrhosis, the use of vasodilators may be dangerous, since these drugs, by enhancing the already existing peripheral vasodilation, further decrease arterial blood pressure and activate endogenous vasoactive systems that may lead to water and sodium retention and renal failure (282).

II. Anti-α-adrenergic agents *Prazosin* is an α_1-adrenergic antagonist that markedly reduces HVPG in patients with cirrhosis. This reduction is associated with an increased hepatic blood flow, suggesting a reduction in hepatic vascular resistance (283,284). However, chronic prazosin administration was associated with a significant reduction in arterial pressure and systemic vascular resistance and with an activation of endogenous vasoactive systems, leading to plasma volume expansion, sodium retention, and, in some cases, accumulation of ascites (284). These findings have discouraged its use. Recent data suggest that the adverse effects of prazosin on the systemic circulation and renal functions may be attenuated by the combined administration of prazosin and propranolol (284,285).

Clonidine is a centrally acting α_2-adrenergic agonist that results in reduced peripheral adrenergic output. Its hemodynamic effects are reminiscent of both β- and α-adrenergic blockade. In the systemic circulation, clonidine causes reductions in heart rate, cardiac index, and arterial blood pressure, while in the splanchnic circulation, it reduces the HVPG by decreasing portohepatic resistance and splanchnic inflow (286–289). Despite the marked fall in arterial pressure following clonidine administration, hepatic blood flow and liver function are maintained and renal function and sodium handling do not appear to be altered. The magnitude of the fall in HVPG is slightly greater than that achieved with propranolol (289).

Carvedilol is a nonselective β blocker with intrinsic anti-α-adrenergic activity, recently introduced in the treatment of arterial hypertension, ischemic heart disease, and heart failure. In a recent study, acute administration of carvedilol induced a marked decrease in HVPG which was significantly greater than that achieved by propranolol, despite both agents causing a similar reduction in splanchnic blood flow (290). This suggests that carvedilol reduced the hepatic and collateral resistance due to its anti-α1-adrenergic activity. However, the greater portal hypotensive effect of carvedilol was accompanied by a more pronounced reduction in mean arterial pressure, which is a matter of concern in patients with cirrhosis (290).

III. BLOCKADE OF THE RENIN-ANGIOTENSIN SYSTEM Activation of the renin-angiotensin system is a frequent finding in patients with cirrhosis, especially in those with more advanced disease. This is thought to represent a homeostatic response to counterbalance the systemic and splanchnic vasodilation and arterial hypotension observed in PH. In a recent study in patients with PH, losartan, a nonpeptide antagonist of angiotensin receptor type I, was reported to cause a dramatic reduction in portal pressure without producing significant changes in arterial pressure (291). If these impressive results can be confirmed, angiotensin receptor type 1 antagonists would have a potential for clinical use.

Up to now, there has been no study evaluating the clinical efficacy of prazosin, clonidine, carvedilol, or losartan in preventing variceal hemorrhage. Their theoretical potential makes it likely that some of them will be tested in clinical trials. Other drugs such as molsidomine, calcium channel blockers, or other blockers of the renin-angiotensin system have undergone hemodynamic testing, with disappointing results (279).

b. Drugs That Decrease Splanchnic Blood Flow Most attempts at pharmacological treatment of PH have been aimed at correcting the increased portal blood inflow with splanchnic vasoconstrictors. The hemodynamic profile and clinical application of these drugs have been extensively reviewed recently (279). Some of these drugs, such as nonselective β blockers, can be given orally and are appropriate for long-term treatment of PH, while others, such as somatostatin or terlipressin, require parenteral administration and are only used for short-term administration, as in the treatment of acute variceal hemorrhage.

I. NONSELECTIVE β BLOCKERS Nonselective β blockers, such as propranolol, nadolol, and timolol, reduce portal pressure by reducing portal venous inflow as a result of a decrease in cardiac output (due to the blockade of cardiac β_1-adrenoceptors) and of splanchnic vasoconstriction (due to the blockade of the vasodilating β_2-adrenoceptors in the splanchnic vasculature) (292,293). This dual effect explains why cardioselective β blockers have less portal pressure reducing effect than nonselective β blockers (294,295). The beneficial effect of reduced portal pressure is accompanied by a significant reduction of pressure in the esophageal varices and of azygous blood flow (296,297), an index of blood flow through esophageal varices (298). Propranolol is given orally. In general, the dose is increased every 2 days until the heart rate decreases by approximately 25%, but not below 55 beats/min. Nadolol is easier to administer because of a more prolonged half-life that allows administration once a day, and it is eliminated by the kidneys, which makes its dosage easier than that of propranolol. Also, since it does not cross the blood-brain barrier, it is less likely to cause central effects and side effects.

II. VASOPRESSIN AND ITS ANALOGUES *Vasopressin* is thought to be the most powerful splanchnic vasoconstrictor. In pharmacological doses, it reduces blood flow to all splanchnic organs, and thereby decreases portal blood flow and portal pressure. Vasopressin is also effective in reducing collateral blood flow and variceal pressure (299). Adverse hemodynamic effects of vasopressin derive from systemic vasoconstriction with increased peripheral vascular resistance and reduced cardiac output, heart rate, and coronary blood flow. These effects may result in serious complications such as myocardial ischemia or infarction, arrhythmias, mesenteric ischemia, limb ischemia, and cerebrovascular accidents. In 25% of cases, vasopressin therapy has to be withdrawn because of these complications (300).

The association of nitroglycerin with vasopressin enhances the reduction in portal pressure, while attenuating the systemic side effects of vasopressin (301). This is achieved because nitroglycerin, which acts by delivering NO, reduces the vascular resistance in the liver microcirculation (which has insufficient endogenous production of NO) and in the portal venous system and improves myocardial performance. Several RCTs and meta-analyses have shown that this drug combination is more effective and safer than vasopressin alone in controlling bleeding from ruptured esophageal varices (300).

Terlipressin is a synthetic vasopressin analogue (triglycyl lysine vasopressin) that is slowly converted *in vivo* into vasopressin after its intravenous injection by enzymatic cleavage of the triglycyl residues. Terlipressin has a longer biological activity than vasopressin, which makes its continuous infusion unnecessary (302). The preferred schedule of administration is as intravenous injections of 2 mg every 4 h until a bleeding-free period of 24–48 h is achieved. Therapy may then be maintained at a reduced dose (1 mg/4 h) up to 5 days to prevent early rebleeding. Available data on the use of terlipressin indicate that it is effective in controlling bleeding and in reducing mortality (300).

III. SOMATOSTATIN AND ITS ANALOGUES *Somatostatin* was introduced for the treatment of variceal hemorrhage because of its capacity to decrease portal pressure without the adverse effects of vasopressin on the systemic circulation (303,304). Somatostatin causes selective splanchnic vasoconstriction and thereby decreases portal and collateral blood flow and portal pressure (304). This is probably due to the inhibition by somatostatin of the release of splanchnic vasodilatory peptides, specifically glucagon (305). In addition, somatostatin blocks the postprandial increase in portal blood flow and portal pressure. Bolus injections of somatostatin cause marked vasoconstrictor effects in humans, with rapid and intense, but transient, falls in portal pressure and azygous blood flow that are much greater than those caused by continuous infusions (306). The usual dose for a bolus injection is 250 μg, and 250 μg per hour is given as a continuous infusion. These doses, however, are largely empirical, since hemodynamic studies have shown that to achieve a consistent hemodynamic effect, with significant reductions in HVPG and azygos blood flow, a dose of 500 μg per hour is required. A recent study suggests that this greater hemodynamic effect translates into greater clinical efficacy (307). When successful, therapy is maintained for 2–5 days. The lack of significant side effects from somatostatin represents its major advantage over other agents.

Octreotide and *lantreotide* are cyclic octapeptide analogs of somatostatin with a longer biological half-life (308,309). Somatostatin analogues have been shown to reduce portal pressure in animals; however, their hemodynamic effects in cirrhotic patients are controversial and the efficacy in variceal hemorrhage has not been adequately assessed so far, although it has been shown to improve the results of endoscopic injection sclerotherapy (309–314).

c. Agents That Reduce Splanchnic Blood Volume Splanchnic vasodilation is characteristically associated with peripheral vasodilation, reduced arterial pressure and peripheral resistance, and increased cardiac output (314). Peripheral vasodilation plays a major role in the activation of endogenous neurohumoral systems, leading to sodium retention and expansion of the plasma volume. Expansion of the plasma volume is thought to play a key role in the maintenance of an increased cardiac index, which, in turn, aggravates PH (315). This provides the rationale for using a low-sodium diet and/or diuretics in the treatment of PH. Indeed, low-sodium diet and spironolactone have been shown to reduce portal pressure in patients with cirrhosis (316,317). No study has evaluated the efficacy of spironolactone in preventing variceal hemorrhage.

3. Portal Decompression Procedures

The only definitive therapy for PH is decompression of the portal system by shunting the high-pressure portal blood into the lower pressure systemic venous system. Surgical portal-systemic shunts (PSS) and radiographic transjugular intrahepatic portosystemic shunt (TIPS) are the procedures that accomplish this objective, and they are discussed in detail below.

II. Portal-Systemic Shunt

A. The Eck Fistula

In 1877, Nikolai V. Eck (1849–1908), a 29-year-old military surgeon working in the Military Medical Academy in St. Petersburg, published a brief article describing his experiments and technique for creating a portacaval shunt (Eck fistula) in eight dogs (318). This was not only the beginning of the surgical treatment of PH but also the first vascular anastomosis. In his article, Eck stated: "I am conducting these experiments with the purpose of clarifying some physiologic problems as well as to determine whether it would be possible to treat some cases of mechanical ascites by means of forming such a fistula. I operated on 8 dogs, one recovered completely and lived in the laboratory for 2.5 months. Because of lack of attention, he ran away. I had to postpone further experiments because I was called to join the active army."

Eck's work would probably have remained unknown outside Russia had it not been for Ivan Pavlov (1849–1936), who used the procedure extensively in laboratory studies of liver physiology and named the operation the Eck fistula, giving full credit to Eck for its invention (319,320). The landmark description by Pavlov *et al.* of portal-systemic encephalopathy following feeding meat to dogs with an Eck fistula, which they called "meat intoxication," was part of the work that resulted in Pavlov's receiving the Nobel Prize in 1904 for his contributions on the physiology of digestion (319). Pavlov spent his entire career at the Military Medical Academy in St. Petersburg, the same institution where Eck developed the portacaval shunt. Since its original description, the Eck fistula has been used extensively for a wide range of studies in animals and humans and clinically for the treatment of the life-threatening complications of PH.

B. Experimental Studies

1. Role of Hepatotrophic Factors in Liver Regeneration and Atrophy

The Eck fistula has been used extensively in studies of liver regeneration and atrophy. Liver regeneration has been a subject of study by both basic scientists and clinicians for many years because of its fundamental biologic significance and its bearing on our understanding and treatment of hepatic disease. The adult mammalian hepatocyte shows little turnover of nuclear DNA, rarely undergoes mitosis, and has a life span commensurate with the adult life of the organism, be it the rat or man (321,322). However, destruction or removal of part of the liver gives rise to mitotic activity and cell division of such intensity that the organ is reconstituted within days or weeks, depending upon the species. This precisely regulated response, which begins with a burst of proliferative activity and ceases when the deficit has been restored, has been demonstrated in every animal investigated, including humans (321,323). Following a 68% hepatectomy in the rat, DNA replication is detectable after 12–14 h, and mitoses are seen 6–8 h later, reaching a peak at about 24 h (322). The initial response involves only the hepatocytes but, beginning a day later and thereafter, the bile ducts and littoral cells share in the response (323). Hepatocytes throughout the liver divide synchronously and with equal responsivity (322). The magnitude of the response is proportional to the amount of liver removed (324). All of the mitotic activity involves mature cells, and there is no evidence of progenitor stem cells (325). The rate of doubling of hepatocytes is about once per 24 h, which is similar to that of many embryonic cells and exceeds most neoplasms (326). Restoration of collagen proceeds slowly and is not complete for 6 or 7 months (323). When the cellular deficit has been repleted, cell division stops, and the liver architecture is indistinguishable from the normal. Following removal of two-thirds of the liver, complete restoration requires 10–14 days in the rat, 6–8 weeks in the dog, and about 4–6 months in man (327). An interesting and potentially important aspect of the hepatocyte renewal pattern is the striking zonal localization of the initial and maximal mitotic response. Over 90% of the dividing cells are found in the area surrounding the terminal portal venule (i.e., the site of entrance of portal blood into the smallest parenchymal unit) (328–330). The complex processes involved in cell proliferation undoubtedly are under the control of intracellular mechanisms throughout the body. However, it has been suspected for many years that extracellular mechanisms are responsible for initiating and regulating the remarkable chain of events that occurs in liver regeneration. The exact nature of the regulatory system has been the subject of much research.

Pavlov observed in autopsies of dogs with an Eck fistula that the liver had undergone atrophy and fatty infiltration. These observations were subsequently confirmed by Bollman *et al.* (331,332). More recently, ultrastructural changes consisting of depletion and disruption of the rough endoplasmic reticulum and reduction in membrane-bound polyribosomes have been identified in Eck fistula livers from various animals and from humans (333–341). At the same time, a marked increase in hepatocyte renewal has been observed (333–336,340,341).

In 1920, Rous and Larimore suggested that atrophy of the liver following Eck fistula was due to diversion of essential hepatotrophic factors in portal blood (342). However, that hypothesis was discarded by Mann who, along with others, produced evidence to indicate that the quantity of hepatic blood flow and not the quality or contents of portal blood was responsible for hepatic integrity and prevention of liver atrophy (338–347). The pendulum swung back to the hepatotrophic hypothesis when Weinbren in 1955 challenged all previous work done in Eck fistula animals by pointing out that the basis for studying regeneration (which used as controls the liver mass after hepatectomy in a normal animal) was invalid (348). He showed that decreasing the blood supply to a lobe of the liver by ligating a branch of the PV induced atrophy of that lobe. When he used rats with ligation of a branch of the PV as controls (rather than normal rats), he demonstrated that the liver with a decreased blood supply was capable of regenerating following hepatectomy. Fisher, Lee, *et al.* (349) confirmed Weinbren's work in the Eck fistula rat. They showed that regeneration following partial hepatectomy was good when nonhepatectomized Eck fistula rats were used as controls, that restoration of protein content was good, and that cell division was active as determined by mitotic counts and by incorporation of ^{32}P into DNA. Further challenges to the "blood flow theory" have come from studies demonstrating that liver regeneration can occur when hepatic perfusion is greatly reduced (322,350,351) and that regeneration is not enhanced by increasing the blood flow to the liver above normal (352). Although total blood flow to the liver may have some influence on hepatic regeneration, it does not appear to be a major regulatory factor.

Substantial evidence indicates that humoral factors arising outside of the liver are the major influence responsible for initiating and regulating regeneration following loss of hepatic tissue. Early reports regarding humoral factors were based on experiments involving injections of serum or plasma from partially hepatectomized rats into normal rats or cell cultures (323,353–357) and on studies of normal and hepatectomized rats joined in parabiosis (358–360). Inability to confirm these studies led to initial skepticism about a humoral stimulant (323,361–363). However, subsequently it was demonstrated repeatedly that intact livers of normal rats undergo DNA synthesis and mitoses when cross-circulated with partially hepatectomized rats (324,364,365). The response of the intact liver has been shown to be directly related to the amount of tissue removed from the hepatectomized partner. Furthermore, it has been demonstrated that small vascularized liver autografts implanted in sites remote from the portal venous circulation proliferate in response to partial ablation of the parent organ.

The nature of the extrahepatic humoral factors responsible for liver regeneration has been the subject of investigation in several laboratories, including our own. Using a microvascular technique for heterotopic transplantation of 30% of the liver in inbred rats (366), we demonstrated that in the presence of a whole host liver, the auxiliary isograft required a portal venous blood supply for regeneration (367). Grafts supplied by the hepatic artery alone or by systemic venous blood atrophied. Further studies showed that portal blood was required for DNA synthesis and vigorous mitoses in heterotopic liver isografts (368). In the absence of portal blood, even grafts that received a large afferent flow of both systemic venous and hepatic arterial blood failed to regenerate. We concluded that there is a specific trophic factor in portal blood that controls liver regeneration (369). Additional studies in our laboratory demonstrated that the trophic factor in portal blood is utilized and/or destroyed by both regenerating and normal liver tissue, so that the host liver and the auxiliary graft compete for a finite amount of trophic humoral agent (370). Fisher *et al.*, using an identical experimental preparation, confirmed and extended our findings (371,372). They demonstrated that there is a "portal blood factor" capable of stimulating liver cells and that its effectiveness is inversely related to the number of liver cells present. They showed that the humoral factor is not destroyed in systemic blood so that regeneration takes place in the face of an Eck fistula as long as the shunted blood does not pass through another liver before recirculation. They provided solid evidence against the hepatic origin of both a stimulatory and an inhibitory factor in liver regeneration. Of relevance to the proposal regarding hepatotrophic factors in portal blood is the consistent observation, mentioned previously, that most of the cells involved in replication in the regenerating liver are located in the portal half of the lobule. It has been demonstrated that the site of mitotic activity can be shifted to the centrilobular region by directing the afferent inflow into the hepatic veins in liver autografts (373).

Interest in liver transplantation and, particularly, in the vascular requirements of auxiliary liver grafts focused new attention on the role of blood supply in liver nutrition and integrity. In 1964, Starzl *et al.* observed in dogs that auxiliary homografts with a purely systemic blood supply rapidly underwent atrophy (374,375). Thomford *et al.* observed similar shrinkage of systemically vascularized auxiliary liver allografts in dogs and apparent competition between the host liver and the graft (376). Marchioro *et al.* showed that auxiliary transplants attached to the splanchnic venous system in dogs did not atrophy when portal blood was completely diverted from the host organ, while the host liver underwent shrinkage (377). When the splanchnic portal blood supply was shared between the host and transplanted organ, the effects were variable but they tended to show less atrophy in the graft than when it was completely deprived of access to splanchnic venous blood. In an extension of these studies, Halgrimson *et al.* observed that a portacaval shunt (PCS) had a modest protective effect against shrinkage of systemically vascularized auxiliary grafts (378). Similarly, Tretbar *et al.* reported that end-to-side PCS protected a systemically vascularized auxiliary liver allograft from shrinkage, while the host liver underwent atrophy (379). The results of these studies led Starzl and his group to propose the concept that the host liver and the graft were in competition for a nutritional substrate in portal blood. The above studies were beset by the difficulties associated with graft rejection and immunosuppression therapy, which resulted in a high mortality rate and the necessity to draw conclusions from a small number of animals. In addition, conclusions were based on graft size and weight and not on measurements of cellular activity. Nevertheless, the results were consistent and the proposed concept appears to be valid. Furthermore, the suggestion that the findings might have been a reflection of inadequate quantity rather than quality of blood supplying the graft was disproved by a subsequent study in which blood flow was measured and was usually found to be greater in the graft than in the host liver (380).

Studies regarding a hepatotrophic influence of portal venous blood subsequently were conducted in preparations not requiring immunosuppression therapy. Sigel *et al.* reported that an autotransplanted liver lobe underwent less atrophy, when the portal blood to the parent liver was diverted into the systemic system by a PCS (381,382). Marchioro *et al.* found that when half of the liver was supplied with systemic venous blood by a portacaval transposition and the other half was allowed to retain its normal splanchnic venous supply, the systemically vascularized side underwent atrophy (383). However, Wellborn *et al.*, using a similar experimental model, were unable to confirm these observations (384). Finally, Fisher *et al.* found that in the face of a PCS, constriction of the hepatic venous outflow to one liver lobe prevented atrophy of that lobe, while the rest of the liver underwent atrophy (385). They concluded that atrophy of the whole liver is due to some modification of sinusoidal pressure or blood flow and not to a hepatotrophic humoral factor.

It may be important to draw a distinction between studies of liver regeneration following partial hepatectomy and studies of shrinkage or atrophy of the whole organ following a change in its blood supply. On first examination, it may appear that both regeneration and prevention of atrophy involve the same processes and are dependent on the same hepatotrophic factor in portal blood. Indeed, such may be the case. On the other hand, regeneration requires cell proliferation, while there is no evidence as yet that prevention of atrophy involves DNA synthesis and formation of new cells. It is recognized that ischemia, surgical trauma, and immunologic rejection may so damage an auxiliary allograft as to require new cell formation if atrophy is to be avoided, but there is no proof that this takes place. Moreover, if the hepatotrophic portal blood factor is utilized only by the liver and is not degraded systemically, it is difficult to understand why recirculation of the factor would not prevent the invariable liver atrophy that follows PCS. It is possible that the liver depends on two (or more) trophic factors, one that initiates regeneration when part of the organ is removed, and one that maintains cell size and nutrition of the whole organ under both normal and adverse circumstances.

In 1973, on the basis of animal experiments, we proposed that the hepatotrophic factors in portal blood originate mainly in the pancreas (386). Subsequent experiments in our laboratory added weight to that proposal (387–389). Starzl *et al.* made a similar proposal in 1973 (390). To identify these hepatotrophic factors, we developed a double-liver rat bioassay model for testing candidate substances (389). The assay liver is a 30% isograft that is vascularized entirely by systemic venous blood from the caudal IVC, and that ordinarily exhibits minimal or no regenerative activity. Hepatotrophic material that is perfused through the assay graft subsequently passes through the normal host liver and, thereby, is largely removed from the circulation. Perfusion of the bioassay graft with a crude extract of fresh pancreas stimulated significant regeneration, and perfusion with a mixture of insulin and glucagon was significantly more stimulatory than all of the other test substances (391). Subsequently, we confirmed these findings in dogs with a 70% hepatectomy and pancreatectomy in which replacement of both insulin and glucagon restored peak regenerative activity to the normal range (392). In an extensive series of related experiments, Starzl *et al.* demonstrated an important hepatotrophic role for insulin but also provided evidence that there are multiple hepatotrophic factors which remain to be identified (393).

2. Gastric Acid Secretion and the Intestinal Phase Hormone

Although stimulation of gastric acid secretion by food in the intestine was identified early in the 20th century (394–396) and humoral mediation of this phenomenon was suggested over a half century ago (397–399), it has been recognized only recently that the intestinal phase of gastric secretion plays an important role in acid production during digestion. Moreover, it is only within the past 30 years that research has provided convincing physiologic evidence that the stimulatory intestinal phase is mediated by one or more hormones.

The consistent observation of profound gastric acid hypersecretion in dogs with a PCS was largely responsible for recent interest in the intestinal phase of gastric secretion (400–406) (Fig. 6). Numerous studies have shown that PCS-related hypersecretion is most marked following ingestion of protein (400,405,407) and that it is not related to the cephalic or antral phases of gastric acid secretion, since it is not abolished by truncal vagotomy (403) or antrectomy (400,403,408–411). It has been shown to occur following systemic shunting of venous blood draining the small intestine, but not after hepatic bypass of venous blood from the stomach, proximal duodenum, pancreas, and spleen (412–415). Substantial evidence suggests that the striking acid hypersecretion associated with PCS is due to unmasking of the intestinal phase of gastric secretion by hepatic bypass of a gastric secretory stimulant in portal blood that normally is inactivated to a considerable extent by the liver.

In 1966, we began a series of experiments in dogs directed at answering the question of humoral mediation of PCS-related acid hypersecretion and of the intestinal phase of gastric secretion. The first of these studies involved measurements in antrectomized dogs of the Heidenhain pouch secretory response to an intestinal meal during isovolemic autotransfusion of blood from the PV to the thoracic aorta, to simulate an acute PCS (416). Combination of an intestinal meal with portal-systemic autotransfusion resulted in significantly greater gastric acid secretion than an intestinal meal alone or portal-systemic autotransfusion alone. These results suggested that a humoral agent in portal blood was responsible for PCS-related gastric hypersecretion.

To further examine the question of humoral mediation, we conducted studies using the classic physiologic technique of controlled, isovolemic cross-transfusion (410). Heidenhain pouch acid output was measured during cross-transfusion of systemic blood between an antrectomized "donor" dog with a PCS and an intact "recipient" dog, in the presence and absence of food in the donor's intestine. The intestinal meal in the donor dog with a PCS stimulated marked acid secretion, not only in the donor but also in the intact recipient that received the donor's blood by cross-transfusion (417). These results provided direct evidence for humoral mediation of PCS-related gastric hypersecretion.

We next sought to determine whether the humoral mediator of PCS-related hypersecretion was a secretagogue absorbed from food or a hormone of endogenous origin. To this end, we compared the Heidenhain pouch secretory response to an intestinal meal with the response to balloon distention at physiologic pressures 20 cm distal to the duodenal-jejunal junction before and after PCS (418). Intestinal distention stimulated gastric hypersecretion in shunted animals to the same extent as an intestinal meal. These results suggested that the humoral agent was a hormone that originated in the intestine.

To determine the site of origin of the hormone responsible for PCS-related hypersecretion, our next experiments examined the gastric secretory responses of a Heidenhain pouch to the introduction of food into isolated segments of jejunum, ileum, and colon before and after PCS (418). Food

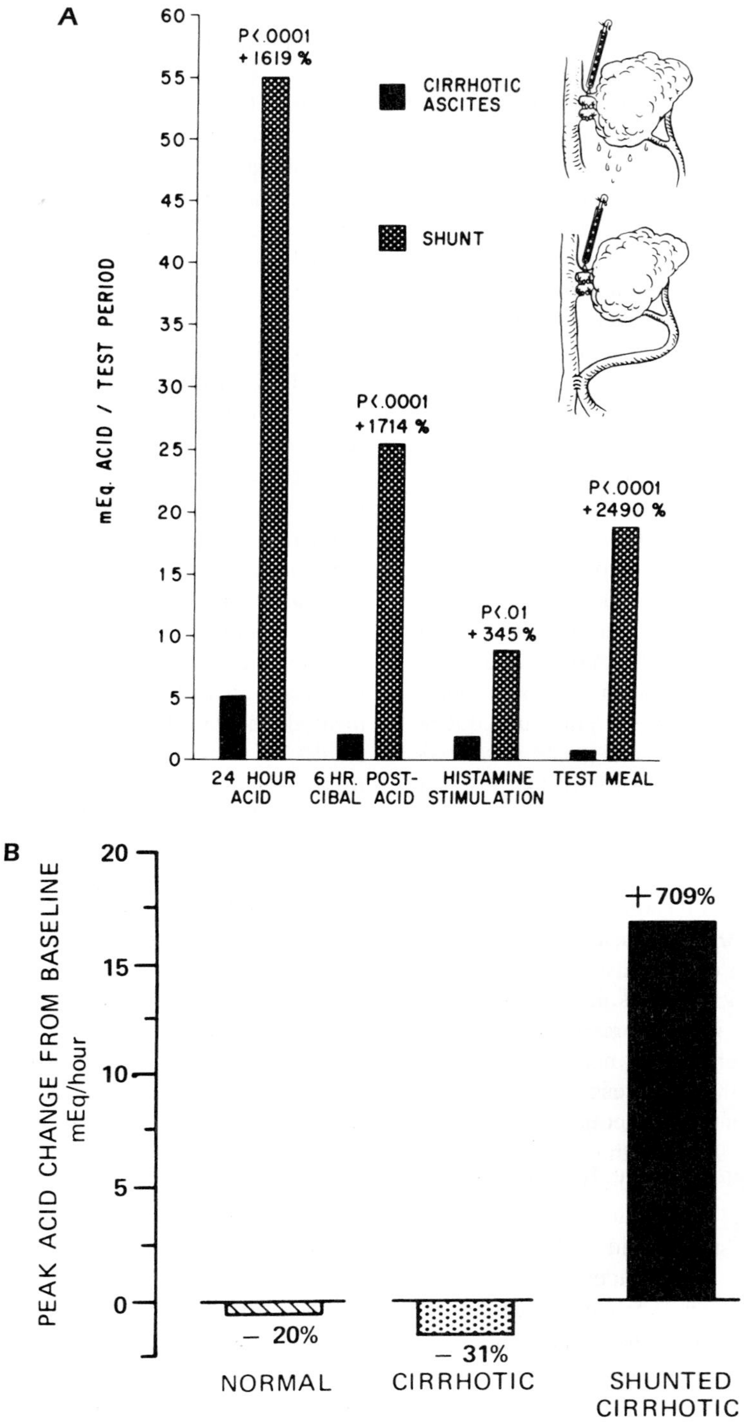

Figure 6 Effect of portacaval shunt on gastric acid secretion in dogs and humans with and without a portacaval shunt (PCS): (A) Heidenhain pouch acid secretion in dogs; (B) gastric acid response to an intestinal meal in 10 normal subjects, 20 patients with cirrhosis, and 15 cirrhotic patients with a PCS. [From Ref. (426), Orloff, M.J., *et al.* (1969). Gastric secretion and peptic ulcer following portacaval shunt in man. *Ann. Surg.* **170,** 515–527.]

in the isolated jejunum produced substantial gastric acid secretion before PCS and sustained acid hypersecretion after PCS. Food in the isolated ileum stimulated modest gastric secretion in unshunted dogs, but PCS did not enhance acid output, and food in the colon failed to produce a gastric secretory response. It was concluded that the jejunum was the major source of the humoral agent responsible for PCS-related acid hypersecretion.

The applicability of the striking findings of dog experiments to humans with PCS was unknown as of 1969. Indeed, up to that time a number of studies of basal and histamine-stimulated gastric secretion in patients with PCS had not shown an increase in acid production (419–425). However, all of these clinical studies suffered from failure to examine the intestinal phase of gastric secretion. Accordingly, we undertook a study of the gastric secretory response to instillation of a liquid meal directly into the upper jejunum in 10 normal subjects, 20 ambulatory patients with compensated cirrhosis, and 15 ambulatory, compensated cirrhotic patients who had undergone PCS (426). The PCS group was subsequently expanded to 52 patients, and 11 patients were studied both before and after PCS. As other workers had reported, patients with PCS were found to have normal levels of basal and histamine-stimulated gastric acid secretion. However, each of the 52 shunted cirrhotic patients responded to an intestinal meal with a marked, prolonged, and highly significant hypersecretion of acid that, at its peak, averaged 709% above the basal level. Food in the intestine of normal subjects and unshunted cirrhotics failed to stimulate gastric secretion. It was concluded that hepatic bypass of portal blood unmasked the intestinal phase of gastric secretion in humans, just as it did in dogs.

As we had done in dog experiments, our next study in humans compared the gastric secretory response to balloon distention of the upper jejunum for 20 min at physiologic pressures with the response to an intestinal meal (427). Studies were performed in normal subjects, unshunted cirrhotic patients, and cirrhotic patients with PCS. Balloon distention of the jejunum did not stimulate acid secretion in normal subjects and unshunted cirrhotic patients but produced a highly significant output of acid in every cirrhotic patient with a PCS, similar in magnitude to the secretory response to an intestinal meal. These results suggested that PCS-related hypersecretion in humans, as in dogs, was mediated by an endogenous hormone rather than by a substance absorbed from food.

Our final study in humans was directed at localizing the intestinal site from which the intestinal phase hormone (IPH) originates. For this purpose, we compared the gastric secretory responses to the instillation of food directly into the jejunum (just beyond the ligament of Treitz) and into the ileum (21/2–3 feet proximal to the ileocecal valve) in cirrhotic patients with and without PCS (428,429). In the patients with PCS, food in the ileum did not stimulate acid secretion but food in the jejunum produced a marked and highly significant hypersecretion of gastric acid. These results suggested that the stimulatory IPH in humans originated mainly in the jejunum, just as it did in dogs.

The nature of the gastric secretory stimulant in portal blood has been the subject of much speculation and considerable study. With our physiologic observations as a background, we have used a classic method for extracting acidic peptides to prepare a hog intestinal mucosa extract (HIME) that has all of the known physiologic properties of an IPH. Specifically, HIME contains a potent stimulant of gastric acid secretion that acts according to a linear dose-response relationship, that is not gastrin in any of its immunoassayable forms, that significantly augments the maximal acid secretory responses to pentagastrin, gastrin, CCK, and histamine, and that is substantially degraded by the liver, in contrast with gastrin and CCK. Efforts at isolating the gastric stimulatory substance in HIME suggest that it is a peptide of low molecular weight. Efforts are being directed at further purification and eventual isolation of IPH from HIME, establishing proof of homogeneity, determination of the primary sequence, and, finally, total synthesis. Once IPH has been isolated and synthesized, efforts can be undertaken to develop a radioimmunoassay and to determine cross-reactivity with the known digestive hormones. Availability of synthetic IPH will make it possible to conduct a wide range of physiologic studies on the actions and metabolism of the hormone. Ultimately, it will be important to demonstrate IPH in humans and to determine its role in normal digestion and in digestive disease.

3. Ascites

Ascites is a common and serious complication of cirrhosis of the liver. In most patients, ascites responds to medical therapy consisting of abstinence from alcohol, dietary sodium restriction, diuretic drugs, and, when necessary, large-volume paracentesis. However, in some patients, approximately 10%, ascites is refractory to these measures. Patients with intractable cirrhotic ascites have a mortality rate that is higher than that of most common cancers, ranging from 20–50% in one year (430–432). It is for these patients that invasive procedures and surgical operations provide the only hope of long-term survival.

The pathogenesis of cirrhotic ascites involves a number of factors, some proved and others postulated. Included among these are increased hydrostatic pressure in the hepatic sinusoids, decreased serum protein osmotic pressure from hypoalbuminemia, renal sodium retention, activation of the sympathetic nervous system, abnormal secretion of several hormones, such as aldosterone, antidiuretic hormone, and atrial natriuretic peptide, and splanchnic vasodilatation caused by various vasodilator substances. The initiating and perpetuating abnormality in many, if not all, cases appears to be sinusoidal hypertension resulting from postsinusoidal outflow obstruction.

The rationale for the use of portal-systemic shunts (PSS) in the treatment of intractable cirrhotic ascites is directly related to the primary role of sinusoidal hypertension in the pathogenesis of ascites and is based on the capacity of the shunt procedure to decompress the liver. Side-to-side PCS (SSPCS) and its equivalents, such as interposition mesocaval H-graft shunt, central splenorenal shunt, and transjugular intrahepatic portosystemic shunt (TIPS), accomplish sinusoidal decompression by shunting splanchnic blood away from the liver and by improving the outflow of hepatic blood through retrograde flow through the valveless portal vein into the low-pressure IVC.

Beginning in 1961, we began a series of studies aimed at determining the effects of PCS on ascites and the associated metabolic abnormalities (433–440). We produced hepatic venous outflow obstruction and massive ascites in dogs by the method we described for direct ligation of the hepatic veins (52–54). The onset and persistence of ascites was determined by physical examination and abdominal paracentesis at regular intervals. In our initial experiments, dogs were divided randomly into three groups: I (n = 14), unaltered controls subjected to sham laparotomy after ascites was well established; II (n = 15), performance of an end-to-side PCS after ascites was well established; and III (n = 16), construction of a SSPCS after ascites was well established. Table IX documents results of our initial experiments on the effect of PCS on intractable ascites produced by hepatic vein ligation in dogs. In the controls, the volume of ascites removed at the time of sham laparotomy ranged from 1.3 to 4.9 L, with a mean of 2.6 L. After sham laparotomy, all 14 surviving dogs reaccumulated large quantities of ascites. In the end-to-side PCS group, the volume of ascites at the time of the shunt was similar to that of the controls, ranging from 1.6 to 4.2 L, with a mean of 2.7 L. After end-to-side PCS, 12 of the 15 surviving dogs (80%) re-formed massive ascites. In the SSPCS group, the volume of ascites at the time of shunt ranged from 1.0 to 5.2 L, with a mean of 2.9 L. In contrast to the other two groups, only 2 (12.5%) of the survivors reaccumulated ascites following SSPCS. One of these 2 was the only dog in the group with thrombosis of the shunt, and the other dog had a large liver abscess, both animals died. From these studies, we concluded that SSPCS was very effective in overcoming hepatic outflow block and relieving severe ascites and that end-to-side PCS was usually ineffective (433,434).

In our second series of experiments, we studied the effect of PCS on thoracic duct lymph flow in dogs with intractable ascites produced by hepatic vein ligation (435–437). The thoracic duct was cannulated with a polyethylene catheter into the neck, and lymph flow was measured in acute experiments lasting 4 h in five groups of dogs: 1 (n = 10), unaltered controls; 2 (n = 20), control dogs subjected to an end-to-side PCS (n = 15) or SSPCS (n = 5) 2 or 3 weeks before the acute experiment; 3 (n = 6), dogs with well-established ascites produced by hepatic vein ligation; 4 (n = 6), dogs that had undergone an end-to-side PCS after ascites was well established; and 5 (n = 8), dogs that had undergone a SSPCS after ascites was well established. Table X shows the results. Unaltered control dogs had a thoracic duct lymph flow rate that ranged from 20 to 42 mL/h (mean 27 mL/h) and was not affected by PCS of either type (mean 30 mL/h). Dogs with massive ascites produced by hepatic vein ligation had a 13-fold increase in lymph flow rate above the controls (range 214 to 682 mL/h, mean 350 mL/h). End-to-side PCS in dogs with massive ascites reduced thoracic duct lymph flow rate substantially (range 76–181 mL/h, mean 129 mL/h), but lymph flow remained almost 5 times above normal. SSPCS not only eliminated massive ascites but also accomplished the greatest reduction in thoracic duct lymph flow rate (range 31–101 mL/h, mean 77 mL/h). In half of the dogs with SSPCS, lymph flow rates were within the normal range. From this study, we concluded that SSPCS often decompressed the liver completely and that it was more effective than end-to-side PCS in overcoming sinusoidal hypertension.

In our third series of experiments, we studied the effects of PCS on the aldosterone secretory response to hepatic venous outflow occlusion in dogs (438–440). The studies consisted of serial measurements of aldosterone in adrenal

Table IX Experimental Effect of Portacaval Shunts on Intractable Ascites Produced by Hepatic Vein Ligation in Dogs[a]

Experimental group	n	Volume of ascites (L)	Reaccumulation of ascites (%)	Shunt patency (%)
Control-sham laparotomy	14	1.3–4.9	100	—
End-to-side portacaval shunt	15	1.6–4.2	80	93
Side-to-side portacaval shunt	16	1.0–5.2	12.5	94

[a]From Ref. (434).

Table X Experimental Effect of Portacaval Shunts on Thoracic Duct Lymph Flow in Dogs with Intractable Ascites Produced by Hepatic Vein Ligation[a]

	Lymph flow rate (mL/h)		
Experimental group	*n*	Mean	Range
Unaltered control	10	27	20–42
Control with portacaval shunt	20	30	22–48
Intractable ascites	6	350	214–682
Intractable ascites, end-to-side shunt	6	129	76–181
Intractable ascites, side-to-side shunt	8	77	31–101

[a]Reprinted from Ref. (437). *Am. J. Surg.* **114**; M.J.Orloff, B. Goodhead, D.W.O. Windsor, M.E. Musicant, and O.L. Annetts; Effect of portacaval shunt on lymph flow in the thoracic duct. Experiments with normal dogs and dogs with cirrhosis and ascites, pp. 213–221. Copyright 1967, with permission from Excerpta Medica Inc.

vein blood and in peripheral plasma in conscious dogs for 6 h, during which time progressive hepatic venous outflow obstruction was produced by tightening a polyethylene choker around the superior hepatic vein. The superior hepatic vein choker was inserted 2 weeks before the experiment; at this time all other hepatic veins were ligated and divided by a technique we described previously (52–54). The adrenal vein catheter was inserted 1 day before the experiment, and monitoring and sampling catheters were introduced on the day of experiment. Aldosterone analysis was performed by modifications of the double isotope derivative assay method. Four groups of dogs were studied: 1 ($n = 5$), unaltered controls; 2 ($n = 7$), animals subjected to progressive hepatic venous outflow occlusion; 3 ($n = 6$), dogs subjected to progressive hepatic outflow occlusion in the presence of an end-to-side PCS that had been constructed at the time of hepatic vein ligation; and 4 ($n = 6$), dogs subjected to hepatic outflow occlusion in the presence of a previously constructed SSPCS. Table XI gives the results.

Before these experiments, we observed that minimal hepatic outflow occlusion produced a marked rise in adrenal aldosterone secretion and peripheral plasma aldosterone concentration and that dogs with massive ascites produced by hepatic vein ligation developed marked and persistent elevations of aldosterone excretion rate in urine and aldosterone concentrations in plasma (438). In the experiments described in Table XI, hepatic venous outflow obstruction produced a great increase in adrenal aldosterone secretion and in plasma concentration. The elevations were highly significant ($p < 0.0001$), appeared rapidly after the superior hepatic vein choker was minimally tightened, and occurred without any changes in vital signs, behavior, or blood volume. End-to-side PCS resulted in less marked, although significant ($p < 0.0001$), increases in aldosterone levels and was unable to prevent hypotension and an additional rise in aldosterone secretion when hepatic outflow occlusion was complete. SSPCS prevented significant elevations of aldosterone secretion ($p = 0.368$), even when hepatic outflow occlusion was complete. From these experiments, we concluded again that SSPCS was completely effective in decompressing the obstructed hepatic vascular bed and relieving sinusoidal hypertension.

4. Portal-Systemic Encephalopathy

Hepatic encephalopathy is a neuropsychiatric disorder that results from impaired liver function. It occurs in two distinct forms: (1) in acute or fulminant hepatic failure it takes the form of a neurological disorder that progresses from altered mental status to coma, generally within hours or days, and is associated with increased intracranial pressure caused by massive brain edema; (2) portal-systemic encephalopathy (PSE), which commonly occurs in cirrhosis, in which there are spontaneous or created portal-systemic shunts that permit toxins of intestinal origin to bypass the liver into the systemic circulation. Neurologically, PSE develops slowly, starting with sleep abnormalities, shortened attention span, and muscular incoordination, progressing through lethargy, ataxia, stupor, and coma. PSE is often precipitated by events such as gastrointestinal bleeding, ure-

Table XI Experimental Effect of Portacaval Shunts on the Aldosterone Secretory Response to Hepatic Venous Outflow Occlusion in Dogs[a]

		Aldosterone mean peak percent rise above baseline	
Experimental group	*n*	Adrenal secretion	Plasma concentration
Unaltered control, no outflow occlusion	5	43	13
Hepatic outflow occlusion alone	7	1695[b]	336[b]
Hepatic outflow occlusion plus end-to-side PCS	6	290[b]	209[b]
Hepatic outflow occlusion plus side-to-side PCS	6	27	24

[a]From Ref. (439).
[b]$p = 0.0001$ compared to unaltered control. *n*, number.

mia, hypokalemia, or ingestion of excessive amounts of protein. Neuropathologically, PSE is characterized by astrocytic rather than neuronal changes, and brain edema and intracranial hypertension are not found.

Since the description in 1893 of "meat intoxication" in the Eck fistula dog by the Pavlov group, animals with a PCS have been used extensively for research studies of the pathogenesis and treatment of PSE (319). The PCS rat has been consistently reported to have neurobehavioral abnormalities when subjected to sophisticated testing (441,442). One of the best animal models of chronic recurrent PSE is the dog with a congenital or surgically created PCS (443). Animal and human studies have demonstrated that chronic liver failure and spontaneous or created PSS result in the accumulation of neurotoxic substances in the brain. Two such substances are ammonia and manganese.

Ammonia derived from colonic bacteria as well as from the deamination of glutamine in the small bowel is absorbed by passive diffusion and normally undergoes a high first-pass extraction by the liver (444). In chronic liver failure, hepatic urea synthesis declines and this, in addition to portal-systemic shunting, results in increased blood ammonia concentrations. Furthermore, cirrhotic patients are hypersensitive to ammoniagenic conditions such as an oral protein load or gastrointestinal hemorrhage. An illustration of this hypersensitivity is provided by a report of studies in the 1950s in which attempts were made to treat ascites in cirrhotic patients with ion-exchange resins that absorbed sodium but released ammonium ions (445). This treatment led to a significant reduction in ascitic volume but precipitated severe PSE in many of the patients treated. If present in high concentrations, ammonia has the potential to adversely affect central nervous system (CNS) function by several mechanisms, which include a direct effect of the ammonium ion [NH_4^+] on inhibitory and excitatory neurotransmission as well as inhibition of the tricarboxylic acid cycle enzyme ketoglutarate dehydrogenase, with potential impairment of brain energy metabolism (446,447). However, brain energy metabolism does not appear to be impaired in chronic liver failure until very late stages associated with isoelectric electroencephalography (EEG) traces (448). On the other hand, increases of cerebrospinal fluid lactate have been described both in cirrhotic patients with PSE (449) and in experimental animals with chronic liver failure and ammonia-precipitated encephalopathy (450), findings that are consistent with an inhibitory effect of ammonia on cerebral glucose oxidation.

Other effects of ammonia on cerebral function include a stimulatory effect on L-arginine uptake by brain preparations resulting in increased production of nitric oxide (451) and inhibition of the capacity of astrocytes to accumulate glutamate (452,453), a major excitatory neurotransmitter.

In 1963, we performed a study that subsequently influenced the use of PCS in the treatment of PH and variceal hemorrhage. We examined the influence of the stomal size of the portacaval anastomosis, and in turn of the blood flow rate through the anastomosis, on peripheral blood ammonia levels (454). Induced ammoniemia was studied in two groups of dogs, one of which had large end-to-side PCS measuring at autopsy 2.0–4.2 cm in greatest diameter, and the other of which had small end-to-side PCS measuring 0.5–1.8 cm in greatest diameter. A third group of intact dogs served as controls. Ammoniemia was induced by three standardized methods that consisted of the administration by gavage of ammonium citrate (0.5 g/kg), gavage of fresh whole blood (30 mL/kg) plus urease (4 U/mL), and gavage of fresh whole blood (30 mL/kg) alone. All three techniques of ammonium loading resulted in significantly higher mean peak blood ammonia levels in the dogs with large shunts than in those with small shunts. Furthermore, in the animals with large shunts, markedly elevated blood ammonia concentrations persisted for longer periods of time. Measurements of the pressure gradients across the shunts at operation revealed a mean gradient of 31.0 mm saline in the small-shunt group as compared to only 3.0 mm in the large-shunt group. A consistent inverse relationship was demonstrated between the height of the blood ammonia level and the magnitude of the pressure gradient across the portacaval anastomosis. Application of Gorlins' hydraulic formula to these studies provided support for the presumption that the magnitude of ammoniemia was directly related to the blood flow rate through the shunt. We concluded that the stomal size of end-to-side PCS, and in turn the rate of blood flow through the shunts, have a definite influence on the concentration of ammonia in the peripheral blood of the dog. These results suggested the possibility of a relationship between shunt size and postshunt PSE. The results of this study served as the basis for the subsequent use of reduced-caliber PCS in the treatment of variceal bleeding (455,456).

In addition to ammonia, chronic liver failure and portal-systemic shunting result in increased blood and brain concentrations of manganese (18,22–24). Manganese is neurotoxic, affecting both neuronal and astrocytic integrity. In the case of astrocytes, exposure to manganese results in altered expression of several key astrocytic proteins (457,458) and Alzheimer Type II changes (459).

Other toxins in addition to ammonia and manganese are known to increase in the systemic circulation in chronic liver failure. Such toxins include mercaptans, phenols, and short-chain fatty acids (460). While there is no convincing evidence that these toxins alone cause cerebral dysfunction in chronic liver failure, they could combine with ammonia or manganese to act synergistically (461).

Recently, attention has been focused on changes in brain neurotransmitter systems as the likely mediators of the neuropsychiatric manifestations of PSE in chronic liver failure. Recent studies using molecular biological approaches continue to confirm that, when liver fails, brain responds with significant alterations in gene expression. In many cases, these alterations involve genes that code for neurotransmitter-related proteins, many of which are essential for CNS function. Many of the symptoms of early PSE in chronic liver failure, such as altered personality, depression, and inverted sleep patterns, are symptoms that have classically been associated with alterations in biogenic amine function. RNA extracts of brain tissue obtained at autopsy from cirrhotic patients who died in hepatic coma have been found to show increased expression of the neuronal isoform of the monoamine-metabolizing enzyme MAO-A (462). This increase in MAO-A gene expression was found to be associated with increased activities of the enzyme and increased densities of catalytic sites on the enzyme protein (462). Moreover, studies of the same brain extracts revealed increased concentrations of homovanillic and 5-hydroxyindoleacetic acids, the final metabolites of dopamine and serotonin, respectively (463). Increased concentrations of 5-hydroxyindoleacetic acid were also reported in cerebrospinal fluid from patients (464) and experimental animals (465) with chronic liver failure. On the basis of these findings, it has been suggested that altered monoaminergic function may be responsible for the early neuropsychiatric symptoms of PSE in chronic liver disease (465,466).

The *"peripheral-type" benzodiazepine receptor (PTBR)* is a heterooligomeric protein complex located (like MAO-A) on the outer mitochondrial membrane of the astrocyte. Increased PTBR gene expression has been reported in brain extracts from rats with PCS (467). This increased gene expression resulted in increased receptor sites in the brains and peripheral tissues of these animals as revealed by quantitative receptor autoradiography and the highly selective PTBR ligand [^{3}H] PK 11195 (468,469). Increased [^{3}H] PK 11195 binding sites were also reported in autopsied brain tissue from cirrhotic patients who died in hepatic coma (470). There is evidence to suggest that the increased expression of PTBRs in brain in chronic liver failure is the consequence of exposure to ammonia and/or manganese. The precise mechanism whereby increased expression or activation of PTBRs results in altered brain excitability characteristic of PSE has not been established. PCS in the rat results in increased gene expression of the constitutive (neuronal) isoform of nitric oxide synthase (nNOS) in brain (471). Increased nNOS mRNA is accompanied by increased nNOS protein (471) and by increased nNOS enzyme activities (420) Recent evidence suggests that, in addition to an induction in nNOS gene expression, increased nNOS activities may also result from a stimulatory effect of ammonia on L-arginine uptake by neuronal preparations shown both *in vitro* and *in vivo* (472). Increased production of NO as a consequence of increased nNOS activities could contribute to the alterations of cerebral perfusion observed in chronic liver disease (473).

The appearance of extrapyramidal symptoms, particularly rigidity, in cirrhotic patients with end-stage liver disease has prompted, by analogy with the well-established dopamine deficit in Parkinson's disease, evaluations of the dopamine system in relation to PSE. Studies in autopsied brain tissue from cirrhotic patients(463) and from rats with PCS(465) reveal severalfold increases in concentration of the dopamine metabolite homovanillic acid, a finding that could result from increased activities of monoamine oxidase reported in the same material (462). In another study, densities of the postsynaptic dopamine D_2 receptor were significantly reduced in pallidum/putamen from cirrhotic patients (474), a finding that could have resulted from manganese deposition in the brains of these patients (475).

Strategies aimed at the prevention and treatment of PSE in chronic liver failure are of two major types, namely, ammonia-lowering strategies and approaches aimed directly at the CNS (444,476). Since PSE is frequently precipitated by ammoniagenic situations such as an oral protein load or a gastrointestinal hemorrhage, various treatment modalities are aimed at the gut. Such strategies include reduction of the absorption of nitrogenous substances arising from bacterial action in the colon. Colonic cleansing reduces the luminal ammonia content and lowers blood ammonia content in cirrhotic patients (477).

Nonabsorbable disaccharides are routinely used to decrease ammonia production in the gut. The action of the most popular substance in this class, lactulose, involves increased fecal nitrogen excretion by facilitation of the incorporation of ammonia into bacteria as well as a cathartic effect (444). Lactulose administered orally reaches the cecum, where it is metabolized by enteric bacteria, causing a fall in pH (478). The dose is adjusted to produce two or three soft bowel movements daily (444).

Antibiotics such as neomycin are also useful for lowering blood ammonia, mainly by an effect on ammonia production by intestinal bacteria. However, neomycin therapy may be associated with some toxic side effects (444).

Restriction of dietary protein remains a cornerstone of therapy for PSE in cirrhotic patients (477). However, long-term nitrogen restriction is potentially harmful and a positive nitrogen balance is necessary to promote liver regeneration as well as to increase the capacity of skeletal muscle to remove ammonia in the form of glutamine (479). Protein intake of 1 g/kg per day may be required in order to maintain an adequate nitrogen balance (480).

An alternative strategy for the lowering of blood ammonia is the stimulation of ammonia fixation (476). Under normal physiological conditions, ammonia is removed by the formation of urea in periportal hepatocytes and by glutamine synthesis in perivenous hepatocytes, skeletal muscle, and brain. In cirrhosis, both urea cycle enzymes and glutamine synthetase in liver are decreased in activity. Strategies to stimulate residual urea cycle activities and/or glutamine synthesis have been tried over the past 20 years. One of the most successful agents to be used so far is L-ornithine-L-aspartate (OA). RCTs with OA demonstrate significant ammonia lowering and concomitant improvement in psychometric test scores in cirrhotic patients with PSE (481). Studies in experimental animals suggest that the metabolic basis for the beneficial effect of OA on blood ammonia in chronic liver failure resides in its ability to stimulate residual hepatic urea cycle function and also to promote glutamine synthesis, particularly in skeletal muscle (482).

Benzoate is also effective in reducing blood ammonia both in patients with inherited urea cycle disorders and in cirrhotic patients (471). In a RCT with sodium benzoate versus lactulose, improvement in neuropsychiatric performance was found to be comparable using both treatments (483).

In contrast to the multiple strategies used successfully to lower blood ammonia and improve neurological status in patients with chronic liver failure (above), drugs that act directly on neuronal excitability have not been widely applied in this patient group. The major reason for this is that the precise neurotransmitter changes responsible for PSE in chronic liver failure are still being elucidated. Some attempts to treat PSE in cirrhotic patients with benzodiazepine receptor antagonists and dopamine agonists have occurred, but with limited success.

Several RCTs have been performed to assess the efficacy of the benzodiazepine receptor antagonist flumazenil in cirrhotic patients with various degrees of severity of PSE (476). Spectacular improvements in neuropsychiatric status were recorded in a subset of patients receiving flumazenil (484,485). However, enthusiasm for this approach has been tempered by the possible confounding effects of prior exposure to benzodiazepines and the seeming lack of correlation between clinical response and blood levels of substances with benzodiazepine receptor agonist properties in these patients (486).

C. Clinical Studies

1. Types of Portal-Systemic Shunt (PSS)

Because the portal venous system contains no valves, it is possible to decompress it at various points provided the anastomosis with the low-pressure systemic venous system is of sufficient size to accommodate a large flow of blood. Several types of PSS are available for relief of PH (Fig. 7). Descriptions of these shunts follow.

a. Direct Portacaval Shunt (PCS) The most commonly used shunt procedures are the direct end-to-side and side-to-side anastomoses between the PV and IVC. The *end-to-side PCS* accomplishes splanchnic decompression by shunting all splanchnic venous blood into the IVC; at the same time, it decompresses the liver sinusoid by eliminating the contribution of portal venous blood to hepatic inflow and pressure. However, it rarely lowers hepatic sinusoidal pressure to normal, and sinusoidal hypertension often persists because hepatic arterial blood continues to encounter difficulty in leaving the liver through the obstructed hepatic venous outflow system. The *side-to-side PCS* (SSPCS) produces splanchnic decompression equivalent to the end-to-side anastomosis, but it accomplishes significantly greater hepatic decompression by allowing egress of liver blood in a retrograde direction through the PV into the low-pressure IVC. SSPCS converts the PV into an outflow tract, and portal blood does not continue to perfuse the liver. An important question about the SSPCS concerns the theoretical possibility that it creates an intrahepatic arteriovenous fistula in which hepatic arterial blood leaves the liver via the PV without having made contact with the hepatic cells and having contributed to hepatic nutrition and metabolism. Our studies in experimental animals suggest that arteriovenous shunting occurs to some degree but is compensated for by an increase in afferent hepatic arterial blood flow, so that hepatic nutrition is not compromised (487).

Although the two types of direct PCS produce similar splanchnic decompression and are equally effective in relieving and preventing variceal hemorrhage, the overall hemodynamic effects of the two procedures are distinctly different. Hence, there has been a continuing controversy regarding the comparative advantages and disadvantages of end-to-side PCS and SSPCS (488–491). In a series of studies, we compared the effects of the two types of shunt (1) on hepatic blood flow, liver function, liver morphology, and ammonia tolerance in dogs with experimental cirrhosis and (2) on hepatic function, ammonia tolerance, the 5-year incidence of PSE, and the 5-year survival rate in cirrhotic humans who were operated on for bleeding esophageal varices (492,493). There were no significant differences between end-to-side PCS and SSPCS in any of the parameters evaluated. We have concluded that there is no demonstrable advantage to one type of direct PCS over the other under most circumstances. The one exception may be the unusual patient with severe hepatic outflow obstruction manifested by a pressure on the hepatic side of a clamp occluding the PV (hepatic occluded portal pressure, or HOPP) that is higher than the free portal pressure (FPP). Such patients may have reversal of portal flow, and they have been known to develop intractable ascites following an end-to-side PCS, which eliminates the PV as an outflow tract and thereby may increase sinusoidal hypertension (494). SSPCS is the procedure of choice in such cases.

b. Conventional Splenorenal Shunt (SRS) The *splenorenal anastomosis* is a variant of SSPCS. It utilizes tributaries of the PV and IVC that, obviously, are of smaller size than the parent vessels. It is followed by a lower incidence of protein-related PSE than direct PCS because it shunts a small volume of nitrogen-containing portal blood into the systemic circulation. At the same time, it does not decompress the portal bed as effectively as direct PCS, is associated with a significant incidence of variceal rebleeding, and has a high incidence of

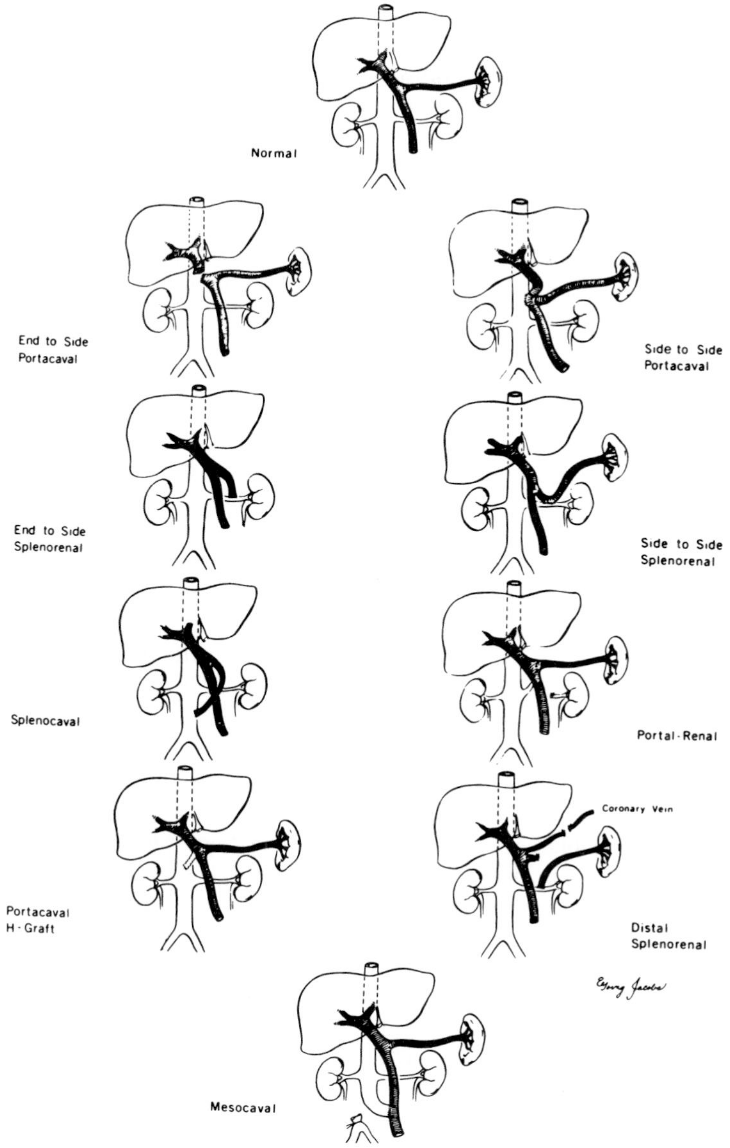

Figure 7 Types of portal-systemic venous shunts used to relieve portal hypertension. [From Orloff, M.J. (1981). The liver *In* Davis–Christopher Textbook of Surgery (Sabiston, D.C., Jr., Ed.), 12th ed., pp. 1131–1194. Saunders, Philadelphia.]

thrombosis. In the author's opinion, SRS is the procedure of choice only in rare instances when severe and intractable hypersplenism complicates PH and requires splenectomy or when previous operations in the right upper quadrant of the abdomen make it technically difficult to perform a direct PCS. Also, SRS is indicated when it is desirable to avoid dissection of the PV and IVC because orthotopic liver transplantation at some time in the future is being contemplated. The most commonly used type of SRS involves removal of the spleen and anastomosis of the end of the splenic vein to the side of the left renal vein. However, a central side-to-side SRS can be done in continuity without splenectomy and is our choice of operation whenever a SRS must be done. This variant has been said to permit continued portal venous perfusion of the liver, but it is doubtful that such is the case, since the principles that govern the hemodynamics of a valveless system dictate that flow is in the direction of the area of lower pressure, i.e., the splenorenal anastomosis.

c. Mesocaval Shunt (MCS) and Mesocaval H-Graft *Mesocaval shunt* is an anastomosis between the superior end of the divided IVC and the side of the superior mesenteric vein. In principle, it is hemodynamically similar to the side-to-side PCS. In patients with extrahepatic PH due to occlusion of the PV, this type of shunt is very effective. However, in adult cirrhotic patients it is doubtful that this procedure represents a first choice. Cirrhotic patients retain salt and water, and division of the IVC may lead to intractable edema of the lower extremities.

The use of H-grafts between the intact PV or superior mesenteric vein and IVC, introduced in 1959, attracted renewed interest in the 1970s (495–502). Synthetic prostheses of Dacron and Teflon, autogenous jugular vein, and homologous vena cava have been used for this purpose. The *interposition mesocaval or portacaval H-graft* is a relatively minor technical variation of direct SSPCS and, despite claims to the contrary, the two procedures are hemodynamically identical. The major advantage claimed for the H-graft procedure is that it is technically less difficult to perform than conventional shunts. The major potential disadvantage is the possibility of thrombosis, particularly of the synthetic prostheses. In general, use of synthetic grafts in the venous system has a long history of failure, so there is justifiable skepticism about the possibility of consistent long-term patency of the H-graft. Short-term results of interposition shunts involving a collective total of some 400 patients have been reported from 15 centers. The operative mortality rate in this heterogeneous collection of patients has been about 15%, which is not lower than that associated with conventional PCS. The short-term incidence of thrombosis has ranged from 5 to 20%, which is unacceptable when compared with the less than 2% long-term occlusion rate of direct PCS in experienced hands. The incidence of postshunt PSE has been similar to that following direct PCS, as expected.

d. Selective Distal Splenorenal Shunt (DSRS) An unsettled issue of great importance regarding the use of PCS concerns its effect both on liver cell function, presumably related to liver blood flow, and on PSE, presumably related to hepatic bypass of nitrogenous substances absorbed from the intestines. When portal blood is completely shunted away from the liver, further liver damage might be anticipated unless there is a compensatory increase in hepatic arterial blood flow. It is not possible by any currently available, practical method to predict the adequacy of hepatic arterial compensation prior to performance of a PCS. It has been proposed that a worsening of liver function or outright hepatic failure following PCS is due to a sudden diversion of needed blood away from the liver. The familiar hepatic dysfunction that follows creation of a PCS (Eck fistula) in the dog with a normal liver is cited as evidence for this proposal. The absence of significant hepatic dysfunction in patients with extrahepatic occlusion of the PV, either before or after PSS, is thought to result from the combination of a long period of adaptation to diminished portal flow and an initially normal hepatic parenchyma.

On the basis of preoperative and intraoperative measurements made in a small group of subjects, it was proposed that cirrhotic patients with normal or near-normal portal blood flow, who often appear to be the best-risk patients with the least severe liver disease, are intolerant of sudden shunting of portal blood and often die of progressive hepatic failure. On the other hand, it was proposed that patients with substantially reduced portal blood flow tolerate a PCS well because the bypass produces little further reduction in the blood supply to the liver. Finally, it was suggested that calculations of maximal portal perfusion pressure from intraoperative pressure measurements reflect portal blood flow and permit a prediction of the response to PCS. The logic of this simple hypothesis is attractive, even though it ignores the vital role of the hepatic arterial blood supply in compensating for portal diversion and the complex nature of the hepatic circulation. However, substantial data obtained by five separate groups from preoperative and intraoperative measurements of both pressure and blood flow in the PV in large numbers of patients failed to show a correlation between any hemodynamic measurements performed prior to PCS and survival, hepatic function, or development of PSE after PCS (503–507). There was no statistically significant correlation between preshunt maximum perfusion pressure and postshunt survival, liver function, hepatic failure, or development of PSE. Contrary to the hypothesis, patients with the lowest preshunt maximum perfusion pressure had the lowest survival rate, whereas patients with the highest preshunt maximum perfusion pressure had the highest survival rate and the lowest incidence of PSE following PCS. The only hemodynamic parameter that has been shown to correlate with the response to PCS is the magnitude of compensatory increase in hepatic artery flow, determined in retrospect after performance of the shunt. In a significant study, Burchell *et al.* (106) demonstrated, by direct intraoperative blood flow measurements immediately after PCS, that survival and incidence of PSE were directly related to the amount of increase in hepatic artery flow. Unfortunately, there is no currently available practical method of predicting this increase preoperatively.

On the presumption that PCS injures the liver and increases PSE in patients with a large hepatopedal portal flow, Warren and his associates proposed in 1967 a modified shunting procedure that they believed would selectively decompress esophageal varices while, at the same time, preserving blood flow to the liver and avoiding systemic shunting of intestinal blood (508). The operation consists of a *distal splenorenal shunt (DSRS)*, in which the splenic side of the divided splenic vein is anastomosed to the intact left renal vein, and *gastrosplenic isolation* aimed at diverting the gastroesophageal venous flow through the shunt. Gastrosplenic isolation is accomplished by ligating the coronary, right gastric, and right gastroepiploic veins and by dividing the gastrohepatic, gastrocolic, and splenocolic ligaments.

The objectives of DSRS were to produce better results than those achieved with direct PCS by (1) preventing recurrent bleeding (and death from such bleeding) as effectively as direct PCS; (2) improving the immediate and long-term survival rates by decreasing the number of deaths from liver failure; and (3) improving the quality of life by reducing the incidence of PSE. Interest in DSRS has been widespread since its introduction in 1967. Table XII shows some results of the operation (509–525).

DSRS has been used mainly as an elective procedure in patients who have survived one or more episodes of varix hemorrhage. By and large the operation has been reserved for good-risk subjects with various forms of mild-to-moderate liver disease, good hepatic function, and excellent liver blood flow. Ascites has been considered a contraindication to the operation by most surgeons, although ascites that promptly responds to diuretic therapy has recently been removed by some workers from the list of contraindications. It is important to recognize that the highly selected patients who have undergone DSRS are not representative of the spectrum of bleeding cirrhotics admitted to a general hospital.

Has the DSRS accomplished the objectives that Warren and his colleagues (508) believed it would accomplish? There have been at least seven RCTs comparing DSRS with PCS or other total shunts, but it is still not possible to draw firm conclusions (510,513,520,524,525). Nevertheless, available data provide the following impressions: (1) The operation effectively prevents bleeding from varices in most patients. However, compared with direct end-to-side PCS or SSPCS performed electively in similar patients, it appears to be associated with higher incidences of recurrent variceal hemorrhage, persistence of varices, and occlusion of the shunt. In three series, rebleeding occurred in 29, 26, and 18% of patients, respectively (512,517,524). (2) Although the operative mortality rate in almost every institution has been high during the initial phase when the procedure was being learned, it has declined progressively as experience with the operation has increased. Nevertheless, the operative mortality rate appears to be somewhat higher than that of direct end-to-side PCS or SSPCS performed electively in comparable good-risk patients. It is generally agreed that DSRS is technically the most difficult of all the commonly used shunt procedures. (3) The 5-year survival rate does not appear to be different from that associated with direct PCS in similar patients; if anything, the long-term survival rate is somewhat lower following DSRS, but available data are inconclusive. (4) The incidence of PSE during the first few years after DSRS is lower than the incidence following direct PCS, and PSE tends to be milder. Thus, the advantage or disadvantage of DSRS compared with direct PCS during the first 5 years postoperatively depends on the relative importance given to a lower incidence and severity of PSE on the one hand versus apparently higher rates of recurrent variceal hemorrhage, shunt occlusion, operative mortality, and, perhaps, long-term mortality on the other hand.

There is reason to raise the possibility that, with the passage of time following DSRS, the incidence of PSE will increase and the survival rate will decrease compared with statistics for direct PCS. Accumulating evidence from detailed studies during prolonged follow-up shows that liver function deteriorates, the incidence of death from liver failure increases, hepatic blood flow decreases, collateral vessels connecting the portomesenteric and gastrosplenic sides of the portal circulation develop, and portal perfusion of the liver is lost with diversion of portomesenteric blood through the splenorenal shunt (522,523,525). Furthermore, reports of studies in patients with DSRS have identified a substantial incidence of thrombosis of the PV, which, of course, eliminates the main objective of the operation, namely, continued perfusion of the liver (522,525). The theoretical attractiveness of DSRS for a selected segment of the bleeding cirrhotic population is undeniable, but its value remains to be established by long-term studies from several centers of survival rates, incidence of shunt thrombosis, frequency of rebleeding, and incidence of liver failure and PSE.

e. Portacaval Shunt with Arterialization In the hope of improving liver blood flow after end-to-side PCS, in 1968 Maillard *et al.* proposed a procedure that *combined PCS with arterialization of the hepatic stump of the PV* (526,527). In 1974, Maillard *et al.* summarized the experience of others using this approach in 46 patients and described in detail their own experience with 36 patients (527). Maillard *et al.* used the splenic artery to arterialize the hepatic stump of the PV and performed the procedure electively in good-risk patients (Child's groups A and B). The operative mortality rate was 17% and 1 month postoperatively 30% of the arteriovenous anastomoses had thrombosed. After 1 year, the majority of the patients studied had developed thromboses of either the anastomosis or the intrahepatic branches of the PV. The incidence of PSE in the patients with patent anastomoses was 17%. On the basis of these results, there is little to recommend serious consideration of this operation.

f. Other (Uncommon) Shunts None of the several other techniques for creating connections between the portal and systemic venous systems are used widely or are established therapy for PH. The left gastric-vena caval shunt developed by Inokuchi and his colleagues (528) in Japan is based on the concept of selectively decompressing esophageal varices through the left gastric (coronary) vein while maintaining portal perfusion of the liver similar to the DSRS. The small left gastric vein is connected to the IVC by an interposed graft of autogenous saphenous vein or superficial femoral vein. Splenectomy, ligation of the tributaries of the splenic vein, and ligation of the connections between the right and

Table XII Results of Elective Therapeutic Distal Splenorenal Shunt in Highly Selected Patients with Liver Disease

Authors	Year of report	Type of series	Number of patients	Underlying disease	Child's risk class	Operative mortality rate (%)	Years of follow-up	Total mortality rate (%)	Encephalopathy (%)	Rebleeding (%)	Known shunt occlusion (%)
Vang *et al.* (517)	1976	Retrospective, selected patients	25	Cirrhosis of various types	A13, B9, C2	16	2.4–5.5	58	56	29	8
Martin *et al.* (512)	1978	Retrospective, selected patients	50	Cirrhosis of various types	A12, B32, C6	10	Variable	24 (3 years)	18	26	2
Zeppa *et al.* (519)	1978	Retrospective, selected patients	91	Cirrhosis (52 alcoholic, 39 nonalcoholic)	Mostly A	1	0.5–6	43 (5-year actuarial)	?	?	?
Rikkers *et al.* (513)	1978	Prospective, randomized, selected patients	26	Cirrhosis of various types	A	12	2–6	38 (3 years)	13	13	10
Bhalerao *et al.* (509)	1978	Retrospective, selected patients	52	Liver disease of various types	?	40	0.5–4	52	0	11	16
Langer *et al.* (510)	1980	Prospective, randomized, selected patients	27	Cirrhosis of various types	A6, B16, C5	19	1–7	33	14	9	10
Turcotte and Eckhauser (516)	1980	Retrospective, selected patients	55	Cirrhosis of various types	?	16	1–7	31	?	?	?
Fischer *et al.* (520)	1981	Prospective, randomized, selected patients	23	Cirrhosis (22 alcoholic, 1 nonalcoholic)	A13, B8, C2	4	1–5	22	9	14	27
Warren *et al.* (521)	1982	Retrospective, selected patients	348	Cirrhosis (198 alcoholic, 150 nonalcoholic)	86% A and B	4	1–10	41 (5-year actuarial)	4	?	?
Grace *et al.* (524)	1988	Prospective, randomized, selected patients	43	Cirrhosis (38 alcoholic)	A23, B19, C1	9	3–10	46	51	18	17

left gastric veins are added to the shunt procedure. By 1978, Inokuchi *et al.* had performed the operation electively in 103 patients with postnecrotic or posthepatitic cirrhosis, 32 patients with idiopathic PH, and 5 patients with extrahepatic PH. The shunt was done as a therapeutic procedure for bleeding varices in 97 patients and as a prophylactic operation in 43 patients. In the therapeutic shunt group, the operative mortality rate was 5%, the cumulative mortality rate during 3 months to 5 years of follow-up 29%, the incidence of shunt occlusion 1 month postoperatively 11%, and the frequency of rebleeding 10%. That none of the patients was observed to have PSE after operation is remarkable in light of the consistent observation that many cirrhotic patients who are not operated upon have PSE. The results of left gastric-vena caval shunt have not been confirmed by other workers.

The portarenal shunt is a form of in-continuity shunt similar to the SSPCS (529). The left renal vein is transected, and the vena caval end is anastomosed to the side of the PV, superior mesenteric vein, or splenic vein. Alternatively, the PV may be divided and its splanchnic end anastomosed to the end of the transected renal vein, which is hemodynamically similar to an end-to-side PCS. Under most circumstances, the portarenal shunt has no advantages over conventional PCS.

Shunts have been devised that utilize the reopened umbilical vein which connects with the PV, but they are not promising because of the small size of the vessel. Included in this category are the omphalocaval shunt and the saphenoumbilical shunt (530).

2. Portal-Systemic Shunt for Portal Hypertension Related Bleeding

a. Clinical Research Much of the research in the field of PH has been conducted in patients. Since PH-related bleeding is a highly lethal disorder that demands treatment that can only be assessed in patients, much of existing information has come from clinical observations. Clinical research takes many forms and the results vary in validity. The least valid, and yet most common, type of study is the retrospective review of medical records in the absence of a study protocol. Of greater validity is the prospective nonrandomized clinical trial in which data are collected prospectively according to a well-defined and rigorously applied protocol. Of greatest validity is the prospective, randomized clinical trial (RCT) in which two or more treatments are compared with each other or a treatment is compared with no treatment or placebo. For a RCT to be valid, and such is not always the case, the protocol must spell out specific rules and criteria regarding selection or nonselection of patients, end points, escape clauses, data recording, and data analysis. The well-designed and conducted RCT is the gold standard of clinical research.

Meta-analysis (MA), the process of combining the results of multiple similar investigations, was devised by G. V. Glass and is being used with increasing frequency (531). A well-done MA is a complex, labor-intensive process that requires a carefully designed search strategy, establishment of the high quality of the many components of the RCTs, and meticulous standardized analysis and recording of many clinical and methodological aspects of the disorder and patients under analysis (532). A MEDLINE search is the usual starting point for almost all MAs. It can be supplemented by searches of pharmaceutical and appropriate societal registers of RCTs (533). The RCTs to be included must be carefully screened. The inclusion of non-peer-reviewed reports, such as abstracts, theses, chapters, workshops, and correspondence, diminishes the validity of the analysis. RCTs to be included should be truly randomized, they should be analyzed on an intent-to-treat basis, and the recording of adverse events should be blindly performed. Only the first treatment period from crossover trials can be included, and no RCT selected for inclusion can retrospectively be excluded. All details of the disease and its treatment must be recorded along with those patients lost-to-follow-up, and the reasons for loss or exclusion must be available to the analysts for blind, independent analysis. Retrospective examination indicates that the five most critical criteria for a sound MA are

1. The existence of a detailed protocol
2. Contact by the analysts with the primary investigators to obtain additional information and to clarify ambiguities
3. Analysis according to intent-to-treat principle
4. Sensitivity analysis
5. Publication of the results of the MA in a peer-reviewed journal

Avoidance of bias of all sorts is essential, as is the need to identify all RCTs on the subject. Heterogeneity of results should be investigated by sensitivity analyses. A recently published analysis of five large, published MAs on important investigative subjects, by an experienced, dedicated analyst showed that these MAs contained many serious, often inexplicable, flaws and biases (534), reached conclusions that may not have been justified, reported heterogeneous results, managed data inconsistently, and omitted needed subgroup analyses (535). MA represents a potentially important statistical advance in the combining of data from similar trials. Because it is so simple in concept and appears so easy to conduct, particular attention must be paid to assure objective, well-conceived analyses.

b. Emergency Treatment PSS is the only available definitive treatment for PH-related bleeding. Numerous studies have shown that a technically satisfactory PSS will permanently solve the problem of bleeding in the vast majority of patients. The obvious potential advantage of performing this procedure under emergency circumstances is that, unlike other forms of treatment, it can be expected to provide both immediate and prolonged control of hemorrhage. The question is, can cirrhotic patients tolerate an operation of this magnitude when it is performed as an emergency in the face of bleeding? To answer this question, we have conducted seven *prospective* studies of emergency PCS (EPCS) over the past 37 years (536–549), as follows: (1) an unrandomized study of 400 unselected patients who underwent EPCS; (2) a RCT of EPCS versus emergency medical therapy involving 43 patients at our Veterans Administration Hospital; (3) an unrandomized study of 94 unselected, consecutive patients with Child's class C cirrhosis; (4) an unrandomized study of unselected patients bleeding from gastric varices; (5) an unrandomized study in 12 patients with uncontrollable bleeding from portal hypertensive gastropathy; (6) a NIH grant supported RCT of EPCS versus emergency endoscopic sclerotherapy (EST) that enrolled 201 patients whose follow-up is being completed; and (7) a RCT of TIPS versus EPCS that is in progress and has enrolled 110 patients thus far. The unique features of our studies that, together, make them different from other reported investigations are as follows: (1) EPCS was undertaken within 8 h of initial contact of the patient with our institution; (2) the patients were unselected, which means that all patients with bleeding varices, regardless of their condition, were entered in the studies and treated; (3) the studies were prospective, which means that the patients were managed according to a well-defined and consistently applied protocol, and specific data were collected at the time of diagnosis, treatment, and follow-up; and (4) the patients were followed up monthly for the first year and every 3 months thereafter for life, such that the 1-, 5-, and 10-year follow-up rates were 100, 98, and 97%, respectively. A total of 860 patients have been involved in these studies.

Our first study was a prospective, unrandomized evaluation of EPCS that involved 400 patients who were divided into two groups for analysis: an early group of 180 treated from 1968 to 1978, and a recent group of 220 treated from 1978 to July 1990 (536,539,540,547). The characteristics of the two groups were similar but the outcome was much better in the recent group. All of the patients underwent EPCS more than 5 years ago. Proof of acute variceal bleeding and of cirrhosis of the liver (alcoholic in 95%) was obtained in every patient. Child's risk classes determined quantitatively were A in 11% of the patients, B in 65%, and C in 24%. All patients had a direct PCS, side-to-side in 85%, which reduced the mean PV-to-IVC pressure gradient from 271 to 21 mm saline solution. All but 4 patients, 99%, had immediate and permanent control of variceal bleeding. Thrombosis of the shunt occurred in only 2 patients (0.5%). Survival rates at 30 days, 5 years, 10 years, and 15 years in the early group were 58, 40, 30, and 30%, respectively, while in the recent group they were 85, 78, 71, and 57%, respectively ($p < 0.0001$) (Fig. 8). Other striking gains in the recent group were abstention from alcohol, improvement in liver function, and improvement in Child's class, all in 70% of patients. Recurrent PSE occurred in 9% of the early group and 8% of the recent group. EPCS substantially improved survival and quality of life of patients with cirrhosis of the liver and bleeding varices. We attributed our results to rapid and simplified diagnosis, prompt operation, an organized system of care, and rigorous, lifelong follow-up evaluation that emphasized abstinence from alcohol and dietary protein control. Our results showed that transplantation of the liver is infrequently required in patients whose bleeding is permanently controlled.

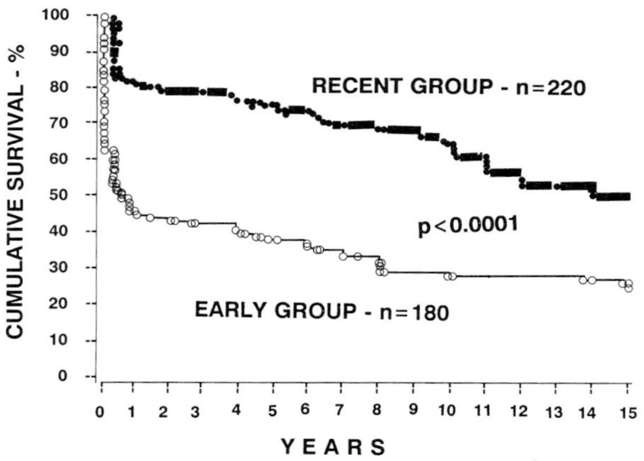

Figure 8 Fifteen-year Kaplan–Meier plots after emergency portacaval shunt in the early group and recent group unadjusted by age and gender for the California population. *n*, number of patients. From Ref. (547). Reprinted with permission from the American College of Surgeons (Journal of the American College of Surgeons, 1955, Vol. 180, pp. 257–272).

Our second study was a prospective RCT conducted from 1978 to 1982 at our Veterans Administration Hospital in which we compared EPCS and emergency medical therapy in unselected patients with alcoholic cirrhosis and bleeding esophageal varices (546). If the patients survived emergency medical therapy, they underwent an elective PCS within 2–6 weeks. The study was planned in 1977, when standard emergency medical therapy consisted of esophageal balloon tamponade and intravenous vasopressin. Endoscopic sclerotherapy had not yet been widely adopted and was not included in emergency medical treatment. All patients underwent exactly the same diagnostic workup and received the same initial therapy. Randomization was done after the diagnosis of bleeding varices was made by the sealed envelope method. Twenty-one patients were randomized to EPCS and 22 patients were randomized to emergency medical therapy followed by elective PCS. The follow-up rate was 100% in both groups. The two groups of patients were similar in every respect. Results of laboratory studies were also similar in the two groups, as was the incidence of significant risk factors. EPCS permanently controlled variceal hemorrhage in every patient, but emergency medical therapy permanently controlled bleeding in only 45%. The requirement for blood transfusion was almost 3 times greater in the medical treatment group than in the EPCS group, a highly significant difference in this day when every blood transfusion carries a substantial risk. Eighty-one percent of the patients treated by EPCS survived to leave the hospital, while only 45% of the patients who received emergency medical therapy survived. There were highly significant, more than 2- to 3-fold higher, 1-, 3-, 5-, and 10-year survival rates in patients treated by EPCS than in patients who received emergency medical therapy followed by elective PCS (Fig. 9). The results of EPCS in this RCT were similar to those obtained in the much larger unrandomized study.

Our third study of EPCS was a prospective unrandomized study of 94 unselected patients treated from 1978 to 1990 who were classified on initial contact in Child's class C, according to the point scoring system of Campbell *et al.* (545). All reports of Child's class C patients describe a very high mortality rate during the acute bleeding episode and a negligible long-term survival rate, regardless of treatment. Many clinicians have understandably concluded that PSS is not worthwhile in Child's class C cirrhosis. The characteristics of the 94 patients included ascites in 97%, jaundice in 86%, PSE on admission *or* in past history in 71%, and severe muscle wasting in 96%. Ninety-three percent were alcoholics and 16% had delirium tremens on admission. All 94 patients had varices on endoscopy, cirrhosis on liver biopsy, elevated serum bilirubin, serum albumin of 2.9 g/100 mL or less, and marked ICG retention. Ninety-eight percent had a hyperdynamic state. Sixty percent had a SGOT level of 100 or more IU/L, indicating acute alcoholic hepatitis superimposed on cirrhosis. Mean Child's point score for the group was 13.7 of a maximum of 15 points. All 94 patients had PH with a PV-IVC pressure gradient that averaged 286 mm saline. Emergency PCS reduced the PV-IVC pressure gradient to a mean 23 mm saline (<2 mm Hg). Eighty-five patients had a SSPCS and 9 an end-to-side PCS. The bleeding was promptly and permanently controlled in every patient. Blood transfusions averaged 9.6 units and ranged from 0 in a Jehovah's Witness to 42 units. Seventy-five of the 94 patients survived more than 30 days and left the hospital alive, an early survival rate of 80%. Survival rates for the first and fifth years after emergency shunt were 72 and 64%, respectively (Fig. 10). The bulk of deaths occurred in and around the acute bleeding episode. The survival rate declined only 8% between the first and fifth years. Once patients survived 6 months, their chances of prolonged survival were very good (545).

Our fourth study was a prospective unrandomized evaluation of EPCS in treatment of bleeding gastric varices (BGV) in 80 unselected patients with cirrhosis (84% alcoholic) (549). According to recent literature, BGV account for 20% of PH-related bleeding in cirrhosis, bleed more severely and are more lethal than esophageal varices, and respond inconsistently to medical treatment, including endoscopic sclerotherapy or band ligation. Little has been reported or is known about surgical treatment of BGV. As in our first study, the patients were divided into two groups: an early group of 30 treated from 1963 to 1978, and a recent group of 50 treated from 1978 to 1990. All patients were operated on more than 5 years ago. Follow-up rates were 97% at 10 years and 95% at 15 years. Sixty percent of the patients had undergone previous endoscopic sclerotherapy for bleeding esophageal varices, and 39% had failed attempts at sclerotherapy of BGV. All patients had proof of BGV by endoscopy and/or radiography and of cirrhosis by liver biopsy. The gastric varices were classified according to the method of Sarin *et al.* (550). BGV of the types known to be of greatest risk for hemorrhage and death (Sarin types GOV2, IGV1, and IGV2) were found in 87%. Incidence of serious risk factors was as follows:

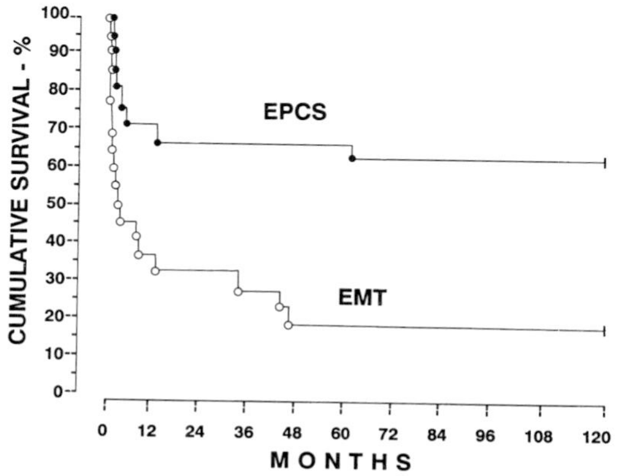

Figure 9 Ten-year Kaplan–Meier survival plots for emergency portacaval shunt (EPCS) and emergency medical therapy (EMT) followed by elective portacaval shunt. There is a statistically significant difference between the two curves at every time interval beginning with 1 month. [From Ref. (546), Orloff, M.J., *et al.* (1994). *Hepatology* **20**, 863–872.]

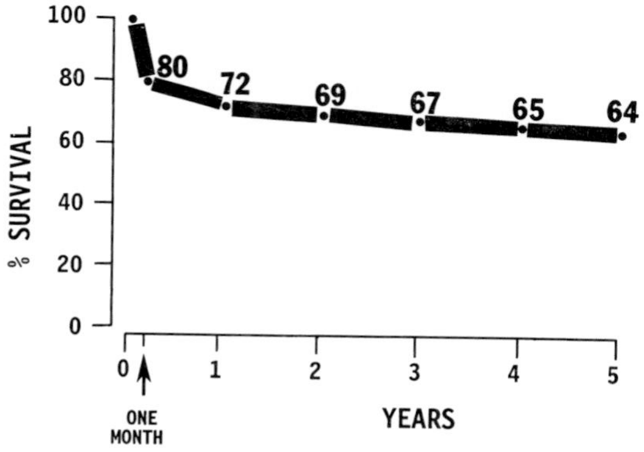

Figure 10 Cumulative survival rate calculated by the actuarial method of 94 unselected cirrhotic patients in Child's class C treated by emergency portacaval shunt. [From Ref. (545), Orloff, M.J., *et al.* (1992). Is portal-systemic shunt worthwhile in Child's class C cirrhosis? Long-term results of emergency shunt in 94 patients with bleeding varices. *Ann. Surg.* **216**, 256–268.]

ascites, 49%; jaundice, 43%; severe muscle wasting, 40%; past or present PSE, 35%; hyperdynamic state, 78%; past delirium tremens, 17%. Quantitative Child's risk classes were A, 10%; B, 60%; and C, 30%. All patients had a direct PCS, side-to-side in 95%, which reduced the mean PV-IVC pressure gradient from 257 to 20 mm saline. Survival to leave the hospital was 60% in the early group and 85% in the recent group. Long-term survival in the recent group of 50 patients was 84% after 1 year, 69% after 5 years, 62% after 10 years, and 56% after 15 years. Shunt patency was demonstrated every 1–2 years in all but 2 patients (98%), and only these (2%) had recurrent BGV. Rigorous follow-up and dietary protein restriction resulted in recurrent PSE in only 8%, compared to 35% pre-PCS. Sixty-four percent abstained from alcohol and their 5-year survival rate was 90%. After 5 years, LFTs were improved in 79%, Child's risk class compared to pre-PCS was 77% (vs 10%) for class A and 5% (vs 30%) for class C, and 64% who were not of retirement age had resumed work. Only 1 of 72 patients (1%) who left the hospital alive became a candidate for liver transplantation. In the largest and longest experience reported to date, we concluded that PCS resulted in prolonged survival and life of satisfactory quality in two-thirds of cirrhotic patients with BGV.

Our fifth study was a prospective unrandomized evaluation of EPCS in 12 unselected patients with massive bleeding from portal hypertensive gastropathy (PHG), which is a vascular disorder of the gastric mucosa distinguished by ectasia of the mucosal capillaries and submucosal veins without inflammation. During 1988 to 1993, 12 patients with biopsy-proven cirrhosis (10 alcoholic, 2 posthepatitic) were evaluated and treated prospectively by PCS for active bleeding from severe PHG (548). Eleven patients had been hospitalized for bleeding three to nine times previously, and one was bleeding uncontrollably for the first time. Requirement for blood transfusions ranged from 11 to 39 units cumulatively, of which 8 to 30 units were required specifically to replace blood lost from PHG. Admission findings were ascites in 9 patients, jaundice in 8, severe muscle wasting in 10, and hyperdynamic state in 9. Child's risk class was C in 7, B in 4, and A in 1. Ten of the 12 patients had previously received repetitive endoscopic sclerotherapy for esophageal varices, which has been reported to precipitate PHG. Eight patients had failed propranolol therapy for bleeding. PCS permanently stopped bleeding in all patients by reducing the mean PV-IVC pressure gradient from 251 to 16 mm saline. There were no operative deaths, and there were two unrelated late deaths after 13 and 24 months. During 6 to 12 years of follow-up, all shunts remained patent by ultrasonography, the gastric mucosa reverted to normal on serial endoscopy, and there was no gastrointestinal bleeding. Recurrent PSE developed in only 8% of patients. Quality of life was generally good. We concluded that PCS provides definitive treatment of bleeding PHG by eliminating the underlying cause and makes possible prolonged survival with an acceptable quality of life.

Our sixth study is a NIH grant supported prospective RCT comparing EPCS versus emergency and long-term repetitive endoscopic sclerotherapy (EST) in unselected patients, "all comers" included. Patient enrollment has been completed and consists of 201 patients. Follow-up and data analysis are near completion. Follow-up is 100%. The study is known as the San Diego Bleeding Esophageal Varices Study. Outcome criteria being compared are (1) mortality; (2) duration and quality of life; (3) direct and indirect economic costs; and (4) treatment failure, defined as rebleeding requiring 6 units of blood transfusion in the first week or 8 units of blood transfusion in any subsequent 12-month period. When treatment failure has been declared, and only then, the patient receives rescue crossover therapy. The study is a community-wide endeavor in which 65 community gastroenterologists and 65 emergency physicians are sending their acute bleeding patients to us. The investigators and external advisory committee agreed at the beginning that until the study is completed, the data will not be analyzed, published, or presented publicly. However, certain results are obvious without statistical analysis, particularly recurrence of bleeding and direct economic costs. Both EPCS and EST have been very effective in controlling acute variceal hemorrhage. Over 90% of the patients in both groups have left the hospital alive. None of the patients treated by EPCS had recurrent bleeding and met the criteria for treatment failure. In contrast, 68% of the patients in the EST group developed recurrent bleeding that met the criteria for treatment failure. The direct costs of care were significantly higher in the EST group than in the EPCS group, largely because of the requirement for repeated sessions of EST to achieve variceal obliteration and the readmissions to the hospital caused by recurrent bleeding.

Our seventh and final study is currently in progress. It is a prospective RCT comparing EPCS versus transjugular intrahepatic portal-systemic shunt (TIPS) in unselected patients with PH-related bleeding, "all comers" included. To date, 110 patients have been enrolled. The target is 200 patients. It is too early to draw conclusions, and none have been reported.

c. Elective Treatment Elective surgical treatment directed at overcoming PH is indicated in patients who have not undergone an EPCS and have recovered from an episode of bleeding esophageal varices provided there is a reasonable likelihood that the patient will survive the elective operation. Table XIII shows the results of two prospective studies of the fate of cirrhotic patients who recovered from a bleeding episode and qualified for surgical therapy but were deliberately not subjected to operation (551,552). Over 90% bled again from esophageal varices and died. In our study, all of the patients were dead within 2 years of their first bleeding episode. The only consistently effective treatment

Table XIII Prospective Studies of the Fate of Cirrhotic Patients Who Survived an Episode of Bleeding Esophageal Varices and Did Not Undergo Portacaval Shunt

Author	Number of patients	Criteria for inclusion in prospective study	Rebleeding from varices (8)	Mortality rate (%)	
				2 years	5 years
Mikkelson (551)	35	Child's risk class A; recovered from one or more bleeding episodes, qualified for shunt	95	50	100
Orloff (552)	27	Unselected, all child's risk classes; recovered from one (first) bleeding episode; qualified for shunt	93	100	—

for PH is PSS, which, when performed properly, will protect more than 95% of patients against subsequent varix hemorrhage (553). Therefore, a single episode of varix bleeding is an indication for elective shunt therapy in all cirrhotic patients unless they have hepatic decompensation. Unfortunately, only 50% of bleeding cirrhotic patients survive nonsurgical emergency therapy and recover sufficient hepatic function to become eligible for elective shunt.

What criteria can be used to predict the likelihood of a patient surviving an elective shunt procedure without serious sequelae? The answer is not known with any degree of certainty and is particularly difficult because the decision not to operate is tantamount to accepting a lethal outcome. Extensive efforts have been directed toward identifying biochemical, hemodynamic, morphologic, and clinical criteria for selecting patients for elective PSS (105,106,541,554–566). The results of liver function tests, such as the level of serum albumin or bilirubin, the amount of bromsulphthalein or indocyanine green dye retention, or the magnitude of prothrombin deficiency, do not correlate with the response to shunt except at the extremes. Hemodynamic studies involving angiography and pressure measurements have been of little predictive value, mainly because of the lack of a practical technique for measuring the capacity of hepatic arterial blood flow to compensate for the diversion of portal venous flow. It has been proposed that the presence of acute alcoholic hepatitis, acute hyaline necrosis, or many Mallory bodies on liver biopsy is a contraindication to operation (552,557,560). However, in our study of liver biopsies from 164 patients with alcoholic cirrhosis who underwent EPCS, there was no correlation between survival and the finding of any or all of these features of acute alcoholic hepatitis (567). In the final analysis, the decision to operate or not is based on a composite of many clinical features of a patient's disease, determined during a period of intensive medical treatment in the hospital. Certain features are ominous; thus, the presence of persistent jaundice, of ascites that cannot be stabilized, of repeated bouts of PSE, of advanced muscle wasting, and of a poor appetite indicates that operation carries a high risk. If these general criteria have been followed, the operative mortality rate has been in the acceptable range of 10% or less.

In the 40 years between 1958 and 1998, we performed 2083 portal-systemic shunts (Table XIV). By 1998 we had performed 622 emergency shunts. Another 1148 patients were referred to us after their bleeding was controlled at another hospital, and these highly selected patients underwent elective therapeutic PCS and were studied prospectively. Elective shunts were also performed in 34 patients with cirrhosis and truly intractable ascites, about 1 patient per year, and in 46 patients with Budd–Chiari syndrome. Finally, elective portal-systemic shunts were performed in 176 patients for bleeding varices due to extrahepatic PH.

Table XV shows our results of elective therapeutic PCS for variceal hemorrhage in 1000 patients who were operated on more than 5 years ago and were studied prospectively (553). All of them had biopsy-proven cirrhosis, alcoholic in 89%. Follow-up rate was 99.6%. SSPCS was done in 92% of patients and end-to-side PCS in 8%. Quantitative Child's risk class was A in 11%, B in 58%, and C in 31% of the patients. The incidence in percent of serious risk factors on admission or in past history was as follows: ascites, 63; jaundice, 55; PSE, 33; severe muscle wasting, 39; hyperdynamic cardiac output of 6 L/min or greater, 74; past delirium tremens, 16. The mean corrected portal pressure in millimeters of saline was 254 before shunt and 21 after shunt. Mean operative blood transfusion was 2.1 units and mean operative time was 3.1 h.

Table XIV Author's Experience with Portal-Systemic Shunt, 1958–1998

Indication for shunt	Number of patients
Emergency therapeutic PCS for bleeding varices due to cirrhosis	622
Elective therapeutic PCS for	
Bleeding varices due to cirrhosis	1148
Bleeding varices due to other liver diseases	57
Ascites due to cirrhosis	34
Budd–Chiari syndrome	46
Elective therapeutic shunt for bleeding varices due to extrahepatic portal hypertension	176
Total	2083

Table XV Results of Elective Therapeutic Portacaval Shunt for Variceal Bleeding in 1000 Patients with Liver Disease Followed Up for More Than 5 years in Author's Series

	Number of patients	Percentage of group
Total group	1000	100
Operative (30-day) mortality	16	1.6
1-year survival	950	95
5-year survival	710	71
10-year survival (actuarial)	—	65
15-year survival (actuarial)	—	61
5-year survival in 621 abstainers	565	91
Shunt thrombosis	3	0.3
Variceal rebleeding	3	0.3
Encephalopathy		
Preoperative	330	33
Postoperative (recurrent)	70	7

The operative mortality rate in the author's series was 1.6%, and 98.4% of the patients left the hospital alive. Survival rates were 95% at 1 year, 71% at 5 years, 65% at 10 years (actuarial), and 61% at 15 years (actuarial). Two-thirds of the deaths were due to continued alcoholism. Long-term shunt patency was demonstrated in 99.7% of patients by yearly angiography and/or Doppler ultrasonography. Only 3 patients (0.3%) had recurrent variceal bleeding, all due to shunt occlusion. PSE occurred recurrently in 7% of patients, compared to 33% before shunt. Sixty-five percent of patients abstained from alcohol for 5 or more years, and their 5-year survival rate was 95%. Sixty-five percent of survivors who were not of retirement age resumed full- or part-time work. After 5 years, liver function had improved in 75% and deteriorated in only 5% of patients.

Table XVI shows some results of elective PSS performed by other surgeons for varix bleeding in patients with cirrhosis (553,568–576). Beyond any doubt, PSS prevents subsequent varix bleeding in almost all patients. Moreover, about two-thirds of highly selected patients subjected to elective treatment have survived 5 years. For those who abstain from alcohol, 5-year survival is substantially greater than that reported for liver transplantation, with much lower morbidity and cost.

The crucial question regarding the value of elective, therapeutic PSS concerns whether a comparable, selected group of patients who are treated medically rather than surgically will survive as long or as well. Unfortunately, despite use of the shunt operation for 55 years, this question has not yet been fully answered. Four prospective clinical trials have been reported, three of them suggesting an advantage of shunt operations and one indicating no advantage (551,572–581). However, all four trials involved small numbers of highly selected patients and had a number of serious shortcomings in design and conduct, so that the results do not warrant a conclusive answer. Moreover, they were reported some years ago. On the basis of our results in 1000 patients and until conclusive information to the contrary is available, the elective PCS is indicated in patients who have bled one or more times from esophageal varices.

3. Transjugular Intrahepatic Portal-Systemic Shunt (TIPS)

TIPS is a radiological procedure performed percutaneously through the internal jugular vein that creates a blunt intrahepatic parenchymal tract between the portal and

Table XVI Results of Elective Portal-Systemic Shunt Performed by Other Surgeons in Highly Selected Patients with Cirrhosis

Authors	Number of patients	Type of shunt	Operative mortality rate (%)	Varix rebleeding (%)	5-year survival (%)
Voorhees *et al.* (573)	404	324 portacaval, 80 splenorenal and other	12	7	51
McDermott *et al.* (571)	237	166 splenorenal, 71 portacaval	23	15	54
Barnes *et al.* (568)	173	103 portacaval, 70 splenorenal	13	14	39
Mikkelson *et al.* (572)	173	All portacaval	12	7	44
Linton *et al.* (570)	169	122 splenorenal, 47 portacaval	12	19	50
Turcotte and Lambert (566)	147	All portacaval	21	—	35
Ottinger (575)	140	All splenorenal	12	10	41
Bismuth *et al.* (569)	120	72 central splenorenal, 48 portacaval	2	3	66
Wantz and Payne (576)	97	All portacaval	11	5	68 (4 years)
Walker *et al.* (574)	50	All portacaval	6	12	70
Orloff *et al.* (553)	1000	All portacaval	1.6	0.3	71

hepatic veins, followed by reinforcement of the tract with a metallic stent. Hemodynamically, it is similar to a SSPCS. The first TIPS was done without a stent in pigs by Rösch, Hanafee, and Snow (582,583), and the procedure was first applied to humans with only limited success by Colapinto *et al.* in 1983 (584). A major advance was made in 1986 by Palmaz *et al.* (585,586), who adapted an expandable metal stent previously used in arteries to keep the hepatic parenchymal tract patent in dogs. In 1989, Richter, Palmaz, and Noeldge (587) applied the Palmaz stent to a TIPS procedure in humans, and in subsequent modifications achieved successful stent placement with regularity (588–590). TIPS was further refined in 1992 by Ring *et al.* (591,592), who substituted the flexible Wallstent (Schneider U.S. Stent Division, Pfizer Hospital Products Group, Plymouth, MN) for the Palmaz stent. Currently, both the Wallstent and Palmaz stent are used for TIPS.

In the short period of time that the stented TIPS has been used clinically, more than 400 reports of TIPS have been published. Many of these have been reports of uncontrolled anecdotal observations involving small numbers of patients followed for short periods of time. The technical success rate of placing TIPS is ≥90%, with good initial control of bleeding (593,594). The major problems with TIPS are a high rate of stenosis and/or thrombosis and an increased incidence of PSE. TIPS stenosis occurs in 50–70% of patients within the first year (595–601), requires a systematic follow-up with use of Doppler ultrasound and recatheterization for its identification and management, and is the major cause for TIPS rebleeding rates of 15–30%. In addition, the need for reintervention raises cost and is a factor in diminishing quality of life. PSE following TIPS is reported as a 30% increased incidence (602–604). In approximately one-quarter, PSE is incapacitating, and the others can be managed with diet and medications. In some patients, accelerated liver failure is associated with the PSE. RCTs comparing TIPS with endoscopic therapy have shown significantly better control of bleeding with TIPS, but significantly lower PSE rates with endoscopic therapy (602,605–607). Meta-analysis of these trials in which both TIPS and sclerotherapy were used as primary therapy to prevent rebleeding shows no difference in mortality.

RCTs are required to compare TIPS with surgical shunts in both the emergency and elective situations. The mechanism of TIPS dysfunction and its detection, treatment, and prevention are research priorities. TIPS is a potentially important new area in managing patients with PH-related bleeding that requires extensive further clinical and basic study.

4. Prophylactic Treatment

Because of the very high mortality rate associated with varix bleeding, some workers have advocated prophylactic PSS in patients with demonstrable varices who have never bled. Although a patient who has bled from esophageal varices is almost certain to bleed again, nothing suggests that the mere demonstration of varices in a patient with no history of bleeding permits one to predict the likelihood of varix rupture. In fact, recent statistics indicate that only one-third to one-half of patients with esophageal varices who have no history of bleeding will subsequently have variceal hemorrhage. Thus, one-half to two-thirds of the patients subjected to prophylactic PCS would undergo an operation to prevent a complication that would not have developed had they not received surgical therapy. Herein lies the fallacy of prophylactic shunt.

Prophylactic PCS has been compared with medical therapy in three prospective studies conducted 25 years ago in selected cirrhotic patients with esophageal varices that had not bled (608–611). All three studies showed that while protecting the patients against bleeding, prophylactic PCS had no influence on survival. These results are not surprising. When a major operation is performed in seriously ill patients to prevent a complication that might develop in only one-half of these patients if they did not have the operation, the results can hardly be expected to be good. Although a different conclusion might result from similar studies performed today, available data indicate that there is no use for the prophylactic operation. However, it is important to emphasize that the results of prophylactic PCS are in no way applicable to the treatment of bleeding esophageal varices by therapeutic PCS because these patients have already developed the complication of bleeding, which is almost certain to recur unless the PH is relieved.

5. Treatment of Extrahepatic Portal Hypertension

Almost all patients with extrahepatic portal hypertension (EHPH) have portal vein thrombosis (PVT). This condition is strikingly different from intrahepatic PH resulting from cirrhosis. The patients are usually much younger and often are children. They have normal liver function, are otherwise in good health, and tolerate variceal bleeding without the development of hepatic decompensation, coagulopathy, PSE, and exsanguination. Except in infancy, they rarely have ascites, and hepatic coma resulting from liver cell failure does not develop. Because the PV is obliterated, a direct anastomosis from the PV to the IVC cannot be performed for portal decompression. Finally, age and the related technical matter of adequate vessel size influence treatment.

Patients with EHPH come to medical attention usually because of bleeding from esophagogastric varices or splenomegaly. Exsanguinating hemorrhage does not occur nearly as often as in cirrhosis. On physical examination, splenomegaly is almost always found, but the liver is not palpable. Dilated collateral veins in the abdominal wall may be striking. Liver function tests are usually normal, but hematologic studies often reveal peripheral cytopenia that reflects hypersplenism. The hypersplenism is infrequently severe. Esophagogastroscopy and upper gastrointestinal contrast radiographs demonstrate varices. Because the obstruction is presinusoidal, hepatic vein catheterization shows a normal WHVP. Ultrasonography of the abdomen regularly shows occlusion of the PV. Splenic or superior mesenteric arteriography, with indirect portography, is the most important diagnostic procedure and provides crucial information about the site of the portal obstruction and the size of the vessels available for portal decompression. Splenoportography with manometry is equally effective, and sometimes more effective, in demonstrating the obstruction, but it is a diagnostic procedure of second choice because of the small risk of bleeding from the spleen.

The definitive treatment of EHPH is PSS. However, emergency shunt operations are rarely necessary. Emergency treatment of variceal hemorrhage consists of blood transfusions and, if the bleeding does not subside spontaneously, pharmacologic therapy with intravenous somatostatin analogues or vasopressin. Failure to control bleeding promptly is an indication for EST or variceal banding. Esophageal balloon tamponade is indicated if other nonoperative measures are unsuccessful. Subsequent rebleeding after these temporizing measures is the rule, but it is usually well tolerated and controllable while diagnostic studies are undertaken and definitive operative shunt therapy is being planned.

For all the reasons stated above, patients with EHPH resulting from PVT should be excellent candidates for definitive operations that relieve PH and prevent recurrent hemorrhage. Nevertheless, there is widespread reluctance to operate on these patients because of a number of reports of series of PSS, often involving retrospective data pooled from several hospitals or many surgeons, that have described a high incidence of shunt occlusion and rebleeding (612–622). Moreover, conventional wisdom holds that many children with PVT ultimately "outgrow" their variceal bleeding if they can be tided over into adulthood by nonoperative, nondefinitive measures. Our experience does not support these contentions.

From 1958 to 1999, we conducted a prospective, unrandomized study of PSS treatment of 200 unselected, consecutive children and adults with PVT who had bled two or more times from esophagogastric varices (623,624). All patients have undergone regular follow-up and 93% have been observed for 5 or more years. Etiology of PVT was neonatal omphalitis in 15%, peritonitis in 7%, umbilical or PV catheterization in 7%, trauma in 4%, thrombotic coagulopathy in 3%, and unknown in 65% of the patients. Liver function test results and liver biopsies were normal in all patients, and none had stigmata of liver disease. All patients with an intact spleen had hypersplenism. Esophagogastric varices were demonstrated by angiography, endoscopy, and contrast X-rays. Previous therapy had failed to stop recurrent bleeding in 95% of patients; splenectomy had been tried and failed in 58 (29%) and repetitive EST or variceal banding had been tried and failed in 106 (53%). Ninety-one percent had three or more bleeding episodes. The extent of occlusion and the veins available for PSS were determined by angiography. Thrombosis involved PV alone in 134 patients (67%), PV and splenic vein in 56 (28%), and PV and superior mesenteric vein in 10 (5%) (Fig. 11). Accordingly, central side-to-side splenorenal shunt without splenectomy was done in 94 patients (47%), conventional central splenorenal shunt with splenectomy was done in 40 (20%), and mesocaval (SMV–IVC) shunt was done in 66 (33%) (Fig. 12). PSS reduced the mean PV–IVC pressure gradient (mm saline) from 296 to 25.

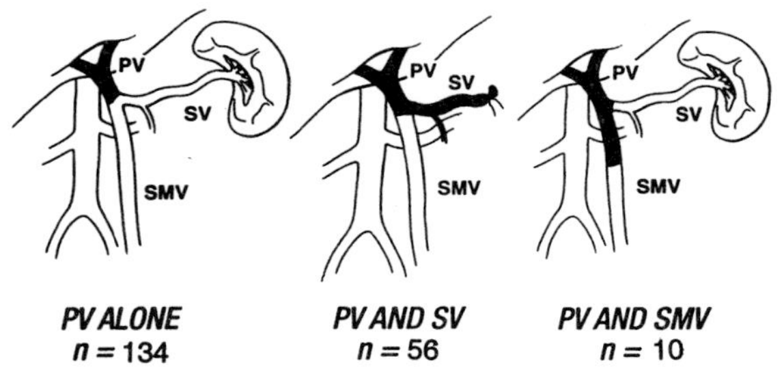

Figure 11 Sites of portal vein thrombosis in 200 patients with extrahepatic portal hypertension.

Postoperative survival to leave the hospital was 100%. Five-, 10-, and 15-year actuarial survival rates were 99, 97, and 96%, respectively. Figure 13 shows a Kaplan–Meier survival plot for 15 years. Angiography and/or Doppler ultrasonography every 1–2 years demonstrated thrombosis of the PSS in 5 patients (2.5%), all of whom developed rebleeding. All other patients remained free of bleeding with patent shunts, normal liver function tests, and no instance of PSE. Hypersplenism was corrected and the platelet count was restored to a level above 100,00/mm^3 in all patients.

The excellent results of PSS in our series are not unique. Bismuth *et al.* (625) reported no operative or late deaths, shunt thrombosis in only 6%, and recurrent bleeding in only

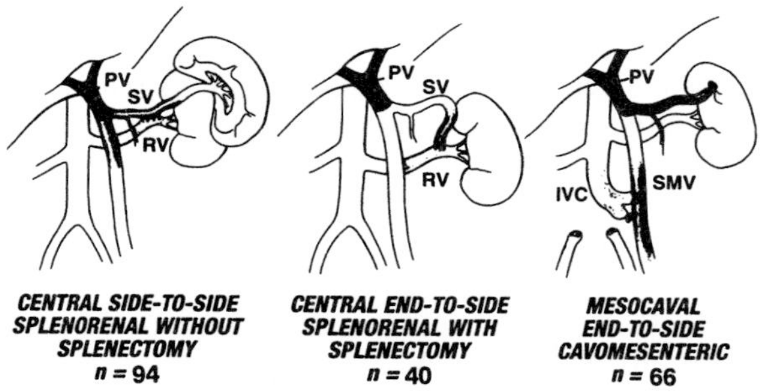

Figure 12 The three types of elective therapeutic portosystemic shunt procedures performed in 200 patients with extrahepatic portal hypertension caused by portal vein thrombosis.

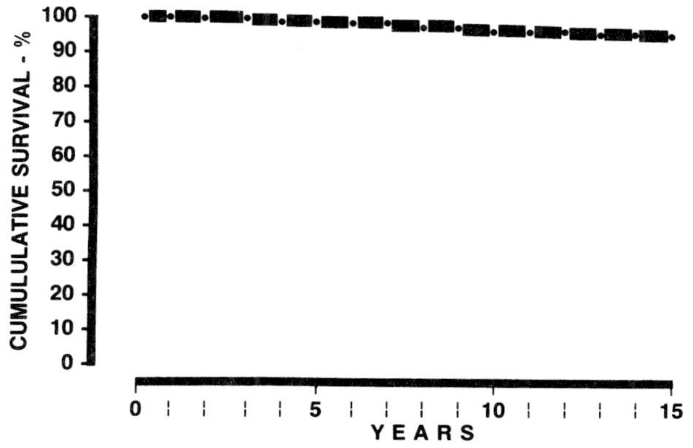

Figure 13 Kaplan–Meier survival plot for 15 years after portosystemic shunt in 200 patients with extrahepatic portal hypertension.

2% of 52 children who underwent PSS for bleeding esophageal varices resulting from EHPH. Tocornal and Cruz (626) reported no operative mortality, a 9% rate of late deaths, and a 9% incidence of shunt thrombosis and rebleeding in 23 children with EHPH who were treated for bleeding varices by PSS. Alvarez *et al.* (627) performed PSS in 72 children with EHPH, 12 of them prophylactically and 64 for variceal hemorrhage, with no early or late mortality and incidences of shunt thrombosis and a recurrent bleeding rate of only 8%. Pande *et al.* (628) reported a more than 90% 5-year survival rate in 102 children and adults with EHPH who had elective therapeutic PSS, with no operative deaths, a 4% rate of late mortality, and a 9% incidence of rebleeding. Gauthier *et al.* (629) reported no operative or late deaths, shunt thrombosis in 8% of patients, and recurrent bleeding in 7% of 59 children with EHPH, most of whom received PSS for variceal bleeding.

Based on our 40-year experience with 100% follow-up of 200 patients, we conclude that PSS is consistently effective in bleeding varices due to PVT and EHPH, resulting in long survival, freedom from rebleeding, and no PSE. No other therapy, including endoscopic therapy, drugs, and TIPS, is consistently effective in this disorder.

6. Ascites

Intractable ascites, refractory to medical therapy, occurs in approximately 10% of patients with ascites from cirrhosis and is almost always fatal. Sinusoidal hypertension resulting from hepatic venous outflow obstruction plays a primary role in the pathogenesis of cirrhotic ascites and provides the rationale for decompression of the liver by SSPCS in treatment of intractable ascites (Fig. 14). In our experimental studies, described previously, SSPCS permanently relieved severe ascites, reduced the 13-fold increase in thoracic duct lymph flow rate to almost normal, and abolished the aldosterone hypersecretory response to minimal hepatic venous outflow obstruction. From 1963 to 1993, on the basis of our experimental observations, we conducted a prospective unrandomized study of SSPCS in 34 carefully selected patients with cirrhosis (91% alcoholic) who had failed medical therapy, including hospitalization for 5–24 months (mean 13.8 months) (630–634). The effects on ascites, survival, metabolic abnormalities, and quality of life were studied prospectively during follow-up that was longer than 5 years in all patients. At the time of admission, quantitative Child's risk classes were A in 0 patients, B in 68%, and C in 32%.

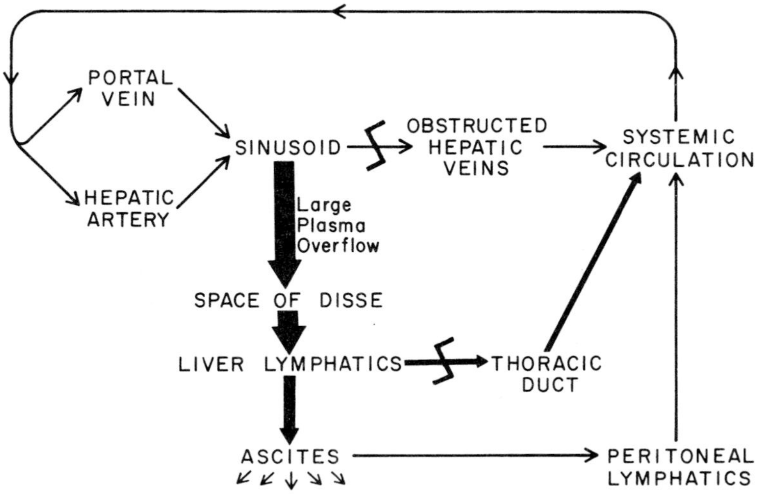

Figure 14 The chain of events in ascites formation. Hepatic venous outflow obstruction and the resultant sinusoidal hypertension play a primary role in causing transudation of ascitic fluid from the hepatic lymphaties. [From Ref. (630), Orloff, M., (1970). *Ann. NY Acad. Sci.* **170**, 213–238.]

SSPCS reduced the mean PV–IVC pressure gradient from 282 mm saline to 4 mm and permanently relieved all patients of ascites, without subsequent requirement of diuretic therapy. Thirty-day mortality rate was 6%, and long-term survival rates at 5, 10, and 15 years were 75, 74, and 73%, respectively. Figure 15 shows a 15-year survival plot following SSPCS and compares it with the survival curve of 1155 patients hospitalized with cirrhosis and ascites reported by D'Amico *et al.* in which the 2-year survival rate was less than 50% (430).

Metabolic balance studies were performed for 10–28 days preoperatively and again 3 weeks after SSPCS while the patients were on a daily sodium intake of 44 mEq. Preoperatively, all patients showed the characteristic pattern of sodium and fluid retention, with low urine volume and sodium excretion, and a dilutional hyponatremia. No patient excreted more than 2.7 mEq/day of sodium. In addition, 29 of the 34 patients (85%) had hypokalemia, a common finding in cirrhosis. All 10 patients in whom urinary aldosterone excretion was measured had evidence of marked hyperaldosteronism, excreting 5–10 times the normal amount of aldosterone. SSPCS produced marked diuresis and natriuresis in all 33 survivors. Urine volume increased markedly and negative fluid balance developed. Within 3 weeks, sodium excretion reached normal levels. Urinary aldosterone excretion returned to the normal range and intermittent determinations for 3 years showed that it remained normal.

Quality of life was generally improved as a result of a low incidence of recurrent PSE (6%), abstinence from alcohol in 91%, improvement in liver function in 81%, and improvement in Child's risk class. Compared to preoperative status, 1 year after PCS 59% of survivors were in Child's class A (versus 0), 34% were in class B (versus 68%), and 6% were in class C (versus 32%). Most patients experienced striking improvements in nutrition in the form of sizeable gains in lean tissue mass and body fat. The PCS remained permanently patent in every patient.

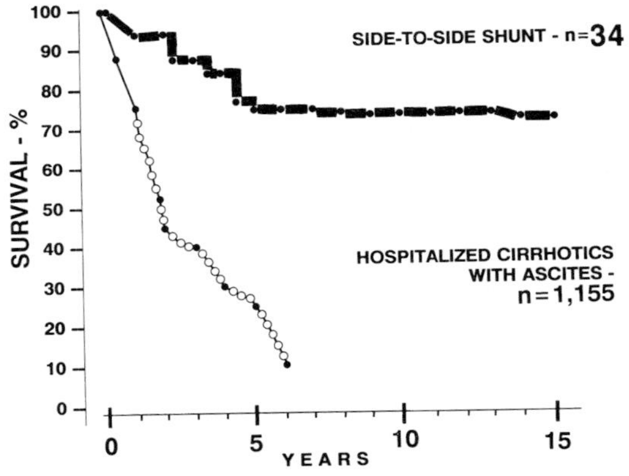

Figure 15 Kaplan–Meier survival plot of 34 patients treated by side-to-side portacaval shunt for intractable cirrhotic ascites compared with survival of 1155 patients hospitalized with cirrhotic ascites reported by D'Amico and associates (430). From Ref. (631). Reprinted with permission from the American College of Surgeons (Journal of the American College of Surgeons, 1997, Vol.184, pp. 557–570).

There are three alternative procedures for treatment of intractable cirrhotic ascites, namely, peritovenous shunt (PVS), TIPS, and orthotopic liver transplantation (OLT). PVS is a palliative procedure that does not treat the underlying cause of ascites. Insertion of a PVS is followed by increases in cardiac output, plasma volume, glomerular filtration rate, renal plasma flow, and creatinine clearance; decreases in plasma or serum levels of catecholamines, renin, and aldosterone; and natriuresis and diuresis (635–638). Diuretics and sodium restriction are usually necessary to initiate and maintain natriuresis after insertion of the shunt, but the responsiveness of the patient to diuretics is enhanced. In the 1980s, PVS was used widely for the treatment of ascites, often in patients who did not have intractable ascites, but enthusiasm diminished considerably with reports of a high incidence of complications, substantial mortality, frequent shunt malfunctions, and recurrence of ascites in many patients (635–653). At least 50% of patients with a PVS have had one or more serious complications (646,648,650,651). Most shunts are reported to develop occlusion in 1 year or sooner (641,646,651). Substantial evidence indicates that the ultimate failure rate of PVS is high (639,640,650,652–654). Ascites has been reported to recur within 1 year in 50% or more of patients whose ascites was relieved initially. Moreover, prospective RCTs have shown no influence of PVS on survival or hepatic function, compared with medical therapy (652–654). The 1-year mortality rate has exceeded 50%. Many authorities have concluded that PVS is not frequently indicated in cirrhotic ascites.

Theoretically, TIPS should have the same hemodynamic effects as a surgical SSPCS. TIPS lowers sinusoidal pressure in the liver, although not to the same extent as the surgical shunt because the intrahepatic veins are of considerably smaller diameter than the main PV and IVC. In patients with refractory ascites, TIPS has produced diuresis and natriuresis, decreased serum aldosterone levels and plasma renin activity, lowered serum creatinine, increased cardiac output, and decreased systemic vascular resistance (655–658). In patients with variceal hemorrhage who also have ascites, TIPS provided relief of the ascites in short-term observations (659,660). There have been no long-term prospective clinical trials of the use of TIPS in the treatment of intractable ascites. Five short-term studies are of interest. Ochs *et al.* performed TIPS in 50 selected patients with refractory ascites, with elimination of the ascites in 74% at 3 months (661). Survival rate was 54% at 1 year and 38% at 2 years, and the post-TIPS incidence of PSE was 52%. Quiroga *et al.* performed TIPS in 17 patients with refractory ascites (658). Seven to 12 months after TIPS, ascites was mild or absent in 57% of patients. Six patients underwent liver transplantation 1–10 months after TIPS. The 3-month mortality rate was 41%, 75% of patients had PSE, and 56% of survivors developed one or more episodes of TIPS stenosis. Crenshaw *et al.* attempted TIPS in 54 patients with intractable ascites, with successful placement in 50 (662). Nine patients underwent liver transplantation. Ascites was eliminated in 57%. One-year mortality rate was 52% and TIPS stenosis requiring revision occurred in 22% of patients. Lebrec *et al.* compared TIPS and paracentesis in a RCT involving 25 patients, 13 of whom received TIPS (657). Improvement in ascites at 4 months was observed in 69% of the TIPS patients, all of them in Child's class B, but the 1-year survival rate was only 17%. In the most recent study, Rössle *et al.* compared TIPS and paracentesis in a RCT involving 60 patients, 29 of whom received TIPS (663). After 3 months, 61% of patients were free of ascites. Survival rates at 1 and 2 years were 69 and 58%, respectively, and the incidence of PSE was 58%.

As discussed previously, there are two major potential problems with TIPS, shunt occlusion and PSE. The incidence of stenosis and occlusion of the shunt in relatively short-term followup ranges from 22 to 50%. Although it has been possible to reopen many shunts by balloon dilatation and to insert a second TIPS, the likelihood of long-term patency of a foreign body stent that is holding open a parenchymal tract in the venous system is questionable. A major cause of stenosis and occlusion appears to be pseudointimal hypertrophy or hyperplasia that develops as the parenchymal tract heals. Furthermore, there has been a high incidence of PSE after TIPS. It has been suggested that the high incidence is from the lack of an organized program of follow-up treatment of the underlying liver disease in most reported series of TIPS. It is clear that the efficacy of TIPS can be determined only by long-term RCTs.

Orthotopic liver transplantation (OLT) has been used with increasing frequency recently for treatment of alcoholic cirrhosis in selected patients. One-year survival rates after OLT in alcoholic cirrhotic patients have been 66–90%, comparable to survival rates in adult patients undergoing OLT for other hepatic disease (664–665). In short-term follow-up, 20% or more of the transplanted patients have resumed alcohol consumption. On the basis of these promising results, Bismuth *et al.* have suggested that OLT be used regularly for patients with Child's class C cirrhosis who have developed complications, in the absence of any contraindications (669). Data in support of this suggestion are lacking, however. Child's class C cirrhosis does not warrant a prediction of death within 1 year, as we reported in 1992 and 1995 (545,547) and as the high long-term survival rate of the class C patients in our studies demonstrates. Furthermore, in patients with intractable cirrhotic ascites, there is good reason to try SSPCS and, subsequently, to perform OLT if the shunt fails or if liver function deteriorates.

Despite the suggestion that direct PCS should be avoided in potential candidates for OLT, at least six recent studies have shown that previous PSS, regardless of type, had no influence on the outcome of OLT (669–674). Aboujaoude and colleagues emphasized that thrombosis of a PSS may seriously compromise performance of OLT, so that long-term shunt patency should be the main factor that determines the type of shunt selected for the potential OLT candidate (674). It is appropriate to emphasize again that direct PCS has had a thrombosis rate of 0.5% or less in all of our studies, compared with occlusion rates of 24–53% for mesocaval interposition shunts (675–677) and 14–23% for distal splenorenal shunts (678) in RCTs reported in the literature.

There has been no reported experience with the use of OLT specifically for treatment of intractable cirrhotic ascites. OLT must be considered a therapeutic option when other forms of therapy have failed and the patient meets the eligibility criteria for transplantation. There is no doubt that OLT will relieve intractable ascites, but the indications for the use of OLT are related to the severity and progression of the underlying liver disease rather than to the presence of ascites.

It is our conclusion that SSPCS is very effective treatment of intractable ascites from cirrhosis. Our results are attributable to careful selection of patients, an organized system of care, and a program of rigorous, lifelong follow-up that emphasizes abstinence from alcohol and dietary protein restriction.

7. Budd–Chiari Syndrome

Budd–Chiari syndrome (BCS) is a group of disorders in which obstruction to hepatic venous outflow results from occlusion of the hepatic veins and/or the adjacent IVC. Although in many cases of BCS no etiologic or predisposing condition can be identified, in recent years an underlying disorder has been found in more than half of the cases. The most common conditions that predispose to BCS are hematologic disorders with thrombotic tendencies such as polycythemia rubra vera and paroxysmal nocturnal hemoglobinuria, use of oral contraceptives, and pregnancy and the postpartum period. The pathologic lesion of BCS is thrombosis of the major hepatic veins and/or the IVC, which results in hepatic venous outflow obstruction, intrahepatic and PH, dilatation of the liver sinusoids, intense centrilobular congestion of the hepatic parenchyma, and ischemia, pressure necrosis, and atrophy of the parenchymal cells in the center of the liver lobule. Early in the course of BCS, these lesions are reversible if the obstruction is relieved. However, persistence of the high pressure and congestion within the liver results in irreversible damage, hepatic fibrosis, and progression to cirrhosis, often within a matter of months. The two paramount dangers in BCS are development of irreversible liver damage and extension of thrombosis from the hepatic veins into the IVC.

The clinical course of BCS in North America is most commonly acute, with rapid progression of liver disease and its consequences over periods ranging from a few weeks to a few months. In some patients, however, BCS develops insidiously and progresses over months or years. The usual clinical manifestations are abdominal distension due to massive ascites, hepatomegaly, abdominal pain, weakness, wasting and anorexia. When the IVC is obstructed, an important additional sign is edema of the lower extremities and lower trunk. In the chronic forms of BCS, all of the manifestations of cirrhosis of the liver are found. Many patients with BCS die within months of the onset of signs and symptoms. Survivors of the acute phase of BCS usually develop cirrhosis and often die of liver failure or bleeding esophagogastric varices within a few years. Unless the liver is decompressed or replaced, few patients with the types of BCS usually encountered in North America survive more than a few years (679–682).

The diagnosis of BCS in the initial weeks and months is based on finding the typical symptoms and signs combined with abnormal results of several diagnostic studies, the two most important of which are angiographic examination of the IVC and hepatic veins with pressure measurements and percutaneous needle biopsy of the liver. In BCS confined to the hepatic veins, IVC studies show a patent IVC and pressure that is substantially lower than WHVP, whereas in BCS involving the IVC, cavography demonstrates an area of IVC obstruction and IVC pressure is markedly elevated. Hepatic venography shows occlusion of the major hepatic veins. WHVP is markedly elevated. Liver biopsy reveals the typical lesion of obstruction to hepatic venous outflow, namely, intense centrilobular congestion and centrilobular loss of parenchyma and necrosis.

Decompression of the liver by nonoperative measures is rarely, if ever, feasible. The prognosis of BCS with nonoperative therapy is poor. In his large collective review in 1959, Parker wrote: "The majority of cases have proved fatal and there is little evidence to suggest that recovery from occlusion of the major hepatic veins occurs once symptoms have been produced" (679). Similarly, in 1975, Tavill *et al.* wrote: "The prognosis of the Budd–Chiari syndrome is almost uniformly bad . . . " (680) and in 1982, Mitchell *et al.* stated in their collective review: "Spontaneous resolution of hepatic vein occlusion rarely if ever occurs. Conventional medical therapy does little to reverse the pathophysiology in patients with hepatic vein occlusion" (681).

Because of the failure of all forms of nonoperative therapy, we took the problem to the experimental research laboratory. We produced BCS in dogs by our technique of direct ligation of all hepatic veins except the large left hepatic vein, which was loosely surrounded by an ameroid constrictor (51,53). Within 35–53 days, the hygroscopic ameroid constrictor completely occluded the remaining left hepatic vein and produced full-blown BCS. We then studied surgical methods of portal decompression in three groups of dogs with established BCS: group I, sham laparotomy; group II, end-to-side PCS; group III, SSPCS (54). Table XVII summarizes the results. SSPCS, which converts the valveless PV into an outflow tract and allows reversal of portal blood flow, cured BCS in 96% of the dogs. SSPCS relieved ascites, reduced liver size to normal, reversed the pathologic lesions in the liver often to normal, and resulted in long-term survival of many of the dogs (54).

These experimental findings served as the basis for our use of SSPCS in patients with BCS (683–686). From 1972 to 1999, we conducted a prospective unrandomized study of the treatment of 65 patients with BCS divided into three groups: I (n = 32) had occlusion confined to the hepatic veins, and they were treated by direct SSPCS; II (n = 18) had occlusion involving the IVC as well as the hepatic veins, and they were treated by a portal decompressive procedure that bypassed the obstructed IVC; III (n = 15) were patients with advanced cirrhosis and hepatic decompensation who were referred too late for treatment by portal decompression and required liver transplantation (LT). The patients were treated according to a well-defined protocol. Data were collected online and recorded on standard data forms for analysis. Follow-up was 100%. Every year or two in follow-up,

Table XVII Reaccumulation of Ascites in Dogs with BCS Following Sham Laparotomy, End-to-Side Portacaval Shunt, and Side-to-Side Portacaval Shunt[a]

		Ascites at operation			Ascites at autopsy		
			Volume (L)			Volume (L)	
Group	Number of dogs	Percentage of group	Mean	Range	Reaccumulation percentage of group	Mean	Range
I, sham laparotomy	20	100	3.2	2.2–5.3	100	3.4	1.4–7.2
II, end-to-side shunt	20	100	3.0	2.0–5.7	100	3.8	1.6–6.8
III, side-to-side shunt	24	100	3.3	2.5–6.2	4	1.4	1.4

[a]From Ref. (54), M.J. Orloff and K.H. Johansen (1978). Treatment of Budd-Chiari syndrome by side-to-side portacaval shunt:Experimental and clinical results. *Ann. Surg.* **188**, 494–512.

patients underwent liver biopsy and determinations of shunt patency by duplex Doppler ultrasonography and angiography with pressure measurements.

Table XVIII shows long-term results in the 50 patients in groups I and II who underwent portal decompression operations. In 32 patients with BCS due to hepatic vein occlusion alone, SSPCS had an operative mortality rate of 3%, and 94% of the patients are currently alive 3.5–27 years postoperatively. All 31 survivors have remained free of ascites and almost all have normal liver function. No patient with a patent shunt has had PSE. The SSPCS has remained patent in all but one patient. Liver biopsies have shown no evidence of congestion or necrosis, and 48% of the biopsies were diagnosed as normal.

In group II, mesoatrial shunt with a 16-mm ring-reinforced Gore-Tex prosthesis was performed in 8 patients with BCS caused by thrombosis of the IVC. All patients survived the operation, but 5 of 8 (63%) subsequently developed thrombosis of the synthetic graft and died. Others have reported thrombosis of the mesoatrial shunt in 40–70% of patients, an event that is often followed by death (687–692). Because of the poor results, we abandoned mesoatrial shunt and took the problem to the experimental research laboratory in hopes of devising an effective surgical procedure for treatment of BCS due to IVC occlusion (49). We produced BCS by gradual occlusion of the suprahepatic IVC with an ameroid constrictor in rats with massive ascites, hepatomegaly, and portal hypertension that were divided into three groups: group I, sham thoracolaparotomy; group II, mesoatrial shunt; group III, combined SSPCS and caval–atrial shunt (CAS) from the IVC to the right atrium with a 3-mm polytetrafluoroethylene (Gore-Tex) graft. Figure 16 summarizes the results. All control rats in group I reaccumulated ascites and died within 2 months. Nine of 16 rats with mesoatrial shunts in group II reformed ascites and died within 2 months. All of these animals were found at autopsy to have thrombosis of the mesoatrial graft. In contrast, only 2 of 16 rats treated by combined PCS and CAS in group III developed CAS graft thrombosis, reformed ascites, and died. The remaining 14 rats in group III were found to have patent grafts and shunts when they were killed after 3 months. Liver biopsies in all rats prior to IVC constriction were normal and, after BCS was well established, showed intense centrilobular congestion and moderate central necrosis. Severe pathologic changes persisted until death or sacrifice in all control rats in group I and in 11 of 16 rats with mesoatrial shunts in group II. However, combined PCS and CAS in group III reversed the liver pathology in 14 of 16 rats.

These experimental findings led us to introduce the high-flow combination SSPCS with CAS for treatment of 10 patients with BCS due to IVC occlusion (49) (Fig. 17). There have been no operative or long-term deaths, and the shunts have functioned effectively during 4–16 years of follow-up. Permanent anticoagulation therapy has been used in all patients with synthetic grafts.

Table XVIII Long-Term Results of Portal Decompression Operations in 50 Patients with BCS

		IVC and hepatic vein occlusion	
	Hepatic vein occlusion alone, SSPCS	Mesoatrial shunt	Combined SSPCS and CAS
Number of patients	32	8	10
Onset to operation			
<17 weeks (%)	91	88	100
Mean number of weeks	14.5	12	13
Range (weeks)	4–78	7–19	10–15
Follow-up (years)			
Mean	13.6	17	9
Range	3.5–27	15–19	4–16
Ascites (%)	0	3	63
Need for diuretics (%)	3	63	0
Abnormal liver function tests (%)	10	63	0
Portosystemic encephalopathy (%)	3	38	0
Employed or housekeeping (%)	94	25	100
Survival (%)			
30 days	97	100	100
Current	94	38	100

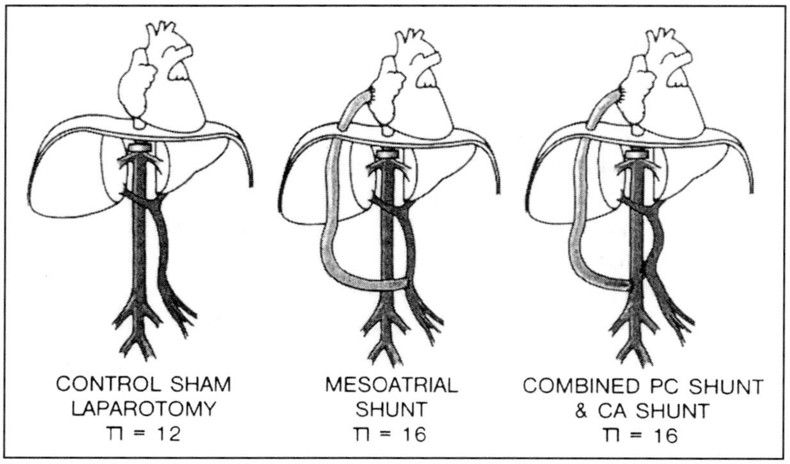

Results of Treatment of Experimental Budd-Chiari Syndrome in Rats Produced by Inferior Vena Cava Occlusion

Group	No. of Rats	Graft or Shunt Thrombosis	Re-formed Ascites	Survived 3 Months	Reversal of Liver Pathology
I. Sham thoracolaparotomy	12	--	12	0	0
II. Mesoatrial shunt	16	9	9	7	5
III. Combined portacaval shunt and caval-atrial shunt	16	2	2	14	14

Figure 16 Results of treatment of experimental BCS produced by suprahepatic IVC occlusion in rats. Reprinted from Ref. (49), *Am. J. Surg.* **163**; Orloff, M.J., Daily, P.O., and Girard, B.; Treatment of Budd-Chiari syndrome due to inferior vena cava occlusion by combined portal and vena caval decompression, pp. 137–143. Copyright 1992, with permission from Excerpta Medica Inc.

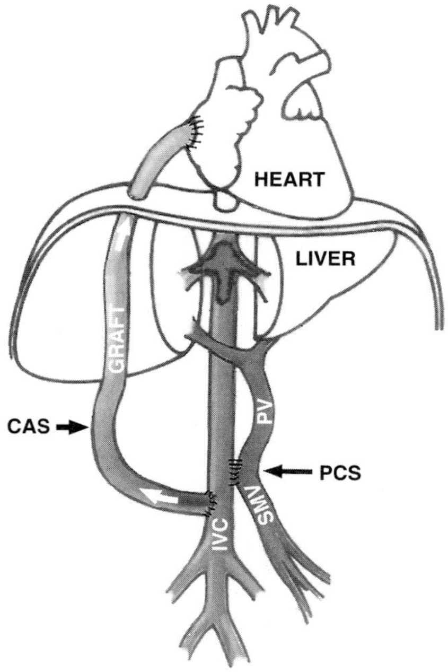

Figure 17 Combined side-to-side portacaval shunt (PCS) and caval–atrial shunt (CAS) with a Gore-Tex graft. Reprinted from Ref. (49), *Am. J. Surg.* **163**; Orloff, M.J., Daily, P.O., and Girard, B.; Treatment of Budd-Chiari syndrome due to inferior vena cava occlusion by combined portal and vena caval decompression, pp. 137–143. Copyright 1992, with permission from Excerpta Medica Inc.

Fifteen patients with advanced cirrhosis in Child's class C were referred too late to benefit from surgical portal decompression, and they were approved and listed for LT. Four patients died from liver failure while on the list awaiting LT, and five patients died after LT. The 5-year survival rate was 40%. The indications for LT that we have adhered to are as follows; (1) cirrhosis with progressive liver failure that has reached the point of permitting a reasonable prediction that the patient will die within 1 year; (2) failure of SSPCS, usually because of thrombosis, with persistence or recurrence of symptoms and signs of BCS; (3) unshuntable PH due to thrombosis of the PV, splenic vein, and much of the superior mesenteric vein, a rare indication that applies if patent blood vessels are available to vascularize the liver allograft; and (4) acute fulminant hepatic failure, a rare indication. It should be emphasized that LT and SSPCS are not competing forms of treatment. SSPCS is the appropriate treatment in the early and middle stages of BCS when portal decompression will sustain life by reversing or stabilizing the liver disease. LT is the appropriate treatment in the late stages of BCS when the liver disease is no longer reversible and when stabilization of progressive hepatic decompensation is not possible. By and large, patients who are candidates for LT should be in Child's class C.

Experience with TIPS in the treatment of BCS is small, most of the reports have been anecdotal, and follow-up generally has been of short duration. The only sizeable series of cases that has been reported is that of the group in Freiburg, Germany (693,694), which included 26 patients, 5 with acute BCS and 21 with chronic BCS. Three of the acute patients died within 10 days (60%) and 3 of the chronic patients died (14%), for an overall mortality rate of 23%. Two patients required LT. During follow-up of 1–6 years (mean 697 days), half of the patients required revision of the TIPS because of stenosis. Although the Freiburg group concluded that TIPS resolves the symptoms and is "safe and effective," the results are not comparable to those of surgical PSS. In the opinion of the author, it is doubtful that TIPS will become an acceptable alternative to surgical treatment of BCS. The key to long survival in BCS is prompt treatment by surgical portal decompression.

References

1. Greenway, C. V., and Stark, R. D. (1971). Hepatic vascular bed. *Physiol. Rev.* **51,** 23–65.
2. Lautt, W. W., and Greenway, C. V. (1988). Hepatic circulation in homeostasis. *In* "The Kidney in Liver Disease" (Epstein, M. Ed.), pp. 244–261. Williams & Wilkins, Baltimore.
3. Groszmann, R. J. (1996). The hepatic venous pressure gradient: Has the time arrived for its application in clinical practice? *Hepatology* **24,** 740–741.
4. Groszmann, R. J., Bosch, J., Grace, N., Conn, H. O., Garcia-Tsao, G., Navasa, M., Albert, J., *et al.* (1998). Hemodynamic events in a prospective randomized trial of propranolol vs. placebo in the prevention of the first variceal hemorrhage. *Gastroenterology* **99,** 1401–1407.
5. Feu, F., García-Pagán, J. C., Bosch, J., Luca, A., Terés, J., Escorsell, A., and Rodés, J. (1995). Relation between portal pressure response to pharmacotherapy and risk of recurrent variceal haemorrhage in patients with cirrhosis. *Lancet* **346,** 1056–1059.
6. Garcia-Tsao, G., Groszmann, R. J., Fisher, R., Conn, H. O., Atterbury, C. E., and Glickmann, M. (1985). Portal pressure, presence of gastroesophageal varices and variceal bleeding. *Hepatology* **5,** 419–424.
7. Viallet, A., Marleau, D., Huet, M., Martin, F., Farley, A., Villeneuve, J. P., and Lavoie, P. (1975). Haemodynamic evaluation of patients with intrahepatic portal hypertension: Relationship between bleeding varices and portohepatic gradient. *Gastroenterology* **69,** 1297–1300.
8. Popper, H. (1977). Pathologic aspects of cirrhosis, a review. *Am. J. Pathol.* **87,** 228–258.
9. Bell, R. H., Jr., Miyai, K., and Orloff, M. J. (1982). Response of cirrhotic patients with acute alcoholic hepatitis to emergency portacaval shunt for bleeding varices. *Gastroenterology* **82,** 1015.
10. Miyai, K., Bell, R. H., Jr., and Orloff, M. J. (1982). Relationship of portal hypertension to hepatic venous outflow obstruction in patients with cirrhosis and bleeding varices. *Gastroenterology* **84,** 1237.
11. Bell, R. H., Miyai, K., and Orloff, M. J. (1984). Outcome in cirrhotic patients with acute alcoholic hepatitis after emergency portacaval shunt for bleeding esophageal varices. *Am. J. Surg.* **147,** 78–84.
12. Groszmann, R. J., and Atterbury, C. E. (1982). The pathophysiology of portal hypertension: A basis for classification. *Semin. Liver. Dis.* **2,** 177–186.
13. Tsukamoto, H., Matsuoka, M., and French, S. W. (1990). Experimental models of hepatic fibrosis: A review. *Semin. Liver Dis.* **10,** 56–65.
14. Proctor, E., and Chatambra, K. (1984). Standardized micronodular cirrhosis in the rat. *Eur. Surg. Res.* **16,** 182–186.
15. McLean, E., McLean, A. E. M., and Sutton, P. M. (1969). Instant cirrhosis: An improved method for producing cirrhosis of the liver in rats by simultaneous administration of carbon tetrachloride and phenobarbitone. *Br. J. Exp. Pathol.* **50,** 502–506.
16. López-Novoa, J. M., Navarro, V., Rodicio, J. L., and Hernando, L. (1976). Cirrosis experimental de instauracion rápida. Cronologia de aparición de las lesiónes hepáticas. *Patología* **9,** 233–240.
17. López-Novoa, J. M., Rengel, M. A., Rodicio, J. L., and Hernando, L. (1977). A micropuncture study of salt and water retention in chronic experimental cirrhosis. *Am. J. Physiol.* **232,** F315-F318.
18. López-Novoa, J. M. (1988). Pathophysiological features of the carbon tetrachloride/phenobarbital model of experimental liver cirrhosis in rats. *In* "The Kidney in Liver Disease" (Epstein, M., Ed.), pp. 309–327. Williams & Wilkins, Baltimore.
19. Levy, M. (1977). Sodium retention and ascites formation in dogs with experimental portal cirrhosis. *Am. J. Physiol.* **233,** F572–F585.
20. Groszmann, R. J., Kravetz, D., Bosch, J., Glickman, M., Briux, J., Bredfelt, J., Conn, H. O., Rodes, J., and Storer, E. H. (1982). Nitroglycerin improves the hemodynamic response to vasopression in portal hypertension. *Hepatology* **2,** 757–762.
21. Shibayama, J., and Nakata, K. (1991). The role of pericentral fibrosis in experimental portal hypertension in rats. *Liver* **11,** 94–99.
22. Fitzhugh, O. G., and Nelson, A. A. (1998). Liver tumors in rats fed thiourea or thioacetamide. *Science* **108,** 626–628.
23. Dashti, H., Jeppsson, B., Hagerstrand, J., Hultberg, B., Srinivas, U., Abdulla, M., *et al.* (1989). Thioacetamide- and carbon tetrachloride-induced liver cirrhosis. *Eur. Surg. Res.* **21,** 83–91.
24. Nuber, R., Teutsch, H. F., and Sasse, D. (1980). Metabolic zonation in thioacetamide-induced liver cirrhosis. *Histochemistry* **69,** 277–288.
25. Perazzo, J., Eizayaga, F., Romay, S., Bengochea, L., Pavese, A., and Lemberg, A. (1999). An experimental model of liver damage and portal hypertension induced by a single dose of monocrotaline. *Hepatogastroenterol* **46,** 432–435.
26. Rubin, E., and Lieber, C. S. (1974). Fatty liver, alcoholic hepatitis and cirrhosis produced by alcohol in primates. *N. Engl. J. Med.* **290,** 128–135.
27. Lieber, C. S., and DeCarli, C. M. (1982). The feeding of alcohol in liquid diets: Two decades of applications and 1982 update. *Alcoholism (NY)* **6,** 523–531.
28. Popper, H., and Lieber, C. S. (1980). Histogenesis of alcoholic fibrosis and cirrhosis in the baboon. *Am. J. Pathol.* **98,** 695–716.
29. Lieber, C. S., DeCarli, C. M., and Rubin, E. (1975). Sequential production of fatty liver, hepatitis, and cirrhosis in subhuman primates fed ethanol with adequate diets. *Proc. Natl. Acad. Sci. U.S.A.* **72,** 437–441.
30. Tsukamoto, H., French, S. W., Benson, N., *et al.* (1985). Severe and progressive steatosis and focal necrosis in rat liver induced by continuous intragastric infusion of ethanol and low fat diet. *Hepatology* **5,** 224–232.
31. French, S. W., Miyamoto, K., and Tsukamoto, H. (1986). Ethanol-induced hepatic fibrosis in the rat: Role of the amount of dietary fat. *Alcoholism (NY)* **10,** 13S–19S.
32. Bras, G., and McLean, E. (1963). Toxic factors in veno-occlusive disease. *Ann. NY Acad. Sci.* **3,** 392–396.
33. Bras, G., Jelliffe, D. B., and Stuart, K. L. (1954). Veno-occlusive disease of the liver with non-portal type of cirrhosis occurring in Jamaica. *Arch Pathol.* **57,** 285–300.
34. Bosch, J., Enriquez, R., Groszmann, R. J., and Storer, E. H. (1983). Chronic bile duct ligation in the dog: Hemodynamic characterization of a portal hypertensive model. *Hepatology* **3,** 1002–1007.
35. Easter, D. W., Wade, J. B., and Boyer, J. L. (1983). Structural integrity of hepatocyte tight junctions. *J. Cell. Biol.* **96,** 745–749.
36. Fernández, M., Pizcueta, P., Garcia-Pagán, J. C., Feu, F., Cirera, I., Bosch, J., and Rodés, J. (1993). Effects of ritanserin, a selective and specific S2-serotoninergic antagonist, on portal pressure and splanchnic hemodynamics in rats with long-term bile duct ligation. *Hepatology* **18,** 389–393.
37. Fernández, M., García-Pagán, J. C., Casadevall, M., Bernadich, C., Piera, C., Whittle, B. J. R., Piqué, J. M., *et al.* (1995). Evidence against a role for inducible nitric oxide synthase in the hyperdynamic circulation of portal-hypertensive rats. *Gastroenterology* **108,** 1487–1495.

38. Fallon, M. B., Abrams, G. A., McGrath, J. W., Hou, Z., and Luo, B. (1997). Common bile duct ligation in the rat: A model of intrapulmonary vasodilatation and hepatopulmonary syndrome. *Am. J. Physiol.* **272,** G779–G784.
39. Nishida, R., Inoue, R., Takimoto, Y., and Kita, T. (1998). Esophageal varices in rat models of liver cirrhosis. *Dig. Dis. Sci.* **43,** 296–1301.
40. Chojkier, M., and Groszmann, R. J. (1981). Measurement of portal-systemic shunting in the rat by using gamma-labeled microspheres. *Am. J. Physiol.* **240,** G371–G375.
41. Lower, R. (1720). "Tractatus du corde, item de motu et colore sanguinis," 6th ed, p. 127. J. Martyn, London.
42. Bolton, C. (1907). Pathology of dropsy produced by obstruction of the superior and inferior venae cavae and the portal vein. *Proc. R. Soc. London* **79,** 267–283.
43. McKee, F. W., Schloerb, P. R., Schilling, J. A., Tishkoff, G. H., and Whipple, G. H. (1948). Protein metabolism and exchange as influenced by constriction of the vena cava. *J. Exp. Med.* **87,** 457–471.
44. Freeman, S. (1953). Recent progress in the physiology and biochemistry of the liver. *Med. Clin. North Am.* **37,** 109–124.
45. Mallet-Guy, P., Devic, G., Feroldi, J., and Desjacques, P. (1954). Étude expérimentale des ascites; sténoses veineuses post-hépatiques et transposition du foie dans le thorax. *Lyon Chir.* **49,** 153–172.
46. Hyatt, R. E., and Smith, J. R. (1954). The mechanism of ascites: a physiologic appraisal. *Am. J. Med.* **16,** 434–438.
47. Gray, H. K. (1951). Clinical and experimental investigation of the circulation of the liver. *Ann. R. Coll. Surg. Engl.* **8,** 354–365.
48. Nix, J. T., Flock, E. V., and Bollman, J. L. (1951). Influence of cirrhosis on proteins of cisternal lymph. *Am. J. Physiol.* **164,** 117–118.
49. Orloff, M. J., Daily, P. O., and Girard, B. (1992). Treatment of Budd-Chiari syndrome due to inferior vena cava occlusion by combined portal and vena caval decompression. *Am. J. Surg.* **163,** 137–143.
50. Orloff, M. J., and Snyder, G. B. (1961). Experimental ascites. I. Production of ascites by gradual occlusion of the hepatic veins with an internal vena caval cannula. *Surgery* **50,** 789–797.
51. Orloff, M. J., Wall, M. H., Hickman, E. G., and Spitz, B. R. (1963). Experimental ascites. III. Production of ascites by direct ligation of the hepatic veins. *Surgery* **54,** 627–639.
52. Orloff, M. J., Baddeley, R. M., Ross, T. H., Nutting, R. O., Thomas, H. S., Halasz, N. A., and Sloop, R. D. (1965). Experimental ascites. V. Production of hepatic outflow block and ascites with an hepatic vein choker. *Ann. Surg.* **161,** 258–262.
53. Sweat, E. R., Musicant, M. D., Annetts, D. L., Goodhead, B., and Orloff, M. J. (1966). Production of hepatic outflow block and ascites with an ameroid constrictor. *Surg. Forum* **17,** 376–378.
54. Orloff, M. J., and Johansen, K. H. (1978). Treatment of Budd-Chiari syndrome by side-to-side portacaval shunt: Experimental and clinical results. *Ann. Surg.* **188,** 494–512.
55. Orloff, M. J., Orloff, M. S., Orloff, S. L., and Girard, B. (1997). Experimental, clinical, and metabolic results of side-to-side portacaval shunt for intractable cirrhotic ascites. *J. Am. Coll. Surg.* **184,** 557–570.
56. Warren, J. V., and Brannon, E. S. (1944). A method of obtaining blood samples directly from the hepatic vein in man. *Proc. Soc. Exp. Biol. Med.* **55,** 144–146.
57. Myers, J. D., and Taylor, W. J. (1951). An estimation of portal venous pressure by occlusive catheterization of an hepatic venule. *J. Clin. Invest.* **30,** 662–663.
58. Paton, A., Reynolds, T. B., and Sherlock, S. (1953). Assessment of portal venous hypertension by catheterization of hepatic vein. *Lancet* **1,** 918–921.
59. Sherlock, S. (1954). Portal circulation in cirrhosis. *Gastroenterologica (Basel)* **81,** 84–85.
60. Reynolds, T. B., Ito, S., and Iwatsuki, S. (1970). Measurement of portal pressure and its clinical application. *Am. J. Med.* **49,** 649–657.
61. Groszmann, R. J., Glickman, M., Blei, A. T., Storer, E., and Conn, H. O. (1970). Wedged and free hepatic venous pressure measured with a balloon catheter. *Gastroenterology* **76,** 254–258.
62. Merkel, C., Bolognese, M., Bellon, S., Zuin, R., Noventa, F., Finucci, G, Sacerdoti, D., *et al.* (1992). Prognostic usefulness of hepatic vein catheterisation in patients with cirrhosis and esophageal varices. *Gastroenterology* **102,** 973–979.
63. Barrett, G., Bosch, J., Garcia-Tsao, G., Groszmann, R. J., Richardson, C. R., Navasa, M., Rodes, J. *et al.* (1990). Hepatic venous pressure gradient (HVPG) as a predictor of survival in patients with cirrhosis. *Hepatology* **12,** 850A.
64. Vorobioff, J., Groszmann, R. J., Picabea, E., Villavicencio, R., Passamonti, M., Lerner, E., and Tanno, H. (1994). Prognostic value of sequential measurement of portal pressure in alcoholic cirrhotic patients. *Hepatology* **20,** 103A.
65. Atkinson, M., and Sherlock, S. (1954). Intrasplenic pressure as an index of portal venous pressure. *Lancet* **1,** 1325–1327.
66. Atkinson, M., Barnett, E., Sherlock, S., and Steiner, R. E. (1955). The clinical investigation of the portal circulation with special reference to portal venography. *O. J. Med.* **24,** 77–94.
67. Turner, M. D., Sherlock, S., and Steiner, R. E. (1957). Splenic venography and intrasplenic pressure measurement in the clinical investigation of the portal venous system. *Am. J. Med.* **23,** 846–859.
68. Boyer, T. D., Triger, D. R., Horisawa, M., Redeker, A. G., and Reynolds, T. B. (1977). Direct transhepatic measurement of portal vein pressure using a thin needle. *Gastroenterology* **72,** 584–589.
69. White, L. P., Phear, S., Summerskill, W. H. J., and Sherlock, S. (1955). Clinical investigation of portal circulation with special reference to portal venography. *O. J. Med.* **24,** 77–82.
70. Summerskill, W. H. J., Davidson, E. D., Sherlock, S., and Steiner, R. E. (1956). Neuropsychiatric syndrome associated with hepatic cirrhosis and extensive portal collateral circulation. *O. J. Med.* **25,** 245–266.
71. Becker, C. D., and Cooperberg, P. L. (1988). Sonography of the hepatic vascular system. *Am. J. Roentgenol.* **150,** 999–1005.
72. Foley, W. D., and Erickson, S. J. (1991). Color Doppler flow imaging. *Am. J. Roentgenol.* **156,** 3–13.
73. Grant, E. G., Schiller, V. L., Millener, P., *et al.* (1992). Color Doppler imaging of the hepatic vasculature. *Am. J. Roentgenol.* **159,** 943–950.
74. Koslin, D. B., Mulligan, S. A., and Berland, L. L. (1992). Duplex assessment of the portal venous system. *Semin. Ultrasound CT MR* **13,** 22–33.
75. Merritt, C. R. B. (1992). Doppler color imaging. *Clin. Diagn. Ultrasound* **27,** 1–6.
76. Ralls, P. W. (1990). Color Doppler sonography of the hepatic artery and portal venous system. *Am. J. Roentgenol.* **155,** 517–525.
77. Ralls, P. W., and Mack, L. A. (1992). Spectral and color Doppler sonography. *Semin. Ultrasound CT MR* **13,** 355–366.
78. Vlamonte, M., Jr. LePage, J., Lunderquist, A., *et al.* (1975). Selective catheterization of the portal vein and its tributaries: Preliminary report. *Radiology* **114,** 457–460.
79. Smith-Laing, G., Camilo, M., Dick, R., and Sherlock, S. (1980). Percutaneous transhepatic portography in the assessment of portal hypertension. Clinical correlations and comparison of radiographic techniques. *Gastroenterology* **78,** 197–205.
80. Smith-Laing, G., Scott, J., Long, R. G., Dick, R., and Sherlock, S. (1981). Role of percutaneous transhepatic obliteration of varices in the management of hemorrhage from gastroesophageal varices. *Gastroenterology* **80,** 1031–1036.
81. Bradley, S. E., Inglefinger, F. J., Bradley, G. P., *et al.* (1945). Estimation of hepatic blood flow in man. *J. Clin. Invest.* **24,** 890–897.
82. Bradley, E. I., III. (1974). Measurements of hepatic blood flow in man. *Surgery* **75,** 783–789.
83. Caesar, J., Shaldon, S., Chianducci, L., Guevara, L., and Sherlock, S. (1961). The use of indocyanine green in the measurement of hepatic blood flow as a test of hepatic function. *Clin. Sci.* **21,** 43–57.

84. Combes, B. (1960). Estimation of hepatic blood flow in man and dogs by ^{131}I-labeled rose bengal: Simultaneous comparison with sulfobromophthalein sodium. *J. Lab. Clin. Med.* **56,** 537–543.
85. Winkler, K., Larsen, J. A., Munkner, T., *et al.* (1965). Determination of the hepatic blood flow in man by simultaneous use of five test substances measured in two parts of the liver. *Scand. J. Clin. Lab. Invest.* **17,** 423–432.
86. Tygstrup, N., and Winkler, K. (1958). Galactose blood clearance as a measure of hepatic blood flow. *Clin. Sci.* **17,** 1–9.
87. Huet, P. M., Lavoie, P., and Viallet, A. (1973). Simultaneous estimation of portal and hepatic blood flows by an indicator dilution technique. *J. Lab. Clin. Med.* **82,** 836–846.
88. Shaldon, S., Chiundussi, L., Guevara, L., *et al.* (1961). The estimation of hepatic blood flow and intrahepatic shunted blood flow by colloidal heat-denatured human serum albumin labeled with ^{131}I. *J. Clin. Invest.* **40,** 1346–1354.
89. Christie, J. H., and Chaudhuri, T. K. (1972). Measurement of hepatic blood flow. *Semin. Nucl. Med.* **2,** 97–107.
90. Cohn, J. N., Khatri, I. M., Groszman, R. J., *et al.* (1972). Hepatic blood flow in alcoholic liver disease measured by an indicator dilution technique. *Am. J. Med.* **53,** 704–714.
91. Dobson, E. L., and Jones, H. B. (1952). The behavior of intravenously injected particulate matter: Its rate of disappearance from the blood stream as a measure of liver blood flow. *Acta Med. Scand.* **373** (144 Suppl), 1–71.
92. Vetter, H., Falkner, R., Neumayr, A. (1954). The disappearance rate of colloidal radiogold from the circulation and its application to the estimation of liver blood flow in normal and cirrhotic subjects. *J. Clin. Invest.* **33,** 1594–1602.
93. Fellinger, K., Gisinger, E., and Vetter, H. (1956). Der Stoffwechsel Fe 59—Markerten Kolloidalen Eisen-Saccharates beim Menschen. *In* "Radioaktive Isotope in Klinik und Forschung" (Fellinger, K., and Vetter, H., Eds.), Vol. II, p. 13. Urban and Schwarzenberg, München.
94. Mundschenk, H., Hromec, A., and Fisher, J. (1971). Phagocytic activity of the liver as a measure of hepatic circulation. A comparative study using ^{198}Au and ^{99m}Tc–sulfur colloid. *J. Nucl. Med.* **12,** 711–718.
95. Torrance, H. B., and Gowenlock, A. H. (1962). Radioactive colloidal clearance techniques to measure liver blood flow in man. *Clin. Sci.* **22,** 413–423.
96. Ueda, H., Unuma, T., Ilio, M., *et al.* (1962). Measurement of hepatic arterial and portal blood flow and circulation time via hepatic artery and portal vein with radioisotope. *Jpn. Heart J.* **3,** 154–166.
97. Reichman, S., Davis, W. D., Storaash, J. P., *et al.* (1950). Measurement of hepatic blood flow by indicator dilution techniques. *J. Clin. Invest.* **37,** 1848–1856.
98. Jacobs, R. R., Schmitz, A., Heydon, W. C., *et al.* (1968). A comparison of the accuracies in the electro-magnetic flowmeter and in the cardiogreen dilution blood flow measurement techniques in a model. *Surg Forum* **19,** 113–115.
99. Visscher, M. B., and Johnson, J. A. (1953). The Fick principle: Analysis of potential errors and its conventional applications. *J. Appl. Physiol.* **5,** 635–638.
100. Popper, H., Elias, H., and Petty, D. E. (1952). Vascular pattern of the cirrhotic liver. *Am. J. Clin. Pathol.* **22,** 717–729.
101. Schenk, W. G., McDonald, J. C., McDonald, K., *et al.* (1962). Direct measurement of hepatic blood flow in surgical patients, with related observations on hepatic flow dynamics in experimental animals. *Ann. Surg.* **156,** 463–471.
102. Reichle, F. A., Sovak, M., Soulen, R. L., *et al.* (1972). Portal vein blood flow determination in the unanesthetized human by umbilicoportal cannulation. *J. Surg. Res.* **12,** 146–150.
103. Graf, W. (1959). Patterns of human temperature. *Acta Physiol. Scand.* **160,** (46 Suppl 1), 1–135.
104. Chiandussi, L., Freco, F., Sardi, G., Vaccarino, A., Ferraris, C. M., and Curti, B. (1968). Estimation of hepatic arterial and portal venous blood flow by direct catheterization of the vena porta through the umbilical vein in man. *Acta Hepato-Splenologica* **15,** 166–171.
105. Burchell, A. R., Moreno, A. H., Panke, W. F., Nealon, T. F. (1974). Hemodynamic variables and prognosis following portacaval shunts. *Surg. Obstet. Gynecol.* **138,** 359–369.
106. Burchell, A. R., Moreno, A. H., Panke, W. F., and Nealon, T. F. (1976). Hepatic artery flow improvement after portacaval shunt—A single hemodynamic clinical correlate. *Ann. Surg.* **184,** 289–302.
107. Mena, I., Bennett, L. R., Reynolds, T. B., Redeker, A. G., and Mellinkoff, S. M. (1960). Analysis of cardioportal circulation time by means of simultaneous direct hepatic venous counting. *N. Engl. J. Med.* **263,** 940–943.
108. Biersack, H. J., Torres, J., Thelen, M., Monzon, O., and Winkler, C. (1981). Determination of liver and spleen perfusion by quantitative sequential scintigraphy: Results in normal subjects and in patients with portal hypertension. *Clin. Nucl. Med.* **6,** 218–220.
109. Rypins, E. G., Fajman, W., Serper, R., Henderson, J. M., Kulner, M. J., Tarcan, Y. A., Galambos, J. T., and Warren, W. D. (1981). Radionuclide angiography of the liver and spleen—Noninvasive method for assessing the ratio of portal venous to total hepatic blood flow and portasystemic shunt patency. *Am. J. Surg.* **142,** 574–579.
110. Bolognesi, M., Sacerdoti, D., Merkel, C., and Gatta, A. (1995). Relationship between portal blood flow measured by image-directed Doppler ultrasonography and hepatic blood flow measured by indocyanine green constant infusion in patients with cirrhosis. *J. Clin. Ultrasound* **23,** 297–303.
111. Taniguchi, H., Oguro, A., Koyama, H., Masuyama, M., and Takahashi, T. (1996). Analysis of models for quantification of arterial and portal blood flow in the human liver using PET. *J. Comput. Assist. Tomog.* **20,** 135–144.
112. Nordlinger, B., Parquet, M., Infante, R., Moreels, R., Blondiau, P., Boschat, M., Groussard, M., and Huguet, C. (1982). Noninvasive measurement of nutrient portal blood shunting: An experimental study with [^{14}C]ursodeoxycholic acid. *Hepatology* **2,** 412–419.
113. Porchet, H., and Bircher, J. (1982). Noninvasive assessment of portal-systemic shunting: Evaluation of a method to investigate systemic availability of oral glyceryl trinitrate by digital plethysmography. *Gastroenterology* **82,** 629–637.
114. Hoefs, J., Sakimura, I., and Reynolds, T. B. (1979). Direct measurement of intrahepatic shunting by portal vein injection of microspheres. *Gastroenterology* **75,** 968A.
115. Bosch, J., and Groszmann, R. L. (1982). Measurement of azygos venous blood flow by a continuous thermal dilution technique: An index of blood flow through gastroesophageal collaterals in cirrhosis. *Hepatology* **2,** 424–429.
116. Popper, H., and Zak, F. G. (1958). Pathological aspects of cirrhosis. *Am. J. Med.* **24,** 593–625.
117. Baldus, W. P., and Hoffbauer, F. W. (1963). Vascular changes in the cirrhotic liver as studied by injection technique. *Am. J. Dig. Dis.* **8,** 689–692.
118. Pinzani, M., Failli, P., Ruocco, C., *et al.* (1992). Fat-storing cells as liver-specific pericytes—Spatial dynamics of agonist-stimulated intracellular calcium transients. *J. Clin. Invest.* **90,** 642–646.
119. Rudolph, R., McClure, W. J., and Woodward, M. (1979). Contractile fibroblasts in chronic alcoholic cirrhosis. *Gastroenterology* **76,** 704–709.
120. Bhathal, P. S., and Grossman, H. J. (1985). Reduction of the increased portal vascular resistance of the isolated perfused cirrhotic rat liver by vasodilators. *J. Hepatol.* **1,** 325–337.
121. Rubanyi, G. M. (1990). Endothelium-derived relaxing and contracting factors. *J. Cell. Biochem.* **46,** 27–36.
122. Vane, J. R., Anggard, E. E., and Botting, R. M. (1990). Regulatory functions of vascular endothelium. *N. Engl. J. Med.* **323,** 27–36.

123. Mittal, M. K., Gupta, T. K., Lee, F. Y., *et al.* (1994). Nitric oxide modulates vascular tone in normal rat liver. *Am. J. Physiol.* **267,** G416-G422.
124. Pannen, B. H., Bauer, M., Zhang, J. X., Robotham, J. L., and Clemens, M. G. (1996). A time-dependent balance between endothelins and nitric oxide regulating portal resistance after endotoxin. *Am. J. Physiol.* **271,** H1953–H1961.
125. Gupta, T. K., Toruner, M., Chung, M. K., and Groszmann, R. J. (1998). Endothelial dysfunction and decreased production of nitric oxide in the intrahepatic microcirculation of cirrhotic rats. *Hepatology* **28,** 926–931.
126. Shah, V., Haddad, F. G., Garcia-Cardena, G., Grangos, J. A., Mennone, A., Groszmann, R. J., *et al.* (1997). Liver sinusoidal endothelial cells are responsible for nitric oxide modulation of resistance in the hepatic sinusoids. *J. Clin. Invest.* **100,** 2923–2930.
127. Rockey, D. C., and Chung, J. J. (1998). Reduced nitric oxide production by endothelial cells in cirrhotic rat liver: Endothelial dysfunction in portal hypertension. *Gastroenterology* **114,** 344–351.
128. Garcia-Cardeña, G., Martasek, P., Siler-Masters, B. S., Skidd, P. M., Couet, J., Li, S., *et al.* (1997). Dissecting the interaction between nitric oxide synthase and caveolin. Functional significance of the NOS caveolin binding domain *in vivo. J. Biol. Chem.* **272,** 25437–25440.
129. Kowalski, H. J., and Abelman, W. H. (1953). The cardiac output at rest in Laennec cirrhosis. *J. Clin. Invest.* **32,** 1025–1033.
130. Siegel, J. H., Goldwyn, P. M., Farrell, E. J., Gallin, P., and Friedman, H. P. (1974). Hyperdynamic states and the physiologic determinants of survival in patients with cirrhosis and portal hypertension. *Arch. Surg.* **108,** 282–292.
131. Del Guercio, L. R. M., Commarawasmy, R. P., Feins, N. R., Wollman, S. B., and State, D. (1964). Pulmonary arteriovenous admixture and the hyperdynamic cardiovascular state in surgery for portal hypertension. *Surgery* **56,** 57–74.
132. Waxman, K., and Shoemaker, W. D. (1983). Physiologic determinants of operative survival after portocaval shunt. *Ann. Surg.* **197,** 72–78.
133. Colombato, L. A., Albillos, A., and Groszmann, R. J. (1992). Temporal relationship of peripheral vasodilatation, plasma volume expansion and the hyperdynamic circulatory state in portal-hypertensive rats. *Hepatology* **15,** 323–328.
134. Genecin, P., Pollo, J., Ferraioli, G., *et al.* (1990). Bile acids do not mediate the hyperdynamic circulation in portal hypertensive rats. *Am. J. Physiol.* **259,** G21–G25.
135. Benoit, J. N., Barrowman, J. A., Harper, S. L., Kvietys, P. R., and Granger, D. N. (1984). Role of humoral factors in the intestinal hyperemia associated with chronic portal hypertension. *Am. J. Physiol.* **247,** E486–E493.
136. Benoit, J. N., Womack, W. A., Hernandez, L., *et al.* (1985). "Forward" and "backward" flow mechanisms of portal hypertension. Relative contributions in the rat model of portal vein stenosis. *Gastroenterology* **89,** 1092–1096.
137. Kravetz, D., Bosch, J., Arderiu, M. T., Pizcueta, M. P., Casamitjana, R., Rivera, F., *et al.* (1988). Effects of somatostatin on splanchnic hemodynamics and plasma glucagon in portal hypertensive rats. *Am. J. Physiol.* **254,** G322–G325.
138. Benoit, J. N., Zimmerman, B., Premen, A. J., Go, V. L., and Granger, D. N. (1986). Role of glucagon in splanchnic hyperemia of chronic portal hypertension. *Am. J. Physiol.* **251,** G674–G678.
139. Gomis, R., Fernández-Alvarez, J., Pizcueta, M. P., Fernández, M., Casamitjana, R., Bosch, J., *et al.* (1994). Impaired function of pancreatic islets from rats with portal hypertension resulting from cirrhosis and partial portal vein ligation. *Hepatology* **19,** 1257–1261.
140. Silva, G., Navasa, M., Bosch, J., Chesta, J., Pizcueta, M. P., Casamitjana, R., *et al.* (1990). Hemodynamic effects of glucagon in portal hypertension. *Hepatology* **11,** 668–673.
141. Pizcueta, M. P., García-Pagán, J. C., Fernández, M., Casamitjana, R., Bosch, J., and Rodés, J. (1991). Glucagon hinders the effects of somatostatin on portal hypertension. A study in rats with partial portal vein ligation. *Gastroenterology* **101,** 1710–1715.
142. Sikuler, E., and Groszmann, R. J. (1986). Hemodynamic studies in long and short term portal hypertensive rats: The relation to systemic glucagon levels. *Hepatology* **6,** 414–418.
143. Rodriguez-Perez, F., Isales, C. M., and Groszmann, R. J. (1993). Platelet cytosolic calcium, peripheral hemodynamics, and vasodilatory peptides in liver cirrhosis. *Gastroenterology* **105,** 863–867.
144. Casadevall, M., Panes, J., Pique, J. M., *et al.* (1993). Involvement of nitric oxide and prostaglandins in gastric mucosal hyperemia of portal-hypertensive anesthetized rats. *Hepatology* **18,** 628–634.
145. Pizcueta, M. P., Piqué, J. M., Fernández, M., Bosch, J., Rodés, J., Whittle, B. J. R., *et al.* (1992). Modulation of the hyperdynamic circulation of cirrhotic rats by nitric oxide inhibition. *Gastroenterology* **103,** 1909–1915.
146. Pizcueta, M. P., Piqué, J. M., Bosch, J., Whittle, B. J. R., and Moncada, S. (1992). Effects of inhibiting nitric oxide biosynthesis on the systemic and splanchnic circulation of rats with portal hypertension. *Br. J. Pharmacol.* **105,** 184–190.
147. Vallance, P., and Moncada, S. (1991). Hyperdynamic circulation in cirrhosis: A role for nitric oxide? *Lancet* **337,** 776–778.
148. Niederberger, M., Martin, P. Y., Gines, P., Morris, K., Tsai, P., Xu, D. L., *et al.* (1995). Normalization of nitric oxide production corrects arterial vasodilatation and hyperdynamic circulation in cirrhotic rats. *Gastroenterology* **109,** 1624–1630.
149. Castro, A., Jiménez, W., Claria, J., Ros, J., Martinez, J. M., Bosch, M., *et al.* (1993). Impaired responsiveness to angiotensin II in experimental cirrhosis: Role of nitric oxide. *Hepatology* **18,** 367–372.
150. Lee, F. Y., Albillos, A., Colombato, L. A., and Groszmann, R. J. (1992). The role of nitric oxide in the vascular hyporesponsiveness to methoxamine in portal hypertensive rats. *Hepatology* **16,** 1043–1048.
151. Sieber, C. C., and Groszmann, R. J. (1992). Nitric oxide mediates hyporeactivity to vasopressors in mesenteric vessels of portal hypertensive rats. *Gastroenterology* **103,** 235–239.
152. Sieber, C. C., Lopez-Talavera, J. C., and Groszmann, R. J. (1993). Role of nitric oxide in the *in vitro* splanchnic vascular hyporeactivity in ascitic cirrhotic rats. *Gastroenterology* **4,** 1750–1754.
153. Ortiz, M. C., Fortepiani, L. A., Martinez, C., Atucha, N. M., and Garcia-Estan, J. (1996). Vascular hyporesponsiveness in aortic rings from cirrhotic rats: Role of nitric oxide and endothelium. *Clin. Sci.* **91,** 733–738.
154. Weigert, A. L., Martin, P. Y., Niederberger, M., Higa, E. M., McMurtry, I. F., Gines, P., *et al.* (1995). Endothelium-dependent vascular hyporesponsiveness without detection of nitric oxide synthase induction in aortas of cirrhotic rats. *Hepatology* **22,** 1856–1862.
155. Heinemann, A., Wachter, C. H., Holzer, P., Fickert, P., and Stauber, R. E. (1997). Nitric oxide-dependent and -independent vascular hyporeactivity in mesenteric arteries of portal hypertensive rats. *Br. J. Pharmacol.* **121,** 1031–1037.
156. Wiest, R., Hori, N., Cadelina, G., Das, S., and Groszmann, R. J. (1997). Increased nitric oxide release in response to vasoconstrictors in the superior mesenteric arterial bed of cirrhotic rats. *Hepatology* **26,** 390A.
157. Hori, N., Wiest, R., and Groszmann, R. J. (1998). Enhanced release of nitric oxide in response to changes in flow and shear stress in the superior mesenteric arteries of portal hypertensive rats. *Hepatology* **28,** 1467–1473.
158. Guarner, C., Soriano, G., Tomas, Z., Bulbena, O., Novella, M. T., Balanzo, J., *et al.* (1993). Increased serum nitrite and nitrate levels in patients with cirrhosis: Relationship to endotoxemia. *Hepatology* **18,** 1139–1143.
159. Lee, F. Y., Colombato, L. A., Albillos, A., Albillos, A., and Groszmann, R. J. (1993). N^{ω}-Nitro-L-arginine administration corrects

peripheral vasodilation and systemic capillary hypotension and ameliorates plasma volume expansion and sodium retention in portal hypertensive rats. *Hepatology* **17,** 84–90.

160. Lee, F. Y., Colombato, L. A., Albillos, A., and Groszmann, R. J. (1993). Administration of N^{ω}-Nitro-L-arginine ameliorates portal-systemic shunting in portal hypertensive rats. *Gastroenterology*. **105,** 1464–1470.
161. García-Pagán, J. C., Fernández, M., Bernadich, C., Pizcueta, P., Piqué, M. J., Bosch, J., and Rodés, J. (1994). Effects of continued nitric oxide inhibition on the development of the portal hypertensive syndrome following portal vein stenosis in the rat. *Am. J. Physiol.* **30,** G984-G990.
162. Fernández, M., Garcia-Pagán, J. C., Casadevall, M., Bernadich, C., Piera, C., Whittle, B. J., *et al.* (1994). Evidences against a role for the inducible NO synthase in the hyperdynamic circulation of portal hypertensive rats. *Gastroenterology* **108,** 1487–1495.
163. Rockey, D. C., and Chung, J. J. (1997). Regulation of inducible nitric oxide synthase and nitric oxide during hepatic injury and fibrogenesis. *Am. J. Physiol.* **273,** G124–G130.
164. Sogni, P., Smith, A. P., Gadano, A., Lebrec, D., and Higenbottam, T. W. (1997). Induction of nitric oxide synthase II does not account for excess vascular nitric oxide production in experimental cirrhosis. *J. Hepatol.* **26,** 1120–1127.
165. Atucha, N. M., Shah, V., Garcia-Cardena, G., Sessa, W. E., and Groszmann, R. J. (1996). Role of endothelium in the abnormal response of mesenteric vessels in rats with portal hypertension and liver cirrhosis. *Gastroenterology* **111,** 1627–1632.
166. Niederberger, M., Gines, P., Martin, P. Y., Tsai, P., Morris, K., McMurtry, I., *et al.* (1996). Comparison of vascular nitric oxide production and systemic hemodynamics in cirrhosis versus prehepatic portal hypertension. *Hepatology* **24,** 947–951.
167. Kanwar, S., Kubes, P., Tepperman, B. L., and Lee, S. S. (1996). Nitric oxide synthase activity in portal-hypertensive and cirrhotic rats. *J. Hepatol.* **25,** 85–89.
168. Van Obbergh, L., Leonard, V., Chen, H., Xu, D., and Blaise, G. (1995). The endothelial and non-endothelial mechanism responsible for attenuated vasoconstriction in cirrhotic rats. *Exp. Physiol.* **80,** 609–617.
169. Sha, V., Wiest, R., Garcia-Cardena, G., Cadelina, G., Groszmann, R. J., and Sessa, W. C. (1999). Hsp90 regulation of endothelial nitric oxide synthase contributes to vascular control in portal hypertension. *Am. J. Physiol.* **277**(2 Pt 19), G463-G468.
170. Rizzo, V., McIntosh, D. P., and Schnitzer, J. E. (1998). *In situ* flow activates endothelial nitric oxide synthase in luminal caveolae of endothelium with rapid caveolin dissociation and calmodulin association. *J. Biol. Chem.* **273,** 3472–3479.
171. Sitzmann, J. V., Bulkley, G. B., Mitchell, M. C., and Campbell, K. (1998). Role of prostacyclin in the splanchnic hyperemia contributing to portal hypertension. *Ann. Surg.* **209,** 322–327.
172. Hamilton, G., Phing, R. C., Hutton, R. A., Dandona, P., and Hobbs, K. E. (1982). The relationship between prostacyclin activity and pressure in the portal vein. *Hepatology* **2,** 236–242.
173. Guarner, C., Soriano, G., Such, J., Teixido, M., Ramis, I., Bulbena, O., *et al.* (1992). Systemic prostacyclin in cirrhotic patients: Relationship with portal hypertension and changes after intestinal decontamination. *Gastroenterology* **102,** 303–309.
174. Fernández, M., García-Pagán, J. C., Casadevall, M., Mourelle, M. I., Piqué, J. M., Bosch, J., *et al.* (1996). Acute and chronic cyclooxygenase blockade in portal hypertensive rats influence on nitric oxide biosynthesis. *Gastroenterology* **110,** 1529–1535.
175. Bruix, J., Bosch, J., Kravetz, D., Mastai, R., and Rodés, J. (1985). Effects of prostaglandin inhibition on systemic and hepatic hemodynamics in patients with cirrhosis of the liver. *Gastroenterology* **88,** 430–435.
176. Fernandez, M., and Bonkovsky, H. J. (1999). Increased heme oxygenase-1 gene expression in liver cells and splanchnic organs from portal hypertensive rats. *Hepatology* **29,** 1672–1679.
177. Sieber, C. C., and Groszmann, R. J. (1992). Nitric oxide mediates hyporeactivity to vasopressors in mesenteric vessels of portal hypertensive rats. *Gastroenterology* **103,** 235–239.
178. Sieber, C. C., and Groszmann, R. J. (1992). *In vitro* hyporeactivity to methoxamine in portal hypertensive rats: Reversal by nitric oxide blockade. *Am. J. Physiol.* **262,** G996–G1001.
179. Ratnoff, O. D., and Patek, A. J., Jr. (1942). Natural history of Laennec's cirrhosis of the liver: Analysis of 386 cases. *Medicine* **21,** 207–268.
180. Garceau, A. I., and the Boston Inter-Hospital Liver Group (1963). The natural history of cirrhosis: I. Survival with esophageal varices. *N. Engl. J. Med.* **268,** 469–473.
181. Atik, M., and Simeone, F. (1954). Massive gastrointestinal bleeding: A study of 296 patients at City Hospital of Cleveland. *Arch. Surg.* **69,** 355–365.
182. Cohn, R., and Blaisdell, F. W. (1958). The natural history of the patient with cirrhosis of the liver with esophageal varices following the first massive hemorrhage. *Surg. Gynecol. Obstet.* **106,** 699–701.
183. Higgins, W. H., Jr. (1947). The esophageal varix: A report of one hundred and fifteen cases. *Am. J. Med. Sci.* **214,** 436–441.
184. Merigan, T. C., Jr. Hollister, R. M., Gryska, P. F., *et al.* (1960). Gastrointestinal bleeding with cirrhosis: Study of 172 episodes in 158 patients. *N. Engl. J. Med.* **263,** 579–585.
185. Nachlas, M. M., O'Neil, J. E., and Campbell, A. J. A. (1955). The life history of patients with cirrhosis of the liver and bleeding esophageal varices. *Ann. Surg.* **141,** 10–23.
186. Taylor, F. W., and Jontz, J. G. (1959). Cirrhosis with hemorrhage. *Arch. Surg.* **78,** 786–790.
187. Orloff, M. J. (1966). Emergency treatment of bleeding esophageal varices in cirrhosis. *Curr. Probl. Surg.* **July,** 13–28.
188. Orloff, M. J., and Thomas, H. S. (1963). Pathogenesis of esophageal varix rupture: A study based on gross and microscopic examination of the esophagus at the time of bleeding. *Arch. Surg.* **87,** 301–307.
189. Liebowitz, H. R. (1961). Pathogenesis of esophageal varix rupture. *JAMA* **175,** 874–879.
190. Ludington, L. G. (1958). A study of 158 cases of esophageal varices. *Surg. Gynecol. Obstet.* **106,** 519–526.
191. Conn, H. O. (1958). Hazards attending the use of esophageal tamponade. *N. Engl. J. Med.* **259,** 701–707.
192. Read, A. E., Dawson, A. M., Kerr, D. N. S., *et al.* (1960). Bleeding oesophageal varices treated by oesophageal compression tube. *Br. Med. J.* **168,** 227–231.
193. Orloff, M. J., Halasz, N. A., Lipman, C. A., *et al.* (1967). The complications of cirrhosis of the liver. *Ann. Intern. Med.* **66,** 165–198.
194. Villanueva, A., and Magnenat, P. (1964). Resultats du traitement des hemorrhagies oesophagogastriques sur varices par la sonde de Sengstaken–Blakemore. *Gastroenterologia (Basel)* **102,** 242–246.
195. Hermann, R. E., and Traul, D. (1970). Experience with the Sengstaken–Blakemore tube for bleeding esophageal varices. *Surg. Gynecol. Obstet.* **130,** 879–885.
196. Pitcher, J. L. (1971). Safety and effectiveness of the modified Sengstaken–Blakemore tube: A prospective study. *Gastroenterology* **61,** 291–298.
197. Johansen, T. S., and Baden, H. (1973). Re-appraisal of the Sengstaken–Blakemore balloon tamponade for bleeding esophageal varices; results in 91 patients. *Scand. J. Gastroenterol.* **18,** 181–183.
198. Novis, B. H., Duys, P., Barbezat, G. O., *et al.* (1976). Fiberoptic endoscopy and the use of the Sengstaken tube in acute gastrointestinal hemorrhage in patients with portal hypertension and varices. *Gut* **17,** 258–263.
199. Teres, J., Cecilia, A., Bordas, J. M., *et al.* (1978). Esophageal tamponade for bleeding varices: Controlled trial between the Sengstaken–

Blakemore tube and the Linton–Nachlas tube. *Gastroenterology* **75,** 566–569.
200. Conn, H. O., and Simpson, J. A. (1967). Excessive mortality associated with balloon tamponade of bleeding varices. A critical reappraisal. *JAMA* **202,** 587–591.
201. Terblanche, J., Kahn, D., Campbell, J. A. H., *et al.* (1983). Failure of repeated injection sclerotherapy to improve long-term survival after oesophageal variceal bleeding. *Lancet* **1,** 1328–1332.
202. The Copenhagen Esophageal Varices Sclerotherapy Project (1984). Sclerotherapy after first variceal hemorrhage in cirrhosis. A randomized multicenter trial. *N. Engl. J. Med.* **311,** 1594–1600.
203. Korula, J., Balart, L. A., Ravdin, G., *et al.* (1985). A prospective, randomized controlled trial of chronic esophageal variceal sclerotherapy. *Hepatology* **5,** 584–589.
204. Huizinga, W. K. J., Angorah, I. B., and Baker, L. W. (1985). Esophageal transection versus injection sclerotherapy in the management of bleeding esophageal varices in patients at high risk. *Surg. Gynecol. Obstet.* **160,** 539–546.
205. Soderlund, C., and Ihre, T. (1985). Endoscopic sclerotherapy v. conservative management of bleeding oesophageal varices. *Acta Chir. Scand.* **151,** 449–456.
206. Westaby, D., MacDougall, B. R. D., and Williams, R. (1985). Improved survival following injection sclerotherapy for oesophageal varices: Final analysis of a controlled trial. *Hepatology* **5,** 827–830.
207. Lopes, G. M., and Grace, N. D. (1993). Gastroesophageal varices: Prevention of bleeding and rebleeding. *Gastroenterol. Clin. North Am.* **22**(4), 801–820.
208. Sanyal, A. J., Purdum, P. P., III, Luketic, V. A., and Shiffman, M. L. (1993). Bleeding gastroesophageal varices. *Semin. Liver Dis.* **13,** 328–342.
209. Health and Public Policy Committee, American College of Physicians: Position paper. (1984). Endoscopic sclerotherapy for esophageal varices. *Ann. Intern. Med.* **100,** 608–610.
210. Alwmark, A., Bengmark, S., Borjesson, B., *et al.* (1982). Emergency and long-term transesophageal sclerotherapy of bleeding esophageal varices. A prospective study of 50 consecutive cases. *Scand. J. Gastroenterol.* **17,** 409–412.
211. MacDougall, B. R. D., Theodossi, A., Westaby, D., Dawson, J. L., and Williams, R. (1982). Increased long-term survival in variceal hemorrhage using injection sclerotherapy. Results of a controlled trial. *Lancet* **1,** 124–127.
212. Barsoum, M. S., Bolous, F. I., El-Rooby, A. A., Rizk-Alla, M. A., and Ibrahim, A. S. (1982). Tamponade and injection sclerotherapy in the management of bleeding oesophageal varices. *Br. J. Surg.* **69,** 76–78.
213. Yassin, Y. M., and Sherif, S. M. (1983). Randomized controlled trial of injection sclerotherapy for bleeding oesophageal varices—An interim report. *Br. J. Surg.* **70,** 20–22.
214. Westaby, D., Polson, R. J., Gimson, A. E. S., Hayes, P. C., Hayllar, K., and Williams, R. (1990). A controlled trial of oral propranolol compared with injection sclerotherapy for the long-term management of variceal bleeding. *Hepatology* **11,** 353–359.
215. Burroughs, A. K., McCormick, P. A., Siringo, S., *et al.* (1989). Randomized trial of long-term sclerotherapy for variceal rebleeding using the same protocol to treat rebleeding in all patients. A final report. *Gut* **30,** A1506.
216. Gregory, P. B., and the VA Cooperative Variceal Sclerotherapy Group (1990). Sclerotherapy for male alcoholics with cirrhosis who have bled from esophageal varices: A randomized controlled trial. *World Cong. Gastroenterol. Proc.* A891.
217. Teres, J., Bosch, J., Bordas, J. M. A., *et al.* (1993). Propranolol versus sclerotherapy in preventing variceal rebleeding: A randomized controlled trial. *Gastroenterology* **105,** 1508–1514.
218. Pugh, S., Lewis, S., and Smith, P. M. (1993). Bleeding oesophageal varices in alcoholic cirrhosis: Long-term follow-up of endoscopic sclerotherapy. *Q. J. Med.* **86,** 241–245.
219. Sarin, S. K. (1992). Long-term management of oesophageal varices. *Drugs* **44,** (Suppl 2), 56–69.
220. Stiegmann, G. V. (1994). Endoscopic management of esophageal varices. *Adv. Surg.* **27,** 209–231.
221. Gregory, P. B., and the Veterans Affairs Cooperative Variceal Sclerotherapy Group (1991). Prophylactic sclerotherapy for esophageal varices in men with alcoholic liver disease. A randomized, single-blind, multi-center clinical trial. *N. Engl. J. Med.* **324,** 1779–1784.
222. DeFranchis, R., Primignani, M., Arcidiacono, P. G., *et al.* (1991). Prophylactic sclerotherapy (ST) in high risk cirrhotics selected by endoscopic criteria: A multicenter randomized controlled trial. *Gastroenterology* **101,** 1087–1093.
223. Pagliaro, L., D'Amico, G., Sorensen, T. I. A., *et al.* (1992). Prevention of first bleeding in cirrhosis: A meta-analysis of randomized trials of nonsurgical treatment. *Ann. Intern. Med.* **117,** 59–70.
224. Piai, G., Cipolletta, L., Claar, M., *et al.* (1984). Prophylactic sclerotherapy of high-risk esophageal varices: Results of a multicenter prospective controlled trial. *Hepatology* **8,** 1495–1500.
225. Potzi, R., Bauer, P., Reichel, W., *et al.* (1989). Prophylactic endoscopic sclerotherapy of oesophageal varices in liver cirrhosis: A multicenter prospective controlled randomised trial in Vienna. *Gut* **30,** 873–879.
226. PROVA Study Group (1991). Prophylaxis of first hemorrhage from oesophageal varices by sclerotherapy, propranolol, or both in cirrhotic patients: A randomized multicenter trial. *Hepatology* **14,** 1016–1024.
227. Santangelo, W. C., Dueno, M. I., Estes, B. L., and Krejs, G. J. (1988). Prophylactic sclerotherapy of large esophageal varices. *N. Engl. J. Med.* **318,** 814–818.
228. Sauerbruch, T., Wotzka, R., Kopcke, W., *et al.* (1988). Prophylactic sclerotherapy before the first episode of variceal hemorrhage in patients with cirrhosis. *N. Engl. J. Med.* **319,** 8–15.
229. Sarin, S. K., Lahoti, D., Saxena, S. P., Murthy, N. S., and Makwana, U. K. (1992). Prevalence, classification and natural history of gastric varices: A long-term follow-up study in 568 portal hypertension patients. *Hepatology* **16,** 1343–1349.
230. Trudeau, W., and Pindiville, T. (1986). Endoscopic injection sclerosis in bleeding gastric varices. *Gastrointest. Endosc.* **32,** 264–268.
231. Korula, J., Chin, K., Ko, Y., and Yamada, S. (1991). Demonstration of two distinct subsets of gastric varices observed during a 7-year study of endoscopic sclerotherapy. *Dig. Dis. Sci.* **36,** 303–307.
232. Orloff, M. J., Orloff, M. S., Orloff, S. L., and Haynes, K. S. (1995). Treatment of bleeding from portal hypertensive gastropathy by portacaval shunt. *Hepatology* **21,** 1011–1017.
233. McCormack, T. T., Simms, J., Eyre-Brooke, I., *et al.* (1985). Gastric lesions in portal hypertension: Inflammatory gastritis or congestive gastropathy? *Gut* **26,** 1226–1232.
234. Quintero, E., Pique, J. M., Bombi, J. A., *et al.* (1987). Gastric mucosal vascular ectasias causing bleeding in cirrhosis. *Gastroenterology* **93,** 1054–1061.
235. Vigneri, S., Termini, R., Piraino, A., *et al.* (1991). The stomach in liver cirrhosis. Endoscopic, morphological, and clinical correlations. *Gastroenterology* **101,** 472–478.
236. Triger, D. R. (1992). Portal hypertensive gastropathy. *Bailliere's Clin. Gastroenterol.* **6,** 481–495.
237. Stiegmann, G. V., Goff, J. S., Michaletz-Onody, P. A., *et al.* (1992). Endoscopic sclerotherapy as compared with endoscopic ligation for bleeding esophageal varices. *N. Engl. J. Med.* **326,** 1527–1532.
238. Hou, M. C., Lin, H. C., Kuo, B. I. T., *et al.* (1995). Comparison of endoscopic variceal injection sclerotherapy and ligation for the treatment of esophageal variceal hemorrhage. A prospective randomized trial. *Hepatology* **21,** 1517–1522.
239. Sung, J. J., Chung, S. C., Yung, M. Y., *et al.* (1995). Prospective randomised study of the effect of octreotide on re-bleeding from esophageal varices after endoscopic ligation. *Lancet* **346,** 1666–1669.

240. Besson, I., Ingrand, P., Person, B., *et al.* (1995). Sclerotherapy with or without octreotide for acute variceal bleeding. *N. Engl. J. Med.* **333,** 555–560.
241. Sarin, S. K., Guptan, R. K., Jain, A. K., and Sundaram, K. R. (1996). A randomized controlled trial of endoscopic variceal band ligation for primary prophylaxis of variceal bleeding. *Eur. J. Gastroenterol. Hepatol.* **8,** 337–342.
242. Lay, C. S., Tsai, A. Y., Teg, C. Y., *et al.* (1997). Endoscopic variceal ligation in prophylaxis of first variceal bleeding in cirrhotic patients with high-risk esophageal varices. *Hepatology* **25,** 1346–1350.
243. Laine, L. (1995). Ligation: Endoscopic treatment of choice for patients with bleeding esophageal varices? *Hepatology* **22,** 663–665.
244. Laine, L., and Cook, D. (1995). Endoscopic ligation compared with sclerotherapy for treatment of esophageal variceal bleeding: A meta-analysis. *Ann. Intern. Med.* **123,** 280–287.
245. Saeed, Z. A., Stiegmann, G. V., Ramirez, F. C., *et al.* (1997). Endoscopic variceal ligation is superior to combined ligation and sclerotherapy for esophageal varices: A multi-center prospective randomized trial. *Hepatology* **25,** 71–74.
246. Sarin, S. K., Covil, A., Jain, A. K., *et al.* (1997). Prospective randomized trial of endoscopic sclerotherapy versus variceal band ligation for esophageal varices: Influence on gastropathy, gastric varices and variceal recurrence. *J. Hepatol.* **26,** 826–832.
247. Avgerinos, A., Armonis, A., Manolakopulos, S., *et al.* (1997). Endoscopic sclerotherapy versus ligation in the long-term management of patients with cirrhosis after variceal bleeding. A prospective randomized study. *J. Hepatol.* **26,** 1034–1041.
248. Cello, J. P. (1997). Endoscopic management of esophageal variceal hemorrhage: Injection, banding, glue, octreotide, or a combination? *Semin. Gastrointest. Dis.* **8,** 179–187.
249. Lunderquist, A., and Vang, J. (1974). Transhepatic catheterization and obliteration of the coronary vein in patients with portal hypertension and esophageal varices. *N. Engl. J. Med.* **291,** 646–649.
250. Passariello, R., Rossi, P., Simonetti, G., *et al.* (1979). Emergency transhepatic obliteration of bleeding varices. *Cardiovasc. Radiol.* **2,** 97–106.
251. Lunderquist, A., Borjesson, B., Owman, T., and Bengmark, S. (1978). Isobutyl-2-cyanoacrylate (Bucrylate) in obliteration of gastric coronary vein and esophageal varices. *Am. J. Roentgenol.* **130,** 1–6.
252. Turner, W. W., Jr., and Ellman, B. A. (1981). Transhepatic embolization in patients with acute variceal hemorrhage. *Am. J. Surg.* **142,** 731–734.
253. Bengmark, S., Borjesson, B., Hoevels, J., *et al.* (1979). Obliteration of esophageal varices by PTP: A follow-up of 43 patients. *Ann. Surg.* **190,** 549–554.
254. Smith-Laing, G., Scott, J., Long, R. G., *et al.* (1981). Role of percutaneous transhepatic obliteration of varices in the management of hemorrhage from gastroesophageal varices. *Gastroenterology* **80,** 1031–1036.
255. Sos, T. A. (1983). Transhepatic portal venous embolization of varices: Pros and cons. *Radiology* **148,** 569–570.
256. Benner, K. G., Keeffe, E. B., Keller, F. S., and Rosch, J. (1983). Clinical outcome after percutaneous transhepatic obliteration of esophageal varices. *Gastroenterology* **85,** 146–153.
257. L'Herminé, C. L., Chastanet, P., Delemazure, O., *et al.* (1989). Percutaneous transhepatic embolization of gastroesophageal varices: Results in 400 patients. *Am. J. Roentgenol.* **152,** 755–760.
258. Boerema, I. (1949). Bleeding varices of oesophagus in cirrhosis of the liver and Banti's syndrome. *Arch. Chir. Neerl.* **1,** 253–260.
259. Ottinger, L. W., and Moncure, A. C. (1974). Transthoracic ligation of bleeding esophageal varices in patients with intrahepatic portal obstruction. *Ann. Surg.* **179,** 35–38.
260. Rothwell-Jackson, R. L., and Hunt, A. H. (1971). The results obtained with emergency surgery in the treatment of persistent haemorrhage from gastroesophageal varices in the cirrhotic patient. *Br. J. Surg.* **58,** 205–215.
261. Wirthlin, I. S., Linton, R. R., and Ellis, D. S. (1974). Transthoracoesophageal ligation of bleeding esophageal varices: A reappraisal. *Arch. Surg.* **109,** 688–692.
262. Orloff, M. J. (1962). A comparative study of emergency transesophageal ligation and nonsurgical treatment of bleeding esophageal varices in unselected patients with cirrhosis. *Surgery* **52,** 102–116.
263. Futagawa, S., Sugiura, M., Hidai, J., and Shima, F. (1979). Emergency esophageal transection with paraesophagogastric devascularization for variceal bleeding. *World J. Surg.* **3,** 229–234.
264. Johnson, G. W. (1977). Treatment of bleeding varices by oesophageal transection with the SPTU gun. *Ann. R. Coll. Surg. Engl.* **59,** 404–408.
265. Pugh, R. N. H., Murray-Lyon, P. M., Dawson, J. L., *et al.* (1973). Transection of the oesophagus for bleeding oesophageal varices. *Br. J. Surg.* **60,** 646–649.
266. Sugiura, M., and Futagawa, S. (1977). Further evaluation of the Sugiura procedure in the treatment of esophageal varices. *Arch. Surg.* **112,** 1317–1321.
267. Yamamoto, S., Hidemura, R., Sawada, M., *et al.* (1976). The late results of terminal esophagoproximal gastrectomy (TEPG) with extensive devascularization and splenectomy for bleeding esophageal varices in cirrhosis. *Surgery* **80,** 106–114.
268. Johnston, G. W. (1982). Six years' experience of oesophageal transection for oesophageal varices using a circular stapling gun. *Gut* **23,** 770–773.
269. Osborne, D. R., and Hobbs, K. E. F. (1981). The acute treatment of haemorrhage from oesophageal varices: A comparison of oesophageal transection and staple gun anastomosis with mesocaval shunt. *Br. J. Surg.* **68,** 734–737.
270. Kirby, R., Burke, F. D., and Jones, J. D. T. (1975). Emergency and elective surgical treatment of portal hypertension. A review of 23 years' experience. *Ann. R. Coll. Surg. Engl.* **57,** 148–158.
271. George, P., Brown, C., Ridgway, G., *et al.* (1973). Emergency oesophageal transection in uncontrolled variceal haemorrhage. *Br. J. Surg.* **60,** 635–640.
272. Wanamaker, S. R., Cooperman, M., and Carey, L. C. (1983). Use of the EEA stapling instrument for control of bleeding esophageal varices. *Surgery* **94,** 620–626.
273. Koyama, K., Takagi, Y., Ouchi, K., and Sato, T. (1980). Results of esophageal transection for esophageal varices: Experience in 100 cases. *Am. J. Surg.* **139,** 204–209.
274. Johnson, G., Jr., Womack, N. A., Gabriele, O. F., Peters, R. M. (1969). Control of the hyperdynamic circulation in patients with bleeding esophageal varices. *Ann. Surg.* **169,** 661–671.
275. Umeyama, K., Yoshikawa, K., Yamoshita, T., *et al.* (1983). Transabdominal oesophageal transection for oesophageal varices: Experience in 101 patients. *Br. J. Surg.* **70,** 419–422.
276. Mir, J., Ponce, J., Juan, M., *et al.* (1982). Esophageal transection and paraesophagogastric devascularization performed as an emergency measure for uncontrolled variceal bleeding. *Surg. Gynecol. Obstet.* **155,** 868–872.
277. Van Beek, D. F., Gleysteen, J. J., Malangoni, M. A., *et al.* (1984). Mortality and rebleeding after hypertensive variceal disconnections. *Arch. Surg.* **119,** 446–449.
278. Bosch, J., and Barcia-Pagan, J. C. (2000). Complications of cirrhosis. I. Portal hypertension. *J. Hepatol.* **32,** 141–156.
279. García-Pagán, J. C., Escorsell, A., Moitinho, E., and Bosch, J. (1999). Influence of pharmacological agents on portal hemodynamics: Basis for its use in the treatment of portal hypertension. *Semin. Liver Dis.* **19,** 427–428.
280. García-Pagán, J. C., Feu, F., Navasa, M., *et al.* (1990). Long-term haemodynamic effects of isosorbide-5-mononitrate in patients with cirrhosis and portal hypertension. *J. Hepatol.* **11,** 189–195.
281. Navasa, M., Bosch, J., Reichen, J., Bru, C., *et al.* (1988). Effects of verapamil on hepatic and systemic hemodynamics and liver function

in patients with cirrhosis and portal hypertension. *Hepatology* **8,** 850–854.

282. Salmeron, J. M., Ruiz del Arbol, L., *et al.* (1993). Renal effects of acute isosorbide-5-mononitrate administration in cirrhosis. *Hepatology* **17,** 800–806.
283. Albillos, A., Liedo, J. L., Bañares, R., *et al.* (1994). Hemodynamic effects of alpha-adrenergic blockage with prazosin in cirrhotic patients with portal hypertension. *Hepatology* **20,** 611–617.
284. Albillos, A., Lledo, J. L., Rossi, I., *et al.* (1995). Continuous prazosin administration in cirrhotic patients: Effects on portal hemodynamics and on liver and renal function. *Gastroenterology* **109,** 1257–1265.
285. Albillos, A., García-Pagán, J. C., Iborra, J., *et al.* (1998). Propranolol plus prazosin compared to propranolol plus isosorbide-5-mononitrate in the chronic treatment of portal hypertension. *Gastroenterology* **115,** 116–123.
286. Willett, I. R., Jennings, G., Esler, M., and Dudley, E. J. (1986). Sympathetic tone modulates portal venous pressure in alcoholic cirrhosis. *Lancet* **2,** 939–941.
287. Moreau, R., Lee, S. S., Hadengue, A., *et al.* (1987). Hemodynamic effects of a clonidine-induced decrease in sympathetic tone in patients with cirrhosis. *Hepatology* **7,** 147–154.
288. Roulot, D., Moreau, R., Gaudin, C., *et al.* (1992). Long-term sympathetic and hemodynamic responses to clonidine in patients with cirrhosis and ascites. *Gastroenterology* **102,** 1309–1318.
289. Albillos, A., Banares, R., Barrios, C., *et al.* (1992). Long-term oral administration of clonidine in patients with alcoholic cirrhosis. Hemodynamic and liver function effects. *Gastroenterology* **102,** 248–254.
290. Bañares, R., Moitinho, E., Piqueras, B., *et al.* (1999). Carvedilol, a new non-selective beta-blocker with intrinsic anti-alpha$_1$-adrenergic activity, has a greater portal hypotensive effect than propranolol in patients with cirrhosis. *Hepatology* **30,** 79–83.
291. Schneider, A. W., Friedrich, J., and Klein, C. P. (1999). Effects of losartan, an angiotensin II receptor antagonist, on portal pressure in cirrhosis. *Hepatology* **29,** 334–339.
292. Mastai, R., Bosch, J., Navasa, M., *et al.* (1987). Effects of alpha-adrenergic stimulation and beta-adrenergic blockade on azygos blood flow and splanchnic haemodynamics in patients with cirrhosis. *J. Hepatol.* **4,** 71–79.
293. Escorsell, A., Ferayorni, F., Bosch, J., *et al.* (1997). The portal pressure response to beta-blockade is greater in cirrhotic patients without varices than in those with varices. *Gastroenterology* **112,** 2012–2016.
294. Mills, P. R., Rae, A. P., Farah, D. A., *et al.* (1984). Comparison of three adrenoceptor blocking agents in patients with cirrhosis and portal hypertension. *Gut* **25,** 73–78.
295. Hillon, P., Lebrec, D., Muñoz, C., *et al.* (1982). Comparison of the effects of a cardioselective and a nonselective beta-blocker on portal hypertension in patients with cirrhosis. *Hepatology* **2,** 528–531.
296. Feu, F., Bordas, J. M., Luca, A., *et al.* (1993). Reduction of variceal pressure by propranolol. Comparison of the effects on portal pressure and azygos blood flow in patients with cirrhosis. *Hepatology* **18,** 1082–1089.
297. García-Pagán, J. C., Navasa, M., Bosch, J., *et al.* (1990). Enhancement of portal pressure reduction by the association of isosorbide-5-mononitrate to propranolol administration in patients with cirrhosis. *Hepatology* **11,** 230–238.
298. Bosch, J., Mastai, R., Kravetz, D., Bruix, J., Rigau, J., and Rodes, J. (1985). Measurement of azygos venous blood flow in the evaluation of portal hypertension in patients with cirrhosis. Clinical and haemodynamic correlations in 100 patients. *J. Hepatol.* **1,** 125–139.
299. Bosch, J., Bordas, J. M., Mastai, R., *et al.* (1988). Effects of vasopressin on the intravariceal pressure in patients with cirrhosis: Comparison with the effects on portal pressure. *Hepatology* **8,** 861–865.
300. D'Amico, G., Pagliaro, L., and Bosch, J. (1995). The treatment of portal hypertension: A meta-analytic review. *Hepatology* **22,** 332–354.
301. Groszmann, R. J., Kravetz, D., Bosch, J., *et al.* (1982). Nitroglycerin improves the hemodynamic response to vasopressin in portal hypertension. *Hepatology* **2,** 757–762.
302. Blei, A. T. (1986). Vasopressin analogs in portal hypertension: Different molecules but similar questions. *Hepatology* **6,** 146–147.
303. Kravetz, D., Bosch, J., Arderiu, M. T., *et al.* (1988). Effects of somatostatin on splanchnic hemodynamics and plasma glucagon in portal hypertensive rats. *Am. J. Physiol.* **254,** G322–G328.
304. Bosch, J., Kravetz, D., and Rodes, J. (1981). Effects of somatostatin on hepatic and systemic hemodynamics in patients with cirrhosis of the liver: Comparison with vasopressin. *Gastroenterology* **80,** 518–525.
305. Kravetz, D., Bosch, J., Arderiu, M. T., *et al.* (1988). Effects of somatostatin on splanchnic hemodynamics and plasma glucagon in portal hypertensive rats. *Am. J. Physiol.* **254,** G322–G325.
306. Cirera, I., Feu, F., Luca, A., *et al.* (1995). Effects of bolus injections and continuous infusions of somatostatin and placebo in patients with cirrhosis and portal hypertension. A double-blind hemodynamic investigation. *Hepatology* **22,** 106–111.
307. Moitinho, E., and the Variceal Bleeding Study Group (1998). Randomized controlled trial comparing different schedules of somatostatin in the treatment of acute variceal bleeding. *Hepatology* **28,** 770A.
308. Eriksson, L. S., Brundin, T., Soderlund, C., and Wahren, J. (1987). Hemodynamic effects of a long-acting somatostatin analogue in patients with liver cirrhosis. *Scand. J. Gastroenterol.* **22,** 919–925.
309. Lin, H. C., Huang, Y. T., Wu, H. L., *et al.* (1999). Effects of sustained-release lantreotide on hemodynamics in rats with portal vein stenosis. *J. Hepatol.* **31,** 482–488.
310. Cerini, R., Lee, S. S., Hadengue, A., *et al.* (1988). Circulatory effects of somatostatin analogue in two conscious rat models of portal hypertension. *Gastroenterology* **94,** 703–708.
311. McKee, R. (1990). A study of octreotide in oesophageal varices. *Digestion* **45,** 60–65.
312. MacCormick, P. A., Dick, R., Siringo, S., *et al.* (1990). Octreotide reduces azygos blood flow in cirrhotic patients with portal hypertension. *Eur. J. Gastroenterol. Hepatol.* **2,** 489–492.
313. Lin, H. C., Tsai, Y. T., Lee, F. Y., *et al.* (1992). Hemodynamic evaluation of octreotide in patients with hepatitis B-related cirrhosis. *Gastroenterology* **103,** 229–234.
314. Bosch, J., Pizcueta, M. P., Feu, F., *et al.* (1992). Pathophysiology of portal hypertension. *Gastroenterol. Clin. North Am.* **21,** 1–14.
315. Zimmon, D. S., and Kessler, R. E. (1974). The portal pressure–blood volume relationship in cirrhosis. *Gut* **15,** 99–101.
316. Okumura, H., Aramaki, T., Katsuta, Y., Satomura, K., *et al.* (1991). Reduction in hepatic venous pressure gradient as a consequence of volume contraction due to chronic administration of spironolactone in patients with cirrhosis and no ascites. *Am. J. Gastroenterol.* **86,** 46–52.
317. García-Pagán, J. C., Salmeron, J. M., Feu, F., *et al.* (1994). Effects of low sodium diet and spironolactone on portal pressure in patients with compensated cirrhosis. *Hepatology* **19,** 1095–1099.
318. Eck, N. V. (1877). K voprosu o pereviazke vorotnoi veni: Predvaritelnoye soobschjenie (Concerning ligation of the vena porta: Preliminary notification). *Voen. Med. Zh.* **130,** 1–2.
319. Hahn, M., Massen, V. N., Nenski, M., and Pavlov, I. P. (1893). Die Eck' sche Fistel zwischen der unteren Hohlvene und der Pfortader und ihre Folgen Fur den Organismus. *Arch. Exp. Pathol. Pharmakol.* **32,** 161–210.
320. Pavlov, I. P. (1893). On a modification of the Eck fistula between the portal vien and the inferior vena cava. *Arch. Sci. Biol. (St. Petersburg)* **2,** 580–585.
321. Becker, F. F. (1970). The normal hepatocyte in division: Regeneration of the mammalian liver. *Prog. Liver. Dis.* **3,** 60–76.
322. Bucher, N. L. R. (1963). Regeneration of mammalian liver. *Int. Rev. Cytol.* **15,** 245–300.
323. Bucher, N. L. R. (1967). Experimental aspects of hepatic regeneration. *N. Engl. J. Med.* **277,** 686–696, 738–746.

324. Bucher, N. L. R., Schrock, T. R., and Moolten, F. L. (1969). An experimental view of hepatic regeneration. *Johns Hopkins Med. J.* **125,** 250–257.
325. Klinman, N. R., and Erslev, A. J. (1963). Cellular response to partial hepatectomy. *Proc. Soc. Exp. Biol. Med.* **112,** 338–340.
326. Brues, A. M., Drury, D. R., and Brues, M. C. (1936). Quantitative study of cell growth in regenerating liver. *Arch. Pathol.* **22,** 658–673.
327. Sigel, B. (1969). The extracellular regulation of liver regeneration. *J. Surg. Res.* **9,** 387–394.
328. Grisham, J. W. (1962). A morphologic study of deoxyribonucleic acid synthesis and cell proliferation in regenerating rat liver: Autoradiography with thymidine-H3. *Cancer Res.* **22,** 842–849.
329. Becker, F. F., and Lane, B. P. (1968). Regeneration of the mammalian liver. VI. Retention of phenobarbital-induced cytoplasmic alterations in dividing hepatocytes. *Am. J. Pathol.* **52,** 211–226.
330. Fabrikant, J. I. (1967). The spacial distribution of parenchymal cell proliferation during regeneration of the liver. *Bull. Hopkins Hosp.* **120,** 137–147.
331. Bollman, J. L., Flock, E. V., Grindlay, J. H., *et al.* (1957). Coma with increased amino acids of brain and cerebrospinal fluid in dogs with Eck's fistula: Prevention by portal-systemic collateral circulation. *Arch. Surg.* **75,** 405–412.
332. Bollman, J. L. (1961). The animal with an Eck fistula. *Physiol. Rev.* **41,** 607–621.
333. Starzl, T. E., Porter, K. A., and Putnam, C. W. (1975). Intraportal insulin protects from the liver injury of portacaval shunt in dogs. *Lancet* **2,** 1241–1242.
334. Starzl, T. E., Porter, K. A., Watanabe, K., *et al.* (1976). The effects of insulin, glucagon and insulin–glucagon infusions upon liver morphology and cell division after complete portacaval shunt in dogs. *Lancet* **1,** 821–825.
335. Fisher, E. R., and Fisher, B. (1963). Ultrastructural hepatic changes following partial hepatectomy and portacaval shunt in the rat. *Lab. Invest.* **12,** 929–942.
336. Oudea, P., and Bismuth, H. (1965). L'Anastomose porto-cave experimentale chez le rat normal. *Pathol. Biol. (Paris)* **13,** 288–296.
337. Rubin, E., Gevirtz, N. R., Cohan, P., *et al.* (1965). Liver cell damage produced by portacaval shunt. *Proc. Soc. Exp. Biol. Med.* **118,** 235–237.
338. Wessel, W., Cerny, J., Segschneider, I., *et al.* (1972). Electronenmikroskopische, morphometrische und histologische Untersuchungen an Rattenlebern nach Unterbindung eines Astes der Vena Portae. *Beitr. Pathol.* **145,** 119–148.
339. Mallet-Guy, Y., Hezez, G., and Feroldi, J. (1972). Anastomose portocave laterolaterale experimentale: Documents histologiques et electro-microscopiques. *Lyon Chir.* **68,** 436–445.
340. Starzl, T. E., Lee, I-Y., Porter, K. A., *et al.* (1975). The influence of portal blood upon lipid metabolism in normal and diabetic dogs and baboons. *Surg. Gynecol. Obstet.* **140,** 381–396.
341. Putnam, C. W., Porter, K. A., and Starzl, T. E. (1976). Hepatic encephalopathy and light and electron micrographic changes of the baboon liver after portal diversion. *Ann. Surg.* **184,** 155–161.
342. Rous, P., and Larimore, L. D. (1920). Relation of the portal blood to liver maintenance: A demonstration of liver atrophy conditional on compensation. *J. Exp. Med.* **31,** 609–632.
343. Mann, F. C. (1940). The portal circulation and restoration of the liver after partial removal. *Surgery* **8,** 225–238.
344. Mann, F. C. (1944). The William Henry Welch Lectures: II. Restoration and pathologic reactions of the liver. *J. Mt Sinai Hosp.* **11,** 65–74.
345. Child, C. G., Barr, D., Holswade, G. R., *et al.* (1953). Liver regeneration following portacaval transposition in dogs. *Ann. Surg.* **138,** 600–608.
346. Fisher, B., Russ, C., Updegraff, H., *et al.* (1954). Effect of increased hepatic blood flow upon liver regeneration. *Arch. Surg.* **69,** 263–272.
347. Fisher, B., Fisher, E. R., and Lee, S. (1967). Experimental evaluation of liver atrophy and portacaval shunt. *Surg. Gynecol. Obstet.* **125,** 1253–1258.
348. Weinbren, K. (1955). The portal blood supply and regeneration of the rat liver. *Br. J. Exp. Pathol.* **36,** 583–591.
349. Fisher, B., Lee, S. H., Fisher, F. R., and Saffer, E. (1962). Liver regeneration following portacaval shunt. *Surgery* **52,** 88–102.
350. Becker, F. F. (1963). Restoration of liver mass following partial hepatectomy: Surgical hepartrophy. *Am. J. Pathol.* **43,** 497–510.
351. Alston, W. C., and Thomson, R. Y. (1963). Humoral and local factors in liver regeneration. *Cancer Res.* **23,** 901–905.
352. Thomson, R. Y., and Clarke, A. M. (1965). Role of portal blood supply in liver regeneration. *Nature* **208,** 392–393.
353. Gentile, J. M., and Grace, J. T., Jr. (1968). A cell growth stimulating factor in partially hepatectomized rat serum. *Surg. Forum* **19,** 62–63.
354. Gentile, J. M., Avila, L., and Grace, J. T., Jr. (1970). Liver regeneration: Old and new concepts. *Am. J. Surg.* **120,** 2–6.
355. Adibi, S., Paschkis, K. E., and Cantarow, A. (1959). Stimulation of liver mitosis by blood serum from hepatectomized rats. *Exp. Cell. Res.* **18,** 396–398.
356. Freedrich-Freksa, H., and Zaki, F. G. (1954). Spezifische Mitose-Auslosung in normaler Rattenleber durch Serum von partiell hepatektomierten. *Ratten Z. Naturforsch.* **98,** 394–398.
357. Hughes, P. E. (1960). Humoral factors in liver regeneration. *Aust. Ann. Med.* **9,** 41–43.
358. Christensen, B. G., and Jacobsen, E. (1949–1950). Studies on liver regeneration. *Acta Med. Scand. Suppl.* **234,** 103–108.
359. Bucher, N. L. R., Scott, J., and Aub, J. C. (1951). Regeneration of liver in parabiotic rats. *Cancer Res.* **11,** 457–465.
360. Wennecker, A. S., and Sussman, N. (1951). Degeneration of liver tissue following partial hepatectomy in parabolic rats. *Proc. Soc. Exp. Biol. Med.* **76,** 683–686.
361. Fisher, B., Fisher, E. R., and Saffer, E. (1963). Investigations concerning the role of a humoral factor in liver regeneration. *Cancer Res.* **23,** 914–920.
362. Islami, A. H., Pack, G. T., and Hubbard, J. C. (1959). The humoral factor in regeneration of the liver in parabiotic rats. *Surg. Gynecol. Obstet.* **108,** 549–554.
363. Rogers, A. E., Sharka, J. A., Pechet, G., and Macdonald, R. A. (1961). Regeneration of the liver. Absence of a "humoral factor" affecting hepatic regeneration in parabiotic rats. *Am. J. Pathol.* **39,** 561–578.
364. Moolten, F. L., and Bucher, N. L. R. (1967). Regeneration of rat liver: Transfer of humoral agent by cross circulation. *Science* **158,** 272–274.
365. Sakai, A. (1970). Humoral factor triggering DNA synthesis after partial hepatectomy in the rat. *Nature* **228,** 1186–1187.
366. Lee, S., and Edgington, T. S. (1968). Heterotopic liver transplantation utilizing inbred rat strains. *Am. J. Pathol.* **52,** 649–669.
367. Lee, S., Edgington, T. S., and Orloff, M. J. (1968). The role of afferent blood supply in regeneration of liver isografts in rats. *Surg. Forum* **19,** 360–362.
368. Lee, S., Keiter, J. E., Rosen, H., Chandler, J. G., and Orloff, M. J. Influence of blood supply on regeneration of liver transplants. *Surg. Forum* **20,** 369–371.
369. Lee, S., Chandler, J. G., Williams, R. J., Rosen, H., and Orloff, M. J. (1971). A trophic factor in portal blood required for liver regeneration. *Gastroenterology* **60,** 688.
370. Chandler, J. G., Lee, S., Krubel, R., Rosen, H., and Orloff, M. J. (1971). The roles of inter-liver competition and portal blood in regeneration of auxiliary liver transplants. *Surg. Forum* **22,** 341–343.
371. Fisher, B., *et al.* (1971). A portal blood factor as the humoral agent in liver regeneration. *Science* **171,** 575–577.
372. Fisher, B., Szuch, P., and Fisher, E. R. (1971). Evaluation of a humoral factor in liver regeneration utilizing liver transplants. *Cancer Res.* **31,** 322–331.

373. Siegel, B., Brightman, S. A., *et al.* (1968). Effect of blood flow reversal in liver autotransplants upon the site of hepatocyte regeneration. *J. Clin. Invest.* **47,** 1231–1237.
374. Starzl, T. E., Marchioro, T. L., Huntley, R. T., *et al.* (1964). Experimental and clinical homotransplantation of the liver. *Ann. NY Acad. Sci.* **120,** 739–765.
375. Starzl, T. E., Marchioro, T. L., Rowlands, D. T., Jr., *et al.* (1964). Immunosuppression after experimental and clinical homotransplantation. *Ann. Surg.* **160,** 411–439.
376. Thomford, N. R., Shorter, R. G., and Hallenbeck, G. A. (1965). Homotransplantation of the canine liver. *Arch. Surg.* **90,** 527–538.
377. Marchioro, T. L., Porter, K. A., Dickinson, T. C., *et al.* (1965). Physiologic requirements for auxiliary liver homotransplantation. *Surg. Gynecol. Obstet.* **121,** 17–31.
378. Halgrimson, C. G., Marchioro, T. L., Faris, T. D., *et al.* (1966). Auxiliary liver homotransplantation: Effect of host portacaval shunt. *Arch. Surg.* **93,** 107–118.
379. Tretbar, L. L., Beven, E. G., and Hermann, R. E. (1967). The effects of portacaval shunt and portal flow occlusion on canine auxiliary liver homotransplants. *Surgery* **61,** 733–738.
380. Daloze, P. M., Huguet, C., Groth, C. G., and Stoll, F. (1969). Blood flow in auxiliary canine liver homografts. *J. Surg. Res.* **9,** 10–12.
381. Sigel, B., Baldia, L. B., and Dunn, M. R. (1965). Effect of portosystemic shunting and decreased blood flow on partial heterotopic liver autotransplants. *Surg. Forum* **16,** 288–290.
382. Sigel, B., Baldia, L. B., and Dunn, M. R. (1967). Studies of liver lobes autotransplanted outside the abdominal cavity. *Surg. Gynecol. Obstet.* **124,** 525–530.
383. Marchioro, T. L., Porter, K. A., Brown, B. I., *et al.* (1965). The specific influence of non-hepatic splanchnic venous blood flow on the liver. *Surg. Forum* **16,** 280–282.
384. Wellborn, M. B., Jr., Lanier, V. C., Jr., and Foster, J. H. (1966). Hepatotropic influence of portal venous blood. *Surg. Forum* **17,** 381–383.
385. Fisher, B., Fisher, E. R., and Lee, S. (1967). Experimental evaluation of liver atrophy and portocaval shunt. *Surg. Gynecol. Obstet.* **125,** 1253–1258.
386. Sgro, J. C., Charters, A. C., Chandler, J. G., *et al.* (1973). Site of origin of the hepatotrophic portal blood factor involved in liver regeneration. *Surg. Forum* **24,** 377–379.
387. Broelsch, C. E., Lee, S., Charters, A. C., *et al.* (1974). Regeneration of liver isografts transplanted in continuity with splanchnic organs. *Surg. Forum* **25,** 394–396.
388. Duguay, L. R., Charters, A. C., Lee, S., *et al.* (1975). Time course of liver regeneration after splanchnic organ ablation. *Surg. Forum* **26,** 408–410.
389. Lee, S., Duguay, L. R., and Orloff, M. J. (1976). Pancreas extract and liver regeneration. *Surg. Forum* **27,** 358–360.
390. Starzl, T. E., Francavilla, A., Halgrimson, C. G., *et al.* (1973). The origin, hormonal nature, and action of hepatotrophic substances in portal venous blood. *Surg. Gynecol. Obstet.* **137,** 179–199.
391. Skivolocki, W. P., Duguay, L. R., and Orloff, M. J. (1977). Effect of pancreatic hormones on liver regeneration in a double-liver rat bioassay. *Surg. Forum* **28,** 385–387.
392. Duguay, L. R., and Orloff, M. J. Role of the pancreas in regulation of liver regeneration in dogs. *Surg. Forum* **28,** 387–389.
393. Starzl, T. E., Porter, K. A., and Francavilla, A. (1983). The Eck fistula in animals and humans. *Curr. Prob. Surg.* **20,** 689–752.
394. Ivy, A. C., Lim, R. K. S., and McCarthy, J. E. (1925). Contributions to the physiology of gastric secretion. II. The intestinal phase of gastric secretion. *Q. J. Exp. Physiol.* **15,** 55–67.
395. Leconte, P. (1900). Fonctions gastro-intestinales. *Cellule* **17,** 283–321.
396. Pavloy, I. P. (1902). "The Work of the Digestive Glands," 1st ed. (Thompson, W. H., translator). Charles Griffin & Co., Ltd., London.
397. Gregory, R. A., and Ivy, A. C. (1941). Humoral stimulation of gastric secretion. *Q. J. Exp. Physiol.* **31,** 111–128.
398. Nagano, K., Johnson, A. N., Jr., Cobo, A., and Oberhelman, H. A., Jr. (1959). The effect of distention of the duodenum on gastric secretion. *Surg. Forum* **10,** 152–155.
399. Sircus, W. (1953). Intestinal phase of gastric secretion. *Q. J. Exp. Physiol.* **38,** 91–100.
400. Clarke, J. S., Ozeran, R. S., Hart, J. C., Cruze, K., and Crevling, V. (1958). Peptic ulcer following portacaval shunt. *Ann. Surg.* **148,** 551–566.
401. Dubuque, T. J., Jr., Mulligan, L. V., and Neville, E. C. (1957). Gastric secretion and peptic ulceration in the dog with portal obstruction and portacaval anastomosis. *Surg. Forum* **8,** 208–211.
402. Gerez, L., and Weiss, A. (1936). Über die magensaftsekretion bei Eckscher fistel. *Z. Gesamte Exp. Med.* **100,** 281–288.
403. Kohatsu, S., Gwaltney, J. A., Nagano, K., and Dragstedt, L. R. (1959). Mechanism of gastric hypersecretion following portacaval transposition. *Am. J. Physiol.* **196,** 841–843.
404. Lebedinskaja, S. I. (1933). Uber die magensekretion bei Eckschen fistulhunden. *Z. Gesamte Exp. Med.* **88,** 264–270.
405. Orloff, M. I., and Windsor, C. W. O. (1966). Effect of portacaval shunt on gastric acid secretion in dogs with liver disease, portal hypertension and massive ascites. *Ann. Surg.* **164,** 69–80.
406. Silen, W., and Eiseman, B. (1959). The nature and cause of gastric hypersecretion following portacaval shunts. *Surgery* **46,** 38–47.
407. Rex, J. C., Code, C. F., and ReMine, W. H. (1964). Gastric secretion of acid and urinary excretion of histamine in dogs with portacaval transposition. *Ann. Surg.* **160,** 193–201.
408. Macpherson, W. A., Miller, I., Nishikawa, W. Y., McKissock, P. K., and Clarke, J. S. (1962). The importance of the antrum in gastric hypersecretion after shunt. *Surg. Forum* **13,** 271–273.
409. Newman, P. H., Reeder, D. D., Davidson, W. D., Schneider, E., Miller, J. H., and Thompson, J. C. (1969). Acid secretion following portacaval shunting: Role of vagus, gastrin, intestinal phase and histamine. *Arch. Surg.* **99,** 369–375.
410. Orloff, M. J., Villar-Valdes, H., Rosen, H., Thompson, A. G., and Chandler, J. G. (1969). Humoral mediation of the intestinal phase of gastric secretion and of acid hypersecretion associated with portacaval shunts. *Surgery* **66,** 118–130.
411. O'Sullivan, W. D., Cantlin, M. I., Sweeney, R. D., Rosteing, H. M., and Foster, W. C. (1960). Role of residual stomach in hypersecretion of Heidenhain pouch after portacaval transposition. *Surg. Forum* **11,** 347–348.
412. Clarke, J. S., McKissock, P. K., and Cruze, K. (1959). Studies on the site of origin of the agent causing hypersecretion in dogs with portacaval shunt. *Surgery* **46,** 48–55.
413. Clarke, J. S., Miller, I., and McKissock, P. K. (1966). Increased acid secretion from Heidenhain pouches by shunting colonic venous blood around the liver. *Arch. Surg.* **92,** 653–656.
414. Hayashi, K., Rheault, M. J., Semb, L. S., (1968). Nyhus, J. M. The effect of splenocaval shunt on gastric secretion and liver function as compared with other shunting procedures in the dog. *Surgery* **64,** 1084–1091.
415. Leger, L., Cachin, M., and Pergola, F. (1960). Ulceres gastroduodenaux apres anastomose portocave. A propos de quelques documents personnels. *Presse. Med.* **68,** 63–66.
416. Brown, G. E., Faustina, G. E., and Orloff, M. J. (1967). Humoral mediation of the intestinal phase of gastric secretion. *Surg. Forum* **18,** 298–300.
417. Villar-Valdes, H., Thompson, A. G., Chandler, J. G., and Orloff, M. J. (1969). Endogenous origin of the humoral agent responsible for gastric hypersecretion associated with portacaval shunt. *Surg. Forum* **20,** 360–362.
418. Orloff, M. J., Villar-Valdes, H., Abbott, A. G., Williams, R. I., and Rosen, H. (1970). Site of origin of the hormone responsible for gastric hypersecretion associated with portacaval shunt. *Surgery* **68,** 202–207.

419. Clarke, J. S., Costarella, R., and Ward, S. (1950). Gastric secretion in the fasting state and after antral stimulation in patients with cirrhosis and with portacaval shunts. *Surg. Forum* **9**, 417–420.
420. Ferrarese, S., and Ronzini, V. (1966). Gastric secretion in cirrhotics after portasystemic shunts. *Gaz. Int. Med. Chir.* **71**, 882–889.
421. Ostrow, J. D., Timmerman, R. J., and Gray, S. J. (1960). Gastric secretion in human hepatic cirrhosis. *Gastroenterology* **38**, 303–313.
422. Schriefers, K. H., Schreiber, H. W., and Esser, G. (1963). Zur frage der magensaftsekretion und des magen-duodenalulcus beim pfortaderhochdruck der lebercirrhose und nach portocavalen shunt-operation. *Arch. Klin. Chir.* **302**, 702–715.
423. Scobie, B. A., and Summerskill, W. H. J. (1964). Reduced gastric acid output in cirrhosis: Quantitation and relationships. *Gut* **5**, 422–428.
424. Tabaqchali, S., and Dawson, A. M. (1964). Peptic ulcer and gastric secretion in patients with liver disease. *Gut* **5**, 417–421.
425. Wilkinson, F. O. W., and Riddell, A. G. (1965). Studies on gastric secretion before and after portacaval anastomosis. *Br. J. Surg.* **52**, 530–535.
426. Orloff, M. J., Chandler, J. G., Alderman, S. J., Keiter, J. E., and Rosen, H. (1969). Gastric secretion and peptic ulcer following portacaval shunt in man. *Ann. Surg.* **170**, 515–527.
427. Orloff, M. J., Abbott, A. G., and Rosen, H. (1970). Nature of the humoral agent responsible for portacaval shunt-related gastric hypersecretion in man. *Am. J. Surg.* **120**, 237–243.
428. Abbott, A. G., Rosen, H., and Orloff, M. J. (1970). Site of origin of the hormone responsible for gastric hypersecretion in humans with portacaval shunts. *Surg. Forum* **21**, 340–343.
429. Orloff, M. J., Abbott, A. G., and Rosen, H. (1971). Jejunal origin of the hormone responsible for the intestinal phase of gastric secretion and portacaval shunt-related hypersecretion in man. *Gastroenterology* **60**, 703.
430. D'Amico, G., Morabito, A., Pagliaro, L., and Marubini, E. (1986). Survival and prognostic indicators in compensated and decompensated cirrhosis. *Dig. Dis. Sci.* **31**, 468–475.
431. Capone, R. R., Buhac, I., Kohberg, R. C., and Balint, J. A. (1978). Resistant ascites in alcoholic liver cirrhosis. *Dig. Dis. Sci.* **23**, 867–871.
432. Gines, P., Arroyo, V., Vargas, V., *et al.* (1991). Paracentesis with intravenous infusion of albumin as compared with peritoneovenous shunting in cirrhosis with refractory ascites. *N. Engl. J. Med.* **325**, 829–835.
433. Orloff, M. J., and Snyder, G. B. (1961). Experimental ascites. II. The effects of portacaval shunts on ascites produced with an internal vena cava cannula. *Surgery* **50**, 220–230.
434. Orloff, M. J., Spitz, B. R., Wall, M. H., Thomas, H. S., and Halasz, N. A. (1964). Experimental ascites. IV: Comparison of the effects of end-to-side and side-to-side portacaval shunts on intractable ascites. *Surgery* **56**, 784–799.
435. DeBenedetti, M. J., Wright, P. W., and Orloff, M. J. (1964). Dynamics of hepatic lymph and blood flow in experimental liver disease and ascites. *Surg. Forum* **15**, 110–111.
436. Orloff, M. J., Wright, P. W., DeBenedetti, M. J., *et al.* (1966). Experimental ascites. VII. The effects of drainage of the thoracic duct on ascites and hepatic hemodynamics. *Arch. Surg.* **93**, 119–130.
437. Orloff, M. J., Goodhead, B., Windsor, D. W. O., Musicant, M. E., and Annetts, O. L. (1967). Effect of portacaval shunt on lymph flow in the thoracic duct. Experiments with normal dogs and dogs with cirrhosis and ascites. *Am. J. Surg.* **114**, 213–221.
438. Orloff, M. J., Ross, T. H., Baddeley, R. M., *et al.* (1964). Experimental ascites. VI. The effects of hepatic venous outflow obstruction and ascites on aldosterone secretion. *Surgery* **56**, 83–98.
439. Orloff, M. J., Baddeley, R. M., Ross, T. H., *et al.* (1964). Regulation of aldosterone secretion by an hepatic receptor. *Surg. Forum* **15**, 74–76.
440. Orloff, M. J., Lipman, C. A., Noel, S. M., *et al.* (1965). Hepatic regulation of aldosterone secretion by a humoral mediator. *Surgery* **58**, 225–247.
441. Bengtsson, F., Nobin, A., Falch, B., *et al.* (1980). Portacaval shunt in the rat: Selective alterations in behaviour and brain serotonin. *Pharmacol. Biochem. Behav.* **24**, 1611–1616.
442. Tricklebank, M. D., Smart, J. L., Bloxam, D. L., *et al.* (1978). Effects of chronic experimental liver dysfunction and L-tryptophan on behavior in the rat. *Pharmacol. Biochem. Behav.* **9**, 181–189.
443. Maddison, J. E., Watson, W. J., Dodd, P. R., and Johnston, G. A. R. (1991). Alterations in cortical [^{3}H]kainate and α-[^{3}H]amino-3-hydroxyl-5-methyl-isoxazolepropionic acid binding in a spontaneous canine model of chronic hepatic encephalopathy. *J. Neurochem.* **56**, 1881–1888.
444. Cordoba, J., and Blei, A. T. (1997). Treatment of hepatic encephalopathy. *Am. J. Gastroenterol.* **92**, 1429–1439.
445. Gabuzda, D., Jr., Philips, G. B., and Davidson, C. S. (1952). Reversible toxic manifestations in 2 patients with cirrhosis of the liver given cation-exchange resins. *N. Engl. J. Med.* **46**, 124–130.
446. Szerb, J. C., and Butterworth, R. F. (1992). Effect of ammonium ions on synaptic transmission in the mammalian central nervous system. *Prog. Neurobiol.* **39**, 135–153.
447. Lai, J. C. K., and Cooper, A. J. L. (1986). α-Ketoglutarate dehydrogenase complex: Kinetic properties, regional distribution and effects of inhibitors. *J. Neurochem.* **47**, 1376–1386.
448. Hindfelt, B., Plum, F., and Duffy, T. E. (1977). Effects of acute ammonia intoxication on cerebral metabolism in rats with portacaval shunts. *J. Clin. Invest.* **59**, 386–396.
449. Yao, H., Sadoshima, S., Fujii, K., *et al.* (1987). Cerebrospinal fluid lactate in patients with hepatic encephalopathy. *Eur. Neurol.* **27**, 182–187.
450. Therrien, G., Giguere, J. F., and Butterworth, R. F. (1991). Increased cerebrospinal fluid lactate reflects deterioration of neurological status in experimental portal-systemic encephalopathy. *Metab. Brain Dis.* **6**, 225–231.
451. Raghavendra Rao, V. L., Audet, R. M., and Butterworth, R. F. (1995). Increased nitric oxide synthase activities and L-[^{3}H]arginine uptake in brain following portacaval anastomosis. *J. Neurochem.* **65**, 677–681.
452. Bender, A. S., and Norenberg, M. D. (1996). Effect of ammonia on L-glutamate uptake in cultured astrocytes. *Neurochem. Res.* **21**, 567–573.
453. Knecht, K., Michalak, A., Rose, C., Rothstein, J. D., and Butterworth, R. F. (1997). Decreased glutamate transporter (GLT-1) expression in frontal cortex of rats with acute liver failure. *Neurosci. Lett.* **229**, 201–203.
454. Orloff, M. J., Wall, M. H., Hickman, E. B., and Neesby, T. (1963). Influence of stomal size of portacaval shunts on peripheral blood ammonia levels. *Ann. Surg.* **158**, 172–181.
455. Sarfeh, J. J., and Rypins, E. B. (1994). Partial versus total portacaval shunt in alcoholic cirrhosis. Results of a prospective, randomized clinical trial. *Ann. Surg.* **219**, 353–361.
456. Zervox, E. E., Goode, S. E., and Rosemurgy, A. S. (1998). Immediate and long-term portal hemodynamic consequences of small-diameter H-graft portacaval shunt. *J. Surg. Res.* **74**, 71–75.
457. Hazell, A. S., Desjardins, P., and Butterworth, R. F. (1999). Exposure of primary astrocyte cultures to manganese results in increased binding sites for "peripheral-type" benzodiazepine receptor ligands. *Neurosci. Lett.* **271**, 5–8.
458. Hazell, A. S., Desjardins, P., and Butterworth, R. F. (1999). Increased expression of glyceraldehyde-3-phosphate dehydrogenase in cultured astrocytes following exposure to manganese. *Neurochem. Int.* **35**, 11–17.
459. Weissenborn, K., Ehrenheim, C. H., Hori, A., Kubica, S., and Manns, M. P. (1995). Pallidal lesions in patients with liver cirrhosis: Clinical and MRI evaluation. *Metab. Brain Dis.* **10**, 219–231.
460. Zieve, L., Doizaki, W. M., and Zieve, J. (1974). Synergism between mercaptans and ammonia or fatty acids in the production of coma: A possible role for mercaptans in the pathogenesis of hepatic coma. *J. Lab. Clin. Med.* **83**, 16–28.

461. Zieve, L. (1989). Role of toxins and synergism in hepatic encephalopathy. *In* "Hepatic Encephalopathy: Pathophysiology and Treatment," (Butterworth, R.F., and Pomier Layrargues, G., Eds.), pp. 141–156. Humana Press; Clifton, NJ. 1989.
462. Mousseau, D. D., Baker, G. B., and Butterworth, R. F. (1997). Increased density of catalytic sites and expression of brain monoamine oxidase A in humans with hepatic encephalopathy. *J. Neurochem.* **68,** 1200–1208.
463. Bergeron, M., Reader, T. A., Pomier Layrargues, G., and Butterworth, R. F. (1989). Monoamines and metabolites in autopsied brain tissue from cirrhotic patients with hepatic encephalopathy. *Neurochem. Res.* **14,** 853–859.
464. Young, S. N., and Lai, S. (1980). CNS tryptamine metabolism in hepatic coma. *J. Neural. Transm.* **47,** 153–161.
465. Bergeron, M., Swain, M. S., Reader, T. A., and Butterworth, R. F. (1995). Regional alterations of dopamine and its metabolites in rat brain following portacaval anastomosis. *Neurochem. Res.* **20,** 79–86.
466. Bergeron, M., Swain, M. S., Reader, T. A., Grondin, L., and Butterworth, R. F. (1990). Effect of ammonia on brain serotonin metabolism in relation to function in the portacaval-shunted rat. *J. Neurochem.* **55,** 222–229.
467. Desjardins, P., Bandeira, P., Raghavendra Rao, V. L., Ledoux, S., and Butterworth, R. F. (1997). Increased expression of the peripheral-type benzodiazepine receptor-isoquinoline carboxamide binding protein mRNA brain following portacaval anastomosis. *Brain Res.* **758,** 255–258.
468. Giguère, J. F., Hamel, E., and Butterworth, R. F. (1992). Increased densities of binding sites for the "peripheral-type" benzodiazepine receptor ligand ^{3}H-PK 11195 in rat brain following portacaval anastomosis. *Brain Res.* **585,** 295–298.
469. Raghavendra Rao, V. L., Audet, R., Therrien, G., and Butterworth, R. F. (1994). Tissue-specific alterations of binding sites for peripheral-type benzodiazepine receptor ligand [^{3}H]PK 11195 in rats following portacaval anastomosis. *Dig. Dis. Sci.* **39,** 1055–1063.
470. Lavoie, J., Pomier Layrargues, G., and Butterworth, R. F. (1990). Increased densities of peripheral-type benzodiazepine receptors in brain autopsy samples from cirrhotic patients with hepatic encephalopathy. *Hepatology* **11,** 874–878.
471. Raghavendra Rao, V. L., Audet, R. M., and Butterworth, R. F. (1997). Increased neuronal nitric oxide synthase expression in brain following portacaval anastomosis. *Brain Res.* **765,** 169–172.
472. Raghavendra Rao, V. L., Audet, R. M., and Butterworth, R. F. (1997). Portacaval shunting and hyperammonemia stimulate the uptake of L-^{3}H-arginine but not of L-^{3}H-nitroarginine into rat brain synaptosomes. *J. Neurochem.* **68,** 337–343.
473. Raghavendra Rao, V. L., and Butterworth, R. F. (1998). Neuronal nitric oxide synthase and hepatic encephalopathy. *Metah. Brain Dis.* **12,** 175–189.
474. Mousseau, D. D., Perney, P., Pomier Layrargues, G., and Butterworth, R. F. (1993). Selective loss of pallidal dopamine D_2 receptor density in hepatic encephalopathy. *Neurosci. Lett.* **162,** 192–196.
475. Pomier Layrargues, G., Spahr, L., and Butterworth, R. F. (1995). Increased manganese concentrations in pallidum of cirrhotic patients. *Lancet* **345,** 735.
476. Ferenci, P., Herneth, A., and Steindl, P. (1996). Newer approaches to therapy of hepatic encephalopathy. *Semin. Liver Dis.* **16,** 329–338.
477. Wolpert, E., Phillips, S. F., and Summerskill, W. H. (1970). Ammonia production in the human colon: Effects of cleansing, neomycin and acetohydroxamic acid. *N. Engl. J. Med.* **283,** 159–164.
478. Brown, R. L., Gibson, J. A., Sladen, G. E., Hicks, B., and Dawson, A. M. (1974). Effects of lactulose and other laxatives on ileal and colonic pH as measured by a radiotelemetry device. *Gut* **15,** 999–1004.
479. Lockwood, A. M., McDonald, J. M., and Rieman, R. E. (1979). The dynamics of ammonia metabolism in men: Effects of liver disease and hyperammonemia. *J. Clin. Invest.* **63,** 449–460.
480. Swart, G. R., van den Berg, J. W. O., van Vuure, J. K., *et al.* (1989). Minimum protein requirements in liver cirrhosis determined by nitrogen balance measurements at three levels of protein intake. *Clin. Nutr.* **8,** 329–336.
481. Kircheis, G., Nilius, R., Held, C., Berndt, H., *et al.* (1997). Therapeutic efficacy of L-ornithine-L-aspartate infusions in patients with cirrhosis and hepatic encephalopathy: Results of a placebo-controlled, double-blind study. *Hepatology* **25,** 1351–1360.
482. Rose, C., Michalak, A., Pannunzio, P., *et al.* (1998). L-Orthinine-L-aspartate in experimental portal-systemic encephalopathy: Therapeutic efficacy and mechanism of action. *Metab. Brain Dis.* **13,** 147–157.
483. Sushma, S., Dasarathy, S., Tandon, R. K., Jain, S., Gupta, S., and Bhist, M. S. (1992). Sodium benzoate in the treatment of acute hepatic encephalopathy: A double-blind randomized trial. *Hepatology* **16,** 138–144.
484. Pomier Layrargues, G., Gigùere, J. E., Lavoie, J., *et al.* (1994). Clinical efficacy of benzodiazepine antagonist RO 15–1788 (flumazenil) in cirrhotic patients with hepatic coma: Results of a randomized double-blind placebo-controlled crossover trial. *Hepatology* **19,** 32–37.
485. Gyr, K., Meier, R., Haussler, J., *et al.* (1996). Evaluation of the efficacy and safety of flumazenil in the treatment of portal systemic encephalopathy: A double blind, randomised, placebo controlled multicentre study. *Gut* **39,** 319–324.
486. Butterworth, R. F., Wells, J., and Pomier Layrargues, G. (1995). Detection of benzodiazepines in hepatic encephalopathy: Reply. *Hepatology* **2,** 605.
487. Tamaki, A., Goldby, M., and Orloff, M. J. (1968). Effects of side-to-side portacaval shunt on hepatic hemodynamics and metabolism. *Surg. Forum* **19,** 324–326.
488. Reynolds, T. B., Hudson, N. M., Mikkelson, W. P., *et al.* (1966). Clinical comparison of end-to-side and side-to-side portacaval shunt. *N. Engl. J. Med.* **274,** 706–710.
489. Iwatsuki, S., Mikkelson, W. P., Redeker, A. G., *et al.* (1973). Clinical comparison of the end-to-side and side-to-side portacaval shunt: Ten year follow-up. *Ann. Surg.* **178,** 65–69.
490. Panke, W. F., Rousselot, L. M., and Burchell, A. R. (1968). A sixteen-year experience with end-to-side portacaval shunt for variceal hemorrhage: Analysis of data and comparison with other types of portasystemic anastomoses. *Ann. Surg.* **168,** 957–965.
491. Turcotte, J. G., Wallin, V. W., Jr., and Child, C. G., III. (1969). End-to-side versus side-to-side portacaval shunts in patients with hepatic cirrhosis. *Am. J. Surg.* **117,** 108–116.
492. Bernstein, J. E., Nutting, R. O., and Orloff, M. J. (1968). Comparison of the effects of end-to-side and side-to-side portacaval shunts on liver function, liver blood flow, and ammonia metabolism in dogs and man. *Surg. Forum* **19,** 328–330.
493. Orloff, M. J., Chandler, J. G., Charters, A. C., *et al.* (1974). Comparison of end-to-side and side-to-side portacaval shunts in dogs and humans with cirrhosis and portal hypertension. *Am. J. Surg.* **128,** 195–201.
494. Charters, A. C., Chandler, J. G., Condon, J. K., *et al.* (1974). Spontaneous reversal of portal flow in patients with bleeding varices treated by emergency portacaval shunt. *Am. J. Surg.* **127,** 25–29.
495. Cameron, J. L., Zuidema, G. D., Smith, G. W., *et al.* (1979). Mesocaval shunts for the control of bleeding esophageal varices. *Surgery* **85,** 275–262.
496. Dowling, J. B. (1979). Ten years' experience with mesocaval grafts. *Surg. Gynecol. Obstet.* **149,** 518–522.
497. Drapanas, T. (1972). Interposition mesocaval shunt for treatment of portal hypertension. *Ann. Surg.* **176,** 435–438.
498. Drapanas, T., LoCicero, J., III, and Dowling, J. B. (1975). Hemodynamics of the interposition mesocaval shunt. *Ann. Surg.* **181,** 523–533.
499. Graziano, J. L., and Sullivan, H. J. (1973). Portal decompression: Clinical experience with the "H" graft. *Ann. Surg.* **178,** 209–214.

500. Thompson, B. W., and Read, R. D. (1974). Proceedings: Interposition "H" grafting for portal hypertension. *Arch. Surg.* **108,** 502–506.
501. Mulcare, R. J., Halleran, D. (1984). Gardine, R. Experience with 49 consecutive Dacron interposition mesocaval shunts. *Am. J. Surg.* **147,** 393–399.
502. Reznick, R. K., Langer, B., Taylor, B. R., *et al.* (1984). Results and hemodynamic changes after interposition mesocaval shunt. *Surgery* **95,** 275–280.
503. Burchell, A. R., Moreno, A. H., Panke, W. F., and Nealon, T. F. (1974). Hemodynamic variables and prognosis following portacaval shunts. *Surg. Gynecol. Obstet.* **138,** 359–369.
504. Burchell, A. R., Moreno, A. H., Panke, W. F., and Nealon, T. F., Jr. (1976). Hepatic artery flow improvement after portacaval shunt: A single hemodynamic clinical correlate. *Ann. Surg.* **184,** 289–302.
505. Charters, A. C., Brown, B. N., Sviokla, S., *et al.* (1975). The influence of portal perfusion on the response to portacaval shunt. *Am. J. Surg.* **130,** 226–232.
506. Price, J. B., Jr., Voorhees, A. B., Jr., and Britton, R. C. (1967). Operative hemodynamic studies in portal hypertension. significance and limitations. *Arch. Surg.* **95,** 843–852.
507. Steegmüller, K. W., Märklin, H-M., and Hollis, H. W., Jr. (1984). Intraoperative hemodynamic investigations during portocaval shunt. *Arch. Surg.* **119,** 269–273.
508. Warren, W. D., and Salam, A. A. (1974). Surgery for the portal hypertension of cirrhosis: The need for change. *Major Probl. Clin. Surg.* **14,** 127–164.
509. Bhalerao, R. A., Pinto, A. C., Bapat, R. D., *et al.* (1978). Selective transplenic decompression of oesophageal varices by distal splenorenal and splenocaval shunt. *Gut* **19,** 831–837.
510. Langer, B., Rotstein, L. E., Stone, R. M., *et al.* (1980). A prospective randomized trial of the selective distal splenorenal shunt. *Surg. Gynecol. Obstet.* **150,** 45–48.
511. Maillard, J., Flamant, Y. M., Hay, J. M., and Chandler, J. G. (1979). Selectivity of the distal splenorenal shunt. *Surgery* **86,** 663–671.
512. Martin, E. W., Jr., Molnar, J., Cooperman, M., *et al.* (1978). Observations on fifty distal splenorenal shunts. *Surgery* **84,** 379–383.
513. Rikkers, L. F., Rudman, D., Galambos, J. T., *et al.* (1978). A randomized, controlled trial of the distal splenorenal shunt. *Ann. Surg.* **187,** 271–282.
514. Rotstein, L. E., Makowka, L., Langer, B., *et al.* (1979). Thrombosis of the portal vein following distal splenorenal shunt. *Surg. Gynecol. Obstet.* **149,** 847–851.
515. Salam, A. A., Warren, W. D., LePage, J., Jr., *et al.* (1971). Hemodynamic contrasts between selective and total portal-systemic decompression. *Ann. Surg.* **173,** 827–844.
516. Turcotte, J. G., and Eckhauser, F. E. (1980). Elective portosystemic shunts. *In* "Gastrointestinal Hemorrhage" (Fiddian-Green, T.G., and Turcotte, J.G., Eds.), PP. 311–326. Grune & Stratton, New York.
517. Vang, J., Simert, G., Hansson, J. A., *et al.* (1976). Results of a modified distal splenorenal shunt for portal hypertension. *Ann. Surg.* **184,** 224–228.
518. Warren, W. D., Salam, A. A., Hutson, D., and Zeppa, R. (1974). Selective distal splenorenal shunt: Technique and results of operation. *Arch. Surg.* **108,** 306–314.
519. Zeppa, R., Hensley, G. T., Levi, J. U., *et al.* (1978). The comparative survival of alcoholics versus nonalcoholics after distal splenorenal shunt. *Ann. Surg.* **187,** 510–514.
520. Fischer, J. E., Bower, R. H., Atamian, S., and Welling, R. (1981). Comparison of distal and proximal splenorenal shunts: A randomized prospective trial. *Ann. Surg.* **194,** 531–544.
521. Warren, W. D., Millikan, W. J., Jr., Henderson, J. M., *et al.* (1982). Ten years' portal hypertensive surgery at Emory. *Ann. Surg.* **195,** 530–542.
522. Henderson, J. M., Millikan, W. J., Jr., Chipponi, J., *et al.* (1982). The incidence and natural history of thrombus in the portal vein following distal splenorenal shunt. *Ann. Surg.* 196: 1–7.
523. Belghiti, J., Grenier, P., Nouel, O., *et al.* (1981). Long-term loss of Warren's shunt selectivity: Angiographic demonstration. *Arch. Surg.* **66,** 1121–1124.
524. Grace, N. D., Conn, H. O., Resnick, R. H., *et al.* (1988). Distal splenorenal vs. portal-systemic shunts after hemorrhage from varices: A randomized controlled trial. *Hepatology* **8,** 1475–1481.
525. Langer, B., Taylor, B. R., and Greig, P. D. (1990). Selective or total shunts for variceal bleeding. *Am. J. Surg.* **160,** 75–79.
526. Maillard, J. N., Benhamou, J. P., and Rueff, B. (1970). Arterialization of the liver with portacaval shunt in the treatment of portal hypertension due to intrahepatic block. *Surgery* **67,** 883–890.
527. Maillard, J. N., Rueff, B., Prandi, D., and Sicot, G. (1974). Hepatic arterialization and portacaval shunt in hepatic cirrhosis: An assessment. *Arch. Surg.* **108,** 315–320.
528. Inokuchi, K. (1978). Selective decompression of esophageal varices by a left gastric venacaval shunt. *Surg. Ann.* **10,** 215–236.
529. Baird, R. J., Tutassaura, H., and Miyagishma, R. T. (1971). Use of the left renal vein for portal decompression. *Ann. Surg.* **173,** 551–553.
530. Sobel, S., Kaplitt, M. J., Popowitz, L., *et al.* (1970). Omphalocaval shunt: A new procedure for portal decompression. *Surgery* **68,** 456–460.
531. Glass, G. V. (1976). Primary, secondary and meta-analysis of research. *Educ. Res.* **5,** 3–90.
532. The Asilomar Working Group on Recommendations for Reporting of Clinical Trials in the Biomedical Literature (1996). Checklist of information for inclusion in reports of clinical trials. *Ann. Intern. Med.* **124,** 741–743.
533. Boissel, J. P., and Bossard, N. (1991). Registry of prospective clinical trials. Eleventh report. *Thromb. Haemost.* **66,** 368–383.
534. Felson, D. T. (1992). Bias in meta-analytic research. *J. Clin. Epidemiol.* **45,** 885–892.
535. Bailar, J. C., III (1995). The practice of meta-analysis. *J. Clin. Epidemiol.* **48,** 149–157.
536. Orloff, M. J. (1967). Emergency portacaval shunt: A comparative study of shunt, varix ligation, and nonsurgical treatment of bleeding esophageal varices in unselected patients with cirrhosis. *Ann. Surg.* **166,** 456–478.
537. Orloff, M. J. (1968). Emergency treatment of bleeding esophageal varices. *In* "The Therapy of Portal Hypertension" (Markoff, N. G., Ed.), pp. 211–219 Thieme, Stuttgart.
538. Orloff, M. J. (1969). Emergency treatment of bleeding esophageal varices in alcoholic cirrhosis. *In* "Biochemical and Clinical Aspects of Alcohol Metabolism" (Sardesai, V. M., Ed.), pp. 288–297, Charles C Thomas, Springfield, IL.
539. Orloff, M. J. Chandler, J. G., Charters, A. C., Condon, J. K., Grambort, D. E., Modafferi, T. R., and Levin, S. E. (1974). Emergency portacaval shunt treatment for bleeding esophageal varices. Prospective study in unselected patients with alcoholic cirrhosis. *Arch. Surg.* **108,** 293–299.
540. Orloff, M. J., Charters, A. C., Chandler, J. G., Condon, J. K., Grambort, D. E., Modafferi, T. R., Levin, S. E., Brown, N. B., Sviokla, S. C., and Knox, D. G. (1975). Portacaval shunt as emergency procedure in unselected patients with alcoholic cirrhosis. *Surg. Gynecol. Obstet.* **141,** 59–68.
541. Orloff, M. J., Bell, R. H., Jr., Hyde, P. V., and Skivolocki, W. P. (1980). Long-term results of emergency portacaval shunt for bleeding esophageal varices in unselected patients with alcoholic cirrhosis. *Ann. Surg.* **192,** 325–340.
542. Orloff, M. J., and Bell, R. H., Jr. (1983). Improved survival of unselected cirrhotic patients with bleeding esophageal varices treated by emergency portacaval shunt. *Gastroenterology* **84,** 388.
543. Bell, R. H., Jr., Hyde, P. V. B., Skivolocki, W. P., Brimm, J. E., and Orloff, M. J. (1981). Prospective study of portal-systemic encephalopathy following emergency portacaval shunt for bleeding varices. *Am. J. Surg.* **142,** 144–150.

544. Orloff, M. J., and Bell, R. H., Jr. (1986). Long-term survival after emergency portacaval shunting for bleeding varices in patients with alcoholic cirrhosis. *Am. J. Surg.* **151,** 176–183.
545. Orloff, M. J., Orloff, M. S., Rambotti, M., and Girard, B. (1992). Is portal-systemic shunt worthwhile in Child's class C cirrhosis? Long-term results of emergency shunt in 94 patients with bleeding varices. *Ann. Surg.* **216,** 256–268.
546. Orloff, M. J., Bell, R. H., Jr., Orloff, M. S., Hardison, W. G. M., and Greenburg, A. G. (1994). Prospective randomized trial of emergency portacaval shunt and emergency medical therapy in unselected cirrhotic patients with bleeding varices. *Hepatology* **20** (Pt 1), 863–872.
547. Orloff, M. J., Orloff, M. S., Orloff, S. L., and Rambotti, M. (1995). Three decades of experience with emergency portacaval shunt for acutely bleeding esophageal varices in 400 unselected patients with cirrhosis of the liver. *J. Am. Coll. Surg.* **180,** 257–272.
548. Orloff, M. J., Orloff, M. S., Orloff, S. L., and Haynes, K. S. (1995). Treatment of bleeding from portal hypertensive gastropathy by portacaval shunt. *Hepatology* **21,** 1011–1017.
549. Orloff, M. J., Orloff, M. S., Orloff, S. L., and Girard, B. (1997). Long-term results of portacaval shunt for bleeding gastric varices in 224 patients with cirrhosis. *Gastroenterology* **112**(4), A3194.
550. Sarin, S. K., Lahoti, D., Saxena, S. P., Murthi, N. S., and Makwane, U. K. (1992). Prevalence and classification and natural history of gastric varices: Long term follow-up study in 568 patients with portal hypertension. *Hepatology* **16,** 1343–1349.
551. Mikkelson, W. P. (1974). Therapeutic portacaval shunt: Preliminary data on controlled trial and morbid effects of acute hyaline necrosis. *Arch. Surg.* **108,** 301.
552. Orloff, M. J. (1980). Elective therapeutic portacaval shunt. *In* "Medical and Surgical Problems of Portal Hypertension" (Orloff, M.J., Stipa, S., and Ziparo, V., Eds.), PP. 127–136. Academic Press, New York.
553. Orloff, M. J., Orloff, M. S., Orloff, S. L., and Girard, B. (1998). Long-term results of elective therapeutic portacaval shunt for bleeding esophagogastric varices in 1000 patients with cirrhosis. *Gastroenterology* **114,** A1318.
554. Campbell, D. P., Parker, D. E., and Anagnostopoulos, C. E. (1973). Survival prediction in portacaval shunts: A computerized statistical analysis. *Am. J. Surg.* **126,** 748–751.
555. Charters, A. C., Brown, B. N., Sviokla, S., *et al.* (1975). The influence of portal perfusion on the response to portacaval shunt. *Am. J. Surg.* **130,** 226–232.
556. Child, C. G., III, and Turcotte, J. G. (1964). Surgery and portal hypertension. *In* "The Liver and Portal Hypertension" (Child, C. G., III, Ed.), PP. 1–85. Saunders, Philadelphia.
557. Eckhauser, F. E., Appelman, H. D., O'Leary, T. J., *et al.* (1980). Hepatic pathology as a determinant of prognosis after portal decompression. *Am. J. Surg.* **139,** 105–112.
558. Kanel, G. C., Kaplan, M. M., Zawacki, J. K., Callow, A. D. (1977). Survival in patients with postnecrotic cirrhosis and Laennec's cirrhosis undergoing therapeutic portacaval shunt. *Gastroenterology* **73,** 679–683.
559. Kessler, R. E., Tice, D. A., Soloway, A. C., and Zimmon, D. S. (1975). Clinical vs. hemodynamic classification of cirrhosis. *Surg. Forum* **26,** 417–419.
560. Mikkelson, W. P., and Kern, W. H. (1974). The influence of acute hyaline necrosis on survival after emergency and elective portacaval shunt. *Major Probl. Clin. Surg.* **14,** 233–242.
561. Orloff, M. I., Duguay, L. R., and Kosta, L. D. (1977). Criteria for selection of patients for emergency portacaval shunt *Am. J. Surg.* **134,** 146–152.
562. Price, J. B., Jr., Britton, R. C., and Voorhees, A. B. Jr. (1967). Operative hemodynamics in portal hypertension: Significance and limitations. *Arch. Surg.* **95,** 843–852.
563. Steegmuller, K. W., Marklin, H.-M., and Hollis, H. W. Jr. (1984). Intraoperative hemodynamic investigations during portocaval shunt. *Arch. Surg.* **119,** 269–273.
564. Siege, J. H., Goldwyn, R. M., Farrell, E. J., *et al.* (1974). Hyperdynamic states and the physiologic determinants of survival in patients with cirrhosis and portal hypertension. *Arch. Surg.* **108,** 282–292.
565. Smith, G. W. (1974). Use of hemodynamic selection criteria in the management of cirrhotic patients with portal hypertension. *Ann. Surg.* **179,** 782–790.
566. Turcotte, J. G., and Lambert, M. J. III. (1973). Variceal hemorrhage, hepatic cirrhosis, and portocaval shunts. *Surgery* **13,** 810–817.
567. Bell, R. H., Jr., Miyai, K., and Orloff, M. J. (1984). Outcome in cirrhotic patients with acute alcoholic hepatitis after emergency portacaval shunt for bleeding esophageal varices. *Am. J. Surg.* **147,** 78–84.
568. Barnes, B. A., Ackroyd, F. W., Battit, G. F., *et al.* (1971). Elective portosystemic shunts: Morbidity and survival data. *Ann. Surg.* **174,** 76–84.
569. Bismuth, H., Franco, D., and Hepp, J. (1974). Portal-systemic shunt in hepatic cirrhosis: Does the type of shunt decisively influence the clinical result? *Ann. Surg.* **179,** 209–218.
570. Linton, R. R., Ellis, D. S., and Geary, J. E. (1961). Critical comparative analysis of early and late results of splenorenal and direct portacaval shunts performed in 169 patients with portal cirrhosis. *Ann. Surg.* **154,** 446–459.
571. McDermott, W. V., Pallazzi, H., Nardi, G. L., and Mondet, A. (1961). Elective portal systemic shunt. *N. Engl. J. Med.* **264,** 419–427.
572. Mikkelson, W. P., Turrill, F. R., and Pattison, A. C. (1962). Portacaval shunt in cirrhosis of the liver. Clinical and hemodynamic aspects. *Am. J. Surg.* **104,** 204–215.
573. Voorhees, A. B., Jr., Price, J. B., Jr., and Britton, R. C. (1970). Portasystemic shunting procedures for portal hypertension: Twenty-six-year experience in adults with cirrhosis of the liver. *Ann. Surg.* **119,** 501–505.
574. Walker, R. M., Shaldon, C., and Vowles, K. D. (1961). Late results of portacaval anastomosis. *Lancet* **2,** 727–730.
575. Ottinger, L. W. (1982). The Linton splenorenal shunt in the management of the bleeding complications of portal hypertension. *Ann. Surg.* **196,** 664–668.
576. Wantz, G. E., and Payne, M. A. (1961). Experience with portacaval shunt for portal hypertension. *N. Engl. J. Med.* **265,** 721–728.
577. Jackson, F. C., Perrin, E. D., Felix, W. R., and Smith, A. G. (1971). A clinical investigation of the portacaval shunt: V. Survival analyses of the therapeutic operation. *Ann. Surg.* **174,** 672–701.
578. Resnick, R. H., Sher, F. L., Ishihara, A. M., *et al.* (1974). A controlled study of the therapeutic portacaval shunt. *Gastroenterology* **67,** 843–857.
579. Rueff, B., Prandi, D., Degos, E., Degos, J. D., *et al.* (1976). A controlled study of therapeutic portacaval shunt in cirrhosis. *Lancet* **1,** 655–659.
580. Conn, H. O. (1974). Therapeutic portacaval anastomosis: To shunt or not to shunt. *Gastroenterology* **67,** 1065–1071.
581. Grace, N. D., Muench, H., and Chalmers, T. C. (1966). The present status of shunts for portal hypertension in cirrhosis. *Gastroenterology* **50,** 684–691.
582. Rösch, J., Hanafee, W. N., and Snow, H. (1969). Transjugular portal venography and radiological portosystemic shunt: An experimental study. *Radiology* **92,** 1112–1114.
583. Rösch, J., Hanafee, W. N., Snow, H., Barenfus, M., and Gray, R. (1971). Transjugular intrahepatic portocaval shunt: An experimental work. *Am. J. Surg.* **121,** 588–592.
584. Colapinto, R. F., Stronell, R. D., Gildiner, M., *et al.* (1983). Formation of an intrahepatic portosystemic shunt using balloon dilatation catheter: Preliminary clinical experience. *Am. J. Roentgenol.* **140,** 709–714.

585. Palmaz, J., Sibbitt, R. R., Reuter, S. R., Garcia, F., and Tio, F. O. (1985). Expandable intrahepatic portocaval shunt stents: Early experience in the dog. *Am. J. Roentgenol.* **145,** 821–825.
586. Palmaz, J., Garcia, E., Sibbitt, R. R., *et al.* (1986). Expandable intrahepatic portocaval shunt stents in dogs with chronic portal hypertension. *Am. J. Roentgenol.* **147,** 1251–1254.
587. Richter, G. M., Palmaz, J. C., and Noeldge, G. (1989). Der transjugulare intrahepatische portosystemische stent-shunt (TIPSS). *Radiologe* **29,** 406–411.
588. Richter, G. M., Noeldge, G., and Palmaz, J. C. (1990). The transjugular intrahepatic portosystemic stent-shunt (TIPSS): Results of a pilot study. *Cardiovasc. Intervent. Radiol.* **13,** 200–207.
589. Rössle, M., Noeldge, G., and Richter, G. M. (1990). The transjugular intrahepatic portosystemic shunt (TIPSS): A 1-year follow-up. *Gastroenterology* **98,** A625.
590. Rössle, M., Noeldge, G., and Pararnau, J. M. (1991). Transjugular intrahepatic portosystemic stent-shunt (TIPSS): Experience with an improved technique. *Hepatology* **14,** 96A. [Abstract]
591. Ring, E. I., Lake, J. R., and Roberts, J. P., *et al.* (1992). Using transjugular intrahepatic portosystemic shunts to control variceal bleeding before liver transplantation. *Ann. Intern. Med.* **116,** 304–309.
592. LaBerge, J. M., Ring, E. L., and Lake, J. R. (1992). Transjugular intrahepatic portosystemic shunts (TIPS): Preliminary results in 25 patients. *J. Vasc. Surg.* **16,** 258–267.
593. LaBerge, J. M., Ring, E. J., Gordon, R., *et al.* (1993). Creation of transjugular intrahepatic portosystemic shunts with the Wallstent endoprosthesis: Results in 100 patients. *Radiology* **187,** 413–420.
594. Rössle, M., Haag, K., Ochs, A., *et al.* (1994). The transjugular intrahepatic portosystemic stent-shunt procedure for variceal bleeding. *N. Engl. J. Med.* **330,** 165–171.
595. LaBerge, J. M., Somberg, K. A., Lake, J. R., *et al.* (1995). Two-year outcome following transjugular intrahepatic portosystemic shunt for variceal bleeding: Results in 90 patients. *Gastroenterology* **108,** 1143–1151.
596. Helton, W. S., Belshaw, A., Althans, S., Port, S., Caldwell, D., and Johansen, K. (1993). Critical appraisal of the angiographic portocaval shunt (TIPS). *Am. J. Surg.* **165,** 566–571.
597. Echenagusia, A. J., Camuñez, F., Simó, G., Peiró, J., Garay, M. G., and Rodriguez Laiz, J. M. (1994). Variceal hemorrhage: Efficacy of transjugular intrahepatic portosystemic shunts created with Strecker stents. *Radiology* **192,** 235–240.
598. McCormick, P. A., Dick, R., Panagau, F. B., *et al.* (1994). Emergency transjugular intrahepatic portosystemic stent shunting as salvage treatment for uncontrolled variceal bleeding. *Br. J. Surg.* **81,** 1324–1327.
599. Sauer, P., Stiehl, A., Hermann, S., Richter, G., Roeren, T., and Theilmann, L. (1994). Stent stenosis after transjugular intrahepatic portosystemic shunt. *Hepatology* **20,** 108A.
600. Peramau, J. M., Mrani, S. M., Sarkis, M., Raabe, U., and Arboqast, J. (1994). TIPS indications are depending on follow up. *Hepatology* **20,** 108A.
601. Caldwell, D. M., Ring, E. J., Rees, C. R., *et al.* (1995). Multicenter investigation of the role of transjugular intrahepatic portosystemic shunt in management of portal hypertension. *Radiology* **196,** 335–340.
602. Sanyal, A. J., Freeman, A., Shiffman, M. L., Purdum, P. P., Luketic, V. A., and Cheatham, A. K. (1994). Portosystemic encephalopathy after transjugular intrahepatic portosystemic shunt: Results of a prospective controlled study. *Hepatology* **20,** 46–55.
603. Somberg, K. A., Riegler, J. L., LaBerge, J. M., *et al.* (1995). Hepatic encephalopathy after transjugular intrahepatic portosystemic shunts: Incidence and risk factors. *Am. J. Gastroenterol.* **90,** 549–555.
604. Piotraschke, J., Haag, K., and Berger, E. (1995). Latent hepatic encephalopathy in outpatients with TIPS. *Hepatology* **22,** 476A.
605. Cabrera, J., Maynar, M., Granados, R., *et al.* (1996). Transjugular intrahepatic portosystemic shunt versus sclerotherapy in the elective treatment of variceal hemorrhage. *Gastroenterology* **110,** 832–839.
606. Riggio, O., Copocaccia, L., and Zipaar, V. (1994). Transjugular intrahepatic portosystemic shunt (TIPS) vs. endoscopic sclerotherapy (Es) in preventing variceal rebleeding. *Hepatology* **20,** 107A.
607. Rössle, M., Deibert, P., Haag, K. *et al.* (1997). Randomized trial of transjugular–intrahepatic–portosystemic shunt versus endoscopic plus propranolol for prevention of variceal rebleeding. *Lancet* **349,** 1043–1049.
608. Conn, H. O., (1969). Prophylactic portacaval shunts. *Ann. Intern. Med.* **70,** 859–864.
609. Conn, H. O. and Lindenmuth, W. W. (1969). Prophylactic portacaval anastomosis in cirrhosis patients with esophageal varices and ascites. Experimental design and preliminary results. *Am. J. Surg.* **117,** 656–661.
610. Jackson, F. C., Perrin, F. B., Smith, A. G. *et al.* (1968). A clinical investigation of the portacaval shunt: II. Survival analysis of the prophylactic operation. *Am. J. Surg.* **115,** 22–42.
611. Resnick, R. H., Chalmers, T. C., Ishihara, A. M., *et al.* (1969). Boston Inter-Hospital Liver Group: A controlled study of the prophylactic portacaval shunt: A final report. *Ann. Intern. Med.* **70,** 675–688.
612. Fonkalsrud, E. W., (1980). Surgical management of portal hypertension in children. *Arch. Surg.* **115,** 1042–1045.
613. Fonkalsrud, D. W., Myers, N. A., and Robinson, M. J. (1974). Management of extrahepatic portal hypertension in children. *Ann. Surg.* **180,** 487–498.
614. Belli, L., Romani, F., Riolo, F., *et al.* (1969). Thrombosis of portal vein in absence of hepatic disease. *Surg. Gynecol. Obstet;* **169,** 46–49.
615. Voorhees, A. B., Jr. and Price, J. B. Jr. (1974). Extrahepatic portal hypertension: A retrospective analysis of 129 cases and associated clinical implications. *Arch. Surg.* **108,** 338–341.
616. Voorhees, A. B. Jr., Harris, R. C. Britton, R. C., Price, J. B. and Santulli, T. V. (1965). Portal hypertension in children: 98 cases. *Surgery* **58,** 540–549.
617. Boles, E. T., Jr., Wise, W. E. Jr., and Birken, G. (1986). Extrahepatic portal hypertension in children: Long-term evaluation. *Am. J. Surg.* **151,** 734–739.
618. Aoyama, K., and Myers, N. A. (1982). Extra-hepatic portal hypertension: The significance of variceal haemorrhage. *Aust Paediatr. J.* **18,** 17–22.
619. Webb, L. J., and Sherlock, S. (1979). The aetiology, pesentation and natural history of extra-hepatic portal venous obstruction. *O. J. Med.* **192,** 627–639.
620. Cohen, D., and Mansour, A. (1977). Extrahepatic portal hypertension—long-term results. *Prog. Pediatr. Surg.* **10,** 129–140.
621. Hamilton, D. W., and Hunt, A. H. (1966). Extrahepatic portal obstruction. *Med. J. Aust.* **1,** 493–499.
622. Mikkelsen, W. P. (1966). Extrahepatic portal hypertension in children. *Am. J. Surg.* **111,** 333–340.
623. Orloff, M. J., Orloff, M. S. and Rambott, M. (1994). Treatment of bleeding esophagogastric varices due to extrahepatic portal hypertension: Results of portal-systemic shunts during 35 years. *J. Pediatr. Surg.* **29,** 142–154.
624. Orloff, M. J., and Orloff, M. S. (1998). Extrahepatic portal hypertension. *In* "Problems in General Surgery" (Sarfeh, I.J. Ed.), pp. 131–148. Lippincott Williams & Wilkins, Philadelphia.
625. Bismuth, H., Franco, D., and Alagille, D. (1980). Portal diversion for portal hypertension in children. The first ninety patients. *Ann. Surg.* **192,** 18–24.
626. Tocornal, J., and Cruz, F. (1981). Portosystemic shunts for extrahepatic portal hypertension in children. *Surg. Gynecol. Obstet.* **153,** 53–56.
627. Alvarez, F., Bernard, O., Brunnelle, F., Hadchouel, P., Odièvre, M. and Alagille, D. (1983). Portal obstruction in children. II. Results of surgical portosystemic shunts. *J. Pediatr.* **103,** 703–743.

628. Pande, G. K., Reddy, V. M., Kar, P., *et al.* (1987). Operations for portal hypertension due to extrahepatic obstruction: Results and 10 year follow up. *B. M. J.* **295,** 1115–1117.
629. Gauthier, F., DeDreuzy, O., Valayer, J., and Montupet, P. H. (1989). H-type shunt with an autologous venous graft for treatment of portal hypertension in children. *J. Pediatr. Surg.* **29,** 1041–1043.
630. Orloff, M. J. (1970). Pathogenesis and surgical treatment of intractable ascites associated with alcoholic cirrhosis. *Ann. NY Acad. Sci.* **170,** 213–238.
631. Orloff, M. J., Orloff, M. S., Orloff, S. I., and Girard, B. (1997). Experimental, clinical, and metabolic results of side-to-side portacaval shunt for intractable cirrhotic ascites. *J. Am. Coll. Surg.* **184,** 557–570.
632. Orloff, M. J., and Orloff, M. S. (1997). Operative procedures: Surgical management of ascites. *In* "Maingot's Abdominal Operations," (Zinner, M.J., Schwartz, S.I., and Ellis, H., Eds.), pp. 1623–1663. Appleton and Lange, Stamford, CT.
633. Orloff, M. J., Orloff, M. S., Orloff, S. L., and Girard, B. (1995). Side-to-side portacaval shunt for intractable cirrhotic ascites: Experimental, clinical and metabolic results. *Gastroenterology* **108,** A1138.
634. Orloff, M. J. (1966). Surgical treatment of intractable cirrhotic ascites. *In* "Current Problems in Surgery, Portal Hypertension" (Longmire, W. P., Jr, Ed.), pp. 28–51. Year Book Medical Publishers, Chicago.
635. Epstein, M. (1982). Peritoneovenous shunt in the management of ascites and the hepatorenal syndrome. *Gastroenterology* **82,** 790–799.
636. Schroeder, E. T., and Anderson, G. H. (1983). Effects of the peritoneovenous shunt on the renin–angiotensin system and renal function in cirrhosis. *In* "The Kidney in Liver Disease" (Epstein, M. Ed.), 2nd ed., pp. 569–582. Elsevier Biomedical, New York.
637. Blendis, L. M., Greig, P. D., Langer, B., *et al.* (1979). Renal and hemodynamic effect of the peritoneovenous shunt for intractable hepatic ascites. *Gastroenterology* **77,** 250–257.
638. Greig, P. D., Blendis, L. M., and Langer, B., *et al.* (1981). Renal and hemodynamic effect of the peritoneovenous shunt. II. Long-term effects. *Gastroenterology* **80,** 119–125.
639. Epstein, M. (1983). Role of peritoneovenous shunt in the management of ascites and hepatorenal syndrome. *In* "The Kidney in Liver Disease (Epstein, M. Ed.), 2nd ed., pp. 583–600. Elsevier Biomedical, New York.
640. Moscovitz, M. (1990). The peritoneovenous shunt: Expectations and reality. *Am. J. Gastroenterol.* **85,** 917–929.
641. Fulenwider, J. T., Galambos, I. D., Smith, R. B., III, *et al.* (1986). Denver peritoneovenous shunts for intractable ascites of cirrhosis. *Arch. Surg.* **121,** 351–355.
642. Norfray, J. F., Henry, H. M., Givens, J. D., *et al.* (1979). Abdominal complications from peritoneal shunts. *Gastroenterology* **77,** 337–340.
643. Schwartz, M. L., Swaim, W. R., and Vogel, S. B. (1979). Coagulopathy following peritoneovenous shunting. *Surgery* **85,** 671–676.
644. Harmon, D. C., Demirjian, Z., Ellman, L., *et al.* (1979). Disseminated intravascular coagulation with the peritoneovenous shunt. *Ann. Intern. Med.* **90,** 774–776.
645. Ragni, M. W., Lewis, J. H., and Spero, J. A. (1983). Ascites-induced Le Veen shunt coagulopathy. *Ann. Surg.* **198,** 91–95.
646. Fulenwider, J. T., Smith, R. B., III, Redd, S. C., *et al.* (1984). Peritoneovenous shunts: Lessons learned from an eight-year experience with 70 patients. *Arch. Surg.* **119,** 1133–1137.
647. Foley, W. J., Elliott, J. P., Jr., Smith, R. F., *et al.* (1984). Central venous thrombosis and embolism associated with peritoneovenous shunts. *Arch. Surg.* **119,** 713–720.
648. Greig, P. D., Langer, B., Blendis, L. M., *et al.* (1980). Complications after peritoneovenous shunting for ascites. *Am. J. Surg.* **139,** 125–131.
649. Wormser, G. P., and Hubbard, R. C. (1981). Peritonitis in cirrhotic patients with LeVeen Shunts. *Am. J. Med.* **71,** 358–362.
650. LeVeen, H. H., Wapnick, S., Grosberg, S., *et al.* (1976). Further experience with peritoneovenous shunts for ascites. *Ann. Surg.* **184,** 574–581.
651. Bernhoft, R. A., Pellegrini, C. A., and Way, L. W. (1982). Peritoneovenous shunt for refractory ascites. *Arch. Surg.* **117,** 631–635.
652. Bories, P., Garcia-Compean, D., *et al.* (1986). The treatment of refractory ascites by the LeVeen shunt: A multi-centre controlled trial (57 patients). *J. Hepatol.* **3,** 212–218.
653. Stanley, M. I. Ochi, S., Lee, K. K., *et al.* (1989). Peritoneovenous shunting as compared with medical treatment in patients with alcoholic cirrhosis and massive ascites. *N. Engl. J. Med.* **321,** 1632–1638.
654. Gines, P., Arroyo, V., Vargas, *et al.* (1991). Paracentesis with intravenous infusion of albumin as compared with peritoneovenous shunting in cirrhosis with refractory ascites. *N. Engl. J. Med.* **325,** 829–835.
655. Somberg, K. A., Lake, J. R., Tomlanovich, S. J., *et al.* (1995). Transjugular intrahepatic portosystemic shunts for refractory ascites: Assessment of clinical and hormonal response and renal function. *Hepatology* **21,** 709–716.
656. Wong, F., Sniderman, K., Liu, P., *et al.* (1995). Transjugular intrahepatic portosystemic stent shunt: Effects on hemodynamics and sodium homeostasis in cirrhosis and refractory ascites. *Ann. Intern. Med.* **122,** 816–822.
657. Lebrec, D., Giuily, N., Hadengue, A., and a group of clinicians. (1994). Transjugular intrahepatic portosystemic shunt (TIPS) versus paracentesis for refractory ascites. Results of a randomised trial. *Hepatology* **20,** (P 2), 201A.
658. Quiroga, J., Sangro, B., Nunez, M., *et al.* (1995). Transjugular intrahepatic portosystemic shunt in the treatment of refractory ascites: Effect on clinical, renal, humoral and hemodynamic parameters. *Hepatology* **21,** 986–994.
659. Rössle, M., Haag, K., Ochs, A., *et al.* (1994). The transjugular intrahepatic portosystemic stent-shunt procedure for variceal bleeding. *N. Engl. J. Med.* **330,** 165–171.
660. LaBerge, J. M., Ring, E. J., Gordon, R. L., *et al.* (1993). Creation of transjugular intrahepatic portosystemic shunts with the Wallstent endoprosthesis: Results in 100 patients. *Radiology* **187,** 413–420.
661. Ochs, A., Rössle, M., Haag, K., *et al.* (1995). The transjugular intrahepatic portosystemic stent shunt procedure for refractory ascites. *N. Engl. J. Med.* **332,** 1192–1197.
662. Crenshaw, W. B., Gordon, F. D., McEniff, N. I., *et al.* (1996). Severe ascites: Efficacy of the transjugular intrahepatic portosystemic shunt in treatment. *Radiology* **200,** 185–192.
663. Rössle, M., Ochs, A., Gülberg, V., *et al.* (2000). A comparison of paracentesis and transjugular intrahepatic portosystemic shunting in patients with ascites. *N. Engl. J. Med.* **342,** 1701–1707.
664. Starzl, T. E., Van Thiel, D. H., and Tzakis, A., *et al.* (1988). Orthotopic liver transplantation for alcoholic cirrhosis. *JAMA* **260,** 2542–2544.
665. Kumar, S., Stauber, R. E., Gavaler, J. S., *et al.* (1990). Orthotopic liver transplantation for alcoholic liver disease. *Hepatology* **11,** 159–164.
666. Lucy, M. R. (1993). Liver transplantation for the alcoholic patient. *Gastroenterol. Clin. North Am.* **22,** 243–256.
667. Bird, G. L. A., O'Grady, J. G., Harvey, F. A., *et al.* (1990). Liver transplantation in patients with alcoholic cirrhosis: Selection criteria and rates of survival and relapse. *BMJ* **301,** 15–17.
668. Bonet, H., Maney, R., Kramer, D., *et al.* (1993). Liver transplantation for alcoholic liver disease: Survival of patients transplanted with alcoholic hepatitis plus cirrhosis as compared with those with cirrhosis alone. *Alcohol Clin. Exp. Res.* **17,** 1102–1106.
669. Bismuth, H., Adam, R., Mathur, S., *et al.* (1990). Options for elective treatment of portal hypertension in cirrhotic patients in the transplantation era. *Am. J. Surg.* **160,** 105–110.
670. Iwatsuki, S., Starzl, T. E., Todo, S., *et al.* (1988). Liver transplantation in the treatment of bleeding esophageal varices. *Surgery* **104,** 697–705.

671. Mazzaferro, V., Todo, S., Tzakis, A. G., *et al.* (1990). Liver transplantation in patients with previous portasystemic shunt. *Am. J. Surg.* **160,** 111–115.
672. Langnas, A. N., Marujo, W. C., Stratta, R. J., *et al.* (1992). Influence of a prior porta-systemic shunt on outcome after liver transplantation. *Am. J. Gastroenterol.* **87,** 714–718.
673. Turrion, V. S., Mora, N. P., Cofer, J. B., *et al.* (1991). Retrospective evaluation of liver transplantation for cirrhosis: A comparative study of 100 patients with or without previous porto-systemic shunt. *Transplant. Proc.* **23,** 1570–1571.
674. Aboujaoude, M. M., Grant, D. R., Ghent, C. N., *et al.* (1991). Effect of portosystemic shunts on subsequent transplantation of the liver. *Surg. Gynecol. Obstet.* **172,** 215–219.
675. Terpstra, O. T., Ausema, B., Bruining, H. A., *et al.* (1987). Late results of mesocaval interposition shunting for bleeding oesophageal varices. *Br. J. Surg.* **74,** 787–780.
676. Smith, R. B., Warren, W. D., Salam, A. A., *et al.* (1980). Dacron interposition shunts for portal hypertension. An analysis of morbidity correlates. *Ann. Surg.* **192,** 9–17.
677. Fletcher, M. S., Dawson, J. L., and Williams, R. (1981). Long term follow-up of interposition mesocaval shunting in portal hypertension. *Br. J. Surg.* **68,** 485–487.
678. Grace, N. D., Conn, H. O., Resnick, R. H., *et al.* (1988). Distal splenorenal versus portal systemic shunts after haemorrhage from varices: A randomized controlled trial. *Hepatology* **8,** 1475–1481.
679. Parker, R. G. F. (1959). Occlusion of the hepatic veins in man. *Medicine* **38,** 369–402.
680. Tavill, A. S., Wood, E. I., Kreel, L., *et al.* (1975). The Budd–Chiari syndrome: Correlation between hepatic scintigraphy and the clinical, radiological and pathological findings in 19 cases of hepatic venous outflow obstruction. *Gastroenterology* **68,** 509–518.
681. Mitchell, M. C., Boitnott, J. K., Kaufmann, S., *et al.* (1982). Budd–Chiari syndrome: Etiology, diagnosis and management. *Medicine* **61,** 199–218.
682. Powell-Jackson, P. R., Melia, W., Canalese, J., *et al.* (1982). Budd–Chiari syndrome: Clinical patterns and therapy. *Q. J. Med.* **201,** 79–88.
683. Orloff, M. J., and Girard, B. (1989). Long-term results of treatment of Budd–Chiari syndrome by side-to-side portacaval shunt. *Surg. Gynecol. Obstet.* **168,** 33–41.
684. Orloff, M. J., Orloff, M. S., and Daily, P. O. (1992). Long-term results of treatment of Budd–Chiari syndrome by portal decompression. *Arch. Surg.* **127,** 1182–1188.
685. Orloff, M. J., and Orloff, M. S. (1994). Budd–Chiari syndrome and veno-occlusive disease. In "Surgery of the Liver and Biliary Tract" (Blumgart, L. H., Ed.), 2nd ed., pp. 1725–1759. Churchill–Livingston, London.
686. Orloff, M. J., Daily, P. O., Orloff, S. L., Girard, B., and Orloff, M. S. (2000). A 27-year experience with surgical treatment of Budd–Chiari syndrome. *Ann. Surg.* **232,** 340–352.
687. Wang, Z., Yu, Z., Wang, S., *et al.* (1989). Recognition and management of Budd–Chiari syndrome: Report of one hundred cases. *J. Vasc. Surg.* **10,** 149–156.
688. Henderson, M. J., Warren, W. D., Millikan, W. J., Jr., *et al.* (1990). Surgical options, hematologic evaluation, and pathologic changes in Budd–Chiari syndrome. *Am. J. Surg.* **159,** 41–50.
689. Klein, A. S., Sitzmann, J. V., and Coleman, J., *et al.* (1990). Current management of the Budd–Chiari syndrome. *Ann. Surg.* **212,** 144–149.
690. Stringer, M. D., Howard, E. R., Green, D. W., *et al.* (1989). Mesoatrial shunt: A surgical option in the management of the Budd–Chiari syndrome. *Br. J. Surg.* **76,** 474–478.
691. Khanna, S. K., Dhaliwal, R. S., Chawla, Y. K., and Dilwari, J. B. (1991). Shunt surgery in Budd–Chiari syndrome: Our experience. *In* "Proceedings of the Second International Symposium on Budd–Chiari Syndrome," p. IL02–5. Japan Cardiovascular Research Foundation, Kyoto, Japan.
692. Slakey, D., Klein, A., and Cameron, J. (1997). Budd–Chiari syndrome: Current management options. *Hepatology* 26;178A.
693. Blum, U., Rössle, M., Haag, K., *et al.* (1995). Budd–Chiari syndrome: Technical, hemodynamic, and clinical results of treatment with transjugular intrahepatic portosystemic shunt. *Radiology.* **197,** 805–811.
694. Huber, M., Siegerstetter, V., Haag, K., *et al.* (1997). Budd–Chiari syndrome: Long-term results after treatment with transjugular intrahepatic portosystemic shunt (TIPS). *Hepatology* **26,** 204A.

50

Animal Models of Liver Regeneration

Jacek Rozga

Department of Surgery, Cedars-Sinai Medical Center, Los Angeles, California 90048

I. Introduction

In Greek mythology, Prometheus, who stole fire from the Gods and passed it to the humans, was punished by being chained to a rock. Each day an eagle devoured his liver and for untold years it regrew each night, until Hercules liberated him. According to Homer, Titus was punished for his attack on Leto by eternal preying of vultures on his liver. These myths suggest that already the ancient Greeks knew about the ability of the liver to regenerate.

In modern times, A. Cuveilhier was probably the first, in 1833, to introduce the idea that regeneration was possible (1). Also, Italian scientists at the end of the nineteenth century systematically studied the effect of damage to the continuity of the liver. They removed small portions of liver tissue and studied the division of liver cells (2). In 1886, K. Podwyssozki created a morphological concept of liver cell proliferation (2, 3). He not only noted the time sequence in hepatocyte mitotic activity, but also observed delayed formation of new bile canaliculi. Later investigators, including H. Tillmans (4), E. Ponfick (5), K. Adler (6), and especially L.S. Milne (7) carried out experiments that formed the foundation of our present-day knowledge of pathomorphology in liver regeneration.

Over the past century, countless investigators have demonstrated that mammalian liver possesses an extraordinary capacity for hypertrophy and compensatory growth in response to conditions that induce cell loss by physical, infectious, or toxic injury. Experimentally, the most dramatic and widely studied example of this phenomenon was the restoration of liver mass after partial (two-thirds) hepatectomy (PH) in rats (8). It is an excellent experimental system to study the reentry of normally quiescent cells into the cell cycle. Moreover, the regenerative process in the rat resembles the regrowth of human liver closely enough to merit its widespread use in all spheres (endocrine, cellular, genetic, molecular) of modern biomedical research.

Liver cell proliferation can also be induced by several chemicals (most notably peroxisome proliferators) without preceding cell loss. This process is defined as direct hyperplasia (9). Somatic growth and other forms of adaptive liver growth are also associated with proliferation of liver cells.

This chapter provides a brief overview of regulatory mechanisms involved in liver growth and repair, followed by a description of the basic *in vivo* experimental animal models used in the study of liver regeneration.

II. Liver Regeneration

Liver regeneration is basically a process of both hypertrophy (increase in cell size or protein content during the prereplicative stage) and hyperplasia (increase in the number of cells). However, these two events are quite separable and hyperplasia can be associated with either atrophy or hypertrophy. The increase in liver mass may be due to cell enlargement, but swelling of reticuloendothelial cells and interstitial space may also play a role.

The extent of liver hypertrophy can be determined by volume, dry weight, morphometric (cell volume and size) measurements, light and electron microscopy, and isotopic techniques. It is of importance to stress that increases in RNA synthesis, as well as change in the energy state of the cell, reflect merely hypertrophy. Hepatocyte division can be assessed by measurement of DNA synthesis and by identifying cells in mitosis.

Regeneration of the liver represents primarily a process of compensatory hyperplasia because the gross morphology of the organ does not return to its original form after partial hepatectomy. The term "regeneration" is, however, widely used in the literature. Although some of the mechanisms that regulate liver growth after partial loss and hepatocyte necrosis caused by ischemia and severe viral or drug-induced hepatitis may vary, this tightly regulated process appears to be governed by functional, rather than anatomic, factors. Most investigators believe that the liver grows by division of existing mature liver cells rather than by stem cell proliferation, and that interplay among many humoral stimulatory and inhibitory influences regulates hepatocyte replication. However, whether reduction in liver mass stimulates production of positive growth factors or lowers the concentration of circulating inhibitor(s) is still a matter of dispute. Two pancreatic hormones (insulin, glucagon) are important modulators of, but not triggers of, liver regeneration (10).

Most of the current knowledge regarding restoration of the liver mass is derived from studies in normal rats undergoing partial (two-thirds) hepatectomy. It is proposed that due to the rapid metabolic adaptations occurring after partial hepatocyte loss, residual hepatocytes enter a state of replicative competence ("priming") in which they can respond to extrahepatic and intrahepatic factors such as hepatocyte growth factor (HGF), epidermal growth factor (EGF), and transforming growth factor (TGF)-α (11). The priming step appears to be mediated by tumor necrosis factor (TNF α) released from nonparenchymal sinusoidal cells and by other cytokines, primarily interleukin-6 (IL-6) (12). It involves activation and DNA binding of nuclear factor (NF)-κB and other transcription factors [e.g., signal transducer and activator of transcription (STAT) proteins, activator protein (AP)-1, and CCAAT/enhancer-binding protein (C/EBP)β], which regulate transcription of multiple growth-associated genes (5, 13). Additionally, IL-6 may increase HGF production by hepatic stellate cells (6, 14). Activation of immediate-early genes (e.g., c-*fos*, c-*jun*, c-*myc*) leads, within the first few hours, to progression through the early to mid-G_1 phase of the cell cycle. Thereafter, stimulation by mitogens (e.g., HGF, TGF-α) and other factors induces early-delayed genes [e.g., cyclins and cyclin-dependent kinases (cdk)], which facilitate transition to DNA synthesis and mitosis (15). Other early events in liver regeneration include an increase in ornithine decarboxylase (polyamine biosynthetic enzyme) activity, and Na^+,K^+-ATPase activities (16, 17) and elevation in cAMP (18). It is also postulated that increased Na^+ flux into the cells is needed to initiate proliferation of hepatocytes of adult animals (19). The initial burst of hepatocyte proliferative activity is followed by secondary waves of mitosis until the original mass of the liver is restored (19, 20). The precise mechanisms responsible for termination of the growth response remain largerly unknown. It seems that multiple factors are involved, including growth factors (e.g., TGF-β1), transcription factors (e.g., Spl and p53), interleukin-1β, and cyclin and cyclin-dependent kinase inhibitors (e.g., $p21^{WAF1/CIP1}$, p19, and p27), to name but a few (15).

III. Regeneration Following Hepatic Injury

A number of toxins may cause injury (hepatitis) and cell death in a large percentage of hepatic parenchyma, resulting in a distinct wave of cell proliferation. However, hepatotoxic models have a limited role in studies of liver regeneration because the local and systemic effects of the toxin used depend on the dose and route of administration, animal species and strain, age and nutritional status, and other factors (21, 22). As a result, the extent of liver necrosis is difficult to predict reliably, there is significant variability from experiment to experiment, the growth response includes both DNA replication and DNA repair, and the toxin may directly interfere with cellular and molecular mechanisms of growth control. The latter may include cellular membrane damage (e.g., interruption of growth factor–receptor interaction), impaired gene expression and protein synthesis, inflammatory response, and activation of nonparenchymal liver cells, resulting, for example, in increased TGF-β1 and matrix production (23). Finally, in toxic models, the two processes—injury (cell death) and repair—are intertwined, which further complicates the study of regeneration (24).

For these reasons, agents such as bromobenzene, carbon tetrachloride (CCl_4), and allyl alcohol are of particular value in studies in which injury to the specific zone of the hepatic acinus is desired. It is assumed that after PH, all the hepatic acini remain intact, whereas most forms of liver disease are manifested by either the periportal (zone I) or centrilobular (zone III) damage. In the studies by Nostrant *et al.* (24), rats given intraperitoneal injection of bromobenzene (3.8 m*M*/kg, dissolved in corn oil) showed centrilobular necrosis in 25% of liver parenchyma 48 hr posttreatment. In contrast, in animals treated with allyl alcohol (0.62 m*M*/kg dissolved in 0.9% NaCl), the volume fraction of periportal necrosis determined 24 hr after treatment was 10%.

After the administration of a single intragastric dose of CCl_4 to rats, DNA synthesis and mitotic activity are delayed (48–72 hr) when compared with the findings after partial hepatectomy (24–30 hr). After intraperitoneal injection of D-galactosamine, the regenerative response is much weaker, although the time course of DNA synthesis and hepatocyte mitosis is similar to that after CCl_4 administration (25). The delayed timing of onset of hepatocyte proliferation in these two animal models suggests that after toxic liver injury, cells may be refractory to entering the cell cycle or that the stimuli to regeneration were either reduced (e.g., lesser extent of cellular loss) or altered.

Only limited data exist about the course of liver regeneration in cholestatic liver injury. After common bile duct ligation, posthepatectomy regeneration was found to be partially inhibited, as shown by measurements of DNA synthetic activity, hepatocyte mitotic index, and the rate of restoration of liver weight (8).

An excellent review of liver regeneration following hepatic injury has been published by Czaja (23). Also, additional information about thioacetamide, D-galactosamine, CCl_4, and acetaminophen hepatotoxicity is available in other chapters of this volume.

IV. Regeneration Following Partial Hepatectomy

Surgical removal of two-thirds of the liver in the white rat represents the most valuable and most extensively studied animal model of liver regeneration. The model is based on seminal experiments by Higgins and Anderson (8), who demonstrated in rat liver, which is composed of six mobile lobes, that resection of the two anterior lobes is easy to perform and creates a highly standardized liver deficit of 68%. Furthermore, the response after standard PH is readily quantifiable and highly reproducible, as shown by Grisham (19) and others (26, 27).

Hepatocytes in adult rodents and humans have a long life span, their basal DNA synthesis is low, and very few (~1/20,000) hepatocytes can be found in mitosis at any time. After two-thirds PH, there is marked stimulation of DNA replication followed by mitosis. Proliferation of nonparenchymal cells lags behind that of hepatocytes. Further cycles of liver cell proliferation are neither as prominent nor as synchronized because a progressively smaller proportion of cells undergoes replication. The original liver mass in rats is restored within 7–10 days. The timing of events after PH is divided into a prereplicative phase (0–12 hr), during which hepatocytes move from a state of quiescence (G_0) toward DNA synthesis (G_1), and a replicative phase (12–30 hr), during which DNA synthesis takes place (S) followed by mitosis (M). Under optimal conditions, the initial peak of DNA synthesis occurs at about 24 hr after two-thirds hepatectomy. Mitotic division follows the same course about 6 hr later, showing distinct diurnal periodicity during the first 6 days with 12-hr intervals (21, 22, 27). Some of the cells divide again within 24 hr before returning to G_0 state, although repeated hepatectomy may stimulate them to new mitosis (28).

The regeneration response is maximal when two-thirds of the liver is resected. When a lesser amount of parenchyma is removed, the restoration proceeds more slowly (26). Resections exceeding two-thirds of the liver mass also retard and diminish both DNA synthesis and mitotic activity (29) and subtotal (90%) hepatectomy invariably results in the death of rats without regeneration (30, 31).

A. Two-Thirds Hepatectomy in the Rat

Liver mass bears a predictable relationship with body weight in humans and in several other species, including rodents. In rats, the liver mass represents approximately 4% of the total body weight and the contributions of each liver lobe to the total liver mass are constant. Thus, the two anterior lobes, the two right liver lobes, and the two omental liver lobes (sometimes viewed as a single caudate lobe) comprise 68, 24, and 8% of the liver, respectively (32). Additionally, each lobe has its own pedicle containing a portal triad (Fig. 1). These unique aspects of rat liver anatomy makes resections of various extents simple and highly reproducible. Only basic surgical skills are needed and when properly executed, liver resections are very well tolerated with no operative mortality.

During standard PH in the rat, the filamentous ligaments (coronary, left lateral, gastrohepatic) should be transected and the liver should be handled with care to avoid excessive damage to the liver remnant. After placing a ligature around the anterior lobe pedicle, the liver should be returned to its normal *in situ* position to avoid engorgement with portal blood. After the ligature is tied off and resection completed, the residual liver parenchyma should be inspected for the presence of a bright red color and lack of congestion with blood. The latter may develop if the ligature was placed too

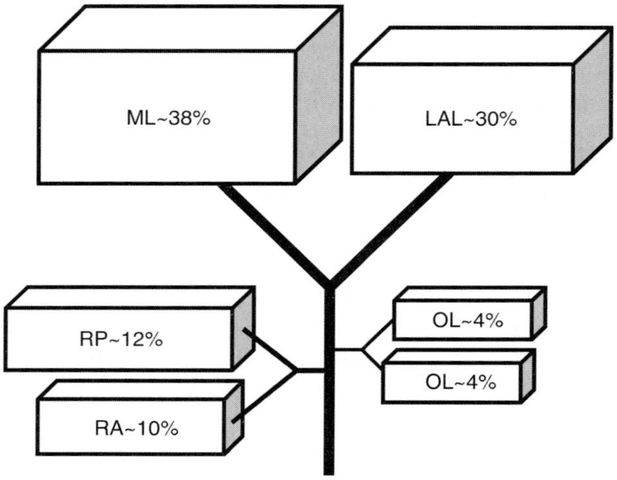

Figure 1 Rat liver anatomy (ML, median lobe; LAL, left anterior lobe; RA, right anterior lobe; RP, right posterior lobe; OL, omental lobe).

low and partially occluded one of the major hepatic veins or even the caval vein.

The duration of the prereplicative stage and both the intensity and timing of maximal DNA synthetic activity and mitosis after PH vary with species used, animal age, nutritional status (diet and feeding schedule), diurnal rhythm, hormonal balance, lighting schedule, and the size of hepatectomy (21, 22, 26–31). Therefore, it is important to standardize all experimental conditions, including 5- to 7-day-long acclimatization periods, housing of rats in a climate-controlled (21°C) room under a 12-hr light/dark cycle, and feeding them with tap water and standard laboratory rat chow (Rodent Chow 5001, Ralston Purina, St. Louis, MO) *ad libitum*. Hepatectomy should be performed between 9 am and noon under general (e.g., methoxyflurane, ether) open-air anesthesia using aseptic surgical technique. At the completion of the surgical procedure, rats should receive a bolus of 10–15 ml of warm physiologic saline subcutaneously (SC) and a single dose of an agent alleviating postoperative pain (e.g., buprenorphine, 0.1–0.5 mg/kg, SC). Until full recovery from anesthesia, the rat should be warmed with a heating lamp. Then, animals should be immediately returned to the vivarium. Properly matched sham-hepatectomized control rats are almost always needed because the surgical stress, in conjunction with liver handling, results in a wave of DNA synthesis in the liver (33).

B. Subtotal (90%) Hepatectomy

In theory, a near-total liver removal may be an ideal model to examine the mechanism of inhibition of hepatic regenerative response in rats with critically low hepatocyte mass. In practice, however, a number of side effects or complications related to this procedure, including portal venous stasis, development of cerebral edema, hypothermia, hypoglycemia, endotoxemia, sepsis, proteinuria, and apoptosis, may all interfere with metabolic, cellular, or molecular measurements under investigation. A fairly detailed description of subtotal hepatectomy in rats is given elsewhere in this volume.

C. Liver Regeneration Studies in Large Animals

Large animals such as dogs and pigs have been used only to a limited extent, because the cost of assessment of DNA synthesis by the standard method of radiolabeled thymidine incorporation is very high. Hepatic thymidine kinase activity has been used by Kahn *et al.* (34) as an inexpensive index of DNA synthesis in pigs.

V. Regeneration Following Portal Branch Ligation

Frerichs (35), as early as 1861, showed that syphilitic obliteration of the portal branch supplying one liver lobe led to atrophy of the affected lobe, whereas the remaining segments were markedly enlarged. This observation was subsequently confirmed by many investigators, who were able to illustrate this phenomenon clinically as well as experimentally (36–40). Thus, it has been shown in several species that ligation of a branch of the portal vein induces atrophy of the portal-deprived liver parenchyma, whereas the residual tissue receiving all the portal flow undergoes compensatory growth. By maintaining a balance between atrophy and growth, the total liver mass remained at the level of sham-operated animals throughout the experimental period.

Rous and Larimore (37) in 1920 were intrigued by the possibility that hyperplastic response after portal branch ligation (PBL) may be stimulated by humoral modulators present in the portal blood. In their unique studies on rabbits, PBL resulted in less atrophy when the bile duct draining the remainder of the liver was also ligated. Less hyperplasia was seen in the lobes receiving the entire portal flow. These observations indicated that atrophy is conditional and dependent on a compensatory growth of the nonoccluded portion of the liver.

Because many studies report varying effects of PBL, particularly in respect to the occurrence of multifocal necrosis in portal-deprived liver parenchyma (35, 37–40), we have found it desirable to reevaluate this model (3, 32). Histologic appearance, DNA synthetic activity, labeling count, and mitotic index were serially evaluated in both portal branch-ligated and nonmanipulated parts of the rat liver after interruption of the portal flow to one-fourth, one-third, and two-thirds of the liver mass. So that hepatic denervation could be avoided and the arterial branch and bile duct could be left intact, PBL was carried out with the use of 7-0 suture under an operating microscope. We confirmed the presence of compensatory hyperplasia induced in the nonligated liver lobe(s) by PBL, and its intensity was roughly proportional to the amount of liver tissue devoid of portal perfusion. Portal-deprived liver tissue underwent rapid and progressive atrophy and, by the end of the first week, the weight of this part had decreased 10-fold. PBL invariably resulted in early centrilobular necrosis, which occupied 15–24% of the ligated lobe(s). However, after 4 days the areas of necrosis were already almost totally resorbed and did not appear *de novo* (3, 32).

In our studies, the hyperplastic response was weaker than that seen after resection of the corresponding liver mass (19, 32). In contrast, in the experiments by Weinbren and Tarsh (40), the difference was minimal. PBL is a useful model to study liver regeneration for several reasons: it is a simple, highly reproducible preparation and unlike partial hepatectomy it is fully reversible; after an initial wave of multifocal necrosis, which eliminates up to one-fourth of the affected liver tissue, the progressive atrophy that follows involves not only shrinkage of hepatocytes and other cell populations but also apoptosis; it is a unique preparation in which two opposite processes take place in the same organ and in the same animal.

VI. Direct Compensatory Hyperplasia

A single intravenous injection of lead nitrate to rats induces proliferation of liver cells without the accompanying liver cell loss (9). The mechanism of this so-called direct hyperplasia is not fully understood. The growth response is not associated with any significant changes in the hepatic levels of known growth factors such as HGF and TGF-α (41, 42). Instead, there is a rapid increase of TNFα in the liver. Treatment with dexamethasone and several TNFα inhibitors (e.g., adenosine, pentoxifylline) inhibits both TNFα expression and liver growth induced by lead nitrate and ethylene dibromide (43). These data support the hypothesis that TNFα may be involved in triggering hepatocyte proliferation by primary mitogens. Lead nitrate (Sigma Chemical Co., St. Louis, MO; 100 μmol/kg) was dissolved in distilled water and injected in male Wistar rats (200 g) through the saphenous vein. After treatment, the peak DNA synthesis occurred after 28–40 hr. The mitotic index was 1.75% at 48 hr posttreatment (43).

References

1. Cuveilhier, A. (1829–1833). "Anatomique Pathologique du Corpus Humain," XII, p. 1. Paris.
2. Harvey, P. (1959). "The Oxford Companion to Clinical Literature," p. 432. Oxford University Press, New York.
3. Rozga, J. (1986). Hepatotrophic effect of portal blood. Ph.D. thesis. Bulletin No.60, pp. 11–14. Department of Surgery, Lund University, Lund, Sweden.
4. Tillmanns, H. (1978). Experimentelle und anatomische Untersuchungen uber Wunden der Leber und Niere. *Virchow's Arch. Pathol. Anat.* **LXXVIII,** 437.
5. Ponfick, E. (1889). Experimentelle Beitr. z. Path. Der Leber, *Virchow's Arch. Pathol. Anat.* **CXVIII,** 209.
6. Adler, K. (1904). Uber helle Zellen in der menschlichen Leber. Beitr. z. path. Anat. v. z. allg. *Pathology* (Jena) **XXXV,** 27.
7. Milne, L. S. (1908–1909). The histology of liver tissue regeneration. *J. Path. Bact.* **13,** 127–147.
8. Higgins, G. M., and Anderson, R. M. (1931). Experimental pathology of the liver I: Restoration of the liver of the white rat following partial surgical removal. *Arch. Pathol.* **12,** 186–202.
9. Columbano, A., and Shinozuka, H. (1996). Liver regeneration versus direct hyperplasia. *FASEB J.* **10,** 1118–1128.
10. McGowan, J. A., Strain, A., and Bucher, N. L. R. (1981). DNA synthesis in primary cultures of adult rat hepatocytes in a defined medium: Effects of epidermal growth factor, insulin, glucagon and cyclic-AMP. *J. Cell Physiol.* **108,** 353–360.
11. Taub, R., Greenbaum, L. E., and Peng, Y. (1999). Transcriptional regulatory signals define cytokine-dependent and - independent pathways in liver regeneration. *Sem. Liver Dis.* **19,** 117–127.
12. Diehl, A. M., and Rai, R. M. (1996). Regulation of signal transduction during liver regeneration. *FASEB J.* **10,** 215–227.
13. Liu, Y., Michalopoulos, G. K., and Zarnegar, R. (1994). Structural and functional characterization of the mouse hepatocyte growth factor gene promoter. *J. Biol. Chem.* **269,** 4152–4160.
14. Russell, D. H., and Snyder, S. H. (1968). Amine synthesis in rapidly growing tissues: Ornithine decarboxylase activity in regenerating rat liver, chick embryo and various tumors. *Proc. Natl. Acad. Sci. U.S.A.* **60,** 1420–1427.
15. Fukada, T., Ohtani, T., Yoshida, Y., *et al.* (1998). STAT3 orchestrates contradictory signals in cytokine-induced G1 to S cell-cycle transition. *EMBO J.* **17,** 6670–6677.
16. Schenk, D., Huber, J., and Leffert, H. (1984). Use of monoclonal antibody to quantify (Na^+,K^+)-ATPase activity and sites in normal and regenerating rat liver. *J. Biol. Chem.* **259,** 14941–14951.
17. Whitfield, J. F., Boynton, A. L., Rixon, R. H., *et al.* (1985). The control of cell proliferation by calcium, Ca^{++}-calmodulin and cyclic AMP. *In* "Control of Animal Cell Proliferation," (A. L. Boynton and H. L. Leffert, eds.), Vol. 1, p.332. Academic Press, Orlando.
18. Leffert, H. L., Koch, K. S., Lad, P. J., *et al.* (1988). Hepatocyte regeneration, replication and differentiation. *In* "The Liver. Biology and Pathobiology," (I.M. Arias, W.P. Jakoby, H. Popper, *et al.*, eds.), pp. 833–844. Raven Press, New York.
19. Grisham, J. W. (1996). A morphologic study of deoxyribonucleic acid synthesis and cell proliferation in regenerating rat liver; autoradiography with thymidine-H3. *Cancer Res.* **22,** 842–849.
20. Terblanche, J., and Hickman, R. (1991). Animal model of fulminant hepatic failure. *Dig. Dis. Sci.* **6,** 15–22.
21. Jaffe, J. J. (1954). Diurnal mitotic periodicity in regenerating rat liver. *Anat. Rec.* **20,** 935–941.
22. LaBrecque, D. R., Feigenbaum, A., and Bachur, N. R. (1978). Diurnal rhythm: Effects on hepatic regeneration and hepatic regenerative stimulatory substance. *Science* **199,** 1082–1084.
23. Czaja, M. J. (1998). Liver regeneration following hepatic injury. *In* "Liver Growth and Repair" (A. J. Strain and A. M. Diehl, eds.), pp. 28–49. Chapman and Hall, London.
24. Nostrant, T. T., Miller, D. L., Appelman, H. D., and Gumucio, J. J. (1978). Acinar distribution of liver cell regeneration after selective zonal injury in the rat liver. *Gastroenterology* **75,** 181–186.
25. Tracy, T. F., Jr., Bailey, P. V., Goerke, M. E., *et al.* (1991). Cholestasis without cirrhosis alters regulatory liver gene expression and inhibits hepatic regeneration. *Surgery* **110,** 176–182.
26. Bucher, N. L. R. , and Swaffield, M. N. (1964). The rate of incorporation of labeled thymidine into the deoxyribonucleic acid of regenerat-

ing rat liver in relation to the amount of liver excised. *Cancer Res.* **24,** 1611–1625.

27. Dallman, P. R., Spirito, R. A., and Siimes, M. (1974). Diurnal patterns of DNA synthesis in the rat: Modification by diet and feeding schedule. *J. Nutr.* **104,** 1233–1237.
28. Dagradi, A., Galanti, G., and Bearby, R. (1964). Regeneration of the liver following multiple resections. *Surgery* **55,** 709–714.
29. Weinbren, K., and Taghizadeh, A. (1965). The mitotic response after subtotal hepatectomy in the rat. *Br. J. Exp. Pathol.* **46,** 413–419.
30. Tuczek, H. V., and Rabes, H. (1971). Vorlest der Proliferationsfahigkeit der Hepatozyten nach Subtotalen Hepatektomie. *Experientia* **27,** 526–530.
31. Eguchi, S., Kamlot, A., Ljubimova, J., *et al.* (1996). Fulminant hepatic failure in rats: Survival and effect on blood chemistry and liver regeneration. *Hepatology* **24,** 1452–1459.
32. Rozga, J., Jeppsson, B., and Bengmark, S. (1986). Portal branch ligation in the rat: Reevaluation of a model. *Am. J. Pathol.* **125,** 300–306.
33. Moolten, F. L., Oakman, N. J., and Bucher, N. L. R. (1970). Accelerated response of hepatic DNA synthesis to partial hepatectomy in rats pretreated with growth hormone or surgical stress. *Cancer Res.* **30,** 2353–2356.
34. Kahn, D., Stadler, J., Terblanche, J., and Hickman, R. H. (1980). Thymidine kinase: An inexpensive index of liver regeneration in a large animal model. *Gastroenterology* **79,** 907–910.
35. Frerichs, F. T. (1861). Klinik der Leberkrankheiten. Braunschweig, Aufl. 2.
36. Benz, E. J., Baggenstoss, A. H., and Wollaeger, E. E. (1952). Atrophy of the left lobe of the liver. *Arch. Pathol.* **53,** 315–330.
37. Rous, P., and Larimore, L. D. (1920). Relation of the portal blood to liver maintenance. A demonstration of liver atrophy conditional on compensation. *J. Exp. Med.* **31,** 609–632.
38. Schalm, L., Bax, H. R., and Mansens, B. J. (1956). Atrophy of the liver after occlusion of the bile ducts or portal vein and compensatory hypertrophy of the unoccluded portion and its clinical importance. *Gastroenterology* **31,** 131–155.
39. Steiner, P. E., and Martinez, J. B. (1961). Effects on the rat liver of bile duct, portal vein and hepatic artery ligations. *Am. J. Pathol.* **39,** 257–289.
40. Weinbren, K., and Tarsh, E. (1964). The mitotic response in the rat liver after different regenerative stimuli. *Br. J. Exp. Pathol.* **45,** 475–480.
41. Shinozuka, H., Kubo, Y., Katyal, S. L., *et al.* (1994). Roles of growth factors and tumor necrosis factor-α on liver cell liver cell proliferation induced in rats by lead nitrate. *Lab. Invest.* **71,** 35–41.
42. Ledda-Columbano, G. M., Columbano, A., Cannas, A., *et al.* (1994). Dexamethasone inhibits induction of liver tumor necrosis factor-α mRNA and liver growth induced by lead nitrate and ethylene dibromide. *Am. J. Pathol.* **145,** 951–958.
43. Kubo, Y., Yasunaga, M., Masuhara, M., *et al.* (1996). Hepatocyte proliferation induced in rats by lead nitrate is suppressed by several tumor necrosis factor a inhibitors. *Hepatology* **23,** 104–114.

51

Animal Models for the Study of Hepatocyte Transplantation

Daniel Inderbitzin, Jacek Rozga, and Achilles A. Demetriou

Department of Surgery, Cedars-Sinai Medical Center, Los Angeles, California 90048

I. Introduction

Whole organ transplantation is the only clinically effective method of treating acute and end-stage chronic liver insufficiency due to specific genetic and other defects of liver function. However, liver transplantation is a very complex undertaking and wider application of this therapeutic modality is limited primarily by shortage of donors, inability to procure organs on short notice, relatively high morbidity, and high cost. In addition, many patients do not qualify for transplantation because of metastatic cancer, concomitant infection, active alcoholism, drug abuse, or concurrent medical problems. As a result of these limitations, 40–60% of patients listed for liver transplantation, including only 10% of those with fulminant hepatic failure, receive a liver graft (1).

In the search for alternative methods of liver support/replacement therapy, investigators have focused on (1) delivery of corrected genes directly to liver cells within the diseased organ, (2) transplantation of genetically corrected liver cells previously obtained from a patient with a genetic liver defect, and (3) transplantation of normal allogeneic hepatocytes. The first two approaches are currently under investigation and are limited primarily by the lack of efficient vectors achieving high levels of sustained genomic integration and expression of the foreign genetic material. The third strategy—allogeneic hepatocyte transplantation—represents a simple, low-risk and possibly more cost-effective option. In addition, it allows efficient use of donor organs (cells from a single donor can be used to treat multiple recipients) and does not deprive recipients of their native liver. The latter applies particularly to patients with inherited defects of liver metabolism, in whom only a small number of normal hepatocytes is needed to replace a single missing function. It would also benefit individuals with acute liver failure, in whom the native liver has potential for regeneration and full recovery. Last, hepatocyte transplantation is a useful tool for investigating liver physiology and pathology (metabolism, immunity, cell proliferation, cell–cell and cell–matrix interaction, etc.).

In the past three decades, a large number of *in vitro* and *in vivo* small and large animal studies of all aspects of hepatocyte transplantation have been carried out to improve our understanding of the process and thus make possible future clinical application of this important tool. Those investigations had the following objectives:

1. Development of optimal methods for isolation, processing, and cryopreservation of mammalian hepatocytes.
2. Development of optimal technique(s) of hepatocyte transplantation.
3. Study of engraftment of transplanted hepatocytes.
4. Study of transplanted hepatocyte proliferation and development of methods to control and modulate this process.
5. Development of appropriate hepatocyte transplantation immunosuppression protocols in small and large animals.

II. Hepatocyte Isolation

Various isolation techniques, including mechanical dissolution by homogenization, pipetting, shaking, and chemical dispersion by citrate, EDTA, EGTA, and sodium tetraphenyl boron have been used in the early stages of hepatocyte harvest development. None of these techniques produced a high yield of viable hepatocytes.

Currently, portal vein collagenase perfusion, as developed by Berry and Friend (2) and Seglen (3), remains the generally accepted method of hepatocyte harvest. In our laboratory, we have modified this technique in the following manner. Under general anesthesia, a donor rat undergoes midline laparotomy and the portal vein is dissected; an 18-gauge catheter is placed in the portal vein and secured with a single 4-0 ligature placed around the catheterized vein and the hepatic artery. The liver is initially perfused with oxygenated 1–2 m*M* EDTA solution to remove blood and to release hepatocytes from their attachments (cleavage of desmosomes). The perfusate is delivered at the rate of 25 ml/min and after 10 min it is changed to calcium-enriched 0.05% type IV collagenase. Collagenase perfusion is carried out at 37°C for another 10 min. Once the liver becomes swollen and breaks under gentle pressure, it is removed and placed in the petri dish containing ice-cold Dulbecco's modified Eagle's medium (DMEM) enriched with bovine calf serum (5–10%). The liver capsule is now incised and the digested liver tissue is passed through a 100-μm nylon mesh. Liver cells are then washed three times in DMEM and centrifuged at 500 rpm. Further filtering through a 50-μm mesh results in a suspension of single hepatocytes. Hepatocyte viability is determined by trypan blue exclusion. The final cell suspension contains >80% viable hepatocytes and is further processed using Percoll density gradient (4). The latter step is carried out to achieve viability of 90% or greater, to remove damaged cells that still excluded the dye, and to remove highly antigenic cells such as endothelial and Kupffer cells.

Rabbit, dog, and porcine hepatocytes should also be harvested using two-step portal vein EDTA/collagenase digestion. In order to decrease the cost of the procedure, recirculation of collagenase rather than single-pass perfusion is recommended. In order to increase the yield and viability of isolated hepatocytes, hepatocyte filtration and enrichment is performed using a three-compartment chamber with meshes of decreased porosity (400, 240, and 100 μm) and a blood cell processor (COBE 2991, Blood Component Technology, Lakewood, CO), as described by Morsiani *et al.* (5).

III. Hepatocyte Cryopreservation

Standard protocols for hepatocyte cryopreservation and rewarming procedures have been described by Fuller and De Loecker (6). Prevention of lethal intracellular ice crystal formation is crucial for the success of hepatocyte cryopreservation. It is, however, a formidable task. The problem is that standard cryoprotectants (e.g., dimethyl sulfoxide) are cytotoxic when used at high concentrations. Perhaps in the future, use of antifreeze proteins and/or development of successful vitrification protocols ("instant" freezing without ice crystal formation) will enable the long-term storage of isolated hepatocytes and liver tissue fragments.

IV. Hepatocyte Transplantation Techniques

For a hepatocyte transplantation method to be useful, the technique must be simple, it should allow early engraftment, it should allow transplantation of an adequate number of hepatocytes, and transplanted hepatocytes should be able to express differentiated functions *in vivo* for prolonged periods of time.

Although significant progress has been achieved in isolated hepatocyte transplantation, the optimal site of implantation has not been determined. In searching for the best transplantation technique and location, hepatocytes have been introduced virtually into every body site, including liver, spleen, thymus, testes, brain, pancreas, lungs, kidneys, peritoneal cavity, subcutaneous tissues, fat pads, and other locations (7).

A. Intrasplenic Hepatocyte Transplantation

Although the spleen and peritoneal cavity have been most frequently used, there are reasons to believe that transplanted hepatocytes, similarly to auxiliary liver (auto)grafts, undergo atrophy when implanted ectopically outside the portal stream. In addition, the intrasplenic route is limited by the relatively small number of cells that can be transplanted without causing spleen infarcts and portal vein thrombosis resulting from massive leakage of transplanted cells into the splenic venous outflow (8). On the other hand, efforts to create a "hepatized spleen" (9) may be justified in patients with intrinsic liver disease such as cirrhosis, where intraportal infusion of cells either may not be feasible or may be associated with high morbidity and mortality resulting from cell aggregates passing into the cardiopulmonary circulation via extra- and intrahepatic portosystemic shunts.

Injection of hepatocytes into the spleen along its long axis is the preferred technique of transplantation in rats. In order to prevent cells from relocating into the liver (10), we have developed a novel hepatocyte transplantation technique, in which the spleen hilum is exposed and three or four out of five or six splenic venous branches are ligated. Next, the splenic artery and the remaining splenic venous branches draining the upper pole of the spleen are cross-clamped and a suspension of isolated allogeneic hepatocytes (2.5×10^7 cells in 1 ml saline) is slowly (2–3 min) injected into the spleen using a 24-gauge Venocath (Becton Dickinson, Sandy, UT). Following hepatocyte transplantation, hemostasis is achieved at the puncture site and after 10–15 min, spleen blood circulation is reestablished. Using this technique we demonstrated in rats rendered anhepatic that cell therapy delayed the onset of encephalopathy and significantly prolonged animal survival. Additionally, transplanted rats had lower blood ammonia levels, improved blood coagulation parameters, and maintained body temperature at near-normal levels. These data indicate that transplanted allogeneic hepatocytes can assume the range of intact whole liver functions (11).

Most studies on intrasplenic hepatocyte transplantation have been carried out in small animals. We therefore carried out a series of experiments to develop a method for large-scale hepatocellular transplantation in large animals, i.e., pigs (12). Allogeneic porcine hepatocytes were transplanted using the following routes: (1) retrograde injection of cells via the splenic vein, (2) intraarterial injection of cells, (3) direct intrasplenic injection of cells after laparotomy, (4) percutaneous intrasplenic injection of cells under laparoscopic control, and (5) laparoscopic intrasplenic injection of cells. The number of cells injected varied from 2×10^9 to 10×10^9 cells. Of all the methods tested, only transplantation of 2 billion cells was found to be compatible with good cell engraftment and animal survival. However, even with this "small" number of cells (2% of the original liver mass), there was a significant risk of spleen infarction, perisplenic adhesion formation, and portal vein thrombosis. The laparoscopic approach was found to be reliable, simple, and safe. We concluded that even though the spleen is considered by many investigators as the optimal site for hepatocellular transplantation, transplantation of the number of cells needed to support the failing liver might be associated with significant complications, morbidity, and mortality.

We further modified our approach to large animal hepatocyte transplantation and transplanted hepatocytes into the pig spleen using multiple (up to 40×) subcapsular injections. After hepatocyte transplantation, none of the pigs developed intracranial hypertension after subsequent induction of total liver ischemia. In addition, transplanted pigs survived longer than sham-transplanted control pigs (13).

B. Intraperitoneal Hepatocyte Transplantation

The peritoneal cavity is an attractive transplantation site because of easy access and potentially large capacity. However, injection of isolated free hepatocytes into the peritoneal cavity results in only transient cell survival and function (14–16). It has been demonstrated that hepatocyte survival and differentiation *in vitro* are enhanced by cell attachment to a collagen matrix (17). We have thus assumed that attachment of isolated hepatocytes to collagen-coated dextran microcarriers prior to transplantation would improve transplanted cell survival and enhance expression of differentiated hepatocyte function *in vivo* (18). In Gunn rats, transplanted cell function was demonstrated by the appearance of bilirubin conjugates and increase in total bilirubin in the bile, accompanied by a decrease in serum bilirubin levels. Similarly, an increase in plasma albumin levels was seen in Nagase analbuminemic rats given intraperitoneal injections of microcarrier-attached normal rat hepatocytes. Large numbers of albumin-staining hepatocytes were found in the peritoneal cavity for up to 6 weeks following transplantation; transmission electron microscopy revealed formation of bile canaliculi-like structures with microvilli. Microcarrier-attached normal rat hepatocytes were also transplanted into rats with subtotal (90%) hepatectomy (19). It is of interest that when hepatocytes were transplanted immediately before or after liver resection, no improvement in animal survival was noted. However, a dramatic improvement in recipient survival and prevention of postoperative hypoglycemia were seen in rats transplanted 4 days prior to hepatectomy. It is presumed that the improved survival, seen in the latter group of animals, was due to the need of several days to allow for transplanted cell engraftment and function.

Other types of matrixes or solid supports (scaffolds) used for hepatocyte attachment include bioabsorbable polymers (20), microcarriers other than dextran particles (21, 22), thin slices of biodegradable type I collagen sponges (23) polyvinyl alcohol (24), and hollow fibers (25), to name but a few. To improve blood supply, leaves of small bowel mesentery have been juxtaposed with polymeric matrices seeded with hepatocytes to create a highly vascularized organoid (26). Attempts have been made to induce neovascularization of matrix-immobilized hepatocytes using vascular endothelial growth factor (27).

Cell microencapsulation has been used to prolong transplanted hepatocyte survival and function (28). The key theoretical advantage of this technique is the selective capsule permeability that allows transport of nutrients and metabolites across the membrane, but excludes antibodies and host cellular elements. Thus theoretically encapsulation should allow free transport of albumin, the major transport protein for hepatotoxins, but exclude immunoglobulins; this requires a molecular weight cut-off at least 60 kDa. In addition, the wall of the capsule should be strong, because destruction of the membrane would result in release of cells into the peritoneal cavity and cell rejection. Furthermore, the wall of the capsule should be inert to prevent significant foreign body reaction leading to fibrosis and impaired transport across the capsule wall.

Transplantation of encapsulated cells has been carried out by many investigators. Most groups use alginate/25-kDa poly(L-lysine) (ALP), as originally described by Cai *et al.* (29). We have carried out a series of experiments using this technique to encapsulate microcarrier-attached hepatocytes (30). We hypothesized that combining microcarrier and encapsulation techniques would allow cell attachment to a matrix, and additionally, immunoisolate the transplanted cells. *In vitro* experiments were first carried out to examine the transport of albumin across the ALP capsule. Encapsulated microcarrier-attached hepatocytes were cultured under standard conditions in defined serum-free media. Albumin release in the media was measured by enzyme-linked immunosorbent assay (ELISA). At 24 hr, nonencapsulated, microcarrier-attached hepatocytes released more albumin into the media than did encapsulated ones (25.0 ± 2.0 vs. 4.1 ± 1.2 ng/ml; $p < 0.02$).

Subsequently, in a series of *in vivo* experiments, analbuminemic rats were transplanted with normal microcarrier-attached allogeneic hepatocytes either with or without encapsulation; no statistically significant differences were noted between the two groups. A very strong inflammatory response was seen in the peritoneal cavity of animals transplanted with allogeneic encapsulated microcarrier-attached hepatocytes. No such reaction was seen in control animals injected with either encapsulated microcarriers alone or transplanted with syngeneic microcarrier-attached encapsulated hepatocytes.

In another experiment, it was noted that treatment of animals transplanted with encapsulated allogeneic microcarrier-attached hepatocytes with cyclosporine A resulted in a very significant reduction in the pericapsular inflammatory reaction. Our data thus suggest that this commonly used encapsulation technique does not ensure prolonged (or indefinite) hepatocyte survival and function *in vivo*. This may be due to inadequate immunoisolation and/or mechanical problems of capsule rupture and material bioincompatibility, which result in significant pericapsular inflammation and fibrosis. However, in spite of its limitations, we believe that this is a valid approach to cell transplantation and further work should be carried out to develop effective encapsulation techniques.

C. Intraportal Hepatocyte Transplantation

In the early 1990s we and other investigators reevaluated the intraportal route of hepatocyte delivery, because it offered several theoretical advantages:

1. Transplanting hepatocytes into the unique hepatic architecture allows interaction with other hepatocytes and nonparenchymal liver cells.
2. Proximity to hepatocyte-specific growth and differentiation factors creates an environment particularly conducive to hepatocyte engraftment.
3. Locally released mitogens and portal-born hepatotrophic factors can increase transplanted cell numbers.
4. The liver may be an immunologically privileged site.
5. Only in the liver would hepatocytes be able to secrete bile into the biliary tree.

Portal vein thrombosis is the most serious potential complication of direct infusion of isolated hepatocytes into the portal system (31–34). In patients, it may cause massive variceal bleeding due to a sudden rise in portal pressure, ascites, coagulopathy, and acute hepatic insufficiency from disseminated liver necrosis (33). In patients with portal hypertension, transplanted cells may escape via extra- and intrahepatic shunts into the systemic circulation, leading to pulmonary embolism. In order to eliminate, or at least significantly reduce, the risk of these complications, we have focused on developing adequate hepatocyte transplantation systems.

Our initial approach was to infuse a hepatocyte suspension selectively into specific liver lobes (Fig. 1) (35). This technique allows maintenance of portal blood flow through the other nonoccluded liver lobes, thus providing portal decompression and prevention of liver injury. In addition, by infusing a single-cell suspension of viable, highly purified hepatocytes without cellular debris and aggregates, integration of transplanted cells with hepatic plates is enhanced and problems associated with pulmonary and/or systemic embolization are avoided. This technique of selective intraportal transplantation was studied in Nagase analbuminemic (NAR) rats and in hyperbilirubinemic Gunn rats. Increase in blood albumin levels (NAR) and bilirubin conjugates in the posttransplantation bile samples and decrease in total serum bilirubin levels (Gunn) were noted, respectively, suggesting the presence of viable and functioning transplanted hepatocytes.

Because only a limited number of hepatocytes can be transplanted using a single intraportal injection without caus-

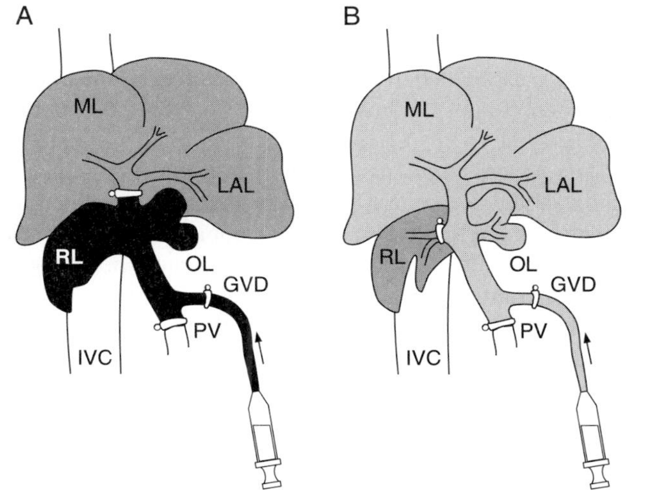

Figure 1 Diagram of hepatocyte transplantation into (A) right and omental liver lobes; (B) anterior and omental liver lobes. The gastroduodenal vein (GDV) is canulated and temporary tourniquets are placed around the portal venous (PV) supply to the nontransplanted lobes. The right and omental lobes represent 30% of the total liver mass; the anterior and omental lobes represent 76% of the liver mass. ML, Median lobe; LAL, left anterior lobe; RL, right lobe; OL, omental lobe; IVC, inferior vena cava. From Ref. (35); M. D. Holzman, J. Rozga, D. F. Neuzil, D. Griffin, A. D. Moscioni, and A. A. Demetriou (1993). Selective intraportal hepatocyte transplantation in analbuminemic and Gunn rats. *Transplantation* **55** (6), 1213–1219.

ing occlusion of numerous portal venules, we have developed a technique that allows repeated infusion of isolated hepatocytes through an implantable portal vein access device (36). Briefly, a small subcutaneous pocket in the left groin is created for placement of a vascular access device (Mini-Port; Pharmacia Deltec Inc., St. Paul, MN). The port is connected to silicone tubing, which is tunneled subcutaneously and brought into the peritoneal cavity through a small puncture in the anterior abdominal wall. It is then placed in the gastroduodenal vein at the junction of the portal vein. During each cell infusion, the Mini-Port chamber is punctured percutaneously (Fig. 2). The catheter and the chamber are subsequently flushed with 2 ml of heparinized saline. Analbuminemic rats subjected to repeated cell infusions showed at 28 days much higher albumin levels than those transplanted with a single dose of normal allogeneic hepatocytes. On light microscopy, NAR rats transplanted with a large single dose of isolated albumin-producing hepatocytes showed albumin-positive cells arranged in small clusters containing 5–20 cells and, in some sections, areas of tissue scarring. In contrast, liver sections from rats subjected to intraportal infusion of six small batches of isolated hepatocytes showed an exceptionally large number of cells that stained positive for albumin and no signs of tissue damage (36).

All methods of hepatocyte transplantation described to date have not demonstrated sustained, long-term liver support or normalization of a genetic liver defect. This has been primarily due to inadequate quantities of hepatocytes transplanted. In order to overcome this problem, several groups of investigators have tried to induce proliferation of intrasplenically transplanted hepatocytes by means of partial hepatectomy (37, 38) or intravenous administration of

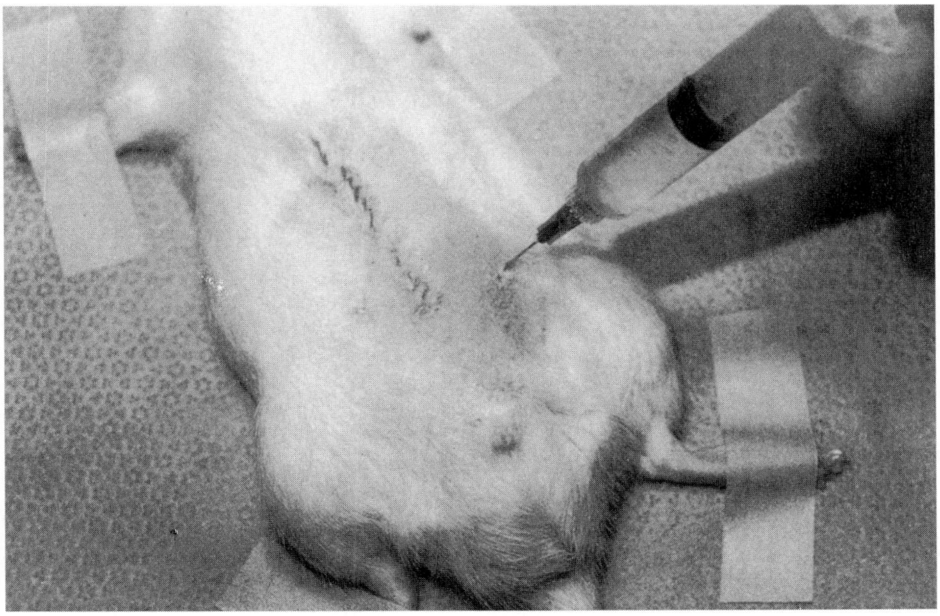

Figure 2 Implantable vascular access device was placed in the left groin. It was punctured percutaneously and isolated rat hepatocytes were infused over a period of 2 min. After injection, the chamber was filled with heparinized saline. From Ref. (36), with permission.

hepatic stimulatory substance (39) or hepatocyte growth factor (40). The results of those studies were not convincing, perhaps due to suboptimal experimental conditions (lack of interaction with liver nonparenchymal cells). We have therefore decided to induce proliferation of hepatocytes transplanted into the liver tissue.

We have previously demonstrated in the rat that by performing portal branch ligation (PBL), in which the two anterior lobes (two-thirds of the liver mass) were permanently excluded from the portal circulation, a regeneration response resulted in the remaining nonoccluded lobes, similar to that seen after standard partial (two-thirds) hepatectomy (41, 42). In contrast to Hamaguchi *et al.* (43), who transplanted hepatocytes shortly after partial hepatectomy, we first allowed hepatocytes, seeded in the posterior liver lobes, to engraft without disturbing liver function and structure, and then by eliminating the portal blood inflow to the nontransplanted anterior liver lobes, we induced hyperplastic response in the transplant-bearing liver parenchyma. Using this approach, we have obtained for the first time a near-total correction of a genetic defect in liver function. At 86 days posttransplantation, five out of eight analbuminemic rats had serum albumin levels between 2.0 and 2.5 g/dl (in normal rat liver cell donors it was 3.5 ± 0.4 g/dl) (44). In addition, we noted a marked increase in the population of albumin-positive cells in the livers of transplanted rats undergoing liver regeneration (approximately 23% of the cell population) (Fig. 3).

Data on intraportal hepatocellular transplantation in large mammals are scarce. Early attempts included treatment of Watanabe hyperlipidemic (WHHL) rabbits using allogeneic and genetically engineered heterologous hepatocytes expressing human low-density lipoprotein receptor (45, 46) and studies in dogs transplanted with allogeneic hepatocytes and autologous retrovirally transduced hepatocytes expressing human α1-antitrypsin cDNA (47). In the latter study, transplantation of 1×10^9 hepatocytes via the portal vasculature resulted in a number of complications, including shock, lethargy, pallor, hypotension, and hematemesis. Although in some dogs the shock episodes appeared to have been vasoactive in origin (reaction to culture medium and fetal calf serum), two out of seven animals died; autopsy revealed small bowel hemorrhage, sanguineous ascites, portal thrombosis, and spleen and liver infarction. In more recent studies by Rivas *et al.* (48), both intrasplenic and portal vein injection of $(1 - 2) \times 10^9$ liver cells in dogs

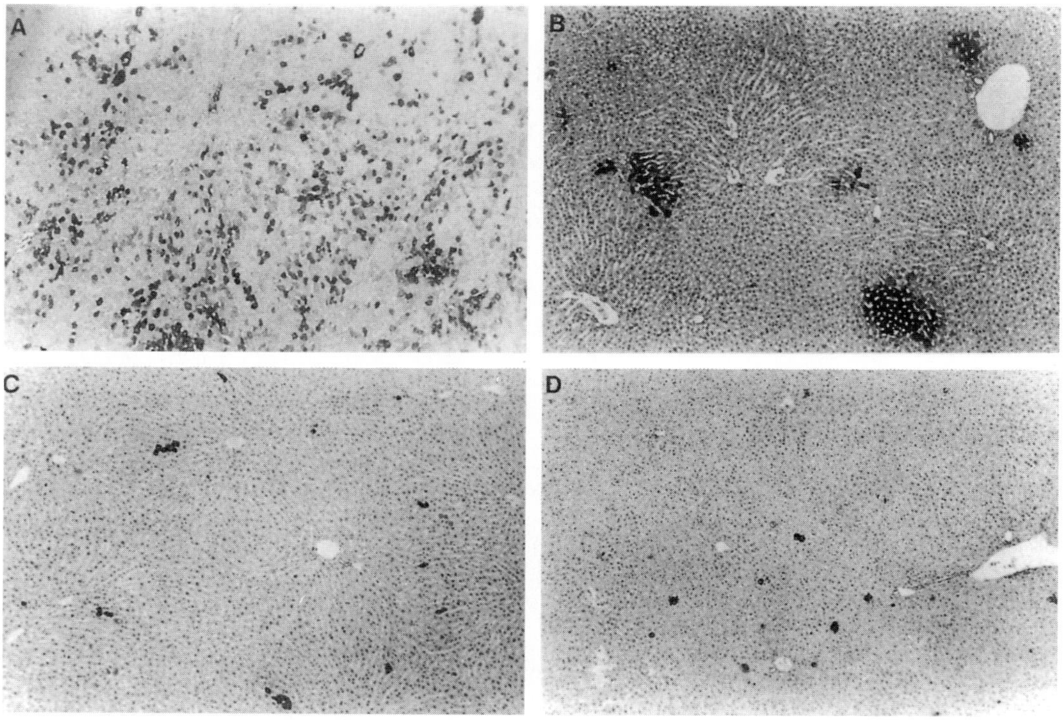

Figure 3 Photomicrographs of liver sections of NAR rats 86 days following selective intraportal hepatocyte transplantation, immunohistochemically probed for albumin-positive hepatocytes. (A) Hepatocyte transplantation of allogeneic hepatocytes and portal branch ligation 4 days after transplatation. (B) Hepatocyte transplantation of allogeneic hepatocytes and sham portal branch ligation. (C) Hepatocyte transplantation of syngeneic hepatocytes from NAR donors and portal branch ligation. (D) Sham hepatocyte transplantation (saline) and sham portal branch ligation. From Ref. (44), with permission.

were associated with embolization of intrahepatic portal branches, causing derangement of hepatic function and histology. Mortality was low, but nevertheless noted.

The success of selective hepatocyte transplantation and subsequent induction of transplanted cell proliferation in Nagase analbuminemic rats encouraged us to use this strategy in WHHL rabbits (49). The genetic defect in these animals is a counterpart of familial hypercholesterolemia in humans. Animals that are homozygous have a mutation in the low-density lipoprotein (LDL) receptor gene and express almost no functional LDL receptors. As a result, intermediate-density lipoproteins and LDLs accumulate in plasma, leading to accelerated atherosclerosis and premature death. Allogeneic New Zealand white rabbit hepatocytes (2×10^8) were infused over a 5-min period selectively into the posterior liver lobes. Before closing the abdomen, the portal venous branch supplying the anterior liver lobe was dissected and a silk thread was placed around it and left untied. One week following cell transplantation, all the animals were reoperated and PBL was completed. Control WHHL rabbits were transplanted with allogeneic hepatocytes and 1 week later were subjected to sham PBL or received an injection of heparinized saline, and 1 week later were subjected to PBL. All rabbits were maintained on daily cyclosporine A (25 mg/kg PO) for the duration of the experiment (150 days). In all WHHL rabbits pretransplant blood cholesterol levels were greater than 800 mg/dl. A marked and sustained reduction of serum cholesterol and LDL levels was recorded in WHHL rabbits in which hepatocyte transplantation was followed by PBL. The functional effect seen in these animals was far more pronounced than in control rabbits receiving hepatocytes + sham PBL (Fig. 4). The livers previously perfused with DiI-labeled LDL contained more LDL-positive hepatocytes in hepatocyte transplantation + PBL animals than in their hepatocyte transplantation + sham PBL partners. Of great importance was the finding of a near total lack of atherosclerotic changes in the aortas of hepatocyte transplantation + PBL WHHL recipients.

While discussing the issue of transplanted hepatocyte proliferation, it is important to mention the work by Rhim *et al.* (50), who demonstrated that a small number of normal adult hepatocytes injected into the spleen can totally repopulate a defective liver in a hepatotoxic transgenic mouse model system (Alb-uPA transgenic mouse). In a series of

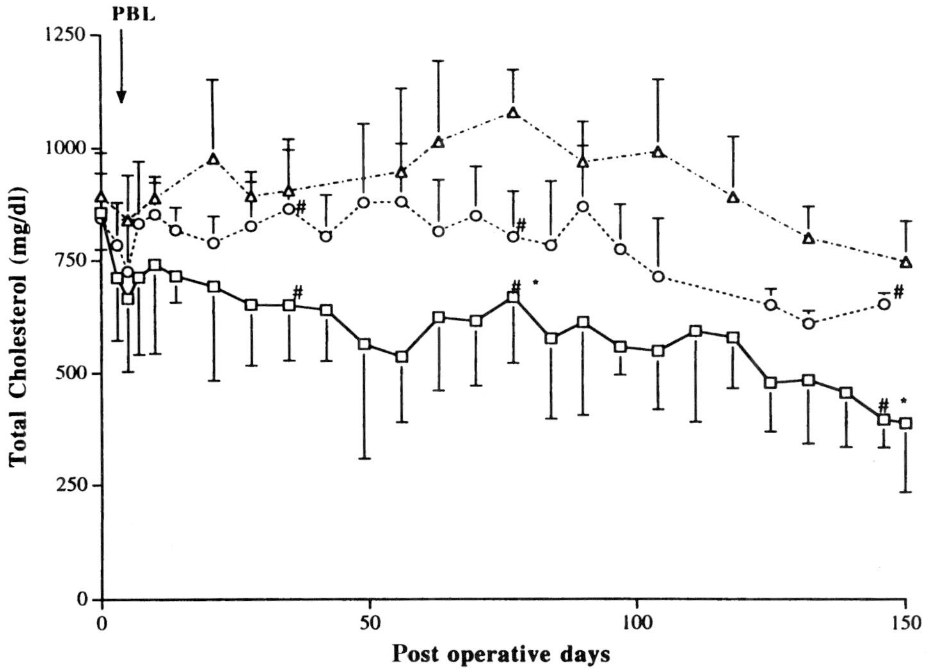

Figure 4 Serum cholesterol levels in the three groups of WHHL rabbits. Group I and II rabbits were transplanted with allogeneic hepatocytes (hepatocyte transplantation). Group III controls received intraportal saline injection only. Portal branch ligation was performed on day 7 after transplantation in group I and III animals. Baseline cholesterol levels were as follows: group I, 855 ± 81 mg/dl; group II, 843 ± 102 mg/dl; and group III, 893 ± 97 mg/dl. Values are given as mean ± SD. *, $P < 0.05$ vs. group II; #, $P < 0.05$ vs. group III. □, group I, hepatocyte transplantation and PBL, $n = 7$; ○, group II, hepatocyte transplantation without PBL, $n = 6$; △, group III, sham hepatocyte transplantation (saline) with PBL, $n = 4$. From Ref. (49); S. Eguchi, J. Rozga, L. T. Lebow, S. C. Chen, C. C. Wang, R. Rosenthal, *et al.* (1996). Treatment of hypercholesterolemia in the Watanabe rabbit using allogeneic hepatocellular transplantation under a regeneration stimulus. *Transplantation* **62** (5), 588–593.

studies, Oren *et al.* (51) have shown that in partially hepatectomized rats, the liver remnant may be repopulated by transplanted hepatocytes when proliferation of native hepatocytes is inhibited. These studies suggest that mature differentiated hepatocytes are capable of proceeding through numerous cell replicative cycles under the influence of a persistent hepatic regenerative stimulus.

D. Identification of Transplanted Hepatocytes

After ectopic (e.g., spleen) hepatocyte transplantation, identification of transplanted cells is relatively simple; it is based on morphologic analysis and Periodic Acid Schiff (PAS) staining for glycogen. After intraportal hepatocyte transplantation, however, integration of transplanted cells with hepatic cell plates is rapid and so complete that their identification requires use of sophisticated techniques. For example, after male-to-female hepatocyte transplantation, the livers can be examined for the presence of parenchymal cells expressing the Y chromosome (*in situ* hybridization of the *sry* region with digoxigenin-labeled DNA probes). In our own studies in analbuminemic rats, transplanted albumin-positive rat hepatocytes were sought on gelatin-coated slides of liver tissue immunostained utilizing rabbit antirat albumin IgG antibodies and an immunoperoxidase avidin–biotin peroxidase complex (Vectastain ABC) method (Fig. 3) (36). Gupta *et al.* (52, 53) analyzed the distribution of transplanted hepatocytes in vascular beds with cells marked by either ^{111}In or ^{99m}Tc or by studying endogenous dipeptidyl peptidase IV (DPPIV) activity in enzyme-deficient F344 rats transplanted with syngeneic hepatocytes isolated from the livers of DPPIV-positive F344 rat donors.

We have developed a method of cellular tagging and *in vivo* identification and quantitation of intraportally transplanted rat, porcine, and rabbit hepatocytes using an intracellular fluorescent dye, 5(6)-carboxyfluorescein diacetate, succinimidyl ester (CSFE) (54). The optimal conditions consisted of a buffered saline suspension of hepatocytes (5×10^6 cells/ml) in 20 m*M* CSFE incubated for 15 min at 37°C. *In vitro*, labeled hepatocytes retained the dye for up to 3 weeks (last day of study). CFSE did not affect hepatocyte viability and there was no evidence of intercellular diffusion of the dye. *In vivo*, inbred Lewis rats underwent selective intraportal infusion of freshly isolated CSFE-labeled syngeneic hepatocytes (2×10^7 cells/2ml saline/rat) into the posterior liver lobes. All recipients were sacrificed 48 and 96 hr later. Transplanted hepatocytes were identified in the recipient liver by fluorescence microscopy and by fluorescence-activated cell sorting (FACS) following liver digestion using portal vein collagenase perfusion. CFSE persisted in a distinct population of viable, engrafted hepatocytes. Flow cytometry demonstrated that 9 ± 3% of the hepatocytes in the posterior liver lobes were labeled at 48 and 96 hr posttransplantation. At 96 hr, multiple engrafted hepatocytes were observed by fluorescence microscopy, predominantly around the central veins. Whether this was an effect of cell migration toward zone 3 of the liver acinus, or merely an effect of excessive pressure during cell infusion, remains to be investigated.

V. Human Hepatocyte Transplantation

Our laboratory has carried out experiments utilizing human hepatocytes in a series of studies resulting in the development of methods of harvesting, testing, and cryopreserving human hepatocytes for future clinical use (55, 56).

A. Hepatocyte Harvest

A biopsy specimen was shaken in EGTA and then digested with collagenase, and a needle biopsy was treated with collagenase only. After liver segmentectomy, hepatocytes were harvested by a multipuncture perfusion method. Briefly, several 14-gauge catheters were introduced into visible vessels on the cut surface of the liver fragment and sutured in place. The liver fragment was first perfused for 15 min at a rate of 10 ml/min per catheter with oxygenated buffer without calcium and then for 20 min with calcium (1.8 m*M* $CaCl_2$)-enriched 0.05% collagenase type I. The pale, digested regions of the liver were excised, minced, and passed through a 100-μm nylon mesh. Hepatocyte-enriched fractions were obtained by repeated (3×) washing with cold 1.8 m*M* calcium buffer. Cell viability was determined by trypan blue exclusion and was rarely found to be satisfactory (>40%). Livers from the Southern California Organ Procurement Center, which were universally (nationally) rejected for transplantation, were transported to our laboratory. The intact liver was transferred to a large 4-liter metal bowl for surgical manipulation. The suprahepatic vena cava was oversewn and the cut end of the infrahepatic vena cava was surrounded with a 4-0 Prolene suture to close it snugly around a size 18 Masterflex tube (Barnant Co., Barrington, IL) inserted to provide the outflow from the liver. The hepatic artery and the common bile duct were closed with a 0 silk ligature. The portal vein was then identified and a size 16 Masterflex tube was inserted and secured with two 0 silk ligatures. This tubing acted as the hepatic inflow for the liver perfusion. The container with the liver was then placed in a water bath set to 42°C. The liver was permitted to float in 2 to 3 liters of warm (37°C) saline. The tubing placed in the portal vein was attached to a roller pump with a loop and was situated in the waterbath, while the end was placed in the reservoir of the perfusate. The roller pump speed was 0.2 ml/min/g liver tissue and the perfusate was placed below the level of the liver. The placement of the end of the outflow tubing from the liver depends on the perfusate step. To begin the perfusion, 4 liters of warm 2 m*M* EDTA solution was flushed through the liver while the outflow was collected in a waste container placed below the level of the liver. On completion of the EDTA perfusion, 200–300 ml of calcium-enriched 0.05% collagenase type P (Boehringer Mannheim, Indianapolis, IN) solution was perfused through the liver and discarded. The outflow tubing from the infrahepatic inferior vena cava was then placed into the container with the collagenase solution, creating a closed recirculation circuit. Approximately 2 liters of the collagenase solution was recirculated through the liver for 15 to 20 min until the liver was palpably digested. Once it was determined that the digestion was satisfactory, the tubing was removed from the liver and the saline was discarded from the bowl. Under sterile technique, 1 liter of 4°C solution containing Williams E (Gibco, Grand Island, NY) and Ham F12 (Gibco) at 1:1 (with 10% fetal bovine serum, 10 mol/liter dexamethasone, 10^{-7} mol/liter insulin) was then slowly added while Glisson's capsule was manually disrupted, allowing the digested liver to fall freely into suspension. The cell suspension was then filtered via custom-made filtration device with filters of decreasing porosity and washed with the Williams-E/Ham F12 medium in a Cobe 2991 blood cell processor, as described above. The cells were then resuspended in Williams-E/Ham F12 and viability was determined by trypan blue exclusion; it was $68 \pm 2\%$ ($n = 8$). These cells, although clearly not optimal (isolated from severely steatotic livers), were subsequently shown to metabolize significant amounts of diazepam and lidocaine.

B. Experimental Studies

Human hepatocyte function was tested by transplanting cells into the peritoneal cavity of athymic (nude) rats with specific inherited defects of liver function (55). These animals served as *in vivo* "test tubes" for evaluating human hepatocyte function. Rat recipients were either hyperbilirubinemic Gunn rats or NAR analbuminemic rats. Rats were made genetically immunodeficient by interbreeding with athymic rats with inherited T cell deficiency. There was no morphologic evidence of rejection in the immunoincompetent recipients, whereas immunocompetent rats demonstrated rejection within 5 days of transplantation. Nude Gunn rat recipients demonstrated excretion of bilirubin glucuronides in bile for up to 30 days and reduction in serum bilirubin levels. In recipient NAR rats, plasma albumin levels increased from a pretransplantation level of 0.025–0.05 mg/ml to 3.9–4.8 mg/ml and remained nearly at that level for 30 days. These experimental studies thus demonstrate that human hepatocytes can perform well-differentiated normal liver functions *in vivo*.

C. Clinical Studies

There is only limited clinical experience with hepatocyte transplantation (57–63). Additionally, convincing evidence of transplanted cell function is lacking, because the number of the transplanted cells was small. It also needs to be pointed out that allogeneic hepatocyte transplantation is hampered by lack of donor organs because harvested normal livers are being used for whole or split organ transplantation. Therefore, the need to develop techniques for isolation of cells from cadaver livers and/or livers rejected from whole organ transplantation exists. Another option would be to transplant liver stem cells. In that case, however, we would need to learn how to isolate them from intact livers, expand them in culture, and then convert them into differentiated mature hepatocytes.

References

1. Shakil, A. O., Mazariegos, G. V., and Kramer, D. J. (1999). Fulminant hepatic failure. *Surg. Clin. North Am.* **79,** 77–108.
2. Berry, M. N., and Friend, D. S. (1969). High-yield preparation of isolated rat liver parenchymal cells: A biochemical and fine structural study. *J. Cell Biol.* **43,** 506–520.
3. Seglen, P. O. (1976). Preparation of isolated rat liver cells. *Methods Cell Biol.* **13,** 29–83.
4. Kreamer, B. L., Staecker, J. L., Sawada, N., *et al.* (1986). Use of a low-speed, iso-density percoll centrifugation method to increase the viability of isolated rat hepatocyte preparations. *In Vitro Cell Dev. Biol.* **22,** 201–211.
5. Morsiani, E., Rozga, J., Scott, H. C., *et al.* (1995). Automated liver cell processing facilitates large scale isolation and purification of porcine hepatocytes. *ASAIO J.* **41,** 155–161.
6. Fuller, B. J., and De Loecker, W. (1997). Hepatocyte cryopreservation. *In* "Hepatocyte Transplantation" (M. Mito and M. Sawa, eds.). Karger Landes Systems, Basel.
7. Rozga, R., Moscioni, A. D., and Demetriou, A. A. (1994). Hepatocyte transplantation; liver transplantation microchip. *In* "Intra-abdominal Organ Transplantation 2000" (L. S. Sher, eds.). R.G.Landes Company, Austin, TX.
8. Vroemen, J. P., Buurman, W. A., Heirwegh, K. P., *et al.* (1986). Hepatocyte transplantation for enzyme deficiency disease in congenic rats. *Transplantation* **42,** 130–135.
9. Kusano, M., and Mito, M. (1982). Observations on the fine structure of long-survived isolated hepatocytes inoculated into rat spleen. *Gastroenterology* **82,** 616–628.
10. Gupta, S., Aragona, E., Vemuru, R. P., *et al.* (1991). Permanent engraftment and function of hepatocytes delivered to the liver: implications for gene therapy and liver repopulation. *Hepatology* **14,** 144–149.
11. Arkadopoulos, N., Lilja, H., Suh, K. S., *et al.* (1998). Intrasplenic transplantation of allogeneic hepatocytes prolongs survival in anhepatic rats. *Hepatology* **28,** 1365–1370.
12. Rosenthal, R. J., Chen, S. C., Hewitt, W., *et al.* (1996). Techniques for intrasplenic hepatocyte transplantation in the large animal model. *Surg. Endosc.* **10,** 1075–1079.

13. Arkadopoulos, N., Chen, S. C., Khalili, T. M., *et al.* (1998). Transplantation of hepatocytes for prevention of intracranial hypertension in pigs with ischemic liver failure. *Cell Transplant.* **7,** 357–363.
14. Sutherland, D. E., Numata, M., Matas, A. J., *et al.* (1977). Hepatocellular transplantation in acute liver failure. *Surgery* **82,** 124–132.
15. Sommer, B. G., Sutherland, D. E., Matas, A. J., *et al.* (1979). Hepatocellular transplantation for treatment of D-galactosamine-induced acute liver failure in rats. *Transplant. Proc.* **11,** 578–584.
16. Baumgartner, D., LaPlante-O'Neill, P. M., Sutherland, D. E., and Najarian, J. S. (1983). Effects of intrasplenic injection of hepatocytes, hepatocyte fragments and hepatocyte culture supernatants on D-galactosamine-induced liver failure in rats. *Eur. Surg. Res.* **15,** 129–135.
17. Reid, L. M., and Rojkind, M., (1979). New techniques for culturing differentiated cells: Reconstituted basement membrane rafts. *Methods Enzymol* **58,** 263-78.
18. Demetriou, A. A., Whiting, J. F., Feldman, D., *et al.* (1986). Replacement of liver function in rats by transplantation of microcarrier-attached hepatocytes. *Science* **233,** 1190–1192.
19. Demetriou, A. A., Reisner, A., Sanchez, J., *et al.* (1988). Transplantation of microcarrier-attached hepatocytes into 90% partially hepatectomized rats. *Hepatology* **8,** 1006–1009.
20. Vacanti, J. P., Morse, M. A., Saltzman, W. M., *et al.* (1988). Selective cell transplantation using bioabsorbable artificial polymers as matrices. *J. Pediatr. Surg.* **23,** 3–9.
21. Nagaki, M., Kano, T., Muto, Y., *et al.* (1990). Effects of intraperitoneal transplantation of microcarrier-attached hepatocytes on D-galactosamine-induced acute liver failure in rats. *Gastroenterol. Jpn.* **25,** 78–87.
22. Dixit, V., Piskin, E., Arthur, M., *et al.* (1992). Hepatocyte immobilization on PHEMA microcarriers and its biologically modified forms. *Cell Transplant.* **1,** 391–399.
23. Demetriou, A. A., Holzman, M., Moscioni, A. D., and Rozga, J., (1993). Hepatic cell transplantation. *Adv. Vet. Sci. Comp. Med.* **37,** 313–332.
24. Kaufmann, P. M., Kneser, U., Fiegel, H. C., *et al.* (1999). Is there an optimal concentration of cotransplanted islets of Langerhans for stimulation of hepatocytes in three dimensional matrices? *Transplantation* **68,** 272–279.
25. Yang, M. B., Vacanti, J. P., and Ingber, D. E., (1994). Hollow fibers for hepatocyte encapsulation and transplantation: Studies of survival and function in rats. *Cell Transplant.* **3,** 373–385.
26. Johnson, L. B., Aiken, J., Mooney, D., *et al.* (1994). The mesentery as a laminated vascular bed for hepatocyte transplantation. *Cell Transplant.* **3,** 273–281.
27. Monney, D. (2000). Personal communication.
28. Dixit, V., Darvasi, R., Arthur, M., *et al.* (1990). Restoration of liver function in Gunn rats without immunosuppression using transplanted microencapsulated hepatocytes. *Hepatology* **12,** 1342–1349.
29. Cai, Z. H., Shi, Z. Q., O'Shea, G. M., and Sun, A. M., (1988). Microencapsulated hepatocytes for bioartificial liver support. *Artif. Organs* **12,** 388–393.
30. Rozga, J., Williams, R. F., Bellew, T., *et al.* (1991). Transplantation of encapsulated microcarrier-attached hepatocytes into analbuminemic rats. *Surg. Forum* **42,** 419–421.
31. Groth, C. G., Arborgh, B., Bjorken, C., *et al.* (1977). Correction of hyperbilirubinemia in the glucuronyltransferase-deficient rat by intraportal hepatocyte transplantation. *Transplant. Proc.* **9,** 313–316.
32. Mehigan, D. G., Bell, W. R., Zuidema, G. D., *et al.* (1980). Disseminated intravascular coagulation and portal hypertension following pancreatic islet autotransplantation. *Ann. Surg.* **191,** 287–293.
33. Walsh, T. J., Eggleston, J. C., and Cameron, J. L., (1982). Portal hypertension, hepatic infarction, and liver failure complicating pancreatic islet autotransplantation. *Surgery* **91,** 485–487.
34. Nieto, J. A., Escandon, J., Betancor, C., *et al.* (1989). Evidence that temporary complete occlusion of splenic vessels prevents massive embolization and sudden death associated with intrasplenic hepatocellular transplantation. *Transplantation* **47,** 449–450.
35. Holzman, M. D., Rozga, J., Neuzil, D. F., *et al.* (1993). Selective intraportal hepatocyte transplantation in analbuminemic and Gunn rats. *Transplantation* **55,** 1213–1219.
36. Rozga, J., Holzman, M., Moscioni, A. D., *et al.* (1995). Repeated intraportal hepatocyte transplantation in analbuminemic rats. *Cell Transplant.* **4,** 237–243.
37. Nordlinger, B., Wang, S. R., Bouma, M. E., *et al.* (1987). Can hepatocytes proliferate when transplanted into the spleen? Demonstration by autohistoradiography in the rat. *Eur. Surg. Res.* **19,** 381–387.
38. Gupta, S., Johnstone, R., Darby, H., *et al.* (1987). Transplanted isolated hepatocytes: effect of partial hepatectomy on proliferation of long-term syngeneic implants in rat spleen. *Pathology* **19,** 28–30.
39. Jiang, B., Sawa, M., Yamamoto, T., and Kasai, S. (1997). Enhancement of proliferation of intrasplenically transplanted hepatocytes in cirrhotic rats by hepatic stimulatory substance. *Transplantation* **63,** 131–135.
40. Kato, K., Onodera, K., Sawa, M., *et al.* (1996). Effect of hepatocyte growth factor on the proliferation of intrasplenically transplanted hepatocytes in rats. *Biochem. Biophys. Res. Commun.* **222,** 101–106.
41. Higgins, G. M., and Anderson, R. M. (1932). Experimental pathology of the liver: restoration of the liver of the white rat following partial surgical removal. *AMA Arch. Pathol.* **1932,** 186–202.
42. Rozga, J., Jeppsson, B., and Bengmark, S. (1986). Portal branch ligation in the rat. Reevaluation of a model. *Am. J. Pathol.* **125,** 300–308.
43. Hamaguchi, H., Yamaguchi, Y., Goto, M., *et al.* (1994). Hepatic biliary transport after hepatocyte transplantation in Eizai hyperbilirubinemic rats. *Hepatology* **20,** 220–224.
44. Moscioni, A. D., Rozga, J., Chen, S., *et al.* (1996). Long-term correction of albumin levels in the Nagase analbuminemic rat: repopulation of the liver by transplanted normal hepatocytes under a regeneration response. *Cell Transplant.* **5,** 499–503.
45. Wiederkehr, J. C., Kondos, G. T., and Pollak, R. (1990). Hepatocyte transplantation for the low-density lipoprotein receptor- deficient state. A study in the Watanabe rabbit. *Transplantation* **50,** 466–471.
46. Tejera, M. L., Cienfuegos, J. A., Maganto, P., *et al.* (1992). Reduction of cholesterol levels following liver cell grafting in hyperlipidemic (WHHL) rabbits. *Transplant. Proc.* **24,** 160–161.
47. Kay, M. A., Baley, P., Rothenberg, S., *et al.* (1992). Expression of human alpha 1-antitrypsin in dogs after autologous transplantation of retroviral transduced hepatocytes. *Proc. Natl. Acad. Sci. U.S.A* **89,** 89–93.
48. Rivas, P. A., Fabrega, A. J., Schwartz, D., *et al.* (1994). Transplantation of hepatocytes: An *in-vitro* and *in-vivo* study in canines. *Cell Transplant.* **3,** 193–201.
49. Eguchi, S., Rozga, J., Lebow, L. T., *et al.* (1996). Treatment of hypercholesterolemia in the Watanabe rabbit using allogeneic hepatocellular transplantation under a regeneration stimulus. *Transplantation* **62,** 588–593.
50. Rhim, J. A., Sandgren, E. P., Degen, J. L., *et al.* (1994). Replacement of diseased mouse liver by hepatic cell transplantation. *Science* **263,** 1149–1152.
51. Oren, R., Dabeva, M. D., Petkov, P. M., *et al.* (1999). Restoration of serum albumin levels in nagase analbuminemic rats by hepatocyte transplantation. *Hepatology* **29,** 75–81.
52. Gupta, S., Lee, C. D., Vemuru, R. P., and Bhargava, K. K. (1994). ^{111}Indium labeling of hepatocytes for analysis of short-term biodistribution of transplanted cells. *Hepatology* **19,** 750–757.
53. Gupta, S., Vasa, S. R., Rajvanshi, P., *et al.* (1997). Analysis of hepatocyte distribution and survival in vascular beds with cells marked by $_{99m}$TC or endogenous dipeptidyl peptidase IV activity. *Cell Transplant.* **6,** 377–386.
54. Fujioka, H., Hunt, P. J., Rozga, J., *et al.* (1994). Carboxyfluorescein (CFSE) labelling of hepatocytes for short-term localization following intraportal transplantation. *Cell Transplant.* **3,** 397–408.

55. Moscioni, A. D., Roy-Chowdhury, J., Barbour, R., *et al.* (1989). Human liver cell transplantation. Prolonged function in athymic-Gunn and athymic-analbuminemic hybrid rats. *Gastroenterology* **96,** 1546–1551.
56. Hewitt, W. R., Corno, V., Eguchi, S., *et al.* (1997). Isolation of human hepatocytes from livers rejected for whole organ transplantation. *Transplant. Proc.* **29,** 1945–1947.
57. Mito, M., Kusano, M., and Kawaura, Y. (1992). Hepatocyte transplantation in man. *Transplant. Proc.* **24,** 3052–3053.
58. Habibullah, C. M., Syed, I. H., Qamar, A., and Taher-Uz, Z. (1994). Human fetal hepatocyte transplantation in patients with fulminant hepatic failure. *Transplantation* **58,** 951–952.
59. Bilir, B., Durham, J. D., Krystal, J., *et al.* (1996). Tranjugular intra-portal transplantation of cryopreserved human hepatocytes in a patient with acute liver failure. *Hepatology* **24,** 308A.
60. Grossman, M., Raper, S. E., Kozarsky, K., *et al.* Successful *ex vivo* gene therapy directed to liver in a patient with familial hypercholesterolaemia [see comments]. *Nature Genet.* **6,** 335–341.
61. Strom, S. C., Fisher, R. A., Thompson, M. T., *et al.* (1997). Hepatocyte transplantation as a bridge to orthotopic liver transplantation in terminal liver failure. *Transplantation* **63,** 559–569.
62. Strom, S. C., Chowdhury, J. R., and Fox, I. J. (1999). Hepatocyte transplantation for the treatment of human disease. *Semin. Liver Dis.* **19,** 39–48.
63. Fox, I. J., Chowdhury, J. R., Kaufman, S. S., *et al.* (1998). Treatment of the Crigler-Najjar syndrome type I with hepatocyte transplantation [see comments]. *N. Engl. J. Med.* **338,** 1422–1426.

52

Biliary Stone Formation

Matthew I. Goldblatt, Attila Nakeeb, and Henry A. Pitt

Department of Surgery, Medical College of Wisconsin, Milwaukee, Wisconsin 53226

I. Introduction

Gallstone disease is a major healthcare concern in the United States. Approximately 12% of the U.S. population, or more than 30,000,000 Americans, have gallstones. As a result, more than 750,000 cholecystectomies are performed each year, and the cost for caring for these patients is estimated to be between 7 and 10 billion dollars annually (1). Gallstones can be classified into three types: cholesterol, black pigment, and brown pigment stones. In Western countries approximately 75% of gallstones are cholesterol, 20% are black pigment, and 5% are brown pigment stones. Stones can be differentiated by the amount of cholesterol they contain. Cholesterol gallstones contain approximately 85% cholesterol by weight, whereas black pigment stones contain only 1–2% cholesterol and are made up of unconjugated bilirubin and calcium phosphate; brown pigment stones are composed of calcium bilirubinate and calcium salts of fatty acids.

Multiple risk factors have been identified for gallstone development. Major factors that impact on gallstones include age, gender, diet, and genetics. Gallstone incidence increases with age. Gallstones are rare in children but in some countries such as Sweden and Chile they occur in 60% of adults reaching the eighth decade (2). In some African countries, on the other hand, gallstones are rare, even in elderly adults, suggesting that both diet and genetics are important risk factors. Hemolytic disorders, ileal disease, ileal resection, cirrhosis, and long-term total parenteral nutrition all increase the incidence of black pigment stones.

The vast majority of patients between the ages of 20 and 60 years with gallstones are female, and most of these women develop cholesterol gallstones. Pregnancy and parity are additional risk factors and the influence of estrogens and progesterone on biliary motility and biliary lipid metabolism likely plays a role. Brown pigment stones are associated with conditions that predispose to biliary tract infections, such as parasitic infections, biliary strictures, biliary cysts, and sclerosing cholangitis.

II. Gallstone Pathogenesis

The primary goal of research in gallstone pathogenesis is the prevention of gallstone formation. Reasons to consider gallstone prevention include (1) the considerable cost of treatment, (2) the morbidity associated with operative intervention, (3) disease complications such as acute cholecystitis, choledocholithiasis, cholangitis, and pancreatitis, (4) treatment complications such as bile duct injury, and (5) increased mortality. In order to achieve the goal of prevention, an understanding of gallstone pathogenesis is necessary.

A. Cholesterol Gallstones

Despite considerable investigation, the pathogenesis of cholesterol gallstones is still not completely understood. However, three factors have been found to be key to the pathogenesis of cholesterol gallstone formation: (1) the supersaturation of cholesterol in bile, (2) the nucleation and growth of cholesterol monohydrate crystals within the gallbladder, and (3) diminished gallbladder motility (Fig. 1). The interrelationship of these three factors ultimately leads to cholesterol gallstone formation.

1. Cholesterol Supersaturation

Cholesterol gallstones form when bile becomes supersaturated with cholesterol. Cholesterol is virtually insoluble in aqueous solutions, but in bile is made soluble by association with bile acids and phospholipids in the form of mixed micelles and vesicles. Micelles are aggregates of lipids with nonpolar hydrocarbon chains directed inward and polar phosphate or hydroxyl groups directed outward toward the aqueous solvent. Vesicles are spherical bilayers of phospholipids with nonpolar hydrocarbon chains hidden inside the bilayer and polar groups directed outward toward the aqueous solvent. Most cholesterol in bile is carried in small (70–100 nm) unilamellar vesicles. As cholesterol saturation increases the vesicles aggregate, enlarge, and fuse to form multivesicular and multilamellar complexes (up to 5000 nm). Cholesterol monohydrate crystals then form on

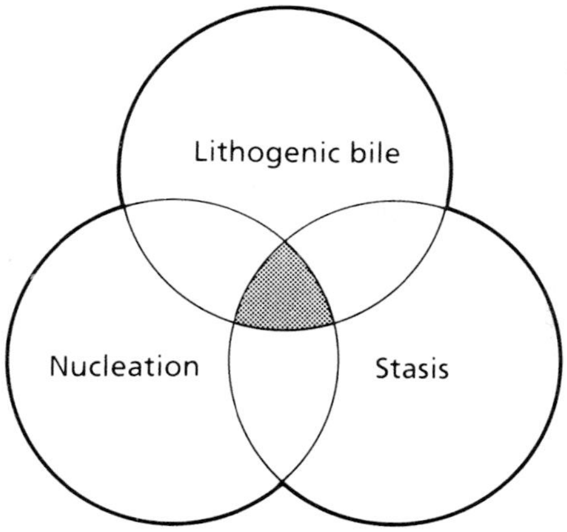

Figure 1 The three interrelated factors involved in gallstone pathogenesis. These three factors also represent the areas in which gallstone research has been focused.

the surface of these vesicles and grow within the mucin gel of the gallbladder.

Cholesterol supersaturation is due principally to an excessive hepatic secretion of cholesterol into bile. This situation results either from increased *de novo* cholesterol synthesis or increased lipoprotein uptake by the liver or from a decreased conversion of cholesterol to bile salts. As a result, a greater fraction of cholesterol is eliminated in the bile. At least three hepatic enzymes that regulate cholesterol metabolism are likely to play a role in cholesterol supersaturation: (1) 3-hydroxy-3-methylglutaryl-CoA (HMG-CoA) reductase, the rate-limiting enzyme of cholesterol secretion into bile, (2) cholesterol 7α-hydroxylase, which regulates the conversion of cholesterol to bile salts, and (3) acyl-CoA:cholesterol acyltransferase (ACAT), which catalyzes the formation of cholesterol esters that are stored in the liver.

Bile composition has been a central focus in research of the formation of cholesterol crystals. The three primary components of bile are cholesterol, bile acids, and phospholipids. In 1968 Admirand and Small (3) demonstrated that it was the relative molar concentrations of cholesterol, phospholipids, and bile salts that defined cholesterol solubility and precipitation (Fig. 2). The balance and relative ratios of these three components were characterized by Carey in 1978 in what are now known as Carey's critical tables (4). By using Carey's critical tables, the relative saturation of cholesterol in bile, or the cholesterol saturation index (CSI), can be calculated. When the CSI is greater than 1, the bile is supersaturated with cholesterol and the environment for cholesterol crystal formation is favorable.

2. Cholesterol Crystal Nucleation

Nucleation refers to the process by which cholesterol monohydrate crystals form and agglomerate into gallstones. Holan and colleagues (5) in 1979 demonstrated that the nucleation time of bile from cholesterol gallstone patients was significantly less than that of control patients. This observation was true despite the fact that cholesterol saturation indices were similar in the study groups. Therefore, factors other than biliary lipids must be present in bile for gallstones to form.

To date, a number of pronucleating and antinucleating factors have been identified. Pronucleators include increased total lipid concentration in bile, increased calcium ion concentration, and high cholesterol to lecithin ratio in bile. More recently, the major area of research in this field has focused on the role of specific proteins in bile as both pro- and antinucleators of cholesterol crystallization. Several glycoproteins have been demonstrated to be pronucleators in that they decrease the amount of time necessary for cholesterol crystals to form in bile. Nonmucin glycoproteins that have pronucleating properties include transferrin, haptoglobin, α1-antichymotrypsin, aminopeptidase N, α1-acid gly-

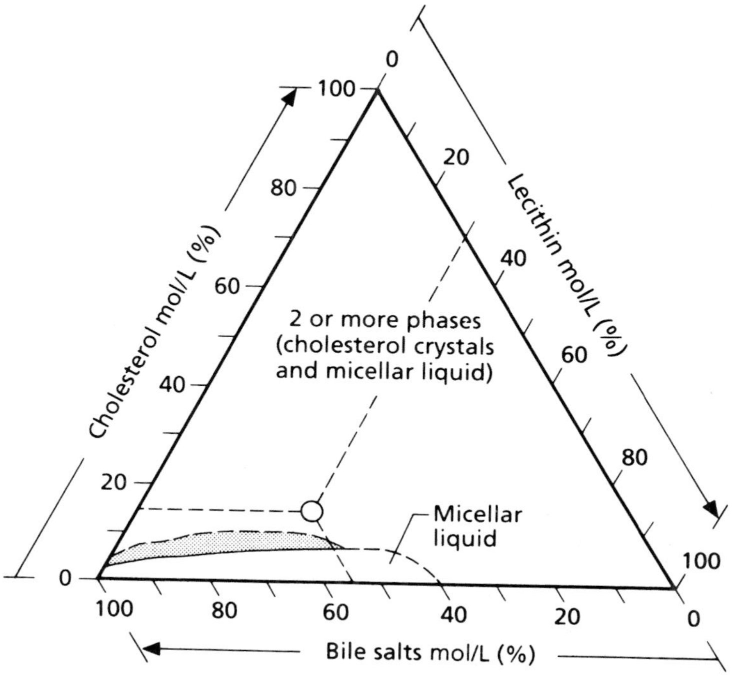

Figure 2 Triphasic diagram representing the three lipid components of bile and their relationship to one another and the cholesterol saturation index. Dashed line, data from Admirand and Small (3); solid line, data from Carey and Small (4a) and Holzbach *et al.* (4b). Shaded area represents a metastable–supersaturated zone.

coprotein, and immunoglobulns of the IgM, IgA, and IgG classes.

3. Biliary Motility

The third critical factor in gallstone pathogenesis is gallbladder hypomotility and biliary stasis. For gallstones to develop there must be sufficient time for cholesterol crystal nucleation to occur within the gallbladder. Biliary stasis also increases the concentration of the bile due to the absorptive effects of the gallbladder mucosa. Over the past 20 years, several studies in both humans and experimental animals have documented stasis of bile within the gallbladder and defects in biliary motility in subjects with gallstones. Gallbladder hypomotility increases as the cholesterol content of gallbladder bile rises (6–8). This finding suggests that cholesterol in some way affects the contractile mechanism controlling gallbladder emptying. When bile is supersaturated with cholesterol, cholesterol can enter gallbladder smooth muscle cells and intercalate within the sarcolemmal membranes, resulting in signal transduction decoupling and subsequent gallbladder hypomotility (9,10). In addition, gallstone formation has been shown to be associated with increased resistance to bile flow across the cystic duct (11) as well as decreased gallbladder emptying. Decreased gallbladder contractility in response to various contractile stimulants such as cholecystokinin (CCK) has also been demonstrated in several animal species (12–14).

Impaired gallbladder emptying has been implicated as a reason for the increased incidence of gallstones reported in patients maintained on long-term parenteral nutrition, following truncal vagotomy, and in pregnant women.

B. Pigment Stones

The pathogenesis of pigment stones is less well understood than that of cholesterol stones. Black pigment stones contain calcium bilirubinate, calcium phosphate, and calcium carbonate in a mucin glycoprotein matrix with only small amounts of cholesterol. The liver takes up bilirubin, where it undergoes conjugation with glucuronic acid. The bilirubin is secreted into bile primarily as the diglucuronide form, but with smaller amounts of the monoglucuronide and unconjugated forms. As for cholesterol, bile salts are necessary for the solubilization of the unconjugated and monoglucuronide forms. The unconjugated form is hydrophobic and may precipitate in bile as calcium salts or bilirubin polymers. An acidic environment enhances calcium and bilirubin solubility. If the gallbladder mucosa is unable to acidify bile, calcium salts will precipitate. In addition, gallbladder mucin can buffer hydrogen ions secreted by the mucosa, resulting in an increased gallbladder pH, which makes bilirubin precipitation more likely.

Ko and Lee (15) have proposed the following hypothesis for the pathogenesis of black pigment gallstones. Bilirubin excretion into bile is increased and gallbladder stasis or infection allows hydrolysis of bilirubin diglucuronide to its less soluble unconjugated forms. Inability of the gallbladder to acidify the bile alters calcium and bilirubin solubility. Mucus secreted by the gallbladder epithelium buffers hydrogen ions and decreases acidity, enabling calcium salts to precipitate and pigment stones to form.

Brown pigment stones result from chronic infection of bile rather than metabolic alterations in bile. Brown pigment stones have only small amounts of calcium phosphates and calcium carbonates and are made primarily of calcium bilirubinate and calcium salts of fatty acids. Bacterial cytoskeletons can be demonstrated in the core of brown pigment stones by electron microscopy. Bacterial β-glucuronidases cleave conjugated bilirubin to the insoluble conjugated form, which precipitates as the calcium salt. Bacterial phospholipases hydrolyze phosphoatidylcholine to form lysolecithin and free fatty acids, which also precipitate out of solution to form stones.

III. Animal Models of Gallstones

Several animal models for the study of gallstone pathogenesis have been developed over the past half-century. These models have been used to study the pathogenesis of both cholesterol and pigment gallstone formation as well as for testing of potential therapeutic and preventive strategies. The ideal animal model for the study of gallstones should possess the following features (16): (1) induction of gallstones should be rapid and reproducible, (2) diets inducing gallstone formation should be simple, similar to human diets, and nutritionally adequate, (3) bile composition, stone composition, and the mechanism of stone formation should resemble the human situation, (4) animals used should be small and easy to maintain to lower costs, (4) adequate amounts of bile, serum, and tissue samples should be easily obtained, (5) the lithogenic stimulus—e.g., cholesterol—should not overwhelm the animals' regulatory mechanisms for the compound, thus maintaining adequate homeostasis, and (6) the experimental group should differ from the control group only with respect to cholelithogenesis.

Unfortunately, no experimental animal model has been identified to date that forms gallstones spontaneously with a frequency similar to that in humans. Therefore, experimental models for gallstones involve some form of dietary manipulation. Although gallstone pathogenesis has been examined in many species, including rabbits, guinea pigs, dogs, swine, ground squirrels, baboons, and spider monkeys, here the focus is on hamsters, prairie dogs, and mice, because these are the most popular models for the study of gallstones.

A. Hamster Models

The Syrian golden hamster *(Mesocricetus auralus)* is one of the most popular animal models for the study of gallstones. In the early 1950s Dam and Christensen (17) developed a dietary model of gallstones in young, rapidly growing hamsters. Their diet consisted of a fat-free diet high in sugar (79% glucose or sucrose) and adequate in proteins, minerals, and vitamins. Ninety percent of hamsters fed this diet for 3 months developed gallstones. In this species the lack of essential fatty acids results in an increase in hepatic cholesterol synthesis and a decrease in bile salts, resulting in a lithogenic bile. Of note, the use of a fat-free diet in hamsters can result in a "wet tail" syndrome, a form of diarrhea that is frequently fatal.

Cohen and Mosbach (18) have developed a semipurified lithogenic diet that is nutritionally complete and results in a 50–70% incidence of cholesterol gallstones in hamsters purchased from Sasco (Charles River Laboratories, Wilmington, MA) after 5 weeks of feeding (Table I). The most important ingredients for the development of cholesterol gallstones in hamsters appear to be the 4% butterfat and 0.3% cholesterol. Interestingly, the incidence of gallstone formation differs according to the source of the hamsters studied. Using Cohen's diet, hamsters purchased from Sasco have the highest incidence of gallstone formation, whereas strains from Harlan Sprague–Dawley and Charles River hamsters do not develop stones.

Pigment gallstones can be induced in hamsters by dietary manipulations as well. Pigment stone diets tend to be high in carbohydrates. A diet consisting of 60% sucrose, 5% lard,

Table I Hamster Cholesterol Gallstone Diet[a]

Ingredient	Weight (gram/kg)
Casein	200
Corn oil	20
Butterfat	40
Cornstarch	434
Dyetrose (soluble starch)	146
Fiber	100
Cholesterol	3
Salt mix	50
Vitamin mix	5
Choline chloride	2

[a]Adapted from Cohen and Mosbach (18).

and 2% cod liver oil will produce pigment stones in hamsters (19). Malet *et al.* (20) produced black pigment crystals in gallbladder bile after 1 week of feeding a diet consisting of 54.3% glucose, 20% starch, and 20% casein. These crystals progressed to pigment stones in 8% of hamsters by 3 weeks and to 23% by 5 weeks. In addition to diet composition, the age and gender of hamsters play a role in the incidence and type of gallstone that develops. Pigment stones form more readily in older hamsters, female hamsters, hamsters treated with progesterone or ethinyl estradiol, and castrated male hamsters than in male hamsters (21).

The advantages of using a hamster model of gallstone pathogenesis include their ready availability, relatively low cost, and a short induction period for gallstone formation with dietary modifications. Disadvantages of using hamsters include their small size and small gallbladders, requiring pooling of bile samples for biliary lipid analysis, and differences in incidence of gallstones among hamsters from various suppliers.

B. Prairie Dog Models

Prairie dogs *(Cynomys ludovicianus)* have been widely used for the study of gallstone pathogenesis. The prairie dog is a good model for studying gallstone pathogenesis because cholesterol gallstones can be induced by administration of a cholesterol-enriched diet in a relatively short period of time and because prairie dog bile resembles human bile with respect to biliary lipids and the types of bile acids present in bile. When animals are fed a semipurified diet high in cholesterol (1.2%), crystalline aggregates of cholesterol form in the gallbladder. These cholesterol aggregates are analogous to pure cholesterol stones in humans. The composition of this high-cholesterol diet is 44% carbohydrate, 41% fat, and 15% protein. The cholesterol is provided as dry egg yolk powder (0.6% cholesterol) plus crystalline cholesterol (0.6%) (22). With this diet, cholesterol crystals can be detected in gallbladder bile after 5 days and stones are found within 2 weeks. These high-cholesterol diets result in a significant increase in the gallbladder bile cholesterol saturation index, with the CSI being greater than 1.0 in cholesterol-fed animals as compared to 0.5–0.6 in controls.

Although 1.2% cholesterol diets are very effective in inducing gallstones, there has been some concern that the large cholesterol load overwhelms the prairie dogs' regulatory mechanisms for the metabolism of cholesterol, resulting in a profound cholesterol and lipid overload and subsequent toxicity. As a result, diets with lower levels of cholesterol have been developed; these do not overwhelm the prairie dogs' homeostatic mechanisms and thus produce a model closer to the human situation. By decreasing the cholesterol content to 0.4%, nearly all prairie dogs will develop gallstones in 8 weeks; if the cholesterol content is further lowered to 0.2%, the induction period will take 6 months (23).

The influence of gender on cholesterol diet-induced gallstones has also been investigated. Female prairie dogs fed a 1.2% cholesterol diet for 21 days had a stone incidence of 79% compared to only 48% for male prairie dogs. This higher stone rate occurred despite there being no difference in cholesterol saturation index or biliary lipids between the males and females (24).

Iron deficiency has been shown to play a role in the development of cholesterol gallstones. Johnston and colleagues (24) have been able to induce cholesterol crystals in adult male prairie dogs fed an iron-deficient diet without the addition of cholesterol. The incidence of cholesterol crystal formation was 80% in the iron-deficient group compared to 20% in the control group. Addition of 0.4% cholesterol to the diet significantly increased the number of crystals in the bile of iron-deficient animals compared to the iron-supplemented group. In addition, 100% of prairie dogs fed the cholesterol-enriched iron-deficient diet developed gallstones. This observation suggests that iron deficiency may play a role in gallstone pathogenesis.

Similar to hamsters, pigment stones can be induced in the gallbladder of prairie dogs by feeding them a high-carbohydrate diet consisting of 35% sucrose, 32% rice, 18% protein, and 4% fat. Stone formation was associated with increased hepatic bile concentrations of phospholipids and calcium and increased gallbladder concentrations of phospholipids, calcium, and bilirubin (25). Further investigations in this model have shown that only 17% of animals developed pigment stones if the diet contained normal amounts of iron, but the incidence could be increased to 67% if animals were rendered iron deficient (26).

Pigment gallstones have also been induced in prairie dogs maintained on total parenteral nutrition (27) and those undergoing ileal resection (28). Forty-four percent of prairie dogs fed a nonlithogenic (low-cholesterol) diet developed pigment stones after ileal resection as opposed to none of the prairie dogs that had a sham laparotomy. Calcium bilirubinate crystals were found in the gallbladders of 94% of the resected animals.

Advantages of using the prairie dog as an animal model for studying gallstone pathogenesis include (1) a bile acid and lipid composition similar to that of humans, (2) small size, (3) sufficient gallbladder volume, allowing bile analysis of individual animals, and (4) a reliable ability to induce gallstones in a short period of time by altering the cholesterol content of the diet. Disadvantages of using prairie dogs as a research model include (1) that they are undomesticated rodents, (2) they are difficult to handle, (3) their seasonal unavailability, (4) their genetic heterogeneity, and (5) that administration of a cholesterol-enriched diet causes a rapid and diffuse systemic lipid overload.

C. Mouse Models

In recent years the mouse has been shown to be a useful model for studying gallstone pathogenesis. As a result of the extensive genetic characterization of the species, the availability of inbred and mutant mouse strains, and the ability to create transgenic and knockout models, mice are especially useful for studying the genetic factors that may be important in the development of gallstones.

Evidence that genetic factors play an important role in gallstone pathogenesis has been provided by several investigators who have documented differences in the susceptibility to gallstone formation in various strains of mice (29–31). In female mice fed a lithogenic diet consisting of 15% dairy fat, 50% sucrose, 20% casein, 1% cholesterol, 0.5% cholic acid, cellulose, vitamins, and minerals for 18 weeks, the incidence of gallstones ranged from 0 to 100% in nine different strains of mice (Table II).

Current research has isolated a number of "Lith" genes present in the inbred strains of mice that are susceptible to gallstone formation. One such gene, termed *Lith1,* has been mapped on chromosome 2 of the mouse genome. *Lith1* has been linked to the "Sister of p-glycoprotein" (Sgrp) gene, which has been shown to transport monovalent bile salts (32). C57L inbred mice have been shown to have a higher CSI and develop gallstones faster on a lithogenic diet than do AKR mice. Also, C57L/AKR cross-bred mice, termed F_1, were shown to develop gallstones as rapidly as the C57L mice, indicating that the Lith gene was dominant. Then the F_1 mice were back-crossed with the AKR mice. Thirty-three back-cross mice without gallstones and 22 with large gallstones showed a highly significant association ($p < 0.0005$) between gallstone formation and a region on chromosome 2. The polymorphic markers *D2Mit11* and *D2Mit66* defined the region on chromosome 2 (31). Using quantitative trait loci (QTL) analysis a gallstone genetic map has been defined in mice (Fig. 3).

Table II Gallstone Incidence in Mice[a]

Strain	Gallstones (%)
C57BL/6J	14
C57L/J	100
SWR/J	67
SM/J	0
A/J	100
AKR/J	0
C3H/HeJ	40
DBA/2J	0
SJL/J	20

[a]Adapted from Paigen (31).

Age, gender, and type of diet also play a role in gallstone pathogenesis in mice. Table III shows three examples of lithogenic diets and their effects on C57BL/6 mice. With some diets, females have a higher incidence of gallstone formation while with other diets male mice have a higher incidence.

IV. Models for Cholesterol Crystal Nucleation

As mentioned earlier, presence of pro- and antinucleating factors in bile plays an important role in gallstone formation. To eliminate potential interactions among various proteins found in bile, a model bile solution can be prepared from cholesterol, egg lecithin, and sodium taurocholic acid to investigate the nucleating properties of different components of gallbladder bile. Depending on what is being studied, the model bile cholesterol saturation index (CSI) can be manipulated by adjusting the concentrations of cholesterol, phospholipids, and bile acids. Once the bile "recipe" has been determined, a potential pronucleator or antinucleator can be added to the model bile and incubated at 37°C. An aliquot of bile is examined by light microscopy and the number of cholesterol crystals per high-power field is counted. Bile samples are examined at regular intervals, usually every 12 hr for a set number of days. The time it takes to identify cholesterol crystals (Fig. 4) in the specimen is called the crystal observation time (COT). The number of cholesterol crystals per time period can also be plotted, and a crystal mass, or area under the crystal growth curve, can be calculated. The slope of the growth curve can be quantified. These measurements describe the ability of a nucleating factor to form crystals compared to bile without the added substance (control). Figure 5 shows an example of a cholesterol crystal growth curve for a pronucleator.

Bile collected from animals or humans can be used to determine the crystal observation time. A control system used for this type of experiment can either be another animal that was, for example, placed on a different diet or otherwise metabolically or genetically altered from the sample group. In this manner, one can determine if the sample bile is different from the control bile. Also, bile analysis performed on the sample bile to determine the cholesterol, phospholipid, and bile acid composition can be used to generate model bile. This model can be used as an additional control. This method, however, only determines if there is a relative increase or decrease in the COT but does not allow one to determine what protein or other factor in the bile is causing the change.

In order to further analyze the contents of bile that may be pronucleators, bile must be processed by the use of either separation columns or gel electrophoresis. Concanavalin A

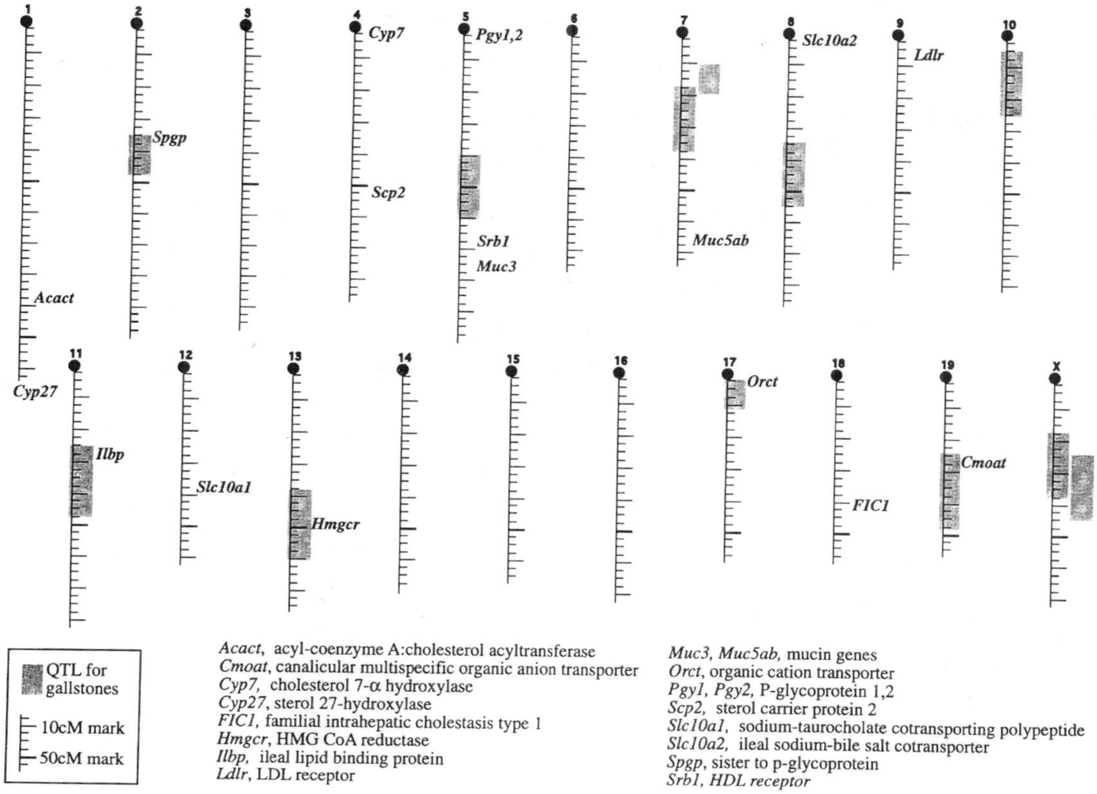

Figure 3 The mouse gallstone genetic map: genetic loci of genes that are potentially related to gallstone pathogenesis in the mouse. QTL, Quantitative trait loci. From Paigen and Carey (31a).

columns have been used to separate nonmucin glycoproteins. Once bile has been separated through a column, the remaining specimen can be run on a sodium dodecyl sulfate–polyacrylamide gel electrophoresis (SDS–PAGE) setup to separate the proteins by size. By then performing Coomasie blue or silver stains and comparing sample bile with control bile, differences can be seen. Bands can then be analyzed for amino acid composition or Western blotting

Table III Lithogenic Diets and Incidence of Gallstones

Diet	Age	Gender	Weeks on diet	Mice with gallstones	Incidence (%)
Lard[a] (29%), cholesterol (1%), cholic acid (0.5%)	7–8 weeks	Male	5	2/3	66
	7–8 weeks	Male	10	7/7	100
	7–8 weeks	Female	5	4/5	80
	7–8 weeks	Female	10	5/5	100
Butter[b] (19%), cholesterol (0.38%), cholic acid (0.5%)	24 weeks	Male	2	64/131	48.9
	24 weeks	Female	2	1/37	2.7
Butter[c] (15%), cholesterol (1%), cholic acid (0.5%)	8 weeks	Female	18	1/6	16.7

[a]Fujihara *et al.* (29).
[b]Alexander and Portman (30).
[c]Khanuja *et al.* (32a).

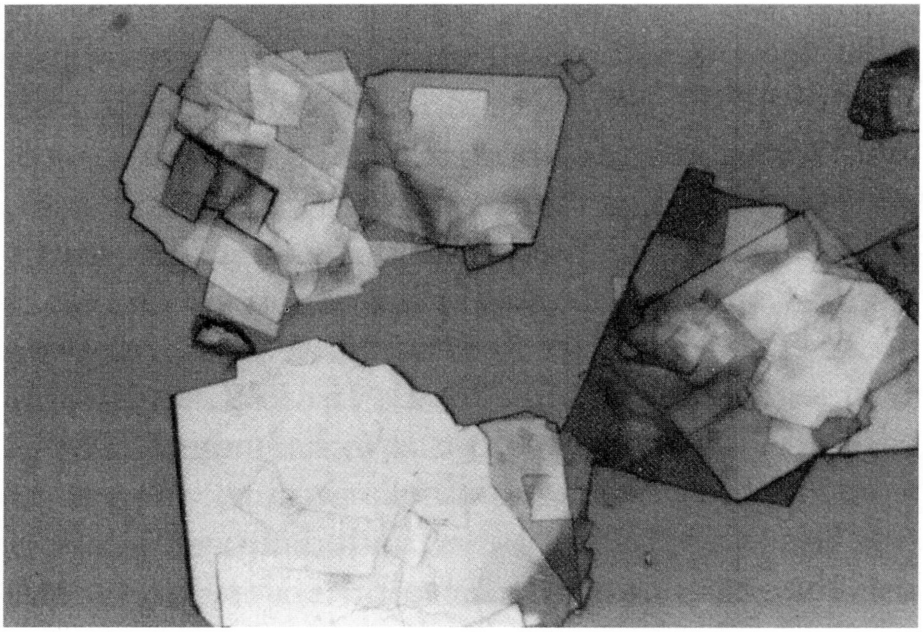

Figure 4 Photomicrograph of cholesterol monohydrate crystals. Note the parallel sides and negative birefringence. From Wang *et al.* (31b).

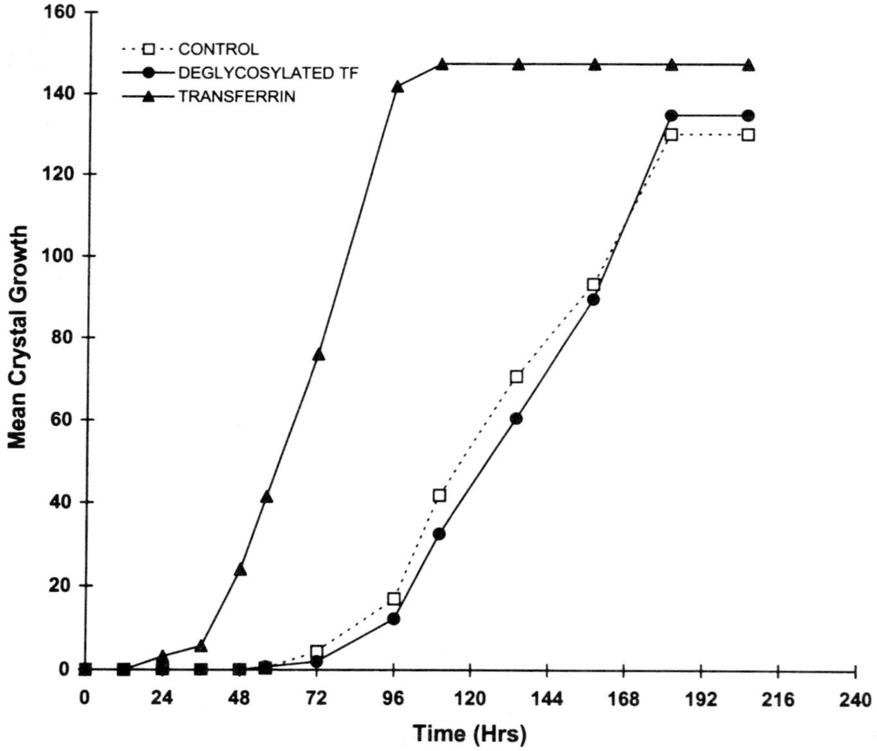

Figure 5 Crystal growth curve. By counting the number of cholesterol crystals in each population, a crystal growth curve can be plotted versus time. Transferrin shifts the curve to the left, but this effect is not achieved by deglycosylated transferrin (TF).

techniques can be used to probe for specific proteins with various antibodies.

Mucin, a glycoprotein produced by the gallbladder epithelium, has been implicated in cholesterol gallstone formation (33). Mucin, though not a cholesterol crystal pronucleator, plays a key role in gallstone matrix formation, thereby accelerating gallstone formation once cholesterol crystals have already formed. Because of this implication in gallstone formation, mucin production by gallbladder epithelial cells has been a focus of study. The relative inaccessibility of an undisturbed gallbladder makes *in vivo* gallbladder epithelial experiments difficult. Therefore, cell cultures of gallbladder epithelial cells have been developed to allow the near-continuous growth of a confluent cell layer in the lab. Oda *et al.* (34) developed a system of isolating gallbladder epithelium from dogs. The isolated epithelial cells retained gallbladder morphology as well as protein synthesis, mucous glycoprotein synthesis, and secretion over time. This model has since been used to alter the cells pharmacologically and physiologically and their mucin production.

V. Models for Studying Biliary Motility

The subject of biliary motility is a complicated one. A number of anatomical structures can be looked at separately as well as together. First, some methods of examining each aspect of the biliary tree separately are described, then the entire system together is covered. The sphincter of Oddi regulates the emptying of bile into the duodenum and has been studied extensively in gallstone pathogenesis. A triple-lumen catheter is just one example of a technique used to measure the contractions of the sphincter. In this model (Fig. 6), a small animal (prairie dog) is anesthetized and a laparotomy is performed. The common bile duct is accessed and a small triple-lumen catheter is advanced distally into the common bile duct (CBD). The catheter is then advanced into the duodenum and a pressure tracing from the middle port is monitored. The catheter is then drawn back into the CBD until a rise in pressure is noted. At this point, the middle port is in the sphincter of Oddi, the distal port is in the duodenum, and the proximal port is in the CBD. Now the experimental protocol can be initiated to examine the effects on the sphincter of either dietary or pharmacologic manipulations.

Gallbladder motility has obviously been an area of active research in gallstone pathogenesis. In an effort to cannulate the gallbladder *in vivo* to ensure that nerves and interactions with the remainder of the biliary tree are intact, the following system has been devised. Briefly, a small silastic catheter is inserted into the gallbladder via a cholecystostomy. The catheter is then perfused with an isotonic solution (lactated Ringer) at a rate of approximately 0.1 ml/min (for the prairie dog), or whatever rate will achieve intracystic pressure of 6–9 mmHg. Drainage from the proximal common bile duct is necessary to avoid overfilling of the gallbladder. At this point, as in the sphincter of Oddi isolation system, experiments can be carried out to examine actions of the gallbladder smooth muscle due to pharmacologic or dietary treatments.

An indirect method of measuring gallbladder stasis is the ratio of specific activity (R_{SA}). The R_{SA} assay takes advantage of the mixing that occurs between gallbladder bile and hepatic bile in a normal organism to measure gallbladder stasis. When stasis occurs, mixing within the gallbladder bile decreases. When a known quantity of ^{14}C-labeled cholic acid is injected intravenously into the animal 12–24 hr prior to laparotomy, the cholic acid is taken up by the liver and either enters the gallbladder or becomes part of the enterohepatic circulation. The following formula is used to calculate the R_{SA}:

$$R_{SA} = SA_{GB} / SA_{HB},$$

where SA_{GB} is the specific activity of gallbladder bile and SA_{HB} is the specific activity of a 1-hr collection of hepatic bile. Specific activity is the total counts of activity of that specimen divided by the bile salt mass of that specimen. Gallbladder bile needs to be assayed for total bile acids (TBAs) and radioactive counts. Common bile duct (CBD) cannulation is required to collect hepatic bile. Hepatic bile is collected for 2 hr and either the first- or second-hour bile is used for the remainder of the equation. When the equation is used, a value of 1 corresponds to equal mixing and any value less than 1 indicates gallbladder stasis.

In addition to R_{SA}, a 2-hr CBD and gallbladder cannulation can be used to calculate the bile salt pool size. The following equation is used to estimate the total body bile salt pool size (BSPS):

$$BSPS = [M_{GB} + M_{H1} + A_0 - (A_{GB} + A_{H1})]/SA_{H2},$$

where M_{GB} is the bile salt mass of the gallbladder, M_{H1} is the bile salt mass of the first-hour hepatic bile collection, A_0 is the total activity of the radiolabeled cholic acid injected, A_{GB} is the activity of the gallbladder bile, A_{H1} is the activity of the first-hour hepatic bile, and SA_{H2} is the specific activity of the second-hour bile collection. Bile salt mass is the concentration of bile acids multiplied by the total volume collected in that specimen.

In some experimental models, it is necessary to examine the effects of various drugs and neurotransmitters in an isolated system. To achieve this goal, *in vitro* tissue baths can be used. The advantages of using an *in vitro* system include ability to divide a tissue into multiple strips to test different drugs at once. Also, it allows the organ (i.e., gallbladder) to

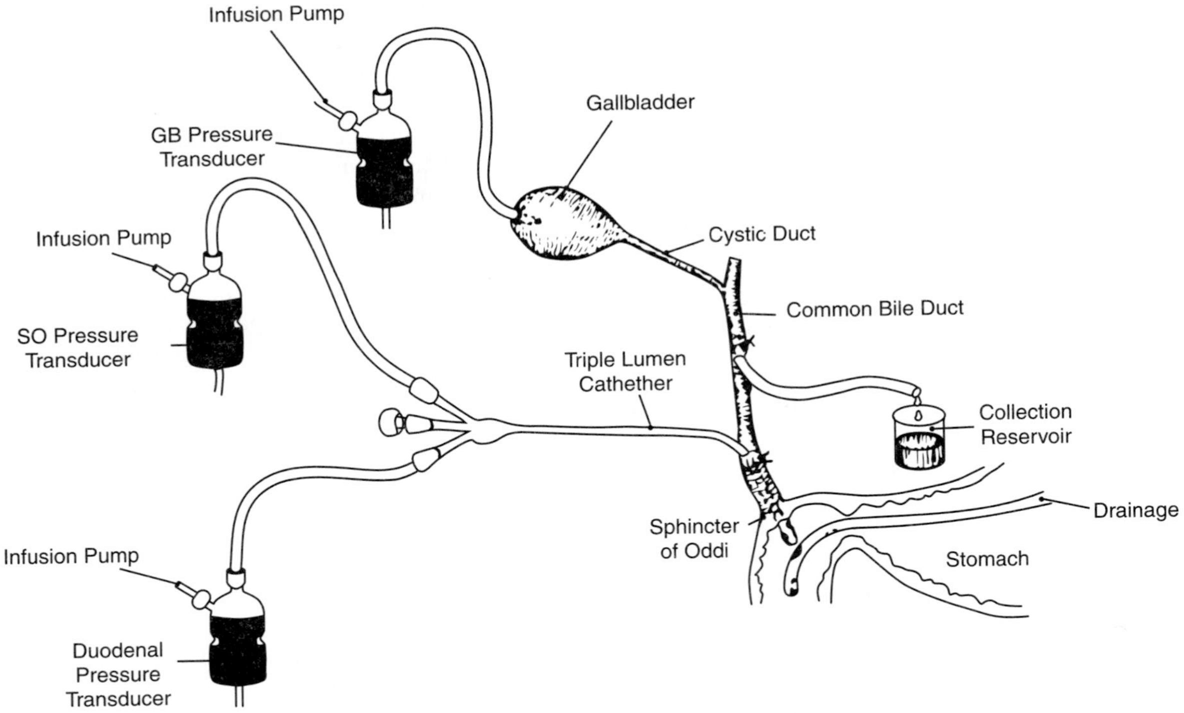

Figure 6 Experimental preparation used to measure gallbladder, sphincter of Oddi (SO), and duodenal pressure. The triple-lumen catheter has a proximal port positioned in the sphincter of Oddi and a distal port in the duodenal lumen.

be isolated from the circulatory and neural inputs of the rest of the animal. Finally, in the case of human tissue, an organ bath allows one to perform experiments that would otherwise be impossible to carry out *in vivo*.

Organ baths come in various sizes, usually ranging from 3 to 5 ml. There are various reviews of *in vitro* tissue systems. A 3-ml bath is described here (Fig. 7). Briefly, a strip of muscle approximately 2 mm by 5 mm in size is used. Sutures are placed at both ends and the muscle strip is strung up. One end is anchored to the bottom while the other is attached to an isometric force transducer. The muscle is placed in the chamber kept at 37°C, with a physiologically buffered solution, usually a modified Kreb's solution, and the bath is bubbled with 95% O_2/5% CO_2. The CO_2 keeps the pH at 7.4 because the buffer in Kreb's is sodium bicarbonate. The muscle is then stretched to an initial length and is allowed to equilibrate (usually 45–90 min). Once the muscle is healthy, the experiments can begin.

To examine the excitatory stimulation of gallbladder smooth muscle, the muscle must be stretched to its optimal length. The Starling curve describes how a muscle that is stretched will exhibit increasing contraction on stimulation up to a point of optimal length. This optimal length needs to be found before experimentation. To achieve this goal an excitatory neurotransmitter, usually acetylcholine (10^{-5} *M*), is added. The force of contraction is determined and the tension on the muscle is increased. After 10–15 min of equilibration, this process is repeated until the force of contraction plateaus or reaches its maximum. This measurement is the optimal length.

VI. Gallbladder Mucosal Absorption

The gallbladder mucosa is second only to the kidney in its absorptive capability. Because of its concentrating ability, the gallbladder removes a large amount of water and ions. This situation allows previously unsaturated bile to reach higher cholesterol saturation indexes. Thus, a number of studies have focused on how various situations can lead to increased or decreased absorption. One method of measuring the ion flux through a tissue is by using an Ussing chamber. In this system, a tissue is placed over a membrane and is used to seal two different physiologic solution reservoirs. At this point isotopes of Na, Cl, or any other ion of interest can be placed in the mucosal side of the tissue if measuring absorption, and in the serosal side if examining secretion. After a given length of time, the solutions are removed and analyzed for the radioactive isotope. Also, various drugs can then be added to assess their effects on absorption or secretion (35).

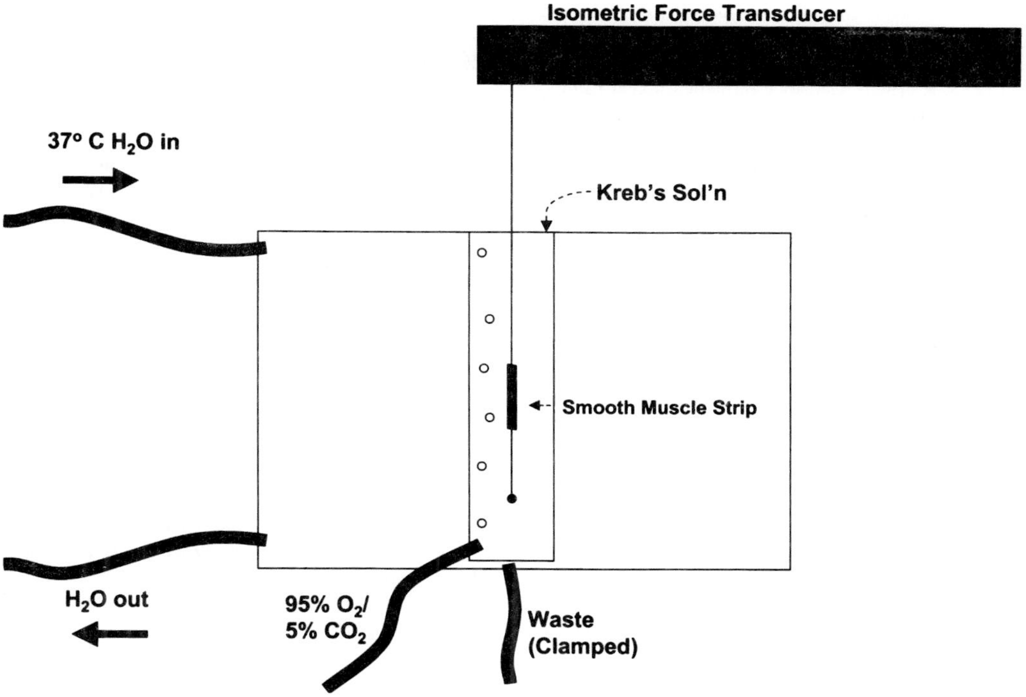

Figure 7 Schematic diagram of muscle bath apparatus: 95% O_2/5% CO_2 is bubbled into a Kreb's solution to keep the muscle strip alive. The muscle strip is attached to an isometric force transducer that measures contractions in response to various excitatory stimuli.

VII. Conclusion

Gallstone disease remains a major healthcare concern in the United States. An understanding of the pathogenesis of both cholesterol and pigment gallstone disease is important in order to develop preventive strategies. To date, the majority of work in gallstone research has been done in small rodent species such as hamsters, prairie dogs, and mice. These models have been useful in determining the effects of biliary lipid metabolism, cholesterol crystal nucleation and growth, and biliary motility on gallstone formation.

References

1. Graves, E. J., and Owings, M. E. (1995). Summary: National Hospital Discharge Survey. Advance data from health statistics; no. 291. National Center of Health Statistics, Washington, D.C.
2. Pitt, H. A. (1995). Gallstone pathogenesis and management: Prospects for the future. *In* "Techniques in the Management of Gallstone Disease" (A. Darzi, P. A. Grace, H. A. Pitt, and D. Bouchier-Hayes, eds.), p. 24. Blackwell Science Ltd., Oxford, England.
3. Admirand, W. H., and Small, D. M. (1968). The physicochemical basis of cholesterol gallstone formation in man. *J. Clin. Invest.* **47**(5), 1043–1052.
4. Carey, M. C. (1978). Critical tables for calculating the cholesterol saturation of native bile. *J. Lipid Res.* **19**(8), 945–955.

4a. Carey, M. C., and Small, D. M. (1978). The physical chemistry of cholesterol solubility in bile. Relationship to gallstone formation and dissolution in man. *J. Clin. Invest.* **61**, 998–1026.

4b. Holzbach, R. T., Kibe, A., Thiel, E., Howell, J. H., Marsh, M., and Hermann, R. E. (1984). Biliary proteins. Unique inhibitors of cholesterol crystal nucleation in human gallbladder bile. *J. Clin. Invest.* **73**, 35–45.

5. Holan, K. R., Holzbach, R. T., Hermann, R. E., Cooperman, A. M., and Claffey W. J. (1979). Nucleation time: A key factor in the pathogenesis of cholesterol gallstone disease. *Gastroenterology* **77**(4, Pt. 1), 611–617.
6. Carey, M. C. (1989). Formation of cholesterol gallstones: The new paradigms. *In* "Trends in Bile Acid Research" (G. Paumgartner, E. Stiehl, and E. Gerok, eds.), p. 259.
7. Van der Werf, S. D. J., Van Berge Henegouwen, G. P., Palsma, D. M. H. *et al.* (1987). Motor function of the gallbladder and cholesterol saturation of duodenal bile. *Neth. J. Med.* **30**, 160.
8. Fisher, R. S., Stelzer, F., Rock, E. *et al.* (1982). Abnormal gallbladder emptying in patients with gallstones. *Dig. Dis. Sci.* **27**, 1019.
9. Behar, J., Lee, K. Y., Thompson, W. R., and Biancani, P. (1989). Gallbladder contraction in patients with pigment and cholesterol stones. *Gastroenterology* **97**, 1479–1484.
10. Yu, P., Chen, Q., Harnett, K. M., Amaral, J., Biancani, P., and Behar, J. (1995). Direct G protein activatiuon reverses impaired CCK signaling in human gallbladders with cholesterol stones. *Am. J. Physiol.* **269**, G659–G665.
11. Pitt, H. A., Roslyn, J. J., Kuchenbecker, S., and DenBesten, L. (1981). The role of increased cystic duct resistance in the pathogenesis of cholesterol cholelithiasis. *J. Surg. Res.* **20**, 508–513.
12. Fridhandler, T. M., Davison, J. S., and Schaffer, E. A. (1983). Defective gallbladder contractility in ground squirrel and prairie dogs during early stages of gallstone formation. *Gastroenterology* **85**, 830–836.
13. Roslyn, J. J., DenBesten, L., Pitt, H. A. *et al.* (1981). Effects of cholecystokinin on gallbladder stasis and cholesterol gallstone formation. *J. Surg. Res.* **30**, 200–204.

14. Li, Y. F., Bowers, R. L., Haley-Russell, D. *el al.* (1990). Actin and myosin isoforms in gallbladder smooth muscle following cholesterol feeding in prairie dogs. *Gastroenterology* **99**, 1460–1466.
15. Ko, C. W., and Lee, S. P. (1999). Gallstone formation: Local factors. *Gastroenterol. Clin. N. Am.* **28**, 99–115.
16. Malet, P. F. (1985). Animal models of gallstone formation. *In* "Gallstones" (S. Cohen and R. Solway, eds.), pp. 309–333. Churchill-Livingstone, New York.
17. Dam, H., and Christensen, F. (1952). Alimentary production of gallstones in hamsters. *Acta Pathol. Microbiol. Scand.* **30**, 236–242.
18. Cohen, B. I., and Mosbach, E. H. (1993). Cholesterol cholelithiasis. *Adv. Vet. Sci. Comp. Med.* **37**, 289–312.
19. Shioda, R. (1965). Experimental studies on gallstone formation. *Arch. Jpn. Chir.* **34**, 571–585.
20. Malet, P. F., Deng, S. Q., and Soloway, R. D. (1989). Gallbladder mucin and cholesterol and pigment gallstone formation in hamsters, *Scand. J. Gastroenterol.* **24**, 1055–1060.
21. Rege, R. V., Dawes, L. G., and Ostrow, J. D. (1993). Animal models of pigment gallstones. *Adv. Vet. Sci. Comp. Med.* **37**, 257–287.
22. Brenneman, D. E., Connor, W. E., Forker, E. L., and DenBesten, L. (1972). The formation of abnormal bile and cholesterol gallstones from dietary cholesterol in the prairie dog. *J. Clin. Invest.* **51**, 1495–1503.
23. DenBesten, L., Safaie-Shirazi, S., Connor, W. E., and Bell, S. (1974). Early changes in bile composition and gallstone formation induced by a high cholesterol diet in prairie dogs. *Gastroenterology* **66**, 1036–1045.
24. Johnston, S. M., Murray, K. P., Martin, S. A., Fox-Talbot, K., Lipsett, P. A., Lillemoe, K. D., and Pitt, H. A. Iron deficiency enhances cholesterol gallstone formation. *Surgery* **122**(2), 354–61.
25. Conter, R. L., Roslyn, J. J., Pitt, H. A., and DenBesten, L. (1986). Carbohydrate diet induced calcium bilirubinate sludge and pigment gallstones in the prairie dog. *J. Surg. Res.* **40**, 580–587.
26. Roslyn, J. J., Conter, R. L., Julian, E., and Abedin, M. Z. (1987). The role of dietary iron in pigment gallstone formation. *Surgery* **102**, 327–333.
27. Muller, E. L., Grace, P. A., and Pitt, H. A. (1986). The effect of parenteral nutrition on biliary calcium and bilirubin. *J. Surg. Res.* **40**(1), 55–62.
28. Pitt, H. A., Lewinski, M. A., Muller, E. L., Porter-Fink, V., and DenBesten, L. (1983). Ileal resection induced gallstones: Altered bilirubin or cholesterol metabolism? *Surgery* **96**, 154–162.
29. Fujihara, E., Kaneta, S., and Ohshima, T. (1978). Strain difference in mouse cholelithiasis and the effect of taurine on the gallstone formation in C57BL/6J mice. *Biochem. Med.* **19**, 211–217.
30. Alexander, M., and Portman, O. (1987). Different susceptibilities to the formation of cholesterol gallstones in mice. *Hepatology* **7**, 257–265.
31. Paigen, B. (1995). Genetic responsiveness to high-fat and high-cholesterol diets in the mouse. *Am. J. Clin. Nutr.* **62**, 458S–462S.
31a. Paigen, B., and Carey, M. C. (2000). Gallstones. *In* "The Genetic Basis of Common Diseases," 2nd Ed. Oxford Univ. Press, NY.
31b. Wang, D. Q., Paigen, B., and Carey, M. C. (1997). Phenotypic characterization of Lith genes that determine susceptibility to cholesterol cholelithiasis in inbred mice: Physical chemistry of gallbladder bile. *J. Lipid Res.* **38**, 1395–1411.
32. Gerloff, T., Stieger, B., Hagenbuch, B., Madon, J., Landmann, L., Roth, J., Hofmann, A. E., and Meier, P. J. (1998). The sister of P-glycoprotein represents the canalicular bile salt export pump of mammalian liver. *J. Biol. Chem* **273**(16), 10046–10050.
32a. Khanuja, B., Cheah, Y. C., Hunt, M., Nishina, P. M., Wang, D. Q. *et al.* (1995). *Lith1,* a major gene affecting cholesterol gallstone formation among inbred strains of mice. *Proc. Natl. Acad. Sci. U.S.A.* **92**, 7729–7733.
33. van den Berg, A. A., van Buul, J. D., Tytgat, G. N., Groen, A. K., and Ostrow, J. D. (1998). Mucins and calcium phosphate precipitates additively stimulate cholesterol crystallization. *J. Lipid Res.* **39**(9), 1744–1751.
34. Oda, D., Lee, S. P., and Hayashi, A. (1991). Long-term culture and partial characterization of dog gallbladder epithelium cells. *Lab. Invest.* **64**(5), 682–692.
35. Moser, A. J., Mohammad, Z. A., Giurgiu, D. I., and Roslyn, J. J. (1995). Octreotide promotes gallbladder absorption in prairie dogs: A potential cause of gallstones. *Gastroenterology* **108**, 1547–1555.

53

Models for the Study of Pancreatitis

Michael L. Steer

Department of Surgery, Beth Israel Deaconess Medical Center, Harvard Medical School, Boston, Massachusetts 02215

I. Introduction

Inflammatory diseases of the pancreas have been divided into two groups: acute pancreatitis and chronic pancreatitis. Although the distinction between these two entities, in the clinical setting, can sometimes be blurred, the two types of pancreatitis appear to differ in respect to their etiologies, their pathologic morphology, and their clinical course. Acute pancreatitis is characterized by an acute inflammatory process within the pancreas with little or no fibrosis. It can be triggered by any one of a number of so-called etiologies, including biliary tract stone disease, trauma, infections, pancreatic duct obstruction, hyperlipidemia, and hypercalcemic states. Once the attack has resolved, the pancreas can and usually does recover both from a morphologic and a functional standpoint and future attacks occur only if the triggering event is repeated. In contrast, chronic pancreatitis is characterized by varying degrees of pancreatic fibrosis along with both chronic and acute inflammation. In developed countries, long-standing abuse of ethanol is the most common cause of chronic pancreatitis, but some patients may develop this disease on a hereditary (i.e., genetic) basis, or in association with cystic fibrosis. In developing countries, nutritional deficiencies and/or exposure to toxins account for many of the cases. On termination of an attack of chronic pancreatitis, the gland remains functionally and/or morthologically abnormal and repeated attacks can occur even without an identifiable precipitating cause.

Ideally, studies designed to examine the etiology, pathophysiology, and treatment of either acute or chronic pancreatitis should be performed using patients with these diseases. Unfortunately, attempts to explore these issues in clinical studies have usually been unsuccessful. The relative inaccessibility of the pancreas and difficulties encountered in sampling the gland during or after an attack have been among the major impediments to clinical studies. In addition, the fact that advanced functional and/or morphological changes are already established before the diagnosis of chronic pancreatitis is established makes clinical studies designed to explore the early events in chronic pancreatitis nearly impossible. Problems encountered in clinical studies dealing with acute pancreatitis are further complicated by the variable, multiple, and for the most part uncontrollable extrapancreatic events that occur during an attack of severe acute pancreatitis.

Experimental models, employing laboratory animals, have been extensively employed to overcome the problems encountered during clinical studies and to permit investigations designed to probe the early events that lead to either acute or chronic pancreatitis, the factors that regulate the severity as well as the course of an attack, and the potential benefit of therapies. Perhaps the earliest such model was that employed in 1856 by Claude Bernard, who injected bile and olive oil, retrogradely, into the pancreatic duct of the dog and noted the appearance of acute pancreatitis shortly thereafter. Since that time, many other models of pancreatitis have been described. Some involve invasive techniques to induce acute pancreatitis and others induce acute pancreatitis by noninvasive means. Attempts to induce chronic pancreatitis by administration of ethanol to laboratory animals have failed but models have been described that explore the effects of long-term ethanol administration on pancreatic function, the short-term toxic effects of ethanol on the pancreas, and the possibility that ethanol administration sensitizes the pancreas to non-ethanol-induced injury.

This review critically describes some of the more commonly used models of pancreatitis. There have been thousands of publications dealing with experimental pancreatitis and a large number of models of pancreatitis have been described. It is not the intention of this review to present an encyclopedic summary of the literature. Rather, a selected sample will be presented and, as a result, many good and potentially important studies will not be discussed. In the spirit of this monograph, the focus is, as much as possible, on methods that may prove useful for future studies, and the advantages as well as the disadvantages of these models are pointed out.

II. Acute Pancreatitis

A. Invasive Models of Acute Pancreatitis

The invasive models of acute pancreatitis (Table I) are, for the most part, assumed to be models of so-called gallstone pancreatitis. Studies by Acosta and Ledesma (1) as well as others have indicated that gallstone pancreatitis is triggered by the passage of a biliary tract stone into or through the terminal biliopancreatic ductal system. Presumably, that stone or stones trigger pancreatitis either by obstructing the flow of pancreatic juice out of the gland or by permitting reflux of bile and/or duodenal juices containing activated digestive enzymes retrogradely into the pancreatic duct. Thus, models have been developed that involve (1) retrograde injection of agents into the pancreatic duct; (2) perfusion of the pancreatic duct with potentially noxious agents; (3) creation of a closed duodenal loop, which leads to reflux of duodenal contents into the pancreas; and (4) obstruction of either the pancreatic or the combined biliopancreatic ductal system outside the pancreas.

Table I Invasive Models of Acute Pancreatitis

Retrograde ductal injection
Closed duodenal loop
Prograde ductal perfusion
Duct ligation

The attractive feature of each of these invasive models of pancreatitis is that it recreates a triggering event that is believed to incite clinical acute gallstone pancreatitis—i.e., obstruction and/or reflux. Furthermore, each of these models has been demonstrated to cause acute pancreatic inflammation with varying degrees of pancreatic necrosis and considerable mortality. Unfortunately, these models have several unattractive features. By definition, they each involve performance of an operative procedure on or around the pancreas. Thus, very small animals such as mice are difficult to use. Anesthesia may be difficult and can result in loss of animals. Postoperative problems, including infection and difficulties in maintaining nutrition, can complicate interpretation of the results. Perhaps the most significant problem with these models is the severity of the pancreatitis that is induced. For the most part, pancreatitis in these models evolves very rapidly, is very severe, and the extent of inflammation is difficult to control. Thus, studies designed to explore the early events in pancreatitis using these models have not been possible because the disease evolves too rapidly to permit study, and studies designed to characterize pancreatic function during pancreatitis have not been possible because of the extensive pancreatic destruction that characterizes these models. The poorly controlled severity seen with these models has led to considerable interinvestigator differences and problems encountered in attempts to duplicate the findings noted by others. On the other hand, these invasive models have clearly been shown to result in severe pancreatic injury, and for that reason they have been of considerable use in studies designed to examine the complications and extrapancreatic events that occur during pancreatitis.

1. Retrograde Ductal Injection

Induction of pancreatitis by retrograde injection of various agents into the pancreatic duct involves cannulation of the duct; therefore, only relatively large animals (dogs, cats, pigs, rats) can be used. Pancreatitis has been observed to follow injection of a variety of agents, including bile (2–5), bile plus trypsin (6,7), sodium taurocholate (8,9), sodium taurocholate plus trypsin (10–13), trypsin alone (14,15), lipase (14), elastase (16), and phospholipase A (17). Injection of fatty acids also can induce severe pancreatitis. The severity of these models is directly related to the pressure used for the injection—pancreatitis can be induced even by injection of sterile buffer (18) if that injection is done at high pressure. Thus, control of the pressure used for injection may be the most important feature of this type of model. For the most part, studies using duct injection to induce pancreatitis have controlled the injection pressure and limited it to the physiologic range of 20–30 cm H_2O.

It is clear that injection of any one of the above-mentioned noxious agents, in high volume and at high pressure, can induce severe pancreatic injury (Table II). Such an approach would be appropriate for the investigator whose goal is to either study systemic events in severe pancreatitis or late complications of pancreatitis. On the other hand, that approach would not be suitable if one wished to study either intrapancreatic events that occur during the evolution of pancreatitis or to examine events that characterize relatively mild pancreatitis. For such studies, the reader is referred to the reports of Aho and co-workers (19,20). They induced pancreatitis in rats by injecting small volumes (0.2 ml) of a solution containing varying concentrations of sodium taurocholate (3.0, 4.5, or 5.0%). Injections were timed to extend over 1 min in an attempt to control the injection pressure. After injection, the duct was allowed to drain freely and the animals were observed by 72 hr. Aho and co-workers noted that pancreatitis, which evolved slowly over 72 hr, could be induced by this method and that the severity of that pancreatitis was related to the sodium taurocholate concentration used.

2. Closed Duodenal Loop

This model of experimental pancreatitis was described in 1957 by Pfeffer and co-workers (21). Using dogs, the duodenum just beyond the pylorus, as well as that just beyond the pancreas, is divided creating a closed segment (7–10 cm long) that communicates with the biliopancreatic ductal system. Bile is excluded by ligation of the bile duct and gastric outflow is reestablished by construction of a gastrojejunostomy. Pfeffer and co-workers noted that pancreatitis characterized by edema, necrosis, and inflammation developed 9–11 hr after the duodenal loop was constructed and suggested that this pancreatitis was the result of pancreatic ischemia. Later studies by others showed that this pancreatitis could be prevented either by pancreatic duct ligation (22) or pancreatic duct cannulation (23), suggesting that the pancreatitis induced by creation of a closed duodenal loop involves reflux of duodenal contents into the pancreatic ductal system. From a clinical standpoint, the closed duodenal loop model of pancreatitis probably simulates the events that couple postgastrectomy, afferent loop obstruction, with the development of pancreatitis.

Several modifications of the closed duodenal loop model of Pfeffer have been described. Nevalainen and Seppa used an intraluminally placed tube to traverse the ligated area and restore intestinal continuity (24). Chetty *et al.* (25) used injection of infected bile into the duodenal loop to worsen the severity of pancreatitis. Orda *et al.* (26) reported the use of this model in rats with the injection of a bile salt–trypsin mixture into the closed loop.

Several features of the closed duodenal loop model make it unattractive for studies of pancreatitis (Table III). As with other invasive models, it involves an operative procedure and should probably be used only with large animals. The pancreatitis that develops evolves over a relatively long period, making studies of pancreatic structure and function during pancreatitis possible, but the severity of the disease induced by this approach is variable and difficult to control. Thus, many animals must be employed to allow for meaningful conclusions. Perhaps the major problem with this model is the uncertainty regarding how it actually causes pancreatic injury and the nature of the injury. Several groups (27,28) have concluded that this model causes pancreatic ischemia and that this is the basis for the pancreatic injury noted. On the other hand, others (25) have suggested that sepsis and duodenal necrosis lead to the pancreatic injury. Most workers who have used this model noted that it is primarily characterized by pancreatic necrosis and intraparenchymal hemorrhage but that fat necrosis and pancreatic inflammation are only infrequently seen. This suggests that the closed duodenal loop model is really a model of pancreatic necrosis rather than a model of acute pancreatitis.

3. Prograde Ductal Perfusion

The pancreatic duct mucosa, much like the mucosa of the gastrointestinal tract, presents a barrier to diffusion. That barrier can be disrupted by prograde perfusion of the

Table II Retrograde Ductal Injection

Advantages	Disadvantages
Clinically relevant	Requires surgery
	Unsuitable for small animals
	Rapid and severe injury
	Difficult to control
	Too destructive for study

Table III Closed Duodenal Loop

Advantages	Disadvantages
Clinically relevant?	Requires surgery
	Unsuitable for small animals
	Clinically relevant?
	Uncertain mechanism
	Necrosis but little inflammation

nonobstructed duct with infected bile, aspirin, hydrochloric acid, ethanol, and certain bile acids (29). Under these conditions, molecules as large as pancreatic digestive enzymes can leak from the ductal space into the pancreatic parenchyma. Perfusion of the duct first with a permeability-increasing agent and then with a solution containing activated digestive enzymes has been shown to result in edematous pancreatitis and, when combined with the administration of a prostaglandin E analog, hemorrhagic pancreatitis (30,31).

For the most part, duct perfusion as a means of inducing acute pancreatitis has involved studies using cats. The tail of the cat pancreas is cannulated and perfused with permeability-inducing agents at low pressure (less than 20 cm H_2O) while drainage into the duodenum remains unobstructed. Subsequently, pancreatitis-inducing agents such as activated digestive enzymes are similarly infused through the cannula while agents regulating the severity of pancreatitis such as prostaglandins are administered systemically.

There are advantages as well as disadvantages to the use of this model (Table IV). Its major advantage appears to be the fact that pancreatitis of differing severity can be induced. Disadvantages include the fact that it involves a rather complex surgical procedure. This model can probably only be used in a large animal whose pancreas includes a single dominant duct suitable for cannulation (i.e., cats, dogs, pigs, primates). Finally, the clinical relevance of this model of pancreatitis has been questioned by those who believe acute gallstone pancreatitis is triggered by pancreatic duct obstruction rather than reflux of bile into the pancreatic ductal system. The complexity and high cost of this model, in all probability, account for the lack of wide usage in studies of acute pancreatitis.

Table IV Prograde Ductal Perfusion

Advantages	Disadvantages
Graded severity	Requires surgery
	Limited to larger animals
	Uncertain clinical relevance
	Used primarily in cats

4. Duct Ligation

The mechanism by which a biliary tract stone, passing into or through the terminal biliopancreatic ductal system, triggers acute pancreatitis is poorly understood. Three competing theories have been proposed. One is based on the concept that a stone passes into the duodenum and, in so doing, stretches the sphincter of Oddi, making it incompetent and permitting reflux of duodenal contents into the pancreatic duct. The second is based on the concept that a stone obstructs a common biliopancreatic channel, allowing bile to reflux retrogradely into the pancreatic duct. The third and most widely accepted theory is based on the concept that a stone, or edema and inflammation caused by the stone, causes pancreatic duct obstruction and that continued secretion into the closed ductal space leads to pancreatic ductal hypertension, rupture of intrapancreatic ducts, and extravasation of pancreatic juice, containing potentially harmful digestive enzymes, into the gland parenchyma.

Given this background, it is not surprising that there have been many attempts to induce pancreatitis by duct ligation in experimental animals. Ligation of the pancreatic duct of most animals, however, does not induce acute pancreatitis. Rather, it stimulates acinar cell apoptosis, leading to atrophy of the exocrine pancreas with little or no acute inflammation. Mild edematous pancreatitis can be induced by combining duct ligation with stimulation of secretion (32,33) and an even more severe form of pancreatitis can be induced by combining duct obstruction, secretory stimulation, and pancreatic ischemia (34). These approaches have only rarely been used in studies of pancreatitis. More common has been the practice of causing pancreatic duct obstruction, usually by duct ligation in rats, and then evaluating the effects of duct obstruction (even without pancreatitis) on pancreatic function, blood flow, and generation of inflammatory mediators within the pancreas.

The American opossum appears to be an exception to the generalization that duct ligation does not cause pancreatitis. The biliopancreatic anatomy of the opossum closely resembles that of humans: a common bile duct is joined, while still extraduodenal, by a single main pancreatic duct. The latter appears to carry secretions from the entire gland into the duodenum. Ligation of either the pancreatic duct or the common biliopancreatic duct results in severe, necrotizing, hemorrhagic pancreatitis (35). Either bile duct obstruction or bile reflux into the pancreatic duct is necessary for induction or progression of this form of pancreatitis (36). This indicates that pancreatitis, in this model, is the result of pancreatic duct obstruction alone. Duct obstruction-induced pancreatitis in the opossum evolves slowly, over several days, and is associated with lung injury that resembles that seen in patients with acute respiratory distress syndrome (ARDS) (37).

The opossum model of severe necrotizing pancreatitis induced by pancreatic duct obstruction is complicated by the fact that wild, trapped animals are used for these studies and a surgical procedure is required. In practice, opossums of either sex weighing about 3–4 kg are obtained from commercial sources. The animals are difficult to handle and are routinely infected with a wide variety of parasites. They survive best if maintained in large cages that permit free range of motion and some concealment. They should be conditioned prior to use and dewormed by administration of an antihelminthic agent. Acute streptococcal bacterial endocarditis is common when these animals are in captivity and, for that reason, they should be given a course of prophylactic antibiotics prior to use. Because of difficulty in handling these animals, almost all procedures must be carried using anesthetized opossums.

The opossum common biliopancreatic duct is quite large and is easily identifiable where it enters the duodenum. At this point it is several millimeters wide and its wall is muscular. On occasion, there may be a septum between the biliary and pancreatic duct and, because of this, ligation of the duct should be accomplished as close to the duodenal wall as possible. The gallbladder should be surgically removed to prevent it from enlarging and acting as a reservoir for bile. Following closure of the laparotomy wound, animals are allowed to recover from anesthesia and are returned to a regular diet. Pancreatitis evolves over a reproducible period with 30–40% of the pancreas noted to be necrotic 5–7 days after duct ligation, and severe lung injury noted at roughly the same time. Early changes of pancreatitis can be detected within 12–24 hr of duct ligation and lung injury is first measurable 2 days after duct ligation.

The advantageous features (Table V) of the opossum duct ligation model include its clinical relevance (i.e., duct obstruction as a cause of pancreatitis) and the severe, necrotizing, nature of the pancreatitis that is induced. The model is also attractive because both the pancreatic and the lung injury evolve slowly over a period of days, and therefore studies characterizing the events that are critical to the evolution of pancreatitis and lung injury in this model are easily performed. This model, however, has considerable limitations. Purchase, housing, and up-keep of these animals can be costly and this is further magnified by the need to condition and deworm the animals as well as the need to give them a course of antibiotics prior to use. The animals are not in-bred and they live in the wild. This results in considerable interanimal variation, making use of large numbers of animals necessary in most experiments.

Acute necrotizing pancreatitis in the opossum, induced by duct ligation, is a diffuse process that is relatively evenly distributed throughout the gland. This feature of this model is useful to the experimentalist because it simplifies issues of tissue sampling and data interpretation. It differs from the clinical setting where, for the most part, severe necrotizing pancreatitis is a focal process involving certain areas of the pancreas while sparing others. Whether this difference between opossum and human pancreatitis is critical is uncertain.

B. In Vivo Noninvasive Models

Three types of noninvasive *in vivo* models of acute pancreatitis have been described (Table VI). They each share the advantages of being easily induced and yielding highly reproducible results (Table VII). Each can be applied to small, low-cost animals such as rats and mice and each can result in the induction of severe necrotizing pancreatitis. Perhaps the most disturbing feature of these noninvasive models is their potential lack of clinical relevance. The models involve administration of either a supramaximally stimulating dose of a secretagogue, a high dose of arginine, or an ethionine-containing diet, but there is no evidence that clinical acute pancreatitis results from excessive secretagogue stimulation, exposure to toxic doses of arginine, or ingestion of ethionine. Thus, results obtained with these models must be interpreted with caution. In spite of these reservations, however, these noninvasive *in vivo* models have been widely used and are popular models currently employed by many investigators. Because of their wide use, at least two of these models (secretagogue and diet induced) have been extensively characterized.

1. Diet-Induced Pancreatitis

The observation that ethionine, the ethyl analog of methionine, could induce pancreatic injury was first reported in 1950 (38,39). Ethionine administration was subsequently used as a means of inducing pancreatitis in a variety of animals, including the rat, cat, dog, and monkey (40). In these studies, pancreatitis was noted to be mild and nonlethal. In 1975, however, Lombardi and co-workers reported that young female mice fed a choline-deficient ethionine-supplemented (CDE) diet developed necrotizing hemorrhagic pancreatitis (41). When mice were fed the CDE diet *ad libitum*, all animals died within 5 days. The severity of this model of pancreatitis is directly related to a number of key features, and the alteration of any either prevents the pancreatitis or reduces its severity. Young female mice (10–11 g) must be used. Ethionine must be administered along with a choline-deficient diet. Reducing the duration of

Table V Duct Ligation

Advantages	Disadvantages
Clinically relevant	Severe pancreatitis in opossums only
Evolves reproducibly	Expense and difficulty using opossums
Evolves slowly	Lesions distributed homogeneously throughout pancreas
Associated lung injury	

Table VI Noninvasive Models of Acute Pancreatitis

Diet induced
Secretagogue induced
Arginine induced

Table VII Noninvasive models

Advantages	Disadvantages
No surgery required	Clinical relavance?
Can use small animals	
Cheap	
Easily induced	
Highly reproducible	
Adjustable severity	
Associated lung injury	
Well characterized	
Extensively used	
Suitable for *in vitro* studies	

CDE diet administration and/or limiting the amount of CDE diet consumed can reduce both the severity of the pancreatitis and the associated mortality. Thus, administration of 3 g/day of the CDE diet to 10- to 11-g female CD-1 mice results in a mortality rate of 40–60%.

From a practical standpoint, mice are purchased from commercial sources, with delivery arranged so that they arrive in the laboratory 2–3 days before the experiment. They are fasted for 24 hr before the start of CDE diet administration and then 3 g of diet is offered. During this time they are given water *ad libitum*. Similarly, they are fasted but given water *ad libitum* for 24 hr after completion of CDE diet administration, before being placed back on a regular diet. Because mice may, on occasion, eat their dead cage mates, mortality rates should be calculated based on the number of surviving live animals rather than by counting the number of dead mice. Finally, it should be noted that the severity and mortality rates of CDE diet-induced pancreatitis can vary considerably between diet mixtures [either made according to published recipes (41) or purchased from commercial sources (Harlan-Teklad Labs, www.harlan.com)] and among animal groups. This should be recognized to allow design of suitably controlled experiments. Thus, when comparing the effects of the CDE diet to other diets, animals from the same purchase group should be randomly assigned to control and experimental groups. Similarly, when evaluating the effects of an intervention or treatment on the progression or outcome of diet-induced pancreatitis, all animals should be fed from the same CDE diet mixture and the control as well as the experimental groups should consist of randomly assigned mice from the same purchase group. In this case, the control and experimental groups should be evaluated simultaneously and replicate experiments performed using similar groups that are also evaluated side by side.

Much has been learned about the cell biological events that couple CDE diet administration to the development of acute pancreatitis. The disease appears to result from a defect in acinar cell stimulus–secretion coupling, which prevents the discharge of newly synthesized digestive enzymes but does not prevent either their synthesis or their intracellular transport and packaging in zymogen granules (42). As a result, digestive enzyme zymogens and zymogen granules accumulate within acinar cells. Within 1 day of the start of CDE diet, some of the accumulated granules fuse with lysosomes, by a process known as crinophagy, resulting in the formation of vacuoles that contain both digestive enzyme zymogens and lysosomal hydrolases (43). It is believed that this colocalization phenomenon permits the lysosomal hydrolase cathepsin B to activate trypsinogen, and trypsin to activate the other zymogens within acinar cells. It is the intraacinar cell activation of these digestive enzymes that subsequently leads to acinar cell injury as well as pancreatitis (44). Mice with diet-induced pancreatitis also develop an acute lung injury, which may resemble that seen in patients with ARDS (45).

The severity of diet-induced pancreatitis can be quantitated by measuring the increase in pancreatic content of myeloperoxidase (i.e., neutrophil sequestration within the pancreas), appearance and extent of acinar cell necrosis (measured by morphometry as a percent of total acinar cell mass), and animal mortality. Because the zymogen and, consequently, the protein contents of the pancreas increase during the evolution of diet-induced pancreatitis, measurements of characteristics, such as myeloperoxidase content, should be expressed per unit DNA rather than per milligram of protein. The severity of pancreatitis-associated lung injury in this model can be characterized by measuring lung myeloperoxidase activity (neutrophil sequestration), leakage of intravenously administered fluoroscein isothiocyanate-labeled albumin into the bronchoalveolar lavage fluid (pulmonary microvascular permeability), and bronchoalveolar lavage fluid lactic dehydrogenase content (Type II pneumocyte injury).

2. Secretagogue-Induced Pancreatitis

Secretion of digestive enzymes by the exocrine pancreas is regulated by secretagogue hormones acting via two second messenger pathways. Secretin and vasoactive intestinal peptide (VIP) act via the cyclic AMP/protein kinase A pathway whereas cholecystokinin and acetylcholine act via the phospholipase C/calcium/protein kinase C pathway. Agents acting via this latter pathway, when given in high concentrations, can induce acute pancreatitis.

The best studied of the secretagogue-induced models of pancreatitis involves administration, to rodents, of the cholecystokinin (CCK) analog cerulein at concentrations above those needed to stimulate a maximal rate of digestive enzyme secretion (46). At these "supramaximally stimulating concentrations," cerulein administration results in inhibition of digestive enzyme secretion.

Acinar cells possess two classes of cholecystokinin A receptors. The high-affinity class mediates the stimulation of enzyme secretion whereas the lower affinity class mediates inhibition of secretion. It is the interaction of cerulein with these low-affinity inhibitory receptors that triggers acute pancreatitis (47), which can be prevented by the coadministration of either a nonspecific CCK antagonist (A364,718) or a specific antagonist of low-affinity receptors (CCK-JMV-180).

When given by constant infusion to rats, supramaximally stimulating doses of cerulein (2–5 μg/kg/hr) induce a transient form of edematous interstitial pancreatitis that becomes apparent within the first hour of cerulein administration, reaches its peak in 3–6 hr after the start of cerulein administration, and begins to resolve within 12 hr of the start of cerulein administration. In rats, secretagogue-induced pancreatitis is characterized by marked hyperamylasemia, massive pancreatic edema, neutrophil sequestration within the pancreas, pancreatic acinar cell necrosis, and pancreatitis-associated lung injury (48,49). Most investigators using this model have chosen to use unrestrained awake animals. Thus, a jugular vein cannula is usually inserted 1 day before the planned experiment. The catheter is tunneled to exit at the base of the tail and then protected by passing through a wire coil until it exits the cage. The animal is allowed to awaken from anesthesia, given water *ad libitum*, and studied the next day, at which time it is free to move about the cage. Catheter patency, prior to the start of cerulein infusion, is maintained by the slow infusion of heparinized saline. An alternative approach is to administer the cerulein by either subcutaneous or intraperitoneal injection at hourly intervals (×4–12) in noncannulated animals. In this case, each injection should deliver roughly 5 μg/kg.

The cerulein model of pancreatitis has also been extensively used in mice (50). In this case, hourly injections (×4–12) are given because cannulation is difficult in such small animals. For the most part, secretagogue-induced pancreatitis in mice appears to be more severe than that noted in rats. There is often extensive necrosis as well as hemorrhage in the pancreas and a fulminant form of lung injury. As noted for rats, the severity of pancreatitis is dependent on the duration of cerulein administration as well as the dose of cerulein given. As in rats, pancreatitis develops with rapidly and easily quantifiable changes in pancreatic morphology and myeloperoxidase content; as well, lung injury can be detected within 3–4 hr after the start of cerulein administration.

The secretagogue-induced model of acute pancreatitis, perhaps because it is so easily created, has been extensively characterized and the cell biological events underlying its development have been described. In addition to inhibiting secretion from acinar cells, cerulein stimulation also causes intracellular calcium levels to rise. By as yet unidentified mechanisms, this combination of elevated intracellular calcium levels and inhibition of secretion causes a derangement of the cytoskeleton and missorting of intracellular proteins. As a result, large vacuoles that contain digestive enzyme zymogens as well as lysosomal hydrolases appear; within these vacuoles, the lysosomal hydrolase cathepsin B activates trypsinogen. Activated trypsin, perhaps along with other activated zymogens, causes acinar cell injury and this triggers a cascade of events that culminate in acute pancreatitis (51).

The secretagogue-induced model has many features that make it attractive for studies dealing with pancreatitis. It can be employed using relatively low-cost laboratory animals (rats, mice), requires no surgical procedure other than jugular vein cannulation (and even this can be avoided if cerulein is given by repeated injection rather than by infusion), evolves rapidly in a highly reproducible fashion, and can be adjusted such that either mild or severe pancreatitis is induced. It is also associated with significant lung injury, which is easily quantifiable. The noninvasive features of this model for induction of both pancreatitis and lung injury also are positive features. On the other hand, secretagogue-induced pancreatitis is usually not a lethal form of pancreatitis, and therefore survival studies are inappropriate. Perhaps the major criticism of this model is its questionable clinical relevance.

3. Arginine-Induced Pancreatitis

Tani and associates, in 1990, described a noninvasive *in vivo* model of acute pancreatitis induced by administration of L-arginine (52). Rats were given a single intraperitoneal injection of 500 mg/100 g body weight of L-arginine. Marked increases in serum amylase and lipase were noted 24 hr later and those elevations regressed to normal values over the next 24–48 hr. Pancreatic protein and digestive enzyme contents decreased over the initial 72 hr but then returned to normal levels by 14 days. Morphologic changes of arginine-induced pancreatitis included the appearance of small vesicles within acinar cells by 6 hr, interstitial edema by 12 hr, and acinar cell necrosis by 24 hr after administration of arginine. Necrosis and intrapancreatic inflammation was noted to be maximal 72 hr after administration of arginine. Recovery appeared to begin at 7 days and to be essentially complete by 14 days after arginine administration. The arginine model has neither been extensively employed nor well characterized. It appears to resemble the CDE diet-induced model but at a lesser level of severity.

C. Miscellaneous Models of Acute Pancreatitis

1. Combined Secretagogue Stimulation and Retrograde Ductal Injection

Schmidt and colleagues combined two previously described models (secretagogue induced and duct injection induced) to develop a model with graded degrees of severity (53,54) (see Table VIII). The rat jugular vein is cannulated and a Teflon catheter is placed in the biliopancreatic duct. After a 5-min period of duct drainage, the bile duct is clamped at the hilus of the liver and a glycodeoxycholic acid solution (pH 8.0, 10 or 34 m*M*) is infused (0.10–0.15 ml, 30 mmHg pressure) into the duct through the catheter. The rats are then started on an intravenous infusion of cerulein (5 μg/kg/hr), which is continued for 6 hr. Either cerulein alone or glycodeoxycholic acid alone was noted to cause mild pancreatitis, but the combination of both agents induced more severe pancreatitis. That severity could be even further increased by either administration of higher concentrations or a greater volume of the bile acid. Pancreatitis, in this model, is characterized by the presence of hyperamylasemia, pancreatic edema, pancreatic inflammation, acinar cell necrosis, and pancreatic hemorrhage.

The advantages of this model include the fact that pancreatitis, varying from mild to severe, can be induced and the severity of the model appears to be more consistently controllable than is the case with most duct injection models. On the other hand, this model requires a more complicated operative procedure and its advantages over the duct injection model described by Aho *et al.* (19,20) would seem to be marginal. Additionally, it has not been extensively used in investigations in the field.

Table VIII Miscellaneous Models of Acute Pancreatitis

Combined secretagogue stimulation and retrograde ductal injection
Immune models
Schwartzman reaction
Arthus reaction
Foreign serum
Antipancreatic antibodies
Ischemia induced
Trauma induced
Infection induced
Ex vivo models

2. Immune Models

A variety of immune models, both invasive and noninvasive, have been described. A Schwartzman-type reaction can be induced in the pancreas of rabbits or goats by an initial intraductal injection of bacterial toxin followed, 24 hr later, by the intravenous administration of the same toxin (55). Under these conditions, hemorrhagic pancreatic necrosis develops. Using an Arthus-type reaction, both edematous and necrotizing pancreatitis can be induced. In this case, rabbits are sensitized to ovalbumin by intravenous and subcutaneous injection of the agent and subsequently ovalbumin is infused into the pancreatic duct (56). Experimental acute pancreatitis can also be induced by intraperitoneal injection of foreign serum (57,58) or by injection of foreign serum into the pancreatic duct (59). Finally, acute pancreatitis can be induced by the intraductal injection of antibasement membrane antibodies (60).

Each of these so-called immune models appears to induce pancreatitis by triggering a local immune reaction within the pancreatic parenchyma. They are all relatively complex and have not been widely utilized. Although these models may be of value in studies focused on local immune processes in pancreatitis, they would appear to be of limited value as general models of pancreatitis.

3. Ischemia, Trauma, and Infection-Induced Models

Clinical pancreatitis can be the result of pancreatic ischemia, direct blunt trauma to the pancreas, or pancreatic infection. It is not surprising, therefore, that each of these approaches has also been used to induce experimental pancreatitis. Ischemia-induced pancreatitis can be elicited either by subjecting animals to transient hypovolemic shock (61) or by transiently clamping the arterial inflow to the pancreas (62). Direct trauma to the pancreas, exerted by placing a crushing clamp on the organ (63), will also result in pancreatic injury. Pancreatitis can also be induced by infecting mice with Coxsackie B virus and, in this case, severe pancreatitis results when the infection is induced in genetically manipulated mice that lack the inducible form of nitric oxide synthase (64). None of these rather specialized models of pancreatitis have been characterized in great detail.

4. *Ex Vivo* Models

Ex vivo models of pancreatitis have been developed to avoid complex and poorly controlled extrapancreatic factors that can occur during the evolution of *in vivo* pancreatitis. Two types of systems have been employed. In one, the gland is totally removed from the animal and mounted in a chamber that permits alteration of the nutritional suspending medium. This approach has been used, for example, to evaluate the effects of ethanol added to the suspending medium, on exocrine pancreatic function (65,66). The other approach involves exteriorization of the pancreas and perfusion with a nutrient solution. The organ can be studied while manipulations of agents flowing into the pancreas or changes in the outflow resistance are made. Either normal arterial inflow and venous outflow can be maintained or the circulation can be interrupted and replaced by pump perfusion with a blood substitute. In early studies using this approach, the *ex vivo* canine pancreas was used (67), but in more recent studies, the *ex vivo* rat pancreas has been used (68).

These *ex vivo* models are complex and difficult to establish. Considerable experience by the staff using these models is required and there is a definite learning curve that must be traversed. The gland is not completely stable during the period of *ex vivo* study and a gradual loss of viability as well as the development of edema complicate interpretation of the data that are obtained under these unstable conditions. The *ex vivo* models are clearly nonphysiologic and their clinical relevance is questionable.

III. Chronic Pancreatitis

Recognized etiologies of chronic pancreatitis include (1) prolonged ethanol abuse, (2) genetic mutations involving cationic trypsinogen, and (3) cystic fibrosis and related genetic conditions. Unfortunately, attempts to induce a chronic pancreatic lesion resembling pancreatitis, characterized by fibrosis as well as inflammation, using approaches based on these etiologies have not been successful. Prolonged feeding of ethanol to rodents does not induce chronic pancreatitis. Genetically modified mice that express the mutant gene found most commonly in hereditary pancreatitis do not spontaneously develop chronic pancreatitis. Finally, knockout mice that lack the cystic fibrosis transmembrane regulator (CFTR) and have the cystic fibrosis phenotype in other organs do not develop chronic pancreatitis. At present, therefore, there is no model that appears to be clinically relevant in terms of a triggering event that results in chronic pancreatitis (Table IX). This lack of a seemingly relevant model has severely hampered research in the field of chronic pancreatitis and has led investigators to seek alternative solutions.

Table IX Models of Chronic Pancreatitis

Partial ductal obstruction
Fibrosis models
Ethanol as a sensitizer

A. Partial Duct Obstruction

Partial obstruction of the feline pancreatic duct leads to chronic inflammation with fibrosis and a form of compartment syndrome in the pancreas distal to the point of obstruction (69). In practice, the main pancreatic duct of cats is partially obstructed with a ligature. Within 3–6 weeks after creation of this incomplete obstruction, fibrosis is clearly evident. This has allowed investigators to study the effect of fibrosis and chronic obstruction on various physiological events such as blood flow, secretagogue-induced secretion, interstitial pH, and interstitial pressure. This model may provide valuable insights into the pathogenesis of pain in chronic pancreatitis and it may also yield useful information regarding the effects of chronic pancreatic inflammation on other pancreatic processes. Unfortunately, because it is induced by partial ductal obstruction rather than by any event believed to trigger clinical chronic pancreatitis, and it is primarily a model of fibrosis with relatively little inflammation, it is unlikely that use of this model will shed light on the events that underlie the pathogenesis of chronic clinical pancreatitis or on those events that modulate its course. It is a complex model involving costly and difficult to handle animals.

B. Models of Fibrosis

Transforming growth factor-β (TGF-β) is a cytokine that plays an important role in wound healing. In liver and pancreas, TGF-β activates stellate cells, stimulates their transformation into myofibroblasts, promotes collagen synthesis, and inhibits collagenolytic enzymes (70–74). Rats that overexpress TGF-β in the pancreas develop pancreatic fibrosis (75). The combination of TGF-β administration along with infusion of a supramaximally stimulating dose of the secretagogue cerulein has been noted to result in chronic pancreatic fibrosis after resolution of acute pancreatitis (76). Similarly, administration of cyclosporin A, which stimulates endogenous TGF-β production, along with repeated cycles of cerulein-induced pancreatitis can lead to chronic pancreatic fibrosis (77).

These models of fibrosis have only recently been reported and their impact on the field of pancreatitis remains uncertain. They may have an important role to play in studies designed to elucidate cell biological events that couple acute and chronic inflammation in the pancreas to fibrosis and atrophy of the gland. It is unlikely, however, that their use will shed light on the mechanisms underlying the initial triggering events in chronic pancreatitis.

C. Models Using Ethanol Sensitization

Although attempts to induce chronic (or even acute) pancreatic injury by administration of ethanol to rodents have failed, investigators have attempted to elucidate potentially harmful effects of ethanol on the pancreas by searching for evidence that ethanol sensitizes the pancreas to injury induced by other agents. Two approaches have been used. In the first, animals are given a short-term exposure to high doses of ethanol either by intravenous ethanol infusion or by placing ethanol in the animals' drinking water. After this short-term exposure to ethanol, pancreatic injury is then induced by another means—most often by exposure to a supramaximally stimulating concentration of secretagogue (78). The second approach involves exposure of the experimental animals, usually rats, to large amounts of ethanol over periods as long as 3–6 weeks. Once again, animals are subjected to an acutely injurious agent after completion of the ethanol exposure phase of the experiment. In both approaches, attempts are made to achieve blood alcohol levels (either acutely or chronically) associated with inebriation and the experimentalist usually searches for evidence that the prior ethanol exposure has made it more sensitive to subsequent injury either by increasing the level of injury resulting from a standard stimulus or by allowing otherwise subinjurious concentrations of the agent to result in acute injury.

Short-term exposure to inebriating doses of ethanol is relatively easily accomplished with administration of ethanol either intravenously or in the drinking water. Long-term exposure to inebriating doses of ethanol, however, is much more problematic. Most strains of rodents are averse to ethanol and, therefore, mere addition of ethanol to the drinking water is usually not enough to achieve adequate ethanol intake. Rather, the animals fail to consume adequate amounts of food and liquid. Thus they lose weight. Furthermore, rodents have relatively high metabolic rates and both mice and rats rapidly metabolize ethanol. This further complicates efforts to achieve high blood alcohol levels in rodents merely by adding the ethanol to either the food or water. The best method of avoiding these problems seems to be the technique developed by Tsukamoto and French (79). These workers surgically placed gastrostomy tubes in rats. The tube was brought out through the back and protected from injury with a wire coil. The animals were allowed to move about freely in their cages and infused with an ethanol-diet mixture via the gastrostomy at a constant rate and in sufficient ethanol concentration such that 36–49% of the calories consumed were from ethanol. Blood alcohol levels were noted to range from 50–450 mg/dl with a periodicity of 5–6 days. After 3–6 weeks of ethanol feeding via the gastrostomy, the animals were exposed to a dose of cerulein that, in non-ethanol-fed animals, did not result in pancreatic injury. Under these conditions, preexposure to ethanol was found to result in enhanced sensitivity to this otherwise noninjurious dose of the secretagogue (80). This approach to the study of ethanol effects on the pancreas and the events underlying ethanol-induced pancreatitis is only now in its infancy. At present, there is no good ethanol model of chronic pancreatitis, thus it is likely that ethanol sensitization models will be more widely employed in the future.

IV. Preparations for in Vitro Study

Not infrequently, contemplated experiments may involve exposure of experimental animals to conditions that lead to the development of pancreatitis as a first phase of the experiment. This is immediately followed by a period in which pancreatic tissue, removed from the animal, is studied under *in vitro* conditions. This approach avoids many of the uncontrollable *in vivo* changes that occur during pancreatitis, including neurohormonal or vascular phenomena. Several *in vitro* systems are available for such studies. They have each been extensively used, primarily for studies of pancreatic acinar cell biology, but they can be applied to characterize events during the evolution of pancreatitis if those events, once triggered *in vivo*, persist under *in vitro* conditions. The most commonly employed *in vitro* pancreas preparations involve (1) isolated pancreatic acinar cells, (2) isolated pancreatic acini, and (3) pancreas fragments (see Table X).

The standard method of preparing isolated acinar cells from rat, guinea pig, or mouse pancreas involves proteolytic digestion of the tissue, chelation of divalent cations, and mechanical disruption (81,82). This method, described in 1974, allows for the study of isolated cells, but the method of preparation is harsh and cell viability may be poor. Even when the normal pancreas is used for preparation of isolated cells, the cells survive for only short periods and their functional integrity, as judged by secretagogue-stimulated secretion, is poor. When tissues taken from animals with pancreatitis are used, these problems are magnified. For this reason, isolated acinar cells are probably not an ideal system for the study of pancreatitis-associated events.

Preparation of suspensions of pancreatic acini requires tissue disruption by proteolytic enzymes such as collagenase, but the chelation step, which is required for preparation

Table X Preparations for in Vitro Study

Single-cell suspensions
Suspensions of acini
Fragments and slices
Long-term culture

of isolated cells, can be avoided (83). The freshly removed pancreas is injected with buffer containing collagenase, incubated to allow for tissue digestion, and then mechanically disrupted usually by vigorous pipetting. The acini are separated from nondissociated tissue and disrupted cells by centrifugation on an albumin cushion, washed, and then studied *in vitro*. For the most part, acini prepared by this method remain viable and healthy for up to 6 hr, during which time they respond vigorously to secretagogue stimulation, exclude markers of cell injury such as propidium iodide and trypan blue, and do not leak LDH. Unfortunately, their long-term viability and functional integrity are poor and, for this reason, their use is limited to short-term experiments.

Pancreas fragments can be prepared by mincing tissue without the need for either divalent ion chelation or exposure to collagenolytic enzymes. Using gentle techniques, these fragments can remain viable, under tissue culture conditions, for up to 24 hr (84), during which time they respond nicely to secretagogue stimulation. Thus, this method of tissue preparation can allow for the *in vitro* study of pancreatitis-associated events over roughly a 24-hr period. At longer times, cell viability diminishes and secretory function is lost.

Ideally, pancreatic acinar cell cultures could be used for the longer term study of pancreatitis-associated events. Unfortunately, attempts to develop methods of culturing acinar cells for prolonged periods have not been promising. With long-term culture, acinar calls frequently dedifferentiate, losing their ability to synthesize digestive enzymes, package digestive enzymes in secretory granules, and discharge stored digestive enzymes in response to secretagogue stimulation. To some extent, growing the cells or artificial basement membranes and supplementing them with growth factors as well as hormones (85) can reduce these problems, but the resulting cell culture preparation remains far from optimal.

V. Conclusions

A large number of experimental models have been developed for studies involving pancreatitis. Each of these models has its advantages as well as its disadvantages (Table XI). To a great extent, choice of an appropriate model for use is determined by the nature of the question being asked. The noninvasive models, because of their simplicity and high level of reproducibility, are ideally suited for studies directed at characterizing cell biological events that lead to cell injury. The *in vivo* invasive models, particularly the duct-injection model of Aho *et al.* (19,20) and the opossum duct ligation model, are attractive because they appear to be clinically relevant in terms of their etiology and they lead to severe pancreatitis, permitting studies evaluating local as well as systemic complications of pancreatitis. It is hoped

Table XI Experimental Pancreatitis Models

Types	Advantages	Disadvantages	Ref.
Acute pancreatitis			
Invasive models			
Retrograde injection	Severe and lethal; clinically relevant basis	Overly destructive; larger animals; difficult to control; requires surgery	19, 20
Closed duodenal loop	Severe; clinically relevant?	Little pancratic inflammation; poorly understood basis; difficult to control; requires surgery; larger animals	
Prograde duct infusion	Graded severity	Complex surgery; larger animals; Clinical relevance?	
Duct ligation	Clinically relevant; severe; slow evolution	Expensive; requires surgery; opossums	35–37
Noninvasive models			
Diet	Cheap and reproducible; well characterized; slow evolution; variable severity	Clinical relevance?	41, 44, 45
Secretagogue	Cheap and reproducible; well characterized; variable severity	Clinical relevance?; nonlethal	46, 48–51
Arginine	Cheap	Poorly characterized	
Miscellaneous			
Combined	Varying severity	Complex	53, 54
Immune	None	Clinical relevance?	—
Ischemia, trauma, infection	None	—	—
Ex vivo	Controllable variables	Complex; poorly charcterized; unstable	66, 67
Chronic pancreatitis			
Partial duct obstruction	Fibrosis 6 inflammation	Clinical relevance?; complex	68
Fibrosis models	Uncertain	Noninvasive	
Ethanol sensitization	Ethanol basis	Sensitization only	78, 79

that models relating long-term ethanol exposure to the development of chronic pancreatitis will be developed because, at present, no adequate model of chronic pancreatitis is available.

References

1. Acosta, J. L., and Ledesma, C. L. (1974). Gallstone migration as a cause for acute pancreatitis. *N. Engl. J. Med.* **290,** 484–487.
2. Beck, I. T., Kahn, D. S., Solyniar, J., *et al.* (1964). The role of proteolytic enzymes in the pathogenesis of acute pancreatitis. *Gastroenterology* **46,** 531–542.
3. Satake, K., Ruzmanith, J. S., Appert, H. E., Carballo, J., and Howard, J. M. (1973). Hypotension and release of kinin-forming enzyme into ascitic fluid exudate during experimental pancreatitis in dogs. *Ann. Surg.* **177,** 497–502.
4. Ohlsson, K., and Eddeland, A. (1975). Release of proteolytic enzymes in bile-induced pancreatitis in dogs. *Gastroenterology* **69,** 668–675.
5. Donaldson, L. A., Williams, R. W., and Schenk, W. G. (1978). Experimental pancreatitis: Effect of plasma and dextran on pancreatic blood flow. *Surgery* **89,** 313–321.
6. Lefer, A. M., Glenn, J. M., O'Neill, T. J., *et al.* (1971). Inotropic influence of endogenous peptides in experimental pancreatitis. *Surgery* **69,** 220–228.
7. Musa, B. E., Nelson A. W., Gillette, E. L., Ferguson, H. L., and Lumb, W. V. (1976). A model to study acute panceatitis in the dog. *J. Surg. Res.* **21,** 51–56.
8. Lankisch, P. G., Winckler, K., Bockermann, M., Schmidt, H., and Creutzfeldt, W. (1974). The influence of glucagon on acute experimental pancreatitis in the rat. *Scand. J. Gastoenterol.* **9,** 725–729.
9. Kivisaari, L. (1979). The effect of experimental pancreatitis and diabetes on the microvasculature of the rat pancreas. *Scand. J. Gastroenterol.* **14,** 520–695.
10. Elliot, D., Williams, R., and Zollinger, R. (1957). Alterations in pancreatic resistence to bile in the pathogenesis of acute pancreatitis. *Ann. Surg.* **146,** 669.
11. Johnson, R. M., Barone, R. M., Newson B. L., Das Gupta, T. K., and Nyhus, L. M. (1973). Treatment of experimental acute pancreatitis with 5-fluorouracil (5-FU). *Am. J. Surg* **125,** 211.
12. Evander, A., Ihse, I., And Lundquist, I. (1981). Influence of hormonal stimulation by caerulein on acute experimental pancreatitis in the rat. *Eur. J. Surg. Res.* **13,** 257.
13. Frey, C. F., Wong, H. N., Hickman, D., and Pullos, T. (1982). Toxicitiy of hemorrhagic ascites fluid associated with hemorrhagic pancreatitis. *Arch. Surg.* **117,** 401–404.
14. Anderson, M. C., Needleman, S. B., Gramatica, L., Toronto, I. R., and Briggs, Dr. (1969). Further inquiries into the role of pancreatic enzymes in the pathogenesis of acute pancreatitis. *Arch. Surg.* **99,** 185.
15. Satake, K., Chung, Y. S., Yoshimoto, T., *et al.* (1982). Radioimmunoreactive serum elastase levels and histologic changes during experimental pancreatitis in rats. *Arch. Surg.* **117,** 777–780.
16. Geokas, M. C., Rinderknecht, H., Swanson, V., and Haverback, B. J. (1969). Role of elastase in acute hemorrhagic pancreatitis. *Lab. Invest.* **19,** 235.
17. Schmidt, H., and Creutzfeldt, W. (1969). The possible role of phospholipase-A in the pathogenesis of acute pancreatitis. *Scand. J. Gastroenterol.* **4,** 39.
18. Condon, R. E., Woods, J. H., Poulin, T. L., Wagner, W. G., and Pissotis, C. A. (1974). Pancreatitis treated with glucagon or lactated Ringers solution. *Arch. Surg.* **109,** 154–158.
19. Aho, H. J., Koskensalo, S. M. L., and Nevalainen, T. J. (1980). Experimental pancreatitis in the rat. Sodium taurocholate-induced haemorrhagic panceatitis. *Scand. J. Gastroenterol.* **15,** 411–416.
20. Aho, H. S., and Nevalainen, T. J. (1980). Experimental pancreatitis in the rat. Ultrastructure of sodium taurocholate-induced pancreatic lesions. *Scand. J. Gastroenterol.* **15,** 417–424.
21. Pfeffer, R. B., Stasior, O., and Hinton, J. W. (1957). The clinical picture of the sequential development of acute hemorrhagic pancreatitis in the dog. *Surg. Forum* **8,** 248–251.
22. McCutcheon, A. D. (1964). Reflux of duodenal contents in the pathogenesis of pancreatitis. *Gut* **5,** 260–265.
23. Paulino-Netto, A., and Dreiling D. A. (1960). Chronic duodenal obstruction: a mechanovascular etiology of pancreatitis. *Am. J. Dig. Dis.* **5,** 1006–1018.
24. Nevalainen, T. J., and Seppa, A. (1975). Acute pancreatitis caused by closed duodenal loop in the rat. *Scand. J. Gastroenterol.* **10,** 521–527.
25. Chetty, V. Gilmour, H. H., and Taylor, T. V. (1980). Experimental acute pancreatitis in the rat—A new model. *Gut* **21,** 115–117.
26. Orda, R., Hadas, N., Orda, S., and Wiznitzer, T. (1980). Experimental acute pancreatitis:inducement by taurocholate sodium-trypsin injection into a temporarily closed duodenal loop in the rat. *Arch. Surg.* **115,** 327–329.
27. Pfeffer, R. B., Stasior, O., and Hinton, J. W. (1957). The clinical picture of the sequential development of acute hemorrhagic pancreatitis in the dog. *Surg. Forum* **8,** 248–251.
28. Rao, S. S., Watt, I. A., Donaldson, L. A., Crocket, A., and Joffe, S. N. (1981). A serial histologic study of the development and progression of acute pancreatitis in the rat. *Am. J. Pathol.* **103,** 39–46.
29. Reber, H. A., Robert, C., and Way, L. W. (1979). The pancreatic duct mucosal barrier. *Am. J. Surg.* **137,** 128–134.
30. Farmer, R. C., Maslin, S. C., and Reber, H. A. (1983). Acute pancreatitis-role of duct permeability. *Surg. Forum* **34,** 224–227.
31. Wedgewood, K. R., Farmer, R. C., and Reber, H. A. (1986). A model of hemorrhagic pancreatitis in rats—The role of 16-16 dimethyl prostglandin E_2. *Gastroenterology* **90,** 32–39.
32. Popper, H. L., and Necheles, H. (1947). Edema of the pancreas. *Surg. Gynec. Obst.* **74,** 123–124.
33. Lium, R., and Maddock, S. (1948). Etiology of acute pancreatitis:an experimental study. *Surgery* **24,** 593–604.
34. Popper, H. L., Necheles, H., and Russell, K. C. (1948). Transition of pancreatic edema into pancreatic necrosis. *Surg. Gyn. Obst.* **87,** 79.
35. Senninger, N., Moody, F. G., Coelho, J. C., and VanBuren, D. H. (1986). The role of biliary obstruction in the pathogenesis of acute pancreatitis in the opossum. *Surgery* **99,** 688–693.
36. Lerch, M. M., Saluja A. K., Runzi, M., Dawra, R., Saluja, M., and Steer, M. L. (1993). Pancreatic duct obstruction triggers acute necrotizing pancreatitis in the opossum (1993). *Gastroenterology* **104,** 853–861.
37. Hofbauer, B., Saluja, A. K., Bhatia, M., Frossard, J. L., Lee, H. S., Bhagat, Z., and Steer, M. L. (1998). Effect of recombinant platelet-activating factor acetylhydrolase on two models of experimental acute pancreatitis. *Gastroenterology* **115,** 1238–1247.
38. Farmer, E., and Popper, H. (1950). Production of acute pancreatitis with ethionine and its prevention by methionine. *Proc. Soc. Exp. Biol. Med.* **74,** 838–840.
39. Goldberg, R. C., Chaikoff, L. L., and Dodge, A. H. (1950). Destruction of pancreatic acinar tissue by *dl*-ethionine. *Proc. Soc. Exp. Biol. Med.* **74,** 869–872.
40. DeAlmeida, A. L., and Grossman, M. I. (1952). Experimental production of pancreatitis with ethionine. *Gastroenterology* **20,** 554–577.
41. Lombardi, B., Estes, L. W., and Longnecker, D. S. (1975). Acute hemorrhagic pancreatitis (massive necrosis) with fat necrosis induced in mice by *dl*-ethionine fed with a choline deficient diet. *Am. J. Pathol.* **79,** 465–480.
42. Powers, R. E., Saluja A. K., Houlihan M. J., Steer, M. L. (1986). Diminished agonist-stimulated inositol trisphoshate generation blocks stimulus-secretion coupling in mouse pancreatic acini during diet-induced experimental pancreatitis. *J. Clin. Invest.* **77,** 1668–1674.

43. Koike, H., Steer, M. L., and Meldolesi, J. (1982). Pancreatic effects of ethionine: Blockade of exocytosis and appearance of crinophagy and autophagy precede cellular necrosis. *Am. J. Physiol.* **242,** G297–G307.
44. Steer, M. L. (1998). Frank Brooks Memorial Lecture: The early intraacinar cell events which occur during acute pancreatitis. *Pancreas* **17,** 31–37.
45. Bhatia, M., Saluja, A. K., Hofbauer, B., Lee, H. S., Frossard, J. L., and Steer, M. L. (1998). The effects of neutrophil depletion on a completely noninvasive model of acute pancreatitis-associated lung injury. *Int. J. Pancreatol.* **24,** 77–83.
46. Lampel, M., Kern, H. F. (1977). Acute interstitial pancreatitis in rats induced by excessive doses of a pancreatic secretagogue. *Virchows Arch. A Pathol. Anat. Histol.* **373,** 97–113.
47. Saluja, A. K., Saluja, M., Printz, H., Zavertnik, A., Sengupta, A., and Steer, M. L. (1989). Experimental pancreatitis is mediated by low-affinity cholecystokinin receptors that inhibit digestive enzyme secretion. *Proc. Natl. Acad. Sci. U.S.A.* **86,** 8968–8971.
48. Grady, T., Saluja, A., Kaiser, A., and Steer, M. (1996). Edema and intrapancreatic trypsinogen activation precede glutathione depletion during caerulein pancreatitis. *Am. J. Physiol.* **271,** G20–G26.
49. Yamanaka, K., Saluja A. K., Brown, G. E., Yamaguchi, Y., Hofbauer, B., and Steer, M. L. (1997). Protective effects of prostaglandin E1 on acute lung injury of caerulein-induced acute pancreatitis in rats. *Am. J. Physiol.* **272,** G23–G30.
50. Gerard, C., Frossard, J. L., Bhatia, M., Saluja, A., Gerard, N. P., Lu, B., and Steer, M. L. (1997). Targeted disruption of the beta-chemokine receptor CCR1 protects against pancreatitis-associated lung injury. *J. Clin. Invest.* **100,** 2022–2027.
51. Saluja, A. K., Bhagat, L., Lee, H. S., Bhatia, M., Frossard, J. L., and Steer, M. L. (1998). Secretagogue-induced digestive enzyme activation and cell injury in pancreatic acini. *Am. J. Physiol.* **276,** G835–G842.
52. Tani, S., Itoh, H., Okabayashi, Y., Nakamura, T., Jujii, M., Fujisawa, T., Koide, M., and Otsuki, M. (1990). New model of acute necrotizing pancreatitis induced by excessive doses of arginine in rats. *Dig. Dis. Sci.* **35,** 367-274.
53. Schmidt, J., Lewandrowski, K., Warshaw, A. L., Compton, C. C., and Rattner, D. W. (1992). Morphometric charcteristics and homogeneity of a new model of acute pancreatitis in the rat. *Int. J. Pancreat.* **12,** 41051.
54. Schmidt, J., Rattner, D. W., Lewandrowski, K., Compton, C. C., Mandavilli, U., Knoefel, W. T., and Warshaw, A. L. (1992). A better model of acute pancreatitis for evaluating therapy. *Ann. Surg.* **215,** 44–56.
55. Thal, A., and Brackney, E. (1954). Acute hemorrhagic pancreatic necrosis produced by local Shwartzman reaction. *JAMA* **155,** 569–574.
56. Thal, A. (1955). Studies on pancreatitis. II. Acute pancreatic necrosis produced experimentally by the Arthus sensitization reaction. *Surgery* **37,** 911–917.
57. Janigan, D. T., Nevalainen, T. J., MacAulay, M. A., and Vethamany, V. G. (1975). Foreign serum-induced pancreatitis in mice. I. A new model of pancreatitis. *Lab. Invest.* **33,** 591–607.
58. Nevalainen, T. J., Fowlie, F. E., and Janigan, D. T. (1977). Foreign serum-induced pancreatitis in mice. II. Secretory disturbances of acinar cells. *Lab. Invest.* **36,** 469–473.
59. Nevalainen, T. J. (1978). Pancreatic injury caused by intraductal injection of foreign serum in rat. *Virchows Arch. B. Cell. Pathol.* **27,** 89–98.
60. Seelig, R., and Seelig, H. P. (1976). Complement-mediated acinar cell necrosis in pancreatitis induced by basement membrane antibodies. *Virchows Arch. A. Pathol. Anat. Histol.* **374,** 69–77.
61. Mithofer, K., Fernandez-Del Costillo, C., Frick, T. W., Foitzik, T., Bassi, D. G., Lewandrowski, K. B., Rattner, D. W., and Warshaw, A. L. (1995). Increased intrapanceatic trypsinogen activation in ischemia-induced experimental panceatitis. *Ann. Surg.* **221,** 364–371.
62. Menger, M. D., Bonkhoff, H., and Vollmar, B. (1996). Ischemia-reperfusion-induced pancreatic microvascular injury. *Dig. Dis. Sci.* **41,** 823–830.
63. Modlin, I. M., Bilchik, A. J., Zucker, K. A., Adrian, J. E., Sussman, J., and Graham S. M. (1989). Cholecystokinin augmentation of "surgical" pancreatitis. Benefits of receptor blockade. *Arch. Surg.* **124,** 574–578.
64. Zaragoza, C., Ocampo, C. J., Saura, M., Bao, C., Leppo, M., Lafond-Walker, A., Thiemann, D. r., Hruban, R., and Lowenstein, C. J. (1999). Inducible nitric oxide synthase protection against coxzackie virus pancreatitis. *J. Immunol.*, 5497–5504.
65. Solomon, N., Solomon, T. E., Jacobson, E. D., and Shanbour, L. L. (1974). Direct effects of alcohol *in vivo* and *in vitro* exocrine secretion and metabolism. *Am. J. Dig. Dis.* **19,** 253–260.
66. Steer, M. L., Glazer, G., and Manabe, T. (1979). Direct effects of ethanol on exocrine secretion from the *in-vitro* rabbit pancreas. *Dig. Dis. Sci.* **24,** 769–774.
67. Sanfey, H., Bulkley, G. B., and Cameron, J. L. (1985). The pathogenesis of acute pancreatitis. The source and role of oxygen-derived free radicals in three different experimental models. *Ann. Surg.* **201,** 633–639.
68. Schonfeld, J. V., Muller, M. K., Augustin, M., Runzi, M., and Goebell, H. (1993). Effect of cysteamine on insulin release and exocrine pancreatic secretion in vitro. *Dig. Dis. Sci.* **38,** 28–32.
69. Karanjia, N. D., Widdison, A. L., Leung, F., Alvarez, C., Lutrin, F. J., and Reber, H. A. (1994). Compartment syndrome in experimental chronic obstructive pancreatitis. Effect of decompressing the main pancreatic duct. *Br. J. Surg.* **81,** 259–264.
70. Gressner, A. M., and Bachem, M. G. (1995). Molecular mechanisms of liver fibrogenesis; a homage to the role of activated fat-storing cells. *Digestion* **56,** 335–346.
71. Bachem, M. G., Sell, K. M., Melchior, R., *et al.* (1993) Tumor necrosis factor alpha (TNFα) and transforming growth factor β1(TGF-β1) stimulate fibronectin synthesis and the transdifferentiation of fat storing cells in the rat liver into myofibroblasts. *Virchows Arch.* **63,** 123-30.
72. Overall, C. M., Wrana, J. L., and Sodek, J. (1989). Independent regulation of collagenase, 72-kDa progelatinase, and metalloendoproteinase inhibitor expression in human fibroblasts by transforming growth factor-beta. *J. Biol. Chem.* **264,** 1860–1869.
73. Edwards, D. R., Murphy, G., Reynolds, J. J., *et al.* (1987). Transforming growth factor beta modulates the expression of collagenase and metalloproteinase inhibitor. *EMBO J.* **6,** 1899–1904.
74. Apte, M. V., Haber, P. S., Darby, S. J., Rodgers, S. C., McCaughan, G. W., Korsten, M. A., Pirola, R. C., and Wilson, J. S. (1999). Pancreatic stellate cells are activated by proinflammatory cytokines: Implications for pancreatic fibrogenesis. *Gut* **44,** 534–541.
75. Lee, M. S., Gu, D., Feng, L., *et al.* (1995). Accumulation of extracellular matrix and developmental dysregulation in the pancreas by transgenic production of transforming growth factor-beta 1. *Am. J. Pathol.* **147,** 42–52.
76. Van Laethem, J.-L., Robberecht, P., Resibois, A., *et al.* (1996). Transforming growth factor β promotes development of fibrosis after repeated courses of acute pancreatitis in mice. *Gastroenterology* **110,** 576–582.
77. Vaquero, E., Molero, X., Tian, X., Salas, A., and Malagelada, J.-R. (1999). Myofibroblast proliferation, fibrosis, and defective pancreatic repair induced by cyclosporin in rats. *Gut* **45,** 269–277.
78. Katz, M., Carangelo, R., Miller, L. J., and Gorelick, F. (1996). Effect of ethanol on cholecystokinin-stimulated zymogen granule conversion in pancreatic acinar cells. *Am. J. Physiol.* **270,** G171–G175.
79. Tsukamoto, H. (1998). Animal models of alcoholic liver injury. *Clin. Liver Dis.* **4,** 739–752.
80. Pandol, S. J., Periskic, S., Gokovsky, I., Zaninovic, V., Jung, Y., Zong, Y., Solomon, T. E., Gukovskaya, A. S., and Tsukamoto, H. (1999). Ethanol diet increases the sensitivity of rats to pancreatitis induced by cholecystokinin octapeptide. *Gastroenterology* **117,** 706–716.
81. Amsterdam, A., and Jamieson, J. D. (1974). Studies on dispersed pancreatic exocrine cells. I. Dissociation technique and morphologic characteristics of separated cells. *J. Cell Biol.* **63,** 1037–1056.

82. Amsterdam, A., and Jamieson, J. D. (1974). Studies on dispersed pancreatic exocrine cells. II. Functional characteristics of separated cells. *J. Cell Biol.* **63,** 1057–1073.
83. Williams, J. A., Korc, M., and Dormer, R. L. (1978). Action of secretagogues on a new preparation of functionally intact, isolated pancreatic acini. *Am. J. Physiol.* **235,** 517–524.
84. Jaffrey, C., Eichenbaum, D., Denham, D. W., and Norman, J. (1999). A novel pancreatic model: The Snip method of pancreatic isolation for *in vitro* study. *Pancreas* **19,** 377–381.
85. Logsdon, C. D. (1986). Stimulation of pancreatic acinar cell growth by CCK, epidermal growth factor, and insulin *in vitro*. *Am. J. Physiol.* **251,** G487–G494.

54

Models of Endocrine Insufficiency

Thomas C. Vary

Department of Cellular and Molecular Physiology, Penn State University College of Medicine, Hershey, Pennsylvania 17033

I. Introduction

Homeostasis in the body is a delicate balance regulated by endocrine, metabolic, and neural influences. All three interact to maintain normal physiologic function. In order to understand the role each plays in maintaining homeostasis, one approach has been to modulate the endocrine, metabolic, and/or neural signal and examine the shift away from homeostasis.

Much of our knowledge regarding the function of the endocrine system derives from disease states in which either the hormone is overexpressed (e.g., hyperthyroid, Cushing's disease) or the gland is destroyed (e.g., type 1 insulin-dependent diabetes mellitus, Addison's disease). A list of the major endocrine glands and their primary effect in maintaining homeostatsis is presented in Table I. Once the physiologic effect of the hormone is established, it is possible to administer the hormones to animals or patients with the hormonal defect to establish the role of that particular hormone in maintaining an important aspect of homeostasis. The unraveling of the role of the pancreas in regulating blood glucose concentrations in the latter half of the nineteenth and first half of the twentieth centuries is the classic example of this approach. This approach has led to the successful treatment of individuals with insufficient endocrine function.

Hormones can be categorized into three types on the basis of their chemical structure. The first type is the peptide hormone. These hormones are composed of amino acids linked together to form a polypeptide chain. A prototype peptide hormone is insulin, a protein synthesized by the β-cells of the pancreas. In general, peptide hormones are incapable of entering the cells directly. Instead, the hormones interact with a receptor on the cell surface, which then signals the cell via a second-messenger cascade system.

The second type is the amine. Amine hormones are derivatives of individual amino acids, such as tyrosine. Two hormones representative of this class are thyroxine, secreted by the thyroid gland, and epinephrine, secreted by the adrenal medulla. Despite being derived from the same amino acid, the mechanism of action of these two hormones differs. Epinephrine and norepinephrine function by binding to a receptor on the cell membrane to activate a second-messenger

Table I Major Endocrine Glands and the Primary Metabolic Effects of Their Hormones

Endocrine gland	Hormone(s) secreted	Primary effects
Adrenal		
Cortex	Aldosterone	Regulates renal Na^+ and K^+ excertion
	Cortisol	Antagonizes action of insulin with regard to carbohydrate, fat, and amino acid metabolism; antiinflammatory and supression of immune function
	Sex hormones	Maintenance of libido
Medulla	Catecholamines	Mimics sympathetic nervous stimulation
Pancreas		
	Insulin	Promotes glucose deposition and anabolism
	Glucagon	Promotes glucose production by liver and kidney
Kidney		
	Renin–angiotensin	Regulates salt and water balance and thereby influences blood pressure; stimulus for aldosterone production by adrenal cortex
Liver		
	Insulin-like growth factor-I	Regulates carbohydrate, protein metabolism, and skeletal growth
Thyroid		
	Thyroxine (T_4)	Regulates metabolic rate; modulates cardiac function
Parathyroid		
	Parathyroid hormone	Regulates Ca^{2+} and phosphate metabolism
Gonads		
Ovaries	Estrogen; progesterone	Reproductive hormones; stimulate secondary sexual characteristics
Testes	Testosterone	Reproductive hormones; stimulate secondary sexual characteristics
Pituitary		
Anterior	Tropic hormones	Stimulates growth and secretion in other endocrine glands
Posterior	Vasopressin (antidiuretic hormone)	Conversion of water by kidneys
	Oxytocin	Promotes uterine contractions

cascade. In contrast, thyroid hormone enters the cell and binds to a receptor on the surface of the nuclear membrane. The hormone–receptor complex then enters the nucleus and interacts with the DNA, enhancing the transcription of specific mRNAs.

The third type is the steroid hormone. Steroid hormones are synthesized from the cholesterol molecule and are secreted by many of the reproductive endocrine glands and the adrenal medulla. Hormones in this category include testosterone, progesterone, and the glucocorticoids. Steroid hormones function by penetrating the cell membranes and binding to a receptor within the cell. This receptor–hormone complex then signals the cell to enhance or repress the expression of specific proteins through control of transcription and translation. It is the alteration in the expression of the cellular proteins under hormonal control that ultimately transmits the cellular effect of the hormone on the target cell.

II. General Approaches to Study of Endocrine Insufficiency

There are several general approaches to creating a relative insufficiency of one or more hormones. First, the endocrine gland producing the hormone can be surgically removed. Over a century ago Minkowski and von Meering removed the pancreas from a dog and created a condition clinically indisquishable from diabetes mellitus in humans. The same animal model was used by Banting and Best and played a crucial role in the discovery of insulin and its first therapeutic trials. Second, the endocrine gland can be destroyed chemically. For example, destruction of the thyroid gland follows injection of radioactive iodine. Third, the ability of the exocrine gland to secrete its hormone can be inhibited. For example, diazoxide or somatamedin inhibit the secretion of insulin by the β-cells of the pancreas, leading to an insulin deficiency. Fourth, the hormone can be prevented from binding to its receptor by antihormones. Antihormones are not antibiosynthetic agents, nor do they work by blocking the transfer of the hormone to its cellular targets. Instead, they act at the receptor level. With high affinities for the receptor, the compounds prevent the natural agonist from binding. Thus, while the hormone concentration in the plasma is within normal values, its ability to elicit its metabolic effects is inhibited. An example of this approach is the use of the glucocorticoid receptor antagonist, RU486, which prevents glucocorticoid from binding to its receptor. Fifth, transgenic techniques designed to knock out vital components of the signaling cascade system render the cell essentially resistant to the effects of the hormone. Although it is recognized that hormone resistance and deficiency are not the same phenomena, the effect on the cell or organism can be similar.

Not all techniques that generate an endocrine insufficiency are applicable to every endocrine gland. Furthermore, care must be exercised when creating an endocrine insufficiency that the experiment has not affected another hormone. Hormones can have secondary effects on other endocrine systems. For example, abolishing β-cell function of the pancreas with alloxan also affects the thyroid, leading to a relative hypothyroid state. The following discussions describe various experimental approaches used to create endocrine insufficiencies for the major hormones of the bodies.

Before discussing various animal models of endocrine insufficiency, however, it is important to understand that extrapolating findings from animals to humans requires the utmost care. The "model" does not necessarily represent a complete reproduction of the human disorder in an animal, neither does it necessarily represent the full range of aberrations or complications observed in the human situation. The potential for animal models lies in the opportunity to investigate specific morphologic, biochemical, immunologic, or metabolic parameters associated with endocine insufficiency not readily amenable in the human by sampling of blood or simple biopsy. Therapeutic measures may be tried in animals models prior to use in humans.

III. Methodology Considerations

In assessing the success of the techniques to generate endocrine insufficiency, one generally compares the manipulation to the normal situation. However, care must be taken in what constitutes a "normal" condition. Studies involving hormone concentrations or responsiveness are dependent on the time of day, degree of agitation, gender, reproductive cycle, and/or nutritional status of the subject.

The secretion of several hormones is dependent on the circadian rhythm of the animal. For example, there are pulsatile secretions of growth hormone throughout the day in children, producing large but short-lived peaks of growth hormone in the blood. Therefore, it is prudent, when designing experiments, to manipulate the subjects, whether animal or human, at the same time each day.

The state of agitation and stress in the subject can also affect the endocrine response. For example, the degree of stress the subject undergoes activates the sympathetic autonomic nervous system, which in turn modulates the secretion of epinephrine by the adrenal gland. Therefore, studies should be performed in a constant and quiet environment. With regard to human studies, distractions such as visitors and/or television should be avoided to ensure a constant experimental stage for each subject. Probably the best location for performing human studies would be in a clinical research center where potential confounding effects such as nursing care, monitoring, and diet can be carefully controlled and standardized from one patient to another. However, clinical research can be performed in the absence of such a facility, as long as care is taken to limit differences in treatment of subjects because of study environment.

When working with animals, most institutions require that virus-free animals be used. If not, it is prudent to do so. Generally, an acclimitization period (1 week) is necessary before the animals can be used for an experiment. In addition, care must be taken with transgenic animals to ensure no viruses contaminate the mice. This can be accomplished by performing serology on one or two mice. Animals should be manipulated under conditions that limit the excitability of the experimental animal to be used as well as the control animals used for the study. For example, Garlick and coworkers (1) have found that wrapping rats in a towel limits their agitation during injection of radioactive phenylalanine to measure rates of protein synthesis in the awake animal.

The secretion of certain hormones involved primarily in the regulation of carbohydrate metabolism is modulated by nutrient input. Insulin secretion is regulated not only by the rise in plasma glucose concentrations but also by amino acids. Therefore, the plasma concentrations of insulin will differ immediately following a meal compared with values obtained 12 hr after feeding. Thus, it is important in designing experimental protocol that the nutritional state of the animal is taken into consideration.

In the subsequent sections, methods are described to create a relative hormone insufficiency of several of the endocrine systems described in Table I. In each case several methods are described and the advantages and disadvantages of using each of the techniques are discussed. This is by no means an exhaustive list but provides a framework for assessing various methods to induce alterations in hormones.

IV. Hypothalamus

The hypothalamus is a neural component of the limbic system. As such, the hypothalamus acts as a signaling organ, adapting the body to various environmental stresses. It is unique because neural projections interface directly with the blood, thereby directly secreting hormones and releasing factors into the bloodstream, ultimately inducing systemic changes. The hypothalamus controls many of the autonomic and endocrine functions of the body.

The hypothalamus regulates endocrine function in two ways. First, endings of nerve axons that arise in the supraoptic and paraventricular nuclei of the hypothalamus project to the posterior pituitary. Generation of action potentials in these nerves results in the release of oxytocin or vasopressin (antidiuretic hormone) directly. Therefore, the hypothalamus functions as an endocrine organ. Second, the hypothalamus synthesizes releasing hormones that are discharged into the capillary network of the median eminence of the hypothalamus. The capillaries then converge into portal veins and empty into the sinusoids of the anterior lobe of the pituitary. The releasing hormones interact with their receptors in the anterior pituitary, where they either stimulate or inhibit the secretion of a particular pituitary hormone. Table II lists the hypothalamic releasing hormones and the known actions of these releasing factors on the anterior pituitary.

As can be garnered from examination of the summary of effects of the hypothalamic releasing hormones, oxytocin and vasopressin, disruption of the normal function of the hypothalamus would generate secondary endocrine insufficiencies by virtue of the lack of trophic actions of the hormones or releasing factors on peripheral endocrine glands or organs. Hypothalamic deficiencies can be created in two ways. First, the animals can undergo a complete hypophysectomy. Hypophysectomized animals are generally purchased at a young age, with this procedure already performed prior to shipment from large breeding firms. The problem with this approach is that all hormones and hormone releasing factors of the hypothalamus are adversely affected. One may wish to induce a growth hormone deficiency, for example, but numerous other endocrine systems would also be affected. Second, areas of neurons within a certain region of the hypothalamus can be lesioned. This would represent a more neurosurgical approach to dissecting out only those hormones or releasing factors that you wish to remove. For example, somatostatin-containing neurons are particularly abundant in the anterior periventricular region, whereas growth hormone-releasing hormone is synthesized in the cell bodies of neurosecretory neurons of the arcuate and ventromedial nuclei of the hypothalamus. The problem with this approach is that it is virtually impossible to eliminate only the selected neurons of interest.

V. Pancreatic Insulin Insufficiency

Secretion of insulin from pancreatic β-cells tightly regulates glucose homeostasis by accelerating the uptake and utilization of glucose by insulin-sensitive peripheral tissues, and by inhibiting glucose production. The cellular response to insulin occurs following binding of insulin to its receptor. Following binding to its receptor, the insulin signal is propagated by phosphorylation of specific intracellular proteins that act in concert to amplify and transmit the signal. Type 1 diabetes mellitus results from the complete destruction of the β-cells of the pancreas, and the ultimate loss of circulating insulin. Type 2 diabetes mellitus, the more common form of the disease, is characterized by an inappropriate circulating insulin concentration for a given plasma glucose concentration. What is described in no way is meant to be an absolute list of all the models for insulin insufficiency, but does provide a description of many of the animal models used.

A. Chemical-Induced Destruction of β Islet Cells

Destroying the β islet cells of the pancreas reduces plasma insulin concentrations. Several chemicals are selectively toxic to the pancreatic β-cells. The principal compounds are alloxan (a pyridine with structural similarity to uric acid and and glucose), streptozotocin (which may be considered as

Table II Hypothalamic Releasing Hormones and Their Effects on the Anterior Pituitary

Hypothalamic releasing hormone	Actions on anterior pituitary	Effect of anterior pituitary hormone on peripheral organs
Corticotropin-releasing factor	Stimulates secretion of ACTH	Stimulates production of cortisol and androgens by adrenal cortex; maintains size of zona fasciculus and zona reticularis of adrenal cortex
Thyrotropin-releasing facctor	Stimulates secretion of thyroid-stimulating hormone	Stimulates production of thyroid hormones T_4 and T_3 by thyroid follicular cells, maintains size of follicular cells
	Stimulates synthesis of prolactin	Essential for milk production by lactating mammary gland
Gonadotropin-releasing hormone, luteinizing hormone releasing factor	Stimulates secretion of follicle-stimulating hormone	Stimulates development of ovarian follicles; regulates spermatogenesis in testes
	Stimulates secretion of luteinizing hormone	Causes ovulation and formation of corpus luteum in ovary; stimulates production of estrogen and progesterone by ovary; stimulates testosterone production by testes
Growth hormone-releasing hormone	Stimulates secretion of growth hormone	Stimulates postnatal body growth; counteracts actions of insulin on carbohydrate and lipid metabolism
Somatostatin	Inhibits release of growth hormone	
Dopamine	Inhibits biosynthesis and secretion of prolactin	

glucose with a highly reactive nitrosourea side chain), and Vacor (a rodenticide).

Alloxan became the first diatogenic chemical agent when Dunn and McLetchie accidently produced islet cell necrosis while investigating the nephrotoxicity of uric acid derivatives. Administration of alloxan produces irreversible functional β-cell damage within minutes and structural changes are observed within hours. Severe insulinopenia is induced by intravenous injection of alloxan (60 mg/kg body weight) in the femoral vein (2). To accomplish this, an incision in the groin is made and the facial surrounding the saphenous vein is removed. The alloxan is injected into the vein using a 26-gauge or smaller needle. Bending the needle approximately 45° facilitates the injection. Within 48 hr, animals show insulin concentrations that are below the level of detection (Table III). By 96 hr postalloxan injection, animals succumb to the effects of severe diabetes. However, alloxan is a toxic compound that destroys β-cells by formation of oxygen free radicals. Alloxan shows specific cytotoxic effects on β-cells, whereas other islet cell types are relatively unaffected. To rule out direct toxic effects of alloxan, animals can be maintained on insulin injections for several days following alloxan injection. The insulin treatment can be suspended 48 hr before the animals are sacrificed. A less severe form of diabetes can be induced by injection of 37.5 mg/kg of alloxan (3). These animals show progressive changes in function and metabolism for periods up to 1 month following injection of the lower doses of alloxan (3). Alloxan is highly unstable in water at physiologic pH, but is reasonably stable at pH 3.

In addition to alloxan, which produces a rapid and severe destruction of the β-cells, streptozotocin can be used to induce diabetes. Streptozotocin is a nitrosourea derivative isolated from the mold *Steptomyces achromogenes*. The diabetogenic action of streptozotocin was discovered during routine testing of antibiotics from this mold. Streptozotocin can induce severe insulinopenia in rats and mice when given either as a single dose (50–100 mg/kg in rats), or as multiple smaller doses. Injection of a single dose (50–60 mg/kg) induces insulin concentrations to fall to 10–30% of normal, resulting in hyperglycemia, polyuria, polydipsia, and weight loss. Severe ketosis does not develop and animals survive for several weeks without insulin replacements. The β-cells appear degranulated, but not necrotic, approximately 4 days following injection of the compound. At higher doses, a more profound depression of insulin concentrations occurs, with spontaneous ketosis and death in the absence of insulin replacement. With the injection of multiple low doses of streptozotocin (5 mg/kg for 5 days in mice), diabetes develops more gradually and appears to have an autoimmune, rather than a toxic, component. The syndrome parallels the human condition in that there is mononuclear cell infiltration of the islets (insulinitis) and β-cell destruction, suggesting the pathogenic involvment of cell-mediated immunity. The model is useful as a tool to study ways in which immune processes may enhance the effects of a β-cell cytotoxic agent, but is not satisfactory for study of spontaneous development of type 1 diabetes mellitus.

The rodenticide, Vicor, was established as a potential diabetogenic agent based on observations of survivors of suicide attempts and intoxication accidents. The diabetes induced has a long-term course resembling type 1 diabetes mellitus and its complications. Unfortunately, Vacor is not siutable for experimental studies because the compound is generally fatal along with causing β-cell destruction.

Table III Comparison of Glucose and Insulin Using Different Methods to Induce Diabetes

Method	Glucose (mg/dl)	Insulin (p*M*)
Nondiabetic	121 ± 6	450 ± 50
Alloxan (60 mg/kg)	883 ± 54	ND[a]
Diazoxide	638 ± 6	43 ± 15
Partial pancreatectomy	227 ± 54	240 ± 50

[a]ND, Below level of detection by RIA.

B. Partial Pancreatectomy

Besides cytotoxic destruction of the β-cells of the pancreas, insulinopenia can be initiated by surgical removal of part of the pancreas. The original description of the partial pancreatectomy procedure was published in 1944 by Foglia (4). Farrell and coworkers (5–7) modified the procedure, using rats weighing 110–140 g as opposed to the weights of 90–110 g, suggested by Foglia. By using small rats, larger percentages (≅88%) of the animals become diabetic following pancreatectomy. The procedure is very difficult to perform in rats weighing more than 140 g because the tissue becomes more fibrous. Rats must be fasted overnight and surgery is done on a heating pad, which maintains the core temperature of the rat. Another modification to the original procedure is the use of a microcauterizer to eliminate small pancreatic blood vessels and to reduce bleeding during surgery. Aseptic conditions are maintained throughout the surgery and we have found that methoxyflurane is a very good anesthetic, although it may no longer be available. Alternatively, ether or a combination of acepromazine and ketamine may be used. The procedure requires the physical removal of pancreatic tissue from the splenic, duodenal, and pyloric regions while leaving major blood vessels intact. A laparotomy is performed and the skin is teased away from the abdominal wall. A sterile drape is used to cover the area around the laparotomy. We start with the area under the duodenum and rub pancreatic tissue away from major blood vessels (leaving blood vessels intact) from just above the hepatic portal vein up to the common bile duct. Pancreatic tissue is also removed from under the spleen and the pylorus. When all that tissue is removed and the pancreatic tissue between the duodenum and the bile duct is left intact, the result is a 90% partial pancreatectomy. Removal of pancreatic tissue is accomplished using sterile cotton-tipped swabs. The abdominal wall is sutured using dissolvable stitches and the skin is sutured using 4-0 silk, with discontinuous sutures. At the conclusion of surgery, rats are given ampicillin (5 mg/100 g body weight, subcutaneaously) to prevent infection. Two weeks after partial pancreatectomy, a tail vein blood sample is obtained in the fed state to determine plasma glucose concentrations. Table III shows the effects of partial pancreatectomy on plasma glucose and insulin concentrations.

This surgical procedure for making rats diabetic has several advantages compared with chemical induction of diabetes. First, partially pancreatectomized rats survive and show classic signs of type 1 insulin-dependent diabetes, including elevated plasma glucose concentrations, insulinopenia, and loss of lean body mass (6, 7). Second, the rats grow at a slightly slower rate than controls, but do not need exogenous insulin for survival. Third, the degree of diabetes can be varied by how fastidious the surgeon is in removing all tissue, with the exception of that located between the common bile duct under the duodenum. Fourth, surgical removal of the pancreas completely avoids cytotoxic effects on other tissues, including the glucagon-secreting cells of the pancreas. In contrast to these positive aspects, this procedure results in the loss of other important cells of the pancreas and the loss of ability to synthesize the couterregulatory hormones glucagon and somatostatin. In addition, there is a loss of pancreatic enzymes necessary for digestion; hence, a diet supplemented with pancreatic enzyme must be considered. The procedure is not without a certain degree of variability. The effectiveness of the pancreatectomy in producing insulinopenia is dependent on the ability to identify the pancreas and to preserve adequate segments of the organ. In animals species such as dogs, pigs, and nonhuman primates, the pancreas is a discrete organ that is readily isolated and resected. This is not the case in rodents, where the pancreas is a relatively diffuse organ. The total resection of the pancreas in rats is very difficult to achieve and the development and severity of the diabetes in partially pancreatectomized rats appear to be strain specific.

C. Diazoxide

An acute insulin deficiency can be produced in fed rats using diazoxide, a specific inhibitor of insulin secretion. In this protocol, diazoxide (20 mg in 3 ml 0.05 *N* sodium hydroxide/100 kg body weight) is injected intraperitoneally. Plasma insulin concentrations are decreased within 1 hr and remain that way for up to 3 hr postinjection. Normally, insulin deficiency is associated with changes in other hormones. However, concentrations of IGF-I, glucagon, and corticosterone were not different than controls given vehicle alone (8). Diazoxide-treated rats also show an increase in plasma nonesterified fatty acids and β-hydroxybutyrate, characteristic of an insulin deficiency. Thus, this procedure is rather specific for reducing plasma insulin concentrations.

There are at least two limitations to this technique to induce a relative insulin deficiency. First, the β islets remain sensitive to insulin secretagogues. Diazoxide blocks insulin secretion without inhibiting its biosynthesis. Therefore, insulin most likely accumulates in β-cells and could be liberated after a bolus injection of secretagogue. For example, infusion of high doses of phenylalanine results in a rapid rise in plasma insulin concentrations (8). A second (15 mg in 2 ml of 0.05 *N* sodium hydroxide/100 g body weight) and/or third dose of diazoxide can be given to prevent the secretion of insulin. Thus, care must be taken when performing metabolic studies with compounds known to modulate insulin secretion. Second, the effects of diazoxide are temporary and are reversed within 5 hr. However, this latter limitation may also be considered unique among models of insulin deficiency. Thus, certain measurements could theoretically be performed in the same animal before, during, and after induction of a transient insulin deficiency. Another advantage to this method is that the plasma concentrations of other hormones (e.g., IGF-I, corticosterone, growth hormone) are not appreciably changed following administration of diazoxide (8).

In addition to diazoxide, LN5330, a benzothiadiazine with structural similarities to diazoxide, also produces a rapid fall in plasma insulin concentrations (9). In contrast to diazoxide, LN5330 also caused a marked increase in plasma glucagon concentrations. Therefore, this compound can effectively induce the hormonal environment observed during diabetes in that both insulin deficiency and hyperglucagonemia are observed.

D. Spontaneous Type 1 Diabetes Mellitus-like Syndromes

Insulitis was observed at autopsy of patients with diabetes shortly after the clinical diagnosis of the disease. This observation along with others led to the role of autoimmunity in the etiology of human type 1 diabetes mellitus. Two animal models in particular, the BB rat and the NOD mouse, show a spontaneous development of insulin deficiency. The BB rats were identified because of their mortality in a colony of Wistar rats at BioBreeding Laboratories in Ottawa, Canada. At about 60–120 days of age (mean, 96 days), there is β-cell loss with a concomitant decrease in plasma insulin concentrations in 50–80% of the inbred rats. Most BB rats are insulin dependent within 2 weeks and remission is exceedingly rare. Breeding of BB rats requires great care because of their vulnerability to infections and the requirement for insulin injection once the diabetes is overt. Although both sexes retain fertility, best results are obtained by mating diabetic males with nondiabetic female siblings. The NOD mouse was raised through inbreeding of subline of mice that developed spontaneous cataracts at the Shionogi Research Laboratories in Japan. The etiology of the insulin deficiency resembles that of the BB rat, with insulinopenia observed at approximately 14 weeks. Affected mice have an absolute requirement for insulin.

E. Transgenic Approaches

Several attempts have been made to modulate the signaling cascade for insulin with the hope of mimicking the response to diabetes. The cellular response following binding of insulin to its receptor is mediated by tyrosine phosphorylation of several cytosolic docking proteins (IRS proteins). IRS proteins serve to couple the insulin receptor to various effector molecules such as phosphotidyl-3 phosphate kinase, Grb2/SOS, SHP2, NCK, and CRK. Disruption of the genes encoding the IRS proteins would be expected therefore to negate the insulin signal despite adequate insulin in the circulation. Thus, a cellular endocrine insufficiency would be anticipated.

These approaches have used the approach of removing or "knocking out" specific substrates of the insulin receptor. The overall strategy to produce a knockout is described below. The gene one wants to knock out is cloned and inserted into a targeting vector. The vector is used to delete the specific gene and is replaced with an another piece of DNA, which allows for selection (e.g., an antibiotic-resistance genes cassette). The recombinant vector is then transfected into embryonic stem cells derived from mouse blastocysts. The embryonic stem cells showing the proper recombination are injected into blastocysts and implanted into pseudopregnant foster mothers. The pups' DNA is screened (tail clips), using Southern blot techniques, for the recombinant transfection. Chimeric male pups are then mated with the strain of mice used to implant the embryonic stem cells into the blastocysts. Germ-line transmission is confirmed by Southern blotting. Heterozygous offspring are intercrossed to produce animals homozygous for the deletion of the gene.

Deletion of the IRS-1 protein retards growth, but diabetes does not develop because insulin secretion increases to compensate for the mild insulin resistance in mice (10). However, disruption of IRS-2 gene impairs both peripheral insulin signaling and the ability of the pancreas to compensate by enhancing insulin secretion (11). The IRS-2-deficient mice can be considered an adequate model for human type 2 non-insulin-dependent diabetes mellitus.

The advantage to such a genetic knockout approach is that the gene encoding for the particular endocrine response is removed from the animal. There is no need for additional chemical or surgical procedures to modify hormone action. The plasma concentration of hormones will change only if the defect initiates a compensatory change. Disruption of the IRS-2 gene causes a compensatory increase in the plasma insulin concentration (11). The progression to type 2 diabetes is accompanied by a rise in the plasma insulin concentration to compensate for the insulin resistance. A similar pattern of β-cell deficiency accompanying a peripheral organ insulin resistance indicates that the IRS-2-deficient mice mimic the disease process observed in humans, providing insights into the pathogenesis of the endocrine disorder. In performing experiments, the mice that do not perpetuate the germ line can be used as negative controls for the experiments. This theoretically limits the variability because the genetic background would be identical except for the gene the had been knocked out.

Although this approach seems very straightforward from a technical standpoint, in reality, the process is fraught with pitfalls. First, some of the genetic knockouts lead to nonviable fetuses. Therefore, no live animals are born, limiting the ability to perform experiments. Second, it can be very difficult to generate the knockout gene because of the nature of the gene. Third, although the knockout of the gene and subsequent breeding are successful, the animal may have redundant systems that compensate adequately for the knockout and no abnormal phenotype is observed.

F. Somatostatin

Somatostatin is a growth hormone releasing–inhibiting hormone in the hypothalamus (see Section IV above). It is a potent inhibitor of insulin and glucagon secretion from the pancreas. Somatostain appears to work directly on the pancreas in a dose-dependent manner. At all doses, glucagon secretion is some 20 times more sensitive to the inhibitory effect of somatostatin than is insulin secretion. Thus this represents another technique to modulate pancreatic hormones to create a relative insulin or glucagon insufficiency. Essentially the preparation results in a "pancreas clamp," whereby the secretion of these hormones is inhibited by somatostatin. Moreover, replacing either and/or both insulin and glucagon intraportally by continuous infusion into the animal model or humans allows for the dissection of the role of these hormones in the regulation of metabolism (12–14).

VI. Adrenal Insufficiency

A. Glucorticoids

Glucocorticoids play an essential role in maintaining basal and stress-induced homeostasis. Cortisol is the major glucocorticoid produced by the adrenal cortex. In resting state, the hypothalamus releases corticotropin-releasing hormone (CRH) and arginine vasopressin (AVP) in a circadian pattern, stimulating the anterior pituitary to secrete adrenocorticotropic hormone (ACTH). ACTH stimulates the adrenal cortex to secrete cortisol. During stress, there is an increased release of ACTH and consequently, an elevated plasma cortisol concentration. Cortisol exerts a negative feedback regulation on the secretion of CRH and ACTH, and to a lesser extent AVP. In tissues, an intracellular glucocorticoid receptor mediates the effects of cortisol. The glucocorticoid receptor is a transcription factor regulating a variety of intracellular enzyme systems by binding to specific glucocorticoid response elements (GREs) of regulatory regions of glucocorticoid target genes. Whether glucocorticoids stimulate or repress a particular gene depends upon the structure of the GREs and the presence of additional other transcription factors.

B. Adrenalectomy

Adrenalectomy remains the mainstay for creating an adrenal insufficiency. The adrenals are exposed by a dorsal approach and are removed. Controls animals should undergo similar surgery and manipulation of the adrenal, but no excision of the gland. Animals undergoing adrenalectomy must be given drinking water containing NaCl (0.9%) to compensate for the loss of mineralcorticoid hormone following removal of the adrenals. Furthermore, stresses may be poorly tolerated in the absence of glucocorticoids, leading to exceedingly high mortality rates. To compensate for this, it may be necessary to supplement animals with corticosterone (10 mg/kg body weight, subcutaneous). Another limitation to using adrenalectomy is that although producing a lowering of the adrenal hormones, the plasma concentrations of other hormones may also be affected. For example, adrenalectomy often causes an insulin deficiency. Thus, it becomes difficult, depending on the endpoint being examined, to know whether there is a primary effect of glucocorticoids or a secondary effect due to alteration of another hormone or metabolite.

C. Steroid Receptor Antagonist

It is possible to block the action of glucocorticoids by preventing the hormone from interacting with its glucocorticoid receptor. In the early 1980s such a steroid receptor antagonist was developed. Originally, the 11β-aminophenyl-substituted 19-norsteroid was named RU38486, but this was shortened to RU486. RU486 blocks the ability of glucocorticoids to bind to their receptor. The compound also has significant antiprogestin activity. RU486 binds strongly and specifically to the glucocorticoid receptor (GR), with an affinity some 18 times greater than cortisol. By blocking the ability of glucocorticoids to bind to its receptor, the transmission of the glucocorticoid signal is abated. Binding of RU486 to the GR causes the receptor to assume a different conformation than occurs when the agonist binds to GR. Thus, the RU486–GR complex cannot interact with the DNA elements or other transcription factors to modulate gene expression. This approach offers a different mechanism to create an endocrine insufficiency.

In Cushing's syndrome caused by adrenal overproduction of glucocorticoids or other tumors secreting ACTH, RU486 can suppress the deleterious effects of hypercortisolism. However, in the case of Cushing's disease under control of the hypothalamus–pituitary system, an increase in ACTH is observed with a compensatory response of increased glucocorticoid production by adrenals.

VII. Thyroid Insufficiency

Thyroidectomy remains one method to generate a thyroid insufficiency. It is important to have animals that are age matched for these studies because the thyroid hormones are known to decrease with age. The strain of animal, time of day, and season are also known to modulate thyroid concentrations in the blood (15). Three days following thyroid removal, serum T4 concentrations are reduced approximately 15% in rats (16). Five days after thyroidectomy, serum T_3 concentrations are reduced over 50% compared with sham-operated rats. The failure to completely eliminate thyroid hormone concentrations most likely indicates that the thyroid gland is not completely removed. This observation reflects technical difficulties in removing the entire thyroid gland. Although the thyroid can be removed, thyroid hormones can be retained within cells for long periods of time. Thyroid hormones are detectable in a variety of tissues for periods up to 4 months (17). Consideration of tissue levels, in addition to serum concentrations, is important in assessing the extent of thyroid insufficiency. Thyroidectomy is known to modulate numerous other physiologic functions of the body that may or may not contribute to the endpoint being measured. Thyroidectomy lowers blood volume, cardiac output, body temperature, and growth hormone. Each of these secondary complications should be addressed by using the appropriate controls.

To compensate for possible damage to the parathyroid gland during thyroidectomy, animals should be given calcium supplements by providing 1% calcium lactate in the drinking water. Despite adding calcium lactate to the drinking water, the plasma calcium concentration remains depressed (18).

In addition to surgical ablation, administration of ^{131}I affords a relatively simple and effective means of destroying the thyroid gland. It can produce the same effects as surgical removal of the thyroid.

VIII. Sex Hormones

A. Male Hormones

Males produce the majority of their testosterone in the testes. The easiest way to assess the role of testosterone is to remove the testes. In males, this process is not life threatening. The timing of the castration will dictate whether the secondary sex characteristics will occur. Moreover, to establish that the effects are mediated by testosterone one can treat females with synthetic testosterone such as dihydrotestosterone (19).

In addition, it is possible to block the testosterone receptor. Flutamide is an acetilid, nonsteroidal active antiandrogen compound. It exerts its antiandrogen effects by inhibiting androgen uptake and binding of androgen to its nuclear receptor in target tissues. Prostatic cancers are known to be androgen senstive and to respond to treatments such as flutamide, which counteract the effects of androgen. Likewise, flutamide improves hepatocellular function and cardiovascular function following trauma with hemorrhagic shock (20). (For a more complete description of the aspects of creating a testosterone insufficiency, see Chapter 30, this volume.)

B. Female Hormones

1. Ovariectomy

The ovaries represent a major source of the hormones estrogen and progesterone in nonpregnant females. As such, ovariectomy represents a simple method to remove the major source of production of estrogen and progesterone. Then either estrogen or progesterone may be added back to investigate which hormone or combination is needed to prove a specific effect of the female hormones. (For a more detailed description of aspects of ovariectomy, see Chapter 30, this volume.)

2. Steroid Receptor Antagonist

RU486, in addition to its ability to bind to the GR, also has the ability to bind to the progesterone receptor, thereby acting as an antiprogesterone. The activity of RU486 is predictable based on the role of progesterone in controlling various aspects of the female cycle. In the hypothalamus–pituitary–ovary system, RU486 causes a decrease in luteinizing hormone (LH). In the uterus, the compound prevents the progesterone-induced maturation of the endometrium as well as the myometrium, the contractility of which is normally depressed by progesterone. In early pregancy, RU486 produces a direct effect on the decidua leading to bleeding, detachment of the blastocyte, a secondary increase in uterine prostaglandin, and an increase in the myocontractibility and opening and softening of the cervix. Secondarily, there is a decrease in human chorionic gonadotropin (hCG) and regression of corpus luteum and its hormonal output. These properties of the RU486 with regard to its antiprogesterone activity have been put forth as a method for birth control.

3. Gonadatropin-Releasing Hormone Antagonists

Gonadatropin-releasing hormone antagonists have the distinct advantage of inducing an immediate decrease in circulating gonadatropin concentrations with rapid reversal of the effect. Initially, these compounds looked promising to limit follicle-stimulating hormone (FSH) and LH (Table II) secretion, however, they suffer from two problems. First, the compounds have a relatively short half-life (6 hr). Second, they induce histamine release by mast cells. However, a member of a new generation of these compounds [GnRH antagonist (Nal^1 Glu^6)] is a potent and long-acting GnRH antagonist. While this solves some of the problem, it remains that these compounds can only suppress gonadotropin secretion by 50–60%.

IX. Conclusion

The approaches described in this chapter represent only a cursory insight into the complexity and sophistication of techniques designed to investigate and probe the function of the endocrine glands. The complexity is imparted in part by the nature of the hypothalamus through releasing and inhibiting factors controlling the secretion of so many hormones. What is clear is that in any investigation in which the goal is to induce a relative endocrine insufficiency, multiple approaches must be applied. Otherwise, important aspects of the regulation of homeostasis can be missed.

Acknowledgments

This work was supported by NIGMS Grant GM-39277 and Grant GM-50919 awarded by the National Institutes of Health.

References

1. Garlick, P. J., McNurlan, M. A., and Preedy, V. R. (1980). A rapid and covenienent technique for measuring the rate of protein synthesis in tissue by injection of [^{3}H]phenylalanine. *Biochem. J.* **192,** 719–723.
2. Vary, T. C., and Neely, J. R. (1982). A mechanism for reduced myocardial carnitine levels in diabetic animals. *Am. J. Physiol. Heart Circ. Physiol.* **243,** H154–H158.
3. Feuvray, D., Idell-Wenger, J. A., and Neely, J. R. (1979). Effects of ischemia on rat myocardial function and metabolism in diabetes. *Circ. Res.* **44,** 322–329.
4. Foglia, V. A. (1944). Charcartistics de la diabetes en la rata. *Rev. Soc. Argent Biol.* **20,** 21–37.
5. Farrell, P. A., Caston, A. L., and Rodd, D. (1991). Changes in insulin response to glucose after exercise training in partially pancreatectomized rats. *J. Appl. Physiol.* **70,** 1563–1569.
6. Farrell, P. A., Fedele, M. J., Vary, T. C., Kimball, S. R., and Jefferson, L. S. (1998). Effects of intensity of acute-resistance exercise on rates of

protein synthesis in moderately diabetic rats. *J. Appl. Physiol.* **85,** 2291–2297.

7. Farrell, P., Fedele, M. J., Vary, T. C., Kimball, S. R., Lang, C. H., and Jefferson, L. S. (1999). Regulation of protein synthesis after acute resistance exercise in diabetic rats. *Am. J. Physiol. Endocrinol. Metab.* **276,** E721–E727.
8. Sinaud, S., Belage, M., Bayle, G., Dardevet, D., Vary, T. C., Kimball, S. R., Jefferson, L. S., and Grizard, J. Diazoxide-induced insulin deficiency greatly reduced muscle protein synthesis in rats: Involvement of eIF4E. *Am. J. Physiol. Endocrinol. Metab.* **276,** E50–E61.
9. Hillaire-Buys, D., Ribes, G., Blayac, J. P., and Loubatieres-Mariani, M. M. (1984). A new benzothiadiazine derivative, LN 5330: Effects on pancreatic hormones. *Diabetologia* **27,** 583–586.
10. Tamento, H. (1994). Insulin resistance and growth retardation in mice lacking insulin receptor substrate-1. *Nature (London)* **372,** 182–186.
11. Withers, D. J., Gutierrez, J. S., Towery, H., Burks, D. J., Ren, J.-M., Previs, S., Zhang, Y., Bernal, D., Pons, S., Shulman, G., Bonner-Weir, S., and White, M. (1998). Disruption of IRS-2 causes type 2 diabetes in mice. *Nature (London)* **391,** 900–904.
12. Cherrington, A. D., Chaison, J. L., Liljenquist, J. E., Lacy, W. W., and Park, C. R. (1978). Control of hepatic glucose output by glucagon and insulin in the intact dog. *Biochem. Soc. Symp.* **43,** 31–45.
13. Cherrington, A. D. (1997). Banting Lecture 1997. Control of glucose uptake and release by the liver *in vivo*. *Diabetes* **48,** 1148–1214.
14. Liljenquist, J. E., Mueller, G. L., Cherrington, A. D., Perry, J. M., and Rabinowitz, D. (1979). Hyperglycemia per se (insulin and glucagon withdraw) can inhibit glucose production in man. *J. Clin. Endo. Metab.* **48,** 171–175.
15. Wong, C. C., Dohler, K. D., Atkinson, M. J., *et al.* (1983). Influences of age, strain, and season on diurnal periodicity of thyroid stimulating hormone, thyroxine, triiodothyronin and parathyroid hormone in serum of male laboratory rats. *Acta Endocrinol.* **102,** 377–385.
16. Moley, J. F., Ohkawa, M., and Chaudry, I. H. (1984). Hypothyroidism abolishes the hyperdynamic phase and increases susceptibility to sepsis. *J. Surg. Res.* **36,** 265–273.
17. Obregon, M. J., Mallol, J., Escobar del Ray, F., and Morrele de Escobar, G. (1981). Presence of L-thyroxine and 3,5,3′-triiodo-L-thyroxine in tissues from thyrectomized rats. *Endocrinology* **109,** 908–913.
18. Hasselgren, P.-O., Chen, I.-W., James, J. H., Sperling, M., Warner, B. W., and Fischer, J. E. (1987). Studies on the possible role of thyroid hormone in altered muscle protein turnover during sepsis. *Ann. Surg.* **206,** 18–24.
19. Angele, M. K., Ayala, A., Cioffi, W. G., Bland, K. I., and Chaudry, I. H. (1998). Testosterone: The culprit for producing splenocyte immune depression after trauma hemorrhage. *Am. J. Physiol. Cell Physiol.* **274,** C1530–C1536.
20. Remmers, D. E., Wang, P., Cioffi, W. G., Bland, K. I., and Chaudry, I. H. (1997). Testosterone receptor blockade after trauma-hemorrhage improves cardiac and hepatic functions in males. *Am. J. Physiol. Heart Circ. Physiol.* **273,** H2919–H2925.

55

Animal Models in Transplantation

I. L. Laskowski,*,† J. B. Ames,* M. Gasser,*,‡ D. Whitley,§ and N. L. Tilney*

**Surgical Research Laboratory, Harvard Medical School and Department of Surgery, Brigham and Women's Hospital, Boston, Massachusetts 02115*
†Department of General and Transplant Surgery, Warsaw Medical University, 02-006 Warsaw, Poland
‡Department of Surgery, University of Wuerzburg, 97080 Wuerzburg, Germany
§University of Alabama, Birmingham, Alabama 35294

I. Introduction

New developments in transplantation have occurred over the past decades through advances in cell physiology, molecular biology, and pharmacology. In parallel, investigations involving engraftment and manipulation of vascularized organs in laboratory animals have been designed for potential clinical application. Most of the early studies in the field were carried out in large animals and were concerned primarily with improvement of surgical techniques and development of treatments directly relevant to transplantation in patients. Such models still remain important in preclinical trials testing newer immunosuppressive agents. To most individual investigators, however, such studies are costly and variations between outbred species often preclude more than relatively cursory descriptions of biological events.

Before the early 1960s, when Sun Lee first established microvascular techniques to transplant vascularized organ grafts in rats, studies in transplantation biology in small animals had been limited to the grafting of skin (1). Medawar's first description of the "homograft response" in 1944 involved the study of morphologic changes during rejection of skin grafts; the original dogmas of the new subject were formulated on this model, particularly the phenomena of host alloresponsiveness leading to immunologic destruction of foreign tissues and host unresponsiveness allowing their indefinite survival (2). Once techniques to transplant vascularized organs became established, however, many of the original rules had to be redefined. The ability to perform such procedures in inbred strains of small laboratory animals as well as in those lacking particular genes and gene products has encouraged more controlled, complex, and reproducible studies. In addition, increasing information from immunohistology and molecular biology are providing an ever-clearer understanding of the cellular and subcellular interactions between the host and a foreign graft.

Thus, the majority of surgical approaches used currently in studies of transplantation biology are carried out in rodents. Some of these have been reviewed elsewhere (3, 4). The rat has become the favored animal for several reasons. A variety of genetically disparate inbred strains that are available allow predictable degrees of alloresponsiveness against tissue allografts for detailed examination of particular host immune mechanisms. The animals are relatively inexpensive and easy to handle. The species is also large enough to allow research fellows and beginning investigators to perform satisfactory microvascular procedures at relatively low magnification after moderate training and perseverance as well as to develop facility with fine surgical instruments and appropriate sutures. Determining the individual roles of particular cell types and inflammatory factors using genetically altered ("knockout") strains of inbred mice has also come into vogue in recent years, particularly for heterotopic heart transplantation. Although a few talented individuals report the engraftment of kidneys and even livers in this species, such microvascular feats are difficult and involve a long learning curve.

Because the vast majority of transplant models involve the rat, the following discussion will concentrate primarily on various operative maneuvers used in that animal. We will first discuss general techniques for cell isolation and manipulations used in transplantation biology and immunology, routes of intravenous access for administration of drugs or cell transfer, and then the microsurgical techniques of tissue and organ transplantation. It is helpful to use male rats weighing between 150 and 200 g as recipients, because the vessels of older and larger rats are not proportionately greater in size and the increased amounts of retroperitoneal fat may hamper easy dissection. The use of larger species such as dogs, pigs, or primates will not be discussed, because relevant experiments involve primarily preclinical testing of immunosuppressive agents and some xenograft studies.

II. General Techniques

A. Harvesting and Separation of Leukocyte Populations

Suspensions of lymphocytes are necessary in a variety of experimental protocols, particularly for fluorescence-activated cell sorting (FACS), for the mixed lymphocyte reaction, for assays of cytotoxicity, and for adoptive transfer. Although splenic lymphocytes are used for many assays, lymph node lymphocytes or the recirculating population drained from the thoracic duct are often more immunologically active and may be preferable. In combination, lymph nodes, thymus, spleen, and circulating lymphocytes comprise a lymphoid organ of considerable size (5).

The anatomy of the lymphoid tissue in the rat has been well defined (Fig. 1). Both somatic and visceral lymph nodes may be isolated and used as a source of lymphocytes. Commonly harvested groups include the superficial and deep cervical, axillary, and brachial nodes. The femoral nodes are usually too small for use. Mesenteric lymph nodes are large and easily obtainable. All nodes are cleaned of surrounding areolar tissue and placed into cold RPMI 1640 medium on ice. They are then expressed through a 60-gauge stainless-steel mesh using a rubber stopper. The cells are placed in approximately 10 ml of medium and washed twice with centrifugation at 1400 rpm for 10 min. The supernatant is removed without disturbing the cell pellet, which is then resuspended in complete medium (RPMI 1640, 5 m*M* HEPES buffer, 2×10^{-5} *M* 2-mercaptoethanol, 100 U/ml penicillin, 100 μg/ml streptomycin, and 10% fetal calf serum). Washed splenocytes are suspended in 0.83% hypotonic (pH 7.21) ammonium chloride and allowed to stand at room temperature for 10 min to lyse erythrocytes. The red cell-free lymphocytes are then washed three times and resuspended in complete medium. Cell number can be determined using a hemacytometer and adjusted as necessary. Cells may be stored on ice until used.

Discrete populations and subpopulations of lymphocytes can be identified and isolated by phenotype ($CD4^+$, $CD8^+$) using monoclonal antibodies. T cells will be enriched by resuspension in complete medium and filtering slowly (1 hr at 37°C) through a nylon wool column (loose nylon wool placed in the barrel of a 20-ml syringe). B cells and macrophages adhere to the nylon wool and are excluded. The nonadherent T cells in the effluent are labeled with the appropriate monoclonal antibody. To remove the $CD8^+$ population, for instance, cells are incubated with a monoclonal antibody directed against the CD8 receptor. The monoclonal antibody coated on Dynabeads (Degalan V26 beads, Degussa, Teterboro, N. J.) recognizes all mouse antirat IgG subclones. The antibody-positive cells, attached to the magnetic beads, at a ratio of 5:1 beads:target cells, are isolated with a magnetic particle concentrator. The purity of the negatively selected population is confirmed by FACS analysis. The cells are then counted and numbers adjusted for use.

Macrophage-rich peritoneal exudate cells are collected from the abdominal cavity of the animal. These are induced by intraperitoneal injection of 5 ml of fetal calf serum on paraffin oil 48 hr previously. From each rat $(20–40) \times 10^6$ cells may be obtained by washing the peritoneal cavity. The population includes 60–70% large mononuclear cells, primarily macrophages, and 15–30% small lymphocytes. After the nonadherent lymphocytes have been washed away, the macrophages sticking to the glass tube or petri dish may be isolated by adding small amounts of procaine to the washing fluid.

B. Harvest of Bone Marrow Cells

Stem cells may be obtained from the bone marrow of both rats and mice. The humerus, femur, and tibia of the animals are collected, the ends removed, and the marrow cavities flushed with RPMI 1640 medium until the color turns white. The cells are dispersed by repeated expression through an 18-gauge needle. These are then percolated

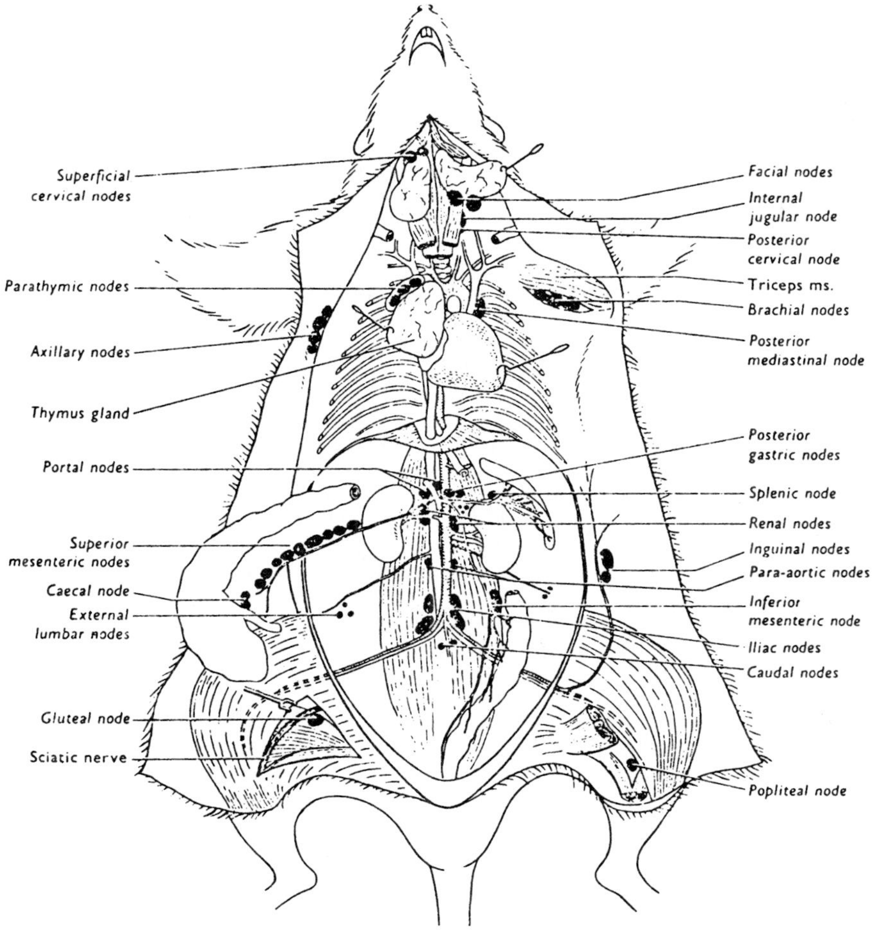

Figure 1 Anatomy of lymphoid tissue in the rat. Adapted from Sanders and Florey (1940) *Br. J. Exp. Path.* **21**, 275, by permission of Blackwell Science Ltd. Adapted figure from Tilney (5).

through a nylon wool column, washed twice, and counted with a hemacytometer. Subpopulations of lymphocytes may be separated using the Dyna bead technique.

C. Intravenous Access

The most convenient intravenous access for administration of either drugs or cell suspensions is the penile vein of male rats. A 25-gauge needle is used for injection of the anesthetized animal. With care, this route can be used several times. Tail veins are an important alternative route, particularly in young animals. Small-gauge needles may be placed in these veins and taped in place for intravenous administration of fluid. The isolated femoral vein is also a dependable access site for prolonged intravenous use (Fig. 2) (5a). A longitudinal incision is made in the groin of the anesthetized animal. After opening the subcutaneous tissues with forceps, the femoral vein is exposed below the inguinal ligament and approximately a 5-mm length is isolated. Two 4-0 silk loops are placed around it. The distal one is ligated and the proximal one is held under slight tension to prevent retrograde blood flow. A small transverse incision made in the anterior portion of the vein is dilated with forceps. Soft polyethylene or silicone tubing (0.965 mm OD) is introduced and advanced for about a centimeter proximally. The tubing is secured in place by ligating the proximal loop. The other end of the cannula is brought out through the buttock of the animal via a large-bore needle for external intravenous administration or attached to an osmotic pump implanted subcutaneously if desired. For continuous intravenous infusion the animal should be placed in a restraining cage.

D. Microsurgery

Appropriate training of the person performing the surgery is of great importance. Although heart transplantation in rats can be carried out under direct vision or with 1.5–2× magnifying loupes, the majority of finer procedures must be performed under a binocular operating microscope with magnification ranging between 5 and 40×. An additional

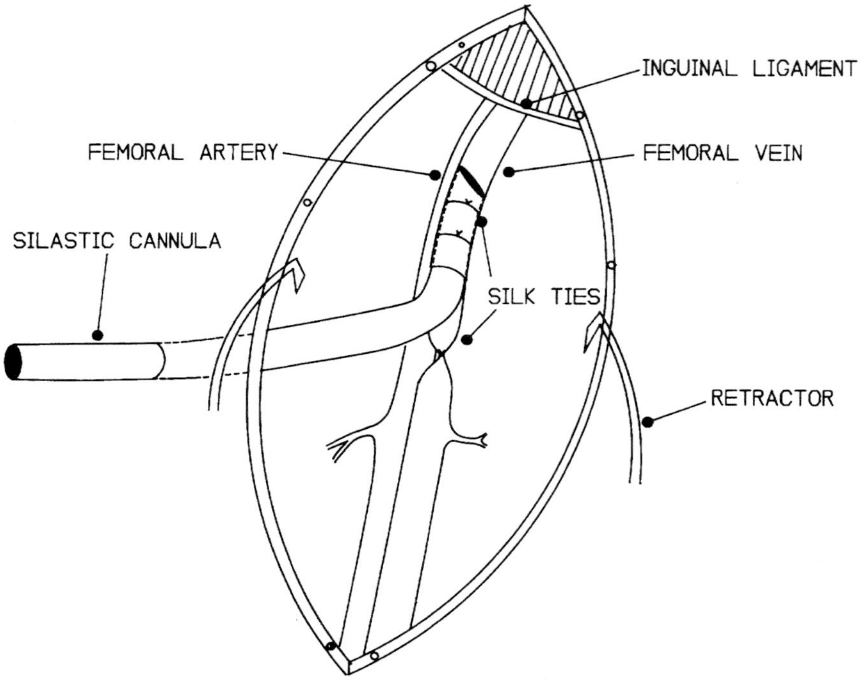

Figure 2 Technique of femoral vein catheter placement in the rat. From Jeppsson (5a). Permission granted by Gordon and Breach Publishers.

monocular head may be useful for teaching purposes or for operations that may require the help of an assistant. To achieve the confidence of movement and stability needed during long operations, the operator should be seated comfortably at the operating table with appropriate support for both forearms. A dedicated operating room for small animal work is optimal (Fig. 3). The light source should be directly focused on the small field. To avoid high costs and unnecessary animal wastage, initial practice for microsurgical suturing should be performed using silicone catheters, rubber

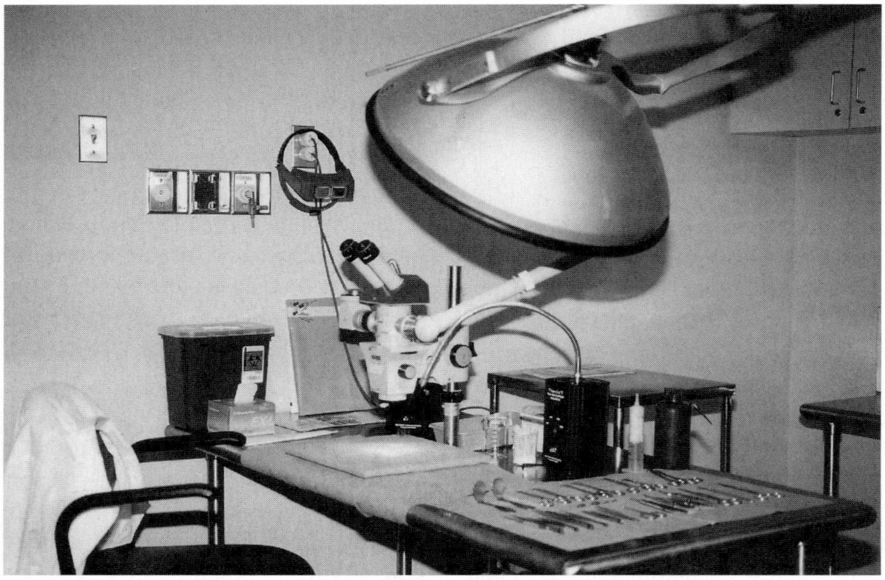

Figure 3 A well-equipped microsurgical laboratory, with standard steel operating table, angle light including a focused light source, and dissecting microscope.

gloves, and other artificial materials. The operator should then practice on dead animals used for other studies and preserved for such a purpose and then perfect individual portions of a given procedure on a living animal. Microsurgical operations involve long minutes of minimal movement and demand a great deal of patience and concentration. Continuous practice and training is required to achieve final success.

The majority of microsurgical instruments used for organ transplantation in small laboratory animals are ophthalmic or fine plastic surgical instruments (Fig. 4) and include the following items:

1. Microsurgical forceps, sizes 3–5 depending on the types of procedures and sizes of the vessels or other structures that require delicate manipulation.
2. Two pairs of straight scissors, small and medium.
3. One pair of 45° angled forceps, sizes 3–5 used for fine dissection.
4. A spring-loaded microsurgical needle holder with or without a lock, depending on the preference of the operator.
5. Several microvascular clamps.
6. A set of retractors of different lengths, preferably made of malleable stainless steel.
7. A pair of small-angled scissors.
8. Small neurosurgical spring clips are often preferred to vascular clamps to occlude the aorta or other vessels.

Good quality microsurgical instruments are expensive and require special care. Immediately after use they should be soaked in warm soapy water and thoroughly cleaned with a toothbrush. They should be handled individually and stored separately in designated boxes with their tips protected with short lengths of rubber tubing. Under no circumstances should they be carried or placed together with larger instruments. Occasionally, they should be oiled to facilitate the movement of their hinges and to protect them from corrosion. Damaged instruments should be repaired or replaced—broken instruments frustrate the operator, affect the surgical performance, and ultimately may result in higher animal mortality and experimental failure.

The optimal suture for microsurgical anastomoses is nonabsorbable monofilament of a size ranging from 7-0 to 10-0, depending on the size of the vessels. The needles should be atraumatic with diameters between 150 and 75 μm; their shape should be three-eighths of a circle. For ligation of larger vessels, 5.0 or 6.0 silk is most suitable and for closure of the chest or abdomen a 3.0 or 4.0 nonabsorbable suture on a straight or curved cutting needle is recommended.

The anesthetized animal can be positioned conveniently on a corkboard using pins placed through small pieces of adhesive tape around the distal extremities. A supply of cotton buds, needles, and syringes of various sizes is necessary (Fig. 5). Surgical incisions are usually not dressed, because the animal will quickly remove the bandage.

E. Anesthesia

Diethyl ether has been important for decades and probably remains the optimal anesthetic for rats, despite increasing pressure from animal committees to use other less flammable agents. However, ether has decided advantages. It is easy to use, relatively safe if standard precautions against flammability are taken, and very effective. It can be administered by ether cone consisting of a large Falcon tube or a

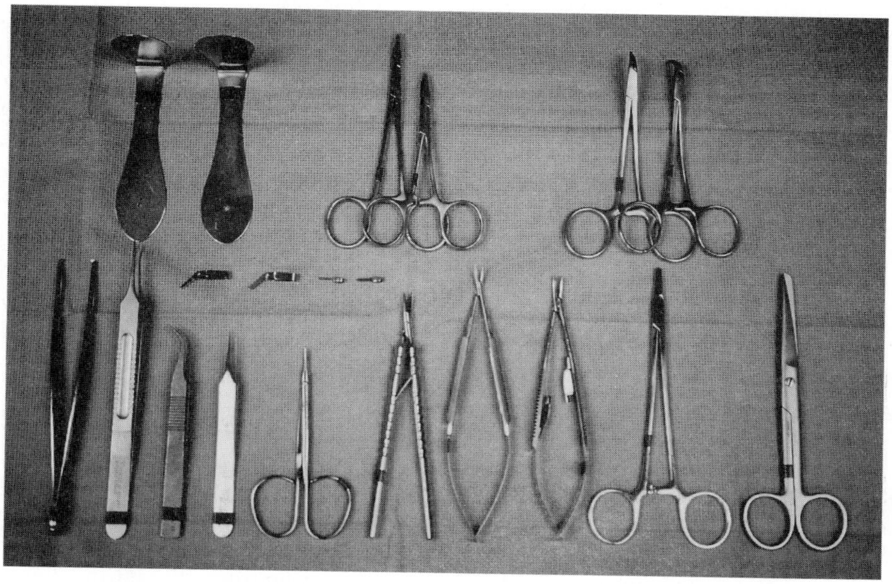

Figure 4 Commonly used microsurgical instruments for organ transplantation.

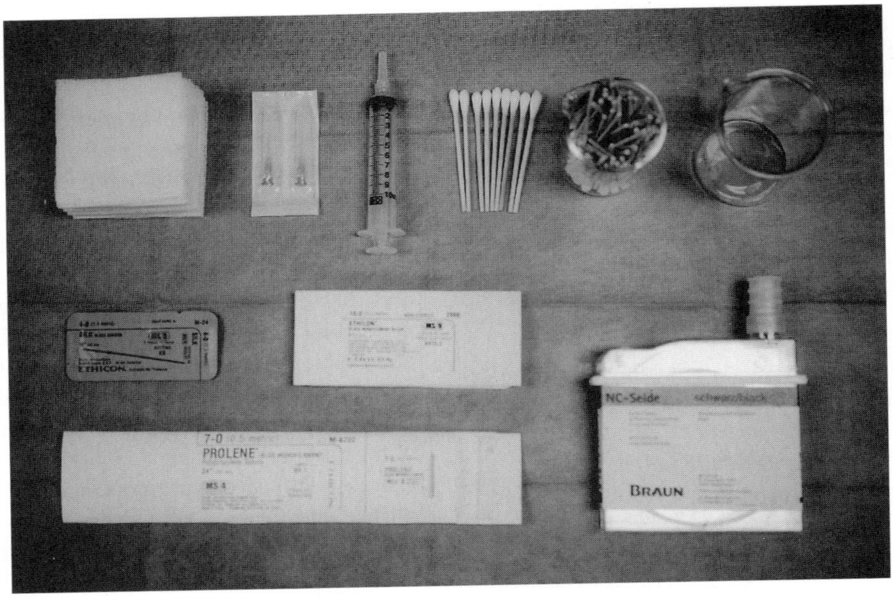

Figure 5 Additional materials used in microsurgery.

syringe cover with gauze packed into the base; this can be moistened intermittently with the anesthetic as necessary. Moving the end of the cone nearer or farther from the animal's muzzle can control the level of anesthesia. If there is a respiratory arrest from overdose, the rat can often be resuscitated by placing a rubber tube over its nose; the operator breathes puffs into the other end. Diethyl ether does not cause changes in cardiac output or peripheral vasoconstriction. This is particularly important because successful kidney transplantation and to a lesser degree heart transplantation in the rats is dependent on optimal hemodynamics both in the donor and the recipient. The kidney is particularly susceptible to vasospasm. If the hemodynamic parameters of the donor rat are depressed, the organ, once transplanted in a vasospastic state, may show initial delayed graft function, which influences markedly the subsequent of host immunological events. Alternatively, long-acting agents such as ketamine or Nembutal injected intramuscularly may give effective anesthesia for the time necessary to perform a transplant operation (6).

III. General Operative Procedures

A. Drainage of the Thoracic Duct

Drainage of the thoracic duct is an alternative method for obtaining high numbers of lymphocytes other than isolating them from lymph nodes, as well as mechanically depleting the animal of circulating T cells for particular experiments (7). Rats or mice are anesthetized and positioned supine with both front legs extended to the right. Access to the left flank is obtained by a short subcostal incision. After the left kidney is isolated and moved medially, the thoracic duct is identified in its subdiaphragmatic portion directly above the cisterna chyli. Surrounding tissues can be cleared from the thoracic duct by careful dissection with damp cotton swabs or blunt forceps. A length of 4-0 silk is placed beneath the duct and a small transverse incision is performed at its junction with the cisterna chyli. After gentle dilatation of this incision with forceps the beveled U-shaped end of a polyethylene cannula (0.61 mm OD), ~25 cm in length filled with heparinized saline, is inserted and tied in place. The other end of the cannula is led out through the skin of the dorsal lumbar area of the subject via a large-bore needle. After closure of the incision, the animal is placed in a restraining cage and the end of the silicone tubing is placed in a cooled collection bottle (Fig. 6). The animal is infused intravenously with Ringer's lactate at the rate of 3ml/hr via an infusion pump. Rats routinely drain over 50 ml of cell-rich lymph/24 hr. Over the first hour, it is important to clear the tubing of small clots that may form; once this transient hypercoaguable state ceases, the lymph will drip freely for 24–48 hr. After that time, however, the output of circulating lymphocytes drops to low and stable levels and the experiment should be terminated.

B. Thymectomy

Thymectomy is performed in young (6-week old) rats by splitting the upper third of the sternum via a midline cervicothoracic incision. The thymus is exposed, grasped gently, teased away from the surrounding tissues, and removed intact. The strap muscles and sternum are reapproximated

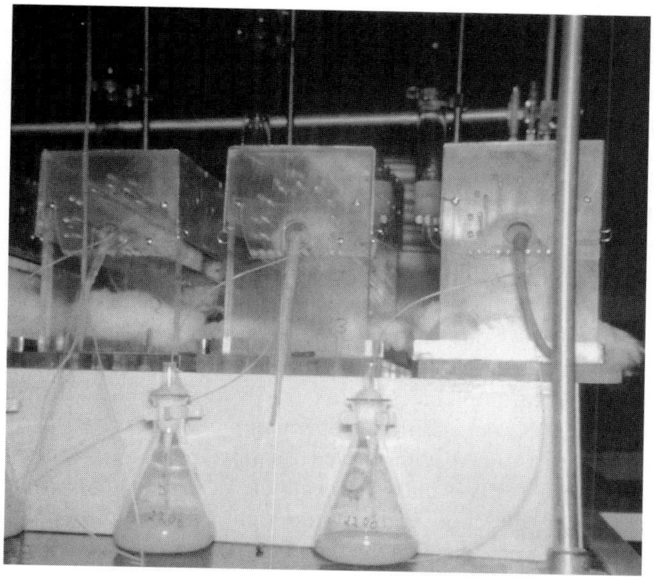

Figure 6 Several rats with thoracic duct fistulas are seen in their restraining cages. The lymph drips dependently into flasks. Intravenous replacement is carried out via the tail veins.

rapidly using a single 4-0 silk suture. The chest should be compressed transiently to remove residual air as the sternal incision is closed. After sacrifice, the animals should be examined for remnants of thymic tissue, and if part of an experiment involving complete thymectomy, those with retained tissue must be excluded. If pure thymocytes are being collected, it is important to remove the parathymic lymph nodes embedded on either side of the gland because they may contaminate the desired cell population. The thymus of mice can be aspirated via a small neck incision.

C. Brain Death

There has been increasing interest over the past few years on the influence of initial injury of an organ on both its short- and long-term behavior following transplantation. Because the effects of the interrelated risk factors of donor brain death and ischemia–reperfusion injury are considered to be important risk factors for the fate of an organ transplant, the techniques for producing such injuries in rats will be described, as a potentially relevant clinical model.

Two kinds of experimental brain death have been described, explosive and gradual onset (8, 9). Much of the earlier work on explosive brain death was performed on large animals and related primarily to resultant functional cardiac changes and morphologic abnormalities in the myocardium; more recent interest in the subject in regard to other organs has centered around controlled studies in rats. Explosive brain death can be produced by rapid balloon inflation (200 μl of saline) of a 3F Fogarty arterial embolectomy catheter introduced into the subdural space through an occipital burr hole. This maneuver suddenly increases intracranial pressure and causes herniation of the brain stem within 20 min. The rats are tracheostomized for intubation with a number 13 blunt-tip cannula and mechanically ventilated for periods up to 6 hr on a rodent ventilator. For gradual-onset brain death, catheter inflation is performed more slowly and under electroencephalographic (EEG) monitoring via an EEG electrode placed on the cranium and a reference electrode attached to the ear. Recordings are performed prior to inflation of the intracranial balloon, during inflation, and for 3 min every hour thereafter. Blood pressure is monitored via a femoral artery catheter. To raise intracranial pressure, the balloon is inflated with 40 μl of saline/min until respiration ceases. The average balloon volume that consistently abolishes all EEG activity is ~200 μl. The balloon is kept inflated during the entire 6-hr follow-up period. In instances in which animals exhibited hypotension and circulatory collapse after induction of brain death, the intracranial balloon volume can be reduced by 10 μl of saline/min until they become normotensive again. The major criterion of herniation of the brain stem and brain death is the development of complete cerebral inactivity confirmed by flatline tracings. The absence of reflexes, apnea, and maximally dilated and fixed pupils confirm the condition.

D. Renal Ischemia–Reperfusion Injury

The abdomen of the anesthetized animal is opened in the midline, the right renal vessels and ureter are ligated and divided, and the right kidney is removed (10). The left kidney, with its artery, vein, and ureter, is isolated from the surrounding fat. The aorta is dissected free proximal and distal to the renal artery and clamped either with small vascular clamps or loops of 4-0 silk held under tension. The ureter is clamped proximally to prevent backflow of blood to the organ via the ureteral vessels. The renal vein is clamped at its junction with the vena cava and a small transverse incision is made in the anterior portion. Cold preservation solution (~5 ml) is then flushed through the kidney by syringe injection into the aorta. This exits via the vent in the vein. Following the flush, the aorta and renal vein are repaired using 10-0 monofilament suture. If cold ischemia studies are to be performed the kidney may then be moved outside the abdomen, wrapped in gauze, and iced for the desired period of study. At the time of reperfusion, the kidney is replaced in the flank, the abdomen is flushed with saline, the clamps are removed, and the abdominal incision is closed.

To produce a warm ischemic injury, the kidney can either be flushed with room temperature preservation solution or the renal vessels can be clamped for the desired period of time. Approximately 45–60 min of warm ischemia will result in significant damage to the kidney, as reflected by elevated serum creatinine levels within the first 24–48 hr and increasing levels of urine protein thereafter. If the ischemic interval is substantially prolonged animals die of acute renal failure. To achieve a similar injury in a perfused kidney, warm ischemia must be continued for 60–75 min and cold ischemia greater than 4 hr. Both warm and cold ischemia–reperfusion types of injury can be studied in isograft and allograft transplant models.

IV. Organ Transplantation

A. Heterotopic Heart Transplantation

This technique of cardiac transplantation in the rat was described in 1964 by Abbot *et al.* (11). A similar method can be used in mice. It remains the most frequently performed organ grafting procedure in transplantation biology. However, due to the heterotopic placement of the organ to the recipient infrarenal great vessels, the heart does not function hemodynamically despite normal ventricular contractions secondary to coronary blood flow. Because the only blood pumped by the heart is from the coronary sinus, this is a nonworking preparation (Fig. 7).

The anesthetized donor is positioned supine (12). The ventral surface is shaved and disinfected appropriately, and the abdominal cavity is opened in the midline. The inferior vena cava (IVC) is exposed by moving the viscera to the right. Heparin (500–700 IU) may be injected intravenously, although many investigators do not anticoagulate either donor or recipient. The diaphragm is incised and the anterior portion of the thorax is opened with a pair of heavy scissors by cutting through the rib cage bilaterally. The adherent pericardium is divided and the musculocostal flap is elevated and fixed to the corkboard to the left of the donor. The remainder of the pericardium is opened, exposing the proximal IVC and both superior vena cavae (SVC). The ascending aorta is dissected free to the brachiocephalic artery. Cold saline or cardioplegic solution (8–10 ml) may be flushed into the IVC depending on operator preference. The three cavae are isolated with curved forceps and are ligated. A length of 3-0 silk is placed beneath the IVC, then guided in a clockwise direction beneath the right SVC, through the transverse sinus beneath the pulmonary artery and aorta, and beneath the left SVC. The length of silk is then looped around the heart and used to mass ligate the pulmonary veins. The heart is gently pulled caudad between the fingers. One blade of a pair of fine blunt-tipped scissors is placed in the transverse sinus and the aorta and pulmonary trunk are transected, leaving as much length of these vessels as possible. The vena cavae are divided distal to their individual ligatures. The heart is removed after division of the pulmonary veins distal to the mass ligature. In a variation of this retrieval technique, the right and left pulmonary veins may be bluntly separated and ligated with the right SVC and left SVC, respectively. Placement of the heart in cold saline completes this step. It is crucial to flush any clots from the aorta and pulmonary artery above their valves.

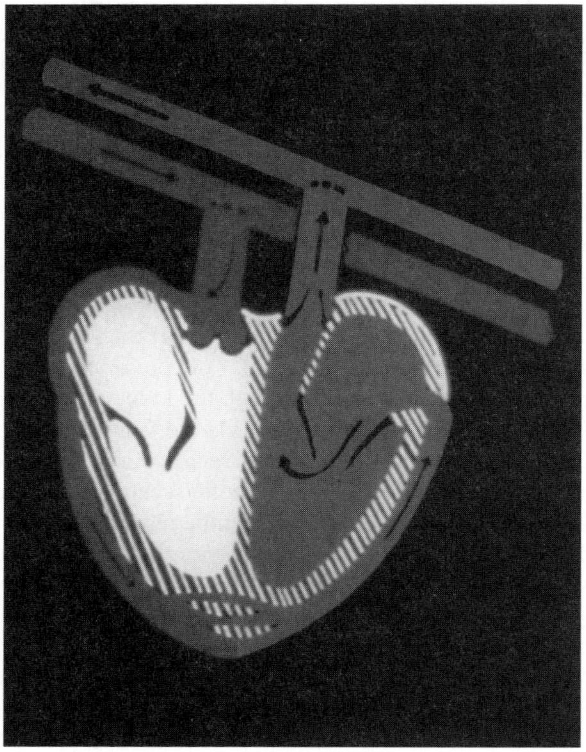

Figure 7 Heterotopic heart transplantation with end-to-side anastomoses of donor aorta and pulmonary artery and recipient abdominal aorta and IVC, respectively.

The abdominal cavity of the anesthetized supine recipient is opened in the midline. The intestines are packed and retracted into the left flank or placed outside the abdomen and wrapped in damp gauze. The IVC and abdominal aorta immediately distal to the renal vessels are exposed by opening the overlying retroperitoneum with forceps or moist cotton swabs. The splanchnic nerves running along the anterior part of these vessels are removed. Because the aorta and IVC are loosely approximated by connective tissue for about 5 mm below the renal vessels, they can easily be separated and isolated. More distally, however, they must be dissected together, because they are tightly adherent and will be damaged if separated. Lumbar veins are ligated *in situ*. The isolated segment of IVC is carefully lifted and the dorsal lumbar vein or veins are dissected free and ligated *in situ*. The distal aorta and vena cava are clamped together and vascular clamps or spring clips are placed individually on the proximal vessels. Alternatively, lengths of 4-0 silk can be looped twice around the distal vessels and the proximal IVC, and held on tension with small mosquito clamps pinned to the corkboard. The proximal aorta is then occluded with a neurovascular spring clip. The corkboard is then rotated so that the left flank of the recipient faces the operator. A small (0.3 mm) longitudinal incision is made in the aortic wall with a tip of an ophthalmic microblade or other sharp blade. Alternatively, a small transverse incision is produced with sharp scissors by lifting up the anterior wall of the aorta with fine forceps. This tiny incision allows the blade of the scissors to enter the aorta and to extend the incision proximally and distally. The aorta is then flushed with saline to remove all clots. The donor heart is positioned on the right of the recipient abdominal cavity with the aorta ventral and wrapped in damp gauze. The end-to-side aortic anastomosis is performed using 7-0 or 8-0 nonabsorbable monofilament suture. Single-armed stay sutures are placed in each end of the arterial incision, outside to inside through the recipient aorta and inside to outside through the donor aorta and tied in place. The nonarmed ends of these sutures are clamped with a mosquito forceps to allow controlled tension on the walls of the collapsed vessels. The anterior wall is then closed from the outside with a running suture, which is tied to the opposite stay suture. Care must be taken not to incorporate the back wall. The board is then turned 180° and the donor heart is flipped to the left to complete the other side of the arterial anastomosis.

A small incision in the anterior wall of the inferior vena cava is then made in similar fashion as in the aorta, or alternatively, a small ellipse can be cut from the wall with scissors. The lumen is flushed to remove all clots. If there is blood leakage into the empty lumen, missed lumbar veins must be identified and ligated. The venous anastomosis is performed with the heart lying on the left of the animal and placed under slight tension via the long end of the pulmonary vein mass ligature. Stay sutures position the donor pulmonary artery end-to-side to the recipient IVC. The distal suture is tied, and the proximal one is kept on slight tension so as to allow perfect visualization of the posterior walls of both vessels. The armed end of the tied suture is then sewn from outside to inside the posterior wall of the recipient vena cava and used to join the back walls of both veins from the inside in a continuous fashion. This posterior suture is then led to the outside of the vessel and can either be tied to the stay suture or continued around the anterior wall and tied to itself. Great care should be taken not to pull the completed suture too tight because this can result in "purse stringing" and stenosis of the anastomosis. The proximal caval clamp or loop and then the distal clamp or loop are slowly released in sequence, followed by removal of the proximal arterial clamp. This maneuver should take 1–2 min to allow sealing of the suture line. Slight pressure held on the venous and then the arterial anastomoses with moist cotton buds ensures hemostasis and prevents blood loss. With revascularization, the heart will enlarge and become pink and well oxygenated; fine ventricular fibrillation will begin within several seconds, which coarsens and is replaced by organized contractions. Significant anastomotic bleeding that persists following application of pressure may be repaired with a single fine suture if necessary after reclamping the proximal aorta. The tiny bronchial artery that runs between the aortic root and the pulmonary artery should be suture-ligated, because this may eventually bleed and can cause death.

A more physiologic model of heterotopic heart transplantation was described in 1995 (13). This technique utilizes a right–left shunt following removal of the atrial septum. The pulmonary artery is ligated, the tricuspid valve is removed, and the heart is anastomosed to the infrarenal portion of the vena cava and the abdominal aorta via the right atrium and ascending donor aorta, respectively. The shunt allows the hemodynamic function of the left ventricle to resemble that of an orthotopic heart more closely than the standard method.

Heterotopic heart transplantation in the mouse is performed in similar fashion except that 10-0 suture is used and the procedure is performed under a microscope.

B. Kidney Transplantation

Although renal transplantation in rats was described in the 1960s, it has been used less in transplantation biology than the heart because of its technical difficulty. On the other hand, unlike the heart, serial functional studies of renal function can be carried out. Two basic techniques are used: orthotopic placement with end-to-end vascular and ureteral anastomoses (Fig. 8), and heterotopic placement with end-to-side vascular anastomoses to the recipient abdominal great vessels and implantation of the donor ureter or a bladder patch to the recipient bladder dome, with or without insertion of a ureteral stent (1, 14).

1. Orthotopic Transplantation

The recipient is anesthetized, prepared, and positioned supine on the corkboard. After opening the abdomen in the midline, the intestines are packed to the right. Appropriate retraction allows access to the left perirenal space. The renal vessels are isolated completely between the great vessels and the hilum of the kidney to their first branch. The ureter is dissected at the renal pelvis, leaving the remainder intact. After placement of vascular clamps on the proximal renal vessels, these are transected, leaving 2–3 mm for anastomosis. The ureter is divided just below the hilus of the kidney and the organ is dissected free from the perinephric fat and removed.

The donor animal is given 500–700 IU of heparin intravenously. Midline laparotomy is followed by horizontal incisions in both flanks. Lateral retraction of the abdominal wall flaps allows access to the renal vessels, IVC, and abdominal aorta. Because of the length of its renal artery, the left kidney is utilized preferentially. The vessels are isolated by blunt and sharp dissection. Ligation of small branches,

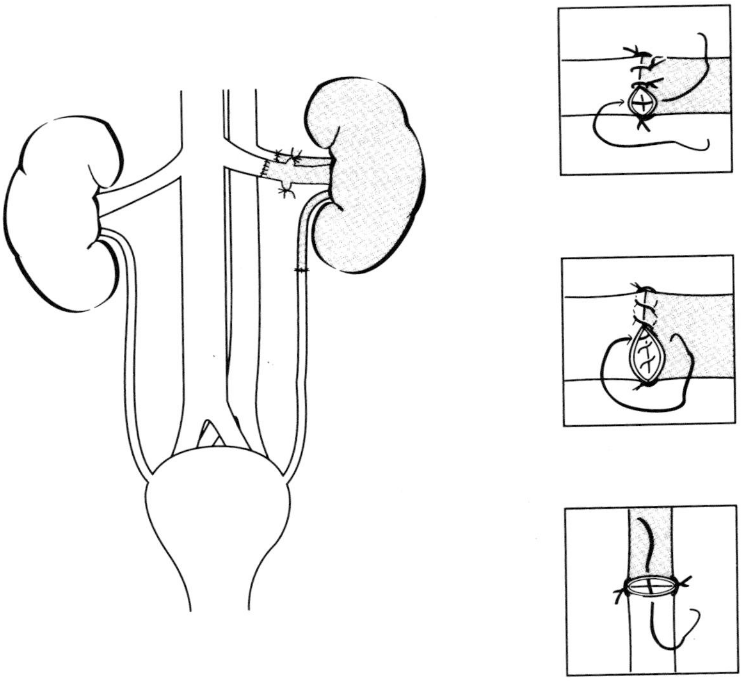

Figure 8 Orthotopic kidney transplantation in a rat with an end-to-end anastomosis technique. Arterial and ureteral anastomoses are performed using single sutures; the venous anastomosis is completed with a running suture. From Ref. (4), "Organ Transplantation in Rats and Mice." W. Timmerman, H. J. Gassel, K. Ulrichs, R. Zhong, and A. Thiede; Fig. 3, p. 77, 1998. Copyright 1998 Springer-Verlag.

particularly to the adrenal gland, may be required for full mobilization. The ureter is isolated with its surrounding fat and transected as far distally as possible without excessive manipulation. The kidney is then separated extracapsularly from the adjacent tissues and adrenal gland. The renal artery, vein, and ureter are transected sequentially and the isolated organ is placed in cold saline.

A microscope is needed for the engraftment procedure. The donor kidney is placed orthotopically in the left flank of the recipient. The renal vessels are positioned appropriately. Stay sutures (10-0) on the opposite edges of the two renal arteries are used to rotate the vessels 180° so that the back wall can be sutured first. The ends of the stay sutures are held under minimal tension with mosquito clamps. Two single sutures are placed in the back wall of the artery and tied before the vessel is rotated back to its original position. After assuring that the arterial lumen is patent, two additional sutures are placed in the front wall of the artery and tied. Ligating the stay sutures completes the arterial anastomosis. For the venous anastomosis, the edges of the donor and recipient renal veins are approximated with a long stay suture held under slight tension. The next suture is positioned on the back wall ~160° from the first. Its unarmed end is clamped with a second mosquito clamp and slight tension is applied. The armed end of the suture is then run around the back wall, tied to the shorter end of the upper stay suture with a single knot, and used to complete the front wall anastomosis. The donor and recipient ureters are trimmed to appropriate lengths and joined with four full-thickness single stitches placed at 90°. The first two sutures are placed 180° apart, tied, then one on the back and one on the front wall. No stent is used. The abdomen is closed routinely.

2. Heterotopic Transplantation

The renal artery and vein of the donor are dissected free of the aorta and vena cava. Adrenal and other small branches are ligated and divided. A patch of aorta or a short aortic segment and a patch of IVC surrounding the orifice are fashioned for end-to-side anastomosis on the appropriate abdominal great vessels of the recipient. The ureter is dissected to its junction with the bladder and a patch of surrounding trigone removed. The bladder patch can be sewn directly to a defect made in the recipient bladder dome, or alternatively, a stent (approximately 0.4 mm OD) is positioned inside the donor ureter and secured with an 8-0 stitch. The other end is inserted through a hole in the recipient bladder and secured with two purse strings around the stent and donor ureter. Although the technically easier vascular anastomoses are similar to those described for heart transplantation, more detailed preparation of the longer vessels

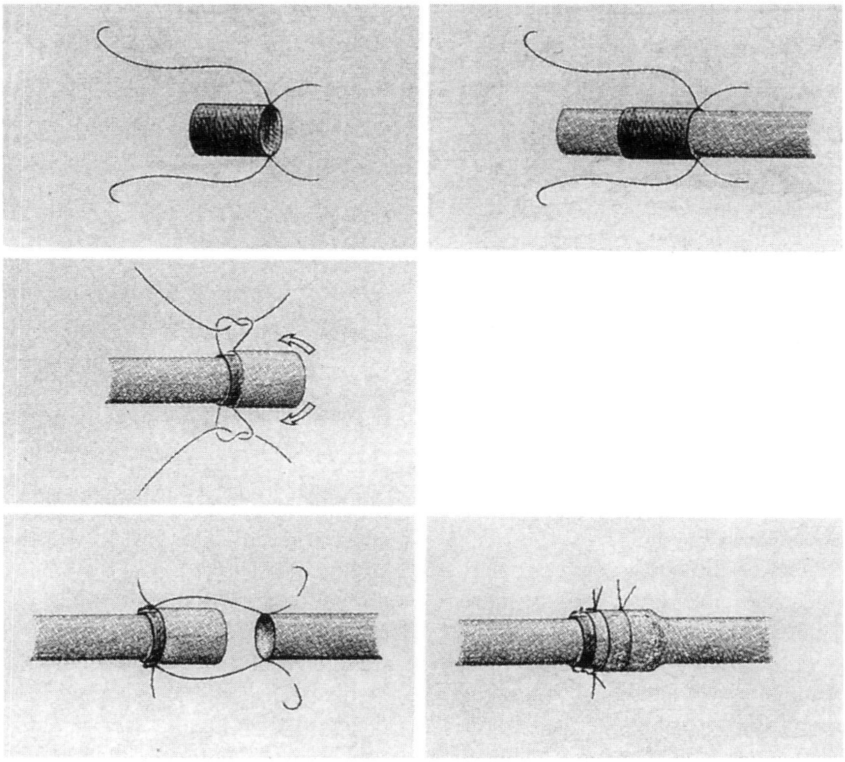

Figure 9 The cuff technique for anastomosis of vessels. From Ref. (4), "Organ Transplantation in Rats and Mice." W. Timmerman, H. J. Gassel, K. Ulrichs, R. Zhong, and A. Thiede; Fig. 1, p. 67, 1998. Copyright 1998 Springer-Verlag.

and ureter is a disadvantage of this technique. With a significant incidence of urine leak, late hydronephrosis, and stone formation, this method is not recommended for long-term studies. A few facile investigators have adapted successfully heterotopic kidney transplantation in mice.

C. Liver Transplantation

Before discussing the method of orthotopic liver transplantation in the rat, a cuff technique for venous anastomosis will be described as an alternative method to the direct running suture (Fig. 9). It can be recommended to decrease the time and complexity of the procedure, or to aid a less experienced surgeon. Use of the cuff technique in liver transplantation may also shorten the time of the procedure, because it can be used to join donor and recipient supra- and infrahepatic vena cavae and the portal vein. A plastic tube of appropriate size is slipped over the vessel to be anastomosed; the vessel end is everted over the tube. Placement of two traction sutures on the opposite edges of the vein is sometimes helpful in this eversion step. The other vein is then pulled over the free end of the tube and the everted end of the opposite vein. This cuff method is simple and undertaken primarily for anastomosing vessels of different diameters.

The technique of hepatic replacement has been well described (Fig. 10) (15, 16). The abdomen of the hepatic donor is opened widely. The intestines are wrapped in damp

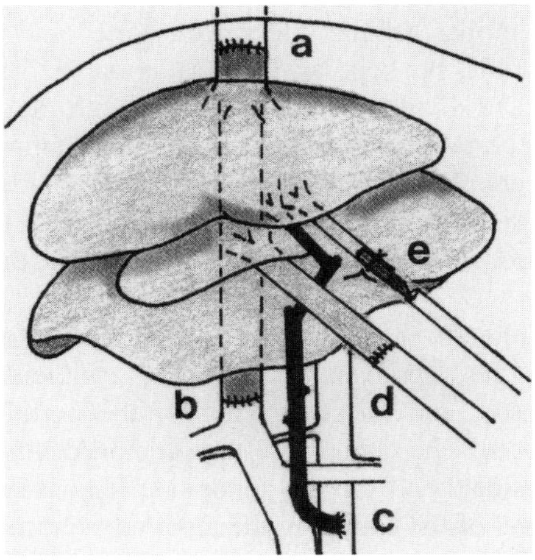

Figure 10 Orthotopic liver transplant in a rat. (a) Suprahepatic anastomosis of the cavae; (b) infrahepatic anastomosis of IVC; (c) aorto–aortoceliac anastomosis; (d) portal vein anastomosis; (e) bile duct anastomosis (stent). From Ref. (4), "Organ Transplantation in Rats and Mice." W. Timmerman, H. J. Gassel, K. Ulrichs, R. Zhong, and A. Thiede; Fig. 1, p. 124, 1998. Copyright 1998 Springer-Verlag.

gauze to reduce fluid loss. The liver is freed from its ligaments; small phrenic vessels are ligated. The caudate lobe is cleared of adjacent structures; small branches of the left hepatic artery and distal esophagus are tied. The infrahepatic IVC is isolated and ligated cephalad to the right renal vein. The right suprarenal vessels and gastroduodenal artery are tied. The portal vein is carefully freed from its connective tissue toward the splenic vein, and the pyloric vein is double ligated and transected. The celiac axis is isolated and all other branches (splenic and left gastric), except the hepatic artery, are ligated. The abdominal aorta is then prepared by ligating all branches except for the superior mesenteric artery. The bile duct is freed to the pancreas and transected; a 0.65-mm outer diameter stent approximately 6 mm long is inserted to its halfway point and tied in the bile duct. The pancreatic end of the duct is tied.

Liver perfusion is carried out as a final step of the retrieval procedure. The abdominal aorta is ligated proximal to the celiac trunk. To maintain the physiologic circulation of the intestine for as long as possible, ligation of the mesenteric artery takes place shortly before the arterial flush of the liver. The infrahepatic IVC is double clamped and transected. The portal vein is canulated *in situ* and flushed with cold saline (4°C). For outflow of the perfusate, the diaphragm is opened and the intrathoracic IVC is transected. The aorta is then cross-clamped at the bifurcation and the aortoceliac segment is flushed via a cannula placed in the distal aorta. The color of the fully perfused liver changes to a homogeneous pale light brown. The proximal end of the aorta is then divided above the ligature; the open distal end will be anastomosed to the recipient aorta. Finally, the portal vein and suprarenal vessels are divided and the liver is removed and stored in 4°C saline.

Access to the recipient liver is achieved via a midline incision. After dissection of the hepatic ligaments, the bile duct and proper hepatic artery are isolated and transected. Those should be kept as long as possible. The IVC is clamped and divided near its junction with the right renal vein. The portal vein is gently isolated and clamped near the splenic vein. The suprahepatic IVC incorporating a small piece of diaphragm is clamped and divided. After ligation and transection of the suprarenal vessels, the liver is removed.

The donor liver is placed in orthotopic position in the recipient; the suprahepatic donor and recipient IVCs are anastomosed, and matching ends of the portal veins are anastomosed. The clamps are then removed, first from the recipient side then from the donor side. This is followed by the removal of the clamp on the repaired suprahepatic IVC, allowing hepatic reperfusion. Next, the infrahepatic IVCs are joined to restore venous outflow from the caudal part of the animal's body. End-to-side anastomosis of the donor aortoceliac segment with the infrarenal portion of the recipient aorta is carried out, allowing arterial perfusion of the organ via the hepatic artery. With complete reperfusion, the liver assumes its normal color. After checking for arterial leaks, donor and recipient bile ducts are joined by advancing the free end of the stent from the donor duct into the recipient duct. Several single stitches are used to complete this anastomosis. The abdominal cavity is then closed.

D. Pancreatic Transplantation

After retracting the intestines of the donor to the right, the omentum is opened to access the pancreas (17, 18). Following the ligation of its vessels, the isolated spleen may be used to maneuver the pancreatic tail without touching it. The pancreatic head is isolated by exposing the regional vessels. The duodenum is freed to the duodenojejunal flexure. The superior mesenteric vessels are isolated and the right gastroepiploic vessels, bile duct, and hepatic artery are ligated and transected. The gastric vessels can be visualized, tied, and divided by retracting the stomach. The pancreas is then turned to the right of the abdominal cavity and the infrahepatic portion of the aorta is cleared to the renal arteries. The right renal artery and other aortic branches are tied and divided. The superior mesenteric artery is ligated and dissected distal to the inferior pancreaticoduodenal artery. The aorta is cross-clamped above the celiac axis and below the left renal artery and the pancreas is flushed via the distal aorta. After tying the distal aorta above the left renal artery, the portion that includes the superior mesenteric artery and celiac axis is removed; the proximal end will be anastomosed to the recipient aorta. The open portal vein is then transected at the liver. Finally, the proximal end of the duodenum is ligated, leaving its distal portion open for end-to-side anastomosis to the recipient bowel. The blood supply of the gland is provided by the portion of abdominal aorta with retained celiac trunk and superior mesenteric artery, with the inferior pancreaticoduodenal artery left opened. Blood drains via the portal vein.

Several alternatives for drainage of the pancreatic duct have been described. Instead of isolating a length of duodenum surrounding the head of the pancreas (Fig. 11), an elliptical duodenal patch surrounding the ostium of the pancreatic duct may be retained for end-to-side anastomosis to the recipient duodenum (Fig. 12). For drainage into the urinary tract, the pancreatic head is completely exposed. The common bile duct is divided and cannulated. The other end of the cannula is inserted either into the recipient ureter or bladder. When the exocrine portion of the gland is not drained, the pancreatic duct can either be ligated or occluded by retrograde injection of various polymeric agents.

To transplant the pancreas graft into the recipient, both systemic and portal venous drainage methods have been used. For drainage into systemic circulation, an infrarenal portion of the recipient IVC and aorta are isolated and

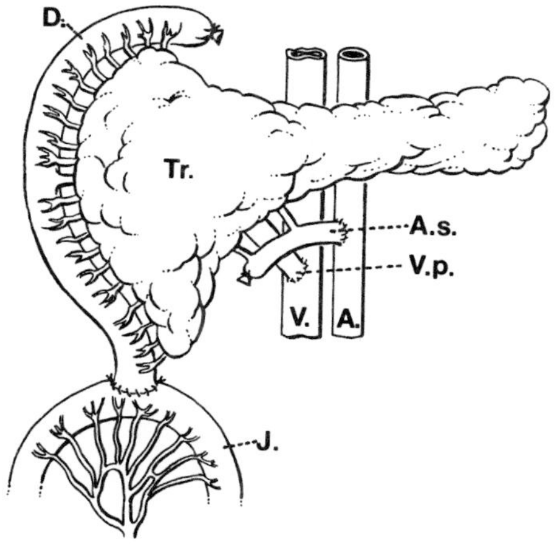

Figure 11 Transplantation of the pancreas in a rat using a pancreatico-duodenal graft Tr, Pancreatic graft; V, IVC; A, abdominal aorta; V. p., portal vein; A. s., aortic segment; D., donor duodenum; J., recipient second jejunal loop. From Ref. (4), "Organ Transplantation in Rats and Mice." W. Timmerman, H. J. Gassel, K. Ulrichs, R. Zhong, and A. Thiede; Fig. 1, p. 106, 1998. Copyright 1998 Springer-Verlag.

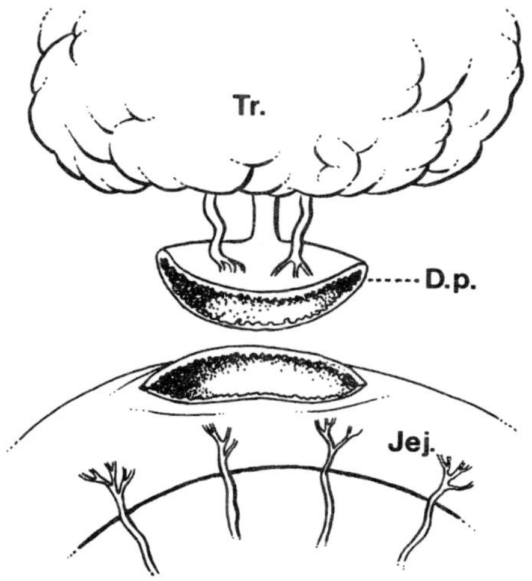

Figure 12 Transplantation of the rat pancreas using a duodenal patch for the intestinal anastomosis. Tr, Pancreatic graft; D.p., duodenal patch; Jej, second jejunal loop. From Ref. (4), "Organ Transplantation in Rats and Mice." W. Timmerman, H. J. Gassel, K. Ulrichs, R. Zhong, and A. Thiede; Fig. 2, p. 107, 1998. Copyright 1998 Springer-Verlag.

clamped. The pancreas is then placed in the left flank of the recipient. An end-to-side anastomosis between the donor portal vein and the recipient IVC is performed with 8-0 monofilament running suture. The end-to-side arterial anastomosis between the proximal end of the donor aortic segment and the host abdominal aorta is then carried out by continuous suture on the front wall of the vessels. To complete the back wall, the transplanted organ is repositioned to the right side of the abdominal cavity. For portal drainage, the recipient portal vein is exposed and cross-clamped. An end-to-side running anastomosis with the donor portal vein is then performed. Maximal length of all vessels should be kept to avoid tension on any anastomosis. Finally, an end-to-side anastomosis of the duodenum or duodenal patch to the second portion of the host jejunum is carried out using full-thickness single 6-0 sutures.

E. Orthotopic Small Bowel Transplantation

Intravenous fluid hydration of the donor is crucial for the success of this procedure. The mesentery of the small intestine from the ligament of Treitz to the terminal portion of the ileum is divided; bleeders are ligated. The portal vein is then gently isolated from the pancreas. Ligation of small branches can be performed with greater ease by tracting the duodenum to the right. The superior mesenteric artery is then isolated as is the celiac axis and its junction with the aorta. The celiac trunk is tied to prevent potential bleeding during bowel preparation. The bowel is flushed with cold Ringer's lactate solution via the distal aorta following ligation of the renal arteries. After dissecting as much length of the portal vein and mesenteric artery as possible, all vessels are divided and the intestine is stored in Ringer's solution at 4°C. Alternatively, a segment of aorta containing the superior mesenteric artery can be used. Intestinal fluid loss is minimized by wrapping the isolated bowel in gauze, which is kept moist throughout the subsequent transplant procedure (19, 20).

Appropriate segments of recipient infrarenal aorta and vena cava are isolated, clamped, and opened. The donor intestine is placed in the left of the abdominal cavity and end-to-side continuous anastomosis between donor mesenteric artery or aorta segment and recipient abdominal aorta is performed (Fig. 13). The portal vein is then joined end-to-side to the recipient IVC. Alternatively, the recipient portal vein can be used for venous drainage. The portal vein is exposed between liver and spleen, and end-to-side anastomosis with the donor portal vein is carried out using a 10-0 continuous suture. After completion of the anastomoses, the venous and arterial clamps are released sequentially and the organ is reperfused. The native bowel is then removed, leaving ~15 mm of jejunum and ileum. The respective segments of donor and recipient bowel are anastomosed end-to-end using full-thickness running 7-0 silk sutures. Optionally, both ends of the graft can be exteriorized in a form of stomas using silk sutures, if the recipient bowel is left in place.

V. Summary

Early experimental progress in transplantation was achieved primarily using large animals, particularly studies on surgical techniques, effectiveness of initial immunosuppressive treatments, and beginning exploration of the host

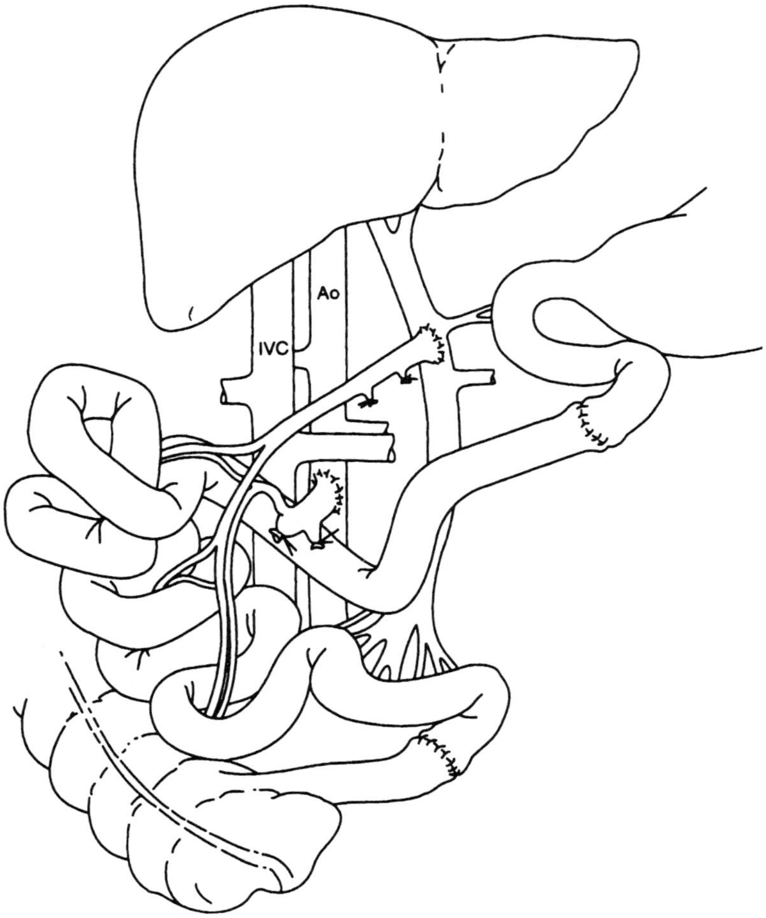

Figure 13 Rat orthotopic small bowel transplantation with portal venous drainage. IVC, Inferior vena cava; Ao, aorta. Note end-to-side porto–portal anastomosis. From Ref. (4), "Organ Transplantation in Rats and Mice." W. Timmerman, H. J. Gassel, K. Ulrichs, R. Zhong, and A. Thiede; Fig. 4, p. 90, 1998. Copyright 1998 Springer-Verlag.

response against solid organs. However, it soon became apparent that variations among individual animals of the same species were a limiting factor for the many biological applications under investigation. Developments in microsurgery opened new possibilities for investigators, allowing them to exploit varieties of inbred strains of small laboratory animals. Such experiments were highly reproducible, of relatively low cost, and resulted in the establishment of many models both in rats and in mice. Developments in related sciences followed. The current availability of new gene knockout strains of mice is opening ever-greater possibilities for relevant experiments, which, with progressing advances in cell and molecular biology and in pharmacology, provide opportunities to use more refined tools in transplant research. It is important to emphasize that despite the many advances in basic science, perfect microsurgical technique and a keen understanding of small animal models are crucial for the success of any experiment in transplant biology, because the correlation between *in vitro* findings and *in vivo* events is not invariable.

Acknowledgment

This work was supported by U.S. PHS Grant 5RO1 1DK 4490-26 and IPOI AI 40152-04.

References

1. Fisher, B., and Lee, S. (1965). Microvascular surgical techniques in research, with special reference to renal transplantation in the rat. *Surgery* **58,** 904.
2. Medawar, P. B. (1944). The behavior and fate of skin autografts and skin homografts in rabbits. *J. Anat.* **78,** 176.
3. Whitley, D., and Tilney, N. L. (1998). Surgical techniques: Transplantation biology allograft models and manipulation of the laboratory rat. *In* "Animal Modelling in Surgical Research" (B. Jeppsson, ed.), pp. 227–238. Norwood Academic Publishers, Amsterdam.

4. Timmerman, W., Gassel, H. J., Ulrichs, K., Zhong, R., and Thiede, A. (1998). "Organ Transplantation in Rats and Mice." Springer-Verlag, Berlin Heidelberg.
5. Tilney, N. L. (1971). Patterns of lymphatic drainage in the adult laboratory rat. *J. Anat.* **109,** 369.
5a. Jeppsson, B., ed. (1998). "Animal Modelling in Surgical Research." OPA, Amsterdam.
6. Jenkins, W. L. (1987). Pharmacologic aspects of analgesic drugs in animals: An overview. *J. Am. Vet. Med. Assoc.* **191,** 1231.
7. Gowans, J. L. (1957). The effect of continuous reinfusion of lymph and lymphocytes on the output of lymphocytes from the thoracic duct of anesthetized rat. *Br. J. Exp. Pathol.* **38,** 67.
8. Takada, M., Nadeau, K. C., Hancock, W. W., Mackenzie, H. S., Shaw, G. D., Waaga, A. M., Chandraker, A., Sayegh, M. H., and Tilney, N. L. (1998). Effects of explosive brain death on cytokine activation of peripheral organs in the rat. *Transplantation* **65,** 1533.
9. Pratschke, H., Wilhelm, M. J., Kusaka, M., Laskowski, I. L., and Tilney, N. L. (2000). A model of gradual onset brain death for transplantation associated studies. *Transplantation* **69**; 427.
10. Takada, M., Nadeau, K. C., Shaw, G. D., Marquette, K. A., and Tilney, N. L. (1997). The cytokine-adhesion molecule cascade in ischemia/reperfusion injury of the rat kidney. Inhibition by a soluble P-selectin ligand. *J. Clin. Invest.* **99,** 2682.
11. Abbott, C., Lindsey, E. S., Creech, O., and Dewitt, C. W. (1964). A technique for heart transplantation in the rat. *Arch. Surg.* **89,** 645.
12. Araneda, D., Padberg, W. M., and Tilney, N. L. (1989). Refined techniques for heterotopic cardiac transplantation in the rat. *Transplant. Proc.* **21,** 2562.
13. Yokoyama, H., Ohmi, M., Murata, S., Nakame, T., Tabayashi, K., and Mohri, H. (1995). Proposal of a working left heart model with a heterotopic transplantation technique in rats. *J. Heart Lung Transplant.* **14,** 706.
14. French, M. E., and Batchelor, J. R. (1969). Immunological enhancement of rat kidney grafts. *Lancet* **2,** 1103.
15. Lee, S., Charters, A. C., Chandler, J. G., and Orloff, M. J. (1973). A technique for orthotopic liver transplantation in the rat. *Transplantation* **16,** 664.
16. Kamada, N., and Calne, R. Y. (1983). A surgical experience with five hundred thirty liver transplants in the rat. *Surgery* **93,** 64.
17. Nolan, M. S., Lindsey, N. J., Savas, C. P., Herold, A., Beck, S., Slater, D. N., and Fox, M. (1983). Pancreatic transplantation in the rat. Long-term study following different methods of management of exocrine drainage. *Transplantation* **36,** 26.
18. Klempnauer, J., and Settje, A. (1989). Vascularized pancreas transplantation in the rat—Details of the microsurgical techniques, results, and complications. *Transpl. Int.* A2:84, 1989
19. Monchik, G. J., and Russell, P. S. (1971). Transplantation of small bowel in the rat: technical and immunological considerations. *Surgery* **70,** 693.
20. Zhong, R., Grant, D., Sutherland, F., Wang, P. Z., Chen, H. F., Lo, S., Stiller, C., and Duff, J. (1991). Refined technique for intestinal transplantation in the rat. *Microsurgery* **12,** 268.

56

Models to Study Surgical Nutrition and Metabolism

Wiley W. Souba* and Douglas W. Wilmore†

**Department of Surgery, The Milton S. Hershey Medical Center, Penn State College of Medicine, Hershey, Pennsylvania 17033*
†Department of Surgery, Brigham and Women's Hospital, Boston, Massachusetts 02115

I. Introduction

"Metabolism" is a broad term that has whole body, regional, cellular, and molecular implications. The study of nutrition and metabolism as related to surgical diseases has been approached using a variety of different models, all which have their inherent strengths and weaknesses. These can generally be classified as whole body techniques, regional/organ models, studies in cultured cells, and research using organelles. Human studies are the most relevant but also the most difficult to perform because there are limits to the types of studies that can be performed and the amount of tissue and/or blood that can be sampled. Moreover, human studies require approval by the Institutional Review Board, informed consent, and proper patient selection. Certain invasive studies are not feasible in human subjects and, therefore, must be done in intact animals, isolated organs, or cultured cells.

Given the sophistication with which biochemical and physiologic events can now be studied, many investigators choose not to study the *in vivo* environment but focus on specific regulatory steps using *in vitro* models. Although the danger of this approach is that the "big picture" can become blurred, an enormous amount of valuable information describing nutrition and metabolism in health and in disease states has been acquired from *in vitro* investigations.

Because no single model is without limitations, caution should be used when extrapolating results from findings in one study to another setting. When results from human, animal, and cellular models are combined and compared in a complementary manner, a powerful story can be developed that integrates metabolic and nutritional findings and draws reliable conclusions.

II. Determining the Initial Metabolic/Nutritional State

In order to understand the impact of a disease or a nutritional therapy on an individual or animal, the initial or basal metabolic state of the individual must be determined (Table I). With long-term nutrition studies this may include a description of initial body composition (see Chapter 58, this volume), or with short-term investigations this may represent dietary intake, body weight, body mass index, basal metabolic rate [usually measured by determining oxygen consumption (see Chapter 59)], and possibly nitrogen balance or protein turnover. When examining specific substrates, basal turnover studies of the metabolites of interest are important (see Chapter 57).

Because surgeons deal with seriously ill patients and seek metabolic and nutritional means to improve their outcome, it is important to quantify their illness. Burn size, injury severity scores, infection severity scores, or other measures help quantitate the degree of stress (see Chapters 28 and 66). The physiologic state of the patient should also be measured by determining cardiac output and oxygen consumption. Measures of the acute-phase response (total white blood cell count, C-reactive protein concentration, body temperature) are important descriptors of the response to inflammation and these measures have been expanded to include plasma cytokine concentrations or those cytokines produced following monocyte harvest and stimulation. Often a battery of immunological tests is included to describe the immunological status of the patient.

If studies are designed to determine the response pattern of organs to a disease or the effect of a treatment on the function of a specific organ, specific tests should be obtained.

Animal studies standardize many of the variables previously discussed (nutritional state; extent of injury, infection, tumor, or other disease) but it is still important to quantitate response patterns and show the range of these responses that can occur when a group of normals undergoes a specific perturbation.

III. Studying Altered Metabolic States

A. Studies in Normals

It is not uncommon to study the effect of a nutrient or a metabolic approach in a normal population before investigating patients. The criteria for a "normal" subject needs to be established and a pool of volunteers screened. The study can be performed using outpatients, but compliance and monitoring are major issues. A more controlled approach is to house subjects in a clinical research center (CRC). This affords consistency in diet and activity and allows constant monitoring. However, with reliable subjects such as motivated hospital workers or volunteers from religious groups, food can be supplied from a CRC kitchen and long-term studies can be performed using outpatients. For acute studies (such as endotoxin injection) we have favored a 24- to 48-hr admission before the experiment to ensure stability of the subject.

Animal studies in these areas should allow for adequate stabilization before study initiation (see Chapter 7). If the animals are to be studied in separate metabolic cages, they should be moved into this environment for at least 3 days before study initiation.

B. Study of Subjects with Illness

These studies usually involve administration of a diet or a metabolically active drug to a group of patients; the effects are compared to responses in similar individuals receiving the standard of care (another diet) or a placebo (nonactive form of the drug). Strict entry criteria are required for such investigations and usually subjects are stratified utilizing

Table I Examinations Used to Determine Nutritional Status

Examination	Types of measurement
Nutritional history screen	Nutritional history; review of dietary habits; 24-hr dietary recall, 3- or 7-day food records; food frequency questionnaire
Physical examination	Examination for nutrient deficiency or protein-calorie malnutrition
Anthropometric	Height–weight measurements; body mass index, head circumference (infants); skinfold thickness; midarm muscle circumference
Body density	Body volume displacement and body weight; calculation of specific gravity
^{40}K analysis (and other isotopic dilution methods)	Disappearance potassium-40 (or other isotopes) from plasma as an index of lean body mass
Radiologic and/or whole body measurements	Area X rays; CAT scan; NMR; gamma neutron activation
Laboratory tests	Tissue biopsy (skeletal muscle, liver); creatinine–height index; serum proteins and amino acids; immunocompetence testing; 3-methyl histidine excretion; measurement of white count C-reactive protein, cytokines and other mediators

block design so that the patient groups match when the study is finally analyzed. Stratification is commonly performed utilizing such factors as age, gender, nutritional state, lifestyle (such as smoking, drug use, and exercise) and disease-related factors (see Chapters 9 and 12 for a more detailed discussion of these issues). An initial characterization of the patients needs to be performed as previously discussed and, finally, primary and secondary outcome criteria (e.g., weight gain, nitrogen balance) also need to be clearly established.

Before the study is initiated (*pre hoc*) dropout criteria should be discussed with all involved investigators. Once these criteria are established, they should be rigidly followed. If the study involves a therapeutic approach, it is important to discuss whether all patients who are randomized should be evaluated at the end of the study (intent to treat) vs. only those who actually received an adequate quantity of the active agent or placebo.

Many of the factors relating to clinical studies are resolved when working with animals, but issues such as dropouts should be discussed before study initiation.

IV. Methodology—General Principles

Studies that determine physiologic responses (3- to 4-hr glucose clamp or endotoxin studies) should be performed in a constant, quiet environment, at the same time of day and under the same nutritional conditions (usually fasting). After placing catheters, the subject should be allowed to achieve near-basal conditions in a semidark room. Distraction such as television or visitors are not permitted and even interactions with investigators are controlled in an attempt to achieve constancy with all subjects. Likewise, animals are manipulated outside the animal husbandry room to minimize the effect of handling a particular animal on other study animals.

Although sampling of blood, urine, or tissue depends on the exact protocol, a constant feature is that samples should be obtained in triplicate, if at all possible. Values obtained from these samples are meant to minimize variation of single samples; if an odd or outlier value is obtained, it is discarded and the remaining two samples are averaged.

V. Expressing Results

Metabolic and nutritional effects are usually related to metabolic mass. Thus, many results are expressed per kilogram of body weight. The assumption of linearity between the measure of interest and body weight is satisfactory if the largest weight is no more than two times the smallest weight (1). With such weight disparity (for example, using children and adults, or normals and massively obese individuals), the assumption that weight is linear with the metabolic measure is no longer appropriate and a weight transform (log or exponential) is needed. One satisfactory resolution of this problem is to use body surface area instead of weight to express metabolic data. Tables are available for both humans and animals to derive these values (2, 3).

If an initial body compositional measurement is available, metabolic data should be expressed as a function of fat-free mass, lean body mass, or body cell mass (e.g., the active protein-containing components of the body).

When studying specific organs, metabolic functions are usually expressed per 100 g or 1 kg of organ weight. When measuring extremity flux, the volume of the extremity should be determined and flux expressed per 100 g of tissue. Organ size (particularly liver and kidney) can now be more precisely measured in humans and large animals utilizing computerized scanning techniques or nuclear magnetic resonance (NMR) methodology. Small animal studies allow the direct measure of organ weight if the protocol indicates that the animal can be sacrificed at the appropriate time period.

VI. Methods in Humans with Application in Animal Models

A. Whole-Body Balance

Two basic approaches exist to measure changes in the components of fat, protein, carbohydrate, and minerals in the body. For long-term studies, the composition of the body is measured (or the amount of a mineral within the body is determined), then the nutritional or metabolic perturbation is imposed on the organism and the compositional analysis is repeated at the end of the study. By quantitating protein, fat, calcium, or other constituents at the start of the study and subtracting the quantity measured at the end of the study, the gain or loss of a substance can be determined (see Chapter 58 for more details). This approach, however, requires that the compositional changes anticipated exceed the error of the compositional measurements and this occurs only with reasonably long-term studies (10 days to 2 weeks in catabolic humans and 4–6 weeks in stable individuals) and moderate metabolic stress (injury, infection, fasting). For the short term (7–10 days in humans), balance studies are required.

Balance techniques are some of the oldest and most widely used measures in nutritional research, and much of our present information is based on body balance. As the term implies, balance is the measure of the intake of a particular substance and the loss of that substance from the body. If carefully performed, the investigator can determine the body's gain or loss of an element over time. Balance is classically determined with nitrogen (which reflects protein metabolism), but this approach can also be performed with carbon, water, sodium, potassium, phosphorous, calcium, and other substances (4).

Several drawbacks to this approach are apparent: (1) it is an exceedingly difficult technique to perform accurately and requires a metabolic unit to monitor food intake and collections of all losses from the body; (2) the approach has inherent errors; and (3) the results do not reflect the mechanisms involved in the metabolism of a substance. Techniques such as regional flux studies and isotopic turnover methodology are needed for more detailed metabolic assessment of a specific element. Nonetheless, this approach has great value, especially when coupled with other methodology.

Nitrogen balance will be discussed as a general approach to most nutrient balance studies. Nitrogen is utilized as the marker of protein balance—e.g., nitrogen in grams equals protein (g)/16.5. Nitrogen balance is nitrogen intake minus nitrogen loss from the body:

$$N_{balance} = N_{in} - N_{out},$$

where N_{in} is the dietary nitrogen (determined from food composition tables or by food analysis) and

$$N_{out} = N_{urine} + N_{stool} + N_{skin} + N_{nasogastric\ and/or\ fistula}.$$

The quantity of nitrogen measured in body fluids and stool is determined by the Kjeldahl or by chemiluminescence techniques. Stool nitrogen rarely exceeds 1–2 g/day if diarrhea is not present. During parenteral feedings, stool losses may be absent. Skin losses range between 0.1 and 0.4 g/m^2/day for most individuals. Although cutaneous losses are much greater in burn patients with abnormal skin or wound losses, skin plus stool nitrogen losses in normals do not exceed 2 g/day. Urea accounts for 75–90% of the urinary nitrogen lost. By adding an additional 20% to urinary urea measurements (urine urea concentration × 24-hr urinary volume), an approximation of urine nitrogen losses can be made, 2 g added for stool and skin losses and nitrogen balance approximated. This is probably useful only in the research setting if nitrogen balance is not a major study endpoint.

The error of nitrogen balance is always in the positive direction, with positive balance favored by accounting for food intake that does not actually occur and by underestimating urine excretion due to sample loss. The quantity of creatinine excreted in the urine should always be measured in each 24-hr collection to ensure adequate collections.

Cumulative nitrogen balance is the addition of the daily balances over a predetermined time period. Because the error of balance determinations always favors a positive nitrogen balance, cumulative nitrogen balance cumulates a constant positive error; the calculated data always appear more favorable for nitrogen retention and protein synthesis than actually exists. The calculation of cumulative balance is rarely advised. Some key points in balance measurements are listed in Table II (see also Fig. 1).

Table II Key Points for Performing Nitrogen Balance

1. Calculate and also measure nitrogen intake. The composition of liquid diets can easily be measured. For meal feeding, make two identical food trays of meals with the exact composition and use a blender and homogenize to make a digest for analysis.
2. Ensure all collections are accurate. Train all personnel associated with the study and reinforce the need for accurate collections. Use creatinine as a measure of adequacy of collection. If individuals receive a nonmeat diet, all excreted creatinine arises from the body and approximately the same quantity of creatinine is excreted daily. Daily creatinine excretion values may reflect inadequate collections. Outlier values can be corrected to the mean value if loss of urinary volume is apparent; this "corrected volume" should be used to correct nitrogen loss.
3. Do not use cumulative balance data, because this technique cumulates positive error.
4. In plotting data, first indicate nitrogen intake above the baseline for each respective day. Then, plot balance for the appropriate day. Some individuals will use different colors or stippling to indicate periods above or below the zero balance line (Fig. 1).

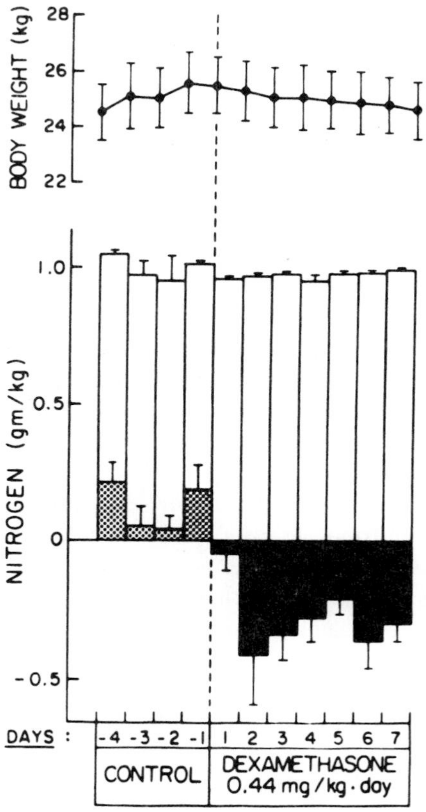

Figure 1 The effect of glucocorticoids on body weight and nitrogen in normal dogs (N = 4, mean ± SEM). Nitrogen intake is plotted upward from zero (0) balance and output is plotted downward from the top of the intake line. Positive nitrogen balance is indicated by the stippled bars, and negative balance is shown by the solid bars. From Muhlbacher *et al.* (31), with permission.

Table III Worksheet for Calculations of Substrate Oxidation, Metabolic Water, and Heat Production[a]

Component	Urinary nitrogen (grams)	Oxygen consumed (liters)	Carbon dioxide (liters)	Sum of values
Protein (g)	+6.25 × ___			
Carbohydrate (g)	−2.54 × ___	−2.91 × ___	+4.12 × ___	= ___
Fat (g)	−1.94 × ___	+1.69 × ___	−1.69 × ___	= ___
Metabolic water (g)	−1.04 × ___	+0.062 × ___	+0.662 × ___	= ___
Metabolic heat (kcal)	−2.98 × ___	+3.78 × ___	+1.16 × ___	= ___

[a]All standardized per unit time. These equations were derived from the following formulas: V_{O_2} = 6.03 nitrogen in the urine + 0.83 carbohydrate in the diet + 2.02 fat in the diet. V_{CO_2} = 4.88 nitrogen in the urine + 0.829 carbohydrate in the diet + 1.43 fat in the diet. Adapted from Consolazio *et al.* (6).

Finally, administered protein or amino acids may be converted to urea but not excreted. The blood urea nitrogen gradually rises and under these conditions balance should be corrected for urea accumulation [total liters of body water × urea nitrogen concentration (grams/liter)]. Retained urea will again suggest a more positive nitrogen balance if this increase is not taken into consideration. It has also been suggested that such an adjustment should be made for changes that occur in the intracellular amino acid pool (5).

Nitrogen balance can be combined with the measurement of respiratory gas exchange and the metabolic components or mixture of substrate utilized calculated (Table III). Other methodology is available for the balance measurement of water and minerals (6). Some of these measurements also allow calculation of gain or loss of muscle protoplasm (Table IV), which can be used for comparison with simultaneously performed compositional measures (7).

B. Organ Balance Using the Arterial–Venous Technique

The balance of a nutrient across an organ with single major venous drainage can be studied utilizing the arterial–venous difference technique. Similar to whole body balance, this technique measures the input (arterial concentration) and output (venous concentration) of a substance across an organ. The difference reflects the loss or gain of a substance in the particular tissue, and when combined with blood flow, the net rates of tissue metabolism can be determined (Fig. 2). This approach can be combined with tracer methodology and/or biopsy techniques and the absolute

Table IV Factors Used in Deriving Certain Components of Muscle Protoplasm from Nitrogen Balance[a]

Components to be derived	Final unit	Factor[b]
Protein in protoplasm	g	6.25
Protoplasm, fat free but not extracellular fluid free	g	32
Protoplasm, fat free and extracellular fluid free ("true muscle")	g	27
Intracellular fluid in protoplasm	ml	19
Extracellular fluid in protoplasm	ml	5
Potassium in intracellular fluid in protoplasm	mEq	2.7
Sodium in extracellular fluid in protoplasm	mEq	0.77
Phosphorus in protoplasm	g	0.066
Sulfur in protoplasm	g	0.069
Fat calorically equivalent to protoplasm	g	2.8
Protoplasm (fat free) minus fat calorically equivalent to protoplasm	g	29.2

[a]From Reifenstein *et al.* (4).
[b]To derive the component, multiply nitrogen in grams by the factor.

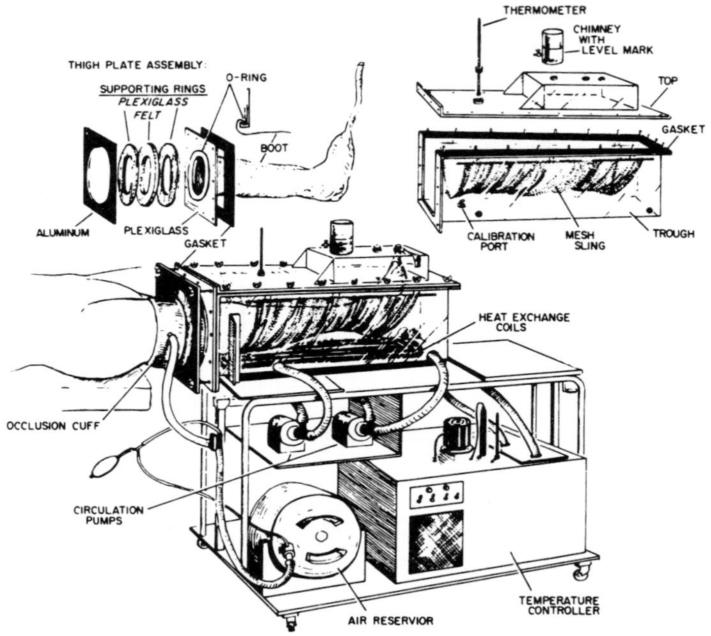

Figure 2 A full-leg water-filled plethysmography; with inflation of the cuff above venous pressure, the leg swells, displacing water from the rigid plethysmography. Water rises in the chimney, and the initial rate of change is related to arterial blood flow. From L. H. Aulick *et al.* (1977). Influence of the burn wound on peripheral circulation in thermally injured patients. *Am. J. Physiol.* **233,** H520–H526.

rates of protein synthesis and breakdown can be determined (Fig. 3). In humans, catheters have been placed in veins draining the liver (8) (splanchnic bed), kidney (9), brain (10), and skeletal muscle of the arm (11) and/or leg (12). Studies performed in individuals undergoing laparotomy have catheterized the portal vein and selected mesenteric veins (13). Blood is drawn simultaneously from an artery (any arterial sample is appropriate) to determine arterial concentration. A site utilized in normal volunteers or patients without an arterial line is a dorsal vein of the hand

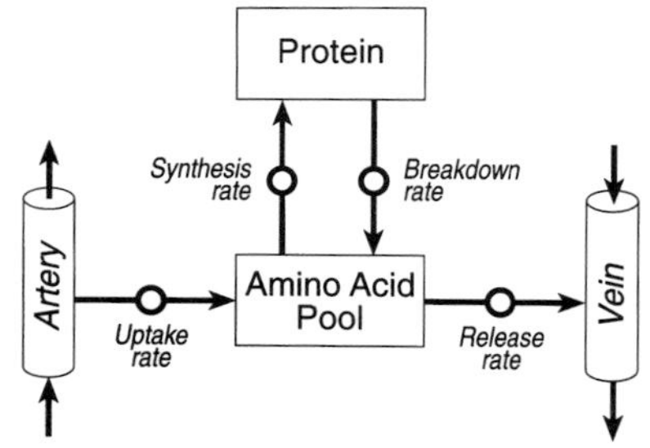

Figure 3 A general model for organ protein metabolism. The $A - V$ differences measure net exchange rates. When coupled with tissue biopsy or tracer techniques, the pool size can be determined and the absolute synthesis and breakdown rates measured.

using the hot hand technique, thus sparing an arterial puncture (14, 15).

To quantitate the rate of substrate flux, blood flow across the specific vascular bed must be measured. These methods are summarized on Table V and are also discussed in Chapter 71. In the case of tissues that are nourished by a single major vessel (i.e., kidney, leg) flux is calculated using the following formula:

$$\text{Flux (exchange)} = ([\text{arterial substrate conc}] - [\text{venous substrate conc}]) \times (\text{blood flow})$$

For organs that have two blood supplies (e.g., the liver; Fig. 4), calculation of flux involves two components of the equation (Fig. 4). In the case of the liver, which receives blood from both the hepatic artery and the portal vein, the following formula is used:

$$\text{Flux} = [(PV_{sub} - HV_{sub})(PV_{FLOW}) + (HA_{sub} - HV_{sub})](HA_{FLOW}),$$

where PV_{sub} is the portal vein substrate concentration, HV_{sub} is the hepatic vein concentration, HA_{sub} is arterial substrate concentration (usually measured in another artery), PV_{FLOW} is the portal vein blood flow, and HA_{FLOW} is the hepatic artery blood flow. Note that measurement of whole blood concentrations of tracers or nutrients is necessary (16, 17). If

Table V Measurements of Blood Flow Utilized for Regional Metabolic Measurements

Region	Humans	Animals
Skeletal muscle (forearm or leg)	Plethysomograph; dye dilution technique; xenon washout from muscle	Electromagnetic flow probes; dye or isotope dilution; radioactive microspheres
Liver	Indocyanine green dye; extraction	Indocyanine green extraction; flow probes; dye or isotope dilution; radioactive microspheres
Kidney	*Para*-amino hippurate acid excretion	*Para*-Amino hippurate acid excretion; isotope extraction
Bowel	Use of flow probes at the time of operation	Flow probes; dye or isotope dilution technique; radioactive microspheres

only plasma measurements are made, then a value reflecting plasma blood flow can be utilized by using the hematocrit to calculate the proportion of blood flow that is plasma.

It is important to realize that such measurements reflect net exchange rates (often expressed in mol/unit body or organ weight/unit time) that represent the sum of the various flux rates by the individual cell populations that comprise the organ. Thus, flux rates do not provide information about absolute unidirectional fluxes or about the relative contributions of the individual cell populations in the tissue to the net

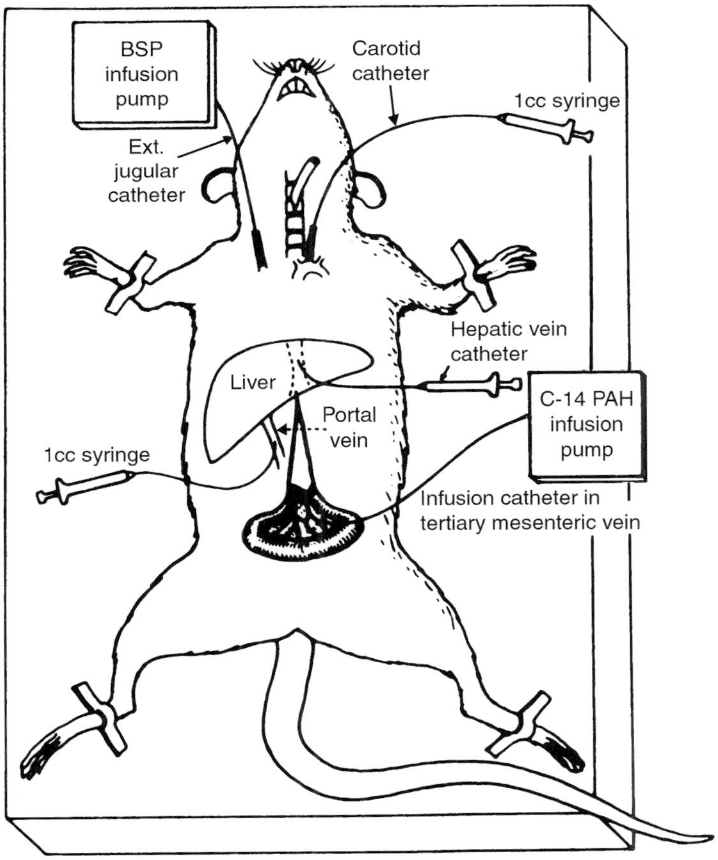

Figure 4 Anesthetized rat model used to measure splanchnic substrate exchange. Catheters are inserted into the indicated blood vessels. Intestinal and hepatic blood flows are quantitated using bromosulfthalein (BSP) and [^{14}C]PAH (*para*-amino hippurate) and exchange is calculated using the formula described in the text. From Souba, W. W. (1992), "Glutamine: Physiology, Biochemistry and Nutrition in Critical Illness." Medical Intelligence Unit, Armstrong Printing Company, Austin, Texas.

overall exchange rate. For example, one cell population may release net amounts of an amino acid, while another may consume amino acids. The net flux measurement across the entire organ (uptake, release, or balance) represents a sum of these individual rates. Because blood flow is always a positive number, the arteriovenous concentration difference ($A - V$ difference) across the organ determines whether the organ is a net consumer (i.e., $A - V$ is a positive number), a net releaser ($A - V$ is a negative number), or is an organ of balance ($A - V$ is not different from zero).

The net fluxes of a variety of substances have been studied in this manner, including glucose, free fatty acids, ketones, and amino acids (18). Oxygen consumption values of organs have also been determined by this technique (19). Because the concentration differences between the arterial and venous measurements are quite small, attention should be focused on analytical methodology—for example, measuring concentrations in each sample in triplicate. Samples should be obtained by simultaneous blood draws from the arterial and venous catheters; venous samples should be withdrawn slowly and should not exceed 15–20% of the rate of blood flow through the catheterized vessel. Triplicate samples should be drawn at each steady-state time point.

One variation on this technique is to study two tissues in the same individual simultaneously, regionally infusing or perturbing one tissue and using the other as a control. This can be done by studying kidneys, arms, legs, or lungs. These studies accommodate systemic reflex changes that may be associated with systemic circulatory adjustments or thermoregulatory drives (20). In unique human investigation, burn patients were studied with one injured and one noninjured lower extremity (21). The findings from the human trial were later confirmed in animals (22). In this manner, the contribution of the wound to injury metabolism could be determined.

Although flux studies do not provide detailed information about the kinetics of synthesis and breakdown within a tissue, they do provide important information about how organs handle a specific nutrient during feeding, starvation, critical illnesses, and other pathophysiologic states. Combined with data obtained from the other models and/or biopsy techniques, much has been learned about organ metabolism in health and disease.

C. Response to Substrate Administration

In addition to studies of whole body balance or regional infusions, investigators are frequently interested in the handling of specific nutrients, their disappearance from the bloodstream, or the effect of a disease on substrate metabolism. Although such investigations have evolved into practical diagnostic tests (such as the oral glucose tolerance test), most of these studies are performed as intravenous infusions, bypassing the problems associated with gastric emptying and the variations associated with intestinal absorption.

Intravenous nutrients can be delivered by two general methods. The first is a bolus injection that is followed by multiple blood sampling to determine the disappearance of the substance from the bloodstream (Fig. 5). From this test, the distribution space and disappearance constant *(k)* are determined. The area under the curve described by the injected substance can be calculated and utilized to describe the kinetics or to evaluate a second response, such as a hormonal elaboration. This approach has been applied to glucose (23), amino acids (24), and drug pharmacokinetics (25, 26).

Another approach is the constant infusion method. Although substrates can be administered at constant rates, their concentrations may change over time, or may vary depending on the disease or study condition. Because differing plasma concentrations create variations in concentration gradients that affect transport, the concept of "clamping" the concentration of a substrate was conceived. The most common "clamp" experiments utilize glucose (27) and insulin (28), but amino acids and lipid emulsion infusions have also been utilized for clamp studies (29). With the hyperglycemic glucose clamp, a constant infusion of glucose is given to achieve a fixed concentration. Plasma samples are measured at 10-min intervals and this immediate determination is utilized to adjust the infusion rate in order to maintain the predetermined or targeted glucose concentration. (A computer algorithm has been devised to aide in making this adjustment (27); alternatively servo pumps, which measure intravascular concentrations and automatically adjust flow rates, can be utilized.) After a relatively steady state has been achieved, the amount of glucose administered over a fixed interval can be determined, and these disposed rates

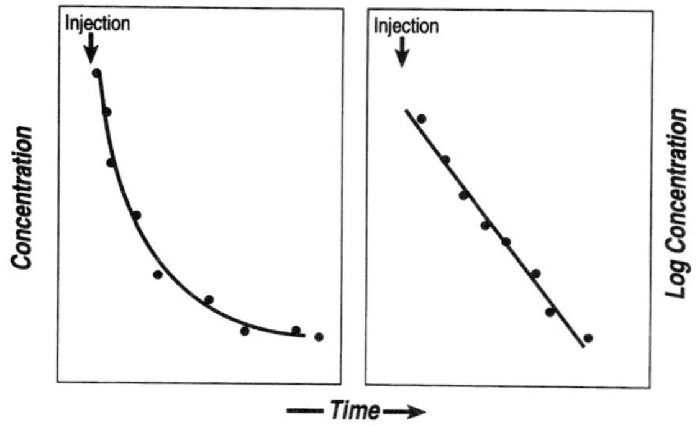

Figure 5 Concentration of an injected substance in the bloodstream over time. The data on the left are plotted on a linear graph, and on the right are transferred to log data. Extrapolation of the concentration at time = 0 allows calculation of the distribution space following injection of a known quantity. The slope derived from the log transform data expresses the rate constant of disappearance from the bloodstream.

can be compared between patient groups, or in the same individual following a specific treatment.

A similar approach is utilized with the euglycemic insulin clamp (Fig. 6). Insulin is infused, glucose is administered to prevent hypoglycemia, and the rate of glucose infused reflects insulin sensitivity (Fig. 7).

Both systems are frequently utilized in patients and methods have also been devised for investigations in small animals (30).

VII. Animal Models

Animal models play a key role in providing information about metabolism and nutrition. There are several advantages to utilizing animals for study: (1) the investigation controls for multiple variables that occur in patients, even when imposing experimental conditions such as injury, tumor growth, or infection; (2) exacting body and tissue analyses can be performed; (3) multiple studies can be performed; and (4) the investigator can study regional and cellular metabolism because tissue can be obtained for study.

The major disadvantages include the relevance of the model to the human condition, cost, and the difficulty of appropriately studying a species in a restricted environment (Table VI). In the acute situation, animals are frequently studied while receiving anesthesia, and a number of faulty conclusions have been made about a particular response because of this approach.

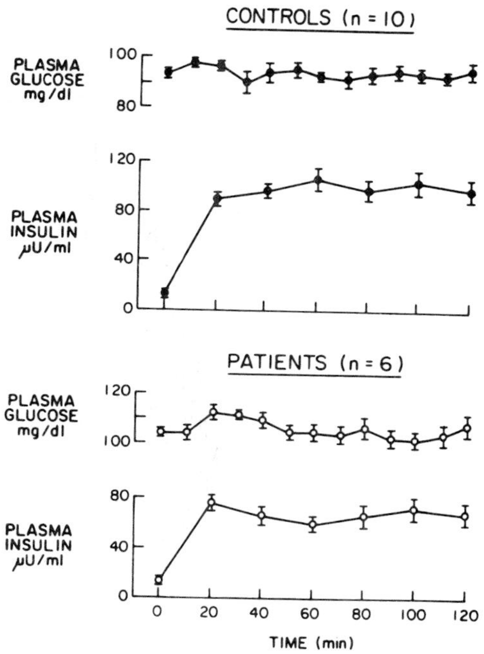

Figure 6 Plasma glucose and insulin concentrations during euglycemia while infusing insulin at a rate of 1.0 mU/kg·min. Values represent mean ± SEM. From Ref. (28), P.R. Black *et al.* (1982). Mechanisms of insulin resistance following injury. *Ann. Surg.* **196**, 420–435.

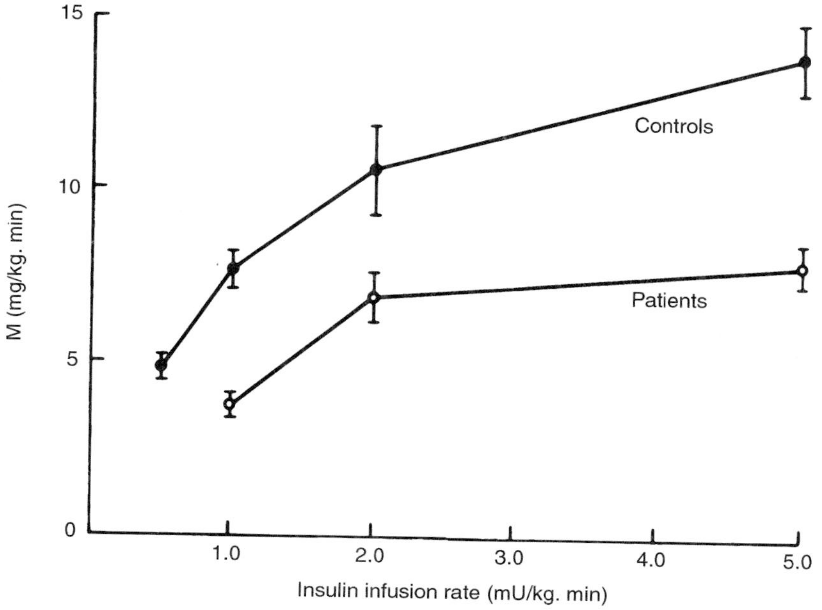

Figure 7 The total amount of glucose infused during euglycemic insulin infusions; this is referred to as the M value (Y axis). When this value is plotted against the various doses of insulin infused, an insulin sensitivity curve can be generated (mean ± SEM). From Ref. (28), P.R. Black *et al.* (1982). Mechanisms of insulin resistance following injury. *Ann. Surg.* **196**, 420–435.

Table VI Common Animal Models

Species	Advantages	Disadvantages
Dog	Good temperament; regional studies and multiple blood sampling possible; studies in puppies possible; moderate past information; germ-free model available.	Large space requirements; moderate public resistance; relevance to humans questionable.
Rat	Low cost—little space; large numbers can be studied simultaneously; rapid growth.	Relevance to humans questionable; blood sampling limited; regional studies difficult; duration of infusion limited.
Primate (monkey)	Simulates humans closely; psychometric studies possible; high intelligence.	High cost; high public resistance; asepsis difficult; bad temperament, large space requirements; restraint usually required; blood sampling limited.

If studies in anesthetized animals are necessary, some effort should be made in the nonstressed, unrestrained setting to confirm these observations. The study of unrestrained animals requires reasonably prolonged training, but important metabolic data can be obtained using this approach (31).

Selection of the appropriate animal model is important, but with cost a major factor, most studies are now performed in rodents. Rats can be chronically infused and tissues can be analyzed (Fig. 8). Mice can be genetically manipulated and thus provide unique study models if sampling throughout the study is not indicated. Dogs are ideal for chronic study; they tolerate individual catheters and long-term infusion (Fig. 9), and can stand or sit for prolonged studies.

Primates are more expensive, but on occasion studies in these animals are necessary. Guinea pigs, miniature swine, sheep, goats, cows, and horses have all been investigated. These models are all important when addressing a specific question, but their cost and the question of applicability of the information to the human condition make these models less useful. Moreover, the ability to perform multiple studies in rodents compared to only limited studies in larger species argues for the use of the small animal model, particularly if large variability in physiologic and biochemical response exists and a large number of studies are required.

A. Dietary Studies

1. Oral Feedings

Normal animals generally consume a standard amount of an appropriate animal chow each day. However, when the animals are perturbed (injured, infected, or subjected to a surgical procedure) intake is altered. This poses a problem when comparing the metabolic response of this group to a normal control group, if metabolic changes are observed and the specific cause is not known (e.g., are the changes due to the perturbation or to altered food intake?). To solve this problem, pair feeding studies are performed. Animals are paired, one experimental animal with one control. If the experimental animal eats less than the control, the food intake for that animal is measured and the next day only that amount is given to the paired control. If the experimental animal eats more than the control, the control animal's food

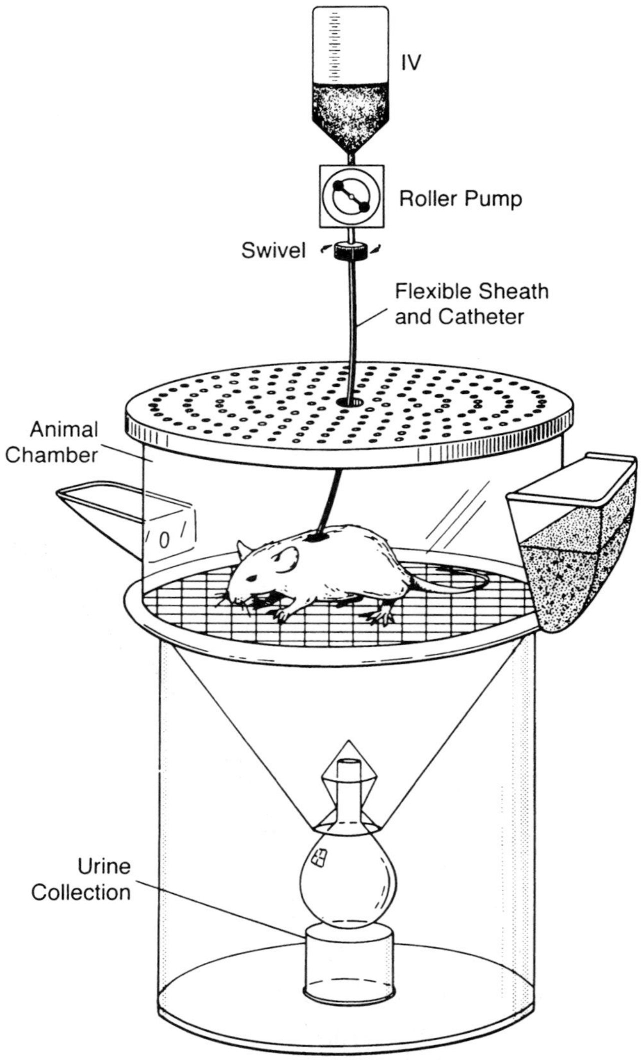

Figure 8 Metabolic studies can be performed in this chronic infusion, which separates urine from stool.

intake is monitored, so that only the amount consumed by the control is given the following day to the experimental animal. Thus, at the end of the experiment, intake between the two groups is the same.

When performing these and other feeding studies wherein intake is monitored, special devices are available to prevent food spillage and wastage and to ensure food consumption. In addition, a variety of food formulas are available for nutritional studies (see list of resources in Section XI, B).

2. Parenteral Feedings or Constant Infusions

A model that has been quite useful is the continuous infusion of nutrients in an unrestrained animal. Specialized cages are necessary for dogs, monkeys, and rats, but a large number of rodents can be infused simultaneously to accrue reasonably large numbers of studies for investigational purposes. The infusion apparatus (see Figs. 8 and 9) is commercially available and the feeding formulas have been well described (32, 33).

These models require some surgical skill and a high degree of maintenance. Catheter infection and malfunction are the primary complications, but with experience approximately 90% of animals should complete a rodent infusion protocol lasting 7–10 days.

3. Gastrostomy Feedings

By performing a laparotomy, the infusion catheter can be placed in the stomach or small bowel and enteral nutritional studies can be performed. The diet should be advanced slowly, and drinking water should be available to the animal. If this approach of gradual adaptation to feeding is followed, diarrhea is infrequent. Alternatively, an oral liquid diet can be provided and is often taken freely by rodents. If adequate time for the study is provided, a constant intake is usually achieved.

B. Other Animal Preparations

1. Indwelling Catheters

Catheters can be placed in large vessels of the venous system and in the arterial tree and utilized in chronic preparations. Because infection is a problem, we have made a

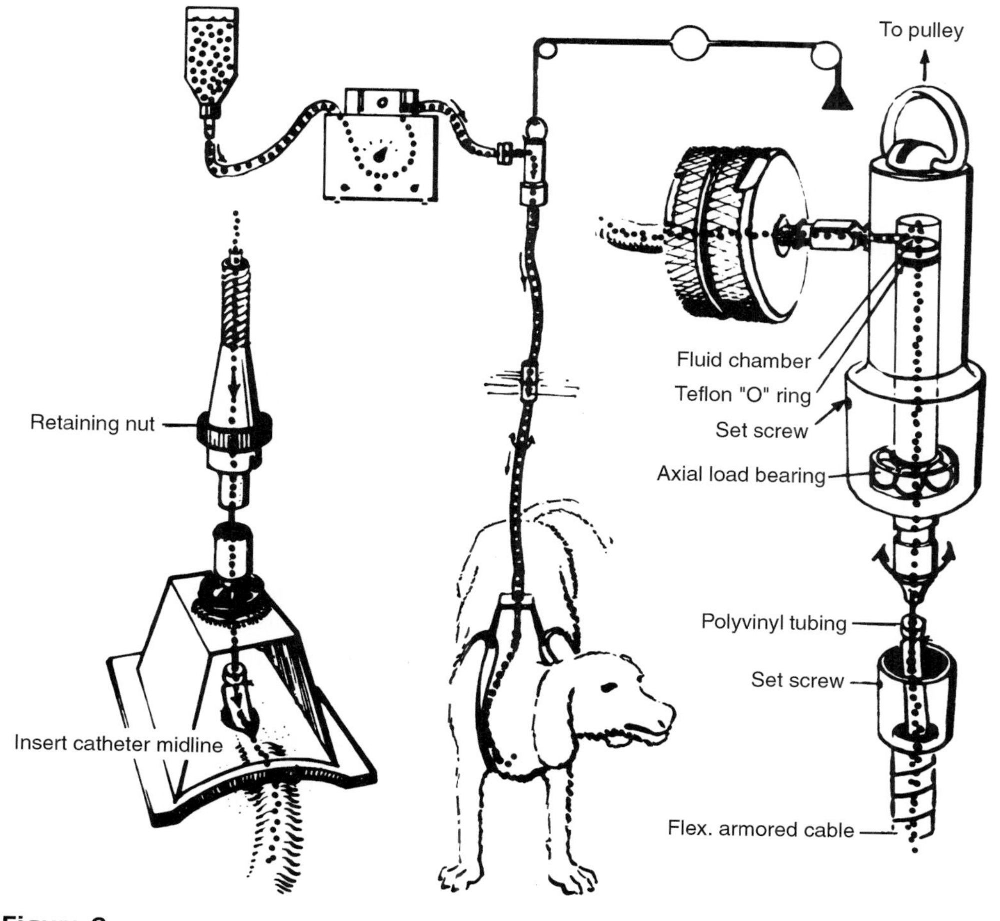

Figure 9 A chronic infusion device used for a large animal model. From Dudrick *et al.* (33), with permission.

subcutaneous port and implanted the distal end under the skin (much like a portacath) (31). The catheters are heparinized and then flushed when utilized.

2. Constant Administration of a Drug or Hormone

Many experiments involve low-dose infusion and implantable pumps (ALZA pumps, Palo Alto, CA, are one example) are frequently utilized for these studies (34). These osmotic pumps are planted subcutaneously or in a body cavity and infuse a fixed amount of fluid hourly. By connecting the pump to a catheter, the substance can be infused into the blood, body cavity, subcutaneously, or into a specific organ such as the brain.

Another approach is to implant time-released pellets containing a hormone or drug (34). This has been a highly satisfactory approach to clamp hormonal responses (following adrenalectomy, a pellet of corticosterone is implanted) before administering a drug. Commercial sources are available to obtain these substances.

3. Models Altering Normal Anatomy

Many nutritional studies have been performed whereby the gastrointestinal tract, in particular, has been altered by resection or rearrangement. These studies have included the nutritional effect on hepatic resection, bowel resection, intestinal transposition, and other experiments. These models can be combined with the feeding techniques previously described to study specific questions.

C. Organ Perfusion and Tissue Studies

1. Regional Perfusion Models

Isolated perfusion of an organ *ex vivo* or in continuity to maintain neural innervation is another commonly used technique to study the net substrate uptake or release by an organ. These studies have generated useful information about the liver (35, 36) and the gut (37). The organ is often studied as an isolated perfused preparation, separated from the rest of the circulation and perfused by an oxygenated perfusate that contains nutrients and other factors such as hormones. The concentration of the compound being studied can be varied and the extraction rate can be calculated as a function of the concentration in the perfusate. From these data whole organ kinetic uptake parameters can be determined. A weakness of this technique is that the relative contributions of the specific cell populations that constitute one portion of the whole organ are not specifically studied.

2. Tissue Uptake of Labeled Substrates

Accumulation of a radiolabeled substrate within an organ following intravascular injection is yet another technique that can be used to quantitate uptake. For example, Windmueller's early studies (38) on gut glutamine metabolism used a radiolabeled injection of glutamine to demonstrate that the majority of glutamine taken up by the small intestine occurred in the mucosal cells. Like the *in vivo* flux measurements described above, the methodology does not specifically measure transport kinetics, but does provide important clues about relative transport rates. Moreover, increased accumulation of the label within the tissue being studied is suggestive of an increase in carrier-mediated transport, but does not provide conclusive data. An increase in diffusion may contribute to differences in the accumulation of label, particularly if the bloodstream delivers large amounts of the substrate. If the amino acid employed is a naturally occurring one, it is not possible to discriminate transport from subsequent intracellular metabolism. Use of nonmetabolizable amino acid analogs [i.e., 2-(methylamine)isobutyric acid (MeAIB), a nonmetabolizable system A-selective substrate] helps to overcome this problem and the resultant steady-state distribution ratio measured represents an index of transport activity. The lack of selective nonmetabolizable substrates limits this technique for a detailed analysis of discrete transport systems.

3. Tissue Biopsies

Tissue biopsies represent another technique that can be used to garner information about regional metabolism. The investigator might treat an animal (or human subject) with one of several diets and subsequently biopsy skeletal muscle or the liver. Some of the early studies on glutamine metabolism in surgical patients used this technique to demonstrate that muscle glutamine depletion is characteristic of catabolic illnesses (39, 40). Most studies of this nature have been done in animals. Following a particular perturbation, tissues can be biopsied or harvested for measurement of enzyme activities, histologic examination, protein synthetic rates, and for concentrations of intracellular amino acids. Because of its accessibility and large contribution to the free amino acid pool, skeletal muscle has been the principal tissue studied.

Other investigators have utilized isotopic infusions to determine the fractional rate of synthesis from organ biopsies. For example, Yang and colleagues (41) have infused L-[U-^{14}C]tyrosine into rats treated with interleukin-1 and measured plasma tyrosine flux, oxidation, and incorporation of tyrosine into protein. This method is attractive because, unlike tracer studies in humans, which measure only whole body protein turnover, specific tissue incorporation rates of tyrosine can be measured.

VIII. Cultured Cells

Cultured cells (and incubations of tissue slices) have been extensively used to study metabolism. Although cell culture studies yield valuable information on substrate consumption, product formation, and signaling mechanisms, they are limited by factors such as cell viability, contamination, and absence of a true physiologic environment. Moreover, these studies do not always quantitatively reflect *in vivo* pathways of metabolism.

Employing cultured cells (primary cultures or established cell lines) to study plasma membrane transport and intracellular metabolism allows the investigator to study the regulation more directly—i.e, apart from other cells, separate from paracrine or endocrine influences, and independent of changes in the microcirculation. Studies have been performed in countless types of cells—maintained in culture, in suspension, adherent to plastic, or attached to special discs that allow access to both apical and basolateral membranes. The use of multiwell cluster trays (42) is an attractive and convenient way to study transport in cultured cells because measurements can be made in many samples at once, which saves on both cost and time. Inhibitors of transcription and translation can be utilized in cultured cells to determine whether alterations in transport or metabolism require *de novo* RNA and/or protein synthesis.

A disadvantage of cell culture studies is that enzyme activity may change during the course of the incubation. Furthermore, some cells require the addition of certain hormones (e.g., insulin or glucocorticoids) to maintain optimal viability. Others can differentiate over time such that their behavior changes from day to day or with multiple serial passages.

Tissue slices incubated in culture or isolated segments of tissue can also be studied. Twenty-five years ago, Goldberg (43) had determined rates of protein synthesis in incubating rat diaphragm by measuring rates of incorporation of [^{14}C]phenylalanine or [^{14}C]tyrosine into muscle protein, after correcting for intracellular-specific activity. Rates of protein degradation were measured by following the net release of tyrosine from cell protein because this amino acid is neither synthesized nor catabolized by muscle. Consequently, its production by isolated muscles reflected net protein breakdown. Many of these methods continue to be used today (see Chapter 59).

IX. Organelle Studies

Subcellular particles and organelles can also be used to study substrate transport and metabolism. Mitochondria have been isolated from cell preparations and studied as intact organelles or prepared as mitochondrial membrane vesicles (mitoplasts) to study amino acid transport. They are easily prepared from fresh tissue using differential and density gradient centrifugation and offer unique advantages over other approaches (44–47). In the case of the gut mucosa, vesicles can be made from the brush border (brush border membrane vesicles, BBMVs) or from the basolateral membrane (BLMVs). Similarly, vesicles from hepatocyte plasma (sinusoidal) membranes (HPMVs) are a useful tool for studying the influence of disease on transport in the liver. Transport activity representative of that occurring in intact cells is adequately preserved in vesicles. Alterations in transport (i.e., following treatment with a hormone, nutrient, or cytokine) reflect the changes that occur *in vivo* and thus may be secondary to direct or indirect effects of mediators. By employing vesicles, it is possible to separate clearly the intrinsic level of membrane transport activity free from other confounding influences (e.g., metabolism, substrate deliver, trans-effects).

Because vesicles are spheres of the cell membrane (they do not contain other organelles), sodium-dependent amino acid transport is driven by a sodium gradient that is artificially created by adding sodium to the transport buffer containing the labeled amino acid of interest. Sodium-dependent amino acid transport by vesicles exhibits a brisk "overshoot" due to rapid Na^+-activated movement of the amino acid into the intravesicular space. With time, as the intra- and extravehicular spaces equilibrate and the sodium gradient is lost, the measured transport velocity approaches zero. Vesicles are cell-free preparations, lacking intracellular organelles and enzymatic pathways, and therefore postreceptor events (i.e., signal transduction) cannot be studied. Mitochondrial transport has been less extensively studied than has plasma membrane transport. Attempts have been hampered by the ability to distinguish transport from metabolism in intact mitochondria. To circumvent this problem, Sastrasinh (48) developed a method of preparing submitochondrial particles (SMPs, membrane vesicles from inner mitochondrial membrane) to study substrate transport. This preparation results in membranes that allow transport to be studied independently of metabolism. In contrast to studies with intact organelles, in which the presence of a specific carrier has never been rigorously demonstrated, the transport of amino acids in SMPs has characteristics indicative of carrier-mediated transport. These features include saturation kinetics, trans-stimulation effects, and substrate specificity. This methodology will allow further studies to be performed to gain insight into how mitochondrial transport is regulated during critical illnesses.

X. Conclusion

No single approach can satisfactorily address nutritional and metabolic questions. The use of multiple approaches provides information that can be utilized to make appropriate conclusions. Alternatively, combining approaches (e.g., flux studies plus tissue biopsy and analysis) is a highly useful technique to describe responses and provide mechanism. The approaches, advantages, and disadvantages are summarized in Table VII.

Table VII An Overview of Various Approaches to the Study of Nutrition and Metabolism

Model/technique	Advantages	Disadvantages
Whole body studies	Easy and relatively inexpensive to perform; provide information describing system as a whole	Do not provide a detailed picture of the status and integration of metabolism within the body
In vivo flux model	Quantitates amino acid flux organ across the entire organ; measurements are made *in vivo*; tissue can be processed for preparation of vesicles or enzyme assays	Does not partition the relative contribution of the various cells in the tissue; does not measure unidirectional fluxes; i.e., is a net measurement
Regional perfusion	Measures whole organ substrate uptake; composition and flow of the perfusate can be controlled	Does not partition the relative contribution of the various cells in the tissue; not an *in vivo* model
Cultured cells	Investigator can study the regulation more directly, separate from paracrine or endocrine influences; inhibitors of transcription and translation can be utilized	Measurements are made separate from other cells in the tissue of origin; transport may be confounded by subsequent metabolism; enzyme activity may change as cells remain in culture; *in vitro* prep—cell viability may be limited or cells may differentiate with multiple passages
Organelle models (membrane vesicles)	Alterations in transport reflect the changes that occur *in vivo*; can discriminate the intrinsic level of membrane transport activity apart from other confounding influences (e.g., metabolism, trans-effects).	Examines only one factor that determines amino acid utilization; transport measurements made in a subcellular membrane; transport changes may be due to direct or indirect effects

XI. Resources

A. General References

The following texts and handbooks provide valuable information on aspects of nutrition and metabolism [see also Kleiber (1), Wilmore (2), Lusk (3), and Consolazio *et al.* (6) in the reference list].

Altman, P. L., and Katz, D. D. (1977). **"Biological Handbooks II. Human Health and Disease."** Federation of American Societies for Experimental Biology, Bethesda.

Bloch, A. S., and Shils, M. E. (1996). **"Nutrition Facts Manual: A Quick Reference."** Williams & Wilkins, Baltimore.

Moore, F. D. (1959). **"Metabolic Care of the Surgical Patient."** W. B. Saunders, Philadelphia.

Munro, H. N., and Allison, J. P. (1964). **"Mammalian Protein Metabolism" [three volumes].** Academic Press, New York.

Peters, J. P., and Van Slyke, D. D. (1932). **"Quantitative Clinical Chemistry."** Williams & Wilkins, Baltimore.

Shils, M. E., Olson, J. A., Shike, M., and Ross, A. C. (1999). **"Modern Nutrition in Health and Disease,"** 9th Ed. Williams & Wilkins, Baltimore.

B. Resources for Studies and Models

1. Food Intake

The appropriate chapters in the Shils *et al.* text on nutrition (see Section XI,A, general references) have helpful information; see also Rimm, E. B., Giovannucci, E. L., Stampfer, M. J., *et al.* (1992). Reproducibility and validity of an expanded self-administered semiquantitative food frequency questionnaire. *Am. J. Epidemiol.* **135,** 1114–1126. In addition, there are many computerized methods for assessing the components of dietary intake. We use the food processor (version 7.0, Esha Research, Salem, OR, 1997).

2. Nitrogen Balances

See Reinfenstein *et al.* (4), Consolazio *et al.* (6), and Byrne *et al.* (7) in the reference list for helpful information.

3. A–V Difference Studies

See studies by Rowell (8), Ahlborg *et al.* (18), Andres *et al.* (19), and Wilmore *et al.* (21).

4. Specialized Rodent Diets

Bio-Serv (One 8th Street, Suite 1, Frenchtown, New Jersey 08825; phone 1-908-996-2155) provides products for rodent studies.

5. Literature on Models

The rat IV model is discussed in Pop and Wagner (32); see also Popp, M. B., and Brennan, M. F. (1981). Long-term vascular access in the rat: Importance of a sepsis. *Am. J. Physiol.* **241,** H606–H612.

The dog chronic catheterization model is discussed in Bessey and Wilmore (30) and Muhlbacher *et al.* (31); see also McGuinness, O. P., Donmoyer, C., Ejiofor, J., McElligot, S., and Lacey, D. B. (1998). Hepatic and muscle glucose metabolism during total parenteral nutrition: Impact of infection. *Am. J. Physiol.* **275,** E763–E769.

6. Animal Research Equipment/Accessories

The following companies provide animal research equipment.

Harvard Apparatus, Inc.
84 October Hill Road
Building No. 7

Holliston, Massachusetts 01746-1371
Phone: 508-655-7000, 800-272-2775

Instech Laboratories, Inc.
5209 Militia Hill Road
Plymouth Meeting, Pennsylvania 19462
Phone: 610-941-0132, 800-443-4227

Lab Products, Inc.
P.O. Box 639
Seaford, Delaware 19973
Phone: 302-628-4300, 800-526-0469

Alza Corporation
950 Page Mill Road
P.O. Box 10950
Palo Alto, California 94303-0802
Phone: 650-494-5000, 800-692-2990

References

1. Kleiber, M. (1961). "The Fire of Life. An Introduction to Animal Energetics." John Wiley and Sons, Inc. New York.
2. Wilmore, D. W. (1977). "The Metabolic Care of the Critically Ill." Plenum Publishing, New York.
3. Lusk, G. (1928). "The Science of Nutrition," 4th ed. Saunders, Philadelphia.
4. Reinfenstein, E. C., Albright, F., and Wells, S. T. (1945). The accumulation, interpretation, and presentation of data pertaining to metabolic balances, notably those of calcium, phosphorous and nitrogen. *J. Clin. Endocrinol.* **5,** 367–395.
5. Welser, M. (1991). Misinterpretation of nitrogen balances when glutamine stores fall or are replenished. *Am. J. Clin. Nutr.* **53,** 1337–1338.
6. Consolazio, C. F., Johnson, R. E., and Pecora, L. J. (1963). "Physiological Measurements of Metabolic Functions in Man." McGraw-Hill, New York.
7. Byrne, T. A., Morrissey, T. B., Gatzen, C., *et al.* (1993). Anabolic therapy with growth hormone accelerates protein gain in surgical patients requiring nutritional rehabilitation. *Ann. Surg.* **218,** 400–416.
8. Rowell, L. B. (1974). Measurements of hepatic splanchnic blood flow in man by techniques. *In* "Dye Curves: The Theory and Practice of Indicator Dilution" (D. A. Bloomfield, ed.) University Park Press, Baltimore.
9. Wilmore, D. W., Goodwin, C. W., Aulick, C. H., *et al.* (1980). Effect of injury and infection and visceral metabolism and circulation. *Ann. Surg.* **192,** 491–504.
10. Owen, O. E., Morgan, A. P., Kemp, H. G., *et al.* (1967). Brain metabolism during fasting. *J. Clin. Invest.* **46,** 1089–1095.
11. Bessey, P. Q., Brooks, D. C., Black, P. R., *et al.* (1983). Epinephrine acutely mediates skeletal muscle insulin resistance. *Surgery* **94,** 172–179.
12. Aulick, L. H., and Wilmore, D. W. (1979). Increased peripheral amino acid release following burn injury. *Surgery* **85,** 560–565.
13. van der Hulst, R. R., von Meyenfeldt, M. F., Deutz, N. E., and Soeters, P. B. (1997). Glutamine extraction by the gut is reduced in depleted patients with gastrointestinal cancer. *Ann. Surg.* **225,** 112–121.
14. Abumrad, N. N., Rabin, D., Diamond, M. P., *et al.* (1981). Use of a heated superficial hand vein as an alternative site for the measurement of amino acid concentrations and for the study of glucose and alanine kinetics in man. *Metabolism* **30,** 936–940.
15. Brooks, D. C., Black, P. R., Arcangeli, M. A., *et al.* (1989). The heated dorsal hand vein: An alternative arterial sampling site. *JPEN* **13,** 102–105.
16. Elwyn, D. H., Launder, W. J., Parikh, H. C., and Wise, E. M. (1972). Roles of plasma and erythrocytes in the intraorgan transport of amino acids in dogs. *Am. J. Physiol.* **222,** 1333–1342.
17. Aoki, T. T., Muller, W. A., Brennan, M. F., and Cahill, G. F., Jr. (1973). Blood cell and plasma amino acid levels across forearm muscle during a protein meal. *Diabetes* **22,** 768–775.
18. Ahlborg, G., Felig, P., Hagenfeldt, L., *et al.* (1974). Substrate turnover during prolonged exercise in man: Splanchnic and leg metabolism of glucose, fatty acids and amino acids. *J. Clin. Invest.* **53,** 1080–1090.
19. Andres, R., Cader, G., and Zierler, K. L. (1956). The quantitatively minor role of carbohydrate in oxidative metabolism by skeletal muscle in intact man in the basal state. Measurements of oxygen and glucose uptake and carbon dioxide and lactate production in the forearm. *J. Clin. Invest.* **35,** 671.
20. Aulick, L. H., Wilmore, D. W., Mason, A. D., Jr., and Pruitt, B. A., Jr. (1982). Depressed reflex vasomotor control of the burn wound. *Cardiol. Res.* **16,** 113–119.
21. Wilmore, D. W., Aulick, L. H., Mason, A. D., Jr., and Pruitt, B. A., Jr. (1977). Influence of the burn wound on local and systemic responses to injury. *Ann. Surg.* **186,** 444–458.
22. Aulick, L. H., Baze, W. B., McLeod, C. G., and Wilmore, D. W. (1980). Control of blood flow to a large surface wound. *Ann. Surg.* **191,** 249–258.
23. Wilmore, D. W., Mason, A. D., Jr., and Pruitt, B. A., Jr. (1976). Insulin response to glucose in hypermetabolic burn patients. *Ann. Surg.* **183,** 314–320.
24. Herndon, D. N., Wilmore, D. W., Mason, A. D., Jr., and Pruitt B. A., Jr. (1978). Abnormalities of phenylalanine and tyrosine kinetics. *Arch. Surg.* **113,** 133–135.
25. McDougal, W. S., Wilmore, D. W., and Pruitt, B. A., Jr. (1977). Glucose-dependent hepatic membrane transport in nonbacteremic and bactermic thermally injured patients. *J. Surg. Res.* **22,** 697–708.
26. Ritshel, W. A. (1983). "Graphic Approach to Clinical Pharmacokinetics." JR Prous Publishers, Barcelona.
27. DeFronzo, R. A., Tobin, J. D., and Andres, J. D. (1979). Glucose clamp technique: A method for quantifying insulin secretion and resistance. *Am. J. Physiol.* **237,** E214–E223.
28. Black, P. R., Brooks, D. C., Bessey, P. Q., *et al.* (1982). Mechanisms of insulin resistance following injury. *Ann. Surg.* **196,** 420–433.
29. Iriyama, K., Tsuchibashi, T., Urata, H., *et al.* (1996). Elimination of fat emulsion particles from plasma during glucose infusion. *Br. J. Surg.* **83,** 946–948.
30. Bessey, P. Q., and Wilmore, D. W. (1983). β-Adrenergic regulation of glucose disposal: A reciprocal retionship with insulin release. *J. Surg. Res.* **34,** 404–414.
31. Muhlbacher, F., Kapadia, C. R., Colpoys, M. F., Smith, R. J., and Wilmore, D. W. (1984). Effect of glucocorticoids on glutamine metabolism in skeletal muscle. *Am. J. Physiol.* **247,** E75–E83.
32. Pop, M. B., and Wagner, S. C. (1984). Nearly identical oral and intravenous nutritional support in the rat: Effects on growth and body composition. *Am. J. Clin. Nutr.* **40,** 107–115.
33. Dudrick, S. J., Steiger, E., Wilmore, D. W., and Vars, H. M. (1970). Continuous long-term intravenous infusion in unrestrained animals. *Lab. Animal Care* **20,** 521–529.
34. Hill, A. G., Jacobson, L., Gonzalez, J., Rounds, J., Majzoub, J. A., and Wilmore, D. W. (1996). Chronic central nervous exposure to interleukin-1β causes catabolism in the rat. *Am. J. Physiol.* **271,** R1142–R11428.
35. Flaim, K. E., Peavy, D. E., Everson, W. V., *et al.* (1982). The role of amino acids in the regulation of protein synthesis in perfused rat liver. I. Reduction in rates of synthesis resulting from amino acid deprivation and recovery during flow-through perfusion. *J. Biol. Chem.* **257,** 2932.

36. Flaim, K. E., Liao, M., Peavy, D. E., *et al.* (1982). The role of amino acids in the regulation of protein synthesis in perfused rat liver. II. Effects of amino acid deficiency on peptide chain initiation, polysomal aggregation, and distribution of albumin mRNA. *J. Biol. Chem.* **257,** 2939.
37. Windmueller, H. G., and Spaeth, A. E. (1974). Uptake and metabolism of plasma glutamine by the small intestine. *J. Biol. Chem.* **249,** 5070–5079.
38. Windmueller, H. G., and Spaeth, A. E. (1974). Uptake and metabolism of plasma glutamine by the small intestine. *J. Biol. Chem.* **249,** 5070–5079.
39. Roth, E., Funovics, J., Muhlbacher, F., *et al.* (1982). Metabolic disorders in severe abdominal sepsis: Glutamine deficiency in skeletal muscle. *Clin. Nutr.* **1,** 25–41.
40. Vinnars, E., Bergstrom, J., and Furst, P. (1975). Influence of the postoperative state on the intracellular free amino acids in human muscle tissue. *Ann. Surg.* 1975, 665–671.
41. Yang, R. D., Moldawer, L. L., Sakamoto, A., *et al.* (1983). Leucocyte endoggenous mediator alters protein dynamics in rats. *Metabolism* **32,** 654.
42. Gazzola, G. C., Dall'Asta, V., Franchi-Gazzola, R., *et al.* (1981). The cluster tray method for rapid measurement of solute fluxes in adherent cultured cells. *Anal. Biochem.* **115,** 368–374.
43. Goldberg, A. L. (1983). Factors affecting protein balance in skeletal muscle in normal and pathologic states. *In* "Amino Acids: Metabolism and Medical Applications" (C.L. Blackburn, J.P. Grant, and V.R. Young, eds.), P. 201. John Wright, Littleton, Massachusetts.
44. Ghishan, F. K., Sutter, W., Said, H., *et al.* (1989). Glutamine transport by rat basolateral membranes. *Biochem. Biophys.* **979,** 77–81.
45. Said, H. M., Van Voorhis, K., Ghishan, F. K., Abumrad, N. N., Nylander, W., *et al.* (1989). Transport characteristics of glutamine in human intestinal brush border membrane vesicles. *Am. J. Physiol.* **256,** G240–G245.
46. Salloum, R. M., Copeland, E. M., and Souba, W. W. (1991). Brush border transport of glutamine and other substrates during sepsis and endotoxemia. *Ann. Surg.* **213,** 401–410.
47. Lohmann, R. G., Souba, W. W., Zakrzewski, K., and Bode, B. P. (1998). Burn-dependent stimulation of rat hepatic amino acid transport. *Metabolism* **47,** 608–616.
48. Sastrasinh, S., and Sastrasinh, M., Glutamine transport in submitochondrial particles. *Am. J. Physiol.* **257,** 1050–1058.

57

Stable Isotopes

Robert R. Wolfe

The University of Texas Medical Branch, Galveston, and Shriners Burns Hospital, Metabolism Unit, Galveston, Texas 77550

I. Isotopes

Many atoms have more than one isotope. Isotopes of an atom are chemically identical elements that differ slightly in weight, a difference that is due to different numbers of neutrons in the atoms. The number of neutrons does not affect the chemical properties of the atom, which are determined by electronic configuration. Thus a commonly used radioactive isotope of carbon (^{14}C) has the same mass as the most abundant isotope of nitrogen (^{14}N), yet these two atoms are chemically distinct. Isotopes can be either radioactive or stable (Table I), and each type has appropriate uses (Table II).

A radioactive nuclide spontaneously disintegrates to form an atom of another element, with the resultant emission of radiation. For example, ^{14}C has 8 neutrons and 6 protons. When undergoing decay, a neutron becomes a proton. In the case of ^{14}C, a neutron becoming a proton results in the formation of nitrogen, which has 7 neutrons and 7 protons, and an electron is released.

In contrast to radionuclides, stable isotopes do not spontaneously disintegrate. Stable isotopes of the same atom vary from each other primarily by mass difference. The most common atoms in biological compounds (C, N, O, H) all have naturally occurring stable isotopes. In the case of carbon, approximately 1.1% of all C has a mass of 13 (^{13}C), with the majority (98.9%) having a mass of 12 (^{12}C). Naturally occurring isotopes of N, O, and H are less abundant, relative to the lowest molecular weight of the atom, than is the case for carbon. In all cases (including C) it is possible to produce or isolate "enriched" isotopes, and then incorporate the heavy isotope into a specific position within a molecule in order to produce a compound distinct from the most commonly occurring form of the molecule by the mass difference at the site of the enriched atom. Such an "enriched" molecule can be used as a metabolic tracer.

II. Tracers

An ideal isotopically labeled tracer is chemically identical to the most abundant form of the molecule, but is detectable in small quantities with high precision. When a tracer is given to an individual, measurement of its fate can enable quantification of the metabolism of its more abundant (naturally occurring) counterpart. An ideal tracer will not affect the metabolism of the molecule being traced (i.e.,

Table I Isotopes Commonly Used in Biological Research

Common forms	Rare stable	Radioactive
^{1}H	^{2}H (0.02%)	^{3}H
^{12}C	^{13}C (1.1%)	^{14}C
^{14}N	^{15}N (0.37%)	^{13}N[a]
^{16}O	^{18}O (0.04%)	^{11}O[a]

[a]Rapid disintegration occurs.

the "tracee"). Thus it is necessary to administer, and therefore be able to detect, small amounts of the tracer. In the case of radioactive isotopes, tracers can readily be detected because of the spontaneous decay of the tracer. In the case of tracers labeled with stable isotopes, it is necessary to determine their abundance by determination of mass differences, because there is no spontaneous decay. Because determination of mass differences is not as precise as detection of radioactivity, it is often necessary to administer considerably more of a stable isotope of a radioactive tracer. This may introduce the possibility of the tracer influencing the metabolism of the tracee. On the other hand, there are several advantages of stable isotope tracers. The most obvious advantage is that they are not radioactive and present little or no risk to human subjects, particularly in tracer doses. Because ^{13}C naturally contributes 1.1% of the carbon pool, and because it has not been possible to demonstrate more than trivial *in vitro* isotopic effects on chemical reactions with carbon-labeled substrates (1, 2), significant side effects *in vivo* are not expected from administration of "tracer" doses of ^{13}C. In fact, Gregg *et al.* (3) fed ^{13}C-enriched algae to mice and raised the ^{13}C content of their total body pool to the 60–70% level with no discernible effect on the animals. Replacement of H_2O with D_2O, however, can affect the growth of microorganisms. To see an effect, however, the deuterated water must be in excess of 20% of the total water (4). Similarly, $H_2{}^{18}O$, ^{13}C, and ^{15}N can be shown to affect certain parameters of cell function at extremely high levels of enrichment, which would never be attained in an *in vivo* study in humans (4, 5). There is no evidence that stable isotope tracers present an identifiable risk to human subjects at the highest levels of enrichment that might reasonably be achieved, with the exception that increasing the enrichment of body water more than 5% with deuterium can cause some neurologic effects.

Whereas isotope effects are not likely at the physiologic level, certain enzymatic effects of stable isotopes have been reported, such that the isotope will be selectively fractionated from its more abundantly occurring counterpart (6–8). Potential isotope effects when carbon, nitrogen, and oxygen are used as tracers are rarely of concern. However, it is possible that isotope effects might occur with ^{3}H or ^{2}H sufficiently to be of physiologic significance. For example, an isotope effect was claimed in the clearance of [3-^{3}H]glucose from blood (9), as well as for [6-^{3}H]glucose and [6,6-$^{2}H_2$]glucose (10). However, it seems likely that these so-called isotope effects can largely, or entirely, be explained by tracer contamination (11) or problems in modeling. Thus, although concern for isotope effects is appropriate, there is little evidence that such errors are a significant problem in *in vivo* studies when the tracer atom is not directly involved in a metabolic reaction. On the other hand, isotope effects are of more potential concern when the tracer in question is directly involved in a metabolic reaction (e.g., loss of ^{13}C from a molecule of $^{13}CO_2$). In any case, with the stable isotope tracers of carbon (^{13}C) and hydrogen (^{2}H), the mass displacement from the most abundant isotope is less than with the corresponding radioactive isotopes (^{14}C and ^{3}H), so less pronounced isotope effects will occur with stable isotopes than with radioisotopes.

In addition to the safety of stable isotopes for human use and the fact that isotope effects should be minimized, there are other advantages of stable isotopic tracers (12). Most obviously, there are no practical radioisotopes of nitrogen (N) or oxygen (O), whereas there are stable isotopes of each element (^{15}N and ^{18}O). Also, when analysis by gas chromatography/mass spectrometry (GCMS) is used, it is often possible to determine enrichment on small samples of blood. Further, there are analytical advantages with stable isotopes. First, by the nature of analysis, identification and purity of the sample are directly confirmed. Also, an internal standard can be added in order to measure the concentration and enrichment simultaneously. Further, the position of a label within a molecule can often be determined. Finally, multiple

Table II Advantages and Disadvantages of Various Approaches to Using Isotopes

Isotope	Advantages	Disadvantages
Stable	No ionizing radiation; safe, nontoxic, can be used in children and repeatedly in adults	Background enrichment requires higher concentrations for measurement; detection less sensitive than for radio isotopes; high costs of isotope, some molecules unavailable; high capital and maintenance cost of detecting equipment, requiring specialized staff
Radioactive	Available, easy to detect, low cost; may still be a preferred tracer in specific groups of adults	Radiation concerns

tracers with the same label can be used simultaneously, because the process of mass spectrometry isolates individual compounds before analysis. For example, several amino acids enriched with ^{13}C can be given simultaneously, and the enrichment of each tracer can be measured independently of the other labeled compounds. On the negative side, because of analytical insensitivity, it is often necessary to give so much "tracer" that the endogenous kinetics of the tracee could be affected.

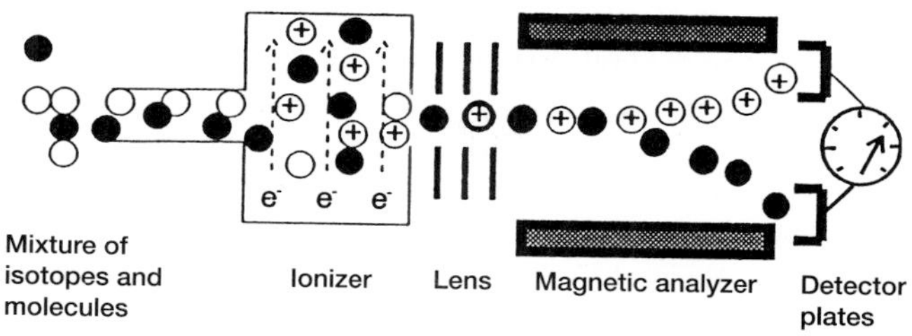

Figure 1 Principles of a gas isotope ratio mass spectrometer.

III. Analysis

A. Gas Isotope Ratio Mass Spectrometer

The use of stable isotopes as tracers dates to the early 1930s and the groundbreaking work of Schonheimer (13). These early studies utilized a mass spectrometer to quantitate abundance of stable isotope tracers in biological samples. The same basic analytical approach is used today, with few conceptual differences. Schoenheimer used a mass spectrometer specifically designed to measure isotope abundance. This kind of mass spectrometer is currently referred to as a gas isotope ratio mass spectrometer (IRMS). Although the isotope ratio of any number of gases can be measured, most instruments designed for use in metabolic studies are set up to conveniently analyze H_2, N_2, or CO_2 gas.

The inlet system to the mass spectrometer is usually a vacuum-line/gas-handling system with holding cells for both a reference gas and the sample gas. The pressures of the reference and sample gases can be equilibrated to eliminate pressure variation as a potential source of error. Capillary "leak" lines are attached to the gas-holding cells and lead to a pair of switching valves that admit the sample and the reference alternately to the ion source. The gas molecules stream from the holding chamber via the molecular "leaks" into the mass spectrometer, which is under high vacuum. This "dual-inlet" system allows for the almost simultaneous analysis of a sample and a reference standard.

Once in the source, the gas molecules are bombarded by electrons that are emitted from a filament wire. As the gas molecules undergo bombardment from the electron beam, some of them lose an outer electron and become positively charged molecular ions. Repelling electrodes force these ions past a series of focusing lenses into the analyzer section of the mass spectrometer (Fig. 1). With IRMS instruments, either a permanent magnet or an electromagnet is used to deflect the molecular ions according to their masses. The radial path of a molecular ion varies with the square root of its mass. Each mass is different enough that the major and minor isotopes of the gaseous molecular ions can simultaneously be collected on spatially separate detector plates. The "double-collector" concept enhances the precision of isotope ratio measurements. As the two ion beams hit the two collectors, they discharge a measurable electron current. For example, $^{12}CO_2$ at mass 44 and $^{13}CO_2$ at mass 45 would each create an ion current. The ratio of these ion currents is then measured so that the isotope ratio is directly related to the current ratio. In an analogous manner, a triple collector allows direct detection of three masses. For example, for CO_2, masses of 44, 45, and 46 ($^{12}C^{16}O_2$, $^{13}C^{16}O_2$, and $^{12}C^{16}O^{18}O$, respectively) would be collected. From the measured ratios obtained before and after administration of tracer, the unit of enrichment needed for calculation of kinetic parameters (tracer/tracee ratio) can be derived.

B. Gas Chromatography/Mass Spectrometry

Whereas the precision and accuracy of the IRMS is outstanding, the necessity to isolate the compound being traced and then convert it (e.g., by combustion) to a gaseous form that can be analyzed is a major limitation. For example, measurement of a ^{13}C-enriched amino acid by IRMS would first require isolation and combustion to CO_2 gas before analysis. Thus, the introduction of gas–liquid chromatography in 1952 (14) and its subsequent interface with mass spectrometry was a major breakthrough in analytical technology. The power of chromatography as a separation technique made it possible to analyze by mass spectrometry biological substances that were otherwise unrealistically difficult to separate. Advances in gas chromatography/mass spectrometry methodology have been the primary reason behind the wider application of stable isotopes in metabolic research.

Gas chromatography provides a simple, rapid, and reproducible method for high-resolution separation of volatile compounds. An inert carrier gas (helium, hydrogen, nitrogen, or methane) passes into the injector. The sample is vaporized in the heated injector and swept through the column by the carrier gas. The separation process on the column occurs in a temperature-controlled oven and the effluent enters the MS interface.

To be separated by gas chromatography, organic compounds must generally be converted to derivatives that are thermally stable, chemically inert, and volatile at temperatures below about 300°C. Derivatization is done in order to increase volatility and, in some circumstances, to improve chromatographic behavior or detectability. Most metabolic substrates in the body are not particularly volatile and therefore require derivatization prior to analysis.

As each compound elutes from the gas chromatograph it enters the ionization chamber of the mass spectrometer. For the analysis of isotopic enrichment, two types of ionization are most widely used, electron impact and chemical. Electron impact (EI) ionization was described for the IRMS. Briefly, the sample molecules pass through a beam of electrons, with the result being removal of an electron from the sample molecule and the formation of a positively charged molecular ion. Further, the energy in excess of that required to ionize the sample molecule is dissipated by fragmentation of the molecular ion. Multiple fragmentations occur with even simple molecules, and the pattern of fragmentation, as reflected by the mass spectrum, is consistently characteristic of that particular sample. Consequently, the mass spectrum of a sample can be considered to be analogous to its "fingerprint" for the purposes of identification and evaluation of the purity of the sample.

In contrast to EI, chemical ionization (CI) is gentle and as a consequence a greater portion of the molecular ions is left intact. CI involves the ionization of a reagent gas, such as methane, at a relatively high pressure. Because CI spectra usually contain abundant ions in the molecular ion region and just a few fragment ions, CI is useful for determining molecular weights, or the total mass enrichment resulting from stable isotope tracers. Also, it is helpful to use CI when analyzing small quantities of a substance, because most of the molecules present are left intact and are detected in a single peak. Due to the reproducible fragmentation pattern with EI, that mode is generally more useful for determining enrichment in specific positions in a molecule.

IV. Calculation of Isotope Enrichment from Mass Spectrometer Data

A. IRMS

The most common expression of data from the IRMS for use in tracer studies is atom percent excess (APE), which is defined as follows:

$$\text{APE} = \frac{r_{sa} - r_r}{(r_{sa} - r_r) - 1} \times 100\%,$$

where r is the isotope ratio signal of the sample (r_{sa}) or reference gas (r_r). For example, in determining $^{13}CO_2/^{12}CO_2$ enrichment, r would be the ratio of mass 45/mass 44 in the sample and reference gases, respectively. Thus, each sample has an APE, expressed in relation to the reference sample. The isotope enrichment resulting from a tracer infusion is then expressed as the difference between the APE of the sample after tracer infusion minus the APE of the background sample drawn before the tracer is given.

The derivation and explanation of APE is somewhat obscure, and in fact although this is generally the data provided by the mass spectrometer, APE is not the most appropriate term for tracer studies. Rather, data should be expressed as the tracee/tracer ratio (*t/T*). The *t/T* ratio is simply the difference between the isotope ratios of the sample and the background ($r_{sa} - r_r$). Using traditional IRMS methodology, this is determined as $t/T = (r_{sa} - r_r) - (r_{bk} - r_r)$.

B. GCMS

The calculation of isotope enrichment using GCMS can be rather complex. A complete description has been given by Wolfe (15). Briefly, the calculation of the *t/T* ratio is the same in principle as for the IRMS, i.e., the ratio of heavy to light isotope samples obtained after tracer infusion minus the same ratio in the background sample. However, the approach for calculating this ratio is different for GCMS. The method involves selection of specific ions to monitor. Generally this will involve determining the relative quantities of ions of different masses of a particular molecular fragment. Because there is a natural abundance of stable isotopes of C, H, O, and N, samples obtained before tracer is given will have a predictable distribution of masses based on the natural occurrence of a heavy stable isotope. For example, if a fragment has three carbon atoms, and 1.1% of all carbon is ^{13}C, then approximately 3.3% of the ions in a background sample will have a ^{13}C molecule. The exact distribution of heavy isotopes in the fragment depends on the structure of the ion, and can be predicted precisely from the known abundance of naturally occurring heavy isotopes (15). When a tracer is given, the ratio of ions with a heavy isotope to the lowest molecular weight of the ion will increase, and the difference between the sample ratio and background ratio is the *t/T* ratio. In the case of the example given above of an ion with three carbons, if 10% of the ions contain a ^{13}C somewhere in the molecule after tracer infusion, then the *t/T* ratio will be $0.10 - 0.033 = 0.067$.

V. Tracer Models

Stable isotope tracers are tools with which to model metabolic processes. The specific models that can be used are limitless. Various books give examples (e.g., 15, 16), but are incomplete because new applications are constantly being described in the current literature. In general, the models can be classified as depending on dilution of tracer by unlabeled tracer, or the direct incorporation of tracer into a product. Some models couple these two types of approaches.

Dilution methods include quantification of the rate of appearance of unlabeled tracee. For example, if a glucose tracer (e.g., ^{2}H-labeled glucose) is infused, then the extent to which the tracer is detected can be used to calculate the rate of appearance of unlabeled glucose. In the absence of glucose intake, the rate of appearance is equivalent to the rate of production (Fig. 2). In a similar manner, the rate of appearance of an unlabeled essential amino acid can be taken as an index of the rate of protein breakdown, because that is the only source of the amino acid. Widely used tracer dilution methods are also available to also quantify lipolysis (17) and free fatty acid flux (18), as well as less commonly used methods for urea (19), acetate (20), and numerous other compounds. More complex tracer dilution methods, when coupled with concentration measurement and regional sampling protocols, can be used to calculate a variety of factors. For example, the rate of muscle protein synthesis, (Fig. 3), breakdown, and amino acid transmembrane transport can be quantified by a dilution method involving sampling from the femoral artery and vein as well as from the tissue free amino acid pool (obtained by biopsy) (21).

The second general category of tracer study involves the quantitation of the rate of incorporation of tracer into a product. For example, the rate of incorporation into product has been used to quantify substrate oxidation (from ^{13}C incorporation into CO_2), protein synthesis, very low-density lipoprotein triglyceride (VLDL-TG) synthesis, and the production of other compounds. The calculation of the rate of synthesis of the product (i.e., protein) requires dividing the isotopic enrichment of the product by the enrichment of the precursor. This is because the extent of incorporation of a tracer into a product will depend not only on the actual rate of synthesis, but also on the abundance of tracer. Thus, for a given rate of synthesis of protein, doubling the tracer infusion rate will double the rate of incorporation of tracer into protein, even though the absolute synthesis rate remains constant.

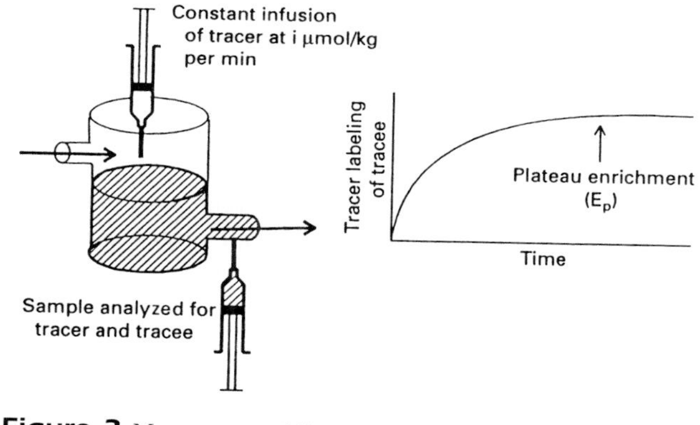

Figure 2 Measurement of flux using the constant infusion technique. Flux through the pool (μmol/kg·min) is determined as i/E_p, where i is the infusion rate of the tracer and E_p is the enrichment reached at plateau (or steady state).

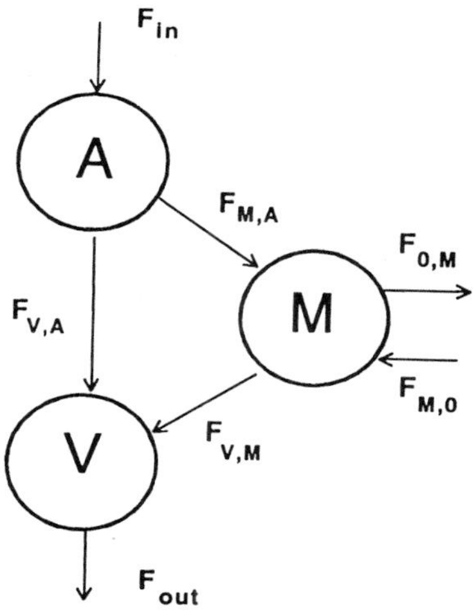

Figure 3 The three-compartment model for measuring protein synthesis in skeletal muscle. *A*, Arterial concentration; *V*, venous concentration; F_{in}, amino acids entering the extremity; F_{out}, amino acids leaving the extremity; $F_{M,A}$ and $F_{V,M}$, inward and outward amino acid flux rates; $F_{0,M}$ and $F_{M,0}$, protein synthesis and breakdown. From Biolo *et al.* (21).

Accurate determination of the precursor enrichment is usually problematic, because it is rarely possible to sample the precursor directly. For example, when ^{13}C-labeled free fatty acids (FFAs) are infused, the rate of FFA oxidation is reflected by the excretion of $^{13}CO_2$ in the breath. However, only plasma ^{13}C-labeled FFAs can be conveniently measured as an indicator of precursor enrichment, but the actual precursor for oxidation is intracellular. Use of plasma FFA enrichment therefore will result in an erroneous rate of oxidation, and the measured value may be as low as 30% of the true value (22). Similarly, charged tRNA is the true precursor for protein synthesis, yet measurement of tRNA enrichment is difficult in any circumstance and particularly difficult in human studies because of the sample size required. Various surrogates for tRNA enrichment can be used (23), and the errors can be minimized. However, by virtue of the fact that by definition any measured "precursor" has not been incorporated into the product, it is uncertain if that "precursor" will in fact reflect the true pool of molecules from which the product will be synthesized. In this regard, a newly described method called mass isotopomer distribution analysis has been developed; this technique examines the pattern of enrichment of the product in order to determine what the enrichment of the precursor had to be to produce that pattern of enrichment in the product. For example, [1-^{13}C]acetate can be used as a precursor to measure the rate of fatty acid synthesis. There are eight "units" of the two-carbon acetate required to produce one molecule of palmitate. The higher the precursor enrichment of acetate, the more likely it is that more than one tracer molecule will be incorporated into the product. Thus, by analyzing the relative number of palmitate molecules that have two versus one [^{13}C]acetate molecules incorporated, it is possible to calculate the precursor enrichment (24). As with any model, this new method has its limitations, but it has the major conceptual advance that the precursor enrichment is determined from measurement of the product rather than from measurement of a surrogate for the true precursor.

VI. Assumptions

Each specific model used has assumptions unique to that model, and these assumptions must be clearly stated and assessed for the particular application. Beyond that, certain general assumptions underlie all tracer studies and all of these must be assessed in the context of any experiment.

1. The tracer does not affect the metabolism of the tracee, or account must be taken of the effect of the tracer on the tracee. This issue may be of concern with stable isotopes that often must be given in large doses because of limitations in instrumental capabilities. In particular, bolus injection studies can be problematical, because in order to measure decaying enrichment the starting enrichment often has to be so high as to significantly affect the total concentration of the compound of interest. This makes the popular approach of compartmental modeling difficult to apply with stable isotopes. Rather, steady-state models requiring only low levels of enrichment are often preferable.

2. The tracer must reflect the metabolism of the tracee. This is the most commonly overlooked assumption. What may seem to be a simple tracer incorporation study may in fact be enormously complicated by a variety of potential sites of isotope exchange. An example of isotope exchange, and how it might be possible to account for such exchange, is provided for the case described above of fatty acid oxidation (25). In this case, isotopic exchange occurs in the Kreb's cycle that results in the underestimation of the true rate of oxidation. Further, the extent of underestimation is variable, and is a function of the rate of V_{CO_2} (25). In this case, identification of the sites of the tracer exchange enabled the application of an appropriate correction factor using carbon-labeled acetate (25). In other cases, correction for isotopic exchange has proved more problematical. In particular, investigators have attempted to overcome the problem of isotopic exchange in the pathway of gluconeogenesis for at least 30 years, and a consensus on the best approach has not yet been achieved. On the other hand, it is possible to capitalize on known pathways of isotope exchange to quantify rates of intracellular reactions. In the case of hepatic glucose metabolism, for example, substrate cycles involving glucose (26) and phosphoenolpyruvate–pyruvate–oxaloacetate (27) have been quantified by capitalizing on known sites of tracer exchange.

3. There is no isotope discrimination. This was discussed briefly above. There are two types of isotope discrimination. In one case, the atom is treated differently because of its mass difference (e.g., ^{2}H vs. ^{1}H). In the other case, molecules labeled with different tracers behave differently. The best examples that can illustrate the latter phenomenon and how it can be capitalized on are the distinct isotope enrichment patterns that follow from the ingestion of ^2H_2O and $H_2{}^{18}O$. The oxygen in H_2O equilibrates with the oxygen in CO_2. Consequently, the label in $H_2{}^{18}O$ will decay after a bolus ingestion not only as a function of water turnover, but also CO_2 turnover. In contrast, ^2H_2O enrichment will decay as a function of water turnover alone. The difference in the decay rates will therefore reflect the rate of CO_2 turnover. This principle has been used to quantify energy expenditure by the so-called doubly-labeled water technique in freely living subjects (28). Other examples of differently labeled tracers yielding distinct kinetic rates, depending on the particular site and atom labeled, are abundant (e.g., 29, 30). It is thus pertinent in selecting a particular tracer (e.g., ^{15}N- or ^{13} C-labeled amino acid) to consider the fate of each atom within the molecule.

4. The site of infusion and site of sampling of the tracer are appropriate for a particular model. This issue has been discussed in a number of publications, and often represents a problem that cannot be overcome. Thus, in general it is necessary to sample downstream of both the site of entry (i.e., infusion) and metabolism of the tracer, and in some cases this may not be practical in human subjects.

VII. If Assumptions Are Not Satisfied

Modeling in human subjects often requires application of models that are known to have certain assumptions that are imprecise, or even completely wrong. For example, the optimal infusion site-sampling site mode is not practical in human subjects. It is necessary to not only acknowledge the general problem, but to attempt to quantify the magnitude of error that might be expected in extreme circumstances. Thus, it is generally possible to calculate upper and lower "bounds" to a model-derived value based on the most extreme errors likely to result from all assumptions made. If differences between treatment groups are large, relative to the upper and lower bounds of the calculated value, then the conclusion is likely valid, even if there is an uncertainty regarding precise quantitation.

Acknowledgment

Supported by Shriners Hospital for Children–Galveston Burns Hospital Grant #8490.

References

1. O'Leary, M. D., Richard, D. T., and Hendrickson, J. (1970). Carbon isotope effects on the enzymatic decarboxylation of glutamic acid. *J. Am. Chem. Soc.* **92,** 4435.
2. Eakin, R. T. (1975). Kinetic properties of an enzyme highly enriched in carbon-13. *Biochim. Biophys. Acta* 377–379.
3. Gregg, C. T., Hutson, J. Y., Prine, J. R., Ott, D. G., and Furchner, J. E. (1973). Substantial replacement of mammalian body carbon with carbon-13. *Life Sci.* **13,** 775.
4. Carpioli, R. M. (1970). Use of isotopes. *In* "Biochemical Applications of Mass Spectrometry" (G. R. Waller, ed.), pp. 735–771. Wiley-Interscience, New York.
5. Uphaus, R. A., Flaumenhaft, E., and Katz, J. J. (1967). A living organism of unusual isotopic composition: Sequential and cumulative replacement of stable isotopes in *Chlorella vulgaris. Biochim. Biophys. Acta* **141,** 625.
6. Krouse, H. R., and Sasaki, A. (1968). Sulfur and carbon isotope fractionation by *Salmonella beidelbens* during an aerobic SO_3^- reduction in trypticase soy broth medium. *J. Microbiol.* **14,** 417–423.
7. Solverman, M. P., and Ouama, V. I. (1968). Automatic apparatus for sampling and preparing for mass spectral analysis in studies of carbon isotope fraction, during methane metabolism. *Anal. Chem.* **40,** 1833–1839.
8. Mahler, H. R., and Douglas, J. (1957). Mechanisms of enzyme-catalyzed oxidation–reduction reactions (1): Yeast alcohol dehydrogenase reaction by the isotope rate effect. *J. Am. Chem. Soc.* **79,** 1159.
9. Bell, P. M., Firth, R. G., and Rizza, R. A. (1986). Assessment of insulin action in insulin-dependent diabetes mellitus using 6-^{14}C-glucose, 3-^{3}H-glucose, and 2-^{3}H-glucose: Differences in the apparent pattern of insulin resistance depending on the isotope used. *J. Clin. Invest.* **78,** 1479–1486.
10. Argound, G. M., Shade, D. S., and Eaton, R. P. (1987). Underestimation of hepatic glucose production of radioactive and stable tracers. *Am. J. Physiol.* **252,** E606–E612.
11. McMahon, M. M., Schwenk, W. F., Haymond, M. W., and Rizza, R. A. (1989). Accumulation in plasma of a radioactive contaminant present in 6-^{3}H but not 6-^{14}C glucose leads to a systematic underestimation of glucose turnover. *Diabetes* **38,** 97–107.
12. Bier, D. M. (1987). The use of stable isotopes in metabolic investigation. *In* "Clinical Endocrinology and Metabolism" (K. G. M. M. Albuti, P. D. Home, and R. Taylor, eds.), Vol. 1, pp. 817–836. Baillieu Tiudal, London.
13. Schoenheimer, R., Ratner, S., and Rittenberg, D. J. (1939). Protein metabolism (II): Synthesis of amino acids containing isotopic N. *J. Biol. Chem.* **130,** 703.
14. James, A. T., and Martin, A. J. P. (1952). Gas–liquid partition chromatography. Separation and microestimation of volatile fatty acids from formic acid to dodecanoic acid. *Biochem. J.* **50,** 679.
15. Wolfe, R. R. (1992). "Radioactive and Stable Isotope Tracers In Biomedicine: Principles and Practice of Kinetic Analysis." Wiley-Liss, New York.
16. El-Khoury, A. (1999). "Methods for Investigation of Amino Acid and Protein Metabolism." CRC Press, Boca Raton, FL.
17. Wolfe, R. R., Herndon, D. N., Jahoor, F., Miyoshi, H., and Wolfe, M. (1987). Effect of severe burn injury on substrate cycling by glucose and fatty acids. *N. Engl. J. Med.* **317,** 403–408.
18. Wolfe, R. R., Evans, J. E., Mullany, C. J., and Burke, J. F. (1980). Measurement of plasma free fatty acid turnover and oxidation using palmitic acid. *Biomed. Mass Spectrom.* **7**(4), 168–171.
19. Wolfe, R. R. (1981). Measurement of urea kinetics *in vivo* by means of a constant tracer infusion of di-^{15}*N*-urea. *Am. J. Physiol.* **240** (*Endocrinol. Metab.* **3**), E428–E434.
20. Mittendorfer, B., Sidossis, L. S., Walser, E., Chinkes, D. L., and Wolfe, R. R. (1998). Regional acetate kinetics and oxidation in human volunteers. *Am. J. Physiol.* **274** (*Endocrinol. Metab.* **35**), E978–E983.
21. Biolo, G., Fleming, R. Y. D., Maggi, S. P., and Wolfe, R. R. (1995). Transmembrane transport and intracellular kinetics of amino acids in human skeletal muscle. *Am. J. Physiol.* **268** (*Endocrinol. Metab.* **31**), E75–E84.
22. Sidossis, L. S., Coggan, A. R., Gastaldelli, A., and Wolfe, R. R. (1995). Pathway of free fatty acid oxidation in human subjects: Implications for tracer studies. *J. Clin. Invest.* **95,** 278–284.
23. Chinkes, D. L., Klein, S., Zhang, X.-J., and Wolfe, R. R. (1996). Infusion of labeled KIC is more accurate than labeled leucine to determine muscle protein synthesis. *Am. J. Physiol.* **270** (*Endocrinol. Metab.* **33**), E67–E71.
24. Aarsland, A., Chinkes, D. L., and Wolfe, R. R. (1996). Contributions of denovo synthesis of fatty acids and lipolysis to VLDL secretion during prolonged hyperglycemia/hyperinsulinemia in normal man. *J. Clin. Invest.* **98,** 2008–2017.
25. Sidossis, L. S., Coggan, A. R., Gastaldelli, A., and Wolfe, R. R. (1995). A new correction factor for use in tracer estimations of plasma fatty acid oxidation. *Am. J. Physiol.* **269** (*Endocrinol. Metab.* **32**), E649–E656.
26. Miyoshi, H., Shulman, G. I., Peters, E. J., Wolfe, M. H., Elahi, D., and Wolfe, R. R. (1988). Hormonal control of substrate cycling in humans. *J. Clin. Invest.* **81,** 1545–1555.
27. Wolfe, R. R., Chinkes, D. L., Hidefumi, B., Rosenblatt, J., and Zhang, X.-J. (1996). Response of phosphoenolpyruvate cycle activity to fasting and to hyperinsulinemia in human subjects. *Am. J. Physiol.* **271** (*Endocrinol. Metab.* **34**), E159–E176.
28. Schoeller, D. A. (1983). Energy expenditure from doubly-labeled water: Some fundamental considerations in humans. *Am. J. Clin. Nutr.* **38,** 995–1005.
29. Yang, R. D., Matthews, D. E., Bier, D. M., Lo, C., and Young, V. R. (1984). Alanine kinetics in humans: Influence of different isotopic tracers. *Am. J. Physiol.* **247,** E634–E638.
30. Matthews, D. E., Bier, D. M., Rennie, M. J., Edwards, R. H. T., Halliday, D., Milward, D. J., and Clugston, G. A. (1981). Regulation of leucine metabolism in man: A stable isotope study. *Science* **214,** 1129–1131.

58

Body Composition

Lindsay D. Plank and Graham L. Hill

University Department of Surgery, Auckland Hospital, Auckland 1001, New Zealand

I. Introduction

Surgical illness is accompanied by fundamental changes in body composition. These are primarily loss of body protein, gain in body water, and erosion of fat stores. The rate at which these processes occur and the balance between them determine the clinical picture observed, and an understanding of them opens the door to intelligent management of many complex disorders. Protein, fat, and water are the nutritionally important components of the body and the measurement of these is an essential and major aspect of the assessment of nutritional state.

II. Definition of Terms

The three compartments, protein, fat, and water, make up around 95% of body weight, the remainder being minerals and carbohydrate. The relative sizes of these compartments, as typically found in health, are shown in Fig. 1 for the "reference man" (1). This is the classic chemical- or molecular-level body composition model. The terms used for these compartments are not always defined consistently or precisely in the body composition literature. This is particularly true for fat.

A. Fat

Total body fat is generally defined as the ether-extractable portion of the body, principally triglyceride or neutral fat, and is the storage form of fat found in adipose tissue. This nonessential fat together with essential or "structural" fat, which includes phospholipids, sphingolipids, and sterols, makes up the total lipid portion of the body (2). The latter are extractable with polar solvents such as acetone and methanol. Limited data are available on the amount of essential fat in the body. As a percentage of the fat-free mass (FFM), analysis of five cadavers shows the amount may vary between 4 and 15% (3).

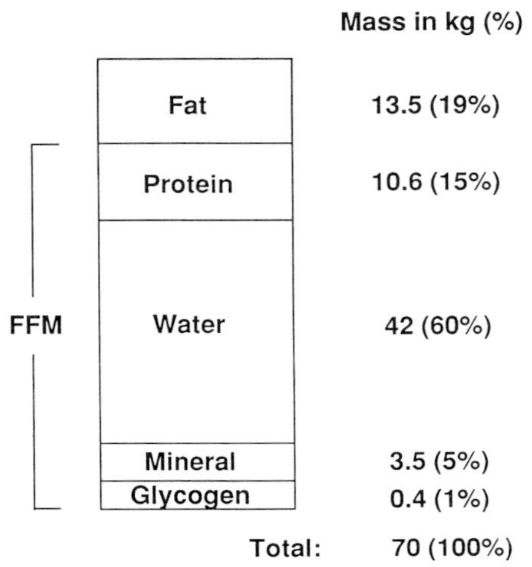

Figure 1 The components of body weight in the "reference man," showing the fat-free mass (FFM).

B. Protein

Total body protein is estimated from measurements of total body nitrogen, all of which is assumed to be incorporated into protein, which on average contains 16% nitrogen (4).

C. Water

Total body water refers to the protein-free component of the total fluid of the body.

D. Minerals and Carbohydrate

Minerals are considered to be the ashed residue of the skeleton together with total nonosseous minerals in the body. Glycogen makes up essentially all the carbohydrate in the body, found predominantly in skeletal muscle and the liver.

III. Methodology

It is now technically feasible to analyze the living human body in a variety of ways. The methodology for body composition assessment may be viewed in a hierarchical manner (Table I) (5). At the highest level is chemical analysis of tissue. The validation of any body composition technique relies ultimately on chemical analysis of tissues from cadaver dissection or biopsies. Unfortunately, only in a very few instances have whole body analyses of cadavers by chemical means been used to check results from other methods (4,6). More generally, published analyses of tissues provide the basis for interpreting *in vivo* measurements. Level II methods allow semidirect quantification of specific body constituents. These include *in vivo* neutron activation analysis (IVNAA) and dual-energy X-ray absorptiometry (DEXA).

Table I Hierarchy of Body Composition Methodology[a]

Level	Methodology
I	Chemical analysis of the whole body and tissues
II	Direct *in vivo* measurement of body constituents
III	*In vivo* estimation of body compartments using modeling approaches
IV	*In vivo* measurement of somatic or physical property calibrated against body constituent derived by methods at levels I–III

[a]After Heymsfield *et al* (5), with permission. © *Am. J. Clin. Nutr.* American Society for Clinical Nutrition.

Level III includes methods based on experimental models requiring assumptions regarding the densities or ratios of measured components—for example, hydrodensitometry for the measurement of body fat. The methods at the lowest level require calibration against criterion measurements from a higher level method. These include skinfold anthropometry and bioimpedance analysis.

A. Hydrodensitometry

This method assumes that the body is composed of two distinct components, fat and FFM, and that it is possible to determine each of these components from a measurement of whole body density. The fat and FFM are each assumed to have known and constant densities. Fat has a lower density than does lean tissue, therefore relatively fatter subjects will have a lower overall density. The equation in widespread use is:

$$\text{body fat }(\%) = 100[(4.95/D) - 4.50],$$

where D is the body density. This equation is based on assumed densities of 0.900 g/cm^3 for fat and 1.100 g/cm^3 for FFM (7). Body density is found by dividing measured body weight by body volume. Body volume is usually determined according to Archimedes' principle by weighing the subject in air and under water and correcting for the volume of air in the lungs (8). Although this method has been used widely to measure the composition of healthy subjects, the requirement for underwater immersion clearly limits its use in clinical investigations. Furthermore, the accuracy with which body fat and changes in body fat can be estimated from body density is grossly impaired by typical pathological changes in the composition of the FFM, as shown by Burkinshaw (9).

B. Dilution Methods

Dilution methods are based on the principle that the amount of a tracer injected into an unknown volume or mass is the same both before and after thorough mixing in that volume or mass. For example, if Q is the mass of tracer administered, with concentration C_1 in a volume V_1, then

$$Q = C_1V_1 = C_2V_2,$$

where V_2 is the volume of dilution and C_2 is the equilibrium concentration of the tracer after mixing. The various techniques for estimation of body fluid volumes are all based on this principle. After an interval has elapsed for equilibration of a known amount of material given to a patient, a sample of plasma, urine, saliva, or exhaled water vapor is obtained for analysis and the dilution volume calculated as

$$V_2 = (Q - Q_{ex})/C_2,$$

where Q_{ex} is the amount of tracer lost during equilibration, usually by excretion in the urine. The volume to be determined has of course been increased by the added volume V_1, but V_1 is usually much smaller than V_2 and can be neglected. The tracer should be nontoxic in the amount used, and mix rapidly and uniformly with the majority of the material to be measured with minimal loss during the equilibration period. Moore and co-workers (10) have provided a detailed discussion of the principles of tracer dilution particularly as they apply in the clinical context.

1. Total Body Water

Undoubtedly the most important dilution method is that involved in the measurement of total body water (TBW), which can be achieved by labeling water with ^3H (tritium), ^2H (deuterium), or ^{18}O (11, 12). Other nonisotopic tracers such as ethanol or urea have also been used, but less successfully. Brodie (13) has given a useful summary of the advantages and disadvantages of these various tracers. The organic solutes, such as urea, merely distribute through the solvent and have metabolism completely distinct from the tracee, whereas the isotopically labeled tracers provide a measure of atomic exchange into the water molecule. As such, the latter measure total exchangeable hydrogen or oxygen (in the case of ^{18}O), which is then converted to a water volume. Tracer equilibration is rapid and essentially complete within 2–3 hr in healthy individuals (11). In patients with significant edema, ascites, pleural effusion, and shock, equilibration may require 4–5 hr (14). In patients receiving continuous infusions of fluid during the equilibration period a correction must be applied to account for these (15). This particularly applies in the case of patients receiving intensive care, because these fluids cannot be withheld over the period of isotope equilibration; their noninstantaneous mixing with body water leads to a dilution effect in plasma water.

For deuterium and tritium, the dilution volume is larger than the body water space because of exchange with nonaqueous hydrogen in water-soluble biochemical components. This overestimation has been shown theoretically to be less than 5.2% (16). The ^{18}O dilution volume is smaller than the ^2H and ^3H spaces but still overestimates the TBW space by about 1%, because of exchange with nonaqueous oxygen (11). Most workers apply a correction of 4–5% to the ^2H and ^3H spaces and 1% to the ^{18}O space to estimate TBW. The actual corrections that should be applied in patients with significant overhydration might be expected to be less than these. Unfortunately, although ^{18}O provides a more accurate estimate of TBW, it is much more expensive than ^2H or ^3H. Like ^2H it is usually assayed by mass spectrometry, whereas ^3H, being a β-emitting radionuclide, is easily measured using scintillation counting (15). The use of ^3H necessitates a small radiation dose to the patient. Effective radiation dose equivalent is 16 μSv/MBq (17). In our laboratory we administer 3.7 MBq (100 μCi) of tritium as tritiated water, which entails a radiation dose of about 60 μSv. The physical half-life of tritium is 12.3 years, but its half-life in the body is typically about 13 days (10).

The precision (coefficient of variation) for a ^3H dilution measurement has been determined by repeated measurements in weight-stable individuals over a 6-week period as 2.5% (18).

Dilution measurements of TBW have been widely used to estimate fat-free mass and hence body fat, based on the assumption that the ratio of TBW to FFM is a constant for all subjects. This hydration constant is usually taken to be 73% for normally hydrated adults (19). This approach is clearly not applicable in the typical surgical patient with an expanded body water compartment.

2. Extracellular Water

A wide variety of tracer substances have been used for estimation of the extracellular water (ECW) volume. None is completely satisfactory owing to the nonhomogeneous nature of the extracellular fluid phase. Further, universal agreement as to what constitutes the extracellular fluid volume is lacking. A reasonable definition (20) considers the extracellular water as made up of (1) plasma water, (2) interstitial-lymph water, (3) dense connective tissue, cartilage, and bone water, and (4) transcellular water, including that found in cerebrospinal fluid and the gut lumen. In a healthy young adult male this water volume constitutes approximately 45% of the total body water and is distributed as shown in Fig. 2 (20). The observation that chloride is almost exclusively extracellular in skeletal muscle led to its use as a measure of extracellular volume. Both ^{38}Cl and ^{36}Cl have been used for this purpose. However, both are radioactive and are inconvenient to use, the former because of its short half-life (37 min) and the latter because of its very long half-life (3×10^5 years), so that it is difficult to prepare with high specific activity. Bromide is distributed very similarly to choride in the body (21) and the "bromide space" is widely used as a measure of extracellular water volume. The advent of high-performance liquid chromatography as a very sensitive technique for assaying stable bromide (22) has effec-

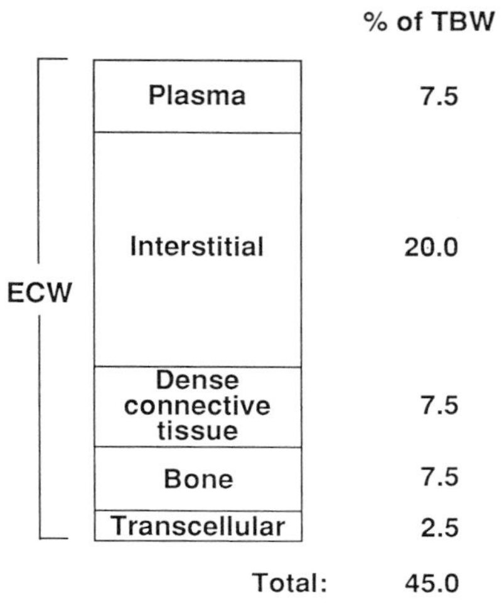

Figure 2 Distribution of the components of extracellular water (ECW) in a normal young adult male as percentages of total body water (TBW).

tively eliminated the need to use the radionuclide ^{82}Br, which again has an inconveniently short half-life (36 hr). Bromide is known to penetrate some tissue cells, especially erythrocytes (20, 23), and a correction should be applied for this. The corrected bromide space (CBS), often assumed to equal the extracellular water volume, is usually given by the following formula (24):

$$\text{CBS} = 0.90 \times 0.95 \times 0.94 \times \text{Br dose}/[\text{Br}]_s,$$

where a known amount of bromide (for example as sodium bromide) is given orally or intravenously and a serum sample is taken after equilibration is reached. In this formula, 0.90 is the correction factor for intracellular penetration, 0.95 is the Donnan equilibrium factor, 0.94 corrects for the protein content of serum, and $[\text{Br}]_s$ is the concentration of bromide in serum after correction for the basal concentration. Basal blood concentration of bromide is normally around 0.06 mmol/liter in adults with no recent abnormal environmental exposure to bromide (25). The half-life for elimination from the body is approximately 12 days (26). Symptoms of bromide toxicity occur at about 9–12 mmol/liter (27), with lower thresholds in those with impaired renal function and the elderly, and researchers need to be mindful of this if repeated doses are given within a short period. In our laboratory, we administer 2.5 g NaBr orally or, when the oral route is unavailable or inconvenient, intravenously. There is no general consensus on the optimal time to allow for equilibration of bromide tracer in the body. In some studies equilibration appeared to be achieved in 2 hr (oral or intravenous administration) in individuals without abnormal fluid collections or distribution (28–30). At least a 5-hr equilibration time has been suggested by other studies (31, 32), especially if edema is present (28, 31). Yet other reports advocate 24 hr as being necessary (18). Limited published data are available concerning equilibration in fluid collections such as ascites and pleural effusions; some evidence suggests 6 hr as adequate (31) and bromide content of pleural and peritoneal fluid was shown to be identical to serum concentration after this time (33). A measurable increase in the bromide space beyond a rapid equilibration phase lasting a few hours may occur because of slow permeation of bromide into CSF particularly (10, 23). The precision (coefficient of variation) for a ^{82}Br dilution measurement has been determined by repeated measurements in weight-stable individuals over a 6-week period as 2.3% (18).

Although bromide has become the most commonly used tracer for ECW measurement, radiosulfate ($^{35}SO_4^{2-}$) has also been widely used, having the advantage of reduced intracellular permeability compared with bromide. Early work on ECW changes in hemorrhagic shock was carried out with radiosulfate (34). Rapid renal excretion of this tracer (biological half-life 4–9 hr) requires that the reverse-extrapolation or slope-intercept method must be used to estimate the dilution space at the time of administration, rather than the plateau method discussed in the preceding paragraphs. Its volume of distribution is about 80% of that measured by bromide because of limited penetration into dense connective tissue and transcellular water spaces (35).

ECW has also been estimated using the saccharides mannitol, sucrose, and inulin to circumvent the problems of cellular permeability to ions. This group of tracers has the disadvantage of slow penetration into dense connective tissue spaces, rapid renal clearance that interferes with reaching a steady state, and some degree of participation in metabolic processes (23).

3. Intracellular Water

A satisfactory dilution method for estimating intracellular water (ICW) volume is not available and this space is usually calculated as the difference between TBW and ECW. The precision errors for the measurements of TBW (2.5%, or about 1.0 kg) and ECW (2.3%, or 0.4 kg) then propagate to about 4.5% for ICW.

4. Blood Volume

The blood volume is traditionally obtained as the sum of independent measurements of red cell volume and plasma volume. Red cell volume is measured by dilution of red cells tagged with radiochromium (^{51}Cr) (36). In the few hours involved with the dilutional measurement, the slow addition of new red cells from the bone marrow and the breakdown of tagged red cells are negligible factors in the volume determination. Evans Blue dye or radioiodinated (^{125}I or ^{131}I) albumin is traditionally used as a dilution marker for estimating the plasma volume (20, 36). The former bonds stoichiometrically with albumin and thus may be considered a tracer for albumin with partition distribution almost identical to radioalbumin.

5. Ratio of Total Exchangeable Sodium to Total Exchangeable Potassium

Dilution of the radioisotopes ^{42}K or ^{43}K together with ^{22}Na yields a determination of the ratio of total exchangeable sodium (Na_e) to total exchangeable potassium (K_e). Sodium is predominantly extracellular, and in fact has been used to estimate extracellular fluid volume, whereas potassium is almost exclusively intracellular and has been used to estimate the total cellular mass of the body (see Section III,E). The ratio Na_e/K_e provides a sensitive index of nutritional state (37) owing to the reciprocal changes that occur in the body cell mass and the extracellular mass with malnutrition and critical illness. ^{42}K and ^{43}K possess short half-lives, which makes their use expensive and logistically difficult. Whole body counting is an alternative for potassium measurement, but these installations are few (see Section III,E). Shizgal *et al.* (38) have described an indirect measurement of K_e based on TBW determination (by tritium dilution) and ^{22}Na dilution entailing a radiation exposure of approximately 2.5 mSv.

C. Anthropometry

Among the range of techniques designed to assess human body composition, anthropometry occupies an important place. It is easily performed at the bedside, has been widely used to assess the nutritional status of an individual, and been extensively applied to the hospitalized patient. In addition to height and weight, the measurements usually performed are skinfold thicknesses and arm circumference.

1. Skinfold Thicknesses

This method involves the measurement of a fold of subcutaneous fat at one or more sites, which can then be interpreted using previously validated prediction equations into an estimate of fat mass. Probably the most widely used prediction equations are those developed by Durnin and Womersley (39) in which the sum of the skinfold thicknesses at one or more sites (up to four) is related to body density in healthy subjects measured by hydrodensitometry by age- and sex-specific equations of the form

$$\text{density} = A - B \log_{10} S,$$

where A and B are empirically derived coefficients and S is the sum of the skinfold measurements. Fat mass is then calculated using the equation of Siri (7) (see Section III,A) and measured body weight. The four sites used by Durnin and Womersly are biceps, triceps, subscapular, and suprailiac. The measurements are made using calipers, which exert a standardized pressure on the measurement site. With a single trained observer the method can yield very reproducible results. Systematic differences are found between skinfold measurements made by different operators on the same subjects. However, these are relatively small (40), although it is often stated that longitudinal studies are best carried out with a single operator. In view of the underlying uncertainty involved in extrapolating from skinfold thickness to body fat, the errors incurred from imprecision in locating the exact site for measurement are also relatively small (41). Accuracy of fat determination will be compromised if the subjects measured are not representative of the subjects whose data were used to establish the equations. Ethnic differences in fat patterning and changes in fat distribution due to disease will confound interpretation of results unless population-specific equations are used. We have shown that skinfold anthropometry is an inaccurate method of assessing total body fat in patients presenting for nutritional support in the surgical ward (42). Body fat was underestimated by about 3 kg in such patients when the reference method was a multicompartment model based on neutron activation and tritium dilution (43). Body fat may be overestimated in the presence of edema partly because of overestimation of the thickness of the skinfold and partly because of the increased body weight due to the excess fluid. In subjects, particularly the elderly, with flabby, easily compressible tissue, skinfold measurements may be difficult. In obese subjects reliable skinfold measurements may not be possible because the thicknesses may exceed the maximum jaw openings of the calipers (Harpenden, 60 mm; Holtain, 50 mm; Lange, 65 mm). Lee and Nieman (44) provide detailed instructions on carrying out the measurements at the various sites.

2. Arm Circumference

Mid-upper arm circumference is in wide use as a component of nutritional status assessment. In combination with measurement of triceps skinfold thickness, attempts have been made to estimate arm muscle circumference and arm muscle area (45).

D. In Vivo Neutron Activation Analysis

Neutron activation techniques allow, in principle, quantitation of all the major elements of the body. Neutrons, which are uncharged nuclear particles, can be produced as controlled beams of varying energy by a number of methods. *In vivo* studies require the irradiation of the subject by fast (or high-energy) neutrons (>10 keV to 20 MeV), which are optimum for tissue penetration. However, most of the interactions of neutrons with nuclei of the target element occur with thermal or low-energy neutrons (<10 keV). By undergoing repeated collisions with nuclei (predominantly hydrogen) the fast neutrons are slowed down rapidly to thermal energies, whereupon they can be captured by an elemental nucleus producing an excited state. The excited nucleus reverts to a stable condition by the emission of one or more gamma (γ) rays either immediately (within $\sim 10^{-15}$ sec, called prompt γ-neutron activation), or after a decay period characteristic of the activation product (delayed γ-neutron activation). Fast neutrons of high enough energy can also undergo inelastic scattering, in which some of the neutron's kinetic energy is converted to internal nuclear energy and in the process excites the incident nucleus with rapid γ-ray release as deexcitation occurs. All neutron activation techniques depend ultimately on the emission of a γ-ray with energy characteristic of the target element and intensity proportional to the amount of that element. Based on these types of neutron–nuclear interactions there are three IVNAA methods in current use. For detailed accounts of these methods several excellent reviews are available (46–49).

1. Prompt γ-Neutron Activation

This is the most widely used technique and its major application is the measurement of body nitrogen. For neutron production, isotopic sources, such as ^{238}Pu–Be or ^{252}Cf, are generally used. The former generates fast neutrons through the interaction with Be of the spontaneously produced α particles from ^{238}Pu whereas ^{252}Cf produces neutrons through spontaneous fission. The prompt gamma spectrum, measured with sodium iodide detectors placed close to the subject and suitable electronic pulse-height analysis equipment, includes a peak due to nitrogen at 10.83 MeV, an energy well removed from potential interferences from other reactions. The conversion of measured counts in the nitrogen region of the spectrum to total body nitrogen requires calibration factors derived using suitable phantoms containing the elements of interest. Such calibration can pose considerable problems and details have been published (50–56). The calibration factors determined are unique to the design of each laboratory's instrument. Total body nitrogen can be measured with a precision close to 2% using this technique with approximately 30 min of scan time (57). Radiation dose is about 0.3 mSv. By direct chemical verification using cadavers, accuracy for total body nitrogen of within 3% has been achieved (4). By virtue of the fact that nitrogen in the body is almost exclusively confined to protein at a mean level of 16%, total body protein is usually calculated from total body nitrogen by multiplying by 6.25 (4). This method has been used also for the measurement of total body chlorine to determine extracellular water volume (58, 59).

2. Delayed γ-Neutron Activation

In this approach the subject is first irradiated with neutrons and then quickly transferred to a whole body counter (see Section III,E) for measuring the induced radioactivity. Although N can also be measured by this technique, it has principally been used for the measurement of Ca, P, Na, and Cl (60, 61). Isotopic sources of neutrons, such as ^{238}Pu–Be, can be used, but some facilities have used a neutron generator. This produces 14-MeV neutrons by the fusion reaction of deuterons accelerated against a tritium target within a small sealed tube. The radiation exposure using this method is more than 10-fold higher than for the prompt technique for similar precision of measurement. Measurement of total body chlorine with good precision (2%) by this approach has been used to estimate the extracellular water space (62). Measurement of total body calcium has been important for the quantification of bone mass (48) and, along with Cl, Na, P, and K [the latter measured by whole body counting (section III,E)], provides an estimate of total body minerals.

3. Inelastic Neutron Scattering

This approach, which has been used to measure total body carbon and oxygen, requires 14-MeV neutrons from a generator operated in pulsed mode (63). With radiation exposure of 0.5 mSv, a precision of 3% is possible for total body carbon. In combination with a measurement of total body nitrogen, total body fat can be derived because carbon is largely present in protein and fat (64).

Although more information can be gained from total body neutron activation analysis than by any other available method, there are few centers worldwide with this capability. This is because of the high cost of installation, the need for skilled operators, the lack of mobility of these instruments, and the radiation exposure entailed.

E. Whole Body Counting

Whole body counters were developed initially to measure the natural radioactivity of the body due to ^{40}K. This radioisotope, which is present in constant proportion (0.012%) in all natural potassium, emits penetrating γ-rays (1.46 MeV) that can be measured by radiation detectors placed around the body. With suitable calibration, the total mass of potassium can be estimated from the measured intensity of the emitted γ radiation. Precision of better than 3% for this measurement in adults is possible, with counting times of 15–30 min, provided that adequate shielding is used to reduce natural background radiation levels (cosmic rays and radioactive contaminants in construction materials). The "shadow-shield" counter design utilizes lead shielding placed directly around the detectors (thallium-activated sodium iodide crystals) and along the sides of the movable scanning table on which the patient is placed (65). An alternative, much heavier, design uses a totally shielded room constructed from materials with low radiocontamination. After adjustment of the measured count in the ^{40}K energy region due to the background contribution, the net counts must be converted to mass of body potassium by the use of calibration factors. Body size and geometry influence the measured counts; the shielding effect of adipose tissue means that fewer counts will be recorded for an obese subject than for a lean one with similar total potassium. One approach to calibration is to measure the gamma spectra from subjects of differing body habitus who have received known amounts of the radioisotope ^{42}K, which will become dispersed in the body similarly to ^{40}K, emitting gamma rays of similar energy. Alternatively, a series of anthropometric phantoms containing a physiologic solution or ground meat of known potassium concentration may be used. Validation based on cadaver analysis has not been performed.

Potassium is not found in stored triglycerides in the body and potassium content per unit of FFM is often assumed to be constant in healthy individuals. Hence a measurement of total body potassium (TBK) has been used as a means of calculating total body fat. The variation in potassium content of FFM observed by different investigators in normal adults (66) suggests that significant error may be associated with fat measurement using this method. TBK has also been assumed to bear a constant relationship to body cell mass (BCM), defined by Moore and associates (67) as "the working, energy-metabolizing portion of the human body in relationship to its supporting structures." Given that TBK is almost wholly (>97%) intracellular, changes in this quantity will tend to reflect changes in cellular mass. However, the relationships between TBK and FFM or BCM will be altered in patients with abnormal body composition, such as dehydration or overhydration.

F. Dual-Energy X-Ray Absorptiometry

Dual-energy X-ray absorptiometry is emerging as one of the most frequently used techniques for body composition measurement owing to the increasing worldwide availability of these scanners. The technique is easily applied in both normals and patients, typically takes less than 30 min for a whole body scan, and involves a very small radiation dose (~1 μSv). This compares with a natural background radiation dose for a single day of ~5 μSv. The underlying concept of this technology and its precursor, single-photon absorptiometry, is that photon attenuation *in vivo* is a function of tissue composition. A rectilinear scan of the supine body is performed, which divides the body into a series of pixels, within each of which the photon attenuation is measured at two different energies. The DEXA body composition approach assumes that humans consist of three components that are distinguishable by their X-ray attenuation properties: fat, bone mineral, and fat-free or "lean" soft tissue. Within any pixel the proportions of only two components can be resolved by the differential absorption of two photon energies. Soft tissues, consisting largely of water and organic compounds, reduce photon flux to a much lesser extent than bone mineral, and pixels containing bone are relatively easily distinguished from those with no bone present. In areas where bone is not present, suitable calibration allows fat and lean fractions to be resolved from soft tissue. The composition of these areas of soft tissue is extrapolated to the soft tissue overlying bone to produce total body fat and lean soft tissue. Technical details of the methodology have been reviewed (68). Bone mineral is the inorganic ash residue of the skeleton. Exactly how much essential lipid is measured by DEXA as fat is not clear and will depend on the "fat standard" used for calibration. Water and protein solids are essentially indistinguishable by absorptiometry and can be grouped together as a single lean component.

The equipment for this technique is currently available from three manufacturers, Hologic, Lunar, and Norland. Technical differences in both hardware and software mean that results from one instrument are not necessarily the same as those from another (69). Some concern has also been reported about consistency between machines from the same manufacturer (70). The size of the scanning area (approximately 190 × 60 cm) is a limiting factor for whole body measurement on these machines. For those subjects whose body dimensions exceed those of the scanning area, measurements have been carried out by scanning one side of the body only (71). Software upgrades that appear from time to time often include changes in the algorithms used for body composition calculation, which can affect the measurements for an individual. Reanalysis of the data using the most recent software is then indicated. Investigators should be aware that subject clothing may contribute to the attenuation and should ideally be standardized. Sheets routinely used to cover subjects during scans do not significantly affect results, whereas pillows that may be used to support patients who have difficulty lying flat can produce systematic errors (72). Concerns have been raised as to the possible confounding effects of large changes in hydration status on the accuracy with which bone mineral and fat can be determined using DEXA. Theoretically, increased extracellular fluid in the fat-free mass would result in underestimation of total body fat (68). In practice any differences in measured composition that can be ascribed to fluid changes are relatively minor (73). Bone density and fat mass measured in hemodialysis patients were found to be unaffected by the fluid changes (74). Paracentesis of ascites did not change total fat mass measurements by DEXA (75). A study we carried out with mincemeat phantoms undergoing increasing degrees of fluid overload, comparable to those seen in critically ill patients, showed a small (2–3%) dependence of total fat measurement on degree of hydration (76). The trend was significant because of the high short-term precision of this measurement (better than 2%).

In vivo precision estimates from repeated measurements over 1 day in the same subject are around 1% for total body bone mineral and for fat-free soft tissue, and 2% for fat (72). Although excellent reproducibility is obtainable with this technique, there are very few data comparing absolute measurements to chemical analysis of cadavers. Cadaver dissection and chemical analysis have not been performed to assess accuracy of whole body fat and lean tissue determinations by DEXA. In comparison with other *in vivo* techniques for fat measurement DEXA compares well on a group basis, although substantial individual differences may occur

(77–79). *In vitro* experiments suggest that accuracy of fat mass measurement may depend on tissue thickness (80).

A significant advantage of this technology is that the tissue content of different regions of the body can also be measured—for instance, measurement of abdominal fat (81) and appendicular muscle mass (82, 83).

G. Bioimpedance Methods

Although studies of the conduction of electrical currents in biological tissues date to the turn of the century, the specific use of electrical impedance to quantify aspects of body composition is relatively recent. The first commercially available, affordable bioimpedance devices for body composition analysis were introduced in the mid-1980s by RJL, Inc. (Clinton Twp., MI). At the simplest level, bioimpedance analysis (BIA) is based on the relationship between the resistance, R, of a cylindrical conductor of length, L, and cross-sectional area, A:

$$R = \rho L/A,$$

where ρ is the resistivity of the conducting fluid. Because the volume, V, of such a conductor is AL, this expression can be rewritten as

$$V = \rho L^2/R.$$

For application to humans, a constant current (800 μA is used by the RJL instrument) is applied, usually between the hand and the foot, and the resistance measured. If the volume of electrolyte, i.e., total body water, is measured by a reference method such as deuterium or tritium dilution, it is found to be highly correlated with H^2/R, where height H of the subject replaces L in the formula above. Of course, the model of the body as a cylindrical volume of fluid of uniform composition is a gross approximation. For this reason, regression relationships have been developed between the criterion measure of TBW and various predictors in addition to H^2/R. These include body weight, age, and sex (84). Essentially devices for assessing electrolyte volume, bioimpedance analyzers have received most attention for their ability to "measure" fat-free mass and hence body fat. The close relationship between fat-free mass and its total water content in normal individuals ensures such a measurement is possible. In practice, empirical equations have been developed relating hydrodensitometrically determined fat-free mass and various predictors (85). The literature on BIA contains an extensive array of equations for predicting total body water and fat-free mass, which tend to be instrument and population specific (86). In particular, in surgical patients in whom expanded extracellular water is the rule, fat-free mass prediction equations developed from normal populations should be used with caution.

Rather than being of uniform composition the human body is composed of cells and various tissue interfaces embedded in extracellular fluid. From an electrical circuit point of view the body may be modeled most simply as shown in Fig. 3, where the extracellular fluid compartment is represented as a pure resistance that is in parallel with a resistance representing the intracellular electrolyte and a capacitor representing the effects of the cellular membranes. This model for living tissue is approximately valid for frequencies of applied current over the range of about 5 kHz to 1 Mhz (87, 88). Capacitors provide an impedance to current flow (called reactance) that is inversely proportional to frequency. At low frequencies, therefore, the current will effectively pass only through the extracellular fluid. At very high frequencies, current flow will not be impeded by the capacitive reactance and current will flow in proportion to the relative sizes of the resistances of the extra- and intracellular fluid spaces. At intermediate frequencies the measured impedance will consist of both resistive and reactive components. Most bioimpedance devices operate at a single intermediate frequency (usually 50 kHz), where the applied current is carried by the extracellular fluid and some component of intracellular fluid (89). Provided the relative proportions of the extra- and intracellular components of total body water are approximately constant, as they are in health, the single-frequency measurement should predict both TBW and ECW reasonably satisfactorily. Reactance has been included as a predictor in some of the published regression equations for these fluid spaces (90) and for fat-free mass (91). Deviations from the normal fluid distribution, as in edema and dehydration, will cause inaccuracy in the bioimpedance predictions, particularly because the resistivity of extra- and intracellular fluids differ (92, 93).

To more directly assess the volumes of total body and extracellular water, prediction equations have been constructed based on bioimpedance measurements at low

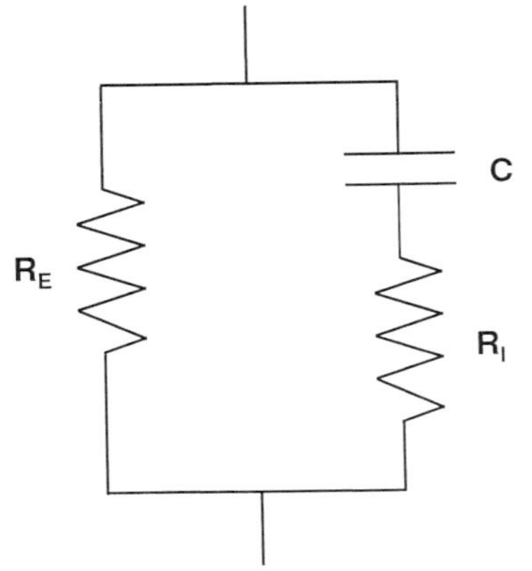

Figure 3 Simple electrical circuit model of the body. Resistor R_E models the electrical resistance of the extracellular fluid; resistor R_I and capacitor C model the impedance to current flowing through intracellular fluid.

(5 kHz) and high frequencies (100 kHz) (94). The first commercially available multifrequency bioimpedance instrument for body composition analysis was introduced by Xitron Technologies (San Diego, CA) in 1991. This provides measurements of resistance and reactance at up to 50 frequencies over the range from 5 kHz to 1 Mhz. By incorporating a more sophisticated electrical circuit model of the body that takes account of the variability in cell size, orientation, and concentration within various tissues, and fitting this model to the measured bioimpedance frequency spectrum, the Xitron software extracts resistance data for the extracellular and intracellular fluids. Based on mixture theory, these resistance values are used to determine the fluid space volumes, given appropriate calibration constants, which are generally derived from bromide and deuterium dilution data in normal subjects (95). This approach (*bioimpedance spectroscopy*) should improve the determination of extra- and intracellular fluid volumes when abnormal fluid shifts occur (96). This has been shown for ECW in surgical patients (97). In critically ill patients, changes in ECW over 3 weeks following admission to intensive care were faithfully reproduced by multifrequency BIA measurements (98).

Whole body measurements are usually performed with a tetrapolar electrode configuration, whereby the current is applied distally through electrodes on the dorsal surfaces of the hand and foot proximal to the metacarpal phalangeal and metatarsal phalangeal joints, respectively, and the voltage-sensing electrodes are applied at the pisiform prominence of the wrist and between the medial and lateral malleoli of the ankle. Standardization of conditions of measurement is essential to obtain meaningful results. A recent consensus statement on BIA (99) provides useful details on the optimal conditions for measurements. Under these circumstances, precision is high, with day-to-day variability in impedance in weight-stable subjects reported to be 2% (85).

In patients who have fluid accumulation in the trunk, such as ascites, whole body BIA is not able reliably to measure the body water spaces (100, 101). In liver disease patients undergoing paracentesis, BIA was not able to measure the water changes (14, 100, 101). Given that more than 70% of the impedance reading derives from the arms and legs and only about 30% derives from the trunk, this is not surprising. The use of segmental electrode placement so that trunk impedance is measured independently of legs and arms has shown promise (102).

As body composition assessment tools, BIA systems are relatively inexpensive, portable, and noninvasive, and little operator training is required. For the estimation of body fat they provide an attractive alternative to skinfold anthropometry, particularly because they are capable of good precision, probably better than skinfolds (78), with better consistency between observers, and they provide reproducible measurements in the obese.

H. Computed Tomography

Computed tomography (CT) scanning provides detailed cross-sectional images of the body in which adipose, muscle, bone, and vascular tissues are resolved. Each cross-sectional image is produced from a series of linear projections of X-ray opacity along strips through the sample of interest. A projection reconstruction computational algorithm is used to form the image from these projections. Slice thickness may vary from as little as 1 mm to typically 10–13 mm. The earliest reports of the use of this technique for body composition analysis investigated muscle area in the thigh (103) and midarm muscle, bone, and fat areas (104). Analysis of CT images provides tissue areas and, with suitable assumptions regarding changes in tissue distribution between slices, tissue volumes. This multislice approach has been used to estimate total adipose tissue volume in the body (105, 106). Conversion to mass of tissue requires an assumption about its density. To date, CT scanning has mostly been used for the measurement of intraabdominal and subcutaneous fat (107). To provide fat mass with which to compare other methods of estimating fat requires knowledge of the fat content of adipose tissue, which may vary with illness and/or degree of obesity. The technique is capable of very high precision (better than 1% for adipose tissue) (106), although validation must rely ultimately on cadaver dissection.

Much interest in the technique lies in its potential to measure total skeletal muscle mass, and a 22-slice protocol has been used to estimate this quantity in groups of healthy men and men with AIDS (108). Good agreement has been obtained between CT-determined cross-sectional areas and volumes of skeletal muscle and cadaver measurements in isolated arms and legs (109). Cadaver dissection to validate whole body skeletal muscle determination using a multislice CT protocol has not been carried out. Close agreement has been obtained in a group of healthy males between measured body weight and CT-derived body weight, whereby a 28-slice whole body scan was used to determine areas of tissues and organs that were converted to weights using published density data (110). The effective radiation dose equivalent to the total body was estimated to be 2.5–5 mSv. The value of CT scanning may lie in its ability to monitor changes in fat distribution and muscularization (111). Radiation exposure is clearly a concern for longitudinal studies, and for studies of pregnant women and children. Also the cost and general availability of CT scanners prohibit the routine use of this technique for body composition assessment.

I. Magnetic Resonance Imaging

Whereas conventional X-ray radiographic and CT images depend on electron density, nuclear magnetic resonance imaging (MRI) depends on the density of hydrogen nuclei and the physical state of the tissue as reflected in the magnetic relaxation times. Tissue contrast is high between fat and muscle and can be enhanced by changing the magnetic relaxation time variable of the MRI instrument. MRI has evolved to the stage where it can provide anatomical detail similar to that of CT (112) and has also been used to measure total adipose tissue in the human body using multiple cross-sectional slices (113, 114). As with CT, a value for the fat content of adipose tissue must be assumed in order to derive fat mass (112). Comparison with the CT technique for adipose tissue estimation suggests that both imaging methods give similar results for subcutaneous fat but that MRI may be less accurate for visceral fat, probably due to movement artifacts in the visceral area coupled with the longer acquisition time for MRI scans (115). The validity of MRI abdominal subcutaneous and visceral adipose tissue estimates has been examined using human cadavers (116). The mean difference between dissection weight and MRI-estimated adipose tissue weights was ~6% (0.076 kg). The reproducibility based on repeated estimates of the adipose tissue mass by MRI was below 14% (CV). Close agreement has been obtained between MRI-determined cross-sectional areas and volumes of skeletal muscle and cadaver measurements in isolated arms and legs, with reproducibility for MRI estimates of around 2% (109). Fast imaging techniques are becoming available and will reduce movement artifacts and allow data acquisition in relatively short periods of time. Whole body imaging is now possible in <30 min. This technique is attractive for longitudinal studies on individuals because no radiation hazards are involved. Restricted availability and high cost of the machines are significant practical limitations for routine body composition measurement.

IV. Body Composition Models

Body composition research involves subdividing the body into two or more compartments. A considerable diversity of approaches to this subdivision is now possible with the advances in technology over the last three decades. Wang *et al.* (117) have considered these to comprise a hierarchical scheme of five levels (Fig. 4). At the most fundamental level is elemental analysis (the atomic model). *In vivo* estimation of the major elements of the body, largely by neutron activation techniques, allows the reconstruction of greater then 98% of the body mass (117).

The cornerstone of body composition research is the chemical (or molecular) model, primarily due to its central role in the study of energy metabolism, protein nutriture, and mineral physiology (118). This model considers the chemical compounds of the body in categories of closely related molecular species. We (43) and others (117) have described a five-compartment model comprising water, protein, glycogen, minerals, and fat. The usefulness of this model is extended by the further subdivision of water into the extra- and intracellular spaces.

In addition to studies of fluid balance based on the intra/extracellular division of body water, investigations into thermogenesis are aided by models based on a cellu-

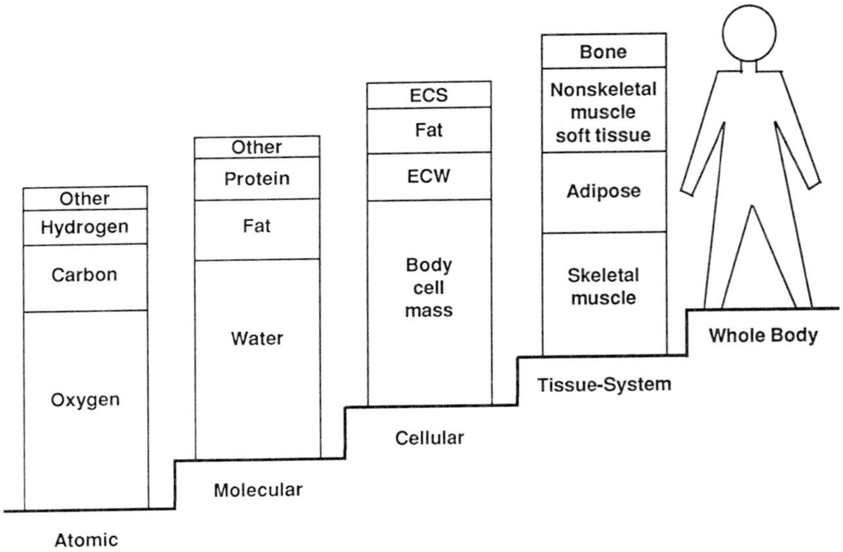

Figure 4 Adapted from Wang *et al.* (117). © *Am. J. Clin. Nutr.* American Society for Clinical Nutrition. Five levels of human body composition. ECS, extracellular solids; ECW, extracellular water.

lar/noncellular compartmentalization. These are exemplified by the breakdown into body cell mass as defined by Moore and colleagues (67), fat, extracellular fluid, and the remaining extracellular solids (cellular model). Almost half of the body protein is an extrusion from cells and spends its life outside cells as structural protein or as soluble protein or as enzymes. These proteins form most of what is called extracellular solids; they include the fibrous supporting structures of the body, including collagen, elastin, the dermis, hair, teeth, cartilage, and joint capsules. These substances probably do not contribute in any way to the active metabolic processes of the body. However, the recent availability of DEXA, MRI, and CT scanners makes it feasible to consider the characterization of the body in terms of tissue groupings such as skeletal muscle, adipose tissue, bone, and nonskeletal muscle soft tissue. At this tissue-system level the measurement of skeletal muscle mass has attracted considerable attention over the years, beginning with anthropometric methods and those based on excretion of metabolites such as creatinine (119) and 3-methylhistidine (120).

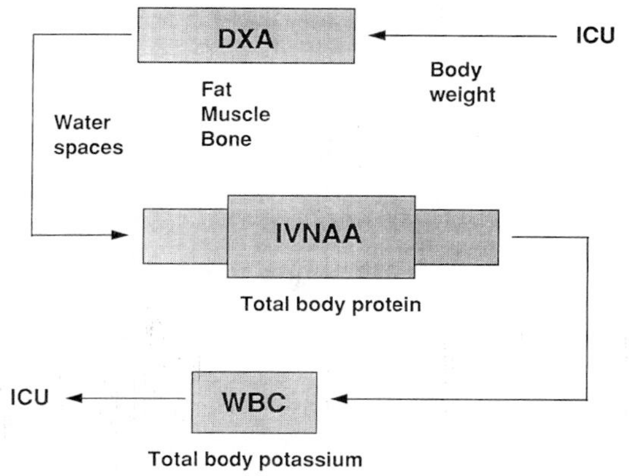

Figure 5 Schematic representation of the body composition facility in the University Department of Surgery at Auckland Hospital designed to accommodate intensive care patients. Patients are transported from the intensive care unit (ICU) to this facility where they are weighed, injected with tritiated water and sodium bromide solution for water spaces determination, and undergo dual-energy X-ray absorptiometry (DXA), *in vivo* neutron activation analysis (IVNAA), and whole body counting (WBC).

V. Practical Problems in Measuring Body Composition in Intensive Care Patients

Critically ill patients in intensive care present formidable problems for the investigator interested in quantifying the body compositional changes associated with severe illness. All the standard methods for body composition measurement must be reevaluated in view of the extreme compositional abnormalities seen in these patients. Body weight is a fundamental measurement that is not generally available in the intensive care unit (ICU) and may require transport of these patients outside of the unit, a significant exercise in itself. Since the early 1980s we have maintained a body composition facility designed for intensive care patients that is located within a short distance of the ICU (Fig. 5). A hoist weighing system (consisting of an electrically operated block and tackle attached to a load cell and to a frame that supports a canvas sheet on which the patient lies) is used to transfer the patient from the bed to the scanning machines, and the body weight is measured during the transfer. Most of these patients undergo dramatic changes in body weight during the course of their illness (121, 122) and most of this change in weight is due to water change (123). Fluid changes in excess of 10 liters are not uncommon in ICU patients. Application of dilution methods for measuring TBW and ECW in these patients requires consideration of the infusion volumes and losses during the equilibration period (see Section III,B) (123). Body fat assessment using skinfold anthropometry leads to large errors, as might be expected (123). The use of simple body composition models or techniques that rely on the assumption of a normally hydrated FFM are inappropriate. Care must be taken in applying bioimpedance methods; we obtain unpredictable results performing bioimpedance spectroscopy measurements on standard hospital beds as used in our ICU. The large fluid changes present potential problems for the accuracy of DEXA (see Section III,F) and IVNAA systems. We have investigated the effect of these changes on total body protein measurements by prompt γ-IVNAA using anthropomorphic phantoms (76). Our state-of-the-art methodology (Fig. 6) has been used to demonstrate the underlying similarity of the metabolic response to the systemic inflammatory response syndrome (SIRS), whether a result of severe sepsis or major blunt injury (124).

VI. Summary

Table II summarizes the characteristics of the body composition methods described in this chapter that may be pertinent to selection of a method that best meets the objectives of the proposed research. An understanding of the limitations of each method and practical considerations, such as cost, ease of operation, technical skills required, and subject cooperation, will influence this selection.

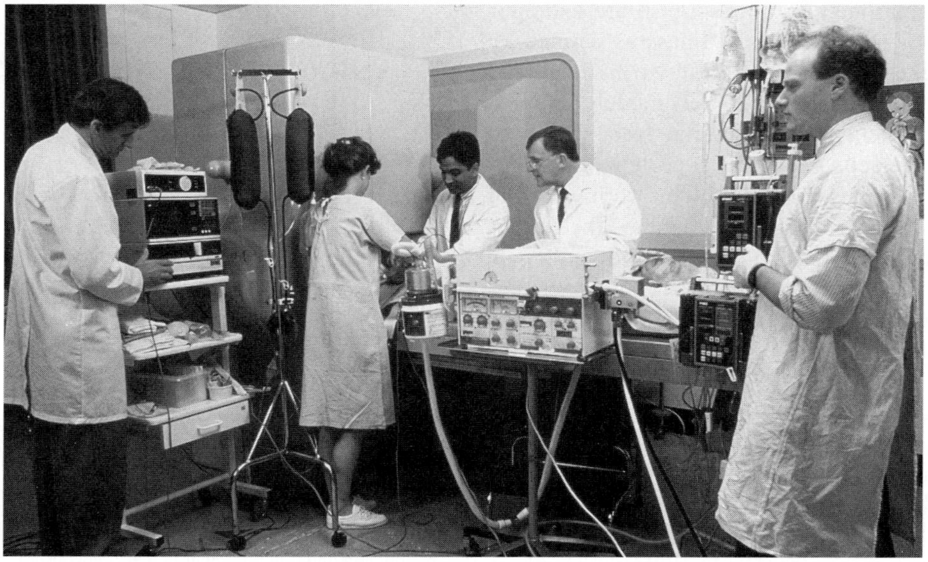

Figure 6 Prompt γ-neutron activation analysis scanner in the University Department of Surgery at Auckland Hospital. A ventilated critically ill intensive care patient is shown being prepared for scanning, with all intravenous lines, drains, and monitors attached. (See color plates.)

Table II Summary of Methods of Determining Body Composition

Method	Total body component measured	Precision	Measurement time[a]	Radiation dose	Cost[b]	Comments
Anthropometry	Fat	2–5%	5 min	Nil	1	Limited application in obese, illness
Hydrodensitometry	Fat	3%	30 min	Nil	3	Impractical in illness
Dilution	Water	2–3%	3–6 hr	Nil (^{2}H, ^{18}O); low (^{3}H)	3 (^{3}H, ^{2}H); 5 (^{18}O)	Immediate results not possible
	Extracellular water	2–3%	3–6 hr	Nil (Br); low (^{35}S)	3	
Neutron activation	Protein	2–3%	30 min	Moderate	5	Limited availability, expensive to install, calibration complex
	Fat	4%	60–90 min	High		
	Bone mineral	2%	30 min	High		
	Extracellular water	2%	30 min	High		
Whole body counting	Potassium	3%	15 min	Nil	4	Limited availability, expensive to install
Dual-energy X-ray absorptiometry	Fat	2%	15–40 min	Very low	4	Regional body composition possible
	Fat-fee soft tissue	1%				
	Bone mineral	1%				
Bioimpedance	Water	2%	5 min	Nil	2	
	Extracellular water	(2%)				
Computed tomography	Skeletal muscle	(1%)	45 min	High	5	Limited availability, instrument expensive
	Adipose tissue	<1%				
Magnetic resonance imaging	Skeletal muscle	(2%)	30 min	Nil	5	Limited availability, instrument expensive
	Adipose tissue	2%				

[a]Excludes time required for data analysis or assay.
[b]Measurement cost ranked from 1 = least to 5 = greatest.

VII. Resources

A. General References

Forbes, G. B. (1987). "Human Body Composition." Springer-Verlag, New York.

Moore, F. D., Olesen, K. H., McMurray, J. D. *et al.* (1963). "The Body Cell Mass and Its Supporting Environment: Body Composition in Health and Disease." WB Saunders, Philadelphia.

Roche, A. F., Heymsfield, S. B., and Lohman, T. G., eds. (1996). "Human Body Composition." Human Kinetics, Champaign, IL.

B. Reviews

Brodie, D. A. (1988). Techniques of measurement of body composition. Part I. *Sports Med.* **5,** 11–40.

Brodie, D. A. (1988). Techniques of measurement of body composition. Part II. *Sports Med.* **5,** 74–98.

Heymsfield, S. B., Wang, Z. M., Baumgartner, R. N., and Ross, R. (1997). Human body composition: Advances in models and methods. *Annu. Rev. Nutr.* **17,** 527–558.

Jebb, S. A., and Elia, M. (1993). Techniques for the measurement of body composition: A practical guide. *Int. J. Obes.* **17,** 611–621.

Lukaski, H. C. (1987). Methods for the assessment of human body composition: Traditional and new. *Am. J. Clin. Nutr.* **46,** 537–556.

Sutcliffe, J. S. (1996). A review of *in vivo* experimental methods to determine the composition of the human body. *Phys. Med. Biol.* **41,** 791–833.

References

1. Snyder, W. S., Cook, M. J., Nasset, E. S., Karhausen, L. R., Parry Howells, G., and Tipton, I. H. (1975). "Report of the Task Group on Reference Man." Pergamon, Oxford.
2. Comizio, R., Pietrobelli, A., Tan, Y. X., Wang, Z., Withers, R. T., Heymsfield, S. B., and Boozer, C. N. (1998). Total body lipid and triglyceride response to energy deficit: Relevance to body composition models. *Am. J. Physiol.* **274,** E860–E866.
3. Clarys, J. P., Martin, A. D., Marfell-Jones, M. J., Janssens, V., Caboor, D., and Drinkwater, D. T. (1999). *Am. J. Hum. Biol.* **11,** 167–174.
4. Knight, G. S., Beddoe, A. H., Streat, S. J., and Hill, G. L. (1986). Body composition of two human cadavers by neutron activation and chemical analysis. *Am. J. Physiol.* **250,** E179–E185.
5. Heymsfield, S. B., Wang, J., Lichtman, S., Kamen, Y., Kehayias, J., and Pierson, R. N., Jr. (1989). Body composition in elderly subjects: A critical appraisal of clinical methodology. *Am. J. Clin Nutr.* **50,** 1167–1175.
6. Nelp, W. B., Denney, R., Murano, R., Hinn, G. M., Williams, J. L., Rudd, T. G., and Palmer, H. E. (1972). Absolute measurement of total body calcium (bone mass) *in vivo*. *J. Lab. Clin. Med.* **79,** 430–438.
7. Siri, W. E. (1956). Body composition from fluid spaces and density: Analysis of methods. University of California Radiation Laboratory Report 3349, University of California, Berkeley.
8. Buskirk, E. R. (1961). Underwater weighing and body density: a review of procedures. *In* "Techniques for Measuring Body Composition" (J. Brozek and A. Henschel, eds.), pp. 90–105. National Academy of Sciences, Washington D.C.
9. Burkinshaw, L. (1985). Measurement of human body composition *in vivo*. *Prog. Med. Rad. Phys.* **2,** 113–137.
10. Moore, F. D., Hartsuck, J. M., Zolinger, R. M. Jr., and Johnson, J. E. (1968). Reference models for clinical studies by isotope dilution. *Ann. Surg.* **168,** 671–698.
11. Schoeller, D. A., van Santen, E., Petersen, D. W., Dietz, W., Jaspan, J., and Klein, P. D. (1980). Total body water measurement in humans with ^{18}O and ^{2}H labelled water. *Am. J. Clin. Nutr.* **33,** 2686–2693.
12. Wong, W. W., Cochran, W. J., Klish, W. J., O'Brian Smith, E., Lee, L. S., and Klein, P. D. (1988). *In vivo* isotope-fractionation factors and the measurement of deuterium- and oxygen-18-dilution spaces from plasma, urine, saliva, respiratory water vapor, and carbon dioxide. *Am. J. Clin. Nutr.* **47,** 1–6
13. Brodie, D. A. (1988). Techniques of measurement of body composition. Part I. *Sports Med.* **5,** 11–40.
14. McCullough, A. J., Mullen, K. D., and Kalhan, S. C. (1991). Measurement of total body and extracellular water in cirrhotic patients with and without ascites. *Hepatology* **14,** 1102–1111.
15. Streat, S. J., Beddoe, A. H., and Hill, G. L. (1985). Measurement of total body water in intensive care patients with fluid overload. *Metabolism* **34,** 688–694.
16. Culebras, J. M., and Moore, F. D. (1977). Total body water and the exchangeable hydrogen. I. Theoretical calculations of nonaqueous exchangeable hydrogen in man. *Am. J. Physiol.* **232:** R54–R59.
17. International Commission on Radiological Protection. (1987). "Radiation Dose to Patients from Radiopharmaceuticals," p. 39. ICRP Publ. 53. Pergamon, Oxford.
18. Price, W. F., Hazelrig, J. B., Kreisberg, R. A., and Meador, C. K. (1969). Reproducibility of body composition in a single individual. *J. Lab. Clin. Med.* **74,** 557–563.
19. Schoeller, D.A (1996). Hydrometry. *In* "Human Body Composition" (A.F. Roche, S.B. Heymsfield, and T.G. Lohman, eds.), pp. 25–43. Human Kinetics, Champaign, IL.
20. Edelman, I. S., and Leibman, J. (1959). Anatomy of body water and electrolytes. *Am. J. Med.* **27,** 256–277.
21. Wallace, G. B., and Brodie, B. B. (1939). The distribution of administered bromide in comparison with chloride and its relation to body fluids. *J. Pharmacol.* **65,** 214–219.
22. Miller, M. E., Cosgriff, J. M., and Forbes, G. B. (1989). Bromide space determination using anion-exchange chromatography for measurement of bromide. *Am. J. Clin. Nutr.* **50,** 168–171.
23. Pierson, R. N., Jr., Price, D. C., Wang, J., and Jain, R. K. (1978). Extracellular water measurements: organ tracer kinetics of bromide and sucrose in man. *Am. J. Physiol.* **235,** F254–F264.
24. Bell, E. F., Ziegler, E. E., and Forbes, G. B. (1984). Letter to the Editor. *Paed. Res.* **18,** 392–393.
25. Olszowy, H. A., Rossiter, J., Hegarty, J., and Geoghegan, P. (1998). Background levels of bromide in human blood. *J. Anal. Toxicol.* **22,** 225–230.
26. Vaiseman, N., Koren, G., and Pencharz, P. (1986). Pharmacokinetics of oral and intravenous bromide in normal volunteers. *J. Toxicol. Clin. Toxicol.* **24,** 403–413.
27. Sourkes, T. L. (1991). Early clinical neurochemistry of CNS-active drugs. Bromides. *Mol. Chem. Neuropathol.* **14,** 131–142.
28. Brodie, B. B., Brand, E., and Leshin, S. (1939). The use of bromide as a measure of extracellular fluid. *J. Biol. Chem.* **130,** 555–563.
29. Howe, C. T., and Ekins, R. P. (1963). The bromide space after the intravenous administration of ^{82}Br. *J. Nucl. Med.* **4,** 469–479.
30. Vaisman, N., Pencharz, P. B., Koren, G., and Johnson, J. K. (1987). Comparison of oral and intravenous administration of sodium bromide for extracellular water measurements. *Am. J. Clin. Nutr.* **46,** 1–4.
31. Nicholson, J. P., and Zilva, J. F. (1957). A 6 hour method for determining the extracellular fluid volume in human subjects. *Clin. Chim. Acta* **2,** 340–344.
32. Leth, A., and Binder, C. (1970). The distribution volume of $^{82}Br^-$ as a measurement of the extracellular fluid volume in normal persons. *Scand. J. Clin. Lab. Invest.* **25,** 291–297.
33. Nicholson, J. P., and Zilva, J. F. (1960). Estimation of extracellular fluid volume using radiobromine. *Clin. Sci.* **19,** 391–398.

34. Middleton, E. S., Mathews, R., and Shires, G. T. (1969). Radiosulphate as a measure of the extracellular fluid in acute hemorrhagic shock. *Ann. Surg.* **170,** 174–186.
35. Barratt, T. M., and Walser, M. (1969). Extracellular fluid in individual tissues and whole animals: The distribution of radiosulphate and radiobromide. *J. Clin. Invest.* **48,** 56–66.
36. McMurrey, J. D., Boling, E. A., Davis, J. M., Parker, H. V., Magnus, I. C., Ball, M. R., and Moore, F. D. (1958). Body composition: simultaneous determination of several aspects by the dilution principle. *Metabolism* **7,** 651–667.
37. Shizgal, H. M. (1976). Total body potassium and nutritional status. *Surg. Clin. North Am.* **56,** 1185–1194.
38. Shizgal, H. M., Spanier, A. H., Humes, J., and Wood, C. D. (1977). Indirect measurement of total exchangeable potassium. *Am. J. Physiol.* **233,** F253–F259.
39. Durnin, J. V. G. A., and Womersley, J. (1974). Body fat assessed from total body density and its estimation from skinfold thickness: measurements on 481 men and women aged from 16 to 72 years. *Br. J. Nutr.* **32,** 77–97.
40. Burkinshaw, L., Jones, P. R. M., and Krupowicz, D. W. (1973). Observer error in skinfold thickness measurements. *Hum. Biol.* **45,** 273–279.
41. Durnin, J. V. G. A., De Bruin, H., and Feunekes, G. I. J. (1997). Skinfold thickness: is there a need to be very precise in their location? *Br. J. Nutr.* **77,** 3–7.
42. Streat, S. J., Beddoe, A. H., and Hill, G. L. (1985). Measurement of body fat and hydration of the fat-free body in health and disease. *Metabolism* **34,** 509–518.
43. Beddoe, A. H., Streat, S. J., and Hill, G. L. (1984). Evaluation of an *in vivo* prompt gamma neutron activation facility for body composition studies in critically ill intensive care patients: results on 41 normals. *Metabolism* **33,** 270–280.
44. Lee, R. D., and Nieman, D. C. (1996). "Nutritional Assessment," 2nd Ed, pp 251–258. Mosby, St. Louis.
45. Heymsfield, S. B., McManus, C., Smith, J., Stevens, V., and Nixon, D. W. (1982). Anthropometric measurement of muscle mass: Revised equations for calculating bone-free muscle area. *Am. J. Clin. Nutr.* **36,** 680–690.
46. Chettle, D. R., and Fremlin, J. H. (1984). Techniques of *in vivo* neutron activation analysis. *Phys. Med. Biol.* **29,** 1011–1043.
47. Cohn, S. H. (1981). *In vivo* neutron activation analysis: state of the art and future prospects. *Med. Phys.* **8,** 145–154.
48. Cohn, S. H., and Parr, R. M. (1985). Nuclear-based techniques for the *in vivo* study of human body composition. *Clin. Phys. Physiol. Meas.* **6,** 275–301.
49. Beddoe, A. H., and Hill, G. L. (1985). Clinical measurement of body composition using *in vivo* neutron activation analysis. *J. Parenter. Enteral Nutr.* **9,** 504–520.
50. Vartsky, D., Prestwich, W. V., Thomas, B. J., *et al.* (1979). The use of body hydrogen as an internal standard in the measurement of nitrogen *in vivo* by prompt neutron capture gamma ray analysis. *J. Radioanal. Chem.* **48,** 243–252.
51. Beddoe, A. H., Zuidmeer, H., and Hill, G. L. (1984). A prompt gamma *in vivo* neutron activation analysis facility for measurement of total body nitrogen in the critically ill. *Phys. Med. Biol.* **29,** 371–383.
52. Ryde, S. J. S., Morgan, W. D., Evans, C. J., Sivyer, A., and Dutton, J. (1989). Calibration and evaluation of a ^{252}Cf-based neutron activation analysis instrument for the determination of nitrogen *in vivo*. *Phys. Med. Biol.* **34,** 1429–1441.
53. Mackie, A., Cowen, S., and Hannan, J. (1990). Calibration of a prompt neutron activation facility for the measurement of total body protein. *Phys. Med. Biol.* **35,** 613–624.
54. Baur, L. A., Allen, B. J., Rose, A., Blagojevic, N., and Gaskin, K. J. (1991). A total body nitrogen facility for paediatric use. *Phys. Med. Biol.* **36,** 1363–1375.
55. Mitra, S., Plank, L. D., and Hill, G. L. (1993). Calibration of a prompt gamma *in vivo* neutron activation facility for direct measurement of total body protein in intensive care patients. *Phys. Med. Biol.* **38,** 1971–1975.
56. Stamatelatos, I. E., Dilmanian, F. A., Ma, R., *et al.* (1993). Calibration for measuring total body nitrogen with a newly upgraded prompt gamma neutron activation facility. *Phys. Med. Biol.* **38,** 615–626.
57. Dilmanian, F. A., Lidofsky, L. J., Stamatelatos, I. E., *et al.* (1998). Improvement of the prompt-gamma neutron activation facility at Brookhaven National Laboratory. *Phys. Med. Biol.* **43,** 339–349.
58. Blagojevic, N., Allen, B. J., and Rose, A. (1990). Development of a total body chlorine analyser using a bismuth germanate detector and a ^{252}Cf neutron source. *In* "Advances in *In Vivo* Body Composition Studies" (S. Yasumura, J.E. Harrison, K.G. McNeil, A.D Woodhead, and F.A. Dilmanian, eds.), pp. 401–408. Plenum, New York.
59. Mitra, S., Plank, L. D., Knight, G. S., and Hill, G. L. (1993). *In vivo* measurement of total body chlorine using the 8.57 MeV prompt de-excitation following thermal neutron capture. *Phys. Med. Biol.* **38,** 161–172.
60. Hill, G. L., King, R. F. G. J., Smith, R. C., *et al.* (1979). Multi-element analysis of the living body by neutron activation analysis—Application to critically ill patients receiving intravenous nutrition. *Br. J. Surg.* **66,** 868–872.
61. Cohn, S. H., and Dombrowski, C. S. (1971). Measurement of total body calcium, sodium, chlorine, nitrogen and phosphorus in man by *in vivo* neutron activation analysis. *J. Nucl. Med.* **12,** 499–505.
62. Yasumura, S., Cohn, S. H., and Ellis, K. J. (1983). Measurement of extracellular space by total body neutron activation. *Am. J. Physiol.* **244,** R36–R40.
63. Kehayias, J. J., and Zhuang, H. (1993). Use of the Zetatron D-T neutron generator for the simultaneous measurement of carbon, oxygen, and hydrogen *in vivo* in humans. *Nucl. Instr. Meth.* **B79,** 555–559.
64. Kehayias, J. J., Heymsfield, S. B., LoMonte, A. F., Wang, J., and Pierson, R. N. Jr. (1991). *In vivo* determination of total body fat by measuring total body carbon. *Am. J. Clin. Nutr.* **53,** 1339–1344.
65. Beddoe, A. H., and Zuidmeer, H. (1986). Design of a shadow shield counter for the measurement of total body potassium. *Australas. Phys. Eng. Sci. Med.* **9,** 173–179.
66. Ellis, K. J. (1996). Whole-body counting and neutron activation analysis. *In* "Human Body Composition" (A. F. Roche, S. B. Heymsfield, and T. G. Lohman, eds.), p.51. Human Kinetics, Champaign, IL.
67. Moore, F. D., Olesen, K. H., McMurray, J. D., Parker, H. V., Ball, M. R., and Boyden, C. M. (1963). "The Body Cell Mass and its Supporting Environment: Body Composition in Health and Disease," p. 19. WB Saunders, Philadelphia.
68. Pietrobelli, A., Formica, C., Wang, Z., and Heymsfield, S. B. (1996). Dual-energy X-ray absorptiometry body composition model: Review of physical concepts. *Am. J. Physiol.* **271,** E941–E951.
69. Tothill, P., Avenell, A., Love, J., and Reid, D. M. (1994). Comparisons between Hologic, Lunar and Norland dual-energy X-ray absorptiometers and other techniques used for whole body soft tissue measurements. *Eur. J. Clin. Nutr.* **48,** 781–794.
70. Tataranni, P. A., Pettitt, D. J., and Ravussin, E. (1996). Dual-energy X-ray absorptiometry: Inter-machine variability. *Int. J. Obes.* **20,** 1048–1050.
71. Tataranni, P. A., and Ravussin, E. (1995). Use of dual-energy X-ray absorptiometry in obese individuals. *Am. J. Clin. Nutr.* **62,** 730–734.
72. Jensen, M. B., Hermann, A. P., Hessov, I., and Mosekilde, L. (1997). Components of variance when assessing the reproducibility of body composition measurements using bioimpedance and the Hologic QDR-2000 DEXA scanner. *Clin. Nutr.* **16,** 61–65.
73. Pietrobelli, A., Wang, Z., Formica, C., and Heymsfield, S. B. (1998). Dual-energy X-ray absorptiometry: Fat estimation errors due to variation in soft tissue hydration. *Am. J. Physiol.* **274,** E808–E816.

74. Formica, C., Atkinson, M. G., Nyulasi, I., McKay, J., Heale, W., and Seeman, E. (1993). Body composition following hemodialysis: Studies using dual-energy X-ray absorptiometry and bioelectrical impedance analysis. *Osteoporosis* **3,** 192–197.
75. Haderslev, K. V., Svendsen, O. L., and Staun, M. (1999). Does paracentesis of ascites influence measurements of bone mineral or body composition by dual-energy X-ray absorptiometry? *Metabolism* **48,** 373–377.
76. Hill, G. L., Monk, D., and Plank, L. D. (1993). Measuring body composition in intensive care patients. *In* "Metabolic Support of the Critically Ill Patient" (D.W. Wilmore and Y.A. Carpentier, eds.), pp. 3–18. Springer-Verlag, Berlin.
77. Heymsfield, S. B., Wang, J., Heshka, S., Kehayias, J. J., and Pierson, R. N., Jr. (1989). Dual-photon absorptiometry: Comparison of bone mineral and soft tissue mass measurements *in vivo* with established methods. *Am. J. Clin. Nutr.* **49,** 1283–1289.
78. Fuller, M. J., Jebb, S. A., Laskey, M. A., Coward, W. A., and Elia, M. (1992). Four-compartment model for the assessment of body composition in humans: Comparison with alternative methods and evaluation of the density and hydration of the fat-free mass. *Clin. Sci.* **82,** 687–693.
79. Van Loan, M. D., and Mayclin, P. L. (1992). Body composition assessment: Dual-energy X-ray absorptiometry (DEXA) compared to reference methods. *Eur. J. Clin. Nutr.* **46,** 125–130.
80. Jebb, S. A., Goldberg, G. R., Jennings, G., and Elia, M. (1995). Dual-energy X-ray absorptiometry measurements of body composition: Effects of depth and tissue thickness, including comparisons with direct analysis. *Clin. Sci.* **88,** 319–324.
81. Schlemmer, A., Hassager, C., Haarbo, J., and Christiansen, C. (1990). Direct measurement of abdominal fat by dual photon absorptiometry. *Int. J. Obes.* **14,** 603–611.
82. Heymsfield, S. B., Smith, R., Aulet, M., *et al.* (1990). Appendicular skeletal muscle mass: Measurement by dual-photon absorptiometry. *Am. J. Clin. Nutr.* **52,** 214–218.
83. Fuller, M. J., Laskey, M. A., and Elia, M. (1992). Assessment of major body regions by dual-energy X-ray absorptiometry (DEXA) with special reference to limb muscle mass. *Clin. Physiol.* **12,** 1–15.
84. Kushner, R. F. (1992). Bioelectrical impedance analysis: A review of principles and applications. *J. Am. Coll. Nutr.* **11,** 199–209.
85. Lukaski, H. C., Johnson, P. E., Bolonchuk, W. W., and Lykken, G. I. (1985). Assessment of fat-free mass using bioelectrical impedance measurements of the human body. *Am. J. Clin. Nutr.* **41,** 810–817.
86. Baumgartner, R. N. (1996). Electrical impedance and total body electrical conductivity. *In* "Human Body Composition" (A. F. Roche, S. B. Heymsfield, and T. G. Lohman, eds.), pp. 79–107. Human Kinetics, Champaign, IL.
87. Kanai, H., Haeno, M., and Sakamoto, K. (1987). Electrical measurement of fluid distribution in legs and arms. *Med. Prog. Technol.* **12,** 159–170.
88. Ackman, J. J., and Seitz, M. A. (1984). Methods of complex impedance measurements in biologic tissue. *Crit. Rev. Biomed. Eng.* **11,** 281–311.
89. Matthie, J., Zarowitz, B., De Lorenzo A., *et al.* (1998). Analytic assessment of the various bioimpedance methods used to estimate body water. *J. Appl. Physiol.* **84,** 1801–1816.
90. Lukaski, H. C., and Bolonchuk, W. W. (1988). Estimation of body fluid volumes using tetrapolar bioelectrical impedance measurements. *Aviat. Space Environ. Med.* **59,** 1163–1169.
91. Lukaski, H. C., Bolonchuk, W. W., Hall, C. B., and Siders, W. A. (1986). Validation of tetrapolar bioelectrical impedance method to assess human body composition. *J. Appl. Physiol.* **60,** 1327–1332.
92. Simons, J. P. F. H. A., Schols, A. M. W. J., Westerterp, K. R., ten Velde G. P. M., and Wouters, E. F. M. (1995). The use of bioelectrical impedance analysis to predict total body water in patients with cancer cachexia. *Am. J. Clin. Nutr.* **61,** 741–745.
93. Jacobs, D. O. (1996). Use of bioelectrical impedance analysis measurements in the clinical management of critical illness. *Am. J. Clin. Nutr.* **64** (Suppl.), 498S–502S.
94. Segal, K. R., Burastero, S., Chun, A., *et al.* (1991). Estimation of extracellular and total body water by multiple-frequency bioelectrical impedance measurement. *Am. J. Clin. Nutr.* **54,** 26–29.
95. De Lorenzo, A., Andreoli, A., Matthie, J., and Withers, P. (1997). Predicting body cell mass with bioimpedance by using theoretical methods: a technological review. *J. Appl. Physiol.* **82,** 1542–1558.
96. Gudivaka, R., Schoeller, D. A., Kushner, R. F., and Holt, M. J. G. (1999). Single- and multifrequency models for bioelectrical impedance analysis of body water compartments. *J. Appl. Physiol.* **87,** 1087–1096.
97. Patel, R. V., Peterson, E. L., Silverman, N., and Zarowitz, B. J. (1996). Estimation of total body and extracellular water in post-coronary artery bypass graft surgical patients using single and multiple frequency bioimpedance. *Crit. Care Med.* **24,** 1824–1828.
98. Finn, P. J., Plank, L. D., Clark, M. A., Connolly, A. B., and Hill, G. L. (1996). Progressive dehydration and proteolysis in critically ill patients. *Lancet* **347,** 654–656.
99. NIH Technology Assessment Statement. (1996). Bioelectrical impedance analysis in body composition measurement. *Nutrition* **12,** 749–759.
100. Guglielmi, F. W., Contento, F., Laddaga, L., Panella, C., and Francavilla, A. (1991). Bioelectric impedance analysis: experience with male patients with cirrhosis. *Hepatology* **13,** 892–895.
101. Zillikens, C. M., van den Berg, J. W., Wilson, J. H. P., and Swart, G. R. (1992). Whole-body and segmental bioelectrical-impedance analysis in patients with cirrhosis of the liver: changes after treatment of ascites. *Am. J. Clin. Nutr.* **55,** 621–625.
102. Tatara, T., and Tsuzaki, K (1998). Segmental bioelectrical impedance analysis improves the prediction for extracellular water changes during abdominal surgery. *Crit. Care Med.* **26,** 470–476.
103. Haggmark, T., Jansson, E., and Svane, B. (1978). Cross-sectional area of the thigh muscle in man measured by computed tomography. *Scand. J. Clin. Lab. Invest.* **38,** 355–360.
104. Heymsfield, S. B., Olafson, R. P., Kutner, M. H., and Nixon, D. W. (1979). A radiographic method of quantifying protein-calorie undernutrition. *Am. J. Clin. Nutr.* **32,** 693–702.
105. Tokunaga, K., Matsuzawa, Y., Ishikawa, K., and Tarui, S. (1983). A novel technique for the determination of body fat by computed tomography. *Int. J. Obes.* **7,** 437–445.
107. Clasey, J. L., Bouchard, C., Teates, C. D., *et al.* (1999). The use of anthropometric and dual-energy X-ray absorptiometry (DEXA) measures to estimate total abdominal and abdominal visceral fat in men and women. *Obes. Res.* **7,** 256–264.
108. Wang, Z. M., Visser, M., Ma, R., Baumgartner, R. N., Kotler, D., Gallagher, D., and Heymsfield, S. B. (1996). Skeletal muscle mass: evaluation of neutron activation and dual-energy X-ray absorptiometry methods. *J. Appl. Physiol.* **80,** 824–831.
109. Mitsiopoulos, N., Baumgartner, R. N., Heymsfield, S. B., Lyons, W., Gallagher, D., and Ross, R. (1998). Cadaver validation of skeletal muscle measurement by magnetic resonance imaging and computerized tomography. *J. Appl. Physiol.* **85,** 115–122.
110. Chowdhury, B., Sjöström, L., Alpsten, M., Kostanty, J., Kvist, H., and Löfgren, R. (1993). A multicompartment body composition technique based on computerized tomography. *Int. J. Obes.* **18,** 219–234.
111. Borkan, G. A., Hults, D. E., Gerzof, S. G., Burrows, B. A., and Robbins, A. H. (1983). Relationships between computed tomography tissue areas, thicknesses and total body composition. *Ann. Hum. Biol.* **10,** 537–546.
112. Thomas, E. L., Saeed, N., Hajnal, J. V., *et al.* (1998). Magnetic resonance imaging of total body fat. *J. Appl. Physiol.* **85,** 1778–1785.
113. Fowler, P. A., Fuller, M. F., Glasbey, C. A., *et al.* (1991). Total and subcutaneous adipose tissue in women: the measurement of

distribution and accurate prediction of quantity by using magnetic resonance imaging. *Am. J. Clin. Nutr.* **54,** 18–25.

114. Ross, R., Shaw, K. D., Martel, Y., de Guise, J., and Avruch, L. (1993). Adipose tissue distribution measured by magnetic resonance imaging in obese women. *Am. J. Clin. Nutr.* **57,** 470–475.
115. Seidell, J. C., Bakker, C. J. G., and van der Kooy, K. (1990). Imaging techniques for measuring adipose-tissue distribution-a comparison between computed tomography and 1.5-T magnetic resonance. *Am. J. Clin. Nutr.* **51,** 953–957.
116. Abate, N., Burns, D., Peshock, R. M., Garg, A., and Grundy, S. M. (1994). Estimation of adipose tissue mass by magnetic resonance imaging: Validation against dissection in human cadavers. *J. Lipid Res.* **35,** 1490–1496.
117. Wang, Z. M., Pierson, R. N., Jr., and Heymsfield, S. B. (1992). The five-level model: A new approach to organizing body-composition research. *Am. J. Clin. Nutr.* **56,** 19–28.
118. Heymsfield, S. B., and Waki, M. (1991). Body composition in humans: Advances in the development of multicompartment chemical models. *Nutr. Rev.* **49,** 97–108.
119. Wang, Z. M., Gallagher, D., Nelson, M. G., Matthews, D. E., and Heymsfield, S. B. (1996). Total body skeletal muscle mass: Evaluation of 24-h urinary creatinine excretion by computerized axial tomography. *Am. J. Clin. Nutr.* **63,** 863–869.
120. Wang, Z. M., Duerenberg, P., Matthews, D. E., and Heymsfield, S. B. (1998). Urinary 3-methylhistidine excretion: Association with total body skeletal muscle mass by computerized axial tomography. *J. Parenter. Enteral Nutr.* **22,** 82–86.
121. Monk, D. N., Plank, L. D., Franch-Arcas, G., Finn, P. J., Streat, S. J., and Hill, G. L. (1996). Sequential changes in the metabolic response in critically injured patients during the first 25 days after blunt trauma. *Ann. Surg.* **223,** 395–405.
122. Plank, L. D., Connolly, A. B., and Hill, G. L. (1998). Sequential changes in the metabolic response in severely septic patients during the first 23 days after the onset of peritonitis. *Ann. Surg.* **228,** 146–158.
123. Streat, S. J., and Hill, G. L. (1987). Nutritional support in the management of critically ill patients in surgical intensive care. *World J. Surg.* **11,** 194–201.
124. Plank, L. D., and Hill, G. L. (2000). Sequential metabolic changes following induction of systemic inflammatory response in patients with severe sepsis or major blunt trauma. *World J. Surg.* **24,** 630–638.

59

Energetics

Danny O. Jacobs and Takeaki Matsuda

Laboratories of Surgical Metabolism, Department of Surgery and Nutrition, Brigham and Women's Hospital, Harvard Medical School, Boston, Massachusetts 02115; and Creighton University Surgical Laboratories for Biomedical Investigation, Omaha, Nebraska 68131

I. Introduction

The human body is an energy machine that converts food or stored body fuels into mechanical work, stored energy, or heat. Following absorption of nutrients, only about one-half of the ingested energy is available for conversion to compounds with high-energy bonds because of biochemical inefficiencies. However, once energy is captured as ATP and other energetic compounds, it is available for mechanical work (such as exercise), transport work (for example, to support membrane pumps), and synthetic work (such as protein synthesis) (1). The quantitation and characterization of this process fall in the general field of energetics.

Calorimetry is the measurement of energy expenditure (EE), whereas specific pathways of energy metabolism can be measured by tissue analysis or utilizing magnetic resonance spectrometry. Discussion of these methods is the main focus of this chapter.

II. Whole Body Measurements

A. Indirect Calorimetry (Respiratory Gas Exchange)

In the steady state, the quantities of oxygen consumed and carbon dioxide produced are related to the release of energy from the body. Because there is a fixed stoichiometric relationship between these two gases and the energy released with the oxidation of a specific food, the gas exchanged in a particular biological reaction can be used to calculate the energy produced from that reaction. This association was established in classic studies of Atwater and Benedict (2), who demonstrated a close relationship between whole body heat production measured directly in a calorimeter or indirectly using respiratory gas exchange. Others have more recently confirmed this observation (3–6).

Indirect calorimetry is the method that measures oxygen consumption (V_{O_2}) and carbon dioxide production (V_{CO_2}) in order to calculate EE and the respiratory quotient (*RQ*). The most common methods for measurement are by closed-circuit and open-circuit techniques. With closed-circuit calorimeters, V_{O_2} is determined by measuring the volumetric change from a reservoir of oxygen over time. With open-circuit calorimeters, V_{O_2} is determined by measuring the difference between inspired and expired gas concentrations and minute ventilation or flow through the system. Open-circuit calorimeters use either a mixing chamber, dilution methodology, or breath-by-breath techniques.

1. Closed-Circuit Calorimetry

This approach allows measurement of oxygen consumption using a facemask or mouthpiece and nose clip. Modification of this technique allows measurements to be obtained in ventilated patients. During measurements, the subject inspires oxygen from a large spirometer and exhales into the same container, which serves as a mixing chamber. The carbon dioxide produced is removed by a soda lime CO_2 absorber. Change in the end-expiratory volume of the spirometer is determined over time and the quantity of V_{O_2} consumed per minute is calculated (Fig. 1). This quantity of oxygen consumed can be expressed as the result, or this quantity can be converted to energy assuming an *RQ* of 0.83 (which is the estimated value for subjects consuming a mixed meal). Under these conditions, 1 liter of oxygen accounts for approximately 4.8 kcal (1).

2. Open-Circuit Calorimetry

a. Mixing-Chamber Method The open-circuit indirect calorimeter has both ends of the system open to atmospheric pressure. The subject's inspired air and expired air are kept separate by means of a three-way respiratory valve or nonrebreathing mask. The expired gases are collected in a Douglas bag or Tissot spirometer for analysis of O_2 and CO_2 content. With the mixing-chamber system, expired gas is directed into the mixing chamber and analyzers sample the gas at factory-selected intervals (at least each minute).

This system is commonly used in a variety of clinical and research settings. There are drawbacks; the subjects must adapt to a mouthpiece or facemask. In untrained subjects, hyperventilation occurs, which may cause inappropriately high levels of O_2 consumption and CO_2 production. The mask or mouthpiece must be frequently checked to assure an airtight seal. Because of mask pressure, it is difficult to study patients with facial injuries. In contrast, this approach is frequently used in bicycle or treadmill exercise studies, or in patients with tracheostomies. Another variation on this approach is the metabolic chamber, an airtight room big enough to live in yet supplied with room air through one port, with exhaust from the room placed on the opposite side. By assuring a constant flow through the room and appropriate gas mixture within the room, the oxygen and gas concentrations can be measured at the input and output ports, this difference multiplied by flow rates, and EE determined (7). In this manner, a relatively free-living subject can be studied over a number of days.

This approach is reasonably accurate, but such chambers are expensive and require fixed space and a large staff to ensure their operation. Chambers in operation are found at Vanderbuilt University, in Louisiana at the Pennington Biomedical University Center, at an NIH center in Phoenix, Arizona, and are associated with direct calorimeters.

b. Dilution Method Dilution systems have been developed to avoid the problems associated with the interface between the subject and the apparatus. Dilution systems usually use a canopy hood to interface with the subject. Expired air is diluted with room air and is collected and discharged from the hood via a single exit port (Fig. 2). Gases may be collected in a mixing chamber for analysis or continuously analyzed (8). One commercially available system (Deltatrac, Instrumentarium Corp., Helsinki, Finland) measures V_{O_2} and V_{CO_2} in spontaneously breathing individuals using a canopy hood, or can be adapted to mechanically ventilated patients. Measurement during spontaneous breathing is made by sucking air through the canopy, and the difference between the inspired and expired oxygen fraction (F_{IO_2}, F_{EO_2}) is measured with a fast-response, paramagnetic differential oxygen sensor. The expired CO_2 fraction (F_{ECO_2}) is also measured continuously using an infrared CO_2 sensor.

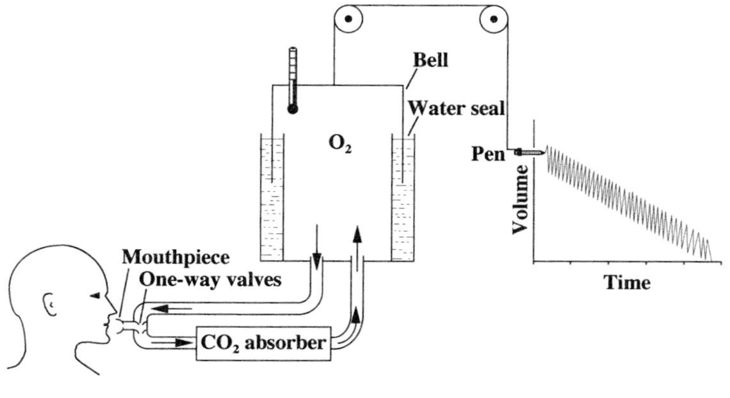

Figure 1 A closed system for measuring oxygen consumption, requiring the use of a mouthpiece and nose clip (not shown).

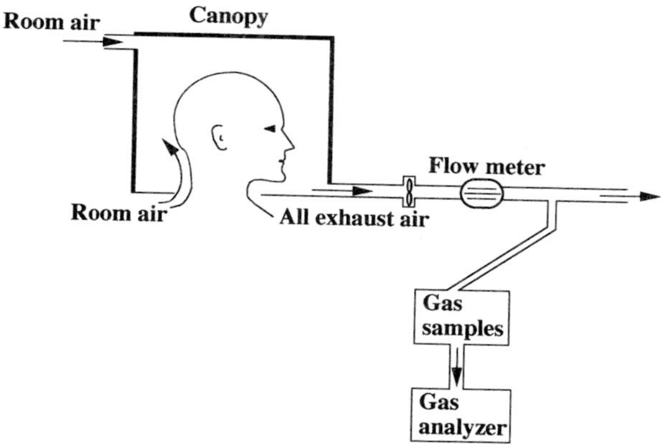

Figure 2 The dilutional method using a canopy system. All expired air must exit through the exit port.

During mechanical ventilation, the device is connected to the outlet port of the ventilator and expired air is collected through a built-in mixing chamber. Similar methods of calculating gas exchange are utilized, although F_{IO_2} is frequently monitored in the inspired gas.

c. Breath-by-Breath Method The mixing-chamber system is also appropriate for the measurement of resting energy expenditure. In contrast, a breath-by-breath approach may be more suitable for the minute-by-minute measurement of EE rather than relying on the mixing-chamber system. The breath-by-breath method samples V_{O_2} and V_{CO_2} at each breath and then averages the data over time. This method may have advantages because it avoids incomplete mixing of inspired gas, unstable F_{IO_2}, and the effects of water vapor and dead space in the measuring devices.

d. Studies in Animals Variations on these methods have been established with small (9) (Fig. 3) and large animals (10, 11).

e. Calculation of Energy Expenditure and Respiratory Quotient Once the total V_{O_2} and V_{CO_2} have been determined, the total energy expenditure can be derived from the de Weir equation (see Table III in Chapter 56).

f. Interpretation of RQ *RQ* is the ratio of the volume of carbon dioxide produced divided by the volume of oxygen consumed during the same time period (V_{CO_2}/V_{O_2}). Measurements of whole body *RQ* reflect substrate utilization at the time of measurement. The physiologic *RQ* ranges between 0.70 and 1.00 and varies with substrate oxidation. The *RQ* of glucose is 1.0; of fat, 0.70; and of protein, 0.79–0.82. An *RQ* above 1.0 usually reflects a nonsteady state of hyperventilation, which is an inaccurate test situation. When calories are given in excess of needs, and fat is produced from excess glucose (lipogenesis), *RQ* will be greater than 1.00 and ranges from 1.00 to 1.30. The *RQ* may decrease to below 0.70 (0.67–0.69) during periods of prolonged ketosis. However, values below 0.70 should be regarded with great suspicion, for they usually reflect methodological error.

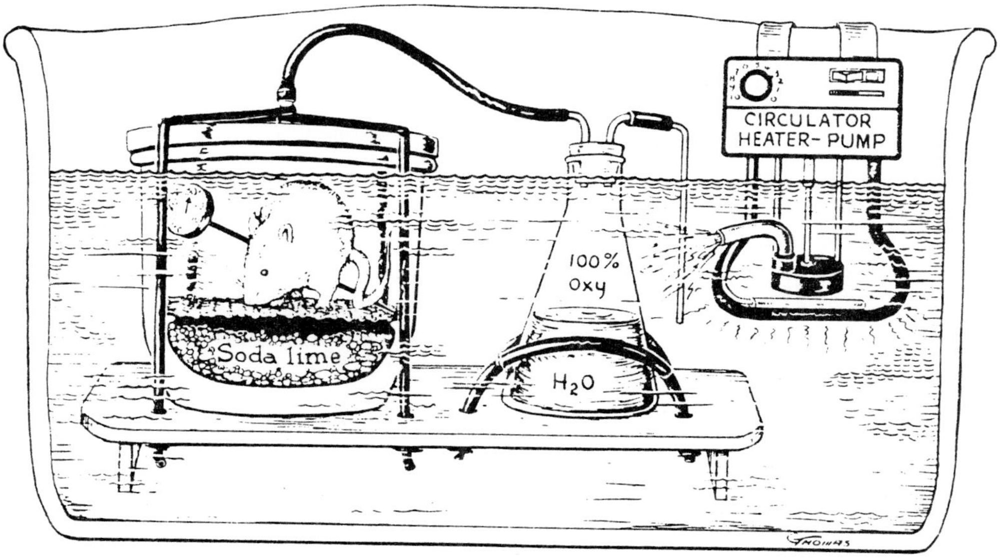

Figure 3 A closed system used to study oxygen consumption in rodents, in a fixed environment determined by bath temperature. As the animals consume oxygen, it is replaced isovolumetrically by water. The amount of water in the flask per unit time is the oxygen consumption of the animal. From Herndon *et al.* (9a).

B. Direct Calorimetry

In patients with a stable body temperature, the heat produced (heat of combustion) is equal to the heat lost from the body. Hence, the direct measurement of heat lost to the surroundings is another method of measuring the energy produced by the body. Devices that measure heat loss directly are large, complex, and expensive, requiring a virtual engineering crew to ensure their proper operation. Initially, such chambers were constructed with a water flowthrough system in the chamber walls (2). By measuring the inflow and outflow temperature of the water and knowing the flow rate, the heat transferred from the subject to the water could be determined. A modern variation of this methodology was the construction of a full-body water-perfused suite that would measure heat loss from the body (3). Other measurement techniques involve chambers with walls made of gradient layers with known conductive properties (4–6). Alternatively, a system using a heat sink can be utilized (12). The most modern calorimeter involves the use of gradient layers to measure heat loss. Multiple thermocouples are placed on the gradient layer (an insulated wall or one that is built so that the outside surface is cooled), which makes up the walls of the chamber. The temperature gradient established across the inside surface, which is exposed to the chamber environment, and the outside surface, which is cooled, generates a voltage potential that is detected by multiple thermocouples. Because the thermal resistance of the walls is constant, the heat flux out of the chamber through the walls is proportional to the voltage output from the thermocouple. With calibration, this electrical signal can be converted to a rate of energy produced.

There are only a few of these complex systems in the world, and in the United States such a device is located at the Diet and Human Performance Laboratory, Beltsville Human Nutrition Center in Maryland. Using direct calorimetry, studies have been performed to measure metabolism in normals and some stable patients (13, 14). The effect of food intake and exercise on heat production has also been studied. Although expense and the enclosed environment limit this approach for studies in ill humans, small chambers are highly desirable for studies in animals (15).

C. Doubly Labeled Water Method

This technique is ideal for measuring EE in humans under free-living conditions over a period of time covering 2–3 weeks, because the subjects may expend more energy in a free-living condition than in a room-sized chamber. This method is valuable for measurements in normal healthy subjects. This technique depends on the exponential disappearance from the body of the stable isotopes ^2H and ^{18}O after administration of a bolus dose of water labeled with both isotopes. The ^2H is lost as water whereas the ^{18}O is lost both as water and as CO_2. The excess disappearance rate of ^{18}O relative to ^2H is a measure of CO_2 production rate. This is then converted to EE using a known or estimated *RQ*. (More on this approach can be found in Chapter 57.)

D. Arterial–Venous O_2 Difference

In critically ill surgical patients who have thermodilution pulmonary artery catheters in place, it is possible to measure V_{O_2} from cardiac output and the arteriovenous oxygen content difference $[(A - V)_{O_2}]$.

Arterial and mixed venous blood samples are obtained simultaneously from an arterial catheter and from the distal port of the pulmonary artery catheter. Rapid injections of iced 5% dextrose in water solution are used to determine cardiac output using the Fick equation:

$$V_{O_2}\ C_O \times (A - V)_{O_2}$$

where C_O (liters/min) is cardiac output and A_{O_2} and V_{O_2} (ml/liters) are arterial and mixed venous total blood oxygen content. These are calculated from the following equation:

$$CA_{O_2} = \text{Hgb} \times 1.37 \times SA_{O_2} + 0.003PA_{O_2},$$

where Hgb (g/liter) is hemoglobin concentration, SA_{O_2} (%) is arterial hemoglobin oxygen saturation, and PA_{O_2} (mmHg) is arterial blood gas level.

Errors abound with this method, in part because cardiac output normally varies, so that multiple measurements must be made. However, this may be an appropriate use of the technology for critically ill patients who are cared for in intensive care units (16).

E. Other Approaches

In normals, heart rate is generally related to oxygen consumption. By determining calibration curves utilizing these two variables, chronic ambulatory monitoring of heart rate can be used to estimate energy production in free-living individuals (17). Changes in thermoregulatory drive will alter this relationship and invalidate this approach. It is also not appropriate in subjects with cardiac disease, large wounds, or infection.

Finally, total energy expenditure can be calculated from studies of body composition. Composition is measured on two occasions separated by a time interval of days or weeks. Food intake is also monitored. The energy received by the body as food is either expended as heat or work or is stored.

The difference between the intake and gain of stored energy is the total energy expenditure (18).

III. Regional Methods

A. $(A - V)_{O_2}$ Difference Technique

This approach involves the measurement of oxygen concentration in arterial and venous blood across an organ, multiplying the difference by the blood flow through the organ (19–21). This approach is discussed in detail in Chapter 56.

Blood oxygen content is measured directly or indirectly. If the patient is febrile, a temperature correction of this measurement may be required. With animal studies, the affinity for hemoglobin differs between model species and humans, and this adjustment must be made when calculating oxygen content from the previously outlined equation. As is emphasized in Chapter 56, multiple samples are necessary to ensure precision of this technique.

This method can also be adapted to perfused organ models by calculating the oxygen required to maintain a normal oxygen content in the perfusate. Alternatively, the $A - V$ difference can be measured and multiplied by flow rate.

B. In Vivo Magnetic Resonance Spectroscopy

The development of magnetic resonance spectroscopy (MRS)—otherwise known as nuclear magnetic resonance spectroscopy, or NMR—has made it possible to examine cellular and organellar energy metabolism noninvasively and, thereby, to improve understanding of the pathophysiologic and clinical changes observed in many disease states (22–24). MRS techniques allow investigators to study intracellular abnormalities in cellular energetics, their biochemical bases, and the mechanisms by which they occur. These responses are important to understand because they may antedate the development of more overt manifestations of disease and end-stage organ failure. Regional organ systems that have been studied include skeletal muscle, heart, brain, and liver.

The advent of MRS has provided tools to determine what "adequacy of oxygenation" actually means on a more fundamental level. Oxidative phosphorylation, which occurs in mitochondria, is the main source of adenosine triphosphate in most mammalian cells. Adenosine diphosphate, inorganic phosphates, and oxygen are the key ingredients used by mitochondria to produce adenosine triphosphate (ATP). Therefore, the adequacy of oxygenation is ultimately defined in terms of mitochondrial function, and the measurement of tissue or cellular bioenergetics likely provides the definitive standard for assessing oxygen delivery and metabolism. Thus, because of the critical role of the respiratory chain in the metabolism of the cell, methods directed at measurement of tissue oxygenation, including measurement of critical intermediates, can be powerful investigative techniques.

1. Limitations of Magnetic Resonance Spectroscopy

Magnetic resonance spectroscopic techniques are continually evolving. Much research effort is expended on new methods that allow the exact area of interest to be more precisely defined. This is important because the researcher typically wants to ensure that the spectrum is obtained from the smallest possible region of interest and not from surrounding and potentially "contaminating" tissues. Other desirable features of an MRS technology used for translational or other applied research activities include equipment and methods that (1) provide the best sensitivity per unit time and volume, (2) obtain the best results in the minimum number of experiments, and (3) are easy to use. A variety of self-contained and self-shielded magnets available from many manufacturers have these features and can be used for MRS experimentation on cells, organelles, and intact animals. Ongoing, on-site support by the manufacturer and dedicated personnel are critically important for success. The spectrometers and their support and maintenance are expensive. For this reason, the intermittent, nondedicated user is best served by access to the resources of a shared MRS facility.

2. Concepts and Techniques

Magnetic resonance techniques are based on the response of certain nuclear species with an odd number of protons or neutrons to static magnetic fields and other energy applied in the radiofrequency range. Some diagnostically relevant nuclei are ^{1}H, ^{2}H, ^{13}C, ^{19}F, ^{23}Na, ^{31}P, and ^{39}K (Table I). These individual nuclei behave like invisible bar "magnets" and will align their "poles" with the direction of an externally applied static magnetic field. When energy is applied to one of these molecules as a radiofrequency pulse, its alignment

Table I Comparisons of Nuclei That Are MRS Visible

Nucleus	Natural abundance	NMR frequency at 1.5 Tesla	Relative sensitivity[a]
^{31}P	100	25.85	6.63
^{1}H	99.98	63.86	100
^{19}F	100	60.08	83
^{13}C	1.11	16.06	1.59
^{23}Na	100	16.89	9.25

[a] At constant field.

with the external magnetic field is perturbed. Once the radiofrequency pulse is discontinued, the nucleus returns to its equilibrium state by dissipating the absorbed energy through interactions with the surrounding environment and with other molecules (25). The computer-assisted capture and analysis of the dissipated energy form the basis for nuclear magnetic resonance spectroscopy (and imaging). Detection is largely dependent on the strength of the NMR signal, which, in turn, is determined by four factors: concentration within the region of interest, natural isotopic abundance, relative sensitivity, and mobility. For example, MRS techniques are only about 1/15th as sensitive to ^{31}P as they are to ^{1}H because the latter are far more abundant in body tissues.

Concentration and mobility are often the most important factors for the investigator. The higher the concentration of the element of interest, the stronger is its signal. Unfortunately, the particular isotope possessing spin may not be the isotope in greatest natural abundance in the body. For example, the predominant isotope of carbon, ^{12}C, is present in reasonably large concentrations in the body. However, ^{12}C has an even number of protons and neutrons, and thus cannot be detected in MRS experiments. The isotope ^{13}C, which is MRS visible, accounts for only 1% of the total carbon in the body. In contrast, ^{31}P is both the naturally occurring isotope and the isotope observable by NMR.

Mobility is also an important determinant of the ability of a given nucleus to generate an effective signal. Mobility is greater if the nucleus is part of a relatively small molecule in the cytoplasm rather than if it is associated with large macromolecules bound to membranes. These factors are particularly important in ^{31}P spectroscopy. *In vivo* ^{31}P magnetic resonance spectroscopy performed using static magnetic fields of the strengths currently available (typical machines used for animal work have magnetic field strengths on the order of 8 Tesla, where 1 Tesla is equal to 10,000 Gauss; the magnet of a refrigerator door is about 100 Gauss), and can detect phosphorus metabolites such as inorganic phosphate and ATP that are present in concentrations greater than 0.5 m*M*. Significant binding to mitochondria and other effects that reduce mobility may decrease the number of ^{31}P nuclei that can be detected to approximately 20% of the total present. However, these are the molecules that are "free" rather than complexed or otherwise bound biochemically and may be more relevant to metabolic regulation and more indicative of the balance between energy supply and demand.

Despite these issues, valuable information on bioenergetic changes in various organs and tissues can be obtained using phosphorus MRS spectroscopy. Phosphorus is a major component of the body and is present at a level that comprises approximately 1% of the lean weight of the healthy human adult. It plays a crucial role in many metabolic processes, e.g., it is present in the sugar phosphate backbone of nucleic acids and forms a part of the polar group of the phospholipids of various cell membranes. In general, however, the phosphorus atoms of DNA and of most phospholipids are not observable by ^{31}P MRS of living tissue, partly because of their relatively low concentration but also because of signal broadening and loss of resolution secondary to the immobility of phosphorus in these compounds (*vide supra*).

Many of the investigations into changes in tissue energetics have been performed in skeletal muscle. ATP is broken down through the activity of various ATPases (including the Na^+,K^+-ATPase) to provide energy for all cellular work:

$$\text{ATP}^* \xrightarrow{\text{ATPases}} \text{ADP} + \text{Pi}^* + \text{energy}$$

$$\text{PCr}^* + \text{ADP} \xrightarrow{\text{Creatine kinase}} \text{ATP}^* + \text{creatine}$$

The compounds that are MRS visible are denoted by an asterisk. As alluded to earlier, ATP is provided by oxidative phosphorylation but is also generated from glycolysis, glycogenolysis, and breakdown of the high-energy phosphate storage compound phosphocreatine (PCr), when this compound is present—as it is in normal myocytes but not hepatocytes and some other cell types.

In the creatine kinase reaction, ADP is rephosphorylated to regenerate ATP. Thus, when ^{31}P compounds are measured in skeletal muscle, the processes associated with the production and utilization of ATP can be followed. Although absolute quantification is possible, changes in the ratios of the phosphate compounds can also be used to estimate changes in energy availability (ATP/Pi), the relationship between high-energy phosphate stores and ATP (PCr/ATP), and thermodynamic capacity (PCr/Pi) (which represents the sum of forward flow through the two pathways illustrated above). The β-ATP peak is used to represent changes in ATP, because other adenine nucleotides or ^{31}P MRS-visible compounds, such as ADP or the oxidized and reduced forms of nicotinamide adenine dinucleotide, do not contaminate its peak, unlike the peaks representing α- and γ-ATP. In skeletal muscle, five major peaks are readily detected representing the three phosphate atoms of ATP, PCr, and inorganic phosphate (Fig. 4). Occasionally, a smaller, broader peak upfield (+ ppm) from the inorganic phosphate peak may be seen, which corresponds to phosphomonoesters (PMEs). Muscle PMEs are believed to be largely composed of glycolytic intermediates such as glucose-6-phosphate. The distance between the PCr and the Pi peaks in skeletal muscle (chemical shift) in ppm can be used to determine intracellular pH because this distance varies linearly with ^{1}H concentration over a wide physiologic range. The intracellular pH value is obtained by comparison with a graph of chemical shifts in ppm versus titrated organic phosphate solutions.

There are two primary aspects that are important in interpreting magnetic resonance spectra correctly. These are the

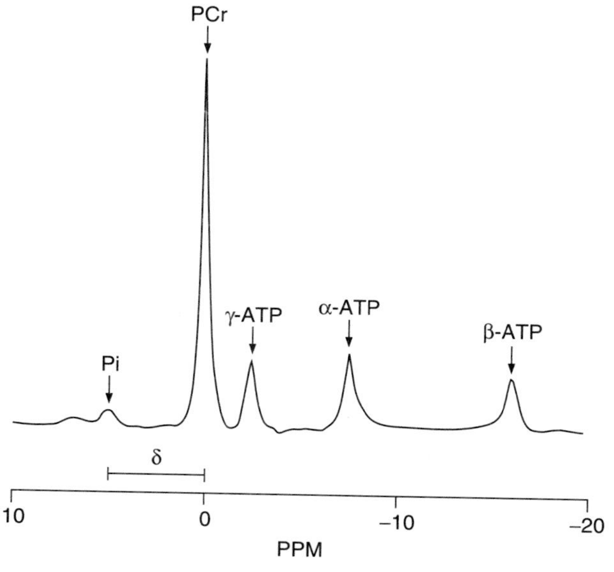

Figure 4 A representative spectrum obtained from rat skeletal muscle at rest using a high-strength magnetic field (8.45 Tesla).

assignment of the peaks, i.e., qualitative analysis, and the measurement of relative or absolute amounts of the various compounds, i.e., quantitative analysis. In general, the amount of tissue from which the signals are obtained varies according to the technique that is used to obtain the signals. Furthermore, determination of the concentration of the MRS-visible metabolites requires the use of internal or external standards, although there are methods that do not require the use of these standards. Many investigators use ATP concentrations, measured *in vitro*, as an internal standard based either on the assumption that the concentration of this metabolite does not vary significantly under the experimental conditions and/or the demonstration that this is true using *in vitro* assays. One potential weakness of this method, especially when it is used to analyze skeletal muscle, is that it assumes that the tissue scanned is relatively homogeneous. Whereas this may be true for the superficial region of the gastrocnemius, if may not be true in other tissues or organ beds.

In addition to the measurement of absolute or relative quantities of phosphorus-containing compounds, e.g., ATP, PCr, and inorganic phosphate, and pH, MRS can also be used to measure chemical reaction rates *in vivo* and *in vitro*. Forsen and Hoffmann (26) first described the use of NMR magnetization transfer to measure chemical fluxes in 1964. In a magnetization transfer experiment a magnetic label is applied to one or more resonances. The transfer of the magnetic label between chemical sites is a reflection of both the chemical reaction rate and the intrinsic NMR relaxation time. In a reaction of the general form

$$AX + B \underset{K_2}{\overset{K_1}{\rightleftharpoons}} BX + A,$$

where A and B transfer a moiety X, which contains a magnetic nucleus, between them; then K_1 and K_2 can be measured separately using magnetization transfer techniques. For example, in skeletal muscle creatine kinase catalyzes the exchange of phosphate between the two distinct MRS-visible sites, PCr and the γ-phosphate of ATP, according to:

$$PCr \underset{k_{rev}}{\overset{k_{for}}{\rightleftarrows}} [\gamma\text{-P}]ATP.$$

Thus, whereas, standard P MRS spectroscopy is used to measure the absolute or relative concentrations of PCr, ATP, or other metabolites, magnetization transfer experiments provide direct estimates of rate constants. In skeletal muscle, selective irradiation and saturation of PCr or [γ-P]ATP with a proportionately long radiofrequency pulse of lower power and of varying durations and measurement of the transfer of magnetic label (e.g., an exponential decrease in the areas under the PCr peak when the pulse is applied at [γ-P]ATP) is used to calculate k_{for} and k_{rev} for the creatine kinase reaction, respectively (Fig. 5). Fluxes through the forward and reverse creatine kinase reactions can be calculated as $k_{for}\cdot$[PCr] and $k_{rev}\cdot$ [ATP], respectively. Furthermore, when the inorganic phosphate signal is well discriminated, saturation at [γ-P]ATP can also be used to measure ATP synthesis from inorganic phosphate *in vivo* because its signal will also decrease exponentially with saturation time.

The measurement of chemical fluxes or the rate constants for the creatine kinase pathway provides useful information about the metabolic status and the physiologic demands being placed on a particular tissue. Such measurements provide more dynamic information than the simpler measurements of high-energy phosphate ratios. The forward rate constant (as a reflection of ATP turnover) is likely a much more sensitive indicator of function or metabolic activity than is the measurement of steady-state PCr and ATP concentration.

3. Importance of the Phosphorylation Potential

All intracellular processes, either directly or indirectly, depend on the ability of the cell to maintain adequate production of ATP. ATP provides the energy necessary for vital cellular functions. Furthermore, many metabolic reactions are controlled changes in the cell "energy status." There are two commonly used indices of cell energy status: Atkinson's energy charge and the phosphorylation potential.

The energy charge is defined as

$$\frac{[ATP] + \frac{1}{2}[ADP]}{[ATP] + [ADP] + [AMP]}.$$

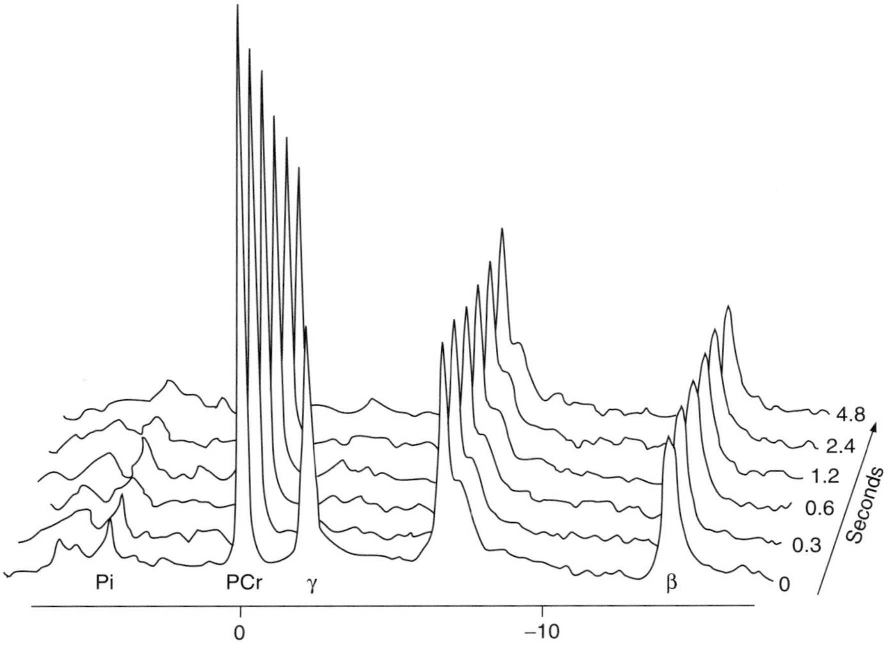

Figure 5 Spectra from a saturation transfer experiment. Spectra were obtained from the gastrocnemius muscle after 0 to 4.8 sec of selective saturation at the γ-ATP peak. Note the changes in the area under the PCr peak.

The phosphorylation ratio, which mirrors changes in Atkinson's energy charge, can be estimated or measured directly using phosphorus MRS. The phosphorylation ratio of a cell is defined as

$$\mathrm{PR} = \frac{[\mathrm{ATP}]}{[\mathrm{ADP}][\mathrm{Pi}]}.$$

The phosphorylation potential is directly related to the free energy available from ATP and, in contrast to Atkinson's energy charge, varies with the concentration of inorganic phosphate. This ratio modulates a variety of metabolic processes, including (1) the efficiency of cardiac work per mole of coronary O_2 delivered, (2) the oxidation–reduction state of cellular cofactors, (3) whether dietary or tissue amino acids will be synthesized into tissue protein or broken down into glucose, (4) the extent of the plasma membrane gradients of the essential electrolytes, (5) the intracellular pH, and (6) the distribution of water between the various cellular compartments.

Normally, the concentration of ADP free in the cytosol (20 to 50 μM) is below the sensitivity of typical MRS equipment. However, the phosphorylation potential in heart, brain, and muscle can be estimated indirectly using the PCr present in these tissues and the creatine kinase equilibrium. Because the reactants of the creatine kinase reaction are in near equilibrium in these tissues, the free ADP concentration can be determined from the intracellular pH, PCr, ATP, and creatine concentrations and the equilibrium constant for the creatine kinase reaction according to

$$[\mathrm{ADP}] = \frac{[\mathrm{ATP}][\mathrm{Cr}]}{[\mathrm{PCr}][\mathrm{H}^+]K_{\mathrm{CK}}},$$

where $[\mathrm{H}^+]$ is derived from the pH measurement and k_{CK} is the equilibrium constant. The creatine concentration may be determined *in vitro* or can be estimated by assuming that any change in this substrate is equimolar to the changes in phosphate. The substrate ratios and the intracellular pH are determined directly from the spectra. The phosphorylation potential, or ratio, can then be derived using the calculated free ADP concentration and the ratio of ATP to inorganic phosphate (Pi) taken directly from the phosphorus MRS spectra.

In spectra of the liver, the three phosphate atoms of ATP and inorganic phosphate are also readily visualized (Fig. 6). The PME peak is prominent and represents phosphomonoesters such as sugar phosphates and membrane phospholipid precursors such as phosphoethanolamine and phosphocholine. This peak area may also include a small contribution from adenosine monophosphate. A peak corresponding to the phosphodiesters (PDEs), i.e., phospholipid catabolites such as glycerophosphocholine and glycerophosphoethanolarnine, is seen between the peaks identifying inorganic phosphate and γ-ATP. Thus, PME and PDE peaks are largely made up by membrane phospholipid precursors and breakdown products. For this reason, changes in the

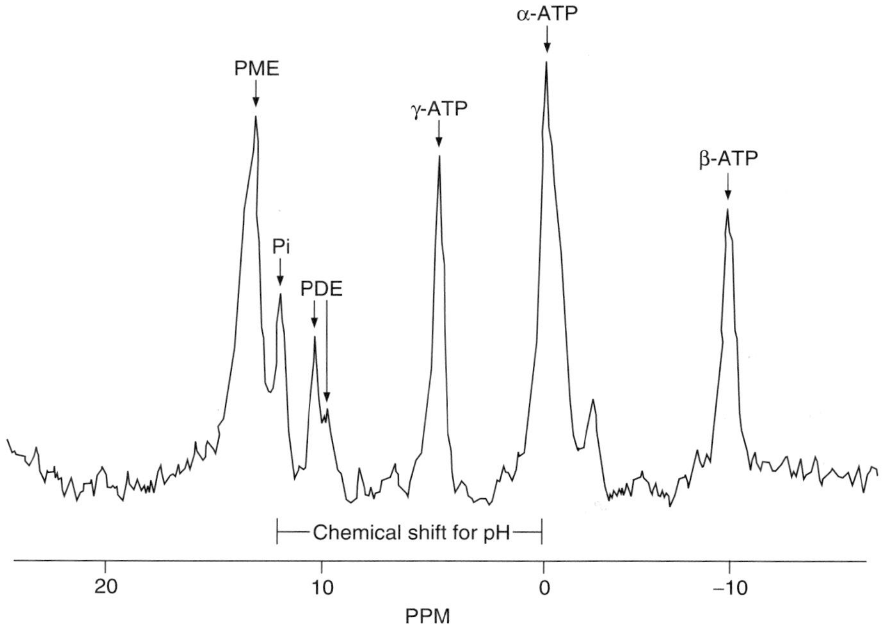

Figure 6 A representative *in vivo* spectrum of the liver. The three phosphate atoms of ATP and inorganic phosphate (Pi) are easily seen. Peaks corresponding to phosphomonoesters (PME) and phosphodiesters (PDE) can also be identified.

PME/ATP and PDE/ATP ratios may correlate with changes in hepatocellular membrane synthesis or degradation if intracellular ATP concentrations do not change significantly.

A PCr peak is not seen in noncontamined hepatic spectra because the liver has no PCr. The same principles apply in studies of the liver that were described for skeletal muscle. Special localization and other techniques can be used to obtain spectra from specific regions within the liver and to quantify the amount of pertinent metabolites directly. These localization techniques can be used to provide "maps" of changes in metabolites in transverse, coronal, or in other anatomical planes. As described previously, one can also derive the ATP/Pi ratio from MRS analysis of the liver by dividing the area under the β-ATP peak by the area under the Pi peak. By convention, this ratio for liver is usually reported as Pi/ATP (rather than ATP/Pi) and is therefore inversely related to cell energy status. Accordingly, as the Pi/ATP ratio increases, cell energy status worsens. The ATP/Pi ratio is an excellent qualitative estimate of the cell's phosphorylation potential because the concentration of ADP is much smaller (less than 5%) than the concentrations of either ATP or Pi, and therefore changes in phosphorylation potential depend largely on changes in ATP and Pi. In MRS scans of the liver, the chemical shift or distance between the Pi and α-ATP peaks is linearly related to intracellular pH.

Phosphorus MRS has been used to study tissue energetics of exercising muscle. During anaerobic (ischemic) contraction, only glycogenolysis and PCr breakdown can regenerate ATP, though the predominant fuel for skeletal muscle in the well-fed state is free fatty acids (30). Under aerobic conditions, especially during the early stages of dynamic exercise, both oxidative and anaerobic reactions contribute to ATP formation. The resynthesis of PCr and the return of the muscle energy state to the equilibrium conditions are thought to be dependent on oxidative processes alone. Furthermore, the maximal mitochondrial metabolic rate can be determined from the time constant of the slope of tile recovery curves. Thus, the restoration of resting PCr concentrations, and the clearance of inorganic phosphate and H^+ after exercise, as measured from the intracellular pH recovery, have characteristic time courses in healthy muscle. The efficiency of the coupling between ATP utilization and work performed can be used to analyze muscle function and metabolic state (31–33). Such studies allow oxidative processes to be modeled under normal conditions and during disease.

C. Tissue Analysis

Instruments have been developed to utilize near-infrared spectroscopy to determine mitochondrial cytochrome *aa* redox shifts, from which oxygenation of a specific tissue can be inferred. Fiber optic technology delivers the appropriate wave form to the tissue and this energy is absorbed, depending on the arterial blood oxygen concentration. The fluorescence that is emitted is detected by a sensor portion of the probe and recorded. Modern single-probe instruments allow specific tissue, such as muscle or gastric mucosa (34), to be monitored over time. Although such an approach is applicable to dynamic states in which relative changes in tissue oxygen tension need to be monitored, the absolute levels measured may be problematic. However, cerebral monitoring, if validated in patient studies, may be quite useful utilizing this approach.

IV. Cells

A. Measurement of Oxygen Consumption

Cells have been placed in suspensions under controlled conditions and the oxygen consumed under these conditions measured. The health of the cells in this changing environment has always been questioned.

Direct measurements of heat loss can be made utilizing more contemporary methodology (e.g., Thermal Activity Monitor, Thermometries AB, Järfallä, Sweden). Using this device, tissue samples are placed in a 5-ml stainless-steel ampule and the container is filled with Ringer's lactate and lowered into the measuring cylinders, which are submerged in a waterbath. All heat generated by the sample is passed to the surrounding bath. Heat flow is measured by a series of detectors and is converted to energy (35).

B. MRS Analysis

A tremendous amount of work has been performed studying the effects of various conditions on bioenergetics of the heart. These are *ex vivo* perfusion studies performed using modifications of the standard Langendorff perfusion apparatus mounted within an NMR spectrometer (36, 37). Similar systems exist for the liver (38).

Standard *in vitro* techniques for measuring ATP content of cells include spectrophotometric and fluoroscopic methods that are well described in standard texts (39, 40). The ATP–luciferase bioluminescence reaction is especially sensitive for measuring small quantities of ATP within cells or small tissue quantities. Spectrophotometric methods can also be used to measure the major metabolites of importance in cellular energy metabolism, including ADP, Pi, and PCr. Measuring small quantities of PCr *in vitro* is extremely difficult and controversial because some PCr may be catabolized (and PCr levels subsequently lowered) regardless of tissue extraction method. When all adenosine metabolites need to be measured, techniques based on high-performance liquid chromatography are advantageous because of their efficiency and sensitivity (41). Protocols for maintaining perfused, respiring tissues slices or cells—typically mounted on beads or otherwise supported in tubes suitable for NMR spectroscopy—have also been reported (42).

Mitochondria can be specifically isolated—usually by differential centrifugation—encapsulated, perfused, and studied (43). Oxygen consumption in isolated mitochondria can also be measured polarographically. Respiratory rates are measured in specialized cuvettes that allow oxygen uptake to be followed. Oxygen uptake can be measured in nanomolar quantities per minute per milligram of tissue. Respiratory control phenomena can be determined by measuring changes in respiration at baseline and in the presence of stimulatants. All of these models are stable for at least 16 hr as long as perfusion and oxygenation are maintained. They also provide an opportunity to study the effects of mediators or other agents on tissue energetics.

References

1. Wilmore, D. W. (1977). "Metabolic Management of the Critically Ill." Plenum Medical Book Co., New York.
2. Atwater, A. O., and Benedict, F. G. (1903). Experiments on the metabolism of matter and energy in the human body. USDA Office of Experimental Stations Bulletin Publication No. 16 [a partial republication of this article (1983) can be found in *Nutr. Rev.* **41,** 353–356].
3. Webb, P., Annis, J. F., and Troutman, S. J., Jr. (1980). Energy balance in man measured by direct and indirect calorimetry. *Am. J. Clin. Nutr.* **33,** 1287–1298.
4. Benzinger, T. H., and Kitzinger, C. (1949). Direct calorimetry by means of the gradient principle. *Rev. Sci. Instrum.* **20,** 849–860.
5. Seale, J. S., and Rumpler, W. V. (1997). Synchronous direct gradient layer and indirect room calorimetry. *J. Appl. Physiol.* **83,** 1775–1781.
6. Seale, J. L., Rumpler, W. V., and Moe, P. W. (1991). Description of a direct-indirect room-sized calorimeter. *Am. J. Phys.* **260,** E306–32.
7. Kavlissin, E., Lillioja, S., Anderson, T. E., Christin, L., and Bogardus, C. (1986). Determinants of 24-hour energy expenditure in man; methods and results using a respiratory chamber. *J. Clin. Invest.* **78,** 1568–1578.
8. Aulick, L. H., Hander, E. H., Wilmore, D. W., Masno, A. D., Jr., and Pruitt, B. A., Jr. (1979). The relative significance of thermal and metabolic demands on burn hypermetabolism. *J. Trauma* **19,** 559–566.

9a. Herndon, D. N., Wilmore, D. W., and Mason, Jr., A. D. (1978). Development and analysis of a small animal model simulating the human postburn hypermetabolic response. *J. Surg. Res.* **25,** 394–403.

9. Herndon, D. W., Hander, E. H., Wilmore, D. W., Mason, A. D., Jr., and Pruitt, B. A., Jr. The relative significance of thermal and metabolic demands on burn hypermetabolism. *J. Trauma* **19,** 559–566.
10. Aulick, L. H., Baze, W. B., Johnson, A. A., Wilmore, D. W., and Mason, A. D., Jr. (1981). A large animal model of burn hypermetabolism. *J. Surg. Res.* **31,** 281–287.
11. Aulick, L. H., Arnhold, H., Handler, E. D., and Mason, A. D., Jr. (1983). A new open and closed respiration chamber. *Q. J. Exp. Physiol.* **168,** 351–357.
12. Webster, J. D., Welsh, G., and, Garrow, J. S. (1986). Description of a human direct calorimeter, with a note on the energy cost of clerical work. *Br. J. Nutr.* **551,** 1–6.
13. Bradham, G. B. (1972). Direct measurement of total metabolism of a burn patient. *Arch. Surg.* **105,** 410–413.
14. Rav, M., Koenig, W., and Lis, S. (1995). Direct calorimetry for the measurement of heat release in preterm infants; methods and applications. *J. Perinatol.* **15,** 379–381.

15. Domenech, T., Rafecas, I., Esteve, M., Argiles, J. M., and Alemany, M. (1988). A sensitive direct calorimeter for small mammals. *J. Biochem. Biophys. Methods* **17,** 35–42.
16. Touho, H., Karasawa, J., Shishido, H., Yamada, K., and Shibamoto, K. (1991). Direct calorimetry using Swan–Ganz catheter for evaluation of general metabolic expenditure in acute cerebrovascular disease—Comparison between direct fick method and indirect calorimetry technique. *Neurol. Med. Chir.* **31,** 691–69.
17. Spurr, G. B., Prentics A. M., Murgatroyd, P. R., Goldberg, G. R., Reina, J. C., and Christman, N. T. (1988). Energy expenditure from minute-by-minute heart-rate recording: Comparison with indirect calorimetry. *Am. J. Clin. Nutr.* **48,** 552–559.
18. Byrne, T. A., Morrissey, T. B., Gatzen, C., Benfell, K., Natrtakom, T. B., Sheltinga, M. R., LeBoff, M. S., Ziegler, T. R., and Wilmore, D. W. (1993). Anabolic therapy with growth hormone accelerates protein gain in surgical patients requiring nutritional rehabilitation. *Ann. Surg.* **218,** 400–416.
19. Andres, R., Cader, G., and Zierler, K. L. (1956). The quantitatively minor role of carbohydrate in oxidative metabolism by skeletal muscle in intact man in the basal state. Measurements of oxygen and glucose uptake and carbon dioxide and lactate production in the forearm. *J. Clin. Invest.* **35,** 671–682.
20. Wilmore, D. W., Aulick, L. H., Mason, D. A., Jr., and Pruit, B. A., Jr. (1977). Influence of the burn wound on local and systemic responses to injury. *Ann. Surg.* **186,** 444–456.
21. Aulick, L. H., Baze, W., McLeod, C. G., and Wilmore, D. W. (1980). Control of blood flow in a large surface wound. *Ann. Surg.* **191,** 249–258.
22. Bruch, M. D. (1996). "NMR Spectroscopy Techniques." Marcel Dekker, Inc., New York.
23. Sohar, P. (1983). Theory of nuclear magnetic resonance spectroscopy. *In*, "Nuclear Magnetic Resonance Spectroscopy," Vol. I. (P. Sohar, ed.), pp. 1–131. CRC Press, Boca Raton.
24. Sohar, P. (1983). NMR spectrometers, recording techniques, measuring methods. *In* Sohar P (ed), "Nuclear Magnetic Resonance Spectroscopy," Vol I. (P. Sohar, ed.), pp. 1–131. CRC Press, Boca Raton.
25. Bore, P. J. (1985). Principles and applications of phosphorus magnetic resonance spectroscopy. *In* "Magnetic Resonance Annual," (H. Y. Kressel, ed.), pp. 45–69. Raven Press, New York.
26. Forsen, S., and Hoffman, R. A. (1963). Study of moderately rapid chemical exchange reactions by means of nuclear magnetic double resonance. *J. Chem. Phys.* **39,** 2892–2901.
27. Rudin, M., and Sauter, A. (1989). The rate constants of the creatine kinase reaction in rat brain: A probe for brain function? Society for Magentic Resonance in Medicine, Eight Annual Scientific Meeting, Vol. 1, p. 489.
28. Atkinson, D. E. (1977). "Cellular Energy metabolism and Its Regulation." Academic Press, Orlando, Florida.
29. Chance, B., and Veech, R. L. (1988). Phosphorus magnetic resonance spectroscopy as a probe of nutritional state. *In* "Nutrition and Metabolism in Patient Care" (J. M. Kinney, K. N. Jeejeebhoy, G. H. Hill, and O. E. Owen, eds.), pp 119–128. WB Saunders, Philadelphia.
30. Fehilg, P., and Warren, J. (1975). Fuel homeostasis in exercise. *N. Engl. J. Med.* **293,** 1078–1081.
31. Argov, S., and Chance, B. (1991). Phosphorus magnetic resonance spectroscopy in nutritional research. *In* "Annual Review of Nutrition," Vol. 11 (R. E. Olson, D. M. Bier, and D. B. McCormick, eds.), pp. 449–464. Annual Reviews Inc., Palo Alto, California.
32. Chance, B., Eleff, S., Leigh, J. S., *et al.* (1981). Mitochondrial regulation of phosphocreatine/inorganic phosphate ratios in exercising human muscle: A gated ^{31}P NMR study. *Proc. Natl. Acad. Sci. U.S.A.* **68,** 6714–6718.
33. Chance, B., Leigh, J. S., Jr., Clark, B., *et al.* (1985). Control of oxidative metabolism and oxygen delivery in human skeletal muscle: A steady state analysis of the work/energy cost transfer function. *Proc. Natl. Acad. Sci. U.S.A.* **82,** 8383–8388.
34. Puyana, J. C., Soller, B. R., Zhang, S., and Heard, S. O. (1999). Continuous measurement of gut pH with near-infrared spectroscope during hemorrhagic shock. *J. Trauma* **46,** 9–14.
35. Bach, F., Singer, D., Schmiedl, A., Bauer, M., and Larsen, R. (1996). High energy phosphates and direct calorimetry as predictive parameters for metabolic recovery of the rat liver following recovery. *Acta Anesthesiol. Scand.* **40,** 940–947.
36. Kaplan, L. J., Blum, H., Bellows, C. F., Banerjee, A., and Whitman, J. R. (1996). Reversible injury: Creatine kinase recovery restores bioenergetics and function. *J. Surg. Res.* **62,** 103–108.
37. Schornack, P. A., Song, S.-K., Hotchkiss, R., and Ackerman, J. J. H. (1997). Inhibition of ion transport in septic rat heart: CS^+ as an NMR active K^+ analog. *Am. J. Physiol.* **272,** c1635–c1641.
38. Colet, J.-M., Makos, J. D., Mallow, C. R., and Sherry, A. D. (1998). Determination of the intracellular sodium concentration in perfused mouse liver by ^{31}P and ^{23}Na magnetic resonance spectroscopy. *Magn. Reson. Med.* **39,** 155–159.
39. Lowry, O. H., and Passonneau, J. V. (1972). "A Flexible System of Enzymatic Analysis," p. 151–153. The New York Academic, New York.
40. Bergmeyer, H. U., ed. (1974). "Methods of Enzymatic Analysis" 2nd Ed., Vols. 1–4. Academic Press, New York.
41. Wiseman, R. W., Moerland, T. S., Chase, P. B., Stuppard, R., and Kushmerick, M. J. (1992). High-performance liquid chromatographic assays for free and phosphorylated derivatives of the creatine analogue β-quanidopropionic acid and l-carboxy-methyl-2-iminoimidezolidine (cyclocreatine). *Anal. Biochem.* **204,** 383–389.
42. Doliba, N. M., Wehrli, S. L., Babsky, A. M., Doliba, N. M., and Osbakken, M. D. (1998). Encapsulation and perfusion of mitochondria in agarose beads for functional studies with ^{31}P-NMR spectroscopy. *Magn. Reson. Med.* **39,** 679–684.
43. Schonfeld, P., Sztark, F., Slimani, M., Dabadie, P., and Mazat, J. P. (1992). Is bupivacaine a decoupler, a protonophore or a proton-leak-inducer? *FEBS Lett.* **304,** 273–276.

60

Models of Protein Metabolism

Per-Olof Hasselgren, David R. Fischer, and Timothy A. Pritts

Department of Surgery, University of Cincinnati College of Medicine, Cincinnati, Ohio 45267

I. Introduction

A number of conditions in surgical patients are associated with changes in protein metabolism. Those conditions include burn and other severe injury, sepsis, shock, ischemia/reperfusion, and cancer (1, 2). Elective major surgery in itself also results in disturbances in protein turnover in various organs and tissues (3). Several changes in protein metabolism are important for the outcome in surgical patients. For example, muscle cachexia in injured and septic patients and in patients with cancer results in muscle wasting and weakness, preventing ambulation and increasing the risk for thromboembolic and pulmonary complications. An appropriate acute-phase response, characterized by increased synthesis of acute-phase proteins in the liver, is important for survival in septic and other critically ill patients (4). Thus, methods to monitor accurately changes in protein metabolism during various disease states and, perhaps more importantly, after different therapeutic interventions are important for investigators involved in surgical research.

In this chapter, we describe methods commonly used to measure protein turnover rates in different tissues from both patients and experimental animals as well as in cell cultures. Technical and practical aspects are emphasized and potential limitations and advantages of different techniques are discussed. Initially, we discuss general aspects involved in the measurement of protein synthesis and degradation. This is followed by a description of specific models used when protein metabolism is studied in intestine and muscle. These tissues are highlighted because they have been the research focus in our laboratory for several years. In addition, they are the site for synthesis of a number of proteins with important biological functions, such as acute-phase proteins and gut hormones in the intestinal mucosa, and the contractile proteins actin and myosin in skeletal muscle. The liver is another organ characterized by high protein turnover rates and production of biologically important proteins. Models of protein metabolism in liver tissue, including isolated and cultured hepatocytes, have been reviewed elsewhere (1, 5, 6).

Different techniques to study protein synthesis and degradation were previously reviewed (7). Some of those methods are summarized in this chapter as well. In addition, more recent methods are discussed here, including the controversy in the literature over the two techniques most commonly used to measure protein synthesis, i.e., the "flooding dose" and "constant infusion" techniques. More extensive reviews of models to measure protein metabolism can be found elsewhere (1, 8, 9).

Protein turnover rates can be measured *in vivo* or *in vitro*. Measurements *in vivo* are important to establish absolute protein synthesis and degradation rates and to study the influence of different physiologic or pathologic conditions on protein metabolism. *In vitro* methods allow for the study of mechanisms and regulation under more controlled and standardized conditions than can be obtained *in vivo*. For example, the effects of different substances, including hormones and cytokines, on protein metabolism can be studied at the tissue or cellular level without the influence of secondary changes caused by the test substances.

One of the limitations of *in vitro* techniques is that protein synthesis rates are lower than they are *in vivo*, and most *in vitro* preparations are in a catabolic state. In most situations, *in vivo* and *in vitro* techniques complement each other and the choice of method is normally based on the hypothesis that is under investigation.

II. Protein Synthesis

Protein balance in any cell and tissue is determined by the rates of protein synthesis and degradation. In some conditions, changes in protein balance are mainly caused by changes in protein breakdown rates, and in other conditions by changes in protein synthesis, but most often, both protein synthesis and degradation are altered simultaneously. Therefore, when experiments are designed to study the influence of different disease states on protein metabolism, techniques to measure both protein synthesis and degradation need to be employed.

Protein synthesis can be measured *in vivo* or *in vitro* in incubated tissues, isolated or cultured cells, or in cell-free systems. The most commonly used techniques to measure protein synthesis involve measurement of the incorporation into protein of a radiolabeled amino acid or an amino acid labeled with a stable isotope, such as ^{13}C or ^{15}N (see also Chapter 57). For measurement of whole body protein synthesis rates, amino acid flux studies are frequently performed. Determination of the ribosomal "profile" (the distribution of ribosomes between monoribosomes and polyribosomes) has been used to assess protein synthesis in different tissues, but this gives only an indirect measure of the biosynthetic capacity at the specific time point when the tissue biopsy was obtained. Amino acid flux over a certain tissue bed (for example, lower extremity) gives information about the net protein balance, but does not give specific information about protein synthesis or degradation rates.

A. Precursor Specific Radioactivity

Many methods used to measure protein synthesis rates are based on the incorporation of radiolabeled amino acids into proteins. When such techniques are used, it is important to understand the concept of precursor specific radioactivity. The specific radioactivity describes the ratio between radiolabeled and unlabeled amino acids and can be expressed as dpm/mole. The amount of radioactivity incorporated into a protein reflects not only the rate of protein synthesis but the specific radioactivity of the precursor amino acid as well. This is illustrated in the simplified scheme in Fig. 1. In this example, the precursor specific radioactivity in panel A is only half of that in panel B, and with identical protein synthesis rates, the amount of radioactivity incorporated into the protein in panel A would be half of that in panel B. Thus, in this example, a different amount of radioactivity incorporated into protein would reflect a difference in precursor specific radioactivity rather than a difference in protein synthesis rate. Although basic, we have found that the concept of specific radioactivity and its importance for interpretation of the results are sometimes confusing for new and young investigators starting in the research laboratory.

One of the most critical issues when radiolabeled amino acids are used to measure protein synthesis rates is to determine the specific radioactivity of the precursor amino acid in the appropriate compartment. The most correct approach is to determine the specific radioactivity in the immediate precursor pool, i.e., the aminoacyl-tRNA pool. Such measurements, however, are technically difficult because of the

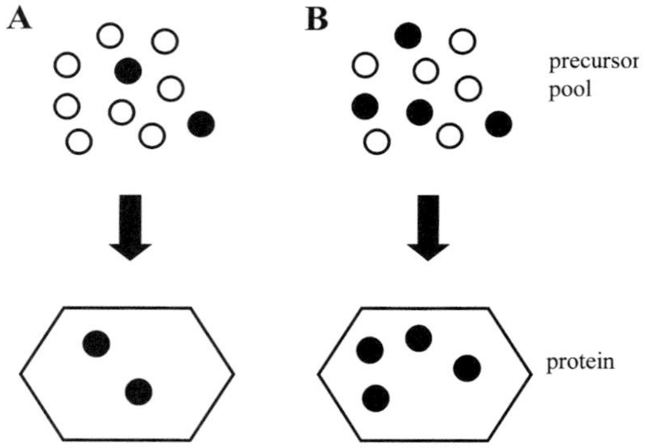

Figure 1 A schematic drawing illustrating the importance of the specific radioactivity in the precursor pool when protein synthesis is measured by determining the amount of radioactivity incorporated into protein, showing labeled amino acids (●) and unlabeled amino acids (○). The specific radioactivity is 2/10 (A) and 4/10 (B). Assuming that 10 amino acids are incorporated into protein per time unit, two radiolabeled amino acids would be incorporated into protein in example A and four radiolabeled amino acids would be incorporated in example B. Thus, in this example, the different amount of radioactivity incorporated into protein would reflect a difference in precursor pool rather than a difference in protein synthesis rate.

small size and rapid turnover of this pool and are not routinely performed by the majority of researchers in the field. Instead, the plasma or intracellular free amino acid pool is frequently used to determine the precursor specific radioactivity. The size of the intracellular amino acid pool is influenced by a number of different factors, including transport of extracellular amino acids across the cell membrane, intracellular proteolysis, and recruitment of amino acids for protein synthesis (8, 10) (Fig. 2). When the intracellular amino acid pool is used to calculate the specific radioactivity, two important conditions should ideally be met: (1) the specific radioactivity should be constant or show only small changes during the period of incorporation of radioactivity into protein and (2) the specific radioactivity should be identical, or at least close, to the specific radioactivity of the aminoacyl-tRNA pool. The techniques most commonly used today to measure protein synthesis *in vivo*, i.e., the flooding dose and the constant infusion methods, were designed to fulfill these criteria.

B. Constant Infusion

In early studies, protein synthesis rates were determined following a single injection of a trace amount of radiolabeled amino acid. Because this method resulted in rapid and pronounced changes in both extracellular and intracellular specific radioactivities, it was necessary to take multiple tissue biopsies during the early period after injection of the precursor, and calculation of protein synthesis rates required complicated mathematical models and calculations (11).

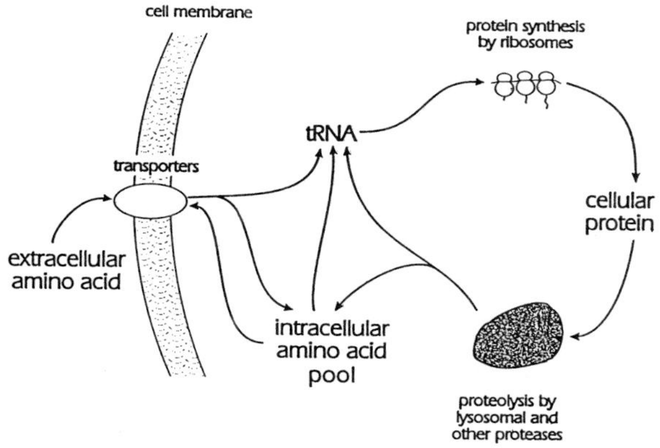

Figure 2 Schematic drawing of different pools from which amino acids can be drawn for protein synthesis. During experiments in which radiolabeled amino acids are used for the study of protein synthesis, isotopic enrichment of tRNA (the immediate precursor pool) depends on relative charging from three different sources: (1) directly from membrane transport at an enrichment similar to that in plasma; (2) from the intracellular pool with an enrichment lower than that in plasma (due to a contribution of unlabeled amino acids from proteolysis); and (3) amino acids directly recycled from proteolysis (without equilibrating with the intracellular pool) with no isotopic enrichment. If source 1 is predominant, enrichment of tRNA will be higher than that of the intracellular pool; if source 3 predominates, amino acid tRNA will be lower than the intracellular pool. From Garlick *et al.* (10), with permission.

With the constant infusion technique, most of these problems are avoided. During the continuous infusion of a radiolabeled amino acid (or amino acid with a stable isotope), the specific radioactivity in plasma reaches a plateau within the first 1–2 hr and remains constant thereafter. The tissue free amino acid specific radioactivity reaches a plateau somewhat more slowly and at a lower level than in plasma, mainly reflecting dilution by amino acids from protein degradation (see Fig. 2). Several studies have shown that the specific radioactivity in the aminoacyl-tRNA pool approaches that of the intracellular amino acid pool or is intermediate between the intracellular and plasma specific radioactivities when a constant infusion of the precursor amino acid is performed. The length of tracer infusion should be long enough to obtain a measurable enrichment of the target proteins but should be short enough to avoid recycling of the precursor amino acid that occurs after degradation of the protein. A constant infusion for 4–6 hr usually fulfills these criteria (12). In humans, a stable isotope is preferably used, and a priming dose of the isotope can be administered to shorten the time to reach equilibrium of labeling in plasma.

Some of the advantages of the constant infusion technique include the fact that protein synthesis rates can be calculated from determination of protein and amino acid specific radioactivity at only one time point, i.e., at the end of infusion. In addition, the amount of precursor amino acid is small (in fact only a tracer is used), thus avoiding the potential influence of a large amount of amino acid on protein synthesis rates, a point pertinent for the comparison between the constant infusion and flooding dose techniques (see below).

One potential drawback of the constant infusion technique is the need for intravenous cannulation, which by itself may induce changes in protein synthesis rates, at least in experimental animals. Another disadvantage of the technique is that changes of protein synthesis rates may not be stable during the length of infusion—therefore, the rate of protein synthesis at a well-defined, specific time point may be difficult to assess. In addition, the rate at which the specific radioactivity reaches steady state varies between different tissues and is also dependent on which precursor amino acid that is used. The experimental conditions therefore need to be established for each individual situation in which the method is used. Among the different amino acids that have been used as precursor during constant infusion, tyrosine offers the advantage of reaching the plateau value of specific radioactivity more rapidly than other isotopes (13). Leucine and phenylalanine are also frequently used for constant infusion.

C. Flooding Dose

The principle behind the flooding dose technique is that administration of a large dose (exceeding the endogenous free pool) of the precursor amino acid results in an equilibration of the specific radioactivity between the different amino acid compartments (10, 14). Thus, by flooding the different amino acid pools, the problem of precursor compartmentalization is minimized and measurement of either the plasma or tissue-free amino acid specific radioactivity can be used for the calculation of protein synthesis rates.

In early studies, the flooding dose technique was used to measure protein synthesis in rat liver and small intestine (15, 16). In those experiments, rats were injected intravenously with 10 μCi of [^{14}C]leucine and 100 μmol of leucine/100 g body weight. With this dose, the whole body free leucine pool was expanded to approximately 10 times the normal size and the specific radioactivity of free leucine was similar in tissue and plasma during the first 10–15 min after administration. The specific radioactivity of protein-bound leucine in tissue was determined 10 min after injection of isotope, and the specific radioactivity of tissue free leucine was determined 2 and 10 min after injection. Because there was a decline in specific radioactivity in the tissue free amino acid pool from 2 to 10 min, the mean specific radioactivity over 10 min was calculated and used for determination of protein synthesis rate. The rate of protein synthesis (K_S), expressed as the proportion of the protein pool replaced each day (percentage/day), was calculated from the equation $K_S = (S_B/S_A)t \times 100$, where S_B is the specific radioactivity of protein-bound leucine, S_A is the mean specific radioactivity of leucine in the precursor pool (tissue free leucine pool), and t is the time expressed in days.

In a modification of the model, the flooding dose of the precursor (150 μmol of phenylalanine and 20 μCi of [^{3}H]phenylalanine/100 g body weight) was administered intraperitoneally instead of intravenously (17). This resulted in a plateau of intracellular specific radioactivity from within 1 min until at least 15 min in liver. In skeletal muscle, the time course of the increase in intracellular specific radioactivity was somewhat slower, with the plateau being reached after 3 min. The time integral for the phenylalanine specific radioactivity in muscle was 0.9 of that which would have been obtained if plateau labeling was immediate. Therefore, in muscle the equation for calculation of protein synthesis rate was modified to $K_S = (S_B/0.9S_A)t \times 100$. With these modifications, protein synthesis rates for both muscle and liver can be calculated from samples obtained at only one time point (15 min) after administration of precursor amino acid.

One of the main advantages of the flooding dose technique is that it avoids the problem of selecting the proper precursor pool for measurement of specific radioactivity because the system is flooded with the precursor amino acid and specific radioactivity equilibrates between different pools. An additional advantage is that protein synthesis is measured over a short period of time. This allows for a more accurate definition of the metabolic and physiologic state of the animal or subject than is possible with a continuous infusion. Finally, because incorporation of precursor into protein is measured over a short time span, potential errors arising because of loss of labeled protein and recycling of precursor amino acid are avoided.

One drawback of the flooding dose technique is that results may be disproportionally influenced by the turnover of short-lived proteins when the synthesis rate is measured over only 10–15 min. The potential limitation of the flooding dose that has attracted most attention, however, is the possibility that the large dose of the precursor amino acid may influence protein synthesis rates, in particular when a flooding dose of leucine is used to measure muscle protein synthesis. This concern has been the subject of recent vivid discussion and disagreement in the literature (see below).

It should be noted that although the flooding dose technique has been described here in the context of *in vivo* experiments, the same principle applies for *in vitro* experiments in which tissues or cells are incubated in the presence of a high concentration of precursor amino acid. Indeed, early *in vitro* experiments validated the concept of the flooding dose with respect to equilibration of specific radioactivity between the extracellular (medium) and intracellular free amino acid pools and the aminoacyl-tRNA pools, making it possible to calculate protein synthesis rates from the specific radioactivity in plasma or in the tissue free amino acid pool (Figs. 3 and 4) (8).

Different techniques used to measure protein synthesis *in vitro* and *in vivo*, in both experimental animals and humans, are summarized in Table I.

D. Constant Infusion vs. Flooding Dose: Conflicting Opinions

Because the constant infusion and flooding dose techniques have given rise to apparent differences in protein synthesis rates, both when applied to animal experiments and studies in patients, controversy has arisen over which method is more accurate. The different opinions regarding the two techniques were discussed in detail in recent review articles written by the major proponents of the two methods, i.e., Rennie *et al.* (12) for the continuous infusion and Garlick *et al.* (10) for the flooding dose. Because both methods are frequently used, an understanding of the conflicting opinions is important for the interpretation of results generated with either technique.

The main focus of the disagreement between the two groups of researchers is whether the two methods give different results for protein synthesis rates and, if so, what the

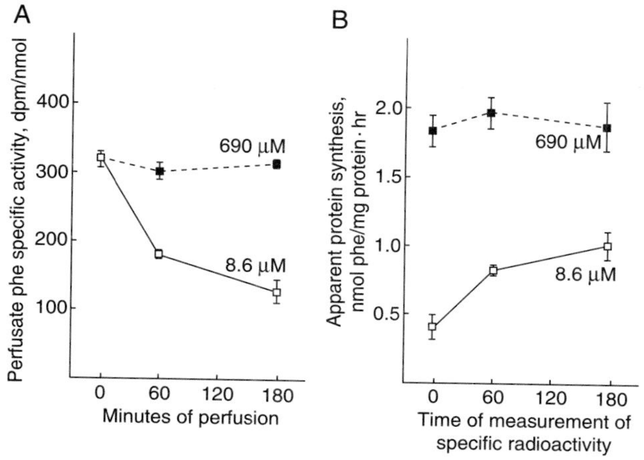

Figure 3 Effect of extracellular phenylalanine concentration on the specific radioactivity of perfusate phenylalanine (A) and apparent rate of protein synthesis (B). Results are from experiments in which protein synthesis was measured in perfused rat lungs. When the concentration of the precursor amino acid in perfusate was increased from 8.6 to 690 μ*M* (the system was flooded with phenylalanine), the precursor specific radioactivity and apparent protein synthesis rate were constant during 180 min of perfusion. Reprinted from (8), *Life Sciences* **30**; D. E. Rannels, S. A. Wartell, and C. A. Watkins. The measurement of protein synthesis in biological systems, pp. 1679–1690. Copyright 1982, with permission from Elsevier Science.

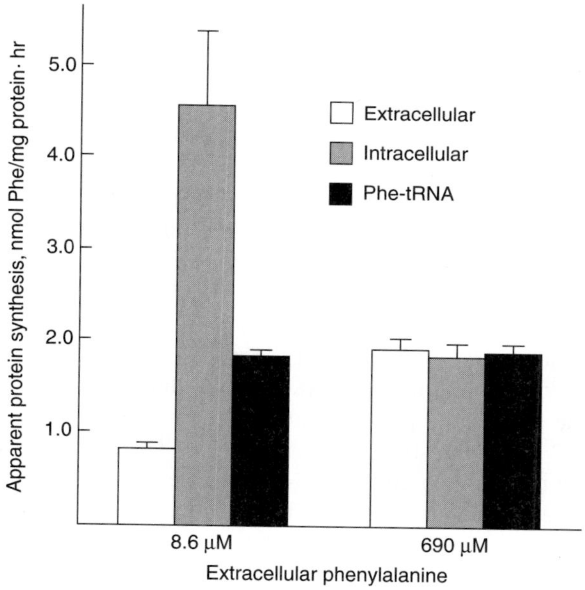

Figure 4 Apparent rate of protein synthesis as a function of the assumed precursor pool (extracellular, intracellular, or tRNA pool) and the concentration of extracellular phenylalanine. Results are from experiments in which protein synthesis was measured in perfused rat lung. When the system was flooded with phenylalanine (690 μ*M*), protein synthesis rates were identical when calculations were based on precursor specific radioactivity in either pool, suggesting that the specific radioactivity equilibrated when the high concentration of precursor amino acid was used. Reprinted from (8), *Life Sciences* **30**; D. E. Rannels, S. A. Wartell, and C. A. Watkins. The measurement of protein synthesis in biological systems, pp. 1679–1690. Copyright 1982, with permission from Elsevier Science.

Table I Methods to Study Protein Synthesis

In vivo
Flooding dose
Constant infusion
Ribosomal "profile"
Amino acid flux studies
In vitro
Perfused organs/tissues
Incubated intact tissue (e.g., muscle)
Isolated/cultured cells
Cell-free systems

reason for the different results may be. The most apparent difference between the two methods has been observed when protein synthesis was measured in skeletal muscle and leucine was used as precursor amino acid. Under other experimental conditions, the differences seem to be less obvious or can be readily explained by the different methods. For example, when experiments were performed in rats, protein synthesis rates for liver were higher with the flooding dose than with constant infusion (15). This difference, however, can be explained by the fact that total hepatic protein synthesis (secreted and nonsecreted proteins) is measured with the flooding dose whereas during the prolonged constant infusion, secreted proteins contribute much less to the protein synthesis rates.

As mentioned above, the most striking difference between the methods has been observed when muscle protein synthesis was measured in skeletal muscle and when leucine was used for the flooding dose technique. Thus, protein synthesis rate in skeletal muscle was 1.1%/day in postabsorptive humans when constant infusion of [^{13}C]leucine was used and was almost double that (2.1%/day) when a flooding dose of [^{13}C]leucine was used. Although the difference between the two techniques was smaller in the fed state (1.8%/day with constant infusion and 2.34%/day with the flooding dose technique), results still indicate that protein synthesis rates are higher with the flooding dose. From these observations it was suggested that the high dose of leucine somehow stimulated protein synthesis in skeletal muscle. Alternatively, the apparent differences could reflect an artifact caused by differences in precursor specific radioactivity in different amino acid pools. It should be noted that the interpretation of the results is complicated by the fact that in dogs an opposite effect was observed (18). Thus, in those experiments, incorporation of [^{14}C]lysine, administered as a constant tracer infusion, was substantially lowered by the flooding dose of leucine.

In order to resolve some of the issues at hand, the two research groups performed joint experiments in which valine or phenylalanine was administered as a constant tracer infusion and a flooding dose of leucine or valine was superimposed (19). The labeling of muscle protein with tracer amino acid (i.e., valine and phenylalanine during a leucine flood or leucine and phenylalanine during a valine flood) was greater during the flooding period whether leucine or valine was used (Fig. 5). Because the data were agreed on by both groups, it seems well established that human muscle protein synthesis rates obtained by using a flooding dose of leucine (or valine) are higher than when constant tracer infusion is used. In more recent experiments, Garlick *et al.* (20) used a flooding dose of [$^2H_5$]phenylalanine and observed a muscle protein synthesis rate substantially lower than when a flooding dose of leucine was used (1.66%/day vs. 2.1%/day), supporting the concept that leucine may stimulate muscle protein synthesis when administered as a flooding dose.

The mechanisms of the stimulatory effect of leucine are not known but may be related to an early observation of increased protein synthesis in rat muscles incubated in the presence of high concentrations of leucine (21). An alternative mechanism may be increased aminoacyl-tRNA stability caused by leucine (22). It is not likely that the relatively small increase in plasma insulin observed after a flooding dose of leucine is large enough to stimulate muscle protein synthesis.

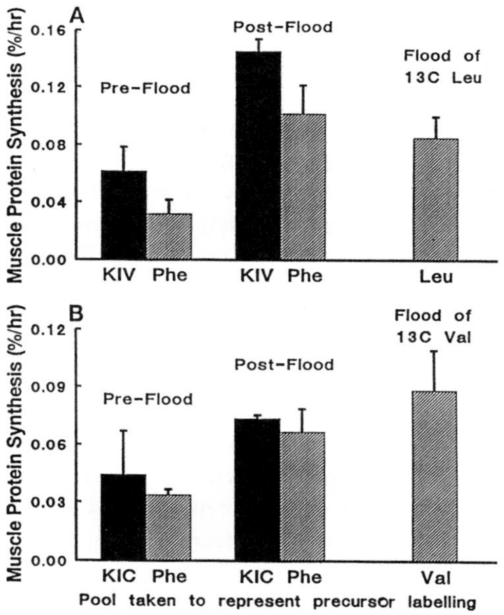

Figure 5 Effect of a flooding dose of [^{13}C]leucine (A) and [^{13}C]valine (B) on muscle protein synthesis rate. Rates were calculated from incorporation of tracer valine and phenylalanine (leucine flood) and tracer leucine and phenylalanine (valine flood), with venous plasma labeling of ketoacid (leucine and valine) or phenylalanine being taken to represent precursor labeling. KIV, α-Keto-isovalerate; KIC, α-keto-isocaproate. From Rennie *et al.* (12), with permission.

In addition to the controversy of whether the two methods give rise to different protein synthesis rates in different tissues, another question that is equally (or perhaps even more) important is whether changes induced by certain pathologic or physiologic conditions are accurately reflected by the two techniques. Also, with regard to this question, the picture is somewhat unclear. For example, when the influence of bacteremia in rats on protein synthesis in liver and skeletal muscle was investigated using a constant infusion of [^{14}C]leucine or a flooding dose of the same precursor, protein synthesis rates were increased to the same extent in liver and gastrocnemius muscle of bacteremic rats (17). In contrast, the influence of starvation and food intake seems to be qualitatively different for each method; results suggest that feeding stimulates human muscle protein synthesis when a constant infusion of [^{13}C]leucine is used (23) whereas when a flooding dose of the same precursor is used, results suggest that feeding does not stimulate muscle protein synthesis (24).

Rennie *et al.* (12) in their review concluded that "the major difficulty in accepting the usefulness of the flooding dose method lies in the fact that the values obtained for the rates of the tissue . . . synthesis are usually higher, than the values obtained by means of the constant infusion protocol." They also state that the controversy is not completely resolved and "urge caution in accepting the results of any of the current methods without vigilant scepticism." In contrast, Garlick *et al.* (10) concluded that "many of the differences between rates obtained by the two methods are minor, are readily explainable (e.g., liver), or do not influence the nature of the response to a stimulus (e.g., bacteremia)." They also list certain practical advantages of the flooding dose technique that may be of particular importance for investigators involved in surgical research, e.g., the fact that acute changes in protein synthesis rates can be monitored as exemplified by changes in human muscle induced by surgery (25). Some of the advantages and limitations of the two techniques are summarized in Table II.

In our laboratory, we have used the flooding dose technique to measure protein synthesis rates *in vivo* in muscle (26, 27) and intestinal mucosa (28, 29). The rationales for using the flooding dose in those experiments are as follows: (1) we are mainly interested in the influence of sepsis and injury on protein metabolism, rather than the absolute protein synthesis rates; (2) the flooding dose is more practical in small animals because it does not require intravenous cannulation; (3) when the flooding dose is administered intraperitoneally, measurements can be performed at only one time point (15 min) after injection of the precursor; (4) although we have not performed a systematic comparison between the flooding dose and constant infusion methods, the relative changes in muscle protein synthesis induced by sepsis were similar when measured *in vivo* using the flooding dose and when measured *in vitro* in incubated muscles; (5) by using a flooding dose of phenylalanine, rather than

Table II Advantages and Limitations of the Flooding Dose and Constant Infusion Techniques

Flooding dose	Constant infusion
Advantages	**Advantages**
Relatively simple	Avoids influence of large dose of amino acid on protein synthesis
Does not require IV cannulation	**Limitations**
Measurement done over short period of time (10–15 min)	Requires long period of time for measurement (3–6 hr)
Equilibration between different amino acid pools	Requires IV cannulation
Limitations	Less efficient equilibration between different amino acid pools
Risk of altered protein synthesis by the flooding dose itself	

leucine, the influence of the flooding dose on protein synthesis in muscle (and perhaps other tissues as well) is probably minimized.

The controversy regarding the flooding dose and constant infusion has been given a relatively large space in this chapter because both methods are used frequently, both in experimental animals and humans. It is obviously important to be aware of the potential limitations of both techniques when experiments are planned and results are interpreted.

III. Protein Degradation

Similar to protein synthesis, protein degradation can be measured *in vivo* or *in vitro*. Methods used to measure protein degradation *in vivo* are associated with more limitations than those used to measure protein synthesis. One way to determine protein breakdown rates *in vivo* is to monitor the loss of radioactivity from proteins previously labeled by the administration of a radiolabeled amino acid. A major concern when this method is used is that radioactive amino acids released during proteolysis enter the precursor pool and are reutilized for protein synthesis, giving rise to an underestimation of protein breakdown rates. Another (practical) concern is that groups of animals need to be studied at different time points after labeling of the proteins and that experiments need to be performed for a relatively extended period of time, depending on which specific protein or proteins are being studied. It is usually recommended that for a single protein, changes in radioactivity should be followed over at least one half-life and for mean turnover rates of mixed proteins measurements should be made over three half-lives or the time it takes for the radioactivity to fall to 10% of its maximal value (30). The long observation times needed for these measurements are a significant limitation when studying the influence of fast-evolving pathologic conditions (such as injury and sepsis) on protein degradation.

Different techniques have been developed to minimize the problem of amino acid recycling when protein degradation is measured *in vivo*. In previous studies, [^{14}C]bicarbonate was used to label hepatic proteins. With this precursor, the majority of radioactivity is incorporated into arginine with approximately 90% of the arginine radioactivity present in the guanidino position (31). Because of the high arginase activity in liver, recycling of radiolabeled arginine is minimized. The validity of this method was tested by comparing protein synthesis and degradation rates under steady-state conditions (when the rates should ideally be identical). Results from those experiments showed that the fractional rate of degradation of liver ornithine aminotransferase, calculated from the decay of radioactivity in amino acids labeled with [^{14}C]bicarbonate, was almost identical to the synthesis rate obtained by the incorporation of [^{3}H]tyrosine (32). The phenylalanine tracer dilution method is an alternative technique for measurement of protein degradation *in vivo* and offers the advantage of not requiring tissue biopsies.

For the measurement of protein breakdown rates *in vitro*, the release of trichloroacetic acid (TCA)-soluble radioactivity from proteins prelabeled with radioactive amino acid is frequently used. The recycling of radioactive amino acid can be prevented either by adding cycloheximide (which blocks protein synthesis) or a large amount of cold amino acid (chasing) to the medium. It should be noted that these methods also have their limitations. For example, cycloheximide not only blocks protein synthesis but also gives rise to inhibition of protein degradation (albeit only to a small extent). Addition of a large amount of cold amino acid may also influence protein degradation rates. These limitations need to be taken into account when the results are interpreted.

In addition to measuring the release of TCA-soluble radioactivity from prelabeled proteins, protein degradation *in vitro* can be determined by measuring the release of a specific amino acid that is not synthesized or metabolized in the specific tissue under study. Phenylalanine and tyrosine are amino acids that fulfill these criteria for muscle tissue whereas the branched-chain amino acids valine and leucine are better suited for measurement of protein degradation rates in liver tissue. Reincorporation of the released amino acids is prevented by the addition of cycloheximide to the incubation or culture medium, with the same limitations to be kept in mind as described above.

In contrast to liver, there is no direct isotope technique available at present to measure muscle protein breakdown *in vivo*. The low levels of arginase in skeletal muscle result in a high degree of recycling of radiolabeled amino acids in muscle tissue after labeling of proteins with [^{14}C]bicarbonate, making this method unsuitable for measurement of muscle protein degradation. In the absence of accurate methods for direct measurements of muscle protein breakdown *in vivo*, different indirect methods are used to assess muscle breakdown. Urinary excretion of 3-methylhistidine (3-MH) has been frequently used to measure muscle protein breakdown, both in experimental animals (33) and humans (34–36). 3-MH is a posttranslationally modified amino acid that is uniquely present in myofibrillar proteins and that is not reincorporated into proteins after its release during proteolysis. The rationale for using urinary excretion of 3-MH was reviewed elsewhere (37). The major portion of total body 3-MH is present in the myofibrillar proteins of skeletal muscle and after its release during proteolysis it is excreted in the urine. It should be noted that the use of urinary excretion of 3-MH as a measure of muscle protein breakdown has been challenged. One reason for this is the fact that although only a small proportion of total body 3-MH is present in tissues other than skeletal muscle, mainly in smooth muscle of the skin and gastrointestinal tract, these tissues can contribute significantly to the urinary excretion of the substance due to high protein turnover rates (38). Indeed, whereas some authors have argued for the continued use of 3-MH excretion as a measure of muscle protein breakdown (39), others consider the method a poor indicator of muscle proteolysis (40). Although results from experiments in which urinary excretion of 3-MH is measured need to be interpreted with caution, we believe the method gives accurate and valuable information regarding changes in muscle protein breakdown rates, at least under certain circumstances.

Additional indirect methods to measure protein breakdown rates *in vivo* include whole body amino acid flux studies as described above for protein synthesis. With this technique, the rate of appearance of a radiolabeled amino acid reflects whole body protein breakdown. It is obvious that one of the major drawbacks of this method is that it does not give information about protein breakdown in a specific tissue. The same critique can be applied to studies in which amino acid balance studies are performed. For example, amino acid flux across an extremity may reflect protein balance not only in skeletal muscle but in other tissues of the extremity as well, including skin, bone, and bone marrow.

An estimation of protein degradation *in vivo* can be obtained by determining the difference in protein synthesis and protein accumulation (or loss) over a period of time. We applied this technique in previous studies to determine the influence of sepsis in rats on muscle protein degradation *in vivo* (27). The major limitation with this method is that changes in protein accumulation (or loss) usually are small and need to be measured over several days, whereas protein synthesis is measured over a period of minutes or hours. Consequently, the calculation of protein degradation has to rely on the assumption that protein synthesis and degradation rates are constant over the time during which protein accumulation is measured.

An additional method, used more frequently in recent years to assess the influence of certain conditions on protein degradation in various tissues, is to determine mRNA levels for proteolytic enzymes and other components of specific proteolytic pathways. For example, in studies from our and other laboratories, the gene expression of ubiquitin and several proteasome subunits as well as key enzymes in the ubiquitin–proteasome proteolytic pathway was increased in skeletal muscle during sepsis and other catabolic conditions (41, 42). Although those studies provide important information about the involvement of different proteolytic mechanisms, the results need to be interpreted with caution for several reasons. First, changes in mRNA steady-state levels do not necessarily reflect changes in gene transcription, but may also be caused by changes in mRNA stability. Second, changes in mRNA levels may or may not be accompanied by changes in enzyme protein levels and, more importantly, by changes in enzyme activities. The role of studying the gene expression for enzymatic enzymes to assess changes in protein breakdown is discussed in more detail in Section IV. Methods used to measure protein degradation *in vivo* and *in vitro* are summarized in Table III.

An interesting method to assess protein turnover is that of determining the "proteome" (compare the term genome). Proteome refers to all the different proteins occurring in an organism, including not only the primary polypeptides created by the individual genes but also the co- and posttranslationally modified forms of a protein. Therefore, the proteome is much more complicated than the genome; whereas the genome refers to all the genes carried by any cell type of an organism, the proteome differs from one cell type to another qualitatively as well as quantitatively and also depends on the course of time, e.g., during development and aging. Two-dimensional gel electrophoresis and two-dimensional immunoblotting have been used to determine the proteome of certain tissues and organs (43, 44).

Table III Methods to Study Protein Degradation

In vivo	
	Decay of radioactivity in labeled tissue proteins (e.g., [^{14}C]bicarbonate for liver tissue)
	Amino acid flux studies
	Loss of tissue protein
	Urinary excretion of nitrogen
	Urinary excretion of 3-methylhistidine
	Monitor tissue levels of mRNA for proteolytic enzymes
In vitro	
	Decay of radioactivity in prelabeled proteins
	Release of TCA-soluble radioactivity from labeled proteins
	Release of certain amino acids from incubated tissues or cells (e.g., valine or leucine from hepatocytes; phenylalanine, tyrosine, or 3-methylhistidine from muscle tissue)

IV. Muscle

Muscle protein turnover rates can be measured *in vivo* or *in vitro*. The methods most commonly used to measure muscle protein synthesis *in vivo* and their potential limitations (the flooding dose and constant infusion techniques) were discussed in detail above. Indirect methods to assess muscle protein breakdown, such as determination of urinary excretion of 3-MH, were also covered in the preceding sections.

In vitro determination of muscle protein synthesis and degradation rates can be performed in a perfused hindlimb or hemicorpus of rats, in incubated intact muscles, in cultured muscle cells, or in cell-free systems. During the past several years we have mainly used incubated muscles from rats or mice and cultured myotubes for measurement of protein turnover rates, and those methods will be the focus of this part of the chapter. Measurements of protein turnover rates in perfused hindlimb or hemicorpus were discussed in previous reviews from this laboratory (1, 7).

A. Incubated Muscle

Different muscles that have been used in previous studies to measure *in vitro* protein turnover rates include the diaphragm, epitrochlearis, plantaris, soleus, and extensor digitorum longus (EDL) muscles of rats and mice. In our laboratory, soleus and EDL muscles have been most frequently used. These muscle offer the advantages of being thin, having well-defined tendons, and representing two different types of skeletal muscle, the soleus muscle being a red, slow-twitch muscle and the EDL muscle being a white, fast-twitch muscle. These are important properties because several studies from our and other laboratories have shown that the response to injury, sepsis, and other catabolic conditions is different in different types of skeletal muscle (with the most pronounced metabolic changes usually occurring in white, fast-twitch muscle).

In addition to being able to measure protein turnover rates specifically in different types of skeletal muscle (i.e., fast twitch vs. slow twitch), the technique also offers the advantage of being rather simple and inexpensive. Muscles are incubated in 25-ml Erlenmeyer flasks in 3 ml of oxygenated medium at 37°C. During incubation, the flasks are oxygenated at regular intervals and are then sealed with a tightly fitting rubber stopper. We usually preincubate the muscles for 30 min whereafter they are transferred to 3 ml of fresh medium and metabolic rates are determined during the subsequent 2-hr incubation. Stable metabolic rates (protein synthesis and degradation rates) and maintained ATP levels suggest that the muscles remain viable during this period of incubation, and other studies suggest that the muscles probably remain viable for even longer periods of time (up to 4–6 hr) (45).

Several studies, both from our and other laboratories, have shown that energy levels and protein balance are better maintained if muscles are incubated at resting length rather than when flaccid (45, 46). We usually incubate the muscles fixed on "racks" that we prepare from paper clips or stainless steel wire and that can be easily adjusted to the resting length of the muscle (Fig. 6). The tendons of the muscle are tied to the rack with 4-0 silk during the dissection of the muscle before the tendons are cut. This prevents the muscles from contracting or being over-stretched, factors that can significantly influence both protein and energy metabolism in the muscles. During dissection of the muscles it is also important to handle the muscle only at the tendons and not to traumatize the muscle fibers. A careful handling of the muscle during dissection and mounting on the racks improves the energy and metabolic status in the tissue and makes results more reproducible.

An additional advantage of using incubated intact muscles is that the technique has been validated in a number of previous studies by demonstrating that changes that occur *in vivo* during various physiologic and pathophysiologic states are accurately reflected by changes in incubated muscles (26, 27). In addition, the muscles are responsive *in vitro* to different hormones and other substances that regulate muscle protein metabolism *in vivo*, such as insulin, insulin-like growth factor I, amino acids, and glucocorticoids (47–49).

Although incubated muscles have several advantages in the study of protein metabolism, it should be noted that the technique has limitations as well, mainly related to oxygenation and viability of the tissue during incubation and to the fact that muscles from small growing rats are used. Because oxygen and nutrients reach the cells of incubated muscles by diffusion, large muscles will develop a central core of hypoxic and undernourished cells. To reduce the risk for a

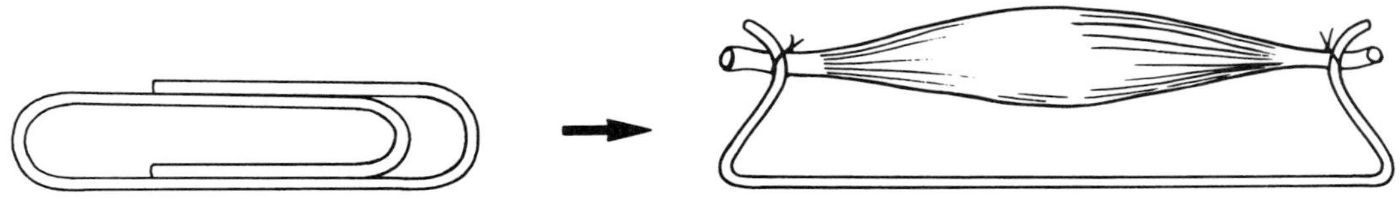

Figure 6 "Racks" for mounting isolated muscles can be made from paper clips. The muscles are tied to the racks at the tendons, and the tension on the muscles can be adjusted by bending the racks. The tendons are tied to the racks with the muscles *in situ*.

large hypoxic core, it is important that the incubated muscles are thin. When EDL and soleus muscles from rats are used, the animals should not weigh more than 60–70 g. When the diaphragm is used, somewhat larger rats can be used (up to 100 g) because the distance from the surface to the central cells is shorter than in EDL and soleus muscles of similar weight. The epitrochlearis muscle is thin enough for *in vitro* incubation even when taken from large rats. One disadvantage of the epitrochlearis muscle is that it lacks well-defined tendons, which makes it difficult to mount the tissue without injuring muscle fibers.

It should be noted that although the development of a central hypoxic core in incubated EDL and soleus muscles is minimized when thin muscles from small rats or from mice are used, it is not completely avoided. In a previous study, we incubated soleus muscles from control and septic rats and assessed the development of a hypoxic core histochemically by staining the muscles for α-glucan phosphorylase activity (26). In addition, protein synthesis rates were measured in the central core and in the periphery of the muscles. Despite the fact that muscles were thin (weighing approximately 25–30 mg) and were from rats weighing 40–60 g, a small central core with loss of α-glucan phosphorylase activity was noted after incubation for 30 min in both control and septic muscles. Despite development of a central core, there was no difference in protein synthesis rates between the periphery and central core of the muscle except when the muscles were incubated in a flaccid (unsupported) state. Importantly, protein synthesis rates in septic muscles were reduced to the same extent, approximately 20%, in the different *in vitro* preparations, both when measured in whole muscle and in the central core or periphery (Table IV). In the same study, the effect of sepsis on muscle protein synthesis was almost identical when measured *in vivo* following a flooding dose of [^{3}H]phenylalanine, further supporting the concept that incubated muscles can be used to study the effects of pathological conditions (at least those of sepsis) on protein metabolism.

One concern when muscles from small growing rats are used is that results may not reflect changes that occur in adult individuals. This concern can be addressed by using epitrochlearis muscles or split muscle preparations (50, 51) from adult rats or muscles from adult mice. Alternatively, EDL or soleus muscles from large rats can be incubated at temperatures lower than 37°C. For example, when rat soleus muscles weighing 70–95 mg were incubated at 20°C, no central hypoxic core developed during incubation for 2.5 hr and protein synthesis rates were the same in the periphery and central portion of the muscles (52). The absolute protein synthesis rates, however, were lower at reduced temperatures.

In a previous study, we compared the influence of sepsis on protein turnover rates in incubated intact muscles from small rats (40–60 g) with protein turnover rates in incubated split muscle preparations from adult rats (51). Although absolute muscle protein turnover rates were higher in muscles from young, growing rats than in muscles from adult rats (as expected), the relative changes induced by sepsis were almost identical in tissue from the young and adult rats. Thus, changes in protein turnover

Table IV Protein Synthesis Rate in Incubated Whole Soleus Muscle and in Core and Periphery of Incubated Soleus Muscles from Control and Septic Rats[a]

Rat	Whole muscle	Central core	Periphery
Control	0.293 ± 0.009	0.315 ± 0.008	0.320 ± 0.013
Septic	0.238 ± 0.014*	0.239 ± 0.019*	0.266 ± 0.019*
Change	−19%	−24%	−17%

[a]Protein synthesis rate is given as μmol phenylalanine/2 hr/g wet weight. *, $p < 0.05$ vs. control. Based on data in Hummel *et al.* (26).

rates observed in incubated muscles from small growing rats seem adequately to reflect changes in adult rats as well, at least changes induced by sepsis. The use of muscles from small growing rats to study the influence of sepsis (and several other catabolic conditions as well) on muscle protein metabolism was further supported by the finding that the gene expression of the ubiquitin–proteasome pathway (the predominant proteolytic pathway in septic muscle) was up-regulated in an almost identical manner in muscles from patients with sepsis (53) as in muscles from small growing rats (41, 54).

When protein synthesis rates are measured, radiolabeled tyrosine or phenylalanine is frequently used as the precursor amino acid, because these amino acids are neither degraded nor synthesized in skeletal muscle. A high concentration of the amino acid is used to ensure equilibration of precursor specific radioactivity between extra- and intracellular compartments. This allows for the calculation of protein synthesis rate from the specific radioactivity of the medium or the intracellular free amino acid pool and the amount of radiolabeled amino acid incorporated into TCA-precipitated proteins at the end of a 2-hr incubation. Protein synthesis rates are constant during incubation for 2–3 hr, as evidenced by linear incorporation of radioactivity into protein (45).

Total and myofibrillar protein breakdown rates are determined by measuring the net release of tyrosine and 3-MH, respectively, from the incubated muscles (Fig. 7). Both amino acids are measured by HPLC (45, 55). In these experiments, reincorporation of released amino acids needs to be blocked in order not to underestimate protein breakdown rates. This can be done by adding cycloheximide (0.5 m*M*) to the incubation medium. Because sepsis, as well as other catabolic conditions, preferentially stimulates the degradation of the myofibrillar proteins actin and myosin (55), it is important to include measurements of 3-MH when incubated muscles are used to study the effect of sepsis on muscle proteolysis. Because the intracellular pool of free amino acids is not stable during a 2-hr incubation, it is important to take changes in the intracellular pool into account when net release of the amino acid is calculated (Fig. 8). For example, the intracellular pool of free 3-MH decreases substantially during incubation of EDL or soleus muscles from small rats (45). Therefore, the accumulation of 3-MH in the medium during incubation reflects both 3-MH generated from myofibrillar protein degradation and 3-MH released from the intracellular pool. To achieve a correct estimate of myofibrillar protein breakdown, the amount of 3-MH released from the intramuscular pool needs to be subtracted from the total amount that has accumulated in the medium during incubation. The conditions for tyrosine are the opposite, i.e., the intracellular concentration of free tyrosine increases to a small extent during incubation, and this increase must be added to the amount of tyrosine that accumulates in the medium when total protein breakdown rates are calculated. In order to allow for the calculation of changes in intracellular amino acids during incubation, EDL (or soleus) muscles from both sides are used. One muscle is used after preincubation for determination of "initial" amino acid levels and the contralateral muscle is incubated for 2 hr whereafter the amino acid (3-MH or tyrosine) is determined in the incubation medium and in the muscle.

B. Assessment of Different Proteolytic Pathways

Intracellular proteolysis is regulated by multiple proteolytic pathways. In general, the different proteolytic mechanisms can be divided into lysosomal and nonlysosomal. Among the nonlysosomal proteolytic mechanisms, the ubiquitin/proteasome- and calcium/calpain-dependent mechanisms are the most important pathways. The role of different proteolytic pathways in the degradation of muscle proteins can be determined by incubating muscles in the absence or presence of specific inhibitors of the individual proteolytic pathways. The difference in protein degradation between muscles incubated in the absence or presence of an inhibitor reflects the contribution of that specific proteolytic mechanism (Fig. 9). For example, incubating muscles in the

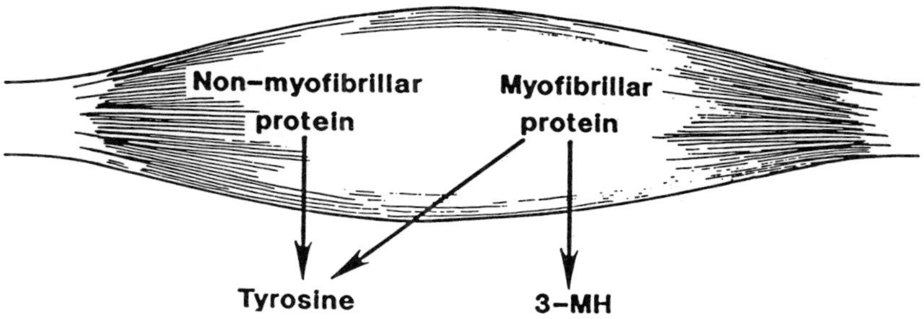

Figure 7 Release of tyrosine from incubated muscles reflects total, i.e., myofibrillar and non-myofibrillar, protein breakdown, whereas release of 3-MH specifically measures myofibrillar protein breakdown. From Hasselgren (1), with permission.

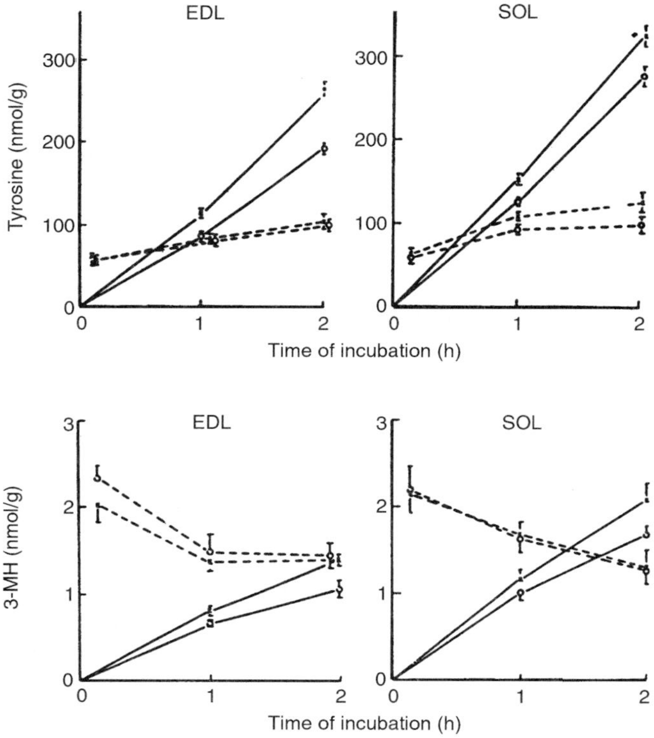

Figure 8 Accumulation of tyrosine (upper panel), and 3-MH (lower panel) in incubation medium (——), and tissue levels of amino acids (– – –) during incubation of rat extensor digitorum longus (EDL) and soleus (SOL) muscles. For calculation of accurate protein breakdown rates, changes in tissue levels of the amino acids must be taken into account. Reproduced with permission from (45), P. O. Hasselgren, M. Hall-Angerås, U. Angerås, D. Benson, J. H. James, and J. E. Fischer (1990). *Biochem. J.* **267**, 37–44. © the Biochemical Society.

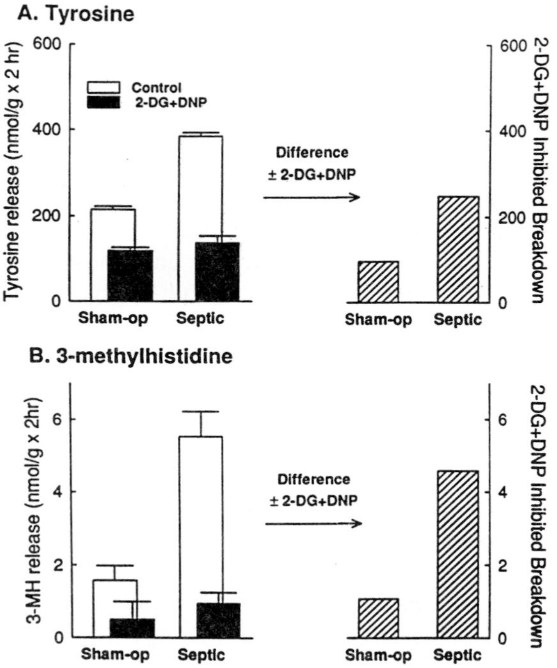

Figure 9 Total protein breakdown (tyrosine release) (A) and myofibrillar protein breakdown (3-MH release) (B) in incubated EDL muscles 16 hr after sham operation or induction of sepsis by cecal ligation and puncture in rats. Muscles were incubated in normal medium (open bars) or in energy-depleting medium containing 5 m*M* 2-deoxyglucose (2-DG) and 2,4-dinitrophenol (DNP) (filled bars). Difference in protein breakdown rates between muscle incubated in normal and energy-depleting medium was calculated and represented the energy-dependent component of protein breakdown (hatched bars). A similar approach can be used to calculate the lysosomal, proteasome-dependent, or calcium-dependent protein breakdown by adding inhibitors of the individual proteolytic pathways to the incubation medium. From Tiao *et al.* (73), with permission.

absence or presence of lactacystin or β-lactone will give information about proteasome-dependent proteolysis (56). Other proteasome blockers that are frequently used in this type of experiment are MG132 and LLnL, but they are less specific than lactacystin and β-lactone. The energy-dependent component of muscle protein breakdown can be determined from the difference in protein breakdown rates between muscles incubated in normal or energy-depleting medium (containing 2-dinitrophenol to block mitochondrial respiration and 2-deoxyglucose instead of regular glucose).

Substances that are commonly used to block lysosomal protein degradation include methylamine, NH_4Cl, and leupeptin. The role of calcium-dependent proteolysis can be determined by incubating muscles in calcium-free medium or by adding a calpain-inhibitor to the medium—for example, E-64 (57). The method described here to assess the role of different proteolytic pathways, i.e., incubating muscle in the absence or presence of inhibitors of the different proteolytic mechanisms, has been used in several previous reports from our (41, 42) and other (58, 59) laboratories. By using specific blockers we have found evidence that sepsis upregulates energy–proteasome-dependent muscle proteolysis with no significant involvement of calcium-dependent or lysosomal protein degradation (41, 60), whereas in severe injury (for example, caused by burn), multiple proteolytic pathways are stimulated (42).

It should be noted that most of the blockers used in this type of experiment are not completely specific in their action, and therefore two or more proteolytic inhibitors are frequently used to determine the role of different proteolytic pathways in any given situation.

C. Cultured Muscle Cells

Cultured muscle cells are frequently used to study the influence of different factors on protein metabolism. Cells can be used at different stages of their differentiation/maturation, i.e., either when they are still myoblasts, when they are isolated as myocytes, or after differentiation into myotubes. A description of different techniques involved in culturing myocytes is beyond the scope of this chapter but can be found in several recent handbooks and reviews (61, 62). (For additional discussion of cell culture methods, see Chapter 18.) We have used cultured L6 myotubes in our laboratory in recent studies designed to determine the mechanisms of glucocorticoid-induced muscle proteolysis and the proteolytic pathways involved in protein breakdown at high temperature (63, 64), and have described the technical aspects of culturing L6 myocytes up to their differentiation into myotubes.

Similar to incubated intact muscles, protein synthesis rates can be determined in cultured myotubes by measuring the incorporation of radiolabeled tyrosine or phenylalanine into protein. A high concentration of the precursor amino acid should be used to provide for flooding of the precursor pools as described above.

Protein degradation rates can be measured as release of free tyrosine or phenylalanine in the presence of cycloheximide (to prevent reincorporation of the released amino acid) or as release of TCA-soluble radioactivity from proteins prelabeled with radioactive tyrosine or phenylalanine. When this method is used to determine protein breakdown rates, recycling of the precursor amino acid is usually prevented by adding a high concentration of cold amino acid to the culture medium (chasing). When release of TCA-soluble radioactivity from prelabeled proteins is used to measure proteolysis, proteins can be labeled for a short time (a few hours) or for a more extended period of time (24–48 hr). Release of radioactive amino acid from proteins labeled for a couple of hours reflects degradation of short-lived proteins, whereas release of radioactive amino acid from proteins labeled for 1–2 days mainly reflects degradation of long-lived proteins. This is an important distinction because the different classes of proteins are degraded at quite different rates and, more importantly, the regulation of the degradation varies between short-lived and long-lived proteins (64).

One of the advantages of cultured myocytes/myotubes as compared to incubated intact muscles is that the effect of different substances, such as hormones and cytokines, on protein turnover can be tested over much longer periods of time. In experiments using incubated muscles, the time is usually limited to 2 hr due to concerns about viability of the tissue after longer incubation times; negative results in experiments using incubated muscles, therefore, will always raise the question whether a specific treatment was too short for an effect to be seen. Another advantage is the fact that degradation of short-lived and long-lived proteins can be measured individually as described above. Cultured muscle cells also provide a "clean" model in which protein turnover rates in muscle cells only are measured. Intact muscles contain several cell types other than myocytes, including satellite cells, endothelial cells, fibroblasts, etc., and the potential contribution of these cells needs to be considered when this technique is used to study protein metabolism. This concern is even greater when other *ex vivo* techniques are used. For example, when protein turnover is studied in perfused hemicorpus or hindlimb, results may be influenced not only by metabolic activity in muscles, but by other tissues as well, including bone, bone marrow, skin, and fat.

An important limitation of cultured myocytes/myotubes is the fact that the model is even more remote from the *in vivo* situation than incubated muscles and perfused hindlimb or hemicorpus. Ideally, cultured myotubes should be used to study mechanisms of metabolic events that are known to occur *in vivo* (this, of course, is true for most *in vitro* experiments). For example, *in vivo* studies in our laboratory have provided evidence that glucocorticoids are an important regulator of muscle proteolysis during sepsis (65, 66). In subsequent experiments we used cultured L6 myotubes to determine which intracellular proteolytic pathway(s) are involved in glucocorticoid-induced protein degradation (63).

Cell-free systems (muscle extracts) can also be used to measure protein synthesis and degradation rates. One advantage of this approach is that the effects of different substances that do not cross the cell membrane can be tested. Important information regarding myofibrillar protein degradation and the role of ubiquitination of proteins in the N-end rule pathway in cachectic muscle has been generated in cell-free systems (67, 68).

D. Indirect Methods

In addition to direct measurements of protein synthesis and degradation rates, other techniques can be used to estimate muscle protein turnover rates. Because of the size of the muscle mass, changes in whole body protein and nitrogen balance and in urinary nitrogen excretion to a great extent reflect changes in muscle protein metabolism (see Chapter 56). The use of urinary excretion of 3-MH as an index of muscle protein breakdown was discussed above.

Muscle biopsy specimens from patients can be used for indirect measurements of protein metabolism. The distribution of ribosomes between polyribosomes and monoribosomes reflects protein synthesis capacity in the tissue. A high proportion of polyribosomes is usually associated with a high protein synthesis rate, whereas increased amounts of monoribosomes indicate reduced protein synthesis rates. Determination of the fractions of poly- and monoribosomes in relation to the total ribosome concentration has been used in previous studies to assess the influence of different conditions on muscle protein synthesis (69). Although this method can provide valuable information, it is important to keep its limitations in mind when results are interpreted. Thus, at best, the method gives a snapshot picture of the synthetic capacity at the translational level without attempting (or claiming) to give information about actual protein synthesis rates.

An additional indirect method to assess the metabolic situation in muscle used frequently during the past couple of years is to determine the gene expression of various catalytic enzymes and other components of proteolytic pathways. In several studies from our and other laboratories, muscle cachexia was associated with increased mRNA levels for ubiquitin and 20S proteasome subunits (41, 42, 54), indicating that ubiquitinproteasome-dependent proteolysis may, at least in part, be responsible for muscle protein breakdown (Fig. 10). Although studies have found a close correlation between ubiquitinproteasome-dependent muscle proteolysis and mRNA levels for ubiquitin and proteasome subunits in various catabolic conditions, including cancer (70), sepsis (41, 53, 54, 66, 71–73), burn injury (42), and fasting and denervation (74), there is not an absolute correlation between the gene expression of the ubiquitinproteasome pathway and protein breakdown rates. For example, we found that treatment of septic rats with IGF-I reduced muscle ubiquitin mRNA levels but did not inhibit protein breakdown rates (75). In other experiments we found that treatment of septic rats with the calcium antagonist dantrolene blocked sepsis-induced muscle proteolysis but did not reduce the increased ubiquitin mRNA levels (unpublished observations). Although this limitation is important to keep in mind when results are interpreted, measurement of mRNA levels for components of the ubiquitin proteasome pathway and other proteolytic pathways as well, including cathepsins and calpains (76), provides important information about potential mechanisms of muscle cachexia in certain disease states. The method has been used in studies in patients with muscle cachexia, including patients with sepsis (53), AIDS (77), severe trauma (78), and cancer (79), and in most instances up-regulated gene expression of the ubiquitinproteasome pathway was found. It will be an important focus of future studies to determine whether the increased mRNA levels of ubiquitin, proteasome subunits, and various proteolytic enzymes reflect up-regulated gene transcription and, more importantly, whether up-regulated transcription of these genes is the cause of muscle breakdown or merely an associated phenomenon.

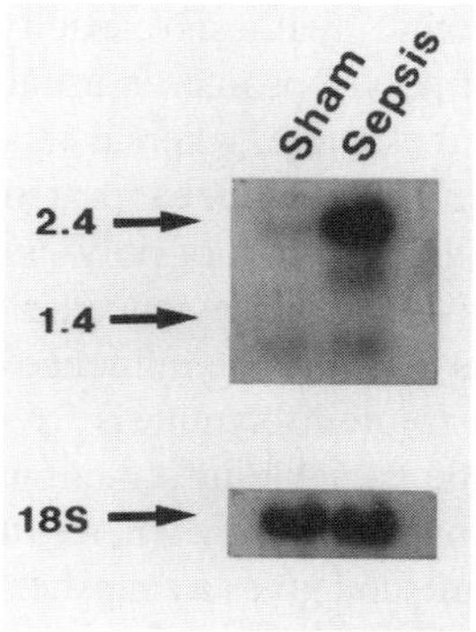

Figure 10 Sepsis in rats induced by cecal ligation and puncture (CLP) results in a substantial up-regulation of the gene expression of ubiquitin in EDL muscles. In other experiments, similar up-regulation of the gene expression of several of the 20S proteasome subunits has been noticed (54). In addition, a similar increase in mRNA levels for ubiquitin and proteasome subunits has been documented in muscles from septic patients (53).

Methods commonly used to measure muscle protein synthesis and breakdown are summarized in Table V.

V. Intestine

The role of the intestine in the metabolic and inflammatory responses to injury and sepsis has attracted great interest in recent years. Protein turnover rates in the gut mucosa are high and it has been estimated that mucosal protein synthesis accounts for 10–15% of whole body protein synthesis (80). It is obvious, therefore, that changes in intestinal protein synthesis rates have an important impact on whole body protein balance. In addition, the mucosa is the production site for several proteins with important biological functions, including cytokines, gut peptides, and at least some of the acute-phase proteins.

Studies on the influence of various disease states on intestinal protein metabolism have mainly focused on changes in protein synthesis rates, and less is known about mucosal protein breakdown. Mucosal protein turnover rates can be measured *in vivo* or *in vitro*. For *in vitro* experiments, freshly isolated or cultured enterocytes, everted "sacs" of intestine, or tissue mounted in Ussing chambers can be used for determination of protein turnover rates.

A. Studies in Vivo

Both the constant infusion and flooding dose techniques have been used to measure mucosal protein synthesis rates in previous reports (15, 81). Compared with the flooding dose technique, the constant infusion method gave a higher protein synthesis rate when the specific activity of the precursor in the tissue was used but a lower rate when the plasma specific radioactivity was used, illustrating the problem of identifying the proper precursor pool. The advantages and limitations of the flooding and constant infusion techniques

Table V Methods to Study Muscle Protein Turnover

Flooding dose
Constant infusion
Urinary excretion of 3-methylhistidine
Muscle levels of mRNA for ubiquitin, proteasome subunits and other proteolytic pathways
Perfused rat hindlimb/hemicorpus
Incubated intact muscles
Cultured myocytes/myotubes
Cell-free systems

were discussed in detail above and will not be elaborated further here.

In experiments in our laboratory, we have used the flooding dose technique to measure mucosal protein synthesis *in vivo* in control and septic rats (28). A minor decline in precursor specific radioactivity was seen in both plasma and tissue during the first 10 min after the intravenous injection of 10 μCi of [^{14}C]leucine and 100 μmol of cold leucine in rats weighing 150–200 g (Fig. 11). The mean specific radioactivity of the precursor during the first 10 min after injection was used to calculate protein synthesis rates. Protein synthesis in jejunal mucosa measured with this technique was approximately 90%/day, similar to other reports in the literature using the flooding dose (15, 16). Protein synthesis rates are higher in mucosa than in the seromuscular layer. Mucosal protein synthesis rates are not uniform along the gastrointestinal tract (for example, mucosal protein synthesis rates are higher in jejunum than in ileum) and, more importantly, the response to various conditions is also not uniform in different parts of the intestine. In previous studies we found evidence that metabolic changes induced by sepsis or endotoxemia are most pronounced in the jejunum (28, 29), an observation that is important to take into account when the influence of different conditions on mucosal protein metabolism is examined.

From a practical standpoint, the flooding dose can be administered intravenously or intraperitoneally. The advantage of intraperitoneal injection is that the tissue specific radioactivity is stable during the first 15 min after injection and only one time point (15 min) needs to be studied for determination of specific radioactivity in both the precursor pool and protein (17). Although previous studies suggest that a flooding dose of leucine does not influence mucosal protein synthesis rates (15, 16), in more recent studies we have routinely used a flooding dose of phenylalanine to measure mucosal protein synthesis. One advantage of this approach is that muscle protein synthesis rates can be measured in the same animals without the concern of muscle protein synthesis being altered by leucine. At 10 or 15 min after injection of the flooding dose, mucosa is harvested by scraping with a microscope slide and can then be stored at −70°C until further analysis. Specific radioactivity of the precursor amino acid in the tissue free amino acid pool and in protein is determined and the protein synthesis rate is calculated using the formula $K_s = (S_B/S_A)t \times 100$, as described above.

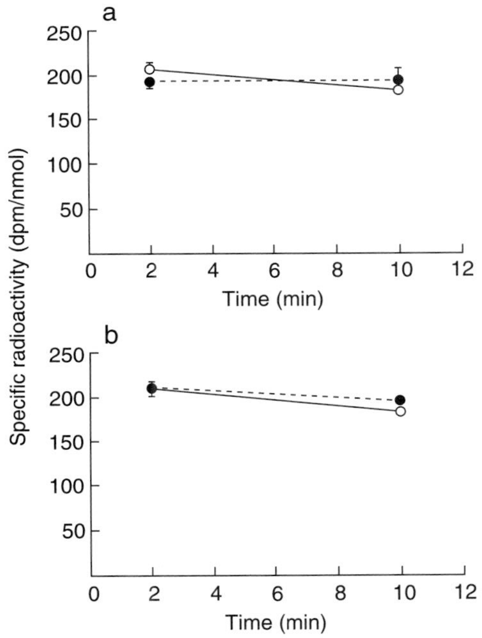

Figure 11 Specific radioactivity of tissue-free leucine 2 and 10 min after an IV flooding dose of [^{14}C]leucine. Determinations were made in (a) mucosa and (b) serosa (seromuscular layer) of sham-operated (○) and septic (●) rats. Reproduced with permission from (28), D. vonAllmen, P. O. Hasselgren, T. Higashiguchi, J. Frederick, O. Zamir, and J. E. Fischer (1992). *Biochem. J.* **286**, 585–589. © the Biochemical Society.

An additional way to assess mucosal protein synthesis *in vivo* is to determine mucosal concentrations of specific protein. In experiments in our laboratory, mucosal concentrations of the proinflammatory cytokine IL-6 and the acute-phase proteins complement component C3 and serum amyloid A (SAA) were increased during sepsis and endotoxemia (82–85). Because mRNA levels for the proteins were increased as well, the results were interpreted as indicating that the local production of IL-6, C3, and SAA was increased. The changes in mucosal IL-6 levels were basically unchanged after perfusion of the intestinal vasculature, suggesting that the cytokine levels did not represent deposition of circulating IL-6. This further supports the concept of local mucosal production of IL-6.

One limitation when changes in protein synthesis are measured in mucosa is that the cell type in which the changes take place is not known. Although the enterocyte is the predominant cell type in the mucosa, other cells, including intraepithelial lymphocytes, submucosal macrophages, and endothelial cells, may contribute to the metabolic changes in mucosa. This question can be addressed in different ways. In previous studies we found that changes in mucosal protein synthesis induced by sepsis and measured *in vivo* were reflected by changes in isolated enterocytes (86), suggesting that the changes observed in mucosa, at least in part, were caused by changes in the enterocyte. When mucosal production of specific proteins is under study, immunohistochemistry can be used to determine in which cell the protein is expressed (83, 84).

The gut mucosa is unique in the sense that amino acids can reach the cells by two different routes, i.e., either from the bloodstream or from the intestinal lumen. This is especially important for the enterocyte because the apical surface brush border and the basolateral membrane are exposed to two different environments, and regulation of metabolism can occur through either of these membranes. Previous studies suggest that intestinal mucosa can incorporate amino acids into protein from either the luminal or basolateral side and that intravenous and luminal routes of tracer administration result in similar protein synthesis rates (87, 88). Adegoke *et al.* described a new method in which a luminal flooding dose of [^{3}H]phenylalanine was used in multiple isolated segments of the small intestine to measure mucosal protein synthesis (89, 90). The method offers the advantage of allowing multiple comparisons between the individual intestinal segments of protein synthesis within the same animal and provides a model to study the acute modulation of mucosal protein synthesis by stimulus in the lumen (Fig. 12). Using this method, the same group found the somewhat surprising result that high concentrations of luminal amino acids acutely decrease intestinal protein synthesis (90).

No methods have been described for direct measurement of mucosal protein degradation *in vivo.* Similar to other tissues, protein degradation rates can be calculated from the difference in protein synthesis rate and changes in protein levels. Protein degradation can also be assessed by measuring mucosal levels of mRNA for different proteolytic systems. In one study, the gene expression for cathepsins B and D, *m*-calpain, and several of the components of the ubiquitin proteasome pathway was up-regulated in intestinal mucosa during fasting, suggesting that a coordinated activation of multiple proteolytic systems contributes to mucosal atrophy in this condition (91). A similar approach to assess mucosal protein degradation was used in a study on the effects of luminal amino acids on protein metabolism (90).

B. Studies in Vitro

In vitro determination of protein turnover rates can be performed in mucosa using everted intestinal sacs or tissue mounted in Ussing chambers. Alternatively, protein turnover rates can be measured in freshly isolated or cultured enterocytes. The different approaches offer obvious advantages and limitations. For example, when everted sacs or tissue in Ussing chambers are used, one is faced with the same problem as in the *in vivo* experiments, i.e., the method does not give direct information about in which cell type the changes occur. Isolated or cultured enterocytes, on the other hand, do not retain the association with other cells in the mucosa. It is not presently known how important this is, but it may be speculated that enterocyte metabolism can be influenced by products from neighboring cells such as intraepithelial lymphocytes and cells (including macrophages) in the lamina propria and submucosa (compare the situation in the liver where cocultures of hepatocytes and Kupffer cells have clearly shown that the cells "cross-talk" and that products released from the Kupffer cells influence protein metabolism in the hepatocyte).

In our laboratory, we have used both isolated and cultured enterocytes to study protein turnover rates. Enterocytes can be isolated from the mucosa by incubating segments of intestine in a calcium-free medium containing a calcium chelator as originally described by Watford *et al.* (92). By gently shaking the tissue, cells are progressively released from the mucosa, and three different fractions of enterocytes can be isolated, i.e., cells from the tips or mid-

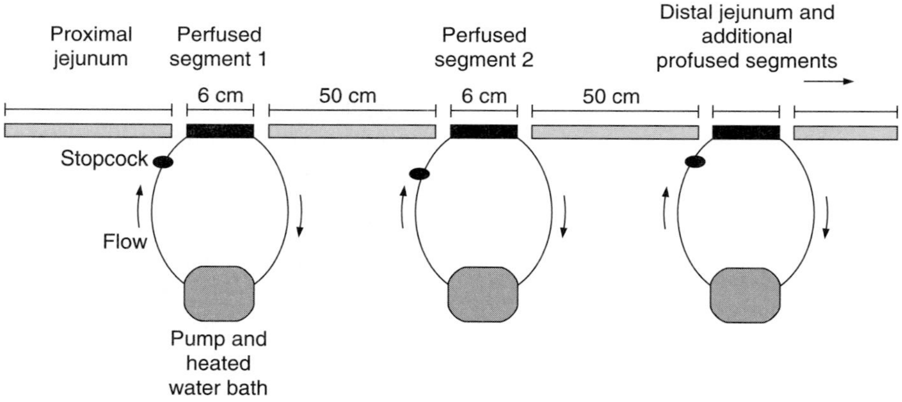

Figure 12 Schematic drawing of a model for measurement of mucosal protein synthesis following a luminal flooding dose. Multiple jejunal segments are cannulated *in situ.* at both ends (inlet at the pyloric end, outlet at the ileal end) with polyethylene tubing. The inlet cannula for the first segment is inserted approximately 15 cm from the ligament of Treitz and subsequent segments are separated by 50 cm of intestine. Each segment is independently perfused at a flow rate of 3 ml/min. Each segment receives a control or test perfusate followed by a 15-min perfusion of the same composition, also containing [^{3}H]phenylalanine for determination of protein synthesis. This system allows multiple comparisons within the same animal and provides a model to study acute modulation of protein synthesis in intestinal mucosa by luminal stimuli. From Adegoke *et al.* (90), with permission. © *J. Nutr.* **129**, 1871–1878, American Society for Nutritional Sciences.

portions of the villi and from the crypts. We have used cells isolated from rat jejunum and measured protein synthesis by determining incorporation of radiolabeled [^{3}H]phenylalanine into protein (82). A major limitation with isolated enterocytes is poor viability of the cells, and this is particularly problematic with rat enterocytes (92). In our experiments, metabolic rates were constant and energy levels were maintained during incubation for up to 30 min, allowing for measurement of protein synthesis and breakdown rates at least during short periods of time. In those experiments, protein synthesis rates were higher in cells from the crypts than in the other cell fractions and the sepsis-induced increase in protein synthesis was also most pronounced in crypt cells (86). Although the short survival time for incubated freshly isolated enterocytes makes it difficult to test the effects of different substances on protein metabolism, we found that protein synthesis was stimulated *in vitro* by glutamine in isolated rat intestinal epithelial cells (86).

Some of the problems with poor viability of isolated enterocytes can be avoided by using cultured cells. Cell cultures can be established from freshly isolated enterocytes, for example, from intestinal specimens obtained from patients. Alternatively, established and commercially available cell lines can be used. In our laboratory, cultured IEC-6 cells, a rat intestinal epithelial cell line, have been used to study the regulation of enterocyte IL-6 production (93, 94). In other and more recent studies we have mainly used cultured Caco-2 cells. This is a human intestinal epithelial cell line originating from a colon cancer that takes on the characteristics of small intestinal epithelial cells during culture (95). Thus, in culture, the cells differentiate into polarized cells with a basolateral membrane and an apical membrane with microvilli, and tight junctions are formed between the cells.

The methods to measure protein synthesis and degradation rates in cultured enterocytes are basically the same as described above for cultured muscle cells. One specific feature of enterocytes that needs to be taken into account is the fact that they are secretory cells. Thus, during culture, newly synthesized proteins will be found both intracellularly (proteins that have not yet been secreted) and in the culture medium. Proteins under study therefore usually need to be measured both in cell lysates and in culture medium. In recent experiments, we have used cultured Caco-2 cells to study the regulation of enterocyte production of IL-6 and complement component C3 (96, 97). The cells can either be used after culture to approximately 90% confluence, which usually takes 2–3 days, or after culture for 2–3 weeks when they form a tight layer of fully differentiated cells resembling small intestinal enterocytes. If the cells are grown on filters in a dual chamber system, the apical and basolateral production of specific proteins and their regulation at the different cellular sites can be determined individually. We have used that approach and found that the production of IL-6 and C3 was differentially regulated by IL-1β at the apical and basolateral membranes of the Caco-2 cell (98). This observation is important considering the situation *in vivo* when the apical surface of the enterocyte is exposed to the contents of the intestinal lumen and the basolateral membrane to the lamina propria. A similar approach can be used in Ussing chambers when cultured cells or mounted mucosa can be treated at the apical or basolateral membrane.

Methods employed to study mucosal and enterocyte protein turnover are summarized in Table VI.

VI. Conclusions

Methods to measure protein turnover rates in various organs and tissues are important for investigators involved in surgical research because many disease states seen in surgical patients are associated with significant changes in protein synthesis and degradation rates. Although this chapter has focused on models of protein metabolism for muscle and intestine (reflecting the major research interests in our laboratory), we have also discussed general aspects of techniques for the measurement of protein turnover rates. Due to space limitations, detailed technical aspects have not been described here but can be found in numerous original articles and handbooks.

The choice between the different methods that are available to measure protein turnover rates should be based on the specific question that is asked, and quite often different techniques need to be employed within the same project. In general, the major role for *in vitro* techniques is to study mechanisms of phenomena that are observed *in vivo*. The sometimes heated debate in the literature regarding the flooding dose versus constant infusion for measurement of protein synthesis *in vivo* is still unresolved and may actually be exaggerated, and has probably attracted greater space and attention than it is worth. After all, the differences between the two techniques are relatively small and mainly pertain to muscle tissue. As long as the limitations of the techniques are appreciated, and in particular if the influence of a certain condition or treatment (rather than the absolute protein turnover rates) is the main focus of the study, either

Table VI Models to Study Intestinal Protein Turnover

Flooding dose
Constant infusion
Luminal flooding dose
Mucosal scraping
Isolated enterocytes
Cultured enterocytes

technique can probably be used. Although a number of previous studies have been performed in experimental animals, the use of stable-isotope-labeled amino acids has dramatically increased the number of human studies and is expected to continue to generate important information about changes in protein metabolism in surgical patients.

Acknowledgments

Supported in part by NIH Grant DK37908, grants from the Shriners of North America, and a Merit Review grant from the Office of Research and Development, Medical Research Service, Department of Veterans Affairs, Washington, D.C. DRF was supported by a Research Fellowship from the Shriners of North America and TAP by NIH Training Grant IT32GM08478.

References

1. Hasselgren, P. O. (1993). "Protein Metabolism in Sepsis." R. G. Landes Co., Austin, Texas.
2. Hill, A. G., and Hill, G. L. (1998). Metabolic response to severe injury. *Br. J. Surg.* **85,** 884–890.
3. Essén, P., McNurlan, M. A., Wernerman, J., Vinnars, E., and Garlick, P. J. (1992). Uncomplicated surgery, but not general anesthesia, decreases muscle protein synthesis. *Am. J. Physiol.* **262,** E253–E260.
4. Dominioni, L., Dionigi, H., Zanello, M., Monico, R., Cremaschi, R, Dionigi, R., Ballabio, A., Marsa, M., Comelli, M., Dal, R. P., and Pisati, P. (1987). Sepsis score and acute phase protein response as predictors of outcome in septic surgical patients. *Arch. Surg.* **122,** 141–146.
5. Miller, L. L. (1983). Role of known hormones in regulating synthesis and secretion of plasma proteins by the isolated perfused rat liver. *In* "Plasma Protein Secretion by the Liver" (T. Glaumann, T. Peters, and C. Redman, eds.), pp. 133–142. Academic Press, New York.
6. Berry, M. N., Edwards, A. M., and Barritt, G. J. (1991). Isolated hepatocytes. Preparation, properties and applications. *In* "Laboratory Techniques in Biochemistry and Molecular Biology" (R. H. Burdon, and P. H. Van Knippenberg, eds.), Vol. 21, pp. 1–460. Elsevier, Amsterdam.
7. Hasselgren, P. O., Pedersen, P., Sax, H. C., Warner, B. W., and Fischer, J. E. (1988). Methods for studying protein synthesis and degradation in liver and skeletal muscle. *J. Surg. Res.* **45,** 389–415.
8. Rannels, D. E., Wartell, S. A., and Watkins, C. A. (1982). The measurement of protein synthesis in biological systems. *Life Sci.* **30,** 1679–1690.
9. Barrett, E. J., and Gelfand, R. A. (1989). The *in vivo* study of cardiac and skeletal muscle protein turnover. *Diab. Metab. Rev.* **5,** 133–148.
10. Garlick, P. J., McNurlan, M. A., Essén, P., and Wernerman, J. (1994). Measurement of tissue protein synthesis rates *in vivo*: A critical analysis of contrasting methods. *Am. J. Physiol.* **266,** E287–E297.
11. Zak, R., Martin, A. F., and Blough, R. (1979). Assessment of protein turnover by use of radioisotopic tracers. *Physiol. Rev.* **59,** 407–447.
12. Rennie, M. J., Smith, K., and Watt, P. W. (1994). Measurement of human tissue protein synthesis: An optimal approach. *Am. J. Physiol.* **266,** E298–E307.
13. Garlick, P. J., Millward, D. J., and James, W. P. T. (1973). The diurnal response of muscle and liver protein synthesis *in vivo* in meal-fed rats. *Biochem. J.* **136,** 935–946.
14. Garlick, P. J., McNurlan, M. A., and Preedy, V. R. (1980). A rapid and convenient technique for measuring the rate of protein synthesis in tissues by injection of [^{3}H]phenylalanine. *Biochem. J.* **192,** 719–723.
15. McNurlan, M. A., Tomkins, A. M., and Garlick, P. J. (1979). The effect of starvation on the rate of protein synthesis in rat liver and small intestine. *Biochem. J.* **178,** 373–379.
16. McNurlan, M. A., and Garlick, P. J. (1981). Protein synthesis in liver and small intestine in protein deprivation and diabetes. *Am. J. Physiol.* **241,** E238–E245.
17. Jepson, M. D., Pell, J. M., Bates, P. C., and Millward, D. J. (1986). The effects of endotoxemia on protein metabolism in skeletal muscle and liver of fed and fasted rats. *Biochem. J.* **235,** 329–336.
18. Jahoor, F., Zhang, X. J., Baba, H., Sakurai, Y., and Wolfe, R. R. (1992). Comparison of constant infusion and flooding dose techniques to measure muscle protein synthesis rate in dogs. *J. Nutr.* **122,** 878–887.
19. Smith, K., Essén, P., McNurlan, M. A., Rennie, M. J., Garlick, P. J., and Wernerman, J. (1992). A multi-tracer investigation of the effect of a flooding dose administered during the constant infusion of tracer amino acid on the rate of tracer incorporation into human muscle protein (abstract). *Proc. Nutr. Soc.* **51,** 109.
20. Calder, A. G., Anderson, S. E., Grant, I., McNurlan, M. A., and Garlick, P. J. (1992). The determination of low d_5-phenylalanine enrichment (0.002–0.09 atom percent excess) after conversion to phenylethylamine in relation to protein turnover studies by gas chromatography/electron ionization mass spectometry. *Rapid Commun. Mass Spectrom.* **6,** 421–424.
21. Buse, M. G., and Reid, S. S. (1975). Leucine: a possible regulator of protein turnover in muscle. *J. Clin. Invest.* **56,** 1250–1261.
22. Morgan, H. E., Chua, B. H., Boyd, T. A., and Jefferson, L. S. (1985). Branched chain aminos acids and the regulation of protein turnover in heart and skeletal muscle. *In* "Metabolism and Clinical Implications of Branded Chain Amino and Ketoacids" (M. Walser and J. R. Williamson, eds.), pp. 217–226. Elsevier, Amsterdam.
23. Halliday, D., Pacy, P. J., Cheng, K. N., Dworzak, F. D., Gibson, J. N. A., and Rennie, M. J. (1988). Rate of protein synthesis in skeletal muscle of normal man and patients with muscular dystrophy; a reassessment. *Clin. Sci.* **74,** 237–240.
24. McNurlan, M. A., Essén, P., Milne, E., Vinnars, E., Garlick, P. J., and Wernerman, J. (1993). Temporal responses of protein synthesis in human skeletal muscle to feeding. *Br. J. Nutr.* **69,** 117– 126.
25. Essén, P., Sonnenfeld, T., Milne, E., Vinnars, E., Wernerman, J., and Garlick, P. J. (1993). Muscle protein synthesis postoperatively - the effects of intravenous nutrition. *Eur. J. Surg.* **159,** 195–200.
26. Hummel, R. P., Hasselgren, P. O., James, J. H., Warner, B. W., and Fischer, J. E. (1988). The effect of sepsis in rats on skeletal muscle protein synthesis *in vivo* and in periphery and central core of incubated muscle preparations *in vitro. Metabolism* **37,** 1120–1127.
27. Hall-Angerås, M., Angerås, U., vonAllmen, D., Higashiguchi, T., Zamir, O., Hasselgren, P. O., and Fischer, J. E. (1991). Influence of sepsis in rats on muscle protein turnover *in vivo* and in tissue incubated under different *in vitro* conditions. *Metabolism* **40,** 247–251.
28. vonAllmen, D., Hasselgren, P. O., Higashiguchi, T., Frederick, J., Zamir, O., and Fischer, J. E. (1992). Increased intestinal protein synthesis during sepsis and following the administration of tumor necrosis factor α or interleukin-1α. *Biochem. J.* **286,** 585–589.
29. Higashiguchi, T., Noguchi, Y., O'Brien, W., Wagner, K., Fischer, J. E., and Hasselgren, P. O. (1994). Effect of sepsis on mucosal protein synthesis in different parts of the gastrointestinal tract in rats. *Clin. Sci.* **87,** 207–211.
30. Waterlow, J. C., Garlick, P. J., and Millward, D. J. (1978). "Protein Turnover in Mammalian Tissues and in the Whole Body." North-Holland, Amsterdam.
31. Swick, R. W., and Ip. M. M. (1974). Measurement of protein turnover in rat liver with ^{14}C-carbonate. *J. Biol. Chem.* **249,** 6836–6841.
32. MacDonald, M. L., Augustine, S. L., Burk, T. L., and Swick, R. W. A. (1979). A comparison of methods for the measurement of protein turnover *in vivo. Biochem. J.* **184,** 473–476.
33. Angerås, U., Jagenburg, R., Lindstedt, G., and Hasselgren, P. O. (1987). Effects of β-adrenergic blocking agents on urinary excretion of 3-methylhistidine during experimental hyperthyroidism in rats. *Eur. Surg. Res.* **19,** 23–30.

34. Adlerberth, A., Angerås, U., Jagenburg, R., Lindstedt, G., Stenström, G., and Hasselgren, P. O. (1987). Urinary excretion of 3-methylhistidine and creatinine and plasma concentrations of amino acids in hyperthyroid patients following preoperative treatment with antithyroid drug or β-blocking agent: Results from a prospective, randomized study. *Metabolism* **36,** 637–642.
35. Neuhäuser, M., Bergström, J., Chao, B., Holmström, J., Nordlund, L., Vinnars, E., and Fürst, P. (1980). Urinary excretion of 3-methylhistidine as an index of muscle protein catabolism in postoperative trauma: The effect of parenteral nutrition. *Metabolism* **29,** 1206–1213.
36. Long, C. L., Birkhahn, R. H., Geiger, J. W., and Blakemore, W. S. (1984). Urinary excretion of 3-methylhistidine before and after major surgical operation. *Metabolism* **33,** 250–256.
37. Young, V. R., and Munro, H. N. (1978). N-methylhistidine (3-methylhistidine) and muscle protein turnover: An overview. *Fed. Proc.* **37,** 2291–2300.
38. Wassner, S. J., and Li, J. B. (1982). N-methylhistidine release: Contributions of rat skeletal muscle, GI tract, and skin. *Am. J. Physiol.* **243,** E293–E297.
39. Ballard, F. J., and Tomas, F. M. (1983). 3-Methylhistidine as a measure of skeletal muscle protein breakdown in human subjects: The case for its continued use. *Clin. Sci.* **65,** 209–215.
40. Rennie, M. J., and Millward, D. J., (1983). 3-Methylhistidine excretion and urinary 3-methylhistidine/creatinine ratio are poor indicators of skeletal muscle protein breakdown. *Clin. Sci.* **65,** 217–225.
41. Tiao, G., Fagan, J. M., Samuels, N., James, J. H., Hudson, K., Lieberman, M., Fischer, J. E., and Hasselgren, P. O. (1994) Sepsis stimulates non-lysosomal energy-dependent proteolysis and increases ubiquitin mRNA levels in rat skeletal muscle. *J. Clin. Invest.* **94,** 2255–2264.
42. Fang, C. H., Tiao, G., James, H., Ogle, C., Fischer, J. E., and Hasselgren, P. O. (1995) Burn injury stimulates multiple proteolytic pathways in skeletal muscle, including the ubiquitin-energy-dependent pathway. *J. Am. Coll. Surg.* **180,** 161–170.
43. Jensen, N. A., and Celis, J. E. (1998). Proteomic changes associated with degeneration of myelin-forming cells in the central nervous system of c-Myc transgenic mice. *Electrophoresis* **19,** 2014–2020.
44. Gauss, C., Kalkum, M., Löwe, M., Lehrach, H., and Kloge, J. (1999). Analysis of the mouse proteome. (I) Brain proteins: Separation by two-dimensional electrophoresis and identification by mass spectometry and genetic variation. *Electrophoresis* **20,** 575–600.
45. Hasselgren, P. O., Hall-Angerås, M., Angerås, U., Benson, D., James, J. H., and Fischer, J. E. (1990). Regulation of total and myofibrillar protein breakdown in rat extensor digitorum longus and soleus muscle incubated flaccid or at resting length. *Biochem. J.* **267,** 37–44.
46. Baracos, V. E., and Goldberg, A. L. (1986). Maintenance of normal length improves protein balance and energy status in isolated rat skeletal muscles. *Am. J. Physiol.* **251,** C588–C596.
47. McGrath, J. A., and Goldspink, D. F. (1982). Glucocorticoid action on protein synthesis and protein breakdown in isolated skeletal muscles. *Biochem. J.* **206,** 641–645.
48. Fang, C. H., Li, B. G., Wang, J. J., Fischer, J. E., and Hasselgren, P. O. (1997). Insulin-like growth factor-I (IGF-I) stimulates protein synthesis and inhibits protein breakdown in muscle from burned rats. *JPEN* **21,** 245–251.
49. Hobler, S. C., Williams, A., Fischer, J. E., and Hasselgren, P. O. (1998). Insulin-like growth factor-I (IGF-I) stimulates protein synthesis but does not inhibit protein breakdown in muscle from septic rats. *Am. J. Physiol.* **274,** R571–R576.
50. Segal, S. S., and Faulkner, J. A. (1985). Temperature-dependent physiological stability of rat skeletal muscle *in vitro*. *Am. J. Physiol.* **248,** C265–C270.
51. Zamir, O., Hasselgren, P. O., Frederick, J. A., and Fischer, J. E. (1992). Is the metabolic response to sepsis in skeletal muscle different in infants and adults? An experimental study in rats. *J. Pediatr. Surg.* **27,** 1399–1403.
52. Essig, D. A., Segal, S. S., and White, T. P. (1985). Skeletal muscle protein synthesis and degradation *in vitro:* Effects of temperature. *Am. J. Physiol.* **249,** C464–470.
53. Tiao, G., Hobler, S., Wang, J. J., Meyer, T. A., Luchette, F. A., Fischer, J. E., and Hasselgren, P. O. (1997). Sepsis is associated with increased mRNAs of the ubiquitin-proteasome proteolytic pathway in human skeletal muscle. *J. Clin. Invest.* **99,** 163–168.
54. Hobler, S. C., Williams, A. B., Fischer, D., Wang, J. J., Sun, X., Fischer, J. E., Monaco, J. J., and Hasselgren, P. O. (1999). The activity and expression of the 20S proteasome are increased in skeletal muscle during sepsis. *Am. J. Physiol.* **277,** R434–R440.
55. Hasselgren, P. O., James, J. H., Benson, D. W., Hall-Angerås, M., Angerås, U., Hiyama, D. T., Li, S., and Fischer, J. E. (1989). Total and myofibrillar protein breakdown in different types of rat skeletal muscle: Effects of sepsis and regulation by insulin. *Metabolism* **38,** 634–640.
56. Lee, D. H., and Goldberg, A. L. (1998). Proteasome inhibitors: Valuable new tools for cell biologists. *Trends Cell Biol.* **8,** 397–403.
57. Sorimachi, H., Ishiura, S., and Suzaki, K. (1997). Structure and physiological function of calpains. *Biochem. J.* **328,** 721–732.
58. Wing, S. S., and Goldberg, A. L. (1993). Glucocorticoids activate the ATP-ubiquitin-dependent proteolytic system in skeletal muscle during fasting. *Am. J. Physiol.* **264,** E668–E676.
59. Price, S. R., England, B. K., Bailey, J. K. van Vreede, K., and Mitch, W. E. (1994). Acidosis and glucocorticoids concomitantly increase ubiquitin and proteasome subunit mRNAs in rat muscle. *Am. J. Physiol.* **267,** C955–C960.
60. Hobler, S. C., Tiao, G., Fischer, J. E., Monaco, J., and Hasselgren, P. O. (1998). The sepsis-induced increase in muscle proteolysis is blocked by specific proteasome inhibitors. *Am. J. Physiol.* **274,** R30–R37.
61. Richler, C., and Yaffe, D. (1970). The *in vitro* cultivation and differentiation capacities of myogenic cell lines. *Dev. Biol.* **23,** 1–22.
62. Yaffe, D. (1971). Developmental changes preceding cell fusion during muscle differentiation *in vitro*. *Exp. Cell Res.* **66,** 33–48.
63. Wang, L., Luo, G. J., Wang, J. J., and Hasselgren, P. O. (1998). Dexamethasone stimulates proteasome- and calcium-dependent proteolysis in cultured L6 myotubes. *Shock* **10,** 298–306.
64. Luo, G. J., Sun, X., and Hasselgren, P. O. (2000). Hyperthermia stimulates energy-proteasome-dependent degradation of short- and long-lived proteins in cultured myotubes. *Am. J. Physiol.* **278,** R749–R756.
65. Hall-Angerås, M., Angerås, U., Zamir, O., Hasselgren, P. O., and Fischer, J. E. (1991). Effect of the glucocorticoid receptor antagonist RU 38486 on muscle protein breakdown in sepsis. *Surgery* **109,** 468–473.
66. Tiao, G., Fagan, J., Roegner, V., Lieberman, M., Wang, J. J., Fischer, J. E., and Hasselgren, P. O. (1996). Energy-ubiquitin-dependent muscle proteolysis during sepsis in rats is regulated by glucocorticoids. *J. Clin. Invest.* **97,** 339–348.
67. Solomon, V., Baracos, V., Sarraf, P., and Goldberg, A. L. (1998). Rates of ubiquitin conjugation increase when muscles atrophy, largely through activation of the N-end rule pathway. *Proc. Natl. Acad. Sci. U.S.A.* **95,** 12602–12607.
68. Solomon, V., Lecker, S. H., and Goldberg, A. L. (1998). The N-end rule pathway catalyzes a major fraction of the protein degradation in skeletal muscle. *J. Biol. Chem.* **273,** 25216–25222.
69. Wernerman, J., von der Decken, A., and Vinnars, E. (1986). Polyribosome concentration in human skeletal muscle after starvation and parenteral or enteral refeeding. *Metabolism* **35,** 447–451.
70. Baracos, V. E., DeVivo, C., Hoyle, D. H. R., and Goldberg, A. L. (1995). Activation of the ATP-ubiquitin-proteasome pathway in skeletal muscle of cachectic rats bearing a hepatoma. *Am. J. Physiol.* **268,** E996–E1006.
71. Hobler, S. C., Wang, J. J., Williams, A. B., Melandri, F., Sun, X., Fischer, J. E., and Hasselgren, P. O. (1999). Sepsis is associated with increased ubiquitin conjugating enzyme $E2_{14k}$ mRNA in skeletal muscle. *Am. J. Physiol.* **276,** R468–R473.

72. Fischer, D. R., Sun, X., Gang, G., Pritts, T., and Hasselgren, P. O. (2000). The gene expression of ubiquitin ligase E3α is upregulated in skeletal muscle during sepsis in rats - potential role of glucocorticoids. *Biochem. Biophys. Res. Commun.* **267,** 504–508.
73. Tiao, G., Lieberman, M. A., Fischer, J. E., and Hasselgren, P. O. (1997). Intracellular regulation of protein degradation during sepsis is different in fast- and slow-twitch muscle. *Am. J. Physiol.* **272,** R849–R856.
74. Medina, R., Wing, S. S., and Goldberg, A. L. (1995). Increase in levels of polyubiquitin and proteasome mRNA in skeletal muscle during starvation and denervation atrophy. *Biochem. J.* **307,** 631–637.
75. Fang, C. H., Li, B. G., Sun, X., and Hasselgren, P. O. (2000). Insulin-like growth factor-I reduces ubiquitin and ubiquitin-conjugating enzyme gene expression but does not inhibit muscle proteolysis in septic rats. *Endocrinology* **141,** 2743–2751.
76. Williams, A., de Courten-Myers, G. M., Fischer, J. E., Luo, G., Sun, X., and Hasselgren, P. O. (1999). Sepsis stimulates release of myofilaments in skeletal muscle by a calcium-dependent mechanism. *FASEB J.* **13,** 1435–1443.
77. Llovera, M., Garcia-Martinez, C., Agell, N., Lopez-Soriano, F. J., Authier, F. J., Gherardi, R. K., and Argiles, J. M. (1998). Ubiquitin and proteasome gene expression is increased in skeletal muscle of slim AIDS patients. *Int. J. Mol. Med.* **2,** 69–73.
78. Mansoor, O., Beaufrere, B., Boierie, Y., Ralliere, C., Taillandier, D., Aurousseau, E., Schoeffler, P., Arnal, M., and Attaix, D. (1996). Increased mRNA levels for components of the lysosomal, Ca^{2+}-activated, and ATP-ubiquitin-dependent proteolytic pathways in skeletal muscle from head trauma patients. *Proc. Natl. Acad. Sci. U.S.A.* **93,** 2714–2718.
79. Williams, A., Sun, X., Fischer, J. E., and Hasselgren, P. O. (1999). The expression of genes in the ubiquitin-proteasome proteolytic pathway is increased in skeletal muscle from patients with cancer. *Surgery* **126,** 744–750.
80. Fanconneau, G., and Michel, M. C. (1970). Role of the gastrointestinal tract in regulation of protein metabolism. *In* "Mammalian Protein Metabolism" (H.N. Munro, ed.), Vol. 4, pp. 480–522. Academic Press, New York.
81. Stein, T. P., Mullen, J. L. Oram-Smith, J. C., Rosato, E. F., Wallace, H. W., and Hargrove, W. C. (1978). Relative rates of tumor, normal gut, liver and fibrinogen protein synthesis in man. *Am. J. Physiol.* **234,** E648–E652.
82. Meyer, T. A., Wang, J., Tiao, G., Ogle, C. K., Fischer, J. E., and Hasselgren, P. O. (1995). Sepsis and endotoxemia stimulate intestinal IL-6 production. *Surgery* **118,** 336–342.
83. Wang, Q., Wang, J. J., Boyce, S., Fischer, J. E., and Hasselgren, P. O. (1998) Endotoxemia and IL-1β stimulate mucosal IL-6 production in different parts of the gastrointestinal tract. *J. Surg. Res.* **76,** 27–31.
84. Wang, Q., Meyer, T. A., Boyce, S., Wang, J. J., Sun, X., Tiao, G., Fischer, J. E., and Hasselgren, P. O. (1998). Endotoxemia in mice stimulates the production of complement component C3 and serum amyloid A in mucosa of small intestine. *Am. J. Physiol.* **275,** R1584–R1592.
85. Wang, Q., Wang, J. J., Fischer, J. E., and Hasselgren, P. O. (1998). Mucosal production of complement C3 and serum amyloid A is differentially regulated in different parts of the gastrointestinal tract during endotoxemia in mice. *J. Gastrointest. Surg.* **2,** 537–546.
86. Higashiguchi, T., Noguchi, Y., Meyer, T., Fischer, J. E., and Hasselgren, P. O. (1995). Protein synthesis in isolated enterocytes from septic or endotoxemic rats: regulation by glutamine. *Clin. Sci.* **89,** 311–319.
87. Weber, F. L., Fresard, K. M., and Veach, G. L. (1989). Stimulation of jejunal mucosa protein synthesis by luminal glucose: effects with luminal and vascular leucine in fed and fasted rats. *Gastroenterology* **96,** 935–937.
88. Nakshabendi, I. M., Obeidat, W., Russell, R. I., Downie, S., Smith, K., and Rennie, M. J. (1995). Gut mucosal protein synthesis measured using intravenous and intragastric delivery of stable tracer amino acids. *Am. J. Physiol.* **269,** E996–E999.
89. Adegoke, O. A. J., McBurney, M. I., and Baracos, V. E. (1999). Jejunal mucosal protein synthesis: Validation of luminal flooding dose method and effect of luminal osmolality. *Am. J. Physiol.* **276,** G14–G20.
90. Adegoke, O. A. J., McBurney, M. I., Samuels, S. E., and Baracos, V. E. (1999). Luminal amino acids acutely decrease intestinal mucosal protein synthesis and protease mRNA in piglets. *J. Nutr.* **129,** 1871–1878.
91. Samuels, S. E., Taillandier, D., Aurousseau, E., Cherel, Y., LeMaho, Y, Arnal, M., and Attaix, D. (1996). Gastrointestinal tract protein synthesis and mRNA levels for proteolytic systems in adult fasted rats. *Am. J. Physiol.* **271,** E232–E238.
92. Watford, M., Lund, P., and Krebs, H. A. (1979). Isolation and metabolic characteristics of rat and chicken enterocytes. *Biochem. J.* **178,** 589–596.
93. Meyer, T. A., Noguchi, Y., Ogle, C., Tiao, G., Wang, J. J., Fischer, J. E., and Hasselgren, P. O. (1994). Endotoxin stimulates IL-6 production in intestinal epithelial cells: A synergistic effect with PGE_2. *Arch. Surg.* **129,** 1290–1295.
94. Meyer, T., Tiao, G., James, J. H., Noguchi, Y., Ogle, C. K., Fischer, J. E., and Hasselgren, P. O. (1995). Nitric oxide inhibits LPS-induced IL-6 production in enterocytes. *J. Surg. Res.* **58,** 570–575.
95. Pinto, M., Robine-Leon, S., Appay, M. D., *et al* (1983). Enterocyte-like differentiation and polarization of the human colon carcinoma cell line Caco-2 in culture. *Biol. Cell* **47,** 323–330.
96. Parikh, A., Salzman, A., Fischer, J. E., and Hasselgren, P. O. (1997). Interleukin-1β and interferon-γ regulate interleukin-6 production in human intestinal epithelial cells. *Shock* **8,** 249–255.
97. Moon, R., Parikh, A. A., Szabo, C., Fischer, J. E., Salzman, A. L., and Hasselgren, P. O. (1997). Complement C3 production in human intestinal epithelial cells is regulated by IL-1β and TNF-α. *Arch. Surg.* **132,** 1289–1293.
98. Moon, M. R., Parikh, A. A., Pritts, T. A., Kane, C., Fischer, J. E., Salzman, A. L., and Hasselgren, P. O. (2000). IL-1β induces complement component C3 and IL-6 production at the basolateral and apical membranes in a human intestinal epithelial cell line. *Shock* **13,** 374–378.

61

Membrane Transport of Nutrients

Bruce R. Stevens

Department of Physiology, College of Medicine, University of Florida, Gainesville, Florida 32610

I. Introduction

A. Transport in Normal and Pathophysiologic States

This chapter concerns the transport of organic nutrients across plasma membranes of cells. The plasma membrane constitutes one of the most important control points in general metabolism within any given cell and between organized cellular systems such as organs: the events of cellular physiology and metabolic biochemical pathways are ultimately related to the exchange of organic molecules between intracellular and extracelluar compartments. Thus, investigations of nutrient membrane transport are essential for a complete understanding of normal physiologic and pathophysiologic states.

Organic nutrients are primarily the focus in this chapter. However, the role of inorganic ions such as Na^+ will also be covered due to their essential role in catalyzing and energizing membrane transport of certain organic solutes. The nutrients primarily served by transporters and/or simple passive diffusion include amino acids, monomer sugars, selected carboxylic acids and bases, and lipids. The methods described for nutrient transport can easily be adapted to study the transport of pharmacologically active compounds into and out of cells; drugs are often structural analogs of natural substrates for nutrient transporters.

B. Importance and Relevance

Ultimately, the functional properties of normal or defective nutrient transporters must be confirmed by cloning putative polypeptides, then the physiologic behavior of the heterologous polypeptide must be reinvestigated in an *in vitro* expression model. Therefore, this chapter provides criteria to characterize cloned putative transporter polypeptides, whether they are derived from normal or pathologic tissues. A current survey of various molecular biology Internet databases indicates that a wide variety of nutrient transporters have been characterized and cloned (1). The most recent surprises concern the recently discovered "FATP" series of nutrient fatty acid transporter proteins (2).

A multitude of clinical disorders are directly attributable to disorders of membrane transport processes (3). In this vein, the discussion here covers epithelia, endothelia, skeletal muscle, and individualized cells. The functions of many epithelial systems are specifically governed by cell membrane transport of organic nutrients, with further subspecialization occurring in the apical and basolateral aspects. These systems include important physiologic events of the gut (especially small intestinal enterocytes), cornea, liver and gall bladder, and kidney (especially the proximal tubule). Endothelial cells associated with peripheral vasculature and the blood–brain barrier display specific nutrient transport mechanisms associated with their localized functions (such as L-arginine transport associated with control of nitric oxide biosynthesis) as well as nutrient delivery to neighboring cell types. Excitable tissues transport organic solutes in the capacity of messengers as well as organic nutrients; their transport events, which are associated with modulation of ion channels, are not covered here. Finally, this chapter covers single cell transport, applicable to not only cell types such as blood cells, but also pertinent to many cell types cultured *in vitro* as single-cell suspensions.

The general principles of membrane transport theory and experimental methods are addressed. The topics described in this chapter are limited to the movement of solute molecules across plasma membranes at the cellular level, rather than mass transport of metabolites between organs via the blood. The latter topic is covered elsewhere in this book, whereby studies largely concern methods for measuring $A - V$ differences, or measuring bulk-phase concentration differences. Inasmuch as different cell types play different metabolic roles in the body, membrane transport mechanism and substrate selectivities have evolved as specialized events in each cell type. At the most fundamental level, nutients enter or leave cells under the influence of electrochemical forces that various cell types exploit for their specific purposes. Thus, this chapter also covers the assessment of thermodynamic coupling to nutrient transport.

II. Survey of Methods

A variety of useful techniques are available to measure nutrient transport. *In vivo* influx/efflux studies by $A - V$ differences in perfused intact organs take the entire organ into consideration, but this is not useful in isolating the localized cellular or membrane sites of transport. Furthermore, metabolism and intraorgan partitioning of the substrate confound interpretation of unidirectional fluxes in intact tissue. Crude partitioning of uptake within an organ can be imaged by positron emmision tomography of ^{18}O-labeled substrates, but this is still unsatisfactory to quantitate accurately transport processes. Bulk-phase transport in the intestine can be followed by breath tests of ingested ^{13}C-labeled nutrients, but changes in motility affect the results. In general, it can be concluded that *in vitro* preparations offer the only means of controlling experimental variables in transport experiments, as expanded below.

In vitro epithelial sheets mounted in Ussing chambers, everted sacs of gut, and perfused intact renal tubules offer some advantages over *in vivo* organ perfusions, primarily due to limiting the exposure and metabolism of a test solute to the tissue of interest. It is now widely accepted that isolated single-cell suspensions, cultured cells, and purified isolated membrane vesicles offer the most control in assessing transport events (4–6). In the case of epithelial cells, transport across apical membranes is easily studied using monolayers grown on plastic, whereas comparisions between apical and basolateral surfaces and transepithelial fluxes can be investigated using cells grown on porous Transwell inserts. To examine rapid kinetic events within the membrane proper, it is often necessary to prepare purified isolated plasma membrane vesicles from either intact tissues or cultures. A variety of putative transporter polypeptides have been cloned (1), but their physiologic properties ultimately must be assessed in a membrane. The most common model of cloned transporter proteins involves heterologous nucleotide expression in *Xenopus* oocytes or in yeast (7). Native or cloned transporter proteins can be reconstituted into liposomes composed of artificial or native lipids for speciality studies on the biophysics of the transporters, but this topic is beyond the scope of the present chapter. The transport methods described below are directly applicable to cultured cells or isolated membrane vesicles derived from native and cultured cells.

III. Experimental Conditions and Interpretations

A. Unstirred Layer Effects

The analysis of a membrane transport event can be confounded by the phenomenon of unstirred layers (USLs), and thus this experimental issue must be addressed. This is especially critical for sheets of epithelia, which are overlayed with endogenous mucus and glycocalyx, or in sheets of endothelial cells. Such organized cell systems can display unstirred layers often >100 μm thick (Fig. 1A). The unstirred water layer arises due to the phenomenon of laminar flow that creates a three-compartment model of solute movement, and USLs thus can profoundly confound membrane transport studies by establishing a concentration of the substrate species that the transporter binding site "sees" (Fig. 1B). This concentration at the membrane surface can be quite different from the bulk phase under certain circumstances. The rate at which a solute diffuses through an unstirred layer is inversly proportional to USL thickness. Furthermore, there is often a pH gradient within the USL that can strongly influence the charge state of the solute species at the membrane binding site proper; this pH can be quite different from the bulk phase as measured by the

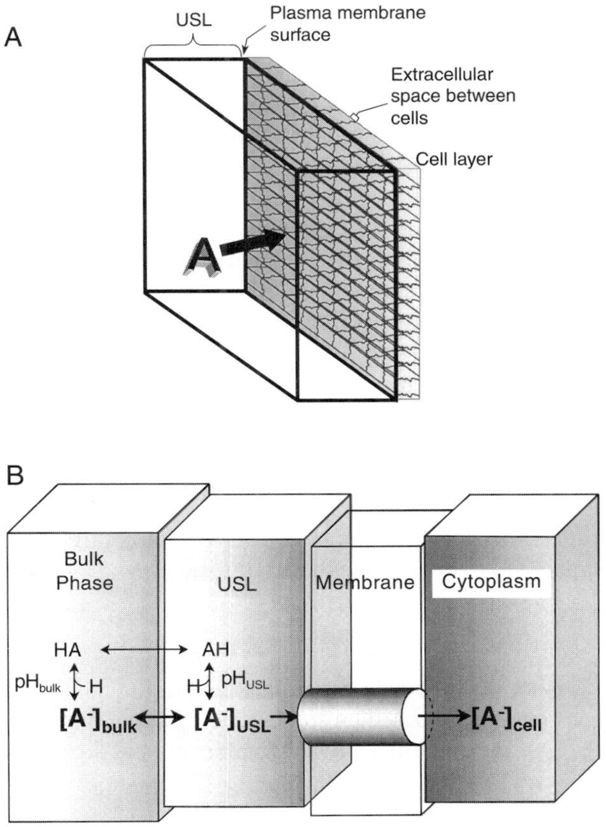

Figure 1 Unstirred layers influence transport experiments. (A) The virtual concentration of solute molecules in the unstirred layer (nominally 100 μm thick) near a sheet of membranes in an organized cell system influences the actual concentration "seen" by the membrane. In some cases of organized cellular systems, the extracellular space between cells comprises an additional fluid compartment that equilibrates with solute. In this example, a single solute molecule denoted "A" existing in the unstirred layer can be transported by the adjacent cell membranes. (B) Laminar properties of fluids near the membrane surface create microscopic gradients in the unstirred layer (USL) that are different from the the bulk-phase concentrations. In the case of ionizable solutes, such as amino acids, the USL pH gradients can influence the concentration of actual species presented to the transporter of a membrane. In this example, a single ionizable solute molecule denoted "A" initially exists in the bulk phase, but must pass through the unstirred layer before it can be transported across the cell membrane into the cytoplasm.

experimenter, and thus can potentially lead to incorect interpretation of the data.

In certain pathophysiologic conditions of the gut, the unstirred layer may represent a true transport barrier to be overcome before enterocyte cell membrane transport proper is even encountered. The USL can arise due to epithelial surface factors such as mucus production, villi and microvilli flattening or elongation, or changes in motility. In cases such as Whipple's disease, amyloidosis, eosinophilic gastroenteritis, tropical sprue, gluten enteropathies, or bowel motility disorders, it is appropriate to investigate models of intestinal transport in the intact epithelium. This is because passive diffusion through the unstirred layer represents the rate-limiting step for net transport from lumen to portal blood.

To reduce USL effects in intact epithelia or in cultured monolayers, experiments must be designed to stir constantly the bulk-phase media. It should be noted, however, that even the most vigorous stirring will not completely eliminate the inherent laminar flow properties of aqueous media covering an epithelial sheet. Nonetheless, cell culture monolayers should be gently rotated during uptake experiments, and media should be constantly moving/stirred across intact epithelial sheet preparations (e.g., intestine, cornea). For single cells or membrane vesicles, the unstirred layer is greater than the diameter of the cell or vesicle, and thus the measured transport data generally represent true events at the membrane proper. Stirring is still required with single cells, however.

B. Extracellular Space as an Uptake Compartment

In some cases, whether measuring uptake *in vitro* or *in vivo*, the extracellular space could constitute a compartment that, if occupied by radiolabel, would potentially confound interpretation of true intracellular uptake (Fig. 1B). Thus, for a given experimental senario, it is necessary at least once to measure the radiolabel that nonspecifically adheres to cells by a double-label experiment using [^{14}C] inulin to estimate the contribution to total uptake by the extracellular space. It is often the case that this space is <1% of the total tissue/culture volume, and can be safely ignored in all subsequent measurements. In some cases, however, such as using whole liver or muscle pieces, the radiolabel entering the extracellular volume must be subtracted from total radioactivity associated with the tissue.

C. Thermodynamic Conditions

To assess and interpret nutrient transport in normal and pathologic cells, the experimental conditions must factor in appropriate thermodynamic conditions that will influence the measurements (8). The most rudimentary experimental condition concerns whether the solute transport involves cellular influx or efflux. Furthermore, transport can be measured under steady-state, pre-steady-state, or equilibrium exchange conditions that can involve either unidirectional influx/efflux or independent bidirectional fluxes, or coupled bidirectional fluxes (9).

D. Assignment of Transport Driving Forces

The movement of solutes across membranes is directly governed by the type of driving forces involved. These are summarized in Fig. 2. Nutrient transport is categorically

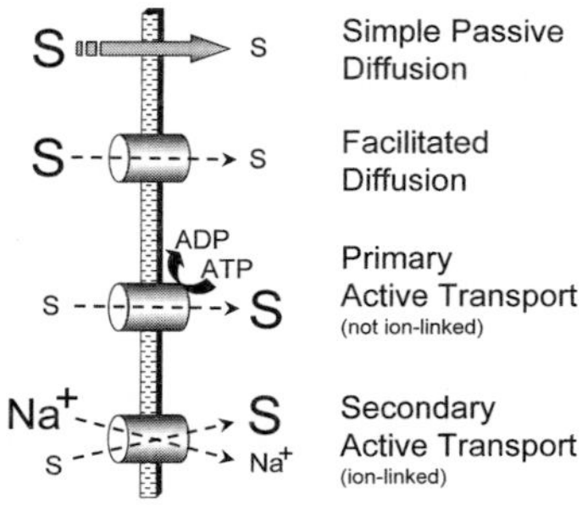

Figure 2 Energetic classification of membrane transport events. The net transmembrane movement of a solute, S, is independent of the transport mechanism, but depends on electrochemical forces. However, specific mechanisms will permit either "downhill" transport or "uphill" active transport depending on the manner by which existing electrical and chemical forces are coupled to the solute electrochemical potential. Simple passive diffusion does not involve a protein carrier, whereas the other cases of transport involve a carrier system. A transport system may be composed of several subunits. Primary active transport of organic solutes primarily concerns the ABC superfamily of carriers that possess an ATP hydrolysis domain. Secondary active transport of organic solutes is a common mode by which solute is accumulated within the cytoplasm, or accumulated across an epithelium. In secondary active transport, ion (often Na^+) electrochemical potentials drive solute transport; the ultimate source of energy is thus an independent ion-ATPase that hydrolyzes ATP. In this figure, the relative size of the solute S denotes relative concentration

linked to the source of its driving force, and thus it is essential to investigate these driving forces to understand fully a given transport process (10). The pathology of nutrient and drug transport is often the consequence of a disruption of the driving force linked to transport. In the case of transport by epithelial cells, multiple driving forces are involved across each membrane as well as via net transepithelial movement. Driving forces can be categorized as either "nonactive" (so-called downhill transport) or "active" (so-called uphill transport). A theoretical treatment of the thermodynamics of solute transport has been covered elsewhere (8).

In the simplest case of nonactive transport, whether movement is catalyzed by a carrier (denoted facilitated diffusion) or if movement occurs by simple passive diffusion, chemical concentration gradients ultimately determine the rate and direction of nutrient transport (Fig. 2). If the nutrient molecule is charged, as for certain amino acids, for example, then the extracellular pH, transmembrane membrane electrical potential, and unstirred layers are each important factors to consider. If energy can be coupled to the transport process for "uphill" concentrative movement, then active transport occurs. The direct coupling of energy from ATP to solute movement is called "primary active transport." Primary active transporters are multiple-subunit ATPases. All dividing cells possess ion-ATPases (e.g., Na^+,K^+-ATPase, Ca^{2+}-ATPase, H^+,K^+-ATPase), which establish the resting membrane potential as well as various electrolyte gradients. Organic solutes, including drugs, can also be pumped out of cells by primary active transporters energized directly by ATP hydrolysis, but unlike the ion-ATPases, they are not energetically or mechanically coupled to ions. Clinically, the most important primary active transporters of organic solutes includes the so-called ABC superfamily of multidrug resistance (MDR) transporters. Complete analysis of the ABC-type primary active transporters is beyond the scope of the present chapter, and the reader is directed to literature covering these systems (1).

By far, the most commonly observed type of uphill nutrient transport concerns indirect coupling to ion electrochemical gradients generated by primary active transporter ion-ATPases. Because the energy is indirectly linked to ATP hydrolysis, this is denoted "secondary active transport," and usually involves coupling to gradients of one or more of the ions Na^+, H^+, K^+, and Cl^-. By coupling to the electrochemical gradients of ions, secondary active transport of nurtients permits a concentration ability of several thousandfold, compared to passive or facilitated diffusion (8).

E. Initial Rates

Most of the following experimental designs and interpretations of data are based on solute unidirectional flux events (Fig. 3A). Meaningful analysis of unidirectional flux of nor-

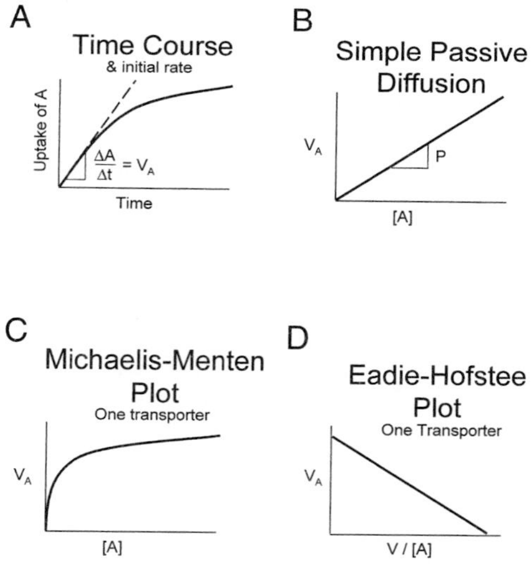

Figure 3 Experimental tools useful in analyzing membrane transport phenomena. Details for each case are described in the text. In these examples, solute species "A" is transported with rates V via solely simple passive diffusion or a single-carrier mechanism. (A) The time course of uptake is used to derive linear initial rates. (B) Simple passive diffusion gives a linear relationship according to the Fick relationship, with the slope equal to the permeability coefficient, P. (C) A hyperbolic Michaelis–Menten relationship indicates the existence of a single transporter for a given substrate. (D) An Eadie–Hofstee plot is a linearization of Michaelis–Menten kinetics. A single straight line indicates the presence of a single transporter, with the V_{max} at the ordinate intercept, and the apparent K_m equal to the negative slope.

mal and pathophysiologic transport events depends critically on obtaining transport initial rates over a range of substrate concentrations. Thus, when undertaking a project to assess nutrient transport, the first measurements undertaken should focus on obtaining time points that represent linear rates of influx (or efflux, if appropriate) at both a high concentration and a low concentration of substrate. This means that a zero time point must also be measured. All subsequent analyses, discussed below, are thus based on linear initial rates.

F. Simple Passive Diffusion: Not Insignificant

When the carrier-mediated components alone are to be considered in kinetic treatments, the contribution by simple passive diffusion must be subtracted from the total flux. Nonetheless, although carrier-mediated transport represents a cell's means to catalyze transmembrane movement of specific solute species, passive diffusion can contribute significantly to net movement at very high solute concentrations, and thus should not be be discounted in the overall assessment of transport. For example, in the gut lumen high concentrations (millimolar) of neutral amino acids can contribute up to 80% of the total uptake, whereas at much lower concentrations (micromolar) the passive diffusion component represents less than 10% of total uptake (11).

The diffusional component can be identified in two ways: either by the residual uptake remaining in an inhibition profile curve (obtained in the presence of large concentrations of substrate), or by kinetically dissecting it out. Simple passive diffusional transport rates are linearly related to concentration (Fig. 3B) by the Fick equation, $V = P[S]$, where P is the passive diffusion permeability coefficient. In the case of ionizable substrates such as amino acids, the pH will influence the concentration of charged and zwitterionic species, and thus pH will influence the relative flux rate, especially in the presence of unstirred layers (see Fig. 1).

G. Kinetic Model of Carrier-Mediated Transport

The most useful simple model of carrier-mediated transport is based on the saturable single binding site theory of transport (4, 12). In this model, initial rates of nutrient solute uptake V provide a hyperbolic function of concentration [S], with an "apparent" half-saturation binding constant denoted K_m (Fig. 3C). That is, $V = (V_{max}[S])/(K_m + [S])$. To verify the presence of a single transport system, a graphical representation of the uptake data plotted using an Eadie–Hofstee plot of V as a function of $V/[S]$ will give a single linear relationship (Fig. 3D). Graphically (Fig. 3D), the V_{max} is obtained from the ordinate intercept and K_m represents the negative slope. If the plotted Eadie–Hofstee data yield a curvilinear relationship (Fig. 4A), it is likely that the sub-

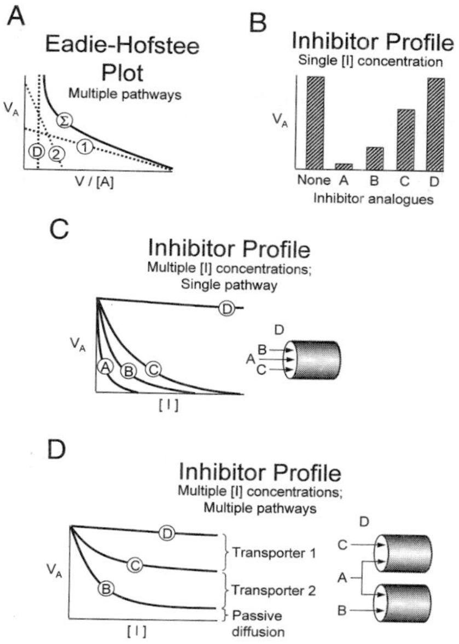

Figure 4 Further experimental tools useful in analyzing membrane transport phenomena. Details for each case are described in the text. In these examples, solute species "A" is transported with rates V via several parallel transport pathways. (A) A curvilinear Eadie–Hofstee relationship represents the sum (Σ) of several parallel pathways that can be dissected by nonlinear regression analysis into discrete components; the V_{max} and K_m kinetic parameters of each transporter 1 and transporter 2 are as described in Fig. 3D; the passive diffusion component (D) is revealed as a vertical line with the abcissa intercept equal to the permeability coefficient, P. (B–D) The pathways can be shared by different structural analogs of substrate "A" (e.g., solutes "B", "C", "D"); shown are various inhibitor profile tools that help to discriminate among the shared pathways.

strate is being transported in parallel by more than one transport system.

H. Kinetics of Multiple Pathways

Often, a given nutrient solute is transported by multiple parallel pathways in a membrane. These can be dissected kinetically based on initial flux rates measured over a range of concentrations. The empirical data give a curvilinear Eadie–Hofstee relationship (Fig. 4A), which is fitted directly to the following equation using nonlinear regression analysis. Figure 4A represents an example in which the solute transport occurs via two different carrier-mediated pathways plus simple passive diffusion:

$$V[S] = [(V^1_{max}[S])/([S] + K^1_m)] + [(V^2_{max}[S])/([S] + K^2_m)] + P[S],$$

where the V_{max} and apparent K_m for independent carrier-mediated pathways 1 and 2 are obtained in addition to the passive diffusion permeability coefficient, P. Graphically (Fig. 4A), V_{max} and K_m are obtained as described above, and the diffusional permeability coefficient P is derived from the abcissa intercept of the vertical line representing the nonsaturable component. Based on statistical argumments, it is usually not practical to assess more than two simultaneous carrier pathways plus simple passive diffusion.

I. Strategy for Transporter Substrate Selectivity Assessment

Transporters are fundamentally defined by which substrates they serve. Nutrient transporter selectivity can be narrow, favoring a single isomer, or it can be rather broad, with several nutrient analogs preferred within a selectivity continuum. For example, in the small intestinal enterocyte apical membrane, SGLT1 displays a relatively narrow preference for naturally occurring D-hexose analogs of glucose or galactose (13), whereas the intestinal system B carrier will serve many aliphatic neutral L-amino acids (12).

The following is a method to discriminate substrate selectivity in single carrier-mediated transport systems that each potentially transport several different structural analog substrates with different affinities. Using the following scheme, adapted from Christensen's (14) classical means to discriminate multiple substrates binding to a single binding site, it is possible to confirm that a single transporter is serving one or multiple substrates. If these criteria do not hold, then the conclusion can be drawn that more than one transport system exists in the same membrane to serve the different chemical species of test substrates. This conclusion is not entirely firm, however, because the substrates could conceivably interact at different binding sites—the arguments presented here pertain to the simple case of competitive inhibition for a single binding site according to the standard hyperbolic kinetic model presented above. Furthermore, this analysis assumes pure competitive inhibition among substrates—a reasonable assumption for substrate analogs. Analyses of noncompetitive deviations from this model are beyond the scope of this chapter. Also, other more complicated models that consider microscopic rate constants at each surface of the membrane are not covered in this chapter. The reader is directed elsewhere (4, 9, 13, 15–17) for advanced treatment of complex or alternative models of transport.

The first step to assigning substrate selectivity to a transporter is to quantify initial rates of uptake of solutes (see Fig. 3A) representing a substrate analog series. This must be conducted in the presence and in the absence of activator ions (e.g., Na^+). This will create a relative ranking of substrate uptake activities for sodium-dependent and sodium-independent uptake; the subsequent steps are then repeated for each of the sodium-dependent components and the sodium-independent components of uptake. As discussed above, the passive diffusion component must be subtracted out so that only the carrier-mediated pathway(s) are under consideration. Figure 4B is an example of a useful simple inhibitor ranking based on single inhibitor concentrations with one substrate concentration.

For a more rigorous description of the interaction of inhibitors with a target substrate binding site, it is necessary to vary the inhibitor concentrations. In the case of a single carrier pathway (Fig. 4C), the analogs may show a relative ranking at low concentrations, but at high concentrations, they will completely inhibit the binding site. If a test nurtient solute is served by more than one transporter, in addition to movement via passive diffusion, then a profile such as Fig. 4D arises.

To extend the degree of interactions of analogs with a given transporter, in the next step it is necessary to screen the analogs for cross-competition inhibition at the transporter binding site(s). This is executed by measuring uptake of a relatively low concentration of a given radiolabeled substrate in the presence of a relatively high concentration (10-fold) of unlabled analog compound. Among the battery of substrates that give the most rapid initial uptake rates, the investigator then choses three analogs—A, B, and C—that suggest good inhibition interactions. Each substrate must be available in the radiolabeled and nonlabeled form.

The K_m is determined (described above) for each of the individual radiolabeled substrates A, B, and C. In each case, a single linear relationship should be obtained using the Eadie–Hofstee criteria described above. The K_i competitive inhibition constant is subsequently determined for unlabeled substrate A inhibiting the uptake of labeled substrate B, and vice versa. The apparent K_i is calculated by nonlinear analysis of the relationship $V^S = V^S_{max}[S]/\{K^S_m[(1 + [I]/K_i) + [S]]\}$, where K^S_m is measured for the labeled substrate S (analog A, B, or C) in the absence of inhibitor I (A, B, or C) and substrate rate V^S is obtained with inhibitor. In practice, the K_i can be obtained by employing a Dixon plot of labeled V^S obtained at several fixed concentrations of unlabeled I, as shown in Fig. 5A. For an ideal transporter, the shared solutes should display mutual K_i values. Hence, $K^A_m = K^B_m$; $K^A_{i,B} = K^B_m$; as well as $K^B_{i,A} = K^A_m$. If this does not hold, then a possible interpretation would be that test substrates A and B are transported by entirely different and independent carrier systems. Note that V^A_{max} could equal V^B_{max}, depending on individual microscopic rate constants describing the interaction of each substrate with the binding site(s) (17).

It is entirely possible that the K_i and K_m values of solutes A and B are coincidently the same for two independent carriers, and therefore an additional step is often undertaken to assess interactions with a third substrate analog, C. This is often (but not necessarily) a synthetic nonmetabolizable analog of A and B. The K_i for C inhibiting the uptake of A should therefore be equal to the K_i for C inhibiting the uptake of B. That is, $K^A_{i,C} = K^B_{i,C}$. The V_{max} values for A, B, and C may be similar, but not necessarily, depending on microscopic rate constants (17). If the given criteria hold, it can be concluded that at least one transporter exists in the

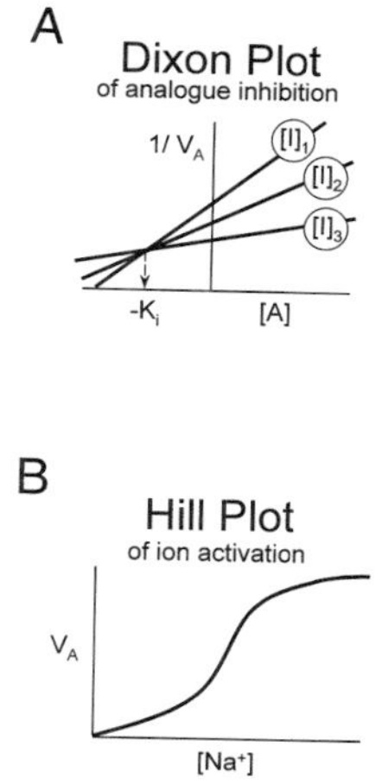

Figure 5 Additional experimental tools useful in analyzing membrane transport phenomena. Each case is described in the text, with solute species "A" transported by rate V. (A) The degree of interaction among solute analogs (e.g., "B", "C", "D") can be quantified by obtaining the K_i for each analog. This parameter is obtained by measuring the uptake kinetics of solute "A" in the presence of at least three fixed concentrations ($[I]_1$, $[I]_2$, $[I]_3$) of a given analog inhibitor; the K_i occurs on a Dixon plot as shown, and is derived mathematicaly as described in the text. (B) Secondary active transport of organic solute "A" can be driven by ion electrochemical gradients. In this example, Na^+ activation of solute "A" transport gives a sigmoid relationship, which is described by the Hill equation. The coupling coefficient is obtained for this activation as described in the text.

membrane that serves A, B, and C with different affinities (Fig. 4C). If single substrate A displays a high affinity surpassing the other substrates, then the transporter system is defined in terms of a "substrate A-preferring" system.

Note that the measurements define uptake function essentially as a black box, and therefore a "transport system" is operationally defined by these means, not a "transporter" protein per se. Assignment as a true transporter protein can occur only if the transport system is characterized in a full-length cloned polypeptide expressed *in vitro* in a membrane (as discussed below).

J. Energy Coupling and Measurement of Ion Coupling Coefficients

Disrupting the coupling of nutrient movement to ion electrochemical gradients can be associated with various pathologic conditions. Thus, it is necessary to assess how the nutrient transporter protein catalyzes the coupling of nutrient movement to ion movement, and to quantiate the relationship between ion electrochemical gradient nutrient transport. One way to assess this is to measure the "coupling coefficient," which is the stoichiometry of ions coupled to each transported nutrient molecule. There are several ways to estimate the coupling coefficient. The most practical laboratory method is to measure initial rates of radiolabeled nutrient transport as a function of activator ion concentration (Fig. 5B). The data are then fit to the Hill equation: $J^S = J^{max}[[Na^+]/(K^S_{0.5} + [Na^+])]^\eta$, for extracellular concentrations of Na^+ at a fixed concentration of nutrient S. The Hill number, η, represents the coupling coefficient (i.e., number of ions that activate nutrient transport in a cotransport system that displays positive cooperativity), and $K^S_{0.5}$ is the concentration of Na^+ that gives the half-maximal rate of nutrient S transport. Often, nutrient transport systems display an $\eta = 2$ or more, indicating that the ratio of nutrient molecule and coupled ions per transport event is at least 2:1.

Another more accurate way to estimate the coupling coefficient is to employ the so-called static head method with membrane vesicle. In practice, this method is not commonly measured because it is considerably more protracted than the Hill activation method. For the static head method, the activator ion gradient conditions are sought whereby net solute flux is zero. Net flux of solute is measured in isolated membrane vesicles (described below) under experimental nonequilibrium conditions with varying membrane voltages experimentally imposed using ions such as potassium with valinomycin ionophore. To employ the static head method, membrane vesicles are first preloaded with sodium gluconate or sodium sulfate [so that the final Na^+ gradient is 1:1 (in:out); assuming that Na^+ is the activator cation], radiolabeled S (at varying gradients of $[S]_i$:$[S]_o$), and also with potassium gluconate or potassium sulfate at fixed in:out ratios to clamp the membrane potential according to the Nernst equation, $\Delta\Psi = (RT/\mathcal{F}) \ln([K]_i/[K]_o)$ (assuming that K^+ does not activate solute transport). The transport rates of radiolabeled nutrient solute are subsequently measured at various clamped $\Delta\Psi$. Under these conditions, the sodium charge stoichiometry equals the coupling coefficient, η, as directly computed from the condition $[S]_i/[S]_o = ([K]_i/[K]_o)^\eta$. A control measurement is made in the absence of Na^+ (by substituting with choline or *N*-methyl-D-glucamine) in order to measure total sodium-independent solute flux. Finally, the actual static head conditions occur at the membrane potential $\Delta\Psi$ that exactly balances the charges carried by the cotransported Na^+. In practical terms, the imposed ratio of $[K]_i/[K]_o$ is experimentally sought that results in a net zero flux of solute (i.e., control). The reader is directed to Turner (9) for additional experimental details.

K. Accumulation of Nutrients Driven by Ion Gradients

The coupling stoichiometry, η, can be used to assess the active accumulation ability of a membrane transport system, according to the rules of nonequilibrium thermodynamics (8). The theoretical maximum concentration gradient of $[S]_i/[S]_o$ driven by Na^+ across a membrane with a potential of $\Delta\Psi$ can be calculated using experimentally obtained values and the following relationship (assuming efficient coupling):

$$[S]_i/[S]_o = [[Na^+]_o/[Na^+]_i \exp(\mathcal{F}\Delta\Psi RT)]^{\eta}$$

IV. Practical Membrane Methods to Assess Solute Transport

A. Single Cell Suspensions

Cells are harvested, counted, assayed for protein, and suspended in appropriate isotonic buffer (about 2×10^7 cells/ml), then preequilibrated at the appropriate uptake temperature. At $t = 0$ an aliquot of cells (25 μl containing about 5×10^5 cells) is mixed with a similar volume of temperature-equilibrated media containing radiolabled substrate and the appropriate activator ion(s) in an Eppendorf tube. Transport in single-cell suspensions can be assayed at room temperature for convenience, or in a 37°C waterbath. The reaction is gently shaken throughout the uptake period. If experience dictates a long incubation period for adequate linear accumulation of substrate (say, 30 min), then an appropriate energy source such as glucose is added to the uptake media. At the designated time point the 50-μl contents are removed and layered on top of 100 μl of a 9:1 (vol:vol) mixture of dibutylphthalate:[phthalic acid-bis(2-ethyl-hexyl ester)] in another 1.8-ml Eppendorf tube. Alternatively, dioctylphthalate or mineral oil could be used instead of the hexyl ester. The tube is immediately centrifuged at full speed for 30 sec, thereby partitioning the cells from radiolabeled media. The liquid layers are aspirated, and 200 μl of 0.5 *N* NaOH is added to the pellet to digest the cells. After several hours of digestion, 250 μl of glacial acetic acid is added to neutralize the NaOH, and an aliquot is sampled for counting of radioactivity in 10 ml of liquid scintillation fluid. Uptake is expressed in units of moles of nutrient taken up per minute per cell, or per milligram of cell protein. Note that in this method, and in all subsequently described methods involving alkaline extraction, the NaOH must be neutralized with acid in order to prevent chemiluminescence of the liquid scintillation fluid.

B. Isolated Plasma Membrane Vesicles

Nutrient transport studies using isolated membrane vesicles offer several advantages over whole tissue or intact cell methods. Most notable is that substrate metabolism is eliminated or reduced. Futhermore, in the case of epithelial cells, the separate events of apical and basolateral transport can be assessed independently. Finally, vesicles offer the experimental advantage of accurately controlling experimental parameters such as transmembrane electrochemical gradients of substrates and cotransported ions, membrane potential, and rapid kinetic manipulations without confounding unstirred layers. As a disadvantage, transport in vesicles examines only membrane phenomena, and thus does not address such *in vivo* parameters as unstirred layer effects, paracellular communication, and regulatory mechanisms and signaling that could influence transporter protein biosynthesis regulation, trafficking, or intracelluar metabolism.

Plasma membranes must be isolated from intracellular organelle membranes, and in the case of epithelial cells, the apical and basolateral membranes are further segregated. The various methods employed in generating membrane vesicles [for a starting point, see Graham and Higgins (6), Findlay and Evans (5), Stevens *et al.* (18), and Stevens and Preston (19)] focus on the means to break open and homogenize the cell components to prevent cross-contamination of intracellular organelle membranes and plasma membrane(s). Ideally, the cell should be disrupted to release physically separated membranes. Commonly employed disruption techniques include (1) osmotic lysis of water-swelled cells, (2) mechanical disruption by glass–glass or glass–Teflon homogenization, (3) rupture of cells by explosive N_2 cavitation employing equilibration with gas followed by sudden release of pressure, sonication, or French press rupture of cells, and (4) Polytron homogenation. The Polytron method appears to be the most practical in preparing plasma membranes, because such homogenization actually combines microsonication and mechanical shearing. Once the cell is disrupted, the membranes are isolated and purified by any number of techniques such as differential centrifugation, density gradient centrifugation, isoelectric focusing, and differential precipitation with divalent cations, or by partitioning with agents such as Percoll. Finally, the isolated membrane fraction must be assessed for purity. This is usually assessed by enzymatic markers, and occasionally electron microscopic examination is required to verify such morphological features as brush borders and inside-out vs right-side out orientation.

The following general plan uses a Polytron to generate and assess apical membrane vesicles from epithelial cells. The reader is directed elsewhere for similar recipes pertaining to preparing plasma membrane vesicles in nonepithelial cells, and for preparing basolateral membranes from epithelial cells (5, 6). In many cases, membrane vesicles can be freshly prepared immediately prior to use. Also presented here is a procedure for storing large quantities of prepared membranes in liquid nitrogen for extensive experiments. This apical membrane preparation concerns small intestinal enterocyte cell membranes, but the procedure has been successfully adapted to virtually any type of epithelium.

First, epithelial cells are gathered, usually by scraping the epithelium from the underlying basement layer with a glass slide. Pooling frozen cells can be employed, although transport activity is often slightly more robust in vesicles prepared from freshly isolated cells. The cells are homogenized for 15 sec in ice-cold buffer containing 300 m*M* mannitol in 1 m*M* HEPES/Tris, pH 7.5, using a Polytron-type homogenizer. The homogenates are pooled in a beaker, and a small aliquot (2 ml) is stored for marker enzyme and protein assays (explained below), while the remaining material is slowly added to concentrated 100 m*M* $MgCl_2$ with gentle stirring to give a final homogenate concentration of 10 m*M* $MgCl_2$. This is stirred for 20 min (4°C). The suspension is centrifuged in 50-ml centrifuge tubes at 1500 *g* (3500 rpm in a Sorvall SS-34 rotor) for 5 min. The loose pellet (containing basolateral and organell membranes) is discarded, and the supernatant is collected and centrifuged again at 1500 *g* for 5 min. The second supernatant is then collected (avoiding the small pellet) and centrifuged in 50-ml polycarbonate centrifuge tubes at 45,000 *g* for 45 min (19,500 rpm using a Sorvall SS-34 rotor). This high-speed supernatant is discarded, and the pellet (containing apical membranes) is washed by adding to a large volume (25 ml) of a buffer appropriate for the final transport assay—often 300 m*M* mannitol in 10 m*M* HEPES/Tris buffer, pH 7.5. Other media containing activator ions, nonradioactive nutrient substrates, or various pH buffers can be used to resuspend the vesicles, depending on the final intended experiment. The washed membranes are then centrifuged again at 45,000 *g* for 45 min, and the final apical membrane-containing pellet is resuspended in the buffer appropriate for the final experiment (e.g., 300 m*M* mannitol in 10 m*M* HEPES/Tris, pH 7.5). The volume of this resuspension is adjusted to give a final membrane protein concentration of about 10–20 mg/ml (assessed by a Lowry protein assay). Resuspension and vesiculation of the final pellet is executed by slowly drawing the membrane suspension several times through a 20- to 22-gauge syringe needle at 22°C. The resulting vesicle diameter is about 100 nm. The membrane vesicles are subsequently cooled on ice for immediate use, or frozen in liquid nitrogen for indefinite storage. The reader is directed elsewhere (18, 19) for references for liquid nitrogen storage.

To ensure that *bona fide* apical membranes are in the final pellet, marker enzyme specific activities are assayed. This involves also measuring the protein concentrations of the orginal homogenate and the final membrane suspension to calculate specific activities. In general, apical membranes of epithelial cells from many organ sources possess at least alkaline phosphatase (assayed as *p*-nitrophenyl phosphatase; EC 3.1.3.1), 5′-nucleosidase, and aminopeptidase N. To confirm the absence of basolateral contamination, the preparation must be tested for negative purification of ouabain-sensitive Na,K-ATPase activity. The Na,K-ATPase activity is localized to basolateral membranes in all known epithelia except choroid plexus, wherein it exists on the apical membrane. Of course, other tissue-specific membrane markers can be employed, depending on the organ of origin. Both the initial homogenate (see above) and the final membrane suspension are assayed for these enzymes. In general, apical membrane marker enzyme specific activities are enriched 10- to 20-fold over the crude homogenate, whereas the Na,K ATPase specific activities are generally decreased compared to the homogenate. The reader is directed elsewhere (5, 6) for these assays. In addition to apical membrane preparations, basolateral membranes can be prepared for similar vesicle uptake studies (5, 6).

C. Uptake in in Vitro Monolayers Grown on Plastic

Measuring unidirectional uptake into *in vitro* monolayers grown on plastic is essentially the same procedure regardless of the cell type, and thus the following protocol can be applied to most monolayers. However, epithelial cells can undergo apical and basolateral membrane differentiation during the formation of the monolayer, and thus this must be considered when growing these cells. The following description of uptake uses monolayers on plastic, exemplified by the Caco-2 human intestinal epithelial cell line. This cell line was originally obtained from a human intestinal adenocarcinoma, and is a useful *in vitro* model for nutrient transport studies of the intact small intestinal epithelium (20). Differention in these cells is controlled by passaging the cells, which spontaneously undergo enterocytic differentiation as they age (12). Generally, cells grown longer than 14 days are considered differentiated, and if grown before 3 days they are considered undifferentiated. The reader is directed to other suitable *in vitro* models of transporting epithelia (21).

Caco-2 cells should be initially obtained from early passages from the American Type Culture Collection. Established Caco-2 stocks are stored in liquid nitrogen or harvested from 100-mm tissue culture dishes (Falcon type 3003) containing 15 ml of Dulbecco's modified Eagle's medium (DMEM) with additives. Cells are grown in a humidified incubator at 37°C in 10% CO_2/90% O_2. The day of seeding is designated as day 0. Caco-2 cells are subcultured by washing with 37°C isotonic calcium-free saline solution containing 0.05% trypsin and 0.02% EDTA, and flooding the dish with 10 ml of the same solution for 5 min. This dissociation fomula appears to be critical. The cell/trypsin mixture is dispersed with a narrow-tip glass pipette, then added to DMEM containing 10% FBS. The dispersed cells are sedimented in a sterile conical centrifuge tube at 1000 *g* for 5 min, and the supernatant is removed. Next, growth medium is added to resuspend the cells (using a narrow-tip glass pipette) until cells are separated. Cell clumps are allowed to settle for a few minutes at 1 *g*, and only the top layer of medium containing single cells is used for subculturing, as confirmed by phase-contrast microscope examination. Cells derived from log-phase growth stocks are seeded in the six-well cluster tissue culture dishes (Falcon type 3046) at a density of 4 × 10^5 cells (in 2 ml) per 35-mm well for transport experiments. The growth medium must be changed daily, and cultures are inspected daily using a phase-contrast microscope to avoid dome formation and contamination by foreign cells such as fibroblasts.

Substrate uptake can be measured in cells 3 days postseeding (undifferentiated state) through 14 days days postseeding (enterocytic differentiated state). At the stated plating density, cultures generally attain confluence by about day 6. Studies designed to compare transport in cells at day 3 postseeding and day 14 postseeding, are conducted using cells started from the same seeding parent cells. Following pretreatment of cells with any desired agents (e.g., growth factors), the medium is aspirated and cells are rinsed three times (23°C) with an appropriate uptake buffer such as 137 m*M* choline chloride, 10 m*M* HEPES/Tris buffer (pH 7.4), 4.7 m*M* KCl, 1.2 m*M* $MgSO_4$, 1.2 m*M* KH_2PO_4, and 2.5 m*M* $CaCl_2$. The uptake is initiated by adding 1 ml of uptake buffer containing 0.5 μ*M* to 1 m*M* unlabeled substrate spiked with L-[^{3}H]-labeled substrate (5 μCi/ml). It is a good general practice to prepare radiolabeled amino acids by first drying aliquots in a stream of nitrogen gas or by using a speed-vac, in order to reduce ^3H_2O present as a common contaminant in the radiolabeled stock. During the uptake time period, culture dishes are continuously shaken by an orbital shaker (about 1 Hz) during the uptake period. At the designated time point, uptake is arrested by aspirating the labeled uptake buffer, then quickly washing three times with ice-cold buffer lacking substrate. Radioactivity of isotope is extracted from the cells by adding 1 ml of 1 *N* NaOH to the washed, aspirated monolayer. After 12 hr, a 200-μl aliquot of the NaOH digest is neutralized with 250 μl of acetic acid, then assayed by liquid scintillation spectrometry. Cell protein in the remaining portion of the NaOH extract is measured using the Bio-Rad protein assay. The specific activity of radiolabeled substrate is measured by sampling 5 μl of labeled uptake media and processing it with NaOH and acetic acid as per the cell digests. Initial rates of transport activity are determined during the linear uptake period, which is generally about 2 min, with additional points obtained at zero time to serve as blanks. As discussed above, it is critical that a complete time course is obtained for each radiolabeled substrate tested, in order to validate the *a priori* assumptions for kinetic analyses. Uptake rates are expressed as moles of substrate per minute per milligram of cell protein.

D. Monolayer Transport Using Porous Filters

In confluent monolayers the rates of transepithelial apical-to-basal or basal-to-apical transport, as well as basal-to-cell and apical-to-cell substrate accumulation, can be measured. This permits assessment of net transepithelial transport or unidirectional movement in a given membrane. The cells are cultured on 3.0-μm pore size 24-mm Transwell-COL-treated microporous polycarbonate membrane filters coated with bovine placenta collagen (Costar), which are inserted in six-well tissue culture dishes (Falcon type 3046). Cells derived from log-phase growth stocks are seeded at a density of 2 × 10^5 cells/ml.

The cells grown on porous filters are allowed to reach confluency, and are stable and useful for up to 20 days. Transport is measured in monolayers that reach a confluent state with tight junctions giving transepithelial electrical resistances ≥300 Ω · cm^2, as measured using an open-circuit potential difference apparatus (World Precision Instrument Inc.). Immediately preceding the uptake measurements, the growth media in the upper and lower chambers are aspirated, and the cells are rinsed three times with uptake buffer containing sodium or choline uptake buffer (described above). Apical → cell amino acid accumulation is initiated by adding uptake buffer containing [^{3}H]-labeled substrate into the upper chamber bathing the apical surface, with the basolateral side (lower chamber) exposed to 3 ml of uptake buffer lacking amino acid. During the uptake period, the cell cultures are continuously shaken by an orbital shaker (1 Hz). Uptake is arrested by aspirating the upper chamber buffer and washing the filter three times with ice-cold uptake buffer. Filters are cut out with a scalpel, and isotope trapped inside the cells is extracted by gently shaking overnight with 2 ml of 1 *N* NaOH. A 200-μl aliquot of NaOH extract is added to 10 ml of scintillation fluid after neutralizing with 250 μl of glacial acetic acid. Isotope trapped in the lower chamber is also measured. Basolateral surface → cell accumulation is measured in a similar manner, with uptake buffer containing [^{3}H]-labeled substrate initiated in the lower chamber.

Apical → basal and basal → apical transcellular amino acid movement across the monolayer is measured by adding uptake buffer with [^{3}H]-labeled substrate to the upper or lower chamber at $t = 0$, and subsequently immersing the filter into 3 ml of buffer (lacking substrate) in the lower chamber at various times. Uptake is stopped by removing filters from the chamber. The isotope accumulated in either the upper or lower chamber buffer is then measured.

E. In Vitro Expression of Cloned Nutrient Transporters in Ooctyes

The expression of heterologous mammalian transporter proteins in *Xenopus laevis* oocytes is a powerful way to investigate cloned transporters (Fig. 6) The oocytes can be used either for "expression cloning" of individual transporter cDNAs, or for measuring the membrane mechanistic properties of functional transporter proteins encoded by cDNA obtained by other means.

Expression cloning is conducted by one of several means (Fig. 6A). The first method concerns using isolated fractions

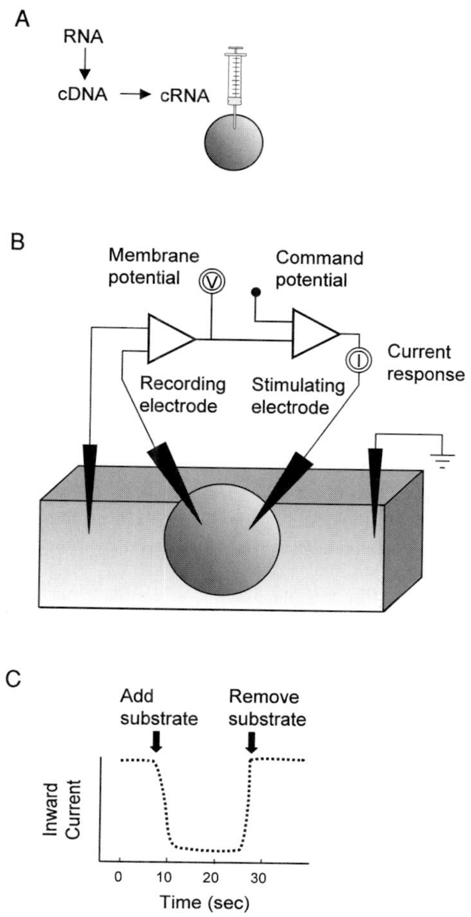

Figure 6 *Xenopus oocyte in vitro* expression of heterologous membrane transporters. (A) Transporter activity derived from mammalian cells can be encoded by a variety of methods, including fractions of RNA or cDNA. Expression of full-length cDNA clones is obtained by preparing the cRNA. In all cases, the appropriate nucleic acid is injected into stages V–VI oocytes in a 50-nl bolus of water. (B) A two-electrode voltage clamp circuit used to assess rheogenic solute transport in an oocyte expressing a heterologous transporter protein. Movement of charge associated with rheogenic solute transport is detected as a change in the transmembrane current. (C) Example of a recording made using the rig described above. Transport can be measured in oocytes expressing nonnative transporter proteins in the membrane. In this example, steady-state inward current (generally in the magnitude of nanoamps) represents solute transporter activity. Rapid (milli- and microsecond) pre-steady-state measurements are also useful in describing the transport mechanism (see text).

of poly(A^+) mRNA obtained from cells that naturally display the nutrient transport phenomenon. The second technique involves injecting selected cDNA obtained from the reverse-transcribed RNA of a mammalian cell that displays functional transport properties. Oocytes are also useful for characterizing clones obtained by means other than expression cloning (7, 22).

Once a putative transporter has been cloned, it is absolutely necessary to characterize the expression product in a membrane to verify that the transport characteristics represent those observed in the native membrane. The expression product is the transcribed cRNA translated into polypeptide properly trafficked to the plasma membrane of *Xenopus* oocytes.

To utilize the oocyte expression system, plasmids containing an appropriate promoter with the full-length putative transporter cDNA are linearized by digestion with the appropriate restriction enzyme. Capped complementary RNA (cRNA) is synthesized *in vitro* by exploiting the appropriate RNA polymerase promoter (e.g., T3) with an mMessage Machine kit (Ambion). *Xenopus laevis* oocytes at stages V–VI are then prepared by standard techniques employing collagenase dissociation and defolliculation (7). Selected oocytes (with uniform color in the animal hemisphere) are injected with 50 ng of the purified target cRNA in a volume of 50 nl of water, delivered via a positive-displacement microinjector. Water-injected oocytes served as controls. Injected oocytes are incubated at 17°C in Barth's saline containing penicillin and streptomycin for 2–5 days, then stored at 14°C up to 10 days before recording. Once the oocytes express transporter protein on the plasma membrane, uptake can then be assessed by either radiolabeled uptake or by electrophysiological means (22).

F. Radiolabled Uptake in Oocytes

Routine transport is measured using modified "ND96" media (96 m*M* NaCl, 2 m*M* KCl, 1 m*M* $MgCl_2$, 1 m*M* $CaCl_2$, 10 m*M* HEPES/Tris, pH 7.5). For radiotracer experiments, the uptake media also contain 5 μCi/ml [^{3}H]-labeled L-amino acids. Uptake experiments are conducted using commonly accepted techniques (7, 13). After exposing oocytes (3–10 per assay) to radiolabeled uptake media in an Eppendorf tube with occasional gentle inversion, the medium is aspirated, and cells are washed three times in ice-cold PBS, solubilized in 0.5 ml 1% SDS, and then assayed for radioactivity in 10 ml of Cytoscint. Initial linear rates of [^{3}H]-labeled L-amino acid uptake can be measured at 22°C during a 30-min interval. Zero time blanks are also executed. Uptake kinetic experiments are executed as described above.

G. Rheogenic Transport in Oocytes

Nutrient transport is often a rheogenic event (current carrying), as described above. This phenomenon can be exploited by measuring transport using electrophysiologic means. For such experiments, oocytes (injected and incubated with cRNA, and expressing transport activity) are placed into a perfusion chamber (0.6-ml volume) and superperfused with media at a rate of about 3 ml/min using a peristaltic pump. Where it is necessary to study possible co- or countertransport of ions, ionic substitutions are with either *N*-methyl-D-glucamine or choline to replace Na^+ or K^+, or with either gluconate or methane sulfonate substitution for Cl^-. Transmembrane inwardly or outwardly directed currents are measured in intact oocytes using a two-electrode voltage clamp (Warner model OC725-B) with agar-bridged bath electrodes, with one configuration described in Fig. 6B. The reader is directed elsewhere for details regarding electrophysiologic measurement techniques and interpretation (4, 7, 13, 22, 23). Uptake (current) is measured under steady-state conditions with this setup (Fig. 6C), and thus data are acquired at modest sampling rates (8 Hz with digitization at 20 Hz) and analyzed with appropriate software such as pClamp. Current–voltage relations are generated using voltage steps or ramps between −100 and +50 mV from a given holding potential (usually −60 mV). Pre-steady-state kinetics can also be assessed (13), but their interpretation is beyond the scope of this chapter. Substrate-dependent currents are obtained by subtracting out control current values measured in the absence of substrate. Endogenous currents (constitutive or elicited by substrates) in water-injected control oocytes are also measured in each batch of injected oocytes, but the values can often be neglected because they are often <1% of target cRNA-associated current values.

V. Conclusions

Nutrient transport can be easily measured by applying the described set of basic tools in a variety of cell types, ranging from *in vitro* single-cell suspensions to *in vivo* preparations. The transport of nutrients obeys the thermodynamic and kinetic rules of general solute movement across a membrane, and thus the described tools exploit these physical and physiologic events to yield meaningful data. Nutrient transport data can describe normal physiologic events of cells and tissues, and are especially useful in describing the physiologic events in the body responding to surgical interventions.

This chapter has provided descriptions and recipes to choose the appropriate model system to investigate nutrient transport events, and has compared and contrasted the menu of tools used to quantify and evaluate data. The importance of investigating solute transport is reflected in the rapid pace of reported discoveries in the literature. Cloning and characterizing new transporters is an especially exciting field in basic biomedical physiology, and the time is ripe to approach nutrient transport from a surgical perspective.

References

1. Griffith, J. E., and Sanson, C. E. (1998). "The Transporter Facts Book." Academic Press, San Diego.
2. Hirsch, D., Stahl, A., and Lodish, H. F. (1998). A family of fatty acid transporters conserved from mycobacterium to man. *Proc. Natl. Acad. Sci. U.S.A.* **95**(15), 8625–8629.
3. Andreoli, T. E., Hoffman, J. F., Fanestil, D. D., and Schultz, S. G. (1986). "Membrane Transport Processes in Organized Systems." Plenum Publishing, New York.
4. Van Winkle, L. J. (1999). "Biomembrane Transport." Acdemic Press, San Diego.
5. Findlay, J. B. C., and Evans, W. H. (1987). "Biological Membranes: A Practical Approach." IRL Press, Oxford.
6. Graham, J., and Higgins, J. (1993). "Methods in Molecular Biology. Biomembrane Protocols. I. Isolation and Analysis," Vol. 19. Humana Press, Totowa, New Jersey.
7. Gould, G. W. (1994). "Membrane Protein Expression Systems. A User's Guide." Portland Press, London.
8. Gerencser, G. A., and Stevens, B. R. (1994). Thermodynamics of symport and antiport catalyzed by cloned or native transporters. *J. Exp. Biol.* **196,** 59–75.
9. Turner, R. J. (1990). Stoichiometry of coupled transport systems in vesicles. *Methods Enzymol.* **191,** 479–494.
10. Byrne, J. H. and Schultz, S. G. (1994). "An Introduction to Membrane Transport and Bioelectricity," 2nd Ed. Raven Press, New York.
11. Stevens, B. R., Kaunitz, J. D., and Wright, E. M. (1984). Intestinal transport of amino acids and sugars: Advances using membrane vesicles. *Annu. Rev. Physiol.* **46,** 417–433.
12. Pan, M., and Stevens, B. R. (1995). Differentiation- and protein kinase C-dependent regulation of alanine transport via system B. *J. Biol. Chem.* **270,** 3582–3587.
13. Wright, E. M., Loo, D. D., Panayotova-Heiermann, M., Hirayama, B. A., Turk, E., Eskandari, S., and Lam, J. T. (1998). Structure and function of the Na^+/glucose cotransporter. *Acta Physiol. Scand. Suppl.* **643,** 257–264.
14. Christensen, H. N. (1985). On the strategy of kinetic discrimination of amino acid transport systems. *J. Membr. Biol.* **84,** 97–103.
15. Stevens, B. R. (1992). Amino acid transport in intestine. *In* "Mammalian Amino Acid Transport: Mechanisms and Control" (M.S. Kilberg and D. Haussinger, eds.), pp. 149–164. Plenum, New York.
16. Stevens, B. R. (1992). Vertebrate intestine apical membrane mechanisms of organic nutrient transport. *Am. J. Physiol.* **263,** R458–R463.
17. Segal, I. H. (1975). "Enzyme Kinetics." Wiley, New York.
18. Stevens, B. R., Fernandez, A., Hirayama, B., Wright, E. M., and Kempner, E. S. (1990). Intestinal brush border membrane Na^+/glucose cotransporter functions *in situ* as a homotetramer. *Proc. Natl. Acad. Sci. U.S.A.* **87,** 1456–1460.
19. Stevens, B. R., and Preston, R. L. (1998). Sodium-dependent amino acid transport is preserved in lyophilized reconstituted apical membranes from intestinal epithelium. *Anal. Biochem.* **265,** 117–122.
20. Souba, W. W., Pan, M., and Stevens, B. R. (1992). Kinetics of the sodium-dependent glutamine transporter in human intestinal cell confluent monolayers. *Biochem. Biophys. Res. Commun.* **188,** 746–753.
21. Smith, M. W., and Sepulveda, F. V. (1989). "Adaptation and Development of Gastrointestinal Function." Manchester University Press, Manchester UK.
22. Feldman, D., Harvey, W., and Stevens, B. R. (2000). A novel electrogenic amino acid transporter is activated by K^+ or Na^+, is alkaline pH-dependent and is Cl^--independent. *J. Biol. Chem.* **275,** 24518–24526.
23. Stuhmer, W. (1992). *In* "Methods in Enzymology," Vol. 207 (R. Bernardo and L.E. Iverson, eds.), pp. 319–339. Academic Press, San Diego.

62

Models of Wound Healing in Growth Factor Studies

Alexandrina Saulis and Thomas A. Mustoe

Division of Plastic and Reconstructive Surgery, Northwestern University Medical School, Chicago, Illinois 60611

I. Introduction

Wounds occur in all living creatures. A wound epitomizes the natural process of breakdown, and an organism's ability to heal a wound is evidence of its complexity and resilience. A malfunction in this intricately balanced process results in abnormal healing. Multiple phases of wound healing have been described, and further research continues to identify undefined aspects of this process, focusing at the molecular level. The force driving research in this field stems from the clinical problem. *In vitro* experiments will always have limitations, and so there is a need for animal models that relate to the clinical problem.

Human wounds can be categorized into three groups. The *acute* wound is defined as a discrete injury followed by a relatively rapid healing phase. Examples include surgical incisions or excisions. In contrast, the *chronic* wound is one that develops either quickly or over a longer period of time, and is characterized by a significant temporal delay in the healing process, usually greater than 2 months. Often the delay in healing is a result of a compromised healing environment. These wounds are then identified as *compromised* wounds. The majority of chronic wounds are compromised wounds and in most cases research has identified the compromise leading to the chronic wound. Perhaps 90% of chronic wounds result from pressure, diabetes, or venous stasis (1). These are all compromised healing environments, as a result of aging and its attendant slower healing rates, resulting in chronic wounds. The identification of the etiologies of chronic wounds alone has, for the most part, not aided us in accelerating the delayed healing process. The need for therapeutic intervention is evident.

Animal models play a critical role in the development of biological therapeutics pertinent to wound healing. They allow testing of a therapy's efficacy and safety in a living model prior to its use in humans. It is important that the model and experimental protocol chosen allow for controlled, reproducible, and quantifiable experimentation. Only under these circumstances can the results be considered valid and subsequently applied to human subjects (2).

Despite the accumulated knowledge of grouped cellular events that occur in wound healing, many of the intricate processes remain unknown. With recent advances in molecular and cellular biology, wound healing can now be studied from an intracellular perspective. The future of wound healing studies lies in therapeutics aimed at specific intracellular and nuclear mechanisms. The study of growth factors and other signaling molecules in wound healing focuses on these cellular/nuclear mechanisms. Ideally, the ability to manipulate the activating factors in this balanced process will allow acceleration or deceleration of the process as needed to reverse abnormal wound healing. Investigations into this aspect of wound healing often combine *in vivo* studies with *in vitro* studies to facilitate investigation at this minute level.

We focus on examples of animal models representing different types of wounds. This will by no means include all existing models, but rather includes the models seen more frequently through the literature and those in which growth factor studies have been undertaken. The positives and negatives in each model will be addressed as well as the model's potential application to the study of growth factors in wound healing. Current methods of quantification of wound healing in these animal models are also addressed. Methods range from direct analysis of actual wound size or tensile strength to more indirect methods such as quantifiying mRNA expression of genes whose products are involved in wound healing.

II. Types of Wounds—Animal Models

A. Acute Wound Models

The simplest of all models, the acute wound model was used by a number of investigators at the beginning of the century to identify the different stages of wound healing (3, 4). Acute wounds were created and were found to heal at normal rates unless in a compromised wound environment. Three main types of acute wounds studied have been incisional wounds, excisional wounds, and burn wounds.

1. Incisional Wounds

Incisional wound models are comparable to surgical wounds. Technically easy to reproduce, these wounds can be performed on practically every type of animal. Healing occurs by reepithelialization within 1–2 days after wounding if edges are reapproximated primarily, but tensile strength increases for several months. This is generally consistent among species (5). In contrast, incisional wounds left to heal by secondary intention will gape. The amount of gape depends on the species used and is associated with the amount of subcutaneous tissue, tensional forces on the wound, and adherence of the dermis to underlying structures. A large gape will be produced in loose-skinned animals such as rodents, guinea pigs, and rabbits, whereas pigs, like humans, will exhibit less gaping due to underlying attachments of the dermis. In general, wounds left to heal by secondary intention will result in increased scarring due to the prolonged inflammation and to the time to complete reepithelialization (6).

The majority of studies of wound healing use incisional models with primary closure. Examples range from full-thickness incisional models assessing wound tensile strength and rate of healing, dating back to the 1920s (7), to more current studies evaluating the efficacy of added growth factors or neutralizing antibodies to growth factors in incisional wounds (8). This easily reproducible and controlled model allows for the manipulation of other aspects of wound healing. Incisional models are often combined with compromised wound environments in an attempt to recreate complicated wounds found in human subjects.

An important factor is the enormous variability in wound healing within incisions, and among different animals, even of the same age, weight, and similar genetic makeup. We have found that paired incisions in the same animal allow reproducible results with 8 to 10 animals per variable being tested, with standard deviations 30% of the mean. If unpaired comparisons are made between different animals, we cannot be confident of the results with less than 30–40 animals with even the simplest incisions. The complexity and variability of wound healing are frequently not comprehended by readers of the many published studies.

Incisional wounds can easily be used to analyze the role of growth factors in wound healing. Ideally, each animal should have both treated and nontreated (control) incisions for direct comparison. Application of the growth factor or antibody should be directly into the dermis by injection within 1 mm of the incision, because the majority of wound healing activity is thought to be limited to this area in normal healing (9). The timing and number of applications, as well as doses applied, need to be taken into account. The point of final analysis also needs to be considered, because the phases of wound healing, even in simple incisional wounds, are spread out over a prolonged period with different crucial events occurring at specific time points (10).

These wounds are ideal for biomechanical analysis of wound strength, and also suitable for histological and immunohistological studies. Molecular biological evaluation is limited by the small amount of tissue directly involved, but careful preservation of the incised area may allow for these analyses. It is often difficult, if not impossible, to separate the wound from the surrounding normal tissue.

2. Excisional Wounds

Excisional wounds can be either partial thickness or full thickness. Both involve the removal of tissue, resulting in a tissue defect. Partial-thickness wounds involve removal of the epidermis and papillary layer of dermis. Left behind is the reticular dermal layer and bases of most epidermal appendages. Reepithelialization is rapid in these wounds and occurs both from the wound edges and from the epidermal appendages. In contrast, full-thickness wounds involve removal of the entire dermis to subcutaneous fat, underlying fascia or cartilage. Healing of these wounds combines wound contraction, granulation tissue formation, and reepithelialization from the wound edges.

Excisional wound defects are generally optimal for producing enough wound tissue to allow for molecular/cellular biological studies, as well as histological studies, to quantify wound healing. Additionally, excisional wounds may be covered with an occlusive dressing, allowing for analyses of soluble factors and cells in the retained wound fluid.

a. The Partial-Thickness Model Pigs are often used in wound studies involving partial-thickness wounds because their skin is similar to human skin in a number of ways. Similarities are a sparse hair coat, a thick epidermis, a dermis with a well-differentiated papillary body, and large elastic tissue content. Furthermore, the kinetics of epidermal proliferation are reported to be similar in pig skin and human skin (11). Partial-thickness wounds are generally created with a dermatome. Appropriate dermatome settings depend on the thickness of the skin, which can vary at different locations on the animal. This variable may be minimized by using same-species animals of the same age and weight and wounding similar sites.

Breuing *et al.* (12) have described a partial-thickness porcine wound model. The wounds are created using a dermatome and multiple wounds can be placed on one animal, allowing for both treatment and control wounds. Quantification of wound healing is done using a sealed vinyl chamber completely covering the wound. This allows monitoring of wound repair through analysis of the collected wound fluid. These investigators used the sealed vinyl chamber to quantify peak levels of various growth factors temporally in partial-thickness wounds. They also used the chamber as a vehicle for delivery of growth factors to the partial-thickness wound surface (12). The outcome measured in the latter experiment was the rate of reepithelialization based on return of wound fluid protein levels back to nonwounded skin protein levels.

b. The Full-Thickness Model These wounds consist of complete removal of the epidermis and dermis. This type of wound can be created using a dermatome, punch biopsy, or scalpel. The depth of the wound is once again dependent on the type of animal used and its skin thickness. Difficulties with this model include more bleeding with wounding and a higher susceptibility to infection due to complete disruption of the protective epidermal/dermal layer. Advantages of this model are involvement of all dermal layers, reepithelialization only from the wound edges, and sufficient tissue to allow for many quantitative studies to assess wound healing.

Healing of full-thickness wounds occurs from the periphery of the wound. A fibrin clot is formed and is replaced initially by granulation tissue and later by migrating epithelium from the wound margins. This process is accelerated by wound contraction, in which wound fibroblasts assume some characteristics of smooth muscle cells, induce contraction of the granulation tissue, and result in a subsequent decrease in wound dimensions (13). Loose-skinned animals may close 90% of their wound area by contraction (14). In contrast, wound contraction contributes only 25–50% of total wound closure in humans (15). To simulate human wounds, wound contraction in animals can be minimized by physical splinting of the wound with foreign materials, or by use of a tight-skinned animal such as a pig as opposed to a loose-skinned animal such as a rabbit or rat. Localizing the wounds to an area with skin that is adherent to underlying structures is another way to avoid wound contraction. The rabbit ear wound model exhibits minimal wound contraction because the dermis on the inner surface of the rabbit ear is tightly adherent to the underlying cartilage. A full-thickness wound in this area heals greater than 90% by the production of granulation tissue and epithelial migration from the wound periphery. This model has been used by our laboratory to analyze cellular and extracellular events selectively in full-thickness wounds with minimal interference of wound contraction (16). It has also been useful in consistently producing scars histologically similar to human hypertrophic scars. The delay in wound reepithelialization, as a result of limited wound contraction, results in excessive granulation tissue production and a hypertrophic scar after complete reepithelialization (17). The wounds are easily reproducible, produce sufficient tissue for wound healing quantification, and also allow for topical delivery of exogenous growth factors to the wound site (18, 19).

3. Burn Wounds

A number of burn wound animal models have been developed for testing of treatment variables such as types of dressings used, infection control, and timing of debridement and skin grafting (20). Inflicted burns can vary between superficial and full-thickness. Superficial burns involve only the epidermal layer. Partial-thickness burns involve damage of the epidermis and part of the dermis, leaving the bases of hair follicles and apocrine glands intact. Healing occurs through reepithelialization from the wound edges and the remaining dermal appendages. Full-thickness burns involve the epidermis and the entire dermis and, like full-thickness excisional wounds, healing involves the triad of granulation tissue formation, wound contraction, and reepithelialization from the wound edge.

Partial-thickness and full-thickness burns can be inflicted using a heated metal object made of a highly conductive metal such as brass or aluminum. To obtain uniform burn wounds in animals, the temperature of the metal object, the amount of pressure applied, and the length of time applied must be kept constant among the wounds created. Because burn injuries evolve over a period of 1–2 days after injury, the depth of the burn should be confirmed histologically at a delayed time point (21).

Kaufman *et al.* (22) describe partial-thickness and full-thickness burn wounds inflicted in guinea pigs. Aluminum templates were heated to 60°C and applied to moistened, clipped, and depilated dorsal skin using minimal hand pressure for 5 sec to obtain partial-thickness burns. The same templates heated to 75°C and applied for 5 sec created full-thickness burns. Burn depth was confirmed with histologic sections at 24 and 36 hr postinjury (22). Using this protocol, burns wounds are easily created and consistent in depth. As a model, guinea pigs are inexpensive to obtain and keep, but only two wounds can be placed on each animal.

Danilenko *et al.* (23) describe a similar protocol for partial-thickness and full-thickness burn wounds in a porcine model. Partial-thickness burns were produced applying 2.5-cm-diameter brass bars heated to 100°C to clipped and scrubbed dorsal pig skin for 20 sec at 2000 *g* pressure. Full-thickness burns were created by applying similar bars, heated to 150°C, to dorsal skin for 20 sec at 1500 *g* pressure. Depth of injury was assessed on days 2, 3, and 4 postburn, using Masson's trichrome stain and immunohistochemical staining for PCNA, to determine depth of collagen denaturation and cell viability, respectively. These investigators inflicted 20 burn wounds per animal (23). In comparison to other burn wound models, the porcine model, as described, exhibits kinetics similar to that of human skin (11), a reproducible burn injury, and allows for numerous wounds per animal.

B. Models of Delayed Healing

In contrast to acute wounds, which are easily reproduced in animal models, models of delayed healing that are more relevant to human chronic wounds require manipulation of the normal wound healing environment seen in domestic and laboratory animals. Chronic wounds do not occur normally in animals, and thus all animal models have limitations. The goal of an animal model is to simulate the wound environment in a human chronic wound, defined as wounds with a delay or halt in the healing process. Human chronic wounds have a number of primary etiologies, often occurring in conjunction with secondary etiologies, resulting in a number of variables that need to be recreated and also controlled for in the specific animal model used. At the primary level, it should be recognized that animal cutaneous anatomy differs considerably from that of human skin, with the exception of perhaps the pig model. Pig skin differs significantly in thickness and biomechanical properties, and open wounds heal substantially by wound contraction unless they are large. Furthermore, the skin changes seen with human aging are a variable almost impossible to control for or recreate in an animal model. The majority of chronic wounds in humans appear to be associated with local ischemia, aging, and pressure. Animal models of these three conditions plus a specific chronic wound model simulating human lower extremity wounds will be discussed in this section.

1. Ischemic Wounds

Reduced tissue perfusion, ischemia–reperfusion injury, or the inability of peripheral tissues to utilize oxygen are perhaps the most significant factors contributing to human chronic wounds. Hypoxic tissue conditions have been associated with an increase in vascular permeability and leukocyte trapping within capillaries, followed by a release of proteolytic enzymes and free radicals, resulting in tissue destruction (24). Additional studies have revealed the importance of molecular oxygen in the posttranslational hydroxylation of proline and lysine residues required for triple helix formation and cross-linking of collagen fibrils in collagen. This step is halted when tissue pO_2 falls below 30 mmHg (25, 26). The lack of oxygen at the molecular level plays a critical role in delayed healing seen in ischemic wounds. Models have been created in different animal species in an attempt to recreate a human hypoxic wound. Models of this nature allow investigators to assess treatments such as hyperbaric oxygen or growth factors in ischemic wounds.

All ischemic models require surgical interruption of the vascular supply to the area to be tested in the animal. Earlier models rendered an entire limb ischemic for studies (27). These models required extensive surgical dissection with ligation of multiple vessels and were time consuming and difficult to reproduce. Current models elegantly localize the ischemia to a small area to be tested and are technically easier to create.

Quirinia *et al.* (28) described a random H-shaped flap as a model for ischemia. The flaps are placed on the dorsum of rats and measure 8 cm in total length, each single flap being 4 cm long and of various widths (1.0, 1.5, 2.0, or 2.5 cm). The hypoxic incisional wound is the distal aspect of the flaps, or the horizontal line of the H between the two flaps. The control wounds are the lateral aspects of the flaps, or the limbs of the H. Using ^{133}Xe clearance to assess perfusion, these investigators described a 93% decrease in perfusion in the ischemic wound on day 1 postwounding. A linear increase in perfusion at this site is detected until normal perfusion is reached by postwounding day 16. The width of the flap does not affect the degree or duration of ischemia in this model (28). Biomechanical properties of the H-flap have also been described and include a 35–67% decrease in biomechanical strength of the ischemic wounds at day 10 postwounding, as compared to controls (29). This model is technically easy to create, because the flaps are random flaps and do not require meticulous dissection and ligation of specific vessels. The short ischemic period, localization of ischemia to only the very edges of the flaps, and limit of one ischemic wound per animal may limit this model in assessing the efficacy of multiple therapeutic agents in an ischemic wound. These investigators have, however, devised a clever model allowing for both a control wound and an ischemic wound within the same incision.

The hairless mouse ear model, described by Kamler *et al.* (30), involves ligation of two of the three main nutritional arteries to the mouse ear in mice with very large ears. Measurements of transcutaneous pO_2 reveal a significant decrease in pO_2 from 24 to 6 mmHg at day 0 after ligation. A linear increase is seen to 15 mmHg by day 15 postwounding (30). This model allows for a nonischemic control wound on the contralateral ear, enabling direct comparison of ischemic and nonischemic wound healing in the same animal. A degree of surgical skill is required to produce this model, but it has been reproduced and used by a different group to look at effects of hyperbaric oxygen on the ischemic wound (31). The size of the animal limits wounding to a maximum of two wounds per ear. There is virtually no connective tissue in these ears, so only epithelialization can be measured and quantified.

The ischemic rabbit ear ulcer model, developed in our laboratory, has been very useful in the analysis of wound healing under ischemic conditions. A circumferential incision is made around the base of the rabbit ear with interruption of all but the caudal artery and three veins (Fig. 1). We confirmed a decrease in tissue perfusion using dermofluorometry, skin temperature, tissue oxygen saturation, and venous blood gas sampling from the ischemic ear. Significant decreases in blood flow were demonstrated out to day 7 postwounding (32). In a subsequent study, the ischemic rabbit ear model was used to demonstrate the efficacy of various topical growth factors on wound healing in ischemic and nonischemic incisional wounds. Significant differences in tissue oxygen tensions were demonstrated between ischemic and control wounds, to day 14 postwounding with a continued trend to day 28 postwounding. Furthermore, a significant decrease in breaking strength was demonstrated in the ischemic wounds as compared to the nonischemic wounds through day 28 postwounding. This model closely simulates human ischemic wounds as demonstrated by the persistent low tissue oxygen tensions and delayed wound healing in the ischemic ears. Rabbit ears are generally large enough to allow for 4–6 wounds per ear, making the model ideal for testing the efficacy of therapeutic agents in hypoxic wounds (33).

2. Aged-Animal Wounds

Aged humans appear to heal wounds at a delayed rate as compared to young humans (34). Surgical wound dehiscence, as a result of decreased inflammation and wound reepithelialization, appears to occur at an increased rate in aged humans (35–37). *In vitro* and *in vivo* animal studies have revealed age-related impairments in inflammation, macrophage function, angiogenesis, fibroblast proliferation, wound contraction, and wound tensile strength (38–43). The direct etiology of the delay in wound healing in aged skin is unknown. Studies have suggested that growth factors may reverse this delay (44, 45) and hold clinical importance for the future of wound healing as the aged population increases rapidly. Aged animal models are important correlates of the aged human.

Ashcroft *et al.* (46) have performed experiments using an aged mouse colony (C57BL/Icrfa pathogen free) with a maximal life-span of 34 months. In validation of the model, these investigators demonstrated the rate of reepithelialization, basement membrane and matrix collagen deposition,

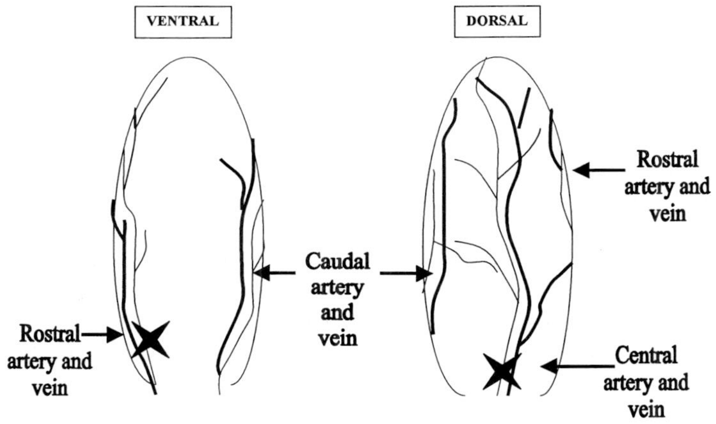

Figure 1 Ischemic rabbit ear model. A circumferential inscision is made at the base of the ear. The rostral and central arteries are ligated, leaving three main veins and the small caudal artery intact.

and subsequent scar formation to be delayed in this particular colony of mice (46). These observations are consistent with wounds in aged humans. Identification of differences in temporal expression and location of growth factors and their receptors were compared between young, middle-aged, and aged mice from this colony. Incisional full-thickness back wounds were created, allowed to heal for a varying number of days, and then analyzed using immunohistochemistry techniques. These investigators identified a delay in the expression of all growth factors evaluated in aged wounds as compared to young wounds, suggesting the need for different temporal therapeutic targets in aged patients (47).

Beck *et al.* (45) describe using an aged group of rats (19 months) to analyze the effects of exogenous TGF-β1 as compared to normal young rats and steroid-impaired rats. Full-thickness incisional wounds were made on the animals' backs and the edges were reapproximated using interrupted stainless-steel sutures. The aged rats exhibited a 27% decrease in wound breaking strength as compared to young rats, confirming aberrant healing in their aged model. The application of TGF-β1 reversed this deficit in breaking strength at day 7 postwounding (44).

Because human aging is often associated with other chronic health problems such as decreased peripheral perfusion, investigators have combined aging models with ischemic models. The H-flap ischemic model developed by Quirinia *et al.* (28), as described earlier, was performed in aged rats (24 months) and compared to young rats (3 months). This group demonstrated similar biomechanical properties between normal young rat and normal aged rat incisional wounds at day 10 and 20 postwounding. However, a 40–64% decrease in biomechanical strength was noted in aged ischemic wounds as compared to young ischemic wounds (48). These investigators concluded that ischemia is the primary cause of delayed healing in aged wounds, as opposed to just the phenomenon of aging alone.

Our laboratory created the ischemic rabbit ear in aged rabbits (43, 49). This combination allowed us to analyze the combined effects of aging and ischemia in wound healing, and the response of each to an exogenous growth factor. The ischemic wounds in aged rabbits demonstrated significant delays in various wound healing parameters that were unresponsive to exogenous TGF-β1 administration, as compared to young ischemic, young nonischemic, and aged nonischemic wounds. The inability to reverse the healing deficit in the aged ischemic wounds suggests an additive effect of aging and ischemia in hindering wound healing. This model may more accurately represent human chronic wounds, which occur most frequently in aged patients with varying degrees of local tissue hypoxia.

A limitation to all aged animal models is the reduced availability and high cost of these animals. Furthermore, the older animals are less resilient to the stresses of anesthesia and wounding. Experiments should be planned anticipating animal losses in the aged groups.

3. Chronic Wounds

Our laboratory has developed a rabbit dermal ulcer model that has some important similarities to human chronic leg ulcers (50). Human chronic leg ulcers are associated with venous stasis, small vessel disease, and arterial insufficiency (51). These ulcers are generally full-thickness and healing has been noted to occur only from the periphery by an interaction between new dermal tissue and new epithelium. Wound contraction appears to contribute little to healing of these ulcers in humans (52, 53).

In this model, young adult rabbits are used. Four 6-mm full-thickness ulcers are created down to bare cartilage on the ventral aspect of the rabbit ear (Figs. 2 and 3). A dissecting microscope is used to dissect the perichondrium off of the cartilage, resulting in an avascular wound base. Because the bare cartilage splints the wound, and the skin and dermis of the ventral surface of the rabbit ear are tightly adherent to the underlying cartilage, little wound contraction is seen and granulation tissue grows in only from the periphery. Histology has confirmed minimal wound contraction, granulation tissue arising solely from the periphery of the wound, no reepithelialization at day 3, with complete reepithelialization by day 10 to day 14. As an adjunct to describing this model, various exogenous growth factors were applied to the dermal ulcers and healing rates were analyzed and quantified histologically. Significantly increased rates of reepithelialization were noted with topical PDGF-BB, bFGF, and EGF, whereas TGF-β1 administration resulted in decreased reepithelialization. However, significantly increased granulation tissue and matrix deposition were noted in PDGF-BB- and TGF-β1-treated wounds.

4. Pressure Ulcer Wounds

Pressure ulcers are the most common chronic wounds seen in the clinical setting. They occur in patients who are unconscious, debilitated, or paralyzed (1). Preventive measures such as regular positioning, pressure-relief bedding, moisture barriers, and adequate nutrition play a large role in avoiding these ulcers. Despite these recommendations, pressure ulcers are prevalent and difficult to heal. The delay in healing is typically due to a continued lack of adherence to a rigid wound care protocol, but in different populations, such as the aging, other factors that may further delay healing come into play. There is a great need for new therapeutics that will accelerate the wound healing process or even change the nature of the healed tissue by perhaps increasing its biomechanical strength and resiliency to future pressure on the site.

Animal models of pressure ulcers date back to before the middle of this century. Some earlier models consisted of

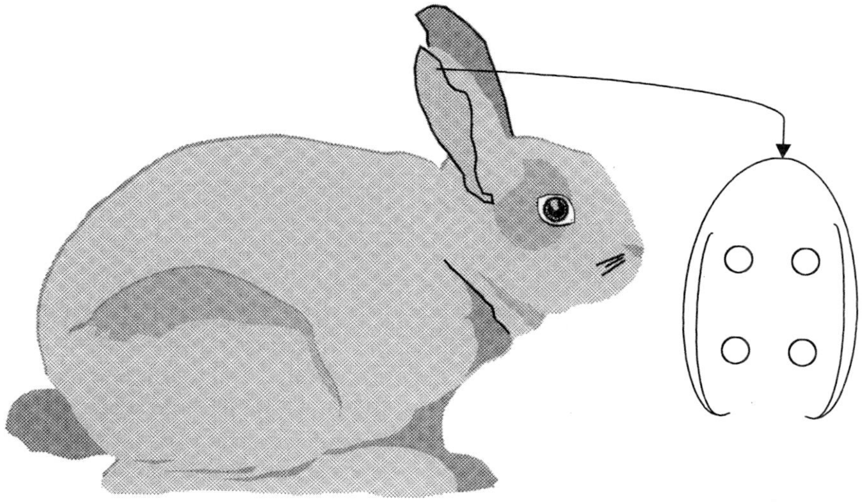

Figure 2 Diagram of the rabbit ear ulcer model. Wound sizes are 6 mm in diameter; both ears can be wounded.

pressure ulcers created in rabbits and dogs (54, 55). The negative aspect of these models is the dissimilarity of the skin of rabbits and dogs and human skin. More recent studies have been undertaken in pigs. A model described by Daniel *et al.* used paraplegic pigs (56). Wounds were created using equal pressure (600 mmHg) for a consistent period of

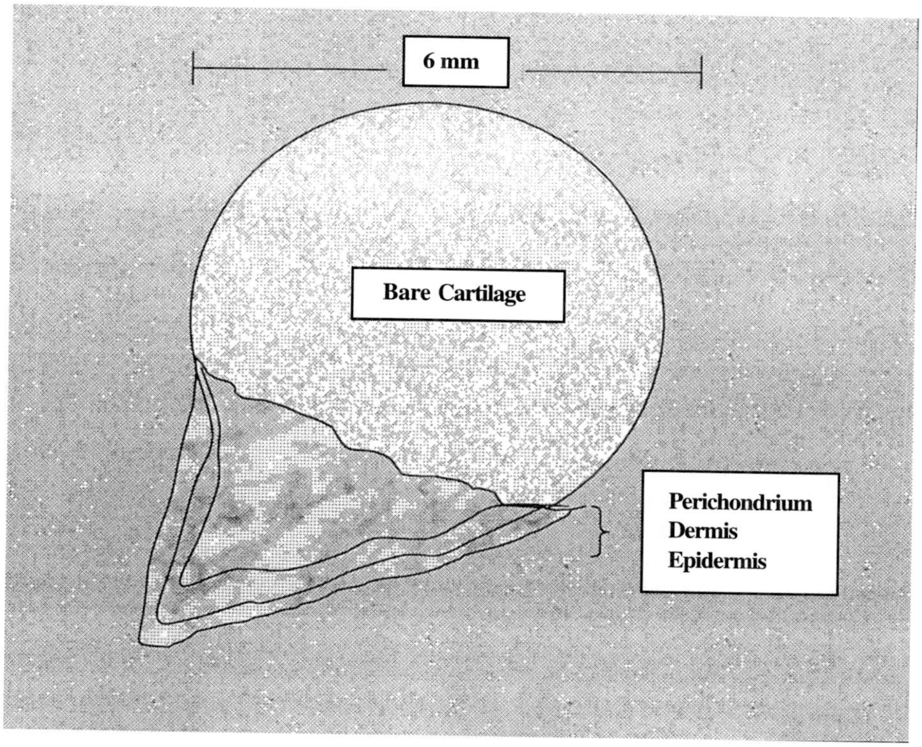

Figure 3 Diagram of the rabbit ear ulcer model depicting removal of epidermis, dermis, and perichondrium, exposing bare cartilage.

time (6 hr) to create a grade III ulcer on an atrophied hind limb. This model required spinal cord transection, an invasive surgical procedure that resulted in bowel and bladder dysfunction with increased rates of complications, morbidity, and mortality among the animals used. Animal rights concerns preclude repetition of this model.

Hyodo *et al.* (57) have described a similar porcine model but with selective surgical resection of unilateral lumbar nerve roots in the spinal canal. This monoplegic model avoids the high morbidity and mortality seen with complete spinal cord transection. These investigators developed custom-made pressure applicators that apply 800 mmHg pressure for 48 hr to create consistent grade IV pressure ulcers. This device is screwed into the cortex of the proximal femoral shaft and the amount of pressure applied is calculated from the calibrated force of a spring acting on a 3-cm-diameter disk applied directly onto the skin surface. The use of this device allows the animal to remain mobile during prolonged application of pressure. Among other limitations, the model is difficult to study in an adequate number of wounds over a long enough period of time to allow testing of various therapeutic strategies.

The greyhound dog has been used as a model for pressure ulcers as well. This animal has very thin skin with little subcutaneous fat. The model described involves placing a limb in a cast designed to apply constant pressure to a site of bony prominence (58). These animals are expensive to obtain and house. Furthermore, there is significant morbidity to the animal because the limb is sensate.

C. Impaired Healing Models

Certain disease processes lend themselves to an increased incidence of surgical wound breakdown or a significant delay in wound healing. Classic human cases of deficient wound healing are patients with long-standing diabetes mellitus and those that have undergone chemotherapy or radiation treatment for cancer. Clinically, these types of wounds cause a significant amount of morbidity and sometimes mortality, and also significantly burden our healthcare system financially. Animal models representing these situations of impaired healing have been developed in an attempt both to identify the deficit these individuals have in their wound healing cascade, and to develop therapeutic agents that either reverse the deficit, or correct the defective process. Despite aggressive attempts to simulate the human impaired wound environment, the criticism of all of these models is that they remain distinctly different from human chronic wounds. Furthermore, the impairment of wound healing is often accomplished in animals by administration of toxic substances that have complicating systemic effects and may alter the natural history of the human disease being simulated. This part will focus on wound healing models for impaired healing due to diabetes mellitus, radiation, steroids, and chemotherapy (adriamycin).

1. Diabetes-Associated Wounds

Patients with long-standing diabetes often suffer from chronic wounds primarily over pressure points in the foot, in what amount to pressure ulcers secondary to ischemia–reperfusion injury. The concept of a diabetic neuropathy as the etiology of these wounds was described by Pryce as early as 1887 (59). These wounds generally occur as a result of a sensory neuropathy that leads to failure to sense and relieve pressure from the weight-bearing areas. Additionally, a motor neuropathy in the feet involving the toe flexors results in unopposed action of the long extensor tendons. This unbalances the foot, resulting in prominence of the metatarsal heads and characteristic deformities such as claw or hammer toes. Autonomic dysfunction in these patients results in dry skin from reduced perspiration and decreased nutrient delivery to peripheral tissues due to arteriovenous shunting. This combination of peripheral sensory neuropathy, a motor neuropathy, and autonomic neuropathy is currently thought to be the cause of increased ulcer formation and deficient healing in diabetics (60).

Two models of diabetic wound healing exist. One employs the use of streptozotocin or alloxan to destroy pancreatic beta cells selectively and the other uses a genetically engineered model of diabetes in mice. These models have been used to identify some aspects of diabetic impaired wound healing such as reduced collagen formation and reduced wound strength (61, 62).

a. Drug Induced Models of Diabetes Intraperitoneal injection of 200 mg/kg of streptozotocin, an antibiotic produced by the bacteria *Streptomyces achromogene* (63), selectively destroys pancreatic Langerhans cells within 7 hr. This model characterizes juvenile diabetes with complete insulin deficiency, increased insulin receptor levels, and hyperglycemia (64). Alloxan is a similar drug inducing pancreatic cell death within 24 hr. Of the two, streptozotocin is preferred for animal experimentation due to its milder toxicity (65). Animals should be fasted for 12 hr prior to treatment and observed for several hours afterward.

Goodson and Hunt induced diabetes in male rats administering 70 mg/kg of streptozotocin intravenously. One week after induction of diabetes, confirmed by blood glucose levels, stainless-steel wire-mesh cylinder wound chambers were implanted in the backs of diabetic and nondiabetic control rats. These investigators demonstrated a significant increase in blood glucose and wound fluid glucose levels, decreased tensile strength of incised wounds, decreased collagen production, and a more acidotic pH in the diabetic rat wound chambers (66). This study intended to examine the effects of insulin-deficient hyperglycemia on wound healing.

Broadly *et al.* (67), using this diabetic model, demonstrated significant defects in wound repair in streptozotocin-induced diabetic rats as well. Tensile strengths of the diabetic rat incisions were 53% of normal on day 7 postwounding and 29% of normal on day 21 postwounding. In this study, TGF-β and bFGF were administered by injection into the incisions, but did not cause significant improvements in tensile strengths of the diabetic incisions as compared to nondiabetic controls (67).

These two studies, among many others, confirm that there is significantly delayed wound healing in animals treated with streptozotocin or alloxan. The negative aspect of the model is the lack of correlation with humans who have chronic diabetes mellitus with the associated neuropathies and chronic wounds that occur over a prolonged period of time. The inflicted wounds in these animals are acute and the delay in healing appears to be secondary to an acutely altered metabolic condition, namely, complete insulin deficiency and hyperglycemia. Additional negative points to this model are the limited availability and cost of the animals, and the high incidence of infection and death in these relatively immunocompromised models. Animal survival under these hyperglycemic conditions is limited to 6 months for rats and 1 year for rabbits. The animals increase their water consumption and urinary output, and generally become severely cachectic, often requiring early euthanasia (6).

b. Genetic Models of Diabetes Genetic engineering has created several rodent strains that develop diabetes within 1 month of birth. These animals include db/db mice and rats, ob/ob mice, and nonobese diabetic (NOD) mice. NOD mice represent an autoimmune model of diabetes similar to human type 1 diabetes mellitus (68). Both db/db and ob/ob are autosomal recessive mutations that characterize type 2 or adult-onset diabetes (69, 70). These animals are obese and demonstrate marked hyperinsulinemia with resistance to endogenous and exogenous insulin. Peak hyperglycemic levels occur during the second and third months of life, and death generally ensues by the tenth month due to progression of disease. This reduced life span requires that animals close in age be used for experimentation.

Goodson and Hunt have undertaken a number of experiments using the ob/ob mouse, demonstrating a consistent deficiency in wound collagen production (71). Interventions such as weight loss and exogenous insulin administration have been tested in this model and their efficacy quantified by measuring wound collagen production (72).

This model is the best available mimic of metabolic conditions seen in type 2 diabetes mellitus. Negative aspects are that the animals are expensive, difficult to obtain, have a short life span and require special care and handling because they are relatively immunocompromised. In addition, the delayed healing of open wounds in these mice appears in part to be due to a deficiency in wound contracture, which does not correlate well to human diabetes. Although the model is a useful model of healing impairment, it has limitations when extrapolated to the problems seen in human diabetic ulcers.

2. Radiation-Induced Wounds

X-Ray radiation of skin at high enough doses creates ulcers that exhibit delayed healing. These ulcers have been used by investigators to represent chronic nonhealing ulcers in humans. The tissue effects of radiation at a cellular level appear to be antiproliferative, closely simulating the delayed process seen in human chronic wounds (73, 74).

Radiation can be administered in two ways: total body radiation or direct surface radiation. Both were tested in a rat model in this lab, exhibiting significantly impaired incisional wound breaking strength in animals treated with either 800 rads total body radiation or 2500 rads surface radiation (75). Animals treated with total-body radiation exhibited significantly depressed bone marrow-derived elements in a dose- and time-dependent manner without altering surface cellular function. Wounds created in these animals were deficient in a normal inflammatory response due to the inability to recruit peripheral cells to the wounds. Surface radiation had no detrimental effect on circulating bone marrow-derived cells but locally delayed healing by inhibiting fibroblast replication in wounds for up to 3 weeks (76). This model allows independent examination of the effects of radiation on cells originating in bone marrow and skin surface cells as they pertain to wound healing. Growth factors PDGF-BB and TGF-β were tested in this model with interesting results (74, 75). Other groups have created similar animal models and tested other treatments such as hyperbaric oxygen on radiated wounds with promising results (77).

Wound healing in radiated models is used to represent human chronic wounds, and some of the parameters of wound healing, such as decreased fibroblast proliferation and collagen production, appear to be similar. Nevertheless, this model may differ from human chronic wounds at the cellular level because radiation may have its effects on a different part of the cell cycle, compared perhaps to aging or hypoxia. Therapeutics directed at radiation wounds may subsequently have little or no effect in human chronic wounds of other etiologies. These models are more correctly used to represent chronic human wounds as a result of radiation treatment. Another important limitation of these models is that they really are acute radiation injuries, whereas human chronic wounds as a result of radiation are due to the late effects of radiation, which include local tissue ischemia and fibrosis.

3. Steroid-Impaired Wounds

Steroid therapy is common in the elderly. Animal models have high clinical relevance. Clinically, steroid-treated patients develop thinning of the skin and a diminished healing capacity. Steroids appear to interfere with the inflammatory phase of wound healing. Monocytes exhibit a diminished capacity to differentiate into growth factor-secreting macrophages, and fibroblasts demonstrate a reduced capacity to produce collagen and other connective tissue components (78, 79). Animal models of steroid-impaired wound healing have been used to elucidate the events that occur early in wound healing during the inflammatory response (80). Experimentation with these models may allow identification of agents that reverse the wound healing defect seen with steroid administration. One important difference is that different species may vary substantially in their steroid sensitivity. Rats are steroid sensitive, exhibiting rapid weight loss and profound effects on circulating inflammatory cells, whereas humans are much less sensitive.

Animals typically receive intraperitoneal injections of the steroid from 2 to 7 days prior to wounding. Dostal and Gamelli looked at the effect of equipotent antiinflammatory doses of dexamethasone sodium phosphate, methylprednisolone sodium succinate, and hydrocortisone sodium succinate on wound healing in mice. They concluded that differences exist between the various types of steroids with regard to their effect on wound healing (81). Karr *et al.* (82) identified in rats the critical dose of methylprednisolone (6.7 mg/kg/day) that caused defective wound healing as measured by breaking strength (82). This information is useful with regard to the animal model, but these concepts can also be extrapolated to the human scenario.

The exogenous application of growth factors in this model has been undertaken by a number of investigators and holds much promise for future therapeutics (83–85). These models are inexpensive and easy to reproduce.

4. Adriamycin-Impaired Wounds

Adriamycin is a potent chemotherapeutic agent used in cancer patients for the treatment of a variety of hematologic and solid cancers. Clincally, this antiproliferative agent depletes bone marrow stem cell populations, resulting in immunosuppression, anemia, and deficient wound healing (86, 87). These animal models are of clinical importance in wound healing and hematologic and oncologic research. Adriamycin-treated animals demonstrate the side effects seen in humans such as weight loss, anemia, cardiotoxicity, and thrombocytopenia. These side effects can alter the results of wound healing studies that use the model as a delayed healing model. Experiments undertaken using this model should be extrapolated primarily to wounds in humans receiving chemotherapy and not generalized to human chronic wounds of other etiologies, such as aging or tissue hypoxia.

Devereux *et al.* (88) describe an animal model in the rat treated with adriamycin. Incisional wounds were inflicted on the backs of rats. These animals received an intravenous injection of adriamycin (6 mg/kg) at various time points before and after wounding. Wound healing was assessed by measuring wound breaking strength and significant differences were noted as compared to controls. Using this model, these investigators drew conclusions as to the optimal time to perform surgical procedures around adriamycin therapy (88). These investigators described alterations in collagen production and maturation in wounds from adriamycin-treated animals and the effect of radiation, in addition to adriamycin, on wound healing (89, 90). These studies are all directly pertinent to patients receiving chemotherapy and useful to the physicians caring for these patients.

A similar model combining adriamycin treatment with a wound chamber model in rats to analyze products of wound healing was described by Lawrence *et al.* (91). Parameters measured in the wound chambers were collagen content, protein content, cellular proliferation rate, and collagen types. Significant decreases were noted in all of these parameters in adriamycin-treated rats. Growth factors applied into the wound chambers shared various degrees of wound healing deficit reversal in response to different growth factors (91).

Most antineoplastic agents create deficiencies in wound healing (92). Adriamycin is the most commonly used antineoplastic agent in wound healing studies. The toxicities of the drug should be appreciated and animal study numbers should take into account possible animal losses due to immunosuppresion, infection, and illness. The model is relatively simple and inexpensive to replicate, but adriamycin is highly toxic, and the model has not been used extensively in recent years.

D. Foreign Body Models

Foreign body models date to 1924 when Sandison described the first rabbit ear wound chamber, allowing the microscopic analysis of growing cells and tissues *in vivo* (93). Many investigators have used this model and modified models not only to examine the events of wound healing, but also to influence these events with the application of various agents directly into the chambers and sponges. These models consist of devices implanted into an animal. Wound chambers allow for external visualization of the events occurring during healing. Implantable sponges allow granulation tissue to grow into the model through pores. The sponges are generally symmetrical in shape, resulting in deposition of the least mature tissue at the core. Both types of foreign body models have demonstrated to be quite useful in identifying important aspects of the wound healing process.

1. Wound Chambers

Wound chambers were first used in rabbit ear wounds. The device consists of a dead-space occluded by coverslips on both sides, permitting the microscopic examination of the process of wound healing. Insertion typically involves a full-thickness punch biopsy made through the tissues with elevation of surrounding skin to allow anchoring of the chamber (94). The artifical dead space fills with plasma, fibrin clot, cells, and extracellular matrix, resulting in granulation tissue. The tissue formed in the chamber is new, vascularized tissue representing the healing response as produced in other wounds (95). The majority of investigators quantify tissue responses by analyzing angiogenesis within the newly formed granulation tissue. This can be done grossly using microscopy and measuring capillary density, or, more analytically, by detecting radioactivity after the injection of radioactive microspheres, or measuring flow with a laser doppler (96–98).

This type of model has been used to assess tissue healing responses to various antiseptic agents, changes in inspired oxygen concentrations, and the administration of exogenous growth factors (91, 96, 99, 100). A modification of this model has been undertaken in humans. Investigators have covered human excisional wounds with transparent occlusive materials, permitting the collection of wound fluid for measurements of cytokines and growth factors and also allowing the administration of exogenous agents directly onto the wound site (101).

2. Dead-Space Models

The use of porous implants placed in subcutaneous tissues allow investigators to isolate the events of connective tissue formation from other events of wound healing, such as epithelialization and wound contraction. Implanted materials such as the Hunt–Shilling stainless-steel mesh chamber, viscose cellulose (VC) and polyvinyl alcohol (PVA) sponges, and polytetrafluoroethylene (PTFE) create tissue dead space into which plasma, fibrin clot, inflammatory cells infuse. An extracellular matrix is deposited, resulting in granulation tissue. The defined dimensions of implants allow quantitative measurements of biochemical parameters such as collagen, glycosaminoglycan, and hyaluronic acid contents, DNA content, and concentrations of cytokines or growth factors in the wound fluid (102–104). A direct correlation between collagen deposition in PVA sponges and incised wound tensile strength has been demonstrated in mice (71). Implants can be removed and embedded in paraffin and sectioned to allow for histologic analysis or processed for light and electron microscopy studies. Growth factors and neutralizing antibodies have been used in such models to assess their efficacy on the early phases of wound healing (105, 106). These models allow not only easy analysis of the healing stages in the acute wound, but also offer the ability to add exogenous agents and quantify the tissue responses.

These models are extensible to humans. PTFE tubing can been implanted underneath the skin using a large needle introducer with an attached stitch to allow easy removal without a significant scar. Hunt *et al.* has used this model extensively to measure collagen content in human wounds and correlate this to issues such as skin oxygenation and body temperature (107, 108).

The major limitation to this model is the lack of correlation with human wounds. The model gives investigators much information about the acute phase of wound healing with regard to the production of granulation tissue, but does not represent the physical interactions of epithelium on wound healing. Additional limitations lie in the materials used. Despite being relatively inert, the materials eventually elicit an inflammatory foreign body response, limiting the relevance of the implant to the first 3–4 weeks of the healing process (6). Furthermore, the sizes of the pores in these materials can affect the degree of collagen deposition and cellular infiltration, making it difficult to draw comparisons between studies unless the exact model is used (109, 110).

III. Methods to Quantify Wound Healing

The ability to quantify properly an outcome difference in a wound healing model is critical. From this information one can determine the efficacy of a therapeutic agent in an animal model and then perhaps extrapolate the results to a human model. Many of these methods involve using *in vitro* techniques, which, although very useful, are one step further removed from the human wound as compared to an animal model. Quantification of wound healing can range from biomechanical assessments, such as the breaking strength of tissue, to detecting differences in mRNA levels of various genes involved in the wound healing process.

A. Biomechanical Measurements

Tensile strength or breaking strength of tissues at various time points during wound healing can be used to determine the rate of healing and the effectiveness of the healing process (7). Tensile strength is measured as applied load per unit of cross-sectional area, described as pounds per square inch or kilograms per square centimeter. Breaking strength is a measurement of the force required to break a wound or tissue without regard to its dimensions. For practical purposes, most surgeons are interested in the breaking strength of wounds, or how much force is required to disrupt a healing wound. Tensile strength more closely describes an intrinsic property of tissue and should be used when comparing different tissues or tissues from different areas on the same animal. Samples tested must be accurately measured in order to calculate tensile strength (111).

Tensiometers, some mechanical and others computer assisted, are typically used to obtain these measurements (112). Tissue samples are attached to grips and pulled. A general consideration to keep in mind when fashioning the sample to be tested is that analysis of wounded tissue should be limited to within 1 mm around the incision, because collagen deposition has been found to be limited to this area in normal healing wounds (9). An increased wound breaking strength has been found to correlate with increased amounts of mature, cross-linked collagen in the healing wound (113)

B. Histology, Immunohistochemistry, and Electron Microscopy

Healing wounds can be excised, embedded in paraffin, sectioned, and stained for various components of the wound. Hemotoxylin and eosin stains are convenient and display general structural features, but are nonspecific in terms of the chemical composition of cell components. Nuclei are stained blue by hematoxylin, and cytoplasm and extracellular material are counterstained pink by eosin. The technique is quick, inexpensive, and easy to master. However, it does not allow detailed analysis of the components found intracellularly or in the extracellular matrix. Special stains are generally used to display structures such as blood vessels, different types of collagen, elastin, bacteria, fats, carbohydrates, melanin, and many others (114).

Our laboratory uses Masson's trichrome staining to differentiate collagen fibers from nuclei and cytoplasm. A more specific collagen stain, the sirius red stain, displays mature collagen fibers as orange-yellowish bifringence and immature granulation tissue collagen fibers as greenish bifringence. Alcian blue stains are used to stain protooglycans such as glycosaminoglycans and hyaluronic acid in the extracellular matrix. Lectin stains or Factor 8 antibodies are used to identify endothelial cells and capillaries by staining for their basement membranes using immunohistochemical methods (115–118).

Quantification of histology in healing wounds encompasses analysis of the types of cells and tissue produced in the healing process. This includes observations such as the number of inflammatory cells per unit area, the degree of angiogenesis or reepithelialization, the amount and organization of components of the extracellular matrix, and many others. Quantification of these histological parameters can be difficult, but is very important when attempting to draw conclusions about an intervention that may affect the healing process. When direct quantification is impossible, our laboratory uses a semiquantitative method consisting of two independent blinded observers, with ratings based on a numerical scale, usually 0 to 4. We have used this method to quantify parameters such as inflammation, angiogenesis, and collagen organization in previous studies (18).

Immunohistochemistry can identify specialized cells or tissues by using antibodies to specific proteins or enzymes found in these cells or tissues. The antibodies are generally conjugated to a fluorescent dye, such as fluorescein, and the reaction between antibody and antigen can be examined, photographed, and later quantified using a fluorescence microscope. Other markers such as gold or ferritin can be attached to the antibody molecule. These markers can be visualized directly using electron microscopy. Immunohistochemistry has also been useful in the analysis of growth factors in wound healing. Using flourescent- or enzyme-conjugated antibodies specific for growth factors, this method has allowed the localization of various growth factors or their receptors in normal and wound tissue (119–121).

Electron microscopy can be used to quantify differences in wound tissue after an intervention as well. A much thinner section is required and embedding is performed with hard epoxy plastic. Once sectioned using a diamond knife, the specimen is collected on small metal grids and the image is obtained using an electron beam and a series of projecting lenses to enlarge the image. Comparisons between collagen fiber size, cell structure, cell–cell junctions, and other properties can be made and quantified (89).

C. Physiologic Biochemistry

Biochemical or physiologic changes that occur as a result of an intervention in a healing wound can be observed and quantified. Tissue perfusion or oxygenation, cell proliferation, and collagen production are the parameters most commonly measured.

Tissue perfusion represents the degree of angiogenesis in the healing wound tissue. Investigators have quantified tissue perfusion microscopically by measuring capillary density. Injection of a radioactive tracer, radioactive microspheres, or sodium fluorescein intravenously allows quantification of tissue perfusion by measuring the amount of radioactivity or fluorescence in the wound. Laser doppler can also be used to quantify tissue perfusion. Tissue oxygenation is an indirect measurement of tissue perfusion.

This parameter can be measured using a transcutaneous oxygen probe. Other indirect measurements of tissue perfusion include venous blood analysis, tissue oxygen saturation, and skin temperature (32, 33, 96–98, 122, 123).

Several methods are available for the evaluation of cell proliferation. The number of mitoses per high-power field can be counted in histologic sections as representative of an increase or decrease in cell proliferation. This method is subject to considerable variation dependent on thickness of the sections, fields chosen, type of microscope used, and the observer's variability in the identification of mitotic figures (124, 125). Immunohistochemical techniques identifying nuclear antigens related to cell growth and division can be used as a more sensitive test for cell proliferation. Bromodeoxyuridine is a thymidine analog that is incorporated into nuclear DNA during the S phase and can be detected using monoclonal antibodies. Proliferating cell nuclear antigen (PCNA), another nuclear antigen elevated in the G_1 and S phases in proliferating cells, can be stained using an antibody (126, 127). Another frequently used and objectively quantifiable method involves *in vitro* labeling of proliferating cells with [^{3}H]thymidine. This radioactive nucleotide is incorporated into the DNA of proliferating cells and allows objective quantification of the number of proliferating cells by measuring radioactivity with a scintillation spectrophotometer (128, 129). A fluorometric assay can also be used to quantify *in vitro* cell proliferation with the assumption that DNA content is proportional to cell number. In this method, Hoechst dye is combined with solubilized cells and the fluorescence is measured using a fluorometer (130). These examples are but a few of many types of studies currently used to analyze cell proliferation.

Collagen production can be assessed semiquantitatively using stains specific for immature collagen fibers, as mentioned above. A more objective method involves *in vitro* pulsation of fibroblasts with [^{3}H]proline. The fibroblasts actively synthesizing collagen will incorporate the radiolabeled proline into the collagen. Objective quantification can be obtained by measuring radioactivity levels in the media and first wash 6 hours after pulsation. This should represent >80% of newly synthesized collagenous proteins (131). Our laboratory has also used a hydroxy-L-proline high-performance liquid chromatography assay to quantify collagen production in samples of solubilized cells (132).

D. Molecular and Cellular Biology

Advancements in biotechnology now allow analysis of cellular responses at the molecular level. Our laboratory and others have utilized competitive reverse-transcription polymerase chain reaction (RT-PCR) techniques to quantify mRNA expression of specific genes pertinent to our field of study (19, 133). This technique involves isolating cellular mRNA and creating cDNA using random primers, followed by PCR using sequence specific primers. Quantification of the desired product is done using nonhomologous DNA as an internal competitor. This competitor, or mimic, is coamplified with the cDNA of interest and the PCR products are separated on an agarose gel. The differential band intensities are then quantified by densitometry imaging (134). Specific primers to a number of growth factors have been created, allowing the detection of increased mRNA levels of these proteins in response to an intervention or treatment. One should keep in mind that although the detection of accumulated mRNA expression suggests up-regulation of a specific gene, it does not indicate the functional activity of the protein once translated from mRNA. Other methods can be used to detect increased functional activity of an enzyme or increased production of a protein after translation, thereby better defining the meaning of increased mRNA levels.

The study of intracellular signaling pathways has allowed us to better understand cellular response to exogenous stimuli such as stress or growth factors. Numerous signaling pathways are made up of a series of kinases controlled by phosphorylation events. With regard to growth factors, kinase activation begins at the cell surface. A growth factor binds to its receptor, typically a tyrosine kinase activates this kinase, which goes on to activate the next kinase, and so forth (135). This cascade of kinase activation ultimately leads to cellular activation, including up-regulation of cellular synthetic mechanisms and cellular proliferation. Some of these kinases have been identified and the amounts of kinase present can be quantified using Western blot techniques. In addition, the activated form of the kinase can be targeted with an antibody and quantified using similar techniques. Examples include the MAP kinases, erk-1, erk-2, and jnk. Erk-1 and erk-2 are activated by growth factors, and jnk, by stress. An up-regulation in activated enzyme typically indicates the cell is responding to the growth factor or stress stimulus. The degree of activation required to create a clinically significant difference in, for example, wound healing, has yet to be determined (136).

IV. Conclusion

The animal models described herein were created by different investigators with different goals, yet all relate to the arena of wound healing. It is difficult to state which model is best overall, because most are suited to a specific type of wound. An important consideration in designing a study is planning appropriately for controls. Our laboratory induces wounds in the ears of animals for a number of reasons, one being the ability to produce a control wound in the same animal, on the contralateral side. This allows the animal to be its own control and strengthens any difference identified statistically. Additional considerations such as cost and availability of the animals should be kept in mind as well.

References

1. Eaglstein, W. H., and Falanga, V. (1997). Chronic wounds. *Surg. Clin. North Am.* **77,** 689–700.
2. Stromberg, K., Chapekar, M. S., Goldman, B. A., Chamber, W. A., and Cavagnaro, J. A. (1994). Regulatory concerns in the development of topical recombinant ophthalmic and cutaneous wound healing biologics. *Wound Rep. Regen.* **2,** 155–164.
3. Howes, E. L., Harvey, S. C., and Hewitt, C. (1939). Rate of fibroplasia and differentiation in the healing of cutaneous wounds in different species of animals. *Arch. Surg.* **38,** 934–945.
4. Levenson, S. M., Geever, E. F., Crowley, L. V., Oates, J. F., Bernard, C. W., and Rosen, H. (1964). The healing of rat skin wounds. *Ann. Surg.* **161**(2), 293–308.
5. Winter, G. D. (1962). Formation of the scab and rate of epithelialization of superficial wounds in the skin of the young domestic pig. *Nature (London)* **193,** 293–294.
6. Davidson, J. M. (1998). Animal models for wound repair. *Arch. Dermatol. Res.* **290** (Suppl.), S1–S11.
7. Howes, E. L., Sooy, J. W., Harvey, and S. C. (1929). The healing of wounds as determined by their tensile strength. *JAMA* **29**(1), 42–45.
8. Shah, M., Foreman, D. M., and Ferguson, M. W. J. (1994). Neutralising antibody to TGF-β1,2 reduces cutaneous scarring in adult rodents. *J. Cell Sci.* **107,** 1137–1157.
9. Bevin, A., and Madden, J. (1969). The localization of collagen synthesis in healing wounds. *Surg. Forum* **20,** 65–66.
10. Lawrence, W. T. (1998). Physiology of the acute wound. *Clin. Plast. Surg.* **25,** 321–339.
11. Bustad, L. K., and McClellan, R. O. (1965). Use of pigs in biomedical research. *Nature (London)* **206,** 531–535.
12. Breuing, K., Andree, C., Helo, G., Slama, J., Liu, P. Y., and Eriksson, E. (1997). Growth factors in the repair of partial thickness porcine skin wounds. *Plast. Reconstr. Surg.* **100,** 657–664.
13. Gabbiani, G., Hirschel, B. J., Ryan, G. B., Statkov, P. R., and Majno, G. (1972). Granulation tissue as a contractile organ. A study of structure and function. *J. Exp. Med.* **135,** 719–734.
14. Kennedy, D. F., Cliff, W. J. (1979). A systemic study of wound contraction in mammalian skin. *Pathology* **11,** 207–222.
15. Catty, R. M. C. (1965). Healing and contraction in experimental full thickness wound in the human. *Bri. J. Surg.* **52,** 542–548.
16. Ahn, S. T., and Mustoe, T. A. (1990). Effects of ischemia on ulcer wound healing: a new model in the rabbit ear. *Ann. Plast. Surg.* **24,** 17–23.
17. Morris, D. E., Wu, L., Zhao, L. L., Bolton, L., Roth, S. I., Ladin, D. A., and Mustoe, T. A. (1997). Acute and chronic animal models for excessive dermal scarring: Quantitative studies. *Plast. Reconstr. Surg.* **100,** 674–681.
18. Zhao, L. L., Davidson, J. D., Wee, S. C., Roth, S. I., and Mustoe, T. A. (1994). Effect of hyperbaric oxygen and growth factors on rabbit ear ischemic ulcers. *Arch. Surg.* **129,** 1043–1049.
19. Bonomo, S. R., Davidson, J. D., Yu, Y., Xia, Y., Lin, X., and Mustoe, T. A. (1998). Hyperbaric oxygen as a signal transducer: Upregulation of platelet derived growth factor-beta receptor in the presence of HBO_2 and PDGF. *Undersea Hyperbar. Med.* **25** (4), 211–216.
20. Nguyen, T. T., Gilpin, D. A., Meyer, N. A., and Herndon, D. N. (1996). Current treatment of severely burned patients. *Ann. Surg.* **223**(1), 14–25.
21. Boykin, J. V., Eriksson, E., and Pittman, R. N. (1991). *In vivo* microcirculation of scald burns and the progression of postburn dermal ischaemia. *Plast. Reconstr. Surg.* **66,** 191–198.
22. Kaufman, T., Lusthaus, S. N., Sagher, U., and Wexler, M. R. (1990). Deep partial skin thickness burns: A reproducible animal model to study burn wound healing. *Burns* **16,** 13–16.
23. Danilenko, D. M., Ring, B. D., Tarpley, J. E., Morris, B., Van, G. Y., Morawiecki, A., Callahan, W., Goldenberg, M., Hershenson, S., and Pierce, G. F. (1995). Growth factors in porcine full thickness burn repair. Differing targets and effects of keratinocyte growth factor, platelet-derived growth factor-BB, epidermal growth factor, and neu differentiation factor. *Am. J. Pathol.* **147** (5), 1261–1277.
24. Coleridge Smith, P. D., Thomas, P., Scurr, J. H., and Dormandy, J. A. (1988). Causes of venous ulceration: a new hypothesis. *Br. Med. J. (Clin. Res. Ed.)* **296,** 1726–1727.
25. Ninikoski, J. (1977). Oxygen and wound healing. *Clin. Plast. Surg.* **4,** 361–374.
26. Udenfriend, S. (1966). Formation of hydroxyproline in collagen. *Science* **152** (727), 1335–1340.
27. Ackerman, N. B., and Brinkley, F. B. (1966). Oxygen tensions in normal and ischemic tissues during hyperbaric therapy. *JAMA* **198** (12), 142–145.
28. Quirinia, A., Jensen, F. T., and Viidik, A. (1992). Ischemia in wound healing I: Design of a flap model—Changes in blood flow. *Scand. J. Plast. Reconstr. Hand Surg.* **26,** 21–28.
29. Quirinia, A., and Viidik, A. (1992). Ischemia in wound healing II: Design of a flap model—Biomechanical properties. *Scand. J. Plast. Reconstr. Hand Surg.* **26,** 133–139.
30. Kamler, M., Lehr, H. A., Barker, J. H., Saetzler, R. K., Galla, T. J., and Messmer, K. (1993). Impact of ischemia on tissue oxygenation and wound healing: Intravital microscopic studies on the Hairless Mouse Ear Model. *Eur. Surg. Res.* **25,** 30–37.
31. Uhl, E., Sirsjo, A., Haapaniemi, T., Nilsson, G., and Nylander, G. (1994). Hyperbaric oxygen improves wound healing in normal and ischemic skin tissue. *Plast. Reconstr. Surg.* **93,** 835–841.
32. Ahn, S. T., and Mustoe, T. A. (1990). Effects of ischemia on ulcer wound healing: A new model in the rabbit ear. *Ann. Plast. Surg.* **24**(1), 17–23.
33. Wu, L., and Mustoe, T. A. (1995). Effect of ischemia on growth factor enhancement of incisional wound healing. *Surgery* **17,** 570–576.
34. Jones, P. L., and Millman, A. (1990). Wound healing and the aged patient. *Nurs. Clins. North Am.* **25,** 263–277.
35. Holt, D. R., Kirk, S. J., Regan, M. C., Hurson, M., Lindblad, W. J., and Barbul, A. (1992). Effect of age on wound healing in healthy human beings. *Surgery* **112,** 293.
36. Goodson, W. H., and Hunt, T. K. (1979). Wound healing and aging. *J. Invest. Dermatol.* **73,** 88–91.
37. Eaglstein, W. H. (1989). Wound healing and aging. *Clin. Geriatr. Med.* **5,** 183–188.
38. Forscher, B., and Cecil, H. C. (1958). Some effects of age on the biochemistry of acute inflammation. *Gerontologia* **2,** 174–175.
39. Cohen, B. J., Danon, D., and Roth, G. S. (1987). Wound repair in mice as influenced by age and antimacrophage serum. *J. Gerontol.* **42,** 295–301.
40. Yamuara, H., and Matsuzawa, T. (1980). Decrease in capillary growth during aging. *Exp. Gerontol.* **15,** 145–150.
41. Bruce, S. A., and Deamond, S. F. (1991). Longitudinal study of *in vivo* wound repair and *in vitro* cellular senescence of dermal fibroblasts. *Exp. Gerontol.* **26,** 17–27.
42. Kennedy, D. F., and Cliff, W. J. (1979). A systematic study of wound contraction in mammalian skin. *Pathology* **11,** 207–222.
43. Holm-Pedersen, P., and Zederfeldt, B. (1971). Strength development of skin incisions in young and old rats. *Scand. J. Plast. Reconstr. Surg.* **5,** 7–12.
44. Wu, L., Brucker, M., Gruskin, E., Roth, S. I., and Mustoe, T. A. (1997). Differential effects of platelet-derived growth factor BB in accelerating wound healing in aged versus young animals: The impact of tissue hypoxia. *Plast. Reconstr. Surg.* **99,** 815–822.

45. Beck, L. S. DeGuzman, L., Lee, W. P., Xu, Y., Siegel, M. W., and Amento, E. P. (1993). One systemic administration of transforming growth factor-B1 reverses age-or glucocorticoid-impaired wound healing. *J. Clin. Invest.* **92,** 2841–2849.
46. Aschcroft, G. S., Horan, M. A., and Ferguson, M. W. (1997). Aging is associated with reduced deposition of specific extracellular matrix components, an upregulation of angiogenesis, and an altered inflammatory response in a murine incisional wound healing model. *J. Invest. Dermatol.* **108,** 430–437.
47. Aschcroft, G. S., Horan, M. A., and Ferguson, M. W. (1997). The effects of ageing on wound healing: Immunolocalisation of growth factors and their receptors in a murine incisional model. *J. Anat.* **190,** 351–365.
48. Quirinia, A., and Viidik, A. (1991). The influence of age on the healing of normal and ischemic incisional skin wounds. *Mech. Ageing Dev.* **58,** 221–232.
49. Wu, L., Xia, Y. P., Roth, S. I., Gruskin, E., and Mustoe, T. A. (1999). Transforming growth factor-beta 1 fails to stimulate wound healing and impairs its signal transduction in an aged ischemic ulcer model: Importance of oxygen and age. *Am. J. Pathol.* **154,** 301–309.
50. Krull, E. A. (1985). Chronic cutaneous ulcerations and impaired healing in human skin. *J. Am. Acad. Dermatol.* **12,** 394–401.
51. Mustoe, T. A., Pierce, G. F., Morishima, C., and Deuel, T. F. (1991). Growth factor-induced accleration of tissue repair through direct and inductive activities in a rabbit dermal ulcer model. *J. Clin. Invest.* **87,** 694–703.
52. Joseph, J., and Townsend, F. J. (1961). The healing of defects in immobile skin in rabbits. *Br. J. Surg.* **48,** 557–564.
53. Zahir, M. (1964). Contraction of wounds. *Br. J. Surg.* **31,** 456–461.
54. Groth, K. E. (1942). Klinische Beobachtungen und esperimentelle Studien uber die Enstehung des Dekubitus. *Acta. Chir. Scand.* **87** (Suppl. 76), 183–200.
55. Kosiak, M. (1959). Etiology and pathology of ischemic ulcers. *Arch. Phys. Med. Rehabil.* **40,** 62–69.
56. Daniel, R. K., Priest, D. L., and Wheatley, D. C. (1981). Etiologic factors in pressure sore: An experimental model. *Arch. Phys. Med. Rehabil.* **62,** 492–498.
57. Hyodo, A., Reger, S. I., Negami, S., Kambic, H., Reyes, E., and Browne, E. Z. (1995). Evaluation of a pressure sore model using monoplegic pigs. *Plast. Reconstr. Surg.* **96,** 421–428.
58. Swaim, S. F., Bradley, D. M., Vaughn, D. M., Powers, R. D., and Hoffman, C. E. (1993). The greyhound dog as a model for studying pressure ulcers. *Decubitus* **6,** 32–40.
59. Pryce, T. D. (1887). A case of perforating ulcers of both feet associated with diabetes and ataxic symptoms. *Lancet* **2,** 11–12.
60. Nwomeh, B. C., Yager, D. R., and Cohen, I. K. (1998). Physiology of the chronic wound. *Clin. Plast. Surg.* **25**(3), 341–355.
61. Levin, M. E. (1993). Diabetic foot ulcers: Pathogenesis and management. *J. ET Nurs.* **20,** 191–198.
62. Rerup, C. C. (1970). Drugs producing diabetes through damage of the insulin secreting cell. *Pharm. Rev.* **22,** 485–518.
63. Junod, A., Lambert, A. E., Orci, L., Pictet, R., Gonet, A. E., and Renold, A. E. (1967). Studies of the diabetogenic action of streptozotocin or by alloxan. *Proc. Soc. Exp. Biol. Med.* **126,** 201–205.
64. Mansford, K. R., and Opie, L. (1968). Comparison of metabolic abnormalities in diabetes mellitus induced by streptozotocin or by alloxan. *Lancet* **1,** 670–671.
65. Covington, D. S., Xue, H., Pizzini, R., Lally, K. P., and Andrassy, R. J. (1993). Streptozotocin and alloxan are comparable agents in the diabetic model of impaired wound healing. *Diabetes Res.* **23**(2), 47–53.
66. Goodson, W. H., and Hunt, T. K. (1977). Studies of wound healing in experimental diabetes mellitus. *J. Surg. Res.* **22,** 221–227.
67. Broadley, K. N., Aquino, A. M., Hicks, B., Ditesheim, J. A., McGee, G. S., Demetriou, A. A., Woodward, S. C., and Davidson, J. M. (1989–1990). The diabetic rat as an impaired wound healing model: Stimulatory effects of transforming growth factor-beta and basic fibroblast growth factor. *Biotechnol. Ther.* **1** (1), 55–68.
68. Lampeter, E. F., Signore, A., Gale, E. A., and Pozzilli, P. (1989). Lessons from the NOD mouse for the pathogenesis and immunotherapy of human type 1 (insulin-dependent) diabetes mellitus. *Diabetologia* **32,** 703–708.
69. Kahn, C. R. (1973). Insulin-receptor interaction in the obese-hyperglycemic mouse. A model of insulin resistance. *J. Biol. Chem.* **273,** 244–250.
70. Soret, M. G., and Dulin, W. E. (1981). Animal models of spontaneous diabetes. *In* "The Islets of Langerhans: Biochemistry, Physiology and Pathology" (S. J. Cooperstein and D. Watkins, eds.), pp.357–385. Academic Press, New York.
71. Goodson, W. H., and Hunt, T. K. (1979). Deficient collagen formation by obese mice in a standard wound model. *Am. J. Surg.* **138,** 692–694.
72. Goodson, W. H., and Hunt, T. K. (1986). Wound collagen accumulation in obese hyperglycemic mice. *Diabetes* **35,** 491–495.
73. Musote, T. A., and Porras-Reyes, B. H. (1993). Modulation of wound healing response in chronic irradiated tissues. *Clin. Plast. Surg.* **20,** 465–472.
74. Cromack, D. T., Porras-Reyes, B., Purdy, J. A., Pierce, G. F., and Mustoe, T. A. (1993). Acceleration of tissue repair by transforming growth factor beta 1 Identification of *in vivo* mechanism of action with radiotherapy-induced specific healing deficits. *Surgery* **113,** 36–42.
75. Mustoe, T. A., Purdy, J. Gramates, P., Deuel, T. F., Thomason, A., and Pierce, G. F. (1989). Reversal of impaired wound healing in irradiated rats by platelet-derived growth factor-BB. *Am. J. Surg.* **158,** 345–350.
76. Vegesna, V., McBride, W. H., Taylor, J. M., and Withers, H. R. (1995). The effect of interleukin-1 beta or transforming growth factor-beta on radiation-impaired murine skin wound healing. *J. Surg. Res.* **59,** 699–704.
77. Schwentker, A., Evans, S. M., Partington, M., Johnson, B. L., Koch, C. J., and Thom, S. R. (1998). A model of wound healing in chronically radiation-damaged rat skin. *Cancer Lett.* **128,** 71–78.
78. Leibovich, S. J., and Ross, R. (1975). The role of the macrophage in wound repair. A study with hydrocortisone and antimacrophage serum. *Am. J. Pathol.* **78,** 71–100.
79. Ehrlich, H. P., and Hunt, T. K. (1968). Effect of cortisone and vitamin A on wound healing. *Ann. Surg.* **167,** 324–328.
80. Hubner, G., Brauchle, M., Smola, H., Madlener, M., Fassler, R., and Werner, S. (1996). Differential regulation of pro-inflammatory cytokines during wound healing in normal and glucocorticoid-treated mice. *Cytokine* **8,** 548–556.
81. Dostal, G. H., and Gamelli, R. L. (1990). The differential effect of corticosteroids on wound disruption strength in mice. *Arch. Surg.* **125,** 636–640.
82. Karr, B. P., Bubak, P. J., Sprugel, K. H., Pavlin, E. G., and Engrav, L. H. (1995). Platelet-derived growth factor and wound contraction in the rat. *J. Surg. Res.* **59,** 739–742.
83. Pierce, G. F., Mustoe, T. A., Lingelbach, J., Masakowski, V. R., Gramates, P., and Deuel, T. F. (1989). Transforming growth factor B reverses the glucocorticoid-induced wound-healing deficit in rats: Possible regulation in macrophages by platelet-derived growth factor. *Proc. Natl. Acad. Sci. U.S.A.* **86,** 2229–2233.
84. Klingbeil, C. K., Cesar, L. B., and Fiddes, J. C. (1991). Basic fibroblast growth factor accelerates tissue repair in models of impaired wound healing. *Prog. Clin. Biol. Res.* **365,** 443–458.
85. Beer, H. D., Longaker, M. T., and Werner, S. (1997). Reduced expression of PDGF and PDGF receptors during impaired wound healing. *J. Invest. Dermatol.* **109,** 132–138.
86. Tan, C., Etcubanas, E., Wollner, N., Rosen, G., Gilladoga, A., Showel, J., Murphy, M. L., and Krakoff, I. H. (1973). Adriamycin, an antitumor antibiotic in the treatment of neoplastic disease. *Cancer* **32,** 9–17.
87. Hortobagyi, G. N. (1997). Anthracyclines in the treatment of cancer. An overview. *Drugs* **54** (Suppl. 4), 1–7.

88. Devereux, D. F., Thibault, L., Boretor, J., and Brennan, M. F. (1979). The quantitative and qualitative impairment of wound healing by adriamycin. *Cancer* **43,** 932–938.
89. Devereux, D. F., Triche, T. J., Webber, B. L., Thibault, L. E., and Brennan, M. F. (1980). A study of adriamycin-reduced wound breaking strength in rats. *Cancer* **45,** 2811–2815.
90. Devereux, D. F., Kent, H., and Brennan, M. F. (1980). Time dependent effects of adriamycin and x-ray therapy on wound healing in the rat. *Cancer* **45,** 2805–2810.
91. Lawrence, W. T., Norton, J. A., Sporn, M. B., Gorschboth, C., and Grotendorst, G. R. (1986). The reversal of an adriamycin induced healing impairment with chemoattractants and growth factors. *Ann. Surg.* **203**(2), 142–147.
92. Cohen, S. C., Gabelnick, H. L., Johnson, R. K., and Goldin, A. (1975). Effects of antineoplastic agents on wound healing in mice. *Surgery* **78** (2), 238–244.
93. Sandison, J. C. (1924). A new method for the microscopic study of living growing tissues by the introduction of a transparent chamber in the rabbit's ear. *Anat. Rec.* **28,** 281–287.
94. Howden, G. F., and Silver, I. A. (1980). The use of an improved rabbit ear chamber technique for the study of dental materials. *Int. Endodont. J.* **14,** 3–16.
95. Edwards, L. C., Pernokas, L. N., and Dunphy, J. E. (1957). The use of plastic sponges to sample regenerating tissue in healing wounds. *Surg. Gynecol. Obstet.* **105,** 303–309.
96. Knighton, D. R., Silver, I. A., and Hunt, T. K. (1981). Regulation of wound-healing angiogenesis—Effect of oxygen gradients and inspired oxygen concentration. *Surgery* **90,** 262–270.
97. Lundberg, C., Campbell, D., Agerup, B., and Ulfendahl, H. (1981). Quantification of the inflammatory reaction and collagen accumulation in an experimental model of open wounds in the rat. *Scand. J. Plast. Reconstr. Surg.* **16,** 123–131.
98. Brennan, S. S., and Leaper, D. J. (1985). The effect of antiseptics on the healing wound: a study using the rabbit ear chamber. *Br. J. Surg.* **72,** 780–782.
99. Viljanto, J. (1980). Disinfection of surgical wounds without inhibition of normal wound healing. *Ann. Surg.* **115,** 253–256.
100. Gruber, R. P., Vistns, L., and Pardoe, R. (1975). The effect of commonly used antiseptics on wound healing. *Plast. Reconstr. Surg.* **55,** 472–476.
101. Breuing, K., Eriksson, E., Liu, P., and Miller, D. R. (1992). Healing of partial thickness porcine skin wounds in a liquid environment. *J. Surg. Res.* **52,** 50–58.
102. Buckley, A., Davidson, J. M., Kamerath, C. D., Wolt, T. B., and Woodward, S. C. (1985). Sustained release of epidermal growth factor accelerates wound repair. *Proc. Natl. Acad. Sci. U.S.A.* **82,** 7340–7344.
103. Ford, H. R., Hoffman, R. A., Wing, E. J., Magee, M., McIntyre, L., and Simmons, R. L. (1989). Characterization of wound cytokines in the sponge matrix model. *Arch. Surg.* **124,** 1422–1428.
104. Sawai, T., Usui, N., Sando, K., Fukui, Y., Kamata, S., Okada, A., Taniguchi, N., Itano, N., and Kimata, K. (1997). Hyaluronic acid of wound fluid in adult and fetal rabbits. *J. Pediatr. Surg.* **32,** 41–43.
105. Mahadevan, V., Hart, I. R., and Lewis, G. P. (1989). Factors influencing blood supply in wound healing granuloma quantitated by a new *in vivo* technique. *Cancer Res.* **49,** 415–419.
106. Barbul, A., Shawe, T., Rotter, S. M., Efron, J. E., Wasserkrug, H. L., and Badawy, S. B. (1989). Wound healing in nude mice: A study on the regulatory role of lymphocytes in fibroplasia. *Surgery* **105,** 764–769.
107. Niinikoski, J., Hunt, T. K., and Dunphy, J. E. (1972). Oxygen supply in healing tissue. *Am. J. Surg.* **123**(3), 247–252.
108. Hunt, T. K., and Pai, M. P. (1972). The effect of varying ambient oxygen tensions on wound metabolism and collagen synthesis. *Surg. Gynecol. Obstet.* **135**(4), 561–567.
109. Pajulo, Q., Vilijanto, J., Lonnberg, B., Hurne, T., Hurme, T., Lonnqvist, K., and Saukko, P. (1996). Viscose cellulose sponge as an implantable matrix: Changes in the structure increase the production of granulation tissue. *J. Biomed. Mater. Res.* **32,** 439–446.
110. Salvatore, J. E., Gimler, Jr., W. S., Kashgaran, M., and Barbee, R. (1961). An experimental study of the influence of pore size of implanted polyurethane sponges upon subsequent tissue formation. *Surg. Gynecol. Obstet.* **112,** 463–468.
111. Peakcock, E. E. (1984). Collagenolysis and the biochemistry of wound healing. *In* "Wound Repair" (E. E. Peakcock, ed.), pp. 102–140. Saunders, Philadelphia.
112. Morin, G., Rand, M., Burgess, L. P., Voussoughi, J., and Graeber, G. M. (1989). Wound healing: Relationship of wound closing tension to tensile strength in rats. *Laryngoscope* **99,** 783–788.
113. McGee, G. S., Davidson, J. M., Buckley, A., Sommer, A., Woodward, S. C., Aquino, A. M., Barbour, R., and Demetriou, A. A. (1988). Recombinant basic fibroblast growth factor accelerates wound healing. *J. Surg. Res.* **45,** 145–153.
114. Ross, M. H., Romrell, L. J., and Kaye, G. I. Methods. *In* "Histology: A Text and Atlas" (M. H. Ross, L. J. Romrell, and G. I. Kaye, eds.), pp. 1–17. Williams & Wilkins, Baltimore.
115. Rosai, J. (1996). "Ackerman's Surgical Pathology," 8th Ed. C. V. Mosby Company, St. Louis.
116. Morotta, M., *et al.* (1985). Sensitive spectrophotometric method for the quantitative estimation of collagen. *Anal. Biochem.* **150**(1), 86–90.
117. Depalma, R. L., Krummel, T. M., Durham, L. A., Michna, B. A., Thomas, B. L., and Nelson, J. M. (1989). Characterization and quantitation of wound matrix in the fetal rabbit. *Matrix* **9**(3), 224–231.
118. Darr, D., McCormack, K. M., Manning, T., Dunston, S., Winston, D. C., Schulte, B. A., Buller, T., and Pinnell, S. R. (1990). Comparison of *Dolichos biflorus* lectin and other lectin-horseradish peroxidase conjugates in staining of cutaneous blood vessels in the hairless mini-pig. *J. Cutan. Pathol.* **17**(1), 9–15.
119. Kane, C. J. M., Hebda, P. A., Mansbridge, J. N., and Hanawalt, P. C. (1991). Direct evidence for spatial and temporal regulation of transforming growth factor B1 expression during cutaneous wound healing. *J. Cell. Physiol.* **148,** 157–173.
120. Nath, R. K., LaRegina, M., Markham, H., Ksander, G. A., and Weeks, P. M. (1994). The expression of transforming growth factor type beta in fetal and adult rabbit skin wounds. *J. Pediatr. Surg.* **29**(3), 416–421.
121. Gold, L. I., Sung, J. J. Siebert, J. W., and Longaker, M. T. (1997). Type I (RI) and type II (RII) receptors for transforming growth factor-B isoforms are expressed subsequent to transforming growth factor-B ligands during excisional wound repair. *Am. J. Pathol.* **150**(1), 209–222.
122. Kamler, M., Lehr, H. A., Barker, J. H., Saetzler, R. K., Galla, T. J., and Messmer, K. (1993). Impact of ischemia on tissue oxygenation and wound healing: intravital microscopic studies on the hairless mouse ear model. *Eur. Surg. Res.* **25,** 30–37.
123. Uhl, E., Sirsjo, A., Haapaniemi, T., Nilsson, G., and Nylander, G. (1994). Hyperbaric oxygen improves wound healing in normal and ischemic skin tissue. *Plast. Reconstr. Surg.* **93,** 835–841.
124. Silverberg, S. G. (1976). Reproducibility of the mitosis count in the histologic diagnosis of smooth muscle tumors of the uterus. *Hum. Pathol.* **7,** 451–454.
125. Donhuijsen, K. (1986). Reproducibility and significance in grading of malignancy. *Hum. Pathol.* **17,** 1122–1125.
126. Gratzner, H. G. (1982). Monoclonal antibodies to 5-bromo- and 5-iododeoxyuridine. A new reagent for detection of DNA replication. *Science* **218,** 474–475.
127. Robbins, B. A., de la Vega, D., Ogata, K., Tan, E. M., and Nakamura, R. M. (1987). Immunohistochemical detection of proliferating cell nuclear antigen in solid human malignancies. *Arch. Pathol. Lab. Med.* **111,** 841–845.

128. Meyer, J. S., Friedman, E., McCrate, M. M., and Bauer, W. C. (1983). Prediction of early course of breast carcinoma by thymidine labeling. *Cancer* **51,** 1879–1886.
129. Tompach, P. C., Lew, D., and Stoll, J. L. (1997). Cell response to hyperbaric oxygen treatment. *Int. J. Oral Maxillofac. Surg.* **26,** 82–86.
130. Hehenberger, K., Brismar, K., Lind, F., and Kratz, G. (1997). Dose-dependent hyperbaric oxygen stimulation of human fibroblast proliferation. *Wound Rep. Regen.* **5,** 147–150.
131. Garner, W. L., Karmiol, S., Rodriguez, J. L., Smith, D. J., and Phan, S. H. (1993). Phenotypic differences in cytokine responsiveness of hypertrophic scar versus normal dermal fibroblasts. *J. Invest. Dermatol.* **101,** 875–879.
132. Siddiqui, A., Galiano, R. D., Connors, D., Gruskin, E., Wu, L., and Mustoe, T. A. (1996). Differential effects of oxygen on human dermal fibroblasts: Acute versus chronic hypoxia. *Wound Rep. Regen.* **4,** 211–218.
133. Wu, L., Siddiqui, A., Morris, D. E., Cox, D. A., Roth, S. I., and Mustoe, T. A. (1997). Transforming growth factor B3 (TGFB3) accelerates wound healing without alteration of scar prominence. *Arch. Surg.* **132,** 753–760.
134. Siebert, P. D., and Larrick, J. W. (1992). Competitive PCR. *Nature (London)* **359,** 557–558.
135. Schillace, R. V., and Scott, J. D. (1999). Organization of kinases, phosphatases, and receptor signaling complexes. *J. Clin. Invest.* **103,** 761–765.
136. Web site: http://stke.org

63

Animal Models of Sepsis and the Multiple Organ Dysfunction Syndrome

Mitchell P. Fink

Departments of Anesthesiology, Critical Care Medicine, and Surgery, University of Pittsburgh Medical School, Pittsburgh, Pennsylvania 15261

I. Rationale

It is reasonable to ask whether the use of animal models for studying sepsis is still necessary or valuable. Certainly, reductionist *in vitro* methods have proved to be enormously powerful for studying immunological processes at the cellular and subcellular levels, and, by using these methods, we have made huge strides in our understanding of the basic biochemical mechanisms underlying inflammation. Furthermore, no animal model, however sophisticated or complex, will ever completely and accurately replicate all the features of a patient being treated for sepsis and multiple organ system dysfunction (MODS) in a modern intensive care unit.

For a number of compelling reasons, however, *in vivo* studies using experimental animal models continue to be an important component of research into the pathogenesis and treatment of sepsis. First, by their very nature, reductionist methods using cultured cells (or parts of cells) grossly oversimplify the complex interactions that are characteristic of the *in vivo* system. Heretofore, progress in science often has been made by choosing the right simplifying assumptions, and one of the goals of experimental design has been to eliminate to as great an extent as possible the confounding influences of uncontrolled variables. But, in the past few years, the advent of potent statistical and mathematical methods and the wide availability of powerful computers have made the analysis of so-called complex systems both feasible and desirable in fields as disparate as engineering and biology (1, 2). The development of rigorous methods for analyzing complex systems has reawakened interest in "integrative biology" and, hence, the need for reasonable animal models of diseases (including sepsis and MODS).

Second, certain experiments—for example, those using *ex vivo* organ preparations or highly invasive monitoring techniques—can only be performed with the use of animal models. Similarly, in order to gain insights into the pathophysiology of sepsis, it often is necessary to obtain samples of tissue (e.g., lung or liver) that are always, or almost always, unavailable in the clinical setting. Only by using animal models is it possible to obtain samples of tissue at various stages in the septic process.

Third, septic humans inevitably receive supportive care (e.g., intravenous fluids, antibiotics, and vasoactive and/or inotropic drugs). Thus, knowledge gained about the pathophysiology of sepsis based on human studies inevitably reflects not the natural history of the syndrome but rather the summation of the effects of the septic process per se and the interventions used to treat it. Animal models provide an opportunity to study the pathophysiology of sepsis in the absence of confounding effects from therapeutic interventions.

Fourth, many insights into the pathogenesis of sepsis have come from using drugs or other reagents, such as antibodies, to antagonize or neutralize selectively the effects of a specific mediator, cell surface receptor, or intracellular signaling molecule. Some of these drugs are known to be toxic, and, thus, are inappropriate for use in clinical studies. Other agents, although not obviously toxic, have not been studied sufficiently in humans to permit their utilization in critically ill patients. Therefore, only by using animal models can investigators ethically take advantage of these compounds to probe the molecular mechanisms responsible for the septic process.

Fifth, although sepsis is a relatively common clinical problem, it is nevertheless a sporadic and unpredictable occurrence. In almost all cases, it is difficult or impossible to determine accurately the time of onset. Premorbid (i.e., "baseline") data obtained before the onset of the septic process are rarely available. In addition, there are numerous precipitating causes of sepsis, such as peritonitis or pneumonia, and literally hundreds of different kinds of pathogens. Furthermore, although previously healthy individuals occasionally fall victim to life-threatening systemic infections, most cases of sepsis occur in people with other serious, unrelated problems. Thus, the biology of sepsis, septic shock, and MODS in humans is inherently "noisy" because of the wide variety of responsible infections and infectious agents and the confounding effects of myriad unmeasured variables. Whereas biological variability is still a problem in studies using animal models, subject-to-subject variation is much less problematic than in the clinical setting, particularly when experiments are performed using highly inbred strains of mice, rats, or guinea pigs. Thus, the minimum sample size needed to obtain a statistically meaningful result is typically much smaller for studies using animal models than is the case for studies using patients.

Sixth, it is always necessary to obtain preliminary data in animals before using experimental drugs or devices in humans. Apart from the obvious regulatory issues, thoughtfully designed preclinical studies in animals can be useful to investigators by helping them to select only the most promising agents for much more costly (and, of course, risky) trials in humans. Preclinical studies also can aid in the development of the best design for a clinical trial. For example, if a new agent works only when it is given as a pretreatment prior to the onset of sepsis, then the compound probably should not be evaluated for the therapy of established sepsis in humans but rather should be tested in a prophylactic fashion in high-risk subjects.

II. The Choice of Species

As noted previously (3), the choice of species for studies of sepsis is dictated by many factors. The most important considerations should be the goals of the study and the constraints imposed by the experimental design. Nevertheless, other considerations are cost and the availability of facilities for the care and housing of the experimental animals. Unfortunately, in some localities, the presence of antivivisectionist groups is another issue that must be considered by the investigator. Studies using certain species, notably cats, dogs, and nonhuman primates, are more likely to engender protests, and even sabotage, than are studies employing mice or rats.

Some of the advantages and disadvantages of various species are summarized in Table I. Being inexpensive to purchase and maintain, small mammals (mice, rats, and guinea pigs) are desirable for many studies, particularly when a large number of conditions (e.g., graded doses of an investigational therapeutic agent) are being evaluated. Studies using survival as a primary endpoint typically require fairly large sample sizes ($N = 12–15$) because of the binary nature of the outcome parameter. Accordingly, smaller (less costly) species, such as mice (4), rats (5), or rabbits (6), are commonly used for survival studies, although larger mammals, such as dogs (7) or baboons (8), also have been employed in selected cases. Smaller animals, notably rats, guinea pigs, and rabbits, are well suited for studies examining organ function *ex vivo*, using, for example, the Langendorf preparation to examine cardiac function (9, 10) or the isolated liver preparation to examine hepatic metabolism (11). Rats are particularly useful for studies using intravital microscopy to examine microvascular function in various organs in the intact animal (12–14).

Extensive inbreeding in certain strains of mice, rats, or guinea pigs tends to minimize subject-to-subject variability. Inbred strains of mice, however, are invaluable in sepsis research for another reason. For many years, inbred strains have been available that manifest special characteristics, such as resistance to the toxic effects of lipopolysaccharide (LPS) in C3H/HeJ mice (15, 16). Now, genetically engineered strains of mice are widely available. Some transgenic strains express or overexpress a specific protein, e.g., human CD14 (17), human copper/zinc superoxide dismutase (18),

Table I Summary of Advantages and Disadvantages of Animal Models of Sepsis

Species	Advantages	Disadvantages
Mouse	Inexpensive; inbred strains available; subject-to-subject variability low; transgenic constructs available; immunologic reagents widely available	Repetitive blood difficult; hemodynamic measurements difficult; moderately resistant to LPS
Rat	Inexpensive; inbred strains available; subject-to-subject variability low; most hemodynamic measurements feasible; chronic instrumentation feasible; fecal flora similar to that of humans	Very resistant to LPS
Rabbit	Inexpensive; chronic instrumentation feasible; most hemodynamic measurements feasible; very sensitive to LPS; acute lung injury reminiscent of human ARDS after bacterial or endotoxic challenge	Gram-positive fecal flora
Sheep	Relatively inexpensive for a large animal; fecal flora similar to that of humans; well-suited for hemodynamic measurements and repetitive blood sampling; acute lung injury reminiscent of human ARDS after bacterial or endotoxic challenge; well-suited for chronic instrumentation; very sensitive to LPS	
Pig	Relatively inexpensive; fecal flora similar to that of humans; well suited for hemodynamic measurements and repetitive blood sampling; acute lung injury reminiscent of human ARDS after bacterial or endotoxic challenge; relatively sensitive to LPS	Chronic instrumentation difficult
Dog	Fecal flora similar to that of humans; well-suited for hemodynamic measurements and repetitive blood sampling; chronic instrumentation feasible	Moderately resistant to LPS; relatively expensive; portal venous hypertension after endotoxic challenge
Baboon	Well-suited for hemodynamic measurements and repetitive blood sampling; antibodies against human proteins (e.g., cytokines) commonly cross react	Very expensive; chronic instrumentation difficult; very resistant to LP

or high-density lipoprotein [19]. Other transgenic constructs, called "knockouts," have been engineered with a targeted mutation in a specific gene that prevents production of a selected protein, such as CD14 (20), STAT1 (21), α-2-macroglobulin (22), neutral endopeptidase (23), interferon-γ (24), metallothionein (25), the inducible isoform of nitric oxide synthase (26), or the 55-kDa tumor necrosis factor receptor (15).

Instrumentation is available that makes it fairly easy to measure cardiac output by thermodilution in rats (27, 28) and even mice (29, 30). Indeed, because of the power and elegance of studies using transgenic mice, physiologists have developed methods for making more and more complex measurements in these small animals. For example, echocardiographic (1, 31) and magnetic resonance imaging (30) techniques have been used in mice to make measurements of left ventricular function. Approaches have been developed for using mice for *in vivo* studies of renal tubular function (32, 33), cerebral blood flow (34), mechanical ventilation (35, 36), and airway pressures and resistance (37).

Although it is remarkable how much physiologic information can be obtained using mice, it is nevertheless true that cardiac output and pulmonary artery pressure are more easily measured in larger animals (e.g., pigs, sheep, dogs, and primates). These larger species also are useful in certain studies because their greater circulating volume permits the investigator to collect multiple blood samples for obtaining cells or for measuring the concentrations of various mediators. Sheep are quite docile. After prior placement under general anesthesia of indwelling catheters and other forms of chronic instrumentation, sheep can be studied in the unanesthetized state over a period of several hours (38, 39) or days (40–43). Although other large animals, including dogs (44–46) and pigs (47), also can be studied in the absence of anesthesia, the techniques required are more involved than is the case with sheep. Renal, cardiovascular, and digestive anatomy and physiology in pigs are thought be quite similar to these aspects in humans (48, 49). Accordingly, pigs have become very popular for physiologic and pharmacologic studies, including those in the area of sepsis research.

Specialized inflammatory cells, called pulmonary intravascular macrophages (PIMs), are embedded within the endothelial lining of pulmonary arterioles in certain species, notably pigs (50) and sheep (51). Probably because of the presence of PIMs, pigs and sheep develop marked pulmonary hypertension and other manifestations of acute lung injury, including pulmonary edema and increased airway resistance, when challenged intravenously with purified LPS or viable gram-negative bacteria (52). In addition, the pulmonary lymphatic anatomy in sheep has been studied extensively (53–55), and a lung lymph fistula preparation, which entails cannulation of the efferent lymphatic vessel from a specific node (the caudal mediastinal lymph node), has been widely employed to investigate the pathophysiology of sepsis-induced acute lung injury (42, 56–59). PIMs are not present in the pulmonary microvasculature of several commonly used laboratory animal species, such as rodents, but may be present in humans (52). However, under pathologic conditions, such as chronic biliary obstruction, PIMs are induced (60); thus, studies using species (such as pigs and sheep) in which PIMs are present constituitively are likely to be pertinent to human acute lung injury.

Nonhuman primates, such as baboons or cynomolgus monkeys, are phylogenetically more similar to humans than are any other species employed for laboratory studies. Thus, primates remain invaluable for certain kinds of studies in the sepsis field. For example, antibodies to certain human cytokines or cell surface receptors (e.g., CD11b) can be very narrowly cross-reactive with the equivalent proteins in other species, and the only appropriate model system for preclinical evaluation may be one using primates. Nevertheless, baboons and other primates are very expensive to acquire and house, and because these animals tend to be both smart and aggressive, working with them requires special skills and training. Thus, primates are best reserved for key experiments that require only relatively small sample sizes.

III. The Ideal Animal Model of Sepsis

Hundreds of different models of sepsis have been described, and new ones are still being developed. Indeed, the sheer number of models is *prima facie* evidence that no single model is perfect or appropriate for all applications—if a perfect sepsis model existed, all investigators would use it, and other models would be unnecessary. If an "ideal" animal model of sepsis existed, it would meet all of the following criteria:

1. Capable of predicting both positive and negative results from clinical trials of new therapeutic agents
2. Inexpensive
3. Reproducible within a given laboratory
4. Reproducible among different laboratories
5. Humane
6. Capable of providing a mortality endpoint
7. Characterized by hemodynamic, hematologic, and biochemical features similar to those observed in human sepsis

Preclinical studies of new therapeutic agents using an "ideal" animal model of sepsis should accurately predict the results of subsequent clinical trials in patients. However, as yet, no new agent for the adjuvant treatment of sepsis has been shown to be effective in a large-scale (phase III) clinical trial. Therefore, it remains to be shown that any existing animal model of sepsis is capable of predicting positive results from a study in patients. Some models (e.g., cecal ligation and perforation in mice) have predicted the negative results obtained in clinical trials with certain new therapeutic interventions [e.g., antibodies to tumor necrosis factor (TNF)] (61–63).

Reproducibility, both within and among laboratories, is an important characteristic of any animal disease model. Unfortunately, clinical verisimilitude and reproducibility are, to some extent, mutually exclusive attributes in sepsis research, because sepsis in humans most commonly occurs in patients with other preexisting serious medical problems. In other words, the underlying substrate for sepsis in humans can be quite variable, whereas in most experimental models, the investigator seeks to maximize reproducibility by employing closely matched young healthy subjects (often from an inbred strain of animals).

In clinical trials of new therapeutic agents for the adjuvant treatment of sepsis, mortality at a specific time point (e.g., 28 or 30 days) has been mandated by the Food and Drug Administration (FDA) as the only acceptable read-out for providing proof of efficacy. A discussion of the relative merits and disadvantages of this view is beyond the scope of the present discussion. Still, it is worth pointing out that changes in mortality rate reflect the summation of all the salutary and deleterious effects of any new therapeutic agent or intervention. In preclinical studies, mortality data provide a similar "integrative" view of the effects of novel therapeutic strategies. Although mortality is not the appropriate read-out for all studies of sepsis using animal models, an "ideal" model should be capable of providing mortality data as necessary.

IV. Specific Animal Models of Sepsis

It would be neither feasible nor desirable to provide here an exhaustive description of every published animal model of sepsis. Nevertheless, certain general categories warrant discussion. A few specific models will be discussed in more detail.

A. Endotoxicosis Models

Administration of lipopolysaccharide (endotoxin) is one of the most commonly employed means for inducing a sepsislike state in experimental animals. The use of lipopolysaccharide (LPS) offers the investigator some important advantages, including convenience, precision in dosing, and reproducibility. For best results, a known quantity of LPS sufficient for all the animals in a given experiment is obtained from a single lot, accurately weighed, and suspended in saline or other physiologic salt solution. Small aliquots are prepared and frozen. The aliquots are thawed for use as needed.

Although inducing "sepsis" by administering LPS is convenient and reproducible, there are important differences between experimentally induced endotoxicosis and clinical sepsis. This important issue has been reviewed recently by O'Reilly *et al.* (64). The key issue is this: In endotoxicosis, the inflammatory response alone, generated by the host, can be deleterious. However, in most cases of clinical sepsis, the host is also confronted by an invasive microbial infection, which can be contained and ultimately eradicated only with the aid of an adequately orchestrated inflammatory response. It is not surprising, therefore, that dramatically different results have been obtained when certain antiinflammatory strategies have been evaluated in pure endotoxicosis models as compared to models characterized by the presence of a true microbial infection. For example, antibodies to TNFα provide dramatic protection in animals challenged with purified LPS (65, 66), but anti-TNFα antibodies generally offer no protection or are even deleterious in animals with a focal source of infection (61, 63, 66, 67). Similarly, treatment with the antiinflammatory interleukin cytokine, IL-10, improves survival in endotoxic mice (68, 69) and neutralization of IL-10 worsens survival in endotoxic mice. In contrast, neutralization of endogenous IL-10 improves survival in mice with a focal infection (70). In other words, IL-10 has a beneficial role when mortality is caused by acute endotoxicosis in the absence of infection, but can be deleterious when mortality is caused by a focal bacterial infection.

There are other differences between experimental endotoxicosis and systemic inflammation triggered by a true invasive infection. At least in models of endotoxicosis induced by injecting a single bolus of LPS, the proinflammatory challenge occurs suddenly and lasts only briefly. In contrast, the inflammatory stimulus in a true infection, like pneumonia or peritonitis, tends to develop more gradually and to persist over hours or days. Circulating concentrations of TNFα are much higher 60–90 min after intravenous or intraperitoneal injection of LPS than they are at any time after the onset of a true focal infection such as fecal peritonitis (61, 71, 72).

The most straightforward means of inducing endotoxicosis in experimental animals is to inject a single bolus of LPS intravenously or intraperitoneally. This approach has been and continues to be widely employed in species ranging from mice (4, 73) to baboons (74–76). Even human volunteers can be safely injected with a tiny intravenous bolus of LPS as a means of modeling some of the hemodynamic, hormonal, and metabolic consequences of sepsis (77–79).

Although simple, a single bolus of LPS fails to replicate the persistent inflammatory stimulus represented by a focus of true infection. Furthermore, in certain species, including rats (80), rabbits (81, 82), and dogs (83, 84), administration of a bolus dose of LPS, particularly in the absence of fluid resuscitation, leads to a hypodynamic circulatory profile (i.e., one characterized by low cardiac output and high calculated systemic vascular resistance), which is quite unlike the usual pattern observed in human sepsis. In an effort to circumvent these criticisms, many laboratories have developed experimental endotoxicosis paradigms, which employ various strategies (often in combination) to achieve a cardiovascular profile similar to the vasodilated, hyperdynamic pattern observed in patients with sepsis or septic shock. Among the strategies employed are aggressive fluid resuscitation (83, 85–87), repetitive injections of small doses of LPS over a period of days (88, 89), continuous infusion of a low dose of LPS (42, 43, 90, 91), or observation several (10–24) hours after a single, sublethal dose of LPS (39, 91, 92). Some of these "hyperdynamic" models are accompanied by significant degrees of organ (e.g., lung and/or kidney) dysfunction (40, 93, 94), although mortality typically has not been employed as a primary read-out.

Humans are exquisitely sensitive to LPS. In human volunteers, LPS doses as low as 2–4 ng/kg produce obvious hemodynamic, hematologic, and hormonal perturbations (77–79). Among commonly employed species of laboratory animals, only rabbits (95), pigs (88), and sheep (89) are as (or nearly as) sensitive to LPS as are humans. Other commonly used laboratory species, such as rodents and baboons, are remarkably resistant to endotoxin. Whereas a lethal dose of LPS is about 5 μg/kg in sheep (96) and an LD_{80} dose is 100 μg/kg in adult rabbits (97), the LD_{70} dose of LPS is 6 mg/kg in baboons (74), and an LD_{100} dose is 20–80 mg/kg in mice (4, 61, 73). A number of techniques can be employed to increase the sensitivity of experimental animals, particularly rodents, to LPS. One commonly employed approach, used mostly in murine endotoxicosis studies, consists of simultaneously injecting animals with LPS and galactosamine (98, 99). D-Galactosamine decreases the lethal dose of LPS in mice by at least 10,000-fold (100). Depletion of uridine in hepatocytes is thought to be responsible for the sensitizing effect of D-galactosamine (99). Although treatment with D-galactosamine dramatically increases the sensitivity of mice to the lethal effects of LPS, the resulting model may be largely irrelevant to the problem of clinical sepsis, because the most prominent pathologic feature of this paradigm is massive hepatic necrosis, a finding that is rarely observed in patients dying as a consequence of overwhelming infections.

A number of other approaches have been developed to increase the sensitivity of rodents to the deleterious effects of LPS. For example, Pickett *et al.* reported that pretreatment of mice with Pluronic F 127, a nonionic polyoxyethylene–polypropylene copolymer, increases sensitivity to the lethal and cytokine-inducing effects of LPS by about 25-fold (101). The mechanism(s) responsible for this effect are unknown. In another report, Ogata *et al.* showed that injecting mice intraperitoneally with carageenan 24 hr prior to challenge with LPS markedly sensitizes the animals to the TNF-releasing and lethal effects of endotoxin (102). Similar findings were previously described by Becker and Rudbach (103). Carageenan is a sulfated polygalactose derivative that is both proinflammatory (104) and cytotoxic to macrophages (105). The mechanisms responsible for the sensitizing effect of carrageenan are unknown. Other agents that have been shown to potentiate the lethal effects of LPS in experimental animals include lead acetate (106), berrylium phosphate (107), and carbon tetrachloride (108).

The sensitivity of mice to the deleterious effects of endotoxin is markedly enhanced if the animals are injected with heat-killed *Proprionibacterium acnes* (109), heat-killed *Corynebacterium parvum* (110), or *Mycobacterium bovis* (BCG) (111) 7–10 days prior to being challenged with LPS. Similar findings have been reported in other species, including rats (112). The mechanisms underlying this phenomenon are complex. Important components include expansion and priming of the pool of hepatic macrophages by the sensitizing agent (110, 111, 113), infiltration of the liver by neutrophils following administration of LPS (114), and complement-stimulated oxidant-mediated damage to hepatocytes resulting from activation of inflammatory cells within the liver parenchyma (112). The production of interferon-γ by T cells is also important, because neutralization of this cytokine ameliorates sensitization (109) and T cell-deficient mice are resistant to the sensitizing effects of agents such as *P. acnes* (115).

Platelet-activating factor (PAF) is another factor that has been shown to sensitize rodents to the deleterious effects of LPS. Rabinovici and colleagues have shown that infusing rats with a very small dose of PAF (1 pmol/kg/min), which alone causes no injurious effects, markedly decreases the dose of intravenous LPS required to induce acute lung injury (116–118). Similarly, combined administration of very small doses of PAF and LPS has been shown to elicit bowel necrosis in rats, whereas either of the agents given alone do not damage the gut (119, 120).

B. Bacterial Infusion Models

In many ways, models of sepsis characterized by the intravenous (or in some instances, intraarterial) infusion of bacteria suffer from many of the same criticisms directed toward acute endotoxicosis models. Indeed, Cross and colleagues have argued that challenging animals with either LPS or an intravenous bolus of bacteria represents "intoxication" rather than "infection" (121). Furthermore, as in the case of acute endotoxemia, the host's inflammatory response to the inciting challenge can have only deleterious consequences. Accordingly, when evaluating antiinflammatory strategies, it may be unwise to extrapolate results obtained in a bacterial infusion model to other forms of infection characterized by the presence of localized tissue invasion by microbes. Despite these legitimate concerns, many laboratories continue to employ bacterial infusion models in a wide variety of species, including rats, nonhuman primates, pigs, and sheep.

For studies using viable bacteria, the organisms are typically grown in culture during a several-hour period prior to being innoculated into the experimental subjects. The number of bacteria in any given preparation is estimated nephilometrically, but accurate quantification can be achieved only retrospectively by enumerating viable colony-forming units on agar plates. Accordingly, it is considerably more difficult to ensure day-to-day reproducibility of the septic challenge when the model employs viable bacteria as compared to purified LPS.

Depending on the experimental conditions employed, infusing rats with viable *Escherichia coli* can result in either a hypodynamic (122, 123) or hyperdynamic (124) circulatory profile. Infusing cortically unconscious rats with viable *E. coli* has been used extensively for studying the effects of hyperdynamic sepsis on microcirculatory blood flow in skeletal muscle (124, 125), kidney (126), and gut (127, 128).

Bacterial infusion has been employed extensively by a number of different laboratories to produce a sepsis in various nonhuman primate species, particularly baboons (75, 129, 130) and cynomolgus monkeys (131–133). One of the most extensively utilized primate bacteremia models was developed by Hinshaw and colleagues at the University of Oklahoma. In this LD_{100} paradigm, baboons are infused intravenously with an enormous dose [about $(2–5) \times 10^{10}$ cfu/kg] of viable *E. coli* over a 2-hr period (134, 135). After the infusion of bacteria is completed, the animals are treated with gentamicin for an additional 10–72 hr (8, 134, 135). Even without massive resuscitation of intravascular volume, this model is characterized by a very transient increase in cardiac output and a more sustained decrease in systemic vascular resistance (136). If baboons infused with viable *E. coli* are adequately resusciatated with intravenous crystalloid solution, it is possible to document a sustained hyperdynamic and vasodilated systemic hemodynamic profile (130).

In contrast to the results obtained in a number of clinical trials in septic patients (137–139), high doses of methylprednisolone provide remarkable protection against mortality in Hinshaw's primate bacteremia model, even when the glucocorticoid is administered after completion of the infusion of bacteria (134, 135). Anti-TNFα monoclonal antibodies also provide dramatic protection against mortality in primates infused with viable *E. coli* (129), a finding that has not been borne out thus far in clinical trials (140–142).

Because nonhuman primates remain invaluable for certain kinds of studies (see above), there has been interest in improving the Hinshaw sepsis model to make it more relevant to the clinical entity. One such effort was described by Schlag and colleagues (143). In this modified version of the Hinshaw model, baboons are infused over a 2-hr period on three successive days (i.e., beginning at 0, 24, and 48 hr) with a much smaller quantity of bacteria (about 1×10^8 cfu/kg per day) than is employed in the classic paradigm. With this approach, mortality is 50%; deaths occur between hours 36 and 72 of observation.

Intravenous infusion of viable bacteria in anesthetized swine has been extensively employed as a model for sepsis-induced adult respiratory distress syndrome (ARDS). The hemodynamic and pulmonary effects observed in this model are dependent on the organism infused. Whereas infusion of viable *Staphylococcus aureus* produces minimal changes, profound physiologic perturbations, including systemic arterial hypotension (due largely to a decrease in cardiac output) and severe acute lung injury, result when pigs are infused with *E. coli* or *Pseudomonas aeruginosa* (144). The most commonly employed version of this model utilizes a 60-min infusion of viable *P. aeruginosa* at a rate of 7.5×10^6 cfu/min (145–147). This is a model of an overwhelming septic insult studied over a relatively short interval (4 to 5 hr), and remains most useful for studying the role of various mediators in the pathogenesis of sepsis-related ARDS. In most respects, the effects of infusing pigs with viable gram-negative bacteria or purified LPS are very similar.

Haberstroh and colleagues have described a more chronic bacterial infusion model using pigs (148). In this paradigm, chronically instrumented unanesthetized pigs are intravenously infused in a continuous fashion for 84 hr with a relatively low dose (8×10^7 cfu/kg/hr) of viable *P. aeruginosa*. The model is characterized by a triphasic hemodynamic response. During the first phase (0–12 hr), the animals develop pulmonary hypertension and a decrease in cardiac output. During the second phase (12–60 hr), pulmonary arterial pressures and cardiac output normalize. The third phase (60–84 hr) is characterized by a secondary rise in pulmonary arterial pressure, moderate systemic arterial hypotension, and a marked increase in cardiac output. Thus, this model successfully reproduces the hemodynamic profile of compensated hyperdynamic sepsis. Lung dysfunction in this sublethal model is relatively minimal.

A similar chronic *Pseudomonas* infusion model also has been described in sheep (149). In this model, chronically instrumented, unanesthetized sheep are intravenously infused in a continuous fashion for 48 hr with a low dose (2.5×10^6 cfu/kg/hr) of viable *P. aeruginosa*. Crystalloid solution is continuously infused during the period of bacterial infusion at a moderate rate (9 ml/kg/hr). This sublethal sepsis model is characterized by the development of a persistent hyperdynamic circulatory state. Mean systemic arterial pressure decreases significantly and cardiac output increases significantly. This ovine bacterial infusion model replicates the physiologic perterbations, such as moderate arterial hypotension and elevated cardiac output, which are observed in ovine models of chronic low-dose LPS infusion (43, 90, 150). Accordingly, the additional complexity incurred by using live bacteria seems likely to be unwarranted, at least for most experimental questions that might be addressed using this type of model.

The majority of bacterial infusion models employ gram-negative organisms, particularly strains of *E. coli* (8, 124) or *P. aeruginosa* (145, 148, 149); nevetheless, a number of studies have been performed using infusions of gram-positive bacteria or even yeast. For example, the effects of intravenously infusing viable *S. aureus* have been evaluated in pigs (144, 151, 152), dogs (153), and baboons (154). Other studies have evaluated intravenous infusions of viable group B *Streptococcus* in pigs (155, 156) or mice (157) as paradigms for neonatal sepsis caused by this organism in human infants. Intravenous injection of mice with 1.8×10^8 cfu of *Streptococcus pyogenes* results in 90–100% mortality over a 72-hr period of observation, with the majority of deaths occuring between 24 and 48 hr (158). Intravenous infusion of viable *Candida albicans* (10^7 cfu) results in 22% mortality over a 72-hr period of observation in normal (i.e., non-neutropenic) rats (159).

Although most bacterial infusion models of sepsis have employed viable organisms, heat-killed microbes have been employed by some investigators. Wakabayashi *et al.* have described two different rabbit models of septic shock, wherein anesthetized animals are infused intravenously over 20 min with either heat-killed *E. coli* (2×10^9 cfu/kg) (6) or heat-killed *Staphylococcus epidermidis* (1×10^{11} cfu/kg) (160). Only maintenance fluid support (5 ml/kg/hr) is provided. Both models are characterized by the development of marked systemic arterial hypotension and preservation of normal cardiac output (at least until minutes before death). Because aliquots of heat-killed organisms suspended in saline can be stored frozen and thawed as needed, models using nonviable bacteria may offer better day-to-day reproducibility than models that require the daily preparation and quantitation of viable microbes. Moreover, being particulate in nature, heat-killed bacteria may trigger responses (e.g., those due to the activation of phagocytic cells), which are not observed with purified LPS (161).

C. Focal Infection Models

In an effort to model the common causes of sepsis and septic shock in patients, a number of different approaches have been developed for creating serious (i.e., potentially life-threatening) focal infections in experimental animals. As noted above, survival in models of sepsis caused by focal infection reflects the net balance between the beneficial aspects of the host's inflammatory response (as a means for localizing and controlling the infectious process) and the deleterious consequences of systemic inflammation. Accordingly, as a means for predicting the outcome of clinical trials of new therapeutic strategies for the adjuvant therapy of sepsis, models of focal infection are likely to provide more meaningful and interpretable results than are models of intoxication induced by intravenous infusion of (viable or nonviable) microbes. For most studies, particularly those designed to be the last step in the development of a new therapeutic agent prior to beginning testing in humans, models of "true" infection should incorporate most or all of the following characteristics:

1. Sepsis should be induced by a relatively small initial inoculum; i.e., the microbes should proliferate *in vivo*, leading ultimately to a potentially lethal burden of bacteria or fungi. Bacteria in the logarithmic phase of growth tend to be more virulent than bacteria isolated after entering the stationary phase (121).
2. The microorganism responsible for the development of sepsis should be a pathogenic strain endowed with features (e.g., presence of a polysaccharide capsule) that interfere with the opsonophagocytic mechanisms of the host (121). It is noteworthy in this regard that of the more than 170 identified O-specific serotypes of *E. coli*, only about 12 or so are commonly identified in patients with bacteremias cause by the microbial species (121). Interestingly, many of the strains of *E. coli*, which have been used commonly in laboratory models of sepsis, lack the virulence factors associated with ability to survive and proliferate *in vivo* (121).
3. The experimental subjects should be treated with appropriate antibiotics, because antimicrobial chemotherapy is a standard component of the management of sepsis in humans.
4. The experimental subjects should be resuscitated (i.e., receive intravenous fluids) so that features of sepsis, such as shock, acidosis, and/or mortality, reflect the septic process per se and not the adverse effects of simple dehydration due to inability to drink fluids.

1. Peritonitis Models Using a Defined Bacterial Innoculum

When a pure culture of bacteria is introduced into the peritoneal cavity of pigs (162, 163) or rats (164–166), the organisms are cleared very rapidly. Moreover, in order to cause lethality by injecting animals intraperitoneally with a pure suspension of bacteria in saline, it typically is necessary to use a very large inoculum. If the dose of bacteria is large enough to cause mortality, death usually occurs within a matter of hours. Accordingly, inoculating animals intraperitoneally with bacteria suspended in saline is virtually equivalent to infusing the organisms intravenously. If, however, the bacteria, rather than being suspended in saline, are mixed with certain substances, called adjuvants, the dose required to induce lethality is markedly diminished. The adjuvant promotes the proliferation of the bacteria *in vivo* (167) and/or interferes with the host defense against the infectious challenge (168–170). Adjuvant substances include sterile feces (5, 67, 171, 172), barium sulfate (173), hemoglobin (165, 167, 169, 169, 174), fibrin (168, 175), agar (176), and mucin (174, 177, 178).

The classic model of adjuvant peritonitis induced by a defined bacterial inoculum was described in 1976 by Onderdonk and colleagues (173). In this model, pure cultures of a single bacterial species (e.g., *E. coli*) or two different bacterial species (e.g., *E. coli* plus *Bacteroides fragilis*) are mixed with barium sulfate and autoclaved rat fecal material. The suspension (0.5 ml final volume) is loaded into a gelatin capsule and implanted intraperitoneally. If rats are innoculated with 5×10^7 cfu of *E. coli*, mortality is 65% and all deaths occur within 48 hr. If *E. coli* (1.3×10^7 cfu) plus *B. fragilis* (2.5×10^7 cfu) are implanted, then there are no deaths, but all animals develop intraabdominal abscesses from which the original species can be cultured.

A number of variations of the standard Onderdonk model have been described. For example, the model described by Dunne *et al.* employs 1.0-ml agar pellets containing 5×10^8 cfu of a pathogenic strain (O18:K1:H7) of *E. coli* (176). Implanting rats intraperitoneally with these infected pellets results in 62% mortality at 48 hr. Vary *et al.* described a model wherein rats are implanted intraperitoneally with 1.5-ml pellets composed of sterile rat feces, agar, and a known number of both *E. coli* (10^2 cfu) and *B. fragilis* (10^8 cfu) (179). This paradigm results in approximately 40% lethality over the first 48 hr; surviving animals develop large intraperitoneal abscesses. Our laboratory has described an antibiotic-treated gram-negative sepsis model wherein rats are implanted intraperitoneally with gelatin capsules containing 0.11 g of a paste consisting of sterile rat fecal material mixed with 6×10^5 cfu of an ampicillin-susceptible, but pathogenic, strain of viable *E. coli* (5). Five doses of ampicillin (85 mg/kg per dose) are administered on an every 12-hr schedule beginning 6 hr after the induction of sepsis. In this model, 7-day mortality is about 70%, and deaths continue to occur over a several-day period of observation.

Saladino *et al.* have described an antibiotic-treated model of gram-negative peritonitis in rabbits, wherein the animals are innoculated intraperitoneally with approximately 3×10^8 cfu of a pathogenic strain (O18:K1) of live *E. coli* suspended in 20 ml of 5% mucin solution (178). A single dose of gentamicin (2.5 mg/kg) is administered 1 hr after the induction of sepsis. Mortality is 90%, and deaths occur rapidly over a 12-hr period.

Our laboratory has described another lapine model of peritonitis (180). In this model, rabbits are chronically instrumented to permit continuous infusion of intravenous fluids and the repetitive administration of antibiotics. Sepsis is induced by implanting within the peritoneal cavity 10 ml of a suspension containing hemoglobin (40 μg/ml), mucin (150 μg/ml), and $1.0 \pm 0.5 \times 10^5$ cfu/kg of viable *E. coli* (O18:K1), a highly pathogenic strain. Beginning at $T = 4$ hr, the rabbits are treated with gentamicin (5 mg/kg every 12 hr) for five doses. Signs of sepsis are evident within 4 hr after the onset of infection. Deaths occur starting at about 18 hr and continue for as long as 5 days after the start of the sepsis protocol. Overall mortality is 95%.

Another well-characterized peritonitis model is derived from an early study by Ahrenholz and Simmons, who reported that immobilization of viable *E. coli* within a fibrin matrix inhibits the early absorption of bacteria, but promotes late abscess formation (175). Extrapolating from these data obtained in rats, Fink *et al.* developed a large animal model of hyperdynamic sepsis, using chronically instrumented dogs implanted intraperitoneally with a bovine fibrin clot containing viable *E. coli* (45). Subsequently, Natanson and colleagues used this canine "fibrin clot" peritonitis model to conduct a series of important and informative studies, addressing questions such as the value of vasopressors and antibiotics for the management of septic shock (181), the efficacy of a monoclonal antibody directed against core-specific epitopes on LPS as adjuvant agent for the treatment of sepsis (7), and the importance of endotoxemia in the pathogenesis of sepsis-related derangements in cardiovascular function (46, 182).

2. Fecal Peritonitis Models

The cecal ligation and perforation (CLP) model developed by Wichterman and colleagues (183) is very widely utilized in sepsis-related research. Although originally described in rats, this model has been extended successfully to other species, notably mice (61) and sheep (41). Irrespective of species, CLP models enjoy several advantages, among which are simplicity and clinical relevance. The CLP model is very straightforward; the cecum is devascularized, ligated in a way that preserves intestinal continuity, and perforated in a standardized fashion (183). Like most cases of secondary peritonitis in humans, sepsis induced by CLP is polymicrobial and is associated with the presence of devitalized tissue. Accordingly, CLP bears close resemblance to clinical entities such as perforated appendicitis, diverticulitis, or colonic anastomotic dehiscence.

The similarity of CLP to the clinical situation, although clearly an obvious virtue, is also a drawback. Just as the degree of peritoneal contamination can vary widely among patients, the magnitude of the septic challenge can be variable in animal models of bowel perforation. Furthermore, the investigator has little control over the microbiology of the resulting infection. In studies using small animals, such as mice or rats, problems related to subject-to-subject variation in the magnitude of the septic challenge can be partially controlled by carefully standardizing the size of the cecal perforation (e.g., a single puncture with an 18-gauge needle) and by increasing the number of replicates for each experimental condition studied.

Some of the problems of controlling the magnitude of the septic insult in fecal peritonitis models can be overcome by inoculating the peritoneal cavity directly with feces rather than allowing fecal material to leak from a perforation in the gut. Various groups have described fecal inoculation models in rats (184–186) and pigs (187, 188).

3. Soft Tissue Infection and Pneumonia Models

Intravascular infusion of bacteria and intraperitoneal contamination are by far the most widely employed means for inducing sepsis in experimental animals. Nevertheless, a number of other sites of infection have been employed. Because bronchopulmonary infection is a major cause of sepsis in the clinical setting, a number of laboratories have established models of pneumonia for studying novel approaches for the management of the systemic consequences of serious infection. Models of pneumonia have been established in rats and mice (70, 189–192), as well as larger species such as dogs (193) and sheep (194).

Experimental soft-tissue infections also have been employed for studying the pathophysiology and/or adjuvant therapy of sepsis. A partial listing of these soft-tissue models includes intramuscular injection of viable *E. coli* in pigs (195), repetitive injections in rats of viable *E. coli* and *B. fragilis* into performed subcutaneous pockets containing gauze sponge (196), implantation of the thigh musclulature of mice with a cotton suture infected with a pathogenic strain of *Klebsiella pneumoniae* (197), and injection of viable *P. aeruginosa* (198) or *Streptococcus pyogenes* (199) into the thigh musculature of mice.

4. Immunosuppressed Host and Sequential Challenge Models

Although life-threatening infections occasionally develop in previously healthy individuals, most cases of sepsis and septic shock occur in patients with serious preexisting underlying medical problems. Common underlying conditions include trauma and hemorrhage, thermal injury, alcoholism, hepatic dysfunction and/or cirrhosis, and treatment of malignancy with myelosuppressive drugs. In contrast, most animal models of sepsis employ young and healthy subjects, a strategy that may minimize variability at the cost of versimilitude. The presence of preexisting conditions can alter the response to sepsis and, possibly, the effectiveness of adjuvant therapies in several ways. First, a smaller initial microbial inoculum is likely to be sufficient to cause full-blown sepsis in immunosuppressed as compared to fully immunocompetent subjects. Second, some of the deleterious effects of the inflammatory response may be blunted when the immune system is already compromised. Third, prior proinflammatory stimuli, such as trauma or hemorrhage or tissue ischemia and reperfusion, may lead to up-regulation or "priming" of aspects of the inflammatory response so that a subsequent septic challenge ("second hit") leads to much greater tissue damage and organ dysfunction than would have been the case in a naive (unprimed) host.

Methods of inducing immunosuppression, which have been employed in studies of exprerimental sepsis, include acute ethanol ingestion in rats (191), carbon tetrachloride-induced cirrhosis in rats (190), hemorrhagic shock in mice (189), cyclophosphamide-induced neutropenia in rats (200, 201), nitrogen mustard-induced neutropenia in rabbits (202, 203), splenectomy in mice (204), and thermal injury in mice (192, 205). As is commonly the case in the clinical setting, sepsis, in some models using immunocompromised animals, develops spontaneously as a result of systemic invasion by endogenous gut-derived microbes. For example, in a model developed by Ziegler and colleagues, rabbits are monoassociated with *E. coli* (strain O4) by having the organisms placed in their drinking water for several days (202). Subsequently, the animals are rendered neutropenic with nitrogen mustard. As the circulating neutrophil count approaches zero at 48–72 hr after treatment with the cytotoxic agent, the rabbits spontaneously develop bacteremia, presumably of enteric origin, caused by strain O4 *E. coli.* More recently, Collins *et al.* described a similar model using rats (201). In this model, the animals are pretreated with cefamandole for several days, rendered neutropenic with two doses of cyclophosphamide (given at 0 and 72 hr), and challenged with a virulent isolate of *P. aeruginosa*. The bacteria are enterally administered using an orogastric tube at 0, 48, and 96 hr after the first dose of the myelosuppressive agent. Mortality (in the absence of therapy with antibiotics or other agents) is 100% during the period from 5 to 8 days after the first dose of cyclophosphamide.

In the past several years, a variety of "two-hit" models of sepsis and sepsis-induced organ system failure have been described. The classic "two-hit" model is the generalized Shwartzman reaction, which is elicited when rabbits are injected with a priming dose of LPS prior to being challenged with a second dose of endotoxin 12–96 hr later (196). The most prominent feature of the generalized Shwartzman reaction is bilateral renal cortical necrosis. Because the presence of circulating leukocytes is necessary for elaboration of the generalized Shwartzman phenomenon (196), it is probable that the initial dose of LPS leads to priming of neutrophils for oxidative burst activity and/or up-regulation of adhesion receptors on the endothelium necessary for the sequestration of neutrophils in the microvasculature of target organs.

Our laboratory described a two-dose model of LPS-induced acute lung injury in pigs (206). In this model, unanesthetized pigs are injected with a small intravenous dose of LPS (20 μg/kg). Eighteen hours later, the animals are anesthetized, instrumented, and then infused intravenously over 60 min with a larger dose of LPS (250 μg/kg). In addition, the animals are resuscitated with Ringer's lactate solution (25 ml/kg/hr) and bolus infusions of 6% dextran-70 solution (in normal saline) titrated to maintain cardiac output at the baseline level. When challenged with a relatively large dose of LPS, primed pigs, as compared to similarly challenged unprimed animals, develop more severe lung injury as manifested by significantly lower arterial oxygen tension and a significantly greater infiltration of neutrophils into alveoli. Our group (207–209) and others (210) have used this model to evaluate a number of agents for the treatment of sepsis-induced acute lung injury.

Another extensively evaluated "two-hit" model was described initially by Koike and colleagues (211). In this model, anesthetized rats are subjected to 45 min of intestinal ischemia. Six hours after reestablishing perfusion of the gut, the animals are challenged with a relatively low dose (for rats) of intravenous LPS (2.5 mg/kg). Whereas this dose of endotoxin does not induce lung injury or mortality in normal (i.e., unprimed) rats, 2.5 mg/kg of LPS increases lung microvascular permeability and causes substantial mortality in rats previously subjected to a short period of intestinal ischemia and reperfusion. Subsequent studies have implicated PAF- and IL-6-mediated priming of neutrophils as being important in the pathogenesis of organ system dysfunction in this particular sequential insult model of sepsis (212). Other two-hit models that have been described include hemorrhagic shock followed by LPS administration 48 (213) or 72 (214) hr later in swine, hemorrhagic shock followed by LPS infusion 24 hr later in rabbits (215), hemorrhagic shock followed by infusion of viable *E. coli* 24 or 72 hr later in rats (216), and LPS administration 7 days after major thermal trauma in sheep (217).

5. Models of MODS

Investigators have had a particularly difficult time developing truly useful models of MODS. Because severe acute lung injury is almost always part of the clinical picture of MODS in humans, and because MODS in patients typically evolves over days, it might be argued that any animal model of MODS is grossly unrealistic if it does not include prolonged mechanical ventilation. Some authors seem to view elevations in circulating liver enzymes (e.g., alanine aminotransferase) and urea following the injection of rats or mice with LPS as evidence of MODS (218, 219). Most investigators view these changes as too acute to be relevant to a clinical syndrome that progresses gradually and is characterized by acute lung injury, noncardiogenic pulmonary edema, ventilator dependence, azotemia, cholestatic jaundice, and often altered mental status and thrombocytopenia.

In 1986, Goris described a rat model of zymosan-induced peritonitis in rats, which replicates many of the features of MODS in humans (220). This model has been adapted for use in mice (221). In the murine version of this model, zymosan is added to liquid paraffin (2.5 g per 100 ml) and the suspension is sterilized by incubation at 100°C for 80 min. To induce peritonitis, mice are injected intraperitoneally with zymosan in paraffin (1 mg/kg of zymosan). The biological response to this challenge is triphasic. In the acute phase, the mice develop shock, lethargy, and anorexia and 20–40% of the animals die. The condition of the surviving animals then improves transiently (second phase). However, beginning around day 8 after the induction of sterile peritonitis, the animals again become lethargic and develop biochemical and histological evidence of MODS. This model has been adapted widely and is generally regarded as the best available model of subacute MODS.

One additional very realistic but very complex and undoubtedly expensive model of MODS has been developed by a surgical research group in Germany (222, 223). In this paradigm, sheep are subjected to hemorrhagic shock and intramedullary femoral nailing on day 0 and then receive an intravenous injection every 12 hr of both LPS (0.75 μg/kg) and zymosan-activated sheep plasma (0.7 ml/kg) for 5 days. This model is characterized by the development of a hyperdynamic circulation, pulmonary edema, cholestatic jaundice, azotemia, and impaired hepatic function.

References

1. Ivanov, P. C., Amaral, L. A., Goldberger, A. L., Havlin, S., Rosenblum, M. G., Struzik, Z. R., and Stanley, H. E. (1999). Multifractality in human heartbeat dynamics. *Nature (London)* **399,** 461–465.
2. Wiechert, W., Mollney, M., Isermann, N., Wurzel, M., and de Graaf, A. A. (1999). Bidirectional reaction steps in metabolic networks: III. Explicit solution and analysis of isotopomer labeling systems. *Biotechnol. Bioeng.* **66,** 69–85.
3. Fink, M. P., and Heard, S. O. (1990). Research review: Laboratory models of sepsis and septic shock. *J. Surg. Res.* **49,** 186–196.
4. Alexander, H. R., Doherty, G. M., Buresh, C. M., Venzon, D. J., and Norton, J. A. (1991). A recombinant human receptor antagonist to interleukin 1 improves survival after lethal endotoxemia in mice. *J. Exp. Med.* **173,** 1029–1032.
5. Aranow, J. S., Zhuang, J., Wang, H., Larkin, V., Smith, M., and Fink, M. P. (1996). A selective inhibitor of inducable nitric oxide synthase prolongs survival in a rat model of bacterial peritonitis: Comparison with two nonselective strategies. *Shock* **5,** 116–121.
6. Wakabayashi, G., Gelfand, J. A., Burke, J. F., Thompson, R. C., and Dinarello, C. A. (1991). A specific receptor antagonist for interleukin 1 prevents *Escherichia coli*-induced shock in rabbits. *FASEB J.* **5,** 338–343.
7. Quezado, Z. M. N., Natanson, C., Alling, D. W., Banks, S. M., Koev, C. A., Elin, R. J., Hosseini, J. M., Bacher, J. D., Danner, R. L., and Hoffman, W. D. (1993). A controlled trial of HA-1A in a canine model of Gram-negative septic shock. *JAMA* **269,** 2221–2227.
8. Creasey, A. A., Chang, A. C. K., Feigen, L., Wün, T. -C., Taylor, F. B., Jr., and Hinshaw, L. B. Tissue factor pathway inhibitor reduces mortality from *Escherichia coli. J. Clin. Invest.* **91,** 2850–2860.
9. Decking, U. K. M., Flesche, C. W., Gödecke, A., and Schrader, J. (1995). Endotoxin-induced contractile dysfunction in guinea pig hearts is not mediated by nitric oxide. *Am. J. Physiol.* **268,** H2460–H2465.
10. Goddard, C. M., Allard, M. F., Hogg, J. C., and Walley, K. R. (1996). Myocardial morphometric changes related to decreased contractility after endotoxin. *Am. J. Physiol.* **270,** H1446–H1452.
11. Dahn, M. S., Lange, M. P., McCurdy, B., and Mahaffey, S. (1995). Metabolic function of the isolated perfused rat liver in chronic sepsis. *J. Surg. Res.* **59,** 287–291.
12. Spain, D. A., Wilson, M. A., and Garrison, R. N. (1994). Nitric oxide synthase inhibition exacerbates sepsis-induced renal hypoperfusion. *Surgery* **116,** 322–331.
13. Steeb, G. D., Wilson, M. A., and Garrison, R. N. (1992). Pentoxyfylline preserves small-intestine microvascular blood flow during bacteremia. *Surgery* **112,** 756–764.
14. Lubbe, A. S., Garrison, R. N., Cryer, H. M., Alsip, N. L., and Harris, P. D. (1992). EDRF as a possible mediator of sepsis-induced arteriolar dilation in skeletal muscle. *Am. J. Physiol.* **262,** H880–H887.
15. Pfeffer, K., Matsuyama, T., Kundig, T. M., Wakeham, A., Kishihara, K., Shahinian, A., Wiegman, K., Ohashi, P. S., Kronke, M., and Mak, T. W. (1993). Mice deficient for the 55 kd tumor necrosis factor receptor are resistant to endotoxic shock, yet succumb to *L. monocytogenes* infection. *Cell* **73,** 457–467.
16. Ayala, A., Perrin, M. M., Wagner, M. A., and Chaudry, I. H. (1990). Enhanced susceptibility to sepsis after simple hemorrhage. Depression of Fc and C3b receptor-mediated phagocytosis. *Arch. Surg.* **125,** 70–74.
17. Ferrero, E., Jiao, D., Tsuberi, B. Z., Tesio, L., Rong, G. W., Haziot, A., and Goyert, S. M. (1993). Transgenic mice expressing human CD14 are hypersensitive to lipopolysaccharide. *Proc. Natl. Acad. Sci. U.S.A.* **90,** 2380–2384.
18. de Vos, S., Epstein, C. J., Carlson, E., Cho, S. K., and Koeffler, H. P. (1995). Transgenic mice overexpressing human copper/zinc-superoxide dismutase (Cu/Zn SOD) are not resistant to endotoxic shock. *Biochem. Biophys. Res. Comm.* **208,** 523–531.
19. Levine, D. M., Parker, T. S., Donnelly, T. M., Walsh, A., and Rubin, A. L. (1993). *In vivo* protection against endotoxin by plasma high density lipoprotein. *Proc. Natl. Acad. Sci. U.S.A.* **90,** 12040–12044.
20. Haziot, A., Ferrero, E., Kontgen, F., Hijiya, N., Yamamoto, S., Silver, J., Stewart, C. L., and Goyert, S. M. (1996). Resistance to endotoxin shock and reduced dissemination of gram-negative bacteria in CD14-deficient mice. *Immunity* **4,** 407–414.
21. Maraz, M. A., White, J. M., Sheehan, K. C., Bach, E. A., Rodig, S. J., Dighe, A. S., Kaplan, D. H., Riley, J. K., Greenland, A. C., Campbell, D., Carver-Moore, K., DuBois, R. N., Clark, R., Aguet, M., and Schreiber, R. D. (1996). Targeted disruption of the Stat1 gene in mice reveals unexpected physiologic specificity in the JAK-STAT signaling pathway. *Cell* **84,** 431–442.
22. Umans, L., Serneels, L., Overbergh, L., Lorent, K., Van Leuven, F., and Van den Berghe, H. (1995). Targeted inactivation of the mouse alpha 2-macroglobulin gene. *J. Biol. Chem.* **270,** 19778–19785.
23. Lu, B., Gerard, N. P., Kolakowski, L. F., Jr., Bozza, M., Zurakowski, D., Finco, O., Carroll, M. C., and Gerard, C. (1995). Neutral endopeptidase modulation of septic shock. *J. Exp. Med.* **181,** 2271–2275.
24. Cowdery, J. S., Chace, J. H., Yi, A. K., and Krieg, A. M. (1996). Bacterial DNA induces NK cells to produce IFN-gamma *in vivo* and increases the toxicity of lipopolysaccharides. *J. Immunol.* **156,** 4570–4575.
25. Rofe, A. M., Philcox, J. C., and Coyle, P. (1996). Trace metal, acute phase and metabolic response to endotoxin in metallothionein-null mice. *Biochem. J.* **314,** 793–797.
26. MacMicking, J. D., Nathan, C., Horn, G., Chartrain, N., Fletcher, D. S., Trumbauer, M., Stevens, K., Quia-wen, X., Sokol, K., Hutchinson, N., Chen, H., and Mudgett, J. S. (1995). Altered responses to bacterial infection and endotoxic shock in mice lacking inducable nitric oxide synthase. *Cell* **81,** 641–650.
27. Zimmer, H. G., and Millar, H. D. (1998). Technology and application of ultraminiature catheter pressure transducers. *Can. J. Cardiol.* **14,** 1259–1266.
28. Irlbeck, M., Iwai, T., Lerner, T., and Zimmer, H. G. (1997). Effects of angiotensin II receptor blockade on hypoxia-induced right ventricular hypertrophy in rats. *J. Mol. Cell Cardiol.* **29,** 2931–2939.

29. Melo, L. G., Veress, A. T., Ackermann, U., Pang, S. C., Flynn, T. G., and Sonnenberg, H. (1999). Chronic hypertension in ANP knockout mice: contribution of peripheral resistance. *Regul. Pept.* **79,** 109–115.
30. Franco, F., Thomas, G. D., Giroir, B., Bryant, D., Bullock, M. C., Chwialkowski, M. C., Victor, R. G., and Peshock, R. M. (1999). Magnetic resonance imaging and invasive evaluation of development of heart failure in transgenic mice with myocardial expression of tumor necrosis factor-alpha. *Circulation* **99,** 448–454.
31. Yang, X. P., Liu, Y. H., Shesely, E. G., Bulagannawar, M., Liu, F., and Carretero, O. A. (1999). Endothelial nitric oxide gene knockout mice: cardiac phenotypes and the effect of angiotensin-converting enzyme inhibitor on myocardial ischemia/reperfusion injury. *Hypertension* **34,** 24–30.
32. Cervenka, L., Mitchell, K. D., Oliverio, M. I., Coffman, T. M., and Navar, L. G. (1999). Renal function in the AT1A receptor knockout mouse during normal and volume-expanded conditions. *Kidney Int.* **56,** 1855–1862.
33. Traynor, T., Yang, T., Huang, Y. G., Krege, J. H., Briggs, J. P., Smithies, O., and Schnermann, J. (1999). Tubuloglomerular feedback in ACE-deficient mice. *Am. J. Physiol.* **276,** F751–F757.
34. Okamoto, H., Meng, W., Ma, J., Ayata, C., Roman, R. J., Bosnjak, Z. J., Kampine, J. P., Huang, P. L., Moskowitz, M. A., and Hudetz, A. G. (1999). Isoflurane-induced cerebral hyperemia in neuronal nitric oxide synthase gene deficient mice. *Anesthesiology* **86,** 875–884.
35. Kolandaivelu, K., and Poon, C. S. (1998). A miniature mechanical ventilator for newborn mice. *J. Appl. Physiol.* **84,** 733–739.
36. De Sanctis, G. T., Mehta, S., Kobzik, L., Yandava, C., Jiao, A., Huang, P. L., and Drazen, J. M. (1997). Contribution of type I NOS to expired gas NO and bronchial responsiveness in mice. *Am. J. Physiol.* **273,** L883–L888.
37. Walker, J. K., Peppel, K., Lefkowitz, R. J., Caron, M. G., and Fisher, J. T. (1999). Altered airway and cardiac responses in mice lacking G protein-coupled receptor kinase 3. *Am. J. Physiol.* **276,** R1214–R1221.
38. Demling, R. H., Lalonde, C., Jin, L. -J., Ryan, P., and Fox, R. (1986). Endotoxemia causes inreased lung tissue lipid peroxidation in unanesthetized sheep. *J. Appl. Physiol.* **60,** 2094–2100.
39. Talke, P., Dunn, A., Lawlis, L., Sziebert, L., White, A., Herndon, D., Flynn, J. T., and Traber, D. (1985). A model of ovine endotoxemia characterized by an increased cardiac output. *Circ. Shock* **17,** 103–108.
40. Hinder, F., Booke, M., Traber, L. D., Matsumoto, N., Nishida, K., Rogers, S., and Traber, D. L. (1996). Nitric oxide synthase inhibition during experimental sepsis improves renal excretatory function in the presence of chronically increased atrial natriuretic peptide. *Crit. Care Med.* **24,** 131–136.
41. Avila, A., Warshawski, F., Sibbald, W., Finley, R., Wells, G., and Holliday, R. (1985). Peripheral lymph flow in sheep with bacterial peritonitis: Evidence for increased peripheral microvascular permeability accompanying systemic sepsis. *Surgery* **97,** 685–695.
42. Demling, R. H., Lalonde, C. C., Jin, L. -J., Albes, J., and Fiori, N. (1986). The pulmonary and sytemic response to recurrent endotoxemia in the adult sheep. *Surgery* **100,** 876–883.
43. Pittet, J. F., and Morel, D. R. (1991). Imbalance between plasma levels of thromboxane B_2 and 6-keto-prostaglandin F_{1a} during subacute endotoxin-induced hyperdynamic sepsis and multiple organ failure syndrome in sheep. *Circ. Shock* **35,** 65–77.
44. Shaw, H. F. S., and Wolfe, R. R. (1984). A conscious septic dog model with hemodynamic and metabolic responses similar to responses of humans. *Surgery* **95,** 553–561.
45. Fink, M. P., Mac Vittie, T. J., and Casey, L. C. (1984). Inhibition of prostaglandin synthesis restores normal hemodynamics in canine hyperdynamic sepsis. *Ann. Surg.* **200,** 619–626.
46. Danner, R. L., Natanson, C., Elin, R. J., Hosseini, J. M., Banks, S., Mac Vittie, T. J., Parrillo, J. E. (1990). *Pseudomonas aeruginosa* compared with *Escherichia coli* produces less endotoxemia but more cardiovascular dysfunction and mortality in a canine model of septic shock. *Chest* **98,** 1480–1487.
47. Fettman, M. J., Hand, M. S., Chandrasena, L. G., Cleek, J. L., Mason, R. A., Brooks, P. A., and Phillips, R. W. (1984). Effects of captopril on hemodynamic and metabolic parameters in awake endotoxemic Yucatan minipigs. *Circ. Shock* **12,** 25–46.
48. Hughes, H. C. Swine in cardiovascular research. *Lab. Anim. Sci.* **36,** 348–350.
49. Swindle, M. M., Smith, A. C., and Hepburn, B. J. (1988). Swine as models in experimental surgery. *J. Invest. Surg.* **1,** 65–79.
50. Morton, D., and Bertram, T. A. (1988). Isolation and preliminary *in vitro* characterization of the porcine pulmonary intravascular macrophage. *J. Leukoc. Biol.* **43,** 403–410.
51. Warner, A. E., Molina, R. M., and Brain, J. D. (1987). Uptake of blood-borne bacteria by pulmonary intravascular macrophages and consequent inflammatory responses in sheep. *Am. Rev. Respir. Dis.* **136,** 683–690.
52. Warner, A. E., and Brain, J. D. (1990). The cell biology and pathogenic role of pulmonary intravascular macrophages. *Am. J. Physiol.* **258,** L1–L12.
53. Landolt, C. C., Matthay, M. A., and Staub, N. C. (1981). Anatomic variations of efferent duct from caudal mediastinal lymph node in sheep. *J. Appl. Physiol.* **50,** 1372–1374.
54. Roos, P. J., Wiener-Kronish, J. P., Albertine, K. H., and Staub, N. C. (1983). Removal of abdominal sources of caudal mediastinal node lymph in anesthetized sheep. *J. Appl. Physiol.* **55,** 996–1001.
55. Matsumoto, N., Koike, K., Yamada, S., and Staub, N. C. (1990). Caudal mediastinal node lymph flow in sheep after histamine or endotoxin infusions. *Am. J. Physiol.* **258,** H24–H28.
56. Brigham, K. L., Bowers, R., and Haynes, J. (1979). Increased sheep lung vascular permeability caused by *Escherichia coli* endotoxin. *Circ. Res.* **45,** 292–297.
57. Kuratomi, Y., Lefferts, P. L., Christman, B. W., Parker, R. E., Smith, W. G., Mueller, R. A., and Snapper, J. R. (1993). Effect of a 5-lipoxygenase inhibitor on endotoxin-induced pulmonary dysfunction in awake sheep. *J. Appl. Physiol.* **74,** 596–605.
58. Bernard, G. R., Lucht, W. D., Niedermeyer, M. E., Snapper, J. R., Ogletree, M. L., and Brigham, K. L. (1984). Effect of *N*-acetylcysteine on the pulmonary response to endotoxin in the awake sheep and upon *in vitro* granulocyte function. *J. Clin. Invest.* **73,** 1772–1784.
59. Wong, C., Fox, R., and Demling, R. H. (1985). Effect of hydroxyl radical scavenging on endotoxin-induced lung injury. *Surgery* **97,** 300–306.
60. Chang, S. W., and Ohara, N. (1994). Chronic biliary obstruction induces pulmonary intravascular phagocytosis and endotoxin sensitivity in rats. *J. Clin. Invest.* **94,** 2009–2019.
61. Eskandari, M. K., Bolgos, G., Miller, C., Nguyen, D. T., DeForge, L. E., and Remick, D. G. (1992). Anti-tumor necrosis factor antibody therapy fails to prevent lethality after cecal ligation and puncture or endotoxemia. *J. Immunol.* **148,** 2724–2730.
62. O'Riordain, M. G., O'Riordain, D. S., Molloy, R. G., Mannick, J. A., and Rodrick, M. L. (1996). Dosage and timing of anti-TNF-alpha antibody treatment determine its effect of resistance to sepsis after injury. *J. Surg. Res.* **64,** 95–101.
63. Echtenacher, B., Falk, W., Mannel, D. N., and Krammer, P. H. (1990). Requirement of endogenous tumor necrosis factor/cachectin for recovery from experimental peritonitis. *J. Immunol.* **145,** 3762–3766.
64. O'Reilly, M., Newcomb, D. E., and Remick, D. (1999). Endotoxin, sepsis, and the primrose path. *Shock* **12,** 411–420.
65. Beutler, B., Milsark, I. W., and Cerami, A. (1985). Passive immunization against cachectin/tumor necrosis factor protects mice from lethal effect of endotoxin. *Science* **229,** 869–871.
66. Remick, D., Manohar, P., Bolgos, G., Rodriguez, J., Moldawer, L., and Wollenberg, G. (1995). Blockade of tumor necrosis factor reduces

lipopolysaccharide lethality, but not the lethality of cecal ligation and puncture. *Shock* **4,** 89–95.

67. Bagby, G. J., Plessala, K. J., Wilson, L. A., Thompson, J. J., and Nelson, S. (1991). Divergent efficacy of antibody to tumor necrosis factor-a in intravascular and peritonitis models of sepsis. *J. Infect. Dis.* **163,** 83–88.
68. Howard, M., Muchamuel, T., Andrade, S., and Menon, S. (1993). Interleukin 10 protects mice from lethal endotoxemia. *J. Exp. Med.* **177,** 1205–1208.
69. Gerard, C., Bruyns, C., Marchant, A., Abramowicz, D., Vandenabeele, P., Delvaux, A., Fiers, W., Goldman, M., and Velu, T. (1993). Interleukin 10 reduces the release of tumor necrosis factor and prevents lethality in expermimental endotoxemia. *J. Exp. Med.* **177,** 547–550.
70. Greenberger, M. J., Strieter, R. M., Kunkel, S. L., Danforth, J. M., Goodman, R. E., and Standiford, T. J. (1995). Neutralization of IL-10 increases survival in a murine model of *Klebsiella* pneumonia. *J. Immunol.* **155,** 722–729.
71. Hadjiminas, D. J., McMasters, K. M., Peyton, J. C., and Cheadle, W. G. (1994). Tissue tumor necrosis factor mRNA expression following cecal ligation and puncture or intraperitoneal injection of endotoxin. *J. Surg. Res.* **56,** 549–555.
72. Cameron, E. M., Zhuang, J., Menconi, M. J., Phipps, R., and Fink, M. P. (1996). Dantrolene, an inhibitor of intracellular calcium release, fails to increase survival in a rat model of intraabdominal sepsis. *Crit. Care Med.* **24,** 1537–1546.
73. Mohler, K. M., Torrance, D. S., Smith, C. A., Goodwin, R. G., Stremler, K. E., Fung, V. P., Madani, H., and Widmer, M. B. (1993). Soluble tumor necrosis factor (TNF) receptors are effective therapeutic agents in lethal endotoxemia and function simultaneously as both TNF carriers and TNF antagonists. *J. Immunol.* **151,** 1548–1561.
74. Fletcher, J. R., and Ramwell, P. W. (1980). Indomethacin treatment following baboon endotoxin shock improves survival. *Adv. Shock Res.* **4,** 103–111.
75. Fischer, E., Marano, M. A., Van Zee, K. J., Rock, C. S., Hawes, A. S., Thompson, W. A., DeForge, L., Kenney, J. S., Remick, D. G., Bloedow, D. C., Thompson, R. C., Lowry, S. F., and Moldawer, L. L. (1992). Interleukin-1 receptor blockade improves survival and hemodynamic performance in *Escherichia coli* septic shock, but fails to alter host responses to sublethal endotoxemia. *J. Clin. Invest.* **89,** 1551–1557.
76. Hawes, A. S., Fischer, E., Marano, M. A., Van Zee, K. J., Rock, C. S., Lowry, S. F., Calvano, S. E., and Moldawer, L. L. (1993). Comparison of peripheral blood leukocyte kinetics after live *Escherichia coli*, endotoxin, or interleukin-1 alpha administration. Studies using a novel interleukin-1 receptor antagonist. *Ann. Surg.* **218,** 79–90.
77. Thompson, W. A., Coyle, S., VanZee, K., Oldenburg, H., Trousdale, R., Rogy, M., Felsen, D., Moldawer, L., and Lowry, S. F. (1994). The metabolic effects of platelet-activating factor antagonism in endotoxemic man. *Arch. Surg.* **129,** 72–79.
78. Martich, G. D., Parker, M. M., Cunnion, R. E., and Suffredini, A. F. (1992). Effects of ibuprofen and pentoxifylline on the cardiovascular response of normal humans to endotoxin. *J. Appl. Physiol.* **73,** 925–931.
79. Michie, H. R., Manogue, K. R., Spriggs, D. R., Revhaug, A., O'Dwyer, S. O., Dinarello, C. A., Cerami, A., Wolff, S. M., and Wilmore, D. W. (1988). Detection of circulating tumor necrosis factor after endotoxin administration. *N. Engl. J. Med.* **23,** 1481–1486.
80. Arden, W. A., Strodel, W. E., Gross, D. R., Anderson, K. W., Oremus, R., Derbin, M., and Schwartz, R. W. (1995). Preincubation of endotoxin with monoclonal anti-lipid A (E5), but not *in vivo* treatment, inhibits circulatory dysfunction. *Shock* **4,** 131–138.
81. Koyama, S., Shibamoto, T., Ammons, W. S., and Saeki, Y. (1995). $rBPI_{23}$ attenuates endotoxin-induced cardiovascular depression in awake rabbits. *Shock* **4,** 74–78.
82. Wyler, F., Neutze, J. M., and Rudolph, A. M. (1970). Effects of endotoxin on distribution of cardiac output in unanesthetized rabbits. *Am. J. Physiol.* **219,** 246–251.
83. Vincent, J.-L., Domb, M., Luypaert, P., De Boelpaepe, C., Van der Linden, P., and Blecic, S. (1987). Endotoxin shock model in the dog: a reevaluation. *Prog. Clin. Biol. Res.* **236A,** 393–399.
84. D'Orio, V., Wahlen, C., Rodriguez, L. -M., Fossion, A., Juchmes, J., Halleux, J., and Marcelle, R. (1987). A comparison of *Escherichia coli* endotoxin single bolus injection with low-dose endotoxin infusion on pulmonary and systemic vascular changes. *Circ. Shock* **21,** 207–216.
85. Breslow, M. J., Miller, C. F., Parker, S. D., Walman, A. T., and Traystman, R. J. (1987). Effect of vasopressors on organ blood flow during endotoxin shock in pigs. *Am. J. Physiol.* **252,** H291–H300.
86. Fink, M. P., Rothschild, H. R., Deniz, Y. F., Wang, H., Lee, P. C., and Cohn, S. M. (1989). Systemic and mesenteric O_2 metabolism in endotoxic pigs: Effect of ibuprofen and meclofenamate. *J. Appl. Physiol.* **67,** 1950–1957.
87. Cholley, B. P., Lang, R. M., Berger, D. S., Korcarz, C., Payen, D., and Shroff, S. G. (1995). Alterations in systemic arterial mechanical properties during septic shock: role of fluid resuscitation. *Am. J. Physiol.* **269,** H375–H384.
88. Klosterhalfen, B., Horstmann-Jungemann, K., Vogel, P., Dufhues, G., Simon, B., Kalff, G., Kirkpatrick, C. J., Mittermayer, C., and Heinrich, P. C. (1991). Hemodynamic variables and plasma levels of PGI_2, TXA_2 and IL-6 in a porcine model of recurrent endotoxemia. *Circ. Shock* **35,** 237–244.
89. Godsoe, A., Kimura, R., Herndon, D., Flynn, J. T., Schlag, G., Traber, L., and Traber, D. (1988). Cardiopulmonary changes with intermittent endotoxin administration in sheep. *Circ. Shock* **25,** 61–74.
90. Traber, D. L., Redl, H., Schlag, G., Herndon, D. N., Kimura, R., Prien, T., and Traber, L. D. (1988). Cardiopulmonary responses to continuous administration of endotoxin. *Am. J. Physiol.* **254,** H833–H839.
91. Traber, D. L., Flynn, J. T., Herndon, D. N., Redl, H., Schlag, G., and Traber, L. D. (1989). Comparison of the cardiopulmonary responses to single bolus and continuous infusion of endotoxin in an ovine model. *Circ. Shock* **27,** 123–138.
92. Fink, M. P., Fiallo, V., Stein, K. L., and Gardiner, W. M. (1987). Systemic and regional hemodynamic changes after intraperitoneal endotoxin in rabbits: Development of a new model of the clinical syndrome of hyperdynamic sepsis. *Circ. Shock* **22,** 73–81.
93. Weber, A., Schweiger, I. M., Poinsot, O., Klohn, M., Gaumann, D. M., and Morel, D. R. (1992). Sequential changes in renal oxygen consumption and sodium transport during hyperdynamic sepsis in sheep. *Am. J. Physiol.* **262,** F965–F971.
94. Fink, M. P., O'Sullivan, B. P., Menconi, M. J., Wollert, P. S., Wang, H., Youssef, M. E., and Fleisch, J. H. (1993). A novel leukotriene B_4-receptor antagonist in endotoxin shock: A prospective, controlled trial in a porcine model. *Crit. Care Med.* **21,** 1825–1837.
95. Greisman, S. E., and Hornick, R. B. (1967). Comparative pyrogenic reactivity of rabbit and man to bacterial endotoxin. *Proc. Soc. Exp. Biol. Med.* **131,** 1154–1158.
96. Esbenshade, A. M., Newman, J. H., Lams, P. M., and Brigham, K. L. (1982). Respiratory failure after endotoxin infusion in sheep: Lung mechanics and lung fluid balance. *J. Appl. Physiol.* **53,** 967–976.
97. Garcia, C., Saladino, R., Thompson, C., Hammer, B., Parsonnet, J., Wainwright, N., Novitsky, T., Fleisher, G. R., and Siber, G. (1994). Effect of a recombinant endotoxin-neutralizing protein on endotoxin shock in rabbits. *Crit. Care Med.* **22,** 1211–1218.
98. Lehmann, V., Freudenberg, M. A., and Galanos, C. (1987). Lethal toxicity of lipopolysaccharide and tumor necrosis factor in normal and D-galactosamine-treated mice. *Exp. Med.* **165,** 657–63.
99. Galanos, C., Freudenberg, M. A., and Reutter, W. (1979). Galactosamine-induced sensitization to the lethal effects of endotoxin. *Proc. Natl. Acad. Sci. U.S.A.* **76,** 5939–5943.

100. Silverstein, R., Johnson, W. M., Bucklin, S. E., and Johnson, D. C. (1996). The protein kinase C activator PMA modulates LPS lethality in normal mice and protects against LPS lethality in D-galactosamine-sensitized mice. *J. Endotoxin Res.* **3,** 29–37.
101. Pickett, W. C., Torley, L. W., Dejoy, S. Q., Gibbons, J. J., Desai, N. R., Oronsky, A. L., and Kerwar, S. S. (1992). Pluronic F 127 liquid sensitizes mice to low doses of *Escherichia coli* lipopolysaccharide. *Crit. Care Med.* **20,** 1448–1453.
102. Ogata, M., Yoshida, S.-I., Kamochi, M., Shigematsu, A., and Mizukami, H. (1991). Enhancement of lipopolysaccharide-induced tumor necrosis factor production in mice by carrageenan pretreatment. *Infect. Immun.* **59,** 679–683.
103. Becker, L. J., and Rudbach, J. A. (1978). Potentiation of endotoxicity by carrageenan. *Infect. Immun.* **19,** 1099–1100.
104. Siegel, M. I., McConnell, R. T., Bonser, R. W., and Cuatracasas, P. (1981). The production of 5-HETE and leukotriene B by neutrophils from carrageenan pleural exudates. *Prostaglandins* **21,** 123–132.
105. Cantanzaro, P. J., Schwartz, H. J., and Graham, R. C. (1971). Spectrum and possible mechanism of carrageenan cytotoxicity. *Am. J. Pathol.* **64,** 387–404.
106. Cheadle, W. G., Ausobsky, J. R., Trachtenberg, L. S., Lamont, P., and Polk, H. C., Jr. (1986). Effects of muramyl dipeptide and lead acetate on carbon clearance and endotoxin-induced mortality in mice. *Am. Surg.* **52,** 613–617.
107. Vacher, J., Delevallee, F., and Deraedt, R. (1977). Mechanism of the hypersusceptibility to the lethal effect of endotoxin (ET) induced in mice by injection of beryllium phosphate. *Toxicol. Appl. Pharmacol.* **40,** 99–108.
108. Chamulitrat, W., Jordan, S. J., and Mason, R. P. (1994). Nitric oxide production during endotoxic shock in carbon tetrachloride-treated rats. *Mol. Pharmacol.* **46,** 391–397.
109. Katschinski, T., Galanos, C., Coumbos, A., and Freudenberg, M. A. (1992). Gamma interferon mediates *Proprionibacterium acnes*-induced hypersensitivity to lipopolysaccharide. *Infect. Immun.* **60,** 1994–2001.
110. Ferluga, J., and Allison, A. C. (1978). Role of mononuclear infiltrating cells in pathogenesis of hepatitis. *Lancet* **2,** 610–611.
111. Ferluga, J. (1981). Tuberculin hypersensitivity hepatitis in mice infected with *Mycobacterium bovis* (BCG). *Am. J. Pathol.* **105,** 82–90.
112. Jaeschke, H., Farhood, A., and Smith, C. W. (1994). Contribution of complement-stimulated hepatic macrophages and neutrophils to endotoxin-induced liver injury in rats. *Hepatology* **19,** 973–979.
113. Arai, M., Mochida, S., Ohno, A., Ogata, I., and Fujiwara, K. (1993). Sinusoidal endothelial cell damage by activated macrophages in rat liver necrosis. *Gastroenterology* **104,** 1466–1471.
114. Sato, T., Shinzawa, H., Abe, Y., Takahashi, T., Arai, S., and Sendo, F. Inhibition of *Corynebacterium parvum*-primed and lipopolysaccharide-induced hepatic necrosis in rats by selective depletion of neutrophils using a monoclonal antibody. *J. Leukoc. Biol.* **53,** 144–150.
115. Tanaka, Y., Takahashi, A., Kobayashi, K., Arai, I., Higuchi, S., Otomo, S., Watanabe, K., Habu, S., and Nishimura, T. (1995). Establishment of a T cell-dependent nude mouse liver injury model induced by *Proprionibacterium acnes* and LPS. *J. Immunol. Methods* **182,** 21–28.
116. Rabinovici, R., Bugelski, P. J., Esser, K. M., Hillegass, L. M., Griswold, D. E., Vernick, J., and Feuerstein, G. (1993). Tumor necrosis factor-a mediates endotoxin-induced lung injury in platelet activating factor-primed rats. *J. Pharmacol. Exp. Ther.* **267,** 1550–1557.
117. Rabinovici, R., Esser, K. M., Lysko, P. G., Yue, T. -L., Griswold, D. E., Hillegass, L. M., Bugelski, P. J., Hallenbeck, J. M., and Feuerstein, G. (1991). Priming by platelet-activating factor of endotoxin-induced lung injury and cardiovascular shock. *Circ. Res.* **69,** 12–25.
118. Rabinovici, R., Bugelski, P. J., Esser, K. M., Hillegass, L. M., Vernick, J., and Feuerstein, G. (1993). ARDS-like lung injury produced by endotoxin in platelet- activating factor-primed rats. *J. Appl. Physiol.* **74,** 1791–1802.
119. Sun, X., Hsueh, W., and Torre-Amione, G. (1990). Effects of *in vivo* "priming" on endotoxin-induced hypotension and tissue injury: The role of PAF and tumor necrosis factor. *Am. J. Pathol.* **136,** 949–956.
120. Gonzalez-Crussi, F., and Hsueh, W. (1983). Experimental model of ischemic bowel necrosis: The role of platelet activating factor and endotoxin. *Am. J. Pathol.* **112,** 127–135.
121. Cross, A. S., Opal, S. M., Sadoff, J. C., and Gemski, P. Choice of bacteria in animal models of sepsis. *Infect. Immun.* **61,** 2741–2747.
122. Pass, L. J., Schloerb, P. R., Pearce, F. J., and Drucker, W. R. (1984). Cardiopulmonary response of the rat to gram-negative bacteremia. *Am. J. Physiol.* **246,** H344–H350.
123. Ammons, W. S., and Mallari, C. (1996). An N-terminal fragment of bactericidal/permeability-increasing protein protects against hemodynamic and metabolic derangements in rat Gram-negative sepsis. *J. Endotoxin Res.* **3,** 57–66.
124. Cryer, H. M., Garrison, R. N., Kaebnick, H. M., Harris, P. D., and Flint, L. M. (1987). Skeletal microcirculatory responses to hyperdynamic *Escherichia coli* sepsis in unanesthetized rats. *Arch. Surg.* **122,** 86–92.
125. Cryer, H. G., Garrison, R. N., Harris, P. D., Greenwald, B. H., and Alsip, N. L. (1990). Prostaglandins mediate skeletal muscle arteriole dilation in hyperdynamic bacteremia. *Am. J. Physiol.* **259,** H728–H734.
126. Cryer, H. M., Unger, L. S., Garrison, R. N., and Harris, P. D. (1988). Prostaglandins maintain renal microcirculatory blood flow during hyperdynamic bacteremia. *Circ. Shock* **26,** 71–88.
127. Whitworth, P. W., Cryer, H. M., Garrison, R. N., Baumgarten, T. E., and Harris, P. D. (1989). Hypoperfusion of the intestinal microcirculation with increased cardiac output during live *Escherichia coli* sepsis in rats. *Circ. Shock* **27,** 111–122.
128. Spain, D. A., Wilson, M. A., Bar-Natan, M. F., and Garrison, R. N. Role of nitric oxide in the small intestinal microcirculation during bacteremia. *Shock* **2,** 41–46.
129. Hinshaw, L. B., Tekamp-Olson, P., Chang, A. C., Lee, P. A., Taylor, F. B., Jr., Murray, C. K., Peer, G. T., Emmerson, T. E., Jr., Passey, R. B., and Kuo, G. C. (1990). Survival of primates in LD100 septic shock following therapy with antibody to tumor necrosis factor (TNF-α). *Circ. Shock* **30,** 279–292.
130. Schlag, G., Redl, H., Hallström, S., Radmore, K., and Davies, J. (1991). Hyperdynamic sepsis in baboons: I. Aspects of hemodynamics. *Circ. Shock* **34,** 311–318.
131. Carroll, G. C., and Snyder, J. V. (1982). Hyperdynamic severe intravascular sepsis depends on fluid administration in cynomolgus monkey. *Am. J. Physiol.* **243,** R131–R141.
132. Schaer, G. L., Fink, M. P., Chernow, B., Ahmed, S., and Parrillo, J. E. (1990). Renal hemodynamics and prostaglandin E_2 excretion in a nonhuman primate model of septic shock. *Crit. Care Med.* **18,** 52–59.
133. Stevens, J. H., O'Hanley, P., Shapiro, J. M., Mihm, F. G., Satoh, P. S., Collins, J. A., and Raffin, T. A. (1986). Effects of anti-C5a antibodies on the adult respiratory distress syndrome of septic primates. *J. Clin. Invest.* **77,** 1812–1816.
134. Hinshaw, L. B., Beller-Todd, B. K., Archer, L. T., Benjamin, B., Flournoy, D. J., Passey, R., and Wilson, M. F. (1981). Effectiveness of steroid/antibiotic treatment in primates administered LD100 *Escherichia coli. Ann. Surg.* **194,** 51–56.
135. Hinshaw, L. B., Archer, L. T., Beller-Todd, B. K., Benjamin, B., Flournoy, D. J., and Passey, R. (1981). Survival of primates in lethal septic shock following delayed treatment with steroid. *Circ. Shock* **8,** 291–300.
136. Hinshaw, L. B., Brackett, D. J., Archer, L. T., Beller, B. K., and Wilson, M. F. (1983). Detection of the "hyperdynamic state" of sepsis in the baboon during lethal *E. coli* infusion. *J. Trauma* **23,** 361–365.
137. Sprung, C. L., Caralis, P. V., Marcial, E. H., Pierce, M., Gelbard, M. A., Long, W. M., Duncan, R. C., Tendler, M. D., and Karpf, M. (1984). The effects of high-dose corticosteroids in patients with septic

shock. A prospective, controlled study. *N. Engl. J. Med.* **311,** 1137–1143.

138. The Veterans Administration Systemic Sepsis Cooperative Study Group. (1987). Effect of high-dose glucocorticoid therapy on mortality in patients with clinical signs of systemic sepsis. *N. Engl. J. Med.* **317,** 659–665.
139. Bone, R. C., Fisher, C. J., Jr., Clemmer, T. P., Slotman, G. J., Metz, C. A., and Balk, R. A. (1987). A controlled clinical trial of high-dose methylprednisolone in the treatment of severe sepsis and septic shock. *N. Engl. J. Med.* **317,** 653–658.
140. Dhainaut, J. -F., Vincent, J. -L., Richard, C., Lejeune, P., Martin, C., Fierobe, L., Stephens, S., Ney, U. M., and Sopwith, M. (1995). CDP571, a humanized antibody to human tumor necrosis factor-α: Safety, pharmacokinetics, immune response, and influence of the antibody on cytokine concentrations in patients with septic shock. *Crit. Care Med.* **23,** 1461–1469.
141. Fisher, C. J., Jr., Opal, S. M., Dhainaut, J. -F., Stephens, S., Zimmerman, J. L., Nightingale, P., Harris, S. J., Schein, R. M. H., Panacek, E. A., Vincent, J. -L., Foulke, G. E., Warren, E. L., Garrard, C., Park, G., Bodmer, M. W., Cohen, J., van der Linden, C., Cross, A. S., and Sadoff, J. C. (1993). The CB0006 Sepsis Syndrome Study Group. Influence of an anti-tumor necrosis factor monoclonal antibody on cytokine levels in patients with sepsis. *Crit. Care Med.* **21,** 318–327.
142. Abraham, E., Wunderink, R., Silverman, H., Perl, T. M., Nasraway, S., Levy, H., Bone, R., Wenzel, R. P., Balk, R., Allred, R., Pennington, J. E., and Wherry, J. C. (1995). Efficacy and safety of monoclonal antibody to human tumor necrosis factor a in patients with sepsis syndrome. A randomized, controlled, double-blind, multicenter clinical trial. *JAMA* **373,** 934–941.
143. Schlag, G., Redl, H., Davies, J., and Haller, I. (1994). Anti-tumor necrosis factor antibody treatment of recurrent bacteremia in a baboon model. *Shock* **2,** 10–18.
144. Dehring, D. J., Crocker, S. H., Wismar, B. L., Steinberg, S. M., Lowery, B. D., and Cloutier, C. T. (1983). Comparison of live bacteria infusions in a porcine model of acute respiratory failure. *J. Surg. Res.* **34,** 151–158.
145. Windsor, A. C. J., Mullen, P. G., Walsch, C. J., Fisher, B. J., Blocher, C. R., Jesmok, G., Fowler, A. A. I., and Sugerman, H. J. (1994). Delayed tumor necrosis factor a blockade attenuates pulmonary dysfunction and metabolic acidosis associated with experimental gram-negative sepsis. *Arch. Surg.* **129,** 80–89.
146. Windsor, A. C. J., Walsch, C. J., Mullen, P. G., Cook, D. J., Fisher, B. J., Blocher, C. R., Leeper-Woodford, S. K., Sugerman, H. J., and Fowler, A. A. I. (1993). Tumor necrosis factor-α blockade prevents neutrophil CD18 receptor upregulation and attenuates acute lung injury in porcine sepsis without inhibition of neutrophil oxygen radical generation. *J. Clin. Invest.* **91,** 1459–1468.
147. Leeper-Woodford, S. K., Carey, P. D., Byrne, K., Fisher, B. J., Blocher, C., Sugerman, H. J., Fowler, A. A. I., and Fowler, A. A. (1991). Ibuprofen attenuates plasma tumor necrosis factor activity during sepsis-induced acute lung injury. *J. Appl. Physiol.* **71,** 915–923.
148. Haberstroh, J., Breuer, H., Lücke, I., Massarrat, K., Früh, R., Mand, U., Hagerdorn, L., and von Specht, B.-U. (1995). Effect of recombinant human granulocyte colony-stimulating factor on hemodynamic and cytokine response in a porcine model of *Pseudomonas* sepsis. *Shock* **4,** 216–224.
149. Brooke, M., Hinder, F., Traber, L. D., McGuire, R., and Traber, D. L. (1995). *S*-Ethylisothiourea, a nonamino acid inhibitor of nitric oxide synthase, reverses septic vasodilation in sheep. *Shock* **4,** 274–281.
150. Meyer, J., Traber, L. D., Nelson, S., Lentz, C. W., Nakazawa, H., Herndon, D. N., Noda, H., and Traber, D. L. (1992). Reversal of hyperdynamic response to continuous endotoxin administration by inhibition of NO synthesis. *J. Appl. Physiol.* **73,** 324–328.
151. Lee, P. A., Matson, J. R., Pryor, R. W., and Hinshaw, L. B. (1993). Continuous arteriovenous hemofiltration therapy for *Staphylococcus aureus*-induced septicemia in immature swine. *Crit. Care Med.* **21,** 914–924.
152. Berg, S., Jansson, I., Hesselvik, F. J., Laurent, T. C., Lennquist, S., and Walther, S. (1992). Hyaluronan: Relationship to hemodynamics and survival in porcine injury and sepsis. *Crit. Care Med.* **20,** 1315–1321.
153. Hinshaw, L. B., Taylor, F. B., Jr., Chang, A. C., Pryor, R. W., Lee, P. A., Straughn, F., Murray, C. K., Flournoy, D. J., Peer, G. T., and Kosanke, S. D. (1988). *Staphylococcus aureus*-induced shock: A pathophysiologic study. *Circ. Shock* **26,** 257–265.
154. Hinshaw, L. B., Emerson, T. E., Jr., Taylor, F. B., Jr., Chang, A. C., Duerr, M., Peer, G. T., Flournoy, D. J., White, G. L., Kosanke, S. D., and Murray, C. K. (1992). Lethal *Staphylococcus aureus*-induced shock in primates: Prevention of death with anti-TNF antibody. *J. Trauma* **33,** 568–573.
155. Gibson, R. L., Redding, G. J., Henderson, W. R., and Truog, W. E. (1991). Group B *Streptococcus* induces tumor necrosis factor in neonatal piglets: Effect of the tumor necrosis factor inhibitor pentoxyfylline on hemodynamics and gas exchange. *Am. Rev. Resp. Dis.* **143,** 598–604.
156. Meadow, W. L., and Meus, P. J. (1986). Early and late hemodynamic consequences of group B beta streptococcal sepsis in piglets: effects on systemic, pulmonary, and mesenteric circulations. *Circ. Shock* **19,** 347–356.
157. Teti, G., Mancuso, G., Tomasello, F., and Chiofalo, M. S. (1992). Production of tumor necrosis factor-α and interleukin-6 in mice infected with Group B streptococci. *Circ. Shock* **38,** 138–144.
158. Wayte, J., Silva, A. T., Krausz, T., and Cohen, J. (1993). Observations on the role of tumor necrosis factor-α in a murine model of shock due to *Streptococcus pyogenes*. *Crit. Care Med.* **21,** 1207–1212.
159. Lechner, A. J., Lamprech, K. E., Potthoff, L. H., Tredway, T. L., and Matushak, G. M. (1994). Recombinant GM-CSF reduces lung injury and mortality during neutropenic *Candida* sepsis. *Am. J. Physiol.* **266,** L561–L568.
160. Wakabayashi, G., Gelfand, J. A., Burke, J. F., Thompson, R. C., and Dinarello, C. A. (1991). *Staphylococcus epidermidis* induces complement activation, tumor necrosis factor and interleukin-1, a shock-like state and tissue injury in rabbits without endotoxemia. Comparison to *Escherichia coli*. *J. Clin. Invest.* **87,** 1925–1935.
161. Ishizaka, A., Hasegawa, N., Sayama, K., Urano, T., Nakamura, H., Sakamaki, F., Soejima, K., Waki, Y., Tasaka, S., Nakamura, M., Matsubara, H., and Kanazawa, M. (1996). Augmentation of endotoxin-induced pulmonary responses by mononuclear cell phagocytosis in the reticuloendothelial system. *Crit. Care Med.* **24,** 1034–1040.
162. Nyström, P.-O., and Skau, T. (1983). Elimination patterns of *Escherichia coli* and *Bacteroides fragilis* from the peritoneal cavity. Studies with experimental peritonits in pigs. *Acta Chir. Scand.* **149,** 383–388.
163. Skau, T., Nyström, P.-O., Öhman, L., and Stendahl, O. (1986). Bacterial clearance and granulocytic response in experimental peritonitis. *J. Surg. Res.* **40,** 13–20.
164. Fink, M. P., Gardiner, M., and Mac Vittie, T. J. (1985). Sublethal hemorrhage impairs the acute peritoneal inflammatory response in the rat. *J. Trauma* **25,** 234–237.
165. Hau, T., Lee, J. T., and Simmons, R. L. (1981). Mechanism of the adjuvant effect of hemoglobin in experimental peritonitis. IV. The adjuvant effect of hemoglobin in granulocytopenic rats. *Surgery* **89,** 187–191.
166. Filler, R. M., and Sleeman, H. K. (1967). Pathogenesis of peritonitis. I. The effect of *Escherichia coli* and hemoglobin on peritoneal absorption. *Surgery* **61,** 385–392.
167. Dunn, D. L., Barke, R. A., Lee, J. T., Jr., Condie, R. M., Humphrey, E. W., and Simmons, R. L. (1983). Mechanisms of the adjuvant effect

of hemoglobin in experimental peritonitis. VII. Hemoglobin does not inhibit the clearance of *Escherichia coli* from the peritoneal cavity. *Surgery* **94,** 487–493.

168. Rotstein, O. D., Pruett, T. L., and Simmons, R. L. (1986). Fibrin in peritonitis. V. Fibrin inhibits phagocytic killing of *Escherichia coli* by human polymorphonuclear leukocytes. *Ann. Surg.* **203,** 413–419.
169. Hau, T., Hoffman, R., and Simmons, R. L. (1978). Mechanisms of the adjuvant effect of hemoglobin in experimental peritonitis. I. *In vivo* inhibition of peritoneal leukocytosis. *Surgery* **83,** 223–229.
170. Sleeman, H. K., Diggs, J. W., Hendry, W. S., Filler, R. M. (1967). Pathogenesis of peritonitis. II. The effect of *Escherichia coli* and adjuvant substances on peritoneal absorption. *Surgery* **61,** 393–398.
171. Flint, L. M., Jr., Calhoun, J. H., Anderson, M. D., and Richardson, J. D. (1981). Studies of peritoneal phagocytes as therapy for fecal peritonitis. *J. Surg. Res.* **30,** 154–158.
172. Sawyer, R. G., Adams, R. B., May, A. K., Rosenlof, L. K., and Pruett, T. L. (1993). Anti-tumor necrosis factor antibody reduces mortality in the presence of antibiotic-induced tumor necrosis factor release. *Arch. Surg.* **128,** 73–78.
173. Onderdonk, A., Bartlett, J. G., Louie, T., Sullivan-Seigler, N., and Gorbach, S. L. (1976). Microbial synergy in experimental intraabdominal abscess. *Infect. Immun.* **13,** 22–26.
174. Marks, M. I., Ziegler, E. J., Douglas, H., Corbeil, L. B., and Braude, A. I. (1981). Induction of immunity against lethal *Haemophilus influenzae* type b infection by *Escherichia coli* lipopolysaccharide. *J. Clin. Invest.* **69,** 742–749.
175. Ahrenholz, D. H., and Simmons, R. L. (1980). Fibrin in peritonitis. I. Beneficial and adverse effects of fibrin in experimental *E. coli* peritonitis. *Surgery* **88,** 41–47.
176. Dunne, J. R., Dunkin, B. J., Nelson, S., and White, J. C. (1996). Effects of granulocyte colony stimulating factor in a nonneutropenic rodent model of *Escherichia coli* peritonitis. *J. Surg. Res.* **61,** 348–354.
177. Shenep, J. L., Barton, R. W., and Mogan, K. A. (1985). Role of antibiotic class in the rate of liberation of endotoxin during therapy for experimental Gram-negative bacterial sepsis. *J. Infect. Dis.* **151,** 1012–1018.
178. Saladino, R., Garcia, C., Thompson, C., Hammer, B., Parsonnet, J., Novitsky, T., Siber, G., and Fleisher, G. Efficacy of recombinant endotoxin neutralizing protein in rabbits with *Escherichia coli* sepsis. *Circ. Shock* **42,** 104–110.
179. Vary, T. C., Siegel, J. H., Nakatani, T., Sato, T., and Aoyama, H. (1986). Effect of sepsis on activity of pyruvate dehydrogenase complex in skeletal muscle and liver. *Am. J. Physiol.* **250,** E634–E640.
180. Camerota, A. J., Creasey, A. A., Patla, V., Larkin, V. A., and Fink, M. P. (1998). Delayed treatment with recombinant human tissue factor pathway inhibitor improves survival in rabbits with gram-negative peritonitis. *J. Infect. Dis.* **177,** 668–676.
181. Natanson, C., Danner, R. L., and Reilly, J. M. (1990). Antibiotics versus cardiovascular support in a canine model of human septic shock. *Am. J. Physiol.* **259,** H1440–H1447.
182. Natanson, C., Danner, R. L., Elin, R. J., Hosseini, J. M., Peart, K. W., Banks, S. M., Mac Vittie, T. J., Walker, R. I., and Parrillo, J. E. (1989). Role of endotoxemia in cardiovascular dysfunction and mortality: *Escherichia coli* and *Staphylococcus aureus* challenges in a canine model of human septic shock. *J. Clin. Invest.* **83,** 243–251.
183. Wichterman, K. A., Baue, A. E., and Chaudry, I. H. (1980). Sepsis and septic shock—A review of laboratory models and a proposal. *J. Surg. Res.* **29,** 189–201.
184. Lorenz, W., Reimund, K.-P., Weitzel, F., Celik, I., Kurnatowski, M., Schneider, C., Mannheim, W., Heiske, A., Neumann, K., Sitter, H., and Rothmund, M. (1994). Granulocyte colony-stimulating factor prophylaxis before operation protects against lethal consequences of postoperative peritonitis. *Surgery* **116,** 925–934.
185. Mourelatos, M. G., Enzer, N., Ferguson, J. L., Rypins, E. B., Burhop, K., and Law, W. R. (1996). The effects of diaspirin cross-linked hemoglobin in sepsis. *Shock* **5,** 141–148.
186. Lang, C. H., Bagby, G. J., Ferguson, J. L., and Spitzer, J. J. (1984). Cardiac output and redistribution of organ blood flow in hypermetabolic sepsis. *Am. J. Physiol.* **246,** R331–R337.
187. Tighe, D., Moss, R., Heywood, G., Al-Saady, N., Webb., A., and Bennett, D. (1996). Goal-directed therapy with dopexamine, dobutamine, and volume expansion: Effects of systemic oxygen transport on hepatic ultrastructure in porcine sepsis. *Crit. Care Med.* **23,** 1997–2007.
188. Antonsson, J. B., Engstrom, L., Rasmussen, I., Wollert, S., and Haglund, U. (1996). Changes in gut intramucosal pH and gut oxygen extraction ratio in a porcine model of peritonitis and hemorrhage. *Crit. Care Med.* **23,** 1872–1881.
189. Abraham, E., and Stevens, P. (1992). Effects of granulocyte colony-stimulating factor in modifying mortality from *Pseudomonas aeruginosa* pneumonia after hemorrhage. *Crit. Care Med.* **20,** 1127–1133.
190. Mellencamp, M. A., and Preheim, L. C. (1991). Pneumococcal pneumonia in a rat model of cirrhosis: Effects of cirrhosis on pulmonary defense mechanism against *Streptococcus pneumoniae. J. Infect. Dis.* **163,** 102–108.
191. Nelson, S., Summer, W., Bagby, G., Nakamura, C., Stewart, L., Lipscomb, G., and Andresen, J. (1991). Granulocyte colony-stimulating factor enhances pulmonary host defenses in normal and ethanol-treated rats. *J. Infect. Dis.* **164,** 901–905.
192. Wilkinson, R. A., and Fishman, J. A. (1999). Effect of thermal injury with *Pseudomonas aeruginosa* infection on pulmonary and systemic bacterial clearance. *J. Trauma* **47,** 912–917.
193. Hanly, P. J., Sienko, A., and Light, R. B. (1988). Role of prostacyclin and thromboxane in the circulatory changes of acute bacteremic *Pseudomonas* pneumonia in dogs. *Am. Rev. Resp. Dis.* **137,** 700–706.
194. Keenan, R. J., Todd, T. R., and Girotti, M. J. (1987). Experimental gram-negative pneumonia produces a hyperdynamic septic profile. *Circ. Shock* **22,** 303–309.
195. Gahos, F. N., Chiu, R. C. J., Bethune, D., Dion, Y., Hinchey, E. J., and Richards, G. K. (1981). Hemodynamic responses to sepsis: Hypodynamic versus hyperdynamic sepsis. *J. Surg. Res.* **31,** 475–481.
196. Mela-Riker, L., Bartos, D., Vlessis, A. A., Widener, L., Muller, P., and Trunkey, D. D. (1992). Chronic hyperdynamic sepsis in the rat. II. Characterization of liver and muscle energy metabolism. *Circ. Shock* **36,** 83–92.
197. Gaar, E., Naziri, W., Cheadle, W. G., Pietsch, J. D., Johnson, M., and Polk, H. C., Jr. (1994). Improved survival in simulated surgical infection with combined cytokine, antibiotic and immunostimulant therapy. *Br. J. Surg.* **81,** 1309–1311.
198. Yasuda, H., Ajiki, Y., Shimozato, T., Kasahara, M., Kawada, H., Iwata, M., and Shimizu, K. (1990). Therapeutic efficacy of granulocyte colony-stimulating factor alone and in combination with antibiotics against *Pseudomonas aeruginosa* infections in mice. *Infect. Immun.* **58,** 2502–2509.
199. Sriskandan, S., Unnikrishnan, M., Krausz, T., and Cohen, J. (1999). Molecular analysis of the role of streptococcal pyrogenic Exotoxin A (SPEA) in invasive soft-tissue infection resulting from *Streptococcus pyogenes. Mol. Microbiol.* **33,** 778–790.
200. Opal, S. M., Cross, A. S., Sadoff, J. C., Collins, H. H., Kelly, N. M., Victor, G. H., Palardy, J. E., and Bodmer, M. W. (1991). Efficacy of antilipopolysaccharide and anti-tumor necrosis factor monoclonal antibodies in a neutropenic rat model of *Pseudomonas* sepsis. *J. Clin. Invest.* **88,** 885–890.
201. Collins, H. H., Cross, A. S., Dobeck, A., Opal, S. M., McClain, J. B., and Sadoff, J. C. (1989). Oral ciprofloxacin and a monoclonal antibody to lipopolysaccharide protect neutropenic rats from lethal infection with *Pseudomonas aeruginosa. J. Infect. Dis.* **159,** 1073–1082.

202. Ziegler, E. J., Douglas, H., Sherman, J. E., Davis, C. E., and Braude, A. I. (1973). Treatment of *E. coli* and *Klebsiella* bacteremia in agranulocytic animals with antiserum to a UDP-Gal epimerase-deficient mutant. *J. Immunol.* **111,** 433–438.
203. Ziegler, E. J., McCutchan, J. A., Herndon, D., and Braude, A. I. (1975). Prevention of lethal *Pseudomonas* bacteremia with epimerase-deficient *E. coli* antiserum. *Trans. Assoc. Am. Physicians* **88,** 101–108.
204. Hebert, J. C., O'Reilly, M., and Gamelli, R. L. (1990). Protective effect of recombinant human granulocyte colony-stimulating factor against pneumococcal infections in splenectomized mice. *Arch. Surg.* **125,** 1075–1078.
205. Silver, G. M., Gamelli, R. L., O'Reilly, M., and Hebert, J. C. (1990). The effect of interleukin la on survival in a murine model of burn wound sepsis. *Arch. Surg.* **125,** 922–925.
206. Wollert, P. S., Menconi, M. J., Wang, H., O'Sullivan, B. P., Larkin, V., Allen, R. C., and Fink, M. P. (1994). Prior exposure to endotoxin exacerbates lipopolysaccharide-induced hypoxemia and alveolitis in anesthetized swine. *Shock* **2,** 362–369.
207. Wollert, P. S., Menconi, M. J., O'Sullivan, B. P., Wang, H., Larkin, V., and Fink, M. P. (1993). LY255283, a novel leukotriene B_4 receptor antagonist, limits activation of neutrophils and prevents acute lung injury induced by endotoxin in pigs. *Surgery* **114,** 191–198.
208. VanderMeer, T. J., Menconi, M. J., O'Sullivan, B. P., Larkin, V. A., Wang, H., Kradin, R. L., and Fink, M. P. (1994). Bactericidal/permeability-increasing protein ameliorates acute lung injury in porcine endotoxemia. *J. Appl. Physiol.* **76,** 2006–2014.
209. VanderMeer, T. J., Menconi, M. J., O'Sullivan, B. P., Larkin, V. A., Wang, H., Sofia, M., and Fink, M. P. (1995). Acute lung injury in endotoxemic pigs: role of leukotriene B_4. *J. Appl. Physiol.* **78,** 1121–1131.
210. Tasaki, O., Goodwin, C., Mozingo, D. W., Cioffi, W. G., Ishihara, S., Brinkley, W. W., Dubick, M. A., Smith, R. H., Srivastava, O., and Pruitt, B. A. (1999). Selectin blockade worsened lipopolysaccharide-induced lung injury in a swine model. *J. Trauma* **46,** 1089–1095.
211. Koike, K., Moore, F. A., Moore, E. E., Poggetti, R. S., Tuder, R. M., and Banerjee, A. (1992). Endotoxin after gut ischemia/reperfusion causes irreversible lung injury. *J. Surg. Res.* **52,** 656–662.
212. Biffl, W. L., and Moore, E. E. (1996). Splanchnic ischaemia/reperfusion and multiple organ failure. *Br. J. Anaesth.* **77,** 59–70.
213. Turnbull, R. G., Talbot, J. A., and Hamilton, S. M. (1995). Hemodynamic changes and gut barrier function in sequential hemorrhagic and endotoxic shock. *J. Trauma* **38,** 705–712.
214. Gavin, T. J., Fabian, T. C., Wilson, J. D., Trenthem, L. L., Pritchard, F. E., Croce, M. A., Stewart, R. M., and Proctor, K. G. (1994). Splanchnic and systemic hemodynamic responses to portal vein endotoxin after resuscitation from hemorrhagic shock. *Surgery* **115,** 310–324.
215. Mileski, W. J., Winn, R. K., Harlan, J. M., and Rice, C. L. (1992). Sensitivity to endotoxin in rabbits is increased after hemorrhagic shock. *J. Appl. Physiol.* **73,** 1146–1149.
216. Spain, D. A., Kawabe, T., Keelan, P. C., Wilson, M. A., Harris, P. D., and Garrison, R. N. (1999). Decreased alpha-adrenergic response in the intestinal microcirculation after "two-hit" hemorrhage/resuscitation and bacteremia. *J. Surg. Res.* **84,** 180–185.
217. Dehring, D. J., Lübbesmeyer, H. J., Fader, R. C., Traber, L. D., and Traber, D. L. Exaggerated cardiopulmonary response after bacteremia in sheep with week-old thermal injury. *Crit. Care Med.* **21,** 888–893.
218. Laubach, V. E., Foley, P. L., Shockey, K. S., Tribble, C. G., and Kron, I. L. (1998). Protective roles of nitric oxide and testosterone in endotoxemia: evidence from NOS-2-deficient mice. *Am. J. Physiol.* **275,** H2211–H2218.
219. Crespo, E., Macias, M., Pozo, D., Escames, G., Martin, M., Vives, F., Guerrero, J. M., and Acuna-Castroviejo, D. (1999). Melatonin inhibits expression of the inducible NO synthase II in liver and lung and prevents endotoxemia in lipopolysaccharide-induced multiple organ dysfunction syndrome in rats. *FASEB J.* **13,** 1537–1546.
220. Goris, R. J. A., Boekholtz, W. K. F., van Bebber, I. P. T., Nuytinck, J. K. S., and Schillings, P. H. M. (1986). Multiple-organ failure and sepsis without bacteria; an experimental model. *Arch. Surg.* **121,** 897–901.
221. Nieuwenhuijzen, G. A., Meyer, M. P., Hendriks, T., and Goris, R. J. (1995). Deficiency of complement factor C5 reduces early mortality but does not prevent organ damage in an animal model of multiple organ dysfunction syndrome. *Crit. Care Med.* **23,** 1686–1693.
222. Dwenger, A., Remmers, D., Grotz, M., Pape, H. C., Gruner, A., Scharff, H., Jochum, M., and Regel, G. (1999). Aprotinin prevents the development of the trauma-induced multiple organ failure in a chronic sheep model. *Eur. J. Clin. Chem. Clin. Biochem.* **34,** 207–214.
223. Pape, H. C., Grotz, M., Remmers, D., Dwenger, A., Vaske, R., Wisner, D., and Tscherne, H. (1999). Multiple organ failure (MOF) after severe trauma—A sheep model. *Intensive Care Med.* **24,** 590–598.

64

The Immuno-Inflammatory Response

Eileen M. Bulger, Avery B. Nathens, and Ronald V. Maier

Department of Surgery, Harborview Medical Center and the University of Washington, Seattle, Washington 98104

I. Introduction

Study of the innate immuno-inflammatory response has implications for the understanding of a number of surgical problems, including intraabdominal sepsis, whole body ischemia/reperfusion injury following hypovolemic shock, and local reperfusion injury following coronary artery bypass grafting and transplantation. The development of an uncontrolled, systemic overexpression of this response has also been implicated in the development of the acute respiratory distress syndrome (ARDS) and multiple organ dysfunction syndrome (MODS), both of which are leading causes of morbidity and mortality in the surgical intensive care unit. There is good clinical and experimental evidence that the biologic responses of the macrophage and the neutrophil are responsible for this inflammatory state. In addition, an immunocompromised state following injury and severe stress appears to be induced by potent biologic modifiers produced by these same cells, and involves alterations in the phenotype of T lymphocytes. There is a shift from a proinflammatory T cell cytokine pattern (Th1) to an immunosuppressive T cell cytokine pattern (Th2). As a result of this shift and direct counterregulatory suppression of the innate immune response, patients are at increased risk for impaired wound healing and nosocomial infection, which will then further drive a dysfunctional inflammatory response.

In this review of models commonly employed for study of the nonspecific immuno-inflammatory response, the focus is primarily on the cell biology of the macrophage and neutrophil. We begin with a summary of the sources of cells used for study and the advantages and disadvantages of harvesting cells from different systems. We then discuss cell stimulation, assays used to assess cellular activation, and techniques used to modulate this response. A review of the techniques used to identify the T helper cell phenotype is also be presented. Extensive research has also focused on the intracellular signaling pathways and molecular biology of these cellular responses. These topics are discussed in greater detail elsewhere in this volume.

II. Monocytes and Macrophages

The tissue-fixed macrophage has been identified as a central regulator controlling the activation and propagation of the inflammatory process (1). Circulating monocytes localize to areas of inflammation or infection or become residents of primary tissue beds where foreign antigens are frequently encountered. Examples include Kupffer cells in the liver and alveolar macrophages in the lung. These monocytes then differentiate to become tissue-fixed macrophages. The macrophage is a component of the local response to infection, serving a key role as a scavenger of bacteria and bacterial products, an antigen-presenting cell, and a coordinator of the inflammatory response via the production of a plethora of cytokines and chemokines. These mediators result in the recruitment and activation of all other components of the inflammatory response, particularly the neutrophil. In addition, activated macrophages produce a number of products, including tissue factor and prostanoids, which have profound effects on the microcirculation, resulting in microvascular thrombosis and local ischemia. Production of toxic reactive oxygen intermediates and proteases by both the macrophage and the neutrophil can result in endothelial cell injury and subsequent capillary leak. Although these processes are necessary to control and contain a local focus of infection, systemic activation of these processes can result in extensive tissue injury and subsequent organ failure. Studies of macrophage activation have thus focused on their responses to a number of inflammatory stimuli (i.e., proinflammatory phenotype) as assessed by the production of cytokines, chemokines, lipid mediators, complement components, and thrombotic agents such as tissue factor. Various strategies to modulate this response have included receptor blockade, alteration of the redox state with antioxidants, interruption of signal transduction with specific inhibitors, inhibition of intracellular calcium mobilization, and metabolism of autocrine mediator production such as platelet-activating factor. This approach has enhanced our understanding of macrophage function and has stimulated a number of clinical trials for the treatment and prevention of the dysfunctional systemic inflammatory response.

A. Source of Monocytes and Macrophages for Study

The source of monocytes or macrophages has important implications concerning the ability to apply the results seen *in vitro* to a clinical situation. A number of transformed cell lines are available for study, including THP-1, U937, Mono-Mac-6, RAW 264.7, and MH-S. THP-1, U937, and Mono-Mac-6 are human monocytic cell lines. THP-1 cells, derived from a patient with acute monocytic leukemia, unlike other leukemic cell lines have a normal diploid karyotype. U937 and THP-1 cells can be differentiated to a macrophage phenotype by treatment with interferon-γ. In addition, culture of these cells with 1α,25-dihyroxyvitamin D_3 results in enhanced membrane expression of CD14, the key receptor involved in macrophage activation by lipopolysaccharide (LPS) (2–4). RAW 264.7 is a transformed murine macrophage line and MH-S is a murine alveolar macrophage cell line transformed by simian virus 40 (5). There are also a number of cell lines derived from transformation of murine peritoneal macrophages. The advantage to using cell lines is that they are easy to maintain, relatively inexpensive compared to animal work, and provide a uniform population of cells. The major disadvantage is that the response of these cells may be significantly altered by their transformed state and thus they may not reflect the human or animal *in vivo* response. In addition, there are likely species differences as well. Thus, definitive conclusions of relevance should be confirmed in normal human-derived tissues.

The alternative to the use of cell lines requires that monocytes or macrophages be harvested from animals or humans. Monocytes are usually obtained by density centrifugation of whole blood. This allows isolation of peripheral blood mononuclear cells (PBMCs), the fraction containing both monocytes and lymphocytes. Monocytes can then be further separated by their innate selective adherence to culture plates. In using this approach it is crucial to recognize that adherence alone can result in significant changes in the activation state of the cells. Monocyte adherence results in alteration in the cytoskeletal structure and increased cytokine production in response to LPS (6). The mechanisms responsible for this process have not been fully elucidated. However, our laboratory has demonstrated that even differentiated alveolar macrophages have a significant increase in LPS-induced tumor necrosis factor (TNF) production when allowed to adhere to culture plates, an effect potentially due to alteration of the intracellular signaling responses (7). Another approach to macrophage isolation that avoids the effects of adherence is reverse immunologic selection (8). For this procedure, mononuclear cells are obtained by Ficoll–Paque density gradient centrifugation. The cells are then resuspended and treated with human IgG as an Fc receptor (FcR) blocking agent and an antibody cocktail, which allows for separation of the lymphocyte component. This results in a 95% pure monocyte fraction.

Tissue-fixed macrophages can be harvested by a variety of techniques. Peritoneal macrophages are prominent in mice and rats and can be obtained by peritoneal lavage. These can either be resident macrophages found in unstimulated animals or elicited macrophages obtained by infusion of an inflammatory agent (thioglycollate) into the peritoneal cavity. The use of thioglycollate allows for a greater number of cells for study; however, these cells are already in an activated (probable proinflammatory) state when obtained, which may significantly alter their responses. For example, thioglycollate-elicted macrophages produce significantly higher levels of tumor necrosis factor in response to endotoxin when compared to resident peritoneal macrophages (9). Humans normally have very few resident peritoneal macrophages and thus these cells are difficult to study.

Alveolar macrophages obtained by means of bronchoalveolar lavage are another commonly studied cell population. The lavage technique commonly requires larger animals, such as rabbits, to obtain sufficient cells for study, and requires sterile cannulation of the trachea followed by repeated gentle lavage with cold (4°C) saline solution. It is important to avoid vigorous lavage because the shear stress may contribute to cellular activation. In addition, the animals used to obtain these cells must be young and housed for minimal times to avoid exposure to respiratory pathogens, which can also lead to cellular activation. The disadvantage to the use of these cells is that activation prior to plating can lead to increased variability in the degree of the measured response. These cells have also been harvested from both normal humans and those with ARDS; however, the genomic variations, particularly in disease states, can make the results difficult to interpret.

A major source of tissue-fixed macrophages from animals includes those within the liver and spleen. These are generally more difficult to isolate. Isolation is usually dependent on the selective avidity of the macrophage to adhere following mechanical and proteolytic disruption of the tissues (10). Artifactual alterations in this process are a significant concern. Another common approach is counterflow centrifugation elutriation. The first step involves *in vivo* perfusion of the organs in anesthetized animals with a cold buffer solution followed by a collagenase digestion. The organs are then harvested and the cell suspension processed via elutriation rather than adherence. Isolation of Kupffer cells via this approach was first described in 1977 and has become a common technique, yielding a fairly pure though heterogeneous population of cells (11). Splenic macrophages can be similarly isolated, but obtaining a sufficient number of cells, particularly from small animals such as mice, can be difficult and requires pooling (12). The spleen possesses four distinct populations of macrophages: the marginal zone macrophages, macrophages of the red pulp, the periarteriolar macrophages, and the marginal metallophils, which have selective responses. Macrophage viability should be verified under each experimental condition and may be assessed by trypan blue or propidium iodide exclusion. Purity of the cell fraction can be determined by autofluorescence gating measured via flow cytometry or expression of nonspecific esterase staining, which is selective for macrophages via light microscopy (12).

B. Macrophage Stimulation

Once a source of cells has been identified, a variety of agents are available to activate the macrophage. The most commonly used are thought to mimic various *in vivo* conditions, including the lipopolysaccharide (LPS) moiety of endotoxin, whole bacteria, cytokines, chemokines, lipid mediators, oxidative stress, and osmotic stress. Cellular activation can occur *in vivo* or *in vitro*. *In vivo* models are generally animal models of sepsis or ischemia/reperfusion (see Chapters 27 and 45, this volume). For the study of sepsis, some models involve the infusion of endotoxin or live bacteria, whereas others more closely mimic specific disease states, such as the cecal ligation and puncture model that effectively models peritonitis. Hemorrhagic shock followed by vigorous resuscitation is a useful model to induce a global ischemia/reperfusion injury. In all these models, macrophages or monocytes can be harvested as described above to assess activation at varying time points. In addition, serum or lavage fluid obtained from the various models can be used to assess levels of various cytokines and other inflammatory mediators in an effort to evaluate the components and extent of the immuno-inflammatory response. The main limitation to this approach is that the mediators either have an endogenously controlled very short half-life, or, although they may have profound paracrine and autocrine effects in the local environment, this may not be reflected by circulating serum or tissue levels.

To avoid these variabilities of animal models, macrophage activation is commonly studied *in vitro*. These studies involve treatment of cultured cells with the agents described above and subsequent analysis of mediator production in the supernatant. Cell-associated products such as tissue factor can also be analyzed via lysis of cell monolayers. The advantage to this approach is that it provides a uniform stimulus to all cells and allows easier detailed study of the steps involved in control, including signal transduction, transcription factor activation, and production and translation of messenger RNA for individual products. The choice of a stimulatory agent depends on the general process under study. For those interested in sepsis, LPS or whole bacteria are commonly used. LPS is preferentially used due to its ability to mimic bacterial interactions while avoiding the difficulty in controlling bacterial load due to variable growth in different experimental conditions. To simulate ischemia/reperfusion *in vitro*, there exist environmentally controlled chambers that allow for a period of hypoxia followed by reoxygenation. This approach involves incubation of the cells in a hypoxic environment, in which the ambient concentration of oxygen is carefully controlled, followed by return of the cells to a normoxic environment. Additional stress responses include altering the osmotic gradient in the media to simulate conditions such as those seen with hypertonic resuscitation and altering the redox state of the cell with oxidant-generating reactions to simulate the oxidative stress of the inflammatory environment.

In addition to primary stimulation with a given agent, there are models of priming and tolerance, both of which are pertinent to an understanding of macrophage biology. Priming involves preexposure of the cell to an agent that may not in itself induce significant cytokine production, but "primes" or reprograms the subsequent response of the cell to a second stimulus. The prior exposure may lead to enhanced or suppressed responsiveness, i.e., cellular tolerance. This has been described in the alveolar macrophage, which when pretreated with platelet-activating factor (PAF) demonstrates a dramatic increase in TNF and tissue factor production following subsequent LPS stimulation (13). This model simulates the proposed two-hit hypothesis of MODS, in which an initial insult is thought to lead to inflammatory cell reprogramming such that a second insult results in excessive inflammatory response, thus contributing to organ injury.

Tolerance results from pretreatment of the macrophage with a low dose of LPS or other agent, resulting in desensitization of the cell such that the response to a subsequent dose of LPS is diminished (14, 15). This model contributes to our understanding of the immunosuppressive state seen following severe stress and extensive disseminated inflammation.

C. Evaluation of Macrophage Activation

1. Cytokine Assays

Assessment of macrophage activation commonly relies on the measurement of the production of cytokines and other secreted products such as prostanoids and chemokines. Cytokine production can be measured in the sera, lavage fluids, or supernatants of cell cultures. The assays used to measure cytokine production include bioassays and immunoassays. Bioassays involve measuring the effect of a cytokine on a target cell culture. The WEHI 164 bioassay for TNF production, for example, measures the cytotoxic effect of TNF on this fibrosarcoma cell line (16). Immunoassays are widely commercially available as enzyme-linked immunosorbent assays (ELISAs) or enzyme immunoassay (EIA) kits. These assays rely on a primary monoclonal antibody to the cytokine of interest. This primary antibody is then recognized by a biotinylated secondary antibody, followed by a streptavidin–enzyme–enzymatic substrate complex. Bioassays are more sensitive, but less specific, compared to immunoassays. Bioassays may also be more biologically relevant because they measure only the active cytokine. Inactive cytokine fragments may bind the primary antibody of an ELISA and spuriously elevate the result. The sensitivity of the ELISA depends on the ability of the primary antibody to bind all of the active cytokine. Several cytokines circulate as complexes bound to serum proteins or soluble receptors, which may be specific to the fluid analyzed and thus may not be detected by all antibodies. ELISAs have the advantage of being easy to perform, with results usually available within hours. Bioassays, on the other hand, are more labor intensive because they require maintenance of the target cells in culture, confirmation of specificity using a cytokine-specific antibody, and interpretation of an S-shaped dose–response curve (17).

There is also debate concerning the optimal specimen for cytokine assays. Blood or body fluids need to be collected rapidly, with cold storage to prevent enzymatic degradation and inactivation or ongoing production of cytokine proteins following isolation. It is not clear whether plasma or serum should be used for optimal results. Leukocytes may be activated during the clotting process (thrombin being a major inflammatory stimulus) and thus release cytokines that do not reflect the *in vivo* situation (18). In addition, patients may have higher circulating levels of endogenous counterregulatory proteases compared to normal controls and so samples obtained from patients may be less stable (17). The general disadvantages to cytokine measurement in blood or body fluids include inaccurate reflection of local cytokine effects, failure to detect membrane-associated cytokines, competition from circulating antibodies and soluble receptors, and variable destruction or ongoing release during processing.

Cytokine levels can also be measured in tissue samples; however, this process requires tissue biopsy and is more labor intensive. Tissue extracts can be processed by ELISA, but this approach does not identify which cells are producing the cytokine or their location. The results should be expressed relative to the total protein content per gram of tissue. Another approach involves the reverse hemolytic plaque assay, which allows visualization of single cytokine-producing cells in tissue samples (19). Alternatively, immunocytochemistry (for protein) and *in situ* hybridization (for mRNA) may be useful techniques for localizing the source of cytokines in tissue specimens. Importantly, the appearance of cytokine mRNA does not necessarily imply the presence of functional protein. TNF and interleukin-1 (IL-1), for example, are synthesized as prohormones that are modified prior to secretion, and thus measurement of mRNA for these cytokines may not reflect their functional activity. Another technique for quantification of cytokine mRNA involves the use of the competitive reverse-transcription polymerase chain reaction as described by O'Garra *et al.* (20). These techniques require that tissues be handled such that degradation of mRNA by endogenous RNase enzymes is avoided. For this reason, newer techniques utilizing *in situ* approaches, with specific antibodies to intracellular levels of specific proteins, are rapidly being developed. These approaches can be combined with fluorescence-activated cell sorter analysis of gated cellular populations to determine specific cell type contents (9). Specific approaches used for assessing the cytokine response *in vivo* and *in vitro*, along with their relative advantages and disadvantages, are summarized in Table I.

2. Measurement of Tissue Factor Activity

Membrane bound enzymes and other mediators can be measured on macrophage cell monolayers following stimulation and lysis. The tissue factor or procoagulant activity assay, for example, is a two-stage amidolytic assay using a

Table I The Monocyte/Macrophage: Methods of Evaluating the Cytokine Response

Cytokine source/method	Advantages	Disadvantages
Supernatant/body fluids		
Immunoassays	Simple; quick; high specificity	May not measure biologically active cytokine; expensive
Bioassays	Measures biologically active cytokine; very sensitive	Lacks specificity; often laborious and time consuming
Cells		
Flow cytometry	Measures cell-associated markers of activation; provides data on both overall expression in a population of cells and magnitude of expression per cell; relatively quick with high sensitivity and high specificity	Equipment may be expensive and not readily accessible
Polymerase chain reaction or Northern blot analysis	Relatively easy; may provide data with relatively few cells (PCR)	Data obtained are limited to mRNA expression; may have little relationship to protein expression
Tissue		
Immunoassays	Simple, quick, quantitative	Limited to tissue extracts; provides no data as to source of cytokine
Polymerase chain reaction or Northern blot analysis	Relatively easy; may provide data with relatively small tissue samples	Limited to tissue extracts; provides no data as to source of cytokine; data are limited to mRNA expression and may have no relationship to protein expression
Immunohistochemistry	Provides information as to source of cytokine protein expression	Laborious; sensitivity/specificity may be dependent on methods of tissue fixation
In situ hybridization	Provides information as to source of cytokine mRNA expression	Difficult; data obtained are limited to mRNA expression; may have little relationship to protein expression

chromogenic substrate (21). In brief, various treated cell monolayers are lysed using sonication, then procoagulant activity is tested against standards of rabbit brain thromboplastin using a reaction mixture containing the chromogenic substrate and Proplex-T (Baxter Healthcare, Garden Grove, CA). Absorbance is then measured at 405 nm.

3. Phagocytosis, Respiratory Burst, and Antigen Presentation

An important antimicrobial function of macrophages involves the ingestion and killing of bacteria and other opsonized particles. Techniques of assessment of macrophage phagocytosis or killing are similar to those used for assessing these same parameters in the neutrophil (22).

Once ingested, foreign antigens can be processed and presented on the cell surface in association with the major histocompatibility complex for activation of the lymphocyte response. There are two common approaches for assessing the macrophage antigen presentation function. The first involves the coculturing of lymphocytes, which have been totally depleted of antigen presenting cells, with macrophages and soluble antigen. The other approach utilizes lymphocytes that have not been rigorously depleted but are cocultured with macrophages that have been previously exposed to the antigen, and thus present it only in a cell-associated form. The endpoint measured in both cases is the degree of lymphocyte proliferation. The downside to the first approach is that it is extremely difficult to isolate a completely pure lymphocyte population. The second approach may also be hampered by residual antigen-presenting cells in the lymphoid population, because some antigen may only loosely adhere to the exposed macrophage population and thus will cross over to the residual antigen-presenting cells (23, 24).

D. Modulation of Macrophage Activation

A number of strategies have been employed both *in vitro* and *in vivo* in an effort to alter macrophage activation and/or specific cytokine production or effect and thus improve outcome. There are multiple steps in the pathway of macrophage activation in which intervention can alter the response (Fig. 1). These include (1) blocking the stimulating agent, (2) blocking the receptor for the stimulus, (3) inhibiting the signal transduction pathway, (4) inhibiting gene transcription, (5) inhibiting protein translation, (6) altering cytokine processing and secretion, and (7) blocking secreted cytokine activity or enhancing its metabolism. Using LPS as the archetypal stimulus of the macrophage, for example, LPS can be bound by monoclonal or polyclonal antiendotoxin antibodies. Other approaches utilize the nonspecific binding of LPS to lipid moieties, such as high-density lipoprotein (HDL). For optimal activation, LPS binds to a serum protein, LPS binding protein (LBP), and this complex interacts with the CD14 receptor on the surface of the macrophage. This process can be interrupted by either depletion of LBP

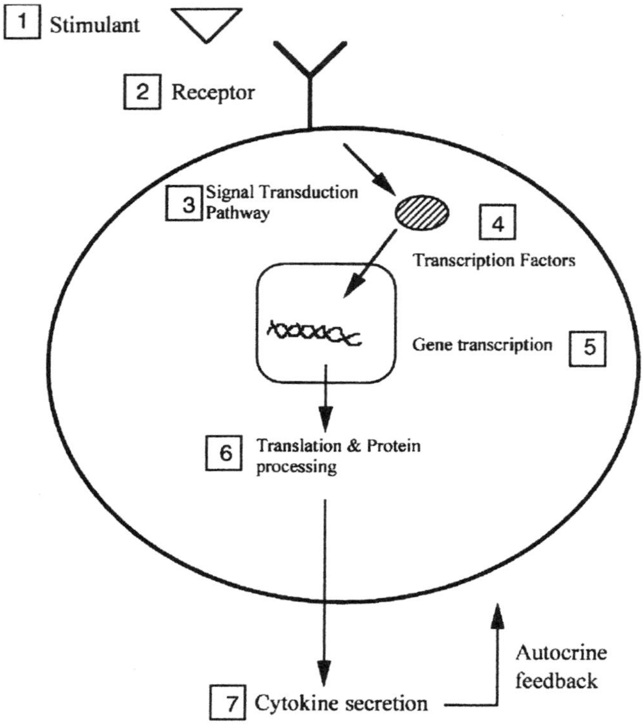

Figure 1 The seven steps involved in macrophage activation. Specific interventions may modulate the process: (1) direct blockade of the inciting stimulant, (2) receptor blockade, (3) inhibition of signal transduction, (4) inhibition of transcription factors, (5) modulation of gene transcription, (6) alteration of translation or protein processing, (7) inhibition of individual inflammatory products.

or blockade of CD14 with a monoclonal antibody or inactive altered endotoxin constructs, such as lipid X or deacylated LPS.

The signal transduction process in response to CD14 activation is complex and a detailed description is beyond the scope of this chapter; however, it involves the activation of a number of protein kinases and the activation of transcription factors, such as nuclear factor κB (NF-κB) and AP-1, which initiate gene transcription. Several strategies have sought to inhibit the activation of the various protein kinases as well as direct inhibition of NF-κB. NF-κB is a redox-sensitive transcription factor, leading many to postulate that intracellular reactive oxygen species may play a role as second messenger in its activation. Therefore, antioxidants have been used as another approach to modulating the activation of NF-κB (25, 26). In considering the use of antioxidants or any other inhibitor of intracellular signal transduction, it is important to select an agent that can incorporate into the cell membrane or intracellular space rapidly and without cytotoxicity. Studies in our laboratory have demonstrated that extracellular antioxidants such as vitamin C and Trolox have no effect on the macrophage response to endotoxin, whereas membrane-incorporated vitamin E and intracellular *N*-acetyl cysteine result in significant inhibition of cytokine production. Another commonly used inhibitor of NF-κB activation is the antioxidant pyrrolidine dithiocarbamate, which can be used both *in vitro* and *in vivo* (27, 28). NF-κB activation is determined by electrophoretic mobility-shift assay or Western blotting of nuclear proteins.

Another approach to modulation of intracellular signaling involves regulation of intracellular calcium concentrations. Calcium channel blockers are used to block the influx of calcium into the cell, whereas TMB-8 or dantrolene inhibits the intracellular release of calcium from the endoplasmic reticulum. Specific inhibitors have also been developed to evaluate the role of calcium/calmodulin-dependent protein kinases (CaMK). W7 and KN-62 are inhibitors of CaMK II and IV, and autocamitide-related inhibitory peptide (AIP) is a specific inhibitor of CaMK II (29, 30). AIP inhibits CaMK II activity independent of calcium and calmodulin by binding to the substrate site for autophosphorylation (31). All these agents can alter the macrophage response to endotoxin (32, 33).

Finally, the effect of inhibition of individual mediators can be evaluated by monoclonal antibodies directed against specific cytokines such as TNF, by the use of soluble receptor antagonists such as the IL-1 receptor antagonist (IL-1ra), or by degrading agents such as platelet-activating factor acetylhydrolase (PAF-AH), which metabolizes platelet-activating factor. This approach can determine the importance of autocrine and paracrine effects of these products. Studies in our laboratory using PAF-AH, for example, have demonstrated marked inhibition of alveolar macrophage activation as measured by the decreased production of a number of inflammatory cytokines in response to endotoxin, thus elucidating the critical role of PAF as an autocrine mediator (E. M. Bulger and R. V. Maier, unpublished data).

These varied approaches allow the careful delineation of the steps involved in macrophage activation in response to a number of stimuli. Further understanding of these mechanisms will eventually guide therapeutic interventions to regulate the immuno-inflammatory response in the critically ill patient.

III. Neutrophils

Neutrophils represent over half of all circulating leukocytes, and as the primary cell involved in the innate immune response, constitute the first line of defense against infectious agents. However, these cells and the inflammatory response they coordinate act as a double-edged sword. Neutrophils have been implicated as the primary inducers of the nonspecific inflammatory response and subsequent tissue injury following trauma, shock, or sepsis (34). Their central role in the pathophysiologic processes that follow both noninfectious and infectious challenges has made neutrophil biology a source of intense study since the time of Metchnikoff (35).

Neutrophil involvement in the inflammatory response is a highly coordinated, multistage process beginning with neutrophil margination and adherence, followed by transendothelial migration, chemotaxis, microbial phagocytosis/-ingestion, and, finally, microbial killing. In the absence of invading microorganisms, the potent effector functions of the neutrophil translate into a nonspecific autodestructive inflammatory response. Methods for measuring these effector functions and their relative advantages and disadvantages are summarized in Table II. The context and rationale behind these assays are described below.

A. Source of Neutrophils for Study

Neutrophils derived from either the peripheral blood or inflammatory sites represent a principal source of cells used for studying the inflammatory response. Neutrophils are highly end-stage differentiated; their degree of differentiation precludes using immortalized cell lines. Peripheral blood neutrophils are isolated from whole blood using dextran sedimentation to remove erythrocytes followed by discontinuous density centrifuguation (36). Neutrophil purity can be assessed by examination of Wright-stained cytospin preparations or by flow cytometry, their size and granularity define a unique cell population. Purity is typically greater than 90%. It is critical to ensure that all media and glassware used for neutrophil isolation are endotoxin-free to prevent inadvertent cell activation in the isolation process. Additionally, adherence of neutrophils polystyrene may activate the cells; polypropylene tubes should be used whenever possible. These precautions should be taken for macrophage or monocyte isolation as well. Even with these precautions, some degree of neutrophil activation is inevitable. For example, increased expression of CD11b, sialyl Lewis^x antigen, IgG receptors, and shedding of L-selectin have all been documented following neutrophil isolation (37–39). Further, it appears that cooling of neutrophils to 4°C, followed by rewarming to 37°C, results in their activation, suggesting that cooling during the preparative process is unnecessary and possibly detrimental (39). These phenotypic and potentially functional alterations should be considered, particularly following *ex vivo* manipulation (e.g., labeling) of neutrophils prior to reinfusion.

Exudative or inflammatory neutrophils represent an additional source for experimental studies. Induction of an alveolar inflammatory response by intratracheal administration of inflammatory cytokines (e.g., TNF-α, IL-1β), chemokines (e.g., IL-8, PAF), or endotoxin followed by lavage of alveolar cells provides an excellent source of neutrophils. Similarly, exudative neutrophils can be obtained from patients with acute lung injury using the technique of bronchoalveolar lavage (40). Alternatively, cells can be obtained following administration of intraperitoneal thioglycollate in rodents or creation of skin blisters in humans (41). These exudative neutrophils are qualitatively different than those obtained from the peripheral blood. Rates of spontaneous apoptosis are lower (41, 42), TNF receptor and L-selectin expression are reduced (41, 43), and intracellular calcium flux, the respiratory burst, and CD11b expression are increased (43).

B. Evaluation of Neutrophil Activation

1. Neutrophil Adherence and Sequestration

The events leading to the influx of neutrophils into inflammatory sites have been well characterized using a combination of approaches, including *in vitro* systems in which conditions of flow are simulated *in vivo* using intravital microscopy (see Chapter 73). The process in its entirety has been referred to as the adhesion cascade, because the individual events appear to be relatively constant and follow a consistent defined sequence, similar in concept to the coagulation cascade (44). This cascade has three stages: (1) neutrophil rolling, (2) neutrophil activation and firm adhesion, and (3) transendothelial migration. These events and the neutrophil and endothelial ligands important for their expression are depicted schematically in Fig. 2. *In vivo*, the relative contributions of these adhesion molecules and their ligands to leukosequestration are evaluated using a variety of methodologies. The most popular of these approaches involves the intravenous administration of antibodies (45–55) or excess ligand (56, 57) prior to or following the induction of the inflammatory cascade to antagonize receptor–ligand interactions competitively at the cellular level. This approach is not without problems; nonspecific binding of the administered antibodies may preclude any assessment of their effectiveness. Animals administered isotypic control antibodies are necessary to assure that any effects are attributable to the antagonism of receptor–ligand interactions.

Targeted deletion of genes encoding adhesion molecules using site-directed mutagenesis might also provide insight into the role of specific receptor–ligand interactions in leukosequestration. Specifically, mice deficient in ICAM-1, selectins, and β_2-integrins have provided valuable data on the importance of these molecules in a variety of inflammatory models (58–61). However, data derived from these models must be interpreted with caution. These animals frequently adapt to the loss of one component of the adhesion cascade by the overexpression of other components (62). For example, mice deficient in ICAM-1 may overexpress ICAM-2 or alternative exons for ICAM-1 and thus may have undetectable, albeit functional, ICAM expression (63).

Table II Methods of Evaluating Neutrophil Activation

Method	Advantages	Disadvantages
Neutrophil adhesion/role of adhesion molecules		
In vivo		
Intravital microscopy	Provides real-time *in vivo* data on effects of an intervention on the adhesion cascade	Technology may not be applicable to all tissues/organs; not readily accessible to most
Administration of blocking antibodies	Relatively simple; approach can be applied to a wide variety of animal models	Antibody specificity may be problematic; requires use of isotypic control antibodies
Site-directed mutagenesis	Often provides great insight into role of neutrophil/endothelial adhesion molecule in inflammatory process; convenient	Mutant strain may not be available for molecule of interest; limited to murine models; animals are not representative of wild type and may have compensatory increases in other adhesion molecules
In vitro		
Adhesion assays (static)	Relatively simple; quantitative; slight adaptation may allow for assessment of transendothelial migration	Absence of flow does not simulate *in vivo* conditions; neutrophil isolation may result in their activation, limiting the ability to extrapolate to *in vivo* conditions
Flow cytometry	Provides data on both overall expression in a population of cells and magnitude of expression per cell; relatively quick with high sensitivity and high specificity; ability to use whole blood obviates need for neutrophil isolation; sensitive and specific	Antibodies may not recognize conformational changes in neutrophil adhesion molecules that may have functional significance (e.g., CD11b/CD18)
Neutrophil deformability/shape change		
Confocal microscopy	Demonstrates (focal/nonfocal) changes in actin polymerization/depolymerization	Actin polymerization/depolymerization may not universally correlate with changes in neutrophil deformability
Neutrophil chemotaxis		
Dual chamber separated by a polycarbonate membrane	Relatively simple and readily available	Cell clumping may lower estimates of chemotactic rates; may also measure adhesion rather than isolated chemotaxis
Leading front	Relatively simple and readily available; measures chemotaxis in isolation; may provide more consistent results	Slightly more difficult to set up than dual-chamber method
Phagocytosis		
Flow cytometry	Provides data on proportion of cells in a population undergoing phagocytoses and quantitates the quantity of phagocytosed particle per cell	Requires quenching to exclude enumeration of extracellular and membrane-associated particles
Microbial killing		
In vivo		
Enumeration of viable organisms in infected tissue	Relatively simple; clinically relevant index of microbial killing	Gross measure; results are sum of neutrophil and nonneutrophil killing
In vitro		
Enumeration of viable organisms in infected tissue	Relatively simple; provides an objective measure of neutrophil killing	Neutrophil/microbe relationship (both quantitative and qualitative)not representative of *in vivo* conditions
Oxidative		
SOD[a]-inhibitable reduction of cytochrome *c*	Simple; relatively specific for superoxide production	Requires neutrophil isolation with potential for inadvertent priming during the process
Chemiluminescence	Provides data on kinetics and magnitude of the response; assay may be adapted to measure different reactive oxygen species; can be performed on whole blood	Luminometer may not be readily available
Flow cytometry	May be performed on whole blood; provides data on both the proportion of cells undergoing a respiratory burst and the magnitude of the response per cell	Kinetics not as easily assessable as with chemiluminescence
Nonoxidative (proteases)		
Immunoassays	Sensitive, specific; convenient	May not correlate with functional protease activity due to presence of inhibitors
Functional assays	Provides good estimate of functional protease activity	Tends to be more cumbersome; may require use of radioactive isotopes or electrophoresis (zymography), depending on the protease of interest

[a]Superoxide dismutase.

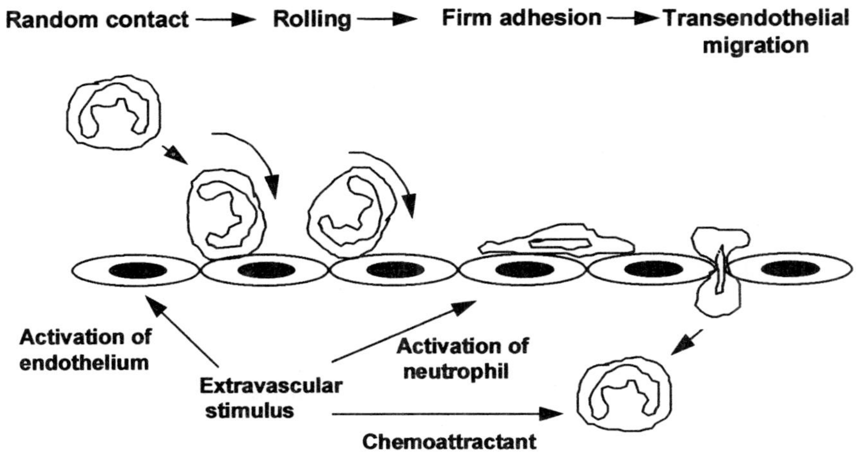

Neutrophil	**-Sialyl Lewis^x & other sialylated, fucosylated structures** **-PSGL-1** **-L-selectin**	**-β_2-integrins**	**-PECAM-1** **- β_2-integrins**
Endothelium	**-P-selectin** **-E-selectin** **-CD34** **-MAdCAM-1**	**-ICAM-1** **-ICAM-2**	**-PECAM-1** **-ICAM-1**

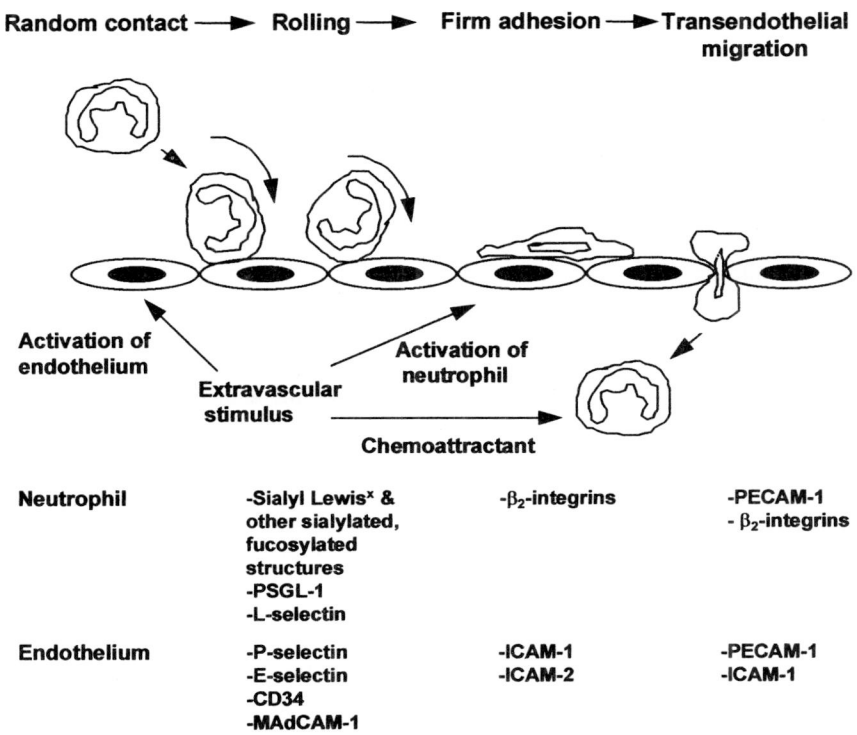

Figure 2 Adhesive interactions leading to neutrophil emigration as identified using intravital microscopy, and the neutrophil and endothelial ligands important for these events.

Alternatively, overexpression of L-selection and/or endothelial ligands for selections may result following deletion of the P- or E-selectin gene.

In vitro adhesion assays may provide more precise assessment of events at the molecular level compared to *in vivo* studies. At a minimum, these systems allow manipulation of the local microenvironment between neutrophils and endothelial cells (64). Endothelial cells derived from a variety of sources, including human umbilical vein (HUVEC), porcine aortic endothelium, and rat heart, have all been used for this purpose (65–67). Cells are plated to confluence and radiolabeled neutrophils are placed atop the endothelial monolayers. After incubation, the nonadherent cells are gently washed off the monolayers and those remaining are quantitated using a scintillation counter (68, 69). If endothelial transmigration is the parameter of interest, then endothelial cells plated atop a microporous polycarbonate filter should be used and quantitation of cells below the filter may be accomplished (70).

Neutrophil expression of adhesion molecules is most commonly evaluated using flow cytometry (71). Almost invariably, increased expression correlates with functional increases in cellular adhesive properties. However, the process of affinity modulation, whereby cell activation induces alterations in conformation of the β_2-integrins, leading to a marked increase in the avidity of the receptor for its endothelial ligand, may account for increased adhesive properties in the absence of increased membrane expression (72–74). Increases in receptor avidity peak within 5 to 10 min of stimulation and decreases peak within 30 min. This process may be initiated by one of two mechanisms—either via activation of the neutrophil by chemokines, endotoxin, or inflammatory cytokines or by cross-linking of L-selectin or the E- and P-selectin ligands. Detection of these conformational changes requires antibodies specific for the different epitopes available for binding in the quiescent and activated conformations.

An alternative means of leukosequestration may be due to alterations in neutrophil deformability. The circulating neutrophil has a mean diameter of approximately 8 μm (75), whereas the average systemic capillary diameter (6.5 μm) or pulmonary capillary (5.5 μm) is significantly smaller. The disparity between the sizes of circulating neutrophils and the capillaries (particularly in the pulmonary circulation) mandates that leukocytes deform during transit through the microvascular bed. The viscoelastic properties of the neutrophil are governed by organizational changes within the actin cytoskeleton (76). Rapid conversion of G-actin to F-actin (polymerization) and/or F-actin to G-actin (depolymerization) in response to several soluble factors permits the neutrophil to reorganize its cytoskeleton rapidly and reversibly, leading to decreases and increases in deformability, respectively (77). The use of confocal microscopy to image this process following labeling of cells using rhodamine phalloidin, an immunostain that binds F-actin, has proved to be useful in evaluating this process (78). Several methods have been used to evaluate cell deformability, including the use of a cell "poker" to assess the degree to which a single cell resists indentation (79), passage of cells through cotton wool or a polycarbonate filter with varying pore sizes (79), or the use of a commercially available cell transit analyzer (CTA) (80). The CTA consists of two fluid reservoirs separated by a thin polycarbonate membrane containing pores of known size. As each cell passes through a pore, it produces a transient change in the electrical resistance of the filter. The apparatus is coupled to a conductimeter and a laboratory computer so that the duration of the change in resistance is calculated. The end result is pore transit time, with an increased transit time reflecting increased neutrophil rigidity. Further support for polymerization of actin in this process can be obtained by prior treatment of cells with cytochalasin D, an agent that prevents actin polymerization (76).

2. Chemotaxis

Chemotaxis, or directional movement of the cell along a concentration gradient, represents another mechanism by which neutrophils reach the site of inflammation or infection. Popular cell migration assays typically measure the net migration of a cell population from an upper chamber across a microporous membrane, to a lower chamber filled with a chemoattractant. Cell migration through the membrane may be quantified by radiolabeling or staining the cells and measuring binding to the lower side of the membrane by scintillation counting or light microscopy, respectively (81). The resulting data are often presented as the proportion of the total number of cells that have traversed the membrane. One limitation of this technique is that artifacts such as cell–cell adhesion atop the filter could give the impression of reduced migration. An alternative measure of chemotaxis is calculation of the leading front (82, 83). This parameter is estimated by fixation of the membrane and measurement of the distance between the starting surface and the point at which at least two cells are found. The latter approach is thought to be susceptible to less variability, although often both parameters are presented. Finally, others have suggested that these assays do not adequately differentiate chemotaxis from chemokinesis, the nondirectional, random movement of cells in response to a stimulus. Using a rather complex mathematical model, Tranquillo *et al.* (84) have described a method for differentiating the two processes using a methodology based on an under-agarose migration assay wherein neutrophils migrate through an agarose gel in response to a chemoattractant. Popular chemoattractants for these studies include *n*-formyl-methionyl-leucyl-phenylalanine (fMLP), leukotriene B4, platelet-activating factor, or interleukin-8. fMLP is used to incite an *in vitro* neutrophil response similar to that seen with microorganisms *in vivo*.

3. Phagocytosis

Invading microorganisms do not undergo phagocytosis until they are opsonized, i.e., coated with antibody, complement, or both. Among other effects, opsonization of bacteria serves to create a binding site for the neutrophil. Neutrophil membranes have receptors for the Fc portion of IgG and the C3b complement component. Activation of the neutrophil by chemotactic factors and bacterial products up-regulates many of the cell surface proteins. The opsonized bacteria bind via these membrane receptors, thus initiating the process of phagocytosis. This process results in the uptake of the organism into a phagosome and eventual microbial death. Traditional methods used to evaluate phagocytosis were based on counting of ingested particles. These methods were limited in that it was often only possible to detect phagocytosed particles when ingested in large quantities. Further, differentiating between ingested and membrane-associated particles is often quite difficult. The preferred methods for evaluating phagocytosis currently rest with the use of flow cytometry (71). Physiologic targets (e.g., bacteria, *Candida albicans*, or zymosan) or latex beads may be used after opsonization and conjugation with a fluorochrome or propidium iodide. Flow cytometric evaluation provides an estimate of both the proportions of cells with intracellular fluorescence and the amount of ingested particles per cell. Quenching, performed with trypan blue or other dyes, is a critical step in flow cytometric evaluation of phagocytosis because it allows the exclusion of the fluorescence emitted by extracellular and membrane-associated (noninternalized) targets (71, 85).

4. Microbial Killing

As the first cellular defense mechanism against potential pathogens, the neutrophil's primary role is to ensure prompt killing of the invading microorganism. *In vivo*, microbial killing requires granulocyte localization to the site of invasion, binding of the organism to the neutrophil, internalization of the organism into the phagosome, and ultimately some combination of oxidative and nonoxidative killing (Fig. 3). *In vitro*, any assessment of microbicidal activity is simply a summary measure of all processes beyond granulocyte localization. Evaluation of microbial killing is relatively straightforward. A predetermined number of live organisms is incubated with cells in a balanced salt solution in the presence of serum as a source of opsonins. At varying time intervals, aliquots of the solution are serially diluted and plated on agar to quantitate the number of viable organisms (40). A similar approach is utilized for *in vivo* assessment of

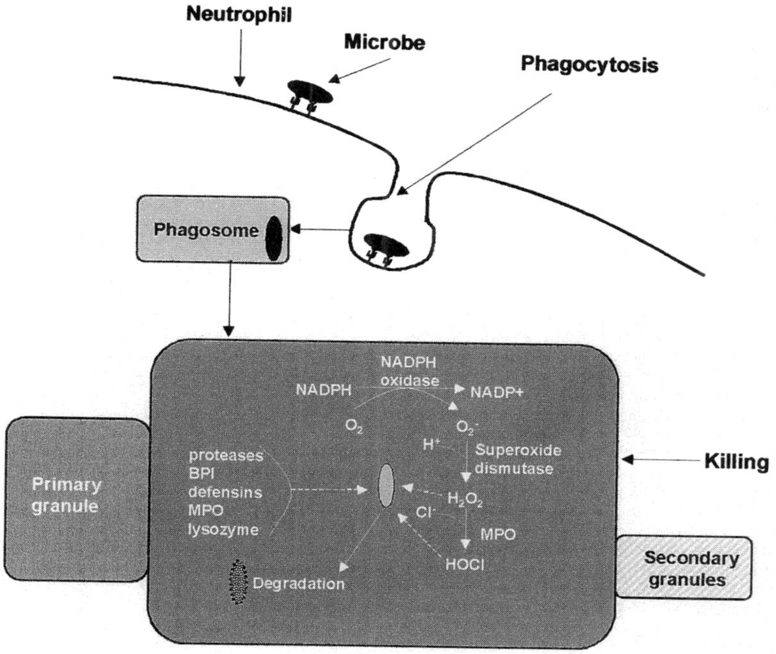

Figure 3 Oxidative and nonoxidative mechanisms of microbial killing.

microbial killing; homogenates of the infected tissue are serially diluted and plated as above (86).

5. Oxidative Killing and Assessment of the Neutrophil Respiratory Burst

Once localized to the inflammatory site, the neutrophil exerts its effector functions through both oxidative and nonoxidative processes. Although neutrophils produce and release a variety of toxic agents directed toward microbial killing, those systems that depend on reactive oxygen species are especially potent. Products of oxidative metabolism have also been incriminated in the development of local tissue injury in the absence of infectious stimuli following trauma, shock, or reperfusion injury. These agents are produced as a consequence of the respiratory burst, a series of events triggered by phagocytosis or exposure to certain inflammatory mediators and featuring a marked increase in oxidative metabolism with direct conversion of molecular oxygen to its univalent reduction product, the superoxide anion. The enzyme directly responsible for this respiratory burst functions as an NADPH oxidase, transferring electrons from cytosolic NADPH across the plasma membrane or phagosome, to oxygen.

Initially, superoxide is formed through the reduction of molecular oxygen by single electrons that originate from NADPH generated via the pentose phosphate pathway. This process is catalyzed by the combined action of a plasma membrane NADPH oxidase and cytochrome b_{558}. Two cytosolic proteins (p47^{phox}, p67^{phox}), a quinone, and a rac-related GTP-binding protein are the other functional components of this electron transport system. The NADPH oxidase system is dissociated and thus inactive in unstimulated neutrophils. Although some components are membrane bound, others are stored in the cytosolic granules (Fig. 3). On activation, the cytosolic components translocate to the plasma membrane to assemble the active oxidase, leading to the production of superoxide. Subsequent reactions lead to the formation of other reactive species, including hydrogen peroxide (H_2O_2), catalyzed by the enzyme superoxide dismutase (SOD) (87), and the superoxide-driven Fenton reaction between H_2O_2 and an appropriate transition metal catalyst (e.g., iron) to form the hydroxyl radical (·OH) (88). Finally, H_2O_2 may be metabolized by a reaction catalyzed by myeloperoxidase, a peroxidase found in abundant quantities within the primary granule of the neutrophil. In the presence of a halide, a hypohalous acid is formed, of which hypochlorous acid (HOCl) is the most common (87). HOCl is generally considered the most bactericidal oxidant produced by the neutrophil.

Induction of the respiratory burst may be induced pharmacologically through activation of protein kinase C using phorbol esters. Alternatively, high concentrations of fMLP, PAF, C5a, and IL-8 may activate the oxidase complex. At lower concentrations, these agents simply prime the system for subsequent activation, presumably through activation of several protein kinases (89–93). Additionally, the process of adhesion to either endothelium or extracellular matrix proteins or simply cross-linking CD11b/CD18, L-selectin, or sialyl Lewis^x moieties may induce a similar priming effect (94–98).

Quantitation of the neutrophil respiratory burst may be achieved using one of several methods. Superoxide anion production is determined by measuring the SOD-inhibitable reduction of cytochrome *c* using a spectrophotometer (99). In this assay, neutrophils are incubated with cytochrome *c* in the presence or absence of superoxide dismutase. Reduction of cytochrome *c* in the presence of SOD is subtracted from the values without SOD to provide an estimate of the rate of superoxide production. Results are typically expressed in nanomoles per minute per million neutrophils.

An alternative means of assessing the neutrophil oxidative burst is the use of chemiluminescence. Chemiluminescence results when electrons from reactive oxygen species revert to their ground state and release a small amount of light energy. This emitted light can be detected using a fluorometer if the sensitivity of the assay is increased sufficiently by a luminigenic probe (e.g., luminol-5-amino-2,3-dihydro-1,4-phthalazinedione). The precise oxidative metabolites (e.g., H_2O_2, HOCl, $O_2^{-}\cdot$) being evaluated are dictated to some extent by the assay conditions and choice of luminigenic probe (100). The advantages of this assay are twofold. First, it is relatively simple and can be performed on whole blood, mitigating the need for neutrophil isolation. Second, if the production of oxidative metabolites is followed for long enough, this technique can provide some assessment of the kinetics of the respiratory burst (Fig. 4).

Finally, flow cytometric assays have become accepted means of assessing production of neutrophil-derived oxidants. Neutrophils can be stained with dihydrorhodamine 123 (DHR). DHR is converted to rhodamine 123, which generates fluorescent light when excited by 488-nm radiation in the presence of reactive oxygen species. Another fluorescent probe, dichlorofluorescein (DCF) diacetate, can enter cells and is trapped intracellularly (by deacylation) in a nonfluorescent reduced form (DCFH). During oxidation by products of neutrophil oxidative metabolism, the probe is converted to a fluorescent molecule that can be detected in a flow cytometer (DCF) (36, 101). Like the chemiluminescent technique described above, these assays can be performed using whole blood (102).

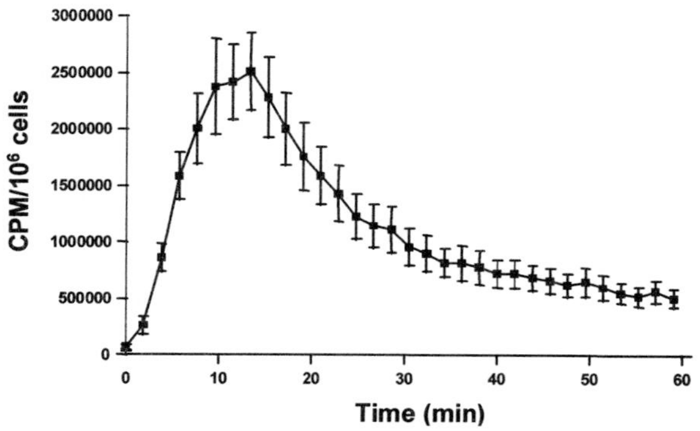

Figure 4 Rat peripheral blood neutrophil chemiluminescence as determined by phorbol ester stimulation of whole blood in the presence of the chemiluminigenic probe, luminol. Chemiluminescence was measured every 60 sec for a period of 60 min following addition of phorbol myristate acetate (12.5 μ*M*).

6. Nonoxidative Killing

Neutrophil nonoxidative killing occurs through the process of degranulation. This process, although important in microbial killing, also causes significant local tissue injury when granule contents are released into the extracellular milieu. Degranulation may be induced *in vitro* by pretreating neutrophils in suspension with cytochalasin B, followed by a variety of neutrophil-activating agents, including PAF, LTB4, and IL-8, or by means of cross-linking the Fc receptor or Cd11b/CD18. Intracellular calcium levels, protein kinase C (PKC) activation, and G-proteins all modulate the processes leading to degranulation, because pertussis toxin, an inhibitor of G-proteins, prevents degranulation (103) and calcium ionophores (104) or phorbol myristate acetate (105), an activator of PKC, induce degranulation.

Three major types of neutrophil granules have been described: primary (azurophilic), secondary, and tertiary (106, 107). Primary granules, identified by their high content of myeloperoxidase, also contain a number of cationic proteins, including lysozyme, bactericidal/permeability-increasing protein (BPI), and defensins, as well as the potent serine protease elastase. The secondary granule, defined by its high content of lactoferrin, also contains cytochrome b_{558} and a FAD flavoprotein important in the respiratory burst, as well as collagenase, a metalloproteinase (107). Lactoferrin, a 80-kDa glycoprotein iron-binding protein, has bactericidal and bacteriostatic effects, presumably by rendering iron inaccessible to bacteria.

Additionally, by scavenging intracellular iron, lactoferrin may also inhibit the formation of the iron-dependent hydoxyl radical. Secondary granules may also be involved in the process of cell adhesion, motility, and cell activation, as their plasma membranes possess receptors for the chemoattractants C5a and fMLP. Gelatinase defines the tertiary granule. Like collagenase, gelatinase is a metalloproteinase. Both are secreted in a latent, inactive form and are activated by chlorinated oxidants such as hypochlorous acid (106). This cross-talk between nonoxidative and oxidative microbicidal pathways may play a significant role in potentiating neutrophil-induced tissue injury. Together, the proteinases elastase, collagenase, and gelatinase may be important effectors of nonoxidative tissue injury by degrading basement membranes and extracellular matrix.

The assessment of protease release may be accomplished using one of two different approaches. Functional assays evaluate enzyme activity and thus provide a reasonable estimate of the potential for tissue injury induced by cell activation. For example, collagenase activity may be assessed by measuring the release of radiolabeled fragments from ^{14}C-labeled type 1 collagen (108) whereas gelatinase activity has been assessed using zymography (109). Elastase activity is frequently measured in an assay using the chromogenic substrate *N*-methoxy-succinyl-Ala-Pro-val *p*-nitroanilide (MEOSAAPVPNA) (110). The alternative approach uses a variety of different immunoassays. These assays may overestimate the quantity of functional enzyme due to binding of proteases with their natural inhibitors, e.g., elastase and α1-antitrypsin (111). Not infrequently, both approaches are used to provide an estimate of both immunoreactive and functional protease expression.

The evaluation of azurophilic (primary) granule exocytosis is typically performed by measuring myeloperoxidase (MPO) activity. This colorimetric assay is based on the oxidation of tetramethylbenzidine in the presence of H_2O_2 (112, 113). With modification, this assay may also be used to objectively quantitate tissue neutrophil content (114).

IV. T Helper Cells

It has been recognized that T helper (Th) cells can be divided into two functional subsets based on the cytokine pattern they produce. These are referred to as Th1 and TH2. The Th1 cells produce predominantly interferon-γ (IFN-γ) and interleukin-2, resulting in stimulation of cellular immunity and enhanced production of opsonizing antibodies. The Th2 clone, on the other hand, down-regulates cellular immunity and augments the production of nonopsonizing antibodies, including IgG_1 and IgE, by the production of interleukins 4, 5, 6, and 10 (Fig. 5). Studies in animal models of burn injury and hemorrhagic shock have demonstrated a shift to a dominant Th2 phenotype in the postinjury period (115, 116). In addition, analysis of cytokine production by the peripheral blood mononuclear cells of burn and trauma patients has also demonstrated increased IL-4 production and decreased IFN-γ production when compared to healthy controls (117). It has been proposed that this shift in favor of the TH2 phenotype explains the immunocompromise seen in these patients following severe stress.

The mechanisms used to study these two T cell phenotypes has involved analysis of the cytokine pattern produced in response to a stimulus such as phytohemagglutinin or concanavalin A. In animal models, lymphocytes are harvested from lymph nodes or spleen and $CD4^+$ T cells isolated by the antibody-mediated lysis of $CD8^+$ cells. Cytokine levels are measured by ELISA and standard proliferation assays performed based on uptake of tritiated thymidine (115). Human studies have involved isolation of peripheral blood mononuclear cells from whole blood, which contains both mononuclear cells and lymphocytes. This fraction is then stimulated *in vitro* and cytokine production is compared between patients and normal controls (117). This approach is cumbersome because it requires several cell culture conditions and the measurement of a number of different cytokines to establish the profile. The identification of a specific cell surface marker to distinguish between Th1 and Th2 cells, or the ability to stain for these cytokines intracellularly, would greatly facilitate the study of these cells because it would allow for sorting via flow cytometry. These techniques are currently under study and several potential surface makers have been evaluated, including CD7, CD27, and CD30 (118). Further studies are needed, however, to establish clearly the markers to define these cell populations.

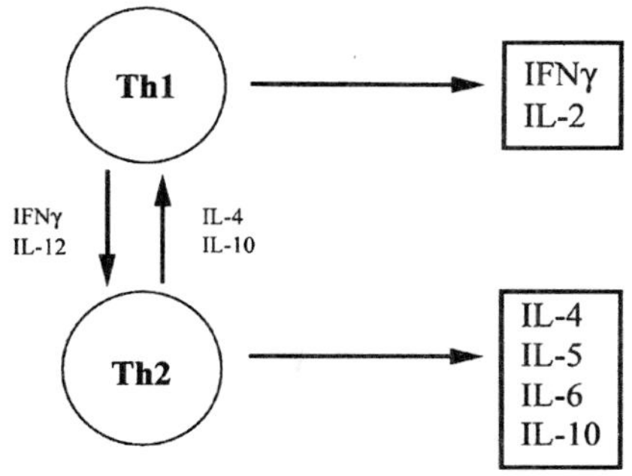

Figure 5 Cytokine profile of Th1 vs. Th2 cells. A regulatory cytokine can shift the phenotype in favor of a given cytokine profile. Interferon-γ (IFN-γ) and IL-12 shift toward the Th2 phenotype, whereas IL-4 and IL-10 shift toward the Th1 phenotype.

References

1. Maier, R. V. The angry macrophage and its impact on host response mechanisms. In: Faist E., Meakins, J., Schildberg F. W., editors. Host Defense Dysfunction in Trauma, Shock, and Sepsis. Heidelberg, Germany: Springer-Verlag, 1993: 191–197.
2. Testa, U., Ferbus, D., Gabbianelli, M., Pascucci, B., Boccoli, G., Louache, F., *et al.* (1988). Effect of endogenous and exogenous interferons on the differentiation of human monocyte cell line U937. *Cancer Res.* **48**(1), 82–88.
3. Tobias, P. S., Soldau, K., Kline, L., Lee, J. D., Kato, K., Martin, T. P., *et al.* (1993). Cross-linking of lipopolysaccharide (LPS) to CD14 on THP-1 cells mediated by LPS-binding protein. *J. Immunol.* **150**(7), 3011–3021.
4. Vey, E., Zhang, J. H., and Dayer, J. M. (1992). IFN-gamma and $1,25(OH)_2D3$ induce on THP-1 cells distinct patterns of cell surface

antigen expression, cytokine production, and responsiveness to contact with activated T cells. *J. Immunol.* **149**(6), 2040–2046.
5. Mbawuike, I. N., and Herscowitz, H. B. (1989). MH-S, a murine alveolar macrophage cell line: Morphological, cytochemical, and functional characteristics. *J. Leukoc. Biol.* **46**(2), 119–127.
6. Rosengart, M., Arbabi, S., Garcia, I., and Maier, R. (1999). Adherence potentiates monocyte lipopolysaccharide-induced tumor necrosis factor-alpha production: A process dependent on Pyk2. *Surg. Forum* **50,** 275–278.
7. Bauer, G. J., Garcia, I., Arbabi, S., and Maier, R. V. (1998). Adherence couples lipopolysaccharide membrane binding to macrophage signal transduction. *Surg. Forum* **49,** 109–110.
8. Bernardo, J., Billingslea, A. M., Ortiz, M. F., Seetoo, K. F., Macauley, J., and Simons, E. R. Adherence-dependent calcium signaling in monocytes: Induction of a CD14-high phenotype, stimulus-responsive subpopulation. *J. Immunol. Methods* **209**(2), 165–175.
9. Othmer, M., and Zepp, F. (1992). Flow cytometric immunophenotyping: Principles and pitfalls. *Eur. J. Pediatr.* **151**(6), 398–406.
10. Maier, R. V., and Hahnel, G. B. (1984). Microthrombosis during endotoxemia: Potential role of hepatic versus alveolar macrophages. *J. Surg. Res.* **36,** 362–370.
11. Knook, D. L., Blansjaar, N., and Sleyster, E. C. (1977). Isolation and characterization of Kupffer and endothelial cells from the rat liver. *Exp. Cell. Res.* **109**(2), 317–329.
12. ten Hagen, T. L., van Vianen, W., and Bakker-Woudenberg, I. A. (1996). Isolation and characterization of murine Kupffer cells and splenic macrophages. *J. Immunol. Methods* **193**(1), 81–91.
13. Maier, R. V., Hahnel, G. B., and Fletcher, R. (1992). Platelet-activating factor augments tumor necrosis factor and procoagulant activity. *J. Surg. Res.* **52,** 258–264.
14. Haas, J., Baeuerle, P., Riethmuller, G., and Ziegler-Heitbrock, H. (1990). Molecular mechanisms in down-regulation of tumor necrosis factor expression. *Proc. Natl. Acad. Sci.* **87,** 9563–9567.
15. Li, M. H., Seatter, S. C., Manthei, R., Bubrick, M., and West, M. A. (1994). Macrophage endotoxin tolerance: Effect of TNF or endotoxin pretreatment. *J. Surg. Res.* **57**(1), 85–92.
16. Espevik, T., and Nissen-Meyer, J. (1986). A highly sensitive cell line, WEHI 164 clone 13, for measuring cytotoxic factor/tumor necrosis factor from human monocytes. *J. Immunol. Methods* **95**(1), 99–105.
17. Whiteside, T. L. (1994). Cytokine measurements and interpretation of cytokine assays in human disease. *J. Clin. Immunol.* **14**(6), 327–339.
18. Cannon, J. G., van der Meer, J. W., Kwiatkowski, D., Endres, S., Lonnemann, G., Burke, J. F., *et al.* (1988). Interleukin-1 beta in human plasma: optimization of blood collection, plasma extraction, and radioimmunoassay methods. *Lymphokine Res.* **7**(4), 457–467.
19. Lewis, C. E., McCracken, D., Ling, R., Richards, P. S., McCarthy, S. P., and McGee, J. O. (1991). Cytokine release by single, immunophenotyped human cells: Use of the reverse hemolytic plaque assay. *Immunol. Rev.* **119,** 23–39.
20. O'Garra, A., and Vieira, P. (1992). Polymerase chain reaction for detection of cytokine gene expression. *Curr. Opin. Immunol.* **4**(2), 211–215.
21. Suprenant, Y., and Zuckerman, S. (1989). A novel microtiter plate assay for the quantitation of procoagulant activity on adherent monocytes, macrophage, and endothelial cells. *Thromb. Res.* **53,** 339–346.
22. Langermans, J. A., Hazenbos, W. L., and Van Furth, R. (1994). Antimicrobial functions of mononuclear phagocytes. *J. Immunol. Methods* **174**(1–2), 185–194.
23. Jenkins, M. K., and Schwartz, R. H. (1987). Antigen presentation by chemically modified splenocytes induces antigen-specific T cell unresponsiveness *in vitro* and *in vivo. J. Exp. Med.* **165**(2), 302–319.
24. Yano, A., Schwartz, R. H., and Paul, W. E. (1978). Antigen presentation in the murine T lymphocyte proliferative response. II. Ir-GAT-controlled T lymphocyte responses require antigen-presenting cells from a high responder donor. *Eur. J. Immunol.* **8**(5), 344–347.
25. Bulger, E. M., Garcia, I., and Maier, R. V. (1996). The differential effects of the membrane antioxidant, vitamin E on macrophage activation. *Surg. Forum* **47,** 92–95.
26. Mendez, C., Garcia, I., and Maier, R. V. (1995). Antioxidants attenuate endotoxin induced activation of alveolar macrophages. *Surgery* **118,** 412–420.
27. Bulger, E. M., Garcia, I., and Maier, R. V. (1998). Dithiocarbamates enhance tumor necrosis factor-alpha production by rabbit alveolar macrophages, despite inhibition of NF-kappaB. *Shock* **9**(6), 397–405.
28. Kovacich, J. C., Boyle, E. M., Jr., Morgan, E. N., Canty, T. G., Jr., Farr, A. L., Caps, M. T., *et al.* (1999). Inhibition of the transcriptional activator protein nuclear factor kappaB prevents hemodynamic instability associated with the whole-body inflammatory response syndrome. *J. Thorac. Cardiovasc. Surg.* **118**(1), 154–162.
29. Enslen, H., and Soderling, T. R. (1994). Roles of calmodulin-dependent protein kinases and phosphatase in calcium-dependent transcription of immediate early genes. *J. Biol. Chem.* **269**(33), 20872–20877.
30. Minami, H., Inoue, S., and Hidaka, H. (1994). The effect of KN-62, $Ca2^{+}$/calmodulin dependent protein kinase II inhibitor on cell cycle. *Biochem. Biophys. Res. Commun.* **199**(1), 241–248.
31. Ishida, A., Kameshita, I., Okuno, S., Kitani, T., and Fujisawa, H. (1995). A novel highly specific and potent inhibitor of calmodulin-dependent protein kinase II. *Biochem. Biophys. Res. Commun.* **212**(3), 806–812.
32. Hotchkiss, R. S., Bowling, W. M., Karl, I. E., Osborne, D. F., and Flye, M. W. (1997). Calcium antagonists inhibit oxidative burst and nitrite formation in lipopolysaccharide-stimulated rat peritoneal macrophages. *Shock* **8**(3), 170–178.
33. West, M. A., Clair, L., and Bellingham, J. (1996). Role of calcium in lipopolysaccharide-stimulated tumor necrosis factor and interleukin-1 signal transduction in naive and endotoxin-tolerant murine macrophages. *J. Trauma* **41**(4), 647–652.
34. Smith, J. A. (1994). Neutrophils, host defense and inflammation: A double-edged sword. *J. Leukoc. Biol.* **56,** 672–686.
35. Palmblad, J. (1984). The role of granulocytes in inflammation. *Scand. J. Rheumatol.* **13,** 163–172.
36. Bass, D. A., Parce, J. W., DeChatelet, L. R., Szejda, P., Seeds, P., Seeds, M. C., *et al.* (1983). Flow cytometric studies of oxidative product formation by neutrophils: A graded response to membrane stimulation. *J. Immunol.* **130,** 1910–1917.
37. Youssef, P. P., Mantzioris, B. X., Roberts-Thomson, P. J., Ahern, M. J., and Smith, M. D. (1995). Effects of *ex vivo* manipulation on the expression of cell adhesion molecules on neutrophils. *J. Immunol. Methods* **186,** 217–224.
38. Macey, M. G., Jiang, X. P., Veys, P., McCarthy, D., and Newland, A. C. (1992). Expression of functional antigens on neutrophils. Effects of preparation. *J. Immunol. Methods* **149,** 37–42.
39. Forsyth, K. D., and Levinsky, R. J. (1990). Preparative procedures of cooling and re-warming increase leukocyte integrin expression and function on neutrophils. *J. Immunol. Methods* **128,** 159–163.
40. Martin, T. R., Pistorese, B. P., Hudson, L. D., and Maunder, R. J. (1991). The function of lung and blood neutrophils in patients with the adult respiratory distress syndrome: Implications for the pathogenesis of lung infections. *Am. Rev. Respir. Dis.* **144,** 254–262.
41. Seely, A. J., Swartz, D. E., Giannias, B., and Christou, N. V. (1998). Reduction in neutrophil cell surface expression of tumor necrosis factor receptors but not Fas after transmigration: Implications for the regulation of neutrophil apoptosis. *Arch. Surg.* **133**(12), 1305–1310.
42. Watson, R. W. G., Rotstein, O. D., Nathens, A. B., Parodo, J., and Marshall, J. C. (1997). Neutrophil apoptosis is modulated by endothelial transmigration and adhesion molecule engagement. *J. Immunol.* **158,** 945–953.
43. Ahmed, N. A., McGill, S., Yee, J., Hu, F., Michel, R. P., and Christou, N. V. (1999). Mechanisms for the diminished neutrophil exudation to

secondary inflammatory sites in infected patients with a systemic inflammatory response (sepsis). *Crit. Care Med.* **27**(11), 2459–2468.
44. Carlos, T. M., and Harlan, J. M. (1994). Leukocyte-endothelial adhesion molecules. *Blood* **84,** 2068–2101.
45. Doerschuk, C. M., Winn, R. K., Coxson, H. O., and Harlan, J. M. (1990). CD18-dependent and independent mechanisms of neutrophil emigration in the pulmonary and systemic microcirculation of rabbits. *J. Immunol.* **144,** 2327.
46. Harlan, J. M., Winn, R. K., Vedder, N. B., Doerschuk, C. M., and Rice, C. L. (1992). *In vivo* models of leukocyte adherence to endothelium. *In* "Adhesion: Its Role in Inflammatory Disease" (J.M., Harlan and D.Y., Liu, eds.), pp. 117–150. Freeman and Company, New York.
47. Mileski, W. J., Winn, R. K., Vedder, N. B., Pohlman, T. H., Harlan, J. M., and Rice, C. L. (1990). Inhibition of CD18-dependent neutrophil adherence reduces organ injury after hemorrhagic shock in primates. *Surgery* **108,** 206–212.
48. Mulligan, M. S., Polley, M. J., Bayer, R. J., Nunn, M. F., Paulson, J. C., and Ward, P. A. (1992). Neutrophil-dependent acute lung injury: Requirement for P-selectin (GMP-140). *J. Clin. Invest.* **90,** 1600–1607.
49. Mulligan, M. S., Varani, J., Dame, M. K., Lane, C. L., Smith, C. W., Anderson, D. C., *et al.* (1991). Role of endothelial-leukocyte adhesion molecule 1 (ELAM-1) in neutrophil mediated lung injury in rats. *J. Clin. Invest.* **88,** 1396.
50. Mulligan, M. S., Smith, C. W., Anderson, D. C., Todd, R. F., Miyasaka, M., Tamatani, T., *et al.* (1993). Role of leukocyte adhesion molecules in complement-induced lung injury. *J. Immunol.* **150,** 2401–2406.
51. Ramamoorthy, C., Sharar, S. R., Harlan, J. M., Tedder, T. F., and Winn, R. K. (1996). Blocking L-selectin function attenuates reperfusion injury following hemorrhagic shock in rabbits. *Am. J. Physiol.* **271,** H1871–H1877.
52. Seekamp, A., Mulligan, M. S., Till, G. O., Smith, C. W., Miyasaka, M., Tamatani, T., *et al.* (1993). Role of beta-2 integrins and ICAM-1 in lung injury following ischemia reperfusion of rat hind limbs. *Am. J. Pathol.* **143,** 464–472.
53. Talbott, G. A., Sharar, S. R., Harlan, J. M., and Winn, R. K. (1994). Leukocyte-endothelial interactions and organ injury: The role of adhesion molecules. *New Horiz.* **2,** 545–554.
54. Winn, R. K., Paulson, J. C., and Harlan, J. M. (1994). A monoclonal antibody to P-selectin ameliorates injury associated with hemorrhagic shock in rabbits. *Am. J. Physiol.* **267,** H2391–H2397.
55. Winn, R. K., Ramamoorthy, C., Vedder, N. B., Sharar, S. R., and Harlan, J. M. (1997). Leukocyte–endothelial cell interactions in ischemia-reperfusion injury. *Ann. N.Y. Acad. Sci.* **832,** 311–321.
56. Mulligan, M. S., Lowe, J. B., Larsen, R. D., Paulson, J., Zheng, Z., DeFrees, S., *et al.* (1993). Protective effects of sialyated oligosaccharides in immune complex-induced acute lung injury. *J. Exp. Med.* **178,** 623–631.
57. Mulligan, M. S., Paulson, J. C., De Frees, S., Zheng, Z. -L., Lowe, J. B., and Ward, P. A. (1993). Protective effects of oligosaccharides in P-selectin dependent lung injury. *Nature* (*London*) **364,** 149–151.
58. Bullard, D. C., Qin, L., Lorenzo, I., Quinlin, W. M., Doyle, N. A., Bosse, R., *et al.* (1995). P-Selectin/ICAM-1 double mutant mice: acute emigration of neutrophils into the peritoneum is completely absent but is normal into pulmonary alveoli. *J. Clin. Invest.* **95,** 1782–1788.
59. Mayadas, T. N., Johnson, R. C., Rayburn, H., Hynes, R. O., and Wagner, D. D. (1993). Leukocyte rolling and extravasation are severely compromised in P-selectin deficient mice. *Cell* **74,** 541–554.
60. Xu, H., Gonzalo, J. A., St. Pierre, Y., Williams, I. R., Kupper, T. S., Cotran, R. S., *et al.* (1994). Leukocytosis and resistance to septic shock in intercellular adhesion molecule 1-deficient mice. *J. Exp. Med.* **180,** 95–109.
61. Mizgerd, J. P., Kubo, H., Kutkoski, G. J., Bhagwan, S. D., Scharffetter-Kochanek, K., Beaudet, A. L., *et al.* (1997). Neutrophil emigration in the skin, lungs and peritoneum: Different requirements for CD11/CD18 revealed by CD18-deficient mice. *J. Exp. Med.* **20,** 1357–1364.
62. Ward, P. A. (1995). Adhesion molecule knockouts: One step forward and one step backward. *J. Clin. Invest.* **95,** 1425–1426.
63. King, P. D., Sandberg, E. T., Selvakumar, A., Fang, P., Beaudet, A. L., and Dupont, B. (1995). Novel isoforms of murine intercellular adhesion molecule-1 generated by alternative RNA splicing. *J. Immunol.* **154,** 6080–6093.
64. Siflinger-Birnboim, A., and Malik, A. B. (1993). Neutrophil adhesion to endothelial cells impairs the effects of catalase and glutathione in preventing endothelial injury. *J. Cell Physiol.* **155,** 234–239.
65. Jaffe, E. A., Nachman, R. L., Becker, C. G., and Minick, C. R. (1973). Culture of human endothelial cells derived from umbilical vein. Identification by morphologic and immunologic critiera. *J. Clin. Invest.* **52,** 2745.
66. Willems, C., Astaldi, G. C., De Groot, P. G., Janssen, M. C., Gonsalves, M. B., Zeijlmaker, W. P., and van Mourik, J. A. (1982). Media conditioned by cultured human vascular endothelial cells inhibit the growth of vascular smooth muscle cells. *Exp. Cell Res.* **139,** 191.
67. Kasten, F. H. (1972). Rat myocardial cells *in vitro*: Mitosis and differentiated properties. *In Vitro* **8,** 128.
68. Fehr, J., and Dahinden, C. (1979). Modulating influence of chemotactic factor-induced cell adhesiveness on granulocyte function. *J. Clin. Invest.* **64,** 8–16.
69. Kubes, P., Niu, X. F., Smith, C. W., Kehrli, M. E., Reinhardt, P. H., and Woodman, R. C. (1995). A novel beta 1 dependent adhesion pathway on neutrophils: a mechanism invoked by dihydrocytochalasin B or endothelial transmigration. *FASEB J.* **9,** 1103–1111.
70. Issekutz, A. C., Chuluyan, H. E., and Lopes, N. (1995). CD11/CD18-independent transendothelial migration of human polymorphonuclear leukocytes and monocytes: Involvement of distinct and unique mechanisms. *J. Leukoc. Biol.* **57,** 553–561.
71. Carulli, G. (1996). Applications of flow cytometry in the study of human neutrophil biology and pathology. *Hematopathol. Mol. Hematol.* **10**(1–2), 39–61.
72. Lo, S. K., Lee, S. L., Ramos, R. A., Lobb, R., Rosa, M., Chi-Rosso, G., *et al.* (1991). Endothelial–leukocyte adhesion molecule-1 stimulates the adhesive activity of leukocyte integrin CR3 (CD11b/CD18, Mac-1) on human neutrophils. *J. Exp. Med.* **173,** 1493.
73. Smyth, S. S., Joneckis, C. C., and Parise, L. V. (1993). Regulation of vascular integrins. *Blood* **81,** 2827–2843.
74. Vedder, N. B., and Harlan, J. M. (1988). Increased surface expression of CD11b/CD18 (MAC-1) is not required for stimulated neutrophil adherence to cultured endothelium. *J. Clin. Invest.* **81,** 676–682.
75. Downey, G. P., Doherty, D. E., Schwab, B., Elson, E. L., Henson, P. M., and Worthen, G. S. (1990). Retention of leukocytes in capillaries: role of cell size and deformability. *J. Appl. Physiol.* **69,** 1767–1778.
76. Worthen, G. S., Schwab, B., Elson, E. L., and Downey, G. P. (1989). Mechanics of stimulated neutrophils: Cell stiffening induces retention in capillaries. *Science* **245,** 183–186.
77. Howard, T. H., and Oresajo, C. O. (1985). The kinetics of chemotactic peptide-induced change in F-actin content, F-actin distribution, and the shape of neutrophils. *J. Cell Biol.* **101,** 1078.
78. Small, J., Rottner, K., Hahne, P., and Anderson, K. I. (1999). Visualizing the actin cytoskeleton. *Microsc. Res. Tech.* **47,** 3–17.
79. Downey, G. P., and Worthen, G. S. (1988). Neutrophil retention in model capillaries: deformability, geometry, and hydrodynamic forces. *J. Appl. Physiol.* **65,** 1861–1871.
80. Drost, E. M., Kassabian, G. E., Meiselman, H. J., Gelmont, D., and Fisher, T. C. (1999). Increased rigidity and priming of polymorphonuclear leukocytes in sepsis. *Crit. Care Med.* **159,** 1696–1702.
81. Nathens, A. B., Marshall, J. C., Watson, R. W. G., Dackiw, A. P. B., and Rotstein, O. D. (1996). Diethylmaleate attenuates endotoxin-induced acute lung injury. *Surgery* **120,** 360–366.

82. Elferink, G. J. R., and de Koster, B. M. (1993). The effect of cyclic GMP and cyclic AMP on migration by electroporated human neutrophils. *Eur. J. Pharmacol.* **246,** 156–161.
83. Zigmond, S. H., and Hirsch, J. G. (1973). Leukocyte locomotion and chemotaxis: New methods for evaluation and demonstration of a cell-derived chemotactic factor. *J. Exp. Med.* **137,** 387–410.
84. Tranquillo, R. T., Zigmond, S. H., and Lauffenberger, D. A. (1988). Measurement of the chemotaxis coefficient for human neutrophils in the under-agarose migration assay. *Cell Motil. Cytoskel.* **11,** 1–15.
85. Fattorosi, A., Nisini, R., Pizzolo, J. G., and D'amelio, R. (1989). New, simple flow cytometry techniques to discriminate between internalized and membrane-bound particles in phagocytosis. *Cytometry* **10,** 320.
86. Jean, D., Rezaigia-Delclaux, S., Delacourt, C., Leclercq, R., Lafuma, C., Brun-Buisson, C., Harf, A., *et al.* (1998). Protective effect of endotoxin instillation on subsequent bacteria-induced acute lung injury in rats. *Am. J. Resp. Crit. Care Med.* **158,** 1792–1708.
87. Klebanoff, S. J. (1980). Oxygen metabolism and the toxic properties of phagocytes. *Ann. Intern. Med.* **93,** 480–489.
88. Halliwell, B. (1978). Superoxide-dependent formation of hydroxyl radical in the presence of iron chelates: Is it a mechanism for hydroxyl radical production in biochemical systems. *FEBS Lett.* **92,** 321–326.
89. Berkow, R. L., Wand, D., Larrick, J. W., Dodson, R. W., and Howard, T. H. (1987). Enhancement of neutrophil superoxide production by preincubation with recombinant human tumor necrosis factor. *J. Immunol.* **139,** 3783–3791.
90. Klebanoff, S. J., Vada, M. A., Harlan, J. M., Sparks, L. H., Gamble, J. R., Agosti, J. M., *et al.* (1986). Stimulation of neutrophils by tumor necrosis factor. *J. Immunol.* **136,** 4220–4225.
91. Roberts, P. J., Pizzey, A. R., Khwaja, A., Carver, J. E., Mire-Sluis, A. R., and Linch, D. C. (1993). The effects of interleukin-8 on neutrophil fMetLeuPhe receptors, CD11b expression and metabolic activity, in comparison and combination with other cytokines. *Br. J. Haematol.* **84,** 586–594.
92. Gaya, J. C. (1986). Modulation of neutrophil oxidative responses to soluble stimuli by platelet activating factor. *Blood* **67,** 931–936.
93. Aida, Y., and Pabst, M. J. (1991). Neutrophil responses to lipopolysaccharide. Effect of adherence on triggering and priming of the respiratory burst. *J. Immunol.* **146,** 1271–1276.
94. Crockett-Torabi, E., Sulenbbarger, B. b., Smith, C. W., and Fantone, J. C. (1995). Activation of human neutrophils through L-selectin and Mac-1 molecules. *J. Immunol.* **154,** 2291–2302.
95. Entman, M. L., Youker, K., Shoji, T., Kukielka, G., Shappell, S. B., Taylor, A. A., *et al.* (1992). Neutrophil induced oxidative injury of cardiac myocytes. A compartmented system requiring CD11b/D18-ICAM-1 adherence. *J. Clin. Invest.* **90,** 1335–1345.
96. Shappell, S. B., Toman, C., Anderson, D. C., Taylor, A. A., Entman, M. L., and Smith, C. W. (1990). Mac-1 (CD11b/CD18) mediates adherence-dependent hydrogen peroxide production by human and canine neutrophils. *J. Immunol.* **144,** 2702–2711.
97. Tsuji, T., Nagata, K., Koike, J., Todoroki, N., and Irimura, T. (1995). Induction of superoxide anion production from monocytes and neutrophils by activated platelets through the P-selectin-sialyl Lewis X interaction. *J. Leukoc. Biol* **56,** 583–587.
98. Waddell, T. K., Fialkow, L., Chan, C. K., Kishimoto, T. K., and Downey, G. P. (1994). Potentiation of the oxidative burst of human neutrophils. A signaling role for L-selectin. *J. Biol. Chem.* **269,** 18485–18491.
99. Metcalf, J. A., Gallin, J. I., Nauseef, W. M., and Root, R. K. (1986). "Labarotory Manual of Neutrophil Function." Raven Press, New York.
100. Allen, R. C. (1986). Phagocytic leukocyte oxygenation activities and chemiluminescence: A kinetic approach to analysis. *Methods Enzymol.* **133,** 449–492.
101. Lundqvist, H., Follin, P., Khalfan, L., and Dahlgren, C. (1996). Phorbol myristate acetate-induced NADPH oxidase activity in human neutrophils; only half the story has been told. *J. Leukoc. Biol.* **59,** 270–279.
102. Richardson, M. P., Ayliffe, M. J., Helbert, M., and Davies, E. G. (1998). A simple flow cytometry assay using dihydrorhodamine for the measurement of the neutrophil respiratory burst in whold blood: comparison with the quantitative nitroblue tetrazolium test. *J. Immunol. Methods* **219,** 187–193.
103. Feister, A. J., Browder, B., Willis, H. E., Mohanakumar, T., and Ruddy, S. (1988). Pertussis toxin inhibits human neutrophil responses mediated by the 42-kilodalton IgG Fc receptor. *J. Immunol.* **141**(1), 228–233.
104. Sengelov, H., Kjeldsen, L., and Borregaard, N. (1993). Control of exocytosis in early neutrophil activation. *J. Immunol.* **150,** 1535–1543.
105. Di Virgilio, F., Lew, D. P., and Pozzan, T. (1984). Protein kinase C activation of physiological processes in human neutrophils at vanishingly small cytosolic Ca^{2+} levels. *Nature (London)* **310,** 691–693.
106. Johnson, K. J., Varani, J., and Smolen, J. E. (1994). Neutrophil activation and function in health and disease. *Immunol. Ser.* **57,** 1–46.
107. Borregaard, N., and Cowland, J. B. (1997). Granules of the human polymorphonuclear leukocyte. *Blood* **89,** 3503–3521.
108. O'Connor, C., Odlum, A., Van Breda, A., Power, C., and Fitzgerald, M. X. (1988). Collagenase and fibronectin in patients with sarcoidosis. *Thorax* **43,** 393–400.
109. Overall, C. M., Wrana, J. L., and Sodek, J. (1989). Independent regulation of collagenase, 72-kDa progelatinase, and metalloproteinase inhibitor expression in human fibroblasts by transforming growth factor beta. *J. Biol. Chem.* **264,** 1860–1869.
110. Delclaux, C., Rezaiguia-Delclaux, S., Delacourt, C., Brun-Buisson, C., Lafuma, C., and Harf, A. (1997). Alveolar neutrophils in endotoxin-induced and bacteria-induced acute lung injury in rats. *Am. J. Physiol.* **273**(1 Pt. 1), L104–L112.
111. Paakko, P., Kirby, M., du Bois, R. M., Gillissen, A., Ferrans, V. J., and Crystal, R. G. (1996). Activated neutrophils secrete stored alpha-1 antitrypsin. *Am. J. Resp. Crit. Care Med.* **154,** 1829–1833.
112. Andrews, P. C., and Krinsky, N. I. (1982). Quantitative determination of myeloperoxidase using tetramethylbenzidine as substrate. *Anal. Biochem.* **127,** 346–350.
113. Suzuki, K., Ota, H., Sasagawa, S., Sakatani, T., and Fujikura, T. (1983). Assay method for myeloperoxidase in human polymorphonuclear leukocytes. *Anal. Biochem.* **132,** 345–352.
114. Nathens, A. B., Bitar, R., Watson, R. W., Issekutz, T. B., Marshall, J. C., Dackiw, A. P., *et al.* (1998). Thiol-mediated regulation of ICAM-1 expression in endotoxin-induced acute lung injury. *J. Immunol.* **160**(6), 2959–2966.
115. Mack, V. E., McCarter, M. D., Naama, H. A., Calvano, S. E., and Daly, J. M. (1996). Dominance of T-helper 2-type cytokines after severe injury. *Arch. Surg.* **131**(12), 1303–1308.
116. Kelly, J. L., O'Suilleabhain, C. B., Soberg, C. C., Mannick, J. A., and Lederer, J. A. (1999). Severe injury triggers antigen-specific T-helper cell dysfunction. *Shock* **12**(1), 39–45.
117. O'Sullivan, S. T., Lederer, J. A., Horgan, A. F., Chin, D. H., Mannick, J. A., and Rodrick, M. L. (1995). Major injury leads to predominance of the T helper-2 lymphocyte phenotype and diminished interleukin-12 production associated with decreased resistance to infection. *Ann. Surg.* **222**(4), 482–490.
118. Lucey, D. R., Clerici, M., and Shearer, G. M. (1996). Type 1 and type 2 cytokine dysregulation in human infectious, neoplastic, and inflammatory diseases. *Clin. Microbiol. Rev.* **9**(4), 532–562.

65

Antibiotic Trials

E. Patchen Dellinger

*Department of Surgery, University of Washington Medical Center,
University of Washington School of Medicine, Seattle, Washington 98195*

I. Introduction

Antibiotic trials in surgical research have most commonly involved the comparison of an antibiotic with either a second antibiotic or a placebo for the treatment or prevention of a surgical infection. The most common source of funding for these trials has been the pharmaceutical industry, and thus the trials have most frequently been either phase 3 or 4 trials designed either to support a new Food and Drug Administration (FDA)-approved indication for use of the sponsor's drug or to provide information useful to the marketing division of the sponsor. The requirement of the pharmaceutical industry to conduct trials of new drugs provides a continuing source of funding that supports antibiotic trials. Unfortunately, it also tends to limit the types of trials that get funded. In addition, the availability of industry funding has resulted in the virtual absence of funding for antimicrobial trials by any of the other research funding sources in the United States, especially the National Institutes of Health. To understand the most common forces behind antibiotic trials, it is useful to review the normal process of antibiotic development in the United States (1). The processes in Europe and other areas in the world are similar but differ in some specific details.

II. Preclinical Studies

Prior to any clinical trials of a new antibiotic, a range of preclinical studies must be completed. First the drug must be tested for *in vitro* antimicrobial activity against a wide variety of standard organisms to determine its antimicrobial spectrum. Organisms tested would include those from standard panels representing gram-positive and gram-negative species, aerobes, facultative anaerobes, and obligate anaerobes. Representative isolates from recent clinical infections would also be included. Minimal inhibitory concentrations (MICs) and minimal bactericidal concentrations (MBCs) would be determined and other characteristics such as postantibiotic effect (PAE) and synergism, additive effect, or antagonism with other classes of antibiotics sought. If an antibiotic looks promising on the basis of this information, then it will be used in animal models to explore pharmacokinetic properties, metabolic pathways, and potential toxicities. Efficacy studies in animal models of infection and investigation of pharmacodynamic properties will then be pursued. Only after all of the above has been completed and information filed with the FDA would human clinical studies be contemplated (1).

III. Regulatory Considerations

Before any human trials can be conducted, the sponsor must file an Investigational New Drug (IND) Application with the FDA. The FDA has 30 days to require new information from the sponsor. If this request is not made, then the sponsor can begin human trials. These trials are categorized as phase 1, 2, 3, or 4 trials, each of which is closely regulated by the FDA. Phase 1 trials are designed essentially to provide information regarding the safety and pharmacokinetic properties of the drug in humans. They may also provide information regarding metabolism of the drug and the effect of increasing doses. The trials are conducted in a limited number of normal, healthy volunteers in most cases (1).

Phase 2 trials begin to use the drug in the treatment of individuals with actual infections. These trials continue to supply information regarding safety and pharmacokinetics, and also demonstrate efficacy or lack of it. Phase 2 studies tend to focus on individuals with relatively straightforward infections and few other serious underlying conditions and receiving few other concomitant medications. All phase 2 protocols are reviewed in advance by the FDA. These trials are usually conducted as comparative studies using a drug that is already licensed and approved for that indication and considered standard treatment, but may occasionally be placebo controlled or rely on historical controls. In many cases the trials are not blinded in order to detect new problems as quickly as possible. Cases in phase 2 trials are generally considered evaluable only if a responsible pathogen susceptible to the study drug has been isolated and definitively identified (1).

Phase 3 studies are conducted after initial evidence of efficacy has been obtained in phase 2 studies and are designed to obtain additional information regarding safety and efficacy in wider categories of patients and for new indications. Much larger numbers of patients are enrolled, and an effort is made to obtain patients characteristic of those encountered in routine clinical practice. In many drug development programs, phase 2 and phase 3 trials blend into one another and the distinction may not be a sharp one. Phase 3 trials form the basis for approved indications that are requested in the New Drug Application (NDA) that the sponsor makes to the FDA. These studies are conducted in a variety of clinical and geographic settings to provide maximum information prior to the licensing of the drug. Phase 3 studies may also be used to refine dosing recommendations and to provide additional information regarding drug metabolism, interactions, and safety. Patient populations should be expanded to include children, pregnant women, and patients with hepatic or renal dysfunction. Phase 3 and phase 4 studies are those most commonly involving surgical indications (1).

Phase 4 studies are those conducted after a drug has received FDA approval for labeling and marketing. Phase 4 studies may be similar in design to phase 3 studies and intended to obtain new indications approved by the FDA. Such trials are conducted in the same manner as phase 3 studies and are subject to the same FDA regulations (1). It is an unfortunate fact that because most pharmaceutical trials are designed to support an indication with the FDA, the sponsor is usually willing to study comparator drugs only in the doses and schedules printed in the FDA-approved package insert. Because these inserts do not necessarily represent best or even usual clinical practice, the studies may lose some degree of clinical relevance. Phase 4 studies may also be conducted in areas that already have approved indications and serve simply to provide additional clinical data, or perhaps to demonstrate comparative efficacy with a commercial competitor. Many of these trials seem designed to establish positioning in a commercial sense rather than to answer important questions of interest to clinical practitioners. Nevertheless, it is in the area of phase 4 trials that independent surgical investigators have some of the best opportunities to conduct interesting and significant antibiotic trials in surgical infections. This will be discussed in more detail later in the chapter.

The FDA is closely involved in all steps of phase 1 through phase 3 trials and many phase 4 trials. The FDA conducts some random and targeted audits to verify accuracy of data, existence of enrolled patients, and appropriate protection of human subjects. A recent survey revealed that many academic surgeons possess deficient knowledge regarding the role of the FDA and the application of federal regulations to protection of human subjects and the conduct of trials (2).

IV. Surgical Trials

Antibiotic trials in surgery share many characteristics with antibiotic trials in other disciplines, but, in addition, have some unique characteristics that strongly influence the design and conduct of trials. The most important aspect is that surgical infections, by definition, involve circumstances in which the identified infectious process is not expected to resolve without surgical intervention in addition to antimicrobial treatment. In many cases, such as an intraabdominal abscess or a necrotizing soft tissue infection, the surgical procedure may be more decisive than the antimicrobial drugs in determining the ultimate course of the infection. This creates a heavy burden for antibiotic trials in surgical infection. Unless the surgical management of the patients is comparable, any comparison between two antibiotic regimens becomes uninterpretable. Many published trials in surgical infection and many trial protocols do not provide the degree of detail regarding this consideration that is required to have confidence in the published outcomes. Indeed, although there is widespread agreement regarding the broad outlines and principles of treatment for surgical infection, there is not agreement on the details of this management in specific cases (3). A brief survey of the literature on the optimal operation for diverticulitis, the advisability of closing skin incisions after contaminated surgical cases, the optimal management strategy for infected necrotizing pancreatitis, the proper role for mandatory reexploration for cases of severe peritonitis, or the proper use of drains after perforated appendicitis demonstrates lack of agreement in each of these areas. One of the challenges for any antibiotic trial in surgical infection is to achieve agreement in advance among all of the investigators and participating clinical surgeons regarding the uniform surgical management of the patients so that any differences observed between trial groups can be attributed to the different antibiotic regimens. This condition is frequently overlooked and often not even commented on.

A. Types of Trials

Antibiotic trials in surgery fall broadly into prophylaxis trials and treatment trials. Prophylaxis refers to the use of an antibiotic (or other treatment modality) to prevent an infection that is not evident at the time of the intervention but for which the patient is at risk. The classic trials in this area have all involved antibiotic administration to patients having scheduled operative procedures. Based on these trials, conducted over the past 35 years, a consensus has evolved regarding most basic aspects of perioperative antibiotic prophylaxis for scheduled surgical procedures (4). Despite this, actual practice differs from recommendations in a number of areas, including duration of prophylaxis after all surgical procedures (5–7), and after orthopedic (8, 9) and cardiac (10–12) surgical procedures specifically. Despite an absence of trials demonstrating any increased efficacy for prolonged prophylactic antibiotic administration, this practice continues, especially for patients with indwelling lines and drains. The field is ripe with opportunity for additional trials to settle this question more definitively.

1. Prophylaxis Trials

Prophylaxis trials with the best chance to obtain a definitive, interpretable result are those focusing on a specific single procedure in a well-defined group of patients. Such trials reduce to a minimum the variability inherent in combining different procedures and thus increase the power of the study. Examples of this include trials examining colectomy (13, 14), cholecystectomy (15), gastric bypass (16), and hip replacement (8). Trials that combine different specific procedures in a class of operations such as clean, clean-contaminated, or contaminated have the advantage of being able to accumulate adequate numbers of patients more quickly, but complicate the analysis. These studies, even when they achieve a statistically significant result, can generate significant controversy regarding the applicability of the results to the range of procedures studied (17–21).

2. Trauma

Another area of controversy in trials of antibiotic prophylaxis has been the classification of antibiotic trials in trauma patients. The earliest animal trials in antibiotic prophylaxis demonstrated the importance of providing antibiotic levels in the wound at or before bacterial contamination (22–24). Subsequent trials in humans confirmed this principle (7, 25, 26). Because most injuries cause tissue contamination before the patient reaches medical care, the opportunity to achieve antibiotic levels before contamination is lost for trauma patients. This has led some to declare definitively that all antibiotic administration to trauma patients is "therapy" and not "prophylaxis." The issue is actually one more of definition than of substance. Numerous trials in trauma patients have demonstrated that the incidence of diagnosed infections that follow injury can be significantly (clinically and statistically) reduced by the administration of appropriate antibiotics as part of the early care of the injured patient (25, 27–29) and that brief courses of antibiotics (≤24 hr) are equal in efficacy to much longer durations (30–34). Whether this antibiotic administration is called "presumptive therapy" or "prophylaxis" is less important than understanding its correct use to reduce infection risk in these patients.

3. Therapeutic Antibiotic Trials

Therapeutic antibiotic trials for established surgical infection have been most commonly carried out in the area of intraabdominal infection. The term "intraabdominal infection" usually is applied to cases of peritonitis or intraabdominal abscess. However, in its broadest sense it includes a wide variety of conditions, including diverticulitis, pyelonephritis, infected pancreatic necrosis, cholangitis, salpingitis or tuboovarian abscess (pelvic inflammatory disease, PID), peritonitis associated with chronic ambulatory peritoneal dialysis, and sometimes severe incisional infections following coeliotomy.

B. Confounding Issues

Combining a variety of different "intraabdominal" infections in a single antibiotic trial creates difficulties in analysis. Patients typically have different underlying conditions, undergo different operative procedures or no procedure at all, and have quite different microbial pathogens recovered. Most investigators agree that patients requiring operative management of an infection should not be combined in a trial with patients who do not require operative intervention. The currently accepted term for patients who require either operative or percutaneous intervention for intraabdominal infection is "complicated intraabdominal infection" (35). Some definitions of complicated infection also include percutaneous or endoscopic drainage of an obstructed biliary tree. A distinct advantage of studying complicated intraabdominal infections is that a definitive culture is available for each entered patient. This avoids the problem associated with the clinical diagnosis of diverticulitis, pelvic inflammatory disease, or nonoperative cellulitis when no culture material is available. With complicated, operative intraabdominal infections, many protocols specify that the patient becomes unevaluable if definitive, culture-positive evidence for infection is not found at the time of operative intervention. A consequence of this is that most antibiotic trials in surgical infection have a rather high number of unevaluable patients due to the uncertainty of the diagnosis prior to operative intervention. This makes the intent-to-treat analysis an important element of all of these trials.

Antibiotic trials for the treatment of "medical" infections nearly always exclude patients who have received prior antibiotics before enrollment in the trial. The exclusion may apply to patients who have received any antibiotics or have received more than a specified amount or duration (usually 24–48 hr) of antibiotics. This is done to reduce confusion regarding whether an antibiotic success is due to the study antibiotic or to the antibiotic given prior to study entry. This particular exclusion is not needed for a trial of complicated intraabdominal infection for two reasons. First, when a patient is enrolled only if operative intervention is required, the patient is, by definition, a failure of the prior antibiotic treatment and thus is a valid candidate to receive the study drug and be evaluable. In addition, because the patient will be operated (or drained percutaneously) there will be good culture material available to document the pathogens present at the time of study entry. One technique to reduce the number of patients declared unevaluable due to lack of documented infection at the time of operation is to perform the randomization after the operation. In this scheme, a patient with a preoperative clinical diagnosis of intraabdominal infection is evaluated and consented preoperatively but not randomized. If, during the operation, no infection is found, the patient is not randomized. If infection is found, the patient is randomized after obtaining operative culture specimens, and only then is the blinded study drug administered.

Another element that complicates interpretation of trials in intraabdominal infection is interpretation of failures. The most common manifestation of a failure after treatment of peritonitis or intraabdominal abscess is a recurrent abscess requiring drainage or a wound infection that must be opened. However, if a continued source of infection such as a leaking anastomosis is not controlled or a second abscess is not located and drained at the index procedure, or if a wound dehiscence occurs even without infection, the investigator is presented with a situation that looks the same as an antibiotic failure but that could not possibly have been prevented by the antibiotic. This situation has led to a call for standardization of "source control," or the mechanical, anatomic, surgical methods performed to eliminate the anatomic cause of a surgical infection.

Two studies have demonstrated a strong relationship between source control and treatment outcome for surgical infections (36, 37). On the other hand, workshops and symposia conducted by the Surgical Infection Society (SIS) have highlighted the fact that there is not even an accepted vocabulary for describing the operative treatment of intraabdominal infection, let alone agreement as to which elements are important or necessary and which should be recorded and standardized in an antibiotic trial (38). This is an area of intense interest at the current time. Until the SIS and/or other societies produce standards for conducting and describing source control, at a minimum, future protocols studying intraabdominal infection should standardize and describe the procedures used in that trial as much as possible (39, 40). In the absence of prospective standards for source control, some trials have established blinded committees of surgeons and others experienced in the conduct of antibiotic trials and in managing surgical infection to review apparent treatment failures (41). Cases that have been judged to have inadequate source control by the blinded evaluation committee are then evaluated and analyzed separately in comparisons of treatment outcome. If a trial is large enough, and the randomization was carried out appropriately, such cases should balance out in the treatment groups, but a study is stronger if known sources of bias such as inadequate source control can be controlled explicitly.

C. Outcomes

Determination of outcome in an antibiotic trial of surgical infections can be complex. Ideally success is defined as recovery to baseline health after one operation and one course of study antibiotics. Patients with intraabdominal infection can be quite sick, and their postoperative course complex, affected by factors not influenced by antibiotics. Other infections, away from the abdomen, such as pneumonia, urinary tract infections, or intravenous catheter-related infections may occur, and patients may manifest fever not caused by infection, tempting the treating clinician to prescribe additional empiric antibiotics that confuse the primary comparison. If prescription of an additional, nonstudy antibiotic is defined as a failure in the absence of evidence for persistent or recurrent intraabdominal infection, then trivial failures become mixed in with significant ones such as recurrent subphrenic abscess. Ideally a clinical trial of patients with intraabdominal infection should prospectively categorize infectious failures into major failures such as recurrent peritonitis or a new intraabdominal abscess, and minor failures such as prescription of additional antibiotics without documentation of persistent/recurrent infection or the occurrence of an incisional infection in the subcutaneous space without fascial dehiscence, managed without a return to the operating room (39). A careful description of failures and analysis of the potential causes for failure often provide the most important information from a clinical trial of antibiotic use.

A well-designed study should minimize the number of failures attributed to additional antibiotic prescription in the absence of failure at the primary site of interest. Commonly, the protocol will allow the administration of another antibiotic for infection at a different anatomic site after an interval such as 5 days. The primary site is evaluated clinically at the time that the additional antibiotic is started, and if the clinical evidence supports resolution of the infection, the patient can be a success provided that new evidence of infection in the abdomen does not occur during the follow-up period. In part, the decision on how to evaluate such patients depends on the primary goal of the study. If the intent is to answer a scientific question regarding the unequivocal comparison of two antibiotics, the answer may be cleaner if such patients are excluded. On the other hand, if the primary goal is to determine the best treatment in real life, then the administration of other antibiotics simply mirrors real life. All patients should be compared in an intent-to-treat analysis, thus testing the effectiveness of initial empiric treatment with the study drug.

Because the evaluation and comparison of outcomes is so complex in trials of intraabdominal infection and most other examples of surgical infection, the value of conducting these trials in a double-blind manner is magnified. No matter how carefully rules for evaluability and outcome are written in a protocol, such trials will inevitably present the investigators with patients and circumstances that were not fully anticipated (E. P. Dellinger, personal observation). Disagreements will arise among investigators, and subjective judgments will have to be made. It is critically important for these decisions to be made with the participants blind to the treatment regimens and to the effect of their decisions on the trial comparison. A rich literature attests to the importance of blinding at every phase of a clinical trial, from the randomization itself, to the decisions regarding evaluability, and the categorization of success or failure. Failure to carry out appropriate blinding and randomization has been associated with unequal distribution of risks between treatment groups (42) and distortion of ultimate results (43). Questions regarding evaluability can be minimized, of course, if every randomized patient is fully followed to the end of the trial and given an outcome, and the primary report is conducted as an intent-to-treat analysis.

During the 1970s and 1980s many antibiotic trials were conducted with comparisons of an antibiotic against a placebo for prophylaxis trials (13, 14, 44, 45), but as more and more trials demonstrated efficacy, a consensus developed that for operations with proved efficacy of antibiotic prophylaxis, placebo control trials should no longer be done (46). In the area of therapy, placebo-controlled trials have not been done. However, during the 1970s and early 1980s a number of comparative treatment trials as well as comparative prophylaxis trials were conducted that demonstrated significant differences between antibiotic regimens. These were, by and large, comparisons of antibiotic regimens that had obvious differences in their antibacterial spectra (13, 27, 47–50). These trials have been very influential in developing our concepts regarding the important characteristics of an antibiotic regimen chosen for either prophylaxis or treatment. In the past two decades we have seen many more trials designed at the outset to demonstrate *equivalence* of two antibiotics or antibiotic regimens. In these the concept is that the new antibiotic is demonstrated to be as effective as the prior standard used for that indication, and a case for its use is then made based on convenience of dosing, adverse event profile, cost, route of administration, or other characteristic. Too often, the difference between a trial designed to show *superiority* of one agent to another and one designed to show equivalence is not fully appreciated. In a superiority trial, the null hypothesis is that no difference exists and the power calculations are performed to ensure an adequate chance to see a true difference, if it exists. In a superiority trial, the most conservative analysis employs an intent-to-treat analysis as a safeguard against declaring a difference that is not real.

In an equivalence trial, on the other hand, the null hypothesis is that there is a difference between the two treatments. Here, the statistical noise induced by analyzing all patients in an intent-to-treat analysis actually has the potential effect of obscuring a true difference between two regimens and thus increasing the odds of declaring two treatments to be equivalent when in fact they are not. Thus, in an equivalence study, the analysis of "evaluable" patients is in some ways a more conservative one than the intent-to-treat analysis (51, 52). In addition, one must realize that the numbers of patients needed for a valid equivalence trial are often considerably larger than in a superiority trial. Of course, one can never prove that two regimens are equal. One can only prove that the likely difference between two regimens (with 95% certainty) is not larger than Δ. It is critical in the design of an equivalence trial that a clinically meaningful delta be specified prior to the beginning of the trial. The clinically significant difference is not a statistical concept. It is a clinical concept and must be plausible to those reading the trial report, but it drives the statistics, including the number of patients who must be enrolled to draw meaningful conclusions. When the trial is concluded, the results of an equivalence trial are better presented as confidence limits demonstrating the likely range of statistically plausible differences rather than the p value for a difference between treatment groups (51, 53).

The maximum benefit from any clinical trial is obtained if clinicians can use the results to influence patient care. For this to be valid, the clinician must be able to understand the type of patients studied and the clinical circumstances in order to know if they apply to his/her patients and practice. For this reason, it is important for a trial report to specify not only the clinical characteristics of the patients studied, but to provide information regarding the patients not studied and to specify if there were any important differences between these groups (54). If a medical center sees 750 patients a year with a specific diagnosis, but a trial that is conducted over 18 months enrolls 150 patients, these may not be representative of all patients with that diagnosis, and the results of the trial may not be generalizable to all such patients. This question can be evaluated if the investigator reports the number of eligible patients either not approached or approached and not enrolled in the trial, and enough demographic information about the patients to evaluate the comparability of the groups (39).

Most antibiotic trials report separately the clinical and the microbiological response. The clinical response is discussed above. The microbiological response is determined by the persistence of bacteria cultured at the time of study entry (a failure) or the proved eradication of the bacteria based on posttreatment cultures. In most clinically successful cases of intraabdominal infection, there is no material available for posttreatment cultures. In such cases, the pathogens are categorized as "presumed eradicated" (1). The microbiological response is reported by pathogen rather than by patient and provides a useful measure of potential antibiotic weaknesses (41, 55).

The prospects for a definitive trial improve significantly if a narrower spectrum of diagnoses is studied. Probably the most consistently successful antibiotic trials in intraabdominal infection involve patients with perforated or gangrenous appendicitis. The advantages of these trials are that the diagnosis is usually more accurate, the surgical management of the disease is more standardized than other sources of peritonitis and abscess, and definitive "source control" can usually be achieved with the initial procedure. The result is that differences between treatment groups are more likely to be due to differences in antibiotic activity and less likely to be obscured by failures related to underlying anatomic problems that could not be solved in the initial operation (47–49, 56). The disadvantage of studying appendicitis alone is that it is a much less serious infection than other causes of peritonitis and abscess (57). The mortality and morbidity are much lower, and the question often remains for studies done only or primarily on patients with appendicitis as to whether the conclusions can be generalized to patients with more severe infections, such as perforated colon cancers, leaking anastomoses, or severe diverticulitis. There has been a tendency in the past for antibiotic trials to emphasize low-risk patients with a low mortality and a high success rate (58), but more recent trials have studied more complex and seriously ill patients (41, 55, 59–61).

D. Exclusion Criteria

There are some types of intraabdominal infections or inflammatory conditions that have usually been excluded from trials of general intraabdominal infections. Uncomplicated early acute appendicitis and cholecystitis are usually cured by a simple operation and with a single dose of perioperative antibiotics administered primarily for prophylaxis against wound infection. Their inclusion with more serious intraabdominal infections dilutes the effects that might be seen in the larger trial. Trials involving these diagnoses are more appropriately regarded as trials of prophylaxis. Early traumatic bowel injury and peptic ulcer perforations less than 24 hr old are also usually excluded from treatment trials because these both respond to 12 hr or less of antibiotics and frequently are sterile on initial culture of peritoneal fluid. Necrotizing pancreatitis is usually excluded because the nature of the disease even without infection can be so overwhelming, and when infection does occur, it quite frequently cannot be managed with a single operative intervention. For a similar reason, patients with severe peritonitis, for which the operating surgeon is committed during the first operation to reoperate on a planned schedule or to pursue the "open abdomen" management plan, are also excluded. Patients with small or large bowel infarction are usually excluded because a surprising number of those patients actually have sterile abdominal cultures despite their "septic" physiologic picture, and failures that do occur are often due to the underlying pathology that led to the infarction rather than to the activity of the antibiotics used. Any of the conditions listed above could be studied alone if a sufficient number of patients could be found to complete the study, but they are poor candidates for inclusion in a general study of intraabdominal infection.

E. Risk Factors

No matter how carefully a protocol is written and carried out, any trial of patients with intraabdominal infection will include patients with a wide range of underlying risk factors and severity of illness at the time of enrollment. These risk factors will affect outcome independently of the treatment regimen chosen, and it is important to record and report these so that the comparability of the treatment groups can be evaluated. These factors include age, underlying health, duration of infection before diagnosis and treatment, and, most importantly, the severity of the disease being studied (39). Since the early 1980s a large number of papers have verified the importance of objectively scored severity indices in defining risk of death and/or failure for patients with intraabdominal infection. The most widely used score is the APACHE II score that utilizes 12 items of physical exam and lab values combined with age and health status to derive a numeric score between 0 and 71. In all studies examined to date where it has been tested, the APACHE II score was one of the most significant determinants associated with treatment failure and death. If the APACHE II score is not used, one of the other validated and published objective scores should be reported (39, 40, 62–64).

Because most trials record multiple risk factors, underlying diseases, and treatment variations for each patient, there is a large and complex set of data to analyze. It is tempting to ask multiple questions of the data. However, multiple queries of a large data set pose serious statistical questions and alter the significance usually associated with statistical tests that are designed to give the statistical significance for a single question.

It is quite important in the design of a clinical trial to specify one primary question at the outset. This question drives the study design and the numbers of subjects needed to answer it with sufficient power. Further exploratory analyses of the entire data set can be quite rewarding for developing new hypotheses that can be tested in future trials. Such explorations, however, can never carry the statistical weight associated with the primary endpoint (40). Another temptation in data analysis is to look for effects within subgroups. Again, this must be done with great care unless the original trial design was performed with subgroup analysis as part of the analysis plan (65). It is imperative to have a statistician involved in the design of clinical trials and not simply the performance of statistical tests at the end on data already gathered that do not now permit the analyses that the investigators wish to do.

For FDA and pharmaceutical industry purposes, soft tissue infections are usually termed skin and skin structure infections. These include subcutaneous abscesses, incisional wound infections or superficial surgical site infections (SSI), infected ischemic ulcers, infected full-thickness burns, and necrotizing soft tissue infections. Subcutaneous abscesses generally respond to surgical drainage without antibiotic administration and are probably not a good choice for an antibiotic study. Most surgical site infections also respond to opening the wound without antibiotics, although the more severe ones may benefit from antibiotics and could be included in a trial if enough can be enrolled to complete a study. Infected ischemic ulcers can be the subject of an antibiotic trial, but only if the degree of ischemia and methods pursued to relieve ischemia are carefully documented and standardized between treatment arms. Full-thickness burn infections will be confined to burn centers and generally will require burn wound biopsies to identify responsible pathogens and to monitor treatment response. Necrotizing soft tissue infections have the advantage that all require operative debridement and thus will have good microbiology. However, these infections are so uncommon that no center is likely to enroll enough patients to conduct a meaningful study, and even a large multicenter study is likely to experience difficulties in enrolling sufficient patients. Here, as in the case of intraabdominal infections, timing of intervention and the details of the surgical management are so important to the outcome that analysis of any results would be quite difficult, especially if the study is conducted at multiple centers, each with only a few cases and with different management styles at different institutions.

V. Current FDA Guidelines

The current system for conducting antibiotic trials has the result that the overwhelming majority of trials are conducted with funding from the pharmaceutical industry. Most of these trials are driven by the manufacturer's obligation to fulfill FDA requirements to demonstrate safety and efficacy and are conducted as phase 1 through phase 4 trials as described earlier. The FDA has established very specific requirements for the design and conduct of these trials that limit the flexibility of an industry sponsor and of clinical investigators. These have been published in a special supplement to *Clinical Infectious Diseases* (66). The prior guidelines had not been revised since 1977. The FDA gave a contract to the Infectious Diseases Society of America (IDSA) in 1988 to review and update the guidelines and this was completed in 1992. Working groups within IDSA and with the assistance of SIS for surgical topics provided suggested guidelines for each type of infection commonly studied in antibiotic trials. This included general guidelines for any clinical antibiotic trials (1) and more specific guidelines for intraabdominal (35), acute pelvic infections in hospitalized women (67), acute pelvic inflammatory disease (68), skin and skin structure infections (69), and prophylaxis of surgical infections (70). The guidelines are suggestions and have never been adopted by the FDA as formal government rules. However, in the absence of other guidelines, they have become the standard that the industry looks to for trial design, and investigators will find it difficult to convince an industry sponsor to stray from them in a trial that will be used to support an indication with the FDA. The IDSA is currently exploring the idea of an update for these guidelines with the FDA. The SIS and others have also published guidelines for the conduct of antibiotic trials in surgical patients (39, 40).

Once a new antibiotic has been licensed and its primary indications approved by the FDA, the manufacturer can fund additional trials that will not necessarily be used to obtain new indications. The manufacturer always has the obligation to collect safety information and to inform the FDA of any new findings, but if a new indication is not being sought, it has greater leeway in designing a new trial. This presents the academic investigator with the opportunity to introduce a trial that asks a clinically interesting question that might not be relevant to an application for a new indication. On the other hand, the pharmaceutical sponsor normally turns over all decisions regarding antibiotic trials to the marketing division of the company once the initial approval for marketing is obtained. Here, business decisions have priority over clinical questions. The sponsor's first priority is to conduct and publish studies that will display their drug in a favorable light. They will be interested in a trial that studies a question of interest to clinicians because this will make any subsequent publications more interesting and more likely to be read by the clinicians the sponsor would like to influence. However, when considering a comparison drug, they will be most interested in comparing their drug with one that is considered a market competitor even if it is not the most logical or interesting comparison from a practicing clinician's point of view.

From the standpoint of an academic investigator interested in conducting clinical antibiotic trials, it is helpful to understand the normal cycle of drug funding. When a drug is in its preclinical phases, all efforts and resources by the company are devoted to completing the trials necessary to obtaining marketing approval from the FDA for the maximum number of appropriate clinical indications in those areas that represent significant clinical and commercial demand and use. Once a drug has been marketed, resources are devoted in some cases to the development and approval of new indications, and also to studies that will position the new drug in relation to competitor's drugs that are heavily used in the market that the company wants to penetrate. Each drug has a patent life of 17 years from the time of patent filing, during which time the company has exclusive rights to market the drug. Normally, 10–12 years of that life are expended in getting to the market. The manufacturer is willing to invest resources in clinical trial research only during the premarketing period and the early portion of the marketed life, when it has a reasonable expectation of recovering the research investment in increased sales.

VI. The Clinical Investigator

A resourceful and successful clinical investigator will learn to propose studies that ask important clinical questions and do so using a drug that is early enough in its patent life that the manufacturer is willing to invest money in additional clinical trials. Some examples of such studies include a comparison of ceforanide with cephalothin for prophylaxis of open heart procedures, which demonstrated the superiority of a long-half-life cephalosporin over a short-half-life drug (71); a comparison of cefonicid with placebo for prophylaxis in hernia and breast operations, which demonstrated the efficacy of prophylaxis in these clean operations (17); the comparison of kanamycin and cephalothin with kanamycin and clindamycin in patients with old penetrating abdominal injuries, which demonstrated the importance of antibiotic activity against obligate anaerobic bacteria in cases with bowel injury (27); and the study of penetrating abdominal injuries, which compared cefoxitin with cefotetan and 1 day of treatment with 5 days and demonstrated that comparable antibiotics given for the same time had comparable results and that 1 day was equivalent to 5 days of treatment (30). Each of these trials employed one drug that was in the new, fundable part of its patent life to conduct a trial that asked a question more significant than simply the superiority (or equivalence) of drug A or drug B for a particular clinical indication. Much of what we have learned about antibiotic principles over the years has been gained in this manner and by deduction and extrapolation from existing studies. Informed industry representatives charged with designing and conducting clinical trials in cooperation with clinical investigators recognize these differing goals, and the best will work with a conscientious investigator to design a study that answers the needs both of the industry sponsor and of the clinical investigator. This is more likely to be achievable for phase 4 than for phase 3 studies.

VII. Pitfalls and Publication Issues

There are some traps in the design of antibiotic trials that the clinical investigator must be aware of and avoid. It is possible, and sometimes in the commercial interest of an industry sponsor, to propose a clinical trial that mixes and matches questions in such a way that a legitimate question cannot actually be answered in the trial. Some examples occurred in the prior decade when the standard prophylactic antibiotic was cefazolin but many surgeons had not accepted the fact that one or at most two doses were sufficient for the great majority of prophylactic indications. Many surgeons continued to administer 48 hr or more of prophylactic drug. As some second- and third-generation cephalosporins with long half-lives were developed (ceforanide, cefonicid, and ceftriaxone, for example), trials were proposed and in some cases carried out comparing one dose of the long-half-life drug (12–24 hr of drug activity) against 48 hr or more of cefazolin. Such a trial does not allow a clean comparison either of one drug to the other or of one duration to the other. In contrast, studies that include treatment arms comparing different drugs given for the same duration or the same drug given for different durations allow valid comparisons both between drugs and between different durations (30, 34, 72).

The management of data and publishing rights are two issues that should be negotiated and clearly agreed on prior to the initiation of any clinical trial. Both the principal clinical investigator and the sponsor of a clinical trial have a legitimate interest in the quality of the data and the resulting publication. However, the motivation to publish the results may be quite different if the results fail to show the sponsor's drug in a favorable light. Academic investigators can only ethically participate in a clinical trial if they have full control of the data from their clinical site and full rights to publish. It is customary for the sponsor to require the submission of any manuscript for inspection and comment prior to submission for publication. A responsible investigator will naturally listen carefully to concerns and suggestions regarding the presentation of data. In the end, however, the investigator must be free to publish without restriction. No trial agreement should be negotiated without this guarantee (73). If the results of a trial do not result in a significant difference between treatment groups, the investigator may be discouraged and may fail to write and submit the results. This practice has the potential for creating publication bias, whereby only positive studies get published (74). Theoretically, a comparison of two equally effective treatments tested in 20 trials would emerge once with a p value of 0.05. If the "negative" trials are not submitted, but the twentieth trial is published, a serious bias in available information will result. A trial important enough to design and conduct should be published.

The reporting of clinical trials is another area where there is great room for improvement (65, 75–77). Several recent workshops of journal editors have resulted in the publication of recommendations for the reporting of clinical trials that, if followed, would greatly improve the quality of information conveyed and allow the discriminating reader to test the quality of the authors' conclusions and to form his own if desired (77). One can only hope that journal editors will insist on these standards in the future.

References

1. Beam, T. R., Jr., Gilbert, D. N., and Kunin, C. M. (1992). General guidelines for the clinical evaluation of anti-infective drug products. Infectious Diseases Society of America and the Food and Drug Administration. *Clin. Infect. Dis.* **15** (Suppl. 1), S5–S32.
2. Rutan, R. L., Deitch, E. A., and Waymack, J. P. (1997). Academic surgeons' knowledge of Food and Drug Administration regulations for clinical trials. *Arch. Surg.* **132,** 94–98.
3. Bohnen, J. M., and Meakins, J. L. (1984). Treatment of intra-abdominal sepsis. *Can. J. Surg.* **27,** 222–223, 225.
4. Dellinger, E. P., Gross, P. A., Barrett, T. L., *et al.* (1994). Quality standard for antimicrobial prophylaxis in surgical procedures. *Clin. Infect. Dis.* **18,** 422–427.
5. Currier, J. S., Campbell, H., Platt, R., and Kaiser, A. B. (1991). Perioperative antimicrobial prophylaxis in middle Tennessee, 1989–90. *Rev. Inf. Dis.* **12,** S874–S878.
6. Shapiro, M., Townsend, T. R., Rosner, B., and Kass, E. H. (1979). Use of antimicrobial drugs in general hospitals: Patterns of prophylaxis. *N. Engl. J. Med.* **301,** 351–355.
7. Classen, D. C., Evans, R. S., Pestotnik, S. L., Horn, S. D., Menlove, R. L., and Burke, J. P. (1992). The timing of prophylactic administration of antibiotics and the risk of surgical-wound infection [see comments]. *N. Engl. J. Med.* **326,** 281-26.
8. Evrard, J., Doyon, F., Acar, J. F., Salord, J. C., Mazas, F., and Flamant, R. (1988). Two-day cefamandole versus five-day cephazolin prophylaxis in 965 total hip replacements. Report of a multicentre double blind randomised trial. *Int. Orthoped.* **12,** 69–73.
9. Norden, C. W. (1991). Antibiotic prophylaxis in orthopedic surgery. *Rev. Infect. Dis.* **10,** S842–S846.
10. Kaiser, A. B., Petracek, M. R., Lea, J. Wt., *et al.* (1987). Efficacy of cefazolin, cefamandole, and gentamicin as prophylactic agents in cardiac surgery. Results of a prospective, randomized, double-blind trial in 1030 patients. *Ann. Surg.* **206,** 791–797.
11. Soteriou, M., Recker, F., Geroulanos, S., and Turina, M. (1989). Perioperative antibiotic prophylaxis in cardiovascular surgery: A prospective randomized comparative trial of cefazolin versus ceftriaxone [see comments]. *World J. Surg.* **13,** 798–801; discussion 801–802.
12. Kreter, B., and Woods, M. (1992). Antibiotic prophylaxis for cardiothoracic operations. Meta-analysis of thirty years of clinical trials. *J. Thorac. Cardiovasc. Surg.* **104,** 590–599.
13. Washington, J. A., 2d, Dearing, W. H., Judd, E. S., and Elveback, L. R. (1974). Effect of preoperative antibiotic regimen on development of infection after intestinal surgery: Prospective, randomized, double-blind study. *Ann. Surg.* **180,** 567–572.
14. Clarke, J. S., Condon, R. E., Bartlett, J. G., Gorbach, S. L., Nichols, R. L., and Ochi, S. (1977). Preoperative oral antibiotics reduce septic complications of colon operations: Results of prospective, randomized, double-blind clinical study. *Ann. Surg.* **186,** 251–259.
15. Grant, M. D., Jones, R. C., Wilson, S. E., *et al.* (1989). Single dose cephalosporin prophylaxis in high-risk patients undergoing surgical treatment of the biliary tract. *Surg. Gynecol. Obstet.* **174,** 347–354.
16. Forse, R. A., Karam, B., MacLean, L. D., and Christou, N. V. (1989). Antibiotic prophylaxis for surgery in morbidly obese patients. *Surgery* **106,** 750–756.
17. Platt, R., Zaleznik, D. F., Hopkins, C. C., *et al.* (1990). Perioperative antibiotic prophylaxis for herniorrhaphy and breast surgery. *N. Engl. J. Med.* **322,** 153–160.
18. Rutkow, I. M., and Robbins, A. W. (1990). Antibiotic prophylaxis for herniorrhaphy and breast surgery (letter). *N. Engl. J. Med.* **322,** 1884.
19. Ergina, P. L., Gold, S., and Meakins, J. L. (1990). Antibiotic prophylaxis for herniorrhaphy and breast surgery (letter). *N. Engl. J. Med.* **322,** 1884.
20. Byrd, R. D., Brown, B. W., and Hohn, D. C. (1990). Antibiotic prophylaxis for herniorrhaphy and breast surgery (letter). *N. Engl. J. Med.* **322,** 1884–1885.
21. Lewis, R. T., Weigand, F. M., Mamazza, J., Lloyd-Smith, W., and Tataryn, D. (1995). Should antibiotic prophylaxis be used routinely in clean surgical procedures: A tentative yes. *Surgery* **118,** 742–746; discussion 746–747.
22. Burke, J. (1961). The effective period of preventive antibiotic action in experimental incisions and dermal lesions. *Surgery* **50,** 161–168.
23. Alexander, J., and Altemeier, W. (1965). Penicillin prophylaxis of experimental staphylococcal wound infections. *Surg. Gynecol. Obstet.* **120,** 243–255.
24. Edlich, R., Smith, Q., and Edgerton, M. (1973). Resistance of the surgical wound to antimicrobial prophylaxis and its mechanisms of development. *Am. J. Surg.* **126,** 583–591.
25. Fullen, W., Hunt, J., and Altemeier, W. Prophylactic antibiotics in penetrating wounds of the abdomen. *J. Trauma* **12,** 282–289.
26. Stone, H. H., Haney, B. B., Kolb, L. D., Geheber, C. E., and Hooper, C. A. (1979). Prophylactic and preventive antibiotic therapy: Timing, duration and economics. *Ann. Surg.* **189,** 691–699.
27. Thadepalli, H., Gorbach, S., Broido, P., *et al.* (1973). Abdominal trauma, anaerobes, and antibiotics. *Surg. Gynecol. Obstet.* **137,** 270–276.
28. Braun, R., Enzler, M. A., and Rittman, W. W. (1987). A double-blind clinical trial of prophylactic cloxacillin in open fractures. *J. Orthoped. Trauma* **1,** 12–17.

29. Boxma, H., Broekhuizen, T., Patka, P., and Oosting, H. (1996). Randomised controlled trial of single-dose antibiotic prophylaxis in surgical treatment of closed fractures: the Dutch Trauma Trial. *Lancet* **347,** 1133–1137.

30. Fabian, T. C., Croce, M. A., Payne, L. W., Minard, G., Pritchard, F. E., and Kudsk, K. A. (1992). Duration of antibiotic therapy for penetrating abdominal trauma: a prospective trial. *Surgery* **112,** 788–795.

31. Dellinger, E. P., Wertz, M. J., Lennard, E. S., and Oreskovich, M. R. (1986). Efficacy of short-course antibiotic prophylaxis after penetrating intestinal injury. A prospective randomized trial. *Arch. Surg.* **121,** 23–30.

32. Dellinger, E., Caplan, E., Weaver, L., *et al.* (1988). Duration of preventive antibiotic administration for open extremity fractures. *Arch. Surg.* **123,** 333–339.

33. Dellinger, E. P. (1991). Antibiotic prophylaxis in trauma: penetrating abdominal injuries and open fractures. *Rev. Infect. Dis.* **13**(Suppl. 10), S847–S857.

34. Bozorgzadeh, A., Pizzi, W. F., Barie, P. S., *et al.* (1999). The duration of antibiotic administration in penetrating abdominal trauma. *Am. J. Surg.* **177,** 125–131.

35. Solomkin, J. S., Hemsell, D. L., Sweet, R., Tally, F., and Bartlett, J. (1992). Evaluation of new anti-infective drugs for the treatment of intraabdominal infections. Infectious Diseases Society of America and the Food and Drug Administration. *Clin. Infect. Dis.* **15**(Suppl. 1), S33–S42.

36. Johnson, S. B., MacArthur, R. D., Maki, D., Albertson, T. E., Panacek, E. A., and Black, G. W. (1996). Impact of surgical source control on outcome from gram negative sepsis, Sixteenth Annual Meeting of the Surgical Infection Society, Milwaukee, Wisconsin, April 25–27, 1996, Vol. 16. Surgical Infection Society.

37. Hau, T., Ohmann, C., Wolmershauser, A., Wacha, H., and Yang, Q. (1995). Planned relaparotomy vs relaparotomy on demand in the treatment of intra-abdominal infections. The Peritonitis Study Group of the Surgical Infection Society—Europe. *Arch. Surg.* **130,** 1193–1196; discussion 1196–1197.

38. Bohnen, J. M., Marshall, J. C., Fry, D. E., Johnson, S. B., and Solomkin, J. S. (1999). Clinical and scientific importance of source control in abdominal infections: Summary of a symposium. *Can. J. Surg.* **42,** 122–126.

39. Dellinger, E. P. (1991). Design and evaluation of clinical trials of antimicrobial agents in surgery. *Surg. Gynecol. Obstet.* **172,** (Suppl.), 65–72.

40. Solomkin, J. S., Dellinger, E. P., Christou, N. V., and Mason, A. D., Jr. (1987). Design and conduct of antibiotic trials. A report of the Scientific Studies Committee of the Surgical Infection Society. *Arch. Surg.* **122,** 158–164.

41. Solomkin, J. S., Reinhart, H. H., Dellinger, E. P., *et al.* (1996). Results of a randomized trial comparing sequential intravenous/oral treatment with ciprofloxacin plus metronidazole to imipenem/cilastatin for intra-abdominal infections. The Intra-Abdominal Infection Study Group. *Ann. Surg.* **223,** 303–315.

42. Chalmers, T., Celano, P., Sacks, H., and Smith, H., Jr. (1984). Bias in treatment assignment in controlled clinical trials. *N. Engl. J. Med.* **310,** 24–31.

43. Kunz, R., and Oxman, A. D. (1998). The unpredictability paradox: review of empirical comparisons of randomised and non-randomised clinical trials. *Br. Med. J.* **317,** 1185–1190.

44. Polk, H. C., Jr., and Lopez-Mayor, J. F. (1969). Postoperative wound infection: A prospective study of determinant factors and prevention. *Surgery* **66,** 97–103.

45. Kaiser, A. B., Clayson, K. R., Mulherin, J. L., Jr., *et al.* (1978). Antibiotic prophylaxis in vascular surgery. *Ann. Surg.* **188,** 283–289.

46. Baum, M. L., Anish, D. S., Chalmers, T. C., Sacks, H. S., Smith, H., Jr., and Fagerstrom, R. M. (1981). A survey of clinical trials of antibiotic prophylaxis in colon surgery: Evidence against further use of no-treatment controls. *N. Engl. J. Med.* **305,** 795–799.

47. Berne, T. V., Yellin, A. W., Appleman, M. D., and Heseltine, P. N. (1982). Antibiotic management of surgically treated gangrenous or perforated appendicitis. Comparison of gentamicin and clindamycin versus cefamandole versus cefoperazone. *Am. J. Surg.* **144,** 8–13.

48. A Danish multicenter study. (1984). Cefoxitin versus ampicillin + metronidazole in perforated appendicitis. *Br. J. Surg.* **71,** 144–146.

49. Yellin, A. E., Heseltine, P. N., Berne, T. V., *et al.* (1985). The role of *Pseudomonas* species in patients treated with ampicillin and sulbactam for gangrenous and perforated appendicitis. *Surg. Gynecol. Obstet.* **161,** 303–307.

50. Morris, D. L., Wilson, S. R., Pain, J., *et al.* (1990). A comparison of aztreonam/metronidazole and cefotaxime/metronidazole in elective colorectal surgery: Antimicrobial prophylaxis must include Gram-positive cover. *J. Antimicrob. Chemother.* **25,** 673–678.

51. Makuch, R., and Johnson, M. (1986). Some issues in the design and interpretation of 'negative' clinical studies. *N. Engl. J. Med.* **315,** 91–96.

52. Jones, B., Jarvis, P., Lewis, J. A., and Ebbutt, A. F. (1996). Trials to assess equivalence: the importance of rigorous methods [see comments] *Br. Med. J.* **313,** 36–39 [published erratum appears in *BMJ* **313**(7056), 550].

53. Detsky, A., and Sackett, D. (1986). When was a "negative" clinical trial big enough? How many patients you needed depends on what you found. *N. Engl. J. Med.* **314,** 889–892.

54. Britton, A., McKee, M., Black, N., McPherson, K., Sanderson, C., and Bain, C. (1999). Threats to applicability of randomised trials: Exclusions and selective participation. *J. Health Serv. Res. Policy* **4,** 112–121.

55. Barie, P. S., Vogel, S. B., Dellinger, E. P., *et al.* (1997). A randomized, double-blind clinical trial comparing cefepime plus metronidazole with imipenem-cilastatin in the treatment of complicated intra-abdominal infections. Cefepime Intra-abdominal Infection Study Group. *Arch. Surg.* **132,** 1294–1302.

56. Lau, W. Y., Fan, S. T., Chu, K. W., Suen, H. C., Yiu, T. F., and Wong, K. K. (1985). Randomized, prospective, and double-blind trial of new beta-lactams in the treatment of appendicitis. *Antimicrob. Agents Chemother.* **28,** 639–642.

57. Dellinger, E. P., Wertz, M. J., Meakins, J. L., *et al.* (1985). Surgical infection stratification system for intra-abdominal infection. Multicenter trial. *Arch. Surg.* **120,** 21–29.

58. Solomkin, J. S., Meakins, J. L., Jr., Allo, M. D., Dellinger, E. P., and Simmons, R. L. (1984). Antibiotic trials in intra-abdominal infections. A critical evaluation of study design and outcome reporting. *Ann. Surg.* **200,** 29–39.

59. Christou, N. V., Barie, P. S., Dellinger, E. P., Waymack, J. P., and Stone, H. H. (1993). Surgical Infection Society intra-abdominal infection study. Prospective evaluation of management techniques and outcome. *Arch. Surg.* **128,** 193–198; discussion 198–199.

60. Lennard, E. S., Minshew, B. H., Dellinger, E. P., *et al.* (1985). Stratified outcome comparison of clindamycin-gentamicin vs chloramphenicol-gentamicin for treatment of intra-abdominal sepsis. *Arch. Surg.* **120,** 889–898.

61. Solomkin, J. S., Dellinger, E. P., Christou, N. V., and Busuttil, R. W. (1990). Results of a multicenter trial comparing imipenem/cilastatin to tobramycin/clindamycin for intra-abdominal infections. *Ann. Surg.* **212,** 581–591.

62. Dellinger, E. P. (1988). Use of scoring systems to assess patients with surgical sepsis. *Surg. Clin. North Am.* **68,** 123–145.

63. Meakins, J. L., Solomkin, J. S., Allo, M. D., Dellinger, E. P., Howard, R. J., and Simmons, R. L. (1984). A proposed classification of intra-abdominal infections. Stratification of etiology and risk for future therapeutic trials. *Arch. Surg.* **119,** 1372–1378.

64. Nystrom, P. O., Bax, R., Dellinger, E. P., *et al.* (1990). Proposed definitions for diagnosis, severity scoring, stratification, and outcome for trials on intraabdominal infection. Joint Working Party of SIS North America and Europe. *World J. Surg.* **14,** 148–158.
65. Pocock, S. J., Hughes, M. D., and Lee, R. J. (1987). Statistical problems in the reporting of clinical trials. A survey of three medical journals. *N. Engl. J. Med.* **317,** 426–432.
66. Beam, T. R., Jr., Gilbert, D. N., and Kunin, C. M. (1992). Guidelines for the evaluation of anti-infective drug products. *Clin. Infect. Dis.* **15**(Suppl. 1), S1–S346.
67. Hemsell, D. L., Solomkin, J. S., Sweet, R., Tally, F., and Bartlett, J. G. (1992). Evaluation of new anti-infective drugs for the treatment of acute pelvic infections in hospitalized women. Infectious Diseases Society of America and the Food and Drug Administration. *Clin. Infect. Dis.* **15**(Suppl. 1), S43–S52.
68. Sweet, R. L., Bartlett, J. G., Hemsell, D. L., Solomkin, J. S., and Tally, F. (1992). Evaluation of new anti-infective drugs for the treatment of acute pelvic inflammatory disease. Infectious Diseases Society of America and the Food and Drug Administration. *Clin. Infect. Dis.* **15,** S53–S61.
69. Calandra, G. B., Norden, C., Nelson, J. D., and Mader, J. T. (1992). Evaluation of new anti-infective drugs for the treatment of selected infections of the skin and skin structure. Infectious Diseases Society of America and the Food and Drug Administration. *Clin. Infect. Dis.* **15,** S148–S154.
70. Gorbach, S. L., Condon, R. E., Conte, J. E., Jr., Kaiser, A. B., Ledger, W. J., and Nichols, R. L. (1992). Evaluation of new anti-infective drugs for surgical prophylaxis. Infectious Diseases Society of America and the Food and Drug Administration. *Clin. Infect. Dis.* **15**(Suppl. 1), S313–S338.
71. Platt, R., Munoz, A., Stella, J., *et al.* (1984). Antibiotic prophylaxis for cardiovascular surgery. Efficacy with coronary artery bypass. *Ann. Intern. Med.* **101,** 770–774.
72. Dellinger, E. P., Caplan, E. S., Weaver, L. D., *et al.* (1988). Duration of preventive antibiotic administration for open extremity fractures. *Arch. Surg.* **123,** 333–339.
73. Condon, R. E. (1992). Industry–investigator relationships. *Arch. Surg.* **127,** 765.
74. Dickersin, K., Chan, S., Chalmers, T. C., Sacks, H. S., and Smith, H., Jr. (1987). Publication bias and clinical trials. *Controlled Clin. Trials* **8,** 343–353.
75. Pocock, S. J. (1985). Current issues in the design and interpretation of clinical trials. *Br. Med. J. (Clin. Res. Ed.)* **290,** 39–42.
76. DerSimonian, R., Charette, L. J., McPeek, B., and Mosteller, F. (1982). Reporting on methods in clinical trials. *N. Engl. J. Med.* **306,** 1332–1337.
77. Begg, C., Cho, M., Eastwood, S., *et al.* (1996). Improving the quality of reporting of randomized controlled trials. The CONSORT statement [see comments]. *JAMA* **276,** 637–639.

66

Scoring Systems for Sepsis and the Multiple Organ Dysfunction Syndrome

John C. Marshall

Department of Surgery, University of Toronto, and University Health Network, Toronto, Ontario, Canada M5G 2C4

I. Introduction

A hospital's intensive care unit (ICU) environment generates enormous amounts of often contradictory data. Continuous monitoring systems record changes in physiologic status on a second-to-second basis, and other clinical and laboratory parameters are measured every hour or two. Automated laboratory equipment and standardized ICU protocols result in the measurement of a host of variables whose diagnostic or prognostic significance is unknown. The inherent biologic volatility of critical illness results in the capture of data that are transient, rapidly changing, and, not infrequently, erroneous. The blood pressure that was dangerously low hours ago has now stabilized with a combination of fluids and vasopressors, but the oxygen requirements are increasing. The core temperature is normal, but the white blood cell count is 23,000, and the platelet count is falling. How can we possibly make sense of such a cacophony of discordant information, so that we can characterize the basal state of a patient at the onset of a study, or describe his or her clinical trajectory over time? And how can we reconcile the distinctly individual patterns of homeostatic derangement that occur in the individual patient following a unique threat, so that we can group patient data to frame and answer a research question? A popular albeit imperfect approach to this challenge has been the development of scoring systems.

A scoring system is a quantitative measure of a state or process that is produced by assigning numeric weights to component variables based on their correlation with an outcome of interest. By converting discrete variables to numeric values based on the intervals of the score, a scoring system permits evaluation of the combined influence of a number of factors on a single outcome. Scoring systems have three main uses:

1. Prognostication and severity stratification [for example, Acute Physiology and Chronic Health Evaluation (APACHE) or Simplified Acute Physiology Score (SAPS) as predictors of ICU outcome, Trauma and Injury Severity Score (TRISS) as a predictor of outcome following trauma, or Ranson's criteria as a predictor of outcome in acute pancreatitis].

2. Description of a process at a point in time, or over time [for example, the Therapeutic Intervention Scoring System (TISS) score as a measure of ICU resource utilization, sepsis scores, or the Crohn's disease activity index].

3. Outcome measurement [for example, the Multiple Organ Dysfunction Score (MODS) as a measure of organ dysfunction, or the SF-36 scale as a measure of quality of life].

Scoring systems serve numerous roles in surgical research. An objective composite measure of illness severity at the onset of a study provides information on the nature of the study population, and permits assessment of the baseline comparability of two or more patient groups. Prognostic scores such as APACHE (1, 2) or SAPS (3) yield reproducible mortality estimates; documentation that mortality rates in a study population are similar to those experienced in other groups of patients with similar disease severity increases confidence in the conclusions of the research, and their relevance to the wider world of ICU care.

Generic severity scoring systems can also be used to define entry criteria for a study, eliminating patients who are either too healthy or too ill to benefit from an intervention. Establishing a minimum APACHE score for entry into a trial of antibiotic therapy for intraabdominal infection, for example, will increase the likelihood that patients studied will truly have serious infection (4). Similarly, if we wish to undertake a study of patients with severe pancreatitis, we could define the population of interest as being all patients with three or more Ranson's criteria (5). Finally, a baseline severity score can be used to stratify patients at the outset of a trial, if it is anticipated that the response to therapy might differ in patients with milder or more severe disease (6).

Severity scores are discussed in greater detail elsewhere in this volume. The focus of this chapter is the use of scores as specific descriptors of the clinical syndrome of sepsis, and as measures of the outcome of organ dysfunction or failure in the critically ill patient.

II. Composite Descriptors: Methodologic Principles

The detailed methodologic principles underlying the development of outcome measures are beyond the scope of this chapter, although excellent discussions are available to the interested reader (7). In general terms, however, an outcome measure that will provide interpretable information in clinical research must be valid, responsive, and reliable.

Validity refers to the ability of a variable to actually measure the events or processes that it is purported to measure. Validity is not an absolute property of a measure, but rather a reflection of its performance in several discrete domains. Construct validity is the extent to which a novel variable reflects the process of interest from the perspective of the primary user of the information. For example, the Childs–Pugh classification of cirrhosis reflects disease severity from the perspective of the clinician; however, for the patient with end-stage liver disease, the serum albumin is of far less importance than the impact of the disease on the ability to enjoy life. Thus a valid patient-centered measure of chronic liver disease will reflect functional status in domains such as fatigue, activity, emotional function, abdominal symptoms, systemic symptoms, and worry (8). An aggregate measure of the severity of sepsis might show similar context-dependent validity. A measure of the severity of sepsis viewed from the perspective of cytokine activation would use as its variables the levels of key individual mediators (9). To evaluate the interaction of infection and the host septic response, we developed a sepsis score with variables restricted to clinical manifestations of systemic inflammation (10), whereas other sepsis scores have used variables reflecting both the microbial stimulus and the host response to provide a comprehensive measure of sepsis as the response to infection (11). Maximal construct validity, then, is a matter of perspective, and the investigator must decide whose perspective the measure is to record, based on the nature of the research question being asked.

Content validity refers to the degree to which a measure reflects the entire spectrum of the domain that it is designed to measure. The evaluation of content validity is also dependent on the purposes to which the score is to be applied. APACHE II, for example, would be a less appropriate measure of the physiologic manifestations of sepsis than would a dedicated sepsis score, because its variables include parameters not normally perceived as manifestations of a septic response, including the serum sodium concentration and the hematocrit.

Finally, criterion validity is a measure of the extent to which the new measurement tool correlates with a "gold standard" measure of the domains it is measuring. In assessing the criterion validity of a sepsis score, for example, we could measure its performance against the presence of culture-proved infection, against an expert's clinical assessment that a patient is septic, or against ICU mortality; the selection of the gold standard, in turn, affects the conclusions that can be drawn using the measurement tool.

A responsive measure is one that will detect a clinically important change when such change has occurred, and conversely, will measure stability when no change is occurring.

A reliable measure is one that yields consistent information when applied in differing populations, at different times, and under variable circumstances, and that can reproducibly differentiate subjects of study groups. Responsiveness and reliability reflect the ability of the measure to detect a signal, and to discriminate that signal from the random noise inherent in any study: they evaluate the signal-to-noise ratio of a measurement tool (12).

Outcome measures can be further characterized as discriminative instruments (those developed to differentiate patients or patient groups at a single point in time) and evaluative instruments (those developed to detect longitudinal changes occurring over a period of time) (7). The signal-to-noise ratio of a discriminative instrument can be summarized as a reliability coefficient, whereas that of an evaluative instrument is reflected in a responsiveness coefficient (12).

III. Scoring Systems for Sepsis

Sepsis is defined as the systemic host response to invasive infection (13). It is a complex, common, and important clinical syndrome, yet it is poorly described as a clinical entity. Although there are several published approaches to quantifying sepsis using aggregate scores, none of these scores was developed using rigorous methodologic approaches, and none has emerged as a standard method for grading the severity of sepsis.

The most widely used diagnostic criteria for sepsis that have been used in clinical trials are those of sepsis syndrome: clinical evidence of infection in association with tachycardia of greater than 90/min, tachypnea of greater than 20 breaths per minute (or the need for mechanical ventilation), temperature changes (≤35.6°C or ≥38.3°C), and evidence of altered organ perfusion (14). These criteria were developed by investigators conducting a multicenter randomized trial of the efficacy of high-dose corticosteroids in patients with sepsis (15). They have not been formally evaluated outside the context of a clinical trial, and have been criticized as being both nonspecific and overly exclusive, precluding enrollment of patients who fail to meet the temperature or heart rate criteria, but who otherwise have a clinical diagnosis of sepsis (16). Criteria for the systemic inflammatory response syndrome (SIRS) are more broad-based (Table I), but like those of sepsis syndrome, lack specificity, and describe the majority of patients admitted to an intensive care unit (17). It is noteworthy that clinical trials that have used sepsis syndrome or SIRS criteria have been largely unsuccessful in demonstrating evidence of clinical benefit for novel therapeutic interventions, and there is an emerging consensus that better models are needed to identify patients who might be appropriate candidates for such studies (18, 19).

Table I The Systemic Inflammatory Response Syndrome

Criterion	Measurement
Tachycardia	>90 beats per minute
Temperature	>38.0°C or <36.0°C
Tachypnea	>20 breaths per minute (or mechanical ventilation)
White cell count	<4000/ml or >11,000/ml

Despite the current lack of reliable diagnostic criteria for sepsis as an entity, scoring systems to quantify its severity have helped to shed light on its natural history.

A. The Sepsis Severity Score (Elebute and Stoner)

The first scoring system for sepsis was published in 1983 by Elebute and Stoner (11) (Table II). The score combines descriptors of local infection with blood culture results, changes in temperature and white cell count, and evidence of organ dysfunction. It was developed in a small cohort of 15 patients, and variable selection and weights were derived through the expert judgment of the authors.

The Elebute and Stoner score has been used as a severity of illness measure in a number of studies of sepsis. Dominioni and colleagues (20), for example, showed that a score above 20 was associated with a 92% mortality, although its predictive power was improved by incorporating circulating levels of complement factor B and α1-acid glycoprotein. It has also found use as an objective measure of sepsis severity to define entry criteria for a multicenter study of high-dose IgG: patients with a sepsis score of 20 who were randomized to receive IgG had a significantly lower mortality than did their placebo controls (38 vs. 67%) (21).

B. The Sepsis Score (Marshall and Sweeney)

A different approach to quantifying the severity of sepsis was used by our group. In order to evaluate the interactions of the clinical syndrome of sepsis with the presence of microbiologically documented invasive infection, we undertook a cohort study of 211 consecutive admissions to a surgical ICU (10). Infection was defined using microbiologic, radiographic, and operative criteria, without reference to the clinical manifestations of the patient. Sepsis was quantified by a score evaluating five cardinal manifestations of sepsis—temperature elevation, leukocytosis, changes in mentation, elevation of cardiac output and reduction in systemic vascular resistance, and insulin requirements—without reference to culture data (Table III).

Table II The Sepsis Severity Score of Elebute and Stoner

Local effects of tissue infection	Score	Secondary effects	Score
Wound infection		Jaundice	2
Daily dressing changes	2	Metabolic acidosis	
More frequent changes, suction	4	Compensated	1
Peritonitis		Uncompensated	2
Localized	2	Renal failure	3
Generalized	6	Altered sensorium	3
Chest infection		Bleeding diathesis	3
Clinical/X-ray signs without productive cough	2	Blood culture	
Clinical/X-ray signs with productive cough	4	Single	1
Bronchopneumonia	6	Two or more, or invasive procedure	3
Deep-seated infection	6	Leukocyte count	
Pyrexia (maximal daily temperature)		12–30,000	1
36.0–37.4	0	>30,000	2
37.5–38.4	1	<2500	3
38.5–39.0	2	Hemoglobin	
>39.0 or <36.0	3	7.0–10.0 g/dl	1
Add if		<7.0 g/dl	2
Minimum temperature >37.5°C	1	Platelets	
Two or more peaks >38.4°C	1	100–150,000	1
Rigors	1	<100,000	2
		Albumin	
		31–35 g/liter	1
		25–30 g/liter	2
		<25 g/liter	3
		Bilirubin	
		>25 μmol/liter	1

Discrimination of the relative influences of infection and the host response allowed us to show that survival is influenced by the magnitude of the septic response in infected patients, but that in patients with an exaggerated response, neither the site, the bacteriology, nor even the presence of infection will influence survival status (Fig. 1). Thus the use of a score permitted separation of the microbial and host response components of sepsis, and facilitated an evaluation of the relative importance of each.

Table III The Sepsis Score

Variable	0	1	2	3
Maximum temperature (°C)	<38.0	38.0–38.9	39.0–39.9	≥40.0
White blood cell count (× 10^9/liter)	<12.0	12.0–18.0	18.1–25.0	>25.0
Decrease in Glasgow Coma Score (from baseline)	0	1	2	≥3
Insulin requirements (units/hour)	0	1–2	3	≥4
Cardiac output or systemic	<7.0	7.0–8.9	9.0–10.9	≥11.0
vascular resistance	>800	600–800	400–600	<400

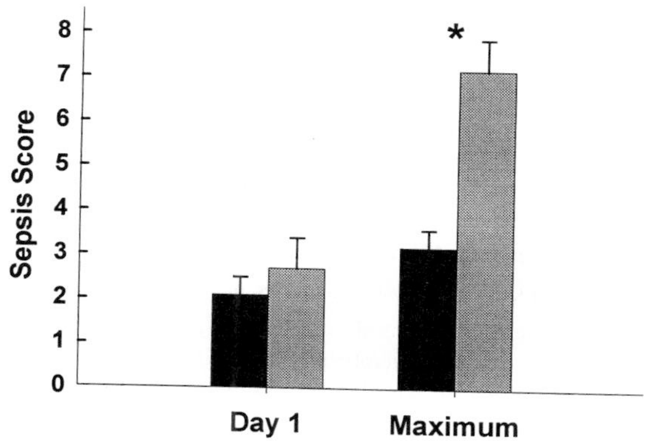

Figure 1 A comparison of sepsis scores in survivors (black bars) and nonsurvivors (shaded bars) among a cohort of 211 critically ill surgical patients. Patients showed similar degrees of clinical sepsis at the time of ICU admission; however, nonsurviving patients had higher maximal sepsis scores. * $p< 0.01$. From Marshall and Sweeney, (10), *Arch. Surg.* (1990) **125**, pp. 17–23. Copyrighted 1990, American Medical Association.

C. The Systemic Inflammatory Response Syndrome Score

Yet another approach to scoring the severity of sepsis has been to use the four criteria for the Systemic Inflammatory Response Syndrome (SIRS) (13) as elements of a score (Table I). Talmor and colleagues (22), for example, used a SIRS score to assess the association of systemic inflammation with adverse outcome in critical surgical illness, and found that SIRS scores were persistently higher in nonsurvivors over the first 7 days of ICU admission, and that a score that remained unchanged or that increased on the second ICU day was associated with increased mortality.

D. Use of Generic Severity Scores to Quantify Severity of Sepsis

Finally, generic severity of illness measures such as SAPS and APACHE II have been used as indices of the severity of sepsis. Gogos and colleagues evaluated the association of circulating cytokine levels with SAPS II scores, and found that the strongest association was between SAPS and the serum concentration of interleukin-10 (23). Versions of SAPS (24) and APACHE (25) customized for patients with sepsis have been developed. These use the variables of the parent score; their major difference lies in the weighting given to the diagnosis of sepsis.

E. Uses of Sepsis Scores

Measures of the severity of sepsis can play a number of roles in ICU-based research. Sepsis scores permit severity stratification at the outset of a study, and provide a basis for discriminating differing levels of risk in subsequent subgroup analyses. They provide a measure of illness severity at baseline, and so permit evaluation of the comparability of two patient populations. They have a largely unexplored role in studies of the natural history of inflammation in critical illness—for example, in evaulating the relationship between clinical inflammation and infection, circulating inflammatory mediators, the development of organ dysfunction or other ICU morbidity, and, ultimately, survival and quality of life. They could also be used to evaluate therapeutic outcomes. An investigator may choose to study whether percutaneous abscess drainage is associated with a lesser degree of sepsis compared to operative drainage, or whether early excision and grafting of burns, or early fracture stabilization, reduce the subsequent severity of the inflammatory response.

IV. Scoring Systems for Multiple Organ Dysfunction Syndrome

The concept that survival in critical illness was determined not by a single disease or event, but rather by multiple physiologic derangements, was first articulated during the 1960s (26, 27); however, it remained for Baue in 1975 to suggest that the concomitant failure of two or more organ systems constituted not only a common pathway to death, but a syndrome that defined the limits of intensive care (28). A spate of largely retrospective studies of the syndrome appeared over the ensuing decades, but it is only quite recently that more formal attempts have been made to measure the syndrome using composite scores.

A. The Multiple Organ Failure Score (Goris)

The first scoring system for multiple organ failure was developed by Goris and colleagues (29) (Table IV). The Goris score measures derangements in seven organ systems—respiratory, cardiovascular, renal, neurologic, hepatic, hematologic, and gastrointestinal—on a scale from 0 to 2, so that the maximum score is 14. It has been quite widely used as an outcome measure in European studies.

B. The Multiple Organ Dysfunction Score

The Multiple Organ Dysfunction (MOD) score (30) is a refinement of a scoring system for organ dysfunction that we originally published in 1988 (31). Its most recent iteration (Table V) involves an explicit developmental process designed to maximize the methodologic rigor of the score (32), using precepts discussed earlier.

The MOD score measures the deranged physiology of organ dysfunction, rather than the clinical interventions used to support failing organs: all of its variables are recorded without consideration of the degree or means of physiologic support. It is designed to reflect stable, postresuscitation

Table IV The Multiple Organ Failure Score (Goris)

System	0	1	2
Pulmonary	No mechanical ventilation	PEEP ≤10; Fi_{O_2} ≤0.40	PEEP >10 ± Fi_{O_2} >0.40
Cardiac	Normal BP	Volume, or dopamine ≤10 μg/kg/min	Dopamine >10 μg/kg/min
Renal	Creatinine <2 mg/dl	Creatinine ≥2.0 mg/dliter	Dialysis
Hepatic	Bilirubin <2 mg/dl; AST <25 U/liter	Bilirubin 2–6 mg/dl; AST 25–50 U/liter	Bilirubin ≥6 mg/dl; AST ≥50 U/liter
Hematologic	Normal WBC, platelets	Platelets <50,000, or WBC 30,000–60,000	Bleeding diathesis, or WBC >60,000 or <2.5
Gastrointestinal	Normal function	Acalculous cholecystitis or stress ulcer	Stress ulcer bleeding >2 units/24 hr; necrotizing enterocolitis, pancreatitis, spontaneous perforation of gall bladder
CNS	Normal function	Diminished responsiveness	Severely disturbed responsiveness or neuropathy

physiology, rather than transient acute derangements in organ function. Because of this, a representative value (usually the first morning value) is recorded daily for each of the six variables in the score; missing data are either imputed normal, or the previous day's value is recorded.

Construct validity was maximized through a systematic review of published organ failure scores that identified 30 published sets of criteria for organ dysfunction/failure (32). Seven organ systems—respiratory, renal, cardiovascular, gastrointestinal, hepatic, hematologic, and neurologic—were included in at least 50% of these, and thus these systems were evaluated for inclusion in the MOD score. The lack of a reliable descriptor variable for the gastrointestinal (GI) system, and the observation that the classic manifestation of gut failure in critical illness—acute erosive gastritis—is becoming uncommon (33), led us to exclude the GI system from the MOD score, leaving six systems in the final score.

Content validity was maximized by developing a list of 12 criteria that defined the optimal descriptor of organ dysfunction, and measuring the performance of candidate variables against these (32). No existing variable that adequately described cardiovascular dysfunction was identified, and therefore we developed a novel descriptor, termed the "pressure-adjusted heart rate" (PAR). The PAR is calculated as the ratio of the central venous pressure (CVP) to mean arterial pressure (MAP), multiplied by the heart rate:

Table V The Multiple Organ Dysfunction Score

Organ system	0	1	2	3	4
Respiratory[a] (PO_2/Fi_{O_2} ratio)	>300	226–300	151–225	76–150	≤75
Renal,[b] serum creatinine					
μmol/liter	≤100	101–200	201–350	351–500	>500
mg/dl	≤1.0	1.1–2.0	2.1–3.5	3.5–5.0	>5.0
Hepatic,[c] serum bilirubin					
μmol/liter	≤20	21–60	61–120	121–240	>240
mg/dL	≤1.0	1.1–3.0	3.1–6.0	6.1–12.0	>12.0
Cardiovascular[d] Pressure-adjusted heart rate (PAR)	≤10.0	10.1–15.0	15.1–20.0	20.1–30.0	>30.0
Hematologic[e] Platelet count/ml	>120	81–120	51–80	21–50	≤20
Neurologic[f] Glasgow Coma Score	15	13–14	10–12	7–9	≤6

[a]The P_{O_2}/Fi_{O_2} ratio is calculated without reference to the use or mode of mechanical ventilation and without reference to the use or level of PEEP.

[b]The serum creatinine level is measured without reference to the use of dialysis.

[c]The serum bilirubin level is measured in μmol/liter or mg/dl.

[d]The pressure-adjusted heart rate (PAR) is calculated as the product of the heart rate and right atrial (central venous) pressure, divided by the mean arterial pressure: PAR = (Heart rate × RAP)/MAP.

[e]The platelet count is measured in platelets/ml × 10^{-3}.

[f]The Glasgow Coma Score in the patient receiving sedation or muscle relaxants is assumed normal unless there is evidence of intrinsically altered mentation.

$$PAR = \frac{\text{Heart rate} \times \text{CVP}}{\text{MAP}}.$$

Similar to the P_{O_2}/Fi_{O_2} ratio to describe pulmonary dysfunction, the PAR is a physiologic measure that reflects the success or failure of therapy. Normal values are less than 10; increasing values reflect increasingly deranged dysfunction. Thus if the heart rate and mean arterial pressure respond normally to fluid challenge, the value of the PAR will remain low; if they do not, it will increase. Similarly, vasoactive agents that cause tachycardia will also increase the value of the PAR.

Finally, criterion validity was maximized by calibrating each variable against ICU mortality. ICU, rather than hospital, mortality was used to reflect the notion that organ dysfunction is synonymous with the need for ICU care. To calibrate the score, the worst daily value for each variable over the ICU stay was recorded, and a 5-point scale (ranging from 0 to 4 points for each) was constructed so that for each variable considered in isolation, a score of 0 reflected normal physiologic function, and was associated with an ICU mortality of less than 5%; a score of 4 was associated with markedly deranged function, and an ICU mortality of greater than 50% (30). Intervening intervals were set to create roughly equal ranges with sensible, whole number boundaries. Calibration was successful for each of the six variables; the association of increasing derangements with ICU mortality for the PAR is illustrated in Fig. 2. The score development and calibration were performed using the first half of a database of 692 surgical patients, and the performance was then evaluated using the second half of the database.

The resulting score has a range from 0 to 24 points; it has been calibrated against the worst value for each variable, and the sum of these—the aggregate MOD score—shows a strong correlation with ICU mortality. Mortality is negligible at a score of 2 or less, and is essentially 100% for a score of greater than 20; a 50% mortality occurs at a score of approximately 12 (Fig. 3).

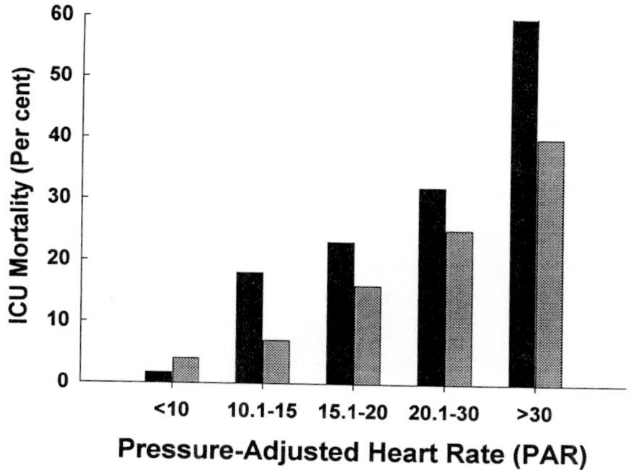

Figure 2 Intervals for the MOD score were established so that 0 represented normal function, and was associated with an ICU mortality of 5% or less; 4 represented severe derangement and an ICU mortality of 50% or more, and the intervening values were whole number, sensible intervals. The graph shows this process for the calibration of the cardiovascular variable, the pressure-adjusted heart rate (see text) in the development (dark bars) and validation (grey bars) sets. From Ref. (30), J. C. Marshall, D. J. Cook, N. V. Christou, G. R. Bernard, C. L. Sprung, and W. J. Sibbald (1995). Multiple organ dysfunction score: A reliable descriptor of a complex clinical outcome. *Crit. Care Med.* **23**, 1638–1652.

C. The Sequential Organ Failure Assessment Score

The Sequential Organ Failure Assessment (SOFA) score was developed using a consensus-based process by an expert committee of the European Society of Intensive Care Medicine in 1994 (34) (Table VI). It measures organ dysfunction in the same six systems as the MOD score, using a 5-point scale. Its major differences lie in the variable used to describe cardiovascular dysfunction (the dose of vasoactive agents administered), its use of urine output as a descriptor for renal dysfunction, and its use of worst, rather than representative, daily values.

D. Modeling Organ Dysfunction for ICU-Based Research

The development of reliable and validated measures of the severity of organ dysfunction provides the ICU-based investigator with new tools to quantify critical illness and to describe its course. Models of potential use in ICU-based research are summarized in Table VII (35).

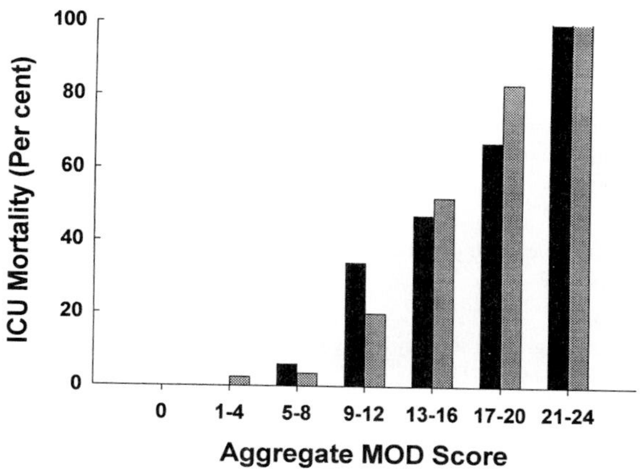

Figure 3 ICU mortality as a function of the aggregate MOD score, created by summing the worst daily values for each organ system over the ICU stay. Development (dark bars) and validation (grey bars) sets. From Ref. (30), J. C. Marshall, D. J. Cook, N. V. Christou, G. R. Bernard, C. L. Sprung, and W. J. Sibbald (1995). Multiple organ dysfunction score: A reliable descriptor of a complex clinical outcome. *Crit. Care Med.* **23**, 1638–1652.

Table VI The SOFA Score

Variable	0	1	2	3	4
Respiration					
Pa_{O_2}/Fi_{O_2} (mmHg)	>400	≤400	≤300	≤200 (with respiratory support)	≤100
Coagulation					
Platelets × 10^3/ml	>150	≤150	≤100	≤50	≤20
Liver					
Bilirubin	<1.2	1.2–1.9	2.0–5.9	6.0–11.9	>12.0
mg/dl mol/liter	<20	20–32	33–101	102–204	>204
Cardiovascular					
Hypotension	No hypotension	MAP <70 mmHg	Dopamine ≤5 dobutamine (any dose)[a]	Dopamine >5 or epinephrine ≤0.1 or norepinephrine ≤0.1[a]	Dopamine >15 or epinephrine >0.1 or norepinephrine >0.1[a]
Central nervous system					
Glasgow Coma Score	15	13–14	10–12	6–9	<6
Renal					
Creatinine	<1.2	1.2–1.9	2.0–3.4	3.5–4.9	>5.0
mg/dl mol/liter	<110	110–170	171–299	300–440	>440
Urine output	—	—	—	<500 ml/day	<200 ml/day

[a]Adrenergic agents administered for at least 1 hr (doses given are in μg/kg/min).

E. MODS as a Baseline Risk Factor and Severity Measure: Admission Scores

The severity of organ dysfunction present at the time of ICU admission is strongly predictive of the ultimate risk of ICU mortality (30, 34, 36). Organ dysfunction scales are not primarily prognostic indices: a valid organ dysfunction scale should fail to predict the demise of a patient who succumbs to an acute myocardial infarction, hypertensive crisis, exsanguinating hemorrhage, or any acute process that is not customarily thought of using the construct of organ dysfunction. Nonetheless, because it has been estimated that 80% or

Table VII Models for the Description of the Outcome of Critical Illness Using the Construct of Organ Dysfunction

Objective	Approach	Uses
To quantify the baseline severity of organ dysfunction	Calculate organ dysfunction score on day of admission (admission MODS)	To establish baseline severity, e.g., for entry criteria for a clinical trial, or to ensure comparability of study groups
To quantify severity of organ dysfunction at a point in time	Calculate score on a particular ICU day (daily MODS)	To determine the intensity of resource utilization, or the evolution or resolution of organ dysfunction at a discrete point in time
To measure aggregate severity of organ dysfunction over ICU stay	Sum the individual worst scores for each organ system over a defined time interval (aggregate MODS)	To determine severity of physiologic derangement over a defined time interval (e.g., ICU stay)
To quantify new organ dysfunction arising following ICU admission	Calculate difference between aggregate and admission scores (Delta MODS)	To measure organ dysfunction attributable to events occurring following ICU admission
To provide a combined measure of morbidity and mortality	Adjust aggregate score so that all patients dying receive maximal number of points (mortality-adjusted MODS)	To create a single measure that integrates impact of morbidity in survivors and mortality for nonsurvivors

more of deaths in a contemporary ICU occur in association with organ dysfunction (37), a measure of the severity of organ dysfunction becomes, by definition, a prognostic measure.

Organ dysfunction scores calculated at the time of ICU admission, or at the time of entry into a clinical study, accomplish several purposes. They provide a composite picture of the severity of organ dysfunction early in the course of illness, and so can serve as entry criteria for a study, and as a tool to ensure comparable severity of illness between study groups. Moreover they can aid in severity stratification, permitting the investigator to exclude patients who are either too well to be at significant risk of a morbid outcome, or too sick to have a reasonable chance of benefiting from therapy.

F. MODS as a Serial Measure of Illness Severity: Daily Scores

Calculation of daily organ dysfunction scores can provide an objective assessment of changes in physiologic status occurring over time. Net clinical improvement or deterioration of a patient or a study population can be followed, and, by tracking the course of individual score components, additional information regarding the nature of the biologic changes associated with clinical improvement can be gleaned. This approach has been used, for example, to demonstrate the impact of pentoxifylline on global organ dysfunction, and on respiratory and cardiovascular dysfunction in a population of septic patients (38), or to compare the clinical courses of survivors and nonsurvivors of ruptured abdominal aortic aneurysms (39) (Fig. 4). Daily scores also provide a measure of the intensity of resource utilization, analogous to the TISS score (40).

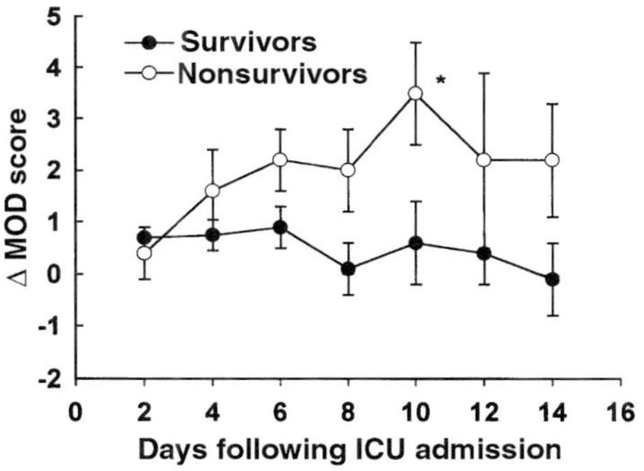

Figure 4 Following rupture of an abdominal aortic aneurysm, nonsurviving patients show progressive deterioration in organ function, whereas survivors show stability or clinical improvement. Divergence of clinical trajectories is apparent over the first week of the ICU stay. From Maziak *et al.* (39), with permission from Springer-Verlag.

G. MODS as a Measure of Morbidity over Time: Aggregate Scores

An aggregate score is calculated by summing the worst daily values for each of the component variables of the score—for example, the respiratory score from day 1, the cardiovascular score from day 3, and the renal score from day 9. An aggregate score provides a measure of the composite morbidity that has developed over a defined time interval such as the ICU stay, or the 28 days of follow-up for a clinical trial. The aggregate score shows the strongest association with ICU mortality (30, 41) (Fig. 3), and so can serve as a sensitive outcome for clinical studies in the ICU (6, 42).

Morbidity over time can be modeled using other approaches. Organ dysfunction can be quantified as serial daily scores, as a cumulative score (daily aggregate scores), as the sum of daily scores, or as the area under the curve over a period of time; the merits of these differing aproaches have not been evaluated.

H. Attributable ICU Morbidity: The Delta Score

The focus of clinical research in the ICU is the understanding and modulation of morbidity arising following ICU admission. Patients are admitted with varying degrees of organ dysfunction; this organ dysfunction has a significant impact on the probability of ultimate survival, but, because it has already occurred, is not amenable to prevention. The clinician, therefore, is interested in preventing *de novo* organ dysfunction, and in hastening the resolution of existing dysfunction. This component of ICU attributable morbidity can be measured by calculating a delta score—the difference between the aggregate score and the admission score. Delta scores correlate well with survival (30, 41, 43) and are able to detect clinically important differences in treatment effect in clinical trials (6).

I. Aggregate Measures of Morbidity and Mortality: The Mortality-Adjusted Score

Finally, morbidity and mortality can be combined into a single quantitative outcome measure by calculating mortality-adjusted organ dysfunction scores and assigning a maximal number of points to patients who die over the study interval and the measured number of points to survivors. The mortality adjustment can also be used with the delta score; because the use of a mortality outcome results in a skewed data distribution, differences must be evaluated using nonparametric statistics.

V. Limitations in the Use and Interpretation of Scores

It is important to realize that the use of a scoring system does not provide the investigator with new information, but only allows combining existing data into a more useful format. The apparent objectivity of a numeric score can provide a patina of authority that obscures its limitations, and it is therefore important for the investigator to understand these.

First, the demonstration of an association between increasing score severity and mortality merely confirms that the score is measuring severity; it does not provide any information about causality, nor does it imply a plausible relationship between the score and the clinical problem to which it is being applied. A hypothetical score that includes, for example, age, degree of baldness, serum glucose, EKG evidence of S-T elevation, and CT findings of liver metastases will show a graded association with mortality, but clearly provides no useful information about any particular disease process. It has been suggested, for example, that the clinical syndrome of SIRS demonstrates measurable progression from mild to severe forms, suggesting that early preemptive therapy may alter outcome (44). However, an alternative interpretation of these data is that it will, on average, take longer to demonstrate the presence of four rather than two criteria, because of the inherent delay in compiling the data.

The presence of shared variables between two scores may also create an artifactual impression of association. SIRS, for example, would be expected to be associated with the development of organ dysfunction, because the tachypnea and tachycardia included in the SIRS criteria are also manifestations of the respiratory and cardiovascular dysfunction that is measured by an organ dysfunction score.

Finally, both random and systematic error can be introduced into a score during the recording of the component varaibles. Random error will result from the limitations of the raw measures, and from errors in transcribing and recording data. Systematic error can arise from differences in the frequency of measurement, from differences in the calibration of measuring devices between centers, and from differing approaches to calculation of scores. These sources of error render comparisons of centers difficult, unless the potential for artifact is recognized and explicit steps are taken to minimize it.

VI. Conclusions

Severity of illness measures such as APACHE and SAPS have become integral components of the design and implementation of ICU-based research. Specific measures of sepsis and organ dysfunction can provide additional tools for the investigator, and can aid in studies of biology, natural history, and therapy. However, the use of such measures is in its infancy. Further refinement of the scores and of the techniques used to apply them should increase their utility in the future.

References

1. Knaus, W. A., Draper, E. A., Wagner, D. P., and Zimmerman, J. E. (1985). APACHE II: A severity of disease classification system. *Crit. Care. Med.* **13,** 818–829.
2. Knaus, W. A., Wagner, D. P., Draper, E. A., Zimmerman, J. E., Bergner, M., Bastos, P. G., Sirio, C. A., Murphy, D. J., Lotring, T., Damiano, A., and Harrell, F. E. (1991). The APACHE III prognostic system. Risk prediction of hospital mortality and critically ill hospitalized adults. *Chest* **100,** 1619–1636.
3. Le Gall, J.-R., Lemeshow, S., and Saulnier, F. (1993). A new simplified acute physiology score (SAPS II) based on a European/North American multicenter study. *JAMA* **270,** 2957–2963.
4. Solomkin, J. S., Reinhart, H. H., Dellinger, E. P., Bohnen, J. M., Rotstein, O. D., Vogel, S. B., Simms, H. H., Hill, C. S., Bjornson, H. S., Haverstock, D. C., Coulter, H. O., and Echols, R. M. (1996). Results of a randomized trial comparing sequential intravenous oral treatment with ciprofloxacin plus metronidazole to imipenem cilastatin for intra-abdominal infections. *Ann. Surg.* **223,** 303–315.
5. Luiten, E. Jt., Hop, W. C. J., Lange, J. F., and Bruining, H. A. (1995). Controlled clinical trial of selective decontamination for the treatment of severe acute pancreatitis. *Ann. Surg.* **222,** 57–65.
6. Hebert, P. C., Wells, G., Blajchman, M. A., Marshall, J., Martin, C., Pagliarello, G., Tweeddale, M., Schweitzer, I., Yetisir, E., and the Transfusion Requirements in Critical Care Investigators for the Canadian Critical Care Trials Group (1999). A multicentre randomized controlled clinical trial of transfusion requirements in critical care. *N. Engl. J. Med.* **340,** 409–417.
7. Guyatt, G. H., Feeny, D. H., and Patrick, D. L. (1993). Measuring health-related quality of life. *Ann. Intern. Med.* **118,** 622–629.
8. Younossi, Z. M., Guyatt, G., Kiwi, M., Boparai, N., and King, D. (1999). Development of a disease specific questionnnaire to measure health related quality of life in patients with chronc liver disease. *Gut* **45,** 295–300.
9. Casey, L. C., Balk, R. A., and Bone, R. C. (1993). Plasma cytokines and endotoxin levels correlate with survival in patients with the sepsis syndrome. *Ann. Intern. Med.* **119,** 771–778.
10. Marshall, J. C., and Sweeney, D. (1990). Microbial infection and the septic response in critical surgical illness. Sepsis, not infection, determines outcome. *Arch. Surg.* **125,** 17–23.
11. Elebute, E. A., and Stoner, H. B. (1983). The grading of sepsis. *B. J. Surg.* **70,** 29–31.
12. Guyatt, G. H., Kirshner, B., and Jaeschke, R. (1992). Measuring health status: What are the necessary measurement properties? *J. Clin. Epidemiol.* **45,** 1347–1351.
13. Bone, R. C., Balk, R. A., Cerra, F. B., Dellinger, R. P., Fein, A. M., Knaus, W. A., Schein, R. M. H., and Sibbald, W. J. (1992). ACCP/SCCM Consensus conference. Definitions for sepsis and organ failure and guidelines for the use of innovative therapies in sepsis. *Chest* **101,** 1644–1655.
14. Bone, R. C., Fisher, C. J., Clemmer, T. P., Slotman, G. J., Metz, C. A., Balk, R. A., and The Methylprednisolone Severe Sepsis Study Group (1989). Sepsis syndrome: A valid clinical entity. *Crit. Care Med.* **17,** 389–393.
15. Bone, R. C., Fisher, C. J., Clemmer, T. P., Slotman, G. J., Metz, C. A., and Balk, R. A. (1987). A controlled clinical trial of high dose methyl-

prednisolone in the treatment of severe sepsis and septic shock. *N. Engl. J. Med.* **317,** 654–658.
16. Sibbald, W. J., Marshall, J. C., Christou, N. V., Girotti, M. J., McCormack, D. G., Rotstein, O. D., Martin, C., and Meakins, J. L. "Sepsis"—Clarity of existing terminology ⋯ or more confusion? *Crit. Care Med.* **19,** 996–998.
17. Vincent, J. L. (1997). Dear SIRS, I'm sorry to say that I don't like you. *Crit. Care Med.* **25,** 372–374.
18. Marshall, J. C. (1999). Rethinking sepsis: From concepts to syndromes to diseases. *Sepsis* **3,** 5–10.
19. Abraham, E., Matthay, M. A., Dinarello, C. A., Vincent, J. L., Cohen, J., Opal, S. M., Glauser, M., Parsons, P., Fisher, C. J., Jr., and Repine, J. E. (2000). Consensus conferences definitions for sepsis, septic shock, acute lung injury, and acute respiratry distress syndrome: Time for a re-evaluation. *Crit. Care Med.* **28,** 232–235.
20. Dominioni, L., Dionigi, R., Zanello, M., Monico, R., Cremaschi, R., Ballabio, A., Massa, M., Comelli, M., Dal Ri, P., and Pisati, P. (1987). Sepsis score and acute phase protein response as predictors of outcome in septic surgical patients. *Arch. Surg.* **122,** 141–146.
21. Dominioni, L., Dionigi, R., Zanello, M., Chiaranda, M., Dionigi, R., Acquarolo, A., Ballabio, A., and Sguotti, C. (1991). Effect of high-dose IgG on survival of surgical patients with sepsis scores of 20 or greater. *Arch. Surg.* **126,** 236–240.
22. Talmor, M., Hydo, L., and Barie, P. S. (1999). Relationship of systemic inflammatory response syndrome to organ dysfunction, length of stay, and mortality in critical surgical illness: Effect of intensive care unit resuscitation. *Arch. Surg.* **134,** 81–87.
23. Gogos, C. A., Drosou, E., Bassaris, H. P., and Skoutelis, A. (2000). Pro- versus anti-inflammatory cytokine profile in patients with severe sepsis: A marker for prognosis and future therapeutic options. *J. Infect. Dis.* **181,** 176–180.
24. Le Gall, J.-R., Lemeshow, S., Leleu, G., Klar, J., Huillard, J., Rue, M., Teres, D., Artigas, A., and the Intensive Care Unit Scoring Group (1995). Customized probability models for early severe sepsis in adult intensive care patients. *JAMA* **273,** 644–650.
25. Knaus, W. A., Harrell, F., Fisher, C. J., *et al.* (1993). The clinical evaluation of new drugs for sepsis: A prospective study design based on survival analysis. *JAMA* **270,** 1233–1241.
26. Maclean, L. D., Mulligan, W. G., Mclean, A. P. H., and Duff, J. H. (1967). Patterns of septic shock in man—A detailed study of 56 patients. *Ann Surg.* **166,** 543–562.
27. Skillman, J. J., Bushnell, L. S., Goldman, H., and Silen, W. (1969). Respiratory failure, hypotension, sepsis, and jaundice. A clinical syndrome associated with lethal hemorrhage and acute stress ulceration in the stomach. *Am. J. Surg.* **117,** 523–530.
28. Baue, A. E. (1975). Multiple, progressive, or sequential systems failure. A syndrome of the 1970s. *Arch. Surg.* **110,** 779–781.
29. Goris, R. J. A., te Boekhorst, T. P. A., Nuytinck, J. K. S., and Gimbrere, J. S. F. (1985). Multiple organ failure. Generalized autodestructive inflammation? *Arch. Surg.* **120,** 1109–1115.
30. Marshall, J. C., Cook, D. J., Christou, N. V., Bernard, G. R., Sprung, C. L., and Sibbald, W. J. (1995). Multiple organ dysfunction score: A reliable descriptor of a complex clinical outcome. *Crit. Care Med.* **23,** 1638–1652.
31. Marshall, J. C., Christou, N. V., Horn, R., and Meakins, J. L. (1988). The microbiology of multiple organ failure. The proximal GI tract as an occult reservoir of pathogens. *Arch. Surg.* **123,** 309–315.
32. Marshall, J. C. (1995). Multiple organ dysfunction syndrome (MODS). *In* "Clinical Trials for the Treatment of Sepsis" (J. W. Sibbald and J.-L. Vincent, eds.), pp. 122–138. Springer-Verlag, Berlin.
33. Cook, D. J., Fuller, H., Guyatt, G. H., Marshall, J. C., Leasa, D., Hall, R., Winton, T., Rutledge, F., Royy, P., and Willan, A. (1994). Risk factors for gastrointestinal bleeding in critically ill patients. *N. Engl. J. Med.* **330,** 377–381.
34. Vincent, J. L., Moreno, R., Takala, J., Willatts, S., De Mendonca, A., Bruining, H., Reinhart, K., Suter, P., and Thijs, L. G. (1996). The sepsis-related organ failure assessment (SOFA) score to describe organ dysfunction/failure. *Intens. Care Med.* **22,** 707–710.
35. Marshall, J. C. (1999). Charting the course of critical illness: Prognostication and outcome description in the intensive care unit. *Crit. Care Med.* **27,** 676–678.
36. Le Gall, J. R., Klar, J., Lemeshow, S., Saulnier, F., Alberti, C., Artigas, A., and Teres, D. (1996). The logistic organ dysfunction system—A new way to assess organ dysfunction in the intensive care unit. *JAMA* **276,** 802–810.
37. Deitch, E. A. (1992). Multiple organ failure. Pathophysiology and potential future therapy. *Ann. Surg.* **216,** 117–134.
38. Staubach, K. H., Schröder, J., Stüber, F., Gehrke, K., Traumann, E., and Zabel, P. (1998). Effect of pentoxifylline in severe sepsis. Results of a randomized, double-blind, placebo-controlled study. *Arch. Surg.* **133,** 94–100.
39. Maziak, D. E., Lindsay, T. F., Marshall, J. C., and Walker, P. M. (1998). The impact of multiple organ dysfunction on mortality following ruptured abdominal aortic aneurysm repair. *Ann. Vasc. Surg.* **12,** 93–100.
40. Keene, A. R., and Cullen, D. J. (1983). Therapeutic intervention scoring system: Update 1983. *Crit. Care Med.* **11,** 1–3.
41. Moreno, R., Vincent, J. L., Matos, R., Mendonca, A., Cantraine, F., Thijs, L., Takala, J., Sprung, C., Antonelli, M., Bruining, H., and Willatts, S. (1999). The use of maximum SOFA score to quantify organ dysfunctio/failure in intensive care. Results of a prospective, multicentre study. *Intens. Care Med.* **25,** 686–696.
42. Sloan, E. P., Koenigsberg, M., Gens, D., Cipolle, M., Runge, J., Mallory, M. N., and Rodman, G., Jr. (1999). Diaspirin cross-linked hemoglobin (DCLHb) in the treatment of severe traumatic hemorrhagic shock: A randomized controlled efficacy trial. *JAMA* **282,** 1857–1864.
43. Jacobs, S., Zuleika, M., and Mphansa, T. (1999). The multiple organ dysfunction score as a descriptor of patient outcome in septic shock compared with two other scoring systems. *Crit. Care Med.* **27,** 741–744.
44. Rangel-Frausto, M. S., Pittet, D., Costigan, M., Hwang, T., Davis, C. S., and Wenzel, R. P. (1995). The natural history of the systemic inflammatory response syndrome (SIRS): A prospective study. *JAMA* **273,** 117–123.

67

Cytokine Biology

Rebecca M. Minter, Frank J. Wessels, and Lyle L. Moldawer

Department of Surgery, University of Florida College of Medicine, Gainesville, Florida 32610

I. Introduction

The field of cytokine biology is rapidly expanding, as are its applications to surgical disease. The roles played by cytokines in the development of inflammation in processes such as wound healing, ischemia/reperfusion injury, and the development of septic shock are only now being fully appreciated. Cytokine biology is infiltrating all aspects of surgical science as it becomes evident that these mediators are intimately involved in the inflammatory response. With the current sequencing of the human genome, the number of cytokines discovered has increased dramatically. For example, there are at least 15 members of the tumor necrosis factor α (TNFα) superfamily known to date (1), and the number of chemokines in the interleukin-8 superfamily has passed 20 (2). More importantly, as our understanding of cytokine biology has progressed, we have become more successful in employing cytokines and cytokine inhibitors as biological response modifiers. The use of interferon-α/β (IFN) in chronic hepatitis C infections (3), erythropoietin for end-stage renal disease-induced anemia (4), and granulocyte colony-stimulating factor (G-CSF) for chemotherapy-induced neutropenia (5) are just three examples of how cytokine therapies have revolutionized treatment regimens for their respective diseases.

In addition, as our understanding of cytokine biology has increased concordant with the development of molecular biology, newer approaches in modifying cytokine activity have developed. For example, studies from our laboratory have demonstrated that the extracellular domains of specific cytokine receptors are often shed from the cell surface (6, 7). Once released into the extracellular compartment, these soluble cytokine receptors can bind to and neutralize the cytokine, preventing it from triggering a receptor-mediated response. These soluble receptors then act as specific inhibitors of their respective cytokine ligand. Recombinant DNA technology has fused these extracellular domains to the Fc and hinge regions of human immunoglobulin and created chimeric "immunoadhesins" with the pharmacodynamics of an antibody, but with the specificity of receptor binding. Immunoadhesins directed against TNFα, interleukin-1 (IL-1), and interferon-γ have been developed (8–10), and the anti-TNFα immunoadhesin developed by Immunex Inc. has been approved for use in patients with rheumatoid arthritis.

Immunoadhesins and antibodies are just two examples of anticytokine-based therapies. The study of cytokine biology has also revealed how some cytokines can counteract the action of other cytokines. This takes advantage of the property that the synthesis of most proinflammatory cytokines is tightly regulated at the level of gene transcription, and they often induce the synthesis of other cytokines that act in an allosteric manner to suppress their synthesis. For example, cytokines such as interleukin-10 (IL-10) inhibit the synthesis of more proximal cytokines such as TNFα and IL-1, and in so doing, act primarily as antiinflammatory agents and/or immunosuppressants. These cytokines have been explored as possible therapeutic modalities for patients in whom suppression of inflammation and/or the immune response is desirable. Other examples include TGF-β, IL-6, IL-13, and IL-4.

These anticytokine-based therapies as well as the administration of exogenous, bioactive cytokines such as IFN-γ, G-CSF, and erythropoietin have been the subject of many phase II and phase III clinical trials in recent years. A better understanding of the complex interactions between pro- and antiinflammatory cytokines, chemokines, acute-phase proteins, glucocorticoids, and the innate and acquired immune system is critical if we hope to develop effective therapies in the future for inflammatory diseases.

II. Cytokine Response to Inflammation

With the recent explosion in the number of identified cytokines, it is recognized that cytokines can rarely be classified according to their biologic function. Rather, most cytokines have overlapping, pleiotropic biologic activities, dependent on what other cytokines and mediators are present in the milieu at that time. What is generally agreed on, however, is that cytokines are protein messengers that convey information between and within cells via specific receptor molecules. Furthermore, cytokines signal to immune and somatic tissues the presence of inflammation, and in doing so, regulate key components of the innate and acquired immune responses.

Cytokine signaling can occur in an endocrine, paracrine, autocrine, and/or juxtacrine fashion, dependent on the cytokine and the current environment in which the cytokine is produced (Table I). This is an important consideration when attempting to measure cytokines in biologic fluids, such as the blood, bronchoalveolar lavage, or cerebrospinal fluid. Some cytokines do behave in a primarily endocrine fashion, but they are a distinct minority. Interleukin-6 (IL-6) is a good example of a cytokine that can act in a typical stress-induced, endocrine fashion. IL-6 can be readily detected in the plasma in a variety of inflammatory conditions, and concentrations usually reflect disease severity and prognosis (11–13). Distant inflammatory processes stimulate the release of IL-6, and on entry into the systemic circulation IL-6 induces a glucocorticoid and hepatic acute-phase protein response (14–16) following binding to specific receptor complexes in the liver (17) and via the hypothalamic–pituitary–adrenal axis. We demonstrated that in response to a local inflammatory challenge produced by a turpentine abscess, local production of IL-1 stimulated the release of IL-6, which acted in an endocrine fashion to produce anorexia and stimulate an hepatic acute-phase response (18, 19). IL-1 could not be detected in the circulation whereas IL-6 levels increased concomitant with the induction of the acute-phase protein response. IL-10 is another cytokine whose plasma concentrations are labile and appear to increase with the severity of the inflammatory insult (20). In this case, plasma appearance of IL-10 plays a significant role in the development of a systemic compensatory antiinflammatory response that is commonly seen in sepsis syndromes (21, 22).

In both these cases, the cytokines routinely found in the circulation during inflammatory processes are those that function primarily to regulate gene expression in a specific organ, such as induction of the hepatic acute-phase protein response by IL-6, or act globally to suppress an acquired immune response, such as IL-10. However, most cytokines act more in a local or immediate microenvironment, and are not usually detected in the circulation. The proinflammatory cytokines IL-1, TNFα, and IL-8 are examples of cytokines that function primarily in this paracrine and autocrine fashion, acting on immediately neighboring cells or on the same cells that produce them, respectively. Additionally, IL-1 and TNFα can be found expressed on the membranes of cells, and can act in a juxtracrine fashion by signaling via cell–cell contact. Cytokines such as IL-1 and TNFα, which act primarily in a paracrine and juxtacrine manner, are only

Table I Patterns of Cytokine Signaling

Cytokine signaling	Definition	Example
Autocrine	Cytokine self-signaling	IL-2-induced proliferation of T lymphocytes
Juxtacrine	Cytokine signaling via cell-to-cell contact	Membrane-associated TNFα-mediated killing of tumor cells by $CD8^+$ T cells
Paracrine	Signaling in local tissue microenvironment	IL-8 recruitment of neutrophils into a wound environment
Endocrine	Distant signaling	IL-6 induction of a hepatic acute-phase response

occasionally detected in the systemic circulation. The systemic appearance of these cytokines may occur when their local production is actually within the vasculature, or when there is excessive production of these cytokines within tissue compartments, with escape of the cytokine into systemic circulation. The former occurs when either endotoxin or live gram-negative or gram-positive bacteria are administered intravenously (23, 24). In this case, the rapid and transitory appearance of cytokines is due in part to the local production by inflammatory cells in the blood as well as by the vascular endothelium. However, even in these examples when the stimulus is intravascular, the bulk of cytokine appearance appears to be from organs and tissues, with release into the systemic circulation. For example, Fong and Lowry demonstrated that following an intravenous endotoxin administration in human volunteers, 40% of the TNFα that appeared in the systemic circulation was derived from the splanchnic bed (23). In infections derived from a single nidus, as may occur in early adult respiratory distress syndrome, the concentrations of proinflammatory cytokines in the local inflamed compartment (the bronchoalveolar lavage fluid in this case) are often 100- to 1000-fold higher than the concentrations in the plasma compartment (25).

Structurally, cytokines are small proteins, usually ranging in size from 5 to 50 kDa. Active forms of the cytokine may exist as individual monomeric cytokine proteins (interleukin-1β) (26, 27), homodimers (IL-8, IL-10) (28–30) or homotrimers (TNFα) (31, 32), or even higher oligomers (platelet factor-4, PF-4). Though unusual, some cytokines are also active as heteromers, such as lymphotoxin (TNFβ) and interleukin-12 (33). Most cytokines are rendered inactive by enzymatic degradation, which further confirms the essential nature of their three-dimensional structure in their spatial interactions with their receptors. Because of their complexity in secondary and tertiary structures, interpreting measurements of their concentration is frequently difficult. This is particularly true for heterodimeric cytokines such as IL-12, which are composed of hetero- and homodimeric complexes of p35 and p40 proteins. Enzyme-linked immunosorbent assays (ELISAs), which recognize only the p40 protein, for example, may not be able to distinguish between the biologically active p70 heterodimer and p40 homodimers, which may actually be receptor antagonists (34, 35).

Cytokines produce their biologic activities by binding to specific, high-affinity receptors on the exterior surface of target cells. These interactions are often complex and may require receptor-associated proteins that either increase the responsiveness of a cell to its ligand (as in the case of IL-1 and IL-1 receptor-associated protein) or are absolutely required for signal transduction (as in the case of IL-6, the IL-6 receptor, and gp130). Thus, the mere presence of a cytokine does not necessarily indicate the responsiveness of a cell. The biologic response to a cytokine is dependent on the concentration of the ligand, the presence of protein cofactors that may either serve as receptor antagonists or as ligand passers, and the number and dissociation constants of the receptors. The number of a particular receptor type on a cell's surface is usually quite low, ranging from 100 to 1000 receptor molecules per cell. The binding affinity of cytokine ligands for their receptors is usually quite high, with dissociation constants (K_d) ranging from 10^{-9} to 10^{-12} M (nanomolar to picomolar). Structurally, most cytokine receptors (and other receptors) consist of three distinct structural and functional domains, as demonstrated in Fig. 1. Considerable structural and functional heterogeneity exists among cytokine receptor families; however, discussion of these variations is well beyond the scope of this chapter.

The number of cell surface receptors for cytokines is regulated by their expression and by internalization and proteolytic cleavage from the cell surface. This is a critical point for analytical efforts to detect cytokines or their receptors in biologic fluids. Many cytokine receptors, such as those in the TNFα, Fas ligand (CD95/Apo 1), and IL-6 familes, can undergo proteolytic cleavage from the cell surface by a class of matrix metalloproteases or disintegrins/adamolysins (36). These enzymes, which may also be cell associated (37), cleave the receptor at specific sites, and yield a biologically and immuologically active peptide. This shedding of the extracellular domain of cellular receptors serves to reduce the cell's responsiveness to the cytokine, and additionally the shed receptor maintains its ability to bind the specific cytokine and modulate its biologic activities (6, 7). These shed receptors can act as both natural inhibitors or facilitators of the cytokine ligand's action, as demonstrated in Fig. 2.

Cytokine signaling ultimately defines the innate and acquired immune responses that develop during an inflammatory process. The innate immune response does not require antigen specificity as the acquired immune system does. The innate immune response is the first line of defense against invading microbes, and is a multiorgan system effort by the host to decrease tissue injury and cell death, promote recovery of the host, and reduce the likelihood of secondary or opportunistic infections (38). The innate immune response is a rapid but less efficient antimicrobial system that is aimed at containing microbial pathogenesis until the more specific acquired immune response develops. Cytokines serve as the primary communicators of the innate immune response, and additionally define the nature of the developing acquired immune response. TNFα, IL-1, and IL-6 are three cytokines that appear to play important roles in initiating and regulating the innate immune response, and in development and propagation of the acquired immune responses. IL-1 is a comitogen for T lymphocytes, TNFα propagates the T helper cell type 1 (TH1), and IL-6 is a growth factor for B lymphocytes. As demonstrated in Fig. 3,

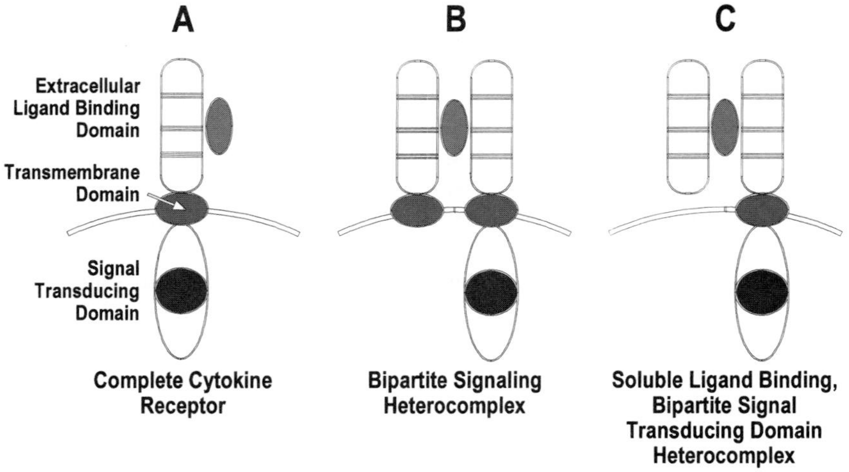

Figure 1 Schematic structure of cytokine receptors. Cytokine receptors are characterized by an extracellular ligand binding domain, a transmembrane domain, and an intracellular signaling domain. A single receptor may possess all three domains (A), may be composed of a bipartite cell membrane-associated ligand binding domain heterocomplexed to a signal transducing domain (B), or may be composed of a soluble ligand binding domain complexed to a receptor containing a binding domain, a transmembrane domain, and a signal transducing domain (C). From Dinarello and Moldawer (35a). Reprinted with permission of Amgen Inc. All other rights reserved to Amgen Inc.

the overlap in functions of TNFα, IL-1, and IL-6 emphasizes the tight interrelationship of the innate and acquired immune responses.

In surgery-related disciplines, catastrophic consequences can develop from the inappropriate activation of the innate immune system, as is seen in overwhelming bacteremia or endotoxemia. Exaggerated production of TNFα, IL-1, and other proinflammatory cytokines leads to vascular collapse, shock, and death (39–41). Similarly, it is now recognized that persistent activation of the innate immune system occurs in several chronic inflammatory processes, such as a chronic nonhealing wound, inflammatory bowel disease,

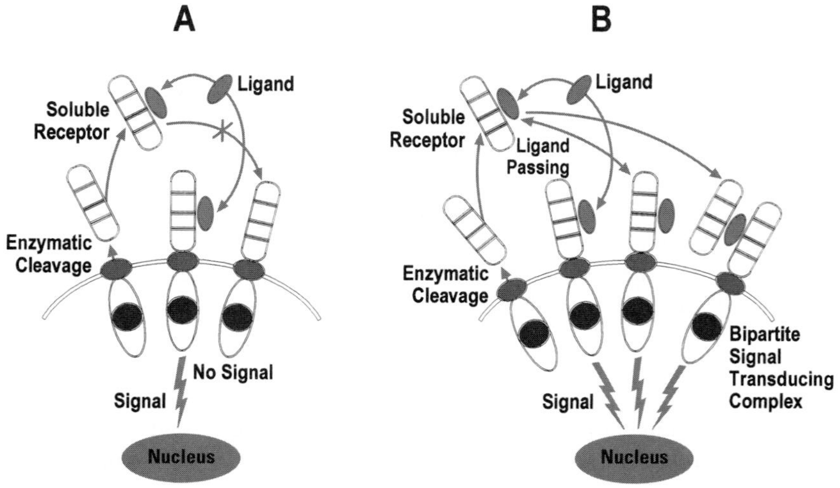

Figure 2 Shedding of cytokine receptors. The extracellular domain of several cytokine receptors can be cleaved enzymatically and released into the extracellular space. The extracellular domain retains ligand binding capability, and the soluble receptor can act either as an inhibitor by preventing ligand binding to the cellular receptor (A) or as a ligand passer by delivering the ligand to the receptor or to its bipartite signal transduction complex (B). From Dinarello and Moldawer (35a). Reprinted with permission of Amgen Inc. All other rights reserved to Amgen Inc.

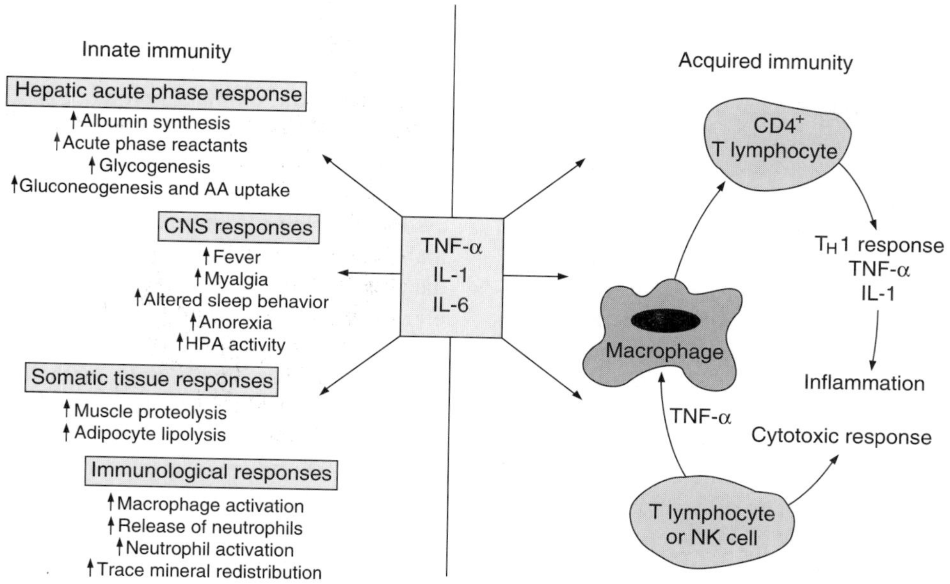

Figure 3 TNFα, IL-1, and IL-6 regulation of innate and acquired immunity. TNFα, IL-1, and IL-6 play central roles in the communication between innate and acquired immunity. Produced by a variety of cells of both lymphoid and myeloid lineage, as well as by somatic tissues, these cytokines play pivotal roles in the induction of the innate immune response as well as in determining the magnitude and nature (TH1 vs. TH2) of the acquired immune response. From Dinarello and Moldawer (35a). Reprinted with permission of Amgen Inc. All other rights reserved to Amgen Inc.

and rheumatoid arthritis. These are appropriate target areas for anticytokine-based therapies.

Although the innate immune response is relatively inflexible, the acquired immune response is infinitely adaptive, allowing the host fine control over its responses to a variety of specific pathogens. Large numbers of cytokines are required to achieve the expansion, differentiation, and activation of diverse populations of effector cells that are involved in the acquired immune response. For example, interleukin-2 drives the activation, proliferation, and differentiation of naive T cells into armed effector T cells. IL-2 is produced by activated T cells and acts in an autocrine fashion. The differentiation of native $CD4^+$ T cells into an armed TH1 or TH2 cells is primarily determined by the cytokines present during the initial T cell proliferation phase of activation. A predominantly TH1 response, or cell-mediated immune response, is dominated by macrophage activation and production of TNFα, IL-1, and IL-18. Production of these proinflammatory cytokines is induced by stimulation of T cells in the presence of IL-12 and IFN-γ. Additionally, IFN-γ inhibits the TH2 cell development. In contrast, stimulation of naive T cells in the presence of IL-4, IL-6, and IL-10 leads to a predominantly TH2, or humoral, immune response. IL-6 and interleukin-11 directly stimulate the differentiation of plasma cells, whereas IL-4 and IL-10 inhibit the generation of TH1 cells. This balance between cytokine signals determines the overall pattern of the acquired immune response to invading pathogens, as well as autoimmune disease.

III. Exogenous Delivery of Cytokines

Much of the early work to identify the functions of individual cytokines was based on an experimental approach. A purified or recombinant cytokine was administered to an animal and its biologic response was determined. Such studies were inherently straightforward from a methodological point of view, but interpretation of results was often complex and misleading. Before the molecular biology revolution in the mid-1980s, initial studies were conducted with only partially purified proteins. The cytokine nomenclature was not yet established and investigators were exploring biologic responses to crude protein preparations with functional monikers such as "leukocyte pyrogen," "leukocyte endogenous mediator," "lymphocyte activating factor," "catabolin," and "osteoclast activating factor" (all original names given to IL-1, prior to its isolation) (42). Because these protein preparations were not pure, interpretation of results was complicated by the lack of any working knowledge of the specific activity of the preparations, synergistic or antagonistic actions of contaminating proteins, or nonspecific responses to administration of large amounts of foreign proteins. Furthermore, because many of the proinflammatory cytokines share overlapping biologic functions, it became evident that one investigator's "leukocyte pyrogen" could be structurally different from another's. One classic example of this confusion was the original finding of Clowes and Baracos that IL-1-like products of activated peripheral blood mononuclear cells could stimulate skeletal muscle protein catabolism (43, 44). These studies were conducted with partially purified preparations thought to contain primarily IL-1, and the studies clearly showed that this product of activated leukocytes was responsible for the increased protein degradation. However, when studies were conducted with recombinant IL-1 or TNFα, similar results could not be obtained (45). In fact, these studies have in general not been repeated with any recombinant protein to date. Clearly, activated leukocytes produce mediators that either alone or in combination can stimulate protein degradation, but they resist identification at the present time.

In many ways, the molecular biology revolution in the 1980s solved the problems associated with biologically derived material. With cloning and the development of both prokaryotic and eukaryotic expression systems, recombinant protein became readily available, and the incertitudes associated with using biologically derived material became a problem of the past.

However, with the ready availability of recombinant proteins came a wealth of experimental studies in which recombinant derived cytokine was administered to healthy and diseased animals, and to human volunteers and hospitalized patients. The importance of these studies should not be underemphasized. Much of what we have learned about the functions of individual cytokines has been obtained from simple and straightforward studies in which recombinant proteins have been administered to a rodent, and a response is observed. However, interpretation of such studies is often more complex than the data obtained. In fact, in some very notable cases, data obtained from studies in which recombinant protein has been administered have been misleading.

Prior to administration of a recombinant or exogenous cytokine to an animal, several considerations must be addressed regarding study designs. These are summarized in Tables II and III. Some of these considerations are merely technical, but others address more fundamental aspects of cytokine biology. Along technical issues, one must ensure that the cytokine being delivered has species specificity for the animal being studied. Human IL-10 (hIL-10), for example, is bioactive in both mice and humans, but mIL-10 is bioactive only in the mouse (46–48). Conversely, human and mouse IFN-γ are active only in their respective species. Recombinant hTNFα is bioactive in both mice and humans, although hTNFα binds only to the type I TNFα receptor in mice (49, 50), whereas, murine TNFα signals through both mouse type I and type II receptors. In fact, this differential responsiveness between human and mouse TNFα has been exploited by several groups to distinguish responses due to TNF signaling through the type I and type II receptors.

Other technical considerations exist. Recombinant cytokines tend to be sticky and adhere readily to plastic and glass surfaces. Because of their high specific activity and affinity for their receptors, frequently only small quantities of protein are administered. With recombinant cytokines, carrier proteins that are biologically inactive and reduce nonspecific adherence must frequently be used, especially when the concentration of the administered cytokine is less than 1.0 μg/ml. Any biologically inactive protein can be used, and albumin has been frequently used in the past. In our rodent studies, we routinely use 0.1% normal mouse or rat serum as a carrier protein source when we administer small quantities of recombinant cytokine. We have generally not recommended using albumin or other purified carrier proteins unless it can be assured that they are endotoxin free.

Table II Technical Considerations for Administration of Cytokines to Animals

Is there species specificity for the cytokine to be administered?

How will the cytokine be administered? Intraperitoneally, intravenously? Is the technician skilled at the procedure?

What will the cytokine be diluted in?
- Has it been thawed repeatedly? Has it been stored appropriately?
- Is it diluted in pH-neutral solutions? Avoid low or high pH, detergents, reducing agents
- Has a carrier protein been used to avoid protein adherence to glass or plastic? Avoid purified proteins that are not assuredly endotoxin-free

Is the dose appropriate?

Table III Theoretical Considerations for Administration of Cytokines to Animals

What is the normal physiologic state of the cytokine *in vivo*? What are the usual peak levels and concentrations of the cytokine in the disease state being studied?

What is the half-life of the cytokine being delivered *in vivo*?

What does and when should the cytokine be delivered to ensure that peak cytokine levels occur at the desired time point?

Typically, following intravenous or intraperitoneal delivery, high peak levels are seen early on, followed by slowly decreasing tissue and plasma levels

Is systemic or targeted delivery more appropriate? Targeted delivery can be achieved using delivery systems such as intradermal, intrathecal, and intratracheal administration

Are the biological responses being measured direct or indirect effects of the cytokine being delivered?

Proteins obtained from commercial sources are often contaminated with trace amounts of endotoxin, which can lead to misleading results. However, we have used intravenous albumin or immunoglobulin preparations from the hospital pharmacy, which are United States Pharmacopeia recognized and endotoxin reduced. It should be recognized, however, that these are human proteins and they will elicit an immune response in rodents or other species if studied over several days. For these reasons, we have generally recommended using normal serum from the species being studied, and of course using equivalent amounts of normal serum in the control or placebo-treated groups.

Because cytokines are proteins, they are susceptible to degradation by substances or processes that destroy their tertiary structure. These include repeated freeze–thaw cycles, dissolution in low- or high pH solutions, reducing agents such as dithiothreitol, ionic detergents such as sodium dodecyl sulfate, or bacterial contamination. Most of our cytokines are stored in sterile physiologic saline at 4°C, or at −70°C. We routinely aliquot our stock solutions in small vials that can be thawed a single time and then stored in a sterile manner at 4°C.

Investigators should also be aware that administration of recombinant proteins to the mouse and rat by intravenous challenge may elicit some stress response independent of the administered protein. We and others have shown that psychologic stress alone can induce an IL-6 and acute-phase protein response (51), which can either accentuate or attenuate responses to the recombinant protein. This is frequently the case when recombinant proteins are intravenously administered to a mouse or rat by someone who is not fully experienced with the procedure. The temptation is to use intraperitoneal administrations as an alternative, because they are less stressful and require less technical skill. However, caution should be used when interpreting data from intraperitoneal injections, because there is clearly a local response by the peritoneal cavity to the administered cytokine, and first-pass effects may be seen when the protein is absorbed and circulated through the portal or lymphatic systems.

Additionally, some cytokines have dose-dependent activities. Human IL-10 has been shown to have profound antiinflammatory effects at lower doses, whereas higher levels of human IL-10 have actually caused inflammation (52, 53).

Although these technical hurdles can be overcome, studying cytokine biology by administering recombinant protein has several conceptual limitations that often need to be considered (Table III). Frequently, we administer cytokines not as therapeutic agents, but to recapitulate the local production of cytokines by their exogenous administration. However, replicating endogenous production with exogenous administration is not possible for most cytokines. Intravenous or intraperitoneal administration of a recombinant cytokine is a purely nonphysiologic state. The early peak in concentration is frequently much greater than the peak concentration seen in most disease processes. For example, administering TNFα or IL-1 to produce shock and hypotension in an otherwise healthy animal results in plasma concentrations almost three logs higher than peak levels seen in rodents and primates administered live bacteria (24, 54, 55), and five to six logs higher than the plasma concentrations in patients dying from septic shock (56, 57). The plasma or tissue concentration of these cytokines is also rapidly changing, generally decreasing as a function of time. The responses seen to exogenous administration of a cytokine are therefore an integration of the responses to a very brief period of high exposure followed by a much longer period when concentrations are low and declining. Therefore, knowledge regarding the half-life of the cytokine *in vivo* is a critical piece of information, if available. If this is known it will help plan the dose and timing of the administration to ensure that peak cytokine levels coincide with tissue injury.

However, even with this knowledge, it must be recognized that because many cytokines are primarily paracrine agents, systemic administration is a nonphysiologic approach. As discussed previously, a large majority of cytokine activities take place at the local level within a tissue compartment. Tissue concentrations are frequently logs higher than systemic levels. Therefore, trying to induce lung injury, for example, by targeted delivery to the lung of a proinflammatory cytokine such as IL-8 may be more desirable than systemic delivery. It is also important to note, however, that even with targeted delivery systems such as intradermal, intrathecal, and intratracheal approaches, the problem of non-steady-state concentrations after a single administration is not obviated.

Multiple delivery modes are possible and all should be explored prior to carrying out the experiment. Some alternative approaches have been to use osmotic minipumps, time-release matrices, or extending the half-life of the protein by pegylation, but many of these are limited by the need for some surgical intervention.

There are two additional limitations associated with protein administration as a means to assess the functions of individual cytokines. The first is that it is frequently not possible to discriminate between biologic responses that are directly attributable to the administered cytokine from those secondary responses that are the result of the subsequent endogenous expression of other cytokines. This has been particularly a problem for many of the proximal proinflammatory cytokines such as TNFα and IL-1, which are potent inducers of downstream cytokines such as IL-6 and IL-8. For example, we have shown that in primates, both IL-1 and TNFα induce hypotension, similar changes in leukocyte kinetics, and an acute-phase protein response (55, 58). However, TNFα is a potent inducer of IL-1, and both IL-1 and TNFα induce IL-6. Thus, it becomes very difficult to ascribe specific functions to TNFα when its effects may be due ultimately to the IL-1 or IL-6 response. Although these results do not negate the value of learning the response to exogenous TNFα administration, such an analytical approach makes it difficult to distinguish direct and indirect effects.

More problematic is how we interpret the results. Ultimately, the goal of these studies is to better understand how individual cytokines contribute to physiologic and pathologic responses, and how as physician-scientists the responses can be modified by cytokine or anticytokine therapies. Thus, studies that have examined how an animal (whether healthy or sick) responds to an exogenously administered cytokine fail to consider the interactions among different cytokines and the endocrine milieu in which cytokines act. They can only illuminate a fraction of the complexity of cytokine biology *in vivo*. It is naive to consider on our part that the response of a sick animal to an endogenously produced cytokine will be similar to the response of a healthy or similarly sick animal to exogenous administration, without determining it experimentally. Thus, this approach, even when optimally designed and performed, only gives a partial and incomplete understanding of cytokine biology.

With that said, however, it is clear that studies using the delivery of exogenous cytokines have given way to a much better understanding of cytokine biology *in vivo*. The administration of recombinant TNFα to a healthy organism recapitulates the physiologic and cytokine responses to endotoxemic or bacteremic shock, including the release of IL-1, IL-6, IL-8, IL-10, p55, p75, and IL-1 receptor antagonist (IL-1ra) (54, 59–63). A great deal of information about IL-1 has been learned from studies in which primates and human subjects were injected with recombinant IL-1α and IL-1β (55). Preclinical studies suggested that IL-1 could play a role in the recovery from bone marrow suppression after chemotherapy; therefore, the infusion of IL-1 was evaluated in human clinical trials in patients who were neutropenic secondary to anticancer chemotherapy. Though there was no reduction in tumor size, increased bone marrow recovery was reported with IL-1 treatment (64). However, in patients receiving IL-1 for bone marrow stimulation, even at low doses on the order of 30–50 ng/kg, all patients developed fever, hypotension, and profound flulike symptoms (64). Additionally, the data from this trial provided information about the potential for IL-1 to induce myalgia, headache, and loss of appetite, which could not be obtained from animal trials. The exquisite sensitivity of humans to systemic administration of IL-1 was also not appreciated in animal studies.

IV. Inhibition of Cytokine Production or Action

Much of what we know today about the functions of individual cytokines has come from studies in which the actions of individual cytokines have been either blocked or inhibited. We have used the term "anticytokine therapies" broadly to refer to therapeutic approaches that can either suppress the synthesis of cytokines, block their posttranscriptional processing, or inhibit their actions. Corticosteroids are an example of an inhibitor of cytokine gene transcription, matrix metalloproteases (for TNFα processing) or caspase-1 inhibitors (for IL-1β or IL-18) are examples of inhibitors of cytokine processing, and monoclonal antibodies are an example of an inhibitor of cytokine action. These "anticytokine therapies" can be generally subdivided further into two approaches, general or specific. General approaches are aimed at blocking the actions of broad classes of cytokines rather than a single cytokine. Corticosteriods are a classic example of a general approach, and they have long been the mainstay of antiinflammatory therapies for several disease processes. Table IV lists some examples of general cytokine inhibitors. In addition, antiinflammatory cytokines such as IL-10, TGF-β, and IL-13 have been employed as nonspecific inhibitors of proinflammatory cytokines. However, the nonspecific nature of steroids or these antiinflammatory cytokines, which target broad biologic mechanisms for inflammation, rather than specific proinflammatory cytokines, can result in unwanted effects such as suppressed T cell function. Naturally occurring IL-4, IL-10, IL-11, IL-13, and TGF-β act to inhibit the transcription and translation of proinflammatory chemokines and cytokines. IL-10 infusion in humans results in a marked suppression of endotoxin-induced IL-1α, TNFα, IL-6, and IFN-γ production (65, 66). Although the precise pathways of action differ among

Table IV Inhibitors of Cytokine Function

Type of inhibitor	Example
General cytokine inhibitor	Corticosteroids
Antiinflammatory cytokines	IL-4, IL-10, IL-11, IL-13, and TGF-β
Inhibitors of cytokine processing	Caspase-1 inhibitors (YVAD), TNFα converting enzyme inhibitor (matrix metalloproteinase inhibitors)
Specific inhibitors of cytokine function	Monoclonal antibodies, soluble receptors, and receptor antagonists

each of the antiinflammatory cytokines, their net effect is the nonspecific reduction of TNFα, IL-1β and IFN-γ levels. Each of the antiinflammatory cytokines possesses other distinct biologic properties, with IL-4, IL-10 and IL-13 acting as B cell growth factors, TGF-β acting as a stimulant of matrix formation, and IL-11 acting as a platelet growth factor and stimulant of hepatic acute-phase protein synthesis. The inherent lack of specificity of these antiinflammatory agents often results in a narrow therapeutic window. This is in contrast to the cytokine-specific modalities (such as IL-1ra and TNFα monoclonal antibodies), which demonstrate a clear dose-dependent therapeutic response and are generally not accompanied by toxicities or side effects associated with increased administration.

Experimental approaches aimed at blocking the biologic effects of singular proinflammatory cytokines include monoclonal antibodies, soluble receptors, and receptor antagonists (see Table IV). Monoclonal antibodies have been generated against TNFα, IL-6, and IL-8, and function by directly binding these cytokines, and thus preventing receptor signaling. Monoclonal antibodies have also been developed against cytokine receptors, the only concern being that some of these receptors have shown agonist rather than antagonist properties. In fact, some of the early monoclonal antibodies developed against the TNF receptors proved to be useful tools as specific receptor agonists (67). Early monoclonal antibodies against TNFα were manufactured from murine immunoglobulins and potentiated immunogenic responses in patients. Newer preparations and advances in genetic engineering have reduced these risks by creating chimeric and humanized proteins that appear to have reduced immunogenicity. Given parenterally, monoclonal antibodies against TNFα have been found to reduce the effects of TNFα-mediated processes. Preclinical studies have demonstrated effectiveness in murine and primate models for endotoxic shock (68), inflammatory bowel disease (69), acute pancreatitis (70), and graft-versus-host-disease (71). Clinical trials with anti-TNFα antibodies demonstrate the most utility in inflammatory bowel disease (72, 73) and rheumatoid arthritis (74), and are currently in development for congestive heart disease.

Receptor Binding Proteins and Receptor Antagonists

One of the most significant advances in the development of specific cytokine inhibitors was the realization that the shed receptors for cytokines maintained their ability to bind ligand and could inhibit the cytokine action. The advantage of this approach was that the specificity of the soluble receptors for their ligand was comparable to monoclonal antibodies, but because the proteins were endogenously produced, they were frequently nonimmunogenic. We were the first to demonstrate that administration of soluble TNF receptors prevents TNFα binding and resultant bioactivity *in vivo*, which could protect animals from TNFα-mediated pathology (7). However the relatively short half-life of these native monomeric proteins required large infusions continuously, and precluded their clinical applications.

There have been two different approaches employed to circumvent the relatively short half-life of these shed receptors. The first has been to create soluble receptor immunoadhesins, which combine the ligand binding specificity of the receptor with the pharmacokinetics and intravascular delivery of an antibody. Immunoadhesins composed of the extracellular domains of the two major TNF receptors (TNF-RI and TNF-RII) exhibit greater affinity and neutralization capacity for TNFα than either monomeric soluble receptors or monoclonal antibodies (75, 76). Unfortunately, clinical trials in sepsis using both TNF immunoadhesins have failed to reveal significant survival benefit (77, 78), whereas these agents have been greatly successful in the treatment of rheumatoid arthritis (79).

An alternative approach has been to employ polyethylene glycol. Polyethylene glycol bound to soluble TNF receptors effectively extends their biological half-life from 20–30 min to almost 2 days (80). These proteins have proved effective in reducing TNFα-mediated injury in primates and rodents (80, 81).

Another example of a specific cytokine inhibitor is the IL-1 receptor antagonist (IL-1ra). Identified *in vivo* and later cloned into a recombinant molecule, IL-1ra is structurally similar to IL-1α and IL-1β, and competitively binds to the type I IL-1 receptor (IL-1RI). However, with IL-1ra binding, there is no subsequent recruitment of IL-1 receptor accessory protein (IL-1rap). Unlike with IL-1α binding to the type I receptor, the net result is a lack of IL-1 receptor-associated kinase recruitment and subsequent absence of IL-1 signal transduction (82). IL-1ra thus acts to block IL-1α and IL-1β binding and subsequent signal transduction. Studies in healthy humans have found that even at doses a 1,000,000-fold greater than IL-1α or IL-1β, IL-1ra acts without agonist activity (83, 84). A number of animal models have demonstrated that IL-1ra reduces the proinflammatory actions of IL-1 and thus the severity of disease. Specifically, studies have found that transgenic mice overexpressing IL-1ra were resistant to lethal effects of endotoxin while expressing markedly attenuated IL-6 and hepatic acute-phase protein response to turpentine abscess (85, 86). Similarly, transgenic mice deficient in IL-ra showed increased mortality with endotoxin injection and turpentine abscess.

To better understand the effects of anticytokine therapy in endotoxemia and sepsis, soluble TNF and IL-1 receptors, and IL-1ra, were administered to healthy human subjects prior to intravenous challenge with low-dose endotoxin. Although the endotoxin model does not represent a pure cytokine model because endotoxin has its own receptors and may induce inflammatory responses distinct from the cytokine production, certain components mimic the systemic inflammatory response syndrome. IL-1ra and soluble IL-1 receptors did not reduce fever or systemic symptoms (87–89). TNF-RII immunoadhesin administration resulted in blunted increases in tissue plasminogen activator, von Willebrand factor, and plasminogen activator inhibitor-1 without affecting thrombocytopenia (90).

V. Measuring Cytokine Expression and Activities

Accurate measurement of cytokines in blood and tissues depends on many factors, including sample collection technique, the presence of natural agonists and antagonists, and determination of the bound versus free state of the cytokine. Multiple assays exist for the measurement of cytokines, and it is important to recognize the pitfalls of each, and to always use appropriate controls.

The systemic levels of some cytokines may have predictive value for patient outcome (91), and therefore an accurate measurement of blood levels of cytokines is critical. It is important to note that plasma (clotting factors present) and serum (clotting factors absent) can have differing physicochemical properties that affect the performance of an immunoassay or bioassay. These potential differences must be vigorously explored in the development of the assay. In considering optimal sample collection, one should take all possible steps to avoid *ex vivo* cytokine secretion from lymphocytes and monocytes in the blood sample. Some commercially available blood collection tubes are contaminated with endotoxin and significant quantities of cytokines can be produced *ex vivo* in under 2 hr if blood is left at room temperature (92, 93). Currently, for immunoassays, we recommend that blood be drawn into a tube containing an anticoagulant (preferably EDTA); immediately centrifuge the blood at 0–4°C and separate the plasma from the cells. This should minimize *ex vivo* cytokine secretion (92, 94–96). EDTA is the preferred anticoagulant for immunoassays because it reportedly inhibits TNFα production in the blood collection tube if there is contamination (92, 95). When performing bioassays, however, EDTA can inhibit cell function and is therefore contraindicated. Heparinized plasma or serum should be used for bioassays and care should be taken to use collection tubes that are endotoxin free. Additionally, the blood should be processed as quickly as possible.

The presence of specific binding proteins for cytokines in the plasma can dramatically alter the cytokine level measured by a particular assay. There are several types of naturally existing binding proteins in plasma, including IgG autoantibodies, α_2-macroglobulin, and soluble receptors that are shed from a cell's surface (97). The concentration of these various binding proteins fluctuates in inflammatory and diseased states, and in fact the levels of soluble shed receptors in the plasma have been used to follow the progression of disease.

Cytokine measurements can be divided into two broad categories: assays based on a biologic response (bioassays) and assays based on the immunologic detection of peptides (immunoassays) (98, 99). Immunoassays rely on at least one antibody that has specificity for the cytokine being measured, and the immunoassay may be in the form of either a radioimmunoassay (RIA) or an enzyme-linked immunosorbent assay. ELISAs have an advantage over RIAs in that they do not require radioactivity and can be read using a 96-well ELISA plate reader, which can be directly interfaced with a computer. One advantage of immunoassays over bioassays is that many are available commercially, and therefore it is not necessary to maintain cell lines or prepare multiple reagents. In addition, many immunoassays use monoclonal antibodies, which have exquisite specificity. One potential disadvantage of immunoassays, however, is that the antibody will recognize only a small portion of the total protein and will possibly measure a degraded fragment of the protein rather than the biologically active material. Additionally, many immunoassays will detect cytokines that are bound to inhibitory substances that render them biologically inactive and maintain them in the circulation for a prolonged period of time (99). This has historically been a problem for the ELISA detection of TNFα. Many of the commercial ELISAs for TNFα cannot distinguish circulating TNFα that has been bound to its soluble receptors. Results obtained with that ELISA give only an estimate of free TNFα. In contrast, we developed two different ELISAs for TNFα, one that could detect TNFα regardless of its bound state, and another that could detect only free TNFα (100). This was based on epitope mapping, and utilizing antibodies that either recognized a region of the TNFα molecule that was blocked during binding to its shed receptor, or a region that remains exposed even when bound to soluble TNFRI and TNFRII. By employing both ELISAs, we could simultaneously determine total and free TNFα, data that were complementary and that provided a more detailed description of not only the total appearance of TNFα, but also its physical state.

Bioassays require that some measure of biologic activity be recorded, such as cell lysis or proliferation. Therefore, cell lines must usually be maintained in order to perform these assays. Similar to ELISAs, these assays can be performed in 96-well plates and read on an automated plate reader, which facilitates the collection of data. Bioassays are often more sensitive than immunoassays, yet may lack their specificity. For example, the thymocyte proliferation assay (lymphocyte activation factor) has been used in the past to measure IL-1. It has since been shown that these cells also respond to TNFα, IL-2, IL-6, and IL-10, and therefore this assay does not provide a very accurate measure of IL-1 levels (99). Similarly, the B9 proliferation assay for IL-6 also responds to other members of the superfamily, including IL-11, LIF, and CNTF. Even the WEHI 164 clone 13 assay, which is highly specific for TNFα, will respond to lymphotoxin or TNFβ. In order to address the lack of specificity in a bioassay, it is best to utilize a cell line that responds only to the cytokine being measured. Recognizing that cytokines that have yet to be identified could be responsible for the response in a bioassay, it is best to repeat positive samples using a neutralizing antibody specific for the cytokine in question. This provides the best confirmation that the cytokine has been measured and obviates some of the difficulties associated with the use of bioassays. Bioassays measure only the cytokine that is biologically active; they do not measure degraded cytokine proteins or cytokines bound to inhibitors in the plasma or serum.

There is controversy in the field of cytokine biology regarding whether immunoassays or bioassays are superior for the detection of cytokines. Some investigators argue that only bioassays should be used, because it is the biological activity of the cytokine that is important, not just the presence of the cytokine. Other investigators feel that the total amount of cytokine should be measured because it will measure the total immune response (99). Additionally, it is argued that cytokine production is pulsatile, and measuring the total cytokine present (using an immunoassay) is more likely to produce positive results because the cytokine will be present for longer periods of time. Figure 4 demonstrates the differing levels of a cytokine that can be measured over time for both an immunoassay and a bioassay. As shown, the bioassay detects early production of the cytokine, but these levels drop off as endogenous inhibitors are produced, even though the cytokine may still be present. Conversely, the immunoassay seems to detect much higher levels of the cytokine for longer periods of time, but these levels represent total cytokine levels in the plasma or serum, which may represent protein bound to shed receptors or protein that is otherwise inactive.

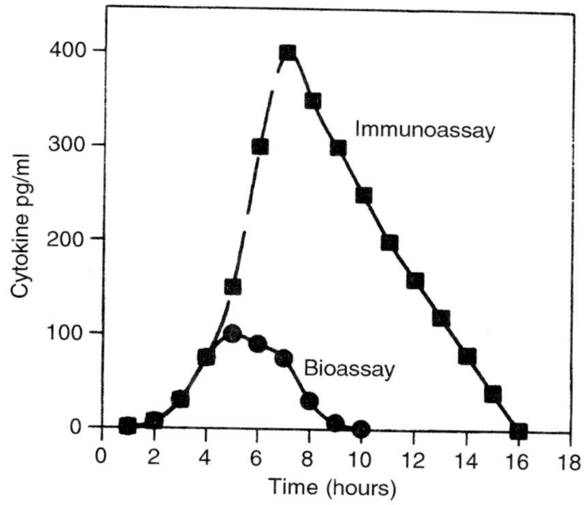

Figure 4 Comparison of immunoassays and bioassays. The immunoassay will generally detect more of the cytokine than will the bioassay, but the cytokine may not be biologically active. With permission, from Ref. (37a), D. G. Remick (1995). Cytokines: A primer for plastic surgeons. *Ann. Plast. Surg.* **35,** 549–559.

Currently, there is not one ideal method for measuring cytokine levels and activity. We can expect that there will be development of better assays as our understanding of cytokine biology increases. In the interim, it is important to understand the various pitfalls associated with the different assays that currently exist, and to strive to find the most appropriate assay for the cytokine being studied. Once this assay is identified, there should be consistent methodology and use of appropriate positive and negative controls.

A brief comment should also be made regarding efforts to detect cytokine mRNA expression. One of the major arguments proposed in this review is that many cytokines are paracrine in nature, and it is often desirable to examine rates of expression in individual tissues or cells rather than blood concentration. Protein levels in tissues can be frequently criticized because of blood contamination and compartmentalization of cytokine between blood, interstitial fluids, and cell-associated proteins. Although a general review of the merits of different approaches to measure mRNA levels is well beyond the scope of this chapter, there are some pertinent points that require discussion. Firstly, Northern analyses and reverse transcription and polymerase chain reactions (RT-PCR) measure only the presence and relative amounts of cytokine mRNA. It is tempting to extrapolate these measurements to rates of expression, but such an effort would be fallacious. A major issue regarding steady-state levels of cytokine mRNA that needs to be considered is the presence of AU sequences in the 3′ untranslated region of cytokine mRNA. These repetitive units appear to promote the degradation of the mRNA and often account for the short half-life of cytokine mRNA. Nuclear run-on and run-off experiments are required to determine rates of expression and half-life.

With those comments made, mRNA levels can be of importance to the understanding of cytokine expression in specific tissues. We have had some difficulty using Northern analyses for detecting TNFα mRNA levels in organs from rodents after inflammation (101). The problem appears to rest with the relatively low abundance of TNFα mRNA in organs where inflammatory cells are a minor component. Although Northern analyses have proved effective for quantitating cytokine mRNA expression in cells and cell lines, we have also employed a PCR-based approach. Another approach that has been successfully employed is the nuclease protection assay.

Once again, a critical discussion of the use of RT-PCR for quantitating cytokine mRNA levels in tissues is well beyond the scope of this chapter, but several points should be considered. RT-PCR is generally a poor technique to quantitate mRNA levels, and is best employed when the presence or absence of a cytokine mRNA is being determined. With that said, however, we have used RT-PCR semiquantitatively, and have gone to considerable lengths to assure that the amount of starting material and the number of PCR cycles were chosen so that the amplicon product was linear to the amount of starting mRNA (102). Other approaches to obtain some quantitative data for mRNA levels have been to use a competitive RT-PCR, using internal Mimics. In some regards, the recent development of Real-Time RT-PCR using the TaqMan technology (Perkin-Elmee/Cetus, Norwalk, CT) has made this argument moot. It should be recognized, however, that the startup costs and learning curve for Real-Time RT-PCR can be considerable.

VI. Conclusion

Our current knowledge of cytokines and their receptors is the product of decades of research by literally hundreds of investigators. Several cytokines and many of their receptors are now well characterized as molecular entities. The roles of many of these cytokines in maintaining health have been described, and increasingly their actions and interactions in the pathogenesis of disease have been defined. However, despite this large body of knowledge, there is often difficulty in translating therapeutic findings to humans from mice and nonhuman primates. Current and future investigators will continue to explore and unravel the complexities of cytokine biology and their role in human disease.

References

1. Bazzoni, F., and Beutler, B. (1996). The tumor necrosis factor ligand and receptor families *N. Engl. J. Med.* **334,** 1717.
2. Taga, T., and Kishimoto, T. (1997). Gp130 and the interleukin-6 family of cytokines. *Annu. Rev. Immunol.* **15,** 797.
3. Lawrence, S. P. (2000). Advances in the treatment of hepatitis C. *Adv. Intern. Med.* **45,** 65.
4. Henry, D. H., and Spivak, J. L. (1995). Clinical use of erythropoietin. *Curr. Opin. Hematol.* **2,** 118.
5. Johnston, E. M., and Crawford, J. (1998). Hematopoietic growth factors in the reduction of chemotherapeutic toxicity. *Semin. Oncol.* **25,** 552.
6. Pruitt, J. H., Welborn, M. B., Edwards, P. D., Harward, T. R., Seeger, J. W., Martin, T. D., Smith, C., Kenney, J. A., Wesdorp, R. I., Meijer, S., Cuesta, M. A., Abouhanze, A., Copeland, 3rd, E. M., Giri, J., Sims, J. E., Moldawer, L. L., and Oldenburg, H. S., (1996). Increased soluble interleukin-1 type II receptor concentrations in postoperative patients and in patients with sepsis syndrome. *Blood* **87,** 3282.
7. Van Zee, K. J., Kohno, T., Fischer, E., Rock, C. S., Moldawer, L. L., and Lowry, S. F. (1992). Tumor necrosis factor soluble receptors circulate during experimental and clinical inflammation and can protect against excessive tumor necrosis factor alpha *in vitro* and *in vivo. Proc. Natl. Acad. Sci. U.S.A.* **89,** 4845.
8. Ashkenazi, A., Marsters, S. A., Capon, D. J., Chamow, S. M., Figari, I. S., Pennica, D., Goeddel, D. V., Palladino, M. A., and Smith, D. H. (1991). Protection against endotoxic shock by a tumor necrosis factor receptor immunoadhesin. *Proc. Natl. Acad. Sci. U.S.A.* **88,** 10535.
9. Pitti, R. M., Marsters, S. A., Haak-Frendscho, M., Osaka, G. C., Mordenti, J., Chamow, S. M. and Ashkenazi, A. (1994). Molecular and biological properties of an interleukin-1 receptor immunoadhesin. *Mol. Immunol.* **31,** 1345.
10. Means, R. T., Jr., Krantz, S. B., Luna, J., Marsters, S. A., and Ashkenazi, A. (1994). Inhibition of murine erythroid colony formation *in vitro* by interferon gamma and correction by interferon receptor immunoadhesin. *Blood* **83,** 911.
11. Hack, C. E., De Groot, E. R., Felt-Bersma, R. J., Nuijens, J. H., Strack Van Schijndel, R. J., Eerenberg-Belmer, A. J., Thijs, L. G., and Aarden, L. A. (1989). Increased plasma levels of interleukin-6 in sepsis [see comments]. *Blood* **74,** 1704.
12. Robak, T., Gladalska, A., Stepien, H., and Robak, E. (1998). Serum levels of interleukin-6 type cytokines and soluble interleukin-6 receptor in patients with rheumatoid arthritis. *Mediators Inflamm* **7,** 347.
13. Holt, I., Cooper, R. G., and Hopkins, S. J. (1991). Relationships between local inflammation, interleukin-6 concentration and the acute phase protein response in arthritis patients. *Eur. J. Clin. Invest.* **21,** 479.
14. Mastorakos, G., Chrousos, G. P., and Weber, J. S. (1993). Recombinant interleukin-6 activates the hypothalamic–pituitary–adrenal axis in humans. *J. Clin. Endocrinol. Metab.* **77,** 1690.
15. Spath-Schwalbe, E., Born, J., Schrezenmeier, H., Bornstein, S. R., Stromeyer, P., Drechsler, S., Fehm, H. L., and Porzsolt, F. (1994). Interleukin-6 stimulates the hypothalamus–pituitary–adrenocortical axis in man. *J. Clin. Endocrinol. Metab.* **79,** 1212.
16. Benigni, F., Fantuzzi, G., Sacco, S., Sironi, M., Pozzi, P., Dinarello, C. A., Sipe, J. D., Poli, V., Cappelletti, M., Paonessa, G., Pennica, D., Panayotatos, N., and Ghezzi, P. (1996). Six different cytokines that share GP130 as a receptor subunit, induce serum amyloid A and potentiate the induction of interleukin-6 and the activation of the hypothalamus–pituitary–adrenal axis by interleukin-1. *Blood* **87,** 1851.
17. Gauldie, J., Northemann, W., and Fey, G. H. (1990). IL-6 functions as an exocrine hormone in inflammation. Hepatocytes undergoing acute phase responses require exogenous IL-6. *J. Immunol.* **144,** 3804.
18. Gershenwald, J. E., Fong, Y. M., Fahey, T. J. D., Calvano, S. E., Chizzonite, R., Kilian, P. L., Lowry, S. F., and Moldawer, L. L. (1990). Interleukin 1 receptor blockade attenuates the host inflammatory response. *Proc. Natl. Acad. Sci. U.S.A.* **87,** 4966.
19. Oldenburg, H. S., Rogy, M. A., Lazarus, D. D., Van Zee, K. J., Keeler, B. P., Chizzonite, R. A., Lowry, S. F., and Moldawer, L. L. (1993). Cachexia and the acute-phase protein response in inflammation are regulated by interleukin-6. *Eur. J. Immunol.* **23,** 1889.
20. Sherry, R. M., Cue, J. I., Goddard, J. K., Parramore, J. B., and DiPiro, J. T. (1996). Interleukin-10 is associated with the development of sepsis in trauma patients. *J. Trauma* **40,** 613.
21. Ayala, A., Lehman, D. L., Herdon, C. D., and Chaudry, I. H. (1994). Mechanism of enhanced susceptibility to sepsis following hemorrhage. Interleukin-10 suppression of T-cell response is mediated by eicosanoid-induced interleukin-4 release. *Arch. Surg.* **129,** 1172.
22. Steinhauser, M. L., Hogaboam, C. M., Kunkel, S. L., Lukacs, N. W., Strieter, R. M., and Standiford, T. J. (1999). IL-10 is a major mediator of sepsis-induced impairment in lung antibacterial host defense. *J. Immunol.* **162,** 392.
23. Fong, Y. M., Marano, M. A., Moldawer, L. L., Wei, H., Calvano, S. E., Kenney, J. S., Allison, A. C., Cerami, A., Shires, G. T., and Lowry, S. F. (1990). The acute splanchnic and peripheral tissue metabolic response to endotoxin in humans. *J. Clin. Invest.* **85,** 1896.
24. Fischer, E., Marano, M. A., Van Zee, K. J., Rock, C. S., Hawes, A. S., Thompson, W. A., DeForge, L., Kenney, J. S., Remick, D. G., Bloedow, D. C., *et al.* (1992). Interleukin-1 receptor blockade improves survival and hemodynamic performance in *Escherichia coli* septic shock, but fails to alter host responses to sublethal endotoxemia. *J. Clin. Invest.* **89,** 1551.

25. Suter, P. M., Suter, S., Girardin, E., Roux-Lombard, P., Grau, G. E., and Dayer, J. M. (1992). High bronchoalveolar levels of tumor necrosis factor and its inhibitors, interleukin-1, interferon, and elastase, in patients with adult respiratory distress syndrome after trauma, shock, or sepsis. *Am. Rev. Respir. Dis.* **145,** 1016.
26. Rosenwasser, L. J., Webb, A. C., Clark, B. D., Irie, S., Chang, L., Dinarello, C. A., Gehrke, L., Wolff, S. M., Rich, A., and Auron, P. E. (1986). Expression of biologically active human interleukin 1 subpeptides by transfected simian COS cells. *Proc. Natl. Acad. Sci. U.S.A.* **83,** 5243.
27. Auron, P. E., Rosenwasser, L. J., Matsushima, K., Copeland, T., Dinarello, C. A., Oppenheim, J. J., and Webb, A. C. (1985). Human and murine interleukin 1 possess sequence and structural similarities. *J. Mol. Cell. Immunol.* **2,** 169.
28. Walter, M. R., and Nagabhushan, T. L. (1995). Crystal structure of interleukin 10 reveals an interferon gamma-like fold. *Biochemistry* **34,** 12118.
29. Zdanov, A., Schalk-Hihi, C., Gustchina, A., Tsang, M., Weatherbee, J., and Wlodawer, A. (1995). Crystal structure of interleukin-10 reveals the functional dimer with an unexpected topological similarity to interferon gamma. *Structure* **3,** 591.
30. Clore, G. M., Appella, E., Yamada, M., Matsushima, K., and Gronenborn, A. M. (1989). Determination of the secondary structure of interleukin-8 by nuclear magnetic resonance spectroscopy. *J. Biol. Chem.* **264,** 18907.
31. Banner, D. W., D'Arcy, A., Janes, W., Gentz, R., Schoenfeld, H. J., Broger, C., Loetscher, H., and Lesslauer, W. (1993). Crystal structure of the soluble human 55 kd TNF receptor-human TNF beta complex: Implications for TNF receptor activation. *Cell* **73,** 431.
32. Lewit-Bentley, A., Fourme, R., Kahn, R., Prange, T., Vachette, P., Tavernier, J., Hauquier, G., and Niers, W. (1988). Structure of tumour necrosis factor by X-ray solution scattering and preliminary studies by single crystal X-ray diffraction. *J. Mol. Biol.* **199,** 389.
33. Mapara, M. Y., Bargou, R. C., Beck, C., Heilig, B., Dorken, B., and Moldenhauer, G. (1994). Lymphotoxin-alpha/beta heterodimer is expressed on leukemic hairy cells and activated human B lymphocytes. *Int. J. Cancer* **58,** 248.
34. Wilkinson, V. L., Warrier, R. R., Truitt, T. P., Nunes, P., Gately, M. K., and Presky, D. H. (1996). Characterization of anti-mouse IL-12 monoclonal antibodies and measurement of mouse IL-12 by ELISA. *J. Immunol. Methods* **189,** 15.
35. Gillessen, S., Carvajal, D., Ling, P., Podlaski, F. J., Stremlo, D. L., Familletti, P. C., Gubler, U., Presky, D. H., Stern, A. S., and Gately, M. K. (1995). Mouse interleukin-12 (IL-12) p40 homodimer: A potent IL-12 antagonist. *Eur. J. Immunol.* **25,** 200.
35a. Dinarello, C. A., and Moldawer, L. L. (1999). "Proinflammatory and Anti-inflammatory Cytokines in Rheumatoid Arthritis—A Primer for Clinicians." Amgen, Inc., Thousand Oaks, CA:
36. Chandler, S., Miller, K. M., Clements, J. M., Lury, J., Corkill, D., Anthony, D. C., Adams, S. E., and Gearing, A. J. (1997). Matrix metalloproteinases, tumor necrosis factor and multiple sclerosis: An overview. *J. Neuroimmunol.* **72,** 155.
37. Maskos, K., Fernandez-Catalan, C., Huber, R., Bourenkov, G. P., Bartunik, H., Ellestad, G. A., Reddy, P., Wolfson, M. F., Rauch, C. T., Castner, B. J., Davis, R., Clarke, H. R., Petersen, M., Fitzner, J. N., Cerretti, D. P., March, C. J., Paxton, R. J., Black, R. A., and Bode, W. (1998). Crystal structure of the catalytic domain of human tumor necrosis factor-alpha-converting enzyme. *Proc. Natl. Acad. Sci. U.S.A.* **95,** 3408.
37a. Remick, D. G. (1995). Cytokines: A primer for plastic surgeons. *Ann. Plast. Surg.* **35,** 549–559.
38. Fearon, D. T., and Locksley, R. M. (1996). The instructive role of innate immunity in the acquired immune response. *Science* **272,** 50.
39. Tracey, K. J., and Cerami, A. (1994). Tumor necrosis factor: A pleiotropic cytokine and therapeutic target. *Annu. Rev. Med.* **45,** 491.
40. Dinarello, C. A. (1996). Cytokines as mediators in the pathogenesis of septic shock. *Curr. Top. Microbiol. Immunol.* **216,** 133.
41. Dinarello, C. A. (1997). Proinflammatory and anti-inflammatory cytokines as mediators in the pathogenesis of septic shock. *Chest* **112,** 321S.
42. Dinarello, C. A. (1984). Interleukin-1 and the pathogenesis of the acute-phase response. *N. Engl. J. Med.* **311,** 1413.
43. Baracos, V., Rodemann, H. P., Dinarello, C. A., and Goldberg, A. L. (1983). Stimulation of muscle protein degradation and prostaglandin E2 release by leukocytic pyrogen (interleukin-1). A mechanism for the increased degradation of muscle proteins during fever. *N. Engl. J. Med.* **308,** 553.
44. Clowes, G. H., Jr., George, B. C., Villee, Jr., C. A., and Saravis, C. A. (1983). Muscle proteolysis induced by a circulating peptide in patients with sepsis or trauma. *N. Engl. J. Med.* **308,** 545.
45. Moldawer, L. L., Svaninger, G., Gelin, J., and Lundholm, K. G. (1987). Interleukin 1 and tumor necrosis factor do not regulate protein balance in skeletal muscle. *Am. J. Physiol.* **253,** C766.
46. Liu, Y., Wei, S. H., Ho, A. S., de Waal Malefyt, R., and Moore, K. W. (1994). Expression cloning and characterization of a human IL-10 receptor. *J. Immunol.* **152,** 1821.
47. Ho, A. S., and Moore, K. W. (1994). Interleukin-10 and its receptor. *Ther. Immunol.* **1,** 173.
48. Vieira, P., de Waal-Malefyt, R., Dang, M. N., Johnson, K. E., Kastelein, R., Fiorentino, D. F., deVries, J. E., Roncarolo, M. G., Mosmann, T. R., and Moore, K. W. (1991). Isolation and expression of human cytokine synthesis inhibitory factor cDNA clones: Homology to Epstein–Barr virus open reading frame BCRFI. *Proc. Natl. Acad. Sci. U.S.A.* **88,** 1172.
49. Brouckaert, P. G., Everaerdt, B., Libert, C., Takahashi, N., and Fiers, W. (1989). Species specificity and involvement of other cytokines in endotoxic shock action of recombinant tumour necrosis factor in mice. *Agents Actions* **26,** 196.
50. Brouckaert, P., Libert, C., Everaerdt, B., and Fiers, W. (1992). Selective species specificity of tumor necrosis factor for toxicity in the mouse. *Lymphokine Cytokine Res.* **11,** 193.
51. Deak, T., Meriwether, J. L., Fleshner, M., Spencer, R. L., Abouhamze, A., Moldawer, L. L., Grahn, R. E., Watkins, L. R., and Maier, S. F. (1997). Evidence that brief stress may induce the acute phase response in rats. *Am. J. Physiol.* **273,** R1998.
52. Minter, R. M., Rectenwald, J. E., Fukuzuka, K., Tannahill, C. L., La Face, D., Tsai, V., Ahmed, I., Hutchins, E., Moyer, R., Copeland, 3rd, E. M., and Moldawer, L. L. (2000). TNF-alpha receptor signaling and IL-10 gene therapy regulate the innate and humoral immune responses to recombinant adenovirus in the lung. *J. Immunol.* **164,** 443.
53. Hess, P. J., Seeger, J. M., Huber, T. S., Welborn, M. B., Martin, T. D., Harward, T. R., Duschek, S., Edwards, P. D., Solorzano, C. C., Copeland, E. M., and Moldawer, L. L. (1997). Exogenously administered interleukin-10 decreases pulmonary neutrophil infiltration in a tumor necrosis factor-dependent murine model of acute visceral ischemia. *J. Vasc. Surg.* **26,** 113.
54. Van Zee, K. J., Stackpole, S. A., Montegut, W. J., Rogy, M. A., Calvano, S. E., Hsu, K. C., Chao, M., Meschter, C. L., Loetscher, H., Stuber, D., *et al.* (1994). A human tumor necrosis factor (TNF) alpha mutant that binds exclusively to the p55 TNF receptor produces toxicity in the baboon. *J. Exp. Med.* **179,** 1185.
55. Fischer, E., Marano, M. A., Barber, A. E., Hudson, A., Lee, K., Rock, C. S., Hawes, A. S., Thompson, R. C., Hayes, T. J., Anderson, T. D., *et al.* (1991). Comparison between effects of interleukin-1 alpha administration and sublethal endotoxemia in primates. *Am. J. Physiol.* **261,** R442.
56. Waage, A., and Espevik, T. (1988). Interleukin 1 potentiates the lethal effect of tumor necrosis factor alpha/cachectin in mice. *J. Exp. Med.* **167,** 1987.
57. Marano, M. A., Fong, Y., Moldawer, L. L., Wei, H., Calvano, S. E., Tracey, K. J., Barie, P. S., Manogue, K., Cerami, A., Shires, G. T., *et al.*

(1990). Serum cachectin/tumor necrosis factor in critically ill patients with burns correlates with infection and mortality. *Surg. Gynecol. Obstet.* **170,** 32.

58. Tracey, K. J., Lowry, S. F., and Cerami, A. (1987). Physiological responses to cachectin. *Ciba Found. Symp.* **131,** 88.
59. Welborn, M. B., 3rd, Van Zee, K., Edwards, P. D., Pruitt, J. H., Kaibara, A., Vauthey, J. N., Rogy, M., Castleman, W. L., Lowry, S. F., Kenney, J. S., *et al.* (1996). A human tumor necrosis factor p75 receptor agonist stimulates *in vitro* T cell proliferation but does not produce inflammation or shock in the baboon. *J. Exp. Med.* **184,** 165.
60. Tracey, K. J., Lowry, S. F., Fahey, T. J. D., Albert, J. D., Fong, Y., Hesse, D., Beutler, B., Manogue, K. R., Calvano, S., Wei, H., *et al.* (1987). Cachectin/tumor necrosis factor induces lethal shock and stress hormone responses in the dog. *Surg. Gynecol. Obstet.* **164,** 415.
61. Van der Poll, T., Romijn, J. A., Endert, E., Borm, J. J., Buller, H. R., and Sauerwein, H. P. (1991). Tumor necrosis factor mimics the metabolic response to acute infection in healthy humans. *Am. J. Physiol.* **261,** E457.
62. van der Poll, T., Jansen, J., Levi, M., ten Cate, H., ten Cate, J. W., and van Deventer, S. J. (1994). Regulation of interleukin 10 release by tumor necrosis factor in humans and chimpanzees. *J. Exp. Med.* **180,** 1985.
63. van der Poll, T., Jansen, P. M., Van Zee, K. J., Welborn, 3rd, M. B., de Jong, I., Hack, C. E., Loetscher, H., Lesslauer, W., Lowry, S. F., and Moldawer, L. L. (1996). Tumor necrosis factor-alpha induces activation of coagulation and fibrinolysis in baboons through an exclusive effect on the p55 receptor. *Blood* **88,** 922.
64. Smith, J. W. D., Longo, D. L., Alvord, W. G., Janik, J. E., Sharfman, W. H., Gause, B. L., Curti, B. D., Creekmore, S. P., Holmlund, J. T., Fenton, R. G., *et al.* (1993). The effects of treatment with interleukin-1 alpha on platelet recovery after high-dose carboplatin. *N. Engl. J. Med.* **328,** 756.
65. Chernoff, A. E., Granowitz, E. V., Shapiro, L., Vannier, E., Lonnemann, G., Angel, J. B., Kennedy, J. S., Rabson, A. R., Wolff, S. M., and Dinarello, C. A. (1995). A randomized, controlled trial of IL-10 in humans. Inhibition of inflammatory cytokine production and immune responses. *J. Immunol.* **154,** 5492.
66. Fuchs, A. C., Granowitz, E. V., Shapiro, L., Vannier, E., Lonnemann, G., Angel, J. B., Kennedy, J. S., Rabson, A. R., Radwanski, E., Affrime, M. B., Cutler, D. L., Grint, P. C., and Dinarello, C. A. (1996). Clinical, hematologic, and immunologic effects of interleukin-10 in humans. *J. Clin. Immunol.* **16,** 291.
67. Sheehan, K. C., Ruddle, N. H., and Schreiber, R. D. (1989). Generation and characterization of hamster monoclonal antibodies that neutralize murine tumor necrosis factors. *J. Immunol.* **142,** 3884.
68. Tracey, K. J., Fong, Y., Hesse, D. G., Manogue, K. R., Lee, A. T., Kuo, G. C., Lowry, S. F., and Cerami, A. (1987). Anti-cachectin/TNF monoclonal antibodies prevent septic shock during lethal bacteraemia. *Nature* (*London*) **330,** 662.
69. Neurath, M. F., Fuss, I., Pasparakis, M., Alexopoulou, L., Haralambous, S., Meyer zum Buschenfelde, K. H., Strober, W., and Kollias, G. (1997). Predominant pathogenic role of tumor necrosis factor in experimental colitis in mice. *Eur. J. Immunol.* **27,** 1743.
70. Hughes, C. B., Grewal, H. P., Gaber, L. W., Kotb, M., El-din, A. B., Mann, L., and Gaber, A. O. (1996). Anti-TNF alpha therapy improves survival and ameliorates the pathophysiologic sequelae in acute pancreatitis in the rat. *Am. J. Surg.* **171,** 274.
71. Hattori, K., Hirano, T., Miyajima, H., Yamakawa, N., Tateno, M., Oshimi, K., Kayagaki, N., Yagita, H., and Okumura, K. (1998). Differential effects of anti-Fas ligand and anti-tumor necrosis factor alpha antibodies on acute graft-versus-host disease pathologies. *Blood* **91,** 4051.
72. Targan, S. R., Hanauer, S. B., van Deventer, S. J., Mayer, L., Present, D. H., Braakman, T., DeWoody, K. L., Schaible, T. F., and Rutgeerts, P. J. (1997). A short- term study of chimeric monoclonal antibody cA2 to tumor necrosis factor alpha for Crohn's disease. Crohn's Disease cA2 Study Group. *N. Engl. J. Med.* **337,** 1029.
73. Stack, W. A., Mann, S. D., Roy, A. J., Heath, P., Sopwith, M., Freeman, J., Holmes, G., Long, R., Forbes, A., and Kamm, M. A. (1997). Randomised controlled trial of CDP571 antibody to tumour necrosis factor-alpha in Crohn's disease [see comments]. *Lancet* **349,** 521.
74. Elliott, M. J., Maini, R. N., Feldmann, M., Kalden, J. R., Antoni, C., Smolen, J. S., Leeb, B., Breedveld, F. C., Macfarlane, J. D., Bijl, H., *et al.* (1994). Randomised double-blind comparison of chimeric monoclonal antibody to tumour necrosis factor alpha (cA2) versus placebo in rheumatoid arthritis. *Lancet* **344,** 1105.
75. Scallon, B. J., Trinh, H., Nedelman, M., Brennan, F. M., Feldmann, M., and Ghrayeb, J. (1995). Functional comparisons of different tumour necrosis factor receptor/lgG fusion proteins. *Cytokine* **7,** 759.
76. Loetscher, H., Gentz, R., Zulauf, M., Lustig, A., Tabuchi, H., Schlaeger, E. J., Brockhaus, M., Gallati, H., Manneberg, M., and Lesslauer, W. (1991). Recombinant 55-kDa tumor necrosis factor (TNF) receptor. Stoichiometry of binding to TNF alpha and TNF beta and inhibition of TNF activity. *J. Biol. Chem.* **266,** 18324.
77. Abraham, E., Glauser, M. P., Butler, T., Garbino, J., Gelmont, D., Laterre, P. F., Kudsk, K., Bruining, H. A., Otto, C., Tobin, E., Zwingelstein, C., Lesslauer, W., and Leighton, A. (1997). p55 Tumor necrosis factor receptor fusion protein in the treatment of patients with severe sepsis and septic shock. A randomized controlled multicenter trial. Ro 45-2081 Study Group. *JAMA* **277,** 1531.
78. Fisher, C. J., Jr., Agosti, J. M., Opal, S. M., Lowry, S. F., Balk, R. A., Sadoff, J. C., Abraham, E., Schein, R. M., and Benjamin, E. (1996). Treatment of septic shock with the tumor necrosis factor receptor:Fc fusion protein. The Soluble TNF Receptor Sepsis Study Group [see comments]. *N. Engl. J. Med.* **334,** 1697.
79. Moreland, L. W., Baumgartner, S. W., Schiff, M. H., Tindall, E. A., Fleischmann, R. M., Weaver, A. L., Ettlinger, R. E., Cohen, S., Koopman, W. J., Mohler, K., Widmer, M. B., and Blosch, C. M. (1997). Treatment of rheumatoid arthritis with a recombinant human tumor necrosis factor receptor (p75)-Fc fusion protein [see comments]. *N. Engl. J. Med.* **337,** 141.
80. Solorzano, C. C., Kaibara, A., Hess, P. J., Edwards, P. D., Ksontini, R., Abouhamze, A., McDaniel, S., Frazier, J., Trujillo, D., Kieft, G., Seely, J., Kohno, T., Cosenza, M. E., Clare-Salzler, M., MacKay, S. L. D., Martin, S. W., Moldawer, L. L., and Edwards, 3rd, C. K. (1998). Pharmacokinetics, immunogenicity, and efficacy of dimeric TNFR binding proteins in healthy and bacteremic baboon. *J. Appl. Physiol.* **84,** 1119.
81. Bendele, A., McAbee, T., Woodward, M., Scherrer, J., Collins, D., Frazier, J., Chlipala, E., and McCabe, D. (1998). Effects of interleukin-1 receptor antagonist in a slow-release hylan vehicle on rat type II collagen arthritis. *Pharm. Res.* **15,** 1557.
82. Dripps, D. J., Verderber, E., Ng, R. K., Thompson, R. C., and Eisenberg, S. P. (1991). Interleukin-1 receptor antagonist binds to the type II interleukin-1 receptor on B cells and neutrophils. *J. Biol. Chem.* **266,** 20311.
83. Smith, J. W. D., Urba, W. J., Clark, J. W., Longo, D. L., Farrell, M., Creekmore, S. P., Conlon, K. C., Jaffe, H., and Steis, R. G. (1991). Phase I evaluation of recombinant tumor necrosis factor given in combination with recombinant interferon-gamma. *J. Immunother.* **10,** 355.
84. Granowitz, E. V., Porat, R., Mier, J. W., Pribble, J. P., Stiles, D. M., Bloedow, D. C., Catalano, M. A., Wolff, S. M., and Dinarello, C. A. (1992). Pharmacokinetics, safety and immunomodulatory effects of human recombinant interleukin-1 receptor antagonist in healthy humans. *Cytokine* **4,** 353.
85. Hirsch, E., Irikura, V. M., Paul, S. M., and Hirsh, D. (1996). Functions of interleukin 1 receptor antagonist in gene knockout and overproducing mice. *Proc. Natl. Acad. Sci. U.S.A.* **93,** 11008.
86. Michael, D., Josephs, C. C. S., Taylor, M., Rosenberg, J. J., Topping, D., Abouhamze, A., MacKay, S. L. D., Hirsch, E., Hirsh, D., Labow,

M., and Moldawer, L. L. (2000). Modulation of the acute phase response by altered expression of the IL-1 type 1 receptor or IL-1ra. *Am. J. Physiol.* **278.**

87. Granowitz, E. V., Porat, R., Mier, J. W., Orencole, S. F., Callahan, M. V., Cannon, J. G., Lynch, E. A., Ye, K., Poutsiaka, D. D., Vannier, E., *et al.* (1993). Hematologic and immunomodulatory effects of an interleukin-1 receptor antagonist coinfusion during low-dose endotoxemia in healthy humans. *Blood* **82,** 2985.
88. Van Zee, K. J., Coyle, S. M., Calvano, S. E., Oldenburg, H. S., Stiles, D. M., Pribble, J., Catalano, M., Moldawer, L. L., and Lowry, S. F. (1995). Influence of IL-1 receptor blockade on the human response to endotoxemia. *J. Immunol.* **154,** 1499.
89. Preas, H. L., 2nd, Reda, D., Tropea, M., Vandivier, R. W., Banks, S. M., Agosti, J. M., and Suffredini, A. F. (1996). Effects of recombinant soluble type I interleukin-1 receptor on human inflammatory responses to endotoxin. *Blood* **88,** 2465.
90. DeLa Cadena, R. A., Majluf-Cruz, A., Stadnicki, A., Tropea, M., Reda, D., Agosti, J. M., Colman, R. W., and Suffredini, A. F. (1998). Recombinant tumor necrosis factor receptor p75 fusion protein (TNFR:Fc) alters endotoxin-induced activation of the kinin, fibrinolytic, and coagulation systems in normal humans. *Thromb. Haemost.* **80,** 114.
91. Waage, A., Halstensen, A., and Espevik, T. (1987). Association between tumour necrosis factor in serum and fatal outcome in patients with meningococcal disease. *Lancet* **1,** 355.
92. Riches, P., Gooding, R., Millar, B. C., and Rowbottom, A. W. (1992). Influence of collection and separation of blood samples on plasma IL-1, IL-6 and TNF-alpha concentrations. *J. Immunol. Methods* **153,** 125.
93. Leroux-Roels, G., Offner, F., Philippe, J., and Vermeulen, A. (1988). Influence of blood-collecting systems on concentrations of tumor necrosis factor in serum and plasma. *Clin. Chem.* **34,** 2373.
94. Cannon, J. G., van der Meer, J. W., Kwiatkowski, D., Endres, S., Lonnemann, G., Burke, J. F., and Dinarello, C. A. (1988). Interleukin-1 beta in human plasma: optimization of blood collection, plasma extraction, and radioimmunoassay methods. *Lymphokine Res.* **7,** 457.
95. Engelberts, I., Moller, A., Schoen, G. J., van der Linden, C. J., and Buurman, W. A. (1991). Evaluation of measurement of human TNF in plasma by ELISA. *Lymphokine Cytokine Res.* **10,** 69.
96. Thavasu, P. W., Longhurst, S., Joel, S. P., Slevin, M. L., and Balkwill, F. R. (1992). Measuring cytokine levels in blood. Importance of anticoagulants, processing, and storage conditions. *J. Immunol. Methods* **153,** 115.
97. Cannon, J. G., Nerad, J. L., Poutsiaka, D. D., and Dinarello, C. A. (1993). Measuring circulating cytokines. *J. Appl. Physiol.* **75,** 1897.
98. Eskandari, M. K. R. D. (1992). "Quantitation of the Biological Activities of Cytokines." Marcel Dekker, New York.
99. Remick, D. G. (1995). Cytokines: A primer for plastic surgeons. *Ann. Plast. Surg.* **35,** 549.
100. Van Zee, K. J., Moldawer, L. L., Oldenburg, H. S., Thompson, W. A., Stackpole, S. A., Montegut, W. J., Rogy, M. A., Meschter, C., Gallati, H., Schiller, C. D., Richter, W. F., Loetscher, H., Ashkenazi, A., Chamow, S. M., Wurm, F., Calvano, S. E., Lowry, S. F., and Lesslauer, W. (1996). Protection against lethal *Escherichia coli* bacteremia in baboons (*Papio anubis*) by pretreatment with a 55-kDa TNF receptor (CD120a)-Ig fusion protein, Ro 45-2081. *J. Immunol.* **156,** 2221.
101. Keogh, C., Fong, Y., Marano, M. A., Seniuk, S., He, W., Barber, A., Minei, J. P., Felsen, D., Lowry, S. F., and Moldawer, L. L. (1990). Identification of a novel tumor necrosis factor alpha/cachectin from the livers of burned and infected rats. *Arch. Surg.* **125,** 79.
102. Tannahill, C. L., Fukuzuka, K., Marum, T., Abouhamze, Z., MacKay, S. L., Copeland, 3rd, E. M., and Moldawer, L. L. (1999). Discordant tumor necrosis factor-alpha superfamily gene expression in bacterial peritonitis and endotoxemic shock. *Surgery* **126,** 349.

68

Biology of Nitric Oxide: Measurement, Modulation, and Models

Joy L. Collins, Yoram Vodovotz, and Timothy R. Billiar

Department of Surgery, University of Pittsburgh, Pittsburgh, Pennsylvania 15261

I. Introduction

Once thought to be merely an environmental pollution by-product of industrial processes, nitric oxide (NO) is now known to be a potent biologic mediator. The discovery that NO is produced by a number of mammalian cells and that it has roles in events such as vasodilatation, neurotransmission, and immune-mediated cytotoxicity has sparked an explosion of scientific studies within the past two decades. In fact, there have been more than 30,000 publications on NO in the past 10 years, and over 3000 of these are review articles. NO has been found to have particular relevance in clinical conditions of great interest to surgeons, such as infection and sepsis, regulation of vascular tone in endotoxic and hemorrhagic shock, intestinal motility, and tissue remodeling and wound repair.

This chapter focuses on the role of NO in surgical disease, current methods for measuring the expression of the enzymes that produce NO and other end products of enzymatic NO synthesis, as well as models for elucidating the effects of NO. First, we give a brief overview of the biosynthesis of NO and its biology, both of which are crucial to the understanding of how the production and actions of NO are regulated. This overview is followed by a discussion of various methods for the detection of NO, and a summary of the currently available ways of manipulating the synthesis, concentration, and availability of NO using pharmacologic and genetic techniques.

The scientific study of NO relies on an array of approaches, based on various *in vitro* and *in vivo* models. The most useful studies of NO have utilized cultured cells, isolated organs, and intact animal models. As we get closer to determining specific mechanisms of NO-based pathophysiology, efforts will be directed toward exploiting substances that either increase or decrease NO as therapeutic strategies to manage some of the above-mentioned conditions.

II. History

Only within the past two decades has the biologic importance of NO become clear, and the history of this discovery is an interesting and complex one. The fact that nitroglycerine has been used in humans for over 100 years indicates that physicians have understood the biological importance of nitrates for some time. However, the suggestion by Mitchell and colleagues in 1916 that humans synthesize nitrates of oxygen (1) was not given serious attention until decades later. In the late 1970s and early 1980s, work by Tannenbaum *et al.* (2, 3) provided the first real evidence that mammalian cells produce nitrates. In their studies of dietary nitrates as a source of carcinogenic nitrosamines, Tannenbaum and associates found that both germ-free rats and humans are capable of excreting more nitrate (NO_3^-) than they ingest (2, 3). This production of NO_3^- is enhanced by infection in humans as well as by endotoxin treatment in rodents, which suggests a role for inflammatory processes as the source (4, 5).

In 1985, Stuehr and Marletta first reported synthesis of nitrogen oxides by a specific cell type when they demonstrated NO_3^- production by activated murine macrophages (6). Two years later, Palmer *et al.* and Ignarro *et al.* showed independently that the endothelium-derived relaxing factor (EDRF), first described by Furchgott and Zawadzki in 1980, was NO (7–9). In 1987, Hibbs published a seminal paper demonstrating that L-arginine was a substrate for NO production (10). Nathan and Hibbs subsequently elucidated the role of NO as a mediator of macrophage actions (11) and Garthwaite showed that NO acts as a second messenger in brain tissue (12, 13).

Since these momentous discoveries, NO has been identified in essentially every eukaryotic cell type, both in vertebrates and in invertebrates such as insects. Aside from its "classic" roles of endothelium-dependent relaxation, neurotransmission, and cell-mediated immune response, NO mediates a vast array of biological processes that are as diverse as the tissues that produce it. These include inhibition of platelet adhesion (14), apoptosis (15, 16), long-term synaptic depression and long-term potentiation of synaptic excitation (17, 18), penile erection (19, 20), ventilation–perfusion matching (17, 21), prevention of pylorospasm in infantile hypertrophic pyloric stenosis (22), angiogenesis and tumor metastasis (23–25), and wound healing (26, 27).

III. Biology of Nitric Oxide in Mammals

Nitric oxide is one of the smallest molecules produced by mammalian cells and is composed of one atom of nitrogen and one atom of oxygen. Because it is an uncharged, lipophilic molecule, NO can diffuse across membranes freely. Nitric oxide has an unpaired electron, and is relatively unstable compared to other free radicals. It has a short half-life (on the order of 2 to 30 sec) and shortly after it is produced it is oxidized into the stable end-products nitrite (NO_2^-) and nitrate (NO_3^-) (28, 29).

Nitric oxide is synthesized by a family of NADPH-dependent flavoprotein enzymes known as the NO synthases (NOSs). Three distinct isoforms of NOS have been isolated, and NO produced by each of these isoforms is differentially regulated and has different physiologic roles. The reaction catalyzed by each of the NOS enzymes involves the synthesis of NO from the 5-electron oxidation of one of the chemically equivalent guanidino nitrogens of L-arginine to form citrulline (Fig. 1). The reaction occurs in two steps, with the first appearing to be a classic P450-dependent N-hydroxylation of L-arginine, leading to the formation of *N*-hydroxy-L-arginine (NOHA) (30). The second step involves the oxidative cleavage of NOHA to release NO and L-citrulline (31). Overall, the two-step reaction utilizes the cosubstrates L-arginine, molecular oxygen, and NADPH, which functions as an electron donor. Flavin adenine dinucleotide (FAD), flavin mononucleotide (FMN), heme (iron–protoporphyrin IX), and tetrahydrobiopterin (BH_4) are required as cofactors

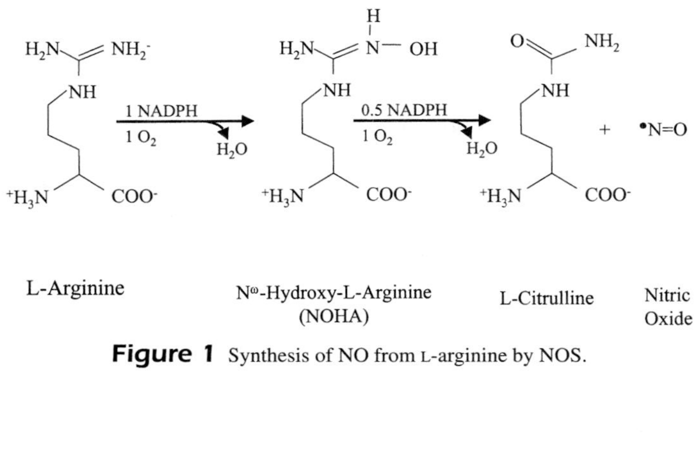

Figure 1 Synthesis of NO from L-arginine by NOS.

(17, 32), and NO, L-citrulline, and water are co-products. It has been demonstrated that the oxygen atom incorporated into NO and L-citrulline originates from molecular oxygen and not from water (33, 34).

In general, the NO synthases fall into one of two groups: constitutive or inducible, though recent developments have blurred this distinction somewhat. Two of the NOS isoforms are continuously present, and are thus called constitutive NO synthases (cNOSs). One of these cNOS enzymes is localized to the endothelium of blood vessels and is mostly membrane bound. This isoform, NOS-III, alternatively known as endothelial NOS (eNOS), has roles in vascular smooth muscle cell relaxation and angiogenesis. This isoform is regulated posttranslationally by the availability of its cofactors and by fluxes of Ca^{2+}, as well as by phosphorylation and translocation to caveolae. Furthermore, studies have demonstrated that the expression of eNOS can be regulated at the transcriptional level by cytokines as well as by physical factors such as shear stress (35, 36). The other constitutive NOS, NOS-I, is found in neurons in the central and peripheral nervous system, as well as in extraneuronal sites such as pancreas, adrenal, kidney, and skeletal muscle. Because of its localization to the brain and its role in neurotransmission, this isoform is referred to as neuronal NOS (nNOS) (37). Similar to eNOS, studies have demonstrated that the "constitutive" expression of nNOS can be modulated in cerebral injury models in animals (38, 39).

The constitutive NOS isoforms are dependent on the binding of Ca^{2+} to calmodulin (CaM) and are involved in cellular signaling. A variety of molecules such as acetylcholine, bradykinin, substance P, thrombin, and ATP are capable of increasing intracellular free Ca^{2+}, thereby activating the constitutive NOS isoforms (40, 41). Constitutive NO synthases produce picomolar quantities of NO when Ca^{2+}/CaM binding permits electron transfer from NADPH via flavin groups within the enzyme to a heme-containing active site (29, 32).

Contrasted with the cNOS isoforms is the Ca^{2+}/CaM-independent inducible NO synthase (iNOS or NOS-II). As its name suggests, iNOS is typically expressed by cells that have been induced by certain stimuli, such as cytokines, hypoxia, microbes, and microbial products. Even in the absence of Ca^{2+}, calmodulin is bound tightly to the active 250-kDa dimer. Thus, unlike eNOS and nNOS, this enzyme is not sensitive to free calcium concentration fluctuations (42, 43). Inducible NOS expression is controlled mainly at the transcriptional level, and its activation results in sustained production of nanomolar quantities of NO throughout the life span of the enzyme. NO production by iNOS occurs in a sustained manner lasting hours to days (44). Perhaps for this reason, iNOS has been found to be expressed in apparently unstimulated tissues such as the lung (45) and kidney (46), although this expression is likely mediated by constant exposure to inducing stimuli. The NO produced by iNOS generally has been found to have both cytostatic/cytotoxic and cytoprotective actions in mammalian cells and tissues, as well as antimicrobial activity toward certain bacterial and viral pathogens. Inducible NOS can be expressed in a large number of cell types. Sustained production of NO at high levels in cells that are also capable of generating reactive oxygen species may lead to the production of numerous reactive nitrogen oxide species (RNOS) that can mediate a broad spectrum of physiologic and pathologic effects (47). Due to the possibility of deleterious effects to the host as a consequence of prolonged exposure to such RNOS, iNOS must be regulated carefully (44).

Each isoform of NOS represents a distinct gene product, and differs from the others based on amino acid sequence, subcellular as well as cellular or organ localization, and sensitivity to calcium stimulation. All three genes have been localized to separate chromosomes, and in humans the genes for all three isoforms have been cloned (48–50).

Although there are many differences among the isoforms, all of them are similar in that they exist as homodimers in the active state, and they are similar in size, ranging from 130 to 161 kDa. Stuehr and colleagues have shown that two monomers containing calmodulin and the cofactors FAD and FMN must interact with two heme and two BH_4 molecules to form the active dimer (30). In addition, the carboxy-terminal end of each isoform shares a large homology with mammalian P450 reductase (51). This C-terminal domain contains consensus sequences for NADPH, FAD, and FMN binding (51, 52), whereas a calmodulin binding site exists toward the N terminus. The N-terminal domain also contains threonine and serine phosphorylation sites, a heme binding site, and probable binding sites for BH_4 and L-arginine, which are not well defined. The N-terminal end of eNOS contains a myristoylation site, which accounts for the fact that this isoform is largely membrane bound (53). For a more complete comparison of the characteristics of the three NOSs, see Table I.

IV. Methods for Detection of NO and Measurement of NOS Activity

The direct measurement of NO concentration in various experimental models and biological systems has proved to be a significant challenge, largely due to its short half-life. Methods vary from direct measurement of NO to indirect quantification through measurement of its reactive metabolites. In biological systems, the amount of NO present is sometimes inferred based on its known physiologic effects. These effects include relaxation of smooth muscle and activation of guanylyl cyclase activity (54). In addition, because eNOS and nNOS have been reported to be inducible under certain special circumstances (55), it is possible that to some extent all isoforms of NOS may be under transcriptional or

Table I Isoforms of NOS

NOS isoform	Chromosome (human)	Protein size	NO production	Subcellular localization	Tissue localization	Activated by	Function/action
Type I—neuronal	12	160–161 kDa (1433 aa)	Constitutive, short-acting, picomolar quantities	Cytosolic, binds to specific proteins; also particulate	Neuronal cells, skeletal muscle, adrenal medulla	Acetylcholine, bradykinin, glutamate, histamine	Cell signaling, neurotransmission
Type II—inducible	17	130–135 kDa (1144 aa)	Inducible, long-lasting, nanomolar quantities	Cytosolic, "nitroxysomal," peroxisomal	Macrophages, liver, lung, aorta, PMNs, and others	Endotoxins, cytokines	Cytotoxicity, immunoregulation
Type III—endothelial	7	133–134 kDa (1200 aa)	Constitutive, short-acting, picomolar quantities	Cytosolic, membrane bound (caveolae)	Epithelial cells, endothelial cells, platelets, cardiac myocytes	Acetylcholine, bradykinin, glutamate, histamine	Cell signaling, vasomotor tone regulation

posttranscriptional control. In addition, the cellular localization of NOS protein can be determined through subcellular fractionation followed by assay of enzyme activity or western blot, whereas the localization in intact cells of the mRNA and protein of the various isoforms of NOS can be determined with *in situ* hybridization and immunohistochemistry, respectively.

Various instruments for measuring NO have been devised, and methods of NO detection are grouped into two general categories: spectroscopic methods and electrochemical methods. Spectroscopic methods include chemiluminescence spectrometry, ultraviolet (UV)visible spectroscopy, and electron spin resonance spectroscopy (ESR; also called electron paramagnetic resonance, or EPR) (32, 56). These methods detect NO indirectly and involve the generation of a product following a reaction with NO. The concentration of NO is then extrapolated based on the formation of these products, such as NO_2^- or NO_3^- (56).

In contrast, electrochemical methods allow direct, *in situ* measurement of NO and are based on electron exchange between NO and a modified oxygen electrode (first known as the Clark electrode). Because electrochemical methods allow the direct detection of NO, these methods are more suited for *in situ* and *in vivo* monitoring of the kinetics of NO release than are spectroscopic methods. Spectroscopic methods are more useful for the determination of an amount of NO by a certain number of cells in culture or a given amount of tissue (56). Other methods, including mass spectrometry and gas chromatography, have been used occasionally, but these will not be discussed in this chapter due to their lack of sensitivity compared to the methods mentioned above. The methodology for the detection of NO is a sufficiently vast and complex topic to be the subject of an entire chapter. Because of the limited scope of this review, the pertinent points of each method are described briefly and comparisons are made among the various modalities based on parameters measured, specificity, sensitivity, and limits of detection (Table II).

A. Spectroscopic Methods

1. Chemiluminescence

A luminescent process is one in which significant numbers of molecules, generated in an excited state, release light. The chemiluminescence assay takes advantage of the reaction of NO with ozone (O_3). This reaction involves the gas-phase oxidation of NO by O_3, and the product of interest in this reaction is an excited molecule of nitrogen dioxide (NO_2^*), which in turn can dissipate energy in the form of a photon (57, 58), as shown in reactions (I) and (II).

$$NO + O_3 \rightarrow NO_2^* + O_2$$
(I)

$$NO_2^* \rightarrow NO_2 + \text{light}$$
(II)

This reaction is useful for the assessment of NO because the number of photons emitted can be measured, and at constant O_3 concentration the number of photons emitted is proportional to the concentration of NO in a given sample (56). In 1970, Fontijn *et al.* (59) first measured the amount of light emitted from the chemical oxidation of NO by O_3 and utilized this measurement to calculate the amount of NO present based on the observation that light emission is linearly related to the NO content of the sample (32, 59, 60). This finding allowed Fontijn and co-workers to develop the chemiluminescence assay that was later used by Ignarro *et al.* and Palmer *et al.* to show that endothelium-derived relaxing factor was NO (8, 9). One clinically relevant application of this method is the measurement of NO in exhaled air from animals or even human patients (61).

Table II Methods for Detection of NO

Method	Parameter measured	Detection limit	Notes
Chemiluminescence	NO_2^*	100 n*M*	Analyzer must be calibrated with pure NO gas; samples should be analyzed soon after collection
Griess reaction assay	NO_2^-	50 n*M*	Must convert NO_3^- in samples back to NO_2^-; better for analyzing cell culture supernatants than plasma or serum
Electron paramagnetic resonance	"Trapped" NO	1–4 μ*M*	
Clark electrode	NO	20–500 n*M*	Electrode is sensitive to NO_2 as well as NO
Porphyrinic microsensor	NO	10 n*M*	Electrode may be sensitive to tyrosine as well as NO
Measurement of NOS mRNA	Isoform-specific NOS mRNA		Quantitative and semiquantitative methods require the use of radioactive isotopes
In situ hybridization	RNA in tissues		Allows localization within tissues; requires the use of radioactive isotopes
Western blotting	NOS protein		Quantitative; easy and inexpensive to perform
Immunohistochemistry	NOS		Allows localization of protein within tissues and cells

Because the chemiluminescence assay requires that NO be in its gaseous phase, NO in the liquid phase can be measured only after being converted back to a gas via a two-step process (54, 61). Nitric oxide in the liquid phase rapidly becomes oxidized to NO_2^- and NO_3^-; therefore, a two-step method is required. Nitrite and nitrate are first converted back to NO, and the liquid NO is then driven into the gas phase by a process known as "stripping." Stripping involves bubbling the liquid solution containing NO with an inert gas such as helium under a vacuum, thereby creating a volume of NO gas above the liquid, called "head space." Stripping is performed in a purge chamber within the chemiluminescence analyzer, and once this process is complete the gaseous specimen is drawn into a reaction chamber, where ozone is mixed with NO in front of a cooled, red-sensitive photomultiplier tube (54). A light detector then collects the emitted energy and transforms this light to an electrical signal, which is picked up by an analog–digital recorder (61).

The detection limit of the chemiluminescence method is approximately 100 n*M* (32). A plot of signal versus NO concentration has two linear regions with different slopes: 20 to 200 n*M* and 300 n*M* to 3 μ*M* (56). Several authors disagree regarding the levels of NO at which the signal–concentration plot is linear [see Archer (54) and Kiechle and Malinski (32) for a more thorough discussion of this subject].

This method has the advantages of high speed of reaction, the ability to measure NO in extremely small sample volumes, and a relatively high sensitivity, but the main limitation is lack of specificity. Substances other than NO, such as DMSO, sulfur, ammonia, and nitrosylated agents (such as NO donors commonly used in cell culture systems), can also cause inaccurate reading of the chemiluminescence signal, making interpretation of data difficult. Other gases, such as NO_2, and pollutants, such as CO_2, C_2H_4, CO, NH_3, SO_2, and H_2O, however, react much more slowly with O_3 than NO and therefore do not affect the chemiluminescence reaction (59, 61). An additional point to remember is that NO can be adsorbed by solid materials such as glass, falsely lowering the measured concentration (32). One additional disadvantage of the chemiluminescence method is the possibility of introducing error with each of the two preparation steps. This method is highly user dependent, and unexplainable variation has been seen in our laboratory and those of others.

2. Measurement of Nitrite and Nitrate

One commonly used, simple method of assessing NO production involves the measurement of nitrite (NO_2^-) and nitrate (NO_3^-), the stable reaction products of NO. This is an especially efficient method when several samples are to be processed at one time. Commonly, NO_2^- alone is measured, especially in cell culture supernatants, because this is the first stable metabolite to be formed from the oxidation of NO and because of the ease of measuring this single metabolite. Some investigators feel that it is important to measure both NO_2^- and NO_3^-, however, because up to 60% of the NO can be converted to NO_3^- in cell culture and over 90% of circulating metabolite in biologic systems is in the form of NO_3^-. Therefore, measurement of NO_2^- alone should be viewed only as an estimate of NO production.

The measurement of the combination of NO_2^- and NO_3^- requires a two-step procedure. The first step involves conversion of the NO_3^- in a sample to NO_2^- via one of three methods. The total NO_2^- then undergoes a stoichiometric diazotization reaction (the Griess reaction) to form a purple azo product that emits a signal at 548 nm (8, 32, 62). This signal can be read on a UV/visible light spectrophotometer, and the NO_2^- + NO_3^- concentration is calculated from comparison to a standard curve. The signal emitted at 548 nm is proportional to the concentration of NO (32, 62) and analysis of NO_2^- in this way is reliable and easy to perform. The detection limit of this method is 50 nM and the signal–concentration curve is linear from 50 nM to 500 mM (32).

The oldest method used for conversion of NO_3^- to NO_2^- is the nonenzymatic conversion using cadmium (Cd), which has been known for over a century and which can be carried out in a semiautomated fashion (63). Modifications of this assay (64) have allowed for determination of $NO_2^- + NO_3^-$ in various biofluids, including the hemolymph of insects (65) in a volume as small as 2–5 μl. The advantages of this method include simplicity and lack of need for standardization of enzyme lots; disadvantages include the toxicity of Cd and the possible interference from other chemical species (63). Several manufacturers offer kit versions of this assay.

A second method for converting NO_3^- to NO_2^- for subsequent measurement with the Greiss reaction involves the use of the enzyme NADPH-nitrate reductase. This method, first described in 1992 by Wu and Brosnan (66), uses NADPH to reduce NO_3^- to NO_2^-. One early problem with this method was that high concentrations of $NADP^+$ were formed during the reduction of NO_3^- to NO_2^- and interfered with color development in the Griess reaction (62). A modification of the nitrate reductase reaction involving the inclusion of a glucose-6-phosphate/glucose-6-phosphate dehydrogenase NADPH-regenerating system resolved this problem (31, 62) [reactions (III) and (IV)].

$$NO_3^- + NADPH + H^+ \rightarrow NO_2^- + NADP^+ + H_2O$$
(**III**), Nitrate reductase

$$G\text{-}6\text{-}P + NADP^+ + H_2O \rightarrow 6\text{-}PG + NADPH + H^+$$
(**IV**, Glucose-6-phosphate dehydrogenase

A third method of converting NO_3^- to NO_2^- utilizes formate–nitrate reductase to reduce FMN, a supplemental electron carrier, to $FMNH_2$ (62, 67). The $FMNH_2$ then reduces NO_3^- to NO_2^-, which can then be measured using the Greiss reagent (62, 67) [reactions (V) and (VI)].

$$FMN + HCOO^- + H_2O \rightarrow FMNH_2 + CO_2 + OH^-$$
(**V**), Formate dehydrogenase

$$FMNH_2 + NO_3^- \rightarrow NO_2^- + FMN + H_2O$$
(**VI**), Nitrate reductase

The main advantage of the enzymatic conversion of NO_3^- to NO_2^- is its lack of use of toxic Cd; its main disadvantage is the need for standardization of enzyme lots. It should be noted, however, that the recent introduction of assay kits using the enzymatic method reduces some of this concern.

A final point to remember is that whether samples are collected for analysis of nitrite via the Griess reaction or via assessment of NO via chemiluminescence, sample handling and storage can be complex. It has been reported that there is no appreciable loss of NO_2^- in samples that are stored at −70°C for up to 6 months (68), but at least one study has called this assumption into question. Kaiser and Williams (69) measured aliquots of NO_2^--containing medium both immediately and after storage at −20°C or −70°C for 5 weeks. They demonstrated that samples stored frozen in either glass or plastic tubes have significantly greater NO_2^- measurements than do the same samples that are measured immediately after collection (69). In addition, Kaiser and Williams showed that samples that underwent four or more freeze–thaw cycles had increased NO_2^- compared with samples analyzed immediately. No explanation for these findings has been offered; however, it is recommended that NO_2^- measurements be conducted as soon after sample collection as possible to ensure reliable results.

3. Electron Paramagnetic Resonance

This method is also known as electron spin resonance, and is based on the principle that NO has an unpaired electron and is therefore paramagnetic and can absorb radiation and undergo transition from a ground state to an excited state (70). This principle is similar to that on which magnetic resonance imaging (MRI) is based, because both MRI and EPR involve assigning a value based on the position of spin compared to a magnetic field. Because NO is unstable with a short half-life, a spin-trapping agent such as hemoglobin, a nitroxide, or a metal-chelator complex such as *N*-methyl-D-glucamine dithiocarbamate ferrous iron [$(MGD_2)/Fe^{2+}$] (71–73), is used to stabilize NO. The magnetic interaction between the electron spin of NO and the applied magnetic field is measured and the amount of NO can be calculated. According to Ohnishi (70), the sensitivity of the EPR method for detecting NO in tissues is approximately 1 μM, and Kiechle and Malinski (32) report a similar sensitivity of 4 μM. Kotake *et al.* (74) have reported that NO/NO_2^- measurement via spin trapping and EPR can detect cellular NO generation into the surrounding medium at a rate as low as 10 pmol/min. Advantages of EPR over the Griess reaction assay include superior sensitivity, and more authentic measurement of NO, because NO is confirmed to be the actual source of detected species due to the characteristics of the EPR spectrum (74). The details of instrumentation needed and protocols have been outlined (70).

B. Electrochemical Methods

Electrochemical methods allow for direct measurement of NO in biological samples. It should be noted that these sensors measure authentic NO concentration, unlike the methods described previously, and should be used to measure amounts of NO in real time. These methods utilize an electrochemical sensor based on a modification of the Clark electrode, which consists of a platinum wire as the anode and a silver wire as the cathode (32, 75). The platinum and silver wires are mounted in a capillary tube filled with an electrolyte solution consisting of sodium chloride and hydrochloric acid. This solution is separated from an analytic solution by a gas-permeable chloroprene rubber membrane (32). A constant potential of 0.9 V is applied and a direct current is generated from the electrochemical oxidation of NO on the platinum anode. This current is proportional to the concentration of NO outside the membrane (76). The Clark-type sensor has a detection limit of ~20 n*M* (76) to 500 n*M* (32), with a linear response from 1 μ*M* to 100 m*M* (32). Although this electrochemical method has the disadvantage of having a sensitivity threshold approximately 10-fold higher than that of chemiluminescence or EPR, it is much less expensive because the latter two methods require complex equipment. In addition to being relatively inexpensive, Clark-type electrodes are commercially available and easy to use (76). One potential limitation is the fact that although the electrode is insensitive to O_2, N_2, CO, and CO_2, it is sensitive to NO_2, which may be generated by the interaction of NO and small amounts of O_2 that traverse the membrane (32, 76). However, this seems to be a problem only for gas-phase NO measurements, because NO_2 is quickly degraded in solution to nitrite and nitrate, which are not detected by the sensor (76). Thus, use of these electrodes requires careful calibration and well-controlled experiments in order to obtain reliable, reproducible results.

Malinski and associates (77–80) have developed an oxygen microsensor that can detect as little as 10^{-20} mol of NO released from a single cell. As with the Clark electrode, the porphyrinic microsensor is based on the electrochemical oxidation of NO and a measurement of the current generated from this reaction. The oxidation of NO is catalyzed on polymeric metalloporphyrin, which is deposited along with the cationic exchanger Nafion (Aldrich Chemical Co., Milwaukee, WI) on the thermally sharpened carbon fiber sensor (32, 77). The porphyrinic microsensor can rapidly detect NO, via its reaction with O_2, *in situ* produced by a single cell. The tip of the sensor is very small (0.2–0.5 μm), allowing this measurement of NO from single cells as well as in small mesenteric resistance arteries in a rat model (80). The microsensor is highly efficient and has a linear response from 10 n*M* to 3 m*M* (32, 77) and a detection limit of 10 n*M*. Because of the low detection limit, the sensitivity, and the efficiency of the porphyrinic sensor, this is a useful tool for studying the kinetics of NO release.

The main advantage of the Clark-type sensor over the porphyrinic microsensor is its commercial availability. However, it is possible to fashion porphyrinic microsensors from commercially available products, and many investigators have done this, often incorporating their own modifications (80, 81). One reported potential limitation of the porphyrinic microsensor is lack of specificity in brain. Stingele *et al.* (82) reported that the porphyrinic microsensor used for detection of NO also detects biologically relevant concentrations of tyrosine in dog brain.

C. Measurement of NOS and NOS Activity

1. Detection of NOS mRNA

Because all isoforms of NOS can be under transcriptional control, the detection of NOS mRNA has an important role in the study of NO and its physiology. Though many cell types are capable of producing NO, they may produce it in such small amounts that it is undetectable by currently available methods. The isolation and detection of NOS mRNA by reverse transcription polymerase chain reaction (RT-PCR) is a powerful tool that allows detection of very small amounts of the mRNA of different isoforms of NOS. The RT-PCR method can indicate the capability of a cell type to produce NO via specific isoforms and, if the amount of NOS mRNA changes under various conditions, can provide invaluable information about the regulation of the different isoforms of NOS. As mentioned earlier, once NOS enzymes are formed, they are only active in the presence of certain necessary cofactors and are subject to a variety of posttranslational modifications. Although the amount of NOS mRNA present does not necessarily correlate with the amount of NO produced (83, 84), the presence of NOS mRNA is a prerequisite for the production of NOS protein.

Another useful way to analyze NOS mRNA is the *in situ* hybridization (ISH) method, which allows the demonstration and subcellular localization of the different isoforms of NOS mRNA within tissues (85). For the appropriate level of sensitivity, a radioisotopic method is recommended. One other important point is that appropriate controls must be included with each experiment, including RNase-treated slides and preabsorption experiments with antisense and irrelevant oligonucleotides as described by Taylor and Cook (85). Although this method is a useful tool allowing the subcellular localization of the various isoforms of NOS, it is important to keep in mind that this method is time consuming, technically challenging, and expensive.

2. Detection of NOS Protein

The amount of NOS in tissues and cells is commonly determined by Western blotting. Antibodies that recognize each of the three NOS isoforms exist and are commercially available. These antibodies are specific and show no cross-reactivity with the other isoforms. The method of Western blotting is inexpensive and easy to perform. Quantitative results can be obtained within 2 days of protein extraction, and this method can detect as little as 1 pg of protein (86).

Another method of analyzing NOS protein in cells or in tissues is via immunohistochemical localization. Immunohistochemistry involves the visualization of an antigen by use of a specific antibody, similar to the antibodies used for Western blotting, and can be applied to cells and tissues (87). Frozen tissue or paraffin-embedded cells are cut into thin slices (approximately 5–7 μm) and placed on glass slides. The cells or tissues are then stained with primary and secondary antibodies in a fashion similar to that used for Western blotting. Antibodies to rat and mouse NOSs, especially iNOS, are readily available and have been used extensively by our lab and those in collaboration with us.

This method is extremely useful for identifying the presence and localization of NOS, but does not allow specific quantification of protein. The antibodies and reagents are inexpensive and the necessary antibodies are commercially available. If immunofluorescence is used, however, a rather expensive immunofluorescence microscope is needed to detect the fluorescently tagged secondary antibody. This technique does require a significant amount of skill, because the preparation of slides must involve carefully controlled methods of fixation, appropriate controls of specificity, and minimization of background staining. One of the most important points to remember is the necessity of a preparing a primary delete slide, in which the primary antibody is omitted and secondary antibody is added alone in order to control for background binding of the secondary antibody. Additional controls are slides to which a specific blocking reagent (e.g., the peptide to which the original antibody was raised) or an isotype-matched control primary antibody has been added. Cattel and Mosley (87) provide a thorough and helpful review of this method, as well as a sample protocol and troubleshooting guide.

Another method for detection of iNOS protein is the enzyme-linked immunosorbent assay (ELISA) (88). This method may have utility as an adjunct to quantification of Western blots.

3. Assessment of NOS Activity

One assay of NOS activity involves a spectrophotometric method based on the rapid oxidation of oxyhemoglobin to methemolobin by NO (89) [reaction (VII)].

$$\mathrm{Hb(II)O_2 + NO \rightarrow Met(III)Hb + NO_3^-}$$
(VII)

Methemoglobin produces a high-absorbance band at 401 nm called a Soret band, which can be measured spectrophotometrically. The detection limit of this method has been reported to be 1 n*M* (32), or 20 pmol/min/g tissue (90), and the signal–concentration response is linear from the nanomolar to the micromolar range (32). This method has been modified to allow NOS activity both *in vitro* and *in vivo*, when NOS inhibitors are used (90). This method is applicable to a variety of preparations except those in which the samples contain large amounts of hemoglobin. The major advantages of this method are that it is suitable for continual monitoring for the enzyme nNOS and perhaps eNOS, and that it is simple and relatively inexpensive to perform. Salter and Knowles (90) outline the materials needed and the protocols for this method.

Another method that can be used to measure NOS activity is based on the fundamental reaction outlined in Fig. 1, in which NOS catalyzes the conversion of L-arginine to L-citrulline (91). This assay involves the determination of the NOS inhibitor-sensitive conversion of ^{14}C- or ^{3}H-radiolabeled arginine to citrulline, with separation of the labeled product from substrate by ion-exchange column (91, 92). This method has been modified and simplified to make it applicable to the study of NOS activity in a variety of settings, including purified enzymes to crude-tissue homogenates (91). Using the modified protocol as described by Knowles and Salter (91), the limit of detection for this method is approximately 50 pmol/min/g tissue or 0.7 pmol/min/mg protein (93).

An additional method used to measure the conversion of ^{14}C-labeled L-arginine to citrulline utilizes either a Dowex cation-exchange chromatography system (91) or high-pressure liquid chromatography (HPLC) separation. The Dowex method is convenient and applicable in cases in which NOS is the predominant arginine-metabolizing enzyme present in a preparation (94). When other pathways of arginine metabolism are present, this method fails to distinguish additional products that may be formed in the reaction (such as ornithine or urea) from arginine and citrulline, respectively (94).

A more specific separation method using HPLC can be used to identify the various products of arginine metabolism directly and accurately when pathways other than that of citrulline formation are present (94). This method is relatively simple to perform and involves the identification of radiolabeled arginine-derived citrulline, ornithine, and urea, thereby allowing the quantification of relative activities of NOS and arginase in cell and tissue preparations (94). This method can be used not only to monitor NOS activity in a particular cell or tissue, but also to assess the contribution of pathways other than those catalyzed by NOS (94). A thorough description of materials and methods for performing sample preparation and HPLC separation of arginine analogs based on a protocol has been provided by Cunningham and Rayne (94) and Vallance *et al.* (95).

One final commonly used method for detecting NOS activity is based on the observation that NO is a potent and effective activator of soluble guanylyl cyclase (GC-S). Although some aspects of the mechanism of this activation are not yet totally clear, it appears that NO binds to GC-S, thereby inducing a conformational change in its heme moiety to form guanosine 3′,5′-cyclic monophosphate (c-GMP) (96–98). This conformational change then either leads to deinhibition or activation of the catalytic site of GC-S (99). In the presence of a phosphodiesterase inhibitor, the levels of cGMP produced following activation of GC-S by NO are stable and quantifiable. This reaction can therefore be used to determine the production and levels of NO in cells or tissues in the form of a bioassay (100). Variations on the methods used for NO-stimulated cGMP production exist, but the most commonly used assay method is a radioimmunoassay (RIA), which is a competitive-binding assay that relies on antibodies specific for cGMP (100, 101).

There are variations on the methodology of RIA, but commonly the cells or tissues to be examined are incubated with a phosphodiesterase inhibitor, which will allow nucleotides to accumulate (100). The cell membranes are then fractured by a method such as sonication, and cGMP is separated from the other nucleotides and purified via ion-exchange chromatography. The recovered cGMP is then concentrated and cGMP samples, in addition to cGMP used to generate a standard curve, are acetylated with triethylamine and acetic anhydride immediately before RIA analysis. The RIA utilizes ^{125}I-labeled cGMP succinyl methyl ester in a competitive-binding assay, and the percentage of ^{125}I-labeled cGMP bound to the antibody in the RIA is used to generate a standard curve against which the samples can be compared (100).

V. Methods of Manipulating NO in Experimental Models

In order to study the effects of NO, it is necessary to be able to control the presence and concentration of NO in various models. Here we discuss ways to increase and decrease NO in a system via either exogenous or endogenous modifications. Exogenous methods of increasing NO are based on the addition of compounds that donate NO, whereas methods of decreasing NO involve the use of NO scavengers, which are compounds that bind or inactivate free NO. Methods of altering endogenous NO in a system rely on manipulation of NOS, the enzyme that synthesizes NO. NOS can be genetically introduced into a cell line or animal, thereby increasing the production of NO. Also, NOS can be either genetically inhibited, as in NOS-deficient animals, or chemically inhibited with pharmacological substances that are either isoform selective or nonselective. As is always the case, neither method of manipulating NO activity or formation in a system should be used as a stand-alone technique, but rather to corroborate other methods.

A. Pharmacologic Methods

As mentioned above, one way to manipulate NO in a cell culture or animal model is through the addition of substances that either generate NO when added or scavenge/inactivate NO. Such compounds are widely available commercially from a number of companies and are relatively inexpensive. The decision of which to choose is based on the experimental model being used and the desired level of selectivity.

1. Chemical Donors of NO

Since the explosion of discoveries regarding the role of NO in various disease processes, investigators have realized the necessary role of NO as a physiologic molecule. Although some conditions, such as hemorrhagic shock, seem to be worsened by an increase in NO, other disorders are characterized by a detrimental loss of NO. Such diseases are primarily related to the circulatory system and examples include ischemia–reperfusion of the heart (102, 103), hypertension (104), atherosclerosis and bowel ischemia (105), pulmonary hypertension of the newborn, and the ventilation/perfusion mismatching seen in adult respiratory distress syndrome (106). Indeed, in the last two conditions, addition of inhaled NO gas seems to be beneficial (107–109). Nitric oxide provided via exogenous NO donors can enhance neutrophil cytotoxicity (110) and inhibit platelet activation in whole blood (111). Because NO donors have such effects, they hold great potential as therapeutic agents to treat those conditions in which a subphysiological level of NO is the cause (109, 112, 113).

An NO donor is a compound that releases NO under physiologic conditions; to date, there are many donors available (see Table III). Different NO sources have been found to release varying proportions of the nitrogen oxides, and over different time courses. Solutions of NO and NO gas have proved inadequate as sources for the exogenous delivery of NO, because these give rise to relatively high NO concentrations initially followed by rapid decline. In contrast, NO donor compounds, many of which are stable in solutions of varying pH and which decompose in a first-order reaction, may release constant amounts of NO after dilution in physiologic buffers (47). The exact concentration of NO cannot be predicted at any given time point; however, due to the confounding event of NO autooxidation, which increases with increasing concentrations of NO (47).

The various groups of NO donors include organic nitrates, inorganic nitrites, inorganic nitroso compounds, and *S*-nitrosothiols (47, 114). These compounds differ in their mechanisms of NO release and in their need for specific cofactors (114, 115). Organic nitrates, such as glyceryl trinitrate (GTN), are metabolized by both enzymatic and nonenzymatic pathways, and all require the presence of thiols in order to become activated. The enzymatic pathways are believed to involve glutathione-*S*-transferase and cytochrome P450-related enzymes. Nonenzymatic pathways are thought to involve thiols present in the cytosol (47, 111, 114). These compounds can be used in biologic models, but when used clinically, tolerance is developed (114, 116).

Inorganic nitrites are potent NO donors, and include drugs such as isoamyl nitrite. They are thought to react with

Table III NO Donors

Class	Donor compound	Mechanism of action	Notes
Organic nitrates	Glyceryl trinitrate	Metabolized by enzymatic and nonenyzymatic pathways	—
	Isosorbide dinitrate	Releases NO on reaction with certain mercapto-group *SH-containing compounds	Used in humans to treat coronary ischemia; may act as a platelet suppressant
	Pentaerithrityl tetranitrate	Unknown	Long-acting NO donor; free of tolerance
Organic nitrites	Amyl nitrite	Requires thiol groups for NO release; nitrosothiols are active intermediates	—
Sydnonimines	Molsidomine	Metabolized to SIN-1 (below)	Inactive *in vitro*; must be converted to active form (SIN-1) by liver esterases; active *in vivo* and used in humans; forms superoxide ions and may also form peroxynitrite and hydroxyl radicals; NO release enhanced by superoxide dismutase
	3-Morpholinosydnonimine (SIN-1)	Hydrolyzed to yield open-ring form, SIN-1A, which releases NO	
S-Nitrosothiols	*S*-Nitroso-*N*-acetyl-D,L-penicillamine (SNAP)	Rapidly decomposes to disulfide and NO	May form thiol radicals
	S-Nitrosoglutathione	As above	As above
NONOates	DETA NONOate	Generates NO spontaneously, independent of tissue; releases NO in a first-order reaction at physiologic pH	High thiol concentrations decrease NO release; alkaline conditions decrease NO release
	Spermine NO	As above	—
	Diethylamine/NO	As above	—
	PYRRO-NO	As above	Liver-specific release
Iron nitrosyls	Sodium nitroprusside	Enzymatic and photochemical NO release	Produces cyanide

available thiol groups and to form *S*-nitrosothiols, which decompose to release NO (114). Their extent of generation of NO, and therefore their duration of action, depends on the rate of formation and subsequent decomposition of *S*-nitrosothiols (114). *S*-Nitroprusside, an inorganic nitroso compound used widely *in vivo*, spontaneously liberates NO via an unknown mechanism. It has a very short half-life (approximately 2 min in humans) and therefore must be administered continuously in order for it to exert a consistent effect (114). Disadvantages of *S*-nitroprusside include tolerance and the formation of the toxic by-product cyanide.

Molsidomine is a sydnonimine that must be metabolized by liver esterases to yield the active form, 3-morpholinosydnonimine (SIN-1). SIN-1 is then hydrolyzed to yield an open-ring form, called SIN-1A, which releases NO and superoxide anions. The formation of superoxide may give rise to oxidative side reactions, generating hydrogen peroxide and hydroxyl radicals as well as peroxynitrite (47). However, Singh *et al.* demonstrated that SIN-1 releases NO preferentially in the presence of electron acceptors, such as hemoglobin *in vivo* or in tissue homogenates, and in the presence of low levels of oxygen (117). The release of superoxide anions by SIN-1 should still be kept in mind by investigators, as should the knowledge that the sydnonimines are susceptible to light and oxygen (114). *S*-Nitrosothiols such as *S*-nitrosoglutathione (GSNO) release NO spontaneously by breakage of their S–NO bonds (115, 118). This NO donor is particularly interesting due to the high likelihood that it is formed *in vivo* through interaction with intracellular pools of glutathione (47).

An NO donor that we have found particularly useful in our laboratory is O_2-vinyl 1-(pyrrolidin-1-yl)diazen-1-ium-1,2-diolate (V-PYRRO/NO), due to the fact that this compound is metabolized to NO by both cultured hepatocytes and hepatocytes *in vivo*, triggering cGMP synthesis and protecting from induced apoptotic cell death and hepatotoxicity (119).

Although NO donors are invaluable in studying NO function, it should be noted that different NO donors have different potencies, half-lives, activation thresholds, and mechanisms of NO release. Because of this, each NO donor should be assessed in each system to ensure that the desired physiologic concentrations are used (47, 120).

2. Chemical Scavengers of NO

Because of the interaction of NO with certain compounds, including metals and hemoglobin, the addition of such materials to a system scavenges free NO and renders it unavailable in the culture media or tissue of interest. Some of the commonly used NO scavengers in experimental models include oxyhemoglobin, carboxy-PTIO, methoxy-PTIO, glutathione, and *N*-methyl-D-glucamine dithiocarbamate-Fe^{2+} (NOX). NOX is one of the most well-known NO scavengers, and is able to trap NO in solution to form a stable and water-soluble $[(MGD)_2–Fe^{2+}–NO]$ complex (71). The complex formed by NOX and trapped NO gives rise to a characteristic three-line EPR spectrum of a mononitrosyl-Fe^{2+} complex that can be measured, and this has been accomplished *in vivo*. This method of spin trapping and EPR measurement of NO production in the blood circulation of live, conscious mice has been described by Komarov and colleagues (71). Our laboratory has demonstrated that treatment of rats with NOX in a hemorrhagic shock model is associated with decreased hepatic injury and improved 24-hr survival following severe hemorrhage (121).

Another common NO scavenger is oxyhemoglobin, as found in red blood cells. This NO scavenger is naturally present in animals, but in cell culture models, red blood cells can be added to a system to scavenge NO reliably. An additional NO scavenger that also has antioxidant effects, methylene blue, has been found to attenuate partially the development of streptozotocin-induced diabetes in rats (122).

Glutathione, a potent endogenous antioxidant that neutralizes free radicals in the body, is also a scavenger of NO (see discussion above regarding GSNO). A deficiency of glutathione has been shown to worsen the severity of organ dysfunction after hemorrhagic shock, which is a condition known to be associated with a significant increase in NO produced by iNOS (123).

Two additional NO scavengers are carboxy-PTIO and methoxy-PTIO. Carboxy-PTIO is an NO scavenger that inactivates free radical NO (124). It inhibits responses to exogenous NO in the rat and mouse anococcygeus muscle and in the porcine anococcygeus muscle and retractor penis muscle (125).

3. NOS Inhibitors

Just as NO donors give valuable information, inhibitors of NOS add another tool for the elucidation of the role of NO in any given system. Inhibitors of NOS generally fall into two categories: the arginine analogs and the nonamino acid inhibitors. The majority of these inhibitors are not selective for any specific isoform of NOS. Isoform-selective NOS inhibitors exist, but it is important to note that their selectivity is only relative at best. All of the NOS inhibitors behave differently, both *in vitro* and *in vivo*. It is expected that each inhibitor will exhibit differences in uptake by cells and in *in vivo* distribution, but most inhibitors also exhibit some nonspecific or indirect effects. For this reason, choice of inhibitors and data interpretation should be made with caution. In addition, more than one inhibitor should be tested in a model when feasible; additional controls include the use of the D stereoisomers of the L-arginine analogs (which should be inactive), as well as competition with additional L-arginine. Nonselective inhibitors include L^G-monomethyl-L-arginine (L-NMMA), N^G-aminoarginine, and N^G-nitro-L-arginine methyl ester (L-NAME). In general, the simple L-arginine analogs inhibit both constitutive and inducible NOS isoforms. Isoform-specific NOS inhibitors mainly exhibit selectivity for nNOS and iNOS, and each may exhibit nearly equal selectivity for two of the NOS isoforms relative to a third. "Selective" nNOS inhibitors include 7-nitroindazole and its analogs, whereas selective iNOS inhibitors include aminoguanidine, L-N^6-(1-iminoethyl) lysine (L-NIL), and S-alkylated isothiourea derivatives (126, 127). It should be noted that aminoguanidine also suppresses spermine production independently of any effects on iNOS (128). N^G-Nitro-L-arginine (L-NA) is relatively selective for both eNOS and nNOS (129) and is one of many NOS inhibitors selective for more than one isoform. The majority of recent efforts have been aimed at developing iNOS-selective inhibitors, due to the implication of this isoform in conditions such as septic and hemorrhagic shock. For many of the isoform-selective inhibitors, the range of fold selectivity is rather large (see Table IV). The investigator must keep in mind that potency and relative selectivity of each NOS inhibitor varies greatly depending on differences in NOS preparations and conditions of specific models and experiments. An accurate summary of the comparative characteristics of the NOS inhibitors is beyond the scope of this chapter; however, several elegant and comprehensive articles have been devoted to this subject (127, 130–136).

B. Genetic Methods

1. Use of NOS-Deficient Animals

Although NO can be decreased significantly with pharmacologic NOS inhibitors, blockade with drugs does not completely distinguish between the three isoforms of NO. The recent development and commercial availability of mice with targeted disruption of the genes for the various isoforms of NOS offer a useful approach to studying the roles of each isoform and examining the effects of their deletion in intact animals (137). Huang *et al.* first made targeted deletions in the nNOS gene (138) and in the eNOS gene (139), and MacMicking *et al.* (140), Wei *et al.* (141), and Laubach *et al.* (142) introduced mice with a disruption of the iNOS gene. Such an approach circumvents the lack of specificity of NOS inhibitors. Since the early 1990s, when the NOS isoform-deficient (also known as NOS knockout) mice were developed, several studies in these animals have shown particular phenotypes for each knockout mouse (see Table V). Many characteristics of each NOS knockout mouse may be irrelevant to a particular study, but it is helpful to be aware of the various phenotypes.

Mice lacking the neuronal nitric oxide synthase gene were generated via homologous recombination by Huang *et*

Table IV Commonly Used NOS Inhibitors

Isoform inhibited	Compound	Class of compound	Type of inhibition	Relative selectivity	Ref.
Neuronal NOS (NOS-1)	L-NA (N^G-nitro-L-arginine)	L-Arginine analog	Reversible, competitive	nNOS = eNOS > iNOS (~10-fold)	129
	7-Nitroindazole (7-NI)	Indazole analog	Reversible, competitive	nNOS > eNOS and iNOS	173–176
	S-Ethyl-L-thiocitrulline	Thiourea analog	Potent, reversible, competitive	nNOS > eNOS (25- to 50-fold)	132
	S-Methyl-L-thiocitrulline	Thiourea analog	Potent, reversible, competitive	nNOS > eNOS (10- to 17-fold)	132, 136
Inducible NOS (NOS-2)	1400W [(aminomethyl) benzyl] acetamidine	Modified bisisothiourea	Slow, tight binding, essentially irreversible	iNOS > eNOS (5000-fold) iNOS > nNOS (200-fold)	177
	AET [*S*-(2-Aminoethyl)-isothiourea]	Bisisothiourea	Reversible by L-arginine, competitive	iNOS > eNOS (~30-fold)	133
	Aminoguanidine	Nonamino acid arginine analog	Reversible by L-arginine, competitive	iNOS > eNOS (50- to 500-fold)	131, 133, 178
	L-NIL [L-N^6-(1-iminoethyl)-lysine]	L-Arginine analog	Slow-binding, competitive iNOS inhibitor; rapid nNOS and eNOS inhibitor	iNOS > eNOS and nNOS (~30-fold)	179, 180
	S-Ethyl-isothiourea (SEITU)	Bisisothiourea (L-arginine analog)	Reversible, competitive	iNOS > nNOS (2- to 20-fold) iNOS > nNOS (2- to 40-fold)	135, 181, 182
	SMT (*S*-methyl-isothiourea)	Bisisothiourea (L-arginine analog)	Reversible, competitive	iNOS > eNOS and nNOS (2-fold)	133, 135, 136, 181
Endothelial NOS (NOS-3)	L-NIO	L-arginine analog	Irreversible, slow binding, potent	eNOS > iNOS and nNOS (5-fold)	136
All isoforms	L-NMMA (N^G-monomethyl-L-arginine)	L-Arginine analog	Reversible, competitive	Nonselective	4, 133
	L-NNA (N^G-nitro-L-arginine)	L-Arginine analog	Reversible inhibitor of eNOS and iNOS Irreversible inhibitor of nNOS in rat cerebellum	Relatively nonselective, but more potent for constitutive isoforms	130, 133, 134, 183
	L-NMA (N^G-methyl-L-arginine)	L-Arginine analog	Irreversible	Nonselective	130, 134, 184, 185
	L-NAME (N^G-nitro-L-arginine methyl ester)	L-Arginine analog	Reversible, competitive	Nonselective Cleaved by esterases to become active as L-NA	133
	L-Thiocitrulline	Thiourea analog	Reversible, competitive	Nonselective	186, 187

al. in 1993 (138). These mice were made by targeting the first translated exon of the nNOS gene, including the protein initiation codon ATG. These mutant mice do not express nNOS mRNA as detected by Northern blot analysis, or nNOS protein as detected by Western blot analysis (138). There is some level of NOS activity in the brain, due to the presence of other isoforms, most likely eNOS. Some of this activity may also be due to the existence of low-level natural splicing variants that remain in the knockout animals (143). Despite this finding, there is substantial evidence that significant NO production is absent in the brains of nNOS knockout animals (144–146). The nNOS mutant mice are fertile and surprisingly show no gross neuroanatomic abnormality. However, nNOS null mice are predisposed to violent, sexually aggressive behavior (147). The majority of experiments utilizing nNOS knockout mice involve the investigation of brain and neural tissue. Kano *et al.* (148) compared the role of NO as an amplifier of neurotransmitter release in the cor-

Table V Phenotypes of NOS Mutant Mice

NOS Isoform	Phenotype[a]	Ref.
Neuronal NOS	Pyloric stenosis and gastric dilatation	138
	Loss of slow IJP responses	137
	Resistance to focal and global cerebral ischemia	144, 188
	Increased aggressive behavior	147
	Preserved hippocampal LTP	143
Inducible NOS	Increased susceptibility to intracellular pathogens	140, 141
	Increased susceptibility to tumors	137
	Resistance to sepsis-induced and hemorrhage-induced hypotension	140
	Increased mortality secondary to polymicrobial abdominal sepsis	151
	Increased susceptibility to acute cardiac allograft rejection; decreased susceptibility to chronic rejection	152, 153
Endothelial NOS	Hypertension (elevated MABP)	139
	Absence of EDRF activity in aorta	137
	Increased susceptibility to global ischemia	189
	Impaired wound healing and angiogenesis	27

[a]Abbreviations: IJP, inhibitory junction potentials; LTP, long-term potentiation; MABP, mean arterial blood pressure; EDRF, endothelial-derived relaxing factor; Ach, acetylcholine.

tex, striatum, and hippocampus of wild-type versus nNOS- and eNOS-deficient mice. Using knockout mice, in addition to the NO donor SNAP and the selective NO inhibitor 7-NI, Kano and colleagues demonstrated that nNOS and eNOS appear to modulate different excitatory and inhibitory pathways of transmission, depending on brain region. Neuronal NOS may promote neuronal damage after cerebral ischemia by amplifying pathologic glutamate release, whereas eNOS activity might be beneficial by enhancing potentially neuroprotective release of GABA.

Targeted disruption of the eNOS isoform was performed in 1995 and has had tremendous impact on the study of vascular tone and vascular injury. Mice lacking the gene for eNOS are viable and fertile. However, Drazen *et al.* (149) demonstrated abnormalities in the reproductive function of eNOS null mice, which may account for their small litter size. These mice have no detectable eNOS mRNA or protein (139), and aortic rings from eNOS mutant mice fail to relax in response to acetylcholine, which is an NO-mediated event (138). The most notable characteristic expressed by eNOS knockout mice is hypertension, with animals having mean arterial blood pressures approximately 30% higher than wild-type littermates (139). Studies in these mice reveal that the absence of the endogenous vasodilator NO leads to elevated baseline blood pressure.

Three separate groups independently created unique targeted disruptions of the mouse iNOS gene in 1995 (140–142). Although each knockout mouse was created in a different manner, iNOS cannot be detected in any of these animals. Each of the mutants demonstrates normal growth and fertility. Characteristic to all three reported iNOS mutant mice is the absence of NO and nitrite production by peritoneal macrophages. This finding demonstrates the importance of NO produced by iNOS in immune-mediated actions. In fact, iNOS knockout mice have been demonstrated to have increased susceptibility to bacterial translocation (150) as well as to tumors and intracellular pathogens, and are relatively resistant to sepsis-induced hypotension (138). Cobb *et al.* (151), however, have made a seemingly counterintuitive discovery. In a model of cecal ligation and puncture, Cobb and associates showed that iNOS-deficient mice demonstrate increased mortality compared to wild-type controls. This finding suggests the possibility that iNOS gene function may provide a survival benefit in septic mice, despite previous reports that iNOS has a detrimental effect in septic and hemorrhagic shock. Inducible NOS appears to have an equally complex role in cardiac allograft rejection. Using a model of cardiac transplantation in iNOS-deficient mice, Koglin *et al.* demonstrated that iNOS appears to promote acute rejection but protects against chronic rejection and transplant arteriosclerosis (152–154).

Another particularly interesting finding in eNOS- and iNOS-deficient animals has been demonstrated by Kanno *et al.* in a study of myocardial ischemia/reperfusion injury in wild-type, eNOS, and iNOS knockout mice (155). The investigators found that in eNOS-deficient mice, ischemia/reperfusion in a Langendorff isolated heart model induced the superinduction of iNOS expression, and consequently significant NO production. In addition, eNOS was induced by ischemia/reperfusion in iNOS-deficient mice, but the amount of NO produced (as measured by nitrite levels) was much less than that produced from iNOS induction. This study supports others (156) that have demonstrated that compensation via alternative isoform use occurs in animals deficient in a particular NOS isoform.

It is clear that the development of animals deficient in the various NOS isoforms is an invaluable tool in NO research. Findings from NOS knockout mice are particularly useful when combined with studies involving the alternative scenario of NO overproduction, induced by gene transfer of various NOS. Because targeted mutations of each isoform of NOS have been performed and these animals studied extensively, NOS knockout mice of various types are available either commercially or via collaboration. Currently, mice deficient in both iNOS and eNOS (the iNOS/eNOS "double knockout") are being developed. However, all experiments in genetically modified animals should be approached with caution, because alterations in basal levels of various genes may affect the outcomes of treatments of these mice. As an example, the heat-shock protein 72 gene is higher at baseline in iNOS null animals, and this protein was associated with the resistance of these animals to renal ischemia/reperfusion injury (157).

2. NOS Gene Transfer

With the advent of recombinant DNA and gene transfer technologies, delivery of specific NOS genes makes local overexpression of NO possible. The advantage of using genetic manipulation rather than pharmacologic agents to increase NO is based on the fact that, unlike pharmacologic NO donors, gene transfer allows relatively long-term production of endogenous NO. Additionally, iNOS can be "induced" without treatment with proinflammatory cytokines and/or microbial products, thereby avoiding potentially confounding effects that are independent of NO production. Commonly employed gene transfer vectors in the scope of research in general include the adenovirus, adeno-associated virus, retrovirus, and herpes virus as well as other nonviral gene transfer methods such as cationic liposomes and the hemagglutinating virus of Japan (HVJ). The most commonly used vectors for NOS gene transfer are the adenovirus, the retrovirus, and HJV. Nonviral vectors are not routinely used in NOS transfer, and therefore will not be discussed in this chapter. (For a comparison of the gene transfer vectors mentioned above, see Chapter 38, this volume.)

The most commonly used method of NOS gene transfer involves the adenoviral vector, which has gained popularity because of its potent gene transfer efficiency. The adenovirus is a complex DNA virus, and its genome contains many overlapping sequences that code not only for the gene of interest, but also for viral proteins. New adenovirus is formed within approximately 30–40 hr postinfection and is released through host cell lysis (158). The adenovirus does not integrate into host genomic DNA, instead existing in the nucleus as an episome. This characteristic allows these viruses to target both actively dividing and quiescent cells. Such a characteristic makes the adenovirus a good vector for infecting those cells that replicate slowly or not at all, such as myocytes, vascular smooth muscle cells, and endothelial cells. In addition, the adenovirus has a particular affinity for human tissues, making it especially useful for human genetic therapies.

A potential limitation of the adenoviral vector is the transient nature of expression of the foreign gene of interest, due to the nonintegrated nature of the adenoviral DNA. There are certain circumstances—for example, in acute disease processes such as intimal hyperplasia secondary to injury—wherein transient gene expression may be sufficient or even ideal. Such transient expression is usually sufficient for studies involving iNOS and eNOS, however, because such models usually involve induced injury of some sort, in which the window of NOS effect is limited. A disadvantage of the adenoviral vector is the induction of a significant host inflammatory response to the transcribed foreign viral proteins, which is deleterious to both the host and to the success of the treatment. Currently, work is being done to develop second-generation adenoviruses that will express fewer viral products, thereby reducing the inflammatory response and potentially prolonging transgene expression.

Transfer of iNOS and eNOS to the wall of artery or vein has been utilized extensively in the study of various diseases (see Table VI). In our laboratory, the adenovirus has been used to transfer iNOS to knockout mice, leading to the discovery that a lack of NO produced by iNOS delays wound healing (26). Also, adenovirus-mediated iNOS gene transfer has been shown effective in blocking spontaneous and induced apoptotic hepatocyte death *in vitro* (159). Endothelial cells, such as hepatocytes, seem to be protected from apoptotic death by vascular adenoviral iNOS transfer (160). In the vasculature, Kibbe *et al.* (161) demonstrated in an *ex vivo* model using internal jugular veins and carotid arteries from domestic pigs that adenoviral iNOS can efficiently transduce vein segments. In addition, cotransfer with an adenovirus carrying the cDNA encoding guanosine triphosphate cyclohydrolase 1 produced maximal NO production compared to transfection with AdiNOS alone.

There is a paucity of literature available on the gene transfer of nNOS. However, successful adenoviral transfer of rat nNOS cDNA to human vascular smooth muscle cells (VSMCs) and human umbilical vein endothelial cells (HUVECs) has been performed (162). Cells infected with adenoviral nNOS (AdnNOS) expressed increased levels of nNOS protein and exhibited marked NO production in response to A-23187, acetylcholine (Ach), or bradykinin. The same investigators extended these observations in an *in vivo* model, in which they delivered a low titer of AdnNOS in a rabbit model of atherosclerotic carotid artery disease, thereby attenuating impaired Ach-induced relaxation in atherosclerotic arteries (162).

Table VI Use of NOS Gene Transfer Vectors in the Study of Various Disease Processes

Disease process	Model	Gene	Vector used	Effect	Ref.
Atherosclerosis	Carotid artery of cholesterol-fed rabbits	Rat nNOS	Adenovirus	Near complete correction of impaired Ach-induced arterial relaxation	162
Arterial injury	Rat carotid artery	Bovine eNOS	HVJ-modified liposomes	70% reduction in neointima/media ratio postinjury	169
	Rat carotid artery	Human iNOS	Adenovirus	97% reduction in I/M area ratio	190
	Porcine iliac artery	Human iNOS	Adenovirus	52% reduction in I/M area ratio	191
	Rat carotid artery	Human eNOS	Adenovirus	72% reduction in intima/media ratio	172
	Transfected RASMCs seeded onto rat carotid artery	Human eNOS	Retrovirus	37% reduction in neointimal area	168
	Porcine coronary artery following angioplasty	Human eNOS	Adenovirus	28% reduction in maximal neointimal thickness	171
Vein graft intimal hyperplasia	Dog model of balloon-induced femoral vein injury	Bovine eNOS	HVJ–liposomes	55% reduction in neointimal area	192
Transplant arteriosclerosis	Rat aortic allograft	Human iNOS	Adenovirus	Inhibited allograft arteriosclerosis	190
Pulmonary hypertension	Rat lung	Human eNOS	Recombinant adenovirus	Attenuated hypoxia-induced pulmonary hypertension	193
Hepatic transplant failure	Cold-preserved rat liver grafts	Human iNOS	Adenovirus	Successful gene induction into hepatocytes	194
Portal hypertension	Cirrhotic rat liver	Rat eNOS	Adenovirus	Reduction in mean portal pressures	195
Wound healing	Wounding in iNOS knockout mice	Human iNOS	Adenovirus	Attenuation of delayed wound healing	26
Cancer	Human carcinoma cells injected into athymic nude mice	Human iNOS	Retrovirus	Reduced tumor growth in athymic nude mice injected with human carcinoma cells	196
	Human renal carcinoma cells	Murine iNOS	Retrovirus	Suppression of tumorigenicity and abrogation of lung metastasis	197
Erectile dysfunction	Aged rats	Rat iNOS	Expression plasmid containing iNOS cDNA	Mitigation of age-associated erectile dysfunction	198

Another more recently developed vector is the adeno-associated virus (AAV), which is a member of the parvovirus family. Much of the research on AAV gene transfer has involved the transfer of NOS into the vascular system (163, 164). Advantages of the AAV include the fact that it has a relatively long duration of expression and produces little viral antigenic protein, thereby eliciting little to no inflammatory response in the host and lengthening the duration of transgene expression. Another attractive characteristic of AAV is its ability to infect a broad range of host cell types and species successfully, including humans, in which its use appears to be quite safe. Disadvantages of the AAV vector include its limited capacity to accommodate the insertion of small transgenes (less than 4.9 kb), and the fact that approximately 80% of humans carry preformed antibodies secondary to prior exposure to this vector, which may bind to AAV and clear it prior to cellular infection (165).

Retroviruses are eukaryotic RNA viruses that contain two single-stranded RNA molecules and viral proteins in an icosahedral viral core. Unlike the larger adenoviruses, these vectors have smaller, less complex genomes. Following viral internalization reverse transcription occurs, and the transferred genetic material becomes integrated into the host genome in a semipermanent fashion, permitting prolonged expression and becoming an inheritable trait. This long-term expression of the NOS gene is the primary advantage of retroviral vectors. Retroviral vectors are associated with very little inflammatory response, due to the possibility of deletion of essentially all of the coding sequences of the viral genome, resulting in elimination of viral protein production (166). Many investigators have used retroviruses to transfer a variety of genes. A discovery in our laboratory by Ceneviva *et al.* (167) utilized the retroviral gene transfer of human iNOS to cultured sheep pulmonary artery endothelial cells (SPAECs). After retroviral gene transfer of iNOS, SPAECs become resistant to lipopolysaccharide (LPS)-stimulated apoptosis. This study was an extension of work done previously by Tzeng *et al.* (160) in which SPAECs were found to be resistant to LPS-induced apoptosis after constitutive synthesis of NO following adenoviral transfer of iNOS or exposure to the NO donor SNAP. Chen *et al.* (168) used a retrovirus to deliver human eNOS to syngeneic rat arterial smooth muscle cells. The investigators then seeded these transfected smooth muscle cells onto the lumenal surface of balloon-injured rat carotid arteries and found that 2 weeks later, vessels seeded with the transfected SMCs displayed a significant reduction in neointimal formation and a threefold increase in vessel diameter.

The final vector used for gene transfer that will be discussed here is the HVJ–liposome complex. This vector is synthesized by the fusion of the DNA/liposome complex with UV-inactivated HVJ (166). Studies using HVJ–liposomes demonstrate much greater levels of successful gene transfer than with liposomes alone. This finding, combined with the fact that there has been no evidence of cellular toxicity with the HVJ–liposome complex, makes this an attractive vector. Endothelial NOS cDNA was first delivered into carotid arteries intralumenally by von der Leyen (169) using this method. This transfection resulted in enhanced arterial relaxation to the calcium ionophore A-23187 4 days after injury and infection, and a 70% reduction in the neointima/media area ratio at 14 days postinjury. Following publication of these results, other investigators used this and other vectors to deliver the eNOS gene to the vasculature to study the development of neotintimal formation (170–172).

VI. Conclusions

Nitric oxide is certainly among the most important signaling and effector molecules in biologic systems, as is demonstrated by the vast field of study surrounding it. In the 1980s, pioneers in the field of NO research dissected out the basic concepts of the synthesis and biology of NO, and new discoveries regarding the myriad functions of NO continue to be made on a daily basis. Despite two decades of intensive study, however, the role of NO in many biologic functions and disease processes remains elusive. By utilizing the currently available tools fully and by developing new innovative techniques for the detection and manipulation of NO in biologic systems, we will be able to delineate the many biologic functions of NO and NOS. It is hoped that this knowledge will allow us to develop new strategies and treatments for those diseases that involve either pathologic overproduction or underproduction of NO.

References

1. Mitchell, H. H., Shonle, H. A., and Grindley, H. S. (1916). The origin of the nitrates in the urine. *J. Biol. Chem.* **24,** 461–490.
2. Green, L. C., Ruiz, D. L., Wagner, D. A., Rand, W., Istfan, N., Young, V. R., and Tannenbaum, S. R. (1981). Nitrate biosynthesis in man. *Proc. Natl. Acad. Sci. U.S.A* **78,** 7764–7768.
3. Green, L. C., Tannenbaum, S. R., and Goldman, P. (1981). Nitrate synthesis in the germfree and conventional rat. *Science* **212,** 56–58.
4. Rees, D. D., Palmer, R. M., Hodson, H. F., and Moncada, S. (1989). A specific inhibitor of nitric oxide formation from L-arginine attenuates endothelium-dependent relaxation. *Br. J. Pharmacol.* **96,** 418–424.
5. Shaffer, J. E., Han, B. J., Chern, W. H., and Lee, F. W. (1992). Lack of tolerance to a 24-hour infusion of *S*-nitroso *N*-acetylpenicillamine (SNAP) in conscious rabbits. *J. Pharmacol. Exp. Ther.* **260,** 286–293.
6. Stuehr, D. J., and Marletta, M. A. (1985). Mammalian nitrate biosynthesis: Mouse macrophages produce nitrite and nitrate in response to *Escherichia coli* lipopolysaccharide. *Proc. Natl. Acad. Sci. U.S.A* **82,** 7738–7742.
7. Furchgott, R. F., and Zawadzki, J. V. (1980). The obligatory role of endothelial cells in the relaxation of arterial smooth muscle by acetylcholine. *Nature (London)* **288,** 373–376.
8. Ignarro, L. J., Buga, G. M., Wood, K. S., Byrns, R. E., and Chaudhuri, G. (1987). Endothelium-derived relaxing factor produced and released from artery and vein is nitric oxide. *Proc. Natl. Acad. Sci. U.S.A* **84,** 9265–9269.
9. Palmer, R. M., Ferrige, A. G., and Moncada, S. (1987). Nitric oxide release accounts for the biological activity of endothelium-derived relaxing factor. *Nature (London)* **327,** 524–526.
10. Hibbs, J. B., Jr., Taintor, R. R., and Vavrin, Z. (1987). Macrophage cytotoxicity: Role for L-arginine deiminase and imino nitrogen oxidation to nitrite. *Science* **235,** 473–476.
11. Nathan, C., and Hibbs, J. B., Jr. (1991). Role of nitric oxide synthesis in macrophage antimicrobial activity. *Curr. Opin. Immunol.* **3,** 65–70.
12. Garthwaite, J., Charles, S. L., and Chess-Williams, R. (1988). Endothelium-derived relaxing factor release on activation of NMDA receptors suggests role as intercellular messenger in the brain. *Nature (London)* **336,** 385–388.
13. Garthwaite, J. (1991). Glutamate, nitric oxide and cell-cell signalling in the nervous system. *Trends Neurosci.* **14,** 60–67.
14. Moncada, S., and Higgs, A. (1993). The L-arginine-nitric oxide pathway. *N. Engl. J. Med.* **329,** 2002–2012.
15. Kim, Y. M., de Vera, M. E., Watkins, S. C., and Billiar, T. R. (1997). Nitric oxide protects cultured rat hepatocytes from tumor necrosis factor-alpha-induced apoptosis by inducing heat shock protein 70 expression. *J. Biol. Chem.* **272,** 1402–1411.
16. Li, J., Billiar, T. R., Talanian, R. V., and Kim, Y. M. (1997). Nitric oxide reversibly inhibits seven members of the caspase family via *S*-nitrosylation. *Biochem. Biophys. Res. Commun.* **240,** 419–424.
17. Nathan, C. (1992). Nitric oxide as a secretory product of mammalian cells. *FASEB J.* **6,** 3051–3064.
18. Izumi, Y., Clifford, D. B., and Zorumski, C. F. (1992). Inhibition of long-term potentiation by NMDA-mediated nitric oxide release. *Science* **257,** 1273–1276.
19. Kim, N., Azadzoi, K. M., Goldstein, I., and Saenz de Tejada, I. (1991). A nitric oxide-like factor mediates nonadrenergic-noncholinergic neurogenic relaxation of penile corpus cavernosum smooth muscle. *J. Clin. Invest* **88,** 112–118.
20. Rajfer, J., Aronson, W. J., Bush, P. A., Dorey, F. J., and Ignarro, L. J. (1992). Nitric oxide as a mediator of relaxation of the corpus cavernosum in response to nonadrenergic, noncholinergic neurotransmission. *N. Engl. J. Med.* **326,** 90–94.
21. Blomqvist, H., Wickerts, C. J., Andreen, M., Ullberg, U., Ortqvist, A., and Frostell, C. (1993). Enhanced pneumonia resolution by inhalation of nitric oxide? *Acta Anaesthesiol. Scand.* **37,** 110–114.
22. Vanderwinden, J. M., Mailleux, P., Schiffmann, S. N., Vanderhaeghen, J. J., and De Laet, M. H. (1992). Nitric oxide synthase activity in infantile hypertrophic pyloric stenosis [see comments]. *N. Engl. J. Med.* **327,** 511–515 [published erratum appears in *N. Engl. J. Med.* **327**(17), 1252].
23. Fukumura, D., and Jain, R. K. (1998). Role of nitric oxide in angiogenesis and microcirculation in tumors. *Cancer Metastasis Rev.* **17,** 77–89.

24. Thomsen, L. L., and Miles, D. W. (1998). Role of nitric oxide in tumor progression: Lessons from human tumours. *Cancer Metastasis Rev.* **17,** 107–118.
25. Lala, P. K., and Orucevic, A. (1998). Role of nitric oxide in tumor progression: Lessons from experimental tumors. *Cancer Metastasis Rev.* **17,** 91–106.
26. Yamasaki, K., Edington, H. D., McClosky, C., Tzeng, E., Lizonova, A., Kovesdi, I., Steed, D. L., and Billiar, T. R. (1998). Reversal of impaired wound repair in iNOS-deficient mice by topical adenoviral-mediated iNOS gene transfer. *J. Clin. Invest* **101,** 967–971.
27. Lee, P. C., Salyapongse, A. N., Bragdon, G. A., Shears, L. L., Watkins, S. C., Edington, H. D., and Billiar, T. R. (1999). Impaired wound healing and angiogenesis in eNOS-deficient mice. *Am. J. Physiol.* **277,** H1600–H1608.
28. Lowenstein, C. J., Dinerman, J. L., and Snyder, S. H. (1994). Nitric oxide: A physiologic messenger. *Ann. Intern. Med.* **120,** 227–237.
29. Geller, D. A., and Billiar, T. R. (1998). Molecular biology of nitric oxide synthases. *Cancer Metastasis Rev.* **17,** 7–23.
30. Stuehr, D. J., Kwon, N. S., Nathan, C. F., Griffith, O. W., Feldman, P. L., and Wiseman, J. (1991). *N*-Omega-hydroxy-L-arginine is an intermediate in the biosynthesis of nitric oxide from L-arginine. *J. Biol. Chem.* **266,** 6259–6263.
31. Vadon-LeGoff, S., and Tenu, J. -P. (1997). Nitric oxide biosynthesis in mammals. *In* "Nitric Oxide Research From Chemistry to Biology: EPR Spectroscopy of Nitrosylated Compounds" (Y. A. Henry, A. Guissani, and B. Ducastel, eds.), pp. 175–192. R.G. Landes Company, Austin.
32. Kiechle, F. L., and Malinski, T. (1993). Nitric oxide. Biochemistry, pathophysiology, and detection. *Am. J. Clin. Pathol.* **100,** 567–575.
33. Kwon, N. S., Nathan, C. F., Gilker, C., Griffith, O. W., Matthews, D. E., and Stuehr, D. J. (1990). L-Citrulline production from L-arginine by macrophage nitric oxide synthase. The ureido oxygen derives from dioxygen. *J. Biol. Chem.* **265,** 13442–13445.
34. Leone, A. M., Francis, P. L., Palmer, R. M., Ashton, D. S., and Moncada, S. (1991). Thermospray tandem mass spectrometric analysis of oxygen incorporation into citrulline by nitric oxide synthase. *Biol. Mass Spectrom.* **20,** 759–762.
35. Sessa, W. C. (1994). The nitric oxide synthase family of proteins. *J. Vasc. Res.* **31,** 131–143.
36. Sase, K., and Michel, T. (1995). Expression of constitutive endothelial nitric oxide synthase in human blood platelets. *Life Sci.* **57,** 2049–2055.
37. Bredt, D. S., and Snyder, S. H. (1992). Nitric oxide, a novel neuronal messenger. *Neuron* **8,** 3–11.
38. Fiallos-Estrada, C. E., Kummer, W., Mayer, B., Bravo, R., Zimmermann, M., and Herdegen, T. (1993). Long-lasting increase of nitric oxide synthase immunoreactivity, NADPH-diaphorase reaction and c-JUN co-expression in rat dorsal root ganglion neurons following sciatic nerve transection. *Neurosci. Lett.* **150,** 169–173.
39. Herdegen, T., Brecht, S., Mayer, B., Leah, J., Kummer, W., Bravo, R., and Zimmermann, M. (1993). Long-lasting expression of JUN and KROX transcription factors and nitric oxide synthase in intrinsic neurons of the rat brain following axotomy. *J. Neurosci.* **13,** 4130–4145.
40. Furchgott, R. F., and Vanhoutte, P. M. (1989). Endothelium-derived relaxing and contracting factors. *FASEB J.* **3,** 2007–2018.
41. Moncada, S. (1992). The 1991 Ulf von Euler Lecture. The L-arginine: Nitric oxide pathway. *Acta Physiol. Scand.* **145,** 201–227.
42. Cho, H. J., Xie, Q. W., Calaycay, J., Mumford, R. A., Swiderek, K. M., Lee, T. D., and Nathan, C. (1992). Calmodulin is a subunit of nitric oxide synthase from macrophages. *J. Exp. Med.* **176,** 599–604.
43. Iida, S., Ohshima, H., Oguchi, S., Hata, T., Suzuki, H., Kawasaki, H., and Esumi, H. (1992). Identification of inducible calmodulin-dependent nitric oxide synthase in the liver of rats. *J. Biol. Chem.* **267,** 25385–25388.
44. Nathan, C., and Xie, Q. W. (1994). Regulation of biosynthesis of nitric oxide. *J. Biol. Chem.* **269,** 13725–13728.
45. Guo, F. H., De Raeve, H. R., Rice, T. W., Stuehr, D. J., Thunnissen, F. B., and Erzurum, S. C. (1995). Continuous nitric oxide synthesis by inducible nitric oxide synthase in normal human airway epithelium *in vivo. Proc. Natl. Acad. Sci. U.S.A.* **92,** 7809–7813.
46. Klahr, S., and Morrissey, J. (1995). Renal disease: The two faces of nitric oxide [editorial; comment]. *Lab. Invest.* **72,** 1–3.
47. Wink, D. A., Feelisch, M., Vodovotz, Y., Fukuto, J., and Grisham, M. B. (1999). The chemical biology of nitric oxide. *In* "Reactive Oxygen Species in Biological Systems: An Interdisciplinary Approach" (C.A. Colton, and D.L. Gilbert, eds.), pp. 245–291. Kluwer Academic/Plenum Publishing, New York.
48. Kishimoto, J., Spurr, N., Liao, M., Lizhi, L., Emson, P., and Xu, W. (1992). Localization of brain nitric oxide synthase (NOS) to human chromosome 12 *Genomics* **14,** 802–804 [published erratum appears in *Genomics* **15**(2), 465].
49. Chartrain, N. A., Geller, D. A., Koty, P. P., Sitrin, N. F., Nussler, A. K., Hoffman, E. P., Billiar, T. R., Hutchinson, N. I., and Mudgett, J. S. (1994). Molecular cloning, structure, and chromosomal localization of the human inducible nitric oxide synthase gene. *J. Biol. Chem.* **269,** 6765–6772.
50. Marsden, P. A., Heng, H. H., Scherer, S. W., Stewart, R. J., Hall, A. V., Shi, X. M., Tsui, L. C., and Schappert, K. T. (1993). Structure and chromosomal localization of the human constitutive endothelial nitric oxide synthase gene. *J. Biol. Chem.* **268,** 17478–17488.
51. Bredt, D. S., Hwang, P. M., Glatt, C. E., Lowenstein, C., Reed, R. R., and Snyder, S. H. (1991). Cloned and expressed nitric oxide synthase structurally resembles cytochrome P-450 reductase. *Nature (London)* **351,** 714–718.
52. Xie, Q. W., Cho, H. J., Calaycay, J., Mumford, R. A., Swiderek, K. M., Lee, T. D., Ding, A., Troso, T., and Nathan, C. (1992). Cloning and characterization of inducible nitric oxide synthase from mouse macrophages. *Science* **256,** 225–228.
53. Sessa, W. C., Barber, C. M., and Lynch, K. R. (1993). Mutation of *N*-myristoylation site converts endothelial cell nitric oxide synthase from a membrane to a cytosolic protein. *Circ. Res.* **72,** 921–924.
54. Archer, S. (1993). Measurement of nitric oxide in biological models. *FASEB J.* **7,** 349–360.
55. Dawson, T. M., and Snyder, S. H. (1994). Gases as biological messengers: Nitric oxide and carbon monoxide in the brain. *J. Neurosci.* **14,** 5147–5159.
56. Malinski, T., Kubaszewski, T., and Kiechle, F. (1996). Electrochemical and spectroscopic methods of nitric oxide detection. *In* "Nitric Oxide Synthase: Characterization and Functional Analysis" (M.D. Maines, ed.), pp. 14–33. Academic Press, San Diego.
57. Aoki, T. (1990). Continuous flow determination of nitrite with membrane separation/chemiluminescence detection. *Biomed. Chromatogr.* **4,** 128–130.
58. Archer, S. L., and Cowan, N. J. (1991). Measurement of endothelial cytosolic calcium concentration and nitric oxide production reveals discrete mechanisms of endothelium-dependent pulmonary vasodilatation. *Circ. Res.* **68,** 1569–1581.
59. Fontijn, A., Sabadell, A. J., and Ronco, R. J. (1970). Homogenous chemiluminescent measurement of nitric oxide with ozone. *Anal. Chem.* **42,** 575–579.
60. Zafiriou, O. C., and McFarland, M. (1980). Determination of trace levels of nitric oxide in aqueous solution. *Anal. Chem.* **52,** 1667.
61. Michelakis, E. D., and Archer, S. L. (1998). The measurement of NO in biological systems using chemiluminescence. *In* "Nitric Oxide Protocols" (M.A. Titheradge, ed.), pp. 111–128. Humana Press, Totowa, NJ.
62. Titheradge, M. A. (1998). The enzymatic measurement of nitrate and nitrite. *In* "Nitric Oxide Protocols" (M.A. Titheradge, ed.), pp. 83–92. Humana Press, Totowa, NJ.
63. Green, L. C., Wagner, D. A., Glogowski, J., Skipper, P. L., Wishnok, J. S., and Tannenbaum, S. R. (1982). Analysis of nitrate, nitrite, and [15N]nitrate in biological fluids. *Anal. Biochem.* **126,** 131–138.

64. Vodovotz, Y. (1996). Modified microassay for serum nitrite and nitrate. *Biotechniques* **20,** 390-2, 394.
65. Luckhart, S., Vodovotz, Y., Cui, L., and Rosenberg, R. (1998). The mosquito *Anopheles stephensi* limits malaria parasite development with inducible synthesis of nitric oxide. *Proc. Natl. Acad. Sci. U.S.A.* **95,** 5700–5705.
66. Wu, G. Y., and Brosnan, J. T. (1992). Macrophages can convert citrulline into arginine *Biochem. J.* **281**(Pt. 1), 45–48 [published erratum appears in *Biochem. J.* **283**(Pt. 3), 919].
67. Taniguchi, S., Takahashi, K., and Sumihare, N. (1985). Nitrate. *In* "Methods of Enzymatic Analysis" (U. Bergmeyer, J. Bergmeyer, and M. Grassl, eds.), pp. 578–585. VCH Publishers, Deerfield Beach, FL.
68. Farrell, A. J., Blake, D. R., Palmer, R. M., and Moncada, S. (1992). Increased concentrations of nitrite in synovial fluid and serum samples suggest increased nitric oxide synthesis in rheumatic diseases. *Ann. Rheum. Dis.* **51,** 1219–1222.
69. Kaiser, L., and Williams, J. F. (1997). Possible problems in measuring nitric oxide. *JAVMA* **210,** 1584–1586.
70. Ohnishi, S. T. (1998). Measurement of NO using electron paramagnetic resonance. *In* "Nitric Oxide Protocols" (M.A. Titheradge, ed.), pp. 129–154. Humana Press, Totowa, NJ.
71. Komarov, A., Mattson, D., Jones, M. M., Singh, P. K., and Lai, C. S. (1993). *In vivo* spin trapping of nitric oxide in mice. *Biochem. Biophys. Res. Commun.* **195,** 1191–1198.
72. Komarov, A. M., and Lai, C. S. (1995). Detection of nitric oxide production in mice by spin-trapping electron paramagnetic resonance spectroscopy. *Biochim. Biophys. Acta* **1272,** 29–36.
73. Pieper, G. M., and Lai, C. S. (1996). Evaluation of vascular actions of the nitric oxide-trapping agent, *N*-methyl-D-glucamine dithiocarbamate-Fe^{2+}, on basal and agonist-stimulated nitric oxide activity. *Biochem. Biophys. Res. Commun.* **219,** 584–590.
74. Kotake, Y., Tanigawa, T., Tanigawa, M., Ueno, I., Allen, D. R., and Lai, C. S. (1996). Continuous monitoring of cellular nitric oxide generation by spin trapping with an iron-dithiocarbamate complex. *Biochim. Biophys. Acta* **1289,** 362–368.
75. Shibuki, K. (1990). An electrochemical microprobe for detecting nitric oxide release in brain tissue. *Neurosci. Res. (N.Y.)* **9,** 69–76.
76. Schmidt, K., and Mayer, B. (1998). Determination of NO with a Clark-type electrode. *In* "Nitric Oxide Protocols" (M.A. Titheradge, ed.), pp. 101–110. Humana Press, Totowa, NJ.
77. Malinski, T., and Taha, Z. (1992). Nitric oxide release from a single cell measured *in situ* by a porphyrinic-based microsensor [see comments]. *Nature* (*London*) **358,** 676–678.
78. Taha, Z., Kiechle, F., and Malinski, T. (1992). Oxidation of nitric oxide by oxygen in biological systems monitored by porphyrinic sensor. *Biochem. Biophys. Res. Commun.* **188,** 734–739.
79. Malinski, T., Bailey, F., Zhang, Z. G., and Chopp, M. (1993). Nitric oxide measured by a porphyrinic microsensor in rat brain after transient middle cerebral artery occlusion. *J. Cereb. Blood Flow Metab.* **13,** 355–358.
80. Tschudi, M. R., Mesaros, S., Luscher, T. F., and Malinski, T. (1996). Direct *in situ* measurement of nitric oxide in mesenteric resistance arteries. Increased decomposition by superoxide in hypertension. *Hypertension* **27,** 32–35.
81. Birder, L. A., and De Groat, W. C. (1998). Contribution of C-fiber afferent nerves and autonomic pathways in the urinary bladder to spinal c-fos expression induced by bladder irritation. *Somatosens. Mot. Res.* **15,** 5–12.
82. Stingele, R., Wilson, D. A., Traystman, R. J., and Hanley, D. F. (1998). Tyrosine confounds oxidative electrochemical detection of nitric oxide. *Am. J. Physiol.* **274,** H1698–H1704.
83. Weinberg, J. B., Misukonis, M. A., Shami, P. J., Mason, S. N., Sauls, D. L., Dittman, W. A., Wood, E. R., Smith, G. K., McDonald, B., and Bachus, K. E. (1995). Human mononuclear phagocyte inducible nitric oxide synthase (iNOS): Analysis of iNOS mRNA, iNOS protein, biopterin, and nitric oxide production by blood monocytes and peritoneal macrophages. *Blood* **86,** 1184–1195.
84. Luss, H., Li, R. K., Shapiro, R. A., Tzeng, E., McGowan, F. X., Yoneyama, T., Hatakeyama, K., Geller, D. A., Mickle, D. A., Simmons, R. L., and Billiar, T. R. (1997). Dedifferentiated human ventricular cardiac myocytes express inducible nitric oxide synthase mRNA but not protein in response to IL-1, TNF, IFNgamma, and LPS. *J. Mol. Cell Cardiol.* **29,** 1153–1165.
85. Taylor, G. M., and Cook, H. T. (1998). A practical protocol for the demonstration of NOS using *in situ* hybridization. *In* "Nitric Oxide Protocols" (M.A. Titheradge, ed.), pp. 191–204. Humana Press, Totowa, NJ.
86. Smith, F. S., and Titheradge, M. A. (1998). Detection of NOS isoforms by Western-blot analysis. *In* "Nitric oxide Protocols" (M.A. Titheradge, ed.), pp. 171–180. Humana Press, Totowa, NJ.
87. Cattel, V., and Mosley, K. (1998). Immunohistochemical localization of NOS isoforms. *In* "Nitric Oxide Protocols" (M.A. Titheradge, ed.), pp. 181–190. Humana Press, Totowa, NJ.
88. Zhang, H. Y., and Phan, S. H. (1999). Inhibition of myofibroblast apoptosis by transforming growth factor beta(1). *Am. J. Respir. Cell Mol. Biol.* **21,** 658–665.
89. Feelisch, M., and Noack, E. A. (1987). Correlation between nitric oxide formation during degradation of organic nitrates and activation of guanylate cyclase. *Eur. J. Pharmacol.* **139,** 19–30.
90. Salter, M., and Knowles, R. G. (1998). Assay of NOS Activity by the measurement of conversion of oxyhemoglobin to methemoglobin by NO. *In* "Nitric Oxide Protocols" (M.A. Titheradge, ed.), pp. 61–66. Humana Press, Totowa, NJ.
91. Knowles, R. G., and Salter, M. (1998). Measurement of NOS activity by conversion of radiolabeled arginine to citrulline using ion-exchange separation. *In* "Nitric Oxide Protocols" (M.A. Titheradge, ed.), pp. 67–74. Humana Press, Totowa, NJ.
92. Knowles, R. G., Palacios, M., Palmer, R. M., and Moncada, S. (1989). Formation of nitric oxide from L-arginine in the central nervous system: A transduction mechanism for stimulation of the soluble guanylate cyclase. *Proc. Natl. Acad. Sci. U.S.A* **86,** 5159–5162.
93. Thomsen, L. L., Miles, D. W., Happerfield, L., Bobrow, L. G., Knowles, R. G., and Moncada, S. (1995). Nitric oxide synthase activity in human breast cancer. *Br. J. Cancer* **72,** 41–44.
94. Cunningham, J. M., and Rayne, R. C. (1998). Radiochemical measurement of NOS activity by conversion of [^{14}C]L-arginine to citrulline using HPLC separation. *In* "Nitric Oxide Protocols" (M.A. Titheradge, ed.), pp. 75–82. Humana Press, Totowa, NJ.
95. Vallance, P., Leone, A., Calver, A., Collier, J., and Moncada, S. (1992). Accumulation of an endogenous inhibitor of nitric oxide synthesis in chronic renal failure. *Lancet* **339,** 572–575.
96. Kerwin, J. F., Jr., Lancaster, J. R., Jr., and Feldman, P. L. (1995). Nitric oxide: A new paradigm for second messengers. *J. Med. Chem.* **38,** 4343–4362.
97. Schmidt, H. H., Lohmann, S. M., and Walter, U. (1993). The nitric oxide and cGMP signal transduction system: Regulation and mechanism of action. *Biochim. Biophys. Acta* **1178,** 153–175.
98. Murad, F. (1994). The nitric oxide-cyclic GMP signal transduction system for intracellular and intercellular communication. *Recent Prog. Horm. Res.* **49,** 239–248.
99. Ignarro, L. J., Wood, K. S., and Wolin, M. S. (1984). Regulation of purified soluble guanylate cyclase by porphyrins and metalloporphyrins: A unifying concept. *Adv. Cyclic Nucleotide Protein Phosphorylation Res.* **17,** 267–274.
100. Laychock, S. G. (1998). Determination of NOS activity using cyclic-GMP formation. *In* "Nitric Oxide Protocols" (M.A. Titheradge, ed.), pp. 93–100. Humana Press, Totowa, NJ.

101. Steiner, A. L., Kipnis, D. M., Utiger, R., and Parker, C. (1969). Radioimmunoassay for the measurement of adenosine 3′,5′-cyclic phosphate. *Proc. Natl. Acad. Sci. U.S.A* **64,** 367–373.
102. Johnson, G., III, Tsao, P. S., and Lefer, A. M. (1991). Cardioprotective effects of authentic nitric oxide in myocardial ischemia with reperfusion. *Crit. Care Med.* **19,** 244–252.
103. Lefer, A. M., and Lefer, D. J. (1993). Pharmacology of the endothelium in ischemia–reperfusion and circulatory shock. *Annu. Rev. Pharmacol. Toxicol.* **33,** 71–90.
104. Luscher, T. F., Raij, L., and Vanhoutte, P. M. (1987). Endothelium-dependent vascular responses in normotensive and hypertensive Dahl rats. *Hypertension* **9,** 157–163.
105. Lefer, A. M., and Ma, X. L. (1991). Endothelial dysfunction in the splanchnic circulation following ischemia and reperfusion. *J. Cardiovas. Res.* **17,** S186–S190.
106. Frostell, C., Fratacci, M. D., Wain, J. C., Jones, R., and Zapol, W. M. (1991). Inhaled nitric oxide. A selective pulmonary vasodilator reversing hypoxic pulmonary vasoconstriction *Circulation* **83,** 2038–2047 [published erratum appears in *Circulation* **84**(5), 2212].
107. Rossaint, R., Falke, K. J., Lopez, F., Slama, K., Pison, U., and Zapol, W. M. (1993). Inhaled nitric oxide for the adult respiratory distress syndrome [see comments]. *N. Engl. J. Med.* **328,** 399–405.
108. Rossaint, R., Pison, U., Gerlach, H., and Falke, K. J. (1993). Inhaled nitric oxide: Its effects on pulmonary circulation and airway smooth muscle cells. *Eur. Heart J.* **14**(Suppl. I), 133–140.
109. Thebaud, B., Arnal, J. F., Mercier, J. C., and Dinh-Xuan, A. T. (1999). Inhaled and exhaled nitric oxide. *Cell. Mol. Life Sci.* **55,** 1103–1112.
110. Andonegui, G., Trevani, A. S., Gamberale, R., Carreras, M. C., Poderoso, J. J., Giordano, M., and Geffner, J. R. (1999). Effect of nitric oxide donors on oxygen-dependent cytotoxic responses mediated by neutrophils. *J. Immunol.* **162,** 2922–2930.
111. Yoshimoto, H., Suehiro, A., and Kakishita, E. (1999). Exogenous nitric oxide inhibits platelet activation in whole blood. *J. Cardiovasc. Pharmacol.* **33,** 109–115.
112. Shah, N. S., Nakayama, D. K., Jacob, T. D., Nishio, I., Imai, T., Billiar, T. R., Exler, R., Yousem, S. A., Motoyama, E. K., and Peitzman, A. B. (1997). Efficacy of inhaled nitric oxide in oleic acid-induced acute lung injury [see comments]. *Crit. Care Med.* **25,** 153–158.
113. Rossaint, R., Falke, K. J., Lopez, F., Slama, K., Pison, U., and Zapol, W. M. (1993). Inhaled nitric oxide for the adult respiratory distress syndrome [see comments]. *N. Engl. J. Med.* **328,** 399–405.
114. Tullett, J. M., and Rees, D. D. (1998). Use of NO donors in biological systems. *In* "Nitric Oxide Protocols" (M.A. Titheradge, ed.), pp. 205–214. Humana Press, Totowa, NJ.
115. Feelisch, M. (1998). The use of nitric oxide donors in pharmacological studies [see comments]. *Naunyn Schmiedebergs Arch. Pharmacol.* **358,** 113–122.
116. Feelisch, M. (1993). Biotransformation to nitric oxide of organic nitrates in comparison to other nitrovasodilators. *Eur. Heart J.* **14**(Suppl.I), 123–132.
117. Singh, U. P., Obayashi, E., Takahashi, S., Iizuka, T., Shoun, H., and Shiro, Y. (1998). The effects of heme modification on reactivity, ligand binding properties and iron-coordination structures of cytochrome P450 nor. *Biochim. Biophys. Acta* **1384,** 103–111.
118. Bauer, J. A., Booth, B. P., and Fung, H. L. (1995). Nitric oxide donors: Biochemical pharmacology and therapeutics. *Adv. Pharmacol.* **34,** 361–381.
119. Saavedra, J. E., Billiar, T. R., Williams, D. L., Kim, Y. M., Watkins, S. C., and Keefer, L. K. (1997). Targeting nitric oxide (NO) delivery *in vivo*. Design of a liver-selective NO donor prodrug that blocks tumor necrosis factor-alpha- induced apoptosis and toxicity in the liver. *J. Med. Chem.* **40,** 1947–1954.
120. Ferrero, R., Rodriguez-Pascual, F., Miras-Portugal, M. T., and Torres, M. (1999). Comparative effects of several nitric oxide donors on intracellular cyclic GMP levels in bovine chromaffin cells: Correlation with nitric oxide production. *Br. J. Pharmacol.* **127,** 779–787.
121. Menezes, J., Hierholzer, C., Watkins, S. C., Lyons, V., Peitzman, A. B., Billiar, T. R., Tweardy, D. J., and Harbrecht, B. G. (1999). A novel nitric oxide scavenger decreases liver injury and improves survival after hemorrhagic shock. *Am. J. Physiol.* **277,** G144–G151.
122. Haluzik, M., Nedvidkova, J., and Skrha, J. (1998). The influence of NO synthase inhibitor and free oxygen radicals scavenger—methylene blue—on streptozotocin-induced diabetes in rats. *Physiol. Res.* **47,** 337–341.
123. Robinson, M. K., Rounds, J. D., Hong, R. W., Jacobs, D. O., and Wilmore, D. W. (1992). Glutathione deficiency increases organ dysfunction after hemorrhagic shock. *Surgery* **112,** 140–147.
124. Akaike, T., Yoshida, M., Miyamoto, Y., Sato, K., Kohno, M., Sasamoto, K., Miyazaki, K., Ueda, S., and Maeda, H. (1993). Antagonistic action of imidazolineoxyl *N*-oxides against endothelium-derived relaxing factor/NO through a radical reaction. *Biochemistry* **32,** 827–832.
125. Li, C. G., and Rand, M. J. (1999). Effects of hydroxocobalamin and carboxy-PTIO on nitrergic transmission in porcine anococcygeus and retractor penis muscles. *Br. J. Pharmacol.* **127,** 172–176.
126. Muscara, M. N., and Wallace, J. L. (1999). Nitric oxide. V. therapeutic potential of nitric oxide donors and inhibitors. *Am. J. Physiol.* **276,** G1313–G1316.
127. Southan, G. J., and Szabo, C. (1996). Selective pharmacological inhibition of distinct nitric oxide synthase isoforms. *Biochem. Pharmacol.* **51,** 383–394.
128. Gahl, W. A., and Pitot, H. C. (1978). Reversal by aminoguanidine of the inhibition of proliferation of human fibroblasts by spermidine and spermine. *Chem. Biol. Interact.* **22,** 91–98.
129. Furfine, E. S., Harmon, M. F., Paith, J. E., and Garvey, E. P. (1993). Selective inhibition of constitutive nitric oxide synthase by L-*N*G-nitroarginine. *Biochemistry* **32,** 8512–8517.
130. Vargas, H. M., Cuevas, J. M., Ignarro, L. J., and Chaudhuri, G. (1991). Comparison of the inhibitory potencies of *N*(G)-methyl-, *N*(G)-*n*. *J. Pharmacol. Exp. Ther.* **257,** 1208–1215.
131. Wolff, D. J., and Lubeskie, A. (1995). Aminoguanidine is an isoform-selective, mechanism-based inactivator of nitric oxide synthase. *Arch. Biochem. Biophys.* **316,** 290–301.
132. Furfine, E. S., Harmon, M. F., Paith, J. E., Knowles, R. G., Salter, M., Kiff, R. J., Duffy, C., Hazelwood, R., Oplinger, J. A., and Garvey, E. P. (1994). Potent and selective inhibition of human nitric oxide synthases. Selective inhibition of neuronal nitric oxide synthase by *S*-methyl-L-thiocitrulline and *S*-ethyl-L-thiocitrulline. *J. Biol. Chem.* **269,** 26677–26683.
133. Jang, D., Szabo, C., and Murrell, G. A. (1996). *S*-Substituted isothioureas are potent inhibitors of nitric oxide biosynthesis in cartilage. *Eur. J. Pharmacol.* **312,** 341–347.
134. Marletta, M. A. (1994). Approaches toward selective inhibition of nitric oxide synthase. *J. Med. Chem.* **37,** 1899–1907.
135. Garvey, E. P., Oplinger, J. A., Tanoury, G. J., Sherman, P. A., Fowler, M., Marshall, S., Harmon, M. F., Paith, J. E., and Furfine, E. S. (1994). Potent and selective inhibition of human nitric oxide synthases. Inhibition by non-amino acid isothioureas. *J. Biol. Chem.* **269,** 26669–26676.
136. Boucher, J. L., Moali, C., and Tenu, J. P. (1999). Nitric oxide biosynthesis, nitric oxide synthase inhibitors and arginase competition for L-arginine utilization. *Cell Mol. Life Sci.* **55,** 1015–1028.
137. Huang, P. L., and Fishman, M. C. (1996). Genetic analysis of nitric oxide synthase isoforms: Targeted mutation in mice. *J. Mol. Med.* **74,** 415–421.
138. Huang, P. L., Dawson, T. M., Bredt, D. S., Snyder, S. H., and Fishman, M. C. (1993). Targeted disruption of the neuronal nitric oxide synthase gene. *Cell* **75,** 1273–1286.

139. Huang, P. L., Huang, Z., Mashimo, H., Bloch, K. D., Moskowitz, M. A., Bevan, J. A., and Fishman, M. C. (1995). Hypertension in mice lacking the gene for endothelial nitric oxide synthase [see comments]. *Nature (London)* **377,** 239–242.
140. MacMicking, J. D., Nathan, C., Hom, G., Chartrain, N., Fletcher, D. S., Trumbauer, M., Stevens, K., Xie, Q. W., Sokol, K., and Hutchinson, N. (1995). Altered responses to bacterial infection and endotoxic shock in mice lacking inducible nitric oxide synthase *Cell* **81,** 641–650 [published erratum appears in *Cell* **81**(7), following 1170].
141. Wei, X. Q., Charles, I. G., Smith, A., Ure, J., Feng, G. J., Huang, F. P., Xu, D., Muller, W., Moncada, S., and Liew, F. Y. (1995). Altered immune responses in mice lacking inducible nitric oxide synthase. *Nature (London)* **375,** 408–411.
142. Laubach, V. E., Shesely, E. G., Smithies, O., and Sherman, P. A. (1995). Mice lacking inducible nitric oxide synthase are not resistant to lipopolysaccharide-induced death. *Proc. Natl. Acad. Sci. U.S.A* **92,** 10688–10692.
143. O'Dell, T. J., Huang, P. L., Dawson, T. M., Dinerman, J. L., Snyder, S. H., Kandel, E. R., and Fishman, M. C. (1994). Endothelial NOS and the blockade of LTP by NOS inhibitors in mice lacking neuronal NOS. *Science* **265,** 542–546.
144. Huang, Z., Huang, P. L., Panahian, N., Dalkara, T., Fishman, M. C., and Moskowitz, M. A. (1994). Effects of cerebral ischemia in mice deficient in neuronal nitric oxide synthase. *Science* **265,** 1883–1885.
145. Darius, S., Wolf, G., Huang, P. L., and Fishman, M. C. (1995). Localization of NADPH-diaphorase/nitric oxide synthase in the rat retina: An electron microscopic study. *Brain Res.* **690,** 231–235.
146. Irikura, K., Huang, P. L., Ma, J., Lee, W. S., Dalkara, T., Fishman, M. C., Dawson, T. M., Snyder, S. H., and Moskowitz, M. A. (1995). Cerebrovascular alterations in mice lacking neuronal nitric oxide synthase gene expression. *Proc. Natl. Acad. Sci. U.S.A* **92,** 6823–6827.
147. Nelson, R. J., Demas, G. E., Huang, P. L., Fishman, M. C., Dawson, V. L., Dawson, T. M., and Snyder, S. H. (1995). Behavioural abnormalities in male mice lacking neuronal nitric oxide synthase [see comments]. *Nature (London)* **378,** 383–386.
148. Kano, T., Shimizu-Sasamata, M., Huang, P. L., Moskowitz, M. A., and Lo, E. H. (1998). Effects of nitric oxide synthase gene knockout on neurotransmitter release *in vivo. Neuroscience* **86,** 695–699.
149. Drazen, D. L., Klein, S. L., Burnett, A. L., Wallach, E. E., Crone, J. K., Huang, P. L., and Nelson, R. J. (1999). Reproductive function in female mice lacking the gene for endothelial nitric oxide synthase. *Nitric Oxide* **3,** 366–374.
150. Mishima, S., Xu, D., Lu, Q., and Deitch, E. A. (1997). Bacterial translocation is inhibited in inducible nitric oxide synthase knockout mice after endotoxin challenge but not in a model of bacterial overgrowth. *Arch. Surg.* **132,** 1190–1195.
151. Cobb, J. P., Hotchkiss, R. S., Swanson, P. E., Chang, K., Qiu, Y., Laubach, V. E., Karl, I. E., and Buchman, T. G. (1999). Inducible nitric oxide synthase (iNOS) gene deficiency increases the mortality of sepsis in mice. *Surgery* **126,** 438–442.
152. Koglin, J., Glysing-Jensen, T., Mudgett, J. S., and Russell, M. E. (1998). NOS2 mediates opposing effects in models of acute and chronic cardiac rejection: insights from NOS2-knockout mice. *Am. J. Pathol.* **153,** 1371–1376.
153. Koglin, J., Granville, D. J., Glysing-Jensen, T., Mudgett, J. S., Carthy, C. M., McManus, B. M., and Russell, M. E. (1999). Attenuated acute cardiac rejection in NOS2 $-/-$ recipients correlates with reduced apoptosis. *Circulation* **99,** 836–842.
154. Koglin, J., Glysing-Jensen, T., Mudgett, J. S., and Russell, M. E. (1998). Exacerbated transplant arteriosclerosis in inducible nitric oxide-deficient mice. *Circulation* **97,** 2059–2065.
155. Kanno, S., Lee, P. C., Zhang, Y., Chien, H., Griffith, B. P., Shears II, L. L., and Billiar, T. R. (2000). Attenuation of myocardial ischemia/reperfusion injury by superinduction of nitric oxide synthase. *Circulation* **101**(23), 2742–2748.
156. Meng, W., Ma, J., Ayata, C., Hara, H., Huang, P. L., Fishman, M. C., and Moskowitz, M. A. (1996). ACh dilates pial arterioles in endothelial and neuronal NOS knockout mice by NO-dependent mechanisms. *Am. J. Physiol.* **271,** H1145–H1150.
157. Ling, H., Edelstein, C., Gengaro, P., Meng, X., Lucia, S., Knotek, M., Wangsiripaisan, A., Shi, Y., and Schrier, R. (1999). Attenuation of renal ischemia-reperfusion injury in inducible nitric oxide synthase knockout mice. *Am. J. Physiol.* **277,** F383–F390.
158. Hitt, M. M., Addison, C. L., and Graham, F. L. (1997). Human adenovirus vectors for gene transfer into mammalian cells. *Adv. Pharmacol.* **40,** 137–206.
159. Tzeng, E., Billiar, T. R., Williams, D. L., Li, J., Lizonova, A., Kovesdi, I., and Kim, Y. M. (1998). Adenovirus-mediated inducible nitric oxide synthase gene transfer inhibits hepatocyte apoptosis. *Surgery* **124,** 278–283.
160. Tzeng, E., Kim, Y. M., Pitt, B. R., Lizonova, A., Kovesdi, I., and Billiar, T. R. (1997). Adenoviral transfer of the inducible nitric oxide synthase gene blocks endothelial cell apoptosis. *Surgery* **122,** 255–263.
161. Kibbe, M. R., Nie, S., Yoneyama, T., Hatakeyama, K., Lizonova, A., Kovesdi, I., Billiar, T. R., and Tzeng, E. (1999). Optimization of *ex vivo* inducible nitric oxide synthase gene transfer to vein grafts. *Surgery* **126,** 323–329.
162. Channon, K. M., Qian, H., Neplioueva, V., Blazing, M. A., Olmez, E., Shetty, G. A., Youngblood, S. A., Pawloski, J., McMahon, T., Stamler, J. S., and George, S. E. (1998). *In vivo* gene transfer of nitric oxide synthase enhances vasomotor function in carotid arteries from normal and cholesterol-fed rabbits. *Circulation* **98,** 1905–1911.
163. Maeda, Y., Ikeda, U., Ogasawara, Y., Urabe, M., Takizawa, T., Saito, T., Colosi, P., Kurtzman, G., Shimada, K., and Ozawa, K. (1997). Gene transfer into vascular cells using adeno-associated virus (AAV) vectors. *Cardiovasc. Res.* **35,** 514–521.
164. Arnold, T. E., Gnatenko, D., and Bahou, W. F. (1997). *In vivo* gene transfer into rat arterial walls with novel adeno-associated virus vectors. *J. Vasc. Surg.* **25,** 347–355.
165. Verma, I. M., and Somia, N. (1997). Gene therapy—Promises, problems and prospects [news]. *Nature (London)* **389,** 239–242.
166. Kibbe, M., Billiar, T., and Tzeng, E. (1999). Nitric oxide synthase gene transfer to the vessel wall. *Curr. Opin. Nephrol. Hypertens.* **8,** 75–81.
167. Ceneviva, G. D., Tzeng, E., Hoyt, D. G., Yee, E., Gallagher, A., Engelhardt, J. F., Kim, Y. M., Billiar, T. R., Watkins, S. A., and Pitt, B. R. (1998). Nitric oxide inhibits lipopolysaccharide-induced apoptosis in pulmonary artery endothelial cells. *Am. J. Physiol.* **275,** L717–L728.
168. Chen, L., Daum, G., Forough, R., Clowes, M., Walter, U., and Clowes, A. W. (1998). Overexpression of human endothelial nitric oxide synthase in rat vascular smooth muscle cells and in balloon-injured carotid artery. *Circ. Res.* **82,** 862–870.
169. von der Leyen, H. E., Gibbons, G. H., Morishita, R., Lewis, N. P., Zhang, L., Nakajima, M., Kaneda, Y., Cooke, J. P., and Dzau, V. J. (1995). Gene therapy inhibiting neointimal vascular lesion: *In vivo* transfer of endothelial cell nitric oxide synthase gene. *Proc. Natl. Acad. Sci. U.S.A.* **92,** 1137–1141.
170. Cable, D. G., O'Brien, T., Schaff, H. V., and Pompili, V. J. (1997). Recombinant endothelial nitric oxide synthase-transduced human saphenous veins: Gene therapy to augment nitric oxide production in bypass conduits. *Circulation* **96,** II–8.
171. Varenne, O., Pislaru, S., Gillijns, H., Van Pelt, N., Gerard, R. D., Zoldhelyi, P., Van de, W. F., Collen, D., and Janssens, S. P. (1998). Local adenovirus-mediated transfer of human endothelial nitric oxide synthase reduces luminal narrowing after coronary angioplasty in pigs. *Circulation* **98,** 919–926.
172. Janssens, S., Flaherty, D., Nong, Z., Varenne, O., Van Pelt, N., Haustermans, C., Zoldhelyi, P., Gerard, R., and Collen, D. (1998). Human endothelial nitric oxide synthase gene transfer inhibits vascu-

lar smooth muscle cell proliferation and neointima formation after balloon injury in rats. *Circulation* **97,** 1274–1281.

173. Wolff, D. J., Lubeskie, A., and Umansky, S. (1994). The inhibition of the constitutive bovine endothelial nitric oxide synthase by imidazole and indazole agents. *Arch. Biochem. Biophys.* **314,** 360–366.

174. Moore, P. K., Wallace, P., Gaffen, Z., Hart, S. L., and Babbedge, R. C. (1993). Characterization of the novel nitric oxide synthase inhibitor 7-nitro indazole and related indazoles: Antinociceptive and cardiovascular effects. *Br. J. Pharmacol.* **110,** 219–224.

175. Babbedge, R. C., Bland-Ward, P. A., Hart, S. L., and Moore, P. K. (1993). Inhibition of rat cerebellar nitric oxide synthase by 7-nitro indazole and related substituted indazoles. *Br. J. Pharmacol.* **110,** 225–228.

176. Mayer, B., Klatt, P., Werner, E. R., and Schmidt, K. (1994). Molecular mechanisms of inhibition of porcine brain nitric oxide synthase by the antinociceptive drug 7-nitroindazole *Neuropharmacology* **33,** 1253–1259 [published erratum appears in *Neuropharmacology* **34**(2), 243].

177. Garvey, E. P., Oplinger, J. A., Furfine, E. S., Kiff, R. J., Laszlo, F., Whittle, B. J., and Knowles, R. G. (1997). 1400W is a slow, tight binding, and highly selective inhibitor of inducible nitric-oxide synthase *in vitro* and *in vivo*. *J. Biol. Chem.* **272,** 4959–4963.

178. Misko, T. P., Moore, W. M., Kasten, T. P., Nickols, G. A., Corbett, J. A., Tilton, R. G., McDaniel, M. L., Williamson, J. R., and Currie, M. G. (1993). Selective inhibition of the inducible nitric oxide synthase by aminoguanidine. *Eur. J. Pharmacol.* **233,** 119–125.

179. Moore, W. M., Webber, R. K., Jerome, G. M., Tjoeng, F. S., Misko, T. P., and Currie, M. G. (1994). L-*N*6-(1-iminoethyl)lysine: A selective inhibitor of inducible nitric oxide synthase. *J. Med. Chem.* **37,** 3886–3888.

180. Connor, J. R., Manning, P. T., Settle, S. L., Moore, W. M., Jerome, G. M., Webber, R. K., Tjoeng, F. S., and Currie, M. G. (1995). Suppression of adjuvant-induced arthritis by selective inhibition of inducible nitric oxide synthase. *Eur. J. Pharmacol.* **273,** 15–24.

181. Southan, G. J., Szabo, C., and Thiemermann, C. (1995). Isothioureas: Potent inhibitors of nitric oxide synthases with variable isoform selectivity. *Br. J. Pharmacol.* **114,** 510–516.

182. Tracey, W. R., Nakane, M., Basha, F., and Carter, G. (1995). *In vivo* pharmacological evaluation of two novel type II (inducible) nitric oxide synthase inhibitors. *Can. J. Physiol. Pharmacol.* **73,** 665–669.

183. Gross, S. S., Stuehr, D. J., Aisaka, K., Jaffe, E. A., Levi, R., and Griffith, O. W. (1990). Macrophage and endothelial cell nitric oxide synthesis: Cell-type selective inhibition by NG-aminoarginine, NG-nitroarginine and NG- methylarginine. *Biochem. Biophys. Res. Commun.* **170,** 96–103.

184. Olken, N. M., and Marletta, M. A. (1993). NG-methyl-L-arginine functions as an alternate substrate and mechanism- based inhibitor of nitric oxide synthase. *Biochemistry* **32,** 9677–9685.

185. Hibbs, J. B., Jr., Taintor, R. R., and Vavrin, Z. (1987). Macrophage cytotoxicity: Role for L-arginine deiminase and imino nitrogen oxidation to nitrite. *Science* **235,** 473–476.

186. Frey, C., Narayanan, K., McMillan, K., Spack, L., Gross, S. S., Masters, B. S., and Griffith, O. W. (1994). L-Thiocitrulline. A stereospecific, heme-binding inhibitor of nitric- oxide synthases. *J. Biol. Chem.* **269,** 26083–26091.

187. Narayanan, K., and Griffith, O. W. (1994). Synthesis of L-thiocitrulline, L-homothiocitrulline, and *S*-methyl-L-thiocitrulline: A new class of potent nitric oxide synthase inhibitors. *J. Med. Chem.* **37,** 885–887.

188. Hara, H., Huang, P. L., Panahian, N., Fishman, M. C., and Moskowitz, M. A. (1996). Reduced brain edema and infarction volume in mice lacking the neuronal isoform of nitric oxide synthase after transient MCA occlusion. *J. Cereb. Blood Flow Metab.* **16,** 605–611.

189. Huang, Z., Huang, P. L., Ma, J., Meng, W., Ayata, C., Fishman, M. C., and Moskowitz, M. A. (1996). Enlarged infarcts in endothelial nitric oxide synthase knockout mice are attenuated by nitro-L-arginine. *J. Cereb. Blood Flow Metab.* **16,** 981–987.

190. Shears, L. L., Kawaharada, N., Tzeng, E., Billiar, T. R., Watkins, S. C., Kovesdi, I., Lizonova, A., and Pham, S. M. (1997). Inducible nitric oxide synthase suppresses the development of allograft arteriosclerosis. *J. Clin. Invest.* **100,** 2035–2042.

191. Shears, L. L., Kibbe, M. R., Murdock, A. D., Billiar, T. R., Lizonova, A., Kovesdi, I., Watkins, S. C., and Tzeng, E. (1998). Efficient inhibition of intimal hyperplasia by adenovirus-mediated inducible nitric oxide synthase gene transfer to rats and pigs *in vivo*. *J. Am. Coll. Surg.* **187,** 295–306.

192. Matsumoto, T., Komori, K., Yonemitsu, Y., Morishita, R., Sueishi, K., Kaneda, Y., and Sugimachi, K. (1998). Hemagglutinating virus of Japan-liposome-mediated gene transfer of endothelial cell nitric oxide synthase inhibits intimal hyperplasia of canine vein grafts under conditions of poor runoff. *J. Vasc. Surg.* **27,** 135–144.

193. Janssens, S. P., Bloch, K. D., Nong, Z., Gerard, R. D., Zoldhelyi, P., and Collen, D. (1996). Adenoviral-mediated transfer of the human endothelial nitric oxide synthase gene reduces acute hypoxic pulmonary vasoconstriction in rats. *J. Clin. Invest.* **98,** 317–324.

194. Chia, S. H., Murase, N., Taylor, B. S., Billiar, T. R., Starzl, T. E., and Geller, D. A. (1999). Adenoviral-mediated gene delivery to liver isografts: Improved model of *ex vivo* gene transfer. *Transplant. Proc.* **31,** 475–476.

195. Fevery, J., Roskams, T., Van de, C. M., Omasta, A., Janssens, S., Desmet, V., and Nevens, F. (1998). NO synthase in the liver: prospects of *in vivo* gene transfer. *Digestion* **59**(Suppl. 2), 58–59.

196. Ambs, S., Merriam, W. G., Ogunfusika, M. O., Bennett, W. P., Ishibe, N., Hussain, S. P., Tzeng, E. E., Geller, D. A., Billiar, T. R., and Harris, C. C. (1998). p53 and vascular endothelial growth factor regulate tumor growth of NOS2-expressing human carcinoma cells. *Nature Med.* **4,** 1371–1376.

197. Juang, S. H., Xie, K., Xu, L., Shi, Q., Wang, Y., Yoneda, J., and Fidler, I. J. (1998). Suppression of tumorigenicity and metastasis of human renal carcinoma cells by infection with retroviral vectors harboring the murine inducible nitric oxide synthase gene. *Hum. Gene Ther.* **9,** 845–854.

198. Garban, H., Marquez, D., Magee, T., Moody, J., Rajavashisth, T., Rodriguez, J. A., Hung, A., Vernet, D., Rajfer, J., and Gonzalez-Cadavid, N. F. (1997). Cloning of rat and human inducible penile nitric oxide synthase. Application for gene therapy of erectile dysfunction. *Biol. Reprod.* **56,** 954–963.

69

Endothelial Cell and Smooth Muscle Cell Biology in Vascular Disease

Richard D. Kenagy and Alexander W. Clowes

Department of Surgery, University of Washington, Seattle, Washington 98195

I. Introduction

Cells of the vascular wall—endothelial cells, smooth muscle cells, and fibroblasts—are central to normal function of the vessel as a conduit for blood. Endothelial cells provide a nonthrombogenic surface and mediate the effects of shear forces and blood-borne growth factors and cytokines. Smooth muscle cells and adventitial fibroblasts play a dynamic role in the structure and tone of the vessel, thus regulating luminal area. These cells, which are coupled through complex autocrine and paracrine interactions, also play critical roles in the pathogenesis of atherosclerotic and aneurysmal degeneration of the vessel wall (1–3). Stroke, angina, myocardial infarction, and claudication result from atherosclerotic disease, which is thought to be the result of recurrent endothelial cell injury. Ironically, the surgical- and catheter-based interventions available for treatment of diseased arteries (endarterectomy, bypass grafting, percutaneous transluminal coronary angioplasty, directional and rotational atherectomy, and stents) are themselves injurious and have significant failure rates because of luminal narrowing. Thus, understanding how the arterial wall and its component cells respond to injury and the regulatory factors involved in these responses will ultimately lead to better treatments for vascular disease. This chapter reviews *in vivo* and *in vitro* methods that can be used to address various questions regarding the vascular response to injury.

II. General Areas of Vascular Cell Research

The tools of biochemistry, biophysics, cell biology, physiology, pharmacology, and pathology can be used to study the vascular response to injury and other vascular diseases. We discuss some general categories of research that are relevant to the study of atherosclerosis, restenosis, and aneurysmal degeneration.

A. Flow, Pressure, and Stretch Effects

The natural development of atherosclerosis in areas of low or turbulent shear led researchers to propose that patterns of blood flow were important (4). Changes in blood flow cause arteries to alter in diameter (5, 6), and changes in flow in rigid synthetic grafts lead to changes in intimal volume (7, 8). Perfusion pressure (i.e., wall tension) has been shown to have effects independent of flow rates (4, 5, 9, 10). In addition, stretch of vessels and of cultured cells regulates growth factor release, collagen and fibronectin synthesis, proteinase production, proliferation, and ion channel flux (11–14).

B. Thrombosis

The regulation of the clotting cascade and clot lysis is the subject of a separate chapter of this volume (Chapter 70), but it deserves specific mention here because thrombosis is the cause of acute myocardial infarction (15–17) and may represent the mechanism of the nonlinear growth of atherosclerotic lesions (18). The endothelial cell normally is a nonthrombogenic surface, but under some circumstances becomes procoagulant (19). Plasminogen activator inhibitor-1, which inhibits fibrinolysis by inhibiting plasminogen activators, is an independent risk factor for myocardial infarction (20). In addition, the rupture, or in some cases erosion without rupture (21), of the atherosclerotic plaque cap exposes the thrombogenic contents of the plaque (22) [see Fuster and colleagues (23)].

C. Cell Proliferation/Movement/Death

The cellular composition of the vascular wall is dictated by the balance between cell proliferation, movement, and death. An atherosclerotic plaque is thought to arise from the migration of medial smooth muscle cells (SMCs) into the intima to form an area of diffuse intimal thickening, which can occur within the first few months of life (2, 24, 25). Monocytes also accumulate in specific regions of the arterial bed (bifurcations and areas of flow disturbance) by migration into the wall, probably stimulated by the induction of monocyte-binding integrins on endothelial cells by oxidized low-density lipoprotein (LDL) or infectious agents (2). SMCs and macrophages can then accumulate by proliferation in the plaque. In an advanced plaque, SMCs die, leaving fewer SMCs in the media beneath the plaque and fewer SMCs in the plaque core and cap (26). Macrophage death is even more pronounced than SMC death (27). Decreased SMC proliferation and increased death are also observed in aneurysms (28, 29). Among the factors that regulate cell proliferation, migration, and death are numerous growth factors and cytokines.

D. Growth Factors/Cytokines

The list of growth factors and cytokines that are relevant to vascular biology is long and growing, but fibroblast growth factors, platelet-derived growth factor (PDGF), and transforming growth factor β have received considerable attention. In addition to studies aimed at understanding the effects of these factors on cell function at the cell, tissue/organ, and whole animal levels, an enormous literature exists on the subcellular signaling pathways activated by growth factors and cytokines (30–35). Particular emphasis has been aimed at understanding the cellular signals governing cell cycle (36–42) and cell death (43, 44) pathways. An additional area of interest is the effects of these factors on the extracellular matrix (ECM).

E. ECM Synthesis/Degradation/Remodeling

The ECM not only is the critical structural element in the wall, but it also modifies cell function. The ECM can regulate cell death, cell proliferation, and cell differentiation (45). Aneurysmal and atherosclerotic plaque rupture result from the degradation and weakening of the ECM. In animal models, matrix metalloproteinases (MMPs) play a key role in the formation of aneurysms (46, 47) and the loss of medial elastin beneath atherosclerotic lesions (48). At present no animal models of plaque rupture are available. In addition, although MMPs are present in human abdominal aortic aneurysm (AAA) and in vulnerable regions of atherosclerotic plaques (49–52), the role of MMPs in human arterial disease remains to be definitively established (53).

It has become clear that restenosis (loss of lumen size gained after intervention) after angioplasty or atherectomy is more the result of the remodeling, or rearrangement, of existing matrix and cells rather than the accumulation of intima (54–56). This remodeling effect has been observed in nonhuman primates (57), pigs (58), and rabbits (59, 60). Constrictive remodeling appears to be mediated, in part, by the PDGFβ receptor (61). The arterial dilation that occurs after increasing blood flow is blocked by MMP inhibition (62) and overexpression of MMP9 increases arterial area and lumen size (63), suggesting that remodeling involves the degradation of existing matrix and synthesis of new matrix proteins. It is of interest that MMP inhibition also blocks collagen synthesis after injury of the rabbit iliac (64), further indicating a linkage between synthesis and degradation of ECM. Thus, there is considerable interest in matrix-degrading proteinases and their inhibitors.

F. Proteinases/Proteinase Inhibitors

Interest has focused on the matrix metalloproteinases, a family of at least 17 members in humans (65, 66), and on the plasminogen activators and plasminogen (67, 68). Inhibitors of these two families of proteinases are the tissue inhibitors of metalloproteinases (TIMP)-1, -2, -3, and -4 and plasminogen activator inhibitors (PAI)-1 and -2 (69, 70). Members of both of these families have a role in endothelial cell and SMC migration, proliferation, and matrix degradation in various model systems (63, 71–78), including knockout mice (79–81).

G. Mediators of ECM/Cell Interactions

A major class of proteins that connects the extracellular matrix to the cytoskeleton is the integrins. The integrins provided the first example of cellular membrane proteins that transmit signals to the cell (see Fig. 1) after binding matrix proteins (82). Various functions have been assigned to integrins, including regulation of cell migration, growth, and death. Other classes of proteins important as mediators of cell-to-cell interactions are the cell adhesion molecules (CAMs) and cadherins (83). More recently a class of membrane-bound tyrosine kinases, the discoidin domain receptors, was found to bind collagens and cause delayed, but sustained, tyrosine kinase activity (84). Thus, tyrosine kinases appear to mediate both soluble growth factor and insoluble matrix protein signaling to the cell.

H. Interactions between These General Categories

There are several interesting examples of interaction between the categories discussed above:

1. The creation of neoepitopes from ECM proteins by proteinases can have multiple effects. Collagenase-digested gelatin causes arteriolar dilation via $\alpha v\beta 3$ (85) and MMP2-cleaved laminin 5 has a promigratory neoepitope (86). The ability of RGD peptides to directly activate cathepsin 3 opens the possibility that protease cleavage products containing the RGD sequence could promote cell death (87). Finally, the angiogenesis inhibitors, angiostatin and endostatin, are proteolytic

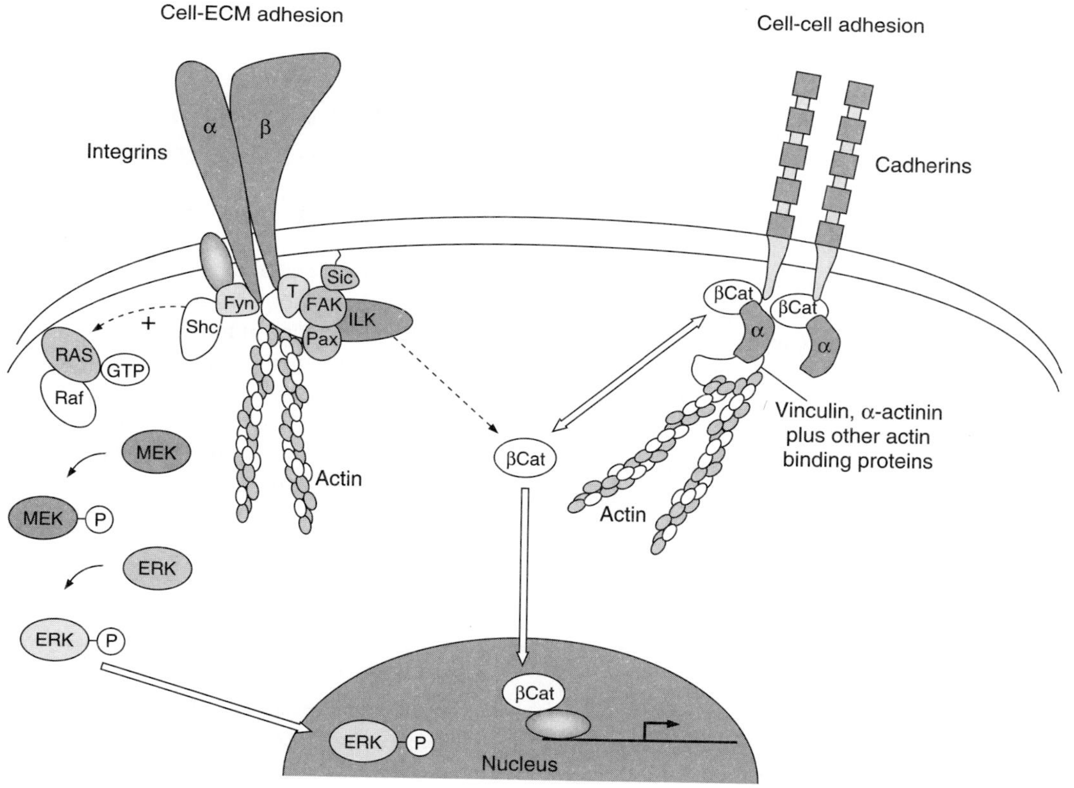

Figure 1 Interactions between integrins, cadherins, and cellular signaling molecules. Pax, Paxillin; ILK, integrin-linked kinase; FAK, focal adhesion kinase; T, talin; βCat, β-catenin, α, α-catenin. Adapted from Ref. (236), *Current Opinion Cellular Biology* **11**; A.E. Aplin, A.K. Howe, and R.L. Juliano; Cell adhesion molecules, signal transduction and cell growth; pp. 737-744. Copyright 1999, with permission from Elsevier Science. Data from Giancotti and Ruoslatti (82).

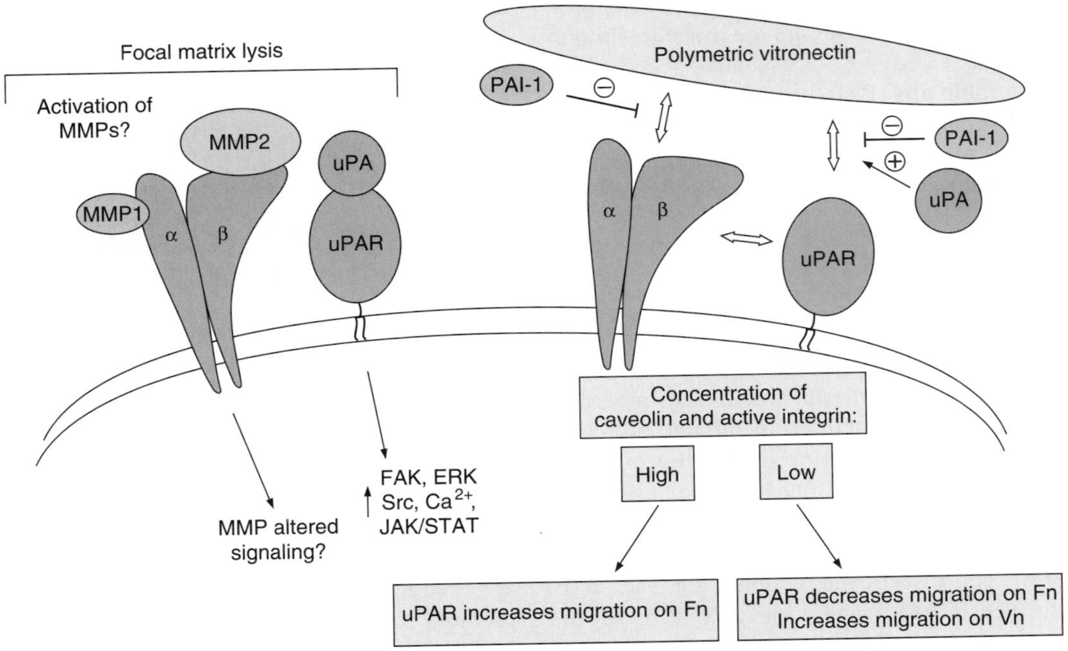

Figure 2 Localization of proteinases by integrins and uPAR and the complex relationship among uPAR, uPA, PAI-1, integrins, and vitronectin. Adapted from Chapman and colleagues (237, 238), Preissner and co-workers (239), and Koshelnick *et al.* (240).

cleavage products of plasminogen and collagen XVIII, respectively (88). MMP2 is the proteinase responsible for angiostatin production (89).

2. The interaction between proteinases and integrins localizes activity (see Fig. 2). MMP2 is specifically bound to αvβ3 (90) and β1 integrins (B. Levkau, R. D. Kenagy, A. W. Clowes, R. Ross, and E. W. Raines, unpublished data). In the case of β1 integrin this association appears to be dependent on integrin activation status (B. Levkau, R. D. Kenagy, A. W. Clowes, R. Ross, and E. W. Raines, unpublished data). It is possible that interaction between the zymogen and integrin activates the enzyme; for example, binding of single-chain urokinase plasminogen activator (uPA) by the uPA receptor increases uPA activity (91). Urokinase, the urokinase receptor, plasminogen activator inhibitor-1 (PAI-1), vitronectin, and αvβ3 are interrelated through overlapping binding sites, and the outcome of these competitive interactions modulates migratory signals (92–94).

3. One protein may have multiple activities. All TIMPs, for example, inhibit MMP activity, but TIMP3 is proapoptotic (95) and TIMP1 and TIMP2 have growth inhibitory or stimulatory properties (96–98). PAI-2 inhibits apoptosis (99) intracellularly and inhibits plasminogen activators extracellularly.

III. Experimental Models of Atherosclerosis, Aneurysm, and Restenosis

A. Animal Models

A few general statements can be made regarding animal models of atherosclerosis, aneurysm, and restenosis. First, atherosclerotic lesions in most animals (large and small) are found only after hypercholesterolemia is achieved by dietary or genetic manipulation (an exception being homocystine-induced arteriosclerosis). Second, arterial injury accelerates atherosclerotic lesion formation. Third, arterial models of aneurysm are mostly limited to small animals. Finally, restenosis, defined as loss of the initial gain achieved in lumen area of atherosclerotic arteries after interventions such as angioplasty (100), is modeled by various reinjury ("double injury") protocols in large and small animals.

1. Large Animal Models

In general, large animals, such as pigs, nonhuman primates, and sheep, offer a size that permits the use of clinical instruments such as intravascular ultrasound in the coronary arteries. A general drawback is the cost of obtaining and maintaining the animals and of the increased amounts of reagents needed. In addition, there is a large animal-to-animal variation.

a. Pig The pig has proved to be a very good model of human atherosclerotic disease. Pigs and humans have a similar coronary artery anatomy. Pigs show spontaneous lesion development, and, with hypercholesterolemia, the development of complicated plaques in the coronary bed (101). Balloon catheter injury of the coronary arteries produces intimal lesions about the thickness of the media. Although the pig is prone to develop ventricular fibrillation during surgery, this complication can be controlled with oral administration of Sotalol (a beta adrenergic blocker) and sublingual nifedipine (calcium channel blocker). Pigs also have a small artery (the saphenous artery, ~1.5 mm) close to the surface of the leg that is useful for catheter-induced arterial injury without compromising blood flow.

An interesting variation on the fat-fed atherosclerosis model is the addition of diabetes, a major risk factor for atherosclerosis (102, 103). Two groups of investigators (M. Sturek and colleagues at the University of Missouri—Columbia and R. Gerrity and colleagues at Emory University) are conducting studies of the combined effects of diabetes (achieved by treatment with alloxan or streptozotocin) and hypercholesterolemia in the pig. More than one treatment with streptozotocine may be needed because enough islet cells may survive initial treatments to maintain euglycemia. These animals develop advanced lesions more quickly than with cholesterol feeding alone and myocardial infarction has been observed (R. Gerrity, personal communication, 1999).

A model of abdominal aortic aneurysm commonly used in large animals is to create a pouch with abdominal facia (104) or venous tissue (105). However, the utility of this model with nonvascular tissue is limited to testing surgical techniques and devices.

Drawbacks with the pig are that (1) prosthetic grafts tend to become infected, (2) their carotid arteries are difficult to access because of neck size and shape, (3) the animals (except minipigs) grow so quickly that artificial grafts or devices may no longer fit the size of the artery, (4) abdominal vascular surgery is difficult, (5) aortic anatomy is unlike that of humans and nonhuman primates and poses some challenges, and (6) hemostatic parameters differ significantly from those in humans (106, 107).

b. Nonhuman Primates Nonhuman primates have been considered to be a superior experimental animal because of the close phylogenetic connection with humans. This is true for the hematological system, which is similar to the human system (108). These animals are low responders to arterial injury in terms of intimal lesion development when compared to the rat (109). Spontaneous atherosclerotic lesions are rarely observed. Types IV–V lesions were observed in 12- to 20-year-old squirrel monkeys, but not in cebus monkeys (110) [see Stary *et al.* (111, 112) for definitions of the types of lesions]. With cholesterol feeding and increased plasma cholesterol, various nonhuman primates develop advanced (type V) lesions. However, long periods (2–5 years) are required to produce these lesions (113–116). In addition, there are hypo- and hyperresponders to cholesterol feeding (117). This means that animals may need to be prescreened for responsiveness, depending on the experimental protocol. In addition, to maintain plasma cholesterol at desired levels the diet may need to be adjusted after determining plasma cholesterol values.

Clarkson has reviewed several variables, including age and gender, that are important in working with nonhuman primates, although these are not specific to nonhuman primates (118). Postpubertal monkeys are more susceptible to development of diet-induced atherosclerotic lesions than are prepubertal monkeys. Unpublished data (N. O. Carragher, R. D. Kenagy, A. W. Clowes, and E. W. Raines, 1999) indicate there is a difference between the arterial smooth muscle cell $\beta 1$ integrin activation state of pregeriatric/geriatric (15–18 years) and juvenile/mature (4–8 years) *Macaque nemistrina* monkeys *in vivo.* Because rats also show differences in function of smooth muscle cells from newborns, young adults, and old adults (119), special attention should be given to the age of the nonhuman primate to be used for experiments. Nonhuman primates with diet-induced atherosclerosis demonstrate constrictive arterial remodeling in response to balloon injury, and so provide a model for aspects of restenosis (57, 120).

Zarins *et al.* (121, 122) have described a model of aneurysm development during regression of diet-induced atherosclerosis. These authors noted that along with a loss of intimal plaque there was a twofold increase in abdominal aortic luminal and arterial area after lowering plasma cholesterol levels for 6 months. Medial wasting is observed beneath human atherosclerotic plaques and some plaques do regress (123), but the relevance of this mechanism for the development of aneurysms is not known.

Drawbacks to using nonhuman primates are that they are expensive, sometimes difficult to find and purchase, difficult to handle, and require long periods of time for diet-induced atherosclerosis studies. The response of coronary vessels to injury has not been studied. These animals are also a biohazard. Fatal infections can be caused by herpes B (about 65% of *Macaque* spp. are positive (124), Marburg virus, and *Shigella* spp. A particular advantage of nonhuman primates is the availability of antibodies to human antigens that cross-react with nonhuman primate antigens.

c. Sheep Sheep are useful for prosthetic grafts and vein grafts. In particular, the venous anastomosis of an arterial–venous fistula in sheep models very well the human response in vascular access grafts (125), whereas that in baboons, pigs, or dogs does not (T. Kirkman, personal communication, 1999). An aneurysm model has also been developed by replacing a section of the the abdominal aorta with the internal jugular vein (126). Unlike other large animals, sheep are docile and do not have to be anesthetized to assess the patency of a graft. A disadvantage is that vascular procedures involving the abdominal cavity are difficult and prone to infection. Like the pig, the aortic anatomy differs significantly from that in the human.

d. Dog Although dogs are used extensively for studies of thrombosis and myocardial infarction, they have not generally been favorable for arterial injury studies because of a low hyperplastic response (127). However, a severe injury by crushing will lead to a significant intimal hyperplasia (128). Drawbacks of the dog are the highly active thrombolytic system and resistance to development of atherosclerosis. As with pig and nonhuman primate, aneurysms have been created surgically in the dog using abdominal fascia (129) or venous tissue (105). In this venous pouch model the dog showed poor neointima formation compared with the pig.

2. Small Animal Models

Small animals, in contrast to large animals, offer (1) lower cost, (2) easy availability, (3) reduced amounts of experimental reagents needed, and (4) often a defined genetic background. Drawbacks to the rat and mouse, until the advent of knockout technology, are the very different lipoprotein profile compared to humans and resistance to diet-induced atherosclerosis.

a. Rat I. BALLOON CATHETER INJURY TO THE RAT CAROTID This model has provided the bulk of information about the arterial response to injury (130, 131). Passage of a balloon catheter with twisting will strip off the endothelium and injure the underlying media. Because individual investigators produce varying degrees of injury, it is important for consistency to have one investigator perform the balloon injuries for an entire experiment. Removal of the endothelium without medial injury can be accomplished using a loop of nylon suture as described by Fingerle (132). This removes the effect of SMC injury and death from the model. A reinjury model in the rat employs two balloon injuries to the carotid, the first via the femoral artery and the second via the external carotid (133, 134). This model has helped define critical differences between intimal and medial SMCs, such as responsiveness to growth factors.

An advantage of the rat carotid artery is that there are no preexisting intimal SMCs in young animals. This allows for the study of SMC migration by measuring movement from the media to the intima. The easiest method is to count luminal cells *en face* 4 days after injury (135), which is before significant proliferation has occurred in the intima. An alternative is to count nondividing SMCs in the intima after continuously labeling the rat with [3H]thymidine (136).

II. VASCULAR GENE TRANSFER EXPERIMENTS Cultured SMCs can be transfected with a retroviral vector containing the gene of interest, selected for gene expression, and then seeded onto the luminal surface of a denuded artery (137–139). Thus, all cells reintroduced into the animal are expressing the gene of interest to test for an effect on the arterial injury process. Direct transduction of cells in the artery wall is also possible with plasmids, adenoviral vectors, or adeno-associated viral vectors, but the fraction of cells expressing the transgene is small (140–147). A weakness of this approach is that control cells with empty vectors (e.g., LXSN) or a marker gene such as that for green fluorescent protein (GFP) probably integrate into the genome at a different location and may exhibit different characteristics. For this reason it is important to test more than one pair of control and experimental cells. Specific inhibitors of the gene product can also be used—for example, MMP inhibitors with MMP9 overexpression (63). In addition, a built-in control can be achieved when a foreign protein is introduced into the animal. For example, when cells expressing baboon TIMP-1 are seeded into the rat carotid, antibodies to the baboon TIMP-1 are made within 2 weeks (148). Thus, when the remaining carotid is injured and seeded with TIMP-1-expressing cells, the TIMP-1 no longer suppresses neointima formation because endogenous antibodies are blocking its activity (149). A specific point to note for this method is that after infusing cells into the carotid, the animal is placed on its stomach for 2 min followed by 13 min on its back. This leads to an even seeding around the lumen. Finally, cells may also be seeded in the adventitia of the artery. One application is to kill endogenous cells by freezing, and then seeding transfected cells on the adventitia to study migration into the media of the vessel (63). Migration can also be followed by labeling SMCs with BrdU *in vitro* before seeding the cells into the animal (150).

Transgenic rats have been used for the study of hypertension (151), but this technology has not yet been applied to rats for the study of restenosis, atherosclerosis, or aneurysm formation. It is clear that differences exist among rat strains in the response to arterial injury (152).

III. MODELS OF AORTIC ANEURYSMAL DEGENERATION There are two main models available now: the elastase injection model (153) and the guinea pig-to-rat aortic xenograft model (154, 155). Each models the human disease in that elastin is lost from the media, there is an inflammatory infiltrate, matrix-degrading proteinases are induced, and there is aneurysmal dilatation. An advantage of the xenograft model in rats preimmunized with an extract of guinea pig aorta is that vessels will rupture. An advantage of the nonpreimmunized xenograft model is the similarity between the inflammatory infiltrate between it and human

AAA (~5% B lymphocytes; E. Alaire, personal communication, 1999). In addition, the slow development of the aneurysm over weeks should be sufficient to test the efficacy of drugs or gene overexpression on reversal or stabilization of the aneurysm. The cell-seeding protocol has been used in the guinea pig-to-rat xenograft model to demonstrate the protective effects of TIMP-1 (155) and PAI-1 (139) toward aneurysm development.

b. Mouse The primary advantage of the mouse is the hundreds of inbred lines of mice and the knowledge about susceptibility to atherosclerosis among these lines. A separate chapter in this volume addresses transgenic and knockout technology (see Chapter 17), and several reviews have discussed mouse models of atherosclerosis and restenosis (156, 157). The primary atherosclerosis models utilize the apoE or LDL receptor knockouts with special diets (158). With the advent of knockout technology has come the impetus to create more antibodies to mouse proteins, thus reversing what has been a drawback to mouse work. However, drawbacks to using the mouse model include genetic distance (the distance between a rat and a mouse is greater than that between a rat and a human), the greater difficulty of working with a mouse because of its size (e.g., the smaller mouse cannot be bled multiple times), the greater difficulty in maintaining in mice a constant anesthesia level and body temperature during surgery (compared with rats), and, as compared with humans, the fact that mice age after maturity about 30 times faster.

Several models of arterial injury in the mouse have been described. These are electric injury (159), wire injury (160), and carotid tie-off injury (161). Electric injury leads to the complete loss of SMCs and is followed by an inflammatory response. Wire injury has generally given a variable and relatively small (about three layers of SMCs) intimal response. However, a report using C57BL/6 mice demonstrated a hyperplastic response to injury of the femoral arteries that resembles that of the rat carotid (162). The tie-off model is more reproducible and easier, but a drawback is that data can only be derived from a very small part of the artery near the tie. Thus, a robust model of arterial injury has not yet been created in the mouse. Nevertheless, these models have provided important information on the role of various gene products in vascular injury [e.g. uPA in the electric injury model (80); nitric oxide synthases in the tie-off model (163)].

There are several possibilities for investigations on aneurysm in the mouse. The blotchy (Blo) mouse, which has a genetic defect in elastin and collagen cross-linking, develops aortic aneurysms leading to rupture (164). Underexpression of fibrillin-1 also induces aneurysm formation (165). Finally, Carmeliet *et al.* (156, 166) have reported in apoE knockout mice the spontaneous formation of aneurysms that is reversed by crossing these animals with uPA knockout mice.

c. Rabbit The rabbit provides a very widely used model of atherosclerosis based on dietary or genetic (e.g., the Watanabe heritable hyperlipidemic rabbit) means of increasing plasma cholesterol. Atherosclerotic lesions progress to type V lesions, but 6 months to 5 years are required for these lesions to develop depending on the protocol (167). Drawbacks to the cholesterol-fed rabbit models include a lipoprotein profile different from that of humans (the major cholesterol carrier is β-VLDL, not LDL). A result of this is cholesteryl ester accumulation in the liver and other organs (168), which is not seen in humans. These effects can be avoided by using a casein-rich diet without cholesterol, but this takes much more time to develop arterial lesions that are less advanced (169, 170).

Double-injury models have been developed to model clinical restenosis, which occurs after angioplasty (second injury) to a primary atherosclerotic lesion. For example, arteries injured by air drying and a high-cholesterol diet lead to focal femoral artery atherosclerosis, which can then be balloon injured. However, the air-drying injury is not necessary to observe luminal narrowing after arterial balloon injury in the atherosclerotic rabbit (171). These models have been useful for looking at the effect of thrombosis and atherosclerotic lesions on the response to injury (172, 173).

B. Summary of Animal Models

Johnson *et al.* (174), Bocan (167), and Wolf (175) have effectively summarized the utility of various animal models for restenosis and atherosclerosis (see also Table I). Several points can be made.

1. Atherosclerosis, aneurysm, and restenosis are modeled to varying degrees by different animal models.
2. Models of intimal hyperplasia do not necessarily model clinical restenosis. Remodeling is the primary issue after angioplasty, whereas intimal hyperplasia remains the primary issue in stented vessels (176–178).
3. The importance of adequate dose–response studies should be emphasized. A 2-day administration of hirudin has no effect on intimal hyperplasia in the pig, whereas 14-day administration does (179). The antiproliferative and antithrombotic effects of heparin differ markedly, depending on the type of arterial injury and the mode of drug administration to the rabbit (180). Low doses of a bFGF–toxin conjugate increased, whereas high doses inhibited, intimal hyperplasia (181).
4. A major limitation at this time is the lack of an animal that shows atherosclerotic plaque rupture. The utility of the model of rupture designed by Rekhter and colleagues (182), which involves chronic placement of a balloon

Table I Advantages and Disadvantages of Various Model Systems

Model	Advantages	Disadvantages
Pig	Size allows use of clinical instruments; coronary anatomy is similar to that in humans; show spontaneous atheroslcerotic lesions and complicated plaques with cholesterol feeding, robust intimal response to injury; lipoprotein profile is similar to human profile	Tendency to develop ventricular fibrillation during surgery; prosthetic grafts tend to become infected; carotid arteries are difficult to access; rapid growth; aortic access; aortic anatomy is dissimilar to that in humans; hemostatic parameters differ from human parameters
Nonhuman primate	Most similar to humans phylogenetically; hemostatic system similar to that in humans; many antibodies to human antigens cross-react	Expensive; sometimes difficult to obtain, hard to handle; present a biohazard; relatively low response to arterial injury (coronary response not studied); spontaneous atherosclerosis rare and development of advanced lesions with cholesterol feeding takes years
Sheep	Easy to handle, useful for prosthetic grafts and vein grafts	Abdominal surgery difficult and prone to infection; aortic anatomy differs from that in humans; arterial response to injury not established
Dog	Coronary anatomy similar to that in humans and use of clinical devices possible	Resistant to diet-induced atherosclerosis, low intimal response to arterial injury; fibrinolytic system differs from the human system significantly
Rat	Well-characterized response to arterial injury, low cost, easy to obtain and handle, ability to study SMC migration *in vivo*	Resistant to diet-induced atherosclerosis; significant differences between human and rat hemostatic systems
Mouse	Low cost, many strains available, easiest for development of transgenics and knockouts	Compared to the rat, mice are more genetically distant from humans, are harder to handle, and arterial injury models are less robust
Rabbit	Diet-induced atherosclerosis and advanced lesions are well described; thrombus is present after balloon injury	Cholesterol-fed atherosclerosis differs from human atherosclerosis in seeing cholesteryl ester in organs and in the lipoprotein profile; advanced lesions require months to years to develop
Vascular organ culture	Can study the artery independently of neural and humoral factors under *in vivo* flow and pressure conditions	Labor intensive, difficult to reproduce *in vivo* redox conditions
Vascular tissue culture	Can study vascular cells in native matrix independent of neural and humoral factors; can study different compartments of the vessel wall and their interactions	The lack of flow and pressure may create artifactual results; difficult to reproduce *in vivo* redox conditions
Vascular cell culture	Easy to manipulate and extract cells	Cells lack all normal matrix and mechanical forces of *in vivo* situation; difficult to reproduce *in vivo* redox conditions

catheter in the aorta of an atherosclerotic rabbit so that a plaque grows over the balloon, is not yet apparent. However, it may allow investigation of factors affecting plaque strength.

5. One aspect of SMC function not yet studied in large animals *in vivo* is migration. Because the arteries of large animals have SMCs in the intima, the internal elastic lamina does not provide a starting point to measure migration.

C. In Vitro Models

The strength of *in vitro* models is the ability of the investigator to isolate and control variables. Although none of these experimental systems can completely model atherosclerosis, aneurysm, or restenosis, specific aspects of each pathology may be modeled quite well. For example, the kinetics of the proliferative, migratory, urokinase, and MMP9 responses of baboon arterial explants replicates the kinetics of these responses to arterial injury *in vivo* (183, 184). However, other aspects, such as the redox conditions of the artery *in vivo*, are very difficult to duplicate *in vitro*. Nonetheless, *in vitro* systems can offer valuable information that can lead to a more informed design of experiments *in vivo*. In addition, *in vitro* experiments can complement *in vivo* protocols by using tissues or cells derived from the experimental animals.

1. Organ Culture

a. No-Flow Conditions Several variations of culturing whole wall artery have been used. Rectangular pieces of rat (185, 186), rabbit (187), pig (188, 189), and human aorta (190, 191) and saphenous vein (192) have been placed in culture dishes with standard culture medium with or without serum. Serum causes necrosis to occur (187, 188), whereas in serum-free conditions cell morphology remains normal. A significant intima is developed in culture. Nicosia and colleagues (193) have suspended rat aortic rings in collagen gels and then placed these in standard culture dishes as a model of angiogenesis. Because the density of cells in the tissue is high, the medium is generally changed frequently (187). For example, a 1-cm^2 segment of rabbit aorta requires 10 ml of medium, changed every 2 days (J. Fingerle, personal communication, 1999).

Adenoviral vectors have been used to overexpress genes of interest—for example, TIMP-1 (194)—in the saphenous vein model. This is of particular interest because of the possibility of treating vessels before use in bypass grafting procedures. An extension of the elastase-induced aneurysm model *in vivo* has been made to organ culture by incubating porcine aorta in elastase *in vitro*. Following this treatment there is a progressive loss of elastin (195).

One aspect of these organ cultures, particularly vein organ cultures, that requires attention is determining the origin of neointimal cells. Cut edges could allow adventitial cells to migrate around and onto the intimal surface. This issue is not entirely settled. Adventitial fibroblasts have been shown to populate the intima of human saphenous veins *in vitro* (196) and porcine saphenous veins *in vivo* (197), so each investigator should put some effort into understanding the origin of intimal cells if this is pertinent to their goals.

b. Flow Conditions Several methods have been used to put arteries under flow *in vitro*. Porter *et al.* (198) have pinned, opened sections of saphenous vein onto the inner wall of silicon tubing through which medium is pumped at venous or arterial pressure, flow rates, and shear stress. Tedgui and colleagues (9, 199) and Fingerle and colleagues (200) have devised an adjustable clamp that allows the researcher to cannulate and remove an artery from the animal without interrupting flow or altering the stretch and pressure on the vessel. Interrupting flow or allowing the vessel to relax, even for a moment, will lead to a loss of endothelial cell integrity (199, 200). The vessels, if mishandled, can lose their "*in vivo*" characteristics. Criteria for a good artery, whether perfused or not, should be as follows: (1) ATP level is preserved, (2) contractility is maintained, although for larger arteries this is difficult to demonstrate, and (3) morphological characteristics of the tissue do not change. Injury (endothelial cell removal) to arteries subjected to 80 mmHg pressure and flow showed increased DNA synthesis, whereas nonperfused, nonpressurized vessels did not (9). This result confirms results from other researchers using static organ culture (201, 202). The rat carotid is especially suitable for perfusion because it lacks side branches. A major drawback for perfused artery systems is that they are labor intensive.

2. Tissue Culture

Explants of arterial media have been used by many investigators. The general method has been described (191, 203), but the use of a tissue chopper improves the reproducibility of explant size (204). In addition, we find it best to tease apart the media and the adventitia at a corner of the opened artery and to continue completely around the perimeter of the opened vessel before stripping the media from the adventitia in one piece to put on the chopper platform. Ostia of any arterial branches should be removed to avoid endothelial cell contamination. Plastic pipettes can be used to distribute explants to 25-cm^2 flasks (prewetted), or forceps can be used for the thinner saphenous vein explants, which tend to get stuck in the plastic pipettes. A variation on the use of explants is coculture of adventitia and media with (205) or without (73) an intervening membrane.

3. Cell Culture

The strength of cell culture is also its weakness—the isolation of cells from tissue. Cultured cells can be manipulated and exposed to factors in ways not possible in tissue or *in vivo*. However, once cells are put into culture they are grown on nonnative matrices and lose any interactions with other cells types found in the vessel wall. In culture SMCs change phenotype dramatically with increased endoplasmic reticulum and protein synthesis, for example (206). In addition, the phenotype of cells changes with increasing population doublings (207, 208), with aneuploidy often occurring at high doubling levels. Also, Schwartz and colleagues (130, 209) have discussed the hypothesis that the artery contains two kinds of SMCs. The definition of an SMC is not firm (210). For example, a classic marker for smooth muscle is smooth muscle α-actin, but fibroblasts and endothelial cells can express this protein at times, making the identification of SMCs an issue. Pauly *et al.* (211) have reviewed markers for SMCs.

a. Cell Isolation Endothelial cells, smooth muscle cells, and fibroblasts can be obtained from arterial samples in two basic ways. Both ways require physically separating the adventitia, media, and endothelial lining. The first method is letting cells grow from explants of medial or adventitial tissue (191, 203). This first requires removing the endothelial cells by scraping them off. Then media is stripped in layers from adventitia and cut into small (1 mm^2) pieces, which are allowed to adhere to the plastic culture flask before adding only enough serum containing growth medium to keep them wet. It is important to keep the explants from being dislodged by the movement of medium, because cells will not move onto the plastic if the explant is floating. The same method is used for isolating fibroblasts from adventitial explants. Cells are trypsinized and passaged before the cells become overconfluent around the explants.

The second method is the enzymatic digestion of the explants. Most methods for the arterial wall include bacterial collagenase with porcine elastase. Pauly *et al.* (211) present a good method for digesting rat aorta that approximates methods used in our laboratory. Predigesting the aorta makes the adventitia separate from the media easier. Pauly *et al.* use slightly higher concentrations of collagenase (2 vs. 1.25 mg/ml) without soybean tripsin inhibitor (we use

0.4 mg/ml) and incubate vessels overnight in culture medium after the predigest, but before the final digest of the media, claiming that the cell viability is improved. We have not used the overnight incubation. Because of variations between lots of collagenase optimal conditions should be determined by each laboratory group. Finally, the predigestion period to remove the adventitia (30 min for adult rats) can be shortened for younger rats. For 1-month-old rats 15 min is sufficient, and no predigestion is required for newborns. The key to success with either of these methods is starting with a cleanly separated media and adventitia. This is easy with large arteries, because when medial tissue is desired, part of the media can be left attached to the adventitia (183). With small arteries or veins the media must be stripped from adventitia at the border between the two layers, which may leave small amounts of adventitia on the media and vice versa.

For endothelial cells, a fast way of isolation is to simply wash the scraper off in endothelial cell growth medium when removing the endothelial cells for preparation of medial explants. The medium should be left undisturbed for a week, which should be time for colonies to be seen. We have used this for bovine, baboon, and human aortic endothelial cells with some success. Endothelial cells can also be obtained from baboon and bovine aortas by digesting closed vessels with collagenase as originally described for umbilical veins by Jaffe (212). McGuire and Orkin (213) described an explant method with collagenase to obtain rat aortic endothelial cells. Hewett and Murray (214) have described methods of isolation of human microvessel endothelial cells. For human and baboon endothelial cell medium we use RPMI-1640 with 20% fetal bovine serum, 90 μg/ml heparin, and 100 μg/ml ECGS (Collaborative Research).

Fluorescence-activated cell sorting (FACS) or magnetic bead technology (215) can be used with specific cell markers to obtain a pure population of cells expressing the selected marker. For example, endothelial cells can be obtained using the acetylated LDL receptor as a marker (216). In this case endothelial cells derived from different vascular beds exhibited different characteristics, illustrating the heterogeneity among endothelial cells [see Garlanda and Dejana (217)]. Finally, the state of differentiation of human umbilical vein endothelial cells changes well before complete senescence, making the reproducibility of experiments difficult (218). This should be kept in mind when doing experiments.

A significant change in vascular cell culture over the past 5 years has been the appearance of commercially available SMCs and endothelial cells from various venous and arterial beds and various species (humans, cows, pigs, rats, and chickens). Commercial sources include Clonetics Cell Systems (San Diego, CA), Cascade Biologics, Inc. (www.cascadebio.com), and Cell Applications, Inc. (San Diego, CA, www.cellapplications.com). This can simplify the workload for an investigator, especially if cell culture is not an ongoing aspect of research in the laboratory.

b. Medium and Serum Issues The use of serum for vascular cell culture does not raise any issues particular to vascular cells. Just as with other cells there are lot-to-lot variations in ability to stimulate growth or alter characteristics of cells. There are sometimes differences described when comparing the effects of serum from different species. For example, heparin is not growth inhibitory in the presence of human serum, but is with bovine serum (219). For a general review on sera and media, see Mather (220). Serum-free medium developed specifically for endothelial cell (221). fibroblast, and smooth muscle cell culture is available from various sources (Clonetics Cell Systems, San Diego, CA; Cascade Biologics, Inc., Cell Applications, Inc., San Diego, CA; HyClone Laboratories, Logan, UT).

c. Flow Experiments The effects of shear forces on cultured cells have been studied using a cone and plate apparatus for many years (222). This has been used to study laminar flow effects, but more recently a rectangular bar has been placed in the system (223), which causes flow disturbances downstream so that the effect of shear gradients can be studied. Parallel plate laminar flow chambers have also been used for many years, and have been combined with coculture to address the effect of flow on endothelial cell effects on SMC function (224–226).

d. Cell Migration Assays Several methods have been used to study migration of cells.

1. Scraping a confluent layer of cells (endothelial cells, SMCs, or fibroblasts) is the easiest. There are several variations on this method: (a) For endothelial cells there is the multiscratch assay using a set of wires as a "broom" to rake at right angles, leaving squares of cells on the dish (227). (b) A razor blade can be used to make a mark on the culture dish and a cotton-tipped swab used to wipe cells from one side of the blade. The dish can be turned 180° and the procedure repeated. This will leave a thin strip of cells down the middle of the dish. We have built a device to hold razor blades steady so that only one scratch is made on the plastic. (c) A section of cells is lifted from the plate with a piece of filter membrane (77). (d) Using a rake shaped like an electrophoresis comb, with the length equal to the radius of a culture dish, the investigator can make multiple scrapes in a confluent culture of SMCs, making biochemical measurements more feasible because a larger proportion of the population is injured.

2. Modified Boyden chambers have been described by Pauly *et al.* (211). Microchemotaxis chambers (48-well chambers; Neuroprobe) are used in essentially the same manner (228, 229). Using chemotaxis chambers with thick

layers of extracellular matrix proteins can a difficult, but useful, protocol. We have used two methods of drying a protein (either Vitrogen, types I and III collagen, or Matrigel, a basement membrane matrix) layer on the membrane. The first is to add the protein solution to the well of the chamber and leave it overnight in a laminar flow hood to dry. The second is to cover the whole membrane with the solution and leave it overnight in a laminar flow hood to dry. Both methods are designed to give the same concentration of protein/cm^2. In our experience, and according to other investigators who have published reports describing using the thick matrix methods and with whom we have discussed these methods, this is a difficult method. Multiple replicates (≥4 per condition) should be used for each experiment, because of variability. Cells are either counted visually or can be determined by quantitation of protein (230).

3. Invasion of collagen gels has been used with success, especially when the short time frame of a Boyden assay may preclude seeing effects of a treatment. For example, we found that MMP9-overexpressing cells in a tetracycline regulatable system invaded collagen twice as much as did control cells in 48 hr. In contrast, these cells migrated only about 30% more than control cells through a Matrigel layer in a microchemotaxis chamber (63). This was because little MMP9 accumulated during the 5-hr Boyden assay. Invasion of a collagen (Vitrogen) gel can be made into a chemotaxis assay by layering the collagen over a PDGF-containing Pluronic gel (10% F-127 Pluronic gel is made by putting the dry Pluronic gel in cold, sterile water and leaving it at 4°C until it is in solution) (63).

e. Three-Dimensional Culture Three-dimensional collagen matrices have a dramatic effect on the phenotype of SMCs (231). This effect appears to be at least in part the result of interaction with polymeric collagen (232). Cell proliferation and protein synthesis are inhibited by polymeric collagen. Coculture of endothelial cells and SMCs can be used to create more complex models to study—for example, changes in monocytes that occur after invasion of the cell layer (233). Another variation on this theme is to put a membrane of varying porosity between the SMCs and the endothelial cells (234, 235).

References

1. Ross, R. (1993). The pathogenesis of atherosclerosis: A perspective for the 1990s. *Nature (London)* **362,** 801–809.
2. Ross, R. (1999). Mechanisms of disease—Atherosclerosis—An inflammatory disease. *N. Engl. J. Med.* **340**(2), 115–126.
3. Davies, M. J. (1998). Aortic aneurysm formation: Lessons from human studies and experimental models. *Circulation* **98**(3), 193–195.
4. Galgov, S. (1973). Mechanical stresses on vessels and the non-uniform distribution of atherosclerosis. *Med. Clin. North Am.* **57**(1), 63–77.
5. Bevan, J. A. (1991). Pressure and flow: Are these the true vascular neuroeffectors. *Blood Vessels* **28,** 164–172.
6. Langille, B. L., and O'Donnell, F. (1986). Reductions in arterial diameter produced by chronic decreases in blood flow are endothelium-dependent. *Science* **231,** 405–407.
7. Geary, R. L., Kohler, T. R., Vergel, S., Kirkman, T. R., and Clowes, A. W. (1993). Time course of flow-induced smooth muscle cell proliferation and intimal thickening in endothelialized baboon vascular grafts. *Circ. Res.* **74,** 14–23.
8. Mattsson, E. J. R., Kohler, T. R., Vergel, S. M., and Clowes, A. W. (1997). Increased blood flow induces regression of intimal hyperplasia. *Arterioscler. Thromb. Vasc. Biol.* **17**(10), 2245–2249.
9. Bardy, N., Karillon, G. J., Merval, R., Samuel, J. -L., and Tedgui, A. (1995). Differential effects of pressure and flow on DNA and protein synthesis and on fibronectin expression by arteries in a novel organ culture system. *Circ. Res.* **77,** 684–694.
10. Bevan, J. A., Garcia-Roldan, J. L., and Joyce, E. H. (1990). Resistance artery tone is influenced independently by pressure and by flow. *Blood Vessels* **27**(25), 202–207.
11. Williams, B. (1998). Mechanical influences on vascular smooth muscle cell functions. *J. Hypertens.* **16,** 1921–1929.
12. Li, Q., Muragaki, Y., Hatamura, I., Ueno, H., and Ooshima, A. (1998). Stretch-induced collagen synthesis in cultured smooth muscle cells from rabbit aortic media and a possible involvement of angiotensin II and transforming growth factor-beta. *J. Vasc. Res.* **35,** 93–103.
13. Kolpakov, V., Rekhter, M. D., Gordon, D., Wang, W. H., and Kulik, T. J. (1995). Effect of mechanical forces on growth and matrix protein synthesis in the *in vitro* pulmonary artery—Analysis of the role of individual cell types. *Circ. Res.* **77,** 823–831.
14. Bardy, N., Merval, R., Benessiano, J., Samuel, J. L., and Tedgui, A. (1996). Pressure and angiotensin II synergistically induce aortic fibronectin expression in organ culture model of rabbit aorta—Evidence for a pressure-induced tissue renin–angiotensin system. *Circ. Res.* **79,** 70–78.
15. Fuster, V., Badimon, L., Badimon, J. J., and Chesebro, J. H. (1992). The pathogenesis of coronary artery disease and the acute coronary syndromes—Part 1. *N. Engl. J. Med.* **326,** 242–250.
16. Fuster, V., Badimon, L., Badimon, J. J., and Chesebro, J. H. (1992). The pathogenesis of coronary artery disease and the acute coronary syndromes. *N. Engl. J. Med.* **326,** 310–318.
17. Davies, M. J. (1996). The contribution of thrombosis to the clinical expression of coronary atherosclerosis. *Thromb. Res.* **82**(1), 1–32.
18. Kiechl, S., Willeit, J., and Bruneck, S. G. (1999). The natural course of atherosclerosis—Part I: Incidence and progression. *Arterioscler. Thromb. Vasc. Biol.* **19**(6), 1484–1490.
19. Cines, D. B., Pollak, E. S., Buck, C. A., Loscalzo, J., Zimmerman, G. A., McEver, R. P., Pober, J. S., Wick, T. M., Konkle, B. A., Schwartz, B. S., Barnathan, E. S., McCrae, K. R., Hug, B. A., Schmidt A. M., and Stern D. M. (1998). Endothelial cells in physiology and in the pathophysiology of vascular disorders. *Blood* **91**(10), 3527–3561.
20. Fujii, S. PAI-1 in thrombosis and arteriosclerosis. *Fibrinolysis* **11,** 137–140.
21. Farb, A., Burke, A. P., Tang, A. L., Liang, Y., Mannan, P., Smialek, J., and Virmani, R. (1996). Coronary plaque erosion without rupture into a lipid core. A frequent cause of coronary thrombosis in sudden coronary death. *Circulation* **93,** 1354–1363.
22. Falk, E. (1992). Why do plaques rupture. *Circulation* **86**(Suppl.), 30–42.
23. Fuster, V., Badimon, J. J., and Chesebro, J. H. (1998). Atherothrombosis: mechanisms and clinical therapeutic approaches. *Vasc. Med.* **3**(3), 231–239.
24. Ikari, Y., McManus, B., Kenyon, J., and Schwartz, S. M. (1999). Neonatal intima formation in the human coronary artery. *Arterioscler. Thromb. Vasc. Biol.* **19**(9), 2036–2040.
25. Schwartz, S. M. (1999). The intima. A new soil. *Circ. Res.* **85**(10), 877–879.

26. Best, P. J. M., Hasdai, D., Sangiorgi, G., Schwartz, R. S., Holmes, D. R., Jr., Simari, R. D., Lerman, A. (1999). Apoptosis—Basic concepts and implications in coronary artery disease. *Arterioscler. Thromb. Vasc. Biol.* **19**(1), 14–22.
27. Daemen, M. J. A. P., Lutgens, E., de Muinck, E. D., Kitslaar, P. J. E. H. M., Tordoir, J. H. M., Wellens, H. J. J., and Daemen, M. J. A. P. (1999). Biphasic pattern of cell turnover characterizes the progression from fatty streaks to ruptured human atherosclerotic plaques. *Cardiovasc. Res.* **41,** 473–479.
28. Henderson, E. L., Gang, Y. J., Sukhova, G. K., Whittemore, A. D., Knox, J., and Libby, P. (1999). Death of smooth muscle cells and expression of mediators of apoptosis by T lymphocytes in human abdominal aortic aneurysms. *Circulation* **99**(1), 96–104.
29. Holmes, D. R., López-Candales, A., Liao, S. X., and Thompson, R. W. (1996). Smooth muscle cell apoptosis and p53 expression in human abdominal aortic aneurysms. *Ann. N.Y. Acad. Sci.* **800,** 286–287.
30. Beck, L., Jr., and D'Amore, P. A. (1997). Vascular development: Cellular and molecular regulation. *FASEB J.* **11**(5), 365–373.
31. Zimmerman, C. M., and Padgett, R. W. (2000). Transforming growth factor beta signaling mediators and modulators. *Gene* **249**(1-2), 17–30.
32. Soskic, V., Görlach, M., Poznanovic, S., Boehmer, F. D., and Godovac-Zimmermann, J. (1999). Functional proteomics analysis of signal transduction pathways of the platelet-derived growth factor β receptor. *Biochemistry* **38**(6), 1757–1764.
33. Fambrough, D., McClure, K., Kazlauskas, A., and Lander, E. S. (1999). Diverse signaling pathways activated by growth factor receptors induce broadly overlapping, rather than independent, sets of genes. *Cell* **97**(6), 727–741.
34. Dikic, I., and Blaukat, A. (1999). Protein tyrosine kinase-mediated pathways in G protein-coupled receptor signaling. *Cell Biochem. Biophys.* **30**(3), 369–387.
35. Combettes-Souverain, M., and Issad, T. (1998). Molecular basis of insulin action. *Diabetes Metab* **24**(6), 477–489.
36. Roberts, J. M. (1999). Evolving ideas about cyclins. *Cell* **98**(2), 129–132.
37. Yang, J., and Kornbluth, S. (1999). All aboard the cyclin train: Subcellular trafficking of cyclins and their CDK partners. *Trends Cell. Biol.* **9**(6), 207–210.
38. Chernoff, J. Protein tyrosine phosphatases as negative regulators of mitogenic signaling. *J. Cell. Physiol.* **180**(2), 173–181.
39. Martelli, A. M., Sang, N., Borgatti, P., Capitani, S., and Neri, L. M. (1999). Multiple biological responses activated by nuclear protein kinase *C. J. Cell Biochem.* **74**(4), 499–521.
40. Friesel, R. E., and Maciag, T. (1995). Molecular mechanisms of angiogenesis: Fibroblast growth factor signal transduction. *FASEB J.* **9**(10), 919–925.
41. Heldin, C. H., and Westermark, B. (1999). Mechanism of action and *in vivo* role of platelet-derived growth factor. *Physiol. Rev.* **79**(4), 1283–1316.
42. Zhang, Y., and Deryck, R. (1999). Regulation of Smad signaling by protein associations and signaling crosstalk. *Trends Cell Biol.* **9**(7), 274–279.
43. Ashkenazi, A., and Dixit, V. (1998). Death receptors: signaling and modulation. *Science* **281,** 1305–1308.
44. Thornberry, N. A., and Lazebnik, Y. (1998). Caspases: Enemies within. *Science* **281,** 1312–1316.
45. Lukashev, M. E., and Werb, Z. (1998). ECM signalling: Orchestrating cell behaviour and misbehaviour. *Trends Cell Biol.* **8,** 437–441.
46. Moore, G., Liao, S., Curci, J. A., Starcher, B. C., Martin, R. L., Hendricks, R. T., Chen, J. J., and Thompson, R. W. (1999). Suppression of experimental abdominal aortic aneurysms by systemic treatment with a hydroxamate-based matrix metalloproteinase inhibitor (RS 132908). *J. Vasc. Surg.* **29**(3), 522–532.
47. Bigatel, D. A., Elmore, J. R., Carey, D. J., Cizmeci-Smith, G., Franklin, D. P., and Youkey, J. R. (1999). The matrix metalloproteinase inhibitor BB-94 limits expansion of experimental abdominal aortic aneurysms. *J. Vasc. Surg.* **29**(1), 130–138.
48. Prescott, M. F., Sawyer, W. K., Von Linden-Reed, J., Jeune, M., Chou, M., Caplan, S. L., and Jeng, A. Y. (1999). Effect of matrix metalloproteinase inhibition on progression of atherosclerosis and aneurysm in LDL receptor-deficient mice overexpressing MMP3, MMP12, and MMP13 and on restenosis in rats after balloon injury. *Ann. N.Y. Acad. Sci.* **878,** 179–190.
49. Thompson, R. W., Holmes, D. R., Mertens, R. A., Liao, S., Botney, M. D., Mecham, R. P., Welgus, H. G., and Parks, W. C. (1995). Production and localization of 92-kilodalton gelatinase in abdominal aortic aneurysms. An elastolytic metalloproteinase expressed by aneurysm-infiltrating macrophages. *J. Clin. Invest.* **96,** 318–326.
50. Herron, G. S., Unemori, E., Wong, M., Rapp, J. H., Hibbs, M. H., and Stoney, R. J. (1991). Connective tissue proteinases and inhibitors in abdominal aortic aneurysms. Involvement of the vasa vasorum in the pathogenesis of aortic aneurysms. *Arterioscler. Thromb.* **11,** 1667–1677.
51. Galis, Z. S., Sukhova, G. K., Lark, M. W., and Libby, P. (1994). Increased expression of matrix metalloproteinases and matrix degrading activity in vulnerable regions of human atherosclerotic plaques. *J. Clin. Invest.* **94,** 2493–2503.
52. Nikkari, S. T., O'Brien, K. D., Ferguson, M., Hatsukami, T., Welgus, H. G., Alpers, C. E., and Clowes, A. W. (1995). Interstitial collagenase (MMP-1) expression in human carotid atherosclerosis. *Circulation* **92,** 1393–1398.
53. Thompson, R. W., and Baxter, B. T. (1999). MMP inhibition in abdominal aortic aneurysms. Rationale for a prospective randomized clinical trial. *Ann. N.Y. Acad. Sci.* **878,** 159–178.
54. Faxon, D. P., Coats, W., and Currier, J. (1997). Remodeling of the coronary artery after vascular injury. *Prog. Cardiovasc. Dis.* **40,** 129–140.
55. Glagov, S. (1994). Intimal hyperplasia, vascular modeling, and the restenosis problem. *Circulation* **89,** 2888–2891.
56. Schwartz, R. S. (1998). Pathophysiology of restenosis: Interaction of thrombosis, hyperplasia, and/or remodeling. *Am. J. Cardiol.* **81**(7A), 14E–17E.
57. Geary, R. L., Williams, J. K., Golden, D., Brown, D. G., Benjamin, M. E., and Adams, M. R. (1996). Time course of cellular proliferation, intimal hyperplasia, and remodeling following angioplasty in monkeys with established atherosclerosis—A nonhuman primate model of restenosis. *Arterioscler. Thromb. Vasc. Biol.* **16,** 34–43.
58. Post, M. J., Borst, C., and Kuntz, R. E. (1994). The relative importance of arterial remodeling compared with intimal hyperplasia in lumen renarrowing after balloon angioplasty: A study in the normal rabbit and the hypercholesterolemic Yucatan micropig. *Circulation* **89,** 2816–2821.
59. Lafont, A., Guzman, L. A., Whitlow, P. L., Goormastic, M., Cornhill, J. F., and Chisolm, G. M. (1995). Restenosis after experimental angioplasty: Intimal, medial, and adventitial changes associated with constrictive remodeling. *Circ. Res.* **76,** 996–1002.
60. Kakuta, T., Currier, J. W., Haudenschild, C. C., Ryan, T. J., and Faxon, D. P. (1994). Differences in compensatory vessel enlargement, not intimal formation, account for restenosis after angioplasty in the hypercholesterolemic rabbit model. *Circulation* **89,** 2809–2815.
61. Bilder, G., Wentz, T., Leadley, R., Amin, D., Byan, L., O'Conner, B., Needle, S., Galczenski, H., Bostwick, J., Kasiewski, C., Myers, M., Spada, A., Merkel, L., Ly, C., Persons, P., Page, K., Perrone, M., and Dunwiddle, C. (1999). Restenosis following angioplasty in the swine coronary artery is inhibited by an orally active PDGF-receptor tyrosine kinase inhibitor, RPR101511A. *Circulation* **99,** 3292–3299.
62. Abbruzzese, T. A., Guzman, R. J., Martin, R. L., Yee, C., Zarins, C. K., and Dalman, R. L. (1998). Matrix metalloproteinase inhibition limits arterial enlargement in a rodent arteriovenous fistula model. *Surgery* **124**(2), 328–334.

63. Mason, D. P., Kenagy, R. D., Hasenstab, D., Bowen-Pope, D. F., Seifert, R. A., Coats, S., Hawkins, S. M., and Clowes, A. W. (1999). Matrix metalloproteinase-9 overexpression enhances vascular smooth muscle cell migration and alters remodeling in the injured rat carotid artery. *Circ. Res.* **85,** 1179–1185.
64. Strauss, B. H., Robinson, R., Batchelor, W. B., Chisholm, R. J., Ravi, G., Natarajan, M. K., Logan, R. A., Mehta, S. R., Levy, D. E., Ezrin, A. M., and Keeley, F. W. (1996). *In vivo* collagen turnover following experimental balloon angioplasty injury and the role of matrix metalloproteinases. *Circ. Res.* **79**(3), 541–550.
65. Ye, S., Humphries, S., and Henney, A. (1998). Matrix metalloproteinases: Implication in vascular matrix remodeling during atherogenesis. *Clin. Sci.* **94,** 103–110.
66. Nagase, H., and Woessner, J. F., Jr. (1999). Matrix metalloproteinases. *J. Biol. Chem.* **274**(31), 21491–21494.
67. Saksela, O., and Rifkin, D. B. (1988). Cell-associated plasminogen activators: Regulation and physiological functions. *Ann. Rev. Cell Biol.* **4,** 93–126.
68. Vassalli, J. -D., Sappino, A. -P., and Belin, D. (1991). The plasminogen activator/plasmin system. *J. Clin. Invest.* **88,** 1067–1072.
69. George, S. J. (1998). Tissue inhibitors of metalloproteinases and metalloproteinases in atherosclerosis. *Curr. Opin. Lipidol.* **9**(5), 413–423.
70. Andreasen, P. A., Georg, B., Lund, L. R., Riccio, A., and Stacey, S. N. (1990). Plasminogen activator inhibitors: Hormonally regulated serpins. *Mol. Cell. Endocrinol.* **68,** 1–19.
71. Southgate, K. M., Davies, M., Booth, R. F. G., and Newby, A. C. (1992). Involvement of extracellular-matrix-degrading metalloproteinases in rabbit aortic smooth-muscle cell proliferation. *Biochem. J.* **288,** 93–99.
72. Kenagy, R. D., Vergel, S., Mattsson, E., Bendeck, M., Reidy, M. A., and Clowes, A. W. (1996). The role of plasminogen, plasminogen activators, and matrix metalloproteinases in primate arterial smooth muscle cell migration. *Arterioscler. Thromb. Vasc. Biol.* **16**(11), 1373–1382.
73. Shi, Y., Patel, S., Niculescu, R., Chung, W. S., Desrochers, P., and Zalewski, A. (1999). Role of matrix metalloproteinases and their tissue inhibitors in the regulation of coronary cell migration. *Arterioscler. Thromb. Vasc. Biol.* **19**(5), 1150–1155.
74. Kanse, S. M., Benzakour, O., Kanthou, C., Kost, C., Lijnen, H. R., and Preissner, K. T. (1997). Induction of vascular SMC proliferation by urokinase indicates a novel mechanism of action in vasoproliferative disorders. *Arterioscler. Thromb. Vasc. Biol.* **17**(11), 2848–2854.
75. Stepanova, V., Bobik, A., Bibilashvily, R., Belogurov, A., Rybalkin, I., Domogatsky, S., Little, P. J., Goncharova, E., and Tkachuk, V. (1997). Urokinase plasminogen activator induces smooth muscle cell migration: Key role of growth factor-like domain. *FEBS Lett.* **414**(2), 471–474.
76. Herbert, J. M., Lamarche, I., Prabonnaud, V., and Dol, F. (1994). Tissue-type plasminogen activator is a potent mitogen for human aortic smooth muscle cells. *J. Biol. Chem.* **269,** 3076–3080.
77. Wijnberg, M. J., Nieuwenbroek, N. M. E., Slomp, J., Quax, P. H. A., and Verheijen, J. H. (1996). Urokinase and tissue-type plasminogen activator stimulate human vascular smooth muscle cell migration. *Fibrinolysis* **10,** 75–78.
78. Kenagy, R. D., Hart, C. E., Stetler-Stevenson, W. G., and Clowes, A. W. (1997). Primate smooth muscle cell migration from aortic explants is mediated by endogenous platelet-derived growth factor and basic fibroblast growth factor acting through matrix metalloproteinases 2 and 9. *Circulation* **96**(10), 3555–3560.
79. Carmeliet, P., Moons, L., Lijnen, R., Janssens, S., Lupu, F., Collen, D., and Gerard, R. D. (1997). Inhibitory role of plasminogen activator inhibitor-1 in arterial wound healing and neointima formation—A gene targeting and gene transfer study in mice. *Circulation* **96**(9), 3180–3191.
80. Carmeliet, P., Moons, L., Herbert, J. M., Crawley, J., Lupu, F., Lijnen, R., and Collen, D. (1997). Urokinase but not tissue plasminogen activator mediates arterial neointima formation in mice. *Circ. Res.* **81**(5), 829–839.
81. Lijnen, H. R., Lupu, F., Moons, L. C. P., Goulding, D., and Collen, D. (1999). Temporal and topographic matrix metalloproteinase expression after vascular injury in mice. *Thromb. Haemost.* **81,** 799–807.
82. Giancotti, F. G., and Ruoslatti, E. (1999). Integrin signaling. *Science* **285,** 1028–1032.
83. Elangbam, C. S., Qualls, C. W., Jr., and Dahlgren, R. R. (1997). Cell adhesion molecules—An update. *Vet. Pathol.* **34**(1), 61–73.
84. Shrivastava, A., Radziejewski, C., Campbell, E., Kovac, L., McGlynn, M., Ryan, T. E., Davis, S., Goldfarb, M. P., Glass, D. J., Lemke, G., and Yancopoulos, G. D. (1997). An orphan receptor tyrosine kinase family whose members serve as nonintegrin collagen receptor. *Mol. Cell.* **1**(1), 25–34.
85. Mogford, J. E., Davis, G. E., Platts, S. H., and Meininger, G. A. (1996). Vascular smooth muscle $\alpha_v\beta_3$ integrin mediates arteriolar vasodilation in response to RGD peptides. *Circ. Res.* **79**(4), 821–826.
86. Giannelli, G., Falk-Marzillier, J., Schiraldi, O., Stetler-Stevenson, W. G., and Quaranta, V. (1997). Induction of cell migration by matrix metalloproteinase-2 cleavage of laminin-5. *Science* **277,** 225–228.
87. Buckley, C. D., Pilling, D., Henriquez, N. V., Parsonage, G., Threlfall, K., Scheel-Toellner, D., Simmons, D. L., Albar, A. N., Lord, J. M., and Salmon, M. (1999). RGD peptides induce apoptosis by direct caspase-3 activation. *Nature (London)* **397**(6719), 534–539.
88. Cao, Y. (1998). Endogenous angiogenesis inhibitors: Angiostatin, endostatin, and other proteolytic fragments. *Prog. Mol. Subcell. Biol.* **20,** 161–76.
89. O'Reilly, M. S., Wiederschain, D., Stetler-Stevenson, W. G., Folkman, J., and Moses, M. A. (1999). Regulation of angiostatin production by matrix metalloproteinase-2 in a model of concomitant resistance. *J. Biol. Chem.* **274**(41), 29568–29571.
90. Brooks, B. P., Stromblad, S., Sanders, L. C., von Schalscha, T. L., Stettler-Stevenson, W. G., Quigley, J. P., and Cheresh, D. A. (1996). Localization of matrix metalloproteinase MMP-2 to the surface of invasive cells by interaction with integrin $\alpha_v\beta_3$. *Cell* **85,** 683–693.
91. Vassalli, J. -D. (1994). The urokinase receptor. *Fibrinolysis* **8**(Suppl. 1), 172–181.
92. Wei, Y., Lukashev, M., Simon, D. I., Bodary, S. C., Rosenberg, S., Doyle, M. V., and Chapman, H. A. (1996). Regulation of integrin function by the urokinase receptor. *Science* **273,** 1551–1555.
93. Waltz, D. A., Natkin, L. R., Fujita, R. M., Wei, Y., and Chapman, H. A. (1997). Plasmin and plasminogen activator inhibitor type 1 promote cellular motility by regulating the interaction between the urokinase receptor and vitronectin. *J. Clin. Invest.* **100**(1), 58–67.
94. Deng, G., Curriden, S. A., Wang, S. J., Rosenberg, S., and Loskutoff, D. J. (1996). Is plasminogen activator inhibitor-1 the molecular switch that governs urokinase receptor-mediated cell adhesion and release? *J. Cell Biol.* **134**(6), 1563–1571.
95. Baker, A. H., Zaltsman, A. B., George, S. J., and Newby, A. C. (1998). Divergent effects of tissue inhibitor of metalloproteinase-1, -2, or -3 overexpression on rat vascular smooth muscle cell invasion, proliferation, and death *in vitro*—TIMP-3 promotes apoptosis. *J. Clin. Invest.* **101**(6), 1478–1487.
96. Murphy, A. N., Unsworth, E. J., and Stetler-Stevenson, W. G. (1993). Tissue inhibitor of metalloproteinase-2 inhibits bFGF induced human microvascular endothelial cell proliferation. *J. Cell Physiol.* **157,** 351–358.
97. Valente, P., Fassina, G., Melchiori, A., Masiello, L., Cilli, M., Vacca, A., Onisto, M., Santi, L., Stetler-Stevenson, W. G., and Albini, A. (1999). TIMP-2 over-expression reduces invasion and angiogenesis and protects B16F10 melanoma cells from apoptosis. *Int. J. Cancer* **75,** 246–253.
98. Guedez, L., Stetler-Stevenson, W. G., Wolff, L., Wang, J., Fukushima, P., Mansoor, A., and Stetler-Stevenson, M. (1998). *In vitro* suppression of programmed cell death of B cells by tissue inhibitor of Metalloproteinases-1. *J. Clin. Invest.* **102,** 2002–2010.

99. Dickinson, J. L., Bates, E. J., Ferrante, A., and Antalis, T. M. (1995). Plasminogen activator inhibitor type 2 inhibits tumor necrosis factor alpha-induced apoptosis: Evidence for an alternate biological function. *J. Biol. Chem.* **270,** 27894–27904.
100. Schwartz, R. S., Topol, E. J., Serruys, P. W., Sangiorgi, G., and Holmes, D. R., Jr. (1998). Artery size, neointima, and remodeling: time for some standards. *J. Am. Coll. Cardiol.* **32**(7), 2087–2094.
101. Reddick, R. L., Read, M. S., Brinkhous, K. M., Bellinger, D., Nichol, T., and Griggs, T. R. (1990). Coronary atherosclerosis in the pig. Induced plaque injury and platelet response. *Arteriosclerosis* **10**(4), 541–550.
102. Howard, C. F. (1985). Atherosclerosis and insulin in primates with diabetes mellitus. *Metabolism* **34**(12, Suppl. 1), 60–66.
103. Howard, C. F., Jr., Vesselinovitch, D., and Wissler, R. W. (1984). Correlations of aortic histology with gross aortic atherosclerosis and metabolic measurements in diabetic and nondiabetic *Macaca nigra. Atherosclerosis* **52**(1), 85–100.
104. Jordan, W. D., Jr., Sampson, L. K., Iyer, S., Anderson, P. G., Lyle, K., Brown, R. J., Luo, J., and Roubin, G. S. (1998). Abdominal aortic aneurysm repair via percutaneous endovascular stenting in the swine model. *Am. J. Surg.* **64**(11), 1070–1073.
105. Raymond, J., Venne, D., Allas, S., Roy, D., Oliva, V. L., Denbow, N., Salazkin, I., and Leclerc, G. (1999). Healing mechanisms in experimental aneurysms. I. Vascular smooth muscle cells and neointima formation. *J. Neuroradiol.* **26**(1, Suppl.], 7–20.
106. Schwartz, R. S. (1994). Neointima and arterial injury: dogs, rats, pigs, and more. *Lab. Invest.* **71**(6), 789–791.
107. Gross, D. R., Thromboembolic phenonmena and the use of the pig as an appropriate animal model for research on cardiovascular devices. *Int. J. Artif. Organs* **20,** 195–203.
108. Hanson, S. R., and Harker, L. A. (1987). Baboon models of acute arterial thrombosis. *Thromb Haemost.* **58**(3), 801–805.
109. Hart, C. E., Kraiss, L. W., Vergel, S., Gilbertson, D., Kenagy, R., Kirkman, T., Crandall, D. L., Tickle, S., Finney, H., Yarranton, G., and Clowes, A. W. (1999). PDGFβ receptor blockade inhibits intimal hyperplasia in the baboon. *Circulation* **99**(4), 564–569.
110. Hoover, G. A., Nicolosi, R. J., Camp, R. R., and Hayes, K. C. (1982). Characteristics of the aortic intima in young and old cebus and squirrel monkeys. *Arteriosclerosis* **2**(3), 252–265.
111. Stary, H. C., Bleakley, Chandler, A., Glagov, S., Guyton, J. R., Insull, W., Jr., Rosenfeld, M. E., Schaffer, S. A., Schwartz, C. J., Wagner, W. D., and Wissler, R. W. (1994). A definition of initial, fatty streak, and intermediate lesions of atherosclerosis: A report from the Committee on Vascular Lesions of the Council on Arteriosclerosis, American Heart Association. *Arterioscler. Thromb.* **14,** 840–856.
112. Stary, H. C., Chandler, A. B., Dinsmore, R. E., Fuster, V., Glagov, S., Insull, W., Jr., Rosenfeld, M. E., Schwartz, C. J., Wagner, W. D., and Wissler, R. W. (1995). A definition of advanced types of atherosclerotic lesions and a histological classification of atherosclerosis—A report from the Committee on Vascular Lesions of the Council on Arteriosclerosis, American Heart Association. *Arterioscler. Thromb. Vasc. Biol.* **15,** 1512–1531.
113. Masuda, J., Ross, R. Atherogenesis during low level hypercholesterolemia in the nonhuman primate. I. Fatty streak formation. *Arteriosclerosis* **10**(2), 164–177.
114. Masuda, J., and Ross, R. (1990). Atherogenesis during low level hypercholesterolemia in the nonhuman primate. II. Fatty streak conversion to fibrous plaque. *Arteriosclerosis* **10**(2), 178–187.
115. Faggiotto, A., Ross, R., and Harker, L. (1984). Studies of hypercholesterolemia in nonhuman primate. I. Changes that lead to fatty streak formation. *Arteriosclerosis* **4,** 323–340.
116. Faggiotto, A., and Ross, R. (1984). Studies of hypercholesterolemia in the nonhuman primate. II. Fatty streak conversion to fibrous plaque. *Arteriosclerosis* **4,** 341–356.
117. Clarkson, T. B., Lofland, H. B., Jr., Bullock, B. C., and Goodman, H. O. (1971). Genetic control of plasma cholesterol. Studies on squirrel monkeys. *Arch. Pathol.* **92**(1), 37–45.
118. Clarkson, T. B. (1998). Nonhuman primate models of atherosclerosis. *Lab. Anim. Sci.* **48**(6), 569–572.
119. Bochaton-Piallat, M. -L., Gabbiani, F., Ropraz, P., and Gabbiani, G. (1993). Age influences the replicative activity and the differentiation features of cultured rat aortic SMC populations and clones. *Arterioscler. Thromb.* **13**, 1449–1455.
120. Geary, R. L., Nikkari, S. T., Wagner, W. D., Williams, J. K., Adams, M. R., and Dean, R. H. (1998). Wound healing: A paradigm for lumen narrowing after arterial reconstruction. *J. Vasc. Surg.* **27**(1), 96–106.
121. Zarins, C. K., Xu, C. P., and Glagov, S. (1992). Aneurysmal enlargement of the aorta during regression of experimental atherosclerosis. *J. Vasc. Surg.* **15**(1), 90–98.
122. Zarins, C. K., Glagov, S., Vesselinovitch, D., and Wissler, R. W. (1990). Aneurysm formation in experimental atherosclerosis: relationship to plaque evolution. *J. Vasc. Surg.* **12**(3), 246–256.
123. Brown, G., Albers, J. J., Fisher, L. D., Schaefer, S. M., Lin, J. T., Kaplan, C., Zhao, X. Q., Bisson, B. D., Fitzpatrick, V. F., and Dodge, H. T. (1990). Regression of coronary artery disease as a result of intensive lipid-lowering therapy in men with high levels of apolipoprotein *B. N. Engl. J. Med.* **323**(19), 1289–1298.
124. Sato, H., Arikawa, J., Furuya, M., Kitoh, J., Mannen, K., Nishimune, Y., Ohsawa, K., Serikawa, T., Shibahara, T., Watanabe, Y., Yagami, K., Yamamoto, H., and Yoshikawa, Y. (1998). Prevalence of herpes B virus antibody in nonhuman primates reared at the National University of Japan. *Exp. Anim.* **47**(3), 199–202.
125. Kohler, T. R., and Kirkman, T. R. (1999). Dialysis access failure: A sheep model of rapid stenosis. *J. Vasc. Surg.* **30,** 744–751.
126. Boudghene, F. P., Sapoval, M. R., Bonneau, M., LeBlanche, A. F., Lavaste, F. C., and Michel, J. B. (1998). Abdominal aortic aneurysms in sheep: prevention of rupture with endoluminal stent-grafts. *Radiology* **206**(2), 447–454.
127. Schwartz, R. S., Edwards, W. D., Bailey, K. R., Camrud, A. R., Jorgenson, M. A., and Holmes, D. R., Jr. (1994). Differential neointimal response to coronary artery injury in pigs and dogs: Implications for restenosis models. *Arterioscler. Thromb.* **14,** 395–400.
128. Scheinowitz, M., Shou, M., Banai, S., Gertz, S. D., Lazarous, D. F., and Unger, E. F. (1994). Neointimal proliferation in canine coronary arteries. A model of restenosis permitting local and continuous drug delivery. *Lab. Invest.* **71**(6), 813–819.
129. Wilson, G. J., Klement, P., Kato, Y. P., Martin, J. B., Khan, I. J., Alcime, R., Dereume, J. P., MacGregor, D. C., and Pinchuk, L. (1996). A self-expanding bifurcated endovascular graft for abdominal aortic aneurysm repair. An initial study in a canine model. *ASAIO J.* **42**(5), M386–M393.
130. Schwartz, S. M., DeBlois, D., and O'Brien, E. R. M. (1995). The intima—Soil for atherosclerosis and restenosis. *Circ. Res.* **77,** 445–465.
131. Allaire, E., and Clowes, A. W. (1997). The intimal hyperplastic response. *Ann. Thorac. Surg.* **64**(4), S38–S46.
132. Fingerle, J., Au, Y. P. T., Clowes, A. W., and Reidy, M. A. (1990). Intimal lesion formation in rat carotid arteries after endothelial denudation in absence of medial injury. *Arteriosclerosis* **10,** 1082–1087.
133. Koyama, H., and Reidy, M. A. (1997). Reinjury of arterial lesions induces intimal smooth muscle cell replication that is not controlled by fibroblast growth factor 2. *Circ. Res.* **80**(3), 408–417.
134. Koyama, H., and Reidy, M. A. (1998). Expression of extracellular matrix proteins accompanies lesion growth in a model of intimal reinjury. *Circ. Res.* **82**(9), 988–995.
135. Bendeck, M. P., Zempo, N., Clowes, A. W., Galardy, R. E., and Reidy, M. A. (1994). Smooth muscle cell migration and matrix metalloproteinase expression after arterial injury in the rat. *Circ. Res.* **75,** 539–545.

136. Clowes, A. W., and Schwartz, S. M. (1985). Significance of quiescent smooth muscle migration in the injured rat carotid artery. *Circ. Res.* **56,** 139–145.
137. Lynch, C. M., Clowes, M. M., Osborne, W. R. A., Clowes, A. W., and Miller, A. D. (1992). Long-term expression of human adenosine deaminase in vascular smooth muscle cells of rats: A model for gene therapy. *Proc. Natl. Acad. Sci. U.S.A.* **89,** 1138–1142.
138. Clowes, M. M., Lynch, C. M., Miller, A. D., Miller, D. G., Osborne, W. R. A., and Clowes, A. W. (1994). Long-term biological response of injured rat carotid artery seeded with smooth muscle cells expressing retrovirally introduced human genes. *J. Clin. Invest.* **93,** 644–651.
139. Allaire, E., Hasenstab, D., Kenagy, R. D., Starcher, B., Clowes, M. M., and Clowes, A. W. (1998). Prevention of aneurysm development and rupture by local overexpression of plasminogen activator inhibitor-1. *Circulation* **98,** 249–255.
140. Shears, L. L., Kibbe, M. R., Murdock, Billiar, T. R., Lizonova, A., Kovesdi, I., Watkins, S. C., and Tzeng, E. (1998). Efficient inhibition of intimal hyperplasia by adenovirus-mediated inducible nitric oxide synthase gene transfer to rats and pigs *in vivo. J. Am. Coll. Surg.* **187,** 295–306.
141. Iaccarino, G., Smithwick, L. A., Lefkowitz, R. J., and Koch, W. J. (1999). Targeting $G_{\beta gamma}$ signaling in arterial vascular smooth muscle proliferation: A novel strategy to limit restenosis. *Proc. Natl. Acad. Sci. U.S.A.* **96**(7, Pt.2), 3945–3950.
142. Lynch, C. M., Hara, P. S., Leonard, J. C., Williams, J. K., Dean, R. H., and Geary, R. L. (1997). Adeno-associated virus vectors vascular gene delivery. *Circ. Res.* **80**(4), 497–505.
143. Isner, J. M. (1998). Arterial gene transfer of naked DNA for therapeutic angiogenesis: early clinical results. *Adv. Drug Deliv. Rev.* **30**(1–3), 185–197.
144. DeYoung, M. B., and Dichek, D. A. (1998). Gene therapy for restenosis—Are we ready? *Circ. Res.* **82**(3), 306–313.
145. Clowes, A. W. (1997). Vascular gene therapy in the 21st century. *Thromb. Haemost.* **78**(1), 605–610.
146. Nabel, E. G., Plautz, G., and Nabel, G. J. (1990). Site specific gene expression *in vivo* by direct gene transfer into the arterial wall. *Science* **249,** 1285–1288.
147. Nabel, G. J. (1999). Development of optimized vectors for gene therapy. *Proc. Natl. Acad. Sci. U.S.A.* **96**(2), 324–326.
148. Forough, R., Hasenstab, D., Koyama, N., Lea, H., Clowes, M., and Clowes, A. W. (1996). Generating antibodies against secreted proteins using vascular smooth muscle cells transduced with replication-defective retrovirus. *Bio Techniques* **20**(4), 694–701.
149. Forough, R., Koyama, N., Hasenstab, D., Lea, H., Clowes, M., Nikkari, S. T., and Clowes, A. W. Overexpression of tissue inhibitor of matrix metalloproteinase-1 inhibits vascular smooth muscle cell functions in vitro and in vivo. *Circ. Res.* **79**(4), 812–820.
150. Hasenstab, D., Lea, H., Hart, C. E., Lok, S., and Clowes, A. W. (2000) Tissue factor overexpression in rat arterial neointima models thrombosis and progression of advanced atherosclerosis. *Circulation* **101,** 2651–2657.
151. Pinto-Sietsma, S. J., and Paul, M. (1997). Transgenic rats as models for hypertension. *J. Hum. Hypertens.* **11**(9), 577–581.
152. Assadnia, S., Rapp, J. P., Nestor, A. L., Pringle, T., Cerilli, G. J., Gunning, W. T., III, Webb, T. H., Kligman, M., and Allison, D. C. (1999). Strain differences in neointimal hyperplasia in the rat. *Circ. Res.* **84**(11), 1252–1257.
153. Moore, G., Liao, S. X., Curci, J. A., Starcher, B. C., Martin, R. L., Hendricks, R. T., Chen, J. J., and Thompson, R. W. (1999). Suppression of experimental abdominal aortic aneurysms by systemic treatment with a hydroxamate-based matrix metalloproteinase inhibitor (RS 132908). *J. Vasc. Surg.* **29**(3): 522–532.
154. Allaire, E., Forough, R., Wang, T., Clowes, M. M., and Clowes, A. W. (1997). Tissue metalloproteinase inhibitor-1 (TIMP-1) overexpression prevents arterial rupture and dilation in a xenograft model. *FASEB J.* **10**(6), 782.
155. Allaire, E., Forough, R., Clowes, W., Starcher, B., and Clowes, A. W. (1998). Local overexpression of TIMP-1 prevents aortic aneurysm degeneration and rupture in a rat model. *J. Clin. Invest.* **102**(7), 1413–1420.
156. Carmeliet, P., Moons, L., and Collen, D. (1998). Mouse models of angiogenesis, arterial stenosis, atherosclerosis and hemostasis. *Cardiovasc. Res.* **39**(1), 8–33.
157. Smith, J. D., and Breslow, J. L. (1997). The emergence of mouse models of atherosclerosis and their relevance to clinical research. *J. Intern. Med.* **242,** 99–109.
158. Cybulsky, M. I., Lichtman, A. H., Hajra, L., and Iiyama, K. (1999). Leukocyte adhesion molecules in atherogenesis. *Clin. Chim. Acta* **286**(1–2), 207–218.
159. Carmeliet, P., Moons, L. S. J. M., De Mol, M., Bouche, A., Van den, Oord J. J., Kockx, M., and Collen, D. (1997). Vascular wound healing and neointima formation induced by perivascular electric injury in mice. *Am. J. Pathol.* **150**(2), 761–776.
160. Lindner, V., Fingerle, J., and Reidy, M. A. (1993). Mouse model of arterial injury. *Circ. Res.* **73,** 792–796.
161. Kumar, A., and Lindner, V. (1997). Remodeling with neointima formation in the mouse carotid artery after cessation of blood flow. *Arterioscler. Thromb. Vasc. Biol.* **17**(10), 2238–2244.
162. Roque, M., Fallon, J. T., Badimon, J. J., Zhang, W. X., Taubman, M. B., and Reis, E. D. (2000). Mouse model of femoral artery denudation injury associated with the rapid accumulation of adhesion molecules on the luminal surface and recruitment of neutrophils. *Arterioscler. Thromb. Vasc. Biol.* **20,** 335–342.
163. Yamashita, T., Kawashima, S., Ozaki, M., Ohashi, Y., Takeuchi, S., Ishida, T., and Inoue, N. (1999). Nitric oxide overproduced by endothelial cells prevents vascular remodeling in the mouse carotid artery. *Circulation* **100**(18, Suppl.), 1–3.
164. Andrews, E. J., White, W. J., and Bullock, L. P. (1975). Spontaneous aortic aneurysms in blotchy mice. *Am. J. Pathol.* **78**(2), 199–210.
165. Pereira, L., Lee, S. Y., Gayraud, B., Andrikopoulos, K., Shapiro, S. D., Bunton, T., Biery, N. J., Dietz, H. C., Sakai, L. Y., and Ramirez, F. (1999). Pathogenetic sequence for aneurysm revealed in mice underexpressing fibrillin-1. *Proc. Natl. Acad. Sci. U.S.A.* **96**(7), 3819–3823.
166. Carmeliet, P., Moons, L., Lijnen, R., Baes, M., Lemaitre, V., Tipping, P., Drew, A., Eeckhout, Y., Shapiro, S., Lupu, F., and Collen, D. (1997). Urokinase-generated plasmin activates matrix metalloproteinases during aneurysm formation. *Nature Genet.* **17,** 439–444.
167. Bocan, T. M. A. (1998). Animal studies of atherosclerosis and interpretation of drug intervention studies. *Curr. Pharmaceut. Des.* **4,** 37–52.
168. Ho, K. J., Pang, L. C., and Taylor, C. B. (1974). Mode of cholesterol accumulation in various tissues of rabbits with prolonged exposure to various serum cholesterol levels. *Atherosclerosis* **19**(3), 561–566.
169. Daley, S. J., Herderick, E. E., Cornhill, J. F., and Rogers, K. A. (1994). Cholesterol-fed and casein-fed rabbit models of atherosclerosis. Part 1: Differing lesion area and volume despite equal plasma cholesterol levels. *Arteriosclerosis* **14**(1), 95–104.
170. Daley, S. J., Klemp, K. F., Guyton, J. R., and Rogers, K. A. (1994). Cholesterol-fed and casein-fed rabbit models of atherosclerosis. Part 2: Differing morphological severity of atherogenesis despite matched plasma cholesterol levels. *Arterioscler. Thromb.* **14**(1), 105–141.
171. Barry, W. L., Wiegman, P. J., Gimple, L. W., Gertz, S. D., Powers, E. R., Owens, G. K., and Sarembock, I. J. (1997). A new single-injury model of balloon angioplasty in cholesterol- fed rabbits: Beneficial effect of hirudin and comparison with double-injury model. *Lab Invest.* **77**(1), 109–116.
172. Jang, Y. S., Guzman, L. A., Lincoff, A. M., Gottsauner-Wolf, M., Forudi, F., Hart, C. E., Courtman, D. W., Ezban, M., Ellis, S. G., and Topol, E. J. (1995). Influence of blockade at specific levels of the

coagulation cascade on restenosis in a rabbit atherosclerotic femoral artery injury model. *Circulation* **92,** 3041–3050.
173. Courtman, D. W., Schwartz, S. M., and Hart, C. E. (1998). Sequential injury of the rabbit abdominal aorta induces intramural coagulation and luminal narrowing independent of intimal mass—Extrinsic pathway inhibition eliminates luminal narrowing. *Circ. Res.* **82**(9), 996–1006.
174. Johnson, G. J., Griggs, T. R., and Badimon, L. (1999). The utility of animal models in the preclinical study of interventions to prevent human coronary artery restenosis: Analysis and recommendations. *Thromb. Haemost.* **81,** 835–843.
175. Wolf, Y. G., Gertz, D., and Banai, S. (1999). Animal models in syndromes of accelerated arteriosclerosis. *Ann. Vasc. Res.* **33**(3), 328–338.
176. Dussaillant, G. R., Mintz, G. S., Pichard, A. D., Kent, K. M., Satler, L. F., Popma, J. J., Wong, S. C., and Leon, M. B. (1995). Small stent size and intimal hyperplasia contribute to restenosis: A volumetric intravascular ultrasound analysis. *J. Am. Coll. Cardiol.* **26,** 720–724.
177. Bauters, C., Van Belle, E., Meurice, T., Letourneau, T., Lablanche, J. M., and Bertrand, M. E. (1997). Prevention of restenosis—Future directions. *Trends Cardiovasc. Med.* **7**(3), 90–94.
178. Post, M. J., De Smet, B. J. G. L., Van der Helm, Y., Borst, C., and Kuntz, R. E. (1997). Arterial remodeling after balloon angioplasty or stenting in an atherosclerotic experimental model. *Circulation* **96**(3), 996–1003.
179. Gallo, R., Padurean, A., Toschi, V., Bichler, J., and Fallon, J. T. (1998). Prolonged thrombin inhibition reduces restenosis after balloon angioplasty in porcine coronary arteries. *Circulation* **97**(581), 588.
180. Rogers, C., Karnovsky, M. J., and Edelman, E. R. (1993). Inhibition of experimental neointimal hyperplasia and thrombosis depends on the type of vascular injury and the site of drug administration. *Circulation* **88**(3), 1215–1221.
181. Yu, C., Cunningham, M., Rogers, C., Dinbergs, I. D., Edelman, E. R. (1998). The biologic effects of growth factor-toxin conjugates in models of vascular injury depend on dose, mode of delivery, and animal species. *J. Pharm. Sci.* **87**(11), 1300–1304.
182. Rekhter, M. D., Hicks, G. W., Brammer, D. W., Work, C. W., Kim, J. S., Gordon, D., K. J. A., and Ryan, M. J. (1999). Animal model that mimics atherosclerotic plaque rupture. *Circ. Res.* **83**(7), 705–713.
183. Kenagy, R. D., Vergel, S., Mattsson, E., Bendeck, M., Reidy, M. A., and Clowes, A. W. (1996). The role of plasminogen, plasminogen activators and matrix metalloproteinases in primate arterial smooth muscle cell migration. *Arterioscler. Thromb. Vasc. Biol.* **16,** 1373–1382.
184. Kenagy, R. D., and Clowes, A. W. (1997). Proliferation response after angioplasty. *In* "Inflammatory and Thrombotic Problems in Vascular Surgery" (R.M. Greenhalgh and J.T. Powell, eds.), pp. 257–266.
185. Fishman, J. A., Ryan, G. B., and Karnovsky, M. J. (1975). Endothelial regeneration in the rat carotid artery and the significance of endothelial denudation in the pathogenesis of myointimal thickening. *Lab Invest.* **32,** 339–345.
186. Cowan, K. N., Jones, P. L., and Rabinovitch, M. (1999). Regression of hypertrophied rat pulmonary arteries in organ culture is associated with suppression of proteolytic activity, inhibition of tenascin-C, and smooth muscle cell apoptosis. *Circ. Res.* **84,** 1223–1233.
187. Ehrlich, H. P. (1980). Culture of aorta. *Methods Cell Biol.* **21A,** 117–134.
188. Gotlieb, A. I., and Boden, P. (1999). Porcine aortic organ culture: A model to study the cellular response to vascular injury. *In Vitro* **20**(7), 535–542.
189. Daley, S. J., and Gotlieb, A. I. (1996). Fibroblast growth factor receptor-1 expression is associated with neointimal formation *in vitro*. *Am. J. Pathol.* **148**(4), 1193–1202.
190. Barrett, L. A., Mergner, W. J., and Trump, B. F. (1979). Long-term culture of human aortas. Development of atherosclerotic-like plaques in serum-supplemented medium. *In Vitro* **15,** 957–966.
191. Kocan, R. M., Moss, N. S., and Benditt, E. P. (1980). Human arterial wall cells and tissues in culture. *Methods Cell Biol.* **21A,** 153–166.
192. Soyombo, A. A., Angelini, G. D., Bryan, A. J., and Newby, A. C. (1993). Surgical preparation induces injury and promotes smooth muscle cell proliferation in a culture of human saphenous vein. *Cardiovasc. Res.* **27,** 1961–1967.
193. Nicosia, R. F. (1998). Rat model of angiogenesis and its applications. *In* "Microvascular Morphogenesis *in Vivo, in Vitro*, and *in Menta*" (V. Mironov, C. Little, and H. Sage, eds.), pp. 111–139. Birkhauser Publ., Boston.
194. George, S. J., Johnson, J. L., Angelini, G. D., Newby, A. C., and Baker, A. H. (1998). Adenovirus-mediated gene transfer of the human TIMP-1 gene inhibits smooth muscle cell migration and neointimal formation in human saphenous vein. *Hum. Gene. Ther.* **9**(6), 867–877.
195. Wills, A., Thompson, M. M., Crowther, M., Brindle, N. P., Nasim, A., Sayers, R. D., and Bell, P. R. (1996). Elastase-induced matrix degradation in arterial organ cultures: An *in vitro* model of aneurysmal disease. *J. Vasc. Surg.* **24**(4), 667–679.
196. Slomp, J., Gittenberger-deGroot, A. C., Van Munsteren, J. C., Huysmans, H. A., Van Bockel, J. H., van Hinsbergh, V. W., and Poelmann, R. E. (1996). Nature and origin of the neointima in whole vessel wall organ culture of the human saphenous vein. *Virchows Arch.* **428**(1), 59–67.
197. Shi, Y., O'Brien, J. E., Jr., Mannion, J. D., Morrison, R. C., Chung, W. S., Fard, A., and Zalewski, A. (1997). Remodeling of autologous saphenous vein grafts—The role of perivascular myofibroblasts. *Circulation* **95**(12), 2684–2693.
198. Porter, K. E., Nydahl, S., Dunlop, P., Varty, K., Thrush, A. J., and London, N. J. M. (1996). The development of an *in vitro* flow model of human saphenous vein graft intimal hyperplasia. *Cardiovasc. Res.* **31,** 607–614.
199. Tedgui, A., and Lever, M. J. Filtration through damaged and undamaged rabbit thoracic aorta. *Am. J. Physiol. Heart Circ. Physiol.* **247**(16), H784–H791.
200. Faulmuller, A. (1996). Modulation of the proliferative behavior of vascular smooth muscle cells *in vitro*: Studies on the rat common carotid in perfusion organ culture. Eberhard-Karls University, Ph.D. thesis, Tübingen, Germany.
201. Boonen, H. C. M., Schiffers, P. M. H., Fazzi, G. E., Janssen, G. M. J., Daemen, M. J. A. P., and De Mey, J. G. R. (1991). DNA synthesis in isolated arteries. Kinetics and structural consequences. *Am. J. Physiol. Heart Circ. Physiol.* **260,** H210–H217.
202. Schiffers, P. M. H., Janssen, G. M. J., Fazzi, G. E., Struijker-Boudier, H. A. J., and De Mey, J. G. R. (1992). Endothelial modulation of DNA synthesis in isolated arteries of the rat. *J. Cardiovasc. Pharmacol.* **20**(Suppl. 12), S124–S127.
203. Ross, R., and Kariya, B. (1980). Morphogenesis of vascular smooth muscle in atherosclerosis and cell culture. *In* "Handbook of Physiology—The Cardiovascular System II" (D. Bohr, ed.), pp. 69–91. *Am. Physiol. Soc.*, Bethesda.
204. McMurray, H. F., Parrott, D. P., and Bowyer, D. E. (1991). A standardised method of culturing aortic explants, suitable for the study of factors affecting the phenotypic modulation, migration and proliferation of aortic smooth muscle cells. *Atherosclerosis* **86,** 227–237.
205. Betz, E., Fallier-Becker, P., Wolburg-Buchholz, K., and Fotev, Z. (1991). Proliferation of smooth muscle cells in the inner and outer layers of the tunica media of arteries: An *in vitro* study. *J. Cell Physiol.* **147,** 385–395.
206. Thyberg, J., Hedin, U., Sjölund, M., Palmberg, L., and Bottger, B. A. (1990). Regulation of differentiated properties and proliferation of arterial smooth muscle cells. *Arteriosclerosis* **10,** 966–990.
207. Murphy-Ullrich, J. E., Pallero, M. A., Boerth, N., Greenwood, J. A., Lincoln, T. M., and Cornwell, T. L. (1996). Cyclic GMP-dependent protein kinase is required for thrombospondin and tenascin mediated focal adhesion disassembly. *J. Cell Sci.* **109**(10), 2499–2508.

208. Cahill, P. A., and Hassid, A. (1993). Differential antimitogenic effectiveness of atrial natriuretic peptides in primary versus subcultured rat aortic smooth muscle cells: Relationship to expression of ANF-C receptors. *J. Cell Physiol.* **154,** 28–38.
209. Adams, L. D., Lemire, J. M., and Schwartz, S. M. (1999). A systematic analysis of 40 random genes in cultured vascular smooth muscle subtypes reveals a heterogeneity of gene expression and identifies the tight junction gene zonula occludens 2 as a marker of epithelioid "Pup" smooth muscle cells and a participant in carotid neointimal formation. *Arterioscler. Thromb. Vasc. Biol.* **19**(11), 2600–2608.
210. Schwartz, S. M. (1999). The definition of cell type. *Circ. Res.* **84**(10), 1234–1235.
211. Pauly, R. R., Bilato, C., Cheng, L., Monticone, R., and Crow, M. T. (1998). Vascular smooth muscle cell cultures. *Methods Cell Biol.* **52,** 133–154.
212. Jaffe, E. A., Nachman, R. L., Becker, C. G., and Minick, C. R. (1973). Culture of human endothelial cells derived from umbilical veins. Identification by morphologic and immunologic criteria. *J. Clin. Invest.* **52,** 2745–2756.
213. McGuire, P. G., and Orkin, R. W. (1987). Methods in laboratory investigation. Isolation of rat aortic endothelial cells by primary explant techniques and their phenotypic modulation by defined substrata. *Lab Invest.* **57,** 94–105.
214. Hewett, P. W., and Murray, J. C. (1993). Human microvessel endothelial cells: Isolation, culture and characterization. *In Vitro Cell Dev. Biol. Anim.* **29A**(11), 823–830.
215. Sinclair, R. (1998). To bead or not to bead. Applications of magnetic bead technology. *The Scientist* **12**(13), 17–21.
216. Craig, L. E., Spelman, J. P., Strandberg, J. D., and Zink, M. C. (1998). Endothelial cells from diverse tissues exhibit differences in growth and morphology. *Microvasc. Res.* **55**(1), 65–76.
217. Garlanda, C., and Dejana, E. (1997). Heterogeneity of endothelial cells. Specific markers. *Arterioscler. Thromb. Vasc. Biol.* **17**(7), 1193–1202.
218. Watson, C. A., Camera-Benson, L., Palmer-Crocker, R., and Pober, J. S. (1995). Variability among human umbilical vein endothelial cultures. *Science* **268**(5209), 447–448.
219. Underwood, P. A., Mitchell, S. M., and Whitelock, J. M. (1998). Heparin fails to inhibit the proliferation of human vascular smooth muscle cells in the presence of human serum. *J. Vasc. Res.* **35,** 449–460.
220. Mather, J. P. (1998). Making informed choices: medium, serum, and serum-free medium. How to choose the appropriate medium and culture system for the model you wish to create. *Methods Cell Biol.* **57,** 19–30.
221. Battista, P. J., and Soderland, C. (1998). Serum-free culture of human arterial and microvascular endothelial cells. *Focus* **17**(3), 106–108.
222. Bussolari, S. R., Dewey, C. F., Jr., and Gimbrone, Jr., M. A. (1982). Apparatus for subjecting living cells to fluid shear stress. *Rev. Sci. Instrum.* **53,** 1851–1854.
223. Nagel, T., Resnick, N., Dewey, C. F., Jr., and Gimbrone, M. A., Jr. (1999). Vascular endothelial cells respond to spatial gradients in fluid shear stress by enhanced activation of transcription factors. *Arterioscler. Thromb. Vasc. Biol.* **19**(8), 1825–1834.
224. Nackman, G. B., Fillinger, M. F., Shafritz, R., Wei, T., and Graham, A. M. (1998). Flow modulates endothelial regulation of smooth muscle cell proliferation: A new model. *Surgery* **124**(353), 361.
225. Nerem, R. M., Alexander, R. W., Chappell, D. C., Medford, R. M., Varner, S. E., and Taylor, W. R. (1998). The study of the influence of flow on vascular endothelial biology. *Am. J. Med. Sci.* **316**(3), 169–175.
226. Raab, L. (1998). Maximize *in vitro* culture possibilities. *The Scientist* **12**(21), 15–16.
227. Selden, S. C., 3d, Rabinovitch, P. S., and Schwartz, S. M. (1981). Effects of cytoskeletal disrupting agents on replication of bovine endothelium. *J. Cell. Physiol.* **108**(2), 195–211.
228. Koyama, N., Koshikawa, T., Morisaki, N., Saito, Y., and Yoshida, S. (1990). Bifunctional effects of transforming growth factor-β on migration of cultured rat aortic smooth muscle cells. *Biochem. Biophys. Res. Commun.* **169,** 725–729.
229. Koyama, N., Hart, C. E., and Clowes, A. W. (1994). Different functions of the platelet-derived growth factor-α and -β receptors for the migration and proliferation of cultured baboon smooth muscle cells. *Circ. Res.* **75,** 682–691.
230. Grotendorst, G. R. (1987). Spectrophotometric assay for the quantitation of cell migration in the Boyden chamber chemotaxis assay. *Methods Enzymol.* **147,** 144–152.
231. Yamamoto, M., Nakamura, H., Yamato, M., Aoyagi, M., and Yamamoto, K. (1996). Retardation of phenotypic transition of rabbit arterial smooth muscle cells in three-dimensional primary culture. *Exp. Cell Res.* **225,** 12–21.
232. Koyama, H., Raines, E. W., Bornfeldt, K. E., Roberts, J. M., and Ross, R. (1996). Fibrillar collagen inhibits arterial smooth muscle proliferation through regulation of Cdk2 inhibitors. *Cell* **87,** 1069–1078.
233. Takaku, M., Wada, Y., Jinnouchi, K., Takeya, M., Takahashi, K., Usuda, H., Naito, M., Kurihara, H., Yazaki, Y., Kumazawa, Y., Okimoto, Y., Umetani, M., Noguchi, N., Niki, E., Hamakubo, T., and Kodama, T. (1999). An *in vitro* coculture model of transmigrant monocytes and foam cell formation. *Arterioscler. Thromb. Vasc. Biol.* **19**(10), 2330–2339.
234. Fillinger, M. F., Sampson, L. N., Cronenwett, J. L., Powell, R. J., and Wagner, R. J. (1997). Coculture of endothelial cells and smooth muscle cells in bilayer and conditioned media models. *J. Surg. Res.* **67**(2), 169–178.
235. D'Amore, P. A. (1992). Capillary growth: A two-cell system. *Semin. Cancer Biol.* **3**(2), 49–56.
236. Aplin, A. E., Howe, A. K., and Juliano, R. L. (1999). Cell adhesion molecules, signal transduction and cell growth. *Curr. Opin. Cell Biol.* **11,** 737–744.
237. Chapman, H. A. (1997). Plasminogen activators, integrins, and the coordinated regulation of cell adhesion and migration. *Curr. Opin. Cell Biol.* **9**(5), 714–724.
238. Chapman, H. A., Wei, Y., Simon, D. I., and Waltz, D. A. (1999). Role of urokinase receptor and caveolin in regulation of integrin signaling. *Thromb. Haemost.* **82**(2), 291–297.
239. Preissner, K. T., Kanse, S. M., Chavakis, T., and May, A. E. (1999). The dual role of the urokinase receptor system in pericellular proteolysis and cell adhesion: Implications for cardiovascular function. *Basic Res. Cardiol.* **94,** 315–321.
240. Koshelnick, Y., Ehart, M., Stockinger, H., and Binder, B. R. (1999). Mechanisms of signaling through urokinase receptor and the cellular response. *Thromb. Haemost.* **82**(2), 305–311.

70

Coagulation Biology

Daniel D. Myers, Jr.,[†] Shirley K. Wrobleski,* Peter K. Henke,* and Thomas W. Wakefield,*[,‡]

*Jobst Vascular Research Laboratory, Section of Vascular Surgery, *Department of Surgery,*
[†]Unit for Laboratory Animal Medicine, University of Michigan Medical Center, Ann Arbor, Michigan 48109
[‡]Ann Arbor Veterans Administration Medical Center, Ann Arbor, Michigan 48109

I. Introduction

In this chapter, we present several models and techniques we have had success with in evaluating the pathobiology of venous thrombosis as well as coagulation–anticoagulant pharmacology. Our laboratory has applied animal models and techniques to better define two broad areas in coagulation biology: (1) heparin anticoagulation and its reversal with protamine sulfate and protamine-like agents and (2) the inflammatory response associated with venous thrombosis. This chapter focuses on these two topics, the animal models used and their usefulness, reliability and limitations, and the techniques employed to generate and evaluate experimental data.

II. Hemodynamic Animal Model for Anticoagulant/Antagonist Evaluation

Currently, protamine sulfate reversal of standard unfractionated heparin and low-molecular-weight heparin (LMWH) anticoagulation may cause adverse side effects such as decreased mean arterial blood pressure (MAP), decreased cardiac output (CO), decreased oxygen consumption (V_{O_2}), and thrombocytopenia (1–3). Due to the unpredictable toxic effects of protamine sulfate, there is a need to develop nontoxic protamine variants that can effectively reverse the anticoagulant effects of heparin and its LMWH fragments (4, 5).

In our investigation of polycationic compounds, it has been necessary to develop an animal model to evaluate the hemodynamic and physiologic effects of these compounds used alone and in combination with heparin and LMWH. The dog (*Canis familiaris*) has proved to be an excellent animal model to evaluate hemodynamic and hematologic toxicity of anticoagulation reversal and antithrombotic agents (6). The surgical procedure using the canine animal model has been previously described in detail (1, 7). The hemodynamic effects of heparin, LMWH, and protamine reversal in dogs are very similar to those in humans, but magnified on a scale that allows thorough evaluation. Additionally, the same coagulation tests used in humans may be used in dogs.

We have typically measured hemodynamic parameters such as systemic arterial blood pressure, heart rate, cardiac output, oxygen saturations, oxygen consumptions, and calculated systemic and pulmonary vascular resistances. Hematologic parameters evaluated have included standard coagulation tests, antifactor Xa and IIa levels, and platelet and leukocyte counts.

III. Venous Thrombosis Animal Models

Deep venous thromboembolism (DVT) is a national health problem, occurring at a constant rate over the past 20 years, with an annual incidence of 250,000 cases. It is estimated that deep venous thrombosis and pulmonary embolism are associated with approximately 300,000 to 600,000 hospitalizations and as many as 50,000 deaths per year. Chronic venous insufficiency, the sequela of venous thrombosis, affects approximately 400,000 to 500,000 patients with skin ulceration and 6 to 7 million patients with skin stasis changes (8, 9). Recent studies have shown that there is a marked interrelationship between the thrombotic process and inflammation, with inflammation augmenting the thrombotic response. Human specimens are not available to study DVT, unlike with neoplasia, so reliable animal models are essential for investigating the basic pathophysiology of DVT and coagulation biology.

A. Rat IVC Stasis Model

1. Rat Stasis

Rats (*Rattus norvegicus*) make an excellent animal model of stasis-induced venous thrombosis. They are easy to handle, relatively inexpensive, tolerate surgery well, and can be used in adequate numbers for statistical purposes. Rats (250–300 g) are anesthetized with isoflurane gas (1–2%) mixed with oxygen (100%) by a nose cone. Isoflurane gas has minimal adverse effects on systemic mean arterial blood pressure, heart rate, and respiratory rate. It is also rapidly absorbed from the lungs and only a minute amount is metabolized in the liver, leading to a more consistent and rapid postanesthetic recovery than that seen when using injectable anesthetics such as ketamine/xylazine (10). We have found that rats with ligated inferior vena cavas have a higher mortality rate when using the ketamine/xylazine anesthetic protocol. Control and experimental animals are administered test agents in 0.1- to 1-ml aliquots via the lateral tail vein (11). A midline laparotomy is then made, the small bowel is moved slightly to the left of the animal, and the inferior vena cava (IVC) is directly approached by careful blunt dissection (Fig. 1). Ligation of the IVC occurs just below the level of the renal veins. The IVC side and back branches are also carefully isolated and ligated. It is imperative that all side and back branches of the IVC be ligated to ensure blood stasis and consistent thrombus formation, which occurs in over 90% of cases when done by this method (12).

This animal model induces approximately a 1-cm segment of thrombus, which begins to form immediately. We have evaluated the thrombus as early as 1 hr after IVC ligation. The thrombus is large and loosely adherent at days 1 to 4, becomes more adherent to the vein wall by day 8, and decreases in size in association with a contracted, fibrosed vein by day 12. Gradual reestablishment of blood flow occurs by formation of microcollaterals in the thrombus (neovascularization) over several weeks and thrombus organization and contraction (13). It is relatively easy to harvest tissue samples for a number of investigative techniques. Investigators must take into consideration that skilled microsurgical techniques and surgical instruments are necessary for developing this model. Standard aseptic techniques are appropriate and few wound infections occur. We have not used prophylactic antibiotics in this model.

2. Rat Stasis Transfection Model

This rat model is a well characterized method for reproducible transfection of genetic material into the vein wall (14). Rats (250–300 g) are anesthetized as previously described. On day 1, aseptic laparotomy is performed and the IVC is dissected to allow temporary proximal and distal occlusion with microvascular clips (Fig. 2). After occlusion, the IVC is cannulated with a 30-gauge needle catheter, the blood is aspirated, and the IVC is then flushed with dilute heparinized saline solution. After this, 0.15 ml instillation of an adenoviral vector is performed for 30 min. The vector solution is then aspirated, the vascular clips are removed to reestablish blood flow, and the midline incision is closed. Two days after the transfection, the rats are anesthetized in the same fashion and a repeat laparotomy is performed. The IVC is then ligated below the renal veins for establishment of thrombosis along with ligation of draining side branches. The thrombosed IVC segment may be harvested as described previously.

For both stasis models, at the time of sacrifice, the thrombosed IVC segment is weighed (milligrams) and corrected to the vein length (centimeters). The vein segment is then usually halved, the proximal portion is placed in a tissue cassette and kept in 10% buffered formalin for 24 hr followed by 70% EtOH for subsequent permanent section processing, and the distal segment is snap frozen in liquid nitrogen and kept at -70°C until homogenized for various tissue assays. This allows histologic, immunohistochemical, and biochemical/molecular biological analyses of a single clotted rat vein segment. Determining success of transfection is most easily done by enzyme-linked immunosorbent assay (ELISA) for gene product or reverse transcriptase polymerase chain reaction RT-PCR for gene analysis.

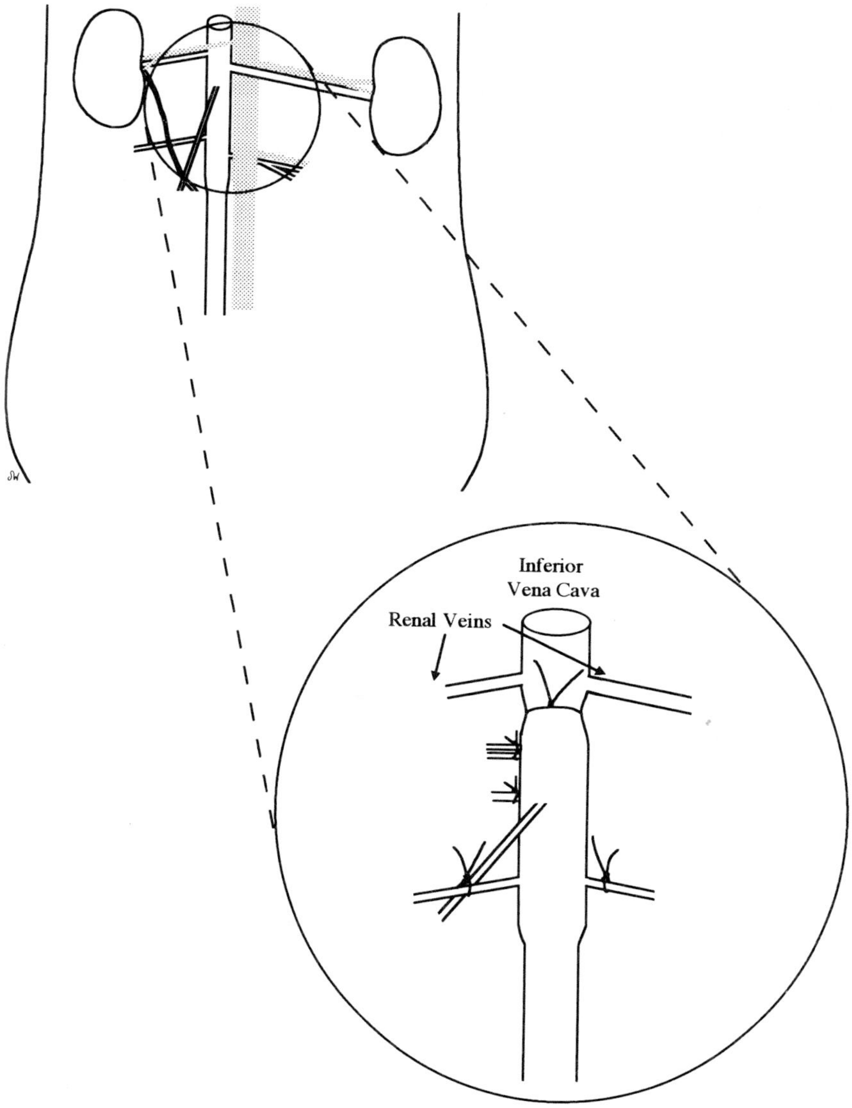

Figure 1 Deep vein thrombosis model in the rat.

3. Distal Venous Pressure Measurements

Rat IVC ligation with distal venous pressure measurements is also easily performed with this model. The rat is prepped down through both groins. A small oblique groin incision is made and the femoral vein is isolated and looped proximal and distally for a segment of 1 cm. The vein is pulled taut and is carefully cannulated with a 21-gauge IV cannula. This is then hooked up to a preflushed water (saline) manometer and measurement is made at cardiac level, allowing approximately 60 sec to equilibrate. The rat then undergoes the earlier described ligation and the pressure is again measured. Once the cannula and ligature are removed, a cotton-tipped applicator is used to apply direct pressure to the femoral vein cannula site until hemostasis is achieved in approximately 30–60 seconds. One should see baseline readings of 2 to 4 cm H_2O and 20 to 30 cm H_2O immediately after ligation. At harvest 2 days later, we have then performed contralateral groin femoral vein measurements and generally the pressure measured was between 8 and 20 cm H_2O.

B. Mouse IVC Stasis Model

The mouse (*Mus musculus*) animal model is similar to the rat model for the investigation of stasis-induced venous thrombosis. There are several advantages in using this animal model. It allows administration of very small volumes of limited availability test agents, reducing costs dramatical-

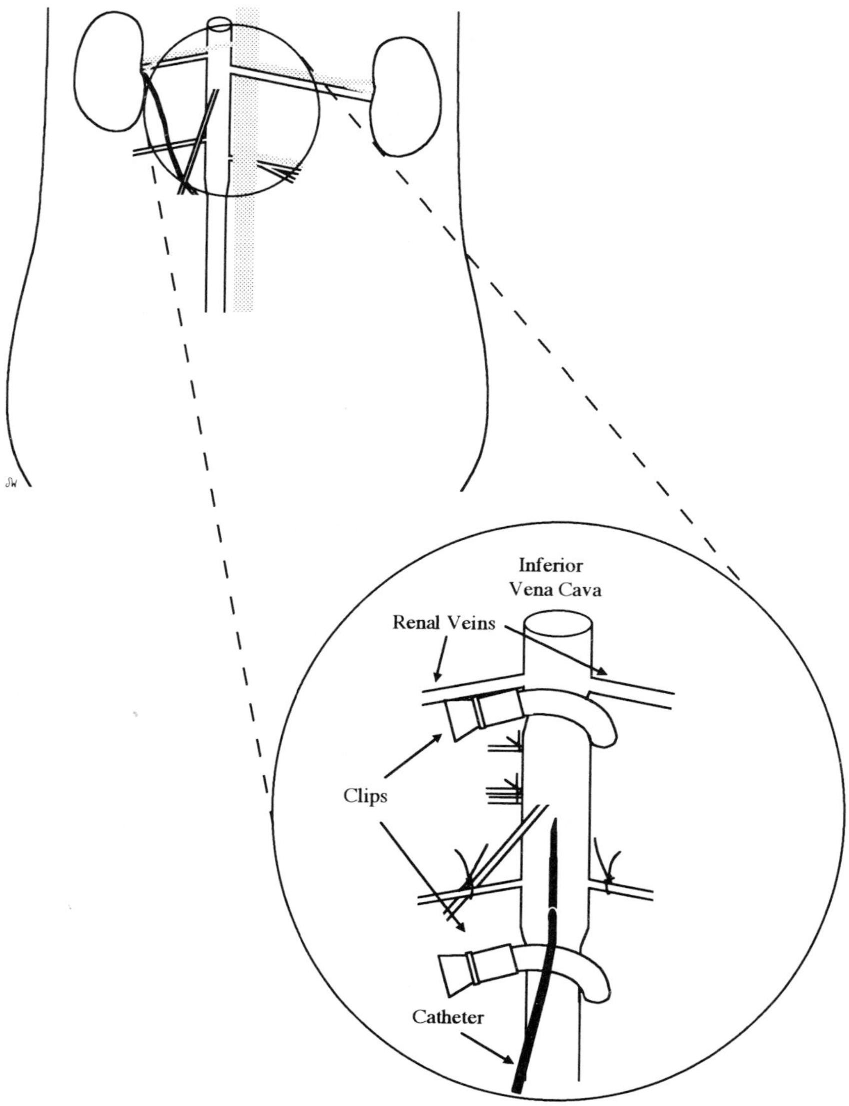

Figure 2 Transfection model in the rat.

ly. Most promising is the potential for mice with gene knockouts, allowing specific inflammatory and coagulation factor functions to be delineated. However, major concerns involving this model are the operative size constraints and the friability of the vessels. Also, due to the small IVC sample weight (mean 0.005 g) it may be necessary to increase animal numbers to pool samples for tissue analysis such as polymerase chain reaction and ELISA assays.

Mice weighing 20 to 30 g are anesthetized with an inhalation mixture of isoflurane gas (1–2%) and oxygen (100%) during the procedure. A midline laparotomy is made, the small bowel is exteriorized from the body cavity and moved slightly to the left of the animal, and then, as in the rat, the IVC is directly approached by careful blunt dissection (Fig. 3). Blunt dissection is facilitated using a sterile applicator swab and extra delicate iris half-curved tissue forceps. Care must be taken in handling mouse tissues because they are extremely fragile. Periodically the exteriorized bowel is moistened with sterile saline to prevent its desiccation. Another advantage of the mouse model over the rat model is that for consistent thrombus formation, only ligation of the IVC below the renals is necessary, without ligation of the side and back venous branches, thus simplifying the operative technique. However, ligation of large venous side branches may be necessary to increase the percentage of thrombus formation. We have found consistent thrombus formation without the need for ligation of the IVC side venous branches unless an extremely large side

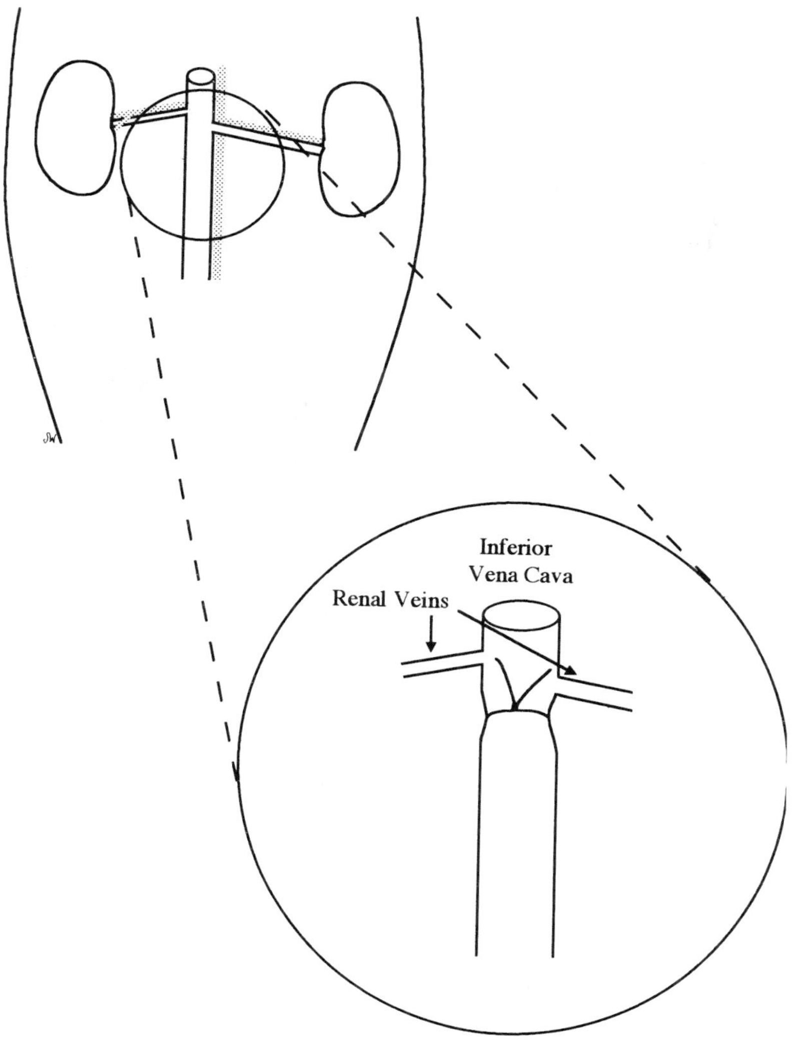

Figure 3 Deep vein thrombosis model in the mouse.

branch is present. The laparotomy incision is closed in a two-layer fashion using a 4-0 or 5-0 nonreactive suture material. Harvest protocol of the IVC is similar to the protocol for the rat.

C. Primate Balloon Occlusion IVC Stasis Model

The male juvenile baboon (*Papio anubis*) is used as an animal model of venous stasis–thrombosis induced by balloon occlusion in the IVC. The advantages of using the baboon are numerous. Anatomically the vascular anatomy of the baboon is similar to that of humans. The baboon is an upright animal, like humans, and the lower extremity venous physiology is reasonably equivalent to the venous physiology in humans. The baboon also has a valve in the iliac vein, which can be examined for competency. Baboons that have been infused experimentally with human plasma proteins and fibrinogen do not mount an immune response, thus demonstrating this similarity to humans (15). Also, the coagulation system of baboons closely resembles that of humans (16). Therefore, the same coagulation tests and reagents used in humans can be used in baboons.

Due to the size of the baboon vasculature, it is possible to study the vein wall by using noninvasive evaluation techniques such as venous duplex ultrasound imaging and magnetic resonance venography (MRV), and invasive techniques such as standard contrast phlebography. Our current primate animal model of venous stasis has been previously described in detail (17). Vein wall endothelium is disrupted at the points of balloon catheter contact with the vessel wall, and thrombus can also form around the catheter and associate with the vessel wall. However, the area of pure stasis between balloons is very similar to the initiation of clinical DVT in which direct vessel wall injury does not occur. In general, most clinical cases of DVT are associated with stasis and local hypercoagulability, both aspects of the area of stasis thrombosis between the balloons in this model. Direct vein wall damage causing venous thrombosis is less common. In this model, thrombus will form in the IVC between balloons in approximately 60 to 70% of the cases and at the balloon sites and the right iliac vein in 75 to 100% of cases (17, 18).

The primate is anesthetized with Telazol (Tiletamine HCL/Zolazepam HCL), 10 mg/kg, IM injection and atropine sulfate, 0.02 mg/kg IM and intubated. Telazol combines the dissociative properties of Tiletamine with the tranquilizer Zolazepam, which provides excellent chemical restraint and anesthesia of the baboon for 45–90 min (19). This allows the laboratory time to transport the primate to facilitate various imaging studies. Bilateral saphenous vein 22-gauge catheters are placed for the administration of fluids, contrast agents, and emergency medications. The animal is maintained in a surgical plane of anesthesia with isoflurane gas, 2.5–3% mixed with 100% oxygen. A 1.5-cm incision is made over the right femoral vein and the right internal jugular vein for the insertion of balloon catheters (Fig. 4). The surgical approach to the femoral vein is just lateral to the femoral artery, and the surgical approach to the internal jugular vein is midneck, just lateral to the carotid artery (20). Catheter placement at the iliac bifurcation and just below the level of the renal veins is facilitated by the use of fluoroscopic imaging. A guidewire is helpful to thread the catheter through the right heart. The position of the catheters is evaluated by inflating the balloons under fluoroscopic imaging using a contrast agent (50% saline/50% hypaque) for balloon inflation. Inflating the proximal balloon first, waiting 30 sec, then inflating the distal balloon allow IVC distension with blood.

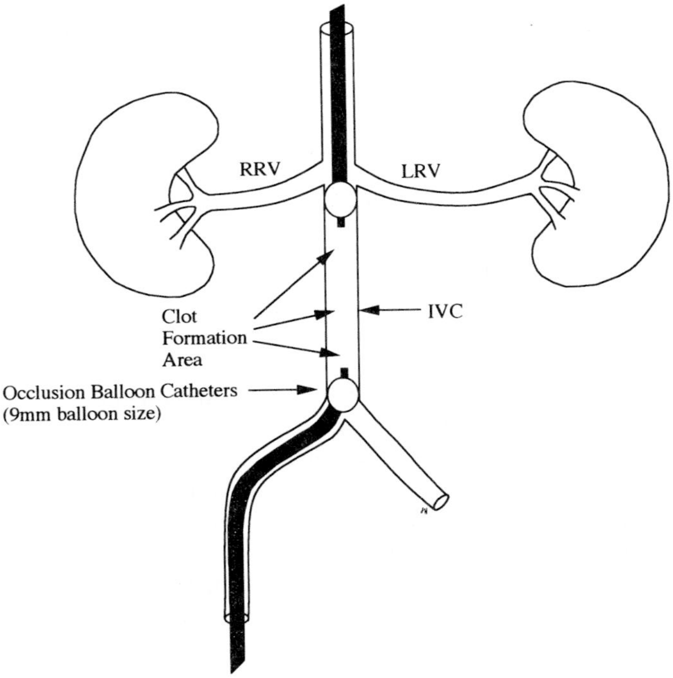

Figure 4 Deep venous thrombosis model in a primate.

Six hours of balloon-induced stasis successfully initiate a thrombus. The internal jugular vein is ligated and the femoral vein incision site is repaired with a two-layer closure of tissue eliminating dead space after the femoral vein is repaired with prolene suture. As seen in the rhesus monkey, the internal jugular vein of the baboon carries the main blood flow from the face and intracranial area (21). Therefore, mild postoperative venous congestion may be noted around the face and eyes for 24–48 hr, although the patent contralateral jugular vein will minimize these changes. Test compounds such as novel anticoagulants can be evaluated, and histologic and coagulation parameters can be measured (17, 18, 22). Finally, the baboon venous stasis model allows investigators to evaluate the age of thrombus, because the time of thrombus initiation is during the period of balloon catheter occlusion.

The disadvantages of using nonhuman primates are the high cost, limited availability of primates, the need for specialized housing and trained staff, and decreased statistical power as opposed to rat or mice animal models, due to the smaller number of experimental observations possible.

D. Alternative Animal Models of Thrombosis

Alternative models of venous thrombosis have been described. Examples of these alternative models include jugular vein thrombosis in the cat (23), IVC thrombosis in the rat using the injection of thrombin or other irritants along with stasis (24), and the graded narrowing of the IVC using an occluding device placed on the IVC just at the infrarenal vein location (25). In all models of venous thrombosis, at least two of Virchow's triad elements must be fulfilled to initiate thrombosis. The triad includes stasis, vein wall injury of some type, and hypercoagulability of the blood.

IV. Biochemical/Molecular Biologic/Immunologic/ Evaluation Techniques

A. Coagulation Tests, Hematologic Analysis, and Thromboelastography

In order to evaluate the efficacy of any anticoagulant or antiinflammatory therapy, evaluation of the full coagulation profile perioperatively is necessary. The integrity of the bloodstream is maintained by the reactions in the clotting cascade. These reactions provide a system of carefully controlled checks and balances. Any pathologic state that disturbs the careful balance of the coagulation cascade can lead to either a hypercoagulability state or a bleeding disorder.

Briefly, there are three stages in the response to vascular injury. The first stage is the vascular component, in which the blood vessels constrict and cause blood flow to slow in the area of injury. The second stage, also known as primary hemostasis, is the formation of a primary platelet hemostatic plug. Platelet contraction and adherence cause the release of adenosine diphosphate (ADP) and thromboxane A_2, and both act as aggregating agents to recruit additional platelets (26). The third stage, also known as secondary hemostasis, requires plasma coagulation factors and leads to the deposition of fibrin strands to reinforce the platelet plug. Activation of factors occurs by a series of proteolytic enzymes. *In vivo*, secondary hemostasis can be initiated through either the intrinsic or extrinsic pathway. The intrinsic pathway is activated by contact with foreign surfaces and the extrinsic pathway is activated by tissue thromboplastin (Fig. 5) (22, 27).

Common measures of coagulation have been described (1, 3) and include the following tests:

1. Activated partial thromboplastin time (aPTT) evaluates the function of coagulation factors in both the intrinsic coagulation pathway (Factors VIII, IX, XI, and XII) and the common coagulation pathway (Factor V, X, prothrombin, and fibrinogen).

2. Activated clotting time (ACT) evaluates the function of coagulation factors in the intrinsic coagulation pathway (Factors VIII, IX, XI, and XII) and the common coagulation pathway (Factor V, X, prothrombin, and fibrinogen). However, the ACT relies on platelet phospholipid to support the reaction. A decrease in platelet counts below 10,000/μl can lead to a prolonged ACT. The aPTT is not affected in this manner by thrombocytopenia.

3. Prothrombin time (PT) evaluates the function of coagulation factors in the extrinsic coagulation pathway (Factor VII) and the common coagulation pathway (Factor V, X, prothrombin, and fibrinogen).

4. Thrombin clotting time (TCT) directly measures functional fibrinogen. This test evaluates the final stage of the clotting process. The only mechanisms to prolong the TCT include a decrease in fibrinogen or the anticoagulant effect of heparin.

5. Fibrinogen is a direct measurement of quantitative circulating fibrinogen (mg/dl). Quantitative fibrinogen determination is performed by converting fibrinogen to fibrin with thrombin (26). Fibrinogen levels are important in the final stage of the clotting cascade.

6. Fibrin degradation products (FDPs) detect the presence of levels of circulating fibrinogen or fibrin broken down by plasmin. However, the test cannot determine the difference between these two products. The test combines detection of primary and secondary fibrinolysis. FDPs evaluate the third stage of the clotting cascade (28):

Fibrinogen → Thrombin/$CaCl_2$ → Fibrin monomer → XIII → Cross-linked fibrin polymers
Plasminogen → Activator → Plasmin

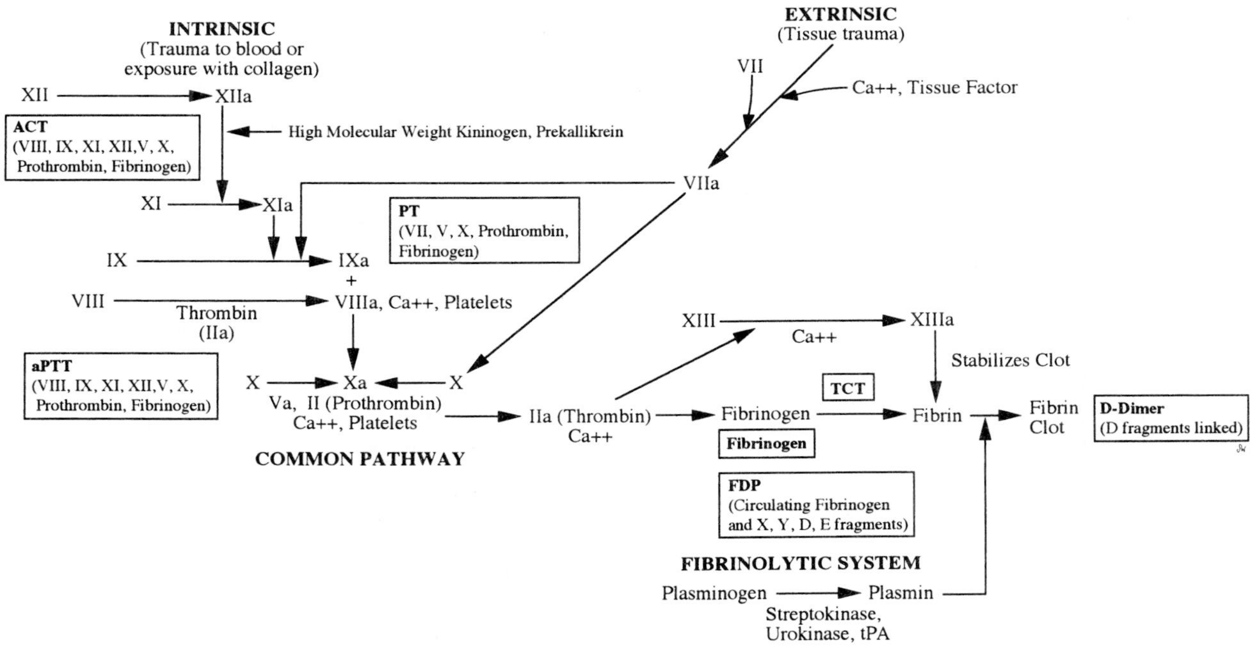

Figure 5 Common coagulation tests and coagulation parameters.

7. The D-dimer test measures the amount of fibrin cleaved by plasmin. The test is an indication of secondary (the breakdown of formed clot) rather than primary fibrinolysis, such as seen with the administration of thrombolytic agents. This test rules out diffuse intravascular coagulation (DIC), in which formed clot and secondary fibrinolysis occur.

8. Bleeding time (BT) is a sensitive measure of primary capillary hemostatic and platelet function (29, 30).

Both canine and primate models allow performance of reliable hematologic studies such as ACT, TCT, aPTT, heparin antifactor Xa activity, heparin antifactor IIa activity, and white blood cell (WBC) and platelet counts that are similar to studies in humans (15).

LMWHs are glycosaminoglycans containing alternating residues of *d*-glucosamine and uronic acid (31). The mechanisms of action of standard fractionated heparin and LMWH differ in that LMWH selectively inhibits more factor Xa than factor IIa (thrombin). When evaluating the effects of LMWH-based anticoagulation quantitatively, it is necessary to perform antifactor Xa and antifactor IIa assays. In brief, the antifactor Xa and antifactor IIa assays use citrated blood samples stored on ice, cold centrifuged at 2900 rpm for 20 min at 4°C to yield a platelet-poor plasma (PPP) supernatant. In the antifactor Xa assay, excess antithrombin followed by factor Xa is added to PPP and reacted with the chromogenic substrate S-2222 (Coatest Heparin; Kabi Vitrum, Stockholm, Sweden). The antifactor IIa assay is performed by adding thrombin, followed by the chromogenic substrate S-2238, to PPP previously incubated with excess antithrombin. Heparin antifactor Xa or antifactor IIa activity is inversely proportional to absorbance at 405 nm, indicating the quantity of uninhibited factor Xa or IIa (thrombin) remaining (7). The evaluation of white blood cell and platelet populations can easily be determined using a manual hemocytometer. Platelet aggregation studies can be performed using citrated venous blood samples centrifuged at 25°C, 150–200 *g* for 10 min, to obtain platelet-rich plasma (PRP).

Thrombelastography (TEG) is a test method for evaluation of clot elasticity and may be used to evaluate many aspects of the coagulation mechanism. A whole blood sample is taken from the animal and immediately transported to a TEG machine. The time of sample collection to the time the sample is tested in the TEG machine should be minimal and consistent due to the clotting properties of whole blood, because clotted blood samples invalidate the test. The test produces a tracing with various parameters (Fig. 6). The *r* value is very sensitive to changes in thromboplastic plasma procoagulants. The *k* value and the α angle measure the speed of clot strengthening. The *ma* value provides a measure of the dynamic properties of fibrin and platelets, and the *ma*-30 is a measure of fibrinolysis. A major advantage of TEG relates to its unique assessment of the interaction of the platelet surface with the coagulation cascade. Interaction between platelet and coagulation factors may provide significant clinical information lacking with measurement of individual components of coagulation, because assays such as PT, aPTT, and TCT neglect possible *in vivo* interactions between platelets and the coagulation cascade.

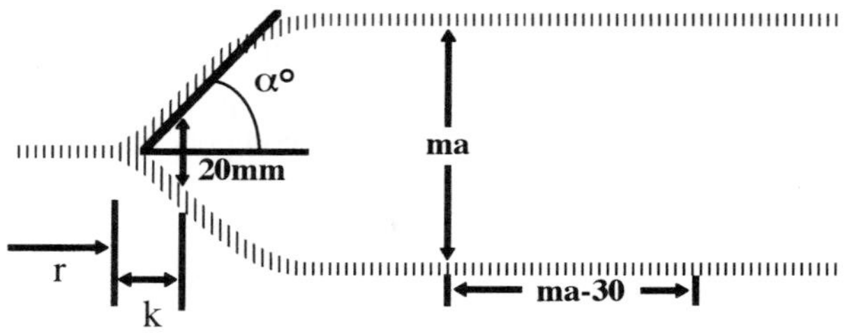

Figure 6 Schematic diagram representing the thrombelastographic parameters, where *r* describes the interval prior to initial evidence of fibrin formation, *k* describes the time from initial fibrin formation until a transverse amplitude of 20 mm is obtained, angle α descibes the angle of maximum rise of the curve, *ma* describes the maximum amplitude of graph deflection, and *ma*-30 is 30 min postmaximum amplitude. Modified from Brothers *et al.* (32).

The thrombelastographic parameters *r*, *k*, and *ma* are extremely sensitive to the presence of heparin, making this test useful for monitoring low-dose heparin administration. However, in the dosage range of heparin required for arterial reconstruction or cardiopulmonary bypass, thrombelastography is too sensitive, with no discrimination between adequate and inadequate anticoagulation. Despite this limitation, TEG has proved to be a significantly better predictor of postoperative hemorrhage and the need for reoperation following cardiopulmonary bypass than has the activated clotting time, PT, aPTT, platelet count, fibrinogen level, or FDP (32).

B. Histology

1. Vein Wall Morphometrics

We utilize histologic methods to study both cellular kinetics and pathologic vein wall changes. Standard methods for tissue fixation with paraffin-embedded sections are used for analysis. Veins are examined under high-power oil immersion light microscopy. Sections are stained with hematoxylin and eosin from paraffin-embedded tissues. Five representative high-power fields (oil immersion, 1000×) are examined around the thrombus in equidistant locations and the cell count of the vein wall is analyzed; cells are identified as either neutrophils, monocytes/macrophages, or lymphocytes based on standard histologic criteria, including nuclear size, cytoplasmic content, and total cell size, or based on immunohistochemical staining for the inflammatory cell types (12, 33). Results from five high-power fields are added together and the mean ± SE is calculated for each vein studied. In each experimental group, veins are added together and then a mean ± SE is calculated to provide a measure of the cellularity of the group as a whole.

2. Immunohistochemical Staining

This technique allows localization of cytokines, chemokines, and inflammatory cells in the vein wall or clot. Immunohistochemical staining is performed as previously described and after special modifications (14). Furthermore, this technique may be used to localize specific cell types (i.e., monocytes/neutrophils) in the thrombus as well as to identify clot endothelial-lined channels with antibody staining against von Willebrand factor (vWF) and laminin. Depending on the antigen, fresh or paraffin-embedded sections are used. Also, testing various antibodies is required to determine the best visualization as well as substrate incubation periods.

3. Trichrome Staining

This technique utilizes special processing to visualize collagen in the histologic section with an intense blue stain. We have used this technique with good success to document clot and vein wall fibrosis over time. Though qualitative, this staining technique is a nice accompaniment to biochemical/genetic methods of determining postthrombotic venous fibrosis.

C. Biochemical Mediator Analysis

1. ELISA Protein Analysis for Cytokines/Chemokines

The enzyme-linked immunosorbent assay technique facilitates detection of either antigen or antibody in a test sample. ELISA techniques are used to quantitate protein levels of cytokines/chemokines in samples of vein wall. Tissue homogenization (utilizing a complete buffer with antiproteases) of a vein wall segment is performed and in this technique well-detailed, immunoreactive cytokine and chemokine levels are quantitated using a double-ligand method (12, 17, 18). Plates are read at 490 nm in an ELISA plate reader. Standards are one-half log dilutions of the cytokines and chemokines from 1 pg/ml to 100 ng/ml. The sensitivity of the ELISA method is $\geq$50 pg/ml. Levels of total protein are determined by a modified Bradford assay, usually from a commercial kit. The cytokine/chemokine levels are standardized by dividing the obtained value by total protein in the sample to assure uniformity.

2. Reverse Transcriptase Polymerase Chain Reaction

The RT-PCR technique is used to synthesize cDNA from mRNA for the identification of specific genes of interest. This technique is cost effective and expedient. RT-PCR is extremely sensitive and requires only small amounts of starting material. Therefore, it is highly recommended that the RT-PCR products are verified by DNA hybridization techniques and/or product sequences when using new or unproved primers (34, 35).

Generally, we find that about 150 mg of rat vein yields enough RNA for analysis and further PCR runs. As for other applications, better results are obtained when RNA purity is high ($A_{260}/A_{280} \geq 1.8$). Poly(A) mRNA (1 μg) from specific samples can be reverse transcribed into cDNA utilizing a reverse transcription kit and oligonucleotide (dt) 22–30 primers. A general RT-PCR protocol takes primers from published sequences that have been evaluated by a computer-assisted system (such as from GenBank) that allows prediction of primer interactions to give a single amplified product. After amplification, the sample (20 μl) can be separated on a 2% agarose gel containing 0.3 μg/ml of ethidium bromide and the band is visualized and photographed using a translucent UV source (35).

D. Ultrasound Analysis

Interior vena cava thrombosis can be quantitated by using venous duplex ultrasound imaging. Such imaging is used to evaluate venous thrombosis in both rats and nonhuman primates (17, 18, 36, 37). Techniques of examination include compression imaging, flow analysis with and without the addition of color, direct imaging of thrombus, and tissue doppler imaging (TDI).

Using the baboon balloon occlusion model of venous thrombosis as an example, duplex ultrasound imaging is performed throughout the experimental period. Ultrasound examinations are performed using a Toshiba Power Vision 6000 (Toshiba Medical Systems, Tustin, CA) and an ATL 3000 (Advanced Technologies Laboratory, Bothell, CA). A linear multihertz (5 to 10 MHz) transducer is utilized, as well as the ATL 10-MHz linear intraoperative transducer.

Ultrasound imaging is performed at baseline, after balloon catheter placement, hourly throughout the 6-hr IVC balloon occlusion period, and after balloon removal. At baseline the IVC and iliac veins are imaged and assessed for patency. After balloon catheter placement the animal is imaged and assessed for correct balloon placement, assessing continued flow in the renal veins. The animal is then scanned hourly to assess venous thrombosis formation within the IVC; continued balloon inflation, position and occlusion; and for confirmation that no prograde blood flow remains in the IVC. After balloon catheter removal at the 6-hr time point, the IVC and iliac veins are again imaged, assessing for flow and thrombus formation. Imaging is also performed, as frequently as dictated by the particular experimental protocol, until the time of sacrifice. Each exam is recorded using premium-grade videocassette tape as well as the printing of images online. Tissue doppler imaging is utilized to allow earlier identification of venous thrombosis. TDI detects slow tissue movement versus fast blood movement. TDI assists in identifying early intraluminal filling defects such as thrombus versus an echogenic artifact.

Ultrasound imaging is performed prior to and at the time of sacrifice using the ATL 3000. All of the above images are obtained presacrifice, with the exception of the TDI, which is not available with the ATL. At the time of sacrifice, an intraoperative duplex image is performed using the 10-MHz intraoperative probe. The probe is placed in a sterile probe cover and scanning is performed directly on the IVC. The entire IVC and iliac segments are evaluated.

E. Assessment of Vein Wall Damage

1. Magnetic Resonance Venography with Gadolinium

This technique is used in both rats and nonhuman primates and has been previously described in detail (17, 18, 38). Imaging is performed on a 1.5 T Clinical MR imaging system (Singa Horizon LX, General Electric Medical Systems, Milwaukee, WI) with 8.1 software. Magnetic resonance venography (MRV) is performed with and without gadolinium. Gadolinium is a heavy metal chelate that prolongs the T1 relaxation time of blood, and extravasates selectively into areas with capillary leak. Postgadolinium images are acquired of the entire IVC as well as the iliac bifurcation and left and right iliac veins. Analysis involves drawing a region of interest (ROI) around the area of gadolinium enhancement and measuring the area (in square millimeters) along with measuring the size of the IVC (17, 18). Additionally, thrombus resolution may be quantitated by this technique on time-of-flight (TOF) imaging (18).

2. Permeability Assay

This technique evaluates vein wall injury as measured by microvascular permeability (39–41). Extravasation of Evans blue dye into the vein wall is used as a quantitative measure of changes in vein wall permeability. Results are reported both nonnormalized and normalized to vein wall length, and compared to Evans blue in the plasma. Three vein wall segments are added together for each vein wall permeability assay when performed in the rat.

F. Colloidal Carbon and Thrombus Fluorescence

Thrombus neovascularization may be evaluated using colloidal carbon perfusion and thrombus fluorescence in the rat IVC ligation model (13). Just prior to sacrifice, colloidal carbon (5 ml in 5 ml NaCl) is perfused via the left ventricle and allowed to circulate for approximately 30 sec. The IVC is then harvested with animal sacrifice as previously mentioned. The presence of colloidal carbon in newly formed vascular channels is measured with a computer imaging program and normalized to total clot area (% neovascularization = area colloidal carbon/total area). Thrombus fluorescence is evaluated by injection of a fluorescent marker via the tail vein at the time of sacrifice. The thrombus is then harvested and divided into two segments. One clot segment is prepared as a homogenate in phosphate buffered saline (PBS), incubated for 24 hr at 4°C, plated, and read on a fluorometer and expressed in relative fluorescence units. The second segment of clot is formalin fixed and placed into paraffin blocks and cut into slides for visual evaluation of fluorescein by fluorescent microscopy. Although reliable, colloidal carbon may underestimate thrombus neovascularity because many more channels are often seen than are found with intraluminal colloidal carbon.

V. Summary

We have utilized whole animal physiologic preparations, small animal rat and mouse preparations, and nonhuman primate models for the investigation of heparin anticoagulation reversal and the evaluation of the inflammatory response associated with venous thrombosis (Table I). With these

Table I Summary of Research Animal Models of Deep Venous Thrombosis

Model	Advantages	Disadvantages	Estimated cost
Nonhuman primates Stasis model	Large vasculature, homologous to humans; no need to pool samples; human physiology similar; ability to perform full coagulation panels	Special housing requirements; trained staff needed; uncertain availability in 4- to 6-kg size; decreased statistical power; expensive	Baboon (n = 1), \$8000–10,000
Rats Stasis model Transfection model	Availability; increased statistical power; decreased costs as compared to primates	Small sample size of tissue, need to pool IVC samples for tests; need to ligate back branches of IVC; coagulation tests limited to blood volume	Rats (n = 10), \$750–800
Mice Stasis model	Availability of gene-targeted animals; increased statistical power; decreased cost (excluding gene-targeted animals); only ligate IVC in the vast majority of animals	Small sample size of tissue, may need to pool IVC samples for tests; friable vessels; increased mortality; coagulation tests limited to blood volume	Mice (n = 20), \$300–400[a]

[a]Gene-targeted animals not included.

models, tests for analysis have ranged from basic hematologic and coagulation assays to sophisticated imaging protocols and techniques in molecular biology. Future investigation will likely involve additional techniques in molecular biology and computer simulations. The use of animal models to simulate human disease will continue to be necessary due to the multiplicity of mechanisms that play a role in normal and abnormal coagulation biology.

Acknowledgment

Supported in part by NIH Grants HL#53355 and HL#63148.

References

1. Hulin, M. S., Wakefield, T. W., Andrews, P. C., Wrobleski, S. K., Kadell, A. M., Downing, L. J., and Stanley, J. C. (1997). Comparison of the hemodynamic and hematologic toxicity of a protamine variant after reversal of low-molecular-weight heparin anticoagulation in a canine model. *Lab. Anim. Sci.* **47,** 153–160.
2. Wakefield, T. W., Wrobleski, S. K., Nichol, B. J., Kadell, A. M., and Stanley, J. C. (1992). Heparin-mediated reductions of the toxic effects of protamine sulfate on rabbit myocardium. *J. Vasc. Surg.* **16,** 47–53.
3. Wakefield, T. W., Bouffard, J. A., Spaulding, S. A., Petry, N. A., Gross, M. D., Lindblad, B., and Stanley, J. C. (1987). Sequestration of platelets in the pulmonary circulation as a consequence of protamine reversal of the anticoagulant effects of heparin. *J. Vasc. Surg.* **5,** 187–193.
4. Harris, R. B. (1999). Design, synthesis, and testing of HepArrest™; a clinically viable alternative to protamine. Presented at "Beyond Heparin, Novel Anticoagulants & Emerging Applications," May 5–7, La Jolla, San Diego.
5. Horrow, J. C. (1999). Neutralase™ reversal of heparin anticoagulation. Presented at "Beyond Heparin, Novel Anticoagulants & Emerging Applications," May 5–7, La Jolla, San Diego.
6. DeLucia, A., 3d, Wakefield, T. W., Andrews, P. C., Nichol, B. J., Kadell, A. M., Wrobleski, S. K., Downing, L. J., and Stanley, J. C. (1993). Efficacy and toxicity of differently charged polycationic protamine-like peptides for heparin anticoagulation reversal. *J. Vasc. Surg.* **18,** 49–60.
7. Wakefield, T. W., Andrews, P. C., Wrobleski, S. K., Kadell, A. M., Fazzalari, B. S., Nichol, B. J., Vanderkooi, T., and Stanley, J. C. (1994). Reversal of low-molecular-weight heparin anticoagulation by synthetic protamine analogues. *J. Surg. Res.* **56,** 586–593.
8. Coon, W. W. (1977). Epidemiology of venous thromboembolism. *Ann. Surg.* **186,** 149–164.
9. Anderson, F. A., Jr., Wheeler, H. B., Goldberg, R. J., Hosmer, D. W., Patwardhan, N. A., Jovanovic, B., Forcier, A., and Dalen, J. E. (1991). A population-based perspective of the hospital incidence and case-fatality rates of deep vein thrombosis and pulmonary embolism. The Worcester DVT Study. *Arch. Int. Med.* **151,** 933–938.
10. Wixson, S. K., and Smiler, K. L. (1997). Anesthesia and analgesia in rodents. *In* "Anesthesia and Analgesia in Laboratory Animals" (D.F. Kohn, S.K. Wixson, W.J. White, and G.J. Benson, eds.), p. 172. Academic Press, San Diego.
11. Waynforth, B. A., and Flecknell, P. A. (1992). Administration of substances. *In* "Experimental and Surgical Technique in the Rat," 2nd Ed. (H.B. Waynforth and P.A. Flecknell, eds.), p. 3. Academic Press, San Diego.
12. Wakefield, T. W., Strieter, R. M., Wilke, C. A., Kadell, A. M., Wrobleski, S. K., Burdick, M. D., Schmidt, R., Kunkel, S. L., and Greenfield, L. J. (1995). Venous thrombosis-associated inflammation and attenuation with neutralizing antibodies to cytokines and adhesion molecules. *Arterioscler. Thromb. Vasc. Biol.* **15,** 258–268.
13. Wakefield, T. W., Linn, M. J., Henke, P. K., Kadell, A. M., Wilke, C. A., Wrobleski, S. K., Sarkar, M., Burdick, M. D., Myers, D. D., and Strieter, R. M. (1999). Neovascularization during venous thrombosis organization: A preliminary study. *J. Vasc. Surg.* **30,** 885–893.
14. Henke, P. K., Debrunye, L. A., Strieter, R. M., Bromberg, J. S., Prince, M. R., Kadell, A. M., Sarkar, M., Londy, F., and Wakefield, T. W. (2000). Viral IL-10 gene transfer decreases inflammation and cell adhesion molecule expression in a rat model of venous thrombosis. *J. Immunol.* **164,** 2131–2141.
15. Feingold, H. M., Pivacek, L. E., Melaragno, A. J., and Valeri, C. R. (1986). Coagulation assays and platelet aggregation patterns in human, baboon, and canine blood. *Am. J. Vet. Res.* **47,** 2197–2199.
16. Kelly, C. A., and Gleiser, C. A. (1986). Selected coagulation reference values for adult and juvenile baboons. *Lab. Anim. Sci.* **36,** 173–175.
17. Downing, L. J., Wakefield, T. W., Strieter, R. M., Prince, M. R., Londy, F. J., Fowlkes, J. B., Hulin, M. S., Kadell, A. M., Wilke, B. A., Brown, S. L., Wrobleski, S. K., Burdick, B. S., Anderson, D. C., and Greenfield, L. J. (1997). Anti P-selectin antibody decreases inflammation and thrombus formation in venous thrombosis. *J. Vasc. Surg.* **25,** 816–828.
18. Wakefield, T. W., Strieter, R. M., Schaub, R., Myers, Jr., D. D., Prince, M. R., Wrobleski, S. K., Londy, F. J., Kadell, A. M., Brown, S. L., Henke, P. K., and Greenfield, L. J. (2000). Venous thrombosis prophylaxis by inflammatory inhibition without anticoagulation. *J. Vasc. Surg.* **31,** 309–324.
19. Popilskis, S. J., and Kohn, D. F. (1997). Anesthesia and analgesia in nonhuman primates. *In* "Anesthesia and Analgesia in Laboratory Animals" (D.J. Kohn, S.K. Wixson, W.J. White, and G.J. Benson, eds.), pp. 234–254. Academic Press, San Diego.
20. Howell, A. B., and Straus, Jr., W. L. (1936). The muscular system. *In* "Anatomy of the Rhesus Monkey" (C.G. Hartmen and W.L. Straus, Jr., eds.), pp. 96–100. Williams and Wilkins Company, New York.
21. Lineback, P. (1936). The vascular system. *In* "Anatomy of the Rhesus Monkey" (C.G. Hartmen and W.L. Straus, Jr., eds.), pp. 262–263. Williams and Wilkins Company, New York.
22. Wrobleski, S. K., Peterson, M. T., and Linn, M. J. (1999). The basics of coagulation. *Lab. Anim. Practit.* **32,** 18–21.
23. Eppihimer, M. J., and Schaub, R. G. (1999). Role of selectin inhibitors on the pathogenesis of deep vein thrombosis (Abstract). XVIIth Congress of the International Society of Thrombosis and Haemostasis, August 14–21, Washington, D. C. *Circulation* **100,** I471.
24. See-Tho, K., and Harris, E. J. (1998). Thrombosis with outflow obstruction delays thrombolysis and results in chronic wall thickening of rat veins. *J. Vasc. Surg.* **28,** 115–123.
25. Northeast, A., and Burnand, K. G. (1992). The response of the vessel wall to thrombosis: The *in vivo* study of venous thrombolysis. *N. Y. Acad. Sci.* **667,** 127–140.
26. Green, R. A., and Thomas, J. S. (1995). Hemostatic disorders: Coagulopathies and thrombosis. In "Textbook of Veterinary Internal Medicine," 4th Ed. (S.J. Ettinger and E.C. Feldman, eds.), Vol. II, pp. 1946–1963. W. B. Saunders Company, Philadelphia.
27. Wakefield, T. W. (2000). Hemostasis. *In* "Surgery: Scientific Principles and Practice," 3rd Ed. (L. Greenfield, K. Lillemoe, M. Mulholland, K. Oldham, and G. Zelenock, eds.). Lippincott Williams & Wilkins, Philadelphia.
28. Greenberg, C. S. (1994). Fibrin formation and stabilization. *In* "Thrombosis and Hemorrhage" (J. Loscalzo and A.I. Schafer, eds.), pp. 107–126. Blackwell Scientific Publications, Boston.
29. Sodikoff, C. H. (1995). Simple coagulation Tests. *In* "Laboratory Profiles of Small Animal Disease, A guide to Laboratory Diagnosis," 2nd Ed. (C.H. Sodikoff, ed.), pp. 86–89. Mosby, St. Louis.
30. Guyton, A. C. (1991). Hemostasis and blood coagulation. *In* "Textbook of Medical Physiology," 8th Ed. (A.C. Guyton, ed.), pp. 390–399. W. B. Saunders, Co., Philadelphia.

31. Weitz, J. I. (1997). Drug therapy: Low-molecular-weight heparins. *N. Engl. J. Med.* **337,** 688–698.
32. Brothers, T. E., Wakefield, T. W., McLaren, I. D., Bockenstedt, P., and Greenfield, L. J. (1993). Coagulation status during aortic aneurysm surgery: Comparison of thrombelastography with standard tests. *J. Invest. Surg.* **6,** 527–534.
33. Downing, L. J., Strieter, R. M., Kadell, A. M., Wilke, C. A., Austin, J. C., Hare, B. D., Burdick, M. D., Greenfield, L. J., and Wakefield, T. W. (1998). IL-10 regulates thrombus-induced vein wall inflammation and thrombosis. *J. Immunol.* **161,** 1471–1476.
34. Kaufman, P. B., Wu, W., Kim, D., and Cseke, L. J. (1995). PCR techniques and applications. *In* "Handbook of Molecular and Cellular Methods in Biology and Medicine" (P.B. Kaufman, W. Wu, D. Kim, and L.J. Cseke, eds.), pp. 244–262. CRC Press, Boca Raton.
35. Watson, J. D., Gilman, M., Witkowski, J., Zoller, M. (1992). The polymerase chain reaction. *In* "Recombinant DNA," 2nd Ed. (J.D. Watson, M. Gilman, J. Witkowski, and M. Zoller, eds.), pp. 79–98. Scientific American Books, New York.
36. Fowlkes, J. B., Strieter, R. M., Downing, L. J., Brown, S. L., Saluja, A., Salles-Cunha, S., Kadell, A. M., Wrobleski, S. K., and Wakefield, T. W. (1998). Ultrasound echogenicity in experimental venous thrombosis. *Ultrasound Med. Biol.* **24,** 1175–1182.
37. Fenn, R. C., Fowlkes, J. B., Moskalik, A., Zhang, Y., Roubidoux, M. A., Adler, R. S., and Carson, P. L. (1997). A hand-controlled, 3-D ultrasound guide and measurement system. 23rd International Symposium on Acoustical Imaging, April 13–16, Boston.
38. Londy, F. J., Kadell, A. M., Wrobleski, S. K., Prince, M. R., Strieter, R. M., and Wakefield, T. W. (1999). Detection of perivenous inflammation in a rat model of venous thrombosis using MRV. *J. Invest. Surg.* **12,** 151–156.
39. Linderkamp, O., Mader, T., Butenandt, O., and Riegel, K. P. (1977). Plasma volume estimation in severely ill infants and children using a simplified evans blue method. *Eur. J. Pediatr.* **125,** 135–141.
40. Murohara, T., Horowitz, J. R., Silver, M., Tsurumi, Y., Chen, D., Sullivan, A., and Isner, J. M. (1998). Vascular endothelial growth factor/vascular permeability factor enhances vascular permeability via nitric oxide and prostacyclin. *Circulation* **97,** 99–107.
41. Downing, L. J., Strieter, R. M., Kadell, A. M., Wilke, C. A., Greenfield, L. J., Wakefield, T. W. (1998). Low-dose low-molecular-weight heparin is anti-inflammatory during venous thrombosis. *J. Vasc. Surg.* **28,** 848–854.

71

Endovascular Research: Stents

Darwin Eton,* Kyung M. Ro,† and Samuel S. Ahn†

**Division of Vascular Surgery, University of Miami School of Medicine, Miami, Florida 33136*
†*Division of Vascular Surgery, UCLA School of Medicine, Los Angeles, California 90095*

I. Introduction

The need to perform vessel reconstruction without disruption of tissue planes has led to a variety of innovative alternatives to conventional open surgical bypass procedures. The emergence of endovascular surgery over the past two decades has led to developments in the available technology associated with the procedure. As technology improves, so must the necessary standardization of research techniques used to evaluate biocompatibility, tissue reaction, and patency following the procedure. Any new clinical intervention must first be thoroughly investigated at the laboratory level. Flow models may be employed to examine the feasibility of a new technique, followed by animal models to assess safety and clinical trials to help evaluate the efficacy for widespread use.

The biological reaction to endoprosthesis is a phenomenon that occurs when host tissue responds to the presence of foreign material. The characteristics of endoprosthetic biomaterials determine the nature and extent of immediate and long-term responses. In stents, a thin layer of metal oxide, which varies depending on the composition of the material and industrial processing used in the surface finishing, provides the ultimate interface between the stent and host tissue (1). Examples of such materials are evident in the Palmaz stent and Z stent, and in numerous inferior vena cava filters, which are composed of stainless steel; nitinol is used in Wallstents and Mediloy is used in the Medivent stent (2). The reactivity of the metal surface placed in contact with the circulating blood depends on the physical characteristics of the surface, which can be influenced by the manufacturing process. As the irregularity of the surface increases, the device becomes more thrombogenic. However, the interface reactions and thrombogenicity can be dampened by properly embedding the endoprosthesis within the vascular wall.

When a prototype is completed, the design should be carefully tested in flow models for ease of deployment and technical feasibility. Flow models ideally allow for a realistic assessment of the ease of deployment in a given luminal area, as well as the capability of the endoprosthesis to allow adequate flow. Once the flow models prove successful, animal models can be used. The initial phase in animal testing requires having a design that will be able to compare the endovascular model with traditional repair. Evaluation of a new endoprosthesis should be compared to the standard of care for the same procedure, traditional open revision, or the currently accepted endovascular repair.

II. Protocols

Below are some examples of such preclinical investigations for stents and stent grafts. The goal is to genetically engineer prosthetic vascular conduits to deliver therapeutic enzymes directly into the circulation. Such proteins include thrombolytic enzyme tissue plasminogen activator (tPA) and intimal hyperplasia inhibitor nitric oxide synthase (NOS). Vascular endothelial cells (ECs) and smooth muscle cells (SMCs) can be obtained from the harvested jugular vein of a host animal. Retroviral gene transfer *ex vivo* results in these cells over-producing these enzymes. These cells can then be suffused into grafts, which are implanted into the host animal. The feasibility of this approach *in vivo* has been previously shown (3). The primary aim of this protocol is to improve cell retention and long-term gene expression.

A. Prosthetic Bypass Grafts

Prosthetic (polytetrafluoroethylene or Dacron) grafts are commonly implanted to treat arterial occlusions or vascular trauma, or for vascular access. Their patency is limited by surface thrombogenicity. Seeding the graft surface with endothelial cells has been reported to improve patency rates of small-diameter grafts in animals (4, 5), whereas similar studies in humans have not shown benefit (6). The major problem encountered is that ECs adhere poorly to prosthetic graft material and are readily stripped away when exposed to flowing blood; in addition, significant attrition of these cells during implantation can occur from dehydration and hypothermia.

Gene transfer to stimulate overexpression of thrombolytic enzymes has been reported to enhance the antithrombotic activity of vascular ECs and SMCs (7–11). Seeding of these cells onto grafts can potentially increase graft patency. In addition to direct thrombolysis, other benefits may be appreciated if continuous *in situ* low-level production of a thrombolytic enzyme were possible. Aggregating platelets secrete mitogens that stimulate intimal hyperplasia, and luminal surface clots stimulate a local inflammatory response that contributes to progressive atherosclerosis. Both produce stenoses locally and/or in the outflow vasculature distally and are common causes of graft failure. As such, inhibition of fibrin cross-linked stabilization of the platelet coagulum by *in situ* overexpression of a thrombolytic agent may have the added benefit of slowing the development of these lesions, hence improving graft patency.

B. Tissue Plasminogen Activator

Tissue plasminogen activator is a thrombolytic protease that converts inactive plasminogen into active plasmin, which then degrades fibrin complexes, a major component of a thrombus. This enzyme can be overexpressed by ECs and SMCs following intracellular transfer of the tPA gene (11, 12). Overexpression of tPA has been shown to further decrease retention of seeded ECs on prosthetic grafts. The higher tPA production induces nonspecific proteolysis of the supporting extracellular matrix (ECM), thus reducing the adhesion of ECs to the graft surface (13, 14). A zymogen tPA variant (15) can be used to overcome the adverse effects of tPA on cell adhesion. Wild-type tPA is secreted from cells as an active, single-chained enzyme with a catalytic efficiency only slightly less than that of the proteolytically cleaved form. The zymogen mutant tPA (R275E, A292S, F305H) has been reported to have reduced catalytic efficiency by a factor of 200 in a single-chain form, while retaining full activity in its cleaved form, which is accomplished by binding fibrin. The zymogen tPA mutant can be used to advantage: its low protease activity, once secreted from the cell, will limit digestion of the ECM; therefore, the increased tPA expression will have limited adverse effects on cellular adhesion. After the secreted zymogen tPA is bound to fibrin within the thrombus, the mutant tPA will be cleaved into its active form, which will activate plasminogen as efficiently as wild-type tPA.

C. Endothelial Cell and Smooth Muscle Cell Graft Suffusion

Increasing the amount of ECM (proteoglycan, elastin, collagen) improves cell adhesion. Because SMCs produce ECM (16–18), grafts can be suffused with genetically engineered SMCs in addition to ECs. Furthermore, because SMCs proliferate in multiple layers, more "exogenous gene product forming units" per unit volume will be available; in contrast, ECs grow as a monolayer only. The ECs in turn modulate SMC proliferation (19, 20).

D. Nitric Oxide Synthase

Nitric oxide (NO) is a potent vasodilator, inhibitor of platelet aggregation and adhesion, inhibitor of leukocyte adhesion (21), and inhibitor of SMC proliferation and migration (21–25), NO is synthesized from L-arginine by NOS and acts through cyclic guanosine monophosphate (cGMP). The rise in cGMP results in activation of protein kinases, which decrease intracellular calcium and increase the permeability of the potassium channels. This leads to relaxation of vascular SMCs and inhibition of platelet aggregation and adherence (26, 27). Gene transfer of NOS into ECs, using Sendai virus/liposome *in vivo* (28), retroviral vectors *in vitro* (29), and adenoviral vectors (30), reduces SMC hyperplasia. Inhibition *in vivo* has been less successful (29, 31).

E. Stent Grafts

Stent grafts are minimally invasive devices used to treat aneurysmal and occlusive vascular disease. They are composed of a polymer membrane wrapped around a metal framework (32, 33) and are deployed into the circulation using catheter technology via a small incision in a remote artery, typically the femoral artery.

Stent graft technology offers the opportunity to solve one of the problems of bioengineered graft implantation. During traditional surgery, each end of the graft must be sewn onto the vessel, which takes approximately 30 min. During this time, the graft is exposed to ambient temperatures, which can lead to an 80% attrition of cells from the graft. This attrition may be attributed to hypothermia and dehydration. The rapid positioning of a stent graft onto a balloon catheter (3 min) and then into the circulation (less than 1 min) solves this problem.

Bare stent deployment, without the surrounding polymer membrane, has been shown to decrease the overall rate of restenosis (34, 35). However, acute occlusions due to thrombosis and restenosis from intimal hyperplasia still occur (36–38). Even with restoration of normal EC coverage, underlying SMC hyperplasia takes longer to return to the quiescent state (22). Genetically engineered ECs have been used to cover bare stents (7, 39–41), but seeded cells on the lumenal surface were washed away by blood flow. Covering the bare stent with a membrane to make a stent graft provides a sanctuary for cells genetically engineered to produce tPA and NOS. A stent graft consisting of a metallic stent wrapped with a Dacron membrane (Cordis, Miami, FL) can be suffused with genetically engineered cells. Suffusion signifies the seeding of lumenal, ablumenal, and lateral sides, along with permeation of the cells throughout the inner graft wall matrix. The membrane scaffold will help prevent the genetically engineered cells from being stripped away by the shear stress of flowing blood.

F. Dual-Membrane Dacron Stent Graft

In an effort to combat shear stress, a stent graft composed of two concentric genetically engineered suffused grafts has been developed (3). This design allows the suffused cells to grow through the thin Dacron material, and if cells are stripped from the lumenal surface, a large reservoir of cells still remains behind and within the wall of the inner wall of the graft, to repopulate the entire lumenal surface.

G. Dual-Membrane Graft

Although similar in concept to the dual-membrane stent graft, this novel graft can be surgically implanted using standard suture techniques. Cells are injected between the concentric membranes after implantation. The inner membrane is semipermeable, with pore size smaller than a platelet but large enough to allow passive diffusion of nutrients, gene products of interest, and of waste products of metabolism. Cellular immunity elements such as white blood cells and macrophages are unable to traverse the membrane. This permits use of allogeneic cells, obviating the need to harvest a vein from each patient. The outer tube is made of polytetrafluoroethylene (PTFE). Semipermeable membranes have been reported to protect allografts and xenografts from the host cellular immune response (42–44) and have been used to deliver therapeutic agents in animal studies (45, 46).

III. Experimental Design

A. Improved Cell Retention

Attrition of cells during, and immediately following, implantation results in an acutely diminished benefit. Causes include the proteolytic activity of tPA on the ECM, implantation trauma (hypothermia, dehydration, physical deformation), and the sheer stress of flowing blood. Until the graft is repopulated by the remaining cells, little "endocrine" benefit will be seen. Additionally, *in situ* neointima formation may overwhelm the remaining cells, isolating them from the bloodstream. Consideration of several aspects may increase cell retention.

1. Improved Cell Adhesion

Preliminary data show that dual graft suffusion with ECs and SMCs enhances cell retention compared to ECs alone. This can be attributed to the secretions of the ECM and SMCs (proteoglycans, elastin, and collagen). It is important to study ECM production as a function of time and ECM composition to avoid delays *ex vivo*. Changes in EC and SMC phenotypes as a function of time should also be studied. An optimal balance will be necessary to retain the advantages of ECM production toward cell retention while maintaining EC phenotype. Once optimal intervals are determined, cell retention can be evaluated in an *in vitro* flow model and subsequently tested *in vivo*. ECs and SMCs should be transduced with vectors carrying genes coding for β-galactosidase and green fluorescence, respectively. X-Gal staining and fluorescent microscopy can be used to distinguish layered ECs and SMCs. The seeded grafts should then be exposed to flow *in vitro* within a closed circuit containing culture media pumped at defined rates to generate a shear stress of 5–10 dynes/cm^2. This setting is analogous to physiologic conditions even in high-flow sites, such as in the dog carotid or femoral artery. The flow circuit is housed in a tissue culture incubator. Retention of seeded cells can be determined by X-gal staining and fluorescent microscopic assessment.

2. Decreased Matrix Proteolysis

A zymogen tPA mutant that has diminished protease activity until bound to fibrin is utilized. Genes encoding for wild-type tPA and the tPA variant are transduced in ECs and SMCs via vesicular stomatitis virus G glycoprotein (VSV-G) pseudotyped retroviral vectors. The effect of zymogen tPA compared to wild-type tPA on cell adhesion is tested using the *in vivo* protocol described above.

3. Decreased Implantation Trauma

a. Stent Graft Approach Stent graft technology permits rapid deployment of cell-suffused grafts directly into an artery. The prolonged exposure of suffused cells to ambient conditions during traditional surgical sutured anastomoses and the attendant dehydration and hypothermia are thus avoided. Stent grafts composed of a metallic stent wrapped with Dacron membrane are suffused with cells as determined above. The suffused stent grafts are deployed into PTFE grafts, and exposed to flow in an *in vitro* flow circuit as described above. Retention of seeded cells should be determined and compared to the number of cells on the graft pre- and postdeployment trauma. This should then be compared to the dual-membrane protective Dacron stent graft described above. After completing the *in vitro* optimization steps outlined above, ascertain cell retention *in vivo*. A genetically engineered stent graft is placed in each iliac artery in an acute dog model (50 kg) for 8 hr. Side-by-side comparison of stent grafts of different characteristics and suffusion parameters (as determined from *in vitro* data) can be made. Cell retention and tPA activity are measured on explanted grafts. The lumenal surface is examined for platelet and thrombus accumulation, as well as for presence of acute inflammatory response. Once a suitable configuration is selected, a 24-hr implantation experiment follows. Successive longer implantation experiments follow serially, so long as continued retention and repopulation of the grafts are seen. Once these have reached a plateau in these two variables, the study can proceed onto the evaluation of long-term gene expression. This permits the collective assessment of cell retention, cell repopulation, gene expression, gene product function, and arterial response as a function of time *in vivo*.

b. Surgical Implantation of a Novel Graft An alternative solution to the detrimental effects of prolonged ambient exposure and shear stress on cellular retention is the use of a dual-membrane graft. This has the added benefit of avoidance of catheter deployment trauma. The graft is surgically implanted and cells are injected into the space between the concentric graft membranes after implantation. The lumenal semipermeable membrane described above allows free passage of small proteins but serves as a barrier to cell movement. After *in vitro* characterization is completed, *in vivo* implantation studies follow. Begin with autogenous cells harvested from canine jugular vein. In one iliac artery, graft SMCs transduced with LacZ are injected. In the contralateral iliac artery graft, inject SMCs transduced with tPA. The grafts should be harvested at 24 hr and at 4 days to determine surface characteristics. If cell viability persists *in vivo* and gene expression is observed, perform 1- and 2-week experiments. Once a steady state is achieved in cell survival, but before proceeding to the evaluation of long-term gene expression, examine the immunoisolation feature of the graft. Instead of harvesting the dog's own cells, use allogeneic SMCs. The SMCs are transduced with LacZ and injected into interposition grafts implanted into the dog iliac arteries. Grafts seeded with autogenous LacZ-transduced SMCs serve as controls on the contralateral side. After 1 month, the grafts are harvested and cultured to ascertain viability and phenotype of the seeded cells and X-gal stained to document persistent expression of the transduced reporter gene. The space housing the cells should be examined for elements of cellular immunity (lymphocytes, eosinophils, basophils, and macrophages).

As allogeneic cell survival is confirmed, test the efficacy of increased tPA production on the patency of these double-lumen grafts and the differences between tPA production by allogenic versus autogenous cells.

4. Long-Term Gene Expression

In vivo data on sustained stable gene expression at 3 and 6 months are carried out to address concerns of "gene turn-off," up-regulation of inhibitors, and competitive nonengineered cellular neointima formation. The desired endpoint is chronic overexpression of the genetically engineered protein and therapeutic benefit. One should expect increased levels of tPA antigen and accompanying increased thrombolytic activity. If this is not observed, the following strategies may prove successful:

1. If "gene turn-off" is observed (i.e., no increase in tPA antigen is observed over the long term, modify the gene construct.
2. If antigen concentration is high but activity is low, consider the natural inhibitor of tPA, plasma activator inhibitor.
3. Previous investigators have observed *in vitro* and *in vivo* up-regulation of PAI activity as tPA production increases, albeit to a lesser extent.
4. If competing neointima formation is observed, consider that, depending on the acute attrition of the engineered cells, neointima composed of nongenetically engineered cells can form. This neointima may cover underlying populations of genetically engineered cells and pose a barrier to gene product delivery directly into the circulation. Therefore, consider cotransfection of the tPA gene with the NOS gene, which codes for an enzyme that results in the production of nitric oxide and are inhibitor of intima hyperplasia.

Color flow duplex studies should monitor graft patency at monthly intervals. Occlusion leads to early sacrifice of the animal. Angiography should be performed at sacrifice and compared to the study at deployment. Digital planimetry on the vascular cross-sections can be used to measure variances in intima thickness. The degree of surface thrombus and neointima formation is measured from the recovered grafts using computer-assisted imaging techniques. Culture of the recovered graft is used to study viability of the retained cells and assay protein expression.

IV. Methods

A. Retroviral Vector Construction and Cell Transduction

Both amphotropic and VSV-G pseudotyped MuLV vectors bearing a β-galactosidase reporter gene are generated from a transient three-plasmid transfection system (47). Briefly, 293T/17 cells (10^6 cells in a 100-mm-diameter dish) are transferred by calcium phosphate precipitation with plasmids (10 μg each): pCnBgSN, pHIT60, and pCVG for VSV-G-MuLV or pCAE for ampho-MuLV. Plasmid pCN-BgSN (48) is a retroviral vector containing a LacZ gene encoding nuclear localized β-galactosidase and a neomycin resistance gene (*neo*^{r}) encoding neomycin phosphotransferase. Plasmid pCVG is a CMV-driven VSV-G expression vector. Plasmid pCAE is a CMV-driven plasmid expressing amphotropic envelope from MuLV 4070A (49).

Retroviral vectors LtSN with the wild-type human tPA gene (50) and LCNSN carrying the human eNOS gene (29) are obtained from outside laboratories. Mutated tPA (mt) genes can be cloned into the retroviral vector plasmid G1XsvNa to generate plasmid G1mtSvNa. Respective VSV-G pseudotyped MuLV viral supernatants are generated by transient transfection of 293T cells with three different plasmids: pCVG, pHIT60 and pCnBg5N, and the different vectors LtSN, G1mtSvNA, and LCNSN. Stable producer cell lines are generated by a method similar to that described above, utilizing a 293 packaging cell line with a tetracycline-inducible system (51).

B. Endothelial and Smooth Muscle Cell Harvest and Transduction

An excreta human saphenous vein sample can be obtained from patients undergoing bypass procedures following approval by the Institutional Review Board. The vein is transported in sterile RPMI 1640 medium containing 2 m*M* HEPES, 2 m*M* L-glutamine, 50 units/ml penicillin, 50 μg/ml streptomycin, 2.5 μg/ml gentamycin, and 2.5 μg/ml amphotericin B. In the research laboratory, the samples are flushed with the sterile transport medium, clamped at one end, filled with 0.1% collagenase in Dulbecco's phosphate-buffered saline (DPBS), and incubated for 15 min at 37°C. The dissociated ECs are pelleted by centrifugation at room temperature, 1200 rpm (200 *g*) for 5 min. Cells are resuspended and plated on fibronectin (0.1% in PBS) precoated dishes in MCDB 131 medium (Gibco/BRL, Gaitherburg, MD) supplemented with 20% fetal bovine serum (FBS), 17.5 units/ml porcine intestinal mucosa-derived heparin (Sigma), 50 μg/ml EC growth supplement (Becton Dickinson), 2m*M* L-glutamine, and the antibiotics mentioned above.

Following EC dissociation, the remainder of the vein is used for SMC harvesting. The vein is incised longitudinally and the intimal layer scraped off with a scalpel. The cellular composition of the underlying media is primarily vascular smooth muscle. The opened vein is placed in tissue culture flasks. These tissues are agitated in DPBS containing collagenase I (1.8 mg/ml) and elastase (0.2 mg/ml) for 1 hr at 37°C. Single-cell suspension supernatants are removed and pelleted by centrifugation at 1200 rpm for 5 min. The SMCs are resuspended and cultured in Williams' medium containing 20% FBS, L-glutamine (2 m*M*), and the antibiotics mentioned above.

Confirmation of the EC and SMC identity of each culture should be performed. ECs can be identified by their cellular morphology under phase-contrast microscopy, as well as fluorescent staining for von Willebrand factor and low-density lipoprotein uptake. SMCs are identified by positive reaction in smooth muscle α-actin. Both ECs and SMCs are passed at a 1:5 ratio and used for experiments between passages 3 and 12. Using the same methods as above, dog and pig ECs and SMCs can be harvested from pig jugular veins and cultured for *in vivo* experimentation.

C. Gene Transfer and Analysis

Cultured cells are transduced with retroviral vectors by mixing them with viral supernatants containing 8 μg/ml polybrene. After incubation for 2 hr, fresh medium is added and cells are cultured overnight. On the second day, the medium is replaced with fresh medium containing the neomycin analog G418 for selection of transduced cells. Cells transduced with amphoteric MuLV are selected with G418 to produce a population of cells secreting the targeted gene product. Cells transduced with VSV-G pseudotyped MuLV are used directly without selection, because the transduction efficiency is greater than 90%.

Retroviral vector G1nBgSvNa can be utilized to determine the transduction efficiency of the cultured cells. After incubating cells with G1nBgSvNa supernatants for 2 hr, the cells are cultured with fresh medium for 2 additional days, then a β-galactosidase staining assay is performed as follows. Cells are washed with PBS and fixed with 0.5% glutaraldehyde in PBS. After three washes with PBS for 10 min, each time at room temperature, cells are incubated overnight at 37°C with PBS solution containing 1mg/ml X-gal, 2m*M* $MgCl_2$, 5 m*M* $K_3FE(CN)_6$, and 5 m*M* $K_4FE(CN)_6$. Transduction efficiency is calculated by the ratio of blue cells (transduced) to the total cells contained in a viewing field.

Double transduction can be carried out by incubating cells with vectors carrying different genes, e.g., tPA and LacZ. Cotransduction in general does not affect the efficiency of either vector.

D. Gene Expression Measurements

The enzyme activity and antigen concentration of tPA in medium conditioned with transduced cells are measured using Chromalize tPA and Tintliz tPA assay kits from Biopool (Ventura, CA). To identify the persistence and stability of gene expression in the transduced cells, perform Northern blot analysis of transduced ECs and SMCs. The total cellular RNA is extracted from the cells (52). Electrophoresis of 7–10 μg of each sample through 1.2% formaldehyde agarose gels is performed. The RNA is then blotted onto nitrocellulose membranes (Scleider and Schuell, Inc., Keene, NH), vacuumed dried, and hybridized with a radiolabeled fragment of plasminogen activator cDNA. Membranes are then washed on 0.2 *N* saline citrate and 0.1% sodium dodecyl sulfate (SDS) at 55°C and subsequently exposed to phosphor screens for quantification on a Phosphorimager (Molecular Dynamics, Sunnyvale, CA).

Western blot analyses are performed to determine the tPA and NOS expression (28). The cells from culture or recovered grafts are lysed. The supernatant of the lysis should be separated on denture SDS–polyacrylamide gels. Proteins should be blotted onto nitrocellulose membrane. Blots are blocked overnight at 4°C with 5% nonfat dry milk in TBS-T (20 m*M* Tris-HCL, 137 m*M* NaCl, 0.1% Tween 20). Blots are incubated with the first antibody for 1 hr at room temperature and, after washing, with the second antibody (horseradish peroxidase-conjugated sheep antimouse immunoglobulin antibody) for 1 hr. Specific protein bands (NOS at 135 kDa, tPA at 65 kDa) can be detected using an enhanced chemiluminescence (ECL) kit (Amersham). Prestained markers are used for molecular mass determinations.

E. Cell Seeding/Suffusion of Prosthetic Bypass Grafts

Transduced and control (LacZ-transduced) cells are seeded onto prosthetic grafts 5 mm in diameter. Early in the experimental design, test the cell retention efficiency on PTFE grafts. Cells can be trypsinized from 100-mm tissue culture plates and prepared to achieve a density of approximately 10^5 cells/cm^2 of graft surface area. The prosthetic grafts are precoated with fibronectin (in DPBS) as a tissue adhesive via a squeeze-through method, which forces fibronectin into the interstices of the graft (53). The grafts are then filled with cell suspension, sealed with a heated clamp, and incubated at 37°C for 2 hr. The grafts are then opened; the solution inside the grafts is removed and the grafts are placed into a 100-mm culture dish with media. The grafts are incubated at 37°C under 5% CO_2 for 2 days. The seeded grafts are then transferred into a flow circuit to test the retention of seeded cells after exposure to flow.

To double seed the graft, it is filled with secondary cells (ECs) 1 day after the primary cell (SMCs) seeding and processed as above. The SMCs and ECs, layered over one another, are distinguished by fluorescent microscopy and X-gal staining. The seeded grafts are then transferred into a flow circuit to test the retention of seeded cells or are used for implantation in *in vivo* studies.

F. Cell Suffusion of the Stent Graft

Transduced cells are seeded onto stent grafts. Cells are trypsinized from 100-mm tissue culture plates and suspended in culture medium. Grafts are pretreated by immersion in 100% ethanol for 10 min and then immersion in DPBS (twice, 10 min each time) to wash away the ethanol. The grafts can then be mixed with the cell suspension and incubated with manual rolling every other minute at 37°C for 2 hr. At the end of 2 hr, the grafts are moved into a 60-mm dish for culture at 37°C under 5% CO_2 for 2 days.

G. Preparation of the Semipermeable Membrane Graft

Various semipermeable membrane grafts with concentric outer and inner tubes can be obtained from several manufacturers. The cylindrical semipermeable membrane, made of PTFE, is ~70 μm thick and has an internal diameter of 4.5 mm. The fibril length is approximately 40 μm. The length of the graft is approximately 7 cm; the diameter is 5 mm. Endothelial or smooth muscle cells transduced with LacZ gene (control) or the tPA gene are injected into the space between the two tubes where the cells are housed. The graft is then used for both *in vitro* and *in vivo* studies.

Protein diffusibility through the semipermeable membrane can be assessed using bovine serum albumin (BSA). A predetermined concentration of BSA is injected into the semipermeable membrane compartment and suspended in a buffer solution. At specific time intervals, the buffer solution is changed and the amount of BSA is determined by protein concentration assay.

H. In Vitro Flow Studies

A flow circuit can be housed in a tissue culture incubator. Seeded PTFE grafts and stent grafts deployed within PTFE grafts are separately connected to the flow circuit, and a flow with shear stresses between 5 and 17 dynes/cm^2 is applied. Retention of seeded cells is determined via X-gal staining, fluorescent microscopic assessment, assay for tPA production, and cell number counting. After exposure to flow for periods between 1 and 10 hr, the tPA concentration can be measured from the grafts. One portion of the grafts should be fixed in 70% ethyl alcohol and stained with hematoxylin and eosin. The extent of cell cover on the graft is studied using light and scanning electron microscopy. Seeding efficiency of grafts before flow and cell retention after flow are analyzed by computer-assisted imaging techniques and particle morphometric and numerical analyses using image analysis software (OPTIMAS, Optimas Corp., Bothell, WA).

I. Animal Models for Testing PTFE Grafts

Each animal should undergo three procedures: explant of the jugular vein to isolate cells, implantation of grafts, and retrieval of the grafts. The experimental protocol must be approved by the Animal Rights Committee. For insertion of bypass grafts, the iliac arteries must be isolated. A 3-cm portion is excised and the graft is interposed, using a 7-0 prolene suture to create the end-to-end anastomosis of test and control grafts, one on either side. Histologic examination can be carried out on interposition grafts at different time points to define the cellular response. Resuspension of surviving cells will permit assays for marker and thrombolytic protein expression. Measurement of distal aortic and caval fibrin degradation products and systemic fibrinogen can help determine the presence of an *in vivo* lytic state. Planimetry of the vascular cross-sections is used to measure variances in intimal mass. The data can then be compared to control animals treated in parallel with nongenetically altered cells.

J. Animal Models for Testing the Stent Graft

Stent graft implantation is performed through a femoral arteriotomy. The femoral artery is cannulated and a baseline angiogram is performed. Test and control grafts can be placed on either iliac artery and the pigs are maintained for 1–6 months. The subjects should be given coumadin (1 mg for 4 days pre- and postoperatively) and aspirin (325 mg during the entire postoperative period). Angiography and duplex ultrasound should be performed at sacrifice and at intervals up to 6 months. After the grafts are recovered, assays are performed to identify LacZ, tPA, and NOS expression.

K. Analysis of Recovered Grafts

Patency of the grafts can be assessed using planimetry on the vascular cross-sections to measure variances in lumenal diameter. Histopathology is performed to quantitate the degree of thrombosis and neointima formation, as well as any immunoreactivity. Retention of the seeded cells is determined using X-gal staining or fluoroscopy or hematoxylin and eosin staining and cell counting after trypsinization, or using image assist techniques described before. Gene expression of the resuspended cells can be measured by Western blot analysis.

L. Statistical Analysis

All calculated variables should be tabulated for comparison and statistical analysis. Chi-square statistics can be used to compare proportions and frequency distributions of variables among the different groups. Mean values of continuous variables should be compared with analysis of variance and paired two-tailed Students t tests. Significance is attributed when p values are less than 0.05.

The minimum number of animals required in each experiment to achieve statistical significance is dependent on the differential results of the initial experiments. As preliminary results are obtained, the number of animals should be adjusted as required.

M. Vertebrate Animals

Animals of reasonable size to permit vascular procedures should be used, with no sex preference. All experimental protocols should be in accordance with each institution's Animal Rights Committee. Each animal must undergo three procedures, as described below.

1. Operation I: Harvesting the Vein Segments

The procedure is performed in the operating room under standard sterile conditions. Animals must be fasted overnight and the procedure performed as follows:

1. Initial sedation with tiletamine and zolazepam (IM), medetomidine (IM), and buprenorphine (IM/SQ).
2. Placement of animal to maximize peripheral venous access.
3. Atropine administration and endotracheal intubation, done in the usual fashion.
4. General anesthesia using halothane/isofluorane.
5. Betadine preparation and sterile draping in the usual fashion.
6. Isolation of the external jugular vein. The vein should be ligated, excised, and placed in transport solution (RPMI media, antibiotics, glutamine, and HEPES buffer) and brought to the vascular laboratory in a 37°C bath.

7. Wound assessment for hemostasis; wound closure with 3-0 vicryl sutures. The skin is closed with staples and sterile dressing is placed over the incision site.
8. Extubation in the operating room; transfer to the recovery room.
9. Postoperative analgesia using buprenorphine (IM/SQ).

There should be minimal to no pain during the procedure and the length of the operation should be approximately 30 min.

2. Operation II: Interposition Graft (Iliac) Placement

The procedure is performed in the operating room under standard sterile conditions about 10–14 days after the vein graft segments are harvested.

1. Animals are given 325 mg aspirin and 1.1 mg coumadin (0.05 mg/kg) starting 3 days before surgery for anticoagulation. The animals are fasted overnight.
2. General anesthesia as described above.
3. The iliac arteries are mobilized and a 3-cm segment is excised. On one side a control graft will be placed and on the other side a test graft will be placed. Both end-to-end anastomoses are sewn using 7-0 prolene.
4. The wounds are be irrigated and checked for hemostasis. The wound is closed with 3-0 vicryl and the skin is closed with staples.
5. Animals are extubated in the operating room and transferred to the recovery room. Buprenorphine (IM/SQ) is given to the animals immediately postoperatively for analgesia and they are then transported to their housing location.

The length of the operation is about 2 hr. Animals are maintained up to 6 months. They should be given aspirin (325 mg) during the entire postoperative period and 1.1 mg coumadin (0.05 mg/kg) for 4 days postoperatively.

3. Operation III: Graft Harvest

The following steps are carried out in the operating room under standard sterile conditions:

1. General anesthesia as described above.
2. Angiography should be repeated using the technique described above.
3. Grafts must be harvested and fixed with 10% formalin for histological analysis.
4. In accordance with the Guidelines on the Panel of Euthanasia of the American Veterinary Medical Association, sodium pentobarbital IV injection in an overdose amount (120 mg/kg) can be used.

The length of the procedure is 1 hr. The risk to the animals is the usual risk of general anesthesia, including the risk of death. The risk from harvesting the vein segments are bleeding and infections, which are minimal (<5%). There are small risks associated with intravenous contrast agents, including renal failure and anaphylactic reactions. There should be minimal to no pain during the procedures.

V. Clinical Evaluation

Following successful completion of the animal studies, Food and Drug Administration and Institutional Review Board approval should be obtained to proceed to pilot clinical testing. The next phase involves the performance of a randomized, prospective study comparing the new endoprosthesis to the standard procedure and concomitantly comparing for both primary and secondary characteristics. Primary characteristics include mortality and morbidity, technical success, stent/graft patency, and stent/graft migration; secondary characteristics include the duration of the surgical procedure, amount of blood loss, number of patients requiring blood transfusion, time to unassisted ambulation, time to resumption of normal diet, and length of hospital stay. All patients enrolled in the study should be thoroughly evaluated prior to hospital discharge, at 6 and 12 months, and then annually thereafter. Follow-up should include clinical correlation with the preprocedural studies; if a patient has lower extremity disease, patients should undergo preoperative ankle/arm indices, duplex scan, and/or angiography to ascertain postoperative patency.

VI. Conclusion

The above experimental protocols are just a few examples of how one can conduct research to develop improved stents or stent grafts. Obviously, numerous other procedures have been described previously, but they have not been included here. Furthermore, other techniques have yet to be described, and are limited only by imagination and ingenuity. This field is fertile and awaits creative investigators.

References

1. Palmaz, J. C. (1993). Intravascular stents: Tissue–stent interactions and design considerations. *Am. J. Radiol.* **160,** 613–618.
2. Teitelbaum, G. P., Bradley, W. G., and Klein, B. D. (1988). MR imaging artifacts, ferromagnetism and magnetic torque of intravascular filters, stents, and coils. *Radiology* **166,** 657–664.
3. Eton, D., Terramani, T. T., Wang, Y., *et al.* Genetic engineering of stent grafts with a highly efficient pseudotyped retroviral vector. *J. Vasc. Surg.* **29,** 863–873.
4. Herring, M., Gardner, A., and Glover, J. (1978). A single-staged technique for seeding vascular grafts with autogenous endothelium. *Surgery* **84,** 498–504.

5. Eickhoff, J. H., Broome, A., Ericcson, B. F., *et al.* (1987). Four years' results of a prospective, randomized clinical trial comparing Polytetrafluoroethylene and modified human umbilical vein for below-knee femoro-popliteal bypass. *J. Vasc. Surg.* **6,** 506–511.
6. Jensen, N., Lindblad, B., and Bergqvist, D. (1994). Endothelial cell seeded dacron aortobifurcated grafts: Platelet deposition and long-term follow-up. *J. Cardiovasc. Surg.* **35,** 425–429.
7. Dichek, D. A., Neville, R. F., Zwiebel, J. A., *et al.* (1989). Seeding of intravascular stents with genetically engineered endothelial cells [see comments]. *Circulation* **80,** 1347–1353.
8. Wilson, J. M., Birinyi, L. K., Salomon, R. N., *et al.* (1989). Implantation of vascular grafts lined with genetically modified endothelial cells. *Science* **244,** 1344–1346.
9. Podriazik, R. M., Whitehill, T. A., Ekhterae, D., *et al.* (1992). High-level expression of recombinant human tPA in cultivated canine endothelial cells under varying conditions of retroviral gene transfer. *Ann. Surg.* **216,** 446–452; discussion, 453.
10. Dichek, D. A. (1993). Gene transfer in the treatment of thrombosis. *Thromb. Haemost.* **70,** 198–201.
11. Ekhterae, D., and Stanley, J. C. Retroviral vector-mediated transfer and expression of human tissue plasminogen activator gene in human endothelial and vascular smooth muscle cells. *J. Vasc. Surg.* **21,** 953–962.
12. Shayani, V., Newman, K. D., and Dichek, D. A. (1994). Optimization of recombinant tPA secretion from seeded vascular grafts. *J. Surg. Res.* **57,** 495–504.
13. Huber, T. S., Welling, T. H., Sarkar, R., *et al.* (1995). Effects retroviral-mediated tissue plasminogen activator gene transfer and expression on adherence and proliferation of canine endothelial cells seeded onto expanded polytetrafluoroethylene. *J. Vasc. Surg.* **22,** 795–803.
14. Dunn, P. F., Newman, K. D., Jones, M., *et al.* (1996). Seeding of vascular grafts with genetically modified endothelial cells. Secretion of recombinant tPA results in decreased seeded vell retention *in vitro* and *in vivo* [see comments]. *Circulation* **93,** 1439–1446.
15. Tachias, K., and Madison, E. L. (1995). Variants of tissue-type plasminogen activator which display substantially enhanced stimulation by fibrin. *J. Biol. Chem.* **270,** 1819–1822.
16. Lynch, C. M., Clowes, M. M., Osborne, W. R., *et al.* (1992). Long-term expression of human adenosine deaminase in vascular smooth muscle cells in rats: A model for gene therapy. *Proc. Natl. Acad. Sci. U.S.A.* **89,** 1138–1142.
17. Clowes, M. M., Lynch, C. M., and Miller, A. D. (1994). Long-term biological response of injured rat carotid artery seeded with smooth muscle cells expressing retrovirally introduced human genes. *J. Clin. Invest.* **93,** 644–651.
18. Geary, R. L., Clowes, A. W., Lau, S., *et al.* (1994). Gene transfer in baboons using prosthetic vascular grafts seeded with retrovirally transduced smooth muscle cells: a model for local and systemic gene therapy. *Hum. Gene. Ther.* **5,** 1211–1216.
19. Fillinger, M. F., O'Connor, S. E., Wagner, R. J., *et al.* (1993). The effect of endothelial cell coculture on smooth muscle cell proliferation. *J. Vasc. Surg.* **17,** 1058–1067; discussion, 1067–1068.
20. Powell, R. J., Cronenwett, J. L., Fillinger, M. F., *et al.* (1996). Endothelial cell modulation of smooth muscle cell morphology and organizational growth pattern. *Ann. Vasc. Surg.* **10,** 4–10.
21. Moncada, S., Palmer, R. M., and Higgs, E. A. (1991). Nitric oxide: Physiology, pathophysiology, and pharmacology. *Pharmacol. Rev.* **43,** 109–142.
22. Luscher, T. F., and Tanner, F. C. (1993). Endothelial regulation of vascular tone and growth. *Am. J. Hypertens.* **6,** 283S–293S.
23. Sarkar, R., Meinberg, E. G., Stanley, J. C., *et al.* (1996). Nitric oxide reversibly inhibits the migration of cultured vascular smooth muscle cells. *Circ. Res.* **78,** 22530.
24. Garg, U. C., and Hassid, A. (1989). Nitric oxide-generating vasodilators and 8-bromo-cyclic guanosine monophosphate inhibit mitogenesis and proliferation of cultured rat vascular smooth muscle cells. *J. Clin. Invest.* **83,** 1774–1777.
25. Kariya, K., Kawahara, T., Araki, S., *et al.* (1989). Anti-proliferative action of cyclic GMP-elevating vasodilators in cultured rabbit aortic smooth muscle cells. *Atherosclerosis* **80,** 143–147.
26. Dattilo, J. B., and Makhoul, R. G. (1997). The role of nitric oxide in vascular biology and pathobiology. *Ann. Vasc. Surg.* **11,** 307–314.
27. Moncada, S. (1997). Nitric oxide in the vasculature: Physiology and pathophysiology. *Ann. N.Y. Acad. Sci.* **811,** 60–67; discussion, 67–69.
28. Von der Leyen, H. E., Gibbons, G. H., Morishita, R., *et al.* (1995). Gene therapy inhibiting neointimal vascular lesion: *In vivo* transfer of endothelial cell nitric oxide synthase gene. *Proc. Natl. Acad. Sci. U.S.A.* **92,** 1137–1141.
29. Chen, L., Daum, G., Forough, R., *et al.* (1998). Overexpression of human endothelial nitric oxide synthase in rat vascular smooth muscle cells and in balloon-injured carotid artery. *Circ. Res.* **82,** 862–870.
30. Cable, D. G., O'Brien, T., Schaff, H. V., *et al.* (1997). Recombinant endothelial nitric oxide synthase-transduced human saphenous veins: Gene therapy to augment nitric oxide production in bypass conduits. *Circulation* **96**(9 suppl.) II, 173–178.
31. Radomski, M. W., Palmer, R. M., and Moncada, S. (1987). The anti-aggregating properties of vascular endothelium interactions between prostacyclin and nitric oxide. *Br. J. Pharmacol.* **92,** 639–646.
32. Eton, D., Warner, D. L., Owens, C., *et al.* (1996). Histological response to stent graft therapy. *Circulation* **94**(9 suppl) II, 182–187.
33. Parodi, J. C. (1995). Endovascular repair of abdominal aortic aneurysms and other lesions. *J. Vasc. Surg.* **21,** 549–555.
34. Fischman, D. L., Leon, M. B., Baim, D. S., *et al.* (1994). A randomized comparison of coronary-stent placement and balloon angioplasty in the treatment of coronary artery disease. Stent Restenosis Study Investigators [see comments]. *N. Engl. J. Med.* **331,** 496–501.
35. Serruys, P. W., de Jaegere, P., Kiemeneij, F., *et al.* (1994). A comparison of balloon expandable-stent implantation with balloon angioplasty in patients with coronary artery disease. Benestent Study Group [see comments]. *N. Engl. J. Med.* **331,** 489–495.
36. Serruys, P. W., Strauss, B. H., Beatt, K. J., *et al.* (1991). Angiographic follow-up after placement of self-expanding coronary-artery stent [see comments]. *N. Engl. J. Med.* **324,** 13–17.
37. Schatz, R. A., Baim, D. S., Leon, M., *et al.* (1991). Clinical experience with the Palmaz–Schatz coronary stent. Initial results of a multi-center study. *Circulation* **83,** 148–161.
38. Serruys, P. W., Emanuelsson, H., von der Giessen, W., *et al.* (1996). Heparin-coated Palmaz–Schatz stents in human coronary arteries. Early outcome of the Benestent-II Pilot Study. *Circulation* **93,** 412–422.
39. Flugelman, M. Y., Virmani, R., Leon, M. B., *et al.* (1992). Genetically engineered endothelial cells remain adherent and viable after stent deployment and exposure to flow *in vitro*. *Circ. Res.* **70,** 348–354.
40. Flugelman, M. Y. (1995). Inhibition of intravascular thrombosis and vascular smooth muscle cell proliferation by gene therapy. [Review, 35 refs.] *Thromb. Hemostas.* **74,** 406–410.
41. Scott, N. A., Candal, F. J., Robinson, K. A., *et al.* (1995). Seeding of intracoronary stents with immortalized human microvascular endothelial cells. *Am. Heart J.* **129,** 860–866.
42. Brauker, J., Martinson, L. A., Young, S. K., *et al.* (1996). Local inflammatory response around diffusion chambers containing xenografts. Nonspecific destruction of tiissues and decreased local vascularization. *Transplantation* **61,** 1671–1677.
43. Pollok, J. M., Ibarra, C., and Vacanti, J. P. (1997). A new method of xenotransplantation barrier for the transplantation of xenogeneic islets of Langerhans. *Transplant. Proc.* **29,** 909–911.
44. Lanza, R. P., and Chick, W. L. (1997). Immunoisolation: at turning point. *Immunol. Today* **18,** 135–139.
45. Cotton, C. K. (1996). Engineering challenges in cell-encapsulation technology. *Trends Biotechnol.* **14,** 158–162.

46. Winn, S. R., Hammang, J. P., Emerich, D. F., *et al.* (1994). Polymer-encapsulated cells genetically modified to secrete human nerve growth factor promote the survival of axotomized septal cholinergic neurons. *Proc. Natl. Acad. Sci. U.S.A.* **91,** 2324–2328.
47. Soneoka, Y., Cannon, P. M., Ramsdale, E. E., *et al.* (1995). A transient three-plasmid expression system for the production of high titer retroviral vectors. *Nucleic Acids Res.* **23,** 628–633.
48. Han, J. Y., Cannon, P. M., Lai, K. M., *et al.* (1997). Identification of envelope protein residues required for the expended host range of 10A1 murine leukemia virus. *J. Virol.* **71,** 8103–8108.
49. Morgan, R. A., Nussbaum, O., Muenchau, D. D., *et al.* (1993). Analysis of the functional and host range-determining regions of the murine ecotropic and amphotropic retrovirus envelope proteins. *J. Virol.* **67,** 4712–4721.
50. Dichek, D. A., Lee, S. W., and Nguyen, N. H. (1994). Characterization of recombinant plasminogen activator production by primate endothelial cells transduced with retroviral vectors. *Blood* **84,** 504–516.
51. Chen, S. T., Lida, A., Guo, L., *et al.* (1996). Generation of packaging cell lines for pseudotyped retroviral vectors of the G protein of vesicular stomatitis virus by using a modified tetracycline inducible system. *Proc. Natl. Acad. Sci. U.S.A.* **93,** 1057–1062.
52. Chomczynski, P., and Sacchi, N. (1987). Single-step method of RNA isolation by acid guanidinium thiocyanate-phenol-chloroform extraction. *Anal. Biochem.* **162,** 156–159.
53. Falk, J., Townsend, L. E., Vogel, M., *et al.* (1998). Improved adherence of genetically modified endothelial cells to small-diameter expended polytetrafluoroethylene grafts in a canine model. *J. Vasc. Surg.* **27,** 902–909.

72

Noninvasive Vascular Measurements

Stephen R. Lauterbach, Nancy R. Macdonald, and William M. Abbott

Division of Vascular Surgery, Massachusetts General Hospital, Boston, Massachusetts 02114

I. Introduction

The noninvasive vascular laboratory used today by clinicians caring for patients with vascular disease had its origin in the research laboratory, where investigators developed methods for measuring physiologic parameters of vascular function. In 1970, the American Heart Association's Subcommittee on Peripheral Vascular Disease cited an urgent need for simple, reliable, reproducible instrumental methods to screen for occlusive arterial disease. The quantitative methods should be easy to perform, quick, and have intrinsic standardization (1). During the 1970s vascular laboratories were developed throughout the United States, incorporating newly devised techniques. The instrumentation used in the diagnosis and care of patients with vascular disease was reported by Peripheral Vascular Disease Subcommittees of the American Heart Association in 1972 and in 1976. These reports reflect the rapid development of noninvasive techniques and their effective application to the care of vascular patients by physicians (2, 3).

Over the past several decades, technology has advanced to the point where detection, quantification, and often localization of pathology in the arterial and venous systems of patients can be done in the vascular laboratory. The laboratory also serves an important role in evaluating patients for further invasive studies such as angiography, for documenting the progression or resolution of disease, and for documenting the hemodynamic results of intervention.

The purpose of this chapter is to review the hemodynamics behind the instrumentation of the most commonly used devices in the noninvasive vascular laboratory today and discuss the clinically relevant information they provide. By no means is this a complete summary nor an exhaustive collection of all available techniques to measure vascular function noninvasively. The reader is referred to excellent sources for detailed information on the physical principles of blood flow and the noninvasive vascular technologies of the past and present (4–8).

II. Patient Compliance, Safety, and Limitations

Noninvasive laboratory studies pose minimal medical risk and discomfort to the patient. However, the patient's medical condition, body habitus, and ability to follow directions are factors that potentially alter the technologist's ability to perform studies properly. If patients are unable to walk on a treadmill due to congestive heart failure or osteoarthritis, postexercise lower extremity arterial measurements are not obtainable. Because the patient's hemodynamic picture is not complete, conclusions will not be as valid as the ones based on a complete study. In addition, the studies need to be reproducible so that a change in the test result actually reflects changes in the patient.

The noninvasive laboratory, when properly supervised, is an extremely safe environment. Elderly patients with comorbidities not only need close supervision while visiting the laboratory, but often require cardiac monitoring, pulse oximetric monitoring, and vital sign monitoring, depending on the study and the patient's response to the testing (9). Appropriate personnel competent in advanced cardiac life support (ACLS) need to be on hand in the event of a medical emergency.

The reliability and accuracy of measurements made in the vascular laboratory are directly related to the skill and experience of the technologist performing the study. It is important to obtain accreditation for the laboratory through the Intersocietal Commission for the Accreditation of Vascular Laboratories (ICAVL). As part of this accreditation process, it is mandated that the laboratory staff are, at the very least, supervised by a Registered Vascular Technologist (RVT) and recommend that all staff are RVTs. Because some of the testing is dependent on subjective decisions by the technologist, the experience held by the laboratory staff is invaluable to the patient and clinician.

III. Rationale for Acquiring Quantitative Hemodynamic Data

In patients with vascular disease, the majority of diagnoses can be made based on a careful history and physical examination. The noninvasive laboratory can aid the clinician in determining the significance of disease by providing hemodynamic data and often the location of the disease. In the case of patients with claudication, the laboratory can assess the degree of exercise restriction as well as determine if the cardiopulmonary symptoms are more limiting than the exercise producing the lower extremity symptoms. These objective data are useful because they supplement the subjective data gained by history and physical examination, especially when subjective examination is either not possible or inaccurate. Imaging studies such as contrast arteriography provide an anatomic picture without physiologic data. The noninvasive tools are the most powerful clinical research tools available to assess the significance of vascular pathology and the success or failure of medical or surgical therapy.

IV. Hemodynamic Concepts and Principles

Hemodynamic principles are derived from the concepts of fluid energy. Even though limited, these parameters are helpful in understanding physiology and the testing modalities that were developed to study it.

$$\text{Total fluid energy } (E) = \text{kinetic energy } (E_k) + \text{potential energy } (E_p).$$

Kinetic energy (E_k) is the ability of the fluid to do work based on fluid motion:

$$E_k = \tfrac{1}{2} pv^2,$$

where p = specific gravity of the fluid and v = velocity of the fluid. Potential energy (E_p) is the ability of a volume of fluid to do work based on height of the fluid above a certain level:

$$E_p = P + pgh,$$

where P = intravascular pressure, g = acceleration due to gravity, and h = height. Combining the two equations gives

$$E = \tfrac{1}{2} pv^2 + P + pgh.$$

This represents the total fluid energy per unit volume of blood.

In a system that obeys the laws of ideal flow, Bernoulli's principle states that energy is constant as fluid flows from one point to another. Kinetic energy, potential energy, and pressure are related in this ideal fluid system according to the following equation:

$$P_1 + (E_k)_1 + (E_p)_1 = P_2 + (E_k)_2 + (E_p)_2.$$

Blood flow in the human vascular system is not steady, but rather is pulsatile, and thus energy is lost as blood flows within the vascular system due to branch points, nonlaminar flow, areas of reversed flow, and stenoses. Energy losses are either viscous losses or losses based on a change in velocity or direction, i.e., inertial losses (Fig. 1). Most of the lost energy is dissipated as heat.

Poiseuille's law attempts to describe the laws of fluid flow and can be used to better understand the relationship

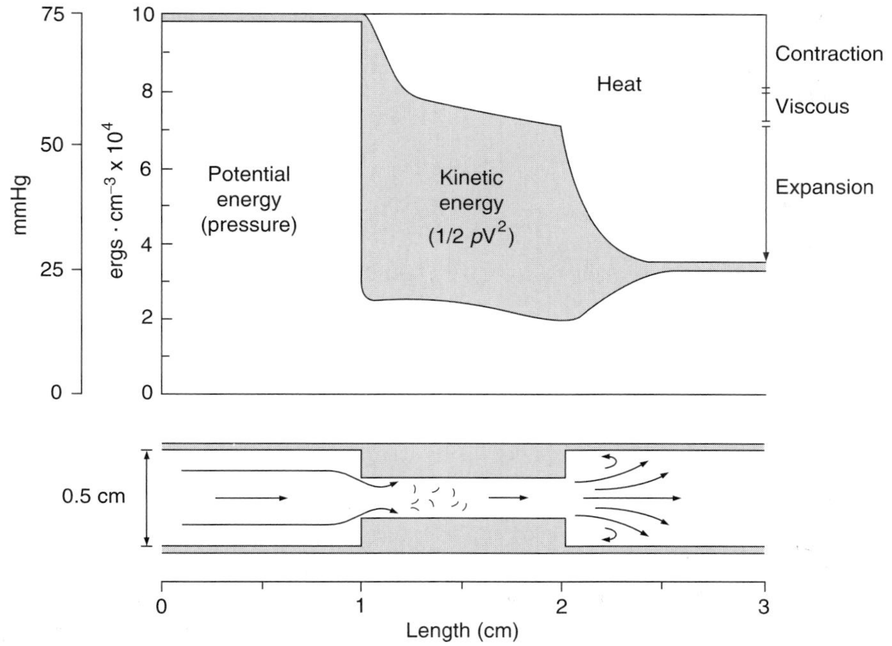

Figure 1 Diagram illustrating energy losses experienced by blood passing through a stenosis 1 cm long. Flow is assumed to be unidirectional and steady. Note that very little of the total energy loss is attributable to "viscous" losses. Thus, applications of Poiseuille's law greatly underestimate the pressure drop across an arterial. From Summer (9a).

between pressure and flow and the viscous energy losses existing in the ideal system:

$$P_1 - P_2 = Q\,(8nL)/(\Pi\, r^4),$$

where Q = flow, L = length of tube, n = viscosity, and r = radius. This principle only directly applies to steady flow through straight rigid tubes and thus has obvious limitations in the human vascular system. It does, however, demonstrate the relationship between several factors and how these factors individually relate to blood flow. It should be emphasized that energy losses are inversely proportional to the fourth power of the radius. This results in sharply curved pressure–flow graphs based on Poiseuille's law (Fig. 2). Reduction in lumen diameter results in very little change in the pressure gradient until a certain point is reached. Beyond this point, the pressure gradient rises sharply.

Inertial losses are based on velocity changes. Because velocity is a vector quantity, directional change results in velocity change. In pulsatile flow, as blood flow accelerates or decelerates, blood flow velocity changes. Velocity also changes as blood flows in response to changing blood vessel size. The direction of flow changes at curves, branch points, and at stenotic entry and exit sites. Also, the direction of flow changes during systole and diastole due to the elastic properties of blood vessels. All of the above conditions exist in the human circulatory system and contribute to the inertial energy loss of flowing blood.

Because inertial losses, like viscous losses, are inversely proportional to the fourth power of the radius, the effect of the vessel radius becomes apparent. Increasing the flow velocity results in greater inertial energy loss than viscous energy loss (Fig. 3). One can see that velocity is squared in the kinetic energy formula and enters Poiseuille's law in the first power.

Human arteries experience turbulent flow due to the anatomy of the circulatory tree and the development of disease. The development of atherosclerosis produces areas of luminal narrowing, resulting in obstructive arterial lesions. Flow through these areas of obstruction becomes more chaotic, random, and nonlaminar i.e., turbulent. Energy losses are great in such circumstances. The Reynolds number (R_e), which defines turbulence, is a dimensionless entity that is related to many factors that describe the transition from laminar flow to turbulent flow.

$$R_e = Vdp/n,$$

where V = mean velocity, d = diameter, p = fluid density, and n = viscosity. This can only be applied to steady flow and is dependent on the experimental conditions in place.

Viscosity is the friction between contiguous layers of fluid due to intermolecular attractions that causes the fluid to resist deformation. Shear stress is the tangential force that a lamina, or unit, of fluid experiences as it travels at a constant velocity within a tube. If the velocity of the lamina changes

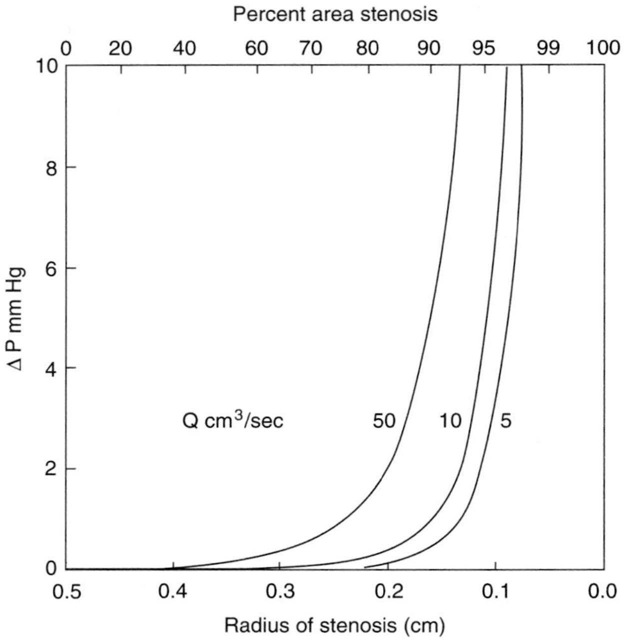

Figure 2 Curves derived from Poiseuille's law. The stenotic segment is assumed to be 1.0 cm long. Viscosity is 0.035 poise. From Summer (9b).

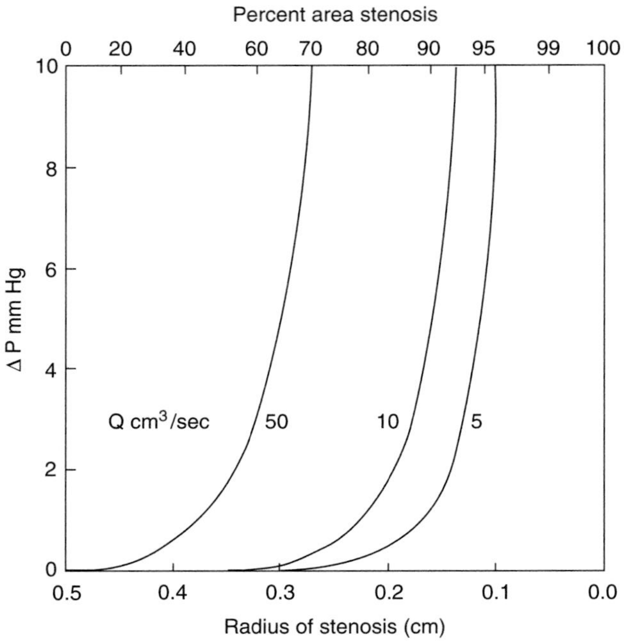

Figure 3 Effect of increasing stenosis and blood flow on inertial losses at the exit of a stenotic segment that leads into a tube with a radius of 0.5 cm. An abrupt exit is assumed. From Summer (9c).

with respect to a neighboring lamina the shear rate or the velocity gradient across the radius of the tube is established. Viscosity is the ratio between shear stress and shear rate. Because density and viscosity are relatively constant, the development of turbulence is mainly dependent on the size of the vessel and the velocity of flow.

Resistance (R) is the ratio of energy drop between two points to mean blood flow. From Ohm's law, $P_1 - P_2 = RQ$, where $P_1 - P_2$ represents the pressure drop across the segment of vessel, R = resistance, and Q = flow. After Poiseuille's law, $R = 8nL/\Pi r^4$. Of all the components of Poiseuille's law, the single most important factor affecting resistance is vessel radius, which enters the equation to the fourth power in the denominator.

V. Doppler Ultrasound

Flow velocity is a vector quantity containing components of speed and direction. The speed is related to a reference point or is corrected for direction. It is one of the most common pieces of information obtained when screening for and evaluating arterial obstruction in the laboratory. In order to measure velocity, the Doppler ultrasound device is employed.

The Doppler principle formulated by the Austrian physicist Christian Johann Doppler states that the frequency of sound (or light) emitted by a moving source is perceived as higher than the transmitted frequency by a stationary observer when the source is moving toward the observer. When the source is moving away from the observer, the perceived frequency is lower than the transmitted frequency. The Doppler equation is

$$\Delta f = (2f_t V \text{Cos} \varnothing)/C,$$

which defines the frequency shift (Δf), where f_t = frequency of the transmitted sound, V = velocity of red blood cells, $\varnothing$ = angle of insonation, and C = velocity of sound in tissue.

As a transmitted ultrasound beam at a known frequency strikes moving particles (such as red blood cells), the ultrasound is backscattered by a frequency shift proportional to the velocity of blood flow (Fig. 4). The detected frequency shift can then be amplified as an audible signal or recorded as an analog waveform, for example. Doppler insonation therefore readily provides a means to measure blood flow velocity. Conveniently, ultrasonic transmission devices used clinically today in the range of 2.0–12 MHz coupled with human blood flow velocities of 3–150 cm/sec generate frequency shifts in the range of 0–10 kHz, which is in the audible frequency range for humans.

The angle of insonation is a critical element of the Doppler equation. If a vessel is insonated at an angle of 90°, a zero frequency shift will be generated, because the cosine of 90 is zero. The greatest frequency shift is observed when the angle of insonation is 0°, because the cosine of 0 is one. A zero degree angle is not possible with extraluminal

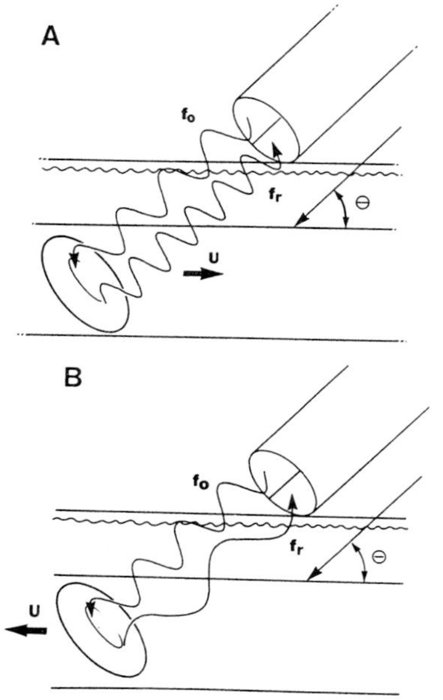

Figure 4 Doppler shifts produced by red blood cells moving toward a probe (A) and away from a probe (B). Transmitted frequency (f_o) is the same in both examples, but backscattered frequency (f_r) is increased when a cell moves toward the probe and is reduced when a cell moves away. Velocity of a red blood cell is represented by U, and the angle at which a sound beam intersects the velocity vector is indicated by θ. From Kempczinski and Yao (6).

insonation obtained transcutaneously or even intraoperatively. Intravascular insonation, made possible with endoluminal devices, allows the angle of insonation to be zero. In clinical use the angle of insonation is 60° because it is relatively easy to accomplish in most anatomic circumstances. When comparing velocity data, the angle of insonation must be known to calculate velocities accurately.

Doppler ultrasound used today is primarily either continuous wave (CW) or pulsed. Depending on the equipment and the task at hand, both have their strengths and weaknesses. CW doppler ultrasound is the most widely used technique to assess the vascular system. It is relatively simple in design and inexpensive. Two separate transducers are contained in the head of the probe. One continuously sends out sound waves while the other awaits the returning echoes. These devices can conveniently be made portable, which can make the evaluation process relatively easy. However, because the CW device insonates all structures in the path of the ultrasound beam, exact site identification is difficult. This range ambiguity can be problematic if the specific anatomy of the desired vessel is not known, or if it is surrounded by other vessels, or it has branches. Additionally, because the angle of insonation cannot be determined, the actual velocity cannot be calculated accurately. Most commonly, a hand-held device is used to document signals in peripheral arteries, to measure blood pressure with the aid of pneumatic cuffs, and to record velocity waveforms, which can be qualitatively analyzed.

Pulsed doppler systems were developed to overcome some of the shortcomings of CW systems—primarily, the ability to detect frequency shifts at a known depth in tissue. Pulsed systems use only one transducer. This alternates between sending and receiving sound waves. There is a delay between cycles of transmission that allows the transducer to receive the returning echoes (Fig. 5). Pulsed doppler provides discrimination of doppler signals from different depths, allowing detection of moving interfaces only from within a well-defined sample volume. Only the data from the desired depth are saved. The pulsed doppler system, when combined with two-dimensional B-mode ultrasound, is called a duplex scan. This instrument provides complementary information: the B-mode can outline

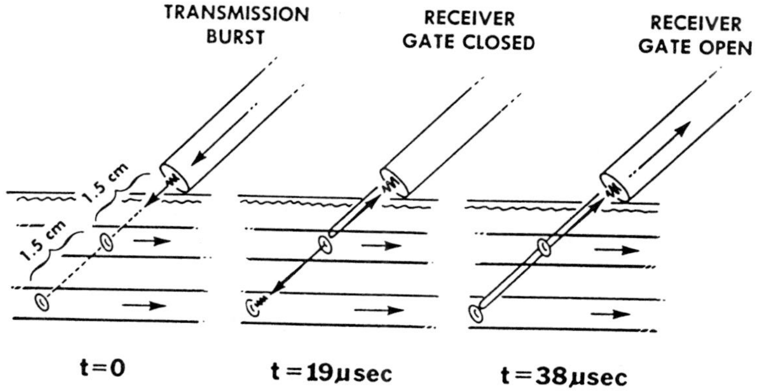

Figure 5 Operation of pulsed doppler flow detector. Red blood cells are shown moving in two vessels 1.5 and 3.0 cm from the probe. Time after transmission of a 1.0-µsec burst of 5-MHz sound is indicated at the bottom of three panels. Initially, the receiver gate is closed, opening at 38 µsec to permit detection of signal from deeper vessel; signals from superficial vessels are not detected (t indicates time). From Kempczinski and Yao (6).

anatomic structures and the doppler yields information about flow patterns. The B-mode image is typically used to localize areas where examination of flow is desired. The technologist controls the position of the cursor, which greatly facilitates the positioning of the doppler sample volume in the area of interest. Because the angle of insonation is specifically calculated, accurate calculation of velocity is obtained. However, there are limitations produced by the pulsed repetition frequency. As one exceeds the Nyquist limit, aliasing of the doppler velocity signal occurs, reducing the ability to obtain the highest peak systolic velocity.

VI. Measurements of Pressure

Noninvasive measurement of blood pressure is one of the most common procedures performed today. The earliest method, the auscultatory technique, involves the use of a stethoscope and a blood pressure cuff. The Korotkoff sounds are auscultated over the desired artery. The first sound during cuff deflation represents the systolic pressure and the onset of muffling is the diastolic pressure. In order to record pressures in the extremities, for example, the CW doppler is placed over an artery distal to the cuff to detect an audible signal. When the doppler signal returns following cuff deflation, systolic pressure is recorded. This flow–velocity detection device is useful for systolic measurements only.

It is important that the cuff size used for indirect pressure measurements is correct. The circumference of the limb determines cuff size. The width of the cuff should be 40% of the circumference of the limb and the length should be twice its width. If a cuff is too small, for instance, erroneously high pressures will be recorded. Also, if the artery is abnormally stiff due, for example, to calcification seen in diabetes mellitus, the pressure may be inaccurately too high. Sometimes the cuff is not able to completely collapse the artery, rendering pressure measurement impossible.

Pressures can be measured at different levels in the lower extremity to gain additional information on localization of arterial obstructive disease (Fig. 6). The thigh, calf, and ankle pressures are measured using different cuff sizes. Measured pressure differences greater than 25 mmHg between sites are diagnostic of occlusive disease in the segment of artery between the cuffs. The thigh measurement cannot differentiate between disease in the common femoral or proximal superficial femoral artery and disease in the aortoiliac segment. To differentiate between these two arterial segments in the thigh, two separate cuffs can be used on the thigh (high and low thigh). It must be remembered to correct for the falsely elevated thigh pressure measurements, given the smaller width cuffs. Approximately 20 to 30 mmHg elevation can be seen when using a 12-cm cuff on the thigh versus the standard 18-cm cuff. For this reason, we use only one cuff at the thigh level in our vascular laboratory.

Pressure measurements generated in the noninvasive laboratory are important both as screening tools as well as a means to assess the results of intervention. The pressure measured at the ankle is compared to the highest brachial systolic pressure, generating an ankle–brachial index (ABI). These indices are helpful because criteria exist for normal versus abnormal values, i.e., for patients with varying degrees of arterial disease. These indices are predictive of functional impairment and can be compared over time to assess the status of the lower limb's circulation. A drop in the ABI of 0.15 or more between tests is considered significant. As noted above, the index can be artifactually elevated when the peripheral arteries are calcified or noncompressible.

VII. Measurements of Flow

Employing the doppler principle and current technology, it is possible to measure blood flow using ultrasound. The cross-sectional area of a vessel can be calculated by measuring its diameter by B-mode ultrasound imaging. The mean velocity within the vessel lumen can be determined as well (Fig. 7). The product of mean velocity and the cross-sectional area will equal volume flow. This technique has been compared to timed blood collections in mammals by cannulating the animal's femoral artery and there was no significant difference between the two methods of calculating volume flow (10).

Another method to measure volume flow is venous occlusion plethysmography. This was one of the earliest techniques developed and its results are reproducible and accurate when compared to direct measurements. Plethysmography measures changes in volume. The different types of plethysmographs differ primarily in the method used to record the change in volume. Air plethysmography, for example, can be used to measure flow in the lower extremity. Briefly, a pneumatic cuff is placed around the lower leg and inflated to a low pressure to ensure occlusion of venous outflow but no obstruction of arterial inflow. As volume changes distal to the cuff, a change in pressure occurs within an air-filled cuff adjacent to the occluding cuff. Integrating the resultant pressure curve allows calculation of blood flow. The system is calibrated by injecting a known volume of air into the cuff and recording the change in pressure

VIII. Pressure–Flow Relationships across Stenosis

There is little change in perfusion pressure and flow in arterial occlusive disease until a relatively high degree of stenosis is reached. The "critical stenosis" is the percent area reduction of the vessel required to produce a measurable decrease in blood flow. This occurs with a greater than 75% reduction in the cross-sectional area or greater than 50%

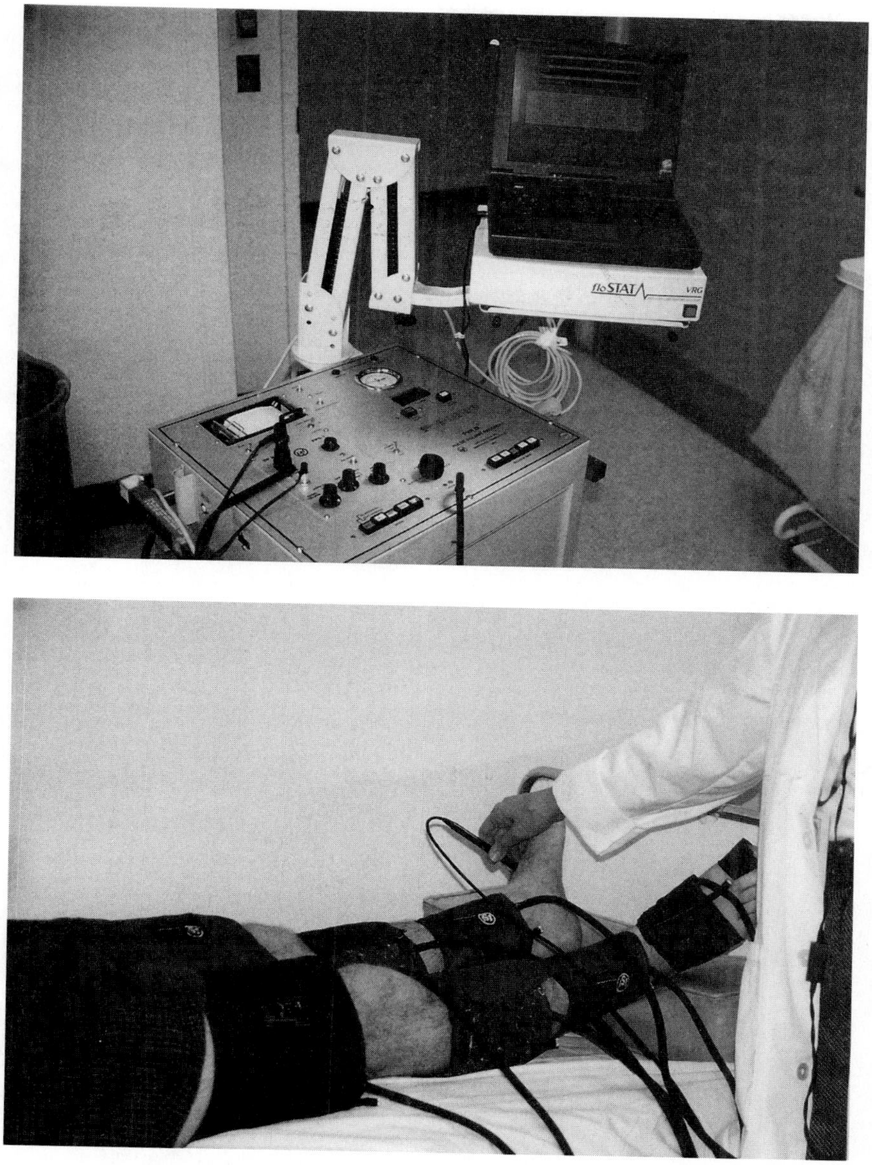

Figure 6 Photos of a PVR machine and segmental cuffs on a patient's legs.

reduction in the diameter of the blood vessel (11, 12). It must be emphasized that a pressure drop caused by an arterial stenosis is dependent on the velocity of blood flow and is not a linear relationship (Fig. 8). "Noncritical" stenoses at rest may become critical with increased blood flow, as seen during exercise, for example. This underscores the importance of obtaining pressure measurements in a patient both at rest and after exercise. The increased flow rate seen with exercise will result in greater energy loss as blood flows through a stenosis, resulting in a greater pressure drop. This explains why a patient with intermittent claudication experiences pain from ischemia only while walking (13). Resting pressures may very well be within near normal ranges but fall to subnormal values after exercise. If patients cannot negotiate the treadmill, reactive hyperemia can be used to obtain these values. This is obtained by inflating a thigh cuff above the brachial systolic pressure to halt arterial inflow in the resting limb and measuring ankle pressures immediately after cuff deflation. This maneuver generates a period of ischemia followed by peripheral vasodilatation. The required 3 min of reactive hyperemia is often too uncomfortable for the patient, precluding meaningful measurements.

Collateral pathways within the circulatory system develop as arterial disease progresses. The patient's symptoms are clearly affected by how effective the collateral vessels are in maintaining adequate circulation to a vascular bed whose

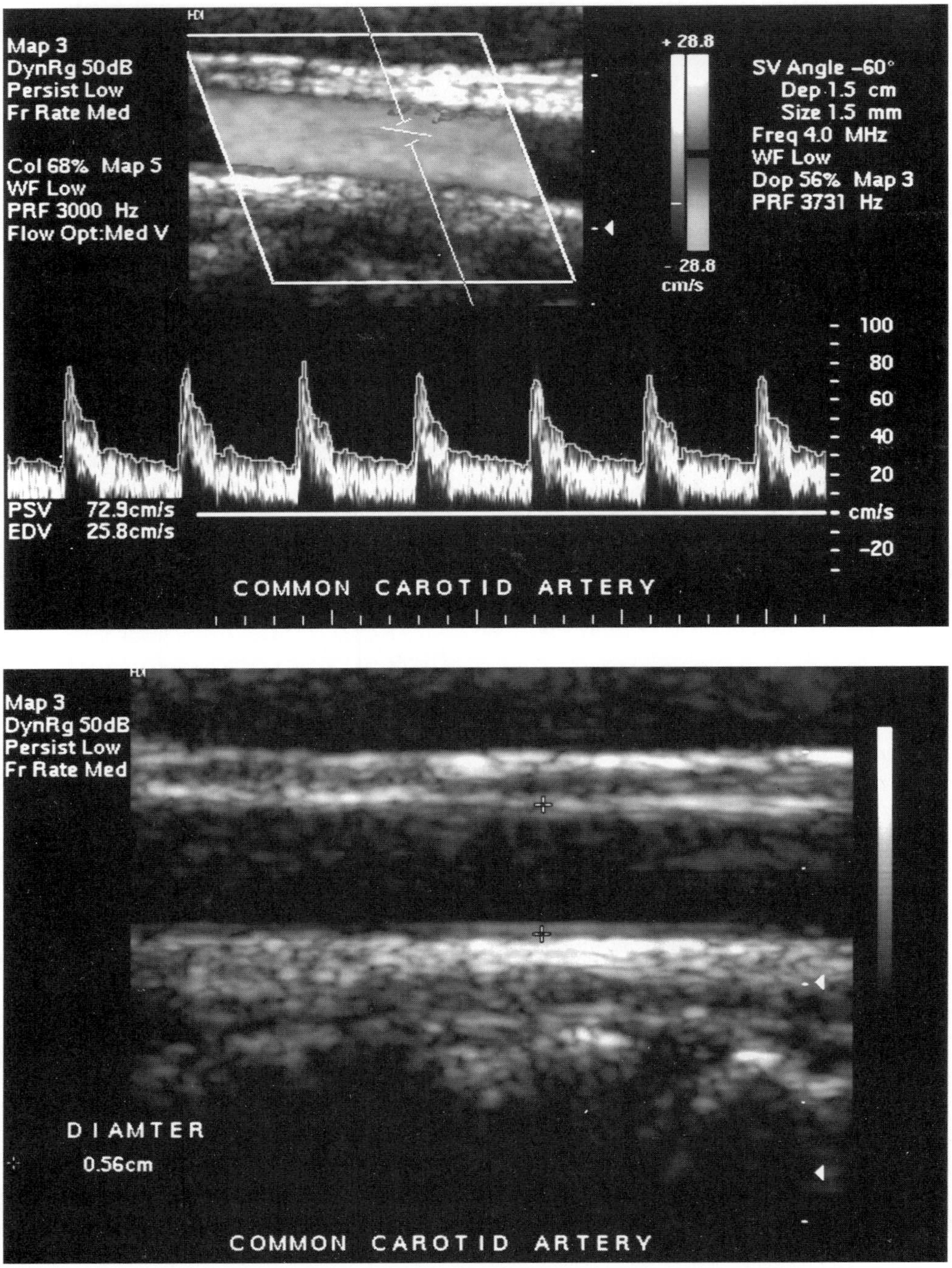

Figure 7 Duplex images of artery and velocity measurement. (See color plates.)

main pathway is diseased. The collateral pathway has been described as a parallel system of vessels bypassing the direct diseased segment of artery and the runoff bed. Stem, midzone, and reentry channels make up this pathway, which is composed of more numerous, smaller vessels with a resistance that is higher than the native vessel they replace (14). The stem vessels are the large distributing branches that are anastamosed to the reentry vessels through the midzone of smaller channels. This system is fundamental to the maintenance of adequate perfusion of organs in the setting of arterial obstructive disease. Pressure drops may be encountered in patients with no symptoms, reflecting adequate collateral circulation. The mechanism driving development of collateral channels has been an interesting topic of investigation.

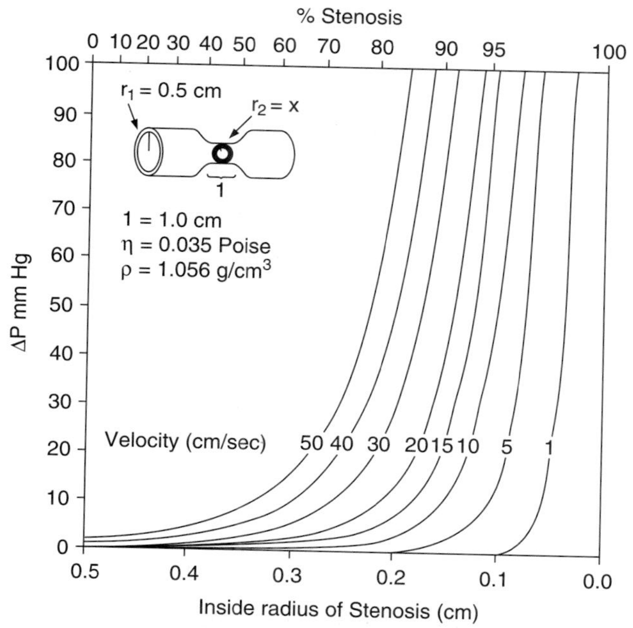

Figure 8 Relationship of pressure drop across a stenosis to the radius of the stenotic segment. Percent stenosis = $(1 - A_2/A_1)(100)$. From Strandness and Sumner (4).

IX. Representative Studies

A. Extracranial Cerebrovascular

1. Duplex Ultrasound

Duplex ultrasound can be used in the management of atherosclerotic disease at the extracranial carotid bifurcation. The location of the bifurcation makes duplex ultrasound an ideal noninvasive means of assessing the anatomy and hemodynamics of the common, internal, external carotid, and vertebral arteries. Duplex provides a B-mode ultrasound image that enables the sonographer to visualize the bifurcation because technical efficiency is enhanced with the addition of color to the image. Vessel identification is improved, thus facilitating the exam. Color power imaging further assists the examiner, especially in cases of vessel tortuosity or in determining vessel occlusion versus very severe stenosis. Plaques can be identified and characterized in the preoperative setting, intraoperatively, and following carotid endarterectomy. Hemodynamic data generated from duplex scans in the form of velocity measurements have been favorably compared to angiographically derived assessments of luminal stenosis (15). Peak systolic velocity, end diastolic velocity, and the ratio of peak systolic velocity in the internal to the common carotid artery are the velocity measurements most commonly used to determine the degree of stenosis. Publication of randomized, controlled trials such as Asymptomatic Carotid Artherosclerosis (ACAS) and North American Symptomatic Carotid Endarterectomy Trial (NASCET), which were performed in an effort to determine which patients should undergo carotid endarterectomy (16–18), precipitated the development of clinical decisions based directly on velocity measurements. A duplex scan is often the only preoperative study a patient will receive prior to surgery. This underscores the importance of standardization as well as the development of reliable and accurate data within an institution.

Duplex scanning is quite accurate in predicting arteriographic findings for severe carotid stenosis and occlusion. The B-mode image has been used to measure the degree of luminal narrowing and was compared to arteriographic measurements. Addition of the velocity data improved prediction in borderline degrees of stenosis (19). In addition, duplex scanning has been used for surveillance after carotid endarterectomy to demonstrate recurrent disease and its progression (20, 21).

2. Transcranial Doppler Ultrasound

Transcranial doppler (TCD) ultrasound technology is a tool used to evaluate the basal cerebral blood vessels that are insonated through the skull. Measurements of velocity, direction, and resistance of blood flow are made in the internal carotid, anterior siphon, the ophthalmic, the M1 and M2 segments of the middle cerebral, the proximal anterior cerebral (A1 segment), the P1 and P2 segments of the posterior cerebral, the distal (intracranial) vertebral, and in the basilar artery. TCD is frequently used in conjunction with carotid duplex ultrasonography to evaluate the hemodynamic effects of extracranial occlusive disease on intracranial flow. It is further utilized to determine intracranial disease/stenosis and vasospasm in the major basal vessels in the Circle of Willis, and to assess the collateral pathways present in various disease presentations.

Using a low-frequency (2-MHz) probe and relying on important known depth of the different arteries determined through angiographic and autopsy studies, the technologist is able to insonate the desired artery transcranially (22) (Fig. 9). There are two methods of performing TCD: direct visualization using a color duplex ultrasound imaging and "blind insonation." The angle of insonation required to measure velocity is assumed to always be zero based on the method of transtemporal insonation.

Intracranial arterial occlusions are not reliably detected by TCD because there are many possible reasons for the lack of a reproducible, traceable signal at a specific depth: vessel size or an incomplete Circle of Willis, for example. Similarly, TCD cannot identify distal branch occlusion. TCD velocity measurements and flow directions must be evaluated in the context of the entire cerebrovascular history and clinical examination because different etiologies for abnormalities exist. There are normal ranges of velocities for the commonly insonated intracranial arteries. These values can be affected by age, sex, hematocrit, P_{CO_2}, brain metabolic function, and intracranial pressure (23).

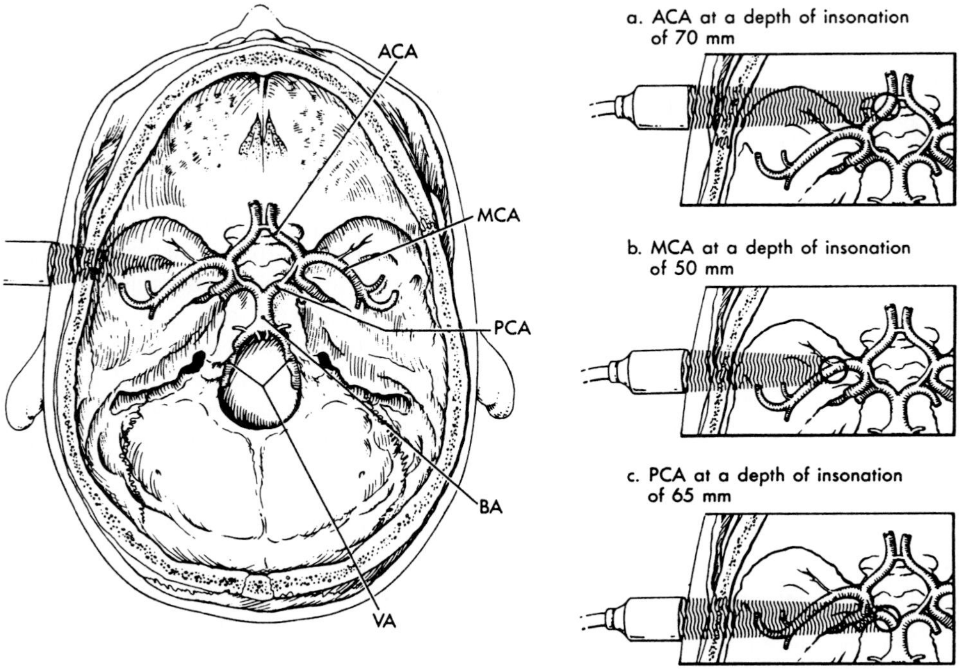

Figure 9 Temporal window. (a) Patient and transducer positioning. (b) Insonated vessels. The middle, anterior, and (c) posterior cerebral arteries (MCA, ACA, and PCA) may be sampled through the thin temporal bone. From Saver and Feldman (22).

TCD has been shown to be very specific in detecting internal carotid arterial stenoses when coupled with the very sensitive carotid duplex study. Investigators from the neurology unit at the Massachusetts General Hospital have studied residual lumen diameters from endarterectomized specimens in an effort to generate TCD criteria for hemodynamically significant internal carotid artery stenoses. Several criteria were identified that had 100% specificity for these stenoses. One criterion, for example, was reversed flow in the ipsilateral ophthalmic artery and a >50% difference in peak systolic velocities in the carotid siphons noted in patients with unilateral internal carotid artery stenosis (24).

B. Renal and Mesenteric Arterial

Duplex ultrasonography, in some laboratories, has become very useful in evaluating the renal and mesenteric arterial systems for occlusive disease. The ratio of renal artery peak systolic velocity to aortic peak systolic velocity has been found to define critical renal artery stenosis, assuming that the renal artery peak systolic velocity will vary with the degree of stenosis (25, 26). Another group found focal renal artery peak systolic velocity greater than 2 m/sec associated with poststenotic turbulence to be the most accurate method in identifying critical renal artery stenosis (27). For accurate measurements, the renal artery must be evaluated from its origin at the aorta to the renal hilum. In experienced centers, this can be done greater than 95% of the time in transcutaneous screening studies (27).

The celiac and mesenteric arteries can also be evaluated by duplex sonography to detect occlusive disease. The velocity measurements have been correlated to degree of stenosis measured by angiography by different investigators and the results have been encouraging (28–30). For example, a peak systolic velocity in the celiac artery of 200 cm/sec or greater, or no flow signal, predicted a 70–100% angiographic stenosis with an 82% accuracy (30). In addition, postprandial velocity measurements can be made in the celiac and superior mesenteric arteries. These measurements reflect the mesenteric arterial response to a food stimulus and can be compared to baseline fasting velocities. The increased mesenteric blood flow after a meal can result in increased velocities within the stenotic arteries. Similarly, normal fasting and postprandial velocities rule out significant disease (31). This is an interesting area of research and may prove useful in aiding in the diagnosis of chronic mesenteric ischemia.

To evaluate the deep, intraabdominal arteries with duplex sonography requires a low-frequency (2.5 or 3.5) transducer, which causes significant reduction in the resolution of the B-mode image. This obviously is a potential source of error in measurement. First, to measure velocity, the vessel has to be visualized by the sonographer for accurate placement of the doppler sample volume. Angulation and tortuosity of the artery, failed placement of the doppler sample volume, and angles of insonation greater than those indicated by the duplex machine all result in erroneous measurements. Bowel gas and body habitus offer significant obstacles to optimum visualization. Successful visualization was accomplished 83% of the time for celiac arteries and 93% of the time for superior mesenteric arteries in one study from a group with significant experience with these techniques (30). Finally, duplex scanning can be used in the operating room to evaluate the arterial reconstruction and postoperatively for surveillance.

C. Lower Extremity Arterial Studies

Data collected in the noninvasive laboratory when evaluating patients with lower extremity vascular disease are most useful in documenting the presence of obstructive vascular disease and in estimating its severity. The ability to compare data from patients with vascular disease to data derived from patients without vascular disease makes the noninvasive laboratory study an excellent screening tool if the history and physical examination are inconclusive. When the clinician knows that vascular disease exists, it is appropriate to document the severity of the disease by obtaining hemodynamic measurements. For example, measuring segmental pressures in the lower limbs and calculating ankle brachial indices will allow patients to be categorized as normal, having claudication, or having critical ischemia. Normal arterial–brachial indices are above 1.0, and values less than 0.9 are abnormal.

Additionally, plethysmographic recorders are used to generate tracings that can be qualitatively assessed. The waveforms at each level can be described as normal, mildly abnormal, moderately abnormal, or severely abnormal. Normal waveform has a sharp rise to peak systole and displays a dicrotic notch. With disease progression, the amplitude becomes reduced, the dicrotic notch is lost, the downslope becomes more gradual and prolonged, and ultimately the tracing becomes a flattened wave representing severe disease (Fig. 10). Pulse volume recordings (PVR) from limbs can be compared before and after vascular intervention, and at different points in time on the same patient to assess the hemodynamic situation. Pulsatile blood flow is necessary and the patient must be able to tolerate the pneumatic cuffs. Plethysmographic data are helpful especially in patients whose arteries are incompressible or if there are no audible doppler signals, because segmental pressures may be inaccurate or may be unobtainable.

After lower extremity arterial reconstructions are performed, noninvasive studies such as PVR, ABI, and duplex sonography can be used as surveillance tools to follow bypass graft potency and to detect stenoses that can be repaired before a graft fails. As in the carotid duplex examination described above, direct visualization of the graft yields specific information anatomically localizing the area of stenosis and thus provides a more sophisticated tool to assess the local hemodynamics at the site of disease. Once a graft fails and the patient requires revision or replacement, the patency and limb salvage rates are reduced (32). Many investigators have studied different methods of vein graft surveillance (33–36). It is clear that the greater saphenous vein is a valuable resource, and if used as an arterial conduit, efforts need to be made to preserve it.

Noninvasive techniques to evaluate the arterial system, such as the pulse volume recorder, ABI calculation, and segmental pressure measurements, provide a global picture that can be correlated with clinical history. In order to answer questions of adequacy of circulation to heal wounds or incisions, an investigator can rely on these accumulated data and their correlation with known clinical outcomes. Additionally, techniques such as transcutaneous P_{O_2} (tcP_{O_2}) have been developed to provide insight as to the level of oxygen at a particular site in the body at a particular time. It is a focused study.

Transcutaneous P_{O_2} differs from doppler ultrasound pressure measurements and limb plethysmographic techniques in that it is based on a metabolic measurement rather than on a hemodynamic representation of the circulation to the limb (37). In addition, tcP_{O_2} determination does not require that blood flow be pulsatile, a condition often seen in low-flow

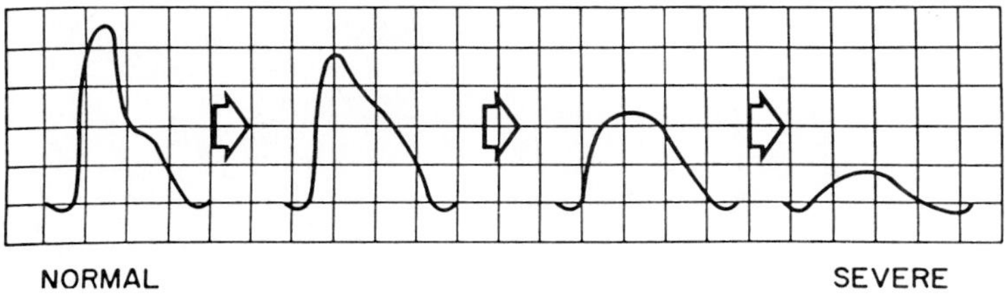

Figure 10 Changes in pulse volume waveforms with progressive arterial narrowing. From Kempczinski and Yao (6).

states such as a chronically ischemic foot. Also, patients who cannot tolerate pneumatic cuffs due to ulceration or pain are not bothered by a small sensor placed on the skin.

Transcutaneous P_{O_2} measures oxygen tension in the skin capillary bed in the region of the transcutaneous sensor. For situations in which arterial flow is obstructed and hemoglobin saturation is normal, tcP_{O_2} reflects the level of regional perfusion. When blood flow is decreased, tissues can increase the oxygen extraction per unit of hemoglobin, thus maintaining an adequate oxygen content to meet metabolic needs. Physiologic function, therefore, is not impaired, despite a hemodynamically significant stenosis that is responsible for reduction in blood flow and pressure. When blood flow is marginal, however, oxygen dissociation is maximized within the capillary bed, P_{O_2} falls, and tcP_{O_2} falls. It is in situations when perfusion is barely adequate to meet metabolic demands that tcP_{O_2} has its greatest utility and sensitivity.

tcP_{O_2} measurement is based on an equilibrium between P_{O_2} in blood and medium adjacent to a transcutaneous sensor. Oxygen reduction occurs at a cathode within the sensor that produces an electrical current proportional to the P_{O_2} within the sensor. The equilibrium depends on several factors. These include capillary oxygen content, oxygen consumption in the skin and at the cathode, and the diffusion barrier provided by the skin, coupling gel, and sensor. Changes in skin temperature will affect blood flow, resulting in different tcP_{O_2} measurements. Changes in the texture of skin may also affect measurements. Measurements therefore need to be standardized within the laboratory by comparing results to measurements obtained from healthy controls (Fig. 11). tcP_{O_2} measurements can be used to provide insight into the metabolic picture of the region in question. This is particularly helpful when hemodynamic data are inconclusive or incomplete. However, due to the physiological variables that affect the measurements, clinical decisions based solely on tcP_{O_2} tension measurements are not justified.

D. Extremity Venous Disease

Plethysmography also plays a role in evaluating patients with venous disease. Patients with chronic venous insufficiency are more numerous than patients with arterial insufficiency and often visit the noninvasive laboratory for evaluation of their lower extremities. Valvular incompetence and obstruction are the two main causes of venous insufficiency. The duplex machine can image veins in the lower extremity to rule out occlusion, and plethysmography can be used to assess valvular incompetence qualitatively and quantitatively.

Photoplethysmography (PPG) uses a small probe that is placed on the calf above the ankle. The probe contains an infrared light-emitting diode and a sensor. The infrared light becomes attenuated by blood in the skin and the arterial pulse wave can be recorded. This technique does not measure volume changes. However, the intensity of the light reflected is proportional to the amount of blood in the skin. As venous volume in the calf increases, the venous volume in the skin increases, resulting in an enhanced recorded pulse wave. To look for venous reflux, the patient contracts the calf quickly and then rests. The recording continues until the tracing returns to the preexercise baseline. The calculated recovery time can be correlated to different severities of reflux. The absence of the initial deflection during exercise

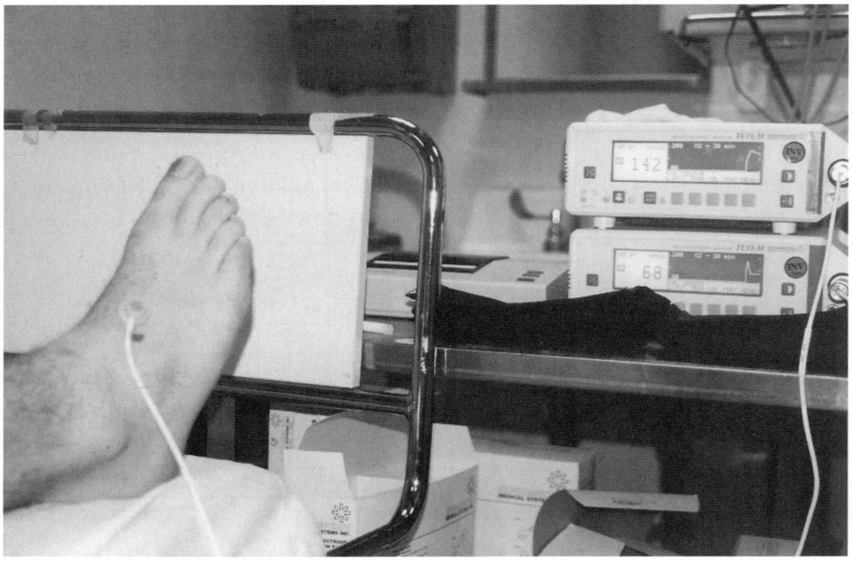

Figure 11 Photo of tcP_{O_2} machine and sensor on patient's foot.

is abnormal because calf muscle contraction results in decreased limb venous volume.

Air plethysmography (APG) provides a global assessment of limb venous hemodynamics. Obstruction, venous valvular insufficiency, and poor calf muscle pump function will result in abnormal measurements based on volume changes in the calf sensed by a pneumatic cuff placed around the lower leg (Fig. 12). By changing the patient's position from supine to standing and performing tiptoe exercises, venous volume, venous filling index, ejection volume, ejection fraction, and residual volume can be measured and calculated (38). These quantitative data can be evaluated in an attempt to distinguish patients with primary obstruction from those with primary reflux because treatment modalities differ. Unfortunately, the picture is not always clear cut. There is significant overlap between the two patient groups and most patients probably have elements of both obstruction and reflux. Regardless, the noninvasive laboratory can provide useful data to better assess the venous limb hemodynamics.

One of the most frequently performed studies in the vascular laboratory is duplex ultrasonography of the lower extremeties for detection of venous thrombosis. The B-mode component images the venous anatomy and the doppler provides the hemodynamic data. When a thrombus is present in the venous system, duplex machinery often demonstrates the thrombus and shows diminished or absent flow that is not augmented by distal limb compression. Additionally, the thrombosed vein is not compressible and phasic flow with respiration is lost. This noninvasive test has replaced phlebography as the study of choice to rule out deep venous thrombosis. As with all noninvasive testing,

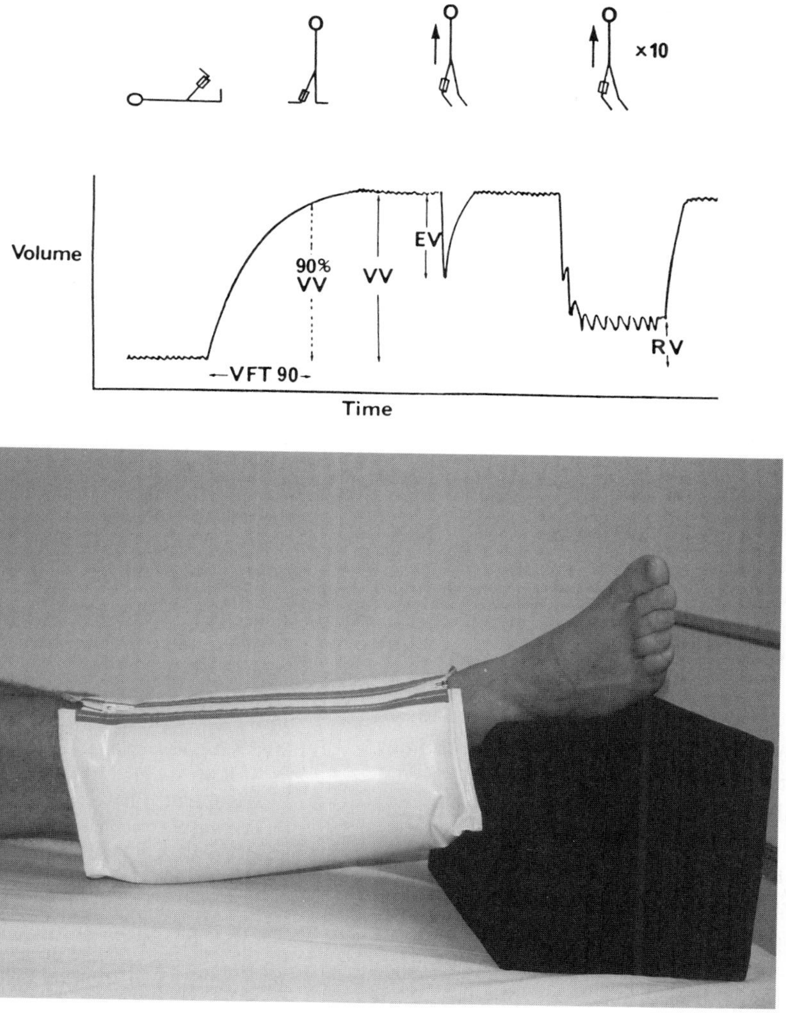

Figure 12 (Top) Pressure changes in the air chamber during standard sequence of postural changes and exercise. The recorded pressure changes are converted to volume changes according to the calibration. From Christopoulous *et al.* (38). (Bottom) Photo of APG cuff around patient's leg.

this study does have limitations. The iliac veins are often difficult to visualize, especially in obese patients. Poor visualization of any of the veins is the most frequent limitation. In this situation, information supplied by doppler analysis of distal veins can often suggest proximal thrombosis. Extrinsic compression in a nonvisualized segment is another potential source of error.

X. New Technology

Diagnostic technology in medicine is continuously developing with the goal of acquiring information more accurately, less invasively, and in less time. The process of evolution of the duplex machine currently used in the noninvasive laboratory is a good example. The issue of cost of testing is important. One device currently under investigation in our vascular unit is an angle-independent doppler system. It has been developed using a special transducer that forms two ultrasound beams at known angles that ultimately can be used to measure blood flow velocity. The basis of the work rests on the development of the diffraction-grating transducers (39). The flowmeter has been tested in *in vivo* models to assess its accuracy in determination of blood flow (40). This device can measure blood flow velocity at reduced cost compared to the currently available duplex machines. Additionally, this system has potential applications intraoperatively and postoperatively as a surveillance tool. It lacks the ultrasound imaging component present in the duplex machine, so examination of deep structures is not possible. However, if it generates velocity data comparable to duplex data, it could become an important tool in the vascular surgeon's armamentarium because it provides more information than is provided by a hand-held CW doppler.

Another technique used by some investigators to study peripheral vascular disease in humans is near-infrared spectroscopy. Hemoglobin's absorption spectrum is in the near-infrared region, allowing noninvasive measurement of tissue oxygenation. One group measured oxygen consumption in the calf muscle of normal controls and patients with peripheral vascular disease subjected to a period of tourniquet-induced ischemia and found oxygen consumption to be reduced in patients with vascular disease (41). Another group used near-infrared spectroscopy to measure tissue oxygenation in the calves of patients with known claudication, in asymptomatic patients with risk factors for the development of peripheral vascular disease, and in normal controls. Measurements were taken before and after exercise and patients with claudication and positive risk factors were found to have lower levels of muscle oxygenation saturation after exercise (42). Near-infrared spectroscopy may be a useful technique for detection of early atherosclerotic disease in addition to assessing metabolic improvement after medical or surgical interventions.

As research and development of new technology advances into the twenty-first century, tecniques are likely to become less invasive, more portable, and more accurate. These new techniques will be developed and tested in the research laboratory. The concept of answering clinical questions by conducting research in the laboratory and applying the new information to patient care is the basis of surgical research. The noninvasive vascular laboratory has been developed to provide information that will ultimately improve the care of patients with vascular disease.

References

1. Spittell, J. A., DeWolfe, V., Hume, M., *et al.* (1970). Prevention and early detection of peripheral vascular disease. *Circulation* **42,** A43–A45.
2. Lippmann, H. I., Winsor, T., and Hume, M. (1972). Medical instrumentation in peripheral vascular disease. *Circulation* **45,** A285–A291.
3. Bergan, J. J., Darling, R. C., DeWolfe, V., *et al.* (1976). Medical instrumentation in peripheral vascular disease. *Circulation* **54,** A1–A9.
4. Strandness, D. E., and Sumner, D. S. (1975). "Hemodynamics for Surgeons." Grune & Stratton, Inc., New York.
5. Bernstein, E. F., ed. (1985). "Noninvasive Diagnostic Techniques in Vascular Disease," 3rd Ed. Mosby, St. Louis.
6. Kempczinski, R. F., and Yao, J. S. T., eds. (1982). "Practical Noninvasive Vascular Diagnosis," 2nd Ed. Year Book Medical Publishers, Inc., Chicago.
7. Rutherford, R. B., ed. (1995). *In* "Vascular Surgery," 4th Ed., Ch. 3–5. W. B. Saunders, Philadelphia.
8. Strandness, D. E. (1993). *In* "Surgical Basic Science" (J. F. Fischer, ed.), pp. 429–470. Mosby, St. Louis.
9. McCabe, C. J., Reidy, N. C., Abbott, W. M., *et al.* (1981). The value of electrocardiogram monitoring during treadmill testing for peripheral vascular disease. *Surgery* **89,** 183–186.

9a. Summer, D. S. (1995). Essential hemodynamic principles. *In* "Vascular Surgery," 4th Ed. (R. Rutherford, ed.), p. 24. W. B. Saunders, Philadelphia.

9b. Summer, D. S. (1995). Essential hemodynamic principles. *In* "Vascular Surgery," 4th Ed. (R. Rutherford, ed.), p. 20. W. B. Saunders, Philadelphia.

9c. Summer, D. S. (1995). Essential hemodynamic principles. *In* "Vascular Surgery," 4th Ed. (R. Rutherford, ed.), p. 21. W. B. Saunders, Philadelphia.

10. Zierler, B. K., Kirkman, T. R., Kraiss, L. W., *et al.* (1992). Accuracy of duplex scanning for measurement of arterial volume flow. *J. Vasc. Surg.* **16,** 520–526.
11. May, A. G., DeWeese, J. A., and Rob, C. G. (1963). Hemodynamic effects of arterial stenosis. *Surgery* **53,** 513–524.
12. May, A. G., Van de Berg, L., DeWeese, J. A., *et al.* (1963). Critical arterial stenosis. *Surgery* **54,** 250–258.
13. Deweese, J. A. (1960). Pedal pulses disappearing with exercise: A test for intermittent claudication. *N. Engl. J. Med.* **262,** 1214.
14. Longland, C. J. (1953). The collateral circulation of the limb. *Ann. R. Coll. Surg. Engl.* **13,** 161–176.
15. Moneta, G. L., Edwards, J. M., Chitwood, R. W., *et al.* (1993). Correlation of North American Symptomatic Carotid Endarterectomy Trial (NASCET) angiographic definition of 70% to 99% internal carotid artery stenosis with duplex scanning. *J. Vasc. Surg.* **17,** 152–157.
16. North American Symptomatic Carotid Endarterectomy Trial Collaborators (1991). Beneficial effect of carotid endarterectomy in symptomatic patients with high-grade stenosis. *N. Engl. J. Med.* **325,** 445–453.
17. Barnett, H. J., Taylor, D. W., Eliasziw, M., *et al.* (1998). Benefit of

carotid endarterectomy in patients with symptomatic moderate or severe stenosis. *N. Engl. J. Med.* **339,** 1415–1425.

18. Executive Committee for the Asymptomatic Carotid Atherosclerosis Study (1995). Endarterectomy for asymptomatic carotid artery stenosis. *JAMA* **273,** 1421–1428.
19. Bebee, H. G., Salles-Cunha, S. X., Scissions, R. P., *et al.* (1999). Carotid arterial ultrasound scan imaging: A direct approach to stenosis measurement. *J. Vasc. Surg.* **30,** 838–844.
20. Ouriel, K., and Green, R. M. (1995). Appropriate frequency of carotid duplex testing following carotid endarterectomy. *Am. J. Surg.* **170,** 144–147.
21. Roth, S. M., Back, M. R., Bandyk, D. F., *et al.* (1999). A rational algorithm for duplex scan surveillance after carotid endarterectomy. *J. Vasc. Surg.* **30,** 453–460.
22. Saver, J. L., and Feldman, E. (1993). Basic transcranial doppler examination: Technique and anatomy. *In* "Transcranial Doppler Ultrasonography" (V.L. Babikian and L.R. Wechsler, eds.), pp. 11–28. Mosby, St. Louis.
23. Brint, S. U. (1999). Transcranial doppler sonography. *In* "Vascular disease: A Multi-Specialty Approach to Diagnosis and Management" (D. Eaton, ed.), pp. 70–76. Landes Bioscience, Austin.
24. Can, U., Furie, K. L., Suwanwela, N., *et al.* (1997). Transcranial doppler ultrasound criteria for hemodynamically significant internal carotid artery stenosis based on residual lumen diameter calculated from en bloc endarterectomy specimens. *Stroke* **28,** 1966–1971.
25. Kohler, T. R., Zierler, R. E., Martin, R. L., *et al.* (1986). Noninvasive diagnosis of renal artery stenosis by ultrasonic duplex scanning. *J. Vasc. Surg.* **4,** 450–456.
26. Taylor, D. C., Kettler, M. D., Moneta, G. L., *et al.* (1988). Duplex ultrasound scanning in the diagnosis of renal artery stenosis: A prospective analysis. *J. Vasc. Surg.* **7,** 363–369.
27. Hansen, K. J., Tribble, R. W., Reavis, S. W., *et al.* (1990). Renal duplex sonography: Evaluation of clinical utility. *J. Vasc. Surg.* **12,** 227–236.
28. Moneta, G. L., Yeager, R. A., Dalman, R., *et al.* (1991). Duplex ultrasound criteria for diagnosis of splanchnic artery stenosis or occlusion. *J. Vasc. Surg.* **14,** 511–520.
29. Bowersox, J. C., Zwolak, R. M., Walsh, D. B., *et al.* (1991). Duplex ultrasonography in the diagnosis of celiac and mesenteric artery occlusive disease. *J. Vasc. Surg.* **14,** 780–788.
30. Moneta, G. L., Lee, R. W., Yeager, R. A., *et al.* (1993). Mesenteric duplex scanning: A blinded prospective study. *J. Vasc. Surg.* **17,** 79–84.
31. Gentile, A. T., Moneta, G. L., Lee, R. W., *et al.* (1995). Usefulness of fasting and postprandial duplex ultrasound examinations for predicting high-grade superior mesenteric artery stenosis, *Am. J. Surg.* **169,** 476–479.
32. Donaldson, M. S., Mannick, J. A., and Whittemore, A. D. (1991). Femoral-distal bypass with *in situ* greater saphenous vein. Long-term results using the Mills valvulotome. *Ann. Surg.* **213,** 457–464.
33. Grigg, M. J., Nicolaides, M. S., and Wolfe, M. S. (1988). Detection and grading of femorodistal vein graft stenoses: Duplex velocity measurements compared with angiography. *J. Vasc. Surg.* **8,** 661–666.
34. Bandyk, D. F., Schmitt, D. D., Seabrook, G. R., *et al.* (1989). Monitoring functional patency of *in situ* saphenous vein bypasses: The impact of a surveillance protocol and elective revision. *J. Vasc. Surg.* **9,** 286–296.
35. Green, R. M., McNamara, J., Ouriel, K., *et al.* (1990). Comparison of infrainguinal graft surveillance techniques. *J. Vasc. Surg.* **11,** 207–214.
36. Buth, J., Disselhoff, B., Sommeling, C., *et al.* (1991). Color-flow duplex criteria for grading stenoses in infrainguinal vein grafts. *J. Vasc. Surg.* **14,** 716–726.
37. Megerman, J., and Abbott, W. M. (1982). *In* "Practical Noninvasive Vascular Diagnosis," 2nd ed. (R. F. Kempczinski and J. S. T. Yao, eds.), pp. 210–228. Year Book Medical Publishers, Inc., Chicago.
38. Christopoulos, D., Nicholaides, A. N., Cook, A., *et al.* (1989). Pathogenesis of venous ulceration in relation to the calf muscle pump function. *Surgery* **106,** 829–835.
39. Vilkomerson, D., Lyons, D., Chilipka, T., *et al.* (1998). Clinical blood flow measurements using diffraction-grating transducers. *In* "Proceedings of 1998 Ultrasonics Symposium," pp. 1501–1508. IEEE Press, Piscataway, NJ.
40. Skladany, M., Vilkomerson, D., Lyons, D., *et al.* (1998). New, angle-independent, low-cost doppler system to measure blood flow. *Am. J. Surg.* **176,** 179–182.
41. Cheatle, T. R., Potter, L. A., Delpy, D. T., *et al.* (1991). Near-infrared spectroscopy in peripheral vascular disease, *Br. J. Surg.* **78,** 405–408.
42. Choudhury, D., Michener, B., Fennelly, P., *et al.* (1999). Near-infrared spectroscopy in the early detection of peripheral vascular disease, *J. Vasc. Tech.* **23,** 109–113.

73

Techniques to Study Microcirculation

David A. Spain and R. Neal Garrison

Department of Surgery, University of Louisville, and Veterans Affairs Medical Center, Louisville, Kentucky 40292

I. Introduction

Inadequate oxygen or nutrient substrate availability leads to an early decrease in ATP, although the cell membrane maintains its metabolic integrity until late in the ischemic process (1, 2). The cell most at risk for dysfunction from lack of ATP is the endothelial cell, in which membrane depolarization occurs early in the shock state (3). Similarly, the endothelial cell is vulnerable to reperfusion injury due to generation of toxic oxygen-derived free radicals (4). In part, injury to the endothelial cell occurs because the same stimuli (ischemia, inflammatory mediators) that induce activation of the endothelial cell also activate neutrophils and render both cells sensitive to adhesion (5).

The endothelial cell has become a primary focus of shock and organ failure research because of four critical functions regulated by the endothelial cell: (1) anticoagulant/procoagulant balance, (2) vascular smooth muscle cell tone, (3) vascular permeability, and (4) leukocyte adhesion/migration into the extracellular matrix (6, 7). Alterations in some or all of these functions occur at different times in the various shock states (hemorrhage, sepsis, ischemia/reperfusion). These changes may lead to disturbances in nutrient blood flow, causing organ ischemia and subsequent organ dysfunction. Therefore, techniques to study the microcirculation provide powerful tools to investigate endothelial and vascular smooth muscle cell function and to determine how alterations in these functions affect organ blood flow, vascular permeability, and endothelial cell–leukocyte interactions.

II. In Vivo Videomicroscopy

A. Technique

In vivo videomicroscopy of small blood vessels is used primarily to assess vascular reactivity of arterioles (Table I) as measured by changes in vessel diameter following either agonist or antagonist stimulation. The two main microscopic

Table I Vessel Types That Can Be Assessed by in Vivo Videomicroscopy

Tissue	Vessels
Striated muscle	Inflow A1 arterioles and outflow V1 venule
	Resistance A3 and A4 arterioles
Small intestine	Inflow A1 arterioles and outflow V1 venule
	Premucosal A3 arterioles
	Serosal A4 arterioles
Kidney	Interlobular arterioles
	Afferent arterioles
	Efferent arterioles
Liver	Sinusoids
Lung	Subpleural arterioles

techniques to study *in vivo* tissue microcirculation utilize transillumination and epiilumination sources of light. During transillumination, light is transmitted through the tissue, generally from a light source below, to a lens and camera system above. This technique can be used only in tissues that are thin enough to allow transmission of light. The most commonly used tissues are small intestine and striated muscle, often the cremaster muscle (8–13). A hydronephrotic kidney preparation also allows visualization of the renal microvasculature with transilluminated light (14–16). Hamster cheek pouch and rabbit ear models have also been studied extensively (17–22). Epiillumination is used for more solid or thicker tissues, such as liver, pancreas, and lung (23–29). Here the light source is from above and the camera uses the reflected light for its signal. With either technique, the signal from the camera is then transmitted to a monitor for real-time visualization and is recorded by a video cassette recorder (example, Panasonic AG 7350E, Osaka, Japan) or a digital image capturer on a personal computer for subsequent analysis (Fig. 1).

A schematic representation of a small intestinal transillumination setup is shown in Fig. 2. We generally use a 100-W quartz–iodide light source, which is passed through an infrared filter to prevent heat damage to the tissue. The light path also contains an interference filter to provide maximal transmission at 545 nm. This wavelength provides maximal contrast between blood and the extravascular tissues. An optical doppler velocimeter (Microcirculation Research Institute, Texas A & M University, College Station, TX) can also be placed between the lens and camera. This allows measurement of blood flow velocity in larger vessels ($\geq$60 μm), which can then be converted to flow by the equation

$$(V/1.6)(0.001\ R^2),$$

where V is centerline velocity, dividing by 1.6 converts centerline velocity to average cross-sectional velocity, R is the intraluminal radius (μm), and multiplying by 0.001 converts to nanoliters/second (30, 31).

Because epiillumination is used from above, this can often be performed *in situ* with little need for direct tissue preparation and manipulation (23, 24, 27–29). Liver microcirculation can be performed *in situ* during either *in vivo* perfusion conditions or with isolated perfusion techniques.

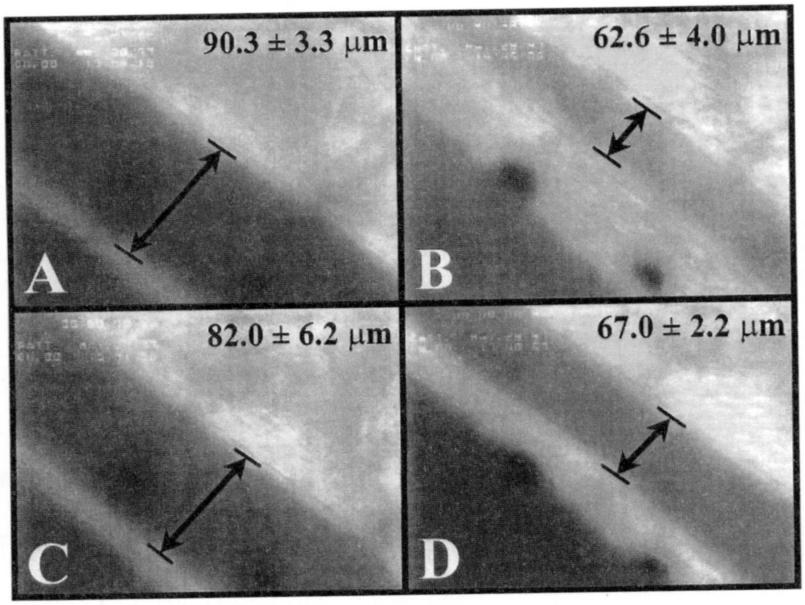

Figure 1 Series of representative images of an intestinal A1 inflow arteriole during the various stages of hemorrhage and resuscitation. (A) Baseline. (B) During hemorrhage. (C) End resuscitation. (D) After resuscitation (2 hr). (See color plates.)

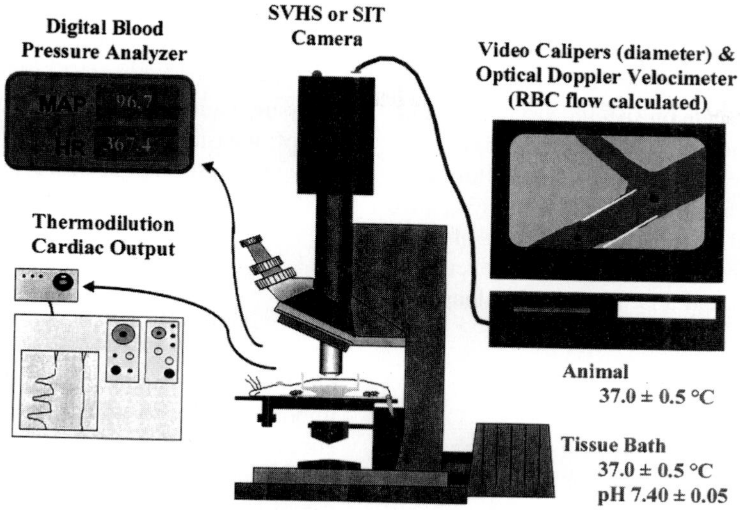

Figure 2 Schematic representation of intestinal intravital videomicroscopy setup. (See color plates.)

Several excellent descriptions of this technique are available (23, 24, 32). Briefly, the preparation is positioned on the microscope stage with the liver under a water-immersion objective. A fiber optic light source can be used to epiilluminate the liver (example, KL 1500, Schott Glaswerke, Wiesbaden, Germany). Fluorescent techniques are very useful in the liver and therefore may require a fluorescent microscope (example, Axiotech Vario 100, Carl Zeiss, Jena, Germany). Digital image processing systems provide on-line enhancement for better resolution (example, Argus-20 Image Processor, Hamamatsu Photonics, Hamamatsu City, Japan) (23, 24).

Study of the lung microcirculation is somewhat more complicated and labor intensive (27–29). First, a thoracotomy must be performed, which results in some physiologic stress. Second, positive pressure ventilation is required, which may alter blood flow and may hinder reliability of measurements due to respiratory movement. Finally, only subpleural vessels can be observed and may not represent the entire microvasculature. Despite these limitations, lung microcirculation studies still provide an excellent means to assess organ blood flow.

Both the small intestine and the cremaster muscle must be exteriorized for transillumination. This requires both specialized surgical preparation and maintenance of physiologic conditions during the microcirculation studies. The surgical techniques for the various tissues (cremaster, intestine, mesentery, kidney) have been described extensively (8, 10, 11, 13–16, 33–35). Briefly, the key to successful study is minimal handling and manipulation of the tissue. Once exteriorized, the tissue is maintained in a physiologic bath (Fig. 3). Temperature is regulated with a heating coil in the bath that is servoregulated by a temperature probe. Carbon dioxide (CO_2) and nitrogen can be bubbled through the tissue bath to maintain pO_2 at 30–55 mmHg, pCO_2 at 35–45 mmHg, and pH at 7.40 ± 0.05. The tissue is bathed in a physiologic solution, generally a Kreb's, that may or may not contain glucose, depending on the tissue type.

In vivo videomicroscopy can also be used to assess vascular permeability and endothelial cell–leukocyte interactions. Briefly, in these techniques a fluorescent light source is used to activate a fluorescence-emitting compound. For vascular permeability, fluorescein isothiocyanate (FITC)-labeled dextran or albumin is often used (10, 27, 28, 33, 35). FITC has an excitation wavelength of 420–490 nm and an emission wavelength of 520 nm. Emitted light can be detected at low light levels with a fluorescent camera (example, model C-2400-08, Hamamatsu Photonics, Hamamatsu, Japan). The degree of perivascular leak is assessed by determining the change in fluorescence in a specific area before and after treatment or by comparing it to unaffected areas

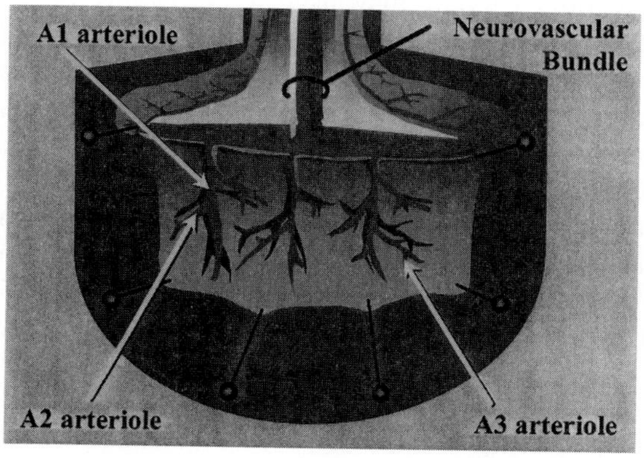

Figure 3 Schematic representation of exteriorized small intestine in tissue bath. (See color plates.)

(27, 28, 35). A variety of image capture systems and analysis software programs (examples; Visionplus AT-OFG, Imaging Technology, Bedford, MA; Optimas, Bioscan, Edmonds, WA) allow one to gate on specific areas and quantify changes based on a standardized grey scale (36).

Fluorescent techniques can also be used to follow neutrophil rolling, adhesion, and tissue migration (37, 38). Leukocytes may be labeled *in vivo* with a variety of compounds, such as Rhodamine-6G, which has an excitation wavelength of 510–560 nm and an emission wavelength of 590 nm (38).

B. Advantages

The main advantage of *in vivo* videomicroscopy techniques is that they allow physiologic assessment of microvascular blood flow. The vessel is perfused with blood in a physiologic environment with an intact neurovascular bundle. Therefore, this represents real-time visualization of the physiology. In addition, microvascular reactivity of both the endothelial cell and vascular smooth muscle cell can be assessed by addition to the tissue bath of vasoactive agonists and antagonists (39, 40). A dose–response curve can be generated by sequential addition of increasing doses of drug. Then, the dose required either to effect or to inhibit a response by a certain percentage (effective dose concentration 50%, EC_{50}, or inhibitory dose concentration 50%, IC_{50}) can be calculated as an index of vascular reactivity.

There are several other advantages. Vascular permeability and endothelial cell–leukocyte interactions can be assessed. Systemic hemodynamics, such as blood pressure and cardiac output, can also be measured simultaneously while tissue conditions in the bath are controlled and manipulated. This allows separate analysis of local microvascular control events from systemic cardiovascular responses.

C. Disadvantages

The main disadvantage of *in vivo* videomicroscopy is the long learning curve. It may take several months for an individual to master the delicate nuances of this technique. Some of the tissue models are pathologic models, such as that for hydronephrotic kidney, or require significant preparation, such as that for lung. Additionally, *in vivo* videomicroscopy is not widely used. A new investigator trying to establish a microcirculation laboratory may have a hard time finding collaborators or consultants who can act as a resource for trouble-shooting problems, which are numerous.

The experiments are very time-consuming, generally taking a full day to complete for a single animal. Although one of the advantages of videomicroscopy is the ability to assess *in vivo* physiology, this may also be a disadvantage. Numerous variables in these experiments are hard to control. These include systemic factors, especially cardiovascular function and neurohormonal input, anesthetic effects, and also some local factors. Upstream and downstream vessel feedback and arterial–venous interactions may be difficult to control. Due to tissue manipulation, these techniques allow only a single set of measurements and currently are not amenable to repeated or continuous observation in an animal over time.

III. Isolated Microvessels

Regulation of arteriolar tone is a complex phenomenon dependent on a host of systemic and local factors. Among the local factors, pressure and flow (i.e., shear stress) are important (41). As noted above, controlling systemic influences using *in vivo* techniques can be very difficult. A technique that may overcome some of these shortcomings is the use of isolated microvessels.

A. Technique

The tissue under study is excised and placed into a refrigerated dissecting dish with a physiologic buffer (41, 42, 43). The vessel of interest is then dissected free, generally using an operating microscope. The free ends are then cannulated and secured onto pipettes. The pipettes are connected to pressure transducers to allow measurement of intraluminal pressure. The pipettes can also be attached to servoregulators to regulate and manipulate intraluminal pressures. The vessel chamber can be connected to a fluid reservoir and a perfusion pump, which allows manipulation and control of flow conditions. The pipette system is mounted under a closed-circuit videomicroscopy system, similar to that described for *in vivo* videomicroscopy. The system is allowed to equilibrate, usually for 30–60 min. After this time, the vessel is assessed for suitability of use. The criteria include return of spontaneous tone, reactivity to vasoactive mediators, and myogenic responsiveness (42–44). A key issue in preparing these tissues is to ensure that the endothelium has not been injured.

Under this system, vessel diameter changes can be measured as a function of changes in either flow or pressure as they are manipulated (41–43). Addition to the perfusate of vasoactive mediators or pharmacologic agonists and antagonist, or variations in electrolyte concentrations such as calcium, can be used to assess endothelial and vascular smooth muscle cell responsiveness (11, 41–43, 45).

The endothelium of a microvessel can be removed, either by physically denuding (42, 43) or by air perfusion (45). Adequate removal of the endothelium is confirmed by the absence of response to an endothelial-dependent vasodilator such as acetylcholine. The functional capacity of a vessel to dilate can be determined with an endothelial-independent vasodilator, such as adenosine or nitroprusside. This facilitates direct assessment of vascular smooth muscle cell responsiveness. Comparing responses before and after removal of the endothelium provides a method to investigate the influence of the endothelium on vascular smooth cell responses.

B. Advantages

The isolated microvessel technique overcomes some of the disadvantages of *in vivo* videomicroscopy. All systemic and neurohumoral influences are eliminated, which removes them as confounding variables. The investigator has strict control over baseline conditions, which can be reliably reproduced. Therefore, responses can be more directly attributed to intrinsic properties of the vessel. This is very important when investigating conditions such as hypertension, diabetes, or endotoxemia, which may alter both systemic hemodynamics and intrinsic microvascular reactivity.

C. Disadvantages

Conversely, the disadvantages of this system are that it is nonphysiologic and often nonperfused, at least not pulsatile. Only a single vessel can be studied at a time and thus repeated or chronic measurements on the same vessel cannot be done. There are size limitations mostly based on the ability to dissect the vessel without injury and the size of the mounting pipette. Many of these technical limitations can be overcome by the ability to strictly control and manipulate the vessel and its environment.

IV. Laser Doppler Flowmetry

A. Technique

With this technology, a laser signal is emitted from a probe. Laser Doppler flowmetry relies on the Doppler effect, whereby the frequency of the returned light signal is shifted by moving objects. The depth of penetration is determined by the wavelength of emitted light, and the shape is determined by the probe configuration. Therefore, this system measures red blood cell movement in a fixed volume of tissue, which is then an indirect measure of red blood cell flow or flux. There is a small zone of injury around the tip of the probe, but the penetration of the signal is greater and therefore is measuring flux in normal tissues. A variety of probes can be used. Surface probes are frequently used in the liver and can also be placed on the gastric or rectal mucosa (46, 47, 48). Implantable probes can also be used in the parenchyma of solid organs, including liver, kidney, and brain (49–51).

B. Advantages

The main advantage is the simplicity of use and relative low cost. Multiple probes can be used in the same animal, therefore it is possible to assess regional changes in blood flow. Also, different wavelength lasers can be used within one organ to measure blood flow at various tissue depths (52–54).

C. Disadvantages

The laser Doppler measures only movement and therefore is not directional. Calibration may be difficult and probe function is position dependent. Therefore, results are usually only given in nondescript, relative perfusion units, not absolute values (55). For this reason it is very difficult to compare baseline flow among groups of animals and results are generally given as a percent change from a somewhat arbitrary baseline. Laser Doppler scanning, which integrates the signal over a given area, may improve reproducibility compared to single-point laser Doppler flowmetry (56).

D. Clinical Utility

Clinical applicability of microcirculation techniques has been limited by several factors, including equipment, access to organs or tissue of interest, and reproducibility. Most clinical studies have relied on indirect techniques such as gastric tonometry (57, 58). Laser Doppler technology, however, has made significant progress in several clinical arenas.

Assessment of gut perfusion using gastric laser doppler flowmetry or scanning has been used in several clinical circumstances, including septic shock (58, 59) and during cardiopulmonary bypass (57). It has also been used to document gastric blood flow following mobilization during esophagectomy (55). Laser Doppler has proved to be beneficial in the planning and postoperative monitoring of free flaps (60, 61) and has been used extensively to investigate a variety of ophthalmologic (62, 63) and skin disorders (64, 65).

V. Microspheres

A. Technique

Another well-established method to study microvascular blood flow distribution is through the use of labeled microspheres. In this technique, polysytrene spheres (typically 15 μm in diameter) are injected into the central circulation, usually through the left atrium. The spheres are allowed to circulate under physiologic conditions as a reflection of regional blood flow distribution. Immediately prior to injection, blood is withdrawn from the femoral artery at constant rate; this is continued for at least two cardiac cycles after injection (usually 70–120 sec). This blood serves as a reference sample, allowing quantitation of blood flow.

Microspheres can be labeled by a variety of techniques. Originally the technique employed radiolabeling, but fluorescent and colorimetric microspheres are now commercially available. These new methods correlate very closely with use of radiolabeled microspheres ($r = 0.96$ to 0.99) (66–68). One advantage of the colorimetric spheres is that up to five different colors can be used in the same animal, each representing a different time point (67).

B. Advantages

The main advantage of this technique is its relative simplicity; the only problem in small animals is difficulty in obtaining central access. Microspheres allow simultaneous assessment of blood flow to multiple organs (67, 69). Another major advantage is the ability to measure blood flow in organs and tissues not accessible with other techniques.

C. Disadvantages

The primary disadvantage of micospheres is that they can measure blood flow at fixed time points and are not continuous. The number of time points, however, may be limited by the amount of blood lost with the reference sample technique, especially in small animals. This technique also relies on good central mixing so that recovery accurately reflects blood flow distribution. The difference between the right and left kidneys can be used as an indicator of adequate mixing. Differences should be less than 10%. Originally, there was concern that the microspheres would occlude small vessels and thus cause blood flow redistribution. It appears that most microspheres attach to the sidewall of larger arterioles ($\approx$100 μm) and have little effect on blood flow.

Although the assay for radioactivity is relatively simple, the fluorescent and colorimetric assays are somewhat laborious and time consuming. However, they avoid difficulties associated with handling and disposing of radioactive material.

VI. Indirect Techniques

There are various techniques that indirectly assess organ blood flow. Most rely on clearance of a compound from the organ of interest, usually under conditions in which clearance is determined by blood flow. Examples include renal blood flow and *p*-aminohippuric acid (PAH) (70, 71), hepatic blood flow and indocyanine green, lidocaine or galactose clearance, and cerebral blood flow and hydrogen clearance (72–75). These techniques may also provide insight into the metabolic function of an organ.

VII. Summary

Microcirculatory techniques provide a powerful tool to investigate regional blood flow and to assess microvascular reactivity, vascular permeability, and endothelial cell–leukocyte interactions. This is best accomplished using either *in vivo* videomicroscopy or the isolated vessel technique. The main disadvantages of these techniques are their difficulty and high cost.

Various other less arduous techniques are available to assess regional and microcirculatory blood flow (laser doppler, microspheres, clearance techniques). In general, these are more straightforward and less demanding. Although they are excellent at assessing regional blood flow, they do not allow delineation of vascular reactivity comparable to the videomicroscopy techniques. It is also very difficult to separate changes in central hemodynamic responses from changes in organ-specific blood flow regulation using these indirect clearance techniques. However, they may be very useful adjuncts when combined with direct microcirculation studies.

VIII. Resources

The following resources are available on Internet web sites related to microcirculation research.

A. Research Centers

Microcirculation Research Institute, Department of Medical Physiology, Texas A&M University
http://mphywww.tamu.edu/MRI.html

Microcirculation Division, Arizona Research Laboratories, University of Arizona
http://dept.physiol.arizona.edu/secomb/arlmicro.html

UCSD Department of Bioengineering
http://www-bioeng.ucsd.edu/

B. Research Societies

Microcirculation Society
http://microcirc.org/

The British Microcirculation Society
http://www.microcirculation.org.uk/

European Society for Microcirculation
http://www.medizin.fu-berlin.de/esm/

Asian Union for Microcirculation
http://www.asahi-net.or.jp/~sb9h-nim/index.html

C. Journals

Microcirculation
http://www.stockton-press.co.uk/mn

Microvascular Research
http://darwin.apnet.com/www/journal/mr.htm

Journal of Vascular Research
http://www.karger.ch/journals/jvr/jvr jh.htm

Circulation
http://circ.ahajournals.org/

Circulation Research
http://circres.ahajournals.org/

D. Industry

Moor Instruments
http://www.moor.co.uk/

Carl Zeiss, Ltd.
http://www.zeiss.co.uk/

Hamamatsu Photonics KK
http://www.hamamatsu.co.uk/

KK Research Technology Limited
http://cbr.nc.us.mensa.org/homepages/kktech/index.htm

Polysciences, Inc.
http://www.polysciences.com/

Triton Technology, Inc.
http://www.physiology.com/

References

1. Wang, P., Ba, Z., and Chaudry, I. H. (1993). Endothelial cell dysfunction occurs very early following trauma-hemorrhage and persists despite fluid resuscitation. *Am. J. Physiol.* **265,** H973–H979.
2. Fry, D. E., Silver, B. B., Rink, R. D., VanArsdall, L. R., and Flint, L. M., Jr. (1979). Hepatic cellular hypoxia in murine peritonitis. *Surgery* **85,** 652–661.
3. Palombo, J. D., Blackburn, G. L., and Forse, R. A. (1991). Endothelial factors and response to injury. *Surg. Gynecol. Obstet.* **173,** 505–518.
4. Zweier, J. L., Kuppusamy, P., and Lutty, G. A. (1988). Measurement of endothelial cell free radical generation: Evidence for a central mechanism of free radical injury in postischemic tissues. *Proc. Natl. Acad. Sci. U.S.A.* **85,** 4046–4050.
5. Law, M. M., Cryer, H. G., and Abraham, E. (1994). Elevated levels of soluble ICAM-1 correlate with the development of multiple organ failure in severely injured trauma patients *J. Trauma* **37,** 100–109.
6. Turnage, R. H., Kadesky, K. M., Rogers, T., Hernandez, R., Bartula, L., and Myers, S. I. (1995). Neutrophil regulation of splanchnic blood flow after hemorrhagic shock. *Ann. Surg.* **222,** 66–72.
7. Cain, B. S., Meldrum, D. R., Selzman, C. H., Cleveland, J. C., Jr., Meng, X., Sheridan, B. C., Banerjee, A., and Harken, A. H. (1997). Surgical implications of vascular endothelial physiology. *Surgery* **122,** 516–526.
8. Spain, D. A., Wilson, M. A., and Garrison, R. N. (1994). The role of nitric oxide in regulation of the rat small intestinal microcirculation during bacteremia. *Shock* **2,** 41–46.
9. Fruchterman, T. M., Spain, D. A., Wilson, M. A., Harris, P. D., and Garrison, R. N. Complement inhibition prevents gut ischemia and endothelial dysfunction after hemorrhage and resuscitation. *Surgery* **124,** 782–792.
10. Madorin, W. S., Martin, C. M., and Sibbald, W. J. (1999). Dopexamine attenuates flow motion in ileal mucosal arterioles in normotensive sepsis. *Crit. Care. Med.* **27,** 394–400.
11. Arii, T., Ohyanagi, M., Shibuya, J., and Iwasaki, T. (1999). Increased function of the voltage-dependent calcium channels, without increase Ca^{2+} rlease from the sarcoplasmic reticulum in the arterioles of spontaneous hypertensive rats. *Am. J. Hypertens.* **12,** 1236–1242.
12. Frisbee, J. C., and Lombard, J. H. (1999). Elevated oxygen tension inhibits flow-induced dilation of skeletal muscle arterioles. *Microvasc. Res.* **58,** 99–107.
13. Miller, F. N., and Wegman, D. L. (1977). Anesthesia-induced alterations of small vessel responses to norepinephrine. *Eur. J. Pharmacol.* **44,** 331–337.
14. Steinhausen, M., Snoei, H., Parekh, N., Baker, R., and Johnson, P. C. (1983). A new method to visualize vas afferens, efferens and glomerular networks. *Kidney Int.* **23,** 794–806.
15. Steinhausen, M., Blum, M., Fleming, J. T., Holz, F. G., Parekh, N., and Wiegman, D. L. (1989). Visualization of renal autoregulation in the split hydronephrotic kidney of rats. *Kidney Int.* **35,** 1151–1160.
16. Spain, D. A., Wilson, M. A., Bloom, I. T. M., and Garrison, R. N. (1994). Renal microvascular responses to sepsis are dependent on nitric oxide. *J. Surg. Res.* **56,** 524–529.
17. Mayhan, W. G., and Sharpe, G. M. (1999). Chronic exposure to nicotine alters endothelium-dependent arteriolar dilatation: Effect of superoxide dismutase. *J. Appl. Physiol.* **86,** 1126–1134.
18. Rivers, R. J. (1999). Pharmacologic study of muscarinic receptor subtypes and arteriolar dilations: A comparison of conducted and local responses. *J. Cardiovasc. Pharmacol.* **33,** 388–393.
19. Li, Z., Koman, L. A., Rosencrance, E., Smith, B. P., and Smith, T. L. (1998). Endogenous nitric oxide influences arteriovenous anastomosis adrenergic tone in the conscious rabbit ear. *J. Cardiovasc. Pharmacol.* **32,** 349–356.
20. Li, Z., Koman, L. A., Smith, B. P., Gordon, E. S., and Smith, T. L. (1998). Alpha adrenoceptors in the rabbit ear thermoregulatory microcirculation. *Microvasc. Res.* **55,** 115–123.
21. Ichioka, S., Shibata, M., Kosaki, K., Sato, Y., Harii, K., and Kamiya, A. (1998). *In vivo* measurement of morphometric and hemodynamic changes in the microcirculation during angiogenesis under chronic alpha1-adrenergic blocker treatment. *Microvasc. Res.* **55,** 165–174.
22. Katada, J., Muramatsu, M., Hayashi, M., and Hattori, M. (1999). Role of mast cell chymase in angiotensin-induced vascular contraction of hamster cheek pouch microvessels. *Eur. J. Pharmacol.* **379,** 63–72.
23. Pannen, B. H., Kohler, N., Hole, B., Bauer, M., Clemens, M. G., and Geiger, K. K. (1998). Protective role of endogenous carbon monoxide

in hepatic microcirculatory dysfunction after hemorrhagic shock in rats. *J. Clin. Invest.* **102,** 1220–1228.

24. Pannen, B. H. J., Bauer, M., Zhang, J. X., Robotham, J. L., and Clemens, M. G. (1996). A time-dependent balance between endothelins and nitric oxide regulating portal resistance after endotoxin. *Am. J. Physiol.* **271,** H1953–H1961.
25. Plusczyk, T., Bersal, B., Westermann, S., Menger, M., and Feifel, G. (1999). ET-1 induces pancreatitis-like microvascular deterioration and acinar cell injury. *J. Surg. Res.* **85,** 301–310.
26. von Dobschuetz, E., Hoffmann, T., and Messmer, K. (1999). Diaspirin cross-linked hemoglobin effectively restores pancreatic microcirculatory failure in hemorrhagic shock. *Anesthesiology* **91,** 1754–1762.
27. Carter, M. B., Wilson, M. A., Wead, W. B., Garrison, R. N. (1995). Pentoxifylline attenuates pulmonary macromolecular leakage after intestinal ischemia-reperfusion. *Arch. Surg.* **130,** 1337–1344.
28. Carter, M. B., Wilson, M. A., Wead, W. B., and Garrison, R. N. (1996). Platelet-activating factor mediates pulmonary macromolecular leak following intestinal ischemia–reperfusion. *J. Surg. Res.* **60,** 403–408.
29. Mitsuoka, H., Unno, N., Sakurai, T., Kaneko, H., Suzuki, S., Konno, H., Terakawa, S., and Nakamura, S. (1999). Pathophysiological role of endothelins in pulmonary microcirculatory disorders due to intestinal ischemia and reperfusion. *J. Surg. Res.* **87,** 143–151.
30. Borders, J. L., and Granger, H. J. (1984). An optical Doppler intravital velocimeter. *Microvasc. Res.* **27,** 117–127.
31. Lee, J. S., and Duling, B. R. (1989). Role of flow dispersion in the computation of microvascular flows by dual-slit method. *Microvasc. Res.* **37,** 280–288.
32. Clemens, M. G., and Zhang, J. X. (1999). Regulation of sinusoidal perfusion: *In vivo* methodology and control by endothelins. *Semin. Liver Dis.* **19,** 383–396.
33. Fox-Robichaud, A., Payne, D., and Kubes, P. (1999). Inhaled NO reaches distal vasculatures to inhibit endothelium- but not leukocyte-dependent cell adhesion. *Am. J. Physiol.* **277,** L1224–L1231.
34. Kubes, P. (1997). The role of shear forces in ischemia/reperfusion-induced neutrophil rolling and adhesion. *J. Leukoc. Biol.* **62,** 458–464.
35. Hickey, M. J., Issekutz, A. C., Reinhardt, P. H., Fedorak, R. N., and Kubes, P. (1998). Endogenous interleukin-10 regulates hemodynamic parameters, leukocyte-endothelial cell interactions, and microvascular permeability during endotoxemia. *Circ. Res.* **83,** 1124–1131.
36. Venturoli, D., Crisafulli, B., Del Fsbbbro, M., Negrinr, D., and Miserocchi, G. (1995). Estimation of *in vivo* pulmonary microvascular and interstitial geometry using digital image analysis. *Microcirculation* **2,** 27–40.
37. Massberg, S., Eisenmenger, S., Enders, G., Krombach, F., and Messmer, K. (1998). Quantitative analysis of small intestinal microcirculation in the mouse. *Res. Exp. Med.* **98,** 23–35.
38. Finkenauer, V., Bissinger, T., Funk, R. H., Karbowski, A., and Seiffge, D. (1999). Confocal laser microscopy of leukocyte adhesion in the microcirculation of the inflamed rat knee joint capsule. *Microcirculation* **6,** 141–152.
39. Spain, D. A., Wilson, M. A., Krysztopik, R. J., Matheson, P. J., and Garrison, R. N. (1997). Differential intestinal microvascular dysfunction occurs during bacteremia. *J. Surg. Res.* **67,** 67–71.
40. Tucker, J. J., Wilson, M. A., Wead, W. B., and Garrison, R. N. (1998). Microvascular endothelial cell control of peripheral vascular resistance during sepsis. *Arch. Surg.* **133,** 1335–1342.
41. Sun, D., Huang, A., Koller, A., and Kaley, G. (1995). Flow-dependent dilation and myogenic constriction interact to establish the resistance of skeletal muscle arterioles. *Microcirculation* **3,** 289–295.
42. Falcone, J. C., and Meininger, G. A. (1996). Endothelin mediates a component of the enhanced myogenic responsiveness of arterioles from hypertensive rats. *Microcirculation* **6,** 305–313.
43. Falcone, J. C., Davis, M. J., and Meininger, G. A. (1991). Endothelial independence of myogenic response in isolated skeletal muscle arterioles *Am. J. Physiol.* **260,** H130–H135.
44. Kuo, L., Davis, M. J., and Chilian, W. M. (1988). Myogenic activity in isolated subepicardial and subendocardial coronary arterioles. *Am. J. Physiol.* **255,** H1558–H1562.
45. Koller, A., Sun, D., and Kaley, G. (1993). Role of shear stress and endothelial prostaglandins in flow- and viscosity-induced dilation of arteioles *in vitro. Circ. Res.* **72,** 1276–1284.
46. Klar, E., Kraus, T., Bleyl, J., Newman, W. H., Bowman, H. F., Hofmann, W. J., Kummer, R., Bredt, M., and Herfarth, C. (1999). Thermodiffusion for continuous quantification of hepatic microcirculation—Validation and potential in liver transplantation. *Microvasc. Res.* **58,** 156–166.
47. Seifalian, A. M., Piasecki, C., Agarwal, A., and Davidson, B. R. (1999). The effects of graded steatosis on flow in the hepatic parenchymal microcirculation. *Transplantation* **68,** 780–784.
48. Emmanuel, A. V., and Kamm, M. A. (2000). Laser Doppler flowmetry as a measure of extrinsic colonic innervation in functional bowel disease. *Gut* **46,** 212–217.
49. Garrison, R. N., Wilson, M. A., Matheson, P. J., and Spain, D. A. (1995). Nitric oxide mediates redistribution of intrarenal blood flow during bacteremia. *J. Trauma* **39,** 90–97.
50. Spain, D. A., Wilson, M. A., Theuer, H. H., and Garrison, R. N. (1996). Nitric oxide: A compensatory mediator of bacteremia-induced visceral microvascular hypoperfusion. *In* "Proceeding of the 3rd International Congress on the Immune Consequences of Trauma, Shock and Sepsis" (E. Faist, ed.), pp. 710–714. Pabst Science Publishers, Lengerich, Germany.
51. Zou, A. P., Billington, H., Su, N., and Cowley, A. W., Jr. (2000). Expression and actions of heme oxygenase in the renal medulla of rats. *Hypertension* **35,** 342–347.
52. Forrester, K., Doschak, M., and Bray, R. (1997). *In vivo* comparison of scanning technique and wavelength in laser Doppler perfusion imaging: Measurement in knee ligaments of adult rabbits. *Med. Biol. Eng. Comput.* **35,** 581–586.
53. Malanin, K., Vilkko, P., and Kolari, P. J. (1998). Venoarteriolar response to experimental venous hypertension in legs with chronic venous insufficiency and in healthy legs, measured using a double-wavelength laser Doppler technique. *Angiology* **49,** 729–733.
54. Fabricius, M., Akgoren, N., Dirnagl, U., and Lauritzen, M. (1997). Laminar analysis of cerebral blood flow in cortex of rats by laser-Doppler flowmetry: A pilot study. *J. Cerebr. Blood Flow Metab.* **17,** 1326–1336.
55. Boyle, N. H., Pearce, A., Hunter, D., Owen, W. J., and Mason, R. C. (1999). Intraoperative scanning laser Doppler flowmetry in the assessment of gastric tube perfusion during esophageal resection. *J. Am. Coll. Surg.* **188,** 498–502.
56. Ances, B. M., Greenberg, J. H., and Detre, J. A. (1999). Laser doppler imaging of activation-flow coupling in the rat somatosensory cortex. *Neuroimage* **10,** 716–723.
57. Ohri, S. K., Bowles, C. W., Mathie, R. T., Lawrence, D. R., Keogh, B. E., and Taylor, K. M. (1997). Effect of cardiopulmonary bypass perfusion protocols on gut tissue oxygenation and blood flow. *Ann. Thorac. Surg.* **64,** 163–170.
58. Duranteau, J., Sitbon, P., Teboul, J. L., Vicaut, E., Anguel, N., Richard, C., and Samii, K. (1999). Effects of epinephrine, norepinephrine, or the combination of norepinephrine and dobutamine on gastric mucosa in septic shock. *Crit. Care Med.* **27,** 893–900.
59. Elizalde, J. I., Hernandez, C., Llach, J., Monton, C., Bordas, J. M., Pique, J. M., and Torres, A. (1998). Gastric intramucosal acidosis in mechanically ventilated patients: Role of mucosal blood flow. *Crit. Care Med.* **26**(5), 827–832.

60. Yuen, J. C., and Feng, Z. (2000). Monitoring free flaps using the laser Doppler flowmeter: Five-year experience. *Plast. Reconstr. Surg.* **105,** 55–61.
61. Yoshino, K., Nara, S., Endo, M., and Kamata, N. (1996). Intraoral free flap monitoring with a laser Doppler flowmeter. *Microsurgery* **17,** 337–340.
62. Harris, A., Chung, H. S., Ciulla, T. A., and Kagemann, L. (1999). Progress in measurement of ocular blood flow and relevance to our understanding of glaucoma and age-related macular degeneration. *Prog. Retin. Eye Res.* **18,** 669–687.
63. Chung, H. S., Harris, A., Halter, P. J., Kagemann, L., Roff, E. J., Garzozi, H. J., Hosking, S. L., and Martin, B. J. (1999). Regional differences in retinal vascular reactivity. *Invest. Ophthalmol. Vis. Sci.* **40,** 2448–2453.
64. Tucker, A. T., Pearson, R. M., Cooke, E. D., and Benjamin, N. (1999). Effect of nitric-oxide-generating system on microcirculatory blood flow in skin of patients with severe Raynaud's syndrome: A randomised trial. *Lancet* **354,** 1670–1675.
65. Clark, S., Campbell, F., Moore, T., Jayson, M. I., King, T. A., and Herrick, A. L. (1999). Laser doppler imaging—A new technique for quantifying microcirculatory flow in patients with primary Raynaud's phenomenon and systemic sclerosis. *Microvasc. Res.* **57,** 284–291.
66. Glenny, R. W., Bernard, S., and Brinkley, M. (1993). Validation of fluorescent-labeled microspheres for measurement of regional organ perfusion. *J. Appl. Physiol.* **74,** 2585–2597.
67. Kowallik, P., Schulz, R., Guth, B. D., Schade, A., Paffhausen, W., Gross, R., and Heusch, G. (1991). Measurement of regional myocardial blood flow with multiple colored microspheres. *Circulation* **83,** 974–982.
68. Walter, B., Bauer, R., Gaser, E., and Zwiener, U. (1997). Validation of the multiple colored microsphere technique for regional blood flow measurements in newborn piglets. *Basic Res. Cardiol.* **92,** 191–200.
69. Hakkinen, J. P., Miller, M. W., Smith, A. H., and Knight, D. R. (1995). Measurement of organ blood flow with coloured microspheres in the rat. *Cardiovasc. Res.* **29,** 74–79.
70. Koller-Strametz, J., Wolzt, M., Fuchs, C., Putz, D., Wisser, W., Mensik, C., Eichler, H. G., Laufer, G., and Schmetterer, L. (1999). Renal hemodynamic effects of L-arginine and sodium nitroprusside in heart transplant recipients. *Kidney Int.* **55,** 1871–1877.
71. Laroute, V., Lefebvre, H. P., Costes, G., and Toutain, P. L. (1999). Measurement of glomerular filtration rate and effective renal plasma flow in the conscious beagle dog by single intravenous bolus of iohexol and p-aminohippuric acid. *J. Pharmacol. Toxicol. Methods* **41,** 17–25.
72. Maynard, N. D., Bihari, D. J., Dalton, R. N., Beale, R., Smithies, M. N., and Mason, R. C. (1997). Liver function and splanchnic ischemia in critically ill patients. *Chest* **111,** 180–187.
73. Purcell, P. N., Branson, R. D., Schroeder, T. J., Davis, K., Jr., and Johnson, D. J. (1992). Monoethylglycinexylidide production parallels changes in hepatic blood flow and oxygen delivery in lung injury managed with positive end-expiratory pressure. *J. Trauma* **33,** 482–486.
74. Schirmer, W. J., Townsend, M. C., Schirmer, J. M., Hampton, W. W., and Fry, D. E. (1987). Galactose elimination kinetics in sepsis. Correlations of hepatic blood blow with function. *Arch. Surg.* **122,** 349–354.
75. Joo, E. H., and Lee, Y. B. (1998). No effect of diltiazem on the hepatic clearance of indocyanine green in the rats. *Arch. Pharm. Res.* **21,** 411–417.

74

Blood Substitutes in Surgery

Gus J. Vlahakes

Massachusetts General Hospital and Harvard Medical School, Boston, Massachusetts 02114

I. Introduction

In the 1980s, tremendous public concern was focused on the safety of the national blood supply. Although efforts to create alternatives to homologous blood transfusion have been ongoing for decades, the effort to develop safe and efficacious blood substitutes accelerated in the 1980s. Although the impetus for this rapid development was driven by concerns about disease transmission, it is now recognized that blood transfusions have additional consequences, such as immunosuppression with impaired host defenses, and alloimmunization and its implications for future organ transplantation. In some parts of the world, blood supply has continued to be a problem, either because of lack of an organized national blood bank system, or inadequate supply at times of unexpected demands. Furthermore, despite the significant reduction in the risk of human immunodeficiency virus (HIV) and hepatitis infections, improvements that resulted from antibody and antigen screening, there still remains ongoing public concern over even the low risk of infection. Approximately 60% of blood transfusions (30 million units annually, worldwide) are infused in conjunction with surgical blood loss (1). Consequently, there remains an important place in the field of surgery and its subspecialties for safe and efficacious blood substitutes.

II. General Principles

An ideal blood substitute should be available in large quantity and should not have associated disease transmission risks. It should be nontoxic for administration in large doses, and it should not require typing or cross-matching. It should be readily available for immediate infusion, particularly for use in settings such as trauma, and should be stable under nominal storage conditions. Most importantly, it should carry and release oxygen under average physiologic conditions, and it should help maintain the circulating blood volume.

Within this field, there have developed two major approaches to blood substitution: the perfluorocarbon (PFC) emulsions and hemoglobin-based oxygen-carrying solutions (HBOCs). Each approach has its own interesting history and distinct physiology. Both types of blood substitutes are currently in intense development by various commercial vendors.

III. Perfluorocarbon Emulsions

A. History

The perfluorocarbon compounds used in this setting are liquid organic compounds in which most or all hydrogen atoms have been replaced by fluorine atoms. Although these materials were initially developed for industrial use in applications such as hydraulic fluids and transformer coolants, their potential as oxygen-carrying compounds became apparent when Clark and Gollan demonstrated their enormous oxygen solubility (2). In their landmark study, they demonstrated that mice could be submerged in oxygenated perfluorocarbon and could survive by liquid breathing of an oxygenated PFC material.

PFC organic liquids have weak intermolecular van der Waals forces, leading to their physical properties (low viscosity, low surface tension), as well as gas solubility (3). However, PFCs are nonpolar molecules immiscible with blood, and thus are unable to dissolve the polar salts and solutes necessary for normal cellular metabolism. Accordingly, when the original PFC compounds were injected systemically, they were highly toxic (4). The solution to this problem was to disperse PFCs into aqueous media in the form of emulsions. Multiple reports subsequently emerged showing blood replacement in animal models, and advances in emulsification technology allowed demonstration of experimental, near-complete blood replacement (5). Although this work was exciting, certain important toxicities and limitations emerged. The PFC emulsion particles are taken up by the reticuloendothelial system (RES), which can be saturated, resulting in impaired host defenses (6). The rate of RES uptake is determined by particle size, with large particles being more rapidly phagocytosed than smaller particles. In early blood replacement studies, the PFC compound used had a 900-day half-life and resulted in substantial, prolonged RES functional blockade. Finally, in the late 1970s, the Green Cross Corporation (Osaka, Japan) developed Fluosol-DA, which consists of a small-particle emulsion containing two perfluorocarbon chemicals: perfluorodecalin (tissue half-life 7 days, with fair emulsification properties) and perfluorotripropylamine (half-life 65 days, with excellent emulsification properties). This combination of PFCs, combined with contemporary emulsification technology, led to the development of Fluosol-DA, which entered clinical trials in Japan (7); in 1980, Fluosol-DA began clinical trials in the United States (8). Although this perfluorocarbon emulsion formulation proved to be an effective volume expander and oxygen carrier at high inspired oxygen concentrations, reports from clinical trials began to reveal the shortcomings and limitations of Fluosol-DA. Clinical studies demonstrated that at low levels of inspired oxygen concentration, this perfluorocarbon formulation had virtually no benefit in oxygen transport, functioning only as a plasma expander (9, 10); a significant contribution to oxygen dynamics occurred only at 100% inspired oxygen.

B. Physiology of PFC Emulsions

Unlike hemoglobin, which demonstrates binding cooperativity and a sigmoidal oxygen binding curve, PFCs carry oxygen by simple dissolution. As shown in Fig. 1, oxygen content is linearly related to oxygen tension and contrasts to the relationship shown for hemoglobin, where maximal oxygen-carrying capacity is reached at lower levels of inspired oxygen concentration, certainly within the range of clinical usefulness. One strategy to overcome this shortcoming is to administer larger doses of PFC. However, the total dose of PFC administration is still limited by dose-dependent blockade of the RES. Perfluorocarbon toxicity to macrophages may be related to uptake of the oxygenated emulsion particles by phagocytic cells (11); the delivery of oxygen into the cells may overwhelm the normal macrophage capacity to remove oxygen free radicals, thus resulting in oxidative cell damage. Because of these limitations, PFC development for systemic use as a blood substitute has been relatively slow.

C. Current Clinical Applications of PFC Emulsions

More recently, contemporary PFCs have been proposed for intraoperative use for normovolemic hemodilution prior to anticipated surgical blood loss (12). Because of the need for high inspired oxygen concentration, the intraoperative environment has been targeted for clinical development of PFC emulsions (13). This concept involves use of PFC emulsions in patients while they are intubated under anesthesia, when the inspired oxygen content is 100%. It has been proposed that a significant portion of the red cell mass can be exchanged out and substituted by PFC emulsion; following completion of surgical blood loss, this reserve of fresh autologous blood can be reinfused. Although not for-

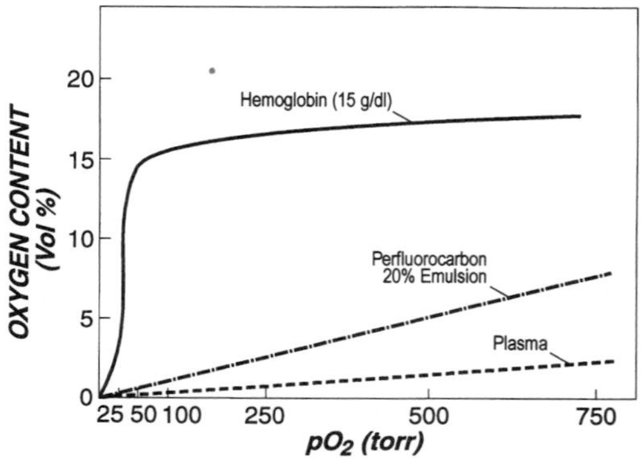

Figure 1 Relationship between oxygen gas tension and oxygen content for hemoglobin, perfluorocarbon emulsions, and the plasma phase.

mally approved for this purpose, a PFC preparation has been studied in a phase II trial (14) and is currently in advanced clinical trials for this application.

Other investigators and commercial vendors have been examining potential applications of PFC emulsions in cardiac surgery, specifically during cardiopulmonary bypass. Patients subjected to extracorporeal circulation, such as that used for cardiac surgery, can experience neuropsychological impairment, and the degree of this impairment is proportional to the length of bypass. Studies using retinal angiography have shown that microemboli occur during bypass and that many of these are gaseous in nature and a natural consequence of having a blood–gas interface in the oxygenator that comprises the extracorporeal circuit. A PFC emulsion has been used in low doses to prevent this, possibly by scavenging microemboli by dissolution into PFC emulsion particles (15).

The current generation of PFC emulsions has overcome some of the earlier concerns about prolonged excretion and emulsion instability. Current-generation materials are in phase III clinical trials for applications in environments where breathing high inspired oxygen concentrations is common, such as during anesthesia, and it is anticipated that if clinical trials are successful, that this will represent the first approved setting for systemic use of perfluorocarbons.

IV. Hemoglobin-Based Oxygen-Carrying Solutions as Blood Substitutes

Most of the current progress in blood substitute development has been in the area of hemoglobin-based oxygen-carrying solutions. Because of its natural oxygen binding and unloading characteristics, the use of stroma-free hemoglobin as a blood substitute has been pursued for well over a century.

A. History

In a 1936 review of the state of blood substitution, attempts at using hemolyzed blood or hemoglobin solutions were noted to date as far back as 1859 (16). Historically, the major obstacle to widespread clinical application of hemoglobin solutions has been the inability to achieve sufficient purification. Early studies using hemoglobin solutions reported frequent toxicities, with the most common toxicities being renal dysfunction and intravascular coagulopathy.

Incremental improvement in techniques used to purify hemoglobin from red blood cells occurred in the 1950s. Despite this, attempts to use these early solutions in patients produced renal failure and coagulopathy; subsequent analysis demonstrated that these early preparations contained substantial stromal phospholipid contamination.

In the 1960s and early 1970s, further advances in hemoglobin purification occurred. In 1967, Rabiner reported a method using hypotonic phosphate buffer to lyse red cells at a slower rate (17). This resulted in larger erythrocyte membrane fragments which could be more completely and easily removed by high-speed centrifugation, the state of the art in purification technology at that time. This led to production of a hemoglobin preparation that, when tested in primates, appeared promising and relatively free of toxicity (18). Using this technology, Savitsky developed a human hemoglobin-based blood substitute, which was tested in a phase I clinical trial in 1978 (19). Unfortunately, the results obtained were unexpected, with temporary but significant adverse changes in renal function, coagulation, and hemodynamics. Further analysis of this hemoglobin preparation demonstrated that it still contained a significant amount of stromal phospholipid (1.2% of that found in raw hemolysate). Thus, even a small amount of phospholipid appeared to produce unacceptable toxicity.

B. Human-Derived Hemoglobin Preparations—The Modern Era

In the early 1980s, as HIV disease was recognized as a major clinical problem, tremendous public attention was directed to the potential risks of disease transmission by transfused blood. Transfusion decision-making was reexamined, and clinicians learned that greater degrees of anemia could be tolerated by most patients, thus decreasing the need for allogeneic transfusions. Despite changes in transfusion practice, antibody screening, and blood conservation techniques, the need for allogeneic transfusions was not eliminated.

During this time, research on blood substitution moved from academic medical centers to commercial laboratories. Modern purification technologies and process engineering were brought to this field. Contemporary ultrafiltration and industrial-scale chromatography were applied to improve hemoglobin purity. Furthermore, because these materials were being used in a manner similar to use of other large-volume parenteral solutions, the same parenteral fluid purity standards, with particular respect to phospholipid and endotoxin contamination, were applied to hemoglobin solutions. The result of this effort was the present generation of HBOCs that are free of the previously observed toxicities. In clinical trials performed with contemporary materials, including materials that reached phase III clinical trials, the previously observed renal and coagulation system toxicities did not occur. Several HBOCs are currently in advanced clinical trials; they differ, in part, because their hemoglobin is derived from different sources.

The most common source of hemoglobin for hemoglobin-based blood substitutes is outdated, banked human blood. Because of its obvious immunologic compatibility in the human circulation, human-derived hemoglobin has been one of the earliest types of hemoglobin tested for potential clinical application. However, when human hemoglobin is removed from erythrocytes and used in the plasma phase, it is in an environment that is devoid of significant amounts of 2,3-diphospoglycerate (DPG). The absence of 2,3-DPG markedly increases hemoglobin affinity for oxygen. In contrast to hemoglobin inside human erythrocytes, the P_{50} decreases from approximately 28 to 12–16 mmHg. Thus, although free hemoglobin in the plasma phase will bind oxygen, it is unable to release it at the tissue level, thus obviating its usefulness as a blood substitute. Because of the relatively short half-life of 2,3-DPG, human hemoglobin cannot be used without chemical modification to adjust its oxygen affinity.

The answer to this problem came with the discovery that allosteric modification of human hemoglobin is relatively easy to achieve. In classic study, Benesh *et al.* (20) demonstrated that pyridoxylation of hemoglobin by covalent binding to pyridoxal phosphate can achieve the same functional effect as 2,3-DPG. This chemical modification solved the problem of excessive oxygen binding of unmodified hemoglobin.

There still remained the other important limitation of a short circulatory half-life of hemoglobin; when hemoglobin was prepared at clinically useful hemoglobin concentrations, the relatively low molecular weight (68,000) resulted in excessive colloid oncotic pressure. Furthermore, the tetrameric hemoglobin molecule is capable is dissociating into α–β hemoglobin dimers, which have a very short circulating half-life and may be associated with significant toxicity. Thus, further modification was needed to achieve physiologic colloid osmotic pressure and to stabilize tetrameric hemoglobin. This was achieved by polymerization with agents such as glutaraldehyde (nonspecific cross-linking) or diaspirin (site-specific cross-linking). Polymerization has two desirable effects: tetrameric hemoglobin is stabilized and does not dissociate into hemoglobin dimers, and larger hemoglobin polymers are produced and decrease oncotic pressure and increase circulating half-life. As a result, polymerized, pyridoxylated human hemoglobin has a physiologic P_{50}, an intravascular persistence time of 24–36 hr, and an acceptable colloid osmotic pressure when prepared at clinically useful hemoglobin concentrations (e.g., 15 g/dl). One such hemoglobin-based blood substitute is currently in phase III clinical trials in the initial management resuscitation of trauma patients (Poly-Heme, Northfield Pharmaceuticals, Chicago, Illinois).

An alternative to using outdated banked blood or selected "pedigree" human volunteer blood donors is recombinant human hemoglobin produced by bacteria or mammals using contemporary genetic engineering techniques and site-specific mutagenesis (21). Hemoglobin generated in this manner can then be subjected to pyridoxylation and subsequent polymerization. It has the theoretical advantage that genetic engineering techniques may allow modification of the primary protein structure to produce alterations in oxygen affinity that will obviate the need for further chemical modification; however, this possibility has not been extensively explored in HBOC development. Although this method of producing human hemoglobin is attractive and is not dependent on the supply of outdated blood, production of recombinant hemoglobin on a large scale remains costly.

C. Bovine-Derived Hemoglobin Preparations

An alternative source material for use in HBOCs is bovine hemoglobin. Bovine hemoglobin differs from human hemoglobin by only 17 amino acids in the hemoglobin α chain and by 24 amino acids in the hemoglobin β chain. Bovine blood is a waste product generated in large quantity in the meatpacking industry. Thus, bovine blood as a source material is readily available at low cost and avoids the potential risks of human disease transmission. Furthermore, bovine hemoglobin has an additional important property. In the cow, hemoglobin affinity is regulated by chloride ions, which control oxygen binding, instead of by 2,3-DPG (22). Thus, for use in humans, bovine hemoglobin does not require further chemical modification: at ambient human plasma chloride levels the resulting hemoglobin P_{50} is 25–30 torr.

A bovine hemoglobin-derived blood substitute is currently in clinical development (Hemopure, Biopure Corp., Cambridge, Massachusetts). This material has completed extensive phase I safety testing and phase II clinical testing in a variety of applications. This material is currently in phase III clinical testing. To date, there have been no findings to suggest human adverse immune responses to bovine hemoglobin.

D. Other Potential Hemoglobin Sources and Approaches

Hemoglobin has been conjugated to other organic molecules, such as polyoxyethylene (23, 24) or polyethylene glycol (25, 26). In addition to increasing vascular persistence time, this approach may also help mask antigenic sites in nonhuman hemoglobin (27).

A novel approach to blood substitution in the early stages of development involves the creation of "synthetic cells" by microencapsulation of hemoglobin. This approach was first described in 1957 (28). In this technology, hemoglobin is encapsulated in one of a variety of synthetic membranes whose permeability can be varied by adjusting membrane chemical composition (29). Furthermore, such artificial cells can also contain other biologically active molecules, such as catalase, methemoglobin reductase, or superoxide dismutase (29, 30). Further contemporary research has also involved the creation of encapsulated hemoglobin using biodegradable polymer microcapsules from polymers such as polylactides and polyglycolides (31).

E. Efficacy Issues in Hemoglobin-Based Oxygen-Carrying Solutions

The majority of experimental and clinical studies using HBOCs have shown that these materials can carry the same amount of oxygen as native erythrocyte-borne hemoglobin at ambient inspired oxygen concentration (1 vol% oxygen per g/dl). Thus, in numerous experimental studies, it has been possible to achieve near-complete replacement of the autologous red cell mass using these materials (32). Furthermore, in addition to tolerability in large blood-replacement doses, the majority of these materials currently in clinical development have an acceptable toxicity profile, with low endotoxin, phospholipid, and pyrogen contaminant contents. The success of these materials in laboratory studies in the 1980s stimulated many industrial vendors to enter this development field.

Following the initial excitement after the introduction of these materials into initial phase I and phase II clinical trials, certain limitations emerged that are influencing the manner in which these materials will be applied in clinical practice. If unpolymerized hemoglobin is introduced into the circulation, it has an exceedingly short half-life, in the range of 6–8 hr. Thus, with the exception of applications in which such an extremely short half-life is adequate, i.e., application for acute stabilization of trauma patients, these types of low-molecular-weight HBOC preparations have limited clinical usefulness as substitutes for traditional blood transfusions. Other types of hemoglobin formulations have been prepared by polymerization, most commonly with glutaraldehyde. This produces a family of polymers, and altering the polymerization process and/or selective molecular weight ultrafiltration can influence the molecular weight distribution. Typically, the average molecular weight of such preparations is in the range of 200,000–250,000. This also results in a decrease in the oncotic pressure for a given hemoglobin concentration. For example, unpolymerized hemoglobin prepared at a clinically useful concentration of 15 g/dl has a colloid oncotic pressure of approximately 60 torr. Polymerization can reduce this to a clinically useful range of 20–25 torr. Nonetheless, polymerization alone still results in a circulatory half-life that is relatively short, especially when compared to traditional red cell transfusions. Furthermore, HBOC solutions can undergo oxidation *in vivo* to methemoglobin, which cannot carry oxygen (33). Under usual physiologic conditions, erythrocyte-borne hemoglobin is maintained in the reduced state by methemoglobin reductase. In the plasma phase, however, there is little methemoglobin reductase activity, and accordingly, HBOCs oxidize to methemoglobin following their administration and oxygenation (Fig. 2). The relatively short circulating half-life of free hemoglobin, even when polymerized, combined with spontaneous oxidation without methemoglobin reductase activity, results in a functional circulating half-life of approximately 24 hr. Accordingly, this important limitation in efficacy must be considered when clinical applications are proposed for these materials.

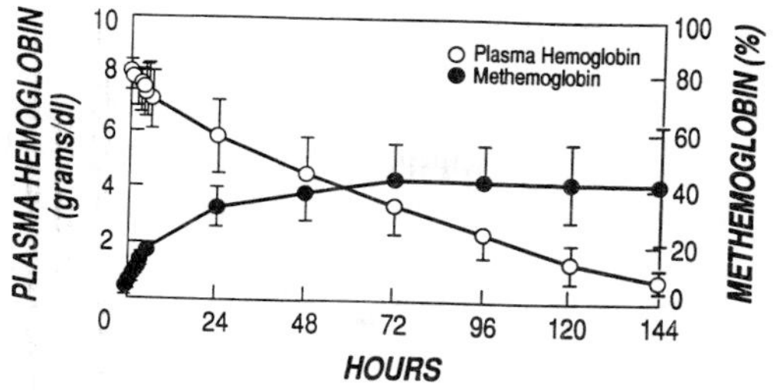

Figure 2 Plasma hemoglobin and methemoglobin levels following near-total blood exchange with a bovine-derived HBOC in a conscious animal model. Note the conversion of up to 40% of the infused HBOC to methemoglobin by 72 hr. With permission, from Lee *et al.* (33).

This conversion to methemoglobin can be accelerated in some clinical settings, such as when these materials are used in extracorporeal circulation, such as cardiopulmonary bypass. In this potential clinical application, exposure of hemoglobin in the plasma phase to the blood–gas interface that is part of cardiopulmonary bypass results in more rapid oxidation of hemoglobin (34) (Fig. 3). For applications in cardiac surgery, this effect limits the effective usefulness of these materials in cardiopulmonary bypass to approximately 2–3 hr, which is adequate for most types of cardiac surgery.

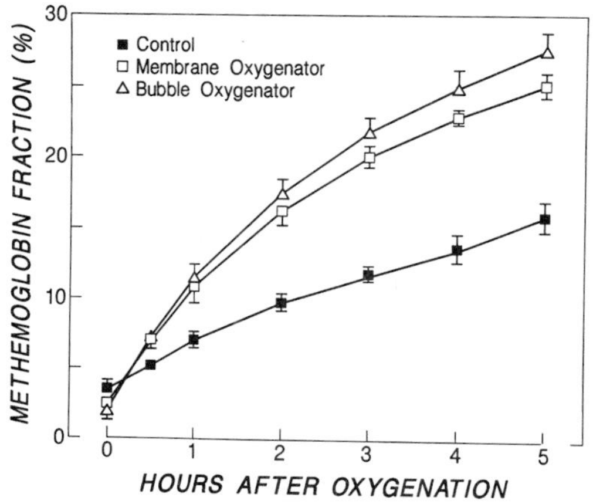

Figure 3 *In vitro* experimental study demonstrating the increased rate of HBOC hemoglobin oxidation when a bovine-derived HBOC is exposed to the blood–gas interface during extracorporeal circulation. Note that *ex vivo*, oxygenated HBOC oxidized rapidly to methemoglobin (■) and that the rate of oxidation is nearly doubled in an extracorporeal circuit. There was a slight advantage to using a membrane oxygenator versus a bubble oxygenator. With permission, from Ref. (34), K. Neya, R. Lee, and G. J. Vlahakes (1998). Hemoglobin-based oxygen carrying solution stability in extracorporeal circulation: An *in vitro* evaluation and implications for clinical use. *ASAIO J.* **44,** 166–170.

F. HBOC Effects in the Circulation

Hemoglobin-based blood substitutes have the important property of being substantially less viscous than blood at normal hematocrit. By comparison, blood at normal hematocrit has a viscosity of approximately 4 cP, as compared to 2 cP for a typical hemoglobin-based blood substitute. This property is of critical importance to understanding how these materials work in the microcirculation.

In a previous study examining the coronary circulation, as progressive hemodilution is performed, decreasing the hematocrit by nearly a factor of 4, there is a gradual increase in maximal vascular conductance through the coronary vascular bed (35). In this study, coronary vascular autoregulation was pharmacologically abolished, resulting in linear pressure–flow relationships with a slope representing maximal vascular conductance through the coronary vascular bed (Fig. 4). As noted, as viscosity is decreased by progressive hemodilution, maximal vascular conductance (the slope of the pressure–flow relation) increases. The result is that the decrement in oxygen-carrying capacity produced by crystalloid hemodilution is offset proportionally by the increase in potential blood flow; thus, over a wide range of hematocrits, there is little change in oxygen delivery by hemodilution alone. Also, as demonstrated in that study, decreasing the hematocrit less than approximately 15–16% does not result in a further decrease in viscosity, and hence no further increase in maximal vascular conductance. As a consequence, at very low hematocrits, oxygen delivery to a vascular bed may potentially be compromised.

In contrast, when hemodilution is carried out with a hemoglobin-based oxygen-carrying solution (36), the same effect on maximal vascular conductance is obtained, due to a decrease in overall blood viscosity (Fig. 5). However, because the hemoglobin solution adds oxygen-carrying capacity, the net effect of decreasing viscosity and adding oxygen-carrying capacity is to increase maximal oxygen delivery. This has a very important implication for the use of these materials, particularly in clinical situations in which there may be significant obstructive vascular disease. This important consequence of hemodilution with this class of materials, namely reduction in viscosity with the addition of oxygen-carrying capacity, has broad implications for a number of potential applications that are different from the traditional "blood substitute" intent for this class of materials. These types of applications are still in the early stages of clinical development.

G. Potential Applications of Hemoglobin-Based Oxygen-Carrying Solutions

1. Use as "Blood Substitutes"

Although hemoglobin-based blood substitutes originally evolved with the intent of replacing traditional blood transfusions, as more has been learned about their properties and

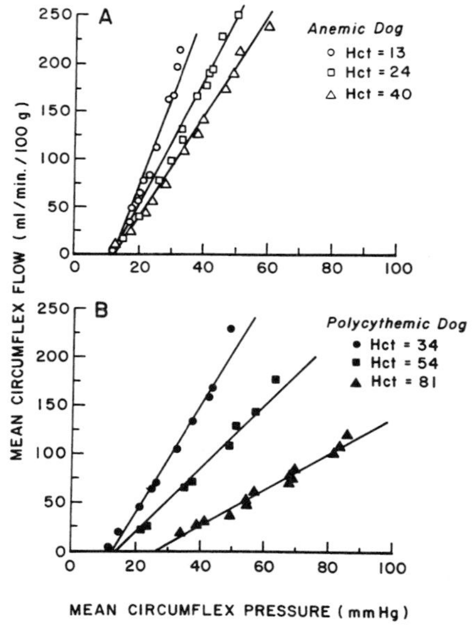

Figure 4 Coronary circulation pressure–flow relations following pharmacologic vasodilation to abolish autoregulation. The resulting linear relations represent maximal vascular conductance through the myocardium. Note the effect of progressive hemodilution with crystalloid solution over a wide range of hematocrits: (A) hematocrit range 13–40%; (B) hematocrit range 34–81%. With permission, from Baer *et al.* (35).

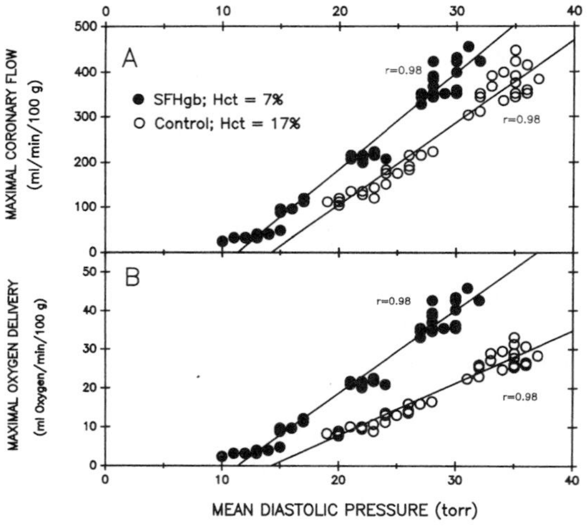

Figure 5 (A) Linear coronary pressure–flow relations obtained following hemodilution with an HBOC (●) and crystalloid (○). Note that the group that was hemodiluted with an HBOC was diluted to a profound degree of anemia not associated with survival. (B) Each pressure–flow relation has been multiplied by the respective oxygen-carrying capacity to yield maximal oxygen delivery. Note that at a canine hematocrit of 7% following hemodilution with HBOC, maximal oxygen-carrying capacity is greater than in control animals hemodiluted with crystalloid to a canine hematocrit of 17%. Reprinted from Hodakowski *et al.* (20), by courtesy of Marcel Dekker Inc.

physiologic consequences, the list of potential applications has grown; they are summarized in Table I.

This class of materials is attractive for use in acute blood loss settings such as trauma, even in the field. These materials have been shown to restore normal hemodynamics and oxygen transport in models of experimental shock where systemic acidosis could be rapidly resolved (37). Furthermore, the vasoconstrictor effect of these materials helps restore blood pressure in this application. In the experimental study referenced, no evidence of end organ damage was found following resuscitation.

For use in more traditional blood-replacement settings, the long-term efficacy limitation of hemoglobin-based blood solutions becomes a significant issue. In phase II and phase III clinical trials, in which these materials are being used in a manner similar to that of autologous red cell transfusions, the doses currently being employed combined with the short half-life have produced limited efficacy in terms of overall blood conservation. A possible exception to this problem is their use to treat postoperative anemia following cardiac surgery employing cardiopulmonary bypass (38). During the first 8–12 hr following cardiopulmonary bypass, cardiac surgical patients usually experience rewarming and arterial and venous vasodilation. The result is a requirement for blood volume replacement and blood volume expansion. During this time, crystalloid or nonheme colloid solutions are administered. As a consequence, hemodilution occurs, producing a low hematocrit within the first few postoperative hours. Transfusion decisions in cardiac surgical patients are generally made at that time (39). In the days that follow a cardiac surgical procedure, as fluid is mobilized and excreted, some hemoconcentration occurs, producing a sharp rise in hematocrit by the fourth or fifth postoperative day. Thus, cardiac surgical patients may benefit from a short-term "oxygen transport bridge" until hemoconcentration occurs. Hemoglobin-based oxygen-carrying solutions may be one possible means of achieving this, as has been suggested in a recent clinical trial (38).

During late recovery, pharmacokinetic studies have suggested that the heme iron in administered hemoglobin-based solutions may produce a hematinic effect to help restore native hematocrit levels at a more rapid rate (40).

One useful technique that has permitted avoidance of allogeneic blood exposure in surgery has been the use of preoperative autologous donation. In some surgical settings, however, patient acuity or lack of physiologic reserves may preclude autologous donation. HBOC solutions, as well as even PFC emulsions, may be used as a novel way to permit extended, acute autologous blood donation immediately prior to surgery. In an experimental model, a hemoglobin-based blood substitute was used to achieve acute donation of approximately 70% of the autologous red cell mass (41). Because of the oxygen-carrying capacity provided by the blood substitute, a high degree of removal of the autologous red cell mass was well tolerated in a subsequent experimental surgical stress. Following surgery and following intraoperative blood loss, the autologous blood may be readministered. In some surgical settings, such as cardiac surgery, the availability of the resulting fresh whole blood may confer an additional benefit for early postoperative hemostasis (42).

Table I Potential Uses of Hemoglobin-Based Oxygen-Carrying Solutions

Stabilization during ongoing acute blood loss; e.g., civilian trauma or military applications
Postoperative treatment of anemia
Extended, acute preoperative autologous blood donation
Intraoperative normovolemic hemodilution
Extracorporeal circulation
Priming solution for cardiopulmonary bypass
Scavenging gaseous microemboli
Carbon monoxide poisoning
Novel applications to improve local tissue oxygenation
Vasoocclusive diseases
Sickle cell crisis
Tumor sensitization to radiation or chemotherapy

2. Novel Applications of Hemoglobin-Based Oxygen-Carrying Solutions

Additional applications for these materials have been suggested and would take advantage of their oxygen-carrying properties in the plasma phase. For example, they may provide short-term oxygen transport capacity in patients who have sustained carbon monoxide poisoning. For this application, HBOCs could potentially be administered in the field.

Because of the low viscosity of these materials, and because they travel in the plasma phase, their behavior in the microcirculation is different than that of erythrocytes. Microcirculation studies using vital microscopy to examine the capillary bed have demonstrated that precapillary sphincters control the transit of erythrocytes, but do not necessarily completely exclude the plasma phase. Thus, if the cell-free hemoglobin-based oxygen-carrying solution is present in the plasma phase, it may reach target tissues with less local regulation than erythrocytes. Using an Eppendorf needle system to measure tissue oxygen tension, Standl demonstrated that addition of even small amounts of HBOC solution into the circulation can substantially change local tissue oxygen tension (43) and that this effect is operative even in the presence of arterial stenosis (44). This has implications for potential applications for management of vasoocclusive diseases, such as peripheral vascular disease producing nonhealing leg lesions. Such applications are presently being tested in clinical trials.

Teicher has suggested in experimental studies another interesting application that may have important therapeutic implications. In experimental models of solid tumors, it has been shown that not only hemoglobin-based oxygen-carrying solutions (45, 46), but also perfluorocarbon emulsions (47), can increase the radiosensitivity and chemosensitivity of tumors. These observations were made with relatively low doses, and hence low plasma concentrations, of these materials. This application is not particularly influenced by the short half-life of hemoglobin solutions, and thus this may be an important area for future clinical development.

H. Issues and Controversies in HBOC Development

Free hemoglobin is known to possess high-affinity nitric oxide binding properties. This area has been explored in the experimental setting for at least a decade, and nitric oxide binding is thought to be mechanism by which many hemoglobin-based blood substitutes exert their so-called vasoconstrictor effect (48). In virtually every clinical study performed to date, some elevation of systemic vascular resistance has been demonstrated. This pressor effect is thought to result from an interaction of hemoglobin with NO; this concept requires diffusion of hemoglobin through the endothelium to the interstitial space, where the physiologic effects of NO are thought to occur. Consistent with this is the observation that if NO synthase inhibitors are simultaneously administered, the pressor effect of HBOCs is diminished (49). Although there may be some applications in which this is of benefit (50), initial concerns were raised about possible deleterious effects.

Proponents of the vasoconstrictor hypothesis have suggested that the vasoconstrictor effect may override or diminish any benefit from improved oxygen delivery. Consistent with this is the observation that when HBOC was administered in a shock animal model, higher lactate levels were observed following resuscitation (51). However, to date, in both experimental and clinical trials, neither vascular bed-specific override of metabolic autoregulation nor ischemic injury has been demonstrated by administration of these materials. Furthermore, the degree of vasoconstrictor activity has been variable from one HBOC preparation to another, and may be related to the molecular weight distribution of hemoglobin entities in each preparation.

More importantly, the decrease of nitric oxide may result in free-hemoglobin-induced oxidant injury of the vascular endothelium. In the setting of reperfusion of ischemic tissue, a common event in surgical fields such as cardiac surgery, concerns have been raised that reperfusion injury may be exacerbated by increasing oxidative stress. The potential for oxidative injury may result from more than one mechanism. Nitric oxide functions as an antioxidant in mammalian physiology (52) via several potential mechanisms. Furthermore, hemoglobin may contribute redox-active iron that can alter the formation of oxygen free radicals in reperfused tissue (53).

These important issues are currently under investigation. As the number of possible clinical applications grows, these issues will need to be explored further. They may be related to the specific hemoglobin preparation under study, and modifications to HBOCs may be required if such effects on vascular biology prove to have deleterious consequences.

References

1. Wallace, E. L., Churchill, W. H., Surgenor, D. M., An, J., Cho, G., McGurk, S., and Murphy, L. (1995). Collection and transfusion of blood and blood components in the United States 1992. *Transfusion* **35,** 802–812.
2. Clark, L. C., and Gollan, F. (1996). Survival of mammals breathing organic liquids equilibrated at atmospheric pressure. *Science* **24,** 755–756.
3. Reiss, J. G., and LeBlanc, M. (1982). Solubility and transport phenomena in perfluorochemicals relevant to blood substitution and other biomedical applications. *Pure Appl. Chem.* **54,** 2383–2406.
4. Sloviter, H. A., and Kamimotot, T. (1967). Erythrocyte substitution for perfusion of brain. *Nature (London)* **216,** 458–460.
5. Clark, L. C., Becattini, F., and Kaplan, S. (1972). The physiologic effects of artificial blood made from inert organic solvents. *Ala. J. Med. Sci.* **9,** 16–29.
6. Lutz, J. (1985). Effect of perfluorochemicals on host defense, especially on the reticuloendothelial system. *Int. Anesthesiol. Clin.* **23,** 63–93.
7. Ohyanagi, H., Toshima, K., Sekita, M., Okamoto, M., Itoh, T., and Mitsuno, T. (1979). Clinical studies of perfluorochemical whole blood substitutes. Safety of Fluosol-DA (20%) in normal human volunteers. *Clin. Ther.* **2,** 306–312.
8. Tremper, K. K., Lapin, R., Levine, E., Friedman, A., and Shoemaker, W. C. (1980). Hemodynamic and oxygen transport effects of a perfluorochemical blood substitute Fluosol-DA (20%). *Crit. Care Med.* **8,** 738–741.
9. Tremper, K. K., Friedman, A. E., Levine, E. M., Lapin, R., and Camarillo, D. (1982). The preoperative treatment of severely anemic patients with a perfluorochemical oxygen-transport fluid, Fluosol-DA. *N. Engl. J. Med.* **307,** 277–283.
10. Gould, S. A., Rosen, A. L., Sehgal, L. R., Sehgal, H. L., Langdale, L. A., Krause, L. M., Rice, C. L., Chamberline, W. H., and Moss, G. S. (1986). Fluosol-DA as a red cell substitute in acute anemia. *N. Engl. J. Med.* **314,** 1653–1656.
11. Bucala, R., Kawakami, M., and Cerami, A. (1983). Cytotoxicity of a perfluorocarbon blood substitute to macrophages *in vitro*. *Science* **220,** 965–967.
12. Keipert, P. E., Faithfull, N. S., Bradley, J. D., Hazard, D. Y., Hogan, J., Levisetti, M. S., and Peters, R. M. (1994). Oxygen delivery augmentation by low-dose perfluorochemical emulsion during profound normovolemic hemodilution. *Adv. Exp. Med. Biol.* **345,** 197–204.
13. Keipert, P. E. (1995). Use of Oxygent, a perfluorchemical-based oxygen carrier, as an alternative to intraoperative blood transfusion. *Art. Cells Blood Substit. Immobil. Biotechnol.* **23,** 381–394.
14. Wahr, J. A., Trouwborst, A., Spence, R. K., Henny, C. P., Cernaianu, A. C., Graziano, A. C., Tremper, K. K., Flaim, K. E., Keipert, P. E., Faithfull, N. S., and Clymer, J. J. (1996). A pilot study of the effects of a Perflubron emulsion, AF0104, on mixed venous oxygen tension in anesthetized surgical patients. *Anesth. Analg.* **82,** 103–107.

15. Spiess, B. D., Braverman, B., Woronowicz, A. W., and Ivankovich, A. W. (1986). Protection from cerebral air emboli with perfluorocarbons in rabbits. *Stroke* **17,** 1146–1149.
16. Amberson, W. R. (1937). Blood substitutes. *Biol. Rev.* **12,** 48–86.
17. Rabiner, S. F., Helbert, J. R., Lopas, H., and Friedman, L. H. (1967). Evaluation of a stroma-free hemoglobin solution for use as a plasma expander. *J. Exp. Med.* **126,** 1127–1142.
18. Birndorf, N. I., and Lopas, H. (1970). Effects of red cell stroma-free hemoglobin solution on renal function in monkeys. *J. Appl. Physiol.* **29,** 573–578.
19. Savitsky, J. P., Doczi, J., Black, J., and Arnold, J. D. (1978). A clinical safety trial of stroma-free hemoglobin. *Clin. Pharmacol. Ther.* **23,** 73–80.
20. Benesh, R. E., Benesh, R., Renthal, R. D., and Maeda, N. (1972). Affinity labeling of the polyphosphate binding site of hemoglobin. *Biochemistry* **11,** 3576–3582.
21. Hoffman, S. L., Looker, D. L., and Roerich, J. M. (1990). Expression of fully functional human hemoglobin by *Escherichia coli. Proc. Natl. Acad. Sci. U.S.A.* **87,** 8521–8525.
22. Fronticelli, C., Bucci, E., and Orth, C. (1984). Solvent regulation of oxygen affinity in hemoglobin. *J. Biol. Chem.* **259,** 10841–10844.
23. Iwashita, Y., Yabuki, A., Yamaji, K., Iwasaki, K., Okami, I., Hirati, C., and Kosaka, K. (1988). A new resuscitation fluid "stabilized hemoglobin." Preparation and characteristics. *Biomat. Art. Cells Art. Organs* **16,** 271–280.
24. Iwashita, Y. (1992). Relationship between chemical properties and biological properties of pyridoxylated hemoglobin-polyoxyethylene. *Biomat. Art. Cells Immobil. Biotechnol.* **20,** 299–308.
25. Conover, C. D., Malatesta, P., Lejeune, L., Chang, C. L., and Shorr, R. G. (1996). The effects of hemodilution with polyethylene glycol bovine hemoglobin (PEG-Hb) in a conscious porcine model. *J. Invest. Med.* **44,** 238–246.
26. Shum, K. L., Leon, A., Viau, A. T., Pilon, D., Nucci, M., and Shorr, R. G. L. (1996). The physiological and histopathological response of dogs to exchange transfusion with polyethylene glycol-modified bovine hemoglobin (PEG-Hb). *Art. Cells Blood Substit. Immobil. Biotechnol.* **24,** 655–683.
27. Chang, T. M. S., Lister, C., Nishiya, T., and Varma, R. (1992). Effects of different methods of administration and effects of modifications by microencapsulation, crosslinkage or PEG conjugation on the immunological effects of homologous and heterologous hemoglobin. *Biomat. Art Cells Immobil. Biotechnol.* **20,** 611–618.
28. Chang, T. M. S. (1988). Hemoglobin corpsucles. *Biomat. Art. Cells Art. Organs* **16,** 1–9.
29. Chang, T. M. S. (1997). Recent and future developments of modified hemoglobin and microencapsulated hemoglobin as red blood cell substitutes. *Art. Cells Blood Substit. Immobil. Biotechnol.* **25,** 1–24.
30. Chang, T. M. S. (1976). Biodegradable semipermeable microcapsules containing enzymes, hormones, vaccines, and other biologicals. *J. Bioeng.* **1,** 25–32.
31. Yu, W. P., and Chang, T. M. S. Submicron biodegradable polymer membrane hemoglobin nanocapsules as potential blood substitutes: Preparation and characterization. *Art. Cells Blood Substit. Immobil. Biotechnol.* **24,** 169–184.
32. Vlahakes, G. J., Lee, R., Jacobs, E. E., Jr., LaRaia, P. J., and Austen, W. G. (1990). Hemodynamic effects and oxygen transport properties of a new blood substitute in a model of massive blood replacement. *J. Thorac. Cardiovasc. Surg.* **100,** 379–388.
33. Lee, R., Neya, K., Svizzero, T. A., and Vlahakes, G. J. (1995). Limitations of the efficacy of hemoglobin-based oxygen-carrying solutions. *J. Appl. Physiol.* **79,** 236–242.
34. Neya, K., Lee, R., and Vlahakes, G. J. (1998). Hemoglobin-based oxygen carrying solution stability in extracorporeal circulation: An *in vitro* evaluation and implications for clinical use. *ASAIO J.* **44,** 166–170.
35. Baer, R. W., Vlahakes, G. J., Uhlig, P. N., and Hoffman, J. I. E. (1987). Maximum myocardial oxygen transport during anemia and polycythemia in dogs. *Am. J. Physiol.* **252,** H1086–H1095.
36. Hodakowski, G. T., Page, R. D., Harringer, W., Jacobs, E. E., Jr., LaRaia, P., Svizzero, T., Guerrero, J. L., Austen, W. G., and Vlahakes, G. J. (1992). Ultra-pure polymerized bovine hemoglobin blood substitute: Effects on the coronary circulation. *Biomat. Art. Cells Immobil. Biotechnol.* **20,** 669–672.
37. Harringer, W., Hodakowski, G. T., Svizzero, T., Jacobs, E. E., Jr., and Vlahakes, G. J. (1992). Acute effects of a bovine hemoglobin blood substitute in a canine model of hemorrhagic shock. *Eur. J. Cardiothorac. Surg.* **6,** 649–654.
38. Levy, J. H., Goodnough, L. T., Greilich, P., Parr, G., Stewart, R. W., Gratz, I., Wahr, J., Williams, J., Comunale, M., and Vlahakes, G. J. (1998). A room-temperature stable hemoglobin (HBOC-201) eliminates allogeneic red blood cell (RBC) transfusion in postoperative cardiac surgery patients. *Circulation* **98**(Suppl. I), 1–132.
39. Stover, E. P., Siegel, L. C., and Parks, R. (1998). Variability in transfusion practice for coronary artery bypass surgery persists despite national consensus guidelines: A 24-institution study. Institutions of the Multicenter Study of Perioperative Ischemia Research Group. *Anesthesiology* **88,** 327–333.
40. Hughes, G. S., Jr., Francom, S. F., Antal, E. J., Adams, W. J., Locker, P. K., Yancey, E. P., and Jacobs, E. E., Jr. (1995). Hematologic effects of a novel hemoglobin-based oxygen carrier in normal male and female subjects. *J. Lab. Clin. Med.* **126,** 444–451.
41. Slanetz, P. J., Lee, R., Page, R. D., Jacobs, E. E., Jr., LaRaia, P. J., and Vlahakes, G. J. (1994). Hemoglobin blood substitutes in extended autologous preoperative blood donation: An experimental study. *Surgery* **115,** 246–254.
42. Mohr, R., Martinowitz, U., Lavee, J., Amroch, D., Ramot, B., and Goor, D. A. (1988). The hemostatic effect of fresh whole blood versus platelet concentrates after cardiac operations. *J. Thorac. Cardiovasc. Surg.* **96,** 530–534.
43. Standl, T. G., Reeker, W., Redmann, G., Kochs, E., Werner, C., and Shulte am Esch, J. (1997). Haemondynamic changes and skeletal muscle oxygen tension during complete blood exchange with ultrapurified polymerized bovine hemoglobin. *Intens. Care Med.* **23,** 865–872.
44. Horn, E. -P., Standl, T., Wilhelm, S., Jacobs, E. E., Freitag, U., Frietag, M., and Schulte am Esch, J. (1997). Bovine hemoglobin increases skeletal muscle oxygenation during 95% artificial arterial stenosis. *Surgery* **121,** 411–418.
45. Teicher, B. A., Ara, G., Herbst, R., Takeuchi, H., Keyes, S., and Northey, D. (1997). PEG-hemoglobin: Effects on tumor oxygenation and response to chemotherapy. *In Vivo* **11,** 301–311.
46. Robinson, M. F., Dupuis, N. P., Kusumoto, T., Liu, F., Menon, K., and Teicher, B. A. (1995). Increased tumor oxygenation and radiation sensitivity in rat tumors by a hemoglobin-based, oxygen-carrying preparation. *Art. Cells Blood Substit. Immobil. Biotechnol.* **23,** 431–438.
47. Teicher, B. A., Herman, T. S., Hopkins, R. E., and Menon, K. (1991). Effects of oxygen level on the enhancement of tumor response to radiation by perfluorochemical emulsions or a bovine hemoglobin preparation. *Int. J. Radiat. Oncol. Biol. Phys.* **21,** 969–974.
48. Vogel, W. M., Dennis, R. C., Cassidy, G., Apstein, C. S., and Valeri, C. R. (1986). Coronary vasoconstrictor effect of stroma-free hemoglobin solutions. *Am. J. Physiol.* **251,** H413–420.
49. Gulati, A., Barve, A., and Sen, A. P. (1999). Pharmacology of hemoglobin therapeutics. *J. Lab. Clin. Med.* **133,** 112–119.
50. Reah, G., Bodenham, A. R., Mallick, A., Daily, E. K., and Przybelski, R. J. (1997). Initial evaluation of diaspirin cross-linked hemoglobin (DCLHb) as a vasopressor in critically ill patients. *Crit. Care Med.* **25,** 1480–1488.
51. Winslow, R. M., Gonzales, A., Gonzales, M. L., Magde, M., McCarthy, M., Rohlfs, R. J., and Vandegriff, K. D. (1998). Vascular resistance and efficacy of red cell substitutes in a rat hemorrhage model. *J. Appl. Physiol.* **85,** 993–1003.

52. Wink, D. A., and Mitchell, J. B. (1998). Chemical biology of nitric oxide: Into regulatory, cytotoxic, and cytoprotective mechanisms of nitric oxide. *Free Radic. Biol.* **25,** 434–456.

53. Goldman, D. W., Breyer, R. J., Yeh, D., Brockner Ryan, B. A., and Alayash, A. I. (1998). Acellular hemoglobin-mediated oxidative stress toward endothelium: A role for ferryl iron. *Am. J. Physiol.* **44,** H1046–1053.

75

Research Models in Pediatric Surgery

Brad W. Warner

Division of Pediatric Surgery, Children's Hospital Medical Center, Cincinnati, Ohio 45229

I. Introduction

The field of pediatric surgery is wide-ranging and the new knowledge afforded by the advent of more sophisticated tools in molecular biology and physiology has heralded an unprecedented effort in pediatric surgical basic science investigation. The aim in this chapter, rather than elucidating specific techniques, is to provide the reader with an overview of several important major conditions that are encountered within the field of pediatric surgery. Many of the techniques used to investigate each specific topic are not unique to the field of pediatric surgery; a detailed outline of the methodology will therefore not be provided. Six topics were chosen on the basis of their relevance to the field, their relatively uncharacterized etiology, as well as the burning need for basic science inquiry. Other vital topics in pediatric surgery, including the bioengineering of artificial organs, congenital diaphragmatic hernia, angiogenesis, and organogenesis, to name but a few, are covered elsewhere in this volume.

II. Biliary Atresia

Biliary atresia is a disorder of infants in which there is obliteration or discontinuity of the extrahepatic biliary system, resulting in obstructed bile flow. Untreated, the cholestasis leads to unconjugated hyperbilirubinemia, cirrhosis, hepatic failure, and death. Biliary atresia has an incidence of one in 10,000 live births and represents the most common indication for liver transplantation in children.

Despite the improved survival of children with biliary atresia following transplantation, the pathogenesis of this condition is poorly understood. Multiple theories have been presented to account for the varied spectrum of pathology seen in these patients, ranging from congenital malformation of the bile ducts to the presence of a causative infectious agent. Because of this lack of understanding, the models utilized to study this disease are varied and diverse.

A. Infectious Models

The inoculation of animals with candidate infectious agents represents a relatively simple model system for studies of the influence of various infections on bile duct embryogenesis, immune responsiveness, and host cellular repair. Multiple viral agents have been implicated to play a role in the pathogenesis of biliary atresia. Following the detection of group C rotavirus RNA using polymerase chain reaction (PCR) in two infants with biliary atresia, Riepenhoff-Talty *et al.* (1) were able to induce extrahepatic biliary obstruction in neonatal BALB/c mice with a single oral inoculation of a more prevalent (group A) strain of rotavirus. Using this model, 42% of infected mice developed hepatobiliary disease. The gross morphology of the biliary tracts demonstrated a wide range of involvement, from mild constrictions to complete luminal obstruction with proximal bile duct dilation. There was histopathologic evidence for an acute inflammatory process and subsequent bile ductule proliferation—an important feature seen in human biliary atresia. These investigators were not able to identify evidence for bile duct atresia. A small proportion of the infected mice recovered clinically. This varied response to the same infectious agent appears to parallel the range of severity seen in humans.

Expanding on this rotavirus model, Petersen *et al.* (2) used scanning electron microscopy to illuminate the gross changes that occur in the biliary tree. Due to the wide spectrum of pathology noted, they were unsuccessful in classifying morphologic changes, but were able to identify the development of atresia of the gallbladder and extrahepatic biliary tree with this model. Hepatobiliary morbidity and lethality appear to be dependent on the mouse strain used, and some protection against the development of cholestasis may be partially prevented by the administration of interferon (3).

Reovirus 3 is another viral agent that has been studied in murine models of biliary atresia. Although the dominant early lesions after inoculation are intrahepatic, the later onset of jaundice coincides with chronic inflammatory lesions of the extrahepatic bile ducts (4, 5). Of particular relevance to human disease is the observation that the virus could no longer be detected by culture or immunocytochemical methods during the stage of obliterative bile duct inflammation and clinical jaundice. This important observation may explain why investigators have not been successful in detecting cytomegalovirus (CMV) (6), reovirus 3 (7), or rotavirus (8) in human infants presenting with jaundice. Alternatively, it is possible that infants presenting with jaundice are well past the stage of viremia (9).

B. Administration of Exogenous Agents

Several agents have been administered to animals at various stages of development to induce bile duct injury and induce histologic features similar to the ones seen in biliary atresia. Vacanti and Folkman suggested that biliary atresia occurred as a result of defective proline metabolism (10). These investigators induced bile duct enlargement in mice given a continuous intraperitoneal infusion of L-proline. They also noted reduced levels of L-proline in the serum of patients with biliary atresia. In a subsequent study, Schier *et al.* were not able to reproduce these observations by the subcutaneous administration of L-proline to pregnant mice (11).

Another agent used to induce bile duct inflammation is the antihelminthic agent 1,4-phenylenediisothiocyanate (PDT) (12, 13). An interesting aspect of PDT is that bile duct pathology appears to be related to the timing of exposure to this agent and the developmental phase of the rat. Using an orogastric gavage of PDT, Ogawa and co-workers observed bile duct enlargement in rats given the agent in the postnatal period. If the PDT was given to pregnant rats, there was no dilation, but fibrosis was seen in the bile ducts of the offspring. If, however, the PDT was given to pregnant rats and a subsequent dose administered to the offspring after delivery, the bile ducts demonstrated wall thickening, along with stenosis and atresia. The relationship between bile duct pathology and developmental exposure to this agent warrants further investigation.

Using subcutaneously implanted miniosmotic pumps, a nonspecific trigger of inflammation (phorbol myristate acetate; PMA) was infused directly into the gallbladder of adult rats (14). Portal fibrosis and neocholangiogenesis were observed following a 28-day infusion. Although PMA is a nonspecific activator of inflammatory and endothelial cells, this agent may offer a starting point for further studies regarding the pathogenic role of inflammation during the development of biliary atresia.

C. The Sea Lamprey

Morphologic studies of the sea lamprey (*Petromyzon marinus*) have revealed an interesting, programmed degeneration of the biliary tract during normal morphogenesis (15). In the ordinary adult lamprey, the biliary tract regresses, resulting in progressive cholestasis and bile pigment accumulation. The liver of the adult lamprey is distinguished from all other vertebrates by the absence of a bile duct system. The spectrum of pathology encountered during bile duct regression resembles the human form of the development of biliary atresia with the accumulation of luminal debris, basement membrane thickening, disorganization of hepatic architecture, extrahepatic bile duct atresia, and either shrinkage or loss of the gallbladder (16, 17). Because these animals live for several years after biliary tract regression they offer unique opportunities to investigate compensatory responses to cholestasis (18) as well as to dissect out the spectrum of changes occurring in the evolution of biliary atresia at the molecular level.

D. Miscellaneous Models

Ligation of the bile duct results in a surgically correctable form of biliary atresia when performed in fetal lambs (19). The bile duct distal to the ligature in this model is atretic and very similar to the human form of biliary atresia. Although it is highly unlikely that biliary atresia results from an acute *in utero* obstruction of the bile duct, this model affords a unique opportunity for studies of the effects of absent bile flow on the developing biliary ductal system. The disadvantages of this model include the complexity of the fetal operative intervention as well as the high cost associated with the care of large animals.

Schreiber *et al.* (20) reported a model of rejection injury to the extrahepatic bile ducts. In this report, segments of the bile duct were removed from fetal, early postnatal, or adult mice and grafted under the renal capsule of congenic mice. Fibrosclerosis developed in the adult grafts by 3 weeks, an effect that was associated with the induction of class I and class II major histocompatibility antigen expression. This effect was attenuated with cyclosporin. This experimental model system may be useful for examination of factors that modulate immune responses directed against biliary duct epithelium.

The observation of increased apoptotic activity in the bile ducts of infants with biliary atresia (21) is noteworthy, because the specific mechanism for bile duct regression is not known. With the inflammatory infiltrate that is often identified in human biliary atresia, the increase in apoptosis may result from local cytokine production. This consideration could guide important future studies regarding the role for cytokines and the regulation of apoptosis during the development of bile duct regression using any of the aforementioned models.

III. Hirschsprung's Disease

Hirschsprung's disease is also referred to as congenital aganglionosis coli and is a defect in intestinal motility associated with absent enteric ganglia in the distal bowel. The overall prevalence of this condition is estimated to be 1 in 5000 live births (22). In virtually all cases, the aganglionic segment extends proximally from the anal sphincter and involves varying amounts of colon and, in some instances, small bowel. The majority of patients with Hirschsprung's disease will be diagnosed during infancy because they present with symptoms of distal intestinal obstruction due to spasmodic contraction of the aganglionic segment of bowel.

The exact etiology of Hirschsprung's disease is presently unknown and the focus of much investigation [see Puri *et al.* (23) for review]. Although it has long been accepted that this condition develops as a result of failure of distal migration of proximal neural crest cells, this notion has been challenged by evidence suggesting the neural cells migrate normally, but for unknown reasons do not differentiate into neurons. Alternatively, there may be abnormalities of the intestinal extracellular matrix, enteric smooth muscle cells, intracellular adhesion molecules, neurotrophic factors, aberrant antigen expression with involvement of the immune system, and genetic factors, all of which may influence both neural migration and/or differentiation. There are experimental model systems to test these various theories.

A. Animal Models

There are several genetically based murine models for Hirschsprung's disease and these provide excellent model systems for elucidation of many of the factors mentioned above. These mouse strains include the *lethal spotted (ls)* (24), *piebald lethal* (s^l) (25), *dominant spotting (Dom)* (26), and *cRET-deficient* (27). Both of the *ls* and s^l are autosomal recessive, the *Dom* is autosomal semidominant, and the *cRET-deficient* is dominant/negative in expression patterns. The *Dom* strain is apparently difficult to maintain and has not been used experimentally. The homozygous *cRET-deficient* mice die soon after birth and have associated renal agenesis.

The majority of experiments have therefore utilized the *ls* and s^l mice. Most homozygous *ls* and s^l mice die at a young age as a consequence of distal colon aganglionosis and are distinguished from nonmutant mice: their normal black-colored coat contains areas that are devoid of pigment due to absent melanocytes. Heterozygous mice are phenotypically identical to the wild-type mice of the same strain. Some homozygous mice survive into adulthood, thus allowing establishment of mutant colonies. The enteric pathology in homozygous *ls* and s^l mice is similar to that seen in human Hirschsprung's disease (28–31).

Enterocolitis is a serious consequence of Hirschsprung's disease and is associated with high morbidity and mortality. The overall etiology of this problem is unknown. In addition to studies of the pathophysiology of enteric nerve migration and development as outlined below, these mutant mice provide excellent models for investigation into the pathophysiology of enterocolitis (32, 33).

Other species have been described with congenital megacolon and may have several advantages over mice. Larger animals allow physiologic studies of motility and also provide a greater volume of tissue for determination of the expression of various factors. In addition, larger animals permit a systematic investigation of various corrective operations for Hirschsprung's disease. The lethal white foal syndrome, a congenital abnormality of overo spotted horses, mimics the human form of aganglionosis (34). Untreated, the foals die from distal intestinal obstruction within a few days of birth.

A naturally occurring mutation of the endothelin receptor type B (EDNRB) gene in spotting lethal (*sl*) rats results in aganglionic megacolon (35). Lipman *et al.* (36) described another mutant rat, which develops severe megacecum and colon with pseudoobstruction and is the familial megacecum and colon strain (36). This rat is unique in that the distal rectum is in spasm, but not aganglionic.

B. Enteric Nerve Migration/Development

The development of molecular probes and retroviral/fluorescent dye techniques for cell lineage analyses has greatly improved our understanding of enteric neurodevelopment. Enteric ganglia are first recognized morphologically in the murine gastrointestinal tract on embryonic day E12.0 (37). Methods for detection of cholinergic neurons involve identifying the synthesis of tritiated acetylcholine combined with immunohistochemistry for acetylcholine. Serotonergic neurons may be distinguished by radioautographic detection of tritiated serotonin uptake as well as immunohistochemical staining for 5-hydroxytryptamine.

Rothman and Gershon were able to study the development of the murine gut *in situ* by placing bowel explants in organotypic tissue culture (37). Using this technique, enteric nerves were observed to develop from tissues harvested at earlier time points, thus indicating that the nerves evolved from nonrecognizable precursors and challenged the proximal-to-distal migration theory of enteric precursor cells.

In addition to tissue culture explants, other model systems for the study of murine enteric nerve development include placing the bowel directly on the chorioallantoic membrane of a developing chick embryo (38). Further, the bowel has been placed below the renal capsule of adult mice (39). In comparing the various methods, Nishijima *et al.* suggested that the subcapsular space was probably the best model because the three-dimensional architecture of the developing bowel was best preserved (39).

A transgenic mouse has been created by Kapur and associates in which the dopamine β-hydroxylase promoter was used to drive the expression of the reporter gene product, β-galactosidase, to enteric neurons and putative embryonic neuroblasts (40). The reporter gene allows selective staining of β-galactosidase in the nuclei of catecholeminergic neurons expressing dopamine β-hydroxylase. This histochemical marker provides a useful model system for studying of neuroblast migration and differentiation in both wild-type and *ls* mice (41).

C. Altered Extracellular Matrix

For normal innervation of the gut, it is intuitive that neural crest cell migration, differentiation, and survival are contingent on a permissive extracellular matrix environment. Models for research on human intestinal specimens from patients with aganglionosis include the determination of expression differences of various extracellular matrix proteins and localization using standard immunostaining methods. Abnormalities in the expression of laminin and collagen type IV (42) as well as tenascin and fibronectin (43) have already been reported in patients with aganglionosis.

Using *ls* mutant mice, abnormalities in the expression and distribution of laminin, type IV collagen, and other extracellular matrix components in the terminal hindgut have been observed as early as E11.5 (44, 45). Using an *in vitro* coculture system, *ls* and wild-type hindguts are obtained from embryos at E9.5 and added to explanted cultures of other sources of enteric neurons, including *ls* and wild-type foregut (46). The disadvantages of the coculture system include the fact that the normal tubular architecture of the intestine is lost and migration that normally occurs in three dimensions is restricted to the flat surface of a culture dish.

D. Other Factors

It has been suggested that neurotrophic factors may play a role in the pathogenesis of Hirschsprung's disease. Using an enzyme-linked immunosorbent assay (ELISA), protein levels of nerve growth factor (NGF) and neurotrophic factor-3 (NT-3) (47) as well as the expression of synapse-associated proteins syntaxin and synaptotagmin (48) in patients with Hirschsprung's disease have been found to be reduced. Along these lines, the reverse transcriptase polymerase chain reaction (RT-PCR) has been utilized to demonstrate reduced levels of transcript for NGF in *piebald lethal* (s^l) mice as well as in patients with Hirschsprung's disease (49). Because NGF-null mice have been designed (50), it would be interesting in future studies to delineate enteric neuron development in them.

Neural cell adhesion molecules (NCAMs) appear to be reduced in the aganglionic segment of the intestine as demonstrated by using immunohistochemical staining methods (51). In addition, expression of neural cell adhesion molecule L1 is reduced in these patients (52). Ectopic expression of major histocompatibility complex (MHC) class II antigens suggests an underlying immune mechanism responsible for Hirschsprung's. Again, immunohistochemical techniques have revealed marked elevations in MHC class II antigens in the aganglionic intestinal segments (53) as well as expression of intracellular adhesion molecule-1 (54).

Although immunohistochemical studies of clinical specimens of aganglionic bowel to determine the expression of assorted factors may provide insight into the pathogenesis of Hirschsprung's disease, it is unclear whether the abnormalities identified are the cause of the aganglionosis or the result of it. The creation of transgenic or knockout mice, which either overexpress or are unable to express a particular candidate gene, will provide a greater insight into the pathogenesis of this process. Cocultures of embryonic intestinal explants with transgenic-, mutant-, or knockout-derived gut or other elements that may influence enteric nerve migration and/or differentiation are also useful.

IV. Necrotizing Enterocolitis

Necrotizing enterocolitis (NEC) represents one of the most common serious acquired gastrointestinal tract problems occurring during the neonatal period and represents the leading cause of death among neonates undergoing surgery. This disease occurs in roughly 1–5% of all infants admitted to neonatal intensive care units; most of them born prematurely (55, 56). The more premature the infant, the greater the risk for NEC (55). The importance of this entity is underscored by the fact that NEC is second only to respiratory distress syndrome (surfactant deficiency of the premature neonate) as the most common cause of death in a large perinatal population (57). Despite the significance of the problem, the underlying cause of this disease is not known and the amount of research dedicated to this particular subject is paltry in comparison with the degree of research in other diseases associated with prematurity, such as surfactant deficiency.

One of the major problems associated with research of NEC is that there is no adequate animal model for this disease [see Crissinger (58) and Topalian and Ziegler (59) for extensive review]. Multiple factors have been implicated in the pathogenesis of NEC and include prematurity, ischemia/reperfusion, cytokines, bacteria, and enteral feeding. Additional components include the multitude of factors associated with immaturity of the intestinal barrier (Fig. 1). Despite the complexity of the problem, there exist several animal models that may provide useful information regarding the pathogenesis of this disease.

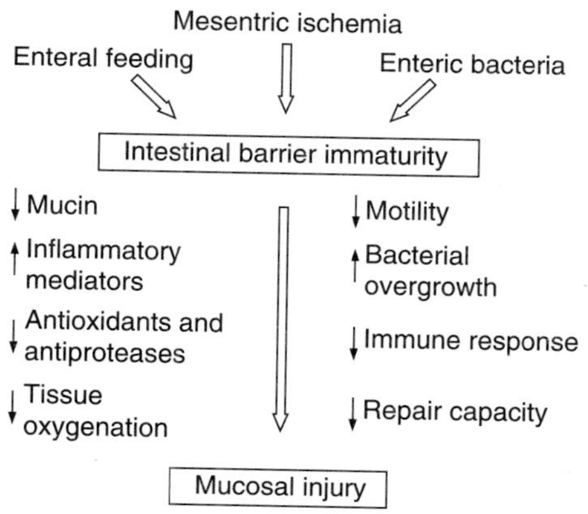

Figure 1 The multiple factors implicated to be associated with mucosal damage in the developing intestine and the onset of necrotizing enterocolitis. From Ref. (58), K.D. Crissinger (1995). Animal models of necrotizing enterocolitis. *J. Pediatr. Gastroenterol. Nutr.* **20**, 17–22.

A. Ischemia/Reperfusion

A classic ischemia/reperfusion model for the intestine involves direct occlusion of mesenteric vessels or the superior mesenteric artery (SMA) for varied periods of time and then allowing time for reperfusion to occur. This has been done in several animal species, but one of the best characterized models is in the neonatal piglet. In one study, the mesenteric vessels were tied off at different points near the distal ileum for 48 hr (60). The closer the occlusion to the ileocecal junction, the greater the likelihood for intestinal injury to occur. The degree of injury was greatest in low-birth-weight piglets (700–1200 g), as measured by ulceration, vascular engorgement, pneumatosis intestinalis, full-thickness necrosis, and ulceration with perforation. In the normal-birth-weight piglets, no injury was observed. This model permits the investigation of differences in intestinal responsiveness to injury as it relates to developmental stages, and the pathologic findings closely mirror what is seen in human NEC.

In mice, the time for the development of ischemic injury following vascular occlusion is substantially less than in low-birth-weight piglets. Occlusion of the superior mesenteric artery for 20 min in adult mice resulted in the development of ischemic intestinal lesions in 50% of the mice by 48 hr (61). A disadvantage of using mice is that their small size makes it technically difficult to evaluate the effect of any developmental variables. The primary advantage of using mice, however, is the ability to utilize various transgenic, mutant, or knockout strains to test directly the importance of the presence or absence of various genes in the pathogenesis of intestinal ischemic injury. Further, exogenous administration of various agents may be done using smaller volumes and with larger numbers of animals (62, 63).

Although ligation or direct occlusion of mesenteric blood vessels does not appear to be the cause of NEC, reduced splanchnic blood flow may result from developmental differences in vascular resistance or collateral circulation. It is interesting that ligation of both the arterial and lymphatic supply results in the development of classic pathologic findings of NEC whereas ligation of the lymphatics alone is associated with a low risk for mucosal damage (64). If the artery alone is ligated, there is mucosal injury, but without pneumatosis intestinalis. Because pneumatosis intestinalis is the radiographic hallmark of NEC, this study strongly implicates an important role for mesenteric lymphatics in the pathogenesis of this condition.

B. Luminal Factors

After evaluation of the intraluminal contents of the intestine of infants with NEC, it was found that the pH was generally <5.0, the protein content >5 g/dl, and sufficient carbohydrate and bacteria were available to ferment the carbohydrate to organic acids (65). Based on these data, investigators created a rabbit model of NEC using a bovine casein formulation that was acidified with propionic acid (65, 66). In weanling rabbits, either saline (control) or a solution of 10 mg/ml casein and 50 mg/ml calcium gluconate acidified with propionate to a pH of 4.0 was instilled into isolated intestinal loops. In this model, intestinal blood flow, mucosal permeability, and histamine release were all increased. Histologically, the villi were blunted, the lymphatics dilated, and edema was observed after 3 hr (67). After 16 hr, 38% of the rabbits had hemorrhagic necrosis and 5 of 8 animals died. Advantages of this model include its simplicity and reproducibility as well as the fact that assorted animals at varied stages of development can be evaluated with regard to their response. A major drawback of this model is the presumption that these intraluminal findings played a role in the development of NEC. It is quite possible that these intraluminal parameters occurred as a result of NEC.

The role for breast milk in preventing the development of NEC has long been debated; however, there are many putative factors within this important source of nutrition which could be explored to test their significance. Several growth factors, including epidermal growth factor, are abundant in breast milk. The effect of supplementation of various formulas with these factors in combination with other NEC models such as ischemia/reperfusion may render some insight into their significance. Indeed, supplementation of standard formulas with IgA has been shown to prevent bacterial translocation in a rabbit model of formula-associated mucosal injury (68). A word of caution is in order with regard to extrapolating the significance of breast milk feeding from various animal models to the human. There are many differences among assorted species with regard to immunologic and absorptive and digestive capacity of the GI tract at various stages of development.

Other luminal nutrients that may be injurious to the gut mucosa include dietary fatty acids. Using piglets at varied stages of development, Crissinger and Tso demonstrated that the lipid component of formula was associated with increased mucosal permeability in an ischemia/reperfusion model (69). Mucosal permeability was calculated in isolated ileal loops by the plasma-to-lumen clearance of [^{51}Cr]ethylenediaminetetraacetic acid. In subsequent studies, these investigators demonstrated that the injurious component of the lipid was related to its luminal concentration and the developmental stage of the animal (i.e., the youngest piglets demonstrated the greatest changes in permeability) (70). A reproducible model of NEC with grossly hemorrhagic and necrotic intestinal lesions was produced after 60 min of mesenteric artery occlusion and another 60 min of reperfusion in 1-day-old piglets (71). The advantages of this model are that the injury is reproducible and more severe in the younger animals. The disadvantages are that the model does not result in pneumatosis intestinalis, which raises questions as to how closely it resembles human NEC.

The importance of luminal bacteria in models of NEC is shown by the work of Musemenche *et al.*, who observed a 75% incidence of gross intestinal necrosis after 48 hr following 30 or 60 min of mesenteric vascular occlusion (72); in germ-free rats, the incidence of intestinal necrosis was 0% after the same interval of vascular occlusion.

C. Inflammatory Mediators

Several inflammatory mediators have been implicated to play a role in the pathogenesis of NEC; however, platelet-activating factor (PAF) has been one of the most extensively studied potential mediators. Intraaortic injection of a low-dose combination of PAF and endotoxin in rats resulted in ischemic intestinal necrosis (73). It was interesting that neither agent affected the gut when administered alone. Also, there were no thrombi seen in the mesenteric arteries, suggesting a mechanism of intestinal injury that is independent of platelet aggregation.

Because hypoxia is considered a predisposing factor for NEC, the effect of hypoxia on PAF formation and intestinal necrosis has been investigated (74). Young male rats were made severely hypoxic by placing them in a 100% N_2 chamber for 2 min; moderate hypoxia was accomplished using 10% O_2 for 15 or 30 min. To evaluate the role of PAF on intestinal perfusion and injury, two PAF antagonists, SRI 63-441 and WEB 2086, were injected 10 min before the hypoxic exposure. Plasma PAF levels were significantly elevated after 2 min of severe hypoxia and after 30 min of moderate hypoxia. This increase in PAF level was not caused by decreased degradation, because neither plasma nor intestinal PAF acetylhydrolase was decreased in the hypoxic rats. Intestinal perfusion was markedly decreased in hypoxic animals. In contrast, all platelet-activating factor antagonist-treated animals had normal intestinal perfusion. Histologic examination of affected bowel from hypoxic animals showed early intestinal necrosis, which was completely prevented by pretreatment with the PAF antagonists. Acidosis alone resulted in moderate increase of plasma PAF but did not produce bowel injury. This study suggests that PAF plays a central role in mediating hypoxia-induced intestinal necrosis. Acidosis may enhance the effect of hypoxia on PAF production. Other investigators have verified the findings with regard to PAF in hypoxia-induced intestinal injury. It is interesting that dietary ω-3 fatty acids suppress intestinal PAF production after hypoxia (75).

Tumor necrosis factor (TNF) is another cytokine that has been implicated to play a role in NEC. Infusion of TNF to healthy rats results in intestinal necrosis, along with other systemic effects (76). This cytokine appears to induce PAF production in intestinal tissue, and TNF-induced intestinal injury is prevented by pretreatment of the animal with PAF antagonists (77). Both endotoxin and PAF appear to induce TNF gene transcription, probably by separate pathways (78). The importance of endotoxin along with either PAF or TNF in inducing intestinal injury was underscored when endotoxin-resistant C3H/HeJ mice were used in the model (79). Control mice had 75% mortality after PAF injection (2.5 μg/kg) as compared with no mortality in the C3H/HeJ mice. Serum TNF levels were elevated in some control mice after PAF, but not in C3H/HeJ mice.

V. Cryptorchidism

Cryptorchidism (undescended testes) is the most common disorder of sexual differentiation and occurs in approximately 2% of human male births (80). The consequences of cryptorchidism include degeneration of the testes with impaired fertility and increased risk for the development of germ cell testicular tumors. Despite the significance of this problem, the cause of cryptorchidism has not been identified in the majority of patients. It is presently unclear whether the peculiar pathologic changes in the cryptorchid testes occur as a result of a primary defect in testicular development or whether normal testes fail to descend and the high body temperature induces a secondary change.

There are multiple animal models of cryptorchidism, but generally they include spontaneous, surgically induced, or testicular undescent caused by drugs or hormones. Evaluation of these models usually involves studying their effects on testicular morphology or development of neoplastic changes. In rodent models, the effects on fertility may be evaluated by determination of the impregnation rate of normal female animals. In large animal models such as the dog or pig, ejaculated semen may be collected for direct analysis.

A. Spontaneously Occurring Models

Several animal species have been recognized as having a finite incidence of cryptorchidism. Boars have a spontaneous rate (6–10%) of unilateral, right-sided cryptorchidism and offer several advantages over other species, including (1) similar hormonal, functional, and morphological characteristics of the ectopic testes when compared with humans, (2) similarity to humans regarding the time of testicular descent (testicular descent influences testicular histology), (3) structural resemblance between human and boar spermatozoa, and (4) similarity in mechanism of testicular thermoregulation (81).

Using the boar model, several stages of testicular descent may be studied. As an example, Hutson *et al.* implanted miniosmotic pumps in the ipsilateral hemiscrotum of the undescended testes to determine which stage of testicular migration was influenced by calcitonin gene-related peptide (CGRP) (82). In that study, only the testes that had been arrested in the inguinal phase of descent responded to the interstitially distributed exogenous CGRP. These results provide a useful model system to study the influence of local hormonal control of testicular descent.

This large animal model also permits capture of ejaculated semen at regular intervals, with a relatively large volume when compared to rodents. In healthy boars, males are allowed to mount a dummy or another female and the ejaculate is collected following stimulation with a gloved hand (81). Using this model, abnormalities of sperm morphology have been characterized (81). These findings may also be correlated with testicular histology.

The Long–Evans cryptorchid rat (LE/ORL) has been described as a spontaneous model of cryptorchidism (83). The incidence of cryptorchidism in this strain is 46% for unilateral cases and is 22% for bilateral cases. One advantage of this model is that surgical placement of the aberrantly located gubernaculum to the bottom of the scrotum at an early age (less than 2 weeks of life) results in a normally descended testes by week 3 or 4 (84). It appears as if gubernaculopexy reverses the histologic changes seen in the ectopic rat testes to a relatively normal architecture (84), thus supporting the value of orchidopexy in the treatment of this condition in humans.

In another mutant rat strain termed TS, 85% of males have either uni- or bilateral cryptorchidism (85). Although originally these rats were believed to have ectopic scrota, closer work with this strain has revealed that the scrota are hypoplastic, not abnormally positioned. In these rats, the testes are situated in a suprainguinal position within the superficial inguinal pouch, thus making this mutant a useful model for studying the abnormalities of inguinoscrotal descent.

Several mutant and knockout murine models of cryptorchidism have been described; these models allow sophisticated molecular dissection of the various genes that coordinate normal testicular descent. Probably one of the most extensively studied model is the androgen-insensitive testicular feminization (*Tfm*) mutant mouse. This mouse lacks androgen receptors and has intraabdominal testes situated at the level of the bladder neck, with no eversion of the scrotal sac (86). This model permits investigation of the androgenic influence of testicular descent. Homozygous mice mutated by homologous recombination for the *Abd*-related *Hoxa-10* gene are viable, but display homeototic transformations of vertebrae and lumbar spinal nerves (87). Mutant males demonstrate uni- or bilateral cryptorchidism—presumably due to developmental abnormalities of the gubernaculum, resulting in abnormal spermatogenesis and sterility. This interesting mouse exploits the influence of *Hox* genes and patterning of posterior body regions on normal testicular descent. Knockout of the Leydig insulin-like hormone (*Insl3*) gene, a member of the insulin hormone superfamily, results in bilateral cryptorchidism due to developmental abnormalities of the guberaculum (88). Although little is known of the specific function of this normally present gene in the developing testes, it would support the notion that testicular decent is dependent on normal gonadal development, as opposed to the influence of high temperatures secondarily affecting the testicle.

B. Surgical Models

Experimental cryptorchidism has been successfully produced in several animal species. Mice are born cryptorchid; however, spontaneously cryptorchid neonatal mice are difficult models due to their small size. Thus cryptorchidism is usually induced in adult mice by surgical fixation of the testes into an abdominal position with the assistance of an operating microscope (89). The model in which the testicle in adult mice is placed into the abdomen does not exactly recapitulate the scenario observed in humans. It does, however, provide a nice model to study the effect of temperature on the already developed testicle. The cryptorchid testes in this model have been well characterized in terms of light microscopy (89) and Leydig cell morphology (90). It is important to underscore that despite the species similarity to the rat, the testicular morphology following surgical cryptorchidism in the mouse is very different (89, 90). Results obtained using this model must therefore be interpreted with caution.

In rats, inguinoscrotal descent does not normally occur until 3–4 weeks postnatally. The rat, therefore, represents a convenient model to elucidate mechanisms of testicular decent. One simple method to induce cryptorchidism in the neonatal rat is to perform wide excision of the scrotal skin (91). In another model, the extraabdominal distal tip of the gubernaculum is exposed via a small transverse inguinal incision and pexed to the fascia of the groin with 7-0 nylon suture (Fig. 2) (92). This procedure may be performed within 48 hr of birth and is considered to be minimally invasive. The gubernaculum may also be surgically divided, resulting in intraabdominal undescended testes in adult rats. The drawback of dividing the gubernaculum is that the intraabdominal testes are subjected to torsion (93) and rats have a relatively high postoperative mortality rate (94).

The gubernaculum, which has an important role to play in testicular descent, is richly supplied by the genital branch of the genitofemoral nerve through its scrotal attachment. In neonatal rats, the genitofemoral nerve overlying the psoas muscle may be safely divided (95). Denervation of the gubernaculum results in an intraabdominal testis. It has been proposed that the genitofemoral nerve, with the neurotransmitter calcitonin gene-related peptide as its second messenger, directs gubernacular migration and inguinoscrotal testicular descent (96). As such, much work has been done

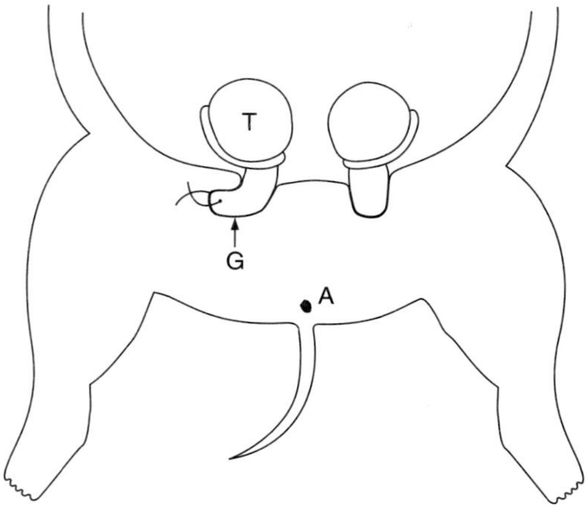

Figure 2 The distal tip of the gubernaculum (G) is exposed extraabdominally within 48 hr of birth in neonatal rats and is pexed on the left side to the fascia of the groin. T, Intraabdominal testes; A, anus. With permission, from Shono *et al.* (92).

using organ cultures of rodent gubernacula to elucidate the role of this neurotransmitter during normal testicular descent (97, 98). Androgens have been proposed to masculinize the normal sexual dimorphism of the genitofemoral nerve spinal nucleus (99). Consistent with this hypothesis is the observation that the normal sexual dimorphism of the genitofemoral nerve spinal nucleus is absent in the mutant TS cryptorchid rat (100).

Other models in the rat include translocation of the normally descended testicle of a mature rat into the abdominal cavity, with closure of the inguinal canal to avoid redescent (101). In other models, the tunica albuginea may be sutured to the abdominal wall (102). The major criticism of both models, however, is that they translocate a normally developed testicle into the abdominal compartment after normal descent has already occurred.

C. Drugs/Hormones

The hormonal control of testicular descent is extremely complex and much information regarding specific hormones and timing of exposure during normal testicular descent remains to be fully characterized. In general, prenatal or postnatal exposure to estrogenic hormones results in cryptorchidism (103–105). Treatment with human chorionic gonadotropin results in testicular descent in some models, without influencing fertility rates (106). Administration of androgenic hormones reverses the effect of estrogenic agents (105). Alternatively, undescended testes are observed in animals after prenatal treatment with the androgen receptor blockade flutamide (105, 107–109) or cyproterone acetate (105). These agents are not effective in preventing cryptorchidism if administered in the postnatal period. Finasteride, an inhibitor of 5α-reductase, has also been associated with testicular undescent (108).

Unfortunately, there are multiple problems associated with many of the aforementioned animal models of cryptorchidism (110). It is therefore important for the investigator to understand the pitfalls of these rodent models. The anatomy of the testicular–gubernacular–cremasteric complex is significantly different in rodents, compared with humans, as are the sequence of appearance and the levels of the various hormones implicated to play a role in this process. Because of these concerns, it has been suggested that the ideal animal model for studies of cryptorchidism would be primates (110). Unfortunately, limited availability, high costs of housing and maintenance, and concerns of institutional animal care committees significantly impact their widespread use for investigational purposes. A thorough understanding of the major differences between rodents and humans coupled with knowledge of the limitations of the rodent studies will pave the way toward an enhanced understanding of this important process.

VI. Intestinal Adaptation Following Massive Small Bowel Resection

The short gut syndrome is a major problem in pediatric surgery. The longer life expectancy of children versus adults and extended duration of need for parenteral nutrition make the likelihood of development of complications associated with this form of nutritional support much greater. Although a substantial proportion of children develop short gut as a result of Crohn's disease, intestinal volvulus, or atresia, the vast majority of cases are due to neonatal necrotizing enterocolitis (NEC). Because survival rates for preterm infants are rising, so too is the incidence of this problem due to NEC. A thorough understanding of the process of gut adaptation and enhancing of this process will facilitate earlier weaning of patients from parenteral nutrition, thereby avoiding much of the associated morbidity.

A. Resection Models

Intestinal resection and subsequent gut adaptation have been well characterized in many animals species, including the pig (111, 112), dog (113–115), rat (116, 117), and mouse (118). There are several advantages in utilizing large animal models of intestinal resection. First, there is a much greater quantity of serum, body fluids, and residual intestine available for analysis during the adaptation phase. Second, the technical aspects of the intestinal resection procedure are more straightforward and easily performed. Finally, the caliber and vascularity of the normal intestine permit the performance of remedial surgical procedures (i.e., valves, lengthening procedures, growth of neomucosa) that are designed to augment absorptive and digestive performance. The major disadvantage of use of the large animal models is the higher cost associated with the purchase and maintenance of the animals. Further, because various hormones and/or growth factors are dosed on a weight basis, larger quantities must be utilized to determine their effects.

Rodent models of intestinal resection and adaptation provide several advantages over large animal models. Their genome is better characterized, thus enabling studies of mutant, transgenic, or knockout strains to test the importance of various factors considered to be involved in adaptation. Further, operative manipulations can be done on greater numbers of animals over shorter periods of time. The animals have short gestation times and the costs for the animals, for the infusion of various substances and for maintenance, are relatively low when compared with other species. The disadvantages of small animal models include the relatively small quantity of tissue and/or serum to study after experimentation. Further, the technical expertise required for the various surgical interventions can be a major limiting factor.

Our laboratory has pioneered an intestinal resection model in the mouse, which we feel is an ideal model system to test various genes considered important for intestinal adaptation (118). All operations are performed under continuous, inhaled isoflurane anesthesia in a sterile operating environment. An operating microscope and microscopic surgical instruments are required to execute the anastomosis. In sham-operated mice, the small bowel is transected 12 cm proximal to the ileocecal valve and a single-layered, interrupted anastomosis is performed. In mice undergoing enterectomy, 50% of proximal intestine is resected and an identical anastomosis is performed, leaving an ileal remnant. A proximal resection is preferred, because adaptive changes are most prominent in the distal intestine. Once the abdomen is closed, the mice are resuscitated with an intraperitoneal injection of normal saline and allowed to recover in a heated incubator. On the day of surgery, mice are given water *ad libitum* and beginning on the first postoperative day, mice from each group are pair-fed a liquid rodent diet (Micro-Stabilized Rodent Liquid Diet LD 101/101A, Purina Mills Inc., Richmond, IN). Pair-feeding of the various groups is important because luminal nutrients have a profound effect on the degree of gut adaptation.

Early experience with this model revealed that mice receiving a solid rodent diet in the postoperative period invariably developed intestinal obstruction and had a high mortality rate. Switching the diet to an isocaloric, isonitrogenous liquid formulation prevented this mortality. This maneuver has had the most profound impact on the success of this model. Another factor that impacted mortality was the size of the suture used for the intestinal anastomosis. The smallest suture was associated with the most ideal outcome and we recommend 9-0 monofilament suture. Initial studies demonstrated that the extent of resection is important. In contrast with other species, 75% resection of the intestine was not well tolerated in the mouse. Therefore, all subsequent studies have been based on a 50% proximal small bowel resection. Immediately following intestinal resection or sham operation, all mice lose weight; however, after 1 week, the mice become anabolic and gain weight.

B. Parameters of Intestinal Adaptation

Several standard parameters of intestinal adaptation must be demonstrated in the various models as internal controls to verify that adaptation has indeed taken place. The increased or decreased expression of various factors in the intestine cannot be considered significant if at least one or two of these factors cannot confirm adaptation. The most basic adaptive parameter includes increase in the wet weight of the remnant intestine, which is normalized to a unit length (such as centimeters). The adaptive response is characterized by both hypertrophy and hyperplasia of all cells within the intestinal wall, but primarily within the mucosa. Increased intestinal remnant DNA and protein content per unit length should be noted. Using these parameters, we have determined that adaptation reaches a peak and is sustained by 1 week in our murine model (Fig. 3).

Structural changes that occur in the remnant intestine during adaptation include increases in villus height and crypt depth. Fixed specimens of ileum are embedded in paraffin and oriented to provide cut sections parallel with the longitudinal axis of the bowel. Slices 5 μm thick are mounted and stained with hematoxylin and eosin. Microscopic measurements are facilitated using a video-assisted integrated computer program (National Institutes of Health, Image 1.57TV). A minimum of 15 villi and crypts are counted per sample. Villi are chosen based on the ability to completely visualize the central lymphatic channel and crypts are chosen based on the ability to visualize the crypt–villus junction on both sides of the crypt.

Because intestinal adaptation represents a mitogenic response, increases in rates of enterocyte proliferation are observed. One method for determination of enterocyte proliferation is to administer 5-bromodeoxyuridine (BrdU) intraperitoneally prior to sacrifice of the animal. This nucleotide analog is incorporated into the nucleus of proliferating crypt cells (S phase). BrdU incorporation is detected in histologic sections of the intestine using a biotinylated monoclonal anti-BrdU antibody system with streptavidin–peroxidase as a signal generator. The staining reagents and methods are provided in kit form (Zymed Laboratories Inc., San Francisco, CA). An index of crypt cell proliferation rates may be derived by counting the number of cells per crypt that incorporated BrdU divided by the total number of cells in the crypt. At least 10 representative crypts should be counted (ability to visualize the crypt–villus junction on both sides of the crypt) from each animal. Investigators should be blinded as to the origin of the tissue section during the scoring procedure.

Another response observed during adaptation is an increase in the rate of enterocyte apoptosis (119). It is presently unclear whether this is simply a physiologic response to the increase in enterocyte proliferation or whether it is a unique event that is regulated by other factors. Initial experiments involving the morphologic study of apoptosis utilized propidium iodide staining as well as labeling of DNA strand breaks with the TdT-mediated dUTP nick-end labeling (TUNEL) method. These methodologies often yielded a great deal of nonspecific background staining, complicating the interpretation of results. Subsequent studies therefore have relied on standard hematoxylin and eosin staining. The rate of apoptosis is quantified by blinded scoring of the number of apoptotic bodies identified within the crypts. Apoptotic bodies are defined as cells containing pyknotic nuclei, condensed chromatin, and nuclear fragmentation (120). Counting the number of apoptotic bodies per crypt and averaging the values of 50 crypts per mouse permits the derivation of an apoptotic index.

C. Testing the Role of Various Factors

Understanding the process of intestinal adaptation is a requisite toward designing therapies to enhance this response. Enhancing adaptation will significantly reduce the need for parenteral nutrition as well as its associated morbidity. Many factors have been proposed to play a role in the genesis of intestinal adaptation and generally include luminal nutrients, pancreaticobiliary secretions, hormones, and growth factors [see Williamson (121) for review].

Many investigators using multiple animal models have recorded the effects of exogenous administration of multiple drugs, hormones, and growth factors on postresection adaptation. It is important to document the optimal route of administration (i.e., orogastric gavage versus subcutaneous versus intraperitoneal), the proper dosage, and timing of administration relative to the time of intestinal resection for each model and substance tested. Evaluating all of these parameters, we demonstrated that the ideal conditions for exogenous epidermal growth factor (EGF) to amplify adaptation in our mouse model of intestinal resection is via the orogastric route at a dosage of 50 μg/kg/day in the immediate period following the enterectomy (122). In that study, higher dosages of EGF actually inhibited adaptation and EGF had minimal effect on adaptation if administered either before the intestinal resection or after the interval of adapta-

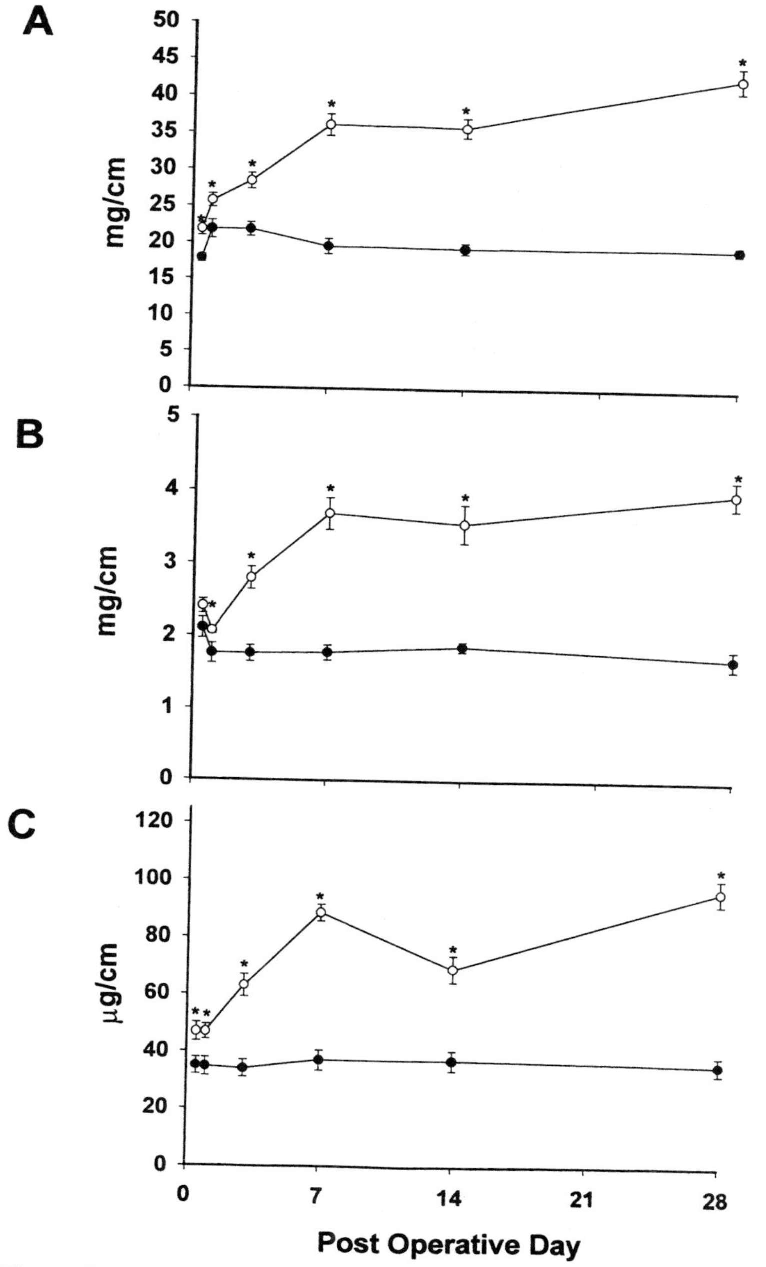

Figure 3 Ileal wet weight (A), protein content (B), and DNA content (C) at various time points following either 50% proximal small bowel resection (SBR, ○) or sham operation (division of the intestine with reanastomosis alone, ●) in mice.

tion had already taken place. Similar data should be ascertained for each candidate factor within the confines of each animal model utilized.

The murine model for intestinal resection allows testing of specific genes considered to be important during intestinal adaptation. In one set of experiments, the importance of a functional EGF receptor was studied using waved-2 mice (123). These commercially available mice have a mutation of the tyrosine kinase domain of the EGF receptor that impairs receptor signaling. Adaptation following intestinal resection in these mice is lethal, because they do not demonstrate an ability to undergo adaptation. Alternatively, we created a transgenic mouse that utilized the intestinal fatty acid-binding promoter to drive the overexpression of EGF specifically within differentiated enterocytes (124). These mice demonstrated a superadaptive response to intestinal resection. By targeting the expression of EGF to the enterocyte, this study affirmed that the beneficial effect of EGF on adaptation was via a direct effect on enterocyte, and not via a secondary effect by some other systemic factor.

The influence of various luminal factors on adaptation may be studied by transposing the distal ileum into a more proximal position within the gastrointestinal tract. Using this model, investigators have documented within the transposed ileum adaptive changes that are very similar to those occurring following massive enterectomy (125, 126). In another model, the effect of pancreaticobiliary secretions on adaptation was evaluated by surgical transposition of the duodenal ampulla into the distal ileum (127). In this anatomic arrangement, mucosal hyperplasia was induced in the ileum distal to the ampulla. The relative contribution of bile alone versus bile plus pancreatic secretions may be studied by diversion of bile above the pancreas into the distal ileum. When this is done and compared with the ampullary transposition model, the combined pancreaticobiliary secretions had the greatest trophic effect on the ileum (128).

Finally, compelling verification of the presence of a systemic factor as an initiator of the process of adaptation has been provided using vascular parabiosis models. In this arrangement, enterectomy in one rat results in proliferative changes in the undisturbed gastrointestinal mucosa of the rat that was sharing a common blood supply (123). This model should foster the development of multiple experiments to determine which specific circulating factor is capable of modulating these changes.

VII. Abdominal Wall Defects

The abdominal wall defects—gastroschisis and omphalocele—occur with a frequency of approximately 1 in every 5000 and 1 in every 6,000–10,000 births, respectively. The cause of these defects is presently unknown, but it likely represents a constellation of chromosomal, environmental, and teratogenic factors. In omphalocele, the intestine and liver are protected from the amniotic fluid by a membrane or sac. The major determinants of morbidity and mortality in these infants are the associated congenital anomalies, rather than the defect. In gastroschisis, the intestine is not covered with a sac and the intestine is exposed to the amniotic fluid. Because infants born with gastroschisis have a much lower incidence of associated anomalies when compared with omphalocele, survival is higher and the major morbidity is associated with the intestinal damage induced by exposure to the amniotic fluid. In addition to embryonic models of abdominal wall defects, most surgical models are designed to investigate what specific component(s) of the amniotic fluid are injurious to the intestine. Additional active investigation has attempted to determine the ideal prosthetic material to use for the closure of large abdominal wall defects.

A. Embryonic Models

Several substances have been administered to pregnant females of various species to induce the development of abdominal wall defects. The results are generally inconsistent and associated with multiple other anomalies. These types of studies, however, may prove of value in terms of elucidating the timing and mechanism for the development of this problem. Aminopyrine was administered to pregnant mice on days 7, 8, and 9 of gestation with resultant development of omphalocele in the offspring (129). This effect appears to be dependent on the strain of mouse utilized, because the incidence of anomalies was greater in C57BL/6N mice when compared with DBA/2N mice. The teratogenic effect of this agent may be enhanced with barbital (130).

In rats, omphalocele and other anomalies have been described in offspring following maternal exposure to DA-125 (anthracycline antineoplastic agent) (131), β-aminopropionitrile (132), or flubendazole (133). In chicken egg embryos, a 15-min infusion of cocaine into eggs at E18 resulted in herniated umbilici in the hatchlings (134). This effect could be blocked by pretreatment with the 5-HT2 antagonist, ritanserin. These data suggest that the vasoconstriction induced by cocaine via 5-HT2 receptors may play a role in the development of abdominal wall defects. In another, nonspecific model (135), placement of pregnant guinea pigs in a hyperthermic environment for 1 hr per day at several periods during gestation was shown to be associated with development of abdominal wall defects, among other abnormalities.

Gastroschisis occurs with a high frequency in the inbred mouse strain HLG with a substantially increased risk after exposure to irradiation during preimplantation development (136). Through backcross breeding studies and genome-wide microsatellite typing, a suggestive linkage for a locus responsible for radiation-induced gastroschisis was identified in a region of the mouse chromosome 7 (137). Future studies with these mice may provide useful information regarding important genomic loci that may be involved in the development of abdominal wall defects.

B. Surgical Models

For surgical models of gastroschisis, sheep, rabbits, and chicken embryos have been utilized. The sheep model of gastroschisis was first described by Haller *et al.* in 1974 (138). In this initial study, fetal lambs underwent operative intervention within a gestational age of 80–100 days (term is 145 days). The caudal half of the fetus was delivered through a uterotomy incision and a full-thickness disk of abdominal wall was excised lateral to the umbilical cord. The disk diameter ranged from 0.5 to 5 cm. With this early model, in over half of the fetuses aborted the exposed intestine in the surviving fetuses displayed the characteristic edema and matted appearance that mimics what is seen in humans.

Langer *et al.* modified this lamb model to include standardizing the abdominal wall defect by the insertion of a 4 × 2-cm oval silastic ring (Fig. 4) (139–141). In addition, the added effect of constricting the base of the exteriorized bowel with umbilical tape could be evaluated. This model was also associated with a relatively high rate of spontaneous abortion (48%). What was learned, however, was that the degree of intestinal damage was directly related to the time of exposure to the amniotic fluid (139, 140). The intestine was evaluated for changes in morphology as well as mucosal enzyme activity. In general, sheep models are associated with high mortality, high cost, only seasonal availability of pregnant ewes, and relatively lengthy gestational period.

Rabbit models of gastroschisis have emerged, providing several advantages over sheep in that they are less costly, have shorter and more frequent gestations, and are associated with lower animal purchase and maintenance costs. This model was initially associated with a success rate of less than 30% (142, 143). With improvements in anesthesia, use of prophylactic antibiotics, and application of basic principles of fetal surgery, success rates have improved to the range of 80–90% (144, 145). One novel technique to test the effect of removal of the amniotic fluid from the exposed intestine was evaluated by suturing the lower half of the experimental fetus to the edges of the uterotomy incision (Fig. 5) (146). Numerous studies with this model have included studies of enterocyte gene expression (147), intestinal nutrient uptake (148), and the influence of intraamniotic dexamethasone infusion (149).

Chicken embryos represent the least costly model for gastroschisis, and much information has been derived from studies using them. The chicken embryo is enveloped in amniotic fluid and a number of membranes (Fig. 6). The egg is first candled to verify fertility, the air pocket is punctured on day 16 of incubation, and 4–5 ml of air is removed. The eggshell is chipped away until a hole with a diameter of roughly 1 cm has been created. After moistening both shell membranes with physiologic saline solution for birds (0.75% NaCl solution), the rich vascular pattern of the chorioallantoic membrane becomes visible. After sharp opening of this membrane, the allantoic cavity is reached. The top end of the umbilical cord is traced after localization

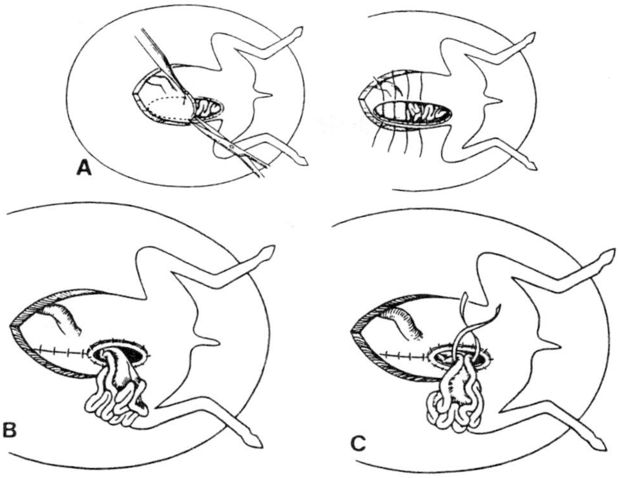

Figure 4 Experimental technique of gastroschisis creation in fetal lambs. (A) Excision of the right side of the abdominal wall and closure of the superior aspect. (B) Insertion of an oval silastic ring to standardize the defect size (4 × 2 cm) and extrusion of the small bowel. (C) Placement of an umbilical tape as a constrictor around the base of the extruded bowel. With permission, from Langer *et al.* (139).

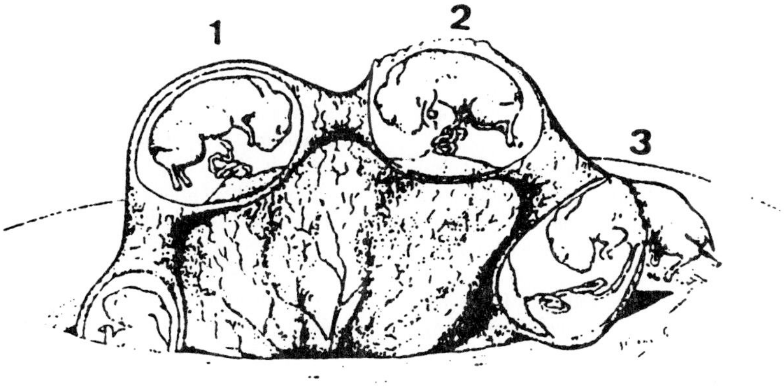

Figure 5 Gastroschisis model designed to remove the effect of the variable of amniotic fluid on the intestinal damage during development. The first rabbit is an unoperated control, the second had a gastroschisis defect created and then returned to the amniotic fluid. The third fetus had a defect created, but the lower half of the body was secured to the periphery of the hysterotomy incision to keep the amniotic fluid away from the exposed intestine. With permission, from Albert *et al.* (146).

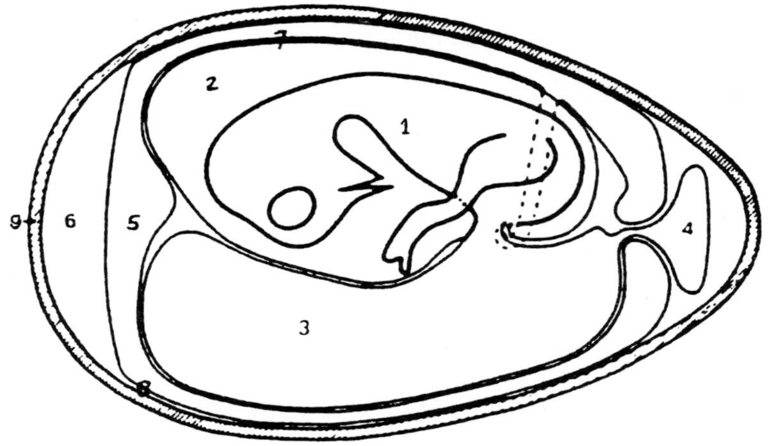

Figure 6 Schematic drawing of the various membranes and cavities in the chicken embryo. 1, Embryo; 2, amniotic cavity; 3, yolk sac; 4, albumin; 5, allantois cavity; 6, air pocket; 7, fusion of allantois and amniotic membranes (seroamniotic fusion); 8, fusion of chorion and allantois membranes; 9, eggshell with outer and inner shell membranes. With permission, from Tibboel *et al.* (150).

of one of the allantoic vessels. Incising into the physiologic umbilical hernia sac creates a gastroschisis (150). The egg is then sealed with a sterile plastic dressing, which allows monitoring of embryo viability. The shells are reopened and embryos studied at the end of day 20.

Using the chick model, investigators have explored the effect of amniotic fluid exchange in an attempt to reduce the severity of intestinal damage (151–153). This work has resulted in better evaluation and management of human fetuses with prenatally diagnosed gastroschisis, with encouraging initial results (154). Additional studies with this model implicate a role for nitric oxide within the exposed intestine as a mediator of intestinal damage (155).

References

1. Riepenhoff-Talty, M., Schaekel, K., Clark, H. F., Mueller, W., Uhnoo, I., Rossi, T., Fisher, J., and Ogra, P. L. (1993). Group A rotaviruses produce extrahepatic biliary obstruction in orally inoculated newborn mice. *Pediatr. Res.* **33,** 394–399.
2. Petersen, C., Grasshoff, S., and Luciano, L. (1998). Diverse morphology of biliary atresia in an animal model. *J. Hepatol.* **28,** 603–607.
3. Petersen, C., Kuske, M., Bruns, E., Biermanns, D., Wussow, P. V., and Mildenberger, H. (1998). Progress in developing animal models for biliary atresia. *Eur. J. Pediatr. Surg.* **8,** 137–141.
4. Phillips, P. A., Keast, D., Papadimitriou, J. M., Walters, M. N., and Stanley, N. F. (1969). Chronic obstructive jaundice induced by Reovirus type 3 in weanling mice. *Pathology* **1,** 193–203.
5. Bangaru, B., Morecki, R., Glaser, J. H., Gartner, L. M., and Horwitz, M. S. (1980). Comparative studies of biliary atresia in the human newborn and reovirus-induced cholangitis in weanling mice. *Lab. Invest.* **43,** 456–462.
6. Jevon, G. P., and Dimmick, J. E. (1999). Biliary atresia and cytomegalovirus infection: A DNA study. *Pediatr. Dev. Pathol.* **2,** 11–14.
7. Brown, W. R., Sokol, R. J., Levin, M. J., Silverman, A., Tamaru, T., Lilly, J. R., Hall, R. J., and Cheney, M. (1988). Lack of correlation between infection with reovirus 3 and extrahepatic biliary atresia or neonatal hepatitis. *J. Pediatr.* **113,** 670–676.
8. Bobo, L., Ojeh, C., Chiu, D., Machado, A., Colombani, P., and Schwarz, K. (1997). Lack of evidence for rotavirus by polymerase chain reaction/enzyme immunoassay of hepatobiliary samples from children with biliary atresia. *Pediatr. Res.* **41,** 229–234.
9. Morecki, R., and Glaser, J. (1989). Reovirus 3 and neonatal biliary disease: Discussion of divergent results. *Hepatology* **10,** 515–517.
10. Vacanti, J. P., and Folkman, J. (1979). Bile duct enlargement by infusion of L-proline: Potential significance in biliary atresia. *J. Pediatr. Surg.* **14,** 814–818.
11. Schier, F., Schier, C., and Szabo, E. (1989). The influence of various amino acids on the extrahepatic bile ducts in newborn mice—An experimental study. *J. Pediatr. Surg.* **24,** 267–270.
12. Ogawa, T., Suruga, K., and Kuwabara, N. (1981). Experimental model of infantile obstructive cholangiopathy using 1,4-phenylenediisothiocyanate. *Jpn. J. Surg.* **11,** 372–376.
13. Ogawa, T., Suruga, K., Kojima, Y., Kitahara, T., and Kuwabara, N. (1983). Experimental study of the pathogenesis of infantile obstructive cholangiopathy and its clinical evaluation. *J. Pediatr. Surg.* **18,** 131–135.
14. Schmeling, D. J., Oldham, K. T., Guice, K. S., Kunkel, R. G., and Johnson, K. J. (1991). Experimental obliterative cholangitis. A model for the study of biliary atresia. *Ann. Surg.* **213,** 350–355.
15. Youson, J. H., and Sidon, E. W. (1978). Lamprey biliary atresia: First model system for the human condition? *Experientia* **34,** 1084–1086.
16. Sidon, E. W., and Youson, J. H. (1983). Morphological changes in the liver of the sea lamprey, *Petromyzon marinus* L., during metamorphosis: I. Atresia of the bile ducts. *J. Morphol.* **177,** 109–124.
17. Youson, J. H. (1993). Biliary atresia in lampreys. *Adv. Vet. Sci. Comp. Med.* **37,** 197–255.
18. Makos, B. K., and Youson, J. H. (1988). Tissue levels of bilirubin and biliverdin in the sea lamprey, *Petromyzon marinus* L., before and after biliary atresia. *Comp. Biochem. Physiol. A* **91,** 701–710.
19. Spitz, L. (1980). Ligation of the common bile duct in the fetal lamb: An experimental model for the study of biliary atresia. *Pediatr. Res.* **14,** 740–748.

20. Schreiber, R. A., Kleinman, R. E., Barksdale, E. M. J., Maganaro, T. F., and Donahoe, P. K. (1992). Rejection of murine congenic bile ducts: A model for immune-mediated bile duct disease. *Gastroenterology* **102,** 924–930.
21. Funaki, N., Sasano, H., Shizawa, S., Nio, M., Iwami, D., Ohi, R., and Nagura, H. (1998). Apoptosis and cell proliferation in biliary atresia. *J. Pathol.* **186,** 429–433.
22. Passarge, E. (1967). The genetics of Hirschsprung's disease. Evidence for heterogeneous etiology and a study of sixty-three families. *N. Engl. J. Med.* **276,** 138–143.
23. Puri, P., Ohshiro, K., and Wester, T. (1998). Hirschsprung's disease: A search for etiology. *Semin. Pediatr. Surg.* **7,** 140–147.
24. Lane, P. W. (1966). Association of megacolon with two recessive spotting genes in the mouse. *J. Hered.* **57,** 29–31.
25. Bolande, R. P. (1975). Hirschsprung's disease, aganglionic or hypoganglionic megacolon. Animal model: Aganglionic megacolon in piebald and spotted mutant mouse strains. *Am. J. Pathol.* **79,** 189–192.
26. Lane, P. W., and Liu, H. M. (1984). Association of megacolon with a new dominant spotting gene (*Dom*) in the mouse. *J. Hered.* **75,** 435–439.
27. Schuchardt, A., D'Agati, V., Larsson-Blomberg, L., Costantini, F., and Pachnis, V. (1995). RET-deficient mice: An animal model for Hirschsprung's disease and renal agenesis. *J. Intern. Med.* **238,** 327–332.
28. Payette, R. F., Tennyson, V. M., Pham, T. D., Mawe, G. M., Pomeranz, H. D., Rothman, T. P., and Gershon, M. D. (1987). Origin and morphology of nerve fibers in the aganglionic colon of the lethal spotted (ls/ls) mutant mouse. *J. Comp. Neurol.* **257,** 237–252.
29. Tennyson, V. M., Pham, T. D., Rothman, T. P., and Gershon, M. D. (1986). Abnormalities of smooth muscle, basal laminae, and nerves in the aganglionic segments of the bowel of lethal spotted mutant mice. *Anat. Rec.* **215,** 267–281.
30. Webster, W. (1974). Aganglionic megacolon in piebald-lethal mice. *Arch. Pathol.* **97,** 111–117.
31. Bolande, R. P., and Towler, W. F. (1972). Ultrastructural and histochemical studies of murine megacolon. *Am. J. Pathol.* **69,** 139–162.
32. Fujimoto, T. (1988). Natural history and pathophysiology of enterocolitis in the piebald lethal mouse model of Hirschsprung's disease. *J. Pediatr. Surg.* **23,** 237–242.
33. Fujimoto, T., Reen, D. J., and Puri, P. (1988). Inflammatory response in enterocolitis in the piebald lethal mouse model of Hirschsprung's disease. *Pediatr. Res.* **24,** 152–155.
34. McCabe, L., Griffin, L. D., Kinzer, A., Chandler, M., Beckwith, J. B., and McCabe, E. R. (1990). Overo lethal white foal syndrome: Equine model of aganglionic megacolon (Hirschsprung disease). *Am. J. Med. Genet.* **36,** 336–340.
35. Gariepy, C. E., Cass, D. T., and Yanagisawa, M. (1996). Null mutation of endothelin receptor type B gene in spotting lethal rats causes aganglionic megacolon and white coat color. *Proc. Natl. Acad. Sci. U.S.A.* **93,** 867–872.
36. Lipman, N. S., Wardrip, C. L., Yuan, C. S., Coventry, S., Bunte, R. M., and Li, X. (1998). Familial megacecum and colon in the rat: A new model of gastrointestinal neuromuscular dysfunction. *Lab. Anim. Sci.* **48,** 243–252.
37. Rothman, T. P., and Gershon, M. D. (1982). Phenotypic expression in the developing murine enteric nervous system. *J. Neurosci.* **2,** 381–393.
38. Meijers, J. H., Tibboel, D., van der Kamp, A. W., Van Haperen-Heuts, I. C., Kluck, P., and Molenaar, J. C. (1987). The influence of the stage of differentiation of the gut on the migration of neural cells: An experimental study of Hirschsprung's disease. *Pediatr. Res.* **21,** 466–470.
39. Nishijima, E., Meijers, J. H., Tibboel, D., Luider, T. M., Peters-van der Sanden, M. M., van der Kamp, A. W., and Molenaar, J. C. (1990). Formation and malformation of the enteric nervous system in mice: an organ culture study. *J. Pediatr. Surg.* **25,** 627–631.
40. Kapur, R. P., Yost, C., and Palmiter, R. D. (1992). A transgenic model for studying development of the enteric nervous system in normal and aganglionic mice. *Development* **116,** 167–175.
41. Coventry, S., Yost, C., Palmiter, R. D., and Kapur, R. P. (1994). Migration of ganglion cell precursors in the ileoceca of normal and lethal spotted embryos, a murine model for Hirschsprung disease. *Lab. Invest.* **71,** 82–93.
42. Parikh, D. H., Tam, P. K., Van Velzen, D., and Edgar, D. (1992). Abnormalities in the distribution of laminin and collagen type IV in Hirschsprung's disease. *Gastroenterology* **102,** 1236–1241.
43. Parikh, D. H., Tam, P. K., Van Velzen, D., and Edgar, D. (1994). The extracellular matrix components, tenascin and fibronectin, in Hirschsprung's disease: An immunohistochemical study. *J. Pediatr. Surg.* **29,** 1302–1306.
44. Payette, R. F., Tennyson, V. M., Pomeranz, H. D., Pham, T. D., Rothman, T. P., and Gershon, M. D. (1988). Accumulation of components of basal laminae: Association with the failure of neural crest cells to colonize the presumptive aganglionic bowel of ls/ls mutant mice. *Dev. Biol.* **125,** 341–360.
45. Tennyson, V. M., Payette, R. F., Rothman, T. P., and Gershon, M. D. (1990). Distribution of hyaluronic acid and chondroitin sulfate proteoglycans in the presumptive aganglionic terminal bowel of ls/ls fetal mice: An ultrastructural analysis. *J. Comp. Neurol.* **291,** 345–362.
46. Jacobs-Cohen, R. J., Payette, R. F., Gershon, M. D., and Rothman, T. P. (1987). Inability of neural crest cells to colonize the presumptive aganglionic bowel of ls/ls mutant mice: Requirement for a permissive microenvironment. *J. Comp. Neurol.* **255,** 425–438.
47. Ohshiro, K., and Puri, P. (1999). Decreased levels of nerve growth factor and neurotropin-3 in the smooth muscle of Hirschprung's disease. The 10th Annual Symposium on Pediatric Surgical Research, October, 1997.
48. Kakita, Y., Ohshiro, K., Puri, P., Kobayashi, H., and O'Briain, D. S. (1998). Lack of a docking mechanism for neurotransmitter release in the aganglionic segment of bowel in patients with Hirschsprung's disease. *Pediatr. Surg. Int.* **13,** 581–583.
49. Kuroda, T., Ueda, M., Nakano, M., and Saeki, M. (1994). Altered production of nerve growth factor in aganglionic intestines. *J. Pediatr. Surg.* **29,** 288–292.
50. Davies, A. M., Wyatt, S., Nishimura, M., and Phillips, H. (1995). NGF receptor expression in sensory neurons develops normally in embryos lacking NGF. *Dev. Biol.* **171,** 434–438.
51. Kobayashi, H., O'Briain, D. S., and Puri, P. (1994). Lack of expression of NADPH-diaphorase and neural cell adhesion molecule (NCAM) in colonic muscle of patients with Hirschsprung's disease. *J. Pediatr. Surg.* **29,** 301–304.
52. Ikawa, H., Kawano, H., Takeda, Y., Masuyama, H., Watanabe, K., Endo, M., Yokoyama, J., Kitajima, M., Uyemura, K., and Kawamura, K. (1997). Impaired expression of neural cell adhesion molecule L1 in the extrinsic nerve fibers in Hirschsprung's disease. *J. Pediatr. Surg.* **32,** 542–545.
53. Hirobe, S., Doody, D. P., Ryan, D. P., Kim, S. H., and Donahoe, P. K. (1992). Ectopic class II major histocompatibility antigens in Hirschsprung's disease and neuronal intestinal dysplasia. *J. Pediatr. Surg.* **27,** 357–362.
54. Kobayashi, H., Hirakawa, H., and Puri, P. (1995). Overexpression of intercellular adhesion molecule-1 (ICAM-1) and MHC class II antigen on hypertrophic nerve trunks suggests an immunopathologic response in Hirschsprung's disease. *J. Pediatr. Surg.* **30,** 1680–1683.
55. Kanto, W. P. J., Wilson, R., Breart, G. L., Zierler, S., Purohit, D. M., Peckham, G. J., and Ellison, R. C. (1987). Perinatal events and necrotizing enterocolitis in premature infants. *Am. J. Dis. Child.* **141,** 167–169.
56. Ryder, R. W., Shelton, J. D., and Guinan, M. E. (1980). Necrotizing enterocolitis: A prospective multicenter investigation. *Am. J. Epidemiol.* **112,** 113–123.

57. Brans, Y. W., Escobedo, M. B., Hayashi, R. H., Huff, R. W., Kagan-Hallet, K. S., and Ramamurthy, R. S. (1984). Perinatal mortality in a large perinatal center: Five-year review of 31,000 births. *Am. J. Obstet. Gynecol.* **148,** 284–289.
58. Crissinger, K. D. (1995). Animal models of necrotizing enterocolitis. *J. Pediatr. Gastroenterol. Nutr.* **20,** 17–22.
59. Topalian, S. L., and Ziegler, M. M. (1984). Necrotizing enterocolitis: A review of animal models. *J. Surg. Res.* **37,** 320–336.
60. Sibbons, P. D., Spitz, L., and Van Velzen, D. (1992). Necrotizing enterocolitis induced by local circulatory interruption in the ileum of neonatal piglets. *Pediatr. Pathol.* **12,** 1–14.
61. Krasna, I. H., Howell, C., Vega, A., Ziegler, M., and Koop, C. E. (1986). A mouse model for the study of necrotizing enterocolitis. *J. Pediatr. Surg.* **21,** 26–29.
62. Krasna, I. H., and Lee, R. T. (1993). Allopurinol protects the bowel from necrosis caused by indomethacin and temporary intestinal ischemia in mice. *J. Pediatr. Surg.* **28,** 1175–1177.
63. Krasna, I. H., and Kim, H. (1992). Indomethacin administration after temporary ischemia causes bowel necrosis in mice. *J. Pediatr. Surg.* **27,** 805–807.
64. Sibbons, P., Spitz, L., and Van Velzen, D. (1992). The role of lymphatics in the pathogenesis of pneumatosis in experimental bowel ischemia. *J. Pediatr. Surg.* **27,** 339–342.
65. Clark, D. A., Thompson, J. E., Weiner, L. B., McMillan, J. A., Schneider, A. J., and Rokahr, J. E. (1985). Necrotizing enterocolitis: Intraluminal biochemistry in human neonates and a rabbit model. *Pediatr. Res.* **19,** 919–921.
66. Miller, M. J., Adams, J., Gu, X. A., Zhang, X. J., and Clark, D. A. (1990). Hemodynamic and permeability characteristics of acute experimental necrotizing enterocolitis. *Dig. Dis. Sci.* **35,** 1257–1264.
67. Clark, D. A., Fornabaio, D. M., McNeill, H., Mullane, K. M., Caravella, S. J., and Miller, M. J. (1988). Contribution of oxygen-derived free radicals to experimental necrotizing enterocolitis. *Am. J. Pathol.* **130,** 537–542.
68. Dickinson, E. C., Gorga, J. C., Garrett, M., Tuncer, R., Boyle, P., Watkins, S. C., Alber, S. M., Parizhskaya, M., Trucco, M., Rowe, M. I., and Ford, H. R. (1998). Immunoglobulin A supplementation abrogates bacterial translocation and preserves the architecture of the intestinal epithelium. *Surgery* **124,** 284–290.
69. Crissinger, K. D., and Tso, P. (1992). The role of lipids in ischemia/reperfusion-induced changes in mucosal permeability in developing piglets. *Gastroenterology* **102,** 1693–1699.
70. Velasquez, O. R., Henninger, K., Fowler, M., Tso, P., and Crissinger, K. D. (1993). Oleic acid-induced mucosal injury in developing piglet intestine. *Am. J. Physiol.* **264,** G576–G582.
71. Crissinger, K. D., Burney, D. L., Velasquez, O. R., and Gonzalez, E. (1994). An animal model of necrotizing enterocolitis induced by infant formula and ischemia in developing piglets. *Gastroenterology* **106,** 1215–1222.
72. Musemeche, C. A., Kosloske, A. M., Bartow, S. A., and Umland, E. T. (1986). Comparative effects of ischemia, bacteria, and substrate on the pathogenesis of intestinal necrosis. *J. Pediatr. Surg.* **21,** 536–538.
73. Gonzalez-Crussi, F., and Hsueh, W. (1983). Experimental model of ischemic bowel necrosis. The role of platelet- activating factor and endotoxin. *Am. J. Pathol.* **112,** 127–135.
74. Caplan, M. S., Sun, X. M., and Hsueh, W. (1990). Hypoxia causes ischemic bowel necrosis in rats: The role of platelet- activating factor (PAF-acether). *Gastroenterology* **99,** 979–986.
75. Akisu, M., Baka, M., Coker, I., Kultursay, N., and Huseyinov, A. (1998). Effect of dietary N-3 fatty acids on hypoxia-induced necrotizing enterocolitis in young mice. N-3 fatty acids alter platelet-activating factor and leukotriene B4 production in the intestine. *Biol. Neonate* **74,** 31–38.
76. Tracey, K. J., Beutler, B., Lowry, S. F., Merryweather, J., Wolpe, S., Milsark, I. W., Hariri, R. J., Fahey, T. J., Zentella, A., and Albert, J. D. (1986). Shock and tissue injury induced by recombinant human cachectin. *Science* **234,** 470–474.
77. Sun, X. M., and Hsueh, W. (1988). Bowel necrosis induced by tumor necrosis factor in rats is mediated by platelet-activating factor. *J. Clin. Invest.* **81,** 1328–1331.
78. Huang, L., Tan, X., Crawford, S. E., and Hsueh, W. (1994). Platelet-activating factor and endotoxin induce tumour necrosis factor gene expression in rat intestine and liver. *Immunology* **83,** 65–69.
79. Sun, X., Caplan, M. S., Liu, Y., and Hsueh, W. (1995). Endotoxin-resistant mice are protected from PAF-induced bowel injury and death. Role of TNF, complement activation, and endogenous PAF production. *Dig. Dis. Sci.* **40,** 495–502.
80. Hutson, J. M., Baker, M., Terada, M., Zhou, B., and Paxton, G. (1994). Hormonal control of testicular descent and the cause of cryptorchidism. *Reprod. Fertil. Dev.* **6,** 151–156.
81. Pinart, E., Camps, R., Briz, M. D., Bonet, S., and Egozcue, J. (1998). Unilateral spontaneous abdominal cryptorchidism: structural and ultrastructural study of sperm morphology. *Anim. Reprod. Sci.* **49,** 247–268.
82. Hutson, J. M., Watts, L. M., and Farmer, P. J. (1998). Congenital undescended testes in neonatal pigs and the effect of exogenous calcitonin gene-related peptide [see comments]. *J. Urol.* **159,** 1025–1028.
83. Mouhadjer, N., Pointis, G., Malassine, A., and Bedin, M. (1989). Testicular steroid sulfatase in a cryptorchid rat strain. *J. Steroid Biochem.* **34,** 555–558.
84. Lugg, J. A., Penson, D. F., Sadeghi, F., Petrie, B., Freedman, A. L., Gonzalez-Cadavid, N. F., Hikim, A. S., and Rajfer, J. (1996). Prevention of seminiferous tubular atrophy in a naturally cryptorchid rat model by early surgical intervention. *J. Androl.* **17,** 726–732.
85. Ikadai, H., Ajisawa, C., Taya, K., and Imamichi, T. (1988). Suprainguinal ectopic scrota of TS inbred rats. *J. Reprod. Fertil.* **84,** 701–707.
86. Hutson, J. M., and Beasley, S. W. (1988). Embryological controversies in testicular descent. *Semin. Urol.* **6,** 68–73.
87. Rijli, F. M., Matyas, R., Pellegrini, M., Dierich, A., Gruss, P., Dolle, P., and Chambon, P. (1995). Cryptorchidism and homeotic transformations of spinal nerves and vertebrae in Hoxa-10 mutant mice. *Proc. Natl. Acad. Sci. U.S.A.* **92,** 8185–8189.
88. Nef, S., and Parada, L. F. (1999). Cryptorchidism in mice mutant for Insl3. *Nature Genet.* **22,** 295–299.
89. Mendis-Handagama, S. M., Kerr, J. B., and de Kretser, D. M. (1990). Experimental cryptorchidism in the adult mouse: I. Qualitative and quantitative light microscopic morphology. *J. Androl.* **11,** 539–547.
90. Mendis-Handagama, S. M., Kerr, J. B., and de Kretser, D. M. (1991). Experimental cryptorchidism in the adult mouse. III. Qualitative and quantitative electron microscopic morphology of Leydig cells. *J. Androl.* **12,** 335–343.
91. Shono, T., and Suita, S. (1995). The effect of the excision of future scrotal skin on testicular descent in neonatal rats: a new experimental model of cryptorchidism. *J. Pediatr. Surg.* **30,** 734–738.
92. Shono, T., Zakaria, O., Imajima, T., and Suita, S. (1996). Extraabdominal fixation of the gubernaculum inhibits testicular descent in newborn rats. *J. Pediatr. Surg.* **31,** 503–506.
93. Beasley, S. W., and Hutson, J. M. (1988). The role of the gubernaculum in testicular descent. *J. Urol.* **140,** 1191–1193.
94. Quinn, F. M. (1991). Evaluation of the scrotal testis before and after orchidopexy in experimental unilateral cryptorchidism. *J. Pediatr. Surg.* **26,** 602–606.
95. Beasley, S. W., and Hutson, J. M. (1987). Effect of division of genitofemoral nerve on testicular descent in the rat. *Aust. N.Z. J. Surg.* **57,** 49–51.
96. Goh, D. W., Momose, Y., Middlesworth, W., and Hutson, J. M. (1993). The relationship among calcitonin gene-related peptide, androgens and gubernacular development in 3 animal models of cryptorchidism. *J. Urol.* **150,** 574–576.

97. Terada, M., Goh, D. W., Farmer, P. J., and Hutson, J. M. (1994). Calcitonin gene-related peptide receptors in the gubernaculum of normal rat and 2 models of cryptorchidism. *J. Urol.* **152,** 759–762.
98. Momose, Y., Goh, D. W., and Hutson, J. M. (1993). Calcitonin gene-related peptide stimulates motility of the gubernaculum via cyclic adenosine monophosphate. *J. Urol.* **150,** 571–573.
99. Kojima, M., and Sano, Y. (1984). Sexual differences in the topographical distribution of serotonergic fibers in the anterior column of rat lumbar spinal cord. *Anat. Embryol. (Berl.)* **170,** 117–121.
100. Goh, D. W., Farmer, P. J., and Hutson, J. M. (1994). Absence of normal sexual dimorphism of the genitofemoral nerve spinal nucleus in the mutant cryptorchid (TS) rat. *J. Reprod. Fertil.* **102,** 195–199.
101. Risbridger, G. P., Kerr, J. B., Peake, R., Rich, K. A., and de Kretser, D. M. (1981). Temporal changes in rat Leydig cell function after the induction of bilateral cryptorchidism. *J. Reprod. Fertil.* **63,** 415–423.
102. Jahnsen, T., Gordeladze, J. O., Haug, E., and Hansson, V. (1981). Changes in rat testicular adenylate cyclase activities and gonadotrophin binding during unilateral experimental cryptorchidism. *J. Reprod. Fertil.* **63,** 381–390.
103. Walker, A. H., Bernstein, L., Warren, D. W., Warner, N. E., Zheng, X., and Henderson, B. E. (1990). The effect of *in utero* ethinyl oestradiol exposure on the risk of cryptorchid testis and testicular teratoma in mice. *Br. J. Cancer* **62,** 599–602.
104. Lein, M., Fahlenkamp, D., Schonberger, B., Prollius, S., and Loening, S. (1996). The pharmacological effect of the gonadotrophin-releasing hormone on experimental cryptorchidism in rats. *Scand. J. Urol. Nephrol.* **30,** 185–191.
105. Spencer, J. R., Vaughan, E. D. J., and Imperato-McGinley, J. (1993). Studies of the hormonal control of postnatal testicular descent in the rat. *J. Urol.* **149,** 618–623.
106. Kogan, B. A., Gupta, R., and Juenemann, K. P. (1987). Fertility in cryptorchidism: Further development of an experimental model. *J. Urol.* **137,** 128–131.
107. van der Schoot, P. (1992). Disturbed testicular descent in the rat after prenatal exposure to the antiandrogen flutamide. *J. Reprod. Fertil.* **96,** 483–496.
108. Spencer, J. R., Torrado, T., Sanchez, R. S., Vaughan, E. D. J., and Imperato-McGinley, J. (1991). Effects of flutamide and finasteride on rat testicular descent. *Endocrinology* **129,** 741–748.
109. Goh, D. W., Middlesworth, W., Farmer, P. J., and Hutson, J. M. (1994). Prenatal androgen blockade with flutamide inhibits masculinization of the genitofemoral nerve and testicular descent. *J. Pediatr. Surg.* **29,** 836–838.
110. Husmann, D. A. (1998). Cryptorchidism—Problems extrapolating experimental animal data to the clinical undescended testicle [editorial; comment]. *J. Urol.* **159,** 1029–1030.
111. Sigalet, D. L., Lees, G. M., Aherne, F., Van Aerde, J. E., Fedorak, R. N., Keelan, M., and Thomson, A. B. (1990). The physiology of adaptation to small bowel resection in the pig: An integrated study of morphological and functional changes. *J. Pediatr. Surg.* **25,** 650–657.
112. Bahr, R., and Flach, A. (1978). Morphological and functional adaptation after massive resection of the small intestine: Experiments using minipigs of the Gottingen strain. *Prog. Pediatr. Surg.* **12,** 107–142.
113. Cuthbertson, E. M., Gilfillan, R. S., Burhenne, H. J., and Mackby, M. J. (1970). Massive small bowel resection in the beagle, including laboratory data in severe undernutrition. *Surgery* **68,** 698–705.
114. Lansky, Z., Dodd, R. M., and Stahlgren, L. H. (1968). Regeneration of the intestinal epithelium after resection of the small intestine in dogs. *Am. J. Surg.* **116,** 8–12.
115. Thompson, J. S., Quigley, E. M., and Adrian, T. E. (1999). Factors affecting outcome following proximal and distal intestinal resection in the dog: An examination of the relative roles of mucosal adaptation, motility, luminal factors, and enteric peptides. *Dig. Dis. Sci.* **44,** 63–74.
116. Dowling, R. H., and Booth, C. C. (1967). Structural and functional changes following small intestinal resection in the rat. *Clin. Sci.* **32,** 139–149.
117. Nygaard, K. (1967). Resection of the small intestine in rats. 3. Morphological changes in the intestinal tract. *Acta Chir. Scand.* **133,** 233–248.
118. Helmrath, M. A., VanderKolk, W. E., Can, G., Erwin, C. R., and Warner, B. W. (1996). Intestinal adaptation following massive small bowel resection in the mouse. *J. Am. Coll. Surg.* **183,** 441–449.
119. Helmrath, M. A., Erwin, C. R., Shin, C. E., and Warner, B. W. (1998). Enterocyte apoptosis is increased following small bowel resection. *J. Gastrointest. Surg.* **2,** 44–49.
120. Arends, M. J., Morris, R. G., and Wyllie, A. H. (1990). Apoptosis. The role of the endonuclease. *Am. J. Pathol.* **136,** 593–608.
121. Williamson, R. C. (1978). Intestinal adaptation (second of two parts). Mechanisms of control. *N. Engl. J. Med.* **298,** 1444–1450.
122. Shin, C. E., Helmrath, M. A., Falcone, R. A. J., Fox, J. W., Duane, K. R., Erwin, C. R., and Warner, B. W. (1998). Epidermal growth factor augments adaptation following small bowel resection: Optimal dosage, route, and timing of administration. *J. Surg. Res.* **77,** 11–16.
123. Helmrath, M. A., Erwin, C. R., and Warner, B. W. (1997). A defective EGF-receptor in waved-2 mice attenuates intestinal adaptation. *J. Surg. Res.* **69,** 76–80.
124. Erwin, C. R., Helmrath, M. A., Shin, C. E., Falcone, R. A. J., Stern, L. E., and Warner, B. W. (1999). Intestinal overexpression of EGF in transgenic mice enhances adaptation after small bowel resection. *Am. J. Physiol.* **277,** G533–G540.
125. Ulshen, M. H., and Herbst, C. A. (1985). Effect of proximal transposition of the ileum on mucosal growth and enzyme activity in orally nourished rats. *Am. J. Clin. Nutr.* **42,** 805–814.
126. Chu, K. U., Tsuchiya, T., Ishizuka, J., Uchida, T., Townsend, C. M. J., and Thompson, J. C. (1995). Trophic response of gut and pancreas after ileojejunal transposition. *Ann. Surg.* **221,** 249–256.
127. Williamson, R. C., Bauer, F. L., Ross, J. S., and Malt, R. A. (1978). Proximal enterectomy stimulates distal hyperplasia more than bypass or pancreaticobiliary diversion. *Gastroenterology* **74,** 16–23.
128. Williamson, R. C., Bauer, F. L., Ross, J. S., and Malt, R. A. (1978). Contributions of bile and pancreatic juice to cell proliferation in ileal mucosa. *Surgery* **83,** 570–576.
129. Takeno, S., Sumita, M., Saito, H., and Sakai, T. (1987). Strain differences in susceptibility to the embryotoxic effects of aminopyrine in mice. *Res. Commun. Chem. Pathol. Pharmacol.* **57,** 409–419.
130. Nomura, T., Isa, Y., Kurokawa, N., Kanzaki, T., Tanaka, H., Tada, E., and Sakamoto, Y. (1984). Enhancement effects of barbital on the teratogenicity of aminopyrine. *Toxicology* **29,** 281–291.
131. Chung, M. K., Kim, J. C., and Roh, J. K. (1995). Teratogenic effects of DA-125, a new anthracycline anticancer agent, in rats. *Reprod. Toxicol.* **9,** 159–164.
132. Barrow, M. V., and Steffek, A. J. (1974). Teratologic and other embryotoxic effects of beta-aminopropionitrile in rats. *Teratology* **10,** 165–172.
133. Yoshimura, H. (1987). Teratogenicity of flubendazole in rats. *Toxicology* **43,** 133–138.
134. Zhang, X., Schrott, L. M., and Sparber, S. B. (1998). Evidence for a serotonin-mediated effect of cocaine causing vasoconstriction and herniated umbilici in chicken embryos. *Pharmacol. Biochem. Behav.* **59,** 585–593.
135. Edwards, M. J. (1969). Hyperthermia and congenital malformations in guinea-pigs. *Aust. Vet. J.* **45,** 189–193.
136. Hillebrandt, S., Streffer, C., and Muller, W. U. (1996). Genetic analysis of the cause of gastroschisis in the HLG mouse strain. *Mutat. Res.* **372,** 43–51.
137. Hillebrandt, S., Streffer, C., Montagutelli, X., and Balling, R. (1998). A locus for radiation-induced gastroschisis on mouse Chromosome 7. *Mamm. Genome* **9,** 995–997.

138. Haller, J. A. J., Kehrer, B. H., Shaker, I. J., Shermeta, D. W., and Wyllie, R. G. (1974). Studies of the pathophysiology of gastroschisis in fetal sheep. *J. Pediatr. Surg.* **9,** 627–632.
139. Langer, J. C., Longaker, M. T., Crombleholme, T. M., Bond, S. J., Finkbeiner, W. E., Rudolph, C. A., Verrier, E. D., and Harrison, M. R. (1989). Etiology of intestinal damage in gastroschisis. I: Effects of amniotic fluid exposure and bowel constriction in a fetal lamb model. *J. Pediatr. Surg.* **24,** 992–997.
140. Langer, J. C., Bell, J. G., Castillo, R. O., Crombleholme, T. M., Longaker, M. T., Duncan, B. W., Bradley, S. M., Finkbeiner, W. E., Verrier, E. D., and Harrison, M. R. (1990). Etiology of intestinal damage in gastroschisis, II. Timing and reversibility of histological changes, mucosal function, and contractility. *J. Pediatr. Surg.* **25,** 1122–1126.
141. Srinathan, S. K., Langer, J. C., Blennerhassett, M. G., Harrison, M. R., Pelletier, G. J., and Lagunoff, D. (1995). Etiology of intestinal damage in gastroschisis. III: Morphometric analysis of the smooth muscle and submucosa. *J. Pediatr. Surg.* **30,** 379–383.
142. Sherman, N. J., Asch, M. J., Isaacs, H. J., and Rosenkrantz, J. G. (1973). Experimental gastroschisis in the fetal rabbit. *J. Pediatr. Surg.* **8,** 165–169.
143. Aoki, Y., Ohshio, T., and Komi, N. (1980). An experimental study on gastroschisis using fetal surgery. *J. Pediatr. Surg.* **15,** 252–256.
144. Phillips, J. D., Kelly, R. E. J., Fonkalsrud, E. W., Mirzayan, A., and Kim, C. S. (1991). An improved model of experimental gastroschisis in fetal rabbits. *J. Pediatr. Surg.* **26,** 784–787.
145. Nelson, J. M., Krummel, T. M., Haynes, J. H., Flood, L. C., Sauer, L., Flake, A. W., and Harrison, M. R. (1990). Operative techniques in the fetal rabbit. *J. Invest. Surg.* **3,** 393–398.
146. Albert, A., Julia, M. V., Morales, L., and Parri, F. J. (1993). Gastroschisis in the partially extraamniotic fetus: Experimental study. *J. Pediatr. Surg.* **28,** 656–659.
147. Srinathan, S. K., Langer, J. C., Wang, J. L., and Rubin, D. C. (1997). Enterocytic gene expression is altered in experimental gastroschisis. *J. Surg. Res.* **68,** 1–6.
148. Shaw, K., Buchmiller, T. L., Curr, M., Lam, M. M., Habib, R., Chopourian, H. L., Diamond, J. M., and Fonkalsrud, E. W. (1994). Impairment of nutrient uptake in a rabbit model of gastroschisis [see comments]. *J. Pediatr. Surg.* **29,** 376–378.
149. Guo, W., Swaniker, F., Fonkalsrud, E. W., Vo, K., and Karamanoukian, R. (1995). Effect of intraamniotic dexamethasone administration on intestinal absorption in a rabbit gastroschisis model. *J. Pediatr. Surg.* **30,** 983–986.
150. Tibboel, D., Molenaar, J. C., and Van Nie, C. J. (1979). New perspectives in fetal surgery: The chicken embryo. *J. Pediatr. Surg.* **14,** 438–440.
151. Aktug, T., Erdag, G., Kargi, A., Akgur, F. M., and Tibboel, D. (1995). Amnio-allantoic fluid exchange for the prevention of intestinal damage in gastroschisis: An experimental study on chick embryos. *J. Pediatr. Surg.* **30,** 384–387.
152. Aktug, T., Ucan, B., Olguner, M., Akgur, F. M., and Ozer, E. (1998). Amnio-allantoic fluid exchange for prevention of intestinal damage in gastroschisis II: Effects of exchange performed by using two different solutions. *Eur. J. Pediatr. Surg.* **8,** 308–311.
153. Aktug, T., Ucan, B., Olguner, M., Akgur, F. M., Ozer, E., Caliskan, S., and Onvural, B. (1998). Amnio-allantoic fluid exchange for the prevention of intestinal damage in gastroschisis. III: Determination of the waste products removed by exchange. *Eur. J. Pediatr. Surg.* **8,** 326–328.
154. Luton, D., de Lagausie, P., Guibourdenche, J., Oury, J., Sibony, O., Vuillard, E., Boissinot, C., Aigrain, Y., Beaufils, F., Navarro, J., and Blot, P. (1999). Effect of amnioinfusion on the outcome of prenatally diagnosed gastroschisis. *Fetal Diagn. Ther.* **14,** 152–155.
155. Dilsiz, A., Gundogan, A. H., Aktan, M., Duman, S., and Aktug, T. (1999). Nitric oxide synthase inhibition prevents intestinal damage in gastroschisis: A morphological evaluation in chick embryos. *J. Pediatr. Surg.* **34,** 1248–1252.

76

Research in Fetal Surgery

Alexander Sasha Krupnick and N. Scott Adzick

Division of Pediatric General, Thoracic and Fetal Surgery, The Children's Hospital of Philadelphia, Philadelphia, Pennsylvania 19104

I. Introduction

Until recently, surgical treatment of a fetus was only theoretical. Minimal information regarding the health of the intrauterine gestation and the difficulty with access to the fetus made therapeutic manipulation impossible. Treatment was limited to chemotherapy for fatal infectious disease and hormonal supplementation for certain endocrine disorders, but the effort was directed primarily toward treatment of the mother, with the fetus benefiting only secondarily (1). With recent expansion in diagnostic modalities such as fetal ultrasound and prenatal screening for genetic and metabolic disorders, diagnosis of anatomic malformations and other life-threatening conditions is routinely made prior to birth. The possibility of prenatal intervention to either save the fetus' life or ameliorate the postnatal morbidity of disease has now become a reality. Animal models for fetal surgery have paved the way for therapeutic intervention in humans.

II. Fetal Wound Healing

Fetal wound healing represents a unique physiologic response characterized by enhanced regeneration rather than scar formation, minimal inflammatory changes, and decreased levels of certain growth factors (2). The study of this phenomenon has improved our understanding of the normal process of adult wound healing as well as pathologic phenomena such as hypertrophic scar formation and non-healing wounds. Further investigation in this field offers promising therapeutic potential for the prevention or amelioration of scar and fibrosis.

A. The Rabbit Model

The rabbit is a widely used animal model for the study of fetal wound healing (3). Its major drawbacks include the short gestation of 31 days, limiting repetition of procedures in one animal, difficulty with fine manipulation due to the small size of the fetus, and high rate of fetal loss, especially early in gestation. In general, most operative procedures can be performed between 22 and 25 days of gestation but surgical manipulation prior to 20 days leads to a high rate of fetal wastage.

Anesthesia in the pregnant doe is difficult due to the narrow margin between surgical anesthesia and respiratory arrest as well as the wide variability in individual response to the anesthetic. Intubation of the rabbit is difficult but rarely necessary. Fasting of maternal rabbits is not necessary because they rarely vomit. Optimal anesthesia in our laboratory has consisted of halothane administered through a plastic cone mask in a semiclosed system with a CO_2 absorber and a rebreathing bag. Halothane has proved to be the ideal anesthetic for fetal manipulation in the rabbit as well as in larger animals due to its effect of uterine relaxation. Induction of anesthesia is accomplished by intramuscular injection of ketamine (Fort Dodge Animal Health, Ford Dodge, Iowa) and xylazine (Phoenix Pharmaceutical, Inc.) in a combination of 35 mg/kg ketamine and 5 mg/kg of xylazine. Penicillin, 200,000 units IM, is given preoperatively. Intravenous access is not usually necessary but can be established through a prominent ear vein.

After adequate muscular relaxation, the rabbit is placed in the supine position on a heating blanket and all four limbs are secured to a small-animal operating board. A plastic nose cone is placed over the nose and mouth and the animal is allowed to breathe the halothane/oxygen mixture spontaneously. Depth of anesthesia throughout the procedure is gauged by the respiratory rate and muscular tone. The coarse abdominal hair is shaved with clippers and a straight-edge razor is used to remove the fine remaining hair. The animal is then prepped with soap, a 70% alcohol solution, and povidine–iodine. The abdomen is draped with sterile towels and strict aseptic technique is followed throughout the procedure. Fine manipulation and visualization are facilitated by strong overhead operating room lights and 3.5×-power magnifying binocular surgical loupes (Design for Vision, Inc., New York, New York).

A midline incision is made from the last pair of nipples to just inferior of the umbilicus with a scalpel and electrocautery. Staying strictly in the midline avoids interrupting the breast tissue. After entering the peritoneum the uterus is palpated to determine the size and number of fetuses. One uterine horn is partially exteriorized for surgical manipulation and kept moist with warm saline. It is imperative to minimize delivery of the gravid uterus from the abdominal cavity in order to prevent compromise of the uterine blood flow. A 4-0 silk pursestring suture is then placed through all layers of the uterine wall as well as the gestational membranes on the antimesometrial portion of the uterus. This site is the watershed area for the uterine blood supply and is relatively avascular. A small uterine incision is then made inside the pursestring suture using fine-tip needle cautery and the amniotic space is entered. The incision is enlarged as necessary using a small hemostat while two Babcock clamps are placed on the edges of the uterine incision. Only the appropriate fetal part for manipulation and not the whole fetus is delivered out of the uterus. After completion of the planned procedure the fetal part is returned to the uterus by applying gentle, steady pressure. The edges of the uterine incision are concurrently held up with two Babcock clamps. The uterine pursestring suture is tied as the Babcock clamps are removed. A running 2-0 Vicryl suture is used to close the peritoneum and fascia and the skin is closed with a 4-0 subcuticular Vicryl suture. A collodion dressing can be applied over the closed incision (3).

The absence of wound contraction in the fetus is unique to the rabbit model (4). Through a minihysterotomy Somasundaram and Prathap (5) excised small 0.5-cm disks of skin from the dorsum of 14- to 25-day gestation rabbit fetuses. Animals were sacrificed at various time points and the wounds examined on days 1, 2, 3, 6, and 11. Throughout the study, and even 11 days after wounding, there was little change in wound morphology or histologic appearance. No wound contraction, granulation tissue formation, or epithelialization could be seen. Further study revealed that excisional wounds bathed in amniotic fluid did not contract or heal secondarily whereas those excluded from contact with amniotic fluid by a silastic patch healed within eight days (5). This observation led to the hypothesis that rabbit amniotic fluid may contain factors that inhibit wound contraction and account for differences between fetal and adult wound healing. Further *in vitro* studies confirmed these initial observations and demonstrated that amniotic fluid inhibits the contraction of fibroblast-populated collagen matrices (6).

B. Sheep Model

The sheep has been extensively utilized for studies of fetal physiology (7) and offers unique advantages for fetal manipulation and study of fetal wound healing. The long gestation of the sheep (145 days) permits comparison of fetal wound healing at different time periods *in utero*. Although exponential in growth, the size of fetal sheep is also comparable to that of fetal humans (Table I) (8), and

Table I Comparison of Fetal Sheep and Fetal Human Gestational Weights[a]

Gestation time	Sheep fetal weight	Human fetal weight
50 days	21 g	—
75 days	163 g	—
100 days	706 g	—
140–145 days	3916 g (term)	—
12 weeks	—	45 g
20 weeks	—	460 g
28 weeks	—	1300 g
38 weeks	—	3400 g (term)

[a]Weight of fetal sheep (8) calculated as body weight (g) = $e^{[\ln \text{age (days)}]509 - 16.88}$. Human fetal weights obtained from Moore and Persaud (8a).

minimal uterine irritability and low rates of abortion, even after an open hysterotomy, decrease animal loss.

Details of possible surgical procedures and the specifics of maternal laparotomy are described in detail elsewhere (9), but will be briefly reviewed here. Animals are generally fasted for 24–48 hr but water is not withheld. Anesthesia is induced with an intramuscular dose of ketamine (2–4 mg/kg) and maintained throughout the procedure with a halothane (2%)–oxygen mixture. Preoperative antibiotics consist of 1000 mg of cefazolin by intravenous access established in the prominent jugular vein of the neck. The maternal abdomen is shaved (this maneuver is facilitated by removing the oily coat with an alcohol solution) and scrubbed with povidone–iodine (Betadine surgical scrub). This is then washed off and the abdomen painted with a povidone–iodine solution (Betadine solution). A lower midline incision is carefully made while avoiding the bilateral nipple lines. The bicornuate uterus is delivered into the surgical field and a hysterotomy is made in the middle of the horn, avoiding the encircling blood vessels (Fig. 1). At the completion of the operation but prior to uterine closure warm saline with 1,000,000 U of penicillin is used to replace the amniotic fluid.

To confirm wound contraction data gathered in the rabbit model, Longaker and colleagues (10) utilized the fetal lamb to study the effects of amniotic fluid on fetal wound contraction. Punch biopsies were created along the back of 100-day gestation fetal lambs and half of the wounds were excluded from contact with amniotic fluid by a silastic patch and half were left exposed to the uterine environment. The wounds excluded from contact with amniotic fluid rapidly decreased in size and were completely healed by 14 days postwounding. Interestingly the wounds directly exposed to amniotic fluid, although exhibiting a slightly decreased initial rate of contraction, were also completely closed by 14 days. These results differ significantly from the rabbit model, indicating that numerous factors other than simple exposure to amniotic fluid account for differences between the fetal and postnatal healing responses.

To evaluate a potential clinical application of scarless fetal healing Longaker and colleagues (11) evaluated the possibility of *in utero* fetal cleft lip repair. Cleft lip and palate defects were surgically created in four 75-day gestation fetal lambs. Two of these defects were then repaired primarily and two were left unrepaired. Harvest of one set of fetuses 14 days after repair and a second set 21 days after

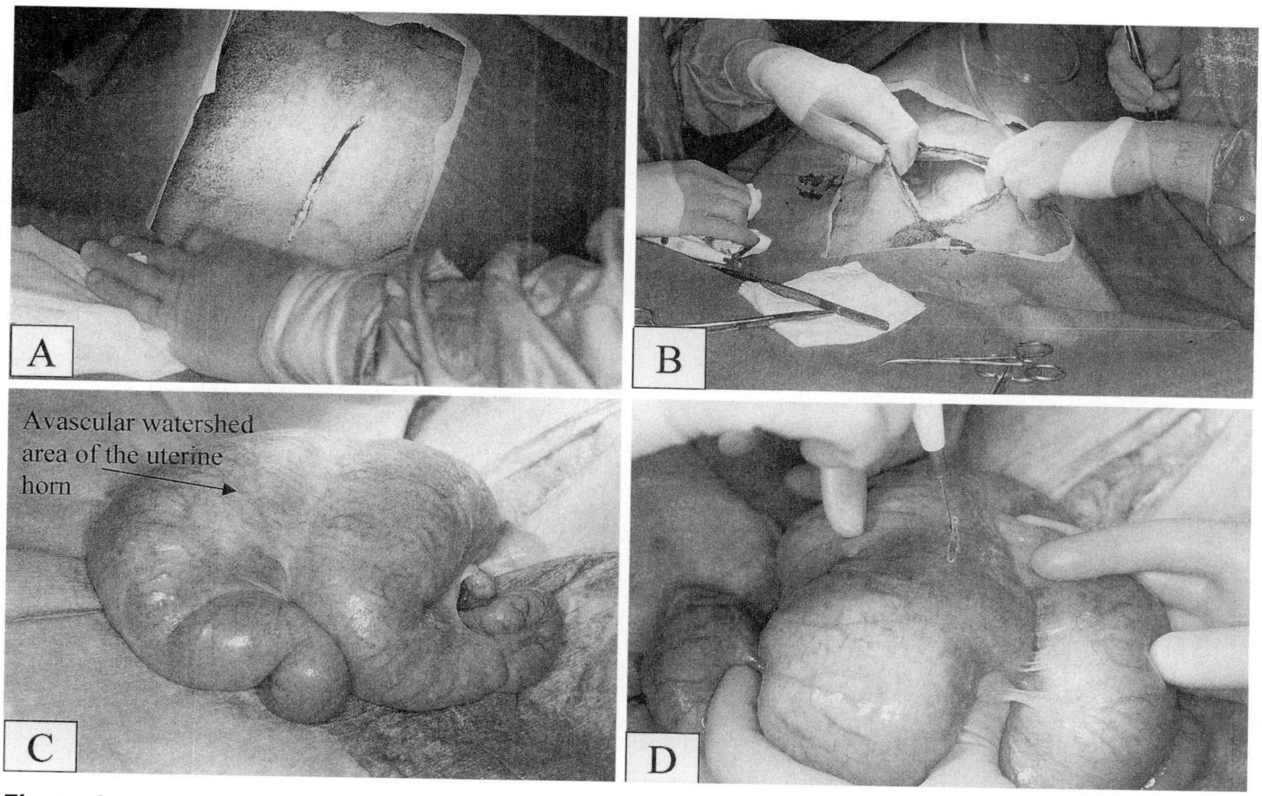

Figure 1 (A, B) Laparotomy in the pregnant sheep involves a lower midline incision, avoiding the bilateral nipple lines. The bicornuate uterus is brought out onto the abdomen (C) and a hysterotomy is made in the relatively avascular midline of the uterine horn, avoiding the encircling blood vessels (D).

repair revealed that the repaired defects primarily healed without scar and could be identified only by the remaining suture. The unrepaired defects, however, demonstrated a persistent cleft lip and oronasal fistula. Extension of these results led to a more clinically relevant sheep model by first creating the defect early in gestation and allowing a 2-week period of abnormal facial growth and development prior to *in utero* repair. This was followed by a third operation to remove and examine the fetus 1 month after the delayed repair (12). Incisional wounds and defects that were repaired primarily healed without scar. Large excisional wounds also healed without excessive scarring, but no true regeneration of skin appendages could be seen. This "transitional wound" may represent the gradual change from fetal wound regeneration to adultlike healing by scar during the course of gestation. The long gestation of the fetal lamb offers a perfect opportunity to study this and other phenomena bridging the fetal-to-adult healing process (2).

C. Mouse Model

There are several advantages to using the mouse model for studying fetal wound healing. Although precise surgical manipulation is hindered by the small size of the fetus, this limitation is outweighed by the low cost of purchasing, decreased cost of housing, and short gestation term (19 days). Numerous transgenic strains, including models of human metabolic, immunologic, and hematologic diseases, are also available for purchase from commercial breeders,* thereby increasing the utility of this animal model. Studies of fetal wound healing in the mouse have relied on numerous available assays for growth factors, collagen deposition, and inflammatory markers. Utilizing previously described techniques, full-thickness lip wounds were made in 14-, 16, and 18-day gestation mice (13). Similar wounds were created in neonatal and adult mice for comparison. Morphological evaluation revealed a gradual transition in the rate and quality of wound healing from fetus to neonate to adult. Whereas reepithelialization was complete in the fetus at 20 hr, the neonatal wound reepithelialized by 48 hr and the adult wound closed by 72 hr. Three days after injury, the fetal wound showed a reticular pattern of type III collagen and was essentially indistinguishable from the surrounding tissue, whereas the adult wound healed with typical scar formation and bands of parallel collagen fibers disrupting normal tissue architecture. The neonatal wound exhibited an intermediate pattern of healing with normal tissue architecture and no scar but loss of hair follicles in the wound.

Staining for endogenous immunoglobulins revealed the presence of IgG and IgM in the neonatal and adult wounds but no immunoglobulins could be detected in the fetal wounds. This ameliorated inflammatory response was supported by the cytokine pattern because platelet-derived growth factor (PDGF) disappeared from the fetal wound by 48 hr and transforming growth factor-β was not detectable in the healing wound at all. Because both cytokines are involved in chemotaxis of fibroblasts and leukocytes as well as collagen matrix synthesis and deposition, their paucity could account for decreased inflammation and scarless fetal wound healing. Further work in this as well as in other animal models (14) is needed in order to better understand the full therapeutic potential of information gained from fetal wound healing studies.

III. Preterm Labor after Fetal Surgery

Preterm labor is the Achilles' heel of fetal surgery and, as stated by Flake and Harrison "preterm labor is to the infantile field of fetal surgery what rejection was to the field of transplantation" (15). Unsuccessful tocolysis and preterm birth after fetal intervention can convert one life-threatening problem to the often more dangerous condition of extreme prematurity. Because preterm labor is not a homogeneous disease but rather one with numerous causes and etiologies, animal models must focus on preterm labor secondary to maternal hysterotomy rather than other factors such as infection or cervical incompetence.

A. Primate Model

Unlike the sheep and other lower animals, in which the uterus is quiescent after a hysterotomy, the primate uterus is extremely sensitive to surgical manipulation. The basis for tocolysis after human fetal surgery was established in the primate with Harrison and colleagues (16) reporting the largest study series in 1982. Twelve cynomolgous (*Macaca fasicularis*) and thirteen rhesus (*Macaca mulatta*) monkeys with a normal gestation period of 160–170 days underwent fetal surgery with creation of experimental obstructive uropathy or bladder drainage. Anesthetic techniques, surgical exposure, and pharmacologic tocolysis were systematically manipulated in order to obtain optimal results and minimize fetal loss. The final regimen consisted of 10 mg/kg of IM ketamine for induction and maintenance of anesthesia with 60% nitrous oxide in oxygen and 0.25–10% halothane. Indomethacin (10 mg) was administered IV prior to the procedure to maintain tocolysis. Dextrose (5%) in a balanced salt solution was infused throughout the procedure (Fig. 2). The monkey was positioned on the table in a left lateral lift in order to avoid aortocaval compression by the gravid uterus and maternal temperature was monitored by a rectal probe while a heating blanket and heat lamps were used to maintain warmth. Maternal hypotension was meticulously

*The Jackson Laboratory, JAX Research Systems, 600 Main St., Bar Harbor, Maine 04609-1500. Telephone: 800-422-MICE. Fax: 207-288-6150. Web site: http://www.jax.org.

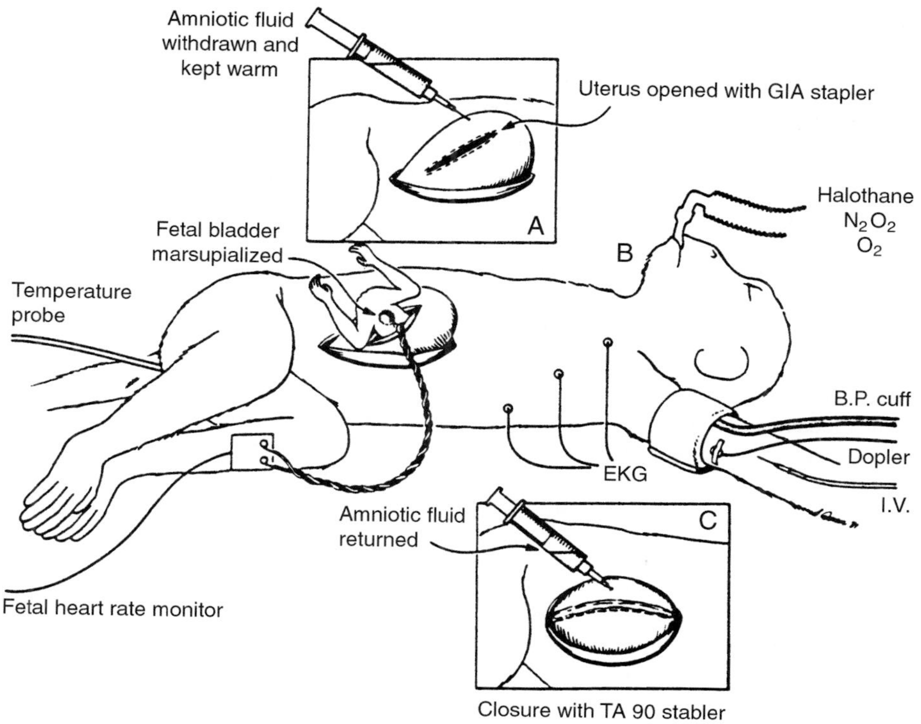

Figure 2 Setup for fetal surgery in the primate. With permission, from Harrison *et al.* (16).

avoided and any decrease in systolic blood pressure below 100 torr was treated by decreasing anesthesia, increasing IV fluids, or giving 1 mg of ephedrine IV.

The gravid uterus was exposed through a midline incision and the site of hysterotomy chosen to avoid the two placental disks with the intervening vessels. A small opening was made in the placenta with cutting electrocautery and the rest of the hysterotomy performed with a gastrointestinal anastomosis (GIA) stapling device (United States Surgical Corporation, Norwalk, CT) that approximated the amniotic membranes to the uterine wall and prevented postoperative membrane separation. A fetal scalp electrode was attached to monitor the fetal heart rate and the appropriate fetal part exteriorized for the operation. At the completion of the procedure the uterus was approximated with two layers of running monofilament suture. After closure of the abdomen, the animal was allowed to wake up by breathing 100% oxygen and 0.5 mg of diazepam given intravenously to prevent postoperative excitation.

The combination of halothane anesthesia to decrease uterine tone during the operation and inhibition of prostaglandin synthesis with one or two doses of intravenous indomethacin significantly increased survival. Although fetal mortality was extremely high during the first half of the series (73.3%), it decreased after the introduction of these techniques. The fetal loss rate of 20% following the last 10 procedures was not statistically different from the 21.4% late gestation and early neonatal mortality in a control group of primates.

Based on the results of this series, a detailed evaluation of uterine electromyographic (EMG) activity after fetal surgery as well as the tocolytic effects on uterine EMG was undertaken (17). Continuous monitoring of uterine electrical activity was established by suturing vinyl-insulated multistrand stainless-steel electrodes to the surface of the uterus as described by Novy (18). The electrodes were tunneled to exit from the animal's flank and chair restraint was employed throughout the experiment to prevent electrode dislodgment and removal by the animal. Two types of uterine electrical activity were recorded. Type I activity consisted of 15- to 75-sec episodes of EMG discharges occurring with a frequency of 10 to 45 per hour. This pattern of activity correlated with uterine contractions producing intraamniotic pressures of more than 20 mmHg. Type II activity consisted of a fragmented series of discharges of lesser frequency and was associated with a minimal rise in the intraamniotic pressure.

All animals undergoing a hysterotomy, with or without fetal manipulation, exhibited frequent coordinated uterine contractions associated with type I activity. This pattern continued throughout the night following the operation, decreased the next morning, but reemerged the following night. The pattern of nocturnal type I activity decreased gradually and disappeared 4 to 10 days postoperatively.

Readministration of halothane eliminated established type I activity in all the animals studied. Surprisingly, preoperative indomethacin (10 mg IV), had no effect on the emergence of type I activity following hysterotomy.

Type I activity was not a prominent EMG pattern after procedures involving minimal uterine manipulation such as amniocentesis or maternal laparotomy alone. When present, this pattern lasted only for a short period of time the night after an operation and was later replaced by type II activity. These procedures resulted in minimal uterine irritability and were associated with a low rate of fetal loss. Overall the chair-restrained primate model provides a powerful tool to evaluate directly the effects of fetal surgery and postoperative tocolytics on uterine electrical activity.

Unlike other surgical therapy, fetal surgery has the potential to jeopardize the health of two individuals, the mother and child. Because the mother benefits only indirectly from an operation focused on saving the life of the fetus, maternal safety as well as future health and reproductive capacity are of paramount importance. With this in mind, we undertook an extensive review to determine the long-term maternal effects of fetal surgery in the nonhuman primate prior to human application (19). A total of 102 fetal surgical procedures were performed by our group between 1979 and 1984 in time-dated pregnant monkeys. Computerized medical records describing postoperative maternal complications as well as the animals' subsequent health and fertility were reviewed. There were three maternal deaths, including a single intraoperative death due to anesthetic mismanagement and one death on postoperative day 8 due to eclampsia and maternal convulsions. Both deaths could have been avoided by meticulous intraoperative anesthetic monitoring and prolonged postoperative evaluation of maternal blood pressure. Based on these two cases an obstetric anesthesiologist monitored all further surgical procedures in the primate and there were no further maternal deaths. More intense postoperative monitoring of the mother was also established. The third mortality resulted from uterine rupture during preterm labor. Overall, there were five cases of uterine rupture during labor after fetal intervention. Based on these results, cesarean delivery is now considered mandatory after fetal surgery in order to avoid rupture of the fresh uterine closure. Interestingly, there were no cases of uterine rupture during later pregnancies, but the long-term strength of the uterine scar still needs to be evaluated.

Animals that underwent metal staple hysterotomy closure exhibited a marked decrease in fertility whereas those whose uteruses were closed with absorbable suture maintained their reproductive capacity. Autopsy 2 to 4 years after fetal surgery revealed that metal staples used to close the uterus had migrated through the uterine wall to the endometrial surface. The presence of this foreign body contributed to the lower fertility rates. Because stapling devices are ideal for expeditiously opening and closing the exceedingly vascular gravid uterus, we developed a stapling device designed to deliver absorbable staples (Premium Poly CS-57, United States Surgical Corporation). This device allows opening of the uterus by placing two rows of absorbable staples while a knife blade cuts between the staple lines. Extended application of this tool, as well as other devices developed for fetal surgery, has proved useful in other applications, such as clinical cesarean section.

B. Rabbit Model

The rabbit offers several advantages over the primate in the study of preterm labor. Although the characteristics and level of uterine irritability after hysterotomy are not similar, care for this animal is less costly and rabbits are readily available at most research facilities. Initial data from experimental groups of large numbers of animals can be gathered in this model prior to advancing trials to the primate.

Although current postoperative tocolysis involves systemic administration of drugs to the mother, future clinical efforts will focus on localized therapy directly targeting myometrial activity. Fauza and colleagues (20) studied the effects of prolonged excitatory blockade of the myometrium on preterm delivery in the rabbit model. Eighteen pregnant New Zealand rabbits at 23 days of gestation were anesthetized with 2–5% halothane after induction with 15 mg/kg of ketamine IM. After antibiotic prophylaxis with 500 mg of cefazolin, a maternal laparotomy was made and the bicornuate uterus exposed. Animals were then divided into three groups. In group I (control) a hysterotomy was performed over the most proximal fetus in both uterine horns. Proximal manipulation of the uterus was chosen because it is more abortifacient than distal hysterotomy. The gestational membranes were then tacked down to the uterine wall with four corner stitches of 6-0 proline in order to prevent membrane separation. The most proximal fetus was then delivered from the womb and subjected to amputation of a forelimb with suture ligation of the stump. The fetus was then returned to the amniotic cavity, the uterus repleted with amniotic fluid, and the hysterotomy closed with a 5-0 double-running propylene suture. After closure of the abdominal wall, the does were returned to their cages. Group II (experimental) underwent the same procedure except the myometrium at the site of incision was injected with 0.5 ml of 0.5% bupivacaine HCL immediately prior to incision. At the completion of the procedure, but before uterine closure, the incised area was infiltrated with 1.5 ml of a novel suspension of a biodegradable poly(lactic–coglycolic) acid microspheres loaded with bupivicaine and incorporated with dexamethasone. This system is designed to deliver the anesthetic in a continuous and controlled manner. Group III (ancillary control) consisted of animals injected with a suspension of the same microspheres but without any drug.

The abortion rates between the groups differed significantly: 83.3% of the mothers in group I aborted and 71.4% of those in group III aborted, but none in group II delivered prematurely. Although the effects of time-release bupivicaine on uterine irritability is encouraging, the fetal death rate in group II was extremely high (87.5%), presumably due to transplacental transfer and toxicity of this drug. Despite the limitations of this particular local anesthetic, this study demonstrated the therapeutic effects of local myometrial conduction blockade on the prevention of premature labor after fetal surgery. Further experimentation using a combination of different drugs and delivery systems can be implemented using this model.

IV. Disease-Based Models

A. Congenital Diaphragmatic Hernia

Congenital diaphragmatic hernia (CDH) is one of the most devastating anomalies afflicting the neonate. The diaphragmatic defect in combination with visceral herniation into the chest and fetal pulmonary hypoplasia carries a 50–60% mortality. Over 1700 babies with congenital diaphragmatic hernia are born annually in the United States, providing a substantial social and economic burden to our health care system.

1. Sheep Model

Pulmonary hypoplasia seen with congenital diaphragmatic hernia has been well documented in the human. Although presumed to result from restriction of *in utero* pulmonary development, an animal model is necessary in order to delineate the exact pathophysiology of this disease, methods of prenatal intervention, and developmental consequences of this intervention. Harrison and colleagues (9) described the necessary characteristics of an animal model of CDH as one that (1) creates a space-occupying lesion in the fetal thorax that progressively enlarges with age and results in severe pulmonary hypoplasia, (2) allows the simulation of CDH correction at birth or during gestation by the removal of the space-occupying lesion, and (3) allows removal of this lesion and assessment of effects of its removal on the pulmonary parenchyma and vascular development. They then created such a model in the fetal sheep.

Using standard surgical techniques, inflatable silicone rubber balloons were inserted in the left hemithorax of fetal lambs at 100 days of gestation. A catheter accessing the intrathoracic balloon as well as fetal subcutaneous EKG electrode wires were tunneled through the hysterotomy plus the maternal abdominal wall and secured in an external Velcro pouch (Fig. 3). At the completion of the procedure, the balloon catheter was filled with 30–50 ml of saline with insufflation monitored on the fetal EKG. If the fetal heart rate dropped with inflation, the balloon was deflated until the heart rate normalized. The ewes were brought back twice a week and the balloon was further insufflated with 10 ml as the EKG was monitored in order to produce a volume of 100 ml at 120 days and 150 ml at 140 days of gestation. These volumes were calculated to parallel lung growth and occupy half of the total lung volume throughout the gestation. The lambs were delivered by a cesarean section between days 141 and 148, intubated, and mechanically ventilated while frequent arterial pH, pO_2, and pCO_2 were recorded. The inflated intrathoracic balloons were deflated in order to simulate neonatal correction of CDH at birth.

The physiologic differences between the two groups were striking. The newborn lambs without balloon placement, or whose balloons were placed but not inflated, were easily resuscitated at birth and weaned off the ventilator to room air. Those lambs with simulated CDH, however, rapidly deteriorated despite maximal resuscitation and succumbed to massive hypoxia and hypercapnia despite balloon deflation at birth. Postmortem physiologic evaluation revealed decreased parenchymal mass, air capacity, and pulmonary vascularity bed in the CDH group.

Although this model did provide a clinical and pathologic picture similar to that in infants with CDH, several differences limit its applicability. Most importantly, the human baby with CDH has a diaphragmatic defect with potential for respiratory failure from both diaphragmatic and pulmonary compromise, whereas this lamb model tests only the effects of a space-occupying mass in the chest. The timing of human CDH is also different than that in this sheep model, because thoracic invasion occurs much earlier in gestation during the pseudoglandular or even embryonic stage of lung development. Balloon placement at 100 days affects only part of the canalicular and most of the saccular and alveolar stages of development (Fig. 4) (21). A more physiologic model of human CDH was subsequently developed (22) by creating a diaphragmatic defect in the fetal sheep between 60 and 63 days of gestation, during the pseudoglandular stage of development. This method allows the herniated viscera rather than an intrathoracic balloon to cause compression of the pulmonary parenchyma and creates pulmonary hypoplasia similar to that seen in the human.

Because neonates with congenital airway obstruction are born with excessive pulmonary mass (23), and normal pulmonary growth has been hypothesized to occur due to the stenting force of produced fetal lung fluid (24), obstruction of the egress of fluid from the fetal lung might be able to reverse the pulmonary hypoplasia associated with CDH. As an extension of the previous models, the effects of tracheal occlusion on correction of pulmonary hypoplasia were studied (25). Time-dated pregnant ewes underwent fetal surgery

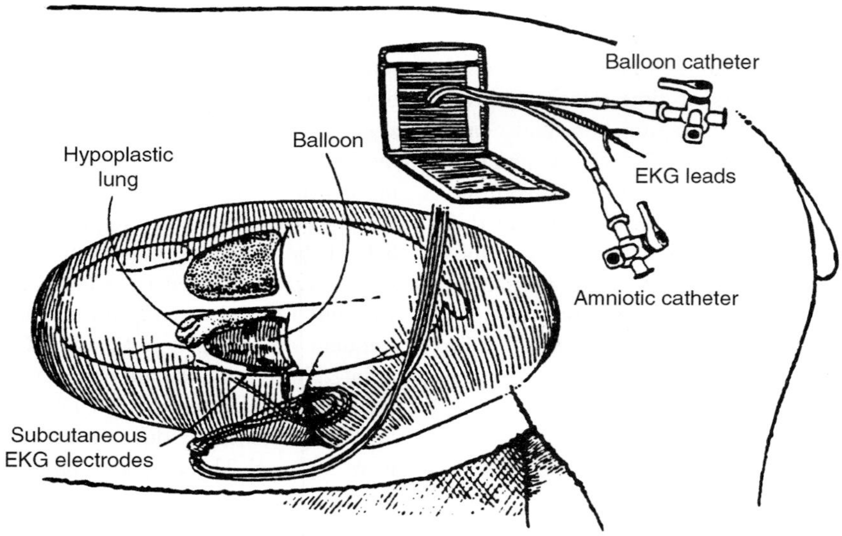

Figure 3 Fetal sheep set up to simulate CDH. A silicone rubber balloon is placed in the left hemithorax at day 100 of gestation and progressively inflated to simulate the herniated viscera. Fetal EKG is monitored during inflation. With permission, from Harrison *et al.* (9).

during the pseudoglandular period of pulmonary development at 75 days of gestation. After maternal hysterotomy the left fetal thorax was exposed through the ninth intercostal space, a small rib spreader was placed, and after retraction of the lung a cruciate incision was made in the tendinous portion of the diaphragm. The stomach and bowel were manually delivered into the chest and the thoracotomy was closed in two layers. The amniotic fluid was restored and hysterotomy was closed with a TA-90 stapler. At 120 days of gestation, after ultrasonographic confirmation of persistent herniation, the fetuses were randomly assigned to the experimental group of tracheal ligation or the unligated control group. Those in the experimental group underwent a repeat maternal hysterotomy and tracheal ligation with umbilical tape and 2-0 prolene suture through a longitudinal neck incision. The unligated controls underwent the same operation except the trachea was exposed, dissected free from surrounding tissue, but left unligated. The skin of the neck, uterus, and maternal abdomen was closed.

At 135–140 days of gestation, fetal lambs were delivered by cesarean section and a 2.5-mm cuffed endotracheal tube was placed by a tracheostomy below the area of tracheal dissection. Under ketamine anesthesia (1 mg/kg IV) the neonate was ventilated for 1 hr while repeat blood gas sam-

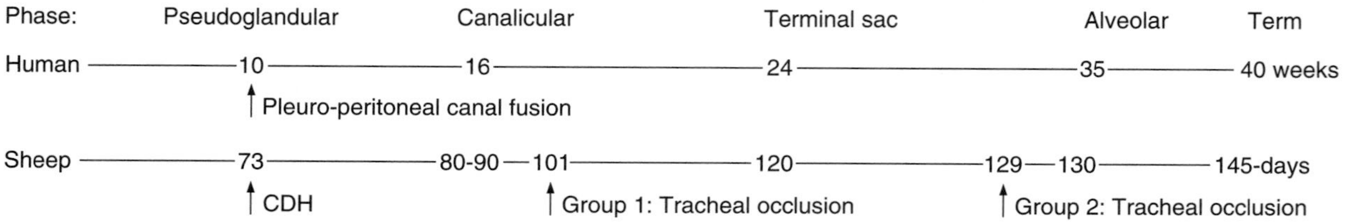

Figure 4 Diagram illustrating the postembryonic stages of lung development in the human and sheep. From Ref. (21), Lipsett *et al.* (1998). Effect of antenatal tracheal occlusion on lung development in the sheep model of congenital diaphragmatic hernia: A morphometric analysis of pulmonary structure and maturity. *Pediatr. Pulmonol.* Copyright ©1998 Wiley-Liss, Inc. Reprinted by permission of Wiley-Liss, Inc., a subsidiary of John Wiley & Sons, Inc.

ples were analyzed. At the end of the hour the animal was sacrificed and the lung tissue analyzed. During necropsy it was noted that all ligated animals had full reduction of the viscera from the chest whereas the unligated controls had the left side of the chest occupied by the abdominal viscera (Fig. 5). The pulmonary dry weight and total lung DNA in the ligated group were significantly higher than those in the unligated group and the volume of pulmonary fluid volume was 15-fold greater. Initial blood gas analysis in both groups revealed fetal hypoxia and hypercarbia but after 1 hr of ventilation the pO_2, pCO_2, and pH normalized in the experimental group but remained pathologic in the unligated CDH controls. This novel group of experiments in the sheep model demonstrated that fetal tracheal ligation can reduce abdominal viscera from the chest, induce growth of hypoplastic lungs, and improve postnatal function (25).

Despite the postmortem morphological evaluation and improved ventilatory status at birth, no useful measurement of pulmonary hemodynamics in CDH was available. Using the sheep model of CDH we set out to develop a minimally invasive measurement of pulmonary vascular resistance *in utero*. Fetal lambs underwent creation of CDH at 80 days of gestation. After an interval of 28 days a portion of the fetuses (CDH + tracheal occlusion group) underwent reoperation and a large Weck clip (Pilling-Weck, Narberth, PA) was placed around the trachea in order to completely prevent the egress of fluid. A second (CDH only) group underwent a creation of CDH but no tracheal ligation and a third group (control group) underwent only a sham operation at 80 days of gestation.

The blood flow in the left pulmonary artery was followed at 2-week intervals by pulsed-wave doppler echocardiography (Acuson 128 XP, Mountain View, CA) using a 5-mHz probe. During the cardiac cycle, the pulsatility index (PI), used to estimate the resistance in the left pulmonary artery vascular bed, was calculated by the formula PI = (peak systolic velocity − end diastolic velocity)/mean velocity. The PI of those sheep with CDH increased dramatically over controls, indicating increased vascular resistance. Two weeks after tracheal occlusion, however, it reversed this trend and by sacrifice at 136 days of gestation the PI of the tracheal occlusion group was the same as that of the controls. The PI in both groups was significantly less than the PI in the CDH group. With maternal hyperoxygenation prior to sacrifice, the fetuses in the control and tracheal occlusion group demonstrated a significant decrease in the PI from

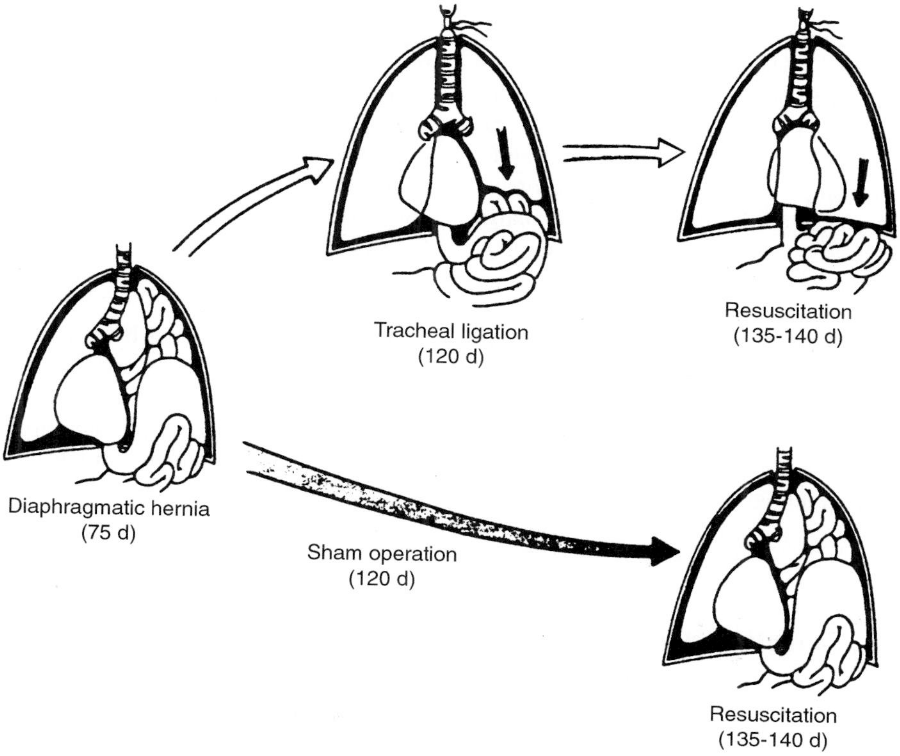

Figure 5 If the creation of a diaphragmatic hernia at 75 days of gestation is followed by tracheal ligation at 120 days, the fetal lungs grow and the viscera are fully reduced at birth. The herniated viscera remain in the chest in the unligated controls. With permission, from Hedrick *et al.* (25).

baseline whereas the PI of the CDH group did not change significantly. This model further supports the role of vascular hypoplasia in the pathogenesis of CDH and the measurement of PI offers a novel method to study *in utero* intervention targeting the pulmonary vascular bed (26).

2. Rat Model

Although the etiology of human congenital diaphragmatic hernia is still undetermined, the rat model of nitrofen-induced spontaneous congenital diaphragmatic hernia closely approximates the human disease. The toxic herbicide 2,4-dichloro-phenyl-*p*-nitrophenyl ether (nitrofen) given as a single dose to time-dated pregnant rats produces a condition remarkably similar to that observed in the human fetus. The timing of nitrofen delivery is critical and administration of a single oral dose of 100 mg on day 9 of gestation produces hernias on the left and/or right side of the diaphragm, whereas administration of a single dose on day 11 produces solely right-sided hernias. The number of fetuses affected varies and is probably a product of teratogen transfer to each fetus (Table II) (27).

Alles and colleagues (28) used this model to study the pattern of nitrofen-induced cell death as a possible etiology of congenital diaphragmatic hernia. Time-dated Sprague–Dawley rats were given 100 mg of nitrofen dissolved in olive oil by gavage on gestational day 9.5 (Wako Bioproducts, Richmont, VA). Control animals received an equal volume of olive oil alone or remained untreated. After 24 (day 10.5) or 48 hr (day 11.5) portions of the embryos were harvested and patterns of cell death analyzed using the supravital dye Nile blue sulfate. This compound accumulates in low-pH cellular compartments such as phagosomes, present at sites of embryonic cell death. Staining and analysis at 24 hr revealed excessive cell death in cervical somites 2, 3, and 4, and at 48 hr cell death was noted in the intermediate mesoderm just ventral to somites 2, 3, and 4. The proportion of embryos showing this pattern of cell death (28.7%) was similar to the incidence of CDH in those embryos that continued in gestation and were harvested at 21.5 days. The destruction of this mesenchyme may reduce its contribution to the diaphragmatic primordia, leaving a paucity of tissue for normal growth and closure of the diaphragm.

Although the pathogenesis of pulmonary hypoplasia as developing from thoracic cavity volume restriction caused by the herniated abdominal viscera is supported by the sheep model, an opposing theory still exists stating that the diaphragmatic malformation is merely a secondary manifestation of pulmonary maldevelopment (29). The nitrofen-induced rat model provides a unique opportunity to study this phenomenon because invasion of the thoracic cavity is a gradual process, occurring with abdominal content expansion and growth. Analysis of lung parameters on day 15 (prior to herniation into the chest) and day 18 (after herniation) revealed that only after day 18 were there significant differences in lung weight, protein content, and DNA content between the CDH animals and the controls. These data further support the theory that lung hypoplasia occurs secondarily to visceral herniation rather than as a primary pulmonary defect (27).

To capitalize on the rat CDH model, efforts in our laboratory have focused on inducing *in utero* pulmonary growth. Because the prevention of the normal egress of pulmonary fluid by tracheal occlusion can accelerate lung growth and development in the sheep, we decided to test the therapeutic applicability of this process in the fetal rat CDH model. Time-dated Sprague–Dawley rats (term is 22 days) were given 100 mg of nitrofen by oral gavage on day 9 of gestation. On day 19 the mother was anesthetized by an intraperitoneal injection of pentobarbital sodium (15 mg/kg) and one of the uterine horns was exposed through a maternal laparotomy. Drops of ritodrine solution (5 mg/ml) were applied to the uterine wall in order to minimize uterine contractions during the dissection. The fetal trachea was exposed under a stereodissection microscope and ligated with a 9-0 nylon suture (Fig. 6). The fetus was returned to the amniotic space, the hysterotomy was approximated with a 6-0 prolene purse-string suture, and the abdominal wall was closed with 5-0 Vicryl running suture.

Fetuses were delivered by cesarean section on day 21.5 of gestation and sacrificed by intraperitoneal pentobarbital sodium (5 mg/fetus). The abdomen and chest were opened to confirm the presence and laterality of the diaphragmatic hernia. The heart and lungs were dissected out below the ligation site and complete tracheal occlusion was confirmed by dye injection into the tracheal stump below the ligature (30).

Table II Incidence of Diaphragmatic Hernias Induced by Nitrofen Administration on Day E9[a]

Total no. of hernias	Normal	Left hernia	Right hernia	Bilateral hernia
181 (17 dams)	86 (48%)	39 (21%)	45 (25%)	11 (6%)

[a]From Allan and Greer (27), with permission.

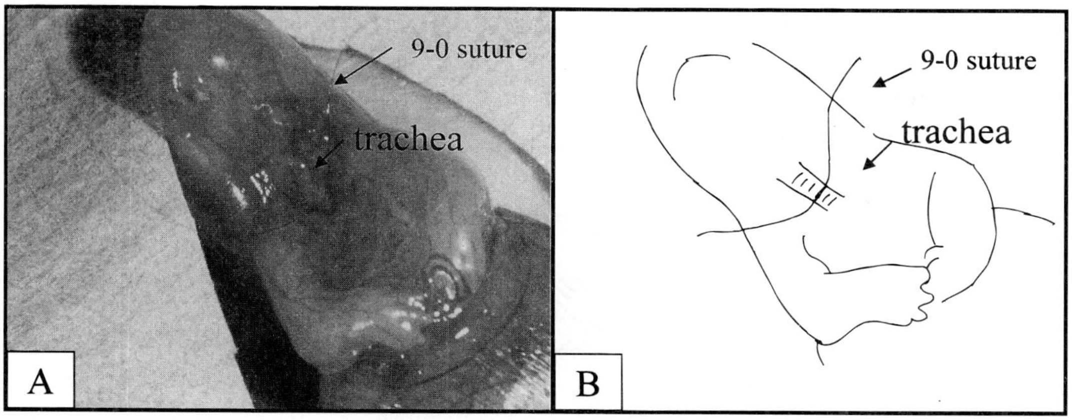

Figure 6 Fetal rat tracheal ligation at 19 days of gestation. Picture courtesy of Dr. Masaki Kanai, The Children's Hospital of Philadelphia.

Only those animals with complete occlusion were included in the experimental group. Pulmonary parameters and architecture were compared to controls, consisting of normal fetuses without CDH and CDH fetuses without tracheal occlusion. Analysis of pulmonary tissue revealed that the decreased lung weight, total lung protein, and DNA content of those animals with left-sided CDH could be reversed by tracheal occlusion and could even be increased above normal controls. Morphometric data supported these findings and revealed an increase in the volume of lung parenchyma and surface area. Future studies using this animal model will focus on reversible tracheal occlusion to allow postnatal survival and functional potential of the developed pulmonary tissue similar to the sheep model (31).

B. Myelomeningocele

Although the paralysis seen in children with myelomeningocele has been attributed to failure of neurulation, a concurrent theory proposes that at least part of the damage is secondary to exposure within the intrauterine environment. This proposal is based on the postmortem anatomic studies of children with myelomeningocele revealing damage and necrosis of the exposed dorsal horns but normal ventral horns (32) and ultrasound studies reporting normal leg movement in fetuses with open spina bifida as late as week 17 of gestation (33).

1. Rat Model

Heffez and colleagues (34) tested the hypothesis that exposure of the developing spinal cord to amniotic fluid results in neurologic damage in a rat model of spinal dysraphism. Time-dated pregnant Sprague–Dawley rats were anesthetized on day 18 (term is 22 days) with acepromazine (0.25–3 mg/kg) and ketamine (60–75 mg/kg), a midline laparotomy was performed, and one horn of the bifid uterus was exteriorized. A single fetus was selected and a small hysterotomy was made, exposing the dorsal midline. The amniotic membrane was opened and a 5-mm incision was made along the dorsal midline of the fetus as the paraspinal muscles were dissected and a two- to three-level laminectomy was performed. The translucent dura was opened using a 26-gauge needle, with extreme care taken not to injure the spinal cord. In the experimental group the skin was left open, exposing the spinal cord to the intrauterine environment, whereas in the control group the skin was approximated over the laminectomy with 9-0 nylon suture. At least one experimental pup and one control pup were operated on in every litter.

The pregnancy continued to term, at which time the pups were either born by cesarean section or spontaneously. Every pup in the experimental group was born with weakness and deformity of the hind limbs and tail. Six of the nine pups in the control group, whose spinal cords were covered by skin, were entirely normal and indistinguishable from the unoperated littermates, but the remaining three pups in the control group had evidence of wound dehiscence and exposure of the underlying spinal cord. These pups manifested varying degrees of weakness or deformity of the hind limbs and tail. Histologic analysis revealed necrosis of the exposed dorsal aspect of the cord but a morphologically normal spinal cord above and below the lesion, adding strength to the theory that cord exposure leads to damage.

2. Sheep Model

Based on these preliminary results we set out to evaluate the possibility of fetal surgery to cover the exposed neural tissue *in utero*. The fetal sheep more realistically model the human disease due to the longer intrauterine gestation.

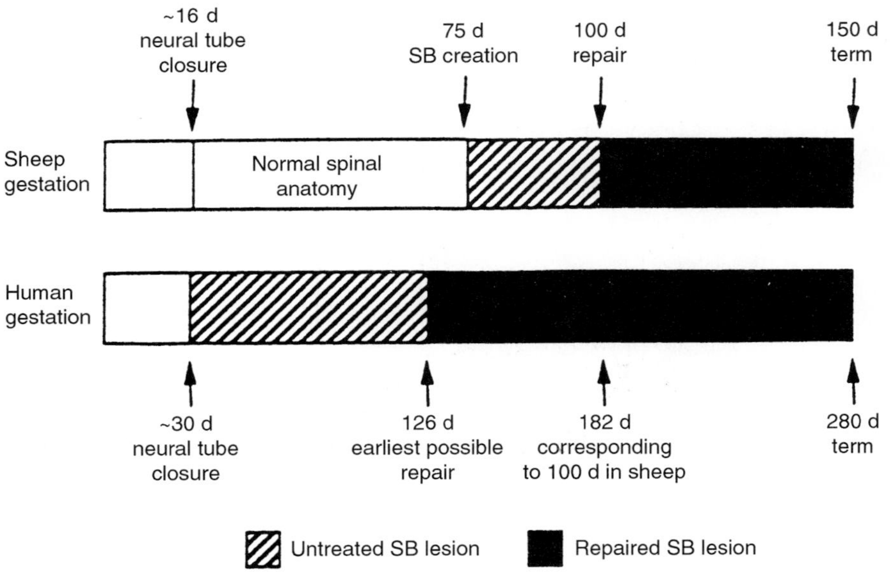

Figure 7 Timeline comparing the experimental creation and repair of myelomeningocele in the fetal sheep to that in the human. From Meuli *et al.* (36), with permission from Nature Medicine and the author.

Spinal dysraphism, created early in gestation, can be followed by a period of exposure to the intrauterine environment, followed by delayed closure simulating human fetal repair (Fig. 7). Efforts at exposure of the spinal canal and creation of the laminectomy at 60 days of gestation resulted in spontaneous healing with near-normal spinal cord pathology and preserved neurologic function. This healing "experiment of nature" furthered the therapeutic potential of *in utero* repair (35). Exposure of the normal spinal cord to the amniotic fluid at 75 days of gestation, however, created a clinical and morphologic picture similar to human myelomeningocele.

Using the standard surgical techniques described previously, 75-day gestation fetal sheep underwent the creation of a spina bifida-type lesion. A circular 4-cm skin excision was made over the lumbar spine as the paraspinal musculature; the posterior parts of the vertebral column, and the dorsal dura, were excised from L_1 to L_4 (Fig. 8). The animals were returned to the uterus and the amniotic fluid volume was restored, with closure of the hysterotomy plus laparotomy in the standard fashion. At 100 days of gestation some of the fetuses were removed for histologic analysis, some continued in gestation to be delivered by cesarean section near term (control group), and the rest (experimental group) underwent *in utero* repair and coverage of the defect with a latissimus dorsi muscle flap. The proximal portion of the latissimus dorsi was mobilized because its origin and the vascular pedicle were transected, leaving the muscle attached to the iliac crest and the distal vascular pedicle. The muscle was then pulled through a subcutaneous tunnel over the lesion, sutured to the surrounding tissue, and the skin incision was closed over the flap. Near term the animals were delivered and assessed.

At birth the unrepaired animals (control group) showed a clinical and pathologic picture similar to that seen in humans. The lambs had complete sensorimotor paraplegia in the hind limbs and were incontinent of urine and stool. Cortical somatosensory-evoked potentials (SEPs) were absent in the hind limbs but normal in the forelimbs. Histology after sacrifice revealed flattening and erosion of the dorsal portions of the spinal cord with complete loss of neural tissue in some specimens. Those animals examined at 100 days revealed lesions intermediate to those at birth, suggesting spina bifida in evolution. The animals that underwent *in utero* repair at 100 days of gestation revealed a different pic-

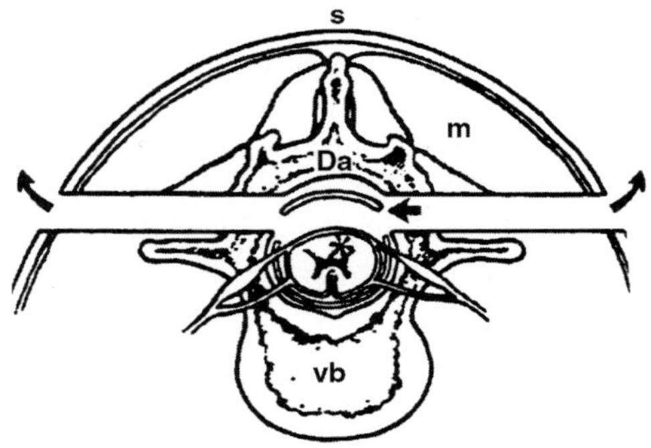

Figure 8 Schematic representation of the parts removed from the fetal spine in order to model the defect of spina bifida. m, Paraspinal muscles; na, neural arch; vb, vertebral body. From Meuli *et al.* (36), with permission from Nature Medicine and the author.

ture, with near-normal hind limb motor function and sensory function confirmed by clinical assessment and SEP. The lambs were continent of both urine and stool and microscopically the cord was flattened, with mild dilation of the central canal, but contained normal cytoarchitecture of the cord and spinal ganglia. These results have paved the way for human *in utero* repair of myelomeningocele (36).

C. In Utero Hematopoietic Stem Cell Transplantation

The fetus offers an ideal opportunity to treat hematopoietic disorders prior to postnatal manifestation of the disease. Advances in prenatal diagnostic tests, genetic screening of families at risk, and molecular analysis have made *in utero* diagnosis of hematopoietic disorders common. The immunologically immature fetus is tolerant of foreign antigens and offers the potential for a high level of hematopoietic stem cell engraftment without immunosuppression, myeloablation, or graft-versus-host (GVH) disease. The widespread availability of high-resolution ultrasound and minimally invasive technology has also decreased the technical difficulties related to access to the fetus.

1. The Sheep Model

To date the most successful animal model of *in utero* hematopoietic stem cell transplantation remains the sheep. Taking advantage of the naturally occurring polymorphism at the β-hemoglobin locus, Flake and colleagues (37) injected liver-derived hematopoietic stem cells (2×10^8 to 5×10^8 nucleated cells/kg) of AA sheep into the peritoneum of 45- to 65-day gestation BB recipients (Fig. 9). Three of the four surviving fetuses demonstrated a high level of engraftment, with 14–29% of the hemoglobin in the host circulation derived from the donor. Chimerism was maintained long term after birth without evidence of GVH disease or immunosuppression.

2. The Mouse Model

The mouse model offers the advantage of numerous available knockout models and models of human hematopoietic disease. Unlike the case with sheep, the level of donor engraftment after *in utero* transplantation has been low. To test the hypothesis that low levels of engraftment are due to the competition between donor and recipient hematopoietic stem cells for available niches we performed in the same animal multiple transplants separated by brief intervals of time. This should allow for the formation of new niches and increase the level of engraftment. Adult bone marrow was harvested from donor C57Pep3B mice, and 14-day fetuses of time-dated C57BL/6 mothers acted as the recipients. Under methoxyflurane anesthesia a midline laparotomy was performed and the uterine horns were delivered into the wound. All fetuses were injected intraperitoneally directly through the transparent uterus with 1×10^6

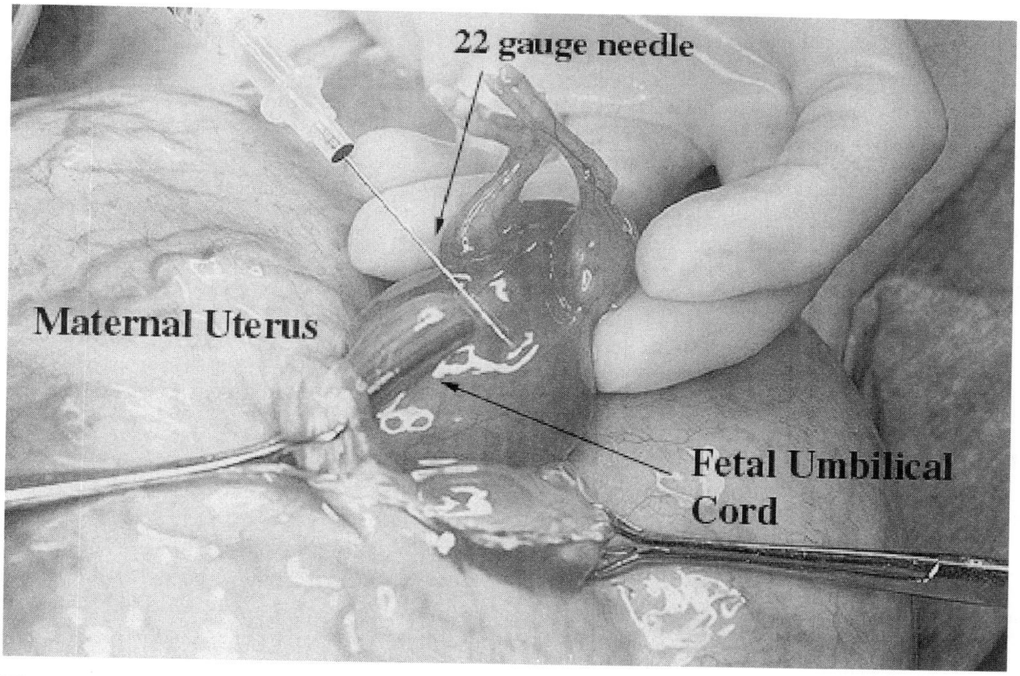

Figure 9 Open intraperitoneal injection of stem cells into a 60-day fetal sheep. The concurrent technique of intraperitoneal injection through the amniotic bubble may be easier and avoids open fetal manipulation (not illustrated).

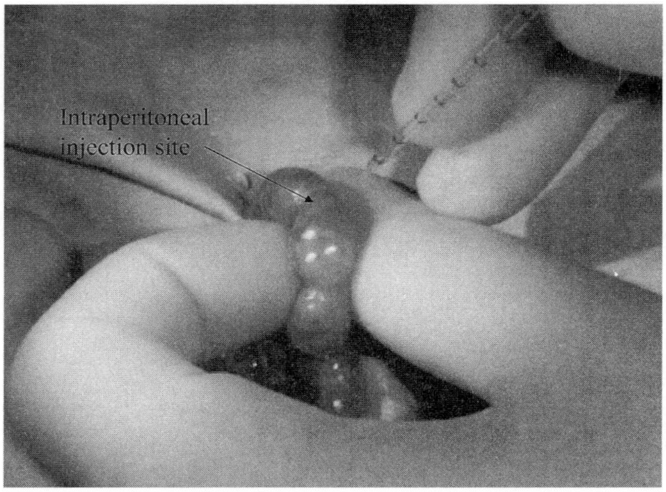

Figure 10 Intraperitoneal injection of adult bone marrow into 14-day gestation fetal mice. Picture courtesy Dr. Aimen Shaaban, The Children's Hospital of Philadelphia.

cells in a 5-μl suspension via a 100-μm beveled glass micropipette (Fig. 10). The abdomen was then closed with two layers of absorbable suture and the pregnancy continued until delivery. Neonates received booster injections using a similar protocol on day of life 2, 4, and 7. The peripheral blood was collected and analyzed for chimerism at 6 weeks, 3 months, and 6 months of age. The mean level of engraftment in the postnatally boosted animals was 3.3 ± 0.8% compared to the 0.69 ± 0.5% in the nonboosted control animals who received only the *in utero* transplant. This level of chimerism was stable for the duration of the study without immunosuppression or evidence of GVH disease. Future work utilizing this model will focus on maximizing engraftment after the establishment of *in utero* donor-specific tolerance (38).

A summary of all of the models used in fetal surgery research is shown in Table III.

Table III Summary of Animal Models in Fetal Surgery Research

Area of research	Advantages	Limitations
Fetal wound healing		
Mouse model	Low cost for experiments involving a large number of animals; numerous transgenic models of human disease; assays for inflammatory markers available from commercial sources	Small size of the fetus can create difficulty with fine manipulation; short gestation creates difficulty in performing multiple procedures
Rabbit model	Low cost for experiments involving a large number of animals	High rate of fetal loss, especially early in gestation
Sheep model	Longer gestation allows repetition of several procedures in the same fetus; low risk of fetal loss; precise manipulation and wounding easier due to the larger size of the animal	High cost of maintaining pregnant sheep
Preterm labor after fetal surgery		
Primate model	Level of uterine irritability similar to that in humans; potential for implantation of long-term indwelling catheters to measure fetal and uterine environment	High cost
Rabbit model	Care for this animal model is less expensive than for the primate; potential to gather data in a large; number of animals prior to advancing to the primate model	Uterine irritability after hysterotomy different from the human condition
Congenital diaphragmatic hernia		
Rat model	Nitrofen-induced model of spontaneous congenital diaphragmatic hernia available	Difficulty in establishing reversible tracheal occlusion in this small animal model
Sheep model	Long gestation allows the creation of hernia with repair or tracheal occlusion during the same gestation; potential for the development of reversible tracheal occlusion device	High cost of maintaining pregnant sheep
Myelomeningocele		
Rat model	Low cost of the rat model; potential to reproduce data in a large number of animals	The short gestation presents difficulty in creating and repairing the spinal cord defect in the same animal
Sheep model	Potential to create and repair spinal cord defect during the same gestation	High cost of maintaining pregnant sheep
***In utero* hematopoietic stem cell transplantation**		
Sheep model	High level of chimerism after *in utero* hematopoietic stem cell transplantation	High cost of maintaining pregnant sheep
Mouse model	Numerous transgenic strains modeling human diseases are available	Low level of chimerism after *in utero* hematopoietic stem cell transplantation

References

1. Adamson, K. (1965). Fetal surgery. *N. Engl. J. Med.* **275**(4), 204–205.
2. Lorenz, H. P., Whitby, D. J., Longaker, M. T., and Adzick, N. S. (1993). Fetal wound healing: The ontogeny of scar formation in the non-human primate. *Ann. Surg.* **217**(4), 391–396.
3. Adzick, N. S., and Harrison, M. R. (1986). Surgical techniques in the fetal rabbit. *In* "Animal Models in Fetal Medicine (V)" (P. W. Nathanielsz, ed.), pp 66-103. Perinatology Press, Ithaca, New York.
4. Somasundaram, K., and Prathap, K. (1970). Intra-uterine healing of skin wounds in rabbit foetuses. *J. Pathol.* **100,** 81–86.
5. Somasundaram, K., and Prathap, K. (1972). The effect of exclusion of amniotic fluid on intrauterine healing of skin wounds in rabbit foetuses. *J. Pathol.* **107,** 127–130.
6. Krummel, T. M., Nelson, J. M., Thomas, B. L., *et al.* (1989). Fetal wounds do not contract *in utero. Surg. Forum* **40,** 613–614.
7. Bell, A. W., Battaglia, F. C., and Meschia, G. (1987). Methods for chronic studies of circulation and metabolism in the sheep conceptus at 70–80 days gestation. *In* "Animal Models in Fetal Medicine (VI)" (P. W. Nathanielsz, ed.), pp 38-54. Perinatology Press, Ithaca, New York.
8. Lumbers, E. R., Smith, F. G., and Stevens, A. D. (1985). Measurement of net transplacental transfer of fluid to the fetal sheep. *J. Physiol.* **364,** 289–299.
8a. Moore, K. L., and Persaud, T. V. N., eds. (1993). "The Developing Human: Clinically Oriented Embryology" (5th Ed.). W. B. Saunders, Philadelphia.
9. Harrison, M. R., Jester, J. A., and Ross, N. A. (1980). Correction of congenital diaphragmatic hernia *in utero*. I. The model: Intrathoracic balloon produces fatal pulmonary hypoplasia. *Surgery* **88**(1), 174–182.
10. Longaker, M. T., Burd, D. A., Gown, A. M., *et al.* (1991). Midgestational excisional fetal lamb wounds contract *in utero. J. Pediatr. Surg.* **26**(8), 942–947.
11. Longaker, M. T., and Kaban, L. B. (1992). Fetal models for craniofacial surgery: Cleft lip/palate and craniosynostosis. *In* "Fetal Wound Healing" (N. S. Adzick and M. T. Longaker, eds.). Elsevier, New York.
12. Hedrick, M. H., Rice, H. E., VanderWall, K. J., *et al.* (1996). Delayed *in utero* repair of surgically created fetal cleft lip and palate. *Plast. Reconstr. Surg.* **97,** 900.
13. Whitby, D. J., and Ferguson, M. W. J. (1991). The extracellular matrix of lip wounds in fetal, neonatal and adult mice. *Development* **112,** 651–668.
14. Ferguson, M. W., and Howarth, G. F. (1992). Marsupial models of scarless fetal wound healing. In Adzick NS, Longaker MT (eds.) "Fetal Wound Healing" (N. S. Adzick and M. T. Longaker, eds.). Elsevier, New York.
15. Flake, A. W., and Harrison, M. R. (1995). Fetal surgery. *Annu. Rev. Med.* **46,** 67–78.
16. Harrison, M. R., Anderson, J., Rosen, M. A., *et al.* (1982). Fetal surgery in the primate I. Anesthetic, surgical, and tocolytic management to maximize fetal–neonatal survival. *J. Pediatr. Surg.* **17**(2), 115–122.
17. Nakayama, D. K., Harrison, M. R., Seron-Ferre, M., *et al.* (1984). Fetal surgery in the primate II. Uterine electromyographic response to operative procedures and pharmacologic agents. *J. Pediatr. Surg.* **19**(4), 333–339.
18. Novy, M. J., Walsh, S. W., and Cook, M. J. (1980). Chronic implantation of catheters and electrodes in pregnant non-human primates. *In* "Animal Models in Fetal Medicine(I)" (P. W. Nathanielsz, ed.), pp. 133–168. Perinatology Press, Ithaca, New York.
19. Adzick, N. S., Harrison, M. R., Glick, P. L., *et al.* (1986). Fetal surgery in the primate III. Maternal outcome after fetal surgery. *J. Pediatr. Surg.* **21**(6), 477–480.
20. Fauza, D. O., Berde, C. B., and Fishman, S. J. (1999). Prolonged local myometrial blockade prevents preterm labor after fetal surgery in a leporine model. *J. Pediatr. Surg.* **34**(4), 540–542.
21. Lipsett, J., Cool, J. C., Runciman, S. I. C., *et al.* (1998). Effect of antenatal tracheal occlusion on lung development in the sheep model of congenital diaphragmatic hernia: A morphometric analysis of pulmonary structure and maturity. *Pediatr. Pulmonol.* **25,** 257–269.
22. Adzick, N. S., Outwater, K. M., Harrison, M. R., *et al.* (1985). Correction of congenital diaphragmatic hernia *in utero* IV. An early gestational fetal lamb model for pulmonary vascular morphometric analysis. *J. Pediatr. Surg.* **20**(6), 673–680.
23. Wigglesworth, J., and Hislop, A. (1987). Fetal lung growth in congenital laryngeal atresia. *Pediatr. Pathol.* **7,** 515–525.
24. Fewell, J. E., Hislop, A. A., Kittermam, J. A., *et al.* (1983). Effect of tracheostomy on lung development in fetal lambs. *J. Appl. Physiol.* **55,** 1103–1108.
25. Hedrick, M. H., Estes, J. M., Sullivan, K. M., *et al.* (1994). Plug the lung until it grows (PLUG): A new method to treat congenital diaphragmatic hernia *in utero*. *J. Pediatr. Surg.* **29**(5), 612–617.
26. Sylvester, K. G., Rasanen, J., Kitano, Y., *et al.* (1998). Tracheal occlusion reverses the high impedance to flow in the fetal pulmonary circulation and normalizes its physiological response to oxygen at full term. *J. Pediatr. Surg.* **33**(7), 1071–1075.
27. Allan, D. W., and Greer, J. J. (1997). Pathogenesis of nitrofen-induced congenital diaphragmatic hernia in fetal rats. *J. Appl. Physiol.* **83**(2), 338–347.
28. Alles, A. J., Losty, P. D., Donahoe, P. K., *et al.* (1995). Embryonic cell death patterns associated with nitrofen-induced congenital diaphragmatic hernia. *J. Pediatr. Surg.* **30**(2), 353–360.
29. Iritani, I. (1984). Experimental study on embryogenesis of congenital diaphragmatic hernia. *Anat. Embryol.* **169**(2), 133–139.
30. Kitano, Y., Yang, E. Y., von Allmen, D., *et al.* (1998). Tracheal occlusion in the fetal rat: A new experimental model for the study of accelerated lung growth. *J. Pediatr. Surg.* **33**(12), 1741–1744.
31. Kitano, Y., Davies, P., von Allmen, D., *et al.* (1999). Fetal tracheal occlusion in the rat model of nitrofen-induced congenital diaphragmatic hernia. *J. Appl. Physiol.* **87**(2), 769–775.
32. Emery, J. L., and Lendon, R. G. (1973). The local cord lesion in neurospinal dysraphism (meningomyelocele). *J. Pathol.* **110,** 83–96.
33. Korenromp, M. J., Van Gool, J. D., Bruinse, H. W., *et al.* (1986). Early fetal leg movements in myelomeningocele. *Lancet* **1,** 917–918.
34. Heffez, D. S., Aryanpur, J., Hutchins, G. M., *et al.* (1990). The paralysis associated with myelomeningocele: Clinical and experimental data implicating a preventable spinal cord injury. *Neurosurgery* **26**(6), 987–992.
35. Meuli, M., Meuli-Simmen, C., Yingling, C. D., *et al.* (1995). Creation of myelomeningocele *in utero*: A model of functional damage from spinal cord exposure in fetal sheep. *J. Pediatr. Surg.* **30**(7), 1028–1033.
36. Meuli, M., Meuli-Simmen, C., Hutchins, G. M., *et al.* (1995). *In utero* surgery rescues neurological function at birth in sheep with spinal bifida. *Nature Med.* **1**(4), 342–347.
37. Flake, A. W., Harrison, M. R., Adzick, N. S., *et al.* (1986). Transplantation of fetal hematopoietic stem cells *in utero*: The creation of hematopoietic chimeras. *Science* **233,** 776–778.
38. Milner, R., Shaaban, A., Kim, H. B., *et al.* (1999). Postnatal booster injections increase engraftment after *in utero* stem cell transplantation. *J. Surg. Res.* **83,** 44–47.

77

Research in Plastic Surgery

Gyu S. Chin,[*] Jason A. Spector,[*] Stephen M. Warren,[†] and Michael T. Longaker[‡]

[*] *Department of Surgery, New York University Medical Center, New York, New York 10016*
[†] *Department of Surgery, Oregon Health Science University, Portland, Oregon 97201*
[‡] *Department of Surgery, Stanford University School of Medicine, Stanford, California 94305*

I. Introduction

Plastic surgery research encompasses a wide range of topics. Because it would be a difficult task to update all related subjects in limited space, we focus here on several specific areas and highlight recent advances and the methods by which they were achieved. With this in mind, we first discuss two areas that may revolutionize the field of plastic surgery. Due to the overlap of topics in the volume, we limit the discussion to the potential of gene therapy and tissue engineering in the field of plastic surgery research, and reference the other chapters for specific methods and techniques. We also discuss contemporary methods of conducting research in the area of craniofacial surgery, concentrating primarily on the different animal models, as they relate to cleft lip and palate repair and craniosynostosis. Where appropriate, advantages and disadvantages of the current procedures are discussed, providing insight into the "tricks and traps" of each methodology.

II. Gene Therapy

Gene therapy is becoming a clinical reality. This has become possible due to the increased understanding of the biomolecular pathogenesis of certain diseases and the advances in gene transfer technology. Plastic surgery researchers have embraced this concept, which may revolutionize the broad spectrum of intricate surgical procedures that are performed, such as skin grafting, nerve and muscle repair, and microvascular tissue transfer, to name a few. Gene therapy has the potential for significant improvement in clinical outcome in these areas by selectively expressing genes of interest at targeted sites. Furthermore, this approach may lead to improvements in the rate and efficiency of the wound repair process, and thus will have a significant impact on the quality of healthcare and the management of healthcare costs (1). This section focuses on the growth factors and their involvement in wound healing, nerve and muscle regeneration, and microvascular thrombosis. We concentrate on recent gene therapy advances and methods of investigation in these areas as well as new approaches for future applications in plastic surgery.

A. Gene Therapy in Cutaneous Wound Healing

Growth factors play a major role in wound healing. Thus, their potential use as gene therapeutic agents is apparent. Using advanced gene transfer techniques (as described in

Chapter 38, this volume), one can transfect a growth factor gene of interest into desired cells, which will ultimately result in the localized expression of their recombinant proteins. In theory, localized overexpression may be ideal, because systemically applied growth factors, which require large doses to produce a biologic effect, may elicit serious side effects.

There are several applications of gene therapy to cutaneous wound healing. One approach may involve use of genetically engineered keratinocytes or fibroblasts to overexpress growth factor genes, which may accelerate healing and regenerate injured tissue. Once the DNA of interest is inserted, genetically modified cells can then be transplanted to the wound area, and will express recombinant proteins for a prolonged time (1, 2). For example, one group has transferred the human epidermal growth factor (hEGF) expression plasmid to porcine partial-thickness wound keratinocytes by particle-mediated DNA transfer (Accell) (3); they found that wounds treated with the hEGF plasmid exhibited a 190-fold increase in EGF concentration and healed 20% earlier than the controls. Such methods could be used to enhance skin regeneration after a burn injury or to accelerate wound healing, including surgical incisions. Similarly, gene therapy may allow scarless healing or total skin regeneration. In addition, others have postulated that gene therapy may be ideal for treating genetic skin diseases. For example, Vogel (4) has hypothesized that adenovirus- or retrovirus-mediated transfer of the normal keratin gene in cultured keratinocytes may reverse the lack of keratin in epidermolysis bullosa simplex, a skin disorder associated with a single mutation of a keratin gene.

Other methods of gene transfer for enhancement of cutaneous wound repair may utilize the introduction of DNA directly into skin, using a gene gun that projects gold particle-coated DNA at high velocity into skin (5), or by direct subcutaneous injection of DNA into skin (6).

B. Gene Therapy for Vessel Thrombosis

Unfortunately, plastic surgeons are occasionally confronted by thrombosis resulting from a microvascular anastomosis. Current protocols for the treatment of thrombosis are systemic and can have major side effects, such as cerebrovascular stroke and hemorrhage (7, 8). Thus, an ideal therapy would involve a local and prolonged application of a thrombolytic agent without systemic side effects. Vascular gene therapy has a potential role in preventing and treating local vessel thrombosis. Specifically, endothelial cells can be targeted to promote the expression of recombinant thrombolytic proteins using viral or nonviral gene transfer techniques (9–11).

A conceptually different *ex vivo* approach to vessel gene therapy involves the use of cultured endothelial cells that are reimplanted *in vivo*. A study by Nabel *et al.* (12) has shown that cultured endothelial cells, transfected with LacZ gene and subsequently reimplanted, expressed β-galactosidase for up to 5 weeks, indicating that the cells were successfully transferred onto the vessel wall.

In the future, constructs carrying thrombolytic agents, such as tissue plasminogen activator, thrombomodulin, streptokinase, and antithrombin III, may be utilized to treat or prevent vessel thrombosis (1).

C. Gene Therapy for Nerve and Muscle Regeneration

Peripheral nerve injuries continue to be a challenging problem confronted by microsurgeons. Even with modern microsurgical techniques, complete regeneration of pheripheral nerves is not achieved. The current direction of research to decrease, or even completely prevent muscle atrophy involves use of neurotrophic factors to enhance pheripheral nerve regeneration.

In addition to targeting nerves, muscle tissues are also being evaluated for neurotrophic factor gene transfer. To date, a number of methods for transferring exogenous genes into skeletal muscle have been described. Wolff *et al.* (13) demonstrated that foreign plasmid DNA was expressed in skeletal muscle for at least 19 months after intramuscular injection. Likewise, plasmids carrying the LacZ reporter gene have also been introduced and were expressed for nearly one year in muscle *in vivo* (5).

Specifically targeting muscle cells, however, may prove a more efficient approach than targeting muscle tissue. In addition, adenoviral-mediated gene transfer to muscle cells may prove to be the most efficient gene transfer technique, as compared with liposome and plasmid-DNA mediated transfer. Certain research groups demonstrated high transfection rates and expression of adenoviral constructs in skeletal muscles (1). More studies are required to confirm that long-term expression of genes delivered by viral and nonviral vectors is possible.

In summary, the main issues facing the clinical application of gene therapy are the need for improvements in the delivery and transfer of genes to the appropriate site and subsequent control of the expression of the gene that has been transferred. Although cDNA complexed to liposomes and retroviral, pseudotyped retroviral, and adenoviral vectors are being used to promote gene transfer, gene delivery systems are still at an early stage of development. Nevertheless, gene therapy will become a clinical reality, and may serve as an adjuvant to conventional therapies in the near future.

III. Tissue Engineering

The loss or failure of body structures can be a devastating and costly problem. The field of tissue engineering applies principles of biology and engineering to the development of structural and functional substitutes for damaged tissue. Thus, tissue engineering provides hope that damaged tissues may someday be replaced without significant donor requirements or need for long-term immunosuppression.

This section discusses the foundations and challenges of this interdisciplinary field and its role in providing solutions to tissue creation and repair. Specifically, we concentrate on recent advances and methods of research in the field of tissue engineering relating to bone, cartilage, and skin.

A. Bone

1. Animal Model

To determine the utility of a bone engineering strategy, an appropriate model must be developed to test the reliability of the construct. This is especially relevant in testing the success of engineered bone constructs because of the different embryologic origins of bone. Because osseous repair in the adult is known to recapitulate bone development (14, 15), the nature of the repair process (direct ossification versus formation of a cartilaginous intermediate) will similarly depend on the embryologic origin of the bone under repair.

The reconstructive plastic surgeon is often faced with large segmental bone defects within the craniofacial skeleton as a result of either surgical resection or trauma. Also, he/she must contend with significant bone hypoplasias secondary to congenital malformations. Thus, a logical place to test the success of bone healing strategies is within the craniofacial skeleton.

The most important assessment of bone repair may be the "critical size defect" parameter, which is defined as the smallest diameter osseous defect (either circular or segmental) that, if left untreated, will form a fibrous union (16). This parameter is useful for determination of the osteoinductive nature of the treatment under consideration, because any therapy that heals this nonhealing defect is by definition osteoinductive. To evaluate the degree to which a material permits growth of osseous tissue, the property of osteoconductivity should be evaluated with subsequent assessment of a noncritical size defect (one that would normally heal) (17).

The dimension of a given critical size defect will vary depending on the location of the wound (e.g., calvarium versus tibia) and the species in which it is being tested. For example, the critical size of a calvarial defect in rats, rabbits, and dogs, respectively, is 8 (18), 15 (19), and 20 mm (16). Aside from the obvious observation that larger animals will necessarily have larger critical size defects, this latter point is an especially relevant one, because certain animals are known to have a much greater capacity to repair and form osseous tissues (16). Thus any successful treatment in one species should be confirmed in others, preferably a species that is genetically closer to the ultimate subject of all of these studies, humans. This concept of successive testing in increasingly "complex" animal species has been suggested by Schmitz and Hollinger in the evaluation of the effects of various treatments on the healing of a critical size calvarial defect (16).

Although the ideal critical size defect would be strictly reproducible, in reality slight variations in technique and instrumentation may result in small, yet important, differences in outcome among investigators. For example, the healing of a circular mandibular defect made by using a drill can be significantly affected by the rate of irrigation that accompanies the drilling. Inadequate irrigation may result in thermal injury and cellular damage or death adjacent to the defect, severely inhibiting the regenerative capacity of the surrounding bone. Such reasoning may account for the variability reported in the literature concerning critical size defects in rat calvaria, which range from 4 to 8 mm (16, 20–23).

Further complicating the study of osseous healing is the fact that there can be significant variability in the capacity of repair among animals of the same species (16, 24). Such variability necessitates the use of adequately large subject populations in which to test the treatment under study. In addition, it is well known that young animals retain a much greater capacity to regenerate osseous tissues (especially in the calvarium), and thus are inadequate subjects for the evaluation of novel healing strategies (16, 24).

Finally, cost considerations also play a role in the determination of the appropriate model to be used. Rodents and rabbits are appealing because of their low cost and ease of care, and thus can be studied easily in large numbers. Unfortunately, however, they suffer from the aforementioned drawbacks associated with studies in "lower" mammalian species (e.g., greater capacity to form bone). Canines and primates are more desirable models, but the increased financial, technical, and ethical burdens associated with their use make them less attractive, at least until the final stages of investigation. In summary, before embarking on the study of novel bone tissue engineering strategies, careful consideration must be given to the choice of a proper model in which to study the treatment in question.

2. Current Therapeutic Strategies

Large segmental bone defects, whether secondary to trauma, surgical resection, or congenital malformation, represent a major biomedical burden. Until this decade, repair of such defects was accomplished largely by use of autogenous tissue grafting. However, this treatment has the disadvantages of limited donor tissue availability and the potential for donor morbidity. Use of allogenic material for grafting carries the risk for transmission of disease and immunologic reaction. Finally, nondegradable materials such as metals can cause stress shielding (deterioration of the bone surrounding the implant secondary to reduced loading of that bone); ceramics can suffer from structural failure and bone cements carry a greater risk of infection (17).

3. Biocompatible Scaffolds

In an effort to circumvent drawbacks associated with current treatment modalities, novel bone tissue engineering approaches are being developed. A central tenet of current bone tissue engineering research is the use of biocompatible and biodegradable scaffold materials. Such scaffolds serve multiple functions. First, they allow localized application, resulting in minimal loss of cells from the target area. Furthermore, most mammalian cells depend on cell–cell or cell–matrix interactions for survival. Attempts to deliver cells without the use of a scaffold have been plagued by such difficulties (25). Second, the pore sizes of the scaffold may be designed to allow "one-way" communication between the construct and the surrounding tissues; small pore sizes would allow outward diffusion of growth factors and other cytokines produced by cells anchored to the scaffold. These constructs would escape immune surveillance, however, because the immunologic cells would be unable to enter the matrix (25). If it is desired that host tissues grow into and eventually replace the construct, a larger pore size would be used (25). Alternatively, a scaffold could be engineered so that it contained factors chemotactic for osteoblasts and their precursors, which would induce the in-growth and subsequent replacement of the synthetic material with mature viable bone. Finally, scaffolds provide a limited measure of mechanical support in that they maintain their shape, although the force that can be withstood is limited with most polymer scaffolds (see below) (25).

Tissue scaffolds can be polymeric or ceramic in nature. Ceramic scaffold materials are composed of either hydroxyapatite or tricalcium phosphate or a combination of the two, and thus they resemble the mineral phase of native bone (17). For example, successful construction of a prefabricated osteomyocutaneous flap utilizing a hydroxyapatite scaffold seeded with human bone marrow stromal cells has been reported in a mouse model (26). The use of a similar technique is under investigation in larger animal models. However, scaffolds constructed from these materials carry the significant disadvantage of having low tensile strength in addition to prolonged (up to years) degradation times, thus preventing their use in locations that experience significant stress, impact, or torque (17).

Polymeric scaffold constructs are built from molecules such as poly(α-hydroxy) esters, each with its own advantages and disadvantages. They are easily synthesized and their physical properties (resorption half-life, porosity, etc.) can be customized as needed (27). Scaffolds composed of α-hydroxy ester molecules such as poly(glycolic acid) and poly(lactic acid) thus far have played a central role in tissue engineering efforts, especially those in bone (25, 28–30). These scaffolds degrade, primarily by passive hydrolysis, to their constituent monomers after implantation, which can potentially result in significant free acid production. However, local acidification is not a concern for most tissue engineering applications because the highly porous structures that are utilized do not release quantities of acid that are as significant as those released by the "solid" α-hydroxy ester polymeric constructs (25).

In vitro studies have demonstrated that osteoblast physiology is not appreciably altered by poly(lactic–coglycolic acid) (PLGA) substrates versus the usual *in vitro* culture substrate, polystyrene (17, 31). Furthermore, osteoblasts placed into three-dimensional PLGA matrices follow the usual progression of differentiation and maturation, demonstrating increased alkaline phosphatase activity followed by matrix deposition and subsequent mineralization of the matrix (17, 32).

An important consideration of any tissue engineering strategy is the interaction between the cell and the surface of the scaffold onto which it is seeded. Although tissue engineering constructs composed of biocompatible substances such as PLGA are not harmful to resident osteoblasts, the potential osteoinductivity of the scaffold can be changed greatly by altering its surface chemistry. Parameters of osteoblast activity such as alkaline phosphatase activity and osteocalcin content can be altered simply by culturing onto smooth versus rough surfaces (17, 33). Current bone engineering strategies must seek to optimize cell–surface interactions in order to encourage maximal osteosynthetic activity.

Still other approaches utilize biodegradable materials that can prevent rapid loss of cells or other macromolecules from a desired area by entrapment within a matrix, such as a polysaccharide (e.g., alginate) or synthetic (e.g., polyphosphazene) gel. Alginate gels have been utilized in strategies for cartilage engineering, but these materials are not suitable for most bone engineering applications.

4. Distraction Osteogenesis

In addition to the "traditional" notion of bone engineering, as just described, there exists another approach to the creation of new bone. Distraction osteogenesis (DO), the formation of new bone between the edges of osteotomized bone by the application of gradual force to separate the two edges, should be thought of as a form of endogenous bone tissue engineering. Though initially attempted at the beginning of this century, this technique did not become widely known until the Russian orthopedic surgeon Ilizarov popularized it more than 50 years later.

Until the beginning of this decade, DO was utilized almost exclusively within the orthopedic community for management of conditions previously treated by bone grafting, such as limb lengthening, nonunions, and repair of bony defects secondary to infection, trauma, or surgery. Extensive study of DO in long bones has demonstrated that the segment of new bone created by DO is similar to the surrounding nondistracted bone in its histology, ultrastructure, and biomechanics (34, 35).

Encouraged by the successful clinical application of this technique to long bone, DO was shown to be feasible for use in the craniofacial skeleton by canine studies in which the mandible was lengthened. McCarthy *et al.* first reported the use of DO on the human mandible in 1992 (36), and less than 5 years later DO had become the preferred treatment for mandibular hypoplasias in the pediatric population, largely obviating the need for complex reconstructive procedures and their associated morbidities.

Studies in several animal models have demonstrated that, as is the case with endochondral bone, distraction of membranous bone results in formation of new bone that is functionally and morphologically equivalent to the nondistracted segments (37–39). Current research is focused on further elucidating the molecular biology underlying DO of the membranous skeleton as well as determination of the optimal rate and rhythm of distraction.

An important consideration for *in vivo* studies of DO is proper choice of the animal model (see above discussion). Our laboratory primarily utilizes a rat model of DO that is technically simple and extremely reproducible, and perhaps most importantly, can be performed in large numbers with relatively low cost. Such a model is useful for biomolecular and biomechanical studies that require large numbers of specimens. Though in much smaller numbers, because of their more humanlike size and anatomy, canine subjects are also utilized to analyze changes in cephalometric variables.

Although animal models for the study of DO are well described, there remains a paucity of suitable *in vitro* studies. It is thought that osteoblast activation during DO is mediated at least in part by strain placed on osteoblasts along the edges of the osteotomy. Most studies analyzing the effects of strain on osteoblast biology have utilized cyclic strain. In DO, osteoblasts experience a constant decaying level of strain between each distraction. Our laboratory is developing a model in which constant equibiaxial strain can be delivered to osteoblasts in culture, thus allowing analysis of osteoblast biology in response to varying amounts of constant mechanical strain alone or in combination with other osteoblast stimulatory elements present within the distraction zone, such as hypoxia and cytokines.

Clinical experience with DO in the craniofacial skeleton is rapidly progressing beyond the mandible. Currently, in preliminary clinical studies, DO is being applied successfully for anterior displacement of the midface (40, 41). Furthermore, in animal studies, our laboratory and others are currently investigating the application of DO to the calvarium (42–44). Trends toward miniaturization of distraction devices may soon obviate the need for external fixation as the devices become small enough to be placed intraorally. Continuing research is leading to the potential for unrestricted use of DO over the entire craniofacial skelton, promising to reshape the future of reconstructive surgery.

B. Cartilage

Currently, the most established strategy for the reconstructive surgeon who is faced with a large-volume cartilage deficit, such as with microtia, is an autograft consisting of cartilage from the patient's rib (45, 46). The morbidities and costs associated with autogenous ear reconstruction and all subsequent procedures required to refine the details of the cartilage framework are significant. Thus, great emphasis has been placed on strategies to allow the bioengineering of new cartilage that would obviate the multiple operations currently required for ear reconstruction.

Engineering new cartilage to replace diseased or deficient tissue presents a problem potentially more challenging than the engineering of new bone. Unlike bone, cartilage is nearly avascular and devoid of a significant pool of progenitor cells. Furthermore, after only a relatively short time in culture, chondrocytes soon cease their production of type II collagen, the matrix protein that defines the phenotype of that cell.

The properties required of the bioengineered cartilage will depend on the anatomic location in which it will be placed. Engineered articular cartilage must be able to withstand the significant loads and stresses that are present within joints, as native hyaline cartilage would. Cartilage destined for external ear reconstruction would theoretically not require the same degree of resilience of engineered articular cartilage. In this section we briefly examine contemporary strategies of cartilage engineering that may be suitable to produce cartilage for use in craniofacial reconstructive procedures.

Scaffold-Based Constructs

The creation of synthetic cartilage constructs has been accomplished with varying degrees of success by numerous investigators. Cao *et al.* (47) demonstrated perhaps the most famous example in 1997 when they reported that they had grown a cartilage construct in the shape of a human ear subcutaneously on the backs of nude mice. In that experiment, chondrocytes obtained from bovine articular cartilage were seeded onto poly(glycolic)–poly(lactic acid) (PGA–PLA) scaffolds formed in the shape of a human auricle. The authors found that 12 weeks after implantation, new cartilage was formed on the scaffold and that the new tissue retained the shape of the PGA–PLA template.

Such an approach to bioengineering of cartilage—the implantation of a biocompatible, biodegradable preformed scaffold seeded with chondoprogenitor cells or chondrocytes—appears to be the most promising strategy. Furthermore, as is the case for similar approaches to bone tissue engineering, this strategy can potentially be augmented by simultaneous addition of growth factors or use of gene therapy techniques to enhance the growth characteristics of the engrafted chondrocytes.

Although cartilage has been engineered into impressively intricate shapes, there remain significant problems associated with such strategies. Most importantly, the long-term stability of these constructs remains in question. Much research is focused on investigating ways to extend the notoriously brief lifetime of engineered constructs. For example, Meinhart *et al.* demonstrated increased stability of fibrin glue-based cartilage constructs that had been treated with inhibitors of fibrinolysis; however, the long-term success of such a strategy remains unclear (48). Furthermore, the immunologic constraints of allotransplantation or xenotransplantation remain significant hurdles to successful application of this strategy.

Finally, a completely novel approach to the engineering of new cartilage is the use of distraction techniques. Just as steady application of force results in the creation of new bone within the gap of an osteotomy, Stelnicki *et al.* have reported the generation of new cartilage within the gap created by a chondrotomy in a rabbit ear subsequently subjected to distraction forces (49). Interestingly, these authors noted the formation of new bone in addition to new cartilage within the chondrotomy gap. These exciting preliminary results demonstrate a potentially viable strategy for "endogenous" engineering of new cartilage. Theoretically, appropriately designed devices could distract and ultimately shape a patient's small microtic cartilage remnant into a relatively normal-appearing appendage. Until the aforementioned problems associated with current scaffold-based cartilage engineering techniques are solved, cartilage distraction may prove a valuable strategic alternative.

C. Skin Substitutes

Over the past decade, major technological advances have been made in the development of skin substitutes for the treatment of cutaneous wounds. The shortcomings of earlier products, including the prolonged amount of time required for expansion of cells, limited handling capability, and the lack of necessary components of human skin to allow wound healing to occur, have prompted investigations into synthetic constructs having increasing structural and biochemical complexity.

1. Apligraf

A bilayered skin construct Graftskin (Apligraf, Organogenesis Inc., Canton, Mass, and Novartis Pharmaceuticals Corporation, East Hanover, NJ) has been developed as a functional skin equivalent. Graftskin incorporates allogeneic cultured human skin cells in a full-thickness skin construct containing a well-differentiated epidermal layer, composed of living keratinocytes, and a dermal layer composed of living human fibroblasts. The dermal matrix is created with a type I bovine-derived collagen matrix. Both the fibroblasts and keratinocytes are derived from neonatal foreskin. Graftskin undergoes thorough and rigorous screening for infectious agents and contaminants at several stages during the manufacturing process, including screening for human immunodeficiency virus, hepatitis A, B, and C viruses, human herpes viruses, and retroviruses. The deficiencies of this graft may be that bovine collagen used to create the dermal matrix may elicit an immune response in certain patients. Furthermore, little is known about the outcome of the allogeneic neonatal cells that are placed into the bilayer matrix (i.e., whether they remain in the wound, and for how long). Nevertheless, several studies support the use of Graftskin in certain wounds.

A study by Falanga *et al.* (50) evaluated the efficacy of Graftskin on patients with hard-to-heal venous leg ulcers of greater than one year duration. Patients received Graftskin plus compression therapy, consisting of a nonadherent primary dressing (Tegapore, 3M Health Care, St. Paul, MN), a secondary gauze pressure bolster, and a self-adherent elastic bandage (Coban, 3M Health Care), or standard compression therapy, and were evaluated for frequency and time to complete wound closure. Adjusting for factors generally thought to influence wound healing (duration, baseline wound area, depth, location, fibrinous wound bed, and infection), Graftskin was found to be twice as likely to complete wound closure by 6 months, and over 60% more effective in achieving wound closure than control. These data indicate that Graftskin may be an effective treatment for venous leg ulcers of greater than one year duration, but more importantly, it is a testament to the major advances in culture techniques and basic science that allow us to create structural platforms and simultaneously target the molecular and cellular deficits of wounds. However, further studies are required to more clearly characterize cellular phenotypes of cutaneous wounds, with the goal of altering and correcting the defects with tissue therapy.

To this end, we feel that there is a need for continued clinical research on the efficacy of skin substitutes to accelerate closure of difficult wounds, such as diabetic ulcers, decubitus ulcers, and burns. More effort must be placed on elucidating the basic biologic mechanisms of wound repair, so as to target specifically the deficiency or overwhelming production of certain growth factors that may be the culprits underlying difficult wound healing problems.

2. Alloderm

It is generally accepted that dermal components are important for successful healing of partial- and/or full-thickness burn wounds (51). The time-honored method for permanent wound closure is split-thickness skin grafts (STSGs). However, the use of STSGs remains imperfect, with undesirable sequelae such as pain, infection, and permanent morbidity of the donor site. Furthermore, use of autologous grafts may be hampered by a deficit of donor tissue.

Although an effective means of wound closure in partial- and full-thickness burns, allografts are temporary and are often rejected as a result of the host immunologic response. In an attempt to reduce allograft rejection and decrease use of autografts, various alternatives have been investigated. One study removed the antigenic epidermis of the cadaver graft, replacing the epidermal layer with autogenous keratinocyte cultures. This process eliminated cells specific for expressing HLA-DR antigens (51). Still others have used immunosuppressive drugs to attenuate the host immunologic response, thereby increasing allograft "take." Nevertheless, a number of complications of the above methods have been reported.

To combat the problems associated with host immune response, researchers have chemically treated cadaver skin grafts, removing the highly antigenic epidermis and cellular components and leaving only an acellular dermal matrix and an intact basement membrane complex. More specifically, the cellular components that may potentially induce rejection, such as epidermal, Langerhans', dendritic, endothelial, and fibroblast cells, are removed. Removal of these cells creates a dermal matrix that is immunologically inert. Thus, products such as AlloDerm (Lifecell Corp., The Woodlands, TX) may have potential for permanent deep partial- and/or full-thickness wound coverage.

IV. Craniofacial Surgery

A. Introduction

Despite obvious differences in human and animal craniofacial characteristics, there is astounding conservation in the molecular specification and assembly of embryonic cranial structures (52). We confine our discussion of craniofacial dysmorpholgy to (1) cleft lip and palate and (2) craniosynostosis. The approach to craniofacial research maybe divided into *in vivo* and *in vitro* paradigms. This artificial division provides didactic clarity, but ultimately these systems are interdependent and their findings complementary. Determining the appropriate craniofacial model for any experimental manipulation or observation is fundamental to successful experimental design. By investigating the fundamental morphogenetic mechanisms of normal craniofacial development, we may understand the etiopathogenesis of craniofacial dysmorphology and devise targeted therapeutic interventions. Ultimately, a combination of minimally invasive techniques and tissue-specific genetic modifications may treat or prevent craniofacial dysmorphogenesis.

B. Data Collection and Analysis

Both qualitative assessment and quantitative analysis are essential for documenting the efficacy of any craniofacial intervention. Craniofacial data are recorded photographically, histomorphologically, biomolecularly, and roentgenographically. Photography provides a tangible (visible) measure of the technical or biological intervention (e.g., scar formation, midface or cranial vault dysmorpholgy). Various types of camera equipment are available, but the authors recommend use of digital technology (Nikon Inc.). Digital equipment provides instant images and allows diligent image manipulation and transmission. In addition, a variety of software programs facilitate minor contrast adjustment for publication-quality prints (Adobe Systems Inc.). This digital equipment can also be fitted to any conventional upright light or stereomicroscope and can be computer-linked for real-time photomicrographic capture (Leica Inc.). Precise histomorphologic documentation is an essential component of most craniofacial comparisons (e.g., epithelial apposition, dermal reconstitution, or cranial suture configuration).

Contemporary craniofacial paradigms demand quantitative biomolecular analysis (for a review of molecular biology, see Chapter 20). Elucidating the mechanisms underlying craniofacial dysmorphology requires the molecular dissection of normal palate and cranial suture assembly. As gene chip technology becomes widely available, we may ultimately decipher the coordinated control of craniofacial assembly.

Cephalometry is the conventional roentgenographic approach to quantitative craniofacial assessment. Head radiographs are obtained using a cephalometer. This device produces standardized radiographs based on a fixed relationship between the X-ray source and the object being analyzed. Craniometric measurements are recorded using a variety of landmarks. Normative data have been published for most animal paradigms. Cephalometry is advantageous because it is a simple method to measure craniofacial dimensions directly. Measurement reliability (intraobserver) and repeatability (interobserver) are quantifiable and, therefore, controllable. The main drawback of cephalometry is the inability to use soft tissue landmarks. Alternatively, computerized tomography and magnetic resonance imaging provide excellent, but expensive, bone and soft tissue analysis.

C. In Vivo Research

1. Small Animal Models

Researchers have developed a variety of small animal models of cleft lip (with or without cleft palate) and models of craniosynostosis. Small animals such as chicks, mice, rats, and rabbits offer the advantages of low cost and large sample size. The early stages of chick embryonic development are arguably the most appealing for craniofacial study; however, the remarkably challenging approach to *in ovo* manipulations prohibits detailed discussion in this text [for an excellent review of avian embryogenesis and operative microtechniques, see Bonner-Fraser (53)]. We limit our small animal discussion to the murine and lagamorph models.

2. Large Animal Models

Although small animals are useful for biomolecular analysis and straightforward surgical procedures, sophisticated craniofacial manipulation remains technically demanding. Animals such as sheep and goats may provide superior surgical models. They permit early gestational manipulation and performance of multiple intrauterine procedures, and enable comparison of bone induction over a wide range of gestational ages. The relative inactivity of the ovine and caprine uterus minimizes preterm labor. In addition, the size of these larger animals facilitates complicated technical intervention, such as multilayered repairs, endoscopic fetal surgery, and extradural dissection of the sutures. Unlike with small animals, expensive operating and husbandry fees, limited spontaneous clefting or craniosynostosis models, and a relative paucity of molecular reagents complicate large animal research (Table I).

D. In Vitro Research

Contemporary *in vitro* cleft lip (with or without cleft palate) and craniosynostosis research requires advanced microsurgical, cell, and organ culture techniques. Sophisticated microdissection is essential for isolating the embryonic and early postnatal palate or cranial suture. Serum-free organ culture is an established technique that provides a chemically defined, well-controlled environment to study the morphogenetic movements of palate and suture assembly. It is important to note that organ culture is predicated on nutrient diffusion; therefore, small tissues exhibit better growth and survival. For example, mouse calvarial explants can be maintained *in vitro* for 30 days, whereas rat calvarial explants do not survive.

E. Cleft Lip and Palate Research

1. *In Vivo* Research

Cleft lip and palate models are based on congenital or surgical clefts. Presently, few spontaneous congenital cleft models exist; however, intensive research has produced teratogenic and novel transgenic constructs. These models are advantageous because epithelial cells naturally line the cleft. Therefore, surgical reconstruction pragmatically reproduces the human experience. In contrast, the conventional surgically created cleft is based on operative excision of the lip and/or palate. This approach is the most commonly described because it affords absolute operator-dependent control of the size and position of the cleft. Furthermore, it permits simultaneous or delayed cleft repair. Critics of this model postulate that the absence of an epithelial lining converts a cleft reconstruction into closure of a surgical wound.

In summary, intrauterine cleft lip and palate repair is important for three reasons: (1) early gestation fetal skin heals without scarring, (2) fetal surgery may circumvent the cascade of midface and maxillary retrusion associated with postnatal repair, and (3) fetal surgery may reduce the number and magnitude of ensuing operations ultimately required to correct the cleft (for a detailed review of fetal surgery, see Chapter 76). Although other paradigms exist, *in utero* creation/repair models dominate the field of experimental cleft lip and palate surgery.

a. Small Animal Models

I. Mouse The mouse model is ideal for biomolecular dissection and presently provides the best environment for deciphering the events of normal palatogenesis. As scientists decode the murine genome, access to novel transgenic and tissue-specific knockout animals will expand; the evolution of these models is essential for sophisticated functional analysis of the master regulatory genes of craniofacial development (for a review of transgenic biology, see Chapter 17). Presently, *in utero* murine craniofacial surgery is confined to late gestational manipulation; this limits the postoperative, intrauterine period, and clinical application of these models. The mouse model is unique because both spontaneous and surgical cleft models are well described.

Table I Craniofacial Animal Paradigms

Paradigm	Advantages	Disadvantages
Small, short-gestational animals	Large sample number; low cost; sophisticated biomolecular analysis	Late gestational manipulation; adult phenotype wound healing; limited clinical application
Large, long-gestational animals	Longer postoperative intrauterine period; intrauterine period; multiple intrauterine procedures; facilitates complex intrauterine procedures	Expensive husbandry; limited spontaneous craniosynostosis/clefting

The most commonly described small animal spontaneous cleft model is the A/J mouse (Jackson Laboratories, Bar Harbor, ME) (54–56). This animal has a spontaneous cleft lip (with or without cleft palate) [CL(P)] formation of 7 to 12% that can be increased to nearly 100% when pregnant mice are treated with teratogens (54, 57, 58, 60, 67, 68). In 1985, Hallock used this model to perform the first *in utero* cleft lip (CL) repair on a gestational day 17 (term, 19 days) A/J fetus (64). The author reported complete epitheliazation with no discernible scarring 48 to 72 hr following the repair. Hallock's success was a considerable technical accomplishment in a 20-mm (crown to rump length) gelatinous embryo and it energized the field of murine craniofacial surgery.

In 1995, Oberg *et al.* (69) introduced an alternative to this spontaneous cleft model. These authors surgically created and simultaneously reconstructed a unilateral cleft involving the lip and alveolus in Swiss–Webster mice (Harlen, Indianapolis, IA). More importantly, this model introduced use of microclip technology, which stimulated performance of advanced intrauterine endoscopic surgery in large animals.

II. Rabbit The rabbit provides an important alternative to mouse cleft lip and palate models. Rabbits are advantageous for surgical research because their larger size facilitates earlier *in utero* cleft reconstruction. In addition, both doe and fetus tolerate anesthesia well and there is an established body of literature on fetal lagamorph wound healing (70, 71). Furthermore, there are excellent cephalometric data documenting the midface deformities associated with postnatal cleft repair (72–75). However, unlike the A/J mouse, spontaneous cleft formation has not been reported in rabbits. In 1977, Bardach *et al.* introduced the first surgical CL rabbit model. In addition to its historical importance, Bardach's work is an excellent reference for identifying lagamorph midface landmarks and measuring craniometric dimensions essential for reconstructive comparisons (72–74, 76–78). Longaker *et al.* (79) have developed the prototypic fetal surgery CL and alveolus model using New Zealand white rabbits (Harlan, Indianapolis, IA). The authors demonstrated that fetal CL creation and reconstruction heals without scar formation, supporting normal early postnatal midface and maxillary growth. Subsequent work validated this model (80, 81).

b. Large Animal Models

I. Sheep Sheep are the most commonly described large animal cleft model (82–88). Preliminary work by Jackson *et al.* (89) and Haller *et al.* (90) provides a useful reference for general ovine management and intraoperative guidelines. Canady *et al.* (91) provide an excellent reference for ovine cephalometric analysis.

Longaker *et al.* (82) created the first intrauterine CL and alveolus model in gestational day 75 lambs (term, 145 days; Torrel Farms, Ukiah, CA). In this study, a 3-mm-wide paramedian section of the fetal lip and premaxilla was excised, creating a full-thickness oronasal fistula. Experimental animals underwent immediate multilayer closure while control animals were left unrepaired. Wounds were photographically and histomorphologically examined at 7, 14, 21, and 70 days following surgery. After 1 week, the CL in the unrepaired fetuses was patent with incomplete reepithelialization. In contrast, the wound in reconstructed animals was grossly imperceptible except for a small indentation of the alveolus. Beyond postoperative day 14 (gestational day 89), the CL in control animals completely reepithelialized, but remained widely patent. In contrast, repaired fetuses demonstrated nearly scarless, symmetric healing of the lip and premaxillary defect. Interestingly, in contrast to the lagamorph model, the anterior segment of the unrepaired ovine maxilla was hypoplastic and deviated toward the cleft.

In vitro evidence suggests that rabbit amniotic fluid contains an inhibitor of fibroblast contraction, whereas lamb amniotic fluid stimulates fibroblast contraction (92). This observation is important when selecting an animal model, because it illustrates fetal wound healing disparities in various animal species.

Estes *et al.* (83, 84) were the first to create and repair CL and alveolus endoscopically in fetal lamb. The authors provide an excellent schematic representation of the endoscopic approach and include the details of CO_2 insufflation and port placement. Their description of materials and methods clearly illustrates the creation of a full-thickness CL using a 5-mm endoscopic hooked scissor. The authors immediately repaired the surgical CL with interrupted 6-0 nylon sutures. Oberg *et al.* (88) extended Estes' model by endoscopically applying microclip technology to repair bilateral full-thickness lip incisions in gestational day 90–95 sheep. After distending the exposed uterus with normal saline, the authors introduced a 10-mm endoscope (Olympus Corp., La Palma, CA) and visualized the fetus with conventional camera equipment (Cabbot Medical Corp., Langhorne, PA). Bilateral CLs were created using a harmonic scalpel (Ultracision, Ethicon Endosurgery, Smithfield, RI) and wounds were reconstructed using an endoscopic multifire clip applier (4-mm VCS clips, U.S. Surgical, Wilton, CT) or an endostitch device (Endostitch, U.S. Surgical). The authors demonstrated a 10-fold reduction in operative time using microclips compared to endoscopic suturing (2.7 $\pm$ 0.5 min compared to 24 $\pm$ 4 min, respectively), but more importantly they showed that sutured repairs generated significantly more scarring and distortion of the lip architecture. Suture-enhanced scarring was likely a consequence of lymphocyte, histiocyte, and giant cell accumulation at the sites of suture penetration. A caveat to consider when applying this model is that scarring on the microclipped CL was more conspicuous than previous open repairs (86). This elevated baseline scarring may have been caused by the application of the harmonic scalpel to create the clefts surgically.

II. GOAT Although sheep provide an excellent animal model, large animal spontaneous cleft formation has not been described. Weinzweig *et al.* (93) described the effects of anabasine on fetal goats, reporting a 100% incidence of CP formation in anabasine-treated goat fetuses. Cleft formation is hypothesized to be due to impairment of jaw opening and tongue protrusion, which inhibits the elevation and fusion of the palatal shelves. These teratogen-treated animals with cleft lip and palate also exhibited midface deficiencies. Initial results from this important model of teratogen-induced cleft suggest that *in utero* repair prevents the midface growth disturbances observed in unrepaired littermates (94).

2. *In Vitro* Research

Without an available *in vitro* primary palate model, researchers have intensively focused on the secondary palate morphogenesis. There are a myriad of secondary palate experimental permutations, but all models share a fundamental, common design. Trowell developed the original model for surface organ culture using a metal grid to support the explanted secondary palate at the gas–fluid interface (95). In 1984, Ferguson and Slavkin modified Trowell's original design by placing the palatal shelves on 0.8-μm Millipore filters (Millipore Corp., Bedford, MA), keeping the medial edge epithelia (MEE) in close apposition (96). The palatal shelves are then cultured in standard serum-free media (Gibco) using conventional Trowell techniques. In addition to facilitating novel heterologous interspecies and genotypic combinations, this model has initiated the temporal and spatial analysis of gene expression in novel transgenic and knockout mice. The potential applications of this model are limitless. For example, this paradigm provides an excellent model for the analysis of homeobox and craniofacial master organizer gene expression. Ultimately, *in vitro* organ culture will facilitate the molecular dissection of the morphogenetic movements that govern normal palate fusion.

F. Craniosynostosis Research

1. *In Vivo* Research

The *in vivo* craniosynostosis models can also be divided into two groups: (1) small, short gestational animals and (2) large, long gestational mammals. Each model is fundamentally predicated on spontaneous or iatrogenic premature cranial suture fusion. Presently there are few spontaneous models available (97–100). Three approaches have been generated to study iatrogenic premature suture fusion: (1) heterotopic placement of cranial suture complex with or without the underlying dura mater, (2) application of a fixative to prevent suture growth, and (3) strip craniectomy inclusive of the cranial suture. These models are important because they produce a dismorphic cranium that recapitulates the human phenotype. In addition, many investigators have used the models to investigate the secondary cascade of midface and cranial base dysmorphology that can accompany syndromic craniosynostosis.

It is important to note that the calvarial, midface, and cranial base biomechanical forces observed in the models discussed below are to a great extent species specific. For example, in the rat, the basioccipital, basisphenoid, and presphenoid lie in a straight line, whereas the cribriform plate of the ethmoid bone is angulated sharply upward. In the rabbit, the cribriform plate lies in the same plane as the three basicranial bones. Finally, in the human, there exists marked kyphosis in the region of the sella turcica, resulting in a marked angular bend between the presphenoid and basisphenoid. The species-specific cranial base phenotype limits interspecies conjecture on the cascade of secondary midface and cranial base deformation (101).

a. Small Animal Models

I. MURINE Rodents are excellent models to study the mechanism of suture fusion because the posterior-frontal cranial suture fuses (between postnatal days 12 and 22 in rats and 25 and 45 in mice), while all other sutures, including the sagittal cranial suture, remain patent (102, 103). A large body of literature suggests that the dura mater acts as an endogenous tissue engineer, guiding the fate of the overlying nascent cranial suture (104–110). Application of molecular biology techniques has enabled researchers to investigate the nature of these dura-derived signals. In addition to the molecular dissection of craniosynostosis, a variety of models have been developed based on the surgical manipulation of the cranial suture complex and underlying dura mater.

Opperman *et al.* introduced the rat transplant model designed to free the calvaria of the putative cranial base biomechanical forces (111). Coronal sutures, with or without underlying dura mater, were transplanted to the center of parietal bones. These transplant experiments suggest that tissue interactions of a biochemical nature, rather than biomechanical forces generated through the cranial base, are required to maintain the (coronal) suture as a nonossified growth center.

Longaker *et al.* developed the prototypic postnatal heterotopic cranial suture models (103, 105, 107, 112–115). Using 2.5× loupe magnification and conventional instruments, the authors were able to separate and rotate the cranial sutures with respect to the subjacent regional dura mater. By molecularly analyzing the cranial suture complexes, they provided significant insights into the mechanisms of cranial suture biology (105, 107–110, 116).

II. RABBIT Using 6- to 8-week-old New Zealand white rabbits, Persson *et al.* developed the first iatrogenic model of lagamorph craniosynostosis (117). These authors also included an excellent anatomic description of lagamorph calvarial and cranial base landmarks necessary for direct cephalometry. After exposing the cranium, Persson *et al.* applied methyl-2-cyanoacrylate (Eastman Kodak Co.) to the entire coronal suture. Bicoronal suture immobilization initiated a temporal dysmorphic cascade from the cranial vault to the cranial base and facial skeleton. The anterior cranial base and midface were significantly foreshortened in the anterior–posterior (AP) dimension. The marked impairment of AP cranial vault growth caused severe alterations in the angular dimensions of the posterior vault. Ultimately, Persson *et al.* produced a brachycephalic skull phenotype (117).

Duncan *et al.* achieved *in utero* premature bicoronal craniosynostosis by performing a strip craniectomy and implanting osteoinductive demineralized bone matrix in gestational day 25 New Zealand white rabbits (118). This experimental design is simple and avoids alloreactivity. Although this model does not shed light on the etiopathogenesis of craniosysnostosis, it does generate a brachycephalic dysmorphology, facilitating analysis of potential secondary midface and skull-based deformities

b. Large Animal Research: Sheep Stelnicki *et al.* have described the first *in utero* large animal craniosynostosis model (119). Using strip craniectomy and demineralized bone matrix, these authors created unilateral craniosynostosis and produced a remarkably authentic plagiocephalic phenotype. These authors have also described a correspondingly obtuse and flattened cranial base. Using this model, Stelnicki *et al.* also reported the first delayed *in utero* repair (120). Twenty-one days after suture fusion was induced, the sheep were treated with a 4-mm × 12-mm strip craniectomy to open the entire synostosed right coronal suture. The edges of the excision were wrapped with 100-μm-thick Gore-Tex (W. L. Gore & Associates, Flagstaff, AZ) sheets to prevent bony refusion. This *in utero* correction led to a marked improvement in the craniofacial morphology when compared with the uncorrected controls (i.e., significant; $p < 0.01$, correction in orbital position, skull length, and shape of the frontal bone).

2. *In Vitro* Research

There are two fundamental approaches to control the myriad of variables inherent in cranial suture biology: (1) organ culture and (2) enriched osteoblast and dura mater cell lines. These models provide a well-controlled environment for gene modification or other therapeutic intervention.

Extirpation of the cranial suture, with or without its underlying dura mater, allows *in vitro* development without extrinsic variables (e.g., tensional forces, cytokines, or endocrine hormones). Opperman *et al.* used this model to demonstrate the dura dependence of embryonic cranial suture complexes (121). Bradley *et al.* have also established a mouse organ culture system. Explanting the cranial suture complex (inclusive of the Posterior-Frontal and Sagittal cranial sutures) into serum-free culture allows *in vitro* suture development without extrinsic influences (e.g., tensional forces transmitted from the cranial base, cytokines, or distant endocrine hormones) (112, 114). The mouse calvarial explants can be maintained *in vitro* for 30 days. Interestingly, the Posterior-Frontal cranial suture, placed in culture with its underlying dura, fuses in a normal fashion, whereas a similarly cultured Sagittal cranial suture remains patent. Importantly, all sutures placed in organ culture without dura remained patent. Using this system, Mehrara *et al.* developed novel approaches to cranial suture biology. For example, the authors altered cranial suture fate by genetically modifying the suture complex with adenoviral vectors (122).

Enriched dura and osteoblast cell lines are an excellent model for deciphering the biomolecular mechanisms of cranial suture biology. These cell lines can be cocultured or grown individually, allowing for innumerable manipulations (123, 124).

References

1. Shenaq, S. M., and Rabinovsky, E. D. (1996). Gene therapy for plastic and reconstructive surgery. *Clin. Plast. Surg.* **23**(1), 157–171.
2. Gallico, G. G., O'Connor, N. E., Compton, C. C., *et al.* (1984). Permanent coverage of large burn wounds with autologous cultured human epithelium. *N. Engl. J. Med.* **311**(7), 448–451.
3. Andree, C., Swain, W. F., Page, C. P., *et al.* (1994). *In vivo* transfer and expression of a human epidermal growth factor gene accelerates wound repair. *Proc. Natl. Acad. Sci. U.S.A.* **91**(25), 12188–12192.
4. Vogel, J. C. (1993). Keratinocyte gene therapy. *Arch. Dermatol.* **129**(11), 1478–1483.
5. Cheng, L., Ziegelhoffer, P. R., and Yang, N. S. (1993). *In vivo* promoter activity and transgene expression in mammalian somatic tissues evaluated by using particle bombardment. *Proc. Natl. Acad. Sci. U.S.A.* **90**(10), 4455–4459.
6. Setoguchi, Y., Jaffe, H. A., Danel, C., and Crystal, R. G. (1994). *Ex vivo* and *in vivo* gene transfer to the skin using replication-deficient recombinant adenovirus vectors. *J. Invest. Dermatol.* **102**(4), 415–421.
7. ISIS-3 Collaborative Group (1992). A randomised comparison of streptokinase vs. tissue plasminogen activator vs. anistreplase and of aspirin plus heparin vs. aspirin alone among 41,299 cases of suspected acute myocardial infarction. Third International Study of Infarct Survival. *Lancet* **339**(8796), 753–770.
8. Grines, C. L. (1992). Thrombolytic, antiplatelet, and antithrombotic agents. *Am. J. Cardiol.* **70**(21), 18I–26I.
9. Nabel, E. G., Plautz, G., and Nabel, G. J. (1991). Gene transfer into vascular cells. *J. Am. Coll. Cardiol.* **17**(6 Suppl. B), 189B–194B.
10. Nabel, E. G., Plautz, G., and Nabel, G. J. (1990). Site-specific gene expression *in vivo* by direct gene transfer into the arterial wall. *Science* **249**(4974), 1285–1288.
11. Nabel, E. G., Pompili, V. J., Plautz, G. E., and Nabel, G. J. (1994). Gene transfer and vascular disease. *Cardiovasc. Res.* **28**(4), 445–455.
12. Nabel, E. G., Plautz, G., Boyce, F. M., *et al.* (1989). Recombinant gene expression *in vivo* within endothelial cells of the arterial wall. *Science* **244**(4910), 1342–1344.
13. Wolff, J. A., Ludtke, J. J., Acsadi, G., *et al.* (1992). Long-term persistence of plasmid DNA and foreign gene expression in mouse muscle. *Human Mol. Genet.* **1**(6), 363–369.

14. Ferguson, C., Alpern, E., Miclau, T., and Helms, J. A. (1999). Does adult fracture repair recapitulate embryonic skeletal formation? [in process citation]. *Mech. Dev.* **87**(1–2), 57–66.
15. Reddi, A. H. (1997). Bone morphogenetic proteins: An unconventional approach to isolation of first mammalian morphogens. *Cytokine Growth Factor Rev.* **8**(1), 11–20.
16. Schmitz, J. P., and Hollinger, J. O. (1986). The critical size defect as an experimental model for craniomandibulofacial nonunions. *Clin. Orthop.* **205,** 299–308.
17. Bostrom, R., and Mikos, A. G. (1997). Tissue engineering of bone. *In* "Synthetic Biodegradable Polymer Scaffolds" (A. Atala, J.P. Vacanti, and R. Langer, eds.), Vol. 1, pp. 215–234. Birkhauser, Boston.
18. Takagi, K., and Urist, M. R. (1982). The reaction of the dura to bone morphogenetic protein (BMP) in repair of skull defects. *Ann. Surg.* **196**(1), 100–109.
19. Frame, J. W. (1980). A convenient animal model for testing bone substitute materials. *J. Oral Surg.* **38**(3), 176–180.
20. Schmitz, J. P., Schwartz, Z., Hollinger, J. O., and Boyan, B. D. (1990). Characterization of rat calvarial nonunion defects. *Acta Anat.* **138**(3), 185–192.
21. Mulliken, J. B., and Glowacki, J. (1980). Induced osteogenesis for repair and construction in the craniofacial region. *Plast. Reconstr. Surg.* **65**(5), 553–560.
22. Marden, L. J., Hollinger, J. O., Chaudhari, A., *et al.* (1994). Recombinant human bone morphogenetic protein-2 is superior to demineralized bone matrix in repairing craniotomy defects in rats. *J. Biomed. Mater. Res.* **28**(10), 1127–1138.
23. Bosch, C., Melsen, B., and Vargervik, K. (1998). Importance of the critical-size bone defect in testing bone- regenerating materials. *J. Craniofac. Surg.* **9**(4), 310–316.
24. Einhorn, T. A. (1999). Clinically applied models of bone regeneration in tissue engineering research [in process citation]. *Clin. Orthop.* **367**(Suppl.), S59–S67.
25. Wong, W., and Mooney, D. J. (1997). Synthesis and properties of biodegradable polymers used as synthetic matrices for tissue engineering. *In* "Synthetic Biodegradable Polymer Scaffolds" (A. Atala, J.P. Vacanti, and R. Langer, eds.), Vol. 1, pp. 51–82. Birkhauser, Boston.
26. Casabona, F., Martin, I., Muraglia, A., *et al.* (1998). Prefabricated engineered bone flaps: An experimental model of tissue reconstruction in plastic surgery. *Plast. Reconstr. Surg.* **101**(3), 577-81.
27. Behravesh, E., Yasko, A. W., Engel, P. S., and Mikos, A. G. (1999). Synthetic biodegradable polymers for orthopaedic applications [in process citation]. *Clin. Orthop.* **367**(Suppl.), S118–S129.
28. Thomson, R. C., Yaszemski, M. J., Powers, J. M., and Mikos, A. G. (1995). Fabrication of biodegradable polymer scaffolds to engineer trabecular bone. *J. Biomater. Sci. Polym. Ed.* **7**(1), 23–38.
29. Whang, K., Healy, K. E., Elenz, D. R., *et al.* (1999). Engineering bone regeneration with bioabsorbable scaffolds with novel microarchitecture. *Tissue Eng.* **5**(1), 35–51.
30. Kenley, R., Marden, L., Turek, T., *et al.* (1994). Osseous regeneration in the rat calvarium using novel delivery systems for recombinant human bone morphogenetic protein-2 (rhBMP-2). *J. Biomed. Mater. Res.* **28**(10), 1139–1147.
31. Ishaug, S. L., Yaszemski, M. J., Bizios, R., and Mikos, A. G. (1994). Osteoblast function on synthetic biodegradable polymers. *J. Biomed. Mater. Res.* **28**(12), 1445–1453.
32. Ishaug, S. L., Crane, G. M., Miller, M. J., *et al.* (1997). Bone formation by three-dimensional stromal osteoblast culture in biodegradable polymer scaffolds. *J. Biomed. Mater. Res.* **36**(1), 17–28.
33. Stanford, C. M., Keller, J. C., and Solursh, M. (1994). Bone cell expression on titanium surfaces is altered by sterilization treatments. *J. Dent. Res.* **73**(5), 1061–1071.
34. Aronson, J. (1993). The biology of distraction osteogenesis. *In* "Operative Orthopaedics" (M. Chapman, ed.). J. B. Lippincott Co., Philadelphia.
35. Ilizarov, G. (1992). "Transosseous Osteosynthesis. Theoretical and Clinical Aspects of the Regeneration and Growth of Tissue." Springer-Verlag, Berlin.
36. McCarthy, J. G., Schreiber, J., Karp, N., *et al.* (1992). Lengthening the human mandible by gradual distraction [see comments]. *Plast. Reconstr. Surg.* **89**(1): 1–8; discussion, 9–10.
37. Karp, N. S., McCarthy, J. G., Schreiber, J. S., *et al.* (1992). Membranous bone lengthening: A serial histological study. *Ann. Plast. Surg.* **29**(1), 2–7.
38. Komuro, Y., Takato, T., Harii, K., and Yonemara, Y. (1994). The histologic analysis of distraction osteogenesis of the mandible in rabbits. *Plast. Reconstr. Surg.* **94**(1), 152–159.
39. Rowe, N. M., Mehrara, B. J., Dudziak, M. E., *et al.* (1998). Rat mandibular distraction osteogenesis: Part I. Histologic and radiographic analysis. *Plast. Reconstr. Surg.* **102**(6), 2022–2032.
40. Cedars, M. G., Linck, D. L., 2nd, and Chin, M., Toth, B. A. (1999). Advancement of the midface using distraction techniques. *Plast. Reconstr. Surg.* **103**(2), 429–441.
41. Toth, B. A., Kim, J. W., Chin, M., and Cedars, M. (1998). Distraction osteogenesis and its application to the midface and bony orbit in craniosynostosis syndromes. *J. Craniofac. Surg.* **9**(2), 100–113; discussion, 119–122.
42. Remmler, D., McCoy, F. J., O'Neil, D., *et al.* (1992). Osseous expansion of the cranial vault by craniotasis. *Plast. Reconstr. Surg.* **89**(5), 787–797.
43. Tung, T. H., Robertson, B. R., Winograd, J. M., *et al.* (1999). Successful distraction osteogenesis across a growing cranial suture without an osteotomy. *Plast. Reconstr. Surg.* **103**(2), 362–370.
44. Losken, H. W., Mooney, M. P., Zoldos, J., *et al.* (1999). Coronal suture response to distraction osteogenesis in rabbits with delayed-onset craniosynostosis. *J. Craniofac. Surg.* **10**(1), 27–37.
45. Brent, B. (1980). The correction of microtia with autogenous cartilage grafts: I. The classic deformity? *Plast. Reconstr. Surg.* **66**(1), 1–12.
46. Brent, B. (1980). The correction of microtia with autogenous cartilage grafts: II. Atypical and complex deformities. *Plast. Reconstr. Surg.* **66**(1), 13–21.
47. Cao, Y., Vacanti, J. P., Paige, K. T., *et al.* (1997). Transplantation of chondrocytes utilizing a polymer-cell construct to produce tissue-engineered cartilage in the shape of a human ear [see comments]. *Plast. Reconstr. Surg.* **100**(2), 297–302; discussion, 303–304.
48. Meinhart, J., Fussenegger, M., and Hobling, W. (1999). Stabilization of fibrin-chondrocyte constructs for cartilage reconstruction. *Ann. Plast. Surg.* **42**(6), 673–678.
49. Stelnicki, E. J. (1999). Tissue engineering of auricular cartilage via the method of distraction chondrogenesis. Submitted.
50. Falanga, V., and Sabolinski, M. (1999). A bilayered living skin construct (APLIGRAF) accelerates complete closure of hard-to-heal venous ulcers. *Wound Rep. Regen.* **7,** 201–207.
51. Cuono, C., Langdon, R., and McGuire, J. (1986). Use of cultured epidermal autografts and dermal allografts as skin replacement after burn injury. *Lancet* **1**(8490), 1123–1124.
52. Schneider, R. A., Hu, D., and Helms, J. A. (1999). From head to toe: conservation of molecular signals regulating limb and craniofacial morphogenesis. *Cell Tissue Res.* **296**(1), 103–109.
53. Bonner-Fraser, M. (1996). "Methods in Avian Embryology" Vol. 51. Academic Press, San Diego.
54. Kalter, H. (1954). Inheritance of susceptibility to the teratogenic action of cortisone in mice. *Genetics* **39,** 185–196.
55. Davidson, J. G., Fraser, F. C., and Schlager, G. (1969). A maternal effect on the frequency of spontaneous cleft lip in the A-J mouse. *Teratology* **2**(4), 371–376.
56. Bornstein, S., Trasler, D. G., and Fraser, F. C. (1970). Effect of the uterine environment on the frequency of spontaneous cleft lip in CL/FR mice. *Teratology* **3**(4), 295–298.

57. Marsk, L., Theorell, M., and Larsson, K. S. (1971). Transfer of blastocysts as applied in experimental teratology. *Nature (London)* **234**(5328), 358–359.
58. Bonner, J. J., and Slavkin, H. C. (1975). Cleft palate susceptibility linked to hisocompatibility-2 (H-2) in the mouse. *Immunogenetics* **2,** 213–218.
59. Kalter, H. (1975). Prenatal epidemiology of spontaneous cleft lip and palate, open eyelid, and embryonic death in A/J mice. *Teratology* **12**(3), 245–257.
60. Biddle, F. G., and Fraser, F. C. (1976). Genetics of cortisone-induced cleft palate in the mouse—Embryonic and maternal effects. *Genetics* **84**(4), 743–754.
61. Juriloff, D. M. (1982). Differences in frequency of cleft lip among the A strains of mice. *Teratology* **25**(3), 361–368.
62. Ciriani, D., and Diewert, V. M. (1986). A comparative study of development during primary palate formation in A/WySn, C57BL/6, and their F1 crosses. *J. Craniofac. Genet. Dev. Biol.* **6**(4), 369–377.
63. Juriloff, D. M. (1986). Major genes that cause cleft lip in mice: progress in the construction of a congenic strain and in linkage mapping. *J. Craniofac. Genet. Dev. Biol. (Suppl.)* **2,** 55–66.
64. Hallock, G. G. (1985). *In utero* cleft lip repair in A/J mice. *Plast. Reconstr. Surg.* **75**(6), 785–790.
65. Sullivan, W. G. (1989). *In utero* cleft lip repair in the mouse without an incision. *Plast. Reconstr. Surg.* **84**(5), 723–730; discussion, 731–732.
66. Wang, K. Y., and Diewert, V. M. (1992). A morphometric analysis of craniofacial growth in cleft lip and noncleft mice. *J. Craniofac. Genet. Dev. Biol.* **12**(3), 141–154.
67. Sulik, K. K., Johnston, M. C., Ambrose, L. J., and Dorgan, D. (1979). Phenytoin (dilantin)-induced cleft lip and palate in A/J mice: A scanning and transmission electron microscopic study. *Anat. Rec.* **195**(2), 243–255.
68. Millicovsky, G., and Johnston, M. C. (1981). Maternal hyperoxia greatly reduces the incidence of phenytoin-induced cleft lip and palate in A/J mice. *Science* **212**(4495), 671–672.
69. Oberg, K. C., Evans, M. L., Nguyen, T., *et al.* (1995). Intrauterine repair of surgically created defects in mice (lip incision model) with a microclip: Preamble to endoscopic intrauterine surgery. *Cleft Palate Craniofac. J.* **32**(2), 129–137.
70. Krummel, T. M., Nelson, J. M., Diegelmann, R. F., *et al.* (1987). Fetal response to injury in the rabbit. *J. Pediatr. Surg.* **22**(7), 640–644.
71. Adzick, N. S., Harrison, M. R., Glick, P. L., *et al.* (1985). Comparison of fetal, newborn, and adult wound healing by histologic, enzyme-histochemical, and hydroxyproline determinations. *J. Pediatr. Surg.* **20**(4), 315–319.
72. Bardach, J., Klausner, E., and Eisbach, K. (1979). The relationship between lip pressure and facial growth after cleft lip repair: An experimental model. *Cleft Palate J.* **16,** 137–146.
73. Bardach, J., Roberts, D. M., and Klausner, E. C. (1979). Influence of two-flap paltoplasty on facial growth in rabbits. *Cleft Palate J.* **16**(4), 402–411.
74. Bardach, J., Roberts, D., Yale, R., *et al.* (1980). The influence of simultaneous cleft lip and palate repair on facial growth in rabbits. *Cleft Palate J.* **17,** 309–318.
75. Bardach, J., Mooney, M., and Giedrojc-Juraha, Z. L. (1982). A comparative study of facial growth following cleft lip repair with or without soft-tissue undermining: An experimental study in rabbits. *Plast. Reconstr. Surg.* **69**(5), 745–754.
76. Bardach, J., and Eisbach, K. (1977). The influence of primary unilateral cleft lip repair on facial growth. Part 1. Lip pressure. *Cleft Palate J.* **14,** 88–97.
77. Bardach, J., Mooney, M., and Giedrojc-Juraha, Z. (1982). A comparative study of facial growth following cleft lip repair with or without soft-tissue undermining: An experimental model study in rabbits. *Plast. Reconstr. Surg.* **69,** 745–753.
78. Bardach, J., Mooney, M., and Bardach, E. (1982). The influence of two-flap palatoplasty on facial growth in beagles. *Plast. Reconstr. Surg.* **69,** 927–936.
79. Longaker, M. T., Dodson, T. B., and Kaban, L. B. (1990). A rabbit model for fetal cleft lip repair. *J. Oral Maxillofac. Surg.* **48**(7), 714–719.
80. Dodson, T. B., Schmidt, B., Longaker, M. T., and Kaban, L. B. (1991). Fetal cleft lip repair in rabbits: Postnatal facial growth after repair. *J. Oral Maxillofac. Surg.* **49**(6), 603–611.
81. Kaban, L. B., Dodson, T. B., Longaker, M. T., *et al.* (1993). Fetal cleft lip repair in rabbits: Long-term clinical and cephalometric results. *Cleft Palate Craniofac. J.* **30**(1), 13–21.
82. Longaker, M. T., Stern, M., Lorenz, P., *et al.* (1992). A model for fetal cleft lip repair in lambs. *Plast. Reconstr. Surg.* **90**(5), 750–756.
83. Estes, J. M., Whitby, D. J., Lorenz, H. P., *et al.* (1992). Endoscopic creation and repair of fetal cleft lip. *Plast. Reconstr. Surg.* **90**(5), 743–746; discussion, 747–749.
84. Estes, J. M., Szabo, Z., and Harrison, M. R. (1992). Techniques for in utero endoscopic surgery. A new approach for fetal intervention. *Surg. Endosc.* **6**(5), 215–218.
85. Canady, J. W., Landas, S. K., Morris, H., and Thompson, S. A. (1994). *In utero* cleft palate repair in the ovine model. *Cleft Palate Craniofac. J.* **31**(1), 37–44.
86. Evans, M. L., Oberg, K. C., Kirsch, W., *et al.* (1995). Intrauterine repair of cleft lip-like defects in lambs with a novel microclip. *J. Craniofac. Surg.* **6**(2), 126–131.
87. Hedrick, M. H., Rice, H. E., Vander Wall, K. J., *et al.* (1996). Delayed *in utero* repair of surgically created fetal cleft lip and palate. *Plast. Reconstr. Surg.* **97**(5), 900–905; discussion, 906–907.
88. Oberg, K., Robles, A., Ducsay, C., *et al.* (1998). Endoscopic excision and repair of simulated bilateral cleft lips in fetal lambs. *Plast. Reconstr. Surg.* **102**(1), 1–9.
89. Jackson, B. T., Egdahl, R. H., and Richmond, V. A. (1960). The performance of complex fetal operations *in utero* without amniotic fluid loss or orther disturbances of fetal–materal relationships. *Surgery* **48**(564), X.
90. Haller, J. A., and Golladay, E. S., J. J. (1979). The performance of complex fetal operations *in utero* without amniotic fluid loss or other disturbances of fetal–maternal relationships. *Res. Ped. Surg.* **12**(41), X.
91. Canady, J. W., Thompson, S. A., and Colburn, A. (1997). Craniofacial growth after iatrogenic cleft palate repair in a fetal ovine model. *Cleft Palate Craniofac. J.* **34**(1), 69–72.
92. Rittenberg, T., Longaker, M. T., Adzick, N. S., and Ehrlich, H. P. (1991). Sheep amniotic fluid has a protein factor which stimulates human fibroblast populated collagen lattice contraction. *J. Cell Physiol.* **149**(3), 444–450.
93. Weinzweig, J., Panter, K. E., Pantaloni, M., *et al.* (1999). The fetal cleft palate: I. Characterization of a congenital model. *Plast. Reconstr. Surg.* **103**(2), 419–428.
94. Weinzweig, J., Panter, K. E., Pantaloni, M., *et al.* (1999). The fetal cleft palate: II. Scarless healing after *in utero* repair of a congenital model. *Plast. Reconstr. Surg.* 104(5), 1356–1364.
95. Trowell, O. A. (1954). modified technique for organ culture in vitro. *Exp. Cell Res.* **6,** 246–248.
96. Ferguson, M. W., Honig, L. S., and Slavkin, H. C. (1984). Differentiation of cultured palatal shelves from alligator, chick, and mouse embryos. *Anat. Rec.* **209**(2), 231–249.
97. Mooney, M. P., Losken, H. W., Tschakaloff, A., *et al.* (1993). Congenital bilateral coronal suture synostosis in a rabbit and craniofacial growth comparisons with experimental models. *Cleft Palate Craniofac. J.* **30**(2), 121–128.
98. Mooney, M. P., Losken, H. W., Siegel, M. I., *et al.* (1994). Development of a strain of rabbits with congenital simple nonsyndromic coronal suture synostosis. Part II: Somatic and craniofacial growth patterns. *Cleft Palate Craniofac. J.* **31**(1), 8–16.

99. Mooney, M. P., Smith, T. D., Burrows, A. M., *et al.* (1996). Coronal suture pathology and synostotic progression in rabbits with congenital craniosynostosis. *Cleft Palate Craniofac. J.* **33**(5), 369–378.
100. Mooney, M. P., Aston, C. E., Siegel, M. I., *et al.* (1996). Craniosynostosis with autosomal dominant transmission in New Zealand white rabbits. *J. Craniofac. Genet. Dev. Biol.* **16**(1), 52–63.
101. Moss, M. L. (1986). Experimental unilateral coronal synostosis in rabbits (discussion). *Plast. Reconst. Surg.* **77**(3), 377.
102. Moss, M. L. (1958). Fusion of the frontal suture in the rat. *Am. J. Anat.* **102,** 141–166.
103. Bradley, J. P., Levine, J. P., Roth, D. A., McCarthy, J. G., and Longaker, M. T. (1996). Studies in cranial suture biology: IV. Temporal sequence of posterior frontal cranial suture fusion in the mouse. *Plast. Reconstr. Surg.* **98**(6), 1039–1045.
104. Bradley, J. P., Levine, J. P., Roth, D. A., *et al.* (1996). Studies in cranial suture biology: IV. Temporal sequence of posterior frontal cranial suture fusion in the mouse. *Plast. Reconstr. Surg.* **98**(6), 1039–1045.
105. Roth, D. A., Longaker, M. T., McCarthy, J. G., *et al.* (1997). Studies in cranial suture biology: Part I. Increased immunoreactivity for transforming growth factor-beta (β1, β2, β3) during rat cranial suture fusion. *J. Bone Miner. Res.* **12,** 311–321.
106. Opperman, L. A., Nolen, A. A., and Ogle, R. C. (1997). TGF-β1, TGF-β2, and TGF-β3 exhibit distinct patterns of expression during cranial suture formation and obliteration *in vivo* and *in vitro. J. Bone Miner. Res.* **12**(3), 301–310.
107. Most, D., Levine, J. P., Chang, J., *et al.* (1998). Studies in cranial suture biology: Up-regulation of transforming growth factor-betal and basic fibroblast growth factor mRNA correlates with posterior frontal cranial suture fusion in the rat. *Plast. Reconstr. Surg.* **101**(6), 1431–1440.
108. Mehrara, B., Greenwald, J., Chin, G., *et al.* (1999). Regional differentiation of rat cranial suture-derived dural cells is dependent on association with fusing and patent cranial sutures. *Plast. Reconstr. Surg.* **104,** 1003–1013.
109. Mehrara, B., Most, D., Chang, J., *et al.* (1999). Basic fibroblast growth factor and transforming growth factor beta-1 expression in the developing dura mater correlates with calvarial bone formation. *Plast. Reconstr. Surg.* **102**(6), 1805–1817; discussion, 1818–1820.
110. Mehrara, B. J., Steinbrech, D. S., Saadeh, P. B., *et al.* (1999). Expression of high-affinity receptors for TGF-beta during rat cranial suture fusion. *Ann. Plast. Surg.* **42**(5), 502–508.
111. Opperman, L. A., Sweeney, T. M., Redmon, J., *et al.* (1993). Tissue interactions with underlying dura mater inhibit osseous obliteration of developing cranial sutures. *Dev. Dyn.* **198**(4), 312–322.
112. Bradley, J. P., Levine, J. P., Blewett, C., *et al.* (1996). Studies in cranial suture biology: *In vitro* cranial suture fusion. *Cleft Palate Craniofac. J.* **33**(2); 150–156.
113. Roth, D. A., Bradley, J. P., Levine, J. P., *et al.* (1996). Studies in cranial suture biology: Part II. Role of the dura in cranial suture fusion. *Plast. Reconstr. Surg.* **97**(4), 693–699.
114. Bradley, J. P., Levine, J. P., McCarthy, J. G., and Longaker, M. T. (1997). Studies in cranial suture biology: Regional dura mater determines *in vitro* cranial suture fusion. *Plast. Reconstr. Surg.* **100**(5), 1091–1099; discussion; 1100–1102.
115. Levine, J. P., Bradley, J. P., Roth, D. A., *et al.* (1998). Studies in cranial suture biology: Regional dura mater determines overlying suture biology. *Plast. Reconstr. Surg.* **101**(6), 1441–1447.
116. Han, V. K., Bradley, J. P., Roth, D. A., *et al.* (1995). Dura mater-suture paracrine signaling during cranial suture fusion: IGF-I, IGF-II *in situ* hybridization and IGF-I, osteocalcin immunolocalization in human and rat cranial sutures. *Surg. Forum,* **46,** 706–708.
117. Persson, K. M., Roy, W. A., Persing, J. A., *et al.* (1979). Craniofacial growth following experimental craniosynostosis and craniectomy in rabbits. *J. Neurosurg.* **50**(2), 187–197.
118. Duncan, B. W., Adzick, N. S., Moelleken, B. R., *et al.* (1992). An *in utero* model of craniosynostosis. *J. Craniofac. Surg.* **3**(2), 70–78.
119. Stelnicki, E. J., Vanderwall, K., Hoffman, W. Y., *et al.* (1998). A new *in utero* sheep model for unilateral coronal craniosynostosis. *Plast. Reconstr. Surg.* **101**(2), 278–286.
120. Stelnicki, E. J., Vanderwall, K., Harrison, M. R., *et al.* (1998). The *in utero* correction of unilateral coronal craniosynostosis. *Plast. Reconstr. Surg.* **101**(2), 287–296.
121. Opperman, L. A., Passarelli, R. W., Morgan, E. P., *et al.* (1995). Cranial sutures require tissue interactions with dura mater to resist osseous obliteration *in vitro. J. Bone Miner. Res.* **10**(12), 1978–1987.
122. Mehrara, B., Fernandez, H., Chau, D., *et al.* (1998). Adenovirus-mediated transmission of a dominant negative truncated transforming growth factor beta receptor inhibits *in vitro* mouse cranial suture fusion. *Surg. Forum* **49,** 492–493.
123. Greenwald, J., Mehrara, B., Spector, J., *et al.* (2000). Biomolecular mechanisms of calvarial bone induction: Immature vs. mature dura mater. *Plast. Reconstr. Surg.* (in press).
124. Greenwald, J. A., Mehrara, B. J., Spector, J. A., *et al.* (2000). Immature vs. mature dura mater II: Differential expression of genes critical to calvarial re-ossification. *Plast. Reconstr. Surg.* (in press).

78

Research Methods in Neurosurgery

Svetlana Ivanova and Kevin J. Tracey

Laboratory of Biomedical Science, North Shore University Hospital, Manhasset, New York 11030

I. Introduction

As recently as a decade ago, it was generally accepted that following cerebral ischemia (stroke), neurons in the oxygen-deficient part of the brain died instantaneously and irreversibly, in a process that was untreatable. Recent scientific and clinical investigation into the pathogenesis of ischemic brain cell death has significantly changed this fatalistic notion. Numerous clinical trials for stroke treatment are currently ongoing, based on a new understanding that the cytotoxic pathways that contribute to brain cell death are active for hours after the onset of stroke, and can be suppressed to reduce brain cell death and ultimate neurological disability. Other longstanding dogmas (e. g., that adults never generate neuronal cells) are also being challenged.

In this chapter, we focus the discussion on research strategies that can be used to answer some fundamental questions in neurobiology. These are presented in the context of a working program in our laboratory that has led to the identification of previously unrecognized molecular mediators of stroke. Methods discussed in this chapter include brain surgical procedures in experimental animals, *in vitro* studies of cultured central nervous system (CNS) cells, as well as multiple other procedures on the boundary of the neurosciences and other disciplines such as cell biology, immunology, and pharmacology. Successful science is a "marriage" of skillful technique with thoughtful design. In order to provide some insight into our use of certain methods, we therefore present the specific methods in the context of the actual experimental program. This gives a general overview of some techniques that can be used in a neuropathologic research program. In the second part of the chapter, we review a range of techniques used in other related neuroscience fields. Finally, we provide a discussion of neural cell cultures used in establishing *in vitro* models for study of the CNS.

II. Neuropathologic Techniques for Study of Cerebral Ischemia and Related Disorders of the CNS

A. Why Study Cerebral Ischemia?

Cerebral ischemia (stroke) is one of the most widely studied neuropathologies, because it is the third leading cause of death in the United States, and the leading cause of neurologic disability. Cerebral ischemia (stroke) is defined as a neurologic deficit that occurs as a result of decreased blood supply to a brain region. This process results in local cell death and the development of neurologic deficits of a varying degree of severity, depending on the size and location of the stroke. Comprehensive research on cerebral ischemic pathogenesis has been critical for the design of novel therapeutics and their implementation into clinical practice. Early investigators presumed that disruption of a continuous supply of glucose and oxygen to neurons caused sudden widespread cell death by an "energy shortage." Subsequent work, however, revealed that ischemic brain areas were actually composed of an ischemic core and an enveloping, partially perfused "penumbra." Whereas cell death in the core occurs within minutes following a critical reduction in blood supply, the process of cell death in the penumbra may not be completed for hours or even days (1, 2). Once triggered by diminished blood flow, the process of cell death thereafter spreads to encompass a larger zone in an essentially self-propagating cytotoxic cascade. Hence, there is a temporal opportunity for an intervention to prevent ischemic penumbral tissue from progressing to infarction, defined as the therapeutic window. Clinical studies suggest that the therapeutic window for acute stroke treatment is most likely confined to the period of 2–4 hr after the onset of ischemic stroke (3, 4). Accordingly, the development of current therapeutic strategies for stroke treatment during this window of opportunity is aimed at (1) recanalization and restoration of blood flow in the occluded vessels and (2) mitigation of the onset and spread of cytotoxicity in the ischemic penumbra.

B. Animal Models of Cerebral Ischemia

To study cytotoxic mechanisms of cerebral ischemia *in vivo*, as well as to assess the efficacy of new therapies, an animal model of cerebral ischemia should be established. The animal model should be based on the specific type of stroke one wishes to study. Strokes are classically divided into two general categories: ischemic (accounting for some 85–90% of the clinical cases), which develop as a result of *in situ* cerebrovascular occlusion, and hemorrhagic (red), which occur as a result of aneurysmal ruptures, or secondary to reperfusion of damaged vessels and tissue. Hemorrhagic strokes occur far less frequently compared to ischemic strokes, hence the more sparse number of animal models for their study (5, 6).

Animal models of cerebral ischemia are generally divided into two types: focal and global occlusive. Animal models of focal cerebral ischemia mimic more closely an acute ischemic episode in human patients, whereas animal models of global cerebral ischemia are more representative of a low-flow state.

1. Animal Models of Focal Cerebral Ischemia

The most commonly employed research technique of inducing focal cerebral ischemia in animals is the rat model of permanent (irreversible) middle cerebral artery occlusion (MCAO) (7–10). Briefly, in this model, the ipsilateral common carotid artery is ligated and divided, the middle cerebral artery is coagulated and divided distal to the lenticulostriate branch, and the contralateral common carotid is occluded for 1 hr. The onset of ischemia in these experiments is defined as the time the middle cerebral artery is severed. The use of this model has proved very effective in the study of experimental therapies that protect the penumbral area at risk. In this model, spread of cytotoxicity evolves with time, offering the additional advantage of assessing experimental interventions for their efficacy following a late postischemic administration during the therapeutic "window of opportunity." The rat, and in some instances the hypertensive rat, is the preferred animal for study in this model. Variations of technique in this model allow a degree of selection of the cerebral infarction area. Thus, a focal cortical cerebral infarct occurs after ligation of the middle cerebral artery distal to the lenticulostriate branch. A larger infarct area that includes the hippocampus can be achieved by ligating the artery proximal to the lenticulostriate artery.

Infusion of tissue plasminogen activator (tPA), a clinically approved thrombolytic agent for acute treatment of stroke, results in reperfusion of the ischemic zone. Hence, animal models of reversible cerebral ischemia have also been developed, whereby damage in the ischemic zone occurs both as a result of ischemia as well as of reperfusion. Occlusion with reperfusion is usually achieved by the use of removable clips or sutures, by passage of an intraluminal filament up through the vessels, or by application of endothelin 1. It is considered that reperfusion/ischemia models most closely mimic the clinical situation after tPA (7, 11, 12).

Disadvantages of focal models of cerebral ischemia relate to the surgical procedure involved, and the substantial number of variations of technique among different operators. Significant variability of infarct size damage among the different animals may also be observed, thus making it necessary to study large groups of animals to achieve statistically significant effects. Experimental therapeutic agents that mitigate the ischemic cytotoxic cascade usually reduce infarct size more significantly in normotensive rats as compared to hypertensive rats, thus pointing to potentially significant differences in animal species selected. Other factors to be considered are the choice of anesthetic, because some sedatives have neuroprotective effects (i.e., the widely used anesthetic ketamine is an antagonist of the NMDA receptor) (13).

2. Animal Models of Global Cerebral Ischemia

There are three commonly used animal models of global cerebral ischemia (7). The gerbil bilateral carotid occlusion model has been used widely because of the simple nature of the surgical procedure involved. This model produces delayed neuronal cell death in the hippocampus, which occurs over several days and is similar to the evolution of hippocampal cell death in humans following cardiac arrest. Disadvantages of this model relate to difficulty of assessing physiological variables in small animals and to significant variations of cerebral arterial anatomy resulting in variable outcomes.

Global ischemia in the rat is achieved by either a two-vessel occlusion plus hypertension, or by a four-vessel occlusion. Advantages of the former are the development of selective cell death, a surgical procedure involving only one step, and ease of measurement of physiologic parameters. Disadvantages are associated with the need for induction of hypertension and the occurrence of occasional postischemic seizures. The four-vessel occlusion model of global ischemia in the rat offers the advantage of inducing ischemia in awake, freely moving animals and has highly reproducible pathology. However, a two-stage operation is needed for this model. Variations of outcome within the same strain are additional disadvantages of this model.

These and a number of other animal models of cerebral ischemia have been established. Unfortunately, the data generated from these animal models have found very little translation into the clinic. Differences in ischemic pathophysiology between humans and animals have been noted (8, 14–17). If an "ideal" animal model of cerebral ischemia could be developed, it would have similarities to humans in regard to vascular anatomy and function, thrombotic pathways, and neuronal and glial cell morphology and function. Rodents have, of course, become the most commonly used model for cerebral ischemia, because of the ease and profuseness of breeding, possibilities for housing large numbers, and cost effectiveness as compared to larger animals (7, 8). Unfortunately, the rodent animal models are far from ideal. Rodents have extensive collateral circulation that differs significantly from that of humans: this limits the extent of tissue injury and increases recovery as compared to human patients. Specific cellular differences have also been noted. For instance, rat thrombocytes are devoid of platelet-activating factor (PAF) receptors, and have notably different interactions with leukocytes as compared to human platelets. Differences in temporal progression of ischemia between different species and animal models have also been noted. These findings should be considered when choosing a particular model of cerebral ischemia. Often, to take advantage of an animal model that most closely mimics the clinical situation, a certain experimental drug and/or pathogenic ischemic mechanism is evaluated in more than one species and in more than one model of ischemia.

C. Pathogenic Mediators of Cerebral Ischemia

A number of molecular substrates of normal brain, as well as extrinsic factors delivered by the circulation, contribute to the development of cell cytotoxicity during ischemia. These include, but are not limited to, glutamate, aspartate, polyamines, nitric oxide, calcium, free radicals, zinc, cytokines, arachidonic acid metabolites, and advanced glycation end-products (AGEs). Additionally, considerable synergy among these cytotoxic mediators has been discovered, i.e., reactive oxygen species are more cytotoxic in the presence of transition metals such as Fe and Cu (18, 19). Thus, the process of cerebral ischemia, which is initially precipitated by diminished regional blood flow, eventually evolves into a complex and essentially self-propagating cascade of metabolic and chemical events that together culminate in regional brain cell death. The precise mechanisms and the roles of yet unidentified cytotoxic mediators of this cascade are subjects of active investigation.

It is thus well beyond the scope of this chapter to provide an overview of all the different techniques that have become available for the study and characterization of all known ischemic cytotoxic mediators. Instead, a brief overview is provided based on the discovery of one mediator of cerebral ischemia, the polyamine catabolite 3-aminopropanal (30). This molecule provides a reference point to discuss the methods used to reveal and characterize a previously unknown cytotoxin in the CNS.

1. Hypothesis Generation: Role of Polyamine Oxidation as a Cytotoxic Pathway in Cerebral Ischemia

Our laboratory's work in this area was based on a series of observations. The polyamines spermine, spermidine, and putrescine are ubiquitous cellular polyamines found in virtually all eukaryotic cells, frequently in millimolar amounts (20). They are released by dying cells during ischemia (21, 22). Inhibition of ornithine decarboxylase (ODC), a biosynthetic polyamine enzyme, prevents accumulation of polyamines in the ischemic brain and leads to a concomitant decrease in infarct size (22). Spermine, and to a lesser degree spermidine, have been implicated in potentiating glutamate-mediated cell damage through agonist binding to the NR1 subunit of the NMDA receptor (23, 24). Following ischemia, however, spermine and spermidine levels decline, and this decline is accompanied by an increase in brain putrescine levels. Further, intracerebral putrescine levels correlate significantly with the volume of dead brain, even though putrescine does not interact with the NMDA receptor and does not potentiate its function (21, 22, 25). 3-Aminopropanal, a by-product of polyamine oxidation formed in equimolar amounts with putrescine, is cytotoxic to cultured cells and mediates tissue necrosis *in vivo* (26). Finally, and most significantly perhaps, administration of aminoguanidine or other inhibitors of polyamine oxidase (PAO) significantly decreases infarct size in experimental animals (10, 27). We reasoned, therefore, that a unifying hypothesis for the observed pathogenicity of polyamines in cerebral ischemia could be found in their catabolic interconversion by the enzyme PAO. We proposed that during ischemia an overactivation of this pathway would lead to metabolic degradation of brain spermine and spermidine, yielding a concomitant increase of the nontoxic metabolite putrescine, and of the cytotoxic by-product 3-aminopropanal, and would thus initiate and propagate ischemic brain damage. We also hypothesized that this cytotoxic 3-aminopropanal by-product generation is a temporally upstream event in the ischemic cytotoxicity cascade, and that 3-aminopropanal initiates a cascade of cytotoxicity involving other cytotoxic mediators. Finally, we hypothesized that the ability to neutralize 3-aminopropanal cytotoxicity results in significant mitigation of ischemic damage in experimental animals. Accordingly, we set up a series of experimental methods to address these hypotheses.

2. Experimental Design

a. Chemical Preparations: Purification and Quantification of 3-Aminopropanal Because 3-aminopropanal is not commercially available, we devised a method for chemical preparation of the aldehyde by hydrolysis of 3-aminopropanal diethyl acetal under mildly acidic conditions. The resultant mixture of 3-aminopropanal diethyl acetal, 3-aminopropanal, and ethyl alcohol was fractionated by Dowex-50 ion-exchange (H^+-form) chromatography using step-gradient elution with 0–3 *M* HCl. Determination of the aldehyde-containing eluted fractions was achieved based on an assay taking advantage of their reactivity with *N*-methyl-2-benzothiazolone hydrazone hydrochloride (NBTH) (28). The reaction complex, when further subjected to reaction with ferric chloride, produced a blue color complex in the aldehyde-containing fractions only. Further quantification of the intensity of blue color by spectrophotometry at 660 nm allowed determination of the most pure fractions. The structure and purity of 3-aminopropanal were next confirmed by ^{1}H-NMR [D_2O and DCl (1:1), 270 MHz].

b. Detection of Aldehyde Concentration To determine the concentration of 3-aminopropanal, a spectrophotometric standard curve was generated against known concentrations of propionaldehyde (Sigma Chemical Co.). The colorimetric assay was based on detecting a dark purple color at $\lambda = 531$ nm, which results from the reaction between aldehydes and 4-amino-3-hydrazino-5-mercapto-1,2,4-triazole (purpald; Aldrich), as described by Dickinson and Jacobsen (29). The concentration of the 3-aminopropanal-containing fractions was determined against the linear part of the generated standard curve for propionaldehyde. To achieve stability of the synthesized and purified product, we further stored it in acidic conditions and at a temperature of −80°C. Aldehydic fractions were stable under the above conditions at all times tested. 3-Aminopropanal was neutralized with NaOH to physiologic pH immediately before use for subsequent experiments. Together, these series of experiments enabled the chemical preparation of 3-aminopropanal, purification by ion-exchange chromatography, confirmation of its structure by ^{1}H-NMR, and determination of its concentration.

c. Derivatization of 3-Aminopropanal We next sought a method to derivatize 3-aminopropanal to a stable product, in order to avoid instability during subsequent analysis in ischemic brains. Further, we sought to develop a method to detect the derivatized product by high-performance liquid chromatography (HPLC), and to separate it from other similarly derivatized compounds in rat brain.

We synthesized a stable derivative of 3-aminopropanal by reacting it with 2,4-dinitrophenyl hydrazine (2,4-DNPH) (31). The reaction produced the stable Schiff base, 3-aminopropionaldehyde-2,4-dinitrophenyl hydrazone (3-AP-2,4-DNP), as confirmed by ^{1}H-NMR [DMSO-d_6 and $CDCl_3$ (1:1), 270 MHz]. The ^{1}H-NMR revealed that two isomers were formed: syn and anti, in a ratio 1:1 as confirmed by integration of the peaks at δ 8.83 and 11.35. The presence of the stable derivative 3-AP-2,4-DNP compound enabled the subsequent development of a chromatographic method for detection of this compound.

d. HPLC A high performance liquid chromatographic method was developed, because this technique offers advantages such as separation and quantitative analysis of a wide range of samples, and efficiency of detection of as little as 200 pg of material (30). We employed reverse-phase chromatography, which is characterized by the use of a nonpolar HPLC column packing, and a solvent of greater polarity with respect to the sample. For the purpose of chromatographic detection by fluorescence, which is characterized by low limits of detection, the 3-AP-2,4-DNP standard samples were subjected to HPLC analysis secondary to derivatization of the primary NH_2 group of the compound with 5-dimethyl-aminonaphthalene sulfonyl-chloride (dansyl chloride). The nonpolar hydrocarbon stationary phases C_4, C_8, and C_{18}, in combination with polar solvent mixtures (water–methanol and water–acetonitrile), were analyzed for optimal detection of dansylated 3-AP-2,4-DNP. The best chromatographic separation profiles were achieved on a C_4 chromatographic column using a solvent mixture of water–methanol (31).

The initial establishment of a chromatographic method was done by analysis of aqueous solutions of dansylated 3-AP-2,4-DNP. To validate the use of this method, an HPLC standard curve of the compound was constructed. Then 3-AP standards were added to brain homogenates and derivatized with 2,4-DNPH. The homogenates were then subjected to HPLC. The aim of these studies was to refine the conditions for separation of 3-aminopropanal from other compounds in a brain homogenate, in terms of appropriate injection volumes, time of elution, and slope of the solvent gradient.

Based on these experiments, the best separation method was defined as follows. A Vydac C_4 column was used for all analyses. The solvent carrier system consisted of distilled water (A) and methanol (B). Using a flow rate of 1.0 ml/min, runs were initiated at 100% A and a linear gradient to 100% B was performed over 45 min., followed by 5 min of 100% B and a return to 100% A over 5 min. This separation method allowed the detection of the two isomers of the compound, as predicted by NMR spectral analysis. Further, a linear standard curve of the dansylated 3-AP-2,4-DNP derivative was constructed for both aqueous and brain samples. These results gave evidence that 3-aminopropanal in rat brain could be derivatized with 2,4-DNPH, separated from other compounds in a brain homogenate, and quantified by HPLC.

e. Measurement of 3-Aminopropanal in Cerebral Ischemic Tissue Having established a reliable method for detection of 3-aminopropanal in brain, we proceeded to investigate whether cerebral ischemia in rats is associated with 3-aminopropanal production. Male Lewis rats were subjected to a standard experimental model of focal cerebral ischemia (9, 10), as described in detail above. This animal model of MCA occlusion has been widely accepted and used for the study of cerebral ischemia.

For detection of brain 3-aminopropanal, the brain region corresponding to the area of ischemia (4 mm thick, located 3 mm caudal to the frontal lobes) was manually homogenized, derivatized in 2,4-DNPH reagent, processed, and analyzed by HPLC, as per the methods defined for the standard curve. Comparable regions from sham-operated animals served as normally perfused controls. To allow for accurate standardization and quantification of brain 3-aminopropanal levels, additional controls were performed by normalizing the results for protein content by the BioRad Protein assay (BioRad) and for the HPLC injection volume by adding the internal standard 1,7-diaminoheptane.

The 3-aminopropanal-derivatized products were not detected in brain homogenates prepared from sham-operated, normally perfused control animals. Significantly, 3-aminopropanal levels were elevated in ischemic tissues within 2 hr after the onset of ischemia (3.8 ± 0.3 μmol/g protein or 0.81 ± 0.06 m*M*, assuming a brain protein content of 213 g/liter). Tissue 3-aminopropanal levels continued to increase for at least 25 hr after the onset of ischemia (12.59 ± 8.39 μmol/g protein or 2.66 ± 1.8 m*M*). These results demonstrate a significant elevation of 3-aminopropanal levels in association with the time of onset of cerebral ischemia (30).

f. EIMS Verification of these HPLC findings was further sought by electrospray ionization mass spectroscopy (EIMS). The HPLC-purified 3-AP-2,4-DNP products from animals subjected to 25 hr of cerebral ischemia were collected on their elution from the HPLC column, and sent for analysis by EIMS. Control samples consisting of the corresponding HPLC-eluted fractions from sham-operated animals, as well HPLC-purified chemical standards of 3-AP-2,4-DNP, were also subjected to this analysis. A mass ion at m/z 251 was detected as a prominent breakup product in both 3-AP-2,4-DNP chemical standards, as well as in the HPLC-purified fractions from ischemic animals. This mass ion was not present in the HPLC-purified fractions from brain homogenates of sham-operated, normally perfused animals. These findings strongly supported the identification of 3-aminopropanal as a prominent compound, which is elevated in the brains of ischemic, but not in brains of normally perfused rats.

g. Stereotactic Microinjecitions and Evaluation of Cerebrodegenerative Changes To assess whether the observed accumulation of 3-aminopropanal after MCA occlusion was associated with cytotoxicity, we administered 3-aminopropanal by stereotactic means directly into the brain cortex of rats. Because stereotactic injections are a widely used technique in neurosurgical research, they are also described in greater detail in Section II,E. The quantity of 3-aminopropanal administered (25 μg/injection) was similar to the amount endogenously produced during ischemia (350 μM), assuming a volume of distribution of a typical middle cerebral artery infarction in this model). Infarct volume was assessed 24 hr later by 2,3,5-triphenyltetrazolium chloride (TTC) staining of coronal brain sections (described in Section II,D), followed by scanning photographic data into an imaging system. Infarct area in each slice was determined by planimetry, and infarct volume was calculated in cubic millimeters by summation of the infarct area in each slice. Data were analyzed statistically by factorial analysis of variance. The outcome of these studies revealed significant cell death following a 3-aminopropanal intracortical (ic) injection, whereas similar administration of vehicle resulted in very minor cell death attributable only to needle tract mechanical injury.

Confirmation of the results of the TTC staining was done by histopathologic examination of brain sections stained with hematoxylin and eosin (HE) and with terminal uridine deoxynucleotide nick-end labeling (TUNEL) 24 hr after 3-aminopropanal injection. (These staining techniques are described in Section II,D.) The staining revealed localized degenerative changes surrounding the zone of injection, with considerable nerve tract necrosis, the appearance of red necrotic neurons, and widely distributed apoptotic cells that stained TUNEL positive. Vehicle injection did not result in histopathologic changes beyond the tip of needle advancement. When considered together with the results indicating increased production of 3-aminopropanal during ischemia, the results of TTC and HE/TUNEL indicate that 3-aminopropanal is a direct molecular mediator of brain damage *in vivo*.

h. Cell Cytotoxicity Assay Although these results are consistent with a role for 3-aminopropanal in mediating cytotoxicity, we wished to obtain direct evidence that 3-aminopropanal could kill cultured CNS cells. Accordingly, 3-aminopropanal cytotoxicity to human glial (HTB14) and neuronal (HTB11) cell lines was tested *in vitro*. After incubating cells in the presence of 3-aminopropanal for 20 hr, we observed that the LD_{50} values for 3-aminopropanal were 160 $\pm$ 10 μM in the glial cell line and 90 $\pm$ 20 μM in the neuronal cell line. 3-Aminopropanal was somewhat more cytotoxic in primary rat astroglial cell cultures (LD_{50} = 80 $\pm$ 9 μM). A time-course study revealed that 3-aminopropanal exposure for as little as 5 min was significantly cytotoxic to neuronal cells, whereas the glial cell line displayed slightly less sensitivity to the compound, and a longer duration of exposure was necessary to elicit cytotoxic effects. In summary, these results established 3-aminopropanal as cytotoxic in physiologic concentrations to cultures of both primary rat astroglial and human glial and neuronal cell lines. The observed cytotoxicity was time and dose dependent. The results from time-course studies suggested that 3-aminopropanal-mediated neuronal cell death most likely occurred through necrosis (lytic cell death), whereas the delayed onset of glial cell death was hypothesized to be most likely attributable to programmed cell death (apoptosis). A detailed discussion of neural cell cultures and the choice of particular cell types is provided in Section IV.

i. Apoptosis vs. Necrosis The mechanism through which 3-aminopropanal induces cell death—apoptosis or necrosis—had not previously been established. These two forms of cell death have certain distinct characteristics and have profoundly different implications for the surrounding tissue. Necrosis is a passive process characterized by cytoplasmic and organelle swelling, rapid disruption of cell membrane integrity, and spillage of cellular contents into the extracellular milieu. This process leads to damage of surrounding tissue, infiltration of inflammatory cells, edema, and eventually fibrosis (32). Apoptosis, on the other hand, is an active process characterized by cellular and nuclear shrinkage, condensation of the chromatin around the nuclear periphery, oligonucleosomal cleavage by endonucleases of DNA into 160- to 200-bp fragments, preservation of cell membrane integrity, and formation of membrane-enclosed apoptotic bodies containing cytoplasmic contents (32, 33). Phagocytic cells recognize and ingest antigenically modified apoptotic cells, but are not activated to produce an inflammatory response. These characteristic features of extensive DNA cleavage and preservation of temporarily intact cell membranes provide the basis for most assays to discriminate between apoptosis and necrosis.

We sought direct biochemical evidence of DNA endonuclease cleavage in 3-aminopropanal-treated glial cells. Cells were exposed for 13 hr to 160 μM 3-aminopropanal, and the DNA was extracted. DNA gel electrophoresis revealed a typical ladder of oligonucleosome-length fragments of DNA characteristic of apoptotic cell death in treated, but not in control, glial cells.

j. FACS for TUNEL and Propidium Iodide Detection of Apoptosis Two alternative methods of flow cytometric detection of apoptosis were employed to verify the finding that 3-aminopropanal induced apoptosis. We used the TUNEL method to detect DNA strand breaks in apoptotic cells by labeling fragmented DNA with dUTP conjugated to fluorescein and terminal dinucleotide transferase (TdT), an enzyme that catalyzes template-independent addition of nucleotide triphosphate to the 3′ OH ends of DNA fragments. Using this procedure, we detected 76% TUNEL-positive cells following 13 hr of exposure of glial cells to 160 μM 3-aminopropanal, whereas vehicle-treated cells were uniformly negative. An additional parameter, which helps distinguish among normal, apoptotic, and necrotic cells, is measurement of cellular forward and side light scatter on a flow cytometer. Our data indicated that treated glial cells exhibited a decrease in forward light scatter and an increase in side scatter compared to controls, which is indicative of apoptotic changes (reflecting cell shrinkage, condensation of chromatin, and fragmentation of nuclei) (33). These morphologic changes were also demonstrated by TUNEL and eosin histological stainings. In separate experiments, these apoptotic changes were further shown to be 3-aminopropanal dose dependent. These data indicate that 3-aminopropanal is cytotoxic to glial cells by stimulating apoptosis.

Further analysis of the cells by subdiploid propidium iodide (PI) staining provided an additional verification by FACS that 3-aminopropanal-treated glial cells underwent apoptosis. A short methanol prefixation was done in order to allow propidium iodide to get inside the cell cytoplasm. It has been established that apoptotic cells leak their degraded low-molecular-weight DNA into the cytoplasm. Labeling of this cytoplasmic DNA with the fluorochrome PI and subsequent analysis by flow cytometry reveals that apoptotic cells exhibit lower PI staining (the peak referred to as subG_1, or A_0), as compared to cells in the G_0/G_1 phase of the cell cycle. By this method, and after electronically gating the flow cytometry results for PI width versus area of fluorescence (which allowed exclusion of doublet cells and debris), we detected 52.3% apoptotic cells after 13 hr of treatment with 160 μM 3-aminopropanal in the A_0 peak, and only 0.43% in control cells. By the separate use of both FACS methods for detection of apoptosis (TUNEL and PI), the effect of a shorter duration of exposure to 3-aminopropanal could be studied. The experiments revealed that within 5 hr apoptosis induced by the cytotoxin was complete. In summary, the use of the above three methods allowed us to establish definitively that 3-aminopropanal is cytotoxic to glial cells by stimulating apoptosis.

Somewhat surprisingly, when we examined neuronal cells (HTB11) similarly exposed for 13 hr to 3-aminopropanal at the LD_{50} concentration (90 μM), we observed the appearance of necrotic cell death, by the use of the above methods. By a histologic HE staining, the 3-aminopropanal-treated cells similarly showed characteristics of dying cells, namely highly eosinophilic cytoplasm, ill-defined nuclear and cytoplasmic membranes, and loss of cell-to-cell contact.

k. FACS for Annexin V/PI Detection of Apoptosis Overall, these results indicated that 3-aminopropanal-induced cell death in the neuronal cell line was necrotic, unless, of course, this was an unusual example of apoptotic cell death not accompanied by DNA cleavage, and therefore not characterized by TUNEL and PI positivity. Indeed, programmed cell death in the nervous system has previously been described in primary cultures of neuronal growth factor (NGF)-deprived sympathetic neurons, and in glucocorticoid-sensitive hippocampal neurons, to occur without the characteristic DNA fragmentation associated with apoptosis (34, 35). Therefore, in order to address this possible mechanism of 3-aminopropanal-induced neurotoxicity, we employed the annexin V/PI assay, which did not rely on apoptotic detection of DNA fragmentation, but on an alternative characteristic feature of apoptotic cells: they develop an early loss of phospholipid asymmetry, resulting in exposure of phosphotidyl serine (PS) on the outer leaflet (36, 37). By adding fluorescein-labeled annexin V to neuronal cells, which binds PS with high affinity, as well as PI, which only binds DNA in cells with compromised membranes, we were able to discriminate between annexin V-positive apoptotic cells and necrotic cells that were positive for both fluorochromes. 3-Aminopropanal-exposed neuronal cells showed no apoptotic changes as compared to controls, whereas the number of necrotic cells increased substantially. To exclude the possibility that neuronal cells died by post-necrotic apoptosis, 90 μM 3-aminopropanal-treated neurons were also analyzed at an early time point (5 hr of exposure) by TUNEL, PI and annexin V/PI staining, and by these studies it was also confirmed that the cells underwent early lytic cell death (necrosis). Finally, we wished to exclude the unlikely possibility that this neuronal cell line was incapable of undergoing apoptosis due to some generalized cell line defect. Accordingly, the neurons were treated with the apoptosis-inducing drug camptothecin (38) (15 μg/ml) for 20 hr, and subsequently were analyzed by the annexin V/PI method. The results revealed that treatment with camptothecin induced apoptosis, indicating that the apoptotic cascade was present in this neuronal cell line. When considered together, these experiments establish 3-aminopropanal as neurotoxic to neuronal cells by inducing early necrotic cell death.

l. Pharmacologic Inhibition of 3-Aminopropanal Formation in Vivo We employed the PAO inhibitor aminoguanidine to test its role in prevention of polyamine oxidative damage in cerebral ischemia. Aminoguanidine, administered after the onset of cerebral ischemia (320 mg/kg IP, 15 min postischemia, then 110 mg/kg IP every 8 hr up to 24 hr), significantly reduced the volume of cerebral damage (10, 27). Consequently, we wished to verify that the observed neuroprotective effect of aminoguanidine was attributable to inhibition of brain 3-aminopropanal production. We administered aminoguanidine by a similar protocol (320 mg/kg IP 2 hr preischemia, then 110 mg/kg IP every 8 hr up to 24 hr). At 25 hr the brain region corresponding to the area of middle cerebral artery occlusion was manually homogenized, processed, and assayed by HPLC for 3-aminopropanal content. Aminoguanidine administered by this established treatment protocol effectively prevented the accumulation of brain 3-aminopropanal, indicating that aminoguanidine protection in cerebral ischemia occurred by preventing PAO-mediated accumulation of 3-aminopropanal. Combined, these studies now indicate that polyamine catabolism and generation of 3-aminopropanal are prominent early events in the ischemic cytotoxicity cascade, and are important therapeutic targets for the treatment of cerebral ischemia (30). The findings of this study provide a logical sequence of experiments that can be used to study neurotoxic mechanisms in the CNS.

D. Methods for Assessment of Cerebral Ischemic Damage

Following euthanasia, the brain is removed from the skull, then fresh brain sections are prepared (1-mm-thick slices). The most commonly utilized method of assessment of the extent of cerebral ischemic damage is by the use of the dye 2,3,5-triphenyltetrazolium chloride (TTC), which stains viable tissue red and leaves the infarcted tissue unstained (white). TTC incubation of brain slices is carried out in 154 m*M* NaCl for 30 min at 37°C. The brain slices are photographed and the pictures of the brain slices are scanned into imaging software. Total cerebral infarct volume is then measured by computerized quantitative planimetry (9, 10, 39).

For verification of the results of the TTC staining, routine histologic staining with hematoxylin and eosin (HE) should be performed in parallel. In this technique, following surgery and decapitation, a coronal slice of the brain is excised (4 mm thick, 3 mm caudal to the frontal poles), corresponding to the area of middle cerebral artery infarct. The brain is then coated with M-1 embedding matrix (Lipshaw, Pittsburgh, PA), and placed on dry ice within 5 min of decapitation. In the next step, frozen brains are sectioned in 5- to 20-μm-thick sections and mounted on uncoated glass slides. These are dried at room temperature, then fixed in 10% formaldehyde solution. At this stage, the slides can be placed (while still wet) into slide boxes and frozen at −70°C until further processing. It should be noted that although this protocol is suitable for most routine stainings, in a number of instances in which the slides are used for immunocytochemistry, the formaldehyde fixation may distort the antigenic sites required for antibody binding. In this instance, alternative fixation methods should be evaluated, such as fixation with 95% ethanol, acetone fixation, or formaldehyde fixation at a different pH.

Certain staining methods, i.e., by the terminal deoxynucleotidyl transferase-mediated dUTP nick end-labeling method (used for assessment of cell death by apoptosis) require quenching of endogenous peroxidase activity. For this purpose slides are placed for 5–10 min in 0.1–1% peroxide in PBS, and subsequently washed twice. An additional consideration when working with frozen tissue, but not with a monolayer of cultured cells, is that it may have relatively high levels of endogenous biotin that can result in high background staining. This problem can be overcome by incubating the sections with an avidin/biotin blocking kit (Vector Laboratories, Inc., Burlingame, CA). For routine histologic staining with HE (as opposed to immunocytochemistry), the steps for quenching peroxidase activity and biotin are omitted. The next step is dehydration, which is performed as follows: soak in 95% ethanol twice for 10 sec each, then 100% ethanol twice for 10 sec each, then xylene three times for 10 sec each. For HE staining, incubation with hematoxylin and then with eosin can be performed at this stage, followed by another series of dehydration procedures. A few drops of a permanent mounting medium (e.g., Permount) are added, and as a last step the slides are covered with glass coverslips. For immunohistochemical staining, there are a number of variations in the steps after dehydration, depending on the choice of antibodies (the conjugation tags on the antibodies requiring different methods for color development/visualization), the different incubation times, and dilutions of the antibodies required. One is advised to seek the manufacturer's recommendations for staining protocols and procedures, as well as to perform experimental testing in parallel of several antibody dilutions and incubation times.

E. Stereotactic Brain Injections

To study the formation and pathogenic significance of cerebral ischemic cytotoxic factors *in vivo*, the investigator can inject the putative cytotoxic factor directly into the cortex (ic injection) of the animal and study the development of pathology. Alternatively, the investigator can study the induction of other factors of pathogenic significance in the cerebrospinal fluid. The latter is best achieved on a practical level by direct injection into the cerebral ventricles [intracerebroventricular (icv) injection]. Stereotactic injections are performed using a stereotactic apparatus. The choice of coordinates from a brain atlas is based on the design of the study and the type of animal. For example, for study of the role of a certain cytotoxin in combination with an MCAO model of cerebral ischemia, we chose coordinates that corresponded to the cerebral cortex perfused by the middle cerebral artery. Intracortical injections are quite suitable to study local degenerative changes, or the diffusion of an injection dye along certain neuronal pathways. Intracerebroventricular injections, on the other hand, are employed in study designs that address mediator effects in the cerebrospinal fluid and/or subarachnoid space.

Intracortical and intracerebroventricular brain injections can be performed by using an animal stereotactic apparatus. Following anesthesia, animals are placed on their ventral surface and a midline skin incision is made from the supraorbital ridge to the level of the external auditory meatus. The junction of the coronal, sagittal, and transverse sutures is exposed. Following determination of the exact coordinates for injection, which is done by using the axial planes of the stereotactic apparatus, entry through the skull is performed by the use of a dental burr. Injection is performed by the use of a precise microliter syringe, by advancing the needle at a steady rate to the required depth (typically 3–3.7 mm for intracortical injections). A very slow rate of injection is advisable to prevent retrograde leak. The maximal volume of injection should not exceed 30 μl. As with any fine technique, an inexperienced user is advised to practice the above steps by initial injection of a histologic stain or ink, in order to verify the correct injection coordinates and procedures.

Intracerebral injections are completed by suturing the skin at the site of incision.

In mice or young rats, entry through the skull does not require the use of a drill to create a craniotomy. The skull in these animals is very thin, and intracerebral injections can be carried out by the direct penetration of the injection needle through the skin and then the skull of the animal. In this and the above instance, intracerebral injections are associated, in general, with very fast postoperative recuperation of the animal. Typically, no overt signs of neurological dysfunction are observed (7).

III. Neuroscience Techniques for Study of the Structure and Function of the CNS

In addition to the above described methods for neuropathologic research, there is in addition a large number of methods used to study the "wiring pattern" of the brain. These methods allow the study of the structure and function of the central nervous system. The most widely used methods in the field are summarized and compared in Table I (40).

IV. Neural Cell Culture

Primary neural cell cultures as well as neural clonal cell lines can be established. Both techniques have advantages and disadvantages. A detailed discussion of the various kinds of both subtypes of neural cell cultures can be found in Banker *et al.* (41). In general, neural clonal cell lines have been used in a wide range of *in vitro* studies in the neurosciences. Cell lines are significantly easier to grow and maintain, as compared to primary cultures. They are also relatively homogeneous and the obtained results can be standardized among different laboratories. Some of the neural cell lines that have been established are permanently differentiated. Among the more commonly used lines are the human neuroblastoma cell line HTB11, and the human glioma/astrocytoma cell line HTB14. The American Type Culture Collection (ATCC) additionally carries a number of other neural tumor cell lines. Rat neuronal cells (PC12), which were derived from an adrenal pheochromocytoma, offer an additional advantage over other neural tumor cell lines in that they can be "differentiated" by exposure to neuronal growth factor. These differentiated cells develop most of the primary characteristic properties of sympathetic neurons, i.e., synthesis of catecholamines, extension of long dendritic arbors, etc.

The disadvantages of neural cell lines primarily relate to their poor state of differentiation and lack of expression of certain neuronal features, such as definitive synapses and myelin sheet formation. Thus, where appropriate, verification of the results should be carried out by the use of primary neural cultures.

Primary neural cell cultures can be obtained from embryonal or early postembryonal neuronal tissue. Under favorable conditions, these cultures can be maintained *in vitro* for weeks or even months. After differentiation, the cells develop dense dendritic arbors, distinct axons, electrically active synapses, and general morphologic and physiologic properties of the tissues of origin. Primary neuronal cultures offer the advantages of individual cell studies of formation of growth cones, propagation of synaptic electrical activity, modes of branching of dendrites, and expression of cell-specific classes of receptors. However, the presence of significant heterogeneity of cell populations has limited the experimental usefulness of primary neuronal cell cultures for pharmacologic and biochemical studies. Certain approaches have been taken to overcome these inherent difficulties. For instance, dissociated cultures of autonomic and sensory glia have become very widely used, because they contain one predominant cell type. Likewise, CNS studies can be accomplished using hippocampal and cerebellar cortical cells, because they also contain a single predominant cell type—pyramidal cells and granule cells, respectively. Elimination of undesirable cell types in heterogeneous cultures has also been achieved by the use of cell-specific cytotoxins and other alternative approaches. Despite these certain successes in achieving more homogeneous types of primary neural cultures, these cultures are still rather difficult to establish and maintain. They require very specific conditions, which necessitate months of establishment and extensive training of the operator. The procedure of cell isolation is also long and elaborate. These cultures cannot be propagated by mitosis, due to the characteristic neuronal feature of permanent differentiation, and cell isolation offers in general only a low and limiting number of cells.

An interesting variance of primary neural cultures has been found in the explant or organotypic culture—a technique established by Gahwiler for neural tissue slices. These originate from embryonal tissue, which is sliced at intervals of 0.4–1.0 mm and subsequently incubated in tissue culture medium in cell culture chambers. Tissue slices offer an unequivocal advantage when preservation of tissue architecture is needed. They would not be useful, however, for studies of drugs directed at specific receptors, because cells buried deep in the explant are generally inaccessible for treatment. Variations of the explant technique (e.g., placement of the tissue culture slice on a slowly rotating device with alternate exposure of the explant to either medium or air) has allowed cultures to be maintained in much thinner slices. These cultures have allowed more sophisticated two- and three-dimensional studies to be performed, with particular usefulness in the study of cellular growth, migration, and cell–cell interaction.

Table I Methods to Study CNS Structure and Function

Method	Application
Nissle staining	Staining of cell bodies used for cytoarchitectonic characterization of the gray matter
Golgi staining	Visualization of a small percentage of all neurons in a given area by impregnation, providing a clear view of neuronal processes
Retrograde degeneration	Following an experimental lesion, shrinkage and disapperance of the perikaryon allows determination of CNS connections
Anterograde degeneration	Following an experimental lesion, axonal changes distal to the cut allow determination of CNS connections
Marchi method	Anterograde degeneration is observed by staining degenerative products of myelin
Transneuronal degeneration	Experimental lesion of a neuronal group sometimes causes other neurons on which the initial group synapsed to also degenerate, thus allowing determination of CNS connections
Silver impregnation	Improved precision in determination of neuronal connectivity; axons can in some cases be followed even to their buttons
Axonal transport	More sensitive than degeneration methods. Tracer substances can be transported along the axon bidirectionally, and subsequently visualialized [i.e., anterograde transport of radioactive amino acids, which can be visualized by autoradiography; or retrograde transport of horseradish peroxidase (HRP), which can be visualized by evaluation of peroxidase activity]
Fluorescent methods	As above, neuronal connections can be visualized by axonal transport, in the case of small molecular fluorescent substances. Double and triple labeling with different fluorescent tracers (each injected in a different place) allows determination of double/triple labeling (connectivity) in a region of interest. Fluorescent methods can also be combined with immunocytochemical methods, which additionally allow visualization of neurotransmitter candidates of the labeled neurons
Radioactive methods	Radioactive labeling of a neurotransmitter, followed by its injection in a region of interest, allows the determination by radiography of groups of neurons with specific uptake mechanisms for this neurotransmitter
Electrophysiology	Electric stimulation of a nucleus is evaluated for causation of change of neuronal activity (connectivity) in other regions (orthodromic stimulation). Measurement of the time from the stimulus to the response allows determination of whether interneuronal connections are monosynaptic or polysynaptic. Antidromic stimulation (involving stimulation of axons within a fiber tract) allows determination of the location of the parent cell bodies
Electron microscopy	Numerous applications for determination of fine structures, synaptic relations, subcellular localization of neurontrasmitters, enzymes, etc.
Immunocytochemistry	Powerful tool for study of transmitter candidates, antigen localization, distribution of molecules, differentiation between cell types, etc. Can be used alone, or in combination with axonal transport techniques for the determination of connections
In situ hybridization	Allows determination of intracellular synthesis vs. uptake, by demonstrating the presence of the specific mRNA
Radioactive binding	Radioactive binding of agonists or antagonists allows determination of the localization of receptors
Lesioning	By observance of functional disturbances that ensue, a determination of function could be made
Electrical stimulation	Use of this method for stimulation of tracts and nuclei allows the mapping of function and behavior control centers
Use of microelectrodes	The activity of single neurons and their processes can be recorded, allowing precise study of synaptic function, response to different stimuli, etc.
Voltage clamp	By manipulation of the membrane potential, properties of synapses are studied
Patch clamp	Allows measurement of ion currents, limited to even single ion channels
Computer tomography	Thin pictures of the brain of a live organism can be obtained by the use of X rays
Magnetic resonance imaging	Signals emitted by protons, when placed in a magnetic field, depending on proton concentration, give clear contrast between, e.g., white and gray matter. Changes in the tissue, e.g., infarction, bleeding, and tumor, can be identified; dynamic processes in the brain can be studied
Positron emission tomography	The distribution of an inhaled or injected radioactive labeled substance of interest is visualized; distribution, metabolic activity, specific binding to certain receptor types, etc., can be studied

References

1. Kirino, T., Tamura, A., and Sano, K. (1984). Delayed neuronal death in the rat hippocampus following transient forebrain ischemia. *Acta Neuropathol. (Berl.)* **64,** 139.
2. Kraig, R. P., Petito, C. K., Plum, F., and Pulsinelli, W. A. (1987). Hydrogen ions kill brain at concentrations reached in ischemia. *J. Cereb. Blood Flow Metab.* **7,** 379.
3. Fisher, M., Pessin, M. S., and Furian, A. J. (1995). ECASS: Lessons for future thrombolytic stroke trials. European Cooperative Acute Stroke Study. *JAMA* **274,** 1058.
4. Haley, E. C., Jr., Levy, D. E., Brott, T. G., Sheppard, G. L., Wong, M.

C., Kongable, G. L., Torner, J. C., and Marler, J. R. (1992). Urgent therapy for stroke. Part II. Pilot study of tissue plasminogen activator administered 91–180 minutes from onset. *Stroke* **23,** 641.

5. McDaniel, W. F., Fjordbak, T., Schmidt, M. S., Tucker, J. C., and Davis, B. K. (1991). The behavioral effects of bilateral middle cerebral artery hemorrhagic ischemia in rat. *Neuroreport* **2,** 699.
6. Kamijyo, Y., Garcia, J. H., and Cooper, J. (1977). Temporary regional cerebral ischemia in the cat. A model of hemorrhagic and subcortical infarction. *J. Neuropathol. Exp. Neurol.* **36,** 338.
7. Waynforth, H. B., and Flecknell, P. A. (1992). "Experimental and Surgical Technique in the Rat." Academic Press Limited, London.
8. Ginsberg, M. D., and Busto, R. (1989). Rodent models of cerebral ischemia. *Stroke* **20,** 1627.
9. Zimmerman, G. A., Meistrell III, M., Bloom, O., Cockroft, K. M., Bianchi, M., Risucci, D., Broome, J., Farmer, P., Cerami, A., Vlassara, H., and Tracey, K. J. (1995). Neurotoxicity of advanced glycation endproducts (AGEs) during focal stroke, and neuroprotective effects of aminoguanidine. *Proc. Natl. Acad. Sci. U.S.A.* **92**(9), 3744.
10. Cockroft, K. M., Meistrell III, M., Zimmerman, G. A., Risucci, D., Bloom, O., Cerami, A., and Tracey, K. J. (1996). Cerebroprotective effects of aminoguanidine in a rodent model of stroke. *Stroke* **27,** 1393.
11. Anonymous (1995). Tissue plasminogen activator for acute ischemic stroke. The National Institute of Neurological Disorders and Stroke rt-PA Stroke Study Group. *N. Engl. J. Med.* **333,** 1581.
12. Wang, Y. F., Tsirka, S. E., Strickland, S., Stieg, P. E., Soriano, S. G., and Lipton, S. A. (1998). Tissue plasminogen activator (tPA) increases neuronal damage after focal cerebral ischemia in wild-type and tPA-deficient mice [see comments]. *Nature Med.* **4,** 228.
13. Brockmeyer, D. M., and Kendig, J. J. (1995). Selective effects of ketamine on amino acid-mediated pathways in neonatal rat spinal cord. *Br. J. Anaesth.* **74,** 79.
14. Camarata, P. J., Heros, R. C., and Latchaw, R. E. (1994). "Brain attack": The rationale for treating stroke as a medical emergency. *Neurosurgery* **34,** 144.
15. del Zoppo, G. J. (1998). Clinical trials in acute stroke: Why have they not been successful? *Neurology* **51,** S59.
16. Hallenbeck, J. M., and Frerichs, K. U. (1993). Stroke therapy: It may be time for an integrated approach. *Arch. Neurol.* **50,** 768.
17. Garcia, J. H. (1984). Experimental ischemic stroke: A review. *Stroke* **15,** 5.
18. Matsuo, Y., Kihara, T., Ikeda, M., Ninomiya, M., Onodera, H., and Kogure, K. (1995). Role of neutrophils in radical production during ischemia and reperfusion of the rat brain: Effect of neutrophil depletion on extracellular ascorbyl radical formation. *J. Cereb. Blood Flow Metab.* **15,** 941.
19. Hall, E. D. (1995). Inhibition of lipid peroxidation in central nervous system trauma and ischemia. *J. Neurol. Sci.* **134**(Suppl. 79–83), 79.
20. Duval, D., Roome, N., Gauffeny, C., Nowicki, J. P., and Scatton, B. (1992). SL82.0715, an NMDA antagoist acting at the polyamine site, does not induce neurotoxic effects on rat cortical neurons. *Neurosci. Lett.* **137,** 193.
21. Paschen, W., Schmidt-Kastner, R., Djuricic, B., Meese, C., Linn, F., and Hossmann, K. A. (1987). Polyamine changes in reversible cerebral ischemia. *J. Neurochem.* **49,** 35.
22. Paschen, W., Rohn, G., Meese, C. O., Djuricic, B., and Schmidt-Kastner, R. (1988). Polyamine metabolism in reversible cerebral ischemia: Effect of alpha-difluoromethylornithine. *Brain Res.* **453,** 9.
23. Dogan, A., Rao, A. M., Baskaya, M. K., Rao, V. L., Rastl, J., Donaldson, D., and Dempsey, R. J. (1997). Effects of ifenprodil, a polyamine site NMDA receptor antagonist, on reperfusion injury after transient focal cerebral ischemia. *J. Neurosurg.* **87,** 921.
24. Baskaya, M. K., Rao, A. M., Donaldson, D., Prasad, M. R., and Dempsey, R. J. (1997). Protective effects of ifenprodil on ischemic injury size, blood–brain barrier breakdown, and edema formation in focal cerebral ischemia. *Neurosurgery* **40,** 364.
25. Traynelis, S. F., Hartley, M., and Heinemann, S. F. (1995). Control of proton sensitivity of the NMDA receptor by RNA splicing and polyamines. *Science* **268,** 873.
26. Morgan, D. M. L., Bachrach, U., Assaraf, G., Harri, E., and Golenser, J. (1986). The effect of purified aminoaldehydes produced by polyamine oxidation on the developtment *in vitro* of *Plasmodium falciparum* in normal and glucose-6-phosphate-dehydrogenase-deficient erythrocytes. *J. Biochem.* **236,** 97.
27. Cockroft, K. M., Meistrell III, M., Zimmerman, G. A., Cerami, A., and Tracey, K. J. (1996). Neuroprotective effects of aminoguanidine in stroke. *J. Invest. Med.* **43**(2), 292A.
28. Bachrach, V., and Reches, B. (1966). Enzymatic assay for spermine and spermidine. *Anal. Biochem.* **17,** 38–48.
29. Dickinson, R., and Jacobsen, N. (1970). A new and sensitive test for detection of aldehydes: Formation of 6-mercapto-3-substituted s-triazolo (4, 3-b-)-s-tetrazines. *Chem. Commun.* 1719.
30. Bidlingmeyer, B. A. (1992). Practical HPLC methodology and applications. John Wiley & Sons, New York.
31. Ivanova, S., Botchkina, G. I., Al-Abed, Y., Meistrell, M., Batliwalla, F., Dubinsky, J. M., Iadecola, C., Wang, H., Gregersen, P. K., Eaton, J. W., and Tracey, K. J. (1998). Cerebral ischemia enhances polyamine oxidation: Identification of enzymatically formed 3-aminopropanal as an endogenous mediator of neuronal and glial cell death. *J. Exp. Med.* **188,** 327.
32. Cotran, R. S., Kumar, V., and Robbins, S. L. (1994). "Pathologic Basis of Disease." W. B. Saunders Company, Philadelphia.
33. Dive, C., Gregory, C. D., Phipps, D. J., Evans, D. L., Milner, A. E., and Wyllie, A. H. (1992). Analysis and discrimination of necrosis and apoptosis (programmed cell death) by multiparameter flow cytometry. *Biochim. Biophys. Acta* **1133,** 275.
34. Martin, D. P., Schmidt, R. E., DiStefano, P. S., Lowry, O. H., Carter, J. G., and Johnson, Jr., E. M. (1988). Inhibitors of protein synthesis and RNA synthesis prevent neuronal death caused by nerve growth factor deprivation. *J. Cell Biol.* **106,** 829.
35. Masters, J. N., Finch, C. E., and Sapolsky, R. M. (1989). Glucocorticoid endangerment of hippocampal neurons does not involve deoxyribonucleic acid cleavage. *Endocrinology* **124,** 3083.
36. Fadok, V. A., Savill, J. S., Haslett, C., Bratton, D. L., Doherty, D. E., Campbell, P. A., and Henson, P. M. (1992). Different populations of macrophages use either the vitronectin receptor or the phosphatidylserine receptor to recognize and remove apoptotic cells. *J. Immunol.* **149,** 4029.
37. Fadok, V. A., Voelker, D. R., Campbell, P. A., Cohen, J. J., Bratton, D. L., and Henson, P. M. (1992). Exposure of phosphatidylserine on the surface of apoptotic lymphocytes triggers specific recognition and removal by macrophages. *J. Immunol.* **148,** 2207.
38. Furuya, Y., Ohta, S., and Ito, H. (1997). Apoptosis of androgen-independent mammary and prostate cell lines induced by topoisomerase inhibitors: Common pathway of gene regulation. *Anticancer Res.* **17,** 2089.
39. Bederson, J. B., Pitts, L. H., Germano, S. M., Nishimura, M. C., Davis, R. L., and Bartkowski, H. M. (1986). Evaluation of 2,3,5-triphenyltetrazolium chloride as a stain for detection and quantification of experimental cerebral infarction in rats. *Stroke* **17,** 1304.
40. Brodal, P. (1992). "The Central Nervous System Structure and Function." Oxford University Press, Cambridge.
41. Banker G., and Goslin, K. (1998). "Culturing Nerve Cells (Cellular and Molecular Neuroscience)." MIT Press, Cambridge, MA.

79

Research in Urologic Surgery

Roger E. De Filippo and Anthony Atala

Laboratory for Tissue Engineering and Cellular Therapeutics, Department of Urology, Children's Hospital and Harvard Medical School, Boston, Massachusetts 02115

I. Introduction

Recent advances in basic science have offered a number of surgical disciplines the opportunity to expand on the armamentarium available for clinical applications. The field of urology is no exception. It is the purpose of this chapter to give the reader a broad overview of some of the techniques and methods of research that are making an impact on the field of urology today, as they relate to the pathophysiology of the genitourinary system.

The focus of this chapter includes areas of basic investigation that have recently provided major contributions to clinical urology, namely, cytogenetics, molecular biology, gene therapy, and tissue engineering. Important data gathered from each of these disciplines are discussed in the context of their impact on certain clinical disorders of the genitourinary tract. The reader will become familiar with some of the techniques commonly used in *in vitro* and *in vivo* models. These model systems have the advantage of a tailored, homogeneous environment influenced by a finite number of factors; however, it becomes a cumbersome task to apply these models to the human condition, wherein a more heterogeneous milieu predominates.

II. Cytogenetics

A. Methodology

Flow cytometry measures the DNA content of cells (1). This technology became particularly useful in the area of oncology when it was discovered that pivotal information about DNA ploidy could be obtained from neoplastic cells and used for both diagnosis and prognosis in cancer patients. Flow cytometry can be used to analyze individual chromosomes, RNA content, cell surface antigens, cell size, and numerous functional characteristics of individual cells (2). This technology has been enhanced to include sample analysis for particular cell cycles and for sorting cells into specific populations (3). This is particularly significant when looking at the mutagenic phenotypes of cells and is the first step toward understanding the mechanisms responsible for a cell's neoplastic conversion.

Cell suspensions can be derived from a viable tumor specimen, or in the case of bladder carcinoma, a bladder washing from voided or Foley catheter-collected urine. Cell suspensions can be prepared using a variety of techniques

(4). Automated cell analysis requires a cell-sorting instrument that employs an optical (laser or fluorescence) device and electrical sensing techniques combined with computer analysis (2). The continuous flow of the samples can be adjusted for a desired cell type as it passes through the flow cytometer. A collection device that converts electrical energy into mechanical energy separates cells into different populations, these can be directly plated onto microscope slides for visual identification or cultured and their genetic material expanded using other techniques, such as the polymerase chain reaction (5). This is a very sensitive technique for cell analysis, although outcome variability stemming from numerous sources, such as sample preparation or cellular debris resulting in nonspecific background, may occur. One method used to avoid nonspecificity is adding to the sample medium a monoclonal antibody that will select for a particular cell by binding to its membrane (6).

B. Bladder Carcinoma

In no other aspect of urology has cytogenetic analysis contributed as much clinically important information than in the study of bladder carcinoma. Bladder cancer is quite suited for flow cytometry because malignant cells, isolated from the patient's urine, can be harvested in a relatively noninvasive manner. The DNA ploidy of these cells indicates the grade of the tumor, which then guides choice of therapeutic options for the patient; these include observation, chemotherapy, or surgical resection. Flow cytometry has proved particularly useful in monitoring the upper urinary tracts for tumor recurrence in patients who have undergone exenterative procedures with orthotopic urinary diversion. Of particular interest is the genetic information gathered from this technology, which lends itself to further investigations involving the isolation of oncogenes expressed in urothelial tumors, and eventually the development of better treatment regimes and drug interventions for patients. Although flow cytometry is a useful tool in patients already diagnosed and treated for bladder tumors, it is not readily applicable as a screening mechanism for new patients presenting with either signs or symptoms of bladder cancer because of cost considerations and lack of specificity.

C. Other Genitourinary Tumors

Cytogenetic analysis has been applied to the investigation of other genitourinary tumors: renal cell carcinoma, prostate cancer, and germ cell tumors of the testis are some examples. Determination of DNA ploidy for these tumors, however, has not yielded the same clinical relevance regarding malignant potential as in the case of bladder cancer. Flow cytometry continues to function more as an investigational tool for these specific tumor types, generating information regarding their genetic makeup and providing important insight into certain genes or tumor markers essential for malignant proliferation.

D. Inflammation

Cytogenetic analysis has played an important role in the study of inflammation in the genitourinary tract. Flow cytometry has been used to study the surface structure of uroepithelial cells to characterize membrane receptors responsible for adherence of pyelonephritogenic *Escherichia coli* (7). This information is useful for detecting high-risk groups among patients with recurrent urinary tract infections who go on to develop renal scarring. This allows a mechanism for screening these patients early so that appropriate intervention can be administered in a timely fashion.

Cytogenetic analysis has revolutionized urologic diagnosis and treatment and has given us the ability to better understand the pathophysiology behind the disease processes commonly encountered in the clinical setting. However, the urologist must bear in mind that the universal use of these techniques in the clinical setting has certain limitations, namely, high cost and limitations in the generation of reliable data of clinical significance for all tumor types.

III. Molecular Biology

A. Methodology for the Characterization of Genes

Basic molecular biology techniques have provided the urologist with an array of data pertaining to the genetic makeup of cells and new insight into possible alterations in cellular DNA that result in aberrant phenotypic expressions. These tools afford investigators the capability to characterize DNA according to a particular disease process and to expand it for both *in vitro* and *in vivo* investigations. In turn, DNA markers may provide the urologist with additional means of identifying certain risky groups of patients and developing new treatment algorithms for their care.

Molecular genetics starts with the isolation of particular sequences of DNA using enzymatic nucleases that cleave the DNA at specific points. DNA fragments can be isolated by gel electrophoresis, transferred to a nitrocellulose membrane, and detected by hybridization with a radiolabeled DNA probe (Southern blotting) (8). Cellular DNA can also be amplified by denaturing the double-stranded DNA into single strands and then replicating these strands with a specific DNA polymerase (9). Finally, individual strands of DNA are rejoined by adjusting to the optimum reannealing temperature. This process is known as the polymerase chain reaction (PCR). The copied DNA can be analyzed by Southern blotting as described above. Samples from a variety of tissue types can be analyzed in this fashion and their specific DNA sequences uncovered.

Similar techniques can be applied to other constituents of the genetic pathway, such as ribonucleic acid (RNA) or proteins. The sample tissue is homogenized in broth containing certain lysates prepared from commercially available ingredients that isolate either RNA or proteins. The RNA or protein fragments can be separated by gel electrophoresis (Northern or Western blotting). In addition, the RNA can be used to expand the genetic information by producing copies of tissue DNA through a process known as reverse transcriptase polymerase chain reaction (RT-PCR).

B. Oncogenes—Animal and Human Models

All of the methods described above have culminated in the discovery of important genetic characteristics in a variety of urologic disorders and diseases. One such discovery was the oncogene, which plays an important role in the homeostasis of cellular growth and development and can confer to a cell its malignant potential (2). The oncogenes of several urologic neoplasms have been characterized, including those of bladder cancer, prostate cancer, renal cell carcinoma, and Wilms' tumor. The discovery of these genes facilitated the detection of tumor suppressor genes, which exert regulatory control over oncogene expression and normally inhibit malignant transformation. Certain mutations in these tumor suppressor genes result in loss of associative control over oncogenes; this subsequently leads to their overexpression and the typical cellular overgrowth that characterizes tumorogenesis (10). This technique is a very powerful tool for investigators in characterizing a variety of chromosomal mutations and deletions responsible for the development of various diseases in urology (11).

Animal models have been used to examine the mechanisms involved in deleterious mutations to human DNA that result in either malignant transformation or congenital disorders (12–15). One such model uses transgenic mice injected *in vivo* as embryos with simian viruses containing a specific gene sequence that will transfect normal mice prostate tissue; with the help of a specific promoter region, these viruses induce a neoplastic transformation. This animal model can be constructed in a similar manner for a variety of neoplasms. Tumor specimens can be processed, and the genetic constituents, DNA or RNA, or products of translation (proteins), can be hybridized through PCR or RT-PCR, identifying which genes are affected by certain mutations, deletions, or translocations to certain segments of a particular chromosome. This same process is applied to research on congenital anomalies such as ambiguous genitalia, hypospadias, cryptorchidism, and Wilms' tumor (16–19).

Often the patient's own blood can be the source of the genetic information, extracted from circulating lymphocytes. Information gathered from these laboratory investigations has resulted in better understanding of certain causal relationships between environmental carcinogens and the development of certain urologic tumors, such as cigarette smoking and bladder cancer. This, in turn, affords opportunities to identify certain patients at risk and to educate the public at large.

C. Immunolabeling

Capitalizing on the abilities of the above technologies to identify certain genes responsible for the malignant transformation of cells, researchers and clinicians have used immunocytochemistry (ICC) to assist in the characterization of tissue specimens according to well-documented mutation types. This information can be used as a guide for analyzing all treatment options for the patient. ICC has become the most common laboratory method employed by clinical urologist today. ICC involves paraffin or frozen fixation of finely sectioned tissues on microscope slides and exposing these tissues to commercially prepared antibodies (biotinylated probes); the probes will bind to a wide variety of cytoplasmic or surface membrane proteins, which serve as the antigenic binding sites (20). In cancer patients, the antibody binds to proteins encoded by either oncogenes or tumor suppressor genes. Following a multistep approach that involves histochemical staining, these antibody-bound proteins react enzymatically with the staining solutions, allowing their visualization under the microscope and quantification of their expression (21).

Immunolabeling has become increasingly useful as a research tool in many aspects of urology, with important ramifications especially for the study of bladder cancer. The tumor suppressor gene p53 is found in a variety of different tissues and is responsible for the normal regulatory cycle of the cell. The p53 gene encodes for a p53 protein that in normal urothelial cells is present in extremely small quantities because of rapid turnover. However, mutated forms of the gene encountered in malignant tissue result in its overexpression; increased nuclear accumulation of p53 protein can be determined by immunohistochemical staining (22–24). Investigations by Stein *et al.* (25) have supported the theory that increased gene mutations of p53 may act as a tumor marker for bladder cancer and may characterize the tumor's increased proclivity for progression. Urologists use this information to examine patients' tissue specimens and identify those with aggressive tumor types in order to develop a better treatment approach; such patients may undergo chemotherapy and extirpative surgery, whereas patients whose tumors display a more benign character histochemically are treated in other ways. There are numerous other tumor markers under investigation, underscoring the importance of ICC techniques in tissue analysis and the direct clinical application of their results.

Tissue *in situ* hybridization, another method for characterizing cells, is often used to complement ICC. This technique involves hybdridizing paraffin-embedded tissue on microscope slides with anitsense oligonucleotide sequences (probes) of DNA (26). These probes bind to the complementary DNA sequences located on the tissue specimens. The DNA can be marked, or illuminated, through a series of peroxidase-based enzymatic reactions, or with a radiolabeled, radioactive tag attached to the tail of an exon. Emulsion autoradiography exposes the results on film and the intensity is then quantified with a densitometer. This technique has been used for the detection of human papilloma virus in bladder specimens of patients with transitional cell carcinoma in an effort to establish its role as a possible precursor for the development of bladder cancer in selected patients (27).

Limitations of ICC include the nonimmunoreactivity of some tumors, the weak immunostaining of different tissue types, the lack of reproducibility from one laboratory to another, and the poor antibody specificity (28). Variability can be reduced by consistently processing the tissues from a reliable laboratory. Nonetheless, ICC still remains one of the few methodologies that has direct translational application to clinical urology today.

D. Multidrug Resistance

Techniques in molecular biology continue to uncover a multitude of important cellular mechanisms that one day may lead to a more efficient therapy for the patient. One such mechanism discovered was multiple drug resistance (MDR) displayed by cancer cells in response to chemotherapeutic agents (29, 30). This mechanism may be mediated by an MDR gene that encodes for transport membrane proteins such as P-glycoprotein (31, 32). Genetic engineering and methods of gene delivery have recently offered scientists new opportunities to explore other methods of combating cellular defense mechanisms such as MDR, along with treating clinical disorders on a cellular genetic level.

E. Gene Therapy

1. Viral Methods

Gene therapy involves the alteration of the phenotypic expression of a targeted cell through the manipulation of the cell's genotypic content, thus achieving a desired therapeutic effect (33). The success of gene therapy depends on the selection of a delivery vector that will allow efficient gene transfer, precise targeting of the desired tissue without causing harm to the surrounding normal tissue, and an appropriate genetic intervention for creating the desired therapeutic effect. The method of recombinant viral reconstruction and the techniques behind recombinant DNA production have allowed researchers to develop the technology for insertion of therapeutic transgenes in place of a virus' endogenous replicative genetic components, thus creating an efficient mechanism for shuttling genes into living tissues (33).

Some of the viral vectors employed include retroviruses, adenoviruses, and adeno-associated viruses. *In situ* construction of the vectors begins with incorporation of a genetically engineered plasmid into the viral genome, facilitated through cleavage enzymes that assist in splicing the plasmid at the desired portion of host DNA or RNA (34–36). In the case of retroviruses, this means replacing that portion of the viral genome responsible for replication and rendering the virus replication deficient. Methods of constructing adenovirus vectors have already been described (37). These viruses can be purchased commercially, genetically altered, and ready for transfection with the plasmid DNA.

Once the vectors are prepared, the next step requires infection of the target cells with the virus vectors. One method of accomplishing this is *ex vivo* transfection. Target tissue cells are cultured outside of the animal or patient, then are incubated with the viral vectors until gene transfer is complete (38, 39). The infected cells, replaced into the animal or patient, effect the desired response, which is encoded by the newly transferred gene. This is the classic model for the creation of a gene-modified tumor vaccine. These genetically altered cells can now stimulate an immune reaction or produce proteins or hormones that were previously absent.

The *in vivo* alternative is infection of the target cells through direct injection into the animal or human of the *in vitro*-prepared vectors, allowing transfection to occur within the body (40). Although direct injection would be ideal, this method has limited practicality over already established, conventional treatments because of the difficulty of specific tissue targeting and transgene insertion into specific host genomic sites, and consequently a lack of consistently reproducible genetic alterations of the host cells. In order to enhance *in vivo* gene transfer, researchers have explored other alternatives to overcome this problem. Production of a tissue-specific promoter encoded within the genome of the vector may be one solution (41, 42). The theory behind a tissue-specific promoter involves genetically engineering a vector to manufacture a protein that is also produced at a unique site in the body—for example, surfactant in the lung, melanin in melanocytes, or prostate-specific antigen in prostate (43–45). This would facilitate attachment of the vector to the particular target cells where transfection is required. Unfortunately, these tissue-specific promoters can also result in cytotoxic consequences for normal tissues, making their application in the clinical setting impractical. Other efforts at overcoming site specificity have been directed toward attaching to the vectors, *in situ*, prior to injection, antibodies or ligands known to bind to specific cell surface receptors (46, 47); however, *in vivo* animal models have resulted in relatively poor tissue-specific targeting.

A novel system for *in vivo* adenovirus-mediated gene transfer to bladder urothelium has been proposed by our laboratory. Adenovirus vectors are very efficient for *in vivo* gene transfer, the process is facilated by their ability to produce high viral titers, and to transfer genes to both dividing and nondividing cells, and to their propensity for attachment to a variety of epithelial cell surfaces, including those in the human respiratory and gastrointestinal tracts. Adenovirus infection also occurs in human bladders, and therefore it was postulated that bladder tissue may make a good target for adenovirus-mediated gene transfer. However, initial data demonstrated that urothelial cells were only occasionally transduced after exposure to the adenovirus intravesically. Researchers have since discovered that hydrochloric acid removal of the polysaccharide glycosaminoglycan (GAG) layer, which is responsible for the antiadherence effect of bladder urothelium, enhanced transfection of recombinant adenovirus to the target cells in the bladder (48).

2. Nonviral Methods

Other methods for gene transfer involve nonviral systems that introduce naked plasmid DNA into target cells. The gene gun, or particle-mediated gene transfer technique, employs a device that can innoculate cells with genetically altered plasmids preloaded into the "gun." The plasmids are then propelled by a variety of means, including electricity or helium, into the host cell, where they are expressed along with the rest of the cell's genome (49).

Another nonviral method is electroporation. Electroporation is a physical method of introducing macromolecules into cells *in vitro* by applying a brief electrical pulse that allows transit of the molecule across the cell membrane (50, 51). Taking this technique a step further, a method that achieves organ-confined gene transfer in urologic organs *in vivo* has been developed in our laboratory. Based on the principle of electroporation, a gene transfer device was constructed for direct *in vivo* electrotransfection (DIVE) in intact kidneys, testes, and bladders (Figs. 1 and 2) (52). The animal model consisted of Sprague–Dawley rats whose kidneys, testes, and bladders were directly injected with recombinant plasmids, then subjected to an electrical current produced by electrolytic capacitors. Histologic examination of the affected organs revealed no evidence of damage. Satisfactory gene activity was confirmed by immunocytochemical and RT-PCR detection of the appropriate protein expression.

Another nonviral modality was investigated in our laboratory using ultrasound energy to enhance transfection of cells both *in vitro* and *in vivo*. Researchers postulate that the mechanism of protein transfer may be achieved through both thermal and nonthermal effects (53, 54). Several investigators believe that nonthermal energy effects, particularly cavitation, may be a major mechanism by which ultrasound enhances permeability of skin, tissue, and cell membranes (55). In our study, ultrasound energy with a frequency of around 1 MHz was used to transfect fibroblasts and urothelial cells with genetically constructed plasmids encoding firefly luciferase (pGL3-Luc) *in vitro*, and vascular endothelial cell growth factor (VEGF) *in vivo* (56). An ultrasound device, or sonicator, was applied directly to the solution containing both plasmids and host cells, or applied directly to the transfected organ, in our case female Sprague–Dawley rat bladders. Posttransfection immunohistochemical analysis revealed enhanced protein expression both *in vitro* and *in vivo* when compared to controls. Histologic examination demonstrated no morphologic changes in the tissues. In addition, there was no evidence of DNA damage to the plasmids from application of ultrasound energy. This study concludes that ultrasound energy can be used safely for gene delivery as a nonviral system with high transfection efficiency, both *in vitro* and *in vivo*.

Both viral and nonviral applications are designed to improve results with *in vivo* gene transfer. These techniques are currently being investigated in clinical trials (Table I).

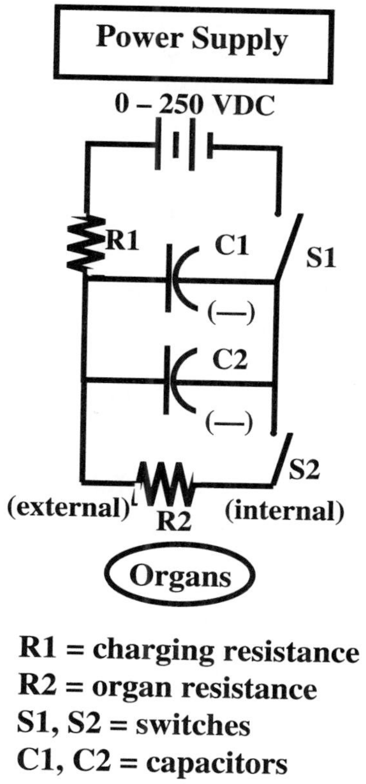

Figure 1 Direct *in vivo* electrotransfection. Diagram of capacitor system and power source.

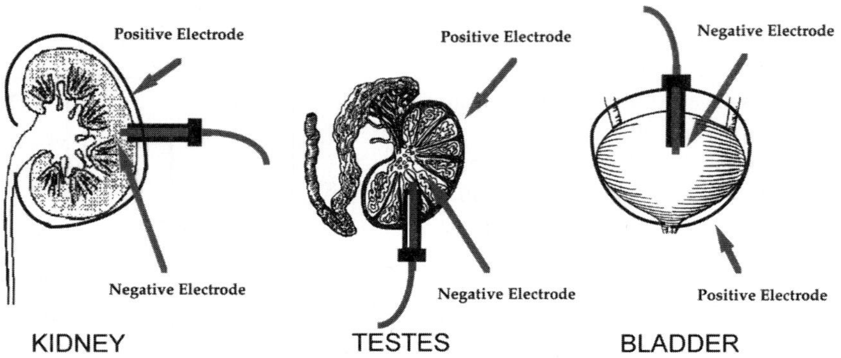

Figure 2 Direct *in vivo* electrotransfection of kidney, testes, and bladder.

Table I Urologic Gene Therapy Clinical Trials[a]

Organ	Strategy	PI	Date	Institution
Ex vivo				
Prostate	Cytokine (GM-CSF) immunotherapy	Simons	8/94	Johns Hopkins
Prostate	Cytokine (GM-CSF) allogeneic immunotherapy	Simons	9/97	Johns Hopkins
Renal	Cytokine (TNF-alpha) immunotherapy	Rosenberg	10/91	NIH
Renal	Cytokine (IL-2) immunotherapy	Rosenberg	10/91	NIH
Renal	Cytokine (IL-2/IFN) with TIL	Economou	4/92	UCLA
Renal	Cytokine (IL-2) allogeneic immunotherapy	Gansbacher	8/92	Memorial Sloan-Kettering Cancer Center
Renal	Cytokine (IL-4) immunotherapy	Lotze	2/93	University of Pittsburgh
Renal	Cytokine (GM-CSF) immunotherapy	Simons	12/93	Johns Hopkins
Renal	Immunotherapy/HLA-B7/β-2 microglobulin	Fox	9/95	Chiles Research Institute
Renal	Immunotherapy/HLA-B7.1/IL-2	Antonia	11/98	University of South Florida
In vivo				
Bladder	Adenovirus RB, intravesical	Small	1/96	UCSF
Bladder	Adenovirus p53, intravesical	Pagliaro	11/97	M.D. Anderson
Prostate	Retrovirus antisense c-myc	Steiner	9/95	Vanderbilt
Prostate	Intradermal vaccinia-PSA	Chen	9/95	Naval Medical Academy
Prostate	Adenovirus ganciclovir/TK	Scardino	1/96	Baylor College of Medicine
Prostate	Intradermal vaccinia-PSA	Kufe	9/96	Dana Farber Cancer Institute
Prostate	Intradermal vaccinia-PSA	Sanda	5/97	University of Michigan
Prostate	Liposome IL-2	Belldegrun	5/97	UCLA
Prostate	Adenovirus ganciclovir/TK	Hall	5/97	Mount Sinai Hospital
Prostate	Adenovirus p53	Belldegrun	9/97	UCLA
Prostate	Adenovirus p53	Logothetis	11/97	M.D. Anderson
Prostate	Adenovirus ganciclovir/TK	Kadmon	2/98	Baylor College of Medicine
Prostate	Intramuscular vaccinia MUC-1-IL-2	Figlin	5/98	UCLA
Prostate	Adenovirus, prostate oncolytic	Simons	6/98	Johns Hopkins
Renal	Liposome HLA-B7/β-2 microglobulin	Chang	8/95	Multicenter
Renal	Liposome HLA-B7/IL-2	Figlin	8/95	UCLA
Renal	Liposome IL-2	Figlin	7/98	UCLA

[a]Abbreviations: PI, Principal investigator; GM-CSF, granulocyte–macrophage colony-stimulating factor; TNF-α, tumor necrosis factor-α; NIH, National Institutes of Health; Il, interleukin; IFN, interferon; TIL, tumor-infiltrating lymphocytes; UCLA, University of California, Los Angeles; UCSF, University of California, San Francisco; PSA, prostate-specific antigen. Both *ex vivo* and *in vivo* trials are shown. Data obtained from the National Institutes of Health Office of Recombinant DNA Activities, last updated December, 1998. Adapted from Rodriguez and Simons (56a).

However, the biggest obstacle to overcome with systemically introduced vectors still remains the patient's own humoral immunity. The immune system is extremely facile at clearing circulating vectors and presents an interesting challenge for researchers.

3. Tumor Vaccines

Gene therapy continues to contribute to many areas of urologic research, including practical human interventions that may lead to wide clinical applications. A great deal of attention has been directed toward the development of tumor vaccines using the previously described techniques of genetic engineering. A major component of the mechanism of action of these vaccines is an intact host immune system. Most tumors are not immunogenic and therefore malignant cells evade recognition by the host's immune surveillance system. The concept behind tumor vaccines is the creation of transfected cells that present cell surface antigens (such as MHC class I antigens) or produce immunostimulatory cytokines [such as IL-2 or granulocyte–macrophage colony-stimulating factor (GM-CSF)], invoking a host immune response against the tumor (57, 58). A rat model for prostate cancer demonstrates how *ex vivo*-engineered prostate cells reinjected into the animal start to secrete GM-CSF, ultimately resulting in tumor regression in some of the animals. Investigators invoke the use of tissue-specific promoters such as prostate-specific antigen to improve targeting of gene therapy to prostate tissue. All of these techniques strive to improve therapy for prostate cancer, especially in patients with advanced metastatic disease for which no effective treatment exists. Other urologic malignancies, such as bladder cancer and renal cell carcinoma, have also been the focus of interest toward developing new treatments for advanced disease using gene therapy (59, 60). Gene therapy continues to be an important area of urologic research with, however, limited clinical application to date.

IV. Tissue Engineering

A. Methodology

Numerous conditions encountered by the urologic surgeon require surgical reconstruction, including epispadias, ambiguous genitalia, traumatic injuries to the external genitalia, and bladder augmentation or lower urinary tract reconstruction. Surgical intervention in some of these patients can be challenging because of the limited availability of tissue. In the past, urologists dealt with this problem by using tissue for coverage from other sites in the body, but not without certain complications (61, 62). Even in cases in which nonurologic tissue is excluded and native urologic tissue is used, as in autoaugmentation or ureterocystoplasty of the bladder, not all patients are ideal candidates for these procedures, and long-term results have not been encouraging (63).

Tissue engineering efforts are currently underway for virtually every tissue type in the genitourinary system, including, kidney, bladder, ureter, urethra, and external genitalia. It is important that laboratory facilities be designed with the proper tools required for sterile cell culture and have personnel who are well trained at techniques of cell harvest, culture, cell expansion, and polymer design. Until recently, it had been difficult to grow and expand benign urothelial cells *in vitro*; however, today several researchers have been successful in culturing and greatly expanding these cells from small biopsies of urothelium (64, 65). Using current methods of cell culture, it is possible to expand bladder, ureter, renal pelvis, and corporal cavernosal muscle cells to sufficient cell yields for tissue regeneration and structuring. It is equally important to develop the proper scaffold, onto which the cells grow and maintain their necessary shape and differentiation for tissue replacement. Resorbable polymers are preferred over other synthetic materials because of decreased risk of infection, calcification, and unfavorable connective tissue response (66). Polymers of lactic and glycolic acid (PLA and PGA) have been extensively used to fabricate tissue-engineering matrices because of their many desirable features; they are biocompatible, processable, biodegradable, and can be readily formed into a variety of structures. Another important feature of PLA and PGA are the relatively small porous films that can be constructed, which are especially desirable in urologic applications in order to prevent leakage of urine from the tissue. The polymers can be manipulated with respect to pore size and total porosity to promote increased vascularization. Collagen scaffolds have also been used successfully both experimentally and clinically (67, 68, 71).

B. Bladder Experimental Models

An elegant model that demonstrates the basic techniques employed with tissue engineering is the *de novo* reconstitution of a functional mammalian urinary bladder. It has already been demonstrated that bladder urothelial and muscle cells can be efficiently harvested from a variety of species, including humans, cultured *in vitro*, and expanded to large quantities (69, 70). In this particular model, beagles underwent either trigone sparing bladder removal or cystectomy. In the study design, a group of dogs received a prefabricated tissue-engineered neoorgan, consisting of a bladder-shaped biodegradable polymer, which delivered autologous urothelial cells attached to the luminal surface and smooth muscle cells attached to the exterior surface.

A 10×10-cm synthetic polymer matrix of PGA with an average fiber diameter of 15 μm and an interfiber distance between 0 and 200 μm was configured into a bladder-shaped mold. The resulting flexible scaffold was coated with a liquefied copolymer (PLGA 50:50, 80 mg/ml methylene chloride), sterilized, and stored in a desiccator. Urothelial and smooth muscle cells were dissociated from bladder biopsies and microsurgically detached from each other and processed separately. Smooth muscle cell cultures were maintained and expanded with Dulbecco's modified Eagle's medium (DMEM) supplemented with 10% fetal calf serum. Urothelial cell cultures were maintained with serum-free keratinocyte growth medium supplemented with epidermal growth factor and bovine pituitary extract. All cells were incubated at 37°C with 5% carbon dioxide. The cells were seeded onto PGA polymers *in vitro*, creating the cell–polymer scaffold that would eventually be augmented onto the bladders. A mean bladder capacity of 95% of the original precystectomy volume was achieved by the tissue-engineered cell–polymer autologous bladder augments. Urodynamic studies showed normal functional parameters. Microscopic inspection revealed maturation toward normal histologic and phenotypic structure, as demonstrated with immunohistochemical techniques using hematoxylin and eosin (HE), trichrome, α-smooth muscle actin, desmin, pancytokeratin, cytokeratin-7, and antiasymmetric unit membrane (AUM) antibodies (Fig. 3). Scaffolds implanted without cells, as controls, failed to form normal bladder reservoirs. This model clearly demonstrates that tissue-engineered organs can readily be applied to *in vivo* models with resulting normal histology and satisfactory function, which are very important in preventing previously described complications of autologous grafts.

C. Other Genitourinary Tissues

Similar experimental protocols have been successfully applied to other conditions and tissue types for genitourinary reconstruction. It has already been demonstrated that urothelial and muscle cells can be expanded *in vitro* and transferred onto a matrix, where sheets of cells are formed. This cell–matrix can then be implanted *in vivo* with encouraging histologic results. The cell–matrix approach was expanded to engineer new functional urologic structures such as ureters in dogs: urothelial and smooth muscle cells were harvested, expanded *in vitro*, and seeded onto biodegradable matrix scaffolds that were tubularized and used to replace ureteral segments in each animal (71). The results suggested that the combination of both smooth muscle and urothelial cell–matrix scaffolds can provide a template wherein a functional ureter may be created *de novo*. The same strategy has been applied for uretheral reconstruction (Fig. 4). In studies involving ureters and urethras, if an entire segment was replaced, cells were needed to prevent contracture, whereas if the area replaced was small in at least one of its dimensions—for example, an onlay graft for urethral replacement—cells were not essential for adequate healing.

In select patients with hypospadias, genital skin may be insufficient for repair and alternative tissues may be needed

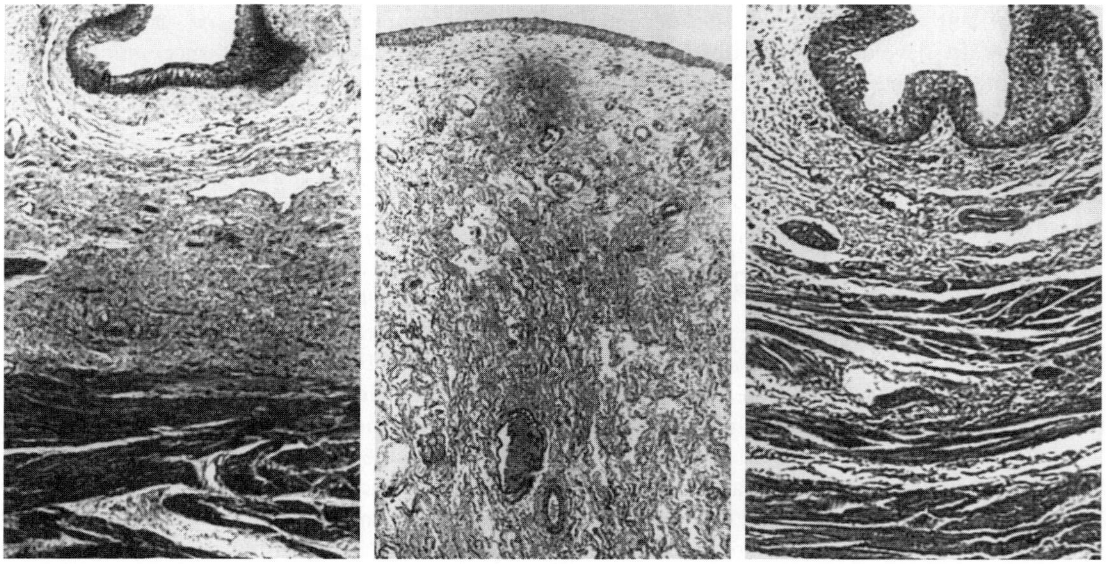

Figure 3 Histologic analysis of scaffold implants 6 months after surgery (hematoxylin and eosin; ×140) are shown for normal canine bladder (left), the bladder dome of a cell-free polymer reconstructed bladder (mostly scar tissue) (middle), and a tissue-engineered neobladder (right).

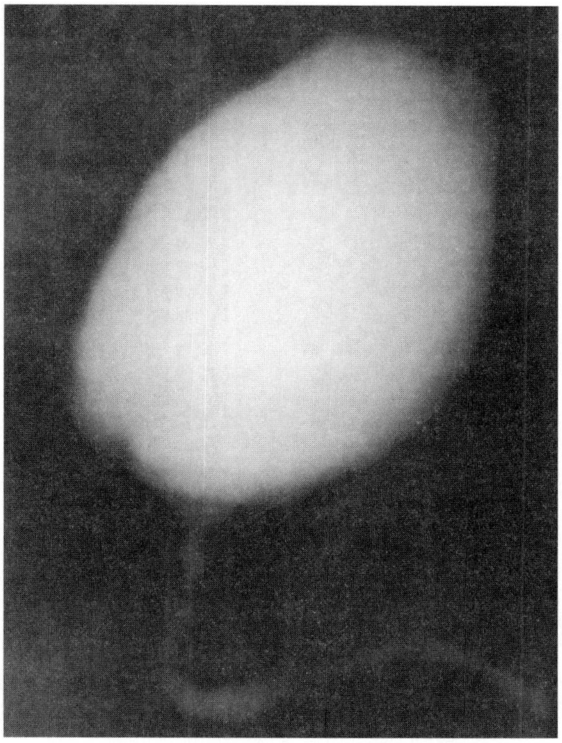

Figure 4 Urethra reconstructed using a collagen matrix. Radiographic urethrogram of reconstructed urethra in a patient using a collagen matrix shows a normal-caliber lumen with no evidence of stricture.

for urethral reconstruction. Clinical results with donor onlay grafts for hypospadias repair have been reported (72). These grafts, composed of microdissected submucosa from donor bladders, are processed in a multistep fashion to produce an acellular matrix that can conform to any desired shape. Long-term follow-up of patients who have undergone repair of their hypospadias with this novel matrix have so far demonstrated successful outcome with regard to cosmesis and function (72a, b). The use of a collagen inert matrix appears to be beneficial in patients who have undergone previous hypospadias repair and may lack genital skin for reconstruction.

Tissue-engineering techniques have also been applied to erectile tissues. Experiments have already demonstrated that human corporal smooth muscle cells can be expanded *in vitro* seeded onto a biodegradable matrix, and transferred *in vivo* where formation of corpus cavernosum muscle occurs (73). Capillary formation was also facilitated by the addition of endothelial cells in composite with the transferred cells. One can envision that corporal cavernosal tissue could be safely and easily obtained under local anesthesia and explanted cultures of autologous human corporal smooth muscle cells, fibroblasts, and endothelial cells could be expanded and delivered with a biodegradable scaffold onto an *in vivo* environment as an autograft for reconstruction. These cells may even be genetically altered to deliver certain local effects, such as production of prostaglandin E, which can lead to resumption of erectile functionality, and this is being explored as a possible treatment for impotency.

There are definite advantages to treating urinary incontinence and vesicoureteral reflux (VUR) endoscopically. However, a major objective has been to find the ideal implant material or bulking agent. The ideal substance should be injectable, nonimmunogenic, nonmigratory, volume stable, and safe for human use. Long-term studies were conducted to determine the effectiveness of injectable chondrocytes *in vivo* (74, 75). Alginate, a liquid solution of glucoronic and mannuronic acid, can be embedded with chondrocytes and delivered through endoscopic injection to the preferred site in the bladder or bladder neck, in the case of incontinence. A biopsy of the ear could easily serve as the autologous source of chondrocytes. Six miniature swine underwent bilateral creation of reflux and served as an animal model. Chondrocytes were harvested from the left auricular surface and expanded *in vitro*. The animals then underwent endoscopic repair of reflux with the injectable chondrocyte solution on the right side only. All animals demonstrated successful cure of reflux in the repaired ureter without evidence of hydronephrosis on excretory urography (75a). This study demonstrates that chondrocytes can be easily harvested and combined with alginate *in vitro* for endoscopic injection to correct VUR without evidence of obstruction. Since its conception, chondrocyte technology has been used in studies sanctioned by the United States Food and Drug Administration in patients with reflux and incontinence. Furthermore, the system of injectable autologous cells may also be applicable for the treatment of other medical conditions, such as rectal incontinence, dysphonia, plastic reconstruction, and whenever an injectable permanent biocompatible material is needed.

With the advent of prenatal ultrasonography, the prenatal diagnosis of patients with bladder disease is now more common. The absence of bladder filling, a mass of echogenic tissue on the lower abdominal wall, or a low-set umbilicus during prenatal sonography may suggest the diagnosis of bladder exstrophy. These findings along with intraluminal intestinal calcifications may also suggest the presence of a cloacal malformation. A prenatal rather than postnatal diagnosis of exstrophy may be beneficial, and there is renewed interest in performing a single-stage reconstruction in some patients. Therefore, having a ready supply of urologic-associated tissue for surgical reconstruction at birth may be advantageous. Theoretically, once the diagnosis of bladder exstrophy is confirmed prenatally, a small bladder and skin biopsy could be obtained via ultrasound guidance. The different cells types could then be expanded *in vitro* and using the tissue-engineering

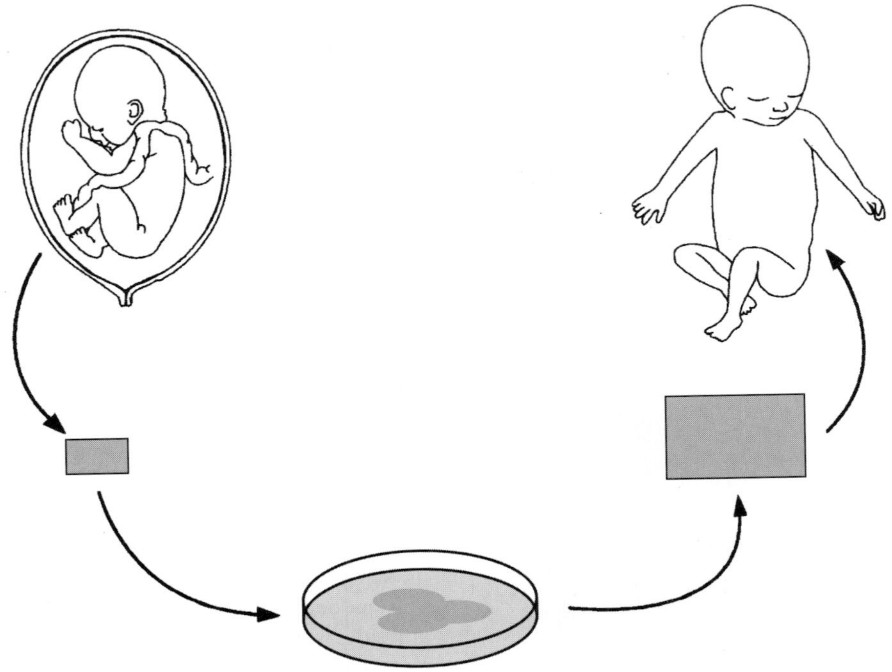

Figure 5 Schematic diagram of fetal tissue harvest and engineering.

techniques previously described, reconstituted bladder and skin structures could be prepared for a one-stage reconstruction at birth, allowing adequate anatomic and functional closure (Fig. 5). Toward this end, bladder exstrophy was created in a group of fetal lambs (76, 77). Small bladder specimens were harvested via fetoscopy. The bladder specimen was separated, and muscle and urothelial cells were harvested and expanded separately. Seven to 10 days before delivery, the expanded bladder muscle cells were seeded on one side, and the urothelial cells on the opposite side, of a PGA polymer. After delivery, surgical closure of the bladders was performed using the tissue-engineered bladder tissue. Cystograms demonstrated that these tissue-engineered augmented bladders were more compliant and had higher capacities when compared to the control group. Histologic analysis also revealed that the engineered tissue demonstrated a normal histologic pattern, indistiguishable from that of native bladders at 2 months. In addition to being able to manage the bladder exstrophy complex *in utero* with tissue-engineering techniques, one could also manage patients after birth in a similar manner. Bladder tissue biopsies could be obtained at the time of the initial operation and the different cell types preserved indefinitely as a repository, which can serve as a resource to elucidate the cellular, molecular, and genetic mechanisms required for the development and future prevention of these anomalies.

V. Conclusion

Cytogenetics, molecular biology, gene therapy, and tissue engineering are just a few examples of some of the expanding areas that continue to make significant contributions to the field of urology. As clinical researchers become more familiar with some of the investigative techniques encountered in the laboratory setting, applications to clinical urology should expand, improving treatment and prevention of disease.

References

1. Hudson, M. A., and Catalona, W. J. (1996). Urothelial tumors of the bladder, upper tracts, and prostate. *In* "Adult and Pediatric Urology" J. Y. Gillenwater, J. T. Grayhack, S. S. Howards, and J. W. Duckett, eds.), p. 1394. Mosby-Yearbook, St. Louis.
2. Whang, I. S., and Benson, M. C. (1992). Flow cytometry in urology, *In* "High Tech Urology: Technical Innovations and Their Clinical Applications" (J.A. Smith, Jr., ed.), p. 234. Saunders, Philadelphia.
3. Shapiro, H. M. (1982). "Pratical Flow Cytometry," 2nd Ed. Alan R. Liss, New York.
4. Pretlow, T. G., and Pretlow, T. P. (1982). "Cell Separation: Methods and Selected Applications." Academic Press, New York.
5. Meyers, F. J., Gumerlock, P. H., Teplitz, R. L., *et al.* (1989). Sequential flow cytometry and single gene analysis by enzymatic amplification and allele specific oligonucleotide hybridization of urothelial cells. *J. Urol.* **142,** 1599–1601.
6. Feitchter, G. E. (1988). DNA flow cytometry in diagnostic cytopathol-

ogy: Methodologic consideration and current state of clinical applications. *In* "New Frontiers in Cytology" (K. Goerttler, G. E. Feichter, and S. Witte, eds.). Springer-Verlag, Berlin.

7. Jacobsen, S., Carstensen, A., Kallenius, G., and Svenson, S. (1986). Fluorescence-activated cell analysis of P-fibriae receptor accessibility on uroepithelial cells of patients with renal scarring, *Eur. J. Clin. Microbiol.* **5**(6), 649–654.
8. Southern, E. M. (1975). Detection of specific sequences among DNA fragments separated by gel electrophoresis. *J. Mol. Biol.* **98,** 503–517.
9. Eisenstein, B. I. (1990). The polymerase chain reaction: A new method of using molecular genetics for medical diagnosis. *N. Engl. J. Med.* **322,** 178–183.
10. Mikkelsen, T., Cavenee, W. K. (1990). Suppressors of the malignant phenotype. *Cell Growth Diff.* **1,** 201–207.
11. Davis, L. M. (1991). Molecular analysis of chromosomal rearrangements using pulsed field gel electrophoresis and somatic cell hybrids. *Environ. Mol. Mutagen.* **18**(4), 263–269.
12. Bell, D. A., Tayor, J. A., Paulson, D. F., Robertson, C. N., Mohler, J. L., and Lucier, G. W. (1993). Genetic risk and carcinogen exposure: A common inhertited defect of the carcinogen (GSTM1) that increases susceptibility to bladder cancer. *J. Nat. Cancer Inst.* **85**(14), 1159–1164.
13. Nishiyama, Y., Suwa, H., Okamoto, K., Fukumoto, M., Hiai, H., and Toyokuni, S. (1995). Low incidence of point mutations in H-, K-, and N-ras oncogenes and p53 tumor suppressor gene in renal cell carcinoma and peritoneal mesothelioma of Wistar rats induced by ferric nitrilotriacetate. *Jpn. J. Cancer Res.* **86**(12), 1150–1158.
14. Bosland, M. C. (1999). Use of animal models in defining efficacy of chemoprevention agents against prostate cancer. *Eur. Urol.* **35**(5–6), 459–463.
15. Nordenskjold, A., Friedman, E., Tapper-Persson, M., Soderhall, C., Leviav, A., Svensson, J., and Anvret, M. (1999). Screening for mutations in candidate genes for hypospadias. *Urol. Res.* **27**(1), 49–55.
16. Melo, K. F., Latronico, A. C., Costa, E. M., Billerbeck, A. E., Medonica, B. B., and Amhold, I. J. (1999). A novel point mutation (R840S) in the androgen receptor in a Brazilian family with partial androgen insensitivity syndrome. *Human Mut.* **14**(4), 353.
17. Kulak, S. C., Kozlowski, K., Semina, E. V., Pearce, W. G., and Walter, M. A. (1998). Mutation in the RIEG1 gene patients with iridogoniodysgenesis syndrome. *Human Mol. Genet.* **7**(7), 113–117.
18. Fagerli, J., Schneck, F. X., Lee, P. A., Bellinger, M. F., and Witchell, S. F. (1999). Absence of microdeletions in the Y chromosome in patients with a history of cryptorchidism and azoospermia or oligospermia. *Fertil. Steril.* **71**(4), 697–700.
19. Kohler, B., Schumacher, V., Schulte-Orerberg, U., Biewald, W., Leunert, T., l'Allenand, D., Royer-Pokora, B., and Graters, A. (1999). Bilateral Wilms tumor in a boy with severe hypospadias and cryptorchidism due to a heterozygous mutation in WT1 gene. *Pediatr. Res.* **45**(2), 187–190.
20. Bratthauer, G. L. (1999). Processing of tissue specimens. *In* "Immunocytochemical Methods and Protocols," 2nd Ed. (L. C. Javois, ed.), pp. 79–84. Humana Press, New Jersey.
21. Nardone, R. M. (1999). *In situ* hybridization to human chromosomes of an alkaline phosphatase-labeled centromeric probe. *In* "Immunocytochemical Methods and Protocols," 2nd Ed. (L. C. Javois, ed.), pp. 365–370. XX, New Jersey.
22. Esrig, D., Spruck, C. H. III, Nichols, P. W., Chaiwun, B., Steven, K., Groshen, S., Chen, S.-C., Skinner, D. G., Jones, P. A., and Cote, R. J. (1993). p53 nuclear protein accumulation correlates with mutations in the p53 gene, tumor grade, and stage in bladder cancer. *Am. J. Pathol.* **143,** 1389.
23. Vet, J. A., Bringuier, P. P., Schaafsma, H. E., Witjes, J. A., Debruyne, F. M., and Schalken, J. A. (1995). Comparison of p53 protein overexpression with p53 mutation in bladder cancer: Clinical and biologic aspects. *Lab. Invest.* **73,** 837.
24. Cordon-Cardo, C., Dalbagni, D., Saez, G. T., Oliva, M. R., Zhang, Z. F., Rosai, J., Reuter, V. E., and Pellicer, A. (1994). p53 mutations in human bladder cancer: Geonotypic versus phenotypic patterns. *Int. J. Cancer* **56,** 347.
25. Stein, J. P., Grossfeld, G. D., Ginsberg, D. A., Esrig, D., Freeman, J. A., Figuero, A. J., Skinner, D. G., and Cote, R. (1998). Prognostic markers in bladder cancer: A contemporary review of the literature. *J. Urol.* **163**(3–1), 645–659.
26. Terada, T., Kato, M., Horie, S., Endo, K., and Kitamura, Y. (1998). Expression of pancreatic alpha-amylase protein and messenger RNA in hilar primitive bile ducts and hepatocytes during human fetal liver organogenesis: An immunohistochemical and *in situ* hybridization study. *Liver* **18**(5), 314–315.
27. Gopalkrishna, V., Srivastara, A. N., Hedau, S., Sharma, J. K., and Das, B. C. (1995). Detection of human papillomavirus DNA sequences in cancer of the urinary bladder by *in situ* hybridisation and polymerase chain reaction. *Genitourin. Med.* **71**(4), 232–233.
28. Eyden, B. (1999). Electron microscopy in tumour diagnosis: Continuing to complement other diagnositc techniques. *Histopathology* **35**(2), 102–108.
29. McGrath, T., and Center, M. S. (1988). Mechanisms of multidrug resistance in HL 60 cells: Evidence that a surface membrane protein distinct from P-glycoprotein contributes to reduced cellular acculmulation of drug. *Cancer Res.* **48,** 3959–3963.
30. Deffie, A. M., Alam, T., Seneviratne, C., *et al.* (1988). Multifactorial resistance to adriamycin: Relationship of DNA repair, glutathione transferase activity, drug efflux, and P-glycoprotein in cloned cell lines of adriamycin-sensitive and resistant P388 leukemia. *Cancer Res.* **48,** 3595–3602.
31. Ueda, K., Cornwell, M. M., Gottesman, M. M., *et al.* (1986). The mdr1 gene, responsible for multidrug-resistance, codes for P-glycoprotein. *Biochem. Biophys. Res. Commun.* **141,** 956–962.
32. Pastan, I., Gottesman, M. M., Ueda, K., *et al.* (1988). A retrovirus carrying an MDR1 cDNA confers multidrug resistance and polarized expression of P-glycoprotein MDCK cells. *Proc. Natl. Acad. Sci. U.S.A.* **85,** 4486–4490.
33. Taneja, S. S., and Belldegrun, A. (1998). Prospects for the application of gene therapy to urologic malignancy. *In* Kirby, Roger S., O'Leary, Michael P. (editors). "Recent Advances in Urology" (R. S. Kirby and M. P. O'Leary, eds.), pp. 151–168. Churchhill Livingstone, New York.
34. Yee, J.-K. (1999). Retroviral vectors. *In* "The Development of Human Gene Therapy" (T. Friedman, ed.), pp. 21–45. Cold Spring Harbor Laboratory Press, New York.
35. Hitt, M. M., Parks, R. J., and Graham, F. L. (1999). Structure and genetic organization of adenovirus vectors. *In* Friedman, T. (editor). "The Development of Human Gene Therapy" (T. Friedman, ed.), pp. 61–86. Cold Spring Harbor Laboratory Press, New York.
36. Samulski, R. J., Sully, M., and Muzyczka, N. (1999). Adeno-associated viral vectors. *In* "The Development of Human Gene Therapy" (T. Friedman, ed.), pp. 131–172. Cold Spring Harbor Laboratory Press, New York.
37. Graham, F., and Prevec, L. (1995). Methods for construction of adenovirus vectors. *Mol. Biotechnol.* **3,** 207–220.
38. Tepper, R. I., Pattengale, P. K., and Leder, P. (1989). Murine interleukin-4 displays potent anti-tumor activiity *in vivo. Cell* **57,** 503.
39. Mehrara, B. J., Saadeh, P. B., Steinbrech, D. S., Dudziak, M., Spector, J. A., Greenwald, J. A., Gittes, G. K., and Longaker, M. T. (1999). Adeovirus-mediated gene therapy of osteoblasts *in vitro* and *in vivo. J. Bone Miner. Res.* **14**(8), 1290–1301.
40. Nabel, G. J., Nabel, E. G., Yang, Z. Y., *et al.* (1993). Direct gene transfer with DNA liposome complexes in melanoma: Expression, biologic activity and lack of toxicity in humans. *Proc. Natl. Acad. Sci. U.S.A.* **90,** 11307.

41. Etienne, J. M., Roux, P., Bourguard, P. *et al.* (1992). Cell targeting by murine recombinant retroviruses. *Bone Marrow Transplant.* **9,** 139.
42. Kasahara, N., Dozy, A. M., Kan, Y. W., *et al.* (1994). Tissue-specific targeting of retroviruses through ligand-receptor interactions. *Science* **266,** 1373.
43. Smith, M. J., Rousculp, M. D., Goldsmith, K. T., Curiel, D. T., and Garver, Jr., R. I. (1994). Surfactant protein A-directed toxin gene kills lung cancer cells *in vitro. Human Gene Ther.* **5,** 29.
44. Vile, R. G., Miller, N., Cernajovsky, Y., *et al.* (1993). *In vitro* and *in vivo* targeting of gene expression to melanoma cells. *Cancer Res.* **53,** 962.
45. Pang, S., Taneja, S., Dardashti, K., *et al.* (1993). Prostate tissue specificity of the prostate-specific antigen promoter isolated from patient with prostate cancer. *Human Gene Ther.* **6,** 1417.
46. Gao, L., Wagner, E., Cotton, M., *et al.* (1993). Direct *in vivo* gene transfer to airway epithelium employing adenovirus–polysine–DNA complexes. *Human Gene Ther.* **4,** 17.
47. Nicolau, C., Le Pape, A., Soriano, P., Fargette, F., and Juhel, M. F. (1983). *In vivo* expression of rat insulin after intravenous administration of the liposome-entrapped gene for rat insulin. I. *Proc. Natl. Acad. Sci. U.S.A.* **80,** 1068.
48. Lin, L., Zhu, G., Yoo, J. J., Sukhatme, V. P., and Atala, A. (2000). A novel system for the enhancement of adenovirus-mediated gene transfer to uroepithelium. Submitted.
49. Mahari, D. M., Sheehy, M. J., Yang, N.-S. (1997). DNA cancer vaccines: A gene gun approach: *Immunol Cell Biol.* **75**(5), 456–460.
50. Weaver, J. C. (1993). Electroporation: A general phenomenon for manipulating cells and tissues. *J. Cell. Biochem.* **51,** 426.
51. Chang, D. C., Gao, P. Q., and Maxwell, B. L. (1992). High efficiency gene transfection by electroporation using a radio-frequency electric field. *Biochim. Biophys. Acta* **1092,** 153.
52. Yoo, J. J., Soker, S., Lin, L. F., Mehegan, K., Guthrie, P. D., and Atala, A. (1999). Direct *in vivo* gene transfer to urologic organs. *J. Urol.* **162,** 1115–1118.
53. Unger, E. C., McCreery, T. P., and Sweitzer, R. H. (1997). Ultrasound enhances gene expression of liposomal transfection. *Invest. Radiol.* **32,** 723.
54. Fechhimer, M., Boylan, J. F., Parker, S., Sisken, J. E., Patel, G. L., and Zimmer, S. G. (1987). Transfection of mammalian cells with plasmid DNA by scrape loading and sonication loading. *Proc. Natl. Acad. Sci. U.S.A.* **84,** 8465.
55. Mitragotri, S., Edwards, D. A., Blankschtein, D., and Langer, R. (1995). A mechanistic study of ultrasound-enhanced transdermal drug delivery. *J. Pharmaceut. Sci.* **84,** 697.
56. Machluff, M., Hirose, K., Soker, S., and Atala, A. (1999). Ultrasound: A novel vector for bladder gene transfection. *J. Urol.* **161**(4) (Suppl.), 171.
56a. Rodriguez, R., and Simons, J. W. (1999). Urologic applications of gene therapy. *Urology* **64**(3), 404.
57. Sanda, M. G., Ayyagari, S. R., Jaffee, E. M., *et al.* (1994). Demonstration of a rational strategey for human prostate cancer gene therapy. *J. Urol.* **151,** 622.
58. Vieweg, J., Rosenthal, F., Banerji, R., *et al.* (1994). Immunotherapy of prostate cancer in the Dunning rat model: Use of cytokine modified tumor vaccines. *Cancer Res.* **54,** 1760.
59. Jaffe, E. M., Dranoff, G., Cohen, L., *et al.* (1993). High efficiency gene transfer into primary human tumor explants without cell selection. *Cancer Res.* **53,** 2221.
60. Werthman, P. E., Drazan, K. E., Rosenthal, J. T., *et al.* (1996). Adenoviral p53 gene transfer to orthotopic and peritoneal murine bladder cancer. *J. Urol.* **155,** 753.
61. Ehrlich, R. M., Reda, E. F., Koyle, M. A., Kogan, S. J., and Levitt, S. B. (1989). Complications of bladder mucosal graft. *J. Urol.* **142,** 626.
62. McDougal, W. S. (1992). Metabolic complications of urinary intestinal diversion *J. Urol.* **147,** 1199–1208.
63. Duel, B. P., Gonzalez, R., and Barthold, J. S. (1998). Alternative techniques for augmentation cystoplasty. *J. Urol.* **159**(3), 999.
64. Cilento, B. J., Freeman, M. R., Schneck, F. X., Retik, A. B., and Atala, A. (1994). Characterization of human bladder urothelia expanded *in vitro. J. Urol.* **152,** 665.
65. Freeman, M. R., Yoo, J. J., Raab, G., *et al.* (1997). Heparin-binding EGF-like growth factor is an autocrine growth factor for human urothelial cells and is synthesized by epithelial and smooth muscle cells in the human bladder. *J. Clin. Invest.* **99,** 1028.
66. Atala, A. (1999). Future perspectives in reconstructive surgery using tissue engineering: *Urol. Clinics N. Am.* **26**(1), 157–165, ix–x.
67. Yoo, J. J., Meng, J., Oberpenning, F., and Atala, A. (1998). Bladder augmentation using allogenic bladder submucosa seeded with cells. *Urology* **54**(2), 221–225.
68. Chen, F., Yoo, J. J., and Atala, A. (1999). Acellular collagen matrix as a possible "off the shelf" biomaterial for urethral repair. *Urology* **54**(3), 407–410.
69. Atala, A., Vacanti, J. P., Peters, C. A., Mandell, J., Retik, A. B., and Freeman, M. R. (1992). Formation of urothelial structures *in vivo* from dissociated cells attached to biodegradable polymer scaffolds *in vitro. J. Urol.* **148,** 658–662.
70. Atala, A., Freeman, M. R., Vacanti, J. P., Shepard, J., and Retik, A. B. (1993). Implantation *in vivo* and retrieval of artificial structures consisting of rabbit and human urothelium and human bladder muscle. *J. Urol.* **150,** 608–612.
71. Yoo, J. J., Satar, N., Retik, A. B., *et al.* (1995). Ureteral replacement using biodegradable polymer scaffolds seeded with urothelial and smooth muscle cells. *J. Urol.* **153,** 4 (Suppl.).
72. Atala, A., Guzman, L., and Retik, A. B. (1999). A novel inert collagen matrix for hypospadias repair. *J. Urol.* **163,** 1148–1150.
72a. Chen, F., Yoo, J. J., and Atala, A. (2000). Experimental and clinical experience using tissue regeneration for urethral reconstruction. *World J. Urol.* **18,** 67–70.
72b. Atala, A., Guzman, L., and Retik, A. B. (1999). A novel inert collagen matrix for hypospadias repair. *J. Urol.* **162,** 1148–1151.
73. Kershen, R. T., Yoo, J. J., Moreland, R. B., *et al.* (1998). Novel system for the formation of human corpus cavernosum smooth muscle tissue *in vivo. J. Urol.* **159,** 156 (Suppl.).
74. Atala, A., Olm, L. G., Kim, W., Paige, K. T., Vacanti, J. P., Retik, A. B., and Vacanti, C. A. (1993). Injectable alginate seeded with chondrocytes as a potential treatment for vesicoureteral reflux. *J. Urol.* **150,** 745.
75. Atala, A., Kim, W., Paige, K. T., Vacanti, C. A., and Retik, A. B. (1994). Endoscopic treatment of vesicouretral reflux with chondrocyte-alginate suspension. *J. Urol.* **152,** 641.
75a. Atala, A., Kim, W., Paige, K. T., Vacanti, C. A., and Retik, A. B. (1994). Endoscopic treatment of vesicoureteral reflux with chondrocyte-alginate suspension. *J. Urol.* **152,** 641–643.
76. Fauza, D. O., Fishman, S., Meheegan, K., and Atala, A. (1998). Videofetoscopically assisted fetal tissue engineering: bladder augmentation. *J. Pediatr. Surg.* **33,** 7.
77. Fauza, D. O., Fishman, S., Meheegan, K., *et al.* (1998). Videofetoscopically assisted fetal tissue engineering: Skin replacement. *J. Pediatr. Surg.* **33,** 357.

80

Research in Cardiac Surgery

Robert M. Mentzer, Jr., Caren M. Mulford, and Robert D. Lasley
Department of Surgery, University of Kentucky College of Medicine, Lexington, Kentucky 40536

I. Introduction

Since the first successful heart operation by Rehn (1) in 1896, cardiac surgery in adults has evolved rapidly from simple closure of heart wounds to complex repairs of congenital and acquired heart diseases (Table I). Major milestones include the ligation of the ductus arteriosus in 1937 (2–4), resection of an aortic coarctation in 1944 (5–7), closed mitral valvulotomies in 1948 (8–11), and, perhaps most importantly, development and application of cardiopulmonary bypass in the 1950s (10, 12, 13). Although coronary artery grafting as we know it today can be traced back to the early experiments by Alexis Carrel in 1910 (14), myocardial revascularization as a therapeutic modality for the treatment of ischemic heart disease began in 1967 (10, 15–17). This year also marks one of the most remarkable achievements in cardiac surgery—the first human heart transplant (18–21).

Perhaps the most significant element linking all of these advances is their foundation in research. Each of these achievements is the result of an investigative process originating in scientific inquiry into surgical problems, continuing with experimentation in laboratory models, and culminating in successful clinical cases. Furthermore, these developments represent the diligence of surgeons and researchers who continually challenged themselves to develop safer and more effective treatments for patients with life-threatening heart disease. These individuals possessed a unique element of adventure, curiosity, perseverance, and courage. Each milestone reflects their ability to apply sound scientific principles and methodologies in a laboratory setting to test hypotheses based on knowledge of cardiac physiology held at the time. Their technological developments and scientific achievements have enabled surgeons to perform more procedures on the heart with relative ease and safety. As a consequence, cardiac surgery is now one of the most commonly performed operations in the United States. Nevertheless, the challenge of surgically treating patients with heart diseases in the future is no less than it was 25 or 50 years ago.

Until recently, many of the most important advances made in cardiac surgery have been technological in nature, primarily developments allowing for new types of operations or improvements on existing procedures. Yet, despite the use of new and creative surgical techniques, patients today still die or experience major complications, requiring therapy after both closed and open-heart procedures. In

Table I Early Developments in Cardiac Surgery Research

Year	Development	Ref.
1882	Block sutures wounds in rabbit hearts	1
1896	Ludwig Rehn, M.D., performs first successful suture in the human heart	1
1905	Harvey Cushing, M.D., experiments with mitral valvulotomy in dogs	8
1905	Alexis Carrel, M.D., conducts early exploration into organ transplantation, involving transplantation of the heart of one dog onto the carotid artery and jugular vein of another	19
1907	John C. Munro, M.D., reports on experiments with ligation of the ductus arteriosus on cadavers of newborn infants	4
1910	Alexis Carrel, M.D., attempts revascularization of the ascending and descending aorta in dogs	14
1916	Jay McLean, M.D., discovers heparin	12
1925	Henry S. Souttar, M.D., performs the first successful mitral valvulotomy	9
1931–1953	John Gibbon, M.D., develops the heart–lung machine	10, 13
1935–1936	Clarence Crafoord, M.D., experiments with correction of aortic coarctation in dogs	5
1937	John W. Streider, M.D., performs ligation of the ductus arteriosus. Patient dies on fourth post-operative day due to acute dilation of the stomach	2
1938	Robert E. Gross, M.D., experiments with correction of aortic coarctation in dogs	6
1938	Robert E. Gross, M.D., performs successful ligation of the ductus arteriosus	3
1944	Clarence Crafoord, M.D., performs successful correction of aortic coarctation	5
1945	Robert E. Gross, M.D., performs successful correction of aortic coarctation	7
1948	Following his own research with the procedure in the 1940s, Charles P. Bailey, M.D., performs a series of mitral valvulotomies. After this point, the procedure becomes more widely used	10, 11
1950	W. G. Bigelow, M.D., reports on use of hypothermia to lengthen the period of total cardiac inflow occlusion in animal models	10
1953	Following years of experimentation in animal models, Claude S. Beck, M.D., performs successful myocardial revascularization	15
1954–1955	C. Walton Lillehei, M.D., uses controlled cross-circulation and a bubble oxygenator for intracardiac surgery in 45 patients	10
1958	Richard Lower, M.D., and Norman Shumway, M.D., begin experimentation with heart transplantation in dogs	21
1962	Vladimir Demikhov, M.D., publishes "Experimental Transplantation of Vital Organs," reporting on his research with organ transplantation in animal models since 1950	20
1967	C. N. Barnard, M.D., performs the first human-to-human heart transplant procedure	18
1967–1969	Following his own experimentation with the procedure, as well as that of other pioneers in myocardial revascularization, W. D. Johnson, M.D., reports on the use of coronary artery bypass grafts in 301 patients, a seminal study marking the beginning of modern CABG surgery	16, 17

patients with ischemic heart disease, the mortality after first-time revascularization [coronary artery bypass grafting (CABG)] ranges between 2 and 3% for low-risk elective patients; it may be as high as 10–20% for high-risk emergent patients. The incidence of perioperative myocardial infarction continues to range between 3 and 7%. In fact, it may be higher depending on the definitions and criteria (22, 23). Finally, myocardial stunning or reversible postischemic myocardial dysfunction often occurs after all types of heart surgery, possibly in as many as 70–90% of the patients. In the setting of depressed left ventricular function, a long aortic cross-clamp time, a repeat coronary artery operation, or an emergent combined valve/CABG procedure, myocardial stunning can contribute significantly to increased morbidity and mortality in high-risk patients (24, 25).

In some respects, solutions to the major challenges facing cardiac surgeons today require less of an emphasis on technological developments and more of an emphasis on experimentation at the basic science level. The next major advance in cardiac surgery may come from a better understanding of the mechanisms of disease in order to manipulate the physiology of the heart to minimize and/or eliminate surgery-related complications. Because surgical reparative procedures usually involve a period of ischemia/reperfusion, there is a great need to elucidate the mechanisms underlying phenomena such as stunning, hibernation, classic ischemic preconditioning, the second window of preconditioning, and pharmacologic preconditioning. We need to identify the cellular and subcellular disturbances that exist among the various sarcolemmal receptors and intercellular signaling pathways and effectors that are involved in limiting both postischemic cardiac dysfunction and myocardial necrosis. Finally, we need to know more about the mechanism(s) underlying apoptosis, or programmed cell death, and the role it plays in the development of myocardial infarction and ventricular remodeling.

This is not to say that investigation into new technological advances that make cardiac surgery safer is not important or necessary. Surgeons and researchers cannot ignore the potential benefits, for example, of developments in robotics, minimally invasive surgical techniques, and the application of computer technology in cardiac surgery. Exploration in these areas will, and should, certainly continue. Presently, however, the main thrust of research in cardiac surgery is at the cellular, subcellular, and molecular levels. The next generation of surgical scientists will need to focus their research on the pathophysiology of myocardial disease in order to develop methods for preventing the complications resulting from cardiac surgery. The purpose of this chapter is to review some of the animal preparations and laboratory techniques that are currently being used to acquire this new knowledge.

II. Myocardial Stunning

Myocardial ischemia is characterized by reduced ventricular function and altered myocardial metabolism. If coronary blood flow is restored within 15–20 min, the injury is reversible, but myocardial contractility may remain depressed for hours to days. This reversible postischemic ventricular contractile dysfunction that occurs despite restoration of normal blood flow is termed myocardial stunning (26, 27) (Table II). There is considerable evidence that the primary mediators of stunning include intracellular calcium overload and oxidative stress induced by reactive oxygen species (ROS) generated at the onset of reperfusion [28, 29]. Although it is known that intracellular calcium may return to normal levels early during reperfusion, transient increases in intracellular calcium can lead to increases in calcium-dependent protein kinase C and proteases, and a concomitant reduction in myofilament calcium sensitivity (28, 30). Likewise, a release of ROS can injure intracellular proteins such as SR calcium ATPase, the ryanodine receptor, and the contractile proteins, the latter most likely being the primary targets. Regardless, although the actual mechanism of stunning is still unknown, there is considerable evidence that the interactions between calcium overload and ROS play important etiologic roles. Because myocardial stunning contributes substantially to postoperative morbidity and mortality after heart surgery, intense efforts are underway to elucidate the phenomenon's relationship to receptor activation, intracellular signaling pathways, and common effectors. This has resulted in the use of numerous experimental preparations, methods, and techniques to study the pathophysiology of stunning both *in vivo* and *in vitro*.

A. Preparations for the Study of Myocardial Stunning

1. Intact Animals

The most commonly used model to study *in vivo* myocardial stunning is a regional myocardial ischemia preparation in which a distal segment of the left anterior descending (LAD) or left circumflex (LCX) coronary artery is occluded. Such regional ischemia stunning experiments can be performed in both large (pig, dog, sheep) and small (rabbit) animal preparations. Large animal models provide the opportunity to simultaneously measure changes in ventricular function, coronary blood flow, and metabolism, in both the stunned and normally perfused myocardium, and each animal can serve as its own control. One of the primary determinants of the degree of stunning is the amount of coronary collateral blood flow during ischemia. Because dogs, but not pigs, have a well-developed native coronary collateral circulation, collateral blood flow during ischemia must be measured in all canine regional ischemia studies. Myocardial stunning can also be studied in global ischemia studies during which animals are placed on cardiopulmonary bypass

Table II Evidence for Ischemic Preconditioning, Stunning, and Chronic Hibernation in Humans

Ischemic Preconditioning	Stunning	Hibernation
Human atrial trabeculae	Unstable angina	Unstable and stable angina
Cultured human cardiac myocytes	Acute myocardial infarction with early reperfusion	Acute myocardial infarction
Warm-up angina	Exercise-induced ischemia	Improved LV function after angioplasty
Preinfarction angina	Open-heart surgery	Improved LV function after coronary artery bypass grafting
Coronary angioplasty	Cardiac transplantation	Congestive heart failure
Cardiopulmonary bypass		
Coronary artery bypass surgery		

and the heart is arrested with or without a cardioplegic solution. Although these studies are technically demanding, they do more closely mimic the patient undergoing heart surgery, compared to regional ischemia studies. The use of hypothermia and cardioplegia permits the ischemic period to be extended beyond the typical 15 min of ischemia used in normothermic regional ischemia studies. Regardless of which stunning model is used, it must be verified that the ischemic time utilized to induce stunning is not associated with myocardial infarction.

In the intact animal, global ventricular function is assessed by measurements of left ventricular developed pressure (LVDP), rate of change of left ventricular pressure ($\pm dP/dt$), LV end-diastolic pressure (LVEDP), and cardiac output. Ventricular pressures are typically measured using a high-fidelity Millar transducer placed through the ventricular wall in the apical region. Cardiac output is measured using a volumetric ultrasonic flow probe placed around the aorta. However, these measurements are inadequate to assess regional ventricular function in regional ischemia studies and are also load dependent. Regional ventricular function is most frequently evaluated by measuring wall thickening (WT) or segment length (SL). Pairs of piezoelectric crystals are normally placed in the LAD and LCX perfused beds such that the distance between either the epicardial and endocardial walls (WT) or a segment of ventricular muscle at a certain depth (SL) is measured during systole and diastole by sonomicrometry. The resulting measurements of systolic WT (SWT) and segment shortening (SS) provide a simple, reliable measurement of regional ventricular function. These piezoelectric crystals can also be used in chronic studies.

The primary limitation to the use of measurements of wall thickening and segment shortening is their sensitivity to changes in heart rate, preload, and afterload. This limitation can be overcome by generating end-systolic pressure thickness and end-systolic pressure length relationships (ESPTR and ESPLR, respectively). Left ventricular pressure thickness/length loops are generated during acute changes in preload or afterload produced by brief (~5–7 sec) occlusions of the vena cava or aorta, respectively. The slope of the line of ESPTR or ESPLR (E_{es}), which is analogous to end systolic elastance (E_{es}) of the end-systolic pressure volume relationship (ESPVR) derived from pressure volume loops, has been shown to be relatively load independent over physiologic pressure ranges. The availability of inexpensive high-speed personal computers and data acquisition software allow for real-time contractility measurements during the experiment. Data collected during the generation of pressure-segment length loops can be further analyzed to measure stroke work (SW), preload recruitable stroke work (PRSW), and preload recruitable stroke work area (PRSWA). Stroke work is afterload sensitive, but PRSW and PRSWA are sensitive and reliable indicators of cardiac contractility independent of preload and afterload. Reportedly, PRSWA is the most sensitive parameter for quantifying regional ischemia-induced ventricular dysfunction (31, 32).

Load-insensitive measurements of cardiac contractility have also been used in global myocardial ischemia studies, based on LV pressure-volume relationships. One technique involves the measurement of LV pressure with a high-fidelity pressure transducer, and ventricular dimensions via the placement of epicardial dimension transducers/crystals along the major and minor axes of the ventricle. Dimension measurements are converted to volume based on the ventricle being modeled as a prolate ellipsoid. An alternative approach is the use of the conductance catheter method to measure electrical conductance of blood in the ventricle (33). Although the cost of this technology has limited its widespread use, recent developments permit the measurement of load-independent cardiac contractility in small animals such as rats and mice.

Because myocardial stunning is defined as reversible postischemic dysfunction on the restoration of coronary perfusion, coronary blood flow must be measured. For the majority of regional and global ischemia studies, the placement of an ultrasonic coronary flow probe on a short segment of dissected coronary artery will suffice. These probes are also designed for use in chronic studies. However, in certain cases, such as in canine models that can exhibit significant coronary collateral blood flow, microsphere techniques must be used to measure residual blood flow during regional ischemia. Microspheres must also be used when measuring blood flow heterogeneity or transmural distribution of blood flow (subepicardial vs. subendocardial). Although this technique has historically relied on the use of radioactive microspheres, the use of fluorescent microspheres has now become accepted.

Metabolic changes that occur in ischemic and stunned myocardium can be assessed by several means. The myocardial biopsy technique is used for obtaining tissue samples of rapidly metabolized compounds such as lactate, ATP, and creatine phosphate (CrP). Transmural tissue samples, which can often be divided into subepicardial and subendocardial layers, are rapidly collected with a standard needle biopsy technique or a rapid-freezing biopsy drill to minimize metabolism and contamination. Samples are then stored in liquid nitrogen until biochemical assays are performed. This method for monitoring myocardial metabolism works well when a limited number of samples are obtained, but multiple biopsies cause tissue trauma and deterioration of the preparation. A noninvasive technique that provides some of the same information as tissue biopsies is nuclear magnetic resonance (^{31}P-NMR) spectroscopy, although this technique is generally not feasible in large animal preparations. Coronary venous or coronary sinus blood samples can be collected to measure the release of numerous metabolites, such as lactate, adenosine, nitric oxide, norepinephrine, and reactive oxygen species, from the area of interest. This technique can be used to supplement metabolic measurements made with tissue biopsies. When used as the sole source for metabolic measurements, however, this technique may not provide an accurate assessment of metabolites from the myocytes or those to which myocytes are exposed. For example, due to the rapid metabolism of adenosine by endothelial cells and erythrocytes, plasma adenosine measurements do not always reflect interstitial fluid levels of adenosine to which the cardiac myocytes are exposed.

A technique that has been used for years to measure neurotransmitter release in the brain, the microdialysis technique, has gained widespread acceptance for estimating interstitial fluid (ISF) metabolites in the heart (34). This technique is based on the principle that small metabolites present in the ISF can diffuse into a small, hollow dialysis fiber inserted into the ventricular muscle. A specified length of dialysis fiber, which is exposed within the muscle wall, is connected to inert silica tubing on both ends. As a physiologic saline solution passes through the fiber, diffusion occurs between the fluid within the dialysis fiber and the ISF surrounding the fiber. The concentration of a compound in the effluent or dialysate collected from the outflow tubing is representative of the intramyocardial ISF concentration of that substance. Because the ISF bathes the cardiac myocytes, the ISF level of a given compound can be used to assess myocyte release rates, substrate utilization, and the presence or absence of exogenously administered agents used to test their cardioprotective effect on stunning. Cardiac microdialysis has been used to measure numerous ISF metabolites such as adenosine, norepinephrine, lactate, and oxygen free radicals (34–37). The advantages of the microdialysis technique are the minimal setup expenses involved and the fact that this technique can provide continuous serial sampling of myocardial ISF metabolites before, during, and after ischemia. The disadvantages of the technique are that it provides only an estimate of ISF concentrations, and there is some tissue trauma incurred during implantation of the fibers.

2. Isolated Perfused Heart Preparations

Another model used to elucidate the detrimental effects of myocardial ischemia on ventricular function is the isolated perfused heart preparation. The standard Langendorff perfused isolated heart is based on the retrograde perfusion of the heart via the aorta and the resultant antegrade coronary perfusion. Hearts in this model can be perfused via either constant flow or constant pressure. However, because left ventricular pressure development is perfusion pressure dependent, ischemia/reperfusion and ventricular function studies in this model should be performed at constant pressure. A variation of this model is the ejecting isolated heart preparation, also referred to as the working heart, which exhibits much higher workloads and O_2 consumption than the Langendorff preparation. In this model, the left atrium is cannulated and connected to a low-pressure reservoir, the aorta is cannulated and connected to a high-pressure reservoir, and the ventricle ejects against this pressure head. Left ventricular output can be altered by adjusting preload, afterload, or both.

Both the Langendorff and ejecting heart preparations are routinely perfused with a buffered physiologic salt solution, e.g., Krebs–Henseleit bicarbonate buffer. The buffer is gassed with 95% oxygen and 5% carbon dioxide to yield P_{O_2} and P_{CO_2} values of ~600 and 40 mmHg, respectively, and pH ~7.4. The buffer must be filtered through a small-pore (~ 0.45-μm) filter to remove small particulate matter that can occlude the capillaries. In the majority of studies glucose (11 m*M*) is the sole energy source, although it is not uncommon to include pyruvate or fatty acids (the latter in the presence of albumin). Extracellular Ca^{2+} concentration should be no greater than 2.0 m*M*, because free plasma Ca^{2+} concentration is in the 1.0–1.5 m*M* range. Although many studies are performed with 2.5 m*M* Ca^{2+}, it has been reported that this extracellular Ca^{2+} concentration accelerates and exacerbates ischemia/reperfusion in this preparation (38). An increasing number of investigators, recognizing the limitations of a blood/protein-free perfusate, now perfuse the Langendorff preparation with erythrocyte-supplemented Krebs buffer or whole blood. This modification increases the O_2-carrying capacity and viscosity of the perfusion medium, which significantly reduces the edema and high coronary flow rates observed in Krebs-perfused hearts.

Ventricular function in the nonejecting preparation is generally measured with a fluid-filled latex balloon, inserted into the left ventricle, that can be filled with varying volumes to generate LV end-diastolic pressures (LVEDP) of 5–10 mmHg. Although pressure–volume curves can be generated prior to and following ischemia, measurement of ventricular function is typically studied using an isovolumetric preparation. The use of the isovolumetric model permits the assessment of ischemia/reperfusion on diastolic function by recording changes in LVEDP. Heart rate can also be controlled by pacing the hearts throughout the study.

The simplicity and high degree of control over experimental conditions with this model permit the study of numerous aspects of ischemia/reperfusion injury on ventricular function. Studies performed in this model are typically performed in rat and rabbit hearts utilizing zero-flow global ischemia, but both low-flow ischemia and hypoxia are also easily studied. These studies are most frequently conducted in the Langendorff preparation with zero-flow global normothermic ischemia, although the ejecting heart preparation is also used. Postischemic ventricular dysfunction in the Langendorff model is assessed by recording changes in systolic and diastolic pressures and/or *dP/dt*. Both normothermic and hypothermic ischemia, with or without cardioplegic arrest, can be studied using this preparation.

Although there have been numerous studies on the effects of global ischemia on ventricular function in isolated perfused hearts, in the vast majority of these cases it is likely that the observed decreases in postischemic function are not due entirely to stunning. This is due to the fact that normothermic ischemia times in isolated rat heart studies are typically 25–30 min in duration, but ischemia times ≥15–20 min are associated with cell death. Deficits in postischemic function thus could be due to stunning, necrosis, or, more likely, to a combination of the two. Based on the numerous studies in the literature, the study of true stunning in the isolated perfused rat heart is difficult, at best. Twenty minutes of global normothermic ischemia in the Krebs-perfused rat heart is associated with a significant increase in reperfusion LVEDP, which is often accompanied by little decrease in systolic LV pressure. However, stunning, as originally defined, is a reversible deficit in systolic function. This limitation needs to be considered when designing stunning experiments.

In order to verify the use of a true stunning model if the ischemic period exceeds 15 min, the extent of irreversible injury or infarction should be determined by one of two methods. The first involves the collection of coronary effluent prior to ischemia and at specific time points throughout reperfusion to measure creatine kinase (CK) release. With this approach, the reperfusion period can be limited to 45–60 min, by which point recovery of LVDP has attained its maximal value. Alternatively, the hearts can be reperfused for 2 hr, after which they are stained with a triphenyltetrazolium chloride (TTC) solution, which stains viable myocardium brick red (due to the presence of dehydrogenase enzymes). If necrosis is to be determined by TTC staining, the hearts must be reperfused for a minimum of 2 hr to obtain valid estimates of necrosis.

3. Other Studies

Many of the same metabolic measurements made in intact animals can be performed in isolated perfused hearts. In global ischemia studies, coronary effluent samples can be readily collected and analyzed for various substrates and catabolites. Tissue samples can be obtained for measurements of cellular metabolites, as described for *in vivo* studies, in both global and regional ischemia studies. The small sizes of rat, rabbit, guinea pig, and mouse hearts are well suited for the use of ^{31}P-NMR spectroscopy. The cardiac microdialysis technique can also be used to estimate ISF metabolites. Metabolic studies with radioactive tracers are routinely used in this preparation.

4. Ventricular Cardiomyocytes

Isolated ventricular cardiomyocyte preparations permit the determination of whether ischemia/reperfusion exerts direct effects on cardiac myocytes. The primary advantage of studying single cardiac myocytes is the ability to determine the role of intracellular pH, Ca^{2+} and other ions, reactive oxygen species (ROS), and other signaling pathways in cardiac myocyte injury. New imaging agents and confocal microscopy permit the measurement of intramitochondrial Ca^{2+} concentrations. The majority of such studies have been performed in ventricular myocytes obtained from rats, guinea pigs, and rabbits, although there are studies in which myocytes have been obtained from canine, porcine, and even human hearts (39, 40).

In general, myocytes are isolated using a Langendorff preparation in which the heart is digested initially with a Ca^{2+}-free physiologic salt solution (PSS), followed by the reintroduction of Ca^{2+} and the enzymes collagenase and hyaluronidase. After various other steps, a relatively homogeneous yield of ventricular myocytes is obtained (41). The quality of the myocyte yield should be verified by determining the percentage of quiescent, rod-shaped cells and/or the number of cells excluding trypan blue. Neonatal ventricular myocytes can be easily cultured, but adult myocytes are typically studied the day of isolation (primary culture). Adult myocytes also do not contract, and thus for contractility studies the myocytes must be electrically stimulated.

There have been numerous studies over the past several years on the effects of simulated ischemia/reperfusion on isolated ventricular myocytes. Although the majority of these studies have investigated mechanisms of cell death, myocardial stunning can also be studied. As in the isolated heart studies, the ischemic or hypoxic insult must be strong enough to induce a contractile deficit but devoid of cell death. Utilizing myocyte suspensions, ischemia is simulated by centrifuging an aliquot of cells into a small pellet and removing the majority of the suspension medium/buffer. The pellet is then covered with a thin layer of mineral oil to prevent myocyte exposure to atmospheric O_2. The packed myocyte pellet in the reduced extracellular volume mimics ischemic conditions. These ischemic incubations are typically performed in the absence of glucose or other energy substrates, and the medium may contain elevated lactate and K^+ to simulate changes that occur during *in vivo* ischemia. After 15–20 min of simulated ischemia, the myocytes are resuspended in an oxygenated medium to simulate reperfusion. Myocyte contractility is measured with a video edge detection system to determine the extent and rate of shortening.

In single myocyte studies, standard fluorescent imaging techniques/systems and various cell-permeable fluorescent dyes permit the measurement of intracellular ions during simulated ischemia/reperfusion. A video edge detection system coupled to the imaging system provides the ability to correlate changes in myocyte contractility with alterations in intracellular metabolites/ions. Myocyte stunning in single cells can be induced with mild hypoxia/reoxygenation or low-flow ischemia.

III. Hibernating Myocardium

Reversible contractile dysfunction that corresponds to or matches a reduction in resting coronary artery blood flow is termed "hibernating myocardium." It represents a balanced reduction in myocardial contraction and myocardial oxygen consumption (42). In general, it is found in patients with severe coronary artery disease and is associated with stable and unstable angina, myocardial infarction, and congestive heart failure. Because it is fully reversible on restoration of normal blood flow, in humans the phenomenon can only be inferred from the findings in clinical studies (43–53) (Table II). Interestingly, human tissue biopsies obtained from hibernating myocardium have shown a dedifferentiation of myocardial cells with the loss of myofibrils, glycogen accumulation, and variable degrees of interstitial fibrosis (42, 54–56). Imaging techniques used to assess hibernating myocardium in humans include the use of positron emission tomography (PET) scanning, thallium redistribution scintigraphy, and dobutamine stress echocardiography. These studies are used to identify the subset of patients with low ejection fractions who would benefit from myocardial revascularization via percutaneous coronary interventions or coronary bypass surgery.

Considerable controversy persists, however, whether the contractile dysfunction is due to an absolute reduction in coronary blood flow or to a reduction in coronary reserve. Likewise, there is controversy whether myocardial hibernation and myocardial stunning may coexist or share a common mechanism (57). Various characteristics of these two phenomena are listed in Table III. It is also unclear whether chronic contractile dysfunction in humans reflects repetitive episodes of stunning or an intrinsic adaptation to ischemia. The latter implies that the heart can alter its phenotype to protect itself from irreversible ischemic injury (52, 58). Consequently, it is not surprising that a number of various animal models have been developed to investigate the perfusion-matching adaptation process. Although the isolated perfused hearts have and can be used to study hibernation, these findings have to be interpreted in the context of denervation, use of crystalloid buffer perfusates, the use of global rather than regional ischemia, and the generally chronic nature of myocardial hibernation. Also, isolated hearts demonstrate little metabolic recovery during prolonged ischemia in contrast to metabolic studies performed *in situ* (43, 59). As a consequence, short-term hibernation is most frequently studied in chronically instrumented dogs, pigs, or miniature swine subjected to regional ischemia. In these short-term hibernation preparations, accumulating evidence suggests that adaptation does occur. If the mechanisms can be elucidated, it may be possible to develop therapeutic strategies that will allow the heart to adapt much more rapidly to ischemia and thus avoid permanent injury (myocardial necrosis) (43, 57).

A. Short-Term Hibernation Models

In the chronically instrumented model described by Sherman *et al.* (60), dogs are sedated and then subjected to general anesthesia. Under sterile conditions, a left thoracotomy is performed in the fifth intercostal space to expose the heart. The dogs are then instrumented for chronic measurements of cardiac and systemic hemodynamics, similar to the parameters described earlier in the *in vivo* myocardial stunning preparation. Following 7 to 10 days of recovery from surgery, the dogs, under light sedation, are subjected to 2 hr of sustained reductions in regional flow sufficient to cause approximately a 50% reduction in regional systolic segment shortening or wall thickening. The heart rate can be maintained constant by atrial pacing to minimize changes in

Table III Characteristics of Reversible Postischemic Myocardial Dysfunction

Stunning	Hibernation
Dysfunctional myocardium with normal or near-normal blood flow	Dysfunctional myocardium with reduced blood flow
Contractile abnormality reversible with time	Contractile abnormality reversible on reperfusion
Absence of irreversible damage	Absence of irreversible damage
Perfusion imaging (PET scan) normal or increased	Perfusion imaging (PET scan) increased
Contractile function decreased	Contractile function decreased
No metabolic deterioration during inotropic stimulation	Recruitment of inotropic reserve is at the expense of metabolic recovery
Disruption of myofibrillar structure in canine model	Disruption of myofibrillar structure in canine model
Heart does not adapt to chronic underperfusion	Heart adapts to chronic underperfusion
Steady state between perfusion and contraction not achieved	Steady state between perfusion and contraction can be reached
Perfusion–contraction mismatching lasts from hours to days to months	Perfusion–contraction matching can be maintained for prolonged periods of time
Lack of evidence for dedifferentiation process in myocytes	Evidence for dedifferentiation process in myocytes

hemodynamics. Measurements are performed before and during the period of reduced blood flow. Depending on the experimental design, the animals can be euthanized at the end of the 2 hr of reduced flow or at a predetermined time point after reperfusion (hours to days). In these studies, measurements of regional myocardial blood flow with microspheres, myocardial oxygen consumption, and regional ventricular function are critical to verify the presence of hibernating myocardium. Measurements of tissue metabolites with biopsies or sampling of the affected bed's coronary venous blood can also be taken to assess metabolic changes.

One disadvantage of this acute preparation is that it deals primarily with short-term changes in hibernating myocardium that, by definition, may not be directly translatable to humans with chronic (months to years) hibernation. The model does, however, meet the traditional definition of hibernating myocardium, i.e., proportionate reductions in systolic function and resting coronary blood flow. More importantly, the use of chronically instrumented conscious dogs or pigs avoids the numerous problems associated with isolated hearts and nonsurvival surgery. It is important to recognize, however, that even in the conscious state, changes in the activity of the animal can lead to an imbalance between myocardial oxygen supply and demand, resulting in a degree of stunning.

B. Long-Term Hibernation Models

In order to study long-term hibernation in animals, a technique described by Fallavollita *et al.* can be utilized to provoke coronary collateral growth in pigs (61, 62). In this model, anesthetized pigs undergo a left lateral thoracotomy in the fourth intercostal space to expose the heart and the proximal LAD coronary artery. The artery is mobilized for a short distance and then instrumented with a 5-mm Delran occluder with a fixed internal diameter ranging between 1.5 and 2.2 mm. After securing the artery within the occluder with a silk ligature, the chest incision is closed. Approximately 3–4 months later, again under general anesthesia, the animals are returned to the laboratory for the performance of hemodynamic studies and procurement of tissue for analysis. To document regional perfusion under resting conditions, colored microspheres can be injected into the left ventricle followed by contrast left ventriculography and selective coronary angiography (63). After completion of the angiography the animals are euthanized and the heart is examined for molecular alterations. Characteristically, this model is associated with depressed anteroapical wall motion, severe proximal stenoses, or total LAD occlusion and angiographic evidence of collaterals.

Regardless of how well the various animal preparations meet the criteria of hibernation, it is important to recognize that all animal experiments are limited by a fixed observation time. In real terms, myocardial hibernation is a clinical phenomenon of contractile dysfunction that exists in patients with coronary artery disease. Although it may exist for months or years, it is fully reversible on reperfusion (64).

IV. Ischemic Preconditioning

A brief period of sublethal ischemia that reduces irreversible tissue injury secondary to a period of subsequent prolonged ischemia is termed ischemic preconditioning (IPC). The attendant reduction in infarct size is associated with a reduced rate of myocardial high-energy phosphate and glycogen catabolism, and reduced accumulation of lactate, hydrogen ions, and catecholamines (65–67). Ischemic preconditioning, which has also been shown to be very effective in reducing ventricular tachycardia and fibrillation, has been shown to occur in every species studied to date, including humans (68–70) (Table II), and in multiple organ systems in addition to the heart. Although the specific triggers and mediators of IPC have not been unequivocally determined, current evidence suggests likely roles for adenosine, nitric oxide, and reactive oxygen species (71). In terms of intracellular signaling mechanisms, the primary focus has been on protein kinase C (PKC), mitogen-activated protein kinases (MAPK), and ATP-dependent K^+ channels (72).

In 1993, Marber *et al.* and Kuzuya *et al.* independently reported that IPC induces a biphasic pattern of protection against myocardial necrosis (73, 74). This form of protection, termed delayed preconditioning or the second window of preconditioning (SWOP), has been confirmed in the rat, rabbit, dog, and pig, including both open-chest and chronically instrumented conscious animals (75–80). Thermal, metabolic, hypoxic, and anoxic delayed preconditioning have also been reported to be protective in cultured rat and rabbit cardiac myocytes (81–86). Unlike acute or classical IPC, however, SWOP requires >6 hr to develop, the protection is conferred around 24 hr later, and it may persist up to 72 hr. It is usually manifested as a reduction in both myocardial stunning and infarct size, and is associated with a decrease in ventricular arrhythmias (73, 79, 87).

In the course of determining the triggers and mechanisms of acute and delayed IPC, it became apparent that preconditioning's protective effects could be mimicked by numerous pharmacologic agents. These agents include, but are not limited to, adenosine and adenosine A_1 and A_3 receptor agonists (88–93), ATP-dependent potassium channel openers, bradykinin, and nitric oxide donors (94–96). This phenomenon is referred to as pharmacologic preconditioning because the heart is typically exposed to a brief drug infusion that is terminated 10–15 min prior to the onset of ischemia. This treatment is distinct from a pretreatment protocol in which the pharmacologic agent is not administered until the onset of ischemia. The ability to pharmacologically precondition the heart may be most applicable to cardiac surgery. In such a scenario, patients could be administered a pharmacologic treatment 24 hr and 5–10 min prior to cross-clamping the aorta during open-heart surgery. The development of pharmacologic preconditioning agents that not only mimic IPC but extend the duration of protection could markedly improve or replace currently employed intraoperative myocardial preservation techniques. Lists of pharmacologic agents used to mimic IPC and those used to inhibit IPC are included in Tables IV and V.

Although all forms of preconditioning are protective against infarction, there are differences with regard to the stunned myocardium. *In vivo* canine and porcine studies indicate that acute ischemic preconditioning does not attenuate myocardial stunning (97, 98). In contrast, delayed preconditioning or SWOP does appear to attenuate stunning in conscious porcine and rabbit models (99, 100). There also appear to be differences in the effects of pharmacologic preconditioning on stunning and infarction. For example, although adenosine preconditioning (in which the infusion is terminated prior to ischemia) reduces infarct size in the rabbit, it does not reduce stunning (101, 102).

A. Preparations for Studying Preconditioning

1. Intact Animals

Ischemic preconditioning has been studied in a variety of intact animals, including rats, rabbits, dogs, pigs, and sheep. These usually involve regional ischemia protocols in which regional ischemia is achieved by tightening a snare (or an occluder in the case of a chronic experiment) to occlude the distal portion of the left anterior descending coronary artery. Five minutes of complete occlusion is usually followed by 5 min of reperfusion before 30–60 min of regional ischemia (depending on the species) and 180 min of reperfusion. Several reports have indicated that *in vivo* myocardium must be reperfused for a minimum of 180 min to provide a reliable

Table IV Tools Used to Study Ischemic Preconditioning: Agents That Mimic Classic and Delayed IPC[a]

Agent	Proposed action
Adenosine (ADO)	ADO A_1, A_3 receptor agonist (classic IPC)
Cyclohexyl adenosine (CHA)	ADO A_1 receptor agonist (classic IPC)
Phenylisopropyl adenosine (PIA)	ADO A_1 receptor agonist (classic IPC)
Chlorocyclopentyladenosine (CCPA)	ADO A_1 receptor agonist (classic IPC)
Phorbol 12-myristate 13-acetate (PMA)	Direct PKC activator
Diacylglycerol (DAG)	Direct PKC activator
Dioctanoyl-*sn*-glycerol (DOG)	Direct PKC activator
Phenylephrine	α_1-Adrenergic receptor agonist and PKC activator
Angiotensin II	AT_1 receptor agonist and PKC activator
Reactive oxygen species (ROS)	PKC activator and phospholipase D stimulator
Bradykinin	Tyrosine kinase, PKC, and NOS activator
Bimakalim	K_{ATP} channel opener
Pinacidil	K_{ATP} channel opener
Nicorandil	K_{ATP} channel opener
Cromakalim	K_{ATP} channel opener
Aprikalim	K_{ATP} channel opener
Diazoxide	K_{ATP} channel opener
Monophosphoryl lipid A (MLA)	K_{ATP} channel opener
Deltorphin	Opioid receptor agonist
DADLE	Opioid receptor agonist
Nitroglycerine	NO donor (delayed IPC)
Diethylenetriamine/NO (DETA-NO)	NO donor (delayed IPC)
S-Nitroso-*N*-penicillamine (SNAP)	NO donor (delayed IPC)

[a]The effects of these agents may vary depending on species studied, experimental design, drug concentration at the site of action, and receptor selectivity. For example, many of these agents can activate more than one pathway depending on the dose used.

Table V Tools Used to Study Ischemic Preconditioning: Agents that Inhibit Classic and Delayed IPC[a]

Agent	Proposed action
Sulfophenyltheophylline (SPT)	Nonspecific ADO antagonist (classic IPC)
8-Cyclopentyl-1, 3 dipropylxanthine(DPCPX)	ADO A_1 receptor antagonist (classic IPC)
Staurosporine (STAU)	PKC blocker
Bisindolylmaleimide (BIS)	PKC blocker
Chelerythrine	PKC blocker
Polymyxin B	PKC blocker
Calphostin C	PKC blocker
Cycloheximide	Protein synthase inhibitor (delayed IPC)
N^{ω}-Nitro-L-arginine (L-NA)	NO-synthase blockers (delayed IPC)
N-Nitro-L-arginine methyl ester (L-NAME)	NO-synthase blockers (delayed IPC)
Aminoguanidine (AG)	Inducible NO-synthase blockers (delayed IPC)
S-methylisothiourea (SMT)	Inducible NO-synthase blockers (delayed IPC)
Genistein	Tyrosine kinase inhibitor
5-Hydroxy decanoate (5-HD)	Mitochondrial K_{ATP} channel blocker
Glibenclamide	Sarcolemmal and mitochondrial K_{ATP} channel blocker
Naltrexone	Opioid receptor antagonist
HOE 140	Bradykinin receptor blocker

[a]The effects of these agents may vary depending on species studied, experimental design, drug concentration at the site of action, and receptor selectivity. Without measuring the activity of the target directly, one must be cautious in interpreting the findings. For example, BIS, a PKC blocker, has been reported to exert a cardioprotective effect under certain conditions (130). BIS and STAU have been reported to not inhibit IPC in the dog and pig (44). Glibenclamide and 5-HD have been reported to have variable results in the rat (131). Furthermore, many of these agents can inhibit more than one pathway, depending on the dose used.

estimate of infarct size. Regional ventricular function can be measured as described earlier for stunning experiments, but in the majority of *in vivo* preconditioning studies this is not done, because the primary objective of IPC experiments is to demonstrate a reduction in infarct size.

As in regional stunning experiments, the area of infarct size and the area at risk (AAR) or ischemic bed size must be measured. Infarct size is then expressed as a percentage of the AAR. The AAR can be determined by perfusing the aortic root with monastral blue dye after ligation of the involved artery at the end of the experiment. The area of the left ventricle supplied by the occluded coronary artery (ischemic bed) is identified by the absence of the dye. In small animals, fluorescent microspheres can also be used to determine AAR. The heart is then cut from the base to the apex into four to five slices, the thickness of which is determined by the particular species being studied. The most frequently used method to differentiate viable from infarcted myocardium is a process whereby the slices are incubated in a 1% solution of triphenyltetrazolium chloride at 37°C for ~ 20 min. The slices are then weighed, photographed, and fixed in a 1% formaldehyde solution. Transparencies are then projected at a 10-fold magnification and traced to delineate nonischemic, ischemic/reperfused, and infarcted regions. The corresponding areas are then measured by videoplanimetry and from these measurements infarct size can be calculated as a percentage of the ischemic bed.

Three key factors must be carefully controlled during *in vivo* animal studies when measuring infarct size (and stunning). Although monitoring and maintenance of normothermic body temperature is often taken for granted, it has been reported that small (<2°C) decreases in body temperature can significantly reduce both infarct size and stunning. Infarct size is also directly dependent on the size of the area at risk. For this reason, it is not always sufficient to merely report infarct size as a percentage of the area at risk, but also as infarct volume. This can be accomplished easily by cutting the heart slices to an exact thickness so that the volume of infarct and risk areas can be determined. Finally, as mentioned earlier, coronary collateral blood flow must be measured in canine regional ischemia studies, because the degree of ischemic injury correlates with the amount of residual collateral flow during ischemia.

Intact animal preparations are also commonly used for delayed ischemic and pharmacologic preconditioning studies. The majority of these studies have been conducted in rabbits and rats, due to the reduced expenses and ease in handling smaller animals, although several studies of this type have been performed in pigs (99, 103). In SWOP ischemic preconditioning infarction protocols, the animals are initially instrumented with a suture or balloon occluder under open-chest, sterile conditions and then allowed up to a week to recover from the surgery prior to performing the preconditioning protocol. In delayed pharmacologic preconditioning studies, the drug being investigated can be administered (IP or IV) in a sedated or anesthetized closed-chest animal. After the preconditioning intervention, the animals are returned to their cages until the prolonged occlusion experiment is performed under open-chest conditions 24–72 hr later. To exclude the effects of anesthesia and the stress of open-chest conditions on the results obtained in intact animal preconditioning studies, conscious rabbit models have been developed (104). Procedures similar to those described above are used, with the exception that the prolonged ischemia is also conducted in conscious animals. Following the prolonged occlusion, the hearts can be reperfused for several days prior to determining myocardial infarct size.

Studies of delayed preconditioning effects on stunning have almost without exception been performed in conscious animals. In these studies, the animal is initially instrumented under sterile conditions with not only a coronary occluder device, but also with either a pulsed doppler ultrasonic epicardial crystal or segment-shortening crystals in the area at risk to measure regional ventricular function. Initial studies of this phenomenon were performed in conscious pigs (103), but subsequent studies have been performed in conscious rabbits (99). Delayed preconditioning is induced by subjecting the heart to six 4-min occlusions interspersed with 4 min of reperfusion. Successful occlusion is verified by changes on the electrocardiogram and the appearance of myocardial wall thinning on the crystal recordings. Regional myocardial function (stunning) is assessed using the doppler probe to measure systolic wall thickening (STw) after each of the brief occlusions and up to 5 hr after the sixth reperfusion. These findings are then compared to the similar measurements obtained after repeating the protocol on days 2 and 3. Improvement in the recovery of STw after the six ischemia/reperfusion cycles are repeated on days 2 and 3 indicates that delayed preconditioning is effective in reducing postischemic stunning. When this preparation is used it is important to demonstrate the absence of infarction using the tissue-staining TTC technique described earlier. This will confirm that the injury associated with the ischemia/reperfusion cycles resulted in reversible injury.

2. Isolated Hearts

Isolated heart models are also frequently used to study delayed preconditioning effects on infarct size. The majority of these experiments have involved pharmacologic preconditioning studies in which the animals, typically rabbits, are treated with the agent being studied 24–72 hr prior to excising the heart. The isolated perfused heart is then submitted to a regional ischemia protocol in which infarct size is measured. To date, there have been relatively few studies in which the effects of delayed preconditioning on ventricular function have been studied in the globally ischemic isolated heart.

3. Cardiomyocytes

The use of ventricular cardiomyocytes (neonatal and adult rats and adult rabbits) facilitates the determination of mechanisms of injury and protection by preconditioning at the myocyte level (84, 85, 105). Myocyte cell suspensions are submitted to simulated ischemia/reperfusion as described earlier for the myocyte stunning model, with the exception that the ischemic period is longer (30 min to 3 hr, depending on the species). Ischemia-induced cell death in aliquots of myocytes is determined by measuring CK or LDH release into the medium or by the percentage of cells that do not exclude trypan blue. A viability curve is then calculated (time versus cell death), and the area under the curve is used to facilitate the comparison of IPC protection with the protection provided by various agents used to mimic or block preconditioning. Preconditioning is induced with 10 minutes of pelleting in glucose-free medium and 15 min of resuspension in oxygenated buffer to most closely mimic IPC. Alternatively, myocytes can be preconditioned with hypoxia or anoxia. Study drugs are selected on the basis of their ability to inhibit or enhance selectively potential mediators of necrosis. To simulate reperfusion, the myocytes can be resuspended in standard oxygenated buffer containing Ca^{2+}. This myocyte suspension model is well suited for the determination of the effects of ischemia and reperfusion and cardioprotective treatments on cardiac myocytes. However, reversible and irreversible injury to cell membranes during ischemia and/or reperfusion and intracellular acidosis may preclude the ability to correlate injury with changes in intracellular ions determined with fluorescent indicators (81, 86, 105, 106).

Although myocyte preparations are best suited for studying the acute effects of preconditioning, they can also be used for delayed preconditioning studies. This is most easily accomplished in myocytes that culture well, such as neonatal rat or fetal chick myocytes (107). However, these cells are typically more resistant to ischemia than are adult myocytes, so longer ischemia times must be used to induce cell death. In addition, results obtained in chick myocytes should be verified in a mammalian species. At least one group has cultured adult rat ventricular myocytes for 24 hr to study delayed preconditioning (83, 85).

4. Human Tissue

The assumption in all experimental animal models is that preconditioning's beneficial effects also apply to humans. This has led to the establishment of several models of preconditioning using human tissue, such as cardiomyocytes and atrial trabeculae obtained from humans at the time of surgery, most frequently tissue obtained from the right atrial cannulation site in patients undergoing coronary artery bypass surgery (68). Studies involving the use of human atrial trabeculae have investigated the effects of IPC on contractility and cell death (70, 89). In the former, one end of the trabecula is attached to a fixed post in an organ bath and the other is attached to a force transducer to measure force generation of stimulated muscles. The muscle is then suspended in an organ bath superfused with an oxygenated physiologic salt solution. Ischemia is simulated with prolonged hypoxic substrate-free superfusion and rapid pacing followed by reperfusion with normal oxygenated buffer. Preconditioning is induced by exposing the trabecula to 3 min of hypoxic substrate-free superfusion with rapid pacing (3 Hz) followed by 7–10 min of reperfusion with oxygenated buffer. Differences in contractile function are assessed after prolonged simulated ischemia. Cell death in these same protocols, or in experiments specifically studying necrosis, is based on measurements of enzyme release (CK, LDH, or troponin I) into the medium.

Although the above studies permit determination of the protective effects of preconditioning on cardiomyocytes, similar observations must be documented in whole heart and/or by *in vivo* studies to verify their physiological relevance. This obviously cannot be done in the case of human tissue when the endpoints are contractility and infarction. Additional limitations of preconditioning studies in human tissue include (1) the limited amount of available tissue, (2) the difference between atrial tissue and myocytes and ventricular myocytes, and (3) the source of ventricular myocytes (when available, they are obtained from diseased hearts, which likely exhibit altered physiology and signaling mechanisms).

Regardless of the model of IPC utilized or species studied, there is the underlying assumption that limiting infarct size is desirable, i.e., a reduction in myocardial necrosis correlates with improved postischemic function. Experimentally, this is not always demonstrable. For example, although it is well established that IPC in the globally ischemic isolated perfused rat heart improves postischemic function, this is generally not the case in the perfused rabbit heart (108, 109). There are some reports, however, that improved functional recovery does correlate with a reduction in infarct size in *in vivo* regional ischemia preparations (109–112). Thus, the investigator needs to take into account not only the species but also the preparation when trying to elucidate the mechanism(s) and effects of preconditioning on infarct size and function.

V. Apoptosis

Apoptosis, or programmed cell death, is now recognized as a possible cause of noninflammatory cardiac myocyte loss and thus cardiac muscle dysfunction in numerous conditions, such as ischemia/reperfusion injury, remodeling, heart failure, hypertrophy, and aging (113–115). Etiologic mechanisms include reperfusion following ischemia, acidosis, ventricular pressure overload, oxidative stress, and activation of several cytokines and receptor agonists (116). Clinically, the phenomenon has been reported in humans with long QT syndrome, hibernation, acute myocardial infarction, and chronic heart failure (117).

Because it is one of the two phenomena responsible for myocyte loss, the characteristics of apoptotic death have been morphologically and biochemically compared to cell death from necrosis (Table VI). Necrosis, or accidental cell death, is associated with significant decreases in energy stores, with swelling, and eventually with rupture of sarcolemmal, mitochondrial, and nuclear membranes and with nuclear chromatin clumping. In contrast, the apoptotic cell, which exhibits near normal energy levels, shrinks, membranes and intracellular organelles remain intact, and the nucleus condenses and breaks into nucleosomes and the DNA fragments. Another major difference between the two causes of cardiomyocyte loss is the difference in the manner in which the cells are removed. Necrotic cells are removed by an inflammatory process, whereas apoptotic cells are phagocytosed by neighboring cells.

Although the exact mechanisms underlying apoptosis are unknown, there is increasing evidence that reactive oxygen

Table VI Myocyte Loss after Ischemia/Reperfusion

Necrosis	Apoptosis
Myocyte swells and ruptures	Myocyte shrinks
Nuclear chromatin clumps into dense masses	Nuclear chromatin condenses and fragments
Nucleus swells	Nucleus condenses and fragments into small nuclear bodies
Mitochondria undergo swelling; cristae fragment and accumulate insoluble calcium-containing phospholipid complexes	Mitochondria and cell membrane remain intact
Dead myocytes removed by inflammatory process	Focal noninflammatory destruction of myocytes
Cytosolic accumulation of calcium and sodium ions	Active, gene-directed process; caspases play a crucial role

species plays an important role. This is based on observations in myocardial ischemia/reperfusion studies that apoptosis commences primarily during reperfusion concomitant with the formation of intracellular ROS and/or intracellular calcium overload (28, 118). This programmed cell death appears to be initiated by the translocation of the proapoptotic proteins Bad and Bax from the cytosol to the mitochondrial membrane. Heterodimerization of Bad or Bax with the antiapoptotic Bcl-2-xl leads to the release of the mitochondrially localized cytochrome *c* into the cytosol (119–121). Formation of a cytosolic complex consisting of cytochrome *c*, apoptosis activating factor-1 (APAF-1), and caspase 9 leads to activation of caspase 3 and the cleavage of poly(ADP)-ribosylating (PARP) protein (36). Activation of PARP appears to be the final step in apoptosis leading to DNA fragmentation (122). The production of ROS and/or intracellular calcium overload also induces mitochondrial permeability transition pore (MPTP) opening (123), which, if not reversed, can result in the loss of mitochondrial proteins and ions.

For years myocardial ischemia/reperfusion injury was generally studied in terms of reversible postischemic dysfunction (stunning and/or hibernation), which progresses to irreversible injury or necrosis with prolonged ischemia times. However, although considerable debate has continued as to whether reperfusion injury truly occurs, it has not been fully understood why a substantial portion of myocardium within the ischemic zone does not show signs of necrosis. With the recognition of the phenomenon of programmed cell death, it now appears that a portion of these cells, which otherwise appear to be normal based on gross morphology, may be undergoing apoptosis. Furthermore, cells in the early stages of apoptosis that are unable to maintain normal oxidative phosphorylation in the face of oxidative stress and decreased antioxidant reserves may eventually die via necrosis. By its very nature, apoptosis, or programmed cell death, may be much more amenable to effective treatments than is accidental or necrotic cell death.

Myocardial apoptosis can be studied in the same *in vivo*, isolated heart, and in isolated myocyte preparations previously described (62, 115, 124–126). Because current evidence suggests that myocardial stunning is associated with minimal apoptosis (114), ischemia times should exceed 20 min to induce programmed cell death. At the conclusion of the *in vivo* and isolated heart regional ischemia experiments the hearts are stained to determine the area at risk and the infarct size. Following this, one or more tissue samples are harvested and frozen in liquid N_2 or in an ultracold freezer (-80°C) prior to preparing specimens for apoptosis assays.

Three techniques are currently utilized to assess apoptosis in intact myocardial tissue: (1) DNA fragmentation via terminal deoxynucleotide transferase-mediated dUTP nick end labeling (TUNEL assay), (2) DNA laddering using SDS gel electrophoresis (SDS-PAGE), and (3) electron microscopy. Many investigators use at least two different methods for the identification of apoptosis in a given experiment to minimize false-positive results. For example, Lim *et al.* demonstrated the presence of apoptosis in an *in vivo* porcine model of hibernating myocardium by TUNEL and electron microscopy (62). Although TUNEL and DNA fragmentation provide qualitative findings, if combined with other techniques the extent of myocyte apoptosis can be quantitated. Thin slices of fixed tissue sections can be appropriately stained and examined under high-magnification light microscopy to demarcate cell membranes and differentiate myocytes from other cell types. The TUNEL assay in combination with epifluorescence permits quantitation of the number of fluorescing nuclei of myocyte origin confirmed by examination at high power (600×). The extent of apoptosis is expressed by normalizing the results to the number of myocyte nuclei per square millimeter.

Electron microscopy can be used to differentiate necrosis from apoptosis. The latter cells have nuclear chromatin margination and condensation in the presence of intact sarcolemmal and mitochondrial membranes. Fresh tissue samples are fixed in glutaraldehyde, postfixed in osmium, and embedded in Embed Araldite mixture using routine procedures. Ultrathin sections are stained with uranyl acetate and lead citrate.

Measurement of apoptosis in intact hearts is typically determined by assessing DNA fragmentation using the TUNEL assay and DNA laddering. The former is most frequently detected using the APOP TAG kit (Oncor, Gaithersburg, MD) in which free 3′-OH DNA ends, generated by DNA fragmentation and typically located in nuclei and apoptotic bodies, are labeled by TdT (an enzyme that catalyzes a template-independent addition of nucleotide triphosphate to the 3′-OH ends of double- or single-stranded DNA) (127). The principle of the method is catalytic addition of residues of digoxigenin-labeled nucleotide to the DNA by TdT. Antidigoxigenin antibody conjugated to peroxidase is then used with chromagen substrate to generate an immunohistochemical signal of the presence of DNA fragmentation, indicating apoptosis.

Apoptosis is also verified by the cleavage of DNA into nucleosomal fragments in multiples of 180 base pairs, which form a laddering pattern on polyacrylamide gels. For DNA laddering, sections are fixed with 10% formalin, embedded in paraffin, sliced into 5-μm sections, and stained with hematoxylin–eosin and trichrome for light microscopy examination. Extraction of DNA is performed using a nonorganic DNA extraction kit (e.g., Oncor). Fresh tissue is minced in phosphate-buffered saline and incubated at 50°C for 3–6 hr with occasional shaking in lysis buffer containing proteinase K and DNase-free RNase A. The DNA solution is then extracted with phenol, precipitated in ethanol, and resuspended in buffer. For analysis of DNA fragmentation, DNA is fractionated by electrophoresis on a 1% agarose gel.

The DNA is visualized by ethidium bromide staining and exposure to ultraviolet light.

Apoptosis in cardiac myocyte preparations can be measured by the TUNEL assay and DNA laddering. There are two advantages to studying apoptosis in isolated cardiac myocytes. One advantage is that because the myocytes are studied in isolation, there is no need to distinguish myocytes from other cell types. A second advantage is the ability to detect apoptosis at a much earlier stage than is detected by the TUNEL assay and DNA laddering. There is evidence that one of the earliest signs of apoptosis is the translocation of phosphatidylserine from the inner surface of the plasma membrane to the cell surface (128, 129). These residues are then accessible to fluorescein isothiocyanate (FITC)-conjugated annexin V, which is a member of a family of proteins that has a strong affinity for phosphatidylserine. Because annexin V fluoresces a bright green when bound to phosphatidylserine on the outer surface of apoptotic cells, this stain can be used to identify early programmed cell death. Viable cells, when excited at 488 nm, fluoresce at 520 nm; however, this fluorescence is of low intensity and can be distinguished from the bright intense fluorescence of FITC-labeled annexin V apoptotic cells.

Apoptotic cells can be distinquished from necrotic cells by the differential staining pattern observed with nuclear dyes such as propidium iodide and Hoechst 33342. Propidium iodide binds to DNA, but does not cross intact cell membranes; thus, it will stain only the nuclei of necrotic cells or those with leaky membranes. When excited at 488 nm, propidium iodide fluorescence is detectable as intense red fluorescence. This method of measuring cell death is thus similar to that determined by using trypan blue exclusion. The Hoechst stain, which is membrane permeable, labels all nuclei; however, under high magnification apoptotic cells exhibit fragmentation of chromatin, degradation of the nuclear envelope, and nuclear blebbing, resulting in the formation of condensed nuclei (micronuclei). Because necrotic cells can also stain positive with FITC-labeled annexin V, cells that stain positive for both dyes are considered necrotic, whereas myocytes that stain positive only for annexin are considered apoptotic.

These staining assays are very simple, because they involve only incubation of aliquots of myocytes or single cells with annexin V and propidium iodide or Hoechst 33342, and visual examination of the cells on an imaging system using the appropriate fluorescent filter combinations. In single-cell studies, it may be possible to measure intracellular Ca^{2+}, ROS, or other metabolites if the dyes used fluoresce at a different wavelength than that of FITC-labeled annexin V. Cell suspension studies are more feasible, and with the use of flow cytometry, cell death in a large sample of cells can be rapidly and reliably determined.

Although the procedures described above determine the presence of apoptotic cell death, they do not provide any information on the mechanisms of this form of cell death. Thus, a complete examination of apoptosis should include measurements of one or more various steps in this program of cell death. These include, but are not limited to, the translocation of cytochrome *c* from the mitochondria to the cytosol, the activation of caspase 3, measurements of the pro- and antiapoptotic proteins Bad/Bax and Bcl-2, and even the intracellular reduced and oxidized glutathione levels, the key metabolite in the cell's antioxidant defenses. It is thought that all of these proteins and metabolites are altered in either their concentration and/or subcellular location prior to the development of DNA fragmentation or laddering. Establishing the time frame for these changes in relation to the development of cell death may be clinically relevant. For example, in current ischemia/reperfusion studies the presence of apoptosis is based on measurements of DNA fragmentation and laddering, which are the final steps in apoptotic cell death. Even the efficacy of antiapoptosis treatments, such as caspase inhibitors, has been based primarily on reduction of infarct size, not reduction of apoptosis. However, once the nucleus is damaged and DNA is fragmented, the cell's ability to synthesize new repair proteins is severely compromised, and damaged cells, even if they survive a first ischemic episode, may die at an accelerated rate during subsequent stress or ischemia. If cell death in ischemic/reperfused myocardium progresses from apoptosis to necrosis, and if the program of cell death in early apoptosis can be interrupted and even possibly reversed, then the most beneficial treatments would be those targeted to early events in apoptosis.

VI. Conclusion

Although research in cardiac surgery has changed dramatically over the past 50 years, the problems facing cardiac surgeons today are just as challenging as those solved by clinician-scientists in the past. This is due to the increasing need to develop and implement therapies to treat the complications that occur after open-heart surgery. The aim is to not only improve survival, but also to enhance the overall quality of life after heart surgery. Research in cardiac surgery, however, is and must continue to be grounded in inquiry at the basic science level. Although cardiac transplantation, replacement of heart valves, performance of complex congenital heart disease operations, and coronary artery bypass grafting represent spectacular accomplishments, fundamentally all these corrective procedures still involve exposing the heart or a region of the heart to a period of ischemia. As a consequence, few, if any, cardiac operations are completely free of significant complications. Heart transplantation is a good example of a procedure in which postischemic myocardial dysfunction plays an important role in outcome. The 30-day mortality after cardiac replacement currently ranges between 5 and 15% and is most frequently related to primary graft dysfunction secondary to prolonged ischemic times and/or inadequate myocardial preservation. Allograft rejection, donor heart ischemia, progressive myocyte loss over time, and the development of graft vasculopathy also have been associated with prolonged ischemic times. Regardless of the cause, the need to improve both the short- and long-term survival is urgent, especially because the 1- and 5-year survival rates after cardiac transplantation still remain at 80 and 60%, respectively. Likewise, although cardiac surgeons can successfully replace heart valves, repair complex congenital heart defects, and revascularize the severely ischemic heart, these operations do not necessarily prevent patients from experiencing myocyte loss over time, which ultimately can progress to heart failure. Thus, it is not surprising that myocardial stunning, myocardial hibernation, ischemic preconditioning, and apoptosis are currently areas of major investigation in cardiac surgery today.

More investigation is needed into myocardial stunning and hibernation in order to comprehend fully the events that take place during both ischemia and reperfusion. Furthermore, research is needed to elucidate how the purported primary mediators, intracellular calcium overload, and oxidative stress caused by ROS generated at the onset of reperfusion result in reversible and irreversible myocardial injury. More specifically, experiments need to be designed to determine how derangements in the various proposed targets of ROS, such as the sarcolemma, the sarcoplasmic reticulum, the mitochondria, and the extracellular collagen matrix, actually result in stunning and hibernation. Likewise, studies are needed to address the role ischemia/reperfusion plays in modulating intracellular acidosis and activation of the sodium/hydrogen exchanger. If the latter is responsible for increased transsarcolemmal calcium influx and intracellular overload, is the evidence strong enough to warrant the use of Na^+/H^+ exchange inhibitors to prevent or reduce the incidence of myocardial infarction or death after open-heart operations? What are the roles, if any, of gene regulation and receptor expression in stunning and hibernation? What are the reparative processes that take place during the recovery process and why does recovery time vary according to the duration and degree of ischemia? When does reversible injury become programmed irreversible injury? Does apoptosis represent just one aspect of a continuum of ischemia, and, if so, is programmed cell death reversible, and at what point in time?

Similarly, there are numerous other questions that need to be answered with respect to both classic and delayed preconditioning. Future research must focus on the triggers, mediators, intracellular signaling pathways, and effectors that actually modulate this powerful endogenous form of myocardial protection. Findings from these types of studies could lead to the development of new pharmacologic preconditioning agents that could be used during cardiac surgery to enhance the heart's tolerance to ischemia and reduce the incidence of stunning, infarction, and heart failure. Currently, several endogenous and exogenous agents are under investigation as potential cardioprotective agents. These include preconditioning mimetics such as adenosine A_1 and A_3 receptor agonists, ATP-dependent potassium channel openers, bradykinin, and nitric oxide donors. Ultimately, elucidation of the mechanisms underlying the potent endogenous cardioprotective effects of IPC and hibernation and the deleterious consequences of stunning and apoptosis depends on focused basic science research that is innovative, hypothesis driven, utilizes modern investigative technology, and is translational in nature.

References

1. Beck, C. S. (1926). Wounds of the heart: The technic of suture. *Arch. Surg.* **13,** 206–227.
2. Graybiel, A., Strieder, J. W., and Boyer, N. H. (1938). An attempt to obliterate the patent ductus arteriosus in a patient with subacute bacterial endarteritis. *Am. Heart J.* **15,** 621–624.
3. Gross, R. E., and Hubbard, J. P. (1939). Surgical ligation of a patent ductus arteriosus. *J. Am. Med. Assoc.* **112,** 729–731.
4. Munro, J. C. (1907). Surgery of the vascular system: Ligation of the ductus arteriosus. *Ann. Surg.* **46,** 335–338.
5. Crafoord, C., and Nylin, G. (1945). Congenital coarctation of the aorta and its surgical treatment. *J. Thorac. Surg.* **14,** 347–361.
6. Gross, R. E., and Hufnagel, C. A. (1945). Coarctation of the aorta: Experimental studies regarding its surgical correction. *N. Engl. J. Med.* **233,** 287–293.
7. Gross, R. E. (1945). Surgical correction for coarctation of the aorta. *Surgery* **18,** 673–678.
8. Cushing, H., and Branch, J. R. B. (1908). Experimental and clinical notes on chronic valvular lesions in the dog and their possible relation to a future surgery of the cardiac valves. *J. Med. Res.* **17,** 471–482.
9. Souttar, H. S. (1925). The surgical treatment of mitral stenosis. *Br. Med. J.* **2,** 603–606.
10. Johnson, S. L. (1970). "The History of Cardiac Surgery, 1896–1955." Johns Hopkins Press, Baltimore.
11. Bailey, C. P. (1949). The surgical treatment of mitral stenosis. *Dis. Chest* **15,** 377–393.
12. McLean, J. (1959). The discovery of heparin. *Circulation* **19,** 75–86.
13. Gibbon, J. H., Jr. (1937). Artificial maintenance of circulation during experimental occlusion of pulmonary artery. *Arch. Surg.* **34,** 1105–1131.
14. Carrel, A. (1910). On the experimental surgery of the thoracic aorta and the heart. *Ann. Surg.* **52,** 83–95.
15. Beck, C. S. (1935). The development of a new blood supply to the heart by operation. *Ann. Surg.* **102,** 801–813.
16. Spencer, F. C. (1983). Intellectual creativity in thoracic surgeons. *J. Thorac. Cardiovasc. Surg.* **86,** 163–179.
17. Johnson, S. L., Flemma, R. J., Lepley, D., and Ellison, E. H. (1969). Extended treatment of severe coronary artery disease. *Ann. Surg.* **171,** 460–469.
18. Barnard, C. N. (1967). A human cardiac transplant: An interim report of a successful operation performed at Groote Schuur Hospital, Cape Town. *S. Afr. Med. J.* **41,** 1271–1274.
19. Carrel, A. (1905). The transplantation of organs: A preliminary communication. *J. Am. Med. Assoc.* **45,** 1645–1646.
20. Demikhov, V. P. (1962). "Experimental Transplantation of Vital Organs." [Translation by B. Haigh.] Consultants Bureau, New York.
21. Lower, R. R., and Shumway, N. E. (1960). Studies on orthotopic homotransplantation of the canine heart. *Surg. Forum* **11,** 18–19.

22. Mentzer, R. M., Jr., Birjinuik, V., Khuri, S., Lowe, J. E., Rahko, P. S., Weisel, R. D., Wellons, H. A., Barker, M. L., and Lasley, R. D. (1999). Adenosine myocardial protection: Preliminary results of a phase II clinical trial. *Ann. Surg.* **229,** 643–650.
23. Mentzer, R. M., Jr., Rahko, P. S., Molina-Viamonte, V., Canver, C. C., Chopra, P. S., Love, R. B., Cook, T. D., Hegge, J. O., and Lasley, R. D. (1997). Safety, tolerance, and efficacy of adenosine as an additive to blood cardioplegia in humans during coronary artery bypass surgery. *Am. J. Cardiol.* **79,** 38–43.
24. Bolli, R. (1998). Basic and clinical aspects of myocardial stunning. *Prog. Cardiovasc. Dis.* **40,** 477–516.
25. Bolli, R. (1998). Why myocardial stunning is clinically important. *Basic Res. Cardiol.* **93,** 169–172.
26. Lasley, R. D., and Mentzer, R. M., Jr. (1982). Protective effects of adenosine in the reversibly injured heart. *Ann. Thorac. Surg.* **60,** 843–846.
27. Braunwald, E., and Kloner, R. A. (1982). The stunned myocardium: Prolonged postischemic ventricular dysfunction. *Circulation* **60,** 1146–1149.
28. Maulik, N., Yoshida, T., and Das, D. K. (1998). Oxidative stress developed during the reperfusion of ischemic myocardium induces apoptosis. *Free Radical Biol. Med.* **24,** 869–875.
29. Bolli, R., and Marban, E. Molecular and cellular mechanisms of myocardial stunning. *Am. J. Physiol.* **79,** 609–634.
30. Urthaler, F., Wolkowicz, P. E., Digerness, S. B., Harris, K. D., and Walker, A. A. (1997). MDL-28170, a membrane-permeant calpain inhibitor, attenuates stunning and PKC epsilon proteolysis in reperfused ferret hearts. *Cardiovasc. Res.* **35,** 60–67.
31. Aversano, T., Maughan, W. L., Hunter, W. C., Kass, D., and Becker, L. (1986). End-systolic measures of regional ventricular performance. *Circulation* **73,** 938–950.
32. Glower, D. D., Spratt, J. A., Snow, N. D., Kabas, J. S., and Davis Rankin, J. S. (1985). Linearity of the Frank–Starling relationship in the intact heart: The concept of preload recruitable stroke work. *Circulation* **71,** 994–1009.
33. Matsuwaka, R., Matsuda, H., Shirakura, R., Kaneko, M., Fukushima, N., Taniguchi K., Nakano, S., and Kawashina, Y. (1994). Changes in left ventricular performance after global ischemia: Assessing LV pressure–volume relationship. *Ann. Thorac. Surg.* **57,** 151–156.
34. Van Wylen, D. G., Willis, J., Sodhi, J., Weiss, R. J., Lasley, R. D., and Mentzer, R. M., Jr. (1990). Cardiac microdialysis to estimate interstitial adenosine and coronary blood flow. *Am. J. Phys. Heart Circ. Physiol.* **258,** H1642–H1649.
35. Delyani, J. A., and Van Wylen, D. G. (1997). Endocardial and epicardial interstitial purines and lactate during graded ischemia. *Am. J. Physiol.* **266,** H1019–1026.
36. Cremers, T. I., Teisman, A. C., van Gilst, W. H., and Westerink, B. H. (1997). Use of microdialysis for monitoring sympathetic and parasympathetic innervation of heart in conscious rats. *Am. J. Physiol.* **273,** H2850–H2856.
37. Obata, T., Tamura, M., and Yamanaka, Y. (1997). Evidence of hydroxyl free radical generation by calcium overload in rat myocardium. *J. Pharm. Pharmacol.* **49,** 787–790.
38. Neely, J. R., and Grotyohann, L. W. (1984). Role of glycolytic products in damage to ischemic myocardium. Dissociation of adenosine triphosphate levels and recovery of function of reperfused ischemic hearts. *Circ. Res.* **55,** 816–824.
39. Hatem, S. N., Benardeau, A., Rucker-Martin, C., Marty, I., de Chamisso, P., Villaz, M., and Mercadier, J. J. (1997). Different compartments of sarcoplasmic reticulum participate in the excitation-contraction coupling process in human atrial myocytes. *Circ. Res.* **80,** 345–353.
40. Buck, E. D., Lachnit, W. G., and Pessah, I. N. (1999). Mechanisms of δ-hexachlorocyclohexane toxicity: I. Relationship between altered ventricular myocyte contractility and ryanodine receptor function. *J. Pharmacol.* **289,** 477–485.
41. Narayan, P., Valdivia, H. H., Mentzer, R. M., Jr., and Lasley, R. D. (1998). Adenosine A_1 receptor stimulation antagonizes the negative inotropic effects of the PKC activator dioctanoylglycerol. *J. Mol. Cell. Cardiol.* **30,** 913–921.
42. Sherman, A. J., Klocke, F. J., Decker, R. S., Decker, M. L., Kozlowski, K. A., Harris, K. R., Hedjbeli, S., Yaroshenko, Y., Nakamura, S., Parker, M. A., Checchia, P. A., and Evans, D. B. (2000). Myofibrillar disruption in hypocontractile myocardium showing perfusion-contraction matches and mismatches. *Am. J. Physiol. Heart Circ. Physiol.* **278,** H1320–H1334.
43. Heusch, G. (1998). Hibernating myocardium. *Am. J. Physiol. Heart Circ. Physiol.* **78,** 1055–1085.
44. Kloner, R. A., Bolli, R., Marban, E., Reinlib, L., and Braunwald, E. (1998). Medical and cellular implications of stunning, hibernation, and preconditioning. *Circulation* **97,** 1848–1867.
45. Rahimtoola, S. (1981). Coronary bypass surgery for chronic angina—1984: A perspective. *Circulation* **69,** 842–848.
46. Rees, G., Bristow, J. D., Kremkau, E. L., Green, G. S., Herr, R. H., Griswold, H. E., and Starr, A. (1971). Influence of aortocoronary bypass surgery on left ventricular performance. *N. Engl. J. Med.* **284,** 1116–1120.
47. Chatterjee, K., Swan, H. J. C., Parmly, W. W., Sustaita, H., Marcus, H. S., and Matloff, J. (1973). Influence of direct myocardial revascularization on left ventricular asynergy and function in patients with coronary disease. *Circulation* **47,** 276–286.
48. Chatterjee, K., Swan, H. J. C., Parmly, W. W., Sustaita, H., Marcus, H., and Matloff, J. (1972). Depression of left ventricular function due to acute myocardial ischemia and its reversal after aortocoronary saphenous vein bypass. *N. Engl. J. Med.* **286,** 1117–1122.
49. Nienaber, C. A., Brunken, R. C., Sherman, C. T., Yeatman, L. A., Gambhir, S. S., Krivokapich, J., Demer, L. L., Ratib, O., Child, J. S., Phelps, M. E., and Schelbert, H. R. (1991). Metabolic and functional recovery of ischemic human myocardium after coronary angioplasty. *J. Am. Coll. Cardiol.* **18,** 966–978.
50. Brundage, B. H., Massie, B. M., and Botvinick, E. H. (1984). Improved regional ventricular function after successful surgical revascularization. *J. Am. Coll. Cardiol.* **3,** 902–908.
51. Rankin, J. S., Newman, G. E., Muhlbaier, L. H., Behar, V. S., Fedor, J. M., and Sabiston, D. C., Jr. (1985). The effect of coronary revascularization on ventricular function in ischemic heart disease. *J. Thorac. Cardiovasc. Surg.* **90,** 818–832.
52. Fallavollita, J. A., Jacob, S., Young, R. F., and Canty, J. M., Jr. (1999). Regional alterations in SR CA^{2+}-ATPase, phopholamban, and HSP-70 expression in chronic hibernating myocardium. *Am. J. Physiol. Heart Circ. Physiol.* **277,** H1418–H1428.
53. Bolli, R. (1998). Basic and clinical aspects of myocardial stunning. *Prog. Cardiovasc. Dis.* **40,** 477–516.
54. Maes, A., Flameng, W., Nuyts, J., Borgers, M., Shivalkar, B., Ausma, J., Bormans, G., Schiepers, C., De Roo, M., and Mortelmans, L. (1994). Histological alterations in chronically hypoperfused myocardium: Correlation with PET findings. *Circulation* **90,** 735–745.
55. Borgers, M., Thone, F., Wouters, L., Ausma, J., Shivalkar, B., and Flameng, W. (1993). Structural correlates of regional myocardial dysfunction in patients with critical coronary stenosis: Chronic hibernation? *Cardiovasc. Pathol.* **2,** 237–245.
56. Schwarz, E. R., Schaper, J., vom Dahl, J., Altehoefer, C., Grohmann, B., Schoendube, F., Sheehan, F. H., Uebis, R., Buell, U., Messmer, B. J., Schaper, W., and Hanrath, P. (1996). Myocyte degeneration and cell death in hibernating human myocardium. *J. Am. Coll. Cardiol.* **7,** 1577–1585.
57. Shen, Y. T., and Vatner, S. F. (1995). Mechanism of impaired myocardial function during progressive coronary stenosis in conscious pigs: Hibernation versus stunning? *Circ. Res.* **76,** 479–488.
58. Canty, J. M., and Fallavollita, J. A. (1999). Resting myocardial flow in hibernating myocardium: Validating animal models of human pathophysiology. *Am. J. Physiol. Heart Circ. Physiol.* **277,** H417–H422.
59. Sommerschild, H. T., Offstad, J., Grund, F., Ilebekk, A., and Kirkeboen, K. A. (1998). Characterization of metabolic responses to low-

flow ischemia in intact pig hearts and isolated blood-perfused neonatal pig hearts. *Basic Res. Cardiol.* **93,** 38–49.
60. Sherman, A. J., Harris, K. R., Hedjbeli, S., Yaroshenko, Y., Schafer, D., Shroff, S., Sung, J., and Klocke, F. J. (1997). Proportionate reversible decreases in systolic function and myocardial oxygen consumption after modest reductions in coronary flow: Hibernation versus stunning. *J. Am. Coll. Cardiol.* **29,** 1623–1631.
61. Fallavollita, J. A., Perry, B. J., and Canty, J. M. (1997). ^{18}F-2-Deoxyglucose deposition and regional flow in pigs with chronically dysfunctional myocardium. *Circulation* **95,** 1900–1909.
62. Lim, H., Fallavollita, J. A., Hard, R., Kerr, C. W., and Canty, J. M. (1999). Profound apoptosis-mediated regional myocyte loss and compensatory hypertrophy in pigs with hibernating myocardium. *Circulation* **100,** 2380–2386.
63. Kowallik, P., Schulz, R., Guth, B. D., Schade, A., Paffhausen, W., Gross, R., and Heusch, G. (1991). Measurement of regional myocardial blood flow with multiple colored microspheres. *Circulation* **83,** 974–982.
64. Wijns, W., Vatner, S. F., and Camici, P. G. (1998). Mechanisms of disease: Hibernating myocardium. *N. Engl. J. Med.* **339,** 173–181.
65. Takasaki, Y., Adachi, N., Dote, K., Tsubota, S., Yorozuya, T., and Arai, T. (1998). Ischemic preconditioning suppresses the noradrenaline turnover in the rat heart. *Cardiovasc. Res.* **39,** 373–380.
66. Murry, C. E., Richard, V. J., Reimer, K. A., and Jennings, R. B. (1990). Ischemic preconditioning slows energy metabolism and delays ultrastructural damage during a sustained ischemic episode. *Circ. Res.* **66,** 913–931.
67. Kida, M., Fujiwara, H., Ishida, M., Kawai, C., Ohura, M., Miura, I., and Yabuuchi, Y. (1991). Ischemic preconditioning preserves creatine phosphate and intracellular pH. *Circulation* **84,** 2495–2503.
68. Speechly-Dick, M. E., Grover, G. J., and Yellon, D. M. (1995). Does ischemic preconditioning in the human involve protein kinase C and the ATP-dependent K^+ channel? Studies of contractile function after simulated ischemia in an atrial *in vitro* model. *Circ. Res.* **77,** 1030–1035.
69. Edwards, R. J., and Marber, M. S. (1998). Myocardial preconditioning mechanisms and man. *Int. J. Clin. Pract.* **52,** 395–401.
70. Tomai, F., Crea, F., Chiariello, L., and Gioffrè, P. A. (1999). Ischemic preconditioning in humans: Models, mediators, and clinical relevance. *Circulation* **100,** 559–563.
71. Downey, J. M., and Cohen, M. V. (1997). Signal transduction in ischemic preconditioning. *Adv. Exp. Med. Biol.* **430,** 39–55.
72. Baxter, G. F., and Yellon, D. M., eds. (1998). Delayed preconditioning and adaptive cardioprotection. *In* "Developments in Cardiovascular Medicine," Series 207. Kluwer Academic Publishers, Boston.
73. Marber, M. S., Latchman, D. S., Walker, J. M., and Yellon, D. M. (1993). Cardiac stress protein elevation 24 hours after brief ischemia or heat stress is associated with resistance to myocardial infarction. *Circulation* **88,** 1264–1272.
74. Kuzuya, T., Hoshida, S., Yamashita, N., Fuji, H., Oe, H., Hori, M., Kamada, T., and Tada, M. (1993). Delayed effects of sublethal ischemia on the acquisition of tolerance to ischemia. *Circ. Res.* **72,** 1293–1299.
75. Baxter, G. F., Marber, M. S., Patel, V. C., and Yellon, D. M. (1994). Adenosine receptor involvement in a delayed phase of protection 24 hours following ischemic preconditioning. *Circulation* **90,** 2993–3000.
76. Baxter, G. F., Goma, F. M., and Yellon, D. M. (1997). Characterisation of the infarct-limiting effect of delayed preconditioning: Timecourse and dose-dependency studies in rabbit myocardium. *Basic Res. Cardiol.* **92,** 159–167.
77. Baxter, G. F., Goma, F. M., and Yellon, D. M. (1995). Involvement of protein kinase C in the delayed cytoprotection following sublethal ischaemia in rabbit myocardium. *Br. J. Pharmacol.* **115,** 222–224.
78. Imagawa, J., Baxter, G. F., and Yellon, D. M. (1997). Genistein, a tyrosine kinase inhibitor, blocks the "second window of protection" 48 h after ischemic preconditioning in the rabbit. *J. Mol. Cell. Cardiol.* **29,** 1885–1893.
79. Yang, X. M., Baxter, G. F., Heads, R. J., Yellon, D. M., Downey, J. M., and Cohen, M. V. (1996). Infarct limitation in the second window of protection in conscious rabbits. *Cardiovasc. Res.* **31,** 777–783.
80. Qiu, Y., Rizvi, A., Tang, X. -L., Manchikalapudi, S., Takano, H., Jadoon, A. K., Wu, W. J., and Bolli, R. (1997). Nitric oxide triggers late preconditioning against myocardial infarction in conscious rabbits. *Am. J. Physiol.* **273,** H2931–H2936.
81. Armstrong, S., Downey, J. M., and Ganote, C. E. (1994). Preconditioning of isolated rabbit cardiomyocytes: Induction by metabolic stress and blockade by the adenosine antagonist SPT and calphostin C, a protein kinase C inhibitor. *Cardiovasc. Res.* **28,** 72–77.
82. Armstrong, S. C., Liu, G. S., Downey, J. M., and Ganote, C. E. (1995). Potassium channels and preconditioning of isolated rabbit cardiomyocytes: Effects of glyburide and pinacidil. *J. Mol. Cell. Cardiol.* **27,** 1765–1774.
83. Yamashita, N., Nishida, M., Hoshida, S., Kuzuya, T., Hori, M., Taniguchi, N., Kamada, T., and Tada, M. (1994). Induction of manganese superoxide dismutase in rat cardiac myocytes increases tolerance to hypoxia 24 hours after preconditioning. *J. Clin. Invest.* **94,** 2193–2199.
84. Cumming, D. V., Heads, R. J., Brand, N. J., Yellon, D. M., and Latchman, D. S. (1996). The ability of heat stress and metabolic preconditioning to protect primary rat cardiac myocytes. *Basic Res. Cardiol.* **91,** 79–85.
85. Zhou, X., Zhai, X., and Ashraf, M. (1996). Direct evidence that initial oxidative stress triggered by preconditioning contributes to second window of protection by endogenous antioxidant enzyme in myocytes. *Circulation* **93,** 1177–1184.
86. Gray, M. O., Karliner, J. S., and Mochly-Rosen, D. (1997). A selective M-protein kinase C antagonist inhibits protection of cardiac myocytes form hypoxia-induced cell death. *J. Biol. Chem.* **272,** 30945–30951.
87. Tang, X. L., Qiu, Y., Turrens, J. F., Sun, J. Z., and Bolli, R. (1997). Late preconditioning against stunning is not mediated by increased antioxidant defenses in conscious pigs. *Am. J. Physiol.* **273,** H1651–H1657.
88. Van Winkle, D. M., Chien, G. L., Wolff, R. A., Soifer, B. E., Kuzume, K., and Davis, R. F. (1994). Cardioprotection provided by adenosine receptor activation is abolished by blockade of the K_{ATP} channel. *Am. J. Physiol.* **266,** H829–H839.
89. Walker, D. M., Walker, J. M., Pugsly, W. B., Pattison, C. W., and Yellon, D. M. (1995). Preconditioning in isolated superfused human muscle. *J. Mol. Cell. Cardiol.* **27,** 1349–1357.
90. Ikonomidis, J. S., Shirai, T., Weisel, R. D., Dorylo, B., Rap, V., Whiteside, C. I., Mickle, D. A. G., and Li, R. -K. (1995). "Ischemic" or adenosine preconditioning of human ventricular cardiomyocytes is protein kinase C dependent. *Circulation* **92,** 1–12.
91. Tsuchida, A., Miura, T., Miki, T., Shimamoto, K., and Iimura, O. (1992). Role of adenosine receptor activation in myocardial infarct size limitation by ischaemic preconditioning. *Pflügers Arch.* **430,** 273–282.
92. Auchsmpach, J. A., and Gross, G. J. (1993). Adenosine A_1 receptors, K_{ATP} channels and ischemic preconditioning in dogs. *Am. J. Physiol.* **264,** H1327–H1336.
93. Kerensky, R. A., Kutcher, M. A., Braden, G. A., Applegate, R. J., Solis, G. A., and Little, W. C. (1995). The effects of intracoronary adenosine on preconditioning during coronary angioplasty. *Clin. Cardiol.* **18,** 91–96.
94. Gross, G. J. (1995). ATP-sensitive potassium channels and myocardial preconditioning. *Basic Res. Cardiol.* **90,** 85–88.
95. Grover, G. J. (1997). Pharmacology of ATP-sensitive potassium channel (K_{ATP}) openers in models of myocardial ischemia and reperfusion. *Can. J. Physiol. Pharmacol.* **75,** 309–315.
96. Parratt, J. R., Vegh, A., and Papp, J. G. (1995). Bradykinin as an endogenous myocardial protective substance with particular reference to ischemic preconditioning—A brief review of the evidence. *Can. J. Physiol. Pharmacol.* **73,** 837–842.
97. Jahania, M. S., Lasley, R. D., and Mentzer, R. M., Jr. (1999). Ischemic preconditioning does not acutely improve load-insensitive parameters

of contractility in *in vivo* stunned porcine myocardium. *J. Thorac. Cardiovasc. Surg.* **117,** 810–817.

98. Bolli, R. (1996). The early and late phases of preconditioning against myocardial stunning and the essential role of oxyradicals in the late phase: An overview. *Basic Res. Cardiol.* **91,** 57–63.

99. Qiu, Y., Tang, X. -L., Park, S. -W., Sun, J. -Z., Kalya, A., and Bolli R. (1997). The early and late phases of ischemic preconditioning. A comparative analysis of their effects on infarct size, myocardial stunning, and arrhythmias in conscious pigs undergoing a 40-minute coronary occlusion. *Circ. Res.* **80,** 730–742.

100. Tang, X. -L., Qiu, Y., Sun, J. -Z., Kalya, A., and Bolli, R. (1996). Time-course of late preconditioning against myocardial stunning in conscious pigs. *Circ. Res.* **79,** 424–434.

101. Sekili, S., Jeroudi, M. O., Tang, X. L., Zughaib, M., Sun, J. Z., and Bolli, R. (1995). Effect of adenosine on myocardial "stunning" in the dog. *Circ. Res.* **76,** 82–94.

102. Lasley, R. D., Konyn, P. J., Hegge, J. O., and Mentzer, R. M., Jr. (1995). Effects of ischemic and adenosine preconditioning on interstitial fluid adenosine and myocardial infarct size. *Am. J. Physiol.* **269,** H1460–H1466.

103. Sun, J. Z., Tang, X. -L., Knowlton, A. A., Park, S. W., Qiu, Y., and Bolli, R. (1995). Late preconditioning against myocardial stunning: An endogenous protective mechanism that confers resistance to postischemic dysfunction 24 hours after brief ischemia in conscious pigs. *J. Clin. Invest.* **95,** 388–403.

104. Bolli, R., Bhatti, Z. A., Tang, X. -L., Qiu, Y. Zhang, Q., Guo, Y., and Jadoon, A. K. (1997). Evidence that late preconditioning against myocardial stunning in conscious rabbits is triggered by the generation of nitric oxide. *Circ. Res.* **81,** 42–52.

105. Critz, S. D., Liu, G. S., Mitsuaki, C., and Downey, J. M. (1997). Pinacidil but not nicorandil opens ATP-sensitive K^+ channels and protects against simulated ischemia in rabbit myocytes. *J. Mol. Cell. Cardiol.* **29,** 1123–1130.

106. Goldberg, M., Zhang, H. L., and Steinberg, S. F. (1997). Hypoxia alters the subcellular distribution of protein kinase C isoforms in neonatal rat ventricular myocytes. *J. Clin. Invest.* **99,** 55–61.

107. Vanden Hoek, T. L., Becker, L. B., Shao, Z. H., Li, C. Q., and Schumacker, P. T. (2000). Preconditioning in cardiomyocytes protects by attenuating oxidant stress at reperfusion. *Circ. Res.* **86,** 541–548.

108. Lasley, R. D., Rhee, J. W., Van Wylen, D. G., and Mentzer, R. M., Jr. (1990). Adenosine A_1 receptor mediated protection of the globally ischemic isolated rat heart. *J. Mol. Cell. Cardiol.* **22,** 39–47.

109. Lasley, R. D., Noble, M. A., Konyn, P. J., and Mentzer, R. M., Jr. (1995). Different effects of an adenosine A_1 analogue and ischemic preconditioning in isolated rabbit hearts. *Ann. Thorac. Surg.* **60,** 1698–1703.

110. Hendrickx, M., Toshim, Y., Mubagwa, K., and Flameng, W. (1993). Improved functional recovery after ischemic preconditioning in the globally ischemic rabbit heart is not mediated by adenosine A_1 receptor activation. *Basic Res. Cardiol.* **88,** 2247–2254.

111. Jenkins, D. P., Pugsley, W. B., and Yellon, D. M. (1995). Ischemic preconditioning in a model of global ischemia: Infarct size limitation, but no reduction of stunning. *J. Mol. Cell. Cardiol.* **27,** 1623–1632.

112. Przyklenk, K., Bauer, B., Ovize, M., Kloner, R. A., and Whittaker, P. (1993). Regional ischemic "preconditioning" protects remote virgin myocardium from subsequent sustained coronary occlusion. *Circulation* **87,** 893–899.

113. Freude, B., Masters, T. N., Kostin, S., Robicsek, F., and Schaper, J. (1998). Cardiomyocyte apoptosis in acute and chronic conditions. *Basic Res. Cardiol.* **93,** 85–89.

114. MacLellan, W. R., and Schneider, M. D. (1997). Death by Design: Programmed cell death in cardiovascular biology and disease. *Circ. Res.* **81,** 137–144.

115. Condorelli, G., Morisco, C., Stassi, G., Notte, A., Farina, F., Sgaramella, G., de Rienzo, A., Roncarati, R., Trimarco, B., and Lembo, G. (1999). Increased cardiomyocyte apoptosis and changes in proapoptotic and antiapoptotic genes *bax* and *bcl-2* during left ventricular adaptations to chronic pressure overload in the rat. *Circulation* **99,** 3071–3078.

116. Anversa, P., Cheng, W., Liu, Y., Leri, A., Redaelli, G., and Kajstura, J. (1998). Apoptosis and myocardial infarction. *Basic Res. Cardiol.* **93,** 8–12.

117. Bartling, B., Holtz, J., and Darmer, D. (1998). Contribution of myocyte apoptosis to myocardial infarction? *Basic Res. Cardiol.* **93,** 71–84.

118. Gottlieb, R. A., Burleson, K. O., Kloner, R. A., Babior, B. M., and Engler, R. L. (1994). Reperfusion injury induces apoptosis in rabbit cardiomyocytes. *J. Clin. Invest.* **94,** 1621–1628.

119. Kirshenbaum, L. A., and de Moissac, D. (1997). The bcl-2 gene product prevents programmed cell death of ventricular myocytes. *Circulation* **96,** 1580–1585.

120. Kluck, R. M., Boss-Wetzel, E., Green, D. R., and Newmeyer, D. D. (1997). The release of cytochrome-c from mitochondria: A primary site for BCL-2 regulation of apoptosis. *Science* **275,** 1132–1136.

121. Yang, J., Liu, X., Bhalla, K., Kim, C. N., Ibrado, A. M., Cai, J., Peng, T. I., Jones, D. P., and Wang, X. (1997). Prevention of apoptosis by BCL-2: Release of cytochrome-*c* from mitochondria blocked. *Science* **275,** 1129–1132.

122. Haunstetter, A., and Izumo, S. (1998). Apoptosis: Basic mechanisms and implications for cardiovascular disease. *Circ. Res.* **82,** 1111–1129.

123. Halestrap, A. P., Kerr, P. M., Javadov, S., and Woodfield, K. Y. (1998). Elucidating the molecular mechanism of the permeability transition pore and its role in reperfusion injury of the heart. *Biochim. Biophys. Acta* **1366,** 79–94.

124. Holly, T. A., Drincic, A., Byun, Y., Nakamura, S., Harris, K., Klocke, F. J., and Cryns, V. L. (1999). Caspase inhibition reduces myocyte cell death induced by myocardial ischemia and reperfusion *in vivo*. *J. Mol. Cell. Cardiol.* **31,** 1709–1715.

125. Faulk, E. A., McCully, J. D., Tsukube, T., Hadlow, N. C., Krukenkamp, I. B., and Levitsky, S. (1995). Myocardial mitochondrial calcium accumulation modulates nuclear calcium accumulation and DNA fragmentation. *Ann. Thorac. Surg.* **60,** 307–310.

126. Yue, T. L., Wang, C., Romanic, A. M., Kikly, K., Keller, P., DeWolf, W. E., Jr., Hart, T. K., Thomas, H. C., Storer, B., Gu, J. L., Wang, X., and Feuerstein, G. Z. (1998). Staurosporine-induced apoptosis in cardiomyocytes: A potential role of caspase-3. *J. Mol. Cell. Cardiol.* **30,** 495–507.

127. Schmitz, G. G., Walter, T., Seibl, R., and Kessler, C. (1991). Nonradioactive labeling of oligonucleotides *in vitro* with the hapten digoxigenin by tailing with terminal transferase. *Anal. Biochem.* **192,** 222–231.

128. van Heerde, W. L., Robert-Offerman, S., Dumont, E., Hofstra, L., Doevendans, P. A., Smits, J. F., Daemen, M. J., and Reutelingsperger, C. P. (2000). Markers of apoptosis in cardiovascular tissues: Focus on Annexin V. *Cardiovasc. Res.* **45,** 549-59.

129. Maulik, N., Kagan, V. E., Tyurin, V. A., and Das, D. K. (1998). Redistribution of phosphatidylethanolamine and phosphatidylserine precedes reperfusion-induced apoptosis. *Am. J. Physiol.* **274,** H242–H248.

130. Vogt, A. M., Htun, P., Arras, M., Podzuweit, T., and Schaper, W. (1996). Intramyocardial infusion of tool drugs for the study of molecular mechanisms in ischemic preconditioning. *Basic Res. Cardiol.* **91,** 389–400.

131. Grover, G. J., and Garlid, K. D. (2000). ATP-sensitive potassium channels: A review of their cardioprotective pharmacology. *J. Mol. Cell. Cardiol.* **32,** 677–695.

81

Research in Orthopedic Surgery

A. Simon Turner

Department of Clinical Sciences, Colorado State University, Fort Collins, Colorado 80523

I. Introduction

The economic cost and social and psycological impact cost of musculoskeletal conditions are substantial. These conditions are responsible for a sizeable amount of health-care use and disability (1). Well-characterized animal models with accuracy and reproducibility have allowed orthopedic surgeons to improve quality of care for their patients. Some of the most successful orthopedic procedures, such as joint replacement, tendon healing, fracture treatment, use of biomaterials, and osteoporosis, to name a few, have relied heavily on animal experiments. There are, however, many orthopedic problems in humans that have not been solved because only relatively advanced stages of the disease can be studied and no proper control group is available (2). Furthermore, the basic mechanisms of some diseases are still unknown because of lack of animal models. Tissue engineering and gene therapy in orthopedics are rapidly emerging as individual disciplines, and the use of animal models will be essential before human clinical trials can be initiated.

This chapter provides an overview of orthopedic research using animal models, with emphasis on approaches that have dominated the field for the past 5–10 years, summarizing various models available to the investigator. Not all animal models or human clinical research could be discussed in a single chapter. Many volumes have been written on this subject of orthopedic research (3), and some researchers will be disappointed because "their model" was seen omitted. Selected for this discussion were published papers in which enough detail was provided to understand the technique (group size, anesthesia/analgesia, surgical approach, endpoints, imaging methods, biomechanical testing, pathologic and histologic techniques, etc.) as well as its strengths and weaknesses (including reported complications). The strengths and weaknesses that the authors felt were relevant to report are discussed.

Unreported complications are likely to exist and may not emerge unless the authors are questioned on a personal level! The advantages in using cadaver material for orthopedic research are obvious. However, emphasis in this chapter has been placed on *in vivo* studies rather than those using animal or human specimens harvested at necropsy. Some references are only in abstract form and readers are encouraged to contact investigators if questions about the model arise.

Like other animal models discussed in this book, the early stages of testing should involve small animals such as mice, rats, or rabbits, because they are less costly. In the later stages of testing, the healing characteristics of the animal should approximate those of humans; therefore, larger models higher up the phylogenetic scale should be used. Nonhuman primates are sometimes necessary before the Food and Drug Administration (FDA) can allow clinical trials to be initiated.

Because orthopedics is now highly specialized, with subspecialties often based on "anatomic location" and "function," the chapter was divided into sections with that in mind. It is well known that animals lower in the phylogenetic scale and immature animals heal faster and more completely compared to aged individuals. For example, skeletal maturity influences the repair of articular cartilage (4). Unless a particular orthopedic problem is specific to neonates and children, orthopedic researchers should use skeletally mature animals. This may entail use of purpose-bred animals of known age, or animals in which skeletal maturity can be radiographically verified by epiphyseal closure. Veterinary anatomy books that document ages of epiphyseal closure are available (5). Some orthopedic research in the past was performed in skeletally immature animals, with falsely optimistic results, when the clinical use was aimed at adult patients. One of the reasons why young animals were used in many studies was availability. Food animals (mainly sheep, cattle, and pigs) are sent to slaughter when they are skeletally immature, to provide consumers with the tenderest meat. Unwanted tissues from these animals (e.g., bones, joints, tendons, ligaments) have provided a very inexpensive and convenient source of research material over the years and are ideal for pilot studies or studies that will eventually be relevant to children or teenagers. However, enthusiasm for the use of specimens from young cadavers should be tempered.

Investigators are encouraged to consult the literature cited in the tables. With the sophistication of modern global communication, it is possible to contact individual researchers who have experience with the model, rather than repeat their experiments. Just as the most dramatic photomicrographs for a publication are selected to support hypotheses, researchers are equally reluctant to report the difficulties they encountered in the development and characterization of a particular model.

A. Networking with Other Disciplines

Scientific research methods have become very refined over time and orthopedic research is no exception. The days in which animal housing, sophisticated surgery, batteries of *in vivo* tests, autopsies, and specimen analyses could be performed in one facility, under one roof, are almost over. As a result, those serious about orthopedic research must collaborate with several other disciplines. With modern technological means of communication, laboratories around the world have no "walls."

B. Veterinary Involvement

Orthopedic surgeons interested in pursuing an idea or hypothesis must first consider the appropriate animal model and understand interspecies differences. This means acquiring sound knowledge not only of the anatomy, biology (including response to different anesthetics and analgesics), biomechanics, and physiology of the various animals, but their general husbandry requirements, including appropriate nutrition and housing, as well. Because ethical constraints associated with use of animals are becoming important worldwide (see Chapter 7 for details), the involvement of a veterinarian familiar with these issues is prudent. Veterinary schools and private research facilities (with a staff veterinarian) provide the best opportunity to engage in collaborative orthopedic research using animals.

C. Engineers and Pathologists

Considerable orthopedic research described in this chapter involves use of a wide variety of sophisticated mechanical testing techniques. Investigators with an interest in this field should contact engineers familiar with handling of autopsy specimens. There is a need for collaborators with a working knowledge of materials testing equipment, electrophysiological monitoring equipment, and other methods necessary to execute successfully most studies that are cited.

There are very few orthopedic research projects that do not require the expertise of a trained pathologist. Veterinary pathologists with training beyond that obtained in veterinary school are available in most countries around the world. Those pursuing osteoporosis research, for example, must work closely with scientists trained in histomorphometry, and those interested in orthopedic implant interfaces must work closely with investigators familiar with specimen preparation and study of bone–implant interfaces.

D. One or Both Limbs?

Due to a wide variability in bone healing and response to treatment among individual animals, the convenience of a model allowing intraanimal control will always exist. This is an issue that will confront all interested in orthopedic research at some point in time. In a canine radial defect model, Johnson and co-workers (6) developed bilateral segmental defects to evaluate the effectiveness of ground cortical autograft as a graft material. Initial attempts to develop this bilateral model using plates and screws were unsuccessful because of "a universal failure of hardware and fixation." External fixation provided adequate strength to avoid the instability experienced with plates. Bilateral defects in large mammalian species have rarely been studied for this reason. Studies such as this allow comparison of an established treatment within the same animal and ultimately use fewer animals for the study. Many Institutional Animal Care and Use Committees (IACUCs), including the IACUC at Colorado State University, do not permit disabling surgery (such as an osteotomy in a weight-bearing bone, e.g., the canine radius) to be performed in both limbs. Ulna defect models in both rabbits and dogs are possible because they are not major weight-bearing bones in the forearm. However, orthopedic surgeons are rarely confronted with a long bone fracture involving segmental bone loss that does not require fixation. Investigators will argue that, after bilateral osteotomies, all animals walk on both limbs with confidence and without fear. This is fallacious reasoning because, in a quadruped, there would be no option but to walk on both forelimbs! Certain bilateral procedures to allow for intraanimal comparison are perfectly acceptable to most IACUCs. These include bilateral arthrotomies and arthroscopies and bilateral defect models in which internal or external fixation is not required.

E. Pain Management in Animal Models

The management of pain and suffering in animals used for research is vital to the preservation of the research community's important privilege to use animal subjects in biomedical research (7). Although most researchers in orthopedic surgery acknowledge the need for postoperative pain medication in animals, careful selection of the most effective analgesic has, for the most, been very limited and at times ignored. Analgesics are often administered based on human studies and one of the limiting factors in the laboratory has been our inability to evaluate pain in animals. An anthropomorphic approach to pain management has serious limitations (8). A working knowledge of interspecies variations in animal behavior is the first step in achieving effective pain control in animals. Schemes for pain assessment and pain scoring are now routinely used in many research laboratories. The ideal analgesic for orthopedic research should be easy to administer without unwanted fear and excessive activity, should provide analgesia without profound sedation or recumbency, and should have minimal or no effect on the experimental condition being studied. Nonsteroidal antiinflammatory drugs (NSAIDs) are useful in alleviating mild to moderate orthopedic pain in large animals; some of the newer NSAIDs, such as flunixin and carprofen, show efficacy comparable to that of opioids (8).

It is the responsibility of scientific journals to ensure that the animals used in studies reported in their pages are properly managed. For example, the *Journal of Bone and Joint Surgery* now requires that information regarding the management of postoperative pain be included in the paragraph dealing with the postoperative care of animals.

II. Long Bones

A. Improvement in Fracture Healing and Distraction Osteogenesis

Of the 33 million individuals in the United States who sustain musculoskeletal injuries, nearly 6.2 million have fractures (9). Fracture healing is a complex physiologic process and mammalian and avian species have played an important role in unraveling the events once thought to be straightforward (10). For an overview of the biology of fracture healing, the reader is directed to other texts and reviews (11–13). There is still a need to develop strategies to expedite the healing process, treat nonunions and delayed unions, and return patients to prefracture life styles. Callus distraction, distraction osteogenesis, and the Ilizarov technique (callotasis) are terms that were not widely understood 15 years ago. Callotasis is now frequently used for the treatment of defects of tubular long bones, leg length deformities, and malignancies (14–15). Study of the biological events associated with callotasis (16) and biological enhancement (17) has become an endeavor for many laboratories around the world. Although distraction osteogenesis is a variation of external fixators, it is included under the heading of fracture healing.

Growth factor regulation of fracture repair is of great interest because herein may lie the key not only for understanding the complexities of the healing process, but for the development of biologic methods for the enhancement of fracture healing (11, 18). For these studies, rats are the models of choice because of their low cost of purchase and upkeep and the ability to use large numbers. The rat femoral shaft fracture repaired by intramedullary (i/m) pinning is probably the most popular of all fracture models when studying biochemical and cellular events. Both limbs are frequently used in rats. Rabbits are more adaptable to fracture repair with plates and screws or external skeletal fixation. However, they are more difficult to manage while under general anesthesia and during the postoperative period. Investigators should expect significant mortality and morbidity when designing such studies. Both rabbits and rats allow use of expensive therapeutic agents compared to larger animals.

Management of fractures in dogs is well established in veterinary orthopedics, and although not show, in Table I, the dog has been a popular animal model when studying internal or external skeletal fixation techniques (10). The ability of dogs to thrive on three legs is well known to the veterinary profession but is often a concern to researchers new to the species (Fig. 1). Sheep have been used for the study of fracture repair (especially in Europe) and were the model of choice of the Association for the Study of Internal Fixation (ASIF) when pioneering the work in primary bone healing in the 1960s. They are becoming more popular in North America because of the changing sentiment toward the use of dogs and cost considerations. Some examples of the animal models used to study the effects of calcitonin on experimental fracture healing have been summarized by Wallach *et al.* (19).

Animal models of fracture healing are also useful in the discovery of how fracture healing can be retarded by adjunctive therapy such as nonsteroidal antiinflammatory drugs (20), bisphosphonates (21), and fluoroquinolones (22). Table I shows various animal models used to investigate improvements in fracture healing and distraction osteogenesis

B. Long Bone Defects and Bone Grafts

Segmental bone loss due to trauma, tumor resection, and nonunion is a challenge to the orthopedic surgeon (Fig. 2). Autograft has traditionally been considered an ideal material in a wide range of orthopedic applications and still remains the "gold standard" (43). In the United States alone, autogenous bone grafting is carried out in about 200,000

Table I Improvement in Fracture Healing and Distraction Osteogenesis

Animal model	Purpose of model	Strength	Weakness	Ref.
Rat	Experimental pseudarthrosis	Standardized model		23
	Expression of cytokines in callus			11, 12
	Effects of ethanol on healing		Fracture malalignment (1 case)	24
	Effects of a bisphosphonate on healing			21
	Effects of ciprofloxacin on healing	Both limbs used		22
Rabbit	Stress shielding by rigid fixation	Both limbs used		25
	Influence of callus deformation time	Repeated harvesting possible		26
	rhBMP-2 in ulnar nonunion	Both limbs used	Postoperative deaths (4 cases)	27
	Indomethacin and bone metabolism		9 out of 20 removed from study	28
	Cyclic compression and distraction			29
	Periosteum and bone marrow in bone lengthening			30
	rhBMP-2 in stable and unstable fractions		Mechanical barrier of carriers	31
	Vitamin D_3 (ED-71) and distraction			32
	Angiogenic response and distraction			33
	Demineralized matrix and lengthening		Death after surgery, or infection and fracture at pin site (9 cases)	34
	Model development and vascular response to distraction		Fracture through pin track	35
	Marrow progenitor cells—distraction	Both limbs used	Intraoperative fractures (3 cases)	17
Dog	Effects of plate luting on vascularity			36
	Fixation and cortical bone blood flow		Some i/m rod loosening	37
	Osteotomy vs. distraction			16
	Fatigue fracture	Naturally occurring		38
	Osteochondral cells from nonunions	Established model for nonunion	Variability between animals	39
Pig	Effect of subcutaneous growth hormone			40
Sheep	Internal fixateur to femur and tibia		Fracture through distal pin (1 case)	41
	Measurement of angiogenic factor			42

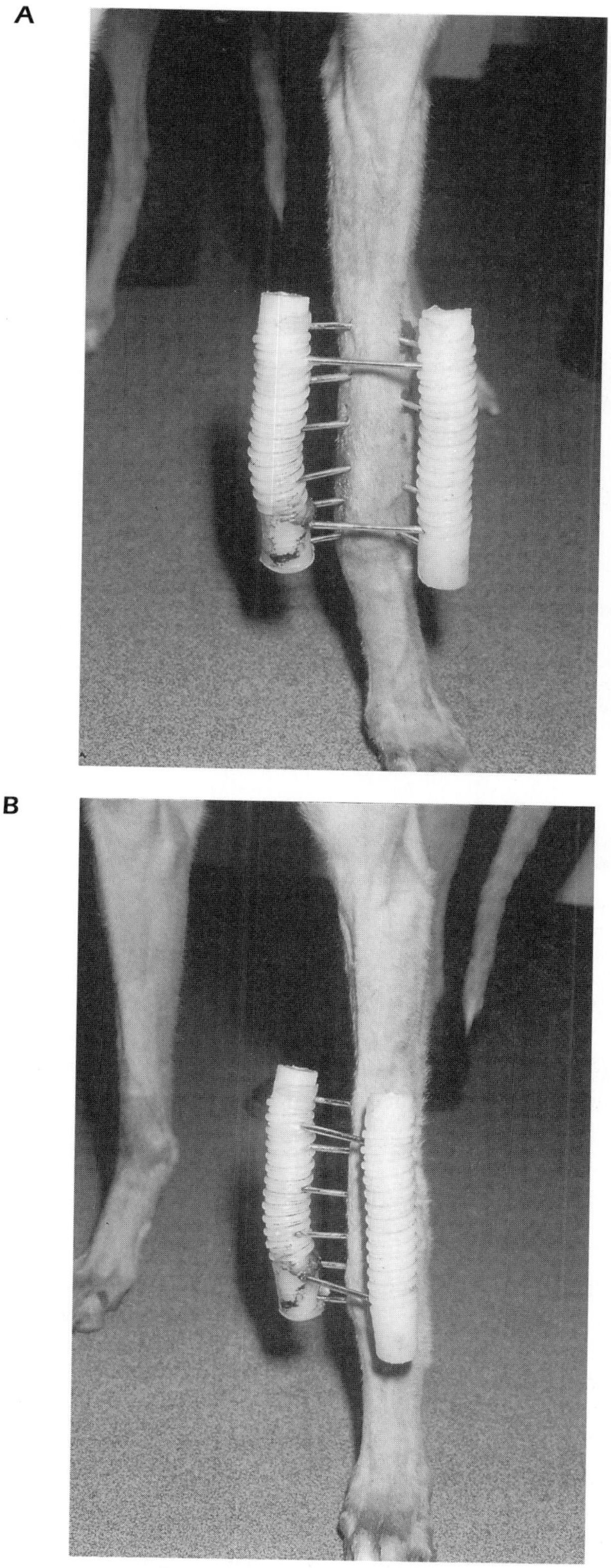

Figure 1 The dog is a popular model for internal and external fixation research (10). Dogs ambulate easily on three limbs but bilateral osteotomies with fracture fixation are not permitted by some IACUCs. Courtesy of Dr. Doug Huber, Colorado State University.

surgical cases annually (44). Increased use of blood products, blood loss, increased operating time, surgical scars, inadequate amounts of bone in young patients, and pain at the donor site are just some of the problems associated with autografts (45–47). Banked allograft, although inferior to autogenous bone, is sometimes available but a serious issue that has emerged over the past decade is the risk of viral transmission (48). This potential complication has stimulated animal research and subsequent clinical application of "graft extenders" and synthetic materials (pellets, pastes, gels, strips, putties, and blocks) in orthopedic, maxillofacial, and dental surgery. Such materials can be readily shaped to suit a defect. The ideal material to be used as a substitute for bone graft is one that is safe, biocompatible, nonallergenic, has good bone-bonding capacity, and provides a favorable scaffold for bone growth (49).

Synthetic material can be placed in bone conduction chambers. These have been designed so that repeated sampling is possible because of the removable inner core of the chamber (50). They can be used in a wide variety of animals, including rats, rabbits, and goats (51, 52). These chambers are typically inserted in the metaphyseal regions of the long bones, where the likelihood of creating a pathologic fracture ("stress-riser effect") is diminished.

The model used to evaluate graft materials should be clinically relevant and should provide a clearly defined and quantifiable measure of outcome (46). Cylindrical cavities in the metaphyses and diaphyses of the long bones (53) or the cranium (54–56) that do not require internal fixation and allow immediate weight-bearing (unloaded) use have been used in many studies in a wide variety of experimental animals and the advantages are obvious. A clear advantage is the ability to use two limbs in the same animal, with minimal pain and suffering, allowing an internal control or comparison between two different treatments within the same animal. Use of either the ipsilateral radius or the ulna of dogs and rabbits has been helpful because weight-bearing is still possible with the defect in only one of the bones (57). This reduces the number of animals that are required to achieve statistical significance. Fracture models heal well in most animals and are not sensitive enough to test the efficacy of bone graft materials. Most investigators have used diaphyseal defect models, which result in nonunion if left untreated (46).

The appropriate defect size is important to show that spontaneous bone repair is unlikely without the bone graft substitute (58) and researchers should be aware of what is known as the critical-sized defect (CSD) for the animal species being used. This is the smallest defect that will heal with less than 10% bony growth. A study may demonstrate an optimistic result if the defect made is too small and would have regenerated spontaneously without treatment.

Materials being tested as fillers of defects include degradable polymers (polylactic acids, polyglycolic acids) as well

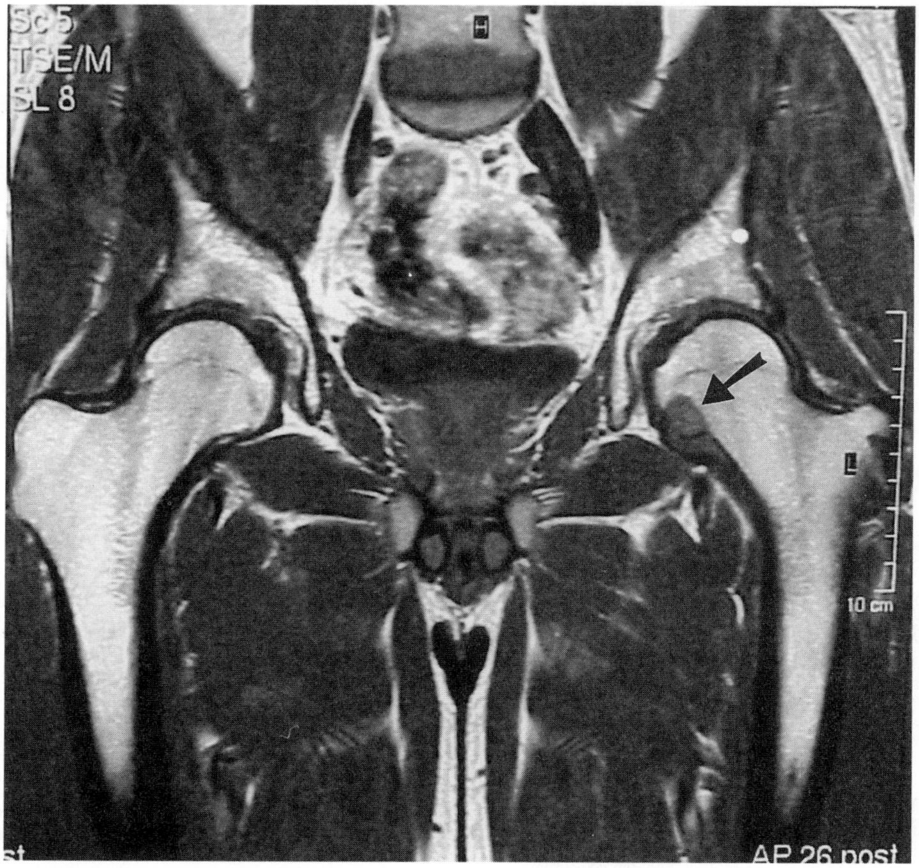

Figure 2 MRI of the left femoral head in a 37-year-old man with 8 months of hip pain. Coronal T1-weighted MR image reveals a cartilagenous lesion later identified as an enchondroma (arrow). The lesion was treated by surgical curettage and grafting using a surgical-grade calcium sulfate preparation mixed with bone marrow aspirate and demineralized bone matrix.

as type I collagen, hydroxyapatite, tricalcium phosphate, and demineralized bone matrix, to name but a few (46, 59, 60). A review of current technology and applications of bone graft and bone graft substitutes concluded that newer materials require a carrier vehicle for optimal expression of conductivity, and collagen may be this "essential" ingredient (49). The discovery of osteoconductive agents to add to an osteoconductive material has been one of the greatest contributions to understanding bone formation (44). The delivery of these signaling molecules, various matrix proteins, and purified growth factors at the correct dose, at an appropriate rate, will eventually produce a composite material that will decrease the morbidity associated with autograft harvest surgery (49). Use of osteoconductive materials as adjuncts to interbody fusion devices is also of interest in spine surgery (61) and is presented elsewhere in this chapter. Expression of these substances through adenovirally mediated gene transfer will likely be another direction this research will take in the future. Suitable animal models for the evaluation of diaphyseal defects in the long bones are summarized in Table II, and examples of suitable models for evaluation of synthetic graft materials are shown in Table III.

C. Evaluation of Pins, Rods, Plates, and Screws

The orthopedic community has been searching for improved fracture fixation devices for centuries. Devices that are implanted into the human body represent an even greater challenge, giving rise to concerns about compatibility, toxicity, carcinogenicity, and mechanical properties. Interest in the biocompatibility of the bioresorbable synthetic polymers used as suture material for several decades has led to the introduction of materials [e.g., polyglycolide (PGA)] for the fixation of fractures. Animal model studies were essential in bringing these devices into clinical use (98). More recently, unwanted foreign-body reaction and osteolysis (99) have stimulated further research in these implants (100).

Table II Long Bone Defects

Animal model	Purpose of model	Strength	Weakness	Ref.
Rat	Repair with rhBMP-2 in PLGA matrix	BMC and BMD measured (DEXA)	Only one time period (9 weeks) studied	62
		Both limbs used		63
	Repair of segmental defects		Short healing time of rodents	64
	Effect of bioactive bone cement			65
Rabbit	TCP/amylopectin paste and $rhTGF\beta_1$		Not a critical-sized defect (1 cm)	66
	Bone formation and rhBMP-2	Critical-sized defect		67
	Porous HA implants—varying density	External fixation not required		68
	Temporal and spatial characterization in limb lengthening	Both tibiae used		14
	Composite injectable bone substitutes	Bilateral implantation	Infection (1 case)	69
	Coral grafting with bone marrow		Ulna fracture	70
	Adsorption and release of IGF-1	Bilateral implantation		71
Dog	Porous coated femoral implants	Both femora used		72
	Porous HA–$CaPO_4$ evaluation		Pin migration (1 case)	73
	rhBMP-7 and ulnar defect	Better Haversian bone		74
	Collagraft in femoral defects		Minor problems (unrelated to graft)	75
	Ground cortical allograft evaluation	Both limbs used	Sepsis (2 cases)	6
	Effect of cisplatin chemotherapy		One death (unrelated)	76
	Bovine-derived bone protein	Both limbs used	Superficial infection (1 case)	77
	Autologous mesenchymal stem cells	No fixation failure		78
	$CaSO_4$ in metaphyseal defects	Both limbs used		79
	$CaSO_4$ in proximal humeral defects	No fixation required (both limbs)		80
	Somatotropin in an unstable gap			81
	Bone–graft substitute for nonunion	Reproducible model	Splint required to avoid ulna fracture	82
Sheep	Effect of rhBMP-2 (femoral defect)		Critical-sized defect	83
	Composite bone substitute		Pathological fracture (1 case)	84
	Influence of size and stability of gap	Repair process similar in humans	Pin loosening, infection, and fracture	85
	Resorbable $CaPO_4$ α-BSM			86
	Defect model development	Bone similar in humans		87
	Resorbable polymeric membranes		Postoperative slinging required	88
	Long bone defect model		Healing at 12 weeks in 2 of 6 cases	89
	Marrow stromal cells and porous HA	Critical-sized defect used (3.5 cm)		90

Plate-induced bone loss late in fracture remodeling has been attributed to stiffness difference between implant and bone. Interference with the blood supply to the bone was another explanation of this phenomenon. Animal models (sheep and dogs) were key to these discoveries (101, 102). Modification of the undersurface of the plate was investigated in dogs (103). Improved fracture fixation by insertion of a space-filling substance, polymethylmethacrylate (PMMA), between the plate and the bone was investigated in horses (104) and dogs (36).

Internal fixation with intramedullary rods, with and without reaming, is more suited to the sheep than to the dog, and the latter is more suited to show the negative effect of reaming (10).

Pin-tract infection is the most common complication of external fixation, with the incidence of infection ranging from 0 to 100% and increasing with the duration of fixation (105–108). Modification of the pin surface or the metal and the addition of various antibacterial agents to decrease infection rate has been tested in *in vitro* studies (109) and extensively in animal models. The bone commonly injured and treated with external fixator pins is the human tibia, and this is the bone in which pin coatings can be conveniently tested in animals. Bilateral procedures are acceptable to most IACUCs if the bone is intact (without the use of an osteotomy or and external fixator). The use of large animals such as goats, sheep, and dogs allows as many as six pins to be placed in each bone, increasing the power of the study and

Table III Bone Grafts

Animal model	Purpose of model	Strength	Weakness	Ref.
Mouse	Angiogenesis and osteogenesis			91
Rat	Fibroblast growth factor—allograft	Bone chamber for sampling		51
	Cell manipulation and TGF-β			92
	Impaction of cancellous bone grafts			93
Rabbit	Revascularization–recirculation	Bone chamber for sampling		94
	Autoclaved bone for defects			95
	Percutaneous marrow grafting			57
	Rigid fixation and only graft survival			54
	Coralline hydroxyapatite	Both femoral condyles used		58
	Polylactide–co-glycolide for repair		Higher animal model warranted	59
Dog	Revascularized bone grafts			96
	Immune response to allografts	Remodeling similar to humans	Assays require specialist laboratory	97
	HA for cranial reconstruction		Nonunions due to movement	56
	Evaluation of plugs to test grafts	Controls graft volume		53
		Can evaluate several materials		
Goat	Allograft incorporation process	Repeated samples possible		50
Primate	Xenogenic implants with carrier	Close anatomy and physiolgy		55

the reduction of number of animals used. (Fig. 3). Stress fracture through one of the pin sites is always a risk if the pins are in diaphyseal bone. The humane aspect of this research in animals must be kept in mind, and pin loosening, development of cellulitis, and lameness must be monitored carefully and considered endpoints for euthanasia. The iliac crest of sheep has also been used to test silver coating of pins (110). Careful experimental planning with microbiologists is essential to ensure the innoculation dose (usually *Staphylococcus aureus*). Clinical and microbiological evaluations of the pins with some semiquantitative grading system are routinely used in such studies. Some examples of animal models used to evaluate pins, rods, plates, and screws are shown in Table IV.

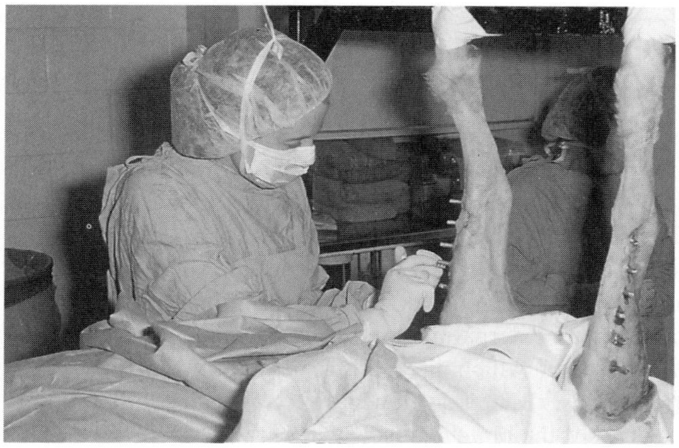

Figure 3 The tibia is a bone in which external fixator pin coatings can be conveniently tested. With the bone intact, bilateral procedures with as many as six pins in each bone are acceptable to most IACUCs.

D. External Fixators

External fixation of fractures is the preferred method of stabilization of severe open fractures. This has resulted in production of new and improved designs of the external fixator (121) and entire texts have been written on the clinical application of external fixators (122). Research in this field of orthopedics has been directed mainly on four fronts: (1) modification of the surfaces to resist infection (discussed above in this chapter), (2) modification of the pin surface to reduce loosening, (3) improving the design to provide stability and withstand activity of patients, and (4) timing the removal of the pins (axial dynamization) to minimize stress protection and optimize remodeling. External fixators are also used for limb lengthening (callotasis) experimentally (34, 42) and clinically, (123) as well as long bone defect models (6).

The mechanical testing of different frame designs, pin diameters, and pin placement lends itself to the use of models or cadaveric bone. In this field of orthopedic research, investigators are encouraged to work closely with engineers with access to facilities that can perform *in vitro* bench work before using live animals. Postmortem measurement of torsional stiffness and strength requires access to a laboratory with experience in potting and mounting the bone ends in a materials testing machine with the appropriate load cell.

Table IV Evaluation of Pins, Rods, Plates, and Screws

Animal model	Purpose of model	Strength	Weakness	Ref.
Rat	Effect of parenteral PTH (1–34)			111
	Memory metal (NiTi) i/m fixation	No immobilization required	Nail migration (4 animals)	112
	HA pins (Ossatite)		Deaths at end of surgery (4 cases)	113
	i/m nails of different rigidity			114
Rabbit	Interface of polyglycolide screws			98
	Infection of HA-coated implants			115
Dog	Modification of plate–bone interface with Silastic			103
	Effect of limited reaming on cortical blood flow			116
	Poly(ortho ester) pins properties		Large variation in mechanical	117
Sheep	Healing after unreamed medullary nailing			118
	"Biological" plate fixation of comminuted femoral fractures			101
	Osteolysis–polyglycolide implants			100
	Intramedullary nail infection			119
	Intramedullary reaming and blood flow using laser doppler flowmetry			120

Transverse osteotomy of the tibia of dogs, sheep, and goats is the most common technique used in this field of external fixator research (Fig. 1). Clinically, the tibia is the bone most frequently requiring external fixation. The tibia in these quadruped models is accessible without compromise to neurovascular structures by the pins, allows wound access for daily pin tract evaluation and cleaning, and has thick cortices to minimize stress fracture during unrestrained activities. The bone is also accessible for radiography and densitometry for assessment of fracture healing. Bilateral procedures have been permitted by the IACUCs of some institutions but have been unacceptable to others.

Improvement in the quality of the bone-to-pin interface has interested researchers and clinicians for some time. Surface modification with osteoconductive materials such as hydroxyapatite (HA) has been the focus of several investigators (124, 125), whereas others have looked at coatings that are more resistant to infection (107). Some examples of animal models used for research on external fixators are shown in Table V.

Table V External Fixators

Animal model	Purpose of model	Strength	Weakness	Ref.
Dog	Effect of external fixation stiffness		Pin loosening—tenotomy required	126
	Effects of axial dynamization	Bilateral osteotomies	Large variation in healing among animals	127
Sheep	Stress protection—external fixation			128
	Plasma-sprayed HA coating on screws	Comparable healing period to that in humans		129
	Effect of HA coating external fixation pins		Collapse and malalignment (6 cases)	124
	HA- and Ti-coated external fixation pins			125
	Strain rate and timing			130
	Stress and strain on bone surfaces			131
	Pin-tract infection model	Osteotomy not required		107
	Fixator stiffness—segmental transport		Variability in animal weightbearing	15
Goat	Pin-tract infection model		Clinical relevance?	106
	Pin infection prevention			132

III. Osteoporosis

Postmenopausal osteoporosis is a major health problem for women, the understanding of which is hindered by the difficulty of studying a disease that is essentially restricted to humans. Osteoporosis is a slowly progressive disease, necessitating a study of several years' duration to allow a response to therapy. Because results are accrued slowly, accumulation of data is time consuming, and maintenance of a study group is made more difficult by natural attrition due to either relocation or death. The high cost and long time frame of clinical testing are other reasons why animal models play a crucial role in osteoporosis research (133). Even a model with a small representation of human functions may be of use for some aspect of the human condition under examination (134). An additional goal for research into osteoporosis is the design of prosthetic devices (with or without biological coatings to promote osseointegration) that will perform optimally in the presence of osteoporotic bone.

A. Small Animal Models

The most commonly used animal model in osteoporosis studies is the rodent (135). The ovariectomized (OVX) rat exhibits many of the characteristics of human postmenopausal osteoporosis. With a fast generation time, rodents are often a starting point for preliminary screenings, efficacy, and toxicity studies of new pharmacologic agents or therapeutic modalities, followed by verification in other species, before undertaking clinical trials in patients (136). The advantages of rodents are numerous; they are inexpensive, easy to house, and the general public is accustomed to the role of rodents for use in research. With intense interest in transgenic animals, availability of strains of mouse mutants with altered bone marrow function, and availability of recombinant murine cytokines, mice will always be a logical starting point for manipulation of the genome (137). A senescence-accelerated mouse (SAM) has been developed as a model for age-related spontaneous osteopenia (138).

There is extensive literature studying the OVX rat, including the histomorphometric changes, biochemical markers, methodology for bone densitometry, and evaluation of bone fragility (139–144). Genetically specific strains can be acquired, thus removing some variability in the studies. Their shorter life span enables studies on the effects of aging on the bone. Because the rodent has been used so extensively in research of all types, much is known about bone turnover and the effect of diet on this process. Cortical thinning and increased fragility are well documented in aging rat and mouse bone, but it is unclear if this results in increased fractures. Weight gain in OVX rats can result in an increase in bone mass with increase in mechanical loading, resulting in protection of OVX animals against age-related loss of bone strength (145); such bone changes are seen as osteopenia rather than osteoporosis.

Rodents do not experience a natural menopause, but OVX has become a time-honored method used to produce an artificial menopause (139–143). Although aged rodents have Haversian systems and OVX results in significant bone loss, the use of this model is hindered because young rats have a limited naturally occurring basic multicellular unit (BMU)-based remodeling. Nevertheless, older rats have lamellar bone (although most is "fine-fibered"), trabecular remodeling, and some secondary osteonal remodeling (141–143). Because older animals more accurately reflect the target population for proposed osteoporosis therapy, the very aged-rat model (30-month old) is an even better choice as a cost-effective animal model (146). The inability to restore bone following OVX in rats is similar to what is seen in human bone (147). Hysterectomy does not impair the ability of estradiol to conserve bone in OVX rats. In other words, estrogen-mediated induction of growth factors from uterine tissue does not play an essential role in mediating the bone-conserving actions of estrogen in the rat (148).

Longitudinal bone growth increases transiently after OVX in long bones of rats, but this can be minimized by the use of either aged rats (9–12 months old) or of skeletal sites where longitudinal growth is greatly reduced (e.g., lumbar vertebrae) (141). Male rats are unsuitable models for osteopenia studies because their growth plates do not close in less than 30 months. The rat is a poor animal to study the effect of OVX on cortical bone because of the lack of Haversian systems, and another limitation is the absence of impaired osteoblast function during the late stages of estrogen deficiency (141). However, rats do show significant elevation of cortical porosity in response to immobilization (149).

In a study designed to investigate the effects of estrogen alone or combined with norethindrone or norgestimate on bone density and compressive mechanical properties in aged rats, both interrupted progestin regimens had a better effect than did estrogen alone (150). The findings of this study showed a reduced modulus of elasticity in the OVX group but an increased flexibility, unlike the brittleness seen in osteopenic women. The authors stated "the rat model may therefore not be appropriate for comparison of mechanical properties with the human," but they also said that "bone mineral density in the aged rat model . . . seems to follow the same pattern as the human in relation to estrogen deficiency and gonadal hormonal replacement" (150). Others (151) have found that the mechanical strength of the femoral neck was a sensitive indicator of bone loss associated with OVX, orchidectomy, and immobilization.

Highly accurate and precise noninvasive measurement of bone mineral content (BMC) and bone mineral density (BMD) in rodents (while under general anesthesia) is now possible using dual-energy X-ray absorptiometry (DXA) with ultra-high-resolution software (Fig. 4). However, for very small animals (<50 g), poor edge detection and accuracy limit the use of DXA (152). To improve resolution in smaller animals, microcomputed tomography (micro-CT), which can provide images of individual trabeculae similar to a histomorphometry slide, has become the industry standard. Micro-CT can image 20-μm isotropic voxels and reconstruct a three-dimensional data set of bone, measuring connectivity, thereby determining the relationship between architecture and strength (153).

As previously mentioned, a stipulation for a model to evaluate implants in osteopenic bone involves suitability for the testing of various prosthetic devices—for example, total

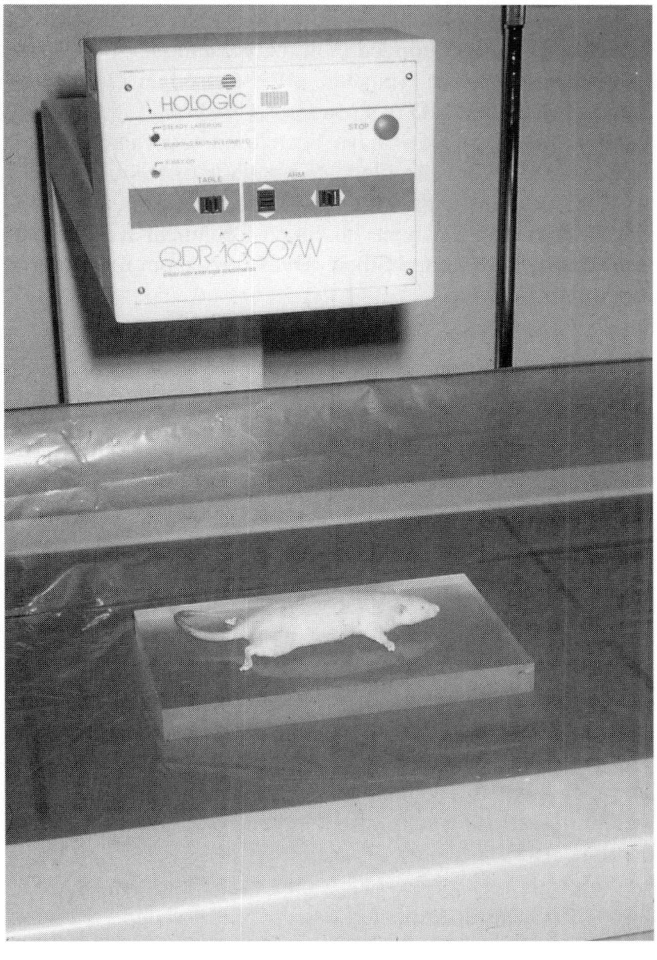

Figure 4 Dual-energy X-ray (DXA) absorptiometry, originally designed for use in humans, is adapted to animals of all sizes and shapes (152). BMC and BMD in rodents are possible using DXA with ultra-high-resolution software, but for very small animals (<50 g), poor edge detection and accuracy limit the use of DXA. Microcomputed tomography (micro-CT), which can provide images of individual trabeculae similar to a histomorphometry slide, has become the industry standard.

hip arthroplasty. Clearly, the size of the rodent, although advantageous for housing, is too small to be suitable for such procedures. However, rats are ideal models to evaluate smaller implants—various matrices or scaffolds, with or without bone-inducing proteins such as the bone morphogenetic proteins—before such implants are used in larger, more expensive animal models. For example, the bone-inductive potential of demineralized bone matrix (DBM), previously taken from OVX rats, was studied in OVX rats (154). Finally, longer term studies that require several biopsies or large blood samples also are very difficult to carry out in animals as small as the rat.

B. Large Animal Models

1. Dogs

For many years, dogs have been used for the study of the human skeleton because of their extensive BMU-based remodeling. A review of the dog as a model for estrogen-depletion bone loss is available (155). Dogs are less expensive than primates, easier to work with, and, like humans, monogastric.

Some studies (156), but not all (157–160), have shown insignificant bone loss in dogs after cessation of ovarian function. The bisphosphonate YM175 was tested in OVX calcium-restricted beagles. BMD, strength and structure, and turnover of bone were evaluated and it was concluded that although calcium restriction increased the sensitivity of bone to OVX in rats and minipigs, such sensitivity was not increased in OVX beagles. Furthermore, it was stated that "the contribution of OVX to the reduction in bone mass and strength at the organ level in the OVX beagle model was small" (161). Group size has been a frequent problem of many studies in dogs but cancellous bone loss may be detectable in studies with large group sizes and with more precise tools (156).

The resistance of the canine skeleton to natural estrogen deficiency or artificial estrogen recession may be related to the infrequent canine estrus cycle. Unlike humans and primates, which are polyestrus, dogs are diestrus, with ovulation occurring twice a year (i.e., spring and fall). Hormone levels remain constant until estrus, at which time they spike. Despite extremely low levels of estrogen throughout most of the year, spontaneous fractures of the appendicular or axial skeleton in dogs are almost unheard of in veterinary practice. Removal of both ovaries and uterus does not appear to be sufficient to create significant bone loss. Furthermore, the histologic response of the dog to loss of ovarian function appears to be heterogeneous, possibly due to the variation in duration of the post-OVX period. The remodeling changes (activation) in cancellous and cortical bone are transient and brief in nature (stabilization within 5–12 months), without sizeable bone loss (155, 156). Furthermore, alterations in skeletal remodeling do not appear sufficiently sustained to have a substantial impact on cancellous bone microstructure and strength. There are millions of dogs without ovaries and uterus, many of them quite old, with sedentary lifestyles, and they do not have fracture rates comparable to those seen in postmenopausal women. Compression tests on trabecular bone samples from vertebral bodies and distal femoral regions were performed 12 months after ovariectomy in beagles (162). There was a decrease in mechanical properties of the vertebrae but femoral properties were conserved.

Dogs, however, have been used for regulatory safety studies to assess the long-term safety of bone-active agents (e.g., bisphosphonates) on bone quality (163–166). A study of the effect of estrogen depletion and parathyroid hormone (PTH) stimulation on ovariohysterectomized dogs found no significant changes in bones (167). It was concluded that "the lack of sizeable responses in histomorphometric, bone mass and biochemical parameters may limit the utility of dogs for the study of cancellous bone loss in ovarian-dysfunction osteoporosis" (167).

Although dogs may be of limited use as a model for estrogen deficiency-related bone loss, they have been extremely useful for evaluation of general aspects of the human skeleton (e.g., fracture healing, effects of immobilization, long-term effects of certain bone-active agents, and allografts). They have also been used extensively for bone ingrowth and joint replacement, as discussed elsewhere in this chapter.

2. Pigs and Minipigs

Previously the size of the pig was a limiting factor in its widespread use as a model for research, but the introduction of the minipig (and the micropig) has eliminated this problem. Although more expensive to acquire, minipigs at maturity weigh 60 kg, whereas the commercial farm pig can weigh in excess of 150 kg. This reduction in size translates into substantially less housing space and greater ease of handling. The reproductive cycle of the pig is similar to that of the human in duration (18–21 days) and, like the human, is continuous. Other important similarities are the omnivorous diet of swine and the anatomy of their gastrointestinal tract; these are their most notable advantages over some other animal models.

Several features of the minipig skeleton are similar to the human skeleton. The skeleton displays extensive BMU-based remodeling in cancellous and metaphyseal cortical bone (168) and pigs possess a definable peak bone mass at 2.5–3 years of age (169). Pigs are one of the few animals species in which a syndrome of spontaneous vertebral fracture has been reported (170). Although pigs are quadrupeds (and therefore have different loading patterns on the bone), they have a higher bone mass and denser trabecular network than do humans (171, 172). On the other hand, like dogs, they are large enough to receive prosthetic implants and withstand repetitive bone biopsies and large-volume blood sampling. Bone removal and deposition of trabecular and cortical bone occur at a rate comparable with that of humans, and swine possess lamellar bone (173).

The skeletal response to OVX in pigs is modulated by dietary calcium. In a study involving OVX Sinclair S-1 minipigs on a 0.75% calcium-restricted diet, there were significant changes in remodeling parameters (e.g., an increase in resorptive cell function at the level of the remodeling unit). This led to significant alterations in bone structure (e.g., trabecular plate perforation) and a significant decline in bone mass and biomechanical competence of vertebral cancellous bone (174, 175). These findings suggest that the OVX calcium-restricted (0.75%) Sinclair S1 minipig has potential as a model for studying the bone remodeling in humans and perimenopausal bone loss in women. The effect of OVX can be confounded in immature animals so skeletally mature sows were evaluated. OVX caused an 11% reduction in vertebral BMD in 12 months (176).

Both pigs and dogs have been used to evaluate bone-active agents. For example, a comparison of the effects of a 1-year treatment with sodium fluoride and the bisphosphonate alendronate on bone quality (mechanical testing) and remodeling (histomorphometry) was carried out in 9-month-old minipigs (177).

3. Sheep

Primary osteopenia in sheep is uncommon. In old age, a limiting factor for survival in sheep is dental health. Wear of teeth and tooth loss lead to gradual wasting and inanition, with bone loss. The changes observed in mandibular bone at various stages of development in sheep from several farms with varying incidence of premature incisor loss have been studied (178). Johnson *et al.* (179) and our work (180, 181) have rekindled interest in the ovine mandible as it relates to estrogen loss.

The effects of various therapeutic drugs, such as fluoride, on bone tissue were investigated by workers in France using sheep (182, 183). The same group used a sheep model to show that OVX induced an increase in bone formation beginning at 10 weeks after surgery and persisting at 6 months (184).

Since those reports, our group (185) and others (184, 186–189) have documented osteopenia in sheep following OVX as well as the response to various agents such as estradiol (189–190), salmon calcitonin (191), and the selective estrogen receptor modulator (SERM) raloxifene (192, 193). Our earlier findings showed a significant decline in cancellous bone volume (BV/TV%) of the iliac crest following OVX (194). Subsequent studies (190) demonstrated bone loss (measured by DXA) in the lumbar vertebrae following OVX (195). These data and findings from other independent laboratories demonstrated that bone loss in the lumbar vertebrae of sheep following OVX was ameliorated by estrogen replacement therapy (ERT).

The skeletal changes seen in the proximal femur following menopause have been studied for many years and we documented a statistically different Singh index in the proximal femur in OVX ewes compared to both young and old sheep (194). Although precise measurements of excised sheep femora using DXA are possible (152), one of the distinct disadvantages of using a quadruped (including dogs) for measuring longitudinal changes in BMD using DXA is the technical difficulties in positioning the animal to examine the femoral neck region. In longitudinal studies, it is critical that an identical region of interest is evaluated repeatedly. Some researchers using DXA have experienced difficulties in edge detection when measuring ovine vertebrae (196), and others have overcome this by scanning only the central portion of the cancellous-rich vertebral body (189) (Fig. 5).

Seasonal changes in bone mass and biochemical markers in elderly women have been reported (197). In a 24-month study in northern New England, significant seasonal changes in BMD, serum 25-hydroxyvitamin D, and parathyroid hormone were seen; the greatest decline in measurable bone mass was in winter. Seasonal fluctuations such as this also occur in sheep and this must be addressed as a potential variable when using sheep in studies of osteopenia (183, 186, 189, 190). Sheep living in more benign climates such as Australia may demonstrate less seasonal variation, although this has not been documented. For these reasons, experiments using sheep should have not only the appropriate control groups, but, if possible, span all four seasons to minimize seasonal changes. Seasonal variation is also related to the periods of seasonal anestrus, which is linked to the environmental photoperiod (198).

To evaluate the effect of salmon calcitonin on bone mass, compression (lumbar vertebrae and femoral neck), torsional stress (femoral neck only), and resonant frequency were measured in excised femoral neck and lumbar vertebral samples from OVX sheep (188, 191). Bone mass was measured using DXA and dual-energy quantitative computed tomography (DEQCT). Sheep were used because "they possess skeletal turnover kinetics similar to humans." OVX resulted in decreased BMD measured by DXA and DEQCT and decreased resistance to rapid compression but not to torsion. Sheep have also been used as a model for glucocorticoid-induced bone loss (187, 189, 199, 200).

Several advantages of sheep include temporal and quantitative similarities between the hormone profiles of ewes and female humans (198). Although some breeds are seasonally polyestrous (cycles begin in the fall season in response to shortening periods of daylight), some breeds (e.g., Merino) can continue to cycle almost year-round (189). An OVX animal model with more frequent estrus cycles than, for example, the dog may prove to be more sensitive to estrogen deficiency. However, sheep, like rats (143) and many of the other animal models, do not have a clear-cut menopause at midlife that is characterized by accelerated bone loss.

One clear disadvantage of the use of sheep is their different gastrointestinal system. Studies in which there is interest in the oral absorption of drugs (avoiding alteration of the drug by rumen microflora) either require surgical insertion of an abomasal fistula, or stimulation of the oropharynx as the medication is delivered (to activate closure of the reticular groove). Another potentially relevant difference in mineral homeostasis between sheep and humans is their phosphorus metabolism. Urinary phosphate excretion is much lower in sheep and the gastrointestinal tract is the major route of phosphate elimination in this species (189).

The cortical bone of sheep is similar to bone of other species of large domestic mammals. The bone of young sheep (less than 3–4 years of age) is plexiform and is a combination of woven and lamellar bone with functional similarities but with distinctly different patterns of deposition and organization (185). Like woven bone, plexiform bone is deposited rapidly but achieves better mechanical properties for large, rapidly growing animals such as the artiodactyls, cows, elephants, and larger breeds of dogs. Plexiform bone is also found in humans in the medial side of the mandibular ramus and in growing children around the time of growth spurts. We have seen Haversian remodeling in sheep 7–9 years of age. As the ovine skeleton ages, one of the first places to see Haversian remodeling is the caudal aspect of the femur; another place of such remodeling is the diaphysis of the radius and humerus (185).

Like dogs and pigs (and most primates), the size of sheep allows researchers to meet other criteria for a model of osteoporosis. Specifically sheep are large enough to accommodate prosthesis implantation, substantial blood and urine sampling, and ample iliac crest biopsies for histomorphometry. This facilitates research to correlate events at the clinical, tissue, cellular, and biochemical levels.

C. Nonhuman Primates

An abundance of literature documents the skeletal effects of ovariectomy in old-world monkeys such as baboons and macaques (rhesus and cynomolgus) as well as the use of different therapies to meet certain regulatory requirements (201–208). These nonhuman primates demonstrate many advanages over other models for osteoporosis because their organ systems most closely resemble the human systems involved, i.e., gastrointestinal tract, endocrine system, and bone

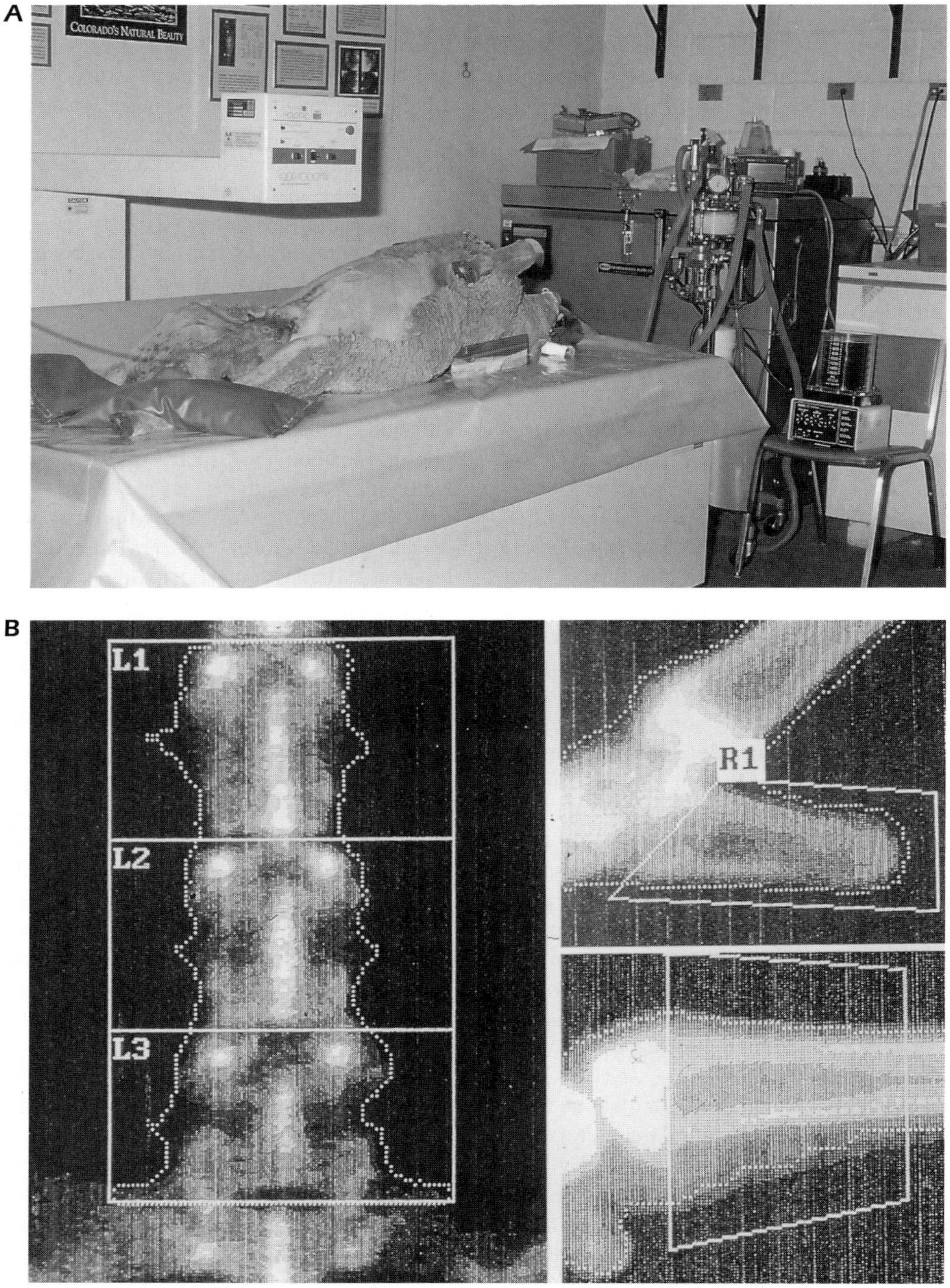

Figure 5 (A) A disadvantage of using a quadruped (including dogs) for measuring longitudinal changes in BMD using DXA is the technical difficulty in positioning the animal to examine the femoral neck region. The lumbar vertebrae of sheep can be scanned with precision (190, 195). (B) DXA scan images of lumbar vertebrae, calcaneus, and distal radius of sheep (195).

metabolism. For example, female macaque monkeys cycle monthly and have hormonal patterns similar to those of humans (201). Most studies in primates have focused on the loss of trabecular bone, and cortical sites have not been examined as extensively. A significant reduction in vertebral cancellous bone volume occurs in response to ovariectomy of the female monkey (202), whereas gonadotropin releasing hormone agonist-treated female rhesus monkeys exhibit decreased BMD at a rate of loss comparable to that of postmenopausal women (203). These data show a similarity between nonhuman primates and humans in the response of bone to cessation of ovarian function.

Menopause occurs in female primates after approximately 20 years of age (204). Both in captivity and in the wild, the live birth rate of primates declines markedly with age, with oligomenorrhea apparent by the early to mid-twenties. They are considered menopausal in the late twenties. Hormonal changes such as increased follicular-stimulating hormone (FSH) and decreased estrogen levels are also noted in monkeys >20 years of age.

Because postmenopausal osteoporosis is clearly hormone related, the similarity in the endocrine system of primates to that of humans is a notable advantage. Unfortunately, peak bone mass is not reached in cynomolgus monkeys until 9 years of age (205), and most studies have used OVX monkeys aged 4–7 years (206). Intuitively, OVX in the skeletally immature primate is an inappropriate model for postmenopausal osteoporosis. However, acquisition of aged female primates is difficult and costly.

The effect of OVX on quality and quantity of cancellous bone using the young cynomolgus monkey was evaluated after a 2-year period (207). The bodies of the second lumbar vertebrae were analyzed for changes in bone mineral quality using density fractionation, chemical analysis, and X-ray diffraction techniques. It was concluded that young OVX female cynomolgus macaques do not appear to be a useful model for the study of postmenopausal bone loss, although they may be a useful animal model to evaluate skeletal pathology after ovariectomy in young human females (207). Biochemical markers of bone turnover have been studied in primates. OVX cynomolgus monkeys had increased serum levels of alkaline phosphatase and acid phosphatase compared with intact and hormone-supplemented animals (208).

Once primates are acquired for study, their handling becomes an issue of concern. Although the sometimes-aggressive primate can be sufficiently controlled by a skilled technician, the risk of zoonotic disease transmission is relatively high. Frequently, primates used for studies are not bred for research but are caught in the wild and are therefore potential reservoirs for a host of zoonotic diseases, including primate retroviruses, which have had a history of jumping host species (185, 209), a consideration that discourages the use of this animal as an experimental model. Other factors when using nonhuman primates are legislated housing and environmental restrictions for the animals. Unfortunately, primates are too potentially dangerous, costly, and difficult to handle for them to be a primary model for the study of therapeutic agents for osteoporosis. Rather, they are of most value as the final step toward clinical trials after rats, and a larger animals, have been used. Some examples of studies using animal models of osteoporosis are shown in Table VI.

IV. Immobilization and the Effects of Exercise

A. Immobilization

The effects of immobilization on the musculoskeletal system are of great interest to the medical profession because immobilization is prescribed for orthopedic treatment of fractures, tendon and ligament damage, and back pain. Immobilization occurs following major surgery and cerebrovascular accidents. More recently, microgravity associated with space flight has stimulated intense research in this field, although animal space flight studies have been limited mainly to rats (229) and chick embryos (230). Humans and laboratory animals (rats) appear to exhibit similar responses to space flight (231, 232), although longer periods using the tail suspension model (discussed below) are needed to achieve some of the changes seen following space flight (229).

Animal models are a convenient way to study biomechanical, biochemical, and histological changes of immobilization, as well as changes at the cellular level (gene expression of matrix proteins and growth factors) (233). These models are also used to study the effects of different drugs that may protect against immobilization-induced bone loss (234). Antiresorptive drugs such as the bisphosphonates are effective in preventing immobilization-induced osteopenia (235).

Methods to provide immobilization in small animal models such as the rat include sciatic neurectomy (235), tenotomy, casting, hind limb taping (234), slinging, hind limb suspension by the tail (232, 233), and space flight (231). Orthopedic casting tape placed along the tail is currently the method of choice for hind limb unloading in rats. The method is well tolerated and is a minimally stressful system (as determined by animal food consumption, weight gain, and corticosteroid levels) that complies with established criteria for animal health and well being (232).

In larger animals, some of the immobilization methods used in the rat raise concern with IACUCs. In dogs, a common method that is well tolerated and routine in veterinary practice is cast immobilization of either the fore limb (236, 237) or hind limb. Casts are well tolerated by dogs and their application is routine in veterinary practice.

Observations from studies of immobilization uniformly show that there is a rapid and early effect on the musculoskeltal system that is difficult to reverse. As a result, some

Table VI Osteoporosis

Animal model	Purpose of model	Strength	Weakness	Ref.
Rat	Effect of naproxen on cancellous bone			210
	Effect of adrenalectomy and OVX			211
	Effects of progesterone on bone loss			212
	OVX and biochemical variables			213
	Ovarian transplantation		Some differences in function	214
	Mechanical strength of bone	Femoral neck a sensitive indicator		151
	Effects of OVX and/or immobilization			215
	Parathyroidectomy and bone loss			216
	Evaluation of calcitonin analog			217
	Magnetic field and PTH			218
	Effect of PTH analog	Site-specific dose response	Remodeling pattern different	219
	Different levels of mechanical strain			220
	Effects of promethazine			221
Dog	Sequential biopsies following OVX	Simulates initiating phase		158
	Effect of calcitonin on torsion		No effect due to OVX	222
	Effects of bisphosphonates		Calcium restriction required	161
	Bone quality and calcitonin			223
Pig	Effect of lactation	Spontaneous fractures		170
	Estimation of trabecular connectivity		Calcium restriction required	174
	Alendronate and sodium fluoride			177
Sheep	Dose response of estradiol	Low cost, easy to handle	No natural menopause	190
	Salmon calcitonin and bone quality			191
	Effects of raloxifene		Seasonal variation	192, 193
Primate	Estrogen and progesterone therapy			205
	Effects of OVX in young	A model for surgical OVX in young		207
	Effect of advancing age on BMC			224
	Effects of androlone decanoate			225
	Oral contraceptives and bone		Immature animals	226
	Effect of aging and natural menopause	Similarity to human effect	Cost	227
	Effect of PFH (1–34)			228

models have also investigated the effects of *remobilization*. We have immobilized one fore limb of sheep (for 12 weeks) and examined changes in BMD measured using DXA. Remobilization after 12 weeks was impossible due to tendon contracture.

Relatively few studies have examined the effect of immobilization on articular cartilage. Hind limb immobilization in dogs was used to characterize the biochemical and structural changes in canine knee cartilage after an initial 11-week immobilization and subsequent remobilization period of 50 weeks (238–240). Immobilization of primates has been used to compare vertebral and peripheral mineral losses in disuse osteoporosis (241, 242), but this model has become less popular largely because of high cost and public opposition. Some examples of studies using animal models of immobilization are shown in Table VII.

B. Effect of Exercise

There is an abundance of literature on the effect of exercise in humans of both genders and all ages participating in almost all types of physical activity and sport, but invasive methods to evaluate bone biology are ethically limited. It is beyond the scope of this chapter to discuss orthopedic manifestations of exercise in human subjects, this section concentrates on animal studies.

The use of physical exercise to enhance bone to treat osteopenia and prevent osteoporosis is well known. Most

Table VII Immobilization

Animal model	Purpose of model	Strength	Weakness	Ref.
Mouse	Sequential changes in bone turnover	Easy to perform		243
Rat	Effect of OVX and immobilization			244
	Torsional strength of tibia	Rapid loss (3 weeks)	Rats still growing	245
	Effect of IGF-1 on trabecular bone			246
	Effect of clodronate on BMD	Well-characterized model		247
	Effect of treadmill running		Older animals required	248
	Effect of TGF-β2 on trabecular bone loss	Well tolerated	Young animals (4 weeks old) used	249
	Molecular responses of bone			250
	Antiresorptive agents and bone mass	Simple to perform	Animals can still walk	251
	Unloading and reloading	Mimics space flight bone loss		233
	Bone and hormonal changes	Cephalad fluid shift		252
	mRNA levels during spaceflight	True representation	Expense; logistical problems	231
Turkey	Mechanical stimuli/remodeling	Functionally isolated ulna		253
	Tissue-wide or specific sites of disuse	Well-characterized model		254
Dog	Pattern of bone loss in older animals		Cast changes required	255
	Effect of tamoxifen citrate	Hind limb cast well tolerated	Young animals (12- to 16-week old)	256
	Changes in bone mass and turnover	Fore limb immobilization	Young animals	257
				237
Sheep	Ultrasonic measurement of bone		Unilateral Achilles tendonectomy	258
	Effect of calcitonin on local disuse	Animal weight closer to human weight	Insufficient dose and frequency	259
				260
Goat	Biochemical/biomechanical changes			261
	Intraosseous prostaglandin E2		Achilles tendonectomy required	262
Primate	Histologic changes in tibia (7 months)	Model for adult osteopenia	Expense	241
				242

studies show that physical activity increases the competence of the skeleton to resist fracture by the maintenance and improvement of BMD and neuromuscular competency, thus reducing skeletal fragility and predisposition to falls and fall impact (263). Animal models have played an important part in determining the optimal amount of exercise (duration, frequency, intensity, etc.) that could be applicable to humans for osteoporosis prevention and treatment. The most common model to study the effect of exercise in postmenopausal women is the OVX rat. Running is the most commonly used exercise stimulus and a wide ranges of exercise protocols using motor-driven treadmills with variable speeds and grades are routinely used for these studies. Most animals require some adaptation to treadmills and some will refuse and can be delegated to the sedentary group (control) group or removed from the study (264). Critics of animal models frequently raise the issue of quadrupedal loading of the axial and appendicular skeleton and whether this relates to the bipedal action in humans. Clearly, conclusions with regards to humans should be drawn with caution (265) but the question of importance is what economically feasible and practical animal models are bipedal.

Controlled loading animal models have been used to measure bone response to precisely quantified loads at distinct skeletal sites. The isolated turkey ulna (266), rat tibia (267–269), rat ulna (270–271), and canine radius (272) are just a few examples. To evaluate if extremely low-magnitude mechanical stimulus (LMMS) can be osteogenic, adult female sheep were separated into two groups—those subjected to LMMS and untreated controls. For 20 min per day, sheep stood confined in a chute such that the hind limbs were subjected to vertical ground-based vibration (273) (Fig. 6). Bone density at various sites was measured using DXA at different time points. Six months exposure to a brief (20-min) extremely low-intensity (<10 microstrain) vibrational loading was osteogenic in sites subjected to transmission of vibration (273). Because of their docile compliant nature, sheep are well behaved and easy to train to stand on this device. Other large animals are less suitable for this type of study. Some examples of studies

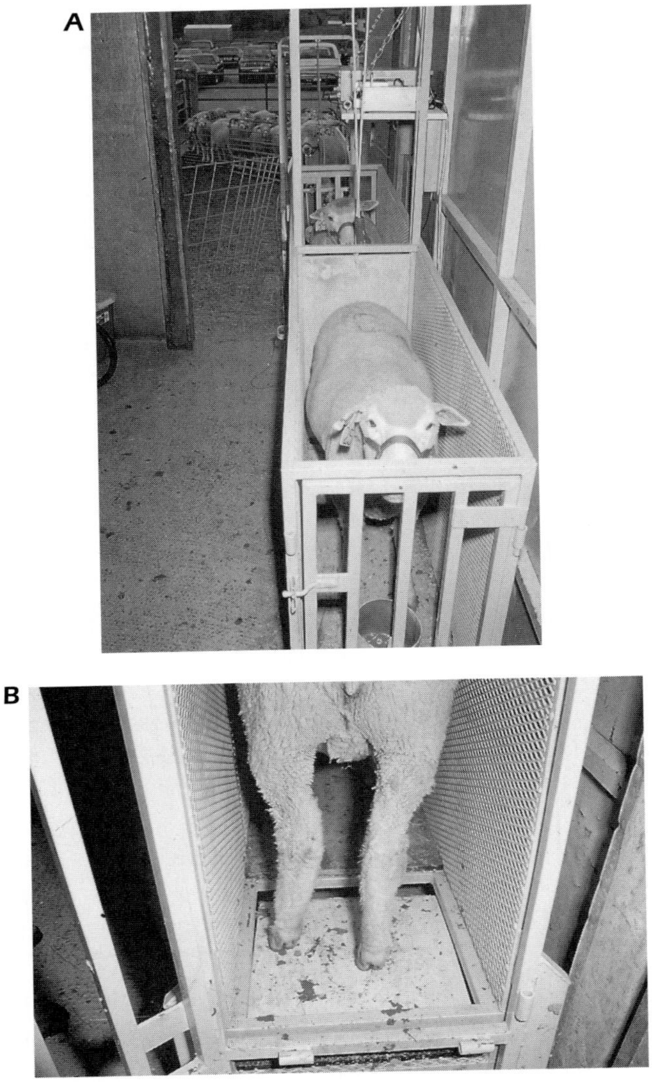

Figure 6 To evaluate if low-magnitude mechanical stimulus can be osteogenic, sheep were confined standing in a chute such that the hind limbs were subjected to vertical ground-based vibration (273). Because of their docile compliant nature, the sheep were easy to train to stand on this device. Other large animals would be less suitable for this type of study.

examining the effect of exercise using animal models are shown in Table VIII.

V. Spine

Both *in vivo* and *ex vivo* animal models have played an important part in studying the biology of normal and diseased spine as well as biomechanics, histology, biological, biochemical, and radiographic responses to surgical spinal fusion with spine implants. Readers interested in this field are directed to reviews on spinal implants (materials and design) (297), the artificial disc (theory, design and materials) (298), and interbody fusion cages (299). The choice of animal model for spine surgery is difficult because very few models (including primates) are bipedal. The author has been approached regarding the suitability of kangaroos for spine research, by investigators unaware of the logistical and societal issues, aside from anesthesia and restraint problems likely to be encountered with this model. The quantitative biomechanical similarities of intact sheep spines and human spines have demonstrated that sheep spines are qualitatively similar, and this model can serve as an alternative for the evaluation of spinal implants (300, 301).

A. Ex Vivo Spine Studies

Cadaveric studies (human and animal) of the biomechanics of normal and surgically instrumented spine have been extensive. The advantages of cadaveric spines are obvious: low cost, good reproducibility, availability, and large numbers of specimens available to be tested to offset the variance seen in biomechanical testing. The disadvantages are that the biological response to the implants and the clinical effects are lacking. Biomechanical testing with these *ex vivo* models requires strong and well-planned collaboration with engineers and spine surgeons. Careful and consistent specimen preparation (fixation jigs, potting methods, maintain specimen hydration, etc.) and a good working knowledge of the material testing apparatus to be used are essential.

Cadaveric calf spine models are widely used and validated for the thoracic and lumbar regions (3, 302) with all the advantages and disadvantages described above. Less interspecimen variability compared with the human cadaveric spine is another advantage of this model (303). Lumbosacral spine specimens from 70- to 83-day-old pigs were used to evaluate the biomechanical properties of the Leeds–Keio artificial ligament (304), and canine rib cage–thoracic spine complexes were used to examine the role of intervertebral disc and costovertebral joint in the stability of the thoracic spine (305). Osteoporotic compression fractures of the vertebrae cause pain, deformity, and poor quality of life (306, 307). Vertebroplasty is discussed in greater detail later in this section.

B. In Vivo Spine Studies

Sheep and dogs have been the most common large animal models for ventral ("anterior") interbody fusion, transpedicular screw fixation, and dorsolateral ("posterolateral") intertransverse process fusion (308, 309). The advantages of larger spine size of sheep, goats, dogs, and pigs for instrumentation procedures compared to rats and rabbits are clear.

Although the rabbit is the most common small animal model for dorsolateral intertransverse process fusion

Table VIII Effect of Exercise

Animal model	Purpose of model	Strength	Weakness	Ref.
Rat	Effect of swimming			274
	Evidence of fatigue microdamage	Low expense		275
	Effects on cancellous bone	Aged females used		276
	17-β-Estradiol and physical activity			277
	Effects of endurance exercise			264
	Effects of nonendurance exercise			278
	BMD and skeletal muscle weight			279
	Castration-induced osteoporosis		Reduced bone turnover	280
	Femoral neck bone mass and strength		Quadrupedal loading pattern	265
	Long-term effect of exercise		Continued growth later in life	281
	Anabolic effect of exercise		Weight gain in OVX rats	282
	Cortical bone mass and turnover			283
	Jump training and bone hypertrophy			284
	Trabecular architecture adaption			285
	Additional weightbearing	Backpack well tolerated	Extrapolation to human bone?	286
	Torsional strength, morphometry, etc.			287
	Intensity and duration of exercise		Body weight gain in OVX animals	288
	Detraining effects in young males			289
	Exercise in mature osteopenic rats	Senile osteoporosis model		290
Rooster	Adaptive changes of growing bone	Low expense	Avian bone	291
Dog	Effects of long-term running	70 weeks well tolerated	Possible secondary amenorrhea	292
Pig	Effects on non-weight-bearing bone		Restraint difficulties	293
Horse	Effect of exercise and inactivity		Expense; small numbers used	294
	Biochemical responses to exercise	Noninvasive monitoring	Expense; seasonal effects (estrus)	295
Primate	Bone mass and cellular variations		Expense; small numbers used	296

(310–317), as mentioned, a common criticism of using quadrupeds is the horizontally positioned spine. Studies using finite-element analysis comparing the forces across the canine spine with the human spine demonstrated a mechanical similarity of the two (318). Sheep have six (occasionally seven) lumbar vertebrae with larger transverse processes and a smaller vertebral diameter. The larger pedicle diameter of sheep is helpful for studies of transpedicular screw fixation because human-sized screws can be used (319). Whatever animal model is chosen, sham animals should not demonstrate spontaneous fusion. Harvesting of iliac bone graft is a frequent technique in animal studies and if bone substitutes to augment spine fusion are being investigated, it is prudent to include a group of animals treated with autograft.

Endpoints for anterior spine fusion studies in animals include macroscopic analysis and flexibility, high-quality ventrodorsal and lateral radiographs, BMD measurement using DXA or CT, and histology and histomorphometry of the vertebral body spanned by the instrumentation (319). Analytical procedures to measure collagen/proteoglycan synthesis are also important in spine research. Biomechanical analysis to characterize stiffness of a motion segment necessitates collaboration with a facility dedicated to this analysis (Fig. 7). Loading modes include lateral bending, flexion, torsion, and axial compression. Removal of rods and wires used for dorsal ("posterior" fusion) before mechanical testing may initiate stress risers in specimens, thus potentiating failure outside the fusion sites (320).

C. Anterior Spine Fusion

Recent interest in performing lumbar interbody arthrodesis is because of the high rate of failure associated with the use of bone graft alone or pedicle–screw instrumentation and the high rate of success associated with anterior fusion (without the use of posterior instrumentation) (299, 321). Animal models have played an important role in the technology, development, biomechanics, and host response.

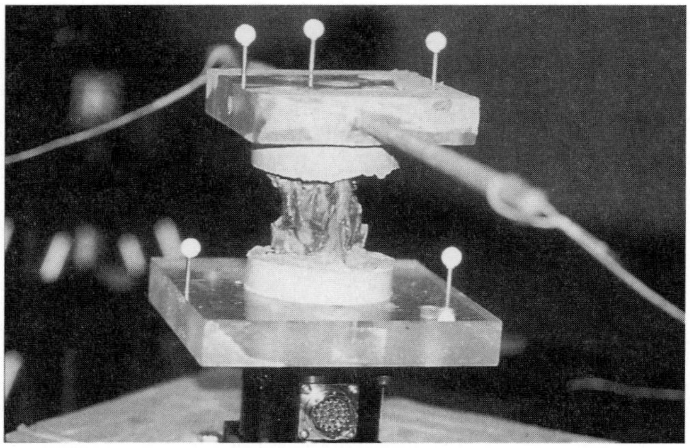

Figure 7 Endpoints for spine fusion studies in animals include stiffness characterzation of the motion segment using a motion analysis system and retroreflective markers attached to the spine (353). Courtesy of Jefferey Toth, Medical College of Wisconsin, Milwaukee, Wisconsin.

Although in humans, anterior lumbar interbody fusion has many positive advantages when compared to posterior fusion techniques, one major problem of anterior fusion has been the lack of a suitable graft (321, 322). This has stimulated a large number of studies to look for different synthetic materials to replace host bone and the use of cages as a vehicle for delivery of osteoconductive materials. More recently, animal models have been used to perfect minimally invasive techniques (laparoscopic spine fusion). Pigs were used successfully for ventral ("anterior") interbody spine fusion at L6/S1. There was no injury to intraperitoneal organs or bleeding from major vessels. This model was also recommended for training before applying the technique to humans. Laparoscopic spine fusion in human patients is associated with a long learning curve but, once mastered, has advantages over current approaches to lumbar fusion (323). Laparoscopic exposure of the lumbosacral spine to insert hollow titanium cylindrical sponges soaked with recombinant bone morphogenetic protein (rhBMP) was performed in monkeys by Boden *et al.* (324). Cunningham *et al.* (325, 326) used endoscopy to insert cages in the thoracic spine of sheep to evaluate osteogenic protein (OP-1). Bioresorbable cages for anterior fusion are likely to replace cages made of metals or alloys (Fig. 8, A and B).

D. Posterior and Posterolateral Fusion

Posterolateral fusion of the treatment of degenerative spinal disorders has been a popular method in spinal surgery (308). The number of animal studies carried out to develop methods to improve the fusion rate, increase the stability of the fusion mass, and decrease the time taken to fuse has been extensive (Fig. 8C). Animal studies have also been used to evaluate a wide variety of bone grafting materials as substitutes for autograft and allograft (320, 327).

E. Vertebroplasty

Loss of vertebral bone is seen due to aging, steroid use, and metastatic disease, and is accentuated in cases of osteoporosis (328–330); the resultant compression fractures of the vertebrae can cause pain and disability. A more invasive approach to strengthen vertebral bodies is sometimes needed in severe cases (331). Percutaneous transpedicular vertebroplasty with PMMA has been used, but a more biological bone cement that has immediate compressive strength and is nonexothermic is yet to be approved for use in human clinical trials at the time of writing. Thermal damage to intraosseous neural tissue caused by cement polymerization has been hypothesized as the reason for the palliative effect of PMMA. *In vitro* studies have shown that this is unlikely but it cannot be ruled out in clinical situations (332).

An animal model to test various compounds for veterbroplasty must be of sufficient size to accommodate large enough volumes of material. The shape of the vertebral bodies of domestic animals is quite different from that of humans. Therefore, biomechanical testing is probably best suited to osteoporotic cadaveric specimens, whereas the biological response of the agent can be tested in the vertebral bodies of pigs, sheep, goats, and large breeds of dogs. Lamghari *et al.* (333, 334) and our team (unpublished data), working independently, have developed a model in the lumbar vertebrae of sheep, suitable for testing biomaterials for bone repair. In this model, a lateral retroperitoneal approach to the vertebral bodies allows the surgeon the option of injecting the biomaterial at hand in three or four vertebral bodies (Fig. 9). The option of using one vertebra, an intervening untreated vertebra, and a second experimental vertebral body allows an animal to act as its own control. The most serious complication of this technique is inadvertent penetration of the floor of the spinal canal with subsequent leakage of material into the dural space. Nacre (mother of pearl from the oyster *Pinctada maxima*) has also been evaluated using this model (333, 334). *In vivo* and *in vitro* studies have provided good evidence for the biocompatibility and osteogenic activity of nacre. Bone loss of the vertebral bodies following ovariectomy in domestic animals is rarely as severe as that seen in elderly female patients with osteoporosis. This limits somewhat the use of estrogen-deficient animals for this type of research.

Figure 8 (A) Anterior fusion of intervertebral lumbar vertebrae in a sheep using a titanium implant (352). (B) Anterior fusion of intervertebral lumbar vertebrae in a sheep using a bioresorbable implant. Such cages for anterior fusion are likely to replace cages made of metals or alloys. (C) Posterior lumbar fusion in a sheep using transpedicular screws and rods. A metal cage was also placed between the vertebral bodies.

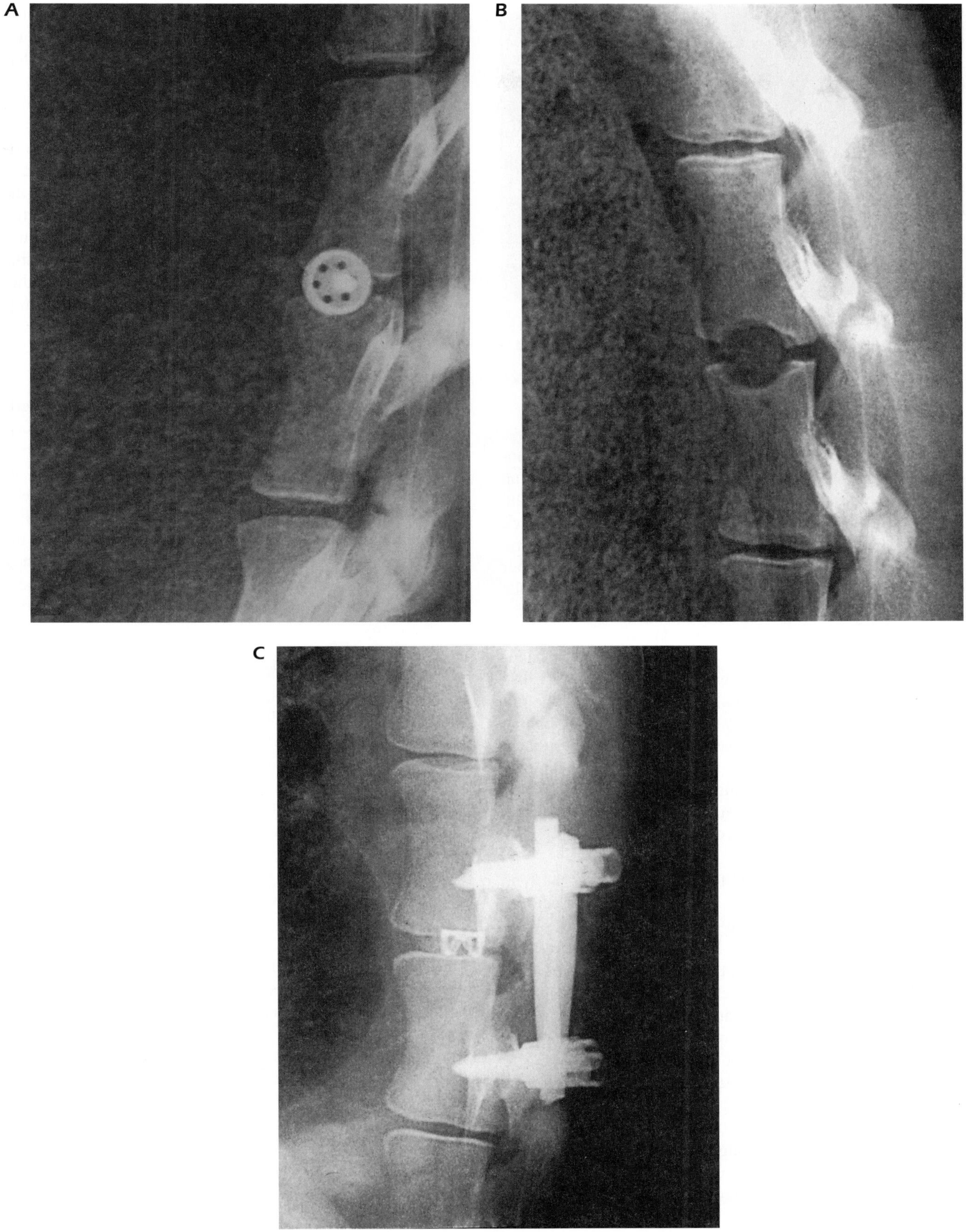
A
B
C

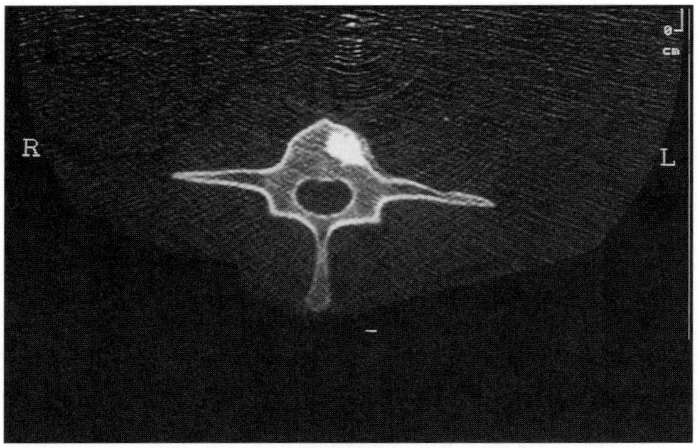

Figure 9 Computerized tomography scan 6 months after vertebroplasty of L3 in a sheep. An osteoconductive biodegradable ceramic was used.

F. Disc Degeneration and Replacement

Low back pain is one of the most common medical conditions in the Western world, and disc degeneration (an inevitable process of aging) is one of the major causes (298, 335). Surgical interventions for the degenerative disc, i.e., discectomy and fusion, have good success in the short term, but biomechanical changes in the spine can result in further deterioration of adjacent discs. Dogs were used to study the healing of the anulus fibrosus with surgically created defects (336), and remodeling of vertebral bone after outer anular injury was studied in sheep (337). Incision in the outer anulus of adult sheep results in degeneration of the lumbar disc within a short time (4 months) despite healing of the cut fibers and does not vary greatly from that seen in the human disc (337, 338). In our experience, the retroperitoneal approach used to create these tears is relatively simple to perform with very low morbidity. Anular tears can also be created in pigs and have been used to elucidate the changes occurring in collagen chemistry in the early phases of disc degeneration (339, 340).

Sheep have also been used to evaluate whether the type of anular incision made at the time of lumbar discectomy plays a role in the subsequent healing and strength of the anulus and the biomechanical flexibility of the corresponding motion segment (341). In these models, access to three disc spaces is offered so different techniques/treatments are possible within the same animal. The retroperitoneal approach has also been used for lumbar intervertebral disc transfer in dogs as well as for evaluation of bioresorbable and metallic cages used for ventral ("anterior") fusion as discussed above.

An artificial disc is an attractive alternative to disc replacement or fusion. Although many challenges remain, including long-term implant fixation, biocompatibility, and particle wear, significant achievements have been made in joint replacement of the hip and knee. However, the search for an artificial disc prosthesis with motion in three planes (flexion–extension, axial rotation, and lateral bending) has been elusive (298). Several laboratories (including our own) have investigated substituting the nucleus, rather than replacing the entire disc.

Monkey models are a logical choice before such materials are used in clinical trials. A less costly large animal model (pig, goat, sheep, or dog) is recommended for the development of the surgical technique and studying the tissue reaction of the implant with the surrounding tissues (biosafety and biocompatibility) (298). The literature on the theory design and materials of the artificial disc and other spinal implants has been reviewed (297).

G. Spinal Cord Trauma

The literature describing the animal models and experimental work used to research the effects of ischemia, injury, and drugs on spinal cord blood flow is considerable. Although a variety of animal models (cats, dogs, rats, rabbits, and ferrets) have been used, their validity has been questioned (342). Some of these animal species have become unpopular for this type of orthopedic research in the eyes of the public. This prompted a detailed anatomic study of the sheep spine and it was determined that it may be a suitable model for studying spinal cord trauma, disorders, and pathophysiology (342, 343).

Chronic compression of the cauda equina and spinal nerve roots in a variety of animal models uses devices such as inflatable balloons, plastic bands, clips, silicone bands, and silicone films (344, 345). Rats are popular because they are easier to manage, more uniform, and economical.

Spinal cord trauma research requires close collaboration with laboratories familiar with blood flow evaluation, including microvasculature techniques, microangiograms, labeled microspheres, photographic equipment, high-resolution scanners, and the appropriate computer-aided image analysis. Some studies require endpoints such as walking duration on a treadmill and paw-withdrawal latencies to thermal stimuli (345). Light microscopic and electron microscopic evaluations of transverse sections are also part of many studies. Some examples of studies using animal models of anterior fusion, posterior/posterolateral fusion, disc degeneration, and replacement and spinal cord trauma are shown in Tables IX–XII.

H. Scoliosis

There have been many reports of experiments, using a wide variety of animals, to induce scoliosis. Research involving adolescent idiopathic scoliosis (AIS) has been hampered by the lack of an appropriate animal model (377).

Table IX The Spine (Anterior Fusion)

Animal model	Purpose of model	Strength	Weakness	Ref.
Dog	Irradiation and vertebral strut grafts	Well tolerated	Corpectomy less destabilizing than many tumors	346
		Well tolerated, easy access to spine, no graft extrusions		347
	Internal fixation/calcium carbonate	No graft dislodgement	Longer postoperative time suggested	348
	Hydroxylapatite (HA) blocks		Block slippage and/or fracture	349
Pig	Laparoscopic fusion at L6/S1	Ideal for training	Tedious until technique is perfected	350
Sheep	Cervical screw-plate locking system	Availability, specimen consistency (*in vitro*)	Anatomic differences to human	351
	Efficacy of osteogenic protein (OP-1)	Minimally invasive (thoroscopy)	Technically demanding	325
				326
	Spinal cord blood flow and function	Results consistent with others		343
	Determine distractive properties		Misplaced cages (2 cases)	352
	Coralline graft substitutes			309
	Direct current electrical stimulation			353
Goat	Three-level cervical fusion	Disc space features, spine loading	Radiographs misleading	354
	Carbon polymer and wear debris		Paraplegia (1 animal), loss of 3 animals due to trauma	355
	Performance of HA versus autograft	Head held erect to load spine	Partial immobilization required	356
			Some graft extrusion due to mobility	
Primate	rhBMP-2 and collagen sponge		Numbers limited (expense)	357

Pinealectomy in chickens after hatching consistently results in scoliosis whereas in young rats or hamsters it does not (377). Machida *et al.* (378) created a bipedal rat model by amputation of fore limbs and tail, forcing the rats to ambulate on their hind limbs. (This model would not be acceptable now to many IACUCs in North America.) Pinealectomy in these rats, but not the quadrupedal rats, resulted in scoliosis and it was speculated that pinealectomy interfered with balance. An intriguing area of research in scoliosis is the elucidation of the role of melatonin (377). Melatonin deficiency secondary to pinealectomy does not produce scoliosis if the quadrupedal condition is maintained (378). It was concluded from these rat experiments that the bipedal condition, such as in humans and chickens, plays an important role in scoliosis. Incidentally induced scoliosis in a series of monkeys used for routine neurovirulence tests was reported but would be impractical (379). Experimental scoliosis has been produced by multiple spinal rhizotomies and by damaging the posterior horn grey matter and adjacent Clark's column in the thoracic spine of primates (379). Experimental scoliosis was also produced in rabbits by direct damage to areas of the spinal cord with laser or stereotactic electromicrocoagulation and longitudinal electrocoagulation (380). More recently, partial resection of approximately 1 cm of the proximal ends of four right lower ribs was performed in rabbits to produce progressive right convex thoracic scoliosis. Kirschner wires were inserted percutaneously and both ends were attached to an external fixator with or without percutaneous discectomy (381). Morbidity was high in this study, with losses due to paresis of the lower limbs and death due to other causes.

VI. Implant Coatings

Intuitively, the success of implants in the axial and appendicular skeleton (as well as the maxillofacial region) depends on good biological fixation of the implant by bone apposition (382–384). Well-osseointegrated implants can transfer the mechanical loads directly to surrounding bone, thereby reducing stress shielding of the bone (385). Implant as well as non-implant-related factors would affect the success of adequate bone–implant interface. Non-implant-related factors include implant location (trabecular versus cortical bone), bone mineral density (e.g., osteopenia/osteoporosis), the surgical technique used to place the implant, implant loading conditions, and the general health of the patient. Important implant-related factors that affect the quality of the fixation of the implant include the implant design, implant material, surface quality, surface roughness, and orientation of surface irregularities, to name but a few (383). Orthopedic research in this field has expanded in response to the long-

Table X The Spine (Posterior and Posterolateral Fusion)

Animal model	Purpose of model	Strength	Weakness	Ref.
Rat	Powdered demineralized bone matrix	Lower cost than larger animals	Further verification in large animals	358
Rabbits	Coralline HA as bone graft substitute	More challenging than the rat	Caution when extrapolating to humans	359
			Ingrowth may increase for up to 1 year	
	Addition of autologous bone marrow			311
	Effect of ketorolac and BMP-2		High perioperative morbidity, lumbar "plexopathy"	312
	Efficacy of a carrier for BMP-2	A well-validated model of intertransverse process arthrodesis	Infection and lumbar plexus palsy	313 314
	Bone graft and direct current stimulation		Single time point (remodeling effect?)	315
	Different formulations of rabbit DBM	Justification for a primate study	Does not predict success in humans	316
	Bioactive bone cement		Stress-shielding effect of cerclage	317
Dog	Evaluation of rhBMP-2 and carriers	Larger model than rabbit; a challenging environment		360
	Comparison of autogenous or synthetic bone grafting materials	Allows testing of 3 materials, well tolerated, no immobilization	Demanding procedure	361
				320
	Direct current electrical stimulation	Utilizes an adult model		362
	Pulsed electromagnetic fields (PEMF)	No clinical complications	Longer follow-up needed	363
Sheep	Effect of spine fusion and kyphosis	Vertebrae closer to human size	Postop. period (16 weeks) too short	364
		Spontaneous fusion unlikely after surgical exposure		
	Instrumentation role during fusion	Two techniques in one animal		365
	Coral porites and biphasic ceramic		Fracture of epiphyseal plate, graft failure	366
	Efficacy of interconnected porous HA		Radiologic fusion assessment difficult	321
	Quantify load-sharing capacity	Greater pedicle diameter compared to dogs		308
	Changes in load sharing/fusion mass			319
	Coralline graft substitutes	Similar biomechanical properties		309
Primate	A ceramic as rhBMP-2 carrier	Laminectomy and arthrodesis	Low numbers (expense), hence no biomechanical testing	367
			Bone formation detection difficult	

term loosening problems associated with cemented total joints (385).

In the operating room, the method of stabilization of joint replacement components remains the widely accepted acrylic cement polymethylmethacrylate. This technique of stabilization has been used successfully in older, less active, patients with low incidence of failure due to loosening (386). With patients living longer and healthier lives and with higher activity levels, there has seen a need to develop implants that will perform well long term. Biologic fixation has proved a viable alternative to acrylic bone cement (382), and the most extensively studied and understood coating both experimentally (387–397) and clinically (398–400) has been hydroxyapatite ($Ca_{10}[PO_4]_6[OH]_2$) and fluoroapatite ($Ca_5[PO_4]_3F$). Consequently, largely the industrial community has supported research to find ways to enhance growth of bone into metal implants.

Prior to choosing an animal model to evaluate implant coatings, certain pretesting must be considered. The coating should be well characterized and analyzed with various *in vitro* tests; a discussion of the details of these tests as suggested by the American Society for Testing Materials is beyond the scope of this chapter. The preimplantation of the coating should be standardized and well controlled, including purification, sterilization, and implant cleaning procedures. The characterization of calcium phosphate materials has been a topic of a workshop (401).

There are many animal models available to study the safety and efficacy of various implant surfaces in search of the optimal coating, and some examples of these are shown in Table XIII. Most models involve either a transcortical or transmetaphyseal location of the implant and therefore are best-suited for animals of a physical size that allows multiple implants in each bone. Bilateral implantation (e.g., both

Table XI The Spine (Disc Degeneration and Replacement)

Animal model	Purpose of model	Strength	Weakness	Ref.
Rat	Compression and immobilization	Similar changes as humans Well controlled loading	Does not simulate loading in humans	368
Rabbit	Cathepsin L for chemonucleolysis	No harm on vertebral body	Biochemical examination needed too Dose for clinical trials undetermined	369
	ChondroitinaseABC and nucleus pulposus transplantation	No palsy after transplantation		370
	Effect of FGF on herniated disc		Muscle weakness, hypersensitive	313
Dog	Effect of running on proteoglycans	Depletion of proteoglycans and anulus enlargement		371
	Study of defects in anulus fibrosus			336
	Disc transplantation	Sufficient size for this surgery	Ventral displacement of discs	372
Pig	Monitor healing process of annulus	Reproducible and simple to induce	Predominant collagen is type I in pigs Different loading pattern than in bipeds	339 340
Sheep	Disc changes following annular tear	Technically simple to perform, reproducible, changes in 4 months		338
	Changes in facet joints and subchondral bone architecture	Well-characterized model of lumbar disc degeneration	Longer study recommended	337 373
	Healing strength after incision			341

femora or both tibiae) or the combination of the bone of a fore limb (e.g., humerus or radius) and the bone of a hind limb (e.g., femur or tibia) are well tolerated by animals, and with the appropriate postoperative care and analgesia, is acceptable to many IACUCs (Fig. 10). Placing multiple implants in the same animal is statistically sound (internal control) and has the advantage of using less animals. Special fixtures for the standardized insertion and mechanical testing of implants have been described (419). Such fixtures are essential to a well-designed characterization of osseointegration of implants because of the inherently large variance typical of mechanical studies.

Mechanical evaluation of transcortical and transmetaphyseal models is used to characterize the behavior of implant coating in cortical and metaphyseal bone, respectively. The location of the test implant will depend on the location of the prosthesis and its coating in human clinical trials. In the animal model, randomization with respect to implant placement and implant location (e.g., proximal versus distal and left versus right) is necessary for optimal study design when evaluating implants. For example, there was a significant effect due to proximal versus distal placement within the canine femur (420).

Several issues arise when using multiple transcortical implants within the same animal. The risk of bone fracture ("stress-riser effect") with such models is real (383, 413), because postoperative compliance in animals is often impossible to control. Researchers must be aware of this, especial-

Table XII The Spine (Spinal Cord Trauma)

Animal model	Purpose of model	Strength	Weakness	Ref.
Rat	Microangiography after methylprednisolone and vitamin E	Economical, easy to manage		344
	Pathophysiology of chronic cauda equina compression	Paralysis, paw ulceration, fecal or urinary incontinence observed	Anatomical differences	345
	Effect of a hydroxyl radical scavenger (EPC-K1)			374
Dog	Intraoperative monitoring of neural injury	Acute study without recovery	Unable to document clinical effects	375
Pig	Measurement of CSF markers of nerve tissue damage	Disc herniation model	Possible immune reaction to nucleus pulposus	376
Sheep	Effect of blood flow with incomplete cord injury	A reproducable injury, comparable anatomy	Not an ideal reproduction of clinical practice	343 342

Table XIII Implant Coatings

Animal model	Purpose of model	Strength	Weakness	Ref.
Rat	Effect of aging on bone formation	Availability of old animals		394
	Hydrofluoro-acid-etched Ti rods	Both limbs used		384
	Screws in medullary cavity (femur)		Unloaded	382
Rabbit	Pore cross-sectional shape	Control of amplitude and frequency Repeated harvesting		402
	Three different HA coatings			388
	TiO_2-blasted and HA-coated implants	Three implants in both limbs		403
	HA-fixation in loaded implants	Load-bearing model		404
	Alkali- and heat-treated Ti alloys	Both limbs used		405
Dog	Dense sintered HA vs. HA coated			390
	Role of different loading conditions	Well-characterized model using a dynamic implant device		406
	Solid and porous materials	Load-bearing conditions (femora)	Pathology in opposing tibiae	407
	HA-coating on arc-sprayed implants	No fractures seen	Unloaded	392
	HA vs. fluoroapatite	Weight-loaded implants		396
	Porous-coated vs. grit-blasted HA	Both limbs used		395
	Intramedullary HA coating	Simulates the clinical implant site	Unloaded	393
	HA coating vs. dense HA implant	Four implants per dog		397
Minipig	Influence of surface characteristics	Tibia or femur (3 implants/site)	Some implants in cortical bone	408
	Effect of surface topology	Eight implant sites/knee		385
Sheep	Dacron velour evaluation	Bilateral cases, low morbidity		386
	HA response in mandible	Five implants in both rami	Wound infection (1 case)	409
	Effect of age on bone formation	Old and young animals used	Unloaded	410
	Characterization of response to HA	Ten implants per limb	Skeletally immature (1-year old)	411
Goat	Different plasma-sprayed coatings	Four implants (femur and humerus)		412
	Tensile test of HA and fluoroapatite	Pull-off model	Limb fracture (1 case)	413
	Effect of warfarin on attachment	Five implants used in both femora		414
	Trabecular bone response to Ca-P	Two implants in both distal femora		415
	Implants in cortical bone	Four implants in both tibiae	Limb fracture (2 cases)	383
	Subperiosteal implantation (tibia)	Six implants in both tibiae		416
Primate	Intramuscular coral-derived HA	Bone similar to human bone	Impractical model in some countries	417
	Comparison of canine and primate	Phylogenetic similarity	Expense	418

ly using transcortical implants beyond a certain size, relative to the diameter of the diaphysis of the long bone they are implanting. Transmetaphyseal implants are less prone to pathologic fracture but the numbers of implants per animal are sometimes limited, especially when larger implants are used. The surgical approach is generally more difficult compared to transcortical implantation because of the proximity of collateral ligaments, joint capsules, and tendons. Eight trabecular bone sites were used in the knees of miniature pigs (385), but the number is clearly dependent on the size of the animal and implant.

To measure dynamic histomorphometric parameters (e.g., remodeling activity), *in vivo* fluorochromes that adsorb to bone mineral during the time they are in the circulation are necessary. These markers are administered at timed intervals. Some fluorochromes produce spectacular colors when viewed under ultraviolet light but they are either too expensive or toxic to the animal, or both. Two labels that are cost effective in large animals are tetracycline (LA-200; Pfizer), which produces a yellow label, and calcein (Sigma), which produces a green label.

A wide variety of endpoints and parameters are measured in models to evaluate implant coatings and, as previously emphasized, this means a good working collaboration with other disciplines such as engineers, pathologists, histomorphometrists, and biochemists. Mechanical push-out data are calculated by dividing the load to failure by the interface area and are reported as shear strength. Pull-out strength is sometimes measured. Analysis of explanted devices is also part of such studies and includes the long-term attachment of the coating and any changes in crystallinity, density, microstructure, strength, and color. There are many textbooks, review papers, and symposia proceedings in the field of coating analysis (401).

Preparation of samples for histomorphometry measurements is a tedious procedure when metal or ceramic implants are being evaluated. A relatively small number of dedicated laboratories around the world have perfected the embedding, sectioning, polishing, and application of certain dyes and stains. Samples are typically fixed in a 4% buffered formaldehyde solution and then dehydrated by a graded series of ethanol before embedding in PMMA. At least three representative sections should be taken at different levels of the same implant because of the significant variance in trabecular bone response (415). Images for sterology can be captured on video and sterology measurements made to measure the percentage coverage (affinity index) of the implants with bone and the bone mass around the implants (Fig. 11). Scanning electron micrographs (SEMs) are used to qualitate and quantitate surface roughness of implant surface (profilometry) (403). Other methods to characterize bone response at the ultrastructural level include transmission electron microscopy (TEM), X-ray diffraction, and energy-dispersive X-ray analysis (411).

When the safety and efficacy of the implant coating prove optimal, these coatings are then tested in animal models in a more realistic loading regimen in total hip replacement (THA) and total knee arthroplasty (TKA) before going into clinical trials. These are discussed in the next section.

VII. Joint Prostheses

Total hip replacement (THR) and total knee arthroplasty (TKA) are among the most successful orthopedic procedures and have revolutionized the management of joint fail-

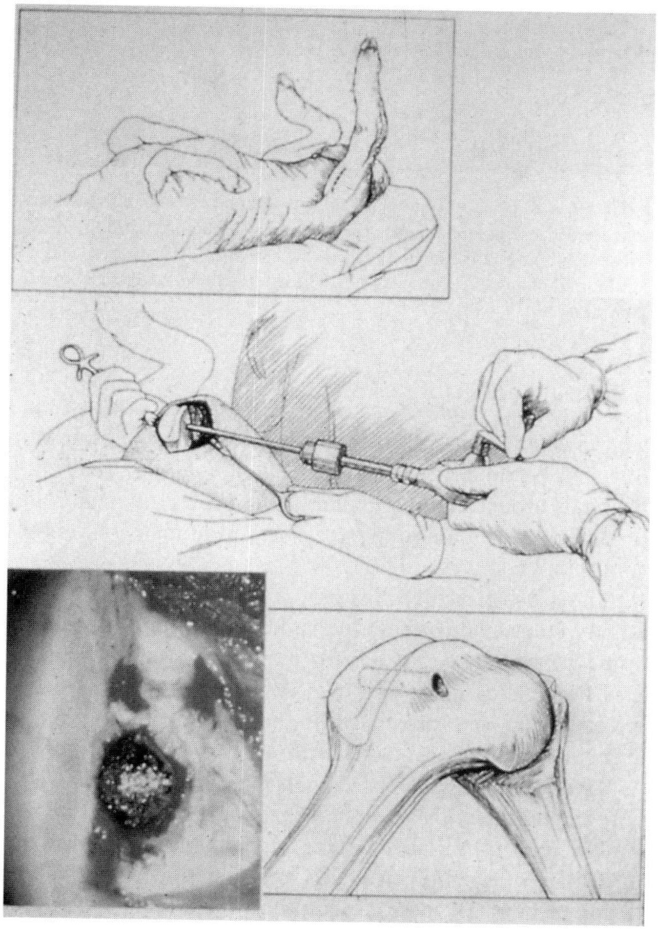

Figure 10 The transcondylar implantation of cylindrical implants (plugs) in the subtrochlear region of both distal femora in a sheep. The risk of pathologic fracture is less compared with the diaphyseal regions of the bone.

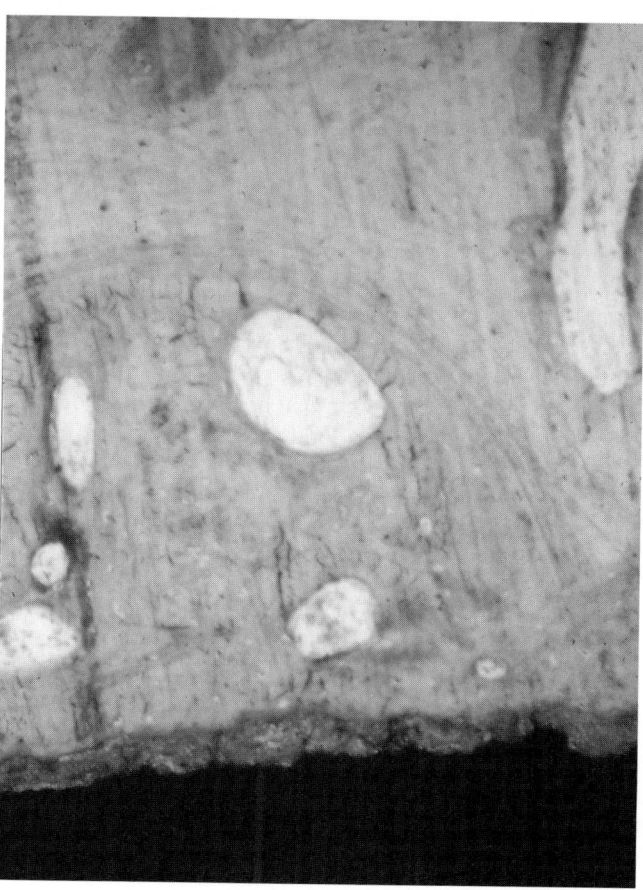

Figure 11 The bone mass around the implant is one of the endpoints for implant coatings. Images for sterology can be captured on video and sterology measurements can be made to measure the percentage coverage (affinity index).

ure due to osteoarthritis (421). *In vitro* tests for evaluating implant design features and material characteristics will not be discussed here; rather, the focus is on *in vivo* studies using mainly large animals, because these will continue to play a significant role in the long and expensive pathway from the laboratory to clinical cases. Although their relevance to human testing can be questioned, well-designed animal testing is sometimes less costly than long-term clinical studies, which have many variables, including age at implantation, hormonal status, quality of bone stock, concurrent illnesses, surgical technique, and preferences of the surgeon.

A. Total Hip Replacement

More than 120,000 artificial hip joints are being implanted annually in the United States. Primary THR is most commonly used for joint failure due to osteoarthritis. Other indications include, but are not limited to, rheumatoid arthritis, traumatic arthritis, benign and malignant bone tumors, arthritis associated with Paget's disease, ankylosing spondylitis, and juvenile rheumatoid arthritis (NIH Consensus Development Panel on Total Hip Replacement, 1995). The most challenging patient populations for THR are young patients with disabling hip disease and patients with a diagnosis of avascular necrosis (AVN) (399).

Optimization of the bone–implant interface remains an important area of research in this field. Newer fixation techniques include noncemented components, which rely on bone growth into porous or roughened surfaces. Other surface modifications of implants are aimed at direct attachment to bone. Several types of calcium phosphate ceramics [e.g., hydroxyapatite (HA)] have been added to THR surfaces. Here, cylindrical alloys with variations in coating are implanted in trabecular or cortical bone and are subjected to mechanical testing (usually torsion alone or in combination with push-out).

Bone resorption (osteolysis), although sometimes pain free, is always of concern because the potential exists for aseptic loosening or fracture (Fig. 12), and wear debris may contribute to osteolysis. There is considerable orthopedic research literature on the subject and much energy has been directed to the study of "particle disease." Particles of polyethylene (from the polyethylene socket) and the resulting inflammatory process have been suspected to play a role in resorption. Analyses of tissues harvested from periprosthetic areas from patients undergoing revision surgery (422) or from animal models (423) have answered many questions (e.g., size) about wear debris. The presence of intracellular particles with the discovery of cytokines and other mediators of inflammation has been a focus of study for many laboratories (424, 425).

Although a quadruped, the dog is still the animal model of choice for *in vivo* research in the field of THR and is the best available model because of its internal and external anatomy (426–442). Furthermore, total hip replacement in dogs has become routine for many well-equipped veterinary hospitals around the world and has a success rate and relief of suffering matching the experience in humans (443–445) (Fig. 13).

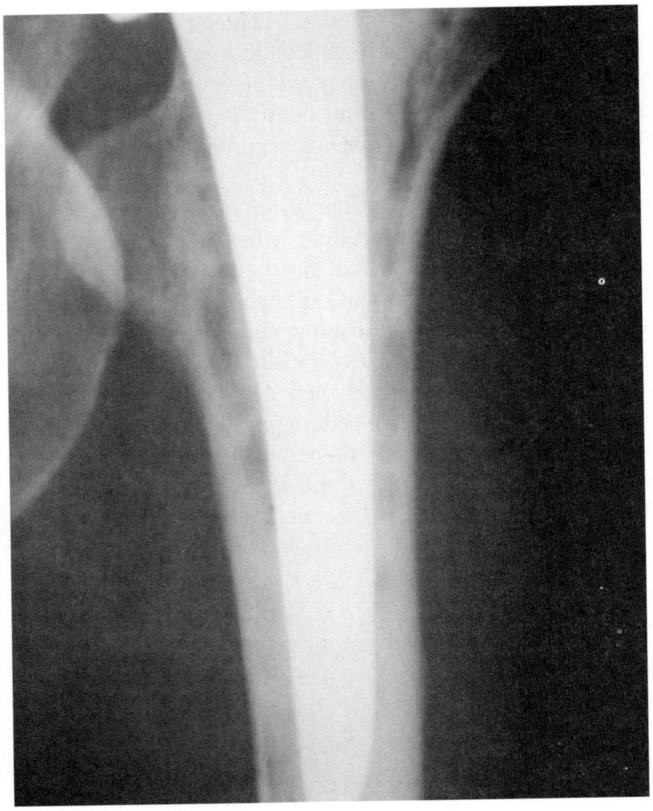

Figure 12 Bone resorption (osteolysis) around an implant is always of concern because potential exists for aseptic loosening or fracture. Particles (wear debris) of polyetheylene (from the polyetheylene socket) and the resulting inflammatory process have been suspected to have a role in resorption.

An issue that investigators in this field may face is whether to use one or both limbs. Implanting prostheses into both limbs has been reported by some (446, 447), but is unacceptable to many IACUCs. A staged insertion (e.g., 6 weeks apart) of a prosthesis in a dog is an option and is acceptable at some research facilities.

Several investigators used sheep and goats to study THR, but the complication rate is higher than in dogs (448–451). Commercially available canine hip prostheses are for the most part unsuitable for sheep and goats because of their larger medullary cavity. Shortening of the canine femoral stem for use in sheep has been reported (448). The cortical bone of the proximal third of the femur in sheep and goats is thinner than in dogs and is prone to fracture at the tip of the implant (449–451). Hip prostheses should be manufactured

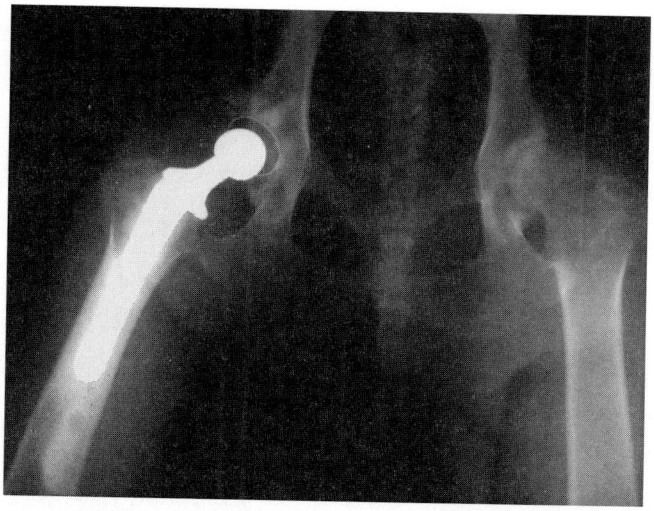

Figure 13 The dog is the animal model of choice for *in vivo* research in the field of THR (426–442). Total hip replacement in dogs has become routine for many well-equipped veterinary hospitals, with a success rate and relief of suffering matching the human experience. Courtesy of Randy Fitch, Colorado State University, Ft. Collins, Colorado.

specifically for these animals with the different femoral geometry in mind. The bone of the acetabular region in sheep and goats is also relatively thinner and does not support the acetabular cup of the prosthesis. Postoperative laxation of the implant has prompted some researchers to immobilize sheep or goats in slings (452).

Reduced cortical thickness and increased porosity are seen in most patients with noncemented total hip arthroplasty (453), and the seven delineated sections around the femoral component for zonal evaluation of progressive loosening are known as Gruen zones (454–457). The zonal classification is also applicable to animal studies (mainly dogs). Dual-energy X-ray absorptiometry using the "metal removal" software program is used routinely in patients to evaluate proximal femoral stress shielding and can be adapted to explanted canine femora (458). Radiostereometric analysis (RSA) is used to measure migration of knee implants and predict later aseptic motion (459) clinically, this not known to be undocumented by research studies in animals. Three-dimensional finite element (FE) models are also an important part of this field and have been useful in predicting proximal bone loss and distal bone densification in animal models (453).

B. Total Knee Arthroplasty

Research in TKA has paralleled THR and has some common goals (e.g., improved cementless fixation and enhancing biological fixation; reduction of wear debris) (460). Complications of TKA are well known to orthopedic surgeons who specialize in arthroplasties (461), and research unique to the anatomy and biomechanics of this complicated joint continues in many laboratories. Failure of fixation and prosthetic wear emerged as the major concern for TKA failure in the 1990s (460, 462). Controversy still exists regarding retention or sacrifice of the posterior cruciate ligament (PCL) (463). Although complications peculiar to TKA such as patellofemoral pain, stiffness, and supracondylar fracture of the distal femur are of great concern, animal models (rabbits, goats, sheep, and dogs) to study TKA (464–467) are uncommon compared to those used to evaluate THR. Knee replacement in pet dogs is not likely to achieve the success enjoyed by THR because of the large variation in breed size and the ability of dogs to function well as pets following amputation. Like THR research, *ex vitro* (468–470) and *in vitro* models (471) also represent an important facet of TKA research and the literature on these studies is extensive.

Quantitative evaluation of the bone–implant interface of THR and TKA has become costly and sophisticated over time. The removed components (animal or human) must gradually be dehydrated in graduated ethyl alcohol solutions ranging from 70 to 100% and embedded in methylmethacrylate. Serial sections 750–1000 μm thick are cut using high-speed diamond cutting and grinding techniques with great care, and the ultimate goal of avoiding artifacts at the interface. Microradiographs using high-resolution film followed by further grinding to 50 μm and then staining (e.g., toluidine blue, basic fuchsin) (472) are routinely used by many laboratories specializing in implant-interface analysis. Sections are qualitatively and quantitatively examined in transmitted and polarized light for determination of the percentage of bone ingrowth into the implant surface and the type of tissue ingrowth. Light microscopy is used to identify submicron polyethylene (PE) particles using a fine, diffuse birefringence (when viewed under polarized light) in the cytoplasm of phagocytic cells around THRs. High-quality optics with magnification up to 2000× using oil immersion are essential to visualize the faint birefringence needed to assess the presence of intracellular material (473). Careful examination of standard stained hematoxylin and eosin sections with polarized light is useful to identify wear debris from ultra-high-molecular-weight polyethylene (UHMWPE) (474). Technology such as backscatter electron imaging-scanning electron microscopy (BEI-SEM) coupled with digital image processing (469, 475) also necessitates collaboration with engineers, pathologists, and laboratories devoted to this type of analysis. Tribology (the study of lubrication and wear and friction of joints) utilizes SEM (476, 477).

The perioperative complication of deep vein thrombosis (DVT) is well recognized in human joint replacement. For example, the incidence of DVT after TKA can reach 85% without prophylaxis (421, 461). There are limited animal models of this condition.

A novel approach to evaluate bone biology (including bone graft materials and extenders) is the use of bone chambers in animals (478–481). These chambers have been used in rabbits, sheep, dogs, and pigs and details of their design are well described. These have become popular because they allow repeated sampling without sacrificing the animal and the morbidity is low. All aspects of bone biology and implantology have been studied in these chambers, including micromotion (482), fluctuating fluid pressures (483, 483), growth factors and polyethylene particles (482), proinflammaory mediator release (480), enzyme activities (481), and concurrent therapies (486, 487), to name but a few.

Relative motion between the prosthesis and the bone is important because of potential effects on ingrowth and remodeling. Several *in vivo* models are available to study the skeletal response to motion, and most utilize the distal femoral metaphyseal region of dogs (488–491); others have used bone chambers implanted in the proximal medial rabbit tibia to evaluate the amplitude of micromotion (492).

C. Endoprostheses

Massive prostheses for malignant bone tumors of the limbs are also of interest to surgeons treating primary bone tumors (493). Like THR and TKA, loosening secondary to stress shielding or osteolysis secondary to particulate debris have been major late complications (494). Our laboratory used the middiaphysis of the sheep femur to study high force compression, loading spring washers to promote strong biologic fixation and avoid stress shielding (494–496) (Fig. 14A). This idea was later tested in TKAs in sheep before initiating clinical trials (Fig. 14B). In a somewhat related load-bearing model to evaluate implants of different stiffness, segmental resection of 15 mm of the midshaft of the caprine tibia was performed (452). Some examples of studies using animal models to study different facets of joint prostheses are shown in Table XIV.

VIII. Articular Cartilage

A. General Considerations

The limited capacity of articular cartilage to regenerate has stimulated many research laboratories around the world to search for cells, tissues, and implants with chondrogenic potential. This poor healing capacity of articular cartilage has led to a search for greater understanding of the pathogenesis and treatment of a leading cause of long-term disability, of osteoarthritis (OA) (505–507). Studies of the early stages of osteoarthrosis in patients are difficult because the course of the disease is slow and ethical constraints preclude the possibility of biopsies (508). This has prompted a search for animal models directed at two main areas: (1) models of osteoarthritis and (2) models to evaluate resurfacing of partial- and full-thickness defects. Table XV presents examples

A

B

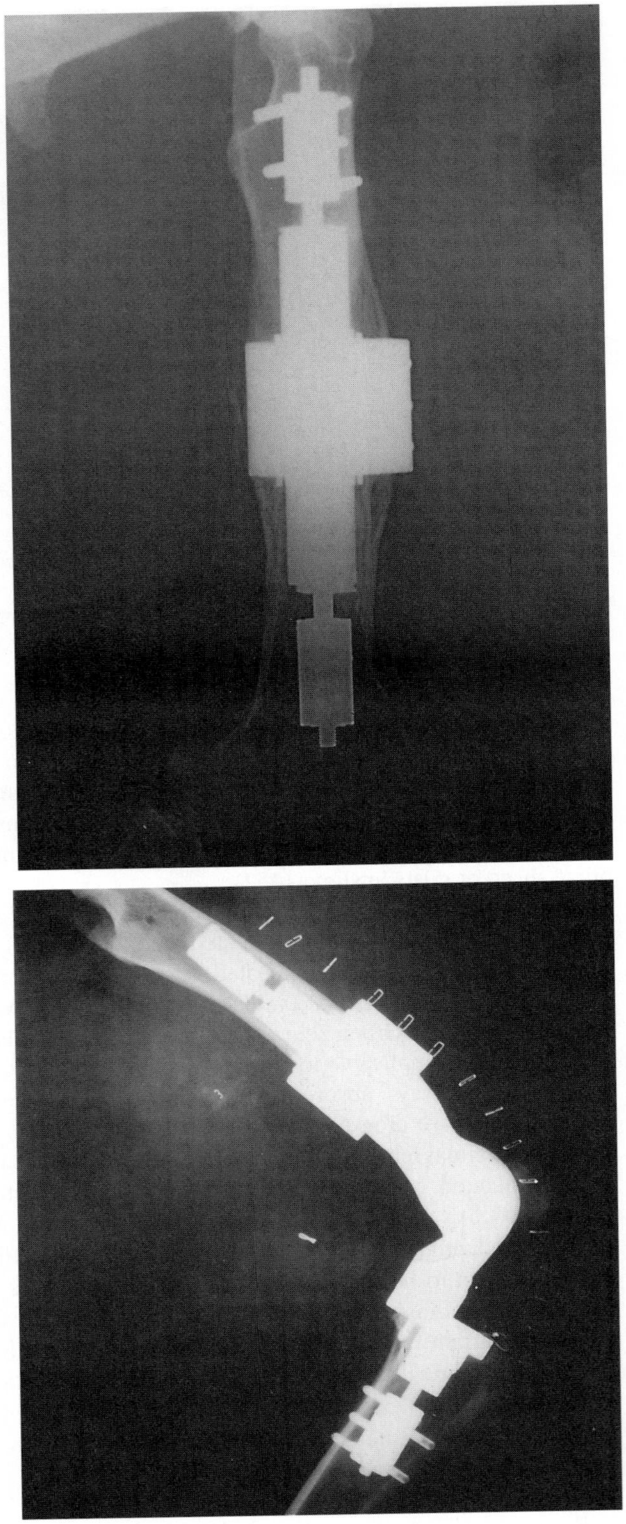

Figure 14 (A) The middiaphysis of the sheep femur to study high-force compression, loading spring washers to promote strong biologic fixation and avoid stress shielding (494–496). (B) The high-force spring washers used in the model shown in (A) were used in a TKA in sheep, before being used in clinical trials in humans.

Table XIV Joint Prostheses

Animal model	Purpose of model	Strength	Weakness	Ref.
Rat	Bisphosphonate effect on instability	Histomorphometry	Clinical relevance?	487
Rabbit	Indomethacin effect on cortical bone	Bone harvest chamber		486
	Tibial hemiarthroplasty	Parallel findings in humans		467
	Micromotion vs. polymer particles	Micromotion chamber		482
	Adaption and ingrowth and stiffness	Well characterized model for THA	Different femoral geometry	497
	Fluid pressure induction of osteolysis	Low morbidity		483
	Healing and stability (2 surface designs)		Unloaded	498
Dog	Ingrowth into tibial component		Complicated radiographic evaluation	464
	Tibial hemiarthroplasty		Implant subsistance	466
	Tibial mass after THA	Combined with THA study		499
	Stability (cemented vs. cementless)	Gait analysis performed		500
	Response of cartilage to metal		Patellar dislocation (1 case)	501
	Tissue ingrowth (stable vs. unstable)		Lameness (1 case)	488, 489
	Vascular effects of reaming			433
	Co-Cr spheres vs. Ti fiber mesh			435
	Radiographic assessment of THA	Clinical material		444
	Revision without cement	Model of aseptic loosening	Infection (1 case)	436
	Ingrowth of acetabular component			502
	Bio-active glass ceramic coating		Dislocation (1/group)	434
	Arc-deposited titanium surface	Bilateral (staged) model	Dislocation (3 cases)	446
	Bioactive bone cement vs. PMMA	Bilateral (unstaged) model	Loosening (1 case)	447
	Skeletal response to induced motion			491
	Less stiff stem in THA			438
	Polyethylene-zirconia wear		External fixator used (3 weeks)	440
	Effect of femoral stem flexibity			441
	Bioactive bone cement and THA	Bilateral (staged) model	Infection (2 cases)	442
Sheep	Changes in bone–cement interface		Femoral fracture	450
	Production of wear debris			423
	Technique and results of THA		Luxation (2) and femoral fracture (5)	449
	Hip joint forces		Quadrupedal loading variability	503
	Bone and nacre interface	Low morbidity		504
Goat	Implants of different stiffness	Agrees with finite element studies	Sling immobilization required (2 days)	452
	Intramedullary morsellized grafting	Normal loading after surgery	Loosening and/or fracture (4 cases)	451

of animal models in these two areas. Animal models of rheumatoid arthritis and infectious arthritis are available, but have been omitted in this chapter.

B. Osteoarthritis Models

Animals have played an important role in the discovery of disease-modifying osteoarthritic drugs. Models of OA can be divided into three categories: spontaneous, chemically induced, and mechanically/surgically induced. A popular model of mechanical/surgical induction involves resection of the cranial cruciate ligament (anterior; ACL) in the dog (518–520, 522, 535). This has become known as the Pond–Nuki model, although the first description of the model was by Marshall (536). Arthroscopic transection of the ligament has advantages over opening the joint with transection or transection through a stab wound.

Other models of instability-induced OA have utilized medial menisectomy in sheep (525, 537–540), rabbits (541), and guinea pigs (511) and collateral ligament transection of the metacarpophalangeal (fetlock) joint in horses (531). Immobilization and denervation have also been used (542). There are a number of spontaneous animal models of OA, but the best described are certain mouse strains, the

Table XV Articular Cartilage

Animal model	Purpose of model	Strength	Weakness	Ref.
Mouse	Role of NO in cartilage destruction	NO synthase-deficent model		509
Rat				
	Effect of chitosan on knee cartilage		Low pH—cartilage destruction	510
Guinea pig	Serological study—bone and cartilage	Model of primary OA	High prevalence, low variability	501
		Like spontaneous OA in humans		
	Subchondral bone changes			511
Rabbit	Bioactive glass vs. hydroxylapatite			512
	Inflammatory arthritis—immobilization			513
	Subfracture insult to knee joint	Early stages of posttraumatic OA	No acute microfractures observed	514
	Repair of defects with fabric	Use of skeletally mature animals		515
	Allogeneic tissue-engineered implants			516
	Quality of repair with rhBMP-2			517
Dog	Long-term observations	Well-characterized model	Per diem expense for 3 years	518
	Mechanical and biochemical changes	Arthroscopic ACL transection		519
	Effect of Tenidap sodium	Well-characterized model		520
	Cultured chondrocytes—regeneration		Suturing required, loupe required	521
	Tibial articular surface changes			522
	Synthesis and distribution of enzymes			523
	Femoral head cartilage composition	Not a surgically induced model		524
Sheep	Intraarticular hyaluronan	Matrix changes similar to humans		525
	Regeneration of fetal cartilage			526
	Transplantation of dowel allografts			527
Goat	Biological implants for defects		Need matching animals for allografts	528
	Resurfacing with marrow chondrocytes			529
	Chondroctes and fibrin glue			530
Horse	Instability model of OA			531
	Compacted cancellous bone grafting			532
Primate	Age, gender, and subchondral bone		Availability	533
	Estrogen replacement and IGF system	Phylogenetically related to human	Cost (per diem + 2 years of therapy)	534

Dunkin–Hartley guinea pig, and the cynomolgus macaque (543). The Dunkin–Hartley guinea pig develops a slowly progressive arthropathy that resembles human primary OA (501). Osteoarthritis is a consequence of canine hip dysplasia and dogs with this disease can serve as a model of human OA (524). Joint instability with hip dysplasia, as with ACL-transection models, alters the distribution of the load within the joint, causing damage to articular cartilage and underlying bone.

Joint injuries can occur following automotive accidents without observable fracture of bone. To better understand the relationship between a single blunt insult to a joint and the pathogenesis of osteoarthrosis, blunt insults were delivered to rabbit patellofemoral joints without producing fractures (while under general anesthesia). Biomechanical and histological studies were performed on the joint tissues at various times after the insults (514). Overlying cartilage showed signs of degeneration and the mechanical stiffness of the cartilage did not change until 12 months after the insult.

Experimental canine arthritis induced with complete Freund's adjuvant causes an increase in body temperature, edema of the injected stifle (knee), and no weight bearing until 2 to 3 days after induction (544). Models of this degree of severity may be unacceptable to many IACUCs. Other inducing agents include intraarticular iodoacetate, papain, callagenase, TGF-β, and hypertonic saline (542).

Women have a higher prevalence of OA after the age of 50. The role of estrogen loss and development of OA and the possible protective effect of estrogen replacement therapy have been elucidated using a number of animal models, including female sheep (545) and monkeys (534). Further research using these models is likely to emerge with emphasis on growth factor and cytokine production such as interlukin-6 (IL-6) and insulin-like growth factor 1 (IGF-1).

The role of cytokines has been investigated in knockout mice (509) and the practical reasons for manipulation of the genome using such small short-lived animals are obvious

C. Resurfacing Partial- and Full-Thickness Defects

Traumatic injuries to articular cartilage can lead to chronic pain, joint dysfunction, and disability. The obvious treatment is to fill the defect in the articular cartilage and allow the joint to return to normal activities. Small defects of uniform depth produced in rats and rabbits simply do not mimic the larger defects of varying size and depth seen in clinical practice. Clinically encountered problems with damaged articular cartilage are mostly related to large defects in partly osteoarthritic cartilage (530). Therefore, the greatest challenge for cartilage resurfacing is the management of large defects in adult cartilage that are of nonuniform depth (Fig. 15). This means that the animal model should be one with a joint closer to the size of those of human, with the appropriate size defect. Enhances cartilage regeneration is a recognized phenomenon in immature smaller animals (530), which have been used in cartilage resurfacing experiments. Results from these studies are often optimistic but do not replicate the thin cartilage seen in the clinical setting. The other challenges to the researcher are that the cartilage of rabbits, goats, sheep, and dogs is usually thinner than that in humans, subchondral and medullary bones differ, and voluntary cooperation with immobilization and no weight bearing or limited weight bearing is almost nonexistent (532). The mechanical environment during convalescence will always challenge researchers using animal models for cartilage resurfacing (Fig. 16). It is difficult to immobilize an animal following surgery in these studies. Thicker cartilage is available in horses (e.g., medial femoral condyle), but the expense of this animal model and the cost of housing limit it to studies of small groups (546).

Full-thickness defects have advantages over partial-thickness defects because they have healing surfaces exposed to a wide variety of cytokines and pluripotential cells conducive to some attempt for cartilage healing. If any scaffold or periosteum is to be used, then a certain amount of depth is essential to avoid unwanted shear forces from opposing joint surfaces (547). Resurfacing of partial-thickness defects represents the extreme challenge for both the orthopedic surgeon and the researcher in search of solutions. Constructs consisting of chondrocytes cultured on suitable scaffolds produced from nonresorbable or resorbable materials have been an attractive solution to resurfacing large articular cartilage defects. Production of these scaffolds has been successful *in vitro* (548). The challenge to both the researcher and the orthopedic surgeon is to keep these constructs in place.

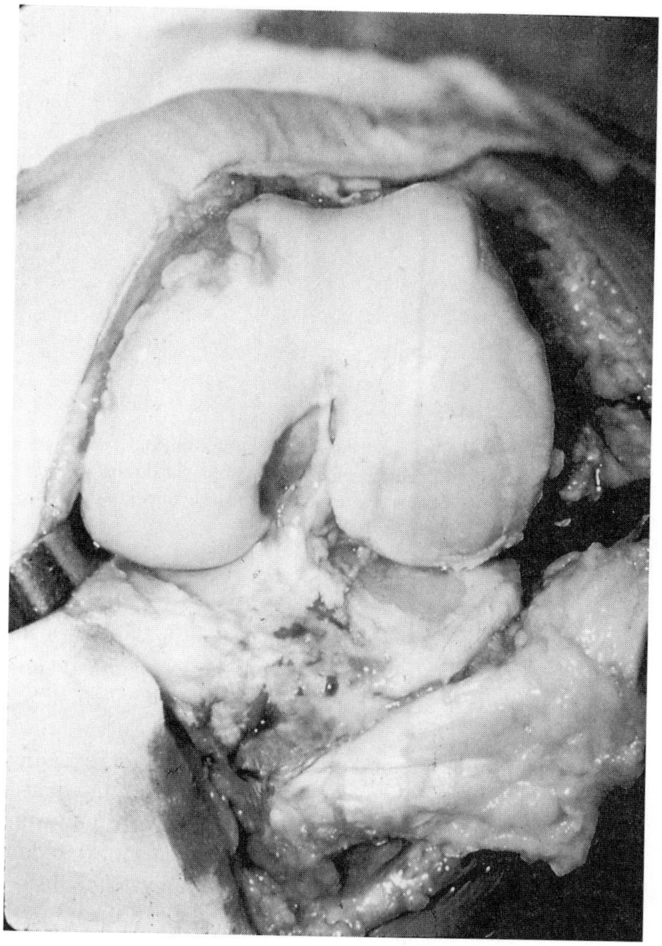

Figure 15 Small defects of uniform depth produced in rats and rabbits do not mimic the larger defects of varying size and depth seen in the knee of the distal femur of this human patient. Resurfacing large defects such as the one shown here is one of the greatest challenges to orthopedic research.

D. Analyzing Cartilage Repair or Effects of Therapies

A wide variety of approaches can be used to analyze cartilage repair. Gross morphology and histopathology are essential. The widely used semiquantitative histologic/histochemical Mankin scoring system and its modifications have become popular in different animal models (523, 530, 537,

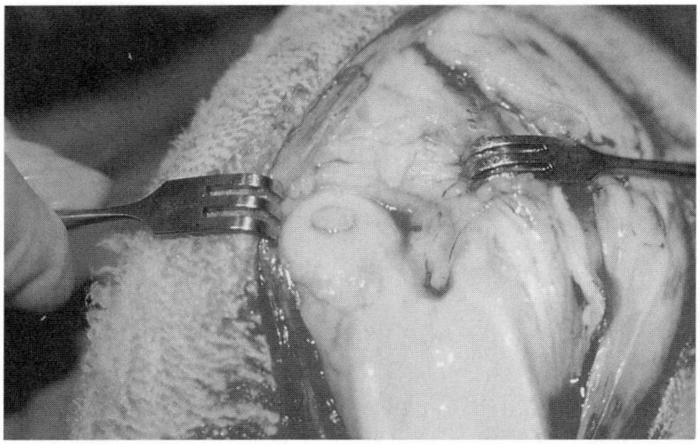

Figure 16 Resurfacing the distal femur of a full-thickness cartilage in a sheep using a scaffold. The mechanical environment during convalescence of some animal models creates unwanted shear forces, with disruption of the construct.

549, 550). Quantitative evaluation of staining intensity by various histochemical stains and immunohistochemical antibodies using image analysis plays an important role in articular cartilage research (529, 550).

Synovial membrane and articular cartilage, are receiving great attention in cartilage research. Tissue levels and distribution of interlukin-1β (IL-1β), collagenase-1, stromelysin-1, cyclooxygenase-2 (COX-2), inducible nitric oxide (iNOS), and nitrotyrosine through immunohystochemistry and morphometric analysis have been studied (535).

Engineering considerations of the biphasic, viscoelastic articular cartilage are important (551, 552). Histological, histochemical, and biochemical evaluations, although important, provide endpoints that may not be relevant to the loading of the joint during weight-bearing activities. Engineered tissue replacement of articular cartilage must be able to replicate the normal load carriage mechanism within articular cartilage and withstand the high stresses (20 Mpa). Important tests of a load-bearing material such as articular cartilage are permeation (flow) and confined compression (553). Regional variations of indentation stiffness and thickness have been reported in rabbit knees, and therefore different parts of the joint may react differently to injury and repair (554) (Fig. 17).

Force plate analysis of gait in dogs provides important means for testing new therapies for osteoarthritis (555). Videotaping of horses to evaluate compacted cancellous bone grafting of bone defects has been used (556).

Examples of other analyses and assays of articular cartilage include immunohistochemistry (523), glycosaminoglycan (GAG) analysis (557), morphometry (523), $^{35}SO_4$ incorporation into proteoglycans (525), metalloprotease assay, RNA extraction and Northern blotting (520), and IGF-1, IGF-2, and IGFBP determinations (534).

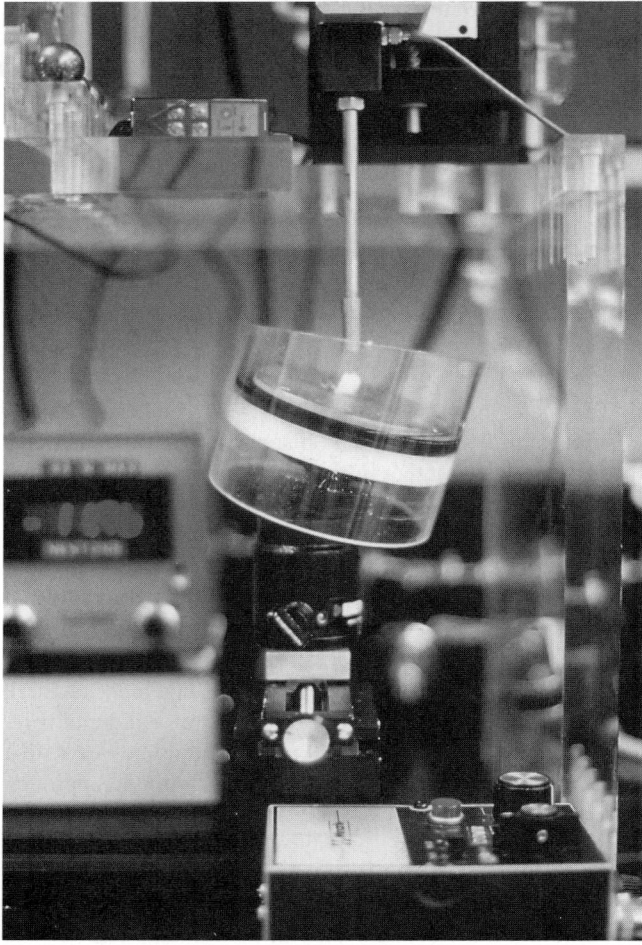

Figure 17 Automated creep indentation apparatus for mechanical testing of articular cartilage (545, 551, 553). Courtesy of Kerry Athanasiou, Rice University, Houston, Texas.

IX. Meniscus

A. Biology

The menisci are fibrocartilaginous structures consisting of interlacing collagen fibers and cells; they were once thought to be functionless structures. It is now well established and documented that they are vital to normal knee function with respect to shock absorption and lubrication of the joint (551), and the indications for repair have been well defined (558). What is also known is that they are vulnerable to trauma or overuse, disuse and degeneration, and the consequences of these conditions. The meniscus is a complex tissue and has been the subject of a wide variety of *in vitro* and *in vivo* studies. Details of the microanatomy, extracellular matrix, functional roles (load bearing, shock absorption, joint stability, lubrication), and the mechanical effects of meniscectomy have been reviewed (559, 560). A more detailed study of the ultrastructure and biochemistry of the meniscus is also available (561).

B. In Vitro Studies

In vitro studies using cadaveric material provide researchers with a good starting point for examining basic histology, biochemistry, biomechanical properties, cell types (meniscal cells, fibroblasts, mesenchymal stem cells), and matrix composition. Explanted menisci from various animals have played an important role in the study of both the normal and reparative properties of the meniscus. The biomechanical properties of human, bovine, ovine, canine, porcine, and nonhuman primate menisci were studied with uniaxial confined compression tests on 1-mm-thick, 4-mm-diameter meniscal discs. Sheep menisci exhibited an aggregate modulus (H_A) and permeability (k) most similar to properties of human menisci. It was concluded that the interspecies variations found in the material properties of the menisci indicate the need for caution when extrapolating biomechanical data (562). Histologic and biochemical studies are also needed to fully substantiate the use of a particular model.

Menisci from animals anatomically similar to humans (12-month-old pigs) were used to compare the load-to-failure of a biodegradable meniscus arrow versus a meniscal suture (563). Like much of the orthopedic research work described in this chapter, the biomechanical testing for such small pieces of tissue requires specially designed clamps. Quantification of the biomechanical properties of the medial bovine meniscus using a creep indentation technique was investigated because of its relevance to loading configuration (564). This study discovered differences between the anterior (cranial), central, and posterior (caudal) aspects of this animal model. In spite of obvious advantages of *in vitro* studies, the biological behavior of repair, especially in avascular parts of the meniscus, and the response of the meniscus to the implant cannot be determined without *in vivo* studies.

C. In Vivo Studies

The two most popular animal models for meniscal research are the rabbit and the dog. Rabbits are useful to document the histologic changes and response to tears of different configuration (565), or agents to promote healing such as HA (566). The size of the rabbit knee makes arthroscopic surgery possible but difficult (567, 568). One of the concerns about research on meniscal tears and the healing response is that the tear does not appear to simulate what is seen clinically (569).

Some of the first meniscus research was performed in dogs as early as 1936 (570). The normal vascular anatomy of canine menisci and their response to injury were studied in detail by Arnoczky and Warren using histology and tissue clearing (Spalteholz) techniques (571). This landmark study provided the orthopedic community a clear explanation as to why certain injuries (in avascular portions) failed to heal. It stimulated more studies of the meniscus in dogs to investigate the vascular response to different types of injury and repair (571), the effect on healing of a fibrin clot (572), synovial flaps (573,574), implants to guide vascular tissue (575), allografts (576), and gene transfer (577). The mechanical function of the meniscus was studied using dogs (578). Medial or lateral meniscetomy, with or without cruciate ligament transection, is a very useful technique to induce OA in an animal model.

New meniscal repair devices have been tested in animals before going into clinical trials. Because of their size, animals used to evaluate these are large-breed dogs, goats, sheep, or pigs. Two basic surgical approaches are used to implant devices for evaluation in animals, open and arthroscopic. One open approach involves a parapatellar incision with subluxation of the patella to the side of the limb away from the incision. Good retraction is essential to view adequately the proximal (superior) surface of the menisci. The other open approach involves detaching the medial collateral ligament along with a block of femoral epiphysis and partially dislocating the patella (572,576). This approach provides an excellent view of the meniscus and has been used for meniscus transplantation (576) and by the author for repair with bioresorbable tacks and arrows (Fig. 18). Closure requires reattachment of the bone plug to the femur with an orthopedic screw. It is essential to use systemic and intraarticular analgesia.

Arthroscopic meniscal repair is a well-established procedure in humans (579). Arthroscopic surgery of the knee in dogs, sheep, goats, and pigs is an attractive way to perform meniscal research because it avoids the postoperative morbidity associated with the open techniques discussed above, it allows the opposite limb to be used as a control (i.e., bilateral surgery that otherwise might not be allowed by most IACUCs), and it allows repair evaluation by second-look arthroscopy. Second-look arthroscopy is useful in patients as well (580).

After the importance of preservation of the meniscus was established, meniscal repair using various "enhancing" techniques, such as fibrin clot, fibrin glue, synovial grafting, suture patterns, and biodegradable tacks and arrows, stimulated many animal studies. The experience from these models was ultimately used in clinical cases with the aid of the arthroscope (581). However, meniscal replacement and tissue engineering are two new directions for current meniscal research and animal models will play important roles in preclinical testing in these areas (582–584). Entire medial meniscus replacement with allograft was investigated in dogs (576) and sheep (585, 586), and autologous perichondral tissue was investigated also using sheep (587). Porous

A
B
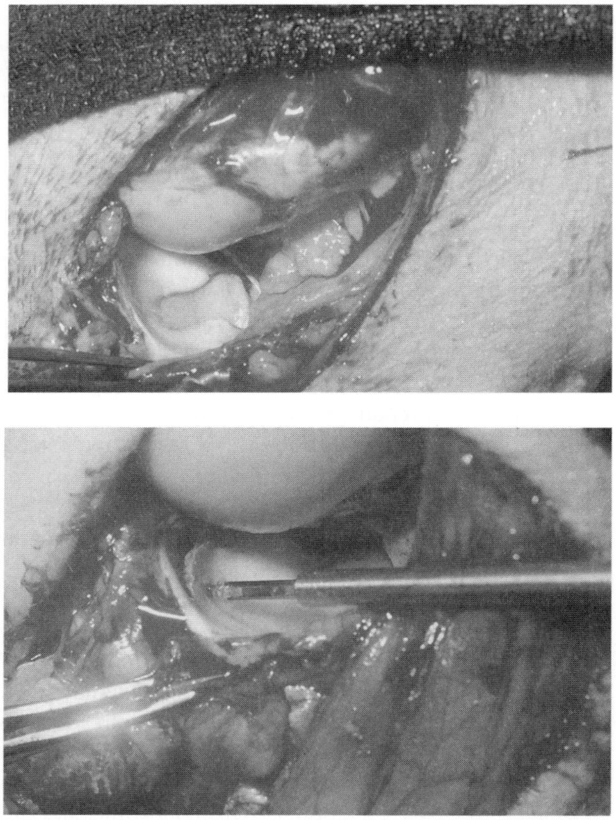

Figure 18 An open approach (first described in dogs) to the medial meniscus in sheep. This approach involves detaching the medial collateral ligament along with a block of femoral epiphysis, partially dislocating the patella (572). It provides an excellent view of the meniscus (A) and has been used for meniscus transplantation (576) or repair using bioresorbable tacks (B).

polyurethane was used for meniscal reconstruction and complete replacement in dogs. Tearing-out of sutures and dislocation of the prosthesis were problems because the tear resistance of the material was low. A more complex suturing technique was recommended (588). The reader is directed to a review of 5 years of experimental investigations using Dacron and Teflon implants (589).

Biocompatible and biodegradable synthetic polymers such as the polylactides and polyglycolides have been approved for use in suture material for many years. These polymers are now popular for developing matrices to support growth of meniscal tissue. Small intestinal submucosa shows promise as a biologic scaffold capable of promoting a reconstructive healing response rather than a nonspecific scar. Segmental replacements of meniscal defects were created in dogs (583). Resorbable collagen meniscus implants to support new tissue regeneration as the scaffold is resorbed are now in clinical trials in humans (590).

The biologic considerations involved in creating a tissue-engineered meniscus require attention to many issues, including cell type, matrix scaffold, and environmental conditions (583). Some of these materials can be readily obtained *in vitro* but the final construct must have long-term functional capabilities and this is still a big step to take from the research lab to the operating room.

D. Specimen Preparation, Testing, and Data Acquisition in Meniscal Research

Gross appearance of the meniscofemoral side is a very simple but important part of data collection. Photography with quantification with a color image processor connected to a personal computer is also of use in evaluating the healing menisci (567,568). Vascular patterns of normal and healing menisci can be studied using histologic analysis by perfusing the arterial tree with dilute India ink (modified Spalteholz technique) (571,591). Automated creep indentation apparatus has been used to study meniscal biomechanics *in vitro* with isolated bovine menisci (564). This type of evaluation will play an important role in assessing a tissue-engineered meniscus that must provide shock absorption, joint congruity, and stabilization, and protect the knee from degenerative changes. Table XVI provides a list of some of the studies in which animal models have been of use in evaluating the meniscus, with emphasis on *in vivo* models.

X. Tendons and Ligaments

Injuries to tendons and ligaments (tendonitis, bursitis, epicondylitis, and complete tendon or ligament rupture) represent a great cost to society (602). The deceleration maneuvers of sports such as football and skiing create valgus and external rotation or varus and internal rotation forces with isolated or combined injuries of the anterior cruciate ligament (ACL), posterior cruciate ligament (PCL), medial collateral ligament (MCL), lateral collateral ligament (LCL), meniscus, and joint capsule. Lateral or anterior blows to the knee are common mechanisms of injury for those playing football or involved in motor vehicle accidents (603). Injuries to the flexor tendons of the hand and the Achilles tendon are also common. Injury to the supraspinatus tendon of the rotator cuff is discussed in the next section.

Biomechanical studies using human (604–607) or animal (608–615) cadavers to mimic the clinical condition have played a vital role in tendon and ligament research. However, animal models are essential in the manipulation of the healing tissue, the addition of biological or genetic factors, and the evaluation of biological or synthetic grafts. As with previous discussions, the emphasis is on *in vivo* models.

Tendons and ligaments of the appropriate animal model lend themselves to gross and histologic acquisition of semi-quantitative data, but mechanical testing is an essential part of most studies. The mechanical properties of various mam-

Table XVI The Meniscus

Animal model	Purpose of model	Strength	Weakness	Ref.
Rabbit	Surgical excision of peripheral rim			565
	Effect of suture vs. no suture			592
	Effect of hyaluronic acid on healing	Opposite limb as a control	Menisci too cellular?	593
	Cell-based meniscus regeneration			594
	Healing of attachments			595
	Histology of repair		Longer evaluation required	596
	Fibrin glue containing marrow cells		Technically difficult with arthroscope	567, 568
	Apoptosis and NO production			597
	Response to laser meniscectomy			598
	Effect of meniscal rasping		Deep flexion of rabbit knee	599
Dog	Healing potential of meniscal tears		Not comparable to clinical injuries	569
	Vascular anatomy	Similar vasculature as human		571
	Fibrin clot to support repair	Opposite limb as a control	Needs biomechanical evaluation	572
	Vascularized synovial tissue		External fixator required	600
	Mechanics of healed meniscus		Lack of protection from hoop stresses	578
	Repair using synovial flap		Groin to ankle cast required	573
	Implant guided vascular tissue	No immobilization		591
	Porous polyurethane replacement		Prosthesis dislocation	575
				588
	Effect of free synovium on healing	Opposite limb as a control	Dislocation of implanted synovium	574
	Transplantation of meniscal allograft		Infection, patellar dislocation	576
	Gene transfer to a meniscal lesion			577
Pig	Effect of suture vs. no suture	No immobilization	Incision extension to periphery	592
	Meniscal arrow vs. meniscal suture	Meniscus size close to human	*In vitro* study only	563
Sheep	Effect of synovial implantation			592
	Transplantation of meniscal allograft		Calcaneal tendon resection required	585
	Effect of abrasion therapy	Meniscus size close to human	Difficult access to posterior region	601
	Autologous perichondral tissue		Tenotomy (calcaneal tendon) required	587
	Autograft vs. allograft transplantation			586
Primate	Healing potential of meniscal tears		Not comparable to clincal injuries	569

malian tendons have been described (616). The bony attachment of tendons or ligaments provides a relatively easy anchor for the attachment of the testing apparatus, even in small specimens. However, gripping a tendon or ligament without a bony attachment is quite complex and this is discussed in more detail in Section XI (Fig. 19).

There are very few comparative studies of morphology, physiology, and biochemistry of animal tendons and ligaments in the different animal species. The physiologic response of healing and remodeling of autografts and allografts in a variety of animal models suggests that the response can be extrapolated to humans (617). As with most *in vivo* studies discussed here, the advantages of smaller animals are cost and ease of care, but larger animals (mainly dogs, sheep, and goats) represent the human condition more closely and allow for more accurate tissue manipulation (602).

A. Ligament Repair

Ligaments are intraarticular (e.g., ACL and PCL) or extraarticular (e.g., MCL) and to model the human condition it is recommended that these be treated as different entities. Smaller animals, particularly rabbits, have been commonly used as models for extraarticular ligaments such as the MCL, whereas larger animals (mostly the dog) are the models of choice for ACL injuries.

In studies of extraarticular ligaments, the medial collateral ligament of the knee joint is the most commonly used model for ligament healing, especially in rabbits (618–621).

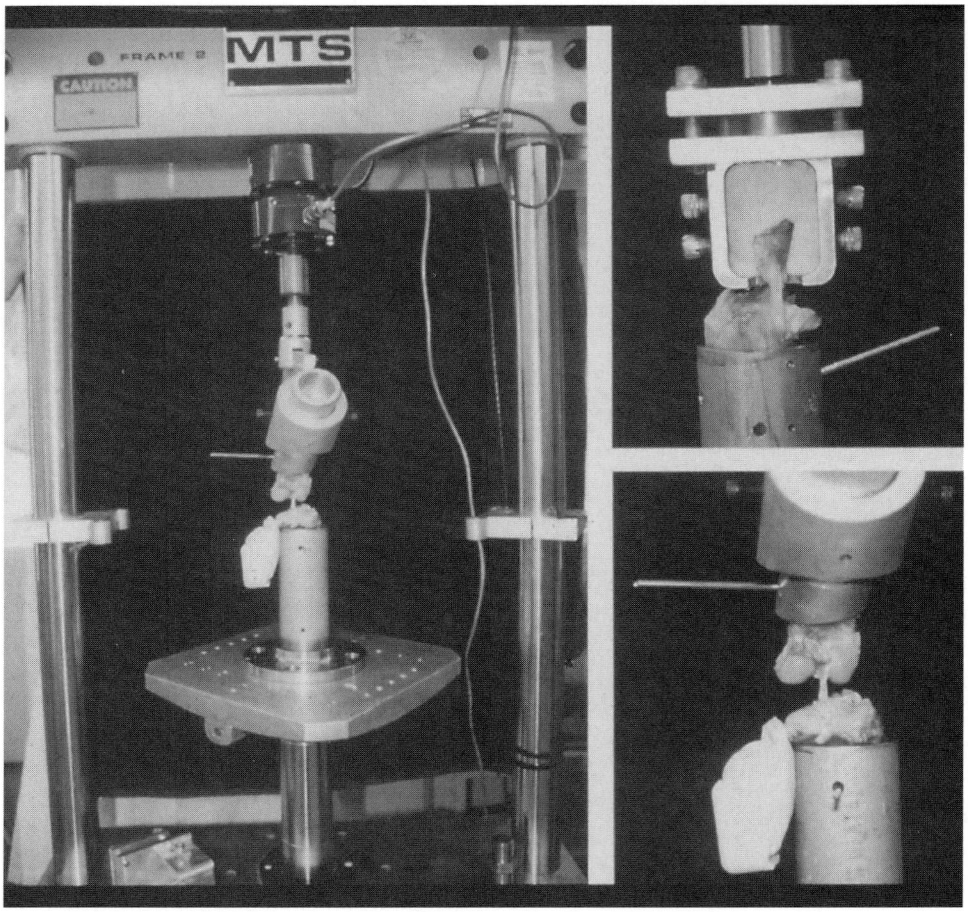

Figure 19 Before testing specimens harvested from an expensive *in vivo* study, the test apparatus should be perfected with cadaver material. Courtesy of Sabrina Strickland, Hospital for Special Surgery, New York.

The molecular biology and biomechanics of normal and healing ligaments in a rabbit model have been reviewed (622). Sheep have been used to study various ligament prostheses for the replacement of both the MCL (and the ACL) (623–625). In studies of intraarticular ligaments, injury to the ACL [known as cranial cruciate ligament (CCL) in quadrupeds] is of major clinical significance in humans because of its limited ability to heal without surgical intervention. Because cruciate ligament rupture in the dog is one of its most common orthopedic injuries, the dog quickly established itself as a popular animal for ligament research (617, 626–628), although sheep (625, 629–633) and goats (634–638) have also been used to study responses to various repair techniques. The structure of the sensory nerve endings of the ACL was studied in sheep (639). The use of nonhuman primates for evaluation of ACL repair (640) is unlikely ever to become popular because of ethical considerations, high cost, and the success of other more practical, less costly and well-established large animal models such as dogs, goats, and sheep.

Smaller animals such as the rabbit are less popular models for ACL reconstruction because of size, although rabbits were used to evaluate the ability of a semitendinosus autograft (641) and a flexor tendon allograft (620) for ACL reconstruction. Furthermore, the effect of a notchplasty on the biological and histologic properties of the ACL was also studied in rabbits (642).

B. Tendon Repair

There are two environments in which tendons exist: intrasynovial (in tendon sheaths) and extrasynovial (with fascial covering to limit their adherence to surrounding tissues) (602). Tendonitis is of great clinical importance in the racehorse and this represents one of the few spontaneously occurring animal models of the disease. Enhancing repair and return to racing performance is of great importance to horse owners. Reproduction of this injury in the horse with various chemicals such as collagenase injections can result in a condition that is histologically similar to a natural traumatic injury (643).

1. Intrasynovial Tendons

The study of tendon healing in the tendon sheaths of animals has played an important role in the understanding of healing of flexor tendons in the human hand. Most readers have been taught that tendon healing in a sheath requires an extrasynovial source of cells to support the healing process, although it has been shown that tendons do have some intrinsic capacity to heal (602).

Adhesion formation after surgery or trauma impairs the gliding mechanism of tendons, especially after the repair process. A number of models have been used to study various approaches to reduce adhesion formation. Dogs are chosen because of the similarities between their flexor tendon apparatus and healing responses to humans (644–647). In the dog, the digital sheaths of the second and fifth digits are exposed between the annular pulleys proximal and distal to the proximal interphalangeal joint. The sheath is entered and the appropriate repair on cut tendon ends is performed (648, 649). Postoperative immobilization in a fiberglass shoulder spica cast is required for this model (650). Autogenous donor flexor tendon grafts placed within the synovial sheaths of the medial and lateral forepaw of the dog were used to understand the biologic mechanisms for incorporation (647).

The knee joint of rabbits has been used to demonstrate that suppression of the actions of transforming growth factor β_1 reduced adhesion formation (651). Although this was a model of intraarticular adhesion, it could potentially have application in prevention of adhesions in tendon sheaths.

2. Extrasynovial Tendons

Whether to repair a ruptured human Achilles tendon (largest of the extrasynovial tendons that are injured) is still fiercely debated among orthopedists (652). This controversy has sustained research using animal models to further elucidate the biology of this structure. The tendon is anatomically accessible in all domestic and laboratory animals. The patellar tendon has been used in animal models. Patellar tendon forces were measured using implantable force transducers in goats (653), whereas the effects of restressing on the mechanical properties of stress-shielded patellar tendons was investigated in rabbits (654, 655).

Because the central one-third bone–patella tendon–bone autograft is presently the procedure of choice for many orthopedic surgeons (656), animal models (both large and small) have been used to examine effects of partial removal of the patellar tendon (657–660). In addition, hamstring tendon grafts are being used for ACL reconstructions and the histology of the intraarticular segment of the graft from 4 to 52 weeks after surgery was described in a sheep model (661). In this study, the relatively large ovine knee joint facilitated arthroscopic reconstruction compared to the joint of smaller animals such as rabbits. If arthroscopic reconstruction is the preferred technique to be used in the model, the patellar fat pad must be removed to facilitate adequate visualization of the joint (549). The knee joint of sheep is valid for cruciate ligament studies and the anatomy has been well described (662).

A wide range of musculoskeletal disorders, such as muscle atrophy, osteoporosis, and chronic edema, to name a few, accompanies disuse of joints. Tendons and ligaments are not spared during the various forms of musculoskeletal immobilization and disuse. There are many experimental studies of joint disuse using models such as rats, rabbits, dogs, and monkeys, but it is beyond the scope of this chapter to discuss all these in detail. Readers are directed to a review of the changes in biomechanical properties of tendons and ligaments from joint disuse (663).

C. Reattachment of Tendons to Bone

Secure anchoring of tendons to bone is an essential part of operative reconstruction to achieve full recovery, and a number of studies have focused on the improvement of healing of tendon reattachment. Early investigators used the Achilles tendon in rabbit models (664, 665). More recently, the long digital extensor tendon was implanted in a bony tunnel of the proximal tibia in dogs to characterize the histologic and biomechanical properties after placement under a physiologic load (666). Healing of acute tears of the infraspinatus and other components of the rotator cuff is prone to recurrent failure. This is discussed in the next section.

Strong and functional reattachment of tendons to bone is of great clinical importance to oncologic surgeons. They are faced with removal of large portions of bone and surrounding soft tissue, including tendons and their insertion, to achieve safe surgical margins (667, 668). Healing of detached tendons (reattachment to healthy bone) or healing in association with large endoprostheses is of concern, and enhancement of the healing process is desirable (668–672). To evaluate biologic attachment of an allograft bone and tendon transplant to a titanium prosthesis, the biceps tendon, with its insertion at the glenoid in a sheep model, has been utilized (668).

A relatively new model to repair extended connective tissue defects (secondary to trauma, infection, or congenital or neoplastic conditions) has been presented. In this model, the use of small intestinal submucosal implants for regeneration of large fascial defects was studied (673) (a 5×5 cm window was created in the fascia lata).

Various surgical techniques are used to perform a lateral release procedure to alter patellofemoral biomechanics in various disorders of the human knee. Explanted caprine knees were used to evaluate the efficacy of the holmium:YAG laser for performing lateral release and medial joint capsular tightening and to compare the laser with a scalpel (674).

A qualitative description of the cellularity, vascularity, collagen organization, and crimp pattern is standard for most specimens in tendon and ligament research. Crimp refers to the sinusoidal pattern or periodicity of the collagen bundles as seen under polarized light (661).

D. Tissue Engineering

The roles of cellular and biochemical mediators in the complex process of tendon healing are being elucidated. Evaluation of tissue engineering techniques that manipulate cellular and biochemical mediators to effect protein synthesis and improve current treatment methods relies on the availability of appropriate animal models. Application of growth factors, gene transfer techniques, and cell therapy, or a combination of these techniques, will likely be the future direction of tendon and ligament research (603, 621). The search for the optimal vehicle for growth factor delivery as encountered in other areas of orthopedic research is a likely direction to be taken by researchers in this field.

Currently, there is greater awareness of health and medical issues specific to female athletes (675). Female athletes tear the ACL more frequently than do male athletes participating in similar sports (676). Different hormonal profiles (estrogen, progesterone, and testosterone) between men and women as well as cyclic variations in women may play a role in the different injury susceptibilities. Future research will require animal models for a greater understanding of hormonal milieu and ligament and tendon healing in light of the risk factors known in female athletes (678). Table XVII presents some examples of animal models used for tendon and ligament research.

XI. Shoulder

A. Acute and Chronic Tears

The rotator cuff is a musculotendinous unit that acts in combination with the deltoid to allow elevation of the shoulder (680). Tears usually affect individuals between 40 and 70 years of age (681) and they are a frequent source of pain and disability in athletes. Repair of chronic rotator cuff tears is associated with a high rate of failure (682, 683) and research on this condition has been carried out using both *in vivo* and *in vitro* models. This research has been focused in two principal directions related to enhancing the ability of the rotator cuff tendon defects to heal. These are (1) variations in the technique of repair (e.g., different suture patterns; metallic and absorbable suture anchors) and (2) enhancement of the bone–tendon interface (e.g., use of various scaffolds with or without growth factors, cytokines, or stimulatory factors) (684). Variations in technique of repair can be evaluated both *in vitro* and *in vivo*, but enhancing the bone–tendon interface requires animal testing with an appropriate model in which repeatable and controllable alterations of intrinsic and extrinsic factors can be performed, monitored, and evaluated. Unfortunately, the bony, ligamentous, and muscular shoulder anatomy of animals does not closely resemble that of humans (685). Although the more bipedal biomechanics and greater size of the rhesus monkey (*Macaca mulatta*) may make the primate more useful, high cost and practical concerns make the rat more attractive. The rabbit is less useful (686) in this area but some studies have used it. For example, the rotator cuff of the shoulder of rabbits was used to examine the neural response to experimentally induced inflammation (687).

Most patients with rotator cuff tears are older and have some degree of osteoporosis. Rabbits were used to induce osteoporosis with systemic corticosteroids to evaluate the histologic and biomechanical characteristics of the insertion of the infraspinatus tendon to the proximal humerus (688). Osteoporosis of the proximal humerus was documented using DXA. Surprisingly, the stiffness of the steroid-treated animals was increased, which is contrary to the finding that steroids weaken fibrous tissues due to inhibition of collagen synthesis.

As with most orthopedic research discussed here, these studies involve sophisticated testing apparatus, the most common being the servo-hydraulic testing machine [such as an MTS (Eden Prairie, MN) materials testing machine or an Instron (Canton, MA) testing machine]. Aside from knowledge of the testing apparatus, mounting of test specimens in these devices can be problematic. For example, when performing biomechanical testing in the shoulder, rigid fixation of the humeral head in a suitable alloy (e.g., Low-temperature thermoset resin, Dyna-Cast; Kindt Collins Co., Cleveland, OH) could present a challenge to the engineer. Eliminating slippage between the myotendinous junction and the grip of the test apparatus requires innovation and ingenuity. Rapidly freezing the grip with liquid nitrogen or solid CO_2 after applying pressure without extending into the area of the study is essential for meaningful testing (689) (Fig. 20).

Histologic evaluation of the repair sites is important, especially for implant biocompatibility. Histologic scoring for inflammatory response, degradation scores, and osteogenesis scores can be used. Colleagues blinded to the treatment groups should carry out grading and scoring.

B. Different Techniques of Repair

In vitro testing with fresh-frozen human shoulders is valuable to assess different repair techniques. To evaluate different sites of insertion of the supraspinatus muscle, a

Table XVII Tendons and Ligaments

Animal model	Purpose of model	Strength	Weakness	Ref.
Mouse	Role of peritendinous tissue		Dissecting microscope required	660
Rabbit	Restressing patellar tendons			655
	Medial collateral healing	Combined with ACL injury		620
	Patellar tendon defect after harvest			658
	Forces in flexor digitorum profundus			678
	PDGF and collateral ligament healing			621
	Effects of rigid and functional casts		Body weight loss	679
	Notchplasty in ACL reconstruction		Limitations of the freeze–thaw model	642
Dog	Tendon healing in a bone tunnel			666
	Kinematics of ACL-deficient knees			627
	Elevation of tibial insertion	No immobilization required		628
	Autogenus flexor tendon grafts			647
	Gap formation at repair site		Disruption of adhesions	648
	Small intestine submucosa implants			673
Sheep	Anatomy and biomechanics of the knee	Similarity to human characteristics	Potential for graft abrasion	631
	Three prostheses for ACL replacement		Tendonectomy +/– cast required	625
	Sensory nerve endings of ACL			639
	Tendon–bone allograft attachment			668
	Absorbable and metal screws		Overnight slinging	632
	Histology of hamstring autograft			633
Goat	Bone–patella–bone allografts		Knee effusion (5 cases), 1 death	634
	Biochemistry of ACL autografts			657
	Patellar tendon forces			653
	Effect of tibial attachment location		Three animals dropped from study	635
	Repair after removal of central one-third of patellar ligament			659
	Small intestinal submucosa as a scaffold for ACL repair			637
	Meniscal changes in ACL-deficient joint			638
Primate	ACL and PCL reconstruction		Expense	640

sophisticated magnetic tracking device (with the scapula fixed to a Plexiglass fixture) measures the glenohumeral angle (690).

Although the anatomy of the shoulder of quadrupeds is quite different from that of humans, tenotomy of the infraspinatus of goats (691), sheep (682), and dogs (692) and subsequent reattachment to the proximal humerus are useful to address the biomechanical, histologic, and biochemical processes of rotator cuff repair. Sheep have been selected because the similarity of the infraspinatus tendon to the human supraspinatus tendon (693). Specimen harvesting times have been reported as 6 and 12 (691), 6, 12, and 24 (682), and 3, 6, 9, and 12 (692) postoperative weeks. Some of the earlier problems using the sheep model of rotator cuff repair were related to suture rupture because of failure to protect the repair from full weight bearing. Because slinging was poorly tolerated in sheep, a rubber ball was placed under the hoof of the involved limb to avoid weight bearing; this was removed at 5 weeks. Delayed repair of the released infraspinatus tendon was not recommended because of the difficulty in distinguishing scar tissue from normal tendon at the time of reattachment (682).

C. Suture Anchors

Although open repair of full-thickness tears of the rotator cuff has a documented history of success, combined arthroscopic and open techniques (694) or purely arthroscopic techniques (695) have emerged. As a result, suture anchors

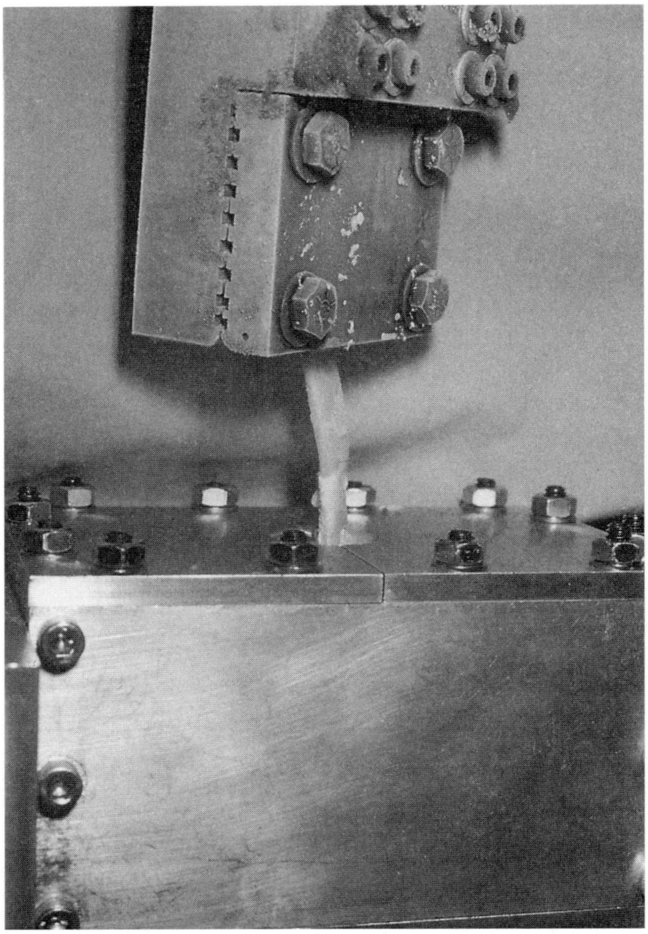

Figure 20 Gripping the tendon of the infraspinatus muscle of the shoulder joint to test attachment strength can be difficult. Different strategies, such as freezing the clamp that grips the tendon with liquid nitrogen or solid CO_2, are useful (689).

to secure tendons and ligaments to bone in the shoulder joint are being used with increasing frequency (696). Their low profile and ease of use with minimally invasive arthroscopic procedures have resulted in a variety of different designs of suture anchor. Both *in vitro* and *in vivo* testing have played a role to bring them into clinical use. *In vitro* testing of suture anchors has played an important role in their development; the advantages are obvious. For example, fatigue properties of suture anchors in anterior shoulder reconstruction using Mitek GII suture anchors were tested to failure using cadaveric glenoids (697), and Burkhart *et al.* (698) compared suture anchor fixation with transosseous bone tunnel fixation, also using fresh-frozen human cadaveric shoulders. In a similar study, static tensile tests and cyclic load tests, using cadaver shoulders, compared three sites of insertion of a suture anchor and compared them with conventional transosseous attachment (699). Roth *et al.* investigated the pullout strength and fatigue properties of a screw design suture anchor with a nonscrew design using cadaveric glenoids (700). *In vitro* testing of suture anchors is not restricted to shoulder joints. Carpenter *et al.* (701) tested five commercially available suture anchor devices in human cadaveric tibiae.

Bioresorbable implants have many advantages over metallic implants (695, 702, 703) and *in vivo* studies in animals have been important for the histologic evaluation of their biocompatibility and degradation. Bone anchors used in the shoulder of humans can be evaluated in other anatomic sites of animals. For example, under general anesthesia and sterile conditions, five samples of four different suture anchors were implanted in the lateral cortex of the left femur of rams (704). Pullout strength (parallel to the axis of the insertion hole) using a servo-hydraulic test system was measured at different time points up to 3 months. Bone anchors consisting of collagen-based bodies, ceramic washers, and polyester sutures were evaluated in the distal femoral condyles (bilaterally) in rabbits (703), whereas a bioresorbable suture anchor for rotator cuff repair was tested in the tibias of dogs (705).

Future research on rotator cuff repair will be directed at enhancement of repair using various proteins, growth factors, and cytokines, delivered by an appropriate scaffold to provide their sustained physiologic release. Studies using mesenchymal stem cells to stimulate tendon-to-bone healing are also likely to appear. The rat has been identified as an appropriate model for such studies (685, 686), especially as a model to evaluate the biological response of interface.

D. Glenohumeral Instability

Glenohumeral instability is a common and recurring problem in the young athletic patient, especially those experiencing repetitive microtrauma, e.g., swimmers and throwing athletes. The need for a simple technique to eliminate capsular redundancy, diminish the joint volume, and help stabilize the shoulder has stimulated *in vivo* and *ex vivo* animal and human cadaver research. Devices to shrink the glenohumeral joint capsule have commonly been nonablative thermal heating generated by the holmium:YAG laser (706–710).

The arthroscope has evolved into an essential tool in the evaluation and treatment of the injured shoulder, thus animals with a joint closer to the size of the human glenohumeral joint are recommended for most studies to simulate operative techniques to be used in clinical practice. Studies using the dissected glenohumeral joint capsules of sheep have been reported (709). However, other joints in animals can be used to evaluate the biological response of procedures to eliminate capsular redundancy, such as the femoropatellar joint of sheep (710). The effect of laser energy on joint capsule properties (ultrastructure, histology, etc.) can be tested in the larger, more voluminous joints of even smaller animals, such as the rabbit femoropatellar joint. This joint was used to evaluate the effect of laser energy at non-ablative levels (711), and tissue shrinkage and tensile stiffness were measured. Ultrastructural alterations in collagenous architecture of the femoropatellar joint capsule in rabbits after application of laser energy have also been analyzed (706). Histology and transmission electron microscopy were used to study the short-term *in vivo* response of nonablative laser energy using the femoropatellar joint of rabbits (707). Some of the animal models used in shoulder research are shown in Table XVIII.

XII. Miscellaneous Conditions

There are additional important orthopedic conditions that are of great clinical importance. These are discussed in the following sections.

A. Lysosomal Storage Diseases

Patients with lysosomal storage diseases have visceral, skeletal, and neurologic abnormalities and a limited life expectancy. Bone marrow transplantation has been used to correct the metabolic defects and leads to improvements (715). One such storage disease is mucopolysaccharidosis type VI (MPS VI; Maroteaux–Lamy syndrome). It is a rare inherited disorder of glycosaminoglycan metabolism that results from a deficiency of the lysosomal hydrolase *N*-acetylgalactosamine 4-sulfatase (716). A range of abnormalities including severely decreased bone length affects clinically severe MPS VI patients. The most popular animal model for the study of MPS VI is the naturally occurring form of the disease in cats. Cats have been studied especially with respect to the skeletal pathology (717–720) (Fig. 21). Cats also have lysosomal storage diseases MPS I (α-iduronidase deficiency) and MPS VII (β-glucuronidase deficiency) (721). Syngeneic bone marrow transplantation has been studied in neonatal mice for the treatment of MPS VII (722).

Table XVIII The Shoulder

Animal model	Purpose of model	Strength	Weakness	Ref.
Rat	Characterization of the model for rotator cuff disease	Distinct capsular and glenoid geometries nearer to human type	Too small for suture anchors	685
			No coracoacromial ligament as in humans	686
Rabbit	Influence of exogenous fibrin clot	Poor healing, similar to human condition		712
	Effect of nonablative laser energy on joint capsule	Opposite knee used as sham-operated control	Uses femoropatellar joint rather than shoulder	707 708
	Effect of corticosteroid-induced osteoporosis in tendon insertion	Simulates uderlying osteoporosis, as seen in many patients	Steroid-treatement elevated the stiffness of tendon–bone construct.	688
	Neural response of mechanoreceptors	Response of sensory nerves to carrageenan-induced inflammation		687
Dog	Evaluation of suture anchors	Can use left and right limb	Many anatomical differences	686
	Healing of rotator cuff		Uses proximal tibia as host bone	705
Pig	Pull-out strength of suture anchors	Low cost		692
			In vitro study using porcine femurs	713
Sheep	Effect of radiofrequency energy on joint capsule	More tissue available for mechanical testing	Anchor insertion difficult in dense bone	714
			In vitro study uses femoropatellar joint	71
		Uses glenohumeral joint, low cost	*In vitro* study	709
	Experimental rotator cuff repair	Similar dimensions of infraspinatus and human supraspinatus	Immobilization in a sling is required	682
			Delayed repair not recommended	
		Size closer to human tendon size		
Goat	Tendon-healing to cortical bone compared to cancellous bone	Size closer to human tendon size		691
Primate	Comparative anatomy with rabbit and rat	Capsule and glenoid anatomy nearer to human	Expense, ethical issues to some	686

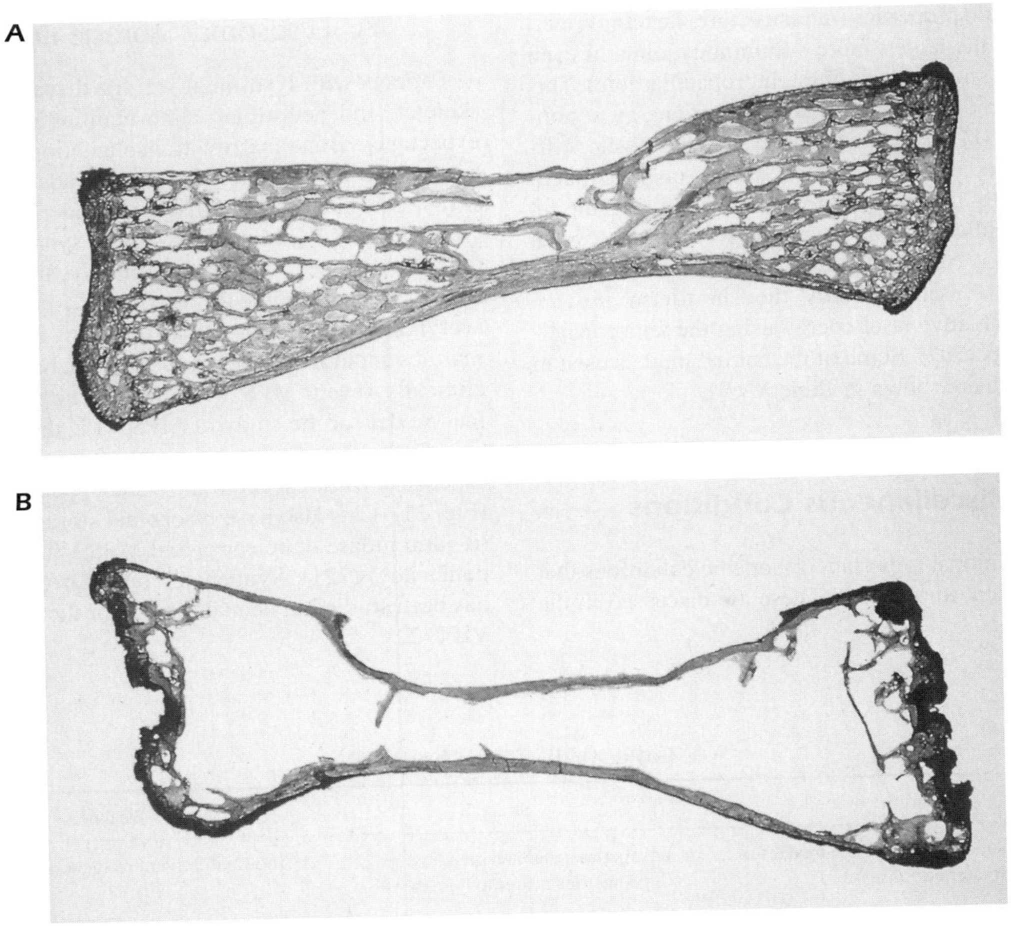

Figure 21 Midsagittal section of L5 in a control cat (A) and a cat with mucopolysaccharidosis VI (B). Toluidine blue stain; original magnification ×8 (718).

B. Marfan Syndrome

Marfan syndrome, a heritable connective tissue disorder caused by an autosomal dominant gene, affects multiple tissues and organs. Bovine Marfan syndrome has all the major pathognomonic, clinical, and pathologic features of the human syndrome, including reduced elastic fiber of the periosteum, capsule, and interosseous ligament, and flexor tendons of the metacarpophalangeal joint (723).

C. Osteogenesis Imperfecta

Osteogenesis imperfecta (OI) is a genetically and biochemically heterogeneous disease marked by frequent and spontaneous fractures (724). The homozygous (*oim/oim*) mutant mouse model of OI was used to investigate bone brittleness by characterizing the material properties of bones with ultrasound critical-angle refractometry (724). It has been speculated that a pluripotential stem cell for mesenchymatous tissues can be isolated from marrow or periosteum and that this cell could provide a vehicle for gene therapy for OI (725).

The literature on the collagen diseases is voluminous; for recent advances in this field, the reader is referred to a review by Kivirikko (726).

D. Dysbaric Osteonecrosis

Dysbaric osteonecrosis is a form of aseptic bone necrosis that can result from hyperbaric exposures during tunnel and caisson work. Sheep have been considered an appropriate animal model for this condition because of the comparable size and architecture, fatty marrow distribution, and blood flow rates in their long bones. Adult sheep have similar body weights and metabolic and tissue perfusion rates that scale to the 3/4 power of the body mass (727). Dysbaric osteonecrosis was induced successfully in adult sheep after

12 to 13 24-hr exposures of compressed air (2.6–2.9 atmospheres absolute) during a 2-month period. All exposed sheep demonstrated extensive bone and marrow necrosis in their long bones (728).

E. Growth Plate

Early orthopedic research to understand the biology of the growth plate was for the underlying purpose of correction of angular limb deformities in children, and such deformities (predominantly in foals and chondrodystrophic dogs) are well known in veterinary medicine. The role of mechanical forces on long bone growth has been studied extensively in rabbits, dogs, calves, and sheep (729, 730). Rabbits are common and convenient animals for *in vivo* studies of the growth plate, although pigs and sheep have been used to study the effects of distraction on the growth plate (731). Rabbits have been used to evaluate the inhibition of primary bony bridge formation by indomethacin on physeal injury (Salter IV fracture) (732). More recently, the role of growth factors, such as basic fibroblast growth factor (bFGF) and acidic FGF, was investigated (also in rabbits) to better understand the coupling of chondrogenesis and osteogenesis (733). Growth plate research has become more sophisticated since the early biomechanical studies of the 1980s. For example, to understand the different cellular processes during the developmental stage of chondrocytes, immunolocalization of c-Myc protein from the growth plate of rabbits was performed (734).

F. Fat Embolism Syndrome

Pulmonary injury may occur after a fracture of a long bone in association with extravasation of marrow fat. The symptoms of fat embolism syndrome may be absent or may be manifest as hypoxemia, cerebral dysfunction, and fever within 24–48 hr after injury (735). Experimental studies have used sheep (736) and dogs (735, 737) to study the pathophysiology of this disease. The canine model of fat embolism was created by pressurization of the medullary canal to study the pulmonary effects of the timing and method of fixation of a fracture (735, 737). Readers interested in this model should consult the literature. The model cannot be applied to the adult respiratory distress syndrome in humans but is useful to study various interventions for the treatment of fractures associated with injury of the lungs secondary to fat embolism (735).

G. Avascular Necrosis of the Femoral Head

Avascular necrosis (AVN) of the femoral head is a complication of treatment of congenital dislocation of the hip, whereas idiopathic avascular necrosis of the femoral head (Perthes disease) of young children is said to be caused by hip joint compression and/or tamponade (738). Various techniques have been used to induce osteonecrosis in animal models to study treatment modalities of the disease. These include multiple peripheral embolization, systemic administration of steroids, alcohol, and a variety of surgically invasive models. None of these exactly reproduce the disease in humans and there is great variability in the pattern of bone repair (739).

Skeletally immature animals are the logical choice for a model of AVN in children. Young puppies (<7 months old) were used to reproduce the disease and the blood flow rate of the femoral head (measured by hydrogen washout technique) was decreased by traction or compression in combination with hip joint tamponade (738). Increasing intracapsular hip pressure with Dextran solution delivered under pressure for 6 hr (using immature pigs) was used to study the reperfusion pattern of the femoral head (740).

Older animals are used to study AVN in the adult population. Using mature beagles, femoral head dislocation with deep freezing and stripping of soft tissues was performed (739). Early MR and histologic changes of AVN were examined in the distal femur of adult beagles following devascularization (741) and in the femoral head of mature mongrels (742) following various devascularization techniques (periosteal stripping, vessel ligation, etc.).

A less practical animal model of AVN is the flightless Australian bird, the emu (*Dromaius novaehollandiae*). With this model, the condition was created by elevation of capsular attachments of the femoral neck and ligation of the medial circumflex artery. Liquid nitrogen was delivered through a transcortical foramen to the metaphyseal and epiphyseal cancellous bone followed by a saline flush (743).

Core decompression is one of the recommended treatment regimens for the early (precollapse) stages of the disease to prevent progression of necrosis and collapse of the femoral head (744). Male sheep were used to study the short- and long-term effects of marrow decompression, and the effects of a biodegradable stent implanted into the drill channel to prolong decompression were also investigated (744). With the increasing popularity of use of osteoconductive matrices for bone regeneration (745–748), future studies of the management of AVN (using animal models) are likely to be directed toward creation of the lesion and replacement of the necrotic bone with these substitutes.

H. Tears of the Triangular Fibrocartilage of the Wrist

The triangular fibrocartilaginous complex (TFCC) of the wrist acts as a stabilizer of the distal radioulnar joint and ulnar carpus. Lesions of the TFCC may be a result of trauma or age-related degenerative changes and are a known cause of ulnar wrist pain (750–751). Studies have shown that there are vascular and structural similarities between the TFCC of dogs and humans (752). The effect of exogenous fibrin clot on regeneration of the TFCC was investigated in this canine model (751).

XIII. The Future Direction of Orthopedic Research

Orthopedic research is likely to progress in a variety of directions with greatest emphasis on tissue engineering, further characterization of cytokines and their role in cell-to-cell interactions within the skeletal tissues, and gene therapy, and various combinations of all of these.

A. Tissue Engineering

Tissue engineering (developing biological substitutes for the repair, reconstruction, regeneration, or replacement of tissues) has wide applications in orthopedics. Research in this area will accelerate in the new millennium and strategies capable of delivering cells, growth factors, and extracellular matrix scaffolds are likely to be used by those treating bone defects and nonunions (753,754). Rat femoral defect models will be useful in regeneration studies.

The difference between the biology and physiology of the young and old has been known for centuries and with tissue-engineered regeneration, this difference may become less of a challenge to the orthopedist. Sports injuries will benefit most in this field, and emphasis will be on improved repair of articular cartilage, the meniscus, ACL, fractures, and skeletal muscle injury.

B. Growth Factors

Research using growth factors is another field of orthopedic research that will continue to expand. The appropriate growth factor to treat the injury, the optimal concentration, and means to deliver the compound will become a challenge to researchers and clinicians. An extensive body of literature devoted to growth factors and the musculoskeletal system is already available (755).

C. Gene Therapy

Gene therapy represents a new approach to deliver therapeutic agents at relatively large concentrations for a longer time in discrete locations (756,757). At the time of writing, adenoviral vectors have shown the most promising results for expression of the transgenic product, although other vectors are being studied.

The clinical use of cytokines is limited because of their short half-lives, so gene delivery offers an alternative administration system. This will avoid administration of the cytokine by daily injections or continuous pumps. In addition, gene delivery offers the possibility of localized targeted delivery, restricted to the tissue of interest, where therapeutic effects may occur without systemic side effects (757).

When perfected, growth factor-based gene transfer will have countless applications for the orthopedic surgeon. Examples include new strategies in acceleration of fracture healing, the treatment of fractures with segmental defects, and nonunions (756). Furthermore, introduction of exogenous therapeutic genes into osteoblasts harvested from cancellous bone will likely lead to novel therapies to treat bone diseases.

Resurfacing of articular cartilage defects and the meniscus are very challenging (725). Cell-based therapy (implantation of cells or engineered cartilage) is likely the direction of cartilage repair (758). Meniscal regeneration may be possible if the scaffold technology is improved in combination with pluripotential cells, specific mesenchymal cells, and activated chondrocytes embedded in the scaffolds combined with gene therapy (759).

Adenoviral-mediated gene transfer of a therapeutic gene to the intervertebral disc has been successful in rabbits and will likely be used in the future to manage degenerative disc disease (760). The use of bone morphogenetic proteins in spine arthrodesis, as discussed previously, has yielded promising results. However, fewer responsive cells and less responsive cells in elderly patients will be fertile ground for local gene therapy to deliver these osteoconductive proteins (761).

Therapy for chronic bone diseases such as osteoporosis may be limited by the transient effects of adenovirally mediated gene transfer unless a convenient method of repeated application can be devised (756). Further animal studies will be essential to investigate the use of gene transfer for the treatment of orthopedic conditions. Mesenchymal stem cells have been shown to be osteogenic and as the technology to purify and deliver these cells is perfected, treatment of diseases such as osteogenesis imperfecta and osteoporosis will be possible (725).

Logistic and regulatory issues will be the biggest barriers to the clinical use of tissue engineering, cytokines, and gene therapy. Reimbursement for the cost of novel and expensive therapies by third-party payers could be an obstacle, unless convincing evidence can show long-term cost savings. Finally, the Food and Drug Administration will have to establish regulatory guidelines to safeguard the best interest and health of the public, yet respond to rapidly changing technologies (753).

Acknowledgments

The author of this chapter is grateful to Lauren Kaufman for entering references.

References

1. Yelin, E., and Callahan, L. F. (1995). The economic cost and social and psychological impact of musculoskeletal conditions. *Arthritis Rheum.* **38**(10), 1351–1362.
2. Roach, H. I., Shearer, J. R., *et al.* (1989). The choice of an experimental model. a guide for research workers. *J. Bone Joint Surg. Br.* **71B,** 549–553.
3. An, Y. H., and Friedman, R. J. (1999). "Animal Models in Orthopaedic Research." CRC Press, Boca Raton.
4. Hasegawa, M., Sudo, A., *et al.* (1999). Biological performance of a three-dimensional fabric as artificial cartilage in the repair of large osteochondral defects in rabbit. *Biomaterials* **20,** 1969–1975.
5. Getty, R. (1975). "The Anatomy of the Domestic Animals." W.B. Saunders Company, Philadelphia.
6. Johnson, K. D., August, A., *et al.* (1996). Evaluation of ground cortical autograft as a bone graft material in a new canine bilateral segmental long bone defect model. *J. Orthop. Trauma* **10**(1), 28–36.
7. Drummond, J. C., Todd, M. M., *et al.* (1996). Use of neuromuscular blocking drugs in scientific investigations involving animal subjects. *Anesthesiology* **85**(4), 697–699.
8. Flecknell, P. A. (1993). Anaesthesia of animals for biomedical research. *Br. J. Anaesth.* **71,** 885–894.
9. Einhorn, T. A. (1998). The cell and molecular biology of fracture healing. *Clin. Orthop.* **355S,** S7–S21.
10. Nunamaker, D. M. (1998). Experimental models of fracture repair. *Clin. Orthop.* **355S:** S56–S65.
11. Einhorn, T. A. (1995). Current concepts review enhancement of fracture-healing. *J. Bone Joint Surg. Br.* **77A**(6), 940–956.
12. Einhorn, T. A., Majeska, R. J., *et al.* (1995). The expression of cytokine activity by fracture callus. *J. Bone Miner. Res.* **10**(8), 1272–1281.
13. Reddi, A. H. (1998). Initiation of fracture repair by bone morphogenetic proteins. *Clin. Orthop.* **355S,** S66–S72.
14. Richards, M., Goulet, J. A., *et al.* (1999). Temporal and spatial characterization of regenerate bone in the lengthened rabbit tibia. *J. Bone Miner. Res.* **14,** 1978–1986.
15. Claes, L., Laule, J., *et al.* (2000). The influence of stiffness of the fixator on maturation of callus after segmental transport. *J. Bone Joint Surg.* **82B**(1), 142–148.
16. Lammens, J., Liu, Z., *et al.* (1998). Distraction bone healing versus osteotomy healing: A comparative biochemical analysis. *J. Bone Miner. Res.* **13**(2), 279–286.
17. Richards, M., Huibregtse, B. A., *et al.* (1999). Marrow-derived progenitor cell injections enhance new bone formation during distraction. *J. Orthop. Res.* **17,** 900–908.
18. Barnes, G. L., Kostenuik, P. J., *et al.* (1999). Growth factor regulation of fracture repair. *J. Bone Miner. Res.* **14,** 1805–1815.
19. Wallach, S., Rousseau, G., *et al.* (1999). Effects of calcitonin on animal and *in vitro* models of skeletal metabolism. *Bone* **25**(5), 509–516.
20. Keller, J. C., Trancik, T. M., *et al.* (1989). Effects of indomethacin on bone ingrowth. *J. Orthop. Res.* **7,** 28–34.
21. Li, J., Mori, S., *et al.* (1999). Effect of bisphosphonate (Incadronate) on fracture healing of long bones in rats. *J. Bone Miner. Res.* **14,** 969–979.
22. Huddleston, P. M., Steckelberg, J. M., *et al.* (2000). Ciprofloxacin inhibition of experimental fracture-healing. *J. Bone Joint Surg.* **82A**(2), 161–173.
23. Ekholm, E. C., Hietaniemi, K., *et al.* (1995). Extended expression of cartilage components in experimental pseudoarthrosis. *Connective Tissue Res.* **31**(3), 211–218.
24. Nyquist, F., Halvorsen, V., *et al.* (1999). Ethanol and its effects on fracture healing and bone mass in male rats. *Acta Orthop. Scand.* **70**(2), 212–216.
25. Låftman, P., Nilsson, O. S., *et al.* (1989). Stress shielding by rigid fixation studied in osteotomized rabbit tibiae. *Acta Orthop. Scand.* **60**(6), 718–722.
26. Aspenberg, P., Goodman, S. B., *et al.* (1996). Influence of callus deformation time. Bone chamber study in rabbits. *Clin. Orthop.* **322,** 253–261.
27. Bostrom, M., Lane, J. M., *et al.* (1996). Use of bone morphogenetic protein-2 in the rabbit ulnar nonunion model. *Clin. Orthop. Res.* **327,** 272–282.
28. Keller, J. C., Trancik, T. M., *et al.* (1989). Effects of indomethacin on bone ingrowth. *J. Orthop. Res.* **7,** 28–34.
29. Matsushita, T., and Kurokawa, T. (1998). Comparison of cyclic compression, cyclic distraction and rigid fixation. *Acta Orthop. Scand.* **69**(1), 95–98.
30. Guichet, J.-M., Braillon, P., *et al.* (1998). Periosteum and bone marrow in bone lengthening. A DEXA quantitative evaluation in rabbits. *Acta Orthop. Scand.* **69**(5), 527–531.
31. Bax, B. E., Wozney, J. M., *et al.* (1999). Bone morphogenetic protein-2 increases the rate of callus formation after fracture of the rabbit tibia. *Calcif. Tissue Int.* **65,** 83–89.
32. Yamane, K., Okano, T., *et al.* (1999). Effect of ED-71 on modeling of bone in distraction osteogenesis. *Bone* **24,** 187–193.
33. Li, G., Simpson, A. H. R. W., *et al.* (1999). Effect of lengthening rate on angiogenesis during distraction osteogenesis. *J. Orthop. Res.* **17,** 362–367.
34. Hagino, T. and Hamada, Y. (1999). Accelerating bone formation and earlier healing after using demineralized bone matrix for limb lengthening in rabbits. *J. Orthop. Res.* **17,** 232–237.
35. DeCoster, T. A., Simpson, A. H. R. W., *et al.* (1999). Biologic model of bone transport distraction osteogenesis and vascular response. *J. Orthop. Res.* **17,** 238–245.
36. Roush, J. K., and Wilson, J. W. (1990). Effects of plate luting on cortical vascularity and development of cortical porosity in canine femurs. *Vet. Surg.* **19**(3), 208–214.
37. Smith, S. R., Bronk, J. T., *et al.* (1990). Effect of fracture fixation on cortical bone blood flow. *J. Orthop. Res.* **8,** 471–478.
38. Muir, P., Johnson, K. A., *et al.* (1999). *In vivo* matrix microdamage in a naturally occurring canine fatigue fracture. *Bone* **25**(5), 571–576.
39. Boyan, B. D., Caplan, A. I., *et al.* (1999). Osteochondral progenitor cells in acute and chronic canine nonunions. *J. Orthop. Res.* **17,** 246–255.
40. Kolbeck, S., Bail, H., *et al.* (2000). Recombinant growth hormone accelerates healing in an osteotomy model in micropigs. 46th Annual Meeting, Orthopaedic Research Society, Orlando, Florida.
41. Seibold, R., Betz, A., *et al.* (1989). Application of an internal fixateur to the femur and tibia. preliminary result or an experimental study. *Vet. Comp. Orthopaed. Traumatol.* **2,** 85–90.
42. Wallace, A. L., Makki, R., *et al.* (1995). Measurement of serum angiogenic factor in devascularized experimental tibial fractures. *J. Orthop. Trauma* **9**(4), 324–332.
43. Goldberg, V. M., and Stevenson, S. (1987). Natural history of autografts and allografts. *Clin. Orthop.* **225,** 7–16.
44. Van Heest, A., and Swiontkowski, M. (1999). Bone-graft substitutes. *Lancet* **353**(Suppl. I), 28–29.
45. Ransford, A. O., Morley, T., *et al.* (1998). Synthetic porous ceramic compared with autograft in scoliosis surgery. *J. Bone Joint Surg.* **80B**(1), 13–18.
46. Muschler, G. F., Negami, S., *et al.* (1996). Evaluation of collagen ceramic composite graft materials in a spinal fusion model. *Clin. Orthop.* **328,** 250–260.
47. Younger, E. M., and Chapman, M. W. (1989). Morbidity at bone graft donor sites. *J. Orthop. Trauma* **3**(3), 192–195.

48. Tomford, W. W. (1995). Transmission of disease through transplantation of musculoskeletal allografts. *J. Bone Joint Surg.* **77A**(11), 1742–1754.
49. Damien, C. J., and Parsons, J. R. (1991). Bone graft and bone graft substitutes: A review of current technology and applications. *J. Appl. Biomater.* **2,** 187–208.
50. Lamerigts, N. M. P. (1998). "The Incorporation Process of Morsellized Bone Graft. Biological and mechanical factors." Feenstra Design/ Advertising Grootebroek, Netherlands.
51. Wang, J. S., and Aspenberg, P. (1994). Basic fibroblast growth factor increases allograft incorporation. bone chamber study in rats. *Acta Orthop. Scand.* **65**(1), 27–31.
52. Lamerigts, N. M. P., Buma, P., *et al.* (1999). Role of growth factors in the incorporation of unloaded bone allografts in the goat. *Clin. Orthop.* **368,** 260–270.
53. Hamson, K. R., Toth, J. M., *et al.* (1995). Preliminary experience with a novel model assessing *in vivo* mechanical strength of bone grafts and substitute materials. *Calcif. Tissue Int.* **57,** 64–68.
54. Lin, K. Y., Bartlett, S. P., *et al.* (1990). The effect of rigid fixation on the survival of onlay bone grafts: An experimental study. *Plast. Reconstr. Surg.* **86**(3), 449–456.
55. Hollinger, J. O., and Kleinschmidt, J. C. (1990). The critical size defect as an experimental model to test bone repair materials. *J. Craniofac. Surg.* **1**(1), 60–68.
56. Holmes, R. E., and Hagler, H. K. (1988). Porous hydroxyapatite as a bone graft substitute in cranial reconstruction: A histometric study. *Plast. Reconstr. Surg.* **81**(5), 662–671.
57. Paley, D., Young, M. C., *et al.* (1986). Percutaneous bone marrow grafting of fractures and bone defects. An experimental study in rabbits. *Clin. Orthop.* **208,** 300–312.
58. Kühne, J.-H., Bartl, R., *et al.* (1994). Bone formation in coralline hydroxyapatite. Effects of pore size studied in rabbits. *Acta Orthop. Scand.* **65**(3), 246–252.
59. Kieswetter, K., Xiong, L., *et al.* (1998). *Polylactide–co-glycolides as biodegradable bone graft substitutes.* 44th Annual Meeting, Orthopaedic Research Society, New Orleans, Louisiana.
60. Winn, S. R., Uludag, H., *et al.* (1999). Carrier systems for bone morphogenetic proteins. *Clin. Orthop.* **367S,** S95–S106.
61. Hadjipavlou, A. G., Simmons, J. W., *et al.* (2000). Plaster of paris as an osteoconductive material for interbody vertebral fusion in mature sheep. *Spine* **25**(1), 10–16.
62. Lee, S. C., Shea, M., *et al.* (1994). Healing of large segmental defects in rat femurs is aided by rhBMP-2 in PLGA matrix. *J. Biomed. Mater. Res.* **28,** 1149–1156.
63. Stevenson, S., Cunningham, N., *et al.* (1994). The effect of osteogenin (a bone morphogenetic protein) on the formation of bone inorthotopic segmental defects in rats. *J. Bone Joint Surg.* **76A**(11), 1676–1687.
64. Chakkalakal, D. A., Strates, B. S., *et al.* (1999). Repair of segmental bone defects in the rat: An experimental model of human fracture healing. *Bone* **25**(3), 321–332.
65. Kobayashi, M., Nakamura, T., *et al.* (1999). Effect of bioactive filler content on mechanical properties and osteoconductivity of bioactive bone cement. *J. Biomed. Mater. Res.* **46,** 447–457.
66. Ongpipattanakul, B., Nguyen, T., *et al.* (1997). Development of tricalcium phosphate/amylopectin paste combined with recombinant human transforming growth factor beta 1 as bone defect filler. *J. Biomed. Mater. Res.* **36,** 295–305.
67. Zegzula, H. D., Buck, D. C., *et al.* (1997). Bone formation with use of rhBMP-2 (recombinant human bone morphogenetic protein-2). *J. Bone Joint Surg.* **79A**(12), 1778–1790.
68. Hing, K. A., Best, S. M., *et al.* (1999). Quantification of bone ingrowth within bone-derived porous hydroxyapatite implants of varying density. *J. Mater. Science* **10,** 663–670.
69. Gauthier, O., Bouler, J. M., *et al.* (1999). Kinetic study of bone ingrowth and ceramic resorption associated with the implantation of different infectable calcium-phosphate bone substitutes. *J. Biomed. Mater. Res.* **47,** 28–35.
70. Louisia, S., Stromboni, M., *et al.* (1999). Coral grafting supplemented with bone marrow. *J. Bone Joint Surg.* **81B,** 719–724.
71. Laffargue, P., Fialdes, P., *et al.* (2000). Adsorption and release of insulin-like growth factor-I on porous tricalcium phosphate implant. *J. Biomed. Mater. Res.* **49,** 415–421.
72. LaBerge, M., Bobyn, J. D., *et al.* (1990). Study of soft tissue ingrowth into canine porous coated femoral implants designed for osteosarcomas management. *J. Biomed. Mater. Res.* **24,** 959–971.
73. Grundel, R. E., Chapman, M. W., *et al.* (1991). Autogeneic bone marrow and porous biphasic calcium phosphate ceramic for segmental bone defects in the canine ulna. *Clin. Orthop.* **266,** 244–258.
74. Cook, S. D., Baffes, G. C., *et al.* (1994). Recombinant human bone morphogenetic protein-7 induces healing in a canine long-bone segmental defect model. *Clin. Orthop.* **301,** 302–312.
75. Zarduacjas, L. D., Teasdall, R. D., *et al.* (1994). Torsional properties of healed canine diaphyseal defects grafted with a fibrillar collagen and hydroxyapatite/tricalcium phosphate composite. *J. Appl. Biomater.* **5,** 277–283.
76. Young, D. R., Shih, L.-Y., *et al.* (1997). Effect of cisplatin chemotherapy on extracortical tissue formation in canine diaphyseal segmental replacement. *J. Orthop. Res.* **15**(5), 773–780.
77. Sciadini, M. F., Dawson, J. M., *et al.* (1997). Evaluation of bovine-derived bone protein with a natural coral carrier as a bone-graft substitute in a canine segmental defect model. *J. Orthop. Res.* **15,** 844–857.
78. Bruder, S. P., Kraus, K. H., *et al.* (1998). The effect of implants loaded with autologous mesenchymal stem cells on the healing of canine segmental bone defects. *J. Bone Joint Surg.* **80**(7), 985–996.
79. Frankenburg, E. P., Goldstein, S. A., *et al.* (1998). Biomechanical and histological evaluation of a calcium phosphate cement. *J. Bone Joint Surg.* **80A**(8), 1112–1124.
80. Turner, T. M., Urban, R. M., *et al.* (1999). Calcium sulfate is as effective as autogenous cancellous bone in healing a large medullary defect at 6 months. 25th Annual Meeting, Transactions Society of Biomaterials, Providence, RI.
81. Millis, D. L., Williams, F. A., *et al.* (1999). The effect of length of treatment with canine recombinant somatotropin on bone healing in an unstable fracture gap model. 45th Annual Meeting, Orthopaedic Research Society, Anaheim, CA.
82. Heckman, J. D., Ehler, W., *et al.* (1999). Bone morphogenetic protein but not transforming growth factor-β enhances bone formation in canine diaphyseal nonunions implanted with a biodegradable composite polymer. *J. Bone Joint Surg.* **81A**(12): 1717–1729.
83. Kirker-Head, C. A. (1995). Recombinant bone morphogenetic proteins: Novel substances for enhancing bone healing. *Vet. Surg.* **24,** 408–419.
84. Gao, T. J., Lindholm, T. S., *et al.* (1996). Enhanced healing of segmental tibial defects in sheep by a composite bone substitute composed of tricalcium phosphate cylinder, bone morphogenetic protein, and type IV collagen. *J. Biomed. Mater. Res.* **32,** 505–512.
85. Augat, P., Margevicius, K., *et al.* (1998). Local tissue properties in bone healing: Influence of size and stability of the osteotomy gap. *J. Orthop. Res.* **16,** 475–481.
86. Wippermann, B. W., den Boer, F., *et al.* (1999). The resorbable calcium phosphate cement alpha BSM in a sheep tibia segmental defect. 45th Annual Meeting, Orthopaedic Research Society, Anaheim, CA.
87. Mathon, D. H., Frayssinet, P., *et al.* (1998). Development of a segmental long-bone defect model in sheep. *Vet. Comp. Orthopaed. Traumatol.* **11,** 1–7.
88. Gugala, A., and Gogolewski, S. (1999). Regeneration of segmental diaphyseal defects in sheep tibiae using resorbable polymeric membranes: A preliminary study. *J. Orthop. Trauma* **13,** 187–195.

89. den Boer, F. C., Patka, P., *et al.* (1999). New segmental long bone defect model in sheep: Quantitative analysis of healing with dual energy x-ray absorptiometry. *J. Orthop. Res.* **17,** 654–660.
90. Kon, E., Muraglia, A., *et al.* (2000). Autologous bone marrow stromal cells loaded onto porous hydroxyapatite ceramic accelerate bone repair in critical-size defects of sheep long bones. *J. Biomed. Mater. Res.* **49,** 328–337.
91. Leunig, M., Demhartner, T. J., *et al.* (1999). Quantitative assessment of aniogenesis and osteogenesis after transplantation of bone. *Acta Orthop. Scand.* **70**(4), 374–380.
92. Liebergall, M., Young, R. G., *et al.* (1994). The effects of cellular manipulation and TGF-β in a composite bone graft. *In* "Bone Formation and Repair," pp. 367–378. J. M. Lane, Brighton, CT.
93. Tagil, M., and Aspenberg, P. (1999). Cartilage induction by controlled mechanical stimulation *in vivo. J. Orthop. Res.* **17,** 200–204.
94. Albrektsson, T. (1980). *In vivo* studies of bone grafts. The possibility of vascular anastomoses in healing bone. *Acta Orthop. Scand.* **51,** 9–17.
95. Köhler, P. (1986). Reimplantation of bone after autoclaving: Reconstruction of large diaphyseal defects in the rabbit. Department of Orthopaedic Surgery, Karolinska Hospital, Stockholm.
96. Donski, P. K., Carwell, G. R., *et al.* (1979). Growth in revascularized bone grafts in young puppies. *Plast. Reconstr. Surg.* **64**(2), 239–243.
97. Stevenson, S. (1987). The immune response to osteochondral allografts in dogs. *J. Bone Joint Surg.* **69A**(4), 573–582.
98. Böstman, O. M., Päivärinta, U., *et al.* (1992). The tissue-implant interface during degradation of absorbable polyglycolide fracture fixation screws in the rabbit femur. *Clin. Orthop.* **285,** 263–272.
99. Böstman, O. M., and Pihlajamäki, H. K. (2000). Adverse tissue reactions to bioabsorbable fixation devices. *Clin. Orthop.* **371:** 216–227.
100. Weiler, A. H., Kirch, H.-J. U., *et al.* (1996). Foreign-body reaction and the course of osteolysis after polyglycolide implants for fracture fixation. experimental study in sheep. *J. Bone Joint Surg.* **78B**(3), 369–376.
101. Baumgaertel, F., Perren, S. M., *et al.* (1994). Tierexperimentelle untersuchungen zur "biologischen" plattenosteosynthese von mehrfragmentfrakturen des femurs. *Unfallchirurg* **97,** 19–27.
102. Field, J. R. (1997). Bone plate fixation: its relationship with implant induced osteoporosis. *Vet. Comp. Orthopaed. Traumatol.* **10,** 88–94.
103. Korvick, D. L., Newbrey, J. W., *et al.* (1989). Stress shielding reduced by a silicon plate-bone interface. A canine experiment. *Acta Orthop. Scand.* **60**(5), 611–616.
104. Nunamaker, D. M., Richardson, D. W., *et al.* (1991). Mechanical and biological effects of plate luting. *J. Orthopaed Trauma* **5,** 138–145.
105. Respet, P. J., Kleinman, P. G., *et al.* (1987). Pin tract infections: A canine model. *J. Orthop. Res.* **5,** 600–603.
106. Warme, W. J., Brooks, D., *et al.* (1998). External fixator pin tract infection model in the caprine tibia. 44th Annual Meeting, Orthopaedic Research Society, New Orleans, Louisiana.
107. Clasper, J. C., Parker, S. J., et al. (1999). Contamination of the medullary canal following pin-tract infection. *J. Orthop. Res.* **17,** 947–952.
108. Ahlborg, H. G., and Josefsson, P. O. (1999). Pin-tract complications in external fixation of fractures of the distal radius. *Acta Orthop. Scand.* **70**(2), 116–118.
109. Arciola, C. R., Montanaro, L., *et al.* (1999). Hydroxyapatite-coated orthopaedic screws as infection resistant materials: *In vitro* study. *Biomaterials* **20,** 323–327.
110. Collinge, C. A., Goll, G., *et al.* (1994). Pin tract infections: Silver vs uncoated pins. *Orthopedics* **17**(5), 445–448.
111. Holzer, G., Majeska, R. J., *et al.* (1999). Parathyroid hormone enhances fracture healing. *Clin. Orthop.* **366,** 258–263.
112. Ryhänen, J., Kallioinen, M., *et al.* (1999). Bone healing and mineralization, implant corrosion, and trace metals after nickel-titanium shape memory metal intramedullary fixation. *J. Biomed. Mater. Res.* **47,** 472–480.
113. Griffet, J., Chevallier, A., *et al.* (1999). Osteosynthesis of diaphyseal fracture by Ossatite® experimental study in rats. *Biomaterials* **20,** 511–515.
114. Probst, A., Jansen, H., *et al.* (1999). Callus formation and fixation rigidity: A fracture model in rats. *J. Orthop. Res.* **17**(256–260).
115. Vogely, H. C., Oosterbos, C. J. M., *et al.* (1999). Direct infection of HA coated and noncoated TI6AL4V implants: Infection susceptibility and implant fixation. 45th Annual Meeting, Orthopaedic Research Society, Anaheim, CA.
116. Hupel, T. M., Aksenof, S. A., *et al.* (1997). The effect of limited reaming on cortical bone blood flow and early strength of union following segmental fracture. 43rd Annual Meeting, Orthopaedic Research Society, San Francisco, CA.
117. Andriano, K. P., Wenger, K. H., *et al.* (1999). Technical note: Biomechanical analysis of two absorbable fracture fixation pins after long-term canine implantation. *J. Biomed. Mater. Res. (Appl. Biomater.)* **48,** 528–533.
118. Runkel, M., Wenda, K., *et al.* (1994). Knochenheilung nach unaufgebohrter marknagelung. *Unfallchirurg* **97,** 1–7.
119. Hill, P. F., Parker, S. J., *et al.* (1999). Contaminated fracture of the tibia: The results of immediate intramedullary nailing in an animal model. *J. Bone Joint Surg.* **81B**(Suppl. 1), 89.
120. Reichert, I. L. H., McCarthy, I. D., *et al.* (1999). Detailed laser doppler flowmetry of reamed and unreamed nail fixation. *J. Bone Joint Surg.* **81B**(Suppl. III), 316–317.
121. Behrens, F., and Searls, K. (1986). External fixation of the tibia. Basic concepts and prospective evaluation. *J. Bone Joint Surg.* **68B**(2), 246–254.
122. Weber, B., and Magerl, F. (1985). "*The External Fixator.*" Springer-Verlag, Berlin.
123. Maffulli, N., Cheng, J. C. Y., *et al.* (1999). Bone mineralization at the callotasis site after completion of lengthening. *Bone* **25**(3), 333–338.
124. Caja, V. L., and Moroni, A. (1996). Hydroxyapatite coated external fixation pins. *Clin. Orthop.* **325,** 269–275.
125. Moroni, A., Toksvig-Larsen, S., *et al.* (1998). A comparison of hydroxyapatite-coated, titanium-coated and uncoated tapered external-fixation pins. *J. Bone Joint Surg.* **80A**(4), 547–554.
126. Gilbert, J. A., Dahners, L. E., *et al.* (1989). The effect of external fixation stiffness on early healing of transverse osteotomies. *J. Orthop. Res.* **7**(3), 389–397.
127. Egger, E. L., Gottsauner-Wolf, F., *et al.* (1993). Effects of axial dynamiztion on bone healing. *J. Trauma* **34,** 185–192.
128. O'Doherty, D. M., Butler, S. P., *et al.* (1995). Stress protection due to external fixation. *J. Biomech.* **28**(5), 575–586.
129. Augat, P., Claes, L., *et al.* (1995). Increase of stability in external fracture fixation by hydroxyapatite-coated bone screws. *J. Appl. Biomater.* **6,** 99–104.
130. Goodship, A. E., Cunningham, J. L., *et al.* (1998). Strain rate and timing of stimulation in mechanical modulation of fracture healing. *Clin. Orthop.* **355**(Suppl.), S105–S115.
131. Claes, L. E., and Heigele, C. A. (1999). Magnitudes of local stress and strain along bony surfaces predict the course and type of fracture healing. *J. Biomech.* **32,** 255–266.
132. Nelson, B. J., DeBerardino, T. M., *et al.* (1999). The efficacy of steel, silver-coated, and chlorhexidine/chloroxylenol-coated external fixator pins in proventing pin tract infections in a caprine model. 45th Annual Meeting, Orthopaedic Research Society, Anaheim, CA.
133. Hartke, J. R. (1999). Preclinical development of agents for the treatment of osteoporosis. *Toxicol. Pathol.* **27,** 143–147.
134. Hazzard, D. G., Bronson, R. T., *et al.* (1992). Selection of an appropriate animal model to study aging processes with special emphasis on the use of rat strains. *J. Gerontol.* **47**(3), B63–64.
135. Barlet, J. P., Coxam, V., *et al.* (1994). Modèles animaux d'ostéoporose postménopausique. *Reprod. Nutr. Dev.* **34,** 221–236.

136. Aerssens, J., Boonen, S., *et al.* (1998). Interspecies difference in bone composition, density and quality: Potential implications for *in vivo* bone research. *Endocrinology* **139,** 663–670.
137. O'Brien, C. A., Jilka, R. L., *et al.* (1997). Generation of mice harboring an IL-6 promoter-luciferase transgene that mimics endogenous IL-6 gene regulation. *J. Bone Miner. Res.* **12**(Suppl.), 435.
138. Okamoto, Y., Takahashi, K., *et al.* (1995). Femoral peak bone mass and osteoclast number in an animal model of age-related spontaneous osteopenia. *Anat. Rec.* **242,** 21–28.
139. Wronski, T. J., Lowry, P. L., *et al.* (1985). Skeletal alterations in ovariectomized rats. *Calcif. Tissue Int.* **37,** 324–328.
140. Wronski, T. J., Walsh, C. C., *et al.* (1986). Histologic evidence for osteopenia and increased bone turnover in ovariectomized rats. *Bone* **7,** 119–123.
141. Wronski, T. J., and Yen, C.-F. (1991). The ovariectomized rat as an animal model for postmenopausal bone loss. *Cells Mater.*(Suppl. 1), 69–74.
142. Frost, H. M., and Jee, W.S.S.(1992). On the rat model of human osteopenia and osteoporoses. *Bone Miner.* **18,** 227–236.
143. Kalu, D. N. (1991). The ovariectomized rat model of postmenopausal bone loss. *Bone Miner.* **15,** 175–192.
144. Dempster, D. W., Birchman, R., *et al.* (1995). Temporal changes in cancellous bone structure of rats immediately after ovariectomy. *Bone* **16,** 157–161.
145. Peng, Z.-Q., Väänänen, H. K., *et al.* (1997). Long-term effects of ovariectomy on the mechanical properties and chemical composition of rat bone. *Bone* **20,**(3), 207–212.
146. Gaumet, N., Seibel, M. J., *et al.* (1996). Influence of ovariectomy on bone metabolism in very old rats. *Calcif. Tissue Int.* **58,** 256–262.
147. Abe, T., Chow, J. W. M., *et al.* (1993). Estrogen does not restore bone lost after ovariectomy in the rat. *J. Bone Miner. Res.* **8,** 831–838.
148. Goulding, A., Gold, E., *et al.* (1996). Effects of hysterectomy on bone in intact rats, ovariectomized rats, and ovariectomized rats treated with estrogen. *J. Bone Miner. Res.* **11,** 977–983.
149. Sietsma, W. K. (1995). Animal models of cortical porosity. *Bone* **17**(Suppl.), 297–305.
150. Vanin, C. M., MacLusky, N. J., *et al.* (1995). Lumbar vertebral density and mechanical properties in aged ovariectomized rats treated with estrogen and norethindrone or norgestimate. *Am. J. Obstet. Gynecol.* **173,** 1491–1498.
151. Peng, Z., Tuukkanen, J., *et al.* (1994). The mechanical strength of bone in different rat models of experimental osteoporosis. *Bone* **15,** 523–532.
152. Grier, S. J., Turner, A. S., *et al.* (1996). The use of dual-energy X-ray absorptiometry(DXA) in animals: A review. *Invest. Radiol.* **31,** 50–62.
153. Hartke, J. R. (1998). Non-primate models of osteoporosis. *Lab. Anim. Sci.* **48,** 623–629.
154. Cesnjaj, M., Stavlijenic, A., *et al.* (1991). Decreased osteoinductive potential of bone matrix from ovariectomized rats. *Acta Orthop. Scand.* **62**(5), 471–475.
155. Kimmel, D. B. (1991). The oophorectomized beagle as an experimental model for estrogen-depletion bone loss in the adult human. *Cells Mater.*(Suppl.), 75–84.
156. Boyce, R. W., Franks, A. F., *et al.* (1990). Sequential histomorphometric changes in cancellous bone from ovariohysterectomized dogs. *J. Bone Miner. Res.* **5**(9), 947–953.
157. Malluche, H. H., Faugere, M.-C., *et al.* (1986). Osteoblastic insufficiency is responsible for maintainence of osteopenia after loss of ovarian function in experimental beagle dogs. *Endocrinology* **119,** 2649–2654.
158. Faugere, M. C., Friedleer, R. M., *et al.* (1990). Bone changes occurring early after cessation of ovarian function in beagle dogs: A histomorphometric study employing sequential biopsies. *J. Bone Miner. Res.* **5**(3), 263–272.
159. Monier-Faugere, M.-C., Friedler, R. M., *et al.* (1993). A new bisphosphonate, BM 21.0955, prevents bone loss associated with cessation of ovarian function in experimental dogs. *Bone Miner. Res.* **9**(11), 1345–1355.
160. Monier-Faugere, M.-C., Geng Z., Qi, Q., *et al.* (1996). Calcitonin prevents bone loss but decreases osteoblastic activity in ovariohysterectomized beagle dogs. *J. Bone Miner. Res.* **11,** 446–455.
161. Motoie, H., Nakamura, T., *et al.* (1995). Effects of bisphosphonate YM175 on bone mineral density, strength, structure, and turnover in ovariectomized beagles on concomitant dietary calcium restriction. *J. Bone Miner. Res.* **10,** 910–920.
162. McCubbrey, D. A., Yian, E. H., *et al.* (1993). The effects of calcitonin on trabecular bone properties in the ovariectomized beagle. Orthop. Res. Soc., San Francisco, CA.
163. Boyce, R. W., Paddock, C. L., *et al.* (1996). Effects of intermittent hPTH (1–34) alone and in combination with 1,25(OH)2D3 or risedronate on endosteal bone remodeling in canine cancellous and cortical bone. *J. Bone Miner. Res.* **11,** 600–613.
164. Forwood, M. R., Burr, D. B., *et al.* (1995). Risedronate treatment does not increase microdamage in the canine femoral neck. *Bone* **16,** 643–650.
165. Grynpas, M. D., Kasra, M., *et al.* (1994). Recovery from pamidronate (APD): A two-year study in the dog. *Calcif. Tissue Int.* **55,** 288–294.
166. Peter, C. P., Cook, W. O., *et al.* (1996). Effect of alendronate on fracture healing and bone remodeling in dogs. *J. Orthop.* **14,** 74–79.
167. Shen, V., Dempster, D. W., *et al.* (1992). Lack of changes in histomorphometric, bone mass, and biochemical parameters in ovariohysterectomized dogs. *Bone* **13,** 311–316.
168. Spurrell, F. A., Felts, W. J. L., and Baudin, L.V. (1965). Osteon development in swine. *In "Swine Biomedical Research,"* pp. 173–192.
169. Bouchard, G. F., Durham, H. E., *et al.* (1995). Determination of the peak bone mass and whole body composition in Sinclair miniature swine. *J. Bone Miner. Res.* **10**(Suppl.), S476.
170. Spencer, G. R. (1979). Animal model: Porcine lactational osteoporosis. *Am. J. Pathol.* **95,** 277–280.
171. Mosekilde, L., Danielsen, C. C., *et al.* (1993). The effect of aging and ovaiectomy on the vertebral bone mass and biomechanical properties of mature rats. *Bone* **14,** 1–6.
172. Mosekilde, L., Weisbrode, S. E., *et al.* (1993). Calcium-restricted ovariectomized Sinclair S-1 minipigs: An animal model of osteopenia and trabecular plate perforation. *Bone* **14,** 379–382.
173. Mosekilde, L., Kragstrup, J., *et al.* (1987). Compressive strength, ash weight and volume of vertebral trabecular bone in experimental fluorosis in pigs. *Calcif. Tissue Int.* **40,** 318–322.
174. Boyce, R. W., Ebert, D. C., *et al.* (1995). Unbiased estimation of vertebral trabecular connectivity in calcium-restricted ovariectomized minipigs. *Bone* **16,** 637–642.
175. Mosekilde, L., Weisbrode, S. E., *et al.* (1993). Evaluation of the skeletal effects of combined mild dietary calcium restriction and ovariectomy in Sinclair S-1 minipigs: A pilot study. *J. Bone Miner. Res.* **8,** 1311–1321.
176. Bouchard, G. F., Boyce, R. W., *et al.* (1997). Standardization of an adult Sinclair miniature swine osteopenia model-preliminary results. *J. Bone Miner. Res.* **12**(Suppl.), T500 (Abstr.)
177. Lafage, M.-H., Balena, R., *et al.* (1995). Comparison of alendronate and sodium fluoride effects on cancellous and cortical bone in minipigs. *J. Clin. Invest.* **95,** 2127–2133.
178. Atkinson, P. J., Spence J. A., Aitchison, G., and Sykes, A. R. (1982). Mandibular bone in aging sheep. *J. Comp. Pathol.* **92,** 51–67.
179. Johnson, R. B., Gilbert, J. A., *et al.* (1997). Alveolar bone loss one year following ovariectomy in sheep. *J. Periodontol.* **68,** 864–871.
180. Turner, A. S., Edgerton, M., *et al.* (1996). Mandibular bone density in the ovariectomized ewe. *Bone* **19**(3), 164.

181. Turner, A. S., Dewell, R. D., *et al.* (1999). Raloxifene (LY 139481) increases bone mineral density of the mandible in aged ovariectomized ewes. 8th World Congress of the International Society of Orthopaedic Research and Traumatology, Sydney, Australia.
182. Chavassieux, P. (1990). Bone effects of fluoride in animal models *in vivo*. A review and a recent study. *J. Bone Miner. Res.* **5**(Suppl. 1), S95–S99.
183. Chavassieux, P., Pastoureau, P., *et al.* (1991). Dose effects on ewe bone remodeling of short-term sodium fluoride administration—A histomorphometric and biochemical study. *Bone* **12,** 421–427.
184. Pastoureau, P., Arlot, M. E., *et al.* (1989). Effects of oophorectomy on biochemical and histological indices of bone turnover in ewes. *J. Bone Miner. Res.* **4**(Suppl. 1), 477.
185. Newman, E., Turner, A. S., *et al.* (1995). The potential of sheep for the study of osteopenia: Current status and comparison with other animal models. *Bone* **16**(4), 277–284.
186. Hornby, S. B., Ford, S. L., *et al.* (1994). Skeletal changes in the ewe after ovariectomy. *J. Bone Miner. Res.* **9**(Suppl. 1), S258.
187. Atley, L. M. (1996). Biochemical markers of bone resorption. Department of Medicine. Melbourne, The University of Melbourne, Australia.
188. Geusens, P. (1992). Photon absorptiometry in osteoporosis. Bone mineral measurements in animal models and humans. Department of Reumatologie Artritis en Metabole Botziekten Onderzoekseenheid. Leuven, Katholieke Universiteit, Fakulteit Geneesekunde.
189. O'Connell, S. L. (1999). The sheep as an experimental model for osteoporosis. Department of Medicine. Melbourne, Melbourne, Australia.
190. Turner, A. S., Alvis, M. R., *et al.* (1995). Changes in bone mineral density and bone-specific alkaline phosphatase in ovariectomized ewes. *Bone* **17**(Suppl.), 395S–402S.
191. Guesens, P., Boonen, S., *et al.* (1996). Effect of salmon calcitonin on femoral bone quality in adult ovariectomized ewes. *Calcif. Tissue Int.* **59,** 315–320.
192. Turner, A. S., Hannan, M. K., *et al.* (1999). Effects of raloxifene (LY139481) on bone density and bone strength in aged, ovariectomized ewes. Proc. Orthop. Res. Soc., Anaheim, CA.
193. Turner, A. S., Dewell, R. D., *et al.* (1999). Raloxifene (LY 139481) increases bone mineral density of the mandible in aged ovariectomized ewes. 8th World Congress of the International Society of Orthopaedic Research and Traumatology, Sydney, Australia.
194. Turner, A. S., Park, R. D., *et al.* (1993). Effects of age and ovariectomy on trabecular bone of the proximal femur and iliac crest in sheep. Orthop. Res. Soc., San Francisco, CA.
195. Turner, A. S., Alvis, M. R., *et al.* (1995). Dual-energy X-ray absorptiometry in sheep: Experiences with *in vivo* and *in vitro* studies. *Bone* **17**(Suppl.), 381–387.
196. Deloffre, P., Hans, D., *et al.* (1995). Comparison between bone density and bone strength in glucocorticoid-treated aged ewes. *Bone* **17,** S409–S414.
197. Rosen, C. J., Morrison, A., *et al.* (1994). Elderly women in northern New England exhibit seasonal changes in bone mineral density and calciotropic hormones. *Bone Miner.* **25,** 83–92.
198. Goodman, R. L. (1994). "Neuroendocrine Control of the Ovine Estrous Cycle." Raven Press, New York.
199. Fortune, C. L., Farrugia, W., *et al.* (1989). Hormonal regulation of osteocalcin plasma production and clearance in sheep. *Endocrinology* **124,** 2785–2790.
200. O'Connell, S. L., Tresham, J., *et al.* (1993). Effects of prednisolone and deflazacort on osteocalcin metabolism in sheep. *Calcif. Tissue Int.* **53,** 117–121.
201. Hodgen, G. D., Goodman, A. L., *et al.* (1977). Menopause in rhesus monkeys. Model for study of disorders in the human climacteric. *Am. J. Obstet. Gynecol.* **127,** 581–584.
202. Miller, L. C., Weaver, D. S., *et al.* (1986). Effects of ovariectomy on vertebral bone in the cynomolgus monkey (*Macaca fascicularis*). *Calcif. Tissue Int.* **38,** 62–65.
203. Mann, D. R., Gould, K. G., *et al.* (1990). Potential primate model for bone loss resulting from medical oophorectomy or menopause. *J. Clin. Endocr. Metab.* **71,** 105–110.
204. Kimmel, D. B. (1996). Animal models for *in vivo* experimentation in osteoporosis research. *In "Osteoporosis"* (R. Marcus, D. Feldman, and K.J., eds.), pp. 671–690. Academic Press, San Diego.
205. Jayo, M. J., Jerome, C. P., *et al.* (1994). Bone mass in female cynomolgus macaques: A cross-sectional and longitudinal study by age. *Calcif. Tissue Int.* **54,** 231–236.
206. Jerome, C. P., Carlson, C. S., *et al.* (1993). Bone functional changes in intact, ovariectomized, and ovariectomized, hormone- supplemented adult cynomolgus monkeys (*Macaca fascicularis*) evaluated by serum markers and dynamic histomorphometry. *J. Bone Miner. Res.* **9**(4), 527–540.
207. Lundon, K., Dumitriu, M., *et al.* (1994). The long-term effects of ovariectomy on the quality and quantity of cancellous bone in young macaques. *Bone Miner.* **24,** 135–149.
208. Jerome, C. P., Lees, C. J., *et al.* (1994). Iliac and lumbar vertebral histomorphometry, bone densitometry and bone biomarker data from raloxifene-treated macaques. *J. Bone Miner. Res.* **12 (Suppl.),** S347.
209. Weiss, R. A. (1998). Retrovial zoonoses. *Nature Med.* **4,** 391–392.
210. Lane, N., Coble, T., *et al.* (1990). Effect of naproxen on cancellous bone in ovariectomized rats. *J. Bone Miner. Res.* **5**(10), 1029–1035.
211. Durbridge, T. C., Morris, H. A., *et al.* (1990). Progressive cancellous bone loss in rats after adrenalectomy and oophorectomy. *Calcif. Tissue Int.* **47,** 383–387.
212. Barengolts, E. I., Gajardo, H. F., *et al.* (1990). Effects of progesterone on postovariectomy bone loss in aged rats. *J. Bone Miner. Res.* **5**(11), 1143–1147.
213. Morris, H. A., Porter, S. J., *et al.* (1992). Effects of oophorectomy on biochemical and bone variables in the rat. *Bone Miner.* **18,** 133–142.
214. Tobias, J. H., Chambers, T. J., *et al.* (1994). The effects of ovarian transplantation on bone loss in ovariectomized rats. *J. Endocrinol.* **142,** 187–192.
215. Bagi, C. M., and Miller, S. C. (1994). Comparison of osteopenic changes in cancellous bone induced by ovariectomy and/or immobilization in adult rats. *Anat. Rec.* **239,** 243–254.
216. Sims, N. A., Morris, H. A., *et al.* (1994). Parathyroidectomy does not prevent bone loss in the oophorectomized rat. *J. Bone Miner. Res.* **9**(12), 1859–1863.
217. McSheehy, P. M. J., Farina, C., *et al.* (1995). Pharmacologic evaluation of the calcitonin analogue SB 205614 in models of osteoclastic bone resorption *in vitro* and *in vivo*. *Bone* **16**(4), 435–444.
218. Ryaby, J. T., Magee, F. P., *et al.* (1996). Combined treatment with magnetic fields and parathyroid hormone to reverse osteopenia in ovariectomized rats. 42nd Annual Meeting, Orthopaedic Research Society, Atlanta, Georgia.
219. Thomsen, J. S., Mosekilde, L., *et al.* (1999). Long-term therapy of ovariectomy-induced osteopenia with parathyroid hormone analog SDZ PTS 893 and bone maintenance in retired breeder rats. *Bone* **25**(5), 561–569.
220. Baldock, P. A. J., Need, A. G., *et al.* (1999). Discordance between bone turnover and bone loss: Effects of aging and ovariectomy in the rat. *J. Bone Miner. Res.* **14**(8), 1442–1448.
221. Rico, H., Gómez, M., *et al.* (1999). Effects of promethazine on bone mass and on bone remodeling in ovariectomized rats: A morphometric, densitometric, and histomorphometric experimental study. *Calcif. Tissue Int.* **65,** 272–275.
222. Lynch, W. R., Goldstein, S. A., *et al.* (1991). The effects of calcitonin on torsional properties of the long bones of ovariohysterectomized

beagles. 37th Annual Meeting, Orthopaedic Research Society, Anaheim, CA.

223. Pienkowski, D., Doers, T. M., *et al.* (1997). Calcitonin alters bone quality in beagle dogs. *J. Bone Miner. Res.* **12**(11), 1936–1943.
224. Champ, J. E., Binkley, N., *et al.* (1996). The effect of advancing age on bone mineral content of female rhesus monkeys. *Bone* **19**(5), 485–492.
225. Baldini, T., Menschik, F., *et al.* (1997). The effect of nandrolone decanoate on the mechanical and physical properties of lumbar vertebrae from ovariectomized monkeys. 43rd Annual Meeting, Orthopaedic Research Society, San Francisco, CA.
226. Register, T. C., Jayo, M. J., *et al.* (1997). Oral contraceptive treatment inhibits the normal acquisition of bone mineral in skeletally immature young adult femal monkeys. *Osteoporos. Int.* **7,** 348–353.
227. Colman, R. J., Kemnitz, J. W., *et al.* (1999). Skeletal effects of aging and menopausal status in female rhesus macaques. *J. Clin. Endocrinol. Metab.* **84,** 4144–4148.
228. Jerome, C. P., Johnson, C. S., *et al.* (1999). Effect of treatment for 6 months with human parathyroid hormone (1–34) peptide in ovariectomized cynomolgus monkeys (*Macaca fascicularis*). *Bone* **25**(3), 301–309.
229. Vico, L., Lafage-Proust, M.-H., *et al.* (1998). Effects of gravitational changes on the bone system *in vitro* and *in vivo*. *Bone* **22**(5, Suppl.), 95S–100S.
230. Suda, T. (1998). Lessons from the space experiment SL-J/FMPT/L7: The effect of microgravity on chicken embryogenesis and bone formation. *Bone* **22**(5, Suppl.), 73S–78S.
231. Backup, P., Westerlind, K., *et al.* (1994). Spaceflight results in reduced mRNA levels for tissue-specific proteins in the musculoskeletal system. *Am. J. Physiol.* **266,** E567–E573.
232. Morey-Holton, E. R., and Globus, R. K. (1998). Hindlimb unloading of growing rats: A model for predicting skeletal changes during space flight. *Bone* **22**(5, Suppl.), 83S–88S.
233. Matsumoto, T., Nakayama, K., *et al.* (1998). Effect of mechanical unloading and reloading on periosteal bone formation and gene expression in tail-suspended rapidly growing rats. *Bone* **22**(5, Suppl.), 89S–93S.
234. Lane, N., Maeda, H., *et al.* (1994). Cancellous bone behavior in hindlimb immobilized rats during and after naproxen treatment. *Bone Miner.* **26,** 43–59.
235. Murakami, H., Nakamura, T., *et al.* (1994). Effects of tiludronate on bone mass, structure, and turnover at the epiphyseal, primary, and secondary spongiosa in the proximal tibia of growing rats after sciatic neurectomy. *J. Bone Miner. Res.* **9**(9), 1355–1364.
236. Schaffler, M. B., and Li, X. J. (1990). Immobilization induced bone loss: Quantitative histological studies of cortical bone resorption. 36th Annual Meeting, Orthopaedic Research Society, New Orleans, Louisiana.
237. Kaneps, A. J., Stover, S. M., *et al.* (1995). Changes in cortical and cancellous bone mechanical properties following immobilization. 41st Annual Meeting, Orthopaedic Research Society, Orlando, Florida.
238. Haapala, J., Arokoski, J. P. A., *et al.* (1996). The effects of 11 weeks immobilization and 50 weeks remobilization on canine knee articular cartilage properties. 42nd Annual Meeting, Orthopaedic Research Society, Atlanta, Georgia.
239. Haapala, J., Arokoski, J. P. A., *et al.* (1999). Remobilization does not fully restore immobilization induced articular cartilage atrophy. *Clin. Orthod. Res.* **362,** 218–229.
240. Haapala, J., Arokoski, J., *et al.* (1999). Incomplete restoration of immobilization induced softening of young beagle knee articualar cartilage after 50-week remobilization. *Int. J. Sports Med.* **20,** 76–81.
241. Cann, C. E., Genant, H. K., *et al.* (1980). Comparison of vertebral and peripheral mineral losses in disuse osteoporosis in monkeys. *Radiology* **134,** 525–529.
242. Young, D. R., Niklowitz, W. J., *et al.* (1986). Immobilization-associated osteoporosis in primates. *Bone* **7,** 109–117.
243. Sakai, A., Nakamura, T., *et al.* (1996). Bone marrow capacity for bone cells and trabecular bone turnover in immobilized tibia after sciatic neurectomy in mice. *Bone* **18**(5), 479–486.
244. Bagi, C. M., Mecham, M., *et al.* (1993). Comparative morphometric changes in rat cortical bone following ovariectomy and/or immobilization. *Bone* **14,** 877–883.
245. Lepola, V., Väänänen, K., *et al.* (1993). The effect of immobilization on the torsional strength of the rat tibia. *Clin. Orthop.* **297,** 55–61.
246. Machwate, M., Zerath, E., *et al.* (1994). Insulin-like growth factor-I increases trabecular bone formation and osteoblastic cell proliferation in unloaded rats. *Endocrinology* **134,** 1031–1038.
247. Tarvainen, R., Arnala, I., *et al.* (1994). Clodronate prevents immobilization osteopenia in rats. *Acta Orthop. Scand.* **65**(6), 643–646.
248. Kannus, P., Sievänen, H., *et al.* (1994). Effects of free mobilization and low- to high-intensity treadmill running on the immobilization-induced bone loss in rats. *J. Bone Miner. Res.* **9**(10), 1613–1619.
249. Machwate, M., Zerath, E., *et al.* (1995). Systemic administration of transforming growth factor-β2 prevents the impaired bone formation and osteopenia induced by unloading in rats. *J. Clin. Invest.* **96,** 1245–1253.
250. Bikle, D. D., Harris, J., *et al.* (1995). The molecular response of bone to growth hormone during skeletal unloading: Regional differences. *Endocrinology* **136**(5), 2099–2109.
251. Ma, Y., Jee, W. S. S., *et al.* (1995). Partial maintenance of extra cancellous bone mass by antiresorptive agents after discontinuation of human parathyroid hormone (1–38) in right hindlimb immobilized rats. *J. Bone Miner. Res.* **10**(11), 1726–1734.
252. Dehority, W., Halloran, B. P., *et al.* (1999). Bone and hormonal changes induced by skeletal unloading in the mature male rat. *Am. J. Physiol.* **276,** E62–E69.
253. Rubin, C. T., and Lanyon, L. E. (1987). Osteoregulatory nature of mechanical stimuli: Functon as a determinant for adaptive remodeling in bone. *J. Orthop. Res.* **5,** 300–310.
254. Gross, T. S., and Rubin, C. T. (1995). Uniformity of resorptive bone loss induced by disuse. *J. Orthop. Res.* **13,** 708–714.
255. Jaworski, Z. F. G., Liskova-Kiar, M., *et al.* (1980). Effect of long-term immobilisation on the pattern of bone loss in older dogs. *J. Bone Joint Surg.* **62B**(1), 104–110.
256. Waters, D. J., Caywood, D. D., *et al.* (1991). Effect of tomoxifen citrate on canine immobilization (disuse) osteoporosis. *Vet. Surg.* **20**(6), 392–396.
257. Lane, N. E., Kaneps, A. J., *et al.* (1996). Bone mineral density and turnover following forelimb immobilization and recovery in young adult dogs. *Calcif. Tissue Int.* **59,** 401–406.
258. Rubin, C. T., Pratt, Jr., G. W., *et al.* (1988). Ultrasonic measurement of immobilization-induced osteopenia: An experimental study in sheep. *Calcif. Tissue Int.* **42,** 309–312.
259. Thomas, T., Skerry, T. M., *et al.* (1995). Ineffectiveness of calcitonin on a local-disuse osteoporosis in the sheep: A histomorphometric study. *Calcif. Tissue Int.* **57,** 224–228.
260. Skerry, T. M., and Lanyon, L. E. (1995). Interruption of disuse by short duration walking exercise does not prevent bone loss in the sheep calcaneus. *Bone* **16**(2), 269–274.
261. Lundy, M. W., Alvis, M. R., *et al.* (1996). Forelimb immobilization in sheep: Bone mineral density, biochemical, and biomechanical changes. *Proc. Am. Soc. Bone Miner. Res.* **11** (Suppl. 1), S323.
262. Welch, R. D., Ashman, R. B., *et al.* (1996). Intraosseous infusion of prostaglandin E2 prevents disuse-induced bone loss in the tibia. *J. Orthop. Res.* **14,** 303–310.
263. Smith, E. L., and Gilligan, C. (1996). Dose-response relationship between physical loading and mechanical competence of bone. *Bone* **18**(Suppl. 1), 45S–50S.

264. Barengolts, E. I., Curry, D. J., *et al.* (1993). Effects of endurance exercise on bone mass and mechanical properties in intact and ovariectomized rats. *J. Bone Miner. Res.* **8**(8), 937–942.
265. Søgaard, C. H., Danielsen, C. C., *et al.* (1994). Long-term exercise of young and adult female rats: Effect on femoral neck biomechanical competence and bone structure. *J. Bone Miner. Res.* **9**(3), 409–416.
266. Rubin, C. T., and Lanyon, L. E. (1987). Osteoregulatory nature of mechanical stimuli: Function as a determinant for adaptive remodeling in bone. *J. Orthop. Res.* **5,** 300–310.
267. Turner, C. H., Woltman, T. A., *et al.* (1992). Structural changes in rat bone subjected to long-term, *in vivo* mechanical loading. *Bone* **13,** 417–422.
268. Forwood, M. R., and Turner, C. H. (1994). The response of rat tibiae to incremental bouts of mechanical loading: A quantum concept for bone formation. *Bone* **15**(6), 603–609.
269. Raab-Cullen, D. M., Akhter, M. P., *et al.* (1994). Bone response to alternate-day mechanical loading of the rat tibia. *J. Bone Miner. Res.* **9**(2), 203–211.
270. Hillam, R. A., and Skerry, T. M. (1995). Inhibition of bone resorption and stimulation of formation by mechanical loading of the modeling rat ulna *in vivo. J. Bone Miner. Res.* **10**(5), 683–689.
271. Mosley, J. R., and Lanyon, L. E. (1998). Strain rate as a controlling influence on adaptive modeling in response to dynamic loading of the ulna n growing male rats. *Bone* **23**(4), 313–318.
272. Mori, S., and Burr, D. B. (1993). Increased intracortical remodeling following fatigue damage. *Bone* **14,** 103–109.
273. Rubin, C., Turner, A. S., *et al.* (1997). Site-specific increase in bone density stimulated non-invasively by extremely low magnitude thirty Hertz mechanical stimulation. Orthop Res. Soc., San Francisco, CA.
274. Swissa-Sivan, A., Azoury, R., *et al.* (1990). The effect of swimming on bone modeling and composition in young adult rats. *Calcif. Tissue Int.* **47,** 173–177.
275. Forwood, M. R., and Parker, A. W. (1992). Repetitive loading, *in vivo,* of the tibia and femora of rats: Effects of a single bout of treadmill running. *Calcif. Tissue Int.* **50,** 193–196.
276. Yeh, J. K., Aloia, J. F., *et al.* (1993). Influence of exercise on cancellous bone of the aged female rat. *J. Bone Miner. Res.* **8**(9), 1117–1125.
277. Yeh, J. K., Liu, C. C., *et al.* (1993). Additive effect of treadmill exercise and 17β-estadiol replacement on prevention of tibial bone loss in adult ovariectomized rat. *J. Bone Miner. Res.* **8**(6), 677–683.
278. Barengolts, E. I., Curry, D. J., *et al.* (1993). Effects of two non-endurance exercise protocols on established bone loss in ovariectomized adult rats. *Calcif. Tissue Int.* **52,** 239–243.
279. Omi, N., Morikawa, N., *et al.* (1994). The effect of voluntary exercise on bone mineral density and skeletal muscles in the rat model at ovariectomized and sham stages. *Bone Miner.* **24,** 211–222.
280. Tuukkanen, J., Peng, Z., *et al.* (1994). Effect of running exercise on the bone loss induced by orchidectomy in the rat. *Calcif. Tissue Int.* **55,** 33–37.
281. Mosekilde, L., Danielsen, C. C., *et al.* (1994). The effect of long-term exercise on vertebral and femoral bone mass, dimensions, and strength-assessed in a rat model. *Bone* **15**(3), 293–301.
282. Peng, Z., Tuukkanen, J., *et al.* (1994). Exercise can provide protection against bone loss and prevent the decrease in mechanical strength of femoral neck in ovariectomized rats. *J. Bone Miner. Res.* **9**(10), 1559–1564.
283. Chen, M. M., Yeh, J. K., *et al.* (1994). Effect of treadmill exercise on tibial cortical bone in aged female rats: a histomorphometry and dual energy x-ray absorptiometry study. *Bone* **15**(3), 313–319.
284. Umemura, Y., Ishiko, T., *et al.* (1995). Effects of jump training on bone hypertrophy in young and old rats. *J. Sports Med.* **16**(6), 364–367.
285. Bourrin, S., Palle, S., *et al.* (1995). Effects of physical training on bone adaptation in three zones of the rat tibia. *J. Bone Miner. Res.* **10**(11), 1745–1752.
286. van der Wiel, Lips, H. E., P., *et al.* (1995). Additional weight-bearing during exercise is more important than duration of exercise for anabolic stimulus of bone: A study of running exercise in female rats. *Bone* **16**(1), 73–80.
287. Wheeler, D. L., Graves, J. E., *et al.* (1995). Effects of running on the torsional strength, morphometry, and bone mass of the rat skeleton. *Med. Sci. Sports Exerc.* **27**(4), 520–529.
288. Peng, Z. Q., Väänänen, H. K., *et al.* (1997). Ovariectomy-induced bone loss can be affected by different intensities of treadmill running exercise in rats. *Calcif. Tissue Int.* **60,** 441–448.
289. Kiuchi, A., Arai, Y., *et al.* (1998). Detraining effects on bone mass in young male rats. *Int. J. Sports Med.* **19,** 245–249.
290. Iwamoto, J., Takeda, T., *et al.* (1998). Effects of exercise on bone mineral density in mature osteopenic rats. *J. Bone Miner. Res.* **13**(8), 1308–1317.
291. Judex, S., and Zernicke, R. F. (2000). Does the mechanical milieu associated with high-speed running lead to adaptive changes in diaphyseal growing bone. *Bone* **26**(2), 153–159.
292. Puustjärvi, K., Karjalainen, P., *et al.* (1991). Effects of long-term running on spinal mineral content in dogs. *Calcif. Tissue Int.* **49**(Suppl.), S81–S82.
293. Tommerup, L. J., Raab, D. M., *et al.* (1993). Does weight-bearing exercise affect non-weight-bearing bone. *J. Bone Miner. Res.* **8**(9), 1053–1058.
294. McCarthy, R. N., and Jeffcott, L. B. (1992). Effects of treadmill exercise on cortical bone in the third metacarpus of young horses. *Res. Vet. Sci.* **52,** 28–37.
295. Price, J. S., Jackson, B., *et al.* (1995). The response of the skeleton to physical training: A biochemical study in horses. *Bone* **17**(3), 221–227.
296. Bourrin, S., Zerath, E., *et al.* (1992). Bone mass and cellular variations after five months of physical training in rhesus monkeys: Histomorphometric study. *Calcif. Tissue Int.* **50,** 404–410.
297. Martz, E. O., Goel, V. K., *et al.* (1997). Materials and design of spinal implants—A review. *J. Biomed. Mater. Res.* **38,** 267–288.
298. Bao, Q.-B., McCullen, G. M., *et al.* (1996). The artificial disc: Theory, design and materials. *Biomaterials* **17,** 1157–1167.
299. McAfee, P. C. (1999). Interbody fusion cages in reconstructive operations on the spine. *J. Bone Joint Surg.* **81A**(6), 859–880.
300. Wilke, H.-J., Kettler, A., *et al.* (1997). Anatomy of the sheep spine and its comparison to the human spine. *Anat. Rec.* **247,** 542–555.
301. Wilke, H.-J., Kettler, A., *et al.* (1997). Are sheep spines a valid biomechanical model for human spines. *Spine* **22,** 2365–2374.
302. Spiegel, D. A., Drummond, D. S., *et al.* (1999). Augmentation of an anterior solid rod construct with threaded cortical bone dowels. *Spine* **24**(22), 2300–2307.
303. Sandhu, H., Kanim, L., *et al.* (1999). Animal models of spinal instability and spine fusion. *"Animal Models in Orthopaedic Research"* (Y. An, ed.), pp. 505–526. CRC Press, Boca Raton.
304. Suzuki, K., Mochida, J., *et al.* (1999). Posterior stabilization of degenerative lumbar spondyolisthesis with a leeds-keio artifical ligament: A biomechanical analysis in a porcine vertebral model. *Spine* **24**(1), 26–31.
305. Takeuchi, T., Abumi, K., *et al.* (1999). Biomechanical role of the intervertebral disc and costovertebral joint in stability of the thoracic spine. a canine model study. *Spine* **24**(14), 1414–1420.
306. Bostrom, M. P. G., and Lane, J. M. (1997). Augmentation of osteoporotic vertebral bodies. *Spine* **22**(24S), 38S–42S.
307. Tohmeh, A. G., Mathis, J. M., *et al.* (1999). Biomechanical efficacy of unipedicular versus bipedicular vertebroplasty for the management of osteoporotic compression fractures. *Spine* **24**(17), 1772–1776.

308. Kotani, Y., Cunningham, B. W., *et al.* (1996). The role of spinal instrumentation in augmenting lumbar posterolateral fusion. *Spine* **21**(3), 278–287.
309. Steffen, T., Marchesi, D., *et al.* (2000). Posterolateral and anterior interbody spinal fusion models in the sheep. *Clin. Orthop.* **371,** 28–37.
310. Boden, S. D., Martin, G. J., *et al.* (1999). Posterolateral lumbar intertransverse process spine arthrodesis with recombinant human bone morphogenetic protein 2/hydroxyapatite-tricalcium phosphate after laminectomy in the nonhuman primate. *Spine* **24**(12), 1179–1185.
311. Curylo, L. J., Johnstone, B., *et al.* (1999). Augmentation of spinal arthrodesis with autologous bone marrow in a rabbit posterolateral spine fusion model. *Spine* **24**(5), 434–439.
312. Martin, G. J., Boden, S. D., *et al.* (1999). New formulations of demineralized bone matrix as a more effective graft alternative in experimental posterolateral lumbar spine arthrodesis. *Spine* **24**(7), 637–645.
313. Minamide, A., Tamaki, T., *et al.* (1999). Experimental spinal fusion using sintered bovine bone coated with type I collagen and recombinant human bone morphogenetic protein-2. *Spine* **24**(18), 1863–1872.
314. Itoh, H., Ebara, S., *et al.* (1999). Experimental spinal fusion with use of recombinant human bone morphogenetic protein 2. *Spine* **24**(14), 1402–1405.
315. Bozic, K. J., Glazer, P. A., *et al.* (1999). *In vivo* evaluation of coralline hydroxyapatite and direct current electrical stimulation in lumbar spinal fusion. *Spine* **24**(20), 2127–2133.
316. Martin, G. J., Boden, S. D., *et al.* (1999). Recombinant human bone morphogenetic protein-2 overcomes the inhibitory effect of ketorolac, a nonsteroidal anti-inflammatory drug (NSAID), on posterolateral lumbar intertransverse process spine fusion. *Spine* **24**(21), 2188–2194.
317. Mousa, W. F., Fujita, H., *et al.* (1999). Bone-bonding ability of bioactive bone cement under mechanical stress. *J. Biomed. Mater. Res. (Appl. Biomater.)* **48,** 726–733.
318. Ashton-Miller, J. A., Phillips, W. A., *et al.* (1989). Musculoskeletal response to an induced scoliosis in the canine spine. *Orthop. Trans.* **13,** 106.
319. Kanayama, M., Cunningham, B. W., *et al.* (1997). Does rigid spinal instrumentation influence the healing process of posterolateral spinal fusion? An in vivo sheep model. 43rd Annual Meeting, Orthopaedic Research Society, San Francisco, CA.
320. Muschler, G. F., Negami, S., *et al.* (1996). Evaluation of collagen ceramic composite graft materials in a spinal fusion model. *Clin. Orthop.* **328,** 250–260.
321. Boden, S. D., Zdeblick, T. A., *et al.* (2000). The use of rhBMP-2 in interbody fusion cages. Definitive evidence of osteoinduction in humans: A preliminary report. *Spine* **25**(3), 376–381.
322. Tan, S. B., Kozak, J. A., *et al.* (1990). A modified technique of anterior lumbar fusion with femoral cortical allograft. *J. Orthop. Surg. Tech.* **5**(3), 83–93.
323. Zucherman, J. F., Zdeblick, T. A., *et al.* (1995). Instrumented laparoscopic spinal fusion. Preliminary results. *Spine* **20**(18), 2029–2035.
324. Boden, S. D., Martin, Jr., G. J., *et al.* (1998). Laparoscopic anterior spinal arthrodesis with rhBMP-2in a titanium interbody threaded cage. *J. Spinal Disord.* **11,** 95–101.
325. Cunningham, B. W., Kotani, Y., *et al.* (1998). Video-assisted thoracoscopic surgery versus open thoracotomy for anterior thoracic spinal fusion a comparative radiographic, biomechanical, and histologic analysis in a sheep model. *Spine* **23,** 1333–1340.
326. Cunningham, B. W., Kanayama, M., *et al.* (1999). Osteogenic protein versus autologous interbody arthrodesis in the sheep thoracic spine. *Spine* **24**(6), 509–518.
327. Baramki, H., Steffen, T., *et al.* (2000). The efficacy of interconnected porous hydroxyapatite in achieving posterolateral lumbar fusion in sheep. *Spine* **25**(9), 1053–1060.
328. Mathis, J. M., Petri, M., *et al.* (1998). Percutaneous vertebroplasty treatment of steriod-induced osteoporotic compression fractures. *Arthr. Rhuem.* **41**(1), 171–175.
329. Cotten, A., Dewatre, F., *et al.* (1996). Percutaneous vertebroplasty for osteolytic metastases and myeloma: Effects of the percentage of lesion filling and the leakage of methyl methacrylate at clinical follow-up. *Radiology* **200,** 525–530.
330. Barr, J. D., Barr, M. S., *et al.* (2000). Percutaneous vertebroplasty for pain relief and spinal stabilization. *Spine* **25**(8), 923–928.
331. Belkoff, S. M., Maroney, M., *et al.* (1999). An *in vitro* biomechanical evaluation of bone cements used in percutaneous vertebroplasty. *Bone* **25**(2), 23S–26S.
332. Deramond, H., Wright, N. T., *et al.* (1999). Temperature elevation caused by bone cement polymerization during vertebroplasty. *Bone* **25**(2), 17S–21S.
333. Lamghari, M., Huet, H., *et al.* (1999). A model for evaluating injectable bone replacements in the vertebrae of sheep: Radiological and histological study. *Biomaterials* **20,** 2107–2114.
334. Lamghari, M., Almeida, M. J., *et al.* (1999). Stimulation of bone marrow cells and bone formation by nacre: *In vivo* and *in vitro* studies. *Bone* **25**(2), 91S–94S.
335. Garfin, S. R. (1998). Degenerative conditions of the spine. *Acta Orthop. Scand.* (Suppl.) **281,** 38–46.
336. Hampton, D., Laros, G., *et al.* (1989). Healing potential of the anulus fibrosus. *Spine* **14**(4), 398–401.
337. Moore, R. J., Vernon-Roberts, B., *et al.* (1996). Remodeling of vertebral bone after outer annular injury in sheep. *Spine* **21**(8), 936–940.
338. Osti, O. L., Vernon-Roberts, B., *et al.* (1990). Anulus tears and intervertebral disc degeneration: An experimental study using an animal model. *Spine* **15**(8), 762–767.
339. Kääpä, E., Holm, S., *et al.* (1994). Collagens in the injured porcine intervertebral disc. *J. Orthop. Res.* **12,** 93–102.
340. Kääpä, E., Han, X., *et al.* (1995). Collagen synthesis and types I, III, IV, and VI collagens in an animal model of disc degeneration. *Spine* **20**(1), 59–67.
341. Ahlgren, B. D., Vasavada, A., *et al.* (1994). Anular incision technique on the strength and multidirectional flexibility of the healing intervertebral disc. *Spine* **19**(8), 948–954.
342. Cain, C. M. J., and Fraser, R. D. (1995). Bony and vascular anatomy of the normal cervical spine in the sheep. *Spine* **20**(7), 759–765.
343. Cain, C. M. J., Langston, P. G., *et al.* (1994). Assessment of spinal cord blood flow and function in sheep after anterolateral cervical interbody fusion in the presence of cord damage. *Spine* **19**(5), 511–519.
344. Daneyemez, M. (1999). Silicone rubber microangiography of injured acute spinal cord after treatment with methylprednisolone and vitamin E in rats. *Spine* **24**(21), 2201–2205.
345. Yamaguchi, K., Murakami, M., *et al.* (1999). Behavioral and morphologic studies of the chronically compressed cauda equina. *Spine* **24**(9), 845–851.
346. Emery, S. E., Brazinski, M. S., *et al.* (1994). The biological and biomechanical effects of irradiation on anterior spinal bone grafts in a canine model. *J. Bone Joint Surg.* **76A**(4), 540–548.
347. Emery, S. E., Fuller, D. A., *et al.* (1996). Ceramic anterior spinal fusion. Biologic and biomechanical comparison in a canine model. *Spine* **21**(23), 2713–2719.
348. Fuller, D. A., Stevenson, S., *et al.* (1996). The effects of internal fixation on calcium carbonate. ceramic anterior spinal fusion in dogs. *Spine* **21**(18), 2131–2136.
349. Cook, S. D., Dalton, J. E., *et al.* (1994). *In vivo* evaluation of osteogenic materials as bone graft substitutes for spine fusions. 20th Annual Meeting of the Society for Biomaterials, Boston, Massachusetts.

350. Hildebrandt, U., Pistorius, G., *et al.* (1996). First experience with laparoscopic spine fusion in an experimental model in the pig. *Surg. Endosc.* **10,** 143–146.
351. Spivak, J. M., Chen, D., *et al.* (1999). The effect of locking fixation screws on the stability of anterior cervical plating. *Spine* **24**(4), 334–338.
352. Sandhu, H. S., Turner, S., *et al.* (1996). Distractive properties of a threaded interbody fusion device. An *in vivo* model. *Spine* **21**(10), 1201–1210.
353. Toth, J. M., Seim, III, H. B., *et al.* (1999). Evaluation of the efficacy of direct current electrical bone growth stimulation of spinal fusion cages: An ovine lumbar interbody fusion model. 45th Annual Meeting, Orthopaedic Research Society, Anaheim, CA.
354. Zdeblick, T. A., Cooke, M. E., *et al.* (1993). Anterior cervical discectomy, fusion, and plating. a comparative animal study. *Spine* **18**(14), 1974–1983.
355. Brantigan, J. W., McAfee, P. C., *et al.* (1994). Interbody lumbar fusion using a carbon fiber cage implant versus allograft bone. an investigational study in the spanish goat. *Spine* **19**(13), 1436–1444.
356. Pintar, F. A., Maiman, D. J., *et al.* (1994). Fusion rate and biomechanical stiffness of hydroxylapatite versus autogenous bone grafts for anterior discectomy. An *in vivo* animal study. *Spine* **19**(22), 2524–2528.
357. Hecht, B. P., Fischgrund, J. S., *et al.* (1999). The use of recombinant human bone morphogenetic protein 2 (rhBMP-2) to promote spinal fusion in a nonhuman primate anterior interbody fusion model. *Spine* **24**(7), 629–636.
358. Guizzardi, S., Silvestre, M. D., *et al.* (1992). Implants of heterologous demineralized bone matrix for induction of posterior spinal fusion in rats. *Spine* **17**(6), 701–707.
359. Boden, S. D., Martin, G. J., *et al.* (1999). The use of coralline hydroxyapatite with bone marrow, autogenous bone graft, or osteoinductive bone protein extract for posterolateral lumbar spine fusion. *Spine* **24**(4), 320–327.
360. David, S. M., Gruber, H. E., *et al.* (1999). Lumbar spinal fusion using recombinant human bone morphogenetic protein in the canine. A comparison of three dosages and two carriers. *Spine* **24**(19), 1973–1979.
361. Muschler, G. F., Huber, B., *et al.* (1993). Evaluation of bone-grafting materials in a new canine segmental spimal fusion model. *J. Orthop. Res.* **11,** 514–524.
362. Kahanovitz, N., and Arnoczky, S. P. (1990). The efficacy of direct current electrical stimulation to enhance canine spinal fusions. *Clin. Orthop.* **251,** 295–299.
363. Kahanovitz, N., Arnoczky, S. P., *et al.* (1994). The effect of electromagnetic pulsing on posterior lumbar spinal fusions in dogs. *Spine* **19**(6), 705–709.
364. Oda, I., Cunningham, B. W., *et al.* (1999). Does spinal kyphotic deformity influence the biomechanical characteristics of the adjacent motion segments. An *in vivo* animal model. *Spine* **24**(20), 2139–2146.
365. Kanayama, M., Cunningham, B. W., *et al.* (1999). Does spinal instrumentation influence the healing process of posterolateral spinal fusion. *Spine* **24**(11), 1058–1065.
366. Guigui, P., Plais, P. Y., *et al.* (1994). Experimental model of posterolateral spinal arthrodesis in sheep. Part 2. Application of the model: Evaluation of vertebral fusion obtained with coral (porites) or with a biphasic ceramic (triosite). *Spine* **19**(24), 2798–2803.
367. Boden, S. D., Martin, Jr., G. J., *et al.* (1999). Posterolateral lumbar intertransverse process spine arthrodesis with recombinant human bone morphogenetic protein 2/hydroxyapatite-tricalcium phosphate after laminectomy in the nonhuman primate. *Spine* **24**(12), 1179–1185.
368. Iatridis, J. C., Mente, P. L., *et al.* (1999). Compression-induced changes in intervertebral disc properties in a rat tail model. *Spine* **24**(10), 996–1002.
369. Kubo, S., Tajima, N., *et al.* (1999). A comparative study of chemonucleolysis with recombinant human cathepsin L and chymopapain. *Spine* **24**(2), 120–127.
370. Ishikawa, H., Nohara, Y., *et al.* (1999). Action of chondroitinase ABC on epidurally transplanted nucleus pulposus in the rabbit. *Spine* **24**(11), 1071–1076.
371. Säämänen, A.-M., Puustjärvi, K., *et al.* (1993). Effect of running exercise on proteoglycans and collagen content in the intervertebral disc of young dogs. *Int. J. Sports Med.* **14:** 48–51.
372. Frick, S. L., Hanley, E. N., *et al.* (1994). Lumbar intervertebral disc transfer. A canine study. *Spine* **19**(16), 1826–1835.
373. Moore, R. J., Crotti, T. N., *et al.* (1999). Osteoarthrosis of the facet joints resulting from anular rim lesions in sheep lumbar discs. *Spine* **24**(6), 519–525.
374. Fujimoto, T., Nakamura, T., *et al.* (2000). Effects of EPC-K1 on lipid peroxidation in experimental spinal cord injury. *Spine* **25**(1), 24–29.
375. Moed, B. R., Hartman, M. J., *et al.* (1999). Evaluation of intraoperative nerve-monitoring during insertion of an iliosacral implant in an animal model. *J. Bone Joint Surg.* **81A**(11), 1529–1537.
376. Skouen, J. S., Brisby, H., *et al.* (1999). Protein markers in cerebrospinal fluid in experimental nerve root injury. A study of slow-onset chronic compression effects or the biochemical effects of nucleus pulposus on sacral nerve roots. *Spine* **24**(21), 2195–2200.
377. O'Kelly, C., Wang, X., *et al.* (1999). The production of scoliosis after pinealectomy in young chickens, rats and hamsters. *Spine* **24**(1), 35–43.
378. Machida, M., Murai, I., *et al.* (1999). Pathogenesis of idiopathic scoliosis. experimental study in rats. *Spine* **24**(19), 1985–1989.
379. Pincott, J. R., and Taffs, L. F. (1982). Experimental scoliosis in primates. A neurological cause. *J. Bone Joint Surg.* **64B**(4), 503–507.
380. Barrios, C., Tuñón, M. T., *et al.* (1987). Scoliosis induced by medullary damage: An experimental study in rabbits. *Spine* **12**(5), 433–439.
381. Abe, J., Nagata, K., *et al.* (1999). Experimental external fixation combined with percutaneous discectomy in the management of scoliosis. *Spine* **24**(7), 646–653.
382. Hazan, R., and Oron, U. (1993). Enhancement of bone growth into metal screws implanted in the medullary canal of the femur in rats. *J. Orthop. Res.* **11**(5), 655–663.
383. Vercaigne, S., Wolke, J. G. C., *et al.* (1998). Histomorphometrical and mechanical evaluation of titanium plasma-spray-coated implants placed in the cortical bone in goats. *J. Biomed. Mater. Res.* **41,** 41–48.
384. Fini, M., Cigada, A., *et al.* (1999). *In vitro* and *in vivo* behaviour of Ca- and P-enriched anodized titanium. *Biomaterials* **20,** 1587–1594.
385. Wong, M., Eulenberger, J., *et al.* (1995). Effect of surface topology on the osseointegration of implant materials in trabecular bone. *J. Biomed. Mater. Res.* **29,** 1567–1575.
386. Walker, P. S., Rodger, R. F., *et al.* (1990). An investigation of a compliant interface for press-fit joint replacement. *J. Orthop. Res.* **8,** 453–463.
387. Ducheyne, P., Hench, L. L., *et al.* (1980). Effect of hydroxyapatite impregnation on skeletal bonding of porous coated implants. *J. Biomed. Mater. Res.* **14,** 225–237.
388. Jansen, J. A., van der Waerden, J. P. C. M., *et al.* (1993). Histological and histomorphometrical evaluation of the bone reaction to three different titanium alloy and hydroxyapatite coated implants. *J. Appl. Biomater.* **4,** 213–219.
389. Jansen, J. A., van der Waerden, J. P. C. M., *et al.* (1993). Histologic investigation of the biologic behavior of different hydroxyapatite plasma-sprayed coatings in rabbits. *J. Biomed. Mater. Res.* **27,** 603–610.
390. Hayashi, K., Inadome, T., *et al.* (1993). Comparison of bone-implant interface shear strength of solid hydroxyapatite and hydroxyapatite-coated titanium implants. *J. Biomed. Mater. Res.* **27,** 557–563.

391. Callahan, B. C., Lisecki, E. J., *et al.* (1995). The effect of warfarin on the attachment of bone to hydroxyapatite-coated and uncoated porous implants. *J. Bone Joint Surg.* **77A**(2), 225–230.
392. Nakashima, Y., Hayashi, K., *et al.* (1997). Hydroxyapatite-coating on titanium arc sprayed titanium implants. *J. Biomed. Mater. Res.* **35,** 287–298.
393. Yang, C. Y., Wang, B. C., *et al.* (1997). Intramedullary implant of plasma-sprayed hydroxyapatite coating: An interface study. *J. Biomed. Mater. Res.* **36,** 39–48.
394. Inoue, K., Ohgushi, H., *et al.* (1997). The effect of aging on bone formation in porous hydroxyapatite: Biochemical and histological analysis. *J. Bone Miner. Res.* **12,** 989–994.
395. Overgaard, S., Lind, M., *et al.* (1997). Improved fixation of porous-coated versus grit-blasted surface texture of hydroxyapatite-coated implants in dogs. *Acta Orthop. Scand.* **68**(4), 337–343.
396. Overgaard, S., Lind, M., *et al.* (1998). Resorption of hydroxyapatite and fluorapatite ceramic coatings on weight-bearing implants: A quantitative and morphological study in dogs. *J. Biomed. Mater. Res.* **39,** 141–152.
397. Ogiso, M., Yamamura, M., *et al.* (1998). Comparative push-out test of dense HA implants and HA-coated implants: Findings in a canine study. *J. Biomed. Mater. Res.* **39,** 364–372.
398. Jaffe, W. L., and Scott, D. F. (1996). Total hip arthroplasty with hydroxyapatite-coated prostheses. *J. Bone Joint Surg.* **78A**(12), 1918–1934.
399. D'Antonio, J. A., Capello, W. N., *et al.* (1997). Hydroxyapatite coated implants. Total hip arthroplasty in the young patient and patients with avascular neorosis. *Clin. Orthop.* **344,** 124–138.
400. Overgaard, S., Lind, M., *et al.* (1998). Resorption of hydroxyapatite and fluorapatite ceramic coatings on weight-bearing implants: A quantitative and morphological study in dogs. *J. Biomed. Mater. Res.* **39,** 141–152.
401. Koeneman, J., Lemons, J., *et al.* (1990). Workshop on characterization of calcium phosphate materials. *J. Appl. Biomater.* **1,** 79–90.
402. Goodman, S., and Aspenberg, P. (1993). Effects of mechanical stimulation on the differentiation of hard tissues. *Biomaterials* **14**(8), 563–569.
403. Gotfredsen, K., Wennerberg, A., *et al.* (1995). Anchorage of TiO2-blasted, HA-coated, and machined implants: An experimental study with rabbits. *J. Biomed. Mater. Res.* **29,** 1223–1231.
404. Maruyama, M. (1995). Hydroxyapatite-clay bone fixation for loaded implants. *J. Biomed. Mater. Res.* **29,** 683–686.
405. Nishiguchi, S., Kato, H., *et al.* (1999). Enhancement of bone-bonding strengths of titanium alloy implants by alkali and heat treatments. *Appl. Biomater.* **48,** 689–696.
406. Overgaard, S., Søballe, K., *et al.* (1996). Role of different loading conditions on resorption of hydroxyapatite coating evaluated by histomorphometric and stereological methods. *J. Orthop. Res.* **14,** 888–894.
407. Chang, Y. -S., Oka, M., *et al.* (1996). Significance of interstitial bone ingrowth under load-bearing conditions: A comparison between solid and porous implant materials. *Biomaterials* **17,** 1141–1148.
408. Buser, D., Schenk, R. K., *et al.* (1991). Influence of surface charactheristics on bone integration of titanium implants. A histomorphometric study in miniature pigs. *J. Biomed. Mater. Res.* **25,** 889–902.
409. Wie, H., Herø, H., *et al.* (1995). Bonding capacity in bone of HIP-processed HA-coated titanium: Mechanical and histological investigations. *J. Biomed. Mater. Res.* **29,** 1443–1449.
410. Eckhoff, D. G., Turner, A. S., *et al.* (1995). Effect of age on bone formation around orthopaedic implants. *Clin. Orthop.* **312,** 253–260.
411. Hemmerlé, J., Önçag, A., *et al.* (1997). Ultrastructural features of the bone response to a plasma-sprayed hydroxyapatite coating in sheep. *J. Biomed. Mater. Res.* **36,** 418–425.
412. Dhert, W. J. A., Klein, C. P. A. T., *et al.* (1993). A histological and histomorphometrical investigation of fluorapatite, magnesiumwhitlockite, and hydroxylapatite plasma-sprayed coatings in goats. *J. Biomed. Mater. Res.* **27,** 127–138.
413. Kangasniemi, I. M. O., Verheyen, C. C. P. M., *et al.* (1994). *In vivo* tensile testing of fluorapatite and hydroxylapatite plasma-sprayed coatings. *J. Biomed. Mater. Res.* **28,** 563–572.
414. Callahan, B. C., Lisecki, E. J., *et al.* (1995). The effect of warfarin on the attachment of bone to hydroxyapatite-coated and uncoated porous implants. *J. Bone Joint Surg.* **77A**(2), 225–230.
415. Caulier, H., van der Waerden, J. P. C. M., *et al.* (1995). Effect of calcium phosphate (Ca-P) coatings on trabecular bone response: A histological study. *J. Biomed. Mater. Res.* **29,** 1061–1069.
416. Wolke, J. G. C., deGroot, K., *et al.* (1998). Subperiosteal implantation of various RF magnetron sputtered Ca-P coatings in goats. *J. Biomed. Mater. Res.* **43,** 270–276.
417. Ripamonti, U. (1996). Osteoinduction in porous hydroxyapatite implanted in heterotopic sites of different animal models. *Biomaterials* **17**(1), 31–35.
418. Shaw, J. A., Wilson, S. C., *et al.* (1994). Comparison of primate and canine models for bone ingrowth experimentation, with reference to the effect of ovarian function on bone ingrowth potential. *J. Orthop. Res.* **12,** 268–273.
419. Brånemark, R., Öhrnell, L. -O., *et al.* (1998). Biomechanical characterization of osseointegration: An experimental *in vivo* investigation in the beagle dog. *J. Orthop. Res.* **16**(1), 61–69.
420. Dalton, J. E., and Cook, S. D. (1995). Influence of implant location on the mechanical characteristics using the transcortical model. *J. Biomed. Mater. Res.* **29,** 133–136.
421. Quinet, R. J., and Winters, E. G. (1992). Total joint replacement of the hip and knee. *Med. Clin. N. Am.* **76**(5), 1235–1251.
422. Schmalzried, T. P., Jasty, M., *et al.* (1994). Polyethylene wear debris and tissue reactions in knee as compared to hip replacement prostheses. *J. Appl. Biomater.* **5,** 185–190.
423. Vidovszky, T. J., Bronk, J. T., *et al.* (1996). Accelerated production of UHMW-PE debris in the sheep: a possible model for bone loss around femoral stems. 42nd Annual Meeting, Orthopaedic Research Society, Atlanta, Georgia.
424. Jasty, M. (1993). Clinical reviews: Particulate debris and failure of total hip replacements. *J. Appl. Biomater.* **4,** 273–276.
425. Huiskes, R. (1993). Failed innovation in total hip replacement. Diagnosis and proposals for a cure. *Acta Orthop. Scand.* **64**(6), 699–716.
426. Turner, T. M., Sumner, D. R., *et al.* (1986). A comparative study of porous coatings in a weight-bearing total hip-arthroplasty model. *J. Bone Joint Surg.* **68A**(9), 1396–1409.
427. Goel, V. K., Drinker, H., *et al.* (1982). Selection of an animal model for implant fixation studies: Anatomical aspects. *Yale J. Biol. Med.* **55,** 113–122.
428. Magee, F. P., Weinstein, A. M., *et al.* (1988). A canine composite femoral stem. an *in vivo* study. *Clin. Orthop.* **235,** 237–252.
429. Maistrelli, G. L., Mahomed, N., *et al.* (1992). Hydroxyapatite coating on carbon composite hip implants in dogs. *J. Bone Joint Surg.* **74B,** 452–456.
430. Sumner, D. R., Turner, T. M., *et al.* (1992). Remodeling and ingrowth of bone at two years in a canine cementless total hip-arthroplasty model. *J. Bone Joint Surg.* **74A,** 239–250.
431. Sumner, D. R., Turner, T. M., *et al.* (1992). Experimental studies of bone remodeling in total hip arthroplasty. *Clin. Orthop.* **276,** 83–90.
432. Bloebaum, R. D., Ota, D. T., *et al.* (1993). Comparison of human and canine external femoral morphologies in the context of total hip replacement. *J. Biomed. Mater. Res.* **27,** 1149–1159.
433. Bouvy, B. M., and Manley, P. A. (1993). Vascular and morphologic changes in canine femora after uncemented hip arthroplasty. *Vet. Surg.* **22**(1), 18–26.
434. Ido, K., Matsuda, Y., *et al.* (1993). Cementless total hip replacement: Bio-active glass ceramic coating studied in dogs. *Acta Orthop. Scand.* **64**(6), 607–612.
435. Jasty, M., Bragdon, C. R., *et al.* (1993). Comparison of bone ingrowth

into cobalt chrome sphere and titanium fiber mesh porous coated cementless canine acetabular components. *J. Biomed. Mater. Res.* **27,** 639–644.
436. Turner, T. M., Urban, R. M., *et al.* (1993). Revision, without cement, of aseptically loose, cemented total hip prostheses. *J. Bone Joint Surg.* **75A**(6), 845–862.
437. Kraemer, W. J., Maistrelli, G. L., *et al.* (1995). Migration of polyethylene wear debris in hip arthroplasties: A canine model. *J. Appl. Biomater.* **6,** 225–230.
438. Turner, T. M., Sumner, D. R., *et al.* (1997). Maintenance of proximal cortical bone with use of a less stiff femoral component in hemiarthroplasty of the hip without cement. *J. Bone Joint Surg.* **79A,** 1381–1390.
439. Kuo, T. Y., Skedros, J. G., *et al.* (1998). Comparison of human, primate, and canine femora: Implications for biomaterials testing in total hip replacement." *J. Biomed. Mater. Res.* **40,** 475–489.
440. Hamada, Y., Horiuchi, T., *et al.* (1999). The wear of a polyethylene socket articulating with a zirconia ceramic femoral head in canine total hip arthroplasty. *J. Biomed. Mater. Res. (Appl. Biomater).* **48,** 301–308.
441. Harvey, E. J., Bobyn, J. D., *et al.* (1999). Effect of flexibility of the femoral stem on bone-remodeling and fixation of the stem in a canine total hip arthroplasty model without cement. *J. Bone Joint Surg.* **81A,** 93–107.
442. Fujita, H., Ido, K., *et al.* (2000). Evaluation of bioactive bone cement in canine total hip arthroplasty. *J. Biomed. Mater. Res.* **49,** 273–288.
443. DeYoung, D. J., and Schiller, R. A. (1992). Radiographic criteria for evaluation of uncemented total hip replacement in dogs. *Vet. Surg.* **21**(2), 88–98.
444. DeYoung, D. J., Schiller, R. A., *et al.* (1993). Radiographic assessment of a canine uncemented porous-coated anatomic total hip prosthesis. *Vet. Surg.* **22,** 473–481.
445. Wylie, K. B., DeYoung, D. J., *et al.* (1997). The effect of surgical approach on femoral stem position in canine cemented total hip replacement. *Vet. Surg.* **26,** 62–66.
446. Walenciak, M. T., Zimmerman, M. C., *et al.* (1996). Biomechanical and histological analysis of an HA coated, arc deposited CPTi canine hip prosthesis. *J. Biomed. Mater. Res.* **31,** 465–474.
447. Matsuda, Y., Ido, K., *et al.* (1997). Prosthetic replacement of the hip in dogs using bioactive bone cement. *Clin. Orthop.* **336,** 263–277.
448. Lanyon, L. E., Paul, I. L., *et al.* (1981). *In vivo* strain measurements from bone and prosthesis following total hip replacement. *J. Bone Joint Surg.* **63A**(6), 989–1001.
449. Bruns, D. P., Olmstead, M. L., *et al.* (1996). Technique and results for total hip replacement in sheep: an experimental model. *Vet. Comp. Orthopaed. Traumatol.* **9,** 158–164.
450. Radin, E. L., Rubin, C. T., *et al.* (1982). Changes in the bone-cement interface after total hip replacement: An *in vivo* animal study. *J. Bone Joint Surg.* **64A,** 1188–1200.
451. Schreurs, B. W., Huiskes, R., *et al.* (1996). Biomechanical and histological evaluation of a hydroxyapatite-coated titanium femoral stem fixed with an intramedullary morsellized bone grafting technique: An animal experiment on goats. *Biomaterials* **17,** 1177–1186.
452. Buma, P., van Loon, P. F. M., *et al.* (1997). Histological and biomechanical analysis of bone and interface reactions around hydroxyapatite-coated intramedullary implants of different stiffness: A pilot study on the goat. *Biomaterials* **18,** 1251–1260.
453. Van Rietbergen, B., Huiskes, R., *et al.* (1993). The mechanism of bone remodeling a resorption around press-fitted THA stems. *J. Biomech.* **26**(4/5), 369–382.
454. Gruen, T. A., McNeice, M. G., *et al.* (1979). "Models of failure" of cemented stem-type femoral components. A radiographic analysis of loosening. *Clin. Orthop.* **141,** 17–27.
455. Kattapuram, S. V., Lodwick, G. S., *et al.* (1990). Porous-coated anatomic total hip prostheses: Radiographic analysis and clinical correlation. *Radiology* **174,** 861–864.
456. D'Antonio, J. A., Capello, W. N., *et al.* (1992). Hydroxylapatite-coated hip implants. Multicenter three-year clinical and roentgenographic results. *Clin. Orthop.* **285,** 102–114.
457. Søballe, K., Toksvig-Larsen, S., *et al.* (1993). Migration of hydroxyapatite coated femoral prostheses. *J. Bone Joint Surg.* **75B,** 681–687.
458. Bobyn, J. D., Mortimer, E. S., *et al.* (1992). Producing and avoiding stress shielding. Laboratory and clinical observations of noncemented total hip arthroplasty. *Clin. Orthop.* **274,** 79–96.
459. Önsten, I., Nordqvist, A., *et al.* (1998). Hydroxyapatite augmentation of the porous coating improves fixation of tibial components. *J. Bone Joint Surg.* **80B**(3), 417–425.
460. Sumner, D. R., and Turner, T. M. (1991). Enhancement of biological fixation in cementless total knee arthroplasty. "*Controversies of Total Knee Arthroplasty*" (V. M. Goldberg, ed.), pp. 105–117. Raven Press, New York.
461. Ayers, D. C., Dennis, D. A., *et al.* (1997). Common complications of total knee arthroplasty. *J. Bone Joint Surg.* **79A,** 278–311.
462. Gustafson, A., Clark, I. C., *et al.* (1993). Catastrophic peri-implant bone loss caused by polyethylene and metallic wear in total knees. *J. Long-term Effects Med. Implants* **3**(2), 91–104.
463. Scuderi, G. R., and Insall, J. N. (1992). Total knee arthroplasty. *Clin. Orthop.* **276,** 26–32.
464. Turner, T. M., Urban, R. M., *et al.* (1989). Bone ingrowth into the tibial component of a canine total condylar knee replacement prothesis. *J. Orthop. Res.* **7,** 893–901.
465. Stulberg, B. N., Watson, J. T., *et al.* (1991). Hydroxylapatite vs. titamium mesh in tibial component fixation: a mechanical and histologic study. Combined Meeting of the Orthopaedic Research Societies of USA, Japan, and Canada, Banff, Alberta.
466. Stulberg, B. N., Watson, J. T., *et al.* (1991). A new model to assess tibial fixation in knee arthroplasty: I. Histological and roentgenographic results. *Clin. Orthop.* **263,** 288–302.
467. Goodman, S. B., Magee, F. P., *et al.* (1993). Radiological and histological study of aseptic loosening using a cemented tibial hemiarthroplasty in the rabbit knee. *Biomaterials* **14**(7), 522–528.
468. Shimagaki, H., Bechtold, J. E., *et al.* (1990). Stability of initial fixation of the tibial component in cementless total knee arthroplasty. *J. Orthop. Res.* **8,** 64–71.
469. Frayssinet, P., Hardy, D., *et al.* (1992). New observations on middle term hydroxyapatite-coated titanium alloy hip prostheses. *Biomaterials* **13**(10), 668–674.
470. Bloebaum, R. D., Mihalopoulus, N. L., *et al.* (1997). Postmortem analysis of bone growth into porous-coated acetabular components. *J. Bone Joint Surg.* **79A**(7), 1013–1022.
471. Kaiser, A. D., and Whiteside, L. A. (1990). The effect of screws and pegs on the initial fixation stability of an uncemented unicondylar knee replacement. *Clin. Orthop.* **259,** 169–178.
472. Cook, S. D., Barrack, R. L., *et al.* (1989). Quantitative histologic analysis of tissue growth into porous total knee components. *J. Arthroplast.* (Suppl.), S33–S43.
473. Guttmann, D., Schmalzried, T. P., *et al.* (1993). Light microscopic indentification of submicron polyethylene wear debris. *J. Appl. Biomater.* **4,** 303–307.
474. Schmalzried, T. P., Jasty, M., *et al.* (1993). Histologic identification of polyethylene wear debris using oil red o stain. *J. Appl. Biomater.* **4,** 119–125.
475. Sumner, D. R., Bryan, J. M., *et al.* (1990). Measuring the volume fraction of bone ingrowth: A comparison of three techniques. *J. Orthop. Res.* **8,** 448–452.
476. Isaac, G. H., Wroblewski, B. M., *et al.* (1992). A tribological study of retrieved hip prostheses. *Clin. Ortho.* **276,** 115–124.
477. Wright, T. M., Rimnac, C. M., *et al.* (1992). Wear of polyethylene in

total joint replacements: Observations from retrieved PCA knee implants. *Clin. Orthop.* **276,** 126–134.

478. Spivak, J. M., Blumenthal, N. C., *et al.* (1990). A new canine model to evaluate the biological effects of implant materials and surface coatings on intramedullary bone ingrowth. *Biomaterials* **11,** 79–82.
479. Stephenson, P. K., Freeman, M. A. R., *et al.* (1991). The effect of hydrocyapatite coating on ingrowth of bone into cavities in an implant. *J. Arthroplast.* **6**(1), 51–58.
480. Trindade, M. C. D., Song, Y., *et al.* (1999). Proinflammatory mediator release in response to particle challenge: Studies using the bone harvest chamber. *J. Biomed. Mater. Res. (Appl. Biomater.)* **48,** 434–439.
481. Röser, K., Johansson, C., *et al.* (2000). A new approach to demonstrate cellular activity in bone formation adjacent to implants. *J. Biomed. Mater. Res.* **51,** 280–291.
482. Goodman, S., Aspenberg, P., *et al.* (1994). Effects of intermittent micromotion versus polymer particles on tissue ingrowth: Experiment using a micromotion chamber implanted in rabbits. *J. Appl. Biomater.* **5,** 117–123.
483. van der Vis, H. M., Aspenberg, P., *et al.* (1998). Short periods of oscillating fluid pressure directed at a titanium-bone interface in rabbits lead to bone lysis. *Acta Orthop. Scand.* **69**(1), 5–10.
484. van der Vis, H. M., Aspenberg, P., *et al.* (1998). Fluid pressure causes bone resorption in a rabbit model of prosthetic loosening. *Clin. Orthop.* **350,** 201–208.
485. Goodman, S. B., Song, Y., *et al.* (1994). Cessation of strain facilitates bone formation in the micromotion chamber implanted in the rabbit tibia. *Biomaterials* **15**(11), 889–893.
486. Sennerby, L., Kälebo, P., *et al.* (1993). Influence of indomethacin on the regeneration of cortical bone within titanium implants in rabbits. *Biomaterials* **14**(2), 156–158.
487. Åstrand, J., and Aspenberg, P. (1999). Alendronate did not inhibit instability-induced bone resorption. *Acta Orthop. Scand.* **70**(1), 67–70.
488. Søballe, K., Hansen, E. S., *et al.* (1992). Tissue ingrowth into titanium and hydroxyapatite-coated implants during stable and unstable mechanical conditions. *J. Orthop. Res.* **10,** 285–299.
489. Søballe, K., Brockstedt-Rasmussen, H., *et al.* (1992). Hydroxyapatite coating modifies implant membrane formation. Controlled micromotion studied in dogs. *Acta Orthop. Scand.* **63**(2), 128–140.
490. Søballe, K., Hansen, E. S., *et al.* (1993). Hydroxyapatite coating converts fibrous tissue to bone around loaded implants. *J. Bone Joint Surg.* **75B**(2), 270–278.
491. Jasty, M., Bragdon, C., *et al.* (1997). *In vivo* skeletal responses to porous-surfaced implants subjected to small induced motions. *J. Bone Joint Surg.* **79A**(5), 707–714.
492. Goodman, S., and Aspenberg, P. (1992). Effect of amplitude of micromotion on bone ingrowth into titanium chambers implanted in the rabbit tibia. *Biomaterials* **13**(13), 944–948.
493. Cannon, S. R. (1997). Massive prostheses for malignant bone tumors of the limbs. *Eur. Instruct. Course Lect.* **3,** 497–506.
494. Johnston, J. O., Martin, D. L., *et al.* (1993). Compliant fixation for segmental bone replacement. 7th International Symposium on Limb Salvage, Singapore.
495. Martin, D. L., Turner, A. S., *et al.* (1993). Spring pre-stress fixation for sgmental bone replacement. 39th Annual Meeting, Orthopaedic Research Society, San Francisco, CA.
496. Martin, D. L., Turner, A. S., *et al.* (1996). Compliant pre-stress offers prosthesis biologic attachment at the sheep femur mid diaphysis. 42nd Annual Meeting, Orthopaedic Research Society, Atlanta, Georgia.
497. Sumner, D. R., Turner, T. M., *et al.* (1998). Functional adaptation and ingrowth of bone vary as a function of hip implant stiffness. *J. Biomech.* **31,** 909–917.
498. Simmons, C. A., Valiquette, N., *et al.* (1999). Osseointegration of sintered porous-surfaced and plasma spray-coated implants: an animal model study of early postimplantation healing response and mechanical stability. *J. Biomed. Mater. Res.* **47,** 127–138.
499. Goethgen, C. B., Sumner, D. R., *et al.* (1991). Changes in tibial bone mass after primary cementless and revision cementless total hip arthroplasty in canine models. *J. Orthop. Res.* **9,** 820–827.
500. Vanderby, R., Jr., Manley, P. A., *et al.* (1992). Fixation stability of femoral components in a canine hip replacement model. *J. Orthop. Res.* **10,** 300–309.
501. LaBerge, M., Bobyn, J. D., *et al.* (1992). Evaluation of metallic personalized hemiarthroplasty: A canine patellofemoral model. *J. Biomed. Mater. Res.* **26,** 239–254.
502. Schiller, T. D., De Young, D. J., *et al.* (1993). Quantitative ingrowth analysis of a porous-coated acetabular component in a canine model. *Vet. Surg.* **22**(4), 276–280.
503. Bergmann, G., Graichen, F., *et al.* (1999). Hip joint forces in sheep. *J. Biomech.* **32,** 769–777.
504. Atlan, G., Delattre, O., *et al.* (1999). Interface between bone and nacre implants in sheep. *Biomaterials* **20,** 1017–1022.
505. McDevitt, C. A., and Marcelino, J. (1994). Composition of articular cartilage. *Sports Med. Arthroscop. Rev.* **2,** 1–12.
506. Buckwalter, J. A., and Mankin, H. J. (1997). Articular cartilage. Part I. Tissue design and chondrocyte-matrix interactions. *J. Bone Joint Surg.* **79A**(4), 600–632.
507. Buckwalter, J. A., and Mankin, H. J. (1997). Articular cartilage. Part II:. Degeneration and osteoarthrosis, repair, regeneration, and transplantation. *J. Bone Joint Surg.* **79A**(4), 612–632.
508. de Bri, E., Reinholt, F. P., *et al.* (1995). Primary osteoarthrosis in guinea pigs: A stereological study. *J. Orthop. Res.* **13,** 769–776.
509. van den Berg, W. B., van de Loo, F., *et al.* (1999). Animal models of arthritis in NOS2-deficient mice. *Osteoarthr. Cart.* **7,** 413–415.
510. Lu, J. X., Prudhommeaux, F., *et al.* (1999). Effects of chitosan on rat knee cartilages. *Biomaterials* **20,** 1937–1944.
511. Pastoureau, P. C., Chomel, A. C., *et al.* (1999). Evidence of early subchondral bone changes in the meniscectomized guinea pig. A densitometric study using dual-energy x-ray absoptiometry subregional analysis. *Osteoarthr. Cart.* **7,** 466–473.
512. Heikkilä, J. T., Aho, A. J., *et al.* (1993). Bioactive glass versus hydroxylapatite in reconstruction of osteochondral defects in the rabbit. *Acta Orthop. Scand.* **64**(6), 678–682.
513. Bogoch, R. R., Moran, E., *et al.* (1995). Arthritis not immobilization causes bone loss in the carrageenan injection model of inflammatory arthritis. *J. Othop. Res.* **13,** 777–782.
514. Newberry, W. N., Zukosky, D. K., *et al.* (1997). Subfracture insult to a knee joint causes alterations in the bone and in the functional stiffness of overlying cartilage. *J. Orthop. Res.* **15,** 450–455.
515. Hasegawa, M., Sudo, A., *et al.* (1999). Biological performance of a three-dimensional fabric as artificial cartilage in the repair of large osteochondral defects in rabbit. *Biomaterials* **20,** 1969–1975.
516. Schreiber, R. E., Ilten-Kirby, B. M., *et al.* (1999). Repair of osteochondral defects with allogeneic tissue engineered cartilage implants. *Clin. Orthop.* **367S,** S382–S395.
517. Sellers, R. S., Zhang, R., *et al.* (2000). Repair of articular cartilage defects one year after treatment with recombinant human bone morphogenetic protein-2 (rhBMP-2). *J. Bone Joint Surg.* **82A**(2), 151–160.
518. Brandt, K. D., Braunstein, E. M., *et al.* (1991). Anterior (cranial) cruciate ligament transection in the dog: A bona fide model of osteoarthritis, not merely of cartilage injury and repair. *J. Rhuematol.* **18,** 436–446.
519. Guilak, F., Ratcliffe, A., *et al.* (1994). Mechanical and biochemical changes in the superficial zone of articular cartilage in canine experimental osteoarthritis. *J. Orthop. Res.* **12,** 474–484.
520. Fernandes, J. C., Martel-Pelletier, J., *et al.* (1995). Effects of tenidap on canine experimental osteoarthritis. I. Morphologic and metalloprotease analysis. *Arthr. Rheumat.* **38**(9), 1290–1303.

521. Shortkroff, S., Barone, L., *et al.* (1996). Healing of chondral and osteochondral defects in a canine model: The role of cultured chondrocytes in regeneration of articular cartilage. *Biomaterials* **17,** 147–154.
522. Chang, Y.-S., Oka, M., *et al.* (1997). Histologic comparison of tibial articular surfaces against rigid materials and artificial articular cartilage. *J. Biomed. Mater. Res.* **37,** 51–59.
523. Fernandes, J. C., Martel-Pelletier, J., *et al.* (1998). Collagenase-1 and collagenase-3 synthesis in normal and early experimental osteoarthritic canine cartilage: An immunohistochemical study. *J. Rheumatol.* **25,** 1585–1594.
524. Burton-Wurster, N., Farese, J. P., *et al.* (1999). Site-specific variation in femoral head cartilage composition in dogs at high and low risk for development of osteoarthritis: Insights into cartilage degeneration. *Osteoarthr. Cart.* **7,** 486–497.
525. Ghosh, P., Read, R., *et al.* (1993). The effects of intraarticular administration of hyaluronan in a model of osteoarthritis in sheep. II. cartilage composition and proteoglycan metabolism. *Semin. Arthr. Rheum.* **22**(6, Suppl. 1), 31–42.
526. Namba, R. S., Meuli, M., *et al.* (1996). Regeneration of superficial articular cartilage defects in a fetal lamb model. 42nd Annual Meeting, Orthopaedic Research Society, Atlanta, Georgia.
527. Schachar, N. S., Novak, K., *et al.* (1999). Transplantation of cryopreserved osteochondral dowel allografts for repair of focal articular defects in an ovine model. *J. Orthop. Res.* **17,** 909–920.
528. Shahgaldi, B. F., Amis, A. A., *et al.* (1991). Repair of cartilage lesions using biological implants. *J. Bone Joint Surg.* **73B**(1), 57–64.
529. Butnariu-Ephrat, M., Robinson, D., *et al.* (1996). Resurfacing of goat articular cartilage by chondrocytes derived from bone marrow. *Clin. Orthop.* **330,** 234–243.
530. van Susante, J. L. C., Buma, P., *et al.* (1999). Resurfacing potential of heterologous chondrocytes suspended in fibrin glue in large full-thickness defects of femoral articular cartilage: An experimental study in the goat. *Biomaterials* **20,** 1167–1175.
531. Simmons, E. J., Bertone, A. L., *et al.* (1999). Instability-induced osteoarthritis in the metacarpophalangeal joint of horses. *Am. J. Vet. Res.* **60,** 7–13.
532. Jackson, W. A., Stick, J. A., *et al.* (2000). The effect of compacted cancellous bone grafting on the healing of subchondral bone defects of the medial femoral condyle in horses. *Vet. Surg.* **29,** 8–16.
533. Carlson, C. S., Loeser, R. F., *et al.* (1996). Osteoarthritis in cynomolgus macaques III: Effects of age, gender, and subchondral bone thickness on the severity of disease. *J. Bone Miner. Res.* **11**(9), 1209–1217.
534. Fernihough, J. K., Richmond, R. S., *et al.* (1999). Estrogen replacement therapy modulation of the insulin-like growth factor system in monkey knee joints. *Arthr. Rheum.* **42**(10), 2103–2111.
535. Pelletier, J.-P., Lascau-Coman, V., *et al.* (1999). Selective inhibition of inducible nitric oxide synthase in experimental osteoarthritis is associated with reduction in tissue levels of catabolic factors. *J. Rheumatol.* **26,** 2002–2014.
536. Marshall, J. L. (1969). Periarticular osteophytes. initiation and formation in the knee of the dog. *Clin. Orthop.* **62,** 37–47.
537. Armstrong, S., Read, R. A., *et al.* (1993). Moderate exercise exacerbates the osteoarthritic lesions produced in cartilage by meniscectomy: A morphological study. *Osteroarthr. Cart.* **1,** 89–96.
538. Ghosh, P., Burkhardt, D., *et al.* (1991). Recent advances in animal models for evalutating chondroprotective drugs. *J. Rheumatol.* **18**(Suppl. 27), 143–146.
539. Ghosh, P., Numata, Y., *et al.* (1993). The metabolic response of articular cartilage to abnormal mechanical loading induced by medial or lateral meniscectomy. *Joint Destruct. Arthr. Osteoarthr.* **AAS39,** 89–93.
540. Ghosh, P., Armstrong, S., *et al.* (1993). Animal models of early osteoarthritis: Their use for the evaluation of potential chondroprotective agents. *Joint Destruct. Arthr. Osteoarthr.* **AAS39,** 195–206.
541. Hashimoto, S., Takahashi, K., *et al.* (1999). Nitric oxide production and apoptosis in cells of the meniscus during experimental osteoarthritis. *Arthr. Rheum.* **42**(10), 2123–2131.
542. Doherty, N. S., Griffiths, R. J., *et al.* (1998). The role of animal models in the discovery of novel disease-modifying osteoarthritis drugs (DMOADs). "Osteoarthritis" (K. D. Brandt, M. Doherty, and L. S. Lohmander, eds.), pp. 439–449. Oxford University Press, New York.
543. Billingham, M. E. J. (1998). Advantages afforded by the use of animal models for evaluation of potential disease-modifying osteoarthritis drugs (DMOADs). *"Osteoarthritis"* (K. D. Brandt, M. Doherty, and L. S. Lohmander, eds.), pp. 429–438. Oxford University Press, New York.
544. Haak, T., Delverdier, M., *et al.* (1996). Pathologic study of an experimental canine arthritis induced with complete freund's adjuvant. *Clin. Exp. Rheumatol.* **14,** 633–641.
545. Turner, A. S., Athanasiou, K. A., *et al.* (1997). Biomechanical effects of estrogen on articular cartilage in ovariectomized sheep. *Osteoarthr. Cart.* **5**(1), 63–69.
546. Jackson, D. W., Felt, J. C., *et al.* (2000). Restoration of large femoral trochlear sulcus articular cartilage lesions using a flowable polymer—An experimental study in sheep. 46th Annual Meeting, Orthopaedic Research Society, Orlando, Florida.
547. O'Driscoll, S. W. (1999). Articular cartilage regeneration using periosteum. *Clin. Orthop.* **367S,** S186–S203.
548. Gugala, Z., and Gogolewski, S. (2000). *In vitro* growth and activity of primary chondrocytes on a resorbable polylactide three-dimensional scaffold. *J. Biomed. Mater. Res.* **49,** 183–191.
549. Turner, A., Tippett, J., *et al.* (1998). Radiofrequency (electrosurgical) ablation of articular cartilage: A study in sheep. *Arthroscopy* **14**(6), 585–591.
550. Sellers, R. S., Zhang, R., *et al.* (2000). Repair of articular cartilage defects one year after treatment with recombinant human bone morphogenetic protein-2 (rhBMP-2). *J. Bone Joint Surg.* **82A**(2), 151–160.
551. Mow, V. C., Fithian, D. C., *et al.* (1990). Fundamentals of articular cartilage and meniscus biomechanics. "Articular Cartilage and Knee Joint Function. Basic Science and Arthroscopy" (J.W. Ewing, ed.), pp. 1–17. Raven Press, New York.
552. Newton, P. M., Mow, V. C., *et al.* (1997). The effect of lifelong exercise on canine articular cartilage. *Am. J. Sports. Med.* **25**(3), 282–287.
553. Mow, V. C., and Wang, C. C.-B. (1999). Some bioengineering considerations for tissue engineering of articular cartilage. *Clin. Orthop.* **367S,** S204–S223.
554. Räsänen, T., and Messner, K. (1996). Regional variations of indentation stiffness and thickness of normal rabbit knee articular cartilage. *J. Biomed. Mater. Res.* **31,** 519–524.
555. Budsberg, S. C., Rytz, U., *et al.* (1999). Effects of accleration on ground reaction forces collected in healthy dogs at a trot. *Vet. Comp. Orthopaed. Traumatol* **12,** 15–19.
556. Jackson, W. A., Stick, J. A., *et al.* (2000). The effect of compacted cancellous bone grafting on the healing of subchondral bone defects of the medial femoral condyle in horses. *Vet. Surg.* **29,** 8–16.
557. Hope, N., Ghosh, P., *et al.* (1993). Effects of intraarticular hyaluronan of matrix changes induced in the lateral meniscus by total medial meniscectomy and exercise. *Semin. Arthr. Rheum.* **22,** 43–51.
558. Rodeo, S. A. (2000). Arthroscopic meniscal repair with use of the outside-in technique. *J. Bone Joint Surg.* **82A**(1), 127–141.
559. DeHaven, K. E. (1990). The role of the meniscus. "Articular Cartilage and Knee Joint Function. Basic Science and Arthroscopy" (J.W. Ewing, ed.), pp. 103–135. Raven Press, New York.
560. Arnoczky, S. P. (1994). Meniscus. "Knee Surgery" (F.H. Fu, C.D. Harner, and K.G. Vince, eds.), Vol. 1, pp. 131–140. William & Wilkins, Baltimore.
561. McDevitt, C. A., Miller, R. R., *et al.* (1992). The cells and cell matrix interactions of the meniscus. "Knee Meniscus: Basic and Clinical

Foundations" (V.C. Mow, S.P. Arnoczky, and D.W. Jackson, eds.), pp. 29–36. Raven Press, New York.

562. Joshi, M. D., Suh, J.-K., *et al.* (1995). Interspecies variation of compressive biomechanical properties of the meniscus. *J. Biomed. Mater. Res.* **29,** 823–828.

563. Song, E. K., and Lee, K. B. (1999). Biomechanical test comparing the load to failure of the biodegradable meniscus arrow versus meniscal suture. *Arthroscopy* **15**(7), 726–732.

564. deHoll, P. D., Burt, D. M., *et al.* (1999). Creep indentation biomechanics of medial bovine meniscus. 45th Annual Meeting, Orthopaedic Research Society, Anaheim, CA.

565. Heatley, F. W. (1980). The meniscus-can it be repaired? An experimental investigation in rabbits. *J. Bone Joint Surg.* **62B**(3), 397–402.

566. Collier, S., Hope, N., *et al.* (1996). Healing of circular defects in the rabbit medial meniscus can occur spontaneously and is not improved by intra-articular hyaluronic acid. *Vet. Comp. Orthopaed. Traumatol.* **9,** 60–65.

567. Ishimura, M., Ohgushi, H., *et al.* (1997). Arthroscopic meniscal repair using fibrin glue. Part I: Experimental study. *Arthroscopy* **13**(5), 551–557.

568. Ishimura, M., Ohgushi, H., *et al.* (1997). Arthroscopic meniscal repair using fibrin glue. Part II: Clinical applications. *Arthroscopy* **13**(5), 558–563.

569. Cabaud, H. E., Rodkey, W. G., *et al.* (1981). Medial meniscus repairs. An experimental and morphologic study. *Am. J. Sports Med.* **9**(3), 129–134.

570. King, D. (1936). The healing of the semilunar cartilages. *J. Bone Joint Surg.* **18,** 333–342.

571. Arnoczky, S. P., and Warren, R. F. (1983). The microvasculature of the meniscus and its response to injury. An experimental study in the dog. *Am. J. Sports Med.* **11**(3), 131–141.

572. Arnoczky, S. P., Warren, R. F., *et al.* (1988). Meniscal repair using an exogenous fibrin clot. An experimental study in dogs. *J. Bone Joint Surg.* **70A**(8), 1209–1217.

573. Kobuna, Y., Shirakura, K., *et al.* (1995). Meniscal repair using a flap of synovium. An experimental study in the dog. *Am. J. Knee Surg.* **8**(2), 52–55.

574. Shirakura, K., Niijima, M., *et al.* (1997). Free synovium promotes meniscal healing. Synovium, muscle and synthetic mesh compared in dogs. *Acta Orthop. Scand.* **68**(1), 51–54.

575. Klompmaker, J., Veth, R. P. H., *et al.* (1996). Meniscal replacement using a porous polymer prosthesis: A preliminary study in the dog. *Biomaterials* **17,** 1169–1175.

576. Mikic, Z. D., Brankov, M. Z., *et al.* (1997). Transplantation of fresh-frozen menisci: An experimental study in dogs. *Arthroscopy* **13**(5), 579–583.

577. Goto, H., Shuler, F. D., *et al.* (1999). Gene transfer to meniscal lesion: TGF-β1 gene retrovirally transduced into meniscal fibrochondrocytes upregulates matrix synthesis. *Arthroscopy* **15**(7, Suppl. 1), S26.

578. Newman, A. P., Anderson, D. R., *et al.* (1989). Mechanics of the healed meniscus in a canine model. *Am. J. Sports Med.* **17**(2), 164–175.

579. Cooper, D. E., Arnoczky, S. P., *et al.* (1990). Arthroscopic meniscal repair. *Clin. Sports Med.* **9**(3), 589–607.

580. Horibe, S., Shino, K., *et al.* (1996). Results of isolated meniscal repair evaluated by second-look arthroscopy. *Arthroscopy* **12**(2), 150–155.

581. Miller, M. D., Ritchie, J. R., *et al.* (1994). Meniscus surgery: Indications for repair. *Operative Tech. Sports Med.* **2**(3), 164–171.

582. Arnoczky, S. P., and Milachowski, K. A. (1990). Meniscal allografts: Where do we stand. "Articular Cartilage and Knee Joint Function: Basic Science and Arthroscopy" (J. W. Ewing, ed.), pp. 129–136. Raven Press, New York.

583. Arnoczky, S. P. (1999). Breakout session 4: Meniscus. *Clin. Orthop.* **367S,** S293–S295.

584. Arnoczky, S. P. (1999). Building a meniscus. Biological considerations. *Clin. Orthop.* **367S,** S244–S253.

585. Milachowski, K. A., Weismeier, K., *et al.* (1989). Homologous meniscus transplantation. Experimental and clinical results. *Int. Orthop. (SICOT)* **13,** 1–11.

586. Szomor, Z. L., Martin, T. E., *et al.* (2000). The protective effects of meniscal transplantation on cartilage. An experimental study in sheep. *J. Bone Joint Surg.* **82A**(1), 80–88.

587. Bruns, J., Kahrs, J., *et al.* (1998). Autologous perichondral tissue for meniscal replacement. *J. Bone Joint Surg.* **80B**(5), 918–923.

588. de Groot, J. H., de Vrijer, R., *et al.* (1996). Use of porous polyurethanes for meniscal reconstruction and meniscal prostheses. *Biomaterials* **17,** 163–173.

589. Messner, K. (1994). The concept of a permanent synthetic meniscus prosthesis: A critical discussion after 5 years of experimental investigations using dacron and teflon implants. *Biomaterials* **15**(4), 243–250.

590. Rodkey, W. G., Steadman, R., *et al.* (1999). A clinical study of collagen meniscus implants to restore the injured meniscus. *Clin. Orthop.* **367S,** S281–S292.

591. Klompmaker, J., Veth, R. P. H., *et al.* (1996). Meniscal repair by fibrocartilage in the dog: Characterization of the repair tissue and the role of vascularity. *Biomaterials* **17,** 1685–1691.

592. Ghadially, F. N., Wedge, J. H., *et al.* (1986). Experimental methods of repairing injured menisci. *J. Bone Joint Surg.* **68B**(1), 106–110.

593. Collier, S., Hope, N., *et al.* (1996). Healing of circular defects in the rabbit medial meniscus can occur spontaneously and is not improved by intra-articular hyaluronic acid. *Vet. Comp. Orthopaed. Traumatol.* **9,** 60–65.

594. Walsh, C. J., Goodman, D., *et al.* (1996). Cell-based meniscus regeneration in a partial meniscectomy model. 42nd Annual Meeting, Orthopaedic Research Society, Atlanta, Georgia.

595. Gao, J. G., and Messner, K. (1996). Natural healing of anterior and posterior attachments of the rabbit meniscus. *Clin. Orthop.* **328,** 276–284.

596. Takeuchi, N., Suzuki, Y., *et al.* (1997). Histologic examination of meniscal repair in rabbits. *Clin. Orthop.* **338,** 253–261.

597. Hashimoto, S., Takahashi, K., *et al.* (1999). Fibrochondrocyte apoptosis and nitric oxide production in the meniscus during experimental osteoarthritis. 45th Annual Meeting, Orthopaedic Research Society, Anaheim, CA.

598. Horan, P. J., Popovic, N. A., *et al.* (1999). Acute and long-term response of the meniscus to partial meniscectomy using the holmium: YAG laser. *Arthroscopy* **15**(2), 155–164.

599. Okuda, K., Ochi, M., *et al.* (1999). Meniscal rasping for repair of meniscal tear in the avascular zone. *Arthroscopy* **15**(3), 281–286.

600. Gershuni, D. H., Skyhar, M. J., *et al.* (1989). Experimental models to promote healing of tears in the avascular segment of canine knee menisci. *J. Bone Joint Surg.* **71A**(9), 1363–1370.

601. Nakhostine, M., Gershuni, D. H., *et al.* (1990). Effects of abrasion therapy on tears in the avascular region of sheep menisci. *Arthroscopy* **6**(4), 280–287.

602. Carpenter, S., Thomopoulos, S., *et al.* (1999). Animal models of tendon and ligament injuries for tissue engineering applications. *Clin. Orthop.* **367S,** S296–S311.

603. Woo, S. L.-Y., Hildebrand, K., *et al.* (1999). Tissue engineering of ligament and tendon healing. *Clin. Orthop.* **367S,** S312–S323.

604. Robertson, D. B., Daniel, D. M., *et al.* (1986). Soft tissue fixation to bone. *Am. J. Sports Med.* **14**(5), 398–403.

605. Caborn, D. N. M., Coen, M., *et al.* (1998). Quadrupled semitendinosus-gracilis autograft fixation in the femoral tunnel: A comparison between a metal and a bioabsorbable interference screw. *Arthroscopy* **14**(3), 241–245.

606. Matthews, L. S., Parks, B. G., *et al.* (1998). Determination of fixation strength of large-diameter interference screws. *Arthroscopy* **14**(1), 70–74.

607. Muellner, T., Reihsner, R., *et al.* (1998). Twisting of patellar tendon grafts does not reduce their mechanical properties. *J. Biomech.* **31,** 311–315.
608. Savage, R. (1985). *In vitro* studies of a new method of flexor tendon repair. *J. Hand Surg.* **10B,** 135–141.
609. Noguchi, M., Seiler, J. G., *et al.* (1993). *In vitro* biomechanical analysis of suture methods for flexor tendon repair. *J. Orthop. Res.* **11,** 603–611.
610. Silfverskiöld, K. L., and Andersson, C. H. (1993). Two new methods of tendon repair: An *in vitro* evaluation of tensile strength and gap formation. *J. Hand Surg.* **18A,** 59–65.
611. Rupp, S., Krauss, P. W., *et al.* (1997). Fixation strength of a biodegradable interference screw and a press-fit technique in anterior cruciate ligament reconstruction with a BPTB graft. *Arthroscopy* **13**(1), 61–65.
612. Abate, J. A., Fadale, P. D., *et al.* (1998). Initial fixation strength of polylactic acid interference screws in anterior cruciate ligament reconstruction. *Arthroscopy* **14**(3), 278–284.
613. Rupp, S., Seil, R., *et al.* (1998). Cortical versus cancellous interference fixation for bone-patellar tendon-bone grafts. *Arthroscopy* **14**(5), 484–488.
614. Weiler, A., Hoffmann, R. F. G., *et al.* (1998). Hamstring tendon fixation using interference screws: A biomechanical study in calf tibial bone. *Arthroscopy* **14**(1), 29–37.
615. Rupp, S., Seil, R., *et al.* (1999). Ligament graft initial fixation strength using biodegradable interference screws. *J. Biomed. Mater. Res.* **48,** 70–74.
616. Bennett, M. B., Ker, R. F., *et al.* (1986). Mechanical properties of various mammalian tendons. *J. Zool. Lond.* **209,** 537–548.
617. Arnoczky, S. P. (1990). Animal model for knee ligament research. "Knee Ligaments: Structure, Function, Injury, and Repair" (D. Daniel, W. Akeson, and J. O'Connor, eds.), pp. 401–417. Raven Press, New York.
618. Woo, S. L. -Y., Gomez, M. A., *et al.* (1987). The biomechanical and morphological changes in the medial collateral ligament of the rabbit after immobilization and remobilization. *J. Bone Joint Surg.* **69A,** 1200–1211.
619. Woo, S. L. -Y., Ohland, K. J., *et al.* (1990). Aging and sex-related changes in the biomechanical properties of the rabbit medial collateral ligament. *Mech. Ageing Dev.* **56,** 129–142.
620. Woo, S. L. -Y., Niyibizi, C., *et al.* (1997). Medial collateral knee ligament healing: Combined medial collateral and anterior cruciated ligament injuries studied in rabbits. *Acta Orthop. Scand.* **68**(2), 142–148.
621. Hildebrand, K. A., Woo, S. L. -Y., *et al.* (1998). The effects of platelet-derived growth factor-BB on healing of the rabbit medial collateral ligament. An *in vivo* study. *Am. J. Sports Med.* **26**(4), 549–554.
622. Frank, C. B., Hart, D. A., *et al.* (1999). Molecular biology and biomechanics of normal and healing ligaments—A review. *Osteoarthr. Cart.* **7,** 130–140.
623. Bolton, C. W., and Bruchman, W. C. (1985). The GORE-TEX™ expanded polytetrafluoroethylene prosthetic ligament: An *in vitro* and *in vivo* evaluation. *Clin. Orthop.* **196,** 202–213.
624. Claes, L., and Neugebauer, R. (1985). *In vivo* and *in vitro* investigation of the long-term behavior and fatigue strength of carbon fiber ligament replacement. *Clin. Orthop.* **196,** 99–111.
625. Dürselen, L., Claes, L., *et al.* (1996). Comparative animal study of three ligament prostheses for the replacement of the anterior cruciate and medial collateral ligament. *Biomaterials* **17,** 977–982.
626. Chiroff, R. T. (1975). Experimental replacement of the anterior cruciate ligament. A histological and microradiographic study. *J. Bone Joint Surg.* **57A**(8), 1124–1127.
627. Korvick, D. L., Pijanowski, G. J., *et al.* (1994). Three-dimensional kinematics of the intact and cranial cruciate ligament-deficient stifle of dogs. *J. Biomech.* **27**(1), 77–87.
628. Keira, M., Yasuda, K. K., *et al.* (1996). Mechanical properties of the anterior cruciate ligament chronically relaxed by elevation of the tibial insertion. *J. Orthop. Res.* **14,** 157–166.
629. Bercovy, M., Goutallier, D., *et al.* (1985). Carbon-PGLA prostheses for ligament reconstruction: Experimental basis and short-term results in man. *Clin. Orthop.* **196,** 159–168.
630. Huguet, D., Faintreny, A., *et al.* (1994). Le mouton: Modèle animal pour les prosthèses ligamentaires. *Chirurgie* **120,** 84–87.
631. Radford, W. J. P., Amis, A. A., *et al.* (1996). The ovine stifle as a model for human cruciate ligament surgery. *Vet. Comp. Orthopaed. Traumatol.* **9,** 134–139.
632. Walton, M. (1999). Absorbable and metal interference screws: Comparison of graft security during healing. *Arthroscopy* **15**(8), 818–826.
633. Goradia, V. K., Rochat, M. C., *et al.* (2000). Natural history of a hamstring tendon autograft used for anterior cruciate ligament reconstruction in a sheep model. *Am. J. Sports Med.* **28**(1), 40–46.
634. Drez, D. J., Jr., DeLee, J., *et al.* (1991). Anterior cruciate ligament reconstruction using bone-patellar tendon-bone allografts. A biological and biomechanical evaluation in goats. *Am. J. Sports Med.* **19**(3), 256–263.
635. Bush-Joseph, C. A., Cummings, J. F., *et al.* (1996). Effect of tibial attachment location on the healing of the anterior cruciate ligament freeze model. *J. Orthop. Res.* **14,** 534–541.
636. Lundberg, W. R., Lewis, J. L., *et al.* (1997). *In vivo* forces during remodeling of a two-segment anterior cruciate ligament graft in a goat model. *J. Orthop. Res.* **15,** 645–651.
637. Badylak, S., Arnoczky, S., *et al.* (1999). Naturally occurring extracellular matrix as a scaffold for musculoskeletal repair. *Clin. Orthop.* **367S,** S333–343.
638. Jackson, D. W., Schreck, P., *et al.* (1999). Reduced anterior tibial translation associated with adaptive changes in the anterior cruciate ligament-deficient joint: Goat model. *J. Orthop. Res.* **17,** 810–816.
639. Halata, Z., Wagner, C., *et al.* (1999). Sensory nerve endings in the anterior cruciate ligament (lig. cruciatum anterius) of sheep. *Anat. Rec.* **254,** 13–21.
640. Clancy, W. G., Narechania, R. G., *et al.* (1981). Anterior and posterior cruciate ligament reconstruction in rhesus monkeys. *J. Bone Joint Surg.* **63A**(8), 1270–1284.
641. Blickenstaff, K. R., Grana, W. A., *et al.* (1997). Analysis of a semitendinosus autograft in a rabbit model. *Am. J. Sports Med.* **25,** 554–559.
642. Asahina, S., Muneta, T., *et al.* (2000). Notchplasy in anterior cruciate ligament reconstruction: An experimental animal study. *Arthroscopy* **16**(2), 165–172.
643. Williams, I. F., McCullagh, K. G., *et al.* (1984). Studies on the pathogenesis of equine tendonitis following collagenase injury. *Res. Vet. Sci.* **36,** 326–338.
644. Gelberman, R. H., Vandeberg, J. S., *et al.* (1985). The early stages of flexor tendon healing: A morphologic study of the first fourteen days. *J. Hand Surg.* **10A,** 776–784.
645. Gelberman, R. H., Manske, P. R., *et al.* (1986). Flexor tendon repair. *J. Orthop. Res.* **4,** 119–128.
646. Rothkopf, D. M., Webb, S., *et al.* (1991). An experimental model for the study of canine flexor tendon adhesions. *J. Hand Surg.* **16A,** 694–700.
647. Seiler, J. G., III., Chu, C. R., *et al.* (1997). Autogenous flexor tendon grafts biological mechanisms for incorporation. *Clin. Orthop.* **345,** 239–247.
648. Gelberman, R. H., Boyer, M. I., *et al.* (1999). The effect of gap formation at the repair site on the strength and excursion of intrasynovial flexor tendons. *J. Bone Joint Surg.* **81A,** 975–982.
649. Bidder, M., Towler, D., *et al.* (2000). Expression of the mRNA for vascular endothelial growth factor at the repair site of canine flexor tendon. *J. Orthop. Res.* **18,** 247–252.

650. Gelberman, R. H., Menon, J., *et al.* (1980). The effects of mobilization on the vascularization of healing flexor tendons in dogs. *Clin. Orthop.* **153,** 283–289.
651. Fukui, N., Tashiro, T., *et al.* (2000). Adhesion formation can be reduced by the supression of transforming growth factor-β1 activity. *J. Orthop. Res.* **18,** 212–219.
652. Maffulli, N. (1999). Rupture of the Achilles tendon. *J. Bone Joint Surg.* **81A**(7), 1019–1036.
653. Korvick, D. L., Cummings, J. F., *et al.* (1996). The use of an implantable force transducer to measure patellar tendon forces in goats. *J. Biomech.* **29**(4), 557–561.
654. Yamamoto, N., Hayashi, K., *et al.* (1996). Effects of restressing on the mechanical properties of stress-shielded patellar tendons in rabbits. *J. Biomech. Eng.* **118,** 216–220.
655. Yamamoto, N., Ohno, K., *et al.* (1993). Effects of stress shielding on the mechanical properties of rabbit patellar tendon. *J. Biomech. Eng.* **115,** 23–28.
656. Molina, M. E., Nonweiller, D. E., *et al.* (2000). Contaminated anterior cruciate ligament grafts: The efficacy of 3 sterilization agents. *Arthroscopy* **16**(4), 373–378.
657. Ng, G. Y. F., Oakes, B. W., *et al.* (1996). Long-term study of the biochemistry and biomechanics of anterior cruciate ligament-patellar tendon autografts in goats. *J. Orthop. Res.* **14,** 851–856.
658. Li, C. K., Maffulli, N., *et al.* (1998). A prospective randomized trial of suture of the patellar tendon defect after harvesting. *Arthroscopy* **14**(7), 682–689.
659. Proctor, C. S., Jackson, D. W., *et al.* (1997). Characterization of the repair tissue after removal of the central one-third of the patellar ligament. *J. Bone Joint Surg.* **79A**(7), 997–1006.
660. Sckell, A., Leunig, M., *et al.* (1999). The connective-tissue envelope in revascularisation of patellar tendon grafts. *J. Bone Joint Surg.* **81B**(5), 915–920.
661. Goradia, V. K., Rochat, M. C., *et al.* (2000). Natural history of a hamstring tendon autograft used for anterior cruciate ligament reconstruction in a sheep model. *Am. J. Sports Med.* **28**(1), 40–46.
662. Allen, M. J., Houlton, J. E. F., *et al.* (1998). The surgical anatomy of the stifle joint in sheep. *Vet. Surg.* **27,** 596–605.
663. Yasuda, K., and Hayashi, K. (1999). Changes in biomechanical properties of tendons and ligaments from joint disuse. *Osteoarthr. Cart.* **7,** 122–129.
664. Whiston, T. B., and Walmsley, R. (1960). Some observations on the reaction of bone and tendon after tunnelling of bone and insertion of tendon. *J. Bone Joint Surg.* **42B**(2), 377–386.
665. Rodeo, S. A., Arnoczky, S. P., *et al.* (1993). Tendon-healing in a bone tunnel a biomechanical and histological study in the dog. *J. Bone Joint Surg.* **75A,** 1795–1803.
666. Forward, A. D., and Cowan, R. J. (1963). Tendon suture to bone an experimental investigation in rabbits. *J. Bone Joint Surg.* **45A,** 807–823.
667. Giurea, A., Paternostro, T., *et al.* (1998). Function of reinserted abductor muscles after femoral replacement. *J. Bone Joint Surg.* **80B**(2), 284–287.
668. Gottsauner-Wolf, F., Egger, E. L., *et al.* (1999). Biologic attachment of an allograft bone and tendon transplant to a titanium prosthesis. *Clin. Orthop.* **358,** 101–110.
669. Gottsauner-Wolf, F., Egger, E. L., *et al.* (1997). Allograft tendon interposition for attachment of muscles to endoprostheses. 43rd Annual Meeting, Orthopaedic Research Society, San Francisco, CA.
670. Gottsauner-Wolf, F., Egger, E. L., *et al.* (1995). Muscle attachment to endoprostheses with tendon allografts. 8th International Symposium on Limb Salvage, Florence, Italy.
671. Gottsauner-Wolf, F., Egger, E. L., *et al.* (1995). Muscle attachment to endoprostheses with tendon allografts. 8th International Symposium on Limb Salvage, Florence, Italy.
672. Gottsauner-Wolf, F., Egger, E. L., *et al.* (1992). Tendon reattachment to a titanium prosthesis. 38th Annual Meeting, Orthopaedic Research Society, Washington, D.C.
673. Dejardin, L. M., Arnoczky, S. P., *et al.* (1999). Use of small intestinal submucosal implants for regeneration of large fascial defects: An experimental study in dogs. *J. Biomed. Mater. Res.* **46,** 203–211.
674. Pluhar, G. E., Manley, P. A., *et al.* (1998). Comparison of three methods of tendon attachment to an allograft/prosthetic composite of the proximal femur in an *in vivo* canine model. 44th Annual Meeting, Orthopaedic Research Society, New Orleans, LA.
675. Arendt, E., and Dick, R. (1995). Knee injury patterns among men and women in collegiate basketball and soccer. *Am. J. Sports Med.* **23**(6), 694–701.
676. Slauterbeck, J., Clevenger, C., *et al.* (1999). Estrogen level alters the failure load of the rabbit anterior cruciate ligament. *J. Orthop. Res.* **17,** 405–408.
677. Huston, L. J., Greenfield, M. L. V. H., *et al.* (2000). Anterior cruciate ligament injuries in the female athlete. *Clin. Orthop.* **372,** 50–63.
678. Malaviya, P., Butler, D. L., *et al.* (1998). *In vivo* tendon forces correlate with activity level and remain bounded: Evidence in a rabbit flexor tendon model. *J. Biomech.* **31,** 1043–1049.
679. Stehno-Bittel, L., Reddy, G. K., *et al.* (1998). Biochemistry and biomechanics of healing tendon: Part I. Effects of rigid plaster casts and functional casts. *Med. Sci. Sports Exerc.* **3,** 788–793.
680. Budoff, J. E., Nirschl, R. P., *et al.* (1998). Débridement of partial-thickness tears of the rotator cuff without acromioplasty. *J. Bone Joint Surg.* **80A**(5), 733–748.
681. Romeo, A. A., Hang, D. W., *et al.* (1999). Repair of full thickness rotator cuff tears. Gender, age, and other factors affecting outcome. *Clin. Orthop.* **367,** 243–255.
682. Gerber, C., Fuchs, B., *et al.* (2000). The results of repair of massive tears of the rotator cuff. *J. Bone Joint Surg.* **82A**(4), 505–515.
683. Gerber, C., Schneeberger, A. G., *et al.* (1999). Experimental rotator cuff repair. *J. Bone Joint Surg.* **81A**(9), 1281–1290.
684. Thomopoulos, S., Lanagan, C. L., *et al.* (1998). The influence of exogenous fibrin clot on healing in a rat supraspinatus tendon defect. 44th Annual Meeting, Orthopaedic Research Society, New Orleans, LA.
685. Soslowsky, L. J., Carpenter, J. E., *et al.* (1996). Development and use of an animal model for investigations on rotator cuff disease. *J. Shoulder Elbow Surg.* **5,** 383–392.
686. Novotny, J. E., Macy, J. C., *et al.* (1999). Comparative anatomy of the human glenohumeral joint to three animal models. 45th Annual Meeting, Orthopaedic Research Society, Anaheim, CA.
687. Yamashita, T., Minaki, Y., *et al.* (1999). Neural response of mechanoreceptors to acute inflammation in the rotator cuff of the shoulder joint in rabbits. *Acta Orthop. Scand.* **70**(2), 137–140.
688. Seneviratne, A. M., Izawa, K., *et al.* (1999). The effect of corticosteroid induced osteoporosis on tendon insertion sites in a rabbit model. 45th Annual Meeting, Orthopaedic Research Society, Anaheim, CA.
689. Riemersma, D., and Schamhardt, H. (1982). The cryo-jaw; a clamp designed for *in-vitro* rheology studies of horse digital flexor tendons. *J. Biomech.* **15**(8), 619–620.
690. Liu, J., Hughes, R. E., *et al.* (1998). Biomechanical effect of medial advancement of the surpraspinatus tendon. *J. Bone Joint Surg.* **80A**(6), 853–859.
691. St. Pierre, P., Olson, E. J., *et al.* (1995). Tendon-healing to cortical bone compared with healing to a cancellous trough a biomechanical and histological evaluation in goats. *J. Bone Joint Surg.* **77A,** 1858–1866.
692. Aoki, M., Isogai, S., *et al.* (1998). Healing of the rotator cuff at tendon insertion to bone: A study using canine infraspinatus. 44th Annual Meeting, Orthopaedic Research Society, New Orleans, LA.
693. Gerber, C., Schneeberger, A. G., *et al.* (1994). Mechanical strength of repairs of the rotator cuff. *J. Bone Joint Surg.* **76B**(3), 371–380.
694. Gartsman, G. M. (1997). Combined arthroscopic and open treatment of tears of the rotator cuff. *J. Bone Joint Surg.* **79A**(5), 776–793.
695. Speer, K. P., and Warren, R. F. (1993). Arthroscopic shoulder stabilization. A role for biodegradable materials. *Clin. Orthop.* **291,** 67–74.

696. Barber, F. A., and Herbert, M. A. (1999). Suture anchors-update 1999. *Arthroscopy* **15**(7), 719–725.
697. Wetzler, M. J., Bartolozzi, A. R., *et al.* (1996). Fatigue properties of suture anchors in anterior shoulder reconstructions: Mitek GII. *Arthroscopy* **12**(6), 687–693.
698. Burkhart, S. S., Pagán, J. L. D., *et al.* (1997). Cyclic loading of anchor-based rotator cuff repairs: Confirmation of the tension overload phenomenon and comparison of suture anchor fixation with transosseous fixation. *Arthroscopy* **13**(6), 720–724.
699. Rossouw, D. J., McElroy, B. J., *et al.* (1997). A biomechanical evaluation of suture anchors in repair of the rotator cuff. *J. Bone Joint Surg.* **79B**(3), 458–461.
700. Roth, C. A., Bartolozzi, A. R., *et al.* (1998). Failure properties of suture anchors in the glenoid and the effects of cortical thickness. *ArthroscopY* **14**(2), 186–191.
701. Carpenter, J. E., Fish, D. N., *et al.* (1993). Pull-out strength of five suture anchors. *Arthroscopy* **9**(1), 109–113.
702. Hofmann, G. O., Kluger, P., *et al.* (1997). Biomechanical evaluation of a bioresorbable PLA dowel for arthroscopic surgery of the shoulder. *Biomaterials* **18,** 1441–1445.
703. Schroeder, J. A., and Brown, M. K. C. (1999). Biocompatibility and degradation of collagen bone anchors in a rabbit model. *J. Biomed. Mater. Res.* **48,** 309–314.
704. Barber, F. A., Cawley, P., *et al.* (1993). Suture anchor failure strength—An *in vivo* study. *Arthroscopy* **9**(6), 647–652.
705. Balch, O. K., Collier, M. A., *et al.* (1999). Bioabsorbable suture anchor (Co-polymer 85/15D,L-lactide/glycolide) implanted in bone: Correlation of physical/mechanical properties, magnetic resonance imaging, and histological response. *Arthroscopy* **15**(7), 691–708.
706. Hayashi, K., Thabit, III, G., *et al.* (1996). The effect of nonalblative laser energy on the ultrastructure of joint capsular collagen. *Arthroscopy* **12**(4), 474–481.
707. Hayashi, K., Nieckarz, J. A., *et al.* (1997). Effect of nonablative laser energy on the joint capsule: An *in vivo* rabbit study using a holmium:YAG laser. *Lasers Surg. Med.* **20,** 164–171.
708. Hayashi, K., Thabit, III, G., *et al.* (1997). The effect of thermal heating on the length and histologic properties of the glenohumeral joint capsule. *Am. J. Sports Med.* **25**(1), 107–112.
709. Obrzut, S. L., Hecht, P., *et al.* (1998). The effect of radiofrequency energy on the length and temperature properties of the glenohumeral joint capsule. *Arthroscopy* **14**(4), 395–400.
710. Lopez, M. J., Hayashi, K., *et al.* (1998). The effect of radiofrequency energy on the ultrastructure of joint capsular collagen. *Arthroscopy* **14**(5), 495–501.
711. Hayashi, K., Markel, M. D., *et al.* (1995). The effect of nonablative laser energy on joint capsular properties: An *in vitro* mechanical study using a rabbit model. *Am. J. Sports Med.* **23**(4), 482–487.
712. Flanagan, C. L., Soslowsky, L. J., *et al.* (1999). A preliminary comparative study on the healing characteristics of fetal and adult sheep tendon. 45th Annual Meeting, Orthopaedic Research Society, Anaheim, CA.
713. Barber, F. A., Herbert, M. A., *et al.* (1995). The ultimate strength of suture anchors. *Arthroscopy* **11,** 21–28.
714. Barber, F. A., Herbert, M. A., *et al.* (1996). Suture anchor strength revisited. *Arthroscopy* **12,** 32–38.
715. Hoogerbrugge, P. M., Brouwer, O. F., *et al.* (1995). Allogeneic bone marrow transplantation for lysosomal storage diseases. *Lancet* **345,** 1398–1402.
716. Neufeld, E. F. (1991). Lysosomal storage diseases. *Annu. Rev. Biochem.* **60,** 257–280.
717. Norrdin, R. W., Moffat, K. S., *et al.* (1993). Characterization of osteopenia in feline mucopolysaccharidosis VI and evaluation of bone marrow transplantation therapy. *Bone* **14,** 361–367.
718. Turner, A. S., Morrdin, R. W., *et al.* (1995). Bone mineral density in feline mucopolysaccharidosis VI measured using dual-energy x-ray absorptiometry. *Calcif. Tissue Int.* **57,** 191–195.
719. Abreu, S., Hayden, J., *et al.* (1995). Growth plate pathology in feline mucopolysaccharidosis VI. *Calcif. Tissue Int.* **57,** 185–190.
720. Nuttall, J. D., Brumfield, L. K., *et al.* (1999). Histomorphometric analysis of the tibial growth plate in a feline model of mucopolysaccharidosis type VI. *Calcif. Tissue Int.* **65,** 47–52.
721. Gitzelmann, R., Bosshard, N. U., *et al.* (1994). Feline mucopolysaccharidosis VII due to β-glucuronidase deficiency. *Vet. Pathol.* **31,** 435–443.
722. Sands, M. S., Barker, J. E., *et al.* (1993). Treatment of murine mucopolysaccharidosis type VII by syngeneic bone marrow transplantation in neonates. *Lab. Invest.* **68**(6), 676–686.
723. Gigante, A., Chillemi, C., *et al.* (1999). Elastic fibers of musculoskeletal tissues in bovine marfan syndrome: A morphometric study. *J. Orthop.* **17,** 624–628.
724. Mehta, S. S., Antich, P. P., *et al.* (1999). Bone material elasticity in a murine model of osteogenesis imperfecta. *Connect. Tissue Res.* **40**(3), 189–198.
725. Caplan, A. I., and Goldberg, V. M. (1999). The principles of tissue engineered regeneration of skeletal tissues. *Clin. Orthop.* **367S,** S1–S5.
726. Kivirikko, K. I. (1993). Collagens and their abnormalities in a wide spectrum of diseases. *Ann. Med.* **25,** 113–126.
727. Lehner, C. E., Adams, W. M., *et al.* (1997). Dysbaric osteonecrosis in divers and caisson workers: An animal model. *Clin. Orthop.* **344,** 320–332.
728. Lin, T. F., Lehner, C. E., *et al.* (1995). Osteonecrosis induced in sheep by a single hyperbaric exposure: a large-animal model of avascular bone necrosis. 41st Annual Meeting, Orthopaedic Research Society, Orlando, Florida.
729. Carvell, J. E. (1983). The relationship of the periosteum to angular deformities of long bones. *Clin. Orthop.* **173,** 262–274.
730. Asimus, E., Collard, P., *et al.* (1997). Effect of low compression on the growth plate. An experimental study in sheep. *Vet. Comp. Orthopaed. Traumatol.* **10,** 16–22.
731. Peltonen, J., Alitalo, I., *et al.* (1984). Distraction of the growth plate. Experiments in pigs and sheep. *Acta Orthop. Scand.* **55,** 359–362.
732. Shindell, R., Lippiello, L., *et al.* (1988). Uncertain effect of indomethacin on physeal growth injury. Experiments in rabbits. *Acta Orthop. Scand.* **59**(1), 46–49.
733. Baron, J., Klein, K. O., *et al.* (1994). Induction of growth plate cartilage ossification by basic fibroblast growth factor. *Endocrinology* **135,** 2790–2793.
734. Aizawa, T., Kokubun, S., *et al.* (1999). c-Myc protein in the rabbit growth plate: Change in immunolocalisation with age and possible roles from proliferation to apoptosis. *J. Bone Joint Surg.* **81B,** 921–925.
735. Schemitsch, E. H., Jain, R., *et al.* (1997). Pulmonary effects of fixation of a fracture with a plate compared with intramedullary nailing: a canine model of fat embolism and fracture fixation. *J. Bone Joint Surg.* **79A,** 984–996.
736. Wenda, K., Runkel, M., *et al.* (1993). Pathogenesis and clinical relevance of bone marrow embolism in medullary nailing-demonstrated by intraoperative echocardiography. *Injury* **24** (Suppl.), S73–S81.
737. Elmaraghy, A. W., Aksenov, S., *et al.* (1999). Pathophysiological effect of fat emobolism in a canine model of pulmonary contusion. *J. Bone Joint Surg.* **81A,** 1155–1164.
738. Naito, M., Schoenecker, P., *et al.* (1992). Acute effect of traction, compression, and hip joint tamponade on blood flow of the femoral head: An experimental model. *J. Orthop. Res.* **10**(6), 800-106.
739. Malizos, K., Quarles, L., *et al.* (1993). An experimental canine model of osteonecrosis: Characterization of the repair process. *J. Orthop. Res.* **11**(3), 350–357.
740. Drescher, W., Schneider, T., *et al.* (1999). Reperfusion pattern of the immature femoral head after critical ischemia. *Acta Orthop. Scand.* **70**(5), 439–445.

741. Brody, A., Strong, M., *et al.* (1991). Avascular necrosis: Early MR imaging and histologic findings in a canine model. *AJR Am. J. Roentgenol.* **157,** 341–345.
742. Nakamura, T., Matsumoto, T., *et al.* (1997). Early magnetic resonance imaging and histologic findings in a model of femoral head necrosis. *Clin. Orthop.* **334,** 68–72.
743. Conzemius, M., Brown, T., *et al.* (2000). Collapse attainment in a new animal model of osteonecrosis. *Proc. Orthop. Res. Soc.* **46,** 206.
744. Simank, H.-G., Graf, J., *et al.* (1997). Long-term effects of core decompression by drilling. *Acta Anat.* **158,** 185–191.
745. Liu, L.-S., Thompson, A., *et al.* (1999). An osteoconductive collagen/hyaluronate matrix for bone regeneration. *Biomaterials* **20,** 1097–1108.
746. Van Heest, A., and Swiontkowski, M. (1999). Bone-graft substitutes. *Lancet* **353** (Suppl. I), 28–29.
747. Lewandrowski, K.-U., Gresser, J. D., *et al.* (2000). Bioresorbable bone graft substitutes of different osteochonductivities: A histologic evaluation of osteointegration of poly(propylene glycol–co-fumaric acid)-based cement implants in rats. *Biomaterials* **21,** 757–764.
748. Lewandrowski, K.-U., Gresser, J. D., *et al.* (2000). Osteoconductivity of an injectable and bioresorbable poly(propylene glycol–co-fumaric acid) bone cement. *Biomaterials* **21,** 293–298.
749. Thiru, R. G., Ferlic, D. C., *et al.* (1986). Arterial anatomy of the triangular fibrocartilage of the wrist and its surgical significance. *J. Hand Surg.* **11A,** 258–263.
750. Bednar, M. S., Arnoczky, S. P., *et al.* (1991). The microvasculature of the triangular fibrocartilage complex: Its clinical significance. *J. Hand Surg.* **16A,** 1101–1105.
751. Whatley, J. S., Dejardin, L. M., *et al.* (2000). The effect of an exogenous fibrin clot on the regeneration of the triangular fibrocartilage complex: An *in vivo* experimental study in dogs. *Arthroscopy* **16**(2), 127–136.
752. Mikic, Z. D., Ercegan, G., *et al.* (1992). Detailed anatomy of the antebrachiocarpal joint in dogs. *Anat. Rec.* **233,** 329–334.
753. Bruder, S. P. (1999). Current and emerging technologies in orthopaedic tissue engineering. *Clin. Orthop.* **367S,** S406–S409.
754. Goldstein, S. A., Patil, P. V., *et al.* (1999). Perspectives on tissue engineering of bone. *Clin. Orthop.* **367S,** S419–S423.
755. Canalis, E. (2000). "Skeletal Growth Factors." Lippincott Williams & Wilkins, Hagerstown.
756. Baltzer, A. W. A., Whalen, J. D., *et al.* (1999). Adenoviral transduction of human osteoblastic cell cultures. A new perspective for gene therapy of bone diseases. *Acta Orthop. Scand.* **70**(5), 419–424.
757. Evans, C. H., and Robbins, P. D. (1999). Genetically augmented tissue engineering of the musculoskeletal system. *Clin. Orthop.* **367S,** S410–S418.
758. Freed, L. E., Martin, I., *et al.* (1999). Frontiers in tissue engineering. *In vitro* modulation of chondrogenesis. *Clin. Orthop.* **367S,** S46–S58.
759. Stone, K. R. (1999). Current and future directions for meniscus repair and replacement. *Clin. Orthop.* **367S,** S273–S280.
760. Nishida, K., Kang, J. D., *et al.* (1999). Modulation of the biologic activity of the rabbit intervertebral disc by gene therapy: An *in vivo* study of advenovirus-mediated transfer of the human transforming growth factor β1 encoding gene. *Spine* **24**(23), 2419–2425.
761. Altman, D. A., Titus, L., *et al.* (1999). Molecular biology and spinal disorders. A survey for the clinician. *Spine* **24**(7), 723–730.

82

Statistical Analysis—Specific Statistical Tests: Indications for Use

David T. Mauger* and Gordon L. Kauffman, Jr.†

**Department of Health Evaluation Sciences and †Department of Surgery, The Milton S. Hershey Medical Center, Penn State College of Medicine, Hershey, Pennsylvania 17033*

I. Introduction

Because a statistic is simply a piece of data, one might logically define the subject of statistics as the study of data. A somewhat more cynical view is that statistics is the study of methods for massaging data to support one's personal agenda. This opinion is well summarized in the following quote attributed to Mark Twain: "Get your facts first, and then you can distort them as much as you please. Facts are stubborn, but statistics are more pliable." At the other extreme, Florence Nightingale apparently held a much more complimentary view of statistics: "To understand God's thoughts we must study statistics, for those are the measure of his purpose." Although it is true that a statistic can be presented in such a way as to be (intentionally) misleading, the careful consumer does have hope. Thomas Carlyle suggested a legitimate, albeit limited, use of statistics: "A judicious man uses statistics, not to get knowledge, but to save himself from having ignorance foisted upon him." A contemporary statistician might define statistics as the "epistemology of science" (*epistemology*: the study or a theory of the nature and grounds of knowledge, especially with reference to its limits and validity). From a practical standpoint, the field of statistics provides a theoretical framework for the development of quantitative methods to make decisions in the face of uncertainty. Statistical inference is the means by which such decisions can be made. This chapter begins with an overview of statistical inference in the clinical research setting followed by methods for analyzing grouped data of different types: continuous, categorical, and censored (also called survival). In the last section correlation analysis is discussed.

Appropriate data reduction and analysis are crucial in the establishment of scientific validity. No investigator would allow her/his scientific integrity to be compromised by publication of conclusions that were drawn from data that were inappropriately tested for statistical significance. As much care must be taken in data analysis as in protocol development and data generation. One need only peruse the surgical literature to realize that inappropriate data reduction and analysis are common. It is all too easy to use standard statistical software to analyze data, without being aware of the principles behind the various options. Each surgical investigator must know the reason why a certain statistical analysis was made on her/his data and understand not only the strengths of that analysis but also its weaknesses. No attempt will be made to describe in detail the more complex mathematics involved in the derivation of formulas, rather, a concise and comprehensive description of the basic theories and their applications is provided in this chapter.

The framework for statistical inference considered here is that observed data (e.g., the results of an experiment) are viewed as one realization from a distribution of potential data. For example, a study into the effect of a new prophylactic drug on the incidence of postoperative infection following routine appendectomy might yield 2 infections out of 100 operations in patients receiving the new drug and 6 infections out of 100 operations in patients not receiving the new drug. If the only goal of the study were to report the rate of postoperative infection in each of these two groups, then descriptive statistics such as the incidence in each group are all that is necessary. If one also wishes to infer something about the expected incidence of infection for future patients who could be given the new drug, however, this requires a framework for relating observed data to potential or as yet unobserved data. A critical part of this framework is the notion of randomness underlying the process giving rise to the observed data. Even if the same experiment were repeated under exactly the same conditions, one would not expect exactly the same results. This uncertainty is due to inherent variability that cannot be explained. The goal of a statistical analysis is to weigh quantitatively this uncertainty against the information contained in the observed data. In this hypothetical example the postoperative infection incidence rate was 2% in the drug group and 6% in the control group. Certainly one would feel more comfortable about concluding that the drug was effective based on data from 200 patients than the same incidence rates in a sample of 100 patients, but how should one quantify the level of belief?

The two most commonly used approaches for quantifying certainty about experimental results are hypothesis testing and confidence intervals. Hypothesis testing reduces the scientific question to a decision between alternative hypotheses. In the example above, the question of drug effectiveness could be stated as a choice between the null hypothesis that the drug has no effect versus the alternative hypothesis that it does. This form of alternative is called a two-sided hypothesis because it states that the drug has an effect, but does not specify the direction of the effect. The one-sided hypothesis would either state that the drug decreases the incidence of postoperative infection or that it increases the incidence of postoperative infection. This corresponds, for example, to a choice between the null hypothesis, that receiving the drug is no better than not receiving it, versus the alternative hypothesis, that it is protective. Thus the one-sided hypothesis is a more narrow form of the same question addressed by the two-sided hypothesis and can therefore be tested more precisely. The choice to use a two-sided or one-sided hypothesis test must be made during study design, not after the data have been collected. In medical research, however, it is generally considered more appropriate to address the two-sided question because answering the one-sided question may lead to ambiguous conclusions. In this example the decision to accept the one-sided null hypothesis, that receiving the drug is no better than not receiving it, would be compatible with the conclusion that receiving the drug may actually be worse than not receiving it. In many cases it may not be acceptable to arrive at an indefinite conclusion. The rule for deciding between hypotheses is based on the p value of the hypothesis test. The p value is a measure of the degree to which the observed data are incompatible with the null hypothesis. A p value ranges between 0 and 1 and can loosely be interpreted as the probability that a future study carried out under the same conditions would yield results at least as incompatible with the null hypothesis as the current study, if the null hypothesis were in fact true. A small p value, say 0.03, indicates that the present results are highly unlikely to have occurred if the null hypothesis were true. Because the present results did in fact occur, the logical decision is to reject the null hypothesis. On the other hand, a large p value indicates that there is little reason to doubt the null hypothesis because the present results are relatively likely to have occurred if the null hypothesis were true.

An oft-cited limitation of the hypothesis testing approach and p values as measures for quantifying evidence is that p values alone are not sufficient to judge the scientific relevance of the study results. In fact, many scientific journals mandate the use of the confidence interval approach. Consider the results of three hypothetical studies enumerated in Table I. The p values of the first two studies corresponding to the test of the null hypothesis, that the drug has no effect, are identical. However, in terms of the magnitude of the apparent drug effect observed, the first study has higher clinical importance than the second. One would be more likely to recommend routine use of the drug based on the first study, even though the statistical significance of the results, as judged by the p value, are equal. This is not to say that statistical significance is unimportant. The magnitudes of the apparent drug effect observed in the first and third studies are identical, but the p value is smaller for the third study than for the first. This is intuitively sensible; one should be more confident of the recommendation for routine use of the

Table I Comparison of Hypothetical Studies

Study	Parameters	Group: Drug	Group: Control	*p* value	Odds ratio	95% confidence interval
1	Total number of patients	100	100			
	Number with postoperative infection	2	6	0.28	3.13	0.54–32.27
	Percent with postoperative infection	2	6			
	Odds of postoperative infection	0.0204	0.0638			
2	Total number of patients	10,000	10,000			
	Number with postoperative infection	563	600	0.28	1.07	0.95–1.21
	Percent with postoperative infection	5.63	6			
	Odds of postoperative infection	0.0597	0.0638			
3	Total number of patients	1000	1000			
	Number with postoperative infection	20	60	<0.01	3.13	1.84–5.20
	Percent with postoperative infection	2	6			
	Odds of postoperative infection	0.0204	0.0638			

drug based on the third study because the amount of evidence (sample size) is greater. The confidence interval approach provides a way to incorporate both statistical significance (measure of the strength of the evidence collected) and scientific relevance (measure of the clinical importance of the result) in a single expression. A confidence interval is associated with a parameter (e.g., mean, incidence rate, odds ratio, correlation) that has clinical relevance and is calculated for a specified confidence level, typically 95%. For example, the postoperative infection odds ratio for the prophylactic drug (odds of infection without drug/odds of infection with drug) based on results from the first hypothetical study is 3.13. The odds of postoperative infection without the drug are 3.13 times higher than the odds of postoperative infection with the drug. The odds ratio based on the third study is also 3.13, but the 95% confidence interval is much wider for the first study than for the third. Obviously one does not know the true value of the parameter of interest (e.g., the odds ratio that would be observed if one knew the postoperative outcomes of all patients that might theoretically be in the study); if so, there would be no point in doing the study. Thus it is impossible to tell whether the observed confidence interval actually captures the true value of the parameter. The statistical theory behind confidence intervals is such that, before the study is actually carried out, the probability that the 95% confidence interval will capture the true value of the parameter is equal to 0.95. Therefore, one can be 95% confident that the observed confidence interval captures the true value of the parameter.

II. Continuous Data

The defining characteristic of continuous data is that there exists some scale underlying the observed data that permits mathematical operations allowing preservation of the scale. For example, pulse rate (beats per minute) is measured on an arithmetic scale. The absolute difference between pulse rates of 65 and 70 (5 beats per minute) is the same as the absolute difference between pulse rates of 82 and 87. The notion of an average or mean value is sensible for continuous data. So, if a patient had pulse rates of 83, 81, 85, 84, and 82 measured at 10-min intervals, it is meaningful to say that the average pulse rate over that time period was 83. By far the model most commonly used to represent continuous data is the normal distribution curve, fully characterized by two parameters, the mean and the standard deviation (typically denoted μ and σ; common statistical parlance is to denote parameters with Greek letters). By "fully characterized" it is meant that there are no other parameters associated with the distribution curve, so knowledge of μ and σ fully specifies the model. For this reason, it is common practice to use the mean and standard deviation to summarize continuous data. This is not to say that other statistics (e.g., minimum, maximum, median) are not useful. Rather, if one accepts the normal distribution model, no other statistics are necessary for understanding the model. The utility of these statistics is as diagnostic tools for assessing the plausibility of the normal model. A complete descriptive analysis of continuous data includes calculation of the sample mean, standard deviation, median, minimum, and maximum. In addition, a graphical summary such as a histogram or box plot should be used to facilitate visual assessment of continuous data.

Figure 1 shows pulse rate data from 30 subjects. The left-hand panel displays a histogram and reports the mean and standard deviation of the data. The heavier line at the bottom of the histogram covers the mean ± 1 standard deviation; the lighter line covers the mean ± 2 standard deviations. If the

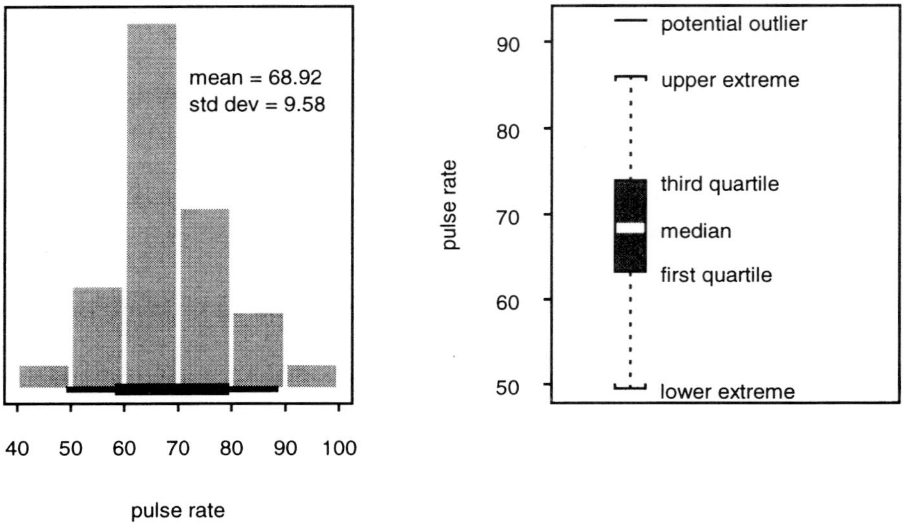

Figure 1 Illustration of descriptive analysis of pulse rates taken from 30 subjects. The left-hand panel shows a histogram, with the heavier horizontal line covering the interval corresponding to the mean ±1 standard deviation and the lighter line covering the mean ±2 standard deviations. The right-hand panel shows a box plot of same data

data followed the normal distribution exactly, one would expect approximately 69% of the distribution to lie within 1 standard deviation of the mean and 95% of the distribution to lie within 2 standard deviations of the mean. If one assumed that pulse rates in the population from which this sample was drawn follow the normal distribution characterized by parameters μ and σ, the observed data could be used to make inference about these parameters. The sample mean and standard deviation (SD) are said to be unbiased estimators of μ and σ, respectively. In statistical language, "unbiased" means that if one were to repeat the experiment an infinite number of times (in this case the experiment is the collection of pulse rates), the average of all the individual sample means would be exactly equal to μ. So even though the sample mean from any particular experiment may or may not be equal to μ, we can expect the sample mean to perform well over the long run. A 95% confidence interval for μ is given by

$$\text{mean} - 1.96\,\frac{\text{SD}}{\sqrt{n}} \text{ - } \text{mean} + 1.96\,\frac{\text{SD}}{\sqrt{n}},$$

where n is the sample size. The multiplier 1.96 is determined by the desired confidence level; a 99% confidence interval would use the multiplier 2.58. The expression, $\text{SD}/\sqrt{n}$, is also called the standard error of the mean (SEM). Unfortunately this is sometimes shortened to just "standard error," leading to confusion with the standard deviation. All other things being equal, the standard error of the mean gets smaller as the sample size gets larger. Thus, the confidence interval gets narrower as the sample size gets larger. Larger samples lead to more precise inference. The magnitude of the sample standard deviation on the other hand, does not depend on the sample size. This is because it is an estimator of the population standard deviation σ, which is irrespective of the sample size. A common misconception, due to the confusion between standard error and standard deviation, is that the sample standard deviation gets smaller as the sample size gets larger. The standard error of the mean is only useful for making inference about the population mean μ. The sample standard deviation is useful for making inference about the distribution of the population, at least in terms of the population standard deviation σ. In a descriptive analysis (an analysis describing the population from which the sample was drawn), it is appropriate to report the sample standard deviation, not the standard error of the mean.

The right-hand panel of Fig. 1 shows a box plot (also called a box-and-whisker plot) of the same data. The box delineates the middle 50% of the data points. That is, 25% of the data points lies below the first quartile and 25% lies above the third quartile. The difference between the third quartile and the first quartile is called the interquartile range (IQR) and is the height of the box. The horizontal line inside the box marks the median, the middle value in a sorted list of the data points. In this example the median is approximately in the middle of the box, but this need not be the case. Most box plot algorithms will identify individual data points that are unusual, compared with the rest of the data, as potential outliers (further discussion on outliers appears at the end of this section). The criteria for identifying outlying data points are based on the IQR. In this example points that lie more than 1.5IQR outside the box are flagged as potential outliers. The standard value of the multiplier is 1.5, but others can be used depending on the situation. The whiskers of the box plot extend out from the ends of the box to the smallest and largest data points, excluding any potential outliers. As a result of this exclusion, whiskers never extend more than 1.5IQR from the ends of the box. Box plots are more useful for identifying particular points in the underlying distribution and can be used with as few as 10 data points. Histograms are more useful for giving an overall impression of the shape of the underlying distribution and should only be used with at least 20 data points, preferably more than 30. The look of a histogram depends on the choice of cutpoints for the individual bars; most computer programs make this choice automatically, and the look of a histogram based on a small sample is extremely sensitive to this choice.

Figure 2 shows a descriptive analysis of a sample from another population. This sample displays right-skewness, meaning that the right-hand tail of the distribution is longer than the left. This can be seen clearly in both the histogram and the box plot. In the box plot, the median is closer to the bottom of the box than to the top, and the upper whisker is longer than the bottom. In the left-hand panel, the mean ±SD bars do not fit the histogram well, an indication that the data are not representative of a normal distribution. Another point to notice is that the median and mean are quite different from each other as compared to Fig. 1. The mean is larger than the median when the distribution is right-skewed. Distributions can also be left-skewed, in which case the mean is smaller than the median, but this is very rare for biomedical data.

A. Two-Group Comparison

In the two-group setting, the goal is to compare the distributions of some outcome measure in two different populations based on a given sample of observations from each population. In an observational study, group membership is determined by some inherent characteristic of the subjects (e.g., age, gender, race); in an intervention study, group membership is determined by the investigator (e.g., received either placebo or active treatment). Consider a controlled randomized clinical trial designed to assess the effect of preoperative treatment with a new drug on postoperative heart rate in hypertensive patients. In this hypothetical study, 40 patients were randomly assigned to receive either placebo or the new drug (20 in each group).

The appropriate statistical analysis for this data depends on the assumptions one is willing to make about the underlying distributions giving rise to the observed data. The two-sample *t* test is called a parametric analysis because it is based on the assumption that postoperative heart rates in each group follow the normal distribution and are characterized by group-specific parameters. In statistical language, it is said that postoperative heart rates are distributed normally with mean μ_P (μ_D) and standard deviation σ_P (σ_D) in the placebo (drug) populations. Statistical analysis allows inference about these parameters. In particular, the null hypothesis that the two means are equal versus the alternative that

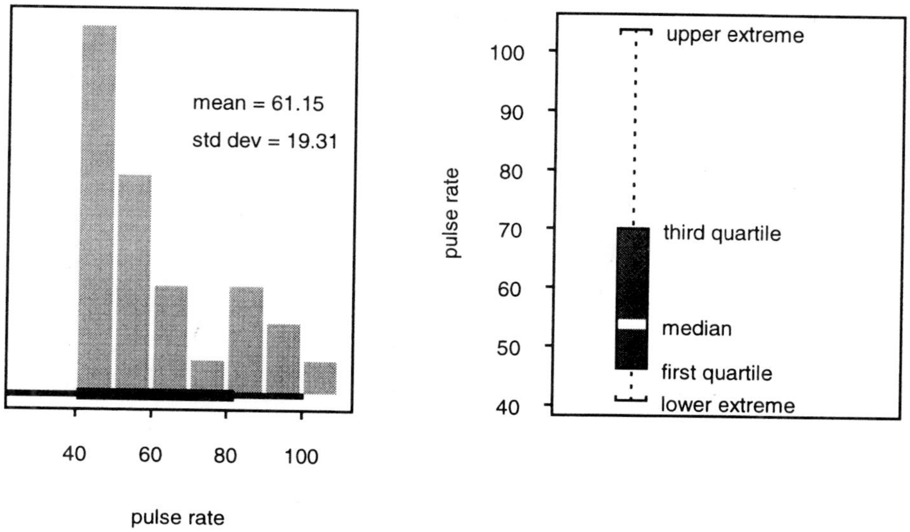

Figure 2 Illustration of descriptive analysis of right-skewed data. Note that the ends of the histogram are not symmetric about the mean (left-hand panel), the median is not in the center of the box (right-hand panel), and the mean is larger than the median.

they are not (H_0: $\mu_P = \mu_D$ versus H_a: $\mu_P \neq \mu_D$) is tested. This set of hypotheses is somewhat imprecise because it does not specify anything about σ_P or σ_D. More precise statements of the hypotheses would be either

$$H_0: \mu_P = \mu_D \text{ and } \sigma_P = \sigma_D \quad \text{versus}$$
$$H_a: \mu_P \neq \mu_D \text{ and } \sigma_P = \sigma_D$$

or

$$H_0: \mu_P = \mu_D \text{ and } \sigma_P > 0 \text{ and } \sigma_D > 0 \quad \text{versus}$$
$$H_a: \mu_P \neq \mu_D \text{ and } \sigma_P > 0 \text{ and } \sigma_D > 0.$$

These sets of hypotheses are illustrated in Fig. 3; the top two panels correspond to the first set of hypotheses and the bottom two panels correspond to the second. The appropriate statistical analysis is the equal variance two-sample *t* test for the first set of hypotheses and the unequal variance two-sample *t* test for the second. The equal variance *t* test is sometimes called the pooled variance *t* test, and the unequal variance *t* test is sometimes called the separate variance *t* test. Use of the term variance is somewhat unfortunate here, because the hypotheses are stated in terms of standard deviation. Variance is equal to standard deviation squared (σ^2), so equal standard deviation implies equal variance and vice versa. Unless otherwise stated, it is generally taken that the assumption is being made that $\sigma_P = \sigma_D$. Likewise, if the reported test is simply called the two-sample *t* test, it is assumed that the equal variance two-sample *t* test was used. Modern statistical software packages routinely report the *p* value associated with either of these tests and the numeric value of the *t* statistic alone is of little use. Because the true values of σ_P and σ_D are not generally known, the choice between the equal and unequal variance *t* tests is typically made empirically based on the sample standard deviations. A common rule of thumb is to use the unequal variance *t* test if the ratio of the larger standard deviation to the smaller is greater than 1.5. A conservative approach is to always use the unequal variance *t* test, regardless of the sample standard deviations. This approach is conservative in the event that σ_P

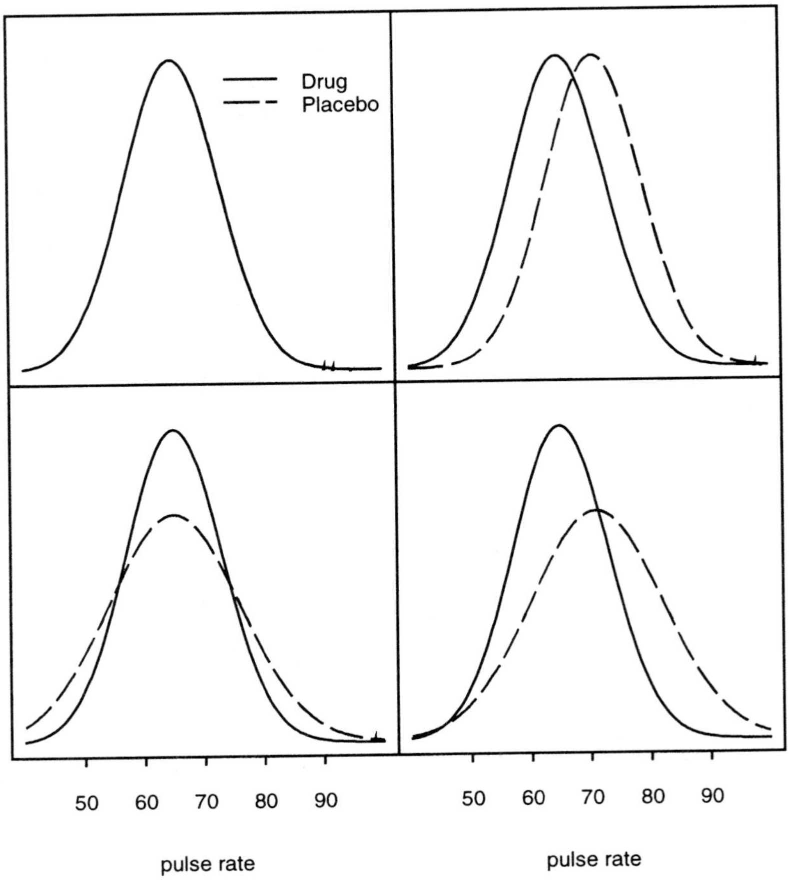

Figure 3 Illustration of alternative hypotheses associated with two-sample *t* test. The top panels (left and right, respectively) represent the null hypothesis of equal means with equal variances and the alternative hypothesis of unequal means with equal variances. The bottom panels (left and right, respectively) represent the null hypothesis of equal means with unequal variances and the alternative hypothesis of unequal means with unequal variances.

is in fact equal to σ_D because the unequal variance *t* test is less efficient than the equal variance *t* test, meaning that it has less power when the null hypothesis is false. The approach of always using the equal variance *t* test is not recommended, because it is anticonservative in the event that σ_P is not equal to σ_D. The term "anticonservative" means that the *p* value is estimated to be smaller than it actually is, potentially leading to erroneous rejection of the null hypothesis. A practical approach with modern software is to apply both tests. If both tests lead to rejection (or acceptance) of the null hypothesis, then it is immaterial what test is used. If the tests do not agree, this is usually because the variances are not equal and so the unequal variance test should be used. The two tests are generally more similar when the variances are equal than when they are not.

If one is unwilling to make specific assumptions about the form of the underlying distribution, the appropriate statistical analysis in the two-group comparison setting is the nonparametric Mann–Whitney test, also called the Wilcoxon Rank Sum test. This analysis is based on a test of the null hypothesis that the distributions of the two populations, although unspecified, are equal, versus the alternative hypothesis that the distributions have the same shape, but are shifted so that the outcomes of one population tend to be larger than the outcomes of the other. This is illustrated in Fig. 4. The alternative hypothesis for the Mann–Whitney test is sometimes written in terms of the population medians so that if the data support rejection of the null hypothesis, the conclusion is that the two populations have different medians. This is in contrast to the two-sample *t* test, which is a comparison of population means. A common misconception with the Mann–Whitney test is that it should be used when the variances are not equal. This is incorrect; unequal variances are not an indication to use the Mann–Whitney test. In fact, the Mann–Whitney test is designed to be used when the variances are equal; this is implied by the assumption that the distributions have the same shape.

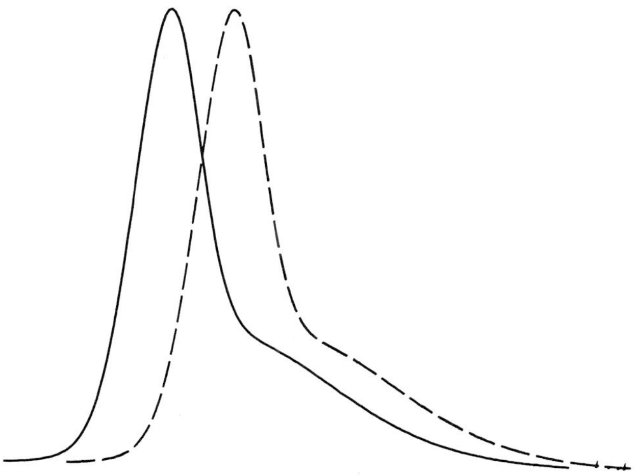

Figure 4 Illustration of two nonnormal distributions that have the same general shape, but are offset so that measurements from one population (dashed line) tend to be larger than measurements from the other (solid line).

As with the decision to use the equal or unequal variance *t* tests, a similar decision must be made between using the parametric *t* test (in either form) or the nonparametric Mann–Whitney test, often empirically. Ideally, one would use a statistical analysis that is optimal for the problem at hand. The Mann–Whitney test is optimal for the setting in which the two populations have arbitrary distributions (not necessarily normal), essentially the most general setting possible. The *t* test is optimal for the setting in which the two populations follow the normal distribution exactly, a special case of the general setting. Unfortunately it is never known for certain whether the normal model holds, although often the observed data can provide evidence as to the plausibility of the normal model.

An instructive approach to this problem is to consider the consequences of using the "wrong" test in each possible setting. If the populations do follow the normal distribution, the only consequence of using the Mann–Whitney test is that it is conservative or inefficient (has less power) relative to the optimal *t* test. This means that if the null hypothesis were false, the type II error rate for the Mann–Whitney test would be higher than it would be for the *t* test (for a discussion of type I and type II error rates, see Chapter 9). On the other hand, if the populations do not follow the normal distribution, the possible consequences of using the *t* test are that the *p* value could be either too large (conservative) or too small (anticonservative), depending on the nature of the deviation from normal. At first it might seem that the Mann–Whitney test should always be used, particularly because anticonservatism is generally considered to be more problematic than conservatism. That is, it is often considered worse to conclude that there is a group difference when there actually is not, compared to concluding that there is not a group difference when there actually is. The salvation of the *t* test however, is its "robustness" to minor departures from normality, which grows stronger with larger sample sizes. Robustness is a statistical term for the extent to which the behavior of a test is preserved even when the assumptions underlying the test are violated. For small samples (less than 15 per group), the *t* test is fairly robust, in terms of anticonservatism, against nonnormality as long as the distributions are reasonably symmetric (not heavily skewed in one direction or the other; see Fig. 2). For moderate and large samples (greater than 15 per group), the *t* test is fairly robust, in terms of anticonservatism, against nonnormality, including skewness. Therefore, at least for large samples, the choice between applying the Mann–Whitney or *t* tests appears somewhat arbitrary. In practice the Mann–Whitney test and *t* test rarely give different answers for large sample sizes, unless there is gross departure from normality in the data. (Possible causes for gross departures from normality will be discussed in the section on pitfalls.) For small sample sizes, on the other hand, there can be important practical differences between the two tests. Choosing the correct test is more critical. Unfortunately, when the sample size is small, there is little direct evidence available for determining whether the normal model is plausible. The conservative approach is to use the Mann–Whitney test because it is never anticonservative. When the normal model does hold, however, the inefficiency of the Mann–Whitney test can be substantial for small samples.

B. Comparing More Than Two Groups

A hypothetical study might have been designed to assess the dose–response effect of preoperative treatment with a new drug on postoperative heart rate in hypertensive patients. In this case, 80 patients might have been randomly assigned to receive either placebo or one of three doses of the new drug (20 in each group). As before, the appropriate statistical analysis for these data depends on the assumptions one is willing to make about the underlying distributions. From a methodological point of view, however, extending to compare more than two groups is relatively straightforward. The multigroup extension of the two-sample t test is analysis of variance (ANOVA), and the Kruskal–Wallis test is the multigroup extension of the nonparametric Mann–Whitney test. The considerations for deciding to use ANOVA or the Kruskal–Wallis test are the same as those for the decision to use the two-sample t test or the Mann–Whitney test. Like the two-sample t test, ANOVA is fairly robust to moderate regarding departures from normality, especially when the sample size is large. Unless otherwise specified, ANOVA is generally taken to be equal variance ANOVA. There are multigroup extensions of the unequal variance two-sample t test (e.g., Welch test and Brown–Forsythe test), but these are not available in the majority of statistical software packages. It may be hoped that these tests will be included in all statistical software packages in the future. ANOVA is susceptible to anticonservatism when the population variances are not equal, just as the equal variance t test is.

From the practical point of view, a shortcoming of ANOVA (and Kruskal–Wallis) is the omnibus nature of the null hypothesis being tested:

$$H_0\colon \quad \mu_1 = \mu_2 = \mu_3 = \cdots = \mu_G$$

versus

$$H_a\colon \quad \text{at least one } \mu \text{ not equal to the others.}$$

The term omnibus means that the ANOVA null hypothesis includes more than one "simple" hypothesis, $\mu_1 = \mu_2$, $\mu_2 = \mu_3$, $\mu_1 = \mu_3$, etc. Rejection of the null hypothesis generally does not provide a complete answer to the research question, What is the nature of the differences between the populations: are they all different from each other, or just some of them? Answering these questions requires further analysis. If the null hypothesis is not rejected, then these additional questions need not be asked. This further analysis is sometimes called a post-hoc analysis because it is done only after the ANOVA (or Kruskal–Wallis), depending on whether the omnibus null hypothesis was rejected. A naive approach to this would be to perform all possible two-sample t tests (or Mann–Whitney tests) to compare each population with all the others one pair at a time. If there are G groups, then there are $G[(G - 1)/2]$ possible pairwise comparisons to be made. For example, if there are five groups (call them A, B, C, D, and E), then there $5(4/2) = 10$ possible pairs (AB, AC, AD, AE, BC, BD, BE, CD, CE, DE).

The major drawback of this approach is the so-called multiplicity of testing problem. If each statistical test has a type I error rate of say 5%, then what is the probability of making one or more type I errors in a series of tests? The answer depends on how many tests are performed and the amount of dependence that exists between the tests. The probability of making one or more type I errors is sometimes called the overall type I error rate, or the experimentwise type I error rate. It is a mathematical result that if all of the tests are independent (i.e., the results of one are unrelated to the results of another), then the overall type I error rate in a series of K tests is $1 - (1 - \alpha)^K$, where α is the type I error rate of each individual test. This expression is approximately equal to $K\alpha$ when α is small, as it usually is, so that the overall type I error rate is approximately equal to $K\alpha$. In other words, the more tests performed, the higher the overall type I error rate. It is intuitively sensible that the more decisions one makes, the more likely it is that one or more errors will be made. When dependence exists between the tests, the overall type I error rate will be less than $K\alpha$. Consider the case in which there is complete dependence between the tests, i.e., all tests give exactly the same result; in this case the overall type I error rate is simple α, the type I error rate for any one of the tests.

Pairwise tests are not independent in the multigroup setting because data from each group appear in more than one test (e.g., the data from group 3 appear in both the test of $\mu_1 = \mu_3$ and $\mu_2 = \mu_3$). Therefore, without knowing exactly how much dependence exists between the tests, the only guarantee is that the overall type I error rate is no greater than $K\alpha$. Even so, there is substantial potential for high overall type I error rates even with moderately sized multigroup designs. For example, with four groups there are $4(3/2) = 6$ possible comparisons. If each pairwise comparison were made at the $\alpha = 0.05$ significance level, the overall type I error rate could be as high as 30% [6(0.05)]. The obvious solution for controlling the overall type I error rate is to reduce α for each of the pairwise comparisons. That is, if the significance level of each pairwise comparison is set at α/K, then the overall type I error rate will be no greater than $K(\alpha/K) = \alpha$. So with four groups and six pairwise comparisons, setting the significance level for each comparison at $0.0083 = 0.05/6$ ensures that the overall type I error rate will not exceed 0.05. This approach is known as the Bonferroni method of multiple comparison adjustment. The major problem with the Bonferroni method is that it becomes overly conservative as the number of groups increases, because the amount of dependence between the tests increases as the number of groups increases. By overly conservative, it is meant that the type II error rate will be larger than necessary due to the fact that the true type I error is smaller than 0.05. The Bonferroni method simply guarantees that the overall type I error rate will be less than 0.05, but it does not control how much less than 0.05.

There are a number of other less conservative methods of adjusting for multiple comparisons that are much more technically complex than Bonferroni, such as the Tukey, Dunnett, Student–Newman–Keuls, and Duncan methods. An historical advantage of the Bonferroni method was its simplicity, but most modern statistical software packages that include ANOVA are capable of performing several different post-hoc multiple-comparison procedures. It must be noted that although all of these methods are less conservative than Bonferroni, not all of them fully control the overall type I error rate. The Dunnett procedure is optimized for the special case of comparing multiple treatment groups to a single control group, but does not allow for comparisons between treatment groups. The Student–Newman–Keuls and Duncan methods partially control the overall type I error rate, but do not ensure that it will not exceed α in all cases and therefore cannot be recommended. The recommended method is the Tukey procedure, which controls the overall type I error rate completely and is less conservative than Bonferroni.

Although the Bonferroni approach is not optimal in the ANOVA setting, it is very useful in other settings. It is important to note that with the exception of the Bonferroni method, these other procedures can only be used in the ANOVA setting. They cannot be used in conjunction with the nonparametric Kruskal–Wallis test. Multiple-comparison adjustment for post-hoc analysis in the nonparametric setting can be made using the Bonferroni method. Most statistical software packages do not do this analysis automatically, so the user must specify the two-sample Mann–Whitney test for each of the various pairwise comparisons and manually adjust the α level of each test to control the overall type I error rate.

C. Repeated Measures

Often measurements of a particular variable in clinical research are taken multiple times on the same subject. In the example study above, the investigators might have measured patient heart rate preoperatively and at various times intraoperatively in addition to the postoperative measurement. This design would allow for an assessment of the within-group effects of the new drug. The original design allowed only for an assessment of the between-group effect of the drug. One advantage of the repeated-measures design, in addition to providing information about intraoperative heart rate, is that in many cases within-subject variability is smaller than between-subject variability, so a smaller sample can be used without sacrificing power. Within-subject variability is the degree to which the outcome, in this case heart rate, varies over time in the same subject, whereas between-subject variability is the degree to which the outcome varies across subjects in the population being studied.

The most simple repeated-measures design (also called the paired design) is one in which all subjects receive the treatment and the outcome is measured both before and after the treatment is given. In this case, the total number of data points is $2N$, where N is the number of subjects. The total number of independently sampled experimental units (subjects) is N. One could use the two-sample t test or Mann–Whitney test to analyze these data: the first group would be the pretreatment measures and the second group would be the posttreatment measures. However, this analysis violates one of the assumptions of the two-group t test, that all of the observations were independently collected. Because of this violation, the two-sample t test can be anticonservative. The appropriate analysis is the paired t test. The null hypothesis being tested by the paired t test is that the population outcome mean is the same at each time point. The nonparametric analog of the paired t test is the Wilcoxon Signed Rank test, which should be used if the data do not follow the normal distribution. Like the two-sample t test, the paired t test is relatively robust to nonnormality, especially for large sample sizes. Both of these tests are available in most modern statistical software packages.

Just as ANOVA is the multigroup extension of the two-sample t test, repeated-measures ANOVA is the multimeasurement extension of the paired t test. This analysis is appropriate for the situation in which all subjects receive the same treatment(s) and are evaluated at more than two time points. As with ANOVA, repeated-measures ANOVA is testing the omnibus null hypothesis that the population outcome means are the same at all time points (e.g., H_0: $\mu_1 = \mu_2 = \mu_3 = \ldots = \mu_T$, where T is total number of time points). If this hypothesis is rejected, then it may be desirable to perform a post-hoc analysis to determine at which time points the population means differ. The Tukey method for multiple comparisons can be used in the repeated-measures setting. The nonparametric analog of repeated-measures ANOVA is called the Freidman test. As with the Kruskal–Wallis test, multiple-comparison adjustment for post-hoc analysis with the Freidman test can only be made using the Bonferroni method. Because software packages do not do this analysis automatically, the user must specify the Wilcoxon Signed

Rank test for each of the various pairwise comparisons and manually adjust the α level of each test to control the overall type I error rate.

One drawback of the repeated-measures design is that the treatment effect is confounded with the time effect, meaning that their individual effects cannot be separated. The time effect is the difference in the population mean outcomes across time points that is not due to the treatment. For example, in the hypothetical heart rate study above, the difference between preoperative and postoperative heart rate might be partially due to the operation and partially due to the drug. In this case the portion of the change in heart rate due to the drug cannot be estimated. A placebo-controlled repeated-measures design would allow estimation of both the treatment effect (in this case the drug) and the time effect (in this case the surgery). Under this design, half the subjects are randomized to receive placebo and half to receive the drug. The heart rate of all patients is measured both preoperatively and postoperatively. The difference between pre- and postoperative heart rates in the placebo group is due entirely to the surgery, whereas the difference between pre- and postoperative heart rates in the drug group is due to the combination of drug and surgery. The effect of the drug can therefore be estimated by the difference between the change in heart rate in the drug group and the change in heart rate in the placebo group. The appropriate analysis for this design is mixed-effects ANOVA. It is referred to as mixed because it is a combination of ordinary ANOVA and repeated-measures ANOVA. The time effect is a within-group effect and the drug effect is a between-group effect. The Tukey method for multiple comparisons should be used for post-hoc analysis in the mixed setting.

There is no nonparametric analog for mixed-effects ANOVA with more than two time points. When there are only two time points, it is appropriate to calculate the individual differences between the two measurements for each subject, rendering one observation per subject (the difference score), and allowing the Kruskal–Wallis test (or Mann–Whitney test if there are only two groups) to be used to test for significance of the treatment effect.

D. Data Transformation and Outliers

The previous discussion has been presented as if the only option is to use a nonparametric analysis when the data do not support the assumption that the normal distribution model is correct. Another possibility is to use a different parametric analysis, one that is not based on the normal distribution. Statistical methods have been developed for models based on, among others, the log-normal, gamma, and weibull distributions. Many of these approaches are relatively recent methodologic advancements made possible only by the advent of superfast computers and have not yet become part of the standard statistical software package.

Instead of changing the model in order to fit the data, another approach is to change the data so that they fit the model. For example, if the data appear to be incompatible with the normal distribution model because of heavy right-skewness, applying a logarithmic transformation may alleviate that problem. Investigators are often hesitant to apply data transformations because they fear that this may be seen as massaging the data in order to manufacture a result or because they believe it will be difficult to interpret any results that are based on transformed data. Data transformation can be used to massage data in order to manufacture a result, but a careful analysis need not be left open to this criticism. The appropriate approach is to choose the transformation based solely on the grounds of meeting distribution assumptions before any analyses are undertaken. An inappropriate approach would be to repeat the analysis on both the transformed and raw data and then choose which one to report based on the results. The problem of interpreting results after data transformation is not easily resolved. If the audience is expecting to see heart rate data presented in beats per minute, the confusion caused by reporting results for log (beats per minute) may outweigh the benefits of meeting the distributional assumptions for the two-sample t test. In the future this problem may be solved by the availability of parametric analyses based on distributions other than normal.

Another common feature of observed data that can cause problems for parametric analyses is the presence of outliers or influential data points. An outlier is an observation that does not follow the pattern of the majority of the data. An influential data point is an observation that unduly influences the results of a parametric analysis. For example, if the p value for a two-sample t test is 0.002 for the complete data and 0.31 when one observation is omitted from the analysis, that observation is highly influential. All influential data points are outliers, but not all outliers are influential. An outlier is much more likely to be influential when the sample size is small than when it is large, because a large sample dilutes the effect of individual data points. Outliers can creep into the data in several ways. If the underlying distribution is highly skewed and the sample size is small, one may observe one or two data points that are disparate from the bulk of the sample. Holes in the sample selection criteria (eligibility criteria) may allow subjects who are not really part of the population of interest to be included in the study. These subjects may be very different from the population of interest. Random measurement errors and/or data recording errors can also lead to the presence of outliers. Outliers that are the result of the last two processes can be appropriately omitted from the analysis if the occasion can be documented. That is, one may leave it out of the data to be analyzed. This action is justified by the fact that the true value of the data point was unobservable and the recorded value is completely uninformative. This is not to say that such cases need not be reported, but they must be carefully documented. A large number of such outliers in a data set may indicate that any analyses should be interpreted with caution. Outliers that cannot be otherwise explained must be assumed to be due to some aspect of the underlying distribution (e.g., heterogeneity or skewness). A parametric analysis may be appropriate even in the presence of outliers if they are not highly influential (e.g., when the sample is large). Influential data points that cannot be justifiably omitted from the analysis are an indication to use a nonparametric procedure.

III. Categorical Data

The defining characteristic of categorical data is that either there is no scale underlying the observed data, or that if there is a scale, it does not permit mathematical operations that preserve the scale. Categorical data of the first type are referred to as nominal, and data of the second type as ordinal. Examples of nominal data are gender, race, medication preference, etc. Examples of ordinal data might be subjective scores such as pain sensation, level of agreement, level of discomfort, etc. A descriptive analysis of categorical data typically includes frequency tables, either numeric or graphical.

It is often difficult to distinguish between ordinal data and continuous data, particularly because ordinal data are often collected numerically. For example, an investigator may ask: "On a scale from one to ten, how uncomfortable are you?" Clearly there is a scale underlying these data, but the issue is whether this scale permits mathematical operations that preserve the scale. One might ask if the difference between a response of 2 versus 3 is the same as the difference between a response of 7 versus 8. Another way of addressing the issue is to consider if it makes sense to calculate a mean (across subjects) for this outcome. If the answer is yes, then the data should be treated as continuous. If the answer is no or uncertain, then the data should be treated as ordinal.

A. Two-Group Comparison

As with continuous data, in the two-group setting the goal is to compare the relative frequencies of some outcome measure in two different populations based on a sample of observations from each population. Consider a controlled randomized clinical trial designed to assess the effect of preoperative treatment with a new drug on preventing postoperative atrial fibrillation (AF) in hypertensive patients. The outcome is clearly nominal in this case. The subject either did or did not experience AF postoperatively. In this setting, the data can be completely summarized in 2 × 2 tables:

Postoperative AF	Group			Postoperative AF	Group	
	Drug	Control	Total		Drug	Control
Yes	1	6	7	Yes	π_D	π_C
No	39	34	73	No	$1 - \pi_D$	$1 - \pi_C$
Total	40	40	80			

The left-hand side shows the observed data and the right-hand side shows the parameters that characterize the population from which the sample was taken; π_D and π_C represent the probability of postoperative AF in the drug and control groups, respectively. The null hypothesis to be tested in the 2 × 2 table is that of no drug effect, H_0: $\pi_D = \pi_C$, versus the alternative that they are not equal. The appropriate statistical analysis for these data is either the Pearson chi-square test or Fisher's exact test. The decision regarding which test to use depends on the number of observations in each cell of the observed table. Fisher's exact test should be used for sparse tables, if the product of the smallest row total and smallest column total is less than 5 times the total number of observations. In this case the product of the smallest row and column totals is $7(40) = 280$ and $5(80) = 400$, so Fisher's exact test should be used. For nonsparse tables Pearson's chi-square test should be used. It is not appropriate to use Pearson's chi-square test for sparse tables and most good computer packages will warn the user when sparseness is a problem. Fisher's exact test can be used for nonsparse tables, but because of the way the test statistic is calculated computer packages may have problems with insufficient computer memory if asked to perform this test with a large table.

These methods can also be used to test for group differences when there are more than two possible outcomes. For example, the outcome in the above trial might have been recorded with four possible values: (1) experienced AF intraoperatively, but not postoperatively, (2) experienced AF postoperatively, but not intraoperatively, (3) experienced AF both intraoperatively and postoperatively, or (4) did not experience AF at any time. These data are summarized in the left-hand 4 × 2 group below.

AF	Group			Group	
	Drug	Control	Total	Drug	Control
Intraoperative	5	12	17	π_{ID}	π_{IC}
Postoperative	1	4	5	π_{PD}	π_{PC}
Both	0	2	2	π_{BD}	π_{BC}
No	34	22	56	$1 - \pi_{ID} - \pi_{PD} - \pi_{BD}$	$1 - \pi_{IC} - \pi_{PC} - \pi_{BC}$
Total	40	40	80		

More parameters are required to characterize the underlying population: π_{ID} is probability of intraoperative AF, π_{PD} is the probability of postoperative AF, and π_{BD} is the probability of both intra- and postoperative AF. The null hypothesis to be tested is that the frequency pattern (the probability of a patient experiencing each of the four possible outcomes) is the same for both groups, i.e., no drug effect. This is an omnibus null hypothesis of the form:

$$H_0\colon\ \pi_{ID} = \pi_{IC} \ \text{ and } \ \pi_{PD} = \pi_{PC} \ \text{ and } \ \pi_{BD} = \pi_{BC}$$

versus

$$H_a\colon\ \pi_{ID} \neq \pi_{IC} \ \text{ and/or } \ \pi_{PD} \neq \pi_{PC} \ \text{ and/or } \ \pi_{BD} \neq \pi_{BC}.$$

The same guidelines for determining sparseness and deciding which test to use in the 2 × 2 table apply here. Rejection of the null hypothesis implies a group difference in the pattern of the outcomes, but does not specify nature of that difference with respect to specific outcomes. By collapsing across rows in the observed table, one can create 2 × 2 subtables that can be used to test specific hypotheses. The previous 2 × 2 table is a subtable of the 4 × 2 table, created by collapsing the row labeled "Postoperative" with the row labeled "Both" and collapsing the row labeled "Intraoperative" with the row labeled "No." One could also test for a drug effect on any AF event by collapsing the three rows labeled "Post-operative," "Intraoperative," and "Both." The Bonferroni method can be used to control the overall type I error rate if multiple post-hoc tests are performed.

B. Comparison of More Than Two Groups

The Pearson chi-square test and Fisher's exact test can also be applied when more than two groups are to be compared, with the same guidelines for determining sparseness. Consider a study designed to compare C different populations with respect to a binary (yes/no) outcome. Data from such a study are summarized in a $2 \times C$ table in which there are two rows for the outcomes and C columns for the groups. The null hypothesis to be tested in the $2 \times C$ table is that the probability of a patient experiencing the outcome of interest is the same for all C of the populations. If this omnibus null hypothesis is rejected, it may be desirable to perform post-hoc analyses to determine which groups differ. This can be accomplished by testing for differences in 2 × 2 subtables created by considering only two columns at a time. The only form of multiple-comparisons adjustment available for this analysis is the Bonferroni method, in which a total of $C[(C - 1)/2]$ possible groupwise comparisons can be made. Most statistical software packages will not do this analysis automatically; the user must manually construct 2 × 2 tables for each of the various pairwise comparisons and adjust the α level of each test to control the overall type I error rate.

The most general setting for categorical data when there are R nominal outcomes and C groups to be compared is called the $R \times C$ table in which there are R rows for the outcomes and C columns for the groups. The null hypothesis to be tested in the $R \times C$ table is that the frequency pattern (the probability of a patient experiencing each of the R possible outcomes) is same for all C of the populations. As with the $2 \times C$ table, it may be desirable to perform post-hoc analyses if the omnibus null hypothesis is rejected. As above, this can be accomplished by collapsing rows and eliminating columns to create 2 × 2 subtables corresponding to specific hypothesis tests.

IV. Survival Data

The term "survival data" is generally used to refer to any data measuring the time until some event occurs. In clinical research the event is often death, but can also be disease recurrence, transplant or graft rejection, discharge from hospital, or resolution of infection, for example. A complication of studying these outcomes is that in some patients the study might end before the event occurs, or some other terminating event (such as death or loss to follow-up) might occur before the event of interest occurs. In this case the observation is "censored" because it was not possible to completely see the outcome of interest. An important assumption here is that the event would have occurred in all subjects if they had been followed over a long enough period of time. Censored data are not the same as missing data because there is partial information on the outcome of interest. For example, in a study of cancer patients, the population of interest might be all those patients who were successfully treated for breast cancer by surgical resection and the event of interest might be cancer recurrence. After surgery the subject leaves the hospital and is followed-up with on a regular basis. However, a subject might move out of the area 2 years later and be lost to follow-up. In this case, the subject is known to be free from cancer 2 years after surgery. All of the statistical methods for analyzing survival data are based on the assumption that censoring, when it occurs, is independent of the event of interest. This assumption is not always easy to confirm. At first it might seem obvious that a subject's decision to move out of the area would be independent of a medical outcome, but it is relatively easy to devise a scenario in which this is not the case. For example, in a study of the elderly the event of interest might be second hip fracture in the population who just had their first hip fracture. More frail subjects might be more likely to move to a retirement facility than would less frail subjects. These subjects would probably also be more likely to suffer a second fracture compared to the others. This scenario would indicate dependence between the censoring mechanism (moving away) and the outcome, because some of those who move away would be more likely to have the event in the near future than those who did not move away. Dependence between censoring and the event is also difficult to detect because there is often more than one censoring mechanism at work.

Unlike continuous data, which can be graphically displayed by histogram or box plot, survival data are typically summarized with a Kaplan–Meier plot of the estimated survival function, which is the probability of surviving (the event not yet occurring) at any given time. Figure 5 displays the estimated survival function from a study comparing the effects of careful preoperative nutritional maintenance on length of postoperative intensive care unit (ICU) stay following renal transplant. The starting point for the survival curve is 100% survival at time zero, i.e., the event cannot occur before the clock starts. Moving from left to right, the survival curve decreases at each observed event time. Censoring times (last observed follow-up for subjects who are censored) are typically indicated by marks (vertical lines or x's) on the survival curve. The estimated survival curve may or may not reach zero at the last observed time point, depending on whether the last observation time is the event of interest (Fig. 5, solid line) or a censoring time (dashed line).

Comparing Groups

Often in trials in which the outcome of interest is the time to an event, the goal is to compare two or more groups. The null hypothesis of interest is that the survival functions are the same for all groups. A typical analysis would use the Kaplan–Meier method to estimate a survival curve for each group and then test the null hypothesis of no group difference using the log-rank test. Most statistical packages will provide the estimates for the survival curve based on the Kaplan–Meier method and the log-rank test in one step. The log-rank test compares the survival curves across the entire time of follow-up. If, *a priori*, one expects the differences to be more evident early in the follow-up, a Wilcoxon test can be used instead. The Wilcoxon test is similar to the log-rank test, but weights the early portion of the follow-up more heavily than the later. It is not appropriate to perform both tests and then decide which to present without using a Bonferroni correction. These methods are robust against fairly heavy censoring (a large fraction of censored observations), particularly if most of the censoring occurs after the observed events. However, they can be very sensitive to dependence between censoring and the event of interest. If there is no censoring, each event time is observed, the data can be treated as continuous and analyzed using the methods discussed above. This should be done with caution because event time data are typically right-skewed and very rarely follow the normal distribution.

V. Correlation

The methods described to this point are appropriate for descriptive analysis and groupwise comparisons of a single-outcome variable. Many important research questions pertain to relationships between two different outcomes, e.g., length of surgery and postoperative pain, muscle strength and cardiomyopathy, or length of time on treadmill and oxygen consumption. The purpose of a statistical correlation analysis is to quantify the relationship between two continuous variables. There is a subtle distinction between everyday

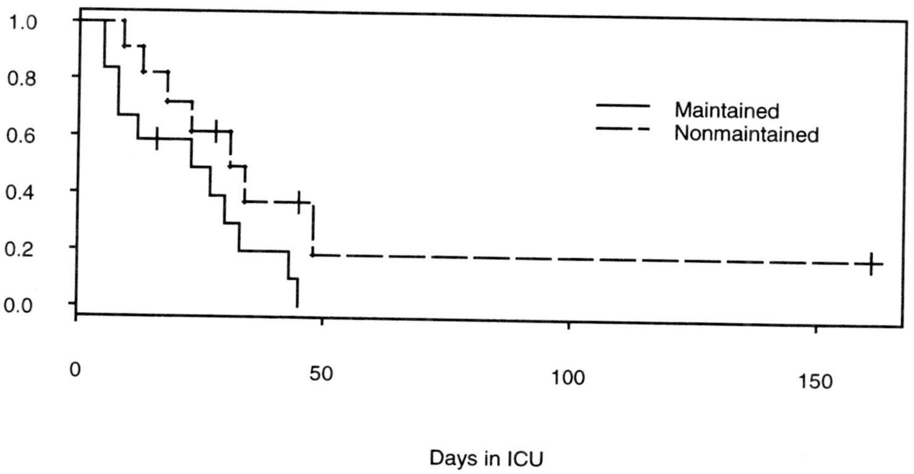

Figure 5 Illustration of Kaplan–Meier survival curves using data from a study comparing the effects of careful preoperative nutritional maintenance (solid line) versus control (dashed line) on length of postoperative ICU stay following renal transplant. Censored observations are denoted with a vertical bar. Note that the survival curve for the control group does not reach zero because the length of ICU stay for the last surviving person was censored.

use of the word "correlation" and its technical definition in statistics. Webster defines correlation quite generally as a "mutual relationship or connection," whereas the statistical correlation coefficient is a measure of the linear relationship. This distinction is demonstrated in Fig. 6. The correlation coefficient can be appropriately used to quantify the association displayed in the left-hand panel because the relationship between the two variables is reasonably described by a straight line. A correlation analysis is not appropriate for the data in the right-hand panel because, although there is clearly a relationship between the two variables, it cannot be reasonably described by a straight line. The first task in any correlation analysis is to plot the data and visually assess the appropriateness of describing the data with a straight line. The correlation coefficient alone is not sufficient to judge the presence or absence of relationships between variables.

The Pearson correlation coefficient (typically denoted r) ranges between -1 and $+1$, with negative values corresponding to a negative relationship, positive values to a positive relationship, and zero to no relationship. The farther the correlation is from zero (in either direction), the stronger the relationship. The numeric value of r does not have a direct interpretation. The square of the correlation coefficient, r^2 (also called the coefficient of determination), does have the direct interpretation as the proportion of the variability in one of the variables that can be explained by the other variable. Thus, a correlation of 0.7 corresponds to an r^2 of approximately 0.5, meaning that 50% of the variation in one variable is accounted for by its association with the other. Hypothesis testing of correlation coefficients is generally done with respect to the null hypothesis of zero correlation: H_0: r = 0 versus H_a: r ≠ 0, where the parameter r is the correlation in the underlying population. The correlation p value printed by default in most software packages corresponds to this test and is based on the value of r and the sample size. The nonparametric analog to the Pearson correlation is the Spearman correlation (r_S) and is also available in most software packages.

A common pitfall in correlation analysis is the possibility for spurious results due to a single outlier. The potential for an outlier to be highly influential in correlation analysis is much greater than for the analyses discussed above. The effect a single outlier can have is demonstrated in Fig. 7. The left-hand panel shows a scenario whereby one observation causes the Pearson correlation to be much larger than the Spearman correlation; the right-hand panel shows a scenario whereby one observation causes the Pearson correlation to be much smaller than the Spearman correlation. The dotted lines demonstrate that the outlier skews the Pearson correlation away from the underlying relationship of the rest of the data. In both cases, the Spearman correlation is a better reflection of the strength of the relationship because it is robust with respect to the effects of observations that are highly influential on the Pearson correlation. A reasonable approach to the detection of this type of problem is to calculate both the Pearson and Spearman correlations and check for discrepancy.

Correlation analysis is one area where the potential for obtaining statistically significant results that are scientifically irrelevant should be remembered. For example, the p value for a correlation coefficient of 0.2 based on a sample of size 100 is 0.048, statistically significant at the 0.05 level. The corresponding r^2 value is 0.04, however, meaning that only 4% of the variation in either variable is accounted for by the relationship. The problem illustrated by this example is that the null hypothesis being tested does not match the scientific question at hand. The clinically relevant question is whether there is a moderate or strong correlation, not whether there is any nonzero correlation. The confidence

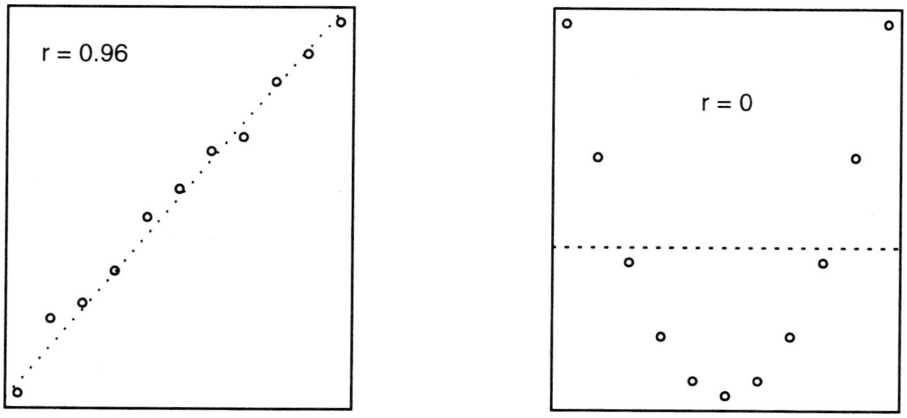

Figure 6 Illustration of correlation analysis. The data in the left-hand panel exhibit a strong linear relationship and the correlation coefficient is close to 1. The data in the right-hand panel exhibit a strong quadratic relationship but the correlation coefficient is 0. Zero correlation does not imply that there is no relationship.

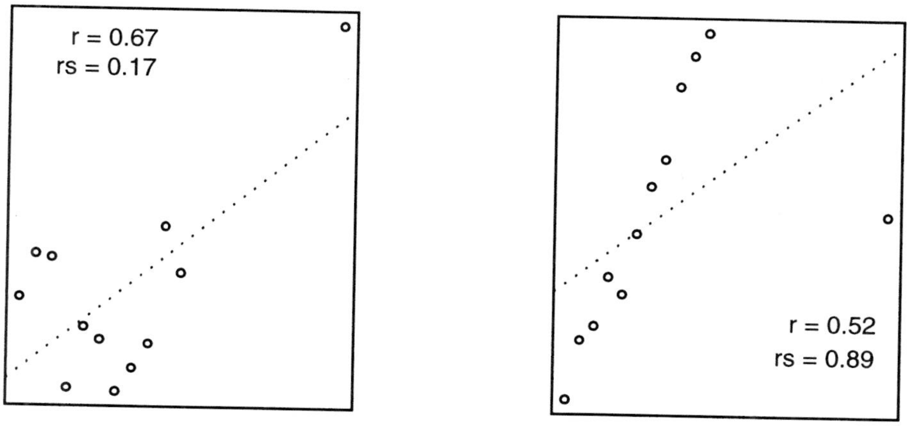

Figure 7 Illustration of the sensitivity of the Pearson correlation coefficient to outliers. In the left-hand panel a single outlier (top right) results in a relatively high Pearson correlation coefficient (0.67), even though the rest of the data do not exhibit a strong relationship. In the right-hand panel a single outlier (middle right) results in a modest Pearson correlation coefficient (0.52), even though the rest of the data exhibit a very strong relationship. In both cases the Spearman correlation coefficient (rs) more accurately reflects the strength of the relationship.

interval approach is more appropriate for reporting the results of a correlation analysis.

VI. Summary

In this chapter, specific statistical tests and the indications for their use have been described with simple examples. Where important, mathematical derivations, again in their simplest terms, were provided for the edification of the reader. The groundwork was established using the fact that it is the null hypothesis that is being evaluated by statistical tests. An attempt has been made to simplify the concepts of confidence intervals, standard error of the mean, and standard deviation using examples. An understanding of these principles is essential if conclusions are to accurately reflect the data. The investigator must be able to assess whether her/his data are normally distributed. If they are, a parametric analysis is appropriate, if not, a nonparametric analysis should be used. The importance of repeated measures and understanding when there may be dependence between observations is emphasized. The reader is cautioned that the number of subjects does not equal the number of observations when there are repeated measures, and that this dependence must be appropriately accounted for. The validity of data transformation was discussed, as was the issue of "outliers." Finally, principles for analyzing survival data, such as the Kaplan–Meier method, were carefully outlined and the pitfalls exposed. The authors anticipate that the citations listed at the end of this chapter will assist the investigator in applying the principles that have been discussed.

References

Altman, D. G. (1991). "Practical Statistics For Medical Research." Chapman & Hall, London.

Bland, M. (1995). "An Introduction To Medical Statistics," 2nd Ed. Oxford University Press, London.

Bowers, D. (1996). "Statistics from Scratch: An Introduction for Health Care Professionals." John Wiley & Sons, New York.

Campbell, M. J., and Machin, D. (1993). "Medical Statistics: A Commonsense Approach," 2nd Ed. John Wiley & Sons, New York.

Clarke, G. M. (1994). "Statistics and Experimental Design." Edward Arnold, London.

Dunn, G., and Everitt, B. (1995). "Clinical Biostatistics: An Introduction to Evidence Based Medicine." Edward Arnold, London.

Fisher, L. D., and Van Belle, G. (1993). "Biostatistics: A Methodology For The Health Sciences." John Wiley & Sons, Inc., New York.

Freidman, L. M., Furberg, C. D., and DeMets, D. L. (1998). "Fundamentals of Clinical Trials," 3rd Ed. Springer-Verlag, New York.

Gonick, L., and Smith, W. (1993). "The Cartoon Guide to Statistics." Harper Perennial, New York.

Katz, M. H. (1999). "Multivariable Analysis: A Practical Guide for Clinicians." Cambridge University Press, New York.

Pocock, S. J. (1983). "Clinical Trials: A Practical Approach." John Wiley & Sons, New York.

Wassertheil-Smoller, S. (1995). "Biostatistics and Epidemiology: A Primer For Health Professionals," 2nd Ed. Springer-Verlag, New York.

Woolson, R. F. (1987). "Statistical Methods for the Analysis of Biomedical Data." John Wiley & Sons, New York.

83

Data Presentation: How to Write and Submit Abstracts and Papers

Nancy R. Ehrlich* and Patricia A. Sheiner*,†

*The Recanati/Miller Transplantation Institute and †The Mount Sinai School of Medicine, New York, New York 10029

I. Introduction

Writing can seem overwhelmingly difficult. Physicians who would efficiently manage the bloodiest emergencies can be frozen into inaction by a blank piece of paper or a blank computer screen. Even for some of the clearest thinkers and most innovative researchers, language barriers or lack of writing experience make the written organization of experimental results a daunting task.

In "How to Write, Speak and Think More Effectively," Rudolph Flesch (1) tells his readers that the most common fault of bad writing is wordiness. He advises prospective writers, "Learn to cut." We encourage you to believe that your training and instincts as a surgeon will serve you well as a writer. The presentation of data is a logical process, best done cleanly, briefly, and directly.

Among the forums for data presentation in academic medicine, the most important are presentations at meetings and publications in journals. Because many researchers present their results at conferences before they present their work for publication, we deal first with abstracts to be submitted for meetings and then with the development and submission of manuscripts. Later, we discuss choosing a journal and responding to reviewers.

Protocols for presentation of data in abstracts and papers are well established. The process is elucidated in the following discussions. For those who find writing difficult, we may be able to show how to make it less of an ordeal. Those who find writing pleasurable may still glean hints to make life easier.

II. What Makes a Good Abstract or a Good Paper?

It is impossible to write a good abstract or paper unless you have done a sound, logical study. When you undertake a study, you should begin by asking questions and by considering why the answers are important. Will a new drug reduce the incidence of postoperative infections? Can we identify a marker that will predict response to chemotherapy? Are tumor size and vascular invasion important prognostic indicators? Do not begin your study with a belief that you know the answer.

Studies may be retrospective or prospective. Although the importance of randomized controlled trials is obvious, other types of studies also have important roles (Fig. 1). Randomized trials tell us whether treatments work, but not how they work. Retrospective studies, particularly those with long-term follow-up, are important for analyzing the natural history of a disease, for example, or when trying to define populations at risk. Case reports may offer valuable information about uncommon occurrences or unusual ways to handle problems. Prospective studies, when properly done, can answer questions about treatments and verify observations made in retrospective studies.

Review the literature and consider earlier work by others before designing a study. Be sure a question has not already been answered conclusively. Journals will not publish papers that report old news. Define the primary and secondary endpoints before beginning to collect data. Then, collect and record as much data as could possibly be relevant. It is difficult, if not impossible, to collect accurate data retrospectively. Involve statisticians in study design and data analysis. Be sure, for example, to include enough subjects and follow them long enough to show statistical significance (2–4).

Do not change the question or start asking new questions after a study has begun. Chi-square tests, *t* tests, and other statistical tests provide a basis for probability statements only when the hypothesis is fully developed before the data are examined (5). If, as you work on your abstract or your paper, your results inspire you to reorganize your data and make unplanned comparisons, your probability statements will not be reliable (5). As you analyze your findings and consider their implications, new questions may occur to you, but these questions must be tested in new studies.

When you have collected your data and analyzed your results, determine what message needs to be conveyed to readers. A review of 100 patients with hepatocellular carcinoma is not meaningful unless it leads to lessons learned, changes in treatment, etc. Did one subset of patients do better than another? Reviewers will ask, "Why is this abstract or paper being written? What is new? What does it add to our knowledge of the subject?"

Avoid the common practices of dividing the results of a single study into one or more papers, or republishing the same material in successive papers that are not identical. These practices are considered dishonorable (6) (see Section VI).

III. Abstracts for Presentation at Meetings

An abstract is a short report of the findings of a study. It is generally no longer than 250 words. It includes a title, a brief introduction, a description of methods, the main results (presented without commentary), and the principal conclusion(s). There is no discussion or literature review. Specula-

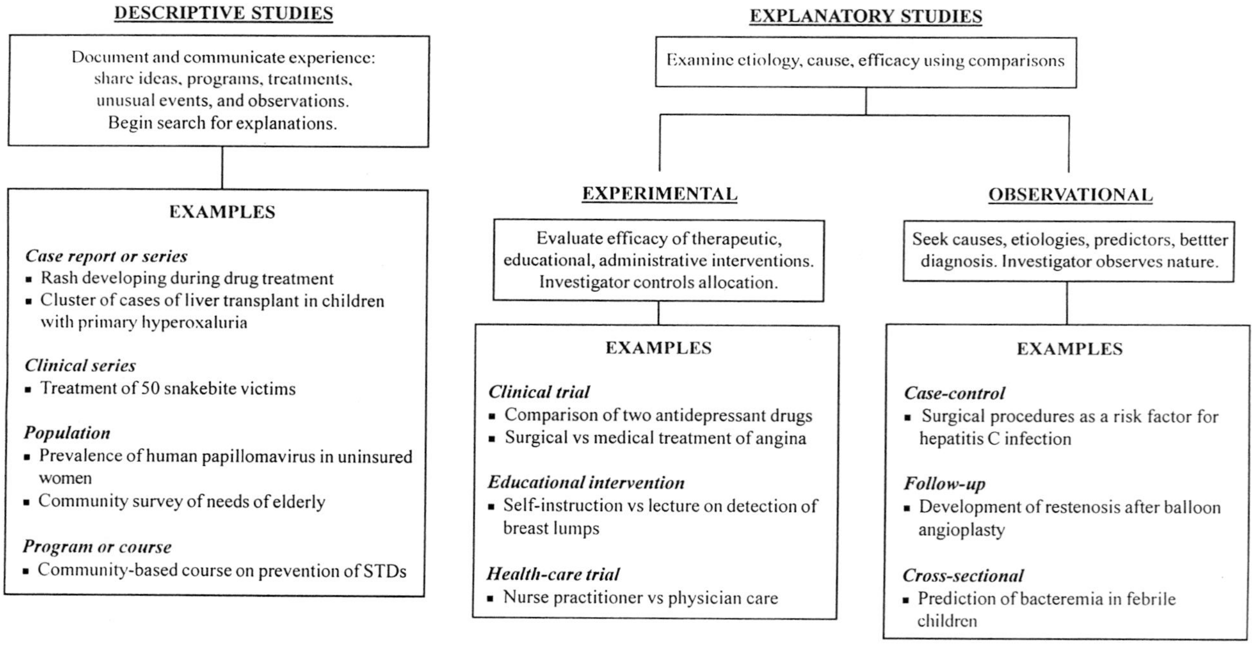

Figure 1 Types of studies. Adapted from Ref. (1a), S. H. Gehlbach (1993). "Interpreting the Medical Literature," 3rd Ed., p. 16. McGraw Hill, New York. Reproduced with permission of The McGraw-Hill Companies. Graphic assistance courtesy of Pamela Guarrera.

tions are kept to a minimum. The facts are presented briefly, with logical conclusions drawn from the available data. For readers who are unfamiliar with abstracts, we have prepared a sample (Exercise 1 and Fig. 2).

The abstract's introduction usually contains a brief historical reference to provide the rationale for the study (e.g., "Esophageal tumors have a poor prognosis"), the observation or hypothesis that inspired the study, and the goal. Try to limit the introduction to two or three sentences. Use abbreviations sparingly.

In the methods section, explain succinctly how the study was done. Was it retrospective, prospective, a chart review, or a randomized trial? Describe the study population. Were subjects divided into groups? On what basis? Was there a control group? What interventions were done? What were the endpoints? Were analysts blinded? What was the time period of the study, and how long was the follow-up? What factors were recorded and analyzed? Define terms that may be interpreted subjectively (e.g., obesity, renal dysfunction, response to treatment). Describe the methods of statistical analysis.

In the results section, do not discuss the results. Merely state findings, with the appropriate statistical analysis. Simple tables and figures may be used, but be sure they are large enough to reproduce clearly. There are strict limitations on abstract length, necessitating a decision on which data need to be included. Certain data, whether significant or not, may be important for the reader. Other findings that do not reach statistical significance may simply be described as nonsignificant (e.g., "there was no significant difference between groups in age, gender, or time of diagnosis"). In the methods section, the specific parameters studied are reported. In the results section, the data should correspond to those parameters. Do not provide data that do not support objectives stated in the methods section.

The conclusions section must be based on the results. Was the hypothesis proved? Do not give answers to questions that were not asked. Keep speculation to a minimum.

It is often easier to write the abstract title after writing the text. The title should be an informative statement that will capture the reviewer's interest (for example, "Lymph node biopsy does not impair survival after . . . " sends a clearer message than "The impact of lymph node biopsy on survival after . . . "). Reviewers read dozens of abstracts. Many will read the abstract's title first, then its conclusions, then its introduction and results, and finally, its methods. Bear this in mind when you are writing the abstract. Avoid abbreviations in the title and in the conclusion, so reviewers who read those parts first will not be frustrated by unfamiliar terms.

On the abstract form for its clinical congress, the American Society for Parenteral and Enteral Nutrition warns of common mistakes that cause abstracts to be rejected: (1) previously reported study or no new information; (2) data presented or published elsewhere; (3) little or no data; (4) inaccurate data; (5) invalid statistics; (6) inadequate controls; (7) inadequate description of methods; (8) insignificant study; (9) abstract did not conform to requirements; (10) poor writing; (11) conclusion not supported by data; (12) product names listed in abstract title (7).

Working with Abstract Forms

In most cases, abstracts must be submitted on a specific form distributed by the affiliated society. Increasingly, medical societies are requesting or demanding that researchers submit abstracts on special electronic forms, via the Internet. If an abstract is to be submitted on a paper form, it is a good idea to contact the sponsoring society in advance to request extra copies of the forms. It is not uncommon for a laser printer to chew up the only copy of the form, or for coffee to spill on it, or for colleagues to beg for extra copies. It is almost never acceptable to submit an abstract on a photocopy or a faxed copy of the original form.

For many researchers, the most challenging problem is the strict limitation on the length of the abstract. On paper forms, the abstract must fit into a small box, the size of which varies from meeting to meeting of sponsoring societies. For electronic submission, a limit is usually placed on the number of characters the abstract may contain. In our experience, the best way to approach the problem of fitting an abstract into the allotted space has been to write a first draft on a regular page with regular margins, without the added pressure of the small borders on the abstract form or the character-count limit. Be as terse and concise as possible, but address each component (see Fig. 2) in a reasonable manner.

If working with a paper form, after preparing a draft (assuming the work is on a computer), move the cursor to the very beginning of the text, before the first word, and reset the page margins to match the margins of the borders on the abstract form. (In Wordperfect, the margins are set under "Format." In Word, the margins are set under "File, Page Setup." In any case, use a ruler; if the left edge of the abstract is 3 inches from the left edge of the page, set the left margin for 3.05 inches, etc.) Then, select a font size that is acceptable according to the instructions on the abstract form. With the margins set to the borders of the allotted space and with the text in an appropriately sized font, scroll down to the end of the text to see how much (if any) of the first draft needs to be trimmed to fit completely into the space. If the instructions state that authors' names and institutions must be included within the space allotted for the text of the abstract, or if the title must be capitalized, or a line must be skipped before the text starts, do not forget to allow the necessary extra lines.

It is not uncommon for the first draft to be twice as long as the allowed finished product. In editing the first draft, remember that the abstract is not a novel. If it is over the word limit, shorter sentences may save space. Delete all expendable adjectives and adverbs. Put long lists into single sentences, when possible, rather than using several

ABSTRACT FORM FOR:
THE AMERICAN SOCIETY OF TRANSPLANT SURGEONS

23rd Annual Scientific Meeting
May 14-16, 1997

DEADLINE FOR RECEIPT OF ABSTRACTS:
JANUARY 22, 1997

(For office use)

A. Topic Categories (Check One)
❑A. Immunogenetics
❑1. T/B macrophage function
❑2. Cytokines
❑3. Immunosuppression
❑4. Tolerance
❑5. Chronic rejection
❑B. Immunogenetics
❑C. Xenotransplantation
❑D. Cell/organ transplantation

	Clinical	Experimental
Kidney	❑	❑
Kidney/pancreas	❑	❑
Islets	❑	❑
Liver	❑	❑
Small bowel	❑	❑
Heart	❑	❑
Lung	❑	❑
Bone marrow	❑	❑
Pediatric	❑	❑

❑E. Organ procurement/preservation/allocation
❑F. Transplant economics
❑G. Ethics
❑H. Transplant coordination
❑I. Others

B. For Human Studies
(check appropriate box):
❑ IRB Approval
❑ Informed consent
❑ Neither

C. Conflict of Interest Statement
I certify that potential conflicts of interest will be disclosed at the time of the oral or poster presentation of the abstract. All potential conflicts of interest will be detailed a separate letter to the ASTS program Committee Chair, 6900 Grove Road, Thorofare, NJ 08086, USA

Signature

D. Disclosure
Will your presentation include discussion of any commercial products or services? ❑Y ❑N
Is your activity supported be a grant from one or more commercial supporters? ❑Y ❑N
Do you have a significant financial interest or other relationships with manufacturer of products or services that would be conflict of interest? ❑Y ❑N
If your answer to any of the above questions is yes, then a letter must accompany your abstract disclosing the name of the product or commercial supporter and describe the nature of the relationship?

E. Young Investigator Award
❑ Check here if this abstract is to be considered for the Young Investigator Award.

PROPHYLACTIC INTERFERON-α2b REDUCES THE INCIDENCE OF RECURRENT HEPATITIS AFTER LIVER TRANSPLANTATION FOR HEPATITIS C.
P.A. Sheiner[1], P. Boros[1], S.N. Thung[2], F.M. Klion[3], S. Emre[1], S.R. Guy[1], L.K. Schluger[3], H.C. Bodenheimer, Jr.[3], I. Fiel[2], M. Yeh[2], E. Mor[4], J.Y.N. Lau[5], M.E. Schwartz[1], C.M. Miller[1]. Depts. of Surgery[1], Pathology[2], and Medicine[3], Mt. Sinai Hospital, NY; Dept. of Transplantation, Rabin Medical Center[4], Israel; Univ. of Florida [5], Gainesville, FL

A: Recurrent hepatitis is an increasing problem after liver transplant (OLT) for hepatitis C, but there is no effective prophylaxis or treatment. We sought to determine whether prophylaxis with interferon-α2b (IFN) would be useful in preventing recurrent hepatitis.

B: __Methods__: In a prospective trial, we randomized 86 patients to either an interferon-α2b group (IFN , 3 million U, 3 times/wk starting within 2 wks post-OLT and continuing at least 1 yr, if tolerated) or a no-IFN group. All patients received OKT3 induction and triple imunosuppression with cyclosporine (CyA), prednisone, and azathioprine. Patients were switched from CyA to tacrolimus for rejection or side effects. We recorded patient demographics, viral genotype, associated alcohol history, rejection episodes, and liver function tests at 1, 3, 6, 9, 12, and 18 mos, as well as serum HCV RNA levels (Chiron branched-chain DNA assay) pretransplant and at 5 days, 1 mo, 3 mos, 6 mos and 1 yr post-OLT. Recurrence was diagnosed either on biopsies performed for abnormal LFTs or on 1-yr protocol biopsies, which were read by a pathologist blinded to treatment group. Protocol biopsies were also reviewed by three pathologists blinded to treatment group and were graded for piecemeal necrosis, portal inflammation, confluent necrosis, lobular activity, bile duct damage, bile duct proliferation, and fat. After randomization, we excluded from further study 3 patients with platelet counts <50,000 by 2 wks and 1 patient who required post-OLT chemotherapy. One patient refused to enter after OLT, and 10 patients (5 IFN; 5 no-IFN) died within 1 mo. We reviewed data

C: on 71 patients who survived 3 mo post-OLT. __Results__: Thirty-one patients received IFN; 40 did not receive any IFN. Mean follow-up was 628±264 days in IFN patients and 594±266 days in no-IFN patients (p=ns). Pre-OLT, groups did not differ in age, gender, associated ETOH, HCV-RNA levels, or genotype. Of the 31 IFN patients, 18 completed the study (433± 121 days on IFN) and 4 are still on drug (216±64 days); in 9, IFN was discontinued (at 105±83 days), usually for a low platelet count. Post-OLT, groups did not differ in number of rejection episodes or serum HCV-RNA levels. Patients on IFN were less likely to develop recurrent hepatitis (8 IFN patients recurred at 194±168 days, vs 22 no-IFN patients at 220±144 days, p=0.017, log-rank analysis; Figure 1). The relative risk of developing recurrent hepatitis in the IFN group was 0.38 (p=0.02, Cox proportional hazards model). On regression analysis, the HCV-RNA level at 1 mo was a significant predictor of recurrent hepatitis(p<.002) that was independent of IFN. Recurrence was not affected by gender, genotype, or number of rejection episodes. Forty-seven 1-yr biopsies (24 IFN; 23 no-IFN) were performed. Piecemeal necrosis was more common in the no-IFN group (12 no-IFN patients vs 4 IFN patients, p<0.02). No other significant histological differences were noted. Among the 71 patients who survived 3 mo post-OLT, 1-and 2-year survival in the IFN group was 96% and 96%, respectively and in the no-IFN group was 91.2% and 87.2%, respectively (p=ns). Two IFN patients lost grafts to recurrence (one during IFN therapy, one after discontinuation of IFN). In the no-IFN group, one patient died of recurrent disease, and another awaits re-OLT.

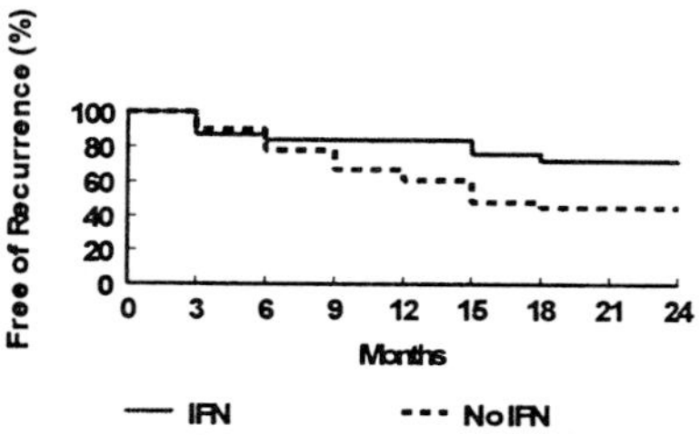

D: __Conclusions__: Prophylactic interferon-α2b reduces the incidence of recurrent hepatitis but does not prevent severe disease after recurrence. This effect seems to be independent of serum HCV-RNA levels, suggesting that IFN may work through alternative mechanisms, which remain to be elucidated. Longer follow-up is necessary to determine appropriate length of treatment; additional agents may be necessary to prevent severe disease.

This research was funded in part by Ortho Biotech, Raritan, New Jersey.
Patricia A. Sheiner, M.D., The Mount Sinai Hospital, Box 1104, One Gustave L. Levy Place, New York, NY 10029; 212-241-8035; fax 212 996-9688

Figure 2 Sample abstract for submission to meetings. In the introduction (A), give a historical reference, the current hypothesis or observation, and the study goal. In the methods section (B), tell how the study was performed. In the results section (C), provide data, with appropriate statistical analysis. In the conclusions section (D), based on the available data, describe the proof of the hypothesis, or the meeting of the goal, or the criteria that were developed—or the failure to do any of the above. Do not give answers to questions that were not asked. Courtesy of the American Society of Transplant Surgeons. Graphic assistance courtesy of Pamela Guarrera.

sentences. Make tables by tabbing columns across the lines, rather than by using the word processor's table function. Tables I–III provide examples of ways to tighten writing without loss of content or meaning. Also, assistance from someone who knows the idiosyncracies of the word processing software is invaluable (in Wordperfect, for example, space is saved by applying "full justification" to the text). Making revisions is discussed further in Section IV,D.

Instructions for abstracts vary from society to society. Some require that titles be in capital letters. Some require authors' full names; others require only first initials and last names. Some forbid abbreviations. Some require payment. Some require the signature of a member of the sponsoring society. Almost all require selection of a category in which the abstract will be considered. Some require that author names and affiliations be blocked out on some of the photocopies. Follow the instructions carefully.

Table I Avoiding Wordiness and Redundancy[a]

Adjectives	**Nouns**
advance planning	doctorate *degree*
awkward predicament	weather *conditions*
close proximity	
definite decision	**Prepositions**
end result	hoist *up*
end product	attach, connect, join, merge *together*
fellow colleagues	follow *after*
first priority	penetrate *into*
good benefit	return *back*
important essentials	sink *down*
joint cooperation	
local resident	**Prepositional phrases**
mutual cooperation	big *in size*
new beginning	biography *of his life*
original source	bisect *into two parts*
passing phase	blue *in color*
past history	classified *into groups*
proposed plan	consensus *of opinion*
retrospective review	few *in number*
root cause	graceful *in appearance*
self-confessed	period *of time*
serious danger	prejudge *in advance*
successful achievements	round *in shape*
surrounding circumstances	surgeon *by occupation*
total annihilation	2 p.m. *in the afternoon*
usual customs	surveyed *a total of* 200 people

[a]Look for words (such as those in italics) that can be deleted without changing the meaning.

IV. Developing the Manuscript

Journals publish information in a variety of formats, including case reports, retrospective reviews, prospective studies, and case-series analyses. With the exception of case reports (Table IV) and reviews, medical papers generally have 10 parts: (1) title, (2) abstract, (3) introduction, (4) methods, (5) results, (6) discussion, (7) conclusions, (8) acknowledgments, (9) references, and (10) tables and illustrations. In "Clinical Trials: Design, Conduct, and Analysis" (8), Meinert and Tonascia include content suggestions for the various parts of a study publication; their suggestions are presented in Table V.

A. The First Draft

Few writers, if any, can produce a perfect manuscript in the first draft. Sir William Osler reportedly revised his manscripts at least three times, and Harvey Cushing reportedly needed as many as nine drafts (9). The point of a first draft is not to have a finished product—the point is to make a start. Roland (10) advises "To write, begin. Don't begin at the beginning; start with any portion of the subject. . . . Ignore grammar and spelling and punctuation, but seize the thought and get it on paper. This is not the time to be concise—that comes later."

To begin the first draft, fill in an outline—introduction, methods, results, etc., without worrying about any specific order. If it is too difficult to write complete sentences, just make notes. In some cases, various members of a team might be responsible for writing the first drafts of different sections. Be careful, however, about where in the outline information is placed. Do not report results in the methods section; do not describe methods in the results section. When the outline seems complete, begin to convert notes into sentences and paragraphs. Edward J. Huth, former editor of *Annals of Internal Medicine*, suggests, "Put the rough outline aside for a few days and then patch some more details into it, perhaps adding mention of more tables (or graphs or illustrations) that will accompany the text and making notations of other papers to be cited. After this patching, sit down to write the first draft" (11).

1. Introduction

The introduction sets the stage for presentation of the study. Many authors make the introduction too long, including material that belongs in the discussion section. The introduction should consist of only a few sentences or paragraphs briefly reviewing (1) the history of the problem the paper addresses, (2) what is most recently known about the problem, (3) the rationale for the study, and (4) what is new in the study, or what was the goal of the study. Do not include data in the introduction. In addition, Huth advises, do not explain what can be found in any textbook in the field, and do not elaborate on terms in the title of the paper,

Table II Avoiding Circumlocutions (Not Ungrammatical, but Wordy)[a]

after the completion of (after)	in the near future (soon)
ahead of schedule (early)	in the vicinity of (near)
am in possession of (have)	in this day and age (today)
at an early date (soon)	it is clear that (clearly)
by the name of (named)	it is often the case that (often)
call a halt (stop)	large numbers of (many)
carry out an investigation (investigate)	made a statement saying (said)
caused injuries to (injured)	present in greater abundance (more abundant)
communicated to (told)	put in an appearance (appear)
during the time that (while)	render assistance to (help)
for the purpose of (for)	retained a position as (remained)
for the reason that (because)	situated on (on)
gathered together (met)	suburban area (suburb)
gave rise to (caused)	succumbed to injuries (died)
give due consideration to (consider)	subsequent to (after)
had occasion to be (was)	take action on (act)
in advance of (before)	take into consideration (consider)
in order to (to)	the patient in question (the patient)
in situations in which (when)	was of the opinion that (believed, thought)
in spite of the fact that (although)	was a witness to (saw)
in the event that (when)	were found to have (had)

[a]Train yourself to look for phrases that could be replaced with a single word.

Table III Wordy and Concise Ways to Say the Same Thing

Wordy:	The antiviral agent lamivudine has been clearly demonstrated to effectively reduce HBV replication with minimal side effects.
Concise:	The antiviral agent lamivudine effectively reduces HBV replication with minimal side effects.
Wordy:	All patients will be evaluated for entrance into the study irrespective of their gender or their race.
Concise:	Entrance into the study will not depend on gender or race.
Wordy:	At least six separate genes are known to be involved in the HLA system.
Concise:	At least six separate genes are involved in the HLA system.
Wordy:	At present, all 10 of the patients in our group of surviving transplant recipients have been weaned off of their steroids.
Concise:	All 10 surviving transplant recipients have been weaned from steroids.
Wordy:	We maintained a record of all infections and other postoperative complications in those patients who were older than 80 years.
Concise:	We recorded postoperative infections and other complications in patients older than 80 years.
Wordy:	It is known that Alagille's syndrome is of autosomal dominant inheritence but with variable penetrance.
Concise:	Alagille's syndrome is of autosomal dominant inheritence but with variable penetrance.
Wordy:	The patient's mother was evaluated for living-related donation. She was a 20-year-old college student.
Concise:	The patient's mother, a 20-year-old college student, was evaluated for living-related donation.
Wordy:	Postperfusion biopsies (which are routinely performed) were also taken and were reviewed for the purpose of this study.
Concise:	Routine postperfusion biopsies were reviewed.
Wordy:	Results of a preliminary trial of lamivudine for patients with chronic hepatitis B infection were recently published. The researchers' conclusions are that 12 weeks of lamivudine therapy was well tolerated and daily doses of 100 and 300 mg reduced HBV-DNA to undetectable levels.
Concise:	In a preliminary trial in patients with chronic hepatitis B infection, a 12-week course of lamivudine in daily doses of 100 or 300 mg was well tolerated and reduced HBV-DNA to undetectable levels.

Table IV Elements of a Case Report

An introduction[a] explaining why the case is worth reading about
A brief, clear case report, with adequate descriptions of relevant test results
A discussion section,[a] with reasons why the case is unusual, explanations for the authors' management approach, and possible alternative explanations for the reported features
Conclusions, including implications for other patients or situations
References

[a]Supported by references.

because "the audience for the paper should be expected to know almost as much as you" (12).

An author should have a collection of reference articles on the topic of research. Refer to these articles in the introduction and discussion sections, to put the study and findings into perspective. (Techniques for literature searches are described in Chapter 92.)

2. Methods

To experienced readers, the methods section can be the most important part of the paper. Methods validate findings. If a study was poorly designed or performed—for example, if the study population was too small, follow-up was too short, statistics were inappropriate—or if the methods are incompletely described, the conclusions, no matter how impressive, are meaningless.

Describe the design and execution of the study (see Table V). The methods, apparatus, and procedures should be described in enough detail to allow other researchers to reproduce the study and obtain the results (13, 14). Have colleagues in other disciplines (e.g., statisticians, pathologists, radiologists, immunologists) describe the methods for which they were responsible. In some cases, when protocols or techniques are well established, it is acceptable merely to cite references for them or to provide only brief descriptions with references. In some cases, editors may request that extensive details on methods appear in an appendix, or they may arrange for the material to be deposited with the National Auxiliary Publications Service, a service that makes copies of appendices available on request at moderate charges.

3. Results

This section is the heart of the paper. All the information revealed by the study goes here (see Table V). If two or more groups have been compared, begin the results section by confirming that they were similar, so that differences in results can be attributed to the study intervention and not to differences in the groups. Be sure to account for all subjects in the study, even those who withdrew or were lost to follow-up (see Fig. 3). Then, report the data, proceeding from old to new; first show results from controls or from the standard intervention, and then present findings in the study group. Include information about statistical significance.

Large amounts of data that require many long or awkward sentences are best presented in tables or figures (15). On the other hand, data that are easily reported in a sentence or two probably belong in the text, not in a table. Graphs should be used to show relationships among sets of numerical data (15). Regardless of the type of study, tables and illustrations must be clear and concise. Readers should be able to interpret them without having to refer to the text of the paper. Do not repeat in the text information that appears in tables, illustrations, or figure legends; only summarize or emphasize important observations (13, 14) (see Section IV,A,7).

Many journals now require that reports of randomized clinical trials conform to the CONSORT (Consolidated Standards of Reporting Trials) recommendations (16). According to the CONSORT statement, the results section in a clinical trial report should include a flowchart diagram summarizing participant flow and follow-up (see Figure 3), as well as the following information:

1. Statements of the estimated effect of interventions on primary and secondary outcome measures, including point estimates and measures of precision (confidence interval).
2. The results in absolute numbers, when feasible (for example, 10/20, not 50%).
3. Summary data and appropriate description and inferential statistics presented in sufficient detail to permit alternative analyses and replication.
4. Descriptions of prognostic variables by treatment group, and any attempt to adjust for them.
5. Descriptions of deviations from the study protocol, together with the reasons.

Be careful not to report finding things that the study was not designed to look for (a finding, reported in the results, requires an explanation in the methods as to how this finding was sought).

4. Discussion

Here is where the most important observations from the study are summarized and their significance is discussed. How do the findings differ from—or agree with—earlier reports by other researchers? Discuss the differences and similarities. If the findings differ from those of others, what might be the explanation? In the discussion, there is some freedom to interpret and to speculate, within reason, on what the new data mean. Do not present any new data or information from the study for the first time in the discussion section. All new information, with statements of statistical significance, should be presented in the results section.

This is the place to explain reasons for an unusual method or approach. What are the advantages of the

Table V Checklist for Content[a]

Abstract

- ☐ Purpose of study
- ☐ Primary outcome measure
- ☐ Test treatment(s)
- ☐ Control treatment(s)
- ☐ Level of treatment masking
- ☐ Number of patients enrolled
- ☐ Method of treatment allocation
- ☐ Results
- ☐ Conclusion(s)

Introduction

- ☐ Historical background
- ☐ Rationale for trial
- ☐ Objective(s)
- ☐ Rationale for choice of test and control treatment(s)
- ☐ Literature review

Methods

- ☐ Study population
  - ☐ Eligibility and exclusion criteria
  - ☐ Method of patient recruitment
- ☐ Treatments
  - ☐ Study treatments used
  - ☐ Method of treatment administration
  - ☐ Level of treatment masking
  - ☐ Treatment proscriptions
  - ☐ Methods of measuring treatment adherence
- ☐ Outcome measures
  - ☐ Primary and secondary outcome measures
  - ☐ Diagnostic criteria for outcome measurements
  - ☐ Methods for coding and classifying outcomes
- ☐ Design specifications
  - ☐ Method of randomization
  - ☐ Safeguards used to ensure the integrity of the allocation process
  - ☐ List of stratification variables
  - ☐ Blocking specifications
  - ☐ Procedures for packaging and dispensing study medications in masked drug trials
  - ☐ Primary outcome measure and rationale for choice
  - ☐ Planned length of patient follow-up and rationale for specification
  - ☐ Planned recruitment goal
  - ☐ Type I and type II error protection level for planned recruitment goal
- ☐ Patient safeguards
  - ☐ Outline of steps for obtaining patient consent
  - ☐ Measures taken to protect patient confidentiality
  - ☐ Procedures used to monitor study results for evidence of treatment effects
- ☐ Data collection schedule
  - ☐ Sequence of baseline and follow-up visits
  - ☐ List of data items collected
  - ☐ Definition of missed visits and dropouts

continues

Table V *continued*

- ☐ Data processing
  - ☐ Cut-off date for data included in manuscript
  - ☐ Approach and supporting rationale for dealing with missing data and departures from the treatment protocol
  - ☐ Literature references for methods used
  - ☐ Description of any special analysis procedures not already described in existing literature
  - ☐ Methods for judging statistical importance of differences observed (e.g., simple p values, adjusted p values, etc.)
- ☐ Quality control procedures
  - ☐ General data editing
  - ☐ Quality control of laboratory tests and for special reading and coding procedures
  - ☐ Checks on data entry, programming, and analysis
  - ☐ Other quality controls, such as site visits to clinics, training and certification, etc.
- ☐ Performance monitoring
  - ☐ Measures for assessing performance of participating clinics and resource centers
  - ☐ Frequency of performance assessments
  - ☐ Methods for reviewing performance monitoring reports and for implementing corrective action
- ☐ Treatment monitoring
  - ☐ Frequency and methods of interim analyses for treatment monitoring
  - ☐ Individual or group responsible for carrying out interim analyses
  - ☐ Procedures for implementing protocol changes based on results from interim analyses
- ☐ Organizational structure
  - ☐ Number and location of participating centers
  - ☐ Location of data center
  - ☐ Location of other resource centers
  - ☐ Standing committees and their membership
  - ☐ Mode of funding (e.g., grant or contract, individual or consortium award)
  - ☐ Policy on investigator conflicts of interests and method used to monitor for potential conflicts of interest
- ☐ Other items
  - ☐ Listing of special actions taken during the trial, including:
    - ☐ Addition or deletion of a treatment
    - ☐ Major modifications of data forms or coding procedures during the course of the trial

Results

- ☐ Number of patients enrolled by treatment group
- ☐ Number of deaths by treatment group
- ☐ Comparison of treatment groups for primary and secondary outcome measures using various analytic techniques
- ☐ Indicators of the completeness of follow-up by treatment group, such as:
  - ☐ Number of missed examinations
  - ☐ Number of dropouts
  - ☐ Number of patients lost to follow-up
- ☐ Indicators of treatment adherence, such as:
  - ☐ Comparison of treatment groups using an adherence score or some laboratory test
  - ☐ Number of patients in each treatment group who received none of the assigned treatment
  - ☐ Number of patients in each treatment group who received an alternative treatment
- ☐ Assessment of the comparability of the treatment groups with regard to baseline characteristics
- ☐ Treatment group comparisons for differences in:
  - ☐ Occurrence of serious side effects
  - ☐ Rate of hospitalization
  - ☐ Other general health indicators
- ☐ Treatment comparisons by selected baseline characteristics
- ☐ Multiple regression analyses using baseline characteristics to provide adjusted treatment comparisons

continues

Table V *continued*

- ☐ Treatment comparisons by level of adherence
- ☐ Treatment comparisons by clinic (in multicenter trials)
- ☐ Other special analyses relating follow-up data for one variable (e.g., cholesterol level) to a primary or secondary outcome measure (e.g., death)

Discussion

- ☐ Discussion of how reported findings relate to previous studies, paying particular attention to findings considered to be new and those that are inconsistent with findings of previous studies
- ☐ Discussion of the implications of the findings
- ☐ Enumeration of questions or areas needing further analysis or research

Conclusions

- ☐ Statement of conclusion
- ☐ Limits on generalizability of the conclusions, including discussion of observed statistical power if no treatment difference is detected

References

- ☐ List of literature references in required journal format, including citations for:
    - ☐ References to previous work
    - ☐ Data analysis methods
    - ☐ Methods not described in the paper
    - ☐ Treatment methods
    - ☐ Study rationale
    - ☐ Discussion
- ☐ List of study documents that may be obtained on request (e.g., study manual of operations, study data forms, data listings, data types)

Appendix

- ☐ Descriptions of special procedures needed to understand results, but too detailed to be included in the body of the publication
- ☐ List of definitions, codes, diagnostic criteria, etc.
- ☐ Special analyses, tabulations, and data listings
- ☐ Sample data forms

[a]Modified from Meinent and Tonascia (8).

approach? What might be the disadvantages? What might have been sources of bias or imprecision in the study? During preliminary research and in preparations for writing, the authors should have been collecting references in support of the rationale for the study and its design. In addition, the reference collection should include articles by other researchers who may not necessarily have the same point of view, to put the study and the findings in perspective. In the discussion section, in covering the points just mentioned, review the relevant literature in greater detail than in the introduction, and discuss how it relates to the report. Finally, what are the implications of the findings for future practice or future lines of research? What are the limitations of the inferences that can be drawn from the results?

If it is difficult to organize the discussion, try this approach: make a list of the important points about the study and its findings. Then, proceed to discuss each of those points in separate paragraphs, in light of other relevant studies conducted by other researchers. Also, analyze the structure of discussion sections in papers that have appeared in the journal to which the paper will be submitted (see Section VII).

5. Conclusions

Restate the most important findings. Were the goals of the study met and the question answered? Reiterate the limitations of the generalizability of the findings (17). Be sure that the conclusions are supported by data in the study. Do not find answers to questions not asked. For example, do not conclude that a given procedure will save money, if the study did not include an analysis of costs.

6. Acknowledgments

According to the Uniform Requirements for Manuscripts Submitted to Biomedical Journals (13, 14), it is appropriate to acknowledge (1) contributions that do not justify authorship (e.g., general support by a departmental chair, scientific advice or review of the paper by a colleague), (2) technical help (e.g., from clinical staff, editors, individuals who assist-

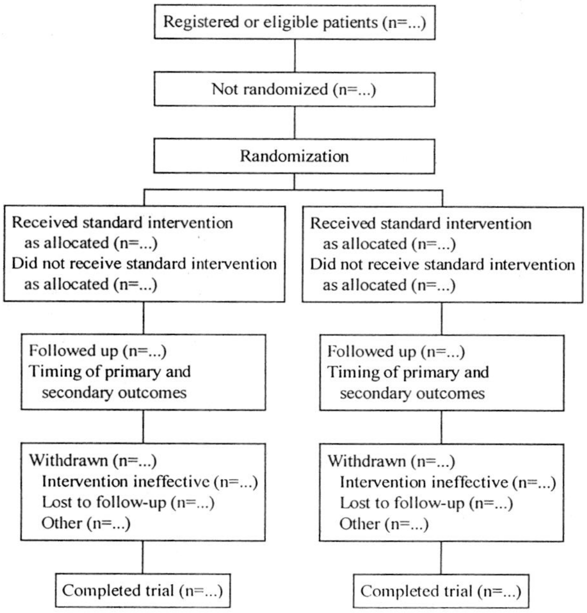

Figure 3 Flow diagram recommended by the CONSORT (Consolidated Reporting of Clinical Trials) Statement. The diagram illustrates progress through the various stages of a trial, including flow of participants, withdrawals, and timing of primary and secondary outcome measures. From Begg *et al.* (16), *JAMA* **276**, 637–639. Copyrighted 1996, American Medical Association. Graphic assistance courtesy of Pamela Guarrera.

ed with data collection), (3) financial and material support, including the nature of such support (e.g., grant support, funds, or supplies from pharmaceutical or equipment companies), and (4) relationships that might pose a conflict of interest. In particular, concealing "ghost authorship" by failing to acknowledge the assistance of a professional writer or editor is considered as inappropriate as awarding authorship to researchers who in fact made no contribution to the work (18) (see Section VI).

It is courteous to obtain written permission from colleagues who will be acknowledged by name, particularly in the case of those who made intellectual contributions, because readers may infer their endorsement of the data and conclusions (13, 14). Some researchers also acknowledge the participation of their study subjects.

7. References

It is preferable to cite original journal articles as references, rather than book chapters or published abstracts. Most journals prefer that authors avoid citing a "personal communication" unless it provides absolutely essential information. Authors should obtain written permission and confirmation from the source of a personal communication.

Do not cite a paper without having reviewed the entire article. Online search services make it easy to review abstracts of published papers without having to go to the library—but unfortunately, abstracts and papers do not always match. A review of articles from *Annals of Internal Medicine*, the *British Medical Journal, The Journal of the American Medical Association, The Lancet, The New England Journal of Medicine*, and the *Canadian Medical Association Journal* found that the proportion of abstracts with information that was either inconsistent with the text or was entirely absent from the paper ranged from 18 to 68% (19, 20).

The individuals who ultimately review papers to determine acceptability for publication are experts who are familiar with the literature. Citing papers incorrectly or inappropriately or omitting the citation of an important paper will be recognized by reviewers and will reflect poorly on an author's credibility.

Do not assign numbers to references cited in the first draft. At this point, it is very likely that references will be rearranged or more references will be added. Therefore, in the first draft merely identify references by what is known as the Harvard system—use the first author's last name and the year of publication. Use of bibliographic management software may simplify this process (21–23). Styling and numbering of references are discussed in Section V.

8. Tables and Illustrations

The purpose of tables and illustrations is to present data more clearly than would be possible with text alone. Do not cite data in several ways in the same paper; rather, text, tables, and illustrations must complement each other, without duplication of information. Tables and illustrations must be designed so that readers can extract data easily, without struggling to understand the format and without having to refer to the text. Look through published papers to find examples of tables and illustrations that could serve as models, or obtain one of the many fine books that provide guidelines for developing tables and illustrations for medical papers (see Table VI).

Each table must have a number and a title. Within each table, columns must have headings that identify the entries below. Rows may need headings that identify the entries to the right. State the units of measure for the data in the column or row just once, in the heading; if the units of measure are too long to include in the heading, put them in a footnote below the table. Abbreviations must be spelled out in a key below the table. When designing a table, bear in mind that it is easier to compare data from column to column than from row to row. Make sure the values in comparable columns are presented in comparable units. Also, be sure that the terminology in the table is comparable with the terms in the text.

Figures should not be titled, but a legend must be written for each figure. Have figures produced as glossy prints or "camera ready" printouts from a laser printer. Do not send original X-rays, EKG tracings, photocopies of illustrations from other sources, etc. If the illustration contains symbols, arrows, etc., explain these in the legend. If figures are photomicrographs, indicate the magnification and stains in the

Table VI Annotated Bibliography

Publication	Comment
"How to Write and Publish Papers in the Medical Sciences," 2nd Ed., E.J. Huth, Williams & Wilkins, Baltimore, 1990	An outstanding book from the former editor of *Annals of Internal Medicine*; topics covered include journal selection, literature searching, preparations for writing, structuring the critical argument in scientific papers, descriptions of different types of papers, writing first drafts, revision of drafts for content and style, development of tables and illustrations, procedures for submission of the manuscript, responding to reviewers, and correcting proofs; also contains useful appendices
"CBE Style Manual," 6th Ed., Council of Biology Editors, Inc., Reston, VA, 1994	Another excellent book covering manuscript preparation, writing the article, scientific prose style, reference citations and style, guidelines for developing illustrations and tables, instructions for checking and correcting proofs; also provides guidelines for reviewers and for author responses; see also the Council of Biology Editors web site, www.cbe.org
"American Medical Association Manual of Style," 8th Ed., C. Iverson, B.B. Dan, P. Glitman, *et al.*, Eds., Williams & Wilkins, Baltimore, 1989	Describes different types of articles, manuscript preparation, authors' legal and ethical responsibilities, journal editorial procedures; also has sections on grammar and punctuation, medical and scientific terminology and nomenclature, and measurements and quantitations; written for authors submitting papers to AMA journals; guidelines occasionally differ from those of other journals
"Words Into Type," Prentice-Hall, Inc.	The publisher's and copyeditor's bible on grammar, word and language usage, and style
"Illustrating Science: Standards for Publication," The Council of Biology Editors, Inc., Bethesda, Maryland, 1988	Includes guidelines for preparation of artwork, graphs and maps, and photographs; also covers ethical and legal issues relating to artwork; contains a particularly useful chapter directed at authors (much of the book is directed at artists), but also contains much that has become obsolete with computer graphics
"How to Write, Speak and Think More Effectively," R. Flesch, Harper & Rowe, Publishers, Inc., New York, 1960	A very entertaining book for anyone—even experienced writers—interested in the principles behind effective communication; Available in paperback

legend as well. Any recognizable face in a photograph requires either a signed release form or masking of the eyes to conceal identity. Type legends on a separate page at the end of the paper (see Section V). Refer to the journal's instructions for authors to determine how many sets of illustrations must be submitted with the paper. Remember that journals charge for each printed page of a manuscript, and they charge extra for color illustrations.

9. Title

Some editors suggest that a writer's first step in developing a paper should be to formulate a title, before writing the outline or the first draft. We believe it is easier to write the paper first and draw the title from the conclusions. An informative title (e.g., "Antibiotics Reduce Hospital Costs") is more useful than a noninformative one (e.g., "Antibiotics and Hospital Costs").

10. Abstract

The abstract is the most widely read part of any research article (24). We recommend writing the abstract after writing a first draft of the paper. Do not use an earlier abstract version that was submitted to a meeting months previously (the information may be outdated, the writing is probably choppy, and the text is probably not structured in accordance with the journal's requirements). Write the paper, and then extract from the up-to-date manuscript the appropriate components for a structured abstract (e.g., introduction, objectives, design or methods, outcome measures, results, and conclusions). Common errors to avoid include inconsistency between data in the abstract and in the text of the paper, data in the abstract that do not appear in tables, and conclusions in the abstract that are not based on information presented in the abstract (24).

B. Permissions and Copyrights

Authors sometimes include documentary evidence from other sources to support their conclusions. Illustrations, photographs, tables, and extensive passages of text [i.e., more than four or five consecutive sentences (25), or about 150 words] are usually protected by copyright and require permission from the copyright holder to reprint the material. The process of obtaining permission can take weeks or more. It is advisable to write for permission during preparation of your draft. Request a sample permission letter from journal editors (see Section VII).

C. Revising the Content

Revision of early drafts is an essential phase of manuscript preparation. Distribute copies of the first draft to coauthors and to nonauthor colleagues, who are likely to review it with a fresh eye. Authors, coauthors, and colleagues should read the manuscript from the perspective of a reviewer. In "How to Write and Publish Papers in the Medical Sciences" (26), Huth suggests that authors ask the following questions as they review their drafts:

1. Is the title accurate, succinct, and effective?
2. Does the abstract represent the content of all the main sections of the paper, within the length allowed by the journal?
3. Does the introduction set the stage adequately but concisely for the main question considered, or for the hypothesis tested? Is that question or hypothesis made clear by the end of the introduction?
4. Is the rest of the text in the right sequence?
5. Is all of the text needed, or can some be discarded? Does any of the text repeat information found elsewhere in the paper?
6. Is any needed content missing?
7. Do data in the text agree with data in the tables?
8. Are all necessary references cited and unnecessary ones omitted?
9. Can any of the tables or illustrations be omitted?

D. Revising Your Writing

Medicine is a fascinating subject. It is wrong to assume that descriptions of medical research must be wordy, dull, and difficult to read. Although it is impossible to teach how to write clearly and directly in the space of a few pages, the following ideas may help improve basic writing. Obtaining one or more of several books available for this purpose is also recommended (see Table VI). In addition, if a paper is to be published in English and English is not your native language, try to have your paper reviewed by a native English speaker before submitting it.

Never forget that the basic goal of a writer is to make it possible for the reader to move effortlessly from one sentence to the next, collecting the information provided by the words. "Reading is really a miracle," writes Rudolph Flesch (27). "Your eyes pick up groups of words in split-second time and your mind keeps these words in delicate balance until it gets around to a point where they make sense." If you write with simple words, avoid redundancy and winding, complicated sentences, the text will make sense to readers quickly, and they will pick up new information with every sentence or paragraph. If you use convoluted sentences and more words than necessary, readers will be forced to reread passages, work harder to move from sentence to sentence, or, worse, skip passages or forget pieces of information that are too twisted or clunky to remember easily.

Here are some principles that can make a paper—and hence a message—clearer.

1. Use as few words as possible. Medical writing is often full of redundancies and circumlocutions (see Tables I–III for examples of ways to trim excess verbiage). Then, go through the text and excise every extraneous word. Cutting the nonessential makes the essential stand out more clearly (28).

2. Try to use the simplest reasonable words, with the fewest syllables (e.g., replace *commence* with *start*, or *utilize* with *use*).

3. Avoid long sentences. If there are many compound sentences (those with *ands* and *buts*) or complex sentences (those with *if, because, as*, etc.), separate some of them into two sentences. Have each sentence express one thought at a time, in as few clauses as possible. (The average sentence length in this chapter is 13 words. The average sentence length in a typical wordy, difficult-to-read medical paper is close to 20 words.)

4. Organize the paragraphs. Each paragraph should begin with a "topic sentence" that prepares the reader for the subject. Then, the sentences that follow should all relate to that first sentence, moving forward in a straight line of thought. (Inexperienced writers often state the point of the paragraph at the end, when it really belongs at the beginning.) There are no firm rules on paragraph length. Huth suggests that 25 lines be the limit (29). We suggest that most paragraphs be limited to no more than two-thirds of a double-spaced page. It may not be possible merely to split a long paragraph in half. Instead, new topic sentences may be required for the two new paragraphs that result from breaking up a larger one.

5. Avoid the passive voice. (Passive voice: "All slides were reviewed by pathologists." Active voice: "Pathologists reviewed all slides.")

6. Avoid using more than two or three prepositions in a single sentence. (Prepositions are words that could fit in the blank spaces in the following sentences: The bird flew _______ the cloud. The boy ran _______ the tree.)

7. Avoid "multiple maybes." You may be reluctant to state that your findings are immutable, but try to avoid excessive hedging, as in the following sentence: "Our results *suggest* that *it may be possible* that this new drug *may be* useful for diabetic patients."

8. Do not succumb to the "Abbreviations Are Great (AAG)" syndrome. Writers with the AAG (WAAG) make up abbreviations to replace any repeated phrase (ARARP). Odd ARARP for words you were tired of typing (TT) annoy serious readers (SRs). TT-induced ARARP by WAAG force SRs to return again and again to the introduction and methods to identify weird abbreviations made up by the writer at his or her whim. Do not invent abbreviations. Editors hate them, and they make a paper difficult to read.

V. Formatting the Manuscript

In the late 1970s, a group of journal editors gathered in Vancouver, British Columbia to set guidelines for the format of manuscripts. This group eventually became known as the

International Committee of Medical Journal Editors, and their guidelines are called the "Uniform Requirements for Manuscripts Submitted to Biomedical Journals." The fifth edition of these guidelines was published in 1997 (13, 14). More than 500 journals have agreed to use the Uniform Requirements.

Most journals, including those that use the Uniform Requirements, publish instructions for authors at the front or back of each issue. Some journals publish their instructions only once or twice a year. The instructions generally provide directions for formatting the title page, listing key words for indexing, formatting abstracts, the maximum word lengths for different types of manuscripts, the order in which the elements of the paper are to appear, the line spacing and margins for the text, the styling of references, how many copies of manuscripts and illustrations should be submitted, and where to send the manuscript. Pay close attention to these instructions to reduce the risk rejection.

A. Title Page

In addition to the title and the authors' names, the title page must usually show each author's degrees and affiliation and the name and address of the author to whom correspondence from the journal and from readers should be sent. If a coauthor participated in the study at one institution but now works elsewhere, include the current affiliation as well. Some journals require that the title page include a "running head," which refers to the abbreviated title that will appear on top of every other page of the published article. The journal may also require that authors' grant support be shown on the title page. Read the instructions for authors to learn what information is required on the title page.

B. Key Words

The National Library of Medicine uses medical subject headings (MeSH terms) for indexing articles from nearly 4000 medical journals, for cataloguing books, and for searching MeSH-indexed databases, including MEDLINE. There are more than 19,000 main MeSH headings. Key words for a paper can be selected using the MeSH browser at the National Library of Medicine's web site (30).

C. References

References must be cited and styled in the manner set forth in the journal's instructions for authors. Whether listed numerically or alphabetically, reference citations generally consist of the authors' last names and initials, the title of the article, the name of the publishing journal, the year of publication, and the volume and page numbers (Table VII). The journal's name is usually abbreviated according to Index Medicus style. A list of these abbreviations is published annually by the National Library of Medicine (31) and can also be viewed online (32).

Most journals require that references be cited sequentially, in the order in which they appear in the text; others require that they be cited in alphabetical order, according to the last name of the first author. If tables include reference citations, check the journal's instructions to see where in the reference list the citations should be placed. Commercially available bibliographic software can number and renumber references, import them from electronic sources, style them according to specific journal guidelines, and build bibliography databases. Reviews of these and other programs have been published (21–23).

D. Tables and Illustrations

In the final review before a paper is submitted, be sure that figures and tables are numbered consecutively and are cited in the text, in the proper order. Editors often receive manuscripts in which there is no indication of where tables or figures are to appear, or with discrepancies between the number of illustrations and tables and the number cited in the paper (9).

Tables generally are placed near the end of the manuscript, after the acknowledgments and references and before the list of figure legends (refer to a journal's instructions for authors). Tables should be typed double-spaced. Abbreviations should be spelled out in a key below the table. Unless a journal specifically indicates otherwise, the proper sequence for footnotes is *, †, ‡, §, ||, ¶, **, ††, ‡‡, §§, etc.

Figure legends should be typed double-spaced on a separate page at the end of the manuscript. The illustrations are sent along with the manuscript in their own envelope. On the back of each copy of each illustration, place a label with the first author's name, the number of the figure, and an arrow pointing to the top of the illustration. Do not write on the illustration, only on the label. If you must write on the back of the illustration, do so with a soft pencil so the impression will not show through the front of the figure. Avoid using ink, which may stain the other illustrations. Do not use paper clips; they may cause indentations that will reproduce in print.

If a paper is not accepted for publication, the journal will return illustrations, but we advise keeping at least one set of duplicates.

VI. The Ethics of Authorship

Whether and where a researcher's name appears in a list of authors is one of the touchiest issues in academic medicine, not least because promotions, tenure, and funding are linked to number of publications (33, 34). The number of authors per article has increased markedly over the past several decades (35). Unfortunately, in many cases authorship has become an activity for which physicians take credit, rather than responsibility. Studies by journal editors show that a substantial proportion of articles have honorary

Table VII Basic Reference Styles[a]

Type of publication	Example
Print	
Journal	Most journal citations are variations of the following: Authorlastname A, Authorlastname B, Authorlastname C. Title of article with only first word capitalized. Index Medicus Abbreviation 199x; vol: pages.
Original paper published in a journal	6. Mor E, Kaspa RT, Sheiner P, Schwartz M. Treatment of hepatocellular carcinoma associated with cirrhosis in the era of liver transplantation. Ann Intern Med 1998; 129: 643–653.
Report by a committee	1. Genetic testing for cystic fibrosis. National Institutes of Health Consensus Development Conference Statement on genetic testing for cystic fibrosis. Arch Intern Med 1999; 159: 1529–1539.
Editorial or letter	1. Sheiner PA. Prostaglandins in liver transplantation [editorial]. Hepatology 1995; 21: 592–593.
	2. Bromberg JS, Baliga PR. Renal transplantation in a noncompliant patient [letter]. N Engl J Med 1994; 330: 371–372.
Chapter in a book with a single author	1. Gehlbach SH. *In* "Interpreting the Medical Literature," 3rd Ed. McGraw-Hill, Inc., New York, 1993, pp. 34–54.
Chapter in a multiauthor book	1. Adler HL. Breast infection. *In* "Surgical Infections: Diagnosis and Treatment." (J. L. Meakins, ed.), pp. 287–290. Scientific American, Inc., New York, 1994.
Electronic[b]	
General website	1. National Library of Medicine. 21 Oct. 1999. Medical Subject Headings (MeSH). <http://www.nlm.nih.gov/mesh/meshhome.html> Accessed 27 Jan 2000.
Online publication	1. Ehrlich N. 6 Dec 1999. Smallpox plagues may have triggered mutation that protects against HIV infection. <http://www.reutershealth.com/PSUser/psfrmqry.htm> Accessed 12 Jan 2000.
File available for downloading from an FTP site	1. E. coli gene protein database project—ECO@DBASE (in NCBI repository). 13 Jan 1995. <ftp://ncbi.nlm.nih.gov/repository/ECO2DBASE/> Accessed 12 Jan 2000.

[a]Each journal seems to have its own reference style. Read the instructions for authors carefully. For special situations (e.g., no author is given, an article has a published erratum, your source is a conference paper), refer to the "Uniform Requirements" (13, 14) or consult the journal to which you are submitting your paper.

[b]There are a variety of styles for citing electronic sources. In "Online! A Reference Guide to Using Internet Sources" (49), Harnack and Kleppinger advise that citations for material on the World Wide Web should include the (1) author's name, if known, (2) date of publication or most recent revision, if known, (3) title of document, (4) title of complete work, if applicable, (5) the URL, in angle brackets, and (6) date on which the site was accessed.

authors who make few or no substantial contributions to the research (36–38). Huth writes, "Abuses of authorship rarely seem to damage the efficiency of science or seriously sap its resources. But they do undermine the ethics of honesty" (6).

The meaning of authorship and the identification of appropriate individuals as authors have been intensely debated (39–42). Several groups, including the International Committee of Medical Journal Editors (ICMJE) (see Table VIII), have published principles for authorship of medical papers and guidelines for applying those principles to specific kinds of articles (42–44). In a position paper published in *Annals of Internal Medicine,* Huth advises that tentative decisions on authorship be made early in the study and that responsibility for subsequent decisions be assigned to the person with the most responsibility for conceiving and designing the study and analyzing and interpreting the results (42). Because author order is assigned in different ways, some groups may wish to explain the order of authorship in a footnote (to state, for example, that the first two authors contributed equally to the project).

The ethics of authorship involve not only the identification of appropriate individuals as authors but also the issue of duplicate publication. The ICMJE defines redundant or duplicate publication as the publication of a paper that overlaps substantially with one already published (13, 14). The editors of six major cardiothoracic journals recently issued a joint statement defining duplicate publication (see Table IX); these journals warn that they will combat duplicate publications by exchanging information with each other (45). Duplicate publications waste the resources of publishers and reviewers and raise costs for subscribers, libraries, and authors. Worse, duplicate publications make literature searches more cumbersome and can misrepresent the incidence of reported conditions or effects.

The practice of slicing data into so-called least publishable units (LPUs) (46), to produce several smaller papers instead of one comprehensive article, is also known perjoratively as "salami" science. If all findings in a study yield a message that can be presented in a single paper of normal length, it is not appropriate to divide these findings into several papers (47).

Table VIII ICMJE Principles for Authorship of Medical Papers

Principle 1. Each author should have participated sufficiently in the work represented by the article to take public responsibility for the content

Principle 2. Participation must include three steps: (1) conception or design of the work represented by the article, or analysis or interpretation of the data, or both; (2) drafting the article or revising it for critically important content; and (3) final approval of the version to be published

Principle 3. Participation solely in the collection of data (or other evidence) does not justify authorship

Principle 4. Each part of the content of an article critical to its main conclusions and each step in the work that led to its publication (steps 1, 2, and 3 in Principle 2) must be attributable to at least one author

Principle 5. Persons who have contributed intellectually to the article but whose contributions do not justify authorship may be named and their contribution described—for example, "advice," "critical review of study proposal," "data collection," "participation in clinical trial"; such persons must have given their permission to be named; technical help must be acknowledged in a separate paragraph

VII. Choosing a Journal

Choosing the appropriate journal for a paper is a process that should begin with the first draft. What question is being addressed? Who would care about the answer? Some journals focus primarily on basic science (e.g., the *Journal of Surgical Research*). Others tend to publish mostly clinical papers (e.g,, the *Journal of the American College of Surgeons*). Be sure the research subject and format are within a journal's scope. Do not submit case reports to journals that never publish them. Do not send a 6000-word paper to a journal that has a 3000-word limit for articles. Do not send a paper to a journal that has recently published a similar paper with similar findings. Copies of journals are available in the library; review several copies to assess a journal's scope. Read the instructions for authors.

Become familiar with specialty journals in specific fields and with journals having broader audiences; note differences in the quality of the writing and recognize the relative importance of the data published. The most formal indicator of a journal's ranking is its so-called "impact factor," calculated by the Institute for Scientific Information and published annually in *Journal Citation Reports*. The impact factor measures the frequency with which the average article in a journal has been cited in a particular year (48). The higher the impact factor, the more prestigious the journal. In fact, promotions committees often consider the impact factors of the various journals when reviewing an individual's curriculum vitae.

Table IX Definition of a Duplicate Publication[a]

1. The hypothesis is similar
2. The numbers or sample sizes are similar
3. The methodology is identical or nearly so
4. The results are similar
5. At least one author is common to both reports
6. No or little new information is made available

[a]All six criteria must be met. Adapted from Tamru *et al.* (45).

Developing a reputation as a good thinker and academician requires publishing well-done studies and reviews, but this does not exclude submitting smaller, less important studies for publication. How can you decide which journal suits which paper, and vice versa? Become familiar with the journals in a field, ask more experienced colleagues for advice, and consider realistically the importance of the information and the quality of a study. A prestigious journal will likely not accept a nice little paper on five cases of arterial thrombosis after liver resection; the same journal might, however, accept a paper that describes a series of 30 such cases with detailed intraoperative and perioperative data and X-ray findings. If a study was retrospective, how many details were missing? Were state-of-the-art tests performed? Even with some missing data, the message may still be important enough to publish in a second-tier journal, but the better journals will reject a paper that has too many missing details.

There is a need to balance the advantage of a journal's high impact factor with the likelihood of acceptance. The most prestigious journals receive thousands of manuscripts a year. How widespread is the problem addressed in a study? How much does the study add to what is already known? Have the study's findings been previously confirmed, or is new ground being broken? The newer the information, the more complete the data, the more state-of-the-art the techniques, and the better the study design and execution, the higher the likelihood that a paper will be accepted at a higher quality journal. If a paper is submitted to a higher level journal first and is not accepted, use the reviewers' criticisms to revise the paper before sending it to the next level journal. A sample submission letter appears in Table X.

VIII. Responding to the Reviewers

A paper has been written, polished and sent off. What next? Expect to receive a letter from the editor within 2 weeks. In some cases, particularly with the more prestigious journals, an editor may reject a paper outright, without sending it off for formal peer review. But if the journal has been selected carefully and appropriately, the editor will acknowl-

Table X Sample Submission Letter

Dear Dr. Editor:

My colleagues and I wish to submit the enclosed manuscript, "The efficacy of prophylactic interferon-α2b in preventing recurrent hepatitis C after liver transplantation," for publication in *Hepatology*.

Portions of this material were presented in May 1997 before the American Society of Transplant Surgeons; otherwise, neither this material nor any portion of it has been published or is under consideration for publication elsewhere.

All listed authors have participated meaningfully in this study and have seen and approved the final manuscript.

A transfer of copyright form, signed by all authors, is enclosed.

Please address all correspondence to:

Patricia A. Sheiner, M.D.
The Mount Sinai Medical Center, Box 1104
One Gustave L. Levy Place
New York, New York 10029

(212) 241-8035; Fax (212) 996-9688
E-mail: patricia.sheiner@mountsinai.org

Thank you for your consideration.

Sincerely,

edge the submission, assign a manuscript number to the paper, and state that the paper has been sent out for review. Review times vary but generally range from 4 to 8 weeks.

Outcomes of submission are shown in Fig. 4. Rarely, a paper will be accepted as it is, with no changes requested. More often, the reviewers will have questions or comments that must be addressed. Sometimes the editor will set a deadline—usually, 4 weeks—for the return of a revised manuscript. (In special circumstances, an extension can be requested.) Sadly, many papers "die" in authors' desk drawers at this point, because the authors are daunted by editorial requests. Do not let that happen! Address the reviewers' comments systematically and appropriately; in most cases the paper will be accepted and published. Furthermore, although nearly all authors find the revision process to be frustrating, nearly all will also admit that after the reviewers' comments are addressed, their paper is better.

When returning the manuscript to the journal, include a letter that describes the changes that were made. Often, the revisions in the manuscript must be underlined. The more specifically the revisions are described, the easier it will be for the editor to realize that the reviewer's comments have been adequately addressed (Table XI).

Exercise 1: The Health Club Dilemma

You are the director of a major medical center. Three months ago, some of the residents were able to persuade their chairman to provide free health club memberships to all 25 residents in their program. Now residents in every program are clamoring for free memberships. Each membership costs $350. You hypothesize that not everyone who has a free membership will actually use it. Before you agree to the residents' request, you want to know whether you can predict which residents are most likely to use the health club regularly.

How would you study this?

First, perform a retrospective review of health club charts over the past three months. You learn that of the 25 residents, 10 never went, 5 went approximately once a week, and 10 went at least twice a week. You feel it would be worthwhile to give free memberships to those residents who would be likely to go at least twice a week. You wish to develop criteria for identifying such residents.

How would you begin?

Divide the study population into two groups: (Group A) Residents who went at least twice a week and *(Group B) Everyone else (i.e., residents who went less often or not at all).* Your secretary has a detailed file on each resident. (She runs a matchmaking service on the side.) You borrow her files and have a medical student review the data for extra credit.

What variables might you have the student record?

1. Age
2. Gender (male vs. female)
3. Body weight (ideal or not)
4. Postgraduate year
5. Call schedule
6. Married or not
7. Children or not
8. Distance from health club to home

You might have chosen other variables, but for the purpose of this exercise we'll use the ones listed above. The student prepares a detailed sheet on each resident and enters the data

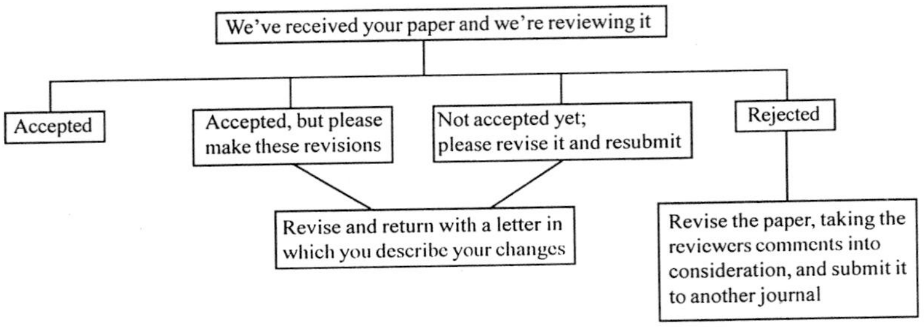

Figure 4 Possible outcomes of manuscript submission.

into a spreadsheet program (Table XII). Statistical analysis reveals that distance from home to health club is the only significant factor determining frequency of use (see Ch. 9). Now prepare an abstract for your report to the residents.

Sample Abstract

Because exercise has been shown to relieve stress, the residents have requested that the medical school provide free health club memberships. Because the dean agreed to give free health club memberships only to residents who would use the club regularly, we attempted to identify factors that would predict regular health club attendance. *Methods:* We reviewed the health club attendance of 25 residents who were given free memberships 3 months ago and identified two separate groups: 10 residents who attended the club at least twice a week and 15 who went less often or not at all. For all residents, we recorded age, gender, postgraduate year (PGY), on-call schedule, marital status, number of children, distance from health club to home, and whether or not they were at their ideal body weight. *Results:* There was no difference between the groups in age, gender, PGY, on-call schedule, marital status, number of children, or weight. Distance from home to health club appeared to be the only sig-

Table XI Sample Response to Reviewer Comments

Dear Dr. Editor:

Enclosed is a modified version of our paper, "Liver transplant recipients are not at increased risk for nonlymphoid solid organ tumors" (manuscript number C1793-97), which we have revised in accordance with your reviewers' comments. Specifically, we have made the following changes to the paper.

Reviewer 1

1. The reviewer wrote, ". . . the conclusion [in the abstract] that there is not an increased risk of solid tumors need have the caveat added that this might change with longer follow-up." We have now added this point to the conclusion of our abstract on page 3.
2. The reviewer requested that we define the mechanism of action of tacrolimus. We now do so, on page 5.
3. We agree that the report from Berlin (Jonas et al.) shows results similar to ours; we now cite this paper (our reference 28) in the Discussion section (on page 15).
4. As requested, Table 2 has been expanded to include patient outcomes.

Reviewer 2

5. As the reviewer points out, our paper is a descriptive analysis of a relatively large number of patients who have undergone liver transplant. The reviewer argues that we do not present data on observed vs expected rates in our results. We now explain in our discussion (page 13) that we did not make more specific comparisons because this was a descriptive study of small numbers of patients. We agree that the proportions of patients with tumors on the different immunosuppressive agents should be provided; in our original manuscript, we included this information for patients with recurrent tumors, and we have now added it to page 9 for patients with *de novo* tumors. In addition, we have added a discussion of this issue to page 14.
6. We agree that patients with hepatocellular carcinoma have a higher recurrence rate and represent a different patient population, as they undergo transplantation with active tumor. We had previously stated that they were excluded from our analysis; now, we explain the reason for their exclusion, on page 11.
7. The reviewer felt that in order to conclude that liver transplantation does not place patients at increased risk for the development of nonlymphoid tumors, a formal comparison to a general population was required. As we note in our response to reviewer comment 5, we believe our study numbers were too small for formal age- and gender-matched comparisons. We did, however, change our conclusion on page 15 to state that liver transplantation does not *appear* to place patients at risk for development of nonlymphoid tumors.

As you requested, 3 copies of the revised manuscript are enclosed. We hope these revisions meet with your approval.

Thank you very much for your consideration.

Sincerely,

Table XII Resident Variables

Subjects		Age	Gender	PGY[a]	On call	Married (Y/N)[a]	Kids (Y/N)	Distance (miles)	Ideal weight (Y/N)
Group 1	1	28	M	2	3	N	N	5	N
	2	35	M	5	4	Y	Y	7	N
	3	25	M	3	2	N	N	2	N
	4	26	F	3	2	N	N	3	N
	5	28	F	4	3	Y	N	2	Y
	6	29	M	4	3	Y	N	4	Y
	7	30	M	2	3	N	N	3	Y
	8	31	F	1	3	N	N	2	N
	9	28	F	3	2	Y	N	7	Y
	10	30	M	4	3	N	N	1	N
	AVG	29	40% F	3	2.8	40% married	10% w/kids	3.6	40% ideal
	STD DEV[a]	2.788	—	1.197	0.63	—	—	2.119	—
Group 2	11	28	M	3	2	Y	Y	2	Y
	12	27	M	3	2	Y	N	15	N
	13	30	F	2	3	N	N	11	N
	14	31	M	2	3	Y	Y	13	N
	15	30	F	4	3	N	N	19	Y
	16	29	M	1	3	Y	Y	5	Y
	17	25	M	5	4	N	N	45	N
	18	26	F	5	4	N	N	30	N
	19	27	F	3	2	Y	Y	12	Y
	20	29	F	3	2	Y	Y	3	Y
	21	25	M	4	3	N	N	18	N
	22	22	M	2	3	Y	N	28	N
	23	33	M	2	3	N	N	30	Y
	24	28	F	2	3	Y	N	35	N
	25	29	M	5	4	N	N	20	Y
	AVG	28	40% F	3	2.9	53% married	33% w/kids	19.1	47% ideal
	STD DEV	2.738	—	1.28	0.70	—	—	12.43	—

[a] PGY, Postgraduate year; Y/N, yes/no; STD DEV, standard deviation

nificant factor determining health club attendance. among the 10 residents who attended more than twice a week, the average distance from home to health club was 3.6 miles (range, 1–7), whereas for the 15 who attended less frequently or not at all, the average distance was 19 miles (range, 2–45). *Conclusion:* Only residents who live near the health club are likely to attend regularly.

Reluctant to provide passes to only some residents, you submit a copy of the abstract to the health club management. You are able to convince them to reduce their membership fees for residents with kids and for those who live greater than 10 miles from the health club, and you are able to provide memberships for everybody. You are named "Physician of the Year" at the residents' annual dinner.

References

1. Flesch, R. (1960). "How to Write, Speak and Think More Effectively." Harper & Rowe, New York.

1a. Gehlbach, S. H. (1993). "Interpreting the Medical Literature," 3rd Ed., p. 16. McGraw-Hill, New York.

2. Olak, J., and Chiu, R. C.-J. (1993). A surgeon's guide to biostatistical inferences. Part I. *Am. Coll. Surg. Bull.* **78**(1), 20–26

3. Olak, J., and Chiu, R. C.-J. (1993). A surgeon's guide to biostatistical inferences. Part II. *Am. Coll. Surg. Bull.* **78**(2), 27–31

4. Olak, J., and Chiu, R. C.-J. (1993). A surgeon's guide to biostatistical inferences. Part III. *Am. Coll. Surg. Bull.* **78**(3), 15–19

5. Bailar, III, J. C. (1986). Science, statistics, and deception. *Ann. Intern. Med.* **104,** 259–260

6. Huth, E. J. (1986). Irresponsible authorship and wasteful publication. *Ann. Intern. Med.* **104,** 257–259.

7. American Society of Parenteral and Enteral Nutrition (1999). Scientific abstract form for the American Society of Parenteral and Enteral Nutrition, 24th Clinical Congress. American Society of Parenteral and Enteral Nutrition, Silver Spring, Maryland.
8. Meinert, C. L., and Tonascia, S. (1986). "Clinical Trials: Design, Conduct, and Analysis," pp. 266–267. Oxford University Press, New York.
9. Harris, M. C., and McGovern, J. P. (1968). Writing for medical journals [editorial]. *Ann. Allerg.* **26,** 644–647.
10. Roland, C. G. (1968). Writing about writing. *JAMA* **204,** 177–178
11. Huth, E. J. (1990). "How to Write and Publish Papers in the Medical Sciences," 2nd Ed., p. 95. Williams & Wilkins, Baltimore.
12. Huth, E. J. (1990). "How to Write and Publish Papers in the Medical Sciences," 2nd Ed., p. 61. Williams & Wilkins, Baltimore.
13. International Committee of Medical Journal Editors (1997). Uniform requirements for manuscripts submitted to biomedical journals. *JAMA* **277,** 927–934
14. International Committee of Medical Journal Editors (1997). Uniform requirements for manuscripts submitted to biomedical journals 19 March, 1997. Web site: http://www.ascp.com/public/pubs/tcp/unireqs.shtml, accessed 31 January, 2000.
15. Hamilton, A. W. (1992). How to write and publish scientific papers: Scribing information for pharmacists. *Am. J. Hosp. Pharm.* **49,** 2477–2484
16. Begg, C., Cho, M., Eastwood, S., Horton, R., Moher, D., Olkin, I., Pitkin, R., Rennie, D., Schulz, K. F., Simel, D., and Stroup, D. F. (1996). Improving the quality of reporting of randomized controlled trials: The CONSORT statement. *JAMA* **276,** 637–639
17. Meinert, C. L., and Tonascia, S. (1986). "Clinical Trials: Design, Conduct, and Analysis," p. 268. Oxford University Press, New York.
18. Flanagin, A., Carey, L. A., Fontanarosa, P. B., Phillips, S. G., Pace, B. P., Lundberg, G. D., and Rennie, D. (1998). Prevalence of articles with honorary authors and ghost authors in peer-reviewed medical journals. *JAMA* **280,** 222–224
19. Pitkin, R. M., Branagan, M. A., and Burmeister, L. F. (1999). Accuracy of data in abstracts of published research articles [see comments]. *JAMA* **281,** 1110–1111.
20. Winker, M. A. (1999). The need for concrete improvement in abstract quality [editorial; comment]. *JAMA* **281,** 1129-30.
21. Hoke, F. (1993). Bibliography-building software eases a 'cruel' task. *The Scientist* **7**(1), 18
22. Hoke, F. (1994). Making the online connection with bibliographic-database software. *The Scientist* **8**(13), 18–19.
23. Finn, R. (1996). Bibliographic software adding new features, becoming web savvy. *The Scientist* **10**(14), 18–19
24. Pitkin, R. M., and Branagan, M. A. (1998). Can the accuracy of abstracts be improved by providing specific instructions? A randomized controlled trial. *JAMA* **280,** 267–269
25. Huth, E. J. (1990). "How to Write and Publish Papers in the Medical Sciences," 2nd Ed., p. 51. Williams & Wilkins, Baltimore.
26. Huth, E. J. (1990). "How to Write and Publish Papers in the Medical Sciences," 2nd ed., pp. 104–107. Williams & Wilkins, Baltimore.
27. Flesch, R. (1960). "How to Write, Speak and Think More Effectively," p. 102. Harper and Rowe, New York.
28. Flesch, R. (1960). "How to Write, Speak and Think More Effectively," p. 321. Harper and Rowe, New York.
29. Huth, E. J. (1990). "How to Write and Publish Papers in the Medical Sciences," 2nd Ed., p. 114. Williams & Wilkins, Baltimore.
30. National Library of Medicine (1999). 21 Medical subject headings (MeSH), October, 1999. Web site: http://www.nlm.nih.gov/mesh/meshhome.html, accessed 27 January, 2000.
31. List of Journals Indexed in Index Medicus (2000). GPO Code: IM2000. Superintendent of Documents, U.S. Government Printing Office, P.O.Box 371954, Pittsburgh, PA 15250-7954.
32. National Library of Medicine (1999). List of journals indexed in Index Medicus, 30 November, 1999. Web site: http://www.nlm.nih.gov/tsd/serials/lji.html, accessed 27 January, 2000.
33. Wilcox, L. J. (1998). Authorship: The coin of the realm, the source of complaints. *JAMA* **280,** 216–217
34. Angell, M. (1986). Publish or perish: A proposal. *Ann. Intern. Med.* **104,** 261–262.
35. Drenth, J. P. H. (1998). Multiple authorship: The contribution of senior authors. *JAMA* **280,** 219–221.
36. Shapiro, D. W., Wenger, N. S., and Shapiro, M. F. (1994). The contributions of authors to multiauthored biomedical research papers. *JAMA* **271,** 438–442.
37. Flanagin, A., Carey, L. A., Fontanarosa, P. B., Phillips, S. G., Pace, B. P., Lundberg, G. D., and Rennie, D. (1998). Prevalance of articles with honorary authors and ghost authors in peer-reviewed medical journals. *JAMA* **280,** 222–224.
38. Slone, R. M. (1996). Coauthors' contributions to major papers published in the AJR: Frequency of undeserved coauthorship. *AJR* **167,** 571–579.
39. Council of Biology Editors (1999). Authroship Task Force: Is it time to update the tradition of authorship in scientific publications?, 30 April 1999. Web site: http://www.cbe.org/ATF.html, accessed 26 November, 1999.
40. Friedman, P. J. (1999). A new standard for authorship, 18 February, 1999. Web site: http://www.cbe.org/AddEvent.html, accessed 12 Jan, 2000.
41. Rennie, D. (1998). Freedom and responsibility in medical publication: Setting the balance right. *JAMA* **280,** 300–302.
42. Huth, E. J. (1986). Guidelines on authorship of medical papers. *Ann. Intern. Med.* **104,** 269–274.
43. International Committee of Medical Journal Editors (1985). Guidelines on authorship. *Br. Med. J.* **291,** 722
44. Rennie, D. (1998). Peer review in Prague [editorial]. *JAMA* **280,** 214–215.
45. Tamru, F. L., Turina, M., Karp, R. B., Ferguson, T. B., Bodnar, E., and Waldhausen, J. A. (1999). Joint statement on redundant (duplicate) publication by the editors of the undersigned cardiothoracic journals. *J. Thorac. Cardiovasc. Surg.* **118,** 210
46. Broad, W. J. (1981). The publishing game: Getting more for less. *Science* **211,** 1137–1139.
47. Huth, E. J. (1990). "How to Write and Publish Papers in the Medical Sciences," 2nd Ed., p. 10. Williams & Wilkins, Baltimore.
48. Institute for Scientific Information (2000). Journal citation reports, 28 January, 2000. Web site: http://www.isinet.com/products/citation/jcr.html#features, accessed 28 January, 2000.
49. Harnack, A., and Kleppinger, E. (1998). "Online! A Reference Guide to Using Internet Sources." Bedford/St. Martin's. Web site: http://www.bedfordstmartins.com/online/index.html, accessed 12 January, 2000.

84

Audiovisual Communications as a Research Skill

Charles M. Balch

Departments of Surgery and Oncology, Johns Hopkins Medical Center, Baltimore, Maryland 21231

I. Introduction

When the analysis of a research project is completed, the work should be considered only half completed! Communicating research results through oral presentations and scientific publications is just as important as conducting the research. A number of surgical scientists who are brilliant in the conception or execution of research ideas never receive the recognition they deserve because they did not develop skills of clearly and effectively communicating their work. Even when research has been well designed, responsibly conducted, and judiciously analyzed, it is all a sterile exercise if the results fail to reach the target audience.

Oral communication is a vital component of research, and its principles must be learned and practiced by the academic surgeon at a high level of sophistication. When the opportunity to speak before colleagues and peers arises, take full advantage of the occasion and treat it as a privilege to share what has been learned. Generally, there is only a short time to convey a message in a way that an audience will understand and incorporate into their fund of knowledge. It is the artful and thoughtful integration of the spoken word and visual images that has the greatest impact. Educational psychologists believe that we retain about 20% of what we hear and 30% of what we see. However, a spoken message augmented by a visual image more than doubles retention. It is a tough job to integrate ideas and images, and the secret of success is preparation, rehearsal, and an approach to communication from the audience's perspective.

In giving a presentation, the goal should be for the audience to hear and understand what is said in a way that it is relevant to their needs and useful enough that they will incorporate key parts of the material into their fund of knowledge.

II. Preparation

When preparing an oral presentation, follow the same approach as in writing an abstract: introduction, methods, results, conclusions. List no more than a few key points at the outset and organize everything around these key points. Most often, the focus should be on the hypothesis being tested and how the results and conclusions are derived from that hypothesis.

A talk should be prepared with a message and theme that is appropriate for the audience. Deliver the talk for the entire audience, including those in the back of the room, who should also be able to read slides, maintain eye contact, and hear the message. It is a simple but vital principle in audio-visual (AV) communication: if the person in the back of the room can see the slides and hear the words, then so can everyone else in the audience.

PowerPoint software (Microsoft) is increasingly becoming a standard approach for preparing presentations. It is recommended to read one or two books on the use of this or similar types of software. PowerPoint allows insertion of images, tables, web hyperlinks, and audio and video clips. Optimal PowerPoint settings are suggested in Fig. 1. Start by formatting the "master slide" (under "View" in the dropdown menu), then select colors (under "Format" in the dropdown menu), and then background settings (also under the "Format" menu). A ramped color gradient on the slide background is recommended; this can be created after clicking on the "Background" menu, under "Fill Effects." Familiarity with the toolbars and other features by using visuals and hyperlinks to web pages will ensure full utilization of current software technology. A period of exploration will uncover an amazing number of resources.

III. Timing and Speaking Style

For a short talk (such as the 10-minute presentation), timing is important. The content of the message must usually be condensed. In this circumstance, it may be appropriate to read from a script so as to ensure staying on time. Remember, the audience (and the next speaker) will be offended if the rules of a timed talk are not observed. It is an expected courtesy to stay within a time limit. Also keep in mind that the language style for a written manuscript is very different from the style and choice of words used in oral communication. So do not cut and paste from an abstract or manuscript, but dictate in a conversational style and then edit the talk from that transcript.

Optimal PowerPoint Settings

- **Balance color: Dark background and light font color**
- **Type face: Times New Roman 32 pt.**
- **Slide surface area: 35mm**
- **Slide layout: Bulleted list**

Figure 1 Tips about the format for a PowerPoint (Microsoft) presentation.

IV. Helpful Principles and Pointers

Here are a few useful pointers:

1. Message: Do not blitz people with excessive data that will bore, confuse, or frustrate. Synthesize data into a few focused messages that the audience should remember. Repeat and reinforce these messages throughout the talk.

2. Audience: Know the audience. If they are familiar with the specialty interest being presented, more details and supporting evidence will be necessary. However, in a setting with an audience outside of the specialty interest, in-depth materials may confuse or frustrate unless details are carefully and logically presented. In other words, speak with an emphasis that is congruent with the perspective and knowledge base of the audience.

3. Slides: Images convey a lot of information. The audience can read much faster than words on the screen can be spoken. Therefore, do not read from a slide verbatim. This may be perceived as a crutch and a lack of knowledge about the material. Project visual images that the audience can grasp in a few seconds and be sure that the spoken message and the images reinforce or complement each other. Pay as much attention to the content and readability of the slides as to the preparation of the spoken words. The two should reinforce each other. Do not overwhelm an audience with either too much data in one image or with too many images. Doing so will cause an audience to focus only on the visual aspect of the presentation and to tune out spoken words! Too many words or details on graphs will turn an audience into readers rather than listeners.

4. Pictures and graphs: These convey more information than text slides—they increase the rate of retention and the overall effectiveness of the message. However, they should not be so self-explanatory that the audience is drawn to the slide and not to the speaker. If the contents of pictures and graphs are used correctly, they cannot be fully interpreted without the speaker's complementary verbal input. Effective visuals allow the audience to better grasp the mental concepts the speaker is communicating.

5. Color and text: When preparing text slides, there are many choices with regard to color of text and background. A ramped, dark blue background with either yellow or white bolded text is preferable. In general, do not use red or green colors; they are not seen as well, especially against a dark background. Remember that about 15% of mates have some degree of red/green color blindness. Keep the content to three to five bulleted points that flow logically within a specific area (e.g., methods, objectives, results, conclu-

sions). The content is summary format, not full text. The size and block style of the letters should project large enough that the audience in the back of the room can easily read the slides. Occasionally, emphasize important points with text highlighted in bright colors, underlining, or changes in font to increase the visual impact. Each slide should complement but not substitute for the spoken word. Above all else, do not read from the slides!

6. Single vs. double slide projection: There are different opinions about this issue. Double projection is useful when the content of a talk requires comparisons and contrasts. Presenting these ideas side by side instead of sequentially enhances the concept. In addition, larger lettering with fewer points per slide has visual impact. Double projection also presents more material in shorter time, but with fewer slides, promoting better attention to, and retention of, verbal material. Double projection also keeps the reading audience interested when the spoken message is exactly the same as the slide material being projected, and the audience also has a visual reminder of the last point (displayed on the parallel slide) that was made in segueing from one issue to another. Use of double projection requires careful attention to the perfect alignment of spoken text content and visual imagery.

7. Laser pointers: These can be used for emphasis, but oftentimes can drive the audience crazy if pointers are used steadily in a circular motion on the slide or around the room. If nervousness is a problem (which it is for many speakers to varying degrees), do not show it visibly with a shaky pointer. Either do not use the pointer or use a podium to steady your arm. Turn the laser pointer on and off as particular parts of the slides are emphasized, but do not draw circles with it or keep it on constantly.

V. Delivery

A great talk requires attention and preparation to all three aspects of delivery: verbal, vocal, and visual content (Fig. 2). All must be in balance. A deficiency in any one of the three can be distracting to the audience.

Here are some of the basic principles to use when giving a talk:

1. Win the interest of the audience and then keep it throughout the talk.

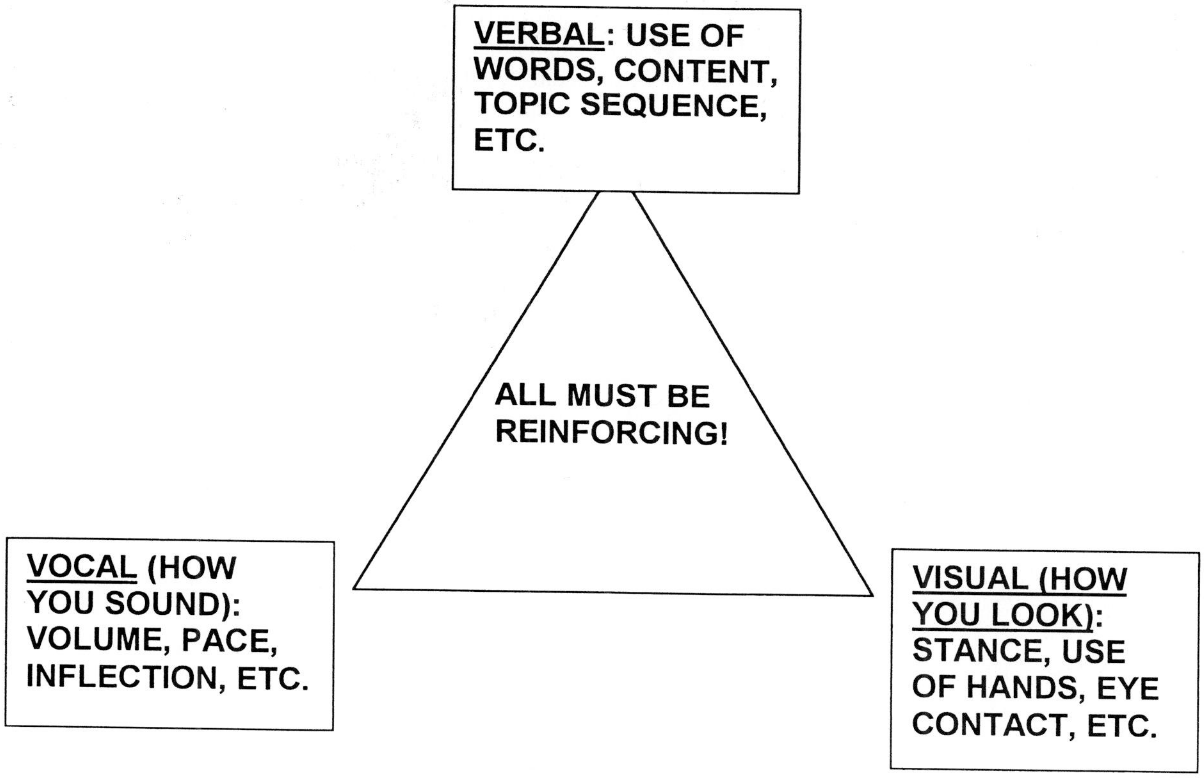

Figure 2 A good talk requires attention and preparation of all three aspects of delivery, plus the integration of complementary slide material.

2. Keep good eye contact throughout the room (people want to be spoken to directly), including those in the last row.

3. Vary vocal pitch and word pace as necessary for emphasis. Do not speak in a monotone and do not read from the slides.

4. Consider asking questions at the outset to keep audience interest.

5. Always check slides after they have been put in the slide tray to be sure they are oriented properly.

6. Go up to the podium before the session starts to become familiar with the microphones, remote controls, and pointers.

7. At the podium, take a moment to remember posture (stand up straight and tall), relax (as much as possible), start off in a conversational tone, and remember that the rhythm developed during rehearsals will come naturally.

Prepare ahead of time. Rehearse in time to change the slides if necessary. Rehearsal and knowledge of material allow greater concentration on delivery. Ask friends or colleagues to listen to a rehearsal. Include someone who is unfamiliar with the content. Check for timing, pace, clarity of message (could they repeat back to you what message they received?). When you think you have the talk down pat, then work on it just a little bit more to polish it up into a really classy talk.

An excellent idea is to rehearse in front of a video camera. There is no better way to see how you come across. You are your best critic on delivery. You will most likely pick up on some distracting gestures, motions, postures, or speech that not everyone would be willing to share with you.

VI. Summary

The following tips are helpful when preparing for an AV presentation:

1. Prepare a talk with a focused theme and a depth of content tailored to the audience.
2. Keep projected data to a minimum, but use slides to distill essential material, along with the *p* values from statistical analyses.
3. Display results so they can easily and quickly be grasped by the audience.
4. Synthesize the results in the broader context of their significance or impact.
5. Summarize the salient points at the end, especially the "take home" messages.
6. Pay equal attention to the verbal, vocal, and visual components of the talk.
7. Stay on time.
8. If the format of the presentation allows, have slides ready for questions from the audience.
9. Above all, keep the presentation as simple and succinct as possible.

An effective lecture or talk requires skill, experience, and, above all, effort. The basic strategy is to have a clear message and conclusion, tailored to an individual audience and delivered in an enjoyable, stimulating, and persuasive manner. Perhaps, Will Mayo summarized it best when he said "Begin with an arresting sentence; close with a strong summary; in between speak simply, clearly, and always to the point; and above all be brief."

Acknowledgment

Ms. Nicole Johnson from the American Society of Clinical Oncology made valuable recommendations about the PowerPoint material.

85

Organizing and Managing Meetings and Conferences

Mary C. Schuerman and P. William Curreri

Strategem, Inc., Daphne, Alabama 36526

I. Introduction

The organization and management of meetings is pivotal for the successful exchange of investigational results among peers and students. Research meetings are rarely satisfying to the attendee if the environment does not promote appropriate interchange between conferees. To be successful, the manager must organize sufficient staff to attend to details both before and during the meeting. In addition, he/she must be a skillful negotiator to obtain fair and reasonable contracts with sufficient protections for the organization in case of cancellation or attrition.

The timeline for the organization activities varies, depending in part on the size of the meeting and in part on the location of the meeting. In general, the larger the attendance, the longer the period of time required for organizational activities (Table I). International meetings held outside the continental United States and Canada may require extra lead time due to limited availability of meeting space and the necessity of giving potential attendees enough notice that they can block extra time required for travel.

Marketing may be used to promote the program. A database of potential attendees should be constructed as soon as the meeting is scheduled and decisions made regarding the subpopulations to target (Table II). Brochures and newsletters should be enclosed in other meeting-related mailings, and may include special features of the scientific program, social/spouse programs, and other local attractions. The list of reference literature at the end of this chapter provides many excellent insights into the requirements for successful planning of meetings and conferences.

Table I Timeline for Organization of Meetings

Number of attendees	Time required
10–30	3–6 months
31–60	6–12 months
61–100	12–18 months
101–200	2 years
201–400	3 years
401–1,000	4 years
>1000	5 years or more

Table II Potential Classes of Attendees for Research Meetings

Physicians	Nurses
Educators	Students
Residents	Exhibitors
Fellows	Spouses

II. Choosing a Site

Depending on the size of the meeting a site must be chosen between 6 months (meetings of 30 or less participants) and 10 years (meetings of greater than 10,000 attendees) prior to the meeting date. A number of factors enter into the consideration of geographic locations, including past meeting sites, ease of transportation, availability of recreational activities for attendees and/or spouses, and cost. The presence of multiple facilities (hotels, convention centers, conference centers) offering adequate meeting space may give the meeting manager a competitive advantage when negotiating room rates. Facilities in any one geographic area may vary considerably from large urban hotels with generous meeting space to small conference centers designed to provide meeting space for 40 of fewer participants. A list of the advantages and disadvantages of each is listed in Table III.

Once a geographical area is chosen, a list of potential facilities should be constructed considering the total number of rooms required, as well as the requirements for meeting and exhibit space. Many of the major hotel chains have web sites that detail meeting space dimensions at each of their properties. In the past, seating capacities published for each room (depending on setup, i.e., schoolroom or theater)* were notoriously inaccurate, although now the Professional Convention Management Association (PCMA) has a verification program in which hotel and convention center meeting space is accurately measured and seating capacity is calculated. Access to these data is available on the PCMA web site at www.pcma.org. This process should narrow down the list of potential properties to a manageable number for evaluation in one or more communities.

A site visit to each of the properties is the next mandatory step. Priority should be given to meeting space and audiovisual (AV) capability, because without the capability of communicating scientific results effectively the meeting will have failed its primary goal. Meeting rooms must be inspected to make certain there are no obstructing columns, unusual wall angles, low-hanging chandeliers, or low ceilings or ceiling overhangs that could dictate the use of less than ideal AV equipment or, worse yet, interfere with attendees' ability to observe screens utilized for slide or computer presentations.

If exhibits or posters are part of the program, sufficient nearby space must be available. Knowledge of local fire marshal regulations is necessary to calculate minimum space requirements. The floor plan and on-site setup is usually delegated at a later date to an exposition company with the appropriate inventory of piping, draping, tables, chairs, carpet, poster boards, etc. to satisfy the needs of poster presenters and exhibitors.

Sleeping rooms should also be inspected to ascertain their acceptability with respect to square footage, amenities, and cleanliness. In addition, various sizes of suites and upgraded rooms should be visited, depending on requirements for officers, invited speakers, or other VIPs. A site inspection of hotel and area restaurants is required to assess the quality of food preparation, the seating capacity of each, and the capability for hosting sponsored meals. Hotel menus should be collected in order to better predict food costs associated with sponsored meal functions.

*Schoolroom design includes 6-foot-long tables and chairs aligned in rows with either two or three participants per table. Theater design has only chairs aligned in rows, allowing increased seating capacity.

Table III Advantages and Disadvantages by Hotel or Center Location

Facility	Meeting space	Cost	Accessibility	Dining facilities	Attractions
Urban hotel	+++	++	+++	++++	+++
Convention center	++++	+	+++	+	+++
Resort	+++	++	+	+++	++++
Conference center	++	++++	++	++	+

Finally, the availability and attractiveness of the site for presentation of special events, such as spouse tours, golf and tennis activities, theme parties, etc., must be evaluated if they are an integral part of the meeting.

III. Contracts

A variety of contracts with suppliers will have to be negotiated, depending in part on the size of the meeting, the number of off-site venues, and the availability of in-house meeting space with adequate dimensions to meet meeting requirements. Larger meetings may require contracts with multiple hotels for sleeping-room blocks, a convention center, audiovisual companies, exposition companies, transportation services providing local mobility, caterers, museums, musicians, restaurants, theme parks, etc. in order to meet the needs of the attendees.

The major contracts will be made with the participating hotel(s) and/or convention centers. After the site visit, proposal agreements should be requested from several properties in order to compare the costs for rooms, food and beverage functions, and utilization of meeting space (often complimentary when participants occupy a majority of hotel sleeping rooms).

Standard hotel contracts commonly include safeguarding clauses for the hotel and relatively few protections for the meeting planner or the sponsoring organization. Virtually everything in the contract can be negotiated and every clause must be carefully scrutinized. Specific attention should be paid to the proposed room block, because failure to fill a minimum of blocked room nights (typically 80–85%) may result in significant attrition fees, which should be clearly expressed in dollar terms within the contract. The hotel may demand monetary remuneration if a meeting is cancelled less than 2–3 years from the anticipated beginning date of the function. Meeting managers should incorporate in the contract similar provisions that provide for compensation from the hotel, should the hotel cancel the meeting as a result of insolvency, renovation, or desire to satisfy a potentially more lucrative client request.

Desired amenities must be included in the contract and may include complimentary use of suites by VIPs, gift baskets, airport–hotel limousine service, reduced room rates for staff, etc. In addition, function space for each scheduled event should be agreed on and attached as an amendment to the contract. A current menu with prices should make up a second amendment with a guarantee in the body of the contract that food and beverage prices will not rise faster than a given rate (generally 3–5% per year). Although hotel meeting space may be offered at a reduced cost or rental fees waived, meeting space obtained by contractual agreement with a conference center or convention center is often expensive, because rental of space is the prime source of income for these entities.

Audiovisual fees are becoming a more significant portion of the meeting budget, as more advanced computer-based presentations are being utilized. Specific lists of AV requirements, including the resolution of each image projector (e.g., XGA, SVGA) for each function, must be constructed along with diagrams outlining the placement of the dais, screens, lectern, microphones, electronic pointers and timers; slide, LCD, overhead, and video projection equipment; and sound system. A bid for the entire scope of the meeting AV needs should be obtained from several AV companies and a final contract negotiated. Most hotels have in-house AV companies, which sometimes offer advantages insofar as they are familiar with property sound systems and often have exclusive use of them. Outside contractors may then have to bring in their own sound systems, often at additional cost.

IV. Establishing a Budget and Setting Appropriate Registration Fees

Probably the most important function of the meeting manager rests with accurately estimating costs and revenue, in order to assure sound fiscal management of the meeting. Estimation of costs per person will assist in establishing appropriate registration fees. During the planning of the event it is necessary for the planners and sponsors to agree on a fiscal philosophy, e.g., the meeting expenses should equal meeting revenues (nonprofit), meeting revenues should exceed meeting costs (profit), or meeting revenues will be subsidized by other revenue streams, such as dues (subsidized). Once these decisions are made, costs is totaled and then divided by expected registrants to estimate a cost per person. Likewise a list of all nonregistrant revenue sources is constructed and the total is divided by the expected number of registrants to arrive at nonregistrant revenue per registrant, and the difference estimates the appropriate registration fee in the break-even (nonprofit) model (Table IV).

V. Food and Beverage

Food and beverage functions are very important cost items at most meetings. With coffee currently priced at \$35.00–50.00 a gallon (1999), a half-hour coffee break twice a day can result in a significant expenditure. Food and beverage functions should be outlined on individual banquet event orders (BEOs), which contain the location, the guaranteed number of people, the room setup, AV requirements, food and beverage orders, and cost (Fig. 1). These are forwarded to the hotel convention or catering manager for

Table IV Setting Appropriate Registration Fees

Variable	Calculation
Revenue, r	c/er = cost/registrant and nrr/er = nonregistration fee revenue/registrant
Costs, c	$c - nrr/er$ = registration fee for nonprofit model
Expected registrants, er	
Nonregistrant revenue, nrr	

approval. If food and beverage costs on hotel-supplied menus appear excessive for the meeting budget, it may be helpful to share budget concerns with the catering manager. Most culinary staffs can suggest alternative menus that could be produced at reduced cost.

A number of strategies may result in significant savings for food and beverage functions as a rule. Coffee and tea should always be ordered by the gallon and restrictions must be placed on refilling service stations. It is recommended that wine and liquor be ordered by the bottle when possible. Conversions of gallons and bottles into cups and drinks are indicated in Table V. When ordering alcoholic or nonalcoholic drinks by the bottle, pre- and postfunction inventories are necessary in order to verify the number of bottles consumed.

VI. Audiovisual

Audiovisual capability plays a major role in the success of a meeting. Clearly the purpose of the meeting is to examine new hypotheses and present results of scientific research. These aims cannot be fulfilled without AV equipment that can provide optimal presentation of the data. AV companies should be sent a request for proposal (RFP) containing all the AV specifications required by the program broken down into audio, lighting, and video requirements, and miscellaneous electronic equipment.

Audio requirements consist of audio sources (microphones, CD players, etc.) a mixing board with enough channels (or inputs) for all the different audio sources, an equalizer (used to adjust sound frequencies to match the acoustics of the meeting space), and an amplifier, which powers the loudness of the audio system.

Lighting requirements are individualized for each meeting. They include simple requests such as a lectern light or more complicated tasks such as spotlighting performers with lights in a colored sequence. If one is going to depend on a projectionist to control house lights, be certain light controls are adjacent to projection equipment.

Video projection varies from the use of simple 35-mm slide projectors to very sophisticated computer presentations. When slide projectors are utilized in large meeting rooms it is frequently necessary to use a high-intensity lamp system (available in a xenon projector) to assure adequate screen illumination. Liquid crystal display (LCD) projectors are required for computerized presentations. LCD portable projectors are completely integrated units that combine the optics of liquid crystal display with the light source of an overhead projector. Such a projector is capable of providing computerized presentations to audiences of 100 or less. Most projectors are integrated ("one-gun") projectors. Resolution must be specified because price differences between systems (XGA, SVGA) are substantial.

Miscellaneous equipment includes electric or laser pointers, timers, screens, and overhead projectors. In general, use the largest screens possible, allowing 4 feet of space between the floor and the bottom of the screen. Finally, always make sure that technicians have available a spare projector and bulbs at all times during the program.

VII. Entertainment

Entertainment at a meeting or conference may take many forms depending on the number of participants attending social functions. For larger meetings, an annual banquet with after-dinner dancing and an invited guest speaker are popular choices. Dance bands range from trios to large groups with 10–12 musicians and singers. Most require a minimum performance time of 4 hours and will require male and female dressing rooms as well as some type of food and beverage. Bands can be hired through local musical agents. Often a list of agencies can be supplied to you by the hotel. Prior to engaging in a contract with a band, preview a number of bands on videotape to gauge their suitability for your attendees and to assess their range of musical presentation. Band expenses will vary between $1000 and $9000, depending on size of the band and their reputation for providing an entertaining performance.

After-dinner speakers or performers must be chosen with care. Even an excellent speaker, who is discussing a serious topic, will find difficulty holding the attention of an audience of researchers following a full-day scientific session, a

Banquet Event Order

Event Date:	**Convention Manager:**	**Page #**
Group Name:		
Billing Address: **Strategem, Inc.** **P. O. Box 1187** **Daphne, AL 36526**	**Meeting Manager:** **Mary Schuerman** **PHONE: (334) 625-2205** **FAX: (334) 625-4439**	
BILL To: MASTER ACCT		
FUNCTION: / **ROOM:**	**Time:**	**#ppl**
SET UP REQUIREMENTS	**MENU DETAIL**	
Audiovisual Services		
Timing Schedule	**Room Arrangements**	

Figure 1 Banquet event orders are used to provide detailed information to the convention manager and his staff for each individual function during the meeting.

reception, and a full-course dinner. Rather, it may be more practical to consider a political comedian, unique singing groups, or an acting group with focus on political satire. Many national booking agents are available for engaging the most popular political, motivational, and comedic speakers, with rates ranging from $5000 to as much as $150,000 for a 1-hour presentation. After reviewing the brochures from several agencies, select several speakers in the budgeted price range to preview by videotape. Local speakers, acting groups, or performing musical groups may often exist, particularly in cities with universities, and may be engaged for lower fees.

Specialized programs for spouses may be designed if there are a sufficient number attending. They may include

Table V Liquid Measurements and Yields

Quantity	Yield
One bottle of wine (24 oz)	6 (4-oz) glasses
One liter (35.6 oz)	33 (1-oz) drinks
One fifth (25.6 oz)	23 (1-oz) drinks
One gallon (4 quarts)	22 (6-oz) cups

lectures (e.g., estate planning), demonstrations (e.g., flower arrangements), area sightseeing trips (e.g., museums or historical points), or shopping tours for local specialty items. Destination management companies (DMC) exist in most cities and can make suggestions for tours and activities and arrange for guides and transportation. If a DMC is utilized, the meeting manager should ask to review the DMC's insurance package, particularly if transportation is involved.

VIII. Registration

A. Premeeting

Many registration software packages are available and can perform a variety of specialized functions (Table VI) to assist with all aspects of meeting management. However, the most sophisticated programs (and also the most expensive) are capable of performing a combination of tasks, including budgeting and financial applications, name badge production, participant meeting room assignments, registration with acknowledgment letter capability, hotel room night tracking, and customized financial reporting programs. Such programs are essential for efficient management of meetings with over 200 participants.

Once a software program has been selected and an association or a potential participant database has been entered into the software, the registration process essentially becomes a one-step process, with the registrant receiving an acknowledging letter informing him of seminars selected, payment submitted, payment due if any, and type of payment (check or credit card). At the same time a name badge is produced for insertion in a registration packet.

Table VI Specialized Functions of Software Packages

Site, destination, and venue selection tools
Budgeting applications
Meeting resumes and specifications
Floor plan design
Name badge programs
Association management software
Registration software
Housing programs
Room scheduling

The design of the registration form is very important. First, it must contain spaces to collect all of the data required by the registration software package. Second, it must clearly outline the registration fee and additional costs and the methods of acceptable payment. Finally, it must describe what food and beverage events are included in the registration fee for each class of participant.

Registration forms should be mailed to potential participants 3–8 months prior to the meeting. International meetings generally require longer lead times to allow for slower mail delivery and the requirement for more complex travel planning. Avoid sending forms during prolonged holiday periods, because the forms are frequently lost or misplaced at these times. Also, it is useful to place both meeting and hotel registration forms on an available web site, in order that they can be completed, downloaded, and then mailed or faxed to the registration office.

B. On Site

As the result of good marketing and with financial incentives for early preregistration, on-site registration should be reduced to a minimum. One may expect to observe preregistration rates of 85–90% even at very large meetings. Nevertheless, personnel are necessary to accommodate those who seek to register on site. In addition, a laptop or conventional personal computer will be required as well as a printer. The registration area at the on-site location should be spacious enough to process on-site registrants and preregistrants in different lines, because on-site registrants would unduly delay distribution of registration packets to preregistrants.

It is beneficial to have the original registration forms on site in addition to the computer-held registrations in order to resolve any disagreements regarding assignment to specific seminars, payment due, or reservations for spouse activities. Experienced meeting managers will be prepared to expect a small percentage of on-site registrants to claim to have preregistered. This often results from miscommunication between the participant and his secretarial staff or the source responsible for providing financial support, e.g., a company or university financial department.

IX. Badges, Signage, and Printing

Badges are an important aspect of successful meetings with more than a few participants. They allow for easy name recognition among participants and provide evidence that the participant has registered for the meeting. Badges generally convey a limited amount of information in order that the lettering can remain large for identification at a distance. Many organizations limit badge content to logo, first and last name, and city and state of residence. Others may add company or university affiliation and/or nickname. Badge holders must be purchased separately and generally are designed in two ways, either as a pocket clip/safety pin combination or as an elastic necklace. The necklace-type holders are more expensive but are generally preferred by attendees.

In order to facilitate movement between meeting rooms and to establish identification of meeting sites, it is imperative to provide signs that direct attendees to their intended destination within the hotel or convention center. A list of potential signs for identification appears in Table VII. In addition, consider using signs with directional arrows. Be certain to check dimensional restrictions imposed by the meeting facility prior to purchasing needed signage.

Printing of marketing brochures, registration forms, stationary and envelopes, and spouse programs may all be accomplished months prior to the meeting. If printing a program containing abstracts, consider getting bids from several printers (local printers are preferred if available, because proof-reading drafts is more convenient and efficient). Do not overlook marketing materials that may be available from the hotel or the convention and visitors' bureau at little or no cost.

X. Exhibits and Posters

Presentation of scientific material by poster board has become more popular in the past decade for a number of reasons. Posters allow presentation of more abstracts in a limited amount of time, because the posters may be viewed during coffee breaks and luncheon breaks, as well as during dedicated program time throughout the meeting. In addition, poster presentation allows one-on-one exchange between the author and the viewer.

Commercial and noncommercial exhibits are common accompaniments to larger meetings. Noncommercial entities use exhibits to promote nonprofit activities and upcoming meetings of interest, whereas commercial exhibitors seek to introduce new and/or current products with the goal of creating enough interest to promote future sales. Charges for space used by commercial exhibitors are usually based on the number of attendees, as well as on the amount of space required (units of 100 ft^2, or 10 × 10-ft booth). To attract commercial exhibitors, two criteria must be satisfied in addition to a fair cost. The attendees must have interest in the exhibitors' products and there must be enough time in the meeting schedule to view the exhibits. Attendance at exhibits may be increased by holding continental breakfasts, coffee breaks, box lunches, and receptions in the exhibit area.

Table VII Potential Areas for Signage

Scientific program	Posters
Committee meetings	Speaker ready room
Food/beverage functions	Registration
Receptions	Press room
Exhibits	Office

Poster boards as well as piping, draping, and furniture can all be obtained by utilizing a regional exposition company. e-Mail addresses of such companies may be searched and obtained on the Internet from the following two web sites: www.mim.com and www.mmaweb.com/meetings. It is desirable to submit RFPs to at least three different companies. RFPs may be submitted online by going to www.plansoft.com on the Internet. Once a proposal has been accepted, the exposition company will provide a proposed diagram of poster and exhibit placement, which may be later modified. The meeting planner should then prepare a resume of exhibit information, including the name of the meeting, the place of the meeting, the number and makeup of the attendees, special events to be held in the exhibit area, the hours of exhibition, the rules to be followed by the exhibitors and the meeting manager, the costs of exhibits, and a numbered site map of proposed exhibit setup. This information is then provided by mail and on a web site to potential exhibitors.

XI. Security Considerations

Internal security provided by hotels may be satisfactory for most meetings, with two exceptions. If commercial exhibits are included in the meeting, outside security should be arranged during nonexhibit hours, because some scientific devices on display may be very expensive. Also, security of meeting room entrances should be considered if research results involving controversial issues are to be discussed, in order to deny entrance by the press and/or protest groups.

XII. Accounting

Appropriate accounting methodology to provide categorization of meeting revenues and expenses is imperative. Not only does it provide detailed explanation of meeting profit or loss, but it provides a framework for budgeting the next meeting. Obtain from the hotel a day-by-day summary of room pickup, in order to better estimate a more accurate room block for a future meeting. If possible, try to estimate revenues to the hotel by participants outside of official meeting expenses. These may include hotel revenue generated from room service, bar and restaurants, gift shops, and fitness facilities. This knowledge may be of benefit during future negotiations with hotels.

XIII. Professional Management

When attendance at a meeting exceeds 200 attendees, contracting a professional management company (PMC) should be considered. Professional management offers many advantages. A PMC provides continuity that ensures that the same personnel who negotiated a contract will also ensure that its terms are honored. Because a PMC manages many meetings on a national or international basis, it can often negotiate more favorable room rates at hotel properties that hope to attract future business. PMCs may be very experienced in exhibit sales and management and often have data files with valuable commercial contacts. Experienced professional managers can more accurately predict attendance at food and beverage functions and thus reduce costs by lowering guarantees.

In summary, PMCs have expertise in site selection, negotiation, amending contracts, budgeting, and accounting. They are also knowledgeable in the procurement of food and beverage and AV services. They own sophisticated software for efficient registration of attendees. A PMC provides sponsoring organizations with historical data, allowing evaluation of past programs and providing a strategy for continuously upgrading meeting format and content.

References

Fox, D. (1998). "Boston Handbook on Meeting Technology," Vol. 1. Professional Convention Management Association, Birmingham, Alabama.

Fox, D., and Atkinson, K. (1999). "Boston Handbook on Meeting Technology," Vol. 2. Professional Convention Management Association, Birmingham, Alabama.

Foster, J. (1995). "Independent Meeting Planning and the Law." Professional Convention Management Association, Birmingham, Alabama.

Foster, J. (1995). "Meetings and Facility Contracts." Professional Convention Management Association, Birmingham, Alabama.

Foster, J. (1995). "Meetings and Liability." Professional Convention Management Association, Birmingham, Alabama.

Polivka, E. G., ed. (1996). "Professional Meeting Management," 3d Ed. Professional Convention Management Association, Birmingham, Alabama.

Price, C. H. (1989). "The AMA Guide for Meeting and Event Planners." American Management Association, New York.

86

The Management and Organization of a Surgical Research Laboratory

David T. Efron, Daniel Most, and Adrian Barbul

Departments of Surgery, Sinai Hospital of Baltimore, and the Johns Hopkins Medical Institutions, Baltimore, Maryland 21215

I. Introduction

The successful surgical laboratory is a happy blending of the desire to pursue scientific questions and attention to the many details that have a major impact on the outcome of any research endeavor. The harmonious integration of new members into the lab and their stimulation by a challenging and cooperative environment, as well as a safe workplace, are key elements to a successful laboratory. Although many of the recommendations that follow may be applied differently depending on the size of a lab, most are necessary for the safe and productive function of all surgical laboratories.

II. Laboratory Personnel

A. Introducing New Lab Members

New members of a laboratory should be given a warm and hospitable welcome. The training and past experiences of the new member should be shared. Discussions should include what the staff member has done in the past, and what they hope for in the way of short- and long-term goals. Their level of training, whether it is the undergraduate volunteer, the technician with a BA/BS, or the Ph.D./M.D. scientist, will help the principal investigator of the laboratory assign responsibilities to these new members, and help mesh their current and past experiences.

It is vital that the principal investigator frame formal duties and responsibilities for new lab members. These may range from continuing projects left by others, to starting one or more new projects. If new members are graduate students or postdoctoral fellows with a finite time commitment, it is important to create projects with a reasonable chance of completion within the limited available time. Some lab members will be present only on a part-time basis, thus limiting the duties/projects they may be assigned. For example, certain types of cell culture and organ culture work require daily maintenance, making them less suitable for someone available only 3 days per week.

We recommend a core of required training for all personnel, regardless of background or experience. Most institutions offer a general laboratory safety course, as well as a simple 1-day course on research ethics. Researchers planning on using radioisotopes or biohazardous materials should also attend safety courses in these areas. If any of these are unavailable at the home facility, local universities and government offices are potential contacts for information and training.

Foreign scholars and international graduate students or postdoctoral fellows present special requirement, and often advantages, over their native counterparts. Language difficulties, cultural barriers, and differences in formal training must be taken into account. Extra language training may be necessary, including formal coursework. On the other hand, these individuals may provide many advantages to a laboratory, including unique perspectives on a project or idea, special techniques brought from previous laboratory experiences, and contacts in other countries. These individuals can bring stimulating insights into other cultures as well as novel methods of approaching science.

An important consideration for visiting foreign scholars is their visa/immigration status. A selected listing of visa classifications, as provided by the United States Immigration and Naturalization Service (INS) is provided in Table I. Note that this listing is not meant to be exhaustive, but merely as a guide to the types of visas most likely to be encountered among surgical laboratory workers. The J-1 visa is by far the likeliest to be encountered (for the most up-to-date information, refer to the INS web site at www.ins.usdoj.gov/graphics/index.htm).

The resource most likely to aid with visa and immigration issues is the institution's credentialing office. This office coordinates visa requirements, and typically has contact persons necessary for approval by the U.S. Immigration and Naturalization Service, such as Designated Program Sponsors. Larger institutions may have a separate Foreign Affairs Office to coordinate these issues. These offices are the pri-

Table I Selected Visas Likely to Be Issued to Researcher Fellows/Assistants

Visa category	Description
B-1	Individuals in the United States for a short period of time for the conduct of business, attending professional conferences, or conducting independent research; may not be paid from U.S. sources; part-time study is allowed
B-2	Prospective student/scholar—individuals who are in the United States for the purposes of academic study, or in the process of applying for J-1 visa status (this process must be completed by the expiration date on their I-94 form); may engage in full-time study, but may not work (volunteer only)
E-1	Treaty trader—dependents of these visa holders may pursue full- or part-time studies, but may not work (volunteer only)
F-1	Individuals in the United States engaged full-time in academic studies at an accredited institution; limited academic-related employment is allowed, but must be authorized through the U.S. State Department. Can be extended with State Department approval
H-1B	Temporary worker in a specialty occupation. Allowed to work in the United States performing specific professional services at a specific institution for a fixed period of time, up to 3 years; one additional renewal of up to 3 years is possible; may also engage in part-time study
H-3	Individuals in the United States for a temporary period of time in order to participate in a specific training program; may engage in part-time study
H-4	Dependents of H-3 visa holders, who may pursue full- or part-time studies, but may not work (volunteer only)
J-1	Exchange visitor (student)—individuals in the United States for the main purpose of studying at an academic institution approved by the United States Information Agency, with a Designated Program Sponsor; limited academic-related employment is allowed, but must be authorized through the U.S. State Department
	Exchange visitor (short-term scholar, specialist, researcher, or professor)—individuals in the United States in an accredited institution approved by the United States Information Agency, with a Designated Program Sponsor; limited academic-related employment is allowed, but must be authorized through the U.S. State Department
J-2	Dependents of J-1 visa holders—individuals may pursue full- or part-time study; may work full-time for any employer, on approval by the U.S. Immigration and Naturalization Service; approval is for a defined time period only (stated on the visa), and employment cannot be needed for the support of the J-1 visa holder
L-1	Employees of an overseas institution who have been transferred for work in a U.S. subsidiary in an executive or specialist position; may also engage in part-time study
O-1	Persons of extraordinary ability in the sciences, arts, education, business, or athletics, who are in the United States as employees of a local sponsoring organization; may engage in part-time study as well
TN	Professionals from Canada or Mexico who enter the United States under the North American Free Trade Agreements (NAFTA), who are authorized to perform specific professional services for a sponsoring institution for a preapproved, fixed period of time; these individuals may also engage in part-time studies

mary interface between institutions abroad, and can facilitate the steps needed to allow foreign workers to perform research in the U.S. surgical laboratory.

B. Role of Masters' Degree Scientists/Doctors of Philosophy in Surgical Research

Medical doctors are often limited by their lack of formal training in techniques of basic science, having received much of their experience on an ad hoc basis. Attempts have been made to overcome these limitations, such as requiring physicians at certain university hospitals to complete one to several years of formal research as part of their residency training. Undergraduate medical education also has made strides in overcoming these deficiencies, ranging from requiring a research project/thesis from their graduates, to formal coursework and involved laboratory benchwork leading to Master's degrees and combined M.D./Ph.D. degrees. Physicians interested in an academic career, who feel they need additional training in science, may complete postdoctoral research fellowships.

In contrast, researchers without medical training, but who have completed a Master's degree or Ph.D. degree in science, are often hampered by their lack of clinical experience. What they can bring to a surgical laboratory, however, is formal expertise in various techniques of basic science and data analysis. Many who have worked in biomedical fields have limited experiences in animal husbandry and surgery, which can be invaluable. If necessary, additional coursework can be completed by the non-M.D. lab member to ground them in medicine and surgery.

III. Collaboration

Competition within a laboratory, although superficially stimulating, is ultimately detrimental to the productivity of the lab. This atmosphere fosters secrecy and inner resentment, and precludes the cooperation and friendliness found in so many successful laboratories. Research projects are hampered at many points by unforeseen variables (such as the failed Northern blot, the inability to clone a gene, etc.), which are often amenable to another's perspective or assistance. A hostile environment saps the morale of staff, often leading to intellectual stagnation and high employee turnover.

Regularly scheduled laboratory meetings among the principal investigator and laboratory staff (at least weekly) are vital to cohesiveness. Having all laboratory members share the results of their work with each other helps to unify their ongoing projects, as well as overcome any difficulties a particular member is having with research. These meetings also force staff to become more involved with each other's projects, helping to develop a synergism of ideas and troubleshooting.

The practice of intralaboratory sharing can be extended further to other laboratories within a given department and institution, and even between different institutions. One of the catalysts of modern scientific progress has been the free intellectual exchange between laboratories, including expertise, recent discoveries, and even reagents, probes, and gene sequences. Forums for exchange can be informal, such as the simple phone call or electronic mail message, or more formal, such as at scientific meetings and conventions.

Unfortunately, this form of intellectual altruism becomes problematic in the areas of commercial research. In pharmaceutical companies and medical device manufacturers, lab personnel are often severely constrained when attempting to collaborate with other researchers, at least until their discoveries are shielded with layers of patents and other legal protections. Conversely, exchange between governmental/university laboratories and commercial laboratories can occasionally be constrained by the former two groups' internal rules limiting involvement with the latter, which is politically sensitive.

IV. Utilization of Laboratory Space

Laboratory space for basic science research is an increasingly rare and precious resource. Young investigators joining the faculties of research institutions have often been lured with the promise of lab space as an incentive. Unfortunately unlimited space is a "pipe dream," and as one prepares to initiate research, there must be some forethought as to the organization and allocation of space within the lab, especially with regard to present and possible future research projects.

A. Design

Rosenlund, in his book "The Chemical Laboratory: Its Design and Operation," notes that the design of laboratory space may occur in three separate situations: (1) at the planning stage of the building, (2) at the construction stage, when preallocated lab space is designated, or (3) after a structure is built and the established rooms are redesignated for laboratory use. Though the first two are not uncommon in university settings, it is rare that surgical research investigators have a great deal of input into the planning of buildings around their own laboratories. More frequently new investigators establishing labs face the third scenario and inherit preexisting lab space or are given rooms to be converted into lab facilities.

Two basic schools of thought govern the interior design of the laboratory. The first prefers large open rooms with centralization of activity and equipment. Such designs promote maximal interaction (and hopefully camaraderie) between research fellows, decrease travel between rooms, and decrease the risk of accidents and spills in hallways. The second school of thought advocates the separation of space into multiple smaller partitions and rooms. Though this may discourage researcher interaction, it allows for the dedication of isolated space to specific activities, and likely lowers the risk of cross-contamination of reagents, cultures, and radioactivity. The advantages and disadvantages of these philosophies are shown in Fig. 1.

Other considerations in room design include workbench islands versus peninsulas, and windowed versus windowless rooms. Windows are often considered a mixed blessing. Though they generally brighten the working areas (and thus potentially raise morale), the presence of a window in a room can significantly alter ambient room temperature, especially if the windows receive direct sunlight. Sunlight causes glare, which may make minute samples difficult to see and process. Additionally, a window often robs the room of potential shelf space, a significant concern in labs in which space is limited.

In some laboratory renovations, alterations in the physical plant can be achieved (i.e., construction or demolition of walls), but structural or utilities considerations may take a hand in limiting design options (for example, load-bearing walls may be unable to be reoriented). If the principal investigator is fortunate enough to have input into future floor plans, those plans must consider the laboratory's current focus as well as the potential for change and expansion in the future. This allows for maximal flexibility for the lab to adapt to new assays, protocols, and equipment.

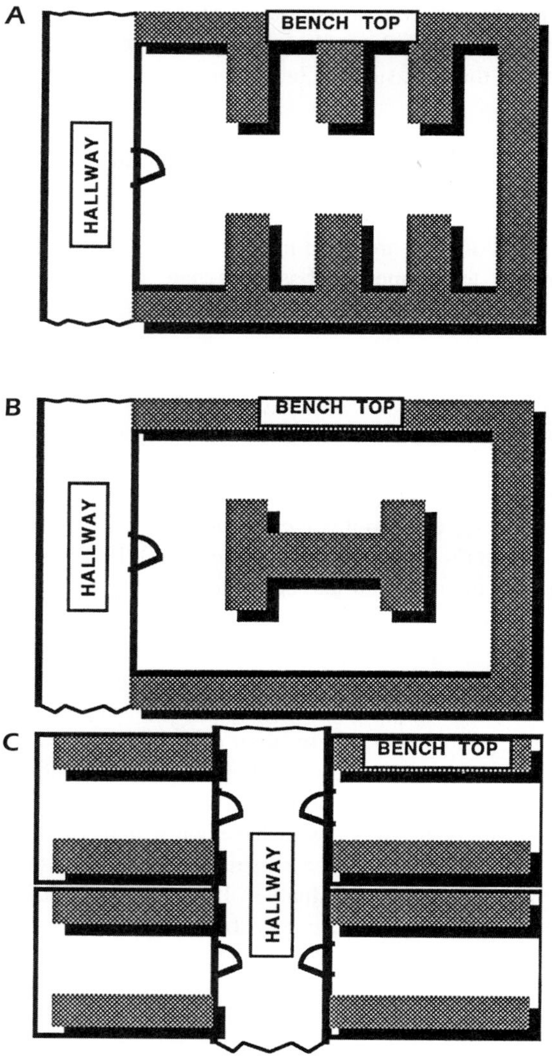

Figure 1 (A) Open room, bench peninsulas. Advantages: Open working area, maximizing researcher interaction; maximal bench surface area; easy extension of utilities from wall conduits. Disadvantages: Disrupted traffic flow; compromised floor space for large equipment. (B) Open room, bench islands. Advantages: Open working area, providing researcher interactions; unimpeded traffic flow. Disadvantages: Difficulty in routing utilities and plumbing through floor. (C) Modular room design. Advantages: Allows for the dedication of room-specific tasks. Disadvantages: Samples may have to be carried from room to room; separates research fellows.

B. Space

For purposes of organization, one can divide the total lab area into three subgroups: active space, conditionally useful space, and dead space. Active space is defined as the space available for the performance of protocols of most types. The best example of this is the benchtop. It is the primary workstation for researchers, and depending on the number of people in the lab, may be a rate-limiting factor in carrying out experiments. When organizing a lab, ample bench surface area must be available.

Although all laboratory space is potentially useful, not all of this is active space. Conditionally active space is space in which certain procedures must be performed, but is otherwise not commonly used for all work. A good example of this is the cell culture hood. All cell culture work is performed within the hood in order to minimize the risk of culture contamination, but other tasks, such as performing various basic chemical assays, should not be performed there. Another example of conditionally active space is the tabletop centrifuge. Vital to many protocols, the latter is not used at all times, yet occupies benchtop space.

If the lab has the luxury of ample space, the notion of conditionally active space may be expanded from simple bench space to include whole rooms. For example, a laboratory may have enough space to dedicate an entire room to cell culture or mRNA work if the risk of devastating cross-contamination is high. This lab structure minimizes the risk of contamination, especially when there are several researchers sharing laboratory space. Dedication of lab space to restricted use is sometimes mandated, such as areas in which animal surgery or radioisotope work is performed, and this should be taken into account when establishing the lab.

The last classification of space in the research lab is the unavoidable "dead space." This includes storage space for supplies, biological samples, hard copy data, journals, catalogues, and books. Drawers, cabinets, and shelves are the best places to store these items, although boxes of reagents and equipment, bought in bulk, often exceed available storage space and may encroach onto active space. Refrigerators, freezers, and file cabinets are all prime generators of dead space and cannot be easily placed out of the way. In order to preserve active space, many storage components are placed in hallways outside of labs. Although this measure is very effective in preserving active space, care must be taken to restrict access to their contents with locks. Additionally, when freezers are in common access areas, it is vital that noninterruptible power sources be provided to prevent accidental sample loss, a potentially devastating event. The ability of a lab to use hallways for extra storage may also be limited by state regulations (such as fire codes) or federal regulations (as from the Joint Committee on the Accreditation of Health Care Organizations, if the lab is adjacent to patient care facilities).

C. Laboratory Inventory

Surgical research ranges from the purely clinical to the purely basic scientific, often with a mixture of the two. The needs of a research lab depend entirely on the nature of research being conducted.

1. Clinical Research

Generally, clinical research laboratories require less space than do those devoted to basic science research. The former may involve a research resident or fellow who is engaged only in chart reviews or meta-analyses and thus may only need desk space and access to computer terminals. Clinical trials of new therapies may require access to an exam room or even a procedure room, with additional space needed for participants' records. Any specimens collected during the process of this research may need a devoted preparation area, where samples may be prepared for courier transport to a central lab (cytology slides dipped in fixative, specimen tubes centrifuged, etc.). The mandated need to ensure the privacy of the patient requires the availability of special locked closets or file cabinets.

If the researcher will be performing assays with information that will be used clinically for patient care, these tests will more than likely come under the jurisdiction of the Clinical Laboratories Improvement Act (CLIA), administered by the U.S. government's Centers for Disease Control and Prevention (CDC). The CLIA is an increasingly complex set of guidelines mandating standards for quality control and assurance of clinical laboratory tests, begun in 1967 and slowly expanded thereafter. Testing centers must be authorized by the CDC, with formal applications, inspections, and licensing procedures. Multiple commercial agencies exist to assist laboratories with gaining and maintaining CLIA certification, although this can be an expensive, time-consuming proposition (for further information, refer to the CLIA and American Society of Clinical Pathology web sites).

2. Basic Science Research

As with clinical research, the requirements for basic science work depend on the type of research being performed. Table II lists some of the general categories of investigational strategies commonly seen in surgical research labs, with some of the equipment likely to be required. A number of items are common to nearly all types of basic science research. A well-equipped lab with a multifaceted approach to research will rapidly fill allocated space. Though several

Table II Procedures and Equipment in Surgical Investigation[a]

Function	Equipment
Sample preservation	4°C refrigerators, −20°C freezers, −80°C freezers, and liquid N_2 storage
Growth	Animal housing, incubators, shakers, tissue culture hoods, and waterbaths
Processing	Surgical areas, homogenizers, centrifuges (ultra and nonultra), ovens (radiant and microwave), hot plates/stirrers, and vortexers
Analysis	Scintillation counters, equipment for high-performance liquid chromatography, polymerase chain reaction,[b] nuclear magnetic resonance, gel electrophoresis, and densitometry; spectrophotometer, microscopes, balances, imaging equipment (X-ray, charge-couple device), pH meter, UV lamps, and computers and related equipment
Miscellaneous	Glassware/other equipment-cleaning areas, autoclaves, hazardous and nonhazardous chemical storage areas, written material storage, and offices for personnel

[a]For cellular and molecular biology, physiology (organ and organ systems), and whole animal (embryology, tumor, microbiology, immunology, and surgical procedures) investigations.

[b]See text for special considerations for PCR experiments.

of the listed instruments are small and may be temporarily moved to produce greater amounts of active space, many are bulky, making their movement impractical. Therefore, careful initial laboratory design is an important consideration for efficient research.

An increasingly important concept in the interest of saving space (and defraying purchase and maintenance costs) is the notion of "common-use" equipment. Many university research centers have established core facilities that not only centralize large expensive pieces of equipment (e.g., fluorescence-assisted cell sorters, electron and confocal microscopes), but that also provide technical support for the appropriate use of these machines. On a smaller level, many labs share the use of centrifuges, scintillation counters, and even freezers. These arrangements are very successful, but require excellent communication about scheduling the use of these machines, especially in the event of equipment failure, because a common-use machine that is out of commission may halt work in multiple labs. Another important aspect is early, clearly communicated agreements for sharing maintenance and repair costs, which occasionally can be quite high.

Assay equipment often needs regular calibration, in order to ensure the quality of research results. Equipment that generates data used for clinical purposes (e.g., arterial blood gas analyzers) may need specialized certification of calibration and accuracy, covered under the Clinical Laboratory Improvement Acts.

3. Data Storage and Ownership

The importance of methodical, regular, legible recording of laboratory data cannot be stressed enough. Traditional forms of data storage, such as the written lab notebook, are perfectly acceptable, albeit laborious. Various software packages exist that are capable of storing data conveniently and efficiently, ranging from various word processor and spreadsheet programs to elaborate database programs. Commercially available software packages, such as HourTrack 98(R) (Decatur Business Systems, Harristown, Illinois), can assist in documenting electronically the date of entry of various data.

Clinical trials engender an entirely new level of stringency on data storage and documentation. Issues of patient confidentiality, as well as accountability in the event of an internal or external (such as a subpoena for a lawsuit) audit gain much more prominence, although these are still potential issues for all types of surgical research laboratories. Consultation with the researcher's legal and medical records department before any project is begun, especially in clinical studies, is mandatory, and can ameliorate or prevent disaster at a later date.

Similarly, careful documentation of all work will prove invaluable in patent or intellectual property issues. It is suggested that all particularly important documents (sequence for a new bioactive peptide drug, design for a new surgical device, etc.) be registered by a notary public, and filed with the local institution's legal department. Confidentiality and discretion are obviously the rule, especially when a new patent may prove lucrative. We suggest early consultation with the researcher's institutional legal department regarding rules for intellectual property, as well as the ownership of data.

V. Laboratory Safety

The primary concern of all principal investigators must be the safety of the researchers in the lab, as well as the safety of the environment. This always takes precedence over laboratory productivity, and safety issues should never be considered an inconvenience. Researchers who disregard safety regulations not only endanger themselves and those around them, they also risk termination of their research funding and/or criminal prosecution. Maintaining a safe environment is simple when researchers understand thoroughly governmental and institutional rules and regulations and recognize the potential hazards associated with their own laboratory's particular research protocols.

Basic scientific research is often fraught with danger, some not readily apparent. A classic example is the discovery of radium; most likely the Curies would have invested heavily in radiation shielding had they known the pitfalls of radiation exposure. Yet hazards can often be markedly reduced with a minimum of effort; the pursuit of knowledge is not an excuse for needless risk taking. A number of governmental agencies have set in place regulations to reduce the risk of injury and accidents. Though it is beyond the scope of this chapter to present a detailed examination of the safe use of hazardous chemical, radioactive, and biological materials, we outline some of the more salient issues and provide a listing of some of the more important available safety resources.

A. Workplace Safety

The Occupational Safety and Health Administration (OSHA) is the branch of the United States Department of Labor charged with overseeing the safety of the workplace. In addition to setting standards and regulations, OSHA has the duty to inspect facilities and the authority to impose penalties on those facilities not in compliance. OSHA regulations require that employees be formally educated with regard to workplace safety issues, including fire and electrical safety, chemical exposures, and how to reduce the risks of work-related injury.

Most hospitals hold annual or biannual seminars regarding occupational safety, and these must be attended by all employees. Safety seminars generally review institutional policies for dealing with emergencies, including the appropriate method of containing spills, evacuating in the event of fires, and, perhaps most importantly, how to initiate action in case such events do occur. Unfortunately, research fellows who often have short stays in the lab may not be required to attend such sessions and may not have access to this valuable and potentially life-saving information. It is the responsibility of the laboratory director to have a thorough knowledge of these regulations, and to see to it that all laboratory personnel are appropriately trained in safety and emergency procedures as dictated by the local institution.

Safety in the lab is ensured at three levels: institutional, laboratory, and personal. Table III summarizes some of the safety measures associated with each level. Though baseline institutionally mandated laboratory safety measures must always be in place, the degree of personal protection employed in the lab may vary with the type of experiment. For example, although gloves should always be worn when performing assays, reactions that do not produce noxious or toxic gases need not be performed in the fume hood. In nearly every type of chemical or biological experiment, proper eye protection must be worn.

The three major categories of hazard, chemical, radiation, and biological, are pertinent to virtually all basic science laboratories and are each separately subject to strict government regulation. Each category presents unique threats to researchers, and injury may be immediate (i.e., lethal or caustic) or delayed (teratogenic or carcinogenic). The absence of immediate injurious potential can lull one into a false sense of security. As a result, regulations are focused on minimizing the risk of accidents and limiting the risk of exposure to noxious substances.

1. Chemical Hazards

It must always be remembered that any chemical substance is potentially harmful. Most surgical research fellows are not formally trained in chemistry and must fall back on undergraduate inorganic and organic chemistry and biochemistry classes taken as requirements for premedical education. Fortunately this education is adequate for understanding most basic chemical reactions, but it may be woefully inadequate for identifying potential by-products of reactions that occur because chemicals were mixed in the wrong order or were disposed of improperly. In addition, though a researcher may be taking appropriate care to protect himself, he may inadvertently neglect the potential exposure danger to a co-worker "across the bench" or in the same room. Thus, it is important for those in the lab to understand the chemical mechanisms behind the assays they use.

OSHA requires that workplaces keep on file a material safety data sheet (MSDS) pertaining to all chemical substances used in a given department. This requirement was originally based on the notion that workers had the right to know what substances they were exposed to in their daily routines. The MSDS contains a complete description of the chemical, its potential to cause injury, how to handle associated emergencies, and the proper method of disposal (Table IV)

A further consideration in the laboratory is the proper labeling of temporary-use containers. Many reagents are prepared in bulk, and are often composed of toxic chemicals, and should be labeled accurately. This is important both for the safe handling of reagents as well as for avoiding costly, experiment-ending mistakes. Additionally, open beakers and containers with unlabeled substances should never be left on the benchtop at the end of the day, because they may place custodial staff at risk.

An often overlooked aspect of safety is the explosion hazard of a chemical. Flash points, volatility, and corrosiveness of the chemicals are all significant to the risk of explosion. Explosion-proof cabinets are available and may be mandated by governmental regulations.

2. Radiation Hazards

Ionizing radiation primarily causes harm by the generation of oxygen radicals that, in turn, disrupt vital chemical bonds. Radioactivity describes a state of energy emission and thus exposure may result from being in proximity with the source and not simply as a result of direct contact. Accordingly, exposure to high-energy radiation sources must be monitored both directly (with biosurveys) and remotely (with dosimetry badges). The degree of protection that is required when working with radiation varies significantly with the type of radioactivity of the substance. Table V summarizes some of the more common sources of ionizing radiation used in contemporary surgical research.

The United States Nuclear Regulatory Commission (NRC) is the federal agency that sets regulations for and licenses and inspects facilities using or producing radioactivity. As with other hazards, the regulations governing the use of radioactive material in the laboratory are designed to protect the health and safety of the users and the environment. Those primarily pertaining to the use of radioactive

Table III Tiers of Pesonnel Safety Assurance

Institutional	Laboratory	Personal
Disaster (i.e., earthquake) plans, fire evacuation plans/drills, radiation accident plans	Fire extinguishers/blankets, chemical showers, eyewashes, first-aid kits, hazard signs, MSDS listings, wipe tests, fume hoods	Safety glasses, lab coats, respirators, gloves, personal bioassays, film badges

Table IV Chemical Information on the Material Safety Data Sheet

1. Chemical identification (name, concentration)
2. Composition/information on ingredients
3. Hazards identification
4. First-aid measures
5. Fire-fighting measures
6. Accidental release measures
7. Handling and storage
8. Exposure controls/personal protection
9. Physical and chemical properties
10. Stability and reactivity
11. Toxicological information
12. Ecological information
13. Disposal consideration
14. Transport information
15. Regulatory information

materials are to be found in Title 10 of the Code of Federal Regulations, Parts 19 and 20. These laws mandate the education of those working with or in proximity to licensed use of radioactive isotopes and require posting of specific notices such as the NRC license, any violation of licensure, and the rights of radiation workers with the responsibility of the employers. Additionally they delineate the NRC standards for personnel exposure limits and outline conduct for monitoring use, storage, receipt, and disposal of radioactive material as well as for keeping records of all activities. Established exposure limits are cumulative, are set at a maximum level measured per annum, and vary with age and pregnancy status as well as the depth of exposure (internal organs or skin).

The long half-lives of radioisotopes and the "silent threat" of ionizing radiation necessitate active monitoring of exposure. This is accomplished with regular wipe tests of surfaces used during the processing of isotopes. Film badges are worn for those likely to be exposed to high-energy sources. Intermittent bioassays via urinalysis or thyroid scan may also be required. Monitoring logs must be kept for at least 3 years in addition to a record of regular calibration of the assay equipment (gamma counters, scintillation counters, etc).

Because of the nature of radioactivity, some exposure to energy emission is inevitable when working with these isotopes. As a result, the NRC's basic philosophy in limiting levels of exposure is summarized by the tenet "as low as reasonably achievable" (ALARA). The use of minimal quantities of isotopes and appropriate shielding combine to keep exposure below the annual dose limits set by the NRC. Experiments must be designed to minimize not only waste, but also the total amount of radioisotopes to be used.

Licensed facilities are required to have a designated radiation safety officer (RSO) who is responsible for assuring compliance with all regulatory and radiation safety policies. The RSO must coordinate inspections of laboratories, keep records of all findings, incidents, and exposures, and submit reports for governmental review. Though the Federal Code of Regulations sets minimal standards for the use of radioactive materials, many states impose stricter regulations, especially with regard to disposal of radioactive waste. As with the institutional safety officer, the RSO is the best source of information on new legislation regarding radioactive materials.

3. Biological Hazards

The manual "Biosafety in Microbiological and Biomedical Laboratories" (4th edition, 1999) is currently the single best source for biological safety issues and can be found at the Internet web site for the National Institutes of Health (NIH), under the publications section of the Office of Research Services link from the Office of the Director link on the home page (www.nih.gov). This document, developed by the NIH and the Center for Disease Control, assigns safety levels to organisms based on their virulence and hazard to human health, and sets guidelines for the safety precautions that are necessary for microbiological containment (Table VI). The manual also gives an excellent description of the various safety cabinets that are appropriate for each biosafety level.

Table V Commonly Used Radioactive Isotopes in Basic Science Research

Isotope	Radioactive emission	Energy (MeV)	Radiation half-life	Required shielding	Target organ
^{3}H	Beta	0.018	12 years	—	Total body water
^{14}C	Beta	0.156	5730 years	—	Total body fat
^{35}S	Beta	0.167	87 days	—	Testes
^{32}P	Beta	1.7	14 days	3/8″ lucite[a]	Bones
^{125}I	Beta and gamma	Beta, 0.030; gamma, 0.035	60 days	1/16″ leaded lucite	Thyroid

[a]Lead shielding is to be avoided with ^{32}P, because the beta energy will be converted with an approximate 10% quantum efficiency into secondary X-ray irradiation via the *bremsstrahlung* effect.

Table VI Summary of Recommended Biosafety Levels for Infectious Agents[a]

BSL	Agents	Practices	Safety equipment (primary barriers)	Facilities (secondary barriers)
1	Not known to cause disease consistently in healthy adults	Standard microbiological practices	None required	Open benchtop sink required
2	Associated with human disease; hazard: percutaneous injury, ingestion, mucous membrane exposure	BSL-1 practice plus Limited access Biohazard warning signs "Sharps" precautions Biosafety manual defining any needed waste decontamination or medical surveillance policies	Primary barriers = Class I or II BSCs or other physical containment devices used for all manipulations of agents that cause splashes or aerosols of infectious materials; PPEs: laboratory coats; gloves; face protection as needed	BSL-1 plus Autoclave available
3	Indigenous or exotic agents with potential for aerosol transmission; disease may have serious or lethal consequences	BSL-2 practice plus Controlled access Decontamination of all waste Decontamination of lab clothing before laundering Baseline serum	Primary barriers = Class I or II BCSs or other physical containment devices used for all open manipulations of agents; PPEs: protective lab clothing; gloves; respiratory protection as needed	BSL-2 plus Physical separation from access corridors Self-closing, double-door access Exhausted air not recirculated Negative airflow into laboratory
4	Dangerous/exotic agents that pose high risk of life-threatening disease, aerosol-transmitted lab infections, or related agents with unknown risk of transmission	BSL-3 practice plus Clothing change before entering Shower on exit All material decontaminated on exit from facility	Primary barriers = All procedures conducted in Class III BSCs or Class I or II BSCs in combination with full-body, air-supplied, positive-pressure personnel suit	BSL-3 plus Separate building or isolated zone Dedicated supply and exhaust, vacuum, and decon systems Other requirements outlined in the text

[a]Adapted from the National Institutes of Health web site: (http://bmbl.od.nih.gov/sect3tab1.htm). From "Biosafety in Microbiological and Biomedical Laboratories," 4th Ed., May 1999. U.S. Dept. of Health and Human Services, Centers for Disease Control and Prevention and the National Institutes of Health, U. S. Gov't Printing Office, Washington, DC, 1999.

a. Recombinant DNA Recombinant DNA represents a unique potential health hazard. Genetic manipulation has given researchers a powerful tool to define the pathogenesis of many diseases as well as to initiate potential therapies. Recombinant DNA is any foreign or altered DNA sequence that has been spliced into cellular DNA, and which may be replicated. One danger unique to recombinant DNA work is the potential for lab personnel to become directly transfected by foreign DNA. Another potential hazard is the production of microbial agents with enhanced virulence, posing a significant environmental threat.

Traditionally gene transfer was accomplished by the introduction of naked plasmid DNA to the cellular target, relying on unassisted recombination to result in its incorporation into the cellular genome. In an effort to improve the efficiency of gene transfer, a number of viral vectors have been designed by incorporating the desired cDNA into the viral genome. The natural history of all viral propagation begins with introduction of the viral genome into the cell. The type of virus determines whether viral DNA will be incorporated into the host DNA and whether cells will be stably transduced. Most viral vectors have been rendered replication incompetent, allowing the introduction of the cDNA into the cell while not permitting propagation of the virus. These vectors have become widely available and their biosafety status may alter previously established laboratory precautions. A clear understanding of the vector (its biology and virulence) and the gene of interest (its protein product and function) is necessary to define the appropriate safety level.

b. Blood-Borne Pathogens OSHA defines "blood-borne pathogens" as "pathogenic microorganisms that are present in human blood and can cause disease in humans. These pathogens include, but are not limited to, hepatitis B virus (HBV) and human immunodeficiency virus (HIV)." Universal precautions were developed recognizing that the safest way to prevent the transmission of blood-borne pathogens is to assume that all persons being treated are potentially infected. Appropriate protection is employed to prevent hazardous exposure to serous and serosanguinous exudates or secretions. Many surgical research labs focus on specimens obtained in the operating room and thus universal precautions must be maintained in the laboratory as well. Fortunately, all surgeons are intimately familiar with universal precautions, although nonmedical laboratory staff may need extra training in these measures.

Most institutions have procedures in place for dealing with exposures to blood-borne pathogens, and often prophylactic treatment with antiretroviral medication is offered as a treatment for potential HIV exposure. An increasing number of institutions offer hepatitis B vaccination to employees, though there is still no vaccination for non-A, non-B hepatitis.

B. Waste Management

In the United States, the Environmental Protection Agency (EPA) is responsible for the regulation of chemical waste, both solid and liquid as well as hazardous chemical vapors. Fortunately, most research laboratories individually produce small amounts of toxic watse, but when combined with the wastes produced by an entire institution, proper disposal becomes a daunting task. The onus is on the researcher to ensure that materials are disposed of properly.

Liquid waste should never be released into storm sewers or simply dumped outside. Some chemicals are suitable for disposal via sanitary sewers (such as salt buffers and neutralized inorganic acids) with large volumes of water. Other hazardous liquids (organic compounds and solvents, alcohols, water laced with heavy metals) must be captured and disposed of professionally. Specially designated areas in the lab should be set up for collection of such wastes. Care must be taken to label exactly what is being disposed of especially so as not to mix incompatible compounds.

Similarly, solid waste that has been contaminated must be considered hazardous waste. Many materials (such as glassware) can be cleaned, decontaminated, or sterilized for reuse and this can reduce the volume of waste. Increasingly there is a push to recycle materials such as plastics and glassware, but this may not be practical depending on the contaminants. One often overlooked waste is nucleic acid gels where ethidium bromide is used. These gels should be collected and disposed of separately from regular waste because of the hazardous ethidium bromide.

Biologically contaminated waste must be disinfected or sterilized before disposal, or disposed of by incineration. Incineration of waste is the preferred method of disposing of biological waste, and most hospitals have on-site incinerators that can handle research laboratory waste. If the autoclave is to be used, a pressure of 15 psi and a temperature of 205°F maintained for at least 15 min should sufficiently sterilize the waste, which may then be disposed of with the ordinary trash. Care must be taken to use autoclavable waste bags, which will not melt under such conditions.

Mixed wastes pose special problems for disposal. Mixed waste is any waste composed of materials in two or more catagories of hazard—for example, radioactive and chemical wastes. Sometimes one of the hazards can be eliminated; for example, mixed waste containing radioactive ^{32}P and biological hazards can be stored until the radiation from the ^{32}P has dissipated (a result of the relatively short half-life of the ^{32}P). The waste can then be incinerated.

Radioactive waste is regulated by both the EPA and the NRC because, unfortunately, most radioactive waste is classified as mixed waste. The radioactivity necessitates collection of all waste, with documentation of the amount of radioactivity. This type of waste must be stored until the radioactivity is gone and as a result disposal is very costly.

Most laboratories do not produce enough gaseous waste to be of consequence to the environment, but an estimate of gaseous emission is important primarily for controlling the exposure of laboratory personel and determining the need for fume hoods. A number of chemicals, such as ozone-threatening refrigerants, are tightly regulated by the EPA and require signed statements from researchers regarding intended use before they may be purchased.

The rules and regulations regarding laboratory and environmental safety are complex and come from all levels of government. Table VII is a list some Internet web

Table VII Relevant Internet Web Sites

Organization	URL
Code of Federal Regulations	www.access.gpo.gov/nara/cfr/index.html
Environmental Protection Agency	www.epa.gov
Immigration and Naturalization Service	www.ins.usdoj.gov/graphics/index.htm
National Institutes of Health	www.nih.gov
Nuclear Regulatory Commission	www.nrc.gov
Occupational Safety and Health Administration	www.osha.gov
Clinical Laboratory Improvement Act	www.phppo.cdc.gov/dls/clia/
American Society of Clinical Pathology	www.ascp.org

sites relevant to the above disscussion. The institutional safety officers and committees remain the best sources for up-to-date information on legislative changes and policy implementation.

Suggested Reading

Coleman, H. S., ed. (1951). "Laboratory Design: National Research Council Report on Design, Construction and Equipment of Laboratories." Reinhold Publishing Co., New York.

Eggleton, E. M., and Rodgers, S. H., eds. (1983). "Ergonomic Design For People at Work." Van Nostrand Reinhold Co., New York.

Reiffel, L. (1956). Beta-ray-excited low-energy X-ray sources. *In* "Handbook of Nuclear Technology." Nucleonics, McGraw-Hill, New York.

Public Health Service Publication No. 1807 (1968). "Health Research Laboratory Design." U.S. Department of Health, Education, and Welfare. NIH, Bethesda, MD.

Purchase, R., ed. (1994). "The Laboratory Environment." Royal Society of Chemistry, Cambridge, U.K.

Rosenlund, S. J., (1987). "The Clinical Laboratory: Its Design and Operation (A Practical Guide for Planners of Industrial, Medical, or Educational Facilities)." Noyes Publications, Park Ridge, NJ.

Stricoff, R. S., and Walters, D. B. (1995). "Handbook of Laboratory Health and Safety." John Wiley & Sons, New York.

White, V. P. (1988). "Handbook of Research Laboratory Management." ISI Press, Philadelphia.

87

History and Philosophy of Surgical Research

Clyde F. Barker

Department of Surgery, University of Pennsylvania, Philadelphia, Pennsylvania 19104

I. History and Philosophy of Surgical Research

A complete history of surgical research would require a very large volume (1); this synopsis is therefore highly selective. However, a short essay on the philosophy of surgical research may be timely because simultaneously with the current explosion in scientific knowledge the capability of surgeons to make contributions in fundamental research has been questioned by basic scientists, medical colleagues, funding agencies, and in some cases by surgeons. This chapter analyzes methods by which several surgeons of the past have done important science and predicts that use of similar strategies will allow the research of future surgeons to be no less important. Central to this argument is that the exposure of surgeons to human disease continuously stimulates them to carry questions from the bedside to the bench for study, and then to carry the solutions back to the bedside. This scenario has led to many of the important scientific discoveries in all of medicine and can be expected to do so in the future.

Several decades ago surgical leaders perceived that surgical research was in decline, in part because it lacked adequate funding. In 1985 representatives from five surgical organizations (The American College of Surgeons, The American Surgical Association, The Society of University Surgeons, the Association for Academic Surgery, and the Society of Surgical Chairmen) formed the Conjoint Council on Surgical Research to study this problem (2). Dr. William Longmire, who chaired this council, noted that in 1984 only 4% of all National Institutes of Health (NIH) grants were awarded to surgeons or surgical specialists, whereas 19% went to departments of medicine or medical specialties. He wrote that

> Surgeons receive such a low percentage of NIH grants because there are few applications and many grant applications are poor. To be a first-rate scientist and a well-qualified physician is a demanding calling. Although this problem affects the entire range of clinical disciplines, maintaining technical skills and at the same time qualifying as a scientist poses a greater challenge to surgery than any other field of medicine.

To consider the reasons for this as related to particular fields of research, Longmire appointed committees in five areas (digestive disease, transplantation, cardiovascular, cancer, metabolism/nutrition, and trauma/burns).

The young surgical scientist's dilemma was summarized by William Silen in his report of the Committee on Digestive Disease (3). Silen quoted Morton Grossman, a famous gastrointestinal physiologist, who had trained many young surgeons. Grossman said

> I have encouraged people in surgery to work with me; first, because the nature of the work I did lent itself to the use of surgical skills. . . . And second, because of my firm belief that the scientific training of surgeons should not be done in the departments of surgery . . . but . . . in other departments. It's very difficult for a surgeon to maintain high scientific standards if he limits himself to the surgical community, because he simply does not get two things. One is the degree of interaction he needs with people working in his field. And second is the high degree of peer review; the surgical journals are not of the same standard as the non-surgical journal.

Silen further analyzed the problem, thus:

> Young surgeons rarely spend sufficient time in preparation for excellent investigation since at least two and occasionally three years of intensive work are necessary in development of sound investigative techniques and scientific inquiry. Six months or a year in the laboratory of a busy surgical faculty member who cannot provide sufficient supervision is clearly inadequate.
>
> Young academic surgeons are confronted with the perennial dilemma of juggling their time among investigation, clinical work and teaching . . . since surgeons are required to maintain clinical expertise in order to retain their identity as surgeons . . . research, teaching and family life often suffer.
>
> Perhaps the biggest problem in surgical research lies with the chairmen of departments who do not plan for adequate investigative training for young surgeons in their departments, who do not protect young surgeons to allow adequate time for research and who may emphasize quantity rather than quality.
>
> [Yet] surgeons bring to research a unique set of qualities which can be enormously productive in the proper setting, as they process attributes which are rarely if ever held by Ph.D.'s. In addition to drive and initiative the strongest of these is the desire to examine clinical phenomena. Where we have failed in the past is that this desire often exceeds the capabilities of the tools at our disposal.

One outcome of the deliberations of Longmire's Conjoint Council on Surgical Research was a biannual conference for young surgical investigators sponsored by the American College of Surgeons. This two day meeting was designed to educate academic surgeons in the first several years of faculty appointment with regard to planning research training, initial activity as independent investigators, funding opportunities, and grant writing. Over the past decade recognition by surgical leaders of the substantial problems facing young surgeon-scientists and initiatives such as this conference may have benefited surgical research, at least as reflected by the somewhat better success of surgeons in obtaining grants. A recent survey indicated that of those attending the ACS meeting for young surgical investigators in 1994 and 1996, 43% submitted research grants and half of these were funded (4). This was a substantially better rate of success than the overall funding ratio of NIH applicants. Between 1990 and 1995 the success of all NIH grants written by surgeons increased substantially both in percent funded and in dollars awarded as compared with those written by members of other clinical departments, including medicine, which plateaued during the same period (5). Contrary to these encouraging data are other indications that not only surgeons but all physician-scientists and even all MDs have become discouraged by the difficulties of obtaining funding for and conducting biomedical research. Leon Rosenberg recently labeled all physician-scientists as an endangered species, citing a recent decrease in numbers of MDs applying for NIH research grants and training grants (6). He also pointed out that the number of MDs applying for their first NIH grant fell by 31% between 1994 and 1997 and that extrapolation of this consistent trend would predict a complete disappearance of MD applicants by the year 2003. Perhaps even more alarming was Rosenberg's finding that the number of graduating medical students expressing a strong interest in research has fallen progressively from 14% in 1989 to only 10% in 1996.

A. Obstacles to Research

The focus of this chapter is surgical research, thus it is appropriate to examine first obstacles to research success that are specific to surgeons.

1. Money

On average, students graduating from medical school have accumulated a debt of $80,000. During the subsequent 6–10 years of postgraduate training in surgery, most surgeons have taken on the financial responsibilities of marriage and children. Further prolongation of a period of low income to obtain extensive training in basic science or to spend major proportions of postresidency life in undercompensated activity such as research is impossible for many young surgeons, and difficult for all. Unless a young surgical faculty member is in a department with a chairman who understands and strongly encourages research and in addition has the financial resources to support it, he or she may be instructed from the beginning to "carry your own weight" by generating surgical fees.

2. Time

That there is insufficient time for surgeons to do research is largely a restatement of the money problem. The salary structure of many departments discourages young surgeons from spending time in non-revenue-generating practice activities, such as research. In addition, young faculty members who have spent many years learning to operate are eager to utilize these skills. They are reluctant to turn down patient referrals to make time for research, fearing that this will prevent them from ever building significant practices. The young surgeon who focuses on building a practice early in his career is unlikely ever to succeed in research.

3. Discrimination

Young academic surgeons who aspire to careers as "triple threats" (clinicians, teachers, and researchers) are soon confronted by discrimination from several quarters: (1) from basic scientists, who tend to believe that the scientific background of surgeons is inadequate and their time commitment insufficient for meaningful research; (2) by academic internists or pediatricians, many of whom share the basic scientists' prejudice because they are in fact basic scientists, only subliminally involved with patient care; (3) by study sections, because even surgery study sections are largely populated by basic scientists (this prejudice is often blamed for unsuccessful grants by surgeons but grants more often fail because they are poorly prepared; (4) by referring doctors, who may label surgical scientists as only "animal doctors," whose clinical skills must therefore be unsuitable for their patients; (5) by fellow surgeons who help spread the word that the surgical scientists do not operate often enough to be skillful; and (6) by promotion committees, which may take the position that publications really do not count if they are in surgical journals rather than in *Nature, Science*, and *Cell*.

Many of our faculty colleagues in "cognitive" disciplines believe that no single individual from any specialty can be expert in both patient care and research. Judith Swain, in her 1996 presidential address to members of the American Society for Clinical Investigation (the medical analog of the Society of University Surgeons), said "for physicians to compete with Ph.D. investigators, they must spend their time engaged in scientific research. I believe it would be a mistake to lead new faculty members to believe that national prominence in research, education, and patient care is an attainable goal. Likewise clinical medicine is not an activity that lends itself any longer to part-time doctors. Clinical physicians should devote their [full] time to the practice of clinical medicine" (7).

4. The Surgical Persona

Finally, according to Folkman, and perhaps even more important than the other deterrents to scientific success by surgeons, is the surgical persona (8). We all recognize and admire, in our surgical role models (and in ourselves), the following characteristics: decisiveness, confidence, and the ability to act promptly, if necessary before complete data can be obtained. The director of a surgical laboratory is likely to exhibit decisiveness, and often impatience, pushing to get things moving and finished. He has deadlines to meet. As a surgical meeting approaches he is tempted to submit an abstract even if the data are not yet complete. The culture of his specialty encourages him to manifest confidence even when there may be considerable reason for doubt. After all, who wants an airline pilot or a surgeon who projects uncertainty? The surgeon is trained to act promptly, almost by reflex, often before definitive studies or proof of an exact diagnosis are possible. This may be necessary at night in the emergency room or trauma bay. And it may save lives. But it is not the formula for doing great science.

Quite obviously the prototype of the surgeon is different than that of the prototypic scientist. The surgeon has little time for thoughtful contemplation or prolonged discussion with his colleagues of alternative hypotheses or failed or incomplete experiments. He rarely has time to attend lunchtime research seminars by visiting scientists presenting obscure topics (even though these presentations may provide crucial insight to the surgeon's own research project). He has no leisure in which to ponder the significance of an unexpected result, to turn over in his mind a tantalizing half-formulated idea and worry it persistently like a dog worries a bone. Clearly if the young surgeon is to be a good scientist he or she needs exposure to scientist role models.

B. Why Should Surgeons Want to Do Research?

Despite these substantial deterrents many young surgeons remain attracted to research. There are several compelling reasons for this: to help mankind by advancing knowledge and improving patient care, for academic advancement, and because research is satisfying and fun. It is probably an unusual surgical neophyte who starts out in research with the expectation of helping mankind. If this were his motivation he might be more likely to enter the priesthood or become a medical missionary. More commonly young surgeons pursue research because of their ambition for academic advancement. This reason is valid because examination of the early careers of department chairmen and other leaders in academic surgery will usually show that recognition outside their own institutions began with their research. But by far the most compelling reason to do research is simply that it is satisfying and fun. Bright people (such as medical students and young surgeons) are curious as to how things work. They are attracted to exploration of any kind and medical research is certainly a form of exploration. Finally, the competitive aspects of biomedical research attract young surgeons, many of whom are competitive by nature.

Although I suspect that the initial goal of most beginning academic surgeons is personal and practical rather than the grand and lofty purpose of helping mankind, research by surgeons has in fact had an impressively positive impact on human health. Consider as examples the impact on human suffering of cardiopulmonary bypass, vascular reconstruction, treatment of shock, and the endocrine treatment of some cancers, all developments that would have been unlikely outcomes of research by nonsurgeons.

II. "Rules" for Successful Research by Surgeons

Because it is presumed that most readers of this textbook are already interested in research or perhaps firmly committed to doing it, the remainder of this chapter is devoted to advising young surgeons on how they might become successful investigators. Examination of the careers and research strategies of successful surgeon-scientists reveals common patterns that suggest useful guidelines. Several analysts of science have set forth guidelines for surgical investigators. In his presidential address of 1996 to the American Surgical Association, Sam Wells suggested several "rules" for young surgeon-scientists: develop laboratory programs during the first 5 years postresidency; focus on projects related to a clinical interest; collaborate with basic scientists; resubmit unfunded grants; work hard (5).

In his lecture to the Young Surgical Investigators at the American College of Surgeons-sponsored meeting in 2000, Haile DeBas advised the following course: To avoid loss of credibility be a competent clinical surgeon first; devote at least 2–3 years (full time) to rigorous scientific training, then strategically manage the first 5 faculty years, avoiding extensive clinical commitments (9).

Sir Peter Medawar, the great transplantation immunologist (who preferred young surgeons as his research fellows), wrote extensively on the philosophy and strategy of scientific discovery (10, 11). Exerpted from Medawar's essays on the subject are these rules:

1. Luck is quite likely to be the most important element; do not overlook an unexpected finding.
2. Take advantage of unexpected findings by following through with definitive experiments.
3. Resist any temptation to manipulate the data.
4. "Original" findings are usually built on earlier work.
5. The scientific paper is a "fraud."

My own rules were heavily influenced by reading Medawar's essays and by working as a member of the basic science department of Medawar's disciple and colleague, Rupert Billingham. My advice to young surgical investigators has been as follows (12):

1. Pick a good mentor.
2. Work with a partner; collaborate.
3. Enjoy competition.
4. Be lucky.
5. Devote just as much effort to presenting your work as to conducting experiments.

A. The Role of Chance in Scientific Discovery

In both Medawar's rules and mine, the role of chance is emphasized. Many other authors have written about the important role of serendipity in science, i.e., accidentally finding something that was not being sought. Some have explained that there are at least several different kinds of luck that can lead to scientific discovery: (1) blind luck, (2) chance favoring the prepared mind, (3) serendipity that follows those with energy and charisma great enough to excite interest in their cause, and (4) bad luck. Totally blind luck is probably an uncommon source of important scientific findings. In fact, Medawar was fond of pointing out that bad luck is much more common than good luck in research. Surprisingly, however, it is bad luck that occasionally positions scientists to make discoveries they would otherwise have missed. In Austin's book "Chase, Chance and Creativity" (13), Austin points out that if an investigator is energetic and active, works hard, and keeps busy doing many experiments, he or she increases the chance of finding something important. Thus, the likelihood increases that two particles in a chamber will collide (using the analogy that a collision of particles represents an important research finding) if the particles move more rapidly, even if their motion is random. Clearly the odds become even better if the motion is not completely random.

Chance favoring the prepared mind (as first emphasized by Pasteur) is probably the most important type of scientific luck. Billingham was fond of quoting William Bateson, who said, "Treasure your exceptions. When there are none the work gets so dull no one cares to carry it further. Exceptions are like the rough brickwork of a growing building, which tells there is more to come and shows where the next construction is to be (14). Medawar and Billingham were always hoping for an unexpected finding, which in their most important experiment led to discovery of transplantation tolerance and Medawar's Nobel Prize. They emphasized the importance of data over hypotheses, thus Medawar's "rule": never manipulate the data. Both scientists considered the data to be sacrosanct and emphasized that data should never be manipulated to fit a hypothesis. Hypothesis, instead, should be discarded or changed to fit the data. After all, hypotheses are only for testing. Medawar in fact believed that research was generally a deductive rather than an inductive process. Thus hypotheses are usually suggested by data rather than important data being generated by testing a hypothesis that was formulated by deep thinking in the absence of some interesting starting point (data).

B. The Importance of Collaboration (Partnerships)

In giving the reasons that nearly all his work was done in collaboration with others, Medawar said "The rationale of collaborative research is the synergism of two or more minds working toward the solution of the same problem. Two or more people working together can accomplish more than the sum of what would have been possible if those same people had been working on their own. More than that, colleagues enhance the satisfaction of having a bright idea or bringing a tricky experiment to a successful conclusion and they make the setbacks that are inevitable in scientific research much more supportable. Loners don't know what they are missing" (15).

C. The Roles of Competition and Presentation

In research, if you have no competition, you are probably not studying anything important. Because it is impossible to avoid it, one should learn to enjoy the excitement and stimulation of competition. Nobel Laureate Macfarlane Burnet put it this way: "Research is essentially intellectual play, to be equated with organized sport and imbued with a competitive spirit. No one can do effective research unless he enthusiastically enjoys it" (16).

The importance of the presentation (oral or written) of research findings cannot be overemphasized. Except to his or her own small group of laboratory co-workers or fellows, an investigator's scientific abilities will be known only by his publications, presentations and grant applications.

III. Successful Surgeon-Scientists

Have successful surgeon-scientists followed the rules? The following discussions examine the careers of several important surgeon-scientists to determine whether they form patterns that either validate or repudiate the several sets of research rules described above.

A. William Longmire

Because Longmire chaired the Conjoint Committee on Surgical Research it is appropriate to begin by reviewing his personal involvement in research and the extent to which he followed the rules. During his early career he was a prominent researcher in transplantation immunology. Shortly after he finished his residency in 1944, Longmire was appointed by his chief Alfred Blalock to direct Plastic Surgery at Johns Hopkins. This was a field in which he had no special training or interest. A question of importance to plastic surgeons of that time was whether skin grafts exchanged between different individuals might ever, through chance histocompatibility of donor and recipient, avoid rejection. One clinical experiment Longmire performed may have been the definitive one to resolve this issue. He transplanted multiple small skin grafts from 71 different donors to the burn wound of a single patient (17). All of the grafts were rejected. When Longmire moved from Johns Hopkins to found a new department at the University of California, Los Angeles, in 1948, he performed other transplant experiments, including one that may have been the first to demonstrate the production of neonatal tolerance (18). In chickens he found that skin allografts transplanted to recipients less than 24 hr old would sometimes (10%) survive permanently, whereas grafts performed later in the recipient's life were all rejected. Also included in the same 1952 report was one of the first demonstrations that immunosuppression (with cortisone) could prolong graft survival.

This experiment of Longmire's illustrates one of Medawar's "rules"; i.e., that "original" findings are usually based on earlier work [Danforth and Foster (19) had done similar studies with chicken skin grafts in 1929]. Nevertheless, Longmire's work on neonatal tolerance could be considered seminal, because it even antedated the 1953 landmark report of Billingham, Brent, and Medawar (20). However, Longmire failed to follow Medawar's even more important advice regarding following up on an important finding by performing the definitive experiments. Instead, Longmire's attention was diverted from his basic research by the consuming task of managing a clinical department in a major new medical school. Thus, Longmire is now known to most surgeons not as the pioneering transplant biologist that he was but as a clinical surgeon and the founding chairman at UCLA. However, in giving up basic research, Longmire became an important mentor of scientists. His continuing interest in transplantation led him to foster the important research of his young department members, such as Paul Terasaki, who developed the methods for histocompatibility testing that are now in universal use for organ transplants.

B. Sir Frederick Banting

Ironically Frederick Banting embodied some of the least suitable characteristics of the prototypic surgeon-scientist (21). He was impatient, overconfident, stubborn, and scientifically untrained. However, luck and persistence allowed him to overcome these disadvantages to become the discoverer of insulin. Although Banting would have strenuously denied that following rules had anything to do with his success, his career illustrates most of the rules listed above. Luck (in fact, blind luck) played a major role. In 1920 Banting, a junior member of the surgical faculty at the medical school in London, Ontario, was assigned to give a lecture to the students on carbohydrate metabolism and diabetes, subjects of which he knew little or nothing. In preparing the lecture he read of the unsuccessful attempts of scientists to extract from the pancreas the hypothesized factor, which was missing in diabetics. One night Banting awoke from sleep with the idea that ligation of the pancreatic duct to promote atrophy of the acinar tissue prior to preparing an extract from the pancreas might allow him to succeed when other experienced scientists had failed. He arose and made a note to himself so he would not forget the idea. There were no large animal laboratory facilities at his medical school and no diabetes experts to advise him on the merits of his idea, so Banting traveled to Toronto to consult the professor of physiology, J. J. Macleod. He asked Macleod to allow him to try his experiment during his approaching summer vacation. Macleod expressed no enthusiasm for Banting's approach, which he said had previously failed. A disappointed Banting went home and applied for a summer job as a doctor for an oil drilling company in the Northern Territories. Later, when this job fell though he returned to Toronto to reexplore the possibility of working in Macleod's laboratory during his vacation. Macleod was about to leave Toronto for his own holiday, but despite his pessimism for the pancreas project he agreed to provide Banting space, animals, and a research fellow for the summer. On the basis of a coin toss, one of Macleod's graduate students, Charles Best, was selected as Banting's partner. By the time Macleod returned from vacation only 2 months later, Banting and Best had succeeded in extracting insulin from the pancreas and had demonstrated that it reversed hyperglycemia in pancreatectomized dogs. The idea that had inspired Banting to begin the research (ligating the pancreatic duct) turned out to be unimportant. The procedure was just as successful when nonmanipulated pancreas was used.

To follow up on this important finding (one of Medawar's rules) Banting and Best needed a collaborator. Therefore, Macleod assigned a young biochemist in his department, James B. Colip, to purify the crude pancreatic extract, a step necessary before it could be given to patients, and one beyond the capabilities of Banting or Best.

Also crucial to the acceptance of the accomplishment of these young, unknown investigators was a prestigious mentor. Ironically Banting discounted Macleod's contribution to the project because he had not been in Toronto when the crucial experiments were done. However, Macleod had provided the space, the necessary financial support, and the services of Best and Collip, the crucial collaborators. More importantly, only through the sponsorship (mentorship) of Macleod, a world famous physiologist, was the work accepted for presentation at an important scientific meeting. There it was immediately accepted as a landmark finding. The earlier essentially identical findings of several less well-known scientists was discounted—overlooked for the lack of a prestigious mentor. Although Banting remained bitter for the rest of his life that Macleod was given any of the credit for the discovery of insulin, the Nobel Committee disagreed and awarded the 1923 Nobel Prize jointly to Banting and Macleod.

C. Sir Alexander Fleming

Some years after Sir Alexander Fleming became famous as the discoverer of penicillin he was offered an honorary fellowship in the Royal College of Surgeons of England (22). He declined, indicating that this would be redundant because he had already earned his Fellow standing through the standard education and examination. Few know that Fleming qualified as a surgeon, because he never practiced this specialty, instead spending his professional life as a bacteriologist. However, his sketch is appropriate for inclusion here not only because of his surgical education but because his scientific career illustrates some important criteria, with regard to the rules for research. Fleming was a prototypic basic scientist—thoughtful, observant, reflective, deliberate, and painstakingly careful. His discovery of penicillin was the product of several kinds of luck. It was blind luck that while Fleming was suffering from a cold a droplet from his nose fell on an agar plate he was studying (23). Where the droplet landed a clear area appeared, caused by the rapid lysis of bacteria, which were being cultured on the plate. Fleming was fascinated by this phenomenon. He gave the name lysozyme to the active agent, which he found to be present in tears, nasal secretions, saliva, eggs of birds and fishes, and seeds of all kinds. His interest in lysozyme diminished only slightly when he found that it had no impact on clinically important bacteria. However, the discovery of lysozyme prepared Fleming's mind for the next important stroke of luck, which came seven years later. The story is widely familiar that in 1929 while cleaning up his cluttered laboratory by discarding old cultures he had finished studying, his attention was drawn to one agar dish he was about to throw out. Appearing on this culture there was one clear area in an otherwise confluent growth of the *Staphylococcus*, which Fleming had plated weeks before. The clear area surrounded a small growth of fungus, which by chance had fallen onto the plate. It was a phenomenon that had probably been observed previously by many bacteriologists. However, the clearing was so reminiscent of that produced by lysozyme that Fleming became quite interested in it. He isolated the product produced by the mold and named it penicillin. In reporting it he suggested that it might have therapeutic possibilities but after a few unsuccessful attempts at purification and concentration of the substance he lost interest in penicillin. He really anticipated that penicillin's only usefulness would be controlling overgrowth in cultures of *Staphylococcus* and other common bacteria, thereby allowing bacteriologists to isolate and study more interesting fastidious bacteria. He never attempted an *in vivo* experiment to assess penicillin's therapeutic potential.

Thus Fleming's prepared mind allowed him to recognize the unexpected (lucky) finding but, because he ignored Medawar's important rule of following up interesting findings, the importance of penicillin went unrecognized for more than a decade. In fact its therapeutic usefulness might have been missed entirely had it not been for Howard Florey and Ernst Chain, who 11 years later, entirely by chance, became aware of Fleming's observation and followed up on it (24). In 1940, Chain, who was working in Flory's department at Oxford, became interested in lysozyme. While looking up an old paper on lysozyme he came across another paper in the same issue of the journal, Fleming's report on penicillin. He decided to study both lysozyme and penicillin. Because Chain and Florey had the expertise to purify and concentrate the product of the penicillium mold, they decided to test its possible therapeutic effect. Ten mice that had been inoculated with a lethal dose of *Staphylococcus* were treated with a small dose of penicillin. Nine of the mice survived. This simplest of experiments immediately demonstrated that penicillin was strikingly therapeutic and virtually free of toxicity.

Had Fleming been a practicing surgeon interested in patient or disease-inspired problems and accustomed to taking them from bedside to bench and back to bedside, it is likely that he would have pursued his chance observation and the world might have had penicillin a decade earlier. As it was Fleming was lucky that his role in penicillin's discovery was not completely overlooked. However, Fleming's career illustrates another important research rule, that of choosing a good mentor. Shortly after Florey and Chain demonstrated the therapeutic effectiveness of penicillin, Fleming's mentor and department chairman, Elmroth Wright, wrote a letter to the *Times of London* proclaiming Fleming as the real discoverer of penicillin. Because public awareness was more influenced by a letter in the *Times* than by Florey and Chain's accounts in scientific journals, Fleming got most of the credit for the discovery of penicillin.

D. Alfred Blalock

Alfred Blalock, one of the twentieth century's most important surgeon scientists, was not blessed with supportive mentors (25). Halsted turned down his application for a position in the surgical residency at Johns Hopkins. After Halsted's death Blalock secured a junior residency there but he was soon dismissed from it over a misunderstanding with the acting chairman, W. M. T. Finney. This "bad luck" at Johns Hopkins turned out to be the making of Blalock's success. His search for a place to finish his surgical residency resulted in his appointment as the first chief resident in a new program starting at Vanderbilt. There was very little clinical activity at the new Vanderbilt Hospital, thus Blalock spent most of his time for the next few years in the laboratory, where he partnered with his friend, Tinsley Harrison, later author of the famous "Textbook of Medicine." Had Blalock become a chief resident and junior faculty member at Johns Hopkins during a period of minimal research interest or activity while Dean Lewis was chairman, it is doubtful that he would ever have begun a research career. Instead, during his formative years at Vanderbilt, Blalock followed one of the most important rules. He greatly increased his chances of making important scientific observations by using his energy and stirring up the environment with a variety of experiments. His research interests included measurement of cardiac output, shock, hypertension, and transplantation of the kidney and adrenal gland. In addition to Harrison he had another important laboratory partner, Vivian Thomas, a young black man who became his technician. Thomas proved to be such a talented experimental surgeon that Blalock soon entrusted him with most of the operative procedures performed in the laboratory. In one experiment they attempted to create a model of pulmonary hypertension by anastomosing the subclavian artery to the pulmonary artery. They were disappointed to find that this procedure failed to increase the pulmonary artery pressure. However, the failed experiment prepared Blalock's mind in an important way. A few years later, after Blalock had returned to Johns Hopkins as chairman, the pediatric cardiologist Helen Tausig asked whether he could find a way to arterialize the pulmonary circulation to treat babies with cyanotic heart disease. This presented Blalock with an unanticipated opportunity to use clinically the very operation that had been so disappointing as a laboratory model of pulmonary hypertension, i.e., subclavian to pulmonary artery anastomosis. The operation, which became famous as the Blalock shunt for Tetrology of Fallot, was a crucial step in the evolution of modern heart surgery.

E. Sir Peter Medawar and Rupert Billingham

Peter Medawar's own remarkably successful research career was surely the inspiration for his advice to young investigators. Completely by chance he and Rupert Billingham, his graduate student (partner), made an unexpected observation (26). Trusting their data rather than the hypothesis, they were able to interpret the data correctly in the light of earlier findings of another scientist. They then promptly followed up on this work by conducting the crucial definitive experiment and by devoting as much time and care to the presentation of the work as to the experiments.

Medawar and Billingham were asked to help a colleague distinguish fraternal from identical twin cattle, an important step in the colleague's research. To accomplish this they exchanged skin allografts between twin pairs, expecting that the grafts from identical twin donors would survive and that grafts from fraternal twin donors would be rejected. Instead all the skin grafts were accepted, a result they puzzled over as they carefully confirmed it by repeated experiments. Eventually they were advised by a colleague that the interpretation of their results might rest on earlier reports of other scientists, which had shown that (1) twin cattle, unlike most other species, have a shared placenta, which allows free exchange of blood *in utero*; (2) in adulthood fraternal twin cattle have red blood cells, not only of their own blood type, but also red blood cells of their twin's blood group (27).

Reasoning that the persistence of blood cells (especially white blood cells, which express histocompatibility antigens) must be the cause of skin graft acceptance, Medawar and his associates quickly followed up on their lucky observation. By inoculating fetuses of another species (mice) with cells from members of a prospective donor strain, they found they could induce specific tolerance. In adulthood these recipients accepted donor strain skin grafts without rejection (20).

In keeping with Medawar's fifth rule (q.v., Section II) the experiments were presented with great care, not in the exact sequence of their conduct but instead to make a fascinating story. Billingham said he learned the rule from Medawar in the following way (26):

> Medawar presented a joint paper on our work. [I was surprised that] his account of our experiments bore no relation to their actual chronology. Some [experiments] we'd carried out had only serendipity as their justification. [But] in the lecture "chance" received no credit . . . hindsight had enabled creditable reasons to be invented. As the story unfolded, it had a beautiful logical sequence, like the plot of a well-contrived detective story. It was obvious that the only things that were sacrosanct or inviolable were actual factual observations . . . Hypotheses could be invented or rejected at will and the chronology of the experiments conducted and the reasons for embarking upon them were altered to make the best possible story.
> It was an important educational event for me. It taught me that to realize one's full potential as a scientist, one must master two quite different arts: a) technique and background knowledge . . . and b) the art of presentation . . . Some talented scientists have never acquired the art of presentation. . . . Their contributions are colorless observations . . . deprived of a story.

Facetiously, Billingham and Medawar referred to the scientific paper as a "fraud." Medawar even published an essay with this title (28). Of course, they never invented or falsified data. But they wove their experimental findings into the fabric of what they always described as "a story." They should instead have described it as an art form, which for them it was.

IV. Surgical Science History

A. Importance of Studying Surgical Research History

Study of the careers of scientists, such as those mentioned here, should encourage young surgeons to believe they could make similar contributions, if they adhere to certain rules, work hard, and have sufficient luck. In his book "Chase, Chance and Creativity," Austin emphasized the importance to young investigators of studying the careers of successful scientists (13). He wrote that these scientists should be remembered: "Not so much for their scientific discoveries but because their stories show us how malleable our own futures are. We can see how many loopholes fate has left us. From their stories we understand that chance can be on our side if we stir it up with our energies" and as Medawar advised, pay attention to the unexpected finding that may allow us to make a meaningful contribution. At the same time we should remember not to take ourselves too seriously, because any success we may have in science is surely based on the findings of our predecessors. And even if we are fortunate enough to make an important new discovery, someone with less luck may have been there before us.

In the previous sections the careers of several scientists of the past are reviewed to illustrate certain guidelines or rules that appear to have helped them generate important contributions. The following section addresses the question whether surgeons of the past have been successful scientists and whether present and future surgeons can be similarly productive.

B. Surgical Science in Remote Times

Any assertion that surgeons were not contributors to early biomedical knowledge is easily refuted by the career of John Hunter (1728–1793). Hunter and his contemporary surgeons were the objects of even more intense bias and discrimination by their more highly educated medical colleagues, than are surgeons of today. However, Hunter was perhaps more responsible than any other individual for bringing a scientific approach not only to surgery but also to all of medicine. Certainly he was the most versatile medical man of his time.

The preface of John Kobler's biography of Hunter provides a summary of his contributions (29):

> To commemorate the bicentenary of Hunter's birth, the Harvard Medical Society held a symposium at which six speakers, each eminent in a different field, acknowledged Hunter's achievements in that field. "What is known as the 'Hunterian method,' " said the brain surgeon, Harvey Cushing, "revolutionized surgery . . . Hunter was the first to teach the science of surgery as Pare two hundred years before had advanced the art."
> Dr. William Pearce Coues, a dermatologist referring to Hunter's treatise on venereal diseases, said: "Much of it could appear in the journals of the last twenty years as the thoughts of the leading urologists of today. . . . John Hunter was an urologist a hundred and fifty years ahead of his time. "Dentistry today," said the Dean of the Harvard Dental School, "is being developed along biological lines with mechanics the servant rather than the master of biological principles. It is clear that Hunter had this idea strongly developed and it seems a pity that it has taken us more than a century to appreciate the truth of what he had to say." Professor Wheeler, an entomologist, declared Hunter to have been "the most important naturalist, between Aristotle and Darwin."
> The remaining eulogists were Dr. Arlie V. Bock, Professor of Internal Medicine, and Dr. Frederick T. Lewis, Professor of Anatomy and an embryologist. The roster could have been extended almost indefinitely to cover pathology, physiology, biology, hematology, military surgery, orthopedics, obstetrics, genetics, artificial insemination, psychology, psychosomatics, sexology, veterinary science, zoology, botany, geology, and paleontology, for in all of these fields Hunter made lasting contributions . . .
> The *Encyclopedia Britannica* devotes more space to Hunter than to Linnaeus, Pare, Harvey, Jenner, Lister, Simpson, Pasteur, Freud or Fleming. What Hunter accomplished . . . however, transcended specific discovery and technical invention. He introduced a new spirit of inquiry, a philosophy, which not only transformed the medical theory and practice of his epoch, but also profoundly influenced scientific thinking everywhere down to our own times.

During the nineteenth century the introduction by surgeons of anesthesia, antiseptic surgery, and aseptic surgery were certainly as important as any innovations in nonsurgical fields. At the turn of the century William Halsted in the United States, in addition to founding the modern surgical residency, was probably this country's first great surgical scientist. He devised new methods of intestinal anastomosis (the submucosal suture), treatment of fractures (the first use of plate and buried screw fixation), and the first successful treatments of breast cancer and inguinal hernia. Other important contributions were made in anesthesia (invention of local and nerve block anesthesia), biliary surgery, endocrine surgery (thyroid), transplantation (parathyroid), and vascular surgery (experimental and clinical treatment of aneurysms) (30). These innovations were all based on extensive laboratory experimentation by Halsted before he applied them to the treatment of patients.

C. Surgical Science of the Past 50 Years

The importance of contributions of the remote past by Hunter and Lister and in the twentieth century by Halsted, Banting, and Blalock does not prove that in a recent and scientifically more sophisticated era surgeons would be capable of important research. However, James Thompson in his 1999 presidential address to the American College of Surgeons argued persuasively that in the past 50 years the contributions of surgeons to medical science were at least as great as those made by members of any other discipline (31). He listed contributions in (1) cardiopulmonary bypass and cardiac surgery, (2) transplantation, (3) vascular surgery, (4) total parenteral nutrition, (5) metabolic response to trauma, sepsis, and burns, (6) controlled trials for cancer, (7) effect of hormones on cancer, and (8) minimally invasive surgery. Interestingly, review of the careers of the surgeon-scientists responsible for these advances reveals that they followed many of the same rules listed at the beginning of this chapter.

1. Cardiopulmonary Bypass and Cardiac Surgery

Chance was quite clearly the inspiration for John Gibbon's research. As a surgical fellow in Edward Churchill's department at the Massachusetts General Hospital, he was assigned to monitor the vital signs of a woman who had suffered a massive pulmonary embolus (32). Throughout a long night Gibbon watched as her condition deteriorated, culminating in cardiac arrest. Because at the time, there had been only nine survivors of pulmonary embolectomy, operative treatment was reserved as a last resort. Although when her heart arrested Dr. Churchill operated on this patient, removing the clot within minutes, she died. Gibbon believed that if her cardiopulmonary function could have been supported artificially for only a short time, she could have survived. He made up his mind to design a machine that would do this. Dr. Churchill regarded the project with skepticism but somewhat reluctantly agreed to provide Gibbon the necessary resources to work on it, including a technician. The technician, Maley Hopkinson, worked with Gibbon on the project for the next 20 years. For the last 19 years of the collaboration, she was also Gibbon's wife. Much of their work was done at the University of Pennsylvania. Gibbon said that his most important mentor there was Eugene Landis, a basic scientist, with whom he studied the physiology of the capillary circulation (33).

At first, the Gibbons were lonely enthusiasts for the heart–lung machine, but in the 1940s other thoracic surgeons saw its possibilities and entered the competition to build a successful pump oxygenator. This group included Blalock, Gross, DeBakey, Bjork, Craford, Kirklin, Lillehei, Glenn, Welch, Lewis, Andresen, and Brukhoneko. At a meeting of the American Surgical Association in 1951, Gibbon reported that his machine had substituted for the cardiopulmonary function of 21 dogs for as long as $1^1/_2$ hr and that 7 of the animals had survived (34). He was followed on the program by Clarence Dennis, who described a machine similar to Gibbon's he had used to provide cardiopulmonary support in nine dogs, with two survivals (35). In addition Dennis reported the use of his machine for closing a septal defect in a patient: however, the patient died during the operation.

Nine months later, Gibbon tested his machine in a human case (32). The infant chosen for his first operation turned out to have a huge patent ductus instead of the anticipated septal defect. This patient died on the table. But in May 1953, Gibbon performed the first successful open-heart operation under cardiopulmonary bypass, closing an atrial septal defect in a young woman. If Dennis' earlier patient had survived it is likely that he rather than Gibbon would be remembered as the father of the heart–lung machine.

Another important chapter in the history of open-heart surgery, which like Dennis' case also took place in Minnesota, is almost forgotten. Although Gibbon's development of the pump-oxygenator yielded great promise, open-heart surgery remained risky, largely because of oxygenator-related complications, which led to a very high mortality rate in early open-heart operations. To avoid such problems, Dr. C. Walton Lillehei decided to connect the heart patients to human "donors" (usually parents), who thus served as living oxygenators (36). Blood flow was routed from the patient's caval system to the donor's femoral vein and lungs. The oxygenated blood was then returned to the patient's carotid artery. In 1954, Lillehei and his team used this technique to correct a ventricular septal defect in an $11^1/_2$-year-old boy. During the next 15 months, they repaired 45 hearts with complex interventricular defects, paving the way for the open-heart surgery era by allowing surgeons to gain experience operating within the heart before heart–lung machines were fully developed.

Cross-circulation was never widely practiced, because it was considered by most too risky for the donor. Meanwhile Dr. Lillehei and Dr. Richard A. DeWall in Minnesota and John Kirklin at the Mayo Clinic continued to improve the pump oxygenator until it had soon become standard, allowing operations for congenital heart disease, acquired valvular disease, and coronary artery bypass.

2. Transplantation

In the first decade of the twentieth century, Alexis Carrel had demonstrated the technical feasibility of organ transplantation (37). Carrel also discovered that an unexplained biological barrier precluded sustained function of allografts, which after days or weeks of normal function would fail. Over the next several decades plastic surgeons, who used skin allografts in treatment of burn wounds, observed that although allografts initially healed in and appeared to be viable and healthy, they were always subsequently destroyed. This phenomenon was explained in the late 1940s by Peter Medawar's detailed study of skin graft rejection in experimental animals. In 1953, the demonstration by Billingham, Brent, and Medawar that tolerance to allografts could be induced in animals encouraged surgeons to persist in studies of experimental organ transplants and to initiate programs in clinical kidney transplantation.

Joe Murray, who was the first to transplant a human organ successfully, appears to have followed all the rules for successful research. An important mentor of his was J. Barrett Brown, who was his commanding officer at Valley Forge Army Hospital during World War II. Brown, a plastic surgeon, in 1936, had been one of the first to demonstrate that identical twins accepted each other's skin grafts and was also one of the first to describe the second-set phenomenon in skin graft rejection. It was Brown who first triggered Murray's interest in transplantation. After the war, Franny Moore, Chief of Surgery at the Peter Bent Brigham Hospital, became an important mentor, encouraging Murray and another young surgeon, David Hume, to do experimental kidney transplants (38). Their initial efforts with human transplants failed because no immunosuppressive agents were available. As luck would have it, in the early 1950s, Hume was drafted to serve in the Korean War, leaving Murray as the head of the Brigham's Transplant Program. In December of 1954, the opportunity came to perform a kidney transplant utilizing an identical twin donor. It succeeded, as did several other identical twin kidney transplants. In 1959, Murray did the first successful kidney allograft in man—using a fraternal twin donor and whole body irradiation for immunosuppression (39). Subsequently Murray had the good fortune to work with partners such as Roy Calne, a young surgeon who brought the first immunosuppressive drug, 5-mercaptopurine, from England to the United States in the early 1960s, and later two basic scientists, the Nobelists George Hitchings and Gertrude Elion, who developed other agents such as Imuran.

Throughout this period Murray had keen competition from other pioneering transplant surgeons, such as Hume and Starzl in the United States and two French groups headed by Hamberger and Kuss. In fact, Hamberger's group successfully transplanted an allograft from a fraternal twin only months after Murray's first successful allograft. However, the Nobel committee chose wisely in 1990 to recognize Joe Murray for the first successful kidney transplant (the identical twin), the first successful allograft, and for pioneering the use of immunosuppressive drugs in animals and human transplants.

The road to success with liver transplants was even more difficult that the story of kidney transplants. Tom Starzl's interest in liver transplantation originated with an unexpected finding. While he was a resident at Hopkins, Starzl assisted Dr. Blalock in an operation on a diabetic patient who, after having a total diversion of the portal blood from the liver, no longer required insulin (40). Starzl hypothesized that diabetes might be a liver disease that could be cured by portacaval shunting. With laboratory experiments, he soon found this hypothesis was wrong, but he remained fascinated by the relationship of the liver to its double blood supply. Utilizing an intricate series of experiments that would certainly have been impossible for anyone but a surgeon (split livers, portacaval shunts, and liver autotransplants), he studied the hepatotropic factor in portal blood, which he eventually defined as insulin. These studies were the origin of his interest in liver transplantation. Starzl's persistence in liver transplantation in the face of many early failures was responsible for the eventual success of the procedure. In 1968, he reported the first survivals of liver transplant patients beyond the first few days, and by 1994, he was able to achieve long-term survivals of greater than 80% (41).

Two early mentors were crucial to Starzl's success (40). The first, his father, was a newspaper editor. Tom grew up helping with his father's paper and later worked as a copyeditor for the *Chicago Tribune*. I believe much of his success as a surgical scientist is due to the excellence of his presentations and publications. Starzl's second important mentor was Horace Magoun, a basic scientist, under whom he studied during an extra year of medical school, thus obtaining a Ph.D. in neurophysiology. Starzl credits Magoun with teaching him the "magic of research." Their joint papers, which defined the reticular activating system, remain classics in neuroscience.

Over the past three decades, Starzl had competition from many other transplant surgeons (42). In the exciting early years of the transplantation era, these included Franny Moore (Starzl's chief competitor during the early canine liver transplant work); Joe Murray and David Hume, who headed the other dominant pioneering kidney transplant groups; Keith Reemtsma, whose early lead in the xenograft field was pursued by Starzl; John Najarian; Roy Calne; Paul Russell; Tony Monaco; Peter Morris; and many others.

The first human heart transplant was done in South Africa by Christian Barnard (43). However, the credit for the initial experimental work in this field and for later establishing it as therapy that could be consistently successful in humans belongs to Norman Shumway (44, 45). Shumway explained the serendipitous nature of his interest in heart transplantation in a 1983 letter (46):

> In 1958 when I started work at Stanford, the idea (cardiac transplantation) grew out of our local cooling experiments, since we had 1 hour of aortic cross clamping during cardiopulmonary bypass. Accordingly, we decided to remove the heart at the atrial level and then to suture it back into position. After several of these experiments, we found it would be easier to remove the heart of another dog and do the actual allotransplant. Something like 20 to 30 experiments were performed before we had a survivor. All of this was done before chemical immune suppression was available.

3. Vascular Surgery

Despite its longer history vascular surgery belongs in this section because only in the last half of the twentieth century did it become a clinical activity. Research in this field began with John Hunter's unexpected finding in a stag: after he had ligated one carotid artery, the antler on the same side became ischemic but then gradually became revascularized via collateral circulation. He then followed up on this finding by successfully treating a man for a popliteal aneurysm by ligation of the femoral artery, finding that collateral circulation maintained the viability of the leg (29). In the ensuing century, progress in vascular surgery was limited to ligation of various arteries to treat aneurysms. Successful vascular anastomoses were not carried out until the time of Jaboulay and his student, Alexis Carrel, 100 years ago. Carrel's early twentieth century research is appropriate for inclusion here because it was so far ahead of his time and because it illustrates many of the rules for research (47).

Alexis Carrel had several important mentors. Mathieu Jaboulay, a pioneer in vascular surgery and the head of surgery in Lyon where Carrel trained, assigned him the project of determining whether anastomosing the carotid artery to the jugular vein in animals would increase cerebral blood flow. To facilitate progress in this experiment Carrel took lessons from another important mentor, Mme. Leroudier, an embroideress of local renown, to whom he later attributed his remarkable skill in sewing.

Carrel is now commonly given credit for most of the important innovations in vascular surgery, but in his day he was not without competitors. While Carrel was still in medical school, Jaboulay had successfully sutured the divided carotid artery, using everting sutures. In 1899 Dorfler, a German surgeon, described the modern method of a running suture incorporating the full thickness of the vessel wall, a technique now commonly attributed to Carrel. Carrel's success actually depended not on his introduction of an entirely new method, but on his recognition that asepsis was of critical importance and on his technical virtuosity in sewing, which he attributed to his lessons from Mme. Leroudier

After Carrel failed examinations that would have qualified him for a position in France, he sought employment in Montreal and shortly thereafter moved to Chicago, where he encountered his first important partner, the physiologist, Charles Guthrie. They collaborated for only 12 months, but during this time described innovations such as interposition grafts of vein to replace arteries and transplantation of the kidney, thyroid, ovary, heart, lung, and small bowel. For this work Carrel received the Nobel Prize in 1912.

After moving to the Rockefeller Institute in New York, Carrel formed an unlikely partnership with a young man who approached him to discuss the possibility of a heart operation on a relative who had rheumatic valvular disease. Carrel responded that open-heart surgery was not possible because it would require a pump-oxygenator. The visitor's offer to build such a device for Carrel must have seemed preposterous, because he was not a scientist, nor even a college graduate. Surprisingly Carrel agreed to provide laboratory space for the project. He was probably influenced by the identity of the stranger, the famous aviator, Charles Lindbergh—only a year after his solo flight of the Atlantic. A 1931 paper in *Science* described the pump. It was published anonymously at Lindbergh's request to avoid the publicity he had come to abhor. The pump was never used for open-heart surgery but rather for perfusion of organs and tissues, the viability of which it could maintain for as long as 3 weeks.

In the early decades of the twentieth century, a few clinical attempts to bridge arterial defects or occlusions with vein grafts were reported. However, not until after the Korean War, when vein grafts were used successfully to repair traumatic lesions, did the use of autogenous saphenous vein for femoral popliteal bypasses become a common treatment for arterial disease of the lower extremities (48, 49).

In the early 1950s the earliest reports of resection of the aorta for occlusion or aneurysm appeared (50, 51). At first the defect in the aorta was bridged with fresh or preserved arterial homografts. However, these were inconvenient to procure and preserve and most ultimately degenerated, sometimes with disastrous results. Thus, extensive application of aortic surgery awaited the development of a suitable fabric prothesis. This development occurred as the result of an accidental observation in 1952 by Arthur Vorhees, then a surgical research fellow at Columbia. Vorhees's account (52) of the discovery follows:

> During one of the early *in vivo* trials I made an error in placing the ventricular suture with the result that the stitch traversed the central part of the ventricular cavity. It would have been too difficult to correct but I did make a note of my error so that several months later, at autopsy, I took pains to find the misplaced suture. To my surprise it was coated with what grossly appeared to be endocardium. It resembled a normal chorda except for the black core of the stitch . . . its appearance was sufficiently startling to make me wonder if a piece of cloth might react in a similar way. From there I speculated that a cloth tube acting as a latticework of threads, might indeed serve as an arterial prosthesis.

Vorhees' discovery was quickly followed by the successful construction of fabric protheses by Vorhees and Blakemore and their successful use in-patients. DeBakey and his group also developed successful fabric prostheses and used them with great success in large numbers of patients. Most credit DeBakey's group with initiating the modern era of clinical vascular surgery.

4. Total Parenteral Nutrition

The landmark work of Jonathan Rhoads and Stan Dudrick on total intravenous nutrition follows all my rules for success in research—mentoring, teamwork, competition, and luck. In this case, the teamwork and mentoring were synonymous. Less well known was the important mentoring of Jonathan Rhoads by his chief, I. S. Ravdin.

As early as 1938, Ravdin and Rhoads studied the detrimental impact of protein malnutrition on wound healing and attempted to correct it by infusing lyophilized plasma. During the next 25 years, they and their associates at Penn pursued the goal of achieving positive nitrogen balance in patients unable to eat (53, 54). A number of strategies were evaluated, including rectal infusions of glucose and alcohol and intravenous gelatin and fat. The culmination of their efforts came after Ravdin had retired and Rhoads had persisted in this line of research for nearly 30 years. Stan Dudrick, a resident working in his laboratory, spearheaded the definitive study. Franny Moore, a chief competitor in this work, tells the story best (55):

> Over thirty years ago, Jonathan became interested in surgical nutrition . . . in fostering nutrition by infusing lots and lots of useful soluble nutrient "goodies" but then getting rid of all that extra water with a solute diuresis. At that time, we were trying to do the same thing providing both calories and a diuresis with intravenous alcohol. So, . . . Jonathan's subjects enjoyed good nutrition, but had to . . . go off down the hall to the bathroom pushing their IV

> poles before them. Meanwhile, our patients enjoyed nutrition and went off blissfully to sleep with smiles on their faces.
> And then finally his team . . . including Dr. Wilmore, Dr. Vars and Dr. Dudrick produced that simple experiment in growing puppies that gave the world modern intravenous nutrition. and that masterly contradiction in terms total parenteral alimentation.
> His were experiments that needed no statistics. There was no complexity. They were simple and direct, right to the point and very, very significant. They did not even need large numbers. They just showed that puppies grown on nothing but intravenous nourishment grew normally in every way. There was a sort of a new phenomenology in this, leaving no doubt in anyone's mind.

In 1972, 3 years after their initial demonstration that puppies could survive and grow normally on intravenous nutrition alone, Stan Dudrick described their experience with the life-saving treatment in 1300 patients (56). In discussion of the paper at the meeting of the American Surgical Association, Clarence Dennis referred to his 30-year experience with intravenous nutrition and Francis Moore to his extensive similar research, thus illustrating that Rhoads and Dudrick had plenty of competition. Luck contributed substantially to their success. First, one of the collaborators, Harry Vars, was not only a great biochemist, but also a great tinkerer, an inventor of gadgets. He designed an ingenious flexible harness for the puppies, without which continuous intravenous infusions could not have been done for several months in the otherwise unfettered pups. Second, rotating through the Hospital of the University of Pennsylvania from an outside institution was a urology resident who knew of a technique for percutaneous catheterization of the subclavian vein. He showed Dudrick how to do this and it proved a key to continuous infusion of intravenous solutions with minimal risk of thrombosis.

5. Metabolic Response to Trauma, Sepsis, and Burns

Many modern surgeon-scientists have studied the physiologic, metabolic, and other changes caused by major injuries, including operative procedures. Not surprisingly scientists in nonsurgical fields appear to be less interested in these phenomena, because they are not required to deal with the clinical management of patients exhibiting them. In earlier eras physiologists and other basic scientists laid the groundwork for understanding these changes.

In the 1800s Claude Bernard proposed that maintenance of internal constancy of body systems was of vital importance. His studies described the digestion of food, the maintenance of blood glucose, and the vasomotor control of circulation, all of which contributed to the constancy of the chemical composition of the body (57). Another major contributor to the understanding of body "homeostasis" (a term he originated) was Walter B. Cannon, a Harvard physiologist. Cannon worked in a number of different areas, including digestion, metabolism, control of hunger and thirst, maintenance of blood glucose tissue energetics, thermoregulation, and maintenance of oxygen supply (58). He noted that homeostatic responses were complex, involving brain, nerves, heart, lungs, kidneys, and spleen. In the latter part of the nineteenth century, Carl Voit and other German scientists studied protein metabolism, nitrogen balance, the thermogenesis of food, and the impact of infection on protein metabolism.

The "modern era" of understanding injury responses has been well reviewed by Wilmore (59). It began in the 1930s with the studies of David Patton Cuthbertson, a clinical chemist working in Scotland. He studied the urinary excretion of calcium and phosphorus in patients with fractures. Cuthbertson noted that the injured patients had increased urinary excretion of phosphorus and exaggerated urinary losses of nitrogen and potassium. He also determined energy requirements using indirect calorimetry in the injured patients and found that increased oxygen consumption accompanied the protein catabolic response. He also described a constant rise in body temperature in uninfected, injured patients and characterized this response as "posttraumatic fever." Alfred Blalock was one of the first surgeons to do important work in this field. His studies on shock in the 1930s indicated that this syndrome was due primarily to loss of blood and fluids rather than to a toxin, as Walter B. Cannon thought (60). In the 1940s and 1950s Francis Moore, a Harvard surgeon, studied the body's homeostatic responses following trauma and surgery. He brought sophisticated scientific techniques to the bedside, used isotopic dilution methodology to measure body composition in patients, and developed an intensive care unit where careful balance studies could be performed in critically ill patients. He evaluated the impact of specific components of the injury response such as bed rest, anesthesia, volume loss, and starvation on metabolic responses and described various stages of convalescence after injury. In his classic book "The Metabolic Care of the Surgical Patient" he translated this information into practical terms that could be applied by the practicing surgeon in treatment of critically ill patients (61).

6. Controlled Trials for Cancer

Although the concept of the controlled clinical trials may not have been totally original with them, surgeons were the first to conduct large-scale multicenter trials to compare treatments of important human diseases. Perhaps the first of these was focused on chemotherapy for breast cancer. I.S. Ravdin was influential in obtaining government support for the earliest trials, which began in the early 1960s and were termed the National Surgical Adjuvant Breast and Bowel Project (NSABP) (62). At an early stage Ravdin involved his trainee, Bernard Fisher, in the trials. Under Fisher's leadership the trial eventually demonstrated that adjuvant chemotherapy and endocrine therapy improved survival. Fisher also believed that the outcome of breast cancer was likely to be determined by genetic factors within tumor cells rather than by anatomic considerations such as spread along lymphatic pathways. When large controlled studies of the NSABP, which he directed, showed that lumpectomy and irradiation were as effective in treating breast cancer as the traditional radical mastectomy, breast conservation became the commonest method of treatment.

Under the auspices of the American College of Surgeons and funded by the NIH, Sam Wells has initiated an extensive series of trials of methods of treating a variety of malignant diseases. There are plans to extend such studies to the treatment of other surgical diseases such as trauma, burns, and transplantation.

7. Effect of Hormones on Cancer

In 1966 Charles Huggins was awarded the Nobel Prize for his recognition in the 1950s of the influence of hormones on cancer (63). Actually, several surgeons noted this relationship much earlier. In 1786, John Hunter had observed that bilateral orchidectomy caused atrophy of the prostate in animals (64). In 1893 J. William White of the University of Pennsylvania reported that castration caused atrophy of the prostate in dogs (65). Two years later White published his experience with castration in 111 patients who had symptoms of prostatic hypertrophy, reporting improvement in 51 (66). About a third of White's patients had carcinoma of the prostate.

Oophorectomy as a treatment for breast cancer, for which Huggins is often credited, was also not new, having been utilized long before Huggins' 1952 report. In 1896, George Beatson of Glasgow was the first to report that the procedure caused regression of metastases (67). This was soon confirmed by others, and by 1905, remissions had been reported in one-third of about 150 patients treated.

However, Huggins' Nobel Prize was based on more than looking up some forgotten old papers. His study of the relationship of tumors to endocrine status was scientifically sophisticated and eventually led to the understanding of estrogen receptors and the modern treatment of breast cancer with inhibitors of these receptors. Huggins was lucky to select the dog for his initial animal studies because this appears to be the only nonhuman species subject to prostatic cancer.

V. Surgical Science: Present and Future

From the preceding section it should be clear that at least throughout the past century research done by surgeons was responsible for many of the important advances in medicine. Nevertheless, it is now a commonly expressed view that science has become so complex that findings of importance can be made only by individuals who spend all of their time in the laboratory. However, surgeons (and other clinically involved physicians) can remain as scientifically productive in the twenty-first century as before. In support of this view is the importance of research being done by several present-day surgeon-scientists.

A. Angiogenesis

Largely responsible for the initiation of this field and subsequent advances in it is a surgeon, Judah Folkman (68). Discovery of substances capable of stimulating the growth of new blood vessels has the potential of revolutionizing treatment of ischemic extremities, hearts, and other vital organs. Of possibly even greater importance is the discovery of antiangiogenic agents, which could be used to treat or prevent cancer. Folkman's work in this field was also seminal. Folkman believes that the recognition of antiangiogenic factors by anyone but a surgeon would have been unlikely. He notes that for many years surgeons have been frustrated and curious over the finding that in some patients who had no discernible metastatic disease preoperatively, the complete excision of a cancer was soon followed by the sudden dissemination of metastatic lesions. This phenomenon and development of a laboratory model of it were the inspirations for an important scientific finding.

In mice, Folkman and O'Reilly found that excision of a primary tumor they had established by transplantation was followed by the rapid appearance of metastasis that had not been evident before the excision (69). They then discovered that the primary tumor produced an antiangiogenic factor that was capable of suppressing metastases by preventing the growth of new blood vessels necessary for their growth. Thus, removal of the primary tumor allowed rapid appearance of metastatic disease. In subsequent experiments they isolated the antiangiogenic factor and showed that its administration could shrink established tumors in other mice. This factor, which they called endostatin, as well as other antiangiogenic agents are now in clinical trials.

B. Genetics, Gene Therapy, and Stem Cell Research

Advances in genetics are among the most important in modern science. Although the molecular aspects of this field are complex, surgeons have been able to contribute importantly to this research and its applications. One example is the work of Sam Wells. For several decades Wells studied the genetic pattern of the MENII syndrome and established the prevalence of thyroid cancer in members of afflicted families. In 1995, Wells reported the cloning of the MENII gene and a screening test for its presence. This allowed him to identify those young children from susceptible families who expressed the gene and thus could be predicted to develop thyroid cancer later in life (5). By performing prophylactic thyroidectomy early in childhood he was able to prevent the development of cancer.

Gene therapy is a fascinating field of great promise in treatment of human diseases. By replacement of a missing or defective gene with a normal one many metabolic diseases and other inheritable diseases might be cured. Cancers caused by genetic mutations might also be prevented or treated by this approach. Two major barriers to the fulfillment of this promise are delivery of vectors carrying the relevant genes and the immune destruction of the new gene or its vector. It is obvious that these are problems analogous to those traditionally confronting surgeons in transplantation. This may account for the prominent involvement of surgeons in the new field of gene therapy.

Stem cell technology is another fascinating new field that promises to allow growth of new organs or other body parts to replace injured or diseased ones. It is highly unlikely that this research can be conducted without important participation by surgeons.

C. Importance of the Surgeon-Scientist (Triple Threat)

Because of the past and recent research contributions of surgeon-scientists, not only will surgeons do important scientific research in the new century, but in many instances their active participation will be indispensable if scientific advances are to achieve clinical importance. Without participation of doctors whose research is stimulated by an active role in clinical care and teaching, scientific advances applicable to human disease will be much less likely. Some of our colleagues in basic science and internal medicine have recently come to the same conclusion. They, too, appear to be recognizing the need for "triple-threat" individuals. In nonsurgical disciplines, such individuals are often called physician-scientists. Alvin Feinstein and G.H. Williams expressed over the disappearance of physician-scientists from the field of internal medicine (70, 71). Feinstein indicates that until the latter part of the past century, advances in medical research were usually based on the principles of physiology. However, in recent years academic leaders in medicine decided that a physiologic approach would not be sufficient to answer fundamental questions as to how processes work at a cellular level. Thus they reasoned that the success of modern medical research would depend on the use of biochemistry and cellular and molecular biology in a reductionist approach to answer fundamental questions. It was anticipated that academic physicians who were trained in basic science because of their medical background would apply their advances in fundamental science to human disease.

It is certainly true that basic scientists and physician-scientists working in the reductionist disciplines of molecular and cellular biology have made extraordinary advances over the past several decades. However, at the same time Feinstein and Williams call attention to an unanticipated problem that has surfaced—the withering of the clinical investigator. Feinstein believes it is now easy to appreciate why this problem occurred:

> It was assumed that physicians who developed expertise in fundamental science would use this knowledge to address clinical problems. In retrospect, this assumption was naïve. The modern physician-scientists were trained to be reductionists. The fundamental research approaches they learned did not lend themselves to an understanding of human physiology or pathophysiology. Physiology and pathophysiology do not readily lend themselves to a reductionist approach. Indeed, by their very nature they use the tools of integration to understand complex processes in living subjects. As a consequence, physiology and pathophysiology as disciplines atrophied. In many medical schools, they became extinct. Furthermore few of the physician-scientists trained in the reductionist environment developed careers in human research. Rather, they became narrowly focused on the fields of the fundamental scientific laboratories in which they were trained, far removed from the bedside. Human diseases after all are disorders of macrobiology not microbiology. They occur at the level of organs and systems, not membranes, cells and molecules. A reductionist is likely to find it hard to relate to such gross phenomena as blockage, spasm, ischemia, and decompensation.

A surgeon-scientist (however well trained in molecular biology) is unlikely to forget these "gross phenomena" because of his or her continuing involvement with patients. Feinstein argues that a major return to integrationist physiology-based training is badly needed. What he neglects to point out is that the surgeon-scientist already has this integrationist training and (if also well trained in modern basic science) is ideally positioned to make major scientific contributions and to apply them in treatment of human disease.

References

1. Wagenstein, O. H., and Wangenstein, S. D. (1978). "The Rise of Surgery from Empiric Craft to Scientific Discipline." University of Minnesota Press, Minneapolis.
2. Longmire, W. P., Jr. (1996). "Conjoint Council on Surgical Research. Reports of the Committee of Special Interest." American College of Surgeons, Chicago.
3. Silen, W. *In* "Conjoint Council on Surgical Research. Reports of the Committee of Special Interest." American College of Surgeons, Chicago.
4. Jonasson, O. Personal communication

5. Wells, S. A., Jr. (1996). The surgical scientist. *Ann. Surg.* **224,** 239–254.
6. Rosenberg, L. E. (1999). Physician-scientists—Endangered and essential. *Science* **283,** 331–332.
7. Swain, J. L. (1996). Is there room left for academics in academic medicine? *J. Clin. Invest.* **98,** 1071–1073.
8. Folkman, J. (1984). Surgical science, a contradiction in terms? *J. Surg. Res.* **36,** 294–299.
9. DeBas, H. (2000). Lecture at American College of Surgeons' Conference for Young Investigators. Chantilly, VA, March 11, 2000.
10. Medawar, P. B. (1992). "Pluto's Republic." Oxford University Press, Oxford and New York.
11. Medawar, P. B. (1996). "The Strange Case of the Spotted Mice and Other Classic Essays on Science." Oxford University Press, New York.
12. Barker, C. F. (1997). Science, specialization, and the American Surgical Association. *Ann. Surg.* **226,** 211–228.
13. Austin, J. H. (1977). "Chase, Chance and Creativity—the Lucky Art of Novelty." Columbia University Press, New York.
14. Bateson, W. (1908). "The Method and Scope of Genetics." Inaugural lecture. Cambridge University Press, London.
15. Medawar, P. B. "Memoirs of a Thinking Radish," pp. 107–108. Oxford University Press, Oxford and New York.
16. Burnet, M. (1969). "Changing Patterns: An Atypical Autobiography." Elsevier, New York.
17. Longmire, W. P., Jr. Personal communication
18. Cannon, J. A., and Longmire, W. P. (1952). Studies of successful skin homografts in the chicken. Description of a method of grafting and its application as a technique for investigation. *Ann. Surg.* **135,** 60.
19. Danforth, C. H., and Foster, F. (1929). Skin transplantation as a means of studying genetic and endocrine factors in the fowl. *J. Exp. Zool.* **52,** 443.
20. Billingham, R. E., Brent, L., and Medawar, P. B. (1953). Actively acquired tolerance of foreign cells. *Nature (London)* **172,** 603–606.
21. Bliss, M. (1984). "Banting, A Biography." McClelland and Stewart Limited, Toronto.
22. Hare, R. (1970). "The Birth of Penicillin." George Allen and Unwin Ltd., London.
23. Ludovici, L. J. (1952). "Fleming, Discoverer of Penicillin." Indiana University Press, Bloomington.
24. MacFarland, G., and Florey, H. (1979). "The Making of a Great Scientist." Oxford University Press, Oxford.
25. Longmire, W. P., Jr. (1991). "Alfred Blalock: His Life and Times," pp. 30–31. Los Angeles, CA.
26. Billingham, R. E. (1991). Reminiscences of a transplanter. *In* "History of Transplantation: Thirty-five Recollections" (P. Terasaki, ed.), p. 80. UCLA Tissue Typing Laboratory, Los Angeles, CA.
27. Owen, R. D. (1945). Immunogenetic consequences of vascular anastomoses between bovine twins. *Science* **102,** 400.
28. Medawar, P. B., ed. (1996). Is the scientific paper a fraud? *In* "The Strange Case of the Spotted Mice and Other Classic Essays on Science," pp. 33–39. Oxford University Press, Oxford.
29. Kobler, J. (1960). "The Reluctant Surgeon, a Biography of John Hunter." Doubleday and Co., Garden City, NY.
30. Cameron, J. L. (1997). "William Stewart Halsted. Our Surgical Heritage." Transactions of the Southern Surgical Association. Lippincott-Raven, Philadelphia.
31. Thompson, J. C. (2000). Gifts from surgical research. Contributions to patients and surgeons. *J. Am. Coll. Surg.* **190,** 509–521.
32. Shoemeker, H. B. (1989). "A Dream of the Heart, the Life of John H. Gibbon, Jr." Fithian Press, Santa Barbara.
33. Romaine-Davis, A. (1991). "John Gibbon and His Heart–Lung Machine," p. 118. University of Pennsylvania Press, Philadelphia.
34. Miller, B. J., Gibbon, J. H., Jr., and Gibbon, M. H. (1951). Recent developments of a mechanical heart and lung apparatus. *Ann. Surg.* **134,** 694–707.
35. Dennis, C., Spreng, D. S., Nelson, G. E., *et al.* (1951). Development of a pump oxygenator to replace the heart and lungs; an apparatus applicable to human patients and application to one case. *Ann. Surg.* **134,** 709–721.
36. Lellihei, C. W. (1994). Cardiopulmonary bypass and myocardial protection. In Stephenson L. W. and Ruggiero R. "Heart Surgery Classics" (L. W. Stephenson and R. Ruggiero, eds.), pp. 121–141. Adams Publishing Group Ltd., Boston.
37. Malinin, T. I. (1979). "Surgery and Life: The Extraordinary Career of Alexis Carrel," pp. 22–29. Harcourt Brace Jovanovich, New York.
38. Moore, F. C. (1972). "Transplant the Give and Take of Tissue Transplantation." Simon and Schuster, New York.
39. Murray, J. E. (1991). "The First Successful Organ Transplants in Man." The Nobel Foundation, Stockholm, Sweden.
40. Starzl, T. E. (1992). "Memoirs of a Transplant Surgeon." University of Pittsburgh Press, Pittsburgh.
41. Todo, S., Fung, J. J., Starzl, T. E., *et al.* (1994). Single center experience with primary orthotopic liver transplantation with FK506 immunosuppression. *Ann. Surg.* **220,** 297–309.
42. Terasaki, P., ed. (1991). "History of Transplantation. Thirty-five Recollections," pp. 61–72. UCLA Tissue Typing Laboratory, Los Angeles, CA.
43. Bernard, C. N. (1967). A human cardiac transplant: An interim report of a successful operation performed at Groote Schuur, Capetown. *S. Africa Med. J.* **41,** 1271–1274.
44. Lower, R. R., and Shumway, N. E. (1960). Studies of on orthotopic homotransplantation of the canine heart. *Surg. Forum* **11,** 18–19.
45. Stinson, E. D., Dong, E., Jr., Schroeder, J. S., Harrison, D. C., and Shumway, N. E. (1968). Initial experience with heart transplantation. *Am. J. Cardiol.* **22,** 791–803.
46. Spencer, F. C. (1983). Intellectual creativity in thoracic surgeons. *J. Thoracic Cardiovasc. Surg.* **86,** 163–179.
47. Edward, W. S., and Edward, D. (1974). "Alexis Carrel, Visionary Surgeon." Charles C. Thomas, Springfield, IL.
48. Spencer, F. (1998). "Presidential Address. American Surgical Association. Past, Present and Future." Transactions of the American Surgical Association. Lippincott Williams and Wilkins, Philadelphia.
49. Jahnke, E. J., Jr., and Howard, J. M. (1953). Primary repair of major arterial injuries. Report of 58 battle casualties. *Arch. Surg.* **66,** 646.
50. Dubost, C., Allary, M., and Oeconomos, N. (1952). Concerning the treatment of aneurysms of the aorta. Ablation of the aneurysm. Reestablishment of continuity by graft of a preserved human aorta. *Arch. Surg.* **64,** 405.
51. DeBakey, M. E., and Cooley, D. A. (1953). Surgical treatment of aneurysm of abdominal aorta by resection and restoration of continuity with homograft. *Surg. Gynecol. Obstet.* **97,** 257.
52. Friedman, S. G. (1989). "A History of Vascular Surgery." Futura Publishing Col, Inc., Mount Kisco, NY.
53. Rombeau, J. L., Muldoon, D., and Rhoads, J. E. (1997). "Quaker Sense and Sensibility in the World of Surgery," pp. 175–214. Hanley & Belfus, Philadelphia.
54. Dudrick, S. J., Wilmore, D. W., Vars, H. M., and Rhoads, J. E. (1968). Long-term parenteral nutrition with growth development and positive nitrogen. *Surgery* **64,** 134–142.
55. Moore, F. C. (1989). In "Jonathan E. Rhoads Eightieth Birthday Symposium" (C. F. Barker and J. M. Daly, eds.). J. B. Lippincott, Philadelphia.
56. Dudrick, S. J., Macfadyen, B. V., VanBuren, C. T., *et al.* (1972). Parenteral hyperalimentation. Metabolic problems and solutions. *Ann. Surg.* **176,** 259–264.
57. Grande, F., and Visscher, M. (1967). "Claude Bernard and Experimental Medicine." Schenkman Publishing Co., Cambridge, Mass.
58. Cannon, W. B. (1925). "Bodily Changes in Pain, Hunger, Fear and Rage." D. Appleton, New York.

59. Wilmore, D. W. (1997). Homeostasis and bodily changes in trauma of surgery. *In* "Sabiston Textbook of Surgery. The Biological Bases of Modern Surgical Practice," Chap. 5. W. B. Saunders and Company, Philadelphia.
60. Brooks, B., and Blalock, A. (1934). Shock with particular reference to that due to hemorrhage and trauma to muscles. *Ann. Surg.* **100,** 728.
61. Moore, F. D. (1959). "The Metabolic Care of the Surgical Patient." W. B. Saunders Company, Philadelphia.
62. Fisher, B. (1959). The evaluation of paradigms for the management of breast cancer. *Cancer Res.* **52,** 2371–2382.
63. Huggins, C., and Hodges, C. V. (1942). Effect of orchidectomy and irradiation on cancer of the prostate. *Ann. Surg.* **116,** 1192–1200.
64. Welbourn, R. B. (1990). "The History of Endocrine Surgery," p. 286. Praeger Publishers, New York.
65. White, J. W. (1893). The present position of the surgery of the hypertrophied prostate. *Ann. Surg.* **17,** 70–75.
66. White, J. W. (1895). The result of double castration in hypertrophy of the prostate. *Ann. Surg.* **22,** 2–80.
67. Beatson, G. T. (1896). On the treatment of inoperable cancer of the mamma: Suggestions for a new method of treatment with illustrative cases. *Lancet* **2,** 104.
68. Folkman, J. (1995). Clinical applications of research on angiogenesis. *N. Engl. J. Med.* **333,** 1757–1763.
69. O'Reilly, M. S., Boehm, T., Shing, Y., Fukai, N., Birkhead, J. R., Olsen, B. R., and Folkman, J. (1997). Endostatin: An endogenous inhibitor of angiogenesis and tumor growth. *Cell* **88,** 277–285.
70. Feinstein, A. R. (1999). Basic biomedical science and the destruction of the pathophysiologic bridge from bench to bedside. *Am. J. Med.* **197,** 461–467.
71. Williams, G. H. (1999). The conundrum of clinical research: Bridges, linchpins and keystones. *Am. J. Med.* **107,** 522–524.

88

The Surgical Research Program as a Business Enterprise

Jeffrey H. Lawson and Robert W. Anderson

Department of Surgery, Duke University Medical Center, Durham, North Carolina 27710

I. Background

Academic departments of surgery have considered it their mission to create an optimal environment for clinical and investigative surgery for students, residents, and faculty. To accomplish this goal, there has been an attempt to balance the clinical care role of the department with education and research. Many academic departments of surgery have depended primarily on the generation of clinical funds to support not only the clinical effort of the faculty and staff, but also the academic component of the department, which includes education and research. Through the 1970s and 1980s, abundant clinical dollars were generated by departments of surgery and it was little problem to retain a portion of the net revenue to support surgical research programs. Many of these research efforts were poorly thought out and had little focus. In many instances, the work was conducted by surgeons who had little training in the scientific method, but were told by enthusiastic chairmen and deans that they needed to conduct some research in order to be eligible for promotion and to demonstrate academic productivity. As patterns of healthcare delivery have changed, with decreasing reimbursement for clinical services and decreasing support by both state and federal sources, the commitment to academic and scholarly productivity has diminished. The emphasis has been on providing clinical training with less commitment to fostering research. Significant changes in the financing of healthcare have led to a diminishing pool of clinical dollars. At the same time, traditional sources of surgical research funding, such as the National Institutes of Health, and the American Heart Association, the American Cancer Society, have become increasingly competitive for research funding, and surgical research has been less supported than in the past because of its traditional emphasis on intact physiology as opposed to the developing areas of molecular biology, genetics, and immunology. Although National Institutes of Health funding has increased over the past few years, competitive granting with a continued push toward basic science has made it difficult for surgical investigators with extensive clinical commitments to continue to be competitive. Many institutions began to question the value of surgical research while others took the approach that departments of surgery made enough money that they could afford to support their own research.

II. A New Look at Surgical Research

These changes have led the Department of Surgery at Duke to consider a more entrepreneurial approach toward planning and funding surgical research programs. When properly formulated, this approach can maintain a strong surgical commitment to research while generating new sources of revenue; we believe we can no longer rely on clinical revenues for sustaining successful research programs. Some academic departments of surgery will decide to focus on clinical care and education and have a very limited research effort. Others will decide to continue both basic and clinical research programs as part of their overall mission. These programs will need to plan to continue to allocate a portion of their revenues toward establishing and building research programs in focused areas, but will also need to develop innovative strategies that can be used to finance these programs over the long term. Program planners who make careful and well-planned investments in research can maintain high-quality research productivity, and, when positioned with the correct intellectual capital, can actually create innovative business opportunities in addition to seeking support through traditional sources such as extramural grants, philanthropy, and clinical revenues. The most important return on research and development investments that will accrue to a department of surgery will be differentiation as innovators in healthcare. The positioning advantage of being a strong research force in the competitive market of healthcare is difficult to validate but is real and sustainable in industry, and should be in healthcare. This approach will require realistic planning, careful prioritization of goals, careful assessment of financial and intellectual resources, and a commitment to implementing the strategy.

How can the knowledge and human resources that reside in academic healthcare centers and, more specifically, in a department of surgery best be used to meet the challenges of the future? This question must be addressed. Regardless of the field of endeavor, only two things are certain: change is essential and inevitable, and that change is now proceeding at a faster rate than ever before. Institutions that are organized and manage to adapt rapidly to change will be the institutions that will prosper in the coming decades. As Michael Hammer has so succinctly stated, "The watchwords of the new decade are innovation, speed, service and quality. Organize around outcomes, not tasks" (1). Success in the future depends on two things—human resources and fiscal resources. How these are managed in a rapidly changing environment is the critical issue and the challenge that must be faced by managers of departments of surgery that wish to maintain a viable research program. The opportunity to create a business opportunity through innovative research programs in departments of surgery exists in a variety of areas, but will differ widely at each institution. No generic process of planning will work and customization and appropriate scaling will be essential as a part of the planning process.

To bring about change in politics, business, and industry, or in a department of surgery, there must be stresses on the organization to motivate behavioral changes before one can bring about institutional change. Although departments of surgery are stressed in a variety of directions, they can and should take pride in their past accomplishments and their special role in society. Departments of surgery have known success, and although there are ominous signs of discontent and problems on the horizon, the forces to bring about change exist if there is a willingness to plan and execute. Those departments of surgery in which culture and basic values do not include a research commitment should place their emphasis in other areas and face reality. For those who are culturally committed to scientific research, the opportunities are great but the challenges are also formidable and success can only be achieved by thoughtful planning and forceful implementation of the plan.

III. Environmental Assessment

Although research dollars continue to grow, a smaller percentage of those dollars is available to the many individual investigators wishing to pursue an idea in the area of their choosing. Society, through its institutions and funding agencies, is saying that we are willing to pay, but we want to direct the areas of research. Hence, we see more rapid growth in research areas involving AIDS, cancer, cardiovascular disease, and aging. In addition, industries now contribute more to university research, but primarily as it benefits their products. Within our institutions, we now see unfunded or underfunded researchers who hold on to scarce resources and demand more support from institutional funds. Other faculty have had large increases in their funding and are demanding institutional responses of more space, facilities, and time to pursue their research efforts. Thus, the ability to respond rapidly to new opportunities for those who "have" while redirecting the efforts of the "have-nots" becomes critical to the expansion and well being of the research enterprise. At present, healthcare that is delivered in academic centers consists of multiple product lines by individuals working in all product lines. As industry knows, this type of organization is disastrous and hence most businesses have organized their human resources by specific product lines, each with responsibilities and authority for outcomes. If research and innovation are going to be an important part of the business of a department of surgery, selected individuals must be given responsibility and authority in research, others in undergraduate education, and still others in graduate education, while still others must direct the clinical effort in meeting patient care expectations and needs. This does not mean that individuals cannot perform in several areas, but it is very difficult, if not impossible, to have the same individuals assuming responsibility for the management of the multiple areas that frequently exist, and that, in reality, represent conflicts of interest. A matrix organization is emerging in which functional and departmental lines are combined to take advantage of each. Unless carefully managed, however, these two can become divisive and confusing, not only to the internal organization, but also to the external environment. Institutes or centers focusing on aging, molecular medicine, cancer, and cardiovascular disease frequently stimulate research and become a focus for patient care or education. However, they also frequently provide conflicting messages as to where an individual should place his efforts and loyalty, and members of academic faculty usually identify with areas that provide their rewards in terms of space, financing of projects, and compensation.

Regardless of the organizational structure used, it is essential to assign responsibility and authority to manage the activity of each product line to assure that institutional goals are met. The performance of each individual must be evaluated by predetermined parameters that are used to evaluate productivity in the multiple areas of endeavor in which they participate and contribute. The percentage of effort in each area must be controlled to assure that the multiple institutional or departmental goals can be met with faculty effort assignments. Faculty are then rewarded both financially and by distribution of resources such as space and equipment on the basis of how well they perform in the areas assigned as a percentage of their total performance evaluation. This change in structure is altering the role of the department chairmen who must now be a leader and facilitator rather than a manager (or micromanager) of the departmental efforts in clinical care, research, and education.

IV. Developing the Financial Plan

In order for an academic department of surgery to develop an overall plan for research and make sound business decisions about the role of research and development, it is necessary to consider the overall effect of financing and investment decisions. This process is called financial planning and the end result is a financial plan. This financial planning is necessary because investment and financing decisions interact and should not be made independently. In other words, the whole may be more or less than the sum of the parts.

This planning process must understand what makes projects work and what could go wrong with them. It must attempt to trace out the possible impact of today's decisions on tomorrow's opportunities. The same approach should be taken when financing or investment decisions are considered in the aggregate. Financial planning must help establish concrete goals to motivate and provide standards for measuring performance. All investments involve risk, whether they concern an individual portfolio or the research portfolio of a department of surgery. The level of financial risk that a department should undertake in order to build its portfolio must be determined by a thoughtful process of planning based on an assessment of strengths and weaknesses, opportunities that are available, the departmental balance sheet of intellectual, financial, and space resources, and, most importantly, the culture and commitment of all of the involved stakeholders, such as the faculty and staff.

Research planning should never be the exclusive preserve of the planners. Unless clinicians, educators, management, and key members of the research and innovation team are involved in the process, there will be lack of faith in the output. The financial plan put forth by a department of surgery must also be closely tied in with the academic medical center's business plan for research and development. Financial planning in not an easy topic to consider and it often attracts empty generalities or ponderous detail. A few important considerations in the financial planning process need to be considered. First, financial planning is a process of analyzing the financing and investment choices open to an entity such as a department of surgery. Second, it is important to project the future consequences of present decisions, in order to avoid surprises and understand the link between present and future decisions. Finally, careful decisions must be made as to which alternatives to undertake, and the measurement of subsequent performance against the goals set in the financial plan must be established. Those department of surgery planners who choose to make investments in research must leverage this investment in clinical areas, which will differentiate them from competitors. Dabbling in research because it has been considered "part of being academic" is no longer justifiable simply because it is no longer an affordable or productive use of resources.

V. Developing the Research Portfolio

Everyone recognizes that the stock market is risky because there is a spread of possible outcomes. The usual measure of this spread is the standard deviation or variance. The risk of any stock can be broken down into two parts: there is a unique risk that is particular to that individual stock and there is a market risk that is associated with market-wide variations. The investor can eliminate unique risk by holding a well-diversified portfolio, but cannot eliminate market risks. All the risk of a fully diversified portfolio is market risk. Investments in research by a department of surgery should be looked at in the same way that stock investments are looked at. A classic article written in 1952 by Markowitz drew attention to the common practice of portfolio diversification and showed how investors in the stock market (or in research projects) can reduce the standard deviation of portfolio returns by making investments that do not move together (2). For a department of surgery, a high-risk portfolio might consist of all the effort and resources being focused on discovery projects in the areas of therapeutics or diagnosis. A low-risk portfolio would involve being a participant only in clinical trials, and more intermediate risk might focus on the development of patient care processes, device testing, or the development of clinical care maps that may have commercial value. What level of risk a department is capable and willing to assume depends on many factors that must be carefully analyzed during the planning process. A second portfolio that must be developed relates to funding resources and how they will be allocated to capitalize research investments.

When one considers the research program for the twenty-first century in a clinically based department, it becomes obvious that the funding of these programs is essential for their continued success. In the past, many investigators were able to concentrate strictly on the academic mission of their science with little regard for the critical nature of funding support to ensure the long-term success of their program. If funding shortfalls arose, they could be readily covered by departmental support while the next funding cycle from a grant was processed. However, as clinical resources have become an ever-diminishing pool of funding for scientific endeavors, it is now imperative that investigators develop a more business-minded approach to the funding of their research program. We have found that it is useful to model research program funding in a model similar to traditional financial portfolios used in both personal and corporate finance (see Fig. 1). In this regard, the funding portfolio for

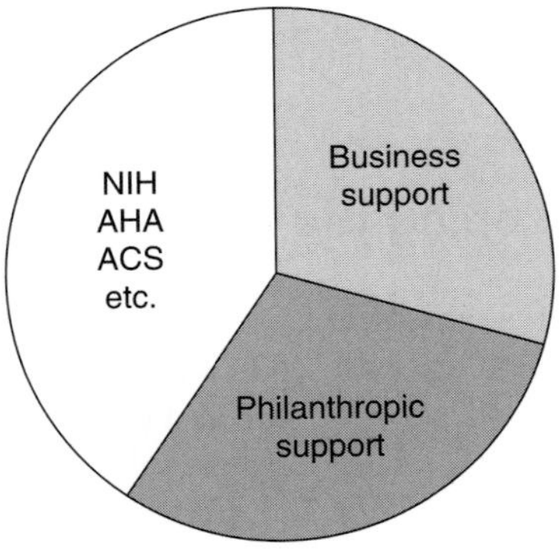

Figure 1 A balanced portfolio of research funding that includes revenue from traditional funding agencies, business, and philanthropy. NIH, National Institutes of Health; AHA, American Heart Association; ACS, American College of Surgeons.

a department of surgery's research program may include research dollars derived from funding agencies such as the National Institutes of Health, the American Heart Association, or the American College of Surgeons. These dollars are competitive and entail the risk of being lost for underperformance at future grant cycles. They are carefully budgeted and require careful oversight and compliance, which require that the appropriate infrastructure be in place. A second source of funding for a complete research portfolio should be that of business and translational research programs. In this regard, surgeons can exploit their intellectual capital by partnering with business to help in the innovative development of products and devices for the surgical arena. Finally, sources of funding through institutional and departmental support and philanthropic donations should be pursued aggressively to allow for the development of startup programs and the maintenance of successful and promising research irrespective of changes in political landscape or corporate interests. If one develops a broad-based portfolio of funding, this can withstand shortfalls that may arise from granting cycles, changes in research agendas, and a fallout of ever-changing corporate support for research. This can allow an investigator to be secure in funding of employees who are important for the success of the laboratory and can allow for a broad-based financial position to endure the constant and fast-paced changes in the scientific landscape. Conversely, there must be a firm resolve to terminate support of programs or investigators that are unsuccessful and have little promise of future success. This is often a painful process, but the failure to recognize "sunk costs" and accept them will lead to pouring resources into a black hole with no chance of success.

A. Federal Funding

The National Institutes of Health (NIH) has expanded its research funding for many areas of basic and translational science in the past few years. There is an ever-increasing number of specific request for applications (RFAs) announced by the National Institutes of Health monthly to support specific areas of funding. To identify these specific programs to which large sums of money are dedicated for research programs, it is essential that a university and/or specific investigator establish mechanisms to identify these novel opportunities when they arise. It was once possible for the surgeon-scientist to stand alone and write grants that focused on scientific problems, related to unique clinical situations. However, the rate of scientific innovation has increased exponentially in the past 10 years with the molecular and genetic revolutions. Thus, for the surgeon to be competitive for peer-reviewed funding from federal sources, a high level of scientific training or partnerships with successful basic scientist coinvestigators are now required. Partnerships with other investigators on the faculty of academic universities should be sought such that strategic alliances between a basic science mission and its translation through a clinically relevant problem can be clearly established and articulated in these competitive NIH grants. If these partnerships can be established, with clear evidence of collaboration and a joint scientific goal, what was once an extremely competitive grant review process can become a much more attainable source of funding because of the outstanding ability to take basic science innovation and apply it directly to a clinically relevant problem. Examples of this would include partnering with basic cancer biologists in the treatment and identification of various solid organ tumors that can be accessed and manipulated directly by surgeons, or the area of cardiovascular medicine in which innovative therapies in angiogenesis or thrombosis developed by the molecular biologist can be directly applied using the skills of the cardiovascular surgeon. Relationships of this type allow the clinician-scientist to bridge the gap between basic science and clinical problems and provide the strongest position possible for the success of grants reviewed in study sections, which all too often criticize the active clinician for his inability to complete the scientifically relevant work necessary to move a grant forward while maintaining certain clinical responsibilities.

B. Corporate and Business Funding

Relationships with business or corporate entities were once scorned by academic investigators as being in violation of the sanctity of the pure nature of the academic mission. However, as medical economics have changed and biotechnology has blossomed, this area of research funding has become an attractive and potentially important source of revenue for even the most basic of research programs. Academic surgeons and scientists hold a high level of intellectual capital, which is valued by industry. This intellectual property has often been undervalued and given to industry at rock-bottom prices to support shortsighted goals of funding some limited research project. The rapid pace of innovative technologies, which are now entering the surgical arena, demands the need for a high-quality interface with universities at both the developmental phase and the clinical trials end of projects. It has been suggested that 9 out of every 10 innovative devices developed by industry and intended for surgical markets fail to make it to market, not because of the lack of good ideas, but rather because of poor insight and input from clinical experts in surgery. Identifying key areas of expertise that add value to the products being developed by industry can result in important funding opportunities for the department of surgery, as well as direct sources of grant support. These relationships can lead to contributions to the research goals of industry. The development of new technologies can be dramatically influenced by the academic partner, resulting in new products that support the needs of the surgical investigator and improve patient care. Once established, these partnerships may also lead to patents and other postdiscovery products, yielding returns to the investigator and/or university in the form of royalties. Partnerships with business that directly impact the positive aspects of research programs should be encouraged to help develop innovative products and technologies that can be used to better patient care. These partnerships can often form a win–win scenario because the investigator can benefit from the sheer financial power that biotechnology and industrial corporations can offer and can foster their own research agenda at the same time. It is imperative, however, in these relationships that academic researchers maintain the highest level of integrity while realizing the important goals of their industrial partners.

Relationships with companies can be formed in two ways; the first is directly related to innovative product development, as discussed above. Second, after a long and trusted relationship is established, many corporations can be encouraged to target specific funds strictly for educational and research grants that are not directly tied to product development, but may simply support the academic mission of an investigator or department. An excellent example of this type of relationship is illustrated at Duke University, where a corporate partnership with U.S. Surgical Corporation established a large educational grant to fund the development of a laparoscopic surgery center. This laparoscopic surgery center has had long-lasting benefits to the university and its investigators in the area of innovative technologies dedicated to laparoscopic surgery. U.S. Surgical has benefited by the training of many surgeons who have been exposed to technologies utilizing their products. Furthermore, this relationship has provided direct funding for educational programs and fellowships that otherwise would have to be eliminated or extracted from the shrinking pool of clinical dollars. Such arrangements must be structured carefully to avoid conflicts of interest and to respect the proprietary and financial interests of both parties. The importance of well-defined guidelines supported by an effective Office of Science and Technology within the university structure that creates win–win situations cannot be overemphasized.

C. Philanthropic Support

Philanthropic support for research programs remains an important potential source of funding for research-driven programs with potential clinical impact. Many investigators struggle to obtain competitive funding from granting agencies for innovative ideas that do not appeal to peer reviewers, who have their own priorities, while millions of dollars circulate in the hands of donors who may be willing to direct their funding to meaningful areas of scientific exploration that they consider important. Philanthropic donations can serve as an important core source of money that can be used from everything from endowing important scientific chairs to establishing startup research packages for innovative young investigators. Unfortunately, these opportunities are often untapped due to a lack of cohesive departmental and university-based effort. Unfortunately, the solicitation of philanthropic donations is often left in the hands of university bureaucrats, who are unable to articulate the important needs of developing research programs. To maximize the potential for philanthropic donations, program-based initiatives should be formed. These would allow groups of lead investigators in specific areas such as cancer biology, cardiovascular medicine, or gene therapies to seek a high level of visibility in both local and national communities. If lead investigators can be identified to prospective donors such that the essential nature of the research mission can be articulated, large sums of dedicated funding can often be obtained. An excellent example of this has been illustrated by the prostate cancer and melanoma research programs at Duke. These programs annually hold updates in which patients who have been treated successfully for these cancers are invited to attend a research forum. In this setting, the key investigators present their important findings to the lay public and stress the need for further research funding that will advance the care of prostate cancer and melanoma. These activities have generated significant donations, which have allowed these research programs to direct research funding to key laboratories in innovative areas. Although many surgeons have been uncomfortable with the notion of lobbying patients for money, there should be no shame in asking patients and/or charitable organizations for money that can further benefit their future care and advance new treatments. The time and effort expended by successful investigators who are active clinicians and scientists are appreciated by donors both at the individual and foundation level. Surgeons enjoy a unique advantage in this regard but frequently are reluctant to take advantage of it.

VI. Research as a Business

Research programs have all too often been viewed as a financial drain on clinical departments of surgery, and their ability to act as a magnet for clinical business has been undervalued. However, as the pool of clinical dollars has continued to shrink, one of the untapped areas of revenue that can be used to drive research support of departments of surgery in the future is the ability to do innovative translational research, such that funds cannot only be used to pay for the research activities, but the extra dollars generated can feed back to the department to fund the educational mission of teaching and expanding programs. With the rise of biotechnology and innovative surgical devices, the need for these novel therapies to be tested both preclinically and clinically is imperative. If one thinks creatively about this as a business opportunity, it is clear that the department of surgery, which can both evaluate the scientific side of a novel technology and access patients in whom these technologies may undergo safe clinical trials, is in an extremely strong position for leveraging those resources to secure competitive contracts with industry. These types of revenue can be separated into three broad categories that are not mutually exclusive, which we will highlight below: first; providing expertise and facilities that allow corporate partners to outsource areas of basic research of mutual interest; second, evaluation of translational device development; and third, providing patients and clinical data management skills for clinical research trials.

A. Outsourcing of Surgical Research Expertise to Corporations

As companies have moved forward in the development of innovative technologies that may be used in the surgical environment, many have been left short in expertise for evaluating basic components of these new therapies. Basic research laboratories, which have a high level of expertise in areas such as cardiovascular medicine, molecular biology, and cancer biology, represent ideal laboratories to generate revenue by providing research expertise to companies that cannot afford the expertise in-house. Although few academic scientists have time to "do research for hire," their laboratories have room for corporate partnerships, which can be used to generate revenue by providing outsourced research with little drain on research programs. In the past, when these relationships have been established with universities, the research expertise of an investigator has often not been adequately compensated. However, if one considers the ability to provide meaningful input and high-quality services to corporations, which lack certain expertise, the value of these services is actually very high. Furthermore, if one realizes what it costs these companies to develop the required expertise in-house, it is easy to see how a reasonable contract can be developed such that research can be performed in concert with a corporate partner while a certain percentage of revenue, in the form of direct compensation, royalties, etc., can actually be used by the investigator and/or department to pay for innovative programs. This requires a change in mindset. Investigators have traditionally felt happy to simply get a grant from a company; a new thought process is more consistent with a small business unit that can provide high-quality services to a company at a fair market price. It is important to stress the intellectual capital that clinician-scientists represent in these relationships. Obvious problems in new technology development, which may be unnoticed by industrial scientists, are easily identified and corrected by the high level of expertise that is often sequestered in the university laboratory. Examples of these can be shown in areas such as assay development, cell biology, and molecular genetics. If these relationships are to be pursued, it is important that an investigator, who previously only thought about the basic needs of their research program, work with more business-minded consultants within the university, such that the true value of the work provided can be determined and not sold short because one simply works for a nonprofit university. Again, the importance of a well-run Office of Science and Technology within the university structure cannot be neglected.

B. Translational Device Development

Universities with large animal facilities and underutilized capacity represent an opportunity for translational device development. If one considers the cost of doing animal studies, it is obvious to most corporate partners that the required expertise in animal facilities represents significant cost to develop and maintain internally. These resources often exist at major universities and have a strong association with the interventional nature of many surgical research programs. These resources can actually form a strategic area for business development such that the margins obtained from a company outsourcing its translational device studies can be used to fund research programs and facilities directly related to the investigator and the department. The value of animal research capabilities as a business opportunity to recruit funding from corporate sources cannot be underestimated. If one samples the industrial leaders in innovative device development, the majority of these companies are in need of skilled personnel and facilities to test and analyze their new devices. This represents a significant business opportunity for the entrepreneurial-minded investigator to not only maintain their own research infrastructure for animal trials, but to do complementary studies for corporations, which can yield significant financial resources. In this setting, investigators must be careful not to spend valuable time supporting bad ideas, but innovative devices and concepts for development should be welcomed to be tested in appropriate animal models in a way that the perceived benefit of the program has value to both the investigator and the corporate sponsor. As highlighted above, the true value of this type of research cannot be underestimated and should not be sold short when one considers the inherent cost to the company of doing their own research. These relationships also allow the academic partner to be linked to the device as it passes from its preclinical evaluation to the clinical trials that will follow should a successful intervention be identified. These relationships can be used to offset the infrastructural costs of a vivarium and the technical staff, which is required to maintain these resources at a university. Furthermore, a reasonable margin or premium can be determined such that these research relationships can actually form a small business enterprise to generate significant revenue that can feed back into the department and university. Some have expressed concern that this will compromise the mission of an academic department, but recent studies have demonstrated that research productivity of investigators is improved by such arrangements (3).

C. Clinical Research Trials

Clinical research trials in the area of surgery represent a potentially important area of clinical research dollars that have not been consumed by clinical research organizations (CROs). If one evaluates for-profit CROs, less than 10% of their business is related to device or surgical trials. This is primarily driven by a lack of expertise in the CRO industry because clinical research trials in surgery have been hard to maintain and difficult to manage. However, if an appropriate infrastructure can be developed such that surgical and/or device-based trials can be run efficiently, this represents a unique opportunity for an academic CRO-type of business to develop. An excellent example of the success of an academic CRO exists at Duke University. The Duke Clinical Research Institute (DCRI) has found a unique niche in running large-scale, high-quality clinical trials for corporations. To date, the majority of these trials have focused on drug therapies; however, success in areas of cardiology device development suggest that the possibility exists to extend these into device development and surgical clinical trials. In this regard, departments of surgery with high clinical volumes represent an ideal business opportunity to develop an academic CRO-based infrastructure that can take part in competitive clinical trials in the evaluation of novel surgical technologies. The majority of surgical trials to date have been fraught with problems related to unique site management and the particular whims of surgical investigators that arise at each site. This has caused many studies to fail, not because the device or technology failed or had no clinical benefit, but rather because clinical protocols and FDA quality data were simply overlooked or bypassed. Furthermore, the cost of developing a small clinical research infrastructure at each unique surgical center is logistically difficult and often cost prohibitive. This provides a unique business opportunity for a surgically based academic CRO to establish linked sites within aligned partners to run efficient clinical trials to investigate new surgical techniques or devices. This can provide significant cost savings for industry and at the same time provide a high level of revenue to fund clinical trial infrastructure and the associated support personnel. This also allows the academic researcher direct access to early clinical information in the development and success of a new technique, as well as providing a unique academic opportunity for publication in the advancement of new knowledge.

VII. Summary

It is reasonable to envision a future in which highly qualified members of an academic surgical department, with an aptitude for basic, translational, and clinical research, will be able to generate significant revenue. This revenue will not only support infrastructure of their own research operation, but can actually generate excess revenue for use in funding the academic mission of a department and/or university. These programs require an innovative mindset that no longer looks at research as a nonpaying portion of a department in need of support by clinical dollars, but rather a true business opportunity that can be used to fuel the engine of surgical programs. It is reasonable to envision a future in which creative business opportunities that exploit the high degree of intellectual capital often found in academic surgical departments can be used to fund many aspects of a department that were once funded from excess revenue related to patient care. At a time when the value of surgical expertise related to patient care has diminished in the eyes of third-party payers and the federal government, this may represent the financial future of surgical departments and may enhance the value of their own faculty in strategic positions that benefit development in novel therapy and patient care.

A final consideration for some departments of surgery is the spin-off of a private company based on work that has been accomplished within the department and has potential commercial value that cannot be realized in an academic setting. This has been successfully accomplished at a number of academic institutions in the United States. This is a complex undertaking that requires extensive planning and cooperation from the parent university and is beyond the scope here, but is discussed in Chapter 100 of this volume

References

1. Hammer, M., and Champy, J. (1993). "Reengineering the Corporation." Harper Collins Publishers, New York.
2. Markowitz, H. M. (1952). Portfolio selection. *J. Finance* **7,** 77.
3. Blumenthal, D., Campbell, E., Causino, N., and Louis, K. (1996). Participation of life-science faculty in research relationships with industry. *N. Engl. J. Med.* 335, 1734–1739.

89

Nobel Laureates in Surgery

Moritz M. Ziegler

Department of Surgery, Children's Hospital Medical Center, Boston, Massachusetts 02115

I. Introduction

The history of the most prestigious award in science and medicine is directly related to the foresight of Alfred Bernhard Nobel, and men and women have been awarded this prize since the turn of the twentieth century. Of the recipients, nine surgeons have won the Nobel Prize in Medicine, and their methods for success have varied from dedicated, life-long work to the unusual "home run" experiment that has characterized several prize winners. This chapter describes the philanthropist Alfred Nobel and the prize awarding process, and selectively identifies and describes the nine surgical Nobel laureate winners.

A. Alfred Bernhard Nobel (1833–1896)

Alfred Bernhard Nobel was born in Stockholm, Sweden on October 21, 1833, the son of an engineer and inventor. After bankruptcy, his father, Immanuel, left Stockholm to begin a new career in Finland and Russia. In 1842, Immanuel moved his family to St. Petersburg, where he was engaged in the production of military equipment, including naval mines consisting of gun powder-filled wooden caskets. After a private education in St. Petersburg, Alfred was sent abroad for further education in chemical engineering. By age 17, he was in Paris to observe Professor Théophile Pelouze, whose student Sobrero had invented nitroglycerine. A decade later Nobel caused nitroglycerine to explode. During experimentation in 1864, his brother Emil was killed by an explosion. At age 30, he patented the blasting cap, and at age 33 he defined "dynamite" as a combination of clay (Kieselguhr) and nitroglycerine, patenting the mixture under two names, "Nobel's Safety Powder" and "Dynamite"; the latter term was coined from the Greek *dynamis*, meaning power. At age 42, Alfred patented the blastine gelatine.

Nobel was known as an inventor, having more than 355 patents, but also as a scientist, pacifist, and writer. A complex man, very successful in business, he had the unusual interest of working with explosive destructive devices. Yet, his philosophy was that the spread of knowledge would promote well being and that the improvement of war materials and the increasing dangers of war would in fact contribute to the pacification of the world. Prior to his death on December 10, 1896 in San Remo, Italy, Nobel documented a last will and testament (1) on November 27, 1895, to state the following:

> The whole of my remaining estate ($9 million dollars) shall be dealt with in the following way: the capital ($9 million dollars), invested in safe securities by my executors, shall constitute a fund, the interest on which shall be annually distributed in the form of prizes to those who, during the preceding year, shall have conferred the greatest benefit on

> mankind. The interest shall be divided into five equal parts, namely, physics, chemistry, physiology or medicine, literature, and the fraternity between nations. The prizes for physiology and medicine shall be awarded by the Royal Caroline Medico-Surgical Institute, Stockholm, and no consideration will be given to the nationality of the candidates, but that the most worthy shall receive the prize, whether he be Scandinavian or not.

This generous act of Nobel initiated the institution of the Nobel Foundation and the Nobel process, the first prize in physiology or medicine being awarded in 1901 after the turn of the century, and on the fifth anniversary of his death.

B. Nobel Prize in Physiology or Medicine

Nominees for the Nobel Prize in physiology or medicine are solicited by the Nobel Assembly members, members of the Royal Academy of Sciences, previous laureates, other Nobel committee members, professors in Sweden, Denmark, Finland, Iceland, and Norway, professors from at least six other centers, and other practitioners of the natural sciences. Typically, candidates are presented to the Nobel Prize Committee, of the Nobel Assembly at the Karolinska Institute in Stockholm, before February 1 of each year. The Committee, with input from selected experts, then makes a candidate recommendation to the Nobel Assembly at the Karolinska Institute, and a vote is taken to confirm the final choice. The announcement of the selection is made soon after the October vote. The prize-awarding ceremony takes place at Concert Hall in Stockholm, Sweden on December 10, the anniversary of Alfred Nobel's death.

A variety of selection criteria are used to select candidates, including the following considerations (2): Was the contribution made in the previous year? Did the contribution culminate years of research? Was the contribution the work of one, two, or three scientists working as a team? Did the discovery of one nominee depend on the work of another nominee working independently?

The prize consists of a cash award of approximately 1 million dollars, a gold medal, and the Nobel diploma. The artist Rune Karlzon designed the medal, the back of which depicts a tunnel blasted by dynamite and a detonator, and the front which depicts a portrait of Nobel and the Latin inscription *Creavit et promovit*, "He created and promoted."

II. Surgical Award Winners

A. Emil Theodor Kocher (1841–1917)

Emil Kocher (Fig. 1) won the Nobel Prize in 1909 "for his work on the physiology, pathology, and surgery of the thyroid gland." Kocher was born in Berne, Switzerland and received his medical doctorate degree from the University of Berne. He was a surgical student of Langenbeck, Virchow, Paget, and Billroth, and he became Professor of Surgery at age 31 in Berne, an appointment not without considerable controversy (3). His contributions encompassed multiple disciplines, including orthopedic surgery, neurosurgery, and abdominal surgery, and he was one of the first surgeons to apply the aseptic principles of Lister. His broad-based surgical contributions included research on the soft tissue impact of high-velocity missiles, acute osteomyelitis, the theory of strangulated hernia, hernia of infancy, gastric resection, transsacral rectal resection, choledochotomy for bile duct stones, spinal injury, traumatic epilepsy, orthopedic malformations, and duodenal mobilization, among other areas (4).

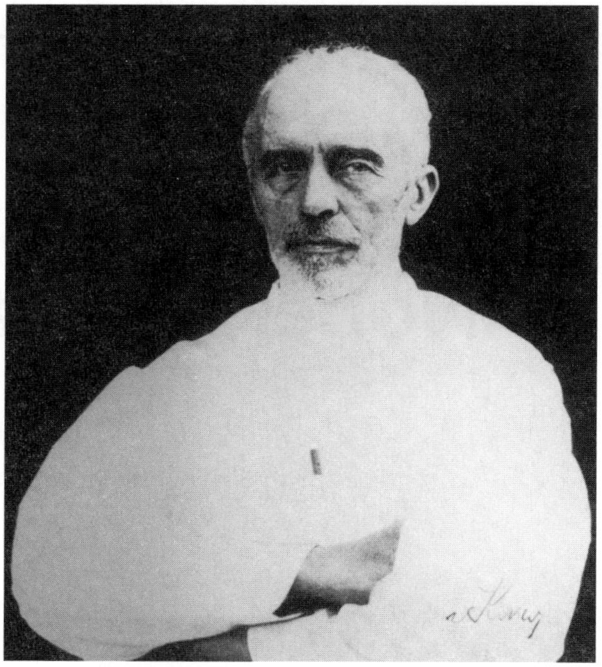

Figure 1 Emil Theodor Kocher (1841–1917). From (5).

In 1872 Kocher did his first thyroidectomy, and within 10 years he had performed 101 thyroidectomies with 13 fatalities (12.8% mortality) (5). This was a remarkable accomplishment in an era when almost three-fourths of all patients did not survive the operation and when recurrent nerve injury and postoperative tetany were commonplace. During this same interval he described cachexia strumipriva, an association of weight gain, slowness of intellect and speech, muscular weakness, hair loss, tongue thickness, and anemia in patients following total thyroidectomy (5) (Fig. 2). He was eventually able to establish the association of these changes with the hypothyroid state and by 1892, oral thyroid supplementation therapy was introduced. He also described the role of the collar incision, meticulous control of blood supply, and refined dissection techniques during thyroidec-

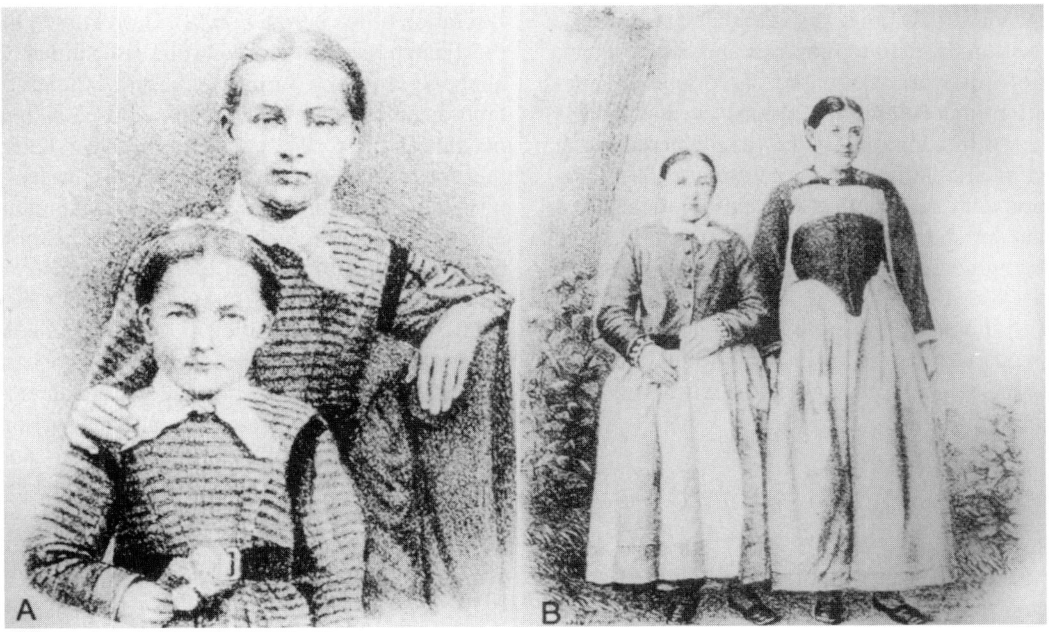

Figure 2 Kocher's patient Maria Richsel. (A) The older and taller patient on whom Kocher had done a total thyroidectomy depicted in a preoperative photograph with her younger sister. (B) Nine years later, the dwarfed and stunted Maria displays the features of cachexia strumipriva when compared with her now taller younger sister. From (14).

tomy. Later in his life, after some 5000–9000 thyroidectomies, he was operating at a mortality rate of 0.5% (3).

Cushing described Kocher as someone who was careful, elaborate, painstaking, and diligent, but one who at times would "dolly unnecessarily" at the operating table. He further compared Kocher's impact on European surgery to be comparable to that of Halsted on American surgery (6). Sauerbruch described Kocher as being overly religious, having a one-track mind, and as being devoted to surgery and surgery alone. Kocher, not known as a classic speaker, coined a series of important surgical thoughts, which included "every ileus ought to be examined at the beginning by both physician and surgeon"; "if two consultants are necessary, it is the surgeon who is indispensable"; and "I cannot admire those itinerant surgeons who place themselves at the service of general practitioners" (3). Emil Kocher succeeded in winning the Nobel Prize for technical surgical achievement and precise clinical observation. He was a master surgeon, "the surgeon's surgeon."

B. Allvar Gullstrand (1862–1930)

Allvar Gullstrand (Fig. 3) won the Nobel Prize in 1911 "for his work on the dioptrics of the eye (science of refracted light of the eye)." He was born in Landskrona, Sweden, and after studies at Uppsala University and Vienna, he received his medical doctorate from Stockholm University. In 1894, Gullstrand became first Professor of Ophthalmology, Uppsala University, at the age of 32. It was there that he made a series of contributions that came to define geometric and physiologic optics. His doctoral thesis in 1890, which

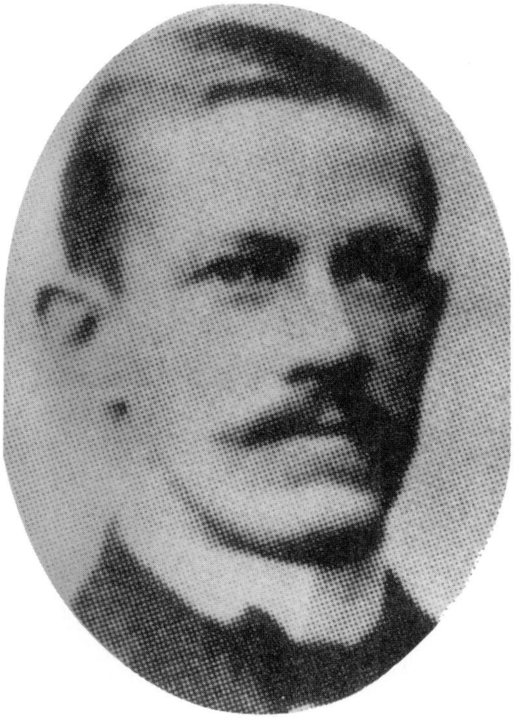

Figure 3 Allvar Gullstrand (1862–1930). From (7).

focused on the theory of astigmatism, stimulated remarkable advancements within the field of dioptrics and optical imaging (7). Much of this work was based on complex mathematical calculations that determined how the eye and its lens focused on objects. In addition, Gullstrand defined the first laboratory of clinical ophthalmology, he initiated an industrial collaboration with Zeiss optical in the development of a lens for astigmatism and aphakia, and he characterized the principles of accommodation. This self-taught ophthalmologist and scientist was a strong administrator, and his inventions significantly impacted the field of ophthalmology. In addition, he is recognized as the inventor of the slit lamp, the corneal microscope, the photometer, and the reflex-free ophthalmoscope (7).

C. Alexis Carrel (1873–1944)

Born in Sainte-Foy-les-Lyon, France, Alexis Carrel (Fig. 4) won the Nobel Prize in 1912 "in recognition of his works on vascular suture and the transplantation of blood vessels and organs." He received his doctorate of medicine in 1900 from Lyon School of Medicine, and he spent the first portion of his career in Lyon. It is reported that Carrel became overwhelmed with sorrow when Sadi Carnot, the prime minister of France, was killed by an assassin's knife

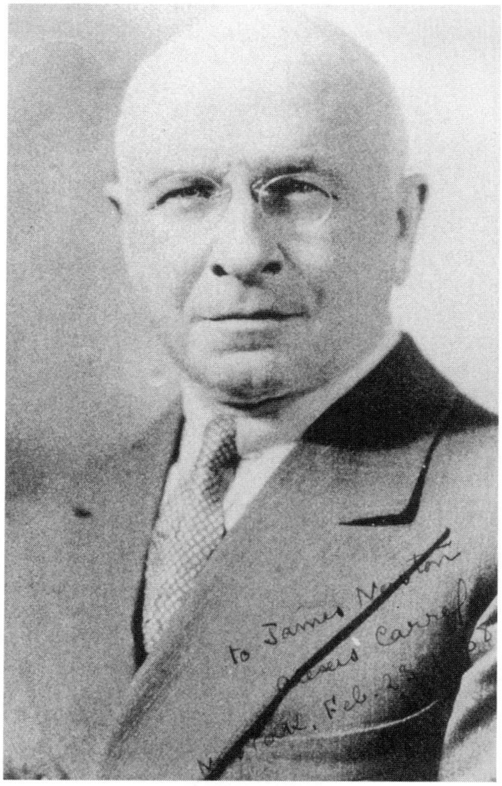

Figure 4 Alexis Carrel (1873–1944). From (11), by permission of the *Texas Heart Institute Journal*.

laceration of his portal vein (8). Carrel noted the inability of the French surgeons to control vessel injury, an event that allegedly inspired him to take sewing lessons from the embroideress Mme. Leroudier and begin the use of finer needles and fine silk suture. Several years later, in 1902, he presented a paper at the Lyon Medical Society on the subject of vascular anastomotic technique (9). Simultaneously, Carrel also became immersed in medical phenomenology, and he traveled to Lourdes to observe various miracles in the making. As a result of his vocal support for this field of study, his outspoken criticism of French medicine, and his failure to pass the entrance exam on two occasions, Carrel fell out of favor with the medical establishment in Lyon, and he was unable to secure an appointment in surgery. Consequently, Carrel moved to Montreal in 1904 and soon thereafter was invited to the University of Illinois in Chicago.

In Chicago, Carrel teamed up with fellow scientists Carl Beck and Charles Guthrie at the University of Chicago. Working collaboratively, the three men utilized fine oiled silk, occlusive ligatures, and the triangulation anastomotic technique, which enabled them to perform vascular anastomoses and associated whole organ and tissue grafting (10). After being invited to lecture at Johns Hopkins by Cushing, a presentation attended by Simon Flexner, Carrel was subsequently recruited by Flexner in 1906 to the Rockefeller Institute. He stayed in that institution until his forced retirement at age 65 in 1939. At the Rockefeller, Carrel changed his focus to tissue culture, whole organ culture and perfusion, and extracorporeal perfusion. In addition, he developed during this time a strong association with the renowned aviator Charles Lindberg, and together they worked to develop an extracorporeal organ perfusion apparatus as a step toward the development of an artificial heart (11).

Carrel's loyalty to his native France was demonstrated during World War I when he established a front-line hospital at Compiègne after being drafted into the French army. There he developed a wound antisepsis technique, and he was aided in this front-line work by Henry Dakin, whom Flexner had dispatched to the hospital specifically to work with Carrel. Soon after, the two men identified the dilute hypochlorite solution, eventually named Carrel–Dakin solution, which they used to treat war wound injuries. The mortality rate in that front-line hospital was the lowest in the history of battle to that point in time (11).

Carrel returned to the United States and the Rockefeller Institute after World War I, but he moved back to France during World War II and established the "Institute of Man" in Paris. Shortly before the end of the war, Carrel was accused of being a Nazi collaborator, and he succumbed to a cardiac illness while being pursued by authorities.

Carrel is a remarkably accomplished Nobel laureate whose prize was awarded early in his career for vascular anastomosis, the triangulation technique (Fig. 5), vessel patch closure, and the Carrel patch vascular pedicle, which

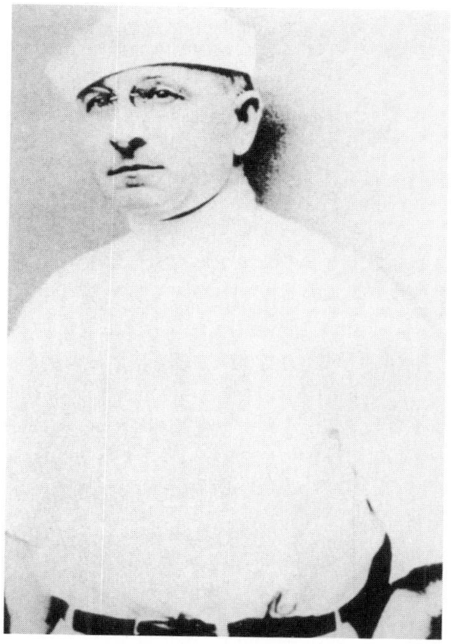

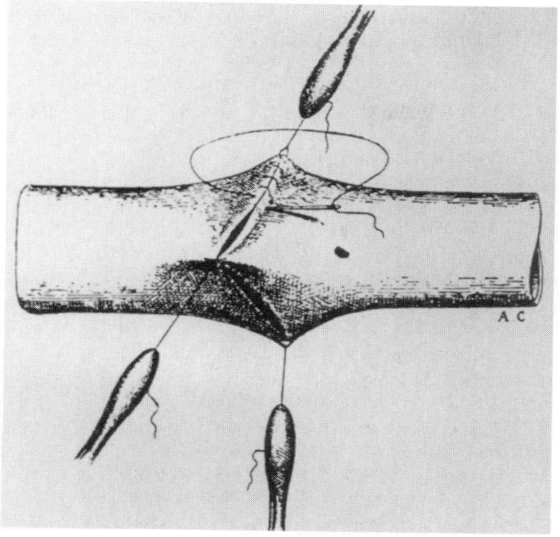

Figure 5 Carrel's triangulation technique defined for end-to-end vessel anastomosis. From (14).

enabled solid organ and limb transplantation. However, Carrel is also the author of such accomplishments as human blood transfusion, cardiothoracic surgery (including coronary artery bypass grafting), endotracheal intubation, wound antisepsis, aortic cross-clamp-induced hind limb paralysis, aorto-aortic bypass, coronary artery bypass, and oxygenated pulsatile organ perfusion, the latter having been developed with Charles Lindberg.

D. Robert Bàràny (1876–1936)

Bàràny (Fig. 6), an otolaryngologist and physiologist, won the Nobel Prize in 1914 "for his work on the physiology and pathology of the vestibular apparatus." Bàràny was born in Vienna and received his medical doctorate at the University of Vienna in 1900. He then studied in Frankfort and Freiburg before returning to Vienna as an otologist. It was then that he did his prize-winning work. During World War I, in 1915, while serving as an Austrian army medical officer, he was captured and imprisoned by Russian officials. While serving as a doctor to fellow prisoners as well as to Russian captors, he learned of his Nobel Prize and he was released to travel to Sweden to receive his award (7). In 1926, after the war and after leaving Vienna, where he felt unwelcomed, Bàràny was made Professor of Otolaryngology at Uppsala, and he remained at that institution until his retirement.

Bàràny's contributions included a definition of the pathophysiology of the human vestibular apparatus, the debridement and closure of war-induced head wounds, work on the thermal–labyrinthine reflex, and a definition of otoneurology and the relationship between the labyrinth and cerebellum (7).

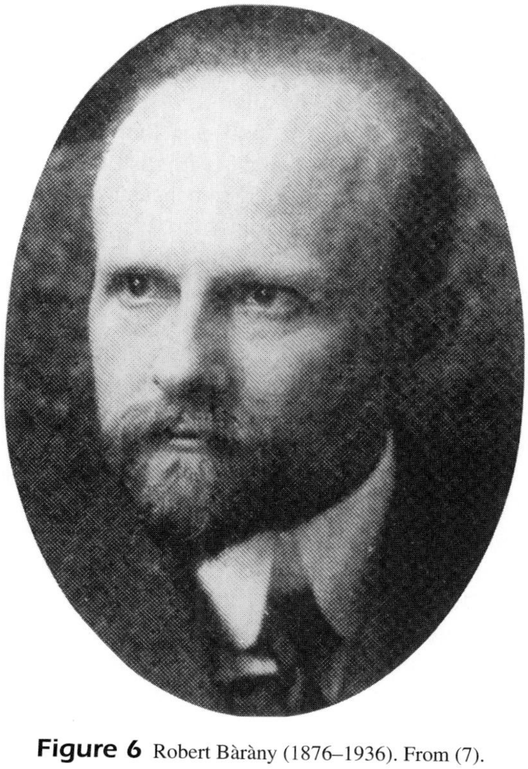

Figure 6 Robert Bàràny (1876–1936). From (7).

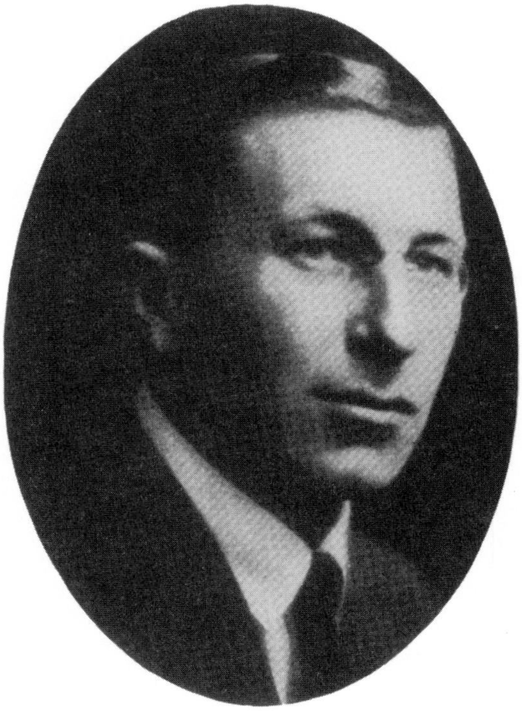

Figure 7 Frederick Grant Banting (1891–1941). From (7).

E. Frederick Grant Banting (1891–1941)

Banting (Fig. 7), born on a farm in Alliston, Ontario, was awarded the Nobel Prize in 1923 with John James Richard MacLeod "for the discovery of insulin." Banting received his medical doctorate degree at Victoria College in Toronto, Canada after first studying divinity at the University of Toronto. In World War I he served in the Royal Canadian Army alongside Clarence Starr, an English orthopedic surgeon who would inspire Banting to consider orthopedic surgery for his career. After a brief stent as a medical practitioner in London, Ontario, Banting began an orthopedic residency at the Hospital for Sick Children, Toronto. As a resident in orthopedics in 1921, Banting was given the opportunity to work on a summer project in the laboratory of J.J.R. MacLeod, Department of Physiology, University of Toronto. Because MacLeod was away for the summer, Banting enlisted the aid of a medical student, Charles H. Best, to participate in experiments of dog pancreatic duct ligation. These investigators then extracted "isletin" from the resected atrophic pancreas, and its administration cured the diabetic coma that was a product of animal pancreatectomy (Fig. 8) (12). These same investigators also isolated fetal bovine pancreatic preparations. When MacLeod returned at the end of the summer, he changed the name of the extracted material to "insulin." The following year, MacLeod invited J.B. Collip to isolate the extracted material from the duct-ligated pancreas. A 12-year-old diabetic patient at the Toronto General Hospital was successfully administered this extract for the treatment of diabetes and the restoration of euglycemia (13).

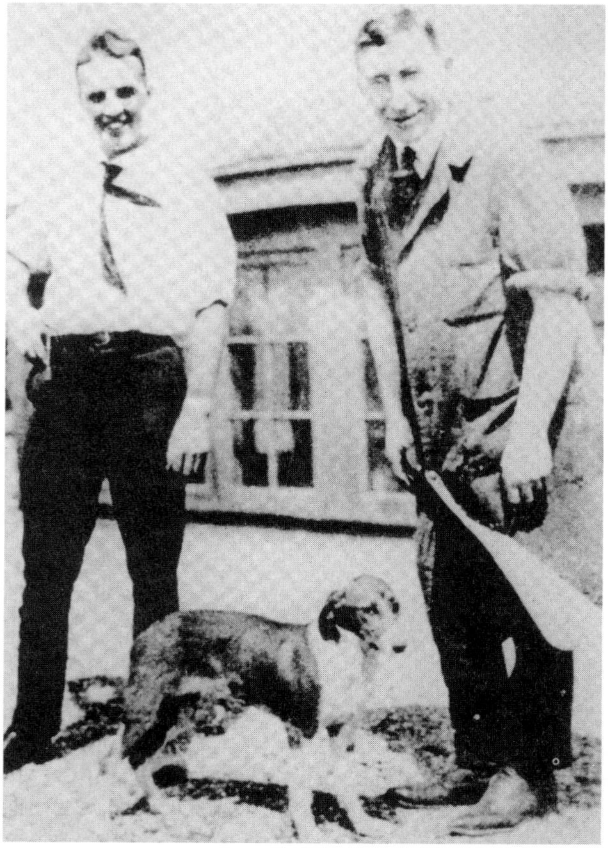

Figure 8 Charles Best (left) and Frederick Banting with a pancreatectomized dog treated with the pancreatic extract "isletin." From (14).

Although Banting is recognized for having made multiple medical advances, the awarding of the Nobel Prize for the discovery of insulin was perhaps the most controversial in history. At the heart of the controversy was the awarding of the prize to Banting and MacLeod, as opposed to the two initial investigators, Banting and Best (14). Furthermore, MacLeod was recognized and Collip was not. In reaction to this injustice neither Banting nor MacLeod was present at the award ceremony in Stockholm; also, Banting shared his award with Best, and MacLeod shared his prize money with Collip. A second aspect of the controversy was Banting's apparent lack of understanding of the work previously done by researchers in the field. In 1912, some 9 years before Banting's summer project, E.L.Scott wrote, "On the influence of intravenous injections of an extract of the pancreas on experimental pancreatic diabetes" a paper that served as his University of Chicago master's thesis. It is unclear whether Banting was aware of that work, or if so, whether he intentionally failed to acknowledge this previous contribution at the time of his discovery (15). Banting had been charged by MacLeod, among others, with neglecting to become more fully informed about previous research in his area of study. Perhaps a more justifiable recognition would have been Banting and Best credited for having produced the pancreatic hormone in a practical and available form utilized to treat diabetes. Banting died in a plane crash over Gander, Newfoundland in 1941, on his way to Europe to test the pressurized flying suit developed in the Banting Institute.

F. Walter Rudolf Hess (1881–1973)

Hess (Fig. 9) received the Nobel Prize in 1949 "for his discovery of the functional organization of the interbrain as a coordinator of the activities of the internal organs." Hess, an ophthalmologist, was born in Frauenfeld, Switzerland to a father who was a physics teacher. He received both his medical doctorate and his ophthalmologic training from the University of Zurich. After practicing ophthalmology, he trained in physiology at the University of Bonn, subsequently returning as Director of the Physiologic Institute, University of Zurich. Numerous Hess contributions included the hemodynamic influence of blood viscosity, the central regulation of respiration, the correlation of psychic and vegetative function, the anatomy and physiology of the diencephalon, brain electrode stimulation topography, and a description of the extrapyramidal system (7). He specifically demonstrated the regulatory role of the hypothalamus in controlling involuntary bodily processes such as blood pressure and heart rate.

G. Werner Theodor Otto Forssmann (1904–1979)

Forssmann (Fig. 10) won the Nobel Prize in 1956 with co-workers Andrè Frèdèric Cournand and Dickinson W. Richards "for their discoveries concerning heart catheterization and pathological changes in the circulatory system." Forssmann was born in Berlin and he was raised by his mother after his father was killed in World War I. He received his medical doctorate degree from the Friedrich-Wilhelms University in that city. He trained in surgery with Richard Schneider at Eberswalde in the Auguste-Viktoria Hospital, and he also trained at the Charite Hospital with Ferdinand Sauerbrach. He received additional training at the Rudolf Virchow Hospital. In 1929, as a 25-year-old first-year surgical resident, Forssmann went to his chairman, Schneider, and proposed an experiment on catheterization of the heart. Forssmann's purpose for the experiment was to identify a direct injection site access to the heart for drug delivery during resuscitation. Forssmann secured the assistance of Peter Romeis, and the two men chose a 35-mm catheter to be inserted through a needle into Forssmann's

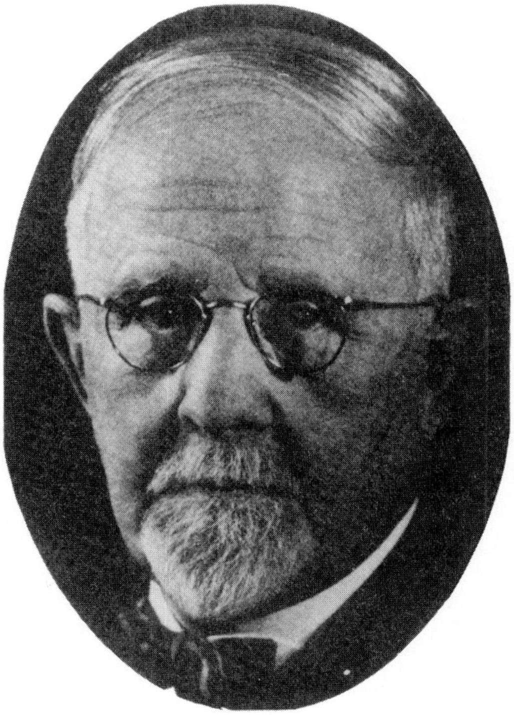

Figure 9 Walter Rudolf Hess (1881–1973). From (7).

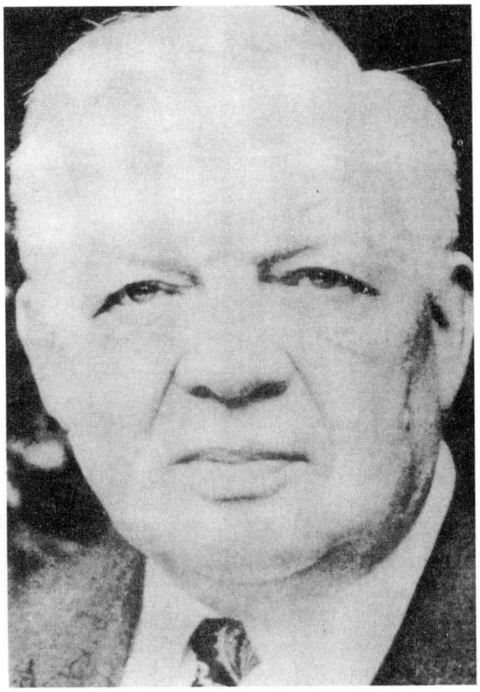

Figure 10 Werner Theodor Otto Forssmann (1904–1979). From (14).

antecubital space. Though Forssmann "knew" that the catheter had passed centrally, the inventors recognized that the catheter was too short to reach the heart, and it was consequently removed. On the following day, Forssmann decided to repeat the experiment on his opposite arm using a cutdown technique and a 65-cm-long catheter. He enlisted the help of a scrub nurse, Gerda Ditzen, but she became agitated when she realized that he would be doing self-experimentation. He therefore bound her and continued with the experiment on himself. Forssmann passed the catheter into his central circulation, walked to a fluoroscopy facility, and then confirmed with radiographic technique that the catheter was in his heart (Fig. 11) (16). He stated "I had the feeling of gentle warmth only during the sliding along the wall of the vein . . . I felt no effect when I injected it, only afterward a slight haziness, a disturbance of consciousness and vision which lasted only a second or two" (16). The experimental results were published in *Klinishce Wochenschrift*, a leading medical journal, and thereafter Forssmann received an appointment to work with Dr. Ferninand Sauerbrach, Germany's leading surgeon. Sauerbrach was heard to say, "You might lecture in a circus about your little tricks, but never in a respectable German university" (17), and Forssmann countered, "Herr Geheimrat Sauerbrach, there are hunters and there are shooters!" Forssman was promptly fired. After returning to work with Schneider and completing further experiments, Forssmann eventually tracked his surgical career to the field of urology. A prisoner of war in World War II, he eventually was released to practice urology in the Black Forest.

H. Charles B. Huggins (1901–1997)

In 1966, Huggins (Fig. 12) received the Nobel Prize "for his discoveries concerning hormonal treatment of prostate cancer," research findings that culminated many years of systematic research. Huggins, born in Halifax, Nova Scotia, was raised in austerity and pragmatism, and by age 18 both parents had died. He received his medical doctorate from the Harvard Medical School and his training in surgery from the University of Michigan. In 1927, though planning to be a community general surgeon, he was recruited to the University of Chicago by Dallas Phemister and appointed Chief of Urology, as the new faculty of the school of medicine was assembled. In 1936, Huggins was made professor of surgery, and in 1950 he was made Director of the Ben May Laboratory for Cancer Research.

Charles Huggins made contributions in both urologic endocrinology and basic laboratory techniques. In urology, he discovered that prostatic secretion is dependent on testicular androgen output, that competitive antagonism occurs between androgens and estrogens, that orchiectomy along with estrogens produces prostate cancer remission, that serum acid phosphatase can be utilized to monitor prostate cancer metastasis, and that adrenalectomy can be used for the therapy of both prostate and breast cancer (18). As a

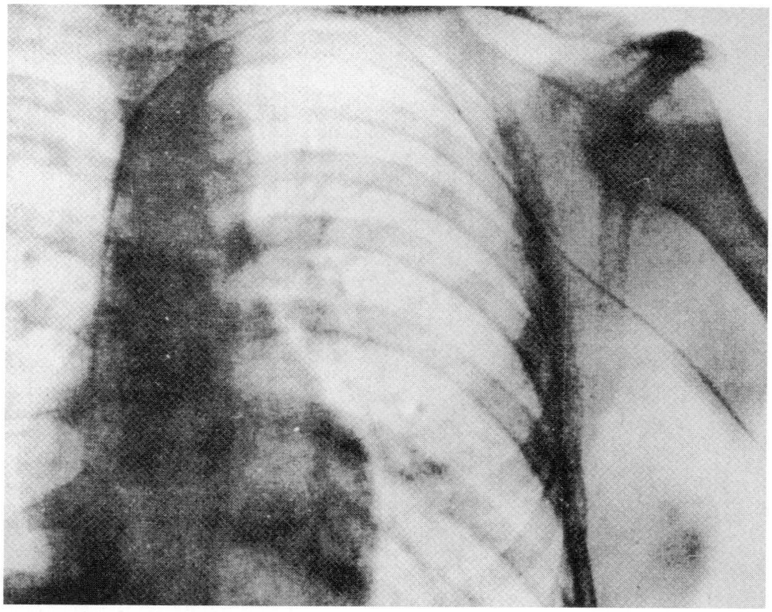

Figure 11 Radiograph depicting Forssmann's self-experimentation in which the catheter he inserted through a left antecubital vein cutdown has its tip in the right heart.

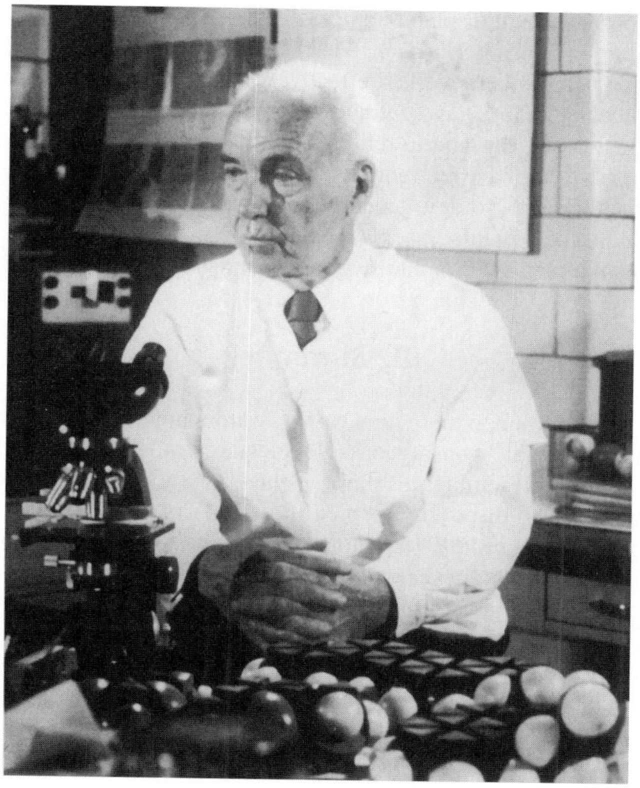

Figure 12 Charles Brenton Huggins (1901–1997). From (20).

result of these observations, Huggins found that certain malignant neoplasms were not autonomous but instead were sustained by normal existing endocrine functions.

The basic laboratory contributions of Huggins included the definition of chromogenic substrates to color enzymatic reactions, and the description of a 1,2-dimethylbenz[*a*]anthracene (DMBA)-induced animal model of breast cancer. Additionally, he defined bone-formation-inducing substances (19). For Huggins, "science is the art of the twentieth century" and "discovery is our business." He defined the basics of a successful research physician as the three Is: imagination, intelligence, and industry. His philosophy of science was most intriguing and included the following philosophic observations: "You practice at experimenting like you practice anything else" . . . "In science one always strives for simplicity which is the elegance of proof: *simplex sigillium veri*" . . . "Always use the carrot, never the stick" . . . "I never hire anyone who is not smarter than myself" . . . "The laboratory bench is the scientist's best friend" . . . "Work on a single scientific problem with a small group of students" . . . "The goal of science is not the acquisition of data . . . but the analysis of facts" . . . "Avoid administration, it attracts only inferior minds" (20). The enthusiasm that Huggins brought to his laboratory, his discovery, and to those around him was legendary. When describing his observations regarding prostate cancer and hormonal interactions, Huggins was quoted to have said, "I was excited, nervous, happy. That night I walked home—one mile—and I had to sit down two or three times, my heart was pounding so. I thought, 'this will benefit man forever' " (13).

I. Joseph E. Murray (1919–)

In 1990, along with E. Donnell Thomas, Joseph Murray (Fig. 13) was awarded the Nobel Prize for "discoveries concerning organ and cell transplantation in the treatment of human disease." Born in Milford, Massachusetts, his father was a lawyer and judge and his mother was a school teacher. Murray graduated from the College of the Holy Cross and then the Harvard Medical School, and he did his surgical training at the Peter Bent Brigham Hospital. After only 9 months as an intern, during World War II, he was assigned to the Valley Forge General Hospital on the service of James Barrett Brown, a plastic surgeon. There he cared for war wounds, burns, and other reconstructive cases and he became fascinated by the slow rejection of foreign skin grafts. Following the war he went to the Memorial Sloan Kettering Hospital in New York, as well as the New York Hospital, for further fellowship plastic surgical training. He

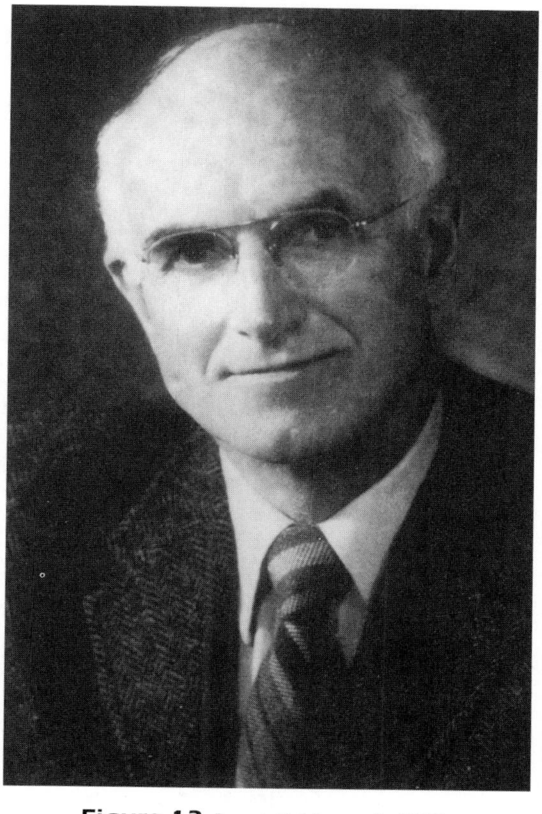

Figure 13 Joseph E. Murray (b. 1919).

then returned to Boston for his plastic surgery career, and his avocation became solid organ transplantation, an extension of the original skin grafting he did at Valley Forge. Many years of experimentation followed in which solid organ grafts were exchanged between animals.

In 1954, Murray and his colleagues did the first kidney transplant between identical twins utilizing the iliac fossa transplant technique (Fig. 14) (21). The transplant operation, which was an overwhelming technical success, demonstrated the genetic interchangeability of large vascular organs of many cell types. Five years later, a fraternal twin kidney transplant was performed, and to assure success, immunosuppression was done by whole body irradiation (22). To continue transplantation across greater barriers of incompatibility, in 1962, a cadaveric kidney transplant was done utilizing pharmacologic immunosuppression with azathioprine. These three sequential transplant donor–host combinations of identical twins, fraternal twins, and unrelated individuals provided the basis for the development of the field of solid organ transplantation and the development of pharmacologic immunosuppression (23). It was these accomplishments in kidney transplantation that resulted in Murray's recognition for the Nobel Prize. Not only did he define the technique of the operation and the role of immunosuppressive therapies, but the concept of the team approach to transplantation was established. The Brigham team of Murray, Harrison, Merrill, Hitchings, Elion, Calne, and many others worked effectively together to assure this success. Dr. Murray continues to be an active contributor to Boston surgery, and in reflection he has said that "my wish would be to have ten more lives to live on this planet—a life each for embryology, genetics, physics, astronomy, geology, and to be a pianist, backwoodsman, tennis player, National Geographic's writer and surgeon-scientist" (24).

III. Summary

In addition to these nine Nobel award winners, there have been several "nonsurgeon" Nobel laureates, including Sir Alexander Fleming, a fellow of the Royal College of Surgeons, who discovered penicillin in 1945. Another is Egas Moniz, who in 1949 (the same year the prize was awarded to Hess) won a Nobel Prize for "therapeutic leucotomy in psychoses," a surgical procedure, though Moniz was a neurologist. Finally, George von Bekesy, a Ph.D., an otolaryngology researcher, won the Nobel Prize in 1961 for defining cochlear function.

There have been 90 years of awards in the twentieth century (none awarded during war years), and 169 awardees

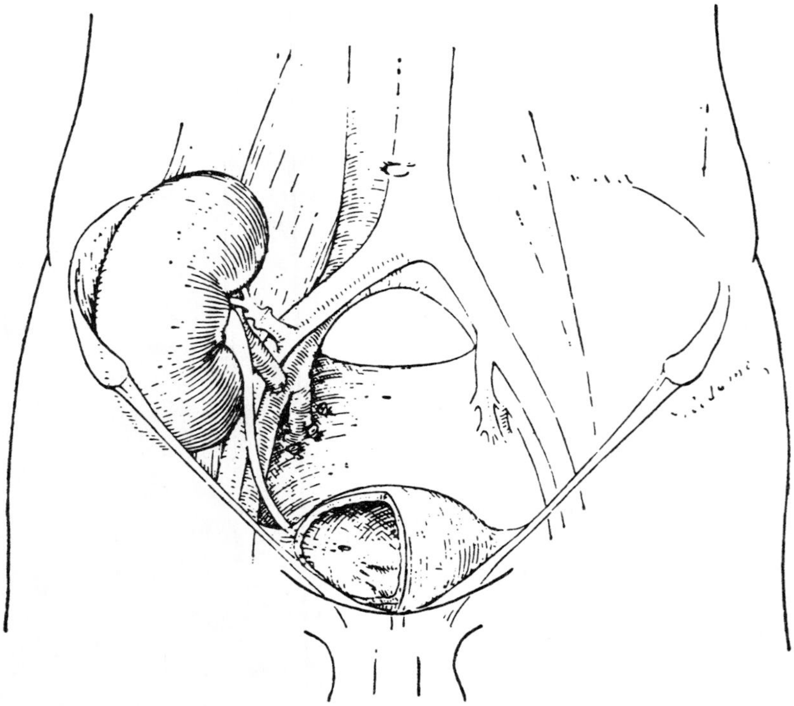

Figure 14 The transplantation technique utilized in the first successful human transplant revascularized the iliac fossa kidney with the iliac vessels. From (22), *Journal of the American Medical Association* **251,** 2566–2571. Copyrighted 1984, American Medical Association.

Table I Nobel Prizes in Physiology and Medicine—1901–1999

Awards[a]	Country
84	United States
24	Great Britain
16	Germany
9	France
6	Sweden
6	Switzerland
5	Denmark
4	Italy
3	Australia, Austria, Belgium
2	Argentina, Netherlands
1	Canada, Hungary, Japan, Luxembourg, Portugal, Romania, Scotland, Spain, USSR

[a]Some winners are represented both in their birth country and the country of their work.

were named through 1999, of which nine were surgeons. The Nobel Prize winners represent numerous nations, as summarized in Table I.

The Nobel Prize in Physiology or Medicine is the most prestigious award for a physician-scientist. The field of surgery is fortunate to have had nine distinguished individuals receive this recognition during the twentieth century. Their accomplishments have varied from clinical to scientific and from the technical to the theoretic. The recipients were most deserving of the recognition of the award; nevertheless, it remains unsettling that other remarkably gifted surgeons have not yet received such Nobel Prize recognition. Examples of such oversight include no winners in the field of cardiac surgery, despite its multiple advances; no recognition in the field of metabolism and nutrition along with the care of the critically ill; no recognition in the field of artifical organs; and no recognition, to date, in the field of angiogenesis and vascular biology.

References

1. Odelberg, W. (1972). "Nobel. The Man and His Prizes." American Elsevier Publishing Co. Inc., New York.
2. Brown, M. C. (1998). Historical background of the Nobel prize. Internet site: www.liblsu.edu/sci/chen/ guides/srs 118-history.htm.
3. McGreevy, P. S., and Miller, F. A. (1969). Biography of Theodor Kocher. *Surgery* **65,** 990–999.
4. Colcock, B. P. (1968). Lest we forget: A story of five surgeons. *Surgery* **64,** 1162–1172.
5. Roses, D. F. (1996). Profile: Theodor Kocher. *Tradit. Surg.* **2,** 2–11.
6. Rutkow, I. M. (1978). William Halsted and Theodor Kocher: An exquisite friendship. *Ann. Surg.* **188,** 630–637.
7. Swan, K. G., and Jain, K. M. (1981). Nobel prize winners in surgery. *Contem. Surg.* **9,** 93–109.
8. Moseley, J. (1980). Alexis Carrel, the man unknown, journey of an idea. *JAMA* **44,** 1119–1121.
9. Carrel, A. (1902). La technique operatoine des anastamoses vasculaires et la transplantation des visceres. *Lyon Med.* **1008,** 859–864.
10. Carrel, A. (1908). Results of the transplantation of blood vessels, organs and limbs. *JAMA* **51,** 1662–1667.
11. Malinin, T. I. (1996). Remembering Alexis Carrel and Charles A. Lindbergh. *Tex. Heart Inst. J.* **23,** 28–35.
12. Banting, G. F., and Best, C. H. (1992). The internal secretion of the pancreas. *J. Lab. Clin. Med.* **8,** 251–266.
13. Banting, G. F., Best, C. H., Collip, J. B., *et al.* (1922). Pancreas extracts in the treatment of diabetes mellitus: Preliminary report. *Can. Med. Assoc. J.* **12,** 141–146.
14. Morris, J. B., and Schirmer, W. J. (1990). The "right stuff": Five Nobel prize-winning surgeons. *Surgery* **108,** 71–80.
15. Hetenyi, G., Jr. (1998). Why can't we get it right? Notes on the discovery of insulin. *Ann. RCPSC* **31,** 237–239.
16. Forssmann, W. (1974). "Experiments on Myself. Memoirs of a Surgeon in Germany," pp. 102–108, St. Martin's Press, New York.
17. Forssman-Falck, R. (1997). Werner Fossmann: A pioneer of cardiology. *Am. J. Cardiol.* **79,** 651–660.
18. Huggins, C. B. (1963). The hormone dependent cancers. *JAMA* **186,** 481–483.
19. Talalay, P. (1965). The scientific contributions of Charles Brenton Huggins. *JAMA* **192,** 1137–1140.
20. Talalay, P. (1997). Charles Brenton Huggins. *Cancer Res.* **57,** cover legend.
21. Merrill, J. P., Murray, J. E., Harrison, J. H., and Guild, W. R. (1956). Successful homotransplantation of the human kidney between identical twins. *JAMA* **160,** 277–282.
22. Merrill, J. P., Murray, J. E., Harrison, J. H., *et al.* (1960). Successful homotransplantation of the kidney between non-identical twins. *N. Engl. J. Med.* **262,** 1251–1260.
23. Murray, J. E., Merril, J. P., Dammin, G. J., *et al.* (1962). Kidney transplantation in modified recipients. *Ann. Surg.* **156,** 337–355.
24. Murray, J. E. (1993). Nobel prize lecture: The first successful organ transplants in man. *In* "Nobel Lectures, Physiology or Medicine, 1981–1990" (T. Frängamy, and J. Lindsten, eds.), pp. 554–570. World Scientific Publishing Co., Singapore.

90

Surgical Education Research

Andreas H. Meier, Paul J. Gorman, and Thomas M. Krummel

Department of Surgery, Stanford University, Stanford, California 94043

I. Introduction

Most medical school faculty . . . are startlingly unaware of research in medical education and of curricular experiments under way at medical schools . . . they almost universally fail to recognize education as a respectable research discipline" (1).

Research on surgical education was formerly of little scientific interest (2); since the late 1980s, however, the number of publications on this topic has markedly increased. More than 800 papers were published over the past decade, compared to roughly 300 articles in the two decades before (3). This increased activity is correlated with recent changes in the American healthcare system, and the rapid expansion of minimally invasive technology. The percentage of papers presenting quantitative data, though, is still small.

Students, residents, and surgeons in practice are the target groups for surgical education (2). Due to rapid changes in both technology and the healthcare environment, optimal surgical education remains a moving target (4). This chapter provides an overview of surgical education and related research. It gives a brief outlook into the challenges and future of surgical education and contains a comprehensive bibliography.

II. Historical Perspective

Research in surgical education started when Billroth published his landmark analysis more than 120 years ago (5). He described the academic system in great detail and envisioned changes for the future. The book was a success with his students, but was criticized sharply by the establishment.

At the end of the nineteenth century the United States desperately needed to develop a large pool of medical practicioners. The focus was therefore more on quantity than quality, leading to a large number of medical schools, most of them substandard (6, 7). Thus, many American surgeons interested in an academic career sought training in Europe (8). Langenbeck, Billroth, and others had established their training programs on a scientific foundation. This concept was so appealing to Halsted that he introduced a similar system at Johns Hopkins University in Baltimore (9, 10).

The standard of training, however, remained poor. Growing concerns about the quality of education highlighted by Flexner in his analysis in 1910 (11) led to widespread activity to improve surgical and general medical training (6, 7). Scientific medical education became a primary focus for the first time (12). In 1912, the Committee on the Standardization of Surgery defined a "minimum standard of requirements . . . to perform independent operations" (6). Over the next 10 years, formal surgical education lengthened. The first approved surgical internships appeared in 1914 and the requirements to enter residency also became more stringent (13).

With the development of specialty examining boards in the 1930s and 40s (12), interest in the analysis of surgical education outcomes increased. In 1934, the Committee on Graduate Training for Surgery began to develop criteria for graduate surgical training (6). Evarts Graham stated that "residency training . . . should be distinctly educational rather than a means of supplying cheaply an assistant to the staff" (14). The foundation of the Residency Review Committee in 1955 marked a further step toward quality control of residency training by introducing an independent oversight committee and a feedback mechanism (10).

Many surgical specialties started to introduce in-service examinations in the 1960s and 1970s to measure the effectiveness of educational programs (7). The results of these exams have been used as a research tool in multiple studies (15). With the establishment of the Liaison Committee in Graduate Medical Education in 1972 and the Association for Surgical Education in 1981, further oversight of the undergraduate and graduate surgical education process materialized. In 1986, the University of Michigan published a comprehensive review on education in surgery (16). With the advent of minimally invasive surgery a few years later and rapid structural and financial change within the American healthcare system, traditional education in surgery has been increasingly scrutinized. Radical changes in the "see one, do one, teach one" methodology of surgical education has been proposed by integrating skill laboratories and surgical trainers into the curriculum (17). Research on surgical education today focuses on evaluating the efficacy and validity of traditional and new teaching methods.

III. Principles, Goals, Variables, Outcomes

Thoughtful research on any subject requires the investigator to characterize goals, identify outcome measures, and define assessable variables. Thus, designing research projects in education can be daunting. Results are commonly open for controversial interpretation, and meaningful outcome analysis frequently requires longitudinal studies that tend to be labor intensive and difficult to design. It is not trivial, and sometimes impossible, to apply probability values to potentially meaningful results (18). Many of the utilized research tools can be criticized for subjectivity, making validation of results difficult. Assessment is easy, but good assessment is not (19)! The analysis of the frequently complex data is time consuming (20).

A. Surgical Education Research Goals

Scientific analysis of surgical education is necessary in order to evaluate the existing training methodologies or to introduce new methods and validate them. Studies have uncovered significant problems with current curricula. These include the lack of continuity from undergraduate to graduate surgical training (21) and lack of supervision when aquiring physical examination skills (22), ultimately resulting in poor performance (23, 24). Suggestions for curricular changes within clerkships and residency programs have been made. Sachdeva and colleagues adjusted the surgical clerkship at Hahnemann, increasing the student's exposure to basic surgical principles (25). Jacobsen proposed a residency program with increased focus on problem-solving skills (26). Recent publications have shown that learning from such analysis and adjusting the training accordingly improves overall performance (27). The economic and organizational challenges present in contemporary medicine have raised concern about the current surgical curriculum (28). Plans for solutions differ widely (29, 30); there is no "gold standard" for surgical education. Further confounding is the disparate group of students who enter residency (21). Another goal is to develop valid methods for applicant screening prior to residency; despite many attempts this search has so far been unsuccessful (31).

B. Variables and Assessment

The definition of variables that can be measured objectively to provide valid and reliable results for surgical education is difficult. Given the complexity of surgical expertise, most isolated variables represent only a very small aspect of the overall picture. However, overall, most agree that the three core areas of surgical competencies are knowledge, operative and technical abilities, and cognitive skills.

1. Knowledge Skills

Assessment of knowledge has been accomplished by evaluating various exam scores (Scholastic Aptitude Test, United States Medical Licensing Exam, American Board of Surgery In-Training Exam, Qualifying Exam). These measures are reliable evaluators of factual knowledge, but their validity regarding overall surgical performance is questionable (32). Oral examinations can validly assess knowledge, but their potential for subjectivity makes them less reliable.

2. Operative Skills

Evaluating operative proficiency remains a challenging task. Psychomotor and dexterity skill testing alone does not correlate well with performance in the operating room (33–35). The best correlation has been established for visuospatial abilities and stress tolerance (36–38). Psychological testing may therefore have some predictive validity for future surgical skills (32, 39). Another valid tool is direct observation of technical skills in the operating room using predefined criteria based on a Likert scale rating (19, 39). Other attempts have been made to develop scoring systems. Recently, the Objective Structured Assessment of Technical Skills (OSATS) score was found to be valid and reliable for senior residents, but less useful for junior housestaff (40, 41). The Structured Technical Skills Assessment Form (STSAF) has demonstrated interrater and construct validity (20). However, at this point we still have not identified a valid, reliable, and sensitive measuring system that is easily administered, allows preemptive evaluation of residency candidates, and analysis of the residents' progress throughout their training.

3. Cognitive Skills

Cognitive abilities are integrative functions and are needed to develop expertise managing patients. Aquiring these skills during residency is necessary for sound surgical judgment. Traditionally, these skills have been analyzed by faculty using performance reviews during clinical rotations. The rating systems have varied significantly. It appears that giving grades is more reliable than a pure pass–fail system (42); a descriptive review with four to five categories seems preferable (43). These evaluations are usually not well suited for research, because they are usually poorly controlled and can be influenced by multiple unrelated factors. Improved reliability can be achieved when the faculty consistently use stringent ranking criteria (44, 45).

Attempts have been made to rate cognitive skills by introducing the Objective Standardized Clinical Exam (OSCE) (21, 46, 47). This approach has shown high reliability and validity (20, 47–50). Some studies have suggested that the OSCE may be useful to predict future resident's performance (51). The disadvantages of this method are its significant costs, logistical demands, and the need for significant faculty time commitment (52). Other investigators developed the Structured Single-Observer Method (SSOM). The scoring system measures patient management skills as well as technical capabilities. In comparison to the traditional observation method, the SSOM showed higher precision and sensitivity, and has correlated well with oral and multiple-choice examinations (53).

Physiologic patient simulation has already been used successfully in anesthesia training programs (54). These simulators allow the teaching and testing of team management skills in crisis situations. Initial results using these simulators within surgery have been published (55). Further investigations will evaluate their potential for surgical resident training and testing.

Although often forgotten, development of interpersonal and communication skills is essential for patient care, effective leadership, and team management. Efforts have been made to measure these skills with checklists (56). Despite ongoing attempts to improve the scientific analysis of surgical education, it is almost certain that some aspects of surgical excellence will remain unmeasured in the near term. As stated by Gardner (57), "Everybody knows that there are other powerful ingredients in successful performance—attitudes, values, motives, non-academic talents—but we have no reliable way of measuring these other ingredients."

C. Outcome Measures

The aim of surgical education research is to optimize surgical training. The question remains: how is optimal surgical training defined, and what does it include? Although this has been the subject of many presidential addresses, no clear answer exists. Surgical excellence contains so many facets that defining meaningful outcome measures remains challenging. Three major target groups need to be considered for outcome measures: medical students, surgical residents, and practicing surgeons; the objectives differ for each of these groups.

1. Medical Students

The surgical core clerkship needs to provide a knowledge base in basic surgical principles, including shock, trauma, nutrition, and sepsis (58). Students should acquire the skill set for basic clinical reasoning (59) and learn to recognize surgical disease processes. Because most students will not pursue a surgical career, it is also important to lay the groundwork for future collegial relationships (60) by helping the students understand basic surgical thinking. The clerkship should teach the ability to combine knowledge and patient information to formulate a strategy for evaluation and management, the foundation for judgment (22). Role modeling, mentoring, and encouragement during the clerkship are essential for students interested in a future career in surgery.

2. Surgical Residents

Optimal surgical education for residents produces technically adept surgeons and caring physicians (61). It provides a sound foundation in basic science (62), allows the trainees to develop communication and management skills (63) and clear thinking and compassionate understanding (26), and encourages the development of leadership and decisiveness (64). The program structure should allow graded responsibility (9). Because a significant aspect of the resident's and future surgeon's activity is spent teaching others, including patients (65, 66), it is important that the training generate future educators and role models (12, 67). In addition, some form of research experience is deemed crucial by most academic programs (13, 68). Finally, residents need to be prepared for the challenging economics of healthcare (62). The best outcome would be a "skilled, safe, technically adept surgeon with keen judgment, dedicated to welfare of the patient" (69).

3. Practicing Surgeons and Educators

The ongoing reeducation of surgeons in practice focuses on assimilation of new medical knowledge and the development of skills in new surgical techniques. Interest in this area has markedly increased since the impact of minimally invasive surgery and our collective inability of effectively teaching it in a timely fashion. Rapidly expanding technology, such as stereotactic breast biopsy or ultrasound evaluation, makes it difficult to provide the necessary continuing education through the traditional continuing medical education (CME) programs. There has been significant effort recently to optimize knowledge delivery utilizing modern information technology. The American College of Surgeons has taken a leadership role, with "hands-on" courses and thoughtful assessment.

Effective surgical educators act as mentors and role models; they should demonstrate enthusiasm and knowledge, allow involvement of the learner in the teaching process, all the while presenting a humanistic orientation (26, 27, 29, 64). Many surgeons trace their career selection to one or two key surgical teachers, whom they consider their main mentors or role models. Our responsibility to the next generation is clear and our commitment cannot waver.

IV. Results of Research in Surgical Education

A. Structuring Surgical Education

Surgeons have always acquired most of their operative and judgment skills through "learning by doing" (70). Due to the nature of surgical practice, this will remain the cornerstone of our education. Studies analyzing learning style preferences of surgical residents show that most of them favor a problem-solving and hands-on approach (71, 72), which may partly explain why this form of teaching has been so successful. However, the validity of these studies remains controversial. The theoretical analysis of the learning process is still in evolution (73).

The "learning by doing" approach *a priori* fails to provide skill acquisition in an organized fashion. Such teaching occurs based on the random opportunity, of patient flow through the office, clinic, emergency room, and operating room. This results in significant variability of educational content provided to the trainees, and precludes any organized curriculum.

Objectives and curricula for medical students and residents in surgical training have been created (74–76). It is crucial that this development process includes residents and students as well as educators. Curricular concerns of the trainees and their feedback regarding changes can then be integrated (77, 78). Such feedback mechanisms are well documented to increase the educational impact of the curriculum (18, 24, 79).

B. Cognitive Aspects

Over the past two decades, educational research has attempted to define the important aspects of adult learning. Adults usually act as self-directed, internally motivated, and experienced students who have a need to know and are attracted to the area of their studies (80). Traditional medical training, however, is rigidly structured, lecture-based, and focuses on memorizing facts. There is little room for self-directed education. Therefore, many medical schools have begun to change their curricula and have introduced principles of problem-based learning (81). Within the past 10 years, these methods have been integrated into surgical education (82). Studies have shown that problem-oriented small groups may perform better compared to lecture-based groups, especially when asked to solve clinical problems (83, 84). Students appear more motivated during the courses (85). It remains to be seen whether this approach actually results in better knowledge transfer (82). The previously mentioned OSCE model has shown promising results. It has been implemented into licensing examinations for family medicine abroad (86, 87), and there are plans underway to integrate the OSCE format into the United States Medical Licensing Exam (USMLE) (88). It still lacks widespread use today, however, due to its high demand on faculty resources.

Over the past years many medical schools have begun to utilize computers in problem-based learning, thereby decreasing the required faculty time. Results with this approach have been promising (89, 90). Studies in other specialties have shown that developing and measuring problem-solving skills with a computerized decision analysis model is feasible (91).

C. Assessing Knowledge

The means to assess knowledge transfer remain quite controversial (78). Oral examinations validly analyze reasoning skills and knowledge base, but have been criticized for possible subjectivity. Multiple-choice tests [e.g., the

American Board of Surgery In-Training Exam (ABSITE)] are objective, and assess recall of knowledge well. Their scores correlate with successful ABS certification (92) and faculty assessments of residents (93). ABSITE analysis serves as a useful tool to validate residency education (15). This form of assessment can also be made available online through computers, which may increase its usefulness by providing immediate scores and feedback (94).

The correlation between knowledge recall and its application in surgical judgment remains controversial. The latter proves to be much more relevant for the development of sound patient management skills. Some groups have thus attempted to create assessment tools to measure application practices directly (95, 96).

D. Teaching and Assessing Surgical Skills

One of the main areas of surgical education research deals with development of surgical technique and its valid assessment. Though an essential portion of surgical practice, most of the instruction occurs by fairly unstructured operating room exposure. In many programs, this hands-on experience excludes the more junior housestaff. Faculty evaluations rarely provide constructive feedback. Ideally, the exposure to operative practice should commence at an early training level in a curricular fashion that allows the breakdown of tasks into simple steps (29). Flexibility of time for this skill training may also be helpful (12). These prerequisites cannot be fulfilled in today's operating rooms. Accurate assessment of the resident's progress poses another significant challenge. Surgical skills training in animal labs has been used successfully for decades (97, 98). The significant amount of faculty time necessary to provide this training, and the increasing critisism from animal rights advocates, does make this approach problematic.

Surgical skills laboratories were first introduced with simple tie and suture boards and pig skin suturing models in the 1960s (99, 100). Multiple tools and materials have since been used (41, 98, 101–103). Introduction of organ perfusion models has allowed operative practice and provides the means to simulate intraoperative complications (17). All these skills laboratories should provide a curriculum and feedback to be effective (104). The overall validity of skills laboratory training has been addressed by Anastakis *et al.* (105), and its increased use has been recommended by others (28).

The need for practicing surgeons to learn minimally invasive techniques has led to a multitude of workshops and training facilities over the past decade. Great efforts have been made to allow gradual learning of the new skills by breaking down complex tasks into simpler ones (106). Another area of interest is the improvement of surgical education within the OR. The use of videotapes followed by debriefing has been successful (19). This method provides good feedback, but again requires significant faculty time. Computer editing technology may make this approach more efficient (107).

The newest addition to surgical skills education has been the development of virtual reality (VR) simulators. The concept of simulating tasks prior to performing them has been integrated into pilot and military education for many years, and has been shown to decrease risks and costs. VR simulation has been appealing to surgeons as well (19), but due to the complexity of human anatomy and problems of interacting directly with computer-generated images, these types of simulators were not available for surgery until the late 1980s. Initially funded by the military to simulate orthopedic injuries, the quality and quantity of these devices have markedly increased (108–111). These devices allow the simulation of tasks on tissues created by high-end graphics workstations. The manipulation is performed through haptic interfaces, thus allowing very precise analysis of the trainee's performance. For the first time, objective data regarding motion, tissue tear forces, precision, and error rates can be acquired and then compiled into a "surgical reportcard" (111, 112).

E. Educating the Educators

Surgeons have educated their colleagues as long as the profession has existed. The educational quality has been dependent on the personal interest and natural skills of the teaching surgeon. Educational research has increased our knowledge in the theory of adult learning. The American College of Surgeons has shown significant interest in implementing this knowledge by providing guidelines for surgical educators. Interested individuals have had the opportunity to participate in various faculty development workshops; the ACS also sponsors a week-long course for surgeons as educators (66, 75, 113).

V. Challenges for Surgical Education in the Future

Medical education has been affected by several technological and financial developments within the healthcare system over the past 10 years. The rapidly evolving technology and knowledge challenged traditional educational concepts (6, 61, 114, 115). The explosion of healthcare costs (62, 70, 116, 117), followed by decreasing Medicare support for medical education (118, 119) has resulted in significant hardship for surgical training. Time in the operating room, the traditional learning ground for surgical residents, has become more precious and costly (19). One study has projected that approximately $53 million per year is spent on additional operating room time in resident teaching (120), most likely a very moderate estimate.

These economic changes have secondary effects as well. Shorter inpatient stays have diminished the traditional learning resources (59, 90). Surgical residents take care of higher acuity in-patients (121), which decreases time for formal teaching (12) and hinders the educational process (9). The educators have been affected as well. Junior faculty members face increasing research requirements to pursue a successful academic career, leaving less time for teaching (58). The lack of faculty supervision has negative impact on student development (22). Surveys have shown that faculty members are aware of these shortfalls (53). The fear of liability and malpractice litigation has also put significant restraints on teaching in the operating room (19, 122).

These changes will continue to impact surgical practice and education. Most likely the situation will continue to worsen. These challenges, however, also create the opportunity to look beyond our current educational models and integrate the increasing knowledge on adult learning with modern information technology. This will allow us to develop the teaching tools for the future and to reinvent surgical education, in a process similar to Billroth's over 100 years ago.

VI. Future Research Opportunities

Further improvement of surgical curricula will require the integration of new teaching modalities (114, 123). The World-Wide Web permits ubiquitous, easily accessible, customizable and potentially interactive information in real time. The Internet is thereby an ideal medium for self-education (124). Its capabilities will continuously increase for years to come. Although we are still at the beginning of this development, the potential for its use in surgical education can already be seen today (125). Statistics for web site access as well as information about user profiles and preferences can be obtained easily. These data are available for research projects, and provide rapid feedback to the educators. The information can then be used to further improve the web-based curriculum. This technology can also be used very effectively for CME programs. Basic familiarity with information technology will be a necessity for the surgeons of the future (126).

The Internet also provides a means of communication for educators and trainees over long distances. Telementoring and teleteaching have become a possibility (127, 128), but their feasibility will require further studies. The continuing increase of computing power will make VR simulators more realistic and applicable for training purposes. Although the initial validation studies have been promising (112), more research is necessary. Eventually, these devices may be used for selection, training, and credentialing (129, 130).

Educational research has been unable so far to define valid predictive parameters for a successful surgical career. A study by Gilligan *et al.* demonstrated significant differences of personality traits of surgical residents and residents in other specialties, but it remains unclear whether these findings have any predictive value (131). Psychologists have successfully used the Strategic Management Simulation to test executive-level competencies in nonmedical professions. This method simulates a well-controlled, real-world-like environment, and allows for reliable and valid analysis of complex functioning (132). Preliminary data using this method with surgical residents revealed good correlation with faculty assessment. Although promising, further research will be necessary to analyze whether this method could aid in the selection of surgical residents.

VII. Conclusion

The challenges facing healthcare require us to rethink all aspects of surgical education. Even though the operating room remains a central part of the training, other teaching arenas will supplement its use. The methods of surgical education are changing rapidly. In 1986 Bartlett stated that "there is no simulator for the patient" (16). However, surgical simulation is now beginning to play a role in surgical residency programs. With increasing computer speed and ongoing bandwidth explosion, web-based education will become commonplace. Scientific evaluation of these new. methods is necessary for validation and improvement.

Surgical education in the United States is still considered one of the best in the world (9, 10). Creative approaches to improve our training will be necessary to keep it that way. There is evidence that programs that dedicate research efforts to educational issues successfully attract superior candidates (133). Research in surgical education will therefore be more important than ever before.

References

1. Rogers, D. E. (1989). Clinical education and the doctor of tomorrow: An agenda for action. *In* "Clinical Education and the Doctor of Tomorrow" (B. Gastel and D. E. Rogers, eds.), pp. 109–113. The New York Academy of Medicine, New York.
2. Greenburg, A. G. (1986). The study of surgical education. *In* "Medical Education—A Surgical Perspective" (R. H. Bartlett, G. B. Zelenock, *et al.*, eds.), pp. 411–419. Lewis Publishers Inc, Chelsea, MI.
3. Calhoun, J. G., Ten Haken, J. D., DaRosa, D., and Zelenock, G. B. (1986). Bibliography of publications in surgical education: 1964–1984. *In* "Medical Education—A Surgical Perspective" (R. H. Bartlett and W. E. Strodel, *et al.*, eds.), pp. 507–523. Lewis Publishers Inc, Chelsea, MI.
4. Schwartz, S. I. (1999). The evolution of medical education. *Surgery* **125**(1), 17–18.

5. Billroth, T. (1876). "Über das Lehren und Lernen der medicinischen Wissenschaften an den Universitäten der deutschen Nation nebst allgemeinen Bemerkungen über Universitäten; eine culturhistorische Studie." C. Gerold, Wien.
6. Sawyers, J. L. (1981). Presidential address. Graduate surgical education. *Am. Surg.* **47**(1), 1–5.
7. Larson, C. B. (1971). History and organization of the traditional orthopaedic residency. *Clin. Orthop.* **75**(1–3), 17–21.
8. Rutkow, I. M., and Hempel, K. (1988). An experiment in surgical education—The first international exchange of residents. The letters of Halsted, Küttner, Heuer, and Landois. *Arch. Surg.* **123**(1), 115–121.
9. Walt, A. J. (1994). The uniqueness of American surgical education and its preservation. *Bull. Am. Coll. Surg.* **79**(12), 8–20.
10. Grillo, H. C. (1999). To impart this art: The development of graduate surgical education in the United States. *Surgery* **125**(1), 1–14.
11. Flexner, A. (1910). "Medical Education in the United States and Canada." Carnegie Foundation, New York.
12. Griffen, W. O., Jr. (1980). Surgical residency: On-the-job training or education? *Am. J. Surg.* **140**(6), 720–723.
13. Folse, R. (1986). Conflicts in accreditation of postgraduate surgical education. *Curr. Surg.* **43**(5), 368–372.
14. Graham, E. A. (1938). Graduate training for surgery from the viewpoint of the American Board of Surgery. *Bull. Am. Coll. Surg.* **23**, 33–34.
15. DaRosa, D. A., Shuck, J. M., Biester, T. W., and Folse, R. (1993). What does the American Board of Surgery In-Training/Surgical Basic Science Examination tell us about graduate surgical education? *Surgery* **113**(1), 8–13.
16. Bartlett, R. H., and University of Michigan, Dept. of Surgery, Section of General Surgery (1986). "Medical Education: A surgical Perspective." Lewis Publishers, Chelsea, MI.
17. Gorey, T. F. (1997). Training in minimally invasive therapy and its impact on traditional surgical education [editorial]. *Ir. J. Med. Sci.* **166**(1), 1–2.
18. Schirmer, W. J., Galat, J. A., Morris, J. B., *et al.* (1991). The impact of a resident-directed survey on the education curriculum of a university surgical training program. *Surgery* **110**(2), 405–410.
19. Reznick, R. K. (1993). Teaching and testing technical skills. *Am. J. Surg.* **165**(3), 358–361.
20. Winckel, C. P., Reznick, R. K., Cohen, R., and Taylor, B. (1994). Reliability and construct validity of a structured technical skills assessment form. *Am. J. Surg.* **167**(4), 423–427.
21. Sachdeva, A. K., Loiacono, L. A., Amiel, G. E., *et al.* (1995). Variability in the clinical skills of residents entering training programs in surgery. *Surgery* **118**(2), 300–308; discussion, 308–309.
22. York, N. L., Niehaus, A. H., Markwell, S. J., and Folse, J. R. (1999). Evaluation of students' physical examination skills during their surgery clerkship. *Am. J. Surg.* **177**(3), 240–243.
23. Endean, E. D., Sloan, D. A., Veldenz, H. C., *et al.* (1994). Performance of the vascular physical examination by residents and medical students. *J. Vasc. Surg.* **19**(1), 149–154; discussion, 155–146.
24. Chalabian, J., Garman, K., Wallace, P., and Dunnington, G. (1996). Clinical breast evaluation skills of house officers and students. *Am. Surg.* **62**(10), 840–845.
25. Sachdeva, A. K., Blair, P. G., Kelliher, G. J., *et al.* (1999). Redesigning the surgery clerkship at MCP Hahnemann School of Medicine to address the educational needs of generalists. *Acad. Med.* **74**(1 Suppl.), S98–S101.
26. Jacobsen, D. C. (1980). The pursuit of excellence in graduate surgical education. Visions of the Arizona experience. *Am. J. Surg.* **139**(5), 673–676.
27. Blue, A. V., Griffith, C. H., 3rd, Wilson, J., *et al.* (1999). Surgical teaching quality makes a difference. *Am. J. Surg.* **177**(1), 86–89.
28. Weigelt, J., Brasel, K., Olson, C., and Thal, E. (1998). Opinions of practicing general surgeons on surgical education. *Am. J. Surg.* **176**(5), 481–485.
29. Barnes, R. W. (1987). Surgical handicraft: Teaching and learning surgical skills. *Am. J. Surg.* **153**(5), 422–427.
30. Pories, W. J., Smout, J. C., Morris, A., and Lewkow, V. E. (1994). U.S. health care reform: Will it change postgraduate surgical education? *World J. Surg.* **18**(5), 745–752.
31. Papp, K. K., Polk, H. C., Jr., and Richardson, J. D. (1997). The relationship between criteria used to select residents and performance during residency. *Am. J. Surg.* **173**(4), 326–329.
32. Schueneman, A. L., Pickleman, J., and Freeark, R. J. (1985). Age, gender, lateral dominance, and prediction of operative skill among general surgery residents. *Surgery* **98**(3), 506–515.
33. Harris, C. J., Herbert, M., and Steele, R. J. (1994). Psychomotor skills of surgical trainees compared with those of different medical specialists. *Br. J. Surg.* **81**(3), 382–383.
34. Watson, D. C., and Matthews, H. R. (1987). Manual skills of trainee surgeons. *J. R. Coll. Surg. Edinb.* **32**(2), 74–75.
35. Squire, D., Giachino, A. A., Profitt, A. W., and Heaney, C. (1989). Objective comparison of manual dexterity in physicians and surgeons. *Can. J. Surg.* **32**(6), 467–470.
36. Gibbons, R. D., Baker, R. J., and Skinner, D. B. (1986). Field articulation testing: A predictor of technical skills in surgical residents. *J. Surg. Res.* **41**(1), 53–57.
37. Steele, R. J., Walder, C., and Herbert, M. (1992). Psychomotor testing and the ability to perform an anastomosis in junior surgical trainees. *Br. J. Surg.* **79**(10), 1065–1067.
38. DesCôteaux, J. G., and Leclère, H. (1995). Learning surgical technical skills. *Can. J. Surg.* **38**(1), 33–38.
39. Schueneman, A. L., Pickleman, J., Hesslein, R., and Freeark, R. J. (1984). Neuropsychologic predictors of operative skill among general surgery residents. *Surgery* **96**(2), 288–295.
40. Faulkner, H., Regehr, G., Martin, J., and Reznick, R. (1996). Validation of an objective structured assessment of technical skill for surgical residents. *Acad. Med.* **71**(12), 1363–1365.
41. Martin, J. A., Regehr, G., Reznick, R., *et al.* (1997). Objective structured assessment of technical skill (OSATS) for surgical residents. *Br. J. Surg.* **84**(2), 273–278.
42. Moss, T. J., Deland, E. C., and Maloney, J. V., Jr. (1978). Selection of medical students for graduate training: Pass/fail versus grades. *N. Engl. J. Med.* **299**(1), 25–27.
43. Ravelli, C., and Wolfson, P. (1999). What is the "ideal" grading system for the junior surgery clerkship? *Am. J. Surg.* **177**(2), 140–144.
44. Curtis, D. J., Amis, E. S., Jr., Cruess, D. F., and Riordan, D. D. (1985). Ranking: A reproducible semiobjective means of evaluating overall resident performance. *Invest. Radiol.* **20**(7), 757–758.
45. Curtis, D. J., Cruess, D. F., Riordan, D. D., and Allman, R. M. (1988). Ranking: A year three follow-up in a different institution. *Invest. Radiol.* **23**(7), 541–544.
46. Harden, R. M., Stevenson, M., Downie, W. W., and Wilson, G. M. (1975). Assessment of clinical competence using objective structured examination. *Br. Med. J.* **1**(5955), 447–451.
47. Sloan, D. A., Donnelly, M. B., Johnson, S. B., *et al.* (1993). Use of an Objective Structured Clinical Examination (OSCE) to measure improvement in clinical competence during the surgical internship. *Surgery* **114**(2), 343–350; discussion, 350–341.
48. Sloan, D. A., Donnelly, M. B., Schwartz, R. W., and Strodel, W. E. (1995). The Objective Structured Clinical Examination. The new gold standard for evaluating postgraduate clinical performance. *Ann. Surg.* **222**(6), 735–742.
49. Schwartz, R. W., Witzke, D. B., Donnelly, M. B., *et al.* (1998). Assessing residents' clinical performance: Cumulative results of a four-year study with the Objective Structured Clinical Examination. *Surgery* **124**(2), 307–312.
50. Cohen, R., Reznick, R. K., Taylor, B. R., *et al.* (1990). Reliability and validity of the objective structured clinical examination in assessing surgical residents. *Am. J. Surg.* **160**(3), 302–305.

51. Rutala, P. J., Fulginiti, J. V., McGeagh, A. M., *et al.* (1992). Predictive validity of a required multidisciplinary standardized-patient examination. *Acad. Med.* **67**(10 Suppl.), S60–S62.
52. Shatzer, J. H., Darosa, D., Colliver, J. A., and Barkmeier, L. (1993). Station-length requirements for reliable performance-based examination scores. *Acad. Med.* **68**(3), 224–229.
53. Dunnington, G., Reisner, L., Witzke, D., and Fulginiti, J. (1990). Structured single-observer methods of evaluation for the assessment of ward performance on the surgical clerkship. *Am. J. Surg.* **159**(4), 423–426.
54. Holzman, R. S., Cooper, J. B., Gaba, D. M., *et al.* (1995). Anesthesia crisis resource management: Real-life simulation training in operating room crises. *J. Clin. Anesth.* **7**(8), 675–687.
55. McLellan, B. A. (1999). Early experience with simulated trauma resuscitation. *Can. J. Surg.* **42**(3), 205–210.
56. Reisner, E., Dunnington, G., Beard, J., *et al.* (1991). A model for the assessment of students' physician-patient interaction skills on the surgical clerkship. *Am. J. Surg.* **162**(3), 271–273.
57. Gardner, J. (1962). "Excellence: Can We Be Equal and Excellent too." Harper Colophon Books, New York.
58. Pelletier, M. P. (1995). Undergraduate surgical education in the twenty-first century. *Can. J. Surg.* **38**(1), 42–44.
59. Provan, J. L. (1995). Surgical education: time for a change? [editorial; comment]. *Can. J. Surg.* **38**(1), 8–9.
60. Smoot, E. C. D., and DaRosa, D. (1993). Effective teaching in the operating room [editorial]. *Plast. Reconstr. Surg.* **92**(1), 133–135.
61. Aufses, A. H., Jr. (1989). Residency training programs then and now: Surgery. *Mt. Sinai J. Med.* **56**(5), 367–369.
62. Ritchie, W. P., Jr. (1997). Graduate surgical education in the era of managed care: A Statement from the American Board of Surgery [editorial]. *J. Am. Coll. Surg.* **184**(3), 311–312.
63. Rocmans, P. (1994). Surgical education revisited: Introduction. *Acta Chir. Belg.* **94**(3), 153–154.
64. Hermann, R. E. (1990). Role models in the education of surgeons. *Am. J. Surg.* **159**(1), 2–7.
65. Seely, A. J., Pelletier, M. P., Snell, L. S., and Trudel, J. L. (1999). Do surgical residents rated as better teachers perform better on in-training examinations? *Am. J. Surg.* **177**(1), 33–37.
66. Folse, R. (1993). Surgeons as educators—College aims to improve teaching skills. *ACS Bull.* (March 1993), 31–33.
67. Ko, C. Y., Whang, E. E., Karamanoukian, R., *et al.* (1998). What is the best method of surgical training?: A report of America's leading senior surgeons. *Arch. Surg.* **133**(8), 900–905.
68. Longmire, W. P., Jr. (1986). Surgical research in graduate surgical education. *Curr. Surg.* **43**(5), 377–381.
69. Schwartz, R. W., Donnelly, M. B., Young, B., *et al.* (1992). Undergraduate surgical education for the twenty-first century. *Ann. Surg.* **216**(6), 639–647.
70. Folse, J. R. (1996). Surgical education—Addressing the challenges of change. *Surgery* **120**(4), 575–579.
71. Drew, P. J., Cule, N., Gough, M., *et al.* (1999). Optimal education techniques for basic surgical trainees: Lessons from education theory. *J. R. Coll. Surg. Edinb.* **44**(1), 55–56.
72. Baker, J. D., Reines, H. D., and Wallace, C. T. (1985). Learning style analysis in surgical training. *Am. Surg.* **51**(9), 494–496.
73. Wang, M. J., Contino, P. B., and Ramirez, E. S. (1997). Implementing cognitive learning strategies in computer-based educational technology: A proposed system. *In* "The Emergence of 'Internetable' Health Care: Systems that Really Work: Proceedings, 1997 AMIA Annual Fall Symposium, Formerly SCAMC." (D. R. Masys, ed.), pp. 703–707. Hanley & Belfus, Philadelphia.
74. Folse, R. J., Andriole, D. P., Debas, H. T., *et al.* (1998). Prerequisite objectives for graduate surgical education: a study of the Graduate Medical Education Committee American College of Surgeons. *J. Am. Coll. Surg.* **186**(1), 50–62.
75. DaRosa, D. A., Dunnington, G. L., Sachdeva, A. K., *et al.* (1992). A model for teaching medical students in an ambulatory surgery setting. *Acad. Med.* **67**(10 Suppl.), S45–S47.
76. Herrmann, J. B. (1987). A self-education program for general surgical residents. *Curr. Surg.* **44**(2), 93–96.
77. York, N. L., DaRosa, D. A., and Folse, R. (1996). The learning needs of first-year surgical residents in the intensive care unit. *Am. J. Surg.* **171**(6), 608–611.
78. Mennin, S. P., and Kalishman, S. (1998). Student assessment. *Acad. Med.* **73**(9 Suppl.), S46–S54.
79. Downing, S. M., English, D. C., and Dean, R. E. (1983). Resident ratings of surgical faculty. Improved teaching effectiveness through feedback. *Am. Surg.* **49**(6), 329–332.
80. Knowles, M. S. (1984). "Andragogy in Action," 1st Ed. Jossey-Bass, San Francisco.
81. Barrows, H. S. (1983). Problem-based, self-directed learning. *JAMA* **250**(22), 3077–3080.
82. McGregor, D. B., Arcomano, T. R., Bjerke, H. S., and Little, A. G. (1995). Problem orientation is a new approach to surgical education. *Am. J. Surg.* **170**(6), 656–658; discussion, 658–659.
83. Dunnington, G., Witzke, D., Rubeck, R., *et al.* (1987). A comparison of the teaching effectiveness of the didactic lecture and the problem-oriented small group session: A prospective study. *Surgery* **102**(2), 291–296.
84. Schwartz, R. W., Donnelly, M. B., Nash, P. P., and Young, B. (1992). Developing students' cognitive skills in a problem-based surgery clerkship. *Acad. Med.* **67**(10), 694–696.
85. Chang, G., Cook, D., Maguire, T., *et al.* (1995). Problem-based learning: Its role in undergraduate surgical education. *Can. J. Surg.* **38**(1), 13–21.
86. Brailovsky, C. A., Grand'Maison, P., and Lescop, J. (1992). A large-scale multicenter objective structured clinical examination for licensure. *Acad. Med.* **67**(10 Suppl.), S37–S39.
87. Allen, J., Evans, A., Foulkes, J., and French, A. (1998). Simulated surgery in the summative assessment of general practice training: Results of a trial in the Trent and Yorkshire regions. *Br. J. Gen. Pract.* **48**(430), 1219–1223.
88. Weidenbach, K. (1999). "Staged Encounters," pp. 8–12. Stanford Medicine.
89. Fletcher-Flinn, C. M., and Gravatt, B. (1995). The efficacy of computer assisted instruction (CAI): A meta-analysis. *J. Ed. Comp. Res.* **12**(3), 219–242.
90. Devitt, P., Cehic, D., and Palmer, E. (1998). Computers in medical education 2. Use of a computer package to supplement the clinical experience in a surgical clerkship: An objective evaluation. *Aust. N.Z.J. Surg.* **68**(6), 428–431.
91. Downs, S. M., Friedman, C. P., Marasigan, F., and Gartner, G. (1997). A decision analytic method for scoring performance on computer-based patient simulations. *In* "The Emergence of 'Internetable' Health care: Systems that Really Work: Proceedings, 1997 AMIA Annual Fall Symposium, Formerly SCAMC" (D. R. Masys, ed.). Hanley & Belfus, Philadelphia.
92. Wade, T. P., and Kaminski, D. L. (1995). Comparative evaluation of educational methods in surgical resident education [see comments]. *Arch. Surg.* **130**(1), 83–87.
93. Wade, T. P., Andrus, C. H., and Kaminski, D. L. (1993). Evaluations of surgery resident performance correlate with success in board examinations. *Surgery* **113**(6), 644–648.
94. Dillon, G. F., and Clyman, S. G. (1992). The computerization of clinical science examinations and its effect on the performances of third-year medical students. *Acad. Med.* **67**(10 Suppl.), S66–S68.
95. Ripkey, D. R., Case, S. M., and Swanson, D. B. (1996). A "new" item format for assessing aspects of clinical competence. *Acad. Med.* **71**(10 Suppl.), S34–S36.

96. Gruppen, L. D., Grum, C. M., Fincher, R. M., *et al.* (1996). Multi-site reliability and validity of a diagnostic pattern-recognition knowledge-assessment instrument. *Acad. Med.* **71**(10 Suppl.), S65–S67.
97. Anders, K. H., Goldstein, B. G., Lesher, J. L., Jr., *et al.* (1989). The use of live pigs in the surgical training of dermatology residents. *J. Dermatol. Surg. Oncol.* **15**(7), 734–736.
98. Heppell, J., Beauchamp, G., and Chollet, A. (1995). Ten-year experience with a basic technical skills and perioperative management workshop for first-year residents. *Can. J. Surg.* **38**(1), 27–32.
99. Boyle, D. E., and Gius, J. A. (1968). Tie and suture training board. *Surgery* **63**(3), 434–436.
100. Oneal, R. M., Dingman, R. O., and Grabb, W. C. (1967). The teaching of plastic surgical techniques to medical students. *Plast. Reconstr. Surg.* **40**(5), 494–498.
101. Bevan, P. G. (1981). The craft of surgery. The anastomosis workshop, March 1981. *Ann. R. Coll. Surg. Engl.* **63**(6), 405–410.
102. Stotter, A. T., Becket, A. J., Hansen, J. P., *et al.* (1986). Simulation in surgical training using freeze dried material. *Br. J. Surg.* **73**(1), 52–54.
103. Reznick, R., Regehr, G., MacRae, H., *et al.* (1997). Testing technical skill via an innovative "bench station" examination. *Am. J. Surg.* **173**(3), 226–230.
104. Barnes, R. W., Lang, N. P., and Whiteside, M. F. (1989). Halstedian technique revisited. Innovations in teaching surgical skills. *Ann. Surg.* **210**(1), 118–121.
105. Anastakis, D. J., Regehr, G., Reznick, R. K., *et al.* (1999). Assessment of technical skills transfer from the bench training model to the human model. *Am. J. Surg.* **177**(2), 167–170.
106. Rosser, J. C., Rosser, L. E., and Savalgi, R. S. (1997). Skill acquisition and assessment for laparoscopic surgery. *Arch. Surg.* **132**(2), 200–204.
107. Beckmann, C. R., Lipscomb, G. H., Ling, F. W., *et al.* (1995). Computer-assisted video evaluation of surgical skills. *Obstet. Gynecol.* **85**(6), 1039–1041.
108. Delp, S. L., Loan, J. P., Hoy, M. G., *et al.* (1990). An interactive graphics-based model of the lower extremity to study orthopaedic surgical procedures. *IEEE Trans. Biomed. Eng.* **37**(8), 757–767.
109. Satava, R. M. (1995). Medical applications of virtual reality. *J. Med. Syst.* **19**(3), 275–280.
110. Johnston, R., Bhoyrul, S., Way, L., *et al.* (1996). Assessing a virtual reality surgical skills simulator. *Stud. Health Technol. Inform.* **29**(1), 608–617.
111. Taffinder, N., Sutton, C., Fishwick, R. J., *et al.* (1998). Validation of virtual reality to teach and assess psychomotor skills in laparoscopic surgery: Results from randomised controlled studies using the MIST VR laparoscopic simulator. *Stud. Health Technol. Inform.* **50**(32), 124–130.
112. O'Toole, R. V., Playter, R. R., Krummel, T. M., *et al.* (1999). Measuring and developing suturing technique with a virtual reality surgical simulator [see comments]. *J. Am. Coll. Surg.* **189**(1), 114–127.
113. DaRosa, D. A., Folse, J. R., Reznick, R. K., *et al.* (1996). Description and evaluation of the Surgeons as Educators course. *J. Am. Coll. Surg.* **183**(5), 499–505.
114. Porter, R. W. (1996). Surgical training and education. *J. R. Coll. Surg. Edinb.* **41**(3), 204–206.
115. Griffen, W. O. (1986). "Back to the future". *Curr. Surg.* **43**(5), 372–376.
116. Bagley, J. S. (1996). The problems of surgeons in training. *J. R. Coll. Surg. Edinb.* **41**(3), 206–207.
117. Thompson, J. C. (1995). Impact of managed care on surgical education and research. Boston, Massachusetts, October 20, 1994. Proceedings. *Arch. Surg.* **130**(9), 925–941.
118. Greenfield, L. G. (1986). Support of graduate medical education. *Curr. Surg.* **43**(4), 271.
119. Debas, H. T. (1993). Impact of the changing economy and new technology on surgical practice and education. *Invest. Radiol.* **28**[Suppl. 3(6)], S23.
120. Bridges, M., and Diamond, D. L. (1999). The financial impact of teaching surgical residents in the operating room. *Am. J. Surg.* **177**(1), 28–32.
121. Bahnson, H. T. (1988). Education of a surgical chairman. *Ann. Surg.* **208**(3), 247–253.
122. Coe, N. P., Hirvela, E., Garb, J. L., and Friedmann, P. (1990). Surgical education: A decade of change. *Curr. Surg.* **47**(5), 317–321.
123. Dunnington, G. L., and DaRosa, D. A. (1994). Changing surgical education strategies in an environment of changing health care delivery systems. *World J. Surg.* **18**(5), 734–737; discussion 733.
124. Liu, D. (1999). Evidence-based surgery and the internet. *Ann. R. Coll. Surg. Engl.* **81**(3 Suppl.), 115–117.
125. Doty, J. R., Liddicoat, J. R., Salomon, N. W., and Greene, P. S. (1998). Surgical education via the Internet: The Cardiothoracic Surgery Network. *Md. Med. J.* **47**(5), 264–266.
126. Lindsey, L. A. (1999). Surgery and the information age. *J. R. Coll. Surg. Edinb.* **44**(1), 34–35.
127. Lee, B. R., Bishoff, J. T., Janetschek, G., *et al.* (1998). A novel method of surgical instruction: International telementoring. *World J. Urol.* **16**(6), 367–370.
128. Kingsnorth, A. N., Campbell, J. K., and Vranch, A. (1999). Teleteaching—A practical and economical method of delivering surgical education. *Ann. R. Coll. Surg. Engl.* **81**(2 Suppl.), 66–70.
129. Bodily, K. C. (1999). Presidential address. Surgeons and technology. *Am. J. Surg.* **177**(5), 351–353.
130. Iserson, K. V. (1999). Simulating our future: Real changes in medical education. *Acad. Med.* **74**(7), 752–754.
131. Gilligan, J. H., Welsh, F. K., Watts, C., and Treasure, T. (1999). Square pegs in round holes: Has psychometric testing a place in choosing a surgical career? A preliminary report of work in progress. *Ann. R. Coll. Surg. Engl.* **81**(2), 73–79.
132. Satish, U., and Streuffert, S. (1997). The measurement of behavioral complexity. *J. Appl. Soc. Psych.* **27**(23), 2117–2121.
133. Horan, S. A. (1988). Decision factors in the choice of a surgical residency program. *J. Med. Educ.* **63**(11), 866–867.

91

Mathematical Modeling

Denise E. Kirschner* and Timothy G. Buchman†

**Departments of Microbiology and Immunology, The University of Michigan, Ann Arbor, Michigan 48109*
†Department of Surgery, Washington University School of Medicine, St. Louis, Missouri 63110

I. Mathematical Modeling

Surgical research embraces many disciplines, ranging from molecular biology to human physiology. Irrespective of the physical scale that characterizes a particular project, most surgical investigators will confront some significant aspect of their research that will benefit from—if not explicitly require—mathematical modeling. In this chapter, we explore fundamental aspects of mathematical modeling to address three questions. Why is mathematical modeling an essential surgical research tool? What is (and what is not) a mathematical model? How is a mathematical model designed and used? Answers to these questions constitute an introduction to mathematical biology and serve to illuminate an interface between that discipline and surgical research.

A. Why Model?

The synthetic answer to the question "Why model?" is that it is to encapsulate knowledge regarding a complicated problem into a simplified representation. Such an answer, however, fails to acknowledge and leverage the practical modeling experience familiar to every young surgeon.

B. Static Models

Common folklore suggests that the young surgeon initially displays technical skills by "building model airplanes." Demonstrations of dexterity aside, creation of such scaled physical models provides for examination of spatial organization and relationships that are not otherwise discernable. For example, the passenger in seat 15-C of a Boeing 737 is unlikely to appreciate that the length and wingspan of her conveyance are nearly identical; moreover, this similarity is echoed throughout the Boeing line. This systematic examination of physical models can lead to knowledge abstraction: "Boeing builds square airplanes."

Abstracted knowledge about an object that can be embedded into a static model is frequently used in surgical care. For example, water in the adult human is commonly modeled to occupy two compartments, an intracellular space and an extracellular space, with the extracellular space also consisting of two compartments, an interstitial space and an intravascular space. Clinical estimates of the magnitudes of fluid and electrolyte deficits rely on such a static model.

C. Dynamic Models

The passenger in 15-C is likely less concerned with dimension than with a safe and swift journey. The journey depends on engineering, and the passenger in 15-C is reassured that a professional team has designed systems and subsystems to interact reliably in highly specific and predictable ways. The key phrase is "designed . . . to interact."

Biomedical engineering excepted, the surgical investigator does not participate in the design of the object under study. In most surgical research projects, the goal is to elucidate the design. The key tool is controlled perturbation of the study object followed by sequential measurement of object parameters. From the measurements—whether the data describe gene expression, bulk flow of blood through the heart, or spread of a particular bacterium through an intensive care unit—surgical investigators make inferences about the relevance of a particular process. The inferences become hypotheses that are experimentally probed, most often by comparing objects that differ in a single feature: the knockout mouse versus its parent; flow at a hematocrit of 20 versus a hematocrit of 40; use of water-based handwashing versus alcohol foam degerming.

Data accumulate much faster than knowledge. The classical, reductionist approach to scientific inquiry requires a full factorial design such that each relevant process ought to be tested across its full range of expected performance in order to understand its role. Organ physiologists a generation ago often performed such systematic studies. Their detailed experiments became the basis for clinically essential models such as cardiac performance as a function of preload, afterload, and contractility. Such experiments on the microscale of cells and molecules and on the macroscale of large populations are difficult to design and even more difficult to perform. The usual approach is that a relatively few observations made under arbitrary but strictly controlled conditions in which the object under study has been intentionally "isolated from confounding influences" are extrapolated to more general, analytically "messier" situations. The potential for error is obvious, the realization all too frequent.

D. The Hidden Hypothesis

The passenger in 15-C is flying in an airplane, the behavior of which over time was predicted on the basis of an explicit design. The surgical investigator pursues the "inverse problem." The design of the object under study is to be extracted from its behavior over time subject to a host of noisome experimental constraints. We have already alluded to the limit of the number of data that may be collected. Biologic objects also limit the types of data that can be collected. The precision of the data obtained from biologic objects is typically less than that obtained from physical objects. And so on. The extrapolation to the more general situation and to behaviors over time is an hypothesis in its own right, an hypothesis that is subject to verification by experiment. Testing this "extrapolation hypothesis" drives modeling such that behaviors are predicted and then experimentally tested. Models are merely collections of hypotheses regarding the mechanisms and magnitudes of processes that influence the object under study.*

II. What Is (and What Is Not) a Mathematical Model?

A mathematical model is a tool with which an investigator encapsulates hypotheses concerning the behavior of an object over time into mathematical relationships, at least some of which refer to measurable parameters. Mathematical models are ubiquitous in surgical care. Some are expressed as informal rules, such as the "three-for-one rule" (which states that three volumes of a balanced salt infusion are required to compensate for each volume of acute blood loss). This rule originates from experiments showing that water and small ions readily equilibrate across blood vessel walls into the interstitial compartment, and from a model that envisions the interstitial compartment to be twice as large as the intravascular compartment.

Other mathematical models are more formal, such as the pharmacokinetic models that guide administration of aminoglycoside antibiotics. The nomograms that surgical residents use to make dose adjustments are simply graphic representations of models of the aqueous compartments and the predicted clearance rate of the drug. Each patient is viewed as an individual experiment, with the model offering continuous predictions about plasma concentrations. Measuring the patient's plasma level of the drug at a particular time is a test of the model, not of the patient. An accurate prediction merely indicates that the dose may be left unchanged. An inaccurate prediction does something more—it not only indicates to the surgeon that the dose must be changed but also suggests that the model contains relations that are inaccurate or incomplete. Indeed, unexpectedly high levels may suggest that there is incipient renal insufficiency whereas unexpectedly low levels may suggest that the patient has a larger than normal volume of distribution.

However useful they may be, memorable "rules" and nomograms are no more than representations of someone else's model. The surgical investigator must ultimately venture into building his own model if he is to make and test hypotheses concerning the design of the object being studied. He must ultimately propose relationships that govern

*As a collection of hypotheses that is also an hypothesis, models can never be proved "correct." Their greatest value lies in illuminating what is "missing" or "wrong."

the measurable parameters, make predictions, perturb the object, and observe the fidelity with which his model describes the behavior of his system. Simply stating the anticipated change in a parameter ("I predict drug D will cause parameter P to decrease") is not a model. It may well be an event predicted by a model, but the prediction is not the model.

A. Model Building: An Example

To illustrate one way that modeling illuminates a problem to focus attention on particular aspects of that problem, consider the following familiar and vexing scenario. Review during rounds of a postoperative patient shows two abnormalities. First, the urine output is decreasing. Second, the serum creatinine concentration is rising. The patient has received appropriate volumes of fluid. The inescapable conclusion is that the patient has acute renal insufficiency. The apparent cause of the kidney failure is identified and reversed. The next day, the serum creatinine level has climbed again. Has the true cause of the renal insufficiency been identified? Why has the serum creatinine risen? Is there another cause for the problem? When will the creatinine concentration peak and start back down? These gnawing questions have cost every surgeon anxious moments.

To apply mathematical modeling to this (or any other) problem, the universe of the problem must be explicitly defined along with the hypothesized relationships among the members of that universe. In the case of the patient with renal insufficiency, it is enough to define the universe to include a source of creatinine (muscle breakdown), a reservoir in which the creatinine is accumulated (in total body water), and sinks into which the creatinine flows (urine).

The graphic representation in Fig. 1 encapsulates not only the universe but also the relationships represented in a "conservation of mass" equation. The graphic emphasizes that we are not particularly interested in the exact source of the creatinine, only that the source continues to pour creatinine into the reservoir by the process of myolysis. The graphic also recognizes that the kidney has two distinct mechanisms by which it removes creatinine from plasma

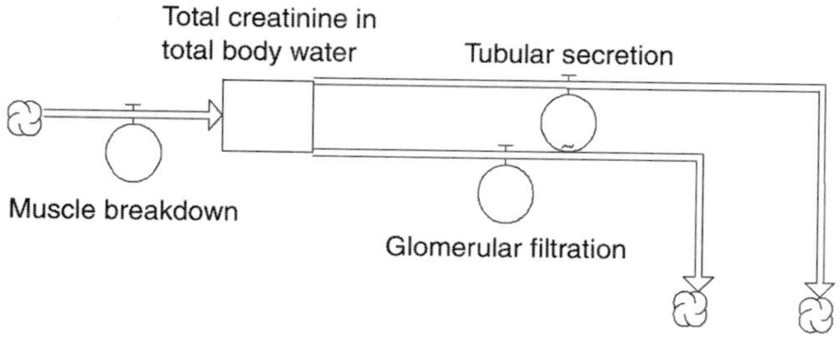

Figure 1 Schematic representation of production and elimination of creatinine. Tubular secretion and glomerular filtration are independent processes that occur in the kidneys and deliver creatinine into the urine.

(and, by extension, from total body water): filtration by the glomerulus and secretion into the renal tubule. Although both mechanisms deliver creatinine into the urine, we can and will treat them as distinct processes. A conservation of mass equation containing these relationships might read:

$$\frac{d([\mathrm{Cr}] \cdot V_{\mathrm{Cr}})}{dt} = \dot{R} - (\dot{S} + \dot{g}\,[\mathrm{Cr}]), \tag{1}$$

where [Cr] is the concentration of creatinine in body water, V_{cr} is the volume of that body water, $\dot{R}$ is the rate of creatinine released by muscle breakdown, $\dot{S}$ is the rate at which creatinine is secreted by the renal tubules, and $\dot{g}$ is the glomerular filtration rate. Only two data series are immediately available to the clinician at the bedside. One is the series of concentrations of creatinine [Cr] and the other is the series of intervals defined by the times between each of the measurements, Δt. What, then, is the appropriate interpretation of the "trend" in creatinine measurements? What (if anything) can be inferred from relationships between the incremental change in creatinine, $\Delta[\mathrm{Cr}]/\Delta t$, and the average value of [Cr] during the change?

Recall the following simple expansion. If m and n are both functions of the variable t, then

$$\frac{d\,(mn)}{dt} = m\,\frac{dn}{dt} + n\,\frac{dm}{dt}.$$

Rearrangement of terms yields

$$\frac{d[Cr]}{dt} = \frac{1}{V_{\mathrm{Cr}}}(\dot{R} - \dot{S}) - \frac{1}{V_{\mathrm{Cr}}}\left(\dot{g} + \frac{dV_{\mathrm{Cr}}}{dt}\right)[\mathrm{Cr}] \tag{2}$$

Inspection shows that so long as V_{cr}, $\dot{R}$, and $\dot{S}$ are constant, the slope of a $d[\mathrm{Cr}]/dt$ vs. [Cr] plot will be a linear function of $\dot{g}$.†

Few of us—surgeons or mathematicians—have the intuition or experience to relate clinical data to this rather unfriendly looking equation. Fortunately, neither are necessary. Desktop microcomputers with appropriate modeling software substitute nicely. Solutions are illustrated using several popular modeling systems.

B. STELLA

STELLA (High Performance Systems, Hanover, NH) is the most intuitive modeling system used in surgical labora-

†Mathematically inclined readers may wish to examine this equation in several special cases. First, if coefficients are constant then an analytic solution is possible. In this case, $\Delta[\mathrm{Cr}]/\Delta t$ can be calculated precisely, and the difference between the measurable and the infinitessimal $d[\mathrm{Cr}]/dt$ can be estimated. Second, behaviors during an acute change in g (step, ramp, and so on) display characteristic plots of $d[\mathrm{Cr}]/dt$ vs. [Cr]. Third, and perhaps most important, the effect of sequential acute changes in g (two steps) is to give characteristic behaviors in the plot.

tories. The simple, graphical approach to defining relationships among elements in the modeling universe and carefully selected defaults invites even the novice to begin modeling within the first hour working with this package. Indeed, STELLA is used in secondary schools and college courses to introduce scientists and nonscientists to systems thinking.

The STELLA workspace is deceptively simple. Modelers define flows among the elements of the model universe and then specify initial values and the mathematical relationships among elements and flows over time. The specifications can take many forms, including formal equations, numerical arrays, and even hand-drawn curves. To set up the clinical problem in STELLA, we used the model shown in Fig. 2. The core of the picture is identical to the representation in Fig. 1. Several variables have been added to the model so that flows can be more precisely specified. For example, glomerular filtration is the product of the glomerular filtration rate and the concentration of creatinine ("measured creatinine") in the plasma. This "measured creatinine" is the ratio of the total creatinine to the total volume of creatinine distribution. The process of tubular secretion is known to be both saturable by and dependent on the concentration of creatinine, so a "ghost" of the measured creatinine is inserted to influence the tubular secretion process.

Exploration of the model requires rational selection of initial values and prediction of model behavior. We chose to study the archetypal 70-kg patient, a young man with normal renal function. We suggested that with a normal diet, exercise, and muscle mass, he would deliver 1.6 g (1600 mg) creatinine to the circulation each 24 hour day. About 60% of his body mass is water, so that the initial volume of distribution of this small molecule is about 42 liters (420 dl). Because a normal creatinine concentration is about 1.0 mg/dl, we set the total creatinine at 420 mg. We set his initial glomerular filtration rate at 80 ml/min (1150 dl/day). We set his initial secretion rate at 150 mg/day. Model parameters are shown in Table I. These settings yield a stable profile over time (Fig. 3). Because the creatinine is stable, a plot of its first derivative versus the creatinine concentration is just a point (Fig. 4).

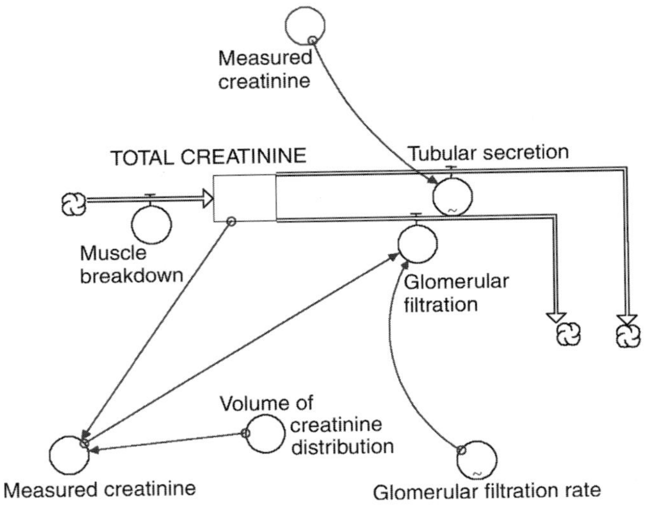

Figure 2 STELLA model of creatinine production and elimination. See text for further details.

Consider the same patient with two modifications. First, the glomerular filtration rate changes with time (Fig. 5). Second, the tubular secretion is a saturable process (Fig. 6). In this setting, the dynamics of creatinine concentration, glomerular filtration, and tubular secretion change markedly over time (Fig. 7). Plotting measured creatinine, [Cr], against its first derivative $d[\mathrm{Cr}]/dt$, a useful dynamic is seen (Fig. 8). This plot provides useful insight to the clinician. Given a "step change" (i.e., instantaneous) decrement in glomerular filtration rate (GFR) followed by a spontaneous (and equally instantaneous) increment back to the GFR baseline, a dynamic plot of daily measurements of [Cr] versus time produces exponential curves. However, a dynamic plot of $\Delta[\mathrm{Cr}]/\Delta t$ versus [Cr] provides direct insight not only into changing glomerular filtration but also into the likely peak value of [Cr] (as a zero-crossing). This can be easily tested with clinical data.

Table I Model Parameters

Parameter	Initial Value	Comment
Body mass	70 kg	Archetype
Total body water	42 liters (420 dl)	60% body mass; may wish to change to a variable in next iteration of the model
Total body creatinine	420 mg	1 mg/dl distributed in 420 dl
Creatinine production rate	1600 mg/day	Typical for young male, normal diet
Glomerular filtration rate	80 ml/min (1150 dl/day)	Low-normal value
Creatinine secretion rate	150 mg day	Low-normal value

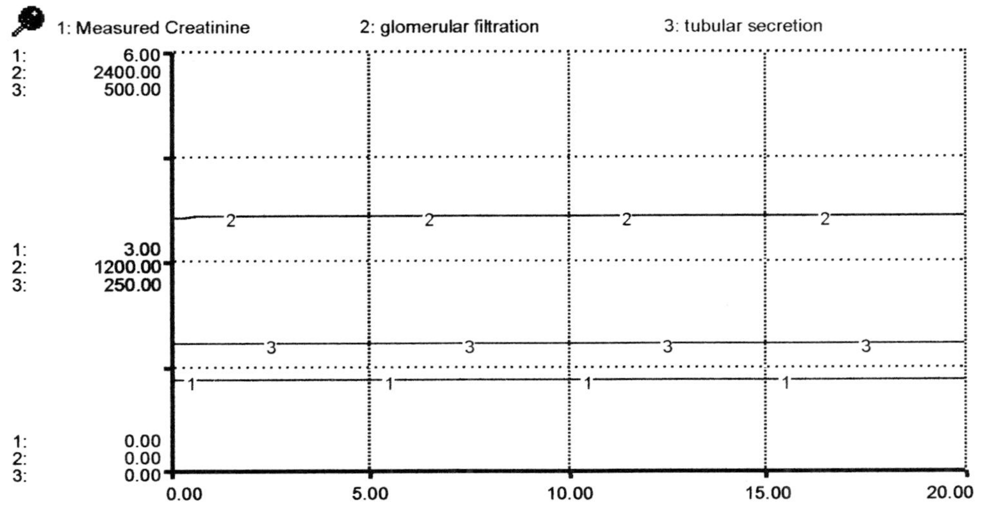

Figure 3 Time plot of stable renal function. Tubular secretion represents <20% of total creatinine clearance.

C. Simulink/MATLAB

MATLAB (The MathWorks, Natick, MA) is an integrated technical computing environment that combines numeric computation, advanced graphics and visualization, and a high-level programming language. It is a widely extensible system that can be used for diverse laboratory computing tasks, including (but not limited to) signal acquisition, processing, and analysis; experiment control; and modeling. At MATLAB's core is a robust, programmable computation engine. MATLAB's architecture promotes the use of tools that sit "on top" of MATLAB. One of these tools, Simulink, facilitates modeling, simulating, and analyzing dynamic systems.

A "conservation of mass" model analogous to that presented in Fig. 2 looks like the representation in Fig. 9 when constructed in Simulink. The elements of the Simulink model do not precisely correspond to the elements of the STELLA model, although they are functionally similar. The reason for the absence of 1:1 correspondence is that Simulink is much more than a modeling environment. Options for data management and flow are more extensive and additional specifications are required.

The Simulink/MATLAB combination is highly recommended for surgeons and investigators who have some prior knowledge of the mathematics behind the modeling (e.g., ordinary differential equations, dynamic systems theory) and will take advantage of the powerful matrix approach

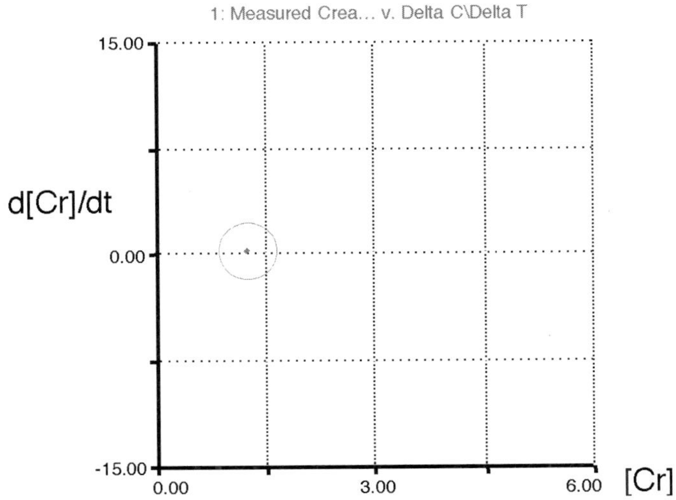

Figure 4 The plot of the first derivative versus creatinine concentration is a single point because the renal function is unchanging.

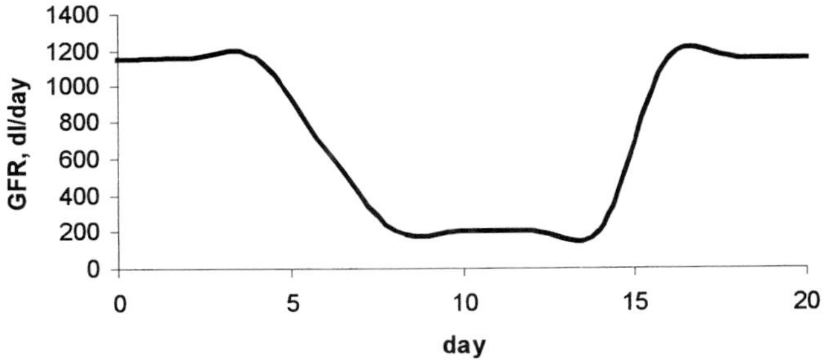

Figure 5 In this scenario, the patient receives a nephrotoxic drug for several days, after which the toxicity is recognized and the drug is removed. Kidney function recovers spontaneously.

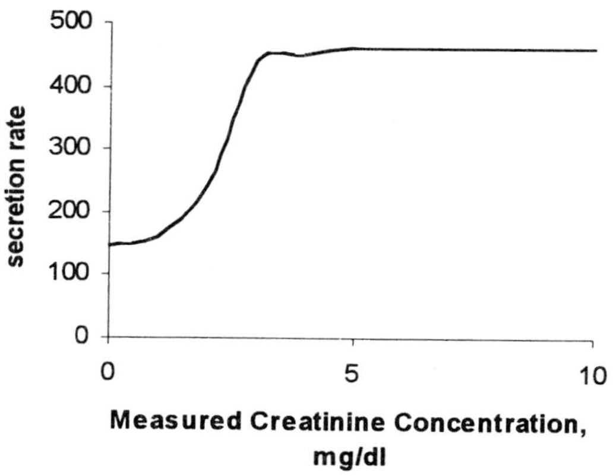

Figure 6 Tubular secretion can partially compensate for the loss of glomerular filtration. The secretion process is here modeled as a saturable process, reaching saturation at about 3 mg/dl.

embedded in MATLAB. The MATLAB environment is ideally suited for problems such as finite element modeling, in which complex interactions among dozens of elements must be accounted for in each processing step.

D. Other Graphical Tools: Madonna

Although run-time and demonstration versions of STELLA and Simulink/MATLAB are available at no cost, authoring versions of these programs may cost hundreds of dollars. An inexpensive but powerful alternative is Berkeley Madonna (Berkeley, CA). Madonna, which was originally designed as an engine to accelerate processing in STELLA, numerically solves ordinary differential equations. The latest release includes a simple graphic authoring interface that is less sophisticated but similar to STELLA. STELLA code can be executed in Madonna at quite breathtaking speeds, a feature that can be useful in complex STELLA models. A shareware download version of Madonna is available for user testing.

E. Computing Tools: Maple and Mathematica

Investigators who are fluent in differential equations are likely familiar with Maple (Waterloo Maple, Waterloo, Ontario, Canada) and Mathematica (Wolfram Research, Champaign, IL), two advanced numerics packages that include powerful solvers. The absence of a graphical interface to modeling (which is a symbol-based method of writing the relevant equations) is offset by highly efficient computation. Investigators working at academic research universities may be able to obtain extremely inexpensive licenses for these packages through their libraries or information systems groups. However, effective use of these tools requires at least some background in modeling and a level of comfort with the relevant mathematics.

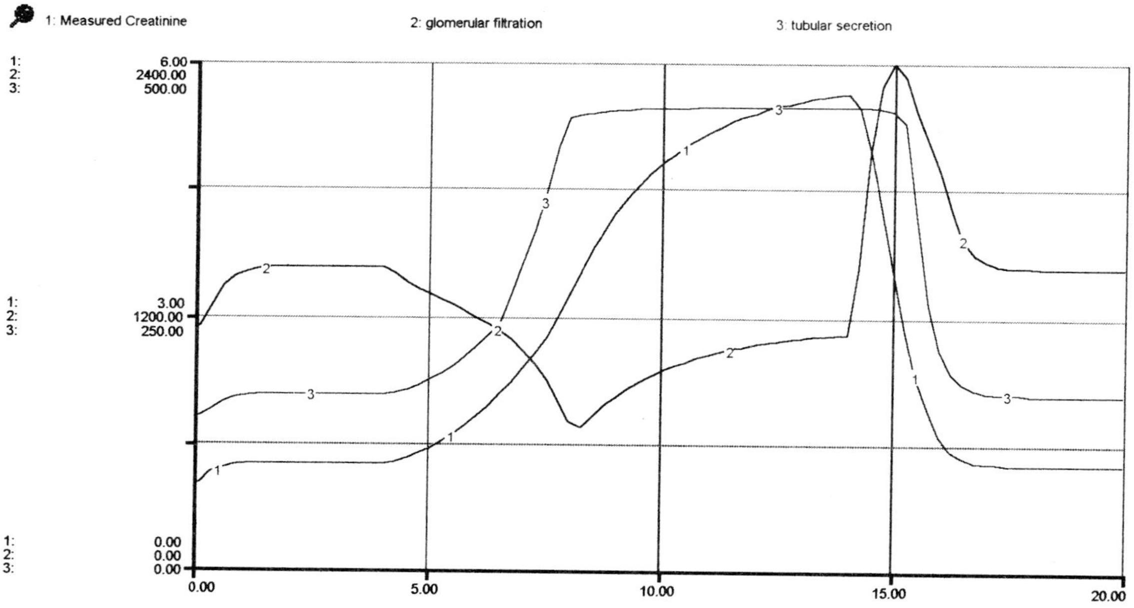

Figure 7 The temporal dynamics of renal failure and recovery. Compare the contributions of glomerular filtration and tubular secretion at different measured creatinine concentrations. Clinically, we measure line 1, creatinine. What we—and our patients!—are interested in, however, is line 2, glomerular filtration. The problem is that line 2 bears no obvious relation to line 1 except that both eventually reach a steady state. How can data from line 1 be used to infer information about line 2?

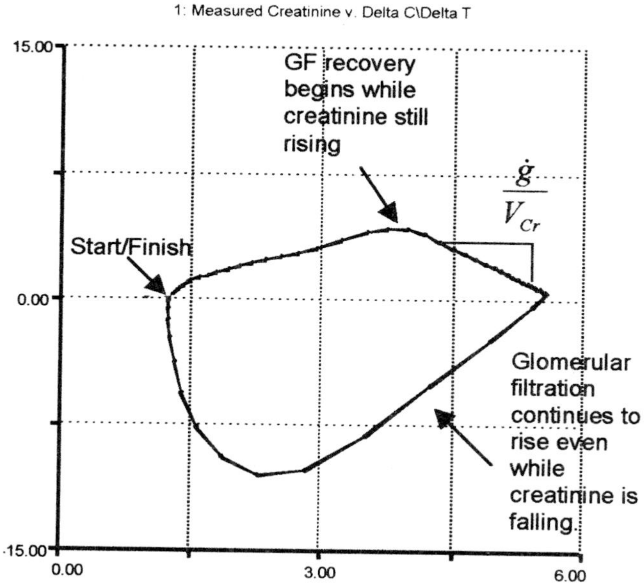

Figure 8 The plot of $d[Cr]/dt$ vs. [Cr] is a loop, returning to the baseline value of [Cr] with no change (a return to stable function). Inflections signal change in glomerular filtration performance. Compare with the Fig. 7.

F. Purpose-Built Modeling Environments

Often the fastest way to develop a model is to adapt a model that has been previously developed by another investigator for a related application. Models are published in books, in journals, and, increasingly, on the Internet. Some models (see, for example, Fig. 10, a general model of cardiac flow) are written in a general-purpose modeling environment (STELLA). Some models are sufficiently complex that they are purpose-built to create a unique environment. For example, mathematical models of cell biology consist of tightly integrated functions describing molecules, subcellular organelles, and membranes defining compartments within the cells. A useful example of such a model is "The Virtual Cell," which is available free to users through a Java Applet interface to the National Resource for Cell Analysis and Modeling at the University of Connecticut (Fig. 11).

III. Summary

Mathematical models can be profitably applied to diverse problems and projects in surgical research. The time invested in constructing and evaluating models pays handsome dividends through explicit hypothesis formulation and testing *in silico*. The results of mathematical models are routinely applied at the bedside. Similar application to routine problems encountered at the bench provides the investigator with insight into the magnitude of the problem and the experimental directions most likely to yield useful data.

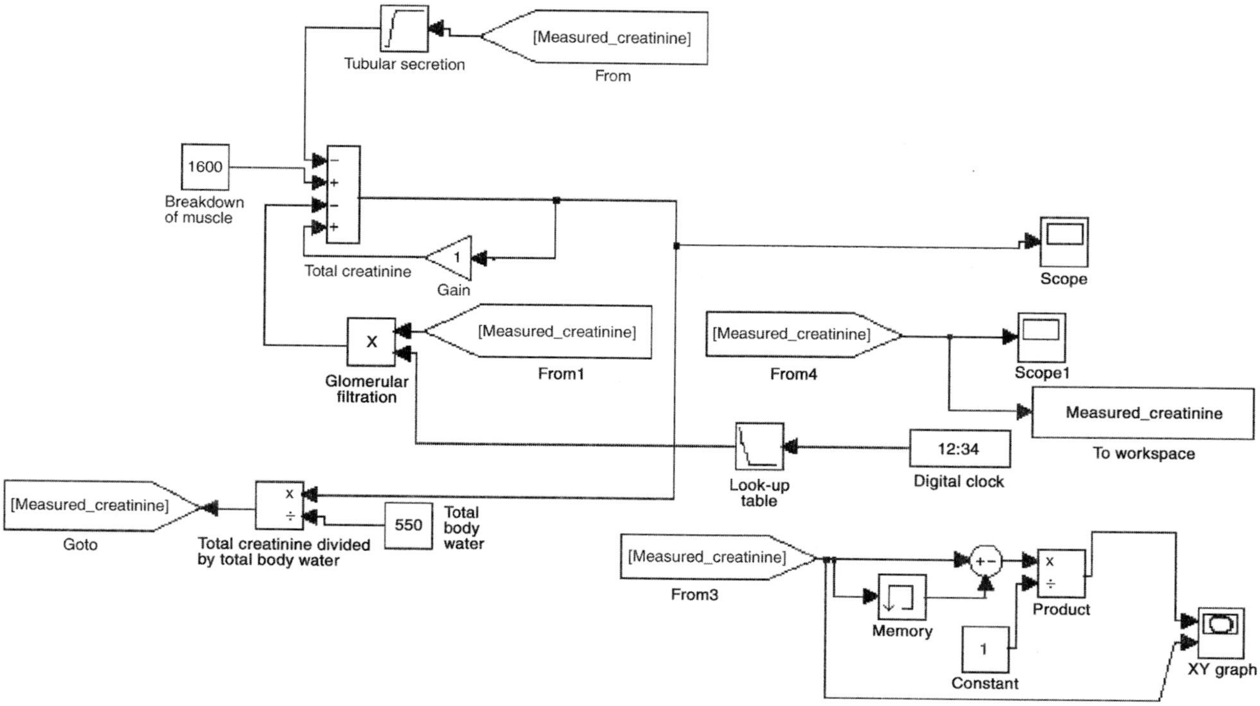

Figure 9 Simulink/MATLAB conservation-of-mass model for renal function. The model is available at the web site (www.mathworks.com).

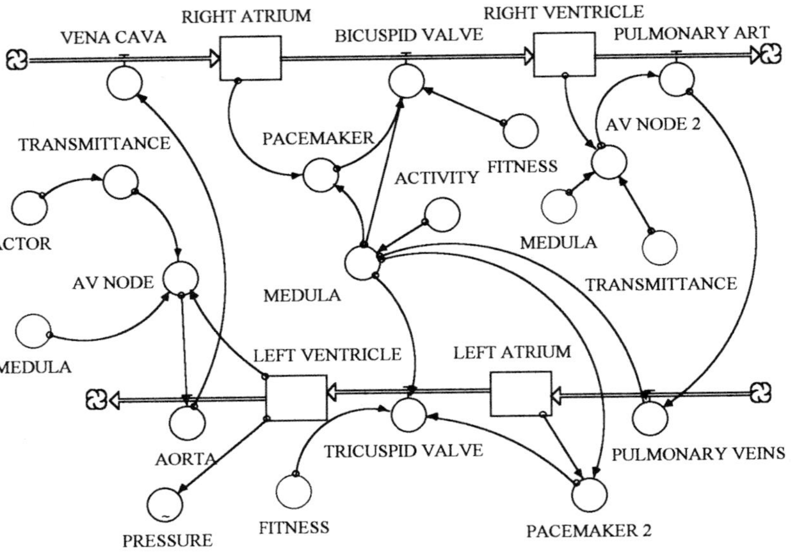

Figure 10 STELLA model of cardiac flow [reproduced with permission from Springer-Verlag, from Hannon and Ruth (1997)]. Medula refers to brainstem regulation of the heart rate. Fitness refers to physical fitness and cardiac efficiency. Activity discriminates resting from active subjects. The I factor is an infarction factor. This model is available at the web site (www.hps-inc.com).

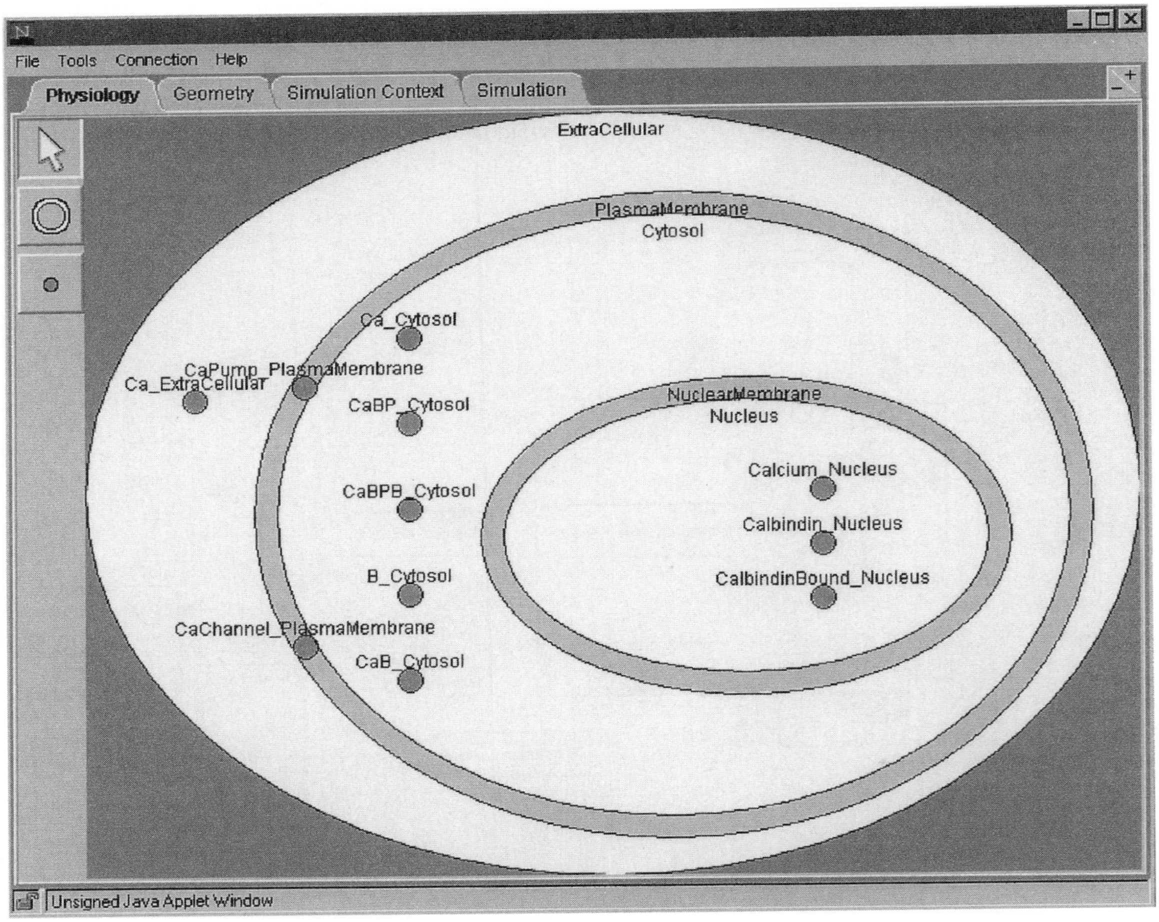

Figure 11 The biological interface to the current version of the Virtual Cell. This purpose-built modeling environment includes tools necessary to describe and test molecular flows within and across membrane-defined compartments.

Suggested Readings, References, and URLs

Edelstein-Keshet, L. (1988). "Mathematical Models in Biology." McGraw Hill, New York.

An especially useful reference text for modeling novices. The clarity of the presentation is excellent and the review of relevant mathematics is done with elegant simplicity.

Hannon, B., and Ruth, M. (1997). "Modeling Dynamic Biological Systems." Springer-Verlag, New York.

This text is based on a variety of STELLA models. The models presented range from the simple to the sophisticated, and several are relevant to physiologic processes. The prose is clear and easily understood even by rank amateur modelers.

Jelliffe, R. W., and Jelliffe, S. M. (1972). A computer program for estimation of creatinine clearance from unstable serum creatinine levels, age sex and weight. *Math. Biosci.* **14,** 17–24.

This classic paper is among the first to report a computational solution to a dynamic model of creatinine kinetics.

Levey, A. S., Perrone, R. D., and Madias, N. E. (1988). Serum creatinine and renal function. *Ann. Rev. Med.* **39,** 465–490.

This is an easily digestible review of the relationship between serum creatinine and renal function. Readers who wish to further develop the model presented in this chapter will wish to incorporate features discussed in this paper.

Madonna: http://www.berkeleymadonna.com/index.html

The Berkeley Madonna web site includes the shareware download of the current version of this software. Links are included to hundreds of models. An authoring version can be purchased online.

Maple: http://www.maplesoft.com/

The Maple web site contains useful information about the capabilities of this suite of symbolic and numerical solvers. Licenses for Maple are often available through university information services departments at nominal cost.

Mathematica: http://www.mathematica.com/

The Mathematica web site is a rich source of information concerning this powerful suite. There is a substantial discount (over 90%) offered to students who are working in accredited programs toward a degree.

MATLAB/Simulink: http://www.mathworks.com/

The MATLAB web site provides enormous help to the end-user through information, help files, and forums. Although there is no direct download, the sales force is very responsive and will typically provide a time-limited trial to potential customers. The power of MATLAB/Simulink needs to be explored first-hand to appreciate its potential.

National Resource for Cell Analysis and Modeling: http://www.nrcam.uchc.edu/

This web site provides Java code and an interface to the purpose-built model of cell dynamics, the Virtual Cell. The general computational framework is unique and especially adaptable to microscopy in which molecular probes have been used to interrogate specific molecules and gradients.

STELLA: http://www.hps-inc.com/

The STELLA web site contains not only run-time versions of the STELLA software but also links to a variety of models that illustrate modeling concepts. The authoring version includes well-written documentation that is readily absorbed even by those with no prior modeling experience. The tutorials are fast and effectively illustrate the capability of the package.

92

Information Resource Discovery for Surgeons: Databases and the Internet

Suzy Conway, Anna Getselman, and Lucretia W. McClure

Francis A. Countway Library of Medicine, Harvard Medical School, Boston, Massachusetts 02115

I. Review of Literature Formats

Surgeons have contributed much to the literature of medicine and its history as well as to the great advances in the field. Nuland (1) describes surgery as a "form of artistry, and the surgeon the personification of the art of medicine." He also reminds that "tissue teaches more then text, pathophysiology more than the printed page. Touching and seeing open the most direct paths to the surgeon's mind." A continuum of learning, whatever the medium, is as necessary to the practitioner as the scalpel or the medication.

A combination of the new developments in science and medicine, the explosion of publishing, and the introduction of electronic devices and resources makes keeping current in one's field a challenge. The sheer number of journals, books, databases, and Internet resources is overwhelming. It calls for a vigorous systematic method for keeping abreast.

How a surgeon, physician, or scientist develops a plan of reading is an individual decision, but it needs to include a variety of resources. For example, as president of Rockefeller University, Joshua Lederberg outlined how he organized his reading: he scanned 50–60 articles in the weekly journals, *New England Journal of Medicine, Science*, and *Nature*; read the publications of his University colleagues; and requested 20–25 reprints or copies each week as well as using a reporting service (2).

The entry point for most individuals in medicine today is the database. With its accessibility from home, laboratory, or library, and the ability to research topics, the database search is key to current information. The values and limitations of a variety of databases as well as Internet resources will be outlined later in this chapter.

Developing a pattern of lifelong learning requires more than finding articles through a database search. The following resources provide different avenues for acquiring essential information.

A. Journals

Reading or scanning surgical journals often introduces the reader to topics or advances not found elsewhere. Serendipity plays an important role in bringing forth new ideas, starting the reader on a path of learning and discovery. The number of titles in surgery and its subspecialties is enormous. The number of titles with surgery either as subject or title word in the Ulrich's International Periodical Directory totals 907. Because the National Library of Medicine (NLM) has established stringent standards of selection for journals indexed in *Index Medicus*, only 136 surgery titles are included.

The standards in general surgery require a surgeon to keep up with the following peer-reviewed titles: *Annals of Surgery, American Journal of Surgical Pathology, Transplantation, Archives of Surgery, British Journal of Surgery, Current Problems in Surgery, World Journal of Surgery*, and *Surgery*. These also are the titles with the highest impact factor. The Institute of Scientific Information (ISI) *Journal Citation Reports* show journals by total number of citations, the cited half-life, and the impact factor. The latter shows the average citation rate of an article and discounts the advantage in citation potential that the larger/older journals have.

Journals carry an array of features of note. They include editorials, often in response to controversial articles, and sparking good debate; book reviews; randomized controlled trials; brief communications, and news of professional organizations. Letters to the editor are invaluable counterbalances, providing corrections to original studies and serving as a starting point for scholarly dialogue.

B. Books

The journal clearly has the advantage in publishing research results as quickly as possible. The textbook or monograph, however, has the advantage of allowing authors to expand on a topic, to explore a broad range of thought and research. Textbooks such as "Principles of Surgery" by S.I. Schwartz or "Current Surgical Diagnosis and Treatment" series are standards that serve as references for both the practitioner and the student.

C. Histories

Although a good book usually provides historical background as an introduction to the topic, there is significant value in reading histories of surgery and medicine. The long and important history of the developments, controversies, discoveries, and failures that constitute the past relate to what is happening in the field today. Oliver Wendell Holmes told how he envisioned these originals: "Willis describes his circle and Fallopius his aqueduct and Varolius his bridge" (3). Minot points out how much "anatomy owes to the method of human dissection; how much pathology owes to the method of staining microscopical preparations; how much surgery owes to the method of antisepsis; how much bacteriology owes to the method of artificial cultures" (4).

D. Reviews

Review articles gather together a plethora of synthesized information, bringing the reader up to date on the state of the art of a subject. Reviews focus on the content of the material and include an extensive bibliography of the literature to date. Reviews are either selective or critical, making a good starting point in a search of the literature. The reader can find the milestones, controversies, and major contributors to the field covered in this format. Publications with the title beginning *Advances in* or *Yearbook of* are examples of the review journal.

E. Citation Indexes

This indexing method uses the cited references in published articles as a means of tracing an author or subject. Citation indexes are used to identify who cites whom or to locate trends in research. The "Science Citation Index" (SCI) is available in both print and electronic formats and provides a structure and capability not found in any other database. The online interface to SCI is the subscription-based Web of Science.

F. Evidence-Based Studies

The Cochrane Controlled Trials Register and Evidence-Based Medicine Reviews bring a cumulation of research on a given topic, providing an array of evidence to the reader. Contributors to the Cochrane collaboration search the world's healthcare journals to create an unbiased source of data for systematic research reviews.

G. Internet Resources

The resources just described are developed through a long-established pattern of publishing. The articles and books are edited and often reviewed by experts. Once in print form, material cannot be manipulated or reordered by readers. This is not true for the materials published on the Internet. There are many valuable and authoritative resources available, published by the National Institutes of Health (NIH) and the Centers for Disease Control and Prevention (CDC), but anyone may post a web page and make unsubstantiated statements. This chapter describes some of the best and most useful web resources currently available, and how to evaluate them.

Minot declared in 1899 that "methods of obtaining knowledge are the means of progress" (5). The methods have greatly expanded since his time, but the purpose remains the same. It is not the "possession of knowledge, of irrefutable truth, that makes the man of science, but his persistent and recklessly critical quest for truth" (6). This statement by Popper defines science and makes clear the need for and the value of the literature that reveals that critical quest.

II. Databases

The variety of resources outlined above are important for continued learning, but the biomedical databases provide the most up-to-date and efficient method of finding relevant literature. The information is from authoritative, refereed journals, accessible any time from any networked computer. There are many reasons the learned surgeon or physician may establish a pattern of searching databases regularly. Historical articles abound, giving current thought on the practices of an earlier day. Comparing techniques and methodologies with those of the past often provides insights to the steps leading to new developments. Who are the leaders, the innovators in a field? What institutions are at the cutting edge of breakthrough research? What are the treatment outcomes of a particular surgical procedure?

Searching the journal literature for information is strategic to lifelong learning, especially given the rate at which information in medicine changes. The reader finds within journals the most relevant research, the most stringent statistical data, the most accurate references. Reading high-quality articles is important to a researcher who plans to write and publish. Mediocre papers stand out in comparison. Reading comprehensively also gives the researcher an edge in identifying what is not being studied and reported. The lack of citations on a subject can serve as an "early warning" to the astute reader, for here is a subject that literally cries out for new ideas and research.

Information seeking is an essential step in the research process, an obligation to all who would diagnose, treat, and care for patients. Paul Weiss describes the importance of this knowledge: "Scientific knowledge grows like an organic tree, not as a compilation of collector's items. Facts, observations, discoveries, as items, are but the nutrients on which the tree of knowledge feeds, and not until they have been thoroughly absorbed and assimilated, have they truly enlarged the body of knowledge" (7). Systematic searching of a variety of databases affects the way medicine is practiced and ensures the best possible treatment outcomes for patients. The best minds, the most specific topics, the latest review articles are just a click away. Some databases, including MEDLINE, are updated daily so that the surgeon can proceed with the latest information.

It takes time and practice to search databases comprehensively and accurately. The surgeon who plans to search must make an investment of time to learn the techniques. Knowing the characteristics of the databases and how to construct the proper strategies will bring highly satisfying results. The best physicians are those who stay ahead in their areas of specialty, read the literature, confer with colleagues, and read specialized textbooks to work within current standards of practice. Four databases (MEDLINE, CancerLit, Current Contents, and SCI) provide the surgeon with the most comprehensive and relevant coverage for information and research. Searching MEDLINE through any gateway [OVID, PubMed, Internet Grateful Med (IGM)] is one way to begin the process.

A. MEDLINE

The MEDLINE database is one place to start the research process, but to be comprehensive and thorough, searching across two or three databases is wise. Databases are as idiosyncratic and unique as individuals. There is overlap of identical information yet each one offers something the other does not. There is always the serendipity of looking in the last place where the scintilla of information reveals itself to make a difference in a patient's life or change the course of a treatment protocol. The truth is that each database is mined for information differently. It is up to the user to learn the strengths and weaknesses of the databases in order to choose the most relevant one and use the best navigation tools germane to it (see Tables I and II).

MEDLINE shines in many ways. It is the oldest database online, with citations going back to 1960. Its forté is clinical medicine and contains those "zebra" case studies that authors are wont to publish. It is a bibliographic database giving the reader information about the full article, but not the full text. About 70% of the 10 million references have English language abstracts attached. As in most databases, the information provided is constructed in fields, so one can search by authors, by the institution of the first author, by subjects, or by key words in the title or the abstract. MEDLINE indicates in the title field when a published paper contains erroneous information, and the source of the correction. This is a formidable strength of the database—the retracted publication.

MEDLINE offers flexibility and pinpoint specificity to match disparate pieces of information. For example, who is publishing in Boston, Houston, or Baltimore on new surgical approaches to the aortic root problems in the Marfan's syndrome patient? Compiled data from search results using these criteria are shown in Figs. 1 and 2.

B. CancerLit

This database is produced by the National Cancer Institute (NCI) and includes information taken not only from the journal literature but from every aspect of cancer reported in proceedings of meetings, government reports, symposia,

Table I Databases I

Interface	Cost	Start date	Update frequency	Boolean operators	Truncation symbol
PubMed—HealthSTAR www.ncbi.nlm.nih.gov/PubMed	Free	1975	Daily	Yes	*
PubMed—MEDLINE www.ncbi.nlm.nih.gov/PubMed	Free	1966	Daily	Yes	*
IGM—BioethicsLine igm.nlm.nih.gov	Free	1973	Bi-monthly	Yes	*
IGM—CancerLit igm.nlm.nih.gov	Free	1983	Weekly	Yes	*
IGM—HealthSTAR igm.nlm.nih.gov	Free	1975	Weekly	Yes	*
IGM—MEDLINE igm.nlm.nih.gov	Free	1966	Weekly	Yes	*
OVID—BioethicsLine gateway.ovid.com	Subscription	1973	Bimonthly	Yes	$
OVID—CancerLit gateway.ovid.com	Subscription	1983	Monthly	Yes	$
OVID Current Contents gateway.ovid.com	Subscription	52-week cumulative rolling file	Weekly	Yes	$
OVID—EBM reviews gateway.ovid.com	Subscription	1991	Quarterly	Yes	$
OVID EMBASE gateway.ovid.com	Subscription	1980	Weekly	Yes	$
OVID—HealthSTAR gateway.ovid.com	Subscription	1975	Monthly	Yes	$
OVID—MEDLINE gateway.ovid.com	Subscription	1966	Weekly	Yes	$
Web of Science—Science Citation Index www.isinet.com	Subscription	1973	Weekly	Yes	*
The Cochrane Library www.cochrane.dk	Subscription	1991	As published	Yes	*

theses, and selected books. Although there is overlap with the journals indexed in MEDLINE, this is the specialized database to search whenever the subject is cancer related. The MeSH vocabulary of the National Library of Medicine is used to search CancerLit, which contains more than 700,000 references, making it a rich source of information for the latest treatment therapies and rare case studies.

C. Current Contents

Current Contents complements MEDLINE in coverage of the biomedical literature, but offers something MEDLINE does not. It brings to the screen the actual Table of Contents of more than 7000 journals. This feature is the singular strength of Current Contents, which has been popular with physicians ever since it was created. It allows a unique way to stay current in a field and to peruse the table of contents of many journals at the desktop. This database does not contain abstracts but it is updated weekly and offers cover-to-cover indexing on each of its journals, another invaluable strength of this resource.

D. MeSH/Key Words and Information Retrieval

The MeSH vocabulary used to retrieve information in MEDLINE, BioethicsLine, HealthSTAR, and CancerLit is a fixed list of subject headings that are attached to each record entered into the database, then in turn used by the end user to retrieve references. There are more than 17,000 searchable MeSH headings. The National Library of Medicine is constantly adding new headings and eliminating those that become obsolete. Subject specialists read each article that is indexed. The indexing is deceptively sophisticated and by virtue of it being done by humans, is also subjective and imperfect. The searcher must understand how indexers think when applying subject headings and realize that no two indexers will index an article exactly the same way. It is an

Table II Databases II

Database	Coverage	Vocabulary	Print counterpart	Publisher
MEDLINE	Journals	MeSH	Index Medicus	National Library of Medicine www.nlm.nih.gov
BioethicsLine	Journals, newspapers, monographs, court decisions, bills/laws	MeSH	Bibliography of Bioethics	Kennedy Institute of Ethics www.georgetown.edu/research/kie
CancerLit	Journals, proceedings, government reports, theses, books	MeSH	None	NCI's International Cancer Information Center www.nci.nih.gov
Current Contents	Journals	Keyword	Current Contents	Institute for Scientific Information www.isinet.com
Science Citation Index	Journals	Keyword	Science Citation Index	Institute for Scientific Information www.isinet.com
Embase	Journals	EMTREE	Excerpta Medica	Elsevier Science www.elsevier.nl
Cochrane Database of Systematic Reviews	Controlled trials	Keyword	None	Cochrane Collaboration www.update-software.com/ccweb/default.html
Evidence-Based Medicine Reviews	Controlled trials	Keyword	ACP Journal Club and Evidence-Based Medicine	American College of Physicians and BMJ Publishing Group www.acponline.org www.bmj.com

art not a science, so the searcher must bring to bear intuition, creativity, imagination, and experience when choosing accurate terminology to construct a search strategy. MeSH is a thesaurus worth mastering. To use it and understand its nuances is to be on the road to becoming an apt and satisfied searcher.

Current Contents is an example of a database that has no thesaurus and is searched only by key words. The computer matches a string of letters to find a word or phrase in or out of context. The word "aids" to a physician means "acquired immunodeficiency syndrome." A machine, however, will retrieve articles on "band aids" or "teaching aids" or "aids to

Medline 1966 to December 1999 Week 4		
#	**Search History**	**Results**
1	boston.in.	66638
2	baltimore.in.	36590
3	houston.in.	33056
4	1 or 2 or 3	136282
5	marfans syndrome/su	214
6	(aortic adj2 root).tw.	2395
7	4 and 5 and 6	17
8	limit 7 to (human and english language and review articles)	1
9	from 8 keep 1	1

Figure 1 Search strategy.

Citation 1

Authors
LeMaire SA. Cioselli JS.
Institution
Department of Surgery, Baylor College of Medicine, Methodist Hospital, **Houston,** Texas, USA.
Title
Aortic root surgery in Marfan **syndrom:** current practice and evolving techniques. [Review] [38 refs]
Source
Journal of Cardiac Surgery. 12(2 Suppl):137-41, 1997 Mar-Apr.

Figure 2 Documented citation.

learning" in addition. Ferreting out information in a huge database of 10 million records with only key words demands a precisely refined search strategy. Knowing how to limit or expand a search strategy, and applying the power of the software will recall the exact kernel of information, no more (see Figs. 3 and 4).

Harness the full capability of the database by using controlled vocabulary. These vocabularies may differ from database to database, but in medicine, MeSH can be used to search several of them. A database with a sophisticated index is easier to search than one that relies on key words. Many databases have pull-down menus, behind which a thesaurus resides. Indeed, the old adage "garbage in, garbage out" still applies. Learn the difference between the two approaches to searching as well as the advantages in combining the two. If the search topic is complex, intricate, and arcane, using a combination of both controlled vocabulary and key words is a necessity (see Figs 5 and 6).

E. PubMed: Free Access to MEDLINE

This interface to MEDLINE provided by the National Library of Medicine (NLM) and the National Center for Biotechnology Information (NCBI) is in a continuous

- Human (or animal study, e.g. transgenic mice)
- English Language
- Age (infant, newborn, adolescent, adult)
- Subheadings
- A subset: Abridged Index Medicus: AIM – 119 core journals
- Focus (making a subject the major focus of the article)
- A more specific term
- Publication type (case study, controlled trials, reviews, etc.)
- Latest several years (two, three, five, etc.)

Figure 3 Keys to limiting a search in MEDLINE.

- Explode a term to pick up related subjects
- Extend the search over more years
- OR synonymous terms together
- Use a broader term
- Include all languages
- Include animal studies along with human
- Repeat the search in other databases

Figure 4 Keys to expanding a search in MEDLINE.

process of growth and change. Because NLM makes PubMed free for all citizens, it is quickly becoming one of the most popular interfaces. The following unique features make PubMed extremely powerful:

1. Journal browser: verifies full journal name and journal abbreviation
2. Citation matcher: verifies a citation
3. Related articles feature: locates precomputed sets of related articles
4. PREMEDLINE file: tracks the most recent references entered daily
5. HealthSTAR: searchable simultaneously with MEDLINE
6. MeSH browser: online controlled vocabulary to search MEDLINE
7. Clinical queries: uses search filters that retrieve key clinical studies cited in MEDLINE

There are help screens and online documentation available at the PubMed homepage (www.ncbi.nlm.nih.gov/PubMed) that explain the functionality of the software and the underlying construct of the database.

F. Science Citation Index

If broader coverage than just biomedicine is needed, Science Citation Index (SCI) provides citations from science journals that are not indexed in MEDLINE. It also allows the searcher to see the number of times a paper has been cited and identify exactly who has cited it. How many times an author has been cited is becoming in itself a science and

- Search across several different databases on any research topic
- If you delegate searching responsibilities, select a trained medical librarian
- Ensure the bibliography reflects quality over quantity: less is more
- Select references that are absolutely relevant to your paper
- Select references that your readers can locate
- Be consistent in how you state your name in publications
- Become expert in one interface to MEDLINE (PubMed, OVID, IGM)
- Document your sources
- Access to it, does not mean you can use it

Figure 5 Tips for searching databases.

- One database covers all the medical literature in the world
- All databases are equally relevant to the information query
- All references are available in full text
- Computers make finding relevant information easy
- If it is in a database it must be right
- All journals are indexed cover to cover
- Everything retrieved is available in the library
- Searching is intuitive and obvious
- All journals indexed in databases are refereed

Figure 6 Myths to remember when searching complex topics.

also a yardstick to judge one's advancement for promotion and tenure. SCI is the only index built on citation indexing rather than on an author or subject approach, although that is possible as well. It cites all references in an author's bibliography, including books or book chapters. This is unique to SCI. If a reference is not indexed anywhere, it might as well not exist because there is no pathway to it.

A powerful feature of SCI Online is the "related articles" feature. If a searcher finds an article that is 100% relevant, with a click on a "related articles" button related references appear. The only other interface with a similar feature is PubMed. It is an extremely popular added value because it saves time and trouble.

Thousands of citations on medical subjects exist in *Index Medicus* and *Current Contents.* Before the electronic resources existed, physicians sat for hours looking through pages of references on penetrating brain injuries before finding one exactly on the mark. Today, using online databases, a skilled searcher can find the few references on Phineas Gage's crowbar incident in seconds.

When searching electronically, it is possible to store a search strategy and rerun it when the database is updated. Some interfaces have links to full-text articles as an added value feature. Others provide document delivery services for a fee. Online databases can be accessed from the office, the patient's bedside, at anytime of the day or night, whether or not a library is open.

A different way of using databases is to think of them as gigantic dictionaries into which you can "throw" any word or phrase that needs unlocking: for example, an acronym that cannot be cracked (MODS), the recipient of a special prize (De Puy Prize), the name of Stonewall Jackson's surgeon, or the spelling of a medical word (squamocolumnar). The ways these information behemoths can be put to use are as endless as the questions you have in a day, or a lifetime.

III. Internet Resources

The Internet and its hypertext graphical medium World Wide Web have significantly changed research practices and scholarly communication. The Internet has connected researchers around the world through time and space, making possible an online discussion, an instant availability of various resources, and timely release of scientific findings. However, as William Hersh noted, "we still have a long way to go toward the ability to easily find and apply online information, especially when that information is intended to be used to improve physician decision making and the outcomes of patient care" (8). In this part of the chapter, benefits of using Internet resources will be discussed, as well as the ways to find quality Internet resources quickly, then evaluate and use them effectively.

A. Organizations and Associations

To check the web sites of scholarly associations dealing with a particular discipline is a good introduction into a research field. Joining an association is a natural way to keep up with peers and subject-specific, time-sensitive information. The Internet and the web development have brought a new meaning and direction to the activities of scholarly associations. It is more than business as usual. While continuing to support conventional types of information (meetings and news updates), many associations have assumed a new role, furnishing means for scholarly communication and publishing on the web. By accessing a web site of a scholarly association a researcher can find out whom it serves and how, who are the leading researchers in the field, what are the themes of the meetings, what the association is publishing, and contact information. By subscribing to a variety of discussion groups and forums that many associations support via their web sites, members and nonmembers alike get a unique opportunity to connect, discuss, and find a solution, find a mentor or become a mentor, and get involved. The discussion groups range from "Listserv" (discussion of clinical cases and other issues) maintained by the American Society of Colon and Rectal Surgeons to "Clinical Case Forum" maintained by the Vascular Surgical Societies.

The associations on the Internet have the ability to put together unique resources and services. Thus, the Society of Thoracic Surgeons provides access to the National Cardiac Surgery Database. In its electronic version of the *Annals of Thoracic Surgery*, this society offers a discussion forum, dating from 1996. The American College of Surgeons provides e-mail delivery of the tables of contents of the future issues of the *Journal of the American College of Surgeons* (*JACS*) to registered e-mail participants (registration is free). *JACS* also has a browsing feature of lead full-text articles for the current year.

There is no way to tell how the information is going to be presented on an association's web site, and how much of it is going to be available over an extended period of time. Nor are there any standards on how restrictive the site is to the nonmember population. These are the uncertainties one has to be prepared for when using associations' web sites (see Table III).

B. E-Mail, Discussion Groups, and Forums

Personal e-mail, online discussion groups and forums have transformed scholarly communication and supplemented meetings and conferences, becoming researchers' primary sources for the latest news, as well as an efficient information exchange. These online interactions offer the power of replying instantaneously with quick entrée to a real person. By participating in a discussion group a researcher can reach a wider audience, be advised by an authority in the subject, and test new ideas. It is good to remember at all times that sending an e-mail message or a response to a discussion group is different from oral communication, because, unlike a conversation, an e-mail message can be cited or forwarded.

The best way to find discussion groups or forums is by reading annotations from refereed medical web services such as Medical Matrix (www.medmatrix.org/) (see also Table IV)

C. Funding Resources

The Internet makes the process of identifying research funds easy and interactive. Besides being able to search available funds, a researcher can explore who is the leading investigator in the field, which institution gets more funds in a particular area of research, who are the reviewers of the grant applications, obtain contact information, read instructions, and apply online.

Major federal funding sources to consider are the NIH, the National Science Foundation (NSF), CDC, and Department of Health and Human Services (see Table V). Each of these agencies has several ways of delivering grant information via the Internet, offering research program descriptions, information about its areas of interest, available funds, and application procedures. NIH Guide for Grants and Contracts, the electronic version of the official document, announces the availability of NIH funds and is accessible from the NIH home page. Other valuable resources from NIH are online Requests for Proposals, Biomedical Research Training and Opportunities, Study Section Rosters, Grant Applications, and Peer Review Notes. The NIH database CRISP (Computer Retrieval of Information on Scientific Projects) searches federally funded biomedical research projects conducted at universities, hospitals, and other research institutions.

The NSF accounts for about 20% of federal support to academic institutions for basic research (www.nsf.gov/home/grants.htm). One of the NSF's electronic grants management initiatives is FastLane, to facilitate business transactions and the exchange of information between the NSF and its client community.

Another venue to explore is private nonprofit foundations. The Internet makes the task of finding an appropriate foundation easier than it used to be. The Foundation Center, for instance, supports Foundation Finder (Inp.fdncenter.org/finder.html) to search basic information about foundations in the United States. Its Foundation Folders give individual foundations an immediate presence on the World Wide Web and make this information available to everyone (fdncenter.org/grantmaker/foldermenu.html). The Foundation's web site offers a refresher course in grantseeking from private foundations and a user-friendly guide to funding research and resources (see Table VI).

The for-profit funding organization, Community of Science (COS), has been publishing on the web since 1994, and it currently works with 500,000 scientists, 800 universities, leading research and development corporations, and government agencies (www.cos.com/aboutcos.shtml). The COS mission is to help the researcher find funding, collaborate

Table III Associations and Societies

Name	Publications	Highlights	Communication
American College of Surgeons www.facs.org	*ACS Scientific American Surgery Bulletin, Journal of the American College of Surgeons* (table of contents, journal archives) www.facs.org:80/about_college/acsdept/jacs/jacshome.html	Information for fellows, clinical resources, meeting and events, online library, surgical research clearing house, and more	Feedback
American Society of Colon and Rectal Surgeons www.fascrs.org	*Diseases of Colon & Rectum* (official journal of the ASCRS) (table of contents and abstracts, author guide, journal information, indices) www.discolrect.com	Practice parameters, membership directory, grants and awards time table, residency programs, meeting calendar, practice registry, core subjects	Listserv (discussion of clinical cases and other issues)
American Association of Neurological Surgeons www.neurosurgery.org/splash.html	Neurosurgical Focus (exclusively online) www.neurosurgery.org/journals/online_j/summary.html *Journal of Neurosurgery* (table of contents and preview articles) www.neurosurgery.org/journals/jneuro/summary.html	Meeting abstract archive, meetings and CME, world directory of neurosurgeons, resident corner, outcomes/guidelines	Mailing lists, bulletin boards, job placement service
American Society of Plastic and Reconstructive Surgery www.plasticsurgery.org	*Plastic and Reconstructive Surgery* (official journal of ASPRS) (abstracts, author instructions, publisher information) www.plasreconsurg.com	Latest statistics and news releases, resident resource guide, calendar of meetings, plastic surgery world, plastic surgeon referral patient advocacy	Plastic surgeons forum (restricted to members only)
American Society of Transplant Surgeons www.asts.org/index.htm	Abstracts Online (23rd, 24th, and 25th Scientific Meetings) www.asts.org/abstracts.htm	Public policy, ethics journal bibliography, meetings, training programs, members directory (restricted to members only)	None
Society of American Gastrointestinal Endoscopic Surgeons www.sages.org	*Surgical Endoscopy: Ultrasound and Interventional Techniques* (official journal of SAGES and E.A.E.S.) (table of contents, abstracts, author instructions) link.springer.de/link/service/journals/00464/index.htm	Statements and standards, resident education, patient information, members database, meeting information, product guide, links and resources	Job board
Society of Laparoendoscopic Surgeons www.sls.org	*JSLS Journal of the Society of Laparoendoscopic Surgeons* (guidelines for authors, index under construction) www.sls.org/JSLS.html	Directory of surgeon members, conferences, programs for surgical residents, discussion group	Discussion group: members helping members
Society of Thoracic Surgeons www.sts.org	*The Annals of Thoracic Surgery* (full-text articles, discussion forums, online manuscript review, and much more) www.sts.org/annals	STS National Cardiac Surgery database, cardiac surgery data analyses	Forums for surgeons (members only), forums for everyone
Vascular Surgical Societies www.vascsurg.org	*Journal of Vascular Surgery* (full-text and abstracts) www.mosby.com/scripts.om.dll.serve?action=searcjDB&searchDBfor=home&id=vs	Research initiatives and grants, physician database, lifeline foundation	Clinical case forum

with colleagues, and promote research. It offers access to COS expertise, COS funding opportunities, Commerce Business Daily, funded research information, the Federal Register, and a COS funding alert. Searching these products requires registration, although it is free to any individual involved with the scientific community.

Table IV Discussion Groups and Forums

Name	Subscription address and message	Highlights
Internet Craniofacial Surgery Discussion	Listserv@cesar.unicamp.br Subscription message: SUBSCRIBE CFSURG-L your name	A discussion group for the discipline; provides notices of new online articles from the OnLine Journal of Plastic and Reconstructive Surgery
Online Facial Plastic Surgery Discussions Mail List	FACEnet-request@tali.uchsc.edu Subscription message: Subscribe (in the subject line)	Devoted to discussion of facial plastic surgery
Society of Laparoendoscopic Surgeons Mail List	majordomo@indra.com Subscription message: Subscribe SLS	Discusses issues regarding diagnostic and therapeutic uses of laparoendoscopic techniques and minimally invasive surgery
Surginet General Surgeons Mail List	www.lsoft.com/scripts/wl.exe?SL1=SURGINET&H=LISTSERV.UTORONTO.CA	Discusses all aspects of general surgery; subscription requires medical credentials; unmoderated, 500+ subscribers

D. Reference Sources

Internet reference sources are composed of four groups: subject indices, directories, electronic full-text books, and online library catalogs (see Table VII). Medical Matrix is one of the few medical subject indices. Its refereed selective nature makes Medical Matrix a unique guide to ranked, peer-reviewed, annotated, and updated clinical medicine resources. First-time users are required to register, but using it is free. Medscape, a new and growing electronic service, aggregates many useful online functions. It is a subject index that provides access to MEDLINE and other databases, offers a variety of full-text electronic journals, and more. One of the most valuable aspects of Medscape is that it gives the user an opportunity to customize a profile such as surgery. Subsequently, the default screen will be loaded with surgery-related resources. Once a week, the Medscape user will get an e-mail alert about surgery news filtered from the major news services, as well as a journal scan, clinical summaries and highlights from *Annals of Surgery, Archives of Surgery, JAMA, Lancet*, and *New England Journal of Medicine*. Similar to Medical Matrix, Medscape requires registration up front, but it is free.

Directories of both people and organizations are posted on the Web. Almost all associations and societies provide access to specialized membership directories. The National Library of Medicine supports DIRLINE, directory of biomedical organizations with summary descriptions and

Table V Federal Funding Sources

Agency/organization	Resource	Highlights
CDC National Prevention Information Network www.cdcnpin.org.start.htm	NPIN Funding Database www.cdcnpin.org/db/public/fundmain.htm	Private and government funding opportunities for community-based and HIV/AIDS, STD, and TB service organizations
Food and Drug Administration www.fda.gov	FDA Grants Opportunities www.fda.gov/oc/ofacs/grants/default.htm	Current RFAs; upcoming RFAs
National Institutes of Health www.nih.gov	CRISP (Computer Retrieval of Information on Scientific Projects) www.nih.gov/grants/award.crisp.htm	Searchable database of federally funded biomedical research projects
National Science Foundation www.nsf.gov	FastLane (electronic business) www.fastlane.nsf.gov	Proposal Review, Panel Review, Panelist Travel System, Panel Pilot, and more
Department of Health and Human Services www.os.dhhs.gov	GrantsNet www.os.dhhs.gov/progorg/grantsnet	A tool for finding and exchanging information
Federal agencies	FEDIX (Federal Information Exchange) web.fie.com/htdoc/fed/all/any/any/menu/any/index.htm	Searchable interface, information on funding opportunities for research

Table VI Nonfederal Funding Sources

Agency/organization	Resource	Highlights
Charles Dana Foundation www.dana.org	Grant Making www.dana.org/grants	Guidelines; summaries of active grant projects; list of publications and peer-reviewed articles
Foundation Center fdncenter.org	Foundation Finder lnp.fdncenter.org/finder.html	Basic information about foundations in the United States
Howard Hughes Medical Institute (HHMI) www.hhmi.org	HHMI Investigators www.hhmi.org/home/research/invest.html	Investigators' names, institutional affiliations, and researcher abstracts for the current year are searchable
W. K. Kellogg Foundation www.wkkf.org	Kellogg Foundation Grants www.wkkf.org/grants/default.htm	Online database of Kellogg Foundation's current grants

contact information. Other directories include best hospitals, medical and research centers, and medical schools in the United States and Canada.

Electronic full-text reference books, with the benefits of instant availability, searching, and browsing functions, are of high value to a researcher. Whereas one has to wait for the new edition of the print book to be published, electronic publications are updated frequently. Harrison's Online Principles of Internal Medicine and Scientific American Medicine Online are examples of reference resources, available by subscription only. Unlike the print version, Harrison's Online has multimedia content, overviews of clinical trials, links to MEDLINE entries, and updated drug and therapy information. MDConsult is an example of a collection of medical textbooks with Sabiston's "Textbook of Surgery" as one of them. The service is equipped with searching and browsing capability, available by subscription only (see Table VIII).

There are full-text handbooks available free on the Web, developed by many institutions, including the University of Iowa, the Naval Aerospace Medical Institute, and the Brigham and Women's Hospital in Boston.

E. Electronic Publishing

Electronic publishing intensified the debate of what is published, how it is reviewed, and how fast it is delivered to the research community. A recent editorial in the *BMJ: British Medical Journal* claims the "burgeoning of the world wide web makes it inevitable that new systems of disseminating research will replace or at least supplement traditional journals" (9). The electronic journals support search/browsing capability and provide instructions for authors, thus continuing a traditional mission of print publishing online (for access points to electronic journals see Table IX). At the same time, publishers and researchers alike create new ways to disseminate information to satisfy special needs of medical researchers. According to an editorial published in *Lancet* "the research with which they must keep up to date is fragmented across many journals" (10). Indeed, the *BMJ* editorial that was quoted earlier suggests, "anybody who has ever attempted a systematic review knows that it's extremely difficult to find all relevant research studies and very expensive to get copies once you do locate them" (9). To address these issues, members of prominent research journals have developed several initiatives:

Table VII Subject Indices, Directories, and Services

Name	Web address	Publisher
Directory of General Clinical Research Centers	www.ncrr.nih.gov/ncrrprog/clindir/content.htm	National Institutes of Health
Directory of Biomedical Technology Resource Centers	www.ncrr.nih.gov/ncrrprog/btrctitl.htm	National Institutes of Health
DIRLINE: Directory of Health Organizations	sis.nlm.nih.gov/dirline	National Library of Medicine: Specialized Information Services
Hardin Meta Directory of Health Sources	www.lib.uiowa.edu/hardin/md/submit.html	Hardin Library for the Health Sciences (University of Iowa)
Health Web	healthweb.org/subjABC.html	Collaborative project of the health science libraries
Medical Matrix	www.medmatrix.org/index.asp	Medical Matrix L.L.C.
Medscape	www.medscape.com	Medscape, Inc.

Table VIII Handbooks and Textbooks

Reference literature	Cost	Author	Notes
Correlapedia—A Correlative Encyclopedia of Pediatric Imaging, Surgery, and Pathology; last revision date, Dec. 15, 1997 www.vh.org/Orivuders/Teachingfiles/CAPHome.html	Free	Michael P. D'Alessandro, M.D.; Steven J. Fishman, M.D.; and Deborah E. Schofield	Internally peer reviewed (Virtual Hospital)
General Surgery (University of Iowa Family Practice Handbook), 3rd Ed., Chapter 9 www.vh.org/Providers/ClinRef/FPHandbook/09html	Free	Mark A. Graber, M.D.	Externally peer reviewed by Mosby
Harrison's Online Principles of InternalMedicine www.harrisonsonline.com	Subscription, $89.00 yearly	Anthony S. Fauci, Eugene Braunwald, Kurt J. Isselbacher, Dennis L. Kasper, Stephen L. Hauser, Dan L. Longo, and J. Larry Jameson	e-mail: harrisons@romnet.com; fax: 1-617-783-4375; telephone: 1-800-448-1237
The Illustrated Encyclopedia of Human Anatomic Variation; creation date, January, 1996; last revision date, May, 1999 www.vh.org/Providers/Textbooks/AnatomicVariants/AnatomyHP.html	Free	Ronald A. Bergman, Ph.D.; Adel K. Afifi, M.D., M.S.; and Ryosuke Miyauchi, M.D.	Internally peer reviewed
Sabiston: "Textbook of Surgery," 15th Ed., W. B. Saunders Company, 1997	Subscription	David C. Sabiston, Jr., M.D.; and H. Kim Lyerly M.D.	MDConsult (e-mail: customer.service@mdconsult.com; telephone: 800-401-9962)
Online Atlas of Surgery www.bgsm.edu/surg-sci/atlas/atlas.html	Free	Carl J. Westcott, M.D., Wake Forest University	Contact for permission to reproduce
Online Laparoscopic Technical Manual (TransMed Network) www/transmed.net/lapnet/lapmenu.htm	Free	From the book "International Laparoscopy" by Philippe J. Quilici, M.D., FACS	e-mail: transmed@transmed.net
Scientific American Medicine Online (SAM Online); updated quarterly www.samed.com	Subscription, $159 yearly	Editor-in-chief, David C. Dale, M.D.	Contact info: 800-291-5489
1997 U.S. Naval Flight Surgeon Manual, 3rd Ed., 1991 www.vnh.org/FSManual/fsm91.html	Free	Naval Aerospace Medical Institute	Internally peer reviewed
The Whole Brain Atlas (Departments of Radiology and Neurology at Brigham and Women's Hospital, American Academy of Neurology) www.med.harvard.edu/AANLIB/home.html	Free	Keith A. Johnson, M.D. (keith@bwh.harvard.edu); J. Alex Becker (jabecker@mit.edu)	Externally reviewed

1. BMJ Publishing Group proposes to set up an eprint server for clinical medicine and health research in partnership with Stanford University libraries.

2. *JAMA*-EXPRESS offers a rapid peer review and publication option for papers of great scientific or public health importance (11).

3. *BMJ* and *Lancet* utilize fast-track systems for publication of papers (12, 13).

4. The *British Journal of Surgery* supports Scientific Surgery, a monthly electronic publication of randomized controlled trials and meta-analyses collated from English language publications.

5. *Lancet* initiates electronic publication of the protocols for proposed or ongoing research (14).

6. The American College of Physicians, American Society of Internal Medicine, and the BMJ Publishing Group publish Evidence-Based Medicine bimonthly.

7. *Annals of Internal Medicine* publishes nontechnical summaries of research articles with a link to the original reports and related editorials.

8. *Archives of Surgery* and *JAMA* publish author instructions on preparing reports of randomized controlled trials (archsurg.ama-assn.org/info/auinst_trial.html).

Table IX Electronic Journals

Name	Cost	Vendor
European Journal of Surgical Oncology www.hbuk.co.uk/wbs/jso	Subscription	Academic/IDEAL www.academicpress.com
European Journal of Vascular and Endovascular Surgery journals.harcourt-international.com/wbs/ejv	Subscription	Academic/IDEAL www.academicpress.com
Journal of Surgical Research www.idealibrary.com/cgi-bin/links/toc/jr?null	Subscription	Academic/IDEAL www.academicpress.com
Microvascular Research www.academicpress.com/mvr	Subscription	Academic/IDEAL www.academicpress.com
Archives of Facial Plastic Surgery archfaci.ama-assn.org	Free	American Medical Association (AMA) pubs.ama-assn.org
Archives of Otolaryngology—Head and Neck Surgery archotol.ama-assn.org	Free	AMA pubs.ama-assn.org
Archives of Surgery archsurg.ama-assn.org	Free	AMA pubs.ama-assn.org
Annals of Thoracic Surgery www.sts.org/annals	Subscription	Elsevier www.elsevier.nl
Cardiovascular Surgery	Subscription	Elsevier www.elsevier.nl
Dermatologic Surgery	Subscription	Elsevier www.elsevier.nl
European Journal of Cardio-thoracic Surgery	Subscription	Elsevier www.elsevier.nl
Journal of the American College of Surgeons www.facs.org:80/about_college/acsdept/jacs/jacshome.html	Subscription	Elsevier www.elsevier.nl
Transplantation Proceedings	Subscription	Elsevier www.elsevier.nl
Surgical Clinics of North America www.wbsaunders.com/catalog/wbs-prod.pl?0889-857X	Subscription	MDConsult home.mdconsult.com
Year Book of Hand Surgery	Subscription	MDConsult home.mdconsult.com
Year Book of Plastic, Reconstructive and Aesthetic Surgery	Subscription	MDConsult home.mdconsult.com
Year Book of Surgery	Subscription	MDConsult home.mdconsult.com
Year Book of Vascular Surgery	Subscription	MDConsult home.mdconsult.com
Journal of Invasive Cardiology, Health Management Publications, Inc. www.medscape.com/HMP/JIC/public/JIC-journal.html	Free	Medscape www.medscape.com
Medscape Oncology: a Medscape eMed Journal, Medscape, Inc. www.medscape.com/Medscape/oncology/journal/public/onc.journal.html	Free	Medscape www.medscape.com
American Journal of Surgery www.elsevier.com/locate/amjsurg	Subscription	OVID gateway.ovid.com
Annals of Surgery www.annalsofsurgery.com	Subscription	OVID gateway.ovid.com
Archives of Otolaryngology—Head and Neck Surgery archotol.ama-assn.org	Subscription	OVID gateway.ovid.com
Archives of Surgery archsurg.ama-assn.org	Subscription	OVID gateway.ovid.com
British Journal of Surgery www.bjs.co.uk	Subscription	OVID gateway.ovid.com
Journal of Bone and Joint Surgery, American	Subscription	OVID gateway.ovid.com

continues

Table IX *(continued)*

Name	Cost	Vendor
Journal of Bone and Joint Surgery, British www.jbjs.org.uk	Subscription	OVID gateway.ovid.com
Transplantation www.transplantjournal.com	Subscription	OVID gateway.ovid.com
Langenbeck's Archives of Surgery link.springer-ny.com/link/service/journals/00423/index.htm	Subscription	Springer link.springer-ny.com
Surgical Endoscopy link.springer-ny.com/link/service/journals/00464/index.htm	Subscription	Springer link.springer-ny.com
World Journal of Surgery link.springer-ny.com/link/service/journals/00268/index.htm	Subscription	Springer link.springer-ny.com
Computer Aided Surgery jws-edcc.interscience.wiley.com/cas	Subscription	Wiley www.wiley.com
Head and Neck www3.interscience.wiley.com/cgi-bin/jtoc?ID=38137	Subscription	Wiley www.wiley.com
Journal of Surgical Oncology www3.interscience.wiley.com/cgi-bin/jtoc?ID=31873	Subscription	Wiley www.wiley.com

F. Evidence-Based Medicine

Ongoing clinical trials and the results of completed trials, as well as the systematic review of them, have become an integral part of research. Dr. Iain Chalmers, director of the United Kingdom Cochrane Centre, argues that "trials should be registered to inform patients and other decision makers about trials in which they could participate, to prevent costly research duplication and to promote multicentre trial collaboration" (15). The Cochrane Collaboration spearheaded an international organization to conduct rigorous reviews of clinical trials "to help people to make informed decisions about health care by preparing, maintaining, and promoting the accessibility of systematic reviews on the effects of health care interventions" (16). Several web sites provide access to registers of controlled trials for both researchers and patients (see Tables X and XI).

Table X Controlled Clinical Trials

Name	Company/Agency	Features
Clinical Trials Databases www.nih.gov/health/trials/index.htm	NIH, e-mail:NIHInfo@OD.NIH.GOV	Eight databases available
BIOMED On-going research projects www.cordis.lu/biomed/src/project.htm	Biomedicine & Health Programme, European Commission, e-mail: biomedicine@dg12.cec.be	Pharmaceuticals research; research on biomedical technology and engineering; brain research; cancer research; research on cardiovascular diseases
Cancer Clinical Trials Directory www.fda.gov/oashi/cancer/trials.html	Food and Drug Administration of Special Health Issues, e-mail: oshi@oc.fda.gov www.fda.gov/oashi/home.html	Clinical trials by tumor type and by general categories; NCI designated cancer centers; pediatrics and U.S. government
Current Controlled Trials (CCT) www.controlled-trials.com	Current Controlled Trials Ltd., e-mail: anne@cursci.co.uk or clairem@cursci.co.uk	MetaRegister of controlled trials (mRCT)
Current Clinical Research Studies clinicalstudies.info.nih.gov	Warren Grant Magnuson Clinical Center (CC), NIH, NIH, phone: 301-496-2563	Collection of research studies conducted at the NIH Clinical Center
HIV/AIDS Clinical Trials Databases www.actis.org/actis.asp?URL=database&VIEW=general	AIDS Clinical Trials Information Service, e-mail: ACTIS@actis.org	AIDSTRIALS database; AIDS clinical trial results database; new and ongoing clinical trials
PDQ Clinical Trials Database cancernet.nci.nih.gov/trialsrch.shtml	National Cancer Institute www.nci.nih.gov	Types of trials, status of trials, locations of trials

Table XI Protocol Submission Guidelines

Resource	Provider
Cochrane Library www.update-software.com/ccweb/cochrane/cdsr.htm	Cochrane Collaboration e-mail: info@update.co.uk
CONSORT guidelines www.thelancet.com/newlancet/any/author/body.consort1.html	The Lancet Interactive www.thelancet.com
Food and Drug Administration information sheets (Guidance for Institutional Review Boards and Clinical Investigators) www.fda.gov/oc/oha/IRB/toc.html	Food and Drug Administration e-mail: webmail@oc.fda.gov
Online PDQ protocol submission instructions cancernet.nci.nih.gov/protosub/proto_instr.html	National Cancer Institute
PDQ clinical trials information cancernet.nci.nih.gov/clinpdq/other/Clinical_trials_information_for_physicians.html	National Cancer Institute
Protocol reviews www.thelancet.com/newlancet/any/author/menu_NOD7.html	The Lancet Interactive www.thelancet.com
Reports of original data archsurg.ama_assn.org/info/auinst_abs.html#reports	Archives of surgery instructions for authors
Preparing reports of randomized controlled trials archsurg.ama_assn.org/info/auinst_trial.html	archsurg.ama_assn.org/info/auinst.html
Scientific surgery: Randomized trials www.bjs.co.uk/random.htm	British Journal of Surgery Tel: +44 1865 206126

G. Getting Published

Choosing the proper journal is an important decision to make before submitting an article for publication, and the Journal Citation Reports is a perfect tool to point the researcher to a cluster of relevant journals. It is also important to establish whether the journal is peer-reviewed and how many databases index it. Ulrich's International Periodicals Directory, available online by subscription only, is a good source for this.

Finding instructions for authors on an electronic journal site is useful and efficient (see Table XII). Another alternative is to use the PubMed journal browser feature that links to the journal publishers' web sites. A third tool needed is style manuals, many of which are available full-text on the web (see Table XII).

H. Evaluating Internet Resources

Editors of leading journals argue that "the same set of quality moorings that help users of medical information navigate in print should apply in the digital world" (17). They list core standards that are applicable in an electronic context as well:

Table XII Author Instructions and Style Manuals

Resource	Provider
How to cite ACP Journal Club www.acponline.org/journals/acpjc/jccite.htm	ACP Journal Club
Instructions to authors in the health sciences www.mco.edu/lib/instr/libnsta.html	Raymon H. Mulford Library, Medical College of Ohio
MLA style www.mla.org/main_stl.htm	Modern Language Association
Uniform requirements for manuscripts submitted to biomedical journals www.acponline.org/journals/annals/01jan97/unifreqr.htm	International Committee of Medical Journal Editors
World Wide Web policy and procedures www.ed.gov/internal/wwwstds.html	U.S. Department of Education
Writing-related resources owl.english.purdue.edu/writers	Purdue University's writing lab

Table XIII Meta-Sites of Selected Internet Resources

Resource	Provider
Countway web resources www.countway.harvard.edu/web_resources	Countway Library of Medicine, Harvard Medical School
Health Web healthweb.org/index.html	Health sciences libraries of the greater midwest region,National Network of Libraries of Medicine, Committee of Institutional Cooperation
MedWeb www.MedWeb.Emory.Edu/MedWeb	Health Sciences Center Library, Emory University
Selected internet resources in biomedicine www.med.yale.edu/library/sir	Cushing/Whitney Medical Library, Yale School of Medicine

1. Authorship: authors and contributors, their affiliations, and relevant credentials should be provided.

2. Attribution: references and sources for all content should be listed clearly, and all relevant copyright information noted.

3. Disclosure: web site "ownership" should be prominently and fully disclosed, as should any sponsorship, advertising, underwriting, commercial funding arrangements or support, or potential conflicts of interest.

4. Currency: dates that content was posted and updated should be indicated (17).

A more complete version of the criteria for accessing the quality of surgical information on the Internet was recently published in the *Journal of the Royal College of Surgeons of Edinburgh*, and these four basic standards are part of the list. The Internet is at its best generating easy access of research material and making it immediately available. It is precisely because there is so much of it, however, that it has the potential for being a minefield of misinformation, according to McKinley *et al.* (18). They caution "it is important to think critically about the 'facts' presented when searching for surgical information on the Net."

Discovering and evaluating Internet resources is a difficult and time-consuming task. Select two or three meta-sites that aggregate well-organized links, using specific ranking and reviewing mechanisms (see Table XIII). The sites created by librarians reflect the quality and logic of traditional library organization. The associations' web sites link to subject specific information, organized in a nontraditional fashion. Each of the above approaches has its limitations, therefore it is wise to select several of them, learn how they work, and use them continuously.

Resource discovery alone is a worthwhile endeavor in a surgeons' long-term strategy to seek knowledge. Information discovery is the other essential component vital to surgeons' intellectual growth and skill. Indeed, T. S. Eliot's words "Where is the wisdom we have lost in knowledge? Where is the knowledge we have lost in information?" still pose the most important questions of all (19).

IV. Suggested Reading

The following list of literature provides general information on resources for surgical research.

Adelhard, K., and Obst, O. (1999). Evaluation of medical internet sites. *Methods Inf. Med.* **38,** 75–79.

Brazier, H., and McCabe, G. (1998). Making the most of MEDLINE. *Hosp. Med.* **59,** 756–758, 760–761.

Clarke, M., Greaves, L., and James, S. (1997). MeSH terms must be used in Medline searches. *BMJ* **314,** 1203.

Conway, S., and Messerle, J. (1990). Searching MEDLINE: Finding needles in the medical haystack. *Group Pract. J.* **39,** 26–28, 30, 32–34.

Garden, D. L., Dronen, S. C., Gehrig, G., and Zalenski, R. J. (1998). Funding strategies for emergency medicine research. *Acad. Emerg. Med.* **5,** 168–176.

Goldstein, J. L., and Brown, M. S. (1997). The clinical investigator: Bewitched, bothered, and bewildered—but still beloved. *J. Clin. Invest.* **99,** 2803–2812.

Greenhalgh, T. (1997). How to read a paper. The Medline database. *BMJ* **315,** 180–183.

Halperin, E. C. (1999) Publish or perish—and bankrupt the medical library while we're at it. *Acad. Med.* **74,** 470–472.

Haynes, R. B., Wilczynski, N., Kibbon, K. A., Walker, C. J., and Sinclair, J. C. (1994). Developing optimal search strategies for detecting clinically sound studies in MEDLINE. *J. Am. Med. Inform. Assoc.* **1,** 447–458.

Horrobin, D. F. (1996) Peer review of grant applications: A harbinger for mediocrity in clinical research? *Lancet* **348,** 1293–1295.

Jadad, A. R., and Gagliardi, A. (1998). Rating health information on the internet. *JAMA* **279,** 611–614

McKinley J., Cattermole H., and Oliver C. W. (1999). The quality of surgical information on the Internet. *J. R. Coll. Surg. Edinb.* **44,** 265–268.

Silberg, W. M., Lundberg, G. D., and Musacchio, R. A. (1997). Assessing, controlling, and assuring the quality of medical information on the internet. *JAMA* **277,** 1244–1245.

Woods, D., and Trewheellar, K. (1999). MedLine and Embase complement each other in literature searches. *BMJ* **316,** 166.

Woods, S. E., and Francis, B. W. (1996). MEDLINE as a component of the objective structured clinical examination: The next step in curriculum integration. *Bull. Med. Libr. Assoc.* **84,** 108–109

References

1. Nuland, S. B. (1994). A surgeon's valedictory. *Perspect. Biol. Med.* **37,** 160.

2. Lederberg, J. (1987). Personal essay. *In* "Medicine: Preserving the Passion" (P.R. Manning and L. DeBakey), p. 69. Springer-Verlag, New York.
3. Monks, G. H. (1928). Selections from the medical writings and sayings of Dr. Oliver Wendell Holmes. *Boston Med. Surg. J.* **197,** 1392.
4. Minot, C. S. (1899). Knowledge and practice. *Science* **10,** 7 [new series].
5. Minot, C. S. (1899). Knowledge and practice. *Science* **10,** 7 [new series].
6. Popper, K. R. (1959). "The Logic of Scientific Discovery," p. 281. Basic Books, New York.
7. Weiss, P. (1960). Knowledge: A growth process. *Science* **131,** 1716.
8. Hersh, W. (1999). A world of knowledge at your fingertips: The promise, reality, and future directions of on-line information retrieval. *Acad. Med.* **74,** 240–243.
9. Delamothe, T., and Smith, R. (1999). Moving beyond journals: The future arrives with a crash. *BMJ* **318,** 1637–1638.
10. Editorial (1999). NIH E-biomed proposal: A welcome jolt. *Lancet* **353,** 1985.
11. Winker, M. A., and Fontanarosa, P. B. (1999). JAMA-EXPRESS: Rapid peer review and publication. *JAMA* **281,** 1754–1755.
12. Goldbeck-Wood S., and Robinson, R. (1999). BMJ introduces a fast track system for papers. *BMJ* **318,** 620.
13. McNamee D., and Horton R. (1997). Fast-track to publication in The Lancet. *Lancet* **349,** 970.
14. Chalmers, I., and Altman, D. G. (1999). How can medical journals help prevent poor medical research? Some opportunities presented by electronic publishing. *Lancet* **353,** 490–493.
15. Yamey, G. (1999). Scientists who do not publish trial results are "unethical." *BMJ* **319,** 939.
16. Jadad, A. R., Cook, D. J., Jones, A., Klassen, T. P., Tugwell, P., Moher, M., and Moher, D. (1998). Methodology and reports of systematic reviews and meta-analyses: A comparison of Cochrane reviews with articles published in paper-based journals. *JAMA* **280,** 278–280.
17. Silberg, W. M., Lundberg, G. D., and Musacchio, R. A. (1997). Assessing, controlling, and assuring the quality of medical information on the internet. *JAMA* **277,** 1244–1245.
18. McKinley J., Cattermole H., and Oliver C. W. (1999). The quality of surgical information on the Internet. *J. R. Coll. Surg. Edinb.* **44,** 265-8.
19. Eliot, T. S. (1971). Chorus from 'The Rock.' *In* "The Complete Poems and Plays 1909–1950," p. 96. Harcourt, Brace & World, New York.

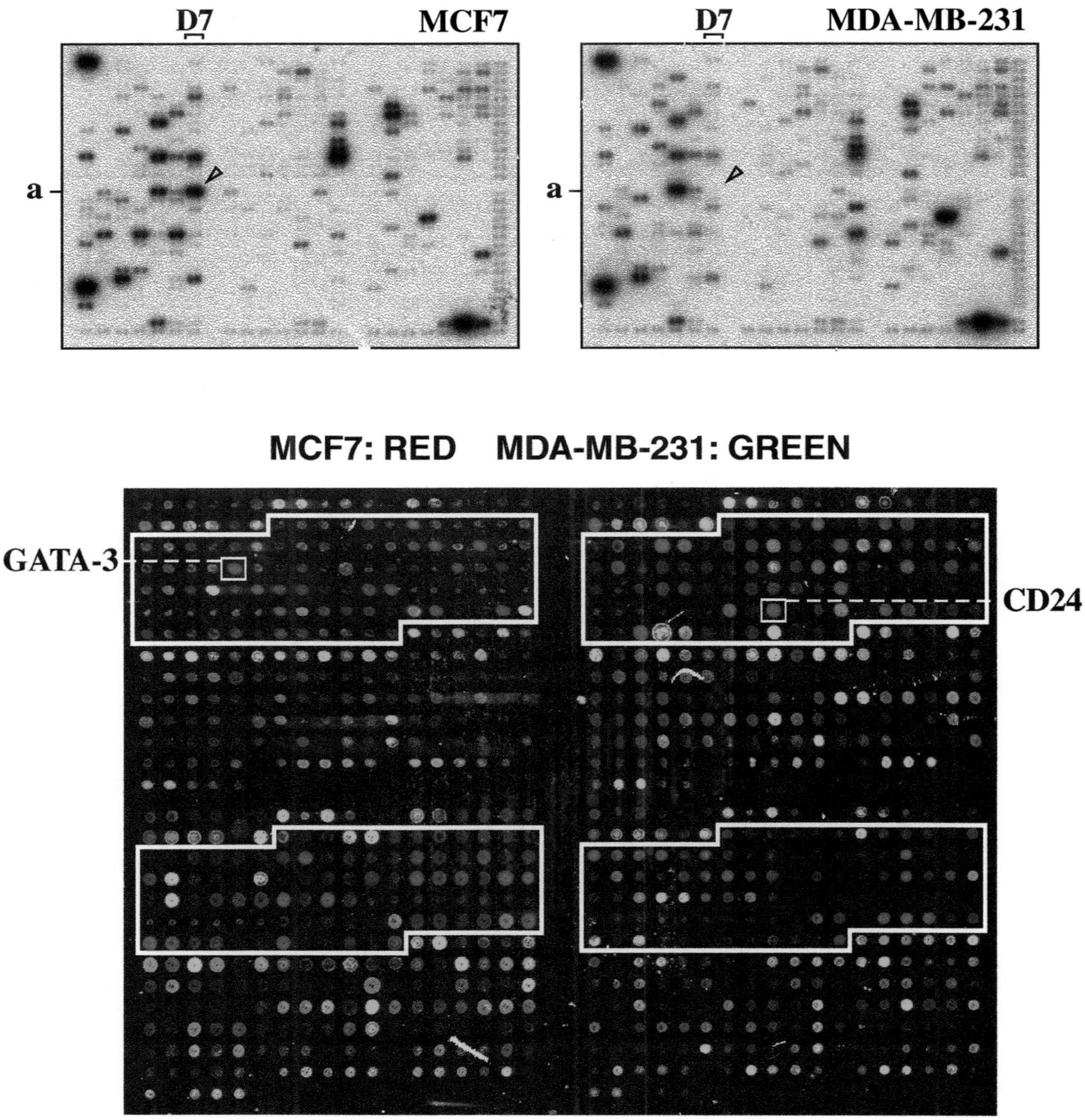

Chapter 21, Figure 6 cDNA arrays. Shown are two examples of conventional arrays (top) and microarrays (bottom) identifying differentially expressed genes comparing MCF7 and MDA-MB-231. In the top figure, the arrow indicates the clone GATA-3 at position D7a. In the bottom figure, GATA-3 is identified on microarrays. The top figure is reprinted from Ref. (22), Hoch, R. V., *et al.* (1999). GATA-3 is expressed in association with estrogen receptor in breast cancer. *Int. J. Cancer* **84**(2), 122–128, copyright © 1999 John Wiley & Sons. Reprinted by permission of Wiley-Liss, Inc., a subsidiary of John Wiley & Sons, Inc. The bottom figure is reprinted from Ref. (24), Yang, G. P., *et al.* (1999). Combining SSH and cDNA microarrays for rapid identification of differentially expressed genes. *Nucleic Acids Res.* **27**(6), 1517–1523, by permission of Oxford University Press.

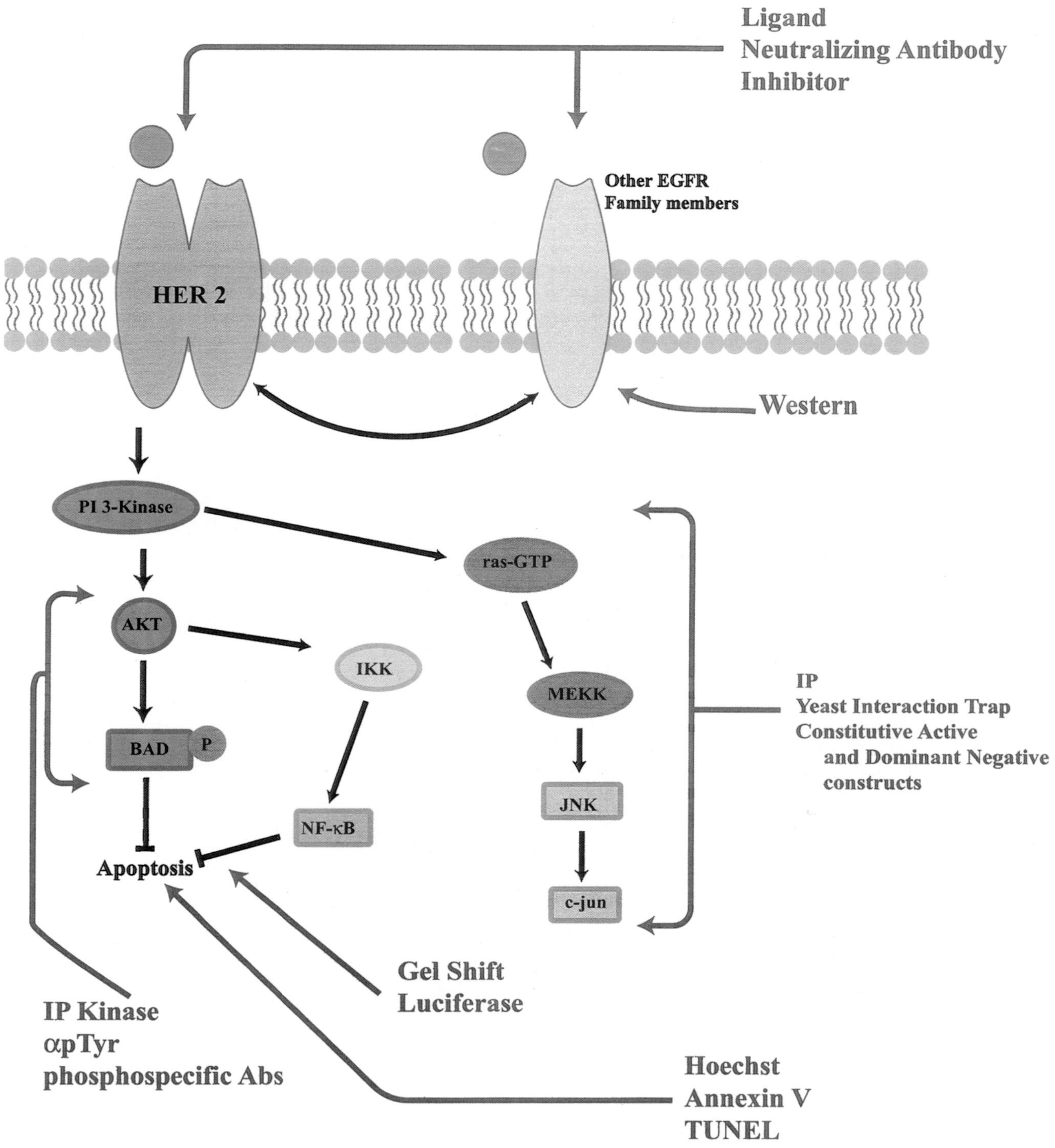

Chapter 22, Figure 1 The Her-2/*neu* signaling cascade. Various signal transduction methodologies can be used to dissect this complex cascade (1).

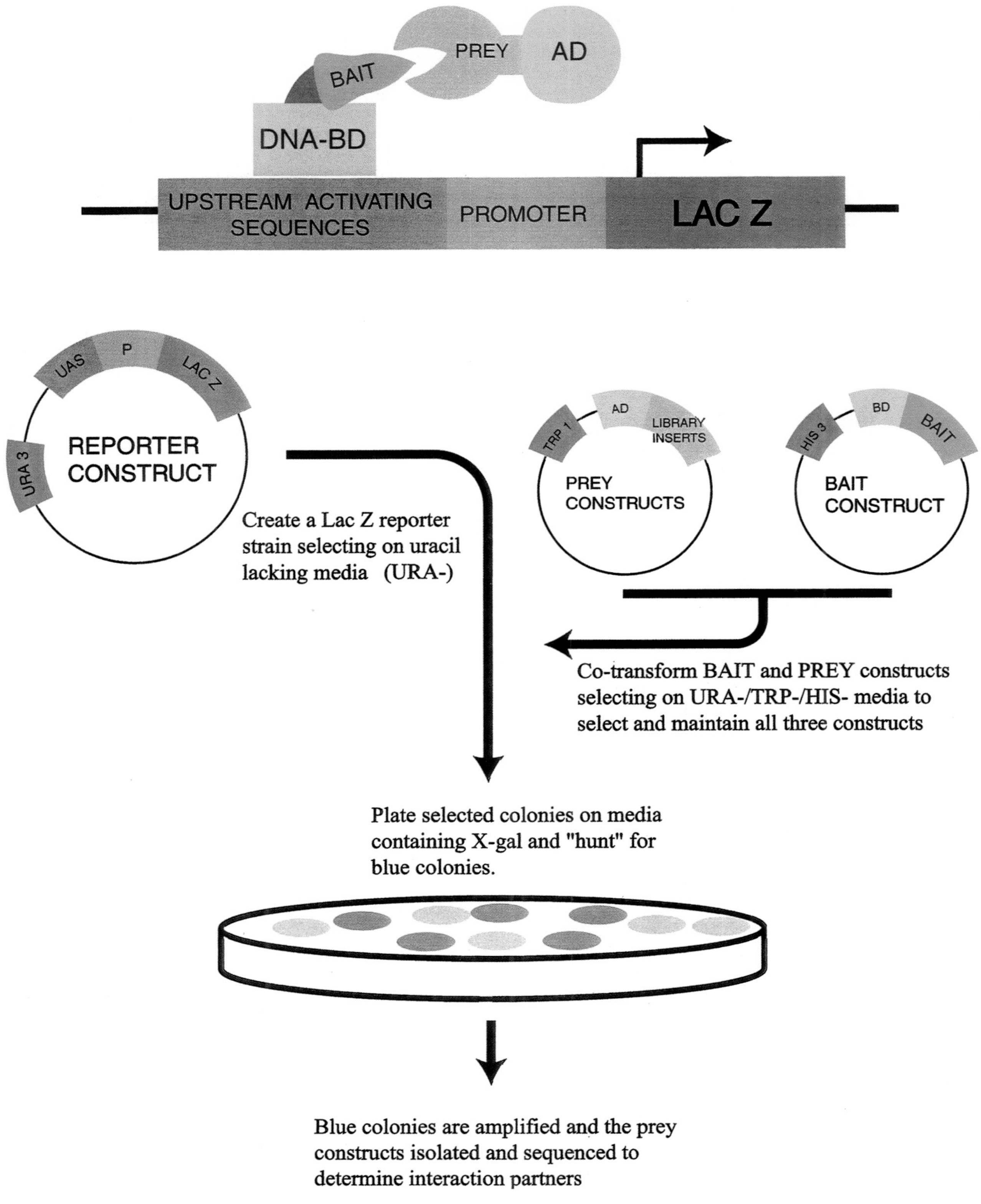

Chapter 22, Figure 8 Yeast two-hybrid system. The prey–AD fusion protein interacts with the bait–DNA BD protein, allowing transcription of *lacZ*. AD, Activation domain; DNA BD, DNA binding domain; UAS, upstream activating sequences; P, promoter.

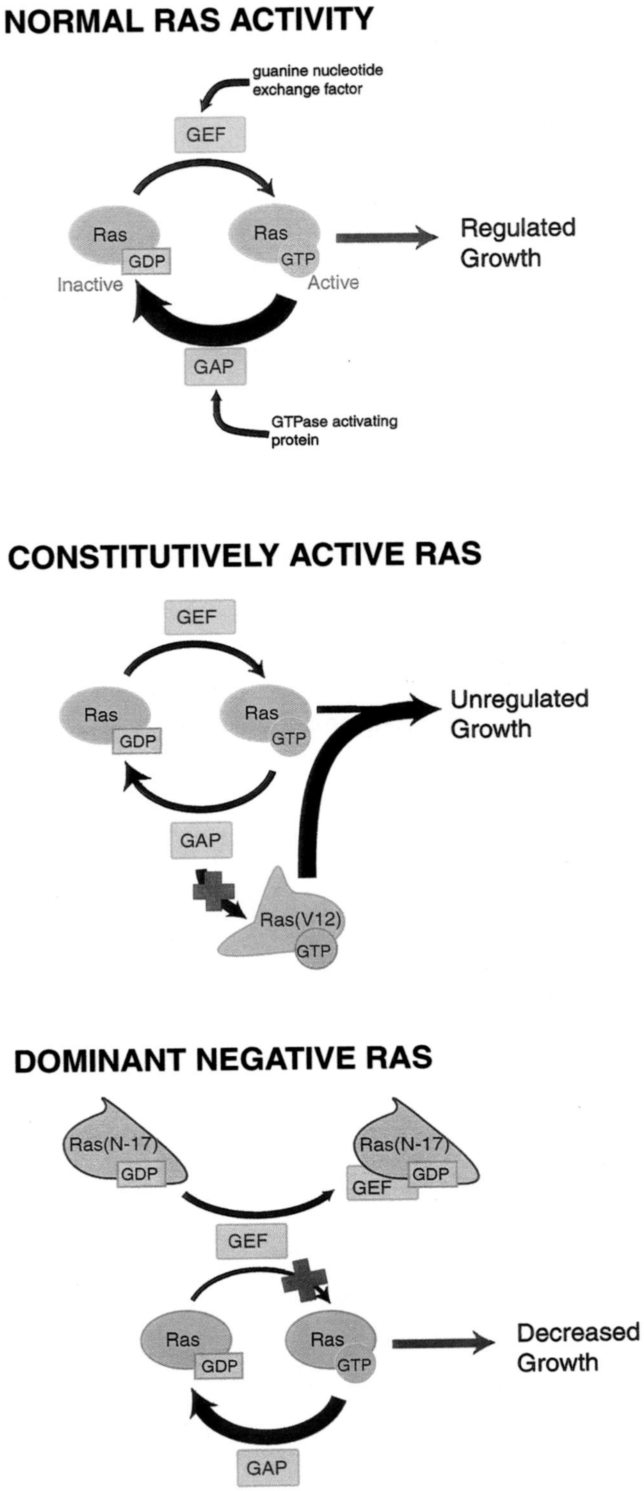

Chapter 22, Figure 13 H-Ras(V12) and H-Ras(N17) are examples of constitutively active and dominant negative proteins. The top panel illustrates wild-type Ras and regulated growth. Ras–GDP is inactive and through the activity of guanidine nucleotide exchange factors (GEFs) the GDP is exchanged for GTP, leading to activation of Ras. GTPase-activating proteins (GAPs) stimulate the intrinsic GTPase activity of Ras, thereby leading to the hydrolysis of GTP to GDP and the deactivation of Ras. H-Ras(V12) contains a single amino acid mutation (Gly to Val at position 12) that renders Ras insensitive to GAPs. So the protein always remains activated because the bound GTP is never hydrolyzed to GDP. H-Ras(N17) contains a different mutation (Ser to Asn at position 17) that gives Ras a preferential affinity for GDP. In this case, Ras(N17)-GDP binds all available GEFs, sequestering them from wild-type Ras. Both mutant Ras(N17) and wild-type Ras remain in the GDP-bound state in this situation, leading to down-regulation of the Ras pathway.

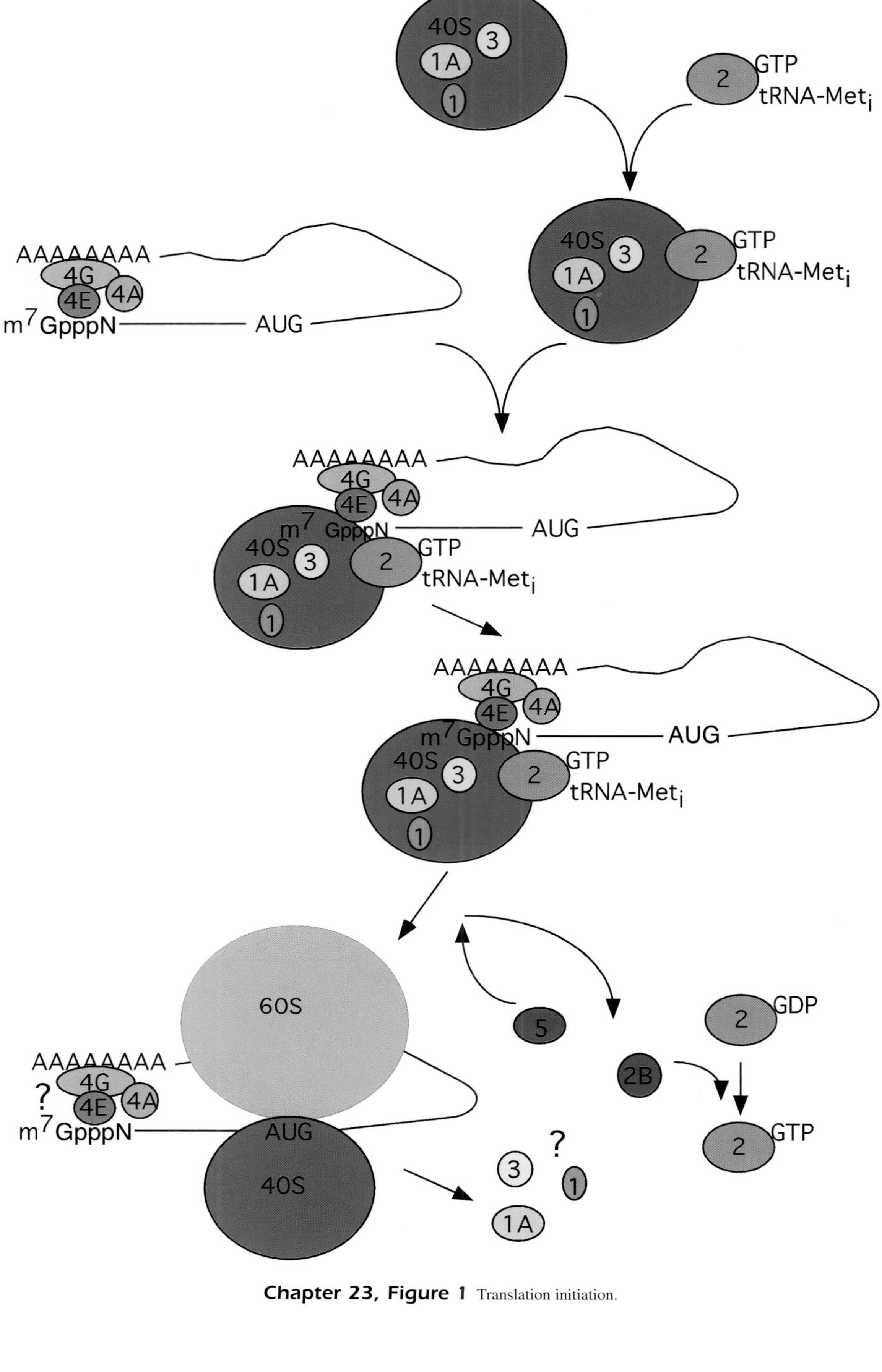

Chapter 23, Figure 1 Translation initiation.

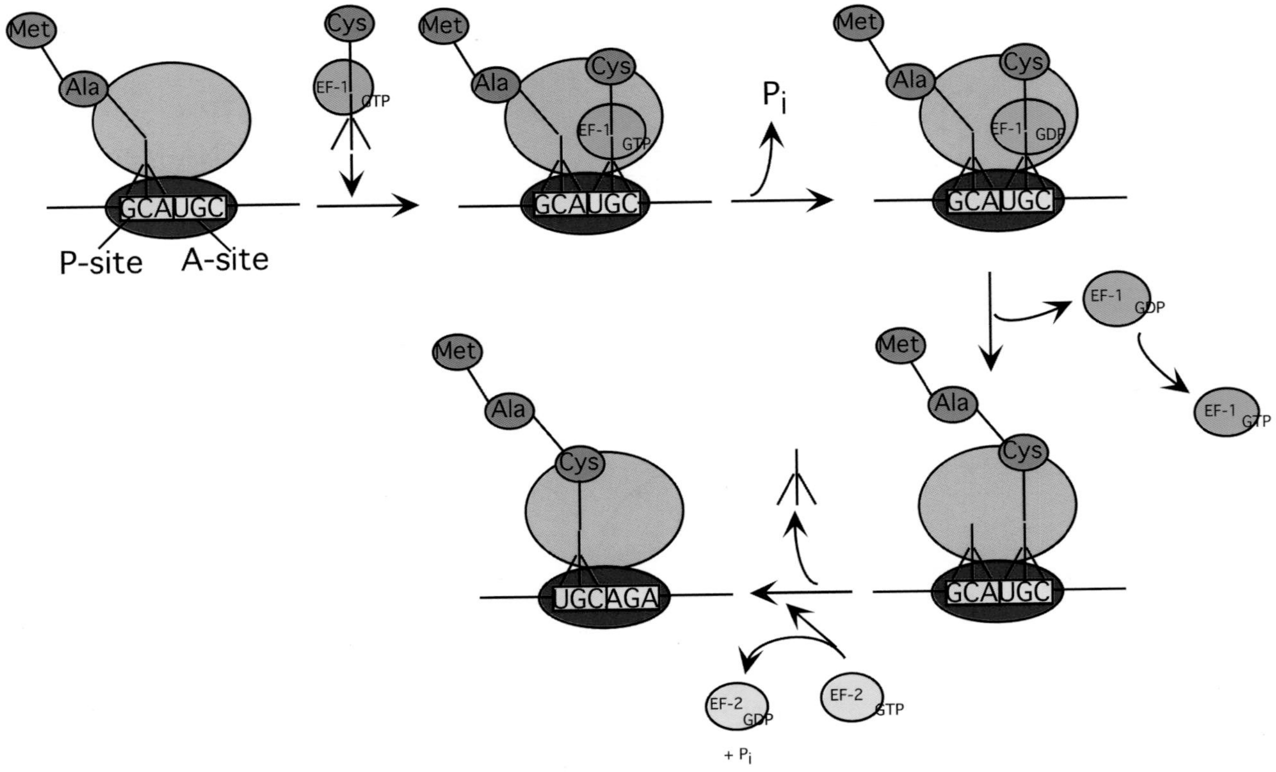

Chapter 23, Figure 2 Translation elongation.

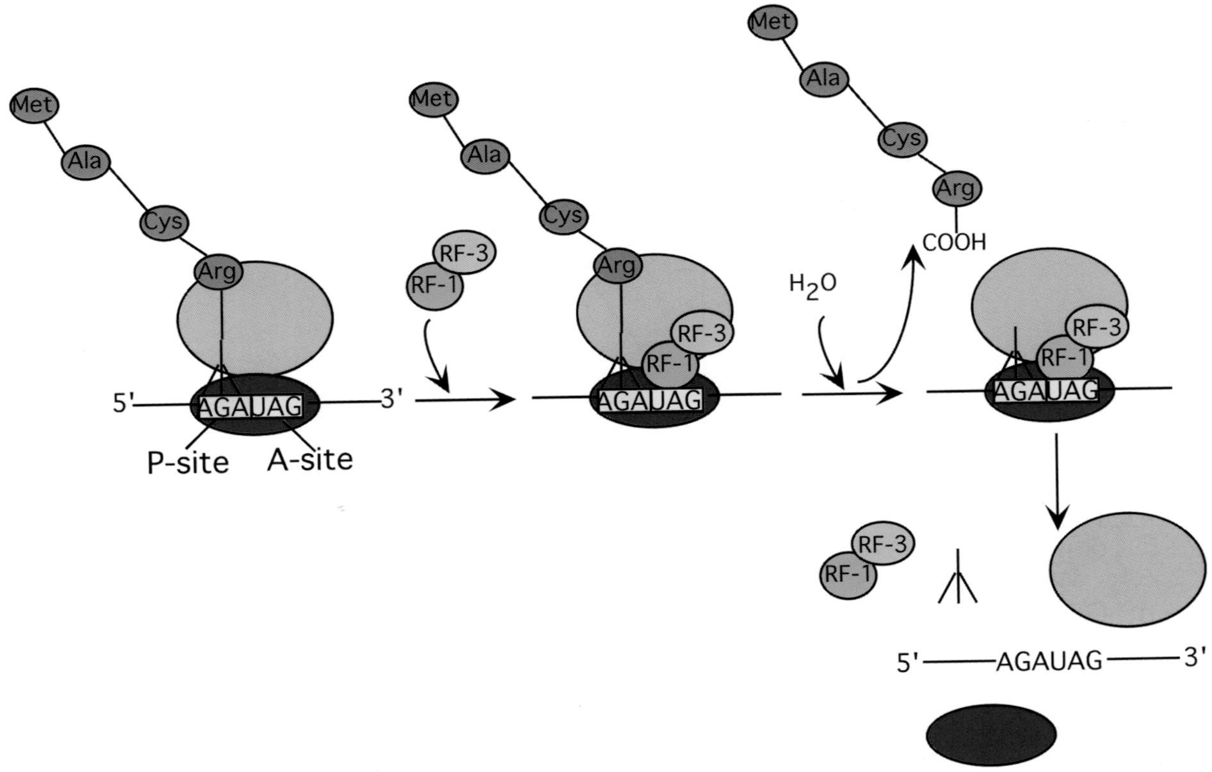

Chapter 23, Figure 3 Translation termination.

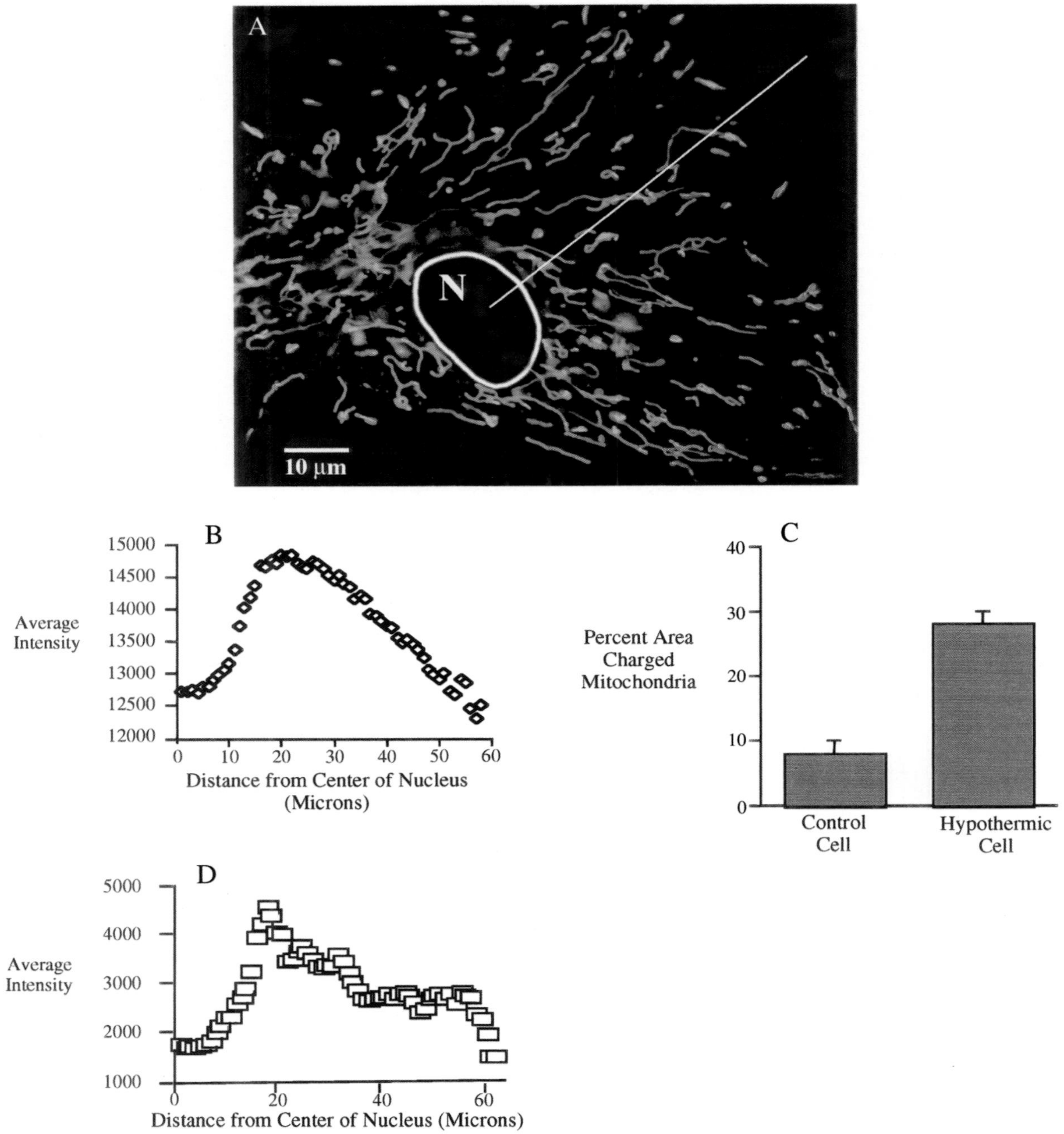

Chapter 24, Figure 5 JC-1-loaded mitochondria show areas of low transmembrane voltage (20 mV. JC-1 monomers only, green) and areas at a high potential (JC-1 aggregates, red). Areas at intermediate potential appear yellow to orange. The nucleus (N) and the cell edge were first found by enhancing the low-intensity autofluorescence. Then the cell body was spanned by a line extending from the nuclear center to 5 μm outside the cell (shown in white). The intensity values for each pixel along the line samples were averaged over 16 lines, each from a different cell, and are presented in panels B and C for the green and red channels, respectively. Generally, all mitochondrial membranes (B) are abundant in the nuclear periphery, and rarer at the cell edge. In contrast, the charged mitochondria plateau (D, note greater density) just near the cell edge. The total number of red pixels (charged mitochondria) can also be expressed as percentage of the total number of green pixels (all mitochondria). (C) Reducing cellular energy demand by cooling to 23°C increases the charged area ($p < 0.01$).

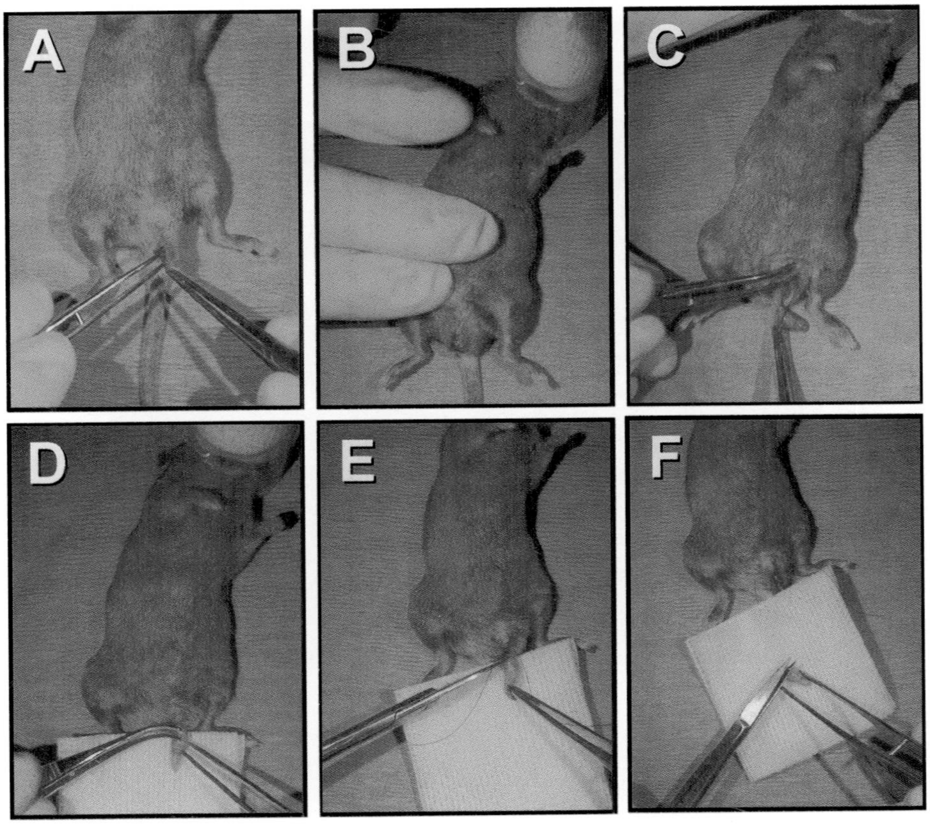

Chapter 30, Figure 1 Surgical castration of the mouse. (A) Scrotal incision. (B) Exposure of the muscular sacs containing the testes. (C) Removal of the testes, epididymis, and vas deferens. (D) Isolation of the testes. (E) Placement of ligature around the blood vessels and vas deferens. (F) Removed testes.

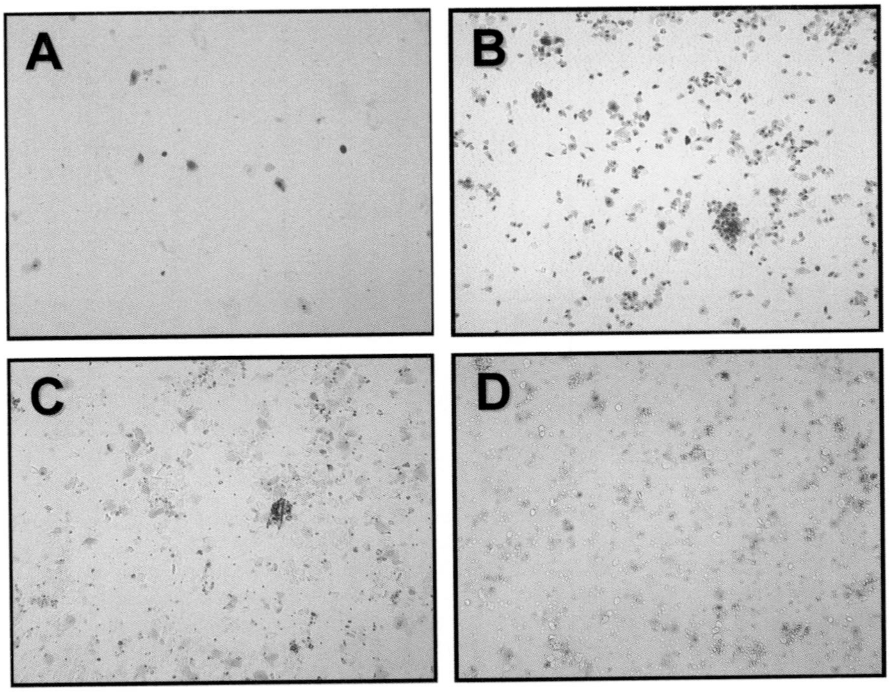

Chapter 30, Figure 2 Vaginal smears from mice at different stages of the estrus cycle. (A) Diestrus, few cells of all types. (B) Proestrus, large numbers of nucleated epithelial cells. (C) Estrus, large numbers of cornified epithelial cells with some nucleated epithelial cells. (D) Postestrus, large numbers of highly refractive polymorphonuclear cells.

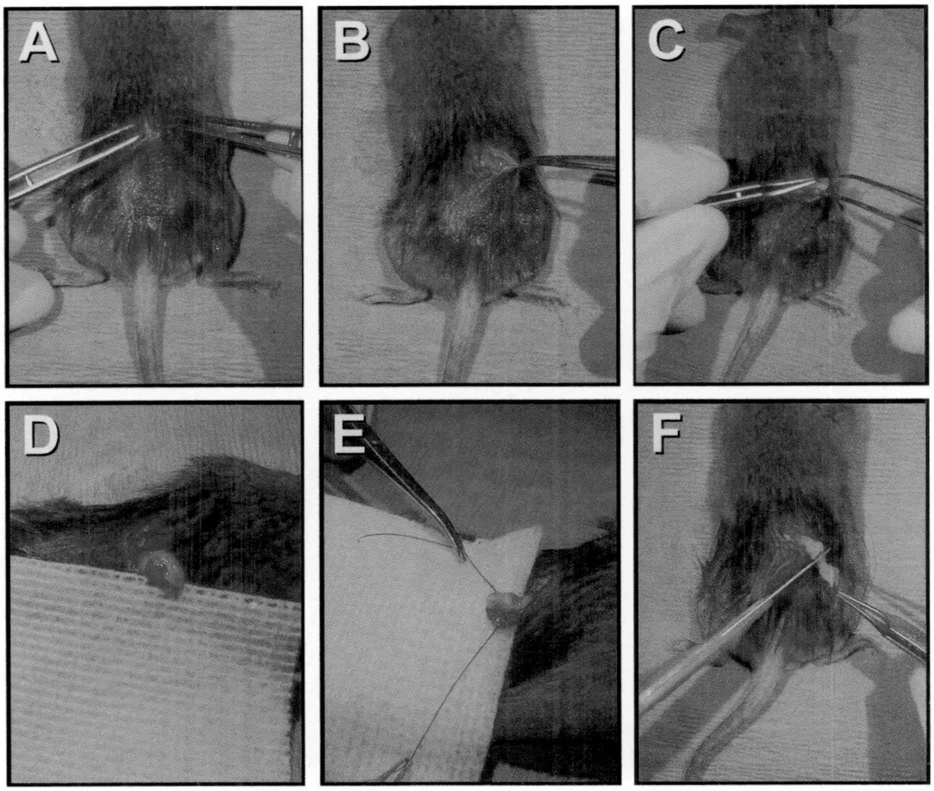

Chapter 30, Figure 3 Surgical ovariectomy of the mouse. (A) Proper placement of midline incision. (B) Retraction of skin incision to one side. (C) Removal of ovary and surrounding fat pad. (D) Isolation of the ovary and fat pad. (E) Placement of ligature around the oviduct and blood vessels. (F) Removal of ovary.

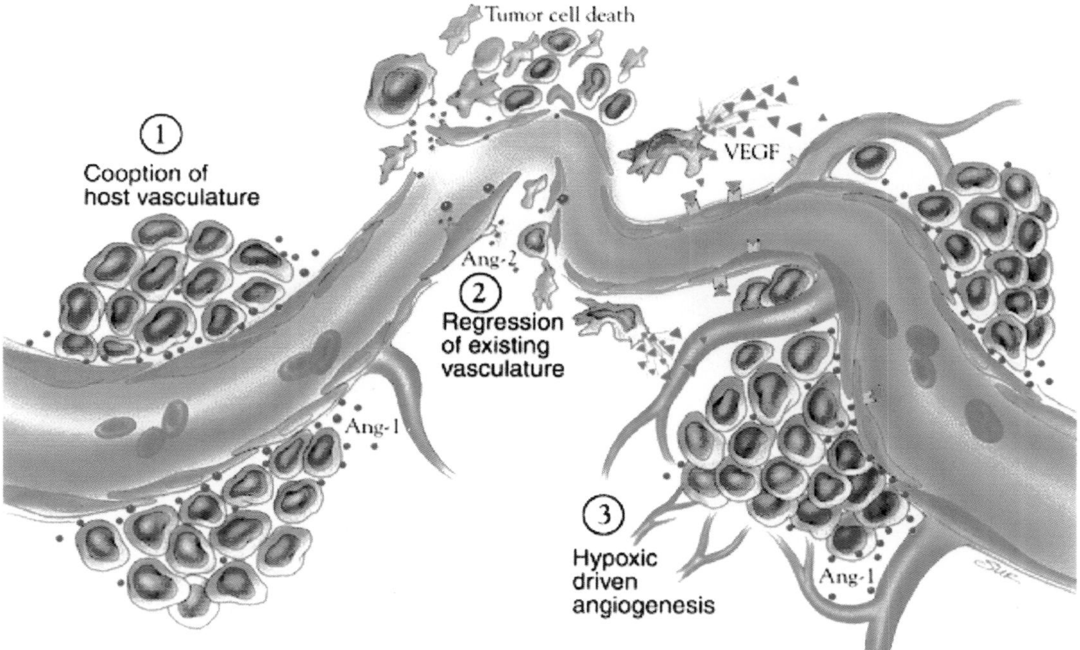

Chapter 34, Figure 1 Host vessel cooption and induction of angiogenesis by tumors. A current hypothesis on tumor angiogenesis suggest that tumors initially use the existing vasculature for a nutrient blood supply. Endothelial cells then release Ang-2, which leads to vessel destabilization and relative hypoxia, which in turn lead to the release of VEGF and robust angiogenesis.

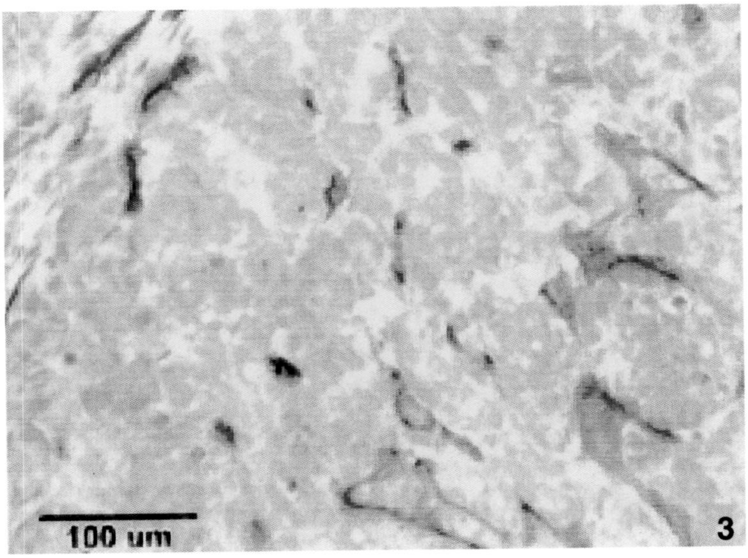

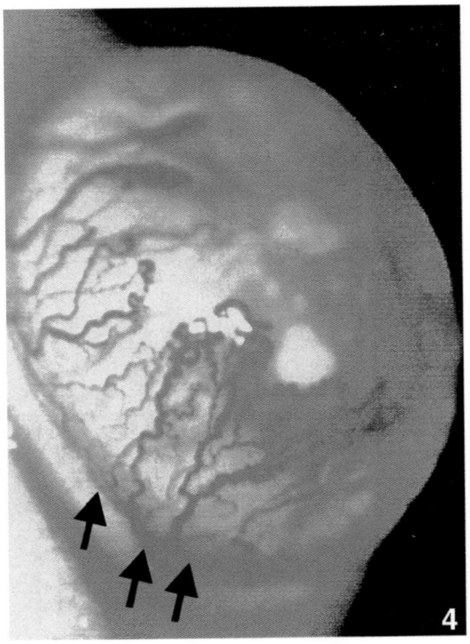

Chapter 34, Figure 3 Examination of tumors for vessel counts. Tumors are harvested and frozen or paraffin embedded. Sections are then stained with an endothelial cell-specific marker and quantified as described in the text. From Shaheen *et al.* (84), with permission.

Chapter 34, Figure 4 Mouse corneal assay for angiogenesis. A micropocket is created in the mouse cornea and a pellet impregnated with an angiogenic factor is implanted therein. Angiogenesis will commence from the corneal margin (arrows). This assay can be used to test systemic inhibitors of angiogenesis by examining the ability of agents to block this neovascularization. From (69) Kenyon *et al.* (1996). A model of the mouse comes. *Invest. Ophthaimol. Vis. Sci.* **37**, 1625–1632, with permission from the Association for Research in Vision and Ophthalmology.

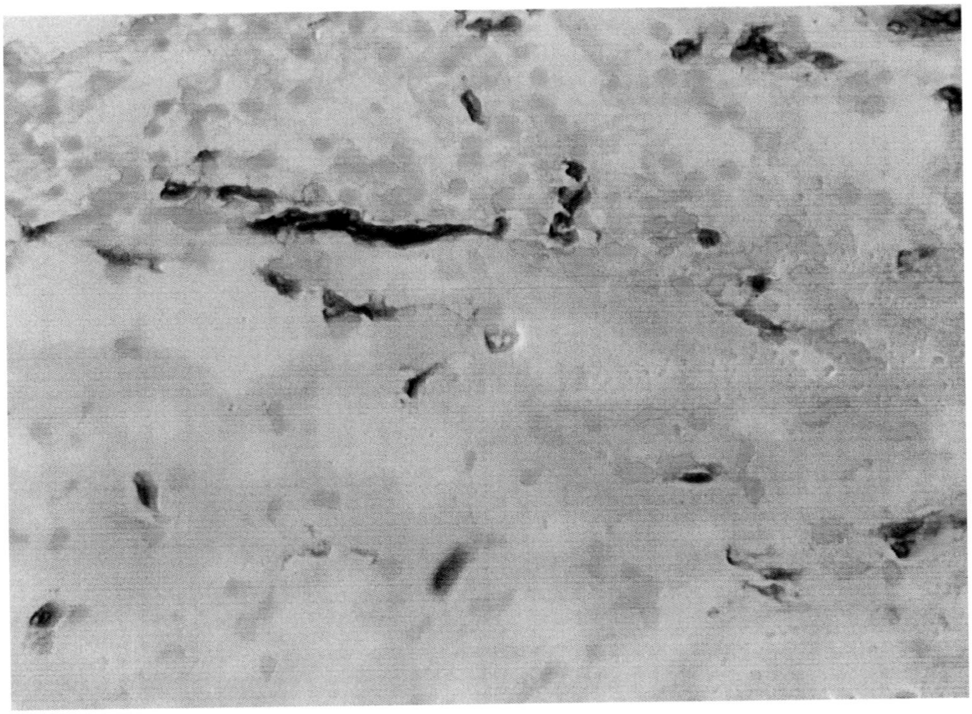

Chapter 34, Figure 5 Matrigel plug assay for angiogenesis. A Matrigel plug (usually mixed with an angiogenic agent) is implanted subcutaneously, harvested (typically 7–10 days later), and processed for immunohistochemistry for the study of newly formed blood vessels. In this specimen, the sample was stained for CD31 (brown) to denote the ingrowth of endothelial cells from the host. Courtesy of Marya McCarty, The University of Texas M. D. Anderson Cancer Center, Houston, Texas.

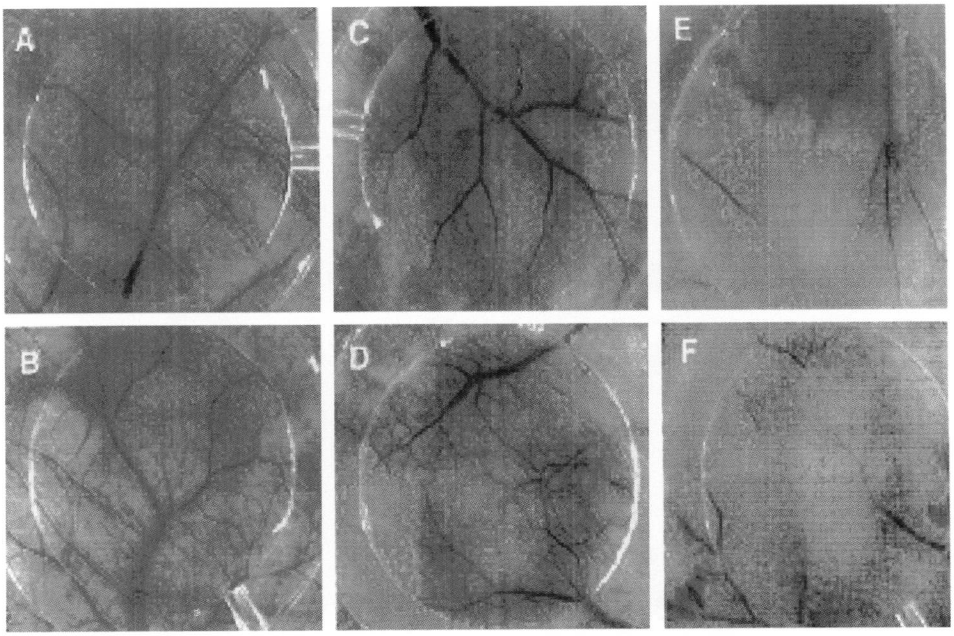

Chapter 34, Figure 6 Dorsal air sac chamber assay for angiogenesis. A subcutaneous pocket is created on the back or flank of mice by repeated injections of air. Cells are then grown on a semipermeable membrane, the membrane is implanted in this pocket, and 7–10 days later the skin flap is retracted and the density of blood vessels observed. In this experiment, the cells on the right (panels E and F) were infected with the wild-type p53 gene, which down-regulated VEGF expression. The cells in panels A–D were controls. From Bouvet *et al.* (58), with permission.

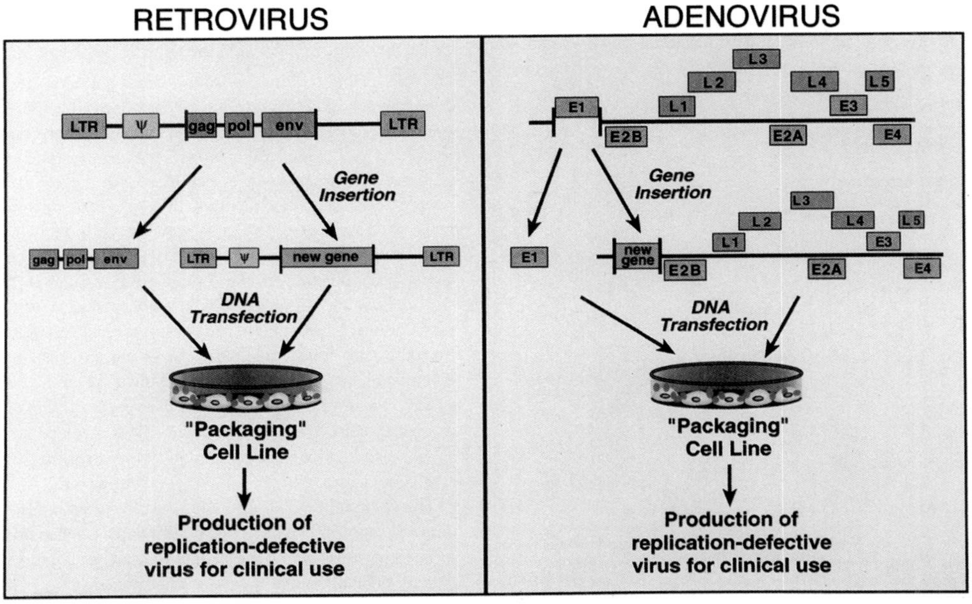

Chapter 38, Figure 1 Replication-defective viral vector systems. (Left) Retroviral vectors are generated by replacing the essential viral genes (*gag, pol,* and *env*) with transgenes. Packaging cell lines have been engineered to express the deleted essential viral genes. Accordingly, introduction of the recombinant retrovirus vector into the packaging cell line results in production of viral particles that can deliver the transgene, but cannot replicate in target cells because they do not express the deleted essential viral genes. (Right) First-generation adenovirus vectors are constructed by replacing the essential *E1* early genes with transgenes. Packaging cells lines have been engineered to express the *E1* gene, and, accordingly, introduction of the recombinant adenovirus vector into the packaging cell line results in production of viral particles that are capable of transgene delivery but incapable of replication in infected target cells. LTR, Long terminal repeat of the retrovirus-encoding gene regulatory sequences; Ψ, the packaging signal required to direct incorporation of viral RNA into the retroviral particles. From (197), G. Dranoff (1998). Cancer gene therapy: Correcting basic research with clinical inquiry. *J. Clin. Oncol.* **16**, 2548–2556.

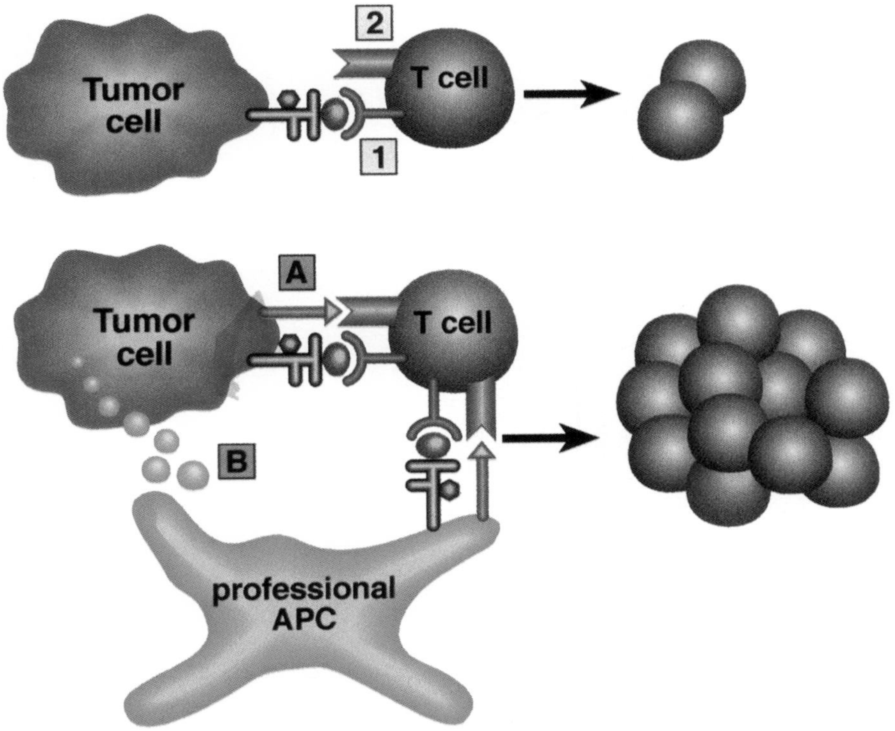

Chapter 38, Figure 2 T cell tolerance occurs when tumor cells present tumor antigens on MHC molecules (1) to T cells without a second costimulatory signal (2). Genetically engineered tumor cells express either costimulatory molecules on their cell surface (A) to activate T cells directly or release cytokines (B) to attract professional APCs, which subsequently activate antigen-specific T cells. (198), T. F. Greten and E. M. Jaffe (1999). Cancer vaccines. *J. Clin. Oncol.* **17**; 1047–1060.

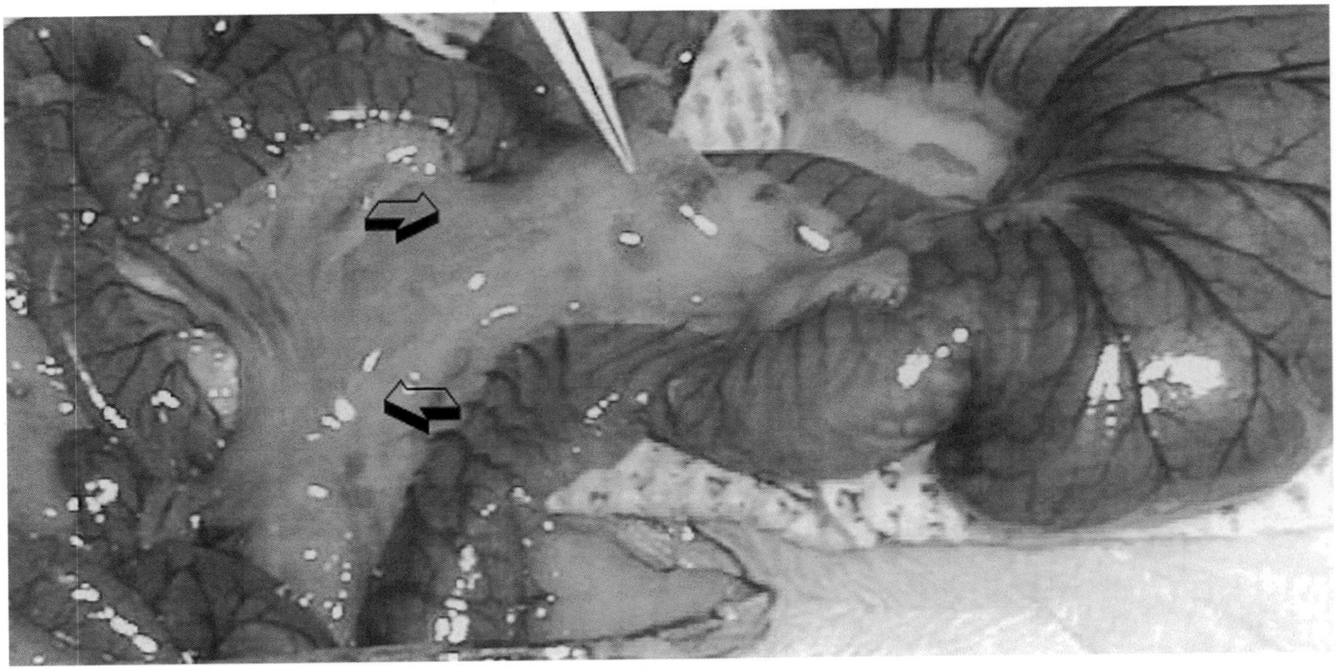

Chapter 46, Figure 1 The mesenteric lymph node complex. The forceps are pointing to segment one of the MLN. The arrows demonstrate the remainder of the MLN chain.

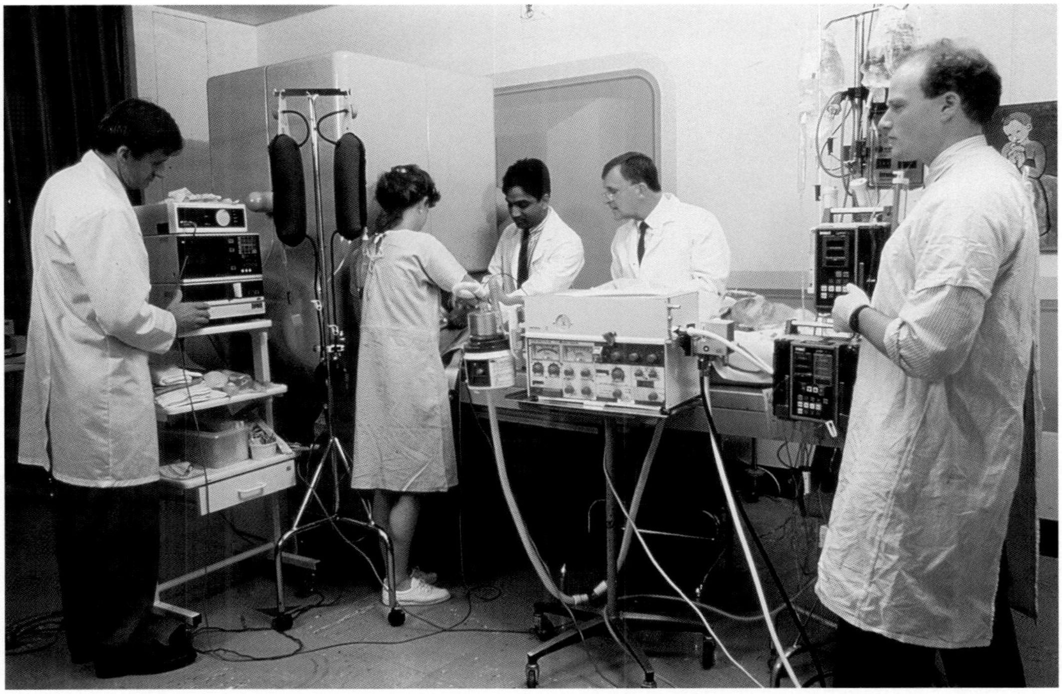

Chapter 58, Figure 6 Prompt γ-neutron activation analysis scanner in the University Department of Surgery at Auckland Hospital. A ventilated critically ill intensive care patient is shown being prepared for scanning with all intravenous lines, drains, and monitors attached.

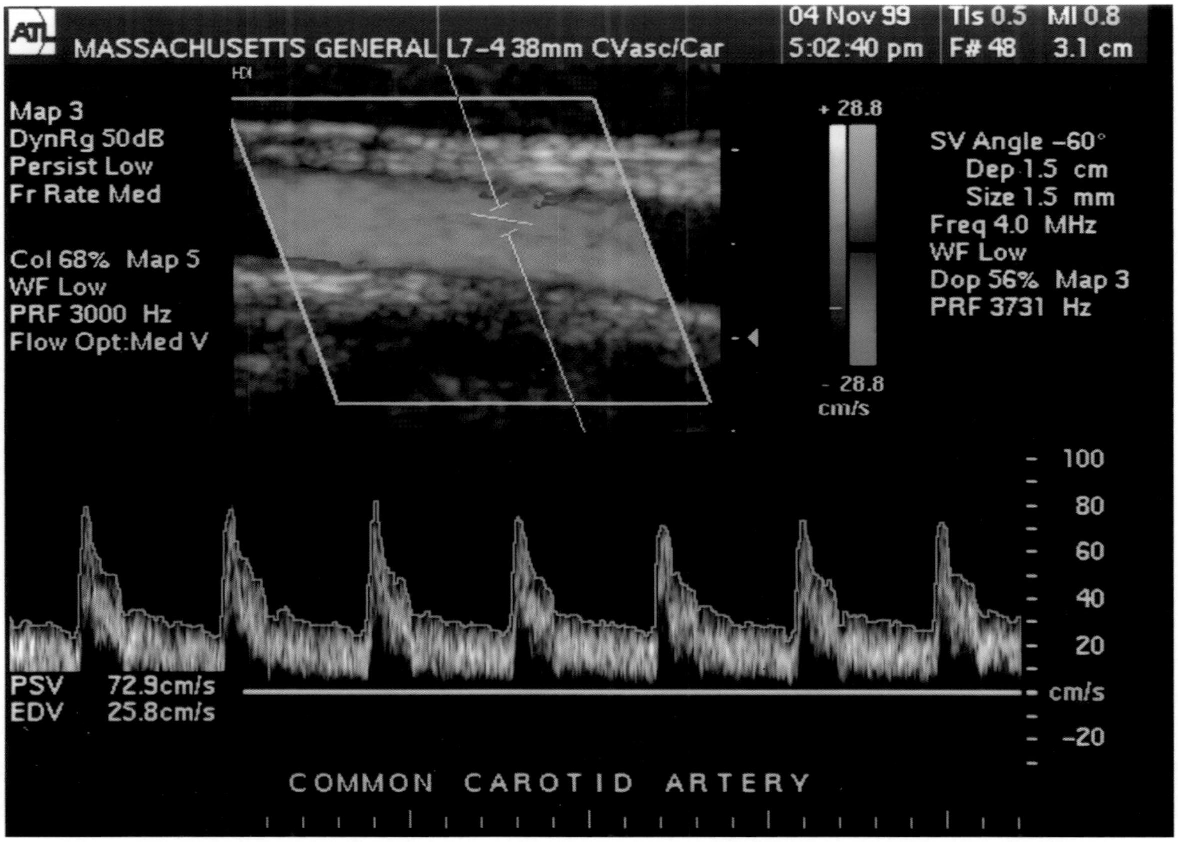

Chapter 72, Figure 7 Duplex images of artery and velocity measurement.

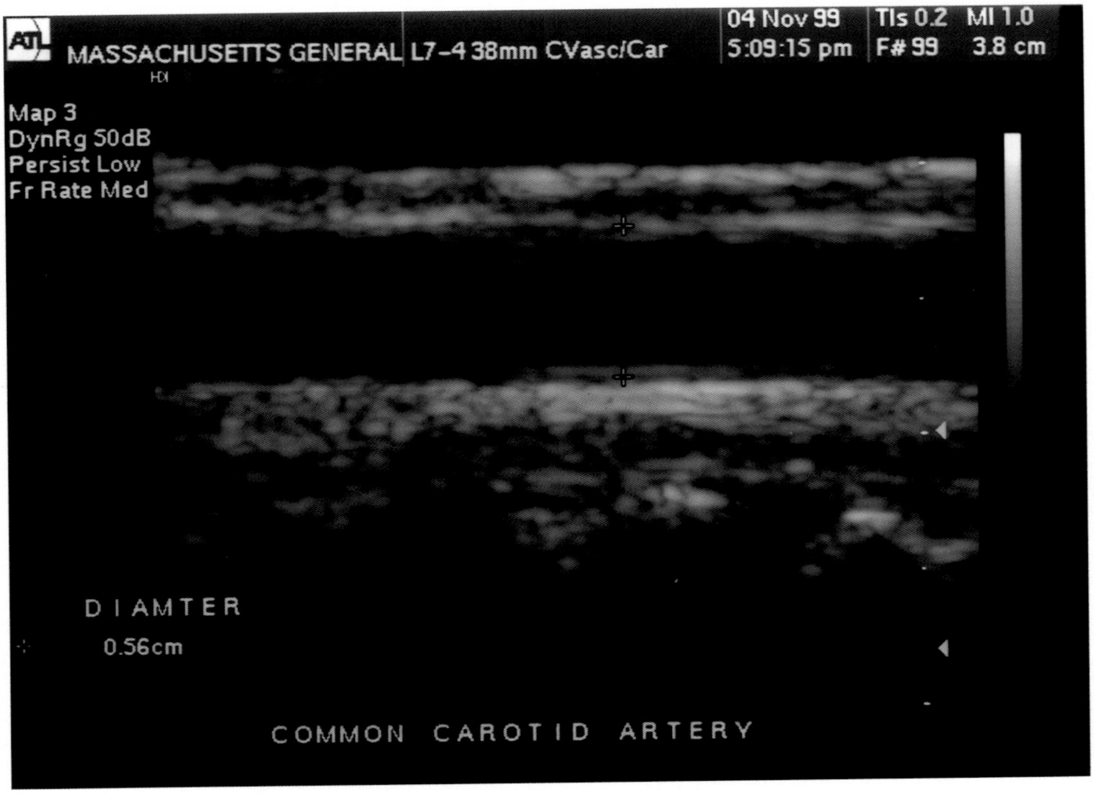

Chapter 72, Figure 7 Continued.

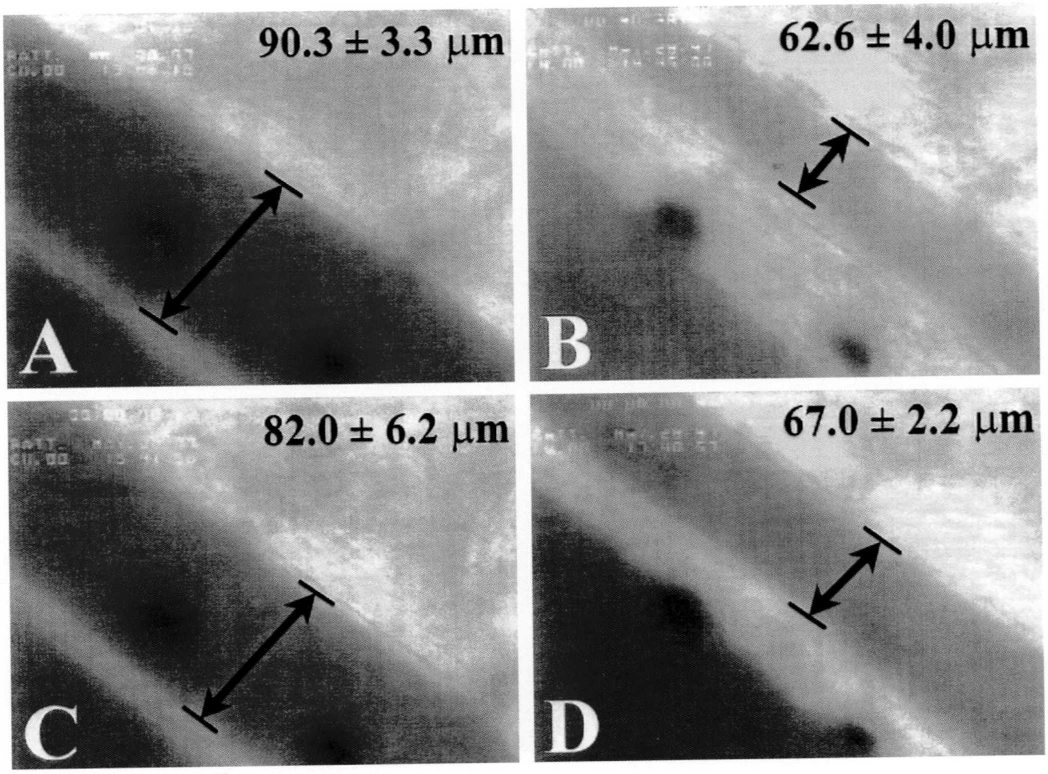

Chapter 73, Figure 1 Series of representative images of an intestinal A1 inflow arteriole during the various stages of hemorrhage and resuscitation. (A) Baseline. (B) During hemorrhage. (C) End resuscitation. (D) After resuscitation (2 hr).

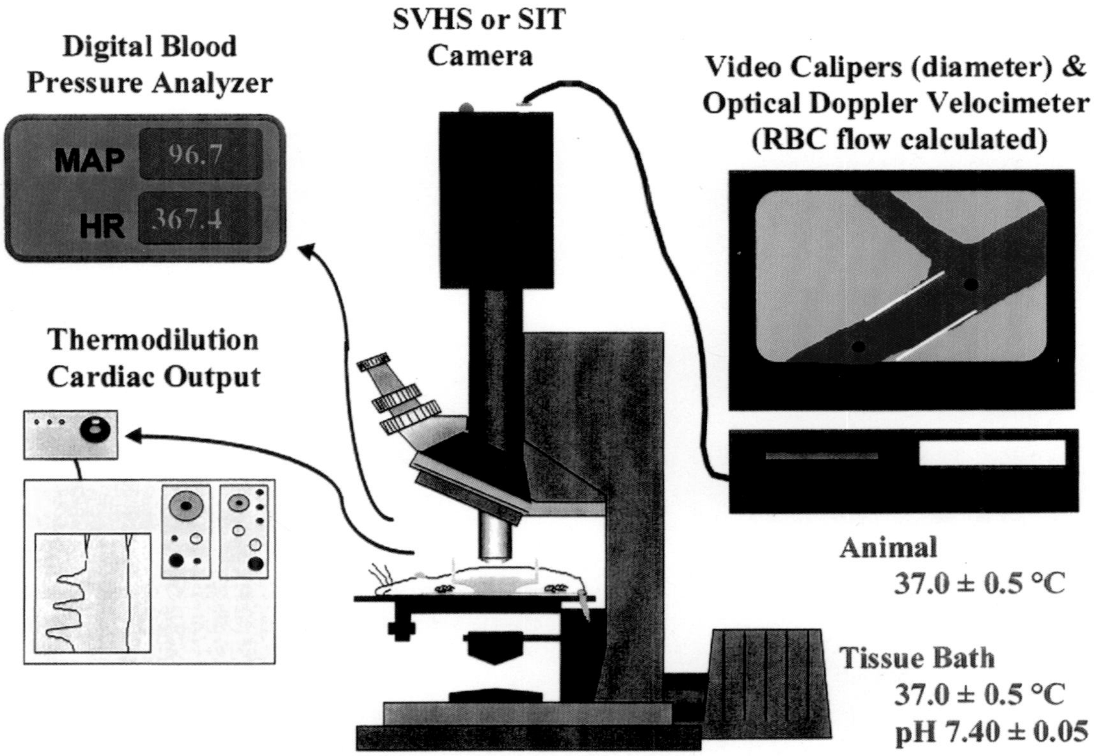

Chapter 73, Figure 2 Schematic representation of intestinal intravital videomicroscopy setup.

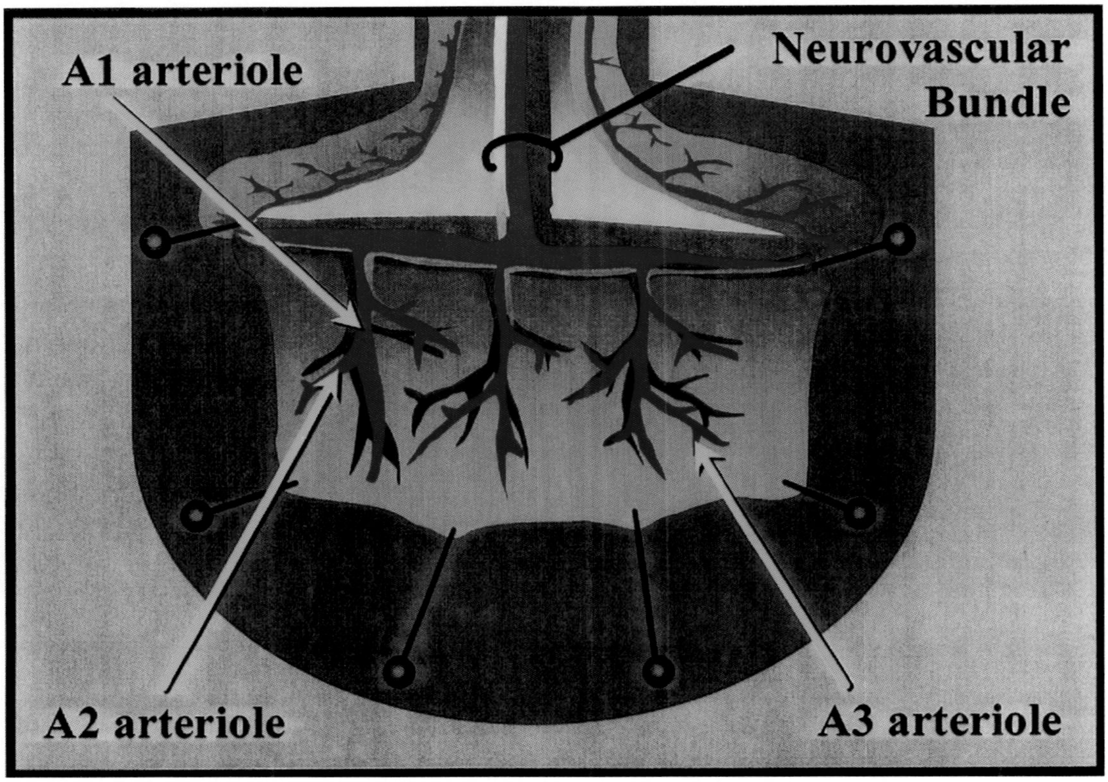

Chapter 73, Figure 3 Schematic representation of exteriorized small intestine in tissue bath.

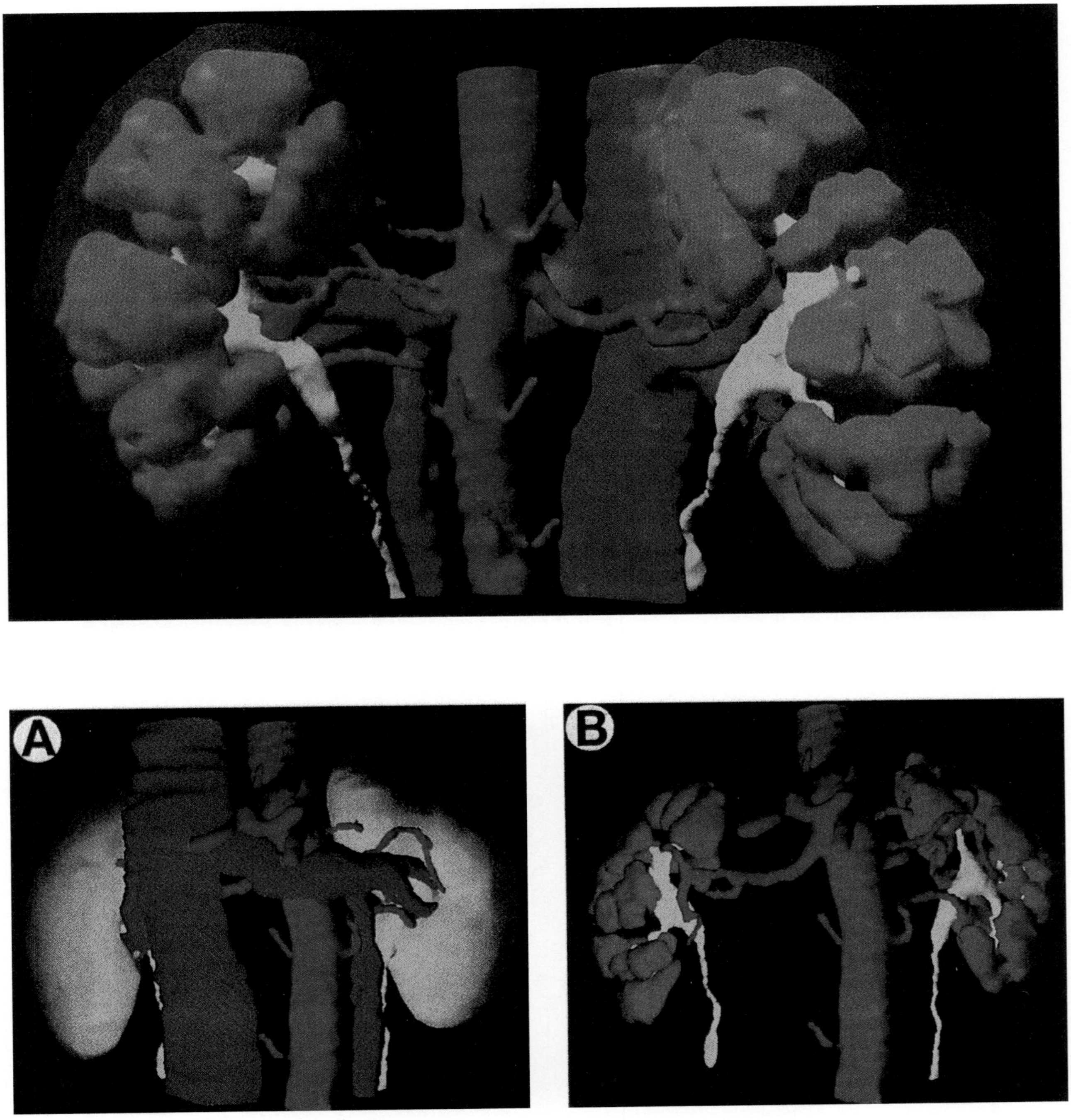

Chapter 98, Figure 1 An anterior view of a 3D reconstruction of the kidney using contrast-enhanced spiral CT data. Courtesy of Lori Lerner.

93

How to Review a Manuscript

Ori D. Rotstein

Departments of Surgery, University Health Network and University of Toronto, Toronto, Ontario, Canada M5G 24C

I. Introduction

Dissemination of information through publication in peer-reviewed journals remains an important means of promulgating advances in the practice of surgery. Clearly, therefore, the review of scientific manuscripts represents a crucial step in the process of popularizing new concepts, because it is the conduit through which most new information passes into the literature. This chapter provides a general approach to reviewing scientific manuscripts, with the expectation that the information might not only assist others in reviewing manuscripts, but might also provide some insight for individuals preparing scientific work for submission to peer-reviewed journals.

II. Why Review Manuscripts?

Serving on an editorial board or being an ad hoc reviewer for a scientific journal can be both time-consuming and tedious. Nevertheless, there are several good reasons to participate in the process. Most importantly, it is an academic responsibility to do so. Manuscript review is a process whereby a specialist can contribute to the development of the specialty. A reviewer therefore owes it to the readership of a journal, to practicing surgeons, as well as to the public to provide a fair, rigorous, and thoughtful review in a timely fashion. In a more direct way, the reviewer also has an opportunity to help authors enhance their research effort by providing comments that might improve and crystallize their ideas. Reviewing manuscripts is also enjoyable, because it is a learning experience. A well-written manuscript "Introduction" succinctly reviews a field of inquiry and updates a reviewer's knowledge of the literature. New experimental models, technical procedures, and the availability of new reagents may be highlighted in the "Methods" section and thus may suggest alternate approaches to testing hypotheses relevant to a reviewer's own area of research. Further, clinical papers describing randomized trials, retrospective reviews, and even case reports may have direct applicability to a reviewer's day-to-day clinical practice, thereby influencing care of patients. The reviewer also gains a sense for writing style and presentation of data, which can be a positive influence. First-hand comparison between a focused, well-designed, and clearly written manuscript and a diffuse rambling submission can unquestionably strengthen a reviewer's personal writing and presentation skills. Finally, it is a privilege to be asked to participate in manuscript review because it represents recognition of interest and expertise in a given field. In summary, the benefits gained from reviewing manuscript submissions, whether scientific or clinical, are substantial.

III. General Issues about Reviewing

Journals vary somewhat regarding how they contact potential reviewers. Although many email or fax individuals regarding their interest in reviewing a particular manuscript, some send the manuscript directly without prior notification of its arrival. Under certain circumstances, it is appropriate and even desirable to decline the request to review a manuscript. These include (1) lack of expertise in the manuscript's subject matter or methodology, (2) competing priorities that preclude timely and thorough review, and (3) conflict of interest regarding authors, products, or other aspects of the work. A prompt Fax or email to the editorial office will permit redirection of the manuscript to the appropriate reviewer. Novice reviewers might view this refusal as a fatal blow to their future opportunities to review, but they should be reassured that editors appreciate this, because poor or delayed reviews significantly hinder their ability to run the journal operations.

Having accepted the task, it is important to carefully review the guidelines for the review process. Some journals have a triage process and request a very rapid opinion regarding suitability of the material for the readership and for the journal. Others provide a timeline ranging from 2 to 6 weeks for the review. One should also examine the criteria for acceptance as well as the readership for the particular journal. The requirements for an original research submission as opposed to a review article or a case report clearly differ. The information regarding this is often included with the reviewer's package, either in the cover letter from the editor or in an accompanying "checklist" format. In addition, most journals now have web sites that can be accessed for information such as readership and acceptable subjects for submission. For example, the site for the *Journal of Surgical Research* provides the following statements:

> *The* Journal of Surgical Research: Clinical and Laboratory Investigation *publishes original articles concerned with clinical and laboratory investigations relevant to surgical practice and teaching. The journal emphasizes reports of clinical investigations or fundamental research bearing directly on surgical management that will be of general interest to a broad range of surgeons and surgical researchers. The articles presented need not have been the products of surgeons or of surgical laboratories. The* Journal of Surgical Research *also features review articles and special articles relating to educational, research, or social issues of interest to the academic surgical community.*

When making ultimate recommendations to the editors regarding suitability of a submission, these criteria should be kept in mind.

Finally, it is worthwhile to underscore the prior comments regarding the importance of the review process. Although the editors are ultimately responsible for determining the acceptance of a particular manuscript, most rely heavily on their reviewers to advise them. With this mandate, the reviewer should feel obliged to give his/her best effort. The reviewer should set aside the time and the place to consider the submission adequately. A review cannot be done while sitting in rounds or conference. This is not only rude to the presenter but does not permit full attention to the manuscript. Further, the practice of asking a surgical resident, a research fellow, or a colleague to perform the review would also seem inappropriate. It is the opinion and expertise of the primary reviewer, rather than a surrogate, that is requested and the responsibility should not be passed on without prior consultation with the editor. It is a separate issue as to whether one might ask for help with respect to reviewing a specific aspect of the manuscript, e.g., choice of statistic tests or specific methodology used. Most cover letters requesting manuscript review indicate the privileged nature of the submission. Some state that consultation with an associate is permitted, whereas others indicate that the manuscript should not be shown to a third party. Direct communication with the responsible editor will help to clarify issues that arise in this regard.

A. Beginning the Review

The comments in this section focus primarily on original research submissions, rather than reviews or case series, although many of the general principles apply to all three types. To begin a review of a manuscript, mentally pose five desirable qualities regarding a paper's acceptability:

1. The scientific justification for the proposed experiments. Is there sound rationale for proposing the studies and has the hypothesis been formulated based on substantive prior knowledge?
2. The originality of the work. Ideally, the research will be totally novel, although an extension of prior knowledge or an improved methodological approach that more definitively answers a question are both acceptable.
3. The importance of the research question. Clearly, this is subjective, but as an expert in the field, the reviewer should be well positioned to provide a credible opinion in this regard.
4. The accuracy and validity of the observations, i.e., whether the applied methods are suitable to address the problem and whether they are used appropriately.
5. The conclusions and their relevance to the major readership of the journal. Specifically, it is important to determine whether the interpretation of the data is appropriate, i.e., the findings and the conclusions are in accord. Although the prime audience of the journal is usually implied in the submission guidelines, occasionally manuscripts with little relevance to the readership are received.

Only after the entire manuscript has been carefully reviewed can one assess the degree to which some or all of these requirements have been fulfilled, and to what extent. Editorial offices provide reviewers with checklists of varying complexity, and these are intended to help organize the review process. For novice reviewers, tabulating this information while reviewing the manuscript can be useful.

An initial rapid read-through of a manuscript provides a general sense of the content. A section-by-section review of the manuscript then follows, with focus on the major components: (1) title and abstract, (2) introduction, (3) methods, (4) results, and (5) discussion.

1. Title and Abstract

The title and abstract should generally reflect the content of the manuscript. If they do not, a comment should be made to the editor and the authors, suggesting the problem and the "fix." This is particularly important information for the authors because the title and abstract represent the screening window for keyword/concept literature searches, determining whether a paper is ultimately read by the relevant audience.

2. Introduction

The introduction should include a clear, succinct statement of the problem and the rationale for the proposed studies. From these, the hypothesis and/or the major objective of the manuscript should be developed and stated. The introduction invariably requires a limited and relevant literature review, although excessive discussion tends to lengthen the paper unnecessarily and often obscures the more important components. By the end of the introduction, there should be a clear sense of the novelty of the work as well as of the scientific justification for proposing the studies. These represent two of the five criteria stated above.

3. Methods

The methods section is a crucial component of any manuscript. In essence, the methodology defines the accuracy of the observations and the conclusions drawn from them. Whether the research is fundamental or clinical in nature, trial design is critically important. General principles of choosing appropriate controls, randomizing of subjects, determining sample size, as well as blinding of treatment and outcomes are applicable to all research. The statistical methods should be clearly stated. Techniques should be clearly stated for each of these, particularly in clinical research, in which greater complexity exists. In general, previously described methodology can be referenced, but new or modified techniques should be described in some detail.

A significant literature has developed regarding the use of the randomized controlled trial (RCT) in the evaluation of surgical therapies. The reader is referred to several articles addressing this subject in detail (1–3). The surgical RCT should include (1) standardization of the surgical procedure (surgeons vary in their technical expertise and thus one might suggest that fewer surgeons in the trial might be desirable; however, this may affect generalizability of the results), (2) timing of the trials (learning curves exist for most new procedures, and clearly this might bias the early results for this procedure compared to the gold standard), and (3) blinding of patients and investigators related to procedures and outcomes. Comparing medical to surgical interventions may preclude adequate blinding. It is therefore desirable to have objective outcome measures to lessen the possibility of bias. In general, clinical randomized controlled trials in surgery appear to be of rather low quality (4, 5). These acknowledged difficulties in performing such trials serve to underscore the importance of careful review of the methods sections of manuscript submissions, because methodological flaws impact directly on the validity and relevance of the reported data.

4. Results

By the time one reaches the stage where review of results is to be done, the rationale, hypothesis, and general methodology should be clearly established in the reviewer's mind. The results section should provide a logical sequence of data designed to guide the reader through a series of arguments, providing support for the hypothesis. In essence, the data make or break a paper. Are the data scientifically valid, with appropriate measurement and statistical analysis? If so, do they support the hypothesis? Specifically, consider whether the research question is addressed directly or whether the data are inferential. Sometimes, the former is impossible due to methodological limitations and one must rely more heavily on the weight of the evidence presented. In this regard, decide whether more data are required to support the argument. This decision can be made after reading the discussion section, because the author will often address these issues.

The figures and tables should be clearly presented, well described in the figure legends and footnotes, respectively, and they should correspond with the description in the text. Assess whether figures and tables are necessary for the flow of the argument or may be better described in the text of the manuscript. Negative data that are supportive of the hypothesis but not central to the development of the argument do not usually benefit from graphic or tabular representation.

It seems self-evident that a manuscript's chance of acceptance would be greatly enhanced if the data were presented in a clear and logical fashion. Nevertheless, this is not uniformly so. Although some manuscripts are frustratingly difficult to read, it is incumbent on the reviewer to sort through the data and render an objective assessment of whether the information appropriately supports the hypothesis. Occasionally, the quality of the presentation is so poor that it precludes review. The reviewer is advised to contact the editor under such circumstance for his/her opinion. Some journals include poor presentation among the criteria for rejection of a manuscript.

5. Discussion

In the discussion section, look for the author to pull together the important findings and to draw conclusions based on this information. Then decide whether the conclusions are supported by the data presented in the manuscript. Several considerations are critical. First, the data must be scientifically valid. The study design must be appropriate, the methodology sound, and the observations accurate. Without these components, no substantial conclusions can be drawn. Second, the conclusions must be consistent with the findings. Usually, the data presented in the paper are sufficient to permit the generation of conclusions. However, the strength of the conclusions may be enhanced when the author puts them in the context of the existing literature. The discussion section is frequently cluttered with unnecessary repetition of the results of the studies, as well as detailed reviews of the literature. Neither is required and both may preclude a clear presentation of the important findings and conclusions.

The discussion section is also strengthened by some speculation as to the significance of the findings and the new avenues of investigation that are suggested by the data. This information makes the discussion more interesting and also helps to underscore the originality and importance of the work. However, it is also important to ensure that the speculation is not exaggerated, beyond what might reasonably be expected from the paper and existing literature.

B. Writing the Review

The format required for the actual written review varies from journal to journal. It usually consists of two sections: a response to the editor and a comment to the author(s). Most journal review forms have a checklist section recommending to the editors the overall acceptability of a manuscript, the recommendations regarding revisions, and the priority of the manuscript. In addition, a narrative is frequently requested to provide relevant details regarding the decision. The reviewer should bear in mind that his/her comments are recommendations to the editor and are frequently pooled with other opinions to make a final decision on the manuscript. Whether the paper is acceptable or unacceptable, one must justify the decision. One should consider the importance of the question, the originality of the work, and the quality of the methodology. Are the conclusions appropriate for the data presented? Is the work of interest to the readership? Based on these issues, the reviewer should also provide direction to the editor as to how an unacceptable manuscript might be revised to make it acceptable. A major revision would consist of a request for more data to support the conclusions of the paper; a minor revision tends to be more stylistic in nature—clarification of methodology, streamlining of data presentation, or alterations of the discussion section. If figures or text require revision or deletion, the request should be made in this section. When one requests new data as part of a major revision, one should be mindful to restrict the request to information that is directly relevant to the existing research question. It is not appropriate to ask for a new set of studies that might be the basis for an entirely new manuscript. Rather, additional studies should be requested to clarify controls, to support the validity of existing data, and to strengthen the conclusions. In the comment to the editors, indicate what information is absolutely required for the manuscript to be acceptable. It should be noted that if a manuscript is truly excellent, it is not a crime to clearly state this. For such papers, there is no obligation to downplay the work or magnify trivial issues in order to show that the review was thorough.

The "Comments to Authors" section should be constructive, with the objective of improving the quality of the article and perhaps providing some alternate insights for the author. Most journals indicate that specific reference to the acceptability of a manuscript should not be made in this section. Rather, it should focus on recommending changes that might improve the quality of the manuscript. This can include focusing the research question, clarifying the methodology, improving the presentation of results, as well as reconsidering interpretation of the data. Additional studies, references, or statements in the text that would help to accomplish these goals should be requested here. If a particularly interesting question or future study comes to mind, it is appropriate to comment on it in this section, without requesting any response from the authors.

Some journals have a section to comment on minor issues such as typographical errors, poor grammar, spelling mistakes, etc. Rather than make a comprehensive listing of these errors, make note of their presence when they are excessive.

C. The Rereview

Revised versions of previously reviewed manuscripts are occasionally returned for reconsideration by the initial reviewers. Almost always, the packet includes the initial review as well as the comments of the other reviewers. For the rereview, focus attention on the author's response to the initial queries. The easiest scenario is one in which the author fully considers each of the points raised and provides a thoughtful response. A positive response can be rapidly provided to the editor. A more difficult circumstance is one in which the initial review raised significant concerns regarding the quality of the manuscript and the author has either rejected or ignored suggestions for changes in the revised version. Take a fresh look at the manuscript in this situation and try to discern whether the author's responses and alterations have made the submission worthy of publication. In essence, return to the fundamental principles underlying the decision for acceptance: importance of the question, rationale for the studies, validity of the findings, significance of the conclusions, and relevance to the journal readership. A narrative response should be provided to the editor so that he/she can collate the gathered reviews and make a final decision. After completion of the assessment, read the other reviewer's comments. This often provides valuable insight into alternate approaches to reviewing. However, the assessment of the specific manuscript should be made independent of other's comments.

IV. Conclusions

Manuscript review is a critical component of the process of knowledge dissemination among surgeons. In this overview, important aspects of the review process have been discussed, and it is hoped that these comments will provide helpful insights into how to review a manuscript and how to prepare one so that it receives a favorable review.

Acknowledgment

The helpful comments of Dr. Andras Kapus are gratefully acknowledged.

References

1. McLeod, R. S. (1999). Issues in surgical randomized controlled trials. *World J. Surg.* **23,** 1210–1214.
2. McLeod, R. S., Wright, J. G., Solomon, M. J., Hu X., and Walters, B. C. (1996). Randomized controlled trials in surgery: Issues and problems. *Surgery* **119,** 483–486.
3. Stirrat, G. M., Farndon, J., Farrow, S. C., and Dwyer, N. (1992). The challenge of evaluating surgical procedures. *Ann. R. Coll. Surg. Engl.* **74,** 80–84.
4. Evans, M., and Pollock, A. V. (1984). Trials on trial. *Arch. Surg.* **119,** 109–113.
5. Emerson, J. D., McPeek, B., and Mosteller, F. (1984). Reporting clinical trials in general surgical journals. *Surgery* **95,** 572–579.

94

Academic Surgical Mentoring

Clay Cothren, Julie Heimbach, Thomas N. Robinson, Casey Calkins, and Alden H. Harken

Department of Surgery, University of Colorado, Denver, Colorado 80262

Wanted: *active, energetic, and insightful individual, willing to share knowledge and connections with impressionable underling. Requires diligence, support, and an occasional "leap of faith." Commitment may be life-long. No financial compensation. Unapproachable, busy, enigmatic boors need not apply.*

What is mentoring? Is it sharing jokes in the locker room after an operative case, or is it something much more profound? How does one build the mentor–mentoree relationship? Or perhaps, how does the relationship begin at all? What are the elements required for its existence? Many questions and perhaps even more answers come to mind, but the resultant conversation is one that affects anyone in the academic realm.

I. Why Mentoring?

Why should mentoring exist? Mentoring has, no doubt, been in existence since our Darwinian ancestors emerged from the primordial ooze. How else did one generation pass its trade and folklore on to the next? Surgical training has long been acknowledged as more an apprenticeship than a residency. From generation to generation, knowledge based on experience is passed down. Without this interaction and exchange, the intricacies and joys of medicine could not be transferred and, hence, experienced in their fullest. In sharing their experience and insight, mentors, in particular, have unique opportunities and responsibilities.

II. The Surgical Mentor

Repeatedly, sociologists have examined factors by which medical students choose a specialty. Lifestyle, financial rewards, esteem, and parental/societal pressures have been subjected to multivariate analysis. Repeatedly, these obviously influential factors have been comfortably ignored in the decision-making process. Consistently, the most robust determinant of career selection is a mentor with whom the student identifies. Interestingly, the academic progeny need not be a clone of the mentor. Students are now conceptually fluent with the wonders of transgenic technology. Students imaginatively splice the "effect" of a socially responsible and rewarding surgical practice with the "affect" of an encouraging, engaging elementary school teacher. Mentors are mosaics. With the evident exception of the authors of this paper, mentors are rarely perfect—even Mary Poppins could not deal with an aortic dissection. Fortunately, a medical school faculty—and society in general—is an *a la carte* menu. We are all obligate role models. Much like our parents, we lead our professional and personal lives either as examples or warnings. However, as academic surgeons, we should delight in taking a more active role in mentoring our residents and students.

So if mentoring is the highest calling, and the goal is to direct the flock into the paths of righteousness, how do we address this challenge? The answer is easy. One must always remember to begin with the ABCs:

A: accessible	**B:** balance	**C:** challenge
advise	backbone	communicate
advocate	boundaries	connect
active		champion

The characteristics espoused by these ABCs are central to the mentor's role. By initiating an advising role and being active in the professional life of one's residents, the mentoring role begins. A mentor is accessible, wishing to further communication and contacts. A mentor should also be an advocate, promulgating ideas and career goals. The mentor provides balance for the resident's efforts and ideas, a type of "sounding-board" with built-in reality checks. When the resident needs extra support or commitment, the mentor can provide some of the backbone needed. Mentors aid residents in realizing their own limits and boundaries, and how best to excel within this framework. Communication is essential between the mentor and mentoree, but the mentor also guides the resident in learning to communicate effectively with others in the professional realm. By knowing when and how much to challenge an individual, combined with the ability to champion their ideas, a mentor will assist them in attaining their goals.

The fundamental basis of the mentor–mentoree relationship has changed over the years. The traditional view of mentors as elder, paternalistic authoritarians has evolved into the view of mentors as inspiring partners. Mentorees no longer see themselves as the subservient underling but rather as a motivated, trusted equal. This evolution has occurred over decades, and at times has been subtle (Fig. 1). It reflects changing attitudes within our society; by fostering our youth, we as a group attain fulfillment.

We have all muttered the phrase, "imitation is the sincerest form of flattery." In mentoring, this rings true. Mentors often lead by example. Residents typically prefer to follow in the footsteps of exemplary mentors. One may model their patient interaction, communication style, and professional attitude after admired staff. Watching success in action is a powerful force that shapes one's future outlook. Residents and faculty alike aspire to a gratifying, rewarding, and stimulating life. So, in order to be the perfect mentor, all you need to do is "live one."

<u>The Mentor's Roles and Responsibilities</u>

Traditional View	**Newer View**
Paternalistic	Empowering
Boss/Authority	Friend/partner
Stern/Strict	Inspiring
In charge	Lets go
Protective	Protective
"Raise" the mentoree	"Develop" the mentoree

<u>The Mentoree's Roles and Responsibilities</u>

Traditional View	**Newer View**
Subservient/obedient	Responsible equal
Favorite son	Mentoree
Company man	Own man
"Made" by mentor	Help " make" yourself
Think alike	Think "outside the box"
Responds to power/orders	Responds to motivation

Figure 1 The evolution of the mentor and mentoree's roles. The subtle shift in character has occurred over decades, in response to individual and societal demands. From Souba (1999), *J. Surg. Res.* **82,** 113–120.

A. Living the Perfect Life (or Eat Your Heart out, Martha Stewart)

In academic surgery, living the perfect life is not as hard as it might, at first blush, appear. When each of us sat in the medical school admissions office and articulated our reasons for going to medical school, we all stated (in unison) that we wanted to contribute to humanity and that we wanted to lead a socially responsible life. Very few specialties (with a National Football League quarterback being the possible exception) enjoy the opportunity of instantaneous fan appreciation afforded the surgeon who removes an inflamed appendix or resects an obstructing sigmoid carcinoma. Unlike the football player, however, our odds of success are far superior, and as a lifetime venture, our knees will not give out as fast. Our patients want to love us. As a fulfilled surgeon with this type of gratification, why would I not want to share this experience with others? As a mentor, one can reveal the possibilities while coaching the next generation to victory.

B. Building the Partnership

Just as learning the alphabet involves steplike progression, the evolution of the mentor–mentoree partnership involves progression from one level to the next (Fig. 2). Each of these steps is characterized by defining moments with individual realization and refinement. The initial steps are small. Merely getting to know individual faculty members and establishing a professional relationship is time consuming for the junior resident. During these early months, the "future mentor" is accessible, setting an example for these impressionable residents and maintaining standards of excellence. Only as the relationship evolves and the shared experience becomes a trusting interaction does the mentoring role come into play. With the mentor's encouragement, the resident begins to define their future role by exploring options. By asking questions, both personal and professional, independent growth and maturation within the workplace

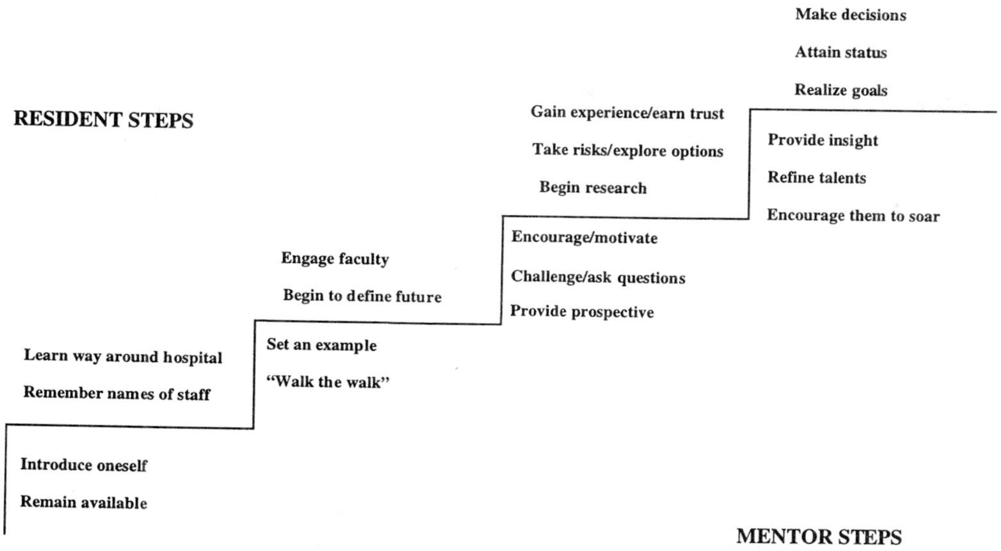

Figure 2 The progression of the mentor–mentoree relationship.

begins. Each of the partners enjoys gratification during the process, and one cannot advance up the ladder without the other. At the end of the journey, each finds fulfillment, the resident in realizing personal and professional accomplishment, the mentor in vicariously sharing successes.

C. Mentors in Surgical Research

The currency of academic activity is the published manuscript. Surgeons are capable of accruing vast amounts of data—and, then we stall. Many successful surgeons never experience the "fun" of academic life because they leave no concrete evidence that they can either read or write. They get hammered by patient care, when they should be hooked on phonics. Here is where a mentor can help.

Surgery is a clinical specialty. After earning "clinical spurs," the academic surgeon must (indeed, can) indulge in the luxury of surgically relevant investigation. Surgical research is best accomplished by those surgeons who want to do it. Coercion is bad. Forcing residents into the laboratory demeans the investigative experience. In Denver, we believe that residents should not be allowed to choose the laboratory experience unless they are doing well clinically. Only by showing proficiency in the clinical realm can one pursue investigation at the laboratory bench. Most residents feel strongly by the end of their third year about "going in the lab." Some are excited about the change of scenery and the pursuit of their research interests; other residents want nothing more than to finish their clinical training. Occasionally a resident will be undecided; to this rare resident a mentor is invaluable. Having established a trusting (and benevolent) relationship, the resident can ask for guidance. The mentor can help the resident ask the right questions, consider multiple options, play out future scenarios, and ultimately lend advice. Experience, of which the resident has little, counts. The mentor provides insight into the research experience and its relevance to the resident's ultimate goals. By knowing the character and mission of a particular resident, the mentor can provide valuable guidance in one of the most important career decisions.

The mentor plays a varied role to the resident interested in research. Mentors do everything from providing encouragement, to instructing basic principles (proofing papers, running gels, mixing solutions), to brainstorming ideas. Allowing for flexibility in collaborating with several different investigators during the lab years vastly broadens a resident's experience. The mentor facilitates the formulation of research goals. Indeed, given the limited research experience of most surgical residents, the responsibility of formulating initial questions for investigation falls largely to the mentor. The first project attempted in the lab ideally would be a continuation of an already established model, or a likely "quick hit" project that teaches the skills necessary to address tightly focused research questions. This avoids the regrettable experience of spending 9 months trying to get a single technique to work, or taking on a question that may in fact better reflect the goals of an entire career. After the eventual success of the initial attempts, a successful mentor will then allow the resident additional liberty in formulating future questions and designing projects.

D. The Lab Experience

Perhaps the most important responsibility of a successful mentor is to be acutely sensitive to the psychology driving the developing academic surgeon. Following 3 years of surgical residency, a surgeon is beginning to feel quite competent in responding to life's daily crises. The morass of critical care information inflicted on the unsuspecting intern is initially daunting, but by the third year, is beginning to fall into place. A single year in the laboratory almost guarantees a dispiriting experience (Fig. 3). More than 2 years in the laboratory risks challenging the aspiring investigator's fundamental surgical identity. The optimum time is 2 years. Thus, the typical surgical resident storms from the clinics (June) into the research laboratory (July) at 5000 rpm and is abruptly shifted into neutral. With the confident promise of solving perplexing problems of biology such as heart disease and cancer, the surgical resident is catapulted into a heady intellectual stratosphere. By the end of August, however, the conscientious resident is beginning to sense the press of inactivity. No leaking aneurysm has surfaced. No one has died. Not even any hassles from an irate X-ray tech. By mid-October, the budding surgical investigator has plummeted into a clinical depression (Fig. 3). In January, the first abstract is accepted and by spring, two manuscripts enjoy early editorial approval. The resident investigator climbs out of the depths of despondency. That June, the research year receives a spotty report card. This is the worst possible time to pack it in; the mentor must encourage perseverance. During the second year, the resident gains comfort with both the process and the pace of research. During this year, the maturing investigator actually evolves interest in the results of his/her labors and, usually for the first time, sees his/her name in print. Cruising in for a landing, at the end of the second year, the resident has become an independent investigator with his/her own projects, some proud publications, and an exciting vision for future work. The temptation is to spend another year in the laboratory. Do not do it. Surgery is ultimately a clinical discipline. The resident must finish off clinical rotations (including board certification), establish a laboratory, and initiate an academic career. This is the proudest moment in mentoring.

E. The Junior Surgical Faculty Challenge

The two biggest jumps in an academic surgical career are hurdling the gulf between the fourth year of medical school and internship, and leaving the Olympian pedestal of Chief Residency into "the real (or seemingly unreal) world." It is frighteningly easy for the overindulgent mentor to jump the gun. Again, surgery is a clinical discipline. The first-year resident and the first-year faculty member need to prove themselves clinically (mostly to themselves) prior to initiating any investigative activities. To our astonishment, even the most promising and accomplished junior faculty mem-

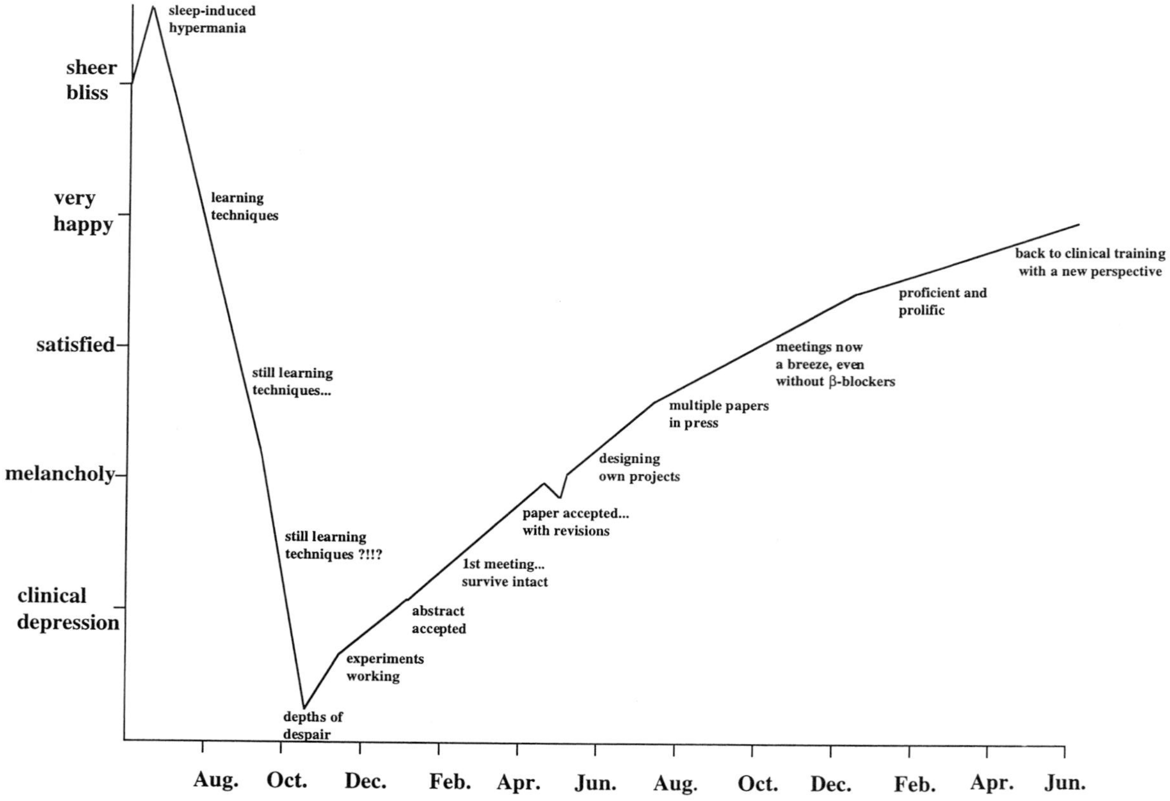

Figure 3 The typical research experience of a surgical resident.

bers need time to settle in clinically. An impatient mentor can ruin everything. The interests, aspirations, and even the relationship between the mentor and the junior faculty member can suffer if not given the required space. Clinical success will come to the junior faculty member; it is then that the mentor may permit and promote time for focused academic activity. Many of the junior faculty members' needs are similar to those of the young resident: encouragement in their newfound role as staff, guidance on their interaction with peers and residents, and of course continued shared experience with their mentor. The mentor may help define a continuation project, complete with structuring their own lab and technicians. And perhaps most importantly, the mentor challenges them to reflect on their own experiences, and how to share these with the next generation of residents. As the junior faculty member accomplishes this, they too will evolve from the motivated mentoree to the trusted and encouraging mentor.

F. Completing the Perfect Academic Surgical Life

Academic surgery incorporates all of the components of a gratifying, rewarding, stimulating, and fun life. Interestingly, however, it is possible to improve on perfection. We are all obligate role models. The primary goal of an academic center is educating future pioneers; academic surgeons must embrace the opportunity to encourage, prod, hassle, and motivate young, industrious, energetic, and intelligent surgeons toward a life that combines the gratification of individual patient care with the rewards of contributing new information to society. A surgeon who is capable of the rigorous discipline of basic science will simply practice superior clinical surgery. That is our goal. In accomplishing this, mentors glory in unique satisfactions. We do not need to resect another diseased gallbladder; nor do we require another published manuscript; the high-octane fuel of our lives is our pride in the photographs on the wall.

Recommended Reading

Ashcraft, K. W. (1998). Seasons, dreams, and mentors. *J. Pediatr. Surg.* **33,** 155–160.

Sandrick, K. (1992). The residency experience: The woman's perspective. *ACS Bull.* **77,** 10–17.

Schwartz, S. I. (1999). The evolution of medical education. *Surgery* **1,** 17–18.

Souba, W. W. (1999). Mentoring young academic surgeons, our most precious asset. *J. Surg. Res.* **82,** 113–120.

95

Ethics and Surgical Research

Timothy M. Pawlik and Lisa Colletti

Department of Surgery, University of Michigan Medical School, Ann Arbor, Michigan 48109

I. Introduction

Although the twentieth century may be remembered for the splitting of the atom and the production of the microchip, the twenty-first century is poised to define itself around such biomedical issues as genetic engineering, cloning, and the mapping of the human genome. Although these advances hold the promise of significant clinical and scientific benefit, they are not without associated ethical and social concerns. Biomedical research increasingly finds itself at the center of ethical issues. The discovery of new biomedical technologies expands not only our scientific horizons, but our moral ones as well. These revolutionary discoveries mandate that biomedical research define guiding principles to direct how this new knowledge should be acquired and used.

In addition to grappling with these societal ethical concerns involving the goals and applications of new technologies, surgical researchers must also contend with the daily ethical challenges found in the individual laboratory. As has been argued elsewhere, the research environment can be an impediment to ethical conduct. Issues of honesty and objectivity, and methods of data collection and analysis, among others, all contribute to a climate that demands particular attention to ethical questions. In his book "The Ethics of Science," David Resnik argues that there are several aspects of the research environment that make it uniquely susceptible to moral strain (1). In striving for success, the surgeon scientist faces constant pressure to "publish or perish." This imperative, whether real or perceived, may tempt some scientists to violate ethical principles, such as manipulating or fabricating certain "details" of their findings. Intimately associated with this drive to succeed scientifically is the stress involved in securing research funding. As funding for research becomes increasingly competitive, surgeon scientists may feel compelled to ignore ambiguous data, negative results, or inconclusive findings. Finally, the structure of the biomedical research laboratory may contribute to unethical behavior. The laboratory, not unlike much of medicine, is often organized in a rigidly hierarchical manner. Those at the "bottom" may find themselves in a compromising position. Students and residents may feel tempted to "massage" data in order to satisfy the expectations of their supervisors. Additionally, ethical issues such as harassment, equality in the work place, and free and open dialogue between co-workers, although not unique to the research laboratory, may be more problematic in an environment in which a hierarchical line of authority has traditionally been established. Given all of this, the ethics of surgical research must not only address the appropriateness of what is happening scientifically, but also the who, how, and where of the scientific endeavor.

An appropriate response to the daily ethical challenges of laboratory work must include the notion of accountability. Science as a profession holds a privileged place in society. It is granted special privileges such as government funding, the right to use hazardous materials, and the use of animals and humans in research. With these privileges comes the implicit trust of the public that science will act on its behalf in a responsible, ethical manner. Science, however, has not always been up to the challenge. Historical incidents such as the Tuskegee (Alabama) experiments, as well as less publicized instances of data fabrication and scientific misconduct, represent deplorable blemishes on the reputation of science. Scientific misconduct is not only of historical interest. A recent *Lancet* article reviewed the handling of scientific dishonesty in Nordic countries. It was found that 22% of the medical scientists surveyed knew about cases of serious misconduct, 3% were aware of falsification or fabrication of data, and 9% admitted to actually contributing to one or more incidents of misconduct (2). The actual incidence of ethical misconduct in the United States may or may not be the same, but the fact that there exists some misconduct is hard to deny. Regardless of the actual numbers, any ethical impropriety in the conduct of medical research is a major threat to the integrity of science and its esteemed scientific method, both of which are grounded in a commitment to honesty and objectivity. In an era of mass media, any scientific misconduct, even by one individual, risks eroding both public and political support for continued research. Given the grave consequences of ethical breeches, scientists must be increasingly aware of their ethical duties and responsibilities, both within the confines of the laboratory, as well as in the clinical setting.

There has been an increasing awareness of the importance of ethics in politics and popular culture. With the human genome project, the cloning of Dolly the sheep, and the birth of gene therapy, the realm of ethics and science has extended beyond the benchtop and into the living rooms of every American. If surgeons wish to maintain a strong voice in the burgeoning ethical debates that surround their research, they must become versed in the terms and the landscape of moral inquiry. Traditionally science has shunned morality and philosophy, believing that science has no role or duty to address moral or ethical questions. Science, it is said, concerns only the objective exploration, discovery, and phenomenological description of the unknown. Science acts; it discovers and invents. Ethicists, not surgeons or scientists, provide moral vision. This view, however, is deeply flawed. By abdicating interest in the moral dimension of research, surgeons will increasingly find that nonscientists are determining the direction and fate of scientific research. The surgeon scientist will come to provide only the "raw material and labor" that ethicists, public pundits, and politicians will analyze, dissect, and utilize to dictate policy. With the recognition by the surgeon scientists of the integral relationship between ethics and science, scientists are empowered to reclaim their voice in these discussions.

II. Guiding Principles of Ethical Surgical Research

There are many approaches to the field of ethics. Moral reasoning is often grounded in appeals to rights, virtues, norms, or principles. A usable and practical scientific ethic will need to be intelligible, pragmatic, and comprehensive. To achieve this, an overdependence on any one ethical theory should be avoided. Instead, a sound scientific ethic will blend themes from different theories to provide a structure for moral deliberation.

Beauchamp and Childress champion an approach to ethics that is widely known as the "principled" approach (3). Principle-based theories emphasize principles of obligation. In the Beauchamp and Childress scheme, these principles are not monistic, but rather pluralistic. That is, there are not one or two absolute principles, which define all of morality. Rather, there are many principles that spring from our sense as a community as to what is moral, ethical, or appropriate. These principles provide a basis for approaching and thinking about ethical problems and dilemmas. They furnish a familiar and structured process to approach and contemplate new complexities. Traditionally, four cardinal principles have been discussed: autonomy, nonmaleficence, beneficence, and justice (3) (Table I). Although these serve well in discussing many ethical issues, including clinical bioethics, a shift to more pragmatic "standards" or principles may be helpful when examining biomedical research ethics. Following largely from David Resnik's work (1), four major categories of principles or standards that guide scientific conduct may be constructed: (1) truth telling or veracity,

Table I "Classic" Principles of Biomedical Ethics[a]

Autonomy
Nonmaleficence
Beneficence
Justice

[a]From Beauchamp T and Childress (3).

(2) dialogue or free exchange, (3) caution or prudence, and (4) social responsibility or civic duty (Table II).

A. Truth Telling/Veracity

Honesty or truth telling is the cornerstone not only of the scientific method, but also of the social contract. In our everyday interactions with those around us we depend on their honesty for almost everything we do. In science the role of truth telling is equally, if not more, important. The very essence of science as a discipline is rooted in its commitment to truthful, objective investigation and reporting. Without honesty, science is unable to accomplish its mission, impotent to even begin the process of discovery and invention. Scientists, therefore, have a duty to be honest, tell the truth, and avoid all fabrication and falsification of data. In order to understand this moral obligation we must make more explicit the definition of dishonesty.

1. Dishonesty: Fabrication, Falsification, or Plagiarism

A rigid and fixed definition of dishonesty remains elusive. Different committees, institutions, and ethical review boards have endorsed varying notions of dishonesty. One interpretation defines scientific dishonesty as any fabrication, falsification, or plagiarism in proposing, performing, and reporting research (4). The National Academy of Sciences, the National Academy of Engineering, and the Institute of Medicine have endorsed such a definition (5). In this definition, dishonesty encompasses a number of areas of untruthfulness, all of which require their own examination.

Fabrication is the baseless creation of data in the absence of empirical experimental results. Although less prevalent, the pure fabrication of data does occur. Examples of researchers falsely claiming to have synthesized certain drugs or perfected certain surgical techniques exist (6, 7).

A less extreme but equally serious form of dishonesty is falsification. Falsification is the manipulation or misrepresentation of data or results that were obtained from experiments. Misrepresentation may include the presentation of false material or the omission of certain facts. Falsification of data can often be more difficult to identify and prove, because it can take on many forms. Falsification can occur in data collection: the "trimming" or "fudging" of data to fit preconceived expectations or to "tighten up" the data. It can occur in the analysis of the data: statistical handling of the data by design, to achieve certain ends. Falsification can also occur in the scientist's omissions: leaving out ambiguous data or outlying, "unexplainable" data points. Unfortunately, it is sometimes difficult to discriminate between intentional falsification and poor methodology on the part of the scientist.

Plagiarism is the taking of undeserved credit for another's ideas or work; it is the claiming of another's words as one's own. Manifestations of plagiarism may range from the reproduction of another scientist's complete manuscript or project to the taking of his or her specific ideas, methods, or specialized techniques without giving proper credit. Although in science it is quite common to base research on earlier work done in the given field, when large segments of another scientist's work (either written, methodological, or theoretical) are going to be used, it is ethically necessary to request permission from that scientist. Furthermore, appropriate credit in the form of authorship or an acknowledgment needs to accompany the work.

2. Consequences of Dishonesty

When dishonesty is discovered action needs to be taken. Dishonesty, whether as fabrication or falsification, erodes both the public's trust and that of other scientists. Fellow researchers depend on the accuracy and integrity of published data to forge ahead in their own research. When dishonesty is recognized, the involved researcher needs to be identified and held accountable, and a retraction of the illegitimate data should be published.

In the end, vigorous definitions of dishonesty are not feasible. When evaluating deviations from good scientific practice, it is often difficult to tell if a scientist is guilty of dishonesty or improper judgment. Whether a given scientist purposefully intended to manipulate and deceive or rather was guilty of an unintended error in scientific judgment can often be difficult to determine. Therefore scientific dishonesty has no discrete, rigorous definition; the establishment of a verdict relies on sound judgment (4). For a complete ethical assessment of a scientist's actions, other

Table II Ethical Conduct

Four ideals to guide scientific conduct	Resnik's standards of ethical conduct[a]
Truth telling—veracity	Honesty
Dialogue—free exchange	Openness, freedom, opportunity, mutual respect, efficiency
Caution—prudence	Carefulness
Social responsibility—civic duty	Social responsibility, legality, respect for subjects, education, efficiency

[a]From Resnik (1).

considerations such as carelessness and judgment will need to be included.

Scientists should hold themselves to the highest standards of truth telling and veracity. At every point in the scientific process, from experimental planning to data collection and analysis, the scientist needs to be vigilant in avoiding the temptation to fabricate or falsify data. The ethical standard of truth telling dictates that the scientist's primary goal is to seek and report only truthful and honest findings, regardless of where they may lead.

B. Dialogue/Free Exchange

Another standard or guiding principle of science is dialogue or free exchange. Accordingly, science needs to foster an atmosphere of openness that encourages cooperation and the sharing of ideas and techniques among all researchers. Science has long been known as a community that promotes the advancement of knowledge through open review and criticism of each researcher's work. The peer review process is based on this very concept. Openness and dialogue contribute to the advancement of science by helping to build an atmosphere of cooperation and trust. This should enable scientists to work together and share data, research sites, and resources (1). Dialogue between researchers can lead to the more efficient use of limited economic, technological, and human resources.

Despite all the aforementioned benefits of cooperation and dialogue, this ideal is often not a reality. Researchers are competing for economic resources, academic positions, and public and professional prestige. This may lead to secrecy and the zealous protection of ideas and techniques. It is understandable that scientists engage in this protective behavior; one example of a fellow researcher or reviewer "stealing" an idea is enough to scare most scientists into silence. Thus, the second standard of good ethical science depends on the first. That is, if science is to foster an open dialogue between its members then each researcher must remain honest in his or her dealings with other investigators. Dialogue can occur only when scientists treat colleagues with mutual respect. No scientist is permitted to steal or take advantage of information that was shared with him or her in a cooperative spirit. This includes both everyday laboratory collaboration as well as the exchange of information involved in the publication peer review process. If this cooperation and trust is abandoned, then dialogue becomes impeded. Without an open and free flow of information, the engines of science slow and everyone suffers.

Scientists should cultivate an open and vital dialogue based on mutual respect with their colleagues. Open dialogue will lead to a more ethical scientific process, promoting more efficient use of resources, more expedient securing of specific objectives, and participation of the scientific community at large. This ethical standard of fostering dialogue demands that the scientist share ideas, methods, and data. It also dictates that scientists be open to review, criticism, and collaboration.

C. Caution/Prudence

With the privileges of science come correlative duties. Science is granted many privileges in society, including the availability of public funds and the use of human and animal subjects. With these benefits come responsibilities. One basic and often overlooked, yet important, responsibility is carefulness. Often ignored in discussions of ethics and science, caution or care needs to be remembered as a critical factor in the practice of science. Caution, like honesty, promotes the goals of science in that errors can hinder the advancement of knowledge as much as outright lies (1). Many scientists, however, do not view error as a serious crime against science, because it does not involve the intent to deceive. Instead errors are seen as honest mistakes.

1. Errors

There are two main types of scientific error: practical and theoretical. Practical error involves mistakes made by people in using instruments, in performing calculations, and in recording data. These types of mistakes are often due to inattention or a disorderliness characteristic of hasty research. In contrast, theoretical error occurs secondary to either self-deception or bias in the analysis of the experiment, either in its construction or results. Self-deception occurs when a scientist is convinced that experimental results have certain significance or validity when the data do not support such an assertion. Because many scientists have spent their entire lives devoted to a specific field of study, it is understandable that they may see what they want to see when evaluating certain data. Perspective and self-criticism can occasionally be lost in enthusiasm for the subject matter.

2. Bias/Conflict of Interest

Bias, unlike self-deception, usually involves an outside force that improperly influences the research scientist. Bias may include social, political, or economic factors. Conflict of interest can also be considered a bias. According to Thompson, a conflict of interest "is a set of conditions in which professional judgment concerning a primary interest tends to be unduly influenced by a secondary interest" (8). In considering scientific ethics, conflict of interest is important because of its potential to damage the trust among physicians, patients, and the public. If a physician-researcher is perceived not to be acting in a patient's best interest, the trust in the medical–scientific profession begins to erode.

Conflict of interest is most commonly recognized around the issues of financial support and reimbursement. Typical examples of conflict of interest are physician self-referrals, the acceptance of recruitment bonuses (i.e., "finders fees" for enrolling patients into research studies), and pharmaceutical support for certain drug research. Here the physician or researcher gains monetarily by virtue of his or her role as a physician-investigator. In these situations, the potential for personal gain is viewed to be so great that most journals require notification of this sort of financial conflict of interest prior to the publication of articles. In the academic community, where monetary gain may not be as large a factor, motivators such as power, tenure, funding, and publications may serve more as potential sources of conflict of interest. By enlisting patients into studies, physicians position themselves to gain secondarily from subsequent publications, recognition, and prestige. Indeed, the dual role of the physician-scientist itself may be problematic. The duty as physician (caretaker, provider, healer) can sometimes conflict with that of the scientist (data collector, academician, researcher). Due to the inherent nature of the physician-scientist role, not to mention the very structure of the entire research enterprise, it is not possible to eradicate completely the potential for conflict of interest (Table III). Positive research will almost always bring secondary gains to the scientist in some form or another. Having a conflict of interest, however, is not in itself grounds for moral repudiation. Rather than implying unethical behavior, the term conflict of interest "merely identifies a context in which diligence may be necessary to ensure that decisions are made appropriately" (9). Having a conflict of interest is not unethical, it is the physician-scientist's actual actions in the context of this particular situation that may be cause for concern. Given this, the scientific community must identify specific ways to recognize conflicts of interest and to address them appropriately.

Acknowledging the importance of this issue, in 1990 the Association of American Medical Colleges (AAMC) formulated guidelines for dealing with conflicts of interest in research (10). In these guidelines, the AAMC stressed that the key to the prevention and resolution of conflicting interests resides in a threefold approach: full disclosure, aggressive monitoring, and misconduct management. Full disclosure should include all relevant information that could potentially restrict or preclude an investigator's activities in a study. To deal effectively with conflict of interest, investigators need to be vigilant in their awareness of conflicts and their potential for harm. As a researcher, one must be cognizant that even the appearance of a conflict of interest may be detrimental. Therefore, researchers are ethically obliged to divulge any and all connections with their research from which they may seem to benefit. This process of disclosure will undoubtedly be carried out differently at varying institutions. Despite this, a policy of full disclosure should always include details of both individual and family financial and professional interests as related to the research under discussion. Disclosure should be reviewed through the appropriate channels. Monitoring for potential conflict of interest will involve supervisors, chairpersons of departments, as well as designated institutional review committees. As the AAMC notes, the institutional committee's role is critical (10). Its first role is evaluative: to review all pertinent information and make a determination as to whether a conflict of interest exists. The second role is adjudicative: to determine the degree of the conflict of interest. Based on the individual case, the conflict of interest may be judged to be prohibitive, thus requiring the removal of the researcher from the project, or at other times, the conflict may be minor, permitting the researcher to continue with his or her research because the conflict does not represent a possible source of bias. Finally, the role of the institutional committee is to develop policy. The committee is charged with the responsibility of formulating standards to determine what constitutes a conflict of interest, and then it must educate the researcher-physician about how to act professionally within these parameters. Any violations of institutional policies regarding conflict of interest need to be dealt with expeditiously and convincingly in order to maintain the integrity of the research environment.

3. Minimizing Errors

Although human error can never be completely eradicated, scientists have a special duty to minimize any and all errors in research. Errors in research, even if not purposeful,

Table III Examples of Conflict of Interest[a]

Type of conflict	Example
Direct economic	Accepting personal gifts from pharmaceutical companies; self-referrals; direct use or promotion of a product (drug/device) in which the researcher has financial stake
Indirect economic	Certain types of research funding by private pharmaceutical companies; recruitment bonuses or "finder fees" for enlisting subjects into research protocols; study of a device or drug by a physician-investigator who designed or holds its patent
Other sources of conflict in physician roles	Physician as academician/researcher: data, publications, tenure, prestige, personal success; physician as healer: patient advocate, care-taker, public health agent, protector

[a]Based on Elks (9).

can be exceptionally dangerous, particularly when applied to human or animal subjects. Errors in basic research lead to a waste of time and resources. Furthermore, errors erode trust and dialogue in the scientific community. Scientists rely on one another's work; they trust that this work has been carefully performed and that it can be the basis of future work. When errors are consistently found in research, scientists begin to mistrust each other and dialogue is hindered.

A number of informal rules for scientific methodology can help in avoiding unnecessary errors, as shown in Table IV; this list is modeled after David Resnik's code of scientific rules (1). First, controlled experiments must be used to study phenomena, and repeated to confirm findings. No data should ever be reported or published based on one experiment. Second, investigators are responsible for using the most reliable instruments available to gather data, and for being able to use these instruments correctly and reliably. Next, all data should be recorded immediately and carefully in a designated laboratory notebook, with at least one copy of this notebook being kept as well. Finally, one should attempt to avoid self-deception and bias by regularly engaging in dialogue with colleagues. Being surrounded by colleagues who are encouraging, yet also skeptical and rigorous about experimental design and interpretation, is invaluable. When uncertain, seek advice and guidance from a laboratory mentor, senior researcher, or other trusted colleague.

Scientists should take measures to avoid errors in research. By using caution or carefulness as a guiding principle of scientific behavior, researchers can avoid most forms of experimental and methodological errors. By emphasizing caution in obtaining and presenting data, researchers can continue to maintain a science that prizes objectivity, accuracy, and rigorous technique.

D. Social Responsibility/Civic Duty

The practice of science has a social responsibility both to those under its care and to society at large. Under this category is the ethical duty to care responsibly for human and animal subjects, to educate the public, to ensure proper use of resources, and to guarantee that research as a whole benefits society and humankind.

1. Human Use in Research

In its use of human subjects, researchers must respect the integrity of life. Various authors have proposed minimal requirements for clinical research (11–13). A representative list is outlined in Table V. Although some research experiments may not hold the hope for direct patient benefit (i.e., chemotherapeutic trials involving patients with advanced cancer), the aggregate benefit to society or future patients must warrant the risk to the current individual patient involved in a study. Endangering subjects to answer unimportant scientific questions is obviously ethically unacceptable.

Attention to all of the standards of ethical research is absolutely mandatory for any clinical research. Scientists must exercise the highest regard for honesty, carefulness, and open dialogue between scientists-physicians and scientists-subjects. Results need to be reported accurately and promptly. In clinical research this is particularly important. Results of ongoing research can directly impact the care of that cohort or that of future subjects. A timely assessment of data may potentially impact clinical and therapeutic decision making and therefore is critical to ethical human studies.

Not only do individual research investigators have a fundamental responsibility to safeguard the welfare of their subjects, but society has also decided by law that an objective review of research activities involving human subjects is necessary to ensure ethically sound research. This independent review usually takes the form of an institutional review board (IRB). IRBs comprise a group of individuals

Table IV Informal Rules for Scientific Methodology[a]

Use controlled experiments
Repeat experiments to confirm findings
Use reliable instrumentation
Be able to use instrumentation correctly and reliably
Carefully record and duplicate laboratory data records
Regularly engage in informal peer review of experimental design and data interpretation

[a]Based on Resnik's code of scientific rules (1).

Table V Minimum Requirements for the Conduct of Human Research

Study design and implementation
The research must be expected to yield significant benefits for the individual patient or society
The risk of research must be proportional to the expected benefit
The question addressed must justify the risk posed to participants
The study must be well designed
The planned experimental procedures must have been previously tested in animal models
The investigations must be conducted honestly
Rights of human subjects[a]
Informed consent
Ability to deny or quit treatment
Privacy and confidentiality
Anonymity

[a]Based on Sharrott (15).

who promote complete and adequate review of research activities commonly conducted by the institution. IRBs evaluate proposed research to guarantee that human subjects are being treated appropriately. IRBs review the design and protocol of the study, the adequacy of the informed consent, and the progression of the study over its course. It is the responsibility of the IRB to (1) approve, disapprove, or approve with modification a protocol; (2) monitor the progress and conduct of a study; and (3) suspend, terminate, restrict, or request modifications to a study as necessary (14). Any research involving human subjects is reviewed by this independent source in order to guarantee that both their autonomy and overall welfare are respected. The Food and Drug Administration (FDA) mandates that for most drug or device studies in which patients could be placed at potential risk that this independent review of the research be part of the overall research protocol. Investigators have a responsibility to ensure that studies are not initiated before final approval by the IRB. Accordingly, investigators are also ethically (and legally) bound to report promptly to the IRB any adverse events due to the research. Furthermore, any revisions or amendments to the research protocol need to meet with IRB approval before being implemented. Finally, all human research protocols must undergo annual review by the IRB (14).

All of these issues highlight the fact that human subjects possess a moral dignity that demands attention. Investigators sometimes find that their obligations to respect this dignity can come into conflict with the goals of their research. To avoid exploiting the human subject, researchers must think constantly of their subjects' rights (Table V). These include, among others, the right of informed consent, the right to deny or quit treatment, the right to privacy, and the right to anonymity (15). Informed consent must include not only the patient's permission, but also the assurance that the subject understands all of the risks and benefits involved. The subject must also be reminded that he or she maintains the right of refusal as well as the right to quit any research protocol whenever he or she so wishes. The right to privacy refers to the subject's right to prevent the researcher from accessing certain information about the subject. Furthermore, the subject also has the right to remain anonymous and his or her identity may not be released as a participant in the study without specific permission. All information gained about subjects in the study is to be used only for the expressed purposes of the study. Because there frequently are so many difficult ethical issues and conflicts around the use of human subjects, researchers are encouraged to enlist the help of the research ethics committee when in doubt.

2. Animal Use in Research

Animals are also frequently used in the research process. Like their human counterparts, animals must be treated with respect. Given that animals continue to be used in research, we must examine the researcher's ethical responsibility when employing them in research. A brief summary of ethical criteria for the use of animals is outlined in Table VI. First, animals should be used only when no other suitable model is available. Many studies can be performed without the use of animal subjects. Every alternative should be sought before employing animals, because the unnecessary use of animal life is never ethically justifiable. Next, animals used in experiments must be treated with dignity and with attention to their suffering. Using animals in research is only justifiable when performed in a controlled environment that ensures adequate anesthesia as well as the absence of excessive pain and suffering. Animals should not be allowed to suffer gratuitously. They must have adequate housing, food, and water. Furthermore, species that experience higher levels of consciousness deserve treatment commensurate with their level of consciousness (1). This implies that animals such as chimpanzees, which exhibit higher levels of awareness, deserve better treatment than cockroaches or mice. Experiments that may be morally licit when performed in mice may be ethically problematic if applied to chimpanzees. The implication is that animals with higher levels of cognition can only be used in experiments sparingly and with exceptional justification. Finally, science has a constant responsibility to seek alternative experimental methodologies that do not utilize animals. Although the use of animal research is currently indispensable, science has an ethical duty to search for ways in which the use of animal subjects in research can be minimized in the future.

3. Ethical Duties to Society at Large

In addition to the social responsibility that scientists have toward their immediate subjects, they also bear an ethical responsibility for society at large. Scientists have a duty to use societal resources efficiently, to avoid causing harm, and to attempt to produce benefits for society. Although scientists cannot always foresee the results of their research, they always need to have in mind the potential application of their work to the public sector.

Table VI Guidelines for the Ethical Use of Animals in Research[a]

Animals should be used only when no other suitable model is available
Animals used in experiments must be treated with dignity and with attention to their suffering
Species that experience high levels of consciousness deserve treatment commensurate with their level of consciousness
Science has a constant responsibility to seek alternative experimental methodologies that do not utilize animals

[a]Based in part on Resnik's code of scientific rules (1).

Scientists bear a social responsibility to educate. To ensure a lasting ethical scientific environment, senior researchers must educate initiate investigators. This often occurs through the process of mentorship, which will be discussed below. Scientists also need to educate the public. Possessing highly specialized and technical knowledge, the scientist needs to reach out and share that knowledge. A public better educated in the sciences can only benefit research. An informed public is more likely to support future research, to encourage its young to study science, and to engage the scientist in his or her work.

Scientists should embrace their ethical duty of civic responsibility (Table VII). The societal responsibility of the scientist includes respecting human and animal subjects, ensuring the social utility of research, and educating prospective generations of scientists. By engaging civic responsibility as a guiding principle of scientific behavior, researchers can foster good relationships with their subjects, build public trust, and ensure the future of the profession.

III. Character as an Ethical Guide in the Research Setting

It has been argued that character must also play a large role in guiding the behavior of the surgeon scientist. Principles or standards are necessary but not always sufficient as an ethical compass. Although principles work well in the realm of the known, they can be insufficient when addressing the unknown. When faced with novel ethical dilemmas, principles can be inadequate and reductionistic. The specific principle that may apply to any truly novel ethical dilemma is not always evident. Even if we could agree on *which* principle did apply, questions of *how* to apply it and whether the agent is capable of applying it would still persist. Thus, scientists must look within the scientific community for a model of ethics that integrates who they are as scientists with who they are as moral agents. The whole of biomedical ethics cannot be found in the formation and observance of principles; rather, a scientific ethic must also engage scientists as both professionals and human beings who are members of a larger society. It must guide not only what they do, but who they should strive to be. An ethics of character helps to accomplish this.

Table VII Social Responsibilities/ Civic Duties of the Ethical Scientist[a]

Use societal resources efficiently
Avoid causing harm
Strive to ensure the social utility and benefit of research
Educate future scientists
Respect the life of research subjects, both human and animal

[a]Based in part on Resnik's code of scientific rules (1).

Character specifically refers to a set of specifiable traits and dispositions that provide a link between intentions and behavior, forming part of the background for our judgments. A rightly formed character cares about a morally appropriate response to a situation. Character understood in this manner implies a scientist's "deliberate disposition to use a certain range of reasons for his or her actions rather than others" (16). Integrity of character is identified with consistency and moral strength. When informed by character, a scientist is not simply following rules of obligation or action guides; rather, the scientist is striving to do what is morally right out of a sense of motivation and desire to perform right actions. Recognizing that rules sometimes do not suffice to determine appropriate conduct, scientists can appeal to their character to play a significant role in deliberating ethical concerns. To have a morally informed character is necessarily to engage in discovery: by our continuing action we strive to discover and discern what is demanded of us ethically. With this understanding, ethics is a dynamic process that continues to expand as we grow as moral agents.

IV. Ethical Issues: Negotiating the Laboratory Experience

Practical issues often arise in the laboratory that can lead to ethical conflicts. Although a full assessment of each of these is not possible, an investigation into three key issues of "laboratory life" that are central to an ethical scientific environment can be achieved. These issues are mentorship, the intricacies of the laboratory hierarchy, and the reporting of observed ethical misconduct.

A. Mentorship

An important component of the laboratory experience for new investigators is finding the right mentor. If young researchers are to develop into ethical scientists, it is crucial that they encounter peers and role models who possess the highest moral integrity. Although this can be difficult to implement, it is absolutely critical because the scientific environment in which we work continually shapes who we are. Mentors play a critical role in educating and shaping the moral character of future scientists. Mentoring involves a one-on-one relationship that provides the mentor a way to pass on scientific standards and traditions to newly initiated scientists. If mentees are surrounded by scientists behaving unethically, they are less likely to develop a moral character or to acquire ethical scientific habits. Senior scientists therefore have a moral responsibility to provide students, residents, and young researchers with more than simple technical or cerebral instruction. Apprenticeship should impart some idea of what constitutes ethically acceptable behavior in the scientific community. Senior researchers should teach young investigators what it means to be honest, how to do careful research, and whom to seek out for advice and criticism. In this way, mentors create an environment in the laboratory that encourages open discussion of ethical issues. They act as role models on how to incorporate scientific research into moral reasoning. The mentee, seeing this, can begin to engage in ethical dialogue from the beginning of the research experience. By practicing ethical reasoning, young researchers are able to create a framework for decision-making that can be used in how they approach their scientific duties.

B. Fitting into the Laboratory Hierarchy

Not unlike other areas of medicine, the research environment is hierarchical in structure. Laboratory personnel includes students, residents, research fellows, junior and senior researchers, and laboratory directors. A line of authority from the director through the junior researchers, down to the fellows and residents, is usually identifiable. In different laboratories the dynamics of how this line of authority is expressed will be different. Some laboratories are loosely structured from an organizational point of view, whereas others are tightly regulated under the authority of the laboratory director. Regardless of the exact details, the relations between members of each group can become ethically complex. Power imbalances between researchers and students may potentially affect how research is performed and how results are reported. Junior research members often feel "under the gun" in their attempts to satisfy their superiors. Because positive results are often rewarded without scrutinizing the method by which they were obtained, and because most residents can anticipate the "right" results, some may be tempted to alter data or manipulate experimental conditions to achieve desirable ends. There are steps that can be taken to minimize this problem. Senior members of the laboratory team should foster an environment that accepts mistakes, ambiguous results, and a deliberate pace of scientific inquiry. It is always ethically improper to pressure fellow researchers for data or to issue ultimatums for experimental reports. Residents and students should be encouraged to work diligently and produce results, but never at the expense of carefulness and honesty. Furthermore, as part of the initiation of new members into the laboratory, the department and institution both have an obligation to define clear mechanisms for identifying and dealing with ethical improprieties. Senior staff needs to provide junior researchers with clear guidelines and rules for how to deal with suspected misconduct. This will facilitate new researchers' participation in the ethical discourse of the laboratory. For their part, junior researchers bear the responsibility of "standing up to" those higher in the hierarchy who may have unreasonable or ethically questionable demands. Although this may be difficult to do, young researchers can be assisted in this process by surrounding themselves with others who possess high ethical standards.

C. Whistle-Blowing: What to Do When Ethical Misconduct Is Identified?

Working in the laboratory, the scientist must be mindful of unethical activity in which he or she may be directly or indirectly involved. A scientist also needs to be aware of any scientific ethical misconduct that is witnessed, regardless of participatory status. Although it is not the job of the researcher to constantly investigate the ethics of every fellow researcher, a close critical eye toward colleagues' conduct in the laboratory is part of a scientist's moral duty. If scientists are to maintain a rigorous objective and ethical environment, everyone must do their part. Despite a widely recognized need, most countries still have no coherent system to deal with scientific misconduct (4). A system to deal with scientific misconduct will primarily have three objectives: (1) assessing the validity of the accusation, (2) formally investigating the grievance, and (3) establishing a punishment or rectifying the situation (Table VIII).

Accusing a fellow researcher of ethical misconduct is a serious matter and should not be taken lightly. Even if later investigations exonerate a researcher, the shadow of the mere accusation may hang over a researcher's work indefinitely, thereby impairing his or her future career. The initiation of a complaint (or "blowing of the whistle") must therefore meet certain criteria (Table IX). First, the complainant should ensure that the information is accurate and based on a thorough understanding of the accused researcher's work. Before lodging an accusation about the ethical impropriety of a fellow scientist's work, the whistle blower should possess a complete understanding of the situation. In some circumstances, the impropriety of an action is readily apparent. When someone witnesses a scientist changing data points or manipulating experimental conditions to suit his or her needs, no other information is usually needed. At other times, however, a full determination of the morality of the given situation cannot be made without a

Table VIII Objectives in Reviewing Accusations of Scientific Misconduct

Assess the validity of the accusation
Formally investigate the grievance: interview members of the research team, review data files, etc.
Enforce appropriate punishment; ensure wrong information is corrected or retracted

Table IX Criteria for "Blowing the Whistle"[a]

Information must be accurate
Individual initiating the complaint must have a thorough understanding of the accused's work
The accuser should first attempt to confront the scientist performing the ethically questionable activity
The accuser should report the suspected ethical misconduct to the appropriate authorities

[a]Based in part on Resnik (1).

certain knowledge of the whole process involved. For example, someone not versed in a statistical method may not be able to assess accurately whether a scientist is "fudging" the data in the statistical manipulations. Only a scientist with this specialized knowledge would be in the position to question the ethics of the other researcher's statistical method. Next, if possible, the accuser should first confront the scientist performing the ethically questionable activity. Most often this is not possible. Fear of retaliation or being "black balled" by the scientific community makes an open confrontation almost always unworkable. In an ideal situation, after identifying an ethically problematic situation, the concerned researcher could approach the scientist in question to allow him or her the opportunity to clarify, even to rectify, what may be an honest, unintended error. By proceeding directly to an institutional review process without first approaching the scientist in question, the opportunity to remedy the situation before it becomes public is lost. Finally, the accuser should report the suspected ethical misconduct to the appropriate authorities. After identifying suspected ethical misconduct, the accuser has an ethical duty not only to be careful and deliberate in the details of the report, but also to ensure that the report gets sent to the proper authorities. It is ethically inappropriate for researchers to give information about suspected ethical misconduct to unsanctioned bodies. By reporting to appropriate authorities such as ethics councils or department review boards, the whistle blower respects the due process that the accused scientist deserves.

On receiving a complaint concerning scientific misconduct, the given authoritative body will usually initiate a full investigation. Depending on the situation, this may range from interviews with laboratory members, review of data files, or even the involvement of legal authorities. A comprehensive review of the investigative process cannot be accomplished here. When ethical impropriety is identified, the investigating committee has a duty to effect the appropriate consequences. Depending on the severity of the ethical misconduct, penalties can range from published retractions, loss of academic positions, withdrawal of funding, removal of licensure, or even a legal sentence.

V. Issues in Publication: Whose Paper Is It, Who Decides, and Who Controls Publication?

One of the main aims of the scientist is to publish his or her work. Publications are important because they serve as the main method by which information is communicated throughout the scientific community. They act as a "measuring stick" of a scientist's productivity, often influencing promotional status as well as overall standing in a particular field. Given the importance of publications, a consideration of the ethical issues involved in publishing is warranted.

A. Authorship

Authorship is a critical issue in the ethics of publication. Authorship dictates largely who receives credit for the work. It decides which members of the scientific community are associated with new findings, and thereby awards prestige, value, and recognition to them. Despite the importance of authorship, no universal definition or criteria of authorship exist. Principle investigators often see authorship as a prerogative, to be decided on a case-by-case basis without any appeal to strict criteria. Different researchers adhere to varying levels of authorship stringency; some scientists easily award honorary authorship to department heads or well-known associates, feeling their research stands a better chance of successful peer review. Other investigators fail to offer authorship to their technicians because they see data collection alone as simply the technician's job. There has been an ever-increasing incline in multiauthored articles that cannot be explained solely by the increased collaboration between centers and funding for research. A multivariable analysis of authorship practices revealed an inflationary trend in the number of authors and centers per article over the past two decades (17). This has caused some to postulate that these "additional" authors of certain published articles have not made significant contributions to them, leading to concerns about the integrity of such research (18).

In deciding what constitutes an ethical approach to authorship it is helpful to review the Vancouver Group's definition (19). Authorship credit should be based on substantial contributions according to the following criteria: (1) conception or design of the experiment; analysis or interpretation of the data, (2) drafting or revising the article for important intellectual content, and (3) final approval of the version to be published, with conditions 1 and 2 being met (Table X). Participation solely in the acquisition of funding or the collection of data does not justify authorship.

In this definition of authorship, the credit that accompanies authorship must be grounded in the researcher's ability to take responsibility for the work. If the author is unable to

Table X Authorship Criteria Based on the Vancouver Group's Definition[a]

Conception or design of the experiment
Analysis or interpretation of the data
Drafting or revising of the article for intellectual content
Final approval of the version to be published, with the preceding three conditions being met

[a]From ICMJE (19).

take responsibility for the work, he or she should not be listed as an author. This definition acknowledges another important function of authorship: accountability. In light of this definition, honorary authorship and "cooperative" authorship deals would be unethical. Scientists can only ethically claim authorship when they have made substantial contributions to the published work; for a contribution to be "substantial" it must mean that the given author is able to assume responsibility for the work that bears his or her name. By adhering to more rigorous criteria for authorship, scientists can reemphasize the credibility and trust of its readership.

B. The Review Process

The peer review of manuscripts represents the gateway to publication. In order for scientific publishing to be an ethical endeavor, the peer-review process must be sound. This process has chiefly been structured in three different manners: single blinded, double blinded, or open. The most prevalent review process is the single-blinded type in which authors are not permitted to know the identity of the reviewer, but the reviewer is aware of the author's identity and institutional affiliation. In the double-blind setting, neither the author nor reviewer knows the other's identity. Much more rare, the open-review process allows for the full disclosure of both parties' identities. Although there remains much discussion around which system may result in the most ethical outcome, at the current time the single-blinded review process predominates. The benefit of this system is that it allows for a more candid assessment of the submitted work without the fear of reprisal or penalty to the reviewer. Others have argued, however, that the single-blinded process is unethical. It may encourage reviewers to favor more famous researchers or institutions, to be more severe and unreasonable in their criticism, and even to possibly steal others' ideas or work.

Given that the single-blinded review process seems likely to continue as the standard of peer review, a number of ethical standards to guide this procedure are necessary. Ethical peer review demands that the reviewer exhibit the highest standards of honesty, carefulness, and expediency. Honesty dictates that reviewers never steal information or ideas from work that has been entrusted to them prior to publication. All information contained in scientific manuscripts should be discussed only in regard to its publication status. No information garnered from submitted manuscripts may be used by the reviewer prior to publication without the explicit consent of the involved investigators. When conducting reviews of manuscripts, reviewers must also exercise the greatest of care. Researchers entrust their work to publishers and deserve a fair, complete, and thorough evaluation. The review process should therefore be educational and productive for the investigators involved. It is ethically unacceptable to produce reviews that attack investigators personally or indiscriminately denigrate their work. The review process should be aimed at increasing dialogue among researchers in the hopes of furthering mutual scientific goals. Finally, the review process should be expeditious. Although care is crucial, the review process also needs to be of a reasonable duration. Scientists depend on publications for promotion, tenure, and funding. The unnecessary delay in the review process unfairly penalizes researchers for submitting their work to a given journal. An ethical review process will therefore stress honesty, integrity, care, and promptness.

VI. Conclusion

Although the future holds the promise of significant advances in the biomedical fields, with attendant clinical and scientific benefits, the magnitude of the associated ethical and social concerns parallels the magnitude of the advances. The daily ethical challenges within the surgical research laboratory equal the more global, societal ethical issues. Issues of honesty, objectivity, and methodology are inherent in all forms of scientific research, both at the bench and in the clinic. Despite the fact that the research environment can be an impediment to ethical conduct, scientists must continue to hold themselves to the highest ethical standards, adhering to the principles of truth telling, free dialogue within the scientific community, caution or prudence, and social responsibility. Only by continuing to be intimately involved with the ethics of research will surgeon-scientists be able to maintain their involvement in the decisions about how new knowledge and technologies will be used within society.

References

1. Resnik, D. (1998). "The Ethics of Science: An Introduction." Routledge, New York.
2. Bekkelund, S. I., and Hegstad, A.-C. Scientific dishonesty in medical research in Norway. *Tidsskr Nor Laegeforen* **115,** 3148–3151 [in Norwegian with English summary].
3. Beauchamp, T., and Childress, J. (1989). "Principles of Biomedical Ethics." Oxford Univ. Press, New York.

4. Nylenna, M., Andersen, D., Dahlquist, G., and Sarvas, M. (1999). Handling of scientific dishonesty in Nordic countries. *Lancet* **354,** 57–61.
5. National Academy of Sciences, National Academy of Engineering, Institute of Medicine (1992). "Responsible Science: Ensuring the Integrity of the Research Process," Vol. 1. National Academy Press, Washington, D.C.
6. Budiansky, S. (1983). False data confessed. *Nature (London)* **301,** 101.
7. Hixson, J. (1976). "The Patchwork Mouse." Doubleday, New Jersey.
8. Thompson, D. F. (1993). Understanding financial conflicts of interests. *N. Engl. J. Med.* **329,** 573–576.
9. Elks, M. L. (1995). Conflict of interest and the physician-researcher. *J. Lab. Clin. Med.* **126,** 19–23.
10. Association of American Medical Colleges Ad Hoc Committee on Misconduct and Conflict of Interest in Research (1990). Guidelines for dealing with faculty conflicts of commitment and conflicts of interest in research. *Acad. Med.* **65,** 487–496.
11. Weijer, C., Dickens, B., and Meslin, E. (1997). Bioethics for clinicians: Research ethics. *Can. Med. Assoc. J.* **156,** 1153–1157.
12. National Commission for the Protection of Human Subjects of Biomedical and Behavioral Research (1979). The Belmont Report: Ethical principles and guidelines for the protection of human subjects of research. *Office Protect. Res. Risks Rep.* **18,** 1–8.
13. Meslin, E., Sutherland, H., Lavery, J., and Till, J. (1995). Principalism and the ethical appraisal of clinical trials. *Bioethics* **9,** 399–418.
14. Skolnick, B. (1998). Ethical and Institutional Review Board issues. *Adv. Neurol.* **76,** 253–262.
15. Sharrott, G. (1985). Ethics of clinical research. *Am. J. Occup. Ther.* **39,** 407–408.
16. Hauerwas, S. (1972). Toward an ethics of character. *In* "Theological Studies," Vol. 33. Theological Studies, Inc., Milwaukee, WI.
17. Khan, K., Nwosu, C., Khan, S., Dwarakanath, L., and Chien, P. (1999). A controlled analysis of authorship trends over two decades. *Am. J. Obstet. Gynecol.* **181,** 503–507.
18. Smith, R. (1997). Authorship: Time for a paradigm shift? *BMJ* **314,** 992.
19. International Committee of Medical Journal Editors (1993). Uniform requirements for manuscripts submitted to biomedical journals. *JAMA* **269,** 2282–2286.

96

The National Institutes of Health: Procedures and Performance

Scott D. Somers

Division of Pharmacology, Physiology, and Biological Chemistry, The National Institute of General Medical Sciences, Bethesda, Maryland 20892

I. Introduction

"Knowledge is of two kinds. We know a subject ourselves, or we know where we can find information on it" (Samuel Johnson, *Letter to Lord Chesterfield,* April 18, 1775). Investigators, new or otherwise, often have many questions about the extramural activities of The National Institutes of Health (NIH):

- What is the NIH?
- What are the individual Institutes? How do I assure that my application goes to the right Institute?
- What are the different types of grants? For which ones am I eligible? What are the advantages and disadvantages of each?
- What happens to my application once it is sent? What is the process timetable? Whom do I talk to and when should I ask? Should I even call?
- What are study sections? Who chooses reviewers? How do study sections work?
- What do reviewers look for in applications?
- What happens after an application is reviewed?
- What should I do if I think the reviewers were wrong?
- What determines funding? Does funding vary from Institute to Institute?
- What do I do if my proposal is not funded?
- What do I do if my proposal is funded?
- Can I take my grant with me to my new position?
- What makes a good proposal?
- Where can I go for help?

The purpose of this chapter is twofold. The first is to provide answers to many of the commonly asked questions. The second, and perhaps more important, purpose is to enable the reader to find the answers to questions, either general or specific in nature, that arise as a routine part of running a research program—in other words, to provide the reader with Dr. Johnson's second kind of knowledge. (Brief answers to the questions listed above will be provided at the end of the chapter.) This chapter may be easily summarized with two separate ideas: search the NIH homepage and contact the NIH via e-mail or telephone. These themes will be repeated often. In fact, most if not all of the information contained within this chapter may be found somewhere on the NIH homepage (http://www.nih.gov).

But why bother to know about the NIH, or any potential source of funds for your research projects? What do scientists need to know to run a successful research program? Obviously, they must know the science—namely, what questions to ask and how to obtain clear definitive answers to those questions. Communication is also a vitally important skill, because scientists must present findings to the scientific community and convince them that both the answers and the wherewithal to obtain further results are possible. With respect to the latter, current medical research is expensive, requiring substantial financial and human resources. Thus successful scientists must be able to convince potential funding sources that their ideas are meritorious. Arguably, there are advantages to knowing as much as possible about the potential funding source to maximize the chances for success and assure appropriate service. Related to the latter is the fact that in-depth knowledge of the funding source will make life easier in the long run (knowing deadlines, who to call, when to call, and the meaning of various informational items, for example). Because the NIH is a major source of funding for biomedical research in this country, there is value to garnering a greater understanding of its operation and practices. Hence this chapter, and hence the above questions, which are legitimate, appropriate, and worthy of detailed answers.

II. Structure of the NIH

The National Institutes of Health is a component organization of the Department of Health and Human Services (DHHS). Accordingly, the yearly budget appropriated by Congress for the NIH is a part of that for the entire DHHS (Fig. 1).

It is important to note that "Institutes" is indeed plural, meaning that the NIH consists of separate administrative and functional entities. The NIH is composed of 25 separate Institutes, Centers, or Offices (given the general abbreviation of IC). Each has responsibility for different areas, delineated by disease process, organ system, scientific endeavors, or administration of various aspects of scientific research administration. Often, research topics are of interest to multiple ICs, giving rise to dual assignments of applications (discussed below). The standard operating procedures for each IC are generally similar, although differences may exist. This again emphasizes the importance of learning as much as possible about the organizations with which the most interactions will occur. There is a huge wealth of information about the whole NIH organization, including links to all the component ICs, on the NIH homepage (http://www.nih.gov). In particular, the homepage contains historical information about the NIH, including data about the budget and funding rates, a search engine, links to other organizations of the DHHS, and information about the intramural program of the NIH. Although this chapter is a general overview of the NIH, some of the material presented will be given from the perspective of a single Institute [the National Institute of General Medical Sciences (NIGMS)].

A longstanding hallmark of the NIH is the determination of the relative scientific merit of grant proposals through the process of peer review. The vast majority of peer review for the NIH falls under the jurisdiction of the Center for Scientific Review (CSR). It is a unique administrative unit of the NIH, separate from the Institutes. In turn, the Institutes have the authority and the resources, both given by Congress, to make grant awards. Thus at the NIH, the review process is separate from the funding and administration of grants.

III. Key Terms and NIH Personnel

A short summary of various terms, acronyms, and definitions used throughout the chapter is found in Table I. Listed in Table II are several key NIH staff having frequent interactions with applicants and grantees. Of course there are many other positions across the NIH in addition to these four general categories; there may exist occasions when communication is required with these other categories of staff. Arguably it is important for any potential grantee to know which of the specific NIH staff are responsible for marshalling applications through the review and funding process. The specific functions for Scientific Review Administrators (SRAs), Program Administrators (PAs), and Grant Management staff will be addressed later in the chapter. It should be noted that although the CSR employs a large number of SRAs, each IC also has a review office and thus SRAs on their staff. As will be discussed, there are some granting mechanisms not reviewed by the CSR, but rather by the individual ICs. The SRAs from the CSR may be responsible for those reviews, but there are occasions when the IC SRAs will handle the responsibilities.

The functions of the Communications and Public Liaison Office deserve a few extra words here. Based on the description in Table II, these NIH staff are of obvious importance to the overall mission and function of the NIH. Each IC has their own office. An additional target audience that these offices will communicate with is Congress. It is crucial that all audiences clearly understand the mission, responsibilities, actions, and accomplishments of the NIH. Grantees share in that responsibility, and should acknowledge NIH support on all publications. Moreover, the yearly progress

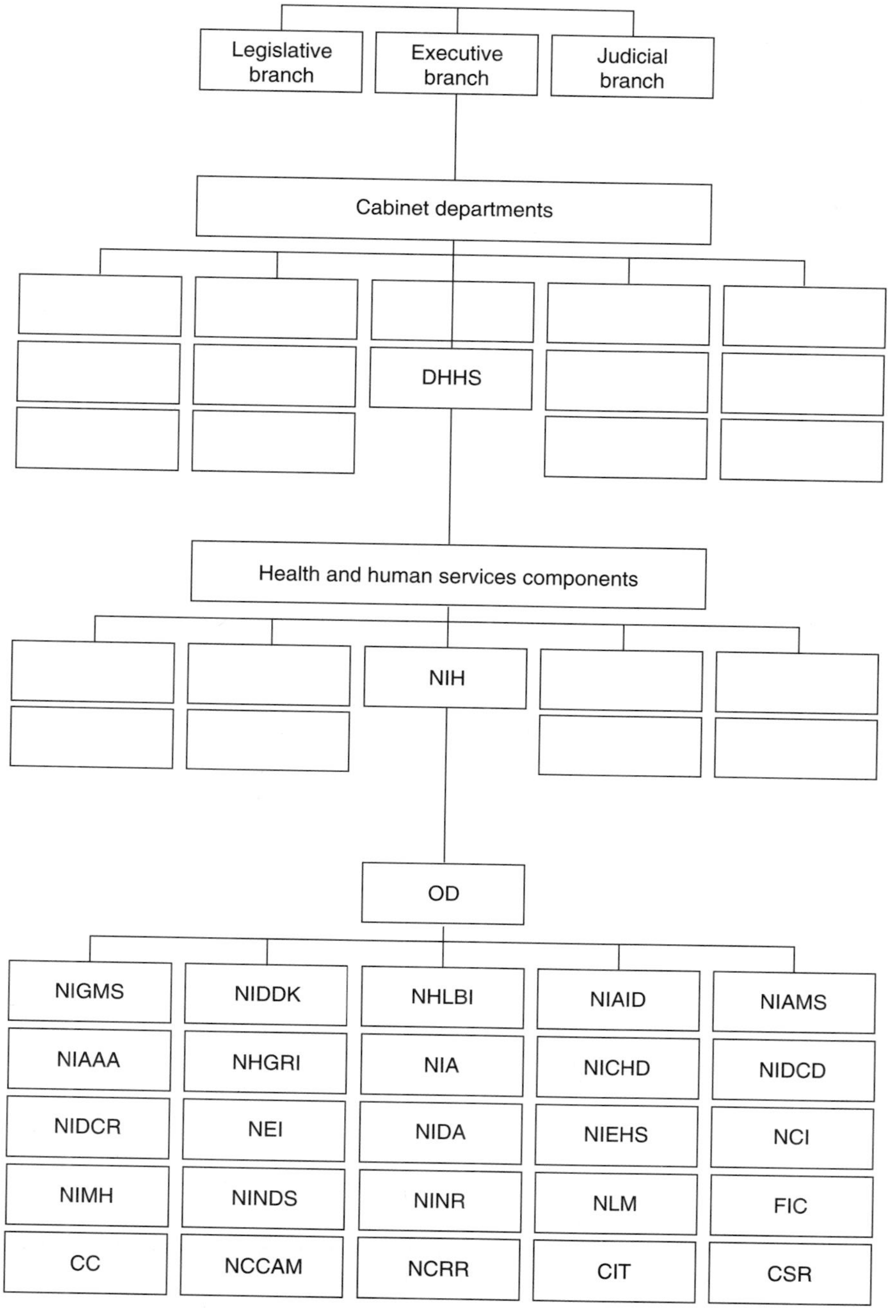

Figure 1 The position of National Institutes of Health within the United States government.

reports are an excellent opportunity to share research advances with program staff. If the advance is highly significant, the PA will share information with staff from the Communications and Public Liaison Office, who then make the findings known to the general public (i.e., possibly a press release). Thus if a staff member from an NIH Communications and Public Liaison Office initiates contact, it is probably important to listen.

IV. Funding Mechanisms

A list of possible funding mechanisms available from the NIH is provided in Table III. Not much additional information will be given here because each IC may use the funding mechanisms in slightly different fashions, and the mechanism may change over time. Again, there are several sites on the NIH homepage that may be worth a bookmark and

Table I Glossary of Key Terms

Term	Definition
Amended application	Resubmission of proposal answering prior critique
Appeal	Process to challenge peer review of application
Center for Scientific Review (CSR)	Organization responsible for administering the majority of peer review
Competitive renewal	Application for ongoing project undergoing peer review
Direct costs	Funds to support research project
Facilities & Administration (F & A) costs	Funds to support institutional costs of research
Grants Management staff	Officials responsible for financial and administrative of awards
Institute/Center (IC)	A component organization of NIH responsible for funding and administration of award
Initial Review Group (IRG)	Cluster of study sections within the CSR
Just in time (JIT)	Information required just before an award is made
Modular grants	New means for budget preparation for requests less than $250,000 in direct costs
National Advisory Council	Group overseeing IC practices
New Investigator	Investigator with no previous research support from the NIH
Noncompetitive renewal	Application for ongoing project not undergoing peer review
Notice of Grant Award (NGA)	Statement sent with award parameters
Office of Protection from Research Risks (OPRR)	Organization responsible for oversight of the welfare of human subjects or animals (http://grants.nih.gov/grants/oprr/oprr.htm)
Principal Investigator (PI)	Individual responsible for research application and project
Program Announcement (PA)	Declaration of NIH interest in a scientific area
Program Administrator (PA)	Official responsible for administration of awards
Request for Application (RFA)	Set-aside funds for research on given topic
Special Emphasis Panel (SEP)	Review group specifically designed for one or more applications
Scientific Review Administrator (SRA)	Official responsible for peer review
Study section	Subset of IRG performing peer review

Table II Key NIH Personnel

Position	Responsibilities
Scientific Review Administrator (SRA)	Referral of applications to appropriate study section; selection of peer reviewers; assignment of applications to reviewers; oversight of the study section meeting; preparation of summary statements; advise applicants about the review process
Program Administrator (PA) or Program Director (PD)	Interact with scientific community and advise about the NIH; develop and administer research program (using program announcements for new areas and yearly review of progress reports, for example); often an observer at study sections, responsible for application after peer review, providing oversight and input through National Advisory Council meeting and funding decisions
Grants Management	Performs financial and administrative evaluation of grants; serves as a source of information for scientific and review staff of DHHS, NIH, and IC regulations and policies; evaluates appropriateness of budgetary requests and effectiveness of grantee's business management systems; monitors grantee performance for compliance with terms and conditions of awards; issues NGAs
Communications and Public Liaison Office	Communicates the goals and results of supported research to the general public and specific target audiences; responds to inquiries from the general public, scientists, students, educators, and the news media; provides information about the IC's mission, programs, activities, and initiatives; information products may include articles, news releases, brochures, newsletters, and the official web site

Table III Partial List of Funding Mechanisms Available from the NIH

Category/code	Title	Review organization[a]
Research		
R01	Research Project Grants	CSR
R15	Academic Research Enhancement Award (AREA)	CSR
R21	Exploratory Studies for High-Risk/High-Impact Research	CSR
R03	Small Grant Program	CSR
P01	Program Project Grants (PPGs)	IC, CSR
P50	Research Center Grants (RCGs)	IC
Fellowship		
F32	Individual National Research Service Awards (NRSAs)	CSR, IC
F33	National Research Service Awards for Senior Fellows (Established Researchers)	CSR, IC
T32	Institutional National Research Service Awards	IC
Career Development		
K08	Mentored Clinical Scientist Development Awards	IC, CSR
K23	Mentored Patient-Oriented Research Career Development Award	IC, CSR
K30	Clinical Research Curriculum Award	IC[b]
Cooperative Agreements		
U01	Cooperative Agreement[c]	IC

[a]The predominant organization responsible for review. Each IC may have different views on how the funding mechanism is to be used, meaning that there may be different review procedures.

[b]The K30 mechanism is reviewed and administered by the National Heart, Lung, and Blood Institute, although most ICs have contributed funds for the program and serve on a steering committee.

[c]Cooperative agreements will have very specific stated goals, and may have different titles.

frequent examination. In particular, a list of most funding mechanisms, complete with descriptions, may be found at http://grants.nih.gov/grants/funding/funding_program.htm. Also, the NIH attempts to be responsive to the needs of the scientific community and the research opportunities that are created by issuing Program Announcements (PAs) or Requests for Applications (RFAs). Another important site is http://grants.nih.gov/grants/forms.htm, where application forms and instructions may be found. These are documents soliciting research applications on specific topics, and are listed in a document published weekly, the *"NIH Guide for Grants and Contracts"* (http://grants.nih.gov/grants/guide/index.html). Check the Guide often and read it carefully. All of these sites are contained on the Grants page, which may be readily found on the NIH homepage.

As a sign of the age in which we live, this chapter relies heavily on potential applicants having access to and some degree of comfort with the Internet. If an individual has neither, the NIH is still accessible. An excellent source of information may well be found at your home institution in an office that is responsible for sponsored research. Additional information could be provided by colleagues and mentors. Either way, work to identify a potential contact individual at the NIH and begin to communicate directly.

The R01 is the standard of NIH funding. New investigators are encouraged to apply for an R01, if of course they have adequate training, a productive track record, a reasonable idea, and sufficient preliminary data. It is important that new investigators identify themselves by marking the appropriate space on the face page of the PHS398 form. By marking this box, the applicant informs the SRA, reviewers, and the PA of their status, meaning that there should be special consideration of the proposal. Other funding mechanisms such as the R21 (High-Risk/High-Impact Research) or the R03 (Small Grant Program) may or may not be appropriate for new investigators, or for established scientists, for that matter. Be aware that not all ICs offer these awards, and each IC may use the mechanism for very different purposes. New investigators may also serve as Principal Investigators (PIs) for subprojects on Program Project Grants (P01) or Research Center Grants (P50). These are, however, large, complex, multicomponent applications that are difficult to construct. The overall PIs for either of these mechanisms are responsible for putting together the entire application. A potential downside to having a project on either a P01 or P50 is that the individual may have lower visibility than if they received an R01.

There are multiple funding mechanisms for individuals not far enough along for an independent research award, i.e., training fellowships and career development awards (see Table III). Again these may be used differently by the ICs, so careful reading of the appropriate PA or RFA and direct contact with the proper contact at the NIH are strongly advised.

As seen in Table III, the funding mechanisms may be reviewed by either the CSR or the IC. The CSR again administers the majority of review for the NIH. There are occasions when the IC desires more oversight of the review process, mainly because the funding mechanism is very specific for the mission and goals of the IC. For example, the NIGMS performs reviews of institutional National Research Service Award applications (the T32 training grants), because these programs have very defined characteristics and requirements. Regardless of which organization is responsible, the peer review process is essentially the same in both practice and quality.

Finally, Fig. 2 presents a generalized timeline of matriculation for academic physicians, complete with some potential funding mechanisms relevant for each career stage. The information presented in the figure is mainly for those individuals interested in the types of scientific research sponsored by NIGMS. The Medical Student Training Program (MSTP), offered only by the NIGMS, allows medical students to receive training leading to dual M.D. and Ph.D. degrees. Beyond that are several other funding mechanisms specific for each career stage. Once again, other ICs might use these mechanisms differently. Thus, contact with program staff is recommended.

V. Life Cycle of an NIH Application

What happens to an application submitted to the NIH is a common yet important question. A graphic depiction of the process flow is shown in Fig. 3, with a general description given in the legend.

Prior to submitting an application, it might be helpful to know whether the NIH supports work of a similar nature. Information about all NIH-funded projects may be found in a searchable database (https://www-commons.cit.nih.gov/crisp) called Computer Retrieval of Information on Scientific Projects (CRISP; see Table IV). From this site, an investigator may gather information about not only what types of research are funded, but also by which IC. The information may be useful for self-referral of an application, meaning requesting assignment to an IC for potential funding as well as a study section for review. A list of study sections, defined by the scientific area covered, and the standing study section roster may be found on the CSR homepage. Sometimes there is also value in contacting the SRA or PA of the identified IC for additional advice. The appropriate IC and the types of unique review expertise that might be required should be put into a cover letter sent with the application.

Within a short time of receiving the application, the referral officers at CSR will assign the application to an IC and Initial Review Group (IRG; i.e., study section). The information will be sent to the applicant in a flyer. Be sure to read and understand the information supplied; assignments can be changed if necessary. The application is assigned a number, the significance of which is explained in Fig. 4.

A major event in an application's life cycle is of course the peer review. The SRA is totally responsible for the study section and thus chooses the reviewers. Applications are assigned to individuals for review, to schedule and oversee meetings, to calculate and record scores, and to prepare the summary statement. Reviewers are chosen to meet several criteria. First and foremost is their knowledge of the particular scientific area. Because individual study sections span a range of techniques, approaches, and disciplines, not every unique subset of specialties is necessarily represented. Thus comes a second important qualification of reviewers, that they must be open-minded and fair with a broad

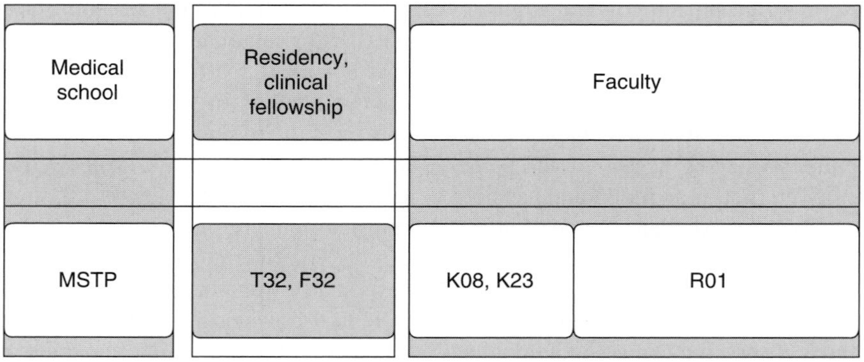

Figure 2 NIGMS award mechanisms available for a typical academic physician applicant (see also Table III).

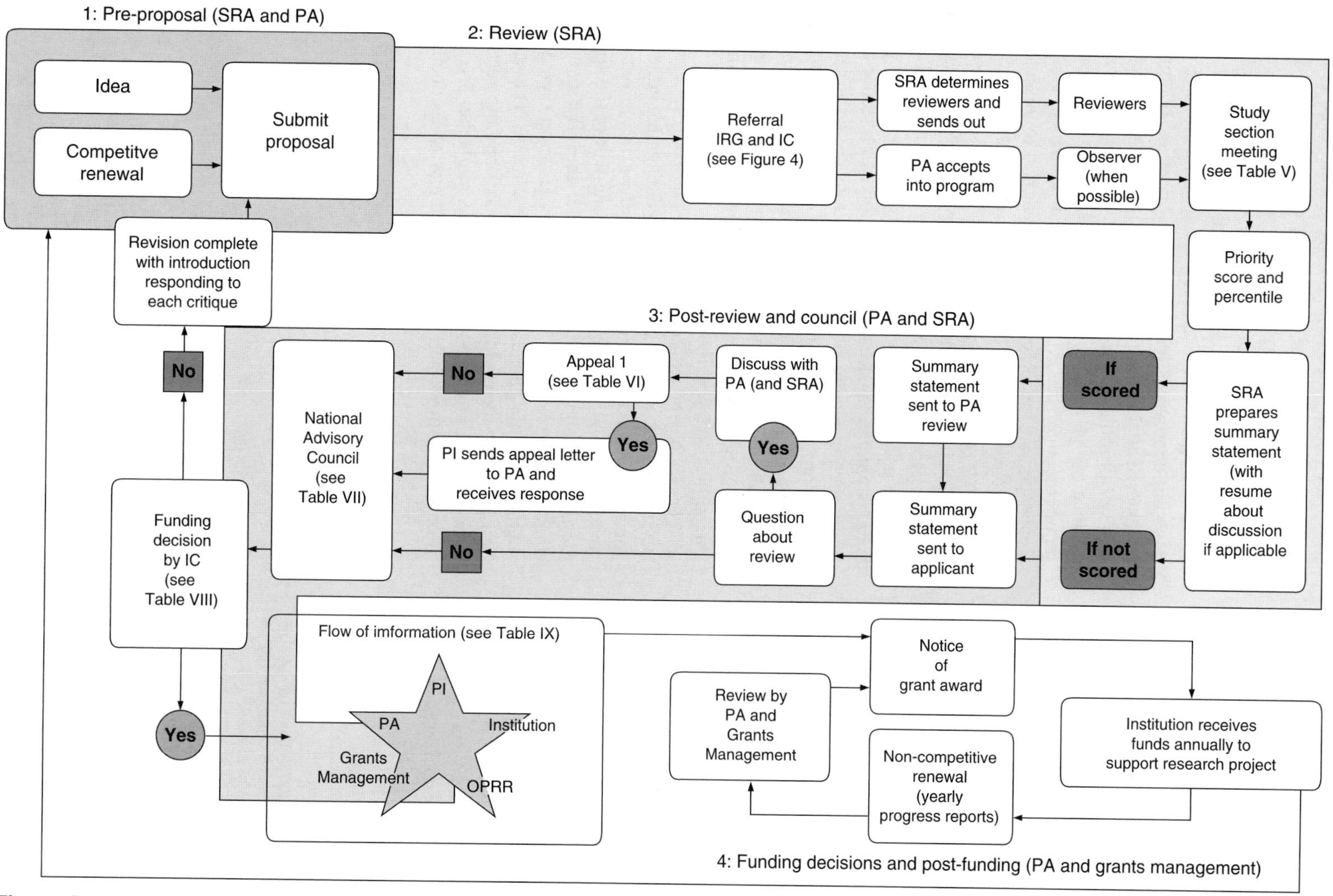

Figure 3 The life cycle of an NIH application. There are four general phases to the life cycle of an application, with the key events and NIH staff to be contacted represented. The preapplication phase should take as long as necessary, and the applicant may contact either the PA or SRA as needed. In the second phase, the application is received at the NIH and assigned to an IC and an IRG. The applicant receives a flyer stating the assignment within 2 months of receipt. Referral of applications is done by CSR staff, including SRAs, who know both the review expertise of the IRG and the scientific interests and responsibilities of the funding components, the ICs. Self-referral is now encouraged, presuming that the applicant has researched the NIH system sufficiently to request a specific study section and IC. Because areas of shared interest exist among the ICs, an application may receive assignment to two or more ICs. The application will be reviewed by a single study section regardless of the assignment. An IC with a secondary assignment might have the opportunity to make an award if the IC holding the primary assignment cannot or does not fund the proposal. This opportunity is not mandatory, however. Study sections meet 3–4 months after receipt of the proposal. The SRA is the primary contact in this phase. The postreview/council phase (phase 3) is usually complete 9–10 months after receipt, and the PA becomes the primary contact person. The SRA calculates the priority score and percentile ranking and completes the summary statement. Any questions about the review should be directed to the PA, who will seek input from the SRA. Finally, if an award is made, phase 4 begins with communication between multiple individuals. An award then begins a yearly cycle of administrative review of the progress report and subsequent funding.

Table IV Computer Retrieval of Information on Scientific Projects[a]

Searchable database of federally funded biomedical research projects
Includes NIH, Food and Drug Administration (FDA), Centers for Disease Control and Prevention (CDCP), Agency for Healthcare Research and Quality (AHRQ), Health Resources and Services Administration (HRSA), and Substance Abuse and Mental Health Services Agency (SAMHSA)
Can search either for funded projects in current fiscal year or historical database
Searchable by key words, PI, funding mechanism, IC, or state
Search will provide abstract of funded project

[a]Internet site: https://www-commons.cit.nih.gov/crisp/.

perspective and interest. This type of individual is usually a seasoned investigator, and most will have NIH funding. Often, however, the SRA will balance a review panel with some younger scientists, especially if a particular expertise is required. Finally, the SRA will attempt as much as possible to assure adequate representation of geographic area, as well as gender and racial diversity. Study section members usually serve a 4-year term. Ad hoc reviewers are often included at a meeting to provide necessary expertise and to assure adequate reviews.

Although each study section is slightly different, there are some general characteristics. Prior to the actual study section meeting, the SRA will have sent to the reviewers the applications for consideration. Each application will be assigned a primary and secondary reviewer who will read and critique the proposal in detail. There will also be at least one other person responsible for reading the application, although some study sections may assign multiple reviewers. The primary and secondary reviewers will provide written comments based on the five criteria listed in Table V. Study sections may have anywhere from several to over 100 applications to review. Thus each reviewer may be responsible for just a few to as many as 10–12 applications per meeting.

The meeting is started by the SRA giving general instructions about the conduct of the meeting, a warning about conflict of interest, and the importance of maintaining confidentiality. With regard to conflict of interest, reviewers collaborating with an applicant or working at the same institution are required to exit the meeting when the application is discussed. Confidentiality is an absolute requirement for the NIH peer review system to function. Reviewers are specifically instructed not to discuss the applications outside of the actual review meeting. The actual review process is presided over by the study section chair, who is responsible for assuring a complete, balanced, and fair process—as well as one that moves along at a reasonable pace. The first order of business is to determine which applications do not fall in the top half of those at that study section meeting. Such applications are considered to be unscored (i.e., triaged) and are not discussed further, allowing the group to focus more time on discussing the proposals in the top half. Be aware that the decision to triage must be unanimous; if one reviewer wishes to discuss the application, it will be done.

For each application to be discussed, the assigned reviewers start by giving a relative level of enthusiasm about the application. If numerical, a score of 1 is the absolute best and 5 is the absolute worst. Because one-half of the applications should be considered unscored, the effective range should reach from 1 to 3. The primary reviewer then gives a summary of the application, then the critique. The secondary reviewer then adds comments, as does the reader or however many other reviewers there might be. A general discussion follows and reviewers attempt to reconcile any

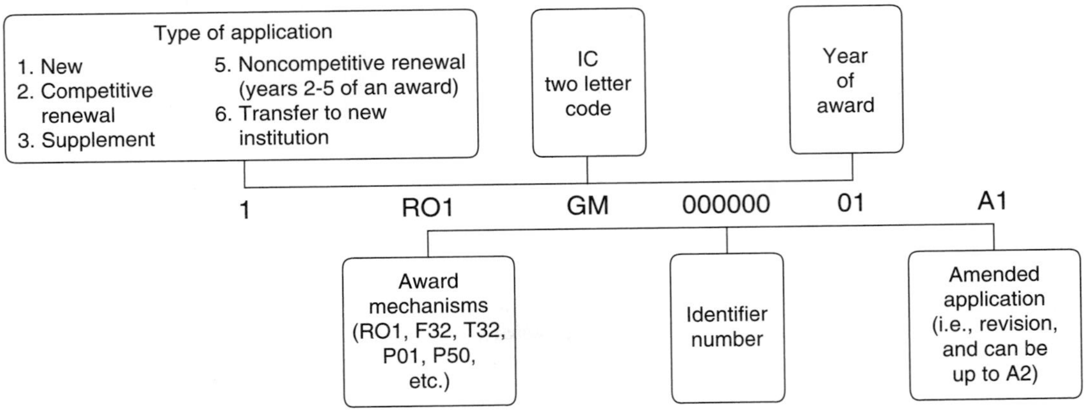

Figure 4 The anatomy of an NIH application number.

Table V Review Criteria[a]

Criterion	Scope
Significance	Does the study address an important problem? How will scientific knowledge be advanced if the aim of the project are achieved? How will the studies effect concepts or methods used in the field?
Approach	Are the conceptual framework, design, methods, and analyses adequately developed, integrated, and appropriate for the project? Does the application identify potential problem areas and propose alternative approaches?
Innovation	Are novel concepts, approaches, or methods used in the proposal? Are the aims original and innovative? Are existing paradigms challenged or new methodologies presented by the application?
Investigator	Is the investigator appropriately trained and capable of the proposed work? Is the proposed work at an appropriate level for the investigator(s)?
Environment	Is the institution supportive of the investigator and the proposed work? Will the environment contribute to the likelihood of success for the project? Does the application take advantage of any unique features of the environment? Do the proposed experiments take advantage of available collaborative arrangements?

[a]The five criteria do not necessarily receive equal weight, nor is the overall score merely a calculated mean. Reviewers apply the criteria to each individual proposal as they see fit. Other review responsibilities that are not factored into the priority score include animal welfare issues (appropriate use of vertebrate animals; numbers used); human subjects (representation of both genders and all racial groups unless there exists a compelling scientific reason for exclusion, and whether pediatric populations should be excluded from the study), and the budget and duration of the project (is the budget and time requested adequate and sufficient to complete project goals?).

differences and come to a consensus about the scientific merit of a proposal, if possible. The SRA takes notes during the discussion in order to prepare a synopsis of the discussion. After a final comment from each assigned reviewer about their degree of enthusiasm, each member of the study section privately records a score based on the discussion and their conscience. There will then be a consideration of whether the requested budget and duration of the project are appropriate, with specific recommendations made. Also, any concerns about animal welfare or human subjects, including using children as subjects, will be addressed. Note that these last points (budget, duration, or concerns) are not factored into the priority score. The reviewers will modify their written comments as necessary and provide them to the SRA for inclusion in the summary statement. Because the study section members were to prepare written comments before the actual meeting, even those unscored applications will receive a summary statement based on peer review.

As often as possible, the PA responsible for an application, or some representative from the IC holding a primary assignment, will attend the study section meeting to listen to the proceedings. Thus, the PA may be able to offer some insight into the reviewer's thoughts about a particular application.

After the meeting, the SRA will calculate the average priority score and a percentile ranking (based on the past performance of that study section or all of the CSR study sections) and a summary of the course of the verbal discussion. The SRA may also do some minor editing of the reviewer's written comments. If unscored, the SRA will release the summary statement to the applicant and the PA at the same time. If scored, the SRA will release the summary statement to the PA, who will review it and then send it to the applicant. All contact between the applicant and the NIH after the study section meeting should go through the PA. Thus, if there are questions concerning the review, the PA should be contacted. Usually, concerns can be handled through consultation between the PA, SRA, and the applicant. If not, there is an appeals process, as shown in Fig. 3 and detailed in Table VI. The key point about appeals is that the process is not for differences in scientific opinion between the reviewers and applicant.

The second layer of peer review occurs at each IC's National Advisory Council (see Fig. 3, and Table VII for a description). These groups of senior, established scientists and lay representatives provide oversight of the review process and give advice to the Institute. They also give the IC authorization to make awards.

Table VI The Appeals Process

Not for differences in scientific opinion!
Means to resolve issues of inappropriate expertise on study section, reviewers missing or misunderstanding information contained in application that was required for fair review, or personal animosity
Program staff, working with the SRA, will try to resolve appeals prior to a National Advisory Council meeting; it is important that the applicant speak with the PA as soon as possible!
National Advisory Council provides final judgment on appeals, with several possible outcomes, including concurence with the study section, recommendation that the application be deferred for review (note—if deferral, the application is reviewed as it stands!), or an offer of advice on funding decisions

Table VII National Advisory Council

All ICs have a unique National Advisory Council
Composed of scientific and lay members with interests and expertise in the IC's mission, as well as a broad perspective of science in general; members usually have 4-year appointments
Offers advice and input on IC activities
Performs second level of peer review; evaluates initial peer review by examination of summary statements
Provides authorization for the IC to make awards on applications
Renders decisions on appeals after considering the summary statement, appeal letter, and any other information provided by the PA or SRA

Actual funding decisions on applications are made by the IC—some with more input from their National Advisory Councils than others. The types of factors taken into account are listed in Table VIII. These are general considerations and may not be all-inclusive. Again, each IC has very different means to arrive at final funding decisions. The factors and means may even change from year to year. And because each IC receives different amounts of money to spend, and might have a multitude of unique demands on that money, funding levels may not be the same across the NIH.

If the IC decides to make an award, there may be considerable exchange of information between several parties (see Fig. 3 and Table IX for more details). Remember from Table II that Grants Management staff are integral to the award process and handle the fiscal information. There is great benefit to becoming familiar with the Grants Management personnel responsible for an award, because they are a wealth of useful and important help. Any study section-initiated concerns over human subjects or animal welfare will also be handled at this stage, often involving OPRR. All impediments because of these issues must be resolved before an award is made.

Table VIII General Factors Considered in Funding Decisions by an IC[a]

Priority score and percentile
Reviewer's comments
Availability of funds
Response to Program Announcement or other special initiatives
Programmatic need or balance
Advice from National Advisory Council
Other considerations, including (but not exclusively) new investigator, underrepresented category of investigators, extent of other research support

[a]In no particular order of importance.

Table IX Types of Postreview Information Needed Prior to Making an Award[a]

Just-in-time information about other research support
Issues of overlap with other funded projects
Issues about overcommitment of principal investigator
Animal usage or human subject concerns or restrictions on funding (work through the OPRR for resolution)
Determine current indirect cost rate
Review financial system (if needed)
Clarify questionable costs request in budget
Confirm start date

[a]In no particular order of importance.

Finally, yearly progress reports are required if an award is made. As previously mentioned, these reports are an excellent way to communicate any and all exciting finds sponsored by that grant. It is worth the effort to prepare clear, concise, and interesting progress reports. Grants Management staff will also examine the fiscal aspects of the award on a yearly basis.

Investigators often change academic appointments during a funding cycle, prompting the question of how grants are moved. The PI should contact their PA and Grants Management staff as soon as a move is finalized. A key point to remember, however, is that the NIH does not make awards to individuals. Rather, the awards are made to the institution. When an investigator moves, the original institution must agree to release the award. Providing this agreement is obtained (and it is exceedingly rare when it is not), and the new institution agrees to accept the award, the PI needs to submit an application, filling in the face page and facility information for the new location. This application is reviewed by the appropriate NIH staff. The review usually proceeds smoothly.

VI. Preparation of a Grant Proposal to the NIH

What makes a successful application for funding from NIH? Obviously there is no simple or magical answer. There are as many ways to obtain the goal as there are successful proposals. Presented below are general suggestions drawn from many NIGMS staff. The points may be of value for an application of any type to any organization, but are offered with the NIH specifically in mind. These suggestions are not, however, totally inclusive, nor are they presented in any particular order of importance. An additional excellent good source of information about grantsmanship may be found at http://www.niaid.nih.gov/ncn/howto$.htm.

Once a good idea is formulated and before the writing begins in earnest, there are several strategic decisions to be made. As previously argued, there is likely merit in getting to know as much as possible about the source of potential funding. With specific reference to the NIH, be aware that competitive pressures have increased the emphasis on hypothesis-based research proposals; "fishing expeditions," "data-gathering exercises," "technique-driven proposals," and "methods development" are in general not favored by reviewers. It may be best to avoid a descriptive research project, unless that is truly the status of the field. There remains a place for observation in the scientific process prior to the formalization of hypotheses. However, once sufficient background information is available, a hypothesis-driven research proposal is far more likely to succeed (at least in peer review).

To be taken seriously, a proposal for a new project in a highly competitive area must demonstrate a unique insight or approach, with data to back it up. Incremental research is not highly valued. In other words, what is the problem that needs solving, why, and who cares? Place the research in context. Do not ignore other work in the field. Do not ignore historical work that may not be currently popular—this is reinventing the wheel.

A plan to propose research on a new organism or a nontraditional experimental system must provide compelling reasons centered on the opportunity to obtain new insights that will be of general significance. Also required are rational arguments why the proposed model is more advantageous than other established models. If at all feasible, use model systems that are recognized as standards in the field.

Finally, before pen is put to paper (or fingers to keyboard, as the case may be), think through the entire project. It is important to provide a biological context for the project, and to give long-term goals, even though they might not be accomplished during the course of the proposed funding cycle.

There are many factors to consider when starting the preparation of an application. If success depends on materials or services from a collaborator, provide letters that clearly spell out what they will provide. Draw clear boundaries between the proposed research and that of a former mentor, complete with documentation of any agreements that have been reached. Evidence of independence (first authorship on papers, separate publications) is highly valued by reviewers. If the most current methods are not being used, state why not, or the reviewers might assume lack of knowledge. If possible, present preliminary data for anything that has not been done before. At the very least, lacking personal data, cite precedents from the literature. Even better, get a statement of intent to collaborate from consultant and have that consultant write a strong and specific (not a generic) letter of collaboration.

The reviewers cannot read minds. If a project is interesting, tell them why. State plans in sufficient detail that reviewers will understand the rationale; assume nothing. Write clearly. The quality of prose in a plan will be assumed to mirror the quality of thought processes. It is always advisable to have a colleague who is not an expert in your field to read the proposal for logical development and clarity of expression. It is YOUR responsibility to get your ideas across. Remember that each reviewer usually has responsibility for a large number of applications, so make every effort to have yours be the exceptional one that captures their fancy. Tell reviewers what you expect to learn from an experiment and how you will interpret your data.

New investigators without a long track record need to provide enough background and preliminary data to give reviewers confidence in the feasibility of the project and in the investigator's ability to carry it out. Established investigators should not rely on their track record of productivity to convince reviewers that the proposed work can be performed.

A crucial addition to any application is to always point out the pitfalls in the experimental plan and detail alternative strategies. Design a project with several aims that are related but not completely interdependent; avoid the appearance that if one experiment or aim fails, the project is doomed. Balance conservative and daring approaches. A common problem for new investigators is to propose too large a project. Be realistic about what can be accomplished in 3 or 4 or 5 years.

Focus—and keep focused. Starting with the title, then the abstract, then the aims, then the experimental plan, make it clear what will be done and why. Do not try to do more than reasonable given the available time and resources. Instead, prioritize and provide a time line for the proposed studies, detailing which specific aims will be performed in which year.

Do not rush to make a specific receipt date. Take time to prepare a truly complete, thorough, and scholarly application. The receipt dates for various award mechanisms, and whether the application is new, a competitive renewal, or revised, are shown in Fig. 5. Also depicted is the corresponding time frame for review and potential award.

When putting the finishing touches on the application, several critical details require attention. Follow all instructions very carefully, including page limits and the recommended type size to use. Do not annoy reviewers by making the proposal difficult to read. Have zero tolerance for typographical errors, mislabeled or poorly legible figures, inconsistencies, etc. Applications may be immediately returned if the rules are violated.

Provide a realistic budget, with careful justifications where needed. Proposing either an excessively large or an overly modest budget could make reviewers wonder if

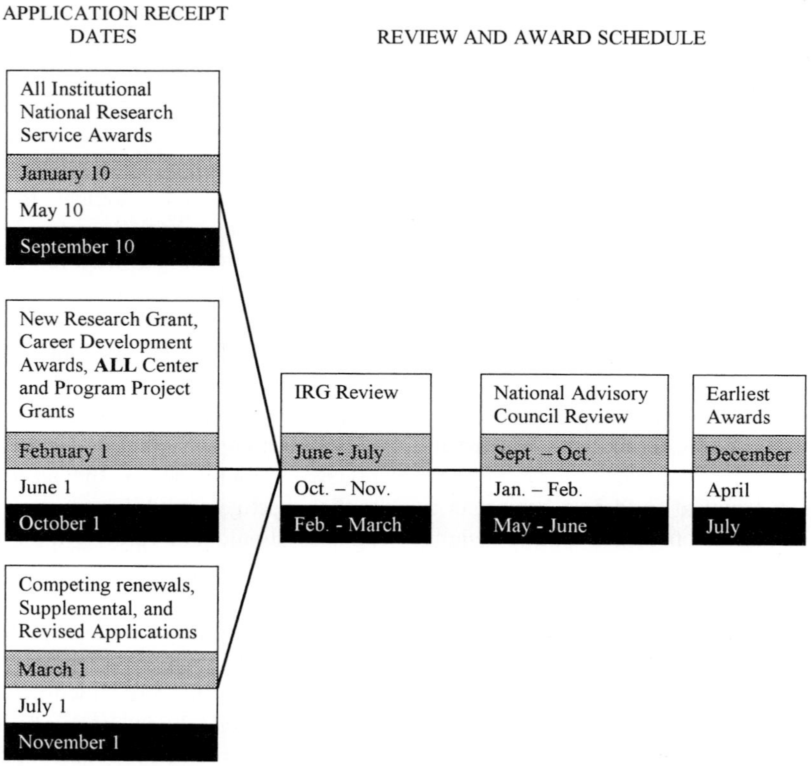

Usual Application Receipt Dates	Initial Review Dates	Funding Component Dates	Earliest Start Date
April 5	**June/July**	**Aug./Sept.**	**Sept.**
August 5	**Oct./Nov.**	**Dec./Jan.**	**Jan.**
December 5	**Feb./March**	**April/May**	**May**

Figure 5 Time line for receipt, review, and award for various types of funding mechanisms. The bottom time line shows the review and award schedule for National Research Service Award Individual Fellowships.

you can manage a grant. Be aware that budget requests under $250,000 are now done in modules of $25,000. There is no escalation in the amount awarded in the out years for grants submitted using the modular format (see http://grants.nih.gov/grants/funding/modular/modular.htm for details).

If the use of vertebrate animals is proposed, provide realistic and adequate information about experimental details and numbers as well as approval and assurance information. Do the same for human subjects; including the necessary considerations for inclusion or exclusion of research subjects based on gender, racial status, and age (i.e., children). This is absolutely mandatory; failure to do so will likely significantly delay an award. Also, include target data for recruitment of human subjects in the application (target numbers broken down by gender and racial status).

Ask the SRA about the possibility of sending an update to the application approximately 1 month before the study section meeting. The update might include a list of published, accepted, and submitted manuscripts. Include manuscripts or reprints of any new items or one to two pages of updated preliminary results if the information is necessary to convince the reviewers of the project's merit. It is crucial, however, to make the actual application as complete and self-contained as possible. It is not wise to depend on supplemental material to improve the application's chances of positive review.

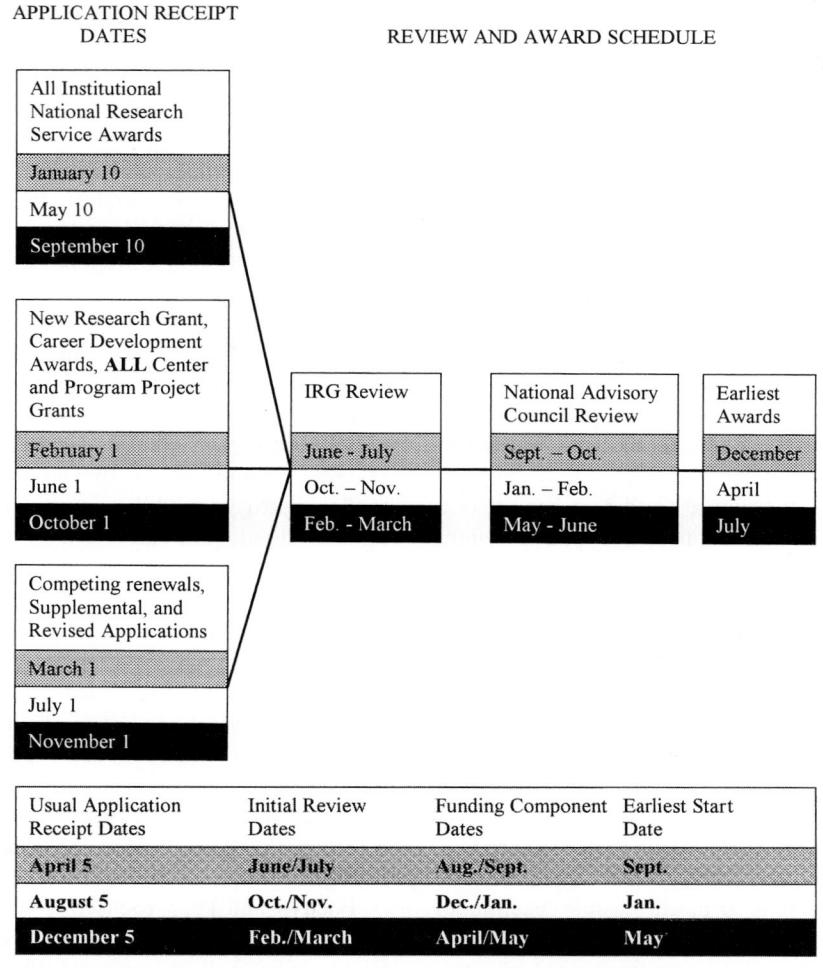

If the application receives a good score and is to be funded, be prepared to interact with the PA, Grants Management staff, and possibly the OPRR to assure prompt processing of the award. Yearly progress reports are then required and should be taken seriously. These reports are a good opportunity to inform the NIH of the progress made during the year, or, alternatively, to communicate any problems, complete with proposed solutions. The reports should contain sufficient but not overwhelming scientific detail concerning the progress. Reprints are useful, but at the very least include a list of publications. Finally, if human subjects are used in the project, provide data about recruitment, broken down by gender and ethnicity.

If, however, the application is not funded, do not panic! Many new proposals do not succeed on their first try, but do so on revision. Talk to the program director about the review before revising. They may have been present at the study section meeting during the discussion. If the application was not scored, the program director may be able to offer insight and interpretation of the summary statement. In revising the application, read the critique carefully to determine the problems with the proposal and how it can be improved. Write a thorough and noncombative introduction to the revised proposal. Make and delineate real changes in the proposal to demonstrate how the criticisms were addressed. If there are questions, consult the appropriate NIH staff, because their job is to provide answers. Your colleagues may not have the most complete and accurate information. Remember that differences in scientific opinion can always occur, meaning that you may not always agree with the reviewer's opinion of the relative merit of your proposal.

VII. Summary

As promised in Section I, here are short answers to the questions asked by many investigators:

- *What is the NIH?* See Fig. 1 and http://www.nih.gov.
- *What are the individual Institutes?* See Section II and the NIH homepage under "Institutes." *How do I assure that my application goes to the right Institute?* Through research and understanding of the NIH system, identify the proper IC for your work and "self-refer" the application in a cover letter.
- *What are the different types of grants?* See Table III. *For which ones am I eligible? What are the advantages and disadvantages of each?* Go to http://grants.nih.gov/grants/funding/funding.htm for more information.
- *What happens to my application once it is sent? What is the process timetable? Whom do I talk to and when should I ask?* See Fig. 3 and Section V. *Should I even call?* YES!
- *What are study sections?* See http://csr.nih.gov. *Who chooses reviewers?* The SRA. *How do study sections work?* See Section V.
- *What do reviewers look for in applications?* See Table V.
- *What happens after an application is reviewed?* See Section V, Fig. 3, and Tables VI–IX.
- *What should I do if I think the reviewers were wrong?* See Table VI.
- *What determines funding?* See Table VIII. *Does funding vary from Institute to Institute?* Yes, funding might differ among Institutes.
- *What do I do if my proposal is not funded?* See Section VI.
- *What do I do if my proposal is funded?* See Section VI.
- *Can I take my grant with me to my new position?* Most likely, yes. See Section V.
- *What makes a good proposal?* Unfortunately, there is no simple answer to this question.
- *Where can I go for help?* Contact NIH staff.

Acknowledgments

The author thanks Laurette Langlois for the figures, and Steward Wang, Paul Bankey, and David Mercer for providing questions that needed answers.

97

Measuring the Performance of Surgical Research[1]

Wiley W. Souba* and Douglas W. Wilmore†

**Department of Surgery, The Milton S. Hershey Medical Center, Penn State College of Medicine, Hershey, Pennsylvania 17033*
†Department of Surgery, Brigham and Women's Hospital, Boston, Massachusetts 02115

What gets measured gets done. What gets measured and fed back gets done well. What gets rewarded gets repeated.

[John E. Jones, in Crane (1)]

I. Introduction

University-based departments of surgery have, for many years, regarded an active research program to be an integral part of their purpose. The creation of new knowledge through basic research or clinical trials is one of the social missions of academic medical centers. Indeed, research has been responsible for many of the improvements in the care of the surgical patient that have occurred over the years.

In the past, departments of surgery were able to use overages from clinical revenues to support research, but this approach is no longer a viable strategy. Mounting pressures to reduce costs together with major reductions in reimbursement have made cross-subsidization of the research program more and more difficult. These challenges have placed the research enterprise in most departments of surgery in jeopardy—achieving the goals of research are inherently more difficult because of these new constraints (Fig. 1). In order to meet these challenges and preserve research in academic departments of surgery, several aspects of the research enterprise will have to change. The department will have to develop expertise in strategic research management.

Because surgical research can be examined as a process with a series of inputs and outputs (Fig. 2), it can be monitored and measured. Departments that are able to leverage their research competencies will be more successful in converting their research "supply chain" into a value chain (2, 3) (Fig. 3), thereby enhancing the efficiency and effectiveness of their academic mission. The performance of the research program will have to be measured to ensure that the results derived from it add value to the department.

[1]An extended version of this chapter is published in *Annals of Surgery* (2000). Vol. 232, pp 32-41,

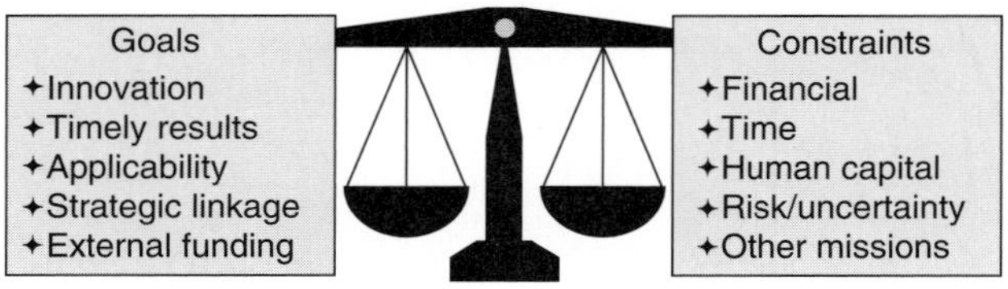
Goals
✦Innovation
✦Timely results
✦Applicability
✦Strategic linkage
✦External funding
Constraints
✦Financial
✦Time
✦Human capital
✦Risk/uncertainty
✦Other missions

Figure 1 Surgical research—goals and constraints.

II. Assessing the Performance of the Research Program

The measurement system used by the department of surgery to evaluate and assess research performance will influence the behavior of its investigators. If the emphasis is on translational research, a strong alignment between basic science and clinical programs is likely to exist. Traditional measures such as productivity (e.g., number of grants awarded/year) can give misleading indices for innovation and growth, the characteristics that will distinguish a successful research program in the future.

In assessing the performance of the research programs in the department, several questions must be answered: What is the purpose of surgical research? How should we evaluate its performance? Is a contemporary research program most effective when it uses the new knowledge it creates to enhance the clinical business?

Because of the difficulties of "quantifying" surgical research, assessment and judgment are often used rather than formal measurement. But reliable tools and performance metrics are necessary if the department is to grow and accomplish more than just publishing papers and securing grants. Performance can be categorized along several dimensions (Table I) (4–6): internal measures, customer satisfaction, market share, and financial indices.

In assessing how well it is achieving its goals, it will be beneficial for the department of surgery to generate a "report card" that evaluates its current research activities and links this performance to future goals (4) (Table II). The grading categories in Table II are listed as being equal but may be ranked (or prioritized) to reflect the importance of each category to the department's (or division's) overall goals. For example, a department of surgery that emphasizes translational research may wish to ascribe more points (say 8–10, rather than the average of 5) to measures such as innovation and profitability and give fewer points to factors such as cost and output (productivity). In contrast, a department whose focus was largely clinical but wanted to ensure a research exposure for the residents might rank productivity above innovation (in all cases the final possible points should add up to 100). A major strength of this grading system is that it allows each department or division to set its own goals.

A. Internal Measures

1. Quality

Quality raises the central question of "How good is the work?" Because the assessment of quality is subjective, it is often judged on the basis of the particular journal in which the work is published. This influences the granting of promotion and tenure at most colleges of medicine.

2. Productivity

Productivity measures output/time (for example, number of publications/year). It does not take into account quality—it focuses on quantity. It precludes us from answering, "Is

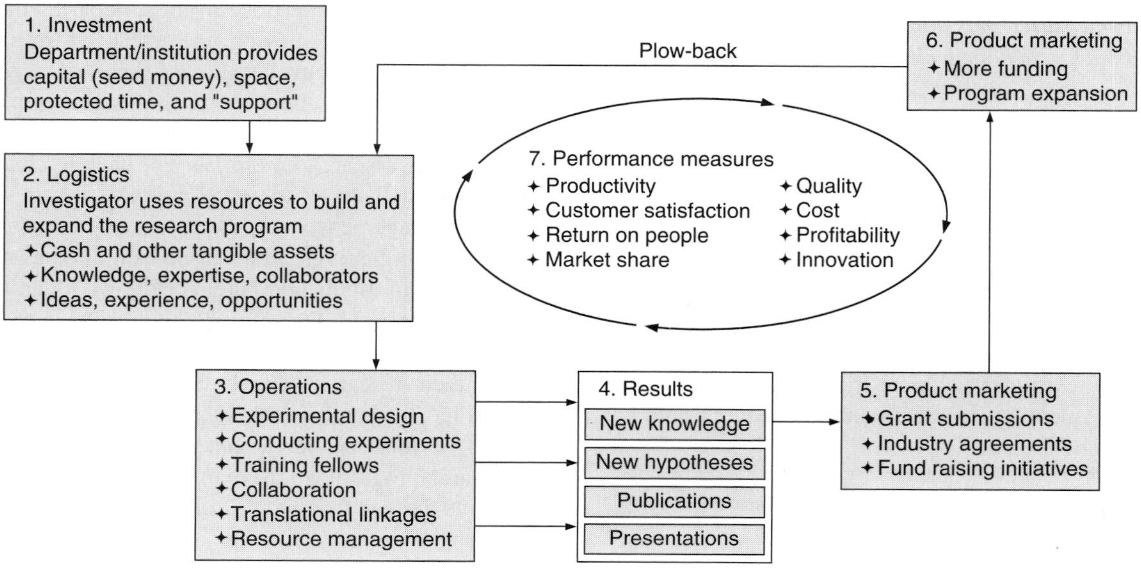

Figure 2 The process of surgical research.

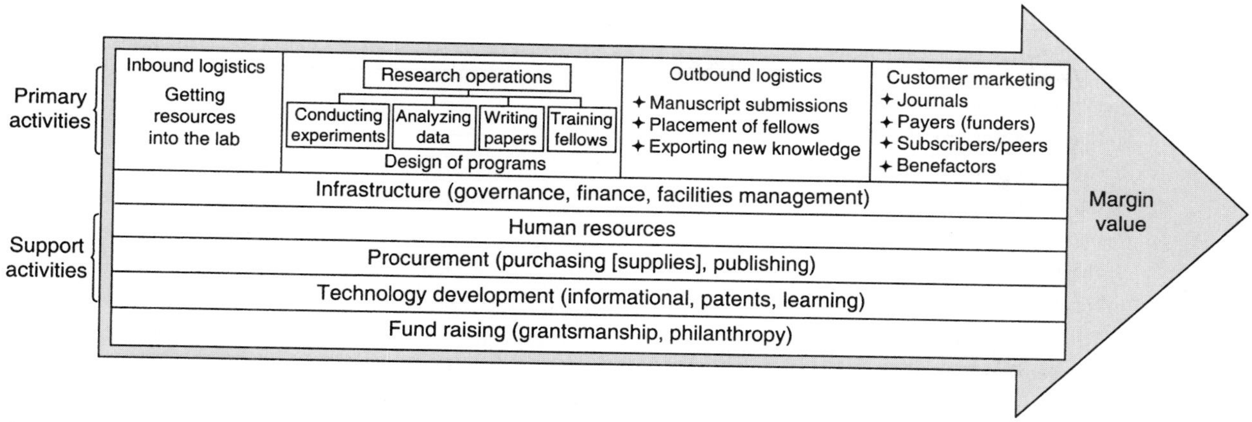

Figure 3 The value chain for a surgical research laboratory. The chain evaluates revenues and expenses but also examines the stream of research activities and ways to improve the processes involved. The activities consist of four primary activities and five secondary activities that must be coordinated to maximize performance and minimize costs. Primary activities represent the sequence of getting resources into the lab (inbound logistics), conducting research (operations), publishing and presenting research results (outbound logistics), and marketing. The support activities that maintain and enable these primary activities include the research infrastructure (e.g., governance, finances, facilities management), human resource management (career development), procurement (customer engagement, acquisition of inputs that support each primary activity), technology development, and fund-raising. Careful analysis of each process requires observation (gathering data), analyzing data, and making revisions with the goal of improving results and adding value. Modified from Porter (2) and Souba and Wilmore (3).

the research group that publishes eight papers a year in surgical journals outperforming the team that publishes two papers a year in basic science journals?"

3. Innovation

Innovation refers to novelty and originality. It asks, "Is the research team producing important new knowledge and/or making breakthrough discoveries?" Innovative research groups are often awarded patents and they may form startup companies. Such creativity is not restricted to the development of new products or devices—the development of novel cost-saving clinical care plans can be just as important.

4. The Development of Young Investigators

The training of young people who subsequently develop their own research program is a critical factor that must be considered in assessing research performance. Most surgical residents seek out positions in laboratories of established scientists and mentors. When young investigators establish a successful independent research program, it is a feather in their cap and a compliment to the department that was responsible for their training.

Table I Measures of Performance in Surgical Research

Performance indicator	Indicator focus
Quality	Asks "How good is the work?" Includes dimensions such as reputation, excellence, publication vehicle, and perceived quality of the work
Productivity	New knowledge generated/unit time; papers published/year; grants awarded/unit time; residents trained/year
Innovation	How much clinically relevant (usable) novel knowledge and technology is created by or derived from the laboratory?
Development of junior investigators	How successful are the residents in the lab? How many of the surgical trainees develop independent research programs?
Customer satisfaction	How satisfied are the various stakeholders (funding agencies, peers) with the research? Is funding renewed?
Market share	What portion of publications (or grants) in the specific field of investigation originates from the laboratory?
Cost	How much does it cost to produce the research? How efficient are the researchers in using resources?
Profitability	What is the return on the investment? How much additional funding, patents, new technology does the research generate?

Table II Departmental Report Card

Parameter	Current score	Goal[a]	Points[b]
1. Quality of research			
(a) Number of papers published/year	_______	_______	_______
(b) Average impact score of publications	_______	_______	_______
(c) Quality index (multiply a × b)	_______	_______	_______
2. Quantification of research			
(a) Number of publications/year	_______	_______	_______
(b) Number of grants awarded/year	_______	_______	_______
(c) Total dollars from grants	_______	_______	_______
(d) Number of trainees in laboratories/year	_______	_______	_______
3. Innovation			
(a) Average citation index of publications	_______	_______	_______
(b) Number of patents issued	_______	_______	_______
(c) Total dollars from industrial support/year	_______	_______	_______
(d) Number of collaborations/spin-offs	_______	_______	_______
(e) Quality of research trainees (0–5; 5 = best)	_______	_______	_______
4. Percent of trainees with grants	_______	_______	_______
5. Customer satisfaction			
(a) Total dollars from NIH/year	_______	_______	_______
(b) Total dollars from industry/year	_______	_______	_______
(c) Total dollars from philanthropy/year	_______	_______	_______
6. Market share			
(a) Number of papers/total number in field	_______	_______	_______
(b) Research dollars/total dollars allocated in field	_______	_______	_______
7. Cost			
(a) Current expenditures (dollars/year)	_______	_______	_______
8. Profitability			
(a) Growth in funding (gain in dollars/year)	_______	_______	_______
(b) Royalties (dollars/year)	_______	_______	_______
(c) Total dollars from consultantships with industry or from gifts	_______	_______	_______
TOTAL			_______

[a]Goals should be established by a neutral group (such as the research committee) or individual (such as the outside consultant).

[b]Points (100% of goal = 5 points; 80% of goal = 4 points; 60% of goal = 3 points; 40% of goal = 2 points; 20% of goal = 1 point; 0% of goal = 0 points). With 20 categories, maximum number of points = 100. The categories may be prorated to emphasize particular aspects of the research enterprise (see text), but the point total should always add up to 100.

B. Customer Satisfaction

The performance of the research program can also be assessed in relation to the expectations of external constituents that judge the program or provide resources to the organization. Stakeholders include funding agencies, philanthropists, industry, and patients. The needs and wants of these customers must be met because loyalty from these clients is crucial. The department of surgery is becoming more dependent on long-standing relationships with industry, continued support from benefactors, and successful renewal of extramural grants. These stakeholders have varying expectations and distinct feedback requirements.

C. Market Share

A research team can judge performance in a particular area of research on the basis of the number of papers (or grants) it generates in that specific field. Expertise and recognition in a particular field stem from frequent, high-quality publications and sustained focused productivity. The relative contribution of an individual research unit to the total output in the field can be calculated.

D. Financial Indices

1. Cost

Cost issues concern the expenses involved in managing the laboratory and generating results. They impact every level of the value chain—to the extent that these expenses can be administered effectively and resources used efficiently, performance will improve. A resource is an asset, skill, or knowledge. Most resources are not strengths or weaknesses, but are necessary for performance. A resource offers an advantage if it provides the research team with a competitive advantage.

Traditional cost-accounting measures determine what it costs to carry out an experiment—expenses would include the use of equipment, people, and supplies. Activity-based costing also takes into account the costs of not using a piece of equipment and the costs associated with repeating experiments because of errors. Opportunity costs are relevant to the surgical investigator as well. Any decision to commit people, money, or time to one project precludes those resources from being committed to another. The trade-off becomes one of estimating the highest return from asset allocation.

2. Profitability

It is difficult to measure a return on investment in surgical research because many of the returns are difficult to quantify. However, in monetary terms, the research enterprise can keep score in terms of additional funding and royalties that have been awarded. From a competitive standpoint, the potential value of a particular research program will be highest where its relative strength is greatest and the strategic importance of the program is core to the department's mission (7) (Fig. 4). As opposed to the "equality zone," where competition is keenest, the "zone of distinction," offers the highest likelihood for sustainable success because the program has differentiated itself from others. These zones differ in terms of funding, skill set requirements, value to the organization, and the role of technology (to include information technology).

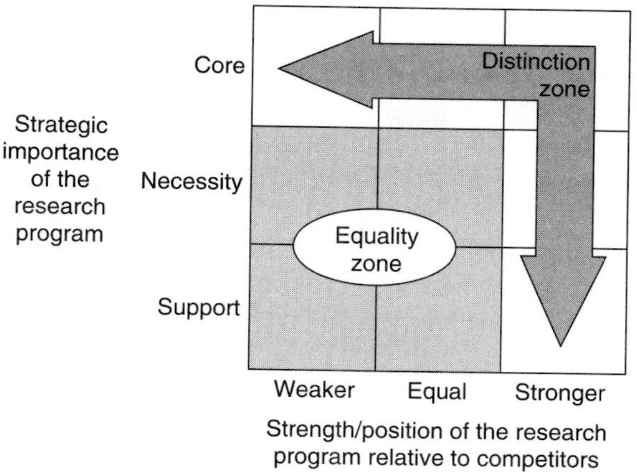

Figure 4 Aligning distinct research capabilities with the strategic importance of the research program. Adapted from Venkatraman (7).

III. A New Research Model in Surgical Research?

The specific research model utilized by a particular department will depend in part on its objectives, culture, and priorities. It is becoming increasingly important for surgery departments to select an alignment perspective between their research and clinical initiatives that best fit the department's goals and identify the appropriate criteria to assess research performance. No single research model fits all departments and there are several levels at which the research enterprise can enhance a department's clinical mission. In general, the greater the degree of transformation of the research program, the greater the potential benefit (Table III). In developing its research strategy, a department can configure its academic programs so they serve one or more of three purposes (4, 8): to support and/or expand existing businesses, to drive new business opportunities, and/or to increase the breadth and depth of existing research and technological capabilities.

A number of departments are actively participating in randomized prospective trials that attract patients and help support clinical research initiatives. Such endeavors frequently increase the size of clinical programs and attract industry sponsors as well. Other departments are using their research capabilities and expertise to create new business ventures. This requires a tighter linkage between biomedical research (whose purpose is the creation of new knowledge), development (the application of this knowledge to achieve practical results), and technology transfer (taking an idea to a product). The research goal is the production of knowledge that will enable the department to participate in the forefront of new technology (devices, treatments) or to lay the scientific foundation for the development of new products or processes. Finally, managing the research enterprise strategically can also enable the department to increase the breadth and depth of existing research and development capabilities. Research collaborations can add value by narrowing proficiency gaps, building critical mass, and increasing efficiency. The recognition of research and development as a competitive advantage to be capitalized on will ensure a rich future for surgical research.

Table III The Spectrum of Relationships between the Research Enterprise and the Clinical Programs

Nature of the research enterprise	Philosophy of the research enterprise	Structure/operations of the research enterprise	Funding of the research enterprise	Strategy of the research enterprise	Performance assessment of the research enterprise
Independent/isolated research programs	Scientists presume that management does not appreciate research; administration assumes that researchers do not understand the clinical business	Independent research ventures; limited constructive dialogue and interchange	Minimal investment by department; research viability dependent on external grants; research programs viewed as cost centers	Minimal linkage between research programs and business strategy; focus is on getting funded and discovery	Traditional measures are stressed: Number of papers published Number of grants awarded Number of presentations made Number of residents trained in the lab
Transitional–unified agenda initiated	Communication and interaction between research programs and clinical programs will enhance organizational productivity and success	Power of collaboration is recognized; steps are taken to identify complementary extradepartmental research initiative and enhance collaboration and openness	Organization recognizes the importance of committing resources to support research efforts	Recognition of role of research in supporting existing businesses, driving new ventures, and increase the scope of existing capabilities; focus is on discovery and innovation	Nontraditional performance measures are developed; for example, how much clinically relevant (exploitable) new knowledge is generated by the research enterprise?
Integrated/unified programs	The organization utilizes research to sustain and drive clinical success; technology-oriented research programs are leveraged to support and drive clinical excellence	Interdisciplinary research programs are created; scientists and physicians regularly interact with each other to achieve goals and enhance performance	Department/hospital allocate resources strategically; industrial support is developed; research programs are viewed as investment centers	Research initiatives fully aligned with the clinical mission; technology transfer drives clinical programs; research results are exploited to improve performance; focus is on invention and application	Impact of research programs on clinical productivity, innovation, cost, and profitability is monitored; returns on invention and application are assessed

References

1. Crane, T. (1999)"The Heart of Coaching." FTA Press, San Diego.
2. Porter, M. E. (1985). "Competitive Advantage: Creating and Sustaining Superior Performance." Free Press, New York.
3. Souba, W. W. (1999). How competitive forces mold strategy in academic surgery. *Surgery* **125;** 616–629.
4. Souba, W. W., and Wilmore, D. W. (2000). Judging surgical research: How should we evaluate performance and measure value? *Ann. Surg.* (in press).
5. Drucker, P. (1998). The information executives truly need. *In* "Harvard Business Review on Measuring Corporate Performance," pp. 1–24. Harvard Business School Press, Boston.
6. Eccles, R. (1998). The performance measurement manifesto. *In* "Harvard Business Review on Measuring Corporate Performance," pp. 25–45. Harvard Business School Press, Boston.
7. Venkatraman, N. (1994). IT-enabled business transformation: From automation to business scope transformation. *Sloan Mgmt. Rev.* **35**, 73–87.
8. Roussel, P, Saad, K, and Erickson, T. (1991)."Third Generation R&D: Managing the Link to Corporate Strategy." Harvard Business School Press, Boston.

98

Virtual Reality and Surgery

Joseph M. Rosen,* Marcus K. Simpson,† and Charles Lucey‡

**Plastic and Reconstructive Surgery, Dartmouth-Hitchcock Medical Center, Lebanon, New Hampshire 03756; and Thayer School of Engineering, Dartmouth College, Hanover, New Hampshire 03755*

†Dartmouth College, Hanover, New Hampshire 03755

‡21st Century Health Concepts, Houston, Texas 77061; and Dartmouth College, Hanover, New Hampshire 03755

I. Introduction

Virtual reality (VR) encompasses a number of surgical research topics, including computer graphics, imaging, visualization, simulation, data fusion, and telemedicine. In this chapter we define VR and each of these areas, focusing on a state-of-the-art review of the research and recent accomplishments. However, first we provide an overview vision of this field and a research agenda to reach it.

This vision comes from work done by Robert Mann in the 1960s (1). We can imagine a patient undergoing a complex operation such as a joint replacement. The surgeon needs to choose from several approaches, a number of different prostheses, and a number of postoperative rehab protocols. The surgeon would like to select each of these choices of treatment and among the various outcomes choose the best for the patient. In reality the surgeon can only select one course.

Mann's vision was to create a virtual patient-specific model of the patient and the procedures, prostheses, and rehab protocols. The physician could then review several different alternatives in a virtual environment. The virtual model would undergo rehab over a 2-year period and would then be assessed to determine what was the best outcome. Once this was accomplished, the surgeon could choose which complex procedure should be performed in reality and carry it out (2). The first steps towards this vision have been realized, especially over the past 10 years in several areas at a number of institutions. Further research in surgery needs to be done in a number of areas, as will be described below.

To accomplish the above goal requires development of a patient model of the actual patient in need of the procedure. The model needs to be "accurate" in a number of ways, including anatomy and physiology. The virtual model not only needs to be accurate with respect to normal anatomy but needs to model the pathology as well. If the patient has degenerative knee joint disease, this needs to be included with regard to effects on muscle function, ligaments, cartilage, and the patient's ability to walk. More difficult is the ability to predict wound healing and subsequent rehabilitation. This involves not just the musculoskeletal system, but it also involves a model that assesses higher functions. There already exist software approaches that simulate some of these aspects, but more modeling approaches need to be developed to better predict mathematically the outcomes and to integrate a number of varying models into one overall master system for the patient. This is similar to what Boeing did using computers to simulate and test completely all of the systems for their new 777 (3). Building all of the parts of a truly realistic virtual medical model still entails much research and experimentation.

As the human virtual model in all its dimensionality is developed, several other areas need further development. These include the tools to interact with the model and the environment, and the ability to overlay the model on the real patient. Finally, there is also an interest in doing all of this at a distance in special cases (telesurgery).

Within the virtual environment where the model exists, a virtual operating room would be created. This operating room should in some cases allow the surgeon to perform the procedure and "see" and "touch" the virtual human. Although this is now possible, the resolution of both of these senses is still limited. The vision component is being actively addressed in other industrial fields, but the detail required in "touch" is more unique to surgery. Force feedback, or haptics, requires machines that use the information from the virtual patient model and transform it into a realistic touch for the surgeon. These instruments have improved recently, but still lack the resolution needed for a surgeon to experience fully and learn from operating in a virtual world. The virtual environment as an operating room can be approached through several "portals." These are usually visual with the addition of haptic devices, all of which at present still lack the ability to provide the fully immersive experience that should be our goal. Each of these approaches will be discussed further below.

When coupling the virtual model to the real patient, invariably a mismatch occurs between the real patient at the time of operation and the patient virtual model. This registration of the real and the virtual is more complex than it first appears. More innovative methods need to be developed to perform this superimposition. Finally, as we attempt to perform telesurgery we must develop solutions for the delays that occur as we move further away from the real patient. There are a number of approaches being developed to address this issue.

II. Definitions and Background

Virtual reality is the use of a computer interface to simulate, in a synthetic environment, a real or imaginary world, through the computer operator's senses (2). These are most commonly visual, tactile (haptic), or auditory senses and allow for an interactive, virtual environment. The terms *virtual reality*, *synthetic environment*, and *virtual environment* are often used interchangeably. The historic ancestors of VR are the flight simulator and the popular videogames (4).

Flight simulators are cost-effective and proved means to train pilots and maintain pilot skills. This technology is now aiding medicine and surgery to train and assess professional medical skills (5). There has been mounting concern that traditional continuing medical education (CME) courses that utilize didactic lectures do not improve physician performance. Interactive CME alone, or combined with didactic instruction, allows an opportunity to practice skills and can change physician performance (6). A review of the literature shows that small group discussions, interactive videos, and simulated patient encounters have been employed. VR has potential to become the natural progression of these methods for teaching and CME.

VR is predicted to very soon play a critical role in credentialing surgeons (7, 8). With its power to allow training and testing in any procedure, it will serve as an objective tool to measure competence, just as it is used in the airline industry. It will offer the additional advantage of avoiding the use of animal models or patients to improve surgical skills (9). VR for teaching and credentialing is an important area for further research.

In the following discussions we explore three-dimensional (3D), multidimensional, and multiuser virtual human modeling applications. We then look to virtual environment representation. The use of virtual tools and manipulation in surgical simulators will also be reviewed. The use of augmented reality to benefit surgical planning and procedures and the roles that telesurgery and cybersurgery may play in the coming years are then examined.

III. Surgical Simulators

Surgical simulators require three fundamental needs to be met (10). The first is a virtual human model. Classical anatomy, ultrasonography (USG), computer tomography (CT), and magnetic resonance imaging (MRI) provide two-dimensional imaging, which may be manipulated by volumetric mathematical computerization to provide detailed 3D imaging, (see Fig. 1). A fourth or multiple dimension may be added with further overlaid information showing function (e.g., liver function tests), time (future growth), predicted healing, operative parameters (blood loss), and so forth. The second requirement is for virtual instrumentation and tracking to perform surgical procedures. This involves solving tactile feedback for incising tissues and detecting abnormal tissue. The third requirement is a virtual environment that can be shown to be effective in training and cost, and is

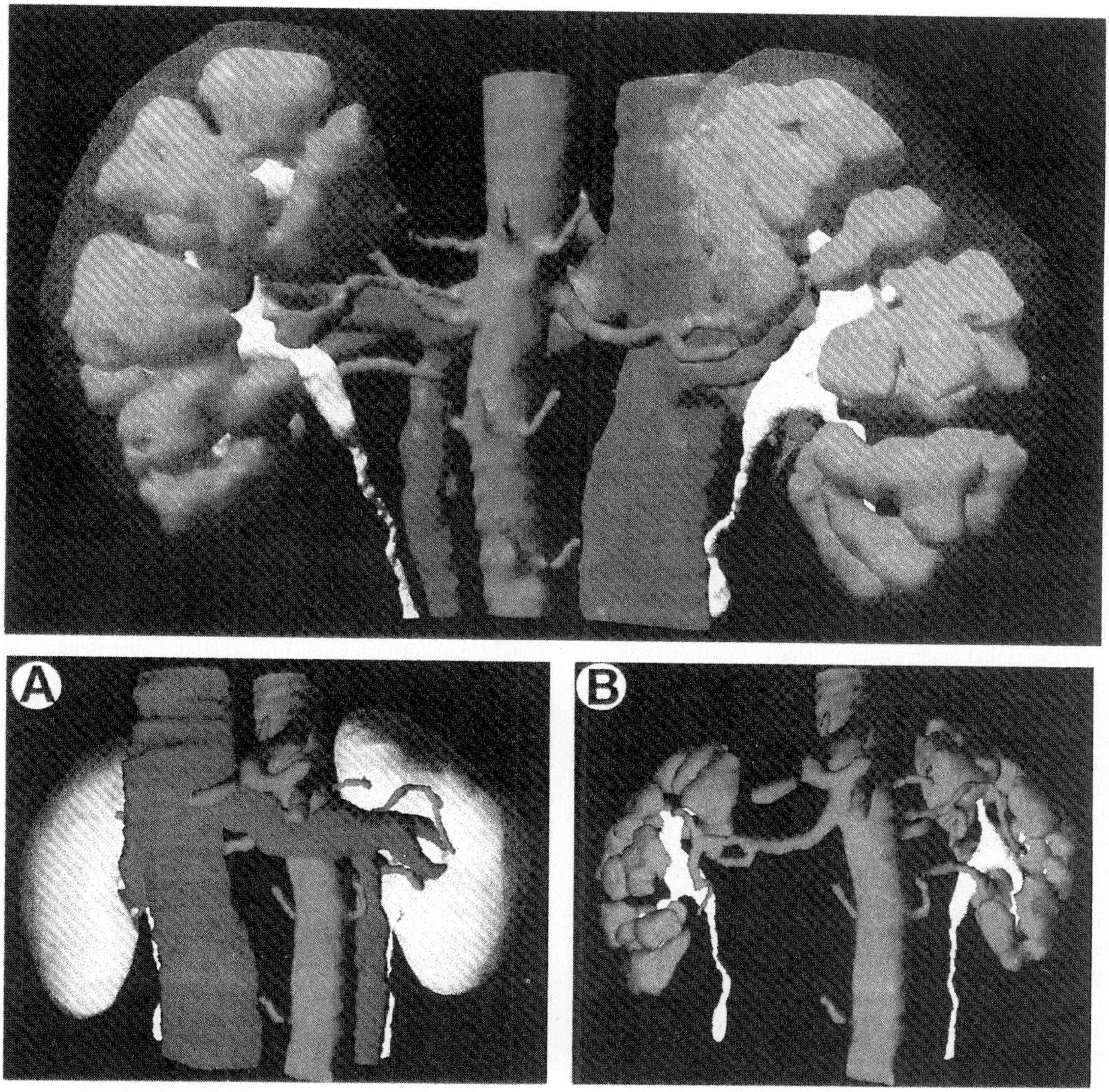

Figure 1 An anterior view of a 3D reconstruction of the kidney using contrast-enhanced spiral CT data. Courtesy of Lori Lerner. (See color plates.)

accepted by users, in terms of comfort and convenience (user friendliness). A virtual environment system consists of the operator, the machine (display) interface, and the computer simulator. A measure of the success of the VR is the degree of sense of being completely immersed within the computer representation.

A. General Approaches

The National Library of Medicine (NLM) at the National Institutes of Health (NIH) sponsored The Visible Human Project to create complete, anatomically detailed, three-dimensional representations of the normal male and female human bodies (see the NIH web site at www.nlm.nih.gov/research/visible). Transverse CT and MRI cryosection images were acquired; the male cadaver was sectioned at 1-mm intervals and the female cadaver was sectioned at 0.33-mm intervals. The Visible Human Project transparently linked visual knowledge forms to symbolic knowledge formats such as the names of body parts (11, 12). These data in turn have been incorporated into various projects, both on the web through links at the NIH site and into the leg bullet wound simulator discussed below.

The VR human model requires accurate patient-specific data to be mapped to the tissue, organ, system, and body region from CT, MRI, and ultrasound imaging. This requires volumetric encoding with reference to an absolute reference frame independent of and exterior to the patient. Mathematical algorithms can be employed to define a finite element mesh (FEM). The FEM allows each point in the VR human to be defined into elements that can be grouped with other points to approximate a tissue or organ and its behavior or its relationship to adjacent elements, for example, skin, muscle, fascia, bone, and organs. This allows a computer to model how a distortion of one set of elements will affect a second—for example, a simulation may predict how lower extremity tendon transfer operations will affect ambulating. How tissues and organ systems behave over time is a future research question (13).

Virtual tools primarily are for seeing and touching, though hearing may be useful as a primary sense, or substituted as an aid for virtual seeing and touching (sonar to find an embedded tumor). Head-mounted displays (HMDs) allow a screen to be placed before an operator's eyes. These displays stem from research done by NASA, and their resolution is currently approaching TV image quality (14). Screens may also be placed on the patient or suspended in front of the surgeon. Virtual retinal display focuses a fine beam of light onto the retina. Further development of this lightweight technology is needed to improve resolution and to broaden the imaging to the entire retina. The University of Illinois has developed the CAVE system where by 3D images are projected within an 8-ft^3 room, allowing physicians to walk between images (for example, neurons from a brain biopsy). Holographic imaging is another area of investigation (14).

The sense of touch includes proprioception, vibration, temperature, kinesthesia, texture, and light and heavy pressure. Haptic input devices currently in use primarily sense pressure. By the resistance, which a probe generates via joystick-type or glove-based devices, a surgeon "feels" contact with different tissues. Current systems, including the Massachusetts Institute of Technology (MIT) Newman Laboratory joystick or the PHANToM interface used by MusculoGraphics Inc., simulate forces on an instrument held in the user's hand (15). However, translating texture is presently a research challenge. A microelectromechanical system (MEMS) employs computer chip fabrication technology and mechanical components to create miniature sensors for pressure, acceleration, and fluid flow. By combining computer chip technology with sensors and actuators, the MEMS promises future progress as more mechanical functions are matched to advances in mirocomputing; this technology is expected to impact future haptic research (16).

Instrument tracking may be done with real-time imaging and processing (fluoroscopy, USG) or may be done with attached sensors. Optical, electromagnetic, ultrasonic sensors can provide continuous spatial localization. Current research is developing a virtual operating tray from which a surgeon can choose virtual instruments, which then may be manipulated to repair soft tissue and bone trauma (17). The instruments actually handling the tissue must have dexterity, force, and precision; they must also give quality sensory output that can reach the surgeon's hands. Daum is investigating the use of a three-fingered grasper that can be controlled by a glove device. Other investigators are using shape memory allow materials to increase the dexterity of the instruments (13). Tactile sensors may be placed in the tips to provide force feedback pressure.

As an example of existing applications of virtual reality simulation, McKenna has developed a biomechanical model and simulator (see Fig. 2) to generate stable standing posture, rising on the toes, and arm movement to reach objects, using a 90-degrees-of-freedom algorithm (18). Using a high-end computer workstation and the Copus computer program, simulation times range from real-time for simplified models to approximately half an hour for complex models. Future research could expand the degrees of freedom to 142 to include all 136 joints found in humans. Importing patient-specific information for surgical planning is a future research goal. Better modeling of the soft tissue components could create a highly sophisticated human figure model.

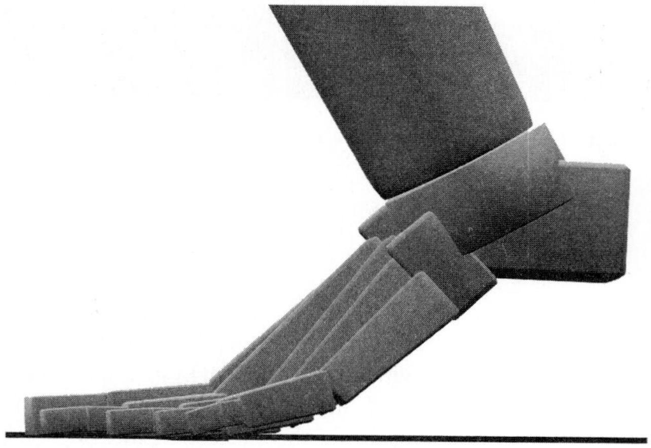

Figure 2 An image of McKenna's fully articulated simulation of the foot. Courtesy of Mike McKenna.

Another simulation predicts the path of a bullet wound through the thigh and the resulting soft tissue injury (Fig. 3) (19). The model accounts for the cylindrical entrance wound, the bullet's breakup into four fragments on striking the femur, the deflection of bone and bullet fragments, and the resulting soft tissue injuries. Future work may more accurately calculate the sizes and positions of the bone fragments from the bullet's parameters. Current imaging resolution is less than that for the virtual human to allow the computer to simulate bleeding, wounding, and instrument interaction. The program can predict functional consequences for the musculoskeletal and circulatory systems and the patient's ability to walk after healing. The circulatory model predicts blood loss, heart rate, and cardiac output as the wound is repaired. These are complex situations to simulate and the model simplifies some functions, which may eventually be incorporated for better accuracy. The purpose of this simulator is to train combat physicians and the application has become part of the training at Special Operations Command Medical Training Center, Ft. Bragg, NC. This type of virtual reality simulator replaces the traditional animal model wound study, a distinct advantage (19).

Endoscopic simulators have been developed for hysteroscopy using a haptic device for hysteroscopic instruments and imported patient-specific anatomy and pathology, allowing surgeons to practice virtual pathology before operating on real patients (35). VR bronchoscopy and colonoscopy using CT, MRI, or USG results in 3D images comparable to videoendoscopy. Future applications can explore areas not accessible to endoscopes, such as the inner ear and celiac ganglion. Satava has created a virtual abdomen that can teach anatomy and operative procedures (20). The user can virtually fly through the organs and systems from the inside and experience anatomical relationships.

Currently, it is too difficult to simulate the complexity of an entire surgical procedure. The future of VR for training and testing has been proposed to start with studying expert surgeons, to analyze and categorize surgical procedures as defined sets of skills and knowledge, tasks and subtasks, the routine and extraordinary, successful and unsuccessful outcomes. VR can make this lifelike, variable, and real time to be realistic. Key elements and tasks could then be targeted and addressed with VR applications. How to best employ VR in this setting is an important question.

B. Representations

Virtual colonoscopy (VC) has been shown to have similar efficacy as conventional colonoscopy (CC) for detecting polyps 6 mm or more in diameter (21). VC uses a helical (spiral) CT scanner to generate images at 2-mm intervals, with a 3-mm slice overlap, with the patient in both the prone

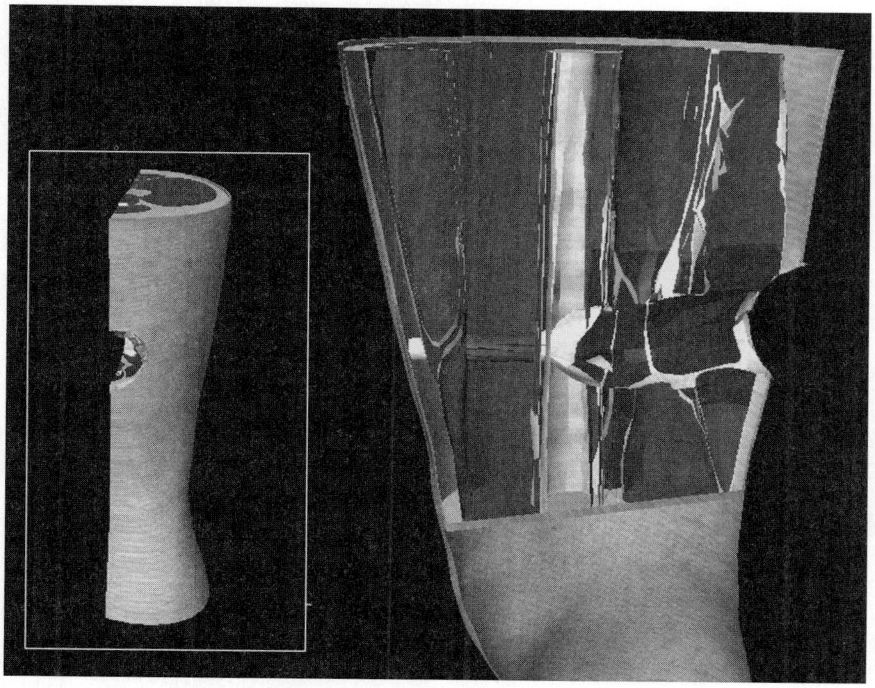

Figure 3 A simulated model of tissue damage caused from cavitation caused by the entry of a high-velocity bullet into the human thigh. Combined with surgical simulation programs, this system is used for wound trauma training. Courtesy of MusculoGraphics Inc., Evanston, IL.

and supine positions. The patient has undergone a very thorough bowel preparation, has had the colon inflated to the maximum level of tolerance, and has an injection of glucagon to minimize smooth-muscle spasm and peristalsis. A radiologist then examines the VC at a computer workstation, using 3D software (www.cs.sunysb.edu/vislab/projects/colonoscopy/colonoscopy.html). It has been pointed out that these are promising results but that more work needs to show that this can replace CC or a barium enema for screening purposes. It remains technically challenging and time-consuming for study review. Sessile 1-cm polyps are regularly missed in the right colon, and because of the gas insufflation, patients may rate CC as more comfortable than VC. This study raises some technical questions, but the most fundamental question concerns whether the viewing process be computerized to find lesions for the physician to then study. This application may also eventually be helpful for VR spiral CT chest screening (22).

One commonly asked question is whether we can afford this new technology or how it can be justifiably used. Although VC may not yet be affordable when compared to conventional treatment, one new VR application does claim to be both cost-effective and clinically better. How does a surgeon decide which kidney to harvest when a patient donates a kidney (23)? Living renal donor transplantation normally requires renal arteriography and, at some institutions, excretory urography (IVP) to evaluate renal function and anatomy. Medical Media Systems has developed computer software to take helical CT scanner data and, with color coding of structures by trained biomedical engineers, construct 3D, multiplanar reformatted images (24) (Fig. 4). Within 72 hr, a floppy disk is available for the surgeon to view the kidneys, ureters, and arterial and venous structures in beautiful, bright colors.

Conventional angiography has a complication rate of 1.4% and includes arterial dissection, thrombosis, groin hematoma, bleeding, contrast reactions, contrast-induced renal failure, angina, and (rarely) neurological injuries. In comparison, CT rarely leads to complications such as contrast reactions. In addition, angiography has been reported to miss up to 8% of living donor vessels and poorly visualizes venous vasculature, whereas 3D modeling of 20 patients did not miss any arterial vasculature, identified plaques and calcifications, and accurately portrayed venous

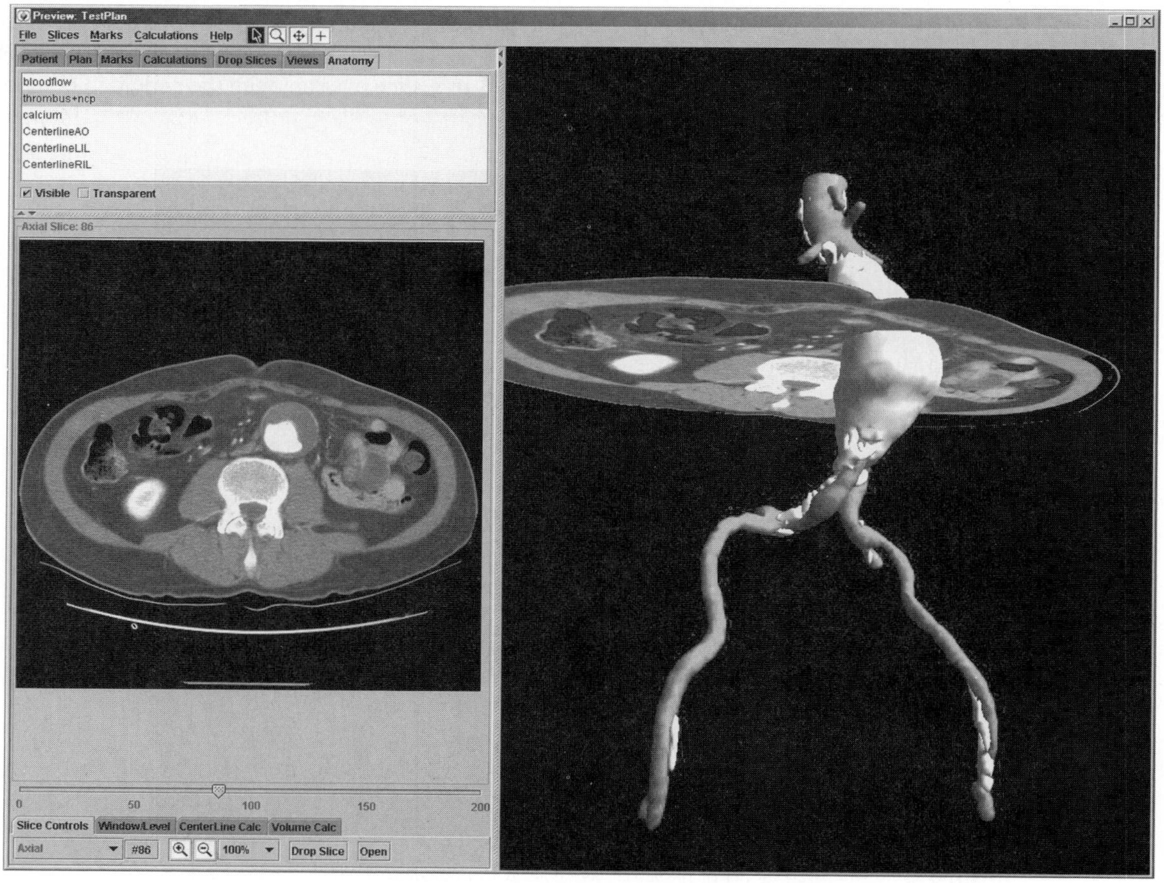

Figure 4 An image from the Preview application by Medical Media Systems. The three-dimensional, patient-specific image is useful to the surgeon in both planning surgery and targeting. Courtesy of Medical Media Systems, West Lebanon, NH.

vasculature. The cost for the VR study is $450 for the CT and 3D imaging, a substantial savings compared to angiography and IVP (25).

IV. Augmented Reality

Augmented reality (AR) systems superimpose virtual information over real structures (Fig. 5). Goggles allow CT, MRI, or USG display of patient-specific data while the surgeon is viewing the patient's abdomen, for example. It has been used to view a pregnant woman's fetus in a 3D manner prior to operation. Novice surgeons may have difficulty visualizing organs in 3D. AR enables viewing the anatomy in 3D to help master this knowledge faster (36). An AR system for neurosurgeons allows for CT or MRI imaging of a brain tumor to be transformed into a 3D image, which is then superimposed on the patient's head to help plan the skin incision and bone flap approach. The surgeons may then use the program in the operating room as a reference map to help assess the surgical margins.

Computer-aided plastic surgery (CAPS) uses a 3D model of the human face with a FEM overlaying soft tissue to estimate the results of tissue ablation and rearrangement (Fig. 6). CAPS allows a surgeon to simulate and plan facial surgery. The FEM technology allows volumetric remodeling after removing or relocating soft tissue, this essential feature of CAPS begins with a videoscan of the face, yielding cylindrical coordinates and documenting skin color. CAPS then translates the cylindrical coordinates into rectangular coordinates, allowing the viewer to manipulate the image from any outside point (26–32). The surgeon uses a mouse to make incisions, flaps, remove tissue, and so forth. The computer then segments the face into triangular or quadrilateral facets, incorporating the incisions as edges. The user designates simple approximation or a double Z-plasty rhomboid-to-W closure. A skin stiffness matrix is referenced to integrate the strain and distortion this reconstruction produces on the skin soft tissue. An algorithm for the displacement data then constructs the CAPS-predicted outcome (31).

V. Robotic Employment of Virtual Reality

Hip replacement surgery has traditionally been planned by overlaying templates on X-ray views to select implant type and size (33). ORTHODOC is a computer workstation that takes a special CT of the hip, after implanting three bone screw reference points; this helps the surgeon plan the operation in 3D. The ROBODOC operation is then performed with ORTHODOC, giving cutting instructions to the robot to form the cavity, using the screws as reference points. The surgeon may stop the robot at any time and revert to customary procedure because the operative field is fully exposed (33).

Robotically assisted heart bypass surgery, using the ZEUS Robotic Surgical System, is undergoing U.S. Food and Drug Administration (FDA)-approved Investigational Device Exemption (IDE) clinical trials. This system enables the surgeon to perform critical suturing through small pencil-sized ports. An endoscope is inserted into the chest and positioned by a voice-controlled robotic arm. While seated

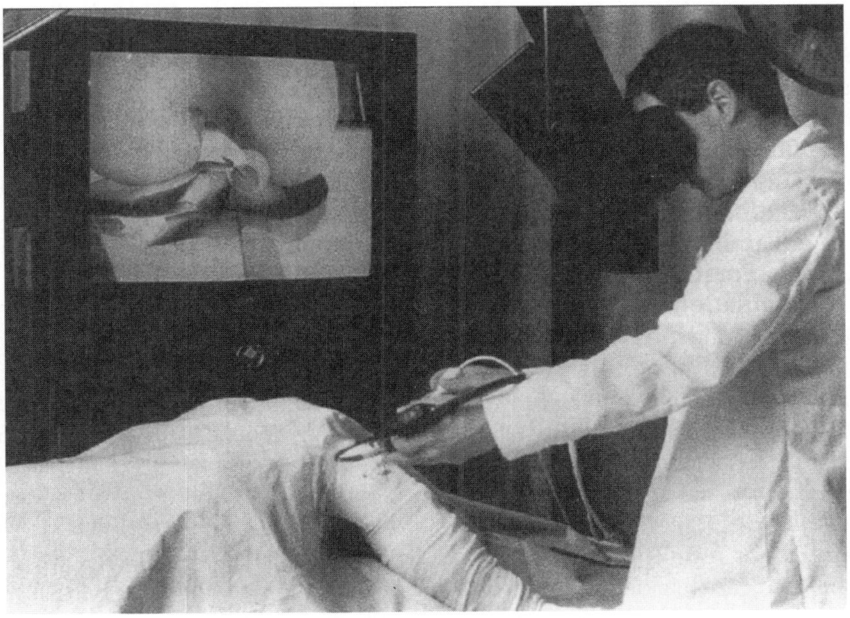

Figure 5 Data fusion by augmented reality.

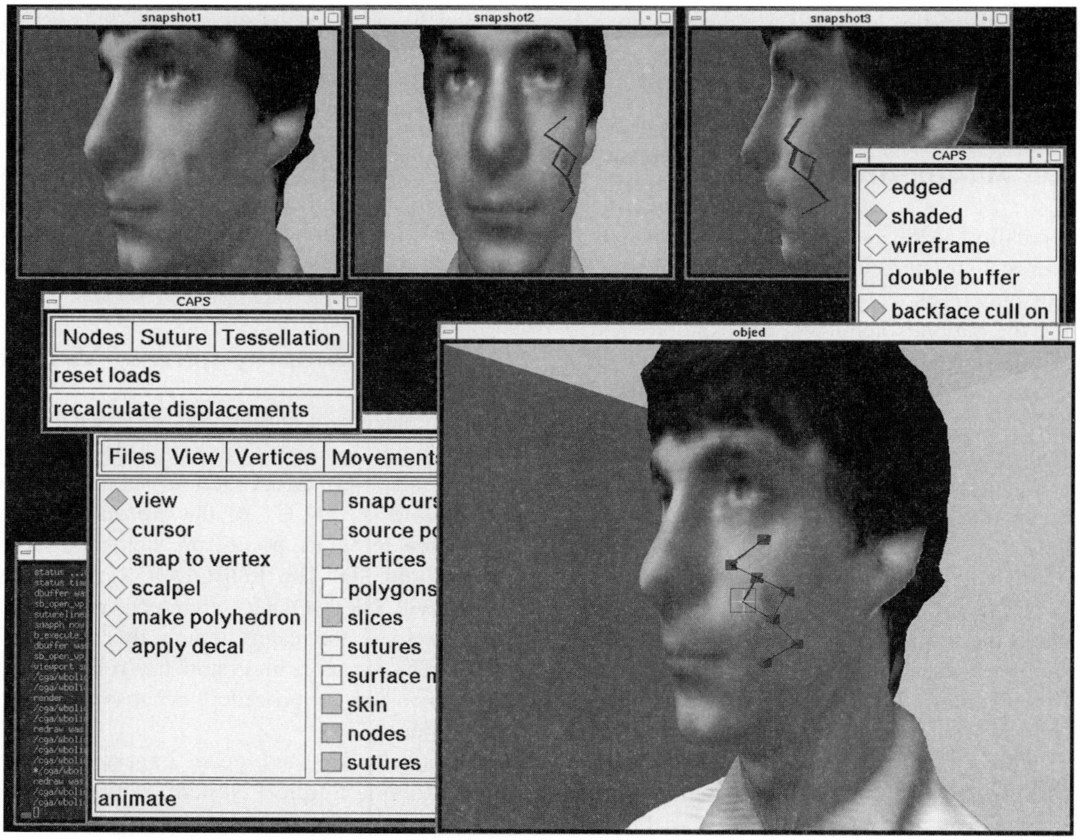

Figure 6 An image from the Computer-Aided Plastic Surgery Program (CAPS) developed to assist the physician in presurgical planning. It allows the surgeon to try a number of approaches before entering the operating room, which is especially useful when aesthetics is a crucial factor, such as this situation in which a small lesion is being removed from the patient's cheek. From Ref. (31), S.D. Peiper, D.R. Laub, Jr., and J.M. Rosen (1995). A finite-element facial model for simulating plastic surgery. *Plast. Reconstr. Surg.* **96**, 1100–1105.

at the console, the surgeon can view the operative site in either 3D or 2D, depending on preference. Movements of the surgical instruments are controlled via handles that resemble conventional surgical instruments. These movements of the handles are scaled, and tremor is filtered to enhance surgical precision (34)

VI. Telesurgery

By using electronic information and communication technologies, surgeons can practice at a distance from a patient (13). A surgeon may telementor a student, to train and educate, or teleproctor an experienced practitioner, to evaluate and certify skills. These techniques have been successfully applied to laparoscopic hernia repairs and other teaching situations. However, questions have been raised about licensing requirements for recipient practitioners of electronically transmitted medical technology. Other concerns include the need for backup plans in the event of communication breakdown, and proper preparation prior to surgery (adequate review of medical documentation and treatment discussion). Wire transmission over 200 miles and wireless transmission greater than 50 km are the limits to performing telesurgery, due to lag-time problems and effects on coordination (telepresence). Satellite transmission cannot be used for this reason.

Telesurgery is a natural extension of the skills younger physicians have learned playing videogames, which requires decoupling of the oculo–vestibular axis from the tactile–proprioceptive axis to manipulate the game consoles. Telepresence surgery attempts to transform the remote feeling of laparoscopic surgery into the more natural feeling of open surgery. With the SRI system (SRI International, Menlo Park, CA), the surgeon views a 3D image from a minimally invasive procedure, which portrays organs and instruments as if the operative field was fully open. The surgeon sits at a console, inside or outside the operating suite, while an assistant stays with the patient, and receives tactile feedback from the instrument tips.

Using this technology the following procedures have been demonstrated with animals: gastrostomy and closure, gastric resection, bowel anastomosis, liver laceration suture, liver lobe resection, splenectomy, aortic graft replacement, and arteriotomy repair (13).

Technology can compensate for human limitations of hand positioning (200 μm), intention tremor, and eye saccade motion (13). The Hunter telepresence system for opthalmological surgery tracks the motion of the eye. It increases instrument scale such that 1 cm of hand motion equals 10 μm of laser movement. Videoimages magnify retina vessels to the size of fingers. Digital signal processing and filtering remove hand tremor. By using these techniques, the limits of human accuracy are improved from 200 to 10 μm.

VII. Conclusions and Future Research

The critical steps toward realizing the promise of virtual reality in surgery involve continued significant development in the fields of human models, interface devices, and system verification. Human modeling by far poses the greatest challenge and will require several generations of improved computer mathematical algorithms to achieve accurate representation of normal humans and pathologic conditions. This is especially true for predicting changes over time (e.g., aging and outcomes). The second critical component, haptic or visual interface tools, will continue to evolve with the help of many industries (e.g., defense contractors) that also benefit from improving this technology. The third requirement, system verification, is key to the acceptance of VR by practicing surgeons and consists of two components. The first is scientific demonstration of how well virtual reality systems provide the "touch" and "feel" of true reality. Second, we will need to prove that a training experience in a virtual reality simulator translates into actual improvement in the performance of the clinician. Just as the incorporation and acceptance of flight simulators in pilot training took many years, a serious, long-term research effort will be necessary before the tools and interfaces of virtual reality become an integral dimension of surgery. The future of VR is exciting and its benefits will soon be within our grasp.

References

1. Mann, R. (1965). The evaluation and simulation of mobility aids for the blind. *In* "Rotterdam Mobility Research Conference." American Foundation for the Blind, New York.
2. Mann, R. (1985). Computer-aided surgery. *In* "Proceedings of RESNA 8th Annual Conference." Rehabilitation Engineering Society of North America, Bethesda, MD.
3. Boeing (1995). Boeing 777 Digital Design Process Earns Technology Award. Accessed Feb. 2, 2000, at http://www.boeing.com/news/releases/1995/news.release.950614a.html.
4. Rosen, J. M., Laub, D. R., Jr., and Pieper, S. D. (1997). Virtual reality and plastic surgery. *Adv. Plast. Reconstr. Surg.* **13**.
5. Isenberg, S. B., McGaghie, W. C., Hart, I. R., *et al.* (1999). Simulation technology for health care professional skills training and assessment. *JAMA* **282**(9), 861–866.
6. Davis, D., Thomson O'Brien, M. A., Freemantle, N., *et al.* (1999). Impact of formal continuing medical education. *JAMA* **282**(9); 867–874.
7. Krummel, T. M. (1998). Surgical simulation and virtual reality: The coming revolution [editorial]. *Ann. Surg.* **228**(5), 635–637.
8. Raibert, M., Playter, R., and Krummel, T. M. (1998). The use of a virtual reality haptic device in surgical training. *Acad. Med.* **73**(5), 596–597.
9. Bodily, K. (1999). Surgeons and technology: Presidential address. *Am. J. Surg.* **177**(5), 351–353.
10. Delp, S. (1993). Surgery simulation: Using computer graphics models to study the biomechanical consequences of musculoskeletal reconstructions. *In* "Proceedings of NSF Workshop on Computer-Assisted Surgery. National Science Foundation, Biomedical Engineering Section and the Robotics and Machine Intelligence Program." NSF, Washington, D.C.
11. NLM (1999). The Visible Human Project. National Library of Medicine web site:http://www.nlm.nih.gov/research/visible/visible_human.html.
12. Ackerman, M. (1995). Accessing the Visible Human Project. *D-Lib Magazine*, October, www.dlib.org/dlib/october95/10ackerman.html, 10/9/00.
13. Satava, R. (1998). "Cybersurgery: Advanced Technologies for Surgical Practice." Wiley-Liss, Inc., New York.
14. Fakespace. (1999). Fakespace Systems Announces Industry First: A Fully Reconfigurable Display System for Immersive Visualization. Accessed at http://www.fakespace.com/press/101599.html, 12/30/99.
15. Adelstein, B. R., and Rosen, J. M. (1992). Design and implementation of a force reflecting manipulandum for manual control research. *In* "Advances in Robotics," pp. 1–12. ASME, New York.
16. Madhani, A., Niemeyer, G., and Salisbury, J. K. (1998). The Black Falcon: A teleoperated surgical instrument for minimally invasive surgery. *In* "International Conference on Intelligent Robots and Systems (IROS)." IEEE/RSJ, Victoria, B.C., Canada.
17. Madhani, A. (1997). Design of teleoperated surgical instruments for minimally invasive surgery. *In* "Mechanical Engineering." Thesis, Massachusetts Institute of Technology, Cambridge.
18. McKenna, M. (1994). "A Physically Based Human Figure Model with a Complex Foot and Low Level Behavior Control." Thesis, Massachusetts Institute of Technology, Cambridge.
19. Delp, S. L., Loan, J. P., Rosen, J. M., *et al.* (1995). Surgical simulation: An emerging technology for military training. *In* "Military Medicine On-Line Today," pp. 29–34. IEEE Press, New Jersey.
20. Satava, R. M. (1993). Virtual reality surgical simulator: The first steps. *Surg. Endosc.* **7**(3), 203–205.
21. Fenlon, H. M. Nunes, D. P., Schroy, P. C., *et al.* (1999). A comparison of virtual and conventional colonoscopy for the detection of colorectal polyps. *N. Engl. J. Med.* **341**(20), 1496–1503.
22. Black, W., M. D., Department of Radiology, Dartmouth College, 11/23/99, personal communication.
23. Lerner L. H., Henriques, H. F., and Harris, R. D. (1999). Interactive 3-dimensional computerized tomography reconstruction in evaluation of the living kidney donor. *J. Urol.* **161**, 403–407.
24. Medical Media Systems (1999). Web site accessed Dec. 20, 1999: http://www.medicalmedia.com/.
25. Fillinger, M. F. (1999). New imaging techniques in endovascular surgery. *Surg. Clin. North Am.* **79**(3), 451–475.
26. Pieper, S. (1989). More Than Skin Deep. Masters thesis (unpublished), Massachusetts Institute of Technology, Cambridge.
27. Pieper, S. (1992). CAPS: Computer Aided Plastic Surgery. Thesis, Massachusetts Institute of Technology, Cambridge.

28. Pieper, S., Rosen, J., and Zeltzer, D. (1992). Interactive graphics for plastic surgery: A task-level analysis and implementation. *In* "Symposium on Interactive 3D Graphics." ACM, New York.
29. Pieper, S., Chen, D., *et al.* (1992). Surgical simulation: From computer-aided design to computer-aided surgery. *In* "Proceedings of Imaging." OCM, Monaco.
30. Pieper, S., McKenna, M., and Chen, D. (1994). Computer animation for minimally invasive surgery: Computer system requirements and preferred implementations. *In* "SSPIE: Stereoscopic Displays and Virtual Reality Systems—The Engineering Reality of Virtual Reality." SPIE, Bellingham, WA.
31. Pieper, S. D., Laub, D. R., Jr., and Rosen, J. M. (1995). A finite-element facial model for simulating plastic surgery. *Plast. Reconstr. Surg.* **96**(5), 1100–1105.
32. Pieper, S.D., Delp, S., Rosen, J. M., and Fisher, S. (1991). A virtual environment system for simulation of leg surgery. *In* "SPIE—The International Society for Optical Engineering, Stereoscopic Displays and Applications II." SPIE, Bellingham, WA.
33. DiGioia, A. J., Jaramaz, B., and Colgan, B. D. (1998). Computer-assisted orthopedic surgery. *Clini Orthop.* **354**, 8–16.
34. Reichenspurner, H. W., Weltz, A., Gulielmos, V., Boehm, D. H., and Reichart, B. (1999). Port-access cardiac surgery using endovascular cardiopulmonary bypass: Theory, practice, and results. *J. Cardiac Surg.* **14**, 275–280.
35. HT Medical Systems (1999). PreOpTM Endoscopy Simulator. Web site: http://www.ht.com/products_endosim.htm.
36. Fuchs, H., Livingston, M. A., Raskar, R., *et al.* (1998). Augmented reality visualization for laparoscopic surgery. *IN* "First International Conference on Medical Image Computing and Computer-Assisted Intervention (MICCAI '98)." Massachusetts Institute of Technology, Cambridge.

99

Surgeons and Health Services Research

Robert S. Rhodes* **and Susan D. Horn**[†]

*University of Pennsylvania School of Medicine, Philadelphia, Pennsylvania 19103
[†]Institute for Clinical Outcomes Research, Salt Lake City, Utah 84109

I. Introduction

Concerns with the cost and quality of healthcare have plagued all industrialized nations for at least the past two decades. Yet there has been a relative paucity of definitive information on which to base changes in healthcare policy. For instance, one study concluded that only about 15% of common medical practices had a documented foundation in any sort of medical research (1). This does not necessarily mean that only 15% of care is effective, but it underscores the lack of hard evidence on the value of the majority of care. The burgeoning field of health services research seeks to fill this void. Broadly defined, this research examines the factors that affect healthcare-seeking behavior, healthcare costs, and healthcare outcomes, and their attendant implications of specific healthcare policies.

Surgical interventions are particularly suitable for such analyses. One reason is the relative ease of such analyses. Surgical illnesses tend to be of relatively short duration, the outcomes are readily quantified, and the costs are often easily identified. There are also quality concerns specifically related to surgery. These include considerable variation in the frequency of surgical procedures among geographically small areas (2–4) and medical record reviews that reveal alarming rates of errors in care (5,6). In both of the latter studies, errors in surgical care accounted for roughly half of the adverse events.

Physicians tend to be reluctant to engage in analyses of quality or the relationship between quality and cost. The prevailing attitude has been that quality is related to appropriateness and that quality and cost are positively related. Any reduction in healthcare expenditures would negatively impact quality. However, these concepts are giving ground to a newer concept that defines quality in terms of structure, process, and outcome (7). Surgeon involvement in these efforts will be important to assure their validity.

This chapter introduces the principles and complexities of health services research as it relates to surgery. Because health services research encompasses many facets of healthcare, Section II addresses specific areas of research. Each discussion contains a short background on the current status of the field and an analysis of the relevant strengths, weaknesses, and pitfalls of research in that area. This is further supplemented with examples from the literature and references to facilitate research productivity. The issues here are too heterogeneous and too diverse to achieve complete analysis. Rather, the overall goals are to help surgeons appreciate the problems of defining quality and the relationship between quality and cost, and to equip them to participate in studies to achieve those ends.

II. Methods

A. General Principles

From the outset, one must appreciate the characteristics that distinguish health services research from the methods that are probably more familiar to the surgical scientist. For instance, "bench" research typically involves continuous variables that are normally distributed. Most parameters are "controlled" and only the variable in question is subject to analysis. In more traditional forms of clinical research, again, many parameters can be controlled. The gold standard of such clinical research is the randomized, controlled trial. Such trials often involve patients from a single institution or a limited number of surgeons.

In contrast, health services research often involves large samples of patients from many surgeons or institutions. The data may be collected retrospectively and the "controls" may be limited. Outcomes assessments often involve categorical variables (e.g., survived vs. died; graft patency). Any continuous variables (e.g., length of stay, cost) are likely to have a skewed rather than normal distribution. Although this appears to lack many of the more traditional features of scientific experiments, outcomes research assesses health services in "real life" conditions. Whereas randomized, controlled trials assess the *efficacy* of a given intervention in close to ideal circumstances, health services research evaluates the *effectiveness* of an intervention as it actually occurs.

Carotid endarterectomy is an excellent example of the difference between efficacy and effectiveness. Randomized, control trials have demonstrated the efficacy of this procedure when performed by surgeons with low perioperative mortality and stroke rates (8,9). Yet the effectiveness of this procedure depends on continued performance with a similarly low incidence of complications. As stroke rates and other complications increase, the effectiveness may decrease or disappear entirely (10–12).

Because health services research usually involves large samples, it often relies heavily on computerized databases. Such databases tend to be associated with administrative or claims data and, compared with more traditional record review, often lack in-depth information on severity and complexity. This can be a catch-22 because the lack of detail confounds analysis and interpretation. Another potential source of bias is that patients, practitioners, hospitals, and healthcare purchasers may each have different perspectives on a given issue. In interpreting reports, the reader must be aware of such potential bias and view the conclusions in relation to the investigator's frame of reference (13,14).

B. Assessing Variations in Use

It is well recognized that there is considerable variation in the frequency of surgical procedures among small geographic areas. Furthermore, this variation has specific characteristics. For instance, procedures with highly specific indications (e.g., repair of hip fracture, inguinal herniorraphy, and appendectomy) tend to have relatively little variation (15). On the other hand, there is considerable variation for procedures such as carotid endarterectomy, hysterectomy, and coronary angiography. Variation also appears related to provider capacity (e.g., availability of services) (16) and a number of physician factors, including physician style, community practice "signatures," and physician uncertainty (17). Many medical decisions appear to be opinion based rather than evidence based (18). This has led to the conclusion that, "marked variability in surgical practices and presumably in surgical judgment and philosophy must be considered to reflect absent or inadequate data by which to evaluate surgical treatment" (19).

Whether areas of high frequency are too high or areas of low frequency are too low is still of concern. The tendency is to believe that high is too high but the association between variation and the ratio of hospital beds to population (20) worries some that low frequency is due to limited access to care. Physician economic incentives, which might seem important, appear to play a relatively small role (21).

C. Assessing Outcomes

Table I shows some traditional outcome measures (22), but the introduction of managed care has made the list dynamic. Lengths of stay, costs, and patient satisfaction are

Table I Outcome Measures

Morbidity/mortality
Recurrence rates
Patient-reported measures of symptoms
Functional status
Length of stay
Charges/cost
Quality-adjusted life years (QALYs)
Emotional consequences of the disease and the treatment
Patient satisfaction

increasingly emphasized. The distribution of variation in these outcomes tends to be skewed with the tail toward the right (Fig. 1). In fact, the skew may be sufficiently great so that for some measures the median is zero (e.g., the frequency of a given procedure among surgeons where the majority of surgeons do not perform the procedure). To circumvent some of the mathematical problems of skewed distributions, the mean may be calculated as the mean of the logarithm of individual values (i.e., geometric mean). This methodology is used to determine diagnosis-related group (DRG) lengths of stay. However, others feel strongly that it is much better to trim outliers and perform analyses on trimmed data (23,24).

Outcome measures also must consider health status and severity of illness prior to treatment (25), but such adjustments can be difficult (26, 27). The data for severity adjustment are usually derived from one of two types of sources—claims and administrative data or medical record review (28). Many more severity factors can be identified from medical record review, but, at least at present, such review is considerably more cumbersome, is more costly, and still cannot account for a major portion of the variation in cost. It is believed that much of the remaining cost variation is due to (nonproductive) variation in treatments (29). Because healthcare purchasers usually make severity adjustments from claims/administrative data and not record review, the validity of such severity adjustment is particularly suspect. In addition, the frequency of miscoding in many claims/administrative databases may exceed 10%.

Patient-related variation may result from age, gender, cultural, ethnic, and socioeconomic factors that are extrinsic to the medical care system (30). Selection bias may also affect reports of outcomes and underscores the need to adjust for patient differences (31). High rates of inadequate functional health literacy are also known to affect compliance (and hence outcomes) adversely (32).

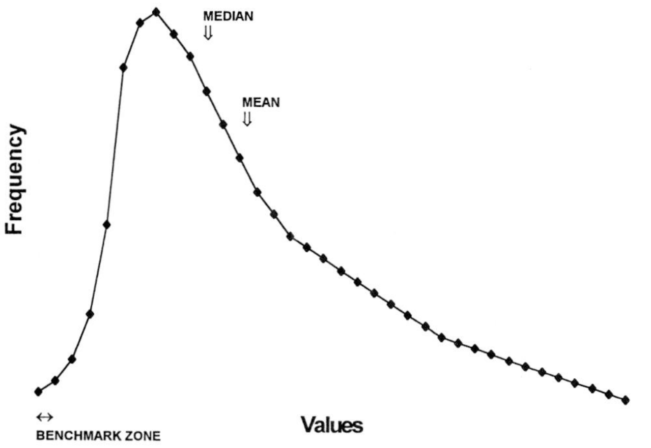

Figure 1 Skewed distribution curve associated with healthcare outcomes such as cost or length of stay.

Healthcare purchasers are well aware of the cost variation among providers and use the low-cost providers as a "benchmark" toward which all providers are expected to strive. Such benchmarks have value in that they may represent "best practice" and are likely to contain lessons for management of similar patients. However, these benchmarks also may represent ideal patients—patients who are exceptions rather than the norm (33). Although use of practice profiles is becoming more widespread, the inability to account fully for severity factors is a significant limitation. Thus, use of these benchmarks as targets for more complicated patients may increase the risk for adverse outcomes among patients who need more care.

Another limitation to practice profiles is that many of the factors that are known to affect variability in cost and length of stay are not under direct control of surgeons (34, 35). On the other hand, protocol-guided decision making has been shown to be of value (36, 37). The validity of outcomes measures as indices for improving the quality of care implies that they must also be intimately related to the processes of care (38).

D. Measuring Quality of Life

Along with continued interest in traditional outcome measures such as morbidity and mortality, there is an increasing emphasis on long-term functional status. The preferred measure of these long-term outcomes is the healthcare quality of life or quality of life years (QALYs) (40, 41). This is a summary measure of the length of time one experiences a given health status. Systems used to quantify this health status (42) may consist of objective measures (such as functional status) and/or use subjective estimates of well being. The latter often involve patient estimates of the meaningfulness of a given functional status. For instance, Patient A may not be able to walk as far as Patient B, but one cannot extrapolate that Patient A has a poorer quality of life unless that functional status is placed in a context that is meaningful to the patient (43).

A given individual's estimate of the future value of an outcome measure may vary with time or with the specific circumstances at the time of measurement. QALYs may also vary among individuals or groups. Elderly (or other) patients might place greater value on quality of life and less value on longevity if the latter were not associated with an independent existence (44). Such differences underscore the impact of socioeconomic status, ethnicity, religious beliefs, and attitudes about healthcare. Outcomes should be based on evidence-based interventions but may be assessed by more than one measure. Patients, providers, and healthcare purchasers may then have different perspectives on which measure should be used to judge the outcome of a given intervention.

E. Relating Outcome to Provider Volume

An increasing number of reports emphasize favorable outcomes associated with increased surgeon and/or hospital volume to outcome (45–50). Similar reports also exist with regard to the issue of surgeon subspecialty training (49, 51). There are also data that indicate an inverse relationship between hospital volume and cost (52). Thus, high-volume institutions may have advantages in both the numerator and the denominator of cost-effectiveness. The empiric relationship between surgical volume and outcome has raised the question of regionalization of care (53). However, it is important to remember that the data represent probabilities and not absolute relationships. Not all "low" volume is associated with poorer outcomes and not all "high" volume is associated with better outcomes. At least one large study of eight common surgical procedures, using medical record data rather than claims data, was unable to establish a correlation between the institutional volume of surgery and postoperative mortality (54). Thus, the relationship between the effects of hospital volume versus surgeon volume may vary with specific procedures. Complex, team-dependent procedures, such as coronary artery bypass grafting, may be more hospital-volume dependent whereas less complicated procedures may be more surgeon-volume dependent.

The issue of whether "practice makes perfect" or "perfect makes practice" needs further investigation (55). Because of potential adverse and/or unintended consequences of drawing conclusions from current studies, it is probably premature to use such data as a final determinant of quality (56). Indeed, patient selection may produce "paradoxical" outcomes (57).

F. Assessing Costs and Cost-Effectiveness

Understanding the basis of costs is extremely important but is not always straightforward. A basic but critical distinction must be made between costs and charges. Charges reflect price structure but poorly reflect the actual cost. Thus, there are often also substantial variations among institutions in the relationship between charges and cost. Even when considering costs, there is often considerable variation among institutions for the costs of apparently similar services. This is in part due to substantial differences in cost accounting. However, such differences are even observed among relatively standardized accounting systems, such as those used by the Health Care Financing Administration (HCFA).

The complexity of calculating costs is also expressed in the statement, "Cost is a noun that never really stands alone" (58). Thus, costs are often categorized in ways to meet decision makers' specific needs (Table II). Traceability is perhaps the most important characteristic of cost in relation to health services research. Variable costs, such as supplies, change as output changes and the change occurs in a constant, proportional manner. In contrast, fixed costs do not change in response to changes in outputs. Semivariable costs (e.g., utilities) include elements of both fixed and variable costs. There will be a fixed basic cost per unit time but there is also likely to be a direct, proportional relationship between output and utility costs. Semifixed, or step, costs may change with respect to changes in output but they are not proportional. Costs will change, but not unless the step threshold is attained. Thus, a semifixed cost might be considered a variable or a fixed cost, depending on the size of the steps relative to the range of output. A protocol may help resolve the complexities of cost analyses that do not report all this information (59).

Cost-effectiveness is generally defined as cost divided by net benefits, with the numerator, or cost, expressed in dollars and the denominator expressed as beneficial outcomes minus adverse outcomes. As such, it also reflects quality in healthcare and is distinct from cost–benefit analysis, which assesses return on investment (with both the numerator and denominator in dollars), and from efficiency, which measures outputs divided by inputs (i.e., productivity). Although theoretically simple, the actual measurement of cost-effectiveness is complicated by both difficulties in measuring cost and difficulties in measuring outcomes. Analyses of cost-effectiveness may vary widely in the costs and the health effects that they consider, and thereby produce very different cost-effectiveness ratios for the same intervention. The investigator's perspective on the attribution of cost and the effects of comorbid conditions on cost and outcome are particularly vexing issues. A recent consensus statement recommended standards to improve study comparability and quality. It also advocated that calculations be based on a societal perspective rather than the perspective of patient, provider, or purchaser (60–62).

Cost-effective analysis, by definition, compares two approaches to a given problem. In some cases it compares two interventions; in others it compares an intervention with no treatment. The numerator is the difference in cost and the denominator is the difference in outcome. As with any ratio, costs (numerator) or quality (denominator) may preferentially affect the calculation. Favorable cost-effectiveness may result from a relatively low cost differential or a relatively high quality differential. QALYs are also a ratio and, when used in the denominator, can affect the quality differential either through a predominant effect on quality or the duration of that quality. Table III demonstrates the relative effect of the numerator and the denominator on the cost-effectiveness of selected surgical procedures. It is also important to recognize that the interval from the intervention to the point of measurement will affect the estimate of cost-effectiveness (63, 64). Moreover, patients, providers, and purchasers may focus on different intervals and, thus, again reach different conclusions.

Table II Categories, Types, and Examples of Hospital Costs

Category	Type	Definition/example
Traceability to the object being costed	Direct	Salaries, supplies, rents, and utilities
	Indirect	Depreciation and employee benefits
Behavior of cost to output or activity	Variable	Supply costs
	Fixed	Depreciation
	Semivariable	Utilities
	Semifixed	Number of full-time equivalents per step in outputs
Management responsibility for control		Often limited to direct, variable costs
Future vs. historical	Avoidable costs	Costs affected by a decision under consideration
	Sunk costs	Costs not affected by a decision under consideration
	Incremental costs	Changes in total costs resulting from alternative courses of action
	Opportunity costs	Value foregone by using a resource in a particular way instead of in its next best alternative way

A particularly powerful form of cost-effectiveness analysis is the use of clinical decision analysis in conjunction with sensitivity analysis (65–67). Such models can predict cost-effectiveness and the criteria that critically affect care decisions. Two examples of such sensitivity analysis are related to management of penetrating colon trauma (68) and carotid endarterectomy in asymptomatic patients (69). Cost-effectiveness analysis may also be well suited to examine the potential impact of delayed referral or an evaluation pathway.

An example of the potential variability in determining cost-effectiveness is the use of computed tomography (CT) in the diagnosis of appendicitis (70). In this study, the clinical likelihood of appendicitis was estimated by the referring surgeon and categorized into four groups based on their estimate of the clinical probability of appendicitis. These estimates were then compared with the estimates of appendicitis by computed tomography. Operation or recovery confirmed the actual pathology. The CT interpretations had 98% sensitivity, 98% specificity, 98% positive predictive value, 98% negative predictive value, and 98% accuracy for diagnosing or ruling out appendicitis. Interestingly, there was lack of agreement between the actual incidence of appendicitis and the initial clinical estimates, emphasizing that surgeon estimates of "outcomes" often differ from the actual data. Although the authors concluded that CT scanning was cost-effective, actual costs (and any savings) are likely to vary with, among other things, surgeon estimates of the clinical likelihood of appendicitis, availability of less expensive options to in-hospital observation, and the use of the

Table III Cost-Effectiveness Studies of Some Surgical Procedures

Procedure	$/QALY	ΔQALY	Comment	Ref.
Carotid endarterectomy in asymptomatic patients	8000	+0.25	The initial cost of endarterectomy is offset by the high cost of care after major stroke. The relative cost of surgical treatment increased substantially with increasing age, increasing perioperative stroke rate, and decreasing stroke rate during medical management	69
Routine radiation therapy following conservative surgery for early breast cancer	28,000	+0.35	The ratio is heavily influenced by the cost of radiation therapy and the quality-of-life benefit that results from decreased risk of local recurrence	98
Total hip arthroplasty for osteoarthritis of the hip—60-year-old woman	117,000 in cost saving	+6.9	The cost savings result from the high cost of custodial care associated with dependency	99
Total hip arthroplasty for osteoarthritis of the hip—85-year-old man	4600	+2	—	99
Endoscopic versus open carpal tunnel release	195	0.235	Cost-effectiveness is very sensitive to a major complication such as median nerve injury	100
Lumbar discectomy	29,200	0.43	Cost-effectiveness results from its substantial effect on quality of life and moderate costs	101

emergency room for triage. In this study, 53% of the patients were proved to have appendicitis. In other institutions, only 30% of patients with an admitting diagnosis of appendicitis eventually have an appendectomy (71). Thus, the value of this approach for other institutions will depend on specific factors in those institutions.

Ambulatory surgery (72) and trauma care (73,74) are two examples of potential cost-saving that may also depend on specific circumstances. Although dollar amounts per outcome provide a framework for healthcare policy decisions, they do not necessarily correspond to an intervention's societal value. Thus, a threshold "amount per outcome" for what is or is not cost-effective remains somewhat arbitrary and relative.

G. Assessing New Technology

The explosive growth in technology has increased the need for technology assessment. An interesting paradox of new technology is that it may lower cost per procedure but, as a result of increases in volume, may increase aggregate costs. Such is the case with laparoscopic cholecystectomy (75). This exemplifies how patients and healthcare purchasers might reach differing opinions as to the "value" of new technology. Another pitfall in assessing technology relates to tests that allow diagnosis at an earlier stage of disease. Earlier diagnosis does not necessarily mean that screening prolongs survival but simply that those patients with "presymptomatic disease" are aware of the condition a longer time. This is referred to as lead-time bias. In general, advances in diagnostic imaging increase the likelihood of such bias and overestimate disease prevalence (76).

III. Clinical Practice Improvement—A New Approach

A. Introduction

Clinical practice improvement (CPI) is a new study methodology designed to develop analytically based protocols to achieve desirable outcomes at the lowest essential cost over the continuum of care (77). Several elements of the clinical practice improvement approach make it attractive to clinicians. First, CPI is a scientific "bottom-up" approach that places accountability for practice improvement and outcomes with clinicians. Clinicians are not told to follow guidelines or protocols developed by others, but instead collect data on outcomes, on treatments, and on patient signs and symptoms that support practice change. CPI supports caregivers in making their own decisions about optimal care on the basis of objective statistical evidence gathered in the routine, everyday practice of medicine. Second, CPI measurement encompasses a comprehensive view of the care management process: patient characteristics, process steps, and outcomes. All three classes of data are considered simultaneously. This comprehensive measurement framework provides a basis for meaningful analyses of significant associations, as well as relationships between process and outcome. Third, the CPI methodology focuses on application. There is a continual emphasis on factors that can be implemented to improve outcomes and the process to achieve these results.

B. CPI: Study Design

A clinical practice improvement study design includes measures of patient factors (physiologic severity of illness and psychosocial derangements presented at each visit or at each admission), medical care process factors (e.g., medications, treatments), and outcome factors. More specific characteristics of each of these three types of factors are as follows:

1. Patient factors. These are key characteristics of the population such as demographics, specific indications for treatment and severity of illness, and psychosocial factors. To have enough detail describing patients and their needs usually requires disease-specific physiologic data, such as those contained in the inpatient and outpatient components of an instrument such as the Comprehensive Severity Index (CSI) (28,29,77–83). This instrument not only measures initial patient severity but can also measure continuous changes in severity during the course of illness. Without such detailed information, clinicians often find it difficult to agree to stabilize their processes of care.
2. Medical care process factors. These are measurable factors that describe each major process step. Examples include which drugs are dispensed, how often prescriptions are filled, what dose is used, and how a ventilator is set.
3. Outcome factors. Outcomes factors commonly assessed in data collection instruments include diagnosis-specific complications, diagnosis-specific long-term medical outcomes (which may be assessed by both clinicians and patients), patient functional status, patient satisfaction, and cost. Outcome factors may be thought of as analogs of the assessment endpoints in a randomized controlled trial.

All three types of data from the care management process are required. If only process and outcome data are available, but not detailed patient data, clinicians cannot tell if the outcomes achieved are due to the process steps or to differences in patient severity levels. The interactions of these three factors are shown in Fig. 2.

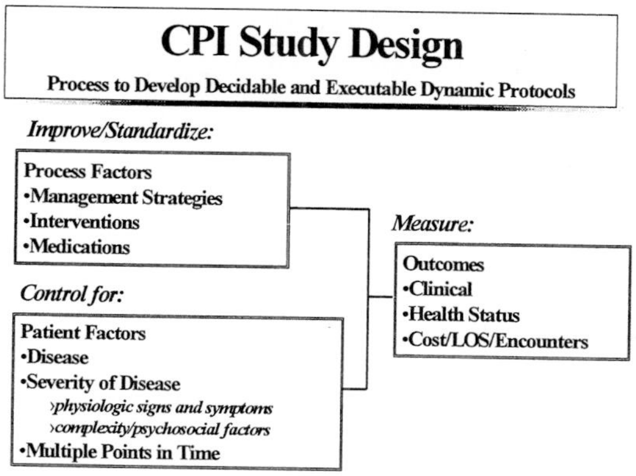

Figure 2 Relationship among process factors in CPI study design.

C. CPI: Analytic Methods

A clinical practice improvement study database usually includes many variables and is so designed to measure patient characteristics, processes of care, and patient outcomes. When more than three or four patient and process (independent) variables must be taken into account, the effects of these factors on the outcome (dependent) variables are modeled using multiple regression analyses. Such multivariate statistical methods allow comparisons of alternative treatments while controlling for other variables that may be driving observed differences between the outcomes of the treatments. These statistical methods allow researchers to examine relationships far more complex than those defined using only one explanatory variable at a time. The coefficients of the independent variables in the regression equations identify key process steps that, when controlling for patient factors, lead to better outcomes.

Another important aspect of CPI is that it uses a systems approach. Thus, in addition to participation by relevant medical specialists, every study should also involve representatives from other applicable services. Such representation might include administration, nursing, pharmacy, medical records, information systems, and dietetics. Working together, these individuals then identify the variables of interest. Although the group has considerable professional knowledge of critical measures, it should include a wide variety of patient, process, and outcome variables to allow for unanticipated findings. The nonphysician participants and the literature on known best practices may be important sources of such variables. The team's participants do not need to represent just one institution but may actually represent multiple institutions within a "network." The final decision on which variables to include often involves an iterative approach.

The measurement instrument, containing critical patient characteristics, process steps, and outcomes, is then circulated until consensus is reached on the variables to be included and their definitions. Data collection is automated by programming the measurement instrument into the CSI or some other software system as a table-driven database, known as an auxiliary data module (ADM). Data from participating surgeons and/or participating sites are harvested and merged for analysis. To start, univariate and bivariate analyses are used to examine means, standard deviations, ranges, rates, frequencies, and correlations between relevant patient or process variables and each of the outcome variables. Logistic regressions are performed for dichotomous outcomes and ordinary least-squares regressions are performed for continuous outcomes, in order to determine which patient and process variables are associated with the various outcomes. Typical outcomes for a surgical study might be length of stay, development of postoperative infection, and increase in severity from admission to maximum.

An example of such a study is one that involved abdominal surgery. Retrospective data were collected on 747 abdominal surgery patients, with about 100 patients from each of eight participating sites. Patient average age varied by more than 20 years across sites, from an average age of 49.0 years at one site to 69.7 years at another. Based on the Comprehensive Severity Index, the percentage of patients in admission severity level 1 varied from 53.7 to 86.7%. Thus, the percentage of sicker patients (admission severity > 1) ranged from 13.3 to 46.3% of the patients at each site. In particular, the percentage of life-threatening or catastrophic patients on admission (level 4) varied from 0 to 6.3%. Controlling for patient severity is essential to distinguish whether different outcomes are related to differences in process steps or to differences in patient severity.

Table IV shows some of the comparisons among factors across sites in this study. Although this particular study involved comparisons across institutions, similar analyses could be performed among surgeons at a single institution. Regression analyses helped the clinical practice improvement team identify critical areas for improvement when all the variables were considered simultaneously. Among the appendectomy DRGs (163–167) the patient factors associated with longer length of stay included higher admission severity, ruptured appendix, having previous abdominal surgery, and preadmission diarrhea. After controlling for these patient differences, several medical process steps were associated with significant differences in length of stay. Delivering the preoperative antibiotic within 2 hr before incision was associated with shorter length of stay; longer anesthesia start-to-incision times and use of drains were associated with longer length of stay. Postoperative care steps associated with longer length of stay included using a patient-controlled analgesia (PCA) pump and discharge to a skilled nursing facility.

For patients in the bowel surgery DRGs (146–149), the continuous CSI admission and maximum scores identified a

Table IV Significant Factors in a Study of Abdominal Surgery

Factor type	Factor	Compliance/variance	Comment
Medical process	Antibiotic prophylaxis within 2 hr of incision	33–60%	Known to be associated with fewer postoperative deep wound infections
Medical process	Patient mobilized from bed	1.18–2.49 days	—
Medical process	Time from anesthesia start to incision[a]	20.88–47.3 min	—
Medical process	Time from incision open to close	84.28–194.59 min	—
Medical process	Time from incision close to anesthesia stop	7.17–17.82 min	—
Medical process	Use of drains	14–66%	—
Outcome	Severity-adjusted length of stay (bowel surgery)	6.75–10.23 days	—
Outcome	Severity-adjusted length of stay (appendectomy)	2.62–5.45 days	—

[a]For CSI severity level I patients in DRGs 146–149.

number of variables that were significant in predicting an increase in severity from admission to maximum throughout the hospital stay. The following patient factors were associated with an increase in severity:higher admission severity score: having had previous abdominal surgery, needing assistance with mobility, and having a higher admission creatinine. After controlling for these patient differences, the following surgical process steps were associated with increasing severity: longer skin-to-skin times and longer anesthesia start-to-incision times. Putting the patient in lithotomy position was found to be beneficial, because it was negatively associated with change in severity. Postoperative care steps associated with increase in severity included not feeding the patient within 48 hr after surgery and longer time to first activity.

Patient factors associated with infection for patients in DRGs 146–149 (bowel surgery) included having chronic obstructive pulmonary disease, using corticosteroids before admission, having a higher body mass index, and having preadmission vomiting. After controlling for these patient differences, we found the surgical process step of skin-to-skin time was positively associated with infection. Finally, a postoperative care step associated with infection was use of a PCA pump.

Although many of the findings of these and similar studies may make "intuitive" sense, the value of CPI studies is often to bring this information to institutional or surgeon attention in an objective and nonjudgmental way. Although there may be initial reluctance to accept some of the findings and to change practice, such reluctance is far less than might occur otherwise. In the above example one might argue that the adverse findings associated with use of drains are actually a patient severity factor rather than a medical process factor. Yet the use of many other severity variables should control for this and help focus the discussion on process. Having identified significant process-related factors, the next steps are for the team to modify these factors and then continue the measurements to confirm that change has been affected.

D. Advantages of CPI

The goal of most clinical practice improvement studies is to help interested clinicians produce research-based dynamic protocols, i.e., protocols based on statistical findings that show the specified process steps that are associated with better outcomes. These protocols have the advantages of being (1) decidable and executable, i.e., they have specific process steps to follow based on deviations of a patient's signs and symptoms from normal values; and (2) based on analyses of data.

A key advantage of clinical practice improvement methodology is the naturalistic view of medical treatment that is provided by retrospective data recorded routinely by medical providers. This view is critical to determine implications of treatment alternatives. In everyday practice, patients are assigned to different treatments based on the provider's medical judgment, patient compliance is not artificially influenced, and monitoring of results is based on the provider's need for information about how a patient is doing. All these factors can impact the effectiveness of medical treatment.

A second key advantage of clinical practice improvement study methodology is cost. Using existing data from medical records and computerized databases is generally much less costly than implementing a prospective randomized controlled trial (RCT). Other advantages of retrospective data include the large number of observations that can be available for analysis and the usefulness of the data for hypothesis generation and refinement. Observational studies do not scientifically prove the causality of any underlying relationships, but they can point to hypotheses that can be clinically evaluated. These advantages of CPI go beyond the value of outcomes research, practice guidelines, and randomized, controlled trials. Outcomes research typically uses large, existing claims databases to find outcome failures. Such failures are often identified as poor outcomes beyond some statistical threshold, e.g., high mortality rates. But most outcomes research does not lead to practice improvement because (1) outcome failures are not scientifically related to detailed process steps that are under a practitioner's control, so it is unclear how to improve the outcome; and (2) patients are described only by diagnosis codes, so the severity of illness is not controlled.

Clinical practice guidelines or pathways are very popular but also have limitations. Thus, the effort to develop clinical guidelines is characterized by several weaknesses that hamper their relevance to local practice reform:

1. The guidelines often focus on the quality and the efficiency of care *after* decisions have been made to admit the patient or perform a procedure.
2. Standardization per se does not equate to quality.
3. The guidelines are developed nationally or centrally, based on expert consensus and literature review/synthesis. Because evidence-based guidelines must be all things to all people, they are often encyclopedic, or too general or inconclusive to be useful to clinicians. Moreover, the patient populations from which the "evidence" comes (usually randomized controlled trials) often differ from that in which the guideline will be used.
4. Not all guidelines adhere to established methodological standards (84, 85).

People now favor "evidence-based" methods of guideline development, rather than consensus-based methods. Good summaries of the process of pathway development, implementation, and trouble-shooting are available (86, 87). However, if guidelines are not decidable and executable at the local level they lose credibility with clinicians, and thus these clinicians are often unwilling to follow them.

Clinical practice improvement also differs from randomized controlled trials. These trials use a protocol document to create an artificial practice environment that allows for valid statistical inference. Although that structure eliminates practice variation, it usually covers a very limited subset of patients and practices. Because participants in randomized controlled trials are screened, selected, and subjected to scrutiny and intervention beyond that occurring in everyday treatment, the trials sometimes report results that are not broadly applicable in everyday medical treatment. Clinical practice improvement addresses the same issues—practice variation and valid statistical inference—from another point of view. It measures process variation, then eliminates it through a combination of statistical analysis, consensus, and feedback. CPI protocols allow valid statistical inference, because groups of similar patients receive the same treatment.

RCTs also tend to be limited in time; in most circumstances, they explicitly modify clinician behavior only for the duration of a study and only for the individuals directly involved in the trial. In contrast, clinical practice improvement establishes a permanent feedback loop aimed at all clinicians in an institution. It integrates research into daily practice, giving individual clinicians the information necessary to understand and modify their own activities at a detailed, operational level. Clinical practice improvement analyses help the team evaluate current practices and use the results to develop fact-based improvements. Changes to the process of care are supported by clinical data rather than by opinion.

The design of clinical practice improvement studies also allows the inclusion of large numbers of patients who are likely to have been excluded from an RCT. This improves their applicability (i.e., external validity). The ability to measure severity and control for confounding variables across multiple domains permits identification of associations rather than causality. The results of sensitivity analyses and the concurrence of findings with other research can further help to determine whether the identified associations are real and are relevant to existing practices (88, 89). Finally, the clinical practice improvement study design also results in an extremely low rate of attrition over time, thus avoiding a persistent problem with RCTs in health services research.

IV. Summary and Future Considerations

Good health services research is the foundation of sound health policy. This chapter has outlined the need for assessment of quality in healthcare as well as the advantages and pitfalls of various approaches to that assessment. Although the current best methods may seem cumbersome because they are typically abstracted by hand from existing paper medical records, this situation is likely to change. In the future, most hospitals will use computerized clinical information systems (CISs). Then, rather than relying on labor-intensive manual data abstraction, the needed patient, process, and outcome data can be found electronically in the hospitals' CIS. The efficiency and logistics of this new data acquisition modality will make it easier and less costly to conduct iterative clinical practice improvement studies to determine best practices. Also, the resulting research-based dynamic protocols can be programmed into the hospitals' CIS to flag for clinicians the appropriate protocol steps for a specific combination of patient signs and symptoms. This should result in more consistent implementation of protocol steps.

Although a number of strategies to control cost and improve quality are currently at work in the healthcare system, which one(s) will prove the best is by no means clear. Consumer report cards have been used but with mixed results (90–93). Individual surgeon self-assessment projects are underway, but it is still too early for results (94). On the other hand, a cooperative venture among cardiovascular surgeons has achieved notable success (95). It is particularly noteworthy that this very successful model used methods very similar to those used in CPI.

Physicians will undoubtedly have a role in the ongoing discussion and debate on the future of healthcare systems. The magnitude of their input in this debate may depend on their ability to address the larger issues of quality. Specifically, they must address two important sources of variation. One is variation in outcomes—which relates to judgment and skills—and the other is variation in rates of intervention. Medical decision-making must increasingly be based on evidence. If wide variations persist, especially for procedures for which there are clearly proved indications (e.g., carotid endarterectomy), healthcare purchasers may choose to reimburse only for proved indications and for surgeons with suitable low morbidity and mortality rates. Such policy was the case with pneumoreductive surgery for end-stage chronic pulmonary obstructive disease. This procedure was increasingly performed but without hard data to support its long-term efficacy. HCFA then announced it would pay for the procedure only if performed as part of a clinical trial to prove its efficacy. Other payers quickly followed suit (96).

Unfortunately, calls for assessing outcomes are met with varying degrees of disinterest or, in some cases, defensiveness. Such was the case roughly 100 years ago in Boston when E. A. Codman crusaded for hospitals and surgeons to publicize their end results (97). Although human nature leads every surgeon to believe that they are among the best, the data clearly show considerable variation in surgical outcomes (94). Surgeons are encouraged to participate in health services research in order to help resolve the important issues related to surgical care.

References

1. Williamson, J. W., Goldschmidt, P. G., and Jillson, I. A. (1979). Medical Practice Information Demonstration Project: Final Report. Office of the Assistant Secretary of Health, DHEW, Contract No. 282-77-0068GS. Baltimore, MD: Policy Research Inc.
2. Wennberg, J., and Gittelsohn, A. (1982). Variations in medical care among small areas. *Scientif. Am.* **246,** 120–134.
3. Chaissin, M. R., Brook, R. H., Park, R. E., *et al.* (1986). Variations in the use of medical and surgical services by the Medicare population. *N. Engl. J. Med.* **314,** 285–290.
4. The Dartmouth Atlas of Health Care. (1998). American Hospital Publishing, Chicago.
5. Leape, L. L., Brennan, T. A., Laird, N., *et al.* (1991). The nature of adverse events in hospitalized patients. Results of the Harvard Medical Practice Study II. *N. Engl. J. Med.* **324,** 377–384.
6. Gawande, A. A., Thomas, E. J., Zinner, M. J., *et al.* (1999). The incidence and nature of surgical adverse events in Colorado and Utah in 1992. *Surgery* **126,** 66–75.
7. Donabedian, A. (1980). "Explorations in Quality Assessment and Monitoring, Volume I: The Definition of Quality and Approaches to its Assessment." Health Administration Press, Ann Arbor, MI.
8. North American Symptomatic Carotid Trial Collaborators. (1991). Beneficial effect of carotid endarterectomy in symptomatic patients with high-grade carotid stenosis. *N. Engl. J. Med.* **325,** 445–453.
9. Executive Committee for the Asymptomatic Carotid Atherosclerosis Study. (1995). Endarterectomy for asymptomatic carotid artery stenosis. *JAMA* **273,** 1421–1428.
10. Tu, J. V., Hannan, E. L., Anderson, G. M., *et al.* (1998). The fall and rise of carotid endarterectomy in the United States and Canada. *N. Engl. J. Med.* **339,** 1441–1447.
11. Wennberg, D. E., Lucas, F. L., Birknmeyer, J. D., *et al.* (1998). Variation in carotid endarterectomy in the Medicare population. Trial hospitals, volumes, and patient characteristics. *JAMA* **279**, 1278–1281.
12. Chassin, M. R. (1998). Appropriate use of carotid endarterectomy. *N. Engl. J. Med.* **339**, 1468–1471.
13. Rhodes, R. S. (1999). How much does it cost? How much can be saved? *Surgery* **125**, 102–103.
14. Roberts, R. R., Frutos, P. W., Ciavarella, G. G., *et al.* (1999). Distribution of variable vs. fixed costs of hospital care. *JAMA* **281**, 644–649.
15. Birkmeyer, J. D., Sharp, S. M., Finlayson, S. R., *et al.* (1998). Variation profiles of common surgical procedures. *Surgery* **124**, 917–923.
16. Wennberg, D. E., Kellett, M. A., Dickens, J. D., *et al.* (1996). The association between local diagnostic intensity and invasive cardiac procedures. *JAMA* **275**, 1161–1164.
17. Eddy, D. M. (1984). Variations in physician practice: the role of uncertainty. *Health Aff. (Millwood)* **3**(2), 74–89.
18. Muir Gray, J. A. (1997). Evidence-based health care: How to make health policy and management decisions: Churchill Livingstone, New York.
19. Bunker, J. P. (1970). Surgical manpower: A comparison of operations and surgeons in the United States and in England and Wales. *N. Engl. J. Med.* **282**, 135–144.
20. Health Services Research Group. (1992). Small area variations: What are they and what do they mean? *Can. Med. Assoc. J.* **146**, 467–470.
21. Ashton, C. M., Petersen, N. J., Souchek, J., *et al.* (1999). Geographic variations in utilization rates in Veterans Affairs hospitals and clinics. *N. Engl. J. Med.* **340**, 32–9.
22. Reemtsma, K., and Morgan, M. (1997). Outcomes assessment: A primer. *Bull. Am. Coll. Surg.* **82**, 34–39.
23. Iezzoni, L. I., Ash, A. S., and Moskowitz, M. A. (1987). Report to HCFA (Cooperative Agreement No. 18-C-98526/1-03).
24. Horn, S. D. (1999). Personal communication.
25. Kreder, H. J., Wright, J. G., and McLeod, R. (1996). Outcomes studies in surgical research. *Surgery* **121**, 223–225.
26. Garvin, D. A. (1990). Afterword: Reflections on the future. *In* "Curing Health Care: New Strategies for Quality Improvement: A Report on the National Demonstration Project on Quality Improvement in Health Care" (D.M. Berwick, A.B. Godfrey, and J. Roessner, eds.), pp. 159–165. Josey-Bass Publishers, San Francisco.
27. Brook, R. H., Kamberg, C. J., and McGlynn, E. A. (1996). Health system reform and quality. *JAMA* **276,** 476–480.
28. Iezzoni, L. I., ed. (1997). Risk Adjustment for Measuring Healthcare Outcomes, 2nd Ed. Health Administration Press, Ann Arbor, MI.
29. Horn, S. D., Sharkey, P. D., Buckle, J. M., *et al.* (1991). The relationship between severity of illness and hospital length of stay and mortality. *Med. Care* **29,** 305–317.

30. Salem-Schatz, S., Moore, G., Rucker, M., *et al.* (1994). The case for case-mix adjustment in practice profiling: When good apples look bad. *JAMA* **272,** 871–874.
31. Melton, J. L. (1985). Selection bias in the referral of patients and the natural history of surgical conditions. *Mayo Clin. Proc.* **60,** 880–889.
32. Williams, M. V., Parker, R. M., Baker, D. W., *et al.* (1995). Inadequate functional health literacy among patients at two public hospitals. *JAMA* **274,** 1677–1682.
33. Rutledge, R. (1998). An analysis of 25 Milliman & Robertson guidelines for surgery: Data-driven versus consensus-driven clinical practice guidelines. *Ann. Surg.* **228,** 579–587.
34. Rhodes, R. S., Sharkey, P. D., and Horn, S. D. (1995). Effect of patient factors on hospital costs for major bowel surgery: Implications for managed health care. *Surgery* **117,** 443–450.
35. Kalman, P. G., and Johnston, K. W. (1996). Sociological factors are major determinants of prolonged hospital stay following abdominal aneurysm repair. *Surgery* **119,** 690–693.
36. Horst, H. M., Mouro, D., Hall-Jenssens, R. A., *et al.* (1998). Decrease in ventilation time with a standardized weaning process. *Arch. Surg.* **13,** 483–489.
37. Thomsen, G. E., Pope, D., East, T. D., *et al.* (1993). Clinical performance of a rule-based decision support system for mechanical ventilation of ARDS patients. *Proc. Annu. Symp. Comput. Appl. Med. Care*, pp. 339–343.
38. Chassin, M. R., Galvin, R. W., *et al.* (1998). The urgent need to improve health care quality: Institute of Medicine National Roundtable on health care quality. *JAMA* **280,** 1000–1005.
39. Reference deleted in proof.
40. Testa, M. A., and Simonson, D. C. (1996). Assessment of quality of life outcomes. *N. Engl. J. Med.* **334,** 835–840.
41. Russell, L. B., Gold, M. R., Siegel, J. E., *et al.* (1996). The role of cost-effectiveness analysis in medicine. *JAMA* **276,** 1172–1177.
42. Velanovitch, V. (1999). Using quality of life instruments to assess surgical outcomes. *Surgery* **126,** 1–4.
43. Leplège, A., and Hunt, S. (1997). The problem of quality of life in medicine. *JAMA* **278,** 47–50.
44. Eiseman, B. (1996). Surgical decision making and elderly patients. *Bull. Am. Coll. Surg.* **81,** 8–11.
45. Sosa, J. A., Bowman, H. M., Tielsch, J. M., *et al.* (1998). The importance of surgeon experience for clinical and economic outcomes from thyroidectomy. *Ann. Surg.* **228,** 320–330.
46. Sosa, J. A., Bowman, H. M., Gordon, T. A., *et al.* (1998). Importance of hospital volume in the overall management of pancreatic cancer. *Ann. Surg.* **228,** 429–438.
47. Birkmeyer, J. D., Finlayson, S. R. G., Tosteson, A. N. A., *et al.* (1999). Effect of hospital volume on in-hospital mortality with pancreaticoduodenectomy. *Surgery* **125,** 250–256.
48. Begg, C. B., Cramer, L. D., Hoskins, W. J., *et al.* (1998). Impact of hospital volume on operative mortality for major cancer surgery. *JAMA* **280,** 1747–1751.
49. Pearce, W. H., Parker, M. A., Feinglass, J., *et al.* (1999). The importance of surgeon volume and training in outcomes for vascular surgical procedures. *J. Vasc. Surg.* **29,** 768–778.
50. Harmon, J. W., Tang, D. G., Gordon, T. A., *et al.* (1999). Hospital volume can serve as a surrogate for surgeon volume for achieving excellent outcomes in colorectal resection. *Ann. Surg.* **230,** 404–413.
51. Porter, G. A., Soskolne, C. L., Yakimets, W. W., *et al.* (1998). Surgeon-related factors and outcome in rectal cancer. *Ann. Surg.* **277,** 157–167.
52. Project Hope (1988). Trends in the Concentration of Six Surgical Procedures Under PPS and Their Implications for Patient Mortality and Medicare Cost. Technical Report #E-87-08. Chevy Chase, MD.
53. Luft, H. S., Bunker, J. P., and Enthoven, A. C. (1979). Should operations be regionalized? The empiric relation between surgical volume and mortality. *N. Engl. J. Med.* **301,** 1364–1369.
54. Khuri, S. F., Henderson, W. G., Hur, K., *et al.* (1999). The relationship of surgical volume to outcome in eight common operations. *Ann. Surg.* **230,** 414–432.
55. Houghton, A. (1994). Variation in outcome of surgical procedures. *B. J. Surg.* **81,** 963–660.
56. Hannan, E. L. (1999). The relation between volume and outcome in health care. *N. Engl. J. Med.* **340,** 1677–1679.
57. Rhodes, R. S., Krasniak, C. J., and Jones, P. K. (1986). Factors affecting length of stay for femoropopliteal bypass: Implications of the DRGs. *N. Engl. J. Med.* **314,** 153–157.
58. Cleverly, W. O. (1986). "Essentials of Healthcare Finance," 2nd Ed., p. 191. Aspen Publishers Inc, Rockville, MD.
59. Balas, E. A., Kretschmer, R. A. C., Gnann, W., *et al.* (1998). Interpreting cost analyses of clinical interventions. *JAMA* **279,** 54–57.
60. Russell, L. B., Gold, M. R., Siegel, J. E., *et al.* (1996). The role of cost-effectiveness analysis in medicine. *JAMA* **276,** 1172–1177.
61. Weinstein, M. C., Siegel, J. E., Gold, M. R., *et al.* (1996). Recommendations of the Panel on Cost-Effectiveness in Health and Medicine. *JAMA* **276,** 1253–1258.
62. Siegel, J. E., Weinstein, M. C., Russell, L. B., *et al.* (1996). Recommendations for reporting cost-effectiveness analyses. *JAMA* **276,** 1339–1341.
63. Schermerhorn, M. L., Birkmeyer, J., Gould, D. A., *et al.* (2000). The impact of operative mortality on cost-effectiveness in the UK small aneurysm trial. *J. Vasc. Surg.* **31,** 217–226.
64. Heudebert, G. R., Marks, R., Wilcox, C. M., *et al.* (1997). Choice of long-term strategy for the management of patients with severe esophagitis: A cost-utility analysis. *Gastroenterology* **112,** 1078–1086.
65. Richardson, W. S., and Detsky, A. S. (1995). Users' guides to the medical literature: VII. How to use a clinical decision analysis. A. Are the results of the study valid? *JAMA* **273,** 1292–1295.
66. Birkmeyer, J. D., and Welch, H. G. (1997). A reader's guide to surgical decision analysis. *J. Am. Coll. Surg.* **184,** 589–595.
67. Millilli, J. J., Philiponis, V. S., and Nusbaum, M. (1998). Predicting surgical outcome using Bayesian analysis. *J. Surg. Res.* **77,** 45–49.
68. Brasel, K. J., Borgstrom, D. C., and Weigelt, J. A. (1999). Management of penetrating colon trauma: A cost-utility analysis. *Surgery* **125,** 471–479.
69. Cronenwett, J. L., Birkmeyer, J. D., Nackman, G. B., *et al.* (1997). Cost-effectiveness of carotid endarterectomy in asymptomatic patients. *J. Vasc. Surg.* **25,** 298–311.
70. Rao, P. M., Rhea, J. T., Novelline, R. A. *et al* (1998). Effect of computed tomography of the appendix on treatment of patients and use of hospital resources. *N. Engl. J. Med.* **338,** 141–146.
71. Gill, B. D., and Jenkins, J. R. (1996). Cost-effective evaluation and management of the acute abdomen. *Surg. Clin. N. Am.* **76**(1), 71–82.
72. Rhodes, R. S. (1994). Ambulatory surgery and the societal cost of surgery. *Surgery* **116,** 938–940.
73. Taheri, P. A., Wahl, W. L., Butz, D. A., *et al.* (1998). Trauma service cost: The real story. *Ann. Surg.* **227,** 720–725.
74. Taheri, P. A., Butz, D. A., Watts, C. M., *et al.* (1999). Trauma services: A profit center? *J. Am. Coll. Surg.* **188,** 349–354.
75. Legorreta, A. P., Silber, J. H., Constantino, G. N., *et al.* (1993). Increased cholecystectomy rate after the introduction of laparoscopic cholecystectomy. *JAMA* **270,** 1429–1432.
76. Black, W. C., and Welch, H. G. (1993). Advances in diagnostic imaging and overestimations of disease prevalence and the benefits of therapy. *N. Engl. J. Med.* **328,** 1237–1243.
77. Horn, S. D. (1997). "Clinical Practice Improvement: Implementation and Evaluation." Faulkner & Gray, New York.
78. Horn, S. D. (1995) Clinical Practice Improvement: Improving quality and decreasing cost in managed care. *Med. Interface* **8**(7), 60–64, 70.
79. Horn, S. D., Sharkey, P. D., and Levy, R. (1995). A managed care pharmacoeconomic research model based on the Managed Care Outcomes Project. *J. Pharm. Prac.* **8**(4), 172–177.

80. Horn, S. D., Sharkey, P. D., Tracy, D. M., *et al.* (1996). Intended and unintended consequences of HMO cost containment strategies: Results from the Managed Care Outcomes Project. *Am. J. Manag. Care* **2**(3), 253–264.
81. Horn, S. D., Sharkey, P. D., and Gassaway, J. (1996). Managed Care Outcomes Project: Study design, baseline patient characteristics, and outcome measures. *Am. J. Manag. Care* **2**(3), 237–247.
82. Horn, S. D., Buckle, J. M., and Carver, C. M. (1988). The Ambulatory Severity Index: Development of an ambulatory case mix system. *J. Ambulat. Care Manage.* **11,** 53–62.
83. Averill, R. F., McGuire, T. E., Manning, B. E., *et al.* (1992) A study of the relationship between severity of illness and hospital cost in New Jersey hospitals. *Health Serv. Res.* **27**(5), 587–617.
84. Shaneyfelt, T. M., Mayo-Smith, M. F., and Rothwangl, J. (1999). Are guidelines following guidelines? The methodological quality of clinical practice guidelines in the peer-reviewed medical literature. *JAMA* **281,** 1900–1905.
85. Cook, D., and Giacomini, M. (1999). The trails and tribulations of clinical practice guidelines. *JAMA* **281,** 1950–1951.
86. Pearson, S. D., Goulart-Fisher, D., and Lee, T. H. (1995). Critical pathways as a strategy for improving care: Problems and potential. **123,** 941–948.
87. Hoyt, D. B. (1997). Clinical practice guidelines. *Am. J. Surg.* **173,** 32–34.
88. Magi, D., Douglas, J. M., Jr., and Schwartz, J. S. (1996). Doxycycline compared with azithromycin for treating women with genital *Chlamydia trachomastis* infections: An incremental cost-effectiveness analysis. *Ann. Intern. Med.* **124**(4), 389–399.
89. Pestotnik, S. L., Classen, D. C., Evans, R. S., *et al.* (1996). Implementing antibiotic practice guidelines through computer-assisted decision support: Clinical and financial outcomes. *Ann. Intern. Med.* **124**(10), 884–890.
90. Hannan, E. L., Kilburn, H., Racz, M., *et al.* (1994). Improving the outcomes of coronary artery bypass surgery in New York State. *JAMA* **271,** 761–766.
91. Green, J., and Winfield, N. (1995). Report cards on cardiac surgeons: Assessing New York State's approach. *N. Engl. J. Med.* **332,** 1229–1232.
92. Chaissin, M. R., Hannan, E. L., and DeBunno, B. A. (1996). Benefits and hazards of reporting medical outcomes publicly. *N. Engl. J. Med.* **334,** 394–398.
93. Schneider, E. C., and Epstein, A. M. (1996). Influence of cardiac surgery performance report cards on referral practices and access to care. *N. Engl. J. Med.* **335,** 251–256.
94. Tunner, W. S., Christy, J. P., and Whipple, T. L. (1997). System for outcomes-based report card. *Bull. Am. Coll. Surg.* **82,** 18–33.
95. O'Connor, G. T., Plume, S. K., Olmstead, E. M., *et al.* (1996). A regional intervention to improve the hospital mortality associated with coronary artery bypass graft surgery. *JAMA* **275,** 841–846.
96. Bodily, K. C. (1999). Surgeons and technology. *Am. J. Surg.* **177,** 351–353.
97. Passaro, E., and Organ, C. H. (1999). Ernest A. Codman: The Improper Bostonian. *Bull. Am. Coll. Surg.* **84,** 16–22.
98. Hayman, J. A., Hillner, B. E., Harris, J. R., *et al.* (1998). Cost-effectiveness of routine radiotherapy following conservative therapy for early-stage breast cancer. *J. Clin. Oncol.* **16,** 1022–1029.
99. Chang, R. W., Pellisier, J. M., and Hazen, G. B. (1996). A cost-effectiveness analysis of total hip arthroplasty for osteoarthritis of the hip. *JAMA* **275,** 858–865.
100. Chung, K. C., Walters, M. R., Greenfield, M. L., *et al.* (1998). Endoscopic versus open carpal tunnel release: A cost-effectiveness analysis. *Plast. Reconstr. Surg.* **102,** 1089–1099.
101. Malter, A. D., Larson, E. B., Urban, N., *et al.* (1996). Cost-effectiveness of lumbar discectomy for the treatment of herniated intervertebral disc. *Spine* **21,** 1048–1054.

100

From Idea to Product: Financing and Regulatory Issues in Product Development

Jonathan Gertler*,† and James Garvey†

*Division of Vascular Surgery, Massachusetts General Hospital, and Harvard Medical School, Boston, Massachusetts 02114
†Schroder Ventures International Life Science Fund, Boston, Massachusetts 02114

I. Introduction

Although the current atmosphere in medicine is characterized by many as unfriendly to the individual physician, there remains tremendous opportunity and respect for technical advances that further improve clinical care. Many of the technical innovations currently changing the methods by which care is delivered in a number of specialties emanate from physician insights, aided in development by appropriate engineering, financial, and development support. This chapter reviews the issues facing the physician/inventor through the lens of the investment community funding the processes of invention and development and provides a detailed description of regulatory processes critical to understanding device development and deployment in the current era.

II. Development of an Idea into an Investment Proposition

Device development in the medical arena is dependent on a variety of support structures. The introduction of a new medical device ideally begins with innovation responding to clinical need, progresses through engineering and development, is fostered by financing from a variety of sources, and reaches the markets through disparate commercial structures. Along the way, the device is subject to scientific, clinical, engineering, and regulatory scrutiny and may be lost to the target community by recognition of a lack of validity, safety, or effectiveness, or by mismanagement of its development.

It is critical to understand the method by which new medical devices are funded in the period between concept and product launch. Broadly termed the investment process, this funding can take the form of small-business grants from the government (SBIRs), so-called angel investment (funding from private individuals), corporate strategic partnership, or venture capital and mezzanine investment. Regardless of the origin of the funds, the diligent process in assessing the attractiveness of the device in question to the investor and to the market, and, most importantly, the potential efficacy for the clinical users, carries certain overlapping responsibilities and methods. The following discussions explore in detail the concerns that must be accounted for in the development of any new technology from the commercial investment perspective, thus emphasizing for the inventor both the strategic needs and the ethical responsibilities in this process.

A. Technology, Products, and Core Competency of the Developing Device Company

The first step in identifying whether a product should be regarded as a serious entry into the medical device marketplace entails determining the credibility of the device in question. Although numerous clever engineering solutions can be arrived at in the production or design of a new medical device, many of these products are severely limited by a misunderstanding of the clinical scenario that they must serve. Invention in search of an application or market either leads to increasing cost in our healthcare system without the benefit of improved quality or safety or leads to investment failure either financially or ethically with regard to promotion of an inappropriately supported device. Devices that exemplify this concept are as follows (with numerous other categories applicable):

1. Coronary angioplasty catheters (capability in noncompliance balloons and catheter component manufacture; competence in understanding disease patterns, risk of misapplied interventional concepts, and market needs of practicing cardiologists; danger of rapid diffusion of invasion without clear clinical justification present).

2. Rapid-throughput pathology-specimen automating machines (capability in specimen staining, pattern recognition, reagent preparation, molded plastic construction; competence in recognition of bottlenecks in pathology processing, diagnostic dilemmas in tailoring special staining, market dynamics in pathology referrals, diagnostic processes in a tertiary care hospital setting; danger of overautomation leading to inaccuracy and diagnosis must be addressed by regulatory process in allowing device to go forward).

3. Coagulation function testing for the point-of-care market (capability in reagent preparation, reporting standards for diagnostic laboratory testing, formulation of kits emphasizing ease of use; competence in understanding the interactions among new pharmacologic interventions for coagulation disorders, mechanism of new drugs, market needs of prescribing physicians for maintenance and titration of said agents; potential for high costs, and pharmacoeconomic analysis of both drugs and their monitoring is necessary for ultimate acceptance of these diagnostic devices).

B. Market Dynamics and Attractiveness

Market dynamics depend on numerous factors. Although clinical needs remain the major drivers of development and diffusion, numerous steps must be evaluated to account for the attractiveness of the device to the medical community at large. Such evaluation determines the investment vehicle funding the project. In the relative order of importance, these factors are as follows:

1. The target population, including risk factors and projected growth or shrinkage of the clinical problem.
2. Current solutions for the clinical problem (as above) and degree of acceptance of various approaches.
3. Opinions and characteristics of the healthcare providers involved in this patient segment.
4. Perceived needs of the patient population as expressed by the patients and as studied and represented by their representative groups.
5. Competitive forces and other projected developments.
6. Previous failures in the same field with attendant analysis of these attempts.
7. Current and projected reimbursement schemes and distribution of payers responsible for the involved patient segment.
8. Distribution channels.
9. International review of all the competitors and world markets.

C. Intellectual Property

Intellectual property rights remain extremely important to maintaining dominance in the field, both with regard to potential entry and infringement on existing patents as well as market entry and protection of an established position. Patent filings with regard to earliest proof of concept, date of provisional filings, date of final filing, breadth of claims, and type of patent (design, materials, manufacturing, use, method, etc.) are all critical in an area in which intellectual property rights will allow market dominance and control of technology diffusion. All too often, inventors do not take adequate steps to ensure their position in the patent landscape. Clear delineation of parent institution's rights or prenegotiated licensing arrangements, early filings with the patent office, and thorough notebook validation of the date of invention are critical to commercializing a product. An early review of the prior art in the field will allow an invention to be developed while preserving the freedom to enhance invention development and reduce risk of patent infringement.

Nonetheless, circumstances exist in which intellectual property is not necessarily the most important aspect of either market penetration or market dominance. The circumstances arise in which either manufacturing capability or distribution is sufficiently idiosyncratic or experience dependent, that being first or largest with regard to any of these aspects of device diffusion will allow the inventor/manufacturer/distributor to dominate in the absence of clear intellectual property rights. Caution must be maintained, however, that there is no infringement on the smaller, less marketable possessors of intellectual property, who could then potentially claim rights to the success of the technology diffusion in question.

D. Evaluation of Current Existing Therapies

From both a marketing and medical perspective, and with the expected clinical response and patient demand in mind, a thorough analysis of existing current therapies must be undertaken. This analysis should include the following evaluations:

1. Current effectiveness of interventional and noninterventional approaches to the disease as published in appropriate randomized studies or meta-analysis of high-level reviews of similar problems. In the absence of such data, review of anecdotal literature may be undertaken with the caveat that current therapies may reflect long-standing clinical assumptions rather than demonstrated effectiveness.
2. Risk–benefit ratio for current therapies; a complete audit of complications, morbidity, and mortality associated with these current therapies must be established.
3. Ease of use, learning curve, quality of life, discomfort level, and required ancillary services for existing therapies must be reviewed and compared to the proposed alternatives.

E. Scientific Due Diligence

The due diligence process, which an inventor should undertake and which will be further developed by any investors supporting the project, must address the data available to assess adequately the technology under development. Data available reflect the stage of development and therefore reflect the stage of the investment as well as the terms of investment. Nonetheless, diligence must demonstrate at least the following parameters, as organized by stage of investment:

1. Seed stage: a logical mechanical, physiologic, and engineering approach to a well-defined clinical problem and need for which current solutions remain imperfect.
2. Early stage: proof of concept as represented by computer modeling, prototype development with *in vitro* testing, or early animal validation.
3. Preclinical stage: demonstrated safety and efficacy in animal models with progression to phase 1 testing demonstrating safety in humans.
4. Prelaunch (premarket approval/510K regulatory) stage: phase 2 and phase 3 trials demonstrating efficacy and ultimately effectiveness under tightly controlled circumstances (see Sections III,D and III,E).

F. Regulatory Structure

Determination of the class of device is critically related to the time of market launch. From both a practical and an ethical perspective, it is imprudent at best and criminal at worst to manipulate the regulatory system as a strategy for early market entry. Full analysis of precedent devices will reveal whether the device in question can be categorized in either class 1, 2, or 3 (see Section III,C), and, in the case of a completely innovative device, analysis of potential risk via expert review and prospective discussions with appropriate Food and Drug Administration (FDA) committees will allow appropriate classification. Subsequent submission of either a 510K or a premarket approval application will depend on internal review, appropriate selection of regulatory consultants, and appropriate preliminary discussions with the relevant FDA subcommittees.

G. Management Capability, Experience, and Integrity

By the time the medical device has reached the maturity to attract outside investors, experienced business development personnel assume management of the project. Inventors, scientists, and clinicians responsible for the original development of the device or technology and question often have been relegated to the role of either chief scientific officer, director of research and development, or head of a scientific advisory board. Structure of companies, even at an early stage, will therefore involve people well schooled and experienced in the process of fund raising, human resource management, overall company vision, and engineering. Clinical or scientific core competence, which supported the company in the beginning, will also continue to drive the project. Therefore, a long track record should be available for all the involved personnel, and this must be examined to determine the capability for execution, work ethic, behavioral code, management, scientific integrity, and previous successes and failures of the assembled team. Direct meetings, review of previous accomplishments, and interviews can accomplish this diligence, with both identified and unidentified referees providing information about the individuals in question.

H. Manufacturing Diligence

Manufacturing standards must be established for the sites involved in producing the device in question. This must include materials testing; appropriate fatigue, deformation, dysfunction, and breakage expectations based on well-engineered *in vitro* stress simulations; and sterility, packaging, labeling, and adherence to ISO 9000 international manufacturing standards.

I. Conclusion

Although viewed as a potential major contributor to spiraling healthcare costs, appropriate development of new technology (scientifically sound, ethically developed, market based, or serving niche patient needs) has the potential to improve quality of life significantly for recipient patient populations while removing cost from the system overall. For this to be accomplished, numerous checks and balances in the development system must be in place (technology assessment), which will necessarily be distributed among the various participants involved in the diffusion of the technologies. Lengthy analyses of the management of the engineering and manufacturing processes, the scientific validation process, the regulatory pathway, intellectual property development, marketing distribution channels, and postintroductions surveillance are needed for organized technology assessment, for which different segments of society should be responsible. Although the investment side traditionally looks to structure and maximization of return on investment as the primary drivers of adoption of technologies, successful investment is predicated as well on responsible due diligence regarding technological, scientific, clinical, and ethical management issues. Examples of successful device development whereby cost reductions have coincided with a migration of techniques from invasive to minimally invasive, with attendant marked improvement in quality and patient care, include pacemakers and implantable defibrillators (originally open thoracotomy procedures), laparoscopic surgical equipment, pulse oximetry, blood glucose monitoring, angioplasty and stents, and computerized tomography and magnetic resonance imaging. The list is long and reflects the marriage of quality enhancement and cost reduction, so critical to successful deployment of new approaches to clinical problems.

III. Regulatory Structure for New Device Products

The definition of a medical device is offered by United States Statue, Section 201H of the Food, Drug, and Cosmetic Act, Title 21, United States code. A medical device is defined as follows:

An instrument apparatus, implement machine, contrivance implant, in-vitro *reagent or other similar or related article including any component part or accessory that is*

1. *Recognized in the official national formula or the U.S. Pharmacopoeia or any supplement to them.*
2. *Intended for use in the diagnosis of disease or other conditions or in the cure, mitigation, treatment or prevention of disease in man or other animals, or*
3. *Intended to affect the structure or any function of the body of man or other animals and which does not achieve its primary intended purposes through chemical action within or on the body of man or other animals and which is not dependent upon being metabolized for the achievement for any of its primary intended purposes.*

This broad-reaching definition is reflected by a dense medical regulatory organization that has its roots in serious omissions with regard to patient safety and serious violations of the spirit of medical invention. The following discussions provide background concerning the shortcomings in American law that led to expanded device regulation and evolution into the current system. In addition, the current organization is fully defined with regard to government structure, classification, and medical devices and recommendations for current strategies for regulatory submissions.

A. Historical Reasons for Device Regulation and Evolution of the Current Structure

Initial efforts to control food and drugs on a federal level reflected only import regulations. Interstate shipping of undesirable food and drugs, and the use of the mail for misrepresentation of health-related entities, were initially only regulated via the United States Post Office, under the postal fraud statues of 1872. However, specific medical devices did not fall under the purview of these acts.

Although the first proposition to regulate food and drugs on a national level was made in 1869, the first act on a federal level was introduced by Theodore Roosevelt in 1906. Known as the Food and Drug Act, this law was aimed at postmarketing enforcement authority over food and drugs but made no mention whatsoever of medical devices. In an annual report in 1917, the administrators of the Food and Drug Act noted the lack of control of medical devices, and although the post office regulations remained in force, there was no essential authority for medical device control. In 1938, the Food, Drug, and Cosmetics Act expanded the earlier regulations by insisting on food ingredient listing and by broadening the FDA's authority to stop marketing on an ineffective therapeutic claim. In addition, medical devices were defined for the first time as

instruments, apparatus, and contrivances, including their components parts and accessories intended;

1. *For use in diagnosis, cure, mitigation, treatment or prevention of diseases in man or other animals or*
2. *To affect the structure as any other function of the body of man or animals.*

The Food and Drug Administration was thus charged with the authority to regulate misbranded, misrepresented, or adulterated medical devices. Nonetheless, this act extended only to postmarketing enforcement authority and there was no premarketing regulatory capability, which proved so important in later legislation.

The first major premarketing enforcement authority over devices came with the medical device amendments of 1976, in the Nixon administration. These were amendments of a previous senate bill introduced by Edward Kennedy. These bills had their roots in a 1955 citizens' advisory committee of the FDA, which recognized that false claims were frequently being made for medical devices and that no real regulatory oversights were provided by current FDA legislation. Nonetheless, despite an evolutionary approach via the Congress, it was not until the Nixon amendments of 1976 that our current system began to take shape.

The 1976 medical device amendments had several impacts:

1. The FDA was authorized to categorize all medical devices into a three-tier classification and regulatory system based on the risk that the devices posed to their intended recipients.

2. Premarketing approval procedures were outlined in detail. New and high-risk devices demanded a detailed submission called a premarket approval (PMA), although devices that were substantially equivalent to those that had been marketed before the enactment of the amendments in 1976 required a less thorough submission. These submissions today are known as 510K submissions, primarily because the premarket notification was detailed in Section 510K of the Food, Drug, and Cosmetics Act, Section 21 of the U.S. Code.

Both of the above regulatory categories are described in detail in Sections III,D and III,E.

The Medical Device Amendments Act of 1976 also introduced concepts that are widely recognized today. Manufacturing practices; FDA authority to ban dangerous products; notification, recall, repair, or refund for defective devices; investigational device exemptions (IDEs); listing of all devices and registration of device manufacturing establishments; and adverse event reporting were all detailed in these amendments.

The authority of the 1976 amendments was further strengthened by the Safe Medical Devices Act of 1990. Although this had the beneficial effect to industry of expediting the review process, the review process was implemented primarily because of a much more rigid postmarketing surveillance protocol. The Safe Medical Devices Act of 1990, which was earmarked for user and distributor medical device recording, postmarketing surveillance, and tracking, included civil penalties, recall authority, and humanitarian device exemptions (compassionate use), and also expanded the purview of the Medical Device Act to include certain drugs. Further amendments in 1992 in the Bush administration again broadened the indications for medical device reporting and gave muscle to postmarket surveillance by providing an enforcement authority for the FDA.

The current structure of the FDA primarily reflects this legislation. Continued amendments to the regulatory process have been introduced and in Congressional Committee and have been the subject of ongoing administrative and legislative activities. However, the structure as it is worked today is not significantly different from that seen in 1992.

B. Structure of the FDA

The Food and Drug Administration is a federal agency of the Public Health Service in the Department of Health and Human Services. It is in the executive branch of government, is considered a cabinet-level department, and is headed by the commissioner of food and drugs. Within the Food and Drug Administration are numerous offices with specific oversight. These are enumerated below:

1. Office of Regulatory Affairs. This office is responsible for evaluation and coordination of compliance with legal actions. It is divided into six regional districts that coordinate routine inspections; investigate complaints; respond to requests by hospitals, patients, or other individuals to investigate potential violations; and handle the premarket approval of Class III medical devices (see Section III,C,3) with regard to auditing of the manufacturing facilities. Manufacturers continue to contact this regional office as the primary link to the FDA, once marketing approval has been accomplished.

2. Center for Devices and Radiological Health (CDRH). The CDRH consists of six offices: Office of Device Evaluations, Office of Science and Technology, Office of Surveillance and Biometrics, Office of Compliance, Office of Systems and Management, and Office of Health and Industry Programs. The Office of Device Evaluations is further divided into the (a) Division of Reproductive, Abdominal, Ear, Nose and Throat, and Radiological Devices, (b) Division of Clinical Laboratory Devices, (c) Division of General and Restorative Devices, (d) Division of Ophthalmic Devices, (e) Division of Cardiovascular, Respiratory, and Neurologic Devices, and (f) Division of Dental Infection Control and General Hospital Devices. Similarly, the Office of Health and Industry Programs is subdivided into a division that aids small Manufacturers, with the goal of ensuring competitiveness and compliance with the sometimes

abstruse FDA regulations, and (a) Division of Communication Media, (b) Division of Device User Programs and Systems Analysis, and (c) Division of Mammography Quality and Radiation Programs. The latter three subdivisions serve the purpose of data collection and surveillance and also provide biostatical, economic, cost-effective, and other device-oriented business and regulatory expertise. The Office of Device Evaluations serves the purposes of classifying devices and reviewing and evaluating premarket approvals, protocols for product development, institutional device exemptions, and 510K submissions. It is also charged with the postmarket surveillance and monitoring of the performance of the devices, once they are in use. The Office of Device Evaluations is obviously divided along clinical lines to facilitate expert development under each of the major clinical categories.

3. Center for Biologics Evaluation and Research. This office is primarily oriented toward the area of blood components and blood products with regard to the medical devices specific to this area. However, blood-related products used for direct therapeutic action, such as blood transfusion devices, do not fall into the purview of this office.

4. Center for Drug Evaluation and Research. This office oversees the "gray area" regarding medical devices that have some drug action.

C. Classification of Devices

A three-tier classification system of medical devices is predicated on risk. The lower the class, the lower the risk and therefore the lower the degree of regulation. Class I, II, and III devices are all associated with general controls, and in addition Class II and III devices are further regulated with performance standards and premarket approval (Class III). The classification of a device is possible based on either the FDA or a manufacturer's initiative and also that of interested third parties. Reclassification of a device is not intended only for a sole manufacturer's device but rather is considered to be a petition for all devices within the category to be reclassified. Devices marketed before the Medical Device Act of 1976 were allowed to maintain continued distribution; however, ultimately the FDA intends to call for premarket approval submissions for all preamendment Class III devices. All devices that have been marketed since the Medical Devices Act of 1976 require a 510K or a PMA submission.

1. Class I Devices

Class I devices are essentially safe devices—tongue depressors, bandages, thermometers, etc. A safe device is defined by the U.S. Government as one for which "the probable benefits for health from the device for its intended uses and conditions of use, when accompanied by adequate directions and warnings against unsafe use, outweigh any probable risk." Similarly, an effective device is defined by the government as one for which "in a significant portion of the target population, the use of a device for its intended uses and conditions for use, when accompanied by adequate directions for use and a warning against unsafe use, will provide clinically significant results."

Class I devices are regulated by general controls that are primarily directed at purity and appropriate labeling of products, and premarket notification, reporting, recall, replacement, refund, and notification requirements. Whereas other classes of devices also require general controls, additional controls are necessary for Class II and III devices. A Class I device is ultimately defined as "not supported or represented to be for use in supporting or sustaining human life and for use which is of substantial importance in preventing impairment of human health and does not present a potential unreasonable risk of illness or injury."

2. Class II Devices

Class II devices are essentially under the same general controls as Class I devices, but performance standards and special controls have been added. Performance standards relate to safe and effective performance, and the Food, Drug, and Cosmetics Act includes provisions concerning "the construction, components, ingredients, and properties of the device and its compatibility at power systems." Class II devices in addition must include appropriate instructions and/or labeling for installation, maintenance, operation, and use, and furthermore must entail postmarket surveillance, patient registries, guidelines, and recommendations, among other dictates. However, Class II devices are subject to the general controls of a Class I device, but any Class II devices relating to critical care, i.e, life support or interventions under acutely life-threatening circumstances, must have special controls identified by the Food and Drug Administration to provide continued assurance of both safety and effectiveness.

3. Class III Devices

Class III device categorization relates to significant indwelling devices used either for invasion of, or subsequent removal of substances from, a body cavity, or indwelling devices that are permanent, such as heart valves. Devices that were marketed prior to the 1976 Food, Drug, and Cosmetics Act have been allowed to stay on the market unless the FDA elected to call for a premarket approval for the devices or unless the devices were reclassified. For devices developed after 1976, 510K submissions (see below) are required, unless the FDA or its local office has elected for a premarket approval classification. The only way for a nonsubstantiated equipment device to not require PMA is for it to be reclassified by the FDA as a Class I or II device.

D. Aspects of Premarket Notification

Premarket notification can be divided into 510K processes and formal premarket approval. The 510K process is designed for the marketing of postamendment (Food, Drug, and Cosmetics Act 1976) Class III devices when they are essentially the same as a previously legally marketed Class II device that predated the amendment (predicate Class III device), for which a PMA has not yet been requested by the FDA. New devices in the Class II category that are not considered equivalent cannot be marketed via a 510K process. The 510K is essentially premarket notification and its intent is to identify those devices that must undergo PMA because of their Class III categorization, or must be reclassified as Class I or Class II devices prior to marketing. In addition, the 510K process is manufacturer friendly in that substantially equivalent new devices are allowed to get to market more rapidly, without facing any greater regulatory burden as a barrier to entry than is faced by manufacturers of devices that have predated the amendment (predicate Class III device).

The 510K process is required for any device being introduced for the first time, regardless of category; for a replica of a device (by a new manufacturer) that is already being manufactured by another manufacturer; for reintroduction of a device; and for significant changes in commercial distribution of a device or evolutionary modifications that could potentially affect device function. Equivalence is considered when a new device has technology characteristics and purposes similar to predicate devices, or different technological characteristics but for which continued safety and efficacy can be readily demonstrated by the manufacturer. The FDA will review any submission for any 510K and issue a letter pronouncing the device substantially equivalent or not substantially equivalent. Equivalence, again, is predicated on intended use, technological characteristics, and descriptive and performance information as the arbiters of substantially equivalent or not substantially equivalent.

E. 510K Medical Device Submissions

The 510K, a premarketing submission made to the FDA, demonstrates the device is safe and effective. In addition, a 510K submission must demonstrate that the device in question is substantially equivalent to a legally marketed device that is not subject to a premarket approval. In order to make a substantial equivalency claim, an applicant for 510K device must compare in their application their own device to a similar device currently being marketed in the United States. A legally marketed device may be a device that is preamendment, i.e., legally marketed prior to May 28, 1976, or a device that has been downgraded from a Class III category to either Class II or Class I. The preamendment or legally marketed devices are known as "predicate" devices. Again, a device is substantially equivalent if it has the same intended use as the predicate device, the same technological characteristics as the predicate device, or different technological characteristics, but does not raise new questions of safety and effectiveness. In this setting the sponsor must demonstrate that the devices are as safe and effective as an already legally marketed device.

It is critical to realize that a claim of substantial equivalence does not mean the new and predicate devices must be identical. Substantial equivalence is established with regard to intended use, design, energy use or delivery, materials, performance, safety, effectiveness, labeling, biocompatibility, standards, and other applicable characteristics.

There are four categories of interested parties who must submit the 510K to the FDA. These include domestic manufacturers who are introducing a new device to the United States market. Component parts of a new device need not undergo a 510K submission unless these are promoted for sale to an end-user as replacement parts. In addition, specification developers, defined by the FDA as persons who develop specifications for a finished device but have them manufactured by a third party, must submit the 510K application. Interestingly, the specification developer, not the contract manufacturer, is responsible for the application. Repackagers and relabelers may be required to submit a PMA if they change the labeling or the condition of any said device. All foreign manufacturers and exporters or United States representatives of foreign manufacturers and exporters who seek to introduce a device to the U.S. market are required to submit a 510K.

The Modernization Act of 1996 attempts to streamline the evaluation of premarket notifications for the reserve Class I devices, Class II devices subject to premarket notification, and preamendment Class III devices for which the FDA has not yet called PMAs.

F. Premarket Approval

Premarket approval is the most stringent device marketing application in the FDA system. A PMA is an FDA application that requests clearance for marketing or continuation of marketing for a Class III medical device. Although the technical review time for PMA is listed as up to 180 days, the review time is normally much longer. The process involves FDA advisory committee review of the PMA at a public meeting and provision of the FDA with the committee's recommendation as to whether approval should be forthcoming. Unlike premarket notification, premarket approval requires that the FDA determine that the application contains decedent's sufficient valid scientific evidence, providing reasonable assurance that the device is safe as well as effective for its intended use or uses. Following notification of the applicant of the FDAs action, a Federal Register notice is published, announcing the data on which the decision was based and providing interested persons an opportunity to petition the FDA within 30 days for reconsideration of the approval/denial decision.

The PMA must be submitted by the person who owns the rights to, or otherwise has some authorized access to, data and information to be submitted in support of the PMA. This "person" may be an individual, a government agency, a scientific or academic establishment, a corporation, a partnership, or any of a number of legal entities. PMA requirements apply to all Class III devices that are commercially distributed or are to be commercially distributed in United States. There are three types of Class III devices: transitional, preamendment, or not substantially equivalent postamendment; there are different requirements for each type:

1. Transitional Class III devices all require an approved PMA before U.S. marketing is allowed. Examples of these devices include soft contact lenses and related lens care products, intraocular lenses, surgical sutures, bone segments, vascular grafts of animal origin, and absorbable hemostatic devices and dressings. These devices were regulated by the FDA as "new drugs" before the May 28, 1976 enactment of the medical device amendment.

2. Preamendment Class III devices and postamendment devices that are determined to be equivalent can be marketed without submission or FDA approval of the PMA until such approval is required by regulation. These devices, other than transitional Class III devices, were all in commercial distribution preamendment. Examples provided by the FDA include heart valves, intrauterine devices, contraceptive tubal occlusion devices, and diaphragmatic or phrenic nerve simulators. A PMA for such a device cannot be required until 30 months after classification as Class III, or 90 days after publication of a final regulation requiring submission of the PMA, whichever is longer.

3. Not substantially equivalent postamendment class III devices must have an approved PMA prior to commercial distribution in United States. These are all devices that were introduced or intended to be introduced after May 28, 1976 and were determined by the FDA to have no predicate devices. Examples include extracorporeal shock wave lithotripsy, percutaneous transluminal coronary angioplasty devices, porous coated orthopedic prostheses for uncemented use, implanted defibrillators, contraceptive cervical caps, synthetic ligaments, and implanted drug delivery systems.

G. Investigational Device Exemptions

The investigational device exemption is a critical portion of the PMA process. An IDE allows manufacturers to distribute for use unapproved medical devices for investigational protocols in human subjects. The IDE regulation is applicable to most clinical studies in United States designed to determine safety and effectiveness of a medical device. There are two types of devices covered by IDE regulations: significant risk devices and nonsignificant risk devices.

Significant risk devices require FDA and institutional review board (IRB) approval prior to initiation of clinical studies, whereas nonsignificant risk devices require only IRB approval. The purpose of the IDE is to allow clinical studies that support PMA or 510K applications. Investigational use may also include clinical evaluation of modification of existing devices, or new intended or projected uses of already established devices. To obtain IDE approval for significant risk device investigation, a sponsor must develop an investigational plan and assemble a report of prior investigations, select qualified investigators and obtain signed agreements from them, submit the investigational plan, report any prior investigation to the IRB at each individual institution where a trial is to be conducted, and, finally, submit a completed IDE application to the FDA for review and obtain approval of the same.

Nonsignificant risk devices are defined simply by the FDA as those not posing a significant risk to human subjects. Examples provided by the FDA include daily-wear contact lenses and associated solutions, ultrasound dental devices, and indwelling Foley bladder catheters.

H. Overview of the FDA Modernization Act of 1997

On November 21, 1997 the Food and Drug Administration Modernization Act of 1997 was signed into law. The following portion of this report summarizes the device-related sections of the modernization act.

1. Investigational Device Exemptions

The modernization act impacts IDEs with regard to protocols and device changes, early collaboration about data requirements for clinical studies, meetings to present evidence of effectiveness for PMAs, expanded humanitarian device (HD) exemption access to investigational devices, and practicing medicine.

Clinical protocols may be changed without FDA approval if the changes do not affect (1) the validity of the data resulting from the study, (2) the risk-to-benefit ratio relied on to approve the protocol, (3) the scientific soundness of the study, and (4) the rights, safety, or welfare of the human subjects. Devices may be altered in the process of a trial, including manufacturing changes, without additional FDA approval, provided that the basic design or principle of operation of the devices is not altered in any way.

2. Early Collaboration about Data Requirements for Clinical Studies

In an effort to streamline the process for risky devices, sponsors who intend to perform a clinical study of any Class III device, or any implanted device in any class, can meet with the FDA to discuss the investigational plan, including the clinical protocol. This will allow agreements to be reached for the investigational plan before the IDE application.

3. Meetings to Present Evidence of Effectiveness for PMAs

In an effort to better inform sponsors planning to submit a PMA, sponsors may submit a written request to meet with the FDA to determine the type of information and the valid scientific evidence that will be necessary to support the effectiveness of their device. The request must include the following information: (1) a detailed description of the device, (2) proposed conditions of use, (3) investigational plan, and (4) if possible, the expected performance of the device.

4. Expanded Humanitarian Device Exemption

The modernization act diminishes the amount of time needed for FDA approval or denial, from 180 to 75 days. The FDA may require a sponsor to demonstrate continued compliance with regard to the humanitarian device as necessary to protect public health, or if the agency has reason to believe the criteria for a humanitarian device are not being fulfilled. Emergency use is also allowed, assuming that approval by an IRB cannot be obtained in time. However, following emergency use, the IRB is notified of the name of the patient, the device used, and the reason for use.

The FDA will permit shipment of an investigational device for diagnosis, monitoring, or therapy of a serious disease or condition in emergency situations. In addition, the act allows any person (in alliance with a physician) to request from a manufacturer or distributor an investigational device as long as the following criteria are met: (1) the licensed physician determines there is no comparable or satisfactory alternative treatment and the risk from the device does not exceed the risk of the disease or condition, (2) no comparable or satisfactory alternative is present, (3) the device is under an approved IDE, or all clinical investigations to support PMA have been completed, (4) the sponsor is actively pursuing a PMA, (5) use will not interfere with patient enrollment in clinical trials, (6) there is already sufficient evidence of safety and effectiveness to support the device's use in treatment, and (7) in the setting of immediately life-threatening situations, the available scientific evidence supports the conclusion that the device may be effective in treatment and will not put the patient at unreasonable risk.

5. Premarket Approval

The modernization act allows for the submission of data from investigations of earlier versions of a device in support of safety and effectiveness. The data are considered valid only if device modifications do not constitute a significant change that would otherwise invalidate the relevance of the data. Under the modernization act, the FDA will also provide special review, which can include expedited processing of a PMA for devices intended to treat or diagnose life-threatening irreversible and debilitating diseases or conditions. Devices may receive special review if they meet the following criteria: (1) the device represents a breakthrough technology, (2) there are no approved alternatives, and (3) the use of the device offers significant advantages over existing approved alternatives or (4) availability is in the best interest of the patients.

Risk-based reclassification of postamendment Class III devices may be requested from an applicant who submits the 510k submission and receives a "not substantially equivalent" determination, placing the device into a Class III category. The device may be reclassified as Class I or II. A request must be sent in writing within 30 days from the receipt of the "not substantially equivalent" determination. The request must include a description of the device, reasons for the recommended reclassification, and information to support the recommendation. If the device is reclassified it may then be used as a predicate device for other 510Ks. If, however, the device must remain in Class III, the applicant must obtain PMA or improve on an approved IDE before proceeding in any fashion.

I. Summary

Full information on regulatory processes is critical to the marketing of any new device, and a revolution is occurring in many aspects of healthcare-related fields with regard to device development. Venture capital and corporate investment in devices have continued to be strong. The modernization act, with its improved access to existing data as well as streamlined mechanisms for entry into the marketplace, will help businesses develop quantum-leap technology while protecting the spirit and the intent of the original legislation directed at medical device proliferation and optimization of patient care.

IV. Overview and Conclusion

Numerous avenues for bringing a new idea to an established product include, but are not limited to, licensing, private benefactor (angel) investment, venture capital investment, and strategic partnerships with device companies. The common denominator, which is reflected in both the regulatory and the financing aspects of new product development, is an understanding of how a product develops value. The physician/inventor must keep in mind both the investment decision process, applicable to all potential partners in product development despite differing financial orientations, and the FDA regulatory process, which can greatly influence the time course and expense of new product development. The FDA Internet web site home page at http://www.fda.gov/ is a source of useful information (see also additional FDA information at fda.gov/opacom/Imodact.html, fda.gov/cdrh/index.html, and fda.gov/medwatch/index.html.

Recommended Reading

Bygrave, W. D., and Timmons, J. A. (1992). "Venture Capital at the Crossroads." Harvard Business School Press, Boston.

Sexton, D. D., and Smilor, R. W., eds. (1986). "The Art and Science of Entrepreneurship." Ballinger, Cambridge, MA.

Timmons, J. A., and Sapienza, H. A. (1990). Venture capital: More than money? *In* "Pratt's Guide to Venture Capital Sources," 14th Ed. (J. Morris and S. M. Pratt, eds. Venture Economics, Inc., Needham, MA.

Index

A

B

C

D

E

F

G

H

J

K

L

M

N

P

Q

R

S

T

U

V

W

X

Y

Z